369 0127999

KU-279-093

Joslin's Diabetes Mellitus

Fourteenth Edition

Joslin's Diabetes Mellitus

Fourteenth Edition

Edited by

C. Ronald Kahn, M.D.

President and Director,
Joslin Diabetes Center;
Mary K. Iacocca Professor of Medicine,
Harvard Medical School,
Boston, Massachusetts

Gordon C. Weir, M.D.

Head of the Section on Islet Transplantation
and Cell Biology and Diabetes Research
and Wellness Foundation
Chair, Joslin Diabetes Center;
Professor of Medicine,
Harvard Medical School,
Boston, Massachusetts

George L. King, M.D.

Director of Research and Head of the
Section on Vascular Cell
Biology, Joslin Diabetes Center;
Professor of Medicine,
Harvard Medical School,
Boston, Massachusetts

Alan M. Jacobson, M.D.

Senior Vice President, Strategic Initiatives Division,
and Head of the Behavioral
and Mental Health Unit,
Joslin Diabetes Center;
Professor of Psychiatry,
Harvard Medical School,
Boston, Massachusetts

Alan C. Moses, M.D.

Former Chief Medical Officer,
Joslin Diabetes Center;
Professor of Medicine (on leave),
Harvard Medical School,
Boston, Massachusetts
Associate Vice President of Medical Affairs,
Novo Nordisk Pharmaceuticals Inc.,
Princeton, New Jersey

Robert J. Smith, M.D.

Director of Medicine and the Hallett Center for
Diabetes and Endocrinology,
Professor of Medicine,
Brown Medical School,
Providence, Rhode Island

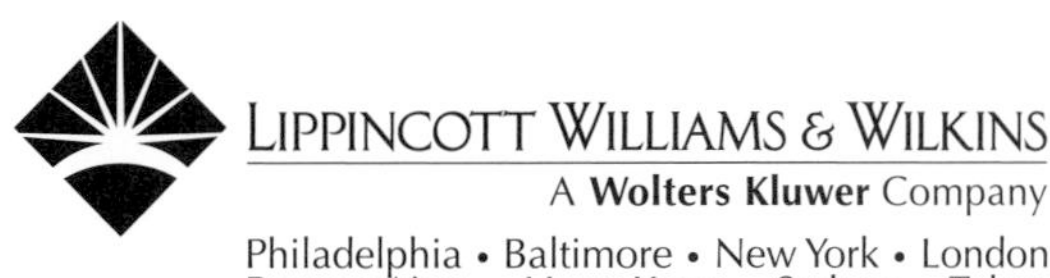

Lippincott Williams & Wilkins
A **Wolters Kluwer** Company
Philadelphia • Baltimore • New York • London
Buenos Aires • Hong Kong • Sydney • Tokyo

Acquisitions Editor: Lisa McAllister
Developmental Editor: Joyce Murphy
Manufacturing Manager: Angela Panetta
Production Service: Nesbitt Graphics, Inc., Bonnie Boehme/Marilyn Dwyer
Director, Medical Production: Charlene Catlett Squibb
Compositor: Nesbitt Graphics, Inc.
Printer: Quebecor World–Taunton

One Joslin Place
Boston, MA 02215
joslin.org

Printed in the USA

Library of Congress Cataloging-in-Publication Data

Joslin, Elliott Proctor, 1869-1962.
Joslin's diabetes mellitus.-- 14th ed. / edited by C. Ronald Kahn ... [et al.].
p. cm.
Includes bibliographical references and index.
ISBN 0-7817-2796-0
1. Diabetes. I. Title: Diabetes mellitus. II. Kahn, C. Ronald. III. Title.
RC660.J6 2005
616.4'62--dc22

2004025662

Care has been taken to confirm the accuracy of the information presented and to describe generally accepted practices. However, the editors, authors and publisher are not responsible for errors or omissions or for any consequences from application of the information in this book and make no warranty, express or implied, with respect to the currency, completeness, or accuracy of the contents of the publication. Application of this information in a particular situation remains the professional responsibility of the practitioner.

The editors, authors and publisher have exerted every effort to ensure that drug selection and dosage set forth in this text are in accordance with current recommendations and practice at the time of publication. However, in view of ongoing research, changes in government regulations, and the constant flow of information relating to drug therapy and drug reactions, the reader is urged to check the package insert for each drug for any change in indications and dosage and for added warnings and precautions. This is particularly important when the recommended agent is a new or infrequently employed drug.

Some drugs and medical devices presented in this publication have Food and Drug Administration (FDA) clearance for limited use in restricted research settings. It is the responsibility of the health care provider to ascertain the FDA status of each drug or device planned for use in clinical practice.

10 9 8 7 6 5 4 3 2

Preface

We are pleased to present this 14th edition of *Joslin's Diabetes Mellitus.* This textbook continues to evolve and address the newest and most important insights into this very old but very challenging disease. Indeed, as this book goes to press, despite multiple medical and scientific advances, we are facing a worldwide epidemic of diabetes. This involves a steady increase in type 1 diabetes and almost an exponential increase in type 2 diabetes. The latter is accompanied by a parallel increase in obesity, the metabolic syndrome, and other closely related disorders. Thus we are at a fascinating point in the evolution of diabetes and a fascinating point in the evolution of a book devoted to this disease.

The first edition of the Joslin textbook was published in 1916, a single-handed contribution by a man of extraordinary dedication, vision, and energy, Dr. Elliott P. Joslin. Dr. Joslin began his practice in 1898 in the pre-insulin era, and in this setting, developed a unique understanding of the natural history of diabetes. This perspective was clearly evident in the first edition, which was published some five years before the discovery of insulin by Banting, Best, Macleod, and Collip.

The third edition, published in 1923 shortly after the discovery of insulin, showed how quickly Joslin grasped the principles of insulin therapy, adopting approaches that would be considered modern even by today's standards. As a student of metabolism, Dr. Joslin was unwavering in his conviction that blood glucose levels should be kept as close to normal as possible, even though the importance and even the existence of chronic complications of diabetes were not appreciated until many years later. He understood the critical role of education for people with diabetes and made it the cornerstone of all treatment programs. His insights into the interaction between diet, exercise, and glucose control were also remarkable, considering how difficult it was to assess control accurately at this time. His descriptions of the symptoms of hypoglycemia are as well defined as can be found anywhere today, and he rapidly determined the small quantity of carbohydrate required to treat insulin reactions. Any serious student of diabetes should spend time with these early editions.

The evolution of the Joslin textbook mirrors the development of the field of diabetes and in some ways the development of Joslin Diabetes Center. Although the book was originally written entirely by Dr. Joslin himself, in subsequent editions he included his colleagues in the task, taking advantage of their special expertise. Eventually, substantial contributions to the book were provided not only by the staff of Joslin Diabetes Center, but also by clinicians from the adjacent New England Deaconess Hospital, where most Joslin patients were hospitalized.

Patients come to Joslin and its affiliated institutions from all over the world, knowing that whatever problems they have can be addressed by someone who understands the full complexity of diabetes. Thus, the Joslin staff consists of adult and pediatric diabetologists, nephrologists, ophthalmologists and optometrists, and mental health professionals, as well as nurse educators and nutrition specialists. Problems in vascular disease, cardiology, neurology, and in virtually all other areas of medicine, are now managed in collaboration with colleagues at the Beth Israel Deaconess Hospital (BIDMC). Women with diabetes also receive coordinated care between Joslin and BIDMC, and sick children often are hospitalized at Children's Hospital Boston.

To meet the challenges of the epidemic of diabetes, Joslin has established Affiliated Centers with 22 sites throughout the United States and our first international Affiliate in Bahrain. Because there are experts at these institutions who have extensive experience in virtually every aspect of diabetes care, some have joined with Joslin staff to write the clinical chapters, describing the characteristics and outcomes of their patients in the context of the broader literature.

Research has always been a fundamental focus at Joslin and as such has been reflected in all of the editions. Dr. Joslin himself was a fine clinical investigator who made astute observations about his patients and recorded the information in meticulous fashion, as can be appreciated in his numerous publications. He also recognized the need for a more organized approach to research and appointed Dr. Alexander Marble as the first head of research in 1934. The research programs were greatly expanded when Dr. Albert Renold took over the leadership in 1957, and further enhanced under the leadership of George Cahill, Stuart Soeldner, C. Ronald Kahn, and now George King.

Thus, the most recent editions of *Joslin's Diabetes Mellitus*, including the current edition, reflect not only the practice and experiences of the physicians of the Joslin Diabetes Center, but also the remarkable body of new scientific information that has had such an impact on the field. In addition, we have called upon former fellows and trainees of Joslin, now numbering over 1,200, and our academic colleagues elsewhere, to help present the latest advances in basic and clinical research.

The 14th edition is very different from the 13th edition published a decade ago. These differences demonstrate the dramatic advances in knowledge and research. Progress in the basic sciences has been explosive in recent years, particularly in the areas of immunology, insulin signaling, cell and molecular biology, and genetics. This has resulted in a remarkable increase in our understanding of the basic processes underlying type 1 and type 2 diabetes, as well as diabetes complications.

Because of this rapid rate of new knowledge, this text, like all modern biomedical texts, must be considered a living document, subject to change and updated regularly. Every reasonable effort has been made to have the 14th edition closely reflect our current understanding of diabetes.

In addition, while less emphasis has been given to the local Joslin experience in describing various aspects of diabetes care and more effort has been made to incorporate the experiences of others described in the literature, an effort has been made to retain the flavor of Joslin's clinical strategies and the emphasis on the importance of the team approach.

The Joslin Diabetes Center stands today as an institution on the front lines of the world epidemic of diabetes, leading the battle to conquer diabetes in all of its forms through cutting-edge research and innovative approaches to clinical care and education. Our task, of course, is to realize our vision of a world without diabetes and its complications. Disseminating the most current diabetes research and approaches to care is part of our vision and mission.

This 14th edition of *Joslin's Diabetes Mellitus* is dedicated to a number of special individuals—first, to Dr. Robert F. Bradley, who arrived at Joslin in 1950 as a young clinician fresh out of the Navy. By 1968, he had become the Medical Director of the Joslin Clinic, and in 1977, he became President of the fully integrated Joslin Diabetes Center. Under his leadership, Joslin grew steadily in both its clinical and research missions.

Perhaps Dr. Bradley's most significant contribution was his role in a major controversy of the mid-1970s over the use of oral drugs in the treatment of diabetes. A large NIH-funded study, the UGDP, suggested that the available oral agents for diabetes, the sulfonylureas, might not be safe. In fact, the study suggested that these agents might cause more deaths by producing certain cardiovascular side effects than they saved through treatment of diabetes. Dr. Bradley found this conclusion contrary to his own experience with thousands of patients with diabetes, and so he challenged this study, not just quietly and privately, but loudly and in the public eye. Consequently the UGDP study was found to be seriously flawed, and thus sulfonylureas, very important drugs for the treatment of type 2 diabetes, remained on the market. As a result, millions of patients with diabetes have benefited from improved diabetes control.

During his tenure, Dr. Bradley also edited the Joslin textbook, gave numerous lectures, and served on the first National Diabetes Advisory Board from 1977 to 1980. Bob retired in 1987 and died on October 12, 2003. He will always be remembered as a soft-spoken, highly dedicated leader and for the wonderful legacy he left for Joslin and people with diabetes throughout the world.

Second, we dedicate this 14th edition of *Joslin's Diabetes Mellitus* to all of the patients with diabetes and their families who have allowed us to care for them over the 106-year history of the Joslin Diabetes Center. They are the reason for our existence and the inspiration for working even harder. They inform our search for knowledge and our efforts to improve the lives of people with diabetes across the globe.

We also dedicate this 14th edition of *Joslin's Diabetes Mellitus* to all of those who have so generously supported Joslin with their efforts and funds to support research, clinical care, and education. Without that support, the institution could not survive and continue to work toward the cure, prevention, and improved treatment of diabetes and its complications.

Last, we wish to thank all of the individuals who worked together to bring this book to fruition. The authors of the various chapters spent untold hours thinking, researching, and writing to reach the level of excellence expected of a book of this stature. Two individuals, with whom it has been a pleasure to work, have made great contributions to the project. Susan Sjostrom, the Director of Publications at Joslin, was remarkably efficient at keeping track of all the manuscripts, disks, correspondence and e-mail. Nancy Voynow, the editorial assistant in Boston, was thoroughly professional, skilled, and efficient throughout, doing a wonderful job editing this enormous amount of complicated material. We also greatly appreciate the efforts and skill of our publisher, Lippincott Williams & Wilkins.

And, of course, most of all, we thank our families for their support and tolerance of the never-ending intrusion of this book into evenings, weekends, and at times even vacations.

Boston, Massachusetts

C. Ronald Kahn
Gordon C. Weir
George L. King
Alan M. Jacobson
Alan C. Moses
Robert J. Smith

Contributors

Martin J. Abrahamson, MD,
Acting Chief Medical Officer,
Joslin Diabetes Center;
Associate Professor of Medicine,
Harvard Medical School,
Boston, Massachusetts

Rexford S. Ahima, MD, PhD,
Attending Endocrinologist,
Hospital of the University of Pennsylvania;
Assistant Professor of Medicine, Division of Endocrinology,
University of Pennsylvania School of Medicine,
Philadelphia, Pennsylvania

Lloyd M. Aiello, MD,
Director, Beetham Eye Institute,
Joslin Diabetes Center;
Massachusetts Eye and Ear Infirmary;
Associate Clinical Professor of Ophthalmology,
Harvard Medical School,
Boston, Massachusetts

Lloyd Paul Aiello, MD, PhD,
Associate Director, Beetham Eye Institute,
Joslin Diabetes Center;
Massachusetts Eye and Ear Infirmary;
Associate Professor of Ophthalmology,
Harvard Medical School,
Boston, Massachusetts

Cameron M. Akbari, MD,
Attending Vascular Surgeon;
Director, Vascular Diagnostic Laboratory,
Washington Hospital Center,
Washington, DC

Stephanie A. Amiel, BSc, MD, FRCP,
Professor of Diabetic Medicine,
King's College Hospital;
R.D. Lawrence Professor of Diabetic Medicine,
Guy's King's and St. Thomas' School of Medicine,
King's College London,
London, United Kingdom

Barbara J. Anderson, PhD,
Pediatric Psychologist,
Department of Pediatric Endocrinology and Metabolism,
Texas Children's Hospital;
Associate Professor,
Department of Pediatrics,
Baylor College of Medicine,
Houston, Texas

Houman Ashrafian, BM, BChir, MA, MRCP,
Specialist Registrar,
Ealing Hospital
Middlesex, United Kingdom

Maha T. Barakat, MBBChir, MA, MRCP, PhD,
Honorary Consultant, Endocrinology,
Hammersmith Hospital;
Clinical Senior Lecturer,
Department of Metabolic Medicine,
Division of Investigative Science,
Imperial College, London, Hammersmith Hospital Campus,
London, United Kingdom

Donald M. Barnett, MD,
Senior Consultant,
Joslin Diabetes Center;
Assistant Clinical Professor of Medicine,
Harvard Medical School,
Boston, Massachusetts

Ananda Basu, MD, MRCP,
Consultant, Endocrinology and Metabolism, Mayo Clinic;
Assistant Professor, Department of Internal Medicine,
Mayo Clinic College of Medicine,
Rochester, Minnesota

Richard S. Beaser, MD,
Medical Executive Director of Professional Education, Strategic Initiatives,
Joslin Diabetes Center;
Assistant Clinical Professor of Medicine,
Harvard Medical School,
Boston, Massachusetts

Peter H. Bennett, MB, FRCP,
Scientist Emeritus, Phoenix Epidemiology and Clinical Research Branch,
National Institute of Diabetes and Digestive and Kidney Diseases,
Phoenix, Arizona

Caroline S. Blaum, MD, MS,
Associate Professor of Internal Medicine, Division of Geriatic Medicine,
University of Michigan Medical School;
Research Scientist,
Ann Arbor DVAMC GRECC,
Ann Arbor, Michigan

Stephen R. Bloom, MBBChir, MA, MD, DSc, FRCP, FRCPath,
Clinical Director of Pathology and Therapy Services,
Endocrinology, Hammersmith Hospitals NHS Trust;
Professor of Medicine, Department of Metabolic Medicine;
Head, Division of Investigative Science,
Imperial College, London, Hammersmith Hospital Campus,
London, United Kingdom

Lisa M. Bolduc-Bissell, RN, CDE,
Diabetes Nurse Clinician,
Department of Endocrinology,
Vermont Regional Diabetes Center,
Fletcher Allen Health Care,
Burlington, Vermont

Susan Bonner-Weir, PhD,
Senior Investigator, Section of Islet Transplantation and Cell Biology,
Joslin Diabetes Center;
Associate Professor of Medicine,
Harvard Medical School,
Boston, Massachusetts

Florence M. Brown, MD,
Senior Staff Physician,
Adult Internal Medicine,
Joslin Diabetes Center;
Instructor in Medicine,
Harvard Medical School,
Boston, Massachusetts

A. Enrique Caballero, MD,
Associate Director of Professional Education,
Director of the Latino Diabetes Initiative,
Joslin Diabetes Center;
Instructor in Medicine,
Harvard Medical School,
Boston, Massachusetts

Jonathan Castro, MD,
Clinical Assistant Instructor,
Division of Endocrinology,
State University of New York Downstate,
Brooklyn, New York

Melissa K. Cavaghan, MD,
Assistant Professor of Clinical Medicine,
Division of Endocrinology and Metabolism,
Indiana University School of Medicine,
Indianapolis, Indiana

Jerry D. Cavallerano, OD, PhD,
Staff Optometrist, Beetham Eye Institute,
Joslin Diabetes Center;
Associate Professor,
New England College of Optometry,
Boston, Massachusetts

Karen Hanson Chalmers, MS, RD, CDE,
Advanced Practice Diabetes Specialist,
Nutrition Services and Insulin Pump Program,
Joslin Clinic,
Joslin Diabetes Center,
Boston, Massachusetts

Alice Y.Y. Cheng, MD, FRCPC,
Endocrinologist, Division of Endocrinology and Metabolism;
Lecturer, Department of Medicine,
University of Toronto,
Toronto, Ontario, Canada

Stuart R. Chipkin, MD,
Professor of Exercise Science,
University of Massachusetts,
Amherst, Massachusetts

Ondine Cleaver, PhD,
Postdoctoral Fellow,
Molecular and Cellular Biology,
Harvard University,
Boston, Massachusetts

Sheila Collins, PhD,
Senior Investigator,
Endocrine Biology Program,
CIIT Centers for Health Research,
Research Triangle Park, North Carolina

Patrick Concannon, PhD,
Director, Molecular Genetics Program,
Benaroya Research Institute;
Affiliate Professor, Department of Immunology,
University of Washington,
Seattle, Washington

Ramachandiran Cooppan, MBChB, FRCP(c)FACE,
Senior Staff Physician, Department of Medicine,
Beth Israel Deaconess Medical Center;
Assistant Clinical Professor of Medicine,
Harvard Medical School,
Boston, Massachusetts

Alessandro Doria, MD, PhD,
Investigator, Section on Genetics and Epidemiology,
Joslin Diabetes Center;
Assistant Professor of Medicine,
Harvard Medical School,
Boston, Massachusetts

Jeffrey S. Dover, MD, FRCPC,
Director, SkinCare Physicians of Chestnut Hill,
Chestnut Hill, Massachusetts;
Professor of Dermatology,
Dartmouth Medical School,
Hanover, New Hampshire;
Professor of Dermatology,
Yale University School of Medicine,
New Haven, Connecticut

Victor J. Dzau, MD,
Chancellor for Health Affairs at Duke University;
President and CEO of Duke University Health System,
Durham, North Carolina

George S. Eisenbarth, MD, PhD,
Director, Barbara Davis Center for Childhood Diabetes,
University of Colorado Health Sciences Center;
Professor of Pediatrics/Immunology/Medicine,
University of Colorado,
Denver, Colorado

George M. Eliopoulos, MD,
Physician, Department of Medicine,
Division of Infectious Diseases,
Beth Israel Deaconess Medical Center;
Professor of Medicine,
Harvard Medical School,
Boston, Massachusetts

Elof Eriksson, MD, PhD,
Chief of Plastic and Reconstructive Surgery,
Division of Plastic Surgery,
Brigham and Women's Hospital,
The Children's Hospital Boston;
Joseph E. Murray Professor of Plastic and Reconstructive Surgery,
Harvard Medical School,
Boston, Massachusetts

Edward P. Feener, PhD,
Investigator, Section on Vascular Cell Biology,
Joslin Diabetes Center;
Assistant Professor of Medicine,
Harvard Medical School,
Boston, Massachusetts

Jeffrey S. Flier, MD,
Chief Academic Officer,
Beth Israel Deaconess Medical Center;
George C. Reisman Professor of Medicine,
Harvard Medical School,
Boston, Massachusetts

Roy Freeman, MD,
Director, Autonomic and Peripheral Nerve Laboratory, Department of Neurology,
Beth Israel Deaconess Medical Center;
Associate Professor of Neurology,
Harvard Medical School,
Boston, Massachusetts

Parham A. Ganchi, MD, PhD,
Assistant Professor of Plastic Surgery,
Division of Plastic and Reconstructive Surgery,
University of Medicine and Dentistry of New Jersey Hospital,
Newark, New Jersey

Om P. Ganda, MD,
Senior Physician,
Joslin Clinic, Joslin Diabetes Center;
Associate Clinical Professor of Medicine,
Harvard Medical School,
Boston, Massachusetts

Michael S. German, MD,
Hormone Research Institute and Diabetes Center,
Department of Medicine,
University of California at San Francisco,
San Francisco, California

John M. Giurini, DPM,
Chief, Division of Podiatry,
Beth Israel Deaconess Medical Center;
Associate Professor of Surgery,
Harvard Medical School,
Boston, Massachusetts

Benjamin Glaser, MD,
Director, Endocrinology and Metabolism Service,
Department of Internal Medicine,
Hadassah-Hebrew University Medical Center,
Jerusalem, Israel

Ann E. Goebel-Fabbri, PhD,
Psychologist,
Mental Health Unit,
Joslin Diabetes Center;
Instructor in Psychiatry,
Harvard Medical School,
Boston, Massachusetts

Allison B. Goldfine, MD,
Research Associate, Cellular and Molecular Physiology and
Clinical Research,
Joslin Diabetes Center;
Assistant Professor of Medicine,
Harvard Medical School,
Boston, Massachusetts

Irwin Goldstein, MD,
Professor of Urology,
Boston University School of Medicine,
Boston, Massachusetts

Laurie J. Goodyear, PhD,
Investigator and Section Head: Metabolism,
Joslin Diabetes Center;
Assistant Professor of Medicine,
Harvard Medical School,
Boston, Massachusetts

Raj K. Goyal, MD,
Staff Physician,
Gastroenterology,
VA Boston Healthcare System;
Mallinckrodt Professor of Medicine,
Harvard Medical School,
Boston, Massachusetts

Daryl K. Granner, MD,
Staff Physician,
VA Tennessee Valley Healthcare System;
Director, Vanderbilt Diabetes Center,
Vanderbilt University Medical Center;
Professor of Molecular Physiology and Biophysics,
Vanderbilt University,
Nashville, Tennessee

Gabriella Gruden, MD, PhD,
Researcher, Internal Medicine,
University of Turin,
Turin, Italy

Joel F. Habener, MD,
Chief, Medicine, Laboratory of Molecular Endocrinology,
Massachusetts General Hospital;
Professor of Medicine,
Harvard Medical School,
Boston, Massachusetts

Philippe A. Halban, PhD,
Professor, Department of Genetic Medicine
and Development,
University of Geneva,
Geneva, Switzerland

Jeffrey B. Halter, MD,
Director, Geriatrics Center and Institute of Gerontology;
Chief, Division of Geriatric Medicine, and
Professor of Internal Medicine,
University of Michigan Medical School,
Ann Arbor, Michigan

Andrew T. Hattersley, BM, BCh, DM,
Consultant Physician, Diabetes,
Royal Devon and Exeter Hospital;
Professor of Molecular Medicine,
Diabetes and Vascular Medicine,
Peninsula Medical School,
Exeter, United Kingdom

Meredith A.M. Hawkins, MD, MS,
Associate Professor,
Department of Medicine,
Diabetes Research and Training Center,
Albert Einstein College of Medicine,
Bronx, New York

Zhiheng He, MD, PhD,
Research Fellow,
Section for Vascular Biology and Complications,
Joslin Diabetes Center,
Boston, Massachusetts

Jean-Claude Henquin, MD, PhD,
Professor and Chairman, Department of Physiology and Pharmacology,
University of Louvain School of Medicine,
Brussels, Belgium

Edward S. Horton, MD,
Vice President and Director of Clinical Research,
Joslin Diabetes Center;
Professor of Medicine,
Harvard Medical School,
Boston, Massachusetts

Barbara V. Howard, PhD,
President, MedStar Research Institute,
Hyattsville, Maryland;
Professor of Medicine,
Georgetown University,
Washington, DC

Wm. James Howard, MD,
Vice President, Academic Affairs,
Washington Hospital Center;
Professor of Internal Medicine,
George Washington University,
Washington, DC

M. Elaine Husni, MD,
Associate Physician,
Rheumatology Department,
Brigham and Women's Hospital;
Instructor in Medicine,
Harvard Medical School,
Boston, Massachusetts

Alan M. Jacobson, MD,
Senior Vice President, Strategic Initiatives Division; Head of the Behavioral and Mental Health Unit,
Joslin Diabetes Center;
Professor of Psychiatry,
Harvard Medical School,
Boston, Massachusetts

Michael D. Jensen, MD,
Professor of Medicine,
Division of Endocrinology,
Mayo Clinic College of Medicine,
Rochester, Minnesota

Michael T. Johnstone, MD,
Staff Cardiologist, Department of Medicine,
Beth Israel Deaconess Medical Center;
Assistant Professor of Medicine,
Harvard Medical School,
Boston, Massachusetts

Alison C. Jozsi, PhD,
Medical Science Liaison,
Bristol-Myers Squibb Company,
Cardiovascular Divison,
Old Greenwich, Connecticut
(formerly Postdoctoral Fellow in Medicine,
Joslin Diabetes Center,
Boston, Massachusetts)

Barbara B. Kahn, MD,
Chief, Division of Endocrinology, Diabetes and Metabolism,
Beth Israel Deaconess Medical Center;
Professor of Medicine,
Harvard Medical School,
Boston, Massachusetts

C. Ronald Kahn, MD,
President and Director,
Joslin Diabetes Center;
Mary K. Iacocca Professor of Medicine,
Harvard Medical School,
Boston, Massachusetts

Timothy J. Kieffer, PhD,
Associate Professor,
Physiology and Surgery,
University of British Columbia,
Vancouver, British Columbia,
Canada

George L. King, MD,
Director of Research and Head of the
Section on Vascular Cell Biology,
Joslin Diabetes Center;
Professor of Medicine,
Harvard Medical School,
Boston, Massachusetts

Dmitri Kirpichnikov, MD,
Chief, Division of Endocrinology,
Lutheran Hospital Center,
Brooklyn, New York

William C. Knowler, MD, PhD,
Chief, Diabetes and Arthritis Epidemiology Section,
National Institute of Diabetes and Digestive and Kidney Diseases,
Phoenix, Arizona

Leo P. Krall, MD†

Andrzej S. Krolewski, MD, PhD,
Senior Investigator and Section Head,
Research Division,
Genetics and Epidemiology,
Joslin Diabetes Center;
Associate Professor of Medicine,
Harvard Medical School,
Boston, Massachusetts

Susan F. Kroop, MD,
Attending Physician,
Department of Medicine,
Vanderbilt University Medical Center;
Assistant Professor, Department of Medicine,
Vanderbilt University School of Medicine,
Nashville, Tennessee

Lori M.B. Laffel, MD, MPH,
Chief, Pediatric and Adolescent Unit,
Joslin Diabetes Center;
Assistant Professor of Pediatrics,
Harvard Medical School,
Boston, Massachusetts

Margaret T. Lawlor, MS, CDE,
Coordinator of Pediatric Research and Education,
Pediatric and Adolescent Unit,
Joslin Diabetes Center,
Boston, Massachusetts

Jack L. Leahy, MD,
Chief, Division of Endocrinology,
Diabetes and Metabolism,
Fletcher Allen Health Care;
Professor of Medicine,
University of Vermont,
Burlington, Vermont

Harold E. Lebovitz, MD,
Professor of Medicine, and Chief,
Section of Endocrinology and Diabetes,
State University of New York Health Science Center at Brooklyn,
Brooklyn, New York

Gil Leibowitz, MD,
Senior Lecturer, Endocrinology and Metabolism Service,
Department of Internal Medicine,
Hadassah-Hebrew University Medical Center,
Jerusalem, Israel

Edward H. Leiter, PhD,
Senior Staff Scientist,
The Jackson Laboratory,
Bar Harbor, Maine

Frank W. LoGerfo, MD,
Chairman, Department of Surgery;
Program Director, The William J. von Liebig Foundation,
Beth Israel Deaconess Medical Center;
The William V. McDermott Professor of Surgery,
Harvard Medical School,
Boston, Massachusetts

Phillip A. Low, MD,
Consultant, Neurologist,
Department of Neurology,
Mayo Clinic;
Professor, Department of Neurology,
Mayo School of Graduate Medical Education,
Rochester, Minnesota

Mark H. Lowitt, MD,
Physician, Annapolis Dermatology Associates, Annapolis;
Clinical Associate Professor,
Department of Dermatology,
University of Maryland School of Medicine,
Baltimore, Maryland

Eleftheria Maratos-Flier, MD,
Adjunct Senior Investigator,
Joslin Diabetes Center;
Associate Professor of Medicine,
Harvard Medical School,
Boston, Massachusetts

† Deceased.

Hiroshi Mashimo, MD, PhD,
Chief of Gastroenterology,
Department of Medicine,
VA Boston Healthcare System;
Assistant Professor of Medicine,
Brigham and Women's Hospital,
Harvard Medical School,
Boston, Massachusetts

Clayton E. Mathews, PhD,
Assistant Professor, Diabetes Institute,
Children's Hospital of Pittsburgh;
Assistant Professor of Pediatrics,
University of Pittsburgh,
Pittsburgh, Pennsylvania

Roger J. May, MD[†]

Karen C. McCowen, MD,
Physician, Department of Medicine, Beth Israel Deaconess Medical Center;
Assistant Professor of Medicine,
Harvard Medical School,
Boston, Massachusetts

Samy I. McFarlane, MD, MPH,
Associate Professor of Medicine and Radiology,
State University of New York Downstate/
King's County Hospital Center,
Brooklyn, New York

Douglas A. Melton, PhD,
Principal Investigator,
Department of Molecular and Cellular Biology,
Harvard University,
Boston, Massachusetts

Alan C. Moses, MD,
Former Chief Medical Officer,
Joslin Diabetes Center;
Professor of Medicine (on leave),
Harvard Medical School,
Boston, Massachusetts;
Associate Vice President of Medical Affairs,
Novo Nordisk Pharmaceuticals Inc.,
Princeton, New Jersey

Ricardo Munarriz, MD,
Assistant Professor of Urology,
Boston University School of Medicine,
Boston, Massachusetts

Martin G. Myers, Jr, MD, PhD,
Assistant Professor,
Department of Internal Medicine and
Department of Physiology,
University of Michigan Medical School,
Ann Arbor, Michigan

K. Sreekumaran Nair, MD, PhD, FRCP,
Consultant in Endocrinology,
Department of Medicine/Endocrinology, Metabolism, and Nutrition,
Mayo Clinic;
Professor of Medicine, David Murdock Dole Professor of Nutrition,
Department of Internal Medicine,
Mayo Clinic College of Medicine,
Rochester, Minnesota

David M. Nathan, MD,
Director, Diabetes Center and General Clinical Research Center,
Massachusetts General Hospital;
Professor of Medicine,
Harvard Medical School,
Boston, Massachusetts

Richard W. Nesto, MD,
Chairman, Department of Cardiovascular Medicine at Lahey Clinic Medical Center,
Burlington;
Associate Professor of Medicine,
Harvard Medical School,
Boston, Massachusetts

Cynthia Pasquarello, BSN, RN, CDE,
Pediatric and Adolescent Diabetes Nurse Specialist, Joslin Clinic,
Joslin Diabetes Center,
Boston, Massachusetts

F. Xavier Pi-Sunyer, MD, MPH,
Chief, Division of Endocrinology, Diabetes, and Nutrition,
St. Luke's–Roosevelt Hospital Center;
Professor of Medicine,
Columbia University,
New York, New York

Kenneth S. Polonsky, MD,
Adolphus Bush Professor and Chairman,
Department of Medicine,
Washington University School of Medicine,
St. Louis, Missouri

Christian Rask-Madsen, MD, PhD,
Research Fellow,
Section for Vascular Biology and Complications,
Joslin Diabetes Center,
Boston, Massachusetts

Helena Reijonen, PhD,
Staff Scientist,
Department of Immunology,
Benaroya Research Institute,
Seattle, Washington

Christopher J. Rhodes, PhD,
Associate Scientific Director,
Professor of Pharmacology (affiliated),
Pacific Northwest Research Institute,
Seattle, Washington

James L. Rosenzweig, MD,
Associate Chief, Section on Adult Diabetes;
Director, Disease State Management Program, Joslin Diabetes Center;
Staff Physician, Department of Internal Medicine,
Beth Israel Deaconess Medical Center;
Assistant Professor of Medicine,
Harvard Medical School,
Boston, Massachusetts

Luciano Rossetti, MD,
Professor of Medicine and Molecular Pharmacology;
Director, Diabetes Research and Training Center,
Albert Einstein College of Medicine,
Bronx, New York

Neil B. Ruderman, MD, DPhil,
Director, Diabetes Unit, Department of Medicine (Endocrinology),
Boston Medical Center;
Professor of Medicine and Physiology,
Boston University School of Medicine,
Boston, Massachusetts

Alan R. Saltiel, PhD,
Director, Life Sciences Institute;
John Jacob Abel Professor, Professor of
Internal Medicine and Physiology, Life Sciences Institute,
Ann Arbor, Michigan

Donald K. Scott, PhD,
Assistant Professor,
Department of Biochemistry and Molecular Biology,
Louisiana State University Health Sciences Center,
New Orleans, Louisiana

Deborah E. Sentochnik, MD,
Chief, Infectious Disease Division,
Bassett Healthcare, Cooperstown;
Assistant Clinical Professor of Medicine,
Department of Internal Medicine,
Columbia University College of Physicians and Surgeons,
New York, New York

Julie Lund Sharpless, MD,
Assistant Professor of Medicine,
Department of Endocrinology,
University of North Carolina,
Chapel Hill, North Carolina

Jonathan Shaw, MD, MRCP,
Director of Research,
International Diabetes Institute,
Caulfield, Victoria;
Senior Lecturer,
Department of Medicine,
Monash University,
Melbourne, Australia

Steven E. Shoelson, MD, PhD,
Associate Director of Research,
Head of Section on Cellular and Molecular Physiology,
Joslin Diabetes Center;
Professor of Medicine,
Harvard Medical School,
Boston, Massachusetts

Gerald I. Shulman, MD, PhD,
Attending Physician, Department of Internal Medicine,
Yale–New Haven Hospital;
Investigator, Howard Hughes Medical Institute;
Professor of Internal Medicine and Cellular and Molecular Physiology,
Yale School of Medicine,
New Haven, Connecticut

Lee S. Simon, MD,
Associate Chief of Medicine,
Beth Israel Deaconess Medical Center;
Assistant Professor of Medicine, Division of Rheumatology,
Harvard Medical School,
Boston, Massachusetts

[†] Deceased.

Robert J. Smith, MD,
Director of Endocrinology and the Hallett Center for Diabetes and Endocrinology, Rhode Island Hospital;
Professor of Medicine and Director, Division of Endocrinology, Brown Medical School,
Providence, Rhode Island

James R. Sowers, MD,
Professor of Medicine and Physiology,
Associate Dean of Clinical Research,
University of Missouri Health Science Center,
Columbia, Missouri

Robert C. Stanton, MD,
Chief, Renal Section,
Joslin Diabetes Center;
Assistant Professor of Medicine,
Harvard Medical School,
Boston, Massachusetts

Jeanne H. Steppel, MD,
Research Associate, Clinical Research,
Joslin Diabetes Center;
Instructor in Medicine,
Harvard Medical School,
Boston, Massachusetts

Craig S. Stump, MD,
Staff Physician, Specialty Service, Endocrinology,
Harry S. Truman VA Hospital;
Assistant Professor of Internal Medicine,
Division of Endocrinology and Metabolism,
University of Missouri–Columbia,
Columbia, Missouri

Roy Taylor, BSc, MB, ChB, MD, FRCP, FRCPE,
Honorary Consultant Physician,
Diabetes Unit, Royal Victoria Infirmary;
Professor of Medicine and Metabolism,
School of Clinical Medical Sciences,
Newcastle University Medical School,
Newcastle upon Tyne, United Kingdom

Keith Tornheim, PhD,
Associate Professor of Biochemistry,
Boston University School of Medicine,
Boston, Massachusetts

Abdulmaged Traish, PhD,
Professor of Urology,
Boston University School of Medicine,
Boston, Massachusetts

GianCarlo Viberti, MD, FRCP,
Honorary Consultant Physician,
Endocrinology and Diabetes,
Guy's Hospital;
Professor of Diabetes and Metabolic Medicine, Division of Cardiovascular Medicine,
Guy's King's and St. Thomas' School of Medicine, King's College London,
London, United Kingdom

James H. Warram, MD, ScD,
Investigator, Research Division,
Genetics and Epidemiology,
Joslin Diabetes Center;
Instructor of Epidemiology,
Harvard School of Public Health,
Boston, Massachusetts

Katie Weinger, EdD, RN,
Director, Office of Research Fellow Affairs;
Director, Center for Innovation in Diabetes Education,
Joslin Diabetes Center;
Assistant Professor of Psychiatry,
Harvard Medical School,
Boston, Massachusetts

Gordon C. Weir, MD,
Head, Section on Islet Transplantation and Cell Biology;
Diabetes Research and Wellness Foundation Chair,
Joslin Diabetes Center;
Professor of Medicine,
Harvard Medical School,
Boston, Massachusetts

Mark E. Williams, MD,
Senior Staff Physician,
Renal Unit,
Joslin Diabetes Center;
Associate Clinical Professor of Medicine,
Harvard Medical School,
Boston, Massachusetts

Howard A. Wolpert, MD,
Section on Adult Diabetes,
Joslin Diabetes Center;
Instructor in Medicine,
Harvard Medical School,
Boston, Massachusetts

Jennifer Wyckoff, MD,
Physician, Section on Adult Diabetes and Endocrinology,
Joslin Diabetes Center;
Instructor in Medicine,
Harvard Medical School,
Boston, Massachusetts

Paul Zimmet, MD, PhD, FRACP, FRCP, FACE, FACN, FAFPHM,
Director, International Diabetes Institute,
Caulfield,Victoria;
Professor, Department of Biochemistry and Molecular Biology,
Monash University,
Melbourne, Australia

Bernard Zinman, MDCM, FRCPC, FACP,
Director, Leadership Sinai Centre for Diabetes,
Mount Sinai Hospital;
Professor of Medicine,
University of Toronto,
Toronto, Ontario, Canada

Contents

† Deceased.

†Deceased.

CHAPTER 1
The History of Diabetes

Donald M. Barnett and Leo P. Krall†

When Elliott Proctor Joslin first published his textbook *The Treatment of Diabetes Mellitus* more than 85 years ago in 1916, it represented the first rendition of its kind in the English language (1). During Joslin's long professional life, he remained the senior editor for 10 editions, maintaining the same enthusiasm as he and his team continued to report the experience of the Joslin Clinic and increasingly that of other investigators. Elliott P. Joslin (1869–1962) (Fig. 1.1) was part of the last generation of physicians who received much of their postgraduate training in Europe (2). After his 1895 graduation from Harvard Medical School, he became inspired by the examples of the French and German medical schools that sought to combine laboratory and clinical medicine. From the start of his practice in 1898, he continued to attract assistants and students to observe and apprentice with him in the treatment of an increasing number of patients with this hitherto poorly defined condition, diabetes.

Fifteen years before the discovery of insulin, Joslin began collaborating with the physiologist Francis Benedict of the Carnegie Institute on studies of metabolic balance (3). Joslin's simultaneous association with the young polymath investigator Frederick Allen at the Harvard Medical School also proved fortunate. Allen, who was observant of all the known literature on the subject up to that time, was able to translate his ideas from his experimental animal models to humans on the wards of the new Rockefeller Institute (4). By 1914, Joslin, desperate to lower the death rate from ketoacidosis in his mostly young patients with diabetes, combined Benedict's balance study format with diets in a wide range of human subjects in near or actual acidosis (2). By 1917, he had become progressively convinced that he had developed a regimen that could extend the life expectancy of these fatally ill patients (5).

In his writings and lectures on diabetes, Joslin was an early proponent of several concepts, with two being especially important. First, as early as 1920 he emphasized the need to contain the "epidemic" of the disease by judicious diet and exercise (6); second, he pioneered patient education as a primary part of treatment. His goals were to prevent the onset of the disease or to retard its progression. To accomplish these aims, he created a freestanding clinic devoted to a single disease.

Joslin's interest in all matters of medicine could be inferred from pictures on the walls of his office, as well as from the bas relief panels on the modern exterior of his institute, where sculptured portraits were displayed of many of his "medical saints," as he phrased it, from Thomas Hunter, the father of comparative anatomy, to Charles Best, the "codiscoverer of insulin." Three investigators of the 19th century particularly influenced Joslin's world: Louis Pasteur, Claude Bernard, and Rudolf Virchow. Two were Frenchmen, Pasteur, who understood the cause-and-effect contributions of microbes in the pathogenesis of infection, and Bernard, who established modern physiologic investigation. The third investigator, Virchow, the leading German pathologist of his time, demonstrated that disease entities were characterized primarily by a disruption of the integrity of normal cellular health (7).

The story of diabetes and dates in the life of Joslin were closely intertwined. In 1869, the year of Joslin's birth, Paul Langerhans,

†Deceased.

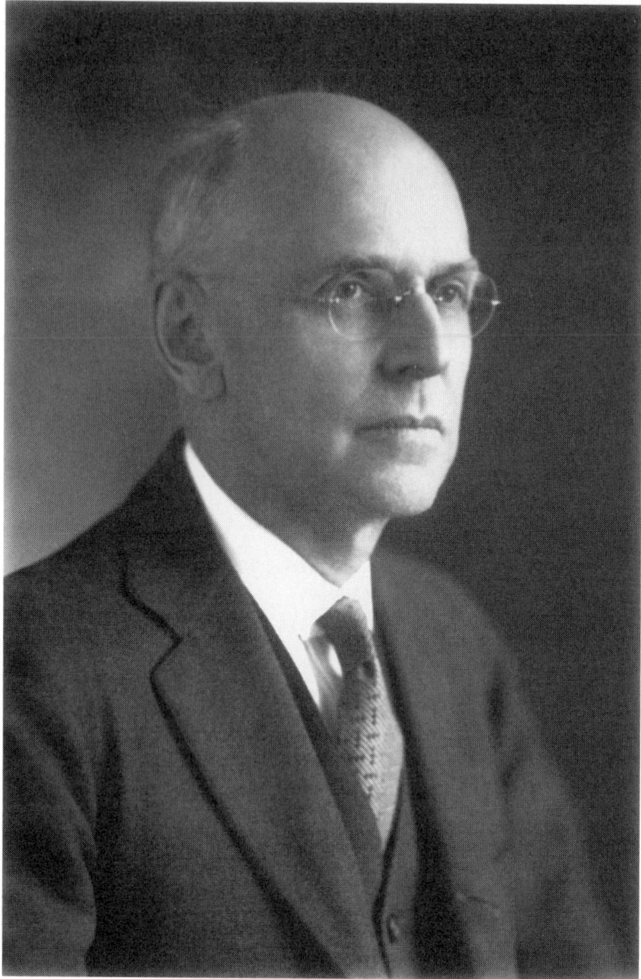

Figure 1.1. Eliott Proctor Joslin at 60.

a senior medical student in Virchow's department, published his medical dissertation on pancreatic histology in which he described "clumps of cells," which were named the *islets of Langerhans* shortly after his premature death in 1888 (8–10). By 1889, the year that Minkowski and Von Mering, in Strassburg, Germany, discovered the central role of the pancreas in diabetes (11,12), Joslin decided to spend a postgraduate year in physiologic chemistry at Yale's Sheffield School of Science, an experience that led to his initial interest in diabetes. It was not until midcareer, when Joslin was in his early 50s, that the discovery of insulin ended years of frustration encountered in caring for desperately ill patients with diabetes.

By 1952 organizational efforts in many countries developed to the point that the International Diabetes Federation was formed to increase awareness of the disease and to promote better investigation and treatment programs worldwide. Elliott Joslin became honorary president of the International Diabetes Federation, confirming his role as the international "dean" in the cause of diabetes. By this time he had initiated the first population survey and follow-up studies demonstrating a surprisingly high prevalence rate of diabetes in a typical U.S. population, the study being carried out in his hometown of Oxford, Massachusetts. In addition, the prevalence rate was nearly equally divided among those people with undetected disease and those with diagnosed diabetes (13). These studies set the stage for early-detection programs countrywide sponsored by the American Diabetes Association.

Joslin and his early associates became identified with the conservative viewpoint that "good" control delayed or prevented microvascular complications, particularly in type 1 diabetes. This position inaugurated an intense nationwide 30-year debate that only ended in 1993 with the publication of the results of the Diabetes Control and Complications Trial (14), which clearly supported Joslin's claim.

THE ROAD TO INSULIN

The story of the earliest recognition of diabetes and the path to the discovery of insulin is filled with marvelous insights as well as egregious errors, serendipity and futile labors, triumphs, and defeats. The best early evidence of a description of the symptoms of diabetes in the world's literature is recorded in the Ebers papyrus that appears to date from 1550 B.C. This links the description of polyuria to Imhotep, a man of medicine, architecture, and magic, who was a high priest and minister to the Pharaoh Zosser in 3000 B.C. (15). Two Greek physicians in the Roman era, Galen (A.D. 130–201), who practiced in Rome, and Arateus of Cappadocia, delineated the disease further. Arateus is credited, despite the survival of only fragments of his documents, with some of the best descriptions of medicine in the ancient literature. In his work *Acute and Chronic Diseases*, he coined the term *diabetes*, meaning "siphon," to explain the "liquefaction of the flesh and bones into urine" (16).

The following masterly description of severe diabetes by Arateus from about A.D. 150 represents the sum of our knowledge up until the second half of the 17th century (17):

> Diabetes is a wonderful affection, not very frequent among men, being a melting down of the flesh and limbs into urine. Its course is of a cold and humid nature, as in dropsy. The course is the common one, namely, the kidneys and the bladder; for the patients never stop making water, but the flow is incessant, as if from the opening of aqueducts. The nature of the disease then, is chronic, and it takes a long period to form: but the patient is short-lived, if the constitution of the disease be completely established; for the melting is rapid, the death speedy.

In 1674, Thomas Willis, a physician, an anatomist, and a professor of natural philosophy at Oxford, discovered (by tasting) that the urine of individuals with diabetes was sweet (18). This was actually a rediscovery, for unbeknownst to him, an ancient Hindu document by Susruta in India in about 400 B.C. had described the diabetic syndrome as characterized by a "honeyed urine" (19). Willis could not pinpoint the chemical nature of the "sweet" substance, because a variety of different chemical substances could be equally sweet to the sense of taste. It was Matthew Dobson of Manchester, England, who demonstrated, in 1776, that persons with diabetes actually excrete sugar in the urine. After boiling urine to dryness, he noted that the residue, a crystalline material, had the appearance and taste of "brown sugar" (20).

Dobson's definitive finding soon began influencing clinicians as to the possible causes of the disease and the bodily organs primarily involved. The prevalent view up to that time was that the kidneys were the major source of the problem, because its most striking signs and symptoms were the frequency and degree of urination. Some clinical observers also noted a tendency toward enlargement of the liver, which we now know to be usually due to intense infiltration of the organ with fat in persons with uncontrolled diabetes. In a case report, which also gave a detailed description of postmortem findings, Thomas Cawley reported in 1788 (without particular comment) on a shriveled pancreas with stones in a diabetic patient at autopsy (21). This may have been the first published reference to the pancreas in relation to human diabetes, but no deductions were drawn regarding etiology.

It was John Rollo, Surgeon General of the Royal Artillery, who in 1797 first applied the discovery of glycosuria by Dobson to the quantitative metabolic study of diabetes. Aided by William Cruickshank, "apothecary and chemist to the ordinance," Rollo devised the first rational approach to the dietary treatment of the disease, shifting the view then current that the primary seat of the disorder was the kidneys to a view of its being the gastrointestinal tract (22). Rollo studied Captain Meredith, a corpulent man with adult-onset diabetes and severe glycosuria. Rollo made daily recordings of the amounts and kinds of food Meredith ate and weighed the sugar cake obtained by boiling Meredith's daily urine output. Rollo noted that the amount of sugar excreted varied from day to day, depending primarily on the type of food ingested. "Vegetable" matter (i.e., breads, grains, fruits) increased glycosuria, whereas "animal" matter (i.e., meat) resulted in a comparatively lower excretion of sugar. Rollo and Cruickshank concluded, therefore, that the glycosuria was secondary to the "saccharification" of "vegetable" matter (i.e., carbohydrate-containing foods in the stomach and the influx of sugar into the body) and concluded that the "morbid" organ in diabetes was not the kidney but the "stomach," which overproduced sugar from "vegetable" matter. The indicated treatment was thus a diet low in carbohydrates and high in fat and protein (22). It was not until the advent of insulin that this dietary prescription was altered significantly.

Although Rollo suspected the presence of excessive sugar in the blood of persons with diabetes, at that time there was no convincing proof of the existence of hyperglycemia. William Wollaston (1766–1828), a renowned chemist and physician, tried to measure "sugar" in the blood but failed to detect it, possibly because he assumed it had the same chemical characteristics as table sugar (19). In 1815, Chevreuil showed that blood sugar behaved chemically as if it were "grape" sugar (i.e., dextrose or glucose) (23). Only in the period 1914 to 1919 were specific methods of analysis devised and used to measure glucose as the major "reducing substance" in the serum and urine (24–26). Rollo's predictions were confirmed—that in diabetes an increase in blood sugar level causes the excretion of sugar and that the "seat" of diabetes was outside the kidneys.

Lavoisier's Legacy

A set of experiments initiated in the late 18th century deepened understanding of the basic metabolic principles of human physiology and had far-reaching consequences for medicine and for diabetes in particular. Antoine Lavoisier (1743–1794) established the concept of the respiratory quotient and with the aid of calorimetric studies measured oxygen consumption at rest and under different conditions, such as during food ingestion and work; however, his studies were interrupted by his death by guillotine during the French Revolution. A generation later, Baron Justus von Liebig (1803–1873) advanced the field of physiologic chemistry by determining that there were three categories of food: protein, carbohydrate, and fat. As described by Rosen (27), Liebig showed how protein was used to build up or repair the organism while carbohydrate and fat were used for fuel. He determined how much oxygen was needed to burn the different classes of food and how much energy was released as heat. Carl Voit, writing in 1865, described his teacher's work in these terms: "Liebig was the first to establish the importance of chemical transformations in the body. He stated that the phenomena of motion and activity which we call life arise from the interaction of oxygen, food and the components of the body. He clearly saw the relation between metabolism and activity and that not only heat but all motion was derived from metabolism. . . ." Voit's work, as carried on by his student Max Rubner in Germany and by his American students Graham Lusk and W. O. Atwater, made it possible to study metabolic activities more precisely and to apply the results to clinical and theoretical problems. Rubner, in 1888 to 1890, finally produced incontrovertible experimental proof that the principle of the conservation of energy held for living systems, a finding confirmed for humans by Atwater and Benedict in 1903 (28). In 1874 the unique respirations seen in diabetic ketoacidosis were described by Adolph Kussmaul as being deep and having long pauses between expiration and inspiration (29).

Turning their attention to the pancreas, clinicians in England, France, and Germany in the mid-1800s described cases of diabetes with postmortem findings of diseased, atrophic, or stone-filled pancreases. Speculations on the role of this organ in diabetes abounded, but the evidence was not at all convincing, because in the vast majority of patients with diabetes, the pancreas was of normal size and appearance at autopsy. With the pancreas being thought of only as a purely exocrine gland, the finding of pathologic lesions in the pancreas in a small group of diabetic individuals was interpreted as only a chance phenomenon.

In France, Claude Bernard was aware of the findings and speculations regarding the possible role of the pancreas in diabetes. To test this hypothesis, he ligated pancreatic ducts of dogs and/or injected them with oil or paraffin to block all secretion, which led to profound atrophy of the gland. Because only a few strands of what appeared to be lifeless scar tissue remained, Bernard assumed that the atrophy was indeed complete. Despite this, the animals showed neither glycosuria nor any other indication of diabetes (30). Such experiments also were performed by Moritz Schiff, with equally negative results. This "antipancreatic" viewpoint was thus immeasurably strengthened by the authoritative voices of the foremost physiologists of the age. Bernard's celebrated findings of glycosuria after "piqûre" of the IVth ventricle drew attention to the possibility that alterations in the central nervous system could be etiologically related to diabetes. A lesion in the brain would cause hyperglycemia by way of the "visceral" nerves acting on the liver.

The Search for the Cause of Diabetes

Between 1840 and 1860, physiologic studies in metabolism as they relate to diabetes began their advance, especially in France under the leadership of Claude Bernard. His epoch-making discovery that blood glucose was derived in part from glycogen as a "secretion" of the liver thus identified the liver as a central organ in diabetes and explained how a diabetic patient whose liver was scarred by the end stages of cirrhosis might be "cured" of his hyperglycemia and glycosuria.

The two strongest forces arguing for a "pancreatic" factor in the etiology of diabetes were Apollinaire Bouchardat and E. Lancereaux. Bouchardat, who trained in organic chemistry and was an early pioneer in the study of fermentation and a professor of public health, did meticulous long-term studies on human diabetes. These began in 1835 and were gathered into his 1875 book, *De la Glycosurie ou Diabète Sucré* (31). He followed the essentials of Rollo's dietary regimen in treating diabetes but added a very important therapeutic arm by encouraging hard physical labor, having observed ameliorative effects of muscular work on glycosuria and hyperglycemia. Yet above all, his clinical experience taught him to distinguish at least two different types of diabetes: the severe type in younger persons who responded poorly to his regimen and the type in older, obese persons for whom the prescribed therapy of diet and physical exertion worked admirably. The clinical behavior of the two types of diabetes and the postmortem findings led Bouchardat to suggest that the more severe form was pancreatic in origin.

Lancereaux and his students came to identical conclusions about etiology and introduced the terms *diabète maigre* (diabetes of the thin) and *diabète gras* (diabetes of the fat) for the two common clinical forms of the disease (32). Because *diabète gras* was the more frequently occurring type, it now became understandable why severe pancreatic damage was found less frequently than expected. A pancreatic etiology for *diabète maigre* thus became an acceptable postulate, even though one could not yet form a sound notion about the mechanisms involved.

The concept that the body possesses glands that deliver their products directly to the blood (ductless or "blood" glands) gained substantial ground through Berthold's study of castration in 1849 (33), the clinical description of Addison disease in 1849 (34), and the experimental ablation of the adrenal gland by Charles Brown-Séquard in 1856 (35).

Pancreatic Diabetes

A decisive turning point in the history of diabetes was marked by the experimental work of Joseph von Mering and Oscar Minkowski in 1889 (11,12). Von Mering was interested in the possible role of the pancreas in the digestion and absorption of fats. From the literature then available, primarily the writings of Claude Bernard, von Mering understood that it was virtually impossible for an animal to survive total removal of the pancreas. He consulted with Minkowski, the assistant to Albert Naunyn, the foremost European clinician in diabetes at that time. Undaunted by the previous experiments, von Mering and Minkowski operated on two dogs, and both animals survived the complete pancreatectomy. Within less than a day, these animals exhibited unexpected behavior—in particular, frequent and voluminous urination. Minkowski's experience with severe human diabetes led him to examine the urine for sugar. During the next 2 years, Minkowski extended this serendipitous finding into an in-depth, now classic, study of experimental diabetes and its metabolic deviations. The study remains a model of scientific physiologic inquiry. He demonstrated clearly that the pancreas was a gland of internal secretion and that a small portion of the gland, when implanted under the skin of a freshly depancreatized dog, prevented the appearance of hyperglycemia until the implanted tissue was removed or had degenerated spontaneously.

Confirmation of these findings came very quickly from Hedon and coworkers in France. In 1893 Laguesse drew proper attention to the almost forgotten original observations of Langerhans and suggested the collections of interacinar cells (which he designated the *islets of Langerhans*) as a gland of secretion within the pancreas (36).

Thus, modern experimental and clinical endocrinology developed during the last decade of the 19th century. The term *hormone* was introduced by William Bayliss and Ernest Starling in 1902 to designate a specific chemical material elaborated by a ductless gland into the blood that is conveyed to other parts of the body and exerts an effect upon its "target" tissues (37). In 1910, Jean de Meyer suggested that the pancreatic secretion that was lacking in the diabetic state should, when found, be called "insulin" to denote its origin from the "insulae" of Langerhans (38).

Between 1895 and 1921, experimental work developed in two directions. One was the careful histologic study of the islets, which led to the finding of several distinct cell types, thus foreshadowing our present knowledge that the islets of Langerhans are the site of production and secretion of several hormones in addition to insulin. Of note was the description of hyalinization in islets of people with diabetes by E. L. Opie in 1900 (39). This hyalinization has since been shown to be the amyloid commonly found in the islets of people with type 2 diabetes, but this observation again linked the islets of Langerhans with diabetes. The other was a search for insulin itself. The requirements for insulin as a potential therapeutic agent were stringent: (a) the preparation had to be of consistent potency; (b) it should reverse the metabolic abnormalities of the depancreatized animal; (c) it should reverse the signs, symptoms, and chemical abnormalities of human diabetes; and (d) it should produce no harmful side effects.

The difficulties in the early attempts to isolate insulin were legion. There was total ignorance of the chemical nature of the postulated antidiabetic substance, making the extraction procedure a hit-or-miss proposition. At that time, quantitative estimates of the blood sugar required inordinate amounts of blood and the procedure was not generally available. Because of ignorance about the profound effects of low blood sugar levels on the nervous system (hypoglycemic convulsions), they were also not recognized as such and were initially attributed to a "toxic" action of the extract. In addition, fever and infections were frequent sequelae of the injections of extracts. In view of the protein nature of the hormone (which, of course, was not yet known), it is obvious that those workers who used oral administration of the extract were bound to fail. Of the many forerunners of Banting and Best, those who came closest to the mark were E. L. Scott, Israel Kleiner, Ludwig Zuelzer, and Nicolas Paulesco, as has been well described by Bliss (40). Indeed, Paulesco, a distinguished Romanian physiologist, produced a pancreatic extract that fulfilled all the criteria for "insulin" in animal experimentation but did not succeed in showing its application in human diabetes (41). Thus, the significance of his contribution was appreciated only much later.

Frederick Banting, a young surgeon; John Macleod, a professor of physiology; Charles Best, a graduate student; and J. B. Collip, a skilled chemist, succeeded during the years 1921 and 1922 in fulfilling all of the criteria for a therapeutically active insulin and produced the first useful and consistently successful insulin preparation for the treatment of human diabetes. Thus, the pancreatic etiology of diabetes was finally established (42).

The Nobel Prize for the Discovery of Insulin

The awarding of the Nobel Prize in Medicine in October 1923, 18 months after the first news of the discovery of insulin, was part of a gripping tale of success, disappointment, and conflict. The story of Banting, Best, Collip, and Macleod brought to light the tensions of a 6-month period that began in the summer of 1921 and intensified when the new extract corrected the metabolic acidosis in the first person to receive the substance in January 1922 (Leonard Thompson, age 14 years, at the Toronto General Hospital in Canada).

The drama started when Frederick Banting, a World War I veteran surgeon who was barely employed, was asked to be an instructor in physiology at the University of Western Ontario in Canada and became inspired by reading an article in the fall of 1920 by the pathologist Moses Barron. The article was entitled "The Relation of Islets of Langerhans to Diabetes with Special Reference to Cases of Pancreatic Lithiasis" (43). Armed with this information, the 29-year-old Banting persuaded Professor Macleod of the University of Toronto to provide him the space and equipment to attempt to extract a pancreatic hormone from dog pancreases. Banting's original idea was to extract the substance, or "ferment," from the dog pancreas after ligating the pancreatic ducts, but this failed. They were successful only with the total extraction of the pancreas from numerous laboratory dogs followed by injection of the resultant crude extract to demonstrate partial correction of the elevated blood sugar level in depancreatectomized dogs. Alone, except for one graduate student (Best), during the first 3 months of the project, because Macleod was in Europe, starting in August 1921, Banting and Best demonstrated a significant lowering of the elevated glucose level in depancreatectomized dogs with their dog pancreas extract.

By November, Macleod felt that biochemical expertise was critical for further refinement of the "hormone," then given the name *isletin* by the young investigators. The following month James Collip, a young professor of biochemistry on a sabbatical leave in Macleod's department, joined the three researchers. Despite Collip's ability in January to prepare an effective extract for the first human recipient, Leonard Thompson, the success did not last. By the spring of 1922, both Banting and Best, as well as Collip, found it impossible to reproduce useful material. The prospects for the production of insulin brightened with the help of a brilliant strategist, George Clowes, the research director at the then small company called Eli Lilly, who developed a favorable contract with the trustees of the University of Toronto to work out conditions for large-scale production (40). Clowes fortunately had employed a rare talent at that time in the person of a chemical engineer by the name of George Walden, who made the critical observation in the fall of 1922 that maintenance of the isoelectric point of insulin afforded a maximum extraction of insulin from beef and pork pancreases (44). This paved the way for production of enough insulin to meet the needs of desperate patients and physicians worldwide.

Apart from the objective merits of the work and the investigators who produced it, the complexity of the Nobel Committee's assignment of merit to only Banting and Macleod requires comment. In 1951 the Nobel Foundation published a historical commentary on its work, which contained information about the selection process in 1923 (45). Banting and Macleod, but not Best, were nominated, an essential requirement for Nobel laureate consideration. Furthermore, the Nobel report admitted that the committee reviewed only three presentations reporting on the insulin discovery. These articles did not include the first Banting and Best article of February 1922 (42), but they did review the seven-authored May 1922 article published in the *Transactions of the Association of American Physicians* (46). From their vantage point of the mid-20th century, the Nobel report concluded that Collip and Best had probably been assumed to be assistants and therefore not prime candidates for recognition (45).

The historian Michael Bliss, after all the principal parties in the case had died, was able to search anew, mainly in the archives at the University of Toronto, and concluded that all four of the investigators were essential to the discovery and could share in what a sage of the early 1920s had remarked was "glory enough for all" (40). Likewise, the scholar investigator Rachmiel Levine gave a good degree of closure on this matter when he commented in the 1993 version of this chapter:

> As such things commonly proceed [the discovery of insulin in 1921], there was a tendency to overdo the interpretation. First, all diabetes was ascribed to insulin deficiency. The role of other hormones in metabolic control and an awareness of the bewildering heterogeneity of the diabetic syndrome belong to the half century and more that has elapsed since that momentous summer in Toronto in 1921. In 1922 Banting and Macleod received a Nobel Prize for this historic discovery. There was immediate controversy about the omission of Best and Collip from the prize—a controversy that has continued to the present day. Recent historical research into the details of the Banting and Best collaboration confirm that J. J. R. Macleod, Professor of Physiology at the University of Toronto, facilitated as much as he could the research suggested by Banting and was probably an appropriate co-recipient of the Nobel Prize [(44)]. It has always been clear that, of the participants, Macleod was certainly the most knowledgeable in the fields of carbohydrate metabolism and diabetes mellitus. The success of the work by Banting and Best was due to Macleod's basic knowledge, Banting's stubborn persistence, and the important specific skills of Best and Collip [(47)].

THE INSULIN ERA

The Years 1922 to 1960

During the period from the discovery of insulin through the 1950s, the effects of the availability of insulin were felt in three notable ways: an improved life expectancy for patients with type 1 diabetes, a surge of interest in understanding the mechanism of action of insulin on intermediary metabolism, and an increasing recognition of the syndromes we have come to appreciate as the chronic complications of diabetes. A combination of factors promoted a longer life span for the beleaguered patient with the disease, beginning with the near elimination of death from diabetic coma that coincided with improved means of treating the complications of diabetes. Hormonal regulation of glucose metabolism was clarified, with progress made in understanding the role of hepatic, adipose, and muscle tissues in the uncontrolled diabetic state. Success in defining the entire endocrine network, especially in demonstrating the importance of the pituitary-adrenal axis, gave the field of endocrinology a specialty status.

The Insulin Timetable

The discovery of insulin changed forever the treatment of diabetes; these and related developments are outlined in Table 1.1 (48).

The arrival of an adequate supply of commercial insulin for patients from 1923 onward was followed by the development of procedures for purifying and standardizing insulin. By 1926 crystalline insulin in concentrations of 10, 20, and 40 units per milliliter became available worldwide. The task of purifying insulin continued for decades, starting with early efforts to avoid contaminants such as glucagon. Starting in 1936 protamine and zinc were used to prolong the action of insulin (49). In the 1970s, self-monitoring of blood glucose became a standard of care. Further changes were made possible with the tools of molecular biology, which allowed the production of human insulin and analogues that change absorption characteristics. These insulin variations, coupled with the arrival of finer, less painful, needles, facilitated multi-injection programs that provide better glucose control. Pump delivery systems also became available. It is difficult for those involved with diabetes today to comprehend fully the changes that have taken place since the introduction of insulin. The first Joslin patient to receive insulin was Elizabeth Mudge, R.N., who was first treated on August 7, 1922, at the New England Deaconess Hospital in Boston. She had not been able to leave her apartment for 9 months, but after 6 weeks of insulin therapy, she could walk 4 miles daily, and she lived for 25 more years. Regarding the preinsulin days, Dr. Joslin noted, "I used to count the days my diabetic children lived" (50). This is emphasized by an episode that took place in the crowded original offices of the Joslin Clinic

TABLE 1.1. Insulin Timetable: 1921 through the Present

1921	Pancreatic extracts demonstrated to lower blood sugar levels in experimental diabetic dogs (Banting, Best, and Macleod, Toronto)
1922	Insulin first used in human (Leonard Thompson, Toronto)
1923	"Isoelectric point" produced larger quantities of higher-potency insulin from animal sources—enough to satisfy commercial supply (Lilly Company)
1925	First international insulin unit defined (1 unit = 0.125 mg of standard material). U40/80 insulins become available
1926	Crystallized amorphous insulin adds to insulin stability (Abel)
1936	Addition of zinc to protamine insulin (PZI) to create a prolonged duration of action of the hormone (Scott, Fisher, and Hagedorn)
1939	Globin insulin with a shorter duration of action than PZI developed
1950	NPH (neutral protamine Hagedorn) insulin developed with controlled amounts of protamine (Nordisk Company)
1951	Lente insulins developed by acetate buffering of zinc insulin (Novo Company, Hallas-Moller)
1955	Structure of insulin delineated (Sanger and coworkers)
1960	Radioimmunoassay of insulin becomes available (Berson and Yalow)
1967	Proinsulin discovered (Steiner)
1967	First pancreas transplant (Kelly, Lillehei, and coworkers)
1971	Insulin receptor defined (Roth, Cuatrecasus, and coworkers)
1972	U100 insulin introduced to promote better accuracy in administration
1973	Small-dose intravenous insulin treatment for acidosis emerges as alternative to large-dose subcutaneous treatment (Alberti and coworkers)
1976	C-peptide becomes clinical tool (Rubenstein et al.)
1977	Insulin gene cloned (Ullrich, Rutter, Goodman, and others)
1978	Purified "single-peak" pork insulin introduced (Lilly Company)
1978	Open-loop insulin delivery system clinically introduced (Pickup and coworkers)
1981	Insulin-receptor kinase activity described (Kahn and coworkers)
1982	Recombinant human insulin becomes available (Lilly Company)
1989	First islet transplants (Lacy and coworkers)
1990s (early)	Insulin pen delivery devices become popular
1996	Short-acting insulin analogue introduced—insulin lispro (Humalog)
2000	"Edmonton Protocol" improved results of islet transplantation
2001	Long-acting insulin analogue introduced—insulin glargine (Lantus, Aventis Company)

Adapted from Haycock P. History of insulin therapy. In: Schade DS, Santiago JV, Skyler JS, Rizza RA. *Intensive insulin therapy*. Princeton, NJ: Excerpta Medica, 1983:1–19.

on Bay State Road in the 1940s, when a child patient became more than a bit noisy. Dr. Joslin came by and said, "Make all the noise you want. We love noisy children around here. For many years there were no normal children. They were very quiet and after a visit or two they did not return" (L. P. Krall, personal communication).

Prior to the use of insulin, most young patients with diabetes died shortly after diagnosis. The Joslin Clinic experience (51) showed the commonest cause of death to be ketoacidosis (63.8% until 1914 and 41.5% until August 1921). The improvement from 1914 to 1921 was probably due to the introduction of Frederick Allen's "semistarvation" therapy in about 1915. Even though patients with type 1 diabetes could sometimes survive for years using this form of starvation therapy, most died sooner. By comparison, in affluent countries, the rate of death due to coma is now a rare event, although in some developing countries, death rates still approach preinsulin levels.

When Joslin wrote the preface to his third edition of *The Treatment of Diabetes Mellitus* late in 1923, the experience he drew upon was based on 3,000 cases and his use of insulin had been extended to 1 year (52). He wrote: "Compared to the last decade, the doctor now has twice as many diabetics to treat. . . . Of the 48 children cared for in this period, 46 remain alive . . . and as for Bouchardat, Cantani, Kulz, Lepine and all the other diabetic saints, how they would have enjoyed this year!"

The Study of Diabetes and the Development of Clinical Care

The original physicians on the first Insulin Committee of the University of Toronto in 1922 were Elliott P. Joslin of Boston; Robert Williams of Rochester, New York; Frederick Allen of Morristown, New Jersey; Rollin Woodyatt of Chicago, Illinois; Russell Wilder of the Mayo Clinic, Rochester, Minnesota; and Richard Geyelin, of New York City (53). These men, each in his own way, were leaders in the new treatment of diabetes in the first decade after the discovery of insulin. They were the first physicians to report on the detailed management of children and adults presenting in metabolic acidosis. With time, new clinical problems emerged in the medical literature as the first decade of insulin use ensured longer-living patients. By the early 1930s, the occurrence of lower extremity neuritis was becoming more common, as was the number of persons with a combination of Bright's disease (nephrotic syndrome) and hypertension. In 1928 Joslin described neuritis on one page of his 500-page fourth edition (54), but by his eighth edition (1946) the subject had been expanded to an entire chapter (55). By World War II the goals were clear: first, prevent death from diabetic coma; and second, train patients to help decrease the appearance and impact of diabetic complications.

Diabetic Manuals and Early Diabetes Education

Most of the leading physicians of the 1920s and 1930s who were interested in diabetes produced instructional guidebooks that covered the use of insulin, care of equipment, and management approaches to hyperglycemia and hypoglycemia. However, the majority of these instructional renditions went through only one edition, with the notable exceptions of the guidebooks of R. D. Lawrence of London and Joslin, which were revised approximately every 4 years. Lawrence titled his book appropriately *The Diabetic Life*, which set a publication record, reaching 17 editions by 1965 (56).

Joslin began to publish his first manuals shortly after the first edition of his diabetes textbook in 1916 (1), and by his third edition in 1923 (52), he had quickly adapted the contents to the arrival of insulin while maintaining the length of the manual to fewer than 200 pages. This practical "reader" for patients reached more people with diabetes in America than any other guide in the immediate decades following the introduction of insulin. The early editions were subtitled *For Mutual Use of Doctor and Patient*, as the practitioner absorbed, along with the patient, the details of the new treatment (57). Each table of contents boldly proclaimed the value of self-care in matters as far reaching as prevention of gangrene and constipation and proper dental care. He maintained that steady care of oneself, with proper treatment defined as a combination of more than one adjustable daily insulin dose (as a rule) and dietary restrictions along with regular, planned exercise, favored a longer life. His life-expectancy predictions for people with diabetes underlined the value of his advice by showing a steady improvement in longevity.

Joslin was a highly organized person who not only was interested in his patients' health but also found time to inquire into the details of their lives. From the first use of "diet therapy," he recognized the value of hospitalization in a hospital "cottage" or "schoolroom" setting that was dedicated to patient treatment *through* education. These cottages later evolved into an ambulatory inpatient ward he termed the *Diabetes Treatment Unit*. Patients were expected, while under supervision in this ambulatory setting, to enter into a team approach with doctor and educator in choice of insulin doses according to exigencies of the particular day's program. However, in recent years, cost-containment restraints on medical insurance have moved diabetes education to outpatient venues.

Recognition of the Complications of Diabetes

Continuous reporting of protocols on treating diabetic coma with improvements in mortality rates was at the core of the most often published communication coming from Joslin's early clinic. Joslin's associate, Howard Root, published a collection of articles in monograph form on diabetes and tuberculosis, a much-feared infection decreasing significantly after 1940 (58).

Classification of neuropathy was to be continuously readdressed in the 30 years following the publication of one of the most definitive reports on the emerging subject by a Joslin associate, W. R. Jordan (59). In this anthology of the many presentations of diabetic neuropathy came one of the earliest notations of severe joint neuropathy, diabetic osteoarthropathy, which is now better known as the Charcot foot phenomenon. A monograph on the visual problems in diabetes published in 1935 by Waite and Beetham (60) was to be a basis for Beetham's later studies on the natural history of retinopathy (61). His extensive experience obtained from a 30-year observation of the Joslin patients allowed him to formulate the potential value of laser photocoagulation in treating diabetic retinopathy. His critical observation was based on the observation that neovascular changes were never seen in the retinas of patients who already had evidence of previous chorioretinitis (62).

In 1936, Kimmelstiel and Wilson's article on a kidney lesion that seemed pathognomonic for diabetes rounded out the early description of diabetic complications (63). Implicit in many of the discussions in these monographs, particularly those on pathology, diabetic coma, and retinopathy, was the concomitant presence of severe macrovascular disease. The suggestion of a high incidence of coronary artery disease emphasized in these publications was clearly substantiated in Bell's monumental study on arteriosclerosis (64).

The Team Approach to the Treatment of Diabetes

The study of clinical diabetes in the early years of insulin use convinced Dr. Joslin of the need for different strategies for delivery of care. A half-dozen initiatives were incorporated into his clinic programs, some of which have gained broad acceptance in the decades since their initiation. The common denominator in his plan was to create teams of subspecialists to maximize the benefit to the patient. He was fond of citing the value of the "fecundity of the aggregation" (65).

The team approach to care was originally an approach to treating diabetic coma. The use of special-duty nurses with expertise regarding fluid replacement, constant observation of signs and symptoms, and the monitoring of laboratory results was championed by Joslin before the replacement of intravenous fluids and electrolytes became routine. In the late 1930s, the addition of a special intravenous nurse team to administer fluids and to act as phlebotomists for the critically ill and often dehydrated patient was a pioneering step.

Along with the publication in 1928 of the first monograph, entitled *Diabetic Surgery*, by the surgeon L. S. McKittrick and the internist H. Root, Joslin created a "foot team" (66). This group acknowledged the need for a special foot-dressing nurse to apply frequent bandages to prevent progression of foot lesions from neuropathic, ischemic, or "mixed" lesions. In addition to the surgeon and internists, importance was placed on the team's schedule of daily and weekly conference rounds, with the inclusion of a chiropodist (podiatrist) to provide preventive foot care with proper booting of the patient.

Always a pioneer, Joslin appointed Priscilla White to his practice team "to study and care for children with diabetes" (65) (Fig. 1.2). She quickly saw the need for good control as a preventive for the growth retardation that plagued children with chronic hyperglycemia. Later, as the teenagers matured, their desire for pregnancy became White's major challenge. She favored the emphasis on "pregnancy complicated by diabetes," not vice versa (67). After working on these problems for more than a decade, by 1937 she had devised a team approach to prenatal care for pregnant women with diabetes. Cesarean sections

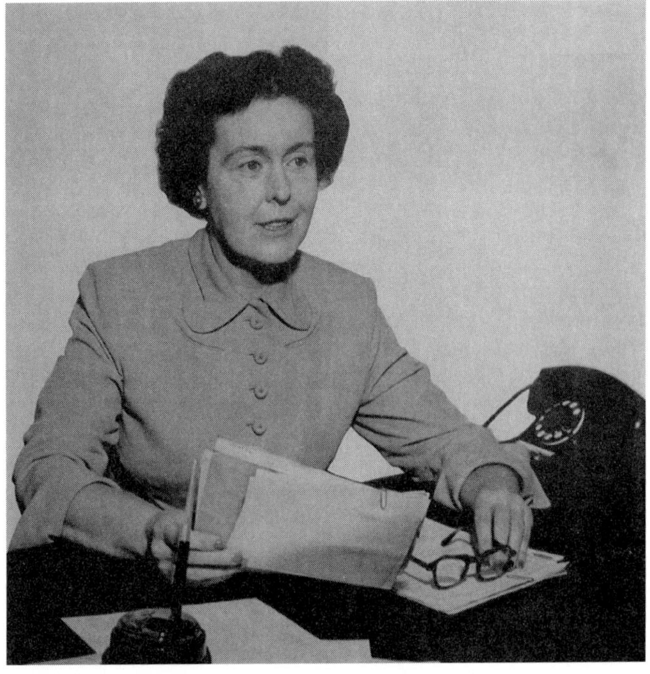

Figure 1.2. Priscilla White at the telephone.

at or near the 37th week of gestation were inaugurated as early as 1928 to avoid the dangers of edema of the fetus on the one hand and respiratory distress on the other. Her experience with variations in the response to pregnancy in these women who had a spectrum of diabetes (from gestational diabetes to pregnancy complicated by the diabetic nephrotic syndrome) allowed her to formulate by 1949 a classification of diabetic pregnancy that was accepted worldwide and still is known as the White classification (68).

A unique venture introduced by Joslin in the management of diabetic youth came at the time insulin was made available in the creation of the "wandering" or "visiting nurse" to join families and adjust the new insulin to the daily activity and the changing dietary needs of the growing child (69). These nurses supervised the initial Joslin diabetes camp effort. In the past three decades, professionals other than doctors and nurses have joined the education team; these have included nutritionists, psychologists, and exercise physiologists. Today, the status of diabetes educators has been strengthened by a rigorous credentialing process that leads to the designation "certified diabetes educators" (CDE) (70). Moreover, diabetes has become a field that lends itself logically to including nurse practitioners and physician assistants as members of the diabetes care team.

The educator mission was to be extended to all settings, from the recovery time after a critical illness all the way to camp programs, starting with the creation in 1932 of the Clara Barton Birthplace Camp for Girls in Oxford, Massachusetts. These summer camp experiences had their diabetes education dimension, as the daily schedule was divided evenly between typical camp activities and instructional opportunities that could be provided by the staff.

Modern Endocrinology Comes of Age

Endocrinology as a medical specialty developed quite late compared with most other fields. Endocrinology had its beginning in the 19th century with reports describing conditions of hormone excess, as in Graves disease, and deficiencies, as in Addison disease. By 1891, the first example of treatment with desiccated thyroid was realized and heralded as effective "replacement" therapy for thyroid "deficiency" (71). However, it was not until the decades embracing the arrival of insulin that impressive advances were seen in the chemistry of and therapy for a full range of the endocrine- and vitamin-related disorders and that they were defined as we presently understand them. As an example, the early 20th century witnessed the first descriptions of an impressive number of nutritional deficiencies, starting with the work in England of Hopkins and Funk with the B vitamins (named the "vital amines" and abbreviated as "vitamins"). Nobel prizes in 1937 went to Szent-Györgyi for elucidating ascorbic acid and in 1934 to three Americans, Minot, Whipple, and Murphy, who spearheaded the spectacular success with liver therapy for pernicious anemia (16). George Minot (1985–1950) was characterized by his doctor, Elliott Joslin, as "saved" by insulin when it fortuitously became available in 1922, preventing an almost certain lethal descent for the young hematologist and assuring him a brilliant research career (72).

By the third decade of the 20th century, there had been sufficient development in topics such as body salt and water balance, digestive functions, and intermediary metabolism to allow recognition of the role of humorally transported integrators, a term originally used to describe hormones (72). The arrival of insulin certainly became one of the main engines of growth for the development of endocrinology over the next 35-year period. A centerpiece of this new age in the study of metabolism was the work of the Nobel laureate Bernardo Houssay of Argentina. His 30-year perspective on the field of metabolism following the discovery of insulin was summarized in Houssay's address at the dedication of the new Banting and Best Institute in Toronto in 1952 (73).

> Working with Biasotti; I found the hypophysectomies diminished the severity of diabetes by pancreatectomy in the dog. Implantation of the pars distalis (anterior lobe of mammals) again increases the severity of diabetes. The diabetogenic effect of the hypophysis was thus demonstrated. The severe symptoms of pancreatic diabetes were due to two factors: (a) presence of a hypophyseal hormone, and (b) a lack of secretion of insulin. The diabetogenic effect of hypophyseal extract in mammals was demonstrated in 1932 simultaneously in three laboratories: in Evan's, in Marine's, and in mine. In 1932, I was able to provoke permanent diabetes by hypophyseal treatment in dogs previously submitted to partial pancreatectomy. Young obtained this effect in dogs with intact pancreas in 1937.

Houssay's work became the needed fulcrum for the advancements in understanding of the whole endocrine network that we appreciate today. In the 10 years following the availability of insulin, Houssay was able to study the action of insulin by applying his earlier investigations on the effects of thyroid, adrenal, and pituitary ablation upon glucose regulation. Diabetes became a convenient and measurable parameter in the study of metabolism for him and his contemporaries.

During the 1930s there was an eruption of information about hormonal regulation of intermediary metabolism. Carl Cori (74) and Hans Krebs (75) were leaders in defining steps in glucose regulation. Developments in the field of pharmacology spearheaded advances in the clinical isolation of hormones. An American pioneer in the field, J. J. Abel (1857–1938), isolated epinephrine and later produced crystalline insulin, an advance that facilitated production of insulin for therapy (76).

The adrenal gland became a continued focus of investigation, aided by Cushing's work on human adrenal pathology earlier in the decade (77). Long's work on the effect of adrenal hormones on carbohydrate metabolism was a significant step in understanding the regulation of blood sugar in health and disease states like diabetes (78).

As Harvey pointed out in his "Classics in Clinical Science," Dana Atchley and Robert Loeb during this time made major contributions to the understanding of the treatment of diabetic acidosis (79).

> In the early 1930's Atchley and Loeb in their metabolic "study unit" in New York conducted studies on the electrolyte changes in diabetic acidosis. Atchley suggested that they bring well-regulated diabetic patients into the hospital and follow the sequential metabolic changes after discontinuing their insulin. They selected three patients: in the first, when insulin was taken away, the diabetes was so mild that little change occurred. The second had more severe diabetes, and the third had very severe diabetes and became seriously ill within a few hours after his insulin was discontinued. Their quantitative observations demonstrated the progressive loss of body water, sodium and potassium. These elegant balance studies represent one of the classic contributions in the evolution of our understanding of the electrolyte changes that occur in diabetes mellitus.

It took another decade and a half before the practical implementation of correct replacement of electrolytes in diabetic acidosis was completed. The better availability of infection-free intravenous solutions was crucial to providing optimal care for the acutely ill diabetic patient. The arrival in 1948 of the flame photometer for more rapid determination of potassium levels focused attention on the need to replace this electrolyte in almost all cases of diabetic acidosis.

From today's perspective the last major advance in the treatment of diabetic coma came with the use of intravenous insulin

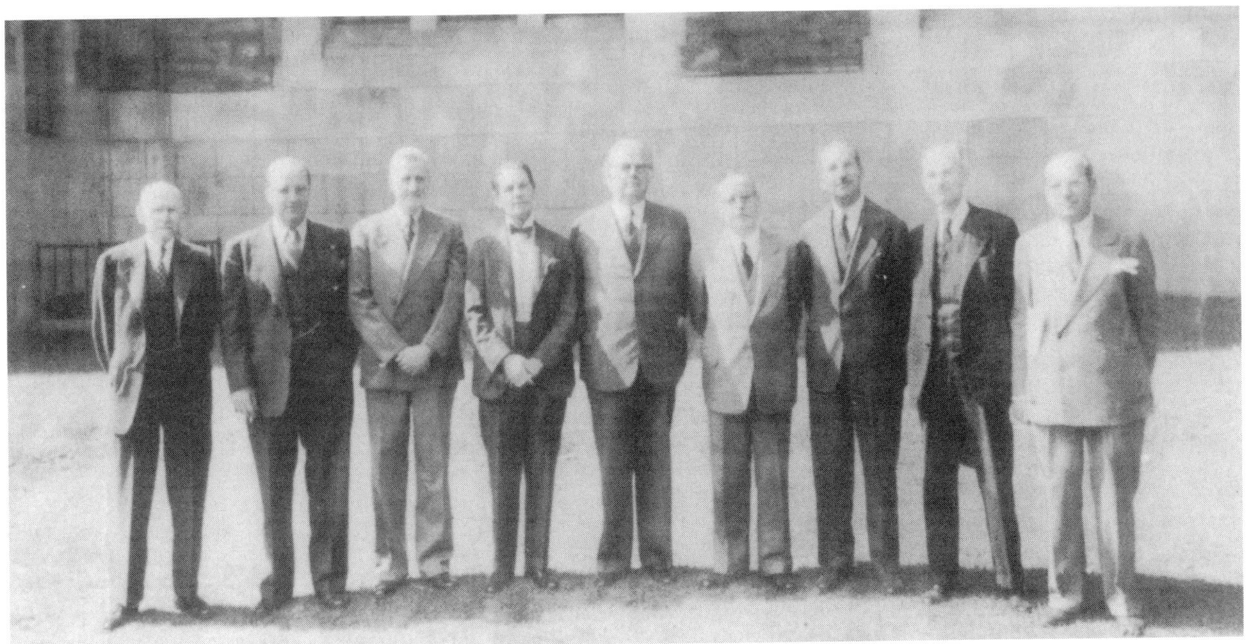

Figure 1.3. Officers and honored guests at the celebration of the 25th anniversary of the discovery of insulin, in Toronto, September 16–18, 1946. Left to right: Elliot P. Joslin, Boston, honorary president, American Diabetes Association; Charles H. Best, Toronto, codiscoverer of insulin; Russell M. Wilder, Rochester, Minnesota, president-elect, American Diabetes Association; Robert D. Lawrence, London, founder, the Diabetic Association; H. C. Hagedorn, Denmark, discoverer of protamine insulin; B. A. Houssay, Buenos Aires, researcher, "Houssay phenomenon"; Joseph H. Barach, Pittsburgh, president, American Diabetes Association; Eugene L. Opie, New York, discoverer, islets of Langerhans pathology; Cecil Striker, Cincinnati, first president, American Diabetes Association.

infusions in the 1970s. Since 1980, the formula for correcting the insulin deficit in patients with ketoacidosis has been contained in a mere half-page of the treatment guidelines of the American Diabetes Association (80). This abbreviation of the treatment of diabetic acidosis parallels the marked decrease in mortality that has been observed over the past several decades.

The principals who marked the celebration of the 25th anniversary of insulin in 1946 are shown in Figure 1.3. This sampling of investigators and their particular fields of interest illustrate the beginning of what has become a virtual army of different scientific disciplines now employed in the study of diabetes. Best, Houssay, and Hagedorn were basic scientists; Wilder was a pioneer clinical endocrinologist; Opie was a pathologist; and Joslin, Lawrence, Barach, and Striker were eminent diabetologists.

Early Work in the Epidemiology of Diabetes

Joslin's interest in epidemiology, pursued with diligence during his 60-year professional life, centered on three areas: first, maintaining vital statistics on his patients with diabetes; second, promoting epidemiologic studies; and third, garnering information from these to translate principles into practice for individual patients.

From the very start of his practice, he devised a registry of patients with diabetes and strove to follow them through their life span. Gradually his "black books" were enlarged into a system of vital statistics on his patients, increasing over decades to become the largest medical record system devoted to diabetes in the world. He collaborated with the medical director of the Metropolitan Life Insurance Company so that his compilations could receive the expertise of actuarial professionals (81).

The rising incidence of diabetes during the past five decades provides one of the best examples in medicine of the emergence of a chronic disease as a threat to world health. Elliott Joslin had an appreciation of epidemiology even in the earliest stages of his career, beginning with his pioneering report in 1898 on the 75-year review of medical records on diabetic patients at the Massachusetts General Hospital (one of the earliest hospital record systems in the United States) (82), which revealed a dismal outlook for patients with diabetes over this time period. As early as 1921, he appreciated the concept of epidemiology and even applied the term "epidemic" to diabetes (6) and made the following prescient comment:

> In a country town in New England . . . on its peaceful, elm-lined Main Street, there once stood three houses, side by side, as commodious and attractive as any in the village. In these three houses lived in succession four women and three men—heads of families—and of this number, all but one has subsequently succumbed to diabetes. . . . Although six of the seven persons dwelling in these adjoining houses died from a single complaint, no one spoke of an epidemic. Contrast the activities of the local and state boards of health if these deaths had occurred from scarlet fever, typhoid fever or tuberculosis. Consider the measure which would have been adopted to discover the source of the outbreak and to prevent a recurrence. Because the disease was diabetes, and because the deaths occurred over a considerable interval of time, the fatalities passed unnoticed (6).

Joslin's registry recorded experience with 1,000 cases of diabetes by the time he was able to assess his own 5-year trial with Allen's "undernutrition" regimen. Therefore, in 1916, armed with evidence showing an increase in the short-term life span for his patients with type 1 diabetes following the Allen undernutrition regimen, he felt justified in publishing a definitive monograph on all the known facts related to the disease, which contained a wealth of epidemiologic information (1).

By 1928, when he had 5 years of experience in the use of insulin treatment, Joslin had started to employ a follow-up plan on the medical status of all his patients. He regularly wrote patients a personalized message on a detailed form letter and recorded their answers about health and disease in his ledgers. By this device, Joslin enhanced an already close relationship that afforded him the most comprehensive set of medical data on diabetes then in existence. By 1980, this resource led to a valuable series of analyses of the complications of three cohorts of patients with type 1 diabetes from the years 1939, 1949, and 1959 (83). This type of investigation clarified the changing appearance of the chronic diabetic syndrome, particularly with the occurrence of renal failure.

In a sense, this textbook was an epidemiologic tract that was to be continually updated in each edition with information garnered from the "follow-up" system of his medical record ledgers. The Oxford Study in 1947, instigated by Joslin, was the first whole-town survey of the incidence of diabetes. It established a 4% prevalence rate for diabetes in the United States, underscoring that the disease was undetected in half the population with the disease (84).

Earlier, Joslin had been involved in some of the original fieldwork on the prevalence of diabetes. He reported on his experience in Arizona in 1940 and corrected the perception that the incidence of diabetes was less than that noted in the eastern United States (85). He did not observe the well-known high prevalence of diabetes in Native Americans, perhaps because a large proportion of the population was probably still active in farming in the 1930s. For example, prevalence data from surveillance of a Pima Indian population in a reservation in New Mexico showed that more than 50% of the population over 35 years of age had diabetes (86).

The Current Era (1960 to the Present)

The past four decades have witnessed major advances in the treatment and understanding of diabetes. The field has been aided greatly by organizational agreement on an upgraded terminology necessary to properly classify the heterogeneity of the diabetes syndrome.

By the 20th century's end, the long-term acrimonious debate over the value of good glycemic control of diabetes became resolved with the results of several large well-designed and well-executed clinical studies. However, despite major improvement in the options for care and the depth of research in affluent areas, this progress is dampened by the challenge seen in an increasing epidemic of diabetes throughout the world among disadvantaged populations both in this country and beyond.

The Classification of Diabetes

A major step in world recognition and confirmation of diabetes as a major health problem was the development of improved criteria for diagnosis and classification of the types of diabetes, particularly for types 1 and 2 diabetes. Table 1.2 charts these developments (55, 87, 88, 89).

Defining diabetes in the past was, at best, a sorting-out process. The father of modern medicine, Sir William Osler (1849–1919), composed a one-authored text of internal medicine in 1893 as he awaited the first class of students at the Johns Hopkins University Medical School in Baltimore, Maryland. He placed diabetes under the topic of "Constitutional Diseases" and implied that it was "familial" (90). The timing of the Osler textbook nearly coincided with the finding of Minkowski and von Mering that the pancreas was central to the disease. Lancereaux, a student of the French clinician Bouchardat, had divided diabetes into a "lean" and a "fat" category (31). Since that time, various adjectives have been employed to classify and describe diabetes (Table 1.2). In the 1960s it became apparent that separate criteria needed to be employed for gestational diabetes (91). By the mid-1970s, these descriptions and the half-dozen diagnostic criteria had become unworkable. The 1979 National Diabetes

TABLE 1.2. Understanding Diabetes: A Century of Effort in Classifying the Disease (1880 to the Present)

Type 1 (insulin-dependent diabetes mellitus; IDDM)	
Preinsulin era	*Diabète maigre (lean)* True diabetes (Naunyn) Asthenic/Unterdruk type
Insulin era	*Juvenile-onset type* (JODY = juvenile-onset diabetes of youth) Ketosis prone Brittle diabetes
Type 2 (non–insulin-dependent diabetes mellitus; NIDDM)	
Preinsulin era	*Diabète gras (big)* Sthenic, Überdruk type
Insulin era	*Adult-onset diabetes* Maturity-onset type diabetes Ketosis-resistant diabetes Stable diabetes (MODY = maturity-onset diabetes of youth)
Gestational diabetes mellitus (GDM)	Established firmly in 1964 (O'Sullivan and Mahan (91)
Impaired glucose tolerance (IGT)	
Impaired fasting glucose (IFG)	
Other types (associated with pancreatic diseases, removal endocrinopathies, genetic syndromes)	Secondary diabetes

From Joslin EP, Root H, White P, et al. *The treatment of diabetes mellitus,* 8th ed. Philadelphia: Lea & Febiger, 1946:310–313; National Diabetes Data Group. Classification and diagnosis of diabetes mellitus and other categories of glucose intolerance. *Diabetes* 1979;28:1039–1057; Fajans SS, Cloutier MC, Crowther R. Banting Memorial Lecture. Clinical and etiologic heterogeneity of idiopathic diabetes mellitus. *Diabetes* 1978;27:1112–1125; Report of the Expert Committee on the Diagnosis and Classification of Diabetes Mellitus. *Diabetes Care* 2002;25[Suppl 1]: S5–S20.

Data Group Committee, with a wide assembly of epidemiologists and students of the disease, agreed upon new definitions (87). Although it was a compromise, it was accepted by the National Institutes of Health, the American Diabetes Association, the European Association for the Study of Diabetes, the International Diabetes Federation, and the World Health Organization.

From a historical perspective, the 1979 classification "institutionalized" the concept that insulin resistance is important (91a). The British investigator H. P. Himsworth should be credited with the initial formulation on the subject 50 years previously (92). Prophetically, Himsworth stated: "Diabetes mellitus is a disease in which the essential lesion is a diminished ability of the tissues to utilize glucose . . . [this disease] is referable either to deficiency of insulin or to insensitivity to insulin, although it is possible that both factors may operate simultaneously." The concept of two forms of diabetes, type 1 [formerly juvenile-onset or insulin-dependent diabetes mellitus (IDDM)] and type 2 [formerly adult-onset or non–insulin-dependent diabetes mellitus (NIDDM)], became accepted and has helped greatly with communication on the subject. Although communication with laymen and professionals was enhanced, this simplistic terminology can overlook the complexity of the diabetic syndrome. The classic review by Fajans et al. in 1978 pointed out the variability of the syndrome that this disease can present to physician and researcher alike (88).

The criteria for the diagnosis and classification of diabetes have continued to evolve with the accumulation of new knowledge. The 1979 report was updated by the Expert Committee on the Diagnosis and Classification of Diabetes Mellitus in 1997 and then modified in 1999 to make some changes in the diagnosis of gestational diabetes (89). The major categories now include types 1 and 2 diabetes described by Arabic numbers rather than Roman numerals. The "other specific types" include various genetic, endocrinopathic, drug-induced, and infectious causes. Gestational diabetes has its separate criteria. A particularly important category is impaired glucose tolerance (IGT) for which the term impaired fasting glucose (IFG) is now often used. One of the major changes in 1997 was the increased emphasis upon fasting plasma glucose levels, with the cut-off for diabetes being lowered to 126 mg/dL (7.0 mM) from the earlier value of 140 mg/dL (7.7 mM).

Efforts have continued to update the classification and clarify diagnostic criteria in a drive to enhance promulgation of information on this topic. Each January, the clinical organ for the American Diabetes Association produces a supplement to the journal *Diabetes Care* entitled "Clinical Practice Recommendations." This issue contains position statements and a summary of revisions to the practice recommendations of the association.

Oral Hypoglycemic Agents

The introduction of sulfonylurea agents in 1955 provided a valuable treatment option for insulin-fearing patients and provided a new tool for research. The earliest sulfonylureas gave way to second-generation and third-generation agents (Chapter 41). In 1957, at a symposium on these agents held at the New York Academy of Sciences, Rachmiel Levine encapsulated the past and predicted the future in the following excerpt from his concluding remarks (93). "To me the most important aspect of the research in this field has been the stimulus it has provided to renewed work on the etiology of diabetes mellitus and on the synthesis of insulin, its storage, and the control of its release. We may say that, in addition to stimulating the B cells, the sulfonylureas have stimulated the investigators." Other oral agents soon followed, with the biguanide metformin succeeding over phenformin, which was discredited because of concerns about lactic acidosis. The α-glucosidase inhibitors (acarbose and miglitol) became more widely used in the 1980s. The thiazolidinediones were introduced in the 1990s, although troglitazone (Rezulin) was rapidly withdrawn because of hepatic toxicity; however, pioglitazone and rosiglitazone are now in widespread use. Other recent additions include the nonsulfonylureas repaglinide and nateglinide that work through pathways similar to those of the sulfonylureas but have shorter half-lives.

The Diabetic Control Controversy

Any history of diabetes since the discovery of insulin would be incomplete without an explanation of the control and complications controversy [see Chapter 48 and (94)]. The first generation of physicians after the discovery of insulin, many of whom had cared for dying patients during the decade before 1923, felt that tight control of diabetes by blood glucose and urine determinations was of paramount importance. In the 1920s, Joslin, having been interested in diabetes as long as any physician at that time, thought that the careful treatment of diabetes would lead to partial remission of the condition. He felt that restricted nutrition had been helpful in prolonging the life of some patients between 1915 and 1923 and that these dietary measures should be extended with modification to the insulin era. Other practitioners, however, felt that with the advent of insulin treatment, the diet could be greatly liberalized. Therefore, the diabetic "diet" became the target of debate in the earliest years of insulin use.

The founding members of the American Diabetes Association quickly became polarized on this issue. For instance, Joslin, along with H. Ricketts of Chicago, often faced off with H. Mosenthal and E. Tolstoi of New York City (95). Indeed, about the time of the 25th anniversary of insulin, Tolstoi wrote a monograph that was a rallying cry for "purely symptomatic" care of diabetes (96). Some of the best summaries can be found in debates published in 1966 (97) and 1974 (98) entitled *Controversies in Internal Medicine*. The earlier dialogue on diabetes—entitled "Are the Complications of Diabetes Preventable?"—had Alexander Marble of the Joslin Clinic and Harvard Medical School paired off with Philip Bondy of Yale Medical School. As usual, these discussions were energetic but inconclusive. All agreed this area would be aided by future prospective studies.

The considerations regarding the value of "loose" or "tight" control led to the development of a well-intended, but flawed, long-term prospective clinical trial with insulin, oral agents, and diet called the University Group Diabetes Program (UGDP). This study that was concluded in 1970 failed to show that "improved control" prevented or slowed the development of complications (99). These findings caught the attention of the entire medical community in 1970 and were subsequently debated and discussed almost ad infinitum in the literature (100,101). Although the UGDP study was a laudable attempt, if it were designed today, the protocol would no doubt be quite different. However, because no effort has been made to repeat the study, the conclusions are largely ignored today, although the package inserts for the sulfonylureas state that they are to be used with some caution.

A decade later, the National Institute of Diabetes, Digestive and Kidney Diseases developed a study called the Diabetes Control and Complications Trial (DCCT), which was focused on insulin therapy only and confined its analysis only to patients with type 1 diabetes (14). In 1993, the results of the DCCT were reported, with the remarkable finding that almost all of the 1,441 patients from 29 centers completed the study. The major conclusion was that intensive control of the blood sugar over a 7-year study interval reduced the progression of diabetic retinopathy, nephropathy, and neuropathy but also resulted in a threefold increased risk of serious hypoglycemia.

The relationship between control and complications in type 2 diabetes was evaluated in the United Kingdom Prospective Diabetes Study (UKPDS) (102,103). This study of 14 years' duration enlisted more than 5,000 patients with newly diagnosed diabetes, who were followed up for an average of a decade. The study concluded that for every 1% decrease in glycosylated hemoglobin A_{1c} (HbA_{1c}) there was a 35% reduction in the risk of microvascular complications. Although the effect of reduction in glucose levels on macrovascular complications was of marginal statistical significance, the importance of blood pressure improvement with regard to cardiovascular events was clearly shown.

These two studies, coming as they did at the end of the 20th century, gave patients with diabetes and their care team solid confirmation of the benefits of good control, thus ending nearly 50 years of divisiveness and confusion on this central matter in the treatment of the disease.

Advances in Diabetes Management

Advances in the medical management of diabetes over the past 50 years have had a major impact on the attainment of better glycemic control. Equally important is the recent effort to provide financial mandates to cover the cost of diabetic medical supplies, including the insulin pump delivery units, along with reimbursement of patient instruction (104). For the past two decades these technical and economic gains have facilitated regimens that more accurately mimic normal insulin action patterns, allowing for some patients to reach near-physiologic control (105).

SELF-MONITORING OF BLOOD GLUCOSE

Replacement of urine testing by self-monitoring of blood glucose (SMBG) beginning in the late 1970s represents the single most important advance in fostering better management of diabetes since the introduction of insulin. The "Benedict" urine test introduced in 1911 by the chemist S. R. Benedict (1884–1936) was time consuming and odorous in preparation. With the advance of glucose oxidase–impregnated paper strips or the "Clinitest" tablets introduced in the 1950s, the use of urine glucose measurements remained, at best, a crude indicator of control. SMBG, introduced first by the glucose oxidase strip method, was a significant advance in management, contributing greatly to the patient's sense of control over treatment. In recent years an array of models have been marketed by more than a half-dozen medical technology firms in the United States and Europe. Some of the improvements include requirements for less blood, faster readings, and computer storage of measurement results. Newer but still unproved approaches to glucose monitoring include a watch-like device that can measure glucose on fluid driven through the skin by the process of iontophoresis (106) and a subcutaneous needle device with a tip impregnated with glucose oxidase that allows continuous measurement of glucose levels (107). Both approaches need frequent calibration and require further refinement.

GLYCOSYLATED HEMOGLOBIN

In the late 1970s, the glycosylated hemoglobin assay gained rapid application. The use of this property of glucose to bind to hemoglobin was noted serendipitously in 1968 when an investigator discerned that a subgroup of subjects with diabetes had a marked difference in the minor hemoglobin fraction during an electrophoresis analysis (108,109). The hemoglobin moiety most often used is HbA_{1c}. This property provides a practical and objective means of assessing average blood glucose levels over a time frame of about 2 months and has proven to be a very useful adjunct to SMBG.

INSULIN DELIVERY

The development of fine needles (up to 29 gauge) has made it easier for many patients to switch to multi-injection insulin therapy, this being especially helpful for children. Continuous subcutaneous insulin infusions (CSII) via pumps had limited popularity after their introduction in the early 1980s (110), but in recent years, along with their becoming smaller and more sophisticated, their popularity has increased.

NEW INSULINS

In the past decade and a half, fierce competition for patient allegiance to a brand name of insulin has intensified. The European company Novo acquired its competitor Nordisk to become Novo Nordisk and entered the American market, vying with Eli Lilly. Both companies attempted to increase their market share by various means, including various "insulin pen" delivery systems with their convenient "dose-dialing" features. Further competition has come from Aventis, which introduced the long-acting insulin glargine, a recombinant insulin analogue that is growing in popularity. Other insulin analogues include lispro and insulin aspart, which are short-acting insulins designed to cover meals. These insulins have made it easier for people to use more intensive approaches with multiple injections when a pump is not suitable or available.

DIET

Despite the growing epidemic of worldwide obesity, dietary options for persons with diabetes have became more diversified, with the steady appearance of a wide variety of foods with fewer calories. Carbohydrate-free soft drinks and low-fat foods have become options for menu planning of health-conscious Americans. The "Mediterranean"-style diet consisting of a preponderance of fish, pasta, and olive oil has gained favor, especially in advancing low-animal-fat substitutions in the so-called "Western" diet. However, recent reviews have highlighted a threefold increase over the past 30 years in childhood obesity, with a concomitant increase in type 2 diabetes. One factor noted is the neglect of the old guide of a "measured" diet, ironically not for its once dreaded "sugar" content of menus of the early insulin era but for an equal emphasis on total caloric intake of each meal (111). Emphasis on "portion control" of all categories of food is now seen as a strategy equal to the need to decrease animal fat in the diet (111). Restaurant and fast-food establishments have made sporadic attempts to offer "heart–healthy" and low-calorie selections, and the food industry has been mandated into providing better food labeling. The use of more intensive insulin regimens, such as "carbohydrate counting," to help plan premeal insulin doses has become more widespread (see Chapter 36).

In summary, in the past decades these advances have given an impetus to a changed role for the person with diabetes from a dependent "patient" to an active participant in control of his or her diabetes management. These improvements in technology have also led to a shift to a "consumer" attitude, as cost and quality comparisons of medical equipment and diet choices became evident. Recent estimates of healthcare expenditures have shown that the costs of caring for persons with diabetes are about three times those for persons without diabetes (112). Despite the rationing of health insurance coverage by managed-care organizations in the past 20 years that usually limited payment for diabetes education and supplies, patients' rights groups have prevailed in many state legislatures, forcing insurance companies to cover these services. Another encouraging trend is the inauguration of standards of care, often developed by the American Diabetes Association, that have been employed by various health plans.

Treatment Advances for Diabetes Complications

Complementing the arrival of practical management aids to help with glycemic control of diabetes has been the progressive improvement in the treatment of complications. Limb salvage arterial bypass operations have continued to become more efficacious, as have coronary bypass and angioplasty procedures. It is now common for octogenarian diabetic patients with cardiac risk factors to undergo femoral artery bypass surgery, with this being facilitated by modern anesthesiology and improved postoperative care. The pharmacologic revolution in the hypertension-cardiovascular area has become a boon to the vascularly compromised patient with diabetes.

Treatment of end-stage renal disease for all age groups is another example of the remarkable advances in the treatment of life-threatening diabetic complications. A very important step was taken in 1972, with the passage of legislation by Congress stipulating that chronic renal failure was to be covered as a disability by Medicare (113), which made it possible for many more people with diabetes to be treated with dialysis or transplantation.

One of the most impressive improvements in the quality of life for the person with diabetes has been the development of laser treatment for diabetic retinopathy. This advance followed earlier complex and less efficacious treatments such as pituitary ablation and the futile use of various medications. Laser therapy moved rapidly from the research phase to acceptance and use. The multicenter Diabetes Retinopathy Study started in 1971 and reached the conclusion by 1975 that laser therapy was very effective in preserving vision and preventing blindness (114). Furthermore, the Early Treatment of Diabetic Retinopathy Study, which was completed in 1990, clearly showed that laser treatment could preserve vision in patients with macular edema (115). Thus, laser treatment, coupled with the new devices and aids that help the visually handicapped, has had a major impact on people with diabetes.

Advances in Diabetes Research (1960 to the Present)

The development of the radioimmunoassay for insulin in 1960 led to important insights about insulin secretion and helped clarify some of the differences between type 1 and 2 diabetes (116). A few years later, it was determined that proinsulin was a biosynthetic precursor for insulin, which provided a fundamental insight into how cells process proteins and led the way to the useful radioimmunoassay for C-peptide. The insulin gene was cloned in 1977, which made human insulin available for clinical use and helped bring diabetes research to the new era of molecular biology. This recombinant technology also has permitted the development of the insulin analogues that are now in widespread use. During the past 40 years, research institutions around the world have been engaged in studies that impact on cause, prevention, and improvement in the treatment of diabetes, providing remarkable advances in many areas.

CELLULAR AND MOLECULAR BIOLOGY

The new technologies in the areas of molecular biology, biochemistry, and cell biology have greatly increased our understanding of how cells work at a basic level. This has led to a much deeper appreciation of such areas as insulin action; glucose transport; the function of muscle, adipose, liver, vascular, and islet cells; cellular growth and differentiation; and the biochemistry of the complications of diabetes.

METABOLISM

There have been important advances in the understanding of whole-body metabolism. Much of this has been made possible with the use of such technologies as stable isotopes, magnetic resonance imaging, positron emission tomography, and sophisticated analyses of biopsy specimens. There is a much improved understanding of fuel fluxes between organs, with delineation of the contributions of gluconeogenesis, glycogenolysis, lipogenesis, and lipolysis. Important new insights have emerged in the areas of exercise and weight maintenance. The complex contributions of the central nervous system, the autonomic nervous system, and the gastrointestinal tract to metabolism are now far better understood.

PATHOPHYSIOLOGY AND GENETICS OF DIFFERENT TYPES OF DIABETES AND OBESITY

Work in only the past 30 years has made it clear that type 1 diabetes is caused by an autoimmune process with strong genetic determinants, particularly from the human leukocyte antigen (HLA) system (117). Antibodies to β-cell antigens have proved to be very useful markers of autoimmunity, allowing the process to be identified years before the onset of hyperglycemia and thus allowing prediction, which opened the way to trials focused on prevention (118). For type 2 diabetes, there is now general appreciation that its development is usually dependent on both of two major processes: insulin resistance that results from a combination of our modern sedentary, food-abundant lifestyle and failure of β-cells to compensate adequately. Genetics is known to play a major role in the susceptibility to type 2 diabetes. In addition to types 1 and 2 diabetes, other discrete forms of diabetes are being defined. These include the MODY (maturity-onset diabetes of the young) forms of diabetes, most of which are now known to be caused by genetic defects in transcription factors that are important in islet development and function. Another form of MODY (MODY 2) is caused by mutations of the glucokinase gene. Another form of diabetes that is better understood at a molecular level is caused by mutations in mitochondrial DNA that lead to defective β-cell function. There has been an explosion of studies of obesity, with the identification of many peptide mediators that appear to be critically important for the control of food intake, including leptin, melanocortin, ghrelin, peptide YY (PYY), and neuropeptide Y (NPY).

VASCULAR CELL BIOLOGY AND COMPLICATIONS

There have been major advances in understanding the molecular basis of large- and small-vessel disease and in understanding the pathogenesis of diabetic nephropathy and neuropathy. The process of atherosclerosis is now better understood, and much is being learned about the abnormalities in vascular reactivity that occur in the early stages of disease. A great deal is now known about lipid metabolism, and the widespread use of statin drugs to lower low-density lipopolysaccharide (LDL) cholesterol appears to be having a significant impact. An important example of the progress made in understanding the pathophysiology and genetics of hypertension is the extensive use of angiotensin-converting enzyme (ACE) inhibitors for the treatment of hypertension, congestive heart failure, and diabetic nephropathy. The roles of vascular endothelial growth factor and protein kinase C in the development of microvascular disease are being defined.

β-CELL REPLACEMENT THERAPY

A great deal of attention is now being focused on the potential of β-cell replacement therapy, which could be important for both types 1 and 2 diabetes. The first successful pancreas transplants were performed in the 1960s, and by the 1980s the treatment had become available at many medical centers. It is hoped that transplantation of islets alone will supersede the transplantation of whole organs because the morbidity associated with islet transplantation is so much lower. After initial success with rodent islet transplants in the 1970s, the first serious islet transplants were carried out in the 1990s, with few of the recipients becoming insulin independent. The greatly improved results reported by workers in Edmonton, Canada, in 2000 have given new energy to the field. This success seems to be due to the use of a steroid-free immunosuppression regimen, the use of rapamycin, and the provision of enough high-quality islets, with two or more donor cadaver pancreases usually being necessary. The major problem facing islet transplantation is the shortage of insulin-producing cells due to the small number of cadaver donors. Many investigators are now joining the search for an abundant supply of insulin-producing cells, with considerable hope being placed in the potential of both adult and embryonic stem cells

THE DIABETES RESEARCH ENTERPRISE

Starting in the late 1990s, the interest of the diabetes community in increasing funding for diabetes research was greatly intensified, resulting in planning and lobbying on many fronts. In 1999 a congressionally established diabetes research group published a report entitled *Conquering Diabetes: A Strategic Plan for the 21st Century* (119). This group described the current state of knowledge about diabetes and developed a plan of priorities for areas of research needing more attention. Recognizing the personal toll of diabetes, the financial costs that exceeded $100 billion annually, and impressive research opportunities, they recommended marked increases in spending for diabetes research from the fiscal year (FY) 1999 National Institutes of Health (NIH) budget figure of $442.8. In FY2001, the NIH expenditures for diabetes reached $720.5 million. The Juvenile Diabetes Research Foundation also reassessed its priorities and fund-raising strategies. While more sharply focusing its goals, it increased contributions to diabetes research from $27.7 million in 1997 to $115 million in 2001. The American Diabetes Association has also placed more emphasis on raising funds for diabetes research, as have an important number of private foundations. In addition to the work being done in academic laboratories in the United States, institutions in many other countries place a high priority on diabetes research. Moreover, industry has made major investments in developing new treatments for people with diabetes.

The Worldwide Epidemic of Diabetes

Today the United States 2000 census serves as an updated warning about race and its relationship to diabetes (120). The Hispanic population in the United States has grown by 61% in the past 10 years to the 25 million level, and there has been a 20% increase in the African-American population. These figures alone predict heavy pressure on healthcare budgets, as the diagnosis of diabetes is more prevalent in these population groups. In addition, people in many countries, especially the United States, are becoming heavier, more sedentary, and older, which further increases the prevalence of type 2 diabetes. The increase in type 2 diabetes in children is an even more startling trend (Fig. 1.4) (111). The reports of the World Health Organization (WHO) in the past decade have seen a march in prevalence of worldwide diabetes from 100 million a decade ago to 135 million in 1995, 151 million by 2000, and a projected number of 221 million by 2010 (121–123).

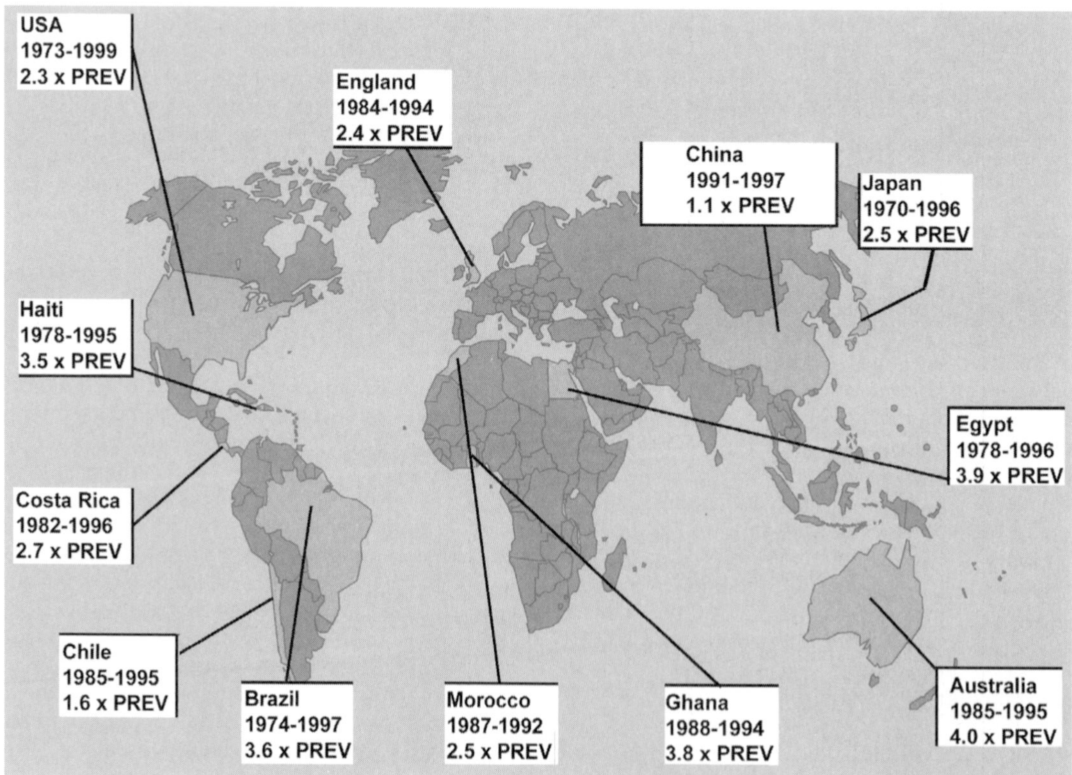

Figure 1.4. Global increase in prevalence (PREV) of childhood obesity—predictor of type 2 diabetes in youth. (Modified from Ebbeling CB, Pawlak DB, Ludwig DS. Childhood obesity: Public-health crisis, common sense cure. *Lancet* 2002; 360: 476.)

Prevention of Diabetes

After World War II, a combination of factors promoted the understanding of diabetes as a rising health problem in the world. Following the example of the British Diabetes Association in 1934, other organizations concerned with diabetes were founded in rapid succession, including WHO in 1948 and the International Diabetes Federation in 1952. These two latter organizations collaborated, and by the 1980s, three international standard reference documents on public health aspects of diabetes became available. Along with this development, a variety of study groups under the auspices of WHO began collecting data on many aspects of diabetic complications. These developments formed the initiative for preventive care programs at the regional level (121). Following the Oxford Study of 1947, the American Diabetes Association launched a nationwide detection drive that became a popular part of the Association's annual goal of lay education.

During the Nixon administration in the 1970s, the United States embarked on "crusades" against important diseases. A congressional mandate led to the National Commission on Diabetes in 1976, which led to a comprehensive report on diabetes and established centers to foster research and translate these findings to the diabetic population (124).

An appreciation of the relation of diabetes to both societal and genetic factors increased. A common denominator accounting for a growing diabetes population is the phenomenon of the migration of agrarian peoples to urban centers during time of war or industrialization. The resultant inactivity, coupled with obesity, has no doubt been responsible for most of the increase in the incidence of diabetes.

Interventions in lifestyle have been recently studied in the "prediabetic" person with IGT. A small reduction in weight and an increase in exercise led to a substantial reduction in the development of diabetes (125,126). The appearance of diabetes was also delayed by the pharmacologic agent metformin (126).

The U.S. Postal Service recently produced a Diabetes Awareness stamp (127) (Fig. 1.5) and publicized the fact that 8% of the current population (18 million) has diabetes (127). Figure 1.5 represents diabetes in the United States at a figure double the 4% estimate found in Joslin's 1947 Oxford, Massachusetts, study (84), underscoring the true extent of the diabetes epidemic in the United States.

Organizational Growth

The organization and mobilization of worldwide resources in the fight against diabetes by researchers, clinicians, and persons with diabetes themselves have been some of the most remarkable advances of the past several decades. In 1935, the British Diabetes Association was established under the sponsorship of two celebrities who had diabetes: H. G. Wells, the writer, and R. D. Lawrence, a physician, who was one of the first persons in the country to receive insulin. The organization was largely a lay endeavor. In 1937, a group of U.S. physicians interested in diabetes met during a meeting of the American College of Physicians in New Orleans (128) and after many discussions started the American Diabetes Association (ADA) in 1941. The first meeting, held in Cleveland, Ohio, on June 1, 1941, was attended by about 300 physicians who discussed the scientific aspects of diabetes. Cecil Striker of Cincinnati was the founder and first president. The ADA grew rapidly, and by 1960, there were more than 25,000 members. The organization, which had started as a physicians-only group, recognized that its many goals could be fulfilled only by including laypersons, particularly those with diabetes, and other interested parties.

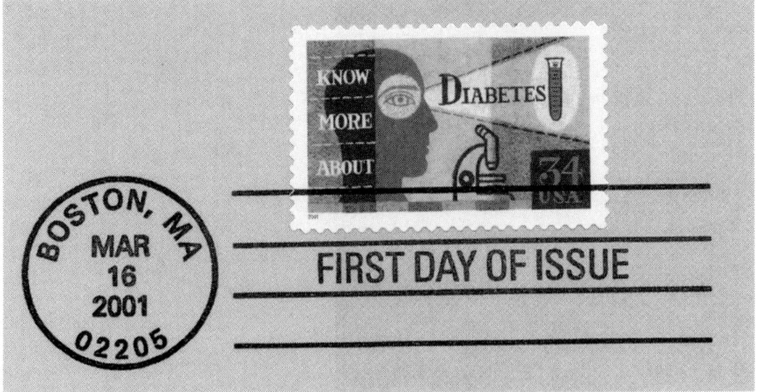

Figure 1.5. Diabetes Awareness Stamp, first issued on March 16, 2001, by U.S. Postal Service. United States, 8% prevalence rate (122); 4% rate in 1947 (84).

Vigorous growth of the ADA has continued, and it is now at the forefront of all issues relating to diabetes, with more than 9,000 professional members and 250,000 general members. The ADA raises money for research, hosts meetings, publishes four journals, and is concerned with every aspect of the well-being of those with diabetes. One of its major publications for the lay public is the journal *Diabetes Forecast*, which started with a circulation of 50,000 in 1948 and now has a worldwide circulation of 275,000.

The need for more emphasis on funding for research also spawned the Juvenile Diabetes Research Foundation in 1970, whose primary goal is the prevention and cure of juvenile diabetes through increased research. This same movement toward research and education was taking place in Europe, where the European Association for the Study of Diabetes was formed for similar purposes in 1965. Paralleling these developments was the organization by diabetes educators of the American Association of Diabetes Educators, which has played a key role in training and certification.

Because diabetes is a problem in virtually all nations, there was recognition of the need for attention to the problem. In June 1949, the president of the Belgian Diabetic Association, J. P. Hoet; his counterpart from England, R. D. Lawrence; and 75 other physicians and patients from 11 countries discussed their mutual problems. Meeting again in Amsterdam in 1950, they started the International Diabetes Federation (IDF) (129), with one lay delegate and one medical delegate from each country. The First Congress of the new organization was held in Leiden, The Netherlands, in 1952, attracting 241 representatives from 20 countries. Recent meetings held in Helsinki (1997) and Mexico City (2000) have hosted more than 8,000 attendees. The IDF is a confederation of some 85 world diabetes associations, the largest of which is the ADA, which has developed many education and service programs worldwide. Increasingly, its direction is moving toward regions that need the most help, with valuable assistance and coordination coming from WHO, the health arm of the United Nations.

CONCLUSION

As we start a new millennium, writers of medical publications, especially texts like this, can reflect on past events that have made "a difference" in the lives of the sick. The *New England Journal of Medicine* has assessed this progress in clinical medicine over the past thousand years and pointed out that most of the advances have occurred in the past century. Specifically, the dozen examples cited that gave the "greatest benefit to mankind" in the form of a longer life included the treatment of diabetes (130).

These advances have coincided with the 87-year interval since the publication of the first edition of Joslin's first monograph in 1916 and help explain the need for a book of this size to describe the condition. When one views the spectrum of progress named in this historical overview, ranging from a greatly increased understanding of the pathophysiology of diabetes all the way to the continued advances in the prevention and treatment of diabetes and its complications, the adage "to know diabetes is to know medicine" becomes axiomatic (47).

The 21st century will continue to focus on the premise that the diabetic state may really be *prevented* or *cured* through the power of modern science, targeting interventions at the genetically prone person that are aimed at correcting core abnormalities before they emerge. Such advances should bring preventive medicine into a realm never envisioned by Elliott Joslin, a true pioneer in the field.

REFERENCES

1. Joslin EP. *The treatment of diabetes mellitus*. Philadelphia: Lea & Febiger, 1916.
2. Barnett DM. Joslin Elliott Proctor. *American national biography*. North Carolina: Oxford University Press, 1999:282–283.
3. Benedict FG, Joslin EP. *The study of metabolism in severe diabetes*. Washington, DC: Carnegie Institution of Washington, 1912:176.
4. Allen FM, Stillman E, Fitz R. *Total dietary regulation in the treatment of diabetes*. Monographs of the Rockefeller Institute for Medical Research, no. 11. New York: Rockefeller Institute, October 15, 1919.
5. Joslin EP. Present-day treatment and prognosis in diabetes. *Trans Assoc Am Physicians* 1915;XXX:2.
6. Joslin EP. The prevention of diabetes mellitus. *JAMA* 1921;76:79–84.
7. Nuland S, Virchow R. *Doctors—the biography of medicine*. New York: Knopf, 1988.
8. Langerhans P. Beitrage zur mikroskopischen Anatomie der Bauchspeicheldruse. Med Diss (Berlin), 1869.
9. Morrison H. Translation and introductory essay. Langerhans P. Contributions to the microscopic anatomy of the pancreas. *Bull Inst Hist Med* 1937;5:259–269.
10. Laguesse GE. Sur la formation des ilots de Langerhans dans le pancreas. *Compte Rendus Societé de Biologie*, 1893.
11. Von Mering J, Minkowski O. Diabetes Mellitus nach Pankreasexstirpation. *Zentralbl Klin Med* 1889;10:393–394.
12. Minkowski O. Historical development of the theory of pancreatic diabetes (introduction and translation by R. Levine). *Diabetes* 1989;38:1–6.
13. Joslin EP, Krall LP. The incidence of diabetes. In: Joslin EP, Root HF, White P, Marble A, eds. *Treatment of diabetes mellitus*, 10th ed. Philadelphia: Lea & Febiger, 1959:35–37.
14. The Diabetes Control and Complications Trial Research Group. The effect of intensive treatment of diabetes on the development and progression of long-term complications in insulin-dependent diabetes mellitus. *N Engl J Med* 1993;329:977–986.
15. Shafrir E. History and perspective of diabetes illustrated by postage stamps. Freund Publishing House Ltd, 1999 [Reprinted by Joslin Diabetes Center, Publication Dept., Boston MA. March 2001].
16. Porter R. *The greatest benefit to mankind, a medical history of humanity*. New York: WW Norton, 1997:71.
17. Major RH. II. Diseases of metabolism. In: *Classic descriptions of disease with biographical sketches of authors*, 3rd ed, 5th printing. Springfield, IL: Charles C Thomas, 1959:235–237.
18. Willis T. Pharmaceutica rationalis sive diatriba de medicamentorum operationibus in humano corpore. 2 vols. London, 1674–1675.
19. Schadewaldt H. The history of diabetes mellitus. In: Van Englehardt D, ed. *Diabetes, its medical and cultural history*. Berlin: Springer Verlag, 1987:43–100.
20. Dobson M. Experiments and observations on the urine in diabetes. In: *Medical observations and inquiries by a society of physicians in London*, Bd. 5, London, 1776:S.298–316.
21. Cawley T. A singular case of diabetes, consisting entirely in the quality of the urine; with an inquiry into the different theories of that disease. *London Med J* 1788;9:286–308.
22. Rollo J. *An account of two cases of the diabetes mellitus, with remarks as they arose during the progress of the cure*. London: Dilly, 1797.
23. Chevreuil ME. Note sur le sucre de diabète. *Ann Chim* (Paris) 1815;95:319.
24. Benedict SR. A modification of the Lew-Benedict method for the determination of sugar in the blood. *J Biol Chem* 1918;34:203–207.
25. Folin O, Wu H. A system of blood analysis. *J Biol Chem* 1919;38:81–110.
26. Epstein AA. An accurate microchemical method of estimating sugar in the blood. *JAMA* 1914;63:1667–1668.
27. Rosen G. The conservation of energy and the study of metabolism. In: Chandler McC, Brooks C, Cranefield PF, eds. *The historical development of physiological thought*. New York: Hafner Publishing Company, 1959;243–263.
28. Shor EN. Benedict, Francis Gano. *American National Biography*. North Carolina: Oxford University Press, 1999:555–556.
29. Major RH. Adolph Kussmaul. In: *Classic descriptions of disease with biographical sketches of authors*, 3rd ed, 5th printing. Springfield, IL: Charles C Thomas, 1959:245–248.
30. Bernard C. Du suc pancréatique et de son rôle dans les phénomènes de la digestion. *C R Soc Acad Sci* (Paris) 1850;1849:99–119.
31. Bouchardat A. *De la glycosurie ou diabète sucré*. Paris, 1875.
32. Lancereaux E. Le diabète maigre: ses symptômes, son évolution, son pronostic et son traitement; ses rapports avec les alterations du pancréas. *Union Med* (Paris) 1880;29:161–168.
33. Chandler McC, Brooks C, Levey HA. Humorally-transmitted integrators of body function and the development of endocrinology. In: Chandler McC, Brooks C, Cranefield PF, eds. *The historical development of physiological thought*. New York: Hafner Publishing Company, 1959:184.
34. Major RH. II. Diseases of metabolism. In: *Classic descriptions of disease with biographical sketches of the authors*, 3rd ed, 5th printing. Springfield, IL: Charles C Thomas, 1959:290–294.
35. Brown-Sequard CE. Recherches expérimentales sur la physiologie et la pathologie des capsules currenales. *C R Acad Sci* 1856:43:422.
36. Laguesse E. Structure et développement du pancréas d'après les travaux récents. *J Anat* (Paris) 1894;30:591–608.
37. Starling EH. The Croonian Lectures on the chemical correlation of the functions of the body. *Lancet* 1905;2:339–341, 423–425, 501–503, 579–583.
38. De Meyer J. Contribution à l'étude de la pathogénie du diabete pancréatique. *Archive Internationale de Physiologie* 1909:121–180.
39. Opie EL. The relation of diabetes mellitus to lesions of the pancreas: hyaline degeneration of the islands of Langerhans. *J Exp Med* 1900;5:527–540.
40. Bliss M. *The discovery of insulin*. Chicago: University of Chicago Press, 1982.
41. Paulesco NC. Action de l'extrait pancréatique injecté dans le sang, chez un animal diabétique. *C R Soc Biol* 1921;85:555–559.
42. Banting FG, Best CH. The internal secretion of the pancreas. *J Lab Clin Med* 1922;7:251–266.
43. Barron M. The relations of the islets of Langerhans to diabetes with special reference to cases of pancreatic lithiasis. *Surg Gynecol Obstet* 1920;31:437–448.
44. Eli Lilly Company. Archives File, Indianapolis, Indiana, McCormick reference 3B, 6.
45. Nobel Foundation. *Nobel, the man and his prizes*. Oklahoma: University of Oklahoma Press, 1951:221–223.
46. Banting FG, Best CH, Collip JB, et al. The effect produced on diabetes by extracts of pancreas. *Trans Assoc Am Physicians* 1922:1–11.
47. Levine R, Krall L, Barnett D. The history of diabetes. In: Kahn CR, Weir GC, eds. *Joslin's diabetes mellitus*, 13th ed. Philadelphia: Lea & Febiger, 1994:1–14.
48. Haycock P. History of insulin therapy. In: Schade DS, Santiago JV, Skyler JS, et al. *Intensive insulin therapy*. Princeton, NJ: Excerpta Medica, 1983:1–19.
49. Deckert T. Protamine insulin. In: *H.C. Hagedorn and Danish insulin*. Hening, Denmark: Poul Kristensen Publishing Co, 2000:175–194.
50. White P. *Diabetes in childhood and adolescence*. Philadelphia: Lea & Febiger, 1932.
51. Marble A, Krall LP, Bradley RF, et al, eds. *Joslin's diabetes mellitus*, 11th ed. Philadelphia: Lea & Febiger, 1971:362.
52. Joslin EP. *The treatment of diabetes mellitus, with observations based upon three thousand cases*, 3rd ed. Philadelphia: Lea & Febiger, 1923.
53. Colwell AR. The Banting memorial lecture 1968: fifty years of diabetes in perspective. *Diabetes* 1968;17:599–610.
54. Joslin EP. Preface. In: *Treatment of diabetes mellitus*, 4th ed. Philadelphia: Lea & Febiger, 1928.
55. Joslin EP, Root H, White P, et al. *The treatment of diabetes mellitus*, 8th ed. Philadelphia: Lea & Febiger, 1946:310–313.
56. Lawrence RD. *The diabetic life, its control by diet and insulin and oral treatment by sulphonyl-urea, a concise practical manual*, 17th ed. London: J. & A. Churchill Ltd, 1965.
57. Joslin E. *A diabetic manual for mutual use of doctor and patient*. Philadelphia: Lea & Febiger, 1918.
58. Root HF. The association of diabetes and tuberculosis: epidemiology, pathology, treatment and prognosis. *N Engl J Med* 1934;210:1–13.
59. Jordan WR. Neuritic manifestations in diabetes mellitus. *Arch Intern Med* 1936;57:307–66.
60. Waite JH, Beetham WP. The visual mechanism in diabetes mellitus: a comparative study of 2002 diabetics, and 457 non-diabetics for control. *N Engl J Med* 1935;212:429–443.
61. Beetham WP. Visual prognosis of proliferating diabetic retinopathy. *Br J Ophthalmol* 1963;611–619.
62. Aiello L, Beetham W, Balodimos, et al. Ruby laser photocoagulation in treatment of diabetic proliferating retinopathy: preliminary report. In: *Symposium on the treatment of diabetic retinopathy. Airlie House Conference*. Public Health Service publication no. 1890. Washington, DC: US Department of Health, Education and Welfare, 1968:437–463.
63. Kimmelstiel P, Wilson C. Intercapillary lesions in the glomeruli of the kidney. *Am J Pathol* 1936;12:83–97.
64. Bell ET. A postmortem study of vascular disease in diabetics. *Arch Pathol* 1952;53:444–455.
65. Barnett DM. *Elliott P. Joslin, MD: a centennial portrait*. Boston: Joslin Diabetes Center, 1998:43–57.
66. McKittrick LS, Root HF. *Diabetic surgery*. Philadelphia: Lea & Febiger, 1928.

67. White P. Pregnancy and diabetes. In: Marble A, White P, Bradley, RF, Krall LP, eds. *Joslin's diabetes mellitus*, 11th ed. Philadelphia: Lea & Febiger, 1971:584–593.
68. White P. Classification of pregnant diabetics in treatment of diabetes mellitus. In: Joslin EP, Root HG, White P, Marble A, eds. *Joslin's diabetes mellitus*, 10th ed. Philadelphia: Lea & Febiger, 1959:702–703.
69. Joslin EP. The nurse and the diabetic. Address reported in the 1924 New England Deaconess Hospital Annual Report, 16–21.
70. American Association of Diabetes Educators, 20 years Yesterday, Today and Tomorrow . . . Diabetes Educators Making a Difference. Chicago: Stenson Publications, 1994.
71. Murray GR. Note on the treatment of myxedema by hypodermic injection of an extract of the thyroid gland of a sheep. *BMJ* 1891;2:796–797.
72. Brooks C. Chandler McC, Levey HA. Humorally-transported integrators of body function and the development of endocrinology. In: Chandler McC, ed. *The historical development of physiological thought*. New York: Hafner Publishing Company, 1959:185–186.
73. Houssay B. Memorable experiences in research. In: Banting and Best Research Institute inaugural dedication program, Toronto, 1952:31–32.
74. Cori CF. Enzymatic reactions in carbohydrate metabolism. *Harvey Lectures* 1945–1946;41:243–272.
75. Krebs HA. The intermediate metabolism of carbohydrates. *Lancet* 1937;2: 736–738.
76. Abel JJ. Crystalline insulin. *National Academy Society Proceedings* 1926;12:132.
77. Cushing H. The basophil adenomas of the pituitary body and their clinical manifestations (pituitary basophilism). *Bull Johns Hopkins Hosp* 1932;50:50–137.
78. Long CNH. The Banting Lecture: the endocrine control of the blood sugar. *Diabetes* 1952;1:11.
79. Harvey AM. Classics in clinical science: the electrolytes in diabetic acidosis and Addison's disease. *Am J Med* 1980;68:322–324.
80. American Diabetes Association. *The physician's guide to type 1 diabetes (IDDM): diagnosis and treatment*. Alexandria, VA: American Diabetes Association, 1988.
81. Joslin EP, Dublin LI, Marks HH. Studies, characteristics and trends in diabetic mortality throughout the world. *Am J Med Sci* 1937;193:8.
82. Fritz RH, Joslin EP. Diabetes mellitus at the Massachusetts General Hospital for 1824 to 1898. A study of the medical records. *JAMA* 1898;31:165–171.
83. Krolewski AS, Warram JH, Christlieb AR, et al. The changing natural history of nephropathy in type I diabetes. *Am J Med* 1985;78:785–794.
84. Wilkerson HLC, Krall LP. Diabetes in a New England town: a study of 3,516 persons in Oxford, Mass. *JAMA* 1947;135:209–216.
85. Joslin EP. The universality of diabetes, a survey of diabetic morbidity in Arizona. *JAMA* 1940;115:2033–2038.
86. Knowler WC, Bennett PH, Hamman RF, et al. Diabetes incidence and prevalence in Pima Indians: a 19-fold greater incidence than in Rochester, Minnesota. *Am J Epidemiol* 1978;108:497–505.
87. National Diabetes Data Group. Classification and diagnosis of diabetes mellitus and other categories of glucose intolerance. *Diabetes* 1979;28:1039–1057.
88. Fajans SS, Cloutier MC, Crowther R. Banting Memorial Lecture. Clinical and etiologic heterogeneity of idiopathic diabetes mellitus. *Diabetes* 1978;27: 1112–1125.
89. Report of the Expert Committee on the Diagnosis and Classification of Diabetes Mellitus. *Diabetes Care* 2002;25[Suppl 1]:S5–S20.
90. Osler W. Diabetes mellitus. In: *The principles and practice of medicine*. New York: D. Appleton and Company, 1893:295–230.
91. O'Sullivan JB, Mahan CM. Criteria for oral glucose tolerance test in pregnancy. *Diabetes* 1964;13:278.
91a. Reaven GM. Banting Memorial Lecture. Role of insulin resistance in human disease. *Diabetes* 1988;37:1595–1607.
92. Himsworth HP. The Goulstonian lectures on the mechanism of diabetes mellitus. *Lancet* 1939;2:1,65,118,171.
93. Levine R. Concluding remarks: the effects of the sulfonyl-ureas and related compounds in experimental and clinical diabetes. *Ann N Y Acad Sci* 1957;71: 291.
94. Nathan DM. The long-term complications of diabetes mellitus. *N Engl J Med* 1993;328:1676.
95. Born DM, ed. *The journey and the dream (a history of the American Diabetes Association)*. Alexandria, VA: American Diabetes Association, 1990;16,57.
96. Tolstoi E. *The practical management of diabetes*. Springfield, IL: Thomas Publications, 1953.
97. Are the complications of diabetes preventable? In: Ingelfinger FJ, Relman AS, Finland M, eds. *Controversies in internal medicine*, Vol 1. Philadelphia: WB Saunders, 1966:489–514.
98. Management of adult-onset diabetes. In: Ingelfinger FJ, Ebert RV, Finland M, Relman AS, eds. *Controversies in internal medicine II*. Philadelphia: WB Saunders, 1974:387–417.
99. University Group Diabetes Program. *Diabetes* 1970;19[Suppl 2]:747–830.
100. Prout TE. A prospective view of the treatment of adult-onset diabetes: with special reference to the University Group Diabetes Program and oral hypoglycemic agents. *Med Clin North Am* 1971;55:1065–1076.
101. Bradley RF. Oral hypoglycemic agents are worthwhile. In: Ingelfinger FJ, Ebert RV, Finland M, Relman AS, eds. *Controversies in internal medicine II*. Philadelphia: WB Saunders, 1974:408–415.
102. UK Prospective Diabetes Study Group. Intensive blood-glucose control with sulfonylureas or insulin compared with conventional treatment and risk of complications in patients with type 2 diabetes (UKPDS 33). *Lancet* 1998;352: 837–853.
103. UK Prospective Diabetes Study Group. Effect of intensive blood-glucose control with metformin on complications in overweight patients with type 2 diabetes (UKPDS 34). *Lancet* 1998;352:854–865.
104. Massachusetts Legislature Acts of 2000. The Diabetes Cost Reduction Act.
105. Beaser RS. Using insulin to treat diabetes—general principles (Chapter 8). In: *Joslin's diabetes deskbook*. Boston: Joslin Diabetes Center, 2001:203–232.
106. Tamada JA, Garg SK, Jovanovic L, et al. Non-invasive glucose monitoring: comprehensive clinical results. *JAMA* 1999;282:1839–1844.
107. Gross TM, Bode BW, Einhorn D, et al. Performance evaluation of the Minimed® continuous glucose monitoring system during patient home use. *Diabetes Technol Ther* 2000;2:49–59.
108. Rahbar S. An abnormal hemoglobin in red cells of diabetics. *Clin Chim Acta* 1968;22:296–298.
109. Bunn HF, et al. Further identification of the nature and linkage of the carbohydrate in hemoglobin A1c. *Biochem Biophys Res Comm* 1975;67:103–109.
110. Pickup JC, Keen H, Parsons JA, et al. Continuous subcutaneous insulin infusion: improved blood-glucose and intermediary-metabolite control in diabetics. *Lancet* 1979;1:1255–1257.
111. Ebbeling CB, Pawlak DB, Ludwig DS. Childhood obesity: public-health crisis, common sense cure. *Lancet* 2002;360:476.
112. Rubin RJA, William M, et al. Health care expenditures for people with diabetes mellitus: 1992. *J Clin Endocrinol Metab* 1994;78:809A–809F.
113. Evans RW, Blagg CR, Bryan FA. Implications for health care policy: a social and demographic profile of hemodialysis patients in the United States. *JAMA* 1981;245:487–491.
114. Preliminary report on effects of photocoagulation therapy. The Diabetic Retinopathy Study. *Am J Ophthalmol* 1976;91:383–396.
115. Photocoagulation for diabetic macular edema. Early Treatment Diabetic Retinopathy Study report no. 4. *Int J Ophthalmol* 1987;27:265–272.
116. Yalow RS. Remembrance project: origins of RIA. *Endocrinology* 1991;129: 1694–1695.
117. Gale EA. The discovery of type 1 diabetes. *Diabetes* 2001;50:217–226.
118. Srikanta S, Ganda OP, Rabizadeh A, et al. First-degree relatives of patients with type 1 diabetes mellitus. Islet cell antibodies and abnormal insulin secretion. *N Engl J Med* 1985;313:461–464.
119. A report of the congressionally established Diabetes Research Group. *Conquering diabetes, a strategic plan for the 21st century*. Washington, DC: National Institutes of Health, publication no. 99-4398, 1999.
120. US Census Report, March 2001.
121. World Health Organization Study Group. *Prevention of diabetes mellitus*. Technical report 844. Geneva: World Health Organization, 1994.
122. Gan D, ed. Regional estimates for diabetes for the year 2000. *Diabetes atlas 2000*. Brussels: International Diabetes Federation, 2000:9,11.
123. Zimmet P, Albert KG, Shaw J. Global and societal implications of the diabetes epidemic. *Nature* 2001;414:782–787.
124. National Commission on Diabetes, United States. The long-range plan to combat diabetes: 1976 update. Bethesda, MD: National Institutes of Health. Department of Health Education and Welfare publication no. NIH 77-1229.
125. Tuomilehto J, Lindstrom J, Eriksson JG, et al. Prevention of type 2 diabetes mellitus by changes in lifestyle among subjects with impaired glucose tolerance. *N Engl J Med* 2001;344:1343–1350.
126. Knowler WC, Barrett-Connor E, Fowler SE, et al. Reduction in the incidence of type 2 diabetes with lifestyle intervention or metformin. *N Engl J Med* 2002;346:393–403.
127. U.S. Postal Service. First day of issue—Diabetes Awareness Stamp. March 16, 2001.
128. Striker C. The American Diabetes Association. *Med Clin North Am* 1947;31: 483–487.
129. Krall LP. A prescription for world diabetes. In: Serrano-Rios M, Lefebvre PJ, eds. *Diabetes 1985*. Amsterdam: Elsevier, 1986:2–24.
130. Looking back on the millennium in medicine [Editorial]. *N Engl J Med* 2000; 342:42–49.

SECTION I

Basic Mechanisms of Islet Development and Function

CHAPTER 2

Development of the Endocrine Pancreas

Ondine Cleaver and Douglas A. Melton

The vertebrate pancreas is an essential organ, responsible for both digestion and glucose homeostasis. The pancreas is also the sole source of insulin production in vertebrates, and impairment leads to a major health problem, diabetes mellitus. Current research on early development of the pancreas is aimed at elucidating the generation of pancreatic cells and the genetic mechanisms underlying the anatomy and physiology of the pancreas. More specifically, the central goals of pancreas developmental studies include mapping of the spatiotemporal origins of endocrine cells and the identification of key genes that determine endocrine character. These studies also examine regulatory factors that direct the proliferation and differentiation of the pancreas from its initial commitment in the endoderm through morphogenesis and growth during postnatal life. The possibility of islet neogenesis *in vitro* and transplantation as a potential treatment for diabetes makes the study of the basis for β-cell development and insulin production particularly significant (1). In addition, the prospect of using pluripotent stem cells to generate an unlimited supply of β-cells underscores our need to understand the regulation of normal endocrine cell generation in the embryo (2).

In this chapter, we will present studies on the development of the pancreas in humans and in model organisms, including mice, rats, chickens, and frogs (3–6). Fundamental genetic mechanisms controlling germ layer and organ development are highly conserved throughout evolution, and conclusions drawn from model organisms can often be extrapolated generally. We will first review the principal landmarks of pancreatic function and anatomy. We define fundamental cell types that comprise the pancreas and examine in detail the commitment, patterning, and morphogenesis of the pancreas. We also discuss cell-lineage relationships among pancreatic cells, providing insights into the origins of endocrine cells. In addition, we introduce current research on putative pancreatic stem cells and the potential for therapeutic applications. Last, we will briefly review some of the important transcriptional regulators and growth factors demonstrated to play critical roles during islet development.

THE PANCREAS

General Anatomy

The human pancreas is a racemose, lobulated gland that weighs 60 to 170 g, is 13 to 25 cm long, and is located just caudal to the stomach and opposite the liver along the gastrointestinal tract (7,8) (Fig. 2.1). Its head (proximal portion) lies in the crook of the duodenum, and its tail (distal portion) contacts the spleen. It is also in juxtaposition to a number of large blood vessels, including the aorta, the inferior vena cava, and the superior mesenteric vein and artery and is in direct contact with the portal and splenic veins (8). The pancreas consists primarily of exocrine, endocrine, and ductal cell types that together with a blood supply coordinate to regulate nutritional equilibrium. The exocrine function of the pancreas is carried out by acinar cells, which secrete digestive enzymes and other nonenzymatic components into the duodenum. Acinar cells are located at the tips of the smaller ducts, which connect to an extensive system of larger ducts and in turn join the primary excretory duct of the pancreas. This duct, also called the canal of Wirsung, extends transversely through the body of the pancreas and connects to the duodenum at the ampulla of Vater, where it joins the common bile duct (9). The endocrine function of the pancreas is carried out by the islets of Langerhans. These are compact, spheroid clusters of cells scattered throughout the more abundant exocrine tissue. Islets consist of four different cell types that secrete hormones into the bloodstream to regulate glucose homeostasis. Islets are therefore penetrated by a network of fenestrated microvasculature and nerve fibers that help administer this regulation (10–13). It has long been observed that both endocrine and exocrine cells originate in the pancreatic endodermal epithelium and then migrate into the surrounding mesenchyme before undergoing differentiation (14–17).

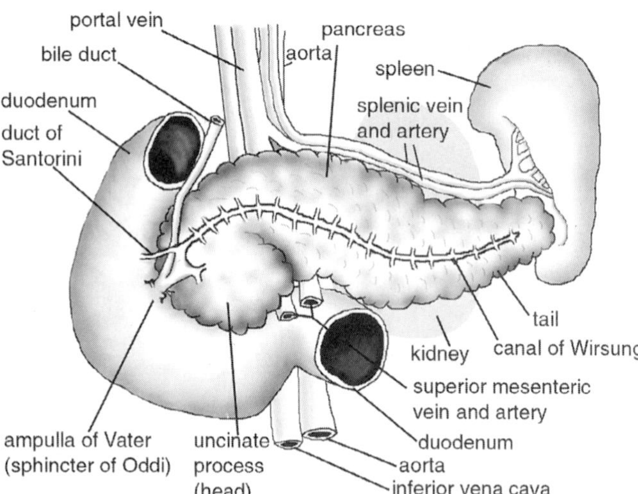

Figure 2.1. Anatomy of the human adult pancreas. Ventral view of pancreas; anterior is toward the top of the page. The body of the pancreas lies posterior to the stomach and extends laterally from the duodenum to the spleen (stomach has been omitted at top of figure). The head of the pancreas is tucked into the curvature of the duodenum, and the tail of the pancreas contacts the spleen and left kidney. The principal excretory duct, or the canal of Wirsung, spans the length of the pancreas and connects to the duodenum via the ampulla of Vater, where it joins the bile duct. The sphincter of Oddi, within the ampulla of Vater, regulates secretions from the pancreas into the gastrointestinal tract. An accessory pancreatic duct, or the duct of Santorini, joins the duodenum more anteriorly. The posterior portion of the pancreas, or the uncinate process, extends behind the superior mesenteric artery and vein. The body of the pancreas lies in proximity to multiple large blood vessels, including the portal vein (connected to the splenic vein and superior mesenteric veins), the aorta (connected to the splenic and superior mesenteric arteries), and the inferior vena cava.

The Exocrine Pancreas

The exocrine pancreas constitutes the bulk of pancreatic tissue and comprises primarily acinar cells. Acinar cells are organized into acini, which are epithelial pouches located at the tips of a branched network of ducts (Fig. 2.2A,D). These secretory cells are linked to each other by large gap junctions and are flanked by centroacinar cells at the neck of the acini. Acinar cells are pyramidal in shape and contain an extensive secretory apparatus at the apical end, including numerous zymogen granules (18). These granules contain digestive enzymes, including amylases, proteases, nucleases, and lipases, which are secreted into the duodenum. Initially, these are produced and secreted as inactive proenzymes, which are then activated by limited proteolysis once they enter the digestive tract. The ducts connect the acini and constitute a tubular epithelial network that is continuous with the gut tube. It is through the ducts that the exocrine secretions are transported into the duodenum. The duct cells produce mucins and a bicarbonate-rich fluid, which is used to neutralize the acidic product of the stomach (19). The ducts contain scattered endocrine cells, and it has been hypothesized that the ducts include a population of precursor cells that can give rise to endocrine and exocrine cells (6,17,20).

The Endocrine Pancreas

The endocrine function of the pancreas is performed by a number of cell types in the islets of Langerhans. These structures were identified by the German physician Paul Langerhans in 1869. Islets are tight aggregations or clusters of cells embedded in the surrounding exocrine tissue. There are four cell types found in pancreatic islets: α-cells, β-cells, δ-cells, and PP-cells (pancreatic peptide; also called γ-cells) (Fig. 2.2A–C). The β-cells are the majority of the endocrine cell population of the pancreas and secrete insulin, the insulin antagonist amylin, and other peptides (21). Insulin release is stimulated by high glucose levels, as well as by glucagon, gastric inhibitory peptide, epineph-

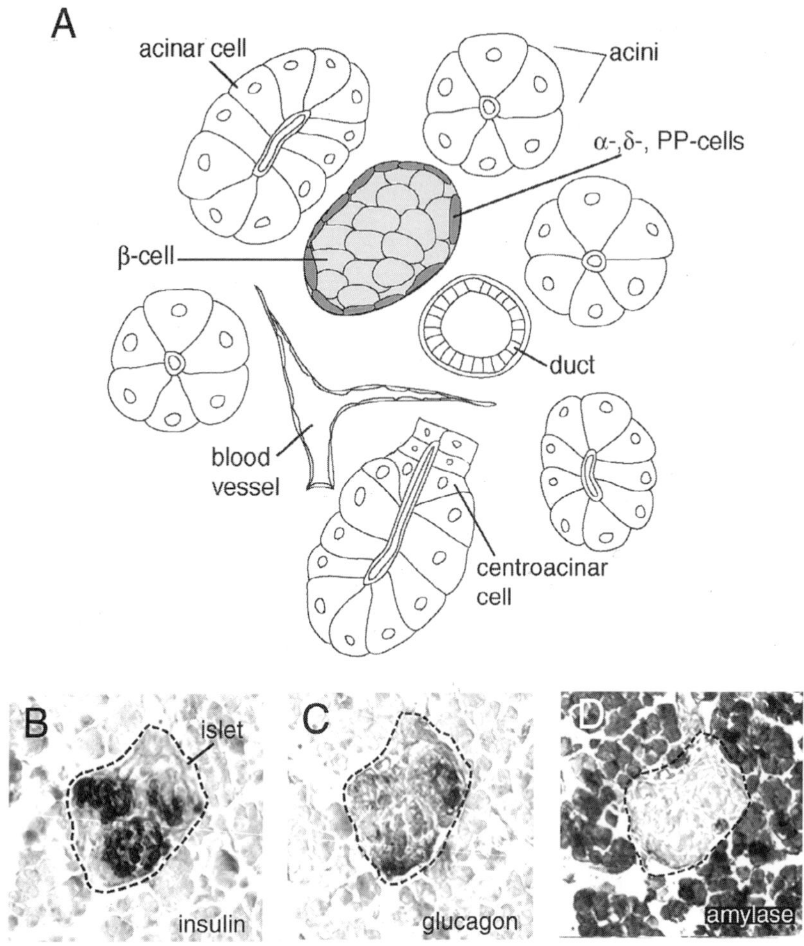

Figure 2.2. Principal pancreatic cell types. **A:** Schematic representation of cell types in the pancreas. An islet is surrounded by more abundant exocrine tissue. β-Cells *(light gray)* and peripheral non–β-cells *(dark gray)* are indicated. Acini are composed of acinar and centroacinar cells. A duct and blood vessel are also represented. Both form extensive networks throughout pancreatic tissue, and usually lie in proximity to islets. **B–D:** Adjacent sections through an islet in pancreatic tissue of an E18.5 mouse embryo stained using antibodies to pancreatic gene products. **B:** β-Cells clustered within the islet. Immunostain for insulin. **C:** β-Cells located at the periphery of the islet. Immunostain for glucagon on adjacent section to B. **D:** Exocrine tissue composed of acinar cells surrounding the islet. Immunostain for amylase on adjacent section to C.

rine, and increased levels of amino acids (see Chapter 6). β-Cells are polyhedral and packed with secretory granules (22). The α-, δ-, and PP-cells secrete glucagon, somatostatin, and pancreatic polypeptide, respectively. In most mammals, the β-cells lie in the middle of the islet and are surrounded by a thin layer of α-, δ-, and PP-cells (one to three cells thick) (23). These peripheral cells are smaller than β-cells and are also well granulated. In humans and other primates, the concentric segregation of cells within the islet is less defined, with islets sometimes taking on oval and cloverleaf patterns (24,25). The endocrine cells that produce some islet hormones are found in other regions of the gut; however, within the endoderm, insulin-expressing cells are found only in the pancreas (26).

In the islets of the mature human pancreas, β-cells constitute approximately 70% to 80% of the islet mass; α-cells, approximately 15% to 20%; δ-cells, approximately 5%; and PP-cells, up to 1%. The pancreas of an adult human of average weight (70 kg) contains between 300,000 and 1.5 million islets (27), adult mice have approximately 100 to 200 islets (JM Wells and DA Melton, unpublished observations), and some fish have a single islet (28). Hormones produced by the islets appear sequentially during development, and the order of appearance varies slightly among different organisms. In the mouse embryonic pancreas, differentiated glucagon cells first appear at E9.5 (9.5 days postconception) followed by insulin-expressing β-cells at E10.5, and finally by somatostatin- and PP-expressing cells at E15.5 (29,30). Endocrine gene transcription, however, can be detected earlier. Somatostatin transcripts are first detectable throughout the foregut epithelium at E8; insulin and glucagon transcripts are found a day later at E9; and last, pancreatic polypeptide is detectable at E10 to 10.5 (31). Transcription of exocrine genes begins slightly later than that of all endocrine genes. Despite the synthesis of endocrine hormones during embryogenesis, it is unclear whether islets are actually functional at this time. In mouse embryos, endocrine cells respond to glucose only after fetal day 18 (32).

Overview of Pancreatic Development

In the early rodent embryo, the pancreas derives from distinct dorsal and ventral endodermal evaginations caudal to the developing stomach (33) (Fig. 2.3A,B). The dorsal bud becomes evident slightly before the ventral bud. The buds then grow and proliferate rapidly into highly branched structures. As the epithelium grows, it depends on its intimate association with a growing cap of mesodermal mesenchyme surrounding it (34,35). The dorsal and ventral anlagen then fuse during gut rotation, when the ventral bud rotates around the duodenum and joins the dorsal bud on the dorsal portion of the gut tube (Fig. 2.3C,D). The dorsal bud will form the largest portion of the pancreas, including part of the head and all of the body and tail of the pancreas, while the ventral bud will form the posterior portion of the head. Exocrine, endocrine, and ductal cell types arise from the endodermal epithelium, whereas the mesenchyme forms smooth muscle and supportive tissue (36).

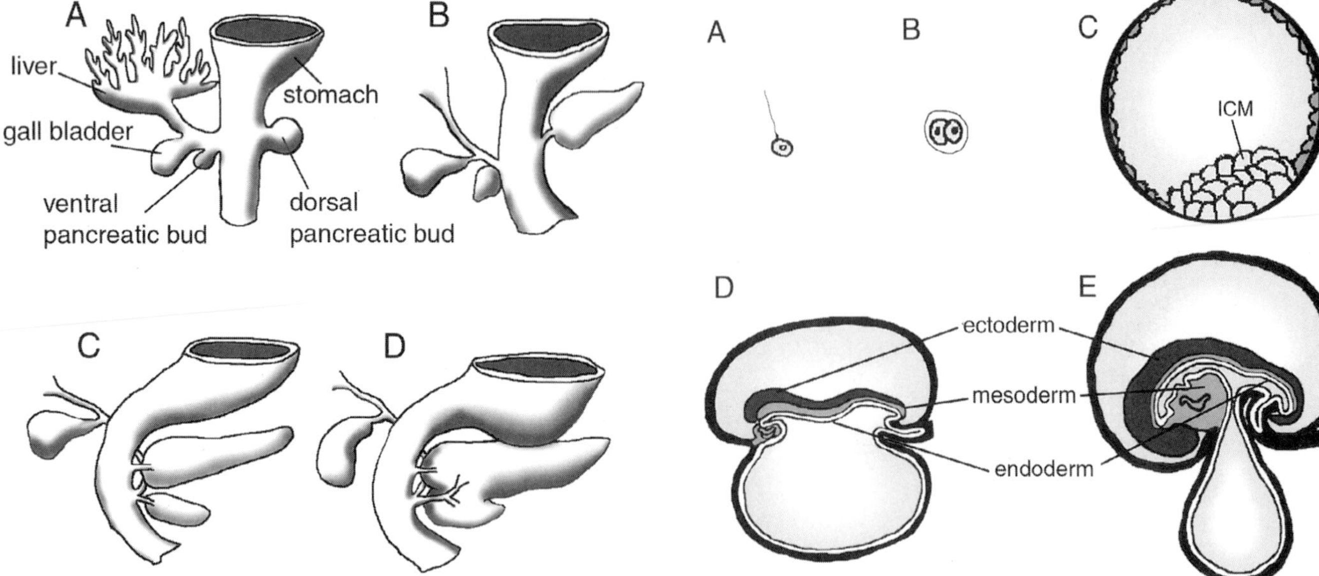

Figure 2.3. Development of the pancreatic primordia. All diagrams are ventrolateral views. **A:** Schematic drawing of the dorsal and ventral pancreatic evaginations located posterior to the stomach along the gut tube. The gallbladder and liver connect to the duodenum via the common bile duct. This stage of pancreatic development is comparable to an E10.5 mouse and to a human in the early 5th week of gestation. **B:** The dorsal pancreas grows and extends dorsally. The ventral pancreas rotates dorsally around the gut tube in the direction of the dorsal pancreas. This stage is comparable to an E11 mouse embryo and to a human in the late 5th week of gestation. **C:** After rotation of the duodenum and migration of the ventral pancreas, the dorsal and ventral pancreata come to rest in proximity. This stage is comparable to an E12.5 mouse embryo and to a human in the early 6th week of gestation. **D:** The dorsal and ventral buds fuse. The dorsal pancreas appropriates the ventral duct and the duct systems anastomose. This is comparable to an E14.5 mouse embryo and to a human in the late 7th week of gestation.

Figure 2.4. Schematic drawing of germ layer development in the early amniote. **A:** Fertilization of egg. Sperm binds to the oocyte zona pellucida. This occurs 12 to 24 hours after ovulation in humans. **B:** Two-cell stage, at approximately 30 hours after fertilization in humans. **C:** Early blastocyst stage embryo, prior to implantation at 5 days post-fertilization. Inner cell mass (ICM) cells give rise to the embryo and are surrounded by trophoblast cells, which give rise to the placenta. **D:** Germ layers of a seven-somite human embryo. Ectoderm *(dark gray)*, mesoderm *(light gray)*, and endoderm *(white)* are indicated. The endoderm lines the developing gut tube. The anterior and caudal intestinal portals are beginning to form. **E:** Embryonic germ layers of a 35-somite embryo. This represents the embryo at the end of the first month of gestation in humans. At this stage the anterior and caudal intestinal portals have met and the yolk stalk is constricting.

Although the key landmarks of pancreatic development have been investigated quite thoroughly, many questions remain. For instance: What are the early events that result in regionalization of the endoderm along the developing gut? What determines the position of committed pancreatic endoderm between the stomach and duodenum? Are there common signals that direct the formation of pancreatic buds on both the dorsal and ventral portions of the gut tube? What is the nature of the signals from the pancreatic mesenchyme to the endoderm that are necessary for later morphogenesis and cell differentiation? Most important for diabetes research, What are the specific combinations of factors that give rise to β-cells?

ENDODERMAL ORIGINS OF ENDOCRINE CELLS

Germ Layers

During gastrulation, three fundamental germ layers are established in the embryo: the ectoderm, the mesoderm, and the endoderm (Fig. 2.4). The ectoderm gives rise to the epidermis and nervous system. The mesoderm develops into the notochord, the muscle, the heart, the kidney, the vasculature, the gut mesenchyme, and the blood. The endoderm gives rise to a variety of organs along the anterior-posterior axis, more specifically that of the gastrointestinal and respiratory tracts (Fig. 2.5). Pharyngeal endoderm gives rise to the pharynx, as well as to portions of the thymus and thyroid gland. Foregut endoderm

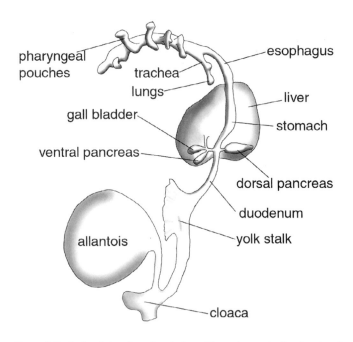

Figure 2.5. Stylized drawing of endoderm illustrating major landmarks of embryonic endoderm. Lateral view; dorsal is to the right and anterior is up. The pancreas develops from two evaginations of the endodermal epithelium that emerge posterior to the stomach and just anterior to the duodenum. The ventral pancreas originates adjacent to the gallbladder and liver along the common bile duct. The dorsal pancreas evaginates opposite the ventral bud on the dorsal side of the gut tube. (Adapted from endodermal derivatives of the 10 mm pig embryo, as drawn in Shumway W. *Vertebrate embryology*, 2nd ed. London: John Wiley and Sons, 1930.)

forms the esophagus, lungs, stomach, liver, gallbladder, and both the endocrine and exocrine cells of the pancreas. The midgut endoderm gives rise to the jejunum, the ileum of the small intestine, and the anterior colon; and the hindgut endoderm forms the caudal large intestine and rectum. In all cases, the endoderm generates primarily the epithelial lining of the organs. Splanchnic mesodermal mesenchyme surrounds the endoderm and is active in inducing and supporting its proliferation and morphogenesis.

Endoderm Formation in Amphibians

The genetic basis for endoderm cell specification is presently not well understood. The signals that determine endodermal cell fate remain largely unknown, although a growing number of candidate molecules are being identified, including members of the transforming growth factor–β (TGF-β), fibroblast growth factor (FGF), and Wnt (small secreted glycoproteins) growth factor families (37,38). It is also unclear at what point embryonic cells become determined to form endoderm. This process appears to be complete by the end of gastrulation because all three germ layers are identifiable at this time.

Studies in amphibians have identified a number of genes that can direct endodermal cell fate. In the frog *Xenopus laevis*, the endoderm arises from the vegetal blastomeres, which invaginate through the blastopore and become internalized. The fate of these blastomeres becomes increasingly restricted to endoderm after the mid-blastula transition, as shown by transplantation experiments (39,40). These experiments have suggested that both cell-autonomous and non–cell-autonomous mechanisms are involved in the initiation of early endodermal gene expression. Several nodal-related molecules (41–43) and two vegetally localized maternal determinants, Vg1 and VegT, have been implicated in the regulation of both mesoderm and endoderm (44,45). In addition, several endoderm-specific factors have been identified that can direct the fate of endodermal cells in a cell-autonomous fashion. For example, the transcription factors Mixer, Mix.1, and Sox 17(α and β) and the ribonucleic acid–binding molecule XBic-C are expressed exclusively in the early endoderm and can direct ectopic endoderm formation when expressed in ectoderm cells, such as animal caps (46–49). Furthermore, when dominant-negative forms of some these molecules are expressed in the endoderm, its formation is disrupted (50). Mammalian and avian orthologues of these endoderm genes have not yet been identified.

Endoderm Formation in Amniotes

In amniotes, the primitive streak is directly involved in endoderm cell fate specification. As cells delaminate from the epiblast and migrate through the primitive streak, they become committed to either a mesodermal or an endodermal cell fate (51). Lineage tracing shows that the definitive endoderm in mice and humans originates from a group of cells at the most distal end of the primitive streak (52). In chick embryos, the endoderm originates from the posterior third of the epiblast (53).

In mice, chimeric embryo experiments demonstrate that TGF-β signaling is required for the specification of the definitive endoderm. In these experiments, *Smad2* mutant embryonic stem (ES) cells extensively colonize ectodermal and mesodermal derivatives of the early embryo but are not recruited into the endoderm lineage during gastrulation (54). This reveals that *Smad2* signals promote recruitment of epiblast cells into the definitive gut endoderm. FGF signaling has also been implicated during endoderm formation. FGF-4 is expressed in the primitive streak, and gene-targeting experiments demonstrate that FGF-4 is required for initial outgrowth of the epiblast (55). FGF-4 is also capable of inducing endoderm differentiation in a concentration-dependent manner and may therefore act as a posterior morphogen for endoderm in the embryo (56). In addition, FGF receptor 1 (FGFR-1) mutant ES cells fail to populate endodermal derivatives in chimeric embryo experiments (57). A direct role for other growth factors in mammalian endoderm formation remains under investigation.

Neural Origin of Endocrine Cells Refuted

For many years, it was postulated that endocrine cells might originate from the neural crest rather than from the endoderm (58–60), a theory based on the shared characteristics of islet and neuronal cells of "amine precursor uptake and decarboxylation" (APUD) (61). The APUD hypothesis received considerable attention because it seemed to be supported by numerous lines of evidence. Endocrine and neural cells express many of the same genes and share cytochemical and ultrastructural characteristics. For instance, pancreatic endocrine cells express the neuronal marker tyrosine hydroxylase, whereas neurons located in the neural tube express the insulin gene (62). In fact, a surprising number of genes are expressed in both tissues, including an L-amino acid decarboxylase (63), a specific acetylcholinesterase (64), a neuron-specific enolase (65), the glycoprotein synaptophysin (66), and the antigens PGP9.5 (67) and A2B5 (68). More recently identified genes that also are found in both tissues include *Pax6*, *Isl1*, *Nkx2.2*, and *HNF-3β* (see discussion below). Endocrine cells will extend neurites when grown in culture under certain conditions (69,70).

In addition to similar gene expression patterns of neural and endocrine cell types, analogies have been drawn between the mechanisms underlying the specification of these cell types. The neurectoderm and pancreatic endoderm are controlled, at least in part, by inductive interactions with the notochord (see below) (71). In addition, comparative studies in vertebrates and invertebrates have reinforced this intriguing link between endocrine and neural cells (33,72). For instance, somatostatin-expressing cells are found in the paired cerebral ganglia of the flatworm *Dugesia lugubris* (73). In hornworm moths and blowflies, all four pancreatic endocrine cell types are detected in the brain and the corpus cardiacum (74,75). In the invertebrate chordates, tunicates and amphioxus, both the brain and the gastrointestinal tract contain somatostatin-, PP-, and glucagon-expressing cells (72).

Despite all the evidence for a similarity and coincidence in gene expression, it is a mistake to conclude that cells expressing similar genes derive from a common precursor. Indeed, the neural origin of pancreatic endocrine cells has no direct support from experimental studies and, in fact, the hypothesis has been rendered untenable on the basis of chick-quail chimera lineage studies. In chick-quail chimera experiments, quail neural tube or neurectoderm is grafted to the endomesoderm of the chick and allowed to develop. Invariably, both pancreas and gut endocrine cells are shown to be of chick origin, thus demonstrating that the endocrine cells of the pancreas do not arise as a result of cellular migration from neural tissues (76,77).

PATTERNING OF THE GUT TUBE

Formation of the Gut Tube

In fish, birds, and mammals, the result of gastrulation is the formation of an endodermal sheet, which must be transformed into a proper gut tube. This sheet overlies the yolk sac and first develops tubelike folds at the anterior and posterior extremities. Once formed, these blind cavities are called the anterior and caudal intestinal portals. As development proceeds, the portals move toward each other and meet at the increasingly constricted yolk stalk, leaving an endodermally lined tube in their wake. Cells originally at the midline of the endodermal sheet now constitute the dorsal midline of the embryonic gut tube. Cells originally at the lateral edges of the sheet are now located on the ventral side of the gut. Gene-targeting experiments reveal that a number of genes are important for this gut folding and closure, including *GATA4*, its Drosophila homologue *Serpent*, the proprotein convertase gene *Furin*, and the bone morphogenic protein genes (*BMP1*, *2*, *4*, *5*, and *7*) (78–82).

Regionalization of the Gut Tube

How is this developing gut endoderm patterned along the anterior-posterior axis? The answer to this question is likely to be complex, and it is only beginning to be addressed. As previously mentioned, it is likely that a certain level of patterning occurs during gastrulation. Immediately after gastrulation, and before formation of the gut tube, the early mouse endoderm already expresses some genes in a regionalized manner. For instance, *cerberus-like*, *Otx1*, and *Hesx1* are expressed in the anterior endoderm at this time, while the posterior endoderm expresses *IFABP* and *Cdx2* (38,83–86). The factors that regulate this early regional expression of genes remain largely unknown, although members of the FGF family have been implicated (38). Numerous studies demonstrate that the endoderm continues to receive signals from adjacent mesoderm and ectoderm long after gastrulation and that these tissues are dependent on reciprocal signaling for proper differentiation (see discussion below). Once the gut tube is formed, it must undergo further anterior-posterior and dorsal-ventral patterning to ensure that prospective organ territories are appropriately assigned and that derivative organs develop at their correct location. Early endoderm regionalization is thus translated into patterning along the gut tube as a requisite prelude to organogenesis. Recent fate-mapping experiments and gene-expression analyses in a number of different organisms indicate that organs have overlapping presumptive domains that become restricted during development (87). The subsequent onset of organogenesis is evident as localized thickening and budding of the endodermal epithelium.

HOX GENES

Hox genes are excellent candidates for patterning molecules in the endoderm. *Hox* genes are expressed in sequential, overlapping patterns in the vertebrate mesoderm and ectoderm, and particular combinations of these genes lead to positional commitment along the anterior-posterior axis in the limb, vertebrae, and neurectoderm. Recent gene-expression studies in the chick embryo reveal that only a small number of *Hox* genes can be detected in the endoderm by *in situ* hybridization (87). However, the anterior expression boundaries of *Hox* gene expression in the surrounding intestinal smooth muscle match anatomic boundaries in the intestinal epithelium (88,89). When a posterior mesodermal *Hox* gene, *Hoxd-13*, is misexpressed in the midgut mesoderm, the underlying endoderm acquires a morphology reminiscent of the hindgut. Therefore, *Hox* gene–directed positional information exists in the visceral mesoderm and this information is transmitted vertically to the underlying endoderm.

MORPHOGENESIS AND DIFFERENTIATION OF THE PANCREAS

Epithelial Budding

During vertebrate embryogenesis, the first morphologic sign of pancreatic development is an evagination of the dorsal endodermal epithelium and a condensation of the dorsal mesenchyme that lies above it. This pancreatic bud formation is evident at the 22- to 25-somite stage or E9.5 in mice (4,34), at the 30-somite stage or stage 15 in chickens (90,91), and during the fourth week of gestation in humans (92). Subsequently, approximately 12 hours later, the ventral bud becomes evident (Fig. 2.6A,B). The dorsal bud arises from the endodermal epithelium caudal to the stomach anlage and slightly caudal to the biliary duct. At this point, the liver has developed into a trilobular structure and is joined to the duodenum via the biliary duct. The ventral bud arises from epithelium at approximately the same anterior-posterior location as the dorsal bud but on the ventral side of the gut tube at the base of the biliary duct. Some organisms (such as the rat and human) have only one ventral bud and others have two (chick and frog) (93). In the mouse, two ventral buds are detectable transiently during bud evagination (93; E Lammert and DA Melton, unpublished observations).

Branching and Bud Fusion

As development proceeds, the dorsal pancreatic bud begins to proliferate and branch, progressively forming a tree-like structure (Figs. 2.7 and 2.8) (5,6). This process begins around the 25- to 35-somite stage in mice (E10.5) and the 26-somite stage in chicks and continues throughout pancreatic development (6,90). Initially, the branching epithelium appears as a solid tissue; however, it actually consists of a compact bulb of highly folded epithelium. It has been hypothesized that branching occurs because the number of cells in the wall of the diverticulum increases while the bud remains the same size (6), causing lateral pressure until the epithelium buckles and produces a digitation. Unlike the branching that occurs in kidney epithelium, including both lateral and terminal bifid branching, or the asymmetric branching of lungs, pancreatic branching is not stereotyped (94,95).

After the 25-somite stage in mice (E10), mesodermal mesenchyme continues to condense around the pancreatic bud and accumulates on the left side of the gut tube, breaking the symmetrical morphology of the pancreatic rudiment (4). At this stage, islet structures begin to protrude from the pancreatic epithelium (14). Bud growth and elaboration is followed by a constriction at the base of the pancreatic diverticulum, near the duodenum, and formation of a narrow stalk (4). As development proceeds, between E11 and E12, the gut tube bends and rotates, swinging the ventral bud dorsally and bringing it into immediate proximity to the dorsal bud (Fig. 2.6C,D). The dorsal and ventral buds then fuse sometime around E13 (96). In humans, mice, and rats, this fusion occurs between a dorsal bud and a single ventral bud, whereas in chicks and amphibians, the dorsal bud fuses with paired ventral buds. At E14.5, acini and ducts become clearly visible as distinct structures embedded within the more abundant exocrine tissue. Subsequently, the pancreas continues to grow and extend into adulthood (Fig. 2.6E,F).

Dorsal and Ventral Bud Derivatives

The dorsal and ventral buds later develop into different portions of the mature pancreas. The dorsal bud connects to the duodenum via the duct of Santorini and forms the upper part

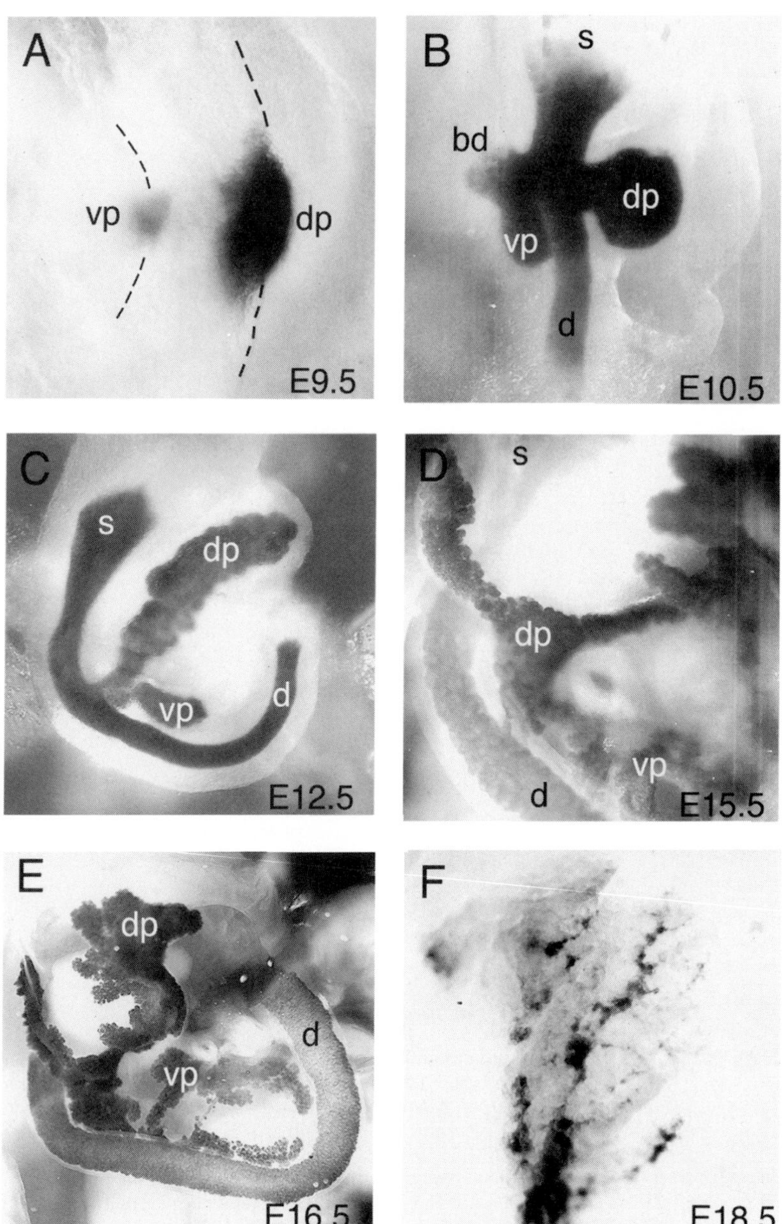

Figure 2.6. Stages of pancreatic bud development in the mouse. Whole-mount β-galactosidase staining of *Pdx1-LacZ* transgenic embryos showing *Pdx1* expression in the pancreas. Series of photographs show pancreatic bud development during embryogenesis. All pancreases shown are cleared with glycerol and dissected away from the embryo. Ventrolateral view; dorsal is toward right and stomach is at top of each panel. **A:** E9.5. Dorsal pancreatic bud is evident along the gut tube *(right)* and ventral bud is appearing at this stage *(left)*. Gut tube is outlined with dashed lines. **B:** E10.5. Dorsal pancreatic bud has grown and connection to the duodenum has narrowed. Ventral bud is evident on the opposite side of the gut tube. **C:** E12.5. Both dorsal and ventral pancreatic bud are in close proximity on the dorsal side of the gut tube. Both buds have branched and elongated, although each remains encased in surrounding mesenchyme. **D:** E15.5. Pancreas continues to grow, and acini are visible at this stage. The mesenchymal layer surrounding each bud is relatively thinner. Dorsal and ventral buds have fused proximally at this stage. Extensions of the pancreas can be seen around the stomach and posteriorly along the duodenum. **E:** E16.5. Branches of the pancreas extend in multiple directions around the stomach and duodenum. Expression of *Pdx1* in pancreatic epithelium can still be seen throughout the pancreatic epithelium. **F:** E18.5. Dorsal pancreatic tissue. Expression of *Pdx1* is declining in most pancreatic tissues, except in δ- and β-cells. Dorsal pancreas (dp), ventral pancreas (vp), stomach (s), duodenum (d), and bile duct (bd) are indicated.

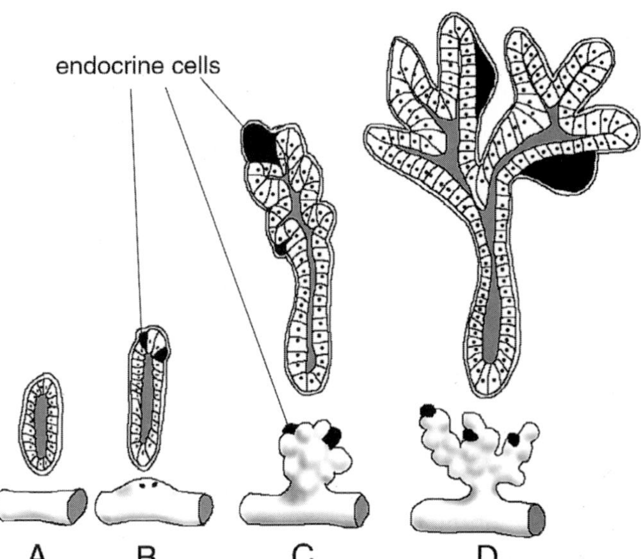

Figure 2.7. Schematic representation of morphologic and functional differentiation of the pancreatic bud during development. **A:** Pancreatic endoderm before budding. Gut tube is drawn both in three dimensions and in cross-section at the position of pancreatic budding. **B:** Initiation of dorsal bud formation. Endocrine cells are evident in the epithelium as scattered cells *(black)*. Representation of ventral bud has been omitted. **C:** Growth and buckling of the pancreatic epithelium and initiation of branching. **D**: Elaboration and extension of pancreatic branching. (Adapted from Rutter WJ. *Handbook of physiology: endocrinology I*. Washington, DC: American Physiological Society, 1972.)

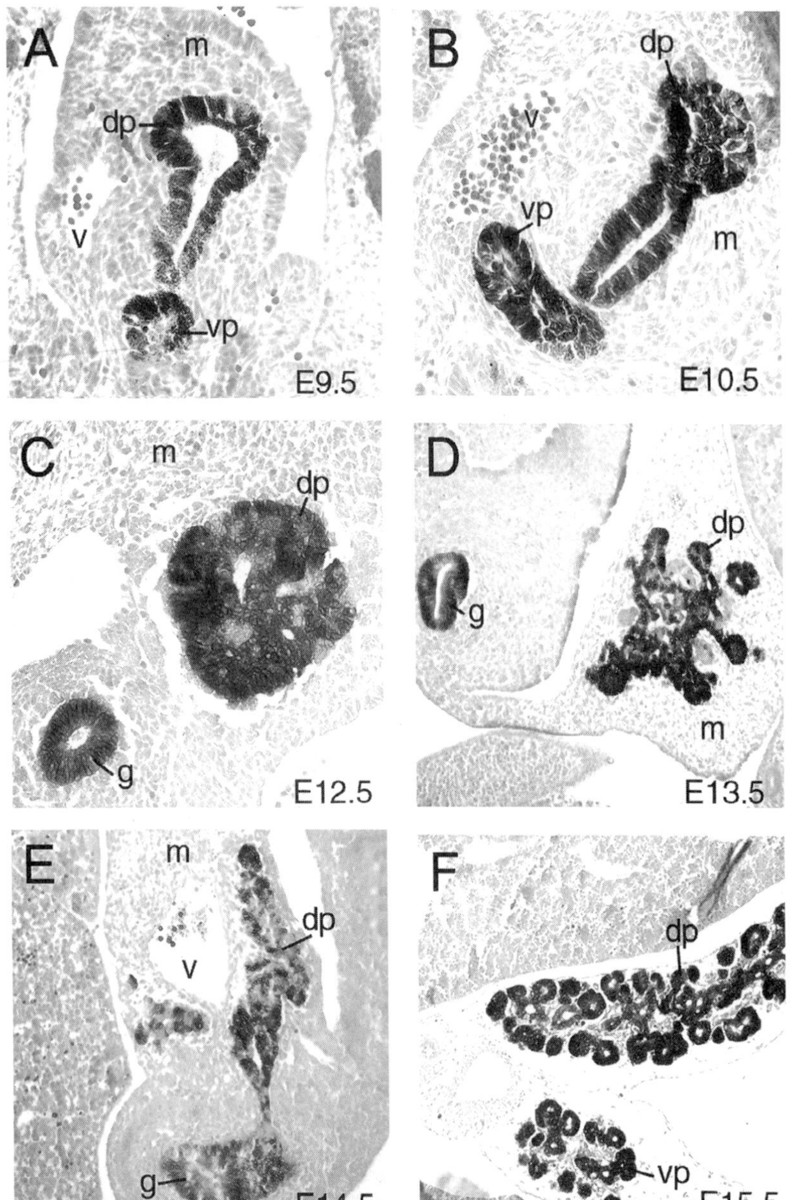

Figure 2.8. Branching morphogenesis of pancreatic primordium in the mouse embryo. Transverse sections through *Pdx1-LacZ* transgenic embryos showing *Pdx1* expression in the pancreas by β-galactosidase staining. All sections are counterstained with eosin. **A:** E9.5. 20× **B:** E10.5. 20× **C:** E12.5. 20× **D:** E13.5. 10× **E:** E14.5. 10× **F:** E15.5. 10× Dorsal pancreatic bud (dp), ventral pancreatic bud (vp), gut tube lumen (g), blood vessels (v), and mesenchyme (m) are indicated.

of the head of the pancreas; the body; and the tail, or splenic portion, of the pancreas. The ventral bud connects to the duodenum via the duct of Wirsung and forms the lower part of the head of the pancreas, or the uncinate process. Generally, after the fusion of the primordia, the dorsal pancreas appropriates the duct of the ventral pancreas proximally and it becomes the primary pancreatic duct, or the duct of Wirsung. More distally, the dorsal pancreas sometimes retains its own connection to the duodenum, or the duct of Santorini. Many of the smaller epithelial ductules anastomose during the fusion process, leading to functional connections between tissue of dorsal and ventral origin (97).

The dorsal and ventral anlagen, as well as their adult derivative portions of the mature pancreas, differ in their component cell types. The dorsal pancreas develops larger insulin-secreting islets that contain more insulin-producing and glucagon-producing cells and fewer PP-producing cells than do those of the ventral pancreas. The ventral pancreas develops mainly into exocrine acinar tissue interspersed with smaller islets that contain many more PP-cells (98). One study determined that the dorsal pancreas is composed of 82% β-cells, 13% α-cells, 4% δ-cells, and 1% PP-cells and that the ventral pancreas is composed of 79% PP-cells, 18% β-cells, 2% δ-cells, and 1% α-cells (99). However, the relative concentration of islets is more or less equivalent in the two tissues (100,101).

Normal Development of Embryonic Islets

Morphologically distinguishable islets of Langerhans arise late during embryogenesis (Fig. 2.9). However, the endocrine cells that will aggregate to form islets appear much earlier. The process by which these endocrine precursors delaminate from the endoderm, migrate, and coordinate to form a functional islet is one that has been noted repeatedly during the past century in fish, amphibians, birds, and mammals. Initially, endocrine precursors are observed as scattered individual cells, often still embedded in the epithelium of the ducts (16,97). These precursors have recently been referred to as islet precur-

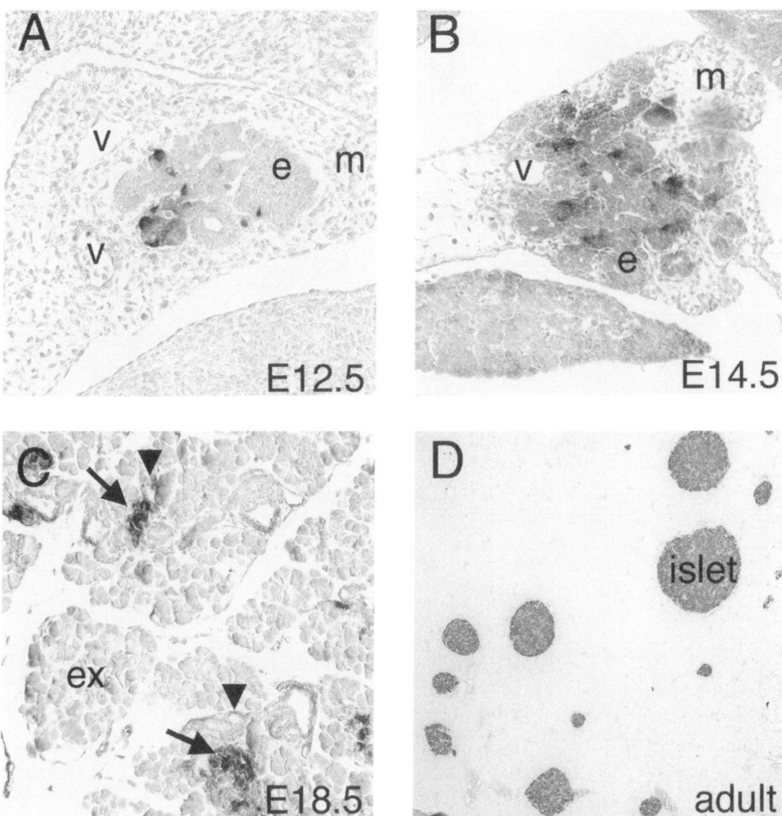

Figure 2.9. Islet development in the mouse. Immunohistochemical staining of sections through the pancreas using an antibody to insulin. **A:** E12.5. A few insulin-positive cells are found scattered in the pancreatic epithelium of the early branching pancreas. **B:** E14.5. The number of insulin cells increases as the pancreas branches and grows. Insulin cells are distributed throughout the epithelium. **C:** E18.5. Insulin cells aggregate into clusters *(arrows)*, closely associated with smaller ducts *(arrowheads)*. **D:** Adult. Insulin cells are located in mature compact islets. Blood vessels (v), mesenchyme (m), pancreatic epithelium (e), and exocrine tissue (ex) are indicated.

sor cells and are thought to be multipotent (102). The first endocrine cells that can be identified in the developing pancreas are the α-cells or glucagon-expressing cells (30). Insulin-expressing cells are detectable soon after. These endocrine precursors remain associated with the ducts as individual cells until well into embryogenesis—as late as E15.5 in the mouse. These cells then begin to dissociate from the duct epithelium, migrate a short distance away from the ducts, and aggregate into small clusters. Shortly before birth, compact islets have formed and are recognizable by their characteristic concentric arrangement of β-cells surrounded by α, δ, and PP endocrine cell types. Studies with aggregation mouse chimeras clearly indicate that islets are not clonally derived but are rather the result of the clustering of individual endocrine cells or clusters of cells that arise independently of each other (103).

INDUCTION OF PANCREATIC CELL FATE

Commitment to Pancreatic Cell Fate

The initiation of pancreatic commitment to a pancreatic cell fate occurs before overt morphogenesis of the pancreas. Mouse pancreatic buds cultured *in vitro* will grow and branch, revealing that foregut epithelial cells of the early pancreatic bud are already programmed to take on a pancreatic fate (4). However, the pancreas is said to be committed even earlier, at the 8- to 12-somite stage in mice, or E8.5 (4), and the 13-somite stage in chickens, or stage 11 (98). This commitment has been shown in experiments involving the culture of isolated mouse foregut tissues. For example, when the pancreatic endoderm and associated mesenchyme are excised from an eight-somite mouse embryo and cultured in isolation, morphologically distinct exocrine tissue develops, with acinar cells filled with distinguishable zymogen granules. This commitment is likely to be influenced by both intrinsic and extrinsic factors. The endoderm alone is said to be committed by the 15-somite stage, at which time it has the capacity to form exocrine tissue in response to signals from heterologous mesenchyme. *In vitro* culture of committed pancreatic endoderm in combination with either pancreatic or heterologous mesenchyme leads to the differentiation of pancreatic cell types; however, culture of isolated endoderm does not (4,34,96,104). This shows that the competence to form pancreas is intrinsic to the pancreatic epithelium but that inductive signals from adjacent mesenchyme or other tissues are required.

Sources of Inductive Signals

Regionalized gene expression in the gut tube is generated by early interactions with adjacent mesoderm, ectoderm, or anterior visceral endoderm. As the dorsal pancreatic anlage develops, it comes in contact with a number of different neighboring tissues that may be sources of inductive or maintenance signals, including the notochord, the dorsal aorta, and the visceral mesenchyme (Fig. 2.10). The notochord, for instance, is embedded in the endodermal epithelium following gastrulation. The notochord remains in contact with the endoderm from the time it becomes morphologically recognizable as a rod of cells until well into embryogenesis (105). The entire endoderm, including the region that will give rise to the pancreas, remains in immediate contact with the notochord throughout the period during which pancreatic fate becomes committed. This contact persists until about the 13-somite stage in mice (E8) and the 22-somite stage in chicks (embryonic day 2.5). Studies of chicks have shown that the notochord sends permissive signals to the pan-

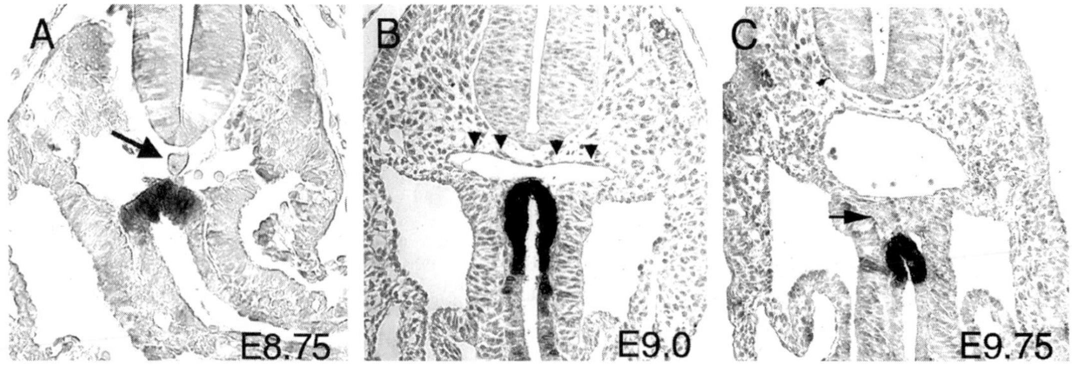

Figure 2.10. Tissues juxtaposed to the developing pancreatic endoderm. **A:** Transverse section through an E8.75 mouse embryo. Prepancreatic *Pdx1* expressing endoderm *(dark gray)* is immediately in contact with the notochord at this stage *(arrow)*. **B:** Transverse section through an E9.0 mouse embryo. Prepancreatic *Pdx1*-expressing endoderm is in direct contact with the dorsal aorta. The paired dorsal aortae have fused at the midline over the dorsal pancreatic bud evagination *(arrowheads)*. **C:** Transverse section through an E9.75 mouse embryo. Dorsal pancreatic bud expresses *Pdx1* and is surrounded by mesenchyme *(thin arrow)*.

creatic endoderm (71). Removal of the notochord in chick embryos leads to the elimination of the expression of insulin, glucagon, and carboxypeptidase A. However, the recombination of notochord with endoderm not fated to become pancreas cannot induce the expression of pancreatic gene expression, suggesting that some patterning of the endoderm has already occurred by the stage at which these experiments are carried out (106). Additional experiments demonstrate that the notochord signal is possibly composed of activin-βB and FGF-2 signaling and participates in repressing *Shh* in the underlying pancreatic endoderm (108). This repression of *Shh* is required for the initiation of the expression of pancreatic gene expression and development. It is interesting that cyclopamine, which acts as an inhibitor of *hedgehog* signaling, can mimic the notochord signal and promote pancreatic development (107).

Epithelial-Mesenchymal Interactions

Reciprocal epithelial-mesenchymal interactions have also been shown to be critical for the regionalization of the gut tube and the development of most endodermally derived organs (108). Generally, gut endoderm signals to the splanchnic mesoderm, recruiting it to surround the gut tube as visceral mesoderm (109,110) and inducing region-specific gene expression in the mesoderm (111). The mesoderm, in turn, signals back to the endoderm and directs its morphologic differentiation (109,112). Heterologous recombination experiments in which mesoderm from different anterior-posterior locations along the gut tube is cultured with endoderm have been carried out in chicks (113), rats (114), and mice (4,115). For instance, when chick foregut mesoderm is recombined with midgut endoderm, the endoderm becomes respecified to take on foregut endoderm morphology (109). Similarly, intestinal mesenchyme can cause the respecification of stomach epithelium into intestinal epithelium (116–119). It has been suggested that the basis for the epithelial-mesenchymal interactions may depend on the formation of distinct basement membrane components at the interface of the two tissues (97).

Development of the pancreas also requires the origination of signals in the surrounding pancreatic mesenchyme. In fact, pancreatic endoderm alone fails to grow and shows only limited differentiation in the absence of pancreatic mesenchyme (34). This mesenchyme accumulates around the growing epithelial bud and is required for proliferation of the epithelium. It is interesting that heterologous mesenchyme derived from other branching organs also can promote the development of pancreatic cells (120,121). When presumptive pancreatic epithelium is recombined with salivary gland mesenchyme, endoderm cells differentiate into morphologically distinct acini that express amylase (33). In addition, this inductive effect occurs across a filter, suggesting that the mesenchyme secretes soluble factors. Despite the many attempts made to identify and purify this mesenchymal factor, its nature remains unresolved (122,123). A number of experiments have shown no effect of basic FGF (bFGF), recombinant human hepatocyte growth factor (rhHGF), insulin-like growth factor-2, platelet-derived growth factor, and nerve growth factor on pancreatic tissue (124), but others suggest that HGF/scatter factor (SF), FGF-2, FGF-7, and follistatin may be involved (125–128).

Mesenchymal signals have also been shown to be important in determining the ratio of exocrine to endocrine cell types. Studies have shown that removal of large portions of the mesenchyme at a certain time will promote differentiation of endocrine cell types (129). It has been concluded that mesenchyme suppresses endocrine cell differentiation and that therefore the default pathway for the pancreatic epithelium is to form islets. In addition, recent studies have begun to shed light on the identity of the factors involved in this ratio determination. Follistatin, for instance, is expressed in the pancreatic mesenchyme and is thought to suppress factors important for endocrine differentiation such as TGF-β1. Follistatin alone can mimic some of the functions of the mesenchyme in culture and promote exocrine cell differentiation (128). However, the development of the pancreas appears to be normal in follistatin-deficient mice (130). TGF-β1, in contrast, is expressed in the pancreatic epithelium, and overexpression of TGF-β1 can inhibit the development of acinar tissue and promote the development of endocrine cells, especially β- and PP-cells (124).

LINEAGE OF ENDOCRINE AND EXOCRINE CELLS

Precursors in the Epithelium

Critical to an understanding of the factors responsible for β-cell development and function is an understanding of the lineage of pancreatic endocrine cells. Where do they come from and what signals do they receive? Does a common progenitor give rise to both endocrine and exocrine cell types? Are there precursors that give rise to multiple endocrine cell lineages? As mentioned previously, there is ample histologic evidence demonstrating that endocrine precursors originate in the pancreatic endodermal epithelium (14). In early experiments, *in vitro* culture of pancreatic rudiments demonstrated that in fact both exocrine and endocrine cells can arise from isolated epithelium and that neither form in isolated mesoderm (6). Recent recombination experiments using genetically marked epithelium and unlabeled mesenchyme support these observations and convincingly demonstrate that all exocrine and endocrine cells originate in pancreatic epithelium (36). However, it is still unclear whether both tissues arise from a single cell type within the epithelium or distinct progenitors exist that give rise exclusively to either endocrine or exocrine cells. In addition, the lineage relationships of the four islet endocrine cell types are just as far from being resolved. Intense interest in questions of endocrine cell lineage continues to demand investigation. Elucidation of these relationships may help shed some light on the parameters that will prove important for the production of islets as a potential therapy for diabetes.

Experimental Approaches to Lineage Analysis

Lineage relationships among pancreatic cell types have been investigated with a variety of experimental approaches. These include analysis of coexpression of genes in pancreatic cells and the phenotypes resulting from gene-ablation experiments and analysis of transgenic animals in which reporter genes, oncogenes, or toxins are driven from endocrine hormone promoters. All these approaches, however, are filled with uncertainties, and thus the conclusions that can be confidently drawn are limited. It is clear that co-localization of gene expression cannot be used for drawing definitive conclusions about lineage relationships. Expression of endocrine genes may be transient, and descendant cells may not give rise to distinct endocrine progeny. Furthermore, all the transgenic approaches used to address questions of lineage depend on the accurate expression of the endocrine promoters that are used and on the cell autonomy of the ablation or oncogenic effects. In more general terms, cell identity is known to depend both on intrinsic factors, such as gene expression, and on extrinsic factors, such as microenvironments consisting of secreted factors, cell-cell interactions, or extracellular matrix (131). Therefore, cells experiencing equivalent extrinsic factors, but having different origins, could initiate similar gene expression patterns that would make lineage impossible to ascertain. However, despite the limitations and uncertainties inherent in any lineage study, pancreatic lineage studies provide tantalizing hints as to the possible common progenitors of endocrine cell types.

Analysis of Endocrine Gene Coexpression and Lineage Tracing

Numerous lineage relationships have been inferred on the basis of coexpression of genes in cells of the developing pancreas. The coexpression of various genes in the pancreatic epithelium, such as insulin and glucagon or glucagon and PP, led to the proposal that these coexpressing cells represent precursors that give rise to multiple endocrine cell types in the islets (62,132–134). Yet another study inferred the existence of common endocrine precursors on the basis of the coexpression of the peptide hormone YY in all islet cell types (135). More recently, the observed coexpression of the homeobox gene *Pdx1* (pancreatic duodenal homeodomain-containing protein 1) in both endocrine and exocrine precursors has led to the suggestion that these tissues may arise from common *Pdx1*-expressing precursors (136). These correlations, however, do not provide indisputable evidence for a common endocrine precursor cell, since cells of different origins may transiently express the same genes.

The assumptions drawn from coexpression studies are nonetheless supported by gene-ablation experiments in mice. In a number of mouse mutants lacking the function of endocrine genes, the absence of multiple lineages suggests the possibility that common precursors may be deleted as a direct result of the gene ablation. For instance, mutant mice lacking the function of the homeobox gene *Pdx1* fail to develop all pancreatic tissues, including both endocrine and exocrine lineages. It could be presumed from these observations that all pancreatic cell lineages originate from *Pdx1* precursors. In addition, the bHLH (basic helix-loop-helix) gene *ngn3* is found to be expressed in endocrine precursors and its expression is required for the development of all four islet endocrine cell types (137,138). Other examples of genes whose absence leads to the failure of multiple endocrine lineage development include *Pax4*, *Pax6*, and *Nkx2.2* (see discussion below). However, once again it is impossible to determine conclusively that common precursors are being lost in these mouse mutants. The effect of these mutations may not be entirely cell autonomous. For instance, endocrine cells may develop from a lineage that is completely separate from exocrine cells. It is also possible that exocrine cells are absolutely required for the proper development of endocrine cells. A mutation in a gene required only for exocrine development would therefore be misinterpreted as also being required for endocrine cell formation because of the failure of endocrine cell formation.

Another approach that has been used to determine cell-lineage relationships is the use of endocrine gene promoters to drive various reporter genes in transgenic mice. When the rat insulin promoter is used to drive expression of the SV40 T antigen (Tag), coexpression of Tag is detectable in all endocrine cell types in the islet (62). Because insulin is not detectable in all endocrine cells, these experimental results imply that all endocrine cells arise from a common insulin-expressing progenitor. A different conclusion is reached in a more recent study. In this experiment, islets are irreversibly "tagged" using the activity of Cre recombinase (139). More specifically, glucagon or insulin promoters are used to drive expression of Cre recombinase, which then activates a reporter gene and marks all descendants of founder cells that express the promoters. In these experiments, adult glucagon- and insulin-expressing cells are shown to derive from cells that have never expressed the reciprocal gene, demonstrating that islet α- and β-cell lineages arise independently during embryogenesis. In addition, further experiments demonstrate that β-cells, but not α-cells, share a common progenitor with PP-expressing cells. Finally, when *Pdx1*-expressing cells are tagged, both adult α- and β-cells are observed to express Cre recombinase. Therefore, it is likely that both insulin- and glucagon-expressing cells arise independently during embryogenesis but that they share a very early common precursor.

Islet Cell Tumors

Another approach to the study of endocrine cell lineage comes from studies of islet cell tumors. This approach is based on the analysis of the heterogeneous cell populations within tumors, which can then be correlated back to an originally transformed founder cell. Islet cell tumors frequently consist of mixed cell populations that produce multiple hormones (140,141). Of course, in most cases it is unclear whether these tumors result from the simultaneous transformation of a number of cell types or from the transformation of a single pluripotent progenitor cell. This uncertainty has been resolved by showing that clonal cell lines derived from a pancreatic islet tumor simultaneously express all four endocrine hormones (142). Subsequently, multiple islet cell types are generated from a single cell clone, suggesting the existence of common precursors. In other experiments, when an oncogenic transgene is targeted to the pancreas using the glucokinase promoter, tumors develop in close association with the duct epithelium that give rise to cells expressing multiple islet hormones when cultured (143). Assuming that these tumors derive from individual transformed cells, this again lends support to the idea that multiple islet cell types can be derived from common progenitors.

Toxigenes

Finally, additional evidence for lineage relationships comes from studies of transgenic mice with the expression of toxic genes in different islet cell populations. One such transgenic study made use of the diphtheria toxin driven behind the insulin, glucagon, or PP promoters (144). At extremely low levels, this toxin blocks protein synthesis, and its effects are cell autonomous, since it is not passed on to neighboring cells. In the resulting transgenic mice, it was found that only one specific cell type was affected in both the insulin- and glucagon-promoter driven lines (either β- or α-cells, respectively). In agreement with lineage-tracing experiments described previously, this strongly argues for independent lineages for β- and α-cells. However, when the diphtheria toxin was driven behind the PP promoter, both insulin- and somatostatin-producing cells were markedly decreased, implying that the lineages of these two cell types share a common progenitor. Additional islet hormone promoter–driven endocrine cell lineage–tracing and ablation experiments should contribute to our understanding of lineage relationships. However, like coexpression and lineage-tracing studies, cell-ablation experiments depend on the accurate expression of promoters used and on the absence of transient expression by unrelated cell types.

POSTNATAL DEVELOPMENT OF THE PANCREAS

Normal Pancreatic Growth

A number of reports indicate that islets in higher vertebrates arise throughout embryogenesis but that the generation of islets decreases precipitously shortly after birth (145). This led to the belief that one acquired all the β-cells one would have during embryonic development. Studies of growth in the postnatal pancreas, however, have identified changes in endocrine cell populations and have described a slow but measurable increase in cell division in all pancreatic cell types after birth and into adulthood. These data are based on studies of mitotic index or of labeling with tritiated thymidine, bromodeoxyuridine, Ki-67, or PCNA (145–150). In the rat, the estimated β-cell mass of the adult (100-day-old animal) is up to 9.8×10^6 cells, and the reported rate of β-cell replication has been calculated to be almost 3% new cells per day (147,151). If an equivalent rate of associated apoptosis is assumed, measurements have estimated that the life span of a β-cell is between 30 and 90 days (147,152–154). The endocrine pancreas is therefore slowly and continuously replacing itself during all of postnatal life.

The process by which new endocrine cells are generated in the growing postnatal and adult pancreas remains unclear. Generally speaking, new endocrine cells might arise in a number of different ways (103,143,151,155). They could arise either from the replication of pre-existing differentiated cells, such as resident islet cells, or from the transdifferentiation of cells from surrounding tissues, such as endothelium or mesenchyme or exocrine tissue. Alternatively, new endocrine cells could arise from the differentiation of duct cells by a process termed neogenesis, which represents a recapitulation of embryonic islet development. Or, finally, the new cells could develop from an entirely separate population of pancreatic stem cells dedicated to replenishing islet endocrine cells and themselves. This question is presently under active investigation, and observations have been made that could support any one of these three possible mechanisms. In particular, the theory of duct origin of endocrine cells has recently gained much attention. However, despite our increasing understanding of pancreatic development and growth, many questions remain regarding the landmarks of the endocrine cell life span. What is the normal source for endocrine precursors in the adult? What regulates the balance of cell proliferation, cell differentiation, and cell loss in pancreatic tissue and how do these processes coordinate to shape the population of endocrine cell types in the islets? Understanding the mechanisms that regulate β-cell generation in the adult will further our understanding of islet cell regeneration and will help in the development of therapies for diabetes mellitus.

Embryonic and Postnatal Pancreatic Cell Populations

There are numerous examples of dynamic changes in endocrine cell populations during islet growth, both before and after birth. In the rat, at gestational day 16, α-cells constitute over 96% of the endocrine cell mass (148). Shortly before birth, however, there is a rapid increase in the mass of all endocrine cells, particularly β-cells. The predominant cell type in islets at birth are β-cells, which constitute more than 65% of the islets, while the percentage of α-cells has decreased to 32% (156). A number of studies also have noted interesting periods of accelerated proliferation of endocrine cells 4 days after birth and just before weaning, possibly indicating remodeling of the pancreas (145,147). Changes in specific endocrine populations in different portions of the human pancreas have also been analyzed. In the posterior part of the head of the pancreas, the percentage of PP- and insulin-expressing cells is constant during fetal life, at approximately 50% and 25%, respectively. However, these percentages increase after birth and surpass 70% and 30% in adults (157–159). In the upper part of the head of the pancreas, the percentage of glucagon-expressing cells increases during gestation to over 30% but then decreases to 20% just before birth, remaining at this level into adulthood (16). The proportion of somatostatin-expressing cells remains stable at 20% during fetal development but decreases to about 10% in adults (157). The relative proportions of different endocrine cell types change dramatically during normal postnatal growth and development.

Postnatal and Adult Neogenesis of β-Cells

New islets are indeed generated postnatally and throughout adulthood. In one study, the number of islets itself was observed to change dramatically during postnatal growth, increasing from over 600 in the rat neonate to over 4,500 in the adult rat (160). The relative proportion of islets to the rest of the pancreas, however, falls from approximately 4% to 1.5% during the first 200 postnatal days (161). That new endocrine cells are produced continuously as pancreatic mass increases during postnatal growth and during maintenance of adult pancreatic tissue is supported by the finding of measurable mitotic activity in adult islet cells and the presence of islet precursors in the adult duct epithelium (162,163). In addition, changes both in β-cell number (hyperplasia) and in β-cell volume (hypertrophy) have been detected in the adult pancreas. Other studies have focused on endocrine cell populations during pancreatic adaptation to changing physiologic demands. Indeed, the number of postnatal β-cells has been shown to be remarkably dynamic. This flexibility and adaptability of β-cells can be observed during pregnancy, obesity, or insulin resistance (164). Pregnant rats show a 50% increase in β-cell mass directly caused by β-cell proliferation induced by placental lactogen (165). Mice that lack the function of the insulin receptor and the insulin receptor substrate 1 (IRS-1) are severely insulin resistant and have a 10- to 30-fold increase in β-cell mass (166). Islet growth and the maintenance of islet mass during normal postnatal growth, however, are under strict regulatory controls and have generally been correlated with body weight (148,151).

Regeneration of the Pancreas under Experimental Conditions

Dramatic changes in β-cell mass in the postnatal pancreas have also been demonstrated under experimental conditions. One of the most striking examples is the regeneration that occurs after partial pancreatectomy of young rats (167–169). Surgically removing all but 10% of the pancreas results in the rapid regeneration of both endocrine and exocrine tissues due both to replication of differentiated tissue and to neogenesis from duct epithelium. Other methods have yielded more limited regeneration. For instance, wrapping the head of the pancreas in cellophane also can induce the formation of new islets (170). Specifically, this manipulation causes a continuous inflammation of the pancreas, which in turn leads to duct proliferation, the reduction of smaller duct secretion, and islet budding from ductules. Similar experimental islet neogenesis is observed with a number of other methods. These include destruction of β-cells by streptozotocin in newborn and neonatal mice (171), administration of alloxan (172), dietary treatment with soybean trypsin inhibitors (173) or ethionine in combination with a protein-free diet (174), ligation of pancreatic arteries (175), or expression of high levels of interferon-γ or specific growth factors (126). Overall, these methods demonstrate that exocrine tissue is capable of rapid and robust regeneration, whereas β-cells are generally resistant to regeneration. Taken together, however, these data point to the existence of endocrine precursor cells, perhaps pancreatic stem cells, with the capacity to differentiate into functional islets.

PANCREATIC STEM CELLS

Islet Cell Expansion and Transplantation

The occurrence of β-cell neogenesis in the adult pancreatic ducts offers the possibility of generation of β-cells for transplantation into patients with diabetes. During the latter part of the 20th century, transplantation of whole pancreases and of purified islets has achieved a certain level of success at stabilizing glucose levels in rodents and humans with diabetes mellitus; however, these procedures are costly, invasive, and require tissue that is of limited availability (149). *In vitro* proliferation of preparations of adult islet has offered some promise but usually has involved a concurrent loss of insulin production, rendering the islets biologically impotent (176,177). The prospect of identifying and expanding putative pancreatic stem cells has stimulated a number of studies aimed at identifying regions of active cell proliferation in the adult pancreas, culturing and expanding pancreatic duct preparations, and possibly isolating stem cells.

Stem Cell Developmental Potential

Stem cells have the capacity to reproduce themselves throughout the life of the organism and to generate multilineage differentiated cells (178,179). Stem cells also are thought to maintain an undifferentiated or embryonic phenotype, to divide very slowly, and to divide asymmetrically, producing daughter cells that can differentiate. If pancreatic stem cells in fact exist in the mature pancreas, they have not yet been identified histologically. Morphologic studies of pancreatic islets find no indication of "undifferentiated" or otherwise distinguishable cell type (180). Nonetheless, there is increasing evidence that stem cells or precursor cells are located in duct epithelium. A number of studies show that culturing duct epithelium can result in the expansion of β-cells (see below). In addition, members of the *Notch* family of genes are expressed in pancreatic duct cells (181). *Notch* genes have been implicated in regulating the balance between cell proliferation and differentiation, and disruption of *Notch* signaling leads to accelerated endocrine differentiation, disrupted pancreatic branching, and exocrine differentiation (182).

It is also possible that pancreatic stem cells may be found within the islets themselves. Recently, the gene *Nestin* was found to be expressed in a small number of cells within islets of postnatal juvenile mice (183). Nestin, an intermediate filament protein, has been called a marker for neural stem cells because it is expressed in central nervous system (CNS) cells that are capable of differentiating into various neural cell lineages. Finally, it is also possible that pancreatic stem cells emerge following the dedifferentiation of committed pancreatic endocrine cells. Human islets are known to lose insulin and *Pdx1* expression when cultured *in vitro* and can become duct-like in appearance when embedded in three-dimensional collagen gels (176,184). However, these may actually result from an expansion of contaminating duct cells.

Pancreatic Duct Expansion

In the past few years, an increasing number of studies have shown the broad potential of stem cells (185–188). These studies show that stem cells not only are found in a wide range of tissues but also have broad differentiation repertoires. For instance, neural stem cells and muscle progenitors have been shown to give rise to blood cells, hematopoietic stem cells can differentiate into myocytes, and bone marrow stem cells can generate astrocytes. Although pancreatic stem cells have not yet been identified, a number of studies have focused on the properties of pancreatic ducts. In one study, immature but functional islets were generated by the culture of islet precursor cells isolated from duct epithelium (189). These cells, kept in long-term cultures, reversed insulin dependence when implanted into diabetic mice (102). Recent studies have demonstrated that preparations of adult tissue composed primarily of duct cells can be expanded and differentiated *in vitro* into functional islets that secrete insulin in response to glucose stimulation (164). Although these recent experiments offer new hope for large-scale generation of islets, an actual pancreatic stem cell has yet to be isolated and the mechanisms by which duct tissue expands remain unclear. The cellular and molecular characterization of stem cells or multipotential precursors in the pancreatic epithelium presents important challenges for the future.

MOLECULAR MARKERS OF THE DEVELOPING PANCREAS

There is increasing evidence that the molecular mechanisms controlling tissue patterning and cellular differentiation are surprisingly conserved throughout evolution—from worms and flies to mice and humans. The genes that regulate these early processes during development of the pancreas and differentiation of endocrine cells are steadily being identified. On the whole, pancreatic genes have proven surprisingly similar in their expression patterns in different species and in their functions in most metazoans, including humans. The study of pancreatic genes and the factors they encode will advance our understanding of differentiation of endocrine cells and of the factors that give the β-cell its functional identity. We summarize below some of the regulatory factors that have been implicated in cell-fate decisions in the development of the pancreas and the morphogenesis of islets.

Pdx1

Pancreatic duodenal homeodomain-containing protein 1, or Pdx1, is expressed in the pancreatic anlagen and plays a critical role in the development of the pancreas. The gene *Pdx1* was originally isolated in the frog *X. laevis* as *XIHbox8* (190,191). Since then, the gene product has undergone intense investigation and is known by a number of different names, including insulin-promoter factor-1, islet/duodenum homeobox-1, somatostatin transactivating factor-1, glucose-sensitive factor, and glucose-sensitive transcriptional factor. Expression of *Pdx1* in mice is initiated at E8.0 in regions of the endoderm that will form the ventral pancreas. Slightly later, at E9.0, expression of *Pdx1* is found in the epithelium that spans the midgut, including both the dorsal and ventral pancreatic anlagen during most of fetal development, and in the caudal stomach and rostral duodenum (136,192). Shortly before birth, expression of *Pdx1* becomes restricted to β- and δ-cells and to the duodenum. *In vitro* experiments demonstrate that Pdx1 can bind specific DNA promoter sequences and activate insulin, somatostatin, glucokinase, glucose transporter 2 (GLUT2), and islet expression of the amyloid polypeptide gene (193–198). Mice or humans with homozygous null mutations of *Pdx1* are born apancreatic because of the arrest in development of pancreatic epithelium during early bud formation (199–201). In these mutant buds, a few insulin cells and glucagon cells appear; however, without Pdx1 function, the epithelium is unable to respond to mesenchymal signals that promote pancreatic branching and growth. However, the pancreatic mesenchyme itself grows and develops both morphologically and functionally, independent of the epithelium (202). Therefore, *Pdx1* acts autonomously in the endoderm, and the failure of pancreatic development is due to defects specifically in pancreatic epithelium.

In adults, *Pdx1* is expressed in pancreatic islets. When *Pdx1* is specifically ablated in mouse β-cells, the mice initially appear healthy but later diabetes mellitus develops (203). Analysis of these mutants reveals that the number of insulin- and amylin-expressing cells decreases by approximately 60%, while the number of glucagon-expressing cells increases almost 250%. *Pdx1* appears to be required for insulin secretion from β-cells, and this requirement is dosage dependent. Heterozygous mutation of *Pdx1* in humans results in maturity-onset diabetes of the young (MODY4), which is characterized by defects in insulin secretion (201). Heterozygous *Pdx1* mice have a reduced number of β-cells, decreased expression of insulin and GLUT2 in those β-cells that remain, a thicker mantle of non–β-cells, and impaired glucose tolerance (204). It has therefore been suggested that normal levels of Pdx1 protein are required for β-cell homeostasis and that reduction of these levels may contribute to type 2 diabetes mellitus (124). Chronic exposure of β-cells to a high concentration of either glucose or fatty acids causes a concomitant decrease in *Pdx1* expression over time (205). Thus, there seems to be a dual function of *Pdx1* during development and later endocrine function. Initially, it is required for early pancreas formation and elaboration, while later its expression in β-cells is required to maintain proper hormone production by β-cells.

ngn3

ngn3 is a basic helix-loop-helix factor (bHLH) that is expressed in both the CNS and the pancreas. Expression of *ngn3* in the pancreas can be seen in scattered cells in the pancreatic duct epithelium (206). Expression of *ngn3* can first be detected at E9.5, reaching its highest levels at E15.5 and decreasing until birth (182); it cannot be detected in the adult pancreas. It is interesting that *ngn3* is never observed in differentiated endocrine cells that express pancreatic hormones and has therefore has been described as a "pro-endocrine" gene that drives islet cell differentiation. ngn3 protein is detected along with early islet differentiation factors Nkx6.1 and Nkx2.2, but not with differentiated islet hormones or the islet transcription factors Isl1, Brn4, Pax6, or Pdx1. The role of *ngn3* has recently been demonstrated in pancreatic endocrine cells. Mice that lack *ngn3* function fail to develop any pancreatic endocrine cells and die of diabetes a few days after birth (138). Specifically, expression of *Isl1*, *Pax4*, *Pax6*, and *NeuroD* is lost, and endocrine precursors are not observed in the mutant pancreatic epithelium. When *ngn3* is overexpressed in pancreatic cells under the control of the *Pdx1* promoter, the pancreas lacks all exocrine cells and develops hyperplastic endocrine cells. Precocious expression can also cause early differentiation of endocrine cells. In the chick, when *ngn3* is ectopically expressed in combination with *Pdx1*, ectopic glucagon cells are induced in most regions of the gut tube (207). *ngn3* is thus required for the formation of all four types of islet cells.

Shh

Sonic hedgehog (*Shh*) and *Indian hedgehog* (*Ihh*) are members of the hedgehog family of potent intercellular signaling molecules. Both these genes are uniformly expressed throughout the mouse gut endoderm, with the striking exception of the dorsal and ventral pancreatic anlagen (208,209). Correspondingly, Patched (*Ptc*), the candidate receptor for *Shh*, is expressed in the mesoderm surrounding the stomach and duodenum; however, it is also absent from the mesenchyme surrounding the pancreas (72). In transgenic mice that ectopically express *Shh* in the pancreatic endoderm, proper pancreas and spleen morphogenesis is completely disrupted, although some endocrine and exocrine cytodifferentiation occurs normally (209). Specifically, pancreatic mesoderm is completely converted into smooth muscle and interstitial cells of Cajal, which are characteristic of the intestine, and the pancreatic epithelium initiates some intestinal gene expression. *In vitro* experiments with explants of pancreatic endoderm cultured in the presence of Shh protein show the same initiation of intestine differentiation. This repression of *Shh* in the pancreatic endoderm is likely mediated by signals from the notochord, possibly activin-βB and FGF-2

(70,104). Removal of the notochord in early chick embryos leads to ectopic expression of *Shh* in the pancreatic epithelium and to the failure of pancreatic development. *In vitro* culture of pancreatic epithelium with activin-βB or FGF-2 restores the repression of *Shh* and the expression of pancreatic genes. In addition, prevention of Shh signaling using antibodies that block *hedgehog* activity has the same results. Therefore, repression of *Shh* in the pancreatic endoderm seems to be required for proper pancreatic development. Recent observations have been made in mice with disrupted hedgehog signaling (210). *Ihh*-null mice exhibit ectopic branching of the ventral pancreas, resulting in a pancreatic annulus encircling the duodenum. *Shh* null mice and *Shh/Ihh* double mutants have a relative increase in pancreas mass and a fourfold increase in endocrine cell numbers.

Hb9

Hlxb9 (*Hb9*) is a homeobox gene expressed in the CNS and transiently in regions of the endoderm that will give rise to the respiratory and gastrointestinal tracts, including the pancreatic anlagen (211). Initially, expression is found in the notochord, the entire dorsal gut endoderm, and the ventral endoderm in the pancreatic region. In the dorsal pancreas, *Hlxb9* expression begins slightly before *Pdx1* expression, while in the ventral pancreas their expression begins concurrently. Later in development, *Hlxb9* expression in the pancreas is restricted to β-cells. In mice lacking *Hlxb9* function, dorsal pancreatic bud development is dramatically inhibited and *Pdx1* expression is completely absent (212,213). The dorsal pancreatic mesenchyme, however, develops normally but lacks expression of *Isl1*. The ventral pancreas develops almost normally, showing some limited disruption in the proportion and spatial organization of endocrine cells. There is a reduction of approximately 20% to 65% in the number of insulin-expressing cells and a threefold increase in the number of somatostatin-expressing cells in the ventral bud. In addition, there is a lack of GLUT2 expression in those insulin cells that remain. *Hlxb9* is therefore required for the initial evagination of the pancreatic epithelium and for subsequent development of the dorsal pancreatic bud. The requirement for *Hlxb9* demonstrates a clear molecular distinction between the dorsal and ventral pancreas.

BETA2/NeuroD

BETA2/NeuroD is a bHLH protein that is expressed in the CNS, pituitary gland, intestine, and pancreatic islets. In the developing pancreas, BETA2 is found in scattered cells in the pancreatic epithelium that coexpress glucagon as early as E9.5 in mice. Later, BETA2 can be found in α-, β-, and δ- cells in the islets. BETA2 has been shown to transactivate insulin, glucagon, *Pdx1*, and secretin genes (30). Examination of *BETA2* expression shows that it partially overlaps that of *ngn3*, and ectopic *ngn3* can induce ectopic *BETA2NeuroD* in *Xenopus* embryos (214). In addition, *in vitro* binding assays have demonstrated that *ngn3* can bind E boxes in the BETA2 promoter directly and is therefore likely to lie upstream in a regulatory pathway during endocrine cell development. When *BETA2* is disrupted by targeted ablation, mutant mice die of diabetes a few days after birth (215). Closer examination of the pancreas in null embryos reveals that endocrine cells fail to organize into mature islets and that their numbers decrease by almost 60% around E17.5 during embryonic development. Specifically, the number of β-cells was strikingly reduced. Decreased *Pdx1* expression is not observed in BETA2 null mice, however. The decrease in the number of endocrine cells is thought to result from increased programmed cell death, because TUNEL (*T*dT-mediated d*U*TP-x *n*ick *e*nd *l*abeling) assay of the mutant pancreas shows an increase in the number of apoptotic cells. BETA2 has therefore been suggested to be important in the proliferation, rather than the differentiation, of endocrine cells in the pancreas (216). It is interesting that, in humans, two mutations in *NEUROD1* have been associated with the development of type 2 diabetes mellitus in the heterozygous state (217).

Isl1

Isl1 is a member of the LIM family of homeodomain proteins and was originally isolated because of its ability to bind insulin gene regulatory sequences (218). *Isl1* is expressed in a wide variety of tissues, including the CNS, lung, kidney, and pancreas. In the pancreas, *Isl1* is expressed in differentiated islet cells that have left the cell cycle during embryonic development, and in the adult, its expression is found in all classes of islet cells in the pancreas (219). *Isl1* also is expressed in the mesenchyme that surrounds the pancreatic dorsal bud (120). Mice lacking *Isl1* function fail to develop any differentiated islet cells or dorsal pancreatic mesenchyme. In addition, there is a failure of exocrine cell differentiation in the dorsal, but not ventral, bud. *In vitro* culture of mutant pancreatic endoderm with wild-type mesenchyme, however, can restore exocrine but not endocrine cell differentiation in these mutants. *Isl1* is therefore required for islet cell development, but it is unclear if this requirement is direct or due to secondary effects mediated by mesenchyme.

Pax Genes

Pax genes encode paired-box transcription factors that regulate multiple aspects of embryonic development and organogenesis. *Pax4* is expressed in the spinal cord and in scattered cells of the pancreatic epithelium starting at E10.5 in the mouse (220,221). Subsequently, around E15.5, *Pax4* becomes expressed in a much larger population of cells, including insulin-positive cells. *Pax4* is then restricted to the β-cells in the adult. Mice lacking *Pax4* function die of diabetes mellitus within 3 days following birth and exhibit a complete loss of mature β- and δ-cells and have an associated increase in the number of α-cells. However, at E10.5, insulin- and glucagon-producing cells can be identified in the pancreatic epithelium in mutant embryos and *Pdx1* expression is normal. It is only later that the expression of both insulin and *Pdx1* decreases precipitously. *Pax4* may therefore be required for the maintenance of β- and δ-cells rather than for their initial formation. Like *Pax4*, *Pax6* also is expressed in the CNS, as well as other tissues, including the pancreas (222). *Pax6* binds to the pancreatic islet cell enhancer sequence that is found in the promoters of insulin, glucagon, and somatostatin genes (223,224). Expression in the pancreatic bud begins at E9.0 and continues in all four endocrine cell types during fetal and postnatal life. In mice lacking *Pax6* function, all α-cells fail to differentiate (223). The decrease first becomes evident at E10.5. In addition, β-, δ-, and PP-cells are present in mutant embryos but fail to aggregate properly to form mature islets; *Pdx1* expression appears normal, however. Mice null for both *Pax4* and *Pax6* fail to develop any mature endocrine cells. Given that endocrine cells are initially present in mice lacking *Pax6* gene function, it seems likely that *Pax* genes are required for the maintenance or maturation endocrine cell fate (221).

Nkx Genes

Another family of genes important during endocrine cell development is the NK homeobox family. *Nkx2.2* is expressed in both the CNS and the pancreatic islets (225). Expression can first be detected broadly in the dorsal pancreatic bud at E9.5, and expression later becomes restricted to α-, β-, and PP-cells. Ablation of the *Nkx2.2* function results in mice that do not synthesize insulin, show severe hyperglycemia, and die a few days after birth (226). Large numbers of disorganized endocrine cells can be found that express some β-cell markers, but no insulin, suggesting that these may represent incompletely differentiated β-cells. In addition, these mutants exhibit a significant general reduction in the number of α-, β-, and PP-cells. *Nkx2.2* is therefore important during the differentiation of a number of endocrine cells. *Nkx6.1*, on the other hand, is widely expressed in the pancreatic epithelium during early pancreas development but becomes restricted exclusively to β-cells by the end of fetal development (227). Targeted ablation of *Nkx6.1* demonstrates that it is specifically required for β-cell differentiation (227). Initially, β-cell commitment appears to proceed normally; however, further differentiation is arrested at around E13.0. In contrast, α-, δ, and PP-cells are not affected. *Nkx6.1* is therefore likely to be important during the β-cell expansion that occurs late in embryogenesis and during the final differentiation of β-cells. *Nkx6.1* is thought to function downstream of *Nkx2.2*, because *Nkx6.1* expression is lost in *Nkx2.2* mutant embryos but the reverse is not true. In addition, recently generated *Nkx2.2Nkx6.1* double mutants exhibit a phenotype identical to that of *Nkx2.2*.

CONCLUSION

Although the morphologic landmarks of pancreatic development have been characterized and studied extensively, we are only beginning to understand the multitude of regulatory factors and intercellular signaling molecules responsible for generating the fates of pancreatic cells. It is likely that a specific combination of gene products exists that determines the character of endocrine cells. Gene expression studies and analysis of lineage relationships have expanded the picture of how endocrine cells are generated in the developing pancreas. Identifying additional cell surface markers of islet cells may eventually prove useful for the characterization and possible purification of pancreatic precursors—possibly pancreatic stem cells. In combination with optimized culture conditions, this would be invaluable for the generation of replacement β-cells for patients with diabetes mellitus.

Acknowledgments

We thank Eckhart Lammert, Guoqiang Gu, and Maya Kumar for critical reading of the manuscript and for useful discussions. Dr. Cleaver is supported by the Cancer Research Fund of the Damon Runyon–Walter Winchell Foundation Fellowship, DRG 1534. Dr. Melton is an investigator of the HHMI. Work in this laboratory is also supported by the Juvenile Diabetes Foundation and the National Institutes of Health.

REFERENCES

1. Dudek RW, Lawrence IE, Hill RS, et al. Induction of cytodifferentiation by fetal mesenchyme in adult pancreatic ductal epithelium. *Diabetes* 1991;40: 1041–1048.
2. Bonner-Weir S, Taneja M, Weir GC, et al. In vitro cultivation of human islets from expanded ductal tissue. *Proc Natl Acad Sci U S A* 2000;97:7999–8004.
3. Githens S. Differentiation and development of the exocrine pancreas in animals. In: Go VLW, Lebenthal E, Reber HA, et al. *The exocrine pancreas biology, pathobiology and diseases.* New York: Raven Press, 1986:21–32.
4. Wesells NK, Cohen JH. Early pancreas organogenesis: morphogenesis, tissue interactions and mass effects. *Dev Biol* 1967;15:237–270.
5. Pictet RL, Clarke WR, Williams RH, et al. An ultrastructural analysis of the developing embryonic pancreas. *Dev Biol* 1972;29:436–467.
6. Pictet R, Rutter WJ. Development of the embryonic endocrine pancreas. In: Steiner DF, Frenkel N, eds. *Handbook of physiology*, section 7, vol 1, American Physiological Society. Washington, DC: Williams and Wilkins, 1972: 25–66.
7. Gray A. *Gray's anatomy*. New York, Vintage Books, 1994.
8. Bockman DE. Anatomy of the pancreas. In: Go VLW, et al. *The pancreas: biology, pathobiology and disease*, 2nd ed. New York: Raven Press, 1993:1–8.
9. Lewis FT. *Development of the pancreas*. In: Keibel F, Mall FP, eds. *Human embryology by Keibel and Mall.* Philadelphia: JB Lippincott, 1912:429–445.
10. Henderson JR, Daniel PM. A comparative study of the portal vessels connecting the endocrine and exocrine pancreas, with a discussion of some functional implications. *Q J Exp Physiol Cogn Med Sci* 1979;64:267–275.
11. Henderson JR, Moss MC. A morphometric study of the endocrine and exocrine capillaries of the pancreas. *Q J Exp Physiol* 1985;70:347–356.
12. Colen KL, Crisera CA, Rose MI, et al. Vascular development in the mouse embryonic pancreas and lung. *J Pediatr Surg* 1999;34:781–785.
13. Sundler F, Bottcher G. Islet innervation, with special reference to neuropeptides. In: Samols E, ed. *The endocrine pancreas*. New York: Raven Press, 1991: 29–52.
14. Laguesse ME. Sur la formation des ilots de Langerhans dans le pancreas. *Mem (Compt Rend) Soc Biol Paris (9 serie)*. 1893:5:19–820.
15. Liegner B. Studien zur Entwicklung des Pankreas, besonders der Langerhanschen Inseln. *Z Mikrosk-anaat Forsch* 1932:494–529.
16. Dubois PM. Ontogeny of the endocrine pancreas. *Horm Res* 1989;32:53–60.
17. Hellerstrom C. The life story of the pancreatic β-cell. *Diabetologia* 1984;26: 393–400.
18. Yamamoto M, Kataoka K. Large particles associated with gap junctions of pancreatic exocrine cells during embryonic and neonatal development. *Anat Embryol (Berl)* 1985;171:305–310.
19. Alumets J, Sundler F, Hakanson R. Distribution, ontogeny and ultrastructure of somatostatin immunoreactive cells in the pancreas and gut. *Cell Tissue Res* 1977;185:465–479.
20. Bonner-Weir S, Smith FE. Islet cell growth and the growth factors involved. *Trends Endocrinol Metab* 1994;5:60–64.
21. Guest PC, Bailyes EM, Rutherford NG, Hutton JC. Insulin secretory granule biogenesis: co-ordinate regulation of the biosynthesis of the majority of constituent proteins. *Biochem J* 1991;274:73–78.
22. Dean PM. Ultrastructural morphometry of the pancreatic β-cell. *Diabetologia* 1973;9:115–119.
23. Orci L, Unger RH. Functional subdivision of islets of Langerhans and possible role of D cells. *Lancet* 1975;2:1243–1244.
24. Orci L. The microanatomy of the islets of Langerhans. *Metabolism* 1976; 25[suppl]:1303–1313.
25. Grube D, Eckert I, Speck PT, et al. Immunohistochemistry and microanatomy of the islets of Langerhans. *Biomed Res* 1983;4[Suppl]:25.
26. Rawdon BB, Andrew A. Origin and differentiation of gut endocrine cells. *Histol Histopathol* 1993;8:567–580.
27. Saito K, Iwama N, Takahashi T. Morphometrical analysis on topographical difference in size distribution, number and volume of islets in the human pancreas. *Tohoku J Exp Med* 1978;124:177–186.
28. Argenton F, Zecchin E, Bortolussi M. Early appearance of pancreatic hormone-expressing cells in the zebrafish embryo. *Mech Dev* 1999;87:217–221.
29. Yamaoka T, Itakura M. Development of pancreatic islets (Review). *Int J Mol Med* 1999;3:247–261.
30. Rall LB, Pictet RL, Williams RH, et al. Early differentiation of glucagon-producing cells in embryonic pancreas: a possible developmental role for glucagon. *Proc Natl Acad Sci U S A* 1973;71:3478–3482.
31. Gittes GK, Rutter WJ. Onset of cell-specific gene expression in the developing mouse pancreas. *Proc Natl Acad Sci U S A* 1992;89:1128–1132.
32. Hellerstrom C, Swenne I. Functional maturation and proliferation of fetal pancreatic β-cells. *Diabetes* 1991;40[Suppl 2]:89–93.
33. Slack JM. Developmental biology of the pancreas. *Development* 1995;121: 1569–1580.
34. Golosow N, Grobstein C. Epitheliomesenchymal interaction in pancreatic morphogenesis. *Dev Biol* 1962;4:242–255.
35. Goldin GV, Wessels NK. Mammalian lung development: the possible role of cell proliferation in the formation of supernumerary tracheal buds and in branching morphogenesis. *J Exp Zool* 1979;208:337–346.
36. Percival AC, Slack JM. Analysis of pancreatic development using a cell lineage label. *Exp Cell Res* 1999;247:123–132.
37. Conlon FL, Lyons KM, Takaesu N, et al. A primary requirement for nodal in the formation and maintenance of the primitive streak in the mouse. *Development* 1994;120:1919–1928.
38. Wells JM, Melton DA. Vertebrate endoderm development. *Annu Rev Cell Dev Biol* 1999;15:393–410.
39. Wylie C, Snape A, Heasman J, et al. Vegetal pole cells and commitment to form endoderm in *Xenopus laevis*. *Dev Biol* 1987;119:496–502.
40. Yasuo H, Lemaire P. A two-step model for the fate determination of presumptive endodermal blastomeres in *Xenopus* embryos. *Curr Biol* 1999;9: 869–879.
41. Alexander J, Rothenberg M, Henry GL, et al. *Casanova* plays an early and essential role in endoderm formation in zebrafish. *Dev Biol* 1999:215; 343–357.

42. Clements D, Friday RV, Woodland HR. Mode of action of VegT in mesoderm and endoderm formation. *Development* 1999;126:4903–4911.
43. Osada SI, Wright CV. *Xenopus* nodal-related signaling is essential for mesendodermal patterning during early embryogenesis. *Development* 1999; 126:3229–3240.
44. Henry GL, Brivanlou IH, Kessler DS, et al. TGF-beta signals and a pattern in *Xenopus laevis* endodermal development. *Development* 1996;122:1007–1015.
45. Joseph EM, Melton DA. Mutant Vg1 ligands disrupt endoderm and mesoderm formation in *Xenopus* embryos. *Development* 1998;125:2677–2685.
46. Henry GL, Melton DA. Mixer, a homeobox gene required for endoderm development. *Science* 1998;281:91–96.
47. Rosa F. Mix.1, a homeobox mRNA inducible by mesoderm inducers, is expressed mostly in the presumptive endodermal cells of *Xenopus* embryos. *Cell* 1998;57:965–974.
48. Wessely O, De Robertis EM. The *Xenopus* homologue of Bicaudal-C is a localized maternal mRNA that can induce endoderm formation. *Development* 2000;127:2053–2062.
49. Hudson C, Clements D, Friday RV, et al. Xsox17-α- and -β- mediate endoderm formation in *Xenopus*. *Cell* 1997;91:397–405.
50. Lemaire PL, Darras S, Caillol D, et al. A role for the vegetally expressed *Xenopus* gene Mix.1 in endoderm formation and the restriction of mesoderm to the marginal zone. *Development* 1998;125:2371–2380.
51. Lawson KA, Meneses JJ, Pedersen RA. Clonal analysis of epiblast fate during germ layer formation in the mouse embryo. *Development* 1991;113:891–911.
52. Rosenquiest GC. The location of the pregut endoderm in the chick embryo at the primitive streak stage as determined by radioautographic mapping. *Dev Biol* 1971;26:323–335.
53. Hatada Y, Stern CD. A fate map of the epiblast of the early chick embryo. *Development* 1994;120:2879–2889.
54. Tremblay KD, Hoodless PA, Bikoff EK, et al. Formation of the definitive endoderm in mouse is a Smad2-dependent process. *Development* 2000;127: 3079–3090.
55. Feldman B, Poueymirou W, Papaioannou VE, et al. Requirement of FGF-4 for postimplantation mouse development. *Science* 1995;267:246–249.
56. Wells JM, Melton DA. Early mouse endoderm is patterned by soluble factors from adjacent germ layers. *Development* 2000;127:1563–1572.
57. Circuna BG, Schwartz L, Kendraprasad H, et al. Chimeric analysis of fibroblast growth factor receptor (FgFR1) function: a role for FGFR1 in morphogenetic movement through the primitive streak. *Development* 1997;124: 2829–2841.
58. Pearse AGE. Common cytochemical properties of cells producing polypeptide hormones, with particular reference to calcitonin and the thyroid C cells. *Vet Rec* 1966;79:587–590.
59. Pearse AGE. The APUD concept and its implications: related endocrine peptides in brain, intestine, pituitary, placenta and anuran cutaneous glands. *Med Biol* 1977;55:115–125.
60. Le Douarin NM. On the origin of pancreatic endocrine cells. *Cell* 1988;53: 169–171.
61. Pearse AG, Takor TT. Neuroendocrine embryology and the APUD concept. *Clin Endocrinol* 1976;5[Suppl]:229S–244S.
62. Alpert S, Hanahan D, Teitelman G. Hybrid insulin genes reveal a developmental lineage for pancreatic endocrine cells and imply a relationship with neurons. *Cell* 1988;53:295–308.
63. Teitelman G, Lee JK, Alpert S. Expression of cell type-specific markers during pancreatic development in the mouse: implications for pancreatic cell lineages. *Cell Tissue Res* 1987;250:435–439.
64. Cochard P, Coltey P. Cholinergic traits in the neural crest: acetylcholinesterase in crest cells of the chick embryo. *Dev Biol* 1983;98:221–238.
65. Schmechel D, Marangos PJ, Brightman M. Neurone-specific enolase is a molecular marker for peripheral and central neuroendocrine cells. *Nature* 1978; 276:834–836.
66. Wiedenmann B, Franke WW, Kuhn C, et al. Synaptophysin: a marker protein for neuroendocrine cells and neoplasms. *Proc Natl Acad Sci U S A* 1986;83: 3500–3504.
67. Thompson RJ, Doran JF, Jackson P, et al. PGP9.5-a new marker for vertebrate neurons and endocrine cells. *Brain Res* 1983;278:224–228.
68. Eisenbarth GS, Shimizu K, Bowring MA, et al. Expression of receptors for tetanus toxin and monoclonal antibody A2B5 by pancreatic islet cells. *Proc Natl Acad Sci U S A* 1987;79:5066–5070.
69. Polak M, Scharfmann R, Seilheimer B, et al. Nerve growth factor induces neuron-like differentiation of an insulin-secreting pancreatic beta cell line. *Proc Natl Acad Sci U S A* 1993;90:5781–5785.
70. Ohnishi H, Ohgushi N, Tanaka S, et al. Conversion of amylase-secreting rat pancreatic AR42J cells to neuronlike cells by activin A. *J Clin Invest* 1995;95: 2304–2314.
71. Kim SK, Hebrok M, Melton DA. Notochord to endoderm signaling is required for pancreas development. *Development* 1997;124:4243–4252.
72. Falkmer S. Comparative morphology of pancreatic islets in animals. In: Volk BW, Arquilla ER, eds. *The diabetic pancreas*, 2nd ed. New York: Plenum Medical Book Co, 1985:17–52.
73. Schilt J, Richoux JP, Dubois MP. Demonstration of peptides immunologically related to vertebrate neurohormones in *Dugesia lugubris* (Tubellaria, Tricladida). *Gen Comp Endocrinol* 1981;43:331–335.
74. El-Salhy M, Falkmer S, Kramer KJ, et al. Immunohistochemical investigations of neuropeptides in the brain, corpora cardiaca, and corpora allata of an adult lepidopteran insect, *Manduca sexta* (L). *Cell Tissue Res* 1983;232:295–317.
75. Duve H, Thorpe A, Lazarus NR. Isolation of material displaying insulin-like immunological biological activity from the brain of the blowfly *Calliphora vomitoria*. *Biochem J* 1979;184:221–227.
76. Andrew A. An experimental investigation into the possible neural crest origin of pancreatic APUD (islet) cells. *J Embryol Exp Morphol* 1976;35:577–593.
77. Fontaine J, Le Douarin NM. Analysis of endoderm formation in the avian blastoderm by the use of quail-chick chimaeras. The problem of the neurectodermal origin of the cells of the APUD series. *J Embryol Exp Morphol* 1977; 41:209–222.
78. Molkentin JD, Lin Q, Duncan SA, et al. Requirement of the transcription factor GATA4 for heart tube formation and ventral morphogenesis. *Genes Dev* 1997;11:1061–1072.
79. Roebroek AJ, Umans L, Pauli IG, et al. Failure of ventral closure and axial rotation in embryos lacking the proprotein convertase Furin. *Development* 1998;125:4863–4876.
80. Suzuki N, Labosky PA, Furuta Y, et al. Failure of ventral body wall closure in mouse embryos lacking a procollagen C-proteinase encoded by Bmp1, a mammalian gene related to Drosophila tolloid. *Development* 1996;122: 3587–3595.
81. Winnier G, Blessing M, Labosky PA, et al. Bone morphogenetic protein-4 is required for mesoderm formation and patterning in the mouse. *Genes Dev* 1995;9:2105–2116.
82. Solloway MJ, Robertson EJ. Early embryonic lethality in Bmp5; Bmp7 double mutant mice suggests functional redundancy within the 60A subgroup. *Development* 1999;126:1753–1768.
83. Biben C, Stanley E, Fabri L, et al. Murine cerberus homologue mCer-1: a candidate anterior patterning molecule. *Dev Biol* 1998;194:135–151.
84. Bouwmeester T, Kim S, Sasai Y, et al. Cerberus is a head-inducing secreted factor expressed in the anterior endoderm of Spemann's organizer. *Nature* 1996;382:595–601.
85. Rhinn M, Dierich A, Shawlot W, et al. Sequential roles for Otx2 in visceral endoderm and neurectoderm for forebrain and midbrain induction and specification. *Development* 1998;25:845–856.
86. Thomas P, Beddington R. Anterior primitive endoderm may be responsible for patterning the anterior neural plate in the mouse embryo. *Curr Biol* 1996; 6:1487–1497.
87. Grapin-Botton A, Melton DA. Endoderm development: from patterning to organogenesis. *Trend Genet* 2000;16:124–130.
88. Roberts DJ, Smith DM, Goff DJ, Tabin CJ. Epithelial-mesenchymal signaling during the regionalization of the chick gut. *Development* 1988;125:2791–2801.
89. Roberts DJ, Johnson RL, Burke AC, et al. Sonic hedgehog is an endodermal signal inducing Bmp-4 and Hox genes during induction and regionalization of the chick hindgut. *Development* 1995;121:2791–2801.
90. Romanoff AL. *The avian embryo: structural and functional development.* New York: Macmillan, 1960:526–531.
91. Dieterlen-Lièvre F. Étude morphologique et experimentale de la differenciation du pancréas chez l'embryo du poulet. *Bull Biol Fr Belg* 1965;99:3–116.
92. Liu CM, Potter EL. Development of the human pancreas. *Arch Pathol* 1962;74: 439–452.
93. Nelsen OE. *Comparative embryology of the vertebrates.* New York: Blakiston, 1963.
94. Al-Awqati Q, Goldberg MR. Architectural patterns in branching morphogenesis in the kidney. *Kidney Int* 1998;54:1832–1842.
95. Warburton D, Schwartz M, Tefft D, et al. The molecular basis of lung morphogenesis. *Mech Dev* 2000;92:55–81.
96. Spooner BS, Walther BT, Rutter WJ. The development of the dorsal and ventral mammalian pancreas in vivo and in vitro. *J Cell Biol* 1970;47:235–246.
97. Githens S. Development of the duct cells. In: Lebenthal E, ed. *Human gastrointestinal development.* New York: Raven Press, 1989:669–683.
98. Beaupain D, Dieterlen-Lievre F. Étude immunocytologique de la differentiation du pancreas endocrine chez l'embryon de poulet. II. Glucagon. *Gen Comp Endocrinol* 1974;23:421–423.
99. Stefan Y, Orci L, Malaisse-Lagae F. et al. Quantitation of endocrine cell content in the pancreas of nondiabetic and diabetic humans. *Diabetes* 1982;31: 694–700.
100. Orci L. Macro- and micro-domains in the endocrine pancreas. *Diabetes* 1982; 31:538–565.
101. deClercq L, Delaere P, Remacle C. The aging of the endocrine pancreas of the rat. I. Parameters of cell proliferation. *Mech Ageing Dev* 1988;43:11–24.
102. Ramiya VK, Maraist M, Arfors KE, et al. Reversal of insulin-dependent diabetes using islets generated in vitro from pancreatic stem cells. *Nat Med* 2000; 6:278–282.
103. Deltour L, Leduque P, Paldi A, et al. Polyclonal origin of pancreatic islets in aggregation mouse chimeras. *Development* 1991;112:115–121.
104. Le Douarin N, Bussonnet C. Early determination and inductive role of the pharyngeal endoderm. *C R Acad Sci Hebd Seances Acad Sci D* 1966;263: 1241–1243.
105. Lamers CB. Clinical and pathophysiological aspects of somatostatin and the gastrointestinal tract. *Acta Endocrinol Suppl (Copenh)* 1987;286:19–25.
106. Hebrok M, Kim S, Melton D. Notochord repression of endodermal sonic hedgehog permits pancreas development. *Genes Dev* 1998;12:1705–1713.
107. Kim S, Melton D. Pancreas development is promoted by cyclopamine a hedgehog signaling inhibitor. *Proc Natl Acad Sci U S A* 1998;95:13036–13041.
108. Haffen K, Kedinger M, Simon-Assmann P. Mesenchyme-dependent differentiation of epithelial progenitor cells in the gut. *J Pediatr Gastroenterol Nutr* 1987;6:14–23.

109. Kedinger M, Simon-Assmann PM, Lacroix B, et al. Fetal gut mesenchyme induces differentiation of cultured intestinal endodermal and crypt cells. *Dev Biol* 1986;113:474–483.
110. Roberts DJ, Johnson RL, Burke AC, et al. Sonic hedgehog is an endodermal signal inducing Bmp-4 and Hox genes during induction and regionalization of the chick hindgut. *Development* 1995;121:3163–3174.
111. Aufderheide E, Ekblom P. Tenascin during gut development: appearance in the mesenchyme, shift in molecular forms, and dependence on epithelial-mesenchymal interactions. *J Cell Biol* 1988;107:2341–2349.
112. Haffen K, Lacroix B, Kedinger M, et al. Inductive properties of fibroblastic cell cultures derived from rat intestinal mucosa on epithelial differentiation. *Differentiation* 1983;23:226–233.
113. Yasugi S. Differentiation of allantoic endoderm implanted into the presumptive digestive area in avian embryos. A study with organ-specific antigens. *J Embryol Exp Morphol* 1984;80:137–153.
114. Fukamachi H, Takayama S. Epithelial-mesenchymal interaction in differentiation of duodenal epithelium of fetal rats in organ culture. *Experientia* 1980; 36:335–336.
115. Fukamachi H, Mizuno T, Takayama S. Epithelial-mesenchymal interactions in differentiation of stomach epithelium in fetal mice. *Anat Embryol (Berl)* 1979;157:151–160.
116. Yasugi S, Mizuno T. Differentiation of the digestive tract epithelium under the influence of the heterologous mesenchyme of the digestive tract in the bird embryos. *Dev Growth Differ* 1978;20:261–267.
117. Yasugi S, Mizuno T. Mesenchymal-epithelial interactions in the organogenesis of the digestive tract. *Zool Sci* 1990;7:159–170.
118. Ishizuya-Oka A, Mizuno T. Intestinal cytodifferentiation in vitro of chick stomach endoderm induced by the duodenal mesenchyme. *J Embryol Exp Morphol* 1984;82:163–176.
119. Andrew A, Rawdon BB. Intestinal mesenchyme provokes differentiation of intestinal endocrine cells in gizzard endoderm. *Differentiation* 1990;43: 165–174.
120. Ahlgren U, Pfaff S, Jessel TM, et al. Independent requirement for ISL1 in the formation of the pancreatic mesenchyme and islet cells. *Nature* 1997;385: 257–260.
121. Wessels NK. Tissue interactions and cell differentiation. In: *Tissue interactions in development*. Menlo Park, CA: Benjamin, 1977:105–121.
122. Ronzio RA, Rutter WJ. Effects of a partially purified factor from chick embryos on macromolecular synthesis of embryonic pancreatic epithelia. *Dev Biol* 1973;30:307–320.
123. Levine S, Pictet R, Rutter WJ. Control of cell proliferation and cytodifferentiation by a factor reacting with the cell surface. *Nature New Biol* 1973;246: 49–52.
124. Sanvito F, Herrera PL, Huarte J, et al. TGF-beta 1 influences the relative development of the exocrine and endocrine pancreas in vitro. *Development* 1994;120:3451–3462.
125. Sonnenberg E, Meyer D, Weidner KM, et al. Scatter factor/hepatocyte growth factor and its receptor, the c-met tyrosine kinase, can mediate a signal exchange between mesenchyme and epithelia during mouse development. *J Cell Biol* 1993;123:223–235.
126. Otonkoski T, Beattie GM, Rubin JS, et al. Hepatocyte growth factor/scatter factor has insulinotropic activity in human fetal pancreatic cells. *Diabetes* 1994;43:947–953.
127. Arany E, Hill DJ. Ontogeny of fibroblast growth factors in the early development of the rat endocrine pancreas. *Pediatr Res* 2000;48:389–403.
128. Miralles F, Czernichow P, Scharfmann R. Follistatin regulates the relative proportions of endocrine versus exocrine tissue during pancreatic development. *Development* 1998;125:1017–1024.
129. Gittes GK, Galante PE, Hanahan D, et al. Lineage-specific morphogenesis in the developing pancreas: role of mesenchymal factors. *Development* 1996;122: 439–447.
130. Edlund H. Transcribing pancreas. *Diabetes* 1998;47:1817–1823.
131. Watt FM, Hogan BLM. Out of Eden: stem cells and their niches. *Science* 2000; 287:1427–1430.
132. Teitelman G, Alpert S, Polak JM, et al. Precursor cells of mouse endocrine pancreas coexpress insulin, glucagon and the neuronal proteins tyrosine hydroxylase and neuropeptide Y, but not pancreatic polypeptide. *Development* 1993;118:1031–1039.
133. Herrera PL, Huarte J, Sanvito F, et al. Embryogenesis of the murine endocrine pancreas: early expression of the pancreatic polypeptide gene. *Development* 1991;113:1257–1265.
134. Hashimoto T, Kawano H, Daikoku S, et al. Transient coappearance of glucagon and insulin in the progenitor cells of the rat pancreatic islets. *Anat Embryol (Berl)* 1988;178:489–497.
135. Upchurch BH, Aponte GW, Leiter AB. Expression of peptide YY in all four islet cell types in the developing mouse pancreas suggests a common peptide YY-producing progenitor. *Development* 1994;120:245–252.
136. Guz Y, Montminy M, Stein R, et al. Expression of murin STF-1, a putative insulin gene transcription factor, in beta cells of pancreas, duodenal epithelium and pancreatic exocrine and endocrine progenitors during ontogeny. *Development* 1995;121:142–146.
137. Schwitzgebel VM, Scheel DW, Conners JR, et al. Expression of neurogenin3 reveals an islet cell precursor population in the pancreas. *Development* 2000; 127:3533–3542.
138. Gradwohl G, Dierich A, LeMeur M, Guillemot F. Neurogenin3 is required for the development of the four endocrine cell lineages of the pancreas. *Proc Natl Acad Sci U S A* 2000;97:1607–1611.
139. Herrera PL. Adult insulin- and glucagon-producing cells differentiate from two independent lineages. *Development* 2000;127:2317–2322.
140. Larsson L-I. Endocrine pancreatic tumors. *Hum Pathol* 1978;9:401–416.
141. Philippe J, Chick WL, Habener JF. Multipotential phenotypic expression of genes encoding peptide hormones in rat insulinoma cell lines. *J Clin Invest* 1987;79:351–358.
142. Madsen OD, Larsson L-I, Rehfeld JF, et al. Cloned cell lines from a transplantable islet cell tumor are heterogeneous and express cholecystokinin in addition to islet hormones. *J Cell Biol* 1986;103:2025–2034.
143. Jetton TL, Moates JM, Lindner J, et al. Targeted oncogenesis of hormone-negative pancreatic islet progenitor cells. *Proc Natl Acad Sci U S A* 1998;95:8654–8659.
144. Herrera PL, Huarte J, Zufferey R, et al. Ablation of islet endocrine cells by targeted expression of hormone promoter-driven toxigenes. *Proc Natl Acad Sci U S A* 1994;91:12999–13003.
145. Kaung HL. Growth dynamics of pancreatic islet cell populations during fetal and neonatal development of the rat. *Dev Dyn* 1994;200:163–175.
146. Muller R, Laucke R, Trimper B, et al. Pancreatic cell proliferation in normal rats studied by in vivo autoradiography with 3H-thymidine. *Virchows Arch Biol Cell Pathol Incl Mol Pathol* 1990;59:133–136.
147. Finegood DT, Scaglia L, Bonner-Weir S. Dynamics of β-cell mass in the growing rat pancreas: estimation with a simple mathematical model. *Diabetes* 1995;44:249–256.
148. Hellerstrom C, Swenne I. Growth pattern of pancreatic islets in animals. In: Volk BW, Arquilla ER, eds. *The diabetic pancreas*. New York: Plenum Medical Book, 1985:53–79.
149. Gu D, Sarvetnick N. Epithelial cell proliferation and islet neogenesis in IFN-γ transgenic mice. *Development* 1993;118:33–46.
150. Gu D, Lee MS, Krahl T, Sarvetnick N. Transitional cells in the regenerating pancreas. *Development* 1994;120:1873–1881.
151. Hellerstrom C, Swenne I, Andersson A. Islet cell replication and diabetes. In: Lefebvre PJ, Pipeleers DG, eds. *The pathology of the endocrine pancreas in diabetes*. Heidelberg: Springer-Verlag, 1988:141–170.
152. Habener JF, Stoffers DA. A newly discovered role of transcription factors involved in pancreas development and the pathogenesis of diabetes mellitus. *Proc Assoc Am Physicians* 1988;110:12–21.
153. Scaglia L, Smith FE, Bonner-Weir S. Apoptosis contributes to the involution of β-cell mass in the postpartum rat pancreas. *Endocrinology* 1995;136: 5461–5468.
154. Scaglia L, Cahill CJ, Finegood DT, et al. Apoptosis is part of the remodeling of the endocrine pancreas in the neonatal rat. *Endocrinology* 1997;138: 1736–1741.
155. Kassem SA, Ariel I, Thornton PS, et al. β-Cell proliferation and apoptosis in the developing normal human pancreas and in hyperinsulinism of infancy. *Diabetes* 2000;49:1325–1333.
156. McEvoy RC, Madson KL. Pancreatic insulin-, glucagon-, and somatostatin-positive islet cell populations during the perinatal development of the rat. I. Morphometric quantitation. *Biol Neonate* 1980;38:248–254.
157. Rahier J, Wallon J, Henquin JC. Cell populations in the endocrine pancreas in human neonates and infants. *Diabetologia* 1981;20:540–546.
158. Orci L, Stefan Y, Malaisse-Lagae F, et al. Instability of pancreatic endocrine cell populations throughout life. *Lancet* 1979;1:615–616.
159. Stephan Y, Grasso S, Perrelet A, et al. A quantitative immunofluorescent study of the endocrine cell population in the developing human pancreas. *Diabetes* 1983;32:293–301.
160. Hughes H. An experimental study of regeneration in the islets of Langerhans with reference to the theory of balance. *Acta Anatomica* 1956;27:1–61.
161. McEvoy RC. Changes in the volumes of the A-, B- and D-cell populations in the pancreatic islets during the postnatal development of the rat. *Diabetes* 1981;30:813–817.
162. Alumets J, Hakanson R, Sundler F. Ontogeny of endocrine cells in porcine gut and pancreas. An immunocytochemical study. *Gastroenterology* 1983;85: 1359–1372.
163. Githens S. The pancreatic duct cell: proliferative capabilities, specific characteristics, metaplasia, isolation and culture. *J Pediatr Gastroenterol Nutr* 1988;7: 486–506.
164. Bonner-Weir S. Perspective: Postnatal pancreatic beta-cell growth. *Endocrinology* 2000;141:1926–1929.
165. Parsons JA, Brelje TC, Sorenson RL. Adaptation of islets to pregnancy: increased islet cell proliferation and insulin secretion correlates with the onset of placental lactogen secretion. *Endocrinology* 1992;130:1459–1466.
166. Bruning JC, Winnay J, Bonner-Weir S, et al. Development of a novel polygenic model of NIDDM in mice heterozygous for IR and IRS-null alleles. *Cell* 1997;88:561–572.
167. Setalo G, Blatniczky L, Vigh S. Development and growth of the islets of Langerhans through acino-insular transformation in regenerating rat pancreas. *Acta Biol* 1972;23:309–312.
168. Bonner-Weir S, Trent DF, Weir GC. Partial pancreatectomy in the rat subsequent defect in glucose-induced release. *J Clin Invest* 1983;71:1544–1553.
169. Bonner-Weir S, Baxter LA, Schupin GT, et al. A second pathway for regeneration of the adult exocrine and endocrine pancreas. A possible recapitulation of embryonic development. *Diabetes* 1993;42:1715–1750.
170. Rosenberg L, Brown RA, Duguid WP. A new approach to the induction of duct epithelial hyperplasia and nesidioblastosis by cellophane wrapping of the hamster pancreas. *J Surg Res* 1983;35:63–72.
171. Dutrillaux MC, Portha B, Roze C, et al. Ultrastructural study of pancreatic B cell regeneration in newborn rats after destruction by streptozotocin. *Virch Arch Biol Cell Pathol Incl Mol Pathol* 1982;39:173–185.

172. Johnson DD. Alloxan administration in the guinea pig. A study of regenerative phase in the islands of Langerhans. *Endocrinology* 1950;47:393–398.
173. Weaver CV, Sorenson RL, Kaung HC. Immunocytochemical localization of insulin-immunoreactive cells in the pancreatic ducts of rats treated with trypsin inhibitor. *Diabetologia* 1985;28:781–785.
174. Fitzgerald PJ, Carol BM, Rosenstock L. Pancreatic acinar cell regeneration. *Nature* 1966;212:594–596.
175. Adams DJ, Harrison RG. The vascularization of the rat pancreas and the effect of ischemia on the islets of Langerhans. *J Anat* 1953;87:257–267.
176. Beattie GM, Itkin-Ansari P, Cirulli V, et al. Sustained proliferation of PDX-1+ cells derived from human islets. *Diabetes* 1999;48:1013–1019.
177. Kerr-Conte J, Pattou F, Lecomte-Houcke M, et al. Ductal cyst formation in collagen-embedded adult human islet preparations. A means to the reproduction of nesidioblastosis in vitro. *Diabetes* 1966;45:1108–1114.
178. Lathja LG. Stem cells. In: Potten CS, ed. *Stem cells: their identification and characterization*. Edinburgh: Churchill Livingstone, 1983:1–11.
179. Weissman IL. Stem cells: units of development, units of regeneration, and units in evolution. *Cell* 2000;100:157–168.
180. Bonner-Weir S. Morphological evidence for pancreatic polarity of β-cell within the islets of Langerhans. *Diabetes* 1988;37:616–621.
181. Lammert E, Brown J, Melton DA. Notch gene expression during pancreatic organogenesis. *Mech Dev* 2000;94:199–203.
182. Apelqvist A, Li H, Sommer L, et al. Notch signalling controls pancreatic cell differentiation. *Nature* 1999;400:877–881.
183. Hunziker E, Stein M. Nestin-expressing cells in the pancreatic islets of Langerhans. *Biochem Biophys Res Comm* 2000;271:116–119.
184. Yuan S, Rosenberg L, Paraskevas S, et al. Transdifferentiation of human islets to pancreatic ductal cells in collagen matrix culture. *Differentiation* 1996;61: 67–75.
185. Bjornson CR, Rietze RL, Reynolds BA, et al. Turning brain into blood: a hematopoietic fate adopted by adult neural stem cells in vivo. *Science* 1999; 283:534–537.
186. Jackson KA, Mi T, Goodell MA. Hematopoietic potential of stem cells isolated from murine skeletal muscle. *Proc Natl Acad Sci U S A* 1999;96: 14482–14486.
187. Gussoni E, Soneoka Y, Strickland CD, et al. Dystrophin expression in the mdx mouse restored by stem cell transplantation. *Nature* 1999;401:390–394.
188. Kopen GC, Prockop DJ, Phinney DG. Marrow stromal cells migrate throughout forebrain and cerebellum and they differentiate into astrocytes after injection into neonatal mouse brains. *Proc Natl Acad Sci U S A* 1999;96: 10711–10716.
189. Cornelius JG, Tchernev V, Kao KJ, et al. In vitro-generation of islets in long-term cultures of pluripotent stem cells from adult mouse pancreas. *Horm Metab Res* 1997;29:271–277.
190. Wright CV, Schnegelsberg P, De Robertis EM. XlHbox 8: a novel *Xenopus* homeo protein restricted to a narrow band of endoderm. *Development* 1989; 105:787–794.
191. Peshavaria M, Gamer L, Henderson E, et al. XIHbox 8 an endoderm-specific *Xenopus* homeodomain protein, is closely related to a mammalian insulin gene transcription factor. *Mol Endocrinol* 1984;8:806–816.
192. Gannon M, Wright CVE. Endodermal patterning and organogenesis. In: Moody SA, ed. *Cell lineage and fate determination*. New York: Academic Press, 1999:583–615.
193. Ohlsson H, Karlsson K, Edlund T. IPF1, a homeodomain-containing transactivator of the insulin gene. *EMBO J* 1993;12:4251–4259.
194. Leonard J, Peers B, Johnson T, et al. Characterization of somatostatin transactivating factor-1, a novel homeobox factor that stimulates somatostatin expression in pancreatic islet cells. *Mol Endocrinol* 1993;7:1275–1283.
195. Miller CP, McGehee RE Jr, Habener JF. IDX-1: a new homeodomain transcription factor expressed in rat pancreatic islets and duodenum that transactivates the somatostatin gene. *EMBO J* 1994;13:1145–1156.
196. Watada H, Kajimoto Y, Kaneto H, et al. Involvement of the homeodomain-containing transcription factor PDX-1 in islet amyloid polypeptide gene transcription. *Biochem Biophys Res Commun* 1996;229:746–751.
197. Waeber G, Thompson N, Nicod P, et al. Transcriptional activation of the GLUT2 gene by the IPF-1/STF-1/IDX-1 homeobox factor. *Mol Endocrinol* 1996;10:1327–1334.
198. Watada H, Kajimoto Y, Umayahara Y, et al. The human glucokinase gene beta-cell-type promoter: an essential role of insulin promoter factor 1/PDX-1 in its activation in HIT-T15 cells. *Diabetes* 1996;45:1478–1488.
199. Jonsson J, Carlsson L, Edlund T, et al. Insulin-promoter-factor 1 is required for pancreas development in mice. *Nature* 1994;371:606–609.
200. Offield MF, Jetton TL, Labosky PA, et al. PDX-1 is required for pancreatic outgrowth and differentiation of the rostral duodenum. *Development* 1996;22: 983–995.
201. Stoffers DA, Zinkin NT, Stanojevic V, et al. Pancreatic agenesis attributable to a single nucleotide deletion in the human IPF1 gene coding sequence. *Nat Genet* 1997;15:106–110.
202. Ahlgren U, Jonsson J, Edlund H. The morphogenesis of the pancreatic mesenchyme is uncoupled from that of the pancreatic epithelium in IPF1/PDX1-deficient mice. *Development* 1996;122:1409–1416.
203. Ahlgren U, Jonsson J, Jonsson L, et al. Beta-cell-specific inactivation of the mouse Ipf1/Pdx1 gene results in loss of the beta-cell phenotype and maturity onset diabetes. *Genes Dev* 1998;12:1763–1768.
204. Dutta S, Bonner-Weir S, Montminy M, et al. Regulatory factor linked to late-onset diabetes? *Nature* 1998;392:560.
205. Gremlich S, Bonny C, Waeber G, et al. Fatty acids decrease IDX-1 expression in rat pancreatic islets and reduce GLUT2, glucokinase, insulin, and somatostatin levels. *J Biol Chem* 1997;272:30261–30269.
206. Sommer L, Ma Q, Anderson DJ. Neurogenins, a novel family of atonal-related bHLH transcription factors, are putative mammalian neuronal determination genes that reveal progenitor cell heterogeneity in the developing CNS and PNS. *Mol Cell Neurosci* 1996;8:221–241.
207. Grapin-Botton A, Majithia AR, Melton DA. Key events of pancreas formation are triggered in gut endoderm by ectopic expression of pancreatic regulatory genes. *Genes Dev* 2001;14:444–454.
208. Bitgood MJ, McMahon AP. Hedgehog and Bmp genes are coexpressed at many diverse sites of cell-cell interaction in the mouse embryo. *Dev Biol* 1995; 172:126–138.
209. Apelqvist A, Ahlgren U, Edlund H. Sonic hedgehog directs specialised mesoderm differentiation in the intestine and pancreas. *Curr Biol* 1997;7:801–804.
210. Hebrok M, Kim SK, St Jacques B, et al. Regulation of pancreas development by hedgehog signaling. *Development* 2000;127:4905–4913.
211. Harrison KA, Druey KM, Deguchi Y, et al. A novel human homeobox gene distantly related to proboscipedia is expressed in lymphoid and pancreatic tissues. *J Biol Chem* 1994;269:19968–19975.
212. Li H, Arber S, Jessell TM, et al. Selective agenesis of the dorsal pancreas in mice lacking homeobox gene Hlxb9. *Nat Genet* 1999;23:67–70.
213. Harrison KA, Thaler J, Pfaff SL, et al. Pancreas dorsal lobe agenesis and abnormal islets of Langerhans in Hlxb9-deficient mice. *Nat Genet* 1999;23: 71–75.
214. Huang HP, Liu M, El-Hodiri HM, et al. Regulation of the pancreatic islet-specific gene BETA2 (neuroD) by neurogenin3. *Mol Cell Biol* 2000;20:3292–3307.
215. Naya FJ, Huang HP, Qiu Y, et al. Diabetes, defective pancreatic morphogenesis, and abnormal enteroendocrine differentiation in BETA2/neuroD-deficient mice. *Genes Dev* 1997;11:2323–2334.
216. Dohrmann C, Gruss P, Lemaire L. Pax genes and the differentiation of hormone-producing endocrine cells in the pancreas. *Mech Dev* 2000;92:47–54.
217. Malecki MT, Jhala US, Antonellis A, et al. Mutations in NEUROD1 are associated with the development of type 2 diabetes mellitus. *Nat Genet* 1999;23: 323–328.
218. Karlsson O, Thor S, Norberg T, et al. Insulin gene enhancer binding protein Isl-1 is a member of a novel class of proteins containing both a homeo- and a Cys-His domain. *Nature* 1990;344:879–882.
219. Thor S, Ericson J, Brannstrom T, et al. The homeodomain LIM protein Isl-1 is expressed in subsets of neurons and endocrine cells in the adult rat. *Neuron* 1991;7:881–889.
220. Sosa-Pineda B, Chowdhury K, Torres M, et al. The Pax4 gene is essential for differentiation of insulin-producing beta cells in the mammalian pancreas. *Nature* 1997;386:399–402.
221. St-Onge L, Sosa-Pineda B, Chowdhury K, et al. Pax6 is required for differentiation of glucagon-producing alpha-cells in mouse pancreas. *Nature* 1997; 387:406–409.
222. Turque N, Plaza S, Radvanyi F, et al. Pax-QNR/Pax-6, a paired box- and homeobox-containing gene expressed in neurons, is also expressed in pancreatic endocrine cells. *Mol Endocrinol* 1994;8:929–938.
223. Sander M, Neubuser A, Kalamaras J, et al. Genetic analysis reveals that PAX6 is required for normal transcription of pancreatic hormone genes and islet development. *Genes Dev* 1997;11:1662–1673.
224. Wrege A, Diedrich T, Hochhuth C, et al. Transcriptional activity of domain A of the rat glucagon G3 element conferred by an islet-specific nuclear protein that also binds to similar pancreatic islet cell-specific enhancer sequences (PISCES). *Gene Expr* 1995;4:205–216.
225. Price M, Lazzaro D, Pohl T, et al. Regional expression of the homeobox gene Nkx-2.2 in the developing mammalian forebrain. *Neuron* 1992;8:241–255.
226. Sussel L, Kalamaras J, Hartigan-O'Connor DJ, et al. Mice lacking the homeodomain transcription factor Nkx2.2 have diabetes due to arrested differentiation of pancreatic beta cells. *Development* 1998;125:2213–2221.
227. Madsen OD, Jensen J, Petersen HV, et al. Transcription factors contributing to the pancreatic beta-cell phenotype. *Horm Metab Res* 1997;29:265–270.

CHAPTER 3
Islets of Langerhans: Morphology and Postnatal Growth

Susan Bonner-Weir

The islets of Langerhans are clusters of endocrine tissue scattered throughout the exocrine pancreas in all vertebrates higher in evolutionary development than the bony fish (teleosts). In the adult mammal, the islets are 1% to 2% of the pancreatic mass and thus comprise approximately 1 g of tissue in the adult human. Islets are complex structures of cells and function both separately as micro-organs and in concert as the endocrine pancreas. Although the direct secretion of insulin and glucagon from islets into the portal vein has obvious advantages with respect to influence on hepatic function, it is not clear why the endocrine pancreas is dispersed throughout the exocrine pancreas. One suggestion is that the local insular-acinar portal system helps regulate the exocrine function of the pancreas, with this function providing some evolutionary advantage (1).

The pancreas of the adult human contains approximately 200 U, or 8 mg, of insulin (2) and that of the adult rat contains about 100 μg of insulin. The size of an islet can range from only a few cells and less than 40 μm in diameter to approximately 10,000 cells and 400 μm in diameter. The average rat islet is 150 μm in diameter and contains approximately 45 ng of insulin. In the rat, and probably in other mammals, islets smaller than 160 μm in diameter represent 75% of the islets in number but only 15% of the islet volume, whereas islets larger than 250 μm in diameter represent only 15% of the islets in number but 60% of the islet volume (3).

Islet mass is dynamic, adjusting to meet the changing needs of the individual, whose size and level of activity vary at different stages of life. When islet mass cannot adjust to meet the demand, diabetes mellitus results.

Although studies of the islets of nonmammalian vertebrates have been useful in extending our knowledge, we have a far more detailed understanding of the structure, function, and changes in mass of mammalian islets. In a text on diabetes, the emphasis should be on the human islet, but our present understanding of islets is based mainly on rodent studies. Thus, the rodent islet will be used as the paradigm.

This chapter will first address the cellular components of the islet and their organization. We now know that islets are not all the same, and this heterogeneity will be discussed. The manner in which the structural organization of an islet defines its function will be addressed. Finally, issues of islet growth after birth, both normal and compensatory, will be discussed. Embryonic development of the endocrine pancreas has been discussed in the previous chapter (Chapter 2).

OVERALL PANCREATIC ANATOMY

The origin of the pancreas as separate primordia is thought to be the basis of the regional distribution of glucagon-producing and pancreatic polypeptide–producing cells (4). The dorsal pancreas, supplied with blood by the celiac trunk via the gastroduodenal and splenic arteries and drained by one main pancreatic duct, contains the glucagon-rich islets with few pancreatic polypeptide–containing cells. The opposite distribution is found in the ventral pancreas, which is supplied with blood from the superior mesenteric artery via the inferior pancreaticoduodenal artery and is drained by a separate exocrine duct. Here the islets contain pancreatic polypeptide–producing cells and few, if any, glucagon-producing cells. The degree of fusion of these ducts differs among species.

The normal organization of the islet, with its central core of β-cells and its peripheral non–β-cells, is observed only after fetal day 18.5 (5). In adult mammals, 70% to 80% of the islet consists of insulin-producing β-cells, 5% is somatostatin-producing δ-cells, and 15% to 20% is either glucagon-producing α-cells or pancreatic polypeptide–producing PP cells. The proportions of the different cell types differ with age because the different islet cells do not have the same pattern of growth. For example, in both rats and humans, the percentage of islet cells that are δ-cells is considerably greater in perinatal than in adult individuals (6). At birth the β-cells are usually only 50% of the islet, and with postnatal replication of the β-cells and increase in cell volume (7), their proportion increases.

Islets differentiate from the pancreatic ductal epithelium as do exocrine cells, but the question of whether they are derived from the same or different precursor/stem cell populations remains unanswered. Embryonic development of the pancreas as ductules that proliferate, branch, and then differentiate was described by Pictet and Rutter (8). Islet hormone-containing cells are first seen as single cells among the exocrine cells of the terminal pancreatic tubules and then as clusters of cells within the exocrine basement membrane. These clusters then become separated from the exocrine tissue to form distinct islets (8). In the adult pancreas, sometimes the only separation between exocrine and islet cells are their respective basement membranes (Fig. 3.1). However, islets are usually surrounded by at least a partial capsule of fibroblasts and collagen fibers.

In the pancreas of adults of many species, islet cells of all types can be immunolocalized in the pancreatic ducts as occasional single cells or small budding islets. An increased occurrence of these cells has been observed under numerous experimental conditions, including dietary treatment with soybean trypsin inhibitor (9), overexpression of interferon-γ in the β-cells of transgenic mice (10), after partial pancreatectomy (11), and after cellophane wrapping of the head of the pancreas (12), as well as with some human diseases, including recent-onset type 1 diabetes mellitus (insulin-dependent) (13) and severe liver disease. Adult ductal epithelium can be stimulated to undergo morphogenic changes that result in a substantial formation of new islets. In the young adult rat, 3 days after a 90% pancreatectomy, 10% to 15% of the pancreatic remnant volume is composed of proliferating ductules, which differentiate into new islets and exocrine tissue within another 3 to 4 days and largely account for the doubling of remnant mass found within 1 week of surgery (11). When adult ductal epithelium was wrapped in fetal mesenchyme and implanted in nude mice, approximately 20% of the grafts were found to contain "islet-like cell clusters" with hormone immunostaining budding from the ducts (13,14). Adult human ductal tissue can be driven to differentiate into islets *in vitro* (15). The differentiation process can be reprogrammed, as seen in adult rats depleted of copper with a resultant destruction of acinar tissue but "normal islets and ducts." After copper repletion, hepatocytes, rather than acinar cells, regenerate in the pancreas, this being an example of transdifferentiation (16).

PHYLOGENETIC CONSIDERATIONS

The comparative aspects of the endocrine pancreas was the focus of much study in the 1970s (17–20). The first step in the development of a separate islet organ is found in the vertebrate class Agnatha, the primitive jawless fish (represented today by hagfish and lampreys). In hagfish all of the β-cells and most of the δ-cells are no longer in the gut mucosa and are restricted to the bile duct and adjacent islet organ, whereas the glucagon/gastrin-producing cells remain in the gut mucosa (17). The first appearance of a pancreas in which β-, α-, δ-, and

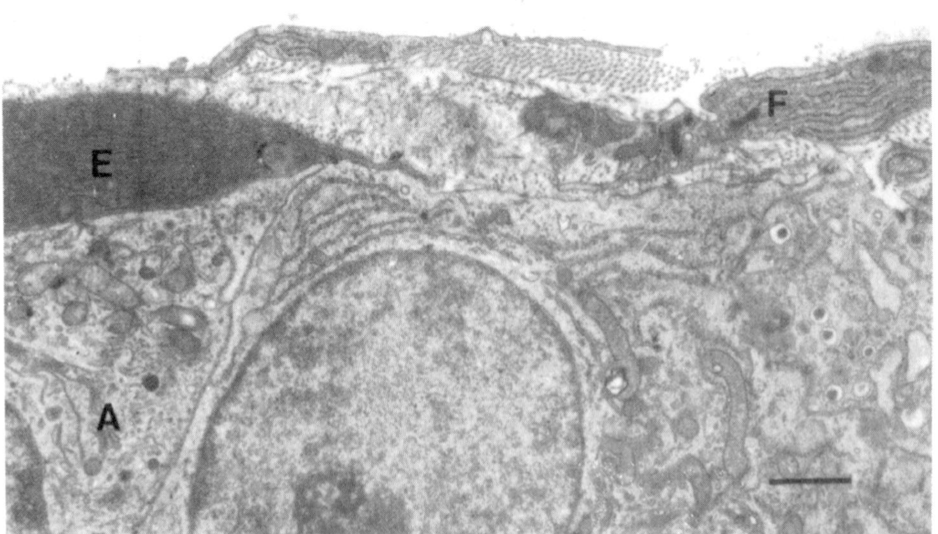

FIGURE 3.1. The periphery of a rat islet showing the capsule of a single layer of fibroblasts (*F*) and collagen fibers laid down by these cells. No capsule is seen between the exocrine cell (*E*) and the endocrine α-cell (*A*); the capsule often incompletely surrounds the islet. Scale bar = 1 μm.

PP-cells are all represented is in the cartilaginous fish (class Chondrichthyes), in which the islet cells are found in the parenchyma, in the pancreatic ducts, or disseminated in the exocrine pancreas (17,21). The bony fish (class Osteichthyes) have large accumulations of endocrine tissue, sometimes called the Brockmann bodies, near the spleen and pylorus and, in addition, have small islets scattered throughout the exocrine tissue, often in association with small ducts. The descriptions of islets in amphibians and reptiles are widely variant, but there seems to be a pattern of three types of islets: large splenic islets with the α-cell population greater than the β-cell population; islets of intermediate size with more β-cells but still a majority of α-cells; and small islets with mostly β-cells. This heterogeneity of islets has been better defined for the birds (class Aves): Dark, or α, islets are composed of α- and δ-cells; and light, or β, islets are composed of β- and δ-cells (PP-cells are often extrainsular). In this class, as in mammals, the regional distribution of islet types has an embryologic origin.

COMPONENTS OF THE ISLETS OF LANGERHANS

Endocrine Cells

There are four major endocrine cell types in mammalian islets: the insulin-producing β-cell, the glucagon-producing α-cell, the somatostatin-producing δ-cell, and the pancreatic polypeptide–producing PP-cell (the latter three will be referred to collectively as the non–β-cells) (Fig. 3.2). Ultrastructural and immunocytochemical techniques are used to distinguish these cell types and have identified other minor cell types (Table 3.1). Numerous other peptides and hormones have been localized to the islet cells with the use of sensitive immunostaining techniques (Table 3.1). Localization of several of these peptides is confusing because the type of cells that are immunostained varies with species. For example, calcitonin gene–related peptide (CGRP) co-localizes with somatostatin in the rat δ-cells but with insulin in mouse β-cells (22). Similarly, an antibody to pancreastatin stains α- and δ-cells in humans but β- and δ-cells in pigs (23,24). An additional level of complexity is introduced by evidence that the hormones thyrotropin-releasing hormone and gastrin are expressed in the islets only during the perinatal period (25,26). It is presently unclear how any of these other hormones/peptides function in the islet. The sensitivity of the techniques and the overlap of antibody recognition may be responsible for some of these confusing data. Another explanation for the overlap may be the sequential differentiation of the islet cell types.

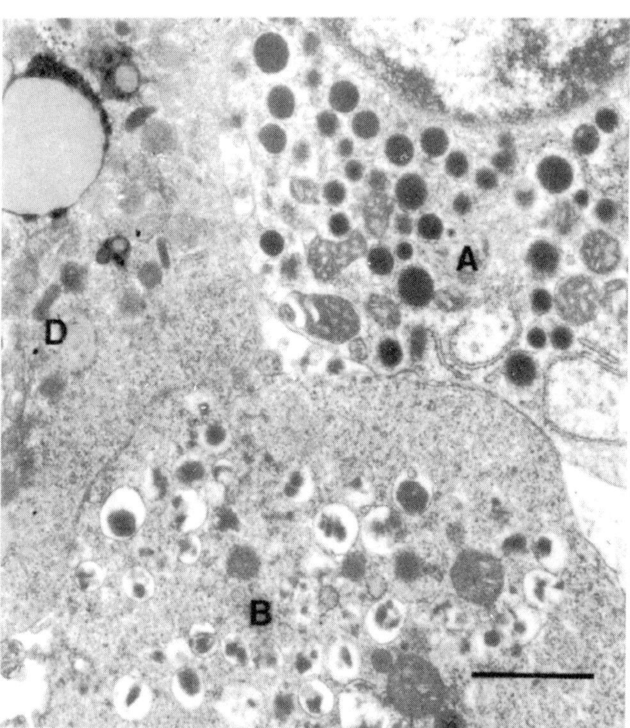

FIGURE 3.2. The secretory granules of the islet endocrine cells have a characteristic morphology. Represented here are those of the β-cell (*B*), the α-cell (*A*), and the δ-cell (*D*) of a human islet. Scale bar = 1 μm.

The β-cells are polyhedral, being truncated pyramids, and are usually well granulated, with secretory granules 250 to 300 nm in diameter (Fig. 3.3). It has been estimated that each mouse β-cell contains approximately 10,000 granules (27). There are

TABLE 3.1. Characteristics of the Endocrine Cells of the Islets of Langerhans[a]

Cell type	Size of secretory granule (nm)	Percentage of islet cells	Hormonal content
β	250–350	60–80	Insulin, IAPP/amylin (thyrotropin-releasing hormone, calcitonin gene–related peptide, gastrin, pancreastatin)
α	200–250	15–20	Glucagon (glicentin, TRH, CCK, endorphin, glucagon-like polypeptide-1, peptide YY, DKP histidyl-proline diketopiperazine, pancreastatin)
δ	300–350 200–300	5–10	Somatostatin (met-enkephalin, CGRP, pancreastatin)
PP	120–160	15–20	Pancreatic polypeptide (met-enkephalin, peptide YY)
δ_1	100–130	<1	Vasoactive intestinal polypeptide
EC	300–350	<1	Substance P, serotonin
G_1	300	<1	Gastrin (adrenocorticotropic hormone-related peptides)

[a]The secretory granules of each cell type have a characteristic size and morphology. The size of δ-cell secretory granules varies with species; hormonal content identified by immunostaining techniques; peptides in parentheses found in at least one species. Some of these peptides, for example, TRH, glucagon-like peptide 1, and gastrin, usually are found only in perinatal islets. The physiologic significance of the islet location is unclear.

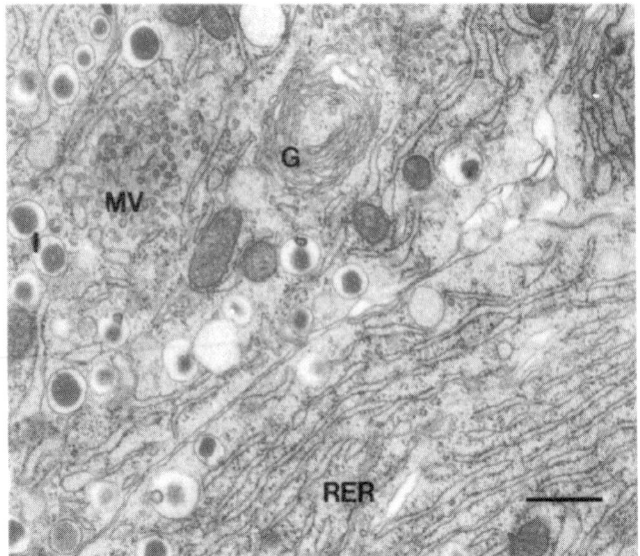

FIGURE 3.3. The synthetic and secretory machinery of the insulin-producing β-cell of a rat islet shown in three adjacent cells. RER, rough endoplasmic reticulum; MV, microvesicles; G, Golgi apparatus; I, insulin secretory granules. Scale bar = 0.5 μm.

two forms of insulin granules: mature granules that have an electron-dense core and a loosely fitting granule-limiting membrane with the appearance of a spacious halo; and immature granules with little or no halo, moderately electron-dense contents, and a clathrin coat. Immature granules have been shown to be the major, if not the only, site of conversion from proinsulin to insulin (28). Other changes, such as the shedding of the clathrin coat, acidification of the granule contents, and crystallization of insulin, occur as the granule matures from a proinsulin-rich granule to an insulin-rich granule (28). In some species the electron-dense core of the mature granule is visibly crystalline. Insulin is not the only peptide in the granules; there are at least 100 other peptides (29).

The α-cells are usually smaller and more columnar than the β-cells and well granulated, with granules 200 to 250 nm in diameter (Fig. 3.2). The granules are electron-dense with a narrow halo of less-dense material and a tightly fitting granule-limiting membrane; there is little species variation.

The δ-cells are usually smaller than either α- or β-cells, are well granulated, and are often dendritic in shape. The electron density of granules within a δ-cell varies greatly (Fig. 3.2). Each granule, 200 to 250 nm in diameter, contains material of homogeneous moderate density that fills the granule-limiting membrane.

PP-cells are the most variable among species. In humans the granules are elongated, very electron dense, and 120 to 160 nm in diameter. In dogs and cats, the granules are spherical, variable in electron density, and approximately 300 nm in diameter (30).

Capsule

The existence of an islet capsule has been a controversial issue, perhaps because the capsule is only a single layer of fibroblasts and the collagen fibers laid down by these fibroblasts (Fig. 3.1). Furthermore, frequently the capsule between islet and exocrine cells is absent. The extant capsule does overlay the efferent blood vessels of the islet and seems to define a subcapsular interstitial space.

Microvasculature

The islet is highly vascularized and has a direct arteriolar blood supply (31). Islet capillaries are fenestrated, whereas fenestration is decreased or absent in capillaries of the surrounding exocrine tissue (32). The fenestrae render these capillaries highly permeable. The passage of horseradish peroxidase into the pericapillary interstitial space of the islet takes only 45 seconds, whereas it takes 5 minutes in cardiac muscle (33). The blood flow to the islets has been found to be disproportionately large (10% to 20% of the pancreatic blood flow) for the 1% to 2% of pancreatic volume (34–37). Factors regulating islet blood flow may affect islet hormone secretion. High concentrations of glucose have been shown to enhance pancreatic blood flow and to preferentially increase islet blood flow (38). In addition, several of the peptides immunochemically localized in islet nerves and/or endocrine cells, for example, CGRP, are vasoactive (39). The relation of the microvasculature to islet endocrine cells is discussed below. Lymphatic vessels, while common in the pancreas, have not been found within the islets (40).

Nerves

The pancreas is innervated by sympathetic fibers from the celiac and superior mesenteric ganglia and by parasympathetic fibers from the vagus nerve (41,42). These parasympathetic fibers synapse in small ganglia dispersed in the pancreas. They may act as pacemakers for the oscillations in hormone secretion (43) that occur without extrinsic nervous connections, as in the isolated perfused canine pancreas (44).

Within the pancreas, nerve fibers terminate in perivascular, periacinar, and peri-insular areas. Within the islets, the nerves follow the blood vessels and terminate within the pericapillary space, within the capillary basement membrane, or closely apposed to the endocrine cells. Because no specialized synapses are found, it has been suggested that neurotransmitters released into the interstitial space may affect a number of neighboring islet cells. In some species, nerve cell bodies are close to or even within the islets (45).

The distribution and number of the different types of nerve fibers differ among species (41,42,45). Cholinergic nerves, identified histochemically by cholinesterase activity or ultrastructurally by the presence of electron-lucent vesicles, are common in rat, cat, and rabbit islets. Adrenergic nerves, as identified immunochemically by antibodies to catecholamine-forming enzymes (including tyrosine hydroxylase) (45) and ultrastructurally by the presence of dense cored vesicles, are common in the hamster, dog, and cat. Peptidergic nerves are less well defined, being identified either immunochemically as containing substance P, enkephalin, vasoactive intestinal polypeptide (VIP), galanin, gastrin-releasing peptide, CGRP, or cholecystokinin, or ultrastructurally by the presence of large granules. A further complication is introduced by the finding of neuropeptide Y and galanin in adrenergic nerves and the identification of VIP in cholinergic nerves (46). Both substance P and CGRP seem to be localized in the sensory fibers. The presence of peptidergic nerve cell bodies in pancreatic ganglia suggests that some of these intrinsic nerves may be involved in the synchronization of islet secretion (45).

The autonomic nervous system modulates islet hormone secretion (41,45,47). Cholinergic stimulation elicits increased secretion of insulin, glucagon, and pancreatic polypeptide. Its effects on somatostatin are less clear but appear to be inhibitory. β-Adrenergic stimulation similarly elicits increased secretion of insulin, glucagon, pancreatic polypeptide, and somatostatin (48). β-Adrenergic stimulation decreases secretion of insulin and somatostatin, but its effect on glucagon secretion varies with species. The effects of stimulation of peptidergic nerves have not been studied as closely, but VIP, cholecystokinin, and galanin can affect islet-cell secretion. VIP causes an increase in insulin secretion that is direct (49). VIP neurons form a peri-insular network in rats (50), but the peptide does not change the islet blood flow as it increases the total pancreatic blood flow (49).

ORGANIZATION OF THE COMPONENTS OF THE ISLETS OF LANGERHANS

The distribution of the endocrine cells is nonrandom, with a core of β-cells surrounded by a discontinuous mantle of non–β-cells one to three cells thick (51,52). The islets of most mammalian species have this pattern, but those of humans and other primates have a somewhat more complex arrangement (Fig. 3.4). Sections of human pancreas show many different islet profiles, including oval and cloverleaf patterns, differences that have resulted in controversy about whether they actually have a mantle-core arrangement (52–54). Nonetheless, in three dimensions, human islets can be considered as composites of several mantle-core subunits or as lobulated with mantle-core lobules (52,55). In sectioned tissue, incomplete fusion of such subunits and penetrations of islet vasculature can appear as invaginations of the islet periphery. Most of the non–β-cells are found along these invaginations and the periphery (52,53), thus maintaining a mantle-core arrangement. Confocal microscopy allows a better appreciation of the three-dimensional organization of islet cells (56). With confocal microscopy, α-cells are seen as a sheet or a peel at the islet periphery and δ-cells are seen as more peripheral to the α-cells in the human but less peripheral in the rat. This pattern of organization is based on intrinsic qualities of the cell surfaces of the different cell types, as shown by reaggregation studies. When single dispersed rat islet cells were allowed to reaggregate, the aggregates showed the same nonrandom organization as native islets, even when the proportions of β-cells and non–β-cells were reversed (57). Both β-cells and non–β-cells have high levels of calcium-dependent cell-adhesion molecules (cadherins), but non–β-cells also contain calcium-independent cell-adhesion molecules (58). It is thought that this differential expression of cell-adhesion molecules may be responsible for the segregation of β-cells and non–β-cells.

The microvasculature forms the infrastructure of an islet. The rat islet has been studied most extensively and will serve as the prototype in this discussion, but this generalization needs to be verified. Afferent vessels to an islet number one to three arterioles, depending on islet size. Each arteriole penetrates the islet through discontinuities of the non–β-cell mantle and enters directly into the β-cell core, where it branches into a number of fenestrated capillaries (3). These capillaries follow a tortuous path, passing first through the β-cell core and then through the non–β-cell mantle. Often the vessels pass along the inside of the mantle before penetrating it. The efferent vessels are collecting or postcapillary venules. It is unclear where the transition from capillary to collecting venule occurs, but collecting venules can often be seen in indentations of the islet. There appears to be a single continuous circulation through the islet. Although each capillary should have functionally different arterial and venous portions, no morphologic differences have yet been found.

The pattern of microvasculature varies, depending on islet size (Fig. 3.5). In large islets, the efferent vessels coalesce into collecting venules within the subcapsular space. In small islets, the efferent capillaries extend into the exocrine tissue for 50 to 100 μm before coalescing into collecting venules. Within the islet, endocrine cells are organized around the microvasculature (Fig. 3.6). In the rat, the β-cells have been found to have two faces on capillaries (59). In cross-section, eight to ten β-cells are seen to form a rosette around one of the capillaries. In three dimensions this pattern would be tubelike. The outer face of each β-cell would be against a capillary, which is probably arterial and orthogonal to the central capillary. In β-cells experimentally degranulated with glyburide, the remaining granules are polarized toward the central "venous" capillary, suggesting an *in situ* polarity of the β-cells. Along the interface of three or more β-cells and extending from capillary face to capillary face are elaborate canaliculi (59). Desmosomes that act as mechanical attachments are preferentially found near these canaliculi. These canaliculi contain large numbers of microvilli (59,60) that have been found to be enriched in glucose transporter 2 (GLUT-2) (61). The presence of these elaborate structures suggests a bulk flow of interstitial fluid through these canaliculi in an arterial-to-venous direction and an uptake of glucose by the β-cells that is carried out mainly by the transporters on these

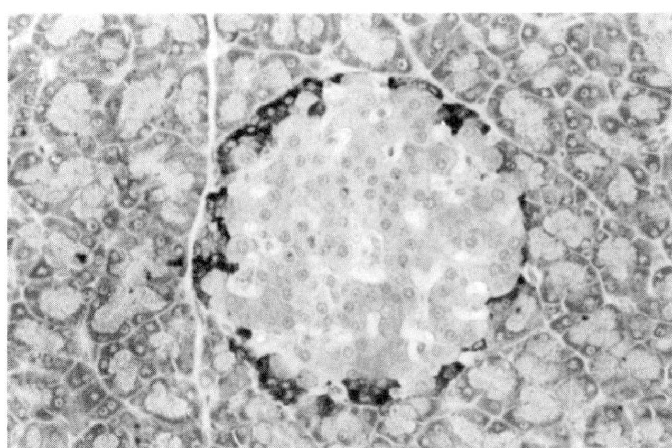

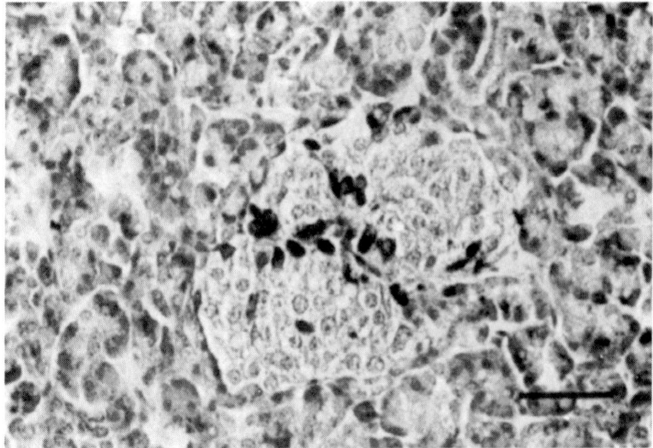

Figure 3.4. The pattern of a mantle of non–β-cells (the glucagon-, somatostatin-, and pancreatic polypeptide–producing cells) around a core of insulin-producing β-cells is seen in the rat *(left panel)* and in the human *(right panel)* with immunostaining of the non–β-cells. Human islets can be considered composites of several subunits and those of the rat, only one subunit. Scale bar = 50 μm.

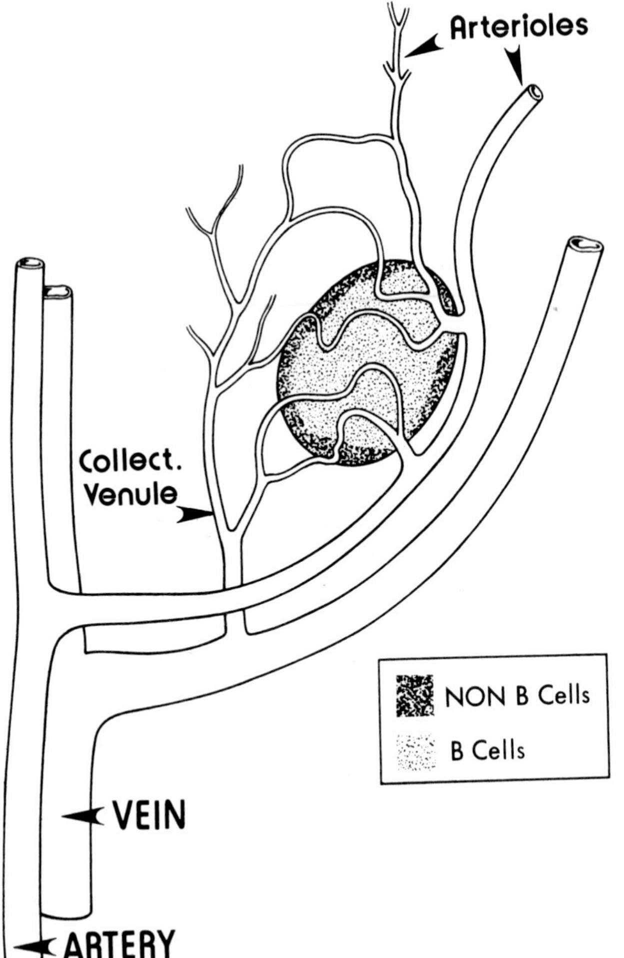

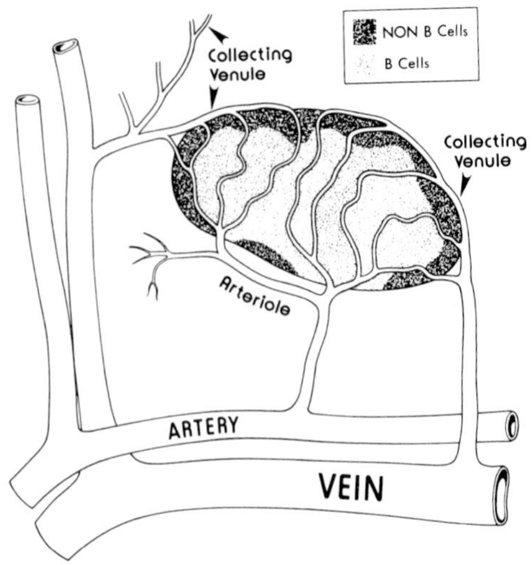

Figure 3.5. Diagrams of the microvasculature of the rat islet based on corrosion casts and serial reconstructions of immunostained paraffin sections. In both small *(left)* and large *(right)* islets, the efferent arteriole enters the islet in a gap or discontinuity of the non–β-cell mantle, such that it enters the β-cell core directly, where it breaks into a number of capillaries. These capillaries (fewer are drawn for diagrammatic purposes) traverse the β-cell core before passing along and through the non–β-cell mantle. In the small islets, the efferent capillaries pass 50 to 100 μm before coalescing into collecting venules, thus providing an insuloacinar portal system. However, in the large islets the efferent capillaries coalesce into collecting venules at the edge of the islet, even within the capsule. Thus, the drainage of large islets is directly into the venous system without passage through the exocrine tissue. (Copyright © 1982 American Diabetes Association. From Bonner-Weir S, Orci L. New perspectives on the microvasculature of the Islets of Langerhans in the rat. *Diabetes* 1982;31:883–889. Reprinted with permission from *the American Diabetes Association*.)

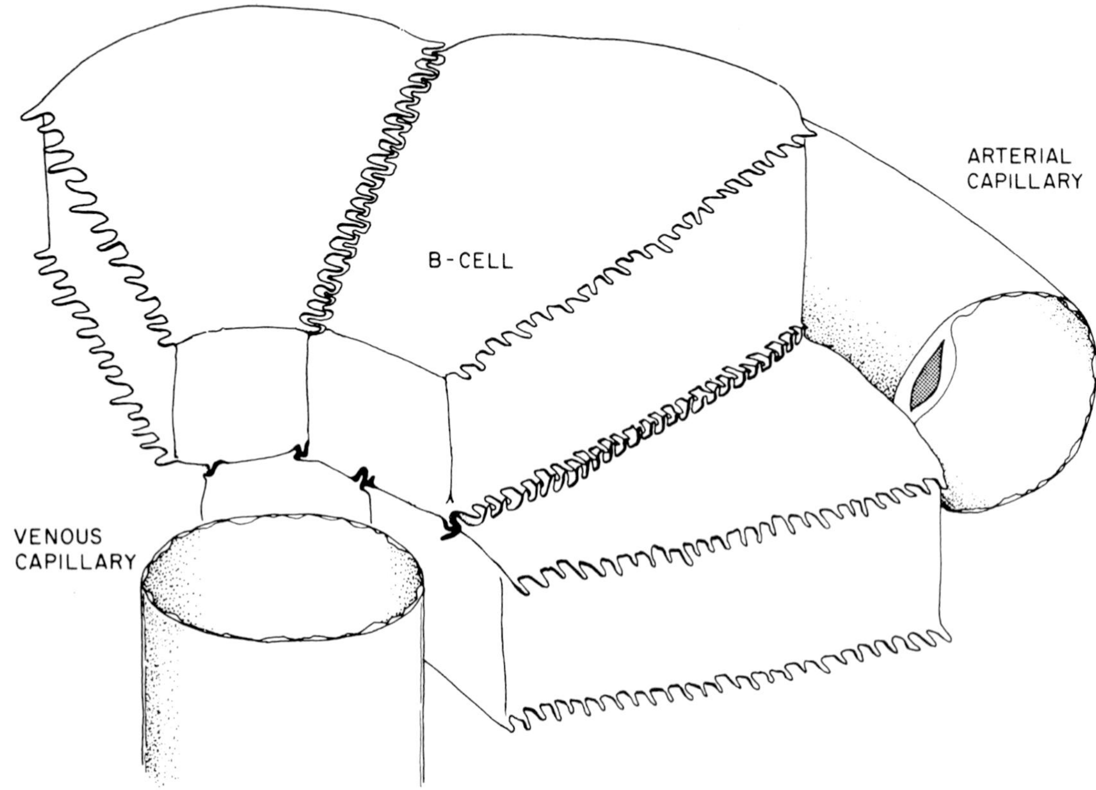

microvilli. Thus, these canaliculi may serve as the initial interface for glucose sensing by the β-cell. Insulin secretory granules appear to be released from the lateral and apical surfaces to enter the venous (central) capillaries.

HETEROGENEITY WITHIN THE ISLETS

We now realize that the islets within one pancreas are not all alike. Islets differ in cellular composition. There is a regional distribution of the glucagon-producing α-cell and the pancreatic polypeptide–producing PP-cell that is based on the embryologic derivation of the pancreas from distinct dorsal and ventral anlage (4). Thus, the splenic or dorsal portion (the tail, body, and superior part of the head) is glucagon-poor and pancreatic polypeptide–rich, while the duodenal or ventral portion (most of the head—sometimes designated as the uncinate process) of the pancreas is glucagon-poor and pancreatic polypeptide–rich. Physiologic data from either islets or perfusion of regions of the pancreas suggest that islets from different regions function differently, with the splenic islets releasing more insulin than the duodenal islets in response to glucose (62,63).

The different vascular relation to the exocrine tissue of islets of difference size was mentioned previously (3). Large islets (those > 250 μm in diameter) are selectively located near the larger ducts and blood vessels. Their efferent vessels coalesce within the islet capsule; thus, they probably have little effect on surrounding exocrine tissue. However, the vascular pattern of the small islets and their abundance would lead to an effective insulo-acinar portal system.

The increasing evidence that not all β -cells within an islet are identical indicates another level of heterogeneity. Older physiologic data from studies of isolated islets suggested different sensitivities for insulin response (64,65). Studies on single islet cells have shown that individual β-cells may have different thresholds for glucose-induced insulin release; thus, with increasing concentrations of glucose, more β-cells are recruited in the response (66,67). This cellular heterogeneity has been extended to include the redox state and the threshold for glucose-induced biosynthesis of proinsulin (68) and glucose-induced cytoplasmic concentration of free calcium (69). However, the question of whether such heterogeneity was artifactual and only the result of isolation as single cells has been raised (70). The recent study comparing the cytoplasmic concentration of free calcium in single and clustered islet cells in the same preparations showed recruitment of both single cells and small cell clusters (2 to 20 cells) with increasing glucose; however, although there was heterogeneity among the clusters, cells within clusters were usually homogeneous (70). With the use of luciferase dye injections, small territories of coupled β-cells, ranging from four β-cells in control conditions to 36 β-cells after treatment with diazoxide, have been shown *in vitro* (71). The increases in coupling (electrical and physical) were correlated with increases in gap junctions. It is likely that there are numerous coupled territories within an islet, each entrained with the β-cell within the cluster with the lowest threshold of response.

It is unclear if the heterogeneous nature of the β-cells as individual cells is intrinsic and constant for a particular cell through its lifetime, is related to the age of the cell, or is imprinted by a factor from the environment. Even the β-cells from the same islet are heterogeneous; in addition, the average insulin secretion per β-cell shows inter-islet variation (72). On the basis of the anatomy of an islet, one can speculate that the environment of a central β-cell is quite different from that of a peripheral one (see below for further discussion). Important questions are raised by this heterogeneity. Are certain populations of β-cells more susceptible than others to autoimmune destruction? Is one population preferentially or selectively lost during the development of non–insulin-dependent diabetes?

STRUCTURAL DEFINITIONS OF ISLET FUNCTION

It is important to understand how the three-dimensional organization of the islet may determine islet function. Experiments in which islet hormones were administered exogenously to isolated islets or to perfused pancreases have provided data indicating that islet hormones are capable of influencing the other islet cells in feedback loops (71,73). Thus, insulin can inhibit both α- and δ-cells, somatostatin can inhibit both α- and β-cells, and glucagon can stimulate both β- and δ-cells. (The role of pancreatic polypeptide or the PP-cell in these potential interactions has not been delineated.) These data have led to the concept that secretion of islet hormones is regulated by specific intra-islet interactions (60). Three levels of interactions are possible: (a) cell-to-cell via junctional communication; (b) bloodborne via the vasculature; and (c) paracrine via the interstitium. What constraints on each of these levels does the anatomy of the islet provide?

Junctional Interactions

The intercellular contacts between the endocrine cells influence their function. Stimulated secretion is enhanced when β-cells have contact with at least one other β-cell (74,75). Gap junctions are the entities that allow cell-to-cell communication and coupling (71,76). Islet hormones would not be expected to pass through these junctions because of molecular-size limitations and, more importantly, because the hormones within a cell would be enclosed within granule membranes. Such junctions have been seen between all types of islet endocrine cells in both heterologous and homologous links. Several connexins, including connexin 43 and connexin 45, are part of gap junctions within the islet (77); recently, connexin 36, a connexin newly identified in mammalian brain and retina, was found to be abundant and selective in the β-cells within the islet (78). The overexpression of connexin 32 in β-cells by transgenesis led to improved electrical synchronization, increased cytosolic calcium, but reduced insulin secretion in response to glucose (79). Contact via gap junctions is thought to be involved, because heptanal, an alcohol that functionally uncouples gap-junction communication, causes paired β-cells to function as if they were

Figure 3.6. Diagram of the intra-islet arrangement of pancreatic β-cells. β-Cells have two capillary faces, one essentially arterial and one venous. The lateral interfaces of β-cells are smooth surfaces; however, where three or more β-cells meet, a canalicular system is found that extends from one capillary to the other. The canaliculi contain microvilli that are enriched in glucose transporters. This specialized arrangement suggests that there is a preferential bulk flow of interstitial fluid through these canaliculi in an arterial to venous direction. (From Weir GC, Bonner-Weir S. Islets of Langerhans: the puzzle of intraislet interactions and their relevance to diabetes. *J Clin Invest* 1990;85:983–798 with permission from the American Society of Clinical Investigation.)

single cells. However, cell adhesion molecules such as integrins may also play a role. Integrins are usually thought to attach the cell to its extracellular matrix, but $\alpha6\beta1$ integrin, found on β-cells and increased with secretagogues, has been associated with increased insulin secretion (80,81).

Bloodborne Interactions

The microvascular pattern of the islet confers a directionality to the blood flow—from the point of arteriolar entry outward through the β-cell core to the peripheral non–β-cell mantle. This directionality has been demonstrated visually by passing a bolus of dye through the islet of a living rabbit (31) and by a video study of blood flow in the living mouse pancreas (82). This pattern of flow would favor insulin having an effect on the α- and δ-cells by its being transported in high concentrations from the core to the mantle. The reverse, that of the β-cells being influenced by local bloodborne somatostatin or glucagon, is not supported by the vascular pattern. Physiologic data from the approach of passive neutralization, using alternating anterograde and retrograde perfusions of dog, rat, monkey, and human pancreas, provide support for a β to α to δ (B-A-D) directional pattern of blood flow (83). The local secretion of insulin is surely important for glucose control over α-cell function (60). This pattern does not preclude the effects of the islet hormones via the systemic circulation. Somatostatin 28, which comes mainly from the gut and reaches the islets via systemic arterial circulation, may have more potent effects than somatostatin 14 on the islet cells of rats but not on those of dogs (84).

Paracrine Interactions

The paracrine effects are defined here as those local events that occur by simple diffusion through the interstitium. Such effects are difficult to evaluate because of the lack of good methods for studying the diffusion of peptides throughout this islet compartment. The pericapillary and subcapsular interstitial space is 6% ± 2% of the islet volume. In contrast, the vascular component (the endothelium and the luminal space) comprises approximately 14% ± 3% of the islet volume (S. Bonner-Weir, unpublished observations). Without having actual measurements, one can guess that the interstitial flow probably would be in the same direction as the blood flow. In such a case, diffusion inward to the core would be severely limited. Thus, in large islets, there would be a central core of β-cells that would be isolated by their distance from the non–β-cells and thus from all but systemically circulating levels of the other islet hormones. On the other hand, the peripheral β-cells could be under the local or paracrine influence of hormones secreted by adjacent or nearby non–β-cells. In small islets, essentially all β-cells might be close enough to the non–β-cells to be influenced by their hormones diffusing into the interstitial fluid and, thus, be regarded as peripheral. In fact, differences have been reported. Central β-cells of large islets have been reported to have smaller nuclei than either the peripheral β-cells of large islets or any β-cells of small islets (85). Furthermore, in rats stimulated *in vivo* with either glucose or glibenclamide, central β-cells degranulate before peripheral β-cells (86). These patterns may reflect the protection of the central β-cells from paracrine secretions or, conversely, the paracrine influence on peripheral β-cells. Presently, we do not know if these differences seen in the whole islets *in vivo* account for the heterogeneity found in single cells *in vitro*.

Somatostatin and glucagon, perfused in the isolated canine pancreas at concentrations that are only a small fraction of their estimated inter-islet concentration, have been shown to have profound effects on the other islet cells (87). The implication of these findings was that at least some cells were protected from the secretory products of their neighbors, and a hypothesis of functional compartmentalization was suggested (87). This hypothesis stated that the interstitial space within the islet was separated functionally into an "exocytotic-venous pathway" and an "arterial-receptor pathway" (87). Tight junctions were suggested as limiting domains of the plasma membrane of islet cells to segregate their sensing and secretory functions. However, although tight junctions have been clearly demonstrated in collagenase-isolated islets (55), they are not common in rodent islets fixed *in situ* (88,89) and therefore do not provide important compartmentalization. A better anatomic basis for compartmentalization probably lies in the polarity of islet cells and the directionality of blood flow (59).

Attention has been given more recently to whether receptors for the different hormones are on the various islet cells since their presence would suggest potential function and specificity of response. Several somatostatin receptor (SSTR) isoforms are expressed in human islets, with SSTR1 being richly expressed in β-cells, SSTR2 in α-cells, and SSTR5 abundant in β- and δ-cells and moderate in α-cells (90). β-Cells can respond to glucagon via either the glucagon or glucagon-like peptide-1 (GLP-1) receptors, allowing detection both at dilute levels in the systemic circulation and at high concentrations in the interstitium (91). However, α-cells expressed neither glucagon nor GLP-1 receptors but did express glucose-dependent insulinotropic polypeptide (GIP) receptors; rat β-cells also expressed GIP receptors (92). The presence of insulin receptors on the β-cells is more controversial. Both purified rat α- and β-cells express receptors for high-affinity insulin-like growth factor (IGF-1) that conveyed a low affinity for insulin binding (93), but an analysis of single rat islet cells by the reverse transcriptase–polymerase chain reaction found that β-cells express insulin receptor mRNA (94). β-Cell–specific insulin receptor knockout mice were generated, but these studies showed that insulin does not have a profound direct effect on the β-cell (95). At 4 months of age, these mice had no profound phenotype, being normoglycemic but hyperinsulinemic, with mildly impaired glucose tolerance and a small reduction in insulin content.

POSTNATAL ISLET GROWTH

Islet mass increases considerably from fetus to adulthood, while the volume of islet tissue relative to that of the pancreas decreases after birth. In newborn humans, islets comprise 20% of the pancreatic tissue; in children (1.5–11 years), 7.5%; and in adults, 1% (96). Similar data have been reported for cattle (97) and rats (98). The relative values are misleading, for by adulthood the islet mass has grown and increased about fivefold from that at birth. In fact, β-cell mass is linearly correlated with body weight in adult mice (99) and rats (100). The relative amount decreases, as the exocrine tissue increases about 15-fold during the same period. Thus, the growth of islet tissue is diluted by the more exuberant postnatal growth of the exocrine tissue after birth.

Islet mass is determined by the number of cells and their cell volume (size). New cells arise by (a) neogenesis or differentiation of islet endocrine cells from ductal epithelium, or (b) replication of existing islet cells. Whereas replication becomes a major mechanism for adding new β-cells (101), both neogenesis and replication continue postnatally (7,100,101). Many new islets are formed in the first few days after birth, and a second wave of neogenesis occurs at about weaning (102). β-Cell replication is significantly higher during late gestation and the neonatal period than following weaning, with little change in replication rates occurring beyond 30 to 40 days of age (7). In rats, β-cells increase in number until the age of 15 months, and afterward they increase in size (hypertrophy) (100). The finding in 6-month-old rats of some pancreatic lobes with high amounts of 5-bromodeoxyuridine (BrdU) incorporation and others with almost no incorporation suggests that whole lobes of pancreas are formed even in adult animals (7).

During the neonatal period, the endocrine pancreas in the neonatal rat is remodeled (103). During the second week after birth, the β-cell mass does not increase even with a high replication of β-cells because a high level of apoptosis occurs simultaneously. This remodeling coincides with marked changes in the levels of messenger RNA for both IGF-I and IGF-II as well as with transient appearances of messenger RNA for IGF binding protein 1 (IGFBP-1) and IGFBP-2 (104), leading to the suggestion that an inadequate availability of survival factors such as the IGFs causes the increased cell loss (103,105). This hypothesis was supported by the suppression of the normal neonatal apoptosis by persistent IGF-II in overexpressing transgenic mice (106).

Cell Replication

What is known about the cell cycle of islets has been determined using isolated rat islets synchronized in culture by temporary exposure to hydroxyurea. A cell cycle of 14.9 hours was calculated and has been assumed to reflect that of the β-cell, the predominant cell of the islet (107). The length of the cell cycle does not change with glucose stimulation or with the age of the animals (107,108). Instead the growth rate is regulated by the number of β-cells that can enter the division phase (G_1) from the resting (G_0) phase. The accuracy of determinations of β-cell replication made by measuring the incorporation of thymidine in whole islets has been questioned because non-endocrine cells found in islets incorporate thymidine at a far greater rate than do islet endocrine cells (109). The measurement of choice is double labeling of insulin-immunostained cells with nuclear labeling (thymidine or BrdU incorporation or immunostaining of various cell cycle proteins such as Ki67, PCNA).

It is now clear that β-cells can replicate: Incorporated BrdU and tritiated thymidine have been localized to cells immunolabeled for insulin, and numerous micrographs of mitotic figures in cells with insulin granules have been published. Yet there may be functional differences between β-cells that can replicate and those that cannot. Nondividing β-cells can be recruited into the cell cycle, and most daughter cells will re-enter the cycle immediately (110). Replicative ability or "age" may be one of the possible bases of the functional heterogeneity of β-cells (111) discussed previously.

Stimuli for Growth

Although there may be numerous stimuli for β-cell growth, three major stimuli are known: prolactin, growth hormone, and glucose. Glucose is a stimulus both *in vivo* and *in vitro*. As early as 1938, Woerner reported an increase in islet tissue in guinea pigs after continuous glucose infusions (112). Such an increase has since been confirmed by several other studies (113–117). Glucose has been shown to stimulate modest growth of both neonatal and adult pancreatic β-cells in culture (118–120). Pregnancy has been shown to cause both increased replication and increased mass of β-cells (121–125). As a parallel finding, *in vitro* studies have shown that prolactin, placental lactogen, and growth hormone can stimulate replication of β-cells (120,126,127). A neural stimulus has been suggested by the increase in islet mass after a ventromedial hypothalamic lesion (128). Possible effects of incretins on islet mass have been suggested by *in vivo* studies using a long-acting GLP-1 agonist, exendin 4, in normal rats. Exendin 4 stimulated β-cell replication as well as neogenesis (129). In addition to these known stimuli, a complex orchestration of, as yet, unidentified factors must be involved. As a means of identifying some of these, peptide growth factors have been studied in islet cultures. The most commonly tested factor has been IGF-I, but results have varied (120,127,130) IGF-I may function more as a survival factor for the islet cells (105). None of the factors studied so far have produced marked stimulation of replication *in vitro*, but the importance of their contribution to growth and development cannot yet be discounted. The coordination of many factors in islet growth promises to be exceedingly complex.

Compensatory Changes

Through a lifetime, there can be compensatory changes in function and mass of β-cells to meet demand and to maintain euglycemia. Functional compensation can be due to changes in β-cell responsiveness by changes in threshold for glucose-induced insulin secretion (131), possibly caused by activation of glucokinase (132), or by recruitment of cells with heterogeneous response thresholds (111). Additionally, the mass of β-cells can be dynamic, with both increases and decreases, to compensate for changing demands, such as pregnancy, obesity, or insulin resistance. Regulation of replication, neogenesis, apoptosis, and the cell size (hypertrophy vs. atrophy) can contribute to these variations in mass (102,133). The physiologic occurrence of β-cell apoptosis is found during the involution of the β-cell mass in the postpartum pancreas (102) and in a remodeling of the endocrine pancreas in the neonatal rat before weaning (103). In addition, substantial β-cell growth has been shown *in vivo* in several animal models (114,134,135). For example, after only 96 hours of glucose infusion, the β-cell mass in adult rats was increased by 50%; both hypertrophy of individual β-cells and hyperplasia contributed to this rapid increase of mass (114).

Because few mitotic figures are seen normally in adult islets and the postnatal proliferation rate of β-cells is low, it has been thought that the capacity for β-cell growth or regeneration is limited. However, the proliferation of differentiated β-cells must not be underestimated; it is adequate to maintain a slowly increasing β-cell mass. Even at the low replicative level of 3% per day, the number of β-cells could double in 30 days if cell death was not appreciable (101). In fact, the β-cell mass in the adult rat does double between the ages of 6 and 10 weeks and continues at a somewhat reduced rate throughout life. Therefore, the β-cell, like most other cell types, must have a finite life span. The frequency of apoptotic β-cells in the adult rat was found to be about 0.5% (100,103); this frequency cannot be equated with a rate because we do not know how long the apoptotic process takes or how long apoptotic bodies are visible. Since the steady-state replication rate is just over 2% a day, the life span of a rat β-cell can be estimated as approximately 58 days (7). The slowly increasing β-cell mass is balanced between cell formation and cell loss, such that the endocrine pancreas must be considered a slowly renewed tissue.

We must assume that the apparently low level of normal β-cell growth in the adult is all that is needed to counterbalance cell loss and to accommodate functional challenges of increased body weight and insulin resistance. Diabetes mellitus results only if increased cell loss or functional demands cannot be met. While the regulation of β-cell mass may be complex, the drive to maintain glucose homeostasis could use glucose as the driving force. As insulin resistance increases, glucose uptake by peripheral tissues would be diminished, with resulting transient postprandial hyperglycemic excursions. Such mild hyperglycemia could signal the β-cells that more insulin is needed, so compensation would occur as enhancement in function, β-cell replication, and cell size. The resulting increased β-cell mass could secrete more insulin that would overcome the insulin resistance and maintain euglycemia. Such a scenario could be repeated numerous times, maintaining compensation as long as the β-cell mass can increase. However, if the hyperglycemia becomes chronic, there can be detrimental secondary effects such as loss of glucose-induced insulin response and even cell death; the term "glucose toxicity" has been used to describe these latter effects. In some strains or species (136,137), β-cells undergo apoptosis when exposed to hyperglycemia, but in other strains, β-cells can have more adaptive responses and maintain a stable mass even in chronic hyperglycemia (138,139). We do not yet know what genes affect renewal or turnover of β-cells or their ability to increase their biosynthetic or secretory capacity.

SUMMARY

The islets of Langerhans are composed of various components that are organized to form micro-organs. The architecture or three-dimensional structure imposes certain constraints on interactions between islet cells. As our knowledge increases about the complex organization of the islet of Langerhans and the changes that islets undergo throughout life, we will be able to develop more meaningful interpretations of the physiologic and pathophysiologic characteristics of islet function.

Islets function both singly and in concert. Yet the diversity in islets appears to be greater than that previously recognized. There is functional heterogeneity among islets and among β-cells within the same islet. Numerous peptides other than the four main islet hormones (insulin, glucagon, somatostatin, and pancreatic polypeptide) have been immunolocalized in islets, but the roles of most are still unknown.

The mass of islets within a pancreas is dynamic and changes both with growth and development and with functional challenges. As we learn more about the regulation of differentiation of islet cell types and the mechanisms of replication, we also may learn how to enhance the growth of islet cells, particularly the β-cells.

REFERENCES

1. Henderson JR. Why are the islets of Langerhans? *Lancet* 1969;2:469–470.
2. Wrenshall GA, Bogosh A, Ritchie RC. Extractable insulin of pancreas: correlation with pathologic and clinical findings in diabetic and nondiabetic cases. *Diabetes* 1952;1:87–107.
3. Bonner-Weir S, Orci L. New perspectives on the microvasculature of the islets of Langerhans in the rat. *Diabetes* 1982;31:883–939.
4. Orci L, Baetens D, Ravazzola M, et al. Pancreatic polypeptide and glucagon: non-random distribution in pancreatic islets. *Life Sci* 1976;19:1811–1816.
5. Hashimoto T, Kawano H, Daikoku S, et al. Transient coappearance of glucagon and insulin in the progenitor cells of the rat pancreatic islets. *Anat Embryol* 1988;178:489–497.
6. Rahier J, Wallon J, Henquin JC. Abundance of somatostatin cells in the human neonatal pancreas. *Diabetologia* 1980;18:251–254.
7. Finegood DT, Scaglia L, Bonner-Weir S. Dynamics of β-cell mass in the growing rat pancreas: estimation with a simple mathematical model. *Diabetes* 1995;44:249–256.
8. Pictet R, Rutter WJ. The endocrine pancreas. In: Steiner D, Freinkel N, eds. *Handbook of physiology.* Baltimore: Williams & Wilkins, 1972:25.
9. Weaver CV, Sorenson RL, Kaung HC. Immunocytochemical localization of insulin-immunoreactive cells in the ducts of rats treated with trypsin inhibitor. *Diabetologia* 1985;28:781–785.
10. Sarvetnick N, Shizuru J, Liggitt D, et al. Loss of pancreatic islet tolerance induced by beta cell expression of IFN-gamma. *Nature* 1990;346:844–847.
11. Bonner-Weir S, Baxter LA, Schuppin GT, et al. A second pathway for regeneration of the adult exocrine and endocrine pancreas: a possible recapitulation of embryonic development. *Diabetes* 1993;42:1715–1720.
12. Rosenberg L, Duguid WP, Vinik AI. The effect of cellophane wrapping of the pancreas in the Syrian golden hamster: autoradiographic observations. *Pancreas* 1989;4:31–37.
13. Gepts W. Pathological anatomy of the pancreas in juvenile diabetes. *Diabetes* 1965;14:619–633.
14. Dudek RW, Lawrence IE, Jr. Morphologic evidence of interactions between adult ductal epithelium of pancreas and fetal foregut mesenchyme. *Diabetes* 1988;37:891–900.
15. Bonner-Weir S, Taneja M, Weir GC, et al. In vitro cultivation of human islets from expanded ductal tissue. *Proc Natl Acad Sci U S A* 2000;97:7999–8004.
16. Ohlsson H, Thor S, Edlund T. Novel insulin promoter- and enhancer-binding proteins that discriminate between pancreatic A- and B-cells. *Mol Endocrinol* 1991;5:897–904.
17. Falkmer S, Ostberg Y. Comparative morphology of pancreatic islets in animals. In: Volk BW, Wellman KF, eds. *The diabetic pancreas.* New York: Plenum Press, 1977:15.
18. Yoshioka N, Kuzuya T, Matsuda A, et al. Serum proinsulin levels at fasting and after oral glucose load in patients with type 2 (non-insulin-dependent) diabetes mellitus. *Diabetologia* 1988;31:355–360.
19. Epple A. The endocrine pancreas. In: Hoar WS, Randall DJ, eds. *Fish physiology*, 2nd ed. New York/London: Academic Press; 1969:275.
20. Epple A, Brinn JE. Islet histophysiology: evolutionary correlations. *Gen Comp Endocrinol* 1975;27:320–349
21. Stefan Y, Falkmer S. Islet hormone cells in cartilaginous fish—the original pancreas? *Diabetologia* 1978;15:272.
22. Petersson M, Ahrén B, Böttcher C, Sundler F. Calcitonin gene related peptide: occurrence in pancreatic islets in the mouse and the rat and inhibition of insulin secretion in the mouse. *Endocrinology* 1986;119:865–869.
23. Schmidt WE, Siegel EG, Lamberts R, et al. Pancreastatin: molecular and immunocytochemical characterization of novel peptide in porcine and human tissues. *Endocrinology* 1986;123:1395–1404.
24. Ravazzola M, Efendic S, Ostenson C-G, et al. Localization of pancreastatin immunoreactivity in porcine endocrine cells. *Endocrinology* 1988;123:227–229.
25. Aratan-Spire S, Wolf B, Czernichow P. Developmental pattern of TRH-degrading activity and TRH content in rat pancreas. *Acta Endocrinol (Copenh)* 1984;106:102–108.
26. Larsson LI, Rehfeld JF, Sundler F, et al. Pancreatic gastrin in fetal and neonatal rats. *Nature* 1976;262:609–610.
27. Dean PM. Ultrastructural morphometry of the pancreatic β-cell. *Diabetologia* 1973;9:115–119.
28. Orci L. The insulin factory: a tour of the plant surroundings and a visit to the assembly line. *Diabetologia* 1985;28:528–546.
29. Guest PC, Bailyes EM, Rutherford NG, et al. Insulin secretory granule biogenesis. *Biochem J* 1991;274:73–78.
30. Larsson L-I, Sundler F, Håkanson R. Pancreatic polypeptide—a postulated new hormone: identification of its cellular storage site by light and electron microscopic immunocytochemistry. *Diabetologia* 1976;12:211–226.
31. Henderson JR, Daniel PM. A comparative study of the portal vessels connecting the endocrine and exocrine pancreas, with a discussion of some functional implications. *Q J Exp Physiol* 1979;64:267–275.
32. Henderson JR, Moss MC. A morphometric study of the endocrine and exocrine capillaries of the pancreas. *Q J Exp Physiol* 1985;70:347–356.
33. Like AA. The uptake of exogenous peroxidase by the beta cells of the islets of Langerhans. *Am J Physiol* 1970;59:225–246.
34. Lifson N, Kramlinger KG, Mayrand RR, et al. Blood flow to the rabbit pancreas with special reference to the islets of Langerhans. *Gastroenterology* 1980; 79:466–473.
35. Jansson L, Hellerstrom C. A rapid method of visualizing the pancreatic islets for studies of islet capillary blood flow using nonradioactive microspheres. *Acta Physiol Scand* 1981;113:371–374.
36. Lifson N, Lassa CV, Dixit PK. Relation between blood flow and morphology in islet organ of rat pancreas. *Am J Physiol* 1985;249:E43–E48.
37. Meyer HH, Vetterlein F, Schmidt G, et al. Measurement of blood flow in pancreatic islets of the rat: effect of isoproterenol and norepinephrine. *Am J Physiol* 1982;242:E298–E305.
38. Jansson L, Hellerstrom C. Stimulation by glucose of the blood flow to the pancreatic islets of the rat. *Diabetologia* 1983;25:45–50.
39. Brain SD, Williams TJ, Tippens JR, et al. Calcitonin gene-related peptide is a potent vasodilator. *Nature* 1985;313:54–56.
40. Brunfeldt K, Hunhammar K, Skouby AP. Studies on the vascular system of the islets of Langerhans in mice. *Acta Endocrinol (Copenh)* 1958;29:473–480.
41. Smith PH, Porte D, Jr. Neuropharmacology of the pancreatic islets. *Ann Rev Pharmacol Toxicol* 1976;16:269–285.
42. Polonsky KS, Given BD, VanCauter E. Twenty-four hour profiles and pulsatile patterns of insulin section in normal and obese subjects. *J Clin Invest* 1988;81:442–448.
43. Lang DA, Matthews DR, Peta J, Turner RC. Cyclic oscillations of basal plasma glucose and insulin concentrations in human beings. *N Engl J Med* 1979;301:1023–1027.
44. Stagner J, Samols E, Weir GC. Sustained oscillations of insulin, glucagon and

somatostatin from the isolated canine pancreas during exposure to a constant glucose concentration. *J Clin Invest* 1980;65:939–942.

45. Sundler F, Böttcher G. Islet innervation, with special reference to neuropeptides. In: Samols E. *The endocrine pancreas*. New York: Raven Press, 1991:29.
46. Ahren B, Bottcher G, Kowalyk S, et al. Galanin is localized with noradrenaline and neuropeptide Y in dog pancreas and celiac ganglion. *Cell Tissue Res* 1990;261:49–58.
47. Ahren B, Taborsky GJ, Porte D, Jr. Neuropeptidergic as cholinergic and adrenergic regulation of islet hormone secretion. *Diabetologia* 1986;29: 827–836.
48. Samols E, Weir GC. Adrenergic modulation of pancreatic A, B and D cells: alpha-adrenergic suppression and beta-adrenergic stimulation of somatostatin secretion, alpha-adrenergic stimulation of glucagon secretion in the perfused dog pancreas. *J Clin Invest* 1979;63:230–238.
49. Jansson L. Vasoactive intestinal polypeptide increases whole pancreatic blood flow but does not affect islet blood flow in the rat. *Acta Diabetol* 1994; 31:103–106.
50. Larsson L-I, Fahrenkrug J, Schaffalitzky de Muckadell OB. Innervation of the pancreas by vasoactive intestinal polypeptide (VIP) immunoreactive nerves. *Life Sci* 1978;22:773–780.
51. Orci L, Unger RH. Functional subdivision of islets of Langerhans and possible role of D-cells. *Lancet* 1975;2:1243–1244.
52. Erlandsen SL, Hegre OD, Parsons JA, et al. Pancreatic islet cell hormones distribution of cell types in the islet and evidence for the presence of somatostatin and gastrin within the D cell. *J Histol Cytol* 1976;24:883–897.
53. Grube D, Eckert I, Speck PT, et al. Immunohistochemistry and microanatomy of the islets of Langerhans. *Biomed Res* 1983;4[suppl]:25–36.
54. Fraser PA, Henderson JR. The arrangement of endocrine and exocrine pancreatic microcirculation observed in the living rabbit. *Q J Exp Physiol* 1991;65: 151–158.
55. Orci L. The microanatomy of the islets of Langerhans. *Metabolism* 1976;25: 1303–1313.
56. Brelje TC, Scharp DW, Sorenson RL. Three dimensional imaging of intact isolated islets of Langerhans with confocal microscopy. *Diabetes* 1989;38: 808–814.
57. Halban PA, Powers SL, George KL, et al. Spontaneous reassociation of dispersed adult rat pancreatic islet cells into aggregates with 3-dimensional architecture typical of native islets. *Diabetes* 1987;36:783–791.
58. Rouiller D, Cirulli V, Halban PA. Uvomorulin mediates calcium-dependent aggregation of islet cells, whereas calcium-independent cell adhesion molecules distinguish between islet cell types. *Dev Biol* 1991;148:233–242.
59. Bonner-Weir S. Morphological evidence for pancreatic polarity of β-cell within the islets of Langerhans. *Diabetes* 1988;37:616–621.
60. Weir GC, Bonner-Weir S. Islets of Langerhans: the puzzle of intraislet interactions and their relevance to diabetes. *J Clin Invest* 1990;85:983–987.
61. Orci L, Thorens B, Ravazzola M, et al. Localization of the pancreatic beta cell glucose transporter to specific plasma membrane domains. *Science* 1990;245: 295–297.
62. Stagner J, Samols E. Differential glucagon and insulin release from the isolated lobes of the in vitro canine pancreas. *Diabetes* 1982;31[suppl 2]:39A.
63. Trimble ER, Halban PA, Wolheim CB, et al. Functional differences between rat islets of ventral and dorsal pancreatic origin. *J Clin Invest* 1982;69:405–413.
64. Grodsky GM. A threshold distribution hypothesis for packet storage of insulin. II. Effect of calcium. *Diabetes* 1972;21[suppl 2]:584–593.
65. Matthews EK, Dean PM. Electrical activity in islet cells. In: Falkmer S, Hellman B, Taljedal I-B, eds. *Structure and metabolism of pancreatic islets*. Oxford, England: Pergamon Press, 1970:305.
66. Pipeleers DG. The biosociology of pancreatic β-cells. *Diabetologia* 1987;30: 277–291.
67. Salomon D, Meda P. Heterogeneity and contact regulation of hormone secretion by individual β-cells. *Exp Cell Res* 1986;162:507–520.
68. Schuit FC, In't Veld PA, Pipeleers DG. Glucose stimulates proinsulin biosynthesis by a dose-dependent recruitment of pancreatic beta cells. *Proc Natl Acad Sci U S A* 1988;85:3865–3869.
69. Jonkers FC, Henquin J-C. Measurements of cytoplasmic Ca^{2+} in islet cell clusters show that glucose rapidly recruits β-cells and gradually increases the individual cell response. *Diabetes* 2001;50:540–550.
70. Bennett BD, Jetton TL, Ying G, et al. Quantitative subcellular imaging of glucose metabolism within intact pancreatic islets. *J Biol Chem* 1996;27: 3647–3651.
71. Meda P, Michaels RL, Halban PA, et al. In vivo modulation of gap junctions and dye coupling between β-cells of the intact pancreatic islet. *Diabetes* 1983; 32:858–868.
72. Hiriart M, Ramirez-Medeles MC. Functional subpopulations of individual pancreatic β-cells in culture. *Endocrinology* 1991;128:3193–3198.
73. Maruyama H, Hisatomi A, Orci L, et al. Insulin within islets is a physiologic glucagon release inhibitor. *J Clin Invest* 1984;74:2296–2299.
74. Bosco D, Orci L, Meda P. Homologous but not heterologous contact increases the insulin secretion of individual pancreatic β-cells. *Exp Cell Res* 1989;184: 72–80.
75. Soria B, Chanson M, Giordano E, et al. Ion channels of glucose responsive and unresponsive β-cells. *Diabetes* 1991;40:1069–1078.
76. Meda P, Perrelet A, Orci L. Gap junctions and cell-to-cell coupling in endocrine glands. *Mod Cell Biol* 1984;3:131–196.
77. Charollais A, Serre V, Mock C, et al. Loss of alpha 1 connexin does not alter the prenatal differentiation of pancreatic beta cells and leads to the identification of another islet cell connexin. *Dev Genet* 1999;24:13–26.
78. Serre-Beinier V, Le Gurun S, Belluardo N, et al. Cx36 preferentially connects beta-cells within pancreatic islets. *Diabetes* 2000;49:727–734.
79. Charollais A, Gjinovci A, Huarte J, et al. Junctional communication of pancreatic beta cells contributes to the control of insulin secretion and glucose tolerance. *J Clin Invest* 2000;106:235–243.
80. Kantengwa S, Baetens D, Sadoul K, et al. Identification and characterization of α3β1 integrin on primary and transformed rat islet cells. *Exp Cell Res* 1997; 237:394–402.
81. Bosco D, Meda P, Halban PA, et al. Importance of cell-matrix interactions in rat islet β-cell secretion in vitro: role of α6β1 integrin. *Diabetes* 2000;49: 233–243.
82. Rooth P, Grankvist K, Tajedal I-B. In vivo fluorescence microscopy of blood flow in mouse pancreatic islets: adrenergic effects in lean and obese-hyperglycemic mice. *Microvasc Res* 1985;30:176–184.
83. Stagner JI, Samols E, Bonner-Weir S. B-A-D pancreatic islet cellular perfusion in dogs. *Diabetes* 1988;37:1715–1721.
84. Klaff LJ, Dunning BE, Taborsky GJ. Somatostatin-28 does not regulate islet function in the dog. *Endocrinology* 1988;123:2668–2674.
85. Hellerstrom C, Petersson B, Hellman B. Some properties of the β-cells in the islets of Langerhans studied with regard to the position of the cells. *Acta Endocrinol (Copenh)* 1960;34:449–456.
86. Stefan Y, Meda P, Neufeld M, et al. Stimulation of insulin secretion reveals heterogeneity of pancreatic β-cells in vivo. *J Clin Invest* 1987;80:175–183.
87. Kawai K, Orci L, Ipp E, et al. Circulating somatostatin acts on the islets of Langerhans via a somatostatin-poor compartment. *Science* 1982;218:477–478.
88. In't Veld PA, Pipeleers D. Evidence against the presence of tight junctions in normal endocrine pancreas. *Diabetes* 1984;33:101–104.
89. Yamamoto M, Kataoka K. A comparative study on the intracellular canalicular system and intercellular junctions in the pancreatic islets of some rodents. *Arch Histol Jpn* 1984;47:485–493.
90. Kumar U, Sasi R, Suresh S, et al. Subtype-selective expression of the five somatostatin receptors (hSSTR1-5) in human pancreatic islet cells: a quantitative double-label immunohistochemical analysis. *Diabetes* 1999;48: 77–85.
91. Moens K, Flamez D, Van Schravendijk C, et al. Dual glucagon recognition by pancreatic beta-cells via glucagon and glucagon-like peptide 1 receptors. *Diabetes* 1998;47:66–72.
92. Moens K, Heimberg H, Flamez D, et al. Expression and functional activity of glucagon, glucagon-like peptide I, and glucose-dependent insulinotropic peptide receptors in rat pancreatic islet cells. *Diabetes* 1996;45:257–261.
93. Van Schravendijk CF, Foriers A, Van den Brande JL, et al. Evidence for the presence of type 1 insulin-like growth factor receptors on rat pancreatic α and β cells. *Endocrinology* 1987;121:1784–1788.
94. Harbeck MC, Louie DC, Howland J, et al. Expression of insulin receptor mRNA and insulin receptor substrate 1 in pancreatic islet beta-cells. *Diabetes* 1996;45:711–717.
95. Kulkarni RN, Bruning JC, Winnay JN, et al. Tissue-specific knockout of the insulin receptor in pancreatic β cells creates an insulin secretory defect similar to that in type 2 diabetes. *Cell* 1999;96:329–339.
96. Witte DP, Greider MH, DeSchryver-Kecskemeti K, et al. The juvenile human endocrine pancreas: normal vs idiopathic hypoinsulinemic hypoglycemia. *Semin Diagn Pathol* 1984;1:30–42.
97. Bonner-Weir S, Like AA. A dual islet population in bovine pancreas. *Cell Tissue Res* 1980;206:157–170.
98. McEvoy RC, Madson KL. Pancreatic insulin-, glucagon- and somatostatin-positive islet cell populations during the perinatal development of the rat. *Biol Neonate* 1980;38:248–259.
99. Bonner-Weir S. Islet growth and development in the adult. *J Mol Endocrinol* 2000;24:297–302.
100. Montanya E, Nacher V, Biarnes M, et al. Linear correlation between beta cell mass and body weight throughout life in Lewis rats: role of beta-cell hyperplasia and hypertrophy. *Diabetes* 2000;49:1341–1346.
101. Hellerstrom C, Swenne I, Andersson A. Islet cell replication and diabetes. In: Lefebvre PJ, Pipeleers DG, eds. *The pathology of the endocrine pancreas in diabetes*. Heidelberg: Springer-Verlag, 1988:141.
102. Scaglia L, Smith FE, Bonner-Weir S. Apoptosis contributes to the involution of β cell mass in the post partum rat pancreas. *Endocrinology* 1995;136: 5461–5468.
103. Scaglia L, Cahill CJ, Finegood DT, et al. Apoptosis participates in the remodeling of the endocrine pancreas in the neonatal rat. *Endocrinology* 1997;138: 1736–1741.
104. Hogg J, Hill DJ, Han VKM. The ontogeny of insulin-like growth factor (IGF) and IGF-binding protein gene expression in the rat pancreas. *J Mol Endocrinol* 1994;13:49–58.
105. Petrik J, Arany E, McDonald TJ, et al. Apoptosis in the pancreatic islet cells of the neonatal rat is associated with a reduced expression of insulin-like growth factor II that may act as a survival factor. *Endocrinology* 1998;139: 2994–3004.
106. Hill DJ, Strutt B, Arany E, et al. Increased and persistent circulating insulin-like growth factor II in neonatal transgenic mice suppresses developmental apoptosis in the pancreatic islets. *Endocrinology* 2000;141:1151–1157.
107. Swenne I. The role of glucose in the in vitro regulation of cell cycle kinetics and proliferation of fetal pancreatic β-cells. *Diabetes* 1982;31:754–760.

108. Swenne I, Andersson A. Effect of genetic background on the capacity for islet cell replication in mice. *Diabetologia* 1984;27:464–467.
109. DeVroede MA, In't Veld PA, Pipeleers DG. Deoxyribonucleic acid synthesis in cultured adult rat pancreatic β cells. *Endocrinology* 1990;127:1510–1516.
110. Brelje TC, Parsons JA, Sorenson RL. Regulation of islet β-cell proliferation by prolactin in rat islets. *Diabetes* 1994;43:263–273.
111. Pipeleers DG. Heterogeneity in pancreatic β-cell population. *Diabetes* 1992;41:777–781.
112. Woerner CA. Studies of the islands of Langerhans after continuous injection of dextrose. *Anat Rec* 1938;71:33–57.
113. Brosky GM, Heuck CC. Der Einfluss von Glukoseinfusionen auf die Proinsulin-und Insulinsynthese in den Langerhansschen Inseln bei der Ratte. *Endokrinologie* 1975;66:46–55.
114. Bonner-Weir S, Deery D, Leahy JL, et al. Compensatory growth of pancreatic β-cells in adult rats after short-term glucose infusion. *Diabetes* 1989;38:49–53.
115. Kinash B, Haist RE. Continuous IV infusion in the rat and the effect on the islets of Langerhans of the continuous infusion of glucose. *Can J Biochem Physiol* 1954;32:428–433.
116. Brosky GM, Kern HF, Logothetopoulos J. Ultrastructure, mitotic activity and insulin biosynthesis of pancreatic beta cells stimulated by glucose infusions. *Fed Proc* 1972;31:250.
117. Logothetopoulos J, Valiquette N. Hormonal and non-hormonal protein biosynthesis in the pancreatic beta cell of the intact rat after prolonged hyperglycemia. *Acta Endocrinol (Copenh)* 1984;107:382–389.
118. Chick WL. Beta cell replication in rat pancreatic monolayer cultures: effects of glucose, tolbutamide, glucocorticoid, growth hormone and glucagon. *Diabetes* 1973;22:687–693.
119. Chick WL, Lauris V, Flewelling JH, et al. Effects of glucose on beta cells in pancreatic monolayer cultures. *Endocrinology* 1973;92:212–218.
120. Nielsen JH. Growth and function of the pancreatic β cell in vitro: effects of glucose, hormones and serum factors on mouse, rat and human pancreatic islets in organ culture. *Acta Endocrinol (Copenh)* 1985;108[suppl. 266]:1.
121. Hellerstrom C. The influence of pregnancy and lactation on endocrine pancreas of mice. *Acta Soc Med Uppsala* 1963;68:17–28.
122. Green IC, Taylor KW. Effects of pregnancy in the rat on the size and insulin secretory response of the islets of Langerhans. *J Endocrinol* 1972;54:317–325.
123. Green IC, El Seifi S, Perrin D, et al. Cell replication in the islets of Langerhans of adult rats: effects of pregnancy, ovarectomy and treatment with steroid hormones. *J Endocrinol* 1981;88:219–224.
124. Marynissen G, Aerts L, Van Assche FA. The endocrine pancreas during pregnancy and lactation in the rat. *J Dev Physiol* 1983;5:373–381.
125. Sorenson RL, Parsons JA. Insulin secretion in mammosomatotropic tumor-bearing and pregnant rats: a role for lactogens. *Diabetes* 1985;34:337–341.
126. Nielsen JH, Linde S, Welinder BS, et al. Growth hormone is a growth factor for the differentiated pancreatic β-cell. *Mol Endocrinol* 1989;13:165–173.
127. Brelje TC, Sorenson RL. Role of prolactin versus growth hormone on islet β-cell proliferation in vitro: implications for pregnancy. *Endocrinology* 1991;128:45–57.
128. Jeanrenaud B. An hypothesis on the aetiology of obesity: dysfunction of the central nervous system as a primary cause. *Diabetologia* 1985;28:502–513.
129. Xu G, Stoffers DA, Habener JF, et al. Exendin-4 stimulates both β-cell replication and neogenesis, resulting in increased β-cell mass and improved glucose tolerance in diabetic rats. *Diabetes* 1999;48:2270–2276.
130. Rabinovitch A, Quigley C, Russell T, et al. Insulin and multiplication stimulating activity (an insulin-like growth factor) stimulate islet β-cell replication in neonatal rat pancreatic monolayer cultures. *Diabetes* 1982;31:160–164.
131. Parsons JA, Brelje TC, Sorenson RL. Adaptation of islets to pregnancy: increased islet cell proliferation and insulin secretion correlates with the onset of placental lactogen secretion. *Endocrinology* 1992;130:1459–1466.
132. Chen C, Hosokawa H, Bumbalo LM, et al. Regulatory effects of glucose on the catalytic activity and cellular content of glucokinase in the pancreatic β cell: study using cultured rat islets. *J Clin Invest* 1994;94:1616–1620.
133. Blume N, Skouv J, Larsson LI, et al. Potent inhibitory effects of transplantable rat glucagonomas and insulinomas on the respective endogenous islet cells are associated with pancreatic apoptosis. *J Clin Invest* 1995;96:2227–2235.
134. Brockenbrough JS, Weir GC, Bonner-Weir S. Discordance of exocrine and endocrine growth after 90% pancreatectomy in rats. *Diabetes* 1988;37:232–236.
135. Bonner-Weir S, Trent DF, Weir GC. Partial pancreatectomy in the rat and subsequent defect in glucose-induced insulin release. *J Clin Invest* 1983;71:1544–1553.
136. Ohneda M, Inman LR, Unger RH. Caloric restriction in obese pre-diabetic rats prevents beta-cell depletion, loss of beta-cell GLUT2 and glucose incompetence. *Diabetologia* 1995;38:173–179.
137. Donath MY, Gross DJ, Cerasi E, et al. Hyperglycemia-induced β-cell apoptosis in pancreatic islets of *Psammomys obesus* during development of diabetes. *Diabetes* 1999;48:738–744.
138. Kaneto H, Kajimoto Y, Fujitani Y, et al. Oxidative stress induces p21 expression in pancreatic islet cells: possible implication in beta-cell dysfunction. *Diabetologia* 1999;42:1093–1097.
139. Kaneto H, Kajimoto Y, Miyagawa J, et al. Beneficial effects of antioxidants in diabetes-possible protection of pancreatic beta-cells against glucose toxicity. *Diabetes* 1999;48:2398–2406.

CHAPTER 4
Genetic Regulation of Islet Function

Michael S. German

Despite their small size and apparent simplicity, pancreatic islets of Langerhans are remarkably sophisticated micro-organs. The four cell types that comprise each islet have in common basic endocrine-cell characteristics and are thought to derive from a common precursor during development. In the mature pancreas, however, each cell type functions quite differently, responding to different signals and producing different secreted products. These marked differences result from the differential expression of a unique set of genes. The mechanisms that control differential gene expression determine the functional characteristics of the islet cells (1–3).

The genes differentially expressed in the islet cells include the peptide hormone genes such as those encoding preproinsulin and proglucagon but also include a variety of genes involved at all levels of cell function, such as glucokinase, glutamic acid decarboxylase, the prohormone convertases, cell surface receptors, and cell adhesion molecules. Clearly, a complex regulatory network is needed to ensure that the complete set of genes is expressed at appropriate levels. This regulatory network in turn must quickly mature as each islet cell type develops from a common cluster of pluripotent progenitor cells. Understanding the genetic control of islet function requires an understanding of both how this network emerges during the differentiation of the islet cells and how it functions in the mature islet cell.

DIFFERENTIATION OF DISTINCT ISLET CELL TYPES DURING DEVELOPMENT

As described in the preceding chapter, the islet cells of the pancreas, along with the exocrine and duct cells, differentiate from a common pool of undifferentiated progenitor cells that form the initial pancreatic buds. This process of differentiation results from serial changes in gene expression as uncommitted precursor cells progress to mature, postmitotic, terminally differentiated cells (1–6).

Several models for the lineage relationships of pancreatic endocrine cells have been proposed, generally based on the order of appearance of cell types during fetal development. For example, because the earliest endocrine cells in the fetal pancreas express glucagon, it has been proposed that α-cells function as precursors for the other islet cell types that appear later (7,8). In the absence of labeling studies, however, order of appearance cannot establish a lineage relationship. In fact, a preponderance of recent evidence strongly suggests that α-cells are not precursors for β-cells. First, the early glucagon-expressing cells are postmitotic and thus cannot provide an explanation for the later appearance of much larger numbers of β-cells without cell replication (9–11). Furthermore, during the peak of formation of new β-cells (around embryonic day [E] 15 in the fetal mouse), no cells representing a transition between α- and β-cells with coexpression of glucagon and insulin can be detected (7,8). Finally, experiments with transgenic mice with toxic genes or *cre* recombinase labeling demonstrate that β-cells do not develop from a precursor in which the glucagon promoter is active (12–14). Together, this evidence supports a model in which islet cell type is determined before the expression of the hormone genes.

Insulin-producing cells may develop via more than one pathway. The earliest insulin-producing cells in the mouse fetus, those appearing before E13, do not express the normal set of β-cell genes, because they lack GLUT2, express low levels of insulin, and may coexpress glucagon. These cells do not replicate, and their numbers are small; thus, it is unlikely that they contribute significantly to the population of β-cells in the mature islet. It still remains to be determined whether all of the β-cells present in the mature pancreas differentiated via a common pathway; but because they express the same restricted set of genes, the mechanisms that control gene expression are likely to be the same.

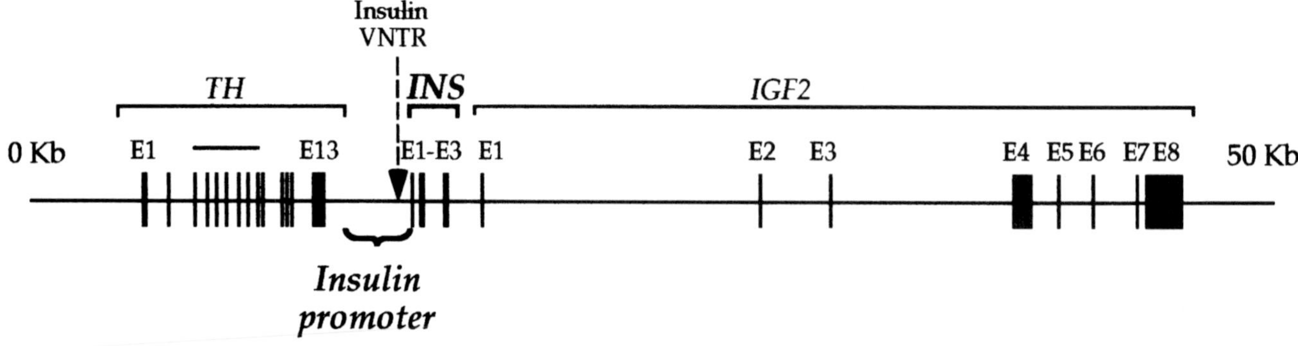

Figure 4.1. The human insulin gene (*INS*) and surrounding loci on chromosome 11. IGF2, insulin-like growth factor-2; TH, tyrosine hydroxylase.

Despite their obvious differences, the four different islet cell types share similar developmental pathways and related functions, and these connections are reflected in similarities in gene-expression mechanisms and in an overlapping set of expressed genes, some of which are also expressed in pancreatic ductal or exocrine cells. Because of its central role in energy metabolism, along with its robust expression and tight restriction to β-cells, the insulin gene has emerged as a paradigm of cell type–restricted expression in the endocrine pancreas.

THE INSULIN-GENE PARADIGM

Humans have a single insulin gene, located on chromosome 2, at 2p21 between the tyrosine hydroxylase (*THI*) gene and the insulin-like growth factor-2 (*IGF-2*) gene (Fig. 4.1) (15). The gene contains two introns, one interrupting the 5′ untranslated sequence and the second interrupting the sequence encoding the C-peptide. This general structure is conserved, with few exceptions, among the other mammalian insulin genes, as well as among the related IGF genes (16).

The sequences upstream of the transcription start site comprise the insulin-gene promoter (17). The promoter directs RNA polymerase II to the correct transcription start site, restricts insulin-gene transcription to the β-cell, and responds to metabolic, hormonal, and neural signals by modulating the rate at which insulin-gene transcription is initiated. These functions of the insulin-gene promoter are relatively independent of chromosomal context: When removed from the remainder of the insulin gene, the promoter can similarly regulate any gene inserted downstream.

The use of such chimeric genes, with the isolated insulin promoter driving the expression of an easily detectable marker gene such as chloramphenicol acetyl transferase, SV40 large T antigen, or firefly luciferase (18–24), provides a simple method of testing the importance of specific sequences within the promoter. When introduced into insulin-producing cells in culture or into transgenic mice, these chimeric genes demonstrate that a relatively small fragment of the insulin promoter, the proximal 250 to 400 base pairs (bp), provides the same regulation of transcription observed with the intact gene, although larger promoters increase the fidelity and the relative level of transcription in transgenic animals (25).

Careful mutational analyses within the proximal promoter have further delineated the specific sequences that contribute to the full activity of the promoter (22–24,26,27). Figure 4.2 outlines the general architecture, including functionally important sequences in the human and rat insulin-gene promoters. In some regards, the insulin-gene promoter is structurally similar to many cellular gene promoters and contains promoter elements that can function in all cell types. These include a consensus TATAA box, the binding site for the TFIID complex, located 30 bp upstream from the transcription start site, a CCAAT box, and one or more cyclic adenosine monophosphate regulatory elements (27–30).

Other portions of the promoter, however, are more unique and give the promoter the specificity that limits its activity to the β-cells. As shown in Figure 4.2, a number of sequence elements along the proximal promoter contribute to this specific activity, but comparison of the available mammalian insulin-gene promoter sequences reveals certain common themes. Most prominently, all of the mammalian insulin-gene promoters con-

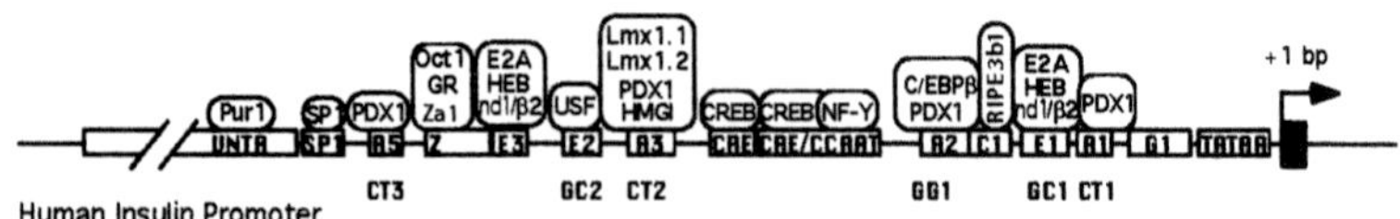

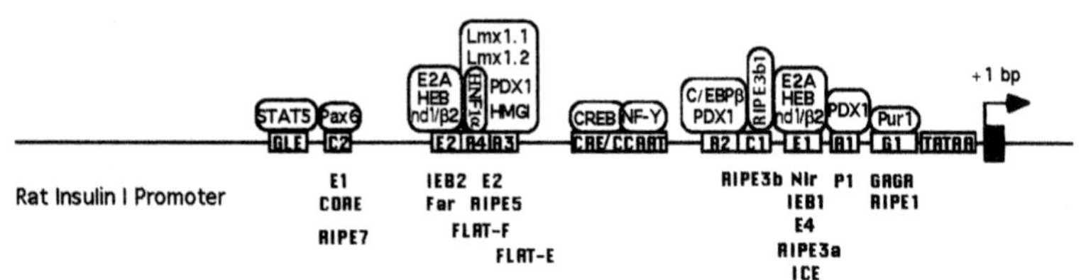

Figure 4.2. The human insulin gene and rat insulin I gene promoters with known sequence elements and binding factors. The boxes represent characterized sequence elements. The binding proteins are circled above the promoter. Older names for the sequence elements are listed below the promoter. GR, glucocorticoid receptor; nd1/β2, neuroD1/BETA2.

tain juxtaposed E and A sequence elements. The E elements contain the core sequence motif CCANCTG, and the A elements contain A/T-rich sequences with one or more copies of the sequence TAAT.

Function of the human and rat insulin promoters depends on the presence of at least one A element and one E element. Mutation of either of the two E elements in the rat insulin I gene results in a 90% loss of promoter activity in insulinoma cells, while mutation of both elements ablates all activity (26). The more proximal E element, E1, is absolutely conserved in all known mammalian insulin genes, and its importance has also been demonstrated in the rat insulin II promoter and the human insulin promoter (23,26,31,32). The A3 and A1 elements are both highly conserved in mammalian insulin genes, and the A3 element has been found to play an important role in both rat insulin-gene promoters and the human insulin promoter (23,26,31,32).

The Basic Helix-Loop-Helix Transcription Factors: NeuroD1

The sequences of the insulin E elements are a subset of the common CANNTG E box elements that play important roles in many cell type–specific promoters, including the promoters for the immunoglobulin genes and muscle-specific genes (33). E boxes are binding sites for proteins of the basic helix-loop-helix (bHLH) family. The bHLH proteins form dimers through their helix-loop-helix domains, and these dimers contact and bind to DNA with the basic domains. Because heterodimerization is permitted, and in most cases favored, a large variety of complexes are possible. Cell type–specific complexes generally result from heterodimerization of one of a limited number of ubiquitously expressed bHLH proteins (class A) with one of a large set of cell type–restricted bHLH proteins (class B).

β-Cells contain several bHLH complexes capable of binding to the insulin E boxes. Nuclear extracts from insulinoma cells demonstrate that the predominant complexes are formed from dimerization of a ubiquitous bHLH protein (the E12 or E47 products of the *E2A* gene or HEB) with the neuroendocrine bHLH protein neuroD1/BETA2 (24,34–39). NeuroD1 is expressed in all of the islet cells, in the endocrine cells of the gut, and in the central nervous system. The carboxyl-terminus of neuroD1 contains a potent transcriptional activation domain (40,41) (Fig. 4.3), and ectopic expression of neuroD1 can activate the insulin promoter in non–β-cells (38).

Mice homozygous for a targeted disruption of the gene encoding neuroD1 have a marked decrease in islet cells due to premature apoptosis and die of diabetes shortly after birth (42,43). In addition, absence of neuroD1 results in losses of enteroendocrine cells and in defects in several aspects of neural development (42–49). Interestingly, insulin is still produced by the remaining β-cells in the pancreas, suggesting either that neuroD1 function is not required for insulin-gene transcription or that other bHLH proteins may be able to substitute for neuroD1 on the insulin promoter (42).

Homeodomain Transcription Factors: PDX1

The A elements function as binding sites for homeodomain proteins, a broad family of transcription factors. Homeodomain proteins have been found in all eukaryotic organisms and are characterized by a conserved stretch of 61 amino acids called the homeodomain, which forms a helix-turn-helix structure that binds to DNA. Homeodomain proteins play critical roles in cell-type determination and differentiation during development, as well as in the regulation of gene expression in the mature cells.

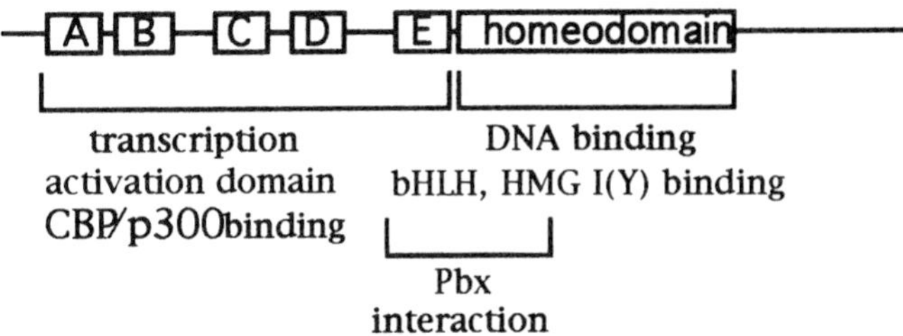

A

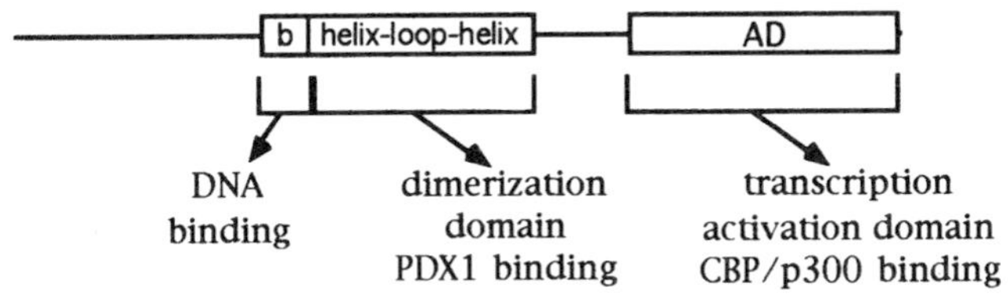

B

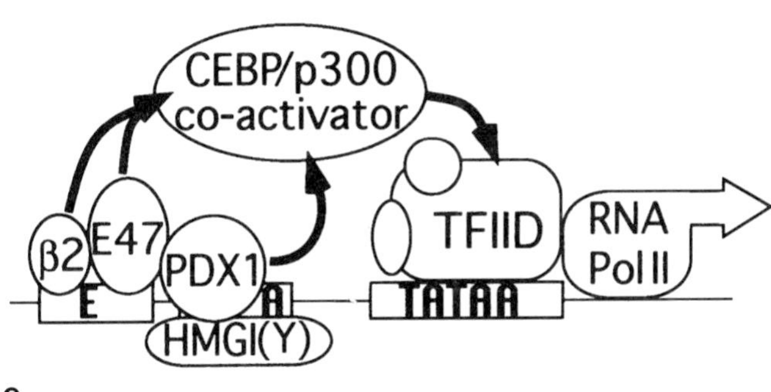

C

Figure 4.3. The insulin promoter transcription complex. **A:** The functional domains of the PDX1 protein are outlined. The regions labeled *A–E* represent conserved domains within the activation domain (90) **B:** The functional domains of the neuroD1/Beta2 protein are outlined. **C:** Interactions are shown among PDX1, the bHLH proteins, HMGI(Y), and p300 that result in transcriptional activation of the E–A mini-enhancer. β2, neuroD1/BETA2.

In extracts from β-cell nuclei, the most abundant protein binding to the A elements is the homeodomain protein PDX1 (also called IPF1, IDX1, STF1, IUF1, and GSF1) (50–56). PDX1 belongs to the parahox family of homeobox genes and is expressed in the antral stomach, duodenum, and pancreas (50,57). Early in development PDX1 is expressed broadly in the pancreatic bud, but after E13 in the mouse, it becomes restricted, with high levels of expression in β-cells and some δ-cells and lower levels of expression in acinar cells and duct cells. PDX1 can bind to all of the A elements in the rat and human insulin promoters and can activate portions of the insulin promoter in cell lines (50–52). Furthermore, forced expression of PDX1 has been reported to activate the endogenous insulin gene in some non–β-cells (58,59).

Mice homozygous for a targeted disruption of the gene encoding PDX1 have a profound defect in pancreatic growth, with essentially no development of the pancreas beyond initial bud formation, and die shortly after birth (60–62). A few hormone-producing cells, including insulin-producing cells, however, can be detected in the remaining dorsal bud (61). If instead the *pdx1* gene is inactivated specifically in β-cells after the pancreas has formed, by using a cre-lox recombination system with the insulin promoter driving the cre recombinase, the differentiated phenotype of the β-cells is partially lost (63). In these animals with a β-cell–specific disruption of the *pdx1* gene, the β-cell mass decreases; and the remaining β-cells coexpress glucagon and have reduced GLUT2 and reduced glucose-stimulated insulin secretion. As in the β-cells lacking neuroD1, however, the β-cells lacking PDX1 continue to produce insulin.

The persistence of insulin-gene transcription in the absence of PDX1 suggests the presence of additional homeodomain proteins in β-cells that can drive insulin-gene expression *in vivo*. Although it is clearly the most abundant nuclear protein capable of binding the A elements in β-cells, PDX1 is not the only homeodomain transcription factor expressed in β-cells nor the only homeodomain protein in β-cells capable of binding and activating transcription through the A elements (54,64–66). Two β-cell homeodomain proteins, Cdx2/3 and lmx1A, have been shown to bind to and activate through the A3 and A4 sites in the rat insulin I promoter (65). In addition, the POU-homeodomain protein HNF1a is also expressed in β-cells, and it binds to and activates the A4 site in the rat insulin I promoter, although the A4 site is not conserved in insulin genes from other species (66). Finally, β-cells express a diverse set of additional homeodomain transcription factors; some of these regulate insulin-gene transcription, but all play some part in β-cell gene expression (54).

Paired-Homeodomain Factors: Pax6

The E and A elements and the protein complexes that bind to them are essential to the function of the insulin promoter but cannot explain all of the activity of the promoter. A G/C rich sequence, C2, in the distal promoter contributes significantly to the activity of the rat insulin promoters both in insulinoma cells and primary-cultured β-cells (26,27,31). Because the C2 element and related elements in the glucagon and somatostatin gene promoters all function in an islet cell–specific manner and bind to an islet-specific complex, this common islet enhancer element has been termed PISCES (pancreatic islet cell-specific enhancer sequence) (67–72).

C2 and the other PISCES elements closely match the consensus binding sequence for the paired-homeodomain transcription factor Pax6, and Pax6 antiserum recognizes the islet-specific complex that binds to all three PISCES elements (73). Pax6 contains a potent transcriptional activation domain and three DNA-binding domains, a paired region composed of the pai and red domains and a homeodomain (74–76). Pax6 protein first appears during development in the nuclei of a few scattered cells in the gut endoderm where the dorsal bud and the first glucagon-producing cells will appear a few hours later (73). From that point on, it is expressed in the nuclei of all the endocrine cells in the pancreas, as well as in a subset of neuroendocrine cells in other tissues.

Mice carrying mutations in the *pax6* gene were previously identified and named small eye because of a defect in eye development in the heterozygous mice. Mice homozygous for the small-eye mutations or a targeted interruption of the *pax6* gene die at birth with multiple craniofacial and neurologic defects. In addition, the homozygous mutant animals have profound defects in islet development, with decreased numbers of all islet cell types (73,77). The remaining β-cells also have a significant decrease in the amount of insulin mRNA and protein per cell. These mice demonstrate that Pax6 is important but not absolutely essential for expression of the insulin gene in mice. The importance of Pax6 in human insulin-gene expression is less certain, however, because the C2 element is not conserved in the human insulin-gene promoter.

Unidentified Factors: RIPE3b1

Immediately upstream of the E1 element lies the C1 element, a cytosine-rich sequence that is conserved in all of the mammalian insulin promoters. The C1 element is critically important for the function of both the human insulin and rat insulin II promoters (31,32,35,78–80). A protein complex found in β-cell nuclei, the RIPE3b1 complex binds specifically to the C1 element and has not been detected in other cell-types, including α-cells (35,81). Although it is known that the RIPE3b1 complex is composed of several proteins of similar molecular mass and that binding to the C1 element requires its phosphorylation, the protein has not been identified (82–84).

Unidentified Factors: Za1

Upstream of the A3 element in the human insulin promoter lies the negative regulatory element (NRE), which strongly inhibits insulin promoter function in β-cell tumor lines (32,85,86). The NRE also inhibits transcription when isolated from the insulin promoter and linked to a heterologous promoter in either β-cell or non–β cell tumor lines (32,85). It has been proposed that the NRE may modulate insulin promoter activity and help restrict insulin expression to the β-cell (85).

The NRE may not always function, however, simply as a silencer of transcription. Walker et al. (18), for example, found that removal of the NRE from the human insulin promoter had no significant effect on the promoter, and Clark et al. (85) found that isolated sequences within the NRE could activate transcription weakly. It is in primary cultured islets, however, that the NRE reveals its most remarkable activity. Removal of the NRE from the human insulin promoter causes a marked loss of activity in cultured fetal rat islet cells (80). Placed upstream of a minimal insulin promoter or a heterologous promoter, the NRE functions as a potent activator of transcription in both fetal and adult islets, whereas in the same constructs it strongly represses transcription in tumor cell lines from β-cells or non–β cells and in primary-cultured fibroblasts (86). Because it appears that the primary function of this region in normal β-cells *in vivo* is to activate transcription, this region has been renamed the Z element. Although a Z element–binding complex that correlates with the positive activity of the Z element can be detected in nuclear extracts from primary cultured islets (86), the proteins in this complex have not been identified.

The Insulin Promoter Transcription Complex

The linear view of the insulin promoter as a series of binding sites and binding proteins, as shown in Figure 4.2, fails to illustrate the complexity and dynamic character of the functioning promoter *in vivo*. Missing from this view is the added dimension provided by the interactions among the transcription factors, DNA structural proteins, co-activators and repressors, intracellular signaling molecules, and the RNA polymerase complex. This view also ignores the role of upstream factors that regulate the expression and function of these proteins. The promoter should be regarded as a large and fluid complex formed by interactions among many different proteins and the chromosome in dynamic equilibrium with forces acting from within and outside the cell.

In this perspective, the bipartite E-A combination represents the minimal functional component of the larger complex and demonstrates the underlying concept of cooperativity. Neither the E elements nor the A elements by themselves have any significant transcriptional activity in β-cells; but together they can dramatically boost the activity of a linked promoter in a β-cell–specific fashion (87,88). The synergy between these elements results from interactions among the proteins that bind to them and non–DNA-binding transcriptional co-activators.

This cooperativity can be demonstrated when PDX1 is coexpressed along with either E47 or E47 plus neuroD1 in non–β-cells: activation of the E-A mini-enhancer depends on the combination of PDX1 bound to the A element and a bHLH dimer bound to the E element (89,90). In addition to both the E and A binding sites, cooperativity between PDX1 and the bHLH dimer requires the DNA-binding domains of all the proteins and the transcriptional activation domains of both PDX1 and at least one of the bHLH proteins (89–93).

Cooperativity results from interactions among the proteins at several levels (Fig. 4.3). First, the proteins cooperate at the level of DNA binding. Physical interaction among the DNA binding domains, the homeodomain of PDX1, and the bHLH domains of E47 and neuroD1/BETA2, stabilizes the complex of all three proteins on DNA. Although DNA binding affinity is increased, with purified proteins *in vitro* the relative increase in binding affinity is small (92). *In vivo*, however, the nuclear environment is very different, with differences in local concentrations of factors and the presence of many other proteins, all of which change the energetic equilibrium of DNA binding. In addition, chromatin structure is quite different from the purified oligonucleotides used to test DNA binding *in vitro*. Chromosome structure is controlled *in vivo* by the binding of histones and of small, abundant DNA-binding proteins, the high-mobility group (HMG) proteins.

The presence of these structural DNA-binding proteins changes the energetic cost of DNA-binding by the transcription factors (for a review, see reference 94). For example, in the presence of HMG I(Y), a small nonhistone DNA-binding protein that can bind to the A3/4 region of the insulin promoter, co-binding of PDX1 and the bHLH dimer is greatly favored *in vitro*. As a result, HMG I(Y) increases PDX-bHLH transcriptional synergy *in vivo*. In insect cells, where HMG I proteins are expressed at very low levels, PDX1 and the bHLH proteins cannot cooperatively activate the E-A mini-enhancer without the addition of HMG I(Y) (92).

At the next level of organization, the insulin promoter activation complex requires non–DNA-binding proteins that form a bridge between the proteins binding at the E and A sites and the basal transcriptional machinery. Just as interactions within the PDX1/bHLH/HMG I(Y) complex stabilize DNA binding and increase the occupancy of the E-A sites on the insulin promoter, multiple protein-protein contacts stabilize the interaction with the basal transcription machinery and ensure efficient transcription initiation. The grouping of transcription factors on adjacent DNA sites, as in the E-A mini-enhancers, creates clusters of protein interaction sites that cooperatively recruit or stabilize binding of the RNA polymerase II transcription initiation complex (95). Non–DNA-binding co-activators promote this process by linking the DNA-bound transcription factors with TFIID complex and the basal transcription machinery. The additional interactions provided by the co-activators provide critical stability and play a linchpin role in the formation and the function of the insulin promoter transcription-activation complex (Fig. 4.3). In support of this model, the E2A proteins, neuroD1, and PDX1 have all been shown to interact with the ubiquitous p300 co-activator (40,41,47,96,97).

If insulin-gene transcription depends on the presence of an active insulin promoter complex and the assembly of that complex depends on the proper interactions of multiple nuclear proteins, then the cell-type specificity of insulin-gene transcription is a product of the uniqueness of the set of proteins that compose the complex. According to this model, the absence of some subset of these proteins in other, non–β-cells, or the presence of proteins that interrupt the interactions that stabilize the complex would block formation of the complex and prevent insulin-gene transcription. The true explanation is not quite this simple, however, as demonstrated by the fact that mice lacking key components of the complex, PDX1, neuroD1, E2A, or HEB, can all continue to transcribe the insulin gene in β-cells (42,63,98). Apparently, the insulin-gene transcription complex has some inherent flexibility and redundancy.

Although the transcription complex certainly provides significant specificity, it cannot by itself provide an explanation for the strict restriction of insulin-gene transcription to the β-cell. Negative regulation in non–β-cells plays a role as well. Non–β-cells contain proteins in their nuclei that interfere with formation of the insulin-gene transcription complex. For example, the homeodomain protein pbx can associate with PDX1 and alter its DNA-binding specificity, thereby preventing it from binding to the insulin promoter A sites (97,99,100). In addition, the physical state of the chromatin surrounding the insulin gene may silence the gene in non–β-cells. Modifications such as methylation or structural changes induced by histone binding can block access to the gene for binding by the transcription complex (101–103). Finally, it must be understood that not only does the physical state of the chromatin at the insulin promoter affect binding of the transcription complex but the proteins of the transcription complex can alter local histone acetylation and binding, thereby opening the chromatin structure of the promoter region and increasing access for the transcription complex. These interactions amplify the effect of small changes in functional levels of the transcription complex, producing a threshold for insulin-gene transcription.

Metabolic Regulation of Gene Expression

In their role as nutrient sensors and metabolic regulators, the islet cells need to alter gene expression in response to the metabolic state of the organism. The paradigm for how the islet cells achieve metabolic regulation of gene expression has been the regulation of the insulin gene by glucose.

Levels of insulin messenger RNA (mRNA) increase in β-cells in response to glucose due to the combined effects of increased insulin-gene transcription, increased insulin pre-RNA splicing, and decreased insulin mRNA degradation (104–106). It has been proposed that the increase in transcription occurs within a few minutes of glucose stimulation (107), but because the half-life of insulin mRNA is 1 to 4 days (105), it is difficult to understand how this rapid change would significantly affect insulin production or secretion in response to a meal. More likely, changes in insulin-gene transcription modulate insulin production in response to long-term dietary changes.

The transcriptional activation induced by glucose in the β-cell is selective for the insulin gene and is due at least in part to activation of the insulin promoter and the E-A mini-enhancer (108) (Fig. 4.4). Glucose regulates the promoter through multiple effects on several of the proteins in the transcription activation complex (27,52,79,80,86,108–110). After glucose stimulation, PDX1 binding to the A elements acutely increases (55,56,109), due in part to phosphorylation of PDX1 through a pathway that involves phosphatidylinositol (PI) 3 kinase and the stress-activated protein kinase 2 (SAPK2) (55,111). Glucose also causes a shift in the cel-

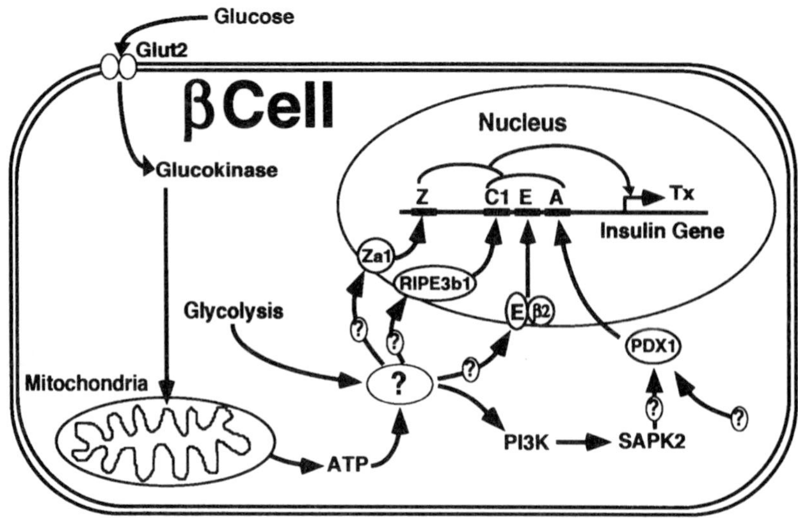

Figure 4.4. Proposed pathways for glucose regulation of insulin gene expression. *IE* represents E2A proteins, and β2 represents the selectively expressed heterodimer partner neuroD1/BETA2. Question marks indicate unknown steps in the pathway or the probable intersection with other pathways. The two objects labeled *IE* and *β2* represent a dimer of the E47 and neuroD1/BETA2 bHLH proteins.

lular distribution of PDX1 to the nucleus (112–114), apparently secondary to its phosphorylation (112,114), and increases the activation potential of the PDX1 activation domain (115).

At the same time, glucose increases the binding of the bHLH dimer to the E elements (27), which in turn cooperate with the activated PDX1 bound at the A site to increase insulin-gene transcription. In addition, sequences outside the E-A elements also contribute to the transcriptional response to glucose, as demonstrated by increased binding of the Za1 (86) and RIPE3b1 (110) protein complexes in response to glucose. All of these effects then combine to produce the overall increase in insulin-gene transcription in response to glucose.

Glucose stimulates insulin-gene transcription indirectly through the end products of its catabolism (116). The rate-limiting step for glycolysis in β-cells is phosphorylation of glucose to glucose-6-phosphate. When the rate of glucose phosphorylation is increased by expressing high levels of hexokinase I in β-cells, glycolysis is accelerated and the insulin promoter is activated. The intermediates of glycolysis are required for this response (116). The intracellular signaling pathways through which glycolysis regulates the insulin-gene activation complex remain elusive, although it has been proposed that insulin secretion may feed back to activate insulin-gene transcription in the β-cell through its receptor, PI 3 kinase, and downstream signaling pathways (117,118).

Application to the Expression of Other Islet Genes

As our understanding of insulin-gene expression has expanded, it has become apparent that many of the lessons learned from studies of the insulin promoter can be applied to the broader problem of islet cell–specific gene expression. The general concept of cooperative protein interactions building an activation complex that is specific to a particular gene and cell type explains the specificity of other islet cell–specific promoters. In addition, many of the proteins that form these complexes are the same. For example, PDX1 binds and activates promoters from the β-cell genes islet amyloid polypeptide, GLUT2, and glucokinase (17,59,119–121) and the δ-cell gene somatostatin (51), as well as the insulin-gene promoter.

The glucagon-gene promoter provides an interesting comparison to the insulin-gene promoter (Fig. 4.5). Like the insulin-gene promoter, the glucagon-gene promoter depends on interactions among several sequence elements. The proximal G1 element is required for function of the promoter and restricts activity to the α-cell, but its activity depends on interactions with at least one of the more distal elements G2 and G3 (122–125), although more distal elements may play important roles as well (126). Like the insulin promoter, many of the sequences found in these elements function as binding sites for homeodomain and bHLH proteins (73,127–133).

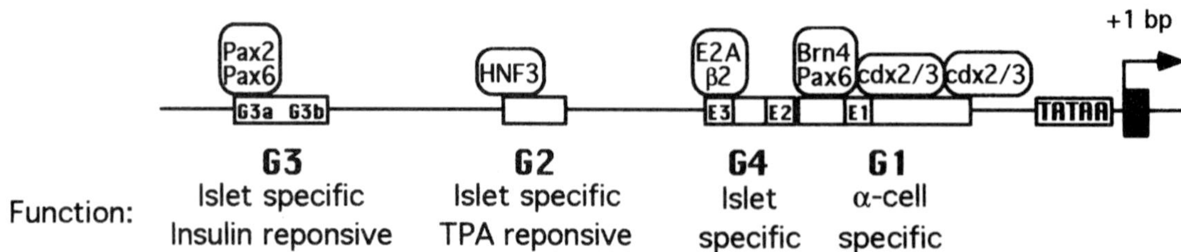

Figure 4.5. The rat glucagon-gene promoter with known sequence elements and binding factors. The boxes represent characterized sequence elements. The four interacting enhancer regions, G1–G4, are labeled below the boxes, and their functional roles are listed underneath. The cloned binding proteins are circled above the promoter. β2, neuroD1/BETA2.

The proximal G1 element contains several adjacent and overlapping binding sites. The pou-homeodomain transcription factor Brn4 binds to an A/T-rich sequence at the 5′ end of the G1 element (133). Within the adult pancreas, Brn4 expression is restricted to the α-cells, and it can activate both an isolated glucagon-gene promoter in a G1-dependent manner (133) and the native glucagon gene (134). Activity of the G1 element also appears to involve two other homeodomain proteins: pax6, which binds to a sequence overlapping the one recognized by brn4, and cdx2/3, which binds to two sites on the 3′ end of the G1 element (129,130,135–138). Pax6 and cdx2/3 then synergize in activating the promoter by cooperatively recruiting the p300 co-activator (136–138).

Full activation of the glucagon promoter results from higher-order interaction between the complex of proteins binding to the G1 element and the complexes on the G2, G3, and G4 elements, each of which depends on additional interactions among proteins binding within each element (71,72,122,123,131, 139–146). Similar to glucose regulation of the insulin promoter, this interdependence of discrete promoter elements and their cognate binding factors allows for regulation of the entire promoter through regulation of individual factors, as exemplified by the regulation of the G3 complex by insulin (143,147,148) and the G2 element by protein kinase C (141).

Upstream Genes in Differentiating and Mature Islet Cells

The preceding discussion yields a model for the expression of islet genes in which gene activation is achieved through multiple protein interactions that combine to produce a unique gene transcription complex on the promoter. Before an active complex can form, however, the genes encoding each of the proteins that comprise the complex must themselves be activated. Studies of the differentiation of islet cells from pluripotent progenitor cells have provided insight into the hierarchy of these factors and the cascade of gene expression events that lie upstream of the activation of the final differentiated genes such as insulin (Fig. 4.6). As a result, islet gene expression is regulated by an entire network of factors directly and indirectly involved in the formation of each gene transcription complex.

ISLET GENE TRANSCRIPTION AND TYPE 2 DIABETES MELLITUS

The determination that mutations in the genes encoding islet transcription factors can lead to diabetes mellitus in mice (Table 4.1) led to the consideration of these genes as candidates in genetic studies of type 2 diabetes mellitus in humans. Type 2 diabetes mellitus in humans is a strongly genetic disorder, but its inheritance is complex, and the identification of the contributing genes has been impeded by the non-Mendelian inheritance of the disease in most families. To simplify genetic studies, efforts to identify diabetes genes initially focused on families with an early onset and autosomal dominant form of the disease termed maturity-onset diabetes of the young (MODY). Of the five causative genes so far identified in families with MODY, four encode islet transcription factors: *HNF4α* (MODY1) (149), *HNF1α* (MODY3) (150), *IPF1* (PDX1, MODY4) (151), and *HNF1β* (MODY5) (152). In addition, mutations in the coding sequence of *isl1* and *neuroD1* have been implicated in families with later-onset diabetes (153,154) (Table 4.1).

How do mutations in these genes cause diabetes mellitus? Even with the availability of mutant mouse lines, answering this question has not been simple. While it is tempting to speculate that these mutations cause diabetes mellitus by affecting the expression of a single key target gene such as insulin or GLUT2, the animal models suggest that the answer is more complex. Given the interdependence of the different islet transcription factors, it is not surprising to find that mutation of a single transcription-factor gene can impair the expression of many islet genes, including many that do not appear to be direct targets of the transcription factor (63,155–159). For that reason, the upstream regulators of islet differentiation and gene expression, the transcription factor genes such as *Nkx2.2*, *Nkx6.1*, *Pax4*, and *neurogenin3*, also

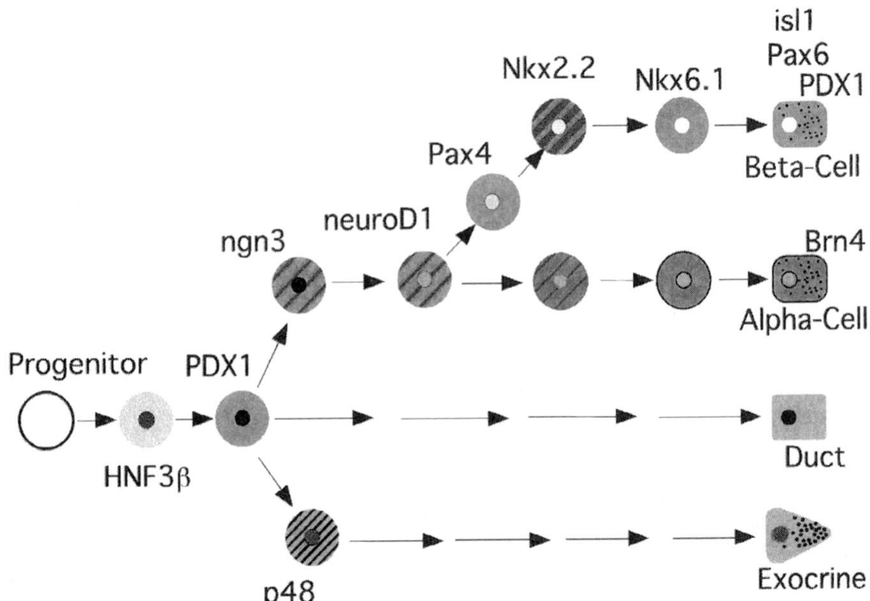

Figure 4.6. A simplified model for the role of islet transcription factors in endocrine differentiation in the developing pancreas. The proposed position for each transcription factor is based on its timing of expression, timing of predominant functional role, or both. Clearly, some factors function at several steps, but a single step is shown for simplicity.

TABLE 4.1. Islet Transcription Factors

Factor	Family	Expression	Downstream islet genes	Mouse mutations[a]	Human mutations	References
Neurogenin 3	bHLH	Fetal pancreas and CNS	NeuroD1/BETA2, Pax4, Nkx2.2	Diabetes, no islet cells		(11,160–163)
NeuroD1/BETA2	bHLH	Islet, gut endocrine cells, CNS	Insulin	Diabetes, decreased islet cells	Het: late-onset diabetes	(38–40,42,47,53)
PDX1/IPF1	Parahox homeodomain	α- and β-cells, duodenum and stomach	Insulin, IAPP, glucokinase, GLUT2	Pancreatic agenesis	Het: MODY4 Hom: pancreatic agenesis	(59–63, 119–121, 151, 164,165)
HB9	Parahox homeodomain	β-cells, gut, lymphoid, CNS	GLUT2	Dorsal pancreatic agenesis	Het: sacral agenesis	(166–168)
Pax2	Paired domain	Islet, urogenital tract and CNS	Glucagon	Defects in optic nerve, CNS and urogenital tract	Het: renal-coloboma syndrome	(169,170)
Pax4	Paired-homeodomain	Fetal pancreas and CNS	Pax4 (autorepression)	Decreased β- and α-cells		(171–173)
Pax6	Paired-homeodomain	Islet, gut endocrine cells, CNS	Glucagon, insulin, somatostatin	Decrease in all islet cells, decreased glucagon	Het: aniridia	(73,77,135)
Nkx2.2	NK-homeodomain	α-, β-, and PP cells and CNS	Nkx6.1, insulin, GLUT2, GK	Diabetes, no insulin		(10,54,174,175)
Nkx6.1	NK-homeodomain	β-cells and CNS		Decreased β-cells, postnatal lethal		(10,54,174,176)
Cdx2/3	Caudal-homeodomain	Islet and gut	Glucagon	Het: gut tumors Hom: embryonic lethal		(65,128–130,177)
Isl1	LIM-homeodomain	Islet and CNS	Somatostatin, glucagon	No islet cells, embryonic lethal		(9,64,154, 178–181)
Lmx1.1	LIM-homeodomain	β-cells and CNS	Insulin	Dreher: roof plate, cerebellum defects		(65,92,182)
Brn4	Pou-homeodomain	α-cells and CNS	Glucagon		Hom: congenital neurogenic deafness	(11,133,183)
HNF1α	Pou-homeodomain	Islet, liver, kidney	Pax4, Ngn3, GLUT2, Rat insulin I	Diabetes, impaired β-cell glucose sensing	Het: MODY3	(66,150,157,159, 171,184,185)
HNF1β	Pou-homeodomain	Islet, pancreatic duct, liver, kidney	Pax4	Embryonic lethal	Het: MODY5	(152,171,186,187)
HNF6	Cut-homeodomain	Pancreatic duct, liver	Neurogenin3	IGT, small islets		(185,188–192)
HNF3α	Winged helix	Islet, gut, liver	Glucagon	Hypoglycemia		(146,193)
HNF3β	Winged helix	Islet, pancreatic duct, gut, liver, CNS	PDX1, neurogenin3	Embryonic lethal		(156,185,190,192, 194–197)
HNF4α	Nuclear receptor	Liver, islet, kidney	HNF1α, glycolytic enzymes, Pax4	Embryonic lethal	Het: MODY1	(149,156,171, 198–200)

CNS, Central nervous system; het, heterozygous; hom, homozygous; MODY, maturity-onset diabetes of the young.
[a]All mouse phenotypes are for homozygous mutant animals unless stated otherwise.

should be considered candidate genes for genetic studies of type 2 diabetes mellitus.

Acknowledgments

I would like to thank the many members of the Rutter and German laboratories who contributed to the work discussed here. The work from our laboratory was supported by NIH grants DK-21344 and DK-48281.

REFERENCES

1. Sander M, German MS. The beta cell transcription factors and development of the pancreas. *J Mol Med* 1997;75:327–340.
2. Edlund H. Transcribing pancreas. *Diabetes* 1998;47:1817–1823.
3. Edlund H. Developmental biology of the pancreas. *Diabetes* 2001;50[Suppl 1]: S5–S9.
4. Slack JM. Developmental biology of the pancreas. *Development* 1995;121: 1569–1580.
5. Edlund H. Pancreas: how to get there from the gut? *Curr Opin Cell Biol* 1999; 11:663–668.
6. St-Onge L, Wehr R, Gruss P. Pancreas development and diabetes. *Curr Opin Genet Dev* 1999;9:295–300.
7. Alpert S, Hanahan D, Teitelman G. Hybrid insulin genes reveal a developmental lineage for pancreatic endocrine cells and imply a relationship with neurons. *Cell* 1988;53:295–308.
8. Teitelman G, Alpert S, Polak JM, et al. Precursor cells of mouse endocrine pancreas coexpress insulin, glucagon and the neuronal proteins tyrosine hydroxylase and neuropeptide Y, but not pancreatic polypeptide. *Development* 1993;118:1031–1039.
9. Ahlgren U, Pfaff SL, Jessell TM, et al. Independent requirement for ISL1 in formation of pancreatic mesenchyme and islet cells. *Nature* 1997;385:257–260.
10. Sander M, Sussel L, Conners J, et al. Homeobox gene Nkx6.1 lies downstream of Nkx2.2 in the major pathway of beta-cell formation in the pancreas. *Development* 2000;127:5533–5540.

11. Jensen J, Heller RS, Funder-Nielsen T, et al. Independent development of pancreatic alpha- and beta-cells from neurogenin3-expressing precursors: a role for the notch pathway in repression of premature differentiation. *Diabetes* 2000;49:163–176.
12. Herrera PL, Huarte J, Zufferey R, et al. Ablation of islet endocrine cells by targeted expression of hormone-promoter-driven toxigenes. *Proc Natl Acad Sci U S A* 1994;91:12999–13003.
13. Herrera PL. Adult insulin- and glucagon-producing cells differentiate from two independent cell lineages. *Development* 2000;127:2317–2322.
14. Herrera PL, Orci L, Vassalli JD. Two transgenic approaches to define the cell lineages in endocrine pancreas development. *Mol Cell Endocrinol* 1998;140: 45–50.
15. Owerbach D, Bell GI, Rutter WJ, et al. The insulin gene is located on chromosome 11 in humans. *Nature* 1980;286:82–84.
16. Steiner DF, Chan SJ. An overview of insulin evolution. *Horm Metab Res* 1988; 20:443–444.
17. German MS, Ashcroft S, Docherty K, et al. The insulin promoter: a simplified nomenclature. *Diabetes* 1995;44:1002–1004.
18. Walker MD, Edlund T, Boulet AM, et al. Cell-specific expression controlled by the 5′ flanking regions of the insulin and chymotrypsin genes. *Nature* 1983;306:557–581.
19. Edlund T, Walker MD, Barr PJ, et al. Cell-specific expression of the rat insulin gene: evidence for role of two distinct 5′ flanking elements. *Science* 1985;230: 912–916.
20. Hanahan D. Heritable formation of pancreatic β-cell tumors in transgenic mice expressing recombinant insulin/simian virus 40 oncogenes. *Nature* 1985;315:115–122.
21. Nir U, Walker MD, Rutter WJ. Regulation of rat insulin 1 gene expression: evidence for negative regulation in nonpancreatic cells. *Proc Natl Acad Sci U S A* 1986;83:3180–3184.
22. Takeda J, Ishii S, Seino Y, et al. Negative regulation of human insulin gene expression by the 5′-flanking region in non-pancreatic cells. *FEBS Lett* 1989; 247:41–45.
23. Whelan J, Poon D, Weil PA, et al. Pancreatic β-cell-type-specific expression of the rat insulin II gene is controlled by positive and negative cellular transcription elements. *Mol Cel Biol* 1989;9:3253–3259.
24. Cordle SR, Henderson E, Masuoka H, et al. Pancreatic β-cell-type-specific transcription of the insulin gene is mediated by basic helix-loop-helix DNA-binding proteins. *Mol Cell Biol* 1991;11:1734–1738.
25. Fromont-Racine M, Bucchini D, Madsen O, et al. Effect of 5′-flanking sequence deletions on expression of the human insulin gene in transgenic mice. *Mol Endocrinol* 1990;4:669–677.
26. Karlsson O, Edlund T, Moss JB, et al. A mutational analysis of the insulin gene transcription control region: expression in β-cells is dependent on two related sequences within the enhancer. *Proc Natl Acad Sci U S A* 1987;84: 8819–8823.
27. German M, Wang J. The insulin gene contains multiple transcriptional elements that respond to glucose. *Mol Cell Biol* 1994;14:4067–4075.
28. Philippe J, Missotten M. Functional characterization of a cAMP-responsive element of the rat insulin I gene. *J Biol Chem* 1990;265:1465–1469.
29. Inagaki N, Maekawa T, Sudo T, et al. c-jun represses the human insulin promoter activity that depends on multiple cAMP response elements. *Proc Natl Acad Sci U S A* 1992;89:1045–1049.
30. Oetjen E, Diedrich T, Eggers A, et al. Distinct properties of the cAMP-responsive element of the rat insulin I gene. *J Biol Chem* 1994;269:27036–27044.
31. Crowe DT, Tsai M-J. Mutagenesis of the rat insulin II 5′-flanking region defines sequences important for expression in HIT cells. *Mol Cell Biol* 1989;9: 1784–1789.
32. Boam DS, Clark AR, Docherty K. Positive and negative regulation of the human insulin gene by multiple trans-acting factors. *J Biol Chem* 1990;265: 8285–8296.
33. Ephrussi A, Church G, Tonegawa S, et al. B lineage-specific interactions of an immunoglobulin enhancer with cellular factors in vivo. *Science* 1985;227: 134–140.
34. Aronheim A, Ohlsson H, Park CW, et al. Distribution and characterization of helix-loop-helix enhancer-binding proteins from pancreatic β-cells and lymphocytes. *Nucl Acids Res* 1991;19:3893–3899.
35. Sheih S, Tsai M. Cell-specific and ubiquitous factors are responsible for the enhancer activity of the rat insulin II gene. *J Biol Chem* 1991;266:16708–16714.
36. German MS, Blanar MA, Nelson C, et al. Two related helix-loop-helix proteins participate in separate cell-specific complexes that bind to the insulin enhancer. *Mol Endocrinol* 1991;5:292–299.
37. Peyton M, Moss LG, Tsai MJ. Two distinct class A helix-loop-helix transcription factors, E2A and BETA1, form separate DNA binding complexes on the insulin gene E box. *J Biol Chem* 1994;269:25936-25941.
38. Naya FJ, Stellrecht CM, Tsai MJ. Tissue-specific regulation of the insulin gene by a novel basic helix-loop-helix transcription factor. *Genes Dev* 1995;9: 1009–1019.
39. Lee JE, Hollenberg SM, Snider L, et al. Conversion of Xenopus ectoderm into neurons by NeuroD, a basic helix-loop-helix protein. *Science* 1995;268: 836–844.
40. Qiu Y, Sharma A, Stein R. p300 mediates transcriptional stimulation by the basic helix-loop-helix activators of the insulin gene. *Mol Cell Biol* 1998;18: 2957–2964.
41. Sharma A, Moore M, Marcora E, et al. The NeuroD1/BETA2 sequences essential for insulin gene transcription colocalize with those necessary for neurogenesis and p300/CREB binding protein binding. *Mol Cell Biol* 1999;19: 704–713.
42. Naya FJ, Huang HP, Qiu Y, et al. Diabetes, defective pancreatic morphogenesis, and abnormal enteroendocrine differentiation in BETA2/neuroD-deficient mice. *Genes Dev* 1997;11:2323–2334.
43. Miyata T, Maeda T, Lee JE. NeuroD is required for differentiation of the granule cells in the cerebellum and hippocampus. *Genes Dev* 1999;13: 1647–1652.
44. Schwab MH, Bartholomae A, Heimrich B, et al. Neuronal basic helix-loop-helix proteins (NEX and BETA2/Neuro D) regulate terminal granule cell differentiation in the hippocampus. [Erratum in: *J Neurosci* 2000 Nov 1;20(21): 8227]. *J Neurosci* 2000;20:3714–3724.
45. Liu M, Pleasure SJ, Collins AE, et al. Loss of BETA2/NeuroD leads to malformation of the dentate gyrus and epilepsy. *Proc Natl Acad Sci U S A* 2000; 97:865–870.
46. Liu M, Pereira FA, Price SD, et al. Essential role of BETA2/NeuroD1 in development of the vestibular and auditory systems. *Genes Dev* 2000;14: 2839–2854.
47. Mutoh H, Naya FJ, Tsai MJ, et al. The basic helix-loop-helix protein BETA2 interacts with p300 to coordinate differentiation of secretin-expressing enteroendocrine cells. *Genes Dev* 1998;12:820–830.
48. Morrow EM, Furukawa T, Lee JE, et al. NeuroD regulates multiple functions in the developing neural retina in rodent. *Development* 1999;126:23–36.
49. Kim WY, Fritzsch B, Serls A, et al. NeuroD-null mice are deaf due to a severe loss of the inner ear sensory neurons during development. *Development* 2001; 128:417–426.
50. Ohlsson H, Karlsson K, Edlund T. IPF1, a homeodomain-containing transactivator of the insulin gene. *EMBO J* 1993;12:4251–4259.
51. Leonard J, Peers B, Johnson T, et al. Characterization of somatostatin transactivating factor-1, a novel homeobox factor that stimulates somatostatin expression in pancreatic islet cells. *Mol Endocrinol* 1993;7:1275–1283.
52. Petersen HV, Serup P, Leonard J, et al. Transcriptional regulation of the human insulin gene is dependent on the homeodomain protein STF1/IPF1 acting through the CT boxes. *Proc Natl Acad Sci U S A* 1994;91:10465–10469.
53. Miller CP, McGehee RE Jr, Habener JF. IDX-1: a new homeodomain transcription factor expressed in rat pancreatic islets and duodenum that transactivates the somatostatin gene. *EMBO J* 1994;13:1145–1156.
54. Rudnick A, Ling TY, Odagiri H, et al. Pancreatic beta cells express a diverse set of homeobox genes. *Proc Natl Acad Sci U S A* 1994;91:12203–12207.
55. MacFarlane W, Read M, Gilligan M, et al. Glucose modulates the binding activity of the beta-cell transcription factor IUF1 in a phosphorylation-dependent manner. *Biochem J* 1994;303:625–631.
56. Marshak S, Totary H, Cerasi E, et al. Purification of the beta-cell glucose-sensitive factor that transactivates the insulin gene differentially in normal and transformed islet cells. *Proc Natl Acad Sci U S A* 1996;93:15057–15062.
57. Peshavaria M, Gamer L, Henderson E, et al. XIHbox 8, an endoderm-specific Xenopus homeodomain protein, is closely related to a mammalian insulin gene transcription factor. *Mol Endocrinol* 1994;8:806–816.
58. Serup P, Jensen J, Andersen FG, et al. Induction of insulin and islet amyloid polypeptide production in pancreatic islet glucagonoma cells by insulin promoter factor 1. *Proc Natl Acad Sci U S A* 1996;93:9015–9020.
59. Watada H, Kajimoto Y, Miyagawa J, et al. PDX-1 induces insulin and glucokinase gene expressions in alphaTC1 clone 6 cells in the presence of betacellulin. *Diabetes* 1996;45:1826–1831.
60. Jonsson J, Carlsson L, Edlund T, et al. Insulin-promoter-factor 1 is required for pancreas development in mice. *Nature* 1994;371:606–609.
61. Ahlgren U, Jonsson J, Edlund H. The morphogenesis of the pancreatic mesenchyme is uncoupled from that of the pancreatic epithelium in IPF1/PDX1-deficient mice. *Development* 1996;122:1409–1416.
62. Offield MF, Jetton TL, Labosky PA, et al. PDX-1 is required for pancreatic outgrowth and differentiation of the rostral duodenum. *Development* 1996;122: 983–995.
63. Ahlgren U, Jonsson J, Jonsson L, et al. Beta-cell-specific inactivation of the mouse Ipf1/Pdx1 gene results in loss of the beta-cell phenotype and maturity onset diabetes. *Genes Dev* 1998;12:1763–1768.
64. Karlsson O, Thor S, Norberg T, et al. Insulin gene enhancer binding protein Isl-1 is a member of a novel class of proteins containing both a homeo- and a Cys-His domain. *Nature* 1990;344:879–882.
65. German MS, Wang J, Chadwick RB, et al. Synergistic activation of the insulin gene by a LIM-homeodomain protein and a basic helix-loop-helix protein: building a functional insulin minienhancer complex. *Genes Dev* 1992;6: 2165–2176.
66. Emens LA, Landers DW, Moss LG. Hepatocyte nuclear factor 1a is expressed in a hamster insulinoma line and transactivates the rat insulin I gene. *Proc Natl Acad Sci U S A* 1992;89:7300–7304.
67. Ohlsson H, Edlund T. Sequence-specific interactions of nuclear factors with the insulin gene enhancer. *Cell* 1986;45:35–44.
68. Ohlsson H, Karlson O, Edlund T. A β-cell-specific protein binds to the two major regulatory sequences of the insulin enhancer. *Proc Natl Acad Sci U S A* 1988;85:4228–4231.
69. Ohlsson H, Thor S, Edlund T. Novel insulin promoter- and enhancer-binding proteins that discriminate between pancreatic alpha- and beta-cells. *Mol Endocrinol* 1991;5:897–904.
70. Knepel W, Jepeal L, Habener JF. A pancreatic islet cell-specific enhancer-like element in the glucagon gene contains two domains binding distinct cellular proteins. *J Biol Chem* 1990;265:8725–8735.

71. Knepel W, Vallejo M, Chafitz JA, et al. The pancreatic islet-specific glucagon G3 transcription factors recognize control elements in the rat somatostatin and insulin-I genes. *Mol Endocrinol* 1991;5:1457–1466.
72. Wrege A, Diedrich T, Hochhuth C, et al. Transcriptional activity of domain A of the rat glucagon G3 element conferred by an islet-specific nuclear protein that also binds to similar pancreatic islet cell-specific enhancer sequences (PISCES). *Gene Expr* 1995;4:205–216.
73. Sander M, Neubuser A, Kalamaras J, et al. Genetic analysis reveals that PAX6 is required for normal transcription of pancreatic hormone genes and islet development. *Genes Dev* 1997;11:1662–1673.
74. Czerny T, Schaffner G, Busslinger M. DNA sequence recognition by Pax proteins: bipartite structure of the paired domain and its binding site. *Genes Dev* 1993;7:2048–2061.
75. Czerny T, Busslinger M. DNA-binding and transactivation properties of Pax-6: three amino acids in the paired domain are responsible for the different sequence recognition of Pax-6 and BSAP (Pax-5). *Mol Cell Biol* 1995;15: 2858–2871.
76. Epstein JA, Glaser T, Cai J, et al. Two independent and interactive DNA-binding subdomains of the Pax6 paired domain are regulated by alternative splicing. *Genes Dev* 1994;8:2022–2034.
77. St-Onge L, Sosa-Pineda B, Chowdhury K, et al. Pax6 is required for differentiation of glucagon-producing alpha-cells in mouse pancreas. *Nature* 1997; 387:406–409.
78. Hwung YP, Gu YZ, Tsai MJ. Cooperativity of sequence elements mediates tissue specificity of the rat insulin II gene. *Mol Cell Biol* 1990;10:1784–1788.
79. Sharma A, Stein R. Glucose-induced transcription of the insulin gene is mediated by factors required for beta-cell-type-specific expression. *Mol Cell Biol* 1994;14:871–879.
80. Odagiri H, Wang J, German MS. Function of the human insulin promoter in primary cultured islet cells. *J Biol Chem* 1996;271:1909–1915.
81. Robinson GLWG, Peshavaria M, Henderson E, et al. Expression of the trans-active factors that simulate insulin control element-mediated activity appear to precede insulin gene transcription. *J Biol Chem* 1994;269:2452–2460.
82. Zhao L, Cissell MA, Henderson E, et al. The RIPE3b1 activator of the insulin gene is composed of a protein(s) of approximately 43 kDa, whose DNA binding activity is inhibited by protein phosphatase treatment. *J Biol Chem* 2000; 275:10532–10537.
83. Matsuoka T, Zhao L, Stein R. The DNA binding activity of the RIPE3b1 transcription factor of insulin appears to be influenced by tyrosine phosphorylation. *J Biol Chem* 2001;276:22071–22076.
84. Harrington RH, Sharma A. Transcription factors recognizing overlapping C1-A2 binding sites positively regulate insulin gene expression. *J Biol Chem* 2001;276:104–113.
85. Clark AR, Wilson ME, Leibiger I, et al. A silencer and an adjacent positive element interact to modulate the activity of the human insulin promoter. *Eur J Biochem* 1995;232:627–632.
86. Sander M, Griffen SC, Huang J, et al. A novel glucose-responsive element in the human insulin gene functions uniquely in primary cultured islets. *Proc Natl Acad Sci U S A* 1998;95:11572–11577.
87. German MS, Moss LG, Wang J, et al. The insulin and islet amyloid polypeptide genes contain similar cell-specific promoter elements that bind identical β-cell nuclear complexes. *Mol Cell Biol* 1992;12:1777–1788.
88. Karlsson O, Walker MD, Rutter WJ, et al. Individual protein-binding domains of the insulin gene enhancer positively activate β-cell-specific transcription. *Mol Cell Biol* 1989;9:823–827.
89. Peers B, Leonard J, Sharma S, et al. Insulin expression in pancreatic islet cells relies on cooperative interactions between the helix loop helix factor E47 and the homeobox factor STF-1. *Mol Endocrinol* 1994;8:1798–1806.
90. Peshavaria M, Henderson E, Sharma A, et al. Functional characterization of the transactivation properties of the PDX-1 homeodomain protein. *Mol Cell Biol* 1997;17:3987–3996.
91. Peshavaria M, Cissell MA, Henderson E, et al. The PDX-1 activation domain provides specific functions necessary for transcriptional stimulation in pancreatic beta-cells. *Mol Endocrinol* 2000;14:1907–1917.
92. Ohneda K, Mirmira RG, Wang J, et al. The homeodomain of PDX-1 mediates multiple protein-protein interactions in the formation of a transcriptional activation complex on the insulin promoter. *Mol Cell Biol* 2000;20:900–911.
93. Glick E, Leshkowitz D, Walker MD. Transcription factor BETA2 acts cooperatively with E2A and PDX1 to activate the insulin gene promoter. *J Biol Chem* 2000;275:2199–2204.
94. Grosschedl R. Higher-order nucleoprotein complexes in transcription: analogies with site-specific recombination. *Curr Opin Cell Biol* 1995;7:362–370.
95. Carey M. The enhanceosome and transcriptional synergy. *Cell* 1998;92:5–8.
96. Eckner R, Yao TP, Oldread E, et al. Interaction and functional collaboration of p300/CBP and bHLH proteins in muscle and B-cell differentiation. *Genes Dev* 1996;10:2478–2490.
97. Asahara H, Dutta S, Kao HY, et al. Pbx-Hox heterodimers recruit coactivator-corepressor complexes in an isoform-specific manner. *Mol Cell Biol* 1999;19: 8219–8225.
98. Sharma A, Henderson E, Gamer L, et al. Analysis of the role of E2A-encoded proteins in insulin gene transcription. *Mol Endocrinol* 1997;11:1608–1617.
99. Dutta S, Gannon M, Peers B, et al. PDX:PBX complexes are required for normal proliferation of pancreatic cells during development. *Proc Natl Acad Sci U S A* 2001;98:1065–1070.
100. Peers B, Sharma S, Johnson T, et al. The pancreatic islet factor STF-1 binds cooperatively with Pbx to a regulatory element in the somatostatin promoter: importance of the FPWMK motif and of the homeodomain. *Mol Cell Biol* 1995;15:7091–7097.
101. Newell-Price J, Clark AJ, King P. DNA methylation and silencing of gene expression. *Trends Endocrinol Metab* 2000;11:142–148.
102. Jenuwein T, Allis CD. Translating the histone code. *Science* 2001;293: 1074–1080.
103. Moazed D. Common themes in mechanisms of gene silencing. *Mol Cell* 2001; 8:489–498.
104. Nielsen DA, Welsh M, Casadaban MJ, et al. Control of insulin gene expression in pancreatic b-cells and in an insulin-producing cell line, RIN-5F cells I. Effects of glucose and cyclic AMP on the transcription of insulin mRNA. *J Biol Chem* 1985;260:13585–13589.
105. Welsh M, Nielsen DA, MacKrell AJ, et al. Control of insulin gene expression in pancreatic b-cells and in an insulin-producing cell line, RIN-5F cells II. Regulation of insulin mRNA stability. *J Biol Chem* 1985;260:13590–13594.
106. Wang J, Shen L, Najafi H, et al. Regulation of insulin preRNA splicing by glucose. *Proc Natl Acad Sci U S A* 1997;94:4360–4365.
107. Leibiger B, Moede T, Schwarz T, et al. Short-term regulation of insulin gene transcription by glucose. *Proc Natl Acad Sci U S A* 1998;95:9307–9312.
108. German MS, Moss LG, Rutter WJ. Regulation of insulin gene expression by glucose and calcium in transfected primary islet cultures. *J Biol Chem* 1990; 265:22063–22066.
109. Melloul D, Ben-Neriah Y, Cerasi E. Glucose modulates the binding of an islet-specific factor to a conserved sequence within the rat I and the human insulin promoters. *Proc Natl Acad Sci U S A* 1993;90:3865–3869.
110. Sharma A, Fusco-DeMane D, Henderson E, et al. The role of the insulin control element and RIPE3b1 activators in glucose-stimulated transcription of the insulin gene. *Mol Endocrinol* 1995;9:1468–1476.
111. Macfarlane WM, Smith SB, James RF, et al. The p38/reactivating kinase mitogen-activated protein kinase cascade mediates the activation of the transcription factor insulin upstream factor 1 and insulin gene transcription by high glucose in pancreatic beta-cells. *J Biol Chem* 1997;272:20936–20944.
112. Macfarlane WM, McKinnon CM, Felton-Edkins ZA, et al. Glucose stimulates translocation of the homeodomain transcription factor PDX1 from the cytoplasm to the nucleus in pancreatic beta-cells. *J Biol Chem* 1999;274:1011–1016.
113. Rafiq I, Kennedy HJ, Rutter GA. Glucose-dependent translocation of insulin promoter factor-1 (IPF-1) between the nuclear periphery and the nucleoplasm of single MIN6 beta-cells. *J Biol Chem* 1998;273:23241–23247.
114. Rafiq I, da Silva Xavier G, Hooper S, et al. Glucose-stimulated preproinsulin gene expression and nuclear translocation of pancreatic duodenum homeobox-1 require activation of phosphatidylinositol 3-kinase but not p38 MAPK/SAPK2. *J Biol Chem* 2000;275:15977–15984.
115. Petersen HV, Peshavaria M, Pedersen AA, et al. Glucose stimulates the activation domain potential of the PDX-1 homeodomain transcription factor. *FEBS Lett* 1998;431:362–366.
116. German MS. Glucose sensing in pancreatic islet beta cells: the key role of glucokinase and the glycolytic intermediates. *Proc Natl Acad Sci U S A* 1993;90: 1781–1785.
117. Leibiger IB, Leibiger B, Moede T, et al. Exocytosis of insulin promotes insulin gene transcription via the insulin receptor/PI-3 kinase/p70 s6 kinase and CaM kinase pathways. *Mol Cell* 1998;1:933–938.
118. Xu GG, Gao ZY, Borge PD Jr., et al. Insulin regulation of beta-cell function involves a feedback loop on SERCA gene expression, Ca(2+) homeostasis, and insulin expression and secretion. *Biochemistry* 2000;39:14912–14919.
119. Watada H, Kajimoto Y, Kaneto H, et al. Involvement of the homeodomain-containing transcription factor PDX-1 in islet amyloid polypeptide gene transcription. *Biochem Biophys Res Commun* 1996;229:746–751.
120. Watada H, Kajimoto Y, Umayahara Y, et al. The human glucokinase gene beta-cell-type promoter: an essential role of insulin promoter factor 1/PDX-1 in its activation in HIT-T15 cells. *Diabetes* 1996;45:1478–1488.
121. Waeber G, Thompson N, Nicod P, et al. Transcriptional activation of the GLUT2 gene by the IPF-1/STF-1/IDX-1 homeobox factor. *Mol Endocrinol* 1996;10:1327–1334.
122. Philippe J, Drucker DJ, Knepel W, et al. Alpha-cell-specific expression of the glucagon gene is conferred to the glucagon promoter element by the interactions of DNA-binding proteins. *Mol Cell Biol* 1988;8:4877–4888.
123. Drucker DJ, Philippe J, Jepeal L, et al. Glucagon gene 5′-flanking sequences promote islet cell-specific gene transcription. *J Biol Chem* 1987;262: 15659–15665.
124. Philippe J, Rochat S. Strict distance requirement for transcriptional activation by two regulatory elements of the glucagon gene. *DNA Cell Biol* 1991;10: 119–124.
125. Morel C, Cordier-Bussat M, Philippe J. The upstream promoter element of the glucagon gene, G1, confers pancreatic alpha cell-specific expression. *J Biol Chem* 1995;270:3046–3055.
126. Nian M, Drucker DJ, Irwin D. Divergent regulation of human and rat proglucagon gene promoters in vivo. *Am J Physiol* 1999;277:G829–G837.
127. Wang M, Drucker DJ. The LIM domain homeobox gene isl-1 is a positive regulator of islet cell-specific proglucagon gene transcription. *J Biol Chem* 1995; 270:12646–12652.
128. Jin T, Drucker DJ. Activation of proglucagon gene transcription through a novel promoter element by the caudal-related homeodomain protein cdx-2/3. *Mol Cell Biol* 1996;16:19–28.
129. Jin T, Trinh DK, Wang F, et al. The caudal homeobox protein cdx-2/3 activates endogenous proglucagon gene expression in InR1-G9 islet cells. *Mol Endocrinol* 1997;11:203–209.

130. Laser B, Meda P, Constant I, et al. The caudal-related homeodomain protein Cdx-2/3 regulates glucagon gene expression in islet cells. *J Biol Chem* 1996; 271:28984–28994.
131. Cordier-Bussat M, Morel C, Philippe J. Homologous DNA sequences and cellular factors are implicated in the control of glucagon and insulin gene expression. *Mol Cell Biol* 1995;15:3904–3916.
132. Dumonteil E, Laser B, Constant I, et al. Differential regulation of the glucagon and insulin I gene promoters by the basic helix-loop-helix transcription factors E47 and BETA2. *J Biol Chem* 1998;273:19945–19954.
133. Hussain MA, Lee J, Miller CP, et al. POU domain transcription factor brain 4 confers pancreatic alpha-cell-specific expression of the proglucagon gene through interaction with a novel proximal promoter G1 element. *Mol Cell Biol* 1997;17:7186–7194.
134. Wang H, Maechler P, Ritz-Laser B, et al. Pdx1 level defines pancreatic gene expression pattern and cell lineage differentiation. *J Biol Chem* 2001;276: 25279–25286.
135. Hill ME, Asa SL, Drucker DJ. Essential requirement for Pax6 in control of enteroendocrine proglucagon gene transcription. *Mol Endocrinol* 1999;13: 1474–1486.
136. Andersen FG, Heller RS, Petersen HV, et al. Pax6 and Cdx2/3 form a functional complex on the rat glucagon gene promoter G1-element. *FEBS Lett* 1999;445:306–310.
137. Hussain MA, Habener JF. Glucagon gene transcription activation mediated by synergistic interactions of pax-6 and cdx-2 with the p300 co-activator. *J Biol Chem* 1999;274:28950–28957.
138. Ritz-Laser B, Estreicher A, Klages N, et al. Pax-6 and Cdx-2/3 interact to activate glucagon gene expression on the G1 control element. *J Biol Chem* 1999; 274:4124–4132.
139. Diedrich T, Furstenau U, Knepel W. Glucagon gene G3 enhancer: evidence that activity depends on combination of an islet-specific factor and a winged helix protein. *Biol Chem* 1997;378:89–98.
140. Philippe J. Hepatocyte-nuclear factor 3 beta gene transcripts generate protein isoforms with different transactivation properties on the glucagon gene. *Mol Endocrinol* 1995;9:368–374.
141. Furstenau U, Schwaninger M, Blume R, et al. Characterization of a novel protein kinase C response element in the glucagon gene. *Mol Cell Biol* 1997;17: 1805–1816.
142. Furstenau U, Schwaninger M, Blume R, et al. Characterization of a novel calcium response element in the glucagon gene. *J Biol Chem* 1999;274:5851–5860.
143. Grzeskowiak R, Amin J, Oetjen E, et al. Insulin responsiveness of the glucagon gene conferred by interactions between proximal promoter and more distal enhancer-like elements involving the paired-domain transcription factor Pax6. *J Biol Chem* 2000;275:30037–30045.
144. Planque N, Leconte L, Coquelle FM, et al. Interaction of Maf transcription factors with Pax-6 results in synergistic activation of the glucagon promoter. *J Biol Chem* 2001;276:35751–35760.
145. Herzig S, Fuzesi L, Knepel W. Heterodimeric Pbx-Prep1 homeodomain protein binding to the glucagon gene restricting transcription in a cell type-dependent manner. *J Biol Chem* 2000;275:27989–27999.
146. Kaestner KH, Katz J, Liu Y, et al. Inactivation of the winged helix transcription factor HNF3alpha affects glucose homeostasis and islet glucagon gene expression in vivo. *Genes Dev* 1999;13:495–504.
147. Philippe J, Morel C, Cordier-Bussat M. Islet-specific proteins interact with the insulin-response element of the glucagon gene. *J Biol Chem* 1995;270: 3039–3045.
148. Philippe J. Insulin regulation of the glucagon gene is mediated by an insulin-responsive DNA element. *Proc Natl Acad Sci U S A* 1991;88:7224–7227.
149. Yamagata K, Furuta H, Oda N, et al. Mutations in the hepatocyte nuclear factor-4alpha gene in maturity-onset diabetes of the young (MODY1). *Nature* 1996;384:458–460.
150. Yamagata K, Oda N, Kaisaki P, et al. Mutations in the hepatocyte nuclear factor-1alpha gene in maturity-onset diabetes of the young (MODY3). *Nature* 1996;384:455–458.
151. Stoffers DA, Ferrer J, Clarke WL, et al. Early-onset type-II diabetes mellitus (MODY4) linked to IPF1 [letter]. *Nat Genet* 1997;17:138–139.
152. Horikawa Y, Iwasaki N, Hara M, et al. Mutation in hepatocyte nuclear factor-1 beta gene (TCF2) associated with MODY [letter]. *Nat Genet* 1997;17:384–385.
153. Malecki MT, Jhala US, Antonellis A, et al. Mutations in NEUROD1 are associated with the development of type 2 diabetes mellitus. *Nat Genet* 1999;23: 323–328.
154. Shimomura H, Sanke T, Hanabusa T, et al. Nonsense mutation of islet-1 gene (Q310X) found in a type 2 diabetic patient with a strong family history. *Diabetes* 2000;49:1597–1600.
155. Stoffel M, Duncan SA. The maturity-onset diabetes of the young (MODY1) transcription factor HNF4alpha regulates expression of genes required for glucose transport and metabolism. *Proc Natl Acad Sci U S A* 1997;94: 13209–13214.
156. Duncan SA, Navas MA, Dufort D, et al. Regulation of a transcription factor network required for differentiation and metabolism. *Science* 1998;281: 692–695.
157. Shih DQ, Screenan S, Munoz KN, et al. Loss of HNF-1alpha function in mice leads to abnormal expression of genes involved in pancreatic islet development and metabolism. *Diabetes* 2001;50:2472–2480.
158. Dukes ID, Sreenan S, Roe MW, et al. Defective pancreatic beta-cell glycolytic signaling in hepatocyte nuclear factor-1alpha-deficient mice. *J Biol Chem* 1998;273:24457–24464.
159. Pontoglio M, Sreenan S, Roe M, et al. Defective insulin secretion in hepatocyte nuclear factor 1alpha-deficient mice. *J Clin Invest* 1998;101:2215–2222.
160. Apelqvist A, Li H, Sommer L, et al. Notch signalling controls pancreatic cell differentiation. *Nature* 1999;400:877–881.
161. Gradwohl G, Dierich A, LeMeur M, et al. Neurogenin3 is required for the development of the four endocrine cell lineages of the pancreas. *Proc Natl Acad Sci U S A* 2000;97:1607–1611.
162. Huang HP, Liu M, El-Hodiri HM, et al. Regulation of the pancreatic islet-specific gene BETA2 (neuroD) by neurogenin 3. *Mol Cell Biol* 2000;20:3292–3307.
163. Schwitzgebel VM, Scheel DW, Conners JR, et al. Expression of neurogenin3 reveals an islet cell precursor population in the pancreas. *Development* 2000; 127:3533–3542.
164. Stoffers DA, Zinkin NT, Stanojevic V, et al. Pancreatic agenesis attributable to a single nucleotide deletion in the human IPF1 gene coding sequence. *Nat Genet* 1997;15:106–110.
165. Guz Y, Montminy MR, Stein R, et al. Expression of murine STF-1, a putative insulin gene transcription factor, in beta cells of pancreas, duodenal epithelium and pancreatic exocrine and endocrine progenitors during ontogeny. *Development* 1995;121:11–18.
166. Harrison KA, Druey KM, Deguchi Y, et al. A novel human homeobox gene distantly related to proboscipedia is expressed in lymphoid and pancreatic tissues. *J Biol Chem* 1994;269:19968–19975.
167. Harrison KA, Thaler J, Pfaff SL, et al. Pancreas dorsal lobe agenesis and abnormal islets of Langerhans in Hlxb9-deficient mice. *Nat Genet* 1999;23: 71–75.
168. Li H, Arber S, Jessell TM, et al. Selective agenesis of the dorsal pancreas in mice lacking homeobox gene Hlxb9. *Nat Genet* 1999;23:67–70.
169. Torres M, Gómez-Pardo E, Gruss P. Pax2 contributes to inner ear patterning and optic nerve trajectory. *Development* 1996;122:3381–3391.
170. Ritz-Laser B, Estreicher A, Gauthier B, et al. The paired homeodomain transcription factor Pax-2 is expressed in the endocrine pancreas and transactivates the glucagon gene promoter. *J Biol Chem* 2000;275:32708–32715.
171. Smith S, Watada H, Scheel D, et al. Autoregulation and maturity onset diabetes of the young transcription factors control the human PAX4 promoter. *J Biol Chem* 2000;275:36910–36919.
172. Smith SB, Ee HC, Conners JR, et al. Paired-homeodomain transcription factor PAX4 acts as a transcriptional repressor in early pancreatic development. *Mol Cell Biol* 1999;19:8272–8280.
173. Sosa-Pineda B, Chowdhury K, Torres M, et al. The Pax4 gene is essential for differentiation of insulin-producing beta cells in the mammalian pancreas. *Nature* 1997;386:399–402.
174. Sussel L, Kalamaras J, Hartigan-O'Connor DJ, et al. Mice lacking the homeodomain transcription factor Nkx2.2 have diabetes due to arrested differentiation of pancreatic beta cells. *Development* 1998;125:2213–2221.
175. Watada H, Mirmira RG, Leung J, et al. Transcriptional and translational regulation of beta-cell differentiation factor Nkx6.1. *J Biol Chem* 2000;275: 34224–34230.
176. Jensen J, Serup P, Karlsen C, et al. mRNA profiling of rat islet tumors reveals nkx 6.1 as a beta-cell-specific homeodomain transcription factor. *J Biol Chem* 1996;271:18749–18758.
177. Chawengsaksophak K, James R, Hammond VE, et al. Homeosis and intestinal tumours in Cdx2 mutant mice. *Nature* 1997;386:84–87.
178. Vallejo M, Penchuk L, Habener JF. Somatostatin gene upstream enhancer element activated by a protein complex consisting of CREB, Isl-1-like, and alpha-CBF-like transcription factors. *J Biol Chem* 1992;267:12876–12884.
179. Leonard J, Serup P, Gonzalez G, et al. The LIM family transcription factor Isl-1 requires cAMP response element binding protein to promote somatostatin expression in pancreatic islet cells. *Proc Natl Acad Sci U S A* 1992;89:6247–6251.
180. Thor S, Ericson J, Brannstrom T, et al. The homeodomain LIM protein isl-I is expressed in subsets of neurons and endocrine cells in the adult rat. *Neuron* 1991;7:1–9.
181. Dong J, Asa SL, Drucker DJ. Islet cell and extrapancreatic expression of the LIM domain homeobox gene isl-1. *Mol Endocrinol* 1991;5:1633–1641.
182. Millonig JH, Millen KJ, Hatten ME. The mouse Dreher gene Lmx1a controls formation of the roof plate in the vertebrate CNS [see comments]. *Nature* 2000;403:764–769.
183. Phippard D, Heydemann A, Lechner M, et al. Changes in the subcellular localization of the Brn4 gene product precede mesenchymal remodeling of the otic capsule. *Heart Res* 1998;120:77–85.
184. Noguchi T, Yamada K, Yamagata K, et al. Expression of liver type pyruvate kinase in insulinoma cells: involvement of LF-B1 (HNF1). *Biochem Biophys Res Commun* 1991;181:259–264.
185. Lee JC, Smith SB, Watada H, et al. Regulation of the pancreatic pro-endocrine gene neurogenin3. *Diabetes* 2001;50:928–936.
186. Coffinier C, Thepot D, Babinet C, et al. Essential role for the homeoprotein vHNF1/HNF1beta in visceral endoderm differentiation. *Development* 1999; 126:4785–4794.
187. Coffinier C, Barra J, Babinet C, et al. Expression of the vHNF1/HNF1beta homeoprotein gene during mouse organogenesis. *Mech Dev* 1999;89:211–213.
188. Lemaigre FP, Durviaux SM, Truong O, et al. Hepatocyte nuclear factor 6, a transcription factor that contains a novel type of homeodomain and a single cut domain. *Proc Natl Acad Sci U S A* 1996;93:9460–9464.
189. Landry C, Clotman F, Hioki T, et al. HNF-6 is expressed in endoderm derivatives and nervous system of the mouse embryo and participates to the cross-regulatory network of liver-enriched transcription factors. *Dev Biol* 1997;192:247–257.

190. Rausa FM, Ye H, Lim L, et al. In situ hybridization with 33P-labeled RNA probes for determination of cellular expression patterns of liver transcription factors in mouse embryos [published erratum appears in Methods 1998 Nov; 16(3):359–360]. *Methods* 1998;16:29–41.
191. Jacquemin P, Durviaux SM, Jensen J, et al. Transcription factor hepatocyte nuclear factor 6 regulates pancreatic endocrine cell differentiation and controls expression of the proendocrine gene ngn3. *Mol Cell Biol* 2000;20: 4445–4454.
192. Rausa F, Samadani U, Ye H, et al. The cut-homeodomain transcriptional activator HNF-6 is coexpressed with its target gene HNF-3 beta in the developing murine liver and pancreas. *Dev Biol* 1997;192:228–246.
193. Shih DQ, Navas MA, Kuwajima S, et al. Impaired glucose homeostasis and neonatal mortality in hepatocyte nuclear factor 3alpha-deficient mice. *Proc Natl Acad Sci U S A* 1999;96:10152–10157.
194. Wu KL, Gannon M, Peshavaria M, et al. Hepatocyte nuclear factor 3beta is involved in pancreatic beta-cell-specific transcription of the pdx-1 gene. *Mol Cell Biol* 1997;17:6002–6013.
195. Rausa FM, Galarneau L, Belanger L, et al. The nuclear receptor fetoprotein transcription factor is coexpressed with its target gene HNF-3beta in the developing murine liver, intestine and pancreas. *Mech Dev* 1999;89:185–188.
196. Gerrish K, Gannon M, Shih D, et al. Pancreatic beta cell-specific transcription of the pdx-1 gene. The role of conserved upstream control regions and their hepatic nuclear factor 3beta sites. *J Biol Chem* 2000;275:3485–3492.
197. Sharma S, Jhala US, Johnson T, et al. Hormonal regulation of an islet-specific enhancer in the pancreatic homeobox gene STF-1. *Mol Cell Biol* 1997;17: 2598–2604.
198. Sladek FM, Zhong WM, Lai E, et al. Liver-enriched transcription factor HNF-4 is a novel member of the steroid hormone receptor superfamily. *Genes Dev* 1990;4:2353–2365.
199. Duncan SA, Manova K, Chen WS, et al. Expression of transcription factor HNF-4 in the extraembryonic endoderm, gut, and nephrogenic tissue of the developing mouse embryo: HNF-4 is a marker for primary endoderm in the implanting blastocyst. *Proc Natl Acad Sci U S A* 1994;91:7598–7602.
200. Miquerol L, Lopez S, Cartier N, et al. Expression of the L-type pyruvate kinase gene and the hepatocyte nuclear factor 4 transcription factor in exocrine and endocrine pancreas. *J Biol Chem* 1994;269:8944–8951.

CHAPTER 5

Insulin Biosynthesis, Processing, and Chemistry

Christopher J. Rhodes, Steven Shoelson, and Philippe A. Halban

Insulin, the major hormonal regulator of glucose metabolism, was first isolated from pancreatic tissue in 1921 by Banting and Best (1). Shortly after the discovery of insulin, the impure extract was used experimentally to treat pancreatectomized dogs (2) and patients with diabetes mellitus (3). As soon as it became clear that the hormone was effective, both the amount of extract isolated and the degree of its purity were increased. Insulin was thus made available to patients with diabetes mellitus. The treatment of such patients underwent a remarkable revolution within 1 to 2 years of the initial discovery of insulin. However, many aspects of insulin biochemistry and chemistry were not understood until years later, and some of these topics remain as areas of intense investigation. This chapter will focus on the biosynthesis of insulin, from insulin gene to secretory granule; the chemistry and structure of insulin; and abnormalities in insulin structure that affect its action or biosynthetic processing.

INSULIN PRODUCTION

In mammals, expression of the insulin gene and insulin biosynthesis are restricted to the β-cells of the endocrine pancreas (4), with the possible exception of the yolk sac and fetal liver (5,6). This exquisite tissue selectivity is conferred upon the insulin gene by a complex interplay between upstream *cis*-elements (short DNA sequences) and cellular *trans*-acting factors (proteins) that bind to the DNA and regulate expression (refer to Chapters 2 and 4). The primary function of the pancreatic β-cell is the production, storage, and regulated secretion of insulin. Under normal circumstances, the β-cell maintains a condition such that there is always a readily available pool of insulin that can be rapidly secreted in response to a stimulus, such as an increase in blood glucose level. Any increase in insulin release is compensated for by a corresponding increase in insulin biosynthesis, so that β-cell insulin stores are constantly maintained. Thus, the biosynthesis and processing of the insulin molecule along the secretory pathway of the β-cell is a highly regulated and dynamic process.

Translation of Preproinsulin and Conversion to Proinsulin

Although the two-chain structure of insulin had been known since 1955 (7), it was not until 1967 that Steiner et al. (8,9) first presented evidence for a single-chain biosynthetic precursor, proinsulin. The identification of a hormone precursor was profound for our understanding not only of insulin synthesis but also of protein synthesis in general. It is now evident that there is also a protein precursor for proinsulin, preproinsulin (10,11) (Fig. 5.1), with (for the human protein) the first 24 amino acids forming a signal peptide. The role of signal peptides in the translocation of nascent proteins to the lumen of the rough endoplasmic reticulum (RER) was first elucidated by Gunter Blobel and colleagues (12), and he was awarded the Nobel Prize for this work in 1999. As preproinsulin is synthesized, the signal peptide is bound by the signal-recognition particle (SRP), which in turn homes to the SRP receptor on the membrane of the RER (13). These events occur after the addition of the first 70 to 80 amino acids to the growing preproinsulin chain (14,15). The signal peptide is rich in hydrophobic residues, facilitating the penetration of the RER membrane. Penetration occurs rapidly, and the rest of the nascent preproinsulin molecule then crosses into the lumen of the RER. A signal peptidase within the RER causes cleavage of the signal peptide from preproinsulin to yield intact proinsulin. This proteolytic event arises for the most part cotranslationally, so that preproinsulin is a very minor constituent of the β-cell (16).

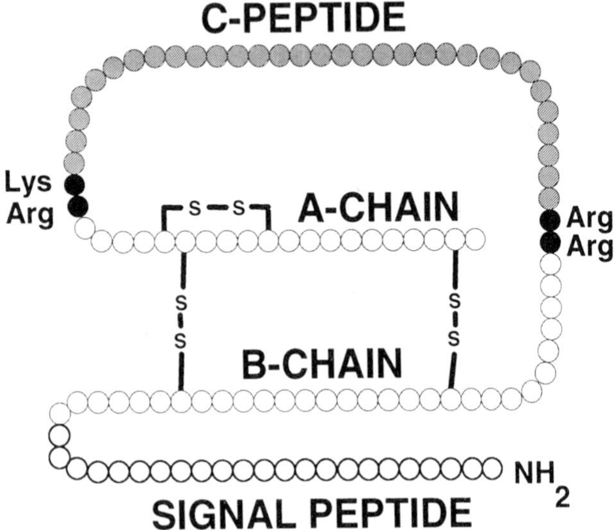

Figure 5.1. Preproinsulin. The initial, high-molecular-weight precursor of insulin consists of four distinct domains. The signal (or pre-) peptide occupies the first (amino-terminal) 24 residues (human preproinsulin) and is cleaved off within the lumen of the rough endoplasmic reticulum to produce proinsulin. Conversion of proinsulin to insulin arises at the pairs of basic residues linking the two insulin (A- and B-) chains to the C- (connecting) peptide, as depicted in Figure 5.3. The two insulin chains are joined together by two disulfide bridges. The molecular mass of insulin is approximately 5,800 daltons.

Regulation of Insulin Biosynthesis in the β-Cell

The rate of proinsulin biosynthesis is controlled by many factors, including nutrients, neurotransmitters, and hormones (17–20). The most physiologically relevant of these is glucose (21). The initial studies on the regulation of biosynthesis were limited to measuring the rate of incorporation of labeled amino acid into insulin or its precursors. The earliest of these studies, dating from the 1960s (22–26), showed that glucose *specifically* stimulated (pro)insulin biosynthesis *in vitro* above that of general protein synthesis in the β-cell. As for insulin secretion, the metabolism of glucose is necessary to generate intracellular signals to stimulate insulin biosynthesis (21,26–29). However, while the threshold concentration of glucose required to stimulate insulin secretion is 4 to 6 mM, that required to stimulate insulin biosynthesis is lower—between 2 and 4 mM (28–31). Maximum proinsulin biosynthesis is reached at a glucose concentration of 10 to 12 mM (21,28,29). As well as glucose (21,30,32–34), other sugars (21,23,27,35) and nutrients, including leucine (36), succinate (37), pyruvate (38), inosine, guanosine, adenosine, and ribose (30,39,40), are capable of stimulating insulin biosynthesis but are generally less effective than glucose. After exposure of pancreatic islet β-cells to a glucose stimulus, there is about a 20-minute lag period before there is any significant increase in proinsulin biosynthesis. By 60 minutes, the rate of proinsulin synthesis is stimulated 10- to 20-fold (28,29,41). Upon removal of the stimulus, downregulation of proinsulin biosynthesis is relatively slow, taking more than 1 hour to return to a basal rate (41).

Certain hormones also specifically stimulate insulin biosynthesis, such as growth hormone (42,43), glucagon (44), and glucagon-like peptide-1 (GLP-1) (45). Glucagon and GLP-1 stimulate insulin biosynthesis via a cyclic adenosine monophosphate (cAMP)–dependent pathway; and indeed, cAMP itself can potentiate glucose-induced proinsulin biosynthesis (30–32,44,46,47). As for insulin secretion, epinephrine inhibits glucose-induced insulin synthesis (46). Whereas somatostatin is a potent inhibitor of insulin secretion, it has no effect on proinsulin biosynthesis (48,49). Relevant to cytokine-mediated β-cell destruction in type 1 diabetes mellitus, it has been shown that interferons can inhibit insulin biosynthesis, but only at extremely high concentrations (50–52). Depending on the concentration used, interleukin-1 can either stimulate or inhibit insulin biosynthesis (52–54). The rate of proinsulin biosynthesis is also increased in pregnancy (55,56) and obesity (57,58) as well as during *in vivo* glucose infusions (59–61), but in these examples, it is in association with increased β-cell mass and islet hyperplasia. On the other hand, in other physiologic or pathophysiologic states, such as aging (62), some animal models of type 2 diabetes mellitus (63,64), or during starvation (38,55,65), there is a degree of inhibition of proinsulin synthesis. However, it is not entirely clear whether this is reflective of decreased β-cell mass.

In general, nutrients that are efficiently metabolized in β-cells stimulate insulin secretion and proinsulin biosynthesis at the translational level in parallel (19,20). This provides an ideal situation where insulin released from the β-cell is rapidly replenished at the biosynthetic level by the same stimulus. However, unlike the metabolic stimulus-response coupling for regulation of insulin secretion (refer to Chapter 6 and references 66–71), information regarding that for proinsulin biosynthesis is lacking. In all likelihood, beyond a requirement for glucose metabolism, the mechanism responsible for stimulus coupling of proinsulin biosynthesis differs from that for insulin secretion.

There are several lines of evidence to suggest this is so. Extracellular Ca^{2+} is essential for glucose-induced insulin release, but proinsulin biosynthesis is independent of Ca^{2+} (66,72). Likewise, inhibitors of Ca^{2+} calmodulin kinase activity (e.g., trifluoperazine) inhibit insulin release (73,74) but have no effect on proinsulin biosynthesis (75). In contrast, Mg^{2+} appears to be a requirement of proinsulin biosynthesis, but not necessarily of insulin release (47). Sulfonylureas, which close the β-cell K_{ATP}-channel in a key step in signal transduction for glucose-induced insulin release (refer to Chapter 6) (69,71), are very effective at inducing insulin release but appear to have little effect on proinsulin biosynthesis (25,76,77). Likewise, diazoxide that keeps the β-cell K_{ATP}-channel open (78) inhibits insulin release (67) but not proinsulin biosynthesis (47). Long-chain fatty acids are marked potentiators of insulin release (79–81) but have a tendency to inhibit glucose-induced proinsulin biosynthesis (38,49). Protein kinase C has been involved in stimulus coupling for insulin secretion (82) but does not appear to be related to the specific regulation of proinsulin biosynthesis (38,49,83,84).

In the early 1970s, Permutt and Kipnis convincingly demonstrated that glucose regulation occurred at both the pretranscriptional and posttranscriptional levels (85–87) and that translation was affected by modulating initiation and, to a lesser extent, by the rate of elongation (87). Such translational regulation by glucose was confirmed by experiments using cell-free systems (88–90). Subsequent studies have found that short-term (less than 4 hours) glucose stimulation of pancreatic islets does not alter the total amount of preproinsulin messenger RNA (mRNA) in a β-cell, even though proinsulin biosynthesis is increased 10- to 20-fold (21,83,91–93). Moreover, short-term glucose-induced proinsulin biosynthesis is unaffected by inhibition of insulin gene transcription (28,85). Thus, short-term proinsulin biosynthesis is principally controlled by translational regulation of preexisting preproinsulin mRNA (19,76). Although total preproinsulin mRNA levels in the β-cell are unchanged, upon an increase in glucose level, preproinsulin mRNA is redistributed from a cytosolic storage pool to polysomes associated with the RER, the major site of proinsulin biosynthesis (4,91,93,94). This reaffirmed that glucose primarily influences the initiation phase of preproinsulin mRNA translation (95–98). The additional glucose-mediated regulation at the elongation phase of translation [below 3 mM glucose; see references (93,99)] and at SRP–SRP-receptor interaction (91,93) is likely adaptive to the primary regulation at the initiation phase of preproinsulin mRNA translation (91,93,100). For general protein synthesis, translational regulation occurs primarily at the initiation phase (98); however, glucose specifically stimulates proinsulin biosynthesis above that of general protein synthesis in the β-cell. Thus, translational control of proinsulin biosynthesis is a relatively exclusive mechanism (21,83,85,100). Although the details of this mechanism have yet to be defined, it is currently thought that there are specific elements within preproinsulin mRNA that control its rate of translation and consequently the biosynthesis of proinsulin (20,100,101). This is analogous to specific translational regulation of ferritin biosynthesis by iron (102).

Under normal physiologic circumstances, where a glucose stimulus lasts no longer than 2 to 3 hours, control of proinsulin biosynthesis is mediated entirely at the translational level (18,28,38,83,93). However, for prolonged exposure to glucose (greater than 4 hours), such as the hyperglycemia in animal models of non–insulin-dependent diabetes mellitus (NIDDM) (103,104), a degree of transcriptional regulation (59,64,105,106) and changes in mRNA stability (107) additionally contribute to the control of proinsulin biosynthesis. During starvation or prolonged hypoglycemia, levels of preproinsulin mRNA are markedly reduced (108,109), in turn reducing proinsulin biosynthesis (55,65). When animals are re-fed after a period of starvation, levels of preproinsulin mRNA rapidly return to normal, allowing proinsulin biosynthesis to recover (108).

Intracellular Trafficking of Proinsulin

From the moment of synthesis, insulin and its precursors, like all secretory proteins, are enveloped in a limiting membrane and as such are protected from the cytosol. The passage from one subcellular compartment to the next occurs by the successive budding and fusion of carrier vesicles, culminating in formation of the mature secretory granule and the ultimate fusion event, exocytosis (Fig. 5.2). These events, initially outlined in pioneering studies by Nobel laureate George Palade (110), provided the point of departure for Orci's seminal studies on the cell biology of the insulin-producing β-cell (4,111,112). Our understanding of these events, and in particular that of the regulated secretory pathway adopted by insulin and its precursors (113–116), has progressed, but remains incomplete in its fine molecular detail.

Once in the RER, proinsulin undergoes appropriate folding so that the disulfide linkage between the A- and B-chains of insulin are correctly aligned. Properly folded proinsulin is then delivered to the *cis*–Golgi apparatus from the RER in transport vesicles in an ATP-dependent process (117,118). The RER to *cis*–Golgi transport mechanism also requires integrity of the β-cell's microtubular network (119), Ca^{2+} (120), guanosine triphosphate (120,121), and certain cytosolic protein factors (120–125). Trafficking of proinsulin from the stacks of *cis*—via the *medial*—to the *trans*–Golgi apparatus is mediated by vesicles reversibly encased by members of the COP family of coatomer-proteins (118,126–128). Intercisternal transport between Golgi stacks also requires several cytosolic factors and various membrane proteins (118,120,125,126,129–134). Once delivered to the *trans*–Golgi network (TGN), proinsulin is separated from other secretory and integral membrane proteins destined for the constitutive pathway and from enzymes destined for lysosomes (116).

Sorting of Proinsulin to the Regulated Secretory Pathway

Secretion of insulin or other proteins can proceed through either constitutive or regulated pathways (113,135,136). All cells use the constitutive secretory pathway, both for secretion and to dispatch integral membrane proteins to their appropriate destinations. Only a few highly differentiated secretory cell types can store products in secretory granules and release them in response to a secretagogue, however. The β-cell is equipped with both these pathways but under normal circumstances directs proinsulin almost exclusively to the regulated pathway (137). The pattern of release using these two pathways is quite different (113). As its name implies, the constitutive pathway is not subject to control by secretagogues. It arises by the rapid transport of proteins from the *trans*-Golgi to the plasma membrane in small vesicles (transit time, approximately 10 minutes). For proteins inserted in the vesicle membrane (i.e., cell-surface receptors), fusion of the vesicle with the plasma membrane results in presentation to the extracellular environment, whereas proteins in solution in the transport vesicles are secreted.

The regulated pathway involves the selective packaging of secretory proteins (for the most part in the form of proproteins, and notably prohormones) into secretory granules, followed by

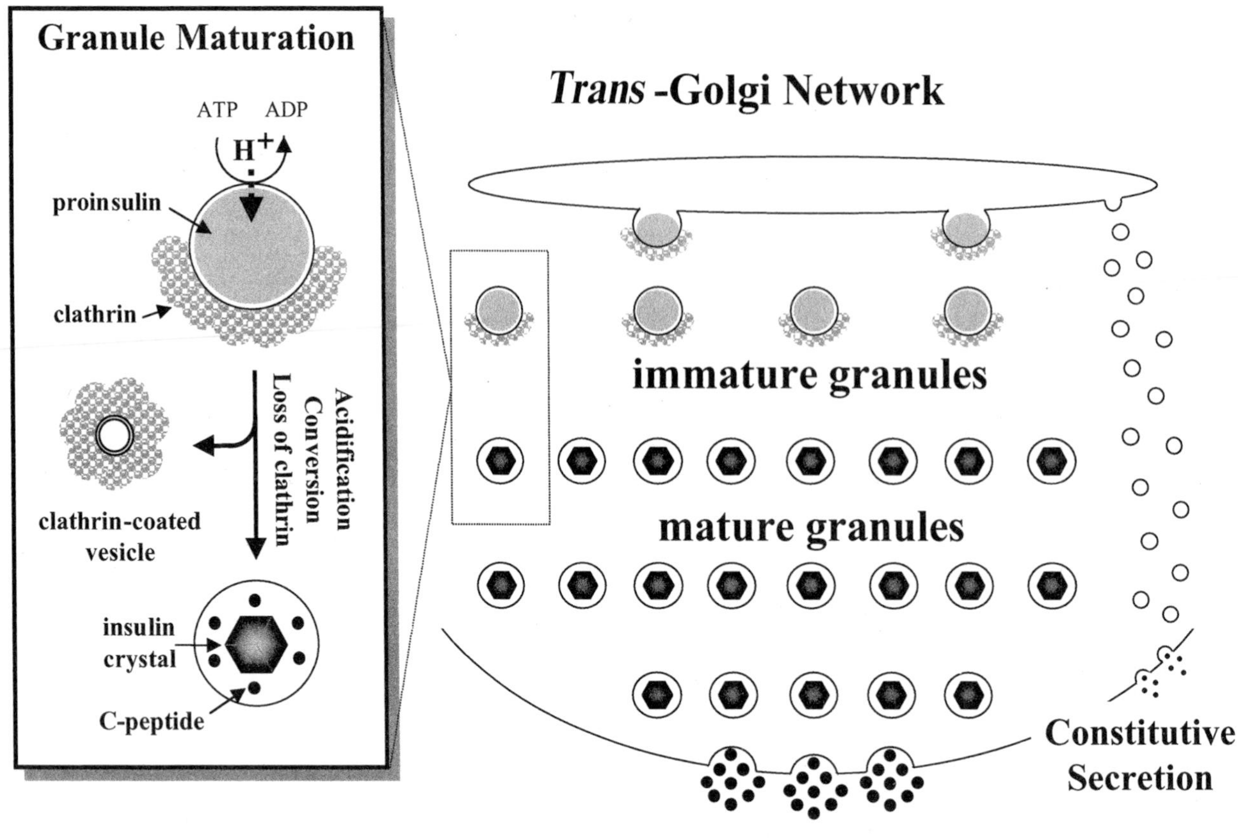

Figure 5.2. Trafficking and processing in the pathway of insulin production by the pancreatic β-cell. Only those steps arising after delivery of proinsulin from the rough endoplasmic reticulum to the *trans*-Golgi network are depicted. For clarity, some steps have been intentionally oversimplified and some critical processes omitted (e.g., granule degradation by crinophagy). The inset shows the major events involved in the maturation of the clathrin-coated, proinsulin-rich immature granule to the uncoated, insulin-rich mature granule. Clathrin-coated vesicles are presumed to bud from maturing granules and to be destined for the endosomal compartment (delivering their contents thereafter to lysosomes or the extracellular space). Little if any proinsulin is released via the constitutive pathway under normal circumstances. ATP, adenosine triphosphate; ADP, adenosine diphosphate.

secretion (exocytosis) in response to a stimulus. Active selection of proinsulin destined for granules is known to take place in the *trans*-most cisternae of the Golgi complex (138). The constitutive pathway, by contrast, is considered to be a default route, accepting any material in the *trans*-Golgi not previously singled out for shipment to a specific destination. In the rat, the sorting process has been shown to be remarkably effective, with more than 99% of newly synthesized proinsulin entering the regulated secretory pathway (137). If this is the case for primary β-cells, sorting to granules appears to be less efficient in transformed cells (139).

The selection process for directing prohormones to granules is not well understood. There is morphologic evidence for an intimate association of proinsulin with the cisternal face of Golgi membranes, suggestive of the presence of receptors (140). If such receptors exist, their unequivocal identification remains elusive. Thus, the postulated role of carboxypeptidase E (also known as carboxypeptidase H), an enzyme involved in the trimming of prohormones following endoproteolytic cleavage (see below), as such a receptor (141–143) has been challenged both in general terms (144) and more specifically in the context of proinsulin sorting (145–147). An alternative sorting mechanism implicates selective protein aggregation in the TGN, leading to concentration/condensation in intimate association with the TGN membrane (116,148–150). It is proposed in this model mechanism that common physicochemical properties of secretory-granule proteins allow them to aggregate (or coaggregate) in the presence of an elevated Ca^{2+} concentration and a mildly acidic pH as encountered in the internal environment of the TGN (116,149–153) and that this event in itself promotes budding of a nascent granule. However, sorting by aggregation is likely to be a complex mechanism, considering that 50 to 100 β-granule proteins (154,155) must be coordinately delivered to the site of secretory granule biogenesis (59,154,156).

Regardless of the true TGN sorting mechanism, it is commonly supposed to be similar in all cells equipped with the regulated pathway. This conclusion is based in part upon the results of experiments in which cells are transfected with genes for foreign proteins. For example, AtT20 (pituitary corticotroph) cells can target foreign secretory peptides such as proinsulin (157) or growth hormone (158) as well as exocrine enzymes such as trypsinogen (159) to secretory granules. Furthermore, a protein normally destined for the constitutive pathway can be rerouted to secretory granules and regulated release if fused to the appropriate sequences of the growth-hormone molecule (160). The last experiment indicates that the targeting machinery must recognize functional domains on the secretory protein. By analogy, there must be functional domains on the proinsulin molecule allowing for its recognition and targeting to the regulated pathway (161). If so, they remain to be identified and characterized experimentally. Although a mutant proinsulin (with aspartate instead of histidine in position 10 of the B-chain) has been shown to be diverted from the regulated to the constitutive pathway (162,163), the reason is not clear. It could be due to perturbation to a "sorting domain," lack of coordination of Zn^{2+} needed for hexamerization [unlikely because another mutant proinsulin unable to form hexamers appears well sorted (164)], or to more esoteric reasons related to the enhanced binding of this particular mutant proinsulin to the insulin receptor (163,165).

The Clathrin-Coated, Immature Secretory Granule

The earliest detectable form of the secretory granule in β-cells is formed from regions of the *trans*-Golgi characterized by the presence of clathrin on their cytosolic face (166), and the immature granule similarly carries a partial coating of clathrin (111). Clathrin consists of two chains, which can associate to form a network of triskelions and cover membranes with a basket-like coat (167–169). The assembly of a clathrin coat depends on associated proteins, and coating of secretory granules involves the adaptor protein AP-1 (149,170) as well as ADP-ribosylation factor-1 (ARF-1) (170,171). It appears increasingly likely that clathrin is involved in the purging of unwanted proteins from granules during their maturation (see next section) rather than in the formation of the immature granule from the TGN (150).

Granule Maturation and Refinement of Granule Constituents

Maturation of the immature granule involves three parallel events: loss of clathrin, progressive acidification, and proinsulin conversion. The loss of clathrin is attributed to the budding of clathrin-coated vesicles from maturing granules (150), as first proposed by Orci (111). They are understood to take with them some soluble granule proteins, with insulin being retained ("sorting by retention") in the granule due to its crystalline state (see below) (172,173). This results in the purging of unwanted proteins that may have been erroneously introduced into the immature granule. A second mechanism, "sorting for exit," operates in parallel to this same end. This involves the selective binding of proteins to the intragranular aspect of mannose-6-phosphate (and possibly other) receptors that participate in coordinating clathrin adaptors via their cytosolic domain. Lysosomal proteases are known to be bound in such a fashion, leading to their sequestration in clathrin-coated vesicles and consequent clearance from maturing granules (150,174,175).

The immature granule is itself mildly acidified, but as it matures and loses its clathrin coat, it becomes progressively more so, reaching a pH as low as 5.0 to 5.5 (176–178). Granule acidification is due to action of an ATP-dependent proton pump and is critical for proinsulin conversion (179).

Conversion of Proinsulin to Insulin

The conversion of proinsulin to insulin and C-peptide occurs in the immature, clathrin-coated secretory granule (4,176,177) and is outlined in Figure 5.3. There are two pairs of basic

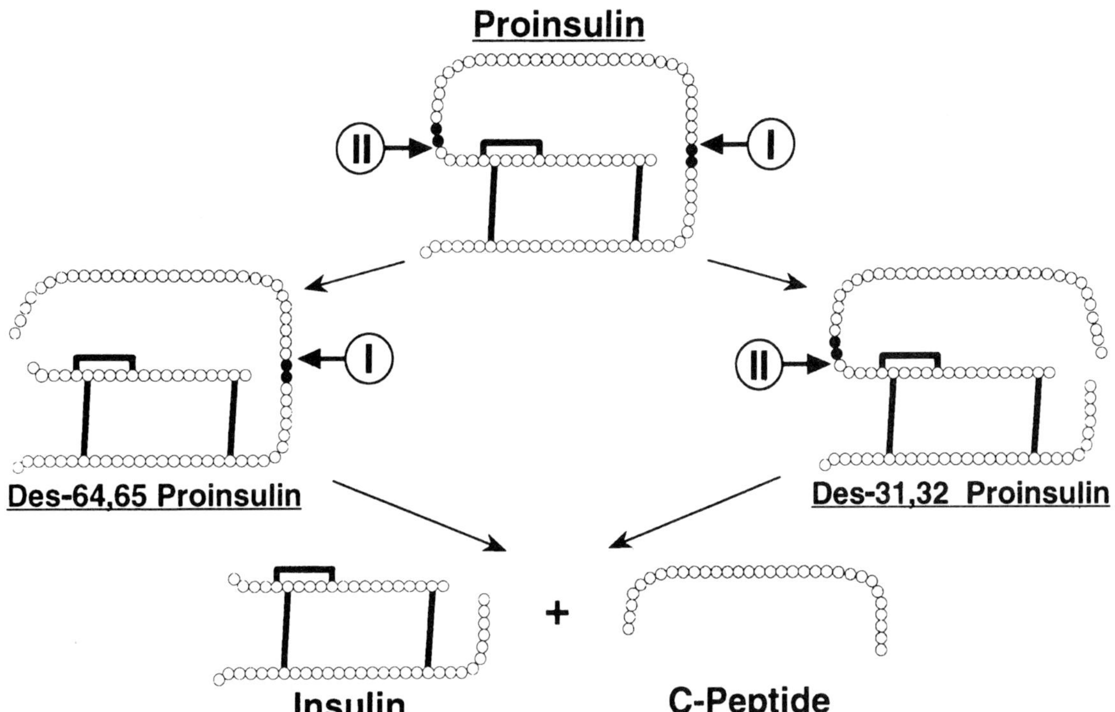

Figure 5.3. Conversion of proinsulin to insulin. Conversion occurs within acidifying secretory granules. The initial event is an endoproteolytic cut on the carboxyl-terminal side of one of the basic residues linking the insulin chains to the C-peptide (in humans, this initial cleavage event occurs predominantly at the B-chain/C-peptide junction). Two endopeptidases are involved: PC3 ("I" in figure), also known as PC1, and PC2 ("II" in figure); each is postulated to display a preference for just one site. The residual basic amino acids left at the carboxyl-terminus of the cleaved proinsulin intermediate are trimmed off by carboxypeptidase H (also known as carboxypeptidase E). These two sequential events lead to one of two proinsulin conversion intermediates: des-31,32-split proinsulin or des-64,65-split proinsulin. A further round of endoproteolytic cleavage and carboxypeptidase trimming of either intermediate generates insulin and C-peptide (as well as the four basic amino acids that originally linked C-peptide to the insulin chains).

residues at which the endoproteolytic conversion event occurs: Arg31-Arg32, linking the insulin B-chain to the C-peptide; and Lys64-Arg65, linking the C-peptide to the insulin A-chain.

The Proinsulin-Processing Enzymes

Endoproteolytic peptide-bond cleavage of proinsulin occurs on the carboxyl side of Arg31, Arg32 and Lys64, Arg65, followed by exopeptidic removal of the newly exposed basic amino acids (180,181) (Fig. 5.3). The proinsulin-processing endopeptidase activity proved elusive and was not discovered until 20 years after that of proinsulin (182). Soon after, it was found that this activity actually consisted of two individual endopeptidases, then named type I and type II (183). Type I cleaved specifically at the Arg31, Arg32 site of proinsulin, and type II preferentially cleaved the Lys64, Arg65 site (Fig. 5.3) (183–187). Soon after, these endopeptidase activities were cloned and found to be members of a family of prohormone processing enzymes (188–191). The type I endopeptidase activity was equivalent to PC3 (also known as PC1) (192–195), and the type II endopeptidase activity was equivalent to PC2 (152,196–198). Cotransfection studies of proinsulin with PC3 and PC2 have confirmed these enzymes as the bona fide proinsulin-processing endopeptidase activities (199).

The third proteolytic enzyme involved in proinsulin processing is an exopeptidase, carboxypeptidase H (CPH) (180,181). CPH [also named CPE (200)] is a Ni^{2+}-requiring exopeptidase with an acidic pH optimum (181). Once proinsulin has been cleaved by PC2 or PC3, CPH specifically and rapidly removes the exposed (C-terminal) basic amino acids (181,183,186).

Regulation of Proinsulin Conversion

PC2 and PC3 are Ca^{2+}-dependent enzyme activities that display an acidic pH optimum of around 5 to 5.5 (183). Maximal activity of these enzymes is appropriately assured by the Ca^{2+}-rich [1–10 mM free Ca^{2+}; see reference (201)] and mildly acidic [pH 5.5; see reference (202)] internal milieu of an immature insulin secretory granule (183,185,194,195), which is also optimal for CPH activity (181). Because these [Ca^{2+}] and acidic pH conditions are not encountered in the secretory pathway of the β-cell until the immature insulin secretory granule compartment is reached, it ensures that insulin is produced only in the intracellular β-granule compartment in which it is stored (183,203). As such, for full PC2, PC3, and CPH activity, activation of the secretory granule proton-pumping ATPase to generate an acidic pH (176,179,202) and Ca^{2+}-translocation proteins to increase [Ca^{2+}] (204) are key regulatory events for controlling proinsulin conversion.

Most members of the proprotein processing endopeptidase family undergo a zymogen-like autocatalytic cleavage activation (205–207). In pancreatic islets, PC2 and PC3 are synthesized initially as inactive proproteins that are subsequently cleaved by limited proteolysis (29,197,208–210). This processing of PC2 and PC3 precursors is thought to be initiated in the RER (152,211) and then completed in the TGN/immature granule compartment (152,211,212). This also ensures that the vast majority of proinsulin is converted to insulin in the secretory-granule compartment (4,203). While it is likely that proteolysis of proPC2 and proPC3 is an autocatalytic process, processing by other endoproteolytic activities has not been ruled out (152,207,211,212). Recently, it has been found that the proteolytic processing of proPC2 is more complex than originally thought because of the transient interaction between proPC2 and its chaperone, 7B2, that inhibits PC2 activity (213,214). Proteolytic cleavage of 7B2 results in subsequent PC2 activation in the *trans*–Golgi region of the secretory pathway (215,216). In part, this may account for the observation that PC2 traverses the secretory pathway more slowly than PC3 and proinsulin (152,208).

As previously outlined, proinsulin biosynthesis is stimulated by glucose at both translational and transcriptional levels (93,106,107). This places an obvious increased demand on the proinsulin conversion mechanism in β-cells. However, proinsulin conversion is adaptable to changes in glucose (217). In the short term (less than 2 hours), the biosynthesis of PC2 and PC3 is stimulated in parallel with that of proinsulin at the translational level (29,58,83). PC2 and PC3 gene expression is also coordinately regulated by long-term exposure to glucose (more than 12 hours) at the level of transcription, along with the preproinsulin gene (218). By contrast, the biosynthesis of CPH in β-cells is not regulated by glucose at either the translational or the transcriptional level (28,83). However, this is believed to be of little consequence, since CPH is much more abundant in the insulin secretory granule compartment relative to PC2 and PC3 (188).

The Efficiency of Proinsulin Conversion

As previously mentioned, in a β-cell of a healthy rat (137), and it is assumed (although not yet demonstrated experimentally) in a healthy human being as well, almost all (more than 99%) newly synthesized proinsulin appears to be destined for secretory granules. Despite this remarkably efficient targeting, there is always a detectable level of proinsulin-like material in the circulation, as became apparent almost as soon as proinsulin had been identified as the immediate precursor of insulin (219–221). With the use of specific antibodies, it has been shown that this material consists not only of intact proinsulin but also of conversion intermediates (222), and this has been confirmed using the higher resolving power of high-performance liquid chromatography (223,224). The major intermediate encountered in the circulation, des-31,32-split proinsulin (223,224), results from cleavage at Arg31, Arg32 (the B-chain/C-peptide junction with trimming of the resulting C-terminal basic residues) leaving the C-peptide joined by its C-terminal extremity to the insulin A-chain (Fig. 5.3). In the fasting state in healthy individuals, proinsulin and this intermediate have been estimated to account for approximately 5% to 10% each of the total insulin-related material in the circulation (222–224). The other major conversion intermediate [des-64,65-split proinsulin (Fig. 5.3), cleaved and trimmed only at Lys64,Arg65, the C-peptide/A-chain junction] is present in much smaller amounts. The relative amounts of proinsulin, intermediates, and insulin in the peripheral circulation reflect not only rates of production by the pancreas but also rates of clearance. Proinsulin is cleared from the circulation less rapidly than insulin (primarily because the insulin receptor displays a lower affinity for proinsulin than for insulin) (225), which explains why the relative concentration of proinsulin in the periphery is higher than that encountered in the portal vein (222). Although the intermediate cleaved at Lys64, Arg65, between the A-chain and C-peptide, may be released in smaller amounts than the other intermediate (223,224), it is also cleared more rapidly (225), which will further reduce its relative concentration in the periphery. Notwithstanding, several lines of evidence have led to the idea that the processing of human proinsulin is sequential, where PC3 cleaves intact proinsulin at Arg31, Arg32 first to generate des-31,32-proinsulin (after CPH trimming), which is then processed by PC2 at

Lys64, Arg65 to generate the final products (after CPH trimming): insulin, C-peptide, and free basic amino acids (185,195,203,226). This preferred route of proinsulin conversion has been observed in human β-cells (227), confirming des-31,32-split proinsulin as the predominant conversion intermediate in humans.

Possible Physiologic Role of C-Peptide

Ever since proinsulin was identified as the biosynthetic precursor of insulin and its structure elucidated, its conversion was known to generate insulin and C-peptide in equimolar quantities. Although it was believed for many years that C-peptide was important only to ensure correct folding of proinsulin, more recent experiments suggest otherwise. C-peptide has thus been shown to exert direct effects on renal function (228,229), to augment glucose utilization (230,231), and to improve autonomic nervous function in insulin-dependent diabetes mellitus (IDDM) (232), as well as to exert direct effects on insulin secretion (233). All these effects could be mediated by a direct impact of C-peptide on $Na^{+}K^{+}$-ATPase activity in various tissues (231, 234,235). Such a physiologic role for C-peptide as a bioactive hormone is still the subject of intense study and debate. The field has been well reviewed by John Wahren, the scientist most responsible for renewed interest in this enigmatic partner of insulin (236–239), and his group, who have demonstrated specific binding of C-peptide to a putative membrane receptor (240), a hotly contested issue (241).

HYPERPROINSULINEMIA IN DISEASE STATES

Diabetes Mellitus

An increased ratio of proinsulin to insulin frequently is found in individuals with NIDDM (224,242–245) and in some individuals with recent-onset IDDM (246–248) and their nondiabetic twins (249) or siblings (250). Proinsulin levels have been found to predict development of NIDDM and as such must be the result (or reflection) of a very early defect in the course of the disease (251).

In most early studies, no attempt was made to distinguish between intact proinsulin and conversion intermediates. When this was achieved (224,243,252,253), des-31,32-split proinsulin was found to contribute significantly toward total "proinsulin-related" immunoreactivity in persons with NIDDM just as in control subjects (see above).

The reasons for elevated ratios of proinsulin to insulin in persons with diabetes mellitus are not known (203,224,254,255). There are two alternative explanations currently under evaluation: (a) proinsulin conversion per se is impaired, and (b) granule turnover is so rapid that a significant amount of proinsulin is released before it can be converted. According to the first explanation, the conversion system (enzymes) itself is at fault. This should lead to an increase not only in the amount of unprocessed proinsulin that leaves the β-cell but also in the amount of any other proprotein normally cleaved within β-cells by the same processing machinery. This has yet to be documented. The second explanation, that hyperproinsulinemia is caused by increased turnover, is based on the suggestion that the rate of turnover of secretory granules might be such that the residence time of some proinsulin molecules within the granules (before release) would be too short to permit conversion. Such might be the case in NIDDM under conditions of increased insulin demand caused by insulin resistance in the face of a partially depleted population of β-cells.

Genetic Defects in Proinsulin Conversion Enzymes

Mice that are PC2-deficient have defective proinsulin processing and increased levels of the conversion intermediate des-31,32-proinsulin, consistent with preferential cleavage by PC2 at the Lys64, Arg65 site on proinsulin (256,257). It is intriguing that these mice have a phenotype of chronic fasting hypoglycemia and a reduced increase in blood glucose levels during an intraperitoneal glucose tolerance test (257). This is not due to increased insulin secretion but rather to a deficiency in circulating levels of glucagon (256,257). This underscores the fact that PC2 and PC3 are involved in the conversion of many other prohormones, in keeping with the limitation of their expression to neuroendocrine cell types (207,258). In mice lacking the PC2-specific chaperone 7B2, no PC2 activity is detected and processing of islet prohormones is defective, resulting in a hypoglycemic, hyperproinsulinemic, and hypoglucagonemic phenotype (259), similar to that in the PC2-deficient mice (256, 257). However, unlike mice with the PC2 null phenotype, these mice also show markedly increased circulating adrenocorticotropic hormone and corticosterone levels, resulting in Cushing syndrome (259).

Deletion of the PC3 gene in mice results in an embryonic lethal phenotype. In humans, mutation in both alleles of the PC3 gene that results in negligible PC3 activity generates a complicated phenotype due to a generalized anomaly in prohormone processing (260). The patient presented with type 2 diabetes mellitus due to abnormal glucose homeostasis, elevated plasma proinsulin concentrations, but very low insulin levels, indicating a severe deficiency in proinsulin processing (260). In addition, marked obesity (developed in childhood), hypogonadotrophic hypogonadism, hypocortisolism, and increased propiomelanocortin concentrations were also apparent, emphasizing the role of PC3 in general neuroendocrine prohormone processing (260).

Obese Cpe(fat)/Cpe(fat) mice have been found to possess a CPH (CPE) mutation that reduces enzyme activity (145). Diarginyl insulin (with residual basic residues at the carboxyl-terminus of the B-chain) rather than insulin itself is the major processed product in β-cells of Cpe(fat)/Cpe(fat) mice, an expected consequence of the absence of active CPH (146). Cpe(fat)/Cpe(fat) mice are, furthermore, hyperproinsulinemic, indicating that loss of CPH activity in some as yet ill-defined fashion results in impaired proinsulin cleavage by PC2 and PC3 (145). As for PC2 and PC3, CPH does not exclusively process proinsulin, being involved in the trimming (subsequent to endoproteolytic cleavage) of many other prohormones in a variety of neuroendocrine cell types (200). The obese phenotype in the Cpe(fat)/Cpe(fat) mouse is not believed to be directly due to inefficient proinsulin processing but is more likely the result of inadequate production of α-melanocyte-stimulating hormone due to defective POMC processing in the pituitary (261,262).

Insulinoma

Aside from the unregulated overproduction of immunoreactive insulin by insulinoma cells, these cells also are characterized by the disproportionate amount of proinsulin secretion (263–266). It is possible, on the basis of the results of studies on human insulinoma tissue (267) or on cell lines derived from animal insulinomas (139,268–270), that their unusually increased production of proinsulin reflects a partial diversion of proinsulin from the regulated to the constitutive pathway. Why such a diversion should be provoked by cellular transformation is unclear. Certainly, tumor cells typically fail to express some of the differentiated features of the native parent cell. The failure to use the regulated pathway to full effect would be an example of such a lesion. Perhaps the need to synthesize unusual quantities of membrane and associated proteins to satisfy accelerated cell division leads to an impaired ability to satisfy luxury pathways such as granule formation. Amyloid deposits often are found in insulinoma tissue (271). As for amyloidosis in islets of individuals with NIDDM, insulinoma amyloidosis also may reflect increased production of pro–islet amyloid polypeptide (the biosynthetic precursor of islet amyloid polypeptide; see below) in association with the observed hyperproinsulinemia.

Other Protein Constituents of the β-Granule

Insulin, C-peptide, and related peptides contribute approximately 80% of the content of the insulin secretory granule protein (154,272) but are not the only proteins present [for a review, see (273)]. As just discussed, proinsulin conversion occurs in the granule itself, which means that the conversion enzymes, PC2, PC3, and CPH, also reside within this organelle. There is another processing enzyme present in β-cell granules, peptidylglycine-amidating monooxygenase (PAM), which converts a peptide carboxyl-terminal glycine to an amide on certain granule peptides (273–275). Granule constituents are categorized into soluble and membrane-bound granule proteins (154). Proinsulin, insulin, C-peptide, and the conversion enzymes are all soluble components of a granule and as such are cosecreted in response to secretagogues (156,273,276–278). It should also be noted that the biosynthesis of the majority of insulin secretory granule proteins is translationally regulated in parallel to proinsulin (29,83,155) to replenish that lost in secretion.

Some of the soluble insulin secretory granule proteins deserve special mention. First, chromogranin A is found in secretory granules of many different secretory cell types, including β-cells (276,279,280). Chromogranin-A is actually a precursor proprotein that is proteolytically processed within the granule by PC2, PC3, and CPH to form a variety of peptides, including β-granin (280,281). Biologic function has yet to be assigned to any of these peptides. However, in the pig, an amidated peptide named pancreastatin is derived from chromogranin A (273,282). In the 1980s, pancreastatin generated some interest as a possible autocrine regulatory factor of insulin secretion, since it was found to inhibit the release of insulin from the β-cell (282,283). However, because of the lack of appropriate processing sites in the corresponding chromogranin A, pancreastatin is not produced in humans (or rodents), and this has downplayed its physiologic relevance (273).

Another insulin secretory granule protein of interest is islet amyloid polypeptide (IAPP) (also known as amylin or diabetes-associated peptide), which displays structural homology with calcitonin gene–related peptide (CGRP) [for reviews, see references (284–287)]. IAPP is generated by PC2/CPH-mediated proteolytic processing of a higher-molecular-weight precursor (pro-IAPP) (285,288,289), then amidated, presumably by PAM (285,286). There is considerable interest in IAPP, since it is the major constituent of islet amyloid deposits (271,286, 287,290,291). These deposits, first reported at the turn of the century, have been found in the pancreases of nearly all individuals with NIDDM (271,292) [and often in insulinoma tissue (271,293)] and are thought to be a major contributor to β-cell dysfunction in NIDDM (254,286,287). Human IAPP can oligomerize to form insoluble fibrils that are characteristic of pancreatic amyloid deposits (294,295). Intriguingly, the varying primary structure of IAPP across mammalian species dictates whether or not it can form fibrils and amyloid deposits (286,290,296). Amyloid deposits are found surrounding islets only in diabetic humans, macaques, and cats, but not in rodents (286,296). However, overexpression of human IAPP in β-cells of transgenic mice can lead to formation of IAPP-fibrils and pancreatic amyloid plaques, accompanied by β-cell dysfunction and symptoms of NIDDM (297–299). In common with other soluble granule constituents, IAPP is cosecreted with insulin (277,278). IAPP has attracted attention because of its reported properties as a diabetogenic agent. IAPP has thus been indicated to inhibit insulin release *in vitro* (300) and to cause insulin resistance (301–303), although these effects are quite controversial (286,287,304,305). IAPP also exerts calcitonin-like effects, but this is probably due to its homology to CGRP (306,307). Despite much research, a convincing physiologic (rather than pharmacologic) function for IAPP remains to be clearly established (286,287). Moreover, it also remains to be shown whether IAPP amyloid formation contributes to the pathogenesis of NIDDM or is merely a consequence of the disease (281,287). Notwithstanding, IAPP, when injected as an adjunct to insulin, may help control glycemia and could thus prove of therapeutic value.

Several insulin secretory granule membrane proteins are also worthy of mention. First, there are the components of the proton-pumping ATPase responsible for lowering the intragranular pH (202,273). There also are certain proteins found in close association with the granule membrane and shown to be involved in promoting insulin exocytosis. These include vesicle-associated membrane protein 2 (VAMP-2) (308,309), synaptotagmin-III (310,311), and rab3A (312–314). Recently, two islet cell autoantigens for type 1 diabetes mellitus, ICA512/IA-2 (315–317) and phogrin (318), have been cloned and located to the insulin secretory granule membrane. Phogrin and ICA512 have homology to tyrosine phosphoprotein phosphatases but actually do not possess phosphatase activity (316–318). As such their biologic function is currently unknown. However, it is interesting that phogrin is phosphorylated in a Ca^{2+}-dependent manner and thus may play a regulatory role in insulin secretory granule transport and/or exocytosis (319).

The Mature Granule and the Insulin Crystal

The combination of granule acidification and conversion of proinsulin to insulin provides the scenario for insulin crystallization within the mature granule. Insulin is known to be able to associate into dimers, and, in the presence of Zn^{2+}, the dimers can associate to form hexamers (320) (Fig. 5.4). The Zn^{2+} is coordinated by the histidine residue at position 10 of the insulin B-chain. The Zn-hexamers can then pack together to form a crystal lattice. Crystallization depends on a very high local concentration of insulin and Zn^{2+}, as well as an acidic milieu, with these conditions being satisfied within the granule (201,273,321). The dense core of the secretory granule observed by electron microscopy is thus taken to be an insulin crystal (119,320). C-peptide does not cocrystallize with insulin to any significant extent and is therefore excluded from the crystal to be found in the clear halo surrounding the dense core of granules (111,322) with other soluble granule constituents, such as PC2, PC3, chromogranin A, and IAPP (323).

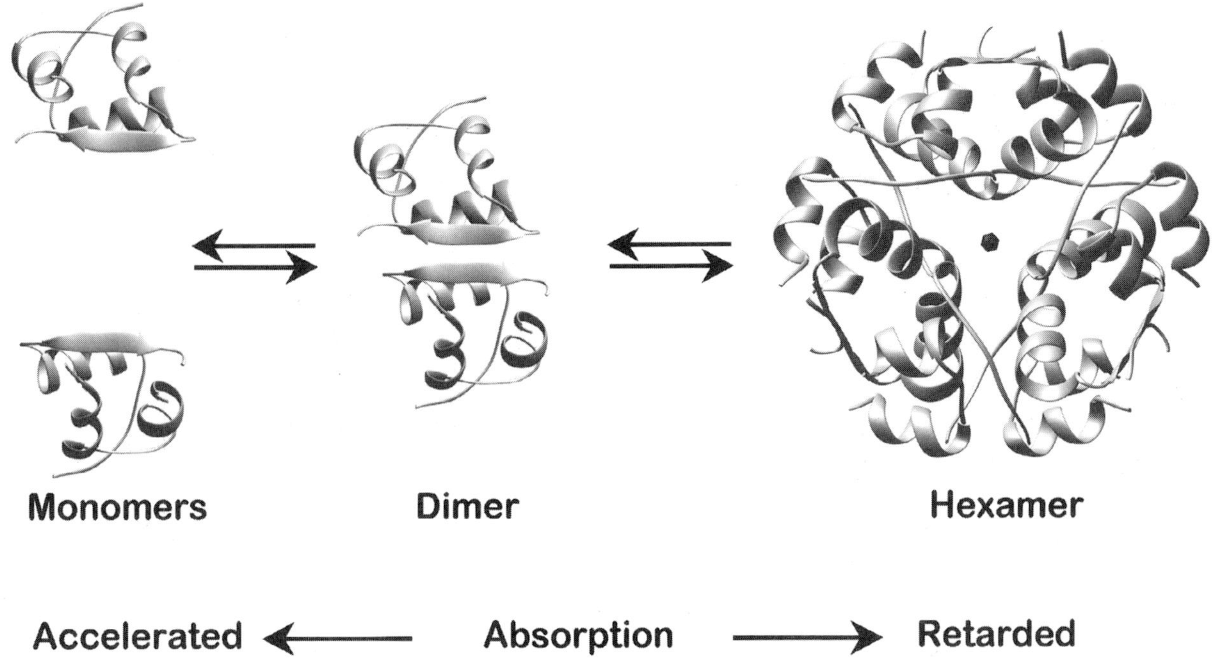

Figure 5.4. Assembly and disassembly of insulin monomers, dimers, and hexamers. Insulin molecules are modeled as ribbon diagrams depicting elements of secondary structure (α helices and β sheets). Monomeric insulins (lispro, aspart) are created by altering residues along the monomer/dimer interface to destabilize dimer formation. This accelerates absorption of the injected insulin. Hexamer formation is stabilized by substitutions in the long-acting insulin, glargine. Enhanced hexamerization retards absorption.

THE FATE OF THE MATURE SECRETORY GRANULE

Insulin is stored in the mature secretory granule until it is either released by exocytosis or degraded by crinophagy.

Transport of Insulin Secretory Granules to the Plasma Membrane

Before the release of insulin via exocytosis, an insulin secretory granule must be transported from an intracellular storage pool to the β-cell surface. The β-cell is polarized (4), and secretory granules appear to be delivered to a certain location on the β-cell plasma membrane (324,325). The directional transport of insulin secretory granules to the plasma membrane is likely mediated via an interaction with the β-cell cytoskeletal framework of microtubules and microfilaments (119,326–329). Granule movement along microtubules is most probably driven by microtubule-associated proteins and motors [e.g., kinesin and dynein (329–334)]. The role of microfilaments [which form a bundled network just beneath and parallel to the plasma membrane of the β-cell called a "cell-web" (335)] is not particularly clear, but they likely provide a proportion of motive force for the transport of insulin secretory granules along microtubules (119,335,336).

The Mechanism of Regulated Insulin Exocytosis

Insulin is stored in the secretory granules of the β-cell in the resting state and is not released from the β-cell to any great extent unless there is a specific signal that stimulates exocytosis (4,137). Insulin exocytosis is triggered by certain intracellular secondary signals, including an increase in cytosolic $[Ca^{2+}]_i$ (as outlined in Chapter 6), and also by several secretory granule, cytosolic, and plasma membrane proteins (337,338). The proteins involved in the mechanism of regulated insulin exocytosis are now becoming better understood, mostly from analogies to the mechanism of synaptic vesicle exocytosis in neurons (312,339–342).

In essence, insulin exocytosis involves docking of the insulin secretory granule with the plasma membrane and subsequent fusion, processes accounted for by the so-called SNARE-hypothesis (118,122,337,338). According to this theory, members of a family of secretory granule proteins called v-SNAREs (vesicle-soluble *N*-ethylmaleimide attachment protein receptors) specifically associate with cognate members of a family of plasma membrane proteins, called target-SNAREs (t-SNAREs). The synaptobrevin family of proteins have been identified as v-SNAREs on secretory vesicles (341,343–345), and the syntaxin family (339,341,343,346,347) and synaptosome-associated protein 25 (SNAP-25, which should not be confused with SNAPs, the soluble NSF attachment proteins) have been identified (132, 343,348,349) as plasma membrane t-SNAREs. VAMP-2, located on insulin secretory granules, is the v-SNARE (308,309,350), and SNAP-25 (350,351) plus syntaxin 1a, 4, and 5 are the t-SNAREs (309,352,353) implicated for insulin exocytosis in β-cells. Syntaxin and SNAP-25 associate with each other to form a high-affinity binding site for VAMP (345). Binding of VAMP to syntaxin/SNAP-25 forms a stable core complex (345,354), allowing a secretory granule to dock with the plasma membrane (341,343). This complex then acts as a receptor for a cytosolic protein, α-SNAP (soluble NSF attachment proteins) (122,132,341,343,349,354), shown to be present in β-cells (355). The α-SNAP association with the complex then promotes association of another cytosolic protein, NSF [*N*-ethylmaleimide sensitive factor (122, 341,343,349,354), also present in β-cells (355)]. A VAMP/syntaxin/SNAP-25/α-SNAP/NSF complex is then formed (341, 354). Upon ATP hydrolysis, catalyzed by an intrinsic ATPase activity of NSF, there is dissociation of this "pre-exocytotic" complex that promotes membrane fusion between the insulin secretory granule and plasma membranes, thus enabling the granule content to be expelled into the surrounding milieu (341,343,354). The involvement of the SNARE complex in regulated insulin exocytosis has recently been highlighted, in that the VAMP/syntaxin/SNAP-25 interaction dissociates during the first phase of glucose-induced insulin exocytosis (356).

However, although the SNARE hypothesis forms a central basis for hormone-regulated exocytosis (122,341,343,349, 357–359), it also applies to most generic vesicular transport membrane fusion events in the cell (339,349), including unregulated constitutive exocytosis (122). While SNARE proteins are an essential part of the mechanics of insulin exocytosis (337,338), the SNARE hypothesis does not account for the tight control of regulated insulin exocytosis (343,349,357,359). As such, other protein factors that interact with SNARE proteins in a regulated manner likely control the insulin exocytotic mechanism (337,338,343,349). For example, a family of secretory granule proteins, named synaptotagmins, act as Ca^{2+} sensors for Ca^{2+}-dependent regulated exocytosis (343,360,361). It has been proposed that synaptotagmins bind to the VAMP/SNAP-25/syntaxin core complex under resting circumstances at low $[Ca^{2+}]_i$, preventing α-SNAP binding. However, when $[Ca^{2+}]_i$ increases in response to a stimulus, synaptotagmin dissociates from the complex, allowing α-SNAP/NSF association, formation of the VAMP/SNAP-25/syntaxin/α-SNAP/NSF complex, and commitment to membrane fusion and exocytosis (343,362). In β-cells, the synaptotagmin-III isoform is found on insulin secretory granules (310,338) and has been postulated to play a regulatory role in controlling insulin exocytosis (310,311). Another example is munc-18, a cytosolic protein that, under resting circumstances, associates with syntaxin, preventing the formation of the VAMP/SNAP-25/syntaxin complex and hence the docking of secretory granules (343,362,363). It is believed that a protein kinase C (PKC)–mediated phosphorylation of munc-18 takes place at a "predocking" step, analogous to synaptic vesicle exocytosis in neurons (364), that results in munc-18/syntaxin dissociation and then allows VAMP/SNAP-25/syntaxin association and secretory granule docking to proceed. Such phosphorylation of munc-18 in β-cells could account in part for a role of PKC in regulating insulin secretion (365,366). One should be aware that synaptotagmin-III and munc-18 represent just two exemplar β-cell proteins that may control the mechanism of insulin exocytosis and that several other factors should also be considered (337,338).

Degradation of Insulin Stores in the β-Cell (Crinophagy)

If not released, insulin can be degraded within the β-cell (367,368). Degradation arises by the fusion of granules with lysosomes (369), an event referred to as crinophagy and that was first shown to occur in pituitary mammotrophic cells (370) and pancreatic β-cells (371). Degradation seems to act in concert with biosynthesis and release to regulate the amount of insulin housed in the β-cell at a given time (367,368). Although the factors regulating crinophagy are not understood, it has been found that when insulin release is inhibited, degradation increases and vice versa (367,368,372,373). Insulin is degraded only slowly, even after its introduction into lysosomes (369,372,374). This is thought to be due to the stability of the insulin crystal in lysosomes, which display an acidic milieu similar to that of the secretory granule. By contrast, both proinsulin and C-peptide (neither of which exists in the crystal state within granules) are degraded rapidly within β-cells (369,372,374).

INSULIN STRUCTURE

Amino Acid Sequence

Although insulin was recognized to be a protein shortly after its discovery (375), the elucidation of its primary structure

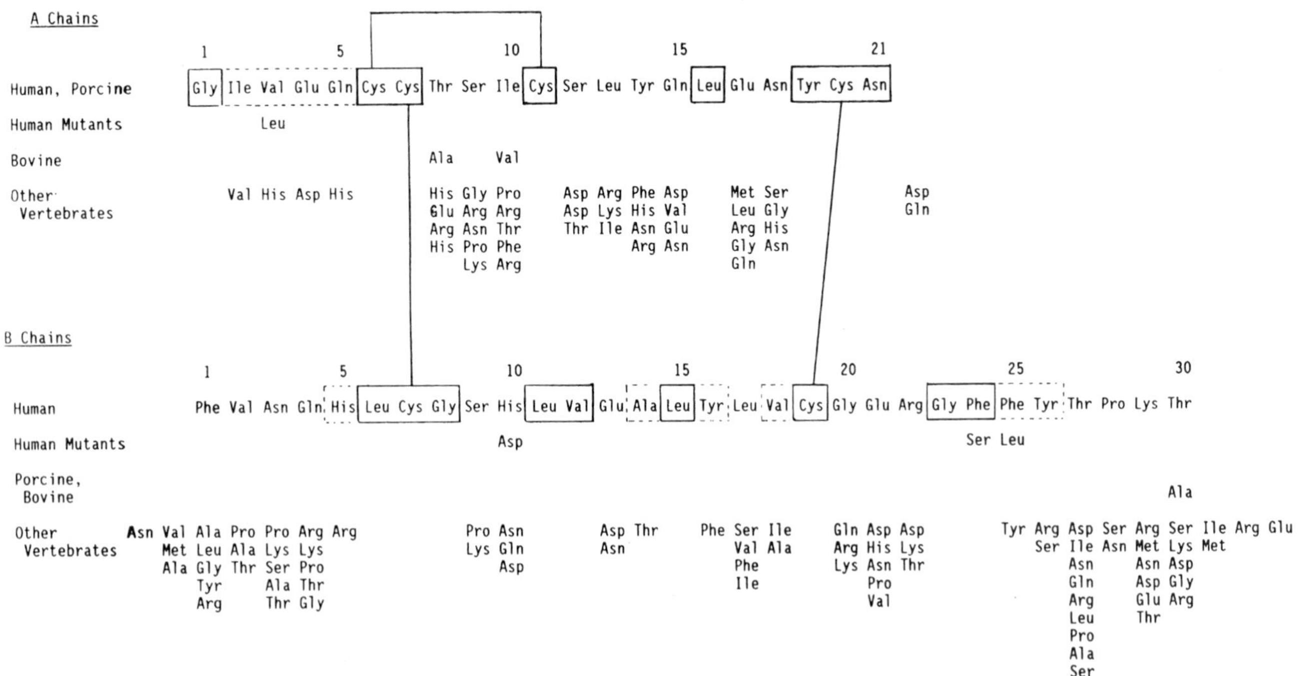

Figure 5.5. Amino acid sequences of therapeutic and mutant human insulins and substitutions occurring in other vertebrate insulins. Solid lines denote disulfide bonds; solid and dashed boxes surround invariant and highly homologous residues, respectively.

came many years later with the development by Sanger and coworkers of methods to determine primary sequences of proteins (7,376). In fact, insulin was the first protein to have its entire primary sequence determined (for which Frederic Sanger received the 1958 Nobel Prize in Chemistry). Figure 5.5 compares the primary sequences of insulins from different animal species. Known insulins are composed of two polypeptide chains that are linked to one another by disulfide bonds. The A- and B-chains of human, porcine, and bovine insulins, like those of most other vertebrate insulins, are composed of 21 and 30 amino acids, respectively. The two peptide chains are covalently linked to one another by two cystine disulfides, one between CysA7 and CysB7 and the other between CysA20 and CysB19. An additional intrachain disulfide connects cysteines A6 and A11. Insulin structure is highly conserved in vertebrate evolution (377). Regions of invariability include the positions of cysteines that form the disulfide bridges, the amino- and carboxyl-terminal regions of the A-chain, and certain hydrophobic residues at the carboxyl-terminus of the B-chain (19,76). Mutations and chemical modifications at invariant or highly conserved positions generally diminish or abolish receptor binding potency and biologic activity, emphasizing the importance of these positions in either creating or maintaining a three-dimensional surface suitable for receptor recognition (378–380).

Three-dimensional Structure of Insulin

The pioneering studies of the x-ray diffraction patterns of insulin crystals, conducted simultaneously by Dorothy Hodgkin (Nobel Prize for Chemistry in 1964) and coworkers (381,382) and the Peking Insulin Structure Group (383), have been the cornerstone for relating the structure and function of insulin. The crystal structure of insulin has been refined to a resolution of 1.5 Å (384). Within each unit cell of two zinc insulin crystals, six insulin molecules compose a hexamer around two zinc atoms; three HisB10 residues (Fig. 5.4) chelate each zinc atom. Two zinc insulin hexamers can be subdivided into three equivalent dimers, with each dimer being composed of two insulin molecules of similar but not identical structure. The hydrophobic core of the insulin monomer is composed of invariant and highly conserved residues, including leucine residues A16, B6, B11, and B15, the A6–A11 cystines, the TyrA19 ring, IleA2, and AlaB14, supporting the notion that core structure must be maintained for insulin action. These core residues with hydrophobic side chains contact additional, more peripheral nonpolar residues, including ValA3, LeuA13, ValB12, ValB18, CysB19, and PheB24, which in turn contact the remaining nonpolar residues (PheB1, ValB3, LeuB17, and PheB25). The more peripheral nonpolar residues that are exposed partially on the monomer surface contribute to the surfaces of insulin involved in protein-protein interactions, including the dimer and hexamer interfaces and possibly the receptor-binding surface as well (378,380,384). Residues from both A- and B-chains comprise the hydrophobic core of insulin and the various binding surfaces. The A-chain forms two helical segments (A1–A8 and A13–A19), which are connected by a turn; the B-chain contains two regions of extended chain (B1–B8, B21–B30) connected by a region of α-helix (B9–B19). The two chains are connected to one another covalently by cystine disulfides (A7-B7, A20-B19), and the overall structure is stabilized by interchain hydrogen bonds (A11-B4, A6-B6, A21-B23, and A19-B25) and ionic interactions between the N-terminus of the A-chain and the C-terminus of the B-chain.

Proinsulin Structure

Structural studies by two-dimensional nuclear magnetic resonance imaging indicated that the insulin portion of proinsulin is similar to that of insulin, whereas the C-peptide portion of proinsulin appears to be unstructured (226). However, there are some perturbations in the insulin moiety of proinsulin that are reverted by cleavage between the A-chain but not by cleavage between the B-chain and C-peptide (226). To account for the reduced biologic potency of proinsulin (385), it has been suggested that the C-peptide obscures a portion of the receptor-binding surface of insulin (386) or, alternatively, prevents movement of the carboxyl-terminus of the B-chain during binding (387). Unlike insulin, the sequence of which is highly conserved, the sequences of the C-peptide portions of different proinsulins show little homology (19). These C-peptides differ markedly both in length and amino acid composition, suggesting that the C-peptide composition itself is not very important. It has been thought that the C-peptide moiety of proinsulin acts as a tether between the A- and B-chains of insulin to guarantee appropriate folding and disulfide pairing during the biosynthetic process (19). However, recent reports suggest that C-peptide might have an endocrine function of its own (388). As previously mentioned, however, the physiologic relevance remains controversial.

Mutant Insulins and Proinsulins

Mutations in the coding sequences of the insulin gene can lead to production of structurally abnormal insulin molecules (389,390). Three different altered forms of insulin with low biologic potency have been associated with diabetes mellitus: PheB25Leu (391,392), PheB24Ser (393,394), and ValA3Leu (395) substitutions. While additional, apparently unrelated, probands have been found who produce the same abnormal insulins from identical insulin gene mutations (396–398), no additional abnormal insulins have yet been identified, although they surely exist. These patients and their families define a clinical syndrome, the insulinopathies, which are characterized by high circulating levels of insulin and a frequent association with mild carbohydrate intolerance (390,398–400). Affected individuals can be distinguished from patients with type 2 diabetes mellitus by a normal or slightly impaired sensitivity to exogenous insulin despite unusually high levels of their own circulating insulin (399). Hyperinsulinemia in these patients is not explained by the presence of circulating antibodies or elevated levels of counterregulatory hormones. In fact, each of these patients produces normal and abnormal forms of insulin in equivalent amounts (391). The more potent normal insulin is cleared more rapidly, resulting in accumulation of the abnormal insulin and in a dramatic degree of hyperinsulinemia. The amounts of normal bioactive insulin in the circulation of these patients are actually inappropriately low, resulting in the observed impaired glucose tolerance and diabetes (395,400).

Mutations in the insulin gene can also result in impaired processing of proinsulin to insulin. Individuals with hyperproinsulinemia caused by impaired processing, like individuals with abnormal insulins, may exhibit carbohydrate intolerance, but not necessarily. For two of the cases studied, large amounts of an insulin molecule with C-peptide still attached at the A-chain/C-peptide junction were found in the circulation. In both cases, impaired processing was due to the mutation of arginine within the Lys64-Arg65 endopeptidase cleavage sequence (401–403).

A third case of familial hyperproinsulinemia results from a HisB10Asp mutation (404,405). It is surprising that a defect in proinsulin structure distant from the paired basic cleavage sites prevents processing. However, transfection of the mutated gene into cells and expression in transgenic mice (163,406) both show that significant proportions of the mutated hormone are secreted from cells via the constitutive pathway. Because proinsulins have substantially less biologic potency than the corresponding insulin molecules, and as much of insulin and proinsulin clearance occurs by receptor-mediated pathways, the proinsulin molecules are cleared more slowly and accumulate in the circulation of affected individuals. The proteolytic product of HisB10Asp proinsulin is HisB10Asp insulin, which unlike other abnormal insulins, exhibits enhanced receptor binding affinity (406,407).

Therapeutic Insulins

Historically, insulin for treating patients with diabetes mellitus was isolated from animals, primarily pigs and cows. However, the human insulin produced today with recombinant DNA methods has the identical sequence and chemical composition as insulin produced in the human pancreas. Use of the human hormone provides a theoretical advantage of lower immunogenicity, compared with use of animal insulins that have slightly different sequences. The use of recombinant techniques to produce insulin also provides the opportunity to modify the insulin sequence to alter both its biologic activity and pharmacokinetic properties. This opportunity has recently been realized, and several modified insulin analogues are available either for clinical use or in clinical trials (408,409).

At the concentrations used for its storage in vials before injection, insulin self-associates to form hexamers. Dissociation of the hexamers into biologically active monomers is slow at the site of injection, and rates of absorption and entry into the circulation are slow because the hexameric complexes are large and diffuse slowly. Insulin monomers, being smaller, diffuse much more rapidly. The rationale for creating fast-acting insulin analogues is based on the desire to decrease the tendency to self-associate but to retain normal receptor binding affinity (Fig. 5.4). This has been accomplished with lispro (Eli Lilly) and aspart (Novo Nordisk) insulins. Positions B28 and B29 of human insulin are proline and lysine, respectively. These residues are reversed in the sequence of insulin-like growth factor 1 (IGF-1), a closely related growth factor that does not self-associate. Thus lispro insulin contains Lys-Pro at the B28–B29 positions, which decreases its tendency to self-associate and increases its rate of absorption following subcutaneous injection. Aspart insulin contains aspartic acid at the B28 position in place of proline. This region at the carboxyl-terminus of the insulin B-chain participates in self-association. The presence of an acidic side chain at this site, and hence a negative charge, diminishes self-association because of charge repulsion. Both lispro and aspart insulins display a rapid onset and a short duration of action, which better matches blood glucose excursions following meals.

Long-acting insulins may be most useful for reducing blood glucose levels during nocturnal periods of fasting, particularly for suppressing hepatic glucose production after 2:00 a.m. to 3:00 a.m. Insulin glargine (Aventis) contains two modifications relative to native human insulin. The addition of two basic arginine residues to the carboxyl-terminus (to create ArgB31 and ArgB32 positions not normally present) shifts the isoelectric point of the protein from a pH of 5.4 to pH 6.7. This renders the molecule more soluble at acidic pH and less soluble at neutral pH. Because the analogue is stored at acidic pH, a second substitution was needed to avoid the undesirable deamidation of asparagine A21 that occurs at low pH. Replacement of AsnA21 with glycine avoids this problem and is otherwise well tolerated. Injected as a clear solution at acidic pH (4.0), insulin glargine forms a microprecipitate at the physiologic pH of the subcutaneous space, which delays its dissolution and absorption from the site of injection. Another method for creating long-acting insulin is linking it covalently to a fatty acid rather than modifying its primary sequence. Insulin detemir (NN304 from Novo Nordisk) is made by acylating the LysB29 side chain of des-B30 insulin with tetradecanoic acid. This modification promotes binding to serum albumin and consequently increases the half-life of insulin at the site of injection and in the circulation. Receptor binding affinities of lispro, aspart, and glargine insulins roughly match that of native human insulin, whereas detemir insulin binds with slightly reduced affinity.

SUMMARY

From the initial seconds of the biosynthesis of its early precursor, preproinsulin, to its release or degradation within the β-cell, insulin is always protected from the cytosol by a limiting membrane. Insulin release reflects a well-orchestrated series of events involving the successive budding, directed movement, and fusion of transport vesicles or granules and intravesicular proteolytic conversion events. The three-dimensional structure and physicochemical properties of insulin and its precursors play an intimate role in this series of events, just as they do for the biologic activity of these molecules.

REFERENCES

1. Banting FG, Best CH. The internal secretion of the pancreas. *J Lab Clin Med* 1922;7:251–266.
2. Banting FG, Best CH. Pancreatic extracts. *J Lab Clin Med* 1922;7:464–472.
3. Banting FG, Best CH, Collip JB, et al. Pancreatic extracts in the treatment of diabetes mellitus. *Can Med Assoc J* 1922;12:141–146.
4. Orci L. The insulin factory: a tour of the plant surroundings and a visit to the assembly line. *Diabetologia* 1985;28:528–546.
5. Muglia L, Locker J. Extrapancreatic insulin gene expression in the fetal rat. *Proc Natl Acad Sci U S A* 1984;81:3635–3639.
6. Giddings SJ, Carnaghi LR. Selective expression and developmental regulation of the ancestral rat insulin II gene in fetal liver. *Mol Endocrinol* 1990;4:1363–1369.
7. Ryle AP, Sanger F, Smith LF, et al. The disulphide bonds of insulin. *Biochem J* 1955;60:541–556.
8. Steiner DF, Oyer PE. The biosynthesis of insulin and probable precursor of insulin by a human islet cell adenoma. *Proc Natl Acad Sci U S A* 1967;57:473–480.
9. Steiner DF, Cunningham D, Spigelman L, et al. Insulin biosynthesis: evidence for a precursor. *Science* 1967;157:697–700.
10. Chan SJ, Keim P, Steiner DF. Cell-free synthesis of rat preproinsulins: characterization and partial amino acid sequence determination. *Proc Natl Acad Sci U S A* 1976;73:1964–1968.
11. Bell GI, Pictet RL, Rutter WJ, et al. Sequence of the insulin gene. *Nature* 1980;284:26–32.
12. Blobel G, Dobberstein B. Transfer of proteins across membranes. I. Presence of proteolytically processed and unprocessed nascent immunoglobulin light chains on membrane-bound ribosomes of murine myeloma. *J Cell Biol* 1975;67:835–851.
13. Walter P, Johnson AE. Signal sequence recognition and protein targeting to the endoplasmic reticulum membrane. *Annu Rev Cell Biol* 1994;10:87–119.
14. Eskridge EM, Shields D. Cell-free processing and segregation of insulin precursors. *J Biol Chem* 1983;258:11487–11491.
15. Okun MM, Eskridge EM, Shields D. Truncations of a secretory protein define minimum lengths required for binding to signal recognition particle and translocation across the endoplasmic reticulum membrane. *J Biol Chem* 1990;265:7478–7484.
16. Patzelt C, Labrecque AD, Duguid JR, et al. Detection and kinetic behavior of preproinsulin in pancreatic islets. *Proc Natl Acad Sci USA* 1978;75:1260–1264.
17. Campbell IC, Hellqvist LNB, Taylor KW. Insulin biosynthesis and its regulation. *Clin Sci* 1982;62:449–455.
18. Shoelson SE, Halban PA. Insulin biosynthesis and chemistry. In: Kahn CR, Weir GC, eds. *Joslin's diabetes mellitus*, 13th ed. Malvern, PA: Lea & Febiger, 1994:29–55.

19. Steiner DF, Bell GI, Tager HS. Chemistry and biosynthesis of pancreatic protein hormones. In: DeGroot LG, ed. *Endocrinology*. Philadelphia: WB Saunders, 1989:1263–1289.
20. Rhodes CJ. Processing of the insulin molecule. In: LeRoith D, Taylor SI, Olefsky JM, eds. *Diabetes mellitus: a fundamental and clinical text*. Philadelphia: Lippincott-Raven Publishers, 1996:27–41.
21. Ashcroft SJH, Bunce J, Lowry M, et al. The effect of sugars on (pro)insulin biosynthesis. *Biochem J* 1978;174:517–526.
22. Taylor KW, Parry DG, Smith GH. Biosynthetic labelling of mammalian insulins in vitro. *Nature* 1964;203:1144–1145.
23. Parry DG, Taylor KW. The effects of sugars on incorporation of [3H]leucine into insulins. *Biochem J* 1966;100:2c–4c.
24. Howell SL, Taylor KW. Effects of glucose concentration on incorporation of [3H]leucine into insulin using isolated mammalian islets of Langerhans. *Biochim Biophys Acta* 1966;130:519–521.
25. Morris GE, Korner A. The effect of glucose on insulin biosynthesis by isolated islets of Langerhans of the rat. *Biochim Biophys Acta* 1970;208:404–413.
26. Lin BJ, Haist RE. Insulin biosynthesis: effects of carbohydrates and related compounds. *Can J Physiol Pharmacol* 1969;47:791–801.
27. Ashcroft SJH. Glucoreceptor mechanisms and the control of insulin release and biosynthesis. *Diabetologia* 1980;18:5–15.
28. Guest PG, Rhodes CJ, Hutton JC. Regulation of the biosynthesis of insulin secretory granule proteins: co-ordinate translational control is exerted on some, but not all, granule matrix constituents. *Biochem J* 1989;257:431–437.
29. Alarcón C, Lincoln B, Rhodes CJ. The biosynthesis of the subtilisin-related proprotein covertase PC3, but not that of the PC2 convertase, is regulated by glucose in parallel to proinsulin biosynthesis in rat pancreatic islets. *J Biol Chem* 1993;268:4276–4280.
30. Pipeleers DG, Marichal M, Malaisse WJ. The stimulus-secretion coupling of glucose-induced insulin release. XIV. Glucose regulation of insular biosynthetic activity. *Endocrinology* 1973;93:1001–1011.
31. Maldonato A, Renold AE, Sharp GWG, et al. Glucose induced proinsulin biosynthesis: role of islet cyclic AMP. *Diabetes* 1977;26:538–545.
32. Tanese T, Lazarus NR, Devrim S, et al. Synthesis and release of proinsulin and insulin by isolated rat islets of Langerhans. *J Clin Invest* 1970;49: 1394–1404.
33. Lin BJ, Nagy BR, Haist RE. Effect of various concentrations of glucose on insulin biosynthesis. *Endocrinology* 1972;91:309–311.
34. Zucker PF, Lin BJ. Differential effect of D-glucose anomers on proinsulin biosynthesis by pancreatic islets. *Can J Physiol Pharmacol* 1977;55:1397–1400.
35. Jain K, Logothetopoulos J, Zucker P. The effects of D- and L-glyceraldehyde on glucose oxidation, insulin secretion and insulin biosynthesis by pancreatic islets of the rat. *Biochim Biophys Acta* 1975;399:384–394.
36. Andersson A. Stimulation of insulin biosynthesis in isolated mouse islets by L-leucine, 2-aminobornane-2carboxylic acid and a-keto-isocaproic acid. *Biochim Biophys Acta* 1976;437:345–353.
37. Malaisse WJ, Rasschaert J, Villanueva-Penacarrillo ML, et al. Respiratory, ionic, and functional effects of succinate esters in pancreatic islets. *Am J Physiol* 1993;264:E428–E433.
38. Skelly RH, Bollheimer LC, Wicksteed BL, et al. A distinct difference in the metabolic stimulus-response coupling pathways for regulating proinsulin biosynthesis and insulin secretion that lies at the level of a requirement for fatty acyl moieties. *Biochem J* 1998;331:553–561.
39. Jain K, Logothetopoulos J. Stimulation of proinsulin biosynthesis by purine-ribonucleosides and D-ribose. *Endocrinology* 1977;100:923–927.
40. Andersson A. Opposite effects of starvation on oxidation of [14C]adenosine and adenosine-induced insulin release by mouse pancreatic islets. *Biochem J* 1978;176:619–621.
41. Kaelin D, Renold AE, Sharp GWG. Glucose-stimulated proinsulin biosynthesis: rates of turn off after cessation of the stimulus. *Diabetologia* 1978;14: 329–335.
42. Whittaker PG, Taylor KW. Direct effects of rat growth hormone on rat islets of Langerhans in tissue culture. *Diabetologia* 1980;18:323–328.
43. Billestrup N, Moldrup A, Serup P, et al. Introduction of exogenous growth hormone receptors augments growth hormone-responsive insulin biosynthesis in rat insulinoma cells. *Proc Natl Acad Sci U S A* 1990;87:7210–7214.
44. Schatz H, Maier V, Hinz M, et al. Stimulation of [3H]leucine incorporation into proinsulin and insulin fraction of isolated pancreatic mouse islets in the presence of glucagon, theophylline and cAMP. *Diabetes* 1973;22:433–441.
45. Fehmann HC, Habener JF. Insulinotropic hormone glucagon-like peptide-I(7-37) stimulation of proinsulin gene expression and proinsulin biosynthesis in insulinoma beta TC-1 cells. *Endocrinology* 1992;130:159–166.
46. Malaisse WJ, Pipeleers DG, Levy J. The stimulus-secretion coupling of glucose induced insulin release. XVI. A glucose-like and calcium-independent effect of cAMP. *Biochim Biophys Acta* 1974;362:121–128.
47. Lin BJ, Haist RE. Effects of some modifiers of insulin secretion and insulin biosynthesis. *Endocrinology* 1973;92:735–742.
48. Olson SE, Andersson A, Peterson B, et al. Effects of somatostatin on the biosynthesis and release of insulin from isolated pancreatic islets. *Diabetes Metab* 1976;2:199–202.
49. Bollheimer LC, Skelly RH, Chester M, et al. Chronic exposure to free fatty acid reduces pancreatic β-cell insulin content by increasing basal insulin secretion that is not compensated for by a corresponding increase in proinsulin biosynthesis translation. *J Clin Invest* 1998;101:1094–11101.
50. Rhodes CJ, Taylor KW. Effect of interferon and double stranded RNA on β-cell function on mouse islets of Langerhans. *Biochem J* 1985;228:87–94.
51. Rhodes CJ, Taylor KW. Effect of lymphoblastoid interferon on insulin synthesis and secretion in isolated human pancreatic islets. *Diabetologia* 1984;27: 601–603.
52. Sandler S, Andersson A, Hellerström C. Inhibitory effects of interleukin-1 on insulin secretion, insulin biosynthesis, and oxidative metabolism of isolated rat pancreatic islets. *Endocrinology* 1987;121:1424–1431.
53. Spinas GA, Hansen BS, Linde S, et al. Interleukin-1 dose-dependently affects the biosynthesis of (pro)insulin in isolated rat islets of Langerhans. *Diabetologia* 1987;30:474–480.
54. Hansen BS, Nielsen JH, Linde S, et al. Effect of interleukin-1 on the biosynthesis of proinsulin and insulin in isolated rat pancreatic islets. *Biomed Biochim Acta* 1988;47:305–309.
55. Bone AJ, Taylor KW. Metabolic adaptation to pregnancy shown by increased biosynthesis of insulin in islets of Langerhans from pregnant rats. *Nature* 1976;262:501–502.
56. Bone AJ, Howell SL. Alterations in regulation of insulin biosynthesis in pregnancy and starvation studied in isolated rat islets of Langerhans. *Biochem J* 1977;166:501–507.
57. Caterson ID, Taylor KW. Islet cell function in gold thioglucose-induced obesity in mice. *Diabetologia* 1982;23:119–123.
58. Martin SK, Carroll R, Benig M, et al. Regulation by glucose of the biosynthesis of PC2, PC3 and proinsulin in (ob/ob) mouse islets of Langerhans. *FEBS Lett* 1994;356:279–282.
59. Alarcón C, Leahy JL, Schuppin GT, et al. Increased secretory demand rather than a defect in the proinsulin conversion mechanism causes hyperinsulinemia in a glucose-infusion rat model of non-insulin-dependent diabetes mellitus. *J Clin Invest* 1995;95:1032–1039.
60. Zucker P, Logothetopoulos J. Persisting enhanced proinsulin-insulin and protein biosynthesis (3H-leucine incorporation) by pancreatic islets of the rat after glucose exposure. *Diabetes* 1975;24:194–200.
61. Heinze E, Hagele U, Fussganger RD, et al. Insulin biosynthesis and release in isolated islets from hyperglycemic male rats. *Horm Metab Res* 1980;12:190–193.
62. Wang SY, Halban PA, Rowe JW. Effects of aging on insulin synthesis and secretion. Differential effects on preproinsulin messenger RNA levels, proinsulin biosynthesis, and secretion of newly made and preformed insulin in the rat. *J Clin Invest* 1988;81:176–184.
63. Portha B. Decreased glucose-induced insulin release and biosynthesis by islets of rats with non-insulin-dependent diabetes: effect of tissue culture. *Endocrinology* 1985;117:1735–1741.
64. Permutt MA, Kakita K, Malinas P, et al. An in vivo analysis of pancreatic protein and insulin biosynthesis in a rat model for non-insulin dependent diabetes. *J Clin Invest* 1984;73:1344–1350.
65. Tjioe TO, Bouman PR. Effect of fasting on the incorporation of [3H]-L-phenylalanine into proinsulin-insulin and total protein in isolated rat pancreatic islets. *Horm Metab Res* 1976;8:261–266.
66. Prentki M, Matchinsky FM. Ca^{2+}, cAMP, and phospholipid-derived messengers in coupling mechanisms of insulin secretion. *Physiol Rev* 1987;67: 1185–1248.
67. Ashcroft FM, Ashcroft SJH. Mechanism of insulin secretion. In: Ashcroft FM, Ashcroft SJH, eds. *Insulin: molecular biology to pathology*. Oxford, UK: Oxford University Press, 1992:97–150.
68. Prentki M. New insights into pancreatic β-cell metabolic signaling in insulin secretion. *Eur J Endocrinol* 1996;134:272–286.
69. Prentki M, Tornheim K, Corkey BE. Signal transduction mechanisms in nutrient-induced insulin secretion. *Diabetologia* 1997;40[Suppl 2]:S32–S41.
70. Newgard CB, McGarry JD. Metabolic coupling factors in pancreatic β-cell signal transduction. *Annu Rev Biochem* 1995;64:689–719.
71. Ashcroft FM, Proks P, Smith PA, et al. Stimulus-secretion coupling in pancreatic beta cells. *J Cell Biochem* 1994;55[Suppl]:54–65.
72. Pipeleers DG, Marichal M, Malaisse WJ. The stimulus coupling of glucose-induced insulin release. XV. Participation of cations in the recognition of glucose by the B-cell. *Endocrinology* 1973;93:1012–1018.
73. Wenham RM, Landt M, Easom RA. Glucose activates the multifunctional Ca^{2+}/calmodulin-dependent protein kinase II in isolated rat pancreatic islets. *J Biol Chem* 1994;269:4947–4952.
74. Ammala C, Eliasson L, Bokvist K, et al. Exocytosis elicited by action potentials and voltage-clamp calcium currents in individual mouse pancreatic B-cells. *J Physiol* 1993;472:665–688.
75. Gagliardino JJ, Harrison DE, Christie MR, et al. Evidence for the participation of calmodulin in stimulus-secretion coupling in the pancreatic β-cell. *Biochem J* 1980;192:919–927.
76. Bailyes EM, Guest PC, Hutton JC. Insulin synthesis. In: Ashcroft FM, Ashcroft SJH, eds. *Insulin: molecular biology to pathology*. Oxford, UK: Oxford University Press, 1992:64–92.
77. Levy J, Malaisse WJ. The stimulus-secretion coupling of glucose induced insulin release. XVII. Effects of sulfonylureas and diazoxide on insular biosynthetic activity. *Biochem Pharmacol* 1975;24:235–239.
78. Gembal M, Gilon P, Henquin J-C. Evidence that glucose can control insulin release independently from its action on ATP-sensitive K^+ channels in mouse β-cells. *J Clin Invest* 1992;89:1288–1295.
79. Stein DT, Stevenson BE, Chester MW, et al. The insulinotropic potency of fatty acids is influenced profoundly by their chain length and degree of saturation. *J Clin Invest* 1997;100:398–403.
80. Stein DT, Esser V, Stevenson B, et al. Essentiality of circulating fatty acids for glucose-stimulated insulin secretion in the fasted rat. *J Clin Invest* 1996;97: 2728–2735.

81. Prentki M, Vischer S, Glennon MC, et al. Malonyl-CoA and long chain acyl-CoA esters as metabolic coupling factors in nutrient-induced insulin secretion. *J Biol Chem* 1992;267:5802–5810.
82. Wollheim CB, Regazzi R. Protein kinase C in insulin releasing cells: putative role in stimulus secretion coupling. *FEBS Lett* 1990;268:376–380.
83. Skelly RH, Schuppin GT, Ishihara H, et al. Glucose-regulated translational control of proinsulin biosynthesis with that of the proinsulin endopeptidases PC2 and PC3 in the insulin-producing MIN6 cell line. *Diabetes* 1996; 45:37–43.
84. Zhou YP, Grill VE. Long-term exposure of rat pancreatic islets to fatty acids inhibits glucose-induced insulin secretion and biosynthesis through a glucose fatty acid cycle. *J Clin Invest* 1994;93:870–876.
85. Permutt MA, Kipnis DM. Insulin biosynthesis: I. On the mechanism of glucose stimulation. *J Biol Chem* 1972;247:1194–1199.
86. Permutt MA, Kipnis DM. Insulin biosynthesis: studies of islet polyribosomes (nascent peptide sucrose gradient analysis gel-filtration). *Proc Natl Acad Sci U S A* 1972;69:505–509.
87. Permutt MA. Effect of glucose on initiation and elongation rate in isolated pancreatic islets. *J Biol Chem* 1974;248:2738–2742.
88. Lomedico PT, Saunders GF. Cell-free modulation of proinsulin synthesis. *Science* 1977;198:620–622.
89. Itoh N, Sei T, Nose K, et al. Glucose stimulation of the proinsulin synthesis in isolated islets without increasing amount of proinsulin mRNA. *FEBS Lett* 1978;93:343–347.
90. Parry DG, Taylor KW. Proinsulin biosynthesis in broken-cell preparations of islets of Langerhans. *Biochem J* 1978;170:523–527.
91. Itoh N, Okamoto H. Translational control of proinsulin synthesis by glucose. *Nature* 1980;283:100–102.
92. Itoh N, Ohshima Y, Nose K, et al. Glucose stimulates proinsulin synthesis in pancreatic islets without a concomitant increase in proinsulin mRNA synthesis. *Biochem Int* 1982;4:315–321.
93. Welsh M, Scherberg N, Gilmore R, et al. Translational control of insulin biosynthesis. Evidence for regulation of elongation, initiation and signal-recognition-particle-mediated translational arrest by glucose. *Biochem J* 1986; 235:459–467.
94. Welsh N, Welsh M, Steiner DF, et al. Mechanisms of leucine- and theophylline-stimulated insulin biosynthesis in isolated rat pancreatic islets. *Biochem J* 1987;246:245–248.
95. Merrick WC. Mechanism and regulation of eukaryotic protein synthesis. *Microbiol Rev* 1992;56:291–315.
96. Clemens MJ. Regulatory mechanisms in translational control. *Curr Opin Cell Biol* 1989;1:1160–1167.
97. Redpath NT, Proud CG. Molecular mechanisms in the control of translation by hormones and growth factors. *Biochim Biophys Acta* 1994;1220:147–162.
98. Pain VM. Inititation of protein synthesis in eukaryotic cells. *Eur J Biochem* 1996;236:747–771.
99. Ashcroft SJH. Protein phosphorylation and beta cell function. *Diabetologia* 1994;37[Suppl 2]:S21–S29.
100. Herbert TP, Alarcón C, Skelly RH, et al. Regulation of prohormone conversion by coordinated control of processing endopeptidase biosynthesis with that of the prohormone substrate. In: Hook VYH, ed. *Proteolytic and cellular mechanisms in prohormone and proprotein processing*. Austin, TX: R.G. Landes Company, 1998:105–120.
101. Knight SW, Docherty K. RNA-protein interactions in the 5′ untranslated region of preproinsulin mRNA. *J Mol Endocrinol* 1992;8:225–234.
102. Klausner RD, Rouault TA, Harford JB. Regulating the fate of mRNA: the control of cellular iron metabolism. *Cell* 1993;72:19–28.
103. Orland MJ, Chyn R, Permutt MA. Modulation of proinsulin messenger RNA after partial pancreatectomy in rats: relationships to glucose homeostasis. *J Clin Invest* 1985;75:2047–2055.
104. Giddings SJ, Chirgwin J, Permutt MA. Effects of glucose on proinsulin mRNA in rats in vivo. *Diabetes* 1982;31:624–629.
105. Brunstedt J, Chan SJ. Direct effect of glucose on the preproinsulin mRNA level in isolated pancreatic islets. *Biochem Biophys Res Comm* 1982;106: 1383–1389.
106. Nielsen DA, Welsh M, Casadaban MJ, et al. Control of insulin gene expression in pancreatic B-cells and in an insulin-producing cell line, RIN-5F cells. I. Effects of glucose and cAMP on the transcription of insulin mRNA. *J Biol Chem* 1985;260:13585–13589.
107. Welsh M, Nielsen DA, MacKrell AJ, et al. Control of insulin gene expression in pancreatic B-cells and in an insulin producing cell line, RIN-5F cells. II. Regulation of insulin mRNA stability. *J Biol Chem* 1985;260:13590–13594.
108. Giddings SJ, Chirgwin J, Permutt MA. The effects of fasting and feeding on preproinsulin mRNA in rats. *J Clin Invest* 1981;67:952–960.
109. Giddings SJ, Carnaghi LR, Shalwitz RA. Hypoglycemia but not hyperglycemia induces rapid changes in pancreatic β-cell gene transcription. *Am J Physiol* 1993;265:E259–E266.
110. Palade G. Intracellular aspects of the process of protein synthesis. *Science* 1975;189:347–358.
111. Orci L. Macro- and micro-domains in the endocrine pancreas. *Diabetes* 1982; 31:528–546.
112. Orci L, Vassalli J-D, Perrelet A. The insulin factory. *Sci Am* 1988;259:85–94.
113. Kelly RB. Pathways of protein secretion in eukaryotes. *Science* 1985;230: 25–32.
114. Halban PA. Differential rates of release of newly synthesized and of stored insulin from pancreatic islets. *Endocrinology* 1982;110:1183–1188.
115. Halban PA. Proinsulin trafficking and processing in the pancreatic β-cell. *Trends Endocrinol Metab* 1990;May:261–265.
116. Halban PA, Irminger J-C. Sorting and processing of secretory proteins. *Biochem J* 1994;299:1–18.
117. Howell SL. Role of ATP in the intracellular translocation of proinsulin and insulin in the rat pancreatic β-cell [letter]. *Nat New Biol* 1972;235:85–86.
118. Rothman JE, Orci L. Molecular dissection of the secretory pathway. *Nature* 1992;355:409–415.
119. Howell SL. The mechanism of insulin secretion. *Diabetologia* 1984;26:319–327.
120. Balch WE. Small GTP-binding proteins in vesicular transport. *Trends Biochem Sci* 1990;15:473–477.
121. Schwaninger R, Plutner H, Bokoch GM, et al. Multiple GTP-binding proteins regulate vesicular transport from the ER to Golgi membranes. *Cell Biol* 1992; 119:1077–1096.
122. Rothman JE, Wieland FT. Protein sorting by transport vesicles. *Science* 1996; 272:227–234.
123. Beckers CJM, Block MR, Glick BS, et al. Vesicular transport between the endoplasmic reticulum and the Golgi stack requires the NEM-sensitive fusion protein. *Nature* 1989;339:397–398.
124. Tisdale EJ, Bourne JR, Khosravi-Far R, et al. GTP-binding mutants of Rab1 and Rab2 are potent inhibitors of vesicular transport from the endoplasmic reticulum to the Golgi complex. *J Cell Biol* 1992;119:749–761.
125. Zerial M, Stenmark H. Rab GTPases in vesicular transport. *Curr Opin Cell Biol* 1993;5:613–620.
126. Orci L, Malhotra V, Amherdt M, et al. Dissection of a single round of vesicular transport: sequential intermediates for intercisternal movement in the Golgi stack. *Cell* 1989;56:357–368.
127. Rothman JE, Orci L. Budding vesicles in living cells. *Sci Am* 1996;274:70–75.
128. Orci L, Glick BS, Rothman JE. A new type of coated vesicular carrier that appears not to contain clathrin: its possible role in protein transport within the Golgi stack. *Cell* 1986;46:171–184.
129. Sollner T. SNAREs and targeted membrane fusion. *FEBS Lett* 1995;369:80–83.
130. Goud B, Zahraoui A, Tavitian A, et al. Small GTP binding protein associated with Golgi cisternae. *Nature* 1990;345:553–556.
131. Clary DO, Griff IC, Rothman JE. SNAPs: a family of NSF attachment proteins involved in intracellular membrane fusion in animals and yeast. *Cell* 1990;61: 709–721.
132. Söllner T, Whiteheart SW, Brunner M, et al. SNAP receptors implicated in vesicle targetting and fusion. *Nature* 1993;362:318–324.
133. Glick BS, Rothman JE. Possible role for fatty acyl-coenzyme A in intracellular protein transport. *Nature* 1987;326:309–312.
134. De Camilli P, Emr SD, McPherson PS, et al. Phosphoinositides as regulators in membrane traffic. *Science* 1996;271:1533–1539.
135. Pfeffer SR, Rothman JE. Biosynthetic protein transport and sorting by the endoplasmic reticulum and Golgi. *Annu Rev Biochem* 1987;56:829–852.
136. Burgess TL, Kelly RB. Constitutive and regulated secretion of proteins. *Annu Rev Cell Biol* 1987;3:243–293.
137. Rhodes CJ, Halban PA. Newly-synthesized proinsulin/insulin and stored insulin are released form pancreatic B-cells via a regulated, rather than a constitutive pathway. *J Cell Biol* 1987;105:145–153.
138. Orci L, Ravazzola M, Amherdt M, et al. The trans-most cisternae of the Golgi complex: A compartment for sorting of secretory and plasma membrane proteins. *Cell* 1987;56:1039–1051.
139. Nagamatsu S, Steiner DF. Altered glucose regulation of insulin biosynthesis in insulinoma cells: mouse βTC3 cells secrete insulin-related peptides predominately via a constitutive pathway. *Endocrinology* 1992;130:748–754.
140. Orci L, Ravazzola M, Perrelet A. (Pro)insulin associates with Golgi membranes of pancreatic B cells. *Proc Natl Acad Sci U S A* 1984;81:6743–6746.
141. Cool DR, Normant E, Shen F, et al. Carboxypeptidase E is a regulated secretory pathway sorting receptor: genetic obliteration leads to endocrine disorders in Cpe(fat) mice. *Cell* 1997;88:73–83.
142. Cool DR, Loh YP. Carboxypeptidase E is a sorting receptor for prohormones: binding and kinetic studies. *Mol Cell Endocrinol* 1998;139:7–13.
143. Normant E, Loh YP. Depletion of carboxypeptidase E, a regulated secretory pathway sorting receptor, causes misrouting and constitutive secretion of proinsulin and proenkephalin, but not chromogranin A. *Endocrinol* 1998;139: 2137–2145.
144. Thiele C, Gerdes HH, Huttner WB. Protein secretion: puzzling receptors [see comments]. *Curr Biol* 1997;7:R496–R500.
145. Naggert JK, Fricker LD, Varlamov O, et al. Hyperproinsulinaemia in obese fat/fat mice associated with a carboxypeptidase E mutation which reduces enzyme activity. *Nat Genet* 1995;10:135–142.
146. Varlamov O, Fricker LD, Furukawa H, et al. Beta-cell lines derived from transgenic Cpe(fat)/Cpe(fat) mice are defective in carboxypeptidase E and proinsulin processing. *Endocrinology* 1997;138:4883–4892.
147. Irminger JC, Verchere CB, Meyer K, et al. Proinsulin targeting to the regulated pathway is not impaired in carboxypeptidase E-deficient Cpefat/Cpefat mice. *Biol Chem* 1997;272:27532–27534.
148. Bauerfeind R, Huttner WB. Biogenesis of constitutive secretory vesicles, secretory granules and synaptic vesicles. *Curr Opin Cell Biol* 1993;5:628–635.
149. Tooze SA. Biogenesis of secretory granules in the trans-Golgi network of neuroendocrine and endocrine cells. *Biochim Biophy Acta* 1998;1404:231–244.
150. Arvan P, Castle D. Sorting and storage during secretory granule biogenesis: looking backward and looking forward. *Biochem J* 1998;332:593–610.
151. Tooze SA, Huttner WB. Cell free protein sorting to the regulated and constitutive secretory pathways. *Cell* 1990;60:837–847.

152. Hutton JC. Insulin secretory granule biogenesis and the proinsulin-processing endopeptidases. *Diabetologia* 1994;37[Suppl 2]:S48–S56.
153. Gerdes H-H, Rosa P, Phillips E, et al. The primary structure of human secretogranin II, a widespread tyrosine-sulfated secretory granule protein that exhibits low pH and calcium-induced aggregation. *J Biol Chem* 1989;264: 12009–12015.
154. Sopwith AM, Hales CN, Hutton JC. Pancreatic β-cells secrete a range of novel peptides besides insulin. *Biochim Biophys Acta* 1984;803:342–345.
155. Guest PC, Bailyes EM, Rutherford NG, et al. Insulin secretory granule biogenesis: co-ordinate regulation of the biosynthesis of the majority of constituent proteins. *Biochem J* 1991;274:73–78.
156. Guest PG, Pipeleers D, Rossier J, et al. Co-secretion of carboxypeptidase H and insulin from isolated rat islets of Langerhans. *Biochem J* 1989;264:503–508.
157. Moore HH, Walker MD, Lee F, et al. Expressing a human proinsulin cDNA in a mouse ACTH-secreting cell. Intracellular storage, proteolytic processing, and secretion on stimulation. *Cell* 1983;35:531–538.
158. Moore HP, Kelly RB. Secretory protein targeting in a pituitary cell line: differential transport of foreign secretory proteins to distinct secretory pathways. *J Cell Biol* 1985;101:1773–1781.
159. Burgess TL, Craik CS, Kelly RB. The exocrine protein trypsinogen is targeted into the secretory granules of an endocrine cell line: studies by gene transfer. *J Cell Biol* 1985;101:639–645.
160. Moore H-PH, Kelly RB. Rerouting of a secretory protein by fusion with growth hormone sequence. *Nature* 1986;321:443–446.
161. Halban PA. Structural domains and molecular lifestyles of insulin and its precursors in the pancreatic beta cell. *Diabetologia* 1991;34:767–778.
162. Gross DJ, Halban PA, Kahn CR, et al. Partial diversion of a mutant proinsulin (B10 aspartic acid) from the regulated to the constitutive secretory pathway in transfected AtT-20 cells. *Proc Natl Acad Sci U S A* 1989;86:4107–4111.
163. Carroll RJ, Hammer RE, Chan SJ, et al. A mutant human proinsulin is secreted from islets of Langerhans in increased amounts via an unregulated pathway. *Proc Natl Acad Sci U S A* 1988;85:8943–8947.
164. Quinn D, Orci L, Ravazzola M, et al. Intracellular transport and sorting of mutant human proinsulins that fail to form hexamers. *J Cell Biol* 1991;113: 987–996.
165. Dodson G, Steiner D. The role of assembly in insulin's biosynthesis. *Curr Opin Struct Biol* 1998;8:189–194.
166. Orci L, Ravazzola M, Amherdt M, et al. Clathrin-immunoreactive sites in the Golgi apparatus are concentrated at the trans pole in polypeptide hormone-secreting cells. *Proc Natl Acad Sci U S A* 1985;82:5385–5389.
167. Hirst J, Robinson MS. Clathrin and adaptors. *Biochim Biophys Acta* 1998;1404: 173–193.
168. Pearse BMF, Robinson MS. Clathrin, adaptors, and sorting. *Annu Rev Cell Biol* 1990;6:151–171.
169. Brodsky FM. Living with clathrin: its role in intracellular membrane traffic. *Science* 1988;242:1396–1402.
170. Dittie AS, Hajibagheri N, Tooze SA. The AP-1 adaptor complex binds to immature secretory granules from PC12 cells, and is regulated by ADP-ribosylation factor. *J Cell Biol* 1996;132:523–536.
171. Austin C, Hinners I, Tooze SA. Direct and GTP-dependent interaction of ADP-ribosylation factor 1 with clathrin adaptor protein, AP-1 on immature secretory granules. *J Biol Chem* 2000;275:21862–21869.
172. Kuliawat R, Arvan P. Protein targeting via the "constitutive-like" pathway in isolated pancreatic islets: passive sorting in the immature granule. *J Cell Biol* 1992;118:521–529.
173. Kuliawat R, Arvan P. Distinct molecular mechanisms for protein sorting within immature secretory granules of pancreatic β-cells. *J Cell Biol* 1994;126: 77–86.
174. Klumperman J, Kuliawat R, Griffith JM, et al. Mannose 6-phosphate receptors are sorted from immature secretory granules via adaptor protein AP-1, clathrin, and syntaxin 6-positive vesicles. *J Cell Biol* 1998;141:359–371.
175. Kuliawat R, Klumperman J, Ludwig T, et al. Differential sorting of lysosomal enzymes out of the regulated secretory pathway in pancreatic beta-cells. *J Cell Biol* 1997;137:595–608.
176. Orci L, Ravazzola M, Amherdt M, et al. Conversion of proinsulin to insulin occurs coordinately with acidification of maturing secretory granules. *J Cell Biol* 1986;103:2273–2281.
177. Orci L, Ravazzola M, Storch M-J, et al. Proteolytic maturation of insulin is a post-Golgi event which occurs in acidifying clathrin-coated secretory vesicles. *Cell* 1987;49:865–868.
178. Orci L, Halban P, Perrelet A, et al. pH-independent and -dependent cleavage of proinsulin in the same secretory vesicle. *J Cell Biol* 1994;126:1149–1156.
179. Rhodes CJ, Lucas CA, Mutkoski RL, et al. Stimulation by ATP of proinsulin to insulin conversion in isolated rat pancreatic islet secretory granules: association with ATP-dependent proton pump. *J Biol Chem* 1987;262:10712–10717.
180. Docherty KD, Hutton JC. Carboxypeptidase activity in the insulin secretory granule. *FEBS Lett* 1983;162:137–141.
181. Davidson HW, Hutton JC. The insulin secretory granule carboxypeptidase-H. Purification and demonstration of involvement in proinsulin processing. *Biochem J* 1987;245:575–582.
182. Davidson HW, Peshavaria M, Hutton JC. Proteolytic conversion of proinsulin into insulin: identification of a Ca^{++}-dependent acidic endopeptidase in isolated insulin secretory granules. *Biochem J* 1987;246:279–286.
183. Davidson HW, Rhodes CJ, Hutton JC. Intraorganellar Ca and pH control proinsulin cleavage in the pancreatic β-cell via two site-specific endopeptidases. *Nature* 1988;333:93–96.
184. Rhodes CJ, Zumbrunn A, Bailyes EM, et al. The inhibition of proinsulin-processing endopeptidase activities by active-site-directed peptides. *Biochem J* 1989;258:305–308.
185. Rhodes CJ, Lincoln B, Shoelson SE. Preferential cleavage of des 31, 32 proinsulin over intact proinsulin by the insulin secretory granule type-II endopeptidase: implications for a favoured route for prohormone processing. *J Biol Chem* 1992;267:22719–22727.
186. Docherty KD, Rhodes CJ, Taylor NA, et al. Proinsulin endopeptidase substrate specificities defined by site-directed mutagenesis of proinsulin. *J Biol Chem* 1989;264:18335–18339.
187. Rhodes CJ, Brennan SO, Hutton JC. Proalbumin to albumin conversion by a proinsulin processing endopeptidase of insulin secretory granules. *Biol Chem* 1989;264:14240–14245.
188. Hutton JC. Subtilisin-like proteinases involved in the activation of proproteins of the secretory pathway of eukaryotic cells. *Curr Opin Cell Biol* 1991;2: 1131–1142.
189. Fuller RS, Sterne RE, Thorner J. Enzymes required for yeast prohormone processing. *Ann Rev Physiol* 1988;50:345–362.
190. Fuller RS, Brake A, Thorner J. Yeast prohormone processing enzyme (KEX2 gene product) is a Ca^{++}-dependent serine protease. *Proc Natl Acad Sci U S A* 1989;86:1434–1438.
191. Julius D, Brake A, Blair L, et al. Isolation of the putative structural gene for the lysine-arginine cleaving endopeptidase for processing yeast prepro-a-factor. *Cell* 1984;37:1075–1089.
192. Smeekens SP, Avruch AS, LaMendola J, et al. Identification of a cDNA encoding a second putative prohormone convertase related to PC2 in AtT20 cells and islets of Langerhans. *Proc Natl Acad Sci U S A* 1991;88:340–344.
193. Seidah NG, Marcinkiewicz M, Benjannet S, et al. Cloning and primary sequence of a mouse candidate prohormone convertase PC1 homologous to PC2, furin, and Kex2: distinct chromosomal localisation and messenger RNA distribution in brain and pituitary compared to PC2. *Mol Endocrinol* 1991;5:111–122.
194. Bailyes EM, Shennan KIJ, Seal AJ, et al. A member of the eukaryotic subtilisin family (PC3) has the enzymic properties of the type-I proinsulin-converting endopeptidase. *Biochem J* 1992;285:391–394.
195. Bailyes EM, Bennett DL, Hutton JC. Proprotein-processing endopeptidases of the insulin secretory granule. *Enzyme* 1991;45:301–313.
196. Smeekens SP, Steiner DF. Identification of a human insulinoma cDNA encoding a novel mammalian protein structurally related to the yeast dibasic processing KEX2. *J Biol Chem* 1990;265:2997–3000.
197. Seidah NG, Gaspar L, Mion P, et al. cDNA sequence of two distinct pituitary proteins homologous to Kex2 and furin gene products: tissue-specific mRNAs encoding candidates for pro-hormone processing proteinases. *DNA Cell Biol* 1990;9:415–424.
198. Bennett DL, Bailyes EM, Nielson E, et al. Identification of the type-II proinsulin processing endopeptidase as PC2, a member of the eukaryotic subtilisin family. *J Biol Chem* 1992;267:15229–15236.
199. Smeekens SP, Montag AG, Thomas G, et al. Proinsulin processing by the subtilisin-related proprotein covertases furin, PC2 and PC3. *Proc Natl Acad Sci U S A* 1992;89:8822–8826.
200. Fricker LD. Carboxypeptidase-E. *Annu Rev Physiol* 1988;50:279–289.
201. Hutton JC, Penn EJ, Peshavaria M. Low molecular weight constituents of isolated insulin secretory granules: bivalent cations, adenine nucleotides and inorganic phosphate. *Biochem J* 1983;210:297–305.
202. Hutton JC. The internal pH and membrane potential of the insulin secretory granule. *Biochem J* 1982;204:171–178.
203. Rhodes CJ, Alarcón C. What β-cell defect could lead to hyperproinsulinemia in NIDDM: some clues from recent advances made in understanding the proinsulin conversion mechanism. *Diabetes* 1994;43:511–517.
204. Formby B, Capito K, Egeberg J, et al. Ca-activated ATPase activity in subcellular fractions of mouse pancreatic islets. *Am J Physiol* 1976;230:441–448.
205. Wilcox CA, Fuller RS. Posttranslational processing of the prohormone-cleaving Kex2 protease in the *Saccharomyces cerevisiae* secretory pathway. *Cell Biol* 1991;115:297–307.
206. Rehemtulla A, Dorner A, Kaufman RJ. Regulation of PACE/furin processing: requirement for a post-endoplasmic reticulum compartment and autoproteolytic activation. *Proc Natl Acad Sci U S A* 1992;89:8235–8239.
207. Steiner DF. The proprotein convertases. *Curr Opin Chem Biol* 1998;2:31–39.
208. Guest PC, Arden SD, Bennett DL, et al. The post-translational processing and intracellular sorting of PC2 in the islets of Langerhans. *J Biol Chem* 1992;267: 22401–22406.
209. Shennan KIJ, Smeekens SP, Steiner DF, et al. Characterization of PC2, a mammalian Kex2 homologue, following expression of the cDNA in microinjected Xenopus oocytes. *FEBS Lett* 1991;284:277–280.
210. Shennan KIJ, Seal AJ, Smeekens SP, et al. Site-directed mutagenesis and expression of PC2 in microinjected Xenopus oocytes. *J Biol Chem* 1991;266: 24011–24017.
211. Steiner DF, Smeekens SP, Ohagi S, et al. The new enzymology of precursor processing endopeptidases. *J Biol Chem* 1992;267:23435–23438.
212. Takagi H, Matsuzawa H, Ohta T, et al. Studies on the structure and function of subtilisin E by protein engineering. *Ann N Y Acad Sci* 1992;672:52–59.
213. Martens GJM, Braks JAM, Eib DW, et al. The neuroendocrine polypeptide 7B2 is an endogenous inhibitor of prohormone convertase PC2. *Proc Natl Acad Sci U S A* 1994;91:5784–5787.
214. Braks JAM, Martens GJM. 7B2 is a neuroendocrine chaperone that transiently interacts with prohormone convertase PC2 in the secretory pathway. *Cell* 1994;78:263–274.

215. Zhu X, Rouille Y, Lamango NS, et al. Internal cleavage of the inhibitory 7B2 carboxyl-terminal peptide by PC2: a potential mechanism for its inactivation. *Proc Natl Acad Sci U S A* 1996;93:4919–4924.
216. Muller L, Zhu X, Lindberg I. Mechanism of the facilitation of PC2 maturation by 7B2: involvement in ProPC2 transport and activation but not folding. *J Cell Biol* 1997;139:625–638.
217. Nagamatsu S, Bolaffi JL, Grodsky GM. Direct effects of glucose on proinsulin synthesis and processing during desensitization. *Endocrinology* 1987;120: 1225–1231.
218. Schuppin GT, Rhodes CJ. Specific co-ordinated regulation of PC3 and PC2 gene transcription with that of preproinsulin in insulin-producing βTC3 cells. *Biochem J* 1995;313:259–268.
219. Rubenstein AH, Cho S, Steiner DF. Evidence for proinsulin in human urine and serum. *Lancet* 1968;1:1353–1355.
220. Horwitz DL, Starr JI, Mako ME, et al. Proinsulin, insulin, and C-peptide concentrations in human portal and peripheral blood. *J Clin Invest* 1975;55: 1278–1283.
221. Robbins DC, Tager HS, Rubenstein AH. Biologic and clinical importance of proinsulin. *N Engl J Med* 1984;310:1165–1175.
222. Sobey WJ, Beer SF, Carrington CA, et al. Sensitive and specific two-site immunoradiometric assays for human insulin, proinsulin, 65-66 split and 32-33 split proinsulins. *Biochem J* 1989;260:535–541.
223. Given BD, Cohen RM, Shoelson SE, et al. Biochemical and clinical implications of proinsulin conversion intermediates. *J Clin Invest* 1985;76:1398–1405.
224. Kahn SE, Halban PA. Release of incompletely processed proinsulin is the cause of the disproportionate proinsulinemia of NIDDM. *Diabetes* 1997;46: 1725–1732.
225. Tillil H, Frank BH, Pekar AH, et al. Hypoglycemic potency and metabolic clearance rate of intravenously administered human proinsulin and metabolites. *Endocrinology* 1990;127:2418–2422.
226. Weiss MA, Frank BH, Khait I, et al. NMR and photo-CIDNP of human proinsulin and prohormone processing intermediates with application to endoprotease recognition. *Biochemistry* 1990;29:8389–8401.
227. Sizonenko S, Irminger J-C, Buhler L, et al. Kinetics of proinsulin conversion in human islets. *Diabetes* 1993;42:933–936.
228. Johansson BL, Sjoberg S, Wahren J. The influence of human C-peptide on renal function and glucose utilization in type 1 (insulin-dependent) diabetic patients. *Diabetologia* 1992;35:121–128.
229. Johansson BL, Kernell A, Sjoberg S, et al. Influence of combined C-peptide and insulin administration on renal function and metabolic control in diabetes type 1. *J Clin Endocrinol Metab* 1993;77:976–981.
230. Wu W, Oshida Y, Yang WP, et al. Effect of C-peptide administration on whole body glucose utilization in STZ-induced diabetic rats. *Acta Physiol Scand* 1996;157:253–258.
231. Ido Y, Vindigni A, Chang K, et al. Prevention of vascular and neural dysfunction in diabetic rats by C-peptide [see comments]. *Science* 1997;277: 563–566.
232. Johansson BL, Borg K, Fernqvist-Forbes E, et al. C-peptide improves autonomic nerve function in IDDM patients. *Diabetologia* 1996;39:687–695.
233. Leclercq-Meyer V, Malaisse WJ, Johansson BL, et al. Effect of C-peptide on insulin and glucagon release by isolated perfused rat pancreas. *Diabetes Metab* 1997;23:149–154.
234. Ohtomo Y, Aperia A, Sahlgren B, et al. C-peptide stimulates rat renal tubular Na^+, $K(^+)$-ATPase activity in synergism with neuropeptide Y. *Diabetologia* 1996;39:199–205.
235. Ohtomo Y, Bergman T, Johansson BL, et al. Differential effects of proinsulin C-peptide fragments on Na^+, K^+- ATPase activity of renal tubule segments. *Diabetologia* 1998;41:287–291.
236. Wahren J, Ekberg K, Johansson J, et al. Role of C-peptide in human physiology. *Am J Physiol Endocrinol Metab* 2000;278:E759–E768.
237. Forst T, Kunt T, Pfutzner A, et al. New aspects on biological activity of C-peptide in IDDM patients. *Exp Clin Endocrinol Diabetes* 1998;106:270–276.
238. Wahren J, Johansson BL, Wallberg-Henriksson H, et al. C-peptide revisited—new physiological effects and therapeutic implications. *J Intern Med* 1996;240: 115–124.
239. Wahren J, Johansson BL, Wallberg-Henriksson H. Does C-peptide have a physiological role? *Diabetologia* 1994;37[Suppl 2]:S99–S107.
240. Rigler R, Pramanik A, Jonasson P, et al. Specific binding of proinsulin C-peptide to human cell membranes. *Proc Natl Acad Sci U S A* 1999;96:13318–13323.
241. Steiner DF, Rubenstein AH. Proinsulin C-peptide—biological activity? [comment]. *Science* 1997;277:531–532.
242. Mako ME, Starr JI, Rubenstein AH. Circulating proinsulin in patients with maturity onset diabetes. *Am J Med* 1977;63:865–869.
243. Temple RC, Carrington CA, Luzio SD, et al. Insulin deficiency in non-insulin-dependent diabetes. *Lancet* 1989;1:293–295.
244. Ward WK, LaCava EC, Paquette TL, et al. Disproportionate elevation of immunoreactive proinsulin in type 2 (non-insulin-dependent) diabetes mellitus and in experimental insulin resistance. *Diabetologia* 1987;30:698–702.
245. Yoshioka N, Kuzuya T, Taniguchi M, et al. Serum proinsulin levels at fasting and after oral glucose load in patients with type 2 (non-insulin-dependent) diabetes mellitus. *Diabetologia* 1988;31:355–360.
246. Heding LG, Ludvigsson J, Kasperska-Czyzykowa T. B-cell secretion in non-diabetics and insulin-dependent diabetics. *Acta Med Scand Suppl* 1981;656: 5–9.
247. Ludvigsson J, Heding L. Abnormal proinsulin/C-peptide ratio in juvenile diabetes. *Acta Diabetol Lat* 1982;19:351–358.
248. Snorgaard O, Hartling SG, Binder C. Proinsulin and C-peptide at onset and during 12 months cyclosporin treatment of type 1 (insulin-dependent) diabetes mellitus [see comments]. *Diabetologia* 1990;33:36–42.
249. Heaton DA, Millward BA, Gray IP, et al. Increased proinsulin levels as an early indicator of B-cell dysfunction in non-diabetic twins of type 1 (insulin-dependent) patients. *Diabetologia* 1988;31:182–184.
250. Hartling SG, Lindgren F, Dahlqvist G, et al. Elevated proinsulin in healthy siblings of IDDM patients independent of HLA identity. *Diabetes* 1989;38: 1271–1274.
251. Kahn SE, Leonetti DL, Prigeon RL, et al. Proinsulin as a marker for the development of NIDDM in Japanese-American men. *Diabetes* 1995;44:173–179.
252. Nagi DK, Hendra TJ, Ryle AJ, et al. The relationships of concentrations of insulin, intact proinsulin and 32-33 split proinsulin with cardiovascular risk factors in type 2 (non-insulin-dependent) diabetic subjects [see comments]. *Diabetologia* 1990;33:532–537.
253. Clark PM, Levy JC, Cox L, et al. Immunoradiometric assay of insulin, intact proinsulin and 32-33 split proinsulin and radioimmunoassay of insulin in diet-treated type 2 (non-insulin-dependent) diabetic subjects. *Diabetologia* 1992;35:469–474.
254. Porte D, Kahn SE. Hyperproinsulinemia and amyloid in NIDDM: clues to etiology of islet β-cell dysfunction. *Diabetes* 1989;38:1333–1336.
255. Kahn SE. Regulation of β-cell function in vivo. *Diabetes Rev* 1996;4:372–389.
256. Furuta M, Carroll R, Martin S, et al. Incomplete processing of proinsulin to insulin accompanied by elevation of des-31,32 proinsulin intermediates in islets of mice lacking active PC2. *J Biol Chem* 1998;273:3431–3437.
257. Furuta M, Yano H, Zhou A, et al. Defective prohormone processing and altered pancreatic islet morphology in mice lacking active SPC2. *Proc Natl Acad Sci U S A* 1997;94:6646–6651.
258. Seidah NG, Chretien M. Eukaryotic protein processing: endoproteolysis of precursor proteins. *Curr Opin Biotechnol* 1997;8:602–607.
259. Westphal CH, Muller L, Zhou A, et al. The neuroendocrine protein 7B2 is required for peptide hormone processing in vivo and provides a novel mechanism for pituitary Cushing's disease. *Cell* 1999;96:689–700.
260. Jackson RS, Creemers JW, Ohagi S, et al. Obesity and impaired prohormone processing associated with mutations in the human prohormone convertase 1 gene. *Nat Genet* 1997;16:303–306.
261. Weigle DS, Kuijper JL. Obesity genes and the regulation of body fat content. *Bioessays* 1999;18:867–874.
262. Fricker LD, Leiter EH. Peptides, enzymes and obesity: new insights from a 'dead' enzyme. *Trends Biochem Sci* 1999;24:390–393.
263. Gorden P, Hendricks CM, Roth J. Circulating proinsulin-like component in man. *Diabetologia* 1974;10:469–474.
264. Melani F, Ryan WG, Rubenstein AH, et al. Proinsulin secretion by a pancreatic beta-cell adenoma: proinsulin and C-peptide secretion. *N Engl J Med* 1970;283:713–719.
265. Gorden P, Sherman B, Roth J. Proinsulin-like component of circulating insulin in the basal state and in patients and hamsters with islet cell tumors. *J Clin Invest* 1971;50:2113–2122.
266. Cohen RM, Given BD, Licinio-Paixao J, et al. Proinsulin radioimmunoassay in the evaluation of insulinomas and familial hyperproinsulinemia. *Metabolism* 1986;35:1137–1146.
267. Creutzfeldt C, Track NS, Creutzfeldt W. In vitro studies of the rate of proinsulin and insulin turnover in seven human insulinomas. *Eur J Clin Invest* 1973;3:371–384.
268. Gold G, Gishizky ML, Chick WL, et al. Contrasting patterns of insulin biosynthesis, compartmental storage, and secretion: rat tumor verses islet cells. *Diabetes* 1984;33:556–561.
269. Gutman RA, Fink G, Shapiro JR, et al. Proinsulin and insulin release with a human insulinoma and adjacent nonadenomatous pancreas. *J Clin Endocrinol Metab* 1973;36:978–987.
270. Wang SY. The acute effects of glucose on the insulin biosynthetic-secretory pathway in a simian virus 40-transformed hamster pancreatic islet beta-cell line. *Endocrinology* 1989;124:1980–1987.
271. Westermark P, Wernstedt C, Wilander E, et al. Amyloid fibrils in human insulinoma and islets of Langerhans of the diabetic cat are derived from a neuropeptide-like protein also present in normal islet cells. *Proc Natl Acad Sci U S A* 1987;84:3881–3885.
272. Hutton JC. Secretory granules. *Experientia* 1984;40:1091–1098.
273. Hutton JC. The insulin secretory granule. *Diabetologia* 1989;32:271–281.
274. Eipper BA, Milgram SL, Husten EJ, et al. Peptidylglycine alpha-amidating monooxygenase: a multifunctional protein with catalytic, processing, and routing domains. *Protein Sci* 1993;2:489–497.
275. Zhou A, Thorn NA. Evidence for presence of peptide-amidating activity in pancreatic islets from newborn rats. *Biochem J* 1990;267:253–256.
276. Hutton JC, Hansen F, Peshavaria M. β-granins: 21kDa co-secreted peptides of the insulin granule related to adrenal medullary chromogranin-A. *FEBS Lett* 1985;188:336–340.
277. Hartter E, Svoboda T, Ludvik B, et al. Basal and stimulated plasma levels of pancreatic amylin indicate its co-secretion with insulin in humans. *Diabetologia* 1991;34:52–54.
278. Moore CX, Cooper GJ. Co-secretion of amylin and insulin from cultured islet beta-cells: modulation by nutrient secretagogues, islet hormones and hypoglycemic agents. *Biochem Biophys Res Commun* 1991;179:1–9.
279. Hutton JC, Davidson HW, Grimaldi KA, et al. Biosynthesis of betagranin in pancreatic β-cells: identification of a chromogranin-A like precursor and its parallel processing with proinsulin. *Biochem J* 1987;244:449–456.

280. Hutton JC, Davidson HW, Peshavaria M. Proteolytic processing of chromogranin-A in purified insulin granules: formation of a 20kDa N-terminal fragment (betagranin) by the concerted action of a Ca^{2+}-dependent endopeptidase and carboxypeptidase H (EC 3.4.17.10). *Biochem J* 1987;244:457–464.
281. Arden SD, Rutherford NG, Guest PC, et al. The post-translational processing of chromogranin A in the pancreatic islet: involvement of the eukaryote subtilisin PC2. *Biochem J* 1994;298:521–528.
282. Tatemoto K, Efendic S, Mutt V, et al. Pancreastatin, a novel pancreatic peptide that inhibits insulin secretion. *Nature* 1986;324:476–478.
283. Ahren B, Lindskog S, Tatemoto K, et al. Pancreastatin inhibits insulin secretion and stimulates glucagon secretion in mice. *Diabetes* 1988;37:281–285.
284. Cooper GJ, Day AJ, Willis AC, et al. Amylin and the amylin gene: structure, function and relationship to islet amyloid and to diabetes mellitus. *Biochim Biophys Acta* 1989;1014:247–258.
285. Nishi M, Sanke T, Nagamatsu S, et al. Islet amyloid polypeptide: a new β-cell secretory product related to islet amyloid deposits. *J Biol Chem* 1990;265: 4173–4176.
286. Nishi M, Sanke T, Ohagi S, et al. Molecular biology of islet amyloid polypeptide. *Diabetes Res Clin Pract* 1992;15:37–44.
287. O'Brien TD, Butler PC, Westermark P, et al. Islet amyloid polypeptide: a review of its biology and potential roles in the pathogenesis of diabetes mellitus. *Vet Pathol* 1993;30:317–332.
288. Nagamatsu S, Nishi M, Steiner DF. Biosynthesis of islet amyloid polypeptide: elevated expression in mouse βTC3 cells. *J Biol Chem* 1991;266:13737–13741.
289. Sanke T, Bell GI, Sample C, et al. An islet amyloid peptide is derived from an 89-amino acid precursor by proteolytic processing. *Biol Chem* 1988;263: 17243–17246.
290. Westermark P, Engström U, Westermark GT, et al. Islet amyloid polypeptide (IAPP) and pro-IAPP immunoreactivity in human islets of Langerhans. *Diabetes Res Clin Pract* 1989;7:219–226.
291. Clark A, de Konig EJ, Hattersley AT, et al. Pancreatic pathology in non-insulin dependent diabetes (NIDDM). *Diabetes Res Clin Pract* 1995;28:39–47.
292. Clark A. Islet amyloid and type 2 diabetes. *Diabet Med* 1989;6:561–567.
293. O'Brien TD, Butler AE, Roche PC, et al. Islet amyloid polypeptide in human insulinomas. Evidence for intracellular amyloidogenesis. *Diabetes* 1994;43: 329–336.
294. Kudva YC, Mueske C, Butler PC, et al. A novel assay in vitro of human islet amyloid polypeptide amyloidogenesis and effects of insulin secretory vesicle peptides on amyloid formation. *Biochem J* 1998;331:809–813.
295. Clark A, Charge SB, Badman MK, et al. Islet amyloid polypeptide: actions and role in the pathogenesis of diabetes. *Biochem Soc Trans* 1996;24:594–599.
296. Betsholtz C, Christmansson L, Engstrom U, et al. Sequence divergence in a specific region of islet amyloid polypeptide (IAPP) explains differences in islet amyloid formation between species. *FEBS Lett* 1989;251:261–264.
297. Fox N, Schrementi J, Nishi M, et al. Human islet amyloid polypeptide transgenic mice as a model of non-insulin-dependent diabetes mellitus (NIDDM). *FEBS Lett* 1993;323:1–2.
298. Verchere CB, D'Alessio DA, Palmiter RD, et al. Islet amyloid formation associated with hyperglycemia in transgenic mice with pancreatic beta cell expression of human islet amyloid polypeptide. *Proc Natl Acad Sci U S A* 1996;93:3492–3496.
299. Janson J, Soeller WC, Roche PC, et al. Spontaneous diabetes mellitus in transgenic mice expressing human islet amyloid polypeptide. *Proc Natl Acad Sci U S A* 1996;93.
300. Ohsawa H, Kanatsuka A, Yamaguchi T, et al. Islet amyloid polypeptide inhibits glucose-stimulated insulin secretion from isolated rat pancreatic islets. *Biochem Biophys Res Commun* 1989;160:961–967.
301. Molina JM, Cooper GJ, Leighton B, et al. Induction of insulin resistance in vivo by amylin and calcitonin gene-related peptide. *Diabetes* 1990;39:260–265.
302. Sowa R, Sanke T, Hirayama J, et al. Islet amyloid polypeptide amide causes peripheral insulin resistance in vivo in dogs. *Diabetologia* 1990;33:118–120.
303. Tabata H, Hirayama J, Sowa R, et al. Islet amyloid polypeptide (IAPP/amylin) causes insulin resistance in perfused rat hindlimb muscle. *Diabetes Res Clin Pract* 1992;15:57–61.
304. Nagamatsu S, Carroll RJ, Grodsky GM, et al. Lack of islet amyloid polypeptide regulation of insulin biosynthesis or secretion in normal rat islets. *Diabetes* 1990;39:871–874.
305. Bretherton-Watt D, Gilbey SG, Ghatei MA, et al. Failure to establish islet amyloid polypeptide (amylin) as a circulating beta cell inhibiting hormone in man. *Diabetologia* 1990;33:115–117.
306. MacIntyre I. Amylinamide, bone conservation, and pancreatic beta cells. *Lancet* 1989;2:1026–1027.
307. Zhu GC, Dudley DT, Saltiel AR. Amylin increases cyclic AMP formation in L6 myocytes through calcitonin gene-related peptide receptors. *Biochem Biophys Res Commun* 1991;177:771–776.
308. Regazzi R, Sadoul K, Meda P, et al. Mutational analysis of VAMP domains implicated in Ca^{2+}-induced insulin exocytosis. *EMBO J* 1996;15:6951–6959.
309. Jacobsson G, Bean AJ, Scheller RH, et al. Identification of synaptic proteins and their isoform mRNAs in compartments of pancreatic endocrine cells. *Proc Natl Acad Sci U S A* 1994;91:12487–12491.
310. Brown H, Meister B, Deeney J, et al. Synaptotagmin III isoform is compartmentalized in pancreatic β-cells and has a functional role in exocytosis. *Diabetes* 2000;49:373–382.
311. Mizuta M, Kurose T, Miki T, et al. Localization and functional role of synaptotagmin III in insulin secretory vesicles in pancreatic beta-cells. *Diabetes* 1997;46:2002–2006.
312. Olszewski S, Deeney JT, Schuppin GT, et al. Rab3A effector domain peptides induce insulin exocytosis via a specific interaction with a cytosolic protein doublet. *J Biol Chem* 1994;269:27987–27991.
313. Regazzi R, Ravazzola M, Lezzi M, et al. Expression, localization and functional role of small GTPases of the Rab3 family in insulin secreting cells. *J Cell Sci* 1996;109:2265–2273.
314. Coppola T, Perret-Menoud V, Luthi S, et al. Disruption of Rab3-calmodulin interaction, but not other effector interactions, prevents Rab3 inhibition of exocytosis. *EMBO J* 1999;18:5885–5891.
315. Kawasaki E, Eisenbarth GS, Wasmeier C, et al. Autoantibodies to protein tyrosine phosphatase-like proteins in type I diabetes: overlapping specificities to phogrin and ICA512/IA-2. *Diabetes* 1996;45:1344–1349.
316. Solimena M, Dirkx RJ, Herme JM, et al. ICA 512, an autoantigen of type I diabetes, is an intrinsic membrane protein of neurosecretory granules. *EMBO J* 1996;15:2102–2114.
317. Lan MS, Wasserfall C, Maclaren NK, et al. IA-2, a transmembrane protein of the protein tyrosine phosphatase family, is a major autoantigen in insulin-dependent diabetes mellitus. *Proc Natl Acad Sci U S A* 1996;93:6367–6370.
318. Kawasaki E, Hutton JC, Eisenbarth GS. Molecular cloning and characterization of the human transmembrane protein tyrosine phosphatase homologue, phogrin, an autoantigen of type 1 diabetes. *Biochem Biophys Res Commun* 1996;227:440–447.
319. Wasmeier C, Hutton JC. Secretagogue-dependent phosphorylation of phogrin, an insulin granule membrane protein tyrosine phosphatase homologue. *Biochem J* 1999;341:563–569.
320. Blundell TL, Dodson GG, Hodgkin D, et al. Insulin: the structure in the crystal and its reflection in chemistry and biology. *Adv Protein Chem* 1972;126: 279–402.
321. Edmin SO, Dodson GG, Cutfield JM, et al. Role of zinc in insulin biosynthesis: some possible zinc-insulin interactions in the pancreatic B-cells. *Diabetologia* 1980;19:174–182.
322. Michael J, Carroll R, Swift HH, et al. Studies on the molecular organization of rat insulin secretory granules. *Biol Chem* 1987;262:16531–16535.
323. Beckers CJM, Keller DS, Balch WE. Semi-intact cells permeable to macromolecules: use in reconstruction of protein transport from the endoplasmic reticulum to the Golgi complex. *Cell* 1987;50:523–534.
324. Bonner-Weir S. Morphological evidence for pancreatic polarity of β-cell within islets of Langerhans. *Diabetes* 1988;37:616–621.
325. Lombardi T, Montesano R, Wohlwend AL, et al. Evidence for the polarization of plasma membrane domains in pancreatic endocrine cells. *Nature* 1985;313: 694–696.
326. Lacy PE, Howell SL, Young DA, et al. New hypothesis of insulin secretion. *Nature* 1968;219:1177–1179.
327. Lacy PE, Walker MM, Fink CJ. Perfusion of isolated islets in vitro: participation of the microtubular system in the phasic mechanism of insulin release. *Diabetes* 1972;21:987–998.
328. Malaisse WJ, Malaisse-Lagae F, Van Obberghen E, et al. Role of microtubules in the phasic pattern of insulin release. *Ann N Y Acad Sci* 1975;253:630–652.
329. Kelly RB. Microtubules, membrane traffic and cell organisation. *Cell* 1990;61:5–7.
330. Cleveland DW. Microtubule MAPping. *Cell* 1990;60:701–702.
331. Vale RD, Goldstein LSB. One motor, many tails: an expanding repertoire of force-generating enzymes. *Cell* 1990;60:883–885.
332. Gelfand VI, Bershadsky AD. Microtubule dynamics: mechanism, regulation and function. *Annu Rev Cell Biol* 1991;7:93–116.
333. Porter ME, Johnson KA. Dynein structure and function. *Annu Rev Cell Biol* 1989;5:119–151.
334. Balczon R, Overstreet KA, Zinkowski RP, et al. The identification, purification, and characterization of a pancreatic β-cell form of the microtubule adenosine triphosphatase kinesin. *Endocrinology* 1992;131:331–336.
335. Orci L, Gabbay KH, Malaisse WJ. Pancreatic β-cell web: its possible role in insulin secretion. *Science* 1972;175:1128–1130.
336. Wang JL, Easom RA, Hughes JH, et al. Evidence for a role of microfilaments in insulin release from purified β-cells. *Biochem Biophys Res Commun* 1990;171: 424–430.
337. Lang J. Molecular mechanism and regulation of insulin exocytosis as a paradigm of endocrine secretion. *Eur J Biochem* 1999;259:3–17.
338. Wollheim CB, Lang J, Regazzi R. The exocytotic process of insulin secretion and its regulation by Ca^{2+} and G-proteins. *Diabetes Rev* 1996;4:276–297.
339. Bennett MK, Scheller RH. The molecular machinery for secretion is conserved from yeast to neurons. *Proc Natl Acad Sci U S A* 1993;90:2559–2563.
340. Kelly RB. Storage and release of neurotransmitters. *Neuron* 1993;10:43–54.
341. Bennett MK, Scheller RH. A molecular description of synaptic vesicle membrane trafficking. *Annu Rev Biochem* 1994;63:63–100.
342. Nuoffer C, Balch WE. GTPases: Multifunctional molecular switches regulating vesicular traffic. *Annu Rev Biochem* 1994;63:949–990.
343. Südhof TC. The synaptic vesicle cycle: a cascade of protein-protein interactions. *Nature* 1995;375:645–653.
344. Cheatham B, Volchuk A, Wang L, et al. Evidence of a functional role for VAMP-2/Cellubrevin in insulin-regulated GLUT4 translocation. *Proc Natl Acad Sci U S A* 1996;93:15169–15173.
345. Hayashi T, McMahon H, Yamasaki S, et al. Synaptic vesicle membrane fusion complex: action of clostridial neurotoxins on assembly. *EMBO J* 1994;13: 5051–5061.
346. Bennett MK, Calakos N, Scheller RH. Syntaxin: a synaptic protein implicated in docking of synaptic vesicles at presynaptic active zones. *Science* 1992;257: 255–259.

347. Bennett MK, García-Arrarás JE, Elferink LA, et al. The syntaxin family of vesicular transport receptors. *Cell* 1993;74:863–873.
348. Horikawa HP, Saisu H, Ishizuka T, et al. A complex of rab3A, SNAP-25, VAMP/synaptobrevin-2 and syntaxins in brain presynaptic terminals. *FEBS Lett* 1993;330:236–240.
349. Söllner T, Rothman JE. Neurotransmission: harnessing fusion machinery at the synapse. *Trends Neurosci* 1994;17:344–348.
350. Wheeler MB, Sheu L, Ghai M, et al. Characterization of SNARE protein expression in B-cell lines and pancreatic islets. *Endocrinology* 1996;137:1340–1348.
351. Sadoul K, Lang J, Montecucco C, et al. SNAP-25 is expressed in islets of Langerhans and is involved in insulin release. *J Cell Biol* 1995;128:1019–1028.
352. Martín F, Moya F, Gutierrez LM, et al. Role of syntaxin in mouse pancreatic β-cells. *Diabetologia* 1995;38:860–863.
353. Nagamatsu S, Fujiwara T, Nakamichi Y, et al. Expression and functional role of syntaxin1/HPC-1 in pancreatic β-cells: syntaxin 1A, but not 1B, plays a negative role in regulatory insulin release pathway. *J Biol Chem* 1996;271:1160–1165.
354. Söllner T, Bennett MK, Whiteheart SW, et al. A protein assembly-disassembly pathway in vitro that may correspond to sequential steps of synaptic vesicle docking, activation and fusion. *Cell* 1993;75:409–418.
355. Kiraly-Borri CE, Morgan A, Burgoyne RD, et al. Soluble N-ethylmaleimide-sensitive-factor attachment protein and N-ethylmaleimide-insensitive factors are required for Ca^{2+}-stimulated exocytosis of insulin. *Biochem J* 1996;314:199–203.
356. Daniel S, Noda M, Straub SG, et al. Identification of the docked granule pool responsible for the first phase of glucose-stimulated insulin secretion. *Diabetes* 1999;48:1686–1690.
357. Morgan A. Exocytosis. *Essays Biochem* 1995;30:77–95.
358. Martin TFJ. The molecular machinery for fast and slow neurosecretion. *Curr Opin Neurobiol* 1994;4:626–632.
359. Edwardson JM, Marciniak SJ. Molecular mechanisms in exocytosis. *J Membr Biol* 1994;146:113–122.
360. DeBello WM, Betz H, Augustine GJ. Synaptotagmin and neurotransmitter release. *Cell* 1993;74:947–950.
361. Geppert M, Goda R, Hammer RE, et al. Synaptotagmin I: a major Ca^{2+}-sensor for transmitter release at a central synapse. *Cell* 1994;79:717–727.
362. Augustine GJ, Burns ME, DeBello WM, et al. Exocytosis: proteins and perturbations. *Annu Rev Pharmacol Toxicol* 1996;36:659–701.
363. Hata Y, Südhof TC. A novel ubiquitous form of munc-18 interacts with multiple syntaxins. *J Biol Chem* 1995;270:13022–13028.
364. de Vries KJ, Geijtenbeek A, Brian EC, et al. Dynamics of munc18-1 phosphorylation/dephosphorylation in rat brain nerve terminals. *Eur J Neurosci* 2000;12:385–390.
365. Howell SL, Jones PM, Persaud SJ. Protein kinase C and the regulation of insulin secretion. *Biochem Soc Trans* 1990;18:114–116.
366. Regazzi R, Li G, Ullrich S, et al. Different requirements for protein kinase C activation and Ca^{++}-independent insulin secretion in response to guanine nucleotides: endogenously generated diacylglycerol requires elevated Ca^{++} for kinase C insertion into membranes. *J Biol Chem* 1989;264:9939–9944.
367. Halban PA, Wollheim CB. Intracellular degradation of insulin stores by rat pancreatic islets in vitro. *J Biol Chem* 1980;255:6003–6006.
368. Halban PA, Renold AE. Influence of glucose on insulin handling by rat islets in culture: a reflection of integrated changes in insulin biosynthesis, release and intracellular degradation. *Diabetes* 1983;32:254–261.
369. Orci L, Ravazzola M, Amherdt M, et al. Insulin, not C-peptide (proinsulin), is present in crinophagic bodies of the pancreatic B-cell. *Cell Biol* 1984;98:222–228.
370. Smith RE, Farquhar MG. Lysosome function in the regulation of the secretory process in cells of the anterior pituitary gland. *J Cell Biol* 1966;31:319–347.
371. Orci L, Junod A, Pictet R, et al. Granulolysis in a cells of endocrine pancreas in spontaneous and experimental diabetes in animals. *J Cell Biol* 1968;38:62–66.
372. Halban PA, Mutkoski R, Dodson G, et al. Resistance of the insulin crystal to lysosomal proteases: implications for pancreatic B-cell crinophagy. *Diabetologia* 1987;30:348–353.
373. Schnell AH, Swenne I, Borg LAH. Lysosomes and pancreatic islet function: a quantitative estimation of crinophagy in the mouse pancreatic β-cell. *Cell Tissue Res* 1988;252:9–15.
374. Halban PA, Amherdt M, Orci L, et al. Proinsulin modified analogues of arginine and lysine and secretion of newly synthesized insulin in isolated rat islets. *Biochem J* 1984;219:91–97.
375. Wintersteiner O, du Vigeaud V, Jensen H. The distribution of nitrogen in crystalline insulin. *J Pharmacol Exp Ther* 1928;32:397–411.
376. Sanger F. Chemistry of insulin: determination of the structure of insulin opens the way to greater understanding of life processes. *Science* 1959;129:1340–1344.
377. Steiner DF, Chan SJ, Welsh JM, et al. Structure and evolution of the insulin gene. *Annu Rev Genet* 1985;19:463–484.
378. Pullen RA, Lindsay DG, Wood SP, et al. Receptor-binding region of insulin. *Nature* 1976;259:369–373.
379. Brandenburg D, Wollmer A. Insulin: chemistry, structure and function of insulin and related hormones. In: *Proceedings of the 2nd international insulin symposium.* Aachen, 1979. Berlin: deGruyter, 1980.
380. Gammeltoft S. Insulin receptors: binding kinetics and structure-function relationship of insulin. *Physiol Rev* 1984;64:1321–1378.
381. Adams MJ, Blundell TL, Dodson EJ, et al. Structure of rhombohedral 2 zinc insulin crystals. *Nature* 1969;224:491–495.
382. Blundell TL, Cutfield JF, Cutfield SM, et al. Atomic positions in rhombohedral 2-zinc insulin crystals. *Nature* 1971;231:506–511.
383. Group PIS. Insulin's crystal structure at 2.5Å resolution. *Peking Rev* 1971;40:11–16.
384. Baker EN, Blundell TL, Cutfield JF, et al. The structure of 2Zn pig insulin crystals at 1.5 Å resolution. *Philos Trans R Soc Lond Biol Sci* 1988;319:369–456.
385. Robbins DC, Tager HS, Rubenstein AH. Biologic and clinical importance of proinsulin. *N Engl J Med* 1984;310:1165–1175.
386. Blundell TL, Bedarkar S, Humbel RE. Tertiary structures, receptor binding, and antigenicity of insulin-like growth factors. *Fed Proc* 1983;42:2592–2597.
387. Renscheidt H, Strassburger W, Glatter U, et al. A solution equivalent of the 2Zn–4Zn transformation of insulin in the crystal. *Eur J Biochem* 1984;142:7–14.
388. Ekberg K, Johansson J, Henriksson M, et al. Role of C-peptide in human physiology. *Am J Physiol Endocrinol Metab* 2000;278:E759–E768.
389. Tager H, Given B, Baldwin D, et al. A structurally abnormal insulin causing human diabetes. *Nature* 1979;281:122–125.
390. Given BD, Mako ME, Tager HS, et al. Diabetes due to secretion of an abnormal insulin. *N Engl J Med* 1980;302:129–135.
391. Shoelson S, Haneda M, Blix P, et al. Three mutant insulins in man. *Nature* 1983;302:540–543.
392. Kwok SC, Steiner DF, Rubenstein AH, et al. Identification of a point mutation in the human insulin gene giving rise to a structurally abnormal insulin (insulin Chicago). *Diabetes* 1983;32:872–875.
393. Shoelson S, Fickova M, Haneda M, et al. Identification of a mutant human insulin predicted to contain a serine-for-phenylalanine substitution. *Proc Natl Acad Sci U S A* 1983;80:7390–7394.
394. Haneda M, Chan SJ, Kwok SC, et al. Studies on mutant human insulin genes: identification and sequence analysis of a gene encoding [SerB24]insulin. *Proc Natl Acad Sci U S A* 1983;80:6366–6370.
395. Nanjo K, Sanke T, Miyano M, et al. Diabetes due to secretion of a structurally abnormal insulin (insulin Wakayama): clinical and functional characteristics of [LeuA3] insulin. *J Clin Invest* 1986;77:514–519.
396. Nanjo K, Miyano M, Kondo M, et al. Insulin Wakayama: familial mutant insulin syndrome in Japan. *Diabetologia* 1987;30:87–92.
397. Iwamoto Y, Sakura H, Ishii Y, et al. A new case of abnormal insulinemia with diabetes. Reduced insulin values determined by radioreceptor assay. *Diabetes* 1986;35:1237–1242.
398. Steiner DF, Tager HS, Chan SJ, et al. Lessons learned from molecular biology of insulin gene mutations. *Diabetes Care* 1990;13:600–609.
399. Haneda M, Polonsky KS, Bergenstal RM, et al. Familial hyperinsulinemia due to a structurally abnormal insulin: definition of an emerging new clinical syndrome. *N Engl J Med* 1984;310:1288–1289.
400. Shoelson SE, Polonsky KS, Zeidler A, et al. Human insulin B24 (Phe–Ser). Secretion and metabolic clearance of the abnormal insulin in man and in a dog model. *J Clin Invest* 1984;73:1351–1358.
401. Robbins DC, Blix PM, Rubenstein AH, et al. A human proinsulin variant at arginine 65. *Nature* 1981;291:679–681.
402. Robbins DC, Shoelson SE, Rubenstein AH, et al. Familial hyperproinsulinemia: two cohorts secreting indistinguishable type II intermediates of proinsulin conversion. *J Clin Invest* 1984;73:714–719.
403. Shibasaki Y, Kawakami T, Kanazawa Y, et al. Posttranslational cleavage of proinsulin is blocked by a point mutation in familial hyperproinsulinemia. *J Clin Invest* 1985;76:378–380.
404. Chan SJ, Seino S, Gruppuso PA, et al. A mutation in the B chain coding region is associated with impaired proinsulin conversion in a family with hyperproinsulinemia. *Proc Natl Acad Sci U S A* 1987;84:2194–2197.
405. Gruppuso PA, Gorden P, Kahn CR, et al. Familial hyperproinsulinemia due to a proposed defect in conversion of proinsulin to insulin. *N Engl J Med* 1984;311:629–634.
406. Schwartz GP, Burke GT, Katsoyannis PG. A superactive insulin: [B10-aspartic acid]insulin(human). *Proc Natl Acad Sci U S A* 1987;84:6408–6411.
407. Weiss MA, Hua QX, Lynch CS, et al. Heteronuclear 2D NMR studies of an engineered insulin monomer: assignment and characterization of the receptor-binding surface by selective 2H and 13C labeling with application to protein design. *Biochemistry* 1991;30:7373–7389.
408. Bolli GB, Di Marchi RD, Park GD, et al. Insulin analogues and their potential in the management of diabetes mellitus. *Diabetologia* 1999;42:1151–1167.
409. Brange J, Volund A. Insulin analogs with improved pharmacokinetic profiles. *Adv Drug Deliv Rev* 1999;35:307–335.

CHAPTER 6

Cell Biology of Insulin Secretion

Jean-Claude Henquin

Under physiologic conditions, the concentration of blood glucose fluctuates only in a narrow range despite alternations in periods of food intake and fasting. This stability is due to a remarkably efficient hormonal system that exerts opposite effects on the organs of glucose storage and production. Whereas several hormones can prevent dangerous declines in blood glucose concentrations by stimulating glycogenolysis and gluconeogenesis, insulin secretion by β-cells of the islets of Langerhans is the only efficient means by which the organism can decrease the blood glucose concentration. Any alteration in the β-cell functioning has thus a profound impact on glucose homeostasis: excessive secretion of insulin causes hypoglycemia, and insufficient secretion leads to diabetes mellitus. It is therefore not surprising that insulin secretion is subject to tight control. This control is ensured by glucose itself and by an array of metabolic, neural, hormonal, and sometimes pharmacologic factors, which necessitates rapid integration by β-cells of a host of signals generating intracellular messengers.

Stimulus-secretion coupling in β-cells is astonishingly complex and still incompletely understood despite continuous investigation. However, its main features are beginning to appear clearly enough to gain wide acceptance. Only these major characteristics will be discussed here, leaving issues that are too controversial and specialized for more specific review articles. Because this chapter is devoted to normal stimulus-secretion coupling, I have given preference to publications of studies performed with normal β-cell models and limited those of studies using insulin-secreting cell lines that often show abnormal properties. Although *in vitro* studies of normal adult human islets are still few, they indicate that the information gained from animal experiments can be extrapolated in large part to humans. Only functionally important specificities of the human β-cell will thus be highlighted.

IDENTIFICATION OF GLUCOSE BY β-CELLS

In most secretory cells, extracellular stimuli bind to membrane receptors and activate stereotyped transduction pathways that eventually trigger specific responses. The existence in the plasma membrane of β-cells of a glucoreceptor that would trigger insulin secretion upon binding of glucose itself has been considered but could never be proved. On the other hand, compelling evidence indicates that glucose must be metabolized by β-cells to induce insulin secretion. Small interferences with glucose metabolism have repercussions on insulin secretion, whereas marked interferences with insulin secretion may be without effect on glucose metabolism in β-cells. The experimental work on which this "fuel-concept" of insulin secretion is based has been discussed in detail in several review articles (1–8).

β-Cells detect blood glucose variations and adjust the rate of insulin secretion to these variations through changes in their metabolism. This ability rests on a peculiar biochemical organization that is summarized in Figure 6.1.

1. In rodent β-cells, as in hepatocytes, glucose entry is mediated by the high-capacity, low-affinity (K_m ~17 mM) glucose

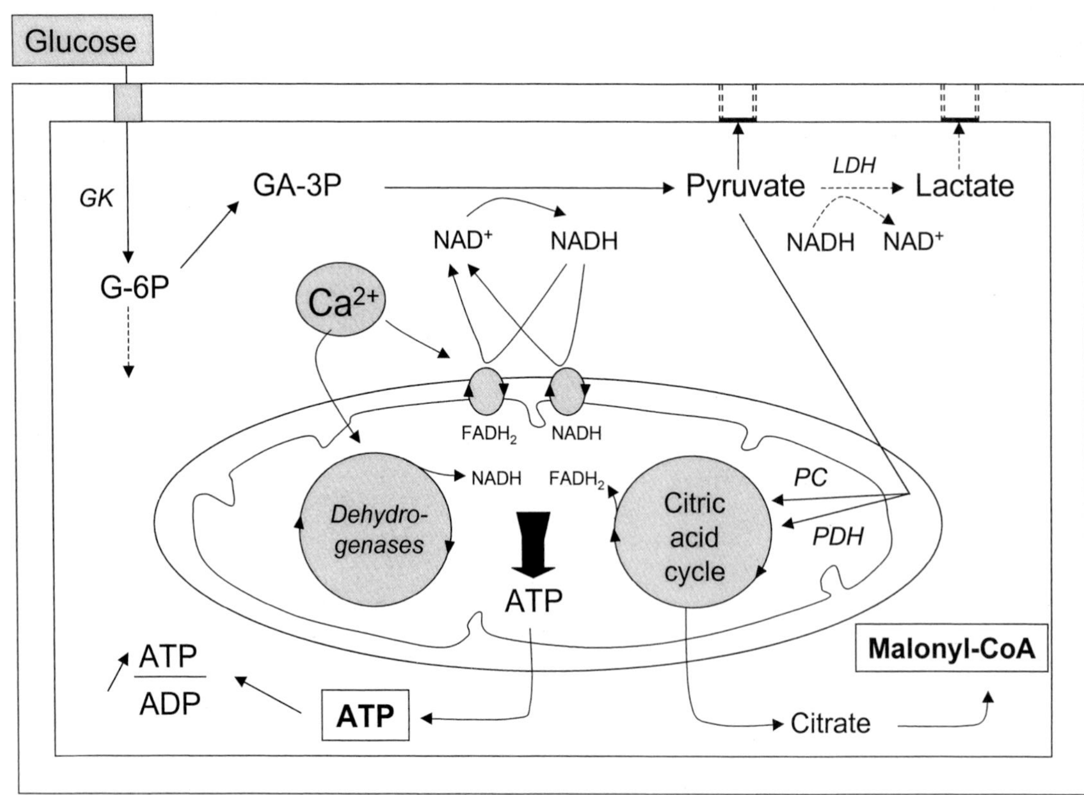

Figure 6.1. Schematic summary of glucose metabolism in the cytoplasm and mitochondria of β-cells. GK, glucokinase; LDH, lactate dehydrogenase; PDH, pyruvate dehydrogenase; PC, pyruvate carboxylase; G-6P, glucose-6-phosphate; GA-3P, glyceraldehyde-3-phosphate; NAD^+ and NADH, oxidized and reduced nicotinamide adenine dinucleotide, respectively; $FADH_2$, reduced flavin adenine dinucleotide; ATP, adenosine triphosphate; ADP, adenosine diphosphate; CoA, coenzyme A.

transporter GLUT2 (9,10). In human β-cells, GLUT2 is less extensively expressed, and GLUT1 predominates (11,12). Nevertheless, whatever the proportion of the different transporters, glucose transport is always efficient enough to permit rapid equilibration between the intracellular and extracellular concentrations of glucose (13,14). The rate of glucose transport exceeds the rate of glucose utilization and is, therefore, not limiting (10,15,16).

2. Phosphorylation of glucose into glucose-6-phosphate is catalyzed by a glucokinase (GK hexokinase IV) similar (15 amino acids shorter) to that present in hepatocytes (17,18). The same gene is controlled by two distinct promoters, permitting differential regulation of the expression—positively by insulin and negatively by glucagon in the liver and positively by glucose in β-cells. The characteristics of GK, a K_m between 6 and 10 mM, sigmoidal dependency on its substrate concentration, and lack of inhibition by its product (glucose-6-phosphate), make it a suitable glucose sensor (15). The view that GK is the flux-determining step of glucose metabolism in β-cells is supported by the fact that its activity is lower than that of the other potentially regulatory enzymes of glycolysis and closely matches glucose usage (10,15,16). Mutations of the GK gene result in the production of either hypoactive isoforms of the enzyme in patients with maturity-onset diabetes of the young (MODY-2) (19) or hyperactive isoforms in glucokinase-linked hyperinsulinemia and hypoglycemia (20). Expression of these mutants in insulin-secreting cell lines produced the expected decreasing and increasing effects on glucose metabolism and insulin secretion (21). Whereas the important role of GK is admitted unanimously, the concept that the enzyme is the sole regulator of glycolysis in β-cells remains disputed (22). The contribution of a high-affinity hexokinase has often been considered, but recent experiments have cast doubt on the presence of this enzyme in β-cells (23).
3. Under physiologic conditions, dephosphorylation of glucose-6-phosphate by glucose-6-phosphatase, storage of glucose as glycogen, and transformation of glucose to sorbitol are quantitatively small (4,5,16,22,24). They play no significant role in the control of normal β-cell function. Glucose metabolism through the pentose phosphate pathway does not exceed 5%, and its relative contribution decreases as the glucose concentration is increased. This pathway also is thought to be unimportant for the control of insulin secretion. Glycolysis is the major route of glucose metabolism in β-cells.
4. β-Cells contain the muscle (PFK1-M) and cerebral (PFK1-C) isoforms of phosphofructokinase (25). The characteristics of the enzyme and of its regulators indicate that PFK adjusts its rate of phosphorylation to that of glucokinase (15,16). Normal β-cells hardly express lactate dehydrogenase (24,26), and plasma membrane monocarboxylate transporters (for lactate and pyruvate) are present in only low amounts (26,27), so that pyruvate generated by glycolysis is channeled (>90%) to the mitochondria. However, the low activity of lactate dehydrogenase is insufficient to regenerate enough oxidized nicotinamide adenine dinucleotide (NAD^+) to sustain a high glycolytic flux. Reoxidation of NADH is thus achieved by two mitochondrial electron shuttles that are unusually active in β-cells: the glycerol-3-phosphate shuttle and the malate-aspartate shuttle (7,26,28,29). The two shuttles appear to be at least partially redundant but, together, play an essential role in β-cell function (30,31).
5. Within mitochondria, pyruvate is transformed approximately equally into acetyl coenzyme A (CoA) by pyruvate dehydrogenase and into oxaloacetate by pyruvate carboxylase (32,33). Acetyl CoA is then used by the citric acid cycle, with formation of NADH and reduced flavin adenine dinucleotide ($FADH_2$), which together with NADH and $FADH_2$ issued from the activity of the shuttles previously described, transfer electrons to the electron-transport chain. This eventually results in hyperpolarization of the mitochondrial membrane and generation of adenosine triphosphate (ATP) (34). The high activity of pyruvate carboxylase in β-cells is unusual for a non-gluconeogenic, non-lipogenic tissue. The enzyme serves to fill the citric acid cycle with intermediates (anaplerosis) (35), which allows some of these intermediates to exit from the mitochondria without compromising the cycle function. These compounds can then be used as precursors of amino acids (24) or, in the case of citrate, produce putative second messengers such as malonyl CoA (36) (see below).
6. When the concentration of glucose is raised, the acceleration of glucose oxidation is greater than that of glycolysis (22). This remarkable feature is attributed to the activation of mitochondrial dehydrogenases. Three of these, pyruvate dehydrogenase, isocitrate dehydrogenase, and α-ketoglutarate dehydrogenase, are activated by the increase in mitochondrial Ca^{2+} that follows the increase in cytoplasmic Ca^{2+} induced by glucose (37) (see below). A fourth dehydrogenase, the FAD-linked mitochondrial glycerol 3-P-dehydrogenase, the key enzyme of the glycerol phosphate shuttle (see point 4 above), is also Ca^{2+}-sensitive, but its activation is achieved by the increase in cytoplasmic Ca^{2+}.
7. The major consequence of this original biochemical organization of β-cells is that the ATP/adenosine diphosphate (ADP) ratio increases with the glucose concentration (38). It is important to emphasize how this situation is exceptional. Thus, most cells, including glucagon-secreting α-cells, adapt their metabolism to maintain a constant ATP/ADP ratio when the concentration of glucose changes (39). The glucose-induced variations in ATP/ADP ratio observed in purified β-cells or in whole islets take place in the cytoplasm. They are often underestimated because of a partial masking by a stable pool of nucleotides within insulin granules, occur over a wide range of glucose concentrations and are rapid, preceding any increase in cytoplasmic $[Ca^{2+}]_i$ (38,40,41). All these characteristics support the proposal that adenine nucleotides serve as second messenger in stimulus-secretion coupling.

This metabolic recognition of glucose by β-cells is then coupled to the process of insulin secretion through the operation of two pathways: a triggering pathway and an amplifying pathway (42). Their major steps are schematized in Figure 6.2.

THE TRIGGERING PATHWAY OF GLUCOSE-INDUCED INSULIN SECRETION

Cytoplasmic Ca^{2+} as Triggering Signal

Direct evidence that cytoplasmic Ca^{2+} triggers exocytosis of insulin granules was obtained from experiments using β-cells of which the plasma membrane was permeabilized. In these cells, the membrane potential is dissipated and the cytosolic concentration of small molecules (e.g., Ca^{2+}, ATP) can be controlled. An increase in free $[Ca^{2+}]_i$ induced insulin release independently from any other change (43,44). More recently, exocytosis of insulin granules was estimated by measuring the capacitance of voltage-clamped single β-cells: increases in capacitance reflect increases in plasma membrane surface caused by the fusion of secretory granules. This technique confirmed that Ca^{2+} directly triggers exocytosis (45,46). Although progressive desensitiza-

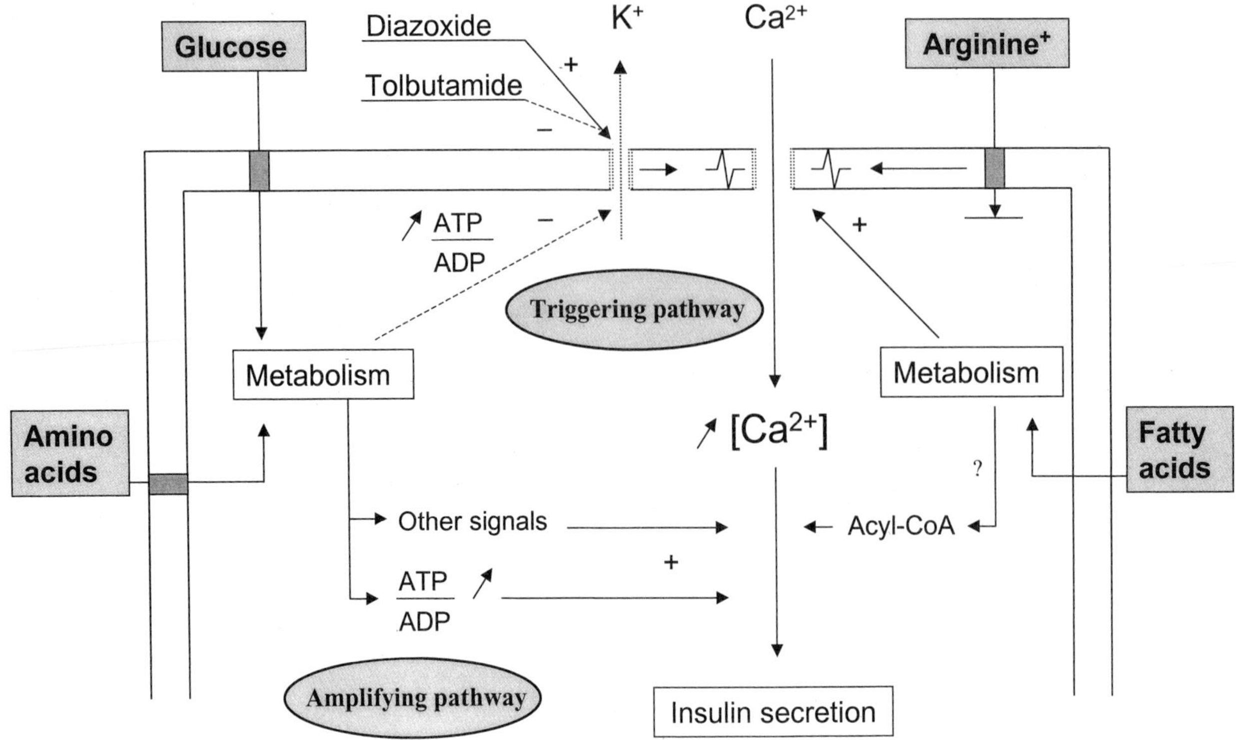

Figure 6.2. Schematic representation of the triggering and amplifying pathways of the stimulation of insulin secretion by glucose, and of the mode of action of other nutrients: +, stimulation; – inhibition; ATP, adenosine triphosphate; ADP, adenosine diphosphate; CoA, coenzyme A.

tion to Ca^{2+} occurs in these preparations, imposed oscillations of $[Ca^{2+}]_i$ were able to entrain oscillations of insulin secretion in permeabilized cells (47), indicating that Ca^{2+} has a minute-to-minute triggering role.

Experiments using permeabilized insulin-secreting cells (47) and capacitance measurements in β-cells (48) have shown that stable derivatives of guanosine triphosphate (GTP) can increase insulin release in a truly Ca^{2+}-independent manner. In intact rat islets, a Ca^{2+}-independent pathway of glucose-induced insulin secretion could be unmasked by strong and combined activation of protein kinases A and C (49). However, the significance of this pathway is unclear (50). Under physiologic conditions, glucose increases the cytoplasmic free Ca^{2+} concentration ($[Ca^{2+}]_i$) in β-cells, and all maneuvers interfering with this increase impair the stimulation of insulin secretion. Although the sequence of events leading to insulin secretion may include Ca^{2+}-independent steps, the physiologic regulation by glucose is achieved through a Ca^{2+}-dependent pathway.

How can cytoplasmic $[Ca^{2+}]_i$ serve as triggering signal? Unstimulated β-cells maintain $[Ca^{2+}]_i$ between 50 and 100 nM by several mechanisms: a low permeability of the plasma membrane to Ca^{2+}, pumping of Ca^{2+} into the endoplasmic reticulum by a sarco(endo)plasmic reticulum Ca^{2+}-ATPase (SERCA) (51,52), and extrusion of Ca^{2+} across the plasma membrane by a calmodulin-sensitive Ca^{2+}-ATPase (53,54) and an Na^+/Ca^{2+} countertransport driven by the electrochemical gradient for Na^+ (55). There thus exist large gradients of Ca^{2+} concentration between the cytoplasm and either the lumen of the endoplasmic reticulum or the extracellular medium. Opening of Ca^{2+} channels in the plasma membrane (e.g., by depolarization) or in the endoplasmic reticulum membranes (e.g., by inositol trisphosphate) allows rapid movements of Ca^{2+} down the electrochemical gradient and causes increases in cytoplasmic $[Ca^{2+}]_i$.

How Does Glucose Increase $[Ca^{2+}]_i$ in β-Cells?

Mobilization of Ca^{2+} from intracellular stores is the major mechanism by which many stimuli increase $[Ca^{2+}]_i$ in electrically non-excitable cells. β-Cells are electrically excitable, and mobilization of intracellular Ca^{2+} by glucose has never been demonstrated by direct measurements in normal β-cells. Although Ca^{2+} handling by intracellular organelles contributes to the fine regulation of $[Ca^{2+}]_i$ during glucose stimulation (56,57), Ca^{2+} influx through voltage-operated Ca^{2+} channels is indisputably the major determinant of the glucose-induced $[Ca^{2+}]_i$ increase (Fig. 6.2).

When the extracellular concentration of glucose increases, β-cell metabolism accelerates (Fig. 6.1). One of the earliest consequences is a decrease in the K^+ conductance of the plasma membrane (58–60). It is due to the closure of the K^+ channels that determine the resting potential of β-cells, the ATP-sensitive K^+ channels (K^+-ATP channels) (61,62). These channels are tetramers of a complex of two proteins: a high-affinity sulfonylurea receptor (SUR 1) and an inwardly rectifying K^+ channel (Kir 6.2) (63–65). The pore of the channel is formed by the four subunits of Kir 6.2 to which ATP binds to close the channel. The four subunits of SUR 1 mediate the opening property of Mg^{2+}-ADP and endow the channel with sensitivity to pharmacologic agents such as sulfonylureas and diazoxide that respectively close and open the channel (Fig. 6.2).

The decrease in K^+ conductance produced by glucose allows a background current of a yet unidentified nature to move the membrane potential away from the equilibrium potential for K^+, that is, to depolarize the membrane (Fig. 6.3). In a mouse β-cell, within an intact islet, the resting potential is about -65 mV in the presence of a non-stimulatory glucose concentration (3 mM). When the concentration of glucose is increased to 10 mM,

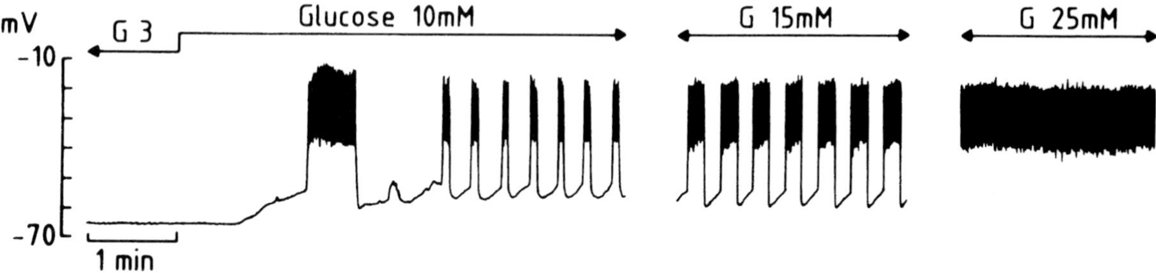

Figure 6.3. Changes in the membrane potential of a mouse β-cell induced by successive increases in the concentration of glucose in the perifusion medium. The three recordings were obtained in the same cell. (Adapted from Henquin JC. Les mécanismes de contrôle de la sécrétion d'insuline. *Arch Int Physiol Biochim* 1990;98:A61-A80, with permission.)

the membrane depolarizes by about 15 mV, to reach the threshold potential for opening of voltage-operated Ca^{2+} channels (66). Depending on the species, these voltage-operated Ca^{2+} channels are predominantly or exclusively of the L-type (67,68). Their opening allows the influx of Ca^{2+}, which manifests itself as a rapid depolarization to a plateau potential on which a burst of Ca^{2+} action potentials appears. The electrical activity then suddenly stops and the membrane repolarizes. The membrane potential then starts to oscillate, thus producing rhythmic openings of Ca^{2+} channels and Ca^{2+} influx. As the glucose concentration increases, the phases of depolarization and Ca^{2+} influx become longer and the intervals become shorter (Fig. 6.3). The membrane eventually remains persistently depolarized at the plateau potential and exhibits continuous electrical activity. This characteristic pattern has been studied primarily in vitro (66) but is also observed when the membrane potential of β-cells is recorded in vivo (69).

Attributing the electrical properties of β-cells only to K^+-ATP channels and voltage-operated Ca^{2+} channels is an oversimplification imposed by the objectives of this chapter. The electrogenic sodium pump and a number of voltage-dependent and voltage-independent ionic channels also participate in the fine tuning of the glucose-induced electrical activity, which is still only partly understood (66,68,70,71). Whether the changes in the ATP/ADP ratio suffice to explain the influence of glucose on the β-cell membrane potential is also uncertain. The fact that the ratio gradually changes between 0 and 20 mM glucose (38) makes the hypothesis at least plausible. Functionally, the decrease in ADP (which acts on SUR 1) is probably more important than the increase in ATP. Other metabolic regulators of the membrane potential have been proposed, but none of these suggestions has gained wide acceptance (63–65).

Characteristics of the Increase in $[Ca^{2+}]_i$ Produced by Glucose

In the presence of a non-stimulatory concentration of glucose, β-cell $[Ca^{2+}]_i$ is low and stable. Upon stimulation with high glucose, $[Ca^{2+}]_i$ changes in three stages (Fig. 6.4A). A small decrease occurs initially, reflecting cytoplasmic Ca^{2+} pumping into the endoplasmic reticulum (72). This Ca^{2+} sequestration might be promoted by the increase in ATP/ADP ratio (73), but its functional significance is unknown. The subsequent $[Ca^{2+}]_i$ increase displays a biphasic pattern. An initial large and sustained increase is followed by a nadir and then by oscillations that persist as long as the glucose stimulation is continued. These changes in $[Ca^{2+}]_i$ are superimposable on those of the membrane potential (compare Fig. 6.4A and Fig. 6.3) (74,75). The initial decrease in $[Ca^{2+}]_i$ occurs during progressive depolarization from the resting to the threshold potential, but the two events do not seem to be causally related (76). In contrast, the long first phase of the $[Ca^{2+}]_i$ increase and the subsequent oscillations not only coincide with but are caused by the influx of Ca^{2+} brought about by the changes in membrane potential. The mechanisms of the oscillations in β-cell membrane potential (66,68,70,71) and $[Ca^{2+}]_i$ (77–79) during steady-state stimulation with glucose remain controversial. They seem to result from a complex interplay between oscillations in metabolic signals and the coordinated opening and closing of ionic channels with distinct time- and voltage-dependent properties. Ca^{2+}-independent, intrinsic oscillations of glucose metabolism (77), Ca^{2+}-induced acceleration of ATP production (80), and Ca^{2+}-induced stimulation of ATP consumption (40) have been proposed. The variability of these oscillations (period from 20 seconds to 4 minutes) between preparations adds to the complexity. Sometimes, glucose-induced electrical activity and $[Ca^{2+}]_i$ oscillations are characterized by a double periodicity in which rapid oscillations are superimposed on slower ones (Fig. 6.4B). It is not unusual that, in the same islet, the oscillatory pattern spontaneously changes from regular, fast oscillations into mixed or slow oscillations. Cyclic adenosine monophosphate (cAMP) increases the rhythm and regularity of the oscillations.

Figure 6.4A also shows that glucose does not increase $[Ca^{2+}]_i$ in the absence of extracellular Ca^{2+}. This is also true when, in the presence of extracellular Ca^{2+}, Ca^{2+} influx is impeded by blocking the voltage-operated Ca^{2+} channels or by preventing the glucose-induced depolarization with diazoxide (see below).

Activation of an Effector System by Ca^{2+}

Insulin is stored in large dense core vesicles. Its secretion in the extracellular space of the islets occurs by a process of regulated exocytosis (81) that involves several steps: recruitment of the granules, followed by their docking, priming, and eventual fusion with the plasma membrane. Extensive description of these complex stages can be found in specialized review articles (82,83).

The importance of the cytoskeleton has been established by the use of drugs capable of interfering with the function of its distinct elements (84,85). The cytoskeleton, composed of microfilaments, microtubules, and intermediary filaments (vimentin, cytokeratin), ensures the transport of the secretory granules to the plasma membrane. Upon β-cell stimulation, tubulin polymerizes to form microtubules that can guide the granules toward the sites of exocytosis. Polymerization of globular actin with formation of microfilaments also occurs. Actin filaments may both facilitate and impede (cortical network) the access of

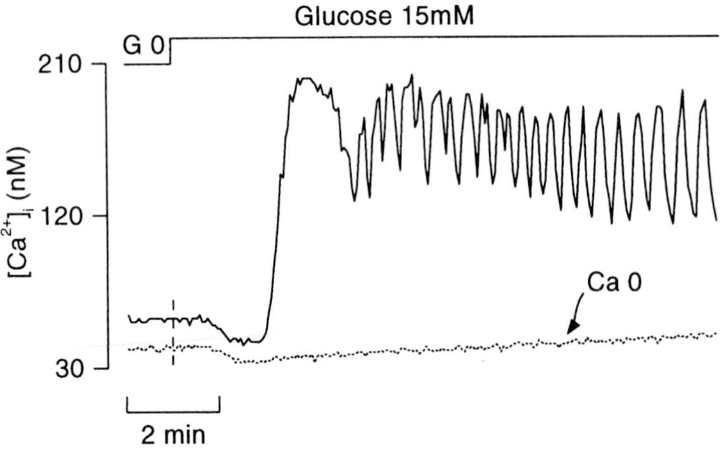

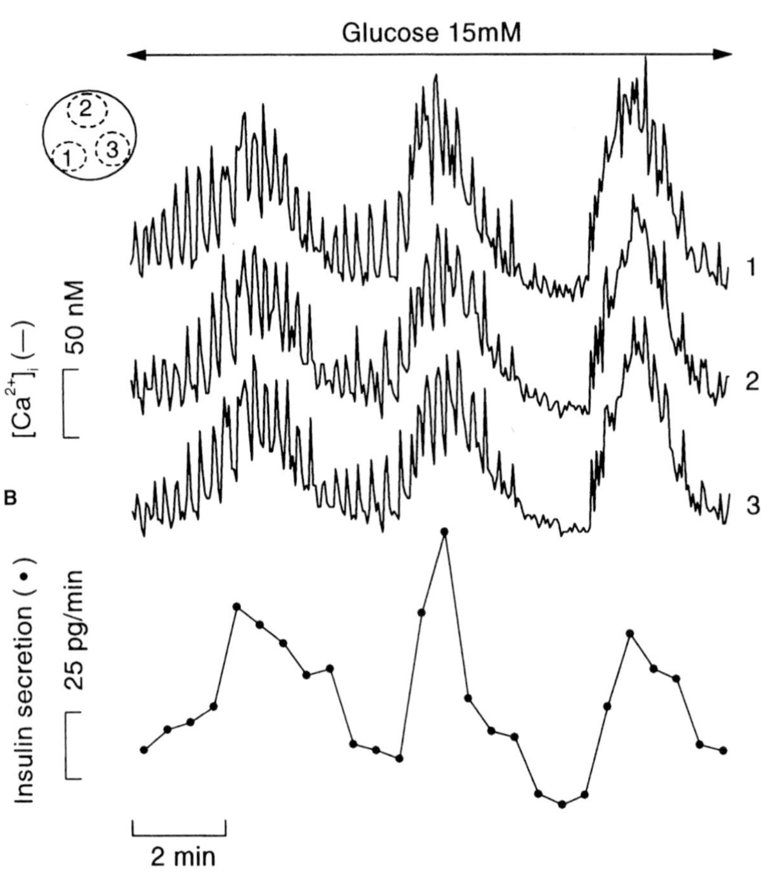

Figure 6.4. Glucose-induced changes in cytoplasmic free Ca^{2+} ($[Ca^{2+}]_i$) in intact mouse islets. **A:** After an initial period of perifusion without glucose (G 0), the islet was stimulated with 15 mM glucose. The medium contained 2.5 mM or 0 mM $CaCl_2$. **B:** $[Ca^{2+}]_i$ and insulin secretion were measured simultaneously in the same mouse islet during continuous stimulation with 15 mM glucose. Traces 1–3 correspond to the $[Ca^{2+}]_i$ signal recorded in the different regions of the islet schematically identified in the upper left corner. They show the excellent synchrony of both slow and rapid oscillations of $[Ca^{2+}]_i$. The lower line shows that insulin secretion (sampling every 30 seconds) oscillates in phase with the slow $[Ca^{2+}]_i$ oscillations. A higher sampling rate would be necessary to show that the fast $[Ca^{2+}]_i$ oscillations also trigger oscillations of insulin secretion (experiments performed by M. A. Ravier).

secretory granules to the plasma membrane. Ca^{2+}-calmodulin protein kinase II (Cam-kinase II), associated with the secretory granules, appears to play an important role in this mobilization of the granules from the Golgi to the exocytotic sites (86). The activation of Cam-kinase II by the increase in $[Ca^{2+}]_i$ that glucose and other secretagogues produce correlates well with insulin secretion. Myosin light-chain kinase also is implicated in granule movements by modulation of actin-myosin interactions (87).

The docking step corresponds to the targeting of the secretory vesicle to the plasma membrane (82,83). It is achieved by the pairing of cognate proteins present on the vesicle membrane (v-SNARE, e.g., synaptobrevin) and the plasma (target) membrane (t-SNARE, e.g., syntaxin). This assembly then recruits several cytoplasmic proteins to reorganize in a multimeric complex through an ATP-dependent process (priming). Finally, Ca^{2+} acts on yet other proteins of the vesicle membrane, among which synaptotagmin is predominant, to induce the fusion of the two membranes. Eventually, the granule content, i.e., insulin, C peptide, other proteins, and nucleotides, is released outside the β-cell.

GTP-binding proteins also control the process of exocytosis (82,83), but it is unclear whether these serve a regulatory role in glucose-induced insulin secretion. As already mentioned, experiments using permeabilized insulin-secreting cells (47) or β-cells patch-clamped in the whole-cell mode (48) (to control the cytosolic composition) have shown that insulin release can be induced by GTP, independently of $[Ca^{2+}]_i$ changes. The G-protein involved in this stimulation often is referred to as G_E (for exocytosis), but its nature is unknown. Heterotrimeric G-proteins can influence insulin secretion independently of their role in membrane receptor–activated signal transduction (88). $G_{\alpha i}$ or $G_{\alpha o}$ mediate an inhibitory effect that abolishes the action of Ca^{2+} (89,90). It has been suggested that the protein phosphatase calcineurin is implicated in this inhibition, but the hypothesis has not been confirmed.

In addition to Cam-kinase II, two other protein kinases have a marked influence on the effector system. The cAMP-dependent protein kinase A and the Ca^{2+}-and phospholipid-dependent protein kinase C strongly amplify the action of Ca^{2+} on exocytosis. Their targets are not known (see below).

Consensus Model of the Triggering Pathway

The entry of glucose in β-cells by facilitated diffusion being not rate limiting, changes in the extracellular (blood) glucose concentration are immediately transduced into changes in β-cell metabolism. The tight coupling between glycolysis and mitochondrial metabolism results in rapid and marked changes in the ATP/ADP ratio that then control K^+-ATP channels in the plasma membrane. These channels serve as transducers of biochemical into biophysical signals. Thus, their closure by an increase in the ATP/ADP ratio leads to membrane depolarization and opening of voltage-operated Ca^{2+} channels. The ensuing Ca^{2+} influx raises $[Ca^{2+}]_i$, which eventually activates an effector system responsible for the exocytosis of insulin granules (Fig. 6.2).

THE AMPLIFYING PATHWAY OF GLUCOSE-INDUCED INSULIN SECRETION

In addition to the generation of a triggering signal, an increase in $[Ca^{2+}]_i$, glucose-induced insulin secretion involves the generation of signals that amplify the action of Ca^{2+} on the exocytotic process (42) (Fig. 6.2). This concept was established by experiments showing that glucose can still increase insulin secretion when K^+-ATP channels cannot be closed (91–93) or are already completely closed (94–96).

Identification of the Pathway

In a control medium, a high glucose concentration increases $[Ca^{2+}]_i$ in β-cells (triggering signal) and stimulates insulin secretion. In a low glucose medium, tolbutamide mimics the effects of glucose. When the drug is used at a maximally effective concentration that closes all K^+-ATP channels (Fig. 6.2), it increases $[Ca^{2+}]_i$ more than does high glucose but has a less potent effect on insulin secretion (Fig. 6.5). Increasing the glucose concentration under these conditions considerably amplifies insulin secretion without affecting $[Ca^{2+}]_i$. However, glucose does not have this effect when the tolbutamide-induced $[Ca^{2+}]_i$ increase has been prevented by omission of extracellular Ca^{2+}.

When K^+-ATP channels are opened by diazoxide (Fig. 6.2), a high glucose concentration is unable to increase $[Ca^{2+}]_i$ and stimulate insulin secretion because it cannot depolarize the β-cell membrane (Fig. 6.5). An increase in $[Ca^{2+}]_i$ can, however, be induced, even in a low glucose environment, by depolarizing the membrane with high extracellular K^+. This is followed by a stimulation of insulin secretion simply because a triggering signal has been produced. Increasing the concentration of glucose in the presence of high K^+, while K^+-ATP channels are held open by diazoxide, leads to a marked increase in insulin secretion without any further increase in $[Ca^{2+}]_i$ (Fig. 6.5). Again, these effects of glucose require that $[Ca^{2+}]_i$ be increased, because they are abolished by omission of extracellular Ca^{2+}.

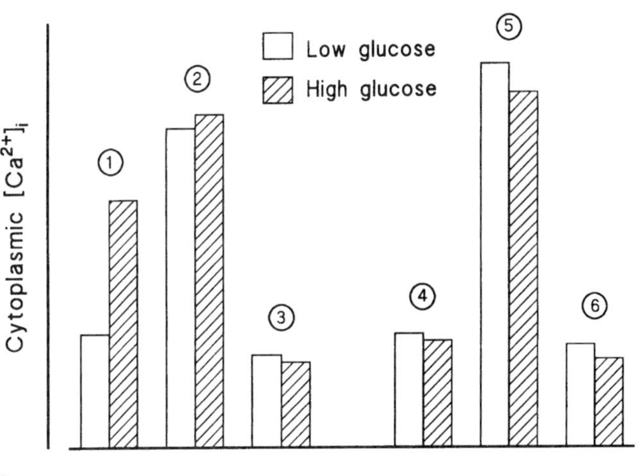

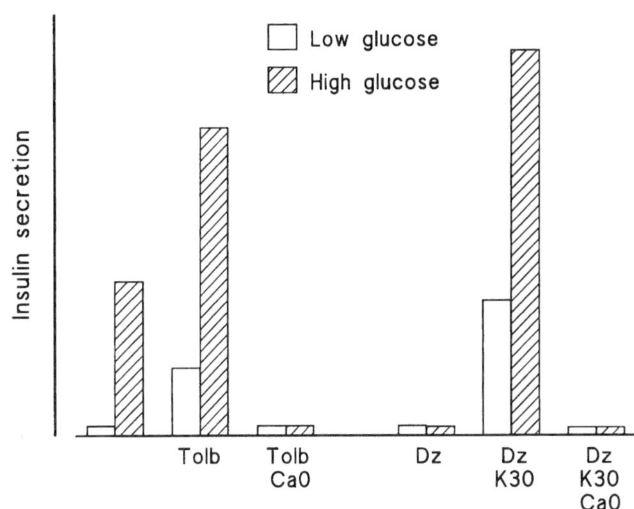

Figure 6.5. Demonstration of the existence of two pathways of control of insulin secretion by glucose. The figure is based on data obtained with mouse islets. Changes in cytoplasmic free Ca^{2+} ($[Ca^{2+}]_i$) **(A)** and in insulin secretion **(B)** under the following conditions are shown: *(1)* In control medium, high glucose raises cytoplasmic $[Ca^{2+}]_i$ and stimulates insulin secretion. *(2)* Blockade of all K^+-ATP channels by a high concentration of tolbutamide (Tolb) in low glucose mimics both effects of high glucose alone, but the stimulation of secretion is smaller in spite of a larger rise in $[Ca^{2+}]_i$. High glucose does not affect $[Ca^{2+}]_i$ but markedly increases insulin secretion. *(3)* The effects of tolbutamide and glucose are abolished when $[Ca^{2+}]_i$ cannot be increased because of omission of extracellular Ca^{2+}. *(4)* Opening of K^+-ATP channels by diazoxide (Dz) prevents the stimulatory effects of high glucose on $[Ca^{2+}]_i$ and insulin secretion. *(5)* Depolarization with high K^+ strongly increases $[Ca^{2+}]_i$ and induces insulin secretion in low glucose. High glucose markedly amplifies the secretory response without changing $[Ca^{2+}]_i$. *(6)* The effects of high K^+ and glucose are abrogated when $[Ca^{2+}]_i$ cannot be raised because of omission of extracellular Ca^{2+}. In conclusion, glucose stimulates insulin secretion by increasing $[Ca^{2+}]_i$ (triggering pathway as shown in 1), and by increasing the efficacy of Ca^{2+} on exocytosis (amplifying pathway as shown in 2 and 5).

Direct comparisons of the relationships between insulin secretion and $[Ca^{2+}]_i$ under various conditions have established beyond doubt that glucose amplifies insulin secretion by increasing the efficacy of cytosolic Ca^{2+} in the secretory process (42,96,97).

Mechanisms of the Amplifying Pathway

The amplifying pathway requires the metabolism of glucose by β-cells (91). The second messenger has not been identified with certainty, but good correlations exist between the ATP/ADP ratio and glucose-induced insulin secretion through this pathway (38,92). Moreover, several experimental approaches have established that ATP influences insulin secretion at steps distal to the increase in $[Ca^{2+}]_i$ (98–100). There is also good evidence that cAMP-dependent protein kinase A and diacylglycerol-activated protein kinase C are not involved (92,101,102). Whether long-chain acyl CoAs participate in this effect is still disputed (101,103). More complete discussion of this question can be found elsewhere (42).

Hierarchy between the Triggering and Amplifying Pathways

Under control conditions, the concentration dependency of glucose-induced insulin secretion displays a sigmoidal shape (Fig. 6.6A). A similar relationship characterizes generation of the triggering signals, electrical activity, and increase in $[Ca^{2+}]_i$ by glucose (104–106). The threshold corresponds to the glucose concentration required to depolarize the β-cell membrane to the potential where voltage-operated Ca^{2+} channels start to open and the triggering signal thus starts to be produced. In contrast, the concentration dependency of the amplifying pathway, which can be established when the triggering signal is kept constant by high K^+ in the presence of diazoxide, is hyperbolic and shifted to the left (Fig. 6.6B). Low concentrations of glucose are thus able to influence insulin secretion, but their influence manifests itself only when a triggering signal has been produced. The similarity of the concentration dependencies of glucose-induced triggering signal and secretory response establishes a clear hierarchy between the two pathways: The amplifying pathway remains functionally silent as long as the triggering pathway has not depolarized the membrane and increased $[Ca^{2+}]_i$, but its role is essential to optimize the secretory response to the triggering signal (42). This hierarchy ensures that no insulin is inappropriately secreted in the presence of low glucose. It may be altered when the function of K^+-ATP channels is perturbed by genetic alterations or by long-acting sulfonylureas (42).

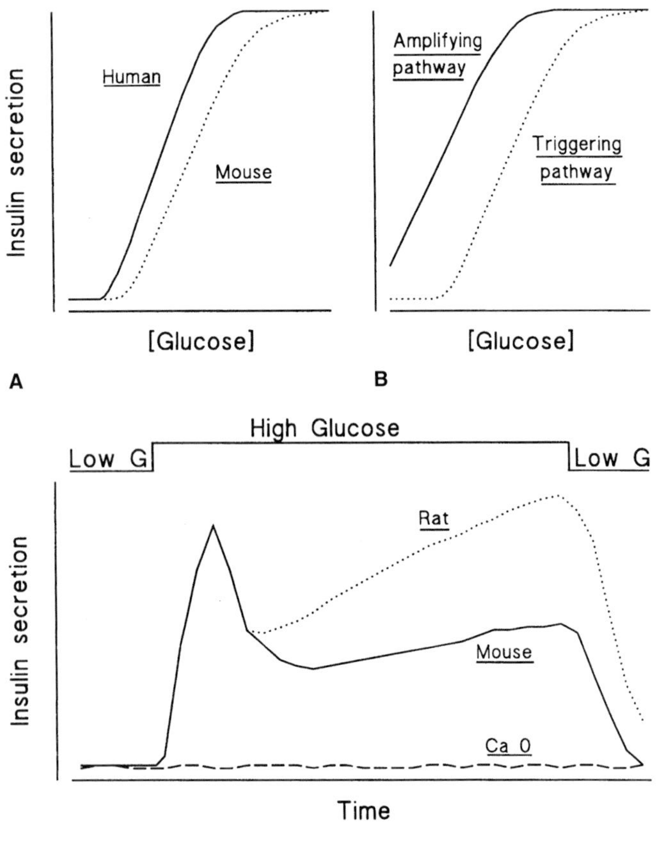

Figure 6.6. Concentration dependence and kinetics of glucose-induced insulin secretion *in vitro*. **A:** The relationship between the glucose concentration and insulin secretion is sigmoidal; it is shifted to the left in humans as compared with the curve in mice; the curve would be intermediate in the rat. **B:** The triggering and amplifying pathways of glucose control of insulin secretion show distinct dependences on the glucose concentration. **C:** An abrupt increase in the glucose concentration triggers a biphasic secretion of insulin. During second phase, the rate of secretion increases more in the rat than in the mouse. Insulin secretion is not stimulated in the absence of extracellular Ca^{2+} (Ca 0).

OTHER PUTATIVE MESSENGERS IN THE β-CELL RESPONSE TO GLUCOSE

As previously discussed, changes in the cytoplasmic ATP/ADP ratio in β-cells are currently thought to be the major coupling factor between glucose metabolism and the biophysical events leading to the generation of the triggering signal. There is also evidence for a role of the ATP/ADP ratio in the amplification pathway (Fig. 6.2). Over the years, however, many other messengers have been considered to play a role in the β-cell secretory response to glucose.

Metabolic Factors

The hypothesis that a specific intermediate of glucose metabolism (e.g., of glycolysis) is directly involved in triggering secretion was abandoned when it became evident that fuel secretagogues metabolized through distinct pathways have largely similar effects.

Reduced pyridine nucleotides (NADPH and NADH) are unlikely to be an essential triggering signal but may play a modulatory role (e.g., by changing the thiol-disulfide equilibrium in various proteins) (107). Fuel-induced insulin secretion is associated with a more reduced state of the cytosol of β-cells (2,108,109).

The GTP/GDP ratio in islet cells increases in parallel with the ATP/ADP ratio upon stimulation with glucose (38,110). This parallelism probably reflects the high activity of the islet nucleotide-diphosphate kinase (111). There exists a good correlation between glucose-induced insulin secretion through either pathway and the GTP/GDP ratio (38), but a specific role of changes in GTP or GDP in stimulus-secretion coupling remains disputed (110,112).

A mitochondrial factor distinct from ATP has been suggested to control exocytosis of insulin granules together with Ca^{2+} and ATP. The proposal that this factor might be glutamate (113) has been challenged (114).

Although protons are produced during glucose metabolism, the cytosolic pH of glucose-stimulated β-cells increases slightly (115) because of the operation of an HCO_3^-/Cl^- exchanger (116). It is possible that this small alkalinization modulates insulin secretion (117).

Malonyl Coenzyme A and Long-Chain Acyl Coenzyme A

The anaplerotic characteristics of glucose metabolism in β-cells lead to the formation of excess citrate that exits mitochondria to serve as a precursor of malonyl CoA in the cytoplasm (36) (Fig. 6.1). Malonyl CoA then inhibits carnitine palmitoyl transferase I and reduces fatty acid uptake by mitochondria, which explains the inhibition by glucose of the oxidation of endogenous (and exogenous) fatty acids (118,119). The result is an increase in cytosolic long-chain acyl CoAs that are proposed to serve as effector signal molecules (36). Because long-chain acyl CoAs open K^+-ATP channels (120), they cannot underlie generation of a triggering signal by membrane depolarization. Long-chain acyl CoA seems to increase the efficacy of Ca^{2+} on exocytosis (121). This attractive model has, however, been challenged by the demonstration that glucose-induced insulin secretion does not correlate with the extent to which lipids are either oxidized or esterified (122). Other signaling functions of glucose-regulated anaplerosis are currently being investigated (123).

Cyclic Adenosine Monophosphate

Glucose increases the concentration of cAMP in β-cells slightly (124), probably secondarily to the increase of $[Ca^{2+}]_i$ and the activation of adenylate cyclase by a Ca^{2+}-calmodulin protein kinase (125). Several phosphodiesterases (PDE) that degrade cAMP are present in β-cells, but the PDE 3 isoform is predominant both quantitatively and functionally (126,127). There is no doubt that an increase in cAMP concentration in β-cells is not a sufficient signal to trigger insulin secretion, but it can amplify the response to various secretagogues. Whereas the role of this amplification during hormonal stimulation of β-cells is well established (see below), its role during stimulation by glucose alone is much less clear. Experiments with isolated β-cells suggest that a minimal concentration of cAMP is necessary for normal stimulation of insulin secretion by glucose (128), and hormones that increase cAMP levels have been suggested to increase the glucose competence of poorly responsive β-cells (129). In contrast, inhibitors of protein kinase A do not impair the effect of glucose in intact islets (130).

Inositol Phosphates and Diacylglycerol

Glucose stimulates both the synthesis and hydrolysis of phospholipids in β-cells (131–134). However, the breakdown of phosphatidylinositol 4,5-bisphosphate and accumulation of inositol 1,4,5-trisphosphate are not primary signals but rather consequences of the increase in $[Ca^{2+}]_i$ (133,134). The acceleration of phospholipid turnover by glucose may serve to optimize the potentiation of insulin secretion by agonists acting via phospholipase C–linked receptors (see below).

Glucose stimulates de novo synthesis of diacylglycerol in β-cells. However, this diacylglycerol is richer in palmitate and poorer in arachidonate than is the diacylglycerol generated by hydrolysis of preexisting glycerolipids and does not significantly increase the total mass of diacylglycerol in islet cells (135). This may explain why glucose is usually (136–138), although not consistently (139,140), found not to translocate and activate protein kinase C in β-cells. It is possible that activation of protein kinase C (by diacylglycerol or another stimulator) contributes to the second phase of insulin secretion in certain species (102), but the bulk of the evidence indicates that its role in glucose-induced insulin secretion is not a major one.

Arachidonic Acid and Other Lipid Derivatives

Glucose stimulation of islet cells increases the release of arachidonic acid from phospholipids. However, decisive arguments that arachidonic acid itself plays a role in stimulus-secretion coupling are still missing (132,138,141). On the other hand, metabolites of arachidonic acid could modulate glucose-induced insulin secretion. The latter is decreased by prostaglandins and increased by certain products formed by lipoxygenation. It has been suggested that phosphatidic acid, formed by activation of phospholipases or by de novo synthesis from glucose, and lysophospholipids formed by activation of phospholipase A_2, might be involved in glucose-induced insulin secretion (138). In no case, however, have the reported effects of these substances carried conviction that their role is critical in stimulus-secretion coupling.

GENERAL CHARACTERISTICS OF GLUCOSE-INDUCED INSULIN SECRETION

Links between Insulin Synthesis and Secretion

The mechanisms of insulin biosynthesis and of its regulation by glucose are dealt with in detail in Chapter 5.

Short-term control of insulin secretion does not depend on insulin synthesis. Pancreatic insulin stores largely exceed the maximal secretory rates (~5% of insulin content per hour). The inhibition of insulin secretion that follows blockade of protein synthesis in β-cells does not reflect requirement of insulin synthesis (142) but results from the loss of other proteins with a short half-life (143). The first alteration is a rapid (1 to 2 hours) impairment of the action of Ca^{2+} on exocytosis followed by a delayed (>5 hours) decrease in the production of the triggering signal (143). Insulin synthesis and secretion can also be dissociated under several conditions. In contrast to glucose and other fuel secretagogues that stimulate both processes, several agents (e.g., arginine, acetylcholine, and hypoglycemic sulfonylureas) increase insulin secretion without increasing its synthesis (2,144). It also is possible to abolish the effects of glucose on secretion without affecting those on synthesis (e.g., by omitting extracellular Ca^{2+}) (2,144).

Insulin synthesis and secretion are, however, not completely independent events. Under certain circumstances, isolated islets release newly synthesized insulin in preference to older stored hormone (145). This may indicate that insulin granules do not undergo exocytosis at random but that a subpopulation of newly formed granules is "marked" to be released rather than to be stored (146). The mechanisms of this marking are not known. Alternatively, the phenomenon of preferential release of newly formed insulin could be due to β-cell heterogeneity within the islets (147). If the rise in glucose concentration recruits the same β-cells to synthesize (148) and to release insulin, and if these cells have low stores of preformed insulin, an apparent preferential secretion of newly formed insulin may be measured.

Kinetics

Insulin secretion depends not only on the ambient concentration of glucose but also on the rate of change of this concentration. When the glucose level increases slowly, the rate of insulin secretion increases in parallel. However, when the concentration of glucose is abruptly increased and then maintained at a high level, insulin secretion follows a biphasic time course (Fig. 6.6C). A nadir and a slowly rising second phase follow a rapid peak (first phase). This pattern, first described in the perfused rat pancreas (149), is commonly observed *in vitro*. It is not seen *in vivo* when the plasma glucose concentration progressively increases after a meal or even after an oral glucose load, but it can be produced by a rapid increase in plasma glucose during intravenous glucose infusion (150). This ability of β-cells to respond rapidly to glucose is thought to be essential for optimal glucose homeostasis. The loss of this ability has long been considered an early sign of β-cell dysfunction characteristic or even predictive of type 2 diabetes mellitus (150,151).

Numerous hypotheses have been put forward to explain the biphasic time course of glucose-induced insulin secretion. Because the glucose dependency of the two phases is similar *in vitro* (152) and *in vivo* (150), there is no evidence that distinct initial steps in glucose recognition are involved. Early suggestions that the nadir between the two phases is due to a negative feedback exerted by insulin secreted during the first phase or to partial inhibition by somatostatin have been abandoned (152,153). The concept that the first phase reflects release of preformed insulin and that the second phase reflects release of newly synthesized insulin is also not correct (152).

According to a "storage-limited" model (152,153), two compartments of insulin granules could exist, the smaller one, in proximity to the plasma membrane, being readily released and responsible for the first phase. The existence of distinct subsets of granules is supported by experiments monitoring insulin release as capacitance changes in single, voltage-clamped β-cells (154,155). It has been suggested that the pool of readily releasable granules is composed of those insulin granules that can be immunoprecipitated by an antibody directed to syntaxin, a plasma membrane protein (156). However, functional evidence indicates that only a fraction of the docked granules is readily releasable (155). This model implies that the second phase reflects the energy-dependent mobilization of granules from a reserve to the readily releasable pool.

According to a "signal-limited" model (153,157), changes in the magnitude or effectiveness of the triggering signal produced by glucose could underlie the biphasic response. Evidence supporting this hypothesis is accumulating. The increase in β-cell $[Ca^{2+}]_i$ produced by glucose is biphasic (74,75), and no first phase of secretion occurs when $[Ca^{2+}]_i$ does not abruptly increase. However, no gradual increase in $[Ca^{2+}]_i$ occurs during sustained glucose stimulation (74,75). Therefore, the slowly increasing second phase of secretion (which is more pronounced in the rat than in the mouse) (Fig. 6.6C) does not depend simply on the concentration of cytoplasmic Ca^{2+} but probably also involves an increase in the efficacy of the Ca^{2+} signal (42,102,158). There is good evidence that the amplifying pathway is implicated, but it is still unclear whether the enlargement of the pool of releasable insulin granules results from a mobilization of granules toward the sites of exocytosis or from a modification of the properties of already adequately situated granules.

Biphasic insulin secretion is not specific to glucose. It can also be induced by other fuel stimuli (159,160). Moreover, the kinetics of the secretory response may be influenced by the concentration of the applied stimulus and by the prevailing concentration of glucose. For instance, the common idea that sulfonylureas simply trigger a first phase of insulin secretion (149) holds true only for stimulation by high concentrations of the drugs in low-glucose environments. When used at a low concentration and in the presence of glucose, sulfonylureas induce a sustained secretion of insulin (161,162). These are further arguments supporting the conclusion that the kinetics of insulin secretion does not depend simply on the existence of different pools of insulin granules.

Either model is probably insufficient. Biphasic secretion of insulin requires immediately releasable and mobilizable granules *and* adequate temporal and quantitative changes in both triggering and amplifying signals. It is also unlikely that an empty pool of releasable granules can explain the lack of first phase in patients with type 2 diabetes mellitus (150,151). If this were the case, why should non-glucose stimuli cause immediate insulin secretion (163,164)? The defect is more likely due to the inability of glucose to induce a rapid increase in $[Ca^{2+}]_i$ in these diseased β-cells.

Concentration Dependency: Recruitment and Increase in the Individual Responses

As previously mentioned, the relationship between the extracellular glucose concentration and the rate of insulin secretion *in vitro* is sigmoidal (1) (Fig. 6.6A). In isolated rat islets or in the perfused rat pancreas, the threshold concentration is around 5 to 6 mM and half-maximal and maximal responses are observed at 9 to 11 mM and 15 to 20 mM, respectively. This relationship is shifted slightly to the left in human islets and to the right in mouse islets, which corresponds well with the differences in blood glucose concentration between the three species. It is also important to bear in mind that circulating nutrients other than glucose, hormones, and neurotransmitters shift the dose-response relationship to glucose to the left *in vivo* (see below).

The sigmoidal shape of the dose-response curve has been attributed to a gaussian distribution of the thresholds for β-cell stimulation (128). Increasing the concentration of glucose would thus recruit more and more β-cells to secrete insulin. Functional heterogeneity between β-cells has been directly demonstrated *in vitro* by measuring (with the reverse hemolytic plaque assay) insulin secretion from single β-cells obtained by dispersion of rat islets (165). The number of secreting cells increases as the concentration of glucose is increased (166,167). The alternative possibility is that the response of each individual cell increases with the concentration of glucose. It has indeed been demonstrated that glucose causes a dose-dependent increase in $[Ca^{2+}]_i$ (106) and in insulin release (166,167) in single isolated β-cells.

The key question is whether the heterogeneity of individual isolated β-cells persists within the islets of Langerhans in which β-cells are preferentially interconnected by gap junctions made of connexin 36 (168). This intercellular coupling and paracrine influences may erase the individual differences to constitute a functionally homogeneous population. Thus, in contrast to the heterogeneous responses produced in isolated β-cells, glucose induces uniform metabolic (NADPH autofluorescence) (169), electrical (69,71,170), and $[Ca^{2+}]_i$ responses (74,75) in β-cells residing within intact islets. The homogeneity and synchrony of complex $[Ca^{2+}]_i$ changes in different regions of an islet are illustrated in Figure 6.4. Recruitment of β-cells can be detected in islets or clusters, but it occurs over a narrow range of glucose concentrations (106). There is no doubt that the triggering signal is not generated in an all-or-none manner; its amplitude increases with the glucose concentration. It is also well established that the secretory performance is greatly improved when contacts are established between β-cells (128,171,172). Through the electrical coupling, the most active β-cells of an islet can entrain the less active ones to generate an increase in $[Ca^{2+}]_i$. Nevertheless, there is indirect evidence that not all β-cells within intact islets secrete insulin at the same rate (173,174). This heterogeneity of secretion in face of a homogeneous triggering signal could be due to a variable production of the amplifying signals (106).

Oscillations

Insulin secretion is pulsatile even during stimulation by a stable concentration of glucose. Simultaneous measurements of $[Ca^{2+}]_i$ and secretion in single mouse islets have shown that $[Ca^{2+}]_i$ oscillations are synchronous in all regions (β-cells) of the islet (74,75) and that each oscillation is accompanied by an oscillation of insulin secretion (175–177). This is illustrated in Figure 6.4 for the slow oscillations but holds true for the fast oscillations, whose detection requires a high temporal resolution (175). The synchrony between $[Ca^{2+}]_i$ and insulin secretion oscillations persists under a variety of experimental conditions (175,178), indicating that the islet behaves as a functional syncytium. Whereas it is widely agreed that $[Ca^{2+}]_i$ oscillations in β-cells induce pulses of insulin secretion, the possibility that pulsatile insulin secretion occurs in the absence of $[Ca^{2+}]_i$ oscillations in β-cells is debated (97,179,180). Although metabolic oscillations could theoretically drive oscillations of secretion through the amplifying pathway, their power is definitely less than that of $[Ca^{2+}]_i$ oscillations (180). It is much more plausible that metabolic oscillations generate oscillations of membrane potential and hence of $[Ca^{2+}]_i$. The latter (triggering pathway) then induce oscillations of exocytosis, the amplitude of which may be increased by metabolism itself (amplifying pathway). The *primum movens* is a metabolic oscillation, but the minute-to-minute regulator is $[Ca^{2+}]_i$.

In healthy human subjects, plasma insulin concentration oscillates at low and high frequencies (181,182). Low-frequency oscillations with a period of about 120 minutes are usually considered to result from feedback loops linking glucose and insulin (183). High-frequency oscillations have a period of 5 to 8 minutes, which is closer to but still substantially longer than the period of the electrical and $[Ca^{2+}]_i$ oscillations in individual islets. Recordings of the β-cell membrane potential within islets of living mice have shown an excellent synchrony between β-cells within the same islet but a lack of synchrony between islets (69). There is at present no evidence that extrinsic signals coordinate the functioning of all islets to generate oscillations of plasma insulin concentration. How these are produced is still unclear.

What can be the functional reasons of the oscillatory behavior of β-cells? The production of pulsatile insulin secretion and oscillations of plasma insulin is the most obvious answer. However, there could also be advantages for the β-cell itself: Oscillations of the signal permit a finer regulation than an amplitude-modulated, sustained signal; oscillations of $[Ca^{2+}]_i$ also may serve to regulate functions other than secretion; oscillations of $[Ca^{2+}]_i$ are less costly for maintenance of cell homeostasis and prevent potentially damaging effects of long-lasting sustained elevations of $[Ca^{2+}]_i$.

THE PREEMINENT ROLE OF GLUCOSE IN THE CONTROL OF INSULIN SECRETION

On the basis of *in vitro* experiments, the numerous agents that increase insulin secretion have traditionally been subdivided into two broad categories: the initiators or primary stimuli that are able to increase insulin secretion in the absence of any other stimulatory agent and the potentiators or secondary stimuli that are ineffective alone but increase insulin secretion in the presence of an initiator, particularly glucose (3). It is, however, essential to emphasize that glucose is by far the most important controller of insulin secretion. One may even consider glucose as the only physiologic initiator of insulin secretion in adult mammals. This concept is illustrated schematically in Figure 6.7.

When insulin secretion is studied *in vitro* with isolated islets or the perfused pancreas and an artificial balanced-salt solution, a stimulatory effect of glucose can already be measured at concentrations within the physiologic range (depicted in hatched area in Fig. 6.7A). In contrast, other initiators, such as amino acids or drugs (e.g., sulfonylureas), must be used at concentrations well above the physiologic or therapeutic range to induce insulin secretion (Fig. 6.7B). Hormones are not initiators; they have no effect when used alone. However, when the incubation or perfusion medium contains a physiologic concentration of glucose, insulin secretion can be increased by amino acids, hormones, or drugs at physiologic or therapeutic concentrations (184–186) (Fig. 6.7B). Glucose thus confers to otherwise ineffective or weakly effective agents the ability to increase insulin

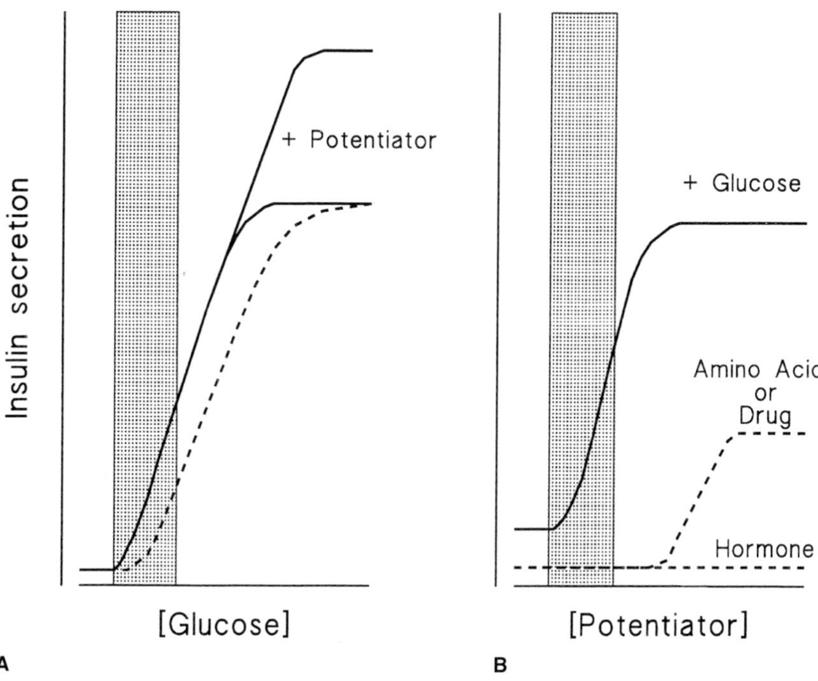

Figure 6.7. Concentration dependence of insulin secretion induced by glucose **(A)** or amino acids, drugs or hormones **(B)**. Hatched areas correspond to the range of physiologic or therapeutic concentrations of the test substance. Broken lines show the effect of the test substance alone. Solid lines show the effect of glucose in the presence of a physiologic or therapeutic concentration of a potentiator **(A)** or the effect of an amino acid, a drug, or a hormone in the presence of a physiologic concentration of glucose **(B)**. Depending on its mode of action, a potentiator may shift the dose-response curve to glucose to the left or increase the maximum response.

secretion, even at low concentrations, a property known as the "permissive action of glucose." If, on the other hand, the medium contains amino acids, hormones, or a drug at physiologic or therapeutic concentrations (potentiator in Fig. 6.7A), the dose-response curve of glucose-induced insulin secretion is shifted to the left. Depending on the mode of action of the potentiator, the sensitivity or the maximum response to glucose, or both, can be increased.

These apparently complex properties can easily be understood by considering how each agent affects the triggering and amplifying pathways. Initiators are those substances that can produce a triggering signal, a rise in $[Ca^{2+}]_i$, independently of glucose. Non-metabolized agents such as sulfonylureas or arginine belong to that category when they are used at high concentrations, but their effect on insulin secretion is usually small or transient because the efficacy of Ca^{2+} on exocytosis is poor in the absence of an amplifying signal (42). When these agents are used at lower concentrations, they become potentiators. They no longer depolarize the β-cell membrane enough to open voltage-dependent Ca^{2+} channels. However, their small effect on the membrane potential is sufficient to increase Ca^{2+} influx and $[Ca^{2+}]_i$ in the presence of a threshold or stimulatory concentration of glucose (187).

Purely potentiating agents do not induce a triggering signal in the absence of glucose but may increase the insulinotropic action of the latter in different ways. The metabolism of a substrate by β-cells may be insufficient to produce enough ATP to depolarize the membrane to the threshold potential at which Ca^{2+} channels open. Ca^{2+} influx, and hence insulin release cannot be stimulated. In the presence of glucose, however, the substrate potentiator increases β-cell metabolism, as if the concentration of glucose had been raised; hence, the larger secretory response. This type of potentiating action has been well characterized for fructose (22) and can probably also explain the potentiation by other fuels, with the reservation that the metabolic usage of different types of substrates is not always simply additive (4). Another mechanism characterizes the action of hormones that may produce a potent amplifying signal such as cAMP but remain ineffective on insulin secretion until a triggering signal has been produced by glucose (or by another initiator).

It is thus evident that the permissive action of glucose (188,189) depends on the β-cell membrane potential. The depolarization induced by glucose permits the small depolarizing action of the potentiators to activate further Ca^{2+} channels (187). However, the amplifying action of glucose augmenting the efficacy of Ca^{2+} also plays a critical role (42).

With this background in mind, it is easy to understand how changes in the glucose concentration below the threshold value measured *in vitro* can influence β-cell function *in vivo*. A small decrease in plasma glucose concentrations (e.g., during fasting) prevents inappropriate insulin secretion in response to non-glucose stimuli. On the other hand, relatively small increases in plasma glucose concentrations (e.g., after meals) lead to larger insulin responses than those expected from dose-response curves defined *in vitro* because of the greater effect of non-glucose stimuli. The marked glucose dependency of the action of various stimuli on β-cells is thus an essential safeguard against both hypoglycemia and hyperglycemia (Fig. 6.7).

THE β-CELL RESPONSE TO NUTRIENTS OTHER THAN GLUCOSE

Sugars and Derivatives

Glucose is the sole sugar of physiologic importance for the control of insulin secretion. Fructose is metabolized slowly by β-cells and causes a modest increase in insulin secretion when it is used at nonphysiologic concentrations and in the presence of glucose (potentiation) (3,22,190). Galactose is not metabolized by β-cells and does not affect insulin secretion. *In vitro*, mannose, glyceraldehyde, dihydroxyacetone, and *N*-acetylglucosamine can increase insulin secretion. The coherent picture that has emerged from a number of studies is that the insulin-releasing capacity of all sugars and derivatives correlates well with their rate of metabolism in β-cells (2,190,191). Their effects are mediated by both the triggering and amplifying pathways. Exogenous pyruvate and lactate are poor insulin-secretagogues even in high concentrations because they are not well taken up and therefore cannot readily be metabolized by β-cells (27,192). Their metabolism by whole islets takes place in non–β-cells which, unlike β-cells, possess plasma membrane transporters for monocarboxylic acids. This also explains why the membrane permeant phenyl-pyruvate is a considerably more potent insulin secretagogue than pyruvate (193).

Amino Acids

The ability of amino acids to increase insulin secretion depends to a marked extent on the ambient concentration of glucose (184) (Fig. 6.7B). At a physiologic concentration, individual amino acids are ineffective, but their combination in proportion to their plasma concentrations is stimulatory (194,195). Their combined action probably involves both metabolic and biophysical mechanisms (Fig. 6.2). Thus, studies using high concentrations of individual amino acids have clearly shown that they distinctly affect stimulus-secretion coupling.

Leucine alone is able to increase insulin secretion, albeit weakly, in the absence of glucose. It is considerably more potent in the presence of glutamine, which itself is ineffective alone. These properties can be explained by changes in β-cell metabolism (196,197). Leucine is degraded by a branched-chain keto acid dehydrogenase to produce acetyl CoA, which is then used by the citric acid cycle. Glutamine is transformed into glutamate by a phosphate-dependent glutaminase. In the presence of leucine, an allosteric activator of glutamate dehydrogenase, glutamate is metabolized into α-ketoglutarate, which eventually fuels the citric acid cycle. Leucine and, even more so, the combination of leucine and glutamine increase the ATP/ADP ratio (92) and stimulate insulin secretion by activating triggering and amplifying pathways similar to those set in motion by glucose (105,198,199) (Fig. 6.2). It is the activation of glutamate dehydrogenase, with subsequent acceleration of the metabolism of endogenous amino acids, that explains the ability of a non-metabolized leucine derivative (BCH, or 2-endoaminonorbornane-2-carboxylic acid) to increase insulin secretion (196,197). Glutamate dehydrogenase may also be indirectly regulated by glucose metabolism (200). Certain mutations of the gene coding for glutamate dehydrogenase increase the activity of the enzyme and provide an explanation for the inappropriate secretion of insulin in the syndrome of leucine-induced hypoglycemia (201).

Alanine is metabolized slowly in islet cells (202) and increases insulin secretion only weakly (203). This effect, which requires the presence of glucose, is probably due to the cotransport of alanine with Na^+ in β-cells (204). The resulting small depolarization slightly augments Ca^{2+} influx and hence the triggering signal $[Ca^{2+}]_i$.

Arginine and other cationic amino acids are only poorly metabolized in islet cells (202,205). Their mode of action markedly differs from that of nutrients that serve as fuels for β-cells. They depolarize the β-cell membrane because of their transport in the cell in a positively charged form (198,206). The depolarization then activates voltage-dependent Ca^{2+} channels, Ca^{2+} influx ensues, and $[Ca^{2+}]_i$ increases (Fig. 6.2). This peculiar mode of action may explain why arginine, unlike glucose, still elicits a rapid secretion of insulin in patients with type 2 diabetes mellitus (163,164). Arginine increases production of nitric oxide (NO) by β-cells (207), but NO is not involved in the stimulation of insulin secretion by the amino acid (207,208).

Fatty Acids

There is wide, albeit incomplete (209), agreement that fatty acids do not acutely increase insulin secretion in the presence of low concentrations of glucose (210–212). This may probably be explained by the fact that fatty acids, although well oxidized by β-cells (118,119), do not increase the ATP/ADP ratio and, therefore, do not depolarize the membrane and increase $[Ca^{2+}]_i$ (212). In the presence of stimulatory concentrations of glucose, fatty acids potentiate Ca^{2+} influx possibly by an action on Ca^{2+} channels. The resulting increase in the triggering signal certainly contributes to the increase in insulin secretion that fatty acids produce under these conditions. However, production of an amplifying signal, long-chain acyl CoAs, also is involved (Fig. 6.2). Thus, malonyl-CoA issued from glucose metabolism (Fig. 6.1) inhibits carnitine palmitoyltransferase 1 and thereby prevents long-chain acyl CoA entry and oxidation in mitochondria (36).

No qualitative differences appear to exist between the effects of saturated, monounsaturated, and polyunsaturated fatty acids, which, however, display distinct potencies (palmitate > stearate ~ oleate > linoleate) (213). It is also evident that the acute effects of fatty acids on β-cell function depend on the unbound fraction rather than on the total concentration. This must be remembered when evaluating the physiologic relevance of *in vitro* studies (213).

Ketone Bodies

Acetoacetate and β-hydroxybutyrate are oxidized by islet cells and slightly increase insulin secretion, at least when used in high concentrations and when the medium also contains glucose (118,214). The available evidence suggests that the effects of ketone bodies on insulin secretion are due to their metabolic degradation in β-cells (214). It is uncertain that these effects observed *in vitro* ever occur *in vivo*, even for maintaining minimum insulin secretion during prolonged fasting.

PHARMACOLOGIC CONTROL OF INSULIN SECRETION

A number of drugs are used in therapeutics with the specific aim of increasing insulin secretion in patients with type 2 diabetes mellitus or, much more rarely, of decreasing insulin secretion in patients suffering from hyperinsulinemic hypoglycemia. Other drugs are used for different purposes but exert side effects in β-cells. Finally, many pharmacologic compounds serve as tools for the study of stimulus-secretion coupling *in vitro*. Only those drugs with a therapeutic potential will be discussed in this section, which is subdivided by site of action rather than by drug family (Fig. 6.8).

Stimulators of Metabolism

No drugs capable of accelerating glucose metabolism have been identified, but synthetic derivatives of glucose or other nutrients that are actively metabolized in β-cells are currently being tested as potential insulin secretagogues (215).

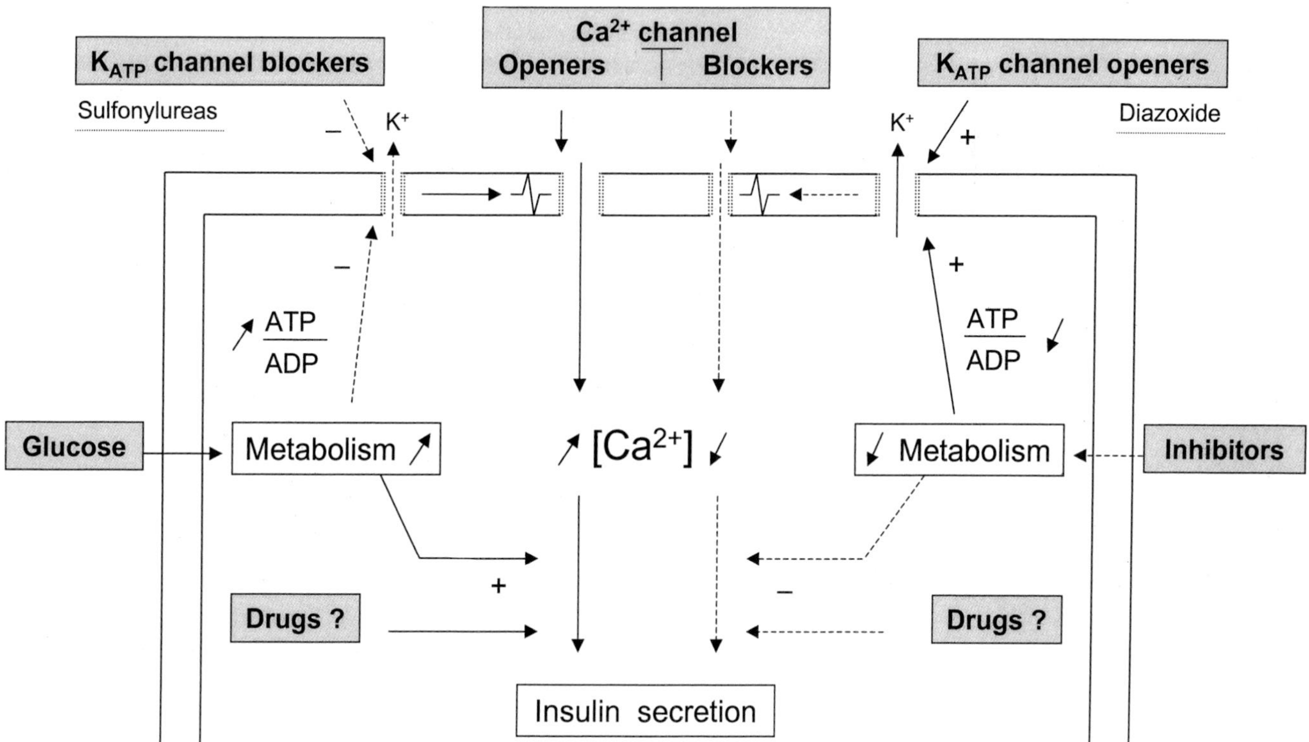

Figure 6.8. Schematic representation of the mechanisms by which pharmacologic agents influence insulin secretion: +, stimulation; –, inhibition; ATP, adenosine triphosphate; ADP, adenosine diphosphate.

K$^+$-Adenosine Triphosphate–Channel Blockers

Hypoglycemic sulfonylureas, commonly used in the treatment of patients with type 2 diabetes mellitus, increase insulin secretion by closing K$^+$-ATP channels. This closure does not involve a change in β-cell metabolism but is the result of a direct interaction with SUR 1, the regulatory subunit of the channel (63–65,216) (Fig. 6.8). The ensuing membrane depolarization opens voltage-operated Ca^{2+} channels, promotes Ca^{2+} influx, and increases $[Ca^{2+}]_i$ (75,162,217). Sulfonylureas thus mimic the biophysical effects of glucose that lead to the production of the triggering signal. All sulfonylureas have a similar mode of action but differ by their affinity for SUR 1. In general, those compounds with the highest affinity for the receptor (glibenclamide >> tolbutamide) show the greatest potency but also the poorest reversibility on the stimulation of insulin secretion (217,218). For example, at equipotent concentrations, tolbutamide has a rapid, stable, and rapidly reversible effect on insulin secretion, whereas glibenclamide exerts a slow, progressively increasing and slowly reversible action. It is also important to bear in mind that sulfonylureas are tightly bound to albumin and that their therapeutic free concentrations are much lower than the free concentrations used in many *in vitro* studies.

Non-sulfonylurea compounds usually derived from glibenclamide (219), the "glinides," have recently become available for the treatment of patients with type 2 diabetes mellitus. The glinides also close K$^+$-ATP channels by binding to SUR 1 (220). In contrast, several imidazoline compounds, including blockers of α_2-adrenoceptors, block the channel by directly closing the pore formed by Kir 6.2 (221,222). Basically, all these substances increase insulin secretion by the same mechanism as sulfonylureas. Some imidazoline compounds may have additional, yet unidentified, sites of action (223–225).

Many other drugs block K$^+$-ATP channels in β-cells (226), and the increase in insulin secretion that they may produce explains the hypoglycemic episodes complicating their clinical use; this is the case for quinine (227) and certain antiarrhythmic agents (228).

Inhibitors of Metabolism

Several substances can interfere with glucose metabolism and, therefore, inhibit secretion of insulin by decreasing both the triggering and amplifying signals (Fig. 6.8). Such substances are used *in vitro* as tools to study stimulus-secretion coupling. It is unlikely that therapeutically useful drugs exert such a side effect.

K$^+$-Adenosine Triphosphate–Channel Openers

Diazoxide inhibits insulin secretion by opening K$^+$-ATP channels (229,230). This opening does not involve a decrease in β-cell metabolism but results from a direct interaction with SUR 1 (Fig. 6.8). The ensuing membrane repolarization closes voltage-operated Ca^{2+} channels, diminishes Ca^{2+} influx, and inhibits insulin secretion (75). Diazoxide thus counteracts the generation of the triggering signal by glucose and other secretagogues that close K$^+$-ATP channels. It is, therefore, understandable that the *genuine* effect of arginine, which acts independently of these channels (Fig. 6.2), is not inhibited by diazoxide *in vivo* (231) and *in vitro* (232). However, one effect of diazoxide is largely misunderstood. The drug can also decrease the insulin-releasing action of agents that do not close K$^+$-ATP channels when these agents are tested in the presence of subthreshold concentrations of glucose. The explanation is that the depolarizing action of these agents (with the exception of high extracellular K$^+$), hence their effect on $[Ca^{2+}]_i$, is diminished when the membrane conductance is increased by opening of K$^+$-ATP channels. In other words, diazoxide counteracts the permissive effect of glucose previously described.

Openers of K$^+$-ATP channels in vascular smooth muscle cells are currently developed as antihypertensive agents (233). The risk that they inhibit insulin secretion is small because the selected drugs have a higher affinity for SUR 2A (the smooth muscle isoform) than SUR 1 (the β-cell isoform).

Ca^{2+}-Channel Openers and Blockers

Blockage of voltage-dependent Ca^{2+} channels by dihydropyridines (e.g., nifedipine) or phenylalkylamines (e.g., verapamil) inhibits Ca^{2+} influx in β-cells (67,68) and, therefore, antagonizes the ability of glucose and other depolarizing agents to increase $[Ca^{2+}]_i$ (234) (Fig. 6.8). This explains why these drugs nonselectively inhibit the secretion of insulin induced by those agents whose effect depends on Ca^{2+} influx, regardless of the mechanisms of depolarization (232). *In vivo*, Ca^{2+}-channel blockers have no or little deleterious influence on insulin secretion and glucose homeostasis (235). There also exist dihydropyridine derivatives that do not block Ca^{2+} channels but act as agonists at the channel level. They are ineffective in unstimulated β-cells, when the membrane potential is high and the voltage-dependent Ca^{2+} channels are closed, but they increase Ca^{2+} influx and insulin secretion in the presence of glucose (226). Unfortunately, these drugs lack a sufficient tissue selectivity to be used as antidiabetic agents.

Drugs Modulating the Amplifying Pathway

Indirect evidence indicates that the amplifying action of glucose is defective in patients with type 2 diabetes mellitus (236). Drugs correcting this defect could thus be useful. It has been suggested that sulfonylureas also amplify the action of Ca^{2+} on exocytosis of insulin granules (237–239), but this view has been challenged (240,241). No currently available drug exerts such an effect to an extent that is significant and beneficial for the patients. Agents aimed at these distal steps of stimulus-secretion coupling may be developed in the future; those that have been proposed thus far (242) appear to be phosphodiesterase inhibitors producing their effect by increasing cAMP in β-cells. The optimal drug should, however, not be so potent that it reverses the normal hierarchy between the triggering and amplifying pathways (42).

Pharmacologic agents may interfere with insulin secretion by acting on the effector system (e.g., the cytoskeleton) (85). However, no therapeutically useful drug is known to impair the amplifying pathway specifically. The proposal that diazoxide interferes with the action of Ca^{2+} is not grounded (240).

NEUROHORMONAL AMPLIFICATION OF INSULIN SECRETION

Insulin secretion is also subject to autocrine, paracrine, neurocrine, and endocrine influences (90,243–245). The list of hormones and neurotransmitters that may modulate the insulinotropic action of glucose and other nutrients is long and easily confusing because of species differences and uncertainties about the physiologic relevance of some of the effects observed with *in vitro* models. It is particularly difficult to establish whether paracrine interactions observed in isolated

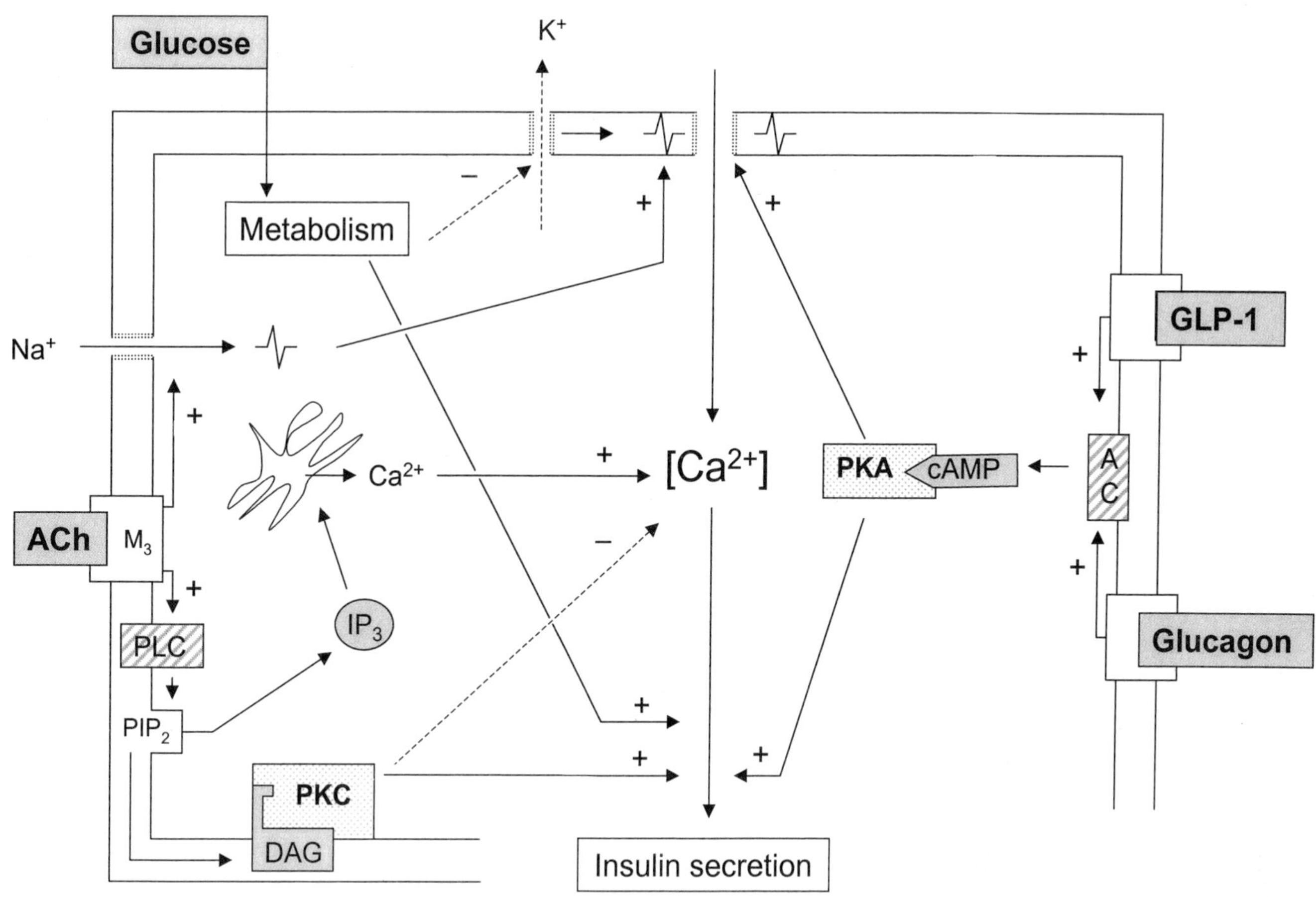

Figure 6.9. Schematic representation of the major mechanisms by which neurotransmitters and hormones amplify insulin secretion: +, stimulation; –, inhibition; ACh, acetylcholine; M_3, muscarinic receptor of the M_3 type; PLC, phospholipase C; PIP_2 , phosphatidylinositol 4,5-bisphosphate; IP_3, inositol 1,4,5-trisphosphate; DAG, diacylglycerol; PKC, protein kinase C; GLP-1, glucagon-like peptide 1 (7–36 amide); AC, adenylate cyclase; PKA, protein kinase A.

islets or dispersed cells really occur *in situ* when secreted products are rapidly cleared by the circulation. In addition, many of these putative regulatory peptides can act on receptors other than their own when they are used, as they often are *in vitro*, at supraphysiologic concentrations.

Neurohormonal agents bind to membrane receptors and activate transduction pathways that are generally not specific to β-cells, but their effects on insulin secretion are tightly conditioned by the prevailing glucose concentration. The major intracellular messengers that amplify insulin secretion are cAMP, inositol phosphates, and diacylglycerol (Fig. 6.9).

The Cyclic Adenosine Monophosphate–Protein Kinase A Pathway

Adenylate cyclase, which synthesizes cAMP from ATP, is linked to several membrane receptors by a stimulatory subtype G_s of the GTP-binding proteins (G-proteins). Once formed, cAMP binds to its target, protein kinase A (PKA), of which the type I and type II isoforms are present in β-cells (137). This binding to the regulatory subunits of the kinase releases the catalytic subunits that catalyze the phosphorylation of distinct proteins, the nature of which has only been partially identified.

Several mechanisms underlie the amplification of insulin secretion by cAMP (125,131,246). The two major ones are depicted in Figure 6.9. Probably by phosphorylating the α_1 subunit of the voltage-operated Ca^{2+} channels (247), PKA slightly increases Ca^{2+} influx triggered by primary secretagogues such as glucose or tolbutamide (248,249) and hence augments the increase in $[Ca^{2+}]_i$ that they produce (131,180). A second, quantitatively more important, mechanism is an amplification of the action of Ca^{2+} on exocytosis. This has been demonstrated by the use of permeabilized (43,137) or voltage-clamped (250) β-cells, in which cAMP increases the amount of insulin secreted in response to a fixed $[Ca^{2+}]_i$. The protein or proteins mediating this effect are not known. It is also unclear whether PKA modulates the action of Ca^{2+} itself or increases the pool of releasable insulin granules or even mediates all cAMP effects. In summary, cAMP potentiates glucose-induced insulin secretion by increasing the triggering signal and by amplifying its efficacy (Fig. 6.9).

The Phosphoinositide–Protein Kinase C Pathway

β-Cells are equipped with different types of receptors that are linked to a phospholipase C-β (PLC-β) by a G-protein of the G_q subtype. On activation of the receptor, the enzyme is stimulated to split phosphatidylinositol 4,5-bisphosphate, a phospholipid present in small amounts in the plasma membrane, into inositol 1,4,5-trisphosphate (IP_3) and diacylglycerol (133, 251) (Fig. 6.9).

Diacylglycerol, which is liposoluble, remains in the plasma membrane, to which it causes translocation of its target, protein kinase C (PKC) (136,252), of which the α-isoform predominates in β-cells (137). This translocation, which also requires Ca^{2+} and phosphatidylserine, activates the kinase, which can then phosphorylate proteins, the nature of which is incompletely known. One of these is the myristoylated alanine-rich C kinase substrate, a protein that binds actin and Ca^{2+}-calmodulin and that has been implicated in vesicle transport (137). The result of these phosphorylations is a sensitization of the releasing machinery to Ca^{2+} (43,253). Experiments using phorbol esters, which activate PKC directly, have shown that this pathway does not increase Ca^{2+} influx and even lowers $[Ca^{2+}]_i$ in normal β-cells (180,249,254), probably by accelerating extrusion of the ion from the cell. Pure activation of the PLC pathway thus potentiates insulin secretion by amplifying the action of the triggering signal (Fig. 6.9).

IP_3, which is hydrosoluble, diffuses in the cytoplasm and binds to receptors present on the membranes of the endoplasmic reticulum, in which Ca^{2+} is present in high concentration because of its active pumping by a Ca^{2+}-ATPase (SERCA pump). IP_3 binding results in the opening of channels through which Ca^{2+} diffuses from the organelle to the cytoplasm (255) (Fig. 6.9). The consequence is an increase in $[Ca^{2+}]_i$ that usually displays two phases: an initial large peak followed by a smaller sustained elevation. The latter not only reflects intracellular Ca^{2+} mobilization, it also depends on Ca^{2+} influx through voltage-independent Ca^{2+} channels (controlled by the repletion state of intracellular Ca^{2+} stores) and through voltage-dependent Ca^{2+} channels (256,257). Actually, the amplitude and pattern of the $[Ca^{2+}]_i$ change are very much dependent on the ambient glucose concentration. In the context of this chapter, one should simply bear in mind that activation of PLC potentiates insulin secretion by both increasing the triggering signal (via IP_3) and amplifying its action (via diacylglycerol).

Physiologic Amplifiers of Insulin Secretion

Glucagon-like peptide-1 [7–36 amide] (GLP-1) is a product of post-translational processing of proglucagon in L-cells from the mucosa of the ileum and colon (244,258).

Glucose-dependent insulinotropic polypeptide (GIP, also known as gastric inhibitory polypeptide) is synthesized by the enteroendocrine K-cells from the duodenojejunal mucosa (244).

These two hormones are important players in the "entero-insular axis." They are released after nutrients are ingested and probably are responsible for the "incretin" effect, that is, the larger increases in plasma insulin levels observed for a given increase in plasma glucose levels when the sugar is absorbed orally rather than administered intravenously (259–261). In humans, the role of GLP-1 is probably more important than that of GIP. GLP-1 and GIP act on G-protein–coupled specific receptors in β-cells (262). They do not affect insulin secretion in the presence of low glucose concentrations but markedly increase it in the presence of threshold or stimulatory glucose concentrations. This amplification is mediated through the cAMP–protein kinase A pathway. Glucose-dependent inhibition of K^+-ATP channels has also been reported (129,263) but is not unanimously accepted (264,265). GLP-1 is currently being evaluated as an antidiabetic agent to increase insulin secretion by mechanisms different from those of sulfonylureas (266).

Amplification of insulin secretion through the phosphoinositide–protein kinase C pathway is physiologically relevant for acetylcholine and cholecystokinin.

Acetylcholine is released by parasympathetic nerve endings in the islets during both the cephalic and intestinal phases of feeding (245). It acts on muscarinic receptors of the M_3 type (267). The effects of acetylcholine are more complex in β-cells than in many other cells (257). In addition to activating PKC (see above), the neurotransmitter activates a phospholipase A_2. More surprisingly, it depolarizes the β-cell membrane by increasing its conductance to Na^+. In the presence of glucose or another primary secretagogue, this additional depolarization augments Ca^{2+} influx through voltage-operated Ca^{2+} channels (Fig. 6.9).

Cholecystokinin (CCK) is released from the duodenum and proximal jejunum during meals but acts primarily as a neurotransmitter at peptidergic synapses present in the islets (245,261). It activates specific (CCK-A) receptors in β-cells (268).

Putative Amplifiers of Insulin Secretion

Glucagon raises cAMP levels in β-cells and amplifies the secretion of insulin induced by various primary secretagogues (124,125). This effect, which is mediated by specific glucagon receptors (not by cross-reaction with GLP-1 receptors) (262), is clear for exogenous glucagon (269), but it is not certain that glucagon released by α-cells of the islets exerts any paracrine action on the neighboring β-cells (270).

Catecholamines have the net effect of inhibiting insulin secretion through α_2-adrenoceptors, but β-adrenergic agonists (stimulating cAMP formation) increase plasma insulin levels *in vivo* (245). They have, however, little or no effect *in vitro*. Functional studies with purified islet cells have suggested that rat β-cells are devoid of β-adrenergic receptors (271). Human β-cells could possess β_2-adrenoceptors (272), but the inhibitory effect of catecholamines remains predominant.

Pituitary adenylate cyclase-activating polypeptide (PACAP), vasoactive intestinal polypeptide, and gastrin-releasing peptide are present in nerve fibers of the pancreas (245,273,274). By activating specific receptors in β-cells, they amplify glucose-induced insulin secretion (245,261). PACAP is particularly potent and acts through the cAMP pathway, as does vasoactive intestinal peptide, whereas gastrin-releasing peptide activates the PLC pathway (245,275). The physiologic importance of these peptides in the control of β-cell function is still unclear.

Vasopressin and oxytocin increase glucose-induced insulin secretion *in vitro* through a stimulation of phosphoinositide metabolism (276,277). This effect does not occur at physiologic concentrations of the hormones in plasma but is compatible with a local control of β-cell function by vasopressin and oxytocin, which are present in the pancreas (278).

The purine nucleotides ATP and ADP amplify insulin secretion, at least in certain species, by activating extracellular P2Y-purinergic receptors in β-cells (279). It is unclear whether ATP, present in secretory granules and released with insulin during exocytosis (280), exerts a direct stimulatory influence on β-cell function by this mechanism. ATP may indeed be rapidly degraded by ecto-ATPases, and adenosine inhibits insulin secretion by acting on A_1 receptors.

Glutamate, at micromolar concentrations, increases insulin secretion from the perfused rat pancreas in a glucose-dependent manner. The effect is mediated by an ionotropic glutamate receptor of the AMPA subtype (281) that has been shown to be present and functional in β-cells by molecular, immunocytochemical, and electrophysiologic techniques (282,283).

NEUROHORMONAL ATTENUATION OF INSULIN SECRETION

Cellular Mechanisms

Attenuation of insulin secretion may be mediated by various types of membrane receptors, which exert their effects by multiple similar mechanisms, the exact nature and relative contribution of which are not completely established (90) (Fig. 6.10).

These receptors are linked to the adenylate cyclase by a pertussis toxin–sensitive, inhibitory subtype (G_i or G_o) of the G-proteins. Activation of the receptor thus leads to a decrease in the concentration of cAMP in β-cells, with consequences opposite to those described above for an increase in cAMP. This mechanism, however, cannot fully account for the attenuation of secretion (125,284). Activation of the receptor also causes partial repolarization of the β-cell membrane, by a mechanism that is still disputed. There is good evidence that opening of K^+ channels is involved (285,286), but it has not been conclusively established whether these are the ATP-sensitive K^+ channels or other K^+ channels (287,288). Direct inhibition of Ca^{2+} channels has also been envisaged. This partial repolarization of the β-cell membrane reduces the influx of Ca^{2+} through voltage-dependent Ca^{2+} channels and thus leads to a small decrease of $[Ca^{2+}]_i$ that is, however, insufficient to account for the abrogation of secretion (175) (Fig. 6.10). Experiments using permeabilized β-cells (289,290) or single β-cells voltage-clamped in the whole-cell mode (240,241,291), in which the composition of the cytoplasm can be controlled, have established the existence of an inhibitory step distal to the generation of cellular messengers (Ca^{2+}, cAMP, diacylglycerol). It involves an heterotrimeric GTP-binding protein implicated in the exocytotic process (290) (see above).

Physiologic Attenuators of Insulin Secretion

These complex mechanisms underlie the physiologically relevant decreases in insulin secretion brought about by catecholamines, galanin, and somatostatin (Fig. 6.10).

Catecholamines are released during exercise and under stress conditions by the adrenal medulla (epinephrine) or by sympathetic nerve terminals in the pancreas (norepinephrine) (245). They exert their inhibitory effect by activating α_2-adrenoceptors (α_{2a} and α_{2c} subtypes) in β-cells (292,293).

Galanin is a 29-residue peptide that is also released by sympathetic nerve endings in the pancreas (294) and acts on specific receptors in β-cells (295).

Somatostatin-28 is released by the gut during absorption of fat-rich meals (296), whereas somatostatin-14 is secreted by islet δ-cells. Somatostatin-28 preferentially binds to β-cells, which express the somatostatin receptor type 5 (297). It is a more potent inhibitor of insulin secretion than is somatostatin-14 (298), which predominantly inhibits glucagon secretion by acting on a receptor type 2 (297). Paracrine control of β-cell function by somatostatin-14 is probably less important than previously thought.

Leptin produced and secreted by adipocytes has generally, although not consistently, been found to inhibit insulin secretion (299,300). Its mode of action differs from that of the previous inhibitors. Upon binding of leptin to its receptor in β-cells, a janus-tyrosine kinase (JAK-2) is activated, which in turn activates phosphoinositide 3-kinase (PI 3-kinase). The final events causing inhibition of insulin secretion are still debated but seem to involve an activation of phosphodiesterase 3B with ensuing decrease in cAMP (301) and an opening of K^+-ATP channels with subsequent membrane repolarization (300,302).

Putative Attenuators of Insulin Secretion

Several other hormones or neuropeptides may attenuate insulin secretion. However, the physiologic relevance of the effects

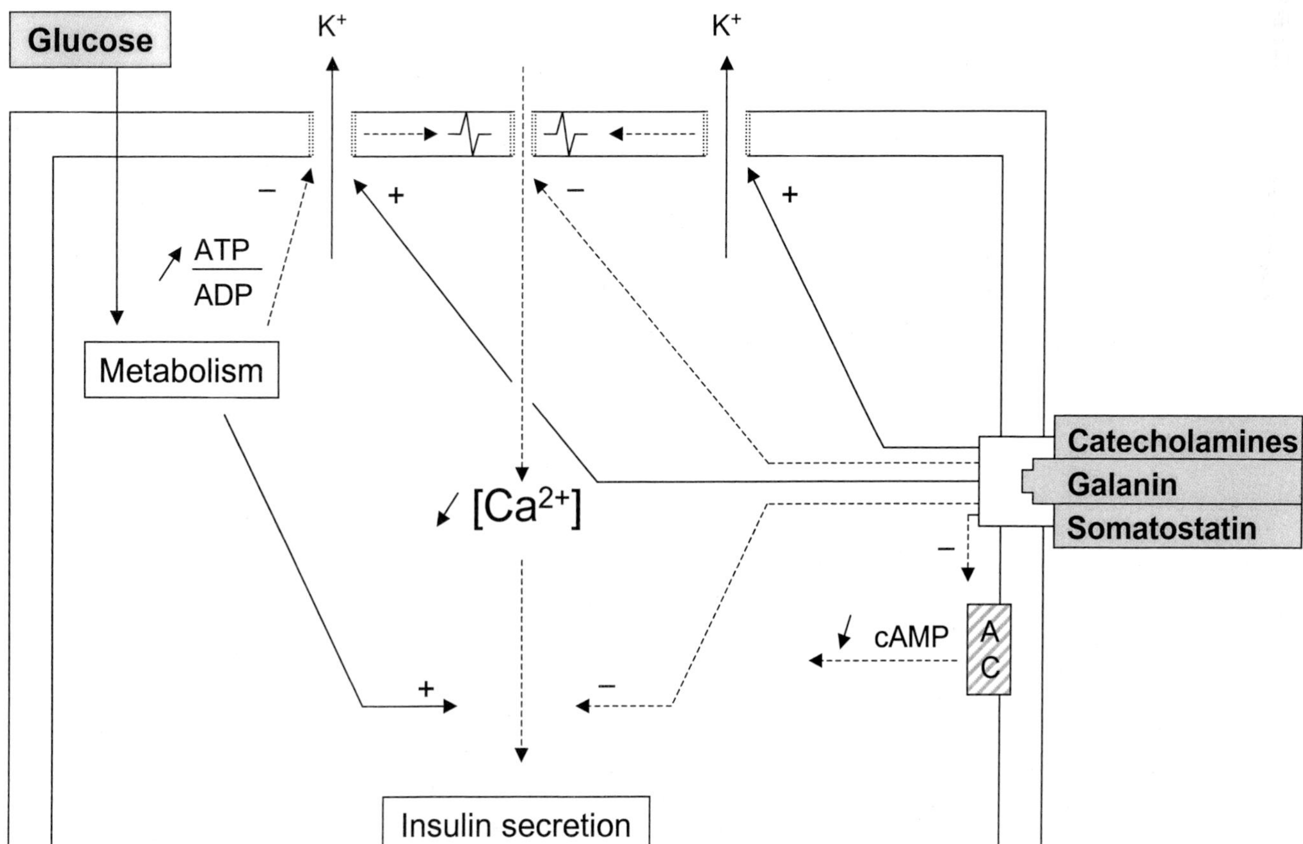

Figure 6.10. Schematic representation of the major mechanisms by which neurotransmitters and hormones attenuate insulin secretion; +, stimulation; –, inhibition; ATP, adenosine triphosphate; ADP, adenosine diphosphate; AC, adenylate cyclase.

observed *in vitro* has yet to be established, and the cellular mechanisms involved are largely unknown.

Insulin-like growth factor-1 (IGF-1) inhibits glucose- and arginine-induced insulin secretion from the perfused rat pancreas (303). This effect occurs at physiologic concentrations, is probably mediated by specific receptors for IGF-1 in β-cells (304), and might involve activation of phosphodiesterase 3B with a subsequent decrease of cAMP (127).

Pancreastatin is a 49-residue peptide produced by proteolytic cleavage of chromogranin A (305,306). It is released by β-cells in parallel with insulin and also by α- and δ-cells. Exogenous pancreastatin causes a modest inhibition of insulin secretion induced by glucose and other secretagogues, but it is unclear whether endogenous pancreastatin causes autocrine inhibition of β-cells (305).

Opioid peptides have inhibitory and stimulatory effects on insulin secretion, depending on the agent used (β-endorphin, type of enkephalin) and on the concentration (307). This may be due to the existence of various types of opioid receptors in β-cells (308).

Calcitonin gene–related peptide (CGRP) is a 37-residue peptide present in intrapancreatic nerve fibers and in δ-cells of the islets (309). Exogenous CGRP inhibits stimulated insulin secretion by decreasing cAMP formation in β-cells.

Islet amyloid polypeptide (IAPP, also known as amylin) is a 37-residue peptide structurally related to CGRP. It is synthesized in β-cells (310) and is secreted with, but in much smaller amounts (<1%), than insulin (311). IAPP in high concentrations has been reported to inhibit insulin secretion (312), but this effect is unlikely to have any physiologic significance (313).

Prostaglandin E2 inhibits glucose-induced insulin secretion by a receptor-mediated, pertussis-toxin–sensitive mechanism (314). Whether prostaglandins are physiologic regulators of β-cell function remains unclear. It is particularly intriguing that only cyclooxygenase type 2 (normally induced by inflammatory events) is expressed in islets (315).

DELAYED CHANGES IN INSULIN SECRETION

Time-Dependent Potentiation

Previous exposure of β-cells to a stimulatory concentration of glucose increases insulin secretion in response to a subsequent challenge by glucose or another secretagogue (153,316,317). This phenomenon has been called "priming," "memory," or "time-dependent potentiation." Its amplitude increases with the magnitude and duration of the first exposure to glucose and decreases with the length of the interval between the end of the first and the start of the second stimulation. Time-dependent potentiation requires glucose metabolism, does not involve cAMP, is not clearly dependent on Ca^{2+}, and does not require exocytosis of insulin granules. It is perhaps linked to phosphoinositide metabolism (102,153,316,317).

A related phenomenon has been called "proemial sensitization." It consists of the enhancement of the β-cell response to glucose by a previous exposure to a neurotransmitter (acetylcholine) or a hormone (cholecystokinin) under conditions in which the latter agents have little or no effect on insulin secretion (318). It has been ascribed to a persistent translocation of protein kinase C to the plasma membrane, where the enzyme can be readily activated by the rise in cytoplasmic Ca^{2+} that occurs on glucose stimulation. This phenomenon could be important to the optimization of the β-cell response to nutrients during a meal (319). Hormones such as GLP-1, GIP, and glucagon might also keep β-cells in a "glucose-competent state" by maintaining adequate cAMP concentrations.

Desensitization

Prolonged stimulation of β-cells with a high concentration of glucose leads to a progressive decrease in the rate of insulin secretion *in vitro*. The phenomenon is already observed after 3 to 4 hours and, at that stage sometimes called the "third phase" (320), does not reflect exhaustion of insulin granules. The underlying mechanisms are still unclear and probably involve time- and Ca^{2+}-dependent decreases in the generation of metabolic signals and efficacy of the triggering signal on the exocytotic process.

β-Cell "desensitization" is best known as a refractory state induced by prolonged exposure (a few days) to high glucose concentrations; it precedes or is associated with poorly reversible β-cell dysfunctions known as "glucose toxicity" (321). However, β-cell refractoriness has often been misinterpreted. It is usually identified as an abnormally small increase in insulin secretion when the preparation is challenged by an acute rise of glucose from expectedly unstimulatory to stimulatory concentrations. This stereotyped approach fails to disclose a marked leftward shift of the dose-response curve, which indicates that the sensitivity to glucose is increased. In fact, β-cells are hypersensitive, not desensitized, to glucose (322–324). This hyperresponsiveness of the β-cells is supported by the observed changes in their membrane K^+ conductance (325). The decrease in the amplitude of the absolute (not fractional) insulin response may be explained by the depletion of the insulin stores. Moreover, a higher proportion of proinsulin is secreted than under control conditions (326).

A similar phenomenon of desensitization can be observed with agents other than glucose (327). After 1 to 2 days of islet exposure to fatty acids, insulin secretion is increased in low glucose and decreased in high glucose (328,329). Whether this reflects changes in glucose metabolism is still debated. Prolonged exposure to glibenclamide also alters the β-cell response to glucose, mainly by preventing the sugar from influencing the membrane potential and changing the triggering signal $[Ca^{2+}]_i$ (330). Here again, the dose responsiveness to glucose is shifted to the left, while the maximum response is decreased.

LONG-TERM INFLUENCES ON INSULIN SECRETION

Neonatal Maturation

Numerous *in vitro* studies have shown that fetal and neonatal islets secrete insulin at a lower rate than do adult islets. The response to glucose is particularly poor, in contrast to that to other secretagogues such as amino acids (331,332). The most striking feature of the functional maturation that β-cells undergo during the perinatal period is the acquisition of a normal responsiveness to glucose in terms of both magnitude and kinetics (332,333). A defect in generation of cAMP has often been thought to contribute to the poor secretory response of fetal and neonatal β-cells, but stimulation of PKA and PKC pathways increases glucose-induced insulin secretion without leading to the appearance of an adult-type, biphasic pattern of release (334). Patch-clamp recordings have shown that K^+-ATP channels are present in fetal β-cells and normally respond to tolbutamide and diazoxide but that they are not closed by glucose (335). Consistent with these findings, glucose, unlike effective insulin secretagogues, does not raise $[Ca^{2+}]_i$ in fetal islets (336). The available evidence indicates that the inability of glucose to induce insulin secretion from fetal and neonatal β-cells is due to an immature metabolism with insufficient production of ATP, hence an inability to produce a triggering signal.

Whether the glucokinase is the site of this immaturity is still disputed (337,338).

Aging

The contribution of impairment in insulin secretion to the deterioration of glucose tolerance with aging is unclear (339,340). It is difficult to isolate the impact of physiologic aging from that of aging-associated diseases. Even *in vitro* studies are fraught with difficulties that explain the major controversies surrounding the specific effects of age on β-cell function (341,342). Impairments of the individual β-cell or islet responses have often been reported. They include diminished insulin secretion associated with or caused by small and inconsistent defects in insulin biosynthesis, glucose metabolism, ionic fluxes, and adenylate cylase activity. At the level of the whole pancreas, however, the insulin secretion capacity does not seem to be altered, possibly because of a compensatory increase in the β-cell mass (343).

Starvation

During starvation, basal plasma insulin levels are lowered and the β-cell secretory response to glucose is impaired. Many *in vitro* studies have shown that glucose-induced insulin secretion is more severely altered than the secretion induced by other fuel or non-fuel secretagogues (344,345). This selective change is generally attributed to a decreased glycolytic rate in β-cells (344,346), which largely, though not exclusively, results from a lower glucokinase activity (5,6,22). Thus, starvation lowers the levels of glucokinase mRNA (347,348) and glucokinase protein (22) in islet cells. During starvation, β-cells also rely on fuels other than glucose, particularly free fatty acids, whose plasma concentration is elevated. It has been proposed that operation of a glucose–fatty acid cycle in β-cells impairs mitochondrial glucose metabolism, and hence insulin secretion, by decreasing the activity of pyruvate dehydrogenase (349). Starvation also reduces the ability of glucose to shift the metabolism of fatty acids from oxidation to esterification in islets (119), an abnormality that could contribute to the alteration of β-cell function, since its correction by 2-bromostearate (an inhibitor of fatty acid oxidation) restores glucose-induced insulin secretion (119). In contrast, positive effects of fatty acids are suggested by experiments showing that a decrease in their concentrations with nicotinic acid in fasted rats impairs the ability of glucose to induce insulin secretion from the pancreas subsequently isolated from these fasted animals (350). Unexpectedly, when studied *in vivo*, β-cells of 48 hour–fasted mice show electrical activity at plasma glucose concentrations that are not stimulatory in living fed mice (351). This paradoxical hyperresponsiveness of the fasted β-cells, which could be ascribed to the high circulating levels of free fatty acid, contrasts with the expectedly low plasma levels of insulin; electrical activity and insulin secretion are thus dissociated. Low concentrations of cAMP usually are found in islets from fasted animals and may contribute to the low insulin secretory responses (345,346). mRNA levels of the voltage-dependent Ca^{2+} channels are also reduced (348), but it is not known whether Ca^{2+} currents are similarly affected.

Exercise Training

Exercise training increases peripheral insulin sensitivity and lowers plasma insulin levels (352) by decreasing the magnitude without affecting the frequency of insulin secretion pulses (353). Isolated islets and the perfused pancreas obtained from trained rats exhibit a diminished glucose- or arginine-induced insulin secretion (354,355). A decrease in islet glucokinase mRNA has been found in islets from trained rats (356), but it is uncertain whether this explains the lower insulin responses, because such islets were found to metabolize glucose at a rate similar to that of islets from sedentary animals (354).

Pregnancy and Lactation

To meet the increased insulin demands during pregnancy, β-cells proliferate, leading to an increased islet size and total mass, and undergo several functional adaptations (357). The major change is an enhancement of glucose-induced insulin secretion with a lowering of the threshold glucose concentration (358,359). It is attributed to the combined increases of glucose metabolism, cAMP concentration, and gap-junctional coupling in β-cells and is compensated for by an increase in insulin synthesis (357–360). Both dietary (increase in food consumption) and hormonal (prolactin and placental lactogen) factors are involved in this functional adaptation of β-cells (357,361).

Plasma glucose and insulin concentrations are relatively low during lactation. Islets from lactating rats have been found to secrete less insulin than islets from nonlactating animals during *in vitro* stimulation with glucose or leucine (362). This decrease in β-cell secretory activity is paradoxically associated with increased activity of adenylate cyclase, protein kinase A, and protein kinase C and increased oxidation of glucose and leucine (362). The β-cell coupling is also increased in islets from lactating rats (363). It should be noted, however, that the suggestion that β-cells of lactating rats have an intrinsically low secretory activity has been challenged (364).

Hormones

Growth-hormone deficiency is associated with decreased plasma concentrations of insulin (365). Glucose metabolism and glucose-induced insulin secretion are lower in islets from hypophysectomized rats than in islets from control animals (366). In most *in vitro* studies, however, growth hormone has no acute impact on β-cell function (367), whereas delayed stimulation of β-cell growth, insulin biosynthesis, and insulin release is well established. These effects appear to be due to a direct action of growth hormone on somatogenic and lactogenic receptors in β-cells (368) rather than to an indirect action mediated by IGF-1 that also stimulates β-cell proliferation (369) but inhibits insulin secretion.

Thyroid hormones in excess decrease the insulin content of the pancreas (370), perhaps by decreasing levels of proinsulin mRNA (371). They also cause a slight and delayed inhibition of insulin secretion in response to glucose but not to other secretagogues in the rat (370). Thyroid hormones do not acutely influence β-cell function (370,372)

Rats deficient in 1,25-dihydroxyvitamin D_3 show impaired insulin secretion *in vivo* and *in vitro* (373). This defect probably reflects both direct effects of the hormone on β-cells and metabolic abnormalities (e.g., hypocalcemia, poor growth) associated with its deficiency. Vitamin D_3 has usually (374), but not always (375), been found to increase insulin secretion *in vitro*. Both genomic and nongenomic pathways have been implicated.

Glucocorticoids indirectly increase insulin secretion through their effects on glucose production and their antagonism of insulin action (370). Paradoxically, their direct effect on β-cells is inhibitory (376,377). This inhibition, mediated by a genomic action, results not from an alteration in glucose recognition or in triggering signal generation but from a decrease in the efficacy of Ca^{2+} on the exocytotic process (376).

Note: The final writing of this chapter was completed in February 2001.

REFERENCES

1. Malaisse WJ, Sener A, Herchuelz A, Hutton JC. Insulin release: the fuel hypothesis. *Metabolism* 1979;28:373.
2. Ashcroft SJH. Glucoreceptor mechanisms and the control of insulin release and biosynthesis. *Diabetologia* 1980;18:5–15.
3. Hedeskov CJ. Mechanism of glucose-induced insulin secretion. *Physiol Rev* 1980;60:442–509.
4. Sener A, Malaisse WJ. Nutrient metabolism in islet cells. *Experientia* 1984;40: 1026–1035.
5. Meglasson MD, Matschinsky FM. Pancreatic islet glucose metabolism and regulation of insulin secretion. *Diabetes Metab Rev* 1986;2:163–214.
6. Lenzen S, Panten U. Signal recognition by pancreatic B-cells. *Biochem Pharmacol* 1988;37:371–378.
7. Malaisse WJ. Glucose-sensing by the pancreatic B-cell: the mitochondrial part. *Int J Biochem* 1992;24:693–701.
8. Newgard CB, McGarry JD. Metabolic coupling factors in pancreatic β-cell signal transduction. *Annu Rev Biochem* 1995;64:689–719.
9. Thorens B, Sarkar HK, Kaback HR, et al. Cloning and functional expression in bacteria of a novel glucose transporter present in liver, intestine, kidney, and β-pancreatic islet cells. *Cell* 1988;55:281–290.
10. Newgard CB. Regulatory role of glucose transport and phosphorylation in pancreatic islet β-cells. *Diabetes Rev* 1996;4:191–206.
11. De Vos A, Heimberg H, Quartier E, et al. Human and rat beta cells differ in glucose transporter but not in glucokinase gene expression. *J Clin Invest* 1995; 96:2489–2495.
12. Ferrer J, Benito C, Gomis R. Pancreatic islet GLUT2 glucose transporter mRNA and protein expression in humans with and without NIDDM. *Diabetes* 1995;44:1369–1374.
13. Matschinsky FM, Ellerman JE. Metabolism of glucose in the islets of Langerhans. *J Biol Chem* 1968;243:2730–2736.
14. Hellman B, Sehlin J, Täljedal I-B. Evidence for mediated transport of glucose in mammalian pancreatic β-cells. *Biochim Biophys Acta* 1971;241:147–154.
15. Matschinsky FM. A lesson in metabolic regulation inspired by the glucokinase glucose sensor paradigm. *Diabetes* 1996;45:223–241.
16. Van Schaftingen E, Schuit F. Signal recognition: glucose and primary stimuli. *Adv Mol Cell Biol* 1999;29:199–226.
17. Meglasson MD, Burch PT, Berner DK, et al. Chromatographic resolution and kinetic characterization of glucokinase from islets of Langerhans. *Proc Natl Acad Sci U S A* 1983;80:85–90.
18. Iynedjian PB, Möbius G, Seitz HJ, et al. Tissue-specific expression of glucokinase: identification of the gene product in liver and pancreatic islets. *Proc Natl Acad Sci U S A* 1986;83:1998–2001.
19. Velho G, Froguel P, Clement K, et al. Primary pancreatic beta-cell secretory defect caused by mutations in glucokinase gene in kindreds of maturity onset diabetes of the young. *Lancet* 1992; 340:444–448.
20. Glaser B, Kesavan P, Heyman M, et al. Familial hyperinsulinism caused by an activating glucokinase mutation. *N Engl J Med* 1998;338:226–230.
21. Burke CV, Buettger CW, Davis EA, et al. Cell-biological assessment of human glucokinase mutants causing maturity-onset diabetes of the young type 2 (MODY-2) or glucokinase-linked hyperinsulinaemia (GK-HI). *Biochem J* 1999; 342:345–352.
22. Malaisse WJ. Metabolic signaling of insulin secretion. *Diabetes Rev* 1996;4: 145–159.
23. Schuit F, Moens K, Heimberg H, et al. Cellular origin of hexokinase in pancreatic islets. *J Biol Chem* 1999;274:32803–32809.
24. Schuit F, De Vos A, Farfari S, et al. Metabolic fate of glucose in purified islet cells—glucose-regulated anaplerosis in β cells. *J Biol Chem* 1997;272: 18572–18579.
25. Yaney GC, Schultz V, Cunningham BA et al. Phosphofructokinase isozymes in pancreatic islets and clonal β-cells (INS-1). *Diabetes* 1995;44:1285–1289.
26. Sekine N, Cirulli V, Regazzi R, et al. Low lactate dehydrogenase and high mitochondrial glycerol phosphate dehydrogenase in pancreatic β-cells. Potential role in nutrient sensing. *J Biol Chem* 1994;269:4895–4902.
27. Ishihara H, Wang HH, Drewes LR, et al. Overexpression of monocarboxylate transporter and lactate dehydrogenase alters insulin secretory responses to pyruvate and lactate in β cells. *J Clin Invest* 1999;104:1621–1629.
28. MacDonald MJ. High content of mitochondrial glycerol-3-phosphate dehydrogenase in pancreatic islets and its inhibition by diazoxide. *J Biol Chem* 1981;256:8287–8290.
29. MacDonald MJ. Evidence for the malate aspartate shuttle in pancreatic islets. *Arch Biochem Biophys* 1982;213:643–649.
30. Eto K, Tsubamoto Y, Terauchi Y, et al. Role of NADH shuttle system in glucose-induced activation of mitochondrial metabolism and insulin secretion. *Science* 1999;283:981–985.
31. Ravier MA, Eto K, Jonkers FC, et al. The oscillatory behavior of pancreatic islets from mice with mitochondrial glycerol-3-phosphate dehydrogenase knockout. *J Biol Chem* 2000;275:1587–1593.
32. MacDonald MJ. Glucose enters mitochondrial metabolism via both carboxylation and decarboxylation of pyruvate in pancreatic islets. *Metabolism* 1993; 42:1229–1231.
33. Khan A, Ling ZC, Landau BR. Quantifying the carboxylation of pyruvate in pancreatic islets. *J Biol Chem* 1996;271:2539–2542.
34. Duchen MR, Smith PA, Ashcroft FM. Substrate-dependent changes in mitochondrial function, intracellular free calcium concentration and membrane channels in pancreatic β-cells. *Biochem J* 1993;294:35–42.
35. Brun T, Roche E, Assimacopoulos-Jeannet F, et al. Evidence for an anaplerotic malonyl-CoA pathway in pancreatic β-cell nutrient signaling. *Diabetes* 1996; 45:190–198.
36. Prentki M, Corkey BE. Are the β-cell signaling molecules malonyl-CoA and cytosolic long-chain acyl-CoA implicated in multiple tissue defects of obesity and NIDDM? *Diabetes* 1996;45:273–283.
37. Rutter GA, Theler JM, Murgia M, et al. Stimulated Ca2+ influx raises mitochondrial free Ca2+ to supramicromolar levels in a pancreatic β-cell line. *J Biol Chem* 1993;268:22385–22390.
38. Detimary P, Van den Berghe G, Henquin JC. Concentration dependence and time course of the effects of glucose on adenine and guanine nucleotides in mouse pancreatic islets. *J Biol Chem* 1996;271:20559–20565.
39. Detimary P, Dejonghe S, Ling Z, et al. The changes in adenine nucleotides measured in glucose-stimulated rodent islets occur in β cells but not in α cells and are also observed in human islets. *J Biol Chem* 1998;273:33905–33908.
40. Detimary P, Gilon P, Henquin JC. Interplay between cytoplasmic Ca2+ and the ADP/ATP ratio: feedback control mechanism in mouse pancreatic islets. *Biochem J* 1998;333:269–274.
41. Kennedy HJ, Pouli AE, Ainscow EK, et al. Glucose generates sub-plasma membrane ATP microdomains in single islet β-cells—potential role for strategically located mitochondria. *J Biol Chem* 1999;274:13281–13291.
42. Henquin JC. The triggering and amplifying pathways of the regulation of insulin secretion by glucose. *Diabetes* 2000;49:1751–1760.
43. Tamagawa T, Niki H, Niki A. Insulin release independent of a rise in cytosolic free Ca^{2+} by forskolin and phorbol ester. *FEBS Lett* 1985;183:430–432.
44. Jones PM, Stutchfield J, Howell SL. Effects of Ca^{2+} and a phorbol ester on insulin secretion from islets of Langerhans permeabilised by high-voltage discharge. *FEBS Lett* 1985;191:102–106.
45. Gillis KD, Misler S. Enhancers of cytosolic cAMP augment depolarization-induced exocytosis from pancreatic B-cells: evidence for effects distal to Ca^{2+} entry. *Pflügers Arch* 1993;424:195–197.
46. Ammala C, Eliasson L, Bokvist K, et al. Exocytosis elicited by action potentials and voltage-clamp calcium currents in individual mouse pancreatic B-cells. *J Physiol* 1993;472:665–688.
47. Jonas JC, Li G, Palmer M, et al. Dynamics of Ca^{2+} and guanosine 5-[gamma-thio]triphosphate action on insulin secretion from alpha-toxin-permeabilized HIT-T15 cells. *Biochem J* 1994;301:523–529.
48. Proks P, Eliasson L, Ammala C, et al. Ca^{2+}- and GTP-dependent exocytosis in mouse pancreatic β-cells involves both common and distinct steps. *J Physiol* 1996;496:255–264.
49. Komatsu M, Schermerhorn T, Noda M, et al. Augmentation of insulin release by glucose in the absence of extracellular Ca^{2+}—new insights into stimulus-secretion coupling. *Diabetes* 1997;46:1928–1938.
50. Sato Y, Nenquin M, Henquin JC. Relative contribution of Ca^{2+}-dependent and Ca^{2+}-independent mechanisms to the regulation of insulin secretion by glucose. *FEBS Lett* 1998;421:115–119.
51. Prentki M, Janjic D, Biden TJ, et al. Regulation of Ca^{2+} transport by isolated organelles of a rat insulinoma. Studies with endoplasmic reticulum and secretory granules. *J Biol Chem* 1984;259:10118–10123.
52. Varadi A, Molnar E, Östenson CG, et al. Isoforms of endoplasmic reticulum Ca^{2+}-ATPase are differently expressed in normal and diabetic islets of Langerhans. *Biochem J* 1996;319:521–527.
53. Pershadsingh HA, McDaniel ML, Landt M, et al. Ca^{2+}-activated ATPase and ATP-dependent calmodulin-stimulated Ca^{2+} transport in islet cell plasma membrane. *Nature* 1980;288:492–494.
54. Varadi A, Molnar E, Ashcroft SJH. A unique combination of plasma membrane Ca^{2+}-ATPase isoforms is expressed in islets of Langerhans and pancreatic β-cell lines. *Biochem J* 1996;314:663–669.
55. Herchuelz A, Plasman PO. Sodium-calcium exchange in the pancreatic B cell. *Ann N Y Acad Sci* 1991;639:642–656.
56. Dukes ID, Roe MW, Worley JF, Philipson LH. Glucose-induced alterations in β-cell cytoplasmic Ca^{2+} involving the coupling of intracellular Ca^{2+} stores and plasma membrane ion channels. *Curr Opin Endocrinol Diabetes* 1997;4: 262–271.
57. Gilon P, Arredouani A, Gailly P, et al. Uptake and release of Ca^{2+} by the endoplasmic reticulum contribute to the oscillations of the cytosolic Ca^{2+} concentration triggered by Ca^{2+} influx in the electrically excitable pancreatic B-cell. *J Biol Chem* 1999;274:20197–20205.
58. Sehlin J, Taljedal IB. Glucose-induced decrease in Rb^{+} permeability in pancreatic β cells. *Nature* 1975;253:635–636.
59. Atwater I, Ribalet B, Rojas E. Cyclic changes in potential and resistance of the β-cell membrane induced by glucose in islets of Langerhans from mouse. *J Physiol* 1978;278:117–139.
60. Henquin JC. D-Glucose inhibits potassium efflux from pancreatic islet cells. *Nature* 1978;271:271–273.

61. Cook DL, Hales CN. Intracellular ATP directly blocks K^+ channels in pancreatic β-cells. *Nature* 1984;311:271–273.
62. Ashcroft FM, Harrison DE, Ashcroft SJH. Glucose induces closure of single potassium channels in isolated rat pancreatic β-cells. *Nature* 1984;312: 446–448.
63. Aguilar-Bryan L, Bryan J. Molecular biology of adenosine triphosphate-sensitive potassium channels. *Endocr Rev* 1999;20:101–135.
64. Ashcroft FM, Gribble FM. ATP-sensitive K^+ channels and insulin secretion: their role in health and disease. *Diabetologia* 1999;42:903–919.
65. Seino S. ATP-sensitive potassium channels: a model of heteromultimeric potassium channel/receptor assemblies. *Annu Rev Physiol* 1999;61:337–362.
66. Henquin JC, Meissner HP. Significance of ionic fluxes and changes in membrane potential for stimulus-secretion coupling in pancreatic B-cells. *Experientia* 1984;40:1043–1052.
67. Plant TD. Properties and calcium-dependent inactivation of calcium currents in cultured mouse pancreatic B-cells. *J Physiol* 1988;404:731–747.
68. Ashcroft FM, Rorsman P. Electrophysiology of the pancreatic β-cell. *Prog Biophys Mol Biol* 1989;54:87–143.
69. Valdeolmillos M, Gomis A, Sánchez-Andrés JV. In vivo synchronous membrane potential oscillations in mouse pancreatic β-cells: lack of co-ordination between islets. *J Physiol* 1996;493:9–18.
70. Satin LS, Smolen PD. Electrical bursting in β-cells of the pancreatic islets of Langerhans. *Endocrine* 1994;2:677–687.
71. Atwater I, Mears D, Rojas E. Electrophysiology of the pancreatic β cell. In: LeRoith S, Taylor SI, Olefsky JM, eds. *Diabetes mellitus.* Philadelphia: Lippincott-Raven Publishers, 1996:78–102.
72. Roe MW, Mertz RJ, Lancaster ME, et al. Thapsigargin inhibits the glucose-induced decrease of intracellular Ca^{2+} in mouse islets of Langerhans. *Am J Physiol Endocrinol Metab* 1994;266:E852–E862.
73. Tengholm A, Hellman B, Gylfe E. Glucose regulation of free Ca^{2+} in the endoplasmic reticulum of mouse pancreatic beta cells. *J Biol Chem* 1999;274: 36883–36890.
74. Santos RM, Rosario LM, Nadal A, et al. Widespread synchronous $[Ca^{2+}]i$ oscillations due to bursting electrical activity in single pancreatic islets. *Pflügers Arch* 1991;418:417–422.
75. Gilon P, Henquin JC. Influence of membrane potential changes on cytoplasmic Ca^{2+} concentration in an electrically excitable cell, the insulin-secreting pancreatic β-cell. *J Biol Chem* 1992;267:20713–20720.
76. Chow RH, Lund P-E, Löser S, et al. Coincidence of early glucose-induced depolarization with lowering of cytoplasmic Ca^{2+} in mouse pancreatic β-cells. *J Physiol* 1995; 485:607–617.
77. Tornheim K. Are metabolic oscillations responsible for normal oscillatory insulin secretion? *Diabetes* 1997;46:1375–1380.
78. Henquin JC, Jonas JC, Sato Y, et al. Regulation of insulin secretion by changes in Ca^{2+} concentration and action in pancreatic β-cells. *Adv Mol Cell Biol* 1999; 29:247–275.
79. Jung SK, Kauri LM, Qian WJ, et al. Correlated oscillations in glucose consumption, oxygen consumption, and intracellular free Ca^{2+} in single islets of Langerhans. *J Biol Chem* 2000;275:6642–6650.
80. Pralong WF, Spät A, Wollheim CB. Dynamic pacing of cell metabolism by intracellular Ca^{2+} transients. *J Biol Chem* 1994; 269:27310–27314.
81. Rhodes CJ, Halban PA. Newly synthesized proinsulin/insulin and stored insulin are released from pancreatic B cells predominantly via a regulated, rather than a constitutive, pathway. *J Cell Biol* 1987;105:145–153.
82. Lang J. Molecular mechanisms and regulation of insulin exocytosis as a paradigm of endocrine secretion. *Eur J Biochem* 1999;259:3–17.
83. Regazzi R. Mechanisms of insulin exocytosis. *Adv Mol Cell Biol* 1999;29: 151–172.
84. Malaisse WJ, Malaisse-Lagae F, Van Obberghen E, et al. Role of microtubules in the phasic pattern of insulin release. *Ann N Y Acad Sci* 1975;253:630–652.
85. Howell SL. The mechanism of insulin secretion. *Diabetologia* 1984;26:319–327.
86. Easom RA. CaM kinase II: A protein kinase with extraordinary talents germane to insulin exocytosis. *Diabetes* 1999;48:675–684.
87. Niki I. Ca^{2+} signaling and the insulin secretory cascade in the pancreatic beta-cell. *Jpn J Pharmacol* 1999;80:191–197.
88. Ullrich S, Wollheim CB. GTP-dependent inhibition of insulin secretion by epinephrine in permeabilized RINm5F cells: lack of correlation between insulin secretion and cyclic AMP levels. *J Biol Chem* 1988;263:8615–8620.
89. Seaquist ER, Walseth TF, Redmon JB, et al. G-protein regulation of insulin secretion. *J Lab Clin Med* 1994;123:338–345.
90. Sharp GW. Mechanisms of inhibition of insulin release. *Am J Physiol Cell Physiol* 1996;271:C1781–C1799.
91. Gembal M, Gillon P, Henquin JC. Evidence that glucose can control insulin release independently from its action on ATP-sensitive K+ channels in mouse B-cells. *J Clin Invest* 1992;89:1288–1295.
92. Gembal M, Detimary P, Gilon P, et al. Mechanisms by which glucose can control insulin release independently from its action on ATP-sensitive K+ channels in mouse B-cells. *J Clin Invest* 1993;91:871–880.
93. Sato Y, Aizawa T, Komatsu M, et al. Dual functional role of membrane depolarization/Ca^{2+} influx in rat pancreatic B-cell. *Diabetes* 1992;41:438–443.
94. Panten U, Schwanstecher M, Wallasch A, et al. Glucose both inhibits and stimulates insulin secretion from isolated pancreatic islets exposed to maximally effective concentrations of sulfonylureas. *Naunyn Schmiedebergs Arch Pharmacol* 1988;338:459–462.
95. Best L, Yates AP, Tomlinson S. Stimulation of insulin secretion by glucose in the absence of diminished potassium ($86Rb^+$) permeability. *Biochem Pharmacol* 1992;43:2483–2485.
96. Sato Y, Anello M, Henquin JC. Glucose regulation of insulin secretion independent of the opening or closure of adenosine triphosphate-sensitive K^+ channels in β cells. *Endocrinology* 1999;140:2252–2257.
97. Jonas JC, Gilon P, Henquin JC. Temporal and quantitative correlations between insulin secretion and stably elevated or oscillatory cytoplasmic Ca^{2+} in mouse pancreatic β-cells. *Diabetes* 1998;47:1266–1273.
98. Detimary P, Gilon P, Nenquin M, Henquin JC. Two sites of glucose control of insulin release with distinct dependence on the energy state in pancreatic β cells. *Biochem J* 1994;297:455–461.
99. Eliasson L, Renström E, Ding WG, et al. Rapid ATP-dependent priming of secretory granules precedes Ca^{2+}-induced exocytosis in mouse pancreatic β-cells. *J Physiol* 1997;503:399–412.
100. Takahashi N, Kadowaki T, Yazaki Y, et al. Post-priming actions of ATP on Ca^{2+}-dependent exocytosis in pancreatic beta cells. *Proc Natl Acad Sci U S A* 1999;96:760–765.
101. Sato Y, Henquin JC. The K+-ATP channel-independent pathway of regulation of insulin secretion by glucose. In search of the underlying mechanism. *Diabetes* 1998;47:1713–1721.
102. Zawalich WS, Zawalich KC. Regulation of insulin secretion via ATP-sensitive K^+ channel independent mechanisms: role of phospholipase C. *Am J Physiol Endocrinol Metab* 1997;272:E671–E677.
103. Komatsu M, Yajima H, Yamada S, et al. Augmentation of Ca^{2+}-stimulated insulin release by glucose and long-chain fatty acids in rat pancreatic islets—free fatty acids mimic ATP-sensitive K+ channel-independent insulinotropic action of glucose. *Diabetes* 1999;48:1543–1549.
104. Meissner HP, Schmelz H. Membrane potential of beta cells in pancreatic islets. *Pflügers Arch* 1974;351:195–206.
105. Gylfe E. Nutrient secretagogues induce bimodal early changes in cytoplasmic calcium of insulin-releasing ob/ob mouse β-cells. *J Biol Chem* 1988;263: 13750–13754.
106. Jonkers FC, Henquin JC. Cytosolic Ca^{2+} measurements in islet cell clusters reveal β cell recruitment and increase of the individual responses by glucose. *Diabetes* 2001;50:540–550.
107. Ammon HPT, Mark M. Thiols and pancreatic β-cell function: a review. *Cell Biochem Funct* 1985;3:157–171.
108. Hedeskov CJ, Capito K, Thams P. Cytosolic ratios of free [NADPH]/[NADP+] and [NADH/NAD+] in mouse pancreatic islets, and nutrient-induced insulin secretion. *Biochem J* 1987;241:161–167.
109. MacDonald MJ. Feasibility of a mitochondrial pyruvate malate shuttle in pancreatic islets. *J Biol Chem* 1995;270:20051–20058.
110. Meredith M, Rabaglia ME, Metz SA. Evidence of a role for GTP in the potentiation of Ca^{2+}-induced insulin secretion by glucose in intact rat islets. *J Clin Invest* 1995;96:811–821.
111. Kowluru A, Metz SA. Characterization of nucleoside diphosphokinase activity in human and rodent pancreatic β cells: evidence for its role in the formation of guanosine triphosphate, a permissive factor for nutrient-induced insulin secretion. *Biochemistry* 1994;33:12495–12503.
112. Detimary P, Xiao CQ, Henquin JC. Tight links between adenine and guanine nucleotide pools in mouse pancreatic islets: a study with mycophenolic acid. *Biochem J* 1997;324:467–471.
113. Maechler P, Wollheim CB. Mitochondrial glutamate acts as a messenger in glucose-induced insulin exocytosis. *Nature* 1999;402:685–689.
114. MacDonald MF, Fahien LA. Glutamate is not a messenger in insulin secretion. *J Biol Chem* 2000;275:34025–34027.
115. Lindstrom P, Sehlin J. Effect of glucose on the intracellular pH of pancreatic islet cells. *Biochem J* 1984;218:887–892.
116. Shepherd RM, Henquin JC. The role of metabolism, cytoplasmic Ca^{2+}, and pH-regulating exchangers in glucose-induced rise of cytoplasmic pH in normal mouse pancreatic islets. *J Biol Chem* 1995;270:7915–7921.
117. Best L. Intracellular pH and B-cell function. In: Flatt PR. ed. *Nutrient regulation of insulin secretion.* London: Portland Press, 1992:157–171.
118. Berne C. The metabolism of lipids in mouse pancreatic islets: the oxidation of fatty acids and ketone bodies. *Biochem J* 1975;152:661–666.
119. Tamarit-Rodriguez J, Vara E, Tamarit J. Starvation-induced changes of palmitate metabolism and insulin secretion in isolated rat islets stimulated by glucose. *Biochem J* 1984;221:317–324.
120. Larsson O, Deeney JT, Bränström R, et al. Activation of the ATP-sensitive K^+ channel by long chain acyl-CoA—a role in modulation of pancreatic β-cell glucose sensitivity. *J Biol Chem* 1996;271:10623–10626.
121. Deeney JT, Gromada J, Hoy M, et al. Acute stimulation with long chain acyl-CoA enhances exocytosis in insulin-secreting cells (HIT T-15 and NMRI β-Cells). *J Biol Chem* 2000;275:9363–9368.
122. Antinozzi PA, Segall L, Prentki M, et al. Molecular or pharmacologic perturbation of the link between glucose and lipid metabolism is without effect on glucose-stimulated insulin secretion—a re-evaluation of the long-chain acyl-CoA hypothesis. *J Biol Chem* 1998;273:16146–16154.
123. Farfari S, Schulz V, Corkey B, et al. Glucose-regulated anaplerosis and cataplerosis in pancreatic β-cells—possible implication of a pyruvate/citrate shuttle in insulin secretion. *Diabetes* 2000; 49:718–726.
124. Sharp GWG. The adenylate cyclase-cyclic AMP system in islets of Langerhans and its role in the control of insulin release. *Diabetologia* 1979;16:287–296.
125. Malaisse WJ, Malaisse-Lagae F. The role of cyclic AMP in insulin release. *Experientia* 1984;40:1068–1075.

126. Shafiee-Nick R, Pyne NJ, Furman BL. Effects of type-selective phosphodiesterase inhibitors on glucose-induced insulin secretion and islet phosphodiesterase activity. *Br J Pharmacol* 1995;115:1486–1492.
127. Zhao AZ, Zhao H, Teague J, et al. Attenuation of insulin secretion by insulin-like growth factor 1 is mediated through activation of phosphodiesterase 3B. *Proc Natl Acad Sci U S A* 1997;94:3223–3228.
128. Pipeleers D. The biosociology of pancreatic B cells. *Diabetologia* 1987;30: 277–291.
129. Holz GG, Kühtreiber WM, Habener JF. Pancreatic beta-cells are rendered glucose-competent by the insulinotropic hormone glucagon-like peptide-1 (7-37). *Nature* 1993;361:362–365.
130. Harris TE, Persaud SJ, Jones PM. Pseudosubstrate inhibition of cyclic AMP-dependent protein kinase in intact pancreatic islets: effects on cyclic AMP-dependent and glucose-dependent insulin secretion. *Biochem Biophys Res Comm* 1997; 232:648–651.
131. Prentki M, Matschinsky FM. Ca^{2+}, cAMP, and phospholipid-derived messengers in coupling mechanisms of insulin secretion. *Physiol Rev* 1987;67: 1185–1248.
132. Turk J, Wolf BA, McDaniel ML. The role of phospholipid-derived mediators including arachidonic acid, its metabolites, and inositoltriphosphate and of intracellular Ca^{2+} in glucose-induced insulin secretion by pancreatic islets. *Prog Lipid Res* 1987;26:125–181.
133. Biden TJ, Wollheim CB. Generation, metabolism and function of inositol phosphates during nutrient- and neurotransmitter-induced insulin secretion. In: Michell RH. Drummond AH, Downes CP, eds. *Inositol lipids in cell signalling*. San Diego: Academic Press, 1989:405–425.
134. Morgan NG, Montague W. Phospholipids and insulin secretion. In: Flatt PR, ed. *Nutrient regulation of insulin secretion*. London: Portland Press, 1992:125–155.
135. Wolf BA, Easom RA, McDaniel ML, et al. Diacylglycerol synthesis de novo from glucose by pancreatic islets isolated from rats and humans. *J Clin Invest* 1990;85:482–490.
136. Wollheim CB, Regazzi R. Protein kinase C in insulin releasing cells: putative role in stimulus secretion coupling. *FEBS Lett* 1990;268:376–380.
137. Jones PM, Persaud SJ. Protein kinases, protein phosphorylation, and the regulation of insulin secretion from pancreatic β-cells. *Endocr Rev* 1998;19: 429–461.
138. Metz SA. Roles of phospholipids and phospholipase activation in β-cell function. *Adv Mol Cell Biol* 1999;29:277–301.
139. Rasmussen H, Isales SM, Calle R, et al. Diacylglycerol production, Ca^{2+} influx, and protein kinase C activation in sustained cellular responses. *Endocr Rev* 1995;16:649–681.
140. Yedovitzky M, Mochly-Rosen D, Johnson JA, et al. Translocation inhibitors define specificity of protein kinase C isoenzymes in pancreatic β-cells. *J Biol Chem* 1997;272:1417–1420.
141. Robertson RP. Arachidonic acid metabolite regulation of insulin secretion. *Diabetes Metab Rev* 1986;2:261–266.
142. Sando H, Grodsky GM. Dynamic synthesis and release of insulin and proinsulin from perifused islets. *Diabetes* 1973;22:354–360.
143. Garcia-Barrado MJ, Ravier MA, Rolland JF, et al. Inhibition of protein synthesis sequentially impairs distinct steps of stimulus-secretion coupling in pancreatic β cells. *Endocrinology* 2001;142:299–307.
144. Permutt MA. Biosynthesis of insulin. In: Cooperstein SJ, Watkins D, eds. *The islets of Langerhans: biochemistry, physiology, and pathology*. New York: Academic Press, 1981:75–95.
145. Sando H, Borg J, Steiner DF. Studies on the secretion of newly synthesized proinsulin and insulin from isolated rat islets of Langerhans. *J Clin Invest* 1972;51:1476–1485.
146. Gold G, Grodsky GM. Kinetic aspects of compartmental storage and secretion of insulin and zinc. *Experientia* 1984;40:1105–1114.
147. Halban PA. Differential rates of release of newly synthesized and of stored insulin from pancreatic islets. *Endocrinology* 1982;110:1183–1188.
148. Schuit FC, in't Veld PA, Pipeleers DG. Glucose stimulates proinsulin biosynthesis by a dose-dependent recruitment of pancreatic beta cells. *Proc Natl Acad Sci U S A* 1988;85:3865–3869.
149. Curry DL, Bennett LL, Grodsky GM. Dynamics of insulin secretion by the perfused rat pancreas. *Endocrinology* 1968;83:572–584.
150. Cerasi E, Luft R, Efendic S. Decreased sensitivity of the pancreatic beta cells to glucose in prediabetic and diabetic subjects. A glucose dose-response study. *Diabetes* 1972;21:224–234.
151. Brunzell JD, Robertson RP, Lerner RL, et al. Relationships between fasting plasma glucose levels and insulin secretion during intravenous glucose tolerance tests. *J Clin Endocrinol Metab* 1976;42:222–229.
152. Grodsky GM. A threshold distribution hypothesis for packet storage of insulin and its mathematical modeling. *J Clin Invest* 1972;51:2047–2059.
153. O'Connor MDL, Landahl H, Grodsky GM. Comparison of storage- and signal-limited models of pancreatic insulin secretion. *Am J Physiol Reg Integr Comp Physiol* 1980;238:R378–R389.
154. Takahashi N, Kadowaki T, Yazaki Y, et al. Multiple exocytotic pathways in pancreatic β-cells. *J Cell Biol* 1997;138:55–64.
155. Rorsman P, Eliasson L, Renström E, et al. The cell physiology of biphasic insulin secretion. *News Physiol Sci* 2000;15:72–77.
156. Daniel S, Noda M, Straub SG, et al. Identification of the docked granule pool responsible for the first phase of glucose-stimulated insulin secretion. *Diabetes* 1999;48:1686–1690.
157. Cerasi E, Fick G, Rudemo M. A mathematical model for the glucose induced insulin release in man. *Eur J Clin Invest* 1974;4:267–278.
158. Aizawa T, Komatsu M, Asanuma N, et al. Glucose action 'beyond ionic events' in the pancreatic β cell. *Trends Pharmacol Sci* 1998;19:496–499.
159. Matschinsky FM, Ellerman J, Stillings S, et al. Hexoses and insulin secretion. In: Hasselblatt A, Bruchhausen FV, eds. *Handbook of experimental pharmacology*. Vol 32. *Insulin II*. New York: Springer-Verlag, 1975:79–114.
160. Panten U, Zielmann S, Langer J, et al. Regulation of insulin secretion by energy metabolism in pancreatic β-cell mitochondria. Studies with a non-metabolizable analogue. *Biochem J* 1984;219:189–196.
161. Joost HG, Hasselblatt A. Insulin release by tolbutamide and glibenclamide: comparative study on the perfused rat pancreas. *Naunyn-Schmiedeberg's Arch Pharmacol* 1979;306:185–188.
162. Henquin JC. Tolbutamide stimulation and inhibition of insulin release: studies of the underlying ionic mechanisms in isolated rat islets. *Diabetologia* 1980; 18:151–160.
163. Palmer JP, Benson JW, Walter RM, et al. Arginine-stimulated acute phase of insulin and glucagon secretion in diabetic subjects. *J Clin Invest* 1976;58: 565–570.
164. Pfeifer MA, Halter JB, Porte D Jr. Insulin secretion in diabetes mellitus. *Am J Med* 1981;70:579–588.
165. Salomon D, Meda P. Heterogeneity and contact-dependent regulation of hormone secretion by individual B cells. *Exp Cell Res* 1986;162:507–520.
166. Hiriart M, Ramirez-Mendeles MC. Functional subpopulations of individual pancreatic B-cells in culture. *Endocrinology* 1991;128:3193–3198.
167. Lewis CE, Clark A, Ashcroft SJH, et al. Calcitonin gene-related peptide and somatostatin inhibit insulin release from individual rat B cells. *Mol Cell Endocrinol* 1988;57:41–49.
168. Serre-Beinier V, Le Gurun S, Belluardo N, et al. Cx36 preferentially connects β-cells within pancreatic islets. *Diabetes* 2000;49:727–734.
169. Bennett BD, Jetton TL, Ying G, et al. Quantitative subcellular imaging of glucose metabolism within intact pancreatic islets. *J Biol Chem* 1996;271:3647–3651.
170. Meissner HP. Electrophysiological evidence for coupling between β-cells of pancreatic islets. *Nature* 1976;262:502–504.
171. Halban PA, Wollheim CB, Blondet B, et al. The possible importance of contact between pancreatic islet cells for the control of insulin release. *Endocrinology* 1982;111:86–94.
172. Bosco D, Orci L, Meda P. Homologous but not heterologous contact increases the insulin secretion of individual pancreatic B-cells. *Exp Cell Res* 1989;184: 72–80.
173. Stefan Y, Meda P, Neufeld M, et al. Stimulation of insulin secretion reveals heterogeneity of pancreatic B cells in vivo. *J Clin Invest* 1987;80:175–183.
174. Jörns A. Immunocytochemical and ultrastructural heterogeneities of normal and glibenclamide stimulated pancreatic beta cells in the rat. *Virchows Arch* 1994;425:305–313.
175. Gilon P, Shepherd RM, Henquin JC. Oscillations of secretion driven by oscillations of cytoplasmic Ca^{2+} as evidenced in single pancreatic islets. *J Biol Chem* 1993;268:22265–22268.
176. Bergsten P, Grapengiesser E, Gylfe E, et al. Synchronous oscillations of cytoplasmic Ca^{2+} and insulin release in glucose-stimulated pancreatic islets. *J Biol Chem* 1994;269:8749–8753.
177. Barbosa RM, Silva AM, Tomé AR, et al. Control of pulsatile 5-HT/insulin secretion from single mouse pancreatic islets by intracellular calcium dynamics. *J Physiol* 1998;510:135–143.
178. Gilon P, Henquin JC. Distinct effects of glucose on the synchronous oscillations of insulin release and cytoplasmic Ca^{2+} concentration measured simultaneously in single mouse islets. *Endocrinology* 1995;36:5725–5730.
179. Westerlund J, Gylfe E, Bergsten P. Pulsatile insulin release from pancreatic islets with nonoscillatory elevation of cytoplasmic Ca^{2+}. *J Clin Invest* 1997;100: 2547–2551.
180. Ravier M, Gilon P, Henquin JC. Oscillations of insulin secretion can be triggered by imposed oscillations of cytoplasmic Ca^{2+} or metabolism in normal mouse islets. *Diabetes* 1999;48:2374–2382.
181. Polonsky KS, Given BD, Van Cauter E. Twenty-four-hour profiles and pulsatile patterns of insulin secretion in normal and obese subjects. *J Clin Invest* 1988;81:442–448.
182. Porksen N, Nyholm B, Veldhuis JD, et al. In humans at least 75% of insulin secretion arises from punctuated insulin secretory bursts. *Am J Physiol Endocrinol Metab* 1997;273:E908–E914.
183. Sturis J, Van Cauter E, Blackman JD, et al. Entrainment of pulsatile insulin secretion by oscillatory glucose infusion. *J Clin Invest* 1991;87:439–445.
184. Pagliara AS, Stillings SN, Hover B, et al. Glucose modulation of amino acid-induced glucagon and insulin release in the isolated perfused rat pancreas. *J Clin Invest* 1974;54:819–832.
185. Gerich JE, Charles MA, Grodsky GM. Characterization of the effects of arginine and glucose on glucagon and insulin release from the perfused rat pancreas. *J Clin Invest* 1974;54:833–841.
186. Weir GC, Mojsov S, Hendrick GK, et al. Glucagon-like peptide I (7–37) actions on endocrine pancreas. *Diabetes* 1989;38:338–342.
187. Hermans MP, Schmeer W, Henquin JC. The permissive effect of glucose, tolbutamide and high K+ on arginine stimulation of insulin release in isolated mouse islets. *Diabetologia* 1987;30:659–665.
188. Efendic S, Cerasi E, Luft R. Role of glucose in arginine-induced release in man. *Metabolism* 1971;20:568–579.
189. Halter JB, Graf RJ, Porte D Jr. Potentiation of insulin secretory responses by plasma glucose levels in man: evidence that hyperglycemia in diabetes compensates for impaired glucose potentiation. *J Clin Endocrinol Metab* 1979;48: 946–954.

190. Zawalich WS. Intermediary metabolism and insulin secretion from isolated rat islets of Langerhans. *Diabetes* 1979;28:252–260.
191. Malaisse WJ, Malaisse-Lagae F, et al. Anomeric specificity of hexose metabolism in pancreatic islets. *Physiol Rev* 1983;63:773–786.
192. Best L, Trebilcock R, Tomlinson S. Lactate transport in insulin-secreting β-cells: contrast between rat islets and HIT-T15 insulinoma cells. *Mol Cell Endocrinol* 1992;86:49–56.
193. Lenzen S, Panten U. Effects of pyruvate, L-lactate and 3-phenylpyruvate on function of ob/ob mouse pancreatic islets: insulin secretion in relation to $45Ca^{2+}$ uptake and metabolism. *Biochem Med* 1981;25:366–372.
194. Sener A, Malaisse WJ. The stimulus-secretion coupling of amino acid-induced insulin release—insulinotropic action of branched-chain amino acids at physiological concentrations of glucose and glutamine. *Eur J Clin Invest* 1981;11:455–460.
195. Bolea S, Pertusa JAG, Martin F, et al. Regulation of pancreatic β-cell electrical activity and insulin release by physiological amino acid concentrations. *Pflügers Arch* 1997;433:699–704.
196. Panten U, Zielmann S, Joost H-G, et al. Branched chain amino and keto acids: tools for the investigation of fuel recognition mechanism in pancreatic B-cells. In: Adibi SA, Fckl W, Langenbeck U, Schauder P, eds. *Branched chain amino and keto acids in health and disease.* Basel: Karger, 1984:134–146.
197. Malaisse WJ. Branched-chain amino and keto acid metabolism in pancreatic islets. *Adv Enzyme Reg* 1986;25:203–217.
198. Henquin JC, Meissner HP. Effects of amino acids on membrane potential and $86Rb^{+}$ fluxes in pancreatic β-cells. *Am J Physiol Endocrinol Metab* 1981;240: E245–252.
199. Ashcroft FM, Ashcroft SJH, Harrison DE. Effects of 2-ketoisocaproate on insulin release and single potassium channel activity in dispersed rat pancreatic β-cells. *J Physiol* 1987;385:517–529.
200. Gao ZY, Li G, Najafi H, et al. Glucose regulation of glutaminolysis and its role in insulin secretion. *Diabetes* 1999; 47:1535–1542.
201. Stanley CA, Lieu YK, Hsu BYL, et al. Hyperinsulinism and hyperammonemia in infants with regulatory mutations of the glutamate dehydrogenase gene. *N Engl J Med* 1998;338:1352–1357.
202. Hellman B, Sehlin J, Täljedal I-B. Effects of glucose and other modifiers of insulin release on the oxidative metabolism of amino acids in micro-dissected pancreatic islets. *Biochem J* 1971;123:513–521.
203. Henquin JC, Meissner HP. Cyclic adenosine monophosphate differently affects the response of mouse pancreatic β-cells to various amino acids. *J Physiol* 1986;381:77–93.
204. Prentki M, Renold AE. Neutral amino acid transport in isolated rat pancreatic islets. *J Biol Chem* 1983;258:14239–14244.
205. Malaisse WJ, Blachier F, Mourtada A, et al. Stimulus-secretion coupling of arginine-induced insulin release. Metabolism of L-arginine and L-ornithine in pancreatic islets. *Biochim Biophys Acta* 1989;1013:133–143.
206. Charles S, Tamagawa T, Henquin JC. A single mechanism for the stimulation of insulin release and $86Rb^{+}$ efflux from rat islets by cationic amino acids. *Biochem J* 1982;208:301–308.
207. Salehi A, Carlberg M, Henningson R, et al. Islet constitutive nitric oxide synthase: biochemical determination and regulatory function. *Am J Physiol Cell Physiol* 1996;270:C1634–C1641.
208. Jones PM, Persaud SJ, Bjaaland T, et al. Nitric oxide is not involved in the initiation of insulin secretion from rat islets of Langerhans. *Diabetologia* 1992;35: 1020–1027.
209. Stein DT, Stevenson BE, Chester MW, et al. The insulinotropic potency of fatty acids is influenced profoundly by their chain length and degree of saturation. *J Clin Invest* 1997;100:398–403.
210. Campillo JE, Valdivia MM, Rodriguez E, et al. Effect of oleic and octanoic acids on glucose-induced insulin release in vitro. *Diabetes Metab* 1979;5: 183–188.
211. Conget I., Rasschaert J, Sener A, et al. Secretory, biosynthetic, respiratory, cationic, and metabolic responses of pancreatic islets to palmitate and oleate. *Biochem Med Metab Biol* 1994;51:175–184.
212. Warnotte C, Gilon P, Nenquin M, et al. Mechanisms of the stimulation of insulin release by saturated fatty acids: a study of palmitate effects in mouse β-cells. *Diabetes* 1994;43:703–711.
213. Warnotte C, Nenquin M, Henquin JC. Unbound rather than total concentration and saturation rather than unsaturation determine the potency of fatty acids on insulin secretion. *Mol Cell Endocrinol* 1999;153:147–153.
214. Malaisse WJ, Lebrun P, Rasschaert J, et al. Ketone bodies and islet function: 86Rb handling and metabolic data. *Am J Physiol Endocrinol Metab* 1990;259: E123–E130.
215. Malaisse WJ. The beta cell in NIDDM: giving light to the blind. *Diabetologia* 1994;37[Suppl 2]:S36–S42.
216. Sturgess NC, Ashford MLJ, Cook DL, et al. The sulphonylurea receptor may be an ATP-sensitive potassium channel. *Lancet* 1985;2:474–475.
217. Panten U, Schwanstecher M, Schwanstecher C. Mode of action of sulfonylureas. In: Kuhlmann J, Puls W, eds. *Oral antidiabetics*. Berlin: Springer, 1996:129–159.
218. Panten U, Burgfeld J, Goerke F, et al. Control of insulin secretion by sulfonylureas, meglitinide and diazoxide in relation to their binding to the sulfonylurea receptor in pancreatic islets. *Biochem Pharmacol* 1989;38:1217–1229.
219. Garrino MG, Schmeer W, Nenquin M, et al. Mechanism of the stimulation of insulin release in vitro by HB 699, a benzoic acid derivative similar to the non-sulphonylurea moiety of glibenclamide. *Diabetologia* 1985;28:697–703.
220. Meyer M, Chudziak F, Schwanstecher C, et al. Structural requirements of sulphonylureas and analogues for interaction with sulphonylurea receptor subtypes. *Br J Pharmacol* 1999;128:27–34.
221. Jonas JC, Plant TD, Henquin JC. Imidazoline antagonists of α_2-adrenoceptors increase insulin release in vitro by inhibiting ATP-sensitive K^{+} channels in pancreatic β-cells. *Br J Pharmacol* 1992;107:8–14.
222. Proks P, Ashcroft FM. Phentolamine block of KATP channels is mediated by Kir6.2. *Proc Natl Acad Sci U S A* 1997;94:11716–11720.
223. Morgan NG, Chan SLF, Mourtada M, et al. Imidazolines and pancreatic hormone secretion. *Ann N Y Acad Sci* 1999;881:217–228.
224. Rustenbeck I, Köpp M, Ratzka P, et al. Imidazolines and the pancreatic B-cell—actions and binding sites. *Ann N Y Acad Sci* 1999;881:229–240.
225. Zaitsev SV, Efanov AM, Raap A, et al. Different modes of action of the imidazoline compound RX871024 in pancreatic β-cells—blocking of K^{+} channels, mobilization of Ca^{2+} from endoplasmic reticulum, and interaction with exocytotic machinery. *Ann N Y Acad Sci* 1999;881:241–252.
226. Henquin JC. Established, unsuspected and novel pharmacological insulin secretagogues. In: Bailey CJ, Flatt PR, eds. *New antidiabetic drugs*. London: Smith-Gordon and Co, 1990:93–106.
227. Henquin JC. Quinine and the stimulus-secretion coupling in pancreatic beta-cells: glucose-like effects on potassium permeability and insulin release. *Endocrinology* 1982;110:1325–1332.
228. Kakei M, Nakazaki M, Kamisaki T, et al. Inhibition of the ATP-sensitive potassium channel by class I antiarrhythmic agent, cibenzoline, in rat pancreatic β cells. *Br J Pharmacol* 1993;109:1226–1231.
229. Henquin JC, Meissner HP. Opposite effects of tolbutamide and diazoxide on $86Rb^{+}$ fluxes and membrane potential in pancreatic B cells. *Biochem Pharmacol* 1982;31:1407–1415.
230. Trube G, Rorsman P, Ohno-Shosaku T. Opposite effects of tolbutamide and diazoxide on the ATP-dependent K^{+} channel in mouse pancreatic β-cells. *Pflügers Arch* 1986;407:493–499.
231. Fajans SS, Floyd JC Jr, Knopff RF, et al. A difference in mechanism by which leucine and other amino acids induce insulin release. *J Clin Endocrinol Metab* 1967;27:1600–1606.
232. Henquin JC, Charles S, Nenquin M, et al. Diazoxide and D600 inhibition of insulin release: distinct mechanisms explain the specificity for different stimuli. *Diabetes* 1982;31:776–783.
233. Quayle JM, Nelson MT, Standen NB. ATP-sensitive and inwardly rectifying potassium channels in smooth muscle. *Physiol Rev* 1997;77:1165–1232.
234. Hellman B, Gylfe E, Grapengiesser E, et al. Cytoplasmic calcium and insulin secretion. In: Flatt PR, ed. *Nutrient regulation of insulin secretion*. London: Portland Press, 1992:213–246.
235. Trost BN, Weidmann P. Effects of calcium antagonists on glucose homeostasis and serum lipids in non-diabetic and diabetic subjects: a review. *J Hypertens* 1987;5[Suppl 4]:S81–S104.
236. Ward WK, Bolgiano DC, McKnight B, et al. Diminished B cell secretory capacity in patients with noninsulin-dependent diabetes mellitus. *J Clin Invest* 1984;74:1318–1328.
237. Eliasson L, Renström E, Ämmälä C, et al. PKC-dependent stimulation of exocytosis by sulfonylureas in pancreatic β cells. *Science* 1996; 271:813–815.
238. Tian YM, Johnson G, Ashcroft SJH. Sulfonylureas enhance exocytosis from pancreatic β-cells by a mechanism that does not involve direct activation of protein kinase C. *Diabetes* 1998;47:1722–1726.
239. Smith PA, Proks P, Moorhouse A. Direct effects of tolbutamide on mitochondrial function, intracellular Ca^{2+} and exocytosis in pancreatic β-cells. *Pflügers Arch* 1999;437:577–588.
240. Mariot P, Gilon P, Nenquin M, et al. Tolbutamide and diazoxide influence insulin secretion by changing the concentration but not the action of cytoplasmic Ca^{2+} in β-cells. *Diabetes* 1998;47:365–373.
241. Kampermann J, Herbst M, Ullrich S. Effects of adrenaline and tolbutamide on insulin secretion in INS-1 cells under voltage control. *Cell Physiol Biochem* 2000;10:81–90.
242. Mukai E, Ishida H, Fujimoto S, et al. The insulinotropic mechanism of the novel hypoglycaemic agent JTT-608: direct enhancement of Ca^{2+} efficacy and increase of Ca^{2+} influx by phosphodiesterase inhibition. *Br J Pharmacol* 2000;129:901–908.
243. Brunicardi FC, Shavelle DM, Andersen DK. Neural regulation of the endocrine pancreas. *Int J Pancreatol* 1995;18:177–195.
244. Fehmann H-C, Göke R, Göke B. Cell and molecular biology of the incretin hormones glucagon-like peptide-I and glucose-dependent insulin releasing polypeptide. *Endocr Rev* 1995;16:390–410.
245. Ahrén B. Autonomic regulation of islet hormone secretion—implications for health and disease. *Diabetologia* 2000;43:393–410.
246. Henquin JC. The interplay between cyclic AMP and ions in the stimulus-secretion coupling in pancreatic B-cells. *Arch Int Physiol Biochim Biophys* 1985; 93:37–48.
247. Leiser M, Fleischer N. cAMP-dependent phosphorylation of the cardiac-type α_1 subunit of the voltage-dependent Ca^{2+} channel in a murine pancreatic β-cell line. *Diabetes* 1996;45:1412–1418.
248. Henquin JC, Meissner HP. The ionic, electrical, and secretory effects of endogenous cyclic adenosine monophosphate in mouse pancreatic B cells: studies with forskolin. *Endocrinology* 1984;115:1125–1134.
249. Henquin JC, Bozem M, Schmeer W, et al. Distinct mechanisms for two amplification systems of insulin release. *Biochem J* 1987;246:393–399.
250. Ammala C, Ashcroft FM, Rorsman P. Calcium-independent potentiation of insulin release by cyclic AMP in single β-cells. *Nature* 1993;363:356–358.
251. Berridge MJ, Irvine RF. Inositol phosphates and cell signalling. *Nature* 1989; 341:197–205.

252. Nishizuka Y. Studies and perspectives of protein kinase C. *Science* 1986;233: 305–312.
253. Vallar L, Biden TJ, Wollheim CB. Guanine nucleotides induce Ca^{2+} independent insulin secretion from permeabilized RJNm5F cells. *J Biol Chem* 1987; 262:5049–5056.
254. Arkhammar P, Nilsson T, Welsh M, et al. Effects of protein kinase C activation on the regulation of the stimulus-secretion coupling in pancreatic β-cells. *Biochem J* 1989;264:207–215.
255. Taylor CW. Inositol trisphosphate receptors: Ca^{2+}-modulated intracellular Ca^{2+} channels. *Biochim Biophys Acta* 1998;1436:19–33.
256. Hamakawa N, Yada T. Interplay of glucose-stimulated Ca^{2+} sequestration and acetylcholine-induced Ca^{2+} release at the endoplasmic reticulum in rat pancreatic β-cells. *Cell Calcium* 1995;17:21–31.
257. Gilon P, Henquin JC. Mechanisms and physiological significance of the cholinergic control of the pancreatic β-cell function. *Endocr Rev* 2001;22:565–604.
258. Drucker DJ. Glucagon-like peptides. *Diabetes* 1998;47:159–169.
259. Elrick H, Stimmler L, Hlad CJ Jr, Arai Y. Plasma insulin response to oral and intravenous glucose administration. *J Clin Endocrinol Metab* 1964;24: 1076–1082.
260. McIntyre N, Holdsworth DC, Turner DS. New interpretation of oral glucose tolerance. *Lancet* 1964;2:20–21.
261. Ebert R, Creutzfeldt W. Gastrointestinal peptides and insulin secretion. *Diabetes Metab Rev* 1987;3:1–26.
262. Moens K, Heimberg H, Flamez D, et al. Expression and functional activity of glucagon, glucagon-like peptide I, and glucose-dependent insulinotropic peptide receptors in rat pancreatic islet cells. *Diabetes* 1996;45:257–261.
263. Gromada J, Holst JJ, Rorsman P. Cellular regulation of islet hormone secretion by the incretin hormone glucagon-like peptide 1. *Pflügers Arch* 1998; 435: 583–594.
264. Britsch S, Krippeit-Drews P, Lang F, et al. Glucagon-like peptide-1 modulates Ca^{2+} current but not K^+ATP current in intact mouse pancreatic B-cells. *Biochem Biophys Res Commun* 1995;207:33–39.
265. Bode HP, Moormann B, Dabew R, et al. Glucagon-like peptide 1 elevates cytosolic calcium in pancreatic β-cells independently of protein kinase A. *Endocrinology* 1999;140:3919–3927.
266. Holst JJ. Glucagon-like peptide 1 (GLP-1): an intestinal hormone, signalling nutritional abundance, with an unusual therapeutic potential. *Trends Endocrinol Metab* 1999;10:229–235.
267. Henquin JC, Nenquin M. The muscarinic receptor subtype in mouse pancreatic B-cells. *FEBS Lett* 1988; 236:89–92.
268. Verspohl EJ, Ammon HPT, Williams JA, et al. Evidence that cholecystokinin interacts with specific receptors and regulates insulin release in isolated rat islets of Langerhans. *Diabetes* 1986;35:38–43.
269. Samols E, Marri G, Marks V. Promotion of insulin secretion by glucagon. *Lancet* 1965;2:415–416.
270. Marks V, Samols E, Stagner J. Intra-islet interactions. In: Flatt PR, ed. *Nutrient regulation of insulin secretion*. London: Portland Press, 1992:41–57.
271. Schuit FC, Pipeleers DG. Differences in adrenergic recognition by pancreatic A and B cells. *Science* 1986;232:875–877.
272. Lacey RJ, Cable HC, James RFL, et al. Concentration-dependent effects of adrenaline on the profile of insulin secretion from isolated human islets of Langerhans. *J Endocrinol* 1993;138:555–563.
273. Bishop AE, Polak JM, Green IC, et al. The location of VIP in the pancreas of man and rat. *Diabetologia* 1980;18:73–78.
274. Knuhtsen S, Holst JJ, Baldissera FGA, et al. Gastrin-releasing peptide in the porcine pancreas. *Gastroenterology* 1987;92:1153–1158.
275. Yada T, Sakurada M, Nakata M, et al. Current status of PACAP as a regulator of insulin secretion in pancreatic islets. *Ann N Y Acad Sci* 1996;805:329–342.
276. Dunning BE, Moltz JH, Fawcett CP. Modulation of insulin and glucagon secretion from the perfused rat pancreas by the neurohypophysial hormones and by desamino-D-arginine vasopressin (DDAVP). *Peptides* 1984;5: 871–875.
277. Gao ZY, Drews G, Nenquin M, et al. Mechanisms of the stimulation of insulin release by arginine-vasopressin in normal mouse islets. *J Biol Chem* 1990;265: 15724–15730.
278. Amico JA, Finn FM, Haldar J. Oxytocin and vasopressin are present in human and rat pancreas. *Am J Med Sci* 1988;296:303–307.
279. Petit P, Loubatières-Mariani MM, Keppens S, et al. Purinergic receptors and metabolic function. *Drug Dev Res* 1996;39:413–425.
280. Hazama A, Hayashi S, Okada Y. Cell surface measurements of ATP release from single pancreatic β cells using a novel biosensor technique. *Pflügers Arch* 1998;437:31–35.
281. Bertrand G, Gross R, Puech R, et al. Evidence for a glutamate receptor of the AMPA subtype which mediates insulin release from rat perfused pancreas. *Br J Pharmacol* 1992;106:354-359.
282. Inagaki N, Kuromi H, Gonoi T, et al. Expression and role of ionotropic glutamate receptors in pancreatic islet cells. *FASEB J* 1995;9:686–691.
283. Weaver CD, Yao TL, Powers AC, et al. Differential expression of glutamate receptor subtypes in rat pancreatic islets. *J Biol Chem* 1996;271:12977–12984.
284. Morgan NG. Regulation of insulin secretion by α_2-adrenergic agonists. *Trends Pharmacol Sci* 1987;8:369–370.
285. Nilsson T, Arkhammar P, Rorsman P, et al. Suppression of insulin release by galanin and somatostatin is mediated by a G-protein: an effect involving repolarization and reduction in cytoplasmic free Ca^{2+} concentration. *J Biol Chem* 1989;264:973–980.
286. Drews G, Debuyser A, Nenquin M, et al. Galanin and epinephrine act on distinct receptors to inhibit insulin release by the same mechanisms including an increase in K^+ permeability of the B-cell membrane. *Endocrinology* 1990; 126:1646–1653.
287. Rorsman P, Bokvist K, Ämmälä C, et al. Activation by adrenaline of a low-conductance G protein-dependent K+ channel in mouse pancreatic B cells. *Nature* 1991;349:77–79.
288. Abel KB, Lehr S, Ullrich S. Adrenaline, not somatostatin-induced hyperpolarization is accompanied by a sustained inhibition of insulin secretion in INS-1 cells. Activation of sulphonylurea K^+ATP channels is not involved. *Pflügers Arch* 1996;432:89–96.
289. Tamagawa T, Niki I, Niki H, et al. Catecholamines inhibit insulin release independently of changes in cytosolic free Ca^{2+}. *Biomed Res* 1985;6:429–432.
290. Ullrich S, Wollheim CB. Galanin inhibits insulin secretion by direct interference with exocytosis. *FEBS Lett* 1989;247:401–404.
291. Renström E, Ding WG, Bokvist K, et al. Neurotransmitter-induced inhibition of exocytosis in insulin-secreting β cells by activation of calcineurin. *Neuron* 1996;17:513–522.
292. Nakaki T, Nakadate T, Kato R. α_2-adrenoceptors modulating insulin release from isolated pancreatic islets. *Naunyn Schmiedeberg's Arch Pharmacol* 1980; 313:151–154.
293. Chan SLF, Perrett CW, Morgan NG. Differential expression of α_2-adrenoceptor subtypes in purified rat pancreatic islet A- and B-cells. *Cell Signal* 1997;9: 71–78.
294. Dunning BE, Taborsky GJ Jr. Galanin—sympathetic neurotransmitter in endocrine pancreas? *Diabetes* 1988;37:1157–1162.
295. Amiranoff B, Servin AL, Rouyer-Fessard C, et al. Galanin receptors in a hamster pancreatic β-cell tumor: identification and molecular characterization. *Endocrinology* 1987;121:284–290.
296. D'Alessio DA, Sieber C, Beglinger C, et al. A physiologic role for somatostatin 28 as a regulator of insulin secretion. *J Clin Invest* 1989;84:857–862.
297. Strowski MZ, Parmar RM, Blake AD, et al. Somatostatin inhibits insulin and glucagon secretion via two receptor subtypes: an in vitro study of pancreatic islets from somatostatin receptor 2 knockout mice. *Endocrinology* 2000;141: 111–117.
298. Mandarino L, Stenner D, Blanchard W, et al. Selective effects of somatostatin-14, -25 and -28 on in vitro insulin and glucagon secretion. *Nature* 1981;291: 76–77.
299. Kulkarni RN, Wang ZL, Wang RM, et al. Leptin rapidly suppresses insulin release from insulinoma cells, rat and human islets and, in vivo, in mice. *J Clin Invest* 1997;100:2729–2736.
300. Kieffer TJ, Habener JF. The adipoinsular axis: effects of leptin on pancreatic β-cells. *Am J Physiol Endocrinol Metab* 2000;278:E1–E14.
301. Zhao AZ, Bornfeldt KE, Beavo JA. Leptin inhibits insulin secretion by activation of phosphodiesterase 3B. *J Clin Invest* 1998;102:869–873.
302. Harvey J, McKay NG, Walker KS, et al. Essential role of phosphoinositide 3-kinase in leptin-induced KATP channel activation in the rat CRI-G1 insulinoma cell line. *J Biol Chem* 2000;275:4660–4669.
303. Leahy JL, Vandekerkhove KM. Insulin-like growth factor-I at physiological concentrations is a potent inhibitor of insulin secretion. *Endocrinology* 1990; 126:1593–1598.
304. Van Schravendijk CFH, Foriers A, Van den Brande JL, et al. Evidence for the presence of type I insulin-like growth factor receptors on rat pancreatic A and B cells. *Endocrinology* 1987;121:1784–1788.
305. Efendic S, Tatemoto K, Mutt V, et al. Pancreastatin and islet hormone release. *Proc Natl Acad Sci U S A* 1987;84:7257–7260.
306. Eiden LE. Is chromogranin a prohormone? *Nature* 1987;325:301.
307. Giugliano D, Torella R, Lefèbvre PJ, et al. Opioid peptides and metabolic regulation. *Diabetologia* 1988;31:3–15.
308. Verspohl EJ, Berger U, Ammon HPT. The significance of μ- and δ-receptors in rat pancreatic islets for the opioid-mediated insulin release. *Biochim Biophys Acta* 1986;888:217–224.
309. Ahren B, Pettersson M. Calcitonin gene-related peptide (CGRP) and amylin and the endocrine pancreas. *Int J Pancreatol* 1990;6:1–16.
310. Nishi M, Sanke T, Nagamatsu S, et al. Islet amyloid polypeptide: a new β-cell secretory product related to islet amyloid deposits. *J Biol Chem* 1990;265: 4173–4176.
311. Kahn SE, D'Alessio DA, Schwartz MW, et al. Evidence of cosecretion of islet amyloid polypeptide and insulin by β-cells. *Diabetes* 1990;39:634–638.
312. Ohsawa H, Kanatsuka A, Yamaguchi T, et al. Islet amyloid polypeptide inhibits glucose-stimulated insulin secretion from isolated rat pancreatic islets. *Biochem Biophys Res Commun* 1989;160:961–967.
313. Nagamatsu S, Carroll RJ, Grodsky GM, et al. Lack of islet amyloid polypeptide regulation of insulin biosynthesis or secretion in normal rat islets. *Diabetes* 1990;39:871–874.
314. Robertson RP, Tsai P, Little SA, et al. Receptor-mediated adenylate cyclase-coupled mechanism for PGE2 inhibition of insulin secretion in HIT cells. *Diabetes* 1987;36:1047–1053.
315. Robertson RP. Dominance of cyclooxygenase-2 in the regulation of pancreatic islet prostaglandin synthesis. *Diabetes* 1998;47:1379–1383.
316. Grill V, Adamson U, Cerasi E. Immediate and time-dependent effects of glucose on insulin release from rat pancreatic tissue. *J Clin Invest* 1978;61: 1034–1043.
317. Nesher R, Praiss M, Cerasi E. Immediate and time-dependent effects of glucose on insulin release: differential calcium requirements. *Acta Endocrinol* 1988;117:409–416.

318. Zawalich WS, Zawalich KC, Rasmussen H. Cholinergic agonists prime the β-cell to glucose stimulation. *Endocrinology* 1989;125:2400–2406.
319. Rasmussen H, Zawalich KC, Ganesan S, et al. Physiology and pathophysiology of insulin secretion. *Diabetes Care* 1990;13:655–666.
320. Grodsky GM. A new phase of insulin secretion: how will it contribute to our understanding of β-cell function? *Diabetes* 1989;38:673–678.
321. Robertson RP, Olson LK, Zhang HJ. Differentiating glucose toxicity from glucose desensitization: a new message from the insulin gene. *Diabetes* 1994;43:1085–1089.
322. Leahy JL. Impaired β-cell function with chronic hyperglycemia: "overworked β-cell" hypothesis. *Diabetes Rev* 1996;4:298–319.
323. Ling Z, Pipeleers DG. Prolonged exposure of human β cells to elevated glucose levels results in sustained cellular activation leading to a loss of glucose regulation. *J Clin Invest* 1996;98:2805–2812.
324. Sreenan SK, Cockburn BN, Baldwin AC, et al. Adaptation to hyperglycemia enhances insulin secretion in glucokinase mutant mice. *Diabetes* 1998;47:1881–1888.
325. Purrello F, Vetri M, Vinci C, et al. Chronic exposure to high glucose and impairment of K+-channel function in perifused rat pancreatic islets. *Diabetes* 1990;39:397–399.
326. Björklund A, Grill V. Enhancing effects of long-term elevated glucose and palmitate on stored and secreted proinsulin-to-insulin ratios in human pancreatic islets. *Diabetes* 1999;48:1409–1414.
327. Kaiser N, Corcos AP, Sarel I, et al. Monolayer culture of adult rat pancreatic islets on extracellular matrix: modulation of B-cell function by chronic exposure to high glucose. *Endocrinology* 1991;129:2067–2076.
328. Zhou YP, Grill VE. Long-term exposure of rat pancreatic islets to fatty acids inhibits glucose-induced insulin secretion and biosynthesis through a glucose fatty acid cycle. *J Clin Invest* 1994;93:870–876.
329. Hosokawa H, Corkey BE, Leahy JL. Beta-cell hypersensitivity to glucose following 24-h exposure of rat islets to fatty acids. *Diabetologia* 1997;40:392–397.
330. Anello M, Gilon P, Henquin JC. Alterations of insulin secretion from mouse islets treated with sulphonylureas: perturbations of Ca^{2+} regulation prevail over changes in insulin content. *Br J Pharmacol* 1999;27:1883–1891.
331. Asplund K, Andersson A, Jarousse C, et al. Function of the fetal endocrine pancreas. *Isr J Med Sci* 1975;11:581–590.
332. Kervran A, Randon J. Development of insulin release by fetal rat pancreas in vitro. Effects of glucose, amino acids, and theophylline. *Diabetes* 1980;29:673–678.
333. Hole RL, Pian-Smith MCM, Sharp GWG. Development of the biphasic response to glucose in fetal and neonatal rat pancreas. *Am J Physiol Endocrinol Metab* 1988;254:E167–E174.
334. Mourmeaux JL, Remacle C, Henquin JC. Effects of stimulation of adenylate cyclase and protein kinase-C on cultured fetal rat B-cells. *Endocrinology* 1989;125:2536–2544.
335. Rorsman P, Arkhammar P, Bokvist K, et al. Failure of glucose to elicit a normal secretory response in fetal pancreatic beta cells results from glucose insensitivity of the ATP-regulated K^+ channels. *Proc Natl Acad Sci U S A* 1989;86:4505–4509.
336. Weinhaus AJ, Poronnik P, Cook DI, et al. Insulin secretagogues, but not glucose, stimulate an increase in $[Ca^{2+}]i$ in the fetal rat β-cell. *Diabetes* 1995;44:118–124.
337. Tu J, Tuch BE. Glucose regulates the maximal velocities of glucokinase and glucose utilization in the immature fetal rat pancreatic islet. *Diabetes* 1996;45:1068–1075.
338. Taniguchi S, Tanigawa K, Miwa I. Immaturity of glucose-induced insulin secretion in fetal rat islets is due to low glucokinase activity. *Horm Metab Res* 2000;32:97–102.
339. Chen M, Bergman RN, Pacini G, Porte D Jr. Pathogenesis of age-related glucose intolerance in man: insulin resistance and decreased β-cell function. *J Clin Endocrinol Metab* 1985;60:13–20.
340. Gumbiner B, Polonsky KS, Beltz WF, et al. Effects of aging on insulin secretion. *Diabetes* 1989;38:1549–1556.
341. Adelman RC. Secretion of insulin during aging. *J Am Geriatr Soc* 1989;37:983–990.
342. Coordt MC, Ruhe RC, McDonald RB. Aging and insulin secretion. *Proc Soc Exp Biol Med* 1995;209:213–222.
343. Reaven EP, Gold G, Reaven GM. Effects of age on glucose-stimulated insulin release by the β-cell of the rat. *J Clin Invest* 1979;64:591–599.
344. Levy J, Herchuelz A, Sener A, et al. The stimulus-secretion coupling of glucose-induced insulin release. XX. Fasting: a model for altered glucose recognition by the B-cell. *Metabolism* 1976;25:583–591.
345. Zawalich WS, Dye ES, Pagliara AS, et al. Starvation diabetes in the rat: onset, recovery, and specificity of reduced responsiveness of pancreatic β-cells. *Endocrinology* 1979;104:1344–1351.
346. Wolters GHJ, Konijnendijk W, Bouman PR. Effects of fasting on insulin secretion, islet glucose metabolism, and the cyclic adenosine 3′, 5′ monophosphate content of rat pancreatic islets in vitro. *Diabetes* 1977;26:530–537.
347. Tiedge M, Lenzen S. Regulation of glucokinase and GLUT-2 glucose-transporter gene expression in pancreatic B-cells. *Biochem J* 1991;279:899–901.
348. Iwashima Y, Kondoh-Abiko A, Seino S, et al. Reduced levels of messenger ribonucleic acid for calcium channel, glucose transporter-2, and glucokinase are associated with alterations in insulin secretion in fasted rats. *Endocrinology* 1994;135:1010–1017.
349. Zhou YP, Priestman DA, Randle PJ, et al. Fasting and decreased B cell sensitivity: Important role for fatty acid-induced inhibition of PDH activity. *Am J Physiol Endocrinol Metab* 1996;270:E988–E994.
350. Stein DT, Esser V, Stevenson BE, et al. Essentiality of circulating fatty acids for glucose-stimulated insulin secretion in the fasted rat. *J Clin Invest* 1996;97:2728–2735.
351. Fernandez J, Valdeolmillos M. Increased levels of free fatty acids in fasted mice stimulate in vivo β-cell electrical activity. *Diabetes* 1998;47:1707–1712.
352. Mikines KJ, Sonne B, Farrell PA, et al. Effect of training on the dose-response relationship for insulin action in men. *J Appl Physiol* 1989;66:695–703.
353. Engdahl JH, Veldhuis JD, Farrell PA. Altered pulsatile insulin secretion associated with endurance training. *J Appl Physiol* 1995;79:1977–1985.
354. Zawalich W, Maturo S, Felig P. Influence of physical training on insulin release and glucose utilization by islet cells and liver glucokinase activity in the rat. *Am J Physiol Endocrinol Metab* 1982;243:E464–E469.
355. Shima K, Hirota M, Sato M, et al. Effect of exercise training on insulin and glucagon release from perfused rat pancreas. *Horm Metab Res* 1987;19:395–399.
356. Koranyi LI, Bourey RE, Slentz CA, et al. Coordinate reduction of rat pancreatic islet glucokinase and proinsulin mRNA by exercise training. *Diabetes* 1991;40:401–404.
357. Sorenson RL, Brelje TC. Adaptation of islets of Langerhans to pregnancy: β-cell growth, enhanced insulin secretion and the role of lactogenic hormones. *Horm Metab Res* 1997;29:301–307.
358. Green IC, Howell SL, Montague W, et al. Regulation of insulin release from isolated islets of Langerhans of the rat in pregnancy. *Biochem J* 1973;134:481–487.
359. Weinhaus AJ, Stout LE, Sorenson RL. Glucokinase, hexokinase, glucose transporter 2, and glucose metabolism in islets during pregnancy and prolactin-treated islets in vitro: mechanisms for long term up-regulation of islets. *Endocrinology* 1996;137:1640–1649.
360. Lipson LG, Sharp GWG. Insulin release in pregnancy: studies on adenylate cyclase, phosphodiesterase, protein kinase, and phosphoprotein phosphatase in isolated rat islets of Langerhans. *Endocrinology* 1978;103:1272–1280.
361. Green IC, Taylor KW. Insulin secretory response of isolated islets of Langerhans in pregnant rats: effects of dietary restriction. *J Endocrinol* 1974;62:137–143.
362. Hubinont CJ, Dufrane SP, Garcia-Morales P, et al. Influence of lactation upon pancreatic islet function. *Endocrinology* 1986;118:687–694.
363. Michaels RL, Sorenson RL, Parsons JA, et al. Prolactin enhances cell-to-cell communication among β-cells in pancreatic islets. *Diabetes* 1987;36:1098–1103.
364. Madon RJ, Ensor DM, Flint DJ. Hypoinsulinaemia in the lactating rat is caused by a decreased glycaemic stimulus to the pancreas. *J Endocrinol* 1990;125:81–88.
365. Kamarudin N, Hew FL, Christopher M, et al. Insulin secretion in growth hormone-deficient adults: effects of 24 months' therapy and five days' acute withdrawal of recombinant human growth hormone. *Metabolism* 1999;48:1387–1396.
366. Parman AU. Effects of hypophysectomy and short-term growth hormone replacement on insulin release from and glucose metabolism in isolated rat islets of Langerhans. *J Endocrinol* 1975;67:1–8.
367. Whittaker PG, Taylor KW. Direct effects of growth hormone on rat islets of Langerhans in tissue culture. *Diabetologia* 1980;18:323–328.
368. Billestrup N, Nielsen JH. The stimulatory effect of growth hormone, prolactin, and placental lactogen on β-cell proliferation is not mediated by insulin-like growth factor-1. *Endocrinology* 1991;129:883–888.
369. Swenne I. Pancreatic beta-cell growth and diabetes mellitus. *Diabetologia* 1992;35:193–201.
370. Lenzen S, Bailey CJ. Thyroid hormones, gonadal and adrenocortical steroids and the function of the islets of Langerhans. *Endocr Rev* 1984;5:411–434.
371. Fernandez-Mejia C, Davidson MB. Regulation of glucokinase and proinsulin gene expression and insulin secretion in RIN-m5F cells by dexamethasone, retinoic acid, and thyroid hormone. *Endocrinology* 1992;130:1660–1668.
372. Ikeda T, Fujiyama K, Hoshino T, et al. Acute effect of thyroid hormone on insulin secretion in rats. *Biochem Pharmacol* 1990;40:1769–1771.
373. Kadowaki S, Norman AW. Dietary vitamin D is essential for normal insulin secretion from the perfused rat pancreas. *J Clin Invest* 1984;73:759–766.
374. Kajikawa M, Ishida H, Fujimoto S, et al. An insulinotropic effect of vitamin D analog with increasing intracellular Ca^{2+} concentration in pancreatic β-cells through nongenomic signal transduction. *Endocrinology* 1999;140:4706–4712.
375. Lee S, Clark SA, Gill RK, Christakos S. 1,25-dihydroxyvitamin D_3 and pancreatic β-cell function: vitamin D receptors, gene expression, and insulin secretion. *Endocrinology* 1994;34:1602–1610.
376. Lambillotte C, Gilon P, Henquin JC. Direct glucocorticoid inhibition of insulin secretion: an in vitro study of dexamethasone effects in mouse islets. *J Clin Invest* 1997;99:414–423.
377. Delaunay F, Khan A, Cintra A, et al. Pancreatic β cells are important targets for the diabetogenic effects of glucocorticoids. *J Clin Invest* 1997;100:2094–2098.

CHAPTER 7
Insulin Secretion In Vivo

Melissa K. Cavaghan and Kenneth S. Polonsky

The classic experiments of Von Mering and Minkowski at the turn of the last century demonstrating that pancreatectomy in dogs resulted in hyperglycemia (1) focused attention on the important role of the pancreas in maintaining glucose homeostasis *in vivo*. Banting and Best (2), by reversing this hyperglycemia with internal secretions of the pancreas, confirmed the belief that the islets of Langerhans were the key cells within the pancreas responsible for maintaining normal blood glucose levels. Although the isolation and purification of insulin rapidly followed, many years passed before sensitive techniques for evaluating β-cell function were devised. Because these techniques are critical to the analysis of insulin secretion *in vivo*, they will be discussed at the outset.

METHODS OF QUANTITATING β-CELL FUNCTION

The development of a sensitive radioimmunoassay for the measurement of insulin levels was the first major advance in our attempts to understand how the β-cell functions *in vivo* (3). For many years afterward, the measurement of peripheral levels of insulin was the gold standard used to evaluate β-cell secretory activity (4–8). This approach, however, is limited by the fact that 50% to 60% of the insulin produced by the pancreas is extracted by the liver without ever reaching the systemic circulation (9,10). While these problems can, in fact, be overcome by hepatic vein catheterization allied to intraportal infusion of insulin, these techniques can only be applied in an investigational setting and, even then, are only of value under steady-state conditions (11). The standard radioimmunoassay for the measurement of insulin concentrations is also limited by its inability to distinguish between endogenous and exogenous insulin, making it ineffective as a measure of endogenous β-cell reserve in the insulin-treated diabetic patient. The problem is further compounded by the development in many of these patients of antibodies to insulin, which interfere in the interpretation of serum levels of immunoreactive insulin. Although insulin-specific assays have been developed, another disadvantage of the conventional insulin radioimmunoassay is its inability to distinguish between levels of circulating proinsulin and true levels of circulating insulin.

Following the discovery of proinsulin, the single-chain precursor of insulin (12), and the identification of the biosynthetic pathway of insulin within the β-cell (13), β-cell secretory products in addition to insulin were found in the circulation. These included proinsulin, proinsulin conversion intermediates (split proinsulins), and connecting-peptide (C-peptide) (see Chapter 5). Within the islet cells, proinsulin undergoes cleavage at the Golgi apparatus (14), a reaction that leads to the formation of insulin, C-peptide, and two pairs of basic amino acids. Insulin is subsequently released into the circulation at concentrations equimolar to those of C-peptide (13–15). In addition, small amounts of intact proinsulin and proinsulin conversion intermediates are released. Although these molecules constitute 20% of the total circulating insulin-like immunoreactivity (16), they are much less potent than insulin biologically. It has been estimated that the biologic potency of proinsulin *in vivo* is only 10% of that of insulin (17,18), whereas the potency of split proinsulin is between that of proinsulin and insulin (19,20). The low concentrations of proinsulin and split proinsulins in serum, however, ensure that *in vivo*, under normal physiologic conditions, their effects are negligible. In contrast to insulin and proinsulin, C-peptide has no known conclusive effects on carbohydrate metabolism (21,22). It has recently been suggested that it may stimulate Na^+/K^+-ATPase and endothelial nitric oxide synthase activities, resulting in a number of biologic activities, including augmented blood flow in skeletal muscle and skin, diminished glomerular hyperfiltration, reduced urinary albumin excretion, and improved nerve function in patients with type 1 diabetes mellitus who lack C-peptide, but not in healthy subjects (23). It has therefore been proposed that replacement of C-peptide together with insulin may prevent or retard the progression of the long-term complications of diabetes mellitus (24,25). Unlike insulin, C-peptide is not extracted by the liver (10,26,27) and is excreted almost exclusively by the kidneys. Its plasma half-life of approximately 30 minutes (28) contrasts sharply with that of insulin, which is approximately 4 minutes.

Because C-peptide is secreted in equimolar concentrations with insulin and is not extracted by the liver, many investigators have used levels of C-peptide as a marker of β-cell function. While C-peptide levels are usually measured in plasma, C-peptide levels in urine have also been used to evaluate endogenous insulin secretion (29–32). This approach is limited, however, because the fraction of the secreted C-peptide that appears in the urine varies considerably among subjects and even in the same subject studied on different occasions (33). The use of plasma C-peptide levels as an index of β-cell function is dependent on the critical assumption that the mean clearance rates of C-peptide are constant over the range of C-peptide levels observed under normal physiologic conditions. This assumption has been shown to be valid for both dogs and humans (10,34), and this approach can be used to derive rates of insulin secretion from plasma concentrations of C-peptide under steady-state conditions (34). However, because of the long plasma half-life of C-peptide, under non–steady-state conditions (e.g., following a glucose infusion), peripheral plasma levels of C-peptide do not change in proportion to the changing insulin secretory rate (34,35). Thus, under these conditions, insulin secretion rates are best calculated with use of the two-compartment model initially proposed by Eaton and coworkers (36). This approach involves nonlinear least-squares regression analysis of C-peptide decay curves to derive model parameters in individual subjects. Once the fractional rate constants and distribution volume are known, the peripheral concentrations of C-peptide can be analyzed mathematically and the corresponding secretion rates derived. Estimates of the secretion rate of insulin in human subjects by this method are quite accurate—reportedly 98% ± 3% of the actual rate as rates of insulin secretion are increasing and 100% ± 2% as they are decreasing (34). Similar findings have been reported for dogs (37). Modifications to the C-peptide model of insulin secretion have recently been introduced. This approach combines the minimal model of insulin action with the two-compartment model of C-peptide kinetics and allows insulin secretion and insulin sensitivity to be derived following either the intravenous or the oral administration of glucose (38–41).

Rates of insulin secretion have also been measured by calculating the difference between arterial and hepatic venous C-peptide and by multiplying this difference by the estimated hepatic plasma flow (42,43), an approach designed to overcome the inherent difficulty of performing portal venous cannulation in humans. Rates of insulin secretion determined by this method are similar to those obtained with other methods, but the technique is invasive and by its nature can only be applied in an investigational setting.

In summary, under steady-state conditions, levels of C-peptide in whole plasma provide an accurate index of the insulin secretory rate, while under non–steady-state conditions, rates of β-cell secretion of insulin can be derived more accurately and easily from mathematical analysis of peripheral C-peptide concentrations with use of a two-compartment model. In interpreting the validity of experimental results evaluating insulin secretion *in vivo*, one should always take into account the limitations of the method used to assess β-cell function.

REGULATION OF INSULIN SECRETION

Carbohydrate Nutrients

The most important physiologic substance involved in the regulation of insulin release is glucose (44–46). The effect of glucose on the β-cell is dose-related. Dose-dependent increases in concentrations of insulin and C-peptide and in rates of insulin secretion have been observed following oral and intravenous glucose loads, with 1.4 units (~50 μg) of insulin, on average, being secreted in response to an oral glucose load as small as 12 g (42,47–49) (Fig. 7.1). The insulin secretory response is greater

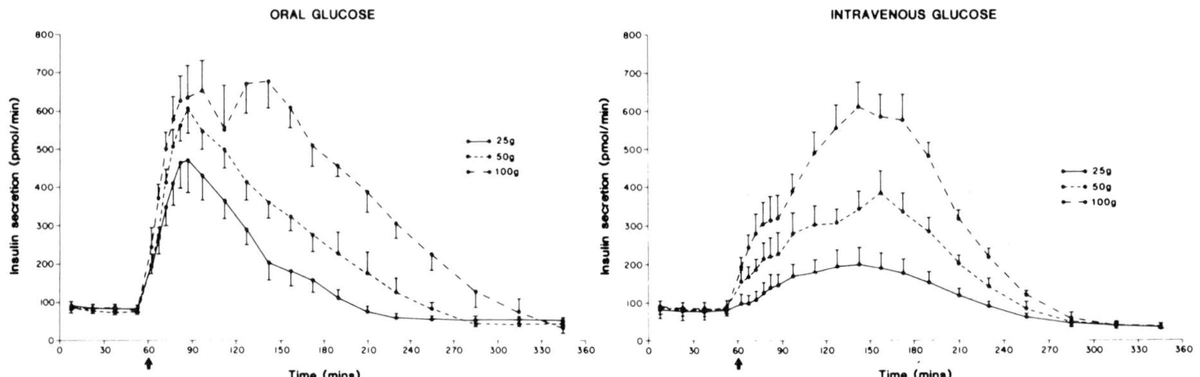

Figure 7.1. Insulin secretory responses to graded glucose doses following oral **(left)** and intravenous **(right)** administration. (From Tillil H, Shapiro ET, Miller MA, et al. Dose-dependent effects of oral and intravenous glucose on insulin secretion and clearance in normal humans. *Am J Physiol* 1988;254: E349–357, with permission. Copyright © 1988 by the American Physiological Society.)

after oral than intravenous glucose administration (49–52). Known as the incretin effect (48,53), this enhanced response to oral glucose has been interpreted as an indication that absorption of glucose by way of the gastrointestinal tract stimulates the release of hormones and other mechanisms that ultimately enhance the sensitivity of the β-cell to glucose (see discussion on hormonal factors below and Chapter 12). In a study involving nine normal volunteers who received a glucose infusion at a rate designed to achieve levels previously attained following an oral glucose load, the amount of insulin secreted in response to the intravenous load was 26% less than that secreted in response to the oral load (52).

Insulin secretion does not respond as a linear function of glucose concentration. The relationship of glucose concentration to the rate of insulin release follows a sigmoidal curve, with a threshold corresponding to the glucose levels normally seen under fasting conditions and with the steep portion of the dose-response curve corresponding to the range of glucose levels normally achieved postprandially (54–56). The sigmoidal nature of the dose-response curve has been attributed to a gaussian distribution of thresholds for stimulation among the individual β-cells (56–58).

When glucose is infused intravenously at a constant rate, an initial biphasic secretory response is observed that consists of a rapid, early insulin peak followed by a second, more slowly increasing, peak (44,59,60). The significance of the first-phase insulin release is unclear but may reflect the existence of a compartment of readily releasable insulin within the β-cell or a transient increase and decrease of a metabolic signal for insulin secretion (61). Despite early suggestions to the contrary (62,63), a subsequent study has demonstrated that the first-phase response to intravenous glucose is highly reproducible within subjects (64). Following the acute response, a second phase of insulin release occurs that is directly related to the level of glucose elevation. *In vitro* studies of isolated islet cells and the perfused pancreas have identified a third phase of insulin secretion commencing 1.5 to 3.0 hours after exposure to glucose and characterized by a spontaneous decline in secretion to 15% to 25% of the amount released during peak secretion—a level subsequently maintained for more than 48 hours (65–68).

The effects of a variety of other sugars, sugar derivatives, and sugar alcohols on the β-cell have also been examined (69). D-glucose, D-mannose, D-glyceraldehyde, dihydroxyacetone, D-glucosamine, *N*-acetylglucosamine, fructose, and galactose have all been shown to be stimulators or potentiators of insulin secretion *in vitro*. *In vivo* studies in dogs and humans suggest that xylitol and sorbitol also enhance β-cell function.

The insulin secretory response to glucose exhibits anomeric specificity, the α-anomer being a more potent stimulator of insulin release than the β-anomer (70). Similar results have been obtained with mannose (71). Because α-anomers are more readily metabolized by the glycolytic pathway than are β-anomers (72,73), it has been suggested that the metabolism of glucose and mannose within the β-cell is a prerequisite for the production of intracellular signals that trigger insulin release in response to these secretagogues. In support of this suggestion is the observation that mannoheptulose, an inhibitor of the glycolytic enzyme glucokinase, blocks the insulin secretory response to glucose. Similarly, iodoacetate, an inhibitor of glyceraldehyde dehydrogenase, blocks the β-cell response to hexoses (74).

Noncarbohydrate Nutrients

Amino acids have been shown to stimulate insulin release in the absence of glucose, the most potent secretagogues being the essential amino acids leucine, arginine, and lysine (75,76). The effects of arginine and lysine on the β-cell appear to be more potent than those of leucine. Although the effects of amino acids on insulin secretion are independent of concomitant changes in glucose levels, the effects are potentiated by glucose (76–78). The response of the islet cells to a series of amino acid metabolites has also been evaluated. Phenylpyruvate, α-ketoisocaproate, α-keto-β-methylvalerate, and α-ketocaproate are potent stimulators of insulin release, and most are effective in the absence of glucose (69,79).

In contrast to amino acids, various lipids and their metabolites appear to have only minor effects on insulin release *in vivo*. Although carbohydrate-rich fat meals stimulate insulin secretion, carbohydrate-free fat meals have minimal effects on β-cell function (80). Ketone bodies and short- and long-chain fatty acids have been shown to acutely stimulate insulin secretion both in isolated islet cells and in humans (81–85). The effects of elevated free fatty acids in the insulin secretory responses to glucose are related to the duration of the exposure. Zhou and Grill first suggested that long-term exposure of pancreatic islets to free fatty acids inhibited glucose-induced insulin secretion and biosynthesis (86). This observation has been confirmed in rats (87). In humans, it was demonstrated that the insulin resistance induced by an acute (90-minute) elevation in free fatty acids was compensated for by an appropriate increase in insulin secretion (88). Following chronic elevation of free fatty acids (48 hours), the β-cell compensatory response for insulin resistance was not adequate. Additional studies have demonstrated that the adverse effects of prolonged elevations in free fatty acids on glucose-induced insulin secretion are not seen in individuals with type 2 diabetes. On the basis of these results, it appears that elevated free fatty acids may contribute to the failure of β-cell compensation for insulin resistance.

Hormonal Factors

The release of insulin from the β-cell following a meal is facilitated by a number of gastrointestinal peptide hormones, including glucose-dependent insulinotropic peptide (GIP), cholecystokinin, and glucagon-like peptide-1 (GLP-1) (53,89–96) (see Chapter 12). These hormones are released from intestinal endocrine cells postprandially and travel in the bloodstream to reach the β-cells, where they act through second messengers to increase the sensitivity of these islet cells to glucose. In general, these hormones are not of themselves secretagogues, and their effects are only evident in the presence of hyperglycemia (89–91). The release of these peptides may explain why the modest postprandial glucose levels achieved in normal subjects *in vivo* have such a dramatic effect on insulin production whereas similar glucose concentrations *in vitro* elicit a much smaller response (96). Similarly, this so-called incretin effect could account for the greater β-cell response observed following oral as opposed to intravenous glucose administration. Whether impaired postprandial secretion of incretin hormones plays a role in the inadequate insulin secretory response to oral glucose and to meals in impaired glucose tolerance (IGT) or diabetes mellitus is controversial (97–104), but pharmacologic doses of these peptides may have future therapeutic benefits. Subcutaneous administration of GLP-1, the most potent of the incretin peptides, lowers glucose levels in patients with type 2 diabetes by stimulating endogenous insulin secretion and perhaps by inhibiting glucagon secretion and gastric emptying (105,106). Because of the short half-life of GLP-1, however, its longer-acting analogue, exendin-4, has greater therapeutic promise (107). Treatment with supraphysiologic doses of GIP during hyperglycemia has been shown to augment insulin secretion in normal (108,109) but not in diabetic humans

(100,109). Although cholecystokinin has the ability to augment insulin secretion in humans, whether it is an incretin at physiologic levels has not been firmly established (110–113). Its effects are also seen largely at pharmacologic doses (114).

The postprandial insulin secretory response may also be influenced by other intestinal peptide hormones, including vasoactive intestinal polypeptide (115), secretin (116–119), and gastrin (116,120), but the precise role of these hormones remains to be elucidated.

The hormones produced by pancreatic α- and β-cells also modulate insulin release. While glucagon has a stimulatory effect on the β-cell (121), somatostatin suppresses insulin release (122). It is currently unclear whether these hormones reach the β-cell by traveling through the islet-cell interstitium (thus exerting a paracrine effect) or through islet-cell capillaries. Indeed, the importance of these two hormones in regulating basal and postprandial insulin levels under normal physiologic circumstances is in doubt. Other hormones that exert a stimulatory role on insulin secretion include growth hormone (123), glucocorticoids (124), prolactin (125–127), placental lactogen (128), and the sex steroids (129). While all of the above hormones may stimulate insulin secretion indirectly by inducing a state of insulin resistance, some also may act directly on the β-cell, possibly to augment its sensitivity to glucose. Thus, hyperinsulinemia is associated with conditions in which these hormones are present in excess, such as acromegaly, Cushing syndrome, and the second half of pregnancy. Furthermore, treatment with placental lactogen (130), hydrocortisone (131), or growth hormone (131,132) is effective in reversing the reduction in insulin response to glucose that is observed *in vitro* after hypophysectomy. Although hyperinsulinemia following an oral glucose load has been observed in patients with hyperthyroidism (133,134), the increased concentration of immunoreactive insulin in this setting may reflect elevations in serum proinsulin rather than a true increase in serum insulin (135).

Neural Factors

The islets are innervated by both the cholinergic and adrenergic limbs of the autonomic nervous system. While both sympathetic and parasympathetic stimulation enhance secretion of glucagon (136,137), the secretion of insulin is stimulated by vagal nerve fibers and inhibited by sympathetic nerve fibers (136–141). Adrenergic inhibition of the β-cell appears to be mediated by the α-adrenoceptor, since its effect is attenuated by the α-antagonist phentolamine (137) and reproduced by the α_2-agonist clonidine (142). There is also considerable evidence that many indirect effects of sympathetic nerve stimulation play a role in regulation of β-cell function via stimulation or inhibition of somatostatin, β_2 adrenoceptors, and the neuropeptides galanin and neuropeptide Y (143). Parasympathetic stimulation of islets results in stimulation of insulin, glucagon, and pancreatic polypeptide directly and via neuropeptides vasoactive intestinal peptide, gastrin-releasing polypeptide, and pituitary adenylate cyclase–activating polypeptide (143). In addition, sensory innervation of islets may contribute to the regulation of insulin secretion. Sensory nerves have been shown to contain calcitonin gene–related peptide (144–146), which may play a inhibitory role, and substance P, whose role is not clearly defined (147,148). The importance of the autonomic nervous system in regulating insulin secretion *in vivo* is unclear. Studies in animals (149,150) and humans (151,152) have emphasized the importance of the cephalic phase of insulin release—that occurring at the sight, smell, and expectation of food—in regulating the postprandial glucose response. It has been suggested that this reflex, which is under vagal control (96,153), may have a key role in minimizing the early increase in glucose levels following meals (152). Because cholinergic agonists increase the response of the β-cell to glucose *in vitro* (154), this may be the mechanism by which vagal stimulation achieves its effect. Decreased glucose tolerance following vagotomy has been reported in human subjects (155,156) and following islet denervation in rats (157,158), whereas the insulin secretory response to meals is delayed in patients who have undergone pancreatic transplantation (159). However, many of these patients remain euglycemic without therapy after transplantation (159–162). Therefore, the importance of the parasympathetic nervous system in maintaining glucose tolerance is unclear. For similar reasons, doubts exist about whether the sympathetic nerve fibers innervating the islets exert a major influence on the basal or postprandial insulin secretory responses. Sympathetic innervation of islets likely accounts for the inhibition of insulin secretion and increased glucagon secretion during exercise and in response to hypoglycemia (163–166). Similarly, inhibition of insulin secretion mediated by the sympathetic nervous system may account in part for the deteriorating glycemic control reported in individuals with diabetes mellitus who are under severe stress (138,167). The relative contributions of the sympathetic and parasympathetic innervation of the pancreas to the hyperinsulinemia of obesity have been studied, but no consistent differences from lean subjects have been found (168–172).

The neural effects on β-cell function cannot be entirely dissociated from the hormonal effects, since some of the neurotransmitters of the autonomic nervous system are in fact hormones. Furthermore, the secretion of insulinotropic hormones such as GIP and GLP-1 postprandially has been shown to be under vagal (173,174) and adrenergic (175,176) control.

TEMPORAL PATTERN OF INSULIN SECRETION

It has been estimated that, in any 24-hour period, 50% of the total insulin secreted by the pancreas is secreted under basal conditions, and the remainder is secreted in response to meals (177,178). The estimated basal insulin secretion rates typically range from 18 to 32 units per 24 hours (0.7 to 1.3 mg) (34,36,42, 177). Moreover, the secretion of insulin is pulsatile, with major pulses being observed every 1.5 to 2 hours (178–182) (Fig. 7.2). These ultradian pulses are present in the basal state but are amplified postprandially (178,179). These pulses have also been observed in subjects receiving glucose intravenously (180,182), suggesting that they are not dependent on food ingestion and are not generated by intermittent absorption of nutrients from the gut. Furthermore, they do not appear to be related to fluctuations in glucagon or cortisol levels (180). Many of these insulin and C-peptide pulses are synchronous with pulses in glucose levels (178,180,182). The ability of an exogenous oscillatory glucose infusion to entrain these pulses in insulin secretion has been shown to indicate normal β-cell function (see Fig. 7.9) (183–185). Experimental evidence from studies of animals and humans suggests that superimposed on these large-amplitude ultradian pulses are more rapid oscillations in β-cell activity that occur at a periodicity of 8 to 16 minutes (186–192). These rapid oscillations in insulin and C-peptide levels do not appear to be coupled as tightly as the ultradian pulses to changes in glucose levels (189,191,193,194). The frequency of these rapid oscillations varies from study to study, and wide variability among subjects is seen even within studies. Accordingly, the physiologic significance of these rapid oscillations in the peripheral circulation is unclear. Although the amplitude of the rapid oscillations is very low in the peripheral circulation, it is much greater in the portal circulation (Fig. 7.3), where these

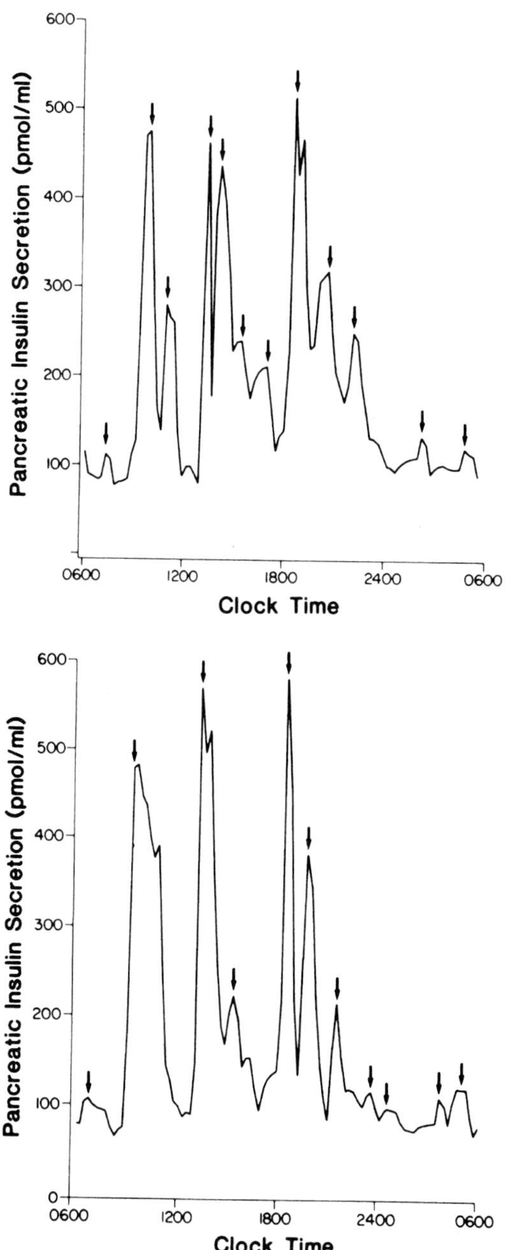

Figure 7.2. Two 24-hour profiles of insulin secretion from normal-weight subjects. Meals were eaten at 0900, 1300, and 1800. Statistically significant pulses of secretion are shown by the arrows. (From Polonsky KS, Given BD, Van Cauter E. Twenty-four-hour profiles and pulsatile patterns of insulin secretion in normal and obese subjects. *J Clin Invest* 1988;81: 442–448, with permission.)

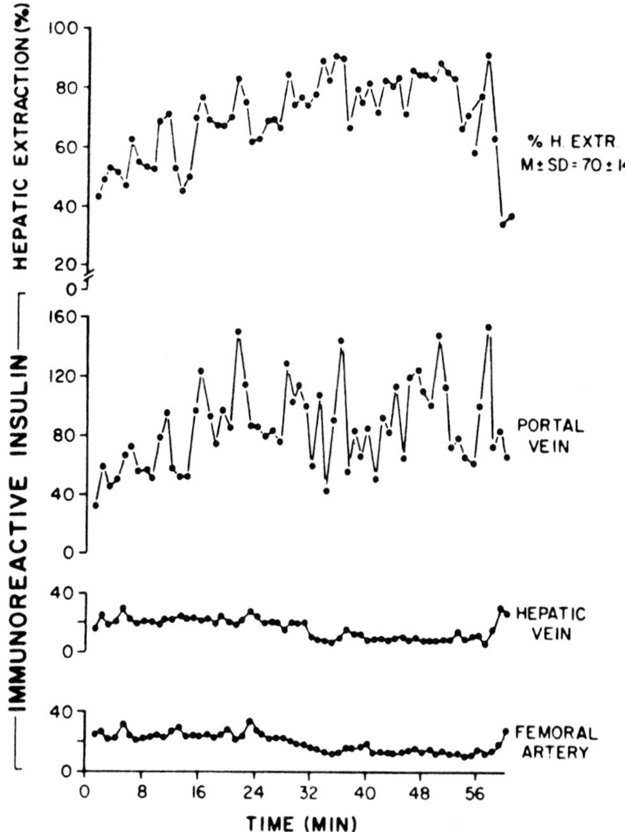

Figure 7.3. Simultaneous minute-to-minute insulin levels in portal vein, hepatic vein, femoral artery, and derived hepatic insulin extraction in one dog. Because of substantial hepatic extraction of insulin, pulsatility in posthepatic circulation is markedly dampened. (From Jaspan JB, Lever E, Polonsky KS, Van Cauter E. In vivo pulsatility of pancreatic islet peptides. *Am J Physiol* 1986;251:E215–E226, with permission. Copyright © 1986 by the American Physiological Society.)

rapid oscillations may have an important biologic function (194). In this regard, it is possible that the liver responds more favorably to insulin delivered in a pulsatile fashion than to insulin delivered at a constant rate (195–197).

Circadian variations in the secretion of insulin have also been reported. When insulin secretory responses are measured during a 24-hour period during which subjects receive three standard meals, the maximal postprandial responses are observed after breakfast (6,178,198). These findings are mirrored by the results of studies in which subjects were tested for oral glucose tolerance at different times of the day and were found to exhibit maximal insulin secretory responses in the morning and lower responses in the afternoon and evening (199–201). These diurnal differences also are noted in tests for intravenous glucose tolerance. Furthermore, although ultradian glucose and insulin oscillations are closely correlated during a constant 24-hour glucose infusion, the nocturnal rise in mean glucose levels is not accompanied by a similar increase in the insulin secretory rate (182). It has been postulated that these diurnal differences may reflect a diminished responsiveness of the β-cell to glucose in the afternoon and evening (201).

INSULIN SECRETION FOLLOWING EXERCISE

The effects of exercise on β-cell function have also been evaluated extensively. Individuals who exercise regularly have reduced fasting levels of insulin and C-peptide (202–204) and also exhibit a reduction in the release of these hormones following a carbohydrate load. This reduction has been seen following a 100-g oral glucose load (205,206) and during hyperglycemic clamping, during which reductions in both first-phase and second-phase secretory responses have been described (202–204,207). Despite these changes, these subjects have normal or even improved glucose tolerance (203,207), consistent with the observation that insulin sensitivity is improved in those who exercise regularly as measured during hyperinsulinemic euglycemic clamping (203,207).

Altered β-cell responses to glucose are apparent even after short periods of exercise and have been observed in individuals subjected to as little as 1 hour of exercise 24 hours before being tested for oral glucose tolerance (208). Similarly, even in well-trained athletes, insulin responses to glucose increase dramatically within 2 weeks of cessation of exercise (202). In this latter study, rates of glucose disposal both before and after cessation of exercise were similar, supporting the view that those who exercise regularly are more sensitive to the action of insulin. The altered β-cell responses to glucose observed in athletic subjects may therefore be a compensatory response to the increased sensitivity to insulin in the periphery. Whatever the mechanism, lack of exercise could be a key factor in the pathogenesis of the insulin resistance associated with aging, because fasting insulin levels and insulin secretory responses to glucose in athletes older and younger than 60 years are similar, the responses in both groups being lower than the corresponding responses in young untrained subjects (205).

INSULIN SECRETION IN THE ELDERLY

Peripheral insulin resistance, impaired glucose tolerance, and postprandial hyperinsulinemia are metabolic changes associated with aging (209–211). Although insulin secretion may be reduced in aging rats (212–214), the results of studies of elderly human subjects have conflicted—with increased, normal, and decreased β-cell responses having been reported (215–217). These discrepancies may be, in part, a reflection of the indirect methods used to quantitate insulin secretion in some of these studies. In experiments that used a direct approach to quantitation of insulin secretory rates from peripheral C-peptide levels by means of the two-compartment model (36), ten elderly subjects demonstrated enhanced insulin secretion under basal conditions, with an accentuation of this response seen postprandially (218). Plotted as a percentage of the basal secretory rate, the secretory response to meals in these elderly subjects was no different from that of younger controls. However, when glucose levels are matched during hyperglycemic clamping, the insulin secretory response—although normal in absolute terms—is disproportionately low in the elderly patients, especially when viewed in relation to the degree of insulin resistance associated with aging. Thus, while elderly subjects have enhanced rates of insulin secretion, the β-cell responses are lower than those predicted when one takes into account the insulin insensitivity associated with this population subgroup. Diminished insulin clearance does not appear to be a contributory factor to the observed hyperinsulinemia in the elderly (218,219).

INSULIN SECRETION IN OBESITY AND INSULIN RESISTANCE

The insulin resistance of obesity is characterized by hyperinsulinemia (220–224). Hyperinsulinemia in this setting reflects a combination of increased insulin production (222,225) and decreased insulin clearance (222–226), but most evidence suggests that increased insulin secretion is the predominant factor (227,228). Both basal and 24-hour insulin secretory rates are three to four times higher in obese subjects and are strongly correlated with body mass index. Insulin secretory responses to intravenous glucose have been studied in otherwise healthy insulin-resistant subjects in comparison to insulin-sensitive subjects by means of a graded glucose infusion (228,229). Figure 7.4 depicts insulin concentrations and insulin secretion rates at each level of plasma glucose achieved, thereby constructing a glucose-insulin or glucose-insulin secretion rate dose-response relationship. Both insulin concentrations and insulin secretion rates are increased in insulin-resistant subjects, resulting from a combination of increased insulin secretion and decreased insulin clearance. For each level of glucose, insulin secretion rates are higher in the insulin-resistant subjects, reflecting an adaptive response of the β-cell to peripheral insulin resistance. Similar compensatory hyperinsulinemia has been demonstrated with other clinical techniques, such as the frequently sampled intravenous glucose tolerance test in obesity and other insulin-resistant states such as late pregnancy (230,231).

The temporal pattern of insulin secretion is unaltered in obese subjects as compared with normal subjects. In the obese, basal insulin secretion accounts for 50% of the total daily production of insulin and secretory pulses of insulin occur every 1.5 to 2 hours (178,227). However, the amplitude of these pulses postprandially is greater in obese subjects. Nevertheless, when these postprandial secretory responses are expressed as a percentage of the basal secretory rate, the postprandial responses in obese and normal subjects are identical (Fig. 7.5). These findings suggest that

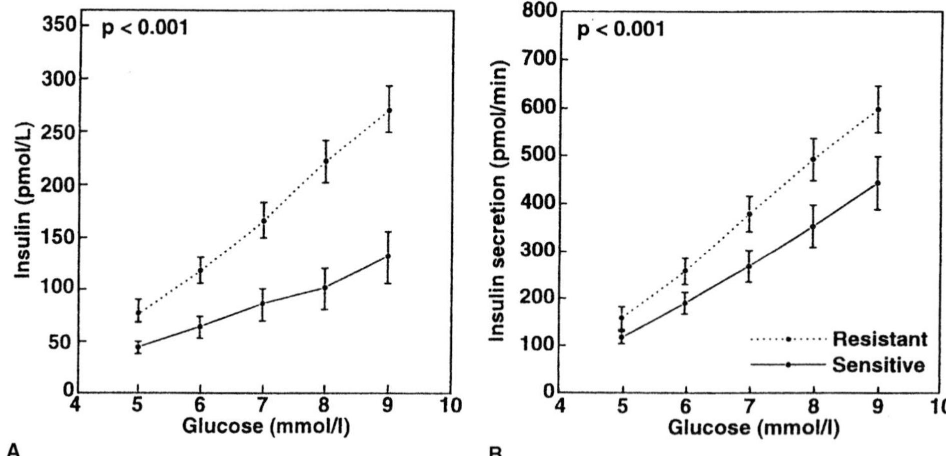

Figure 7.4. Plasma insulin concentrations **(A)** and insulin secretion rates **(B)** in response to molar increments in the plasma glucose concentration during the graded glucose infusion in the insulin-resistant *(dashed line)* and insulin-sensitive *(solid line)* groups. (From Jones CNO, Pei D, Staris P, Polonsky KS, Chen YDI, Reaven GM. Alterations in the glucose-stimulated insulin secretory dose-response curve and in insulin clearance in nondiabetic insulin-resistant individuals. *J Clin Endocrinol Metab* 1997;82: 1834–1838, with permission. Copyright 1997. The Endocrine Society.)

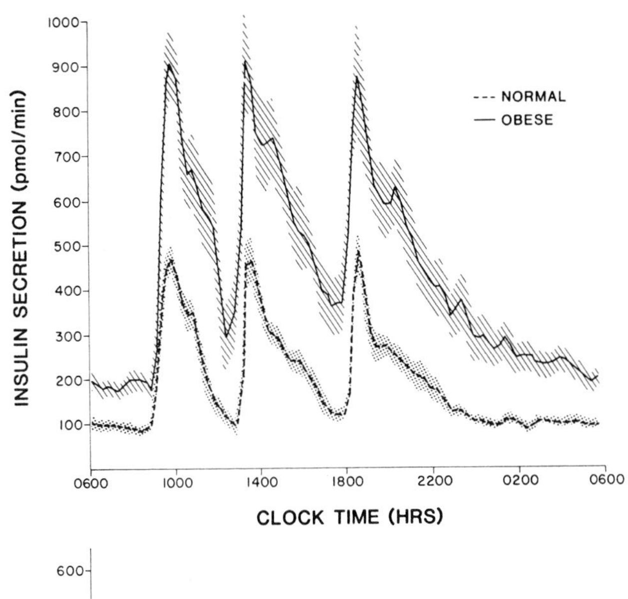

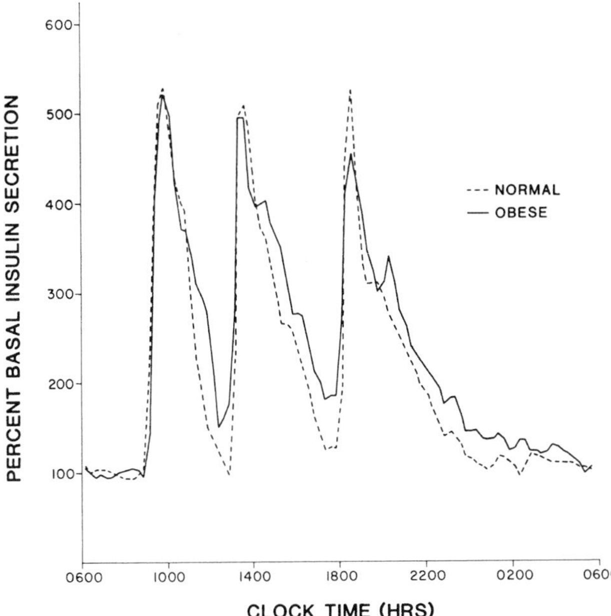

Figure 7.5. Mean 24-hour profiles of insulin secretion rates in normal and obese subjects *(top)*. The hatched areas represent ± SEM. The curves in the lower panel were derived by dividing the insulin secretion rate measured in each subject by the basal secretion rate derived in the same subject. Mean data for normal and obese subjects are shown. (From Polonsky KS, Given BD, Van Cauter E. Twenty-four-hour profiles and pulsatile patterns of insulin secretion in normal and obese subjects. *J Clin Invest* 1988;81:442–448, with permission from the American Society of Clinical Investigation.)

the increase in insulin secretion in the obese is due not to a hyperresponsiveness to secretory stimuli but rather to the presence of an abnormally large functional β-cell mass. This suggestion is consistent with both the earlier pathologic observations of Ogilvie, who described an increased number of islet cells in obese subjects (232), and with animal studies, which confirm the presence of a compensatory increase in β-cell mass in obese insulin-resistant fatty rats that maintain normal glucose tolerance (233). Rapid oscillations in insulin secretion that occur every 10 to 12 minutes and are similar to those in nonobese subjects have also been found in obese patients, although of an amplitude that tended to be lower than that of the corresponding pulses in the nonobese (191). It appears, therefore, that the normal regulatory mechanisms controlling insulin secretion in nonobese controls are also operative in hyperinsulinemic obese subjects and that β-cell function is intrinsically normal in this setting.

INSULIN SECRETION IN TYPE 2 DIABETES MELLITUS

Owing to the common finding of obesity and insulin resistance in type 2 diabetes mellitus, these patients are often hyperinsulinemic but have a degree of hyperinsulinemia inappropriately low for the prevailing glucose concentrations. Nevertheless, many of these patients have sufficient β-cell reserve to maintain a euglycemic state by dietary restriction with or without therapy with an oral agent. It is generally agreed that defects in the β-cell superimposed on a background of insulin resistance converge to cause type 2 diabetes (234–238). In an animal model of type 2 diabetes mellitus, in which obesity, insulin resistance, and hyperinsulinemia are present before the inevitable development of diabetes mellitus, inadequate expansion of β-cell mass is implicated as a significant causative factor (233). Autopsy studies in diabetic humans are consistent with this observation (239–241). Alterations in β-cell gene expression also may play a role (242). Clinically, these patients demonstrate virtually absent first-phase insulin and C-peptide responses to intravenous glucose, a reduced second-phase response (77, 243–246) (Fig. 7.6), and marked flattening of the glucose-insulin secretion dose-response curve (184). This attenuated β-cell response is not confined to glucose; diminished responses to nonglucose secretagogues such as arginine and isoproterenol have also been observed, although the reduction is of a lesser magnitude (77,243). *In vitro* studies using the isolated perfused pancreas have emphasized the importance of hyperglycemia in the mediation of these changes (247,248). However, the abnormal first-phase response to intravenous glucose persists in patients whose diabetic control has been markedly improved (243,244), further supporting the presence of an intrinsic defect in the β-cell in patients with type 2 diabetes mellitus.

Many studies have examined the effects of type 2 diabetes mellitus on levels of proinsulin in serum. These studies have consistently demonstrated elevated levels of proinsulin in association with increases in the molar ratio of proinsulin to insulin (249–254), suggesting that the β-cells of patients with type 2 diabetes mellitus release an excess of immature secretory granules into the circulation. The amount of proinsulin produced in these patients appears to be related to the degree of glycemic control rather than to the duration of the diabetic state. In one series, proinsulin levels contributed almost 50% of the total insulin immunoreactivity in patients with type 2 diabetes mellitus who had marked hyperglycemia (254). Because conventional assays of levels of immunoreactive insulin also measure levels of proinsulin (253), it is possible that the hyperinsulinemia reported in many studies of patients with type 2 diabetes mellitus to some degree represents hyperproinsulinemia rather than true hyperinsulinemia. In support of this view, studies using a sensitive insulin assay that did not cross-react with proinsulin report that insulin levels in both obese and nonobese patients with type 2 diabetes mellitus are lower than those in weight-matched control subjects, although when insulin levels are measured with a conventional insulin assay, differences between patients with diabetes mellitus and control subjects are less apparent (253–255). Furthermore, patients with diabetes in one series had elevated levels of both circulating proinsulin and 32-33 split proinsulin (a proinsulin conversion intermediate molecule) (253).

Abnormalities in the temporal pattern of insulin secretion in patients with type 2 diabetes mellitus have also been demonstrated. In contrast to normal subjects, who secrete equal

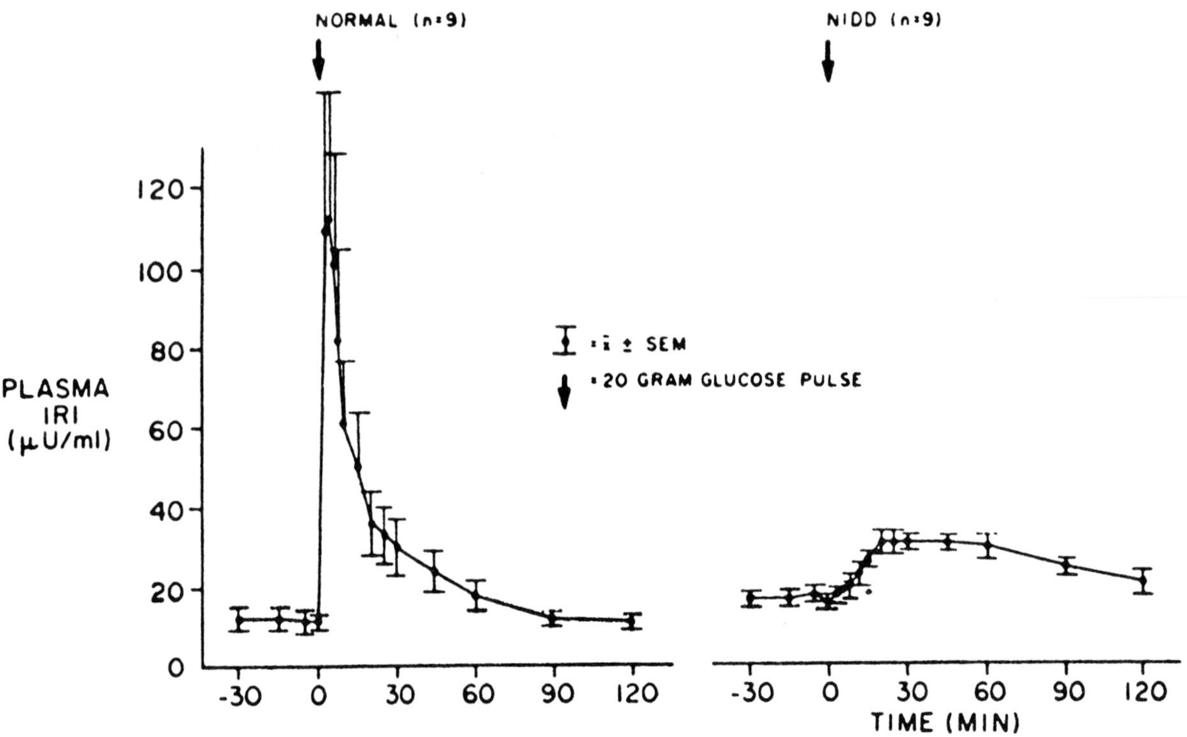

Figure 7.6. Insulin release in response to the intravenous administration of glucose in normal subjects and in patients with non–insulin-dependent diabetes mellitus. Note the lack of first-phase insulin response in the diabetic subjects. (From Pfeifer MA, Halter JB, Porte D Jr. Insulin secretion in diabetes mellitus. *Am J Med* 1981;70:579–588. Copyright 1981 with permission from Elsevier Science.)

amounts of insulin basally and postprandially in a given 24-hour period, patients with type 2 diabetes mellitus secrete a greater proportion of their daily insulin under basal conditions (256). This reduction in the proportion of insulin secreted postprandially appears to be related in part to a reduction in the amplitude of the secretory pulses of insulin that occur after meals rather than to a reduction in the number of pulses. The rapid oscillatory pattern of insulin production by the β-cells is also altered in patients with type 2 diabetes mellitus, who exhibit cycles that are shorter and more irregular than the persistent, regular, rapid oscillations present in healthy subjects (189). The slower ultradian oscillations of insulin secretion described above, which are "entrainable" by exogenous oscillatory glucose infusion in normal subjects, are severely disrupted in diabetic patients, with a nearly complete lack of coordination between pulses of glucose and insulin secretion (257). The effects of therapy on β-cell function in patients with type 2 diabetes mellitus have also been investigated. While interpretation of the results frequently is limited because β-cell function was not always studied at comparable glucose levels before and during therapy (258), the majority of the studies indicate that improvements in diabetic control are associated with an enhancement of β-cell secretory activity (244,259–263). This increased endogenous production of insulin appears to be independent of the mode of treatment and shows a particular association with increases in the amount of insulin secreted postprandially (244,263). The enhanced β-cell secretory activity following meals reflects an increase in the amplitude of existing secretory pulses rather than an increased number of pulses (263). Despite improvements in glycemic control, β-cell function is not normalized with therapy (244,261,263), suggesting that

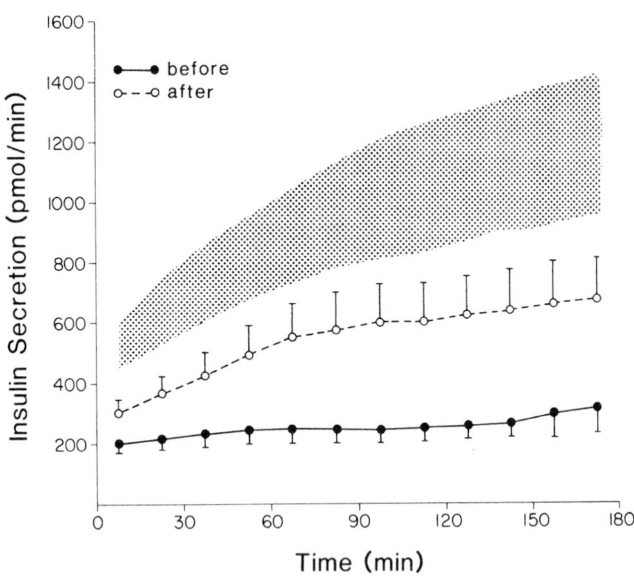

Figure 7.7. Insulin secretion rates (± SEM) during hyperglycemic clamping at 300 mg/dL (16.7 mmol/L) in patients with non–insulin-dependent diabetes mellitus before and during therapy with glyburide. The shaded area represents the secretion rates (± SEM) in a group of nondiabetic subjects. (From Shapiro ET, Van Cauter E, Tillil H, et al. Glyburide enhances the responsiveness of the β-cell to glucose but does not correct the abnormal patterns of insulin secretion in noninsulin-dependent diabetes mellitus. *J Clin Endocrinol Metab* 1989;569:571–576, with permission. Copyright 1989. The Endocrine Society.)

there may be a persistent intrinsic defect in the β-cell in patients with type 2 diabetes mellitus (Fig. 7.7).

INSULIN SECRETION IN IMPAIRED GLUCOSE TOLERANCE

Insulin secretion in subjects with IGT (2-hour glucose >140 mg/dL or 7.8 mmol/L after oral glucose challenge) has been studied to determine at what point measurable defects in β-cell function occur in the deterioration of glucose tolerance. When insulin responses to oral glucose or meals are measured over a range of glucose tolerance, they are found to be highest in subjects with IGT as compared with weight-matched glucose-tolerant controls and diabetic subjects (264). Despite elevated absolute insulin and insulin secretion in IGT, early defects in β-cell function intermediate between normal and diabetic subjects are observed, suggesting that IGT is truly a "prediabetic" state. Detailed study of insulin secretion in patients with IGT has demonstrated consistent quantitative and qualitative defects in this group. During oral glucose tolerance testing, there is a delay in the peak insulin response (265–267). The glucose-insulin secretion dose-response relationship is flattened and shifted to the right (Fig. 7.8), and first-phase insulin responses to an intravenous glucose bolus are consistently decreased in relationship to ambient insulin sensitivity (184,268). Further, there are abnormalities in first-phase insulin secretion in first-degree relatives of patients with type 2 diabetes mellitus who exhibit only mild intolerance to glucose (269) and an attenuated insulin response to oral glucose in normoglycemic co-twins of patients with type 2 diabetes mellitus (270). This pattern of insulin secretion during the so-called prediabetic phase also is seen in subjects with IGT in whom type 2 diabetes develops later (78,271,272) and in normoglycemic obese subjects with a recent history of gestational diabetes mellitus (273), another group at high risk for type 2 diabetes mellitus (274). Abnormalities in β-cells may therefore precede the development of overt type 2 diabetes mellitus by many years.

The temporal pattern of insulin secretory responses is altered in IGT in a manner similar to but not as pronounced as that seen

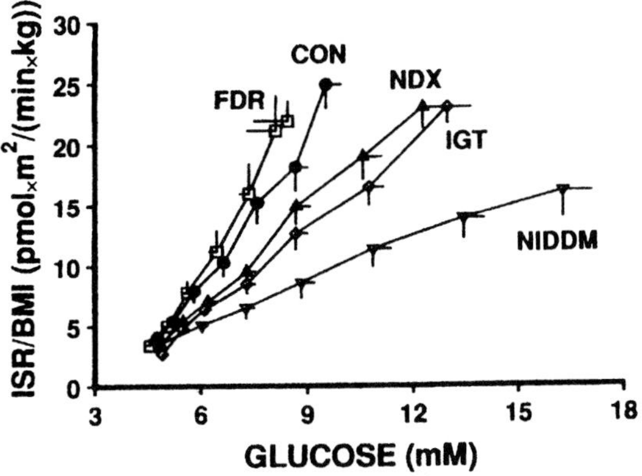

Figure 7.8. Dose-response relationships between glucose and insulin secretory rate (ISR) after an overnight fast in control subjects (CON; *filled circles*), normoglycemic subjects with family history of non–insulin-dependent diabetes mellitus (FDR, first-degree relative; *open squares*), subjects with a nondiagnostic oral glucose tolerance test (NDX; *filled triangles*), subjects with impaired glucose tolerance (IGT; *filled diamonds*), and subjects with non–insulin-dependent diabetes mellitus (NIDDM; *inverted triangles*). BMI, body mass index. (From Byrne MM, Sturis J, Sobel RJ, Polonsky KS. Elevated plasma glucose 2 h postchallenge predicts defects in β-cell function. *Am J Physiol* 1996;270:E572–E579, with permission. Copyright © 1996 by the American Physiological Society.)

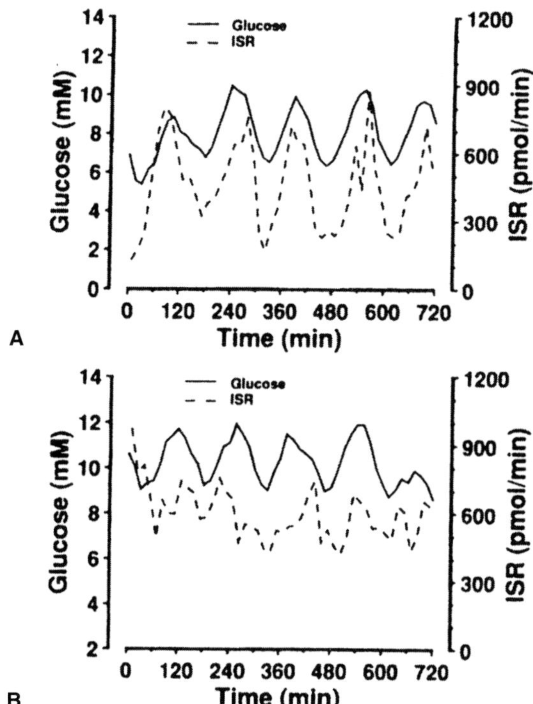

Figure 7.9. Individual glucose and insulin secretion rate (ISR) profiles during oscillatory glucose infusion in a control subject with normal glucose tolerance **(A)** and in a subject with impaired glucose tolerance **(B)**. Note the discordance between glucose and ISR in the subject with impaired glucose tolerance. (From Byrne MM, Sturis J, Sobel RJ, Polonsky KS. Elevated plasma glucose 2 h postchallenge predicts defects in β-cell function. *Am J Physiol* 1996;270:E572–E579, with permission. Copyright © 1996 by the American Physiological Society.)

in diabetic subjects described previously. There is a loss of coordinated insulin secretory responses during oscillatory glucose infusion, indicating that the ability of the β-cell to appropriately sense and respond to parallel changes in the plasma glucose level is impaired (Fig 7.9) (185). Abnormalities in rapid oscillations of insulin secretion have also been observed in first-degree relatives of patients with type 2 diabetes mellitus who have only mild glucose intolerance (275), further evidence suggesting that abnormalities in temporal pattern of β-cell function may be an early manifestation of β-cell dysfunction preceding the development of type 2 diabetes mellitus. Because an increase in serum proinsulin is seen in subjects with diabetes mellitus, the contribution of proinsulin to the hyperinsulinemia of IGT has been questioned. The hyperinsulinemia of IGT has not been found to be accounted for by an increase in proinsulin, although elevations in fasting and stimulated proinsulin or proinsulin/insulin ratios have been found by many, although not all, investigators (252,254,264, 276–278). Correlation of increased proinsulin levels in IGT as a predictor of future conversion to diabetes mellitus has also been observed (279–281).

INSULIN SECRETION IN TYPE 1 DIABETES MELLITUS

In contrast to patients with type 2 diabetes, patients with type 1 diabetes mellitus are insulin-deficient and have practically no β-cell response to glucose and nonglucose stimuli (243). However, the initial period following diagnosis often is associated with an improvement in glucose tolerance to a degree permitting the maintenance of normoglycemia for a self-limiting duration in some patients in the absence of any definitive therapy (282). This so-called honeymoon period is associated with increases in the C-peptide and insulin responses to glucose (8,283–286). Although the secretory capacity of β-cells is improved during this period, it is still less than that observed in healthy subjects. A qualitative defect also is present and is manifested in serum by an increased molar ratio of proinsulin to C-peptide (287–289). Thus, during the honeymoon phase, in addition to secreting less insulin, the pancreas releases greater quantities of immature β-cell granules into the circulation. The subsequent and inevitable deterioration in glycemic control that heralds the end of the honeymoon period is preceded by a gradual reduction in the secretory capacity of the β-cell (8). The assessment of β-cell function in patients with recently diagnosed type 1 diabetes mellitus may be of clinical relevance, in view of the evidence suggesting that the degree of residual β-cell function at this stage is an important prognostic indicator of which patients are most likely to benefit from a period of immunosuppression (290–292).

The β-cell secretory responses during the period before the onset of type 1 diabetes mellitus are also of interest. Studies in normoglycemic, islet cell antibody–positive monozygotic twins in which one twin is already insulinopenic have demonstrated a progressive diminution in the first-phase insulin response to glucose over a number of years before the development of overt diabetes mellitus (293). During this "early" diabetic phase, the β-cell response to other secretagogues, including arginine, tolbutamide, and glucagon, is also impaired, but to a much smaller extent (239). In the future, this identification of β-cell dysfunction in response to intravenous glucose in those at high risk for the development of type 1 diabetes mellitus some years before clinical onset may be of value therapeutically in preventing the onset of type 1 diabetes mellitus in susceptible individuals. Several trials have been designed to determine whether type 1 diabetes mellitus can be prevented in predisposed individuals. The European Nicotinamide Diabetes Intervention Trial (ENDIT) involves the random allocation of patients with type 1 diabetes mellitus to nicotinamide or placebo (294). In the United States, the Diabetes Prevention Trial (DPT-1) (295) recently demonstrated that low-dose parenteral insulin administration failed to delay the onset or progression of type 1 diabetes mellitus.

A number of studies evaluating β-cell function in the transplanted pancreas have been performed (159–162,296,297). Because many of those patients who have undergone pancreatic transplantation remain euglycemic without therapy during the posttransplantation period, the β-cell appears to be functional despite denervation. However, marked alterations in the temporal pattern of insulin secretion have been reported. Although the overall daily number of insulin secretory pulses is not altered following transplantation, basal insulin secretion accounts for up to 75% of the total insulin produced by these patients in a given 24-hour period. Postprandial insulin responses are therefore markedly attenuated (160). Detailed analysis of these postprandial secretory pulses suggests that they are both reduced in amplitude and occur later after meals. This latter factor supports the view that the cephalic phase of insulin secretion mediated by the vagus is an important component of the prompt insulin response to meals usually observed in normal subjects (96,152). In addition to quantitative abnormalities in insulin secretion, qualitative defects in the transplanted β-cell have also been reported, with increased ratios of proinsulin to C-peptide under fasting conditions and a further accentuation of these abnormalities in the postprandial period (161).

INSULIN SECRETION IN PATIENTS WITH INSULINOMA

In the diagnosis of insulinoma, a detailed knowledge and a correct interpretation of the β-cell secretory responses are critical. In distinguishing hypoglycemia caused by an islet cell tumor from hypoglycemia caused by other factors, the measurement of plasma levels of insulin alone may not be sufficient. Under normal physiologic circumstances, β-cell secretion is reduced as glucose levels fall. The hypoglycemia seen in patients with an insulinoma, however, is characterized by low glucose levels with inappropriate levels of insulin (which may be normal or elevated) (298,299). Although hypoglycemia induced by the surreptitious administration of insulin may also be associated with hyperinsulinemia, C-peptide levels will be elevated in patients with an insulinoma whereas administration of exogenous insulin usually suppresses the release of C-peptide from the β-cell (300). Moreover, patients with an insulinoma release a greater proportion of proinsulin into the circulation (301,302). This latter factor could prove to be important in distinguishing patients with an insulinoma from those rare patients with hypoglycemia caused by surreptitious ingestion of oral hypoglycemic agents. Thus, the simultaneous measurement of proinsulin, insulin, and C-peptide levels can be of value in excluding or confirming the presence of an insulinoma in patients who present with hypoglycemia.

EFFECT OF DRUGS ON INSULIN SECRETION

Many pharmacologic agents other than hypoglycemic agents alter insulin secretion *in vivo*. In many instances, the effects of these agents on insulin secretion are associated with a deterioration in glucose tolerance. Some of these agents (e.g., phenytoin, verapamil, diazoxide, pentamidine) exert direct effects on the β-cell to suppress insulin release (303–306). The indirect effects of other drugs may be mediated through alterations in insulin sensitivity (e.g., glucocorticoids) or through potassium depletion (e.g., thiazides), which secondarily alters the resting membrane potential of the β-cell (307,308). Still other pharmacologic agents modulate both insulin secretion and insulin action. Both α- and β-adrenoceptor antagonists are included in this category. Indeed, the effects of this group of drugs on the rapid insulin secretory oscillations (those that occur every 8 to 16 minutes) have also been characterized. α-Adrenoreceptor blocking agents appear to enhance insulin secretion by increasing the amplitude of these rapid pulses, whereas the reduced insulin secretory response in patients receiving α-adrenergic antagonists appears to be in part a reflection of a smaller pulse amplitude (192). Neither α- or β-adrenoceptor antagonists alter the frequency of these rapid oscillations. Other pharmacologic agents that affect both insulin secretion and insulin action include clonidine, prazosin, the benzodiazepine and phenothiazine groups of drugs, and the opiates. In relation to the latter, hyperglycemia has been observed in subjects receiving morphine (309) and hyperinsulinemia has been reported in heroin addicts, who also demonstrate insulin secretory responses to intravenous glucose lower than those in age- and weight-matched control subjects (310). New-onset diabetes mellitus, even diabetic ketoacidosis, has been observed in patients taking clozapine and olanzapine, novel antipsychotic agents, but the underlying mechanism is not yet understood (311–315).

CONCLUDING REMARKS

The study of insulin secretion *in vivo* is greatly facilitated by a clear knowledge of the biosynthetic pathway of insulin within the β-cell and of the factors regulating insulin production and clearance from the circulation. In many clinical situations, the simultaneous measurement of proinsulin and C-peptide levels provides information on β-cell secretory function not possible to obtain by measurement of insulin levels in isolation. In interpreting the concentrations of these peptides, it is necessary to take into account the age and weight of the subjects as well as the glucose level at the time of sampling. The presence of any factor likely to alter insulin sensitivity should also be noted. While glucose is the key stimulus regulating insulin secretion *in vivo*, other nutrients, as well as neural and hormonal factors, interact to modify this response, thus helping to maintain glucose levels within the physiologic range during fasting and postprandial states. This complex regulatory system is disrupted in the early stages of type 1 diabetes mellitus before absolute insulinopenia develops and also in type 2 diabetes mellitus. In both cases, the β-cell is unable to respond appropriately to the prevailing glucose concentration. Future studies of β-cell secretory function *in vivo* are likely to concentrate on the secretory defects present in the β-cell early in the evolutionary phase of diabetes mellitus before the clinical manifestations become apparent. The study of β-cell function and reserve during this period could make a major contribution to our understanding of the pathogenesis of diabetes mellitus and may ultimately lead to the development of suitable approaches for its prevention.

REFERENCES

1. Von Mering J, Minkowski O. Diabetes Mellitus nach Pankreasextirpation. *Arch Exp Pathol Pharmacol*(Leipzig) 1890;26:371–387.
2. Banting FG, Best CH. The internal secretion of the pancreas. *J Lab Clin Med* 1922;7:251–266.
3. Yalow RS, Berson SA. Immunoassay of endogenous plasma insulin in man. *J Clin Invest* 1960;39:1157–1175.
4. Cerasi E, Luft R. Insulin response to glucose infusion in diabetic and non-diabetic monozygotic twin pairs. Genetic control of insulin response? *Acta Endocrinol* 1967;55:330–345.
5. Taylor KW, Sheldon J, Pyke DA, Oakley WG. Glucose tolerance and serum insulin in the unaffected first-degree relatives of diabetics. *BMJ* 1967;4:22–24.
6. Malherbe C, De Gasparo M, Ke Hertogh R, Hoett JJ. Circadian variations of blood sugar and plasma insulin levels in man. *Diabetologia* 1969;5:397–404.
7. Stoffel M, Froguel P, Takeda J, et al. Human glucokinase gene: isolation, characterization, and identification of two missense mutations linked to early-onset non-insulin-dependent diabetes mellitus. *Proc Natl Acad Sci U S A* 1992; 89:7698–7702.
8. Weber B. Glucose-stimulated insulin secretion during "remission" of juvenile diabetes. *Diabetologia* 1972;8:189–195.
9. Polonsky K, Jaspan J, Emmanouel D, et al. Differences in the hepatic and renal extraction of insulin and glucagon in the dog: evidence for saturability of insulin metabolism. *Acta Endocrinol* 1983;102:420–427.
10. Polonsky KS, Jaspan J, Pugh W, et al. Metabolism of C-peptide in the dog: in vivo demonstration of the absence of hepatic extraction. *J Clin Invest* 1983;72: 1114–1123.
11. Ferrannini E, Cobelli C. The kinetics of insulin in man. II. Role of the liver. *Diabetes Metab Rev* 1987;3:365–397.
12. Steiner DF, Oyer PE. The biosynthesis of insulin and a probable precursor of insulin by a human islet cell adenoma. *Proc Natl Acad Sci U S A* 1967;57: 473–480.
13. Rubenstein AH, Clark JL, Melani F, et al. Secretion of proinsulin, C-peptide by pancreatic cells and its circulation in blood. *Nature* 1969;224:697–699.
14. Steiner DF. On the role of the proinsulin C-peptide. *Diabetes* 1978;27[Suppl 1]: 145–148.
15. Horwitz DL, Starr JI, Mako ME, et al. Proinsulin, insulin, and C-peptide concentrations in human portal and peripheral blood. *J Clin Invest* 1975;55: 1278–1283.
16. Melani F, Rubenstein AH, Steiner DF. Human serum proinsulin. *J Clin Invest* 1970;49:497–507.
17. Bergenstal RM, Cohen RM, Lever E, et al. The metabolic effects of biosynthetic human proinsulin in individuals with type I diabetes. *J Clin Endocrinol Metab* 1984;58:973–979.
18. Revers RR, Henry R, Schmeiser L, et al. The effects of biosynthetic human proinsulin on carbohydrate metabolism. *Diabetes* 1984;33:762–770.
19. Peavy DE, Brunner MR, Duckworth WC, et al. Receptor binding and biological potency of several split forms (conversion intermediates) of human proinsulin. Studies in cultured IM-9 lymphocytes and in vivo and in vitro in rats. *J Biol Chem* 1985;260:13989–13994.
20. Gruppuso PA, Frank BH, Schwartz R. Binding of proinsuln and proinsulin conversion intermediates to human placental insulin-like growth factor 1 receptors. *J Clin Endocrinol Metab* 1988;67:194–197.
21. Polonsky KS, Rubenstein AH. C-peptide as a measure of the secretion and hepatic extraction of insulin: pitfalls and limitations. *Diabetes* 1984;33: 486–494.
22. Wojcikowski C, Blackman J, Ostrega D, et al. Lack of effect of high-dose biosynthetic human C-peptide on pancreatic hormone release in normal subjects. *Metabolism* 1990;39:827–832.
23. Wahren J, Ekberg K, Johansson J, et al. Role of C-peptide in human physiology. *Am J Physiol Endocrinol Metab* 2000;278:E759–E768.
24. Johansson BL, Borg K, Fernqvist-Forbes E, et al. Beneficial effects of C-peptide on incipient nephropathy and neuropathy in patients with type 1 diabetes mellitus. *Diabetes Med* 2000;17:181–189.
25. Johansson BL, Borg K, Fernqvist-Forbes E, et al. C-peptide improves autonomic nerve function in IDDM patients. *Diabetologia* 1996;39:687–695.
26. Polonsky KS, Pugh W, Jaspan JB, et al. C-peptide and insulin secretion. Relationship between peripheral concentrations of C-peptide and insulin and their secretion rates in the dog. *J Clin Invest* 1984;74:1821–1829.
27. Bratusch-Marrain PR, Waldhäusl WK, Gasic S, et al. Hepatic disposal of biosynthetic human insulin and porcine C-peptide in humans. *Metabolism* 1984;33:151–157.
28. Faber OK, Hagen C, Binder C, et al. Kinetics of human connecting peptide in normal and diabetic subjects. *J Clin Invest* 1978;62:197–203.
29. Blix PM, Boddie-Willis C, Landau RL, et al. Urinary C-peptide: an indicator of beta-cell secretion under different metabolic conditions. *J Clin Endocrinol Metab* 1982;54:574–580.
30. Gero L, Koranyi L, Tamas GJ Jr. Residual β-cell function in insulin dependent (type 1) and non-insulin-dependent (type 2) diabetics (relationship between 24-hour C-peptide excretion and the clinical features of diabetes). *Diabetes Metab* 1983;9:183–190.
31. Aurbach-Klipper J, Sharph-Dor R, Heding LG, et al. Residual β cell function in diabetic children as determined by urinary C-peptide. *Diabetologia* 1983;24: 88–90.
32. Hoogwerf BF, Goetz FC. Urinary C-peptide: a simple measure of integrated insulin production with emphasis on the effects of body size, diet and corticosteroids. *J Clin Endocrinol Metab* 1983;56:60–67.
33. Tillil H, Shapiro ET, Given BD, et al. Reevaluation of urine C-peptide as a measure of insulin secretion. *Diabetes* 1988;37:1194–1201.
34. Polonsky KS, Licinio-Paixao J, Given BD, et al. Use of biosynthetic human C-peptide in the measurement of insulin secretion rates in normal volunteers and type I diabetic patients. *J Clin Invest* 1986;77:98–105.
35. Shapiro ET, Tillil H, Rubenstein AH, et al. Peripheral insulin parallels changes in insulin secretion more closely than C-peptide after bolus intravenous glucose administration. *J Clin Endocrinol Metab* 1988;67:1094–1099.
36. Eaton RP, Allen RC, Schade DS, et al. Prehepatic insulin production in man: kinetic analysis using peripheral connecting peptide behavior. *J Clin Endocrinol Metab* 1980;51:520–528.
37. Polonsky K, Frank B, Pugh W, et al. The limitations to and valid use of C-peptide as a marker of the secretion of insulin. *Diabetes* 1986;35:379–386.
38. Welch S, Gebhart SS, Bergman RN, et al. Minimal model analysis of intravenous glucose tolerance test-derived insulin sensitivity in diabetic subjects. *J Clin Endocrinol Metab* 1990;71:1508–1518.
39. Breda E, Cavaghan MK, Toffolo G, et al. Oral glucose tolerance test minimal model indexes of beta-cell function and insulin sensitivity. *Diabetes* 2001;50: 150–158.
40. Bergman RN, Phillips LS, Cobelli C. Physiologic evaluation of factors controlling glucose tolerance in man: measurement of insulin sensitivity and beta-cell glucose sensitivity from the response to intravenous glucose. *J Clin Invest* 1981;68:1456–1467.
41. Caumo A, Bergman RN, Cobelli C. Insulin sensitivity from meal tolerance tests in normal subjects: a minimal model index. *J Clin Endocrinol Metab* 2000; 85:4396–4402.
42. Waldhäusl W, Bratusch-Marrain P, Gasic S, et al. Insulin production rate following glucose ingestion estimated by splanchnic C-peptide output in normal man. *Diabetologia* 1979;17:221–227.
43. Waldhäusl W, Bratusch-Marrain P, Gasic S, et al. Insulin production rate, hepatic insulin retention and splanchnic carbohydrate metabolism after oral glucose ingestion in hyperinsulinaemic type 2 (non-insulin-dependent) diabetes mellitus. *Diabetologia* 1982;23:6–15.
44. Porte D Jr, Pupo AA. Insulin responses to glucose: evidence for a two-pooled system in man. *J Clin Invest* 1969;48:2309–2319.
45. Chen M, Porte D Jr. The effect of rate and dose of glucose infusion on the acute insulin response in man. *J Clin Endocrinol Metab* 1976;42:1168–1175.
46. Ward WK, Beard JC, Halter JB, et al. Pathophysiology of insulin secretion in non-insulin-dependent diabetes mellitus. *Diabetes Care* 1984;7:491–502.
47. Eaton RP, Allen RC, Schade DS. Hepatic removal of insulin in normal man: dose response to endogenous insulin secretion. *J Clin Endocrinol Metab* 1983; 56:1294–1300.
48. Nauck MA, Homberger E, Siegel EG, et al. Incretin effects of increasing glu-

cose loads in man calculated from venous insulin and C-peptide responses. *J Clin Endocrinol Metab* 1986;63:492–498.
49. Tillil H, Shapiro ET, Miller MA, et al. Dose-dependent effects of oral and intravenous glucose on insulin secretion and clearance in normal humans. *Am J Physiol* 1988;254:E349–E357.
50. Faber OK, Madsbad S, Kehlet H, Binder C. Pancreatic beta cell secretion during oral and intravenous glucose administration. *Acta Med Scand Suppl* 1979; 624:61–64.
51. Madsbad S, Kehlet H, Hilsted J, et al. Discrepancy between plasma C-peptide and insulin response to oral and intravenous glucose. *Diabetes* 1983;32: 436–438.
52. Shapiro ET, Tillil H, Miller MA, et al. Insulin secretion and clearance: comparison after oral and intravenous glucose. *Diabetes* 1987;93:1120–1130.
53. Creutzfeldt W, Ebert R. New developments in the incretin concept. *Diabetologia* 1985;28:565–576.
54. Pagliara AS, Stillings SN, Hover B, et al. Glucose modulation of amino acid-induced glucagon and insulin release in the isolated perfused rat pancreas. *J Clin Invest* 1974;54:819–832.
55. Gerich JE, Charles MA, Grodsky GM. Characterization of the effects of arginine and glucose on glucagon and insulin release from the perfused rat pancreas. *J Clin Invest* 1974;54:833–847.
56. Grodsky GM. The kinetics of insulin release. In: Hasselblatt A, Bruchhausen FV, eds. *Handbook of experimental pharmacology*. Vol. 32. *Insulin II*. Berlin: Springer-Verlag, 1975:1–19.
57. Salomon D, Meda P. Heterogeneity and contact-dependent regulation of hormone secretion by individual β cells. *Exp Cell Res* 1986;162:507–520.
58. Schmitz O, Pørhsen N, Nyholm B, et al. Disorderly and nonstationary insulin secretion in relatives of patients with NIDDM. *Am J Physiol* 1997;272: E218–E226.
59. Cerasi E, Luft R. The plasma insulin response to glucose infusion in healthy subjects and in diabetes mellitus. *Acta Endocrinol* 1967;55:278–304.
60. Bennett L, Grodsky GM. Multiphasic aspects of insulin release after glucose and glucagon. In: Ostman J, Milner RDG, eds. *Diabetes. Proceedings of the Sixth Congress of the International Diabetes Federation-1967*. Amsterdam: Excerpta Medica, 1969:462–469.
61. Grodsky GM. A threshold distribution hypothesis for packet storage of insulin and its mathematical modeling. *J Clin Invest* 1972;51:2047–2059.
62. Smith CP, Tarn AC, Thomas JM, et al. Between and within subject variation of the first phase insulin response to intravenous glucose. *Diabetologia* 1988; 31:123–125.
63. Bardet S, Pasqual C, Maugendre D, et al. Inter and intra individual variability of acute insulin response during intravenous glucose tolerance tests. *Diabetes Metab* 1989;15:224–232.
64. Rayman G, Clark P, Schneider AE, Hales CN. The first phase insulin response to intravenous glucose is highly reproducible. *Diabetologia* 1990;33:631–634.
65. Bolaffi JL, Heldt A, Lewis LD, et al. The third phase of in vitro insulin secretion: evidence for glucose insensitivity. *Diabetes* 1986;35:370–373.
66. Curry DL. Insulin content and insulinogenesis by the perfused rat pancreas: effects of long term glucose stimulation. *Endocrinology* 1986;118:170–175.
67. Hoenig M, MacGregor LD, Matschinsky FM. In vitro exhaustion of pancreatic β-cells. *Am J Physiol* 1986;250:E502–E511.
68. Grodsky GM. A new phase of insulin secretion: how will it contribute to our understanding of β-cell function? *Diabetes* 1989;38:673–678.
69. Matschinsky FM, Ellerman J, Stillings S, et al. Hexoses and insulin secretion. In: Hasselblatt A, Brudhhausen FV, eds. *Handbook of experimental pharmacology*. Vol. 32. *Insulin II*. Berlin: Springer-Verlag, 1975:79–114.
70. Grodsky GM, Fanska R, Lundquist I. Interrelationships between alpha and beta-anomers of glucose affecting both insulin and glucagon secretion in the perfused rat pancreas. II. *Endocrinology* 1975;97:573–580.
71. Niki A, Niki H, Miwa I. Effect of anomers of D-mannose on insulin release from perfused rat pancreas. *Endocrinology* 1979;105:1051–1054.
72. Malaisse WJ, Sener A, Koser M, et al. Stimulus-secretion coupling of glucose-induced insulin release. Metabolism of α- and β-D-glucose in isolated islets. *J Biol Chem* 1976;251:5936–5942.
73. Malaisse WJ, Malaisse-Lagae F, Lebrun P, et al. Metabolic response of pancreatic islets of the rat to the anomers of D-mannose. *Diabetologia* 1982;23: 185(abst 198).
74. Zawalich WS, Pagliara AS, Matschinsky FM. Effects of iodoacetate, mannoheptulose and 3-O-methyl glucose on the secretory function and metabolism of isolated pancreatic islets. *Endocrinology* 1977;100:1276–1283.
75. Levin SR, Karam JH, Hane S, et al. Enhancement of arginine-induced insulin secretion in man by prior administration of glucose. *Diabetes* 1971;20:171–176.
76. Fajans SS, Floyd JC. Stimulation of islet cell secretion by nutrients and by gastrointestinal hormones released during digestion. In: Steiner DF, Freinkel N, eds. *Handbook of physiology*. Section 7. *Endocrinology*. Vol. 1. Washington, DC: American Physiological Society, 1972:473–493.
77. Ward WK, Bolgiano DC, McKnight B, et al. Diminished β-cell secretory capacity in patients with non-insulin dependent diabetes mellitus. *J Clin Invest* 1984;74:1318–1328.
78. Kadowaki T, Miyake Y, Hagura R, et al. Risk factors for worsening to diabetes in subjects with impaired glucose tolerance. *Diabetologia* 1984;26:44–49.
79. Matschinsky FM, Fertel R, Kotler-Brajtburg K, et al. Factors governing the action of small calorigenic molecules on the islets of Langerhans. In: Mussacchia XJ, Breitenbach KP, eds. *Proceedings of the 8th Midwest Conference on Endocrinology and Metabolism*. Columbia, MO: University of Missouri Press, 1973:63–86.
80. Muller WA, Faloona GR, Unger RH. The influence of the antecedent diet upon glucagon and insulin secretion. *N Engl J Med* 1971;285:1450–1454.
81. Goberna RJ, Tamarit J Jr, Fussganger R, et al. Action of β-hydroxybutyrate, acetoacetate and palmitate on the insulin release from the perfused isolated rat pancreas. *Horm Metab Res* 1974;6:256–260.
82. Crespin SR, Greenough DB, Steinberg D. Stimulation of insulin secretion by long-chain free fatty acids. *J Clin Invest* 1973;52:1979–1984.
83. Crespin SR, Greenough WB 3rd, Steinberg D. Stimulation of insulin secretion by infusion of fatty acids. *J Clin Invest* 1969;48:1934–1943.
84. Paolisso G, Gambardella A, Amato L, et al. Opposite effects of short- and long-term fatty acid infusion on insulin secretion in healthy subjects. *Diabetologia* 1995;38:1295–1299.
85. Boden G, Chen X. Effects of fatty acids and ketone bodies on basal insulin secretion in type 2 diabetes. *Diabetes* 1999;48:577–583.
86. Zhou Y-P, Grill VE. Long term exposure of rat pancreatic islets to fatty acids inhibits glucose-induced insulin secretion and biosynthesis through a glucose fatty acid cycle. *J Clin Invest* 1994;93:870–876.
87. Mason TM, Goh T, Tchipashvili V, et al. Prolonged elevation of plasma free fatty acids desensitizes the insulin secretory response to glucose in vivo in rats. *Diabetes* 1999;48:524–530.
88. Carpentier A, Mittelman SD, Lamarche B, et al. Acute enhancement of insulin secretion by FFA in humans is lost with prolonged FFA elevation. *Am J Physiol* 1999;276:E1055–E1066.
89. Dupre J, Ross SA, Watson D, Brown JC. Stimulation of insulin secretion by gastric inhibitory polypeptide in man. *J Clin Endocrinol Metab* 1973;37:826–828.
90. Andersen DK, Elahi K, Brown JC, et al. Oral glucose augmentation of insulin secretion: interactions of gastric inhibitory polypeptide with ambient glucose and insulin levels. *J Clin Invest* 1978;62:152–161.
91. Schmidt WE, Siegel EG, Creutzfeldt W. Glucagon-like peptide-2 stimulates insulin release from isolated rate pancreatic islets. *Diabetologia* 1985;28: 704–707.
92. Kreymann B, Ghatei MA, Williams G, et al. Glucagon-like peptide-1 7-36: a physiological incretin in man. *Lancet* 1987;2:1300–1304.
93. Zawalich WS, Diaz VA. Prior cholecystokinin exposure sensitizes islets of Langerhans to glucose stimulation. *Diabetes* 1987;36:118–227.
94. Zawalich WS. Synergistic impact of cholecystokinin and gastric inhibitory polypeptide on the regulation of insulin secretion. *Metabolism* 1988;37: 778–781.
95. Weir GC, Mojsov S, Hendrick GK, et al. Glucagon-like peptide 1(7-37) actions on endocrine pancreas. *Diabetes* 1989;38:338–342.
96. Rasmussen H, Zawalich KC, Ganesan S, et al. Physiology and pathophysiology of insulin secretion. *Diabetes Care* 1990;13:655–666.
97. Fukase N, Manaka H, Sugiyama K, et al. Response of truncated glucagon-like peptide-1 and gastric inhibitory polypeptide to glucose ingestion in non-insulin dependent diabetes mellitus. Effect of sulfonylurea therapy. *Acta Diabetologia* 1995;32:165–169.
98. Groop PH. The influence of body weight, age and glucose tolerance on the relationship between GIP secretion and beta-cell function in man. *Scand J Clin Lab Invest* 1989;49:367–379.
99. Creutzfeldt W, Ebert R, Nauck M, et al. Disturbances of the entero-insulin axis. *Scand J Gastroenterol* 1983;83[Suppl]:111–119.
100. Nauck MA, Heimesaat MM, Ørskov C, et al. Preserved incretin activity of glucagon-like peptide 1 (7-36 amide) but not of synthetic human gastric inhibitory polypeptide in patients with type 2 diabetes mellitus. *J Clin Invest* 1993;91:301–307.
101. Ahrén B, Larsson H, Holst JJ. Reduced gastric inhibitory polypeptide but normal glucagon-like peptide 1 response to oral glucose in postmenopausal women with impaired glucose tolerance. *Eur J Endocrinol* 1997;137:127–131.
102. Rushakoff RA, Goldfine ID, Beccaria LJ, et al. Reduced postprandial cholecystokinin (CCK) secretion in patients with noninsulin-dependent diabetes mellitus: evidence for a role for CCK in regulating postprandial hyperglycemia. *J Clin Endocrinol Metab* 1993;76:489–493.
103. Meguro T, Shimosegawa T, Satoh A, et al. Gallbladder emptying and cholecystokinin and pancreatic polypeptide responses to a liquid meal in patients with diabetes mellitus. *J Gastroenterol* 1997;32:628–634.
104. Hasegawa H, Shirohara H, Okabayashi Y, et al. Oral glucose ingestion stimulates cholecystokinin release in normal subjects and patients with non-insulin-dependent diabetes mellitus. *Metabolism* 1996;45:196–202.
105. Nauck MA, Wollschläger D, Werner J, et al. Effects of subcutaneous glucagon-like peptide 1 (GLP-1 [7-36 amide]) in patients with NIDDM. *Diabetologia* 1996;39:1546–1553.
106. Creutzfeldt WO, Kleine N, Willms B, et al. Glucagonostatic actions and reduction of fasting hyperglycemia by exogenous glucagon-like peptide I(7-36) amide in type I diabetic patients. *Diabetes Care* 1996;19:580–586.
107. Young AA, Gedulin BR, Bhavsar S, et al. Glucose-lowering and insulin-sensitizing actions of exendin-4: studies in obese diabetic (ob/ob, db/db) mice, diabetic fatty Zucker rats, and diabetic rhesus monkeys (Macaca mulatta). *Diabetes* 1999;48:1026–1034.
108. Nauck MA, Bartels E, Ørskov C, et al. Additive insulinotropic effects of exogenous synthetic human gastric inhibitory polypeptide and glucagon-like peptide-1-(7-36) amide infused at near-physiological insulinotropic hormone and glucose concentrations. *J Clin Endocrinol Metab* 1993;76:912–917.
109. Elahi D, McAloon-Dyke M, Fukagawa NK, et al. The insulinotropic actions of glucose-dependent insulinotropic polypeptide (GIP) and glucagon-like peptide-1 (7-37) in normal and diabetic subjects. *Regul Pept* 1994;51:63–74.
110. Niederau C, Schwarzendrube J, Luthen R, et al. Effects of cholecystokinin

receptor blockade on circulating concentrations of glucose, insulin, C-peptide, and pancreatic polypeptide after various meals in healthy human volunteers. *Pancreas* 1992;7:1–10.
111. Fieseler P, Bridenbaugh S, Nustede R, et al. Physiological augmentation of amino acid-induced insulin secretion by GIP and GLP-I but not by CCK-8. *Am J Physiol* 1995;268:E949–E955.
112. Reimers J, Nauck M, Creutzfeldt W, et al. Lack of insulinotropic effect of endogenous and exogenous cholecystokinin in man. *Diabetologia* 1988;31: 271–280.
113. Rushakoff RJ, Goldfine ID, Carter JD, Liddle RA. Physiological concentrations of cholecystokinin stimulate amino acid-induced insulin release in humans. *J Clin Endocrinol Metab* 1987;65:395–401.
114. Ahrén B, Holst JJ, Efendic S. Antidiabetogenic action of cholecystokinin-8 in type 2 diabetes. *J Clin Endocrinol Metab* 2000;85:1043–1048.
115. Schebalin M, Said SI, Makhlouf GM. Stimulation of insulin and glucagon secretion by vasoactive intestinal peptide. *Am J Physiol* 1977;232:E197–E200.
116. Dupre J, Curtis JD, Unger RH, et al. Effects of secretin, pancreozymin, or gastrin on the response of the endocrine pancreas to administration of glucose or arginine in man. *J Clin Invest* 1969;48:745–757.
117. Halter J, Porte D Jr. Mechanisms of impaired acute insulin release in adult onset diabetes: studies with isoproterenol and secretin. *J Clin Endocrinol Metab* 1978;46:952–960.
118. Glaser B, Shapiro B, Glowniak J, et al. Effects of secretin on the normal and pathological beta-cell. *J Clin Endocrinol Metab* 1988;66:1138–1143.
119. Bertrand G, Puech R, Maisonnasse Y, et al. Comparative effects of PACAP and VIP on pancreatic endocrine secretions and vascular resistance in rat. *Br J Pharmacol* 1996;117:764–770.
120. Rehfeld JF, Stadil F. The effect of gastrin on basal- and glucose-stimulated insulin secretion in man. *J Clin Invest* 1973;52:1415–1426.
121. Samols E, Marri G, Marks V. Promotion of insulin secretion by glucagon. *Lancet* 1965;2:415–416.
122. Alberti KG, Christensen NJ, Christensen SE, et al. Inhibition of insulin secretion by somatostatin. *Lancet* 1973;2:1299–1301.
123. Felig P, Marliss EB, Cahill GF Jr. Metabolic response to human growth hormone during prolonged starvation. *J Clin Invest* 1971;50:411–421.
124. Kalhan SC, Adam PAJ. Inhibitory effect of prednisone on insulin secretion in man: model for duplication of blood glucose concentration. *J Clin Endocrinol Metab* 1975;41:600–610.
125. Landgraf R, Landgraf-Leurs MM, Weissmann A, et al. Prolactin: a diabetogenic hormone. *Diabetologia* 1977;13:99–104.
126. Gustafson AB, Banasiak MF, Kalkhoff RK, et al. Correlation of hyperprolactinemia with altered plasma insulin and glucagon: similarity to effects of late human pregnancy. *J Clin Endocrinol Metab* 1980;51:242–246.
127. Brelje TC, Sorenson RL. Nutrient and hormonal regulation of the threshold of glucose-stimulated insulin secretion in isolated rat pancreases. *Endocrinology* 1988;123:1582–1590.
128. Beck P, Daughaday WH. Human placental lactogen: studies of its acute metabolic effects and disposition in normal man. *J Clin Invest* 1967;46:103–110.
129. Ensinck JW, Williams RH. Hormonal and nonhormonal factors modifying man's response to insulin. In: Steiner DF, Freinkel N, eds. *Handbook of physiology*. Section 7. *Endocrinology*.Vol. 1. Washington, DC: American Physiological Society, 1972:665–669.
130. Martin JM, Friesen H. Effect of human placental lactogen on the isolated islets of Langerhans in vitro. *Endocrinology* 1969;84:619–621.
131. Curry DL, Bennett LL. Dynamics of insulin release by perfused rat pancreases: effects of hypophysectomy, growth hormone, adrenocorticotropic hormone and hydrocortisone. *Endocrinology* 1973;93:602–609.
132. Malaisse WJ, Malaisse-Lagae F, King S, et al. Effect of growth hormone on insulin secretion. *Am J Physiol* 1968;215:423–428.
133. Randin JP, Scazziga B, Jequier E, et al. Study of glucose and lipid metabolism by continuous indirect calorimetry in Graves' disease: effect of an oral glucose load. *J Clin Endocrinol Metab* 1985;61:1165–1171.
134. Foss MC, Paccola GM, Saad MJ, et al. Peripheral glucose metabolism in human hyperthyroidism. *J Clin Endocrinol Metab* 1990;70:1167–1172.
135. Sestoft L, Heding LG. Hypersecretion of proinsulin in thyrotoxicosis. *Diabetologia* 1981;21:103–107.
136. Nishi S, Seino Y, Ishida H, et al. Vagal regulation of insulin, glucagon, and somatostatin secretion in vitro in the rat. *J Clin Invest* 1987;79:1191–1196.
137. Kurose T, Seino Y, Nishi S, et al. Mechanism of sympathetic neural regulation of insulin, somatostatin, and glucagon secretion. *Am J Physiol* 1990;251: E220–E227.
138. Woods SC, Porte D Jr. Neural control of the endocrine pancreas. *Physiol Rev* 1974;54:596–619.
139. Bloom SR, Edwards AV. Certain pharmacological characteristics of the release of pancreatic glucagon in response to stimulation of the splanchnic nerves. *J Physiol* (Lond) 1978;280:25–35.
140. Porte D Jr, Girardier L, Seydoux J, et al. Neural regulation of insulin secretion in the dog. *J Clin Invest* 1973;52:210–214.
141. Roy MW, Lee KC, Jones MS, et al. Neural control of pancreatic insulin and somatostatin secretion. *Endocrinology* 1984;115:770–775.
142. Skoglund G, Lundquist I, Ahrén B. Selective α2-adrenoceptor activation by clonidine: effects on $45Ca^{2+}$ efflux and insulin secretion from isolated rat islets. *Acta Physiol Scand* 1988;132:289–296.
143. Ahrén B. Autonomic regulation of islet hormone secretion—implications for health and disease. *Diabetologia* 2000;43:393–410.
144. Pettersson M, Ahrén B. Calcitonin gene-related peptide inhibits insulin secretion. Studies on ion fluxes and cyclic AMP in isolated rat islets. *Diabetes Res* 1990;15:9–14.
145. Pettersson M, Ahrén B, Böttcher G, et al. Calcitonin gene-related peptide: occurrence in pancreatic islets in the mouse and the rat and inhibition of insulin secretion in the mouse. *Diabetologia* 1986;119:865–869.
146. Ahrén B, Mårtensson H, Nobin A. Effects of calcitonin gene-related peptide (CGRP) on islet hormone secretion in the pig. *Diabetologia* 1987;30:354–359.
147. Lundquist I, Sundler F, Ahrén B, et al. Somatostatin, pancreatic polypeptide, substance P, and neurotensin: cellular distribution and effects on stimulated insulin secretion in the mouse. *Endocrinology* 1979;104:832–838.
148. Hermansen K. Effects of substance P and other peptides on the release of somatostatin, insulin and glucagon in vitro. *Endocrinology* 1980;107: 256–261.
149. Hommel H, Fischer U, Retzlaff K, et al. The mechanism of insulin secretion after oral glucose administration. II. Reflex insulin secretion in conscious dogs bearing fistulas of the digestive tract by sham-feeding of glucose or tap water. *Diabetologia* 1972;8:111–116.
150. Berthoud HR, Trimble ER, Siegel EG, et al. Cephalic-phase insulin secretion in normal and pancreatic islet-transplanted rats. *Am J Physiol* 1980;238: E336–E340.
151. Taylor IL, Feldman M. Effect of cephalic-vagal stimulation on insulin, gastric inhibitory polypeptide and pancreatic polypeptide release in humans. *J Clin Endocrinol Metab* 1982;55:1114–1117.
152. Bruce DG, Storlein LH, Furler SM, et al. Cephalic phase metabolic responses in normal weight adults. *Metabolism* 1987;36:721–725.
153. Berthoud HR, Bereiter DA, Trimble ER, et al. Cephalic phase, reflex insulin secretion. Neuroanatomical and physiological characterization. *Diabetologia* 1981;20:393–401.
154. Zawalich WS, Zawalich KC, Rasmussen H. Cholinergic agonists prime the β-cell to glucose stimulation. *Endocrinology* 1989;125:2400–2406.
155. Håkanson R, Liedberg G, Lundquist I. Effect of vagal denervation on insulin release after oral and intravenous glucose. *Experientia* 1971;27:460–461.
156. Linquette M, Fourlinnie JC, Lagache G. Etude de la glycemie et de l'insulinemic apres vagotomie et pylor-plastie chez l'homme. *Ann Endocrinol* (Paris) 1969;30:96–102.
157. Louis-Sylvestre J. Relationship between two stages of prandial insulin release in rats. *Am J Physiol* 1978;235:E103–E111.
158. Trimble ER, Siegel EG, Berthoud HR, et al. Intraportal islet transplantation: functional assessment in conscious unrestrained rats. *Endocrinology* 1980;106: 791–797.
159. Pozza G, Bosi E, Secchi A, et al. Metabolic control of type 1 (insulin dependent) diabetes after pancreas transplantation. *BMJ* (Clin Res Ed) 1985;291: 510–513.
160. Blackman JD, Polonsky KS, Jaspan JS, et al. Insulin secretory profiles and C-peptide clearance kinetics at 6 months and 2 years after kidney-pancreas transplantation. *Diabetes* 1992;41:1346–1354.
161. Madsbad S, Christiansen E, Tibell A, et al. Beta-cell dysfunction following successful segmental pancreas transplantation. Danish-Swedish Study Group of Metabolic Effect of Pancreas Transplantation. *Transplant Proc* 1994; 26:469–470.
162. Diem P, Abid M, Redmon J, et al. Systemic venous drainage of pancreas allografts as an independent cause of hyperinsulinemia in type 1 diabetic recipients. *Diabetes* 1990;39:534–539.
163. Havel PJ, Ahrén B. Activation of autonomic nerves and the adrenal medulla contributes to increased glucagon secretion during moderate insulin-induced hypoglycemia in women. *Diabetes* 1997;46:801–807.
164. Havel PJ, Taborski GJ Jr. The contribution of the autonomic nervous system to changes of glucagon and insulin secretion during hypoglycemia stress. *Endocrinol Rev* 1989;10:332–350.
165. Hirsch IB, Marker JC, Smith LJ, et al. Insulin and glucagon in prevention of hypoglycemia during exercise in humans. *Am J Physiol* 1991;260:E695–E704.
166. Järhult J, Holst J. The role of the adrenergic innervation to the pancreatic islets in the control of insulin release during exercise in man. *Pflügers Arch* 1979;383:41–45.
167. Treuting TF. The role of emotional factors in the etiology and course of diabetes mellitus: a review of the recent literature. *Am J Med Sci* 1962;244:93–109.
168. Teff KL, Mattes RD, Engelman K, et al. Cephalic-phase insulin in obese and normal-weight men: relation to postprandial insulin. *Metabolism* 1993;42: 1600–1608.
169. Edvell A, Lindström P. Vagotomy in young obese hyperglycemic mice: effects on syndrome development and islet proliferation. *Am J Physiol* 1998;274: E1034–E1039.
170. Del Rio G, Procopio M, Bondi M, et al. Cholinergic enhancement by pyridostigmine increases the insulin response to glucose load in obese patients but not in normal subjects. *Int J Obes* 1997;21:1111-1114.
171. Ahrén B, Sauerberg P, Thomsen C. Increased insulin secretion and normalisation of glucose tolerance by cholinergic agonism in high fat-fed C57BL/6 J mice. *Am J Physiol* 1999;277:E93–E102.
172. Jeanrenaud B. Energy fuel and hormonal profile in experimental obesities. *Experientia Suppl* 1983;44:57–76.
173. Larrimer JN, Mazzaferri EL, Cataland S, et al. Effect of atropine on glucose-stimulated gastric inhibitory polypeptide. *Diabetes* 1978;27:638–642.
174. Rocca AS, Brubaker PL. Role of the vagus nerve in mediating proximal nutrient-induced glucagon-like peptide-1 secretion. *Endocrinology* 1999;140: 1687–1694.
175. Flaten O, Sand T, Myren J. Beta-adrenergic stimulation and blockade of the

release of gastric inhibitory polypeptide and insulin in man. *Scand J Gastroenterol* 1982;17:283–288.
176. Claustre J, Brechet S, Plaisancie P, et al. Stimulatory effect of beta-adrenergic agonists on ileal L cell secretion and modulation by alpha-adrenergic activation. *J Endocrinol* 1999;162:271–278.
177. Kruszynska YT, Home PD, Hanning I, et al. Basal and 24-h C-peptide and insulin secretion rate in normal man. *Diabetologia* 1987;30:16–21.
178. Polonsky KS, Given BD, Van Cauter E. Twenty-four-hour profiles and pulsatile patterns of insulin secretion in normal and obese subjects. *J Clin Invest* 1988;81:442–448.
179. Simon C, Follenius M, Branderberger G. Postprandial oscillation of plasma glucose, insulin and C-peptide in man. *Diabetologia* 1987;30:769–773.
180. Shapiro ET, Tillil H, Polonsky KS, et al. Oscillations in insulin secretion during constant glucose infusion in normal man: relationship to changes in plasma glucose. *J Clin Endocrinol Metab* 1988;67:307–314.
181. Simon C, Branderberger G, Follenius M. Ultradian oscillations of plasma glucose, insulin and C-peptide in man during continuous enteral nutrition. *J Clin Endocrinol Metab* 1987;64:669–674.
182. Van Cauter E, Desir D, Decoster C, et al. Nocturnal decrease in glucose tolerance during constant glucose infusion. *J Clin Endocrinol Metab* 1989;69: 604–611.
183. Sturis J, Van Cauter E, Blackman JD, et al. Entrainment of pulsatile insulin secretion by oscillatory glucose infusion. *J Clin Invest* 1991;87:439–445.
184. Byrne MM, Sturis J, Sobel RJ, et al. Elevated plasma glucose 2 h postchallenge predicts defects in β-cell function. *Am J Physiol* 1996;270:E572–E579.
185. O'Meara NM, Sturis J, Van Cauter E, et al. Lack of control of ultradian insulin secretory oscillations in impaired glucose tolerance and in non-insulin-dependent diabetes mellitus. *J Clin Invest* 1993;92:262–267.
186. Goodner CJ, Walike BC, Koerker DJ, et al. Insulin, glucagon, and glucose exhibit synchronous, sustained oscillations in fasting monkeys. *Science* 1977; 195:177–179.
187. Lang DA, Matthews DR, Peto J, et al. Cyclic oscillations of basal plasma glucose and insulin concentrations in human beings. *N Engl J Med* 1979;301: 1023–1027.
188. Hansen BC, Pek S, Koerker DJ, et al. Neural influences on oscillations in basal plasma levels of insulin in monkeys. *Am J Physiol* 1981;240:E5–E11.
189. Lang DA, Matthews DR, Burnett M, et al. Brief, irregular oscillations of basal plasma insulin and glucose concentrations in diabetic man. *Diabetes* 1981;30: 435–439.
190. Lang DA, Matthews DR, Burnett M, et al. Pulsatile, synchronous basal insulin and glucagon secretion in man. *Diabetes* 1982;31:22–26.
191. Hansen BC, Jen KC, Belbez Pek S, et al. Rapid oscillations in plasma insulin, glucagon, and glucose in obese and normal weight humans. *J Clin Endocrinol Metab* 1982;54:785–792.
192. Matthews DR, Lang DA, Burnett MA, et al. Control of pulsatile insulin secretion in man. *Diabetologia* 1983;24:231–237.
193. Stagner JI, Samols E, Weir GC. Sustained oscillations of insulin, glucagon and somatostatin from the isolated canine pancreas during exposure to a constant glucose concentration. *J Clin Invest* 1980;65:939–942.
194. Jaspan JB, Lever E, Polonsky KS, et al. In vivo pulsatility of pancreatic islet peptides. *Am J Physiol* 1986;251:E215–E226.
195. Matthews DR, Naylor BA, Jones RG, et al. Pulsatile insulin has greater hypoglycemic effect than continuous delivery. *Diabetes* 1983;32:617–621.
196. Bratusch-Marrain PR, Komjati M, et al. Efficacy of pulsatile versus continuous insulin administration on hepatic glucose production and glucose utilization in type I diabetic humans. *Diabetes* 1986;35:922–926.
197. Ward GM, Walters JM, Aitken PM, et al. Effects of prolonged pulsatile hyperinsulinemia in humans: enhancement of insulin sensitivity. *Diabetes* 1990;39: 501–507.
198. Tasaka Y, Sekine M, Wakatsuki M, et al. Levels of pancreatic glucagon, insulin and glucose during twenty-four hours of the day in normal subjects. *Horm Metab Res* 1975;7:205–206.
199. Jarrett RJ, Baker IA, Keen H, et al. Diurnal variation in oral glucose tolerance: blood sugar and plasma insulin levels morning, afternoon and evening. *BMJ* 1972;1:199–201.
200. Carroll KF, Nestel PJ. Diurnal variation in glucose tolerance and in insulin secretion in man. *Diabetes* 1973;22:333–348.
201. Alparicio NJ, Puchulu FE, Gagliardino JJ, et al. Circadian variation of the blood glucose, plasma insulin and human growth hormone levels in response to an oral glucose load in normal subjects. *Diabetes* 1974;23: 132–137.
202. King DS, Dalsky GP, Clutter WE, et al. Effects of lack of exercise on insulin secretion and action in trained subjects. *Am J Physiol* 1988;254:E537–E542.
203. King DS, Dalsky GP, Staten MA, et al. Insulin action and secretion in endurance-trained and untrained humans. *J Appl Physiol* 1987;63:E537–E542.
204. King DS, Staten MA, Kohrt WM, et al. Insulin secretory capacity in endurance-trained and untrained young men. *Am J Physiol* 1990;259: E155–E161.
205. Seals DR, Hagberg JM, Allen WK, et al. Glucose tolerance in young and older athletes and sedentary men. *J Appl Physiol* 1984;56:1521–1525.
206. Heath GW, Gavin IJR, Hinderliter JM, et al. Effects of exercise and lack of exercise on glucose tolerance and insulin sensitivity. *J Appl Physiol* 1983;55: 512–517.
207. King DS, Clutter WE, Young DA, et al. Effects of exercise and lack of exercise on insulin sensitivity and responsiveness. *J Appl Physiol* 1988;64:1942–1946.
208. LeBlanc J, Nadeau A, Richard D, et al. Studies on the sparing effect of exercise on insulin requirements in human subjects. *Metabolism* 1981;30: 1119–1124.
209. Davidson MB. The effect of aging on carbohydrate metabolism: a review of the English literature and a practical approach to the diagnosis of diabetes mellitus in the elderly. *Metabolism* 1979;28:688–705.
210. DeFronzo RA. Glucose intolerance and aging: evidence for tissue insensitivity to insulin. *Diabetes* 1979;28:1095–1101.
211. Fink RI, Kolterman OG, Olefsky JM. The physiological significance of the glucose intolerance of aging. *J Gerontol* 1984;38:273–278.
212. Reaven EP, Gold G, Reaven GM. Effect of age on glucose-stimulated insulin release by the beta cell of the rat. *J Clin Invest* 1979;64:591–599.
213. Reaven E, Wright D, Mondon CE, et al. Effect of age and diet on insulin secretion and insulin action in the rat. *Diabetes* 1983;32:175–180.
214. Swenne I. Effects of aging on the regenerative capacity of the pancreatic beta-cell of the rat. *Diabetes* 1983;32:14–19.
215. DeFronzo RA. Glucose intolerance and aging. *Diabetes Care* 1981;4:493–501.
216. Palmer JP, Ensinck JW. Acute-phase insulin secretion and glucose tolerance in young and aged normal men and diabetic patients. *J Clin Endocrinol Metab* 1975;41:498–503.
217. Dudl RJ, Ensinck JW. Insulin and glucagon relationships during aging in man. *Metabolism* 1977;26:33–41.
218. Gumbiner B, Polonsky KS, Beltz WF, et al. Effects of aging on insulin secretion. *Diabetes* 1989;38:1549–1556.
219. Chen M, Bergman RN, Pacini G, et al. Pathogenesis of age-related glucose intolerance in man: insulin resistance and decreased β-cell function. *J Clin Endocrinol Metab* 1985;60:13–20.
220. Kissebah AH, Vydelingum N, Murray R, et al. Relation of body fat distribution to metabolic complications of obesity. *J Clin Endocrinol Metab* 1982;54: 254–260.
221. Peiris AN, Mueller RA, Struve MF, et al. Splanchnic insulin metabolism in obesity. Influence of body fat distribution. *J Clin Invest* 1986;78:1648–1657.
222. Meistas MT, Rendell M, Margolis S, et al. Estimation of the secretion rate of insulin from the urinary excretion rate of C-peptide: study in obese and diabetic subjects. *Diabetes* 1982;31:449–453.
223. Faber OK, Christensen K, Kehlet H, et al. Decreased insulin removal contributes to hyperinsulinemia in obesity. *J Clin Endocrinol Metab* 1981;53: 618–621.
224. Savage PJ, Flock EV, Mako ME, et al. C-peptide and insulin secretion in Pima Indians and Caucasians: constant fractional hepatic extraction over a wide range of insulin concentrations and in obesity. *J Clin Endocrinol Metab* 1979; 48:594–598.
225. DeFronzo RA. Insulin secretion, insulin resistance and obesity. *Int J Obes* 1982;6[Suppl 1]:73–82.
226. Rossell R, Gomis R, Casamitjana R, et al. Reduced hepatic insulin extraction in obesity: relationship with plasma insulin levels. *J Clin Endocrinol Metab* 1983;56:608–611.
227. Polonsky KS, Given BD, Hirsch L, et al. Quantitative study of insulin secretion and clearance in normal and obese subjects. *J Clin Invest* 1988;81:435–441.
228. Jones CNO, Pei D, Staris P, et al. Alterations in the glucose-stimulated insulin secretory dose-response curve and in insulin clearance in nondiabetic insulin-resistant individuals. *J Clin Endocrinol Metab* 1997;82:1834–1838.
229. Jones CNO, Abbasi F, Carantoni M, et al. Roles of insulin resistance and obesity in regulation of plasma insulin concentrations. *Am J Physiol* 2000;278: E501–E508.
230. Kahn SE, Prigeon RL, McCulloch DK, et al. Quantification of the relationship between insulin sensitivity and β-cell function in human subjects. Evidence for a hyperbolic function. *Diabetes* 1993;42:1663–1672.
231. Buchanan TA, Metzger BE, Frienkel N, et al. Insulin sensitivity and β-cell responsiveness to glucose during late pregnancy in lean and moderately obese women with normal glucose tolerance or mild gestational diabetes. *Am J Obstet Gynecol* 1990;162:1008–1014.
232. Ogilvie RF. The islets of Langerhans in 19 cases of obesity. *J Pathol Bacteriol* 1933;37:473–481.
233. Pick A, Clark J, Kubstrup C, et al. Role of apoptosis in failure of β-cell mass compensation for insulin resistance and β-cell defects in the male Zucker diabetic fatty rat. *Diabetes* 1998;47:358–364.
234. Weir GC. Non-insulin-dependent diabetes mellitus: interplay between β-cell inadequacy and insulin resistance. *Am J Med* 1982;73:461–464.
235. Reaven GM. Insulin secretion and insulin action in non-insulin dependent diabetes mellitus: which defect is primary? *Diabetes Care* 1984;7[Suppl 1]: 17–24.
236. Cahil GF Jr. Beta-cell deficiency, insulin resistance, or both? [Editorial]. *N Engl J Med* 1988;318:1268–1270.
237. Polonsky KS, Sturis J, Bell GI. Seminars in Medicine of the Beth Israel Hospital, Boston: Non-insulin dependent diabetes: a genetically programmed failure of the beta cell to compensate for insulin resistance. *N Engl J Med* 1996; 334:777–783.
238. Kahn BB. Type 2 diabetes: when insulin secretion fails to compensate for insulin resistance. *Cell* 1998;92:593–596.
239. Kloppel G, Lohr M, Habich K, et al. Islet pathology and the pathogenesis of type 1 and type 2 diabetes mellitus revisited. *Surv Synth Pathol Res* 1985;4: 110–125.
240. Clark A, Wells CA, Buley ID, et al. Islet amyloid, increased α-cells, reduced β-cells, and exocrine fibrosis: quantitative changes in the pancreas in type 2 diabetes. *Diabetes Res* 1988;9:151–159.
241. Stefan Y, Orci L, Malaisse-Lagae F, et al. Quantification of endocrine cell con-

tent in the pancreas of nondiabetic and diabetic humans. *Diabetes* 1982;3: 694–700.
242. Tokuyama Y, Sturis J, DePaoli AM, et al. Evolution of β-cell dysfunction in the male Zucker diabetic fatty rat. *Diabetes* 1995;44:1447–1457.
243. Pfeifer MA, Halter JB, Porte D Jr. Insulin secretion in diabetes mellitus. *Am J Med* 1981;70:579–588.
244. Garvey WT, Olefsky JM, Griffin J, et al. The effect of insulin treatment on insulin secretion and insulin action in type II diabetes mellitus. *Diabetes* 1985; 34:222–234.
245. Ferner RE, Ashworth RL, Tronier B, et al. Effects of short-term hyperglycemia on insulin secretion in normal humans. *Am J Physiol* 1986;250:E655–E661.
246. Nesher R, Della Casa L, Litvin Y, et al. Insulin deficiency and insulin resistance in type 2 (non-insulin-dependent) diabetes: quantitative contributions of pancreatic and peripheral responses to glucose homeostasis. *Eur J Clin Invest* 1987;17:266–274.
247. Leahy JL, Bonner-Weir S, Weir GC. Minimal chronic hyperglycemia is a critical determinant of impaired insulin secretion after an incomplete pancreatectomy. *J Clin Invest* 1988;81:1407–1414.
248. Leahy JL, Weir GC. Evolution of abnormal insulin secretory responses during 48-h in vivo hyperglycemia. *Diabetes* 1988;37:217–222.
249. Duckworth WC, Kitabchi AE. Direct measurement of plasma proinsulin in normal and diabetic subjects. *Am J Med* 1972;53:418–427.
250. Mako ME, Starr JI, Rubenstein AH. Circulating proinsulin in patients with maturity onset diabetes. *Am J Med* 1977;63:865–869.
251. Ward WK, LaCava EC, Paquette TL, et al. Disproportionate elevation of immunoreactive proinsulin in type II (non-insulin-dependent) diabetes mellitus and in experimental insulin resistance. *Diabetologia* 1987;30:698–702.
252. Yoshioka N, Kuzuya T, Matsuda A, et al. Serum proinsulin levels at fasting and after oral glucose load in patients with type 2 (non-insulin-dependent) diabetes mellitus. *Diabetologia* 1988;31:355–360.
253. Temple RC, Carrington CA, Luzio SD, et al. Insulin deficiency in non-insulin-dependent diabetes. *Lancet* 1989;1:293–295.
254. Saad MF, Kahn SE, Nelson RG, et al. Disproportionately elevated proinsulin in Pima Indians with noninsulin-dependent diabetes mellitus. *J Clin Endocrinol Metab* 1990;70:1247–1253.
255. Reaven GM, Chen Y-DI, Jeppeson J, et al. Insulin resistance and hyperinsulinemia in individuals with small, dense, low density lipoprotein particles. *J Clin Invest* 1993;92:141–146.
256. Polonsky KS, Given BD, Hirsch L, et al. Abnormal patterns of insulin secretion in non-insulin-dependent diabetes mellitus. *N Engl J Med* 1988;318: 1231–1239.
257. Sturis J, Polonsky KS, Shapiro ET, et al. Abnormalities in the ultradian oscillations of insulin secretion and glucose levels in type 2 (non-insulin-dependent) diabetic patients. *Diabetologia* 1992;35:681–689.
258. O'Meara NM, Shapiro ET, Van Cauter E, et al. Effect of glyburide on beta cell responsiveness to glucose in non-insulin-dependent diabetes mellitus. *Am J Med* 1990;89[Suppl 2A)]11S–16S.
259. Turner RC, Holman RR. Beta cell function during insulin or chlorpropamide treatment of maturity-onset diabetes mellitus. *Diabetes* 1978;27[Suppl 1]: 241–246.
260. Kosaka K, Kuzuya T, Akanuma Y, et al. Increase in insulin response after treatment of overt maturity-onset diabetes is independent of the mode of treatment. *Diabetologia* 1980;18:23–28.
261. Hidaka H, Nagulesparan M, Klimes I, et al. Improvement of insulin secretion but not insulin resistance after short term control of plasma glucose in obese type II diabetics. *J Clin Endocrinol Metab* 1982;54:217–222.
262. Karam JG, Sanz N, Salamon E, et al. Selective unresponsiveness of pancreatic β-cells to acute sulfonylurea stimulation during sulfonylurea therapy in NIDDM. *Diabetes* 1986;35:1314–1320.
263. Shapiro TE, Van Cauter E, Tillil H, et al. Glyburide enhances the responsiveness of the β-cell to glucose but does not correct the abnormal patterns of insulin secretion in noninsulin-dependent diabetes mellitus. *J Clin Endocrinol Metab* 1989;69:571–576.
264. Reaven GM, Chen YD, Hollenbeck CB, et al. Plasma insulin, C-peptide, and proinsulin concentrations in obese and nonobese individuals with varying degrees of glucose tolerance. *J Clin Endocrinol Metab* 1993;76:44–48.
265. Reaven GM, Bernstein R, Davis B, et al. Nonketotic diabetes mellitus: insulin deficiency or insulin resistance? *Am J Med* 1976;60:80–88.
266. Bergstrom RW, Wahl PW, Leonetti DL, et al. Association of fasting glucose levels with a delayed secretion of insulin after oral glucose in subjects with glucose intolerance. *J Clin Endocrinol Metab* 1990;71:1447–1453.
267. Phillips DI, Clark PM, Hales CN, et al. Understanding oral glucose tolerance: comparison of glucose or insulin measurements during the oral glucose tolerance test with specific measurements of insulin resistance and insulin secretion. *Diabet Med* 1994;11:286–292.
268. Ahrén B, Pacini G. Impaired adaptation of first-phase insulin secretion in postmenopausal women with glucose intolerance. *Am J Physiol* 1997;36: E701–E707.
269. O'Rahilly S, Nugent Z, Rudenski AS, et al. β-Cell dysfunction rather than insulin insensitivity is the primary defect in familial type 2 diabetes. *Lancet* 1986;2:360–363.
270. Barnett AH, Spiliopoulos AJ, Pyke DA, et al. Metabolic studies in unaffected co-twins of non-insulin-dependent diabetics. *BMJ* 1981;282:1656–1658.
271. Kosaka K, Hagura R, Kuzuya T. Insulin responses in equivocal and definite diabetes with special reference to subjects who had mild glucose intolerance but later developed definite diabetes. *Diabetes* 1977;26:944–952.
272. Efendic S, Luft R, Wajngot A. Aspects of the pathogenesis of type 2 diabetes. *Endocr Rev* 1984;5:395–410.
273. Ward WK, Johnston CL, Beard JC, et al. Insulin resistance and impaired insulin secretion in subjects with histories of gestational diabetes mellitus. *Diabetes* 1985;34:861–869.
274. O'Sullivan JB. Body weight and subsequent diabetes mellitus. *JAMA* 1982; 248:949–952.
275. O'Rahilly S, Turner RC, Matthews DR. Impaired pulsatile secretion of insulin in relatives of patients with non-insulin-dependent diabetes. *N Engl J Med* 1988;318:1225–1230.
276. Larsson H, Ahrén B. Relative hyperproinsulinemia as a sign of islet dysfunction in women with impaired glucose tolerance. *J Clin Endocrinol Metab* 1999; 84:2068–2074.
277. Snehalatha C, Ramachandran A, Satyavani K, et al. Specific insulin and proinsulin concentrations in nondiabetic South Indians. *Metabolism* 1998;47: 230–233.
278. Birkeland KI, Torjesen PA, Eriksson J, et al. Hyperproinsulinemia of type II diabetes is not present before the development of hyperglycemia. *Diabetes Care* 1994;17:1307–1310.
279. Inoue I, Takahashi K, Katayama S, et al. A higher proinsulin response to glucose loading predicts deteriorating fasting plasma glucose and worsening to diabetes in subjects with impaired glucose tolerance. *Diabet Med* 1996;13: 330–336.
280. Kahn SE, Leonetti DL, Prigeon RL, et al. Proinsulin levels predict the development of non-insulin-dependent diabetes mellitus (NIDDM) in Japanese-American men. *Diabet Med* 1996;13[9 Suppl 6]:S63–S66.
281. Heine RJ, Nijpels G, Mooy JM. New data on the rate of progression of impaired glucose tolerance to NIDDM and predicting factors. *Diabet Med* 1996;13[3 Suppl 2]:S12–S14.
282. Carlstrom S, Ingemanson CA. Juvenile diabetes with long-standing remission. A case report. *Diabetologia* 1967;3:465–467.
283. Johansen K, Ørskov H. Plasma insulin during remission in juvenile diabetes mellitus. *BMJ* 1969;1:676–678.
284. Block MB, Rosenfield RL, Mako ME, et al. Sequential changes in beta-cell function in insulin-treated diabetic patients assessed by C-peptide immunoreactivity. *N Engl J Med* 1973;288:1144–1148.
285. Park BM, Soeldner JS, Gleason RE. Diabetes in remission. Insulin secretory dynamics. *Diabetes* 1974;23:616–623.
286. Ludvigsson J, Heding LG. Beta-cell function in children with diabetes. *Diabetes* 1978;27[Suppl 1]:230–234.
287. Heding LG, Ludvigsson J, Kasperska-Czyzykowa T. β-Cell secretion in non-diabetics and insulin-dependent-diabetics. *Acta Med Scand Suppl* 1981;656:5–9.
288. Ludvigsson J, Heding L. Abnormal proinsulin/C-peptide ratio in juvenile diabetes. *Acta Diabet Lat* 1982;19:351–358.
289. Snorgaard O, Hartling SG, Binder C. Proinsulin and C-peptide at onset and during 12 months cyclosporin treatment of type 1 (insulin-dependent) diabetes mellitus. *Diabetologia* 1990;33:36–42.
290. Bougneres PF, Carel JC, Castano L, et al. Factors associated with early remission of type I diabetes in children treated with cyclosporine. *N Engl J Med* 1988;318:663–670.
291. Skyler JS, Rabinovitch A. Cyclosporine in recent onset type I diabetes mellitus. Effects on islet beta cell function. Miami Cyclosporine Diabetes Study Group. *J Diabetes Complications* 1992;6:77–88.
292. Yilmaz MT, Devrim AS, Biyal F, et al. Immunoprotection in spontaneous remission of type 1 diabetes: long-term follow-up results. *Diabetes Res Clin Pract* 1993;19:151–162.
293. Srikanta S, Ganda OP, Jackson RA, et al. Type I diabetes mellitus in monozygotic twins: chronic progressive beta cell dysfunction. *Ann Intern Med* 1983; 99:320–326.
294. Knip M, Douek IF, Moore WP, et al. Safety of high-dose nicotinamide: a review. *Diabetologia* 2000;43:1337–1345.
295. The Diabetes Prevention Trial-Type 1 diabetes (DPT-1): implementation of screening and staging of relatives. DPT-1 Study Group. *Transplant Proc* 1995; 27:3377.
296. Osei K, Henry ML, O'Doriso TM, et al. Physiological and pharmacological stimulation of pancreatic islet hormone secretion in type 1 diabetic pancreas allograft recipients. *Diabetes* 1990;39:1235–1242.
297. Östman J, Bolinder J, Gunnarsson R, et al. Metabolic effects of pancreas transplantation: effects of pancreas transplantation on metabolic and hormonal profiles in IDDM patients. *Diabetes* 1989;38[Suppl 1]:88–93.
298. Grunt JA, Pallotta JA, Soeldner JS. Blood sugar, serum insulin and free fatty acid interrelationships during intravenous tolbutamide testing in normal young adults and in patients with insulinoma. *Diabetes* 1970;19:122–126.
299. Marks V. Progress report: diagnosis of insulinoma. *Gut* 1971;12:835–843.
300. Service FJ, Horwitz DL, Rubenstein AH, et al. C-peptide suppression test for insulinoma. *J Lab Clin Med* 1977;90:180–186.
301. Alsever RN, Roberts JP, Gerber JG, et al. Insulinoma with low circulating insulin levels: the diagnostic value of proinsulin measurements. *Ann Intern Med* 1984;82:347–350.
302. Cohen RM, Given BD, Licinio-Paixao J, et al. Proinsulin radioimmunoassay in the evaluation of insulinomas and familial hyperproinsulinemia. *Metabolism* 1986;35:1137–1146.
303. Malherbe C, Burrill KC, Levin SR, et al. Effect of diphenylhydantoin on insulin secretion in man. *N Engl J Med* 1972;286:339–342.
304. Pace CS, Livingston E. Ionic basis of phenytoin sodium inhibition of insulin secretion in pancreatic islets. *Diabetes* 1979;28:1077–1082.

305. De Marinis L, Barbarino A. Calcium antagonists and hormone release. I. Effects of verapamil on insulin release in normal subjects and patients with islet-cell tumor. *Metabolism* 1980;29:599–604.
306. Henquin JC, Meissner HP. Opposite effects of tolbutamide and diazoxide on $86Rb^+$ fluxes and membrane potential in pancreatic β-cells. *Biochem Pharmacol* 1982;31:1407–1414.
307. Gorden P. Glucose intolerance with hypokalemia: failure of short-term potassium depletion in normal subjects to reproduce the glucose and insulin abnormalities of clinical hypokalemia. *Diabetes* 1973;22:544–551.
308. Helderman JH, Elahi D, Andersen DK, et al. Prevention of the glucose intolerance of thiazide diuretics by maintenance of body potassium. *Diabetes* 1983; 32:106–111.
309. Feldberg W, Shaligram SV. The hyperglycemic effect of morphine. *Br J Pharmacol* 1972;46:602–618.
310. Passariello N, Giugliano D, Quatraro A, et al. Glucose tolerance and hormonal responses in heroin addicts. A possible role for endogenous opiates in the pathogenesis of non-insulin-dependent diabetes. *Metabolism* 1983;32: 1163–1165.
311. Koller E, Bennett K, Dubitsky G, et al. Clozapine-associated diabetes. In: *Proceedings of the Endocrine Society's 81st Annual Meeting*. June 1999, San Diego, CA.
312. Hägg S, Joelsson L, Mjörndal T, et al. Prevalence of diabetes and impaired glucose tolerance in patients treated with clozapine compared with patients treated with conventional depot neuroleptic medications. *J Clin Psychiatry* 1998;59:294–299.
313. Lindenmayer J-P, Patel R. Olanzapine-induced ketoacidosis with diabetes mellitus. *Am J Psychiatry* 1999;156:1471.
314. Melkersson KI, Hulting A-L, Brismar KE. Different influences of classical antipsychotics and clozapine on glucose-insulin homeostasis in patients with schizophrenia or related psychoses. *J Clin Psychiatry* 1999;60:783–791.
315. Wirshing DA, Spellberg BJ, Erhart SM, et al. Novel antipsychotics and new onset diabetes. *Biol Psychiatry* 1998;44:778–783.

SECTION II

Hormone Action and the Regulation of Metabolism

CHAPTER 8
Hormone–Fuel Interrelationships: Fed State, Starvation, and Diabetes Mellitus

Neil B. Ruderman, Martin G. Myers, Jr., Stuart R. Chipkin, and Keith Tornheim

BASIC PRINCIPLES

Fuel Reservoirs

Humans have a constant requirement for energy but eat only intermittently. To cope with this problem, we usually ingest food in excess of the immediate caloric needs of our vital organs and store the extra calories in the form of hepatic and muscle glycogen, adipose tissue triglyceride, and to a certain extent, tissue protein. In turn, during starvation and in response to various stresses, we break down these fuel reservoirs to provide energy for organ metabolism and function (Fig. 8.1).

The two principal circulating fuels in humans, glucose and free fatty acids (FFAs), are stored intracellularly as glycogen and triglycerides, respectively. The largest reservoir of glycogen (300 to 500 g) is skeletal muscle (1). However, the principal reservoir of glycogen from which free glucose can be released into the circulation is the liver (Table 8.1) (1). The major site of triglyceride storage is adipose tissue. Adipose tissue triglyceride is the most efficient form of energy storage in humans. Triglyceride contains 9.5 kcal per g and the average caloric content of an adipocyte, including its cytosol, is approximately 8 kcal per g (2). In contrast, glycogen contains 4 kcal per g. Furthermore, because 3 mL of water is needed to maintain the intracellular osmolality of each gram of glycogen *in vivo* (3), in reality glycogen provides only 1 kcal per g. Thus, if the 15 kg of adipose tissue triglyceride in a normal 70-kg man were replaced with an equicaloric quantity of glycogen, the individual would weigh an additional 120 kg!

Body protein, although of considerable mass (Table 8.1), is not, strictly speaking, a fuel reservoir. Protein molecules serve specific roles in maintaining organ structure and function and are less expendable than glycogen or triglycerides. On the other hand, a portion of body protein (e.g., some of the contractile protein of muscle as well as other proteins in liver and muscle) is degraded during starvation and other periods of stress and provides amino acid substrate for gluconeogenesis.

The Brain and Other Vital Organs

The brain has a continuous need for fuel but stores almost no energy as glycogen or fat. Instead, it uses glucose derived from the liver either directly from glycogen or indirectly from other fuel reservoirs through gluconeogenesis. The brain does not use FFAs directly. During prolonged starvation, however, it is able to use energy derived from FFAs after their conversion to ketone bodies. Other vital organs, such as liver, heart, and skeletal muscle, also have a continuous requirement for fuels (Table 8.2), but unlike the brain, these organs can utilize fatty acids directly to meet their energy needs (1,3).

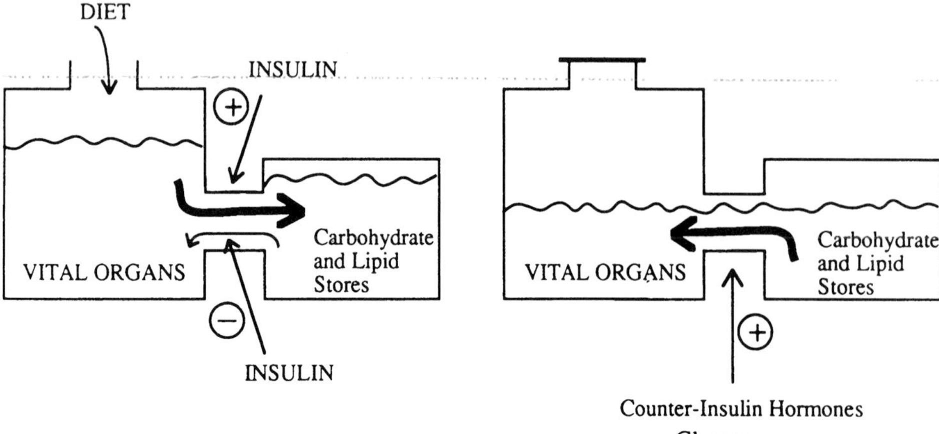

Figure 8.1. Fuel homeostasis in humans. In the fed state, fuels in excess of the needs of vital organs are stored in carbohydrate and lipid reservoirs (i.e., as glycogen and triglycerides and to some extent as protein). During starvation, these stores are broken down to provide fuel for other organs. Changes in circulating levels of insulin and counterinsulin hormones modulate these transitions.

Hormonal Regulators of Fuel Homeostasis

Energy reservoirs in humans are built up and broken down in response to hormonal messages. The principal hormonal messenger is insulin. In the fed state, insulin levels increase, promoting glycogen synthesis in liver and muscle, lipid formation in adipocytes, and amino acid uptake and protein synthesis in most cells. In the postabsorptive state, during starvation and in response to many stresses, decreased insulin levels contribute to glycogen breakdown, lipolysis, hepatic ketogenesis, and decreased synthesis and increased degradation of protein. In the latter situations, a major role of insulin is to act as a restraint on these catabolic events (Fig. 8.1).

Multiple hormones counter the effects of insulin. Glucagon stimulates glycogenolysis, gluconeogenesis, and ketogenesis in the liver (4–7). Glucagon also can stimulate lipolysis in adipose tissue, although the physiologic relevance of this latter effect is unclear. Catecholamines have effects similar to those of glucagon on the liver and are key regulators of lipolysis in adipose tissue and glycogenolysis in muscle and other tissues. In general, the counterinsulin hormones (also called counterregulatory hormones) liberate energy from fuel reservoirs by actions opposite to those of insulin (Fig. 8.1). However, not all of the actions of these counterinsulin hormones are catabolic. For instance, growth hormone, although catabolic in the sense that it stimulates lipolysis in adipose tissue, also has significant anabolic effects and enhances cell growth (8). Similarly, glucagon has the anabolic property of stimulating amino acid uptake by the liver (6). The potential roles of leptin and other hormones released by the adipocyte in regulating fuel homeostasis will be discussed in the section on adipose tissue.

TABLE 8.1. Fuel Reservoirs in Humans

Source	g	kcal
Liver glycogen	75	300
Muscle glycogen	400	1,600
Blood glucose	20	80
Adipose tissue triglyceride	15,000	141,000
Protein	6,000	24,000

Data are estimates for an overnight-fasted man weighing 70 kg.

Nonhormonal Regulation of Fuel Homeostasis

Although fuel homeostasis has been classically envisaged in the context of its regulation by hormones, changes in the concentrations of the fuels themselves may also play a direct role. Thus, increases in circulating glucose levels have been shown to diminish hepatic gluconeogenesis and glycogenolysis and enhance glycogen synthesis independent of their effects on hormone secretion (9,10). In addition, FFAs have been shown to stimulate hepatic gluconeogenesis; indeed recent studies suggest that much of the antigluconeogenic action of insulin in humans and other mammals may be secondary to its antilipolytic action on the fat cell (11).

Glucose Homeostasis

A principal objective of the interplay between insulin and the counterinsulin hormones in humans is the maintenance of normoglycemia. The concentration of glucose in the circulation is more closely controlled than that of any other fuel. Thus, plasma glucose levels are maintained between 4 and 7 mM in normal humans despite varying rates of glucose utilization (Table 8.3), whereas levels of FFAs and ketone bodies may range 10-fold to more than a 100-fold, respectively (12,13). Prevention of hypoglycemia is important because central nervous system (CNS) function is impaired at low plasma glucose concentrations. Likewise, significant hyperglycemia resulting in glycosuria causes a loss of fuel and may contribute to the complica-

TABLE 8.2. Typical Daily Fuel Requirements of Liver, Muscle, and Brain of a Physically Active, Normally Fed Human

Organ	Fuel	~kcal/d
Liver	Amino acids, fat, glucose	280
Muscle	Glucose, fat	880
Brain	Glucose	480

TABLE 8.3. Rates of Glucose Utilization in the Fed and Fasted State

	Glucose utilization (g/d)		
Tissue	12-h fast	8-d fast	Marathon run
Brain	120	45	120
Muscle	30	Very low	500

tions of diabetes mellitus. Whether plasma glucose levels modestly above or below the "normal" range are undesirable remains to be determined.

Insulin lowers plasma glucose levels both by stimulating glucose uptake into muscle and adipose tissue and by inhibiting hepatic glycogen breakdown and gluconeogenesis. The different counterinsulin hormones balance these effects of insulin in order to maintain normoglycemia. Thus, glucagon, epinephrine, and norepinephrine are released into the circulation in response to hypoglycemia (7) and during stresses such as exercise, when glucose utilization is altered by other factors (14,15). In addition to stimulating hepatic glycogenolysis and gluconeogenesis, the catecholamines inhibit insulin-stimulated glucose utilization in muscle and promote lipolysis in adipose tissue (16), thereby providing tissues with an alternative fuel to glucose. Glucocorticoids also are released into the circulation in increased quantities in response to hypoglycemia and other stresses (14,15). Glucocorticoids appear to be necessary for the mobilization of energy stores by catecholamines and glucagon; however, their role may be permissive rather than regulatory (17).

FIVE PHASES OF FUEL HOMEOSTASIS

Immediately after a carbohydrate or mixed meal has been ingested, the concentrations of insulin, glucose, and glucagon in plasma favor fuel storage. Once absorption of the ingested food is complete, the concentrations of these and other hormones and substrates change, causing a shift from energy storage in fuel reservoirs to energy mobilization. Further alterations in fuel homeostasis occur with more prolonged food deprivation. These changes can be broken down into five phases on the basis of the source and quantity of glucose entering the circulation. Figure 8.2 illustrates these changes in a hypothetical human who ingests 100 g of glucose and then begins a prolonged fast (13).

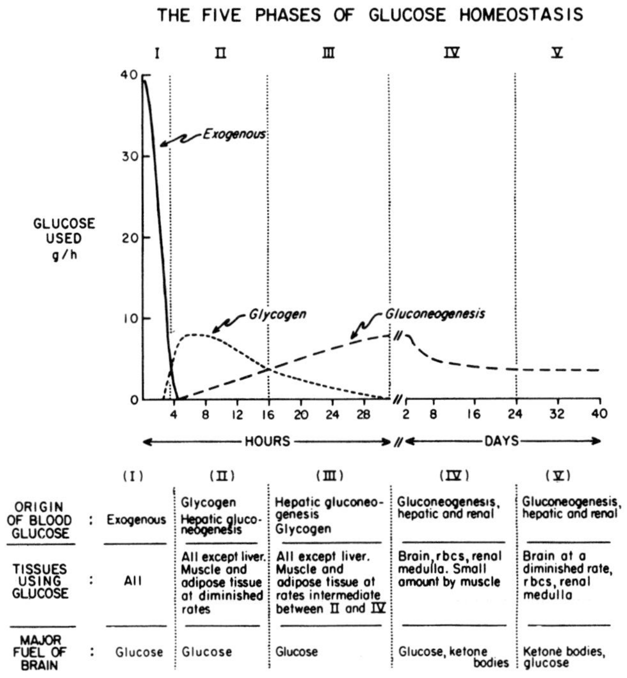

	(I)	(II)	(III)	(IV)	(V)
ORIGIN OF BLOOD GLUCOSE:	Exogenous	Glycogen Hepatic gluconeogenesis	Hepatic gluconeogenesis Glycogen	Gluconeogenesis, hepatic and renal	Gluconeogenesis, hepatic and renal
TISSUES USING GLUCOSE:	All	All except liver. Muscle and adipose tissue at diminished rates	All except liver. Muscle and adipose tissue at rates intermediate between II and IV	Brain, rbcs, renal medulla. Small amount by muscle	Brain at a diminished rate, rbcs, renal medulla
MAJOR FUEL OF BRAIN:	Glucose	Glucose	Glucose	Glucose, ketone bodies	Ketone bodies, glucose

Figure 8.2. The five phases of glucose homeostasis. The figure depicts rates of glucose utilization and the source of glucose entering the circulation in a 70-kg man who ingests 100 g of glucose and then fasts for 40 days.

Fed State

During the first few hours after a carbohydrate meal, glucose absorbed from the gastrointestinal tract provides for the metabolic needs of the brain and other organs (Fig. 8.2, phase I). The absorbed glucose in excess of these needs is used to rebuild fuel reservoirs in liver, muscle, fat, and presumably in other tissues (Fig. 8.3). In this setting, plasma insulin levels are high, plasma glucagon levels are low, and glycogen synthesis is stimulated in liver and muscle. Approximately 75 g of carbohydrate is stored as glycogen in liver, and 300 to 500 g is stored in muscle in a human who has fasted overnight (1) (Table 8.1).

As noted earlier, the major form of lipid storage in humans is triglyceride and the major site for triglyceride storage is adipose tissue (2). Smaller amounts of triglyceride are stored in muscle, liver, and other tissues. Triglycerides also are present in

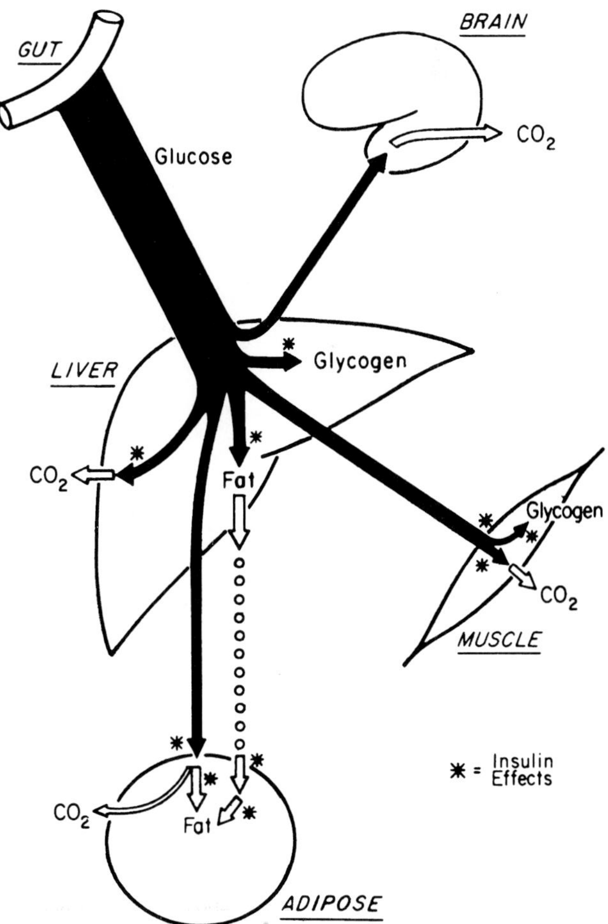

Figure 8.3. Fuel metabolism during a carbohydrate meal. Soon after the ingestion of carbohydrate, insulin levels rise and stimulate the uptake of glucose. Glucose is the major oxidative fuel of all major tissues at this time. Glucose that is present in excess of the oxidative needs of tissues is stored as glycogen or lipid. Asterisks indicate steps enhanced by insulin.

the circulation as constituents of lipoproteins. However, the major circulating lipid fuels are the FFAs. After a carbohydrate meal, high concentrations of insulin favor the use of both glucose and lipoprotein triglycerides for triglyceride synthesis in adipose tissue.

In addition to promoting the synthesis of glycogen and triglycerides in the fed state, insulin inhibits the breakdown of these fuel reservoirs (18) (i.e., it is anticatabolic). The concentrations of insulin that inhibit lipolysis appear to be lower than those that stimulate glucose transport in muscle. Presumably, it is for this reason that patients with mild type 2 diabetes and glucose intolerance are hyperglycemic in the absence of significant elevations of plasma FFAs or ketone bodies.

Early Starvation

With the decrease in plasma insulin and the increase in plasma glucagon that accompany an overnight fast, fuel homeostasis shifts from energy storage to energy production (Fig. 8.4). At this stage, glucose no longer enters the circulation from the gastrointestinal tract but is derived principally from the breakdown of liver glycogen and, via gluconeogenesis, from lactate, amino acids, and glycerol, a process that takes place predominantly in the liver (1) but that also occurs in the kidney (19) and intestines (20). In addition, circulating FFAs, derived from the hydrolysis of adipocyte triglycerides, become a major source of fuel (21). As will be discussed later, by using FFAs, muscle and liver decrease their oxidation of glucose as a fuel, thereby conserving it for the brain.

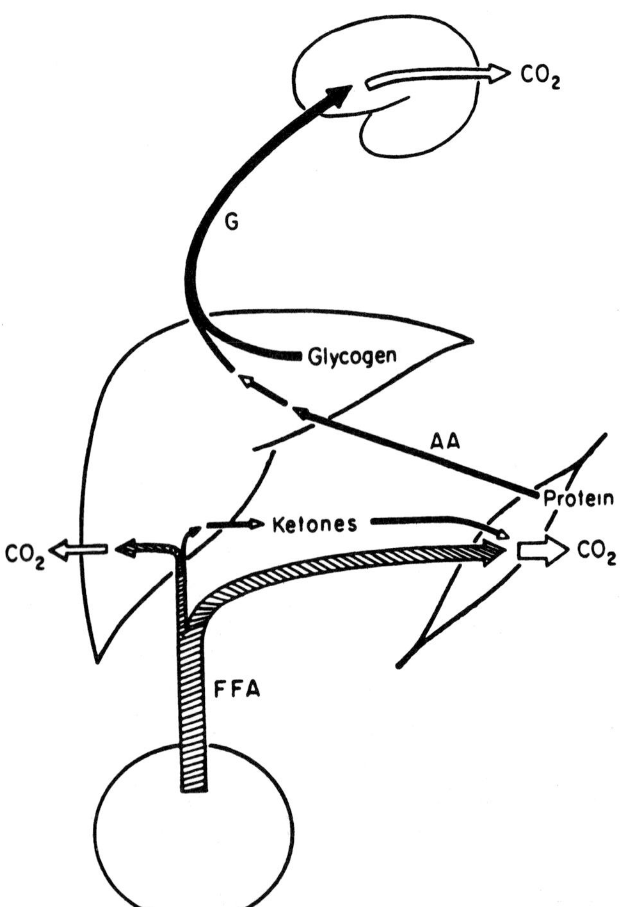

Figure 8.4. Fuel metabolism after an overnight fast (postabsorptive). After approximately 12 hours of starvation, insulin concentrations have returned to basal levels and glucose (G) entering the circulation is derived from both hepatic glycogen and gluconeogenesis. Free fatty acids (FFA) produced from adipocyte lipolysis have become a principal fuel for skeletal muscle. AA, amino acids.

MOBILIZATION OF CARBOHYDRATE AND LIPID STORES

In the earliest phase of starvation (i.e., the postabsorptive state), hepatic glycogen is a major source of the glucose entering the circulation and remains so for 12 to 24 hours (22,23). Glucagon seems to be necessary for hepatic glycogenolysis during this period, although an increase in the level of plasma glucagon does not appear to be the primary stimulus (24–26). After an overnight fast, the average rate of glucose utilization by a healthy human is approximately 7 g per hour (Table 8.3) (1). By extrapolation, the 70 to 80 g of glycogen present in the liver can provide glucose to the brain and peripheral tissues for 12 to 16 hours. Two events allow the maintenance of blood glucose levels beyond this time: (a) Muscle and other tissues begin to oxidize lipid-derived fuels in place of glucose, and (b) hepatic gluconeogenesis, which is also stimulated by fatty acids, replaces glycogenolysis as the principal source of glucose entering the circulation (Fig. 8.4). As will be discussed later, glycogen breakdown in muscle does not yield significant quantities of free glucose, and after an overnight fast, gluconeogenesis by the kidney is of minor importance.

Two factors stimulate the breakdown of adipocyte triglyceride during starvation. First, the concentration of circulating insulin diminishes and, consequently, triglyceride synthesis is decreased and lipolysis is enhanced (2,27). Second, norepinephrine is released from sympathetic nerve endings and directly stimulates lipolysis by raising levels of cyclic adenosine monophosphate (cAMP) in adipocytes (2,27). Epinephrine, which is secreted from the adrenal medulla, appears to play a lesser role. The mechanisms by which FFAs are released into the circulation are discussed in the section "Adipose Tissue." The principal users of FFAs during the early phases of starvation are skeletal muscle and liver.

GLUCONEOGENESIS

Because the brain is unable to use FFAs as a fuel, it must continue to use glucose during the early phases of starvation. Gluconeogenesis is an important source of the glucose that enters the circulation even after an overnight fast (28) and becomes the major source as hepatic glycogen stores become depleted (Fig. 8.2, phase III) (23). Gluconeogenesis is responsible for approximately 35% to 60% of the hepatic glucose output after an overnight fast (12 to 15 hours postabsorptive) and for more than 97% of the output by 60 hours of starvation (23,29,30). At 60 hours, glucose production is limited not by the enzymatic capacity of the liver but by the concentration of gluconeogenic substrate in the circulation (31). During the early phases of starvation, the two principal gluconeogenic precursors are lactate and alanine (Table 8.4) (17,32–34).

TABLE 8.4. Gluconeogenic Substrates in Humans Starved for 24 Hours

Substrate	Amount generated (g/d)
Lactate	60
Amino acids except alanine	25
Alanine only	25
Glycerol	14
Pyruvate	5
Total	129

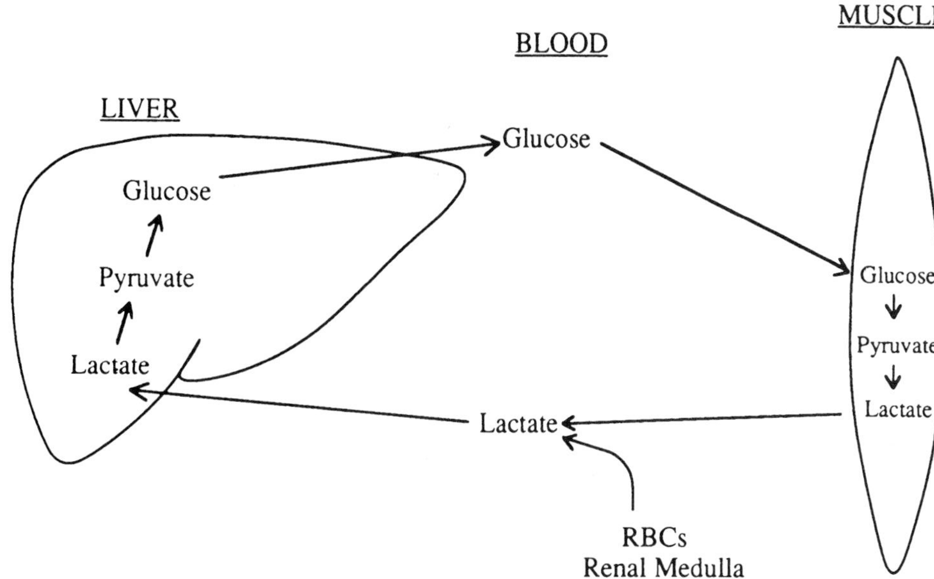

Figure 8.5. The Cori cycle. Lactate derived from glycolysis in skeletal muscle, red blood cells (RBCs), renal medulla, and other tissues is taken up by the liver, which uses it to synthesize glucose. The glucose can then be reused by these same tissues.

Lactate comprises 50% of the gluconeogenic substrate of liver in a human who has fasted overnight and is the major gluconeogenic substrate throughout starvation (Table 8.4) (32). When glucose cannot be metabolized beyond pyruvate in peripheral tissues, much of the pyruvate is reduced to lactate, which is then released into the circulation (Fig. 8.5). In red blood cells and renal medulla, this reduction occurs because there are no mitochondria in which pyruvate can be oxidized. In muscle and other tissues, lactate and pyruvate are released during starvation because the activity of pyruvate dehydrogenase, the enzyme that decarboxylates pyruvate to form acetyl coenzyme A (CoA), is decreased (35). For the most part, lactate generated from glucose in this way is taken up by the liver and reconverted to glucose by the gluconeogenic pathway (33). This recycling of glucose between liver and peripheral tissues via lactate is referred to as the Cori cycle.

A second major group of gluconeogenic substrates is the amino acids. Skeletal muscle is the principal reservoir of amino acids in humans (34). During early starvation, however, the gut and liver also appear to be important sources of the amino acids entering the circulation (36). A major stimulus to protein catabolism (both decreased synthesis and increased degradation) during starvation is the decrease in plasma insulin concentrations (37–39). Glucagon stimulates protein degradation in liver, and glucocorticoids inhibit protein synthesis in muscle and other tissues (34). Although increases in the plasma levels of these counterinsulin hormones almost certainly play a role in modulating protein catabolism in stressful states (e.g., diabetic ketoacidosis and trauma), their concentrations are not dramatically altered during starvation, and their role here is thought to be limited.

The principal amino acids released into the circulation from muscle are alanine and glutamine (Fig. 8.6). Most of the alanine

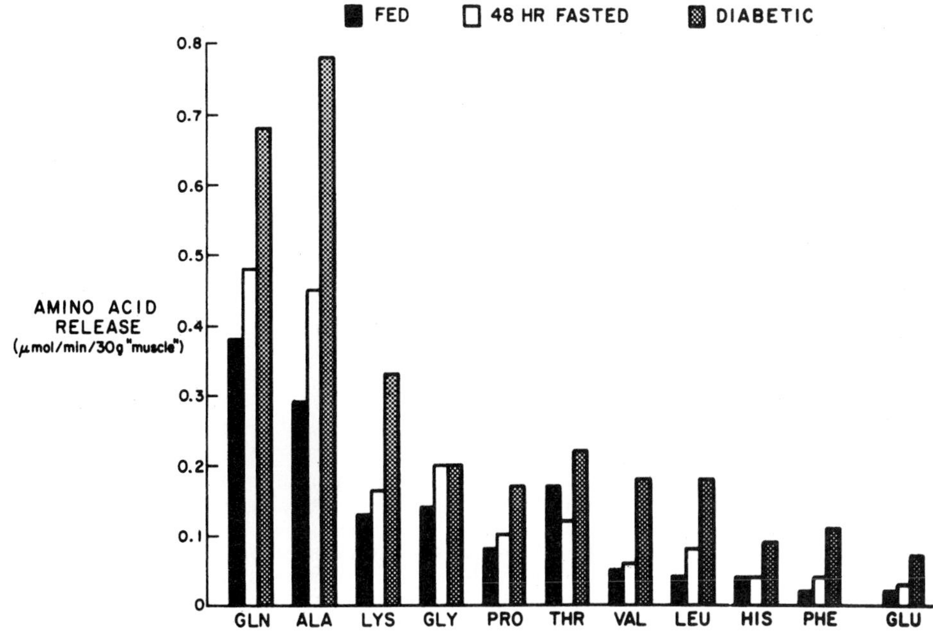

Figure 8.6. Release of amino acids from hind limb muscle of fed, fasted, and streptozotocin-diabetic rats perfused with an amino acid–free medium. The amino acids released in greatest amount are glutamine and alanine. In humans, the pattern of amino acid release is similar except that glutamine is taken up from the circulation.

is taken up directly by the liver, whereas glutamine is metabolized in the gastrointestinal tract, which can use it for gluconeogenesis and to generate alanine (20), and by the kidney, where it is the principal gluconeogenic substrate (19) as well as a major source of the NH_3 used for neutralizing acid in urine. Glutamine and alanine, despite comprising only 15% to 20% of muscle protein (34,39–41), account for 50% of the amino acids released by muscle because these amino acids can be generated from other constituents in muscle as well as from the degradation of protein. Alanine is formed by the transamination of pyruvate by alanine aminotransferase and glutamine by the amidation of glutamate by free ammonia, a reaction catalyzed by glutamine synthetase (41).

The rate of release of alanine increases markedly during starvation and other states of insulin deficiency (34,42). Despite this, the concentration of alanine in plasma is usually diminished in these situations because its uptake by the liver is stimulated to an even greater extent. Since the interorgan relationships of alanine are very much like those of lactate, a "glucose–alanine cycle" similar to the Cori cycle has been proposed (22). Impaired release of alanine from muscle has been postulated as a contributor to impaired gluconeogenesis and hypoglycemia in patients with uremia, maple syrup urine disease, and ketotic hypoglycemia of infancy and in starved women during pregnancy (43).

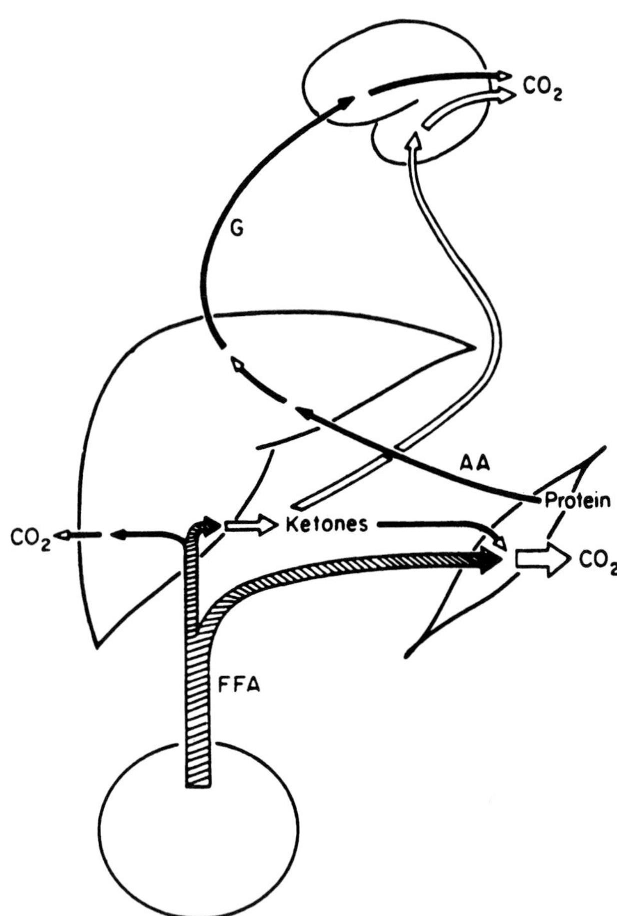

Figure 8.7. Fuel metabolism during prolonged starvation. As fasting continues, insulin levels remain suppressed and the principal source of hepatic glucose (G) production is gluconeogenesis. Skeletal muscle continues to use free fatty acids (FFA) for fuel but also uses ketone bodies produced in the liver. Ketone bodies may also be used by the brain. AA, amino acids.

The other major gluconeogenic substrate is glycerol, which is derived principally from the hydrolysis of adipose tissue triglyceride. In nondiabetic subjects, the rate with which glycerol appears in the circulation correlates with adipose mass (44) and increases during starvation. Glycerol comprises about 10% of total gluconeogenic substrate during early starvation and a much higher percentage during prolonged starvation, when gluconeogenesis from amino acids is markedly diminished (see below).

Prolonged Starvation

KETONE BODIES AND THE BRAIN

With the prolongation of starvation, several events occur that limit the need for gluconeogenesis and thereby conserve body protein (Fig. 8.7). The first of these, as already noted, is an increase in the reliance of muscle and other peripheral tissues on lipid-derived fuels: initially FFAs and later both FFAs and the ketone bodies, acetoacetate and β-hydroxybutyrate. The second is a change in the fuels used by the brain. During early starvation, the CNS continues to use glucose as its exclusive fuel. However, as starvation is prolonged, plasma levels of the ketone bodies increase to values even greater than the level of glucose (Fig. 8.8). Under these circumstances, the brain, or at least parts of it, increases its use of these lipid-derived fuels (1, 45,46). A third factor could be a decrease in plasma leptin, which by diminishing sympathetic nervous system activity, would diminish the basal metabolic rate.

Ketone bodies are produced from acetyl-CoA via the β-oxidation of fatty acids in the liver (Fig. 8.9). This process, termed ketogenesis, is enhanced by glucagon and inhibited by insulin. In contrast to long-chain FFAs, the ketone bodies are water-soluble and cross the blood–brain barrier via specific carrier proteins (47–49). Furthermore, the activity of these carriers is increased in physiologic states associated with sustained hyperketonemia such as diabetic ketoacidosis and starvation (50,51). These physiologic adaptations enhance the use of ketone bodies in place of glucose by the brain and diminish the need to degrade proteins for gluconeogenesis. It is because of

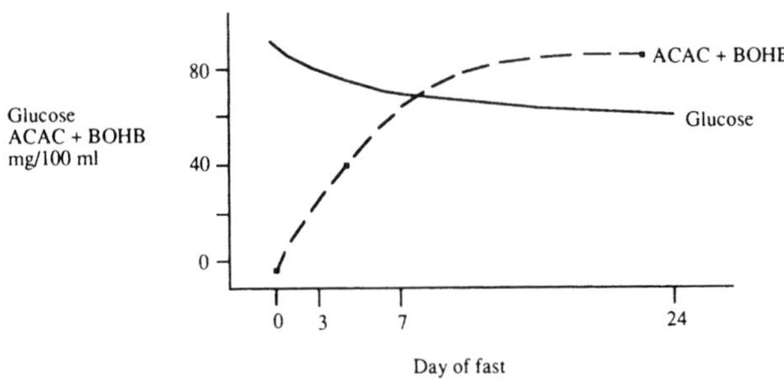

Tissue	Fuel	Quantity Used (g/day)			
Brain	Glucose	120	100		50
	K.B.	0	20		70
Muscle	K.B.	0	100		50
Liver	Glucose	-210	-150	-100	-80

Figure 8.8. Changes in plasma concentrations of fuels during starvation. Blood glucose concentrations decrease during the first 7 days of a fast but then remain relatively stable. As glucose utilization decreases, the concentration and use of ketone bodies increases. After a week of starvation, the concentration of ketone bodies in blood is equal to or greater than the glucose level. K.B., ketone bodies; ACAC, acetoacetate; BOHB, β-hydroxybutyrate.

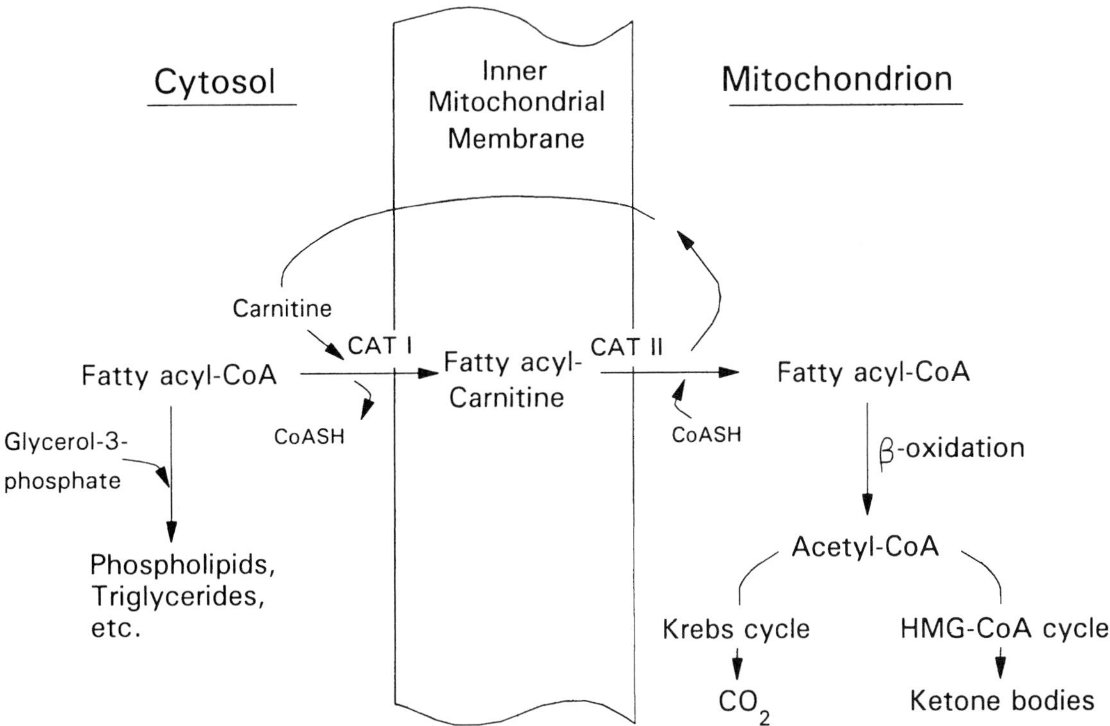

Figure 8.9. Mitochondrial fatty acid transport. Fatty acyl–coenzyme A (CoA) is transported from the cytosol into mitochondria by a series of steps that involves carnitine acyltransferase (CAT) I and II and a carnitine acyltranslocase (not shown). When rates of fatty acid transport into liver mitochondria are high, the hepatocyte obtains most of its fuel needs from the β-oxidation of the fatty acyl-CoA and the Krebs (tricarboxylic acid) cycle is inhibited. By generating malonyl-CoA, an inhibitor of CAT I, insulin inhibits fatty acid transport into mitochondria and, secondarily, ketogenesis. Glucagon has the opposite effect. HMG-CoA, 3-hydroxy-3-methyl glutaryl coenzyme A.

these adaptations that humans of normal weight are able to survive fasts of up to 60 to 70 days.

GLUCONEOGENESIS AND PROTEIN CATABOLISM

The decreased use of glucose by the brain during prolonged starvation is accompanied by a diminished rate of gluconeogenesis in the liver (Fig. 8.2 and Table 8.3). The latter appears to be due to decreases in protein catabolism and secondarily to the release of gluconeogenic amino acids (mostly alanine) from muscle (21,34). Some studies suggest that these adaptations in protein metabolism are related to the increased use of lipid fuels during prolonged starvation (33,52,53). Whatever the mechanism, as one proceeds from early to prolonged starvation, urinary excretion of nitrogen decreases from 12 g per day to 3 to 4 g per day, indicating a decrease in protein catabolism from 75 g per day to 12 to 20 g per day (1).

The relative contribution of the kidney to gluconeogenesis increases from 5% to 10% after an overnight fast to 50% after 3 to 4 weeks of starvation (1,53). However, in absolute amounts, renal production of glucose is still much lower than hepatic production of glucose after 1 to 2 days of fasting. The increase in renal gluconeogenesis during prolonged starvation is linked to an increase in NH_3 generation from glutamine.

Unlike amino acids, the relative importance of glycerol as a gluconeogenic precursor increases during prolonged starvation. This reflects the fact that the release of glycerol from fat is approximately 14 g per day and remains nearly constant during early and late starvation (53). After several weeks of starvation, gluconeogenesis from glycerol hypothetically provides upwards of half of the glucose oxidized by the brain.

Hormonal Controls

The gradual decrease in plasma insulin modulates the orderly breakdown of fuel reservoirs during the early phases of starvation. However, during prolonged starvation, the decreases in protein degradation and in the use of glucose and ketone bodies in muscle (see section titled "Muscle") occur in the absence of further changes in plasma insulin level. Some studies suggest that a decrease in thyroid hormone activity contributes to these adaptations (54). Presumably, the low levels of insulin during prolonged starvation are needed for these adaptations to occur. Thus, patients without any insulin (e.g., during diabetic ketoacidosis) have an impaired ability both to limit the breakdown of their fuel reservoirs and to use glucose and ketone bodies in peripheral tissues. The precise connection between the presence of insulin and these adaptations remains to be determined.

Recent studies suggest that another factor that plays a role in the adaptation of fuel homeostasis during starvation is leptin. As will be discussed in more detail in the next section, during periods of calorie deprivation when plasma insulin levels and adipocyte lipid stores are low, the release of leptin from adipose tissue diminishes, leading to an altered release of neuropeptide Y (NPY) and other CNS peptides and secondarily to a decrease in activity in the sympathetic nervous system. Although the precise interrelation of this chronic regulation of fuel metabolism to that modulated by insulin and counterinsulin hormones is only partially understood, it is highly likely that leptin plays a significant role in the adaptation of mammals to prolonged starvation (55,56).

HORMONE–FUEL INTERRELATIONS AT AN ORGAN LEVEL

Adipose Tissue

THE ADIPOCYTE IN METABOLIC REGULATION

While the adipocyte has classically been viewed as a storage depot for metabolic fuel in the form of lipid, it is now clear that the fat cell plays a central role in the endocrine regulation of energy homeostasis (57). Adipocytes not only respond to numerous hormones to regulate the storage and release of lipids but also secrete hormones (such as leptin, summarized above) that act to control energy balance and endocrine function throughout the rest of the body (57–59). The adipocyte also secretes a number of other protein factors, including resistin (also known as Fizz3) (60); tumor necrosis factor-α (TNF-α), an inflammatory cytokine (61); and Acrp30 (or adiponectin and adipoQ) (62), that may regulate insulin sensitivity elsewhere in the body. Although it was initially suggested that resistin increases with increasing adiposity and plays a role in insulin resistance associated with obesity, a number of subsequent studies failed to support this notion (60,63,64), and more research is necessary to determine the physiologic function of resistin. TNF-α mediates elements of insulin resistance and type 2 diabetes syndromes in some mouse models of obesity and diabetes, although the relevance of TNF-α to obesity and insulin resistance in humans remains unclear (61). In contrast to resistin and TNF-α, Acrp30 appears to mediate insulin sensitization (62). Acrp30 is an adipocyte-derived complement-related protein that is secreted as a high-order multimeric complex. Its production by adipocytes is decreased in obesity and other states of insulin resistance, and exogenously increased levels of this protein enhance numerous insulin actions. Although a great deal remains to be learned about Acrp30 (e.g., the identity of the functional proteolytic product, receptor identity) (62,65), this molecule currently commands a great deal of attention as an insulin sensitizer.

INSULIN ACTION IN ADIPOCYTES

In general, the hormones that regulate energy storage and release in adipocytes are similar to those that regulate these events throughout the body (Figs. 8.10 and 8.11). Insulin pro-

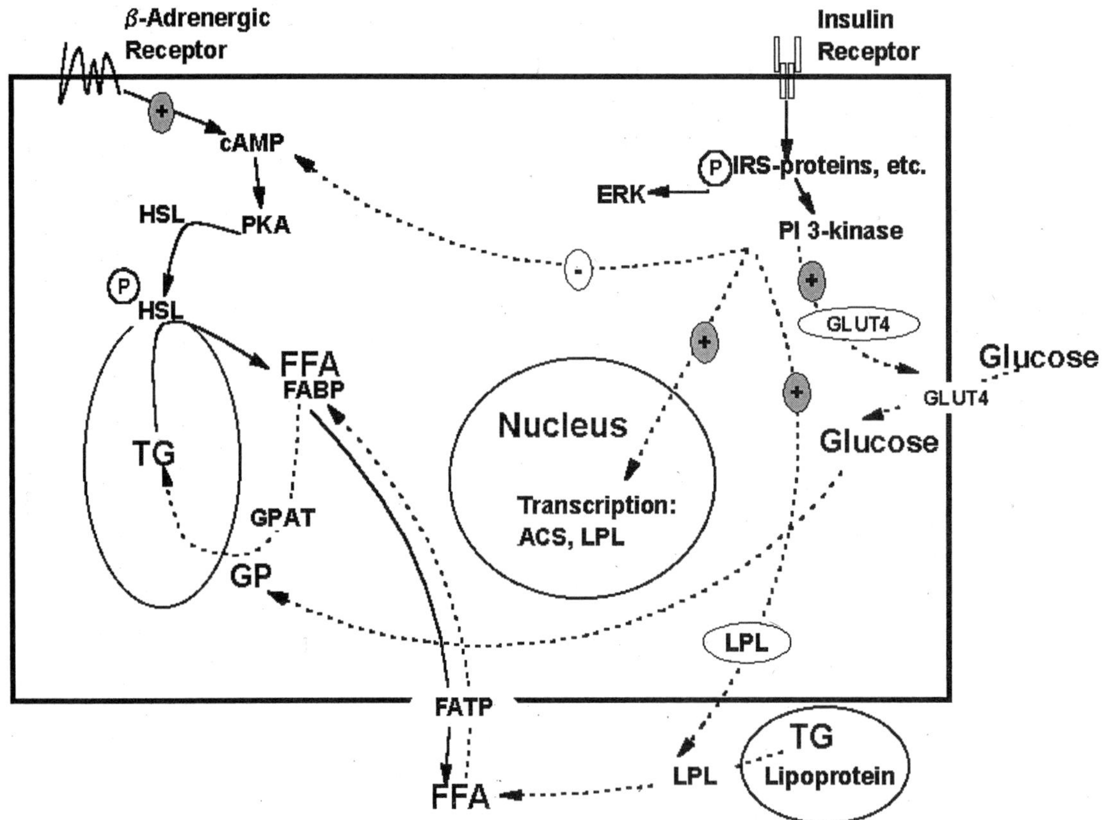

Figure 8.10. Hormonal control of triglyceride metabolism in adipose tissue: signaling and transcriptional events. Insulin stimulation activates its receptor, resulting in the phosphorylation (P) of insulin-receptor substrate (IRS)–proteins and the activation of the extracellular signal–regulated (ERK) kinase and phosphoinositide (PI) 3–kinase pathways. These signals stimulate the movement of GLUT4 from intracellular vesicles to the cell membrane, where they facilitate the uptake of glucose, which is broken down into glycerol-3-phosphate (GP). Insulin also increases the transcription of genes, such as that for lipoprotein lipase (LPL); LPL is secreted from the cell, where it mediates the breakdown of triglyceride (TG) in lipoproteins into free fatty acids (FFAs). FFAs are taken into and moved through the cell by fatty acid–transport and fatty acid–binding proteins (FATP and FABP, respectively). Insulin stimulates the action of glycerol phosphate acyltransferase (GPAT), which mediates the production of intracellular TG from FFA and GP. Receptor binding by counterregulatory hormones such as norepinephrine triggers the accumulation of cyclic adenosine monophosphate (cAMP) and the activation of protein kinase A (PKA), which mediates the phosphorylation of hormone-sensitive lipase (HSL) and its translocation to the lipid droplet, where it mediates the breakdown of TG to FFAs. FFAs are transported through and out of the cell by FABP and FATP. Insulin inhibits the action of HSL by impairing the accumulation of cAMP.

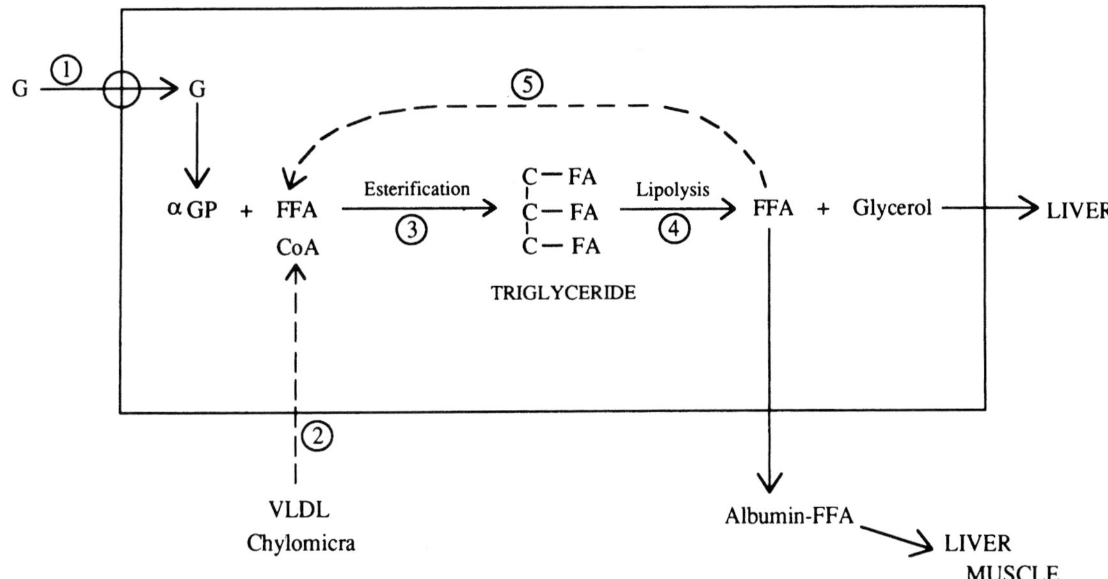

Figure 8.11. Hormonal control of triglyceride metabolism in adipose tissue: regulation by insulin. Insulin stimulates accumulation of triglycerides (TG) by enhancing glucose (G) transport and causing the generation of α-glycerophosphate (α-GP) *(1)*, activating lipoprotein lipase (LPL) *(2)* and glycerol-3-phosphate (GP) acyltransferase *(3)*, and inhibiting hormone-sensitive lipase (HSL) *(4)*. By virtue of its effects on *1* and *3*, insulin also stimulates the reesterification of free fatty acids (FFAs) *(5)* derived from lipolysis of intracellular TG. Hormones, such as norepinephrine, stimulate lipolysis by activating adenyl cyclase and secondarily HSL. Insulin also acts by countering the effects of these hormones. FFAs released from the adipocytes are carried complexed to albumin in the circulation. Principal sites of FFA utilization include muscle and liver (see Fig. 8.12). The glycerol released during lipolysis is not metabolized in the adipocytes, which lack glycerol kinase. Most of this glycerol appears to be used by the liver for gluconeogenesis. VLDL, very-low-density lipoprotein.

motes the uptake of metabolites such as glucose and lipids and their storage as triglyceride. Insulin mediates its effects in adipose and other tissues by binding a cell-surface insulin receptor, activating the tyrosine kinase in the intracellular portion of the receptor (66). The activated insulin receptor then recruits and phosphorylates downstream intracellular substrates, such as the insulin-receptor substrate (IRS)–proteins and Shc. These molecules in turn activate two main intracellular signaling pathways: the phosphoinositide (PI) 3–kinase regulated pathway, and the ras→mitogen-activated protein (MAP) kinase pathway. The counterregulatory hormones, such as catecholamines, oppose the effects of insulin and mediate breakdown and release of stored fats (67,68). In general, the counterregulatory hormones act via seven-transmembrane receptors coupled to heterotrimeric G proteins to stimulate adenylyl cyclase, increasing intracellular levels of cAMP and activating protein kinase A (PKA).

Insulin acts at several levels to promote energy storage. Insulin increases uptake of glucose from the extracellular space by promoting the movement of the insulin-responsive glucose transporter (GLUT4) to the cell surface to increase the rate of glucose flux into the cell (69). Insulin drives the metabolism of glucose to form glycerol 3-phosphate and increases the activity of glycerol phosphate acyltransferase; coupled with the increased FFA uptake also mediated by insulin, the net result is increased triglyceride storage. Insulin increases uptake of FFA by increasing the synthesis and secretion of lipoprotein lipase (LPL) (70,71); LPL degrades triglycerides and phospholipids in adipocyte-bound lipoproteins to FFA. FFAs are then shuttled into the adipocyte by simple diffusion (71a) and/or by specialized fatty acid–transport proteins (FATPs) and fatty acid–binding proteins (FABPs) (72–75), then coupled to CoA by acyl-CoA synthetase (ACS), and finally esterified with glycerol to form triglycerides. Insulin generally acts to increase the production of these and other proteins involved in lipid storage in adipocytes (71,76). Inhibitor studies suggest that most of these effects of insulin require the action of PI 3–kinase but not the ras→MAP kinase pathway (66,77).

NUCLEAR FACTORS IN ADIPOCYTE FUNCTION

The lipid storage function of insulin acts in concert with a number of important nuclear factors that have recently been described. Adipocyte differentiation and determination factor-1/steroid response element binding protein (ADD/SREBP) mediates transcription in response to low levels of cholesterol and other lipids in adipocytes as well as in hepatocytes (78,79). ADD/SREBP is synthesized as an integral membrane protein that is retained in the endoplasmic reticulum (ER). Low cellular levels of cholesterol and other lipids result in the movement of the membrane-bound ADD/SREBP to the Golgi, where it is proteolytically cleaved and released from the membrane. Dissociation from the ER/Golgi allows ADD/SREBP to translocate to the nucleus and increase the transcription of a number of genes required for the synthesis of cholesterol, fatty acids, and triglycerides. The peroxisome proliferator-activator receptor-γ (PPAR-γ) is a so-called orphan nuclear receptor that promotes the differentiation of adipocytes and increases the expression of proteins involved in insulin-stimulated lipid storage, including FATPs, FABPs, ACS, and GLUT4 (80–82). While the endogenous ligand for PPAR-γ remains unknown, the insulin-sensitizing antidiabetic thiazolidinedione compounds act by stimulating PPAR-γ–mediated transcription.

CONTROL OF HORMONE-SENSITIVE LIPASE BY COUNTERREGULATORY HORMONES

The hormone-sensitive lipase (HSL)–mediated breakdown of lipids is one of the best-characterized pathways downstream of counterregulatory hormones such as catecholamines. Although other neutral lipid lipases exist, HSL is the only hormone-regulated neutral lipid lipase (83). HSL is a neutral lipid esterase that mediates the regulated step of triglyceride hydrolysis by removing the first fatty acid moiety from the triglyceride. After generating FFA from triglycerides, FABPs and FATPs transport the FFA through the cytoplasm and out of the cell (73–76). During counterregulatory hormone signaling, PKA mediates the serine phosphorylation of HSL; this phosphorylation event does little to alter the assayable activity of the enzyme, however (84–86). Instead, serine phosphorylation of HSL mediates the translocation of HSL in complex with a protein known as lipotransin from the cytosol to the lipid droplet. Access to the lipid droplet may be increased by the PKA-mediated phosphorylation of the perilipin protein that coats the droplet and by the subsequent dissociation of perilipin from the droplet (87–89). Insulin decreases the phosphorylation of HSL, probably by decreasing intracellular levels of cAMP via increases in phosphodiesterases, but perhaps also by increasing phosphatase activity toward HSL (90,91).

Muscle

FIBER TYPES

Muscle comprises approximately 40% of body mass in a man of normal weight. It accounts for 20% to 30% of the body's consumption of oxygen at rest and for up to 90% during exercise (92). Muscle fibers in the rat are classified as slow-twitch red (type 1), fast-twitch red (type 2a), and fast-twitch white (type 2b) according to their contractile characteristics and their capacity for oxidative metabolism (93,94). The same fiber types are found in human muscle (93). In general, the red fibers have a high oxidative capacity and oxidize fatty acids and other fuels in addition to glucose. White fibers have a lesser ability to oxidize fuels and generate a greater portion of their adenosine triphosphate (ATP) from glycolysis. With respect to exercise, white fibers are those recruited principally during brief periods of intense exercise such as sprinting or weight lifting and red fibers are those recruited during endurance-type activities of low-to-moderate intensity such as walking and running (22,93,95).

All of the fiber types in muscle respond to insulin. However, red fibers have a greater number of insulin receptors (96) and GLUT4 glucose transporters (97) than do white fibers. In addition, muscles rich in red fibers have more capillaries per mass (93,95), which could enhance diffusion of insulin and glucose from the plasma to the muscle cell (98). Perhaps for all of these reasons, glucose uptake in red muscle is more sensitive to insulin than is white muscle both *in vivo* and *in vitro* (99–101). Physical training, which causes white fibers to assume some of the characteristics of red fibers, is associated with an increase in their GLUT4 content (102,103).

FUEL RESERVOIRS

Glycogen

Glycogen in muscle is synthesized from circulating glucose after meals and exercise and is broken down during exercise and starvation. Glycogenolysis in muscle does not result in the release of free glucose into the circulation, since muscle cells are deficient in glucose-6-phosphatase. As a result, the 300 to 500 g of carbohydrate stored as glycogen in muscle is used solely for its own energy needs and for generating lactate and other gluconeogenic substrates for the liver (Fig. 8.12).

The importance of glycogen as a fuel in contracting muscle is underscored by the association of glycogen depletion with the phenomenon of "hitting the wall" in runners (104). Likewise, patients with McArdle syndrome, a hereditary deficiency of muscle phosphorylase, are unable to maintain high-energy phosphate stores during exercise (105). During starvation, mus-

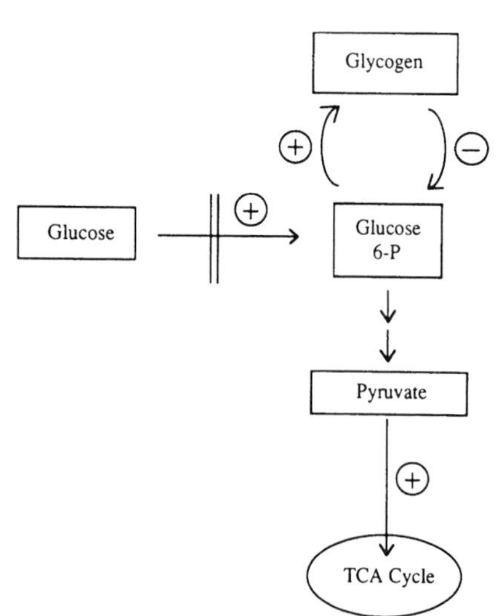

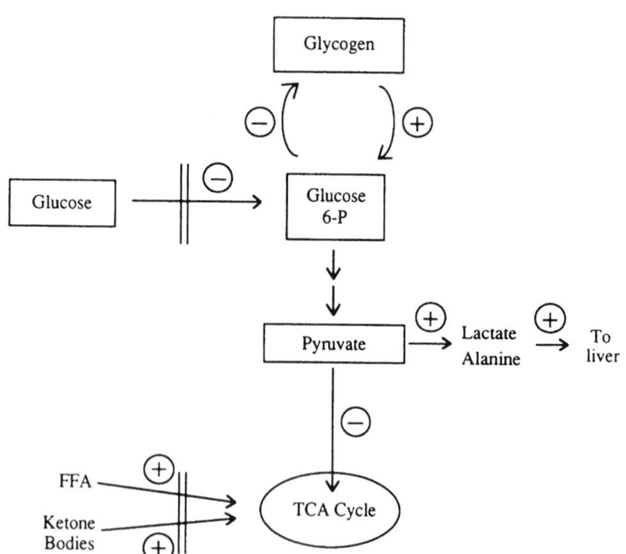

Figure 8.12. Muscle fuel metabolism. **A:** After a carbohydrate meal (high insulin), glucose uptake by the muscle is increased. Within the cell, glycogen synthesis is increased, as is use of glucose by the tricarboxylic acid (TCA) cycle. **B:** After 24 to 48 hours of starvation, glucose uptake by muscle is inhibited and glycogen is broken down. Pyruvate dehydrogenase is inhibited, and pyruvate is converted to lactate and, to a lesser extent, alanine. The + symbols indicate steps enhanced and the – symbols indicate steps diminished in comparison to rates following an overnight fast.

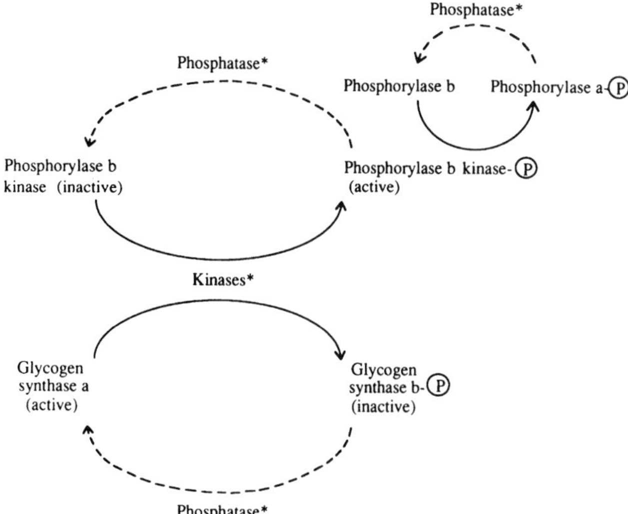

Figure 8.13. Regulation of glycogen synthase and phosphorylase in skeletal muscle. Asterisks, reactions affected by insulin; P, phosphate that alters activity.

cle glycogen in normal individuals diminishes by approximately 33% after 2 to 3 days and then remains constant as muscle switches over more completely to a lipid fuel economy (3,20). During early starvation (phases I and II) and exercise, a considerable portion of the lactate, pyruvate (about 0.1 as much as lactate), and alanine released by muscle is presumably derived from the breakdown of glycogen (34).

The regulation of glycogen synthesis and degradation in muscle by insulin is similar to its regulation of adipocyte triglyceride. Insulin stimulates glycogen synthesis by enhancing glucose transport and activating (dephosphorylating) a key regulatory enzyme, glycogen synthase (106) (Fig. 8.13). Likewise, insulin concurrently diminishes the breakdown of glycogen by inhibiting the conversion (phosphorylation) of phosphorylase *b* to phosphorylase *a* (107). These effects of insulin are thought to be mediated by specific phosphatases that both activate glycogen synthase and eventually inhibit phosphorylase *b* kinase and possibly by the inhibition of a kinase (glycogen synthase kinase 3) that, when active, phosphorylates and inhibits glycogen synthase (108). After exercise, glycogen synthesis is also increased (see Chapter 38), although the responsible mechanism may be different. Catecholamines and exercise per se stimulate the breakdown of muscle glycogen (Fig. 8.14). As in adipose tissue, catecholamines (epinephrine) act by increasing cAMP and secondarily by increasing cAMP-dependent protein kinase, which in turn activates (phosphorylates) phosphorylase *b* kinase (20,109,110).

Lipids

Red muscle fibers, in particular, store some energy as triglycerides, and triglyceride hydrolysis may provide a significant portion of their fuel needs during exercise (111). The question of whether the synthesis and breakdown of triglycerides are regulated in muscle by the same mechanisms as in adipose tissue has not been intensively studied. The activities of lipoprotein lipase in muscle and adipose tissue go in opposite directions during feeding and starvation, suggesting differences between the two tissues with respect to their use of circulating triglycerides (112). A particularly intriguing observation is the strong association of increases in intramuscular triglycerides and insulin resistance (113,114).

Protein

The synthesis and degradation of protein in muscle also are regulated by insulin. Insulin promotes protein synthesis in the fed state and probably acts as a brake on protein degradation during starvation. The mechanisms by which insulin acts on protein metabolism are more complex than those by which it acts on carbohydrate and fat metabolism and have been reviewed elsewhere (115).

Fed State and Starvation

Following a carbohydrate meal or insulin administration, glucose derived from the circulation is the principal oxidative fuel of muscle (116). During early starvation, however, it is placed in this role by fatty acids (116,117) (Fig. 8.12B). As noted earlier, this transition to lipid fuels conserves glucose for use by the

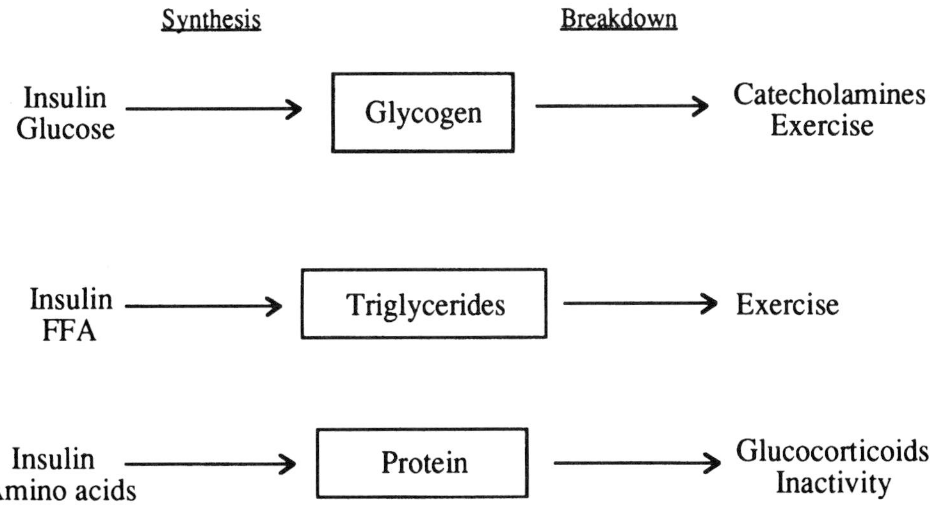

Figure 8.14. Muscle fuel reservoirs and their regulation. Insulin stimulates the synthesis of glycogen, triglycerides, and protein. The breakdown of glycogen and triglycerides is stimulated by catecholamines and by exercise. The breakdown of protein is enhanced by glucocorticoids and inactivity. FFA, free fatty acids.

brain and conserves protein by reducing the need for gluconeogenesis. The precise mechanism by which these events are modulated has not been resolved but is almost certainly related initially to a decrease in circulating levels of insulin to values lower than those in the fed state. Among the changes attributable to the decreased levels of insulin during starvation are (a) diminished glucose transport into muscle; (b) higher plasma levels of FFA; (c) inhibition of pyruvate dehydrogenase in muscle, resulting in a decrease in glucose oxidation and an increase in release of lactate and pyruvate and, secondarily, of alanine; and (d) decreased levels of malonyl-CoA, an inhibitor of carnitine palmitoyltransferase I (CPTI, also referred to as CAT1), which controls the oxidation of fatty acids in muscle and other tissues by regulating the transport of long-chain fatty acyl CoA into the mitochondria (Fig. 8.9). Recent studies have demonstrated that the concentration of malonyl-CoA increases substantially after 1 to 2 hours of refeeding following a fast and that this correlates closely with a decrease in fatty acid oxidation (119).

Another group of fuels used by muscle during starvation is the ketone bodies. Acetoacetate and β-hydroxybutyrate are oxidized by muscle more or less as a function of their concentration in plasma. In rats starved for 48 hours (120) and in humans starved for 1 to 2 weeks (121), the metabolism of these ketone bodies may account for upwards of 70% of the oxygen consumed by muscle. A role for insulin in regulating the utilization of ketone bodies by muscle has been suggested by studies in rats (122) and humans (123,124).

Exercise and Adenosine Monophosphate–Activated Protein Kinase

Exercise can increase oxygen consumption by muscle in excess of 10-fold and, depending on its intensity and duration, may increase both fatty acid and glucose oxidation. It has long been appreciated that the increase in glucose oxidation is the result of increases in glucose transport, glycogenolysis, glycolysis, activation of pyruvate dehydrogenase, and changes in intracellular Ca^{2+} and adenine nucleotides. Recent studies have linked the increase in fatty acid oxidation, at least in part, to activation of an AMP-activated protein kinase (AMPK). Studies in humans and experimental animals have shown that the activity of AMPK is increased within seconds or minutes of the onset of exercise (muscle contraction) and that the activated AMPK phosphorylates acetyl-CoA carboxylase (125,126), which it inhibits, and malonyl-CoA decarboxylase, which it activates (127), leading to a decrease in malonyl-CoA. Abundant evidence suggests that this results in an increase in fatty acid oxidation. It is interesting that treatment with a cell-permeable AMPK-activator, AICAR, also activates glucose transport in the muscle cell, and when administered *in vivo* for several days or longer, increases the expression of the GLUT4, hexokinase 1 and 2, and several mitochondrial enzymes. In other words, it mimics many (although not all) of the effects of exercise, suggesting that activation of AMPK may be an integral component of both the acute- and long-term response of the muscle cell during physical activity. Interestingly, it has recently been shown that the action of the antidiabetic drug metformin (127a) and the adipocyte hormone adiponectin (127b,c) might be mediated by AMPK.

Liver

The liver is the key regulatory site of glucose homeostasis. Blood glucose levels are maintained in a narrow range in great measure because the liver is able to take up glucose in the fed state and to release it in varying amounts into the circulation during starvation, exercise, and other situations in which the ratio of insulin to counterinsulin factors is decreased (Fig. 8.14). Although the liver does not play a key role in determining the rate at which FFAs enter the circulation, it does appear to play a major role in the disposition of FFAs. Thus, the liver can oxidize FFAs for its own energy needs or production of ketone bodies or it can utilize FFAs for the synthesis of triglycerides and phospholipids, which it can export as constituents of very-low-density lipoprotein (VLDL).

FED STATE

High levels of circulating insulin and decreased levels of glucagon, such as occur after a carbohydrate meal, stimulate glycogen synthase and inhibit glycogen phosphorylase in the liver (18,128). These changes in insulin and glucagon also inhibit hepatic gluconeogenesis (25,26,129). However, gluconeogenesis does not appear to cease immediately but may continue for several hours after the termination of a fast with a meal. This persistence of gluconeogenesis after a meal may allow hepatic glycogen synthesis to continue when glucose absorption by the gut is no longer in excess of the needs of other organs. According to this glucose paradox hypothesis (130), dietary glucose is metabolized initially to pyruvate or lactate in peripheral cells; the liver then takes up these gluconeogenic precursors and resynthesizes glucose-6-phosphate, which can be used to synthesize glycogen. Studies in humans suggest that glucose is incorporated into glycogen by this indirect route as well as by the classical direct pathway (131,132). Studies using ^{13}C nuclear magnetic resonance (NMR) spectroscopy suggest that glucose conversion to glycogen via the direct pathway predominates immediately after a standard meal (132).

STARVATION

As starvation proceeds through its different phases (Fig. 8.2), the liver releases fuels into the circulation by three distinct processes: glycogenolysis, gluconeogenesis, and ketone body formation. The breakdown of glycogen in the liver is essentially regulated by insulin and counterinsulin hormones in a manner analogous to that in skeletal muscle (128). A major difference between the two tissues, as previously stated, is that liver can generate free glucose, which is released into the circulation, because of the presence of glucose-6-phosphatase. Another difference is that a primary stimulus of hepatic glycogenolysis is glucagon, which does not act on muscle.

Binding of glucagon to its receptor activates adenylyl cyclase in liver, producing cAMP from ATP (133). Besides initiating glycogenolysis, an increase in liver cAMP suppresses glycogen synthesis and increases gluconeogenesis (4,22,128,133). As noted earlier, liver glycogenolysis is critical in meeting the body's energy requirements in the early stages of starvation. Between one third and two thirds of the glucose released by the liver after an overnight fast is derived from hepatic glycogen (23). Several inherited metabolic disorders of glycogen storage or breakdown have been described. These include von Gierke disease (type I glycogen storage disease), in which glucose-6-phosphatase is deficient and the liver cannot release free glucose into the circulation; Hers disease (type VI glycogen storage disease), in which liver glycogen phosphorylase is absent; and Cori disease (type III glycogen storage disease), in which the debranching enzyme that hydrolyzes the 1,6 linkage of the glycogen molecule is absent (134).

GLUCONEOGENESIS

In humans, the maintenance of euglycemia during starvation depends on the ability of the liver to synthesize glucose from nonhexose precursors (i.e., gluconeogenesis) (Table 8.4 and Fig. 8.15). The molecular mechanisms regulating gluconeogenesis (22,129,135) and the disorders of this pathway in humans have been reviewed elsewhere (13,34,129). Gluconeogenesis uses

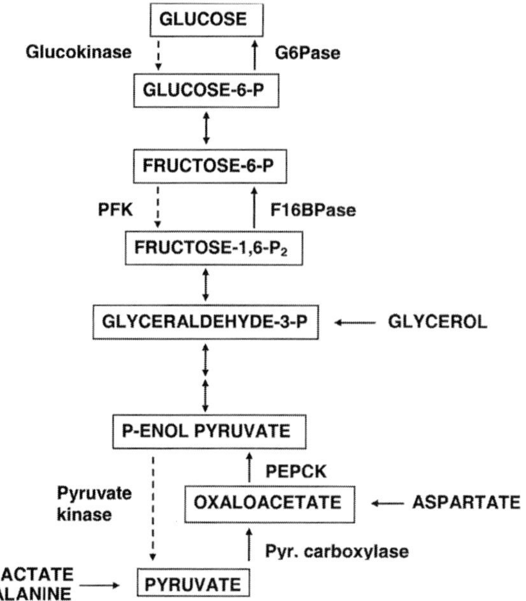

Figure 8.15. Glucose metabolism in the liver during starvation. PEPCK, phosphoenolpyruvate carboxykinase; PFK, phosphofructokinase; F16BPase, fructose 1,6-bisphosphatase.

many of the enzymes involved in glycolysis but requires unique enzymes to circumvent the reactions catalyzed by glucokinase, phosphofructokinase, and pyruvate kinase (Fig. 8.15). As with glycogenolysis, glucagon is a major positive hormonal modulator of gluconeogenesis and insulin is the primary inhibitor. Catecholamines also stimulate gluconeogenesis and may be the principal positive regulator in some patients with long-standing type 1 diabetes in whom glucagon secretion is impaired (7). Glucocorticoids appear to play an important permissive role, since the stimulation of gluconeogenesis by glucagon and catecholamines is diminished in their absence (17).

FORMATION OF KETONE BODIES

Synthesis of ketone bodies occurs almost exclusively within the liver. Mitochondrial acetyl-CoA produced from oxidation of fatty acids either can combine with oxaloacetate and enter the tricarboxylic acid (TCA) cycle or can be used for the synthesis of acetoacetate and β-hydroxybutyrate within the mitochondrion (22,135–138). When rates of FFA–CoA uptake by mitochondria are high, much of the energy needs of the liver are generated by their β-oxidation to acetyl-CoA. Under these conditions, acetyl-CoA preferentially enters the pathway for ketone-body formation and its oxidation in the TCA cycle is diminished (Fig. 8.9). The high ratio of glucagon to insulin and the increase in intrahepatic fatty acids during prolonged starvation stimulate the enzyme CPTI, which is located within the outer leaflet of the inner mitochondrial membrane (Fig. 8.9) (137,138) and is rate-limiting for fatty acid oxidation.

INTERRELATIONS BETWEEN FATTY ACID AND GLUCOSE METABOLISM AND INSULIN RESISTANCE

Glucose in the presence of insulin inhibits the oxidation of fatty acids in muscle, liver, the pancreatic β-cell, and undoubtedly other tissues. Conversely, elevated levels of fatty acids can inhibit the oxidation of glucose. From a functional perspective, such increases in plasma levels of FFA have been linked to events such as the stimulation of hepatic gluconeogenesis and ketogenesis and the maintenance of the low but finite rate of insulin secretion during starvation. The notion that high plasma levels of FFA could also contribute to the insulin resistance (defined as a decrease in the biologic effect of the hormone) in diabetes and obesity was initially given credibility by the studies of Randle et al. (139,140) that led them to propose the existence of a glucose–fatty acid cycle. The Randle mechanism was worked out in a preparation of isolated perfused rat heart, and although it has been difficult to apply it to other tissues, recent studies have strongly suggested a link between abnormalities in fatty acid metabolism and insulin resistance. Thus, the administration of lipids to prevent decreases in plasma FFA levels during an infusion of insulin and glucose (euglycemic–hyperinsulinemic clamp) has been shown to diminish the ability of insulin to increase glucose uptake by muscle and to diminish its production by liver in humans and experimental animals (141,142). Likewise, a close association between insulin resistance (assessed by the clamp procedure) and intramuscular triglycerides, quantified by NMR imagery, has been reported by several groups (113,114). Concurrently, studies in rodents have found that insulin resistance in skeletal muscle in a wide variety of conditions is characteristically associated with increases in the concentrations of malonyl-CoA, long-chain fatty acyl-CoA, diacylglycerol, and triglycerides and alterations in the distribution and activation of certain protein kinase C isoforms (143). Figure 8.16 depicts how increases in PKC activity and other factors linked to insulin resistance (see Chapter 24) might arise in this setting. The possible linkage of this or a similar mechanism to obesity and to the disordered function and metabolism of other tissues in individuals with type 2 diabetes and obesity has been discussed elsewhere (144). An attractive feature of this mechanism is that it could explain why exercise, acting through AMPK, could attenuate insulin resistance and exert effects on multiple tissues.

TYPE 1 DIABETES MELLITUS

The hormone–fuel interrelationships described in healthy humans are abnormal in patients with untreated type 1 diabetes because of the lack of insulin. The precise manifestations of this lack depend on its severity. During the period before the onset of overt type 1 diabetes and during the "honeymoon" phase following its diagnosis, patients may have sufficiently high plasma levels of insulin to maintain a normal fasting concentration of glucose (145,146). Hyperglycemia may be manifest only postprandially, when higher rates of insulin secretion are required to maintain euglycemia. As β-cell destruction progresses, plasma insulin levels fall even during the fasted state, hepatic glucose production increases, and the patient requires insulin therapy (146,147). With more severe insulin deficiency, plasma FFA levels increase in response to enhanced lipolysis, and plasma triglyceride levels may increase because of a decrease in lipoprotein lipase activity (see discussion of lipoprotein lipase in the section titled "Adipose Tissue").

The most extreme form of poorly controlled type 1 diabetes is diabetic ketoacidosis (see Chapter 53). Here the deficiency of insulin and/or the increase in counterinsulin hormones are sufficiently severe to increase glycogen, protein, and lipid catabolism well beyond the fuel needs of the patient. Furthermore, the ability of peripheral tissues to utilize glucose and ketone bodies is impaired and large quantities of these fuels are lost in the

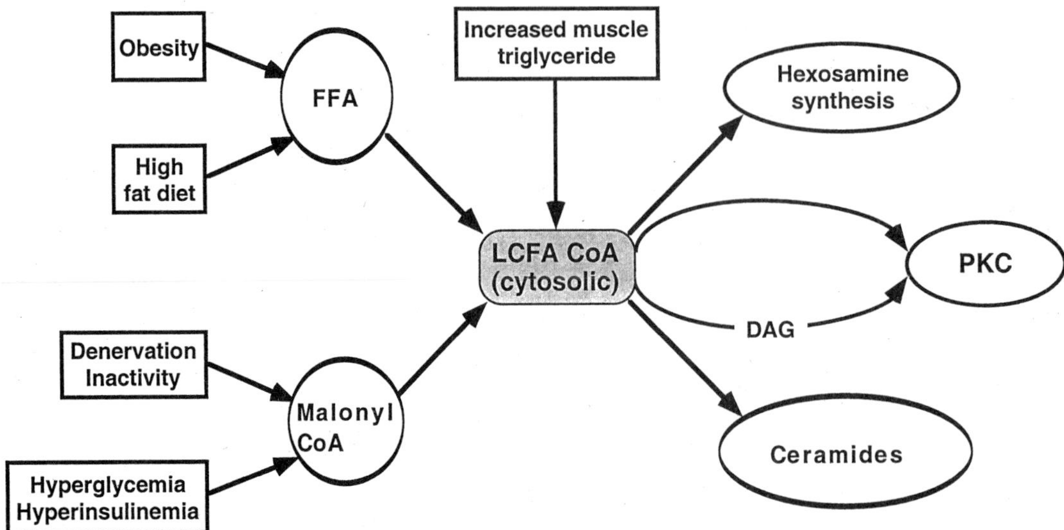

Figure 8.16. Hypothetical interrelations between concentration of cytosolic long-chain fatty acid (LCFA)–coenzyme A (CoA) and development of insulin resistance in muscle. According to this scheme, free fatty acids (FFAs) increase the concentration of LCFA-CoA by mass action and hyperglycemia (in the presence of insulin) by generating malonyl-CoA, which inhibits entrance of LCFA-CoA into mitochondria. By generating α-glycerophosphate, hyperglycemia will also increase fatty acid esterification. Insulin resistance could result from effects on diacylglycerol (DAG)–protein kinase C (PKC) signaling, ceramide synthesis, and so forth. See text for details.

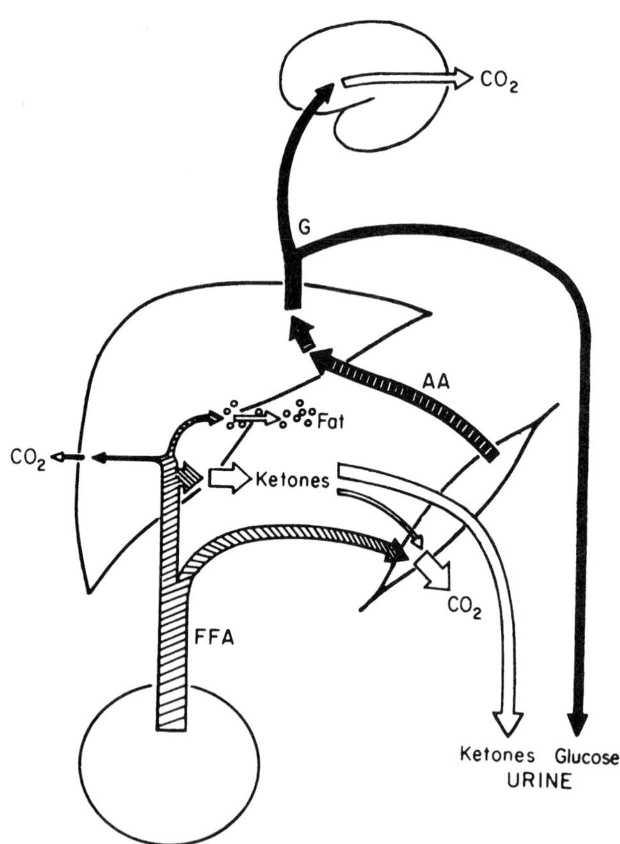

Figure 8.17. Diabetic ketoacidosis. Restraint on catabolism by insulin is lost, and lipolysis, ketogenesis, gluconeogenesis, and protein catabolism are enhanced. In addition, the utilization of ketone bodies and glucose by muscle is impaired. Studies in experimental animals suggest that ketone bodies may be used as a fuel for the brain in this state. G, glucose; AA, amino acids; FFA, free fatty acids.

urine. Some of the metabolic differences between diabetic ketoacidosis and prolonged starvation, in which plasma levels of FFA and ketone bodies are also elevated, are illustrated in Fig. 8.17.

TYPE 2 DIABETES MELLITUS

Whereas the metabolic derangements in type 1 diabetes are readily explained by a lack of insulin, the basis for the metabolic abnormalities in type 2 diabetes is less clear. Nonetheless, type 2 diabetes can be separated into stages according to hormone–fuel interrelationships (Fig. 8.18). An increasing body of evidence suggests that an early abnormality in this disorder is hyperinsulinemia, which is associated with insulin resistance (148–150). Initially, these patients are similar to obese nondiabetic adults, in that they are hyperinsulinemic but usually have normal or near-normal glucose tolerance (Fig. 8.18). In addition, they frequently have higher-than-normal plasma triglyceride levels and elevated blood pressure. Some of them have an upper body (android) pattern of fat distribution with increased intraabdominal fat even if they are not grossly obese (151,152). Current thinking holds that such individuals go on to develop overt type 2 diabetes, hypertension, certain dyslipidemias, and premature atherosclerotic vascular disease, singly or in combination, depending on their genetic makeup and environmental factors such as diet and physical activity (153–155). The insulin-resistant state that antedates these disorders has been referred to as metabolic obesity, the metabolic syndrome, or syndrome X (153).

Type 2 diabetes appears to develop in patients with acquired (diet- or obesity-related) and genetically programmed insulin resistance when the pancreatic β-cells are no longer able to produce enough extra insulin to maintain normoglycemia (155). Changes in plasma insulin and glucose in type 2 diabetes can be depicted, on the basis of published data (148–150), as occurring

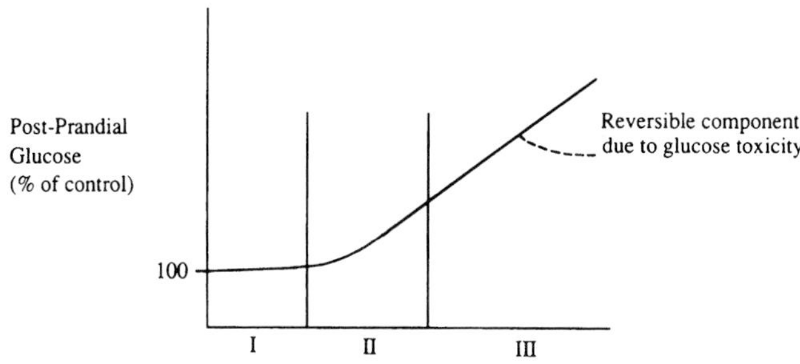

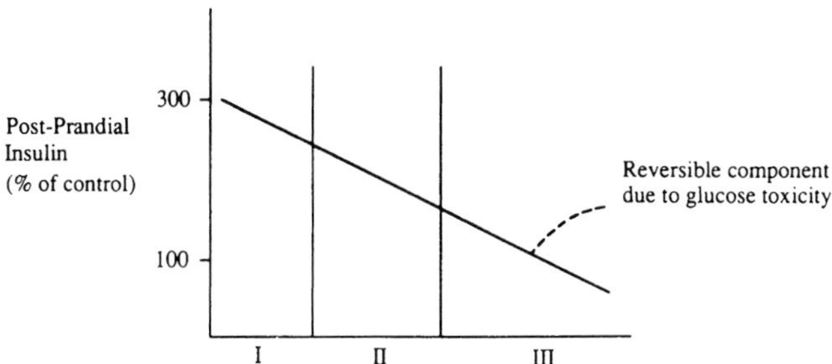

Figure 8.18. Hypothetical changes in postprandial glucose and insulin levels during the evolution of type 2 diabetes mellitus.

in three phases (Fig. 8.18). In phase I, glucose levels are normal but only because hyperinsulinemia compensates for the insulin resistance in muscle, liver, and possibly other tissues. In phase II, insulin levels are somewhat diminished but are generally still higher than those in individuals of normal weight who are not diabetic. On the other hand, the insulin levels in phase II are no longer sufficient to enhance glucose utilization by muscle and/or to restrict hepatic glucose production, and postprandial glucose levels are increased as a result. Finally, in phase III, plasma insulin levels fall even further and overt hyperglycemia occurs both in the fed and fasted states. The inability of the β-cell to secrete insulin at a higher rate indefinitely may therefore determine those who ultimately develop type 2 diabetes. Conversely, the ability of some individuals to maintain hyperinsulinemia might distinguish those who will remain euglycemic and obese. One would predict from this paradigm that therapies designed to diminish insulin resistance and lessen the stress on the β-cell (i.e., diet and regular exercise and insulin-sensitizing drugs) would prevent or at least retard the development of type 2 diabetes (156,157). Thus, it is noteworthy that a lower incidence of progression from impaired glucose tolerance to overt diabetes has recently been reported in individuals undergoing lifestyle modification programs consisting of diet and exercise (158,159) or treatment with metformin (159a). For a more complete discussion of the pathogenesis of type 2 diabetes, see Chapters 24 and 25.

Although the paradigm shown in Figure 8.18 may serve as a model for type 2 diabetes, it provides no insight into either its etiology or its development. Attempts have been made to identify the initial site of insulin resistance. When evaluated with the euglycemic insulin clamp technique, which measures glucose disposal during a continuous infusion of insulin (160), patients with both type 2 diabetes and obesity have been shown to have a significant defect in glucose uptake in skeletal muscle (158), a decrease in glycogen synthesis by muscle (160,161), and an increase in lactate production (161). A decrease in glycogen content has also been observed in skeletal muscle of some patients with type 2 diabetes (162). Some studies suggest that a primary event may be an impairment in the activation of glycogen synthase by insulin in skeletal muscle (163–166). However, investigations in which NMR spectroscopy was used indicate that levels of glucose-6-phosphate and free glucose in muscle are lower in patients with type 2 diabetes than in nondiabetic control subjects during a hyperglycemic–hyperinsulinemic clamp (167), suggesting that a defect in glucose uptake in these individuals is at the level of glucose transport. Yet another metabolic change in muscle in patients with type 2 diabetes is a decrease in pyruvate dehydrogenase activity (168). This presumably contributes to the decrease in glucose oxidation and the increase in muscle lactate release in these individuals. Thus, the mechanisms responsible for the initial insulin resistance in muscle, liver, and adipose tissue and the defect in insulin secretion remain to be absolutely identified.

In addition to the initial site of insulin resistance, the factors that worsen insulin sensitivity and promote transition from one phase to another are not well known. Hyperglycemia may worsen insulin resistance, a phenomenon termed glucose toxicity (169, 170). Persistent hyperglycemia has been shown to inhibit both insulin-stimulated glucose transport and glycogen synthesis in muscle and glucose-mediated insulin secretion (171, 172). In partially pancreatectomized and other rats with hyperglycemia and insulin resistance, increases in insulin sensitivity and the amount of GLUT4 have been shown to occur when the glucose level was made to fall by increasing glycosuria (171, 172). Glycosuria was increased with the use of phloridzin, an inhibitor of renal tubular glucose transport.

Rather than a single specific aberration, type 2 diabetes may prove to be the result of multiple defects in insulin action and insulin secretion. In addition, type 2 diabetes in obese patients may not be due to the same underlying processes as in nonobese patients. In these two groups of patients, the contributions of fasting hyperglycemia (usually attributed to increased hepatic glucose production) and postprandial increases in glucose concentration may also be different. In addition, the abnormalities present in the early stages of type 2 diabetes when blood glucose levels are minimally elevated may not correlate with the factors that perpetuate and worsen the hyperglycemia as time progresses. Interpretation of published studies of fuel homeostasis in patients with type 2 diabetes has been made difficult by the variations in the severity and duration of the diabetes and the unknown impairment of insulin sensitivity. Studies yielding conflicting results may ultimately be reconciled once the magnitude of insulin resistance and impaired insulin secretion has been considered.

REFERENCES

1. Cahill GF Jr. Starvation in man. *Clin Endocrinol Metab* 1976;5:397–415.
2. Renold AE, Cahill GF Jr, eds. In: *Handbook of physiology: a critical comprehensive presentation of physiological knowledge and concepts, V: adipose tissue.* Washington, DC: American Physiological Society, 1965.
3. Ruderman NB, Tornheim K, Goodman MN. Fuel homeostasis and intermediary metabolism of carbohydrate, fat and protein. In: Becker KL, Bilezikian JP, Bremner WJ, et al, eds. *Principles and practice of endocrinology and metabolism.* Philadelphia: JB Lippincott, 2001:1257–1271.
4. Unger RH, Orci L. Glucagon. In: Rifkin H, Porte D, eds. *Ellenberg and Rifkin's diabetes mellitus: theory and practice,* 4th ed. New York: Elsevier, 1990:104–120.
5. McGarry JD, Foster DW. Glucagon and ketogenesis. In: Lefèbvre AM, ed. *Handbook of experimental pharmacology, vol 661: glucagon I.* New York: Springer-Verlag, 1983:383–398.
6. Exton JH. Hormonal control of gluconeogenesis. *Adv Exp Med Biol* 1979;111: 125–167.
7. Cryer PE, Gerich JE. Glucose counterregulation hypoglycemia and intensive insulin therapy in diabetes mellitus. *N Engl J Med* 1985;313:232–241.
8. Merimee TJ, Grant MB. Growth hormone and its disorders. In: Becker KL, Bilezikian JP, Bremner WJ, et al., eds. *Principles and practice of endocrinology and metabolism.* Philadelphia: JB Lippincott, 1990:125–135.

9. Ruderman NB, Herrera MG. Glucose regulation of hepatic gluconeogenesis: *Am J Physiol* 1968;214:1346–1351.
10. Hers H, Hue L. Gluconeogenesis and related aspects of glycolysis. *Annu Rev Biochem* 1983;52:617.
11. Bergman RN. Nonesterified fatty acids and the liver: why is insulin secreted into the portal vein? [Review]. *Diabetologia* 2000;43:946–952.
12. Cahill GF Jr, Herrera MG, Morgan AP, et al. Hormone-fuel interrelationships during fasting. *J Clin Invest* 1966;45:1751–1769.
13. Ruderman NB, Aoki TT, Cahill GF Jr. Gluconeogenesis and its disorders in man. In: Hanson RW, Mehlman MA, eds. *Gluconeogenesis: its regulation in mammalian species.* New York: John Wiley and Sons, 1976:515–532.
14. Richter EA, Ruderman NB, Schneider S. Diabetes and exercise. *Am J Med* 1981;70:201–209.
15. Galbo H. *Hormonal and metabolic adaptation to exercise.* New York: Thieme-Stratton, 1983.
16. Goldstein DS. Physiology of the adrenal medulla and the sympathetic nervous system. In: Becker KL, Bilezikian JP, Bremner WJ, et al., eds. *Principles and practice of endocrinology and metabolism.* Philadelphia: JB Lippincott, 1990: 668–676.
17. Exton JH, Friedmann N, Wong EH-A. Interaction of glucocorticoids with glucagon and epinephrine in the control of gluconeogenesis and glycogenolysis in liver and of lipolysis in adipose tissue. *J Biol Chem* 1972;247:3579–3588.
18. Newsholme EA, Leech AR. Hormones and metabolism. In: Newsholme EA, Leech AR. *Biochemistry for the medical sciences.* New York: John Wiley & Sons, 1983:813–912.
19. Stumvoll M, Meyer C, Mitrakou A, et al. Renal glucose production and utilization: new aspects in humans. *Diabetologia* 1997;40:749–757.
20. Rajas F, Croset M, Zitoun C, et al. Induction of the *PEPCK* gene expression in insulinopenia in rat small intestine. *Diabetes* 2000;49:1165–1168.
21. Owen OE, Reichard GA Jr. Human forearm metabolism during progressive starvation. *J Clin Invest* 1971;50:1536–1545.
22. Felig P. Amino acid metabolism in man. *Annu Rev Biochem* 1975;44:933–955.
23. Rothman DL, Magnusson I, Katz LD. Quantitation of hepatic glycogenolysis and gluconeogenesis in fasting humans with ^{13}C NMR. *Science* 1991;254: 573–576.
24. Sherwin RS, Fisher M, Hendler R, Felig P. Hyperglucagonemia and blood glucose regulation in normal, obese and diabetic subjects. *N Engl J Med* 1976; 294:455–461.
25. Gerich JE, Lorenzi M, Hane S, et al. Evidence for a physiologic role of pancreatic glucagon in human glucose homeostasis: studies with somatostatin. *Metabolism* 1975;24:175–182.
26. Cherrington A, Vranic M. Hormonal control of gluconeogenesis *in vivo.* In: Krauss-Friedman, ed. *Hormonal control of gluconeogenesis.* Boca Raton: FL: CRC Press, 1986:15–37.
27. Cahill GF Jr, Aoki TT, Rossini AA. Metabolism in obesity and anorexia nervosa. In: Wurtman RJ, Wurtman JJ, eds. *Nutrition and the brain.* Vol 3. New York: Raven Press, 1979:1–70.
28. Rothman D, Magnusson I, Katz L, et al. Quantitation of hepatic glycogenolysis and gluconeogenesis in fasting humans with ^{13}C NMR. *Science* 1991; 70:210.
29. Wahren J, Felig P, Cerasi E, Luft R. Splanchnic and peripheral glucose and amino acid metabolism in diabetes mellitus. *J Clin Invest* 1972;51:1870–1878.
30. Consoli A, Kennedy F, Miles J, Gerich J. Determination of Krebs cycle metabolic carbon exchange *in vivo* and its use to estimate the individual contributions of gluconeogenesis and glycogenolysis to overall glucose output in man. *J Clin Invest* 1987;80:1303–1310.
31. Katz H, Homan M, Velosa J, et al. Effects of pancreas transplantation on postprandial glucose metabolism. *N Engl J Med* 1991;325:1278–1283.
32. Ross BD, Hems R, Krebs HA. The rate of gluconeogenesis from various precursors in the perfused rat liver. *Biochem J* 1967;102:942–951.
33. Aoki TT, Toews CJ, Rossini AA, et al. Glucogenic substrate levels in fasting man. *Adv Enzyme Regul* 1975;13:329–336.
34. Ruderman NB. Muscle amino acid metabolism and gluconeogenesis. *Annu Rev Med* 1975;26:245–258.
35. Hagg SA, Taylor SI, Ruderman NB. Glucose metabolism in perfused skeletal muscle: pyruvate dehydrogenase activity in starvation, diabetes and exercise. *Biochem J* 1976;158:203–220.
36. Goodman MN, Ruderman NB. Starvation in the rat, I: effect of age and obesity on organ weights, RNA, DNA and protein. *Am J Physiol* 1980;239: E269–E276.
37. Jefferson LS, Rannels DE, Munger BL, Morgan HE. Insulin in the regulation of protein turnover in heart and skeletal muscle. *Fed Proc* 1974;33:1098–1104.
38. Fulks RM, Li JB, Goldberg AL. Effects of insulin, glucose and amino acids on protein turnover in rat diaphragm. *J Biol Chem* 1975;250:290–298.
39. London DR, Foley TH, Webb CG. Evidence for the release of individual amino-acids from the resting human forearm [Letter]. *Nature* 1965;208: 588–589.
40. Pozefsky T, Felig P, Tobin JD, et al. Amino acid balance across tissues of the forearm in postabsorptive man: effects of insulin at two dose levels. *J Clin Invest* 1969;48:2273–2282.
41. Ruderman NB, Berger M. The formation of glutamine and alanine in skeletal muscle. *J Biol Chem* 1974;249:5500–5506.
42. Felig P, Marliss E, Pozefsky T, et al. Amino acid metabolism in the regulation of gluconeogenesis in man. *Am J Clin Nutr* 1970;23:986–992.
43. Pagliara AS, Karl IE, Haymond M, et al. Hypoglycemia in infancy and childhood: parts I and II. *J Pediatr* 1973;82:365–379, 558–577.
44. Nurjhan N, Consoli A, Gerich J. Increased lipolysis and its consequences on gluconeogenesis in non-insulin-dependent diabetes mellitus. *J Clin Invest* 1992; 89:169–175.
45. Owen OF, Morgan AP, Kemp HG, et al. Brain metabolism during fasting. *J Clin Invest* 1967;46:1589–1595.
46. Bjorkman O, Ahlborg G, Wahren J, Felig P. Changing patterns of brain ketone, glucose and lactate metabolism within 60 hours of fasting in man [abstract]. *Diabetes*1982;31[Suppl 2]:62A.
47. Gjedde A, Crone C. Induction processes in blood-brain transfer of ketone bodies during starvation. *Am J Physiol* 1975;229:1165–1169.
48. Hawkins RA, Biebuyck JF. Ketone bodies are selectively used by individual brain regions. *Science* 1979;205:325–327.
49. Conn AR, Fell DI, Steele RD. Characterization of α-keto acid transport across blood-brain barrier in rats. *Am J Physiol* 1983;245:E253–E260.
50. Oldendorf WH. Carrier-medicated blood-brain barrier transport of short-chain monocarboxylic organic acids. *Am J Physiol* 1973;224:1450–1453.
51. McCall AL, Millington WR, Wurtman RJ. Metabolic fuel and amino acid transport into the brain in experimental diabetes mellitus. *Proc Natl Acad Sci U S A* 1982;79:5406–5410.
52. Sherwin RS, Hendler RG, Felig P. Effect of ketone infusions on amino acid and nitrogen metabolism in man. *J Clin Invest* 1975;55:1382–1390.
53. Owen OE, Felig P, Morgan AP, et al. Liver and kidney metabolism during prolonged starvation. *J Clin Invest* 1969;48:574–583.
54. Goodman MN, Larsen PR, Kaplan MM, et al. Starvation in the rat, II: effect of age and obesity on protein sparing and fuel metabolism. *Am J Physiol* 1980; 239:E277–E286.
55. Flier JS, Spiegelman BM. Obesity and the regulation of energy balance. *Cell* 2001;104:531–543.
56. Ahima RS, Prabakaran D, Mantzoros CS, et al. Role of leptin in the neuroendocrine response to fasting. *Nature* 1996;382:250–252.
57. Flier JS. The adipocyte: storage depot or node on the energy information superhighway. *Cell* 1995;8:15–18.
58. Elmquist JK, Maratos-Flier E, Saper CB, et al. Unraveling the central nervous system pathways underlying responses to leptin. *Nat Neurosci* 1998;1: 445–449.
59. Spiegelman BM, Flier JS. Adipogenesis and obesity: rounding out the big picture. *Cell* 1996;87:377–389.
60. Steppan CM, Bailey ST, Bhat S, et al. The hormone resistin links obesity to diabetes. *Nature* 2001;409:307–312.
61. Hotamisligil GS, Spiegelman BM. Adipose expression of TNFα: direct role in obesity-linked insulin resistance. *Science* 1999;259:87–91.
62. Berg AH, Combs TP, Scherer PE. ACRP30/adiponectin: an adipokine regulating glucose and lipid metabolism. *Trends Endocrinol Metab* 2002;13:84–89.
63. Nagaev I, Smith U. Insulin resistance and type 2 diabetes are not related to resistin expression in human fat cells or skeletal muscle. *Biochem Biophys Res Commun* 2001;285:561–564.
64. Way JM, Gorgun CZ, Tong Q, et al. Adipose tissue resistin expression is severely suppressed in obesity and stimulated by peroxisome proliferator-activated receptor gamma agonists. *J Biol Chem* 2001;276:25651–25653.
65. Fruebis J, Tsao TS, Javorschi S, et al. Proteolytic cleavage product of 30-kDa adipocyte complement-related protein increases fatty acid oxidation in muscle and causes weight loss in mice. *Proc Natl Acad Sci U S A* 2001;98:2005–2010.
66. Myers MG Jr, White MF. Insulin signal transduction and the IRS proteins. *Annu Rev Pharmacol Toxicol* 1996;36:615–658.
67. Lawrence JC Jr, Roach PJ. New insights into the role and mechanism of glycogen synthase activation by insulin. *Diabetes* 1997;46:541–547.
68. Harris RA. Carbohydrate metabolism, I: major metabolic pathways and their control. In: Devlin TM, ed. *Textbook of biochemistry with clinical correlations.* New York: Wiley-Liss, 1997:267.
69. Birnbaum MJ, James DE. The insulin-regulatable glucose transporter GLUT-4. *Curr Opin Endocrinol Diabetes* 1995;2:383–391.
70. Knutson VP. The release of lipoprotein lipase from 3T3-L1 adipocytes is regulated by microvessel endothelial cells in an insulin-dependent manner. *Endocrinology* 2000;141:693–701.
71. Chiappe de Cingalani GE, Goers JW, Giannotti M, et al. Comparative effects of insulin and isoproterenol on lipoprotein lipase in rat adipose cells. *Am J Physiol* 1996;270:C1461–C1467.
71a. Hamilton JA, Kamp F. How are free fatty acids transported in membranes? Is it by proteins or by free diffusion through the lipids? *Diabetes* 1999;48: 2255–2269.
72. Schaffer JE, Lodish HF. Expression cloning and characterization of a novel adipocyte long chain fatty acid transport protein. *Cell* 1994;79:427–436.
73. Storch J, Thumser AE. The fatty acid transport function of fatty acid-binding proteins. *Biochim Biophys Acta* 2000;1486:28–44.
74. Herr FM, Matarese V, Bernlohr DA, et al. Surface lysine residues modulate the collisional transfer of fatty acid from adipocyte fatty acid binding protein to membranes. *Biochemistry* 1995;34:11840–11845.
75. Luxon BA. Inhibition of binding to fatty acid binding protein reduces the intracellular transport of fatty acids. *Am J Physiol* 1996;271:G113–G120.
76. Scheja L, Makowski L, Uysal KT, et al. Altered insulin secretion associated with reduced lipolytic efficiency in aP2−/− mice. *Diabetes* 1999;48:1987–1994.
77. Kraemer FB, Takeda D, Natu V, et al. Insulin regulates lipoprotein lipase activity in rat adipose cells via wortmannin- and rapamycin-sensitive pathways. *Metabolism* 1998;47:555–559.
78. Kim JB, Spiegelman BM. ADD1/SREBP1 promotes adipocyte differentiation and gene expression linked to fatty acid metabolism. *Genes Dev* 1996;10:1096–1107.

79. Brown MS, Goldstein JL. The SREBP pathway: regulation of cholesterol metabolism by proteolysis of a membrane-bound transcription factor. *Cell* 1997;89:331–340.
80. Schoonjans K, Peinado-Onsurbe J, Lefebvre AM, et al. PPARalpha and PPARgamma activators direct a distinct tissue-specific transcriptional response via a PPRE in the lipoprotein lipase gene. *EMBO J* 1996;15:5336–5348.
81. Spiegelman BM. PPARγ: adipogenic regulator and thiazolidinedione receptor. *Diabetes* 1998;47:507–514.
82. Tontonoz P, Hu E, Spiegelman BM. Stimulation of adipogenesis in fibroblasts by PPARγ2, a lipid-activated transcription factor. *Cell* 1994;79:1147–1156.
83. Osuga J, Ishibashi S, Oka T, et al. Targeted disruption of hormone-sensitive lipase results in male sterility and adipocyte hypertrophy, but not in obesity. *Proc Natl Acad Sci U S A* 2000;97:787–792.
84. Syu LJ, Saltiel AR. Lipotransin: a novel docking protein for hormone-sensitive lipase. *Mol Cell* 1999;4:109–115.
85. Anthonsen MW, Ronnstrand L, Wernstedt C, et al. Identification of novel phosphorylation sites in hormone-sensitive lipase that are phosphorylated in response to isoproterenol and govern activation properties *in vitro*. *J Biol Chem* 1998;273:215–221.
86. Clifford GM, Londos C, Kraemer FB, et al. Translocation of hormone-sensitive lipase and perilipin upon lipolytic stimulation of rat adipocytes. *J Biol Chem* 2000;275:5011–5015.
87. Souza SC, de Vargas LM, Yamamoto MT, et al. Overexpression of perilipin A and B blocks the ability of tumor necrosis factor alpha to increase lipolysis in 3T3-L1 adipocytes. *J Biol Chem* 1998;273:24665–24669.
88. Londos C, Gruia-Gray J, Brasaemle DL, et al. Perilipin: possible roles in structure and metabolism of intracellular neutral lipids in adipocytes and steroidogenic cells. *Int J Obes Relat Metab Disord* 1996;20[Suppl 3]:S97–S101.
89. Blanchette-Mackie EJ, Dwyer NK, Barber T, et al. Perilipin is located on the surface layer of intracellular lipid droplets in adipocytes. *J Lipid Res* 1995;36: 1211–1226.
90. Enoksson S, Degerman E, Hagstrom-Toft E, et al. Various phosphodiesterase subtypes mediate the *in vivo* antilipolytic effect of insulin on adipose tissue and skeletal muscle in man. *Diabetologia* 1998;41:560–568.
91. Degerman E, Landstrom TR, Wijkander J, et al. Phosphorylation and activation of hormone-sensitive adipocyte phosphodiesterase type 3B. *Methods* 1998;14:43–53.
92. Astrand PO. Whole body metabolism in exercise. In: Horton ES, Terjung RL, eds. *Exercise, nutrition and energy metabolism*. New York: Macmillan, 1988:1–8.
93. Armstrong RB. Muscle fiber recruitment patterns and their metabolic correlates. In: Horton ES, Terjung RL, eds. *Exercise, nutrition and energy metabolism*. New York: Macmillan, 1988:9–26.
94. Armstrong RB, Phelps RO. Muscle fiber type composition of rat hindlimb. *Am J Anat* 1984;171:259–272.
95. Saltin B, Gollnick PD. Skeletal muscle adaptability: significance for metabolism and performance. In: Peachy LD, Adrian RH, Geiger SR, eds. *Handbook of physiology, 10: skeletal muscle*. Bethesda, MD: American Physiological Society, 1983:555–631.
96. Bonen A, Tan MH, Watson-Wright WM. Insulin binding and glucose uptake differences in rodent skeletal muscles. *Diabetes* 1981;30:702–704.
97. Henriksen EJ, Bourey RE, Rodnick KJ, et al. Glucose transporter protein content and glucose transport capacity in rat skeletal muscles. *Am J Physiol* 1990; 259:E593–E598.
98. Ader M, Poulin RA, Yang YJ, et al. Dose-response relationship between lymph insulin and glucose uptake reveals enhanced insulin sensitivity of peripheral tissues. *Diabetes* 1992;41:241–253.
99. Maizels EZ, Ruderman NB, Goodman MN, et al. Effect of acetoacetate on glucose metabolism in the soleus and extensor digitorum longus muscles of the rat. *Biochem J* 1977;162:557–568.
100. Richter EA, Garetto LP, Goodman MN, et al. Muscle glucose metabolism following exercise in the rat: increased sensitivity to insulin. *J Clin Invest* 1982; 69:785–793.
101. James DE, Jenkins AB, Kraegen EW. Heterogenicity of insulin action in individual muscles *in vivo*: euglycemic clamp studies in rats. *Am J Physiol* 1985; 248:E567–E574.
102. Rodnick KJ, Holloszy JO, Mondon CE, et al. Effects of exercise training on insulin-regulatable glucose-transporter protein levels in rat skeletal muscle. *Diabetes* 1990;39:1425–1429.
103. Houmard JA, Egan PC, Neufer PK, et al. Elevated skeletal muscle glucose transporter levels in exercise-trained middle-aged men. *Am J Physiol* 1991; 261:E437–E443.
104. Bergström J, Hermansen L, Hultman E, et al. Diet, muscle glycogen and physical performance. *Acta Physiol Scand* 1967;71:140–150.
105. Lewis SF, Haller RG. Skeletal muscle disorders and associated factors that limit exercise performance. *Exerc Sport Sci Rev* 1989;17:67–113.
106. Roach PJ. Glycogen synthase and glycogen synthase kinases. *Curr Top Cell Regul* 1981;20:45–105.
107. Chock PB, Rhee SG, Stadtman ER. Interconvertible enzyme cascades in cellular regulation. *Annu Rev Biochem* 1980;49:813–843.
108. Lawrence JC Jr, Roach PJ. New insights into the role and mechanism of glycogen synthase activation by insulin. *Diabetes* 1997;46:541.
109. Exton JH. Mechanisms involved in α-adrenergic phenomena: role of calcium ions in actions of catecholamines in liver and other tissues. *Am J Physiol* 1980; 238:E3–E12.
110. Cohen P. Signal integration at the level of protein kinases, protein phosphatases and their substrates. *Trends Biochem Sci* 1992;17:408–413.
111. Gollnick PD, Saltin B. Fuel for muscular exercise: role of fat. In: Horton ES, Terjung RL, eds. *Exercise, nutrition and energy metabolism*. New York: Macmillan, 1988:72–88.
112. Borensztajn J. Heart and skeletal muscle lipoprotein lipase. In: Borensztajn J, ed. *Lipoprotein lipase*. Chicago: Evener, 1987:133–148.
113. Stein DT, Dobbins RL, Szczepaniak LS, et al. Skeletal muscle triglyceride stores are increased in insulin resistance [abstr]. *Diabetes* 1997;46[Suppl 1]: A23.
114. Krssak M, Falk Petersen K, Dresner A, et al. Intramyocellular lipid concentrations are correlated with insulin sensitivity in humans: a 1H NMR spectroscopy study. *Diabetologia* 1990;276:E529–E535.
115. Kimball SR, Flaim KE, Peavy DE, et al. Protein metabolism. In: Rifkin H, Porte D Jr, eds. *Ellenberg and Rifkin's diabetes mellitus: theory and practice*, 4th ed. New York: Elsevier, 1990:41–50.
116. Kelley DE, Relly JP, Veneman T, et al. Effects of insulin on skeletal muscle glucose storage, oxidation and glycolysis in humans. *Am J Physiol* 1990;258: E923–E929.
117. Andres R, Cader G, Zierler KL. The quantitatively minor role of carbohydrate in oxidative metabolism by skeletal muscle in intact man in the basal state: measurements of oxygen and glucose uptake and carbon dioxide and lactate production in the forearm. *J Clin Invest* 1956;35:671–682.
118. Chien D, Dean D, Saha AK, et al. Malonyl CoA content and distribution and fatty-acid oxidation in rat muscle and liver *in vivo*. *Am J Physiol* 2000;279:1912–1913.
119. McGarry JD, Mills SE, Long CS, et al. Observations on the affinity for carnitine and malonyl-CoA sensitivity, of carnitine palmitoyltransferase I in animal and human tissues: demonstration of the presence of malonyl-CoA in non-hepatic tissues of the rat. *Biochem J* 1983;214:21–28.
120. Ruderman NB, Houghton CRS, Hems R. Evaluation of the isolated perfused rat hindquarter for the study of muscle metabolism. *Biochem J* 1971;124: 639–651.
121. Gammeltoft D. The significance of ketone bodies in fat metabolism, I: concentration of ketone bodies in the arterial and venous blood in human subjects during starvation. *Acta Physiol Scand* 1950;19:270–279.
122. Ruderman NB, Goodman MN. Inhibition of muscle acetoacetate utilization during diabetic ketoacidosis. *Am J Physiol* 1974;226:136–143.
123. Sherwin RS, Hendler RG, Felig P. Effect of diabetes mellitus and insulin on the turnover and metabolic response to ketones in man. *Diabetes* 1976;25: 776–784.
124. Fery F, Balasse EO. Ketone body production and disposal in diabetic ketosis: a comparison with fasting ketosis. *Diabetes* 1985;34:326–332.
125. Vavvas D, Apazidis A, Saha A, et al. Contraction-induced changes in acetyl-CoA Carboxylase and 5′ AMP-activated kinase in skeletal muscle. *J Biol Chem* 1997;272:13255–13261.
126. Winder WW, Wilson HA, Hardie DG, et al. Phosphorylation of rat muscle acetyl-CoA carboxylase and activation of AMP-activated protein kinase and protein kinase. *Am J Appl Physiol* 1997;182:219–225.
127. Saha AK, Schwarsin AJ, Roduit R, et al. Activation of malonyl CoA decarboxylase in rat skeletal muscle by contraction and the AMP-activated protein kinase activator AICAR. *J Biol Chem* 2000;275:24279–24283.
127a. Zhou G, Myers R, Li Y, et al. Role of AMP-activated protein kinase in the mechanism of insulin action. *J Clin Invest* 2001;108:1167–1174.
127b. Yamauchi T, Kamon J, Minokoshi Y, et al. Adiponectin stimulates glucose utilization and fatty acid oxidation by activating AMP-activated protein kinase. *Nat Med* 2002;8:1–8.
127c. Tomas E, Tsao TS, Saha AK, et al. Enhanced muscle fat oxidation and glucose transport by ACRP30 globular domain: Acetyl CoA carboxylase inhibition and AMP-activated protein kinase activation. *Proc Natl Acad Sci U S A* 2002;99:16309–16313.
128. Stalmans W, Bollen M, Mvumbi L. Control of glycogen synthesis in health and disease. *Diabetes Metab Rev* 1987;3:127–161.
129. Kraus-Friedmann N. Hormonal regulation of hepatic gluconeogenesis. *Physiol Rev* 1984;64:170–259.
130. Katz J, McGarry JD. The glucose paradox: is glucose a substrate for liver metabolism? *J Clin Invest* 1981;74:1901–1909.
131. McGarry JD, Kuwajima M, Newgard CB, et al. From dietary glucose to liver glycogen: the full circle round. *Annu Rev Nutr* 1987;7:51–73.
132. Shulman GI, Cline G, Schumann WC, et al. Quantitative comparison of pathways of hepatic glycogen repletion in fed and fasted humans. *Am J Physiol* 1990;259:E335–E341.
133. Exton JH. Mechanisms of hormonal regulation of hepatic glucose metabolism. *Diabetes Metab Rev* 1987;3:163–183.
134. Beaudet AL. The glycogen storage diseases. In: Wilson JD, Braunwald E, Isselbacher KJ, eds. *Harrison's principles of internal medicine*, 12th ed. New York: McGraw-Hill, 1991:1854–1860.
135. Hue L. Gluconeogenesis and its regulation. *Diabetes Metab Rev* 1987;3:111–126.
136. McGilvery RW, Goldstein GW. *Biochemistry, a functional approach*, 3rd ed. Philadelphia: WB Saunders, 1983.
137. McGarry JD, Foster DW. Regulation of hepatic fatty acid oxidation and ketone body production. *Annu Rev Biochem* 1980;49:395–420.
138. McGarry J, Foster D, Ketogenesis. In: Rifkin H, Porte D, eds. *Ellenberg and Rifkin's diabetes mellitus: theory and practice*, 4th ed. New York: Elsevier, 1990:292–298.
139. Randle PJ, Garland PB, Hales CN, et al. The glucose fatty-acid cycle: its role in insulin sensitivity and metabolic disturbances of diabetes mellitus. *Lancet* 1963;1:785–789.

140. Randle PJ, Garland PB, Hales CN, et al. Interaction of hormones and the physiological role of insulin. *Rec Prog Horm Res* 1966;22:1–47.
141. Boden G. Free fatty acids, insulin resistance, and type 2 diabetes mellitus. *Proc Assoc Am Physicians* 1999;111:241–248.
142. Roden M, Price TB, Perseghin G, et al. Mechanisms of free fatty acid induced insulin resistance in humans. *J Clin Invest* 1996;17:2859–2865.
143. Ruderman NB, Saha AK, Vavvas D, et al. Malonyl CoA, fuel sensing and insulin resistance. *Am J Physiol* 1999;276:E1–E18.
144. Ruderman NB, Saha AK, Vavvas D, et al. Lipid abnormalities in muscle of insulin resistance rodents: the malonyl CoA hypothesis. *Ann N Y Acad Sci* 1997;827:221–230.
145. Srikanta S, Ganda OP, Rabizadeh A, et al. First-degree relatives of patients with type I diabetes mellitus: islet-cell antibodies and abnormal insulin secretion. *N Engl J Med* 1985;313:461–464.
146. Palmer JP, Lernmark A. Pathophysiology of type I (insulin-dependent) diabetes. In: Rifkin H, Porte D, eds. *Ellenberg and Rifkin's diabetes mellitus: theory and practice,* 4th ed. New York: Elsevier, 1990:414–435.
147. Eisenbarth GS, Connelly J, Soeldner JS. The "natural" history of type I diabetes. *Diabetes Metab Rev* 1987;3:873–891.
148. Lillioja S, Mott DM, Zawadzki JK, et al. *In vivo* insulin action is familial characteristic in nondiabetic Pima Indians. *Diabetes* 1987;36:1329–1335.
149. Eriksson J, Franssila-Kallunki A, Ekstrand A, et al. Early metabolic defects in persons at increased risk for noninsulin-dependent diabetes mellitus. *N Engl J Med* 1989;321:337–343.
150. Warram JH, Martin BC, Krolewski AS, et al. Slow glucose removal rate and hyperinsulinemia precede the development of type II diabetes in the offspring of diabetic parents. *Ann Intern Med* 1990;113:909–915.
151. Björntorp P. Abdominal obesity and the development of noninsulin-dependent diabetes mellitus. *Diabetes Metab Rev* 1988;4:622–627.
152. Bergstrom RW, Newell-Morris LL, Leonett DL, et al. Association of elevated fasting C-peptide level and increased intra-abdominal fat distribution with development of NIDDM in Japanese-American men. *Diabetes* 1990;39:104–111.
153. Ruderman NB, Schneider SH, Berchtold P. The metabolically obese normal weight individual. *Am J Clin Nutr* 1981;34:1617–1621.
154. Reaven GM. Role of insulin resistance in human diabetes. *Diabetes* 1988;37: 1595–1607.
155. DeFronzo RA, Ferrannini E. Insulin resistance: a multifaceted syndrome responsible for NIDDM, obesity, hypertension, dyslipidemia and atherosclerotic cardiovascular disease. *Diabetes Care* 1991;14:173–194.
156. Ruderman NB, Schneider SH. Exercise in type 2 diabetes. In: Saltin B, Galba H, Richter EA, eds. *Biochemistry of exercise.* Vol 6. Champaign, IL: Human Kinetics Publishers, 1986:255–265.
157. Ruderman NB, Apelian AZ, Schneider SH. Exercise in therapy and prevention of type II diabetes: implications for blacks. *Diabetes Care* 1990;13[Suppl 4]: 1163–1168.
158. Tuomilehto J, Lindstrom J, Eriksson JG, et al. Prevention of type 2 diabetes mellitus by changes in lifestyle among subjects with impaired glucose tolerance. *N Engl J Med* 2001;344:1343–1350.
159. Ruderman NB, Schneider SH, Derlin JF, et al. *Handbook of diabetes in exercise.* Alexandria, VA: American Diabetes Association, 2002:Chapters 8–12.
159a. Diabetes Prevention Program Research Group. Reduction in the incidence of type 2 diabetes with lifestyle intervention or metformin. *N Engl J Med* 1992;346:393–403.
160. DeFronzo RA, Tobin JD, Andres R. Glucose clamp technique: a method for quantifying insulin secretion and resistance. *Am J Physiol* 1979;237:E214–E223.
161. DeFronzo RA. Pathogenesis of type 2 (non-insulin dependent) diabetes mellitus: a balanced overview. *Diabetologia* 1992;35:389–397.
162. DeFronzo RA, Gunnarsson R, Björkman O, et al. Effects of insulin on peripheral and splanchnic glucose metabolism in noninsulin-dependent (type II) diabetes mellitus. *J Clin Invest* 1985;76:149–155.
163. Bogardus C, Lillioja S, Stone K, Mott D. Correlation between muscle glycogen synthase activity and *in vivo* insulin action in man. *J Clin Invest* 1984;73: 1185–1190.
164. Roch-Norlund AE, Bergström J, Castenfors H, et al. Muscle glycogen in patients with diabetes mellitus: glycogen content before treatment and the effect of insulin. *Acta Med Scand* 1970;187:445–453.
165. Schalin-Jäntti C, Härkönen M, Groop LC. Impaired activation of glycogen-synthase in people at increased risk for developing NIDDM. *Diabetes* 1992; 41:598–604.
166. Vaag A, Henriksen JE, Beck-Nielsen H. Decreased insulin activation of glycogen synthase in skeletal muscles in young nonobese Caucasian first-degree relatives of patients with non-insulin-dependent diabetes mellitus. *J Clin Invest* 1992;89:782–788.
167. Rothman DL, Shulman RG, Shulman GI. ^{31}P nuclear magnetic resonance measurements of muscle glucose-6-phosphate: evidence for reduced insulin-dependent muscle glucose transport or phosphorylation activity in non-insulin-dependent diabetes mellitus. *J Clin Invest* 1992;89:1069–1075.
168. Mandarino LJ, Madar Z, Kolterman OG, et al. Adipocyte glycogen synthase and pyruvate dehydrogenase in obese and type II diabetic subjects. *Am J Physiol* 1986;251:E489–E496.
169. Unger RH, Grundy S. Hyperglycaemia as an inducer as well as a consequence of impaired islet cell function and insulin resistance: implications for the management of diabetes. *Diabetologia* 1985;28:119–121.
170. Rossetti L, Giaccari A, DeFronzo RA. Glucose toxicity. *Diabetes Care* 1990;13: 610–630.
171. Kahn BB, Shulman GI, DeFronzo RA, et al. Normalization of blood glucose in diabetic rats with phlorizin treatment reverses insulin-resistant glucose transport in adipose cells without restoring glucose transporter gene expression. *J Clin Invest* 1991;87:561–570.
172. Rossetti L, Smith D, Shulman GI, et al. Correction of hyperglycemia with phlorizin normalizes tissue sensitivity to insulin in diabetic rats. *J Clin Invest* 1987;79:1510–1515.

CHAPTER 9

The Molecular Mechanism of Insulin Action and the Regulation of Glucose and Lipid Metabolism

C. Ronald Kahn and Alan R. Saltiel

More than 18 million people in the United States have diabetes mellitus, and about 90% of these have the type 2 form of the disease. In addition, between 17 and 40 million people have insulin resistance, impaired glucose tolerance, or the cluster of abnormalities referred to variably as the metabolic syndrome, the dysmetabolic syndrome, syndrome X, or the insulin resistance syndrome (1). In all of these disorders, a central component of the pathophysiology is insulin resistance, i.e., reduced responsiveness to insulin in tissues such as muscle, fat, and liver. In type 2 diabetes, the β-cell can no longer secrete sufficient insulin to compensate for insulin resistance, leading to relative insulin deficiency. Insulin resistance is also closely linked to other common health problems, including obesity, polycystic ovarian disease, hyperlipidemia, hypertension, and atherosclerosis. In this chapter, we will attempt to dissect the complexity of the molecular mechanisms of insulin action with a special emphasis on those features of the system that are subject to alteration in type 2 diabetes and other insulin-resistant states.

GLUCOSE HOMEOSTASIS AND INSULIN RESISTANCE

Despite periods of feeding and fasting, in healthy individuals plasma glucose remains in a narrow range between 4 and 7 mM (70 to 120 mg/dL). This tight control of glucose concentration is determined by a balance between glucose absorption from the intestine, glucose production by the liver, and glucose uptake from the plasma (reviewed in detail in Chapters 8, 13 to 16, 24) (Fig. 9.1). In tissues such as muscle, fat, and liver, glucose uptake and/or storage is regulated by insulin, whereas insulin has no apparent role in stimulating glucose metabolism in tissues such as brain, kidney, and erythrocytes. In addition to promoting glucose utilization, insulin inhibits both basal and glucagon-stimulated hepatic glucose production, thus serving as the primary regulator of blood glucose concentration during fasting. Insulin also has a general anabolic role promoting the storage of substrates in fat, liver, and muscle by stimulating lipogenesis and glycogen and protein synthesis; inhibiting lipolysis, glycogenolysis and protein breakdown; and stimulating cell growth and differentiation. In type 1 diabetes, the autoimmune destruction of the pancreatic β-cell leads to severe insulin deficiency with unrestrained hepatic glucose output, unrestrained lipolysis, and increased ketogenesis. In type 2 diabetes, insulin resistance in muscle, adipose tissue, and liver combined with a relative failure of the β-cell leads to increased glucose levels and a variable cluster of metabolic alterations in lipid and protein metabolism. Insulin resistance in patients with type 2 diabetes is usually defined by defects in insulin-stimulated glucose transport, glycogen synthesis, and glucose oxidation, but other pathways of metabolism are clearly altered. The most characteristic feature of the β-cell failure is a specific defect in glucose sensing characterized by loss of first-phase insulin secretion in response to a glucose stimulus, while response to other secretagogues is normal or only mildly depressed.

The control of blood glucose depends upon the balance between glucose production by the liver and glucose utilization by insulin-dependent tissues, such as muscle and fat, and insulin-independent tissues, such as the brain. In mammals, up to 75% of insulin-dependent glucose disposal occurs in skeletal muscle (2–6). This preeminence of muscle, however, has recently been challenged by the finding that mice with a muscle-specific knockout of the insulin receptor exhibit minimal abnormalities in glucose tolerance (7). Adipose tissue accounts for only a small fraction (5% to 15%) of insulin-stimulated glucose disposal. Despite this, knockout of the insulin-sensitive glucose transporter in fat leads to impaired glucose tolerance, apparently by inducing insulin resistance in muscle and liver through a yet undetermined mechanism (see the section Lessons from Knockout Mice about Insulin Action and Insulin Resistance below). Adipose tissue also plays a special additional role in glucose homeostasis through its release of free fatty acids, tumor necrosis factor-α (TNF-α) leptin, Acrp30/adiponectin, and other adipokines that have been shown to contribute to insulin action and insulin resistance (8–12). Furthermore, both obesity (increased fat mass) and lipoatrophy (decreased fat mass) cause insulin resistance and predisposition to type 2 diabetes (13–16).

The liver does not exhibit insulin-stimulated glucose uptake but plays a major role in glucose homeostasis, especially in the fasting state (17). When insulin levels are low, the liver releases glucose into the blood as a result of glycogenolysis

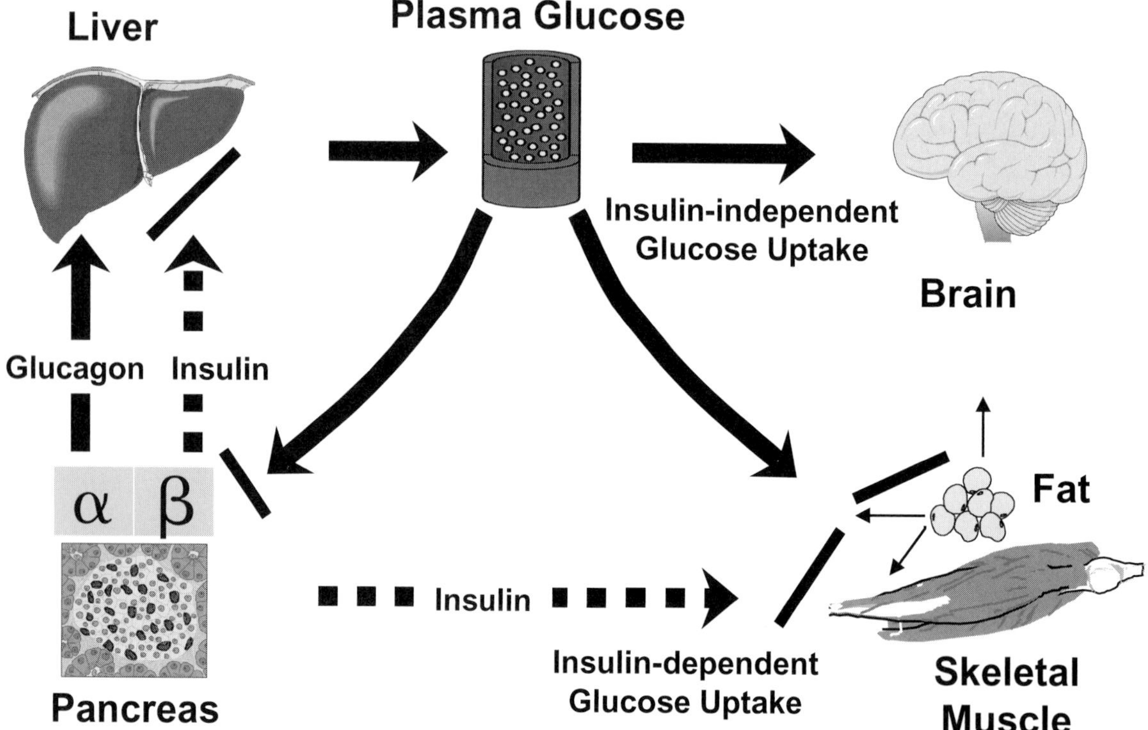

Figure 9.1. Overview of glucose homeostasis and its alterations in type 2 diabetes. In the fasting state, glucose is produced by the liver and utilized by insulin-independent tissues, such as the brain, and insulin-dependent tissues, such as fat and muscle. The balance of glucose production and utilization is controlled by many hormones, but the most important is insulin. In type 2 diabetes, there is insulin resistance in muscle, fat, and liver and relative insulin deficiency.

and gluconeogenesis, providing substrate for tissues with obligate glucose requirements. In the fed state, when insulin levels are high, glucose in the liver is converted to glycogen. Recent studies using knockout and other technologies suggest that insulin action in other tissues, including brain and β-cells, although not major sites of insulin-stimulated glucose uptake, may also play important roles in glucose homeostasis and metabolism (18,19) (see below).

PROXIMAL SIGNALING PATHWAYS

The Insulin Receptor and Its Substrates

The insulin receptor is a tetrameric protein consisting of two α-subunits and two β-subunits that belongs to a subfamily of receptor tyrosine kinases that also includes the insulin-like growth factor-1 (IGF-1) receptor and an orphan receptor called the insulin receptor–related receptor (IRR) (20,21) (Fig. 9.2). Each of these receptors is the product of a separate gene in which the two subunits are derived from a single-chain precursor or proreceptor that is processed by a furin-like enzyme to give a single α-β subunit complex (22,23). Two of the α-β dimers then undergo disulfide linkage to form the tetramer.

The insulin receptor is widely distributed throughout the body, including in tissues classically regarded as "responsive" and "nonresponsive" to insulin. Recent studies suggest that the receptor in most of these tissues has an important functional role, but in some cases this may relate to actions other than the control of glucose or lipid homeostasis. For example, in ovarian granulosa cells, insulin signaling is coupled to regulation of estrogen/androgen balance (24), whereas the role of the insulin receptor in the endothelial cell may be to promote vasodilatation (25,26) or transcytosis of the insulin molecule from the intravascular space to the interstitial space and its target tissues (27–30); in neural or endocrine cells, insulin may have a role regulating hormone production, secretory function, or signal sensing (see below).

Functionally, the insulin receptor behaves as a classical allosteric enzyme in which the α-subunit inhibits the tyrosine kinase activity intrinsic to the β-subunit. Insulin binding to the α-subunit, or removal of the α-subunit by proteolysis or genetic deletion, leads to a derepression, i.e., activation, of the kinase activity in the β-subunit. Following this initial activation, there is transphosphorylation of the β-subunits, i.e., one subunit phosphorylates the other, leading to a conformational change and a further increase in activity of the kinase domain (31,32). The α-β heterodimers of the insulin, IGF-1, and the IRR receptors can form functional hybrids in which occupancy of one receptor's binding domain leads to activation of the other receptor in the heterodimer by this transphosphorylation process. Likewise, a dominant-negative form of one of these receptor subtypes can inhibit the activity of the other receptors by forming heterodimers (33). This may explain in part why individuals with mutations in the insulin receptor exhibit both insulin resistance and growth retardation (33).

The insulin/IGF-1 signaling system is evolutionarily very ancient. Homologues of the insulin/IGF-1 receptor have been identified in *Drosophila*, *Caenorhabditis elegans*, and even metazoan marine sponges of the phylum Porifera that date back over 500 million years (34). In the lower organisms, this system uses many of the same downstream signals used in mammalian cells, i.e., phosphatidylinositol 3-kinase (PI 3-kinase)/Akt/forkhead transcription factors, and may also be involved

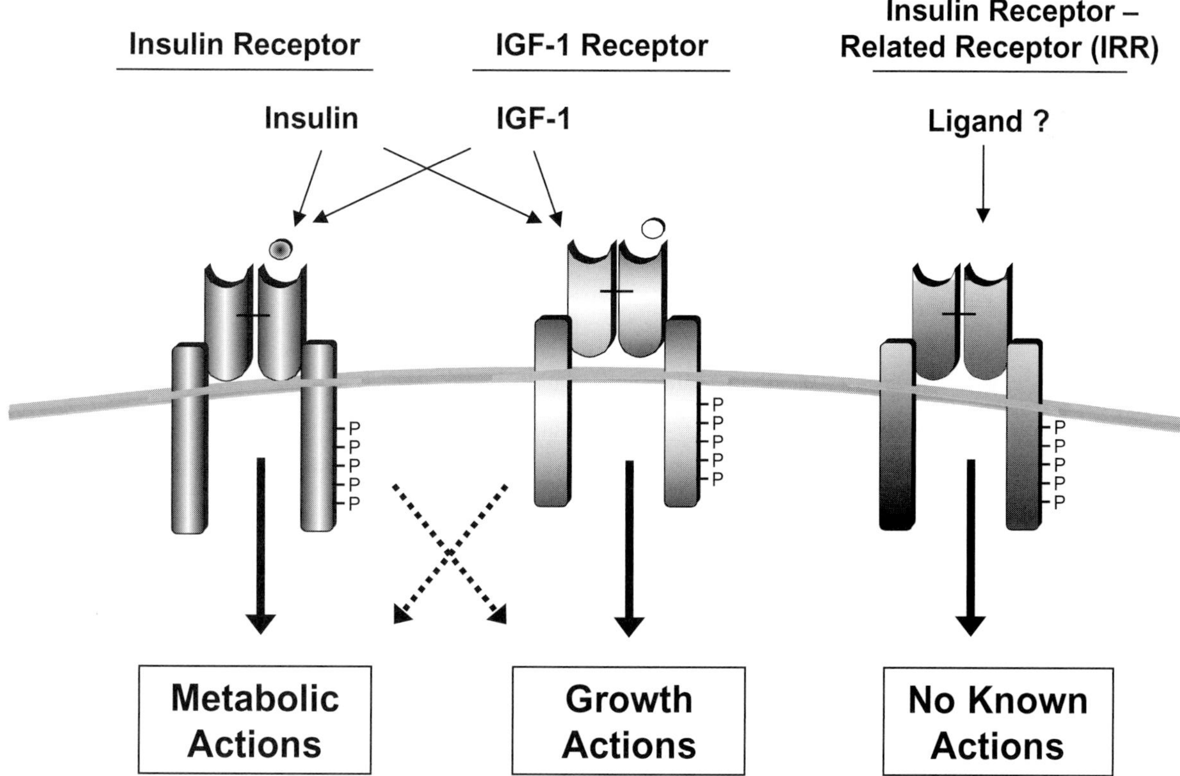

Figure 9.2. The insulin-receptor family, which includes the insulin receptor, the insulin-like growth factor-1 (IGF-1) receptor, and the insulin receptor–related receptor.

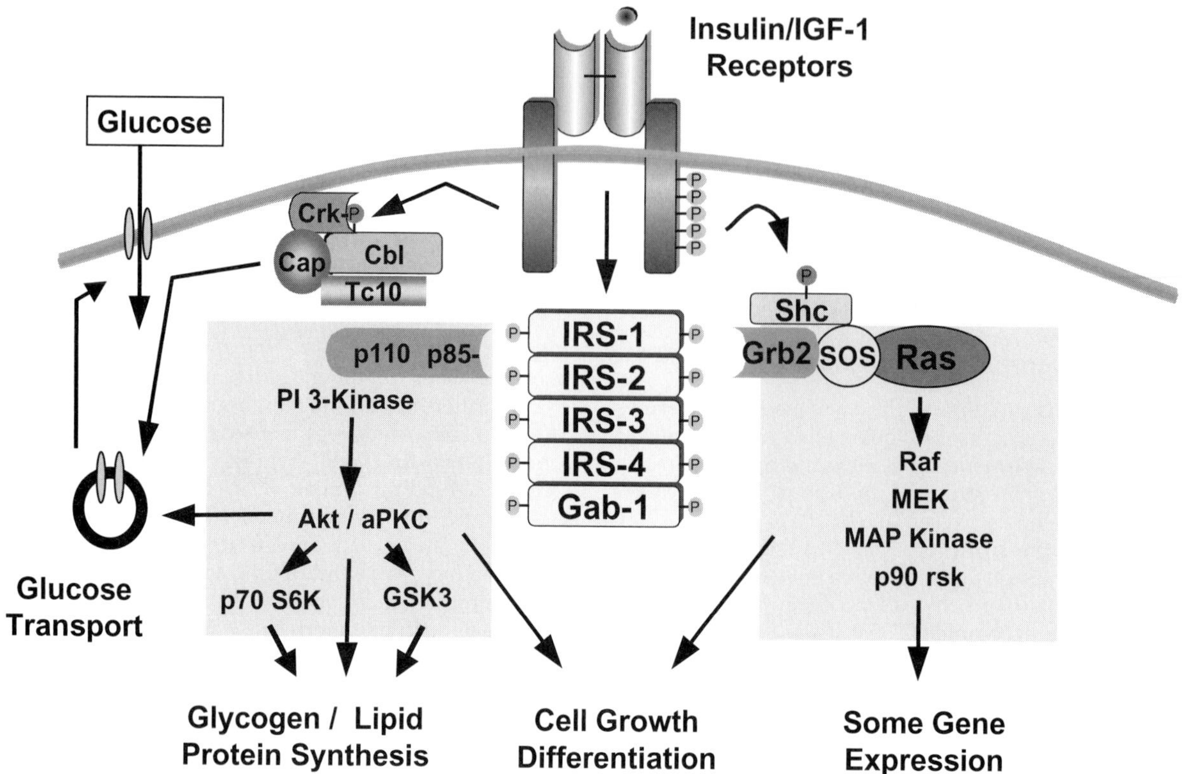

Figure 9.3. The insulin and insulin-like growth factor-1 (IGF-1) signaling network. The two major pathways are the phosphatidylinositol 3-kinase (PI 3-kinase) pathway and the Ras–mitogen-activated protein (MAP) kinase pathway. The PI-3 pathway is the major pathway leading to the metabolic actions of insulin.

in regulation of metabolism (35,36). In *Drosophila*, the insulin-secreting cells are neurons. Ablation of these cells results in changes in the major circulating carbohydrate in flies, trehelose (37). In *C. elegans*, a major effect of the insulin/IGF system is on aging, such that animals with mutations of the receptor that reduce insulin action live much longer than normal animals, whereas mutations in other parts of the pathway may reverse this longevity (38). It is interesting that chronic food restriction and leanness, which are associated with lower circulating insulin levels, increase longevity in rodents (39). This raises a number of interesting questions about the association of hyperinsulinemia and insulin resistance with conditions that shorten life span in humans, such as obesity, diabetes, and accelerated atherosclerosis.

At least nine intracellular substrates of the insulin and IGF-1 receptor tyrosine kinases have been identified (Figs. 9.3 and 9.4). Four of these belong to the family of insulin/IGF-1 receptor substrate (IRS) proteins (40–44). These IRS proteins are characterized by the presence of both pleckstrin homology (PH) and phosphotyrosine binding (PTB) domains near the N-terminus that account for the high affinity of these substrates for the insulin receptor and up to 20 potential tyrosine phosphorylation sites spread throughout the center and C-terminal region of the molecule. The molecular mass of IRS proteins ranges from 60 to 180 kDa. IRS-1 and IRS-2 are widely distributed, whereas IRS-3 and IRS-4 have more limited distributions. IRS-3 is most abundant in adipocytes, and its mRNA is also detected in liver, heart, lung, brain, and kidney (43,45–47). In contrast, the levels of mRNA for IRS-4 are very low, but are detectable, in fibroblasts, embryonic tissues, skeletal muscle, liver, heart, hypothalamus, and kidney (44). Interestingly, in humans the IRS-3 gene appears to be nonfunctional, leaving only IRS-1, -2, and -4 (48). Other direct substrates of the insulin/IGF-1 receptor kinases include Gab-1 (49), $p62^{dok}$ (50), Cbl (51), and the various isoforms of Shc (52,53). Following insulin stimulation, the receptor directly phosphorylates most of these substrates on multiple tyrosine residues. The phosphorylated tyrosines in each of these substrates occur in specific sequence motifs and once phosphorylated serve as "docking sites" for intracellular molecules that contain SH2 (Src-homology 2) domains (44,54). Thus, the insulin-receptor substrates function as key intermediates in insulin-signal transduction.

The SH2 proteins that bind to phosphorylated IRS proteins fall into two major categories. The best studied are adapter molecules, such as the regulatory subunit of PI 3-kinase or the molecule Grb2, which associates with SOS to activate the Ras–mitogen-activated protein (MAP) kinase pathway (54–57). The other major category of proteins that bind to IRS proteins are enzymes, such as the phosphotyrosine phosphatase SHP2 (58,59) and cytoplasmic tyrosine kinases, such as Fyn. A few proteins that bind to phosphotyrosines in the IRS proteins do not contain known SH2 domains; these include the calcium adenosine triphosphatases (ATPases) SERCA 1 and 2 and the SV40 large T antigen (60,61). These pathways are discussed in more detail on page 153.

IRS proteins also undergo serine phosphorylation in response to insulin and other stimuli. In general, serine phosphorylation appears to act as a negative regulator of insulin signaling by decreasing tyrosine phosphorylation of IRS proteins, as well as by promoting interaction with 14-3-3 proteins (62). A number of different intracellular enzymes have been suggested as being involved in this serine phosphorylation, including

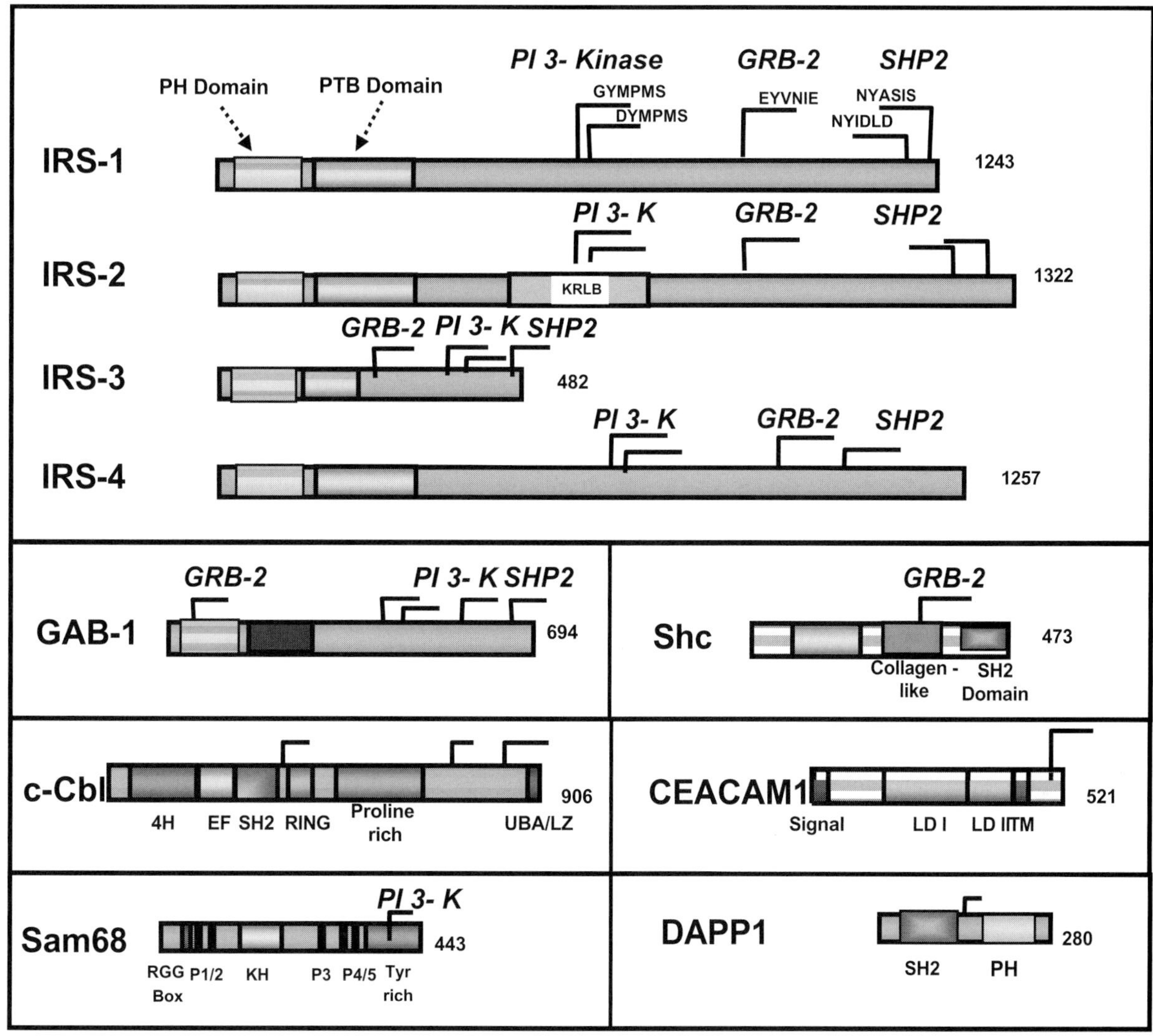

Figure 9.4. The family of insulin-receptor substrates (IRS). The functional domains and major tyrosine phosphorylation sites of each protein are indicated. PH, pleckstrin homology; PTB, phosphotyrosine; PI 3-kinase, phosphatidylinositol 3-kinase.

some in the insulin-signaling pathway, such as Akt (63), JNK kinase (64), and PI 3-kinase (which also has serine kinase activity) (65), thereby providing a form of autoinhibition of signaling, and others that mediate the effects of some inhibitors of insulin action, such as the inhibitor kappa B kinase β (IKKβ) (66,67).

Although the IRS proteins are highly homologous and possess many similar tyrosine phosphorylation motifs, recent studies in knockout mice and knockout cell lines suggest that the various IRS proteins serve complementary rather than redundant roles in insulin and IGF-1 signaling (Fig. 9.5). The IRS-1 knockout mouse exhibits IGF-1 resistance as manifested by prenatal and postnatal growth retardation, as well as insulin resistance, primarily in muscle and fat, resulting in impaired glucose tolerance (68–70). IRS-2 knockout mice also exhibit insulin resistance, but primarily in the liver, and have defects in growth in only selected tissues of the body, including certain regions of the brain, β-cells, and retinal cells (71,72). Likewise at the cellular level, IRS-1 knockout preadipocytes exhibit defects in differentiation (73,74), whereas IRS-2 knockout preadipocytes differentiate normally but fail to respond to insulin-stimulated glucose transport (75).

The β-cell compensatory responses of the IRS knockout mice also differ. In the IRS-1 knockout, although there is some element of β-cell dysfunction, there is sufficient islet hyperplasia such that the animals develop only mildly impaired glucose tolerance. In the IRS-2 knockout mouse, there is a decrease in islet mass due to altered β-cell development. The combination of multifactorial insulin resistance and decreased β-cell mass leads to the development of early-onset diabetes in IRS-2$^{-/-}$ mice (71), although the frequency of this phenotype varies considerably in different laboratories (72). By contrast, IRS-3 knockout mice have normal growth and metabolism, whereas IRS-4 knockout mice exhibit only minimal abnormalities in glucose tolerance (76,77). It is interesting that when IRS-1–deficient mice are crossed with IRS-3–deficient mice to produce a double knockout, the resultant animals exhibit severe hyperglycemia and marked lipoatrophy, indicating that, at least in adipocytes, there is at least some compensation of these two substrates (78).

The differential roles of the IRS proteins may be due to differences in tissue distribution, subcellular localization, and intrinsic activity of the proteins. IRS-1 and IRS-2 are widely distributed, whereas IRS-3 is limited largely to the adipocyte and brain and IRS-4 is expressed primarily in embryonic tissues or

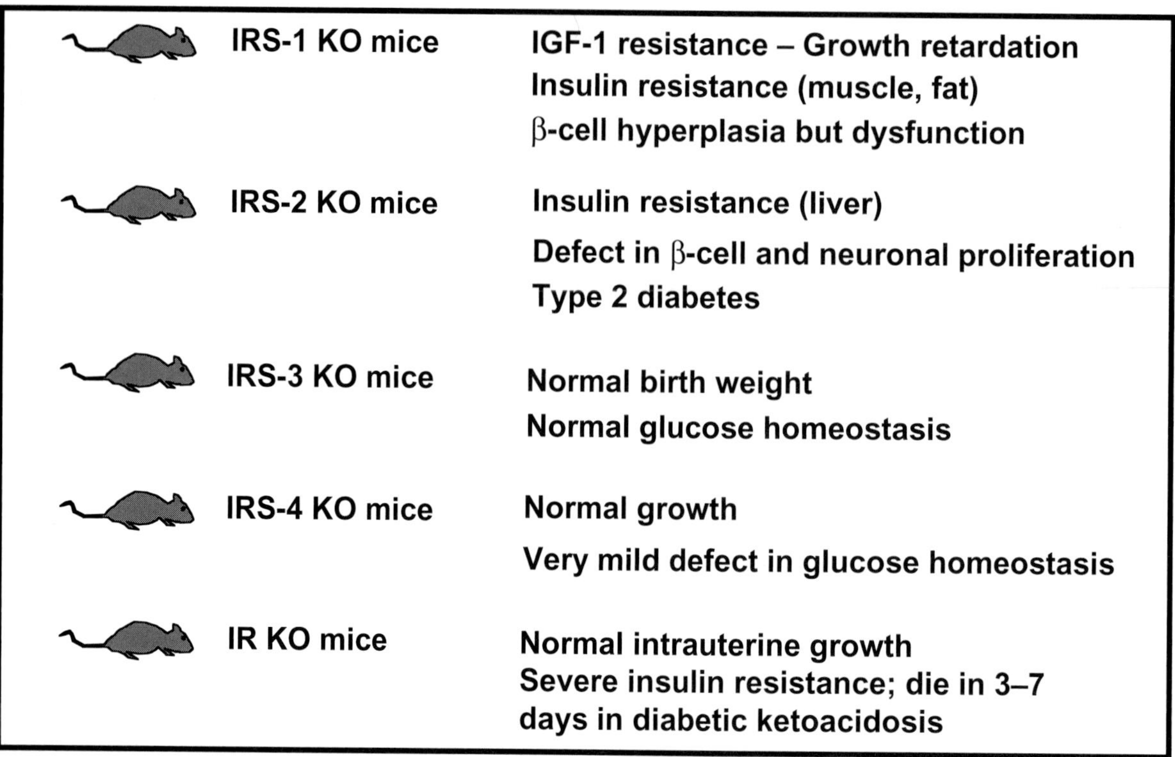

Figure 9.5. Phenotypes of the insulin receptor (IR) and insulin receptor substrate (IRS) knockout (KO) mice. IGF-1, insulin-like growth factor-1.

cell lines (see above). Furthermore, IRS-1 is more closely associated with low-density microsomes, whereas IRS-2 is found in low-density microsomes and in the cytosol (79). IRS-3 is associated more with the plasma-membrane fraction in rat adipocytes (80). In some studies, IRS-1 and IRS-3 appear to translocate to the nucleus (81,82), and IRS-3 has been suggested to possess DNA-binding activity (82).

Turning off the Insulin Signal

Unlike the prolonged actions of steroid and thyroid hormones, insulin action on glucose homeostasis demands a rapid on-and-off response to avoid the dangers of hypoglycemia. Several different mechanisms play a role in turning off the insulin signal (Fig. 9.6). First, insulin may simply dissociate from the receptor and be degraded. Following dissociation of the ligand, phosphorylation of the insulin receptor and its substrates is rapidly reversed by the action of protein tyrosine phosphatases (PTPases). Several PTPases have been identified that are capable of catalyzing dephosphorylation of the insulin receptor *in vitro* or *in vivo*, and some are even upregulated in insulin-resistant states (83–86). Most attention has focused on the cytoplasmic phosphatase PTP-1b. Disruption of the gene encoding this enzyme in mice produces increased insulin-dependent tyrosine phosphorylation of the insulin receptor and IRS proteins in muscle and leads to a state of improved insulin sensitivity (87). PTP-1b knockout mice are also resistant to diet-induced obesity, suggesting an effect of PTP-1b deletion in the brain, with subsequent changes in energy uptake and expenditure. This is opposite the effect of knockout of insulin receptor in the brain (18) (see page 163).

Several other mechanisms may also be involved in turning off the insulin signal in normal or pathologic states. The insulin receptor itself may be internalized and undergo degradation (88,89). As noted above, serine phosphorylation of the insulin receptor and its substrates also inhibits insulin action (90,91). Finally, the phosphorylated receptor may interact with proteins in the cell that block insulin action. This latter mechanism has recently been observed for the SOCS (suppressors of cytokine signaling) proteins in the case of the insulin resistance associated with inflammation and obesity (92).

Phosphatidylinositol 3-Kinase and Downstream Targets

The first SH2 domain protein identified as interacting with IRS-1 was the regulatory subunit of the class Ia form of PI 3-kinase. This enzyme plays a pivotal role in the metabolic and mitogenic actions of insulin and IGF-1 (93,94). Thus, inhibitors of PI 3-kinase or transfection with dominant-negative constructs of the enzyme blocks virtually all of the metabolic actions of insulin, including stimulation of glucose transport, glycogen synthesis, and lipid synthesis. The enzyme itself consists of a regulatory and a catalytic subunit. Activation of the catalytic subunit depends on interaction of the two SH2 domains in the regulatory subunit with specific tyrosine-phosphorylated motifs in the IRS proteins of the sequence pYMXM and pYXXM (95,96).

At least eight isoforms of the regulatory subunits of PI 3-kinase have been identified (Fig. 9.7). These are derived from three genes and alternative splicing (97–99). p85α and p85β represent the "full-length" versions of the regulatory subunits and contain an SH3 domain, a bcr homology domain flanked by two proline-rich domains, two SH2 domains [referred to as the N-terminal (nSH2) and C-terminal (cSH2) domains)], and an inter-SH2 (iSH2) domain containing the p110 binding region (99). The shorter versions of regulatory subunits, AS53 (also known as p55α) (100,101) and p50α (97,101), are splicing variants

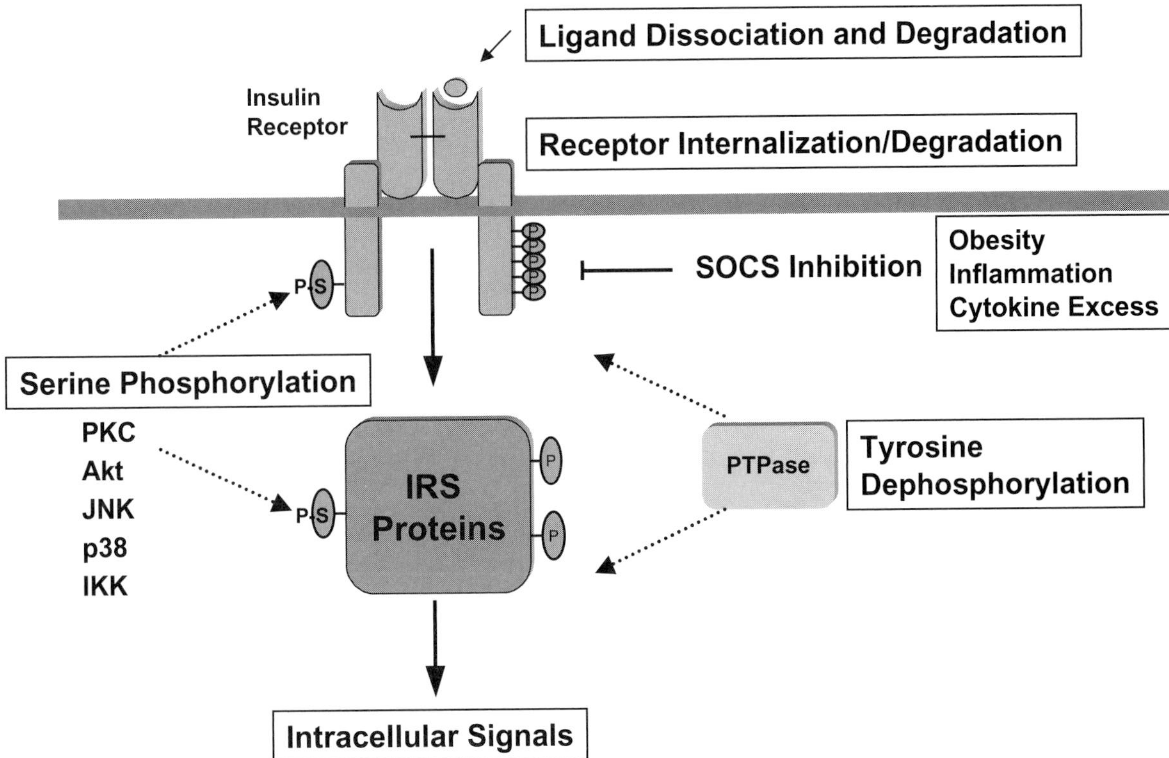

Figure 9.6. Mechanism of turning off the insulin signal. These mechanisms are also activated in a variety of acquired insulin-resistant states. SOCS, suppressors of cytokine signaling; IRS, insulin-receptor substrate; PTPase, protein tyrosine phosphatases.

derived from the same gene encoding p85α (*Pik3r1*) (97). They share the common nSH2-iSH2-cSH2 with p85α but lack the N-terminal half containing the SH3 domain, N-terminal proline-rich domain, and bcr domain and in its place have unique N-terminal sequences consisting of 34 amino acids and 6 amino acids, respectively. Another small version of the regulatory subunit, $p55^{PIK}$, is very similar in structure to p55α/AS53 but is encoded by a different gene (102). Of these isoforms, p85α is predominantly and ubiquitously expressed and is thought to be the major response pathway for most stimuli (94,99); however, the splice variants, p55α/AS53 and p50α, have high levels of potency for PI 3-kinase signaling (100,101,103) and appear to play specific roles in some selected tissues (97,100,101) or in particular states of insulin resistance (104,105). The exact role of the different regulatory subunits of PI 3-kinase in insulin action is unclear. Knockout mice with a disruption of all three isoforms of *Pik3r1* gene die within a few weeks of birth, indicating the importance of p85α and its spliced variants in normal growth and normal metabolism (106). By contrast, mice lacking only the full-length version of p85α (107) or only the shorter spliced forms (107a) can grow to adulthood and exhibit improved insulin sensitivity. One explanation for the increased sensitivity in both cases is the improved stoichiometry of insulin-signaling proteins in the cell (108). Thus, it appears that under normal conditions the concentration of regulatory subunits is in excess of that of the catalytic subunits and phosphorylated IRS proteins. This leads to the binding of free monomeric (and thus catalytically inactive) forms of regulatory subunit to phosphorylated IRS proteins and blocking of the binding of the active heterodimer. Mice with a heterozygous knockout *Pik3r1* gene also have improved stoichiometry of interaction between the regulatory and catalytic subunits. This results in improved sensitivity to insulin and IGF-1 and even protects mice with genetic insulin resistance from developing diabetes (109). Likewise, cell lines derived from heterozygous *Pik3r1*-gene knockout embryos exhibit increased insulin/IGF-1 signaling (108).

The exact mechanisms by which PI 3-kinase transmits the insulin signal appear to be multiple (94,99). PI 3-kinase itself catalyzes the phosphorylation of phosphoinositides on the 3-position to PI-(3)P, PI-(3,4)P_2, and PI-(3,4,5)P_3 (also known as PIP_3). These lipids bind to the PH domains of a variety of signaling molecules and alter their activity or subcellular localization. Three major classes of signaling molecules are regulated by PI 3-phosphates: the AGC superfamily of serine/threonine protein kinases; guanine nucleotide exchange proteins of the Rho family of guanosine triphosphatase (GTPase); and the TEC family of tyrosine kinases, including BTK and ITK. PI 3-kinase also activates the mTOR/FRAP pathway and activates phospholipase D, leading to hydrolysis of phosphatidylcholine and increases in phosphatidic acid (PA) and diacylglycerol (DAG). Insulin also activates the enzyme glycerol-3-phosphate acyltransferase, which increases *de novo* synthesis of PA and DAG by PI 3-kinase–independent mechanisms.

The best characterized pathway involves the AGC kinase known as PDK1. This enzyme is one of the two serine kinases that phosphorylate and activate the serine/threonine kinase Akt (also known as PKB). Akt/PKB is thought to play an important role in the transmission of insulin's metabolic pathways by phosphorylating glycogen synthase kinase-3 (110), and either directly or indirectly the forkhead (FOXO) transcription factors and the cyclic AMP regulatory element binding protein CREB (111–114). However, studies using inhibitors and activators of Akt have not uniformly inhibited or mimicked insulin actions (113). Part of the variability may relate to

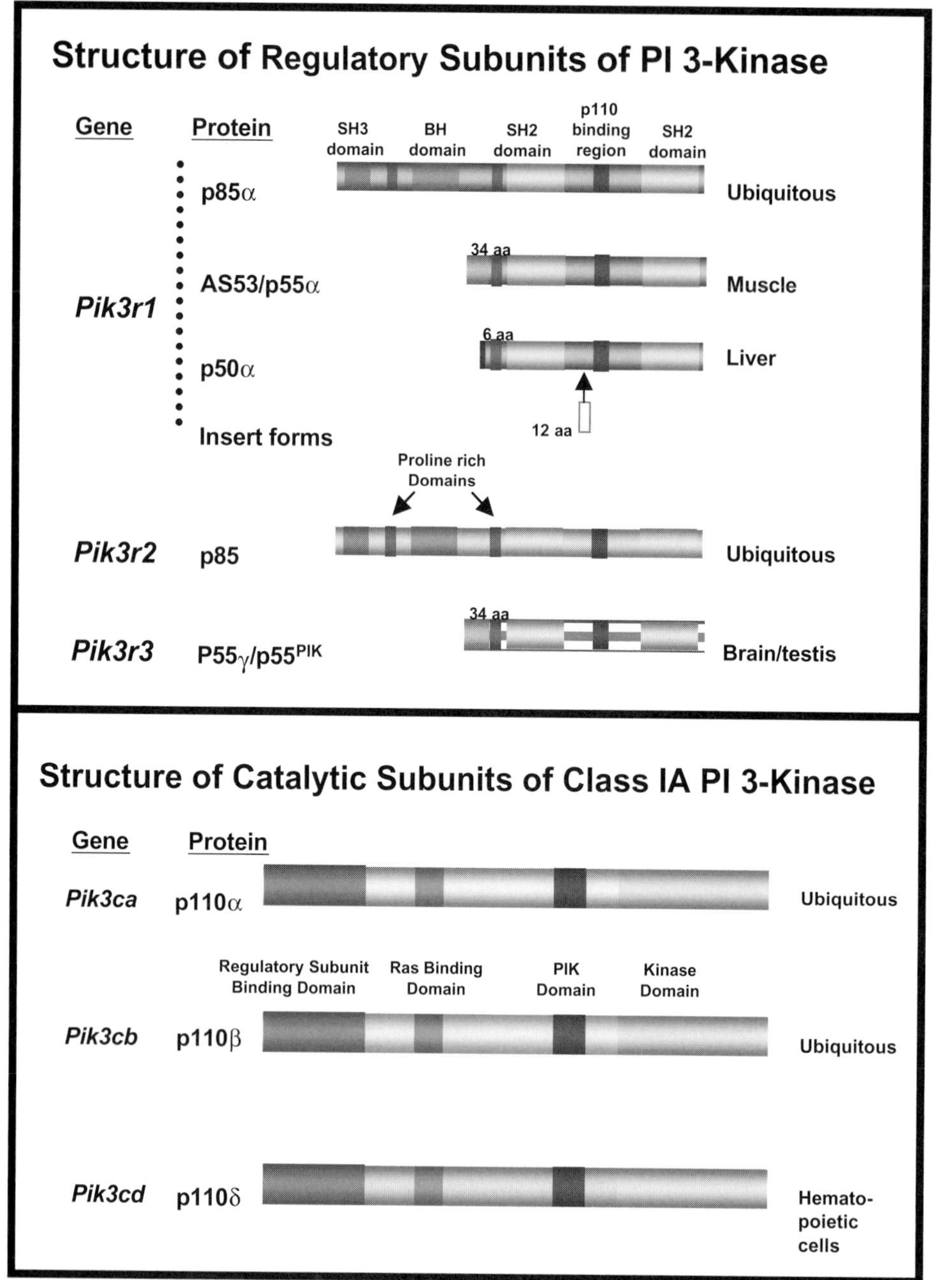

Figure 9.7. The structures of the regulatory and catalytic subunits of phosphatidylinositol 3-kinase (PI 3-kinase).

the fact that there are three isoforms of Akt/PKB (115). Although the major form, Akt1, is clearly important for cell survival and growth, recent data have suggested that Akt2 may be more important in mediating insulin action, at least in the liver (116). Other AGC kinases that are downstream of PI 3-kinase are the atypical forms of protein kinase C (PKC), including PKCζ and PKCλ. Both Akt and the atypical PKCs appear to be required for insulin-induced glucose transport (117). Stable expression of a constitutively active, membrane-bound form of Akt in 3T3L1 adipocytes results in increased glucose transport and persistent localization of GLUT4 to the plasma membrane (118). Conversely, expression of a dominant-interfering Akt mutant inhibits insulin-stimulated GLUT4 translocation. Likewise, overexpression of PKCζ or λ results in GLUT4 translocation (119,120), whereas expression of a dominant-interfering PKCλ blocks the action of insulin (121). PKCζ has been shown to phosphorylate IRS-1 and thus to serve as a potential negative feedback regulator of insulin/IGF signaling (122).

It is important to keep in mind that, although less well studied, PI 3-kinase also has protein kinase activity and that both the regulatory and catalytic subunits of PI 3-kinase possess domains capable of interacting with other signaling proteins. The p85 regulatory subunits possess an SH3 domain, a bcr homology region that interacts with CDC42 and Rac, and two proline-rich regions for which the interacting partners have not yet been defined (99,123). PI 3-kinase also may interact with the PI 5′-kinase PIK-fyve (124) and some G-protein–coupled proteins (125); thus, this enzyme may contribute to insulin signaling in multiple ways.

It should be clear from the above discussion that turning off insulin signaling also involves reducing the level of PIP_3 in the cell. This is achieved through the activity of PIP_3 phosphatases, such as PTEN (126) and SHIP2 (127). PTEN dephosphorylates phosphoinositides on the 3′-position, thus lowering the level of the second messengers. SHIP2 is a 5′-phosphoinositide phosphatase. Disruption of the gene encoding this enzyme yields mice with increased insulin sensitivity (127).

The c-Cbl–Associated Protein/Cbl Pathway and Lipid Rafts

Although PI 3-kinase activity is clearly necessary for insulin-stimulated glucose uptake, several lines of evidence suggest that additional signals may also be required. Indeed, other hormones or growth factors that activate PI 3-kinase, such as platelet-derived growth factor (PDGF) and interleukin-4, do not stimulate glucose transport (51). Likewise, addition of a PIP_3 analogue alone in some studies has no effect on glucose transport (128). In addition, two naturally occurring insulin-receptor mutants that appear to be fully capable of activating PI 3-kinase are unable to mediate full insulin action (129).

Recent studies have suggested that the PI 3-kinase–independent pathway might involve the tyrosine phosphorylation of the Cbl protooncogene (51,130) (Fig. 9.3). This phosphorylation requires the presence of another protein that recruits Cbl to the insulin receptor, the adapter protein APS. In most insulin-responsive cells, Cbl is associated with the adapter protein CAP (c-Cbl–associating protein), which binds to proline-rich sequences in Cbl through its C-terminal SH3 domain (51). CAP expression correlates well with insulin responsiveness, and its expression is increased by treatment of cells with insulin-sensitizing thiazolidinediones (51). CAP belongs to a family of adapter proteins that contain a sorbin homology (SoHo) domain. This allows CAP to interact with one of the components of the lipid raft domain of the plasma membrane, a protein called flotillin. Expression of CAP mutants that cannot bind to Cbl or flotillin inhibit Cbl translocation and insulin-stimulated glucose uptake (51). The translocation of phosphorylated Cbl also recruits the adapter protein CrkII to the lipid raft, which in turn interacts with the guanyl nucleotide exchange protein C3G. C3G catalyzes the exchange of GTP for GDP on TC10, resulting in the activation of this G-protein. TC10 has been suggested to provide the second signal to GLUT4 translocation (131), although the nature of this signal is still unclear.

The Ras–Mitogen-Activated Protein Kinase Cascade and mTOR

The second major pathway activated by insulin is the Ras–MAP kinase cascade. Following the tyrosine phosphorylation of one of the IRS proteins or the alternative substrate Shc, there is binding of the adapter protein Grb2, which in turn recruits the guanyl nucleotide exchange protein SOS to the plasma membrane, thus activating Ras (56,132). Full activation of Ras by insulin requires stimulation of the tyrosine phosphatase SHP2, which also interacts with insulin-receptor substrates such as Gab-1 and IRS1/2 (133). Once activated, Ras operates as a molecular switch, converting upstream tyrosine phosphorylations into a second serine kinase cascade, via the stepwise activation of Raf, the MAP kinase-kinase MEK, and the MAP kinases themselves, ERK1 and ERK2 (134). The MAP kinases, such as ERK1 and 2, can phosphorylate substrates in the cytoplasm or translocate into the nucleus and catalyze the phosphorylation of transcription factors, such as $p62^{TCF}$, initiating a transcriptional program that leads the cell to commit to a proliferative or differentiative cycle. Blockade of the Ras–MAP kinase pathway with dominant-negative mutants or pharmacologic inhibitors can prevent the stimulation of cell growth by insulin but has no effect on any of the anabolic or metabolic actions of the hormone (134).

Yet another component of insulin signaling involved in protein synthesis/degradation and interaction with nutrient sensing is the protein kinase mTOR (mammalian target of rapamycin). mTOR is a member of the PI 3-kinase family but serves primarily as a protein kinase. Stimulation of mTOR appears to involve PI 3-kinase as well as another signal (135,136). mTOR itself helps regulate the mRNA translation via phosphorylation and activation of the p70 ribosomal S6 kinase (p70 S6 kinase), as well as the phosphorylation of the eIF-4E inhibitor, PHAS1 or 4E-BP1 (137). p70 S6 kinase phosphorylates ribosomal S6 protein, thus activating ribosome biosynthesis and increasing translation of mRNAs with a 5′-terminal oligopyrimidine tract. Phosphorylation of PHAS-1 by mTOR results in its dissociation from eIF-2, allowing cap-dependent translation of mRNAs with a highly structured 5′-untranslated region. Although the mechanism of activation of mTOR remains unclear, it appears to require the presence of amino acids and thus may also serve as a nutrient sensor (138).

REGULATION OF GLUCOSE TRANSPORT

The classical effect of insulin on glucose homeostasis is its ability to stimulate glucose transport in fat and muscle. This occurs via a translocation of GLUT4 glucose transporters from intracellular sites to the plasma membrane (Fig. 9.8). The GLUT4 protein consists of 12 transmembrane helices with a characteristic C-terminal tail containing two adjacent leucine residues commonly found in proteins that undergo regulated trafficking. In the basal state, GLUT4 continuously recycles between the cell surface and various intracellular compartments. The GLUT4 vesicle is highly specialized and appears to form from a sorting endosomal population. Insulin markedly increases the rate of GLUT4-vesicle exocytosis and slightly decreases the rate of internalization of the GLUT4 protein. Although the exact domains of the protein involved in localization and trafficking remain controversial, the C- and N-terminal tails of the protein, both of which are oriented on the cytoplasmic side of the vesicle, appear to be required (139). It is likely that the GLUT4 vesicle moves along microtubule tracks to the cell surface, perhaps via kinesin motors (140). These vesicles then fuse with the plasma membrane, allowing for the extracellular exposure of the GLUT4 protein.

Recent evidence also suggests that the actin cytoskeleton plays a critical role in insulin-stimulated GLUT4 translocation. Insulin has been shown to cause a remodeling of actin filaments just below the plasma membrane in a variety of cellular systems, with an induction of actin polymerization and membrane ruffling (141,142). This effect on ruffling is likely to reflect polymerization and depolymerization beneath the membrane, involving lamellipodia and/or filopodia formation. Actin-depolymerizing agents, such as cytochalasin D and the actin monomer–binding toxins latrunculin A and B, inhibit insulin-stimulated GLUT4 translocation (143). The C-terminal tail of GLUT4 in adipocytes has been shown to indirectly interact with F-actin by binding to the glycolytic enzyme aldolase, suggesting a homeostatic mechanism in which glucose metabolism might feedback regulate GLUT4 translocation along the actin cytoskeleton (144).

The docking and fusion of the GLUT4 vesicle at the plasma membrane are subject to regulation by insulin. This involves a series of proteins termed the SNARE proteins. The v-SNARE protein VAMP2 is present on GLUT4-containing vesicles and appears to physically interact with its t-SNARE

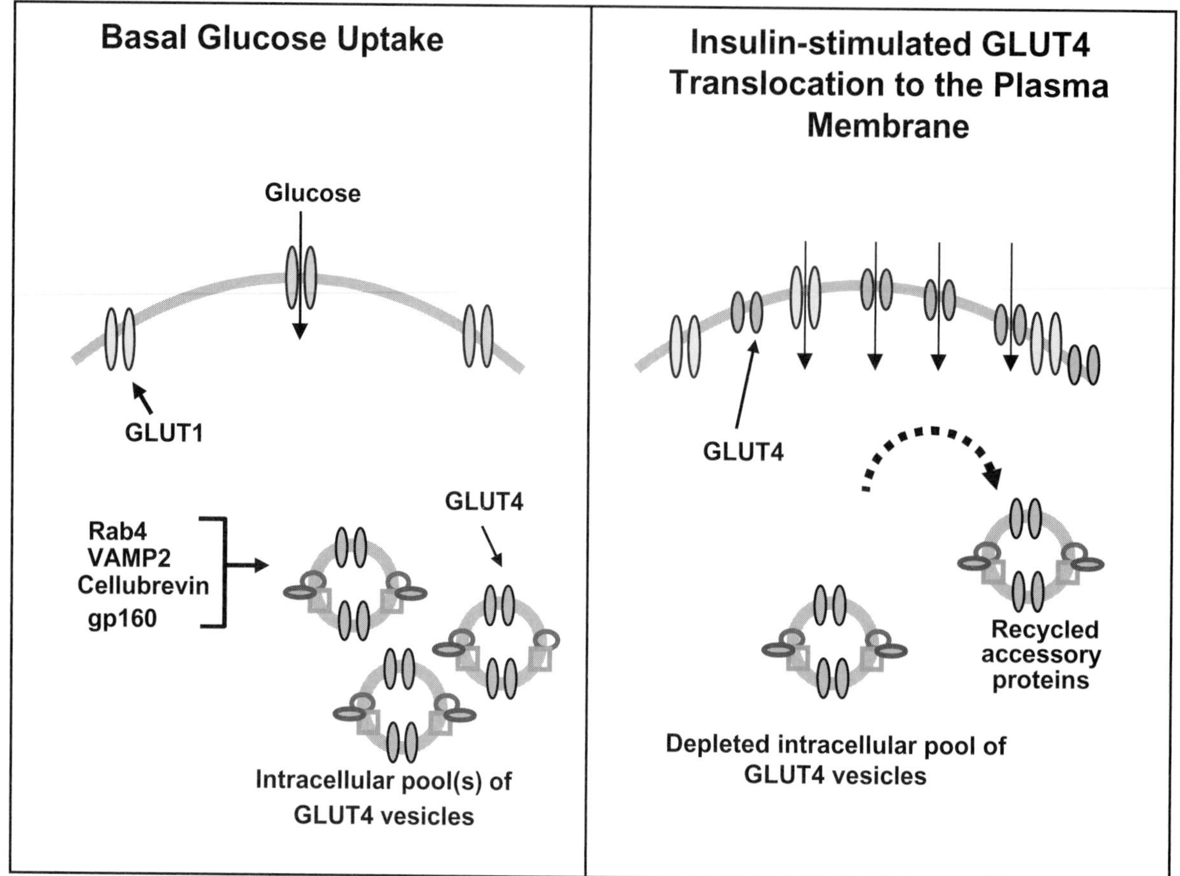

Figure 9.8. The regulation of glucose transport by insulin stimulation of GLUT4 translocation.

counterpart syntaxin 4 during GLUT4-vesicle docking and fusion with the plasma membrane (145), although neither SNARE protein appears to be a direct target of insulin action. However, the SNARE accessory proteins Synip and Munc18c may be involved in the control of GLUT4 docking and fusion in an insulin-dependent, PI 3-kinase–independent manner (146). One interesting possibility is that the PI 3-kinase–independent arm of insulin action may be directed at the docking and fusion step of GLUT4 regulation.

REGULATION OF GLUCOSE AND LIPID SYNTHESIS, UTILIZATION, AND STORAGE

Glucose Oxidation and Storage

Upon entering the muscle cell, glucose is rapidly phosphorylated by hexokinase and either stored as glycogen via the activity of glycogen synthase or oxidized to generate adenosine triphosphate (ATP) synthesis via enzymes such as pyruvate kinase. In the liver and adipose tissue, glucose can also be stored as fat. Some of the enzymes involved in glycolysis, as well as in glycogen and lipid synthesis, are regulated by insulin via changes in their phosphorylation state due to a combination of protein kinase inhibition and phosphatase activation. In addition, some of these enzymes are regulated at the transcriptional level.

Insulin stimulates glycogen accumulation through a coordinated increase in glucose transport and glycogen synthesis. Activation of glycogen synthase involves the promotion of its dephosphorylation via both the inhibition of kinases that can phosphorylate glycogen synthase, such as PKA or GSK3 (137,147), and the activation of phosphatases that dephosphorylate glycogen synthase, such as protein phosphatase 1 (PP1) (148). This process is downstream of PI 3-kinase and involves Akt phosphorylation of GSK-3. This inactivates GSK-3, resulting in a decrease in the phosphorylation of glycogen synthase and an increase in its activity state. However, the inhibition of GSK-3 is not sufficient for full activation of glycogen, because GSK-3 does not phosphorylate all of the residues of glycogen synthase that are dephosphorylated in response to insulin (137).

Activation of PP1 correlates well with changes in glycogen synthase activity (148). However, insulin does not appear to globally activate PP1 but rather to activate specific pools of the phosphatase localized on the glycogen particle. The compartmentalized activation of PP1 by insulin is due to glycogen-targeting subunits that serve as "molecular scaffolds," bringing together the enzyme with its substrates glycogen synthase and glycogen phosphorylase in a macromolecular complex (149). Four different proteins (G_M, G_L, PTG, and R_6) have been reported to target PP1 to the glycogen particle. Overexpression of these scaffolding proteins in cells or *in vivo* by adenovirus-mediated gene transfer results in a dramatic increase in basal cellular glycogen levels (150). Furthermore, glycogen stores in cells overexpressing PTG are refractory to breakdown by agents that raise intracellular cyclic adenosine monophosphate (cAMP) levels, suggesting that PTG locks the cell into a glycogenic mode (149). The mechanism by which insulin activates glycogen-associated PP1 remains unknown. Although it had been proposed that activation of MAP kinase leads to the phosphorylation of the targeting protein G_M and the subsequent release of inhibition of the enzyme by insulin, blockade of this pathway had no effect on the activation of glycogen synthase by insulin and mutation of the identified phosphorylation sites did not impair insulin action. However, inhibitors of PI 3-kinase can block activation of PP1 by insulin, indicating that PIP_3-dependent protein kinases are involved.

Regulation of Gluconeogenesis

Insulin inhibits the production and release of glucose by the liver and, to a lesser extent, by the kidney by blockade of gluconeogenesis and glycogenolysis. Insulin achieves these effects by directly controlling the activities of a subset of metabolic enzymes via the process of phosphorylation and dephosphorylation described above, as well as by regulation of the expression of a number of genes encoding hepatic enzymes. Insulin dramatically inhibits the transcription of the gene encoding phosphoenolpyruvate carboxylase (PEPCK), the rate-limiting step in gluconeogenesis. The hormone also decreases transcription of the genes encoding fructose 1,6-bisphosphatase and glucose 6-phosphatase and increases transcription of those encoding glycolytic enzymes such as glucokinase and pyruvate kinase and lipogenic enzymes such as fatty acid synthase and acetyl CoA carboxylase.

Several transcription factors play a role in this insulin-mediated regulation (Fig. 9.9). Hepatic nuclear factor-3 (HNF3) and HNF4 both appear to be involved in regulation of the PEPCK gene, which is the rate-limiting enzyme of gluconeogenesis (151). Sterol regulatory element-binding protein-1c (SREBP-1c) is regulated by insulin in its phosphorylation and may play a role in the effect of insulin on PEPCK gene transcription (152). The forkhead transcription factor FKHR (now known as FOXO1) also appears to be involved in the regulation of PEPCK and glucose 6-phosphatase, because both PEPCK and glucose 6-phosphatase contain putative FKHR binding sites in their promoter sequences, and overexpression of FKHR in hepatoma cells markedly increases the expression of the catalytic subunit of glucose 6-phosphatase (153). Recently, Yoon et al. (154) showed that both HNF4 and FOXO1 may be modified in their activity by a single co-activator known as PGC-1. PGC-1 levels are increased in insulin-deficient and insulin-resistant diabetes. This creates an attractive hypothesis by bringing together multiple regulators under one common master regulator.

Although there is no doubt that insulin plays a key role in the regulation of the enzymes of gluconeogenesis, insulin can also indirectly influence glucose metabolism. This occurs via changes in the availability of substrates for gluconeogenesis that are being released from muscle and fat (155,156). Thus, when insulin levels are low, there is a breakdown of muscle protein and adipocyte triglycerides, leading to increased levels of gluconeogenic substrates such as alanine and free fatty acids. Careful physiologic experiments in the dog that included time courses and dose responses of insulin action have suggested that under some circumstances this indirect pathway may be the major pathway of insulin regulation of gluconeogenesis (155,156). However, recent experiments with mice with a genetic knockout of the insulin receptor in liver indicate that the direct pathway is more important in that species (157). In any case, in humans the indirect pathway may contribute to the

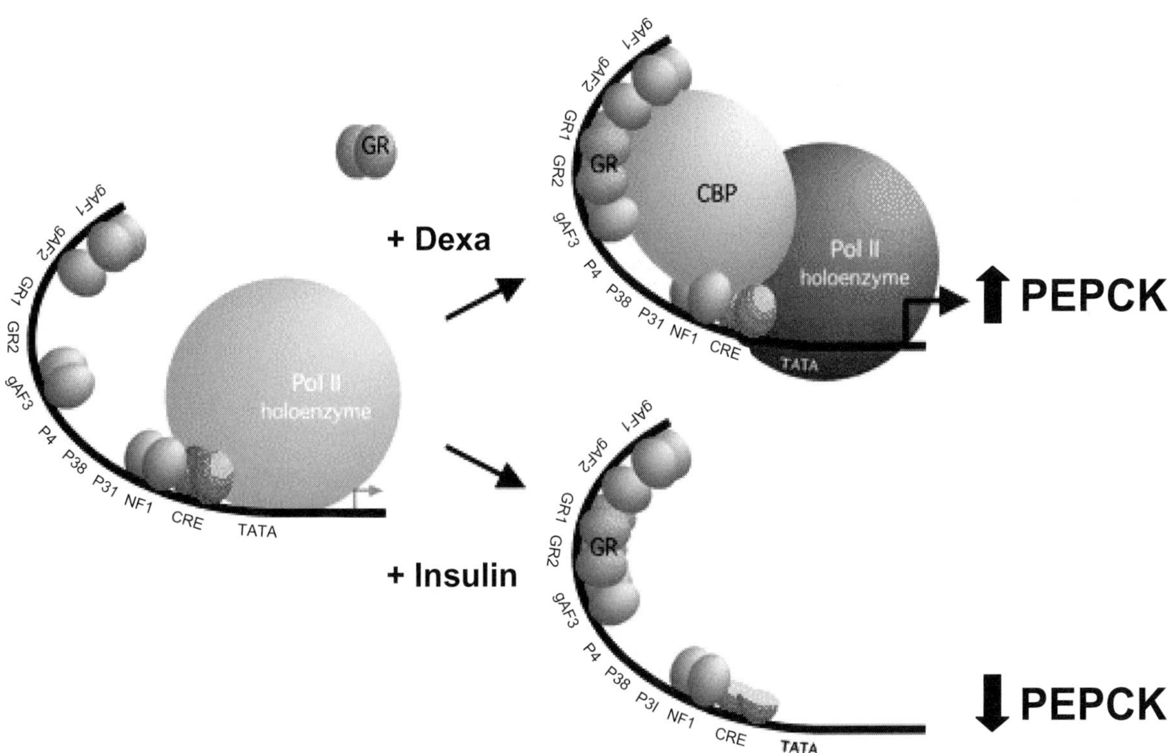

Figure 9.9. Regulation of gluconeogenesis at the molecular level of the promoter of phosphoenolpyruvate carboxylase (PEPCK), the rate-limiting enzyme in gluconeogenesis. (Adapted from Duong DT, Waltner-Law ME, Sears R, et al. Insulin inhibits hepatocellular glucose production by utilizing liver-enriched transcriptional inhibitory protein to disrupt the association of CREB-binding protein and RNA polymerase II with the phosphoenolpyruvate carboxykinase gene promoter. *J Biol Chem* 2002;277: 32234–32242.)

pathogenesis of diabetes, especially in individuals with central obesity, because visceral fat is less sensitive than subcutaneous fat to insulin inhibition of lipolysis, resulting in direct flux of fatty acids derived from these fat cells through the portal vein to the liver.

Regulation of Lipogenesis and Lipolysis

As is the case with carbohydrate metabolism, insulin also promotes the synthesis of lipids and inhibits their degradation. Recent studies suggest that many of these changes also might require an increase in levels of the transcription factor SREBP1-c (158–160). Dominant-negative forms of SREBP1 can block expression of these gluconeogenic and lipogenic genes (159), and overexpression of SREBP-lc can increase their expression (161). Interestingly, hepatic SREBP levels are increased in rodent models of lipodystrophy, and this is associated with coordinated increases in fatty acid synthesis and gluconeogenesis, mimicking the phenotype observed in genetic models of obesity-induced diabetes. These observations led Shimomura et al. (161) to speculate that increased expression of SREBP-1c might lead to the mixed insulin resistance observed in the diabetic liver, with increased rates of both gluconeogenesis and lipogenesis. The pathways that account for the changes in SREBP1-c expression lie downstream of the IRS/PI 3-kinase pathway.

In adipocytes, glucose is stored primarily as lipid. This is the result of increased uptake of glucose and activation of lipid synthetic enzymes, including pyruvate dehydrogenase, fatty acid synthase, and acetyl CoA carboxylase. Insulin also profoundly inhibits lipolysis in adipocytes, primarily through inhibition of the enzyme hormone-sensitive lipase. This enzyme is acutely regulated by control of its phosphorylation state, activated by PKA-dependent phosphorylation, and inhibited owing to a combination of kinase inhibition and phosphatase activation. Insulin inhibits the activity of the lipase primarily via reductions in cAMP levels due to the activation of a cAMP-specific phosphodiesterase in fat cells (162).

WHAT CAUSES INSULIN RESISTANCE?

Defining Insulin Resistance and the Sites of Insulin Resistance

Insulin resistance is said to exist any time a normal amount of insulin produces a less than normal biologic response (163). Insulin resistance can be further divided into states in which there is a rightward shift in the dose response to the hormone but the maximal response remains normal (decreased insulin sensitivity) or states in which the dose response is normal but the maximal response is decreased (decreased responsiveness), or a combination of the two (Fig. 9.10). Insulin resistance is extremely common, occurring both in disease states such as type 2 diabetes, obesity, hypertension, polycystic ovarian disease, and a variety of genetic syndromes and in physiologic conditions such as puberty and pregnancy (164,165). Insulin resistance also is present in many states of stress, in association with infection, and secondary to treatment with a variety of drugs, particularly glucocorticoids.

From a molecular perspective, insulin resistance can occur at multiple levels and be either acquired or genetic. Prereceptor insulin resistance is rare today but formerly was exemplified by patients with high levels of circulating antibodies to insulin that blocked binding of the ligand to its receptor and by patients with what appeared to be increased subcutaneous degradation of injected insulin (166). Insulin resistance at the level of the receptor may be the result of genetic alterations in receptor expression or structure, secondary changes in receptor activity due to serine phosphorylation, or downregulation of receptor concentration. At the postreceptor level, insulin resistance can occur almost anywhere on one of the common or branched pathways of insulin signaling.

In the most common states of insulin resistance, there appear to be defects at multiple levels. For example, in type 2 diabetes, there are decreases in receptor concentration, in receptor kinase activity, in the concentration and phosphorylation of IRS-1 and IRS-2, in PI 3-kinase activity, and in glucose-transporter

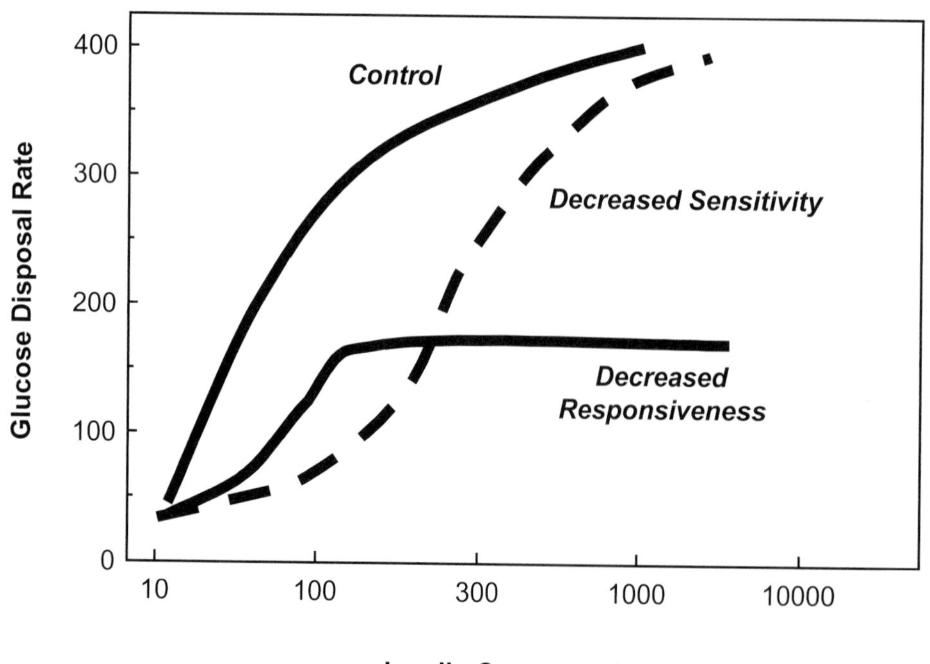

Figure 9.10. Types of insulin resistance. (Adapted from Kahn CR. Insulin resistance, insulin insensitivity, and insulin unresponsiveness: a necessary distinction. *Metabolism* 1978;27:1893–1902.)

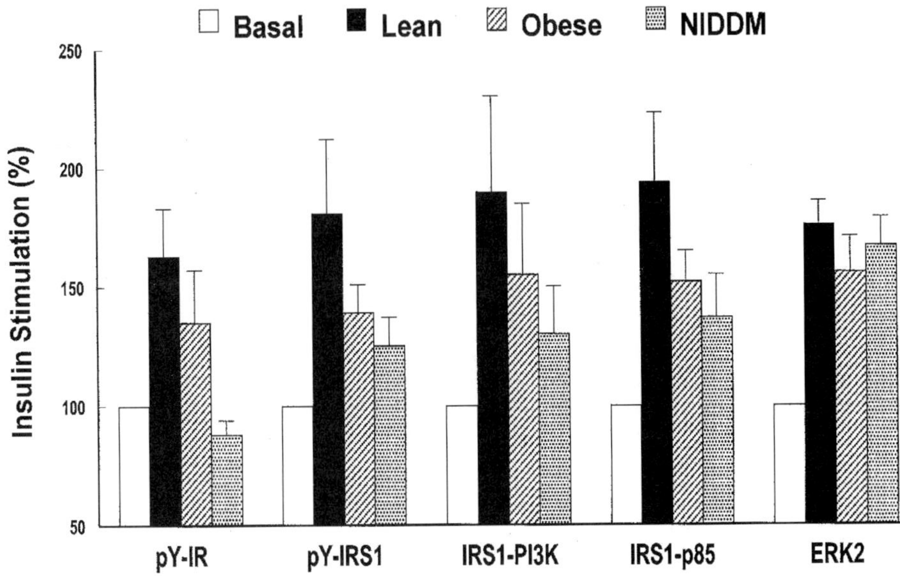

Figure 9.11. Insulin signaling and its alterations in skeletal muscle of obese and type 2 diabetic (NIDDM) Mexican Americans. (Adapted from Cusi K, Maezono K, Osman A, et al. Insulin resistance differentially affects the PI 3-kinase and MAP kinase-mediated signaling in human muscle. *J Clin Invest* 2000; 105:311–320.)

translocation and defects in activity of intracellular enzymes (3,167). Interestingly, in type 2 diabetes, there does not appear to be a reduction in insulin action on the MAP kinase pathway (Fig. 9.11). This blockade of the PI 3-kinase pathway with continued MAP kinase signaling might account for some of the detrimental effects of the chronic hyperinsulinemia on the vasculature (164).

Genetic Forms of Insulin Resistance

Insulin resistance due to genetic defects in insulin-receptor expression or sequence is relatively rare but represents the most severe forms of insulin resistance. In humans, these may present as several different disease syndromes, including two congenital diseases termed leprechaunism and the Rabson-Mendenhall syndrome, in which there is insulin resistance, intrauterine and postnatal growth retardation, and other developmental defects; and the type A syndrome of insulin resistance that appears in childhood, adolescence, or early adulthood (165,168). These are discussed in more detail in Chapter 28.

Although there is some correlation between the severity of the genetic defect in receptor function and the severity of the clinical presentation, the correlation is relatively weak, indicating that other genetic or acquired factors can modify the insulin-resistant state significantly (169). Interestingly, none of these diseases matches the phenotype of the insulin-receptor knockout mouse, which shows normal intrauterine growth but develops diabetic ketoacidosis in the first few days of life and dies (170). This difference in behavior may represent differences in the role of the insulin receptor in different species or the state of development of the human versus that of the mouse at birth. Alternatively, the mutant receptors may produce more complex disease phenotypes as a result of formation of hybrids with IGF-1 or other receptors that also interfere with their function.

Acquired Forms of Insulin Resistance

Acquired forms of insulin resistance may occur as a result of multiple mechanisms (Fig. 9.6). The first of these to be described was that of insulin-receptor downregulation (171,172). In this situation, mild hyperinsulinemia that occurs in response to tissue insulin resistance results in an increase in internalization and degradation of the insulin receptor. This occurs to some extent in the most common insulin-resistant states, i.e., obesity and type 2 diabetes. Recent studies have also shown that hyperinsulinemia can lead to downregulation of insulin-receptor substrates, producing an even greater decrease in insulin signaling (104,173–175). In both humans and rodents, the levels of insulin receptor and IRS-1 in some tissues can each be reduced by more than 50% in some of these insulin-resistant states. Most of the changes in the insulin receptor and its substrates are due to increased protein turnover, but there may also be an element of downregulation at the transcriptional level, especially for IRS-2.

In addition to downregulation, there may be many other factors that contribute to acquired insulin resistance. As noted above, in hyperinsulinemic and other insulin-resistant states, there is increased serine phosphorylation of the receptor and its substrates (174,176). This leads to decreased kinase activity of the receptor and decreased tyrosine phosphorylation of the receptor substrates. Several different serine kinases have been implicated in this serine phosphorylation, including Akt, various isoforms of PKC, and the stress-induced MAP kinases (p38 and JNK) and IKB kinase (64,67,177). The upstream stimulators of these kinases may also be multiple. For example, in obesity and type 2 diabetes, there are increased levels of circulating free fatty acids (FFAs), and in obesity, adipose tissue makes and releases a number of other factors, including TNF-α, leptin, various complement-related peptides, and two recently discovered hormones, resistin and adiponectin (also called Acrp30 and AdipoQ) (see below). Another class of proteins that can act as inhibitors of insulin signaling are the SOCS proteins (92,178,179). These certainly play a role in stress-induced states, such as that created by injection of bacterial lipopolysaccharide, and perhaps in obesity-linked insulin resistance. These SOCS proteins act to inhibit insulin signaling by binding to the phosphorylated insulin receptor and inhibiting phosphorylation of the IRS proteins.

Role of Free Fatty Acids and Intracellular Triglycerides in Insulin Resistance

Circulating FFAs are elevated in many insulin-resistant states and have been suggested to play a central role in the pathogenesis of the insulin resistance. Physiologic increases in plasma FFA levels have been shown to cause insulin resistance by several mechanisms in both diabetic subjects and obese, nondiabetic subjects. FFAs inhibit insulin-stimulated glucose uptake at the level of glucose transport and/or phosphorylation, inhibit insulin-stimulated glycogen synthesis, and inhibit insulin-stimulated glucose oxidation (180–182). As noted above, FFAs might have a special role in the insulin resistance associated with central obesity. Since central adipocytes are more resistant to insulin inhibition of lipolysis, there is an increased delivery of FFAs to the liver. This leads to increased accumulation of triglycerides that could also contribute to increased hepatic glucose output, reduced hepatic extraction of insulin, and hepatic insulin resistance. In experimental lipid-induced insulin resistance, insulin-stimulated IRS-1 phosphorylation and IRS-1–associated PI 3-kinase activity is also reduced. There is also an increase in membrane-bound, i.e., activated, PKCθ that may serve as a mediator of the insulin resistance by increased serine phosphorylation of the insulin receptor and/or IRS-1 (183).

A common link between increased levels of FFAs and the insulin resistance in type 2 diabetes, obesity, and syndrome X could be accumulation of triglycerides in muscle. Recent studies using magnetic resonance spectroscopy have demonstrated that at least some of the lipid accumulation is inside the myocyte itself (184,185). Factors leading to the accumulation of triglycerides are not clear, but it has been speculated that the triglyceride is derived from elevated levels of both circulating FFAs and triglycerides and is also the result of reduced muscle fatty acid oxidation. Whatever the mechanism, there is a close correlation between muscle triglyceride content and whole-body insulin resistance. The notion of a glucose–fatty acid cycle (Randle cycle) has been hypothesized for 40 years as a mechanism by which glucose might autoregulate its own use (186). It is likely that cytosolic accumulation of the long-chain fatty acyl CoAs is involved in the altered insulin signaling. Several mechanisms have been implicated in the inhibition of insulin signaling, including increased serine phosphorylation of the insulin receptor and its substrates or direct inhibition of enzymes such as glycogen synthase. Insulin sensitizers, such as the PPARγ agonists, reduce muscle lipid accumulation and increase insulin sensitivity. Other potent systemic lipid-lowering agents, such as PPARα agonists (e.g., fibrates) or antilipolytic agents (e.g., nicotinic acid analogues), might also improve insulin sensitivity by this mechanism.

Transgenic mice with muscle- and liver-specific overexpression of lipoprotein lipase have recently been developed to help define the roles of muscle FFAs and triglycerides in insulin resistance. Muscle-specific lipoprotein lipase-deficient mice have a threefold increase in muscle triglyceride content and exhibit insulin resistance due to decreases in insulin-stimulated glucose uptake in skeletal muscle and insulin activation of IRS-1–associated PI 3-kinase activity (187). Mice with overexpression of lipoprotein lipase in the liver have increased triglyceride content in the liver and exhibit insulin resistance due to an impaired ability of insulin to suppress endogenous glucose production, along with defects in insulin activation of IRS-2–associated PI 3-kinase activity (187). In both tissues, these defects in insulin action and signaling are associated with increases in intracellular fatty acid–derived metabolites, such as diacylglycerol and fatty acyl CoA.

The Fat Cell as a Secretory Cell and Insulin Resistance

Over the past several years, it has become clear that the adipocyte plays a role in insulin resistance not only by storing

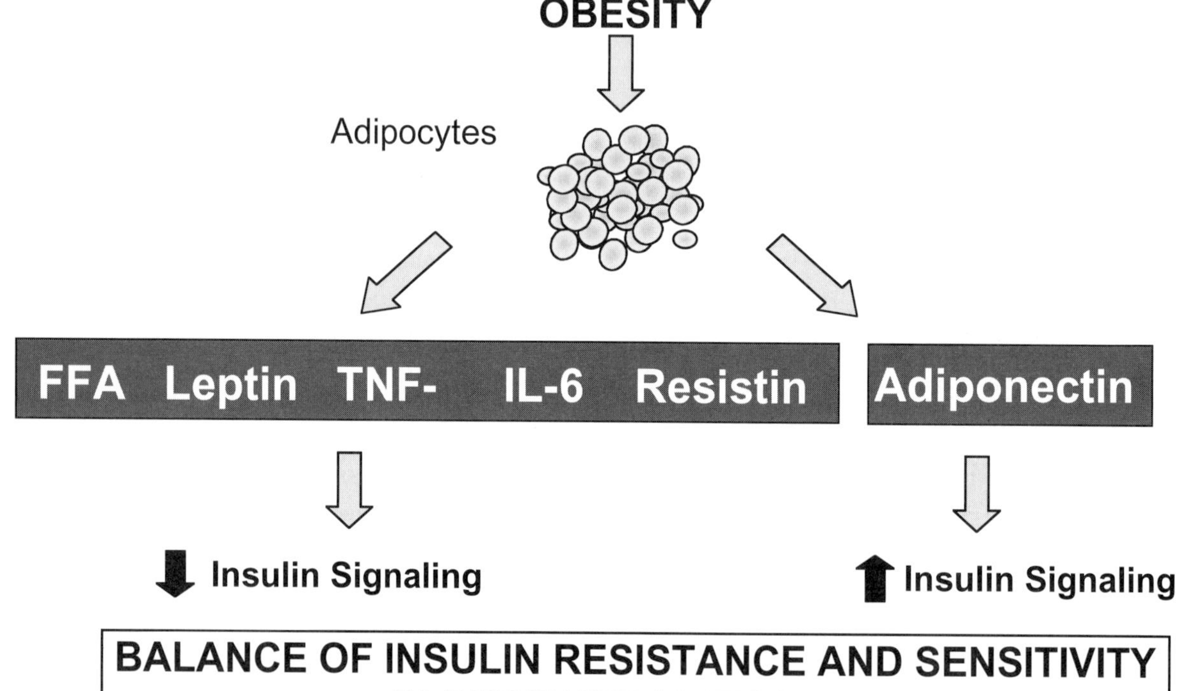

Figure 9.12. Role of adipocyte secretion in insulin resistance. Free fatty acids (FFA), leptin, tumor necrosis factor-α (TNF-α), interleukin-6 (IL-6), and resistin are substrates and adipokines released by fat that increase insulin resistance. Adiponectin, also known as ACRP 30, decreases insulin resistance and increases insulin sensitivity.

fat but also as a secretory cell producing several cytokines and hormones, as well as releasing FFAs (Fig. 9.12). The first of the cytokines to be described as being increased in fat cells of obese animals and humans was TNF-α (188,189). TNF-α could lead to insulin resistance by increasing serine phosphorylation of IRS-1 and decreasing insulin-receptor kinase activity (190). This mechanism is clearly important in rodents, in which anti–TNF-α reagents significantly improve insulin resistance (188). However, the importance of this mechanism in humans is much debated, and limited studies of anti-TNF reagents have shown little or no effect on the insulin-resistant state (191).

Leptin is a member of the cytokine family of hormones that is produced by adipose tissue and acts on receptors in the central nervous system and other sites to inhibit food intake and promote energy expenditure (192,193). Leptin has been shown to interfere with insulin signaling systems *in vitro* (12,194); however, it is not clear if leptin has anti-insulin effects *in vivo*. Indeed, in states of severe leptin deficiency, such as in the ob/ob mouse or several genetic models of lipoatrophic diabetes, administration of exogenous leptin improves glucose tolerance and insulin sensitivity (195). This appears to be primarily the result of an action of leptin at the liver to increase insulin sensitivity, an effect that might be direct or centrally mediated.

Adiponectin (also called Acrp30, adipoQ, APM-1, and GBP28) is a peptide of 247 amino acids that possesses a collagenous domain at the N-terminus and a globular domain that shares significant homology with subunits of complement factor C1q. The expression of adiponectin is highly specific to adipose tissue. Adiponectin is among the most abundant proteins in adipocytes, is secreted into the bloodstream, and is present at very high circulating concentrations (196,197). Several recent studies have pointed to a potentially important role of adiponectin in the insulin resistance of obesity (198,199). First, expression of adiponectin mRNA is decreased in obese humans and mice and in some models of lipoatrophic diabetes (196). Acute treatment of mice with the globular head domain of Acrp30 significantly decreased the elevated levels of plasma FFAs and caused weight loss in mice consuming a high-fat diet. Administration of adiponectin to obese mice also decreases insulin resistance and triglyceride content of muscle and liver. Moreover, insulin resistance in lipoatrophic mice is completely reversed by the combination of physiologic doses of adiponectin and leptin, but only partially by administration of either adiponectin or leptin alone (196). Administration of adiponectin/Acrp30 also lowers glucose levels in normal mice and mouse models of type 1 diabetes, such as NOD mice and streptozotocin-treated mice (200). Recent genome-wide scans have mapped a susceptibility locus for type 2 diabetes and metabolic syndrome to chromosome 3q27, a region where the gene encoding adiponectin is located (196,201). These data suggest that decreased levels of adiponectin are important factors in the insulin resistance of obesity and lipoatrophy and that replacement of adiponectin might provide a novel treatment for some insulin-resistant states.

Resistin is the most recently discovered peptide hormone secreted by adipocytes (202). Resistin belongs to a family of tissue-specific secreted proteins termed resistin-like molecules (RELMs) and the FIZZ (found in inflammatory zone) family (203). Initial studies suggested that resistin levels were increased in both genetic and acquired obesity in mice and reduced by antidiabetic drugs of the thiazolidinedione class. Further, administration of antibody to resistin appeared to improve blood glucose levels and insulin action in mice with diet-induced obesity (202,204). Moreover, insulin-stimulated glucose uptake by adipocytes was enhanced by neutralization of resistin and reduced by resistin treatment. Others have not confirmed these initial studies, finding that resistin expression is significantly decreased in the white adipose tissue of several different models of obesity, including the ob/ob, db/db, tub/tub, and KKA(y) mice, as compared with their lean counterparts (205). Furthermore, treatment of both ob/ob mice and Zucker diabetic fatty rats with several different classes of PPARγ agonists resulted in an increase in resistin expression. The potential role of resistin is further complicated by the fact that the human homologue has relatively poor sequence homology and little difference has been detected in resistin expression by normal, insulin-resistant, or type 2 diabetic subjects (206). Other recent studies have suggested alternative roles for resistin as an adipose sensor for the nutritional state of the animals and an inhibitor of adipocyte differentiation (207).

LESSONS FROM KNOCKOUT MICE ABOUT INSULIN ACTION AND INSULIN RESISTANCE

As noted above, the ability to create genetic knockout of insulin-signaling proteins has allowed us to define the roles of the insulin receptor and its substrates in both whole animals and in cells derived from these animals. The technique of homologous recombination gene targeting has been used to create and characterize mice lacking each of these insulin-signaling proteins. A number of these are described above. In addition, combinatorial knockouts have been produced, both in the homozygous and heterozygous states, as well as tissue-specific knockouts, and these also have provided important insights into the mechanisms of insulin action and the nature of insulin resistance in each tissue.

Mice with Compound Defects

The creation of polygenic models of diabetes was begun by breeding mice heterozygous for deletion of the insulin receptor (IR) with mice heterozygous for deletion of IRS-1 to produce double-heterozygote knockout mice (208). In contrast to the single-heterozygote knockout mice, which appear normal, the IR/IRS-1 double-heterozygote knockout mice manifested marked insulin resistance, with a 10-fold increase in circulating insulin levels and a 5- to 30-fold increase in β-cell mass. Despite this islet hyperplasia, ~50% of these mice developed diabetes by 4 to 6 months of age.

These compound-heterozygote animals have several features of interest. First, despite the genetic nature of the insulin resistance, these mice, like humans, develop diabetes with delayed onset. Second, the 50% incidence of diabetes indicates a marked synergism (epistasis) between the IR defect (which leads to diabetes in <10% of mice) and the IRS-1 defect (which never leads to diabetes). Finally, on a mixed genetic background, only ~50% of the mice develop diabetes, indicating that an additional gene or genes present in the background of these mice contribute to or protect them from the development of diabetes.

Recently, these studies have been extended to produce even more complex compound heterozygous animals and to explore the role of genetic background in the diabetic state. For example, IR/IRS-1/IRS-2 triple-heterozygote knockout mice have been created and shown to have severely impaired glucose tolerance and a doubling of the incidence of diabetes as compared with the double heterozygotes (209). By contrast, IR/IRS-1/p85

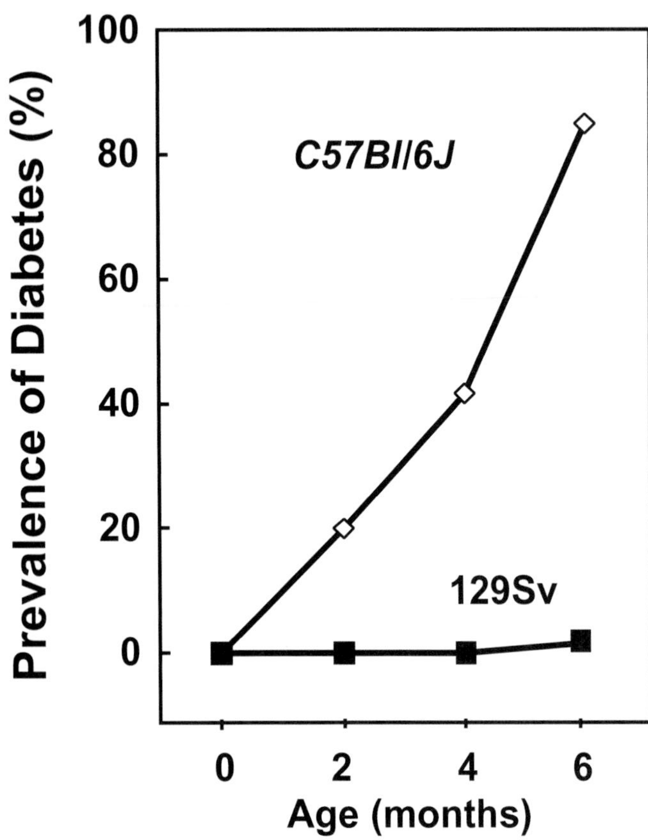

Figure 9.13. Impact of genetic background on the development of type 2 diabetes in mice with genetic insulin resistance. Genetic insulin resistance was created by breeding mice with heterozygous defects in both insulin receptor and insulin-receptor substrate 1 (IRS-1) onto two different genetic backgrounds of mice. On the C57Bl/6J background, about 90% of mice become diabetic within 6 months. On the 129Sv background, fewer than 2% become diabetic at 6 months or even at 18 months. (Redrawn from the data of Kulkarni RN, Almind K, Goren HJ, et al. Impact of genetic background on development of hyperinsulinemia and diabetes in insulin receptor/insulin receptor substrate-1 double heterozygous mice. *Diabetes* 2003;52: 1528–1534.)

triple-heterozyote knockout mice are less severely affected than the IR/IRS-1 double-heterozygote knockout mice owing to the beneficial effect of reduced p85 levels on insulin resistance (109). The phenotype of mice doubly heterozygous (DH) for IR and IRS-1 varies depending on the genetic background (210) (Fig. 9.13). Thus, DH mice on the C57Bl/6J background have a high incidence of diabetes (85% at 6 months of age), whereas the 129Sv strain does not develop diabetes, despite the genetic defects in insulin signaling. DBA mice with the DH mutation show intermediate levels of hyperglycemia and hyperinsulinemia. This illustrates the importance of genetic modifiers of the diabetic state that exist in mice and humans. Genome-wide scans in these mice have identified four loci on three chromosomes that contribute to this difference (211).

CREATION OF TISSUE-SPECIFIC KNOCKOUTS

Two approaches applying mouse genetics have been used to address the role of insulin-receptor signaling in specific tissues. One has used mice that express a dominant-negative mutant of the insulin receptor under control of a tissue-specific promoter, such as the muscle creatine kinase (MCK) or GLUT4 promoters (212,213), and the other has created tissue-specific knockouts using the Cre-*loxP* system to disrupt the insulin-receptor gene in various tissues of the mouse (214). The latter is based on the use of the bacteriophage recombinase Cre to conditionally inactivate genes in mice in which *loxP* sites flanking some critical element have been introduced (215). *LoxP* sites are bacterial DNA sequences of 34 base pairs (bp) that allow for directional recombination of two segments of DNA, eliminating the DNA in between. For tissue-specific knockout of the insulin receptor, *loxP* sites were introduced around exon 4, because deletion of this exon by the Cre recombinase would cause a major deletion and frameshift mutation with a premature stop of translation at amino acid 308 of the insulin-receptor protein. Mice carrying the IR*lox* allele could then be bred with a number of different cre-mice to produce a variety of tissue-specific knockouts of the insulin receptor, depending on the nature of the Cre-transgenic mice with which they are bred. For example, breeding mice carrying the IR*lox* allele with an MCK promoter-Cre mouse would produce a muscle-specific knockout of the insulin receptor (MIRKO) mouse, use of an albumin-Cre mouse would produce a liver-specific insulin-receptor knockout (LIRKO), and use of a P2-Cre mouse would produce a fat-specific insulin-receptor knockout (FIRKO) (Fig. 9.14). This technique has also been used in a more limited way to study the role of GLUT4 in specific tissues (216,217).

MUSCLE-SPECIFIC INSULIN-RECEPTOR KNOCKOUT MOUSE

Because muscle accounts for a large fraction of postprandial glucose uptake and is a site of insulin resistance early in the prediabetic state (218–220), the first tissue-specific knockout to be created was a muscle-specific insulin-receptor knockout. This was created using a Cre transgenic mouse with an MCK gene as promoter/enhancer. The MIRKO mice demonstrated almost complete and specific ablation of insulin-receptor expression in muscle, whereas insulin-receptor expression was unaltered in other tissues. Surprisingly, despite the virtual lack of insulin signaling in muscle, the MIRKO mice were able to maintain euglycemia up to at least the age of 20 months. Moreover, plasma insulin concentrations and insulin tolerance tests were indistinguishable between animals of each group.

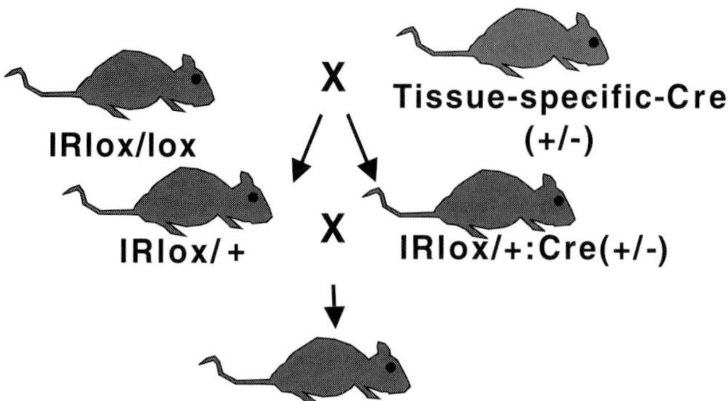

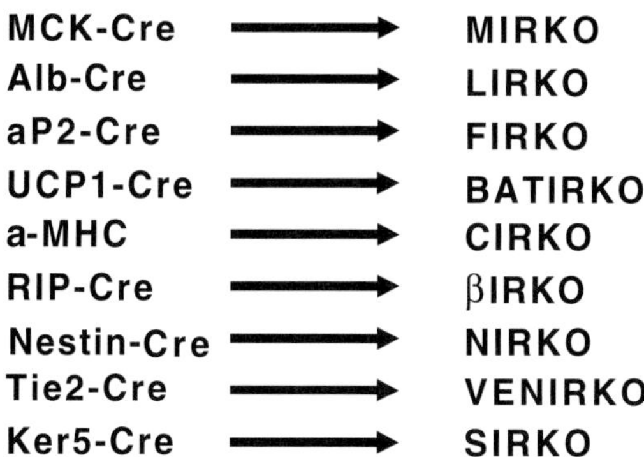

Figure 9.14. Generation of tissue-specific insulin receptor knockout mice using the Cre-lox technology. Mice carrying two alleles of the insulin receptor flanked with lox sites (IRlox/lox) are bred with mice carrying the Cre-recombinase driven by a tissue-specific promoter. After two rounds of breeding, tissue-specific knockout mice are generated. The details of each of the tissue specific knockouts are discussed in the text. MIRKO, muscle-specific insulin-receptor knockout; LIRKO, liver-specific insulin-receptor knockout; FIRKO, fat-specific insulin-receptor knockout; BATIRKO, brown adipose tissue–specific insulin-receptor knockout; CIRKO, cardiac-specific insulin-receptor knockout; βIRKO, β-cell insulin-receptor knockout; NIRKO, neural insulin-receptor knockout; VENIRKO, vascular endothelial cell insulin-receptor knockout; SIRKO, skin-specific insulin-receptor knockout.

On euglycemic clamp studies, however, the rates of insulin-stimulated whole-body glucose uptake were decreased in MIRKO mice, with a 74% decrease in insulin-stimulated muscle glucose transport. What was unexpected, however, was the threefold increase of insulin-stimulated glucose transport in adipose tissue in MIRKO mice. Thus, insulin resistance in muscle produced a shift of substrate to adipose tissue that resulted in increased adipose-tissue mass, hypertriglyceridemia, and a modest increase in FFAs, all features of the metabolic syndrome associated with insulin resistance (221) (Fig. 9.15).

Studies with MIRKO mice demonstrate the utility and value of tissue-specific knockouts for promoting insights into the nature of insulin signaling and testing our concepts of glucose homeostasis and the pathogenesis of type 2 diabetes. They also suggest the presence of some tissue cross-talk between muscle and fat, which, if it also occurs in humans, could contribute to the increase in obesity in people with genetically programmed insulin resistance in muscle, as well as a significant role of muscle insulin resistance in the development of the lipid phenotype of the metabolic syndrome, including elevated plasma triglycerides, FFAs, and central obesity.

MUSCLE-SPECIFIC GLUT4 KNOCKOUT MOUSE

To determine if different types of insulin resistance in a single tissue might produce different alterations in glucose homeostasis, the Cre-*loxP* system also was used to selectively disrupt GLUT4 expression in muscle (216). The muscle-specific GLUT4 knockout (MG4KO) mouse had a greater than 90% reduction of GLUT4 protein in skeletal muscle and no compensatory increase in GLUT1. Basal glucose uptake *in vitro* was reduced 72% to 88% in various muscles of MG4KO mice, and the response to insulin was completely obliterated. In contrast to MIRKO mice, these mice also had increased fasting glucose levels and impaired glucose and insulin tolerance tests. However, they showed no increase in body fat or hyperlipidemia.

LIVER-SPECIFIC INSULIN-RECEPTOR KNOCKOUT MOUSE

The role of the liver in glucose homeostasis has been defined by generating mice with a liver-specific knockout of the insulin receptor using a Cre recombinase under the albumin promoter/enhancer (222). On gross examination, the livers of LIRKO mice were about 50% of normal size, and the insulin-receptor content of the liver was reduced by more than 90%. At 2 months of age, LIRKO mice were hyperglycemic in the fed state as compared with controls and exhibited severely impaired glucose tolerance. Serum insulin levels in LIRKO mice were markedly elevated owing both to an increase in islet size and insulin secretion and to a decrease in insulin clearance. The failure of these mice to respond to insulin in terms of suppression of hepatic glucose output indicates that in mice the direct effect of insulin on this pathway is more important than any indirect effects (157).

FAT-SPECIFIC INSULIN-RECEPTOR KNOCKOUT MOUSE

Mice with a fat-specific knockout of the insulin receptor are perhaps the most interesting of those in the three classical targets of insulin action. Despite the importance of insulin for suppression of lipolysis, FIRKO mice have normal blood glucose levels, normal glucose tolerance tests, and normal levels of FFAs and glycerol (223). In addition, all measures of insulin resistance are within the range of normal controls, including intraperitoneal insulin tolerance tests and fasting and fed serum insulin

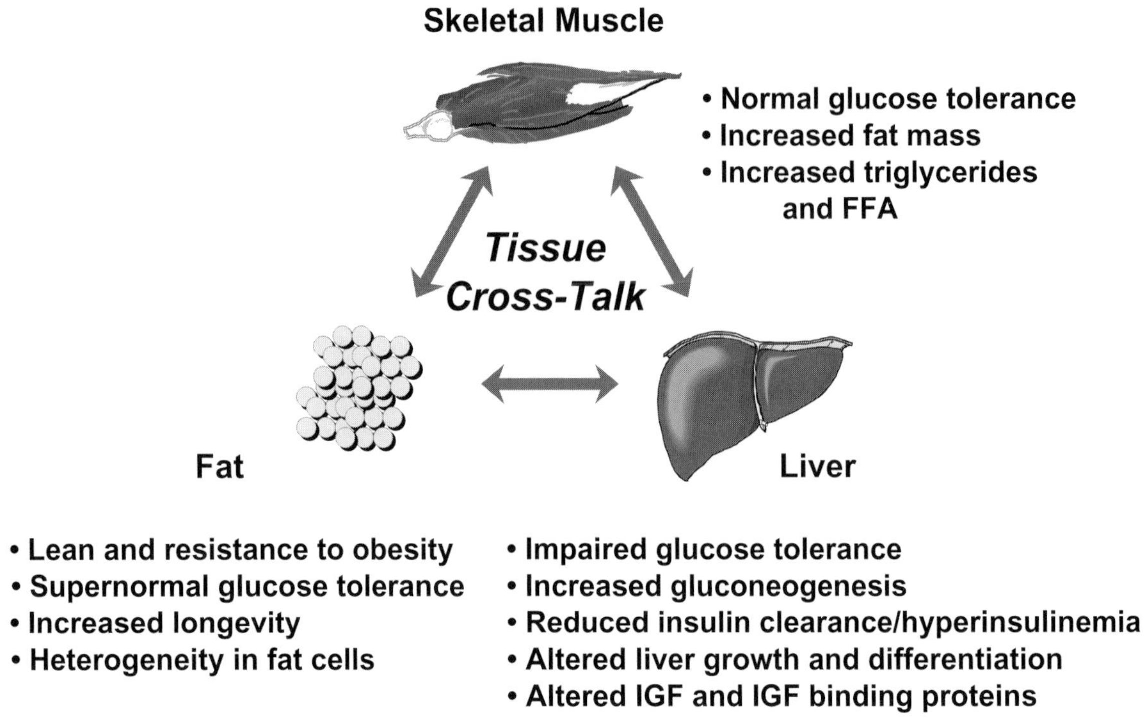

Skeletal Muscle

- Normal glucose tolerance
- Increased fat mass
- Increased triglycerides and FFA

Tissue Cross-Talk

Fat

Liver

- Lean and resistance to obesity
- Supernormal glucose tolerance
- Increased longevity
- Heterogeneity in fat cells

- Impaired glucose tolerance
- Increased gluconeogenesis
- Reduced insulin clearance/hyperinsulinemia
- Altered liver growth and differentiation
- Altered IGF and IGF binding proteins

Figure 9.15. Defects in tissue-specific knockout mice of skeletal muscle, fat, and liver. FFA, free fatty acids; IGF, insulin-like growth factor.

concentrations. The FIRKO mice do, however, demonstrate a ~50% decrease in fat mass by 6 months of age that persists throughout life. FIRKO mice are also resistant to becoming obese as they age and even after treatment with gold thioglucose, an agent that produces a hypothalamic lesion and induces hyperphagia. As a result, these mice are also protected from the development of age- and obesity-related glucose intolerance. Perhaps most interesting is the extended life span of FIRKO mice, indicating the importance of body fat, rather than diet, in longevity (224).

USE OF TISSUE-SPECIFIC KNOCKOUT TO DEFINE INSULIN ACTION IN NONTARGET TISSUES

β-Cell Insulin-Receptor Knockout Mouse

One of the characteristic features of type 2 diabetes is a failure of the β-cell to respond to a glucose stimulus while retaining its response to other secretagogues, such as amino acids (225,226). Although data have conflicted regarding the presence of functional insulin receptors on the β-cell, it has been suggested that insulin regulates its own secretion via regulation of expression of some genes and depolarization of the β-cell (227–229). The Cre-*lox* strategy for tissue-specific gene inactivation was applied to assessing the role of the insulin receptor in the pancreatic (β-cell *in vivo*, taking advantage of mice that carry the Cre transgene on a 668-bp β-cell–specific rat insulin 2 promoter (Rip-Cre) (230–232). This produced a specific recombination and inactivation of the insulin-receptor gene in β-cells but not in non–β-cells. This resulted in a loss of first-phase insulin secretion in response to glucose but not to arginine (19), mimicking the insulin secretory defect in humans with type 2 diabetes (Fig. 9.16). This appeared to be due to a decrease in insulin-stimulated expression of the enzyme glucokinase, which forms a key component of the glucose-sensing machinery. Islet size, morphology, and insulin content was normal at 2 months of age, but by 4 months of age, islet size and insulin content had fallen below that in control mice.

The findings for the β-cell insulin-receptor knockout (βIRKO) mouse demonstrated that β-cells possess functional insulin receptors and suggest the possibility that some of the defects present in type 2 diabetes may represent alterations in the insulin action in β-cells. This is consistent with the recent studies (229,233) demonstrating that insulin may positively regulate insulin biosynthesis and induce the depolarization required for normal insulin secretion. β-cells have also been shown to contain IGF-1 receptors, and IGF-1 has been shown to negatively regulate insulin secretion (234,235). Deletion of the IGF-1 receptor in β-cells also results in a loss of glucose sensing but in no defect in islet growth (236).

Vascular Endothelial Cell Insulin-Receptor Knockout Mouse

Insulin receptors on vascular endothelial cells have been suggested to participate in insulin-regulated glucose homeostasis by facilitating transcytosis of insulin from the intravascular to extracellular space, by promoting vasodilation and enhancing blood flow, and by generating signaling mediators. The role of insulin action in endothelial function was addressed directly by generating mice with a vascular endothelial cell insulin-receptor knockout (VENIRKO) generated by the *Cre-Lox*P system. Despite the previous studies suggesting a role for these receptors in glucose and blood pressure homeostasis, blood glucose and insulin concentrations, and glucose and insulin

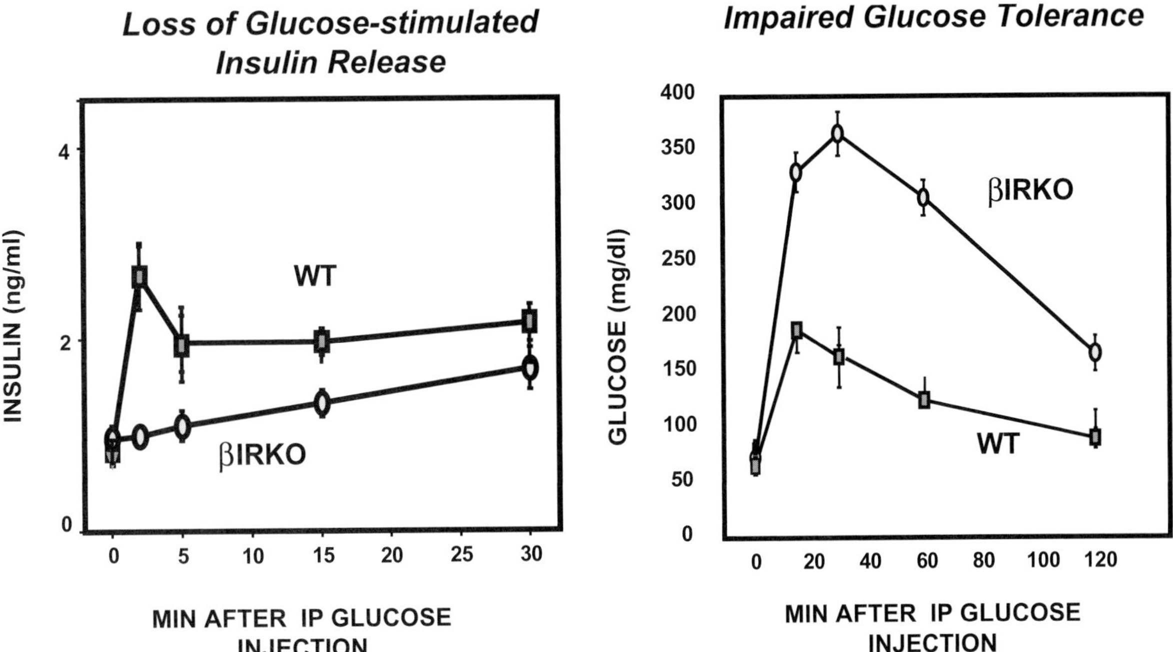

Figure 9.16. The important role of insulin signaling in pancreatic β-cells: studies in the βIRKO (β-cell insulin-receptor knockout) mouse. The left panel illustrates insulin secretion in response to acute intraperitoneal (IP) glucose in βIRKO versus normal mice (WT) and shows the complete loss of first-phase insulin secretion. The right panel shows glucose levels during an intraperitoneal glucose tolerance test in the same mice. Data are for 4-month-old males (19).

tolerance tests, the time course of insulin action on glucose disposal during a euglycemic-hyperinsulinemic clamp and blood pressure were comparable in VENIRKO and control mice (237). However, both endothelial nitric oxide synthase (eNOS) and endothelin-1 mRNA levels were reduced in the endothelial cells of these mice. More important, these mice were protected from the development of neovascularization in a model of retinopathy that mimics diabetes by changing oxygen exposure (238). This is particularly interesting because acute insulin treatment in some patients with poorly controlled diabetes appears to worsen retinopathy over the short term before having its long-term beneficial effects on reducing the progression of retinopathy.

Neural Insulin-Receptor Knockout Mouse: Role of Insulin in the Brain

Insulin receptors have been found to be widely distributed in the brain; however, their function has been highly debated (239). Some studies have suggested a role of insulin in appetite regulation (240,241), and others have suggested a role of insulin in neuron growth (242,243). Again, this problem has been addressed using the tissue-specific knockout technique with the neuron-specific promoter to create the neural insulin-receptor knockout (NIRKO) mouse (18). These mice have normal brain development but exhibit four interesting phenotypes with respect to diabetes and metabolism. First, NIRKO mice are slightly hyperphagic and mildly obese, confirming the role of central nervous system insulin as an appetite suppressant. This also leads to mild insulin resistance and hypertriglyceridemia. Second, NIRKO mice have a defect in the ability of insulin to suppress hepatic glucose output. A role of centrally acting insulin in hepatic metabolism has also been suggested in studies in which insulin has been injected into the third ventricle (244), harkening back to the work 150 years ago of Claude Bernard, who demonstrated that an anatomic lesion to the base of the brain in a rabbit could lead to uncontrolled hepatic release of glucose (245). The third effect of the lack of normal insulin signaling in the brain is a defect in the ability to compensate for hypoglycemia with appropriate rises in catecholamine levels (S. Fisher and C. R. Kahn, unpublished observation, 2003). Finally, the NIRKO mouse also exhibits a form of hypothalamic hypogonadism with reduced fertility (18). Thus, not only does the brain express insulin receptors—these receptors serve a number of important functions.

A UNIFYING HYPOTHESIS OF TYPE 2 DIABETES

Taken together, the studies of these different tissue-specific knockout mice suggest a potential unifying hypothesis for the role of insulin resistance in type 2 diabetes and the metabolic syndrome (Fig. 9.17). In this model, insulin resistance in muscle leads to increased accumulation of fat and secondary insulin resistance, hypertriglyceridemia, and increased levels of FFAs. Insulin resistance in the liver leads to increased hepatic glucose output. Insulin resistance in the brain leads to an increase in appetite, more obesity, and further defects in hepatic glucose output. Finally, insulin resistance in β-cells leads to defects in glucose sensing and thereby to relative insulin deficiency. Thus, insulin resistance in multiple tissues could produce all of the defects associated with type 2 diabetes, and treatments that improve insulin sensitivity would be expected to improve all defects.

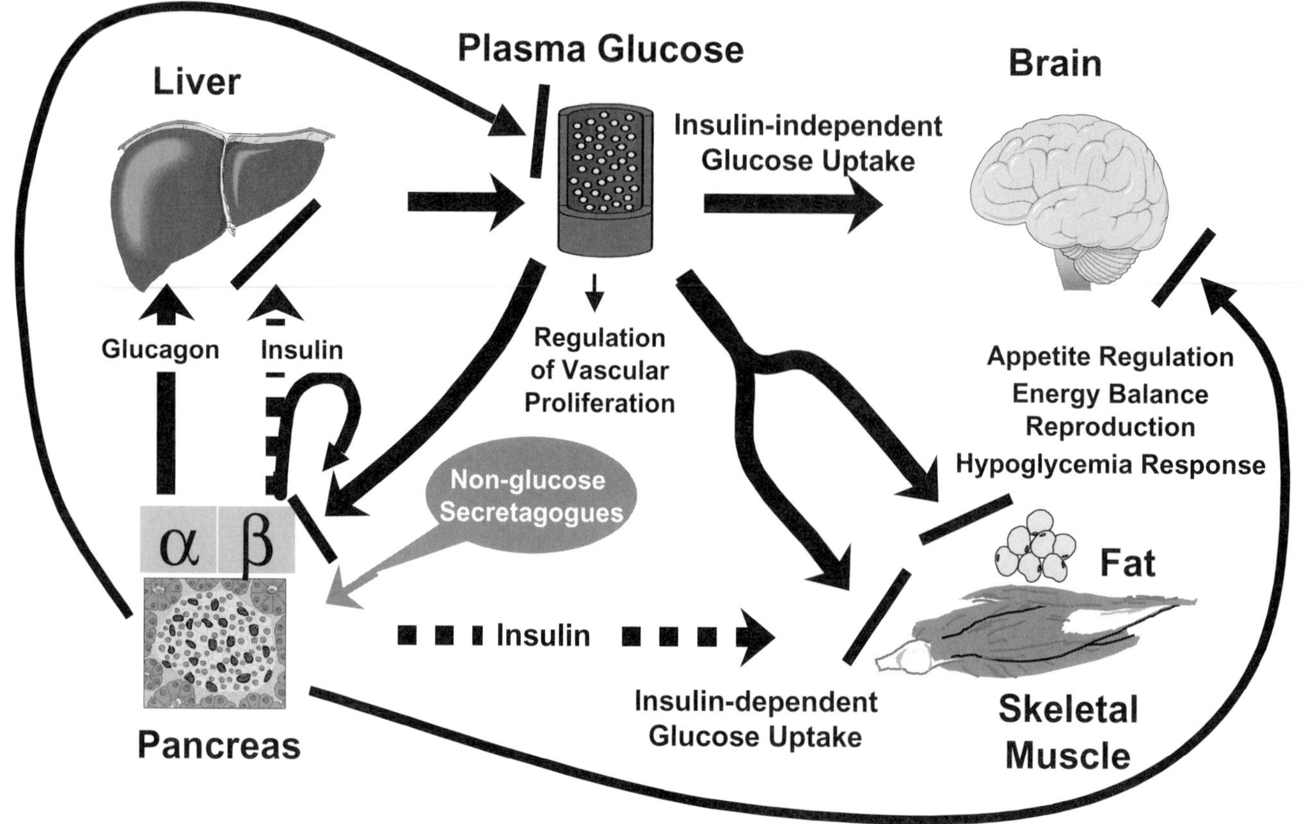

Figure 9.17. A unifying hypothesis for the pathogenesis of type 2 diabetes and insulin resistance based on results from various tissue-specific knockout mice.

REFERENCES

1. Seidell JC. Obesity, insulin resistance and diabetes—a worldwide epidemic. *Br J Nutr* 2000;83[Suppl 1]:S5–S8.
2. Klip A, Paquet MR. Glucose transport and glucose transporters in muscle and their metabolic regulation. *Diabetes Care* 1990;13:228–243.
3. Caro JF, Dohm LG, Pories WJ, et al. Cellular alterations in liver, skeletal muscle, and adipose tissue responsible for insulin resistance in obesity and type II diabetes. *Diabetes Metab Rev* 1989;5:665–689.
4. Bogardus C. Does insulin resistance primarily affect skeletal muscle? *Diabetes Metab Rev* 1979;5:527–528.
5. Beck-Nielsen H. Insulin resistance in skeletal muscles of patients with diabetes mellitus. *Diabetes Metab Rev* 1989;5:487–493.
6. Baron AD, Brechtel G, Wallace, et al. Rates and tissue sites of non-insulin- and insulin-mediated glucose uptake in humans. *Am J Physiol* 1988;255:E769–E774.
7. Brüning JC, Michael MD, Winnay JN, et al. A muscle-specific insulin receptor knockout exhibits features of the metabolic syndrome of NIDDM without altering glucose tolerance. *Mol Cell* 1998;2:559–569.
8. Peraldi P, Spiegelman B. TNF-α and insulin resistance: summary and future prospects. *Mol Cell Biochem* 1998;182:169–175.
9. Hotamisligil GS. The role of TNFalpha and TNF receptors in obesity and insulin resistance. *J Intern Med* 1999;245:621–625.
10. Zavaroni I, Bonini L, Fantuzzi M, et al. Hyperinsulinaemia, obesity, and syndrome X. *J Intern Med* 1994;235:51–56.
11. Groop LC, Saloranta C, Shank M, et al. The role of free fatty acid metabolism in the pathogenesis of insulin resistance in obesity and noninsulin-dependent diabetes mellitus. *J Clin Endocrinol Metab* 1991;72:96–107.
12. Szanto I, Kahn CR. Selective interaction between leptin and insulin signaling pathways in a hepatic cell line. *Proc Natl Acad Sci U S A* 2000;97:2355–2360.
13. Belfiore F, Iannello S. Insulin resistance in obesity: metabolic mechanisms and measurement methods. *Mol Genet Metab* 1998.65:121–128.
14. Kobberling J. Genetic syndromes associated with lipoatrophic diabetes. In: Creutzfeldt W, Kobberling J, Neel JV, eds. *The genetics of diabetes mellitus*. New York: Springer-Verlag; 1976:147–154.
15. Moitra J, Mason MM, Olive M, et al. Life without white fat: a transgenic mouse. *Genes Dev* 1988;12:3168–3181.
16. Shimomura I, Matsuda M, Hammer RE, et al. Decreased IRS-2 and increased SREBP-1c lead to mixed insulin resistance and sensitivity in livers of lipodystrophic and ob/ob mice. *Mol Cell* 2000;6:77–86.
17. Adkins-Marshall BA, Myers SR, Hendrick GK, et al. Interaction between insulin and glucose-delivery route in regulation of net hepatic glucose uptake in conscious dogs. *Diabetes* 1989;39:87–95.
18. Bruning JC, Gautam D, Burks DJ, et al. Role of brain insulin receptor in control of body weight and reproduction. *Science* 2000;289:2122–2125.
19. Kulkarni RN, Bruning JC, Winnay JN, et al. Tissue-specific knockout of the insulin receptor in pancreatic β cells creates an insulin secretory defect similar to that in type 2 diabetes. *Cell* 1999;96:329–339.
20. Zhang B, Roth RA. The insulin receptor-related receptor: tissue expression, ligand binding specificity, and signaling capabilities. *J Biol Chem* 1992; 267:18320–18328.
21. Ward CW, Garrett TPJ, McKern NM, et al. Structure of the insulin receptor family: unexpected relationships with other proteins. *Today's Life Science* 1999;II:26–32.
22. Hedo JA, Kahn CR, Hayoshi M, et al. Biosynthesis and glycosylation of the insulin receptor. Evidence for a single polypeptide precursor of the two major subunits. *J Biol Chem* 1983;258:10020–10026.
23. Lane MD, Ronnett GV, Kohanski RA, et al. Posttranslational processing of the insulin proreceptor. *Curr Top Cell Regul* 1985;27:279–292.
24. Dunaif A, Graf M. Insulin administration alters gonadal steroid metabolism independent of changes in gonadotropin secretion in insulin resistant women with the polycystic ovary syndrome (PCO). *J Clin Invest* 1989;83: 23–29.
25. Baron AD, Steinberg HO, Chaker H, et al. Insulin-mediated skeletal muscle vasodilation contributes to both insulin sensitivity and responsiveness in lean humans. *J Clin Invest* 1995;96:786–792.
26. McVeigh GE, Brennan GM, Johnston GD, et al. Impaired endothelium-dependent and independent vasodilation in patients with type 2 (non-insulin-dependent) diabetes mellitus. *Diabetologia* 1992;35:771–776.
27. King GL, Johnson SM. Receptor mediated transport of insulin across endothelial cells. *Science* 1985;219:865–869.
28. Bergman RN, Yang YJ, Hope ID, et al. The role of the transcapillary insulin transport in the efficiency of insulin action: studies with glucose clamps and the minimal model. *Horm Metab Res* 1990;24[Suppl]:49–56.
29. Dernovsek KD, Bar RS, Ginsberg BH, et al. Rapid transport of biologically intact insulin through cultured endothelial cells. *J Clin Endocrinol Metab* 1984;58:761–765.
30. Steil GM, Ader M, Moore DM, et al. Transendothelial insulin transport is not saturable in vivo. *J Clin Invest* 1996;97:1497–1503.
31. Baron V, Kaliman P, Gautier N, et al. The insulin receptor activation process involves localized conformational changes. *J Biol Chem* 1992;267: 23290–23294.

32. Ablooglu AJ, Kohanski RA. Activation of the insulin receptor's kinase domain changes the rate-determining step of substrate phosphorylation. *Biochemistry* 2001;40:504–513.
33. Fernandez AM, Kim JK, Yakar S, et al. Functional inactivation of the IGF-I and insulin receptors in skeletal muscle causes type 2 diabetes. *Genes Dev* 2001;15:1926–1934.
34. Skorokhod A, Gamulin V, Gundacker D, et al. Origin of insulin receptor-like tyrosine kinases in marine sponges. *Biol Bull* 1999;197:198–206.
35. Oldham S, Stocker H, Laffargue M, et al. The Drosophila insulin/IGF receptor controls growth and size by modulating PtdInsP(3) levels. *Development* 2002;129:4103–4109.
36. Pierce SB. Costa M. Wisotzkey R, et al. Regulation of DAF-2 receptor signaling by human insulin and ins-1, a member of the unusually large and diverse *C. elegans* insulin gene family. *Genes Dev* 2001;15:672–686.
37. Rulifson EJ, Kim SK, Nusse R. Ablation of insulin-producing neurons in flies: growth and diabetic phenotypes. *Science* 2002;296:1118–1120.
38. Kimura KD, Tissenbaum HA, Liu Y, et al. *daf-2*, an insulin receptor-like gene that regulates longevity and diapause in *Caenorhabditis elegans*. *Science* 1997;277:942–946.
39. Roth GS, Lane MA, Ingram DK, et al. Biomarkers of caloric restriction may predict longevity in humans. *Science* 2002;297:811.
40. Sun XJ, Rothenberg PL, Kahn CR, et al. Structure of the insulin receptor substrate IRS-1 defines a unique signal transduction protein. *Nature* 1991;352: 73–77.
41. Sun XJ, Wang LM, Zhang Y, et al. Role of IRS-2 in insulin and cytokine signalling. *Nature* 1995;377:173–177.
42. White MF, Yenush L. The IRS-signaling system: a network of docking proteins that mediate insulin and cytokine action. *Curr Top Microbiol Immunol* 1998;228:179–208.
43. Lavan BE, Lane WS, Lienhard GE. The 60-kDa phosphotyrosine protein in insulin-treated adipocytes is a new member of the insulin receptor substrate family. *J Biol Chem* 1997;272:11439–11443.
44. Fantin VR, Lavan BE, Wang Q, et al. Cloning, tissue expression, and chromosomal location of the mouse insulin receptor substrate 4 gene. *Endocrinology* 1999;140:1329–1337.
45. Myers MG Jr, White MF. New frontiers in insulin receptor substrate signaling. *Trends Endocrinol Metab* 1995;6:209–215.
46. Sciacchitano S, Taylor SI. Cloning, tissue expression, and chromosomal localization of the mouse IRS-3 gene. *Endocrinology* 1997;138:4931–4940.
47. Fantin CR, Lavan BE, Wang Q, et al. Cloning, tissue expression, and chromosomal location of the mouse insulin receptor substrate 4 gene. *Endocrinology* 1999;140:1329–1337.
48. Bjornholm M, He AR, Attersand A, et al. Absence of functional insulin receptor substrate-3 (IRS-3) gene in humans. *Diabetologia* 2002;45:1697–1702.
49. Lehr S, Kotzka J, Herkner A, et al. Identification of major tyrosine phosphorylation sites in the human insulin receptor substrate Gab-1 by insulin receptor kinase in vitro. *Biochemistry* 2000;39:10898–10907.
50. Wick MJ, Dong LQ, Hu D, et al. Insulin receptor-mediated p62dok tyrosine phosphorylation at residues 362 and 398 plays distinct roles for binding GTPase-activating protein and Nck and is essential for inhibiting insulin-stimulated activation of Ras and Akt. *J Biol Chem* 2001;276:42843–42850.
51. Baumann CA, Ribon V, Kanzaki M, et al. CAP defines a second signalling pathway required for insulin-stimulated glucose transport. *Nature* 2000;407: 202–207.
52. Gustafson TA, He W, Craparo A, et al. Phosphotyrosine-dependent interaction of Shc and IRS-1 with the NPEY motif of the insulin receptor via a novel non-SH2 domain. *Mol Cell Biol* 1995;15:2500–2508.
53. Boney CM, Gruppuso PA, Faris RA, et al. The critical role of Shc in insulin-like growth factor-I-mediated mitogenesis and differentiation in 3T3-L1 preadipocytes. *Mol Endocrinol* 2000;14:805–813.
54. Saltiel AR, Kahn CR. Insulin signalling and the regulation of glucose and lipid metabolism. *Nature* 2001;414:799–806.
55. Cheatham B, Kahn CR. Insulin action and the insulin signaling network. *Endocr Rev* 1995;16:117–142.
56. Skolnik EY, Lee CH, Batzer AG, et al. The SH2/SH3 domain-containing protein GRB2 interacts with tyrosine-phosphorylated IRS-1 and Shc: implications for insulin control of ras signalling. *EMBO J* 1993;12:1929–1936.
57. Jhun BH, Rose DW, Seely BL, et al. Microinjection of the SH2 domain of the 85-kilodalton subunit of phosphatidylinositol 3-kinase inhibits insulin-induced DNA synthesis and c-*fos* expression. *Mol Cell Biol* 1994;14:7466–7475.
58. Case RD, Piccione E, Wolf G, et al. SH-PTP2/Syp SH2 domain binding specificity is defined by direct interactions with platelet-derived growth factor β-receptor, epidermal growth factor receptor, and insulin receptor substrate-1-derived phosphopeptides. *J Biol Chem* 1994;269:10467–10474.
59. Kuhne MR, Pawson T, Lienhard GE, et al. The insulin receptor substrate 1 associates with the SH2-containing phosphotyrosine phosphatase Syp. *J Biol Chem* 1993;268:11479–11481.
60. Algenstaedt P, Antonetti DA, Yaffe MB, et al. Insulin receptor substrate proteins create a link between the tyrosine phosphorylation cascade and the Ca2+-ATPases in muscle and heart. *J Biol Chem* 1997;272:23696–23702.
61. Zhou-Li F, D'Ambrosio C, Li S, et al. Association of insulin receptor substrate 1 with simian virus 40 large T antigen. *Mol Cell Biol* 1995;15:4232–4239.
62. Craparo A, Freund R, Gustafson TA. 14-3-3 epsilon interacts with the insulin-like growth factor I receptor and insulin receptor substrate I in a phosphoserine-dependent manner. *J Biol Chem* 1997;272:11663–11670.
63. Li J, De Fea K, Roth RA. Modulation of insulin receptor substrate-1 tyrosine phosphorylation by an Akt/phosphatidylinositol 3-kinase pathway. *J Biol Chem* 1999;274:9351–9356.
64. Hirosumi J, Tuncman G, Chang L, et al. A central role for JNK in obesity and insulin resistance. *Nature* 2002;420:333–336.
65. Tanti JF, Gremeaux T, Van Obberghen E, et al. Insulin receptor substrate 1 is phosphorylated by the serine kinase activity of phosphatidylinol 3-kinase. *Biochem J* 1994;304:17–21.
66. Yuan M, Konstantopoulos N, Lee J, et al. Reversal of obesity- and diet-induced insulin resistance with salicylates or targeted disruption of Ikkbeta. *Science* 2001;293:1673–1677.
67. Gao Z, Hwang D, Bataille F, et al. Serine phosphorylation of insulin receptor substrate 1 (IRS-1) by inhibitor kappaB kinase (IKK) complex. *J Biol Chem* 2002;277:48115–48121.
68. Arak E, Lipes MA, Patti ME, et al. Alternative pathway of insulin signaling in mice with targeted disruption of the IRS-1 gene. *Nature* 1994;372:186–190.
69. Fonseca VA, Valiquett TR, Huang SM, et al. Troglitazone monotherapy improves glycemic control in patients with type 2 diabetes mellitus: a randomized, controlled study. *J Clin Endocrinal Metab* 1998;83:3169–3176.
70. Yamauchi T, Tobe K, Tamemoto H, et al. Insulin signalling and insulin actions in the muscles and livers of insulin-resistant, insulin receptor substrate 1-deficient mice. *Mol Cell Biol* 1996;16:3074–3084.
71. Withers DJ, Gutierrez JS, Towery H, et al. Disruption of IRS-2 causes type 2 diabetes in mice. *Nature* 1998;391:900–904.
72. Kubota N, Tobe K, Terauchi Y, et al. Disruption of insulin receptor substrate 2 causes type 2 diabetes because of liver insulin resistance and lack of compensatory β-cell hyperplasia. *Diabetes* 2000;49:1880–1889.
73. Fasshauer M, Klein J, Kriauciunas KM, et al. Essential role of insulin receptor substrate 1 in differentiation of brown adipocytes. *Mol Cell Biol* 2001;21: 319–329.
74. Miki H, Yamauchi T, Suzuki R, et al. Essential role of insulin receptor substrate 1 (IRS-1) and IRS-2 in adipocyte differentiation. *Mol Cell Biol* 2001;21: 2521–2532.
75. Fasshauer M, Klein J, Ueki K, et al. Essential role of insulin receptor substrate-2 in insulin stimulation of GLUT4 translocation and glucose uptake in brown adipocytes. *J Biol Chem* 2000;275:25494–25501.
76. Liu SC, Wang Q, Lienhard GE, et al. Insulin receptor substrate 3 is not essential for growth or glucose homeostasis. *J Biol Chem* 1999;274:18093–18099.
77. Fantin VR, Wang GE, Lienhard GE, et al. Mice lacking insulin receptor substrate 4 exhibit mild defects in growth, reproduction, and glucose homostasis. *Am J Physiol* 2000;278:E127–E133.
78. Laustsen PG, Michael MD, Crute BE, et al. Lipoatrophic diabetes in Irs1(-/-)/Irs3(-/-) double knockout mice. *Genes Dev* 2002;16:3213–3222.
79. Inoue G, Cheatham B, Kahn CR. Differential subcellular signaling by IRS-1 and IRS-2. *Diabetes* 1997;46(abst).
80. Kaburagi Y, Satoh S, Yamamoto-Honda R, et al. Insulin-independent and wortmannin-resistant targeting of IRS-3 to the plasma membrane via its pleckstrin homology domain mediates a different interaction with the insulin receptor from that of IRS-1. *Diabetologia* 2001;44:992–1004.
81. Lassak A, Del Valle L, Peruzzi F, et al. Insulin receptor substrate 1 translocation to the nucleus by the human JC virus T-antigen. *J Biol Chem* 2002;277: 17231–17238.
82. Kabuta T, Hakuno F, Asano T, et al. Insulin receptor substrate-3 functions as transcriptional activator in the nucleus. *J Biol Chem* 2002;277:6846–6851.
83. Goldstein BJ, Bittner-Kowalczyk A, White MF, et al. Tyrosine dephosphorylation and deactivation of insulin receptor substrate-1 by protein-tyrosine phosphatase 1B. Possible facilitation by the formation of a ternary complex with the Grb2 adaptor protein. *J Biol Chem* 2000;275:4283–4289.
84. Kuhne MR, Zhao Z, Rowles J, et al. Dephosphorylation of insulin receptor substrate 1 by the tyrosine phosphatase PTP2C. *J Biol Chem* 1994;269: 15833–15837.
85. Sugimoto S, Wandless TJ, Shoelson SE, et al. Activation of the SH2-containing protein tyrosine phosphatase, SH-PTP2, by phosphotyrosine-containing peptides derived from insulin receptor substrate-1. *J Biol Chem* 1994;269:13614–13622.
86. Walchli S, Curchod ML, Gobert RP, et al. Identification of tyrosine phosphatases that dephosphorylate the insulin receptor. A brute force approach based on "substrate-trapping" mutants. *J Biol Chem* 2000;275:9792–9796.
87. Zinker BA, Rondinone CM, Trevillyan JM, et al. PTP1B antisense oligonucleotide lowers PTP1B protein, normalizes blood glucose, and improves insulin sensitivity in diabetic mice. *Proc Natl Acad Sci U S A* 2002;99: 11357–11362.
88. Carpentier JL, Paccaud JP, Gorden P, et al. Insulin-induced surface redistribution regulates internalization of the insulin receptor and requires its autophosphorylation. *Proc Natl Acad Sci U S A* 1992;89:162–166.
89. Hari J, Yokono K, Yonezawa K, et al. Internalization and degradation of insulin by a human insulin receptor-v-ros hybrid in Chinese hamster ovary cells. *Biochem Biophys Res Commun* 1989;158:705–711.
90. Aguirre V, Werner ED, Giraud J, et al. Phosphorylation of Ser307 in insulin receptor substrate-1 blocks interactions with the insulin receptor and inhibits insulin action. *J Biol Chem* 2002;277:1531–1537.
91. Greene MW, Sakaue H, Wang L, et al. Modulation of insulin-stimulated degradation of human insulin receptor substrate-1 by serine 312 phosphorylation. *J Biol Chem* 2003;278:8199–8211.
92. Emanuelli B, Peraldi P, Filloux C, et al. SOCS-3 inhibits insulin signaling and is up-regulated in response to tumor necrosis factor-alpha in the adipose tissue of obese mice. *J Biol Chem* 2001;276:47944–47949.

93. Cheatham B, Vlahos CJ, Cheatham L, et al. Phosphatidylinositol 3-kinase activation is required for insulin stimulation of pp70 S6 kinase, DNA synthesis, and glucose transporter translocation. *Mol Cell Biol* 1994;14:4902–4911.
94. Shepherd PR, Withers DJ, Siddle K. Phosphoinositide 3-kinase: the key switch mechanism in insulin signalling. *Biochem J* 1998;333:471–490.
95. Backer JM, Myers MG Jr, Shoelson SE, et al. Phosphatidylinositol 3′-kinase is activated by association with IRS-1 during insulin stimulation. *EMBO J* 1992;11:3469–3479.
96. Myers MG Jr, Grammer TC, Wang LM, et al. IRS-1 mediates PI 3′-kinase and $p70^{s6k}$ signaling during insulin, IGF-1 and IL-4 stimulation. *J Biol Chem* 1994;269:28783–28789.
97. Fruman DA, Cantley LC, Carpenter CL. Structural organization and alternative splicing of the murine phosphoinositide 3-kinase p85α gene. *Genomics* 1996;37:113–121.
98. Antonetti DA, Algenstaedt P, Kahn CR. Insulin receptor substrate 1 binds two novel splice variants of the regulatory subunit of phosphatidylinositol 3-kinase in muscle and brain. *Mol Cell Biol* 1996;16:2195–2203.
99. Carpenter CL, Cantley LC. Phosphoinositide kinases. *Curr Opin Cell Biol* 1996;8:153–158.
100. Antonetti DA, Algenstaedt P, Kahn CR. Insulin receptor substrate 1 binds two novel splice variants of the regulatory subunit of phosphatidylinositol 3-kinase in muscle and brain. *Mol Cell Biol* 1996;16:2195–2203.
101. Inukai K, Funaki M, Ogihara T, et al. p85α gene generates three isoforms of regulatory subunit for phosphatidylinositol 3-kinase (PI 3-kinase), p50α, p55α, and p85α, with different PI 3-kinase activity elevating responses to insulin. *J Biol Chem* 1997;272:7873–7882.
102. Pons S, Asano T, Glasheen EM, et al. The structure and function of $p55^{PIK}$ reveals a new regulatory subunit for the phosphatidylinositol-3 kinase. *Mol Cell Biol* 1995;15:4453–4465.
103. Ueki K, Algenstaedt P, Mauvais-Jarvis F, et al. Positive and negative regulation of phosphoinositide 3-kinase-dependent signaling pathways by three different gene products of the p85alpha regulatory subunit. *Mol Cell Biol* 2000;20:8035–8046.
104. Kerouz NJ, Horsch D, Pons S, et al. Differential regulation of insulin receptor substrates-1 and -2 (IRS-1 and IRS-2) and phosphatidylinositol 3-kinase isoforms in liver and muscle of the obese diabetic (ob/ob) mouse. *J Clin Invest* 1997;100:3164–3172.
105. Anai M, Funaki M, Ogihara T, et al. Altered expression levels and impaired steps in the pathway to phosphatidylinositol 3-kinase activation via insulin receptor substrates 1 and 2 in Zucker fatty rats. *Diabetes* 1998;47:13–23.
106. Fruman DA, Mauvais-Jarvis F, Pollard DA, et al. Hypoglycaemia, liver necrosis and perinatal death in mice lacking all isoforms of phosphoinositide 3-kinase p85alpha. *Nat Genet* 2000;26:379–382.
107. Terauchi Y, Tsuji T, Satoh S, et al. Increased insulin sensitivity and hypoglycaemia in mice lacking the p85 alpha subunit of phosphoinositide 3-kinase. *Nat Genet* 1999;21:230–235.
107a. Chen D, Mauvais-Jarvis F, Bluher M, et al. p50alpha/p55alpha phosphoinositide 3-kinase mice exhibit enhanced insulin sensitivity. *Mol Cell Biol* 2004;24:320–329.
108. Ueki K, Fruman DA, Brachmann SM, et al. Molecular balance between the regulatory and catalytic subunits of phosphoinositide 3-kinase regulates cell signaling and survival. *Mol Cell Biol* 2002;22:965–977.
109. Mauvais-Jarvis F, Ueki K, Fruman DA, et al. Reduced expression of the murine p85a subunit of phosphoinositide 3-kinase improves insulin signaling and ameliorates diabetes. *J Clin Invest* 2002;109:141–149.
110. Rommel C, Bodine SC, Clarke BA, et al. Mediation of IGF-1-induced skeletal myotube hypertrophy by PI(3)K/Akt/mTOR and PI(3)K/Akt/GSK3 pathways. *Nat Cell Biol* 2001;3:1009–1013.
111. Burgering BM, Coffer PJ. Protein kinase B (c-Akt) in phosphatidylinositol-3-OH kinase signal transduction. *Nature* 1995;376:599–602.
112. Downward J. Mechanisms and consequences of activation of protein kinase B/Akt. *Curr Opin Cell Biol* 1998;10:262–267.
113. Lawlor MA, Alessi DR. PKB/Akt: a key mediator of cell proliferation, survival and insulin responses? *J Cell Sci* 2001;114:2903–2910.
114. Pugazhenthi S, Nesterova A, Sable C, et al. Akt/protein kinase B up-regulates Bcl-2 expression through cAMP-response element-binding protein. *J Biol Chem* 2000;275:10761–10766.
115. Datta SR, Brunet A, Greenberg ME. Cellular survival: a play in three Akts. *Genes Dev* 1999;13:2905–2927.
116. Cho H, Mu J, Kim JK, et al. Insulin resistance and a diabetes mellitus-like syndrome in mice lacking the protein kinase Akt2 (PKBβ). *Science* 2001;292:1728–1731.
117. Czech MP, Corvera S. Signaling mechanisms that regulate glucose transport. *J Biol Chem* 1999;274:1865–1868.
118. Kohn AD, Summers SA, Birnbaum MJ, et al. Expression of a constitutively active Akt Ser/Thr kinase in 3T3-L1 adipocytes stimulates glucose uptake and glucose transporter 4 translocation. *J Biol Chem* 1996;271:31372–31378.
119. Bandyopadhyay G, Standaert ML, Zhao L, et al. Activation of protein kinase C (α, β, and zeta) by insulin in 3T3/L1 cells. Transfection studies suggest a role for PKC-zeta in glucose transport. *J Biol Chem* 1997;272:2551–2558.
120. Tremblay F, Lavigne C, Jacques H, et al. Defective insulin-induced GLUT4 translocation in skeletal muscle of high fat-fed rats is associated with alterations in both Akt/protein kinase B and atypical protein kinase C (zeta/lambda) activities. *Diabetes* 2001;50:1901–1910.
121. Kotani K, Ogawa W, Matsumoto M, et al. Requirement of atypical protein kinase C lambda for insulin stimulation of glucose uptake but not for Akt activation in 3T3-L1 adipocytes. *Mol Cell Biol* 1998;18:6971–6982.
122. Weng QP, Kozlowski M, Belham C, et al. Regulation of the p70 S6 kinase by phosphorylation in vivo. Analysis using site-specific anti-phosphopeptide antibodies. *J Biol Chem* 1998;273:16621–16629.
123. Zheng Y, Bagrodia S, Cerione RA. Activation of phosphoinositide 3-kinase activity by CDC42HS binding to p85. *J Biol Chem* 1994;269:18727–18730.
124. Shisheva A, Sbrissa D, Ikonomov O. Cloning, characterization, and expression of a novel Zn2+-binding FYVE finger-containing phosphoinositide kinase in insulin-sensitive cells. *Mol Cell Biol* 1999;19:623–634.
125. Thomason PA, James SR, Casey PJ, et al. A G-protein beta-gamma-subunit-responsive phosphoinositide 3-kinase activity in human platelet cytosol. *J Biol Chem* 1994;269:16525–16528.
126. Nakashima N, Sharma PM, Imamura T, et al. The tumor suppressor PTEN negatively regulates insulin signaling in 3T3-L1 adipocytes. *J Biol Chem* 2000;275:12889–12895.
127. Clement S, Krause U, Desmedt F, et al. The lipid phosphatase SHIP2 controls insulin sensitivity. *Nature* 2001;409:92–97.
128. Jiang T, Sweeney G, Rudolf MT, et al. Membrane-permeant esters of phosphatidylinositol 3,4,5-trisphosphate. *J Biol Chem* 1998;273:11017–11024.
129. Krook A, Moller DE, Dib K et al. Two naturally occurring mutant insulin receptors phosphorylate insulin receptor substrate-1 (IRS-1) but fail to mediate the biological effects of insulin. *J Biol Chem* 19968;271:7134–7140.
130. Ribon V, Saltiel AR. Insulin stimulates tyrosine phosphorylation of the proto-oncogene product of c-Cbl in 3T3-L1 adipocytes. *Biochem J* 1997;324 (Pt3):839–845.
131. Chiang SH, Baumann CA, Kanzaki M, et al. Insulin-stimulated GLUT4 translocation requires the CAP-dependent activation of TC10. *Nature* 2001;410:944–948.
132. Myers MG Jr, Wang LM, Sun XJ, et al. The role of IRS-1/GRB2 complexes in insulin signaling. *Mol Cell Biol* 1994;14:3577–3587.
133. Lima MH, Ueno M, Thirone AC, et al. Regulation of IRS-1/SHP2 interaction and AKT phosphorylation in animal models of insulin resistance. *Endocrine* 2002;18:1–12.
134. Reusch JEB, Bhuripanyo P, Care K, et al. Differential requirement for $p21^{ras}$ activation in the metabolic signaling by insulin. *J Biol Chem* 1995;270:2036–2040.
135. Tremblay F, Marette A. Amino acid and insulin signaling via the mTOR/p70 S6 kinase pathway. A negative feedback mechanism leading to insulin resistance in skeletal muscle cells. *J Biol Chem* 2001;276:38052–38060.
136. Ozes ON, Akca H, Mayo LD, et al. A phosphatidylinositol 3-kinase/Akt/mTOR pathway mediates and PTEN antagonizes tumor necrosis factor inhibition of insulin signaling through insulin receptor substrate-1. *Proc Natl Acad Sci U S A* 2001;98:4640–4645.
137. Lawrence JC Jr, Roach PJ. New insights into the role and mechanism of glycogen synthase activation by insulin. *Diabetes* 1997;46:541–547.
138. Kim DH, Sarbassov DD, Ali SM, et al. mTOR interacts with raptor to form a nutrient-sensitive complex that signals to the cell growth machinery. *Cell* 2002;110:163–175.
139. Haney PM, Levy MA, Strube MS, et al. Insulin-sensitive targeting of the GLUT4 glucose transporter in L6 myoblasts is conferred by its COOH-terminal cytoplasmic tail. *J Cell Biol* 1995;129:641–658.
140. Guilherme A, Emoto M, Buxton JM, et al. Perinuclear localization and insulin responsiveness of GLUT4 requires cytoskeletal integrity in 3T3-L1 adipocytes. *J Biol Chem* 2000;275:38151–38159.
141. Khayat ZA, Tong P, Yaworsky K, et al. Insulin-induced actin filament remodeling colocalizes actin with phosphatidylinositol 3-kinase and GLUT4 in L6 myotubes. *J Cell Sci* 2000;113:279–290.
142. Kanzaki M, Watson RT, Khan AH, et al. Insulin stimulates actin comet tails on intracellular GLUT4-containing compartments in differentiated 3T3L1 adipocytes. *J Biol Chem* 2001;276:49331–49336.
143. Haffner SM, Miettinen H, Gaskill SP, et al. Decreased insulin secretion and increased insulin resistance are independently related to the 7-year risk of NIDDM in Mexican-Americans. *Diabetes* 1995;44:1386–1391.
144. Kao AW, Noda Y, Johnson JH, et al. Aldolase mediates the association of F-actin with the insulin-responsive glucose transporter GLUT4. *J Biol Chem* 1999;274:17742–17747.
145. Randhawa VK, Bilan PJ, Khayat ZA, et al. VAMP2, but not VAMP3/cellubrevin, mediates insulin-dependent incorporation of GLUT4 into the plasma membrane of L6 myoblasts. *Mol Biol Cell* 2000;11:2403–2417.
146. Khan AH, Thurmond DC, Yang C, et al. Munc18c regulates insulin-stimulated GLUT4 translocation to the transverse tubules in skeletal muscle. *J Biol Chem* 2001;276:4063–4069.
147. Cross DA, Watt PW, Shaw M, et al. Insulin activates protein kinase B, inhibits glycogen synthase kinase-3 and activates glycogen synthase by rapamycin-insensitive pathways in skeletal muscle and adipose tissue. *FEBS Lett* 1997;406:211–215.
148. Brady MJ, Bourbonais FJ, Saltiel AR. The activation of glycogen synthase by insulin switches from kinase inhibition to phosphatase activation during adipogenesis in 3T3-L1 cells. *J Biol Chem* 1998;273:14063–14066.
149. Newgard CB, Brady MJ, O'Doherty RM, et al. Organizing glucose disposal: emerging roles of the glycogen targeting subunits of protein phosphatase-1. *Diabetes* 2000;49:1967–1977.
150. Berman HK, O'Doherty RM, Anderson P, et al. Overexpression of protein targeting to glycogen (PTG) in rat hepatocytes causes profound activation of glycogen synthesis independent of normal hormone- and substrate-mediated regulatory mechanisms. *J Biol Chem* 1998;273:26421–26425.
151. Wang JC, Stromstedt PE, Sugiyama T, et al. The phosphoenolpyruvate carboxykinase gene glucocorticoid response unit: identification of the functional domains of accessory factors HNF3 beta (hepatic nuclear factor-3 beta) and

HNF4 and the necessity of proper alignment of their cognate binding sites. *Mol Endocrinol* 1999;13:604–618.

152. Chakravarty K, Leahy P, Becard D, et al. Sterol regulatory element-binding protein-1c mimics the negative effect of insulin on phosphoenolpyruvate carboxykinase (GTP) gene transcription. *J Biol Chem* 2001;27:34816–34823.
153. Barthel A, Schmoll D, Kruger KD, et al. Differential regulation of endogenous glucose-6-phosphatase and phosphoenolpyruvate carboxykinase gene expression by the forkhead transcription factor FKHR in H4IIE-hepatoma cells. *Biochem Biophys Res Commun* 2001;285:897–902.
154. Yoon JC, Puigserver P, Chen G, et al. Control of hepatic gluconeogenesis through the transcriptional coactivator PGC-1. *Nature* 2001;413:131–138.
155. Fisher SJ, Lekas MC, McCall RH, et al. Determinants of glucose turnover in the pathophysiology of diabetes: an in vivo analysis in diabetic dogs. *Diabetes Metab* 1996;22:111–121.
156. Bradley BC, Poulin RA, Bergman RN. Dynamics of hepatic and peripheral insulin effects suggest common rate-limiting step in vivo. *Diabetes* 1993;42:296–306.
157. Fisher SJ, Kahn CR. Insulin signaling is required for insulin's direct and indirect action on hepatic glucose production. *J Clin Invest* 2003;111: 463–468.
158. Kim JB, Sarraf P, Wright M, et al. Nutritional and insulin regulation of fatty acid synthetase and leptin gene expression through ADD1/SREBP1. *J Clin Invest* 1998;101:1–9.
159. Foretz M, Pacot C, Dugail I, et al. ADD1/SREBP-1c is required in the activation of hepatic lipogenic gene expression by glucose. *Mol Cell Biol* 1999;19:3760–3768.
160. Nave BT, Ouwens M, Withers DJ, et al. Mammalian target of rapamycin is a direct target for protein kinase B: identification of a convergence point for opposing effects of insulin and amino-acid deficiency on protein translation. *Biochem J* 1999;344 Pt 2:427–431.
161. Shimomura I, Bashmakov Y, Ikemoto S, et al. Insulin selectively increases SREBP-1c mRNA in the livers of rats with streptozotocin-induced diabetes. *Proc Natl Acad Sci U S A* 1999;96:13656–13661.
162. Stralfros P, Bjorgell P, Belfrage P. Hormonal regulation of hormone-sensitive lipase in intact adipocytes: identification of phosphorylated sites and effects on the phosphorylation by lipolytic hormones and insulin. *Proc Natl Acad Sci U S A* 1984;81:3317–3321.
163. Kahn CR. Insulin resistance, insulin insensitivity, and insulin unresponsiveness: a necessary distinction. *Metabolism* 1978;27:1893–1902.
164. Reusch JE. Current concepts in insulin resistance, type 2 diabetes mellitus, and the metabolic syndrome. *Am J Cardiol* 2002;90:19G–26G.
165. Taylor SI, Arioglu E. Syndromes associated with insulin resistance and acanthosis nigricans. *J Basic Clin Physiol Pharmacol* 1998;9:419–439.
166. Goldstein BJ, Kahn CR. Insulin allergy and insulin resistance. In: Lichtenstein LM, Fauci AS, eds. *Current therapy in allergy, immunology, and rheumatology.* Lewiston: BC Decker, 1988:327–330.
167. Cusi K, Maezono K, Osman A, et al. Insulin resistance differentially affects the PI 3-kinase- and MAP kinase-mediated signaling in human muscle. *J Clin Invest* 2000;105:311–320.
168. Kahn CR, Flier JS, Bar RS, et al. The syndromes of insulin resistance and acanthosis nigricans: Insulin receptor disorders in man. *N Engl J Med* 1976;294: 739–745.
169. Accili D. Molecular defects of the insulin receptor gene. *Diabetes Metab Rev* 1995;11:47–62.
170. Accili D, Drago J, Lee EJ, et al. Early neonatal death in mice homozygous for a null allele of the insulin receptor gene. *Nat Genet* 1996;12:106–109.
171. Gavin JR III, Roth J, Neville DM Jr, et al. Insulin-dependent regulation of insulin-receptor concentration. *Proc Natl Acad Sci U S A* 1974;71:84–88.
172. Bar RS, Harrison LC, Muggeo M, et al. Regulation of insulin receptors in normal and abnormal physiology in humans. *Adv Intern Med* 1979;24:23–52.
173. Turnbow MA, Smith LK, Garner CW. The oxazolidinedione CP-92,768-2 partially protects insulin receptor substrate-1 from dexamethasone down-regulation in 3T3-L1 adipocytes. *Endocrinology* 1995;136:1450–1458.
174. Rui L, Fisher TL, Thomas J, et al. Regulation of insulin/insulin-like growth factor-1 signaling by proteasome-mediated degradation of insulin receptor substrate-2. *J Biol Chem* 2001;276:40362–40367.
175. Zhande R, Mitchell JJ, Wu J, et al. Molecular mechanism of insulin-induced degradation of insulin receptor substrate 1. *Mol Cell Biol* 2002;22:1016–1026.
176. Mothe I, Van Obberghen E. Phosphorylation of insulin receptor substrate-1 on multiple serine residues, 612, 662, and 731 modulates insulin action. *J Biol Chem* 1996;271:11222–11227.
177. Liu YF, Paz K, Herschkovitz A, et al. Insulin stimulates PKCzeta-mediated phosphorylation of insulin receptor substrate-1 (IRS-1). A self-attenuated mechanism to negatively regulate the function of IRS proteins. *J Biol Chem* 2001;276:14459–14465.
178. Emanuelli B, Peraldi P, Filloux C, et al. SOCS-3 is an insulin-induced negative regulator of insulin signaling. *J Biol Chem* 2000;275:15985–15991.
179. Rui L, Yuan M, Frantz D, et al. SOCS-1 and SOCS-3 block insulin signaling by ubiquitin-mediated degradation of IRS1 and IRS2. *J Biol Chem* 2002;277: 42394–42398.
180. Boden G, Shulman GI. Free fatty acids in obesity and type 2 diabetes: defining their role in the development of insulin resistance and beta-cell dysfunction. *Eur J Clin Invest* 2002;32[Suppl 3]:14–23.
181. Groop LC, Bonadonna RC, DelPrato S, et al. Glucose and free fatty acid metabolism in non-insulin-dependent diabetes mellitus. Evidence for multiple sites of insulin resistance. *J Clin Invest* 1989;84:205–213.
182. Roden M, Price TB, Perseghin G, et al. Mechanism of free fatty acid-induced insulin resistance in humans. *J Clin Invest* 1996;97:2859–2865.
183. Griffin ME, Marcucci MJ, Cline GW, et al. Free fatty acid-induced insulin resistance is associated with activation of protein kinase C theta and alterations in the insulin signaling cascade. *Diabetes* 1999;48:1270–1274.
184. Perseghin G, Scifo P, De Cobelli F, et al. Intramyocellular triglyceride content is a determinant of in vivo insulin resistance in humans: a 1H-13C nuclear magnetic resonance spectroscopy assessment in offspring of type 2 diabetic parents. *Diabetes* 1999;48:1600–1606.
185. Virkamaki A, Korsheninnikova E, Seppala-Lindroos A, et al. Intramyocellular lipid is associated with resistance to in vivo insulin actions on glucose uptake, antilipolysis, and early insulin signaling pathways in human skeletal muscle. *Diabetes* 2001;50:2337–2343.
186. Randle PJ. Regulatory interactions between lipids and carbohydrates: the glucose fatty acid cycle after 35 years. *Diabetes Metab Rev* 1998;14: 263–283.
187. Kim JK, Fillmore JJ, Chen Y, et al. Tissue-specific overexpression of lipoprotein lipase causes tissue-specific insulin resistance. *Proc Natl Acad Sci U S A* 2001;98:7522–7527.
188. Hotamisligil GS, Shargill NS, Spiegelman BM. Adipose expression of tumor necrosis factor-α: direct role in obesity-linked insulin resistance. *Science* 1993;259:87–91.
189. Hotamisligil GS, Arne P, Caro JF, et al. Increased adipose tissue expression of tumor necrosis factor-α in human obesity and insulin resistance. *J Clin Invest* 1995;95:2409–2415.
190. Hotamisligil GS, Peraldi P, Budvari A, et al. IRS-1 mediated inhibition of insulin receptor tyrosine kinase activity in TNF-α- and obesity-induced insulin resistance. *Science* 1996;271:665–668.
191. Ofei F, Hurel S, Newkirk J, et al. Effects of an engineered human anti-TNF-α antibody (CDP571) on insulin sensitivity and glycemic control in patients with NIDDM. *Diabetes* 1996;45:881–885.
192. Friedman JM, Halaas JL. Leptin and the regulation of body weight in mammals. *Nature* 1998;395:763–770.
193. Mantzoros CS. The role of leptin in human obesity and disease: a review of current evidence. *Ann Intern Med* 1999;130:671–680.
194. Cohen B, Novick D, Rubinstein M. Modulation of insulin activities by leptin. *Science* 1996;274:1185–1188.
195. Rossetti L, Massillon D, Barzilai N, et al. Short term effects of leptin on hepatic gluconeogenesis and *in vivo* insulin action. *J Biol Chem* 1997;272: 27758–27763.
196. Yamauchi T, Kamon J, Waki H, et al. The fat-derived hormone adiponectin reverses insulin resistance associated with both lipoatrophy and obesity. *Nat Med* 2001;7:941–946.
197. Stefan N, Vozarova B, Funahashi T, et al. Plasma adiponectin concentration is associated with skeletal muscle insulin receptor tyrosine phosphorylation, and low plasma concentration precedes a decrease in whole-body insulin sensitivity in humans. *Diabetes* 2002;51:1884–1888.
198. Maeda N, Shimomura I, Kishida K, et al. Diet-induced insulin resistance in mice lacking adiponectin/ACRP30. *Nat Med* 2002;8:731–737.
199. Hu E, Liang P, Spiegelman BM. AdipoQ is a novel adipose-specific gene dysregulated in obesity. *J Biol Chem* 1996;271:10697–10703.
200. Berg AH, Combs TP, Du X, et al. The adipocyte-secreted protein Acrp30 enhances hepatic insulin action. *Nat Med* 2001;7:947–953.
201. Hara K, Boutin P, Mori Y, et al. Genetic variation in the gene encoding adiponectin is associated with an increased risk of type 2 diabetes in the Japanese population. *Diabetes* 2002;51:536–540.
202. Steppan C, Balley S, Bhat S, et al. The hormone resistin links obesity to diabetes. *Nature* 2001;409:307–312.
203. Steppan C, Brown EJ, Wright CM, et al. A family of tissue-specific resistin-like molecules. *Proc Natl Acad Sci U S A* 2001;98:502–506.
204. McTernan PG, McTernan CL, Chetty R, et al. Increased resistin gene and protein expression in human abdominal adipose tissue. *J Clin Endocrinol Metab* 2002;87:2407.
205. Nagaev I, Smith U. Insulin resistance and type 2 diabetes are not related to resistin expression in human fat cells or skeletal muscle. *Biochem Biophys Res Commun* 2001;285:561–564.
206. Janke J, Engeli S, Gorzelniak K, et al. Resistin gene expression in human adipocytes is not related to insulin resistance. *Obes Res* 2002;10:1–5.
207. Kim KH, Lee K, Moon YS, et al. A cysteine-rich adipose tissue–specific secretory factor inhibits adipocyte differentiation. *J Biol Chem* 2001;276:11252–11256.
208. Bruning JC, Winnay J, Bonner-Weir S, et al. Development of a novel polygenic model of NIDDM in mice heterozygous for IR and IRS-1 null alleles. *Cell* 1997;88:561–572.
209. Kido Y, Burks DJ, Withers D, et al. Tissue-specific insulin resistance in mice with mutations in the insulin receptor, IRS-1, and IRS-2. *J Clin Invest* 2000;105:199–205.
210. Kulkarni RN, Almind K, Goren HJ, et al. Impact of genetic background on development of hyperinsulinemia and diabetes in insulin receptor/insulin receptor substrate-1 double heterozygous mice. *Diabetes* 2003;52:1528–1534.
211. Almind K, Kulkarni RN, Lannon SM, et al. Identification of interactive loci linked to insulin and leptin in mice with genetic insulin resistance. *Diabetes* 2003;52:1535–1543.
212. Chang PY, Benecke H, Le Marchand-Brustel Y, et al. Expression of a dominant-negative mutant human insulin receptor in the muscle of transgenic mice. *J Biol Chem* 1994;269:16034–16040.
213. Moller DE, Chang PY, Yaspelkis BB III, et al. Transgenic mice with muscle-

specific insulin resistance develop increased adiposity, impaired glucose tolerance, and dyslipidemia. *Endocrinology* 1996;137:2397–2405.
214. Gu H, Marth JD, Orban PC, et al. Deletion of a DNA polymerase beta gene segment in T cells using cell type-specific gene targeting. *Science* 1994; 265:103–106.
215. Howe LR, Leevers SJ, Gomez N, et al. Activation of the MAP kinase pathway by the protein kinase raf. *Cell* 1992;71:335–342.
216. Zisman A, Peroni OD, Abel D, et al. Targeted disruption of the glucose transporter 4 selectively in muscle causes insulin resistance and glucose intolerance. *Nat Med* 2000;6:924–928.
217. Abel ED, Peroni O, Kim JK, et al. Adipose-selective targeting of the GLUT4 gene impairs insulin action in muscle and liver. *Nature* 2001;409:729–733.
218. Zierath JR, Wallberg-Henriksson H. From receptor to effector: insulin signal transduction in skeletal muscle from type II diabetic patients. *Ann N Y Acad Sci* 2002;967:120–134.
219. Westermark P, Wilander E. The influence of amyloid deposits on the islet volume in maturity onset diabetes mellitus. *Diabetologia* 1978;15:417–421.
220. Kahn CR. Insulin action, diabetogenes, and the cause of type II diabetes (Banting Lecture). *Diabetes* 1994;43:1066–1084.
221. Reaven GM. Non-insulin-dependent diabetes mellitus, abnormal lipoprotein metabolism and atherosclerosis. *Metabolism* 1987;36:1–8.
222. Postic C, Shiota M, Niswender KD, et al. Dual roles for glucokinase in glucose homeostasis as determined by liver and pancreatic β cell-specific gene knock-outs using Cre recombinase. *J Biol Chem* 1999;274:305–315.
223. Bluher M, Michael MD, Peroni OD, et al. Adipose tissue selective insulin receptor knockout protects against obesity and obesity-related glucose intolerance. *Dev Cell* 2002;3:25–38.
224. Bluher M, Kahn BB, Kahn CR. Extended longevity in mice lacking the insulin receptor in adipose tissue. *Science* 2003;299:572–574.
225. Porte D Jr. 1990 Banting Lecture. β-Cells in type II diabetes mellitus. *Diabetes* 1991;40:166–180.
226. Polonsky KS. 1994. Lilly Lecture: The beta-cell in diabetes: from molecular genetics to clinical research. *Diabetes* 1995;44:705–717.
227. Elahi D, Nagulesparan M, Hershcopf RJ, et al. Feedback inhibition of insulin secretion by insulin: relation to the hyperinsulinemia of obesity. *N Engl J Med* 1982;306:1196–1202.
228. Ammon HP, Reiber C, Verspohl EJ. Indirect evidence for short-loop negative feedback of insulin secretion in the rat. *J Endocrinol* 1991;128:27–34.
229. Leibiger IB, Leibiger B, Berggren PO. Insulin feedback action on pancreatic beta-cell function. *FEBS Lett* 2002;532:1–6.
230. Kuhn R, Schwenk F, Aguet M, et al. Inducible gene targeting in mice. *Science* 1995;269:1427–1429.
231. Metzger D, Clifford J, Chiba H, et al. Conditional site-specific recombination in mammalian cells using a ligand-dependent chimeric Cre recombinase. *Proc Natl Acad Sci U S A* 1995;92:6991–6995.
232. Tsien JZ, Chen DF, Gerber D, et al. Subregion- and cell type-restricted gene knockout in mouse brain. *Cell* 1996;87:1317–1326.
233. Borge PD Jr, Wolf BA. Insulin receptor substrate 1 regulation of sarco-endoplasmic reticulum calcium ATPase 3 in insulin-secreting beta-cells. *J Biol Chem* 2003;278:11359–11368.
234. Van Schravendijk CF, Foriers A, Van den Brande JL, et al. Evidence for the presence of type I insulin-like growth factor receptors on rat pancreatic A and B cells. *Endocrinology* 1987;121:1784–1788.
235. Leahy JL, Vandekerkhove KM. Insulin-like growth factor-1 at physiological concentrations is a potent inhibitor of insulin secretion. *Endocrinology* 1990;126:1593–1598.
236. Kulkarni RN, Holzenberger M, Shih DQ, et al. Beta-cell-specific deletion of the Igf1 receptor leads to hyperinsulinemia and glucose intolerance but does not alter beta-cell mass. *Nat Genet* 2002;31:111–115.
237. Vicent D, Ilany J, Kondo T, et al. The role of endothelial insulin signaling in the regulation of vascular tone and insulin resistance. *J Clin Invest* 2003;111:1373–1280.
238. Vicent D, Ilany J, Kondo T, et al. A tissue-specific knockout of the insulin receptor in vascular endothelial cells. *J Clin Invest* 2003;111:1835–1842.
239. Havrankova J, Roth J, Brownstein M. Insulin receptors are widely distributed in the central nervous system of the rat. *Nature* 1978;272:827–829.
240. Woods SC, Lotter EC, McKay LD, et al. Chronic intracerebroventricular infusion of insulin reduces food intake and body weight of baboons. *Nature* 1979;282:503–505.
241. Baskin DG, Figlewicz Lattemann D, Seely RJ, et al. Insulin and leptin: dual adiposity signals to the brain for the regulation of food intake and body weight. *Brain Res* 1999;848:114–123.
242. Heidenreich KA, Toledo SP, Kenner KA. Regulation of protein phosphorylation by insulin and insulin-like growth factors in cultured fetal neurons. *Adv Exp Med Biol* 1991;293:379–384.
243. Morrione A, Romano G, Navarro M, et al. Insulin-like growth factor I receptor signaling in differentiation of neuronal H19-7 cells. *Cancer Res* 2000;60: 2263–2272.
244. Obici S, Zhang BB, Karkanias G, et al. Hypothalamic insulin signaling is required for inhibition of glucose production. *Nat Med* 2002;8:1376.
245. Bernard C. *Leçons de physiologie expérimentale appliquée à la médecine.* Paris: J.B. Bailliere et Fils, 1855.

CHAPTER 10

Insulin-like Growth Factors

Karen C. McCowen and Robert J. Smith

Insulin-like growth factors (IGFs) belong to a family of peptide hormones with structural and functional similarities to insulin. Initially identified on the basis of their insulin-like glucoregulatory effects, IGFs were given the name *nonsuppressible insulin-like activity*, because hypoglycemia failed to lower their levels in the circulation. Nonsuppressible insulin-like activity was recognized subsequently to consist of various forms of two related proteins, which now are designated insulin-like growth factor-I (IGF-I) and IGF-II. This chapter will focus primarily on IGF-I, a peptide hormone of 7,600 daltons, which is the major mediator of growth-promoting actions of growth hormone. It is present in the circulation at significant levels throughout postnatal life and has glucoregulatory and mitogenic properties that are analogous to those of insulin. IGF-II is related in structure to IGF-I but the product of a separate gene. IGF-II is believed to have important roles in fetal growth and differentiation plus effects on postnatal growth in some tissues. The production of IGF-II by extrapancreatic neoplasms of various types represents an uncommon but well-established cause of tumor-associated hypoglycemia (see Chapter 69 for further discussion).

Unlike insulin, which is derived from a single cell type (pancreatic β-cells) and functions entirely as an endocrine hormone, IGF-I is produced in many different tissues and often acts in a paracrine or autocrine manner. Thus, appreciation of IGF-I function *in vivo* is more difficult than that of a classical endocrine hormone. Insulin and IGFs have common ancestral origins; IGF-I is postulated to have evolved more than 300 million years ago from a single primordial insulin-IGF gene through intron rearrangement followed by gene duplication (1). IGF-I is secreted intact, as it is produced (i.e., not stored intracellularly), and is composed of four domains designated A through D (Fig. 10.1A). The A- and B-domains are analogous to the A- and B-chains of the insulin molecule. The C-domain is retained in mature IGF-I and IGF-II, whereas the equivalent region is excised during processing of proinsulin to insulin. The D-domain also is present in IGF-I and IGF-II but absent from insulin. The potential for cross-reactivity of IGF-I with insulin receptors, as well as insulin binding to IGF-I receptors, may contribute to complications associated with insulin resistance and diabetes. Despite their substantial homology and capacity for activation of similar cellular signaling pathways, IGF-I and insulin have distinct biologic effects on target tissues. However, IGF-I infusions can occasionally be used to decrease blood glucose in cases of extreme insulin resistance, with IGF-I acting either through its own receptor or through the insulin receptor. The major role of IGF-I *in vivo* is most likely its involvement in cell division, growth, and proliferation. IGF-I has been implicated in proliferative aspects of certain complications of diabetes, such as retinopathy and nephropathy, although further research is needed to establish the pathologic importance of IGF-I in diabetes complications, and major therapeutic implications have not been realized.

INSULIN-LIKE GROWTH FACTOR-I STRUCTURE AND REGULATION

Circulating IGF-I is substantially derived from liver parenchymal cells, which are stimulated to synthesize and secrete the hormone in response to growth hormone (GH) acting through

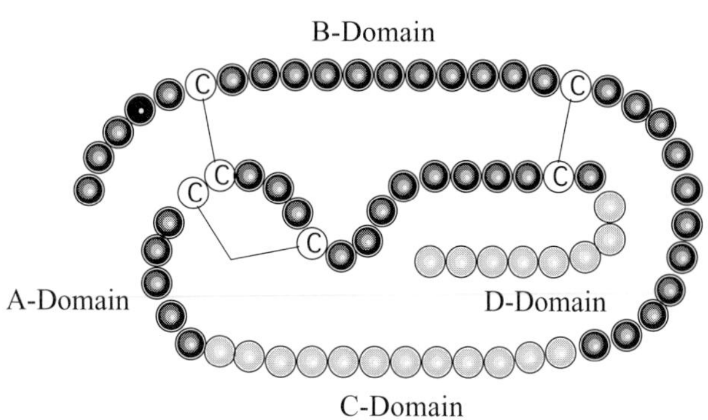

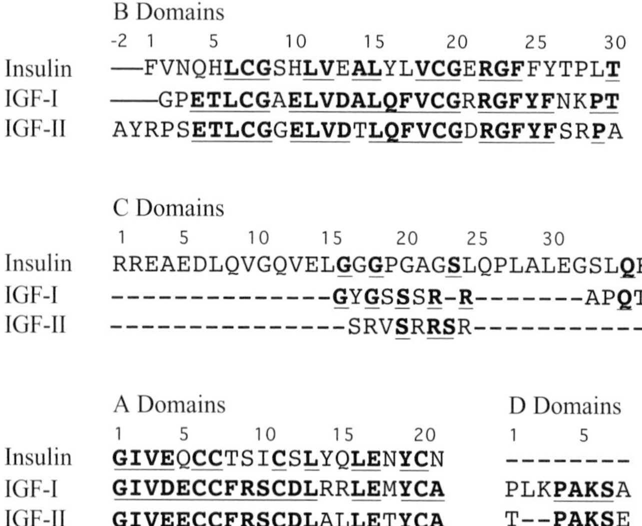

Figure 10.1. A: Domain structure of the insulin-like growth factor-I (IGF-I) protein. The single polypeptide chain extends from the amino-terminal B-domain through the C-domain and A-domain to the carboxy-terminal D-domain. The amino acids labeled C represent cysteines, which are linked by disulfide bonds as shown. **B:** Comparative amino acid sequences of human insulin, IGF-I, and IGF-II. Amino acids that are identical in two or more of these hormones are underlined in bold.

hepatic GH receptors. However, IGF-I can also be synthesized locally in a multitude of different tissues under the influence of GH and, to some extent, independently of GH. As shown in Figure 10.1B, IGF-I is homologous to insulin and, even more so, to proinsulin, which includes the C-domain region. Major structural differences are found in the first 16 amino acids of the B-chain, such that IGF-I has considerable affinity for a family of binding proteins that modulate both its circulating half-life and its accessibility to tissues.

Although GH is an important regulator of IGF-I synthesis and secretion, nutritional status and the presence of hyperglycemia also have important influences on concentrations of IGF-I. GH is secreted in a pulsatile and diurnal variable manner from the anterior pituitary under the influence of both positive and negative hypothalamic peptides. GH concentrations peak in the early morning, and because GH acts as a promoter of insulin resistance, rising levels of GH may contribute to early-morning insulin resistance, the "dawn phenomenon" that occurs commonly in diabetes mellitus. The GH receptor is dimerized upon activation by GH and transmits downstream signals by effecting tyrosine phosphorylation of proteins from both the JAK and STAT families, as well as by activating other signaling intermediates, ultimately leading to changes in expression of genes, including those encoding IGF-I and IGF-binding protein-3 (Fig. 10.2).

Malnutrition, either protein malnutrition or generalized protein-calorie malnutrition (marasmus), also affects IGF-I gene transcription. GH resistance has been reported in malnutrition, with elevated concentrations of GH (2) but low IGF-I mRNA in liver tissue (3,4) and low serum IGF-I (5,6). Fasting has been shown to reduce circulating IGF-I in healthy persons, in association with elevated integrated GH concentrations (7). In rats, GH-binding sites on hepatocytes were reduced following a fast, and GH binding increased in concert with IGF-I plasma concentrations during refeeding (8). In contrast to the effects of overall nutrient restriction, isolated dietary protein depletion results in decreased IGF-I levels in the absence of a change in liver GH-binding capacity, suggesting that postreceptor mechanisms are responsible for the decline in IGF-I in this situation (9–11). Nutritional repletion increases levels of both IGF-I mRNA and protein, and increasing IGF-I concentrations have been shown to predict a return to normal nitrogen balance in ill patients starting nutritional support (12,13). Interestingly, the provision of both energy and protein is required to restore

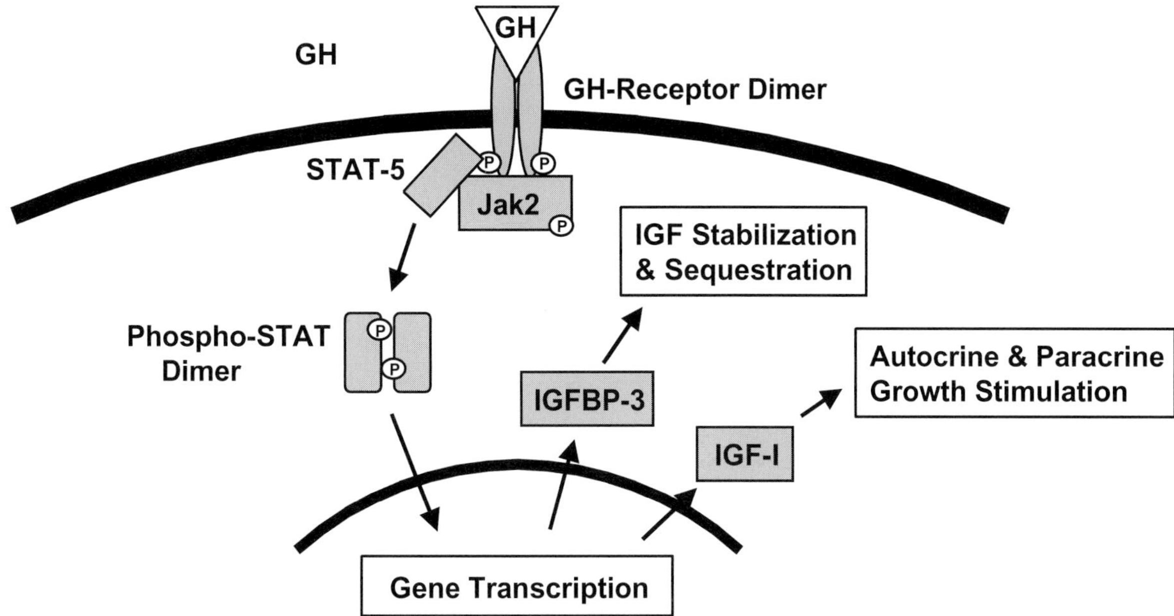

Figure 10.2. Growth hormone (GH) signaling pathways involving initial cytoplasmic events and consequent changes in nuclear gene transcription. IGF, insulin-like growth factor; IGFBP-3, insulin-like growth factor–binding protein-3; P, phosphotyrosine.

IGF-I concentrations. In malnourished laboratory rats, refeeding a eucaloric but low-protein diet was adequate to restore IGF-I, whereas providing protein at 1 g/kg in the face of marked energy restriction was insufficient (14,15). When protein intake is limiting, essential amino acids are more effective at raising IGF-I than is a nonspecific mixture of amino acids (16), although in nutritional support of hospitalized patients, use of essential amino acids has not been associated with improvement in clinical endpoints. As a source of energy, dietary fat appeared to be less effective than carbohydrate in raising IGF-I concentrations and in improving nitrogen balance in a study examining responses to exogenous GH administration in the presence of limited energy intake (15). Hypercaloric nutrition in healthy volunteers has been associated with slight increases in circulating IGF-I, but the effect of overnutrition appears to be much less marked than that of undernutrition (17).

Uncontrolled diabetes is associated with low serum IGF-I concentrations, although whether diabetes has an effect independent of concomitant negative nutritional status has not been determined (18). Insulin-deficient diabetic rats have low IGF-I concentrations, which are restored at least partially with exogenous insulin therapy (19–21). Although nutritional factors confound the relationship between the two hormones, the finding that exposure to insulin *in vitro* increases the number of GH receptors on hepatocytes supports a direct link between insulin status and IGF-I levels (22). Protein restriction in diabetic rats prevents the restoration of IGF-I concentrations following insulin treatment, in contrast to a normalization of IGF-I in insulin-treated diabetic rats given adequate dietary protein (23).

Circulating IGF-I is bound with high affinity to a number of IGF-binding proteins (IGFBPs). Six binding proteins in the range of 20 to 30 kDa have been cloned and sequenced. The bulk (~90%) of measurable IGF-I is bound to IGF-binding protein-3 (IGFBP-3), with only a small fraction (<5%) of total IGF-I being free. IGFBP-3 serves as a reservoir of IGF-I, which retains IGF-I in the circulation, prevents rapid fluctuations in plasma concentrations, and probably functions to prolong the circulating half-life of IGF-I. IGFBP-3 is generally regulated in parallel with IGF-I, with nutrition and GH being major stimulators of IGFBP-3 concentrations. IGFBP-1, forming a smaller complex with IGF-I, can cross capillary endothelium and may participate in the delivery of IGF-I to the cell surface, where IGF-I receptors are accessible. Food intake, in association with rising plasma concentrations of insulin, lowers IGFBP-1 concentrations abruptly, perhaps by inducing its movement out of the vascular lumen (24). Both IGFBP-1 and IGFBP-2 concentrations increase with fasting (25) and, in the presence of diabetes, show opposite regulation from IGFBP-3 and IGF-I (26,27). Assessment of the kinetics of IGF-I action is difficult, because the functions and importance of the IGFBPs have not been fully defined. Synthetic analogues of IGF-I, altered so that binding to IGFBPs is prevented, are more potent than IGF-I when injected into experimental animals (28,29). This suggests that inhibition of IGF-I action is a major function of the binding proteins, although the binding proteins also may have some actions independent of the IGFs (30).

INSULIN-LIKE GROWTH FACTOR-I RECEPTOR

The IGF-I receptor (also designated type I IGF receptor) is present in multiple body tissues, with the notable exceptions of liver parenchymal cells and adipocytes, in which the levels are very low. IGF-I receptor mRNA is most abundant during embryonic life, with significant but much lower levels during adulthood. The functional receptor is a heterotetrameric transmembrane protein containing two types of subunits joined by disulfide bonds in a B-A-A-B configuration (Fig. 10.3). This is closely analogous to the structure of the insulin receptor. The α-subunits (M_r 135 kDa) are entirely extracellular and contain the hormone-binding site; the β-subunits (95–105 kDa, depending on the tissue) span the plasma membrane, and each contains an intracellular tyrosine kinase domain. IGF-I and insulin receptors are encoded by separate genes, but they exhibit approxi-

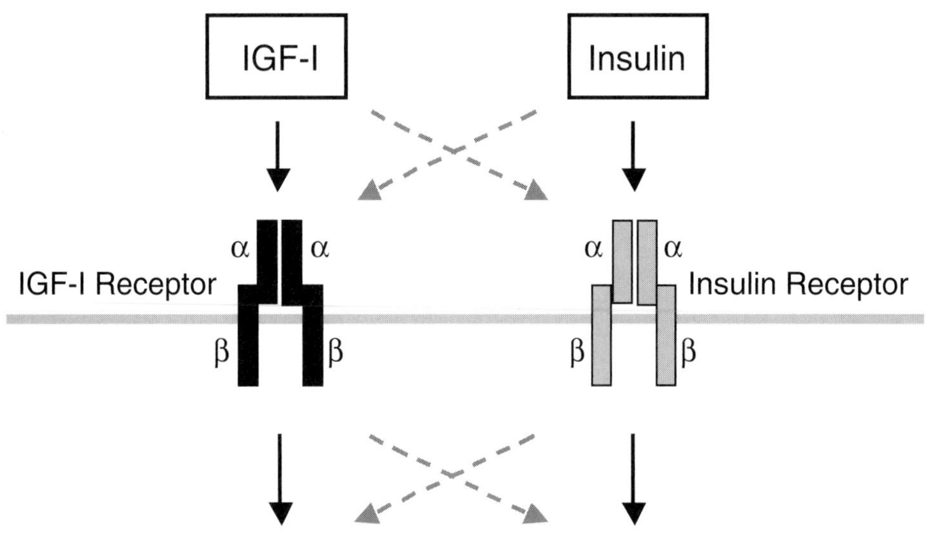

Figure 10.3. Homology in the structures of the insulin-like growth factor-I (IGF-I) and insulin receptors. Each hormone binds with greatest affinity to its own receptor but when present at high concentrations can bind to the other receptor. Both receptors can induce a full complement of cellular signaling responses. However, there is evidence for greater stimulation of cell-growth responses by the IGF-I receptor and greater stimulation of metabolic responses by the insulin receptor.

mately 40% overall amino acid sequence identity, and there is phylogenetic evidence for their emergence from a single precursor receptor. Much higher sequence homology is present in key functional regions, such as the tyrosine kinase domain. In spite of extensive similarities, the critical regions involved in hormone binding establish clear functional differences for insulin and IGF-I receptors. IGF-I and insulin each binds with high affinity to its cognate receptor. There is a potential for binding cross-reactivity related to structural similarities of the ligands and receptors, although such binding generally requires concentrations of the opposing hormone above the normal physiologic range (Fig. 10.3). Thus, the IGF-I receptor binds insulin with much lower affinity than it binds IGF-I.

Hormone-binding specificity depends on key cysteine residues and other structural features in the extracellular receptor α-subunits, whereas the transmembrane β-subunits mediate signal transduction predominantly via their intrinsic tyrosine kinase activity. Binding of IGF-I to its receptors is believed to result in conformational changes that lead to autophosphorylation in a "trans" reaction, in which the tyrosine kinase of one β-chain cross-phosphorylates specific tyrosine residues in the opposite β-chain within the receptor heterotetramer. This positions the active tyrosine kinase domains for the phosphorylation of cellular substrates, such as the insulin receptor substrate (IRS) proteins, which then initiate a cascade of downstream signaling events that result in hormone action (see Chapter 9 for further details on the signaling pathways of the insulin and IGF-I receptors).

INSULIN AND INSULIN-LIKE GROWTH FACTOR-I SPECIFICITY

Although insulin and IGF-I are structurally similar and, at high concentrations, can activate each other's receptors, the receptors provide substantial signaling specificity. IGF-I is approximately 1,000 times less potent than insulin in displacing radiolabeled insulin from its insulin-receptor binding sites. Insulin, in turn, is approximately 500 times less potent than IGF-I in displacing radiolabeled IGF-I from its IGF-I–receptor binding sites. On a molar basis, injected IGF-I is only about 6% as potent as insulin in causing hypoglycemia in humans (31). IGF-I differs from insulin not only in being produced in a wide variety of tissues but in having markedly different diurnal circulating profiles, with an absence of clear peaks for IGF-I. In skeletal muscle biopsies from obese diabetic humans, binding of insulin to its receptors was markedly diminished, but binding of IGF-I was unchanged. IGF-I–stimulated tyrosine kinase activity examined *ex vivo* was also not different in tissue extracts from diabetic and control subjects (32). This suggests discrete downstream pathways with differential regulation of insulin and IGF-I receptors. In another study addressing the same issue, skeletal muscle from nondiabetic individuals demonstrated a twofold increase in glucose transport in response to IGF-I, whereas samples from diabetic patients showed no activation of glucose transport. It was observed, however, that binding of IGF-I to skeletal muscle was normal in the diabetic patients (33). This suggests that there may be changes specific to the insulin receptor in type 2 diabetes but that resistance to both insulin and IGF-I is at a common site downstream of the receptor tyrosine kinases.

Insulin signaling through its receptor activates phosphorylation cascades that lead to both metabolic and mitogenic cellular responses (Fig. 10.3), though the most important actions of insulin are thought to affect metabolic endpoints. Although the binding of IGF-I to its receptors can activate many of the same signaling molecules, IGF-I actions are thought to be primarily mitogenic. In cultured fibroblasts expressing similar numbers of insulin and IGF-I receptors, IGF-I activation of pathways leading to DNA synthesis was more marked, suggesting quantitative differences in the stimulation of different postreceptor pathways by IGF-I and insulin receptors (34). Studies on chimeric receptor proteins containing the receptor-binding portion of a neurotrophin receptor fused to the intracellular domains of either IGF-I or insulin receptors indicate that at least part of receptor signaling specificity lies within the intracellular domains (35). When activated by neurotrophin, the insulin-receptor chimera expressed in cultured fat cells was more effective in stimulating glucose transport and translocation of the GLUT4 glucose transporter. By contrast, when expressed in the same fat cell line, the IGF-I–receptor chimera more effectively activated mitogen-activated protein (MAP) kinase pathways, which are believed to link most strongly to the stimulation of DNA synthesis and cell proliferation.

Investigation of other signaling differences between insulin and IGF-I receptors that confer specificity on each pathway is critically important to our understanding of IGF-I action *in vivo*. Evidence continues to accumulate that differences between these two signaling pathways exist, although there also appears to be substantial overlap. The use of peptides containing four major phosphorylation sites of IRS-1 in kinase assays with each receptor showed identical specificity of insulin and IGF-I receptors for IRS-1 (36). Although the two hormones activate IRS-1 similarly (at least *in vitro*), a specific isoform of phosphoinositide 3-kinase (PI 3-K-C2α), a signaling enzyme activated by IRS-1, was stimulated to a greater extent by insulin receptors than by IGF-I receptors (37). The liver plasma membrane glycoprotein, pp120, also was found to be preferentially phosphorylated by insulin receptors in cultured fibroblasts transfected with insulin as compared with IGF-I receptors (38). By contrast, IGF-I receptors stimulated tyrosine phosphorylation of the signaling adapter Crk II, whereas insulin receptors were substantially less effective (39).

Specificity in IGF-I and insulin action may result from the distinct interactions of these two receptor proteins not only with signal-transducing molecules but also with signaling regulators. For example, Grb10 is a putative adapter protein that has the capacity to bind to IGF-I and insulin receptors through the interaction of motifs in its C-terminal region with phosphotyrosine residues in activated IGF-I and insulin receptors (40–42). Evidence has been presented for both negative and positive effects of Grb10 on IGF-I and insulin signaling. In studies on a specific isoform of Grb10 in mouse tissues (Grb10δ), much stronger interaction was demonstrated with insulin receptors than with IGF-I receptors (43).

cDNA microarray technology has been used to examine the expression levels of genes in cultured fibroblasts overexpressing either insulin or IGF-I receptors (44). IGF-I activation of its receptors led to increased mRNA levels for 30 genes that were not increased as a consequence of insulin activation of insulin receptors. These were mostly genes known to be important in growth and differentiation. A total of nine genes were much more strongly stimulated by insulin receptors than by IGF-I receptors, none of which had previously been noted to be insulin responsive. The implications of this study are yet unclear because the observations were made only in cultured fibroblast cell lines. However, these data add further support to the concept that IGF-I and insulin receptors mediate distinct signaling responses in their target cells.

Insulin and IGF-I receptors are required for normal embryonic growth and development, but their roles early in development are different from those in postnatal life (45). IGF-I receptors mediate the effects of both IGF-I and IGF-II during embryonic development, whereas insulin receptors mediate effects of IGF-II but not those of insulin (46). Humans with homozygous or compound heterozygous mutations of the insulin receptor who present at birth with the leprechaunism syndrome (a severe form of insulin resistance) have severe intrauterine growth retardation and postprandial hyperglycemia, and die in infancy (47). In fibroblasts derived from a patient with this syndrome, IGF-I binding and IGF-I receptor β-subunit tyrosine phosphorylation were normal, as was IGF-I–stimulated thymidine incorporation into DNA, suggesting the potential therapeutic usefulness of IGF-I (48). Clinical investigations in this patient demonstrated low circulating concentrations of IGF-I and IGFBP-3, which were resistant to GH therapy. Administration of recombinant human IGF-I maintained near-normal growth and glycohemoglobin for 6 years. Tonsillar hypertrophy was the only evident complication of IGF-I therapy, as previously has been observed following IGF-I treatment of patients with defects in the GH receptor (Laron dwarfism). Treatment of other patients with insulin-receptor mutations with IGF-I has yielded variable success, with evidence in some patients of combined resistance to both insulin and IGF-I (49). Since IGF-I and insulin receptors exist in part as hybrid constructs composed of one IGF-I and one insulin-receptor αβ-heterodimer, it is possible that some mutated forms of insulin half-receptor could exert a dominant negative effect on the IGF-I half-receptor and thus result in IGF-I resistance.

HYBRID INSULIN-LIKE GROWTH FACTOR-I/INSULIN RECEPTORS

Hybrid IGF-I and insulin receptors (Fig. 10.4) have been described in a number of tissues, and there is some evidence that they have signaling properties more closely related to IGF-I receptors than to insulin receptors. For example, hybrid receptors have a 10-fold lower affinity for insulin than do classical insulin receptors but a preserved sensitivity to IGF-I. It is thought that the fraction of IGF-I or insulin receptors in hybrid constructs in a given tissue reflects the relative abundance of the two receptor types. Thus, in a tissue with much greater abundance of IGF-I receptors than insulin receptors, most insulin receptors would be present in hybrids, whereas there would be a larger fraction of pure IGF-I receptors. The opposite circumstance may characterize skeletal muscle, in which 85% to 90% of IGF-I binding appears to be present in hybrid receptors (50). There is evidence for increased abundance of hybrid receptors in diabetes associated with insulin resistance, although the functional importance of hybrid receptors *in vivo* will require further study (51,52). As noted above for patients with mutations in the insulin receptor and the leprechaunism syndrome, insulin (and IGF-I) resistance may occur in some instances as a consequence of mutant half-receptors for one of the two hormones exerting a dominant-negative effect on the other half-receptor. In rodents with dominant-negative mutations in the IGF-I receptor, both insulin and IGF-I signaling pathways are inhibited in association with the development of insulin-resistant diabetes (53). Significant amounts of the insulin receptor were detected in immunoprecipitates of IGF-I receptor from skeletal muscle homogenates in these animals, and vice versa. The data suggest that expression of a dominant-negative IGF-I receptor in muscle induced the formation of nonfunctioning hybrids containing a normal insulin-receptor αβ pair and a mutant IGF-I receptor αβ. In contrast, knockout of the insulin receptor in muscle was associated with far milder glucoregulatory dysfunction, suggesting that IGF-I receptors can compensate for impaired insulin receptors (54–56).

HUMAN RECEPTOR MUTATIONS

Two individuals with deficient IGF-I function as a consequence of receptor mutations have recently been identified (57). One patient has a distinct substitution mutation in each IGF-I receptor allele (one inherited from each parent). The mutations are located in the receptor α-subunits in the region of the putative IGF-I binding pocket, and the receptors exhibit more than a 10-fold decrease in IGF-I binding affinity. The second individual is heterozygous for a mutation that introduces a stop codon a short distance after the IGF-I–receptor translation start site. The resulting loss of one of two alleles results in a reduction in gene dosage, with a 50% decrease in the abundance of IGF-I

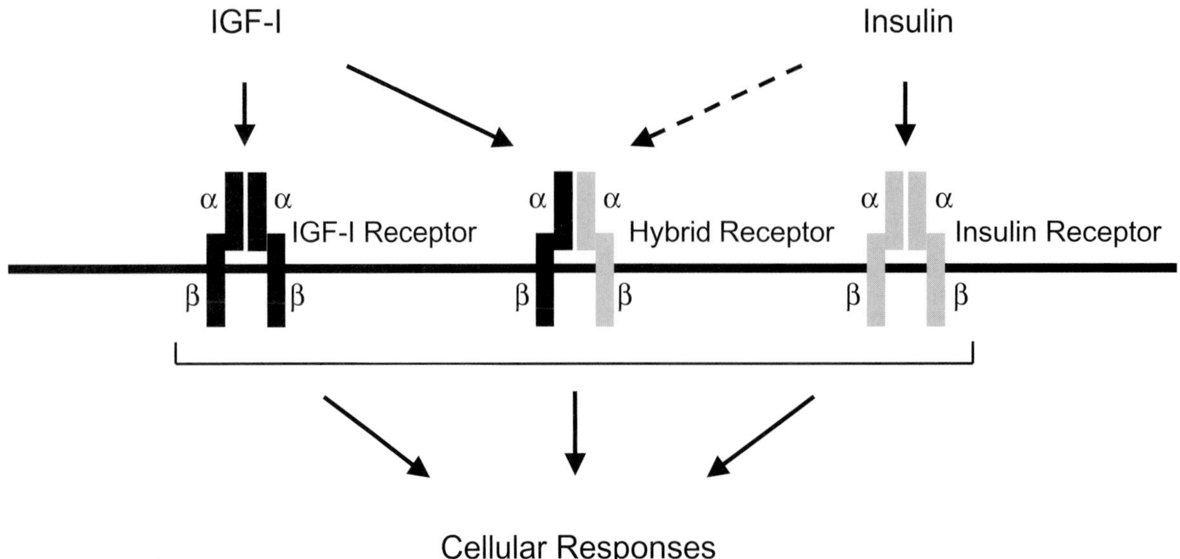

Figure 10.4. Formation of hybrid receptors composed of an insulin-like growth factor-I (IGF-I)–receptor αβ-dimer linked by disulfide bonds to an αβ insulin-receptor dimer. Hybrid formation is believed to occur during synthesis of receptor protein and thus reflects, in general, the relative abundance of newly synthesized IGF-I and insulin receptors in an individual cell. Limited experimental evidence suggests that hybrid receptors may bind IGF-I with higher affinity than they bind insulin. The specific actions of hybrid receptors in stimulating cellular responses to IGF-I and insulin are still under investigation.

receptors demonstrated in cultured skin fibroblasts. The phenotype for both of these individuals includes marked intrauterine and postnatal growth restriction but no abnormalities in glucose or insulin levels (at least in childhood). Additional studies have reported intronic and silent polymorphisms in the IGF-I–receptor gene, but the frequency of these variants was not found to be higher in patients with diabetes than in population controls (58). Taken together, these findings suggest that subtotal loss of IGF-I–receptor signaling in humans is not associated with marked abnormalities in carbohydrate metabolism.

Insulin-receptor mutations are associated with insulin resistance, and a variety of resulting clinical syndromes of insulin resistance have been described. When diabetes mellitus occurs under these circumstances, the effect of the mutations on growth is difficult to interpret because hyperglycemia and other metabolic disturbances associated with deficient insulin action itself will limit growth. Hypoinsulinemia from any cause [e.g., pancreatic agenesis (59) or glucokinase mutations (60)] is associated with growth retardation, suggesting that insulin has a major growth-promoting role in human fetuses. Again, however, it is difficult to separate the direct effects of insulin from its indirect actions via disturbed body fuel metabolism.

RECOMBINANT INSULIN-LIKE GROWTH FACTOR-I AND INSULIN ANALOGUES

Human recombinant IGF-I has been available for use in research studies and for rare clinical conditions (e.g., Laron dwarfism as noted above). The administration of large bolus doses of recombinant IGF-I to experimental animals *in vivo* results in hypoglycemia mediated through increases in glucose uptake by muscle, without effects on hepatic glucose output or suppression of free fatty acid output from adipocytes (61). This is quite different from the effects of bolus insulin injection, suggesting that IGF-I is acting through its own receptor and not merely via cross-reactivity with insulin receptors. In BB/w diabetic rats, which are both insulin deficient and insulin resistant, IGF-I is effective in lowering blood glucose concentrations (62). This occurs in part through decreased hepatic glucose production in response to IGF-I, although the responsible receptor has not been defined. Humans treated with continuous infusions of IGF-I at doses requiring intravenous glucose to maintain normoglycemia show inhibition of circulating free fatty acids and hepatic glucose release, unlike what has been found in the rodent studies of bolus IGF-I administration. Insulin sensitivity as assessed by the insulin/glucose ratio during a glucose tolerance test was increased by an unknown mechanism in humans after IGF-I infusion, possibly through inhibition of release of growth hormone.

The pharmaceutical industry has exploited certain characteristics of the ability of IGF-I to bind the insulin receptor and has investigated the effects of mutation of the insulin molecule to produce insulins with a lower tendency to self-aggregate following subcutaneous injection. One early such compound (B10Asp—referring to substitution with an aspartate on the tenth position on the β-chain of insulin) has mitogenic potential similar to that of IGF-I, and its use in rodents was associated with the development of mammary tumors. Thus, the differential interaction with IGF-I receptors may contribute significantly to the action profile of insulin analogues. In one study, insulin and IGF-I–receptor binding properties and metabolic and mitogenic potencies of insulin aspart (B28Asp insulin), insulin lispro (B28Lys, B29Pro insulin), and insulin glargine (A21Gly, B31Arg, B32Arg insulin) were compared (63). Receptor affinities were measured in purified human receptors, insulin-receptor dissociation rates were determined in Chinese hamster ovary cells overexpressing insulin receptors, metabolic potencies were evaluated using primary mouse adipocytes, and mitogenic potencies were determined in human osteosarcoma cells. Metabolic potencies of the insulin analogues correlated well with insulin-receptor affinities, and mitogenic potencies in general correlated well with IGF-I–receptor affinities. The two rapid-acting insulin analogues, aspart and lispro, resembled human insulin in all parameters except for a slightly elevated affinity of lispro for the IGF-I receptor. In contrast, the long-acting insulin analogue glargine differed significantly from human insulin. The combination of the A21Gly, B31Arg, B32Arg substitutions provided insulin glargine with a six- to eightfold increased affinity for the IGF-I receptor and mitogenic potency as compared with human insulin. The increased growth-stimulating potential of insulin glargine initially raised concern about potential IGF-I receptor–mediated side effects. However, these have not been apparent (64), and insulin glargine is currently available for clinical use in the United States.

GROWTH HORMONE/INSULIN-LIKE GROWTH FACTOR-I AXIS AND DIABETES

A relationship between abnormal GH dynamics and glucose intolerance was first recognized many years ago. This included the observation that hypophysectomy improves glycemic control (65). In uncontrolled diabetes, usual findings include reductions in IGF-I levels, elevated IGFBP-1 levels, and somewhat elevated GH levels, highlighting a GH-resistance state. In general, intensive insulin therapy does not completely reverse these abnormalities.

Elevated circulating levels of GH cause insulin resistance. In acromegaly, this progresses to diabetes in approximately 25% of patients. In experimental animals, infusion of GH is associated with reduced whole-body glucose uptake and decreased sensitivity to insulin in liver and skeletal muscle. GH has been shown to cause downregulation of the insulin signaling cascade in liver and skeletal muscle (66). IGF-I has a negative feedback effect on pituitary release of GH and thus may improve insulin sensitivity by reducing circulating GH concentrations. This observation led to interest in the use of IGF-I therapeutically in type 1 diabetes (67–69). In randomized trials in children, IGF-I (40–80 μg/kg per day) added to usual insulin therapy improved glycemic control compared with placebo (70,71). This appeared to correlate with prevention of the typical early morning rise in GH that contributes to the dawn phenomenon. In a study of 12 adults with type 1 diabetes, IGF-I (40 μg/kg per day) administered in conjunction with a reduced bedtime insulin dose for 7 days resulted in a 50% increase in circulating IGF-I concentrations, a 55% reduction in overnight GH concentrations, and improved insulin sensitivity by hyperinsulinemic euglycemic clamp (72,73). Assuming that the glycemic potency of IGF-I is approximately 8% that of insulin, the IGF-I dosage used was equivalent to an insulin dose of about 0.06 U/kg per day. The reduction in usual insulin dose was 0.11 U/kg per day, which suggests that the hypoglycemic action of IGF-I was not solely due to insulin-like activity. Side effects of recombinant IGF-I therapy include edema and headaches. Administration of IGF-I in combination with IGFBP-3 has been shown to permit the metabolic benefits of IGF therapy with fewer adverse effects (74).

It is likely that improved insulin sensitivity as a result of decreased GH secretion accounts for the improvements in metabolic control. Levels of free fatty acids were noted to be decreased during a hyperinsulinemic clamp after IGF-I administration, which may also have contributed to increased glucose utilization through a reduction in competition of fatty acids with glucose via the glucose–fatty acid cycle. Reduced lipolysis, as a result of IGF-I–induced inhibition of GH secretion, may explain the effect, although not all studies have shown such changes in free fatty acids (75). However, in patients with acromegaly, in whom GH concentrations were stabilized with pegvisomant (a GH-receptor antagonist), administration of IGF-I/IGFBP-3 improved insulin sensitivity, suggesting that mechanisms independent of GH levels also may be important (76).

IGF-I has been used therapeutically in patients with rare forms of diabetes associated with severe insulin resistance. Here the utility probably relates to IGF-I stimulation of glucose uptake and other glucoregulatory responses via activation of the IGF-I receptor. In one study of four adult patients, IGF-I given by subcutaneous injection in a high dose (80 μg/kg) markedly lowered plasma glucose levels (77). In an unusual case of insulin resistance associated with diabetic ketoacidosis in an adolescent patient, IGF-I administration lowered blood glucose levels under circumstances in which insulin was ineffective at extremely high doses. This patient was maintained subsequently on combination therapy with insulin and IGF-I (78). In typical type 2 diabetes, IGF-I therapy by injection can lower plasma glucose levels and improve insulin sensitivity, although it is not clear that this has advantages over the use of insulin alone (79).

Activation of IGF-I receptors by insulin in insulin-resistant states has been associated with untoward effects. For example, in some patients with rare forms of extreme insulin resistance and markedly elevated insulin levels, an acromegalic pattern of body growth has been attributed to insulin cross-reactivity with IGF-I receptors. In polycystic ovary syndrome (PCOS), insulin resistance and secondary hyperinsulinemia are thought to result in activation of ovarian IGF-I receptors, which may contribute to overproduction of androgen and consequent oligomenorrhea and hirsutism. In states of IGF-I excess, IGF-I itself also may lead to IGF-I receptor–mediated production of androgen. For example, in a study of female patients with Laron dwarfism treated with IGF-I, acne and oligomenorrhea developed in parallel with a rise in IGF-I and testosterone levels, and these effects were reversed by interrupting or lowering the dose of IGF-I (80). In cultured theca interstitial cells, both insulin and IGF-I stimulate DNA synthesis in a dose-dependent fashion, with IGF-I having greater potency than insulin (81). An increased number of IGF-I receptors on erythrocytes, irrespective of the patient's body mass index, has been described in patients with PCOS, although serum IGF-I concentrations were similar in the PCOS patients and controls (82). In this study, the degree of hyperinsulinemia, provoked by glucose challenge, correlated as expected with basal insulin but not with the number of IGF-I receptors. However, the number of IGF-I receptors correlated positively with androstenedione levels. This suggests a potential role for altered expression of IGF-I receptors in PCOS and further supports the concept that hyperandrogenism in PCOS may not be a direct result of hyperinsulinemia but a reflection of the ability of either insulin or IGF-I to activate IGF-I receptors. In general, serum IGFBP-1 levels are lower in PCOS, likely because of hyperinsulinemia, and levels of free IGF-I in serum are modestly increased (83). However, many of the findings of links between the IGF system and androgen production from the ovary are confounded by the existence of local production of IGF-I and IGFBPs in both theca cells and stroma of normal as well as cystic ovaries (84,85).

GROWTH HORMONE AND INSULIN-LIKE GROWTH FACTOR-I LINKS TO COMPLICATIONS OF DIABETES

Retinopathy

Activation of the GH/IGF-I axis may contribute to diabetic retinopathy. Early observational studies documented regression of even established retinopathy in patients who developed pituitary failure or underwent hypophysectomy (86). Some studies have reported an association between plasma or intraocular levels of IGF-I and the occurrence or progression of diabetic retinopathy (87,88). However, the general consensus of published work is that levels of IGF-I do not correlate with retinopathy. The observed decrease in retinopathy with hypopituitarism may therefore reflect a role of IGF-I not as a primary causal agent but as a contributor at either normal or elevated levels as a permissive factor in diabetic retinopathy.

In a condition somewhat similar to diabetic retinopathy, ischemia-induced retinopathy, the effects of inhibition of GH have been studied in two experimental model systems. Transgenic mice expressing a GH inhibitor gene and normal mice given a GH antagonist both had marked inhibition of ischemia-induced retinal neovascularization compared with control mice (89). Neovascularization was inhibited in inverse proportion to serum levels of IGF-I, and the protective effect was reversed with systemic administration of exogenous IGF-I. In another study, vascular endothelial cell–specific inactivation of the IGF-I receptor by homologous recombination (tissue-specific gene knockout) resulted in a 34% decrease in neovascularization induced by hypoxia (90). This supports a role for IGF-I action specifically in vascular endothelial cells as a contributing factor, at least in experimental hypoxia-induced retinopathy. In the same model system, inactivation of the insulin receptors of vascular endothelial cells resulted in an even more marked decrease of 57% in retinopathy.

The constellation of data overall suggests that systemic inhibition of the GH/IGF-I system may have therapeutic potential in proliferative diabetic retinopathy. However, beneficial effects of lowering IGF-I levels, either directly or via inhibition of GH action, have not yet been clearly demonstrated. Results following treatment with somatostatin have been inconsistent. The GH antagonist pegvisomant, a mutant form of GH that binds but does not activate GH receptors, also has not been effective in inducing regression of diabetic retinal neovascularization (91). The possibility of decreasing diabetic proliferative retinopathy by specifically suppressing IGF-I pathways in the retina remains a question and a challenge for future study.

Nephropathy

Microalbuminuria in diabetes has been associated with increased urinary and plasma IGF-I concentrations. In a study of adolescents with type 1 diabetes, urinary levels of IGFBP-3 initially appeared to be directly correlated with the rate of urinary albumin excretion (92). However, further analysis demonstrated that an N-terminal fragment of IGFBP-3 was being measured, that intact plasma IGFBP-3 actually was lower in diabetic participants with microalbuminuria than in those without microalbuminuria, and that IGFBP-3 proteolytic activity was enhanced in individuals with microalbuminuria. Subsequent studies have demonstrated elevated IGFBP-3 protease activity in both microalbuminuric and macroalbuminuric patients with type 2 diabetes. In another study of children, urinary IGF-I was strongly correlated with kidney size and subsequent diabetic nephropathy (93). Patients with microalbuminuria had significantly higher levels of both urinary IGF-I and GH. Of interest, only 9% of the variance in urinary IGF-I could be attributed to plasma IGF-I. The precise mechanism that leads to increased urinary IGF-I has not been defined, but these observations suggest that alterations in the bioavailability of IGF-I and the effects of IGF-I on mesangial or tubular-cell proliferation might play a role in diabetic nephropathy (94,95). Hyperglycemia increases sensitivity of mesangial cells in culture to IGF-I, representing another mechanism that may lead to an increased glomerular proliferative response (96).

Therapy with somatostatin analogues to inhibit pituitary GH production has been shown to inhibit renal growth in association with reduced renal medullary concentrations of IGF-I (97). Mice with knockout of the GH receptor that subsequently were rendered diabetic with streptozotocin were protected against diabetic nephropathy (98). Control diabetic mice with an intact GH axis developed glomerulosclerosis, increased glomerular volume, and mesangial expansion, and all of these abnormalities were absent in the knockout mice despite equivalent severity of diabetes.

Neuropathy

In contrast to the potential protective effects of IGF-I deficiency on diabetic retinopathy and nephropathy, there is evidence that IGF-I deficiency in neuronal tissue may contribute to the development and progression of diabetic neuropathy as a consequence of loss of antiapoptotic actions of IGF-I (99,100). Insulin and the IGFs have neurotrophic actions on sensory, sympathetic, and motor neurons, all of which can be affected in diabetic neuropathy (99). IGF activity is reduced in nerve tissue in rodent models of diabetes, and some studies have shown that replacement of IGF-I decreases the occurrence of neuropathy despite ongoing hyperglycemia. In rat superior cervical ganglia studied *in vitro*, hyperglycemia has been shown to induce apoptosis and inhibit neurite growth, similar to what occurs in association with diabetes *in vivo* (101). Treatment with IGF-I prevented these changes. Schwann cells undergo apoptosis after serum withdrawal, and this can be reversed by IGF-I through antiapoptotic pathways involving PI 3-kinase and protein kinase B (102). Further study will be required to determine whether IGF-I deficiency in neuronal tissue is a significant factor in the development of diabetic neuropathy.

At present, there is considerable interest in new pharmacologic approaches to the inhibition of GH and/or IGF action in the prevention or treatment of diabetes complications. As this work progresses, it will be important to carefully evaluate the potential counterbalancing effects of decreased IGF action in protecting against retinopathy and nephropathy and, at the same time, predisposing to neuropathy.

REFERENCES

1. Froesch ER, Zapf J. Insulin-like growth factors and insulin: comparative aspects. *Diabetologia* 1985;28:485–493.
2. Scacchi M, Pincelli AI, Caumo A, et al. Spontaneous nocturnal growth hormone secretion in anorexia nervosa. *J Clin Endocrinol Metab* 1997;82: 3225–3229.
3. Oster MH, Fielder PJ, Levin N, et al. Adaptation of the growth hormone and insulin-like growth factor-I axis to chronic and severe calorie or protein malnutrition. *J Clin Invest* 1995;95:2258–2265.
4. Martinez V, Balbin M, Ordonez FA, et al. Hepatic expression of growth hormone receptor/binding protein and insulin-like growth factor I genes in uremic rats. Influence of nutritional deficit. *Growth Horm IGF Res* 1999;9:61–68.
5. Hintz RL, Suskind R, Amatayakul K, et al. Plasma somatomedin and growth hormone values in children with protein-calorie malnutrition. *J Pediatr* 1978;92:153–156.
6. Oster MH, Levin N, Fielder PJ, et al. Developmental differences in the IGF-I system response to severe and chronic calorie malnutrition. *Am J Physiol* 1996;270:E646–E653.
7. Ho KY, Veldhuis JD, Johnson ML, et al. Fasting enhances growth hormone secretion and amplifies the complex rhythms of growth hormone secretion in man. *J Clin Invest* 1988;81:968–975.
8. Maes ML, Underwood E, Ketelslegers JM. Plasma somatomedin-C in fasted and refed rats: close relationship with changes in liver somatogenic but not lactogenic binding sites. *J Endocrinol* 1983;97:243–252.
9. Maiter D, Maes M, Underwood LE, et al. Early changes in serum concentrations of somatomedin-C induced by dietary protein deprivation in rats: contributions of growth hormone receptor and post-receptor defects. *J Endocrinol* 1988;118:113–120.

10. Bornfeldt KE, Arnqvist HJ, Enberg B, et al. Regulation of insulin-like growth factor-I and growth hormone receptor gene expression by diabetes and nutritional state in rat tissues. *J Endocrinol* 1989;122:651–656.
11. Straus DS, Takemoto CD. Effect of fasting on insulin-like growth factor-I (IGF-I) and growth hormone receptor mRNA levels and IGF-I gene transcription in rat liver. *Mol Endocrinol* 1990;4:91–100.
12. Donahue SP, Phillips LS. Response of IGF-1 to nutritional support in malnourished hospital patients: a possible indicator of short-term changes in nutritional status. *Am J Clin Nutr* 1989;50:962–969.
13. Clemmons DR, Underwood LE, Dickerson RN, et al. Use of plasma somatomedin-C/insulin-like growth factor I measurements to monitor the response to nutritional repletion in malnourished patients. *Am J Clin Nutr* 1985;41:191–198.
14. Isley WL, Underwood LE, Clemmons DR. Changes in plasma somatomedin-C in response to ingestion of diets with variable protein and energy content. *JPEN J Parenter Enteral Nutr* 1984;8:407–411.
15. Snyder DK, Clemmons DR, Underwood LE. Dietary carbohydrate content determines responsiveness to growth hormone in energy-restricted humans. *J Clin Endocrinol Metab* 1989;69:745–752.
16. Clemmons DR, Seek MM, Underwood LE. Supplemental essential amino acids augment the somatomedin-C/insulin-like growth factor I response to refeeding after fasting. *Metabolism* 1985;34:391–395.
17. Forbes GB, Brown MR, Welle SL, et al. Hormonal response to overfeeding. *Am J Clin Nutr* 1989;49:608–611.
18. Strasser-Vogel B, Blum WF, Past R, et al. Insulin-like growth factor (IGF)-I and -II and IGF-binding proteins-1, -2, and -3 in children and adolescents with diabetes mellitus: correlation with metabolic control and height attainment. *J Clin Endocrinol Metab* 1995;80:1207–1213.
19. Bornfeldt KE, Skottner A, Arnqvist HJ. In-vivo regulation of messenger RNA encoding insulin-like growth factor-I (IGF-I) and its receptor by diabetes, insulin and IGF-I in rat muscle. *J Endocrinol* 1992;135:203–211.
20. Cheetham TD, Taylor A, Holly JM, et al. The effects of recombinant human insulin-like growth factor-I (IGF-I) administration on the levels of IGF-I, IGF-II and IGF-binding proteins in adolescents with insulin-dependent diabetes mellitus. *J Endocrinol* 1994;142:367–374.
21. Ekman B, Nystrom F, Arnqvist HJ. Circulating IGF-I concentrations are low and not correlated to glycaemic control in adults with type 1 diabetes. *Eur J Endocrinol* 2000;143:505–510.
22. Tollet P, Enberg B, Mode A. Growth hormone (GH) regulation of cytochrome P-450IIC12, insulin-like growth factor-I (IGF-I), and GH receptor messenger RNA expression in primary rat hepatocytes: a hormonal interplay with insulin, IGF-I, and thyroid hormone. *Mol Endocrinol* 1990;4:1934–1942.
23. Maiter D, Fliesen T, Underwood LE, et al. Dietary protein restriction decreases insulin-like growth factor I independent of insulin and liver growth hormone binding. *Endocrinology* 1989;124:2604–2611.
24. Bar RS, Boes M, Clemmons DR, et al. Insulin differentially alters transcapillary movement of intravascular IGFBP-1, IGFBP-2 and endothelial cell IGF-binding proteins in the rat heart. *Endocrinology* 1990;127:497–499.
25. Takenaka A, Hirosawa M, Mori M, et al. Effect of protein nutrition on the mRNA content of insulin-like growth factor-binding protein-1 in liver and kidney of rats. *Br J Nutr* 1993;69:73–82.
26. Brisma K, Fernqvist-Forbes E, Wahren J, et al. Effect of insulin on the hepatic production of insulin-like growth factor-binding protein-1 (IGFBP-1), IGFBP-3, and IGF-I in insulin-dependent diabetes. *J Clin Endocrinol Metab* 1994; 79:872–878.
27. Radetti G, Paganini C, Antoniazzi F, et al. Growth hormone-binding proteins, IGF-I and IGF-binding proteins in children and adolescents with type 1 diabetes mellitus. *Horm Res* 1997;47:110–115.
28. Ogasawara M, Karey KP, Marquardt H, et al. Identification and purification of truncated insulin-like growth factor I from porcine uterus. Evidence for high biological potency. *Biochemistry* 1989;8:2710–2721.
29. Martin AA, Tomas FM, Owens PC, et al. IGF-I and its variant, des-(1-3)IGF-I, enhance growth in rats with reduced renal mass. *Am J Physiol* 1991;261:F626–F633.
30. Mohan S, Baylink DJ. IGF-binding proteins are multifunctional and act via IGF-dependent and -independent mechanisms. *J Endocrinol* 2002;175:19–31.
31. Guler HP, Zapf J, Froesch ER. Short-term metabolic effects of recombinant human insulin-like growth factor I in healthy adults. *N Engl J Med* 1987;317:137–140.
32. Livingston N, Pollare T, Lithell H, et al. Characterisation of insulin-like growth factor I receptor in skeletal muscles of normal and insulin resistant subjects. *Diabetologia* 1988;31:871–877.
33. Dohm GL, Elton CW, Raju MS, et al. IGF-I–stimulated glucose transport in human skeletal muscle and IGF-I resistance in obesity and NIDDM. *Diabetes* 1990;39:1028–1032.
34. Sasaoka T, Ishiki M, Sawa T, et al. Comparison of the insulin and insulin-like growth factor 1 mitogenic intracellular signaling pathways. *Endocrinology* 1996;137:4427–4434.
35. Urso B, Cope DL, Kalloo-Hosein HE, et al. Differences in signaling properties of the cytoplasmic domains of the insulin receptor and insulin-like growth factor receptor in 3T3-L1 adipocytes. *J Biol Chem* 1999;274:30864–30873.
36. Kruger MS, Klein H, Siddle K, et al. Specificity of insulin and IGF-I receptors for IRS1. *Exp Clin Endocrinol Diabetes* 1996;104:38–39.
37. Urso BR, Brown A, O'Rahilly S, et al. The alpha-isoform of class II phosphoinositide 3-kinase is more effectively activated by insulin receptors than IGF receptors, and activation requires receptor NPEY motifs. *FEBS Lett* 1999;460:423–426.
38. Najjar SM, Blakesley VA, Li Calzi S, et al. Differential phosphorylation of pp120 by insulin and insulin-like growth factor-1 receptors: role for the C-terminal domain of the beta-subunit. *Biochemistry* 1997;36:6827–6834.
39. Beitner-Johnson D, LeRoith D. Insulin-like growth factor-I stimulates tyrosine phosphorylation of endogenous c-Crk. *J Biol Chem* 1995;270:5187–5190.
40. O'Neill TJ, Rose DW, Pillay TS, et al. Interaction of a GRB-IR splice variant (a human GRB10 homolog) with the insulin and insulin-like growth factor I receptors. Evidence for a role in mitogenic signaling. *J Biol Chem* 1996;271:22506–22513.
41. Hansen H, Svensson U, Zhu J, et al. Interaction between the Grb10 SH2 domain and the insulin receptor carboxyl terminus. *J Biol Chem* 1996;271:8882–8886.
42. Morrione A, Valentinis B, Li S, et al. Grb10: a new substrate of the insulin-like growth factor I receptor. *Cancer Res* 1969;56:3165–3167.
43. Laviola, L, Giorgino F, Chow JC, et al. The adapter protein Grb10 associates preferentially with the insulin receptor as compared with the IGF-I receptor in mouse fibroblasts. *J Clin Invest* 1997;99:830–837.
44. Dupont J, Khan J, Qu B, et al. Insulin and IGF-1 induce different patterns of gene expression in mouse fibroblast NIH-3T3 cells: identification by cDNA microarray analysis. *Endocrinology* 2001;142:4969–4975.
45. Rothe KI, Accili D. Role of insulin receptors and IGF receptors in growth and development. *Pediatr Nephrol* 2000;14:558–561.
46. Accili D, Nakae J, Kim JJ, et al. Targeted gene mutations define the roles of insulin and IGF-I receptors in mouse embryonic development. *J Pediatr Endocrinol Metab* 1999;12:475–485.
47. O'Rahilly S, Moller DE. Mutant insulin receptors in syndromes of insulin resistance. *Clin Endocrinol* (Oxf) 1992;36:121–132.
48. Nakae J, Kato M, Murashita M, et al. Long-term effect of recombinant human insulin-like growth factor I on metabolic and growth control in a patient with leprechaunism. *J Clin Endocrinol Metab* 1998;83:542–549.
49. Desbois-Mouthon C, Danan C, Amselem S, et al. Severe resistance to insulin and insulin-like growth factor-I in cells from a patient with leprechaunism as a result of two mutations in the tyrosine kinase domain of the insulin receptor. *Metabolism* 1996;45:1493–1500.
50. Bailyes EM, Nave BT, Soos MA, et al. Insulin receptor/IGF-I receptor hybrids are widely distributed in mammalian tissues: quantification of individual receptor species by selective immunoprecipitation and immunoblotting. *Biochem J* 1997;327:209–215.
51. Federici M, Giaccari A, Hribal ML, et al. Evidence for glucose/hexosamine in vivo regulation of insulin/IGF-I hybrid receptor assembly. *Diabetes* 1999;48:2277–2285.
52. Spampinato D, Pandini G, Iuppa A, et al. Insulin/insulin-like growth factor I hybrid receptors overexpression is not an early defect in insulin-resistant subjects. *J Clin Endocrinol Metab* 2000;85:4219–4223.
53. Fernandez AM, Kim JK, Yakar S, et al. Functional inactivation of the IGF-I and insulin receptors in skeletal muscle causes type 2 diabetes. *Genes Dev* 2001;15:1926–1934.
54. Bruning JC, Michael MD, Winnay JN, et al. A muscle-specific insulin receptor knockout exhibits features of the metabolic syndrome of NIDDM without altering glucose tolerance. *Mol Cell* 1998;2:559–569.
55. Baudry A, Lamothe B, Bucchini D, et al. IGF-1 receptor as an alternative receptor for metabolic signaling in insulin receptor-deficient muscle cells. *FEBS Lett* 2001;488:174–178.
56. Shefi-Friedman L, Wertheimer E, Shen S, et al. Increased IGFR activity and glucose transport in cultured skeletal muscle from insulin receptor null mice. *Am J Physiol Endocrinol Metab* 2001;281:E16–E24.
57. Abuzzahab MJ, Schneider A, Goddard A, et al. Human IGF-I receptor mutations resulting in pre- and post-natal growth retardation. *N Engl J Med* 2003;349:2211–2222.
58. Rasmussen SK, Lautier C, Hansen L, et al. Studies of the variability of the genes encoding the insulin-like growth factor I receptor and its ligand in relation to type 2 diabetes mellitus. *J Clin Endocrinol Metab* 2000;85:1606–1610.
59. Lemons JA, Ridenour R, Orsini EN. Congenital absence of the pancreas and intrauterine growth retardation. *Pediatrics* 1979;64:255–257.
60. Hattersley AT, Beards F, Ballantyne E, et al. Mutations in the glucokinase gene of the fetus result in reduced birth weight. *Nat Genet* 1998;19:268–270.
61. Jacob R, Barrett E, Plewe G, et al. Acute effects of insulin-like growth factor I on glucose and amino acid metabolism in the awake fasted rat. Comparison with insulin. *J Clin Invest* 1989;83:1717–1723.
62. Jacob RJ, Sherwin RS, Bowen L, et al. Metabolic effects of IGF-I and insulin in spontaneously diabetic BB/w rats. *Am J Physiol* 1991;260:E262–E268.
63. Kurtzhals P, Schaffer L, Sorensen A, et al. Correlations of receptor binding and metabolic and mitogenic potencies of insulin analogs designed for clinical use. *Diabetes* 2000;49:999–1005.
64. Ciaraldi TP, Carter L, Seipke G, et al. Effects of the long-acting insulin analog insulin glargine on cultured human skeletal muscle cells: comparisons to insulin and IGF-I. *J Clin Endocrinol Metab* 2001;86:5838–5847.
65. Hansen AP, Johansen K. Diurnal patterns of blood glucose, serum free fatty acids, insulin, glucagon and growth hormone in normals and juvenile diabetics. *Diabetologia* 1970;6:27–33.
66. Thirone AC, Carvalho CR, Brenelli SL, et al. Effect of chronic growth hormone treatment on insulin signal transduction in rat tissues. *Mol Cell Endocrinol* 1997;130:33–42.
67. Dunger DB, Cheetham TD, Crowne EC. Insulin-like growth factors (IGFs) and IGF-I treatment in the adolescent with insulin-dependent diabetes mellitus. *Metabolism* 1995;44:119–123.

68. Savage MO, Dunger DB. Recombinant IGF-I therapy in insulin-dependent diabetes mellitus. *Diabetes Metab* 1996;2:257–260.
69. Lanzetta P, Malara C. Cotherapy with recombinant human IGF-I and insulin improves glycemic control in type 1 diabetes. *Diabetes Care* 2000;23:436–437.
70. Thrailkill K, Quattrin T, Baker L, et al. Dual hormonal replacement therapy with insulin and recombinant human insulin-like growth factor (IGF)-I in insulin-dependent diabetes mellitus: effects on the growth hormone/IGF/IGF-binding protein system. *J Clin Endocrinol Metab* 1997;82:1181–1187.
71. Cheetham TD, Jones J, Taylor AM, et al. The effects of recombinant insulin-like growth factor I administration on growth hormone levels and insulin requirements in adolescents with type 1 (insulin-dependent) diabetes mellitus. *Diabetologia* 1993;36:678–681.
72. Carroll PV, Umpleby M, Alexander EL, et al. Recombinant human insulin-like growth factor-I (rhIGF-I) therapy in adults with type 1 diabetes mellitus: effects on IGFs, IGF-binding proteins, glucose levels and insulin treatment. *Clin Endocrinol* (Oxf) 1998;49:739–746.
73. Carroll PV, Christ ER, Umpleby AM, et al. IGF-I treatment in adults with type 1 diabetes: effects on glucose and protein metabolism in the fasting state and during a hyperinsulinemic-euglycemic amino acid clamp. *Diabetes* 2000;49:789–796.
74. Clemmons DR, Moses AC, McKay MJ, et al. The combination of insulin-like growth factor I and insulin-like growth factor-binding protein-3 reduces insulin requirements in insulin-dependent type 1 diabetes: evidence for in vivo biological activity. *J Clin Endocrinol Metab* 2000;85:1518–1524.
75. Crowne EC, Samra JS, Cheetham T, et al. Recombinant human insulin-like growth factor-I abolishes changes in insulin requirements consequent upon growth hormone pulsatility in young adults with type I diabetes mellitus. *Metabolism* 1998;47:31–38.
76. O'Connell T, Clemmons DR. IGF-I/IGF-binding protein-3 combination improves insulin resistance by GH-dependent and independent mechanisms. *J Clin Endocrinol Metab* 2002;87:4356–4360.
77. Vestergaard H, Rossen M, Urhammer SA, et al. Short- and long-term metabolic effects of recombinant human IGF-I treatment in patients with severe insulin resistance and diabetes mellitus. *Eur J Endocrinol* 1997;136:475–482.
78. Usala AL, Madigan T, Burguera B, et al. Brief report: treatment of insulin-resistant diabetic ketoacidosis with insulin-like growth factor I in an adolescent with insulin-dependent diabetes. *N Engl J Med* 1992;327:853–857.
79. Zenobi, PD, Jaeggi-Groisman SE, Riesen WF, et al. Insulin-like growth factor-I improves glucose and lipid metabolism in type 2 diabetes mellitus. *J Clin Invest* 1992;90:2234–2241.
80. Klinger B, Anin S, Silbergeld A, et al. Development of hyperandrogenism during treatment with insulin-like growth factor-I (IGF-I) in female patients with Laron syndrome. *Clin Endocrinol* (Oxf) 1998;48:81–87.
81. Duleba AJ, Spaczynski RZ, Olive DL. Insulin and insulin-like growth factor I stimulate the proliferation of human ovarian theca-interstitial cells. *Fertil Steril* 1998;69:335–340.
82. Gdansky EY, Diamant Z, Laron Z, et al. Increased number of IGF-I receptors on erythrocytes of women with polycystic ovarian syndrome. *Clin Endocrinol* (Oxf) 1997;47:185–190.
83. Cataldo NA. Insulin-like growth factor binding proteins: do they play a role in polycystic ovary syndrome? *Semin Reprod Endocrinol* 1997;15:123–136.
84. Mason HD, Cwyfan-Hughes SC, Heinrich G, et al. Insulin-like growth factor (IGF) I and II, IGF-binding proteins, and IGF-binding protein proteases are produced by theca and stroma of normal and polycystic human ovaries. *J Clin Endocrinol Metab* 1996;81:276–284.
85. Voutilainen R, Franks S, Mason HD, et al. Expression of insulin-like growth factor (IGF), IGF-binding protein, and IGF receptor messenger ribonucleic acids in normal and polycystic ovaries. *J Clin Endocrinol Metab* 1996; 81:1003–1008.
86. Kohner EM, Hamilton AM, Joplin GF, et al. Florid diabetic retinopathy and its response to treatment by photocoagulation or pituitary ablation. *Diabetes* 1976;25:104–110.
87. Janssen JA, Jacobs ML, Derkx FH, et al. Free and total insulin-like growth factor I (IGF-I), IGF-binding protein-1 (IGFBP-1), and IGFBP-3 and their relationships to the presence of diabetic retinopathy and glomerular hyperfiltration in insulin-dependent diabetes mellitus. *J Clin Endocrinol Metab* 1997;82: 2809–2815.
88. Dills DG, Moss SE, Klein R, et al. Association of elevated IGF-I levels with increased retinopathy in late-onset diabetes. *Diabetes*1991; 40:1725–1730.
89. Smith LE, Kopchick JJ, Chen W, et al. Essential role of growth hormone in ischemia-induced retinal neovascularization. *Science* 1997;276:1706–1709.
90. Kondo TD, Vicent D, Suzuma M, et al. Knockout of insulin and IGF-1 receptors on vascular endothelial cells protects against retinal neovascularization. *J Clin Invest* 2003;111:1835–1842.
91. Growth Hormone Antagonist for Proliferative Retinopathy Study Group. The effect of a growth hormone receptor antagonist drug on proliferative diabetic retinopathy. *Ophthalmology* 2001;108:2266–2272.
92. Cianfarani S, Bonfanti R, Bitti ML, et al. Growth and insulin-like growth factors (IGFs) in children with insulin-dependent diabetes mellitus at the onset of disease: evidence for normal growth, age dependency of the IGF system alterations, and presence of a small (approximately 18-kilodalton) IGF-binding protein-3 fragment in serum. *J Clin Endocrinol Metab* 2000;85:4162–4167.
93. Cummings EA, Sochett EB, Dekker MG, et al. Contribution of growth hormone and IGF-I to early diabetic nephropathy in type 1 diabetes. *Diabetes* 47:1341–1346.
94. Bach LA. IGF-I and IGF binding proteins in diabetes-related kidney growth. *Growth Regul* 1992;2:30–39.
95. Flyvbjerg A. Role of growth hormone, insulin-like growth factors (IGFs) and IGF-binding proteins in the renal complications of diabetes. *Kidney Int Suppl* 1997;60:S12–9:S12-9.
96. Horney MJ, Shirley DW, Kurtz DT, et al. Elevated glucose increases mesangial cell sensitivity to insulin-like growth factor I. *Am J Physiol* 1998;274: F1045–F1053.
97. Gronbaek H, Nielsen B, Frystyk J, et al. Effect of lanreotide on local kidney IGF-I and renal growth in experimental diabetes in the rat. *Exp Nephrol* 1996;4:295–303.
98. Bellush LL, Doublier S, Holland AN, et al. Protection against diabetes-induced nephropathy in growth hormone receptor/binding protein gene-disrupted mice. *Endocrinology* 2000;141:163–168.
99. Zhuang HX, Wuarin L, Fei ZJ, et al. Insulin-like growth factor (IGF) gene expression is reduced in neural tissues and liver from rats with non-insulin-dependent diabetes mellitus, and IGF treatment ameliorates diabetic neuropathy. *J Pharmacol Exp Ther* 1997;283:366–374.
100. Ishii DN. Implication of insulin-like growth factors in the pathogenesis of diabetic neuropathy. *Brain Res Rev* 1995;20:47–67.
101. Russell JW, Feldman EL. Insulin-like growth factor-I prevents apoptosis in sympathetic neurons exposed to high glucose. *Horm Metab Res* 1999;31:90–96.
102. Cheng HL, Steinway M, Delaney CL, et al. IGF-I promotes Schwann cell motility and survival via activation of Akt. *Mol Cell Endocrinol* 2000;170: 211–215.

CHAPTER 11

Glucagon and Glucagon-like Peptides

Joel F. Habener and Timothy J. Kieffer

Investigations during the past 15 years have uncovered a remarkable, unanticipated complexity in the repertoire of biologically active hormones produced by the expression of the proglucagon gene. Because of these new discoveries, an entirely new perspective has arisen regarding the biologic functions and importance of proglucagon-derived peptides in the pathogenesis of diabetes mellitus. The structure of the proglucagon gene, established by DNA cloning approaches, reveals that it encodes a large preproglucagon protein consisting of an N-terminal signal sequence and a prohormone encoding glucagon and several glucagon-like peptides (GLPs). The signal sequence is removed from the prohormone during its synthesis so that the initial completed protein synthesized is the prohormone referred to as *proglucagon*. The structure of proglucagon is representative of prohormones that encode peptide hormones inasmuch as it contains multiple biologically active hormones that are released from the prohormone by tissue-specific proteolytic cleavages. Proglucagon undergoes alternative posttranslational cleavages whereby the hormone glucagon is produced in the α-cells of the endocrine pancreas (islets of Langerhans) and glucagon-like peptides are produced in the L cells of the intestine. Glucagon and the glucagon-like peptides are all members of a superfamily of peptides structurally related to glucagon, including vasoactive intestinal peptide, secretin, gastric inhibitory polypeptide, and growth hormone–releasing hormone, among others. Each of these glucagon-related peptide hormones is involved to some extent in the regulation of nutrient homeostasis, growth, or development, acting via G-protein–coupled receptors that increase the formation of cyclic adenosine monophosphate (cAMP). Glucagon is secreted from α-cells and functions predominantly during the fasting state to maintain blood glucose levels by the mobilization of glucose from glycogen stores in peripheral tissues such as muscle and liver. Excessive production of glucagon contributes to hyperglycemia, and thus approaches that antagonize glucagon action in subjects with diabetes mellitus are being actively investigated. The glucagon-like peptides are secreted in response to feeding. Glucagon-like peptide-1 (GLP-1) and gastric inhibitory polypeptide (GIP) comprise the intestinal "incretin" hormones released from the intestine in response to feeding and augment glucose-stimulated insulin secretion from the β-cells of the islets of Langerhans. GLP-1 also enhances insulin-stimulated glucose uptake in peripheral tissues (muscle, fat, liver), suppresses glucagon secretion, induces satiety, and promotes the growth and differentiation of new β-cells in the pancreas. These antidiabetic properties of GLP-1 have prompted considerable interest in the therapeutic potential of GLP-1 for the treatment of diabetes mellitus. GLP-2 is a potent growth factor for intestinal epithelium and holds promise for the treatment of inflammatory bowel diseases. This chapter provides an overview of the historical advances in the understanding of the biologic and physiologic roles of these proglucagon-derived peptides and their potential importance in the pathogenesis of diabetes mellitus. A recent review describes the biology of glucagon and the GLPs (1). Additional review articles describe the biology of the GLPs in detail (2–10).

EXPRESSION OF THE PROGLUCAGON GENE

Tissue Distribution

The expression of the proglucagon gene (chromosome 2q36-q37 in humans) is restricted to a limited number of tissues. So far, proglucagon or proglucagon messenger RNA (mRNA) has been found in the α-cells of the endocrine pancreas, L cells in the distal small intestine and colon, and localized regions of the brain (hypothalamus and nucleus of the solitary tract). Current evidence indicates that the regulation of expression of the proglucagon gene takes place at two levels of expression: posttranslational processing of proglucagon and the transcription of the preproglucagon gene.

Regulation

ALTERNATIVE POSTTRANSLATIONAL PROCESSING

Proglucagon, synthesized in the α-cells of the islets, is processed by specific proteolytic cleavages in a pattern that differs markedly from the processing in the L cells in the intestine and the peptidergic neurons in the brain (Fig. 11.1). In the α-cells, specific prohormone convertases cleave and liberate glucagon from proglucagon, leaving behind the presumably biologically inert "major proglucagon fragment" and the N-terminal fragment of proglucagon (11). In contrast, in L cells and in peptidergic neurons, cleavages of proglucagon by a different set of prohormone-converting enzymes results predominantly in the formation of GLPs comprising the GLP-1 group of isopeptides and GLP-2.

Much of the new interest and excitement in the field of discovery research on the hormone glucagon produced by the α-cells of the islets of Langerhans arises from the findings that the precursor prohormone, proglucagon, also encodes the GLPs and that these peptides have unanticipated novel biologic activities in the regulation of nutrient metabolism, the growth and differentiation of insulin-producing β-cells of the pancreas, the control of appetite, and the promotion of the growth of intestinal epithelium (5,6,12). These recent findings on the actions of GLPs encoded by the preproglucagon gene have prompted great interest in the pursuance of the biochemistry and mechanism of actions of the GLPs.

The proteolytic cleavages—so-called posttranslational processing—of proglucagon that result in the formation of GLPs are somewhat complex. At least six GLP-1 isopeptides are formed: the largest peptides of 37 and 36 amino acids, C-terminal glycine–extended GLP-1(1–37) and C-terminal–amidated GLP-1(1–36)amide; and the N-terminal–truncated GLP-1s, GLP-1(7–37), GLP-1(7–36)amide, GLP-1(9–37), and GLP-1 (9–36)amide. So far, it appears that the biologic activities of the GLP-1s reside in the peptides GLP-1(7–37) and GLP-1 (7–36)amide; the two peptides have indistinguishable activities. The 1–37/36 and 7–37/36 peptides are cleaved from proglucagon by the actions of the prohormone convertases PC1/3 and PC2, whereas the 9–37/36 peptides are derived from the former peptides by cleavage of two N-terminal amino acids by the enzyme dipeptidyl peptidase IV (DPP-IV), also known as CD26 (13,14). DPP-IV is a ubiquitous enzyme expressed in many tissues and carried in the circulation. Cleavages of the GLP-1s by DPP IV occur at the time of their secretion from the intestinal L cells and within the circulation (15). Notably, the 9–37/36 peptides bind to the GLP-1 receptor but are biologically inactive and are weak antagonists. Most of the GLP-1 in the circulation consists of the apparently inert 1–37/36 and 9–37/36 peptides with no known biologic activities heretofore.

TRANSCRIPTION

A second level of the regulation of the expression of the GLPs is that of gene transcription. The preproglucagon gene consists of a transcribed sequence (Fig. 11.2) and a 5′-flanking promoter sequence (Fig. 11.3). The transcribed sequence in turn consists of six exons separated by five introns (16). Notably, each of the glucagon peptides—glucagon, GLP-1, and GLP-2—are encoded in separate exons (exons 3, 4, and 5), suggesting the occurrence of exonic duplication during evolutionary history (7). Although the peptides are encoded in separate exons, unlike many multi-

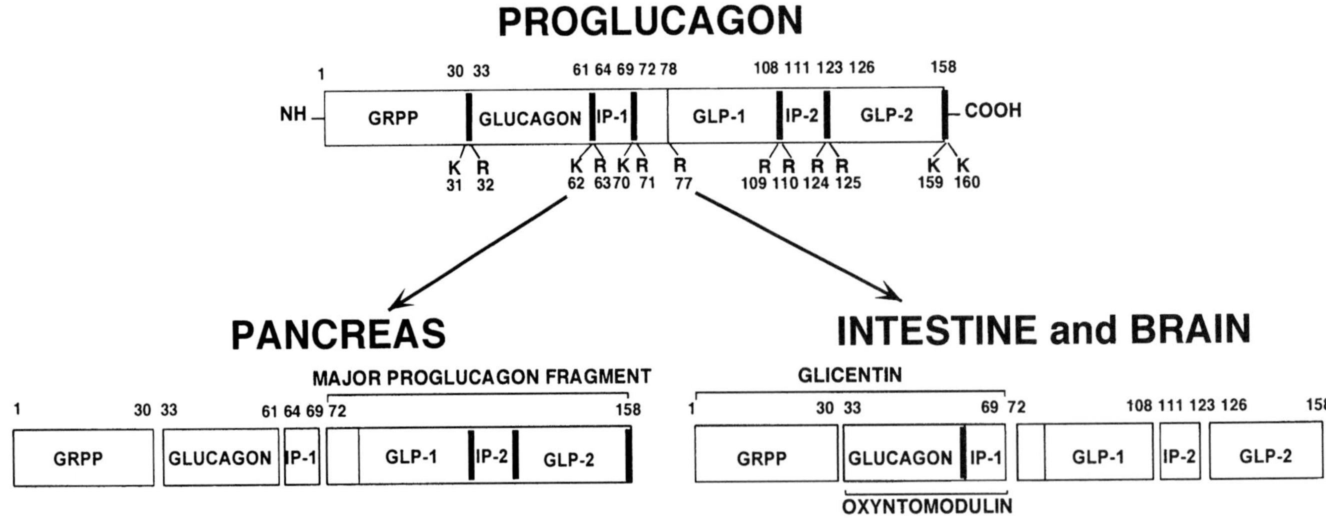

Figure 11.1. Alternative posttranslational processing of proglucagon in pancreas and intestine plus brain. Processing at specific pairs of basic residues produces numerous multifunctional peptide hormones involved in nutrient metabolism. The major bioactive processed hormones are glucagon in the pancreas α-cells and GLP-1 in the intestinal L cells and brain. Numbers on proglucagon denote amino acid positions. K, lysine; R, arginine; GRPP, glicentin-related pancreatic peptide; IP-1 and IP-2, intervening peptides; GLP-1 and GLP-2, glucagon-like peptides. (From Kieffer TJ, Habener JF. The glucagon-like peptides. *Endocr Rev* 1999;20:876–913, with permission. Copyright 1999. The Endocrine Society.)

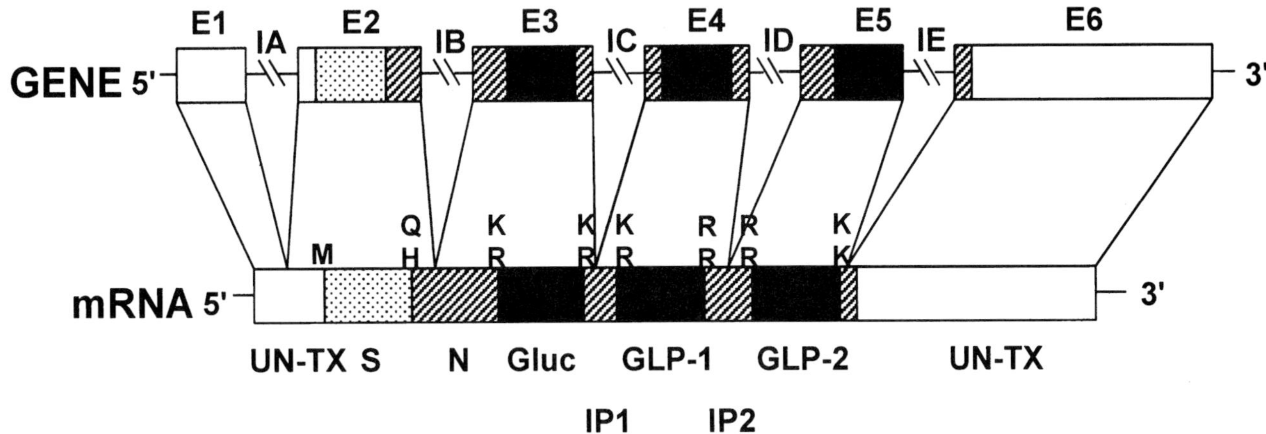

Figure 11.2. Diagram of proglucagon gene and encoded messenger RNA (mRNA). The gene consists of six exons, E1 to E6, and five introns, IA to IE. The exons encode functional domains of the pre-proglucagon. The pairs of basic residues that serve as posttranslational sites of processing of the pre-proglucagon encoded by the mRNA are shown to key in with Figure 11.1. S, signal peptide; N, amino-terminal sequence of proglucagon; Gluc, glucagon; GLP, glucagon-like peptides; IP, intervening peptides; M, methionine encoded by AUG codon that initiates translation; Q, glutamine; H, histidine; and UN-TX, untranslated regions of mRNA. (From Mojsov S, Heinrich G, Wilson IB, et al. Preproglucagon gene expression in pancreas and intestine diversifies at the level of post-translational processing. *J Biol Chem* 1986;261:11880–11889, with permission. Copyright © 1986 by The American Society for Biochemistry and Molecular Biology.)

exonic genes, the expression of these genes in mammals is not regulated by alternative exon splicing of the RNA; pre-proglucagons in both pancreas and intestine appear to be translated from identical mRNAs. However, in lower vertebrates (chickens, fish, and frogs), alternative splicing of exons does occur. The promoter of the preproglucagon gene is bipartite with respect to regions responsible for expression in pancreatic α-cells and intestinal L cells. Promoter sequences within 700 base pairs 5′ flanking the initiation of transcription are sufficient to direct the faithful expression of the preproglucagon gene in α-cells, whereas sequences required for expression in L cells reside more 5′ between nucleotides –3000 to –1000 (5,16, 17). The sequences of these regulatory regions of the promoter contain multiple *cis*-acting control elements that bind proteins termed "transcription factors" that are responsible for activating the transcription of the gene via interactions with the basal promoter consisting of RNA polymerase in association with basal transcription factors. The *cis*-acting control elements and DNA-binding transcription factors responsible for the regulation of expression of the preproglucagon gene in α-cells are much better understood than are those in L cells. The α-cell–specific expression region of the promoter contains at least six clearly identified regions residing within the proximal 300 base pair of the promoter (Fig. 11.3) (16). These regions or elements are designated G1, G2, G3, G4, C/EBP, and CRE (cAMP response element). Each of these elements binds multiple protein complexes consisting of both relatively α-cell–specific proteins and tissue-ubiquitous proteins. These proteins consist of members of the paired homeodomain (Pax), basic helix-loop-helix (bHLH), POU homeodomain, basic leucine zipper (bZip), and hepatocyte nuclear factor (HNF) families of transcription factors. The G1 region of the promoter has been shown to lend

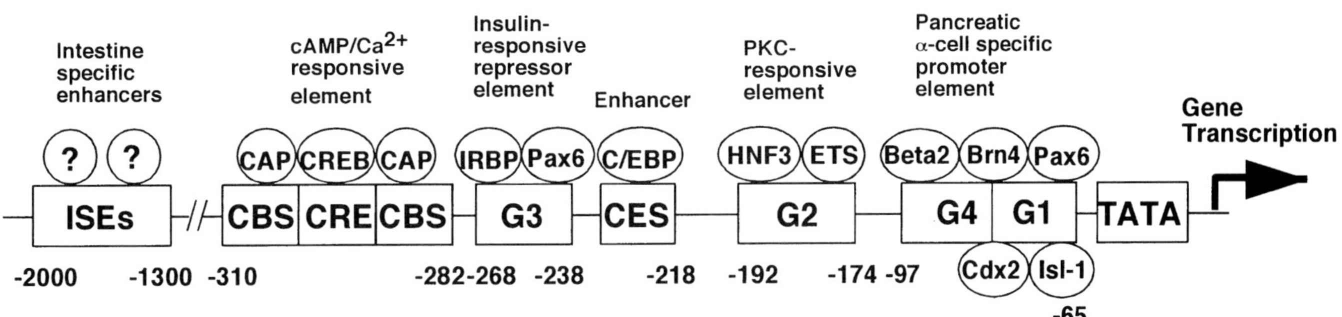

Figure 11.3. DNA control elements and interactive transacting protein factors in the 2,300–base pair promoter of the rat glucagon gene. ISEs, intestinal-specific enhancers (includes the glucagon upstream enhancer); CAP, CREB-associated protein; CBS, CAP-binding site; CREB, cyclic adenosine monophosphate (cAMP) response element binding protein; CRE, cAMP response element; IRBP, insulin responsive binding protein; ?, unknown protein; CES, C/EBP enhancer site; HNF3, hepatic nuclear factor-3; ETS, ubiquitous developmental transcription factors; Beta 2, β2/NeuroD basic helix-loop-helix factor; Isl-1, islet factor-1; Brn4, brain-4; Cdx2, caudal-related homeobox-2; Pax6, paired homeobox-6; G1, G2, G3, major α-cell/islet enhancers; and TATA, TATA box. (From Habener JF. Proglucagon gene structure and regulation of expression. In: Fehmann HC, Göke B, eds. *The insulinotropic gut hormone glucagonlike peptide-1*. Basel: Karger, 1997;15–23, with permission.)

Members of the Super Family of Glucagon-Related Peptides

5 10 15 20 25 30 35 40 45

GLUCAGON.......... H S Q G T F T S D Y S K Y L D S R R A Q D F V Q W L M N T NH2
GLP-1(7-37).......... H A E G T F T S D V S S Y L E G Q A A K E F I A W L V K G R G
GIP...................... Y A E G T F I S D Y S I A M D K I H Q Q D F V N W L L A Q K G K K N D W K H N I T Q
EXENDIN-4.......... H G E G T F T S D L S K Q M E E E A V R L F I E W L K N G G P S S G A P P P S NH2
SECRETIN.............. H S D G T F T S E L S R L R E G A R L Q R L L Q G L V NH2
PHM...................... H A D G V F T S D F S K L L G Q L S A K K Y L E S L M NH2
GLP-2.................. H A D G S F S D E M N T I L D N L A A R D F I N W L I Q T K I T D
PACAP-38.............. H S D G I F T D S Y S R Y R K Q M A V K K Y L A A V L G K R Y K Q R V K N K NH2
GRF...................... Y A D A I F T N S Y R K V L G Q L S A R K L L Q D I M S R Q Q G E S N Q E R G A R A R L NH2
VIP...................... H S D A V F T D N Y T R L R K Q M A V K K Y L N S I L N NH2

Figure 11.4. Amino acid sequences of members of the superfamily of glucagon-related peptides. Sequences include human glucagon, human glucagon-like peptides (GLP-1 and GLP-2), human glucose-dependent insulinotropic polypeptide (GIP), exendin-4 (from *Heloderma horridum*), human secretin, human peptide histidine methionine (PHM), human pituitary adenyl cyclase–activating polypeptide (PACAP-38), human growth hormone–releasing factor (GRF), and human vasoactive intestinal polypeptide (VIP). Residues identical to those of glucagon in the same position are outlined. Standard single-letter abbreviations are used for amino acids [International Union of Pure and Applied Chemistry–International Union of Biochemistry (IUPAC-IUB) Commission on Biochemical Nomenclature]. (From Kieffer TJ, Habener JF. The glucagonlike peptides. *Endocr Rev* 1999;20:876–913, with permission. Copyright 1999. The Endocrine Society.)

α-cell specificity to the expression of the gene (18). The way nutrient signals and hormones regulate the transcription of the proglucagon gene is not completely understood. However, there is convincing evidence that cAMP and insulin signaling are mediated via the CRE and G3 elements of the proglucagon gene promoter, respectively (19,20).

Superfamily of Glucagon-Related Peptide Hormones

The glucagon superfamily of peptide hormones are so designated because of their close similarities in amino acid sequences (Fig. 11.4). They have a diverse number of functions consisting in part of neurotransmitters, growth factors, and regulators of nutrient metabolism. Of these hormones, GLP-1 has the highest degree of similarity to glucagon (48%). The amino acid sequences of the glucagons and GLP-1s have been highly conserved throughout evolution; the human and anglerfish glucagons and GLP-1s are 75% and 79% identical, respectively (5,7). This strong conservation of sequences over 300 million years of evolutionary time attests to the importance of these hormones in physiologic processes.

GLUCAGON

History

In their early studies (1921), Banting and Best (21) suspected the existence of a hyperglycemia-producing hormone in the pancreas. They observed that dogs administered insulin-enriched pancreatic extracts had a biphasic blood glucose response: There was an initial rise in blood glucose followed by a lowering of blood glucose attributable to the expected actions of insulin. They suspected that the initial increase in glucose level was due to a "contaminant" in the crude pancreas extracts, which was later shown to be glucagon. In 1957, Bromer et al. (22) determined the amino acid composition and partial sequence of glucagon and determined that it was a peptide of 29 amino acids. The availability of pure crystalline glucagon led to the establishment of its hyperglycemic properties via the stimulation of glycogenolysis (23) and gluconeogenesis (24) in liver and skeletal muscle and of lipolysis in fat (25). The seminal studies of Sutherland and DeDuve (26) demonstrated that the glycogenolytic and lipolytic actions of glucagon in liver and fat, respectively, were mediated by the stimulation of the formation of the cellular "second messenger" cAMP. The development by Unger et al. (27) of a radioimmunoassay specific for the detection of glucagon in blood plasma paved the way for numerous cellular and physiologic studies showing that glucagon is a hormone critical for the maintenance of blood glucose levels during fasting (28,29). Furthermore, it was soon established that individuals with diabetes have inappropriately elevated levels of glucagon in the circulation, thereby potentially worsening the physiologic derangements of diabetes by driving the overproduction of glucose by the liver (i.e., increasing hepatic glucose output, and raising blood glucose levels) (28,29). The access to a glucagon-specific antiserum and resultant radioimmunoassay also led to the definitive identification of the α-cells of the pancreatic islets as the source of the production of glucagon; the identification of large, immunoreactive, forms of glucagon in the circulation, known then as glucagon-like immunoactivities (GLIs); and the expression of proglucagons in the L cells of the intestine (1).

Chemistry and Structure of Glucagon

Glucagon was crystallized in 1953 (30), and its amino acid sequence was determined in 1957 (22). X-ray analyses of crystallized glucagon provide a tentative structure of the hormone, in which the N-terminal and C-terminal groups consist of α-helices and are in close proximity by virtue of a "hairpin" bend in the molecule (31). However, it is uncertain whether glucagon in solution or bound to its receptor assumes the same secondary structure as it displays in a crystal. Solution nuclear magnetic resonance (NMR) studies are consistent with a largely unstructured and flexible chain (32). Both in crystals and in solution at high concentrations, glucagon self-aggregates in the form of trimers (32). Structure-function studies of N-terminal– and C-terminal–truncated glucagon peptides provide relatively consistent findings. The N-terminal domain of the hormone is critical for the activation of the cAMP-mediated signal transduction pathway, whereas the C-terminal domain is required for high-affinity binding to the glucagon receptor (33). The N-terminal histidine residue, His1 and Asp9 and Ser16, appears to be particularly important for both receptor binding and the activation of cAMP formation (34,35). Removal of the N-terminal histidine and modification of Asp9 result in the formation of a partial antagonist of glucagon actions.

Ontogeny of Pancreatic α-Cells

Although α-cells were identified as being histologically distinct from β-cells in the islets of Langerhans as early as 1907 (36), not until 1962 were α-cells shown to be the source of glucagon (37). The α-cells are one of four recognized hormone-producing cell types in the islets, which also include insulin-producing β-cells, somatostatin-producing δ-cells, and the pancreatic-polypeptide–producing PP cells. In the islets of rodents, the α- and δ-cells are located on the surface, or mantle, of the spherical shaped islets, whereas the β-cells comprise the core of the islets. Glucagon is believed to be the earliest endocrine pancreatic hormone expressed during embryonic development of the pancreas—preceding the expression of insulin (38). The pancreas originates by a dual (dorsal and ventral) outbudding of a specialized endodermal epithelium located in the anterior region of the developing gut tube of the embryonic (E) mouse at day 9 to 9.5 in the mouse (39). Proglucagon mRNA and glucagon immunoreactive positive cells are detected in the early pancreatic buds. From days E10 to E12, the buds undergo branching morphogenesis, forming a ductal tree containing clusters of endocrine cells that express glucagon, insulin, neuropeptide Y, and somatostatin. Between days E13 and E14, a major transition occurs in which the exocrine acinar tissue and aggregating endocrine cells separate into distinct compartments. By days E17 to E19, the morphologic development of the pancreas is essentially completed as the islets condense into spherical structures embedded in the exocrine acinar tissue. For 3 to 6 weeks after birth, the endocrine pancreas undergoes considerable remodeling, as the rate of formation of new endocrine cells by proliferation and differentiation from islet progenitor cells located in the ducts remains high and is associated with comparable rates of apoptosis of existing older endocrine cells.

Regulation of Glucagon Secretion

In the absence of ketosis, glucose is the obligate fuel used by the brain (40). Because the brain cannot synthesize glucose and only has enough glycogen stores to last a few minutes, the glucose required by the brain to maintain viability must be provided by the circulation. The importance of the maintenance of adequate blood glucose levels has resulted in the evolution of insulin counterregulatory hormones, among which glucagon is critical. Impaired formation and action of glucagon results in hypoglycemia. Insulin and glucagon are physiologic antagonists; insulin removes glucose from the circulation by stimulating uptake of glucose into liver, muscle, and fat during meals, whereas glucagon stimulates the formation and release of glucose into the circulation, particularly by the liver. Thus, in direct contrast to insulin secretion, glucagon secretion is increased during periods of fasting and is suppressed by elevated plasma levels of glucose. The balanced counteractions of insulin and glucagon maintain blood glucose levels in a relatively narrow range (~120 mg/dL during feeding and 60 mg/dL during fasting).

The most effective regulator of glucagon secretion is glucose, which suppresses glucagon secretion. However, certain amino acids produced by the digestion of proteins, such as arginine, stimulate glucagon secretion. Notably, carnivores, such as canines, have α-cells in their stomachs, suggesting an adaptive mechanism to provide glucagon early during the digestion of a high-protein meal to defend against insulin-induced hypoglycemia (41). Whether orally ingested fat affects glucagon secretion is unclear, although elevated plasma levels of free fatty acids reduce plasma concentrations of glucagon and inhibit the release of glucagon from the perfused rat pancreas (42). Several hormones regulate α-cell functions and coordinate the secretion of glucagon during changes in nutrient availability. These include the gastrointestinal hormones GLP-1 (5) and GIP (43) and the pancreatic-islet hormones insulin and somatostatin (44). In conditions of metabolic stress, such as hypoglycemia, additional hormones are released (e.g., growth hormone, catecholamines, glucocorticoids, and endorphins) all of which augment the secretion and actions of glucagon on peripheral tissues to ensure the maintenance of adequate blood glucose levels. Glucopenic stress also activates parasympathetic autonomic neural input to the islets that enhances glucagon secretion (45).

The intracellular signaling mechanisms within α-cells that culminate in the secretion of glucagon are complex. In situ hybridization studies of rat α-cells have shown the presence of the mRNAs encoding the K_{ATP} channel subunits Kir6.2 and SUR1 (46). Electrophysiologic studies of mouse α-cells in intact islets have determined that, although the expression of ion channels on α-cells is somewhat similar to that of β-cells and δ-cells, responses to glucose differ. α-Cells are distinguished from β-cells and δ-cells by the presence of a large tetrodotoxin-sensitive Na^+ current, a triethylamine-resistant K^+ current, and two kinetically separable Ca^{2+} currents: low- (T-type) and high-threshold (L-type) Ca^{2+} channels. In contrast to β-cells, α-cells are electrically silent in the presence of insulin-releasing glucose concentrations. The action potentials generated in the absence of glucose are inhibited by tetrodotoxin, nifedipine, and tolbutamide (47). These findings suggest that the electrical activity in and secretion of glucagon from α-cells is dependent on the generation of Na^+-dependent action potentials. Furthermore, the K_{ATP} channel opener diazoxide inhibits the electrical activity and increases the whole-cell K^+ conductance leading to glucagon secretion (46). Thus, glucagon secretion depends on a low activity of K_{ATP} to maintain sufficient negativity of membrane potential to prevent voltage-dependent inactivation of voltage-gated membrane currents. It was postulated that glucose inhibits glucagon release by depolarizing the α-cell, with resultant inactivation of the ion channels that participate in the generation of action potentials (47).

Metabolism and Degradation of Glucagon

Glucagon is cleared relatively rapidly from the circulation, with a half-life of about 5 minutes [metabolic clearance rate (MCR) ~10 $mL \cdot kg^{-1} \cdot min^{-1}$] (48). Both the kidney and the liver remove glucagon from the circulation, accounting for 30% and 20% of disposal, respectively. Notably, the remaining 50% of glucagon is destroyed in the circulation by enzymes, including serine and cysteine proteases, cathepsin B, and primarily DPP-IV, which cleave glucagon into proteolytic fragments. Not all cleavages of glucagon are in the pathway for its disposal. Cleavage after arginines 17 and 18 by an endopeptidase isolated from rat liver membranes results in the formation of glucagon 19–29, so-called *miniglucagon* (49). Remarkably, miniglucagon was found to be a highly potent activator of Ca^{2+} channels in heart and liver cells (49). In heart cells it stimulates the accumulation of Ca^{2+} into sarcoplasmic reticular stores, which are targets for Ca^{2+}-induced Ca^{2+} release by glucagon. Unlike glucagon, miniglucagon does not activate adenylyl cyclase. The cAMP-independent actions of miniglucagon in heart cells are mediated by the release of arachidonic acid, which acts synergistically with glucagon-induced formation of cAMP to trigger inotropic responses (50). There is also evidence that miniglucagon can inhibit glucose-induced insulin secretion from β-cells at picomolar levels (51). The physiologic roles of other potentially biologically relevant truncated glucagon peptides remain to be elucidated.

Physiologic Actions of Glucagon

The most important physiologic action of glucagon occurs during the postabsorptive and fasting states. Through its actions on key enzymes, glucagon induces glycogenolysis, gluconeogenesis, and ketogenesis by the liver, and, to some extent, lipolysis in adipose tissue and glycogenolysis in muscle to mobilize stored energy. In the fasting state, the liver is the essential organ that provides glucose fuel to the brain. In humans the brain requires (utilizes) ~6 g of glucose per hour, whereas all other tissues utilize ~4 g of glucose per hour in the resting state. Collectively, the liver must provide ~10 g of glucose per hour to maintain euglycemia. The actions of glucagon on the liver account for ~75% of the glucose production in the fasting state. Additional fuel is derived from the mobilization of fatty acids from adipose tissue metabolized in the liver to ketone bodies. This process is particularly important during periods of stress or starvation, as these ketones can be used by tissues, particularly the brain, to generate ATP. Other important mediators of this response include catecholamines, growth hormone, and glucocorticoids. The central nervous system senses glucopenia and, in response, triggers neural–sympathoadrenal hormones to counteract hypoglycemia. The ventromedial hypothalamus is proposed to be an important sensor of hypoglycemia and to initiate neural afferent signals to stimulate counterregulatory responses by way of the secretion of catecholamines, growth hormone, and glucocorticoids (52,53).

Glucagon is a major contributor to the immediate responses of the "fight-or-flight" circumstance. During times of sudden and intense physical effort, an instant increase in fuel for skeletal muscle is required without a decrease in fuel delivery to the brain. The skeletal muscles contain a limited supply of glycogen and lipids that can provide energy for the muscles for a short time. Sustained muscular activity requires an increase in circulating glucose and free fatty acids. Catecholamines play a critical role in these fight-or-flight circumstances during which increased fuel in the form of glucose and free fatty acids must be delivered to the circulation. Catecholamines stimulate glucagon secretion and reduce insulin levels during periods of stress and exercise. Notably, the reduction in insulin levels does not limit glucose uptake by exercising skeletal muscle but rather curtails glucose uptake by liver and fat, thereby protecting skeletal muscle from potential deleterious effects of a lowering of blood glucose levels. The increase in glucagon levels, stimulated by increased catecholamines, drives increased glycogenolysis and gluconeogenesis in liver and lipolysis in fat to further augment circulating levels of glucose and free fatty acids.

Mechanisms of Glucagon Action

The glucagon receptor belongs to group IV of the "B" family of seven membrane–spanning G-protein–coupled receptors (54). This family of receptors includes those for the hormones glucagon, GLP-1, GLP-2, GIP, vasoactive intestinal peptide (VIP), pituitary adenylyl activating peptide (PACAP), secretin, calcitonin, parathyroid hormone (PTH), and growth hormone releasing–hormone (GRH). A common feature of the glucagon receptor and these structurally related receptors is their coupling to the G-protein, G_s, that activates adenylyl cyclase and the resultant production of cellular cAMP. A major component of the cAMP-dependent signaling pathway is the activation of protein kinase A (PKA), an enzyme that phosphorylates and activates the functions of many different proteins in cells (55). PKA can activate proteins in the mitogen-activated protein kinase pathways by phosphorylation of Rap-1 that activates B-Raf and the downstream targets MEKKs (MAPK/ERK kinases), including ERK P-42, and ERK P-44. In addition, cAMP can bind directly to and activate a group of cellular mediators known as GEFs (guanine exchange factors). These additional pathways activate phosphoinositol 3-kinase and release of intracellular stores of Ca^{2+}. Thus, the intracellular signaling pathways mediated by the actions of glucagon on its target tissues are highly complex.

The expression of the glucagon receptor has been demonstrated in a large number of different tissues, including not only the generally recognized target tissues of liver, fat, and muscle but also the kidney, heart, lung, brain, intestine, adrenal gland, spleen, ovary, thyroid (56), and the pancreatic islet α-, β-, and δ-cells (57). On the basis of these findings, it seems certain that glucagon has wide-ranging metabolic actions on the functions of many organs in the body. Within the pancreatic islets, the glucagon receptor is expressed in most β-cells and on a substantial subpopulation of the α- and δ-cells (57). It has been suggested that the glucagon receptors on β-cells may stimulate small amounts of insulin during periods of fasting to maintain the β-cells in a primed state awaiting a nutrient challenge and also may provide some insulin to peripheral tissues to facilitate glucose uptake during fasting (57).

Notably, the actions of glucagon may be regulated at the level of the expression of the glucagon receptor. In rats, expression of glucagon receptor in brown adipose tissue is downregulated following exposure to cold under the control of the sympathetic nervous system (58). The hepatic expression of glucagon receptor increases progressively from the first day of life to the adult stage in rodents. However, the expression can be increased under conditions in which intrahepatic glucose metabolism is activated, such as during fasting or in diabetes (59). Glucagon, acting through increased cellular levels of cAMP, is capable of downregulating the expression of hepatocyte glucagon receptors (60). Therefore, regulation at the level of the expression of receptors appears to be another means by which glucagon actions are modulated.

Relevance of Glucagon in Human Diseases

It is generally believed that diabetes mellitus is a bihormonal disease consisting of an absolute or relative deficiency of insulin and a relative excess of glucagon (61). Insulin deficiency results in an impairment in the utilization of glucose, and glucagon excess causes an overproduction of glucose. Both circumstances contribute to the hyperglycemia in diabetic individuals. Therefore, inhibition of the actions of glucagon in diabetes is a rational approach to lowering blood glucose levels in individuals with diabetes. Theoretically, inhibition of glucagon actions could be achieved either by lowering blood glucagon levels or by antagonizing the actions of glucagon on the liver to reduce hepatic output of glucose. The former might be achieved by inhibiting the production/secretion of glucagon by α-cells or by neutralizing circulating glucagon. The latter could be accomplished by administering an effective glucagon-receptor antagonist. Such an antagonist should lower both fasting and postprandial glucagon levels and could theoretically be used in combination with insulin or with agents that increase insulin secretion (e.g., sulfonylureas), inhibit glucose absorption (α-glucosidase inhibitors), or enhance insulin action (thiazolidinediones). Glucagon antagonists consisting of peptide analogues of glucagon have been shown to lower blood glucose levels in diabetic rodents (62). More recently, nonpeptidyl glucagon-receptor antagonists have been developed that may be more amenable to oral delivery (63,64). However, there are yet no proof-of-concept efficacy studies of glucagon antagonists in humans.

Excessive blood levels of glucagon are seen in rare instances of the development of neoplasms of the α-cells of the pancreas (glucagonomas). Glucagonomas are believed to originate from the islet progenitor cells in the pancreatic ducts (65). The clinical manifestations of glucagonoma, known as the "glucagonoma syndrome," are quite distinct, consisting of glucose intolerance, weight loss, anemia, and migratory erythrodermatitis (66); 60% to 80% of glucagonomas are malignant and often metastasize to the liver. The best success for treatment is surgical removal of the tumor from the pancreas before it has metastasized. Thereafter, chemotherapy is required.

Glucagon deficiency is occasionally a consequence of extensive damage of the pancreas, including the islets, caused by inflammatory or neoplastic disease. A panhormonal deficiency may occur in these circumstances. Deficiencies of both insulin and glucagon result in a type 1 insulin-dependent diabetes with a markedly enhanced sensitivity to administered insulin. Clear examples of hereditary α-cell (glucagon) deficiencies are quite rare. Two published cases of isolated glucagon deficiency describe individuals who manifested severe, intractable hypoglycemia incompatible with life (67,68). Other reports describe recurrent hypoglycemia and no detectable plasma glucagon by radioimmunoassay (69). Treatment with glucagon alleviated the hypoglycemia. Glucagon continues to be used therapeutically for acute treatment of hypoglycemia due to insulin overdose, so-called insulin shock. Glucagon also is given to individuals during gastrointestinal radiologic procedures because its actions of reducing gastrointestinal motility and relaxing and dilating the proximal and distal regions of the gut enhance double-contrast imaging (70).

GLUCAGON-LIKE PEPTIDES

History

In 1902, Bayliss and Starling (71) postulated that a gut factor(s) might act on the endocrine pancreas in response to oral nutrients, and in 1906, Moore and colleagues (72) attempted to treat diabetes by injecting extracts prepared from duodenal mucosa. La Barre and Still (73) coined the term *incretin* to describe the hormonal activity released from the intestine that stimulates insulin secretion. The concept that an intestinal incretin factor augments glucose-dependent insulin secretion was set forth by McIntyre et al. (74) in 1964 (Fig. 11.5) and further elaborated on by Unger and Eisentraut (75) to also include nutrients and neuronal pathways originating from the intestine—the so-called enteroinsular axis (Fig. 11.6). For a hormone to be considered an incretin, it must be released from the gut following oral carbohydrate ingestion and stimulate insulin secretion only in the presence of elevated blood glucose levels. The first such incretin hormone to be discovered was *gastric inhibitory polypeptide* (GIP) (76–78), subsequently renamed *glucose-dependent insulinotropic polypeptide* (79). Dupré et al. (80) demonstrated that administration of an infusion of a combination of a semipurified preparation of GIP and glucose into human volunteers stimulated the release of more insulin than did the infusion of glucose alone. Thus, GIP was definitively identified as an intestinal incretin hormone that stimulates insulin release in a glucose-dependent manner. However, subsequent studies using immunoneutralization of GIP with anti-GIP sera indicated that meal-stimulated intestinally derived hormone(s) other than GIP contributed substantially to the incretin effect (81). These findings led to the identification of GLP-1 as the "missing" incretin. GLP-1 was

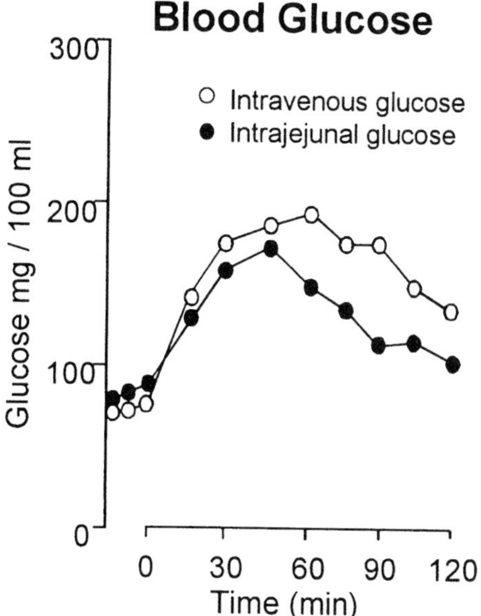

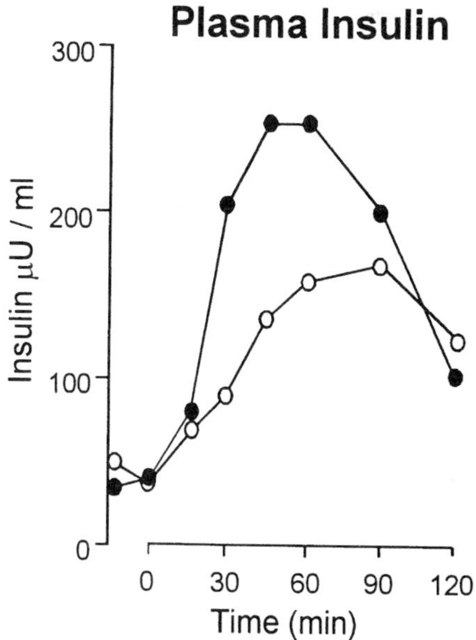

Figure 11.5. Demonstration of the incretin concept. Blood glucose and insulin responses after either intravenous or intrajejunal glucose infusion in healthy subjects. Although plasma glucose levels after intravenous glucose infusion were higher than those after intrajejunal glucose infusion, the latter generated a larger insulin response. On the basis of these results, McIntyre et al. suggested that a humoral substance was released from the jejunum during glucose absorption, acting in concert with glucose to stimulate insulin release from pancreatic β-cells. (Reprinted with permission from Elsevier. From McIntyre N, Holsworth DC, Turner DS. New interpretation of oral glucose tolerance. *Lancet* 1964;2:20–21.)

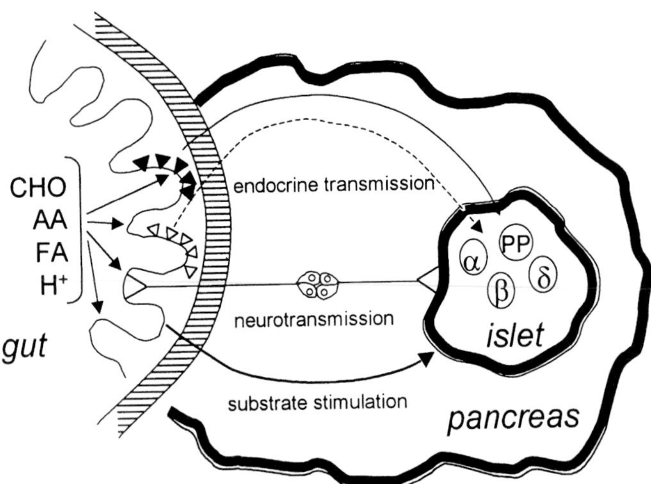

Figure 11.6. The enteroinsular axis. After nutrients are ingested, secretion of hormone from different cell types of the pancreatic islets may be modified by one or more modalities: endocrine transmission; neurotransmission; and direct substrate stimulation. (From Creutzfeldt W. The incretin concept today. *Diabetologia* 1979;16:75–85, with permission. Copyright 1979 by Springer-Verlag.)

first discovered by the cloning of anglerfish preproglucagon complementary DNAs (cDNAs) expressed in the pancreas and the intestine (82). The decoding of the protein-coding sequence of the anglerfish preproglucagon-I cDNA revealed a sequence resembling GIP. This finding led to the postulation that the anglerfish glucagon-related peptide (GRP), resembling GIP, would be a glucagon-like insulinotropic peptide and thus would fulfill the criteria required for an intestinal incretin (82). Mammalian GLP-1s were subsequently cloned (83,84) and found to be insulinotropic in a glucose-dependent manner (85) and released upon ingestion of nutrients (86), thereby fulfilling the criteria of an incretin.

Chemistry and Structure of Glucagon-like Peptide-1

GLP-1 appears to have a structure similar to that of glucagon. When bound to a dodecylphosphocholine micelle, GLP-1 consists of an N-terminal random coil segment (residues 1–7), two helical segments (7–14 and 18–29), and a linker region (15–17) (87). Most of the peptide appears to be necessary for full biologic activity. Thus GLP-1, like glucagon, appears to be folded like a hairpin such that the N- and C-termini must be adjacent to each other to exert optimal biologic actions. Truncation at either the N- or C-terminus drastically reduces biologic activity. Amino acid substitutions throughout the molecule have also identified residues 1 (His), 4 (Gly), 6 (Phe), 7 (Thr), 9 (Asp), 22 (Phe), and 23 (Ile) as important for the binding affinity and biologic activity of GLP-1. These observations explain the difficulty in identifying smaller fragments of GLP-1 that retain potent insulinotropic activity.

Ontogeny of L Cells

The L cells of the intestine that produce proglucagon are reportedly the second most abundant population of endocrine cells in the intestine, outnumbered only by the enterochromaffin cells. They are distributed throughout the distal jejunum, ileum, and colon and have a high density in the rectum. This distribution of L cells is largely distinct from that of the K cells that produce and secrete GIP, which are located predominantly in the stomach, duodenum, and proximal jejunum. The L cells reside throughout the intestinal villi and in the crypts of Lieberkühn. The intestinal L cells are morphologically distinct from the α-cells of the endocrine pancreas (88). The L cells are flask-shaped and open-type. The microvilli of the L cells reach the intestinal lumen, and a domain rich in endocrine granules exists near the basal lamina. The shape of L cells suggests that they can respond to luminal stimuli, resulting in their basal discharge of endocrine granules. L cells first appear in human fetuses at 8 weeks of gestation in the ileum, at the 10th week in the oxyntic mucosa, and at the 12th week in the colon (89). The L cells are believed to arise from pluripotential stem cells located in the crypts that also give rise to enterocytes, goblet cells, and Paneth cells (90).

Regulation of Secretion of Glucagon-like Peptides

GLP-1 and GLP-2 are produced in and secreted from the intestinal L cells located in the distal small intestine, colon, and rectum. Before the processes of formation of hormones and peptides by cleavages from proglucagon were understood, the intestinal products derived from the expression of the proglucagon gene in the intestine were known as GLIs (glucagon-like immunoreactivities), as they were measured in blood plasma by various radioimmunoassays (91). The major intestinal GLI measured at that time was glicentin, a peptide consisting of the N-terminal sequence of proglucagon known as glicentin-related pancreatic peptide, glucagon, and the intervening peptide-1 (Fig. 11.1). Glicentin has no clearly defined biologic activities, and with the discovery of the structure of proglucagon, is generally believed to be a leftover, discarded product of proglucagon after cleavages of GLP-1s and GLP-2s have taken place. The development of radioimmunoassays specific for the detection of the GLPs (GLP-1 and GLP-2) has allowed physiologic assessment of the dynamics and factors controlling GLP secretion (11,92–94).

The regulation of the secretion of GLPs from the L cells is complex and appears to involve a combination of nutrient, hormonal, and neural stimuli. Numerous *in situ* luminal perfusion studies of isolated gut in experimental animals have shown that luminal nutrients, carbohydrate, fat, and to some extent amino acids stimulate the release of GLP-1 into the circulation [reviewed in reference (5)]. However, a paradox arose early in studies of the physiology of GLP-1 secretion (i.e., GLP-1 levels rise in the circulation as early as 15 minutes after a meal or an oral glucose tolerance test, a time much too short for nutrients to reach the distal intestine and colon and mediate luminal stimulation of GLP-1 secretion). The existence of signals arising from the proximal gut to the L cells of the distal gut was proposed to account for the rapid release of GLP-1 in response to ingestion of nutrients (5,95). Indeed, the presence of nutrients in the duodenum of rats can stimulate GLP-1 release, a process that seems to involve the enteric vagal nervous system as well as the duodenal hormone GIP. Thus, L cells that release GIP sense fat and/or glucose in the duodenum, which in turn activates a vagal pathway that ultimately leads to GLP-1 release. Enteric nerves originating in the duodenum may also carry the nutrient signal to the distal L cells.

Given the important actions of GLP-1 in regulating glucose homeostasis, studies have been done to determine whether subjects with type 2 diabetes have impaired GLP-1 secretion. In patients with type 2 diabetes, insulin release is not stimulated more by an oral than by an isoglycemic intravenous glucose load, indicating a loss of incretin-mediated stimulation of insulin secretion (96). However, this issue remains unclear, as there are reports of both decreased (97,98) and increased (99–101) blood levels of GLP-1 in individuals with type 2 diabetes relative to levels in controls. Additional studies are required to clarify these apparent discrepancies. Perhaps approaches that increase the endogenous production of GLP-1 have the therapeutic benefit of improving glucose tolerance. Thus, further investigation into the mechanisms controlling the release of GLP-1 in humans also is required.

Metabolism and Degradation of Glucagon-like Peptides

The rate of removal of GLPs from the circulation is an important determinant of their biologic actions. GLPs are eliminated by at least three processes: renal extraction, hepatic extraction, and proteolytic inactivation within the circulation. The kidney removes GLP-1 from the circulation by a mechanism that involves glomerular filtration and tubular catabolism (102). Thus, circulating levels of GLP-1 are elevated in patients with renal failure and in nephrectomized rats (103,104). Hepatic extraction of GLP-1 also contributes to the clearance of GLP-1 (102). The MCR (the least amount of plasma totally cleared of GLP-1 per unit time) in humans is ~10 mL · kg^{-1} · min^{-1}, providing a half-life of about 5 minutes (105). However, the half-life of biologically active GLP-1 is 1 to 2 minutes because of its inactivation by proteolytic cleavage in the circulation (106). The biologically active forms of GLP-1, GLP-1 (7–36) amide and GLP-1 (7–37) are rapidly cleaved by DPP-IV (CD26) that removes the N-terminal dipeptide, His-Ala, resulting in the formation of the believed-to-be inactive GLP-1 (9–36) amide and GLP-1 (9–37) isopeptides, respectively (107,108). Likewise, GLP-2 is rapidly inactivated by DPP-IV through the conversion of GLP-2 (1–33) to GLP-2 (3–33) (109). Therefore, DPP-IV–mediated inactivation of both GLP-1 and GLP-2 is a critical determinant of the biologic activities of these hormones.

Physiologic Actions of Glucagon-like Peptide-1

GLP-1 exerts several distinct physiologic actions, reflecting the different organ systems in which the GLP-1 receptor is expressed (Fig. 11.7). Receptors have been identified on the pancreatic islet cells (α, β, and δ), stomach, brain, lung, intestine, heart, kidney, and anterior pituitary [reviewed in reference (5)]. There are some findings, predominantly from *in vitro* studies, of GLP-1 actions on liver, fat, and muscle in which GLP-1 stimulates glycogenolysis and lipogenesis. Although GLP-1 binding sites on these tissues appear to exist, attempts to identify expression of the GLP-1 receptor mRNA in these tissues have been unsuccessful (110). This circumstance suggests that an additional GLP-1 receptor(s) may exist. Considerable understanding has accrued about the physiologic relevance of the actions of GLP-1 on pancreatic islets, stomach, and brain. Understandings

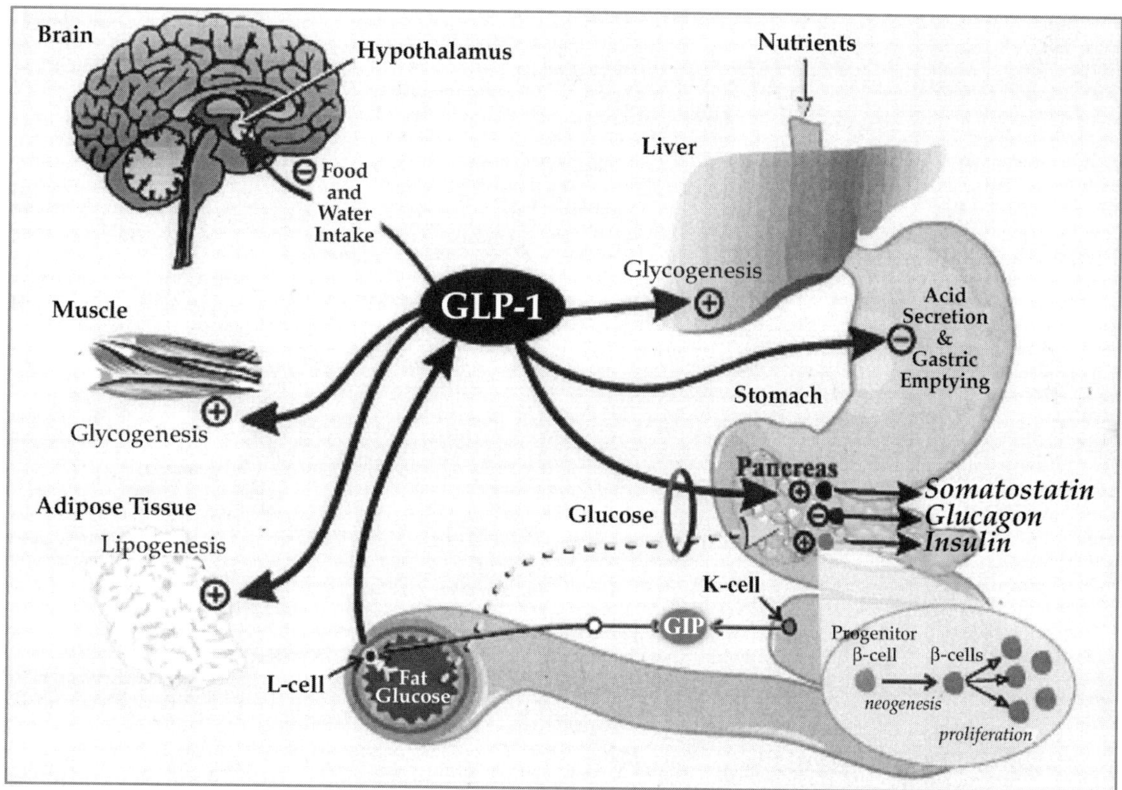

Figure 11.7. Summary of the actions of glucagon-like peptide-1 (GLP-1) showing the currently understood targets of GLP-1 actions. In the endocrine pancreas, GLP-1 stimulates both insulin and somatostatin secretion in a glucose-dependent manner and inhibits glucagon secretion. However, it is uncertain whether GLP-1 inhibits glucagon secretion by direct actions on α-cells or indirectly by the known paracrine-inhibitory effects of insulin and somatostatin on α-cells. The β-cell mass is increased by GLP-1, by the induction of both β-cell neogenesis and proliferation. GLP-1 is an effective inhibitor of gastric motility and emptying and curtails food intake by inducing satiety. Direct "insulinomimetic" actions of GLP-1 on fat, liver, and muscle to induce lipogenesis and glycogenesis have been implied but remain to be definitively established. GLP-1 increases β-cell neogenesis (*lower right*) by stimulating the differentiation of progenitor β-cells (stem cells) and the proliferation of β-cells. (Copyright 1999. The Endocrine Society. From Kieffer TJ, Habener JF. The glucagon-like peptides. *Endocr Rev* 1999;20:876–913, with permission.)

of the physiologic responses of GLP-1 actions on lung, intestine, heart, kidney, and anterior pituitary are incomplete.

The first physiologic action of GLP-1 to be elucidated, after the initial discovery that GLP-1 is a split product of proglucagon derived in the intestinal L cells, was that it is a glucose-dependent stimulator of insulin secretion. GLP-1 is a potent intestinal incretin hormone that acts in concert with GIP to augment glucose-dependent insulin secretion in response to oral nutrients. Although both GLP-1 and GIP augment glucose-mediated insulin secretion, only GLP-1, and not GIP, appears to retain insulinotropic activity in hyperglycemic individuals with type 2 diabetes (111,112). The mechanistic basis for this difference between the dual incretin hormones GLP-1 and GIP remains unknown. Not only is the stimulation of insulin secretion by GLP-1 dependent on a threshold level of plasma glucose (~ >60 mg/dL) but the actions of glucose to stimulate insulin secretion require GLP-1 or other factors that stimulate cAMP formation in β-cells (113). The interdependence of the dual signaling by glucose metabolism and cAMP generation, such as provided by GLP-1, is described as the "glucose competence concept" (114) (Fig. 11.8). The successful achievement of nutrient-stimulated insulin secretion by β-cells depends on the concomitant activations of cAMP and glucose metabolism–driven signaling pathways.

In addition to stimulating insulin secretion, GLP-1 stimulates the biosynthesis of proinsulin and the transcription of the proinsulin gene (115,116). In this manner, GLP-1 contributes to repleting stores of insulin lost from β-cells by secretion. The GLP-1 property of stimulating the formation of insulin distinguishes it from the sulfonylurea drugs, which stimulate the secretion but not the biosynthesis of insulin (117).

Recent studies indicate that GLP-1 and its long-acting agonist exendin-4 stimulate the proliferation and differentiation of progenitor/stem cells in the pancreas into β-cells (118–121). In

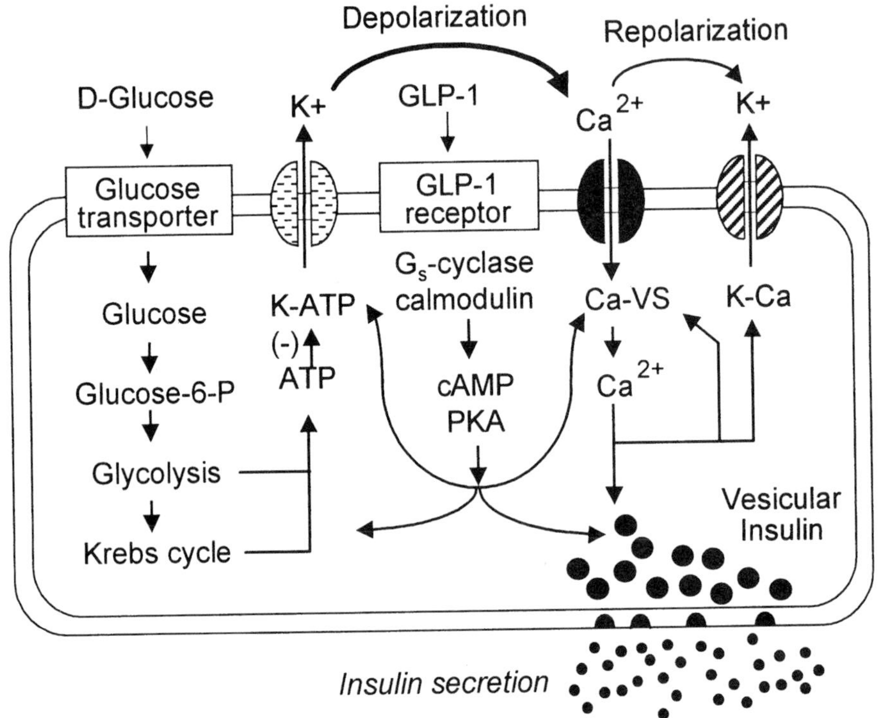

Figure 11.8. Hormonal regulation of glucose-induced insulin secretion from pancreatic β-cells. Essential features of the glucose-regulated adenosine triphosphate (ATP)–dependent signaling system are illustrated on the left. The initial uptake of glucose is facilitated by the type 2 glucose transporter, whereas the conversion of intracellular glucose to glucose-6-phosphate is catalyzed by glucokinase. Stimulation of aerobic glycolysis generates multiple signals, one of which is an increased ratio of intracellular ATP relative to ADP. Binding of ATP to ATP-sensitive K^+ channels (K-ATP) induces closure of the channels, resulting in membrane depolarization, which is necessary for the opening of voltage-sensitive Ca^{2+}-channels (Ca-VS). The opening of Ca^{2+} channels may also be favored by glucose-derived signaling molecules of undetermined origin. Entry of Ca^{2+} across the plasma membrane triggers vesicular insulin secretion by Ca^{2+}-dependent exocytosis. Repolarization of the membrane results from the action of intracellular Ca^{2+} to activate Ca^{2+}-dependent K^+ channels (K-Ca) and to inhibit voltage-sensitive Ca^{2+} channels. Each of these steps in the glucose-regulated ATP-dependent signaling system is viewed as a potential target for modulation by the hormonally regulated cAMP-dependent signaling system. In this example, GLP-1 binds to cell-surface receptors and activates G_s, a heterotrimeric G protein that stimulates adenylate cyclase. Stimulation of adenylate cyclase by GLP-1 is proposed to require the activated form of calmodulin. Since calmodulin is activated by the glucose-induced rise in intracellular Ca^{2+}, the stimulation of adenylate cyclase by GLP-1 is glucose-dependent. The production of cAMP by adenylate cyclase results in the activation of protein kinase A (PKA), which catalyzes the phosphorylation of multiple targets within the glucose-signaling cascade. These targets may include elements of the glucose-sensing mechanism, ion channels, gap junctions, and components of the secretory apparatus that are responsible for mobilization and exocytosis of insulin-containing vesicles. (From Holz GG, Habener JF. Signal transduction crosstalk in the endocrine system: pancreatic beta-cells and the glucose competence concept. *Trends Biochem Sci* 1992;17:388–393, with permission.)

rats and mice, the β-cell mass turns over every 30 to 40 days by processes of apoptosis and the formation of new β-cells, so-called neogenesis of β-cells (122). Progenitors of β-cells reside in the pancreatic ducts, in the centrolobular acini, and within the islets themselves. Receptors for GLP-1 are expressed in β-cells and in localized regions of the ducts, suggesting that these specialized regions of the ducts are a source of the formation of new β-cells by neogenesis. In the clonal β-cell line, INS-1, GLP-1 stimulates the expression of several immediate-early genes encoding transcription factors, such as *c-fos*, *c-jun*, *zif 268*, and *nur-77*, implicated in cell proliferation and differentiation (123). The administration of GLP-1 to glucose-intolerant aged rats improves their glycemic control (124). Therefore, it appears that GLP-1 exerts trophic effects on β-cells and stimulates their growth and differentiation.

The fat-derived satiety hormone, leptin, and GLP-1 exert counterregulatory actions on insulin secretion [reviewed in reference (125)]. Leptin suppresses insulin secretion and gene expression, whereas GLP-1 stimulates insulin secretion and expression. Thus, the enteroinsular axis (GLP-1 secreted from the intestine) and the adipoinsular axis (leptin secreted from adipose tissue) oppose each other (125). Notably, leptin is much more efficient in suppressing insulin secretion in GLP-1 receptor null mice (126). Conversely, GLP-1 is more effective in stimulating insulin release in leptin receptor null mice (*db/db*) and rats (*fa/fa*) (127). GLP-1 overrides the suppressive effect of leptin on insulin secretion, thereby ensuring that β-cells will secrete insulin in response to GLP-1 and glucose during a meal even in the presence of markedly elevated, insulin-suppressive blood levels of leptin. It has been postulated that hypersecretion of insulin in obese individuals may be a consequence of a desensitization of leptin reception by β-cells and a resulting loss of the suppressive affects of leptin on insulin secretion (125).

Receptors for GLP-1 are expressed not only in β-cells of the pancreatic islets but also in α-cells and δ-cells (128,129). GLP-1 stimulates the secretion of somatostatin from δ-cells in a glucose-dependent manner. It is believed that nutrient-dependent stimulation of somatostatin by GLP-1 during meals provides a short-loop feedback suppression of insulin secretion to dampen oversecretion of insulin. A possible role for GLP-I receptors on α-cells is to provide positive autocrine feedback control on glucagon secretion during fasting and/or to dampen the potent paracrine suppression of glucagon secretion by insulin during feeding.

It has long been appreciated that the arrival of the contents of a meal (chyme) in the distal small intestine (ileum) exerts an inhibitory effect on gastric motility, the so-called ileal brake phenomenon (130). This feedback, meal-induced inhibition on the stomach is believed to be due to a combination of neural and hormonal influences. The hormones responsible for the gastric inhibition are now known to be GLP-1 and GIP. The administration of either GLP-1 or GIP to volunteers in amounts that achieve normal meal-induced physiologic blood levels of the hormones inhibits gastric acid secretion, gastric motility, and gastric emptying (131–133). The physiologic purpose of feedback inhibition of gastric motility by hormones (GLP-1 and GIP) produced in the intestine is believed to be one of modulation of the rate of delivery of food from the stomach to the small bowel. In consideration of the use of GLP-1 in the treatment of individuals with diabetes, a delay in gastric emptying is beneficial inasmuch as it helps to dampen the magnitude of the postprandial glucose excursion.

A rather unexpected physiologic action of GLP-1 is promotion of satiety and curtailment of food intake (134). GLP-1 is an anorexigenic hormone, similar in actions to the satiety hormone, leptin, produced by adipose tissue. Receptors for GLP-1 exist at high density in the paraventricular and arcuate nuclei of the ventral medial hypothalamus, the region of the brain responsible for the control of appetite (135,136). The intracerebral administration of GLP-1 to rats and mice markedly inhibits feeding (137,138). GLP-1 rapidly activates the expression of the transcription of *c-fos* in the hypothalamus and inhibits the expression of the hypothalamic orexigenic hormones corticotropin-releasing factor and neuropeptide Y (139). These actions of GLP-1 in the hypothalamus are readily inhibited by the peptide exendin 9–39, a potent, specific antagonist of GLP-1 actions. The administration of GLP-1 to volunteers promotes satiety and suppresses energy intake. Although it was initially controversial whether reduced food intake in response to GLP-1 was due to food aversion secondary to delayed gastric emptying (140) or to a central satiety effect, it now seems clear that GLP-1 administered systemically to volunteers reduces food intake and induces weight loss and does so by suppressing appetite (satiety) (141–144).

The production of GLP-1 is known to occur in localized regions of the brain. The proglucagon gene is expressed in the hindbrain (rhombencephalon) in the nucleus tractus solitarius (NTS), which is the nucleus of the vagal nerve (nerve X) of the autonomic nervous system. The vagus mediates autonomic neural reflexes from the pancreas and intestine, among other organs. Remarkably, the proglucagon produced in the NTS is processed to GLPs (145). Further, injection of the retrograde tracer FluoroGold (Fluorochrome, Inc., Englewood, CO) into the NTS showed that the caudal axons of the neurons project to the paraventricular nucleus of the ventral medial hypothalamus, the site of the satiety center (146). The injection of ^{125}I-labeled GLP-1 peripherally into rats localized to the subfornical organ and the area postrema in sections of the brain (136). These findings provide an attractive mechanism by which vagal efferent signals arising from the ingestion of a meal and resulting in gastric distention and intestinal stimulation can signal the central nervous system that an influx of nutrients is occurring. These findings of combined hormonal and neural mediation of GLP-1 actions on the satiety center of the hypothalamus strongly suggest that GLP-1 plays an important role in signaling the brain to terminate a meal by providing a feeling of satiation.

Mechanism of Action of Glucagon-like Peptide-1

The GLP-1 receptor is a seven membrane–spanning G-protein–coupled receptor and, by similarities in amino acid sequences, belongs to the glucagon family of such receptors [reviewed in (5)]. The binding of GLP-1 to its receptor activates both cAMP and mitogen-activated protein kinase (MAPK) pathways, depending on the particular developmental and environmental status of the cells that express the receptor. In mature β-cells of the islets of Langerhans, the GLP-1 receptor is coupled to G_s and activates adenylyl cyclase and the formation of cAMP. The cAMP signaling acts synergistically with glucose signaling to stimulate the secretion and production of insulin. In immature β-cell progenitor cells, GLP-1 activates proproliferative and anti-apoptotic MAPK pathways, leading to the differentiation of the progenitor cells into insulin-producing β-cells. Interestingly, in extrapancreatic tissues, such as liver, skeletal muscle, and fat, GLP-1 may suppress cAMP levels and stimulate insulin-dependent glucose uptake (147). Because exendin 9–39, a potent antagonist of GLP-1 actions on the recognized GLP-1 receptor, does not antagonize the actions of GLP-1 on these extrapancreatic tissues, it is suggested that a second, as yet unidentified, receptor for GLP-1 must exist.

The importance of GLP-1 in the maintenance of glucose homeostasis further derives from the phenotype of mice in which the GLP-1 receptor (*GLP-1R*) gene is inactivated by targeted disruption (gene knockout). GLP-1 receptor null mice develop glucose intolerance and display an altered morphogenesis of islet development (148). There is no clear effect of the loss of GLP-1 actions in the GLP-1R$^{-/-}$ mice on feeding behavior, perhaps as a result of compensatory mechanisms arising during development that take the place of the inactivated GLP-1R. Nonetheless, the finding that GLP-1 null mice have perturbations in glucose homeostasis lends strong support to the notion that GLP-1 signaling is important for the maintenance of nutrient homeostasis in mammals. However, genetic analyses indicate that the GLP-1R locus (6p21) is not included in chromosomal loci carrying susceptibility for diabetes (149,150).

Relevance of Glucagon-like Peptide-1 to Human Disease

The prevalence of diabetes is increasing at an alarming rate throughout the world. Most remarkable is the occurrence of an epidemic of obesity-related type 2 diabetes, especially in children. Type 2 diabetes now accounts for 95% of cases of diabetes, although the incidence of type 1 autoimmunity-related diabetes (5%) is also rising. The currently available drugs for treatment of diabetes include injected insulin and oral hypoglycemic agents. The oral hypoglycemic agents consist of the sulfonylureas, which inhibit K^+_{ATP} channel activity in β-cells and thereby stimulate insulin secretion; biguanides, which reduce hepatic glucose output; and thiazolidinediones, which increase glucose uptake by peripheral tissues (insulin sensitizers). Without question, the currently available drugs for the treatment of diabetes are useful, but they have several drawbacks. Insulin is administered systemically rather than into the hepatic portal vein where insulin secreted from the pancreas is delivered. Moreover, it is difficult to control for the proper amount of insulin, such that weight gain is often a side effect, as well as hypoglycemia. Insulin also is believed to enhance the development of cardiovascular disease. The sulfonylurea drugs are effective in many individuals with type 2 diabetes, but their actions are not glucose-dependent, causing hypoglycemic episodes. Further, many individuals experience tachyphylaxis at various times after beginning treatment. The biguanides suppress hepatic glucose output but result in lactic acidosis in some.

Metformin is well tolerated with few adverse effects. Mild gastrointestinal symptoms may develop in some individuals but are usually transient and dose-related. Lactic acidosis occurs only rarely and when it occurs is usually associated with significant renal or hepatic insufficiency.

GLP-1 holds substantial promise for the effective treatment of type 2 diabetes, particularly obesity-related diabetes, so-called adipogenic diabetes or diabesity, and may prove effective in the treatment of type 1 diabetes. The desirable and potentially beneficial actions of GLP-1 for the treatment of diabetes are listed in Table 11.1. Like the sulfonylureas, GLP-1 stimulates the secretion of insulin from the β-cells of the pancreas but, unlike sulfonylureas, also stimulates the biosynthesis of insulin. Moreover, the actions of GLP-1 are glucose-dependent. When the blood sugar levels fall below 50 mg/dL, the insulinotropic actions of GLP-1 are lost, thereby avoiding the development of hypoglycemia. GLP-1 also suppresses the secretion of glucagon by the α-cells of the pancreas, thereby inhibiting hepatic glucose output and leading to an enhancement of glycemic control. Other desirable actions of GLP-1 are to delay gastric emptying, thereby dampening postprandial hyperglycemic excursions, and to promote satiety and inhibit energy intake, perhaps preventing weight gain and encouraging weight loss. GLP-1 also augments insulin-stimulated glucose uptake by peripheral tissues (i.e., increases insulin sensitivity) and promotes the growth and differentiation of pancreatic β-cells to increase β-cell mass.

In practice, both subjects with type 2 and type 1 diabetes have been treated successfully with GLP-1 in clinical experimental studies. GLP-1 administered intravenously, subcutaneously, and as oral buccal tablets for periods of several days to 4 weeks lowered blood glucose levels in individuals with type 2 diabetes. An example of the efficacy of GLP-1 in lowering plasma glucose levels in subjects with type 2 diabetes is shown in Fig. 11.9. A 19-hour continuous infusion of GLP-1 beginning at 22:00 effectively lowered elevated plasma glucose to normal within 2 hours after initiation of the infusion and maintained normal levels, both basal and prandial, throughout the next day (151). The blood glucose–lowering effects of GLP-1 administered to individuals with type 1 diabetes who have no functional β-cells, as determined by the absence of circulating C-peptide, is attributable to the GLP-1–mediated inhibition of glucagon secretion and pursuant reduction in hepatic glucose

TABLE 11.1. Actions of Glucagon-like Peptide-1

Stimulates glucose-dependent insulin secretion and synthesis
Promotes β-cell neogenesis and proliferation
Improves glucose disposal
Suppresses glucagon secretion
Delays gastric emptying
Reduces food intake

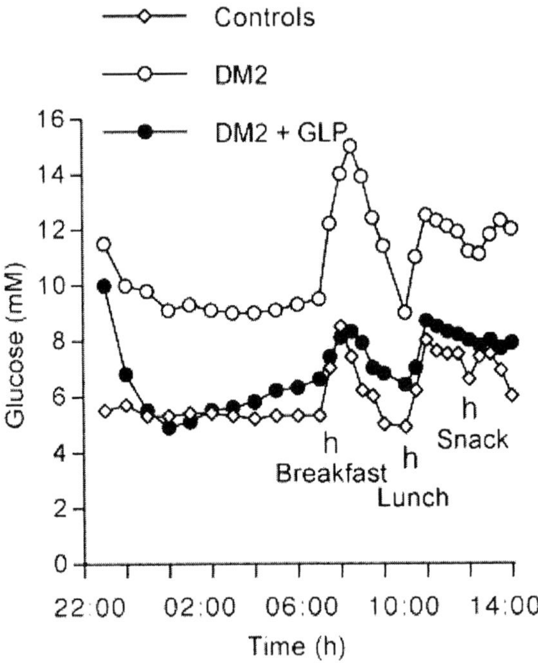

Figure 11.9. Mean diurnal plasma glucose responses in subjects with type 2 diabetes (DM2) in response to continuous 19-hour infusions of saline *(open circle)* or GLP-1 *(closed circle)* compared with subjects without diabetes *(open diamond)*. Note that the administration of GLP-1 "normalizes" both the fasting and prandial (meals) plasma glucose levels. (From Rachmen J, Barrow RB, Levy JC, et al. Near-normalisation of diurnal glucose concentrations by continuous administration of glucagonlike peptide-1 (GLP-1) in subjects with NIDDM. *Diabetologia* 1997;40: 205–211, with permission. Copyright 1997 by Springer-Verlag.)

output, delay of gastric emptying, and consequent dampening of postprandial hyperglycemic excursions and augmentation of glucose uptake by peripheral tissues. Long-term clinical trials of the efficacy of GLP-1 as a treatment of type 2 and type 1 diabetes are under way. Several treatment strategies are under consideration, including the administration of GLP-1 analogues that are resistant to cleavage and inactivation by DPP-IV (CD26), coadministration of inhibitors of DPP-IV activity, delivery of GLP-1 by subcutaneous pumps, development of more effective oral delivery systems for GLP-1, and creation of small-molecule peptide mimetics of GLP-1.

Acknowledgments

We thank T. Budde for help in the preparation of the manuscript and figures. J.F.H. is an investigator with the Howard Hughes Medical Institute. T.J.K. is supported by scholarships from the Canadian Diabetes Association and the Alberta Heritage Foundation for Medical Research and a career development award from the Juvenile Diabetes Research Foundation.

REFERENCES

1. Kieffer TJ, Hussain MA, Habener JF. Glucagon and the glucagon-like peptide production and degradation. In: Jefferson LS, Cherrington AD, eds. *Handbook of physiology, Section 7, the endocrine system; Vol. 2: the endocrine pancreas and regulation of metabolism*. New York: Oxford University Press, 2001:197–265.
2. Drucker DJ. Glucagon-like peptides. *Diabetes* 1998;47:159–169.
3. Habener JF. Glucagon-like peptide-1 agonist stimulation of β-cell growth and differentiation. *Curr Opin Endocrinol Diab* 2001;8:74–81.
4. Holst JJ. Glucagon-like peptide-1, a gastrointestinal hormone with a pharmaceutical potential. *Curr Med Chem* 1999;6:1005–1017.
5. Kieffer TJ, Habener JF. The glucagon-like peptides. *Endocr Rev* 1999;20: 876–913.
6. Perfetti R, Merkel P. Glucagon-like peptide-1: a major regulator of pancreatic β-cell function. *Eur J Endocrinol* 2000;143:717–725.
7. Sherwood NM, Krueckl SL, McRory JE. The origin and function of the pituitary adenylate cyclase-activating polypeptide (PACAP)/glucagon superfamily. *Endocr Rev* 2000;21:619–670.
8. Ahren B. Glucagon-like peptide-1 (GLP-1): a gut hormone of potential interest in the treatment of diabetes. *Bioessays* 1998;20:642–651.
9. Drucker DJ. Glucagon-like peptide-2. *Trends Endocrinol Metab* 1999;10: 153–156.
10. Drucker DJ. Minireview: the glucagon-like peptides. *Endocrinology* 2001;142: 521–527.
11. Mojsov S, Heinrich G, Wilson IB, et al. Preproglucagon gene expression in pancreas and intestine diversifies at the level of post-translational processing. *J Biol Chem* 1986;261:11880–11889.
12. Drucker DJ. Epithelial cell growth and differentiation, I: intestinal growth factors. *Am J Physiol* 1997;273:G3–G6.
13. De Meester I, Korom S, Van Damme J, et al. CD26, let it cut or cut it down. *Immunol Today* 1999;20:367.
14. Yaron A, Naider F. Proline-dependent structural and biological properties of peptides and proteins. *Crit Rev Biochem Mol Biol* 1993;28:31–81.
15. Hansen L, Deacon CF, Ørskov C, et al. Glucagon-like peptide-1-(7–36)amide is transformed to glucagon-like peptide-1-(9–36)amide by dipeptidyl peptidase IV in the capillaries supplying the L cells of the porcine intestine. *Endocrinology* 1999;140:5356–5363.
16. Habener JF. Proglucagon gene structure and regulation of expression. In: Fehmann HC, Göke B, eds. *The insulinotropic gut hormone glucagon-like peptide-1*. Basel: Karger, 1997:15–23.
17. Philippe J. Structure and pancreatic expression of the insulin and glucagon genes. *Endocr Rev* 1991;12:252–271.
18. Philippe J, Drucker DJ, Knepel W, et al. Alpha cell-specific expression of the glucagon gene is conferred to the glucagon promoter element by the interactions of DNA-binding proteins. *Mol Cell Biol* 1988;8:4877–4888.
19. Knepel W, Chafitz J, Habener JF. Transcriptional activation of the rat glucagon gene by the cAMP-response element in pancreatic islet cells. *Mol Cell Biol* 1990;10:6799–6804.
20. Knepel W, Jepeal L, Habener JF. A pancreatic islet cell-specific enhancer-like element in the glucagon gene contains two domains binding distinct cellular proteins. *J Biol Chem* 1990;265:8725–8735.
21. Banting FG, Best CH. The internal secretion of the pancreas. *J Lab Clin Med* 1921;7:25–41.
22. Bromer WW, Sinn LG, Staub A, et al. The amino acid sequence of glucagon 1: amino acid composition and terminal amino acid analyses. *J Am Chem Soc* 1957;79:2794–2798.
23. Cahill GF Jr., Zottu S, Earle ES. *In vivo* effects of glucagon on hepatic glycogen, phosphorylase and glucose-6-phosphatase. *Endocrinology* 1957;60:265–269.
24. Kalant N. The effect of glucagon on metabolism of glycine-1-C^{14}. *Arch Biochem Biophys* 1956;65:469–473.
25. Steinberg DM, Shafrir E, Vaughan M. Direct effect of glucagon on release of unesterified fatty acids (UFA) from adipose tissue. *Clin Res* 1959;7:250.
26. Sutherland EW, DeDuve C. Origin and distribution of the hyperglycemic-glycogenolytic factor of the pancreas. *J Biol Chem* 1948;175:663–674.
27. Unger RH, Eisentraut AM, McCall MS, et al. Glucagon antibodies and their use for immunoassay for glucagon. *Proc Soc Exp Biol Med* 1959;102:621–623.
28. Muller WA, Faloona GR, Aguilar-Parada E, et al. Abnormal alpha-cell function in diabetes: response to carbohydrate and protein ingestion. *N Engl J Med* 1970;283:109–115.
29. Unger RE, Aguilar-Parada E, Muller WA, et al. Studies of pancreatic alpha cell function in normal and diabetic subjects. *J Clin Invest* 1970;49:837–848.
30. Staub A, Sinn L, Behrens OK. Purification and crystallization of hyperglycemic glycogenolytic factor (HGF). *Science* 1953;117:628–629.
31. Saski K, Dockerill S, Adamiak DA, et al. X-ray analysis of glucagon and its relationship to receptor binding. *Nature* 1975;257:751–757.
32. Wagman ME, Dobson CM, Karplus M. Proton NMR studies of the association and folding of glucagon in solution. *FEBS Lett* 1980;119:265–270.
33. Wright DE, Rodbell M. Glucagon 1-6 binds to the glucagon receptor and activates hepatic adenylate cyclase. *J Biol Chem* 1979;254:268–269.
34. Sturm NS, Hutzler AM, David CS, et al. Structure activity studies of hydrophobic amino acid replacements at positions 9, 11, and 16 of glucagon. *J Pept Res* 1997;49:293–299.
35. Unson CG, Gurzenda EM, Iwasa K, et al. Glucagon antagonists: contribution to binding and activity of the amino-terminal sequence 1–5, position 12, and the putative α-helical segment 19–27. *J Biol Chem* 1989;264:789–794.
36. Lane MA. The cytological characteristics of the areas of Langerhans. *Am J Anat* 1907;7:409–422.
37. Baum J, Simons BE Jr, et al. Localization of glucagon in the alpha cells in the pancreatic islet by immunofluorescent techniques. *Diabetes* 1962;11:371–374.
38. Teitelman G, Alpert S, Polak JM, et al. Precursor cells of mouse endocrine pancreas coexpress insulin, glucagon and the neuronal proteins tyrosine hydroxylase and neuropeptide Y, but not pancreatic polypeptide. *Development* 1993;118:1031–1039.
39. Slack JM. Developmental biology of the pancreas. *Development* 1995;121: 1569–1580.
40. Hasselbalch SG, Knudsen GM, Jakobsen J, et al. Brain metabolism during short-term starvation in humans. *J Cereb Blood Flow Metab* 1994;14:125–131.
41. Ohneda A, Kobayashi T, Nihei J. Response of extrapancreatic immunoreactive glucagon to intraluminal nutrients in pancreatectomized dogs. *Horm Metab Res* 1984;16:344–348.
42. Campillo JE, Luyckx AS, Lefebvre PJ. Effect of oleic acid on arginine-induced glucagon secretion by the isolated perfused rat pancreas. *Acta Diabetol Lat* 1979;16:287–293.
43. Taminato T, Seino Y, Goto Y, et al. Synthetic gastric inhibitory polypeptide: stimulatory effect on insulin and glucagon secretion in the rat. *Diabetes* 1977; 26:480–484.
44. Samols E, Stagner JI, Ewart RBL, et al. The order of islet microvascular perfusion is B to A to D in the perfused rat pancreas. *J Clin Invest* 1988;82: 350–353.
45. Havel PJ, Mundinger TO, Taborsky GJJ. Pancreatic sympathetic nerves contribute to increased glucagon secretion during severe hypoglycemia in dogs. *Am J Physiol* 1996;270:E20–E26.
46. Bokvist K, Olsen HL, Hoy M, et al. Characterisation of sulphonylurea and ATP-regulated K^+ channels in rat pancreatic A-cells. *Pflugers Arch* 1999;438: 428–436.
47. Göpel SO, Kanno T, Barg S, et al. Regulation of glucagon release in mouse-cells by K_{ATP} channels and inactivation of TTX-sensitive Na^+ channels. *J Physiol* 2000;528:509–520.
48. Alford FP, Bloom SR, Nabarro JDN. Glucagon metabolism in man: studies on the metabolic clearance rate and the plasma acute disappearance time of glucagon in normal and diabetic subjects. *J Clin Endocrinol Metab* 1976;43: 830–838.
49. Mallat A, Pavoine C, Dufour M, et al. A glucagon fragment is responsible for the inhibition of the liver Ca^{2+} pump by glucagon. *Nature* 1987;325:620–622.
50. Sauvadet A, Rohn T, Picker F, et al. Arachidonic acid drives mini-glucagon action in cardiac cells. *J Biol Chem* 1997;272:12437–12445.
51. Dalle S, Smith P, Blache P, et al. Miniglucagon (glucagon 19–29), a potent and efficient inhibitor of secretagogue-induced insulin release through a Ca^{2+} pathway. *J Biol Chem* 1999;274:10869–10876.
52. Borg W, During M, Sherwin R, et al. Ventromedial hypothalamic lesions in rats suppress counterregulatory responses to hypoglycemia. *J Clin Invest* 1994; 93:1677–1682.
53. Borg MA, Sherwin RS, Borg WP, et al. Local ventromedial hypothalamus glucose perfusion blocks counterregulation during systemic hypoglycemia in awake rats. *J Clin Invest* 1997;99:361–365.
54. Kolakowski LF Jr. GCRDb: a G-protein-coupled receptor database. *Receptor Channels* 1994;2:1–7.
55. Habener JF. The cyclic AMP second messenger signaling pathway. In: De Groot L, Jameson JL, eds. *Endocrinology*. Philadelphia: WB Saunders, 2001: 73–87.
56. Yamato E, Ikegami H, Takekawa K, et al. Tissue-specific and glucose-dependent expression of receptor genes for glucagon and glucagon-like peptide-1 (GLP-1). *Horm Metab Res* 1997;29:56–59.
57. Kieffer TJ, Heller RS, Unson CG, et al. Distribution of glucagon receptors on hormone-specific endocrine cells of rat pancreatic islets. *Endocrinology* 1996; 137:5119–5125.

58. Morales A, Lachuer J, Geloen A, et al. Sympathetic control of glucagon receptor mRNA levels in brown adipose tissue of cold-exposed rats. *Mol Cell Biochem* 2000;208:139–142.
59. Burcelin R, Mrejen C, Decaux JF, et al. *In vivo* and *in vitro* regulation of hepatic glucagon receptor mRNA concentration by glucose metabolism. *J Biol Chem* 1998;273:8088–8093.
60. Abrahamsen N, Lundgren K, Nishimura E. Regulation of glucagon receptor mRNA in cultured primary rat hepatocytes by glucose and cAMP. *J Biol Chem* 1995;270:15853–15857.
61. Unger RH. Diabetes and the alpha cell. *Diabetes* 1976;25:136–151.
62. Van Tine BA, Azizeh BY, Trivedi D, et al. Low level cyclic adenosine 3′,5′-monophosphate accumulation analysis of (des-His1,des-Phe6,Glu9) glucagon-NH2 identifies glucagon antagonists from weak partial agonists/antagonists. *Endocrinology* 1996;137:3316–3322.
63. Cascieri MA, Koch GE, Ber E, et al. Characterization of a novel, non-peptidyl antagonist of the human glucagon receptor. *J Biol Chem* 1999;274:8694–8697.
64. Parker JC, McPherson RK, Andrews KM, et al. Effects of skyrin, a receptor-selective glucagon antagonist, in rat and human hepatocytes. *Diabetes* 2000; 49:2079–2086.
65. Sidhu GS. The endodermal origin of digestive and respiratory tract APUD cells. *Am J Pathol* 1979;96:5–17.
66. Mallison CN, Bloom SR, Warin AP, et al. A glucagonoma syndrome. *Lancet* 1974;2:1–5.
67. Kollee LA, Monnens LA, Cecjka V, et al. Persistent neonatal hypoglycemia due to glucagon deficiency. *Arch Dis Child* 1978;53:422–424.
68. Vidnes J, Oyassaeter S. Glucagon deficiency causing severe neonatal hypoglycemia in a patient with normal insulin secretion. *Pediatr Res* 1977;11: 943–949.
69. Levy L, Spergel G, Bleicher SJ. Glucagon deficient man: model for the role of glucagon in fasting. In: *Proceedings of the 52nd Annual Meeting of the Endocrine Society* 1970:134(abstract).
70. Kozak RI, Bennett JD, Brown TC, et al. Reduction of bowel motion artifact during digital subtraction angiography: a comparison of hyoscine butylbromide and glucagon. *Can Assoc Radiol J* 1994;45:209–211.
71. Bayliss WM, Starling EH. Mechanism of pancreatic secretion. *J Physiol (London)* 1902;28:235–334.
72. Moore B, Edie ES, Abram JH. On the treatment of diabetes mellitus by acid extract of duodenal mucous membrane. *Biochem J* 1906;1:28–38.
73. La Barre J, Still EU. Studies on the physiology of secretin. *Am J Physiol* 1930; 91:649–653.
74. McIntyre N, Holsworth DC, Turner DS. New interpretation of oral glucose tolerance. *Lancet* 1964;2:20–21.
75. Unger RH, Eisentraut AM. Entero-insular axis. *Arch Intern Med* 1969;123: 261–266.
76. Brown JC, Mutt V, Pederson RA. Further purification of a polypeptide demonstrating enterogastrone activity. *J Physiol (London)* 1970;209:57–64.
77. Brown JC, Dryburgh JR. A gastric inhibitory polypeptide, II: the complete amino acid sequence. *Can J Biochem* 1971;49:867–872.
78. Kosaka T, Lim RKS. Demonstration of the humoral agent in fat inhibition of gastric secretion. *Proc Soc Exp Biol Med* 1930;27:890–891.
79. Brown JC, Pederson RA. G.I. hormones and insulin secretion. *Endocrinology* 1976;2:568–570.
80. Dupré J, Ross SA, Watson D, et al. Stimulation of insulin secretion by gastric inhibitory polypeptide in man. *J Clin Endocrinol Metab* 1973;37:826–828.
81. Ebert R, Unger RH, Creutzfeldt W. Preservation of incretin activity after removal of gastric inhibitory polypeptide (GIP) from rat gut extracts by immunoadsorption. *Diabetologia* 1983;24:449–454.
82. Lund PE, Goodman RH, Dee PC, et al. Pancreatic preproglucagon cDNA contains two glucagon-related coding sequences arranged in tandem. *Proc Natl Acad Sci U S A* 1982;79:345–349.
83. Bell GI, Santerre RF, Mullenbach GT. Hamster proglucagon contains the sequence of glucagon and two related peptides. *Nature* 1983;302:716–718.
84. Heinrich G, Gros P, Lund PK, et al. Pre-proglucagon messenger ribonucleic acid: nucleotide and encoded amino acid sequences of the rat pancreatic complementary deoxyribonucleic acid. *J Biol Chem* 1984;115:2176–2181.
85. Mojsov S, Weir GC, Habener JF. Insulinotropin: glucagon-like peptide-I(7–37) co-encoded in the glucagon gene is a potent stimulator of insulin release in the perfused rat pancreas. *J Clin Invest* 1987;79:616–619.
86. Ghatei MA, Uttenthal LO, Christophides ND, et al. Molecular forms of human enteroglucagon in tissue and plasma: plasma responses to nutrient stimuli in health and in disorders of the upper gastrointestinal tract. *J Clin Endocrinol Metab* 1983;57:488–495.
87. Thornton K, Gorenstein DG. Structure of glucagon-like peptide (7–36) amide in a dodecylphophocholine micelle as determined by 2D NMR. *Biochemistry* 1994;33:3532–3539.
88. Ravazzola M, Siperstein A, Moody AJ, et al. Glicentin immunoreactive cells: their relationship to glucagon-producing cells. *Endocrinology* 1979;105:499–508.
89. Leduque P, Moody AJ, Dubois PM. Ontogeny of immunoreactive glicentin in the human gastrointestinal tract and endocrine pancreas. *Regul Pept* 1982;4: 261–274.
90. Potten CS, Loeffler M. Stem cells: attributes, cycles, spirals, pitfalls and uncertainties: lessons for and from the crypt. *Development* 1990;110:1001–1020.
91. Kervran A, Blache P, Bataille D. Distribution of oxyntomodulin and glucagon in the gastrointestinal tract and the plasma of the rat. *Endocrinology* 1987;121: 704–713.
92. Holst JJ. Glucagon-like peptide 1: a newly discovered gastrointestinal hormone. *Gastroenterology* 1994;107:1848–1855.
93. Ørskov C, Rabenhoj L, Wettergren A, et al. Tissue and plasma concentrations of amidated and glycine-extended glucagon-like peptide I in humans. *Diabetes* 1994;43:535–539.
94. Van Delft J, Uttenthal LO, Hermida OG, et al. Identification of amidated forms of GLP-1 in rat tissues using a highly sensitive radioimmunoassay. *Regul Pept* 1997;70:191–198.
95. Rocca AS, Brubaker PL. Role of the vagus nerve in mediating proximal nutrient-induced glucagon-like peptide-1 secretion. *Endocrinology* 1999;140: 1687–1694.
96. Nauck M, Stockmann F, Ebert R, et al. Reduced incretin effect in type-2 (non-insulin dependent) diabetes. *Diabetologia* 1986;29:46–52.
97. Ranganath LR, Beety JM, Morgan LM, et al. Attenuated GLP-1 secretion in obesity: cause or consequence? *Gut* 1996;38:916–919.
98. Vaag AA, Holst JJ, Volund A, et al. Gut incretin hormones in identical twins discordant for noninsulin-dependent diabetes mellitus (NIDDM)—evidence for decreased glucagon-like peptide 1 secretion during oral glucose ingestion in NIDDM twins. *Eur J Endocrinol* 1996;135:425–432.
99. Fukase N, Igarashi M, Takahashi H, et al. Hypersecretion of truncated glucagon-like peptide-1 and gastric inhibitory polypeptide in obese patients. *Diabet Med* 1993;10:44–49.
100. Hirota M, Hashimoto M, Hiratsuka M, et al. Alterations of plasma immunoreactive glucagon-like peptide-1 behaviour in non-insulin-dependent diabetes. *Diabetes Res Clin Pract* 1990;9:179–185.
101. Ørskov C, Jeppesen J, Madsbad S, et al. Proglucagon products in plasma of noninsulin-dependent diabetics and nondiabetic controls in the fasting state and after oral glucose and intravenous arginine. *J Clin Invest* 1991;87:415–423.
102. Deacon CF, Pridal L, Klarskov L, et al. Glucagon-like peptide 1 undergoes differential tissue-specific metabolism in the anesthetized pig. *Am J Physiol* 1996;271:E458–E464.
103. Ørskov C. Glucagon-like peptide-1, a new hormone of the entero-insular axis. *Diabetologia* 1992;35:701–711.
104. Ruiz-Grande C, Alarcón C, Alcántara A, et al. Renal catabolism of truncated glucagon-like peptide-1. *Horm Metab Res* 1993;25:612–616.
105. Ørskov C, Wettergren A, Holst JJ. Biological effects and metabolic rates of glucagon-like peptide-1 7–36 amide and glucagon-like peptide-1 7–37 in healthy subjects are indistinguishable. *Diabetes* 1993;42:658–661.
106. Kieffer TJ, McIntosh CH, Pederson RA. Degradation of glucose-dependent insulinotropic polypeptide and truncated glucagon-like peptide-1 in vitro and in vivo by dipeptidyl peptidase IV. *Endocrinology* 1995;136:3585–3596.
107. Deacon CF, Johnsen AH, Holst JJ. Degradation of glucagon-like peptide-1 by human plasma *in vitro* yields an N-terminally truncated peptide that is a major endogenous metabolite *in vivo*. *J Clin Endocrinol Metab* 1995;80:952–957.
108. Pauly RP, Rosche F, Wermann M, et al. Investigation of glucose-dependent insulinotropic polypeptide (1–42) and glucagon-like peptide-(7–36) degradation *in vitro* by dipeptidyl peptidase IV using matrix assisted laser desorption/ionization-time of flight mass spectrometry. *J Biol Chem* 1996;271:23222–23229.
109. Drucker DJ, Shi Q, Crivici A, et al. Regulation of the biological activity of glucagon-like peptide 2 *in vivo* by dipeptidyl peptidase IV. *Nat Biotechnol* 1997;15:673–677.
110. Bullock BP, Heller RS, Habener JF. Tissue distribution of messenger ribonucleic acid encoding the rat glucagon-like peptide-1 receptor. *Endocrinology* 1996;137:2968–2978.
111. Elahi D, McAloon-Dyke M, Fukagawa NK, et al. The insulinotropic actions of glucose-dependent insulinotropic peptide (GLP) and glucagon-like peptide-1(7–37) in normal and diabetic subjects. *Regul Pept* 1994;51:63–74.
112. Nauck MA, Heimestaat MM, Ørskov C, et al. Preserved incretin activity of glucagon-like peptide 1 (7–36 amide), but not of synthetic human gastric inhibitory polypeptide in patients with type-2 diabetes mellitus. *J Clin Invest* 1993;91:301–307.
113. Holz GG, Kühtreiber WM, Habener JF. Pancreatic beta-cells are rendered glucose-competent by the insulinotropic hormone glucagon-like peptide-1(7–37). *Nature* 1993;361:362–365.
114. Holz GG, Habener JF. Signal transduction crosstalk in the endocrine system: pancreatic beta-cells and the glucose competence concept. *Trends Biochem Sci* 1992;17:388–393.
115. Fehmann HC, Habener JF. Insulinotropic hormone glucagon-like peptide-I(7–37) stimulation of proinsulin gene expression and proinsulin biosynthesis in insulinoma beta TC-1 cells. *Endocrinology* 1992;130:159–166.
116. Drucker DJ, Philippe J, Mojsov S, et al. Glucagon-like peptide I stimulates insulin gene expression and increases cyclic AMP levels in a rat islet cell line. *Proc Natl Acad Sci U S A* 1987;84:3434–3438.
117. Gerich JE. Oral hypoglycemic agents. *N Engl J Med* 1989;321:1231–1245.
118. Xu G, Stoffers DA, Habener JF, et al. Exendin-4 stimulates both β-cell replication and neogenesis resulting in increased β-cell mass and improved glucose tolerance in diabetic rats. *Diabetes* 1999;48:2270–2276.
119. Buteau J, Roduit R, Susini S, et al. Glucagon-like peptide-1 promotes DNA synthesis, activates phosphatidylinositol 3-kinase and increases transcription factor pancreatic and duodenal homeobox gene 1 (PDX-1) DNA binding activity in beta (INS-1) cells. *Diabetologia* 1999;42:856–864.
120. Perfetti R, Zhou J, Doyle ME, et al. Glucagon-like peptide-1 induces cell proliferation and pancreatic-duodenum homeobox-1 expression and increases endocrine cell mass in the pancreas of old, glucose-intolerant rats. *Endocrinology* 2000;141:4600–4605.

121. Stoffers DA, Kieffer TJ, Hussain MA, et al. Insulinotropic glucagon-like peptide-1 agonists stimulate expression of homeodomain protein IDX-1 and increase islet cell size in mouse pancreas. *Diabetes* 2000;49:741–748.
122. Finegood DT, Scaglia L, Bonner-Weir S. Dynamics of beta-cell mass in the growing rat pancreas: estimation with a simple mathematical model. *Diabetes* 1995;44:249–256.
123. Susini S, Roche E, Prentki M, et al. Glucose and glucoincretin peptides synergize to induce *c-fos, c-jun, junB, zif-268*, and *nur-77* gene expression in pancreatic beta (INS-1) cells. *FASEB J* 1998;12:1173–1182.
124. Wang Y, Perfelti R, Greig NH, et al. Glucagon-like peptide-1 can reverse the age related decline in glucose tolerance in rats. *J Clin Invest* 1997;99: 2883–2889.
125. Kieffer TJ, Habener JF. The adipoinsular axis: effects of leptin on pancreatic beta-cells. *Am J Physiol Endocrinol Metab* 2000;278:E1–E14.
126. Scrocchi LA, Brown TJ, Drucker DJ. Leptin sensitivity in nonobese glucagon-like peptide I receptor -/- mice. *Diabetes* 1997;46:2029–2034.
127. Jia X, Elliott R, Kwok YN, et al. Altered glucose dependence of glucagon-like peptide I(7-36)-induced insulin secretion from the Zucker (fa/fa) rat pancreas. *Diabetes* 1995;44:495–500.
128. Fehmann H-C, Habener JF. Homologous desensitization of the insulinotropic glucagon-like peptide-I(7–37) receptor on insulinoma HIT-T15 cells. *Endocrinology* 1991;128:2880–2888.
129. Heller RS, Kieffer TJ, Habener JF. Insulinotropic glucagon-like peptide I receptor expression in glucagon-producing a-cells of the rat endocrine pancreas. *Diabetes* 1997;46:785–791.
130. Spiller RC, Trotman IF, et al. Further characterisation of the `ileal brake' reflex in man—effect of ileal infusion of partial digests of fat, protein, and starch on jejunal motility and release of neurotensin, enteroglucagon, and peptide YY. *Gut* 1988;29:1042–1051.
131. Imeryuz N, Yegen BC, Bozkurt A, et al. Glucagon-like peptide-1 inhibits gastric emptying via vagal afferent-mediated central mechanisms. *Am J Physiol* 1997;273:G920–G927.
132. Schirra J, Katschinski M, Weidmann C, et al. Gastric emptying and release of incretin hormones after glucose ingestion in humans. *J Clin Invest* 1996;97: 92–103.
133. Wettergren A, Wojdemann M, Holst JJ. Glucagon-like peptide-1 inhibits gastropancreatic function by inhibiting central parasympathetic outflow. *Am J Physiol* 1998;275:G984–992.
134. Christophe J. Is there appetite after GLP-1 and PACAP? *Ann N Y Acad Sci* 1998;865:323–325.
135. Merchenthaler I, Lane MA, Shughrue P. Distribution of pre-proglucagon and glucagon-like peptide-1 receptor messenger RNAs in the rat central nervous system. *J Comp Neurol* 1999;403:261–280.
136. Ørskov C, Poulsen SS, Moller M, et al. GLP-1 receptors in the subfornical organ and the area postrema are accessible to circulation glucagon-like peptide 1. *Diabetes* 1996;45:832–835.
137. Rodriquez de Fonseca F, Naavarro M, Alvarez E, et al. Peripheral versus central effects of glucagon-like peptide-1 receptor agonists on satiety and body weight loss in Zucker obese rats. *Metabolism* 2000;49:709–717.
138. Turton DD, O'Shea D, Gunn J, et al. A role for glucagon-like peptide-1 in the central regulation of feeding. *Nature (London)* 1996;379:69–72.
139. Rowland NE, Crews EC, Gentry RM. Comparison of Fos induced in rat brain by GLP-1 and amylin. *Regul Pept* 1997;71:171–174.
140. Thiele TE, van Dijk G, Campfield LA, et al. Central infusion of GLP-1, but not leptin, produces conditioned taste aversions in rats. *Am J Physiol* 1997;272: R726–R730.
141. Gutzwiller J-P, Drewe J, Goke B, et al. Glucagon-like peptide-1 promotes satiety and reduces food intake in patients with diabetes mellitus type 2. *Am J Physiol* 1999;276:R1541–R1544.
142. Naslund E, Barkeling B, King N, et al. Energy intake and appetite are suppressed by glucagon-like peptide-1 (GLP-1) in obese men. *Int J Obes Relat Metab Disord* 1999;23:304–311.
143. Flint A, Raben A, Astrup A, et al. Glucagon-like peptide 1 promotes satiety and suppresses energy intake in humans. *J Clin Invest* 1998;101:515–520.
144. Toft-Nielsen M-B, Madsbad S, Holst JJ. Continuous subcutaneous infusion of glucagon-like peptide-1 (GLP-1) lowers plasma glucose and reduces appetite in type 2 diabetic patients. *Diabetes Care* 1999;22:1137–1143.
145. Larsen PJ, Tang-Christensen M, Jessop DS. Central administration of glucagon-like peptide-1 activates hypothalamic neuroendocrine neurons in the rat. *Endocrinology* 1997;138:4445–4455.
146. Larsen PJ, Tang-Christensen M, Holst JJ, et al. Distribution of glucagon-like peptide-1 and other preproglucagon-derive peptides in the rat hypothalamus and brainstem. *Neuroscience* 1997;77:257–270.
147. Montrose-Rafizadeh C, Yang H, Wang Y, et al. Novel signal transduction and peptide specificity of glucagon-like peptide receptor in 3T3-L1 adipocytes. *J Cell Physiol* 1997;172:275–283.
148. Scrocchi LA, Brown TJ, MacLusky N, et al. Glucose intolerance but normal satiety in mice with a null mutation in the glucagon-like peptide 1 receptor gene. *Nat Med* 1996;2:1254–1258.
149. Stoffel M, Espinoza R, LeBeau MM, et al. Human glucagon-like peptide-1 receptor gene. Localization to chromosome 6p21 by fluorescence *in situ* hybridization and linkage of a highly polymorphic simple tandem repeat DNA polymorphism to other markers on chromosome 6. *Diabetes* 1993;42: 1215–1218.
150. Zhang Y, Cook ITE, Hattersly AT, et al. Non-linkage of the glucagon-like peptide receptor gene with maturity onset diabetes of the young. *Diabetologia* 1994;37:721–724.
151. Rachman J, Barrow RB, Levy JC, et al. Near-normalisation of diurnal glucose concentrations by continuous administration of glucagon-like peptide-1 (GLP-1) in subjects with NIDDM. *Diabetologia* 1997;40:205–211.

CHAPTER 12

Magnetic Resonance Spectroscopy Studies of Liver and Muscle Glycogen Metabolism in Humans

Roy Taylor and Gerald I. Shulman

PRINCIPLES OF MAGNETIC RESONANCE SPECTROSCOPY

Although the vast majority of atoms have no magnetic properties, several atoms have nuclei with spin properties that impart a magnetic component that causes them to behave as miniature bar magnets. Each of these nuclei spins along an axis, which is normally randomly orientated in the weak magnetic field of the earth (50 μ T). In a strong magnetic field (1.5 to 7.0 T for human studies), the axes of spin of the atomic nuclei move into alignment and precess around the axis of spin. It is from this orderly steady state that the magnetic resonance information is gathered. The atomic nuclei relevant to *in vivo* nuclear magnetic resonance spectroscopy (MRS) are listed in Table 12.1, and the sequence of events is illustrated in a two-dimensional fashion in Figure 12.1.

Application of a radio signal at the appropriate frequency for the relevant atom imparts energy to the nucleus, which causes the angle of precession to increase, effectively moving it out of alignment, usually 90 degrees to the direction of magnetic flux. The radio signal is transient, and when it has passed, the atoms move back to their original alignment and release the energy absorbed. This energy is released in the form of radio waves emanating from the atoms themselves, and the radio signal can be detected and analyzed. The two-dimensional display in Figure 12.1 is an oversimplification, because the process actually happens in three dimensions. Each atomic nucleus is not static but rather precesses around its own axis with a frequency that is a characteristic property of each element. It is the angle of precession that changes as the nucleus absorbs the radiofrequency energy.

The principle that the greater the radio signal received the greater the concentration of the relevant atoms in the sample is easy to appreciate. It is rather less obvious how it is possible to tell that a given signal is coming from, say, carbon atoms in one compound rather than from any other that may contain carbon. By drawing analogy with the resonance produced by striking a bell, some features can be simply explained (Fig. 12.2). If several bells of the same size (that is, resonance properties) are struck simultaneously, the resulting resonance will have a greater amplitude than that from only one bell, but the resonance will have the same waveform. On the other hand, if two bells of dif-

TABLE 12.1. Properties of Atomic Nuclei Relevant to *In Vivo* Studies[a]

Atomic nucleus	Natural abundance (%)	Relative sensitivity
^{1}H	99.98	100
^{13}C	1.1	0.016
^{19}F	100	83
^{31}P	100	6.6

MRS, magnetic resonance spectroscopy.
[a]Both natural abundance and magnetic sensitivity determine the ease of detecting signal from each element. The term *relative sensitivity* is the MRS sensitivity of the nucleus relative to that of an equal number of protons multiplied by the natural abundance. It is therefore an index of how readily information may be gathered from each element.

ferent sizes are struck simultaneously, two different waveforms will be superimposed. Thus, the radio waves generated from tissues in a magnetic resonance experiment will consist of many different waveforms, each coming from the ^{13}C atoms in the many different compounds. This is so because the electrochemical environment of a carbon atom in, for example, the $-CH_2$ group of triglycerides differs from that of the carbon atom in, say, the –CO(OH) group of glycerol.

These superimposed different waveforms can be unscrambled and converted to an understandable form by Fourier transformation, a mathematical transformation that results in display of the nuclear magnetic resonance (NMR) signal as a spectrum. This changes the display of an oscillating amplitude to one of separation of different frequencies of oscillation (illustrated on the right of Fig. 12.2). The signals from ^{13}C in different compounds give rise to spatially separated peaks. These are described in arbitrary units of chemical shift or parts per million.

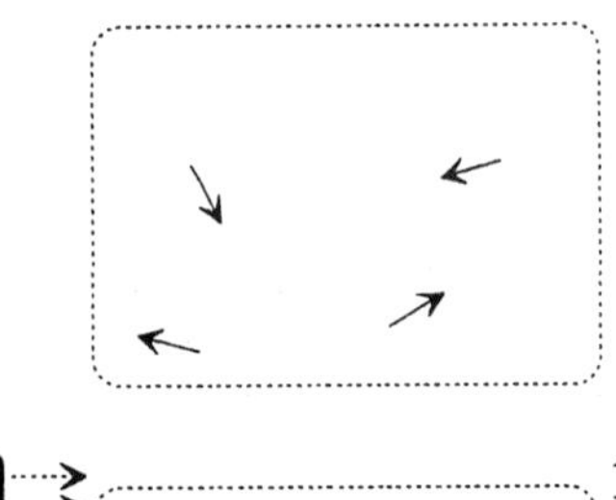

In any volume of tissue ¹³C atomic nuclei are randomly orientated in the earth's relatively weak magnetic field.

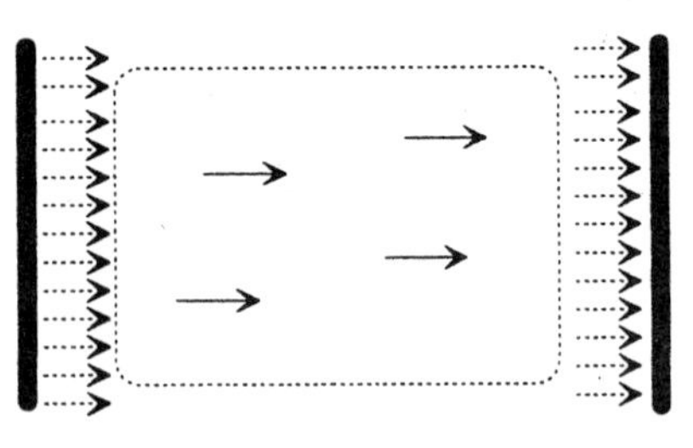

In a strong magnetic field the atomic nuclei become aligned in parallel. This change in orientation has no effect on the substance or tissue they comprise.

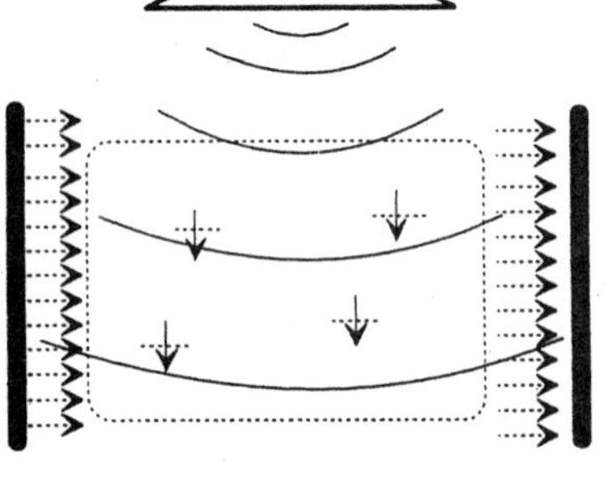

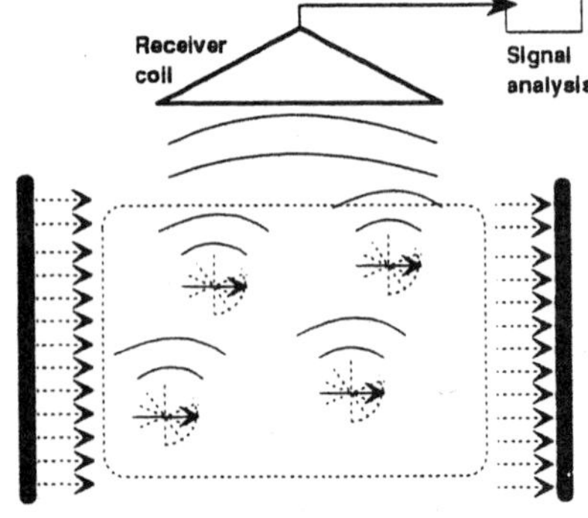

Receiver coil
Signal analysis
The radio-wave is transient, and when it has passed, the atoms oscillate back into their original orientation. In doing so they emit the energy absorbed in the form of radio waves. This signal, originating from the tissue under study, can be detected and analysed.

Figure 12.1. Representation in two dimensions of the behavior under different conditions of atomic nuclei that have magnetic properties. In the relatively weak magnetic field of the earth, they are randomly orientated. In a strong, uniform magnetic field they are aligned and can temporarily be moved out of alignment in synchrony by a radiofrequency pulse. In moving back into alignment, the nuclei emit energy, and this is the signal used in magnetic resonance spectroscopy (MRS) studies. (From Taylor R, Shulman GI. New insights into human carbohydrate metabolism using nuclear magnetic resonance spectroscopy. In: Marshall SM, Home PD, eds. *The diabetes annual*, Vol 8. Amsterdam: Elsevier, 1994:157–175.)

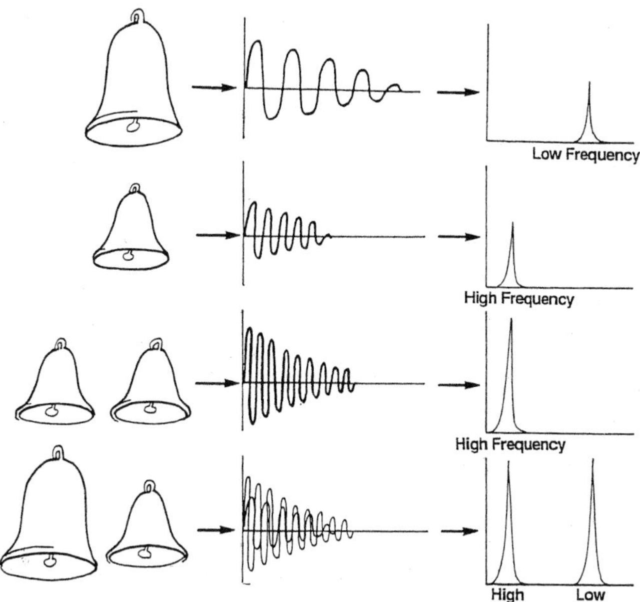

Figure 12.2. Representation of the effect of superimposing similar or dissimilar resonances by analogy with the sound waves produced by bells. A low-frequency note is emitted by the large bell when struck (analogous to the radiofrequency pulse), and a high-frequency note is emitted by the small bell. The oscillating sound wave (radiofrequency wave in the case of magnetic resonance spectroscopy) can be plotted as such or displayed as a frequency display after Fourier transformation (shown on the right). If two small bells are struck (or double the number of nuclei activated), the resulting amplitude of sound is doubled, but this does not change the position of the frequency peak, merely doubling its height). If a large and a small bell are struck simultaneously, a complicated waveform display results, but the frequency display shows two distinct peaks, the position of each being characteristic for each bell. Hence, ^{13}C atoms in different compounds, or in different positions in the same compound, will exhibit a characteristic chemical shift of frequency. (From Taylor R, Shulman GI. New insights into human carbohydrate metabolism using nuclear magnetic resonance spectroscopy. In: Marshall SM, Home PD, eds. *The diabetes annual*, Vol. 8. Amsterdam: Elsevier, 1994:157–175.)

The area under each peak is a measure of concentration of each chemical grouping. To convert such measures to molar terms, it is necessary to place a phantom containing a solution of known concentration into the spectroscope. If the 100 mmol/L solution of glycogen results in a peak of a certain area, then a peak having half that area from an *in vivo* experiment would indicate the presence of 50 mmol/L glycogen in the tissues.

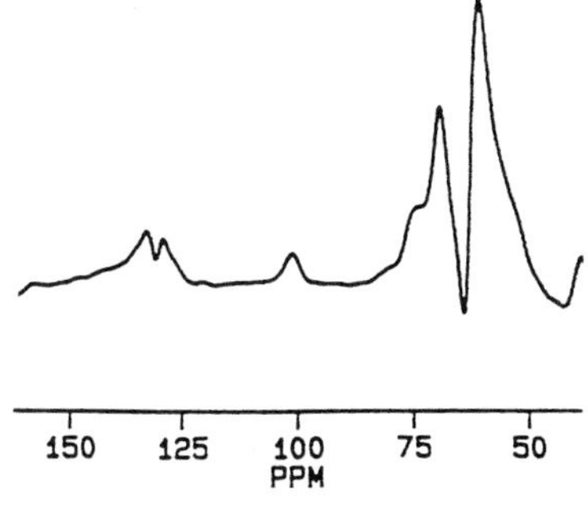

Figure 12.3. ^{13}C-MRS spectrum from the liver of a healthy volunteer. The peak resulting from resonance of the C1 atom of the glycogen molecule is seen at its characteristic position of 100.5 ppm (arbitrary units). Peaks corresponding to lipid and glycerol are seen around 130 and 60 ppm, respectively. The spectrum was kindly provided by Drs. J.-H. Hwang and D. L. Rothman, Yale University, New Haven, CT. (From Taylor R, Shulman GI. New insights into human carbohydrate metabolism using nuclear magnetic resonance spectroscopy. In: Marshall SM, Home PD, eds. *The diabetes annual*, Vol. 8. Amsterdam: Elsevier, 1994:157–175.)

The final spectrum resulting from an NMR acquisition represents the average of many individual radio pulses. Each pulse and resultant signal from the excited atoms lasts only milliseconds and is repeated as rapidly as feasible. For example, routine acquisition of a liver glycogen measurement takes 15 minutes during which time 6,400 signals are accumulated. This allows synthesis of a reliable, reproducible spectrum (Fig. 12.3).

The above explanation is intended to convey a qualitative understanding of NMR spectroscopy. A more quantitative explanation of the technique is found in Gadian (1).

Localization of Signal

If the NMR signals were gathered from the whole body, only limited information could be obtained, as the result would be an average of the signals from liver, muscle, and all other tissues. By having the whole body in a strong magnetic field, but by delivering the radio signal only to a defined volume of tissue, it is possible to be certain how much of which tissue is being studied. In practice, this is achieved by placing a "surface coil" that acts as a radio antenna over the tissue of interest. By altering the power and other parameters of the radio signal, it is possible to know how deeply the signal penetrates. For the study of liver, it is usual to obtain a magnetic resonance image before carrying out spectroscopy to ensure that the organ is entirely within the sensitive volume of the surface coil.

ADVANTAGES OF MAGNETIC RESONANCE SPECTROSCOPY IN METABOLIC RESEARCH

Magnetic resonance spectroscopy allows acquisition of metabolic information in an entirely noninvasive manner. Because multiple measurements may be made, the time course of metabolic reactions and processes can be followed *in vivo*. Use of surface coils and volume-limited techniques permits accurate sampling of the tissues or organs of interest. In contrast, biopsies are limited to, at most, a few time points, so that time-course studies in a particular metabolite concentration are not feasible. In addition, release of stress hormones during biopsies might alter the concentration of the measured metabolites. The time lag between excision and freeze clamping of tissues, but also freeze clamping per se, may result in misestimation of different metabolic effects. Artifactually high concentrations of intracellular free adenosine diphosphate (ADP) can be explained by rapid hydrolysis of high-energy phosphate or by the tight binding of most of the ADP in intact tissue to proteins of myofilaments. In addition, a delay of several seconds during tissue handling already leads to raised intramuscular glucose-6-phosphate concentrations due to increased glycogenolysis (2). Finally, enzyme activities do not necessarily reflect the actual flux through metabolic pathways.

FACTORS LIMITING THE USE OF MAGNETIC RESONANCE SPECTROSCOPY IN METABOLIC RESEARCH

Subjects with magnetic or paramagnetic metal implants of any kind, including plates on bone, surgical clips, and pacemakers, cannot enter the magnet. Also subjects with claustrophobia of any degree may find the examination unbearable. This is typically not problematic if only a limb is to be inserted into the spectrometer.

The ability to detect any compound by NMR spectroscopy depends upon its concentration in the tissue of interest and the properties of the relevant atom (Table 12.1). The hydrogen nucleus has the strongest magnetic atoms, ^{31}P having about 6.6%, and ^{13}C having about 0.02% of the relative magnetic intensity of the hydrogen nucleus. In addition, the natural abundance of the isotope must be considered. ^{1}H and ^{31}P are both effectively 100% abundant, whereas ^{13}C makes up only 1.1% of all carbon, the remainder being ^{12}C. Because ^{31}P has a modest magnetic sensitivity but the ^{31}P isotope accounts for all the phosphorus, a clear signal can be obtained from ATP, inorganic phosphate, and phosphocreatine within cells, even though the concentration of these substances is relatively small. The weaker signal from ^{13}C is suitable for studies of substances present in millimolar concentrations or greater. Hence, glycogen is measurable, as fasting concentrations range from 60 to 140 mmol/L in muscle and from 100 to 500 mmol/L in liver. Substances present in lesser concentrations, such as glycolytic intermediaries, could be measured, but only by enriching the ^{13}C content by infusion of labeled precursor.

A spectrum is acquired by averaging many sequential resonances; hence, the subject must remain in precisely the same position to allow measurement on the same volume of tissue. This is not usually a limitation with studies on adults and is assisted by use of splints to maintain the position of the part of interest relative to the surface coil. Even for natural-abundance studies of ^{13}C requiring total acquisition times of 15 or 20 minutes, comfort and compliance of the subject is not a problem.

VALIDATION OF MAGNETIC RESONANCE SPECTROSCOPY

Validation of the NMR spectroscopy method for determining the concentration of substances *in vitro* was achieved long ago by straightforward chemical analyses on the sample after NMR measurements. For the first studies of the living human body, the assumption was made that the method would be equally precise *in vivo*. However, before embarking on clinical studies of glycogen *in vivo*, it was necessary to define the accuracy and precision of NMR measurements *in vivo*. To accomplish this, a group of subjects underwent measurement of gastrocnemius glycogen concentrated by the NMR method followed by muscle biopsy to allow direct assay of muscle glycogen concentration (3). The NMR glycogen measurements depended on the fact that 1.1% of all carbon in nature (and hence in muscle glycogen) is in the form of ^{13}C, the stable isotope form. For each subject studied, six separate NMR measurements were made and three needle biopsies of the same muscle were taken. There was good agreement between the two methods across a wide range of muscle glycogen concentrations ($r = 0.95$) (Fig. 12.4). Moreover, the NMR method proved to be more precise, the coefficient of variation being 4.3% compared with 9.3% for the biopsy method, despite optimization of the latter technique. Thus, NMR measurement of muscle glycogen in humans *in vivo* is not only precise but also accurate, as judged against direct biochemical measurement. Demonstration of comparability of spectroscopic measurement of liver glycogen with biochemical assay was achieved initially in rabbits (4). In humans, this has been done for triglyceride in subjects who required a diagnostic liver biopsy, and a good correlation with MRS measurement has been demonstrated ($r = 0.89$) (5).

METABOLISM IN THE FASTING STATE

Liver

OVERVIEW

The liver contains the only store of glycogen that is readily available for release into the circulation as glucose. For this reason, estimation of the hepatic concentration of glycogen in healthy and diabetic persons is of considerable importance. By combining ^{13}C-MRS measurements of net hepatic glycogen content with magnetic resonance imaging (MRI) measurements of liver volume, rates of net hepatic glycogenolysis can be determined. The first accurate measurement on healthy young

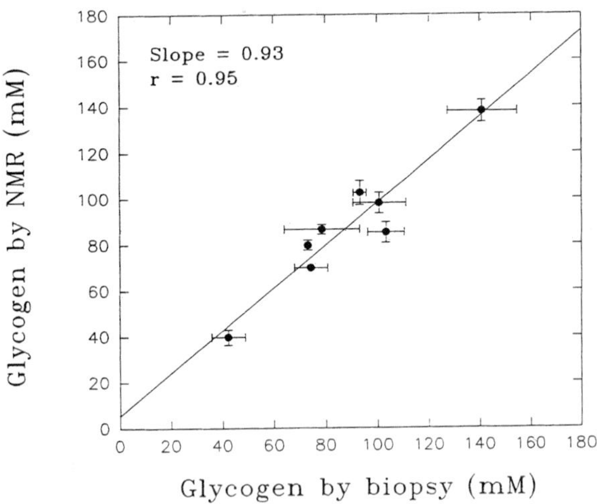

Figure 12.4. Correlation between measurement of muscle glycogen by magnetic resonance spectroscopy (MRS) and by biopsy in a group of healthy volunteers. The vertical and horizontal standard deviation bars for measurement on each subject indicate the greater precision of the MRS measurement. (From Taylor R, Price TB, Rothman DR, et al. Validation of ^{13}C-MRI measurement of human muscle glycogen by comparison with biopsy and direct biochemical measurement. *Magn Reson Med* 1992;27: 13–20, with permission.)

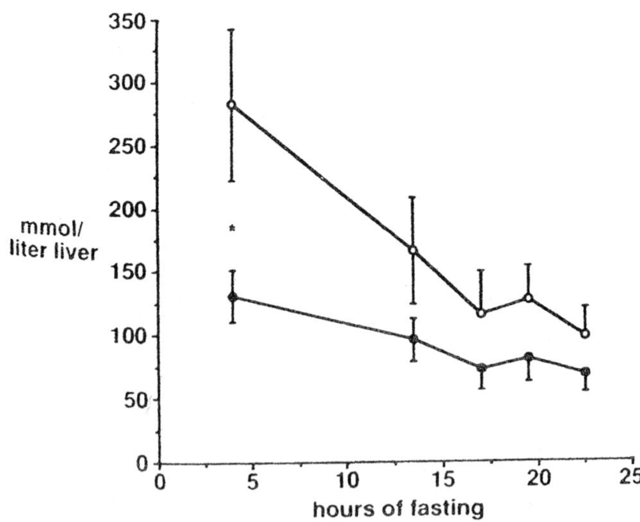

Figure 12.5. Decrease in liver glycogen concentration in healthy subjects (*open symbols*) and subjects with type 2 diabetes during a prolonged fast. The first measurement was made 5 hours after an evening meal, and the overnight-fasted values are shown at 12 hours of fasting. (From Magnussen I, Rothman DL, Katz LD, et al. Increased rate of gluconeogenesis in type II diabetes mellitus. *J Clin Invest* 1992;1323–1327, with permission from the American Society for Clinical Investigation.)

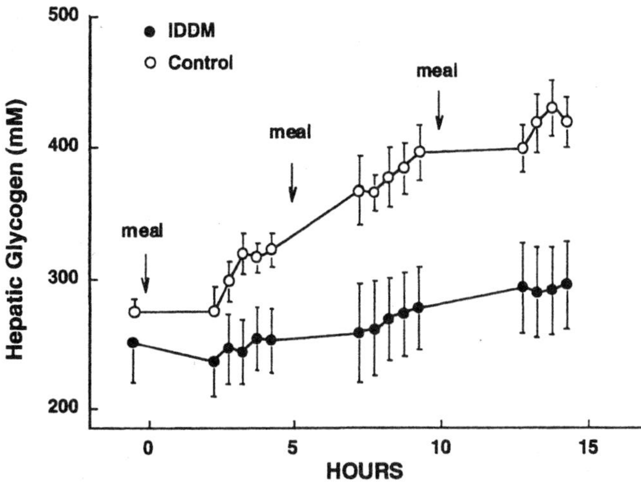

Figure 12.6. Change in hepatic glycogen concentration in healthy subjects (*solid symbols*) and subjects with type 2 diabetes (*open symbols*) during a day in which three isocaloric meals were ingested. (From Hwang J-H, Perseghin G, Rothman DL, et al. Impaired net hepatic glycogen synthesis in insulin-dependent diabetic subjects during mixed meal ingestion. *J Clin Invest* 1995;95:783–787, with permission from the American Society for Clinical Investigation.)

humans demonstrated a glycogen concentration of 251 ± 30 mmol/L of liver after an overnight 15-hour fast (6), and other studies with similar nutritional preparation have observed similar values (7). Subjects with poorly controlled type 2 diabetes (mean fasting blood glucose 14.6 mmol/L) studied after a longer overnight fast were observed to have a significantly lower hepatic glycogen concentration than age- and weight-matched nondiabetic controls (97 ± 18 vs. 169 ± 43 mmol/L) (Fig. 12.5) (8). In subjects with type 1 diabetes, under fairly poor control, fasting concentration of liver glycogen was only slightly lower than in matched nondiabetic subjects (Fig. 12.6) (9).

HEPATIC GLYCOGENOLYSIS

During the overnight period, the hepatic glycogen stores of healthy subjects decrease to around 60% of the level achieved 4 hours after the evening meal (7,9). Direct measurement in two separate groups of healthy subjects has demonstrated that hepatic glycogen concentration decreases in a linear fashion during the night at an average rate of about 6 µmol/kg body weight per minute (10,11). Higher rates of glycogenolysis were associated with higher initial hepatic concentrations of glycogen. In the overnight-fasted state, about 45% of the isotopically measured rate of whole body glucose production can be accounted for by net hepatic glycogenolysis (Fig. 12.7).

GLUCONEOGENESIS

Assessment of this process whereby the three-carbon substrates lactate, pyruvate, and glycerol are converted into glucose is beset with problems. Using hepatic venous catheterization to measure the uptake of gluconeogenic amino acids, pyruvate, and lactate across the splanchnic bed, Wahren et al. (12) estimated that the contribution of gluconeogenesis to total glucose production was only ~20% during the first 12 to 14 hours of a fast. Consoli et al. (13,14) used [2-^{14}C] acetate to calculate the ^{14}C-specific activity of the precursor of glucose produced by gluconeogenesis (phosphoenolpyruvate) to estimate rates of hepatic gluconeogenesis and concluded that hepatic glycogenolysis accounted for 29% ± 2% of overall glucose production after an overnight fast. However, acetate is metabolized in extrahepatic tissues, invalidating this approach (12,15–17). Using [^{14}C]lactate,

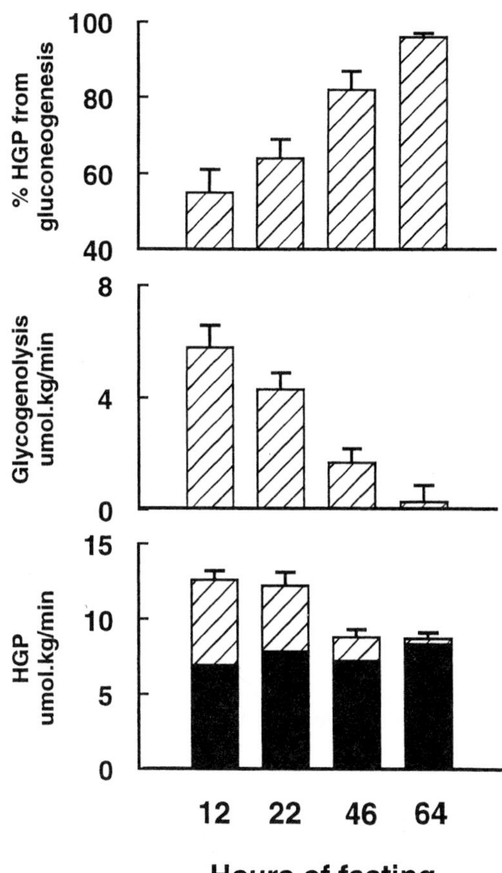

Figure 12.7. Change in hepatic glucose production (HGP), rate of glycogenolysis measured by sequential magnetic resonance spectroscopy, and calculated percentage of HGP due to gluconeogenesis during 64 hours of fasting in healthy subjects. (Data are from Rothman DL, Magnusson I, Katz LD, et al. Quantitation of hepatic glycogenolysis and gluconeogenesis in fasting humans with ^{13}C NMR. *Science* 1991; 254:573–576; and Petersen KF, Price T, Cline GW, et al. Contribution of net hepatic glycogenolysis to glucose production during the early postprandial period. *Am J Physiol* 1996;270(pt 1):E186–E191, with permission. Copyright © 1996 by the American Physiological Society.)

Pimenta et al. (18) estimated that glycogenolysis (from glycogen synthesized by the direct pathway) accounted for ~45.7% ± 4.7% and gluconeogenesis from lactate for a minimum of 18.6% ± 2.4% of overall hepatic glucose production. However, measurements of gluconeogenesis by the incorporation of label from [^{14}C]lactate are complicated by the fact that the specific activity of intracellular lactate cannot be estimated from the specific activity of [^{14}C]lactate in plasma (19).

Rates of gluconeogenesis can be calculated by combining ^{13}C-NMR measurement of liver glycogen concentration with magnetic resonance imaging of liver volume and isotopic measurement of hepatic glucose production (HGP). Net hepatic glycogenolysis was determined by sequential measurement of hepatic glycogen concentrations by ^{13}C-NMR, and rates of net hepatic glycogenolysis were calculated by multiplying this decrease in liver concentration over time by liver volume. Subtraction of these rates from rates of whole-glucose production determined by tracer turnover techniques yields rates of gluconeogenesis (6). Since the labeled carbon in position C6 of glucose is lost during carboxylation of pyruvate into oxaloacetate and during equilibration with dicarboxylic acids, contributions of glucose cycling between glucose and glucose-6-phosphate or between fructose-6-phosphate and fructose-1,6-bisphosphate would not be included in the calculated rate of whole-body glucose production derived from this isotope (20). This approach, therefore, yields a minimum estimate for the rate of whole-body glucose production compared with [2-^{2}H]glucose and [3-^{3}H]glucose and a maximal estimate for the contribution of net hepatic glycogenolysis to the rate of whole body glucose production. Seven healthy volunteers were studied over a 68-hour period, starting with a 1,000-kcal liquid test meal at 5 p.m. Liver glycogen concentration fell from 396 ± 29 mmol/L at 4 hours following the meal to 251 ± 30 mmol/L at 15 hours and to 42 ± 9 mmol/L at 64 hours. Over the first 22 hours of fasting, the rate of decrease of liver glycogen concentration was linear at around 4 mmol/L per minute. After 22 hours of fasting, gluconeogenesis accounted for a mean of 64% of hepatic glucose output (Fig. 12.7).

To estimate the maximum contribution of net hepatic glycogenolysis to whole-body glucose production earlier in the postabsorptive period, studies were performed 5 to 12 hours after the ingestion of a large evening meal. At this time, hepatic glycogen stores were found to be at their maximum daily level (9). [6,6^{2}H]Glucose was used for measuring rates of whole-body glucose production. Under these experimental conditions, net hepatic glycogenolysis contributed 43% ± 5% to whole-body glucose production during the first 12 hours after a meal. This is consistent with earlier NMR data and implies that gluconeogenesis typically contributes ~50% to glucose production even under circumstances when hepatic glycogen stores are at their daily maximal concentration (21,22). This is significantly greater than previous estimates (12,13,18). This result has been confirmed by the more recently developed ^2H_2O method (23).

Because of the methodologic difficulties in measuring hepatic glycogen content *in vivo*, few other studies have directly examined the relative contributions of hepatic glycogenolysis to glucose production in humans. Nilsson and Hultman (24) measured hepatic glycogen concentrations by biopsy in nine subjects 12 hours into a fast and once again 4 hours later and found that the rate of net hepatic glycogenolysis was 288 ± 30 μmol/kg wet liver tissue per minute. This rate is ~30% higher than the MRS-determined rate of 225 μmol/L liver per minute and might be explained by the stress response associated with needle biopsy. These workers, assuming that liver volume was 1.8 L, calculated that net hepatic glycogenolysis contributed ~57% to 67% to the rate of whole-body glucose production (24). If the data of Nilsson and Hultman (24) are recalculated with a liver volume of 1.5 L, as found by NMR imaging, the contribution of net hepatic glycogenolysis would be 47% to 56% of the rate of whole-body glucose production, a figure similar to the findings by NMR spectroscopy.

ADAPTATION TO STARVATION

Since the glycogen stores in the liver are typically limited to approximately 70 g after an overnight fast, and glucose is utilized at a rate of approximately 7 to 10 g per hour, hepatic glycogen stores are largely dissipated early in the course of a prolonged fast (6). Thus, the initial phase of starvation is characterized by an increase in the relative contribution of gluconeogenesis to meet the ongoing demands for glucose by tissues (mainly from the central nervous system). The importance of glucose production from protein is reflected by an increase in urinary excretion of nitrogen in the early phase of starvation (25). During the first 24 hours of a fast, urinary excretion of nitrogen averages 4 to 7 g/m^2 in the absence of nitrogen intake (26). This amounts to approximately 50 to 75 g of protein (~1 g N/6.25 g protein) for the average 70-kg person. Similar results are obtained with isotopic tracer methods for estimating total-body rates of protein oxidation (27). Therefore, regardless of whether simple urinary nitrogen balance is measured or a tracer method is used, the results suggest that about 50 g of protein is oxidized in the 24 hours following a meal. Since the protein content of tissues does not exceed 20% by weight for any tissue, 50 to 75 g of protein translates into 250 to 375 g of tissue or the equivalent of 1% to 1.5% of lean body mass lost on the first day of a fast. In muscle, the release of alanine and other glycogenic amino acids increases in conjunction with an acceleration of proteolysis (27). At the same time, the rate of hepatic conversion of gluconeogenic amino acids into glucose is augmented (6). The increase in glucose synthesis from amino acids is not, however, due solely to increased availability of precursor, since plasma levels of alanine and other glycogenic amino acids decline (28). Taken together, these observations suggest that intrahepatic gluconeogenic mechanisms are stimulated as well, enhancing the efficiency of this process.

The major metabolic changes that occur during the first 60 hours of starvation have been quantified by a combination of MRS and isotopic methods (6,10). Figure 12.7 draws on data from two different studies. The whole-body utilization of glucose falls by 25% from the overnight-fasted state, and the proportion of HGP contributed by gluconeogenesis rises from 55% at 12 hours to 96% at 60 hours.

The metabolic adaptations in the early stages of starvation (namely increased gluconeogenesis, proteolysis, and lipolysis) coincide with and are orchestrated primarily by a decline in insulin secretion to below levels in the overnight fasted condition and by a modest increase in circulating levels of glucagon (6,29). Insulin deficiency promotes all aspects of the metabolic response, whereas the effect of glucagon is confined to the liver. Specifically, the decline in insulin promotes the breakdown of protein and fat and thus the delivery of gluconeogenic amino acids from muscle and glycerol from fat stores to the liver, whereas the activation of intrahepatic gluconeogenic processes is promoted by both the increase in glucagon and the decrease in insulin in the portal circulation. Hypoinsulinemia further contributes to glucose homeostasis by reducing glucose metabolism by extracerebral tissues (e.g., muscle) and by increasing the availability of free fatty acids for oxidative metabolism by muscle and liver and ketones for muscle and the central nervous system.

Liver stores of triglyceride are known to be elevated in type 2 diabetes (30,31), and it is also possible to measure the extent of this accurately with MRS (5). The physiologic relevance of this for management of substrate utilization during fasting in type 2 diabetes remains to be elucidated.

Muscle

In healthy humans, after an overnight fast ~1,600 mmol of glycogen is stored in muscle [calculated from reference (32)] compared with ~420 mmol in the liver. The manner in which glycogen stores are regulated was not easily amenable to study until the development of ^{13}C-NMR spectroscopy made possible accurate measurements *in vivo* (3). By emulation of the energy expenditure of the gastrocnemius muscle during walking, ^{13}C-NMR spectroscopy was able to show that a steady depletion of muscle glycogen occurred during the initial 90 minutes. Thereafter, the glycogen concentration in muscle remained constant at about 70% of the basal level, even though the exercise was continued for many hours (33). This raised the question of whether the steady state during exercise reflected the cessation of utilization of stored glycogen or simultaneous synthesis and degradation. This question was answered by infusing [^{13}C]glucose at a very slowly increasing rate during prolonged low-intensity exercise of the gastrocnemius muscle alone (34). The gradual increase in infusion rate avoided a change in plasma insulin or C-peptide. The accumulation of [^{13}C]glucose in muscle under these conditions demonstrated that simultaneous synthesis and degradation allowed a constant muscle glycogen concentration to be maintained during this intensity of exercise. No such turnover of glycogen was seen in the contralateral, nonexercising muscle, although a very low rate of synthesis and breakdown cannot be excluded. During these studies of single-muscle exercise, plasma levels of insulin, glucagon, and catecholamines remained constant, indicating that autoregulation at the level of the muscle determined this particular aspect of control of glycogen stores and substrate utilization.

In healthy subjects with a normal range of insulin sensitivity a correlation between muscle triglyceride concentration and insulin sensitivity has been observed both by biopsy (35) and by MRS (36). In muscle, triglyceride is stored both as intracellular droplets within the muscle fibers and in adipocytes between the muscle fibers. Measurement of total muscle triglyceride relates less closely to physiologic parameters than does intramyocellular triglyceride, as demonstrated by a biopsy study of normal glucose tolerant women. Intramyocellular triglyceride correlated both with waist: hip ratio and fasting non-esterified fatty acid ($r = 0.47$ and 0.44, $p < 0.01$ and 0.04, respectively), whereas total muscle triglyceride correlated with neither (35). Nonetheless, fat stored within muscle is an indicator of insulin sensitivity, as postprandial muscle glycogen synthase activity correlated both with intramyocellular and total muscle triglyceride ($r = -0.43$ and -0.47, $p < 0.03$ and 0.02, respectively). It has previously been reported that the concentration of triglyceride in muscle of subjects with type 2 diabetes is elevated considerably (37,38). The abnormality also is present in relatives of people with type 2 diabetes (39). The effect of the elevated concentration of triglyceride in muscle in patients with type 2 diabetes on day-to-day muscle metabolism has yet to be precisely assessed.

METABOLISM IN THE POSTPRANDIAL STATE

Liver

OVERVIEW

The liver is central to maintenance of normoglycemia following food ingestion because of suppression of hepatic glucose production and stimulation of hepatic glucose uptake. Insulin is the primary signal that orchestrates the storage and metabolism of glucose (40). Although glucose is the dominant mediator of insulin secretion, stimulation of insulin secretion with meals involves the secretion of multiple incretins from the pancreas and gastrointestinal tract, as well as signals from the central nervous system (parasympathetic innervation of the β-cells of the pancreas) in response to local gastrointestinal stimulation (41). This becomes apparent when comparing the insulin response to identical amounts of glucose given intravenously versus orally (42). Oral glucose raises insulin levels several-fold higher than comparable glycemia achieved by intravenous administration of glucose (43–46). The differences in physiologic response to pure glucose compared with a mixed meal should be noted. The former brings about a decrease in glucagon secretion, whereas the latter stimulates glucagon secretion together with a much brisker insulin secretory response (47–49).

HEPATIC GLYCOGEN STORAGE AFTER EATING

Before the development of ^{13}C-MRS techniques for measuring hepatic glycogen content, data regarding the regulation of hepatic glycogen metabolism in humans were sparse. This technique allows repeated, direct, and noninvasive measurement as a consequence of the natural abundance of ^{13}C (3,50–52). Previous studies of the disposition of glucose following eating have relied upon isotopic methods (53,54), hepatic vein catheterization (55), or both (56), and estimation of change in glycogen stores has not been distinguishable from the rest of splanchnic glucose metabolism. In a group of eight healthy subjects (23.6 ± 1.5 years old; body mass index 23.1 ± 0.7), change in hepatic glycogen concentration was followed with MRS over 7 hours after a liquid mixed meal (7). The meal was representative of an average main meal of a day, containing 824 kcal (67.3% glucose, 18.5% fat, 14.2% protein).

After the test meal, the mean hepatic glycogen concentration increased from 207 ± 22 mmol/L at an average rate of 0.34 mol/L per minute (Fig. 12.8). The mean of the individual peak concentrations was 316 ± 19 mmol/L, and the mean time to peak was just over 5 hours. After reaching a peak value in individual subjects, mean liver glycogen concentration decreased in approximately a linearly fashion ($p < 0.01$) at a rate of 0.26 mmol/L per minute. Over the 260 minutes after the test meal, the average individual increment in glycogen concentration was 79.2 ± 16.2 mmol/L. Multiplying the individual increase in liver glycogen concentration by liver volume yielded net hepatic glycogen synthesis of 28.3 ± 3.7 g, equivalent to approximately 20% of the carbohydrate content of the meal.

Previous estimates of splanchnic glucose uptake after oral loads of pure glucose have ranged from less than 25% to 60% of the administered load (55,56). However, such studies were unable to distinguish between liver glycogen storage and splanchnic glucose metabolism. Most previous studies have

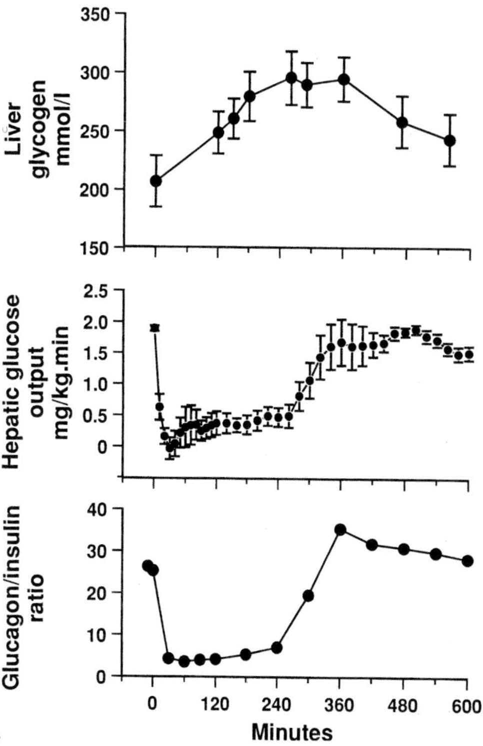

Figure 12.8. Physiologic events following ingestion of a mixed meal in healthy subjects. Change in liver glycogen was tracked by magnetic resonance spectroscopy and hepatic glucose production by the variable rate isotopic method. The plasma molar ratio of glucagon to insulin is shown as a potential controlling influence. (From Taylor R, Magnussen I, Rothman DL, et al. Direct assessment of liver glycogen storage by ^{13}C-nuclear magnetic resonance spectroscopy and regulation of glucose homeostasis after a mixed meal in normal subjects. *J Clin Invest* 1996;97:126–132, with permission from the American Society for Clinical Investigation.)

been terminated at or before 240 minutes (48,55,56), a time when absorption of either glucose or a mixed meal may be incomplete (53,55,57,58) and when liver glycogen storage is submaximal, according to the MRS data. The directly measured 20% of meal carbohydrate present in liver glycogen at peak concentration represents net glycogen synthesis and does not take account of glycogen turnover (59). Hence, to the degree that hepatic glycogen turnover occurs during absorption of meals, the proportion of the meal-derived glucose that becomes at least temporarily incorporated into liver glycogen will be greater than the above net estimates. Liver size would not be expected to exert a major influence on the above estimations, as a 67-hour fast is necessary to decrease liver size by 23% (60).

SOURCE OF GLUCOSE CARBON FOR GLYCOGEN SYNTHESIS

Early work in animals suggested that most liver glycogen is synthesized not from glucose but from three-carbon atom precursors (61,62). More recently, the direct pathway (glucose→glucose-6-phosphate→glucose-1-phosphate→UDP-glucose→glycogen) has been shown to account for 49% of hepatic glycogen synthesis in the fasting state and for 69% following breakfast (63,64). After a [^{14}C]glucose-labeled test meal identical to that used in the MRS study described above, plasma [^{14}C]glucose specific activity rapidly increased over the 30 minutes after the test meal to 87 ± 7 disintegrations per minute (dpm)/μmol then gradually increased to peak at 134 ± 8 dpm/μmol at 160 minutes. In each subject, the highest [^{14}C]glucose specific activity in plasma was very similar to the specific activity in that individual's test meal. By use of acetaminophen labeling of the hepatic glucuronide pool (63), the calculated contribution of the direct pathway to overall glycogen synthesis was 46% ± 5% and 68% ± 8% for each time period, respectively. The measurements between 2 and 4 hours postprandially were made during net hepatic glycogen synthesis and during the second period between 4 and 6 hours were made during little net synthesis but continued turnover. The observed increase in the direct-pathway contribution to hepatic glycogen synthesis from 46% between 2 and 4 hours to 68% between 4 and 6 hours postprandially is consistent with the previous observations that direct-pathway activity is greater after the second meal of the day (63,65). This also is consistent with the observation that glycogen synthesis directly from glucose occurs at a higher rate in primary cultures of hepatocytes isolated from fed rather than from fasted animals (66–68). However, 4 to 6 hours after a meal, rates of net liver glycogen synthesis are low. Hence, less than 10% of the carbohydrate component of a meal is likely to be stored as liver glycogen via the direct pathway between 4 and 6 hours postprandially even though almost 70% of synthesis is via the direct pathway at this time.

LIVER GLYCOGEN CYCLING

The possible occurrence of simultaneous synthesis and breakdown of liver glycogen has been controversial for several decades. That such glycogen cycling occurs in humans has been demonstrated by ^{13}C-MRS pulse-chase studies. In a study of healthy subjects, MRS measurements of the glycogen C1 peak were made continuously during a hyperglycemic hyperinsulinemic clamp (69). [^{13}C]glucose was infused for 90 minutes, and the clamp was continued using [^{12}C]glucose subsequently. In the fasting state, the relative rate of glycogen cycling was 31%, and this increased to 57% in the fed state. The implied autoregulation of hepatic glycogen stores is supported by compilation of data from other studies, which suggests that the higher the glycogen concentration the higher the rate of hepatic glycogenolysis (Fig. 12.6) (6,70).

NORMAL DIURNAL FLUCTUATION IN HEPATIC GLYCOGEN CONTENT

Study of the change of the liver glycogen concentration after a single meal has provided considerable new insight into normal human metabolism. The relatively rapid decline in concentration after attainment of peak levels was particularly striking. However, few people in the Western world eat a single meal per day, and extrapolation from single-meal studies to everyday physiology is unsound. To define the normal diurnal fluctuations in hepatic glycogen concentration, nine healthy subjects (22 ± 1 years; body mass index 23.4 ± 1) and six subjects with type 1 diabetes (34 ± 2 years; body mass index 23.5 ± 2.4) were studied during a day in which three isocaloric meals were eaten at 5-hour intervals (9). Each meal consisted of normal foodstuffs (12 kcal/kg as 60% carbohydrate, 20% fat, 20% protein). The early-morning insulin resistance was reflected in the healthy subjects by considerably higher peak plasma insulin levels after breakfast (107 μU/mL) than after the other two meals (52 and 44 μU/mL, respectively). Thus, in this protocol, insulin stimulation and substrate availability were provided at the time the liver glycogen concentration would be expected, from the results of the single-meal studies, to fall.

The changes in liver glycogen concentration are shown in Figure 12.6. It can be seen that liver glycogen concentration increased sequentially during the day, with no decrease between meals, such that there was a total increase of 144 mmol/L between the fasting level and the postdinner peak in healthy subjects but an increase of only 44 mmol/L in subjects with type 1 diabetes. Overnight, hepatic glycogenolysis both maintains fasting blood glucose concentration and returns the hepatic glycogen concentration to normal fasting levels, whereupon the cycle will recommence. In diabetes, the role of glycogenolysis must be of lesser importance in this process.

Muscle

Postprandial storage of glycogen in muscle has been quantitated by using ^{13}C-MRS to measure the glycogen concentration of the gastrocnemius muscle in young healthy subjects over a 7-hour period following a mixed meal of ordinary foodstuffs (32). Muscle glycogen concentration rose from a mean of 83.3 mM to a peak of 100 mM at 4.9 hours and fell thereafter to a mean of 90.6 mM 7 hours postprandially (Fig. 12.9). It was calculated

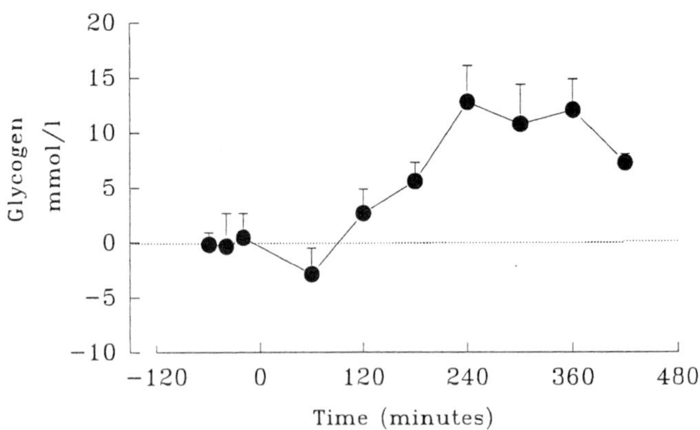

Figure 12.9. Incremental change in gastrocnemius muscle glycogen concentration after breakfast in a group of healthy subjects. Fasting muscle glycogen was 83.3 mmol/L of muscle. (From Taylor R, Price TB, Katz LD, et al. Direct measurement of change in muscle glycogen concentration after a mixed meal in normal subjects. *Am J Physiol* 1993;265: E224–E228, with permission. Copyright © 1993 by the American Physiological Society.)

from measurements of total muscle mass and estimation of rates of carbohydrate absorption that, at peak muscle glycogen concentrations, 26% to 35% of the absorbed carbohydrate was stored as muscle glycogen. The fate of oral glucose has previously been examined by limb balance studies (44,53,71) and indirect calculations based on tracer methodology and hepatic vein catheterization (55,56,72,73). These studies have suggested that up to 70% of ingested carbohydrate is taken up by muscle. Such estimates do not concur with the direct MRS measurements, possibly as a consequence of modeling problems. It should be noted that the MRS measurements were made on a single muscle, rather than on a group of muscles with associated other tissues.

Muscle glycogen concentration did not start to rise until 1 to 2 hours after eating. This slow rise was surprising when viewed in the context of the more rapid time course of arteriovenous difference in plasma glucose measured across forearm or leg after oral glucose (43,54,74,75). Hence, it may be inferred that the predominant fate of glucose taken up by muscle in the immediate postprandial period is oxidation; thereafter, a gradual change to net glycogen synthesis takes place. The observed fall in muscle glycogen concentrations after the fourth postprandial hour when glucose oxidation is likely to be minimal suggests that flux of three-carbon compounds out of muscle may be important in allowing redistribution of excess substrate for storage. The unexpectedly early fall in muscle glycogen concentration suggests that skeletal muscle acts as a dynamic buffer to maintain glucose homeostasis during acute food ingestion, preventing an undue rise in plasma glucose and subsequently permitting substrate redistribution for medium-term storage.

EXERCISE

A study of glycogen depletion following heavy exercise of one gastrocnemius muscle in healthy fasting subjects showed that the process of glycogen reaccumulation exhibited a rapid phase and a subsequent slower phase. A follow-up study using paired somatostatin or control infusions documented the involvement of insulin in the latter but not the former phase (57). The glycogen recovery during the second, slower phase (2.4 mM per hour) was totally abolished during somatostatin infusion, which brought about a decrease in fasting plasma insulin from 12.4 to 5.3 μU/mL (Fig. 12.10). This is of particular metabolic interest as it demonstrates a clear effect of insulin upon muscle at fasting concentrations. Previously, it was thought that such levels of plasma insulin did not exert significant effects on muscle glucose metabolism.

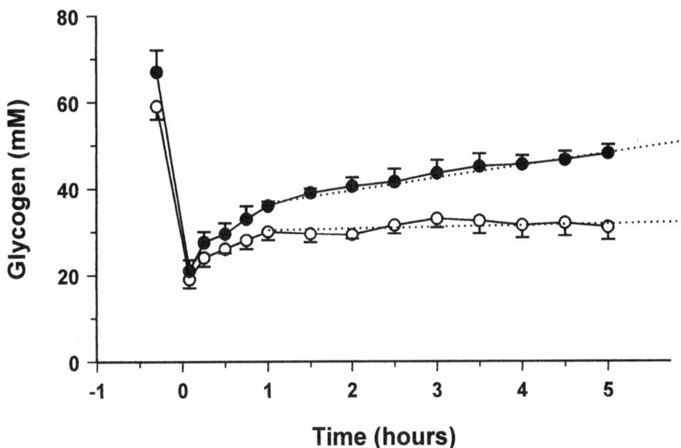

Figure 12.11. Effect of glycogen-depleting exercise and the subsequent rate of recovery of muscle glycogen in control subjects with no family history of diabetes (*solid symbols*) and insulin-resistant relative of subject with type 2 diabetes (*open symbols*). (From Price TB, Perseghin G, Duleba A, et al. NMR studies of muscle glycogen synthesis in insulin-resistant offspring of parents with non-insulin-dependent diabetes mellitus immediately after glycogen-depleting exercise. *Proc Natl Acad Sci U S A* 1996;93:5329–5334, with permission. Copyright 1996 National Academy of Sciences, U.S.A.)

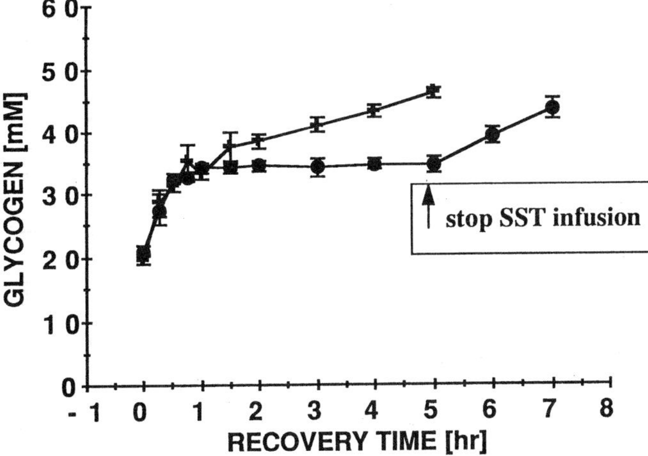

Figure 12.10. Change in muscle glycogen concentration after single-muscle exercise to deplete glycogen stores. The normal two-phase recovery is shown, together with the pattern of recovery during infusion of somatostatin to suppress plasma insulin levels (*round symbols*). The rapid first phase was unaffected whereas the subsequent slower phase was abolished until the somatostatin infusion was stopped. (From Price TB, Rothman DL, Taylor R, et al. Human muscle glycogen resynthesis afer exercise: insulin-dependent and -independent phases. *J Appl Physiol* 1994;76:104–111, with permission.)

The question of whether the insulin resistance characteristic of type 2 diabetes may affect this process of insulin-dependent glycogen repletion has been addressed by study of normoglycemic relatives of people with type 2 diabetes (76). As illustrated in Figure 12.11, the insulin-resistant subjects exhibited subnormal rates of glycogen synthesis, thus demonstrating the practical consequence of low insulin sensitivity even under the condition of basal insulin concentrations. In established type 2 diabetes, it is possible that hyperglycemia provides partial compensation by a mass-action effect of increased muscle glucose uptake (77).

During prolonged exercise in athletes, the depletion of both glycogen and intramuscular triglyceride has been quantified by MRS (78). Heavy exercise (running at 70% of peak oxygen uptake until exhaustion) brought about a 64% decrease in calf-muscle glycogen and a 34% decrease in calf-muscle intramyocellular triglyceride. The exercise capacity of people with type 2 diabetes is not impaired, and further application of MRS studies can be expected to elucidate the dynamics of fuel supply in muscles that are likely to start exercise with lower glycogen and higher triglyceride stores.

MECHANISM OF INSULIN RESISTANCE IN TYPE 2 DIABETES

Insulin resistance is defined as a subnormal change in glucose metabolism in the presence of a given insulin stimulation. Hence, it may be anticipated that specific faulty steps in the cascade of insulin signal transduction may be identified. Defects in glycogen synthase (79–82), hexokinase (83, 84), and glucose transport (85–87) have all been implicated in the subnormal muscle glycogen synthesis in type 2 diabetes. The relative importance of these steps to insulin-stimulated muscle glucose metabolism has been assessed by performing $^{13}C/^{31}P$-MRS studies to measure intracellular concentrations of glucose, glucose-6-phosphate, and glycogen in muscle of patients with type 2 diabetes and age- and weight-matched control subjects (85). Intracellular glucose-6-phosphate is an intermediary metabolite between glucose transport and glycogen synthesis, and hence the relative activities of these two steps will be reflected by its intracellular concentration. In the event of decreased activity of glycogen synthase in diabetes, glucose-6-phosphate in the patients with diabetes would be expected to be increased relative to that in the healthy individuals. When ^{31}P-NMR was used to assess intracellular glucose-6-phosphate under conditions of hyperglycemic-hyperinsulinemia, an increase of approximately 0.1 mM intracellular glucose-6-phosphate was observed in healthy individuals but no change was observed in patients with type 2 diabetes. The blunted incremental change of glucose-6-phosphate concentration in the patients with type 2 diabetes in response to insulin stimulation can therefore be ascribed to either decreased glucose transport activity or decreased hexokinase II activity.

Insulin-resistant offspring of patients with type 2 diabetes were studied in an effort to determine whether this defect in glucose transport or hexokinase II activity was a primary or acquired defect secondary to other factors, such as chronic hyperglycemia. The rate of muscle glycogen synthesis and the muscle concentration of glucose-6-phosphate were measured under the same clamp conditions (88). Although these individuals were lean and normoglycemic, they are known to be at an ~40% increased risk for developing diabetes. The children of parents with diabetes exhibited a 50% decrease in the rate of insulin-stimulated whole-body glucose metabolism compared with age- and weight-matched control subjects, and this was mainly a consequence of decreased rates of muscle glycogen synthesis. The severe blunting of their insulin-stimulated increment of intramuscular glucose-6-phosphate indicated impaired muscle glucose transport or reduced hexokinase activity similar to that seen in patients with fully developed type 2 diabetes. When control subjects were studied at similar insulin levels but at euglycemia, both the rate of glycogen synthesis and the glucose-6-phosphate concentration decreased to values similar to those of offspring of patients with type 2 diabetes. Thus, even before the onset of diabetes, insulin-resistant offspring of patients with type 2 diabetes have decreased rates of muscle glycogen synthesis that are secondary to a defect in muscle glucose transport or hexokinase activity. It can be concluded that defects in one or both of these activities occur early in the pathogenesis of type 2 diabetes.

To determine whether glucose transport or hexokinase II activity is rate controlling for insulin-stimulated muscle glycogen synthesis in patients with type 2 diabetes, a novel ^{13}C-NMR method has been applied to assess intracellular glucose concentrations in muscle under similar hyperglycemic–hyperinsulinemic conditions (89). Intracellular glucose is a transient intermediate between glucose transport and glucose phosphorylation, and its concentration reflects the relative activities of glucose transporters and of hexokinase II. Unlike the standard biopsy method, this approach is noninvasive and is not subject to the errors caused by contamination of biopsy tissue with plasma glucose or by incomplete removal from the biopsy of nonmuscle constituents. If hexokinase II activity was decreased relative to glucose transport activity in patients with diabetes, a substantial increase in intracellular glucose would be predicted, whereas if glucose transport was primarily responsible for maintaining intracellular glucose metabolism, intracellular glucose and glucose-6-phosphate should change proportionately. It was observed that intracellular glucose concentration was far lower in the subjects with type 2 diabetes than the value expected if hexokinase II was the primary rate-controlling enzyme for glycogen synthesis (89). When the rates of muscle glycogen synthesis in the subjects with diabetes were increased by infusing greater amounts of insulin, the changes in the concentrations of intracellular glucose and glucose-6-phosphate indicated that the rates of glucose transport were matched by increases in the rates of glucose phosphorylation and glycogen synthesis. These data indicate the major role of glucose transport in determining muscle glycogen synthesis in diabetes, but they do not rule out the possibility that other abnormal features of glycogen synthesis may be found that do not exert rate-controlling effects under these conditions.

Decreased delivery of substrate or insulin to the tissue bed has been hypothesized to be at least partially responsible for the insulin resistance in type 2 diabetes (90). No difference has been observed in the ^{13}C-NMR–measured ratio of extra- to intracellular water space in the healthy subjects and subjects with diabetes, implying that insulin-mediated vasodilatation could not be responsible. There was no difference in the interstitial insulin concentrations in the two groups during the hyperinsulinemic clamps, and hence the delivery of insulin is not responsible for the insulin resistance in patients with type 2 diabetes. Overall, these data are consistent with the hypothesis that glucose transport is the rate-controlling step for insulin-stimulated muscle glycogen synthesis in patients with type 2 diabetes. These results also suggest that agents that enhance hexokinase II or glycogen synthase activity will not be as effective as any agent that primarily improves glucose transport activity.

Mechanism of Fatty Acid–Induced Insulin Resistance

Increased concentrations of free fatty acids in plasma are typically associated with many insulin-resistant states, including obesity and type 2 diabetes (91–94). An inverse relationship between fasting plasma fatty acid concentrations and insulin sensitivity was found in a cross-sectional study of young, normal-weight offspring of patients with type 2 diabetes, consistent with the hypothesis that altered fatty acid metabolism contributes to insulin resistance in patients with type 2 diabetes (95). Furthermore, recent studies measuring intramuscular triglyceride content by muscle biopsy (35,96) or intramyocellular triglyceride content by ^{1}H-NMR (36,97) have shown an even stronger relationship between accumulation of intramyocellular triglyceride and insulin resistance.

The mechanism originally proposed by Randle et al. (98,99) to explain the insulin resistance was that an increase in fatty acids caused an increase in the intramitochondrial acetyl-CoA/CoA and NADH/NAD^+ ratios, with subsequent inactivation of pyruvate dehydrogenase. This in turn would cause intracellular citrate concentrations to increase, leading to inhibition of phosphofructokinase, a key rate-controlling enzyme in glycolysis. Subsequent accumulation of glucose-6-phosphate would inhibit hexokinase II activity, resulting in an increase in intracellular glucose concentrations and a decrease in glucose uptake.

A recent series of studies have challenged this conventional hypothesis (100–102). In the first study, ^{13}C- and ^{31}P-MRS were used to measure skeletal muscle glycogen and glucose-6-phosphate concentrations in healthy subjects. The subjects were maintained in euglycemic hyperinsulinemic conditions with either low or high levels of plasma fatty acids (100). Increasing the plasma fatty acid concentration for 5 hours caused a reduction of ~50% in rates of insulin-stimulated muscle glycogen synthesis and whole-body glucose oxidation compared with the control studies. In contrast to the predictions of the Randle model, where fat-induced insulin resistance should result in an increase in intramuscular glucose-6-phosphate, the fall in muscle glycogen synthesis was preceded by a decrease in the intramuscular glucose-6-phosphate content. These data suggest that increases in plasma fatty acid concentrations initially induce insulin resistance by inhibiting glucose transport or phosphorylation activity and that the reductions in muscle glycogen synthesis and glucose oxidation follow. The reduction in insulin-activated glucose transport/phosphorylation activity in healthy subjects maintained at high plasma fatty acid levels is similar to that seen in obese individuals (103), patients with type 2 diabetes (85), and lean-normoglycemic insulin-resistant offspring of individuals with type 2 diabetes (88). Hence, accumulation of intramuscular fatty acids (or fatty acid metabolites) appears to play an important role in the pathogenesis of insulin resistance in obese patients and patients with type 2 diabetes. Moreover, fatty acids would seem to interfere with a very early step in insulin-stimulation of GLUT4 transporter activity or hexokinase II activity.

Intracellular concentrations of glucose itself were measured by ^{13}C-NMR to distinguish between possible effects of fatty acids on glucose transport activity and hexokinase II activity (101). Since intracellular glucose is an intermediate between glucose transport and hexokinase II, its concentration reflects the relative activities of these two steps. If a decrease in hexokinase activity is responsible for the lower rate of insulin-stimulated muscle glycogen synthesis, intracellular glucose concentrations should increase. However, if the impairment is at the level of glucose transport, there should be no difference or a decrease in the intracellular glucose concentration. Elevated plasma fatty acid concentrations caused a significant reduction in intracellular glucose concentration in the lipid infusion studies compared with control studies in which glycerol (the other metabolite released by lipolysis) was infused in the absence of any exogenous fatty acid. These data imply that the rate-controlling step for fatty acid–induced insulin resistance in humans is glucose transport.

REFERENCES

1. Gadian DG. *Nuclear magnetic resonance and its applications to living systems.* 2nd ed. Oxford: Clarendon Press, 1982:139–170.
2. Rossetti L, Giaccari A. Relative contribution of glycogen synthesis and glycolysis to insulin mediated glucose uptake: a dose response study. *J Clin Invest* 1990;85:1785–1792.
3. Taylor R, Price TB, Rothman DR, et al. Validation of ^{13}C-NMR measurement of human muscle glycogen by comparison with biopsy and direct biochemical measurement. *Magn Reson Med* 1992;27:13–20.
4. Gruetter R, Magnussen I, Rothman DL, et al. Validation of ^{13}C NMR measurements of liver glycogen *in vivo*. *Magn Reson Med* 1994;31:583–588.
5. Petersen KF, West AB, Reuben A, et al. Noninvasive assessment of hepatic triglyceride content in humans with ^{13}C nuclear magnetic resonance spectroscopy. *Hepatology* 1996;24:114–117.
6. Rothman DL, Magnusson I, Katz LD, et al. Quantitation of hepatic glycogenolysis and gluconeogenesis in fasting humans with ^{13}C NMR. *Science* 1991;254:573–576.
7. Taylor R, Magnussen I, Rothman DL, et al. Direct assessment of liver glycogen storage by ^{13}C-nuclear magnetic resonance spectroscopy and regulation of glucose homeostasis after a mixed meal in normal subjects. *J Clin Invest* 1996;97:126–132.
8. Magnusson I, Rothman DL, Katz LD, et al. Increased rate of gluconeogenesis in type-II diabetes-mellitus—a C-13 nuclear-magnetic-resonance study. *J Clin Invest* 1992;90:1323–1327.
9. Hwang J-H, Perseghin G, Rothman DL, et al. Impaired net hepatic glycogen synthesis in insulin-dependent diabetic subjects during mixed meal ingestion. *J Clin Invest* 1995;95:783–787.
10. Petersen KF, Price T, Cline GW, et al. Contribution of net hepatic glycogenolysis to glucose production during the early postprandial period. *Am J Physiol* 1996;270(Pt 1):E186–E191.
11. Petersen KF, Krssak M, Navarro V, et al. Contributions of net hepatic glycogenolysis and gluconeogenesis to glucose production in normal and cirrhotic subjects. *Am J Physiol* 1998;276:E529–E535.
12. Wahren J, Felig P, Cerasi E, et al. Splanchnic and peripheral glucose and amino acid metabolism in diabetes mellitus. *J Clin Invest* 1972;51:1870–1878.
13. Consoli A, Kennedy F, Miles J, et al. Determination of Krebs cycle metabolic carbon exchange *in vivo* and its use to estimate the individual contributions of gluconeogenesis and glycogenolysis to overall glucose output in man. *J Clin Invest* 1987;80:1303–1310.
14. Consoli A, Nurjhan N, Capani F, et al. Predominant role of gluconeogenesis in increased hepatic glucose production in NIDDM. *Diabetes* 1989;38:550–557.
15. Hetenyi GJ, Lussier B, Ferrarotto C, et al. Calculation of the rate of gluconeogenesis from the incorporation of ^{14}C atoms from labelled bicarbonate or acetate. *Can J Physiol Pharmacol* 1982;60:1603–1609.
16. Petersen KF, Grunnet N. Gluconeogenesis in rat hepatocytes determined with [2-13]acetate and quantitative ^{13}C NMR spectroscopy. *Int J Biochem* 1993;25:1–5.
17. Schumann WC, Magnusson I, Chandramouli V, et al. Metabolism of [2-^{14}C]acetate and its use in assessing hepatic Krebs cycle activity and gluconeogenesis. *J Biol Chem* 1991;266:6985–6990.
18. Pimenta W, Nurjhan N, Jansson P-A, et al. Glycogen: its mode of formation and contribution to hepatic glucose output in postabsorptive humans. *Diabetologia* 1994;37:697–702.
19. Large V, Soloviev M, Brunengraber H, et al. Lactate and pyruvate isotopic enrichments in plasma and tissues of postabsorptive and starved rats. *Am J Physiol* 1995;268:E880–E888.
20. Miyoshi H, Shulman GI, Peters EJ, et al. Hormonal control of substrate cycling in humans. *J Clin Invest* 1988;81:1545–1555.
21. Edwards RHT, Round JM, Jones DA. Needle biopsy of skeletal muscle: a review of 10 years experience. *Musc Nerve* 1983;6:676–683.
22. Jacobs DB, Hayes GR, Lockwood DH. *In vitro* effects of sulphonylurea on glucose transport and translocation of glucose transporters in adipocytes from streptozocin-induced diabetic rats. *Diabetes* 1989;38:205–211.
23. Landau BR, Wahren J, Chandramouli V, et al. Contributions to glucose production in the fasted state. *J Clin Invest* 1996;98:378–385.
24. Nilsson L, Hultman E. Liver glycogen in man: the effect of total starvation or a carbohydrate poor diet followed by carbohydrate refeeding. *Scand J Clin Lab Invest* 1973;32:325–330.
25. Chiasson JL, Liljenquist WW, Lacy WW, et al. Gluconeogenesis: methodological approaches *in vivo*. *Fed Proc* 1977;36:229–235.
26. O'Connell RC, Morgan AP, Aoki TT, et al. Nitrogen conservation in starvation: graded responses to intravenous glucose. *J Clin Endocrinol Metab* 1974; 39:555–562.
27. Fryburg DA, Barrett EJ, Louard RJ, et al. Effect of starvation on human muscle protein metabolism and its response to insulin. *Am J Physiol* 1990;259: E477–E482.
28. Felig P, Marliss E, Owen OE, et al. Role of substrate in the regulation of hepatic gluconeogenesis in fasting man. *Adv Enzyme Regul* 1069;7:41–46.
29. Marliss EB, Aoki TT, Unger RH, et al. Glucagon effects and metabolic effects in fasting man. *J Clin Invest* 1970;49:2256–2270.
30. Turnbull AJ, Mitchison HC, Peaston RTP, et al. The prevalence of hereditary haemochromatosis in a diabetic population in North-East England. *Q J Med* 1997;90:271–275.
31. Ryysy L, Hakkinen A-M, Goto T, et al. Hepatic fat content and insulin action on free fatty acids and glucose metabolism rather than insulin absorption are associated with insulin requirements during insulin therapy in type 2 diabetic patients. *Diabetes* 2000;49:749–758.
32. Taylor R, Price TB, Katz LD, et al. Direct measurement of change in muscle glycogen concentration after a mixed meal in normal subjects. *Am J Physiol* 1993;265:E224–229.
33. Price TB, Rothman DL, Avison MJ, et al. ^{13}C NMR measurements of muscle glycogen during low-intensity exercise. *J Appl Physiol* 1991;70:1836–1844.
34. Price TB, Taylor R, Mason GM, et al. Turnover of human muscle glycogen with low intensity exercise. *Med Sci Sports Exerc* 1994;26:983–989.
35. Phillips DIW, Caddy S, Ilic V, et al. Intramuscular triglyceride and muscle insulin sensitivity: evidence for a relationship in nondiabetic subjects. *Metabolism* 1996;45:947–950.
36. Krssak M, Falk Petersen K, Dresner A, et al. Intramyocellular lipid concentrations are correlated with insulin sensitivity in humans: a ^{1}H NMR spectroscopy study. *Diabetologia* 1999;42:113–116.
37. Falholt K, Jensen I, Jensen SL, et al. Carbohydrate and lipid metabolism of skeletal muscle in type 2 diabetic patients. *Diabet Med* 1988;5:27–31.
38. Szczepaniak LS, Babcock EE, Schick F, et al. Measurement of intracellular triglyceride levels by H spectroscopy: validation *in vivo*. *Am J Physiol* 1999; 276:E977–E989.
39. Jacob S, Machann J, Rett K, et al. Association of increased intramyocellular lipid content with insulin resistance in lean nondiabetic offspring of type 2 diabetic subjects. *Diabetes* 1999;48:1113–1119.
40. Cahill GFJ. Physiology of insulin in man. *Diabetes* 1971;20:785–799.
41. Rasmussen H, Zawalich KC, Ganesan S, et al. Physiology and pathophysiology of insulin secretion. *Diabetes Care* 1990;13:655–666.
42. Tillil H, Shapiro ET, Miller MA, et al. Dose-dependent effects of oral and

intravenous glucose on insulin secretion and clearance in normal humans. *Am J Physiol* 1988;254:E349–357.
43. Radziuk J, Inculet R. The effects of ingested and intravenous glucose and glucogenic substrate in normal man. *Diabetes* 1983;2:977–981.
44. Waldhausl WK, Gasic S, Bratusch-Marrain P, et al. The 75-g oral glucose tolerance test: effect on splanchnic metabolism of substrates and pancreatic hormone release in healthy man. *Diabetologia* 1983;25:489–495.
45. Ishida T, Chou J, Lewis R, et al. Differential effects of oral, peripheral intravenous, and intraportal glucose on hepatic glucose uptake and insulin and glucagon extraction in conscious dogs. *J Clin Invest* 1983;72:590–600.
46. Shulman GI, Rossetti L. Influence of the route of glucose administration on hepatic glycogen repletion. *Am J Physiol* 1989;257:E681–E685.
47. McMahon M, Marsh H, Rizza RA. Comparison of the pattern of postprandial carbohydrate metabolism after ingestion of a glucose drink or a mixed meal. *J Clin Endocrinol Metab* 1989;68:647–653.
48. Elia M, Folmer P, Schlatmann A, et al. Carbohydrate, fat and protein metabolism in muscle and in the whole body after mixed meal ingestion. *Metabolism* 1988;37:542–551.
49. Jones IR, Owens DR, Luzio S, et al. The gastrointestinal inhibitory peptide response to oral glucose and mixed meals is increased in patients with type 2 (NIDDM) diabetes mellitus. *Diabetologia* 1989;32:668–677.
50. Jue T, Rothman DL, Tavitian BA, et al. Natural abundance ^{13}C NMR study of glycogen repletion in human liver and muscle. *Proc Natl Acad Sci U S A* 1989; 86:1439–1442.
51. Shulman GI, Rothman DL, Jue T, et al. Quantitation of muscle glycogen synthesis in normal subjects and subjects with non-insulin dependent diabetes by ^{13}C nuclear magnetic resonance spectroscopy. *N Engl J Med* 1990;322: 223–228.
52. Taylor R, Shulman GI. New insights into human carbohydrate metabolism using nuclear magnetic resonance spectroscopy. In: Marshall SM, Home PD, eds. *The diabetes annual.* Vol 8. Amsterdam: Elsevier, 1994:157–175.
53. Jackson RA, Roshania RD, Hawa MI, et al. Impact of glucose ingestion on hepatic and peripheral glucose metabolism in man: an analysis based on simultaneous use of the forearm and double isotope techniques. *J Clin Endocrinol Metab* 1986;63:541–549.
54. Kelley D, Mitrakou A, Schwenk F, et al. Skeletal muscle glycolysis, oxidation, and storage of an oral glucose load. *J Clin Invest* 1988;81:1563–1571.
55. Katz LD, Glickman MG, Rapoport S, et al. Splanchnic and peripheral disposal of oral glucose in man. *Diabetes* 1983;32:675–679.
56. Ferrannini E, Bjorkman O, Reichard GA, et al. The disposal of an oral glucose load in healthy subjects: a quantitative study. *Diabetes* 1985;34:580–588.
57. Price TB, Rothman DL, Taylor R, et al. Human muscle glycogen resynthesis after exercise: insulin-dependent and -independent phases. *J Appl Physiol* 1994;76:106–111.
58. Collins PJ, Horowitz M, Chatterton BE. Proximal, distal and total stomach emptying of a digestible solid meal in normal subjects. *Br J Radiol* 1988;61: 12–18.
59. Magnusson I, Rothman DL, Jucker B, et al. Liver glycogen turnover in fed and fasted humans. *Am J Physiol* 1994;266:E796–E803.
60. Rothman DL, Magnusson I, Katz LD, et al. Quantitation of hepatic glycogenolysis and gluconeogenesis in fasting humans with ^{13}C NMR. *Science* 1991;254:573–576.
61. Katz J, Golden S, Wals P. Glycogen synthesis by rat hepatocytes. *Biochem J* 1979;180:389–402.
62. Katz J, McGarry JD. The glucose paradox: is glucose a substrate for liver metabolism. *J Clin Invest* 1984;74:1901–1909.
63. Magnusson I, Chandramouli V, Schumann WC, et al. Pathways of hepatic glycogen formation in humans following ingestion of a glucose load in the fed state. *Metabolism* 1989;38:583–585.
64. Shulman GI, Cline G, Schumann WC, et al. Quantitative comparison of pathways of hepatic glycogen repletion in fed and fasted humans. *Am J Physiol* 1990;260:E335–E341.
65. Friedman JE, Caro JF, Pories WJ, et al. Glucose metabolism in incubated human muscle: effect of obesity and non-insulin-dependent diabetes mellitus. *Metab Clin Exp* 1994;43:1047–1054.
66. Agius L, Peak M, Alberti KGMM. Regulation of glycogen synthesis from glucose and gluconeogenic precursors by insulin in periportal and perivenous rat hepatocytes. *Biochem J* 1990;266:91–102.
67. Agius L, Tosh D, Peak M. The contribution of pyruvate cycling to loss of [6-^{3}H]glucose during conversion of glucose to glycogen in hepatocytes: effects of insulin, glucose and acinar origin of hepatocytes. *Biochem J* 1993;289:255–262.
68. Tosh D, Beresford G, Agius L. Glycogen synthesis from glucose by direct and indirect pathways in hepatocyte cultures from different nutritional states. *Biochim Biophys Acta* 1994;1224:205–212.
69. Magnussen I, Rothman DL, Jucker B, et al. Liver glycogen turnover in fed and fasted humans. *Am J Physiol* 1994;266:E796–E803.
70. Magnussen I, Rothman DL, Katz LD, et al. Increased rate of gluconeogenesis in type II diabetes mellitus. *J Clin Invest* 1992;90:1323–1327.
71. Jackson RA, Blix PM, Matthews JA, et al. Comparison of peripheral glucose uptake after oral glucose loading and a mixed meal. *Metabolism* 1983;32: 706–710.
72. Felig P, Wahren J, Hendler R. Influence of oral glucose ingestion on splanchnic glucose and gluconeogenic substrate metabolism in man. *Diabetes* 1975; 24:468–475.
73. Butterfield WJH, Whichelow MJ. Peripheral glucose metabolism in control subjects and diabetic subjects during glucose, glucose-insulin and insulin sensitivity tests. *Diabetologia* 1965;1:45–53.
74. Jackson RA, Hamling JB, Sim BM, et al. Peripheral lactate and oxygen metabolism in man: the influence of oral glucose loading. *Metabolism* 1987;36: 144–150.
75. Mitrakou A, Kelley D, Veneman T, et al. Contribution of abnormal muscle and liver glucose metabolism to postprandial hyperglycemia in NIDDM. *Diabetes* 1990;39:1381–1390.
76. Price TB, Perseghin G, Duleba A, et al. NMR studies of muscle glycogen synthesis in insulin-resistant offspring of parents with non-insulin-dependent diabetes mellitus immediately after glycogen-depleting exercise. *Proc Natl Acad Sci U S A* 1996;93:5329–5334.
77. Kelley DE, Mandarino LJ. Hyperglycemia normalizes insulin-stimulated skeletal muscle glucose oxidation and storage in noninsulin-dependent diabetes mellitus. *J Clin Invest* 1990;86:1999–2007.
78. Krssak M, Petersen KF, Bergeron R, et al. Intramuscular glycogen and intramyocellular lipid utilisation during prolonged exercise and recovery in man: a ^{13}C and ^{1}H nuclear magnetic resonance spectroscopy study. *J Clin Endocrinol Metab* 2000;85:748–754.
79. Bogardus C, Lillioja S, Stone K, et al. Correlation between muscle glycogen synthase activity and *in vivo* insulin action in man. *J Clin Invest* 1984;73: 1185–1190.
80. Johnson AB, Argyraki M, Thow JC, et al. Impaired activation of muscle glycogen synthase in non-insulin dependent diabetes mellitus is unrelated to the degree of obesity. *Metabolism* 1991;40:252–260.
81. Johnson AB, Argyraki M, Thow JC, et al. The effect of sulphonylurea therapy on skeletal muscle glycogen synthase activity and insulin secretion in newly presenting non-insulin dependent diabetic patients. *Diabet Med* 1991;8: 243–253.
82. Wright KS, Beck-Nielsen H, Kolterman OG, et al. Decreased activation of skeletal muscle glycogen synthase by mixed meal ingestion in NIDDM. *Diabetes* 1988;37:436–440.
83. Braithewaite SS, Plazuk B, Colca JR, et al. Reduced expression of hexokinase II in insulin resistant diabetes. *Diabetes* 1995;44:43–48.
84. Kruszynska YT, Mulford MI, Baloga J, et al. Regulation of skeletal muscle hexokinase II by insulin in nondiabetic and NIDDM subjects. *Diabetes* 1998; 47:1107–1113.
85. Rothman DL, Shulman RG, Shulman GI. ^{31}P nuclear magnetic resonance measurements of muscle glucose-6-phosphate: evidence for reduced insulin-dependent muscle glucose transport or phosphorylation activity in non-insulin-dependent diabetes mellitus. *J Clin Invest* 1992;89:1069–1075.
86. Bonadonna RC, Del Prato S, Bonora E. Roles of glucose transport and glucose phosphorylation in muscle insulin resistance of NIDDM. *Diabetes* 1996;45: 915–925.
87. Dohm GL, Tapscott EB, Pories WJ. An *in vitro* human preparation suitable for metabolic studies: decreased insulin stimulation of glucose transport in muscle from morbidly obese and diabetic subjects. *J Clin Invest* 1988;82:486–494.
88. Rothman DL, Magnusson I, Cline G, et al. Decreased muscle glucose transport/phosphorylation is an early defect in the pathogenesis of non-insulin-dependent diabetes mellitus. *Proc Natl Acad Sci U S A* 1995;92:983–987.
89. Cline GW, Petersen KF, Krssak M, et al. Decreased glucose transport as a cause of decreased insulin-stimulated muscle glycogen synthesis in type 2 diabetes. *N Engl J Med* 1999;341:240–246.
90. Yang YJ, Hope ID, Ader M, et al. Insulin transport across capillaries is rate limiting for insulin action in dogs. *J Clin Invest* 1989;84:1620–1628.
91. Frayn KN. Insulin resistance and lipid metabolism. *Curr Opin Lipidol* 1993; 1:197–204.
92. Boden G, Chen X, Ruiz J, et al. Mechanism of fatty acid induced inhibition of glucose uptake. *J Clin Invest* 1994;93:2438–2446.
93. Argyraki M, Wright PD, Venables CW, et al. Study of human skeletal muscle *in vitro*: effect of NEFA supply on glucose storage. *Metabolism* 1989;38: 1183–1187.
94. Johnson AB, Argyraki M, Thow JC, et al. Effect of increased free fatty acid supply on glucose metabolism and skeletal muscle glycogen synthase activity in normal man. *Clin Sci* 1992;82:219–226.
95. Perseghin G, Ghosh S, Gerow K, et al. Metabolic defects in lean nondiabetic offspring of NIDDM parents: a cross-sectional study. *Diabetes* 1997;46: 1001–1009.
96. Pan DA, Lillioja S, Kridetos AD. Skeletal muslce triglyceride levels are inversely related to insulin action. *Diabetes* 1997;46:983–988.
97. Perseghin G, Scifo P, De CF, et al. Intramyocellular triglyceride content is a determinant of *in vivo* insulin resistance in humans: a ^{1}H-^{13}C nuclear magnetic resonance spectroscopy assessment in offspring of type 2 diabetic parents. *Diabetes* 1999;48:1600–1606.
98. Randle PJ, Garland PB, Hales CN, et al. The glucose fatty acid cycle: its role in insulin sensitivity and the metabolic disturbances of diabetes mellitus. *Lancet* 1963;1:785–789.
99. Randle PJ, Kerbey AL, Espinal J. Mechanisms decreasing glucose oxidation in diabetes and starvation: role of lipid fuels and hormones. *Diabetes Metab Rev* 1988;4:623–638.
100. Roden M, Price TB, Perseghin G, et al. Mechanism of free fatty acid-induced insulin resistance in humans. *J Clin Invest* 1996;97:2859–2865.
101. Dresner A, Laurent D, Marcucci M, et al. Effects of free fatty acids on glucose transport and IRS-1-associated phosphatidylinositol 3-kinase activity. *J Clin Invest* 1999;103:253–259.
102. Griffin ME, Marcucci MJ, Cline GW, et al. Free fatty acid-induced insulin resistance is associated with activation of protein kinase C theta and alterations in the insulin signaling cascade. *Diabetes* 1999;48:1270–1274.
103. Petersen KF, Hendler R, Price T, et al. ^{13}C/^{31}P NMR studies on the mechanism of insulin resistance in obesity. *Diabetes* 1998;47:381–386.

CHAPTER 13
Biology of Adipose Tissue

Sheila Collins, Rexford S. Ahima, and Barbara B. Kahn

EVOLVING CONCEPTS ABOUT ADIPOSE TISSUE PHYSIOLOGY

From an evolutionary perspective, the biology of adipocytes begins with the strategies developed by organisms over time to cope with irregular and unpredictable supplies of nutrients. The need for such a mechanism became especially acute in omnivorous mammals and was probably a key survival factor. As *Homo sapiens* developed complex societal rituals that revolved around shared meals and as social status was assessed by the acquisition of resources, to be well endowed with a layer of fat was a clear sign of success, wealth, and social dominance. However, in more recent times, particularly in industrialized societies over the last 40 years, it has been more popular to possess the least amount of body fat. This modern idealism of slimness represents the new prototype of the species, glamorized by fashion and art. Simultaneously, in the medical community, there is also a greater emphasis on a leaner physique because of the growing alarm over the epidemic of overweight and obesity in adults and even children (see Chapter 31 for a detailed definition and discussion of obesity). The most recent statements from the Surgeon General of the United States and the World Health Organization emphasize the need for the general public to lose weight (specifically to reduce percentage of body fat) because of the established associations between excess body fat and increased risk for a host of serious medical complications (1) (http://www.cdc.gov/nccdphp/dnpa/obesity/trend/index.htm), including type 2 diabetes and cardiovascular disease, to name just two. It is also recognized that extreme deficiencies in body fat, such as lipodystrophy, can be as detrimental as excess fat in terms of diabetes risk (2). It is therefore important to understand the development and metabolic functions of adipose tissue and how these processes are regulated.

Until the 1990s, adipose tissue had largely been considered an inert storage depot for excess metabolic fuel. Accumulation of excess calories as triglycerides in adipose tissue is driven largely by insulin, and subsequent access to this stored fuel is gated by the β-adrenergic catecholamine receptors and their ability to stimulate lipolysis. The discovery of leptin as an adipose-derived hormone that can "report" on the status of these energy reserves to other organs of the body, including the central nervous system, gave us a new perspective on the biology of adipose tissue (3). The ensuing years have brought a deeper appreciation of the secretion by adipose tissue of a fairly large number of cytokines and growth factors that may play significant roles in insulin resistance, cell differentiation, and growth (Fig. 13.1). We will review aspects of the biology of adipocytes ranging from general anatomy and cellular and molecular biology to exciting new developments that support the concept that adipose tissue is an endocrine organ and that the adipocyte is a critical player in the regulation of insulin sensitivity as a result of its ability to secrete fatty acids, leptin, various cytokines, and other novel peptides.

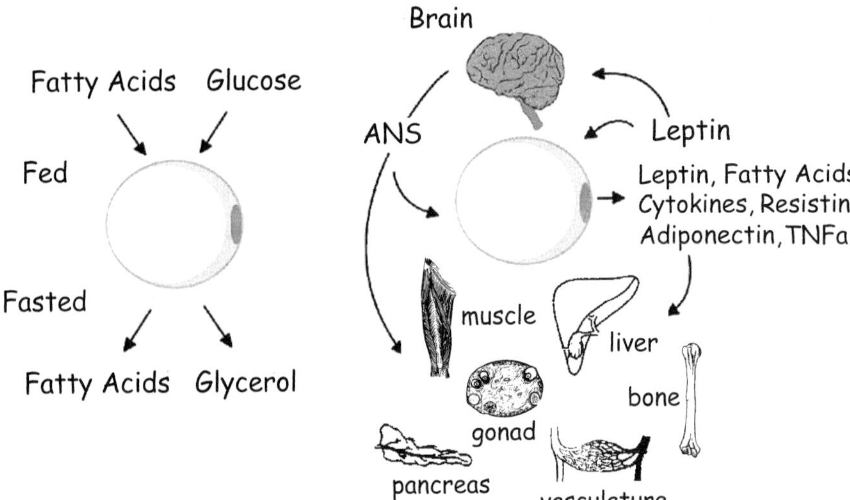

Figure 13.1. Evolving view of the biologic function of the adipocyte. Previously, adipocytes were considered to be inert storage depots releasing fuel as fatty acids and glycerol in times of fasting or starvation. More recently, it has become clear that adipocytes are endocrine glands that secrete important hormones, cytokines, vasoactive substances, and other peptides, with far-reaching effects on other organs and tissues, including the brain. TNF, tumor necrosis factor; ANS, autonomic nervous system; ACRP30, adipocyte complement-related protein–30 kDa (adiponectin). (From Kahn BB, Flier JS. Obesity and insulin resistance. *J Clin Invest* 2000;106:473–481, with permission from the American Society for Clinical Investigation.)

ADIPOSE TISSUE: STRUCTURAL FEATURES AND ANATOMIC DISTRIBUTION

Adipose tissue is present in every mammal and is critical to the maintenance of energy balance. Until the past few years, adipose tissue had been considered a type of loose connective tissue composed of lipid-filled cells (adipocytes) surrounded by a matrix of collagen fibers and a supporting blood supply. However, the current view of adipose tissue is that of a bona fide organ system with distinct tissue types mediating specific functions [e.g., homeostasis of energy reserves, hormone secretion, and immune regulation (4)]. Adipose tissue has been classified into two major forms on the basis of gross appearance, cell type–specific gene expression, and predominant type of adipocytes (5): white adipose tissue and brown adipose tissue.

White Adipose Tissue

White adipose tissue (WAT) is named for its white/yellowish color. It contains adipocytes with a single large lipid inclusion (termed *unilocular*), resulting in displacement of the cytoplasm, flattening of the nucleus to the plasmalemma, and appearance of signet ring–shaped adipocytes. After histologic processing with xylene or other fat solvents, WAT sections lose lipid, such that tissue resembles a meshwork of polygonal or ovoid profiles of variable sizes (20 to 200 μm diameter) when seen under the light microscope (Fig. 13.2). WAT is considered to be less well vascularized than brown adipose tissue (BAT). However, capillaries often are observed at the junctions where adipocytes meet. Heavier connective tissue septa separate WAT depots into lobules of various sizes. Special stains have revealed that the connective tissue surrounding white adipocytes contains precursor cells, fibroblasts, immune cells, reticular fibers, and unmyelinated nerves (6). The nerve fibers have been found to be immunoreactive for tyrosine hydroxylase, calcitonin gene–regulated peptide (CGRP), neuropeptide Y, and substance P (7). The postganglionic tyrosine hydroxylase–positive sympathetic nerves terminate primarily on arterioles and, when stimulated, cause vasoconstriction. In support of earlier anatomic and histologic observations, there is good evidence of a direct sympathetic innervation of white adipocytes originating from the central nervous system (8,9). Electron microscopic examination of white adipocytes shows that they are surrounded by a basal lamina. The cytoplasm is compressed into a thin rim containing a small Golgi complex, endoplasmic reticulum, free ribosomes, and filaments (9–11). Pleomorphic mitochondria are located close to the nucleus. The large lipid inclusion is not surrounded by a membrane but is heavily decorated with a protein called *perilipin* (12). The lipid droplet is also devoid of organelles.

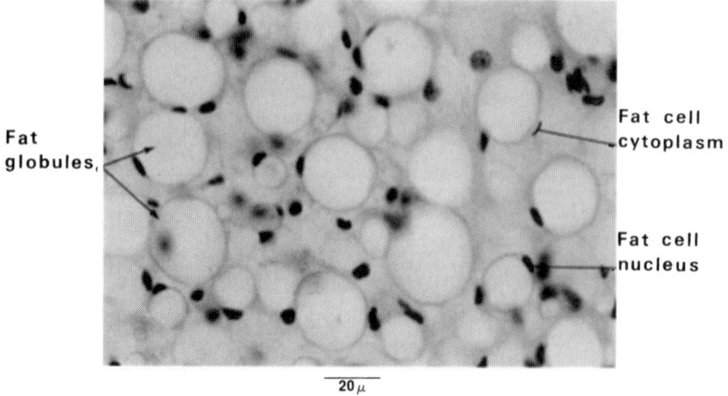

Figure 13.2. White fat cells. The cytoplasm appears as a thin rim at the periphery of the cell. Stored fat is the predominant component of the cell. The nucleus is flattened in the cytoplasm, permitting maximum storage of fat globules. The fat cell lipid is in the form of a single droplet, and these cells are described as unilocular. (From Bergman RA, Afif AK, Heidger PM. *Atlas of microscopic anatomy*, 2nd ed. Philadelphia: WB Saunders, 1974:53 [see color plate], with permission.)

WAT is the predominant type of adipose tissue in adult mammals. In healthy humans it accounts for 15% to 20% of body weight in men and 20% to 25% in women. The majority of WAT is organized into a continuous layer in the subcutaneous tissue called the *panniculus adiposus*. Subcutaneous WAT is especially abundant in the lower abdomen and buttocks, particularly in females. Other WAT depots are located in the omentum, breast, mesentery, and retroperitoneal/perirenal regions in humans, some of which can become pathologically large. WAT also accumulates in the axilla, pericardium, bone marrow, orbits, hands, and soles of the feet and functions as a cushion in these latter regions. In rodents, subcutaneous WAT accumulates around the scapular, axillary, and inguinal regions. Intraabdominal depots are located in the retroperitoneal area and in the mesenteric and perigonadal regions. The sexual dimorphism of body contour in humans is accounted for in large measure by differences in subcutaneous WAT (13). In addition to its abundance in the breasts, WAT is more abundant in the hypodermis of the lower abdomen, buttocks, and thighs in women than in men. These differences are influenced in part by sex hormones, as the female (gynoid) pattern of fat distribution tends to be altered to a central (android) location at menopause. Excessive central adiposity (especially intraabdominal) has been linked to the "metabolic syndrome," which includes insulin resistance, dyslipidemia, and increased risk of cardiovascular disease (14).

In general, the proportion of WAT in healthy adults remains fairly constant over prolonged periods. However, WAT can increase markedly with obesity and decrease with anorexia nervosa, cancer, and other wasting diseases. By weight, WAT comprises between 70% and 90% lipid, 5% to 30% water, and 2% to 3% protein. Most of the lipid content is triglyceride (>90%), although small amounts of diglyceride, cholesterol, and phospholipid are present. As noted above, in all species the ability to store calories efficiently within WAT can confer enormous survival advantage against the threat of starvation. As will be discussed later, fat metabolism is dependent on energy requirements and is regulated by nutrient, neural, and hormonal signals. The postprandial increase in glucose and lipids stimulates insulin release and increases fatty acid transport and lipogenesis in adipocytes. Conversely, reductions in glucose and insulin during fasting and stimulation of the sympathetic nervous system lead to lipolysis and the release of fatty acid for use by other tissues.

The morphology of WAT is affected by nutritional status. Obesity is an increased volume of WAT due to hypertrophy and hyperplasia of adipocytes (15–17). Lipid accumulation is associated with the formation of numerous micropinocytotic invaginations and vesicles, which coalesce into multilocular and finally unilocular lipid inclusions (10,11). By contrast, fasting causes a reduction in the size of the lipid droplet, an irregularity of the plasmalemma associated with numerous micropinocytotic invaginations and vesicles, and a prominent smooth endoplasmic reticulum (18). Prolonged fasting causes white adipocytes to take on the appearance of spindle-shaped fibroblastlike cells containing very few lipid inclusions (19). Moreover, the amount of capillaries is increased during fasting, consistent with the reported rise in blood flow in WAT, to facilitate delivery of oxygen and transport of the hydrolyzed free fatty acids (FFAs) to other tissues (20).

In addition to providing nourishment, proteins secreted by vascular endothelium control adipocyte differentiation and maturation (21). Antiangiogenic factors, e.g., angiopoeitin and TNP-40, inhibit angiogenesis as well as adipogenesis, and deplete adipocyte lipid stores in rodents (22,23). Vascular endothelial growth factor (VEGF) is increased with visceral fat accumulation, stimulated by insulin, and decreased by weight reduction (24,25). Importantly, blockade of VEGF inhibits adipogenesis, suggesting a causal role in adipose tissue development (25). In a recent study, targeting of a novel peptide to prohibitin, a vascular marker of adipose tissue, resulted in destruction of adipose vasculature and rapid reversal of obesity in rodents (26). These findings have generated considerable interest in the use of antiangiogenic agents as treatment for obesity.

The idea that obesity is associated with chronic inflammatory response, e.g., abnormal production of acute-phase reactants, and induction of inflammatory signaling pathways, is an old one (27). Chronic low-grade inflammation had been linked to insulin resistance, diabetes, and cardiovascular disease in obese individuals, although the underlying mechanisms remained unclear until recently. There are remarkable similarities in the patterns of gene expression, activation of complement, and induction of cytokines, among T-cells, macrophages, and adipocytes. Importantly, adipocyte precursors have the capacity to be transformed into phagocytic cells. Futhermore, there is significant overlap between metabolic pathways that mediate lipid metabolism in macrophages and adipocytes. Obesity in rodents and humans triggers a progressive infiltration of the stromovascular compartment of adipose tissue by macrophages (28,29). This process appears to be mediated through production of TNF-α and other cytokines by obese adipocytes, which in turn stimulate preadipocytes and endothelial cells to produce matrix proteins, e.g., monocyte chemoattractant protein (MCP)-1. Macrophage infiltration may be further enhanced by adipocyte hormones, e.g., leptin and adiponectin, as well as oxidative injury to endothelium. A key question is how these local changes eventually lead to diabetes and cardiovascular complications of obesity. Perhaps, cytokines and other chronic inflammatory signals from obese adipose tissue directly regulate glucose metabolism in muscle, liver as well as pancreatic β-cell responses, as shown by the improvement in glucose levels in parallel with inhibition of NF-κB by salicylate (30).

Brown Adipose Tissue

The rich and varied history of BAT as an anatomically discrete type of fat includes early speculations in the 17th century that it was part of the thymus and, a century later, that it was an endocrine organ involved in blood formation or a special form of fat acting as a reservoir for certain nutrients (31). BAT is named for its "brown" color, which is derived from a rich blood supply and an enormous number of mitochondria per cell (5). In overall appearance the adipocytes in BAT are generally smaller than white adipocytes and characterized by numerous small lipid inclusions (termed *multilocular*) (Fig. 13.3). Unlike white adipocytes, the nucleus is eccentric but not flattened.

Only in 1961 was the true function of BAT realized, when it was proposed to be thermogenic (32,33). Since then, an immense body of work has shown that BAT is uniquely capable of responding to various environmental stimuli to generate heat from stored metabolic energy. In response to activation by the sympathetic nervous system, BAT undergoes an orchestrated hyperplastic and hypertrophic expansion, increased blood flow, and recruitment of lipid and carbohydrate fuels for oxidative metabolism (34,35). A unique and critical element of this thermogenic mechanism for dissipation of the proton gradient in brown fat mitochondria was recognized to be due to a brown fat–specific mitochondrial uncoupling protein (UCP) (36), also called *thermogenin* (37). As illustrated in Figure 13.4 and discussed in greater detail by Ricquier and Bouillaud (38), this mitochondrial protein, now known as UCP1, allows controlled proton leakage across the mitochondrial inner membrane for the purpose of generating heat at the expense of respiration-coupled ATP production. This uncoupling activity in brown fat mitochondria is "activated" by FFAs that are released as a result of catecholamine-stimulated lipolysis.

Developmentally, BAT is most abundant in newborn mammals and is principally involved in heat production (5,39). In the human fetus, BAT is located in the dorsal cervical, axillary, suprailiac, and perirenal regions. Smaller amounts are present in the anterior mediastinum, interscapular, intercostal, and retropubic regions. By contrast, BAT is very prominent in the interscapular and axillary areas in mice and rats, with lesser deposits in the dorsal midline of the thorax and abdomen. Light microscopy examination shows that these BAT depots that

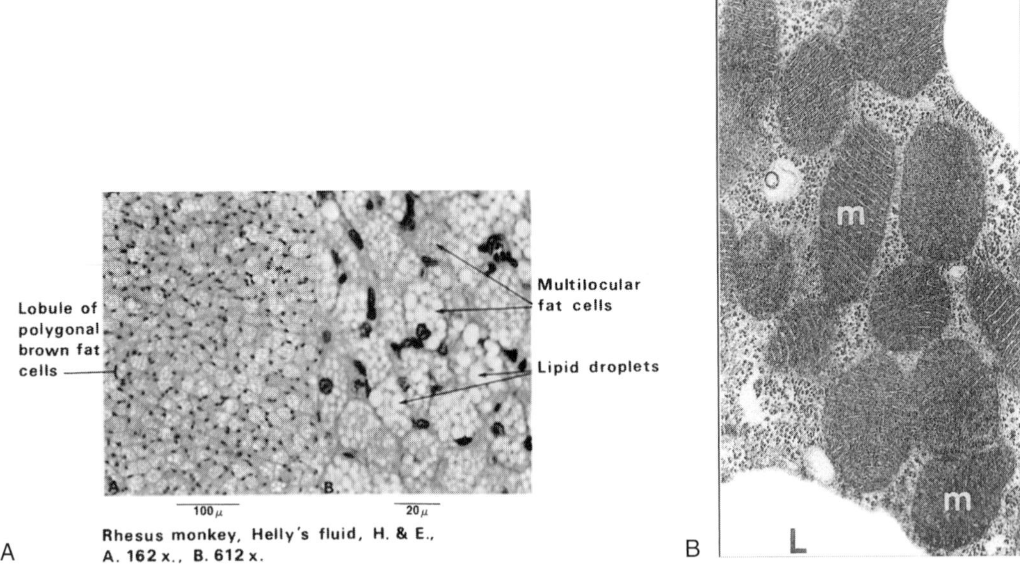

Figure 13.3. A: Brown fat is an uncommon variety of fat found in specific locations in the body. Unlike the more common white fat, brown fat cells contain a number of small lipid droplets; hence the name multilocular fat. **Panel B** illustrates the dense mitochondrial content of brown adipocytes. (From Bergman RA, Afifi AK, Heidger PM. *Atlas of Microscopic Anatomy,* 2nd ed. Philadelphia: WB Saunders, 1989: 54 [see color plate], with permission.)

reside along the midline are partitioned into lobules by dense connective tissue containing numerous blood vessels and nerves. For example, the prominent interscapular BAT in the rat receives two arteries and veins and has abundant capillaries (9). The nerve supply consists of large myelinated fibers, as well as small unmyelinated fibers that stain intensely for neuropeptide Y and tyrosine hydroxylase (9). The latter, which are postganglionic sympathetic fibers, form a periarterial plexus and also innervate brown adipocytes directly. In large mammals such as dogs and primates (including humans), homogenous depots of BAT decline with age beyond infancy but, as in rodents, brown adipocytes can be detected interspersed within typical "white" adipose depots throughout adulthood [reviewed in reference (40)]. Moreover, cold challenge or treatment with a β_3-adrenergic receptor (β_3AR) agonist further provokes the elaboration of such brown adipocytes in all of these animals. Humans with pheochromocytoma exhibit large amounts of BAT as a result of chronic catecholamine stimulation (41).

Development of Adipose Tissue

The origin of adipose tissue was a matter of controversy for a number of years (42,43). Early histologists debated whether adipose tissue was a distinct organ or merely a specialized loose connective tissue with lipid-filled fibroblasts. The current view of adipose tissue as a distinct organ was based on studies showing that adipocyte precursors were derived from mesenchyme and that the blood supply of the so-called primitive fat organ was distinct from the surrounding connective tissue. In humans and most mammals, adipose tissue development begins at midgestation. In rats and mice, WAT does not develop until the perinatal period, but established BAT depots are present in the late stages of gestation. Adipose depots arise from "undifferentiated" cells clustered along blood vessels. Adipocyte precursor cells lack lipid droplets and are associated with a rich supply of proliferating capillaries. The transformation of preadipocytes into white adipocytes is characterized morphologically by the

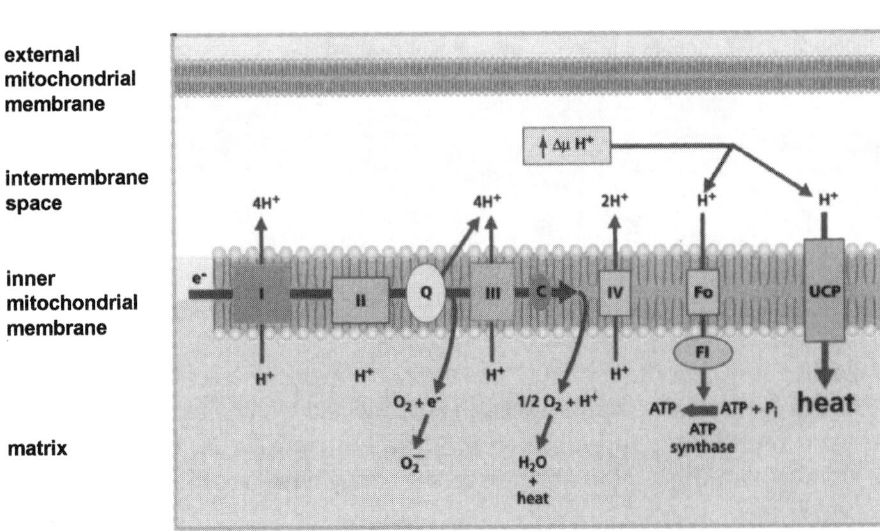

Figure 13.4. Transport of electrons through the respiratory chain complexes (I–IV) is associated with pumping of protons from the mitochondrial matrix into the intermembrane space, creating an electrochemical gradient ($\Delta\mu H^+$) for adenosine triphosphate (ATP) synthesis by the ATP synthase (F0–F1). An uncoupling protein (UCP) provides an alternative route for protons to reenter the matrix, thereby uncoupling the oxidation of fuel from ATP production. (Drawing courtesy of Dr. Antonio Vidal-Puig.)

accumulation of small lipid droplets that eventually coalesce into a single large droplet.

The concept that preadipocytes exist within adipose tissue, even into adulthood, and that they can differentiate into adipocytes under appropriate hormonal stimulation is supported by studies showing that cells isolated by collagenase digestion from the stromal–vascular compartment of fat pads from many sources, including humans, can differentiate into adipocytes when cultured *in vitro* in media enriched with insulin and other serum factors [reviewed in reference (44)]. In addition, studies of obesity in various strains of mice indicate that adipocyte hyperplasia can exist into adulthood (45). The ability of adipocytes to replenish a depot following ablation by gene targeting also supports this idea (46). Our understanding of the biochemistry and genetic program controlling adipocyte differentiation has also benefited enormously from studies of immortalized mouse preadipocyte cell lines such as 3T3-L1 and 3T3-F442A (47). These cells are propagated as fibroblastlike preadipocytes that are capable of differentiating into mature adipocytes under appropriate hormonal stimulation and that for the most part express the same genes as white adipocytes *in vivo*. As a result of extensive studies in these and similar adipogenic cell lines, we know that the adipocyte differentiation program proceeds through a series of well-characterized stages: (a) preconfluent, (b) growth arrest/confluence, (c) clonal expansion, and (d) terminal differentiation. Each stage involves a coordinated expression of transcription factors to culminate in the expression of specific genes for lipid metabolism, hormones, cytokines, and other adipocyte products (44,48).

MOLECULAR EVENTS IN PREADIPOCYTE COMMITMENT AND DIFFERENTIATION

The quest to define the critical required factors and/or temporally specific events in the commitment and differentiation of a given cell type has long fascinated biologists and has driven the field of molecular biology. This line of investigation in general has benefited from the efforts to understand the molecular basis of adipogenesis. The adipogenic cell lines of Green and colleagues (36) provided the technical basis from which to isolate adipocyte-specific genes and identify their regulatory factors. As a result of such approaches, a number of key transcription factors are now known to promote adipogenesis. They include the family of CCAAT/enhancer binding proteins (C/EBP), peroxisome proliferator-activated receptor-γ (PPAR-γ), and the sterol regulatory element binding protein (SREBP) family (SREBP1c, also known as ADD1). As shown in Figure 13.5, during adipocyte commitment and differentiation, the expression of the C/EBPs and PPAR-γ2 occurs in cascade fashion. A large number of studies in cell culture models and in genetically modified animals clearly show that agents or manipulations that interfere with the expression of these factors can inhibit differentiation or result in an incomplete state of differentiation. The genes and signaling pathways that commit cells to the preadipocyte lineage have been less well studied but are now an active area of investigation. In addition, although some of these cell culture models can appear morphologically to differentiate into adipocytes (49), it is now appreciated that in some cases the failure to appropriately express certain transcription factors results in the absence of gene products responsible for critical metabolic activities (50–52).

The PPAR-γ isoform PPAR-γ2 is expressed at high levels in adipose tissue (53,54). Its identification was based on a search for transcription factor(s) implicated in the expression of adipocyte-specific genes (55–57). Fibroblasts such as NIH-3T3 that are genetically engineered to express PPAR-γ2 can be coaxed to differentiate into "adipocytes" by the definition of visual proof of lipid accumulation and the expression of genes related to triglyceride synthesis and storage (53). In agreement with a key role for PPAR-γ2, its failure to be expressed during development prevents adipogenesis (58,59), and deletion of the PPARγ gene from mature adipocytes *in vivo* results in depletion of cells from the depot and decreased adipose mass (46). Provision of PPAR-γ2 by retroviral infection to PPAR-γ–deficient cells fully restores the capacity for differentiation (60,61).

While these results support the primacy of PPAR-γ for adipogenesis, several issues remain unresolved. An "endogenous ligand" for PPAR-γ remains undefined. At present there are two views of this situation. One is that a single, specific, high-affinity ligand is produced in target tissues. A second, based on crystallographic data (62) and comparisons of fatty acid binding and activation, is that the ligand-binding pocket of PPAR-γ can accommodate a variety of ligands, leading to the proposition that the receptor may serve as a general sensor of fatty acid milieu: the so-called PUFA receptor (for *p*oly*u*nsaturated *f*atty *a*cids), with no unique fatty acid ligand. In some sense this latter idea is akin to the ability of the cytochrome P450 family to

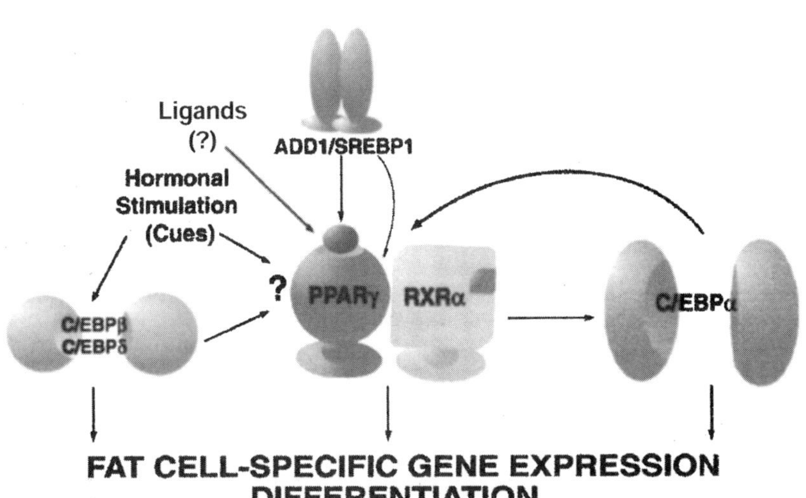

Figure 13.5. The transcriptional control of adipogenesis involves the activation of a variety of transcription factors. These proteins are expressed in cascade fashion, in which C/EBPβ and C/EBPδ are among the earliest seen. These two proteins promote the expression of peroxisome proliferator-activator receptor-γ (PPAR-γ), which in turn activates C/EBPα. C/EBPα feeds back on PPAR-γ to maintain a differentiated state. ADD1/SREBP1 can activate PPAR-γ by inducing its expression, as well as by contributing to the production of an endogenous PPAR-γ ligand. All these factors contribute to the expression of genes that characterize the terminally differentiated phenotype. (From Rosen ED, Spiegelman BM. Molecular regulation of adipogenesis. *Annu Rev Cell Dev Biol* 2000;16:145–171, with permission from the *Annual Review of Cellular and Developmental Biology*, © 2000 by Annual Review.)

accommodate a variety of hydrophobic substrates in the active site of the enzyme, hydroxylating them with turnover numbers that are relatively slow for highly specific enzymes, but nevertheless successfully accomplish the goal of identifying and eliminating xenobiotics (63).

In addition to the endogenous ligand issue, it is clear not only that PPAR-γ is required but also that C/EBPα is critical to the expression of the full complement of genes that define the mature adipocyte phenotype. For example, in NIH-3T3 fibroblasts engineered to express PPAR-γ2 and differentiated into adipocytes (53), even in this so-called differentiated state, these cells lack C/EBPα. As a result, they also lack certain defining features of the adipocyte, such as insulin-stimulated glucose uptake (50,51) and expression of the adipocyte-specific β_3AR (52). These metabolic anomalies are corrected following reintroduction of C/EBPα, confirming the need for C/EBPα in the mature adipocyte, at least for specific adipocyte genes and functions. Interestingly, absence of C/EBPα from adipose tissue in mice prevents the appearance of white, but not brown, fat (64).

Although these models have provided a wealth of information about adipocyte differentiation, it is true that most of these conclusions result from immortalized cell lines grown in isolation from other constituents of the adipose organ. Global targeted disruption of PPAR-γ2 in mice results in embryonic lethality (58,65,66). Consequently, studies of adipogenesis in PPAR-γ-deficient cells were performed in cultured cells derived from these animals. [However, as already noted, mice with adipose-specific "knockout" of PPARγ are viable, lack adipose tissue, and are insulin-resistant (59,67).] In addition, as discussed later in this chapter, the majority of these cell models in culture differentiate into white adipocytes. There have been very few available cell-culture models that differentiate into brown adipocytes, and most do not fully recapitulate the complete characteristics of brown adipocytes *in vivo*. Over the last decade, several immortalized brown adipocyte cell lines have been generated (68–71), providing the opportunity to advance molecular understanding of brown adipocyte differentiation and gene regulation. Several immortalized brown adipocyte cell lines were developed by a strategy called targeted transgenic tumorigenesis. Tissue-specific promoters were used to engineer SV40 T-antigen or oncogenic mutants of p53 to produce brown adipose tumors, from which cell lines were developed. Initially, the characteristics of these cell lines were, in large measure, quite representative of the brown adipocyte *in vivo*, but it is interesting that many of these cells have evolved with continuous passage in culture to express fewer and fewer features of the brown adipocyte: loss of expression of UCP1, depressed expression of other markers of mitochondria, and loss of β_3AR expression [(69,71) and S. Collins and K. W. Daniel, unpublished observations, 1996–1999].

In other cases these brown adipocyte models also lack expression of certain brown adipocyte genes (68,72), or simply have not yet been fully characterized. One theory concerning the loss of phenotypic validity with culture passage is that the more differentiated cells in the culture, expressing UCP1, tend to be at a proliferative disadvantage and over time are lost from the population. In addition, murine preadipocyte cultures do not address the contribution of the connective tissue matrix to the maturation of adipose tissue. Finally, among the various adipose depots *in vivo*, there are significant differences in metabolic characteristics and expression of certain genes that presently cannot be replicated in cell culture. The reader is referred to recent reviews that provide additional details (44,73).

MOLECULAR FEATURES OF WHITE VERSUS BROWN ADIPOCYTES

Despite the wealth of knowledge that has accrued over the past 25 years about the molecular events that set in motion and maintain the phenotype of the differentiated adipocyte, our understanding of the genetic programs that distinguish white from brown adipocytes is still far from complete. Historically, the agreement about the existence of BAT in humans and the importance of brown adipocyte thermogenesis has had a very checkered past. As discussed above, it is clear that a discrete adipose depot of homogeneous brown adipocytes exists at birth but does not remain in adult humans. Nevertheless, one can also readily find "brown adipocytes" in adults, as defined by morphologic and UCP1 histochemical criteria, scattered among white adipocytes in various "white adipose" depots, including perigonadal, perirenal, and pericardial, albeit they appear to be a small percentage of total adipocytes (Fig. 13.6). These BAT depots can undergo significant hypertrophy in adult humans under conditions of chronic catecholamine stimulation, as in pheochromocytoma (41). Similarly, in small rodents that retain *bona fide* BAT depots in adulthood, one finds scattered brown adipocytes in intraabdominal and intrathoracic white adipose depots, but rarely in subcutaneous fat. Part of the difficulty in establishing the extent to which adult humans possess brown adipocytes is that most biopsies are collected from subcutaneous sites. Since this is not the location of brown adipocytes at birth, estimates of residual brown adipocytes in humans, are, indeed, unknown. Thus, several important unanswered questions pertaining to the issue of brown adipocytes in adult humans remain.

First, we need accurate information about the number of brown adipocytes in adult humans. Second, even after we gain an accurate assessment of the number and locations of these scattered brown adipocytes in adult humans, we still must assess whether they are thermogenically active. Finally, we must determine whether these cells can be recruited in greater numbers in response to pharmacologic agents that behave as "thermogenic" drugs in rodent models (discussed in next section).

The unique morphologic differences between brown and white adipocytes (as discussed in an earlier section) are the result of differential gene expression during development and reflect the opposing metabolic functions of these cells: storage of caloric energy versus oxidation of caloric energy as heat. One of the most interesting questions in the field of adipocyte development is how and what molecular "decisions" are made in the mesenchymal precursor cells that give rise to white versus brown adipocytes. As discussed above, our understanding of the molecular events that drive the differentiation of white adipocytes has benefited enormously from the availability of clonal, immortalized cell lines that developmentally and phenotypically recapitulate white adipocytes.

The tissue-specific molecular markers of white and brown adipocytes have traditionally been the fatty acid–binding protein aP2 (also called 442) (55,74) and UCP1 (27), respectively. While aP2 is expressed in both white and brown adipocytes, UCP1 has been the unequivocal defining feature of brown adipocytes. However, for UCP1 to be expressed in such a highly cell type–specific manner, one would expect that other factors in brown adipocytes are required to initiate transcription of the *UCP1* gene. Thus, we still do not know whether there are factors *specifically* expressed in brown adipocytes that are themselves tissue-specific or whether they comprise a set of gene products that are uniquely and coordinately expressed as a result of hormonal cues. Some candidate molecules that are dif-

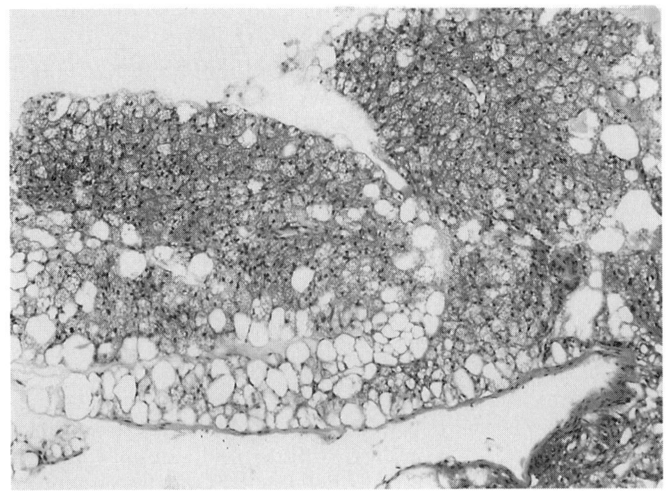
A

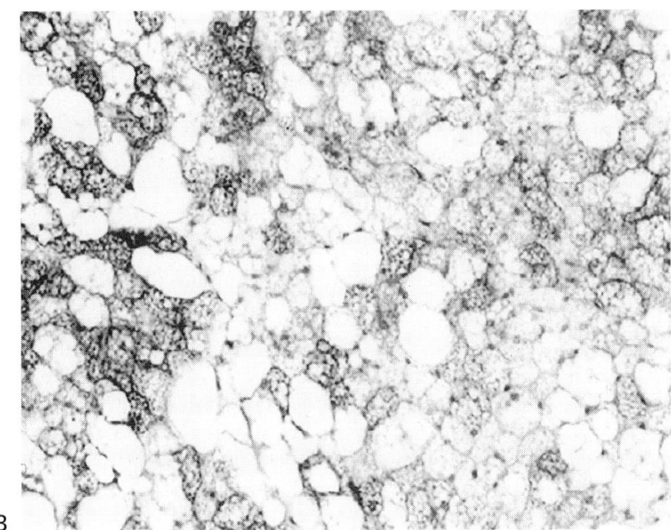
B

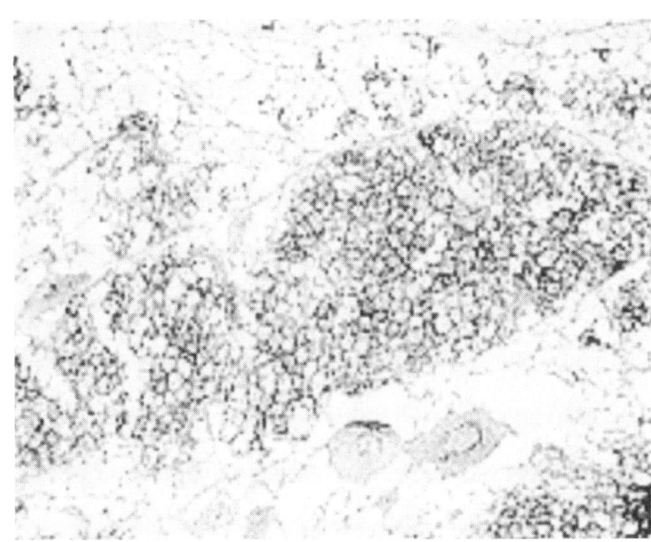
C

Figure 13.6. A: Brown adipocytes within a strip of human adipose tissue from the mediastinum. Hematoxylin and eosin stain. Courtesy of Dr. Laura Hale, Duke University Medical Center. **B:** Section of retroperitoneal adipose tissue from an A/J mouse following treatment with the β_3-adipocyte receptor agonist CL316,243. Brown adipocytes visualized by immunostaining with antisera to uncoupling protein 1 (UCP1). From S. Collins and L. P. Kozak, unpublished observations. **C:** Section of inguinal adipose tissue from an AXB8 mouse after being housed at 5°C for 7 days, showing patches of brown adipocytes as visualized by immunostaining with antisera to UCP1. (From Guerra C, Koza RA, Yamashita H, et al. Emergence of brown adipocytes in white fat in mice is under genetic control: effects of body weight and adiposity. *J Clin Invest* 1998;102:412–420, with permission from the American Society for Clinical Investigation.)

ferentially expressed in brown versus white adipocytes are PPAR-γ-coactivator-1 (PGC1α) and retinoid orphan receptor-γ (RORγ). In particular, PGC1α appears to be an important coordinator and regulator of genes involved in oxidative metabolism (75). For example, when PGC1α is expressed ectopically in white adipocytes, they appear to be "converted" to brown adipocytes where the cells now express UCP1 as well as a panoply of genes required for the genesis of a mitochondrion (75,76). At least in rodent brown adipocytes, the participation of PGC1α also appears to be critical for catecholamine-stimulated expression of UCP1 (77).

IMPORTANT ADIPOCYTE METABOLIC ACTIVITIES AND THEIR REGULATION

As befitting the role of adipose tissue as a "bank" for the deposition and retrieval of stored metabolic energy, it is of paramount importance to understand the hormone systems that control its metabolic processes for whole-body energy homeostasis and for interpreting the malfunctioning of these systems in diseases such as in type 2 diabetes. In this section we review results from several fronts that establish the adipocyte as an endocrine organ that secretes factors that report to other organ systems about the energy reserve status of the organism. One of the pivotal discoveries in this regard that revolutionized our thinking about the overall function of adipose tissue was the identification of the adipocyte-derived hormone leptin. In addition, since the association of obesity with type 2 diabetes is a well-known clinical phenomenon and since obesity has been documented in many instances to be a major contributing factor to insulin resistance, we also discuss obesity and insulin resistance in terms of adipocyte biology. We integrate this new information into current views of the mechanisms by which insulin, catecholamines, and certain cytokines control storage and release of lipid in the adipocyte.

Leptin: An Adipocyte Hormone Regulating Food Intake and Metabolism

Humans and other mammals have an extraordinary ability to match food intake to energy expenditure over long periods so that body weight and adiposity are maintained at near-constant levels. This homeostatic balance is remarkable given the infinite variety of day-to-day physical activity and the great variation in dietary selections and timing of their intake. On the basis of this observation, Kennedy (78) proposed that a signal emanating from adipose tissue informed the brain about the status of energy reserves, leading to alterations in feeding behavior and energy expenditure in an attempt to maintain energy balance. The concept of an "adipostat" was further supported by results of animal experiments in which food deprivation or surgical lipectomy resulted in compensatory hyperphagia and, conversely, acute forced overfeeding led to a reduction in voluntary ingestion until body weight was restored to the previous level.

Despite considerable effort, the identity of a circulating factor linking adiposity to energy homeostasis remained elusive until technical advances in genetics and computational power were made. These developments, combined with the extensive biochemical, physiologic, and genetic studies of the *ob/ob* (*obese*) and *db/db* (*diabetes*) mutant strains of mice, led to the isolation in the mid-1990s of the genes for these loci. Friedman and colleagues (79) determined that the *obese* gene encodes a protein with a relative molecular mass of 16 kDa that is expressed mainly in adipose tissue and circulates in plasma. It has a helical structure similar to that of cytokines and is highly conserved among species. They named this adipocyte-secreted hormone "leptin" (from the Greek *leptos* meaning thin) because it decreased body weight when injected in mice [reviewed in reference (79)]. Moreover, Friedman and others also showed that, as originally postulated by Coleman and colleagues (80,81), the *diabetes* locus encodes the receptor for leptin (82,83). Together these two discoveries were a major step forward in establishing the existence of an "adipostat," and the work led to a deeper appreciation of the endocrine role of adipose tissue (Fig. 13.1). As will be discussed later, this endocrine status of adipose tissue has expanded beyond what was initially implicated from the isolation of leptin.

REGULATION OF LEPTIN PRODUCTION AND KINETICS

There is a strong positive correlation between percent body fat, plasma concentrations of leptin, and expression of the leptin gene in adipose tissue. Moreover, leptin levels are dependent on nutritional status. They are higher in obese individuals and increase with overfeeding. By contrast, leptin levels are lower in lean individuals and decrease during fasting. The reduction in leptin expression and its circulating levels during fasting is rapid and precedes weight loss, suggesting that leptin might serve as a signal for impending energy depletion. Plasma leptin levels are related to the feeding cycle. In humans, concentrations of leptin appear to peak at night and reach a nadir in the morning. By contrast, in rodents concentrations of leptin reach a nadir during the light cycle and peak after the onset of feeding during the dark cycle, consistent with their nocturnal lifestyle. Various studies have suggested that the nutritional regulation of leptin is mediated at least in part by insulin (84), since the postprandial increase in insulin is temporally associated with increased expression of leptin messenger RNA (mRNA). Conversely, leptin decreases in response to insulin deficiency in humans and rodents. Although insulin stimulates the synthesis of leptin in adipocyte culture, and circulating levels of leptin *in vivo,* this effect appears to be due to insulin-stimulated glucose uptake and its metabolism (85,86) rather than to an effect of insulin signal transduction mechanisms per se on gene expression. This concept of insulin regulation is further complicated by the recent observation that mice lacking insulin receptors in fat have reduced fat mass but inappropriately high levels of leptin (87).

Several other hormonal or environmental factors have been noted to modulate leptin levels (84). For example, increases in circulating levels of leptin have been reported in response to acute infection, inflammatory cytokines, and chronic glucocorticoid and estrogen exposure. Although still largely empiric observations, the latter is postulated to be responsible, at least in part, for the higher concentration of leptin in females than in males. Higher expression of leptin in subcutaneous adipose tissue also is thought to play a role. Factors that have been associated with decreases in leptin levels include testosterone, cold exposure, adrenergic stimulation, growth hormone, thyroid hormone, melatonin, smoking, and thiazolidinediones.

ROLE OF LEPTIN IN FEEDING BEHAVIOR AND METABOLISM

At the time of its discovery, there was wide speculation that leptin was the long sought "satiety" and "antiobesity" factor described several decades ago [reviewed in references (35,36, 38)]. This view was based on the following observations. First, *ob/ob* mice with a genetic deficiency in leptin due to a truncated gene product develop early-onset obesity, impaired thermogenesis, and hyperphagia. Similar abnormalities were observed in *db/db* mice and *fa/fa* rats with mutations in the leptin receptor, suggesting that leptin was involved in the negative feedback regulation of feeding and adiposity. Second, administration of leptin peripherally (and, more potently, by the intracerebroventricular route) prevented weight gain in *ob/ob* mice (and to a lesser extent in wild-type mice) through inhibition of food intake and increased energy expenditure, in agreement with the notion that leptin was the missing antiobesity factor in these mice (88–90).

Leptin-mediated weight loss also may involve effects on lipid metabolism and adipocyte survival, as peripheral or intracerebroventricular injection of leptin has been shown to increase fat oxidation and to promote adipocyte apoptosis [discussed in reference (79)]. The increase in energy expenditure following the administration of leptin is mediated by activation of the central sympathetic pathway (91,92) and the predicted downstream stimulation of brown fat–specific uncoupling proteins. Since the receptors and neuroendocrine cells controlling food intake and energy expenditure are situated in the hypothalamus and certain other brain regions (93–95), it must be understood how leptin, produced by adipocytes and released into the general circulation, arrives at these privileged sites within the central nervous system. There is general agreement from the current literature that leptin is delivered from the circulation into the central nervous system by a saturable, facilitated transport mechanism. The so-called long form of the leptin receptor (Ob-Rb), which mediates activation of the JAK-STAT (*J*anus *K*inase—*S*ignal *t*ransducer and *a*ctivator of *t*ranscription) signal transduction pathway, has been colocalized with key neuropeptides and neurotransmitters in these brain regions involved in feeding behavior and energy balance [reviewed in reference (96–98)]. Recent data suggest that in addition to the Jak Stat pathway, leptin also activates the PI3 Kinase pathway and this may play a role in some of its metabolic effects (99,100). In addition, in skeletal muscle leptin activates the AMP-activated protein kinase (AMPK), and this is necessary for its effect on acetyl CoA carboxylase and stimulation of fatty acid oxidation (100a). In the hypothalamus, leptin and other anorexigenic signals inhibit AMPK activity (100b,100c), and this inhibition is necessary for leptin's effect on food intake and body weight (100c).

LEPTIN AS AN ANTIOBESITY HORMONE

The critical role of leptin in regulation of appetite and body weight has been demonstrated in rodents and humans with genetic leptin deficiency or leptin-receptor mutations; however, such mutations are extremely rare [see reference (101)]. The notion of leptin as an antiobesity hormone could be considered to be inconsistent with the empiric observations in both humans and rodent models that high endogenous levels of leptin do not prevent the accumulation of excess adipose tissue (102). However, a counterpoint argument is that the manner in which hyperleptinemia is indicative of "leptin resistance" is markedly similar to hyperinsulinemia in type 2 diabetes. In the latter circumstance it cannot be argued that the phenomenon of "insulin resistance" thus negates the role of insulin in controlling glucose homeostasis. Mechanisms underlying leptin resistance might include impairment of leptin synthesis or secretion, a decrease in transport of leptin across the blood–brain barrier, and abnormal leptin-receptor or postreceptor signaling. Data support both of these latter two possibilities. As expected, leptin treatment reverses hyperphagia, obesity, and hormonal and metabolic abnormalities when administered in *ob/ob* mice (88–90). Similarly, leptin drastically inhibits appetite, reverses obesity and neuroendocrine and immune abnormalities in the few humans with congenital leptin deficiency (103).

Although leptin receptors are present in several tissues, studies indicate that the antiobesity action occurs primarily in the brain. Ob-Rb and downstream leptin signaling molecules, incuding neuropeptide mediators such as neuropeptide Y, agouti-related peptide, proopiomelanocortin (POMC), and cocaine and amphetamine-regulated transcript, are enriched in hypothalamic neurons that mediate feeding, thermogenesis, and hormonal regulation (98). Importantly, targeted ablation of Ob-Rb in neurons recapitulates hyperphagia, abnormal thermoregulation, morbid obesity, hyperinsulinemia, and other metabolic abnormalites in mice (104). In contrast, loss of Ob-Rb in liver has no substantial effects on body weight or hormone levels (104). Reduced leptin-stimulated phosphorylation of STAT3 in the arcuate nucleus of the hypothalamus has been associated with high-fat feeding in mice (104a,104b). To more fully investigate the contribution of STAT3-mediated leptin signaling, Myers and colleagues (105) replaced Tyr 1138 in Ob-Rb with a serine residue, lepr(S1138), which specifically disrupts the Ob-Rb-STAT3 signal. As is the case in *db/db* mice, lepr(S1138) homozygotes were hyperphagic and morbidly obese. However, infertility, impaired linear growth, and diabetes characteristic of *db/db* mice were absent in lepr(S1138) mutants. Whereas hypothalamic expression of neuropeptide Y was increased in *db/db* mice but not lepr(S1138) mutants, POMC, precursor of the anorectic leptin target α-MSH, was suppressed in both *db/db* and lepr(S1138) mice. Thus, it appears that the leptin-Ob-Rb-STAT3 signal is functionally coupled to distinct hypothalamic neuropeptides to control energy homeostasis, growth, reproduction, and glucose levels (105).

Neural-specific disruption of STAT3 in mice resulted in hyperphagia and obesity, consistent with failure of negative feedback regulation by leptin (106). Importantly, STAT3 null mice had reduced energy expenditure and elevated glucocorticoids, and were diabetic and infertile, confirming the importance of STAT3-mediated signaling in the neuroendocrine action of leptin (106). Furthermore, as predicted, loss of STAT3 in neurons resulted in hyperleptinemia associated with marked reduction in POMC and increased levels of neuropeptide Y and agouti-related protein in the hypothalamus (106). The latter features were consistent with lack of leptin feedback in the brain, similar to leptin resistance in *db/db* mice.

Leptin induces suppressors of cytokine signaling (SOCS)-3 levels via JAK-STAT (107,108). Because SOCS-3 inhibits leptin response, it was suggested that this mechanism could explain the failure of elevated endogenous leptin to prevent diet-induced obesity. Recent studies have investigated this possibility in mice (108). Compared to wild-type mice, neuron-specific ablation of SOCS-3 increased leptin response in the hypothalamus, in parallel with induction of STAT3 phosphorylation, increased POMC expression, reduction in feeding, and weight loss (107). Ablation of SOCS3 in neurons also prevented diet-induced obesity and insulin resistance (107). A similar effect of SOC3 was observed in mice with heterozygous SOCS3 deficiency (108). Haploinsufficiency of SOCS3 (+/−) decreased body weight and increased hypothalamic leptin response. Furthermore, SOC3(+/−) mice were protected against diet-induced obesity, insulin resistance, and diabetes (108). Taken together, these data demonstrate important roles for STAT3 and SOCS3 in mediating leptin sensitivity in rodent obesity. However, whether these mechanisms play significant roles in human obesity remains to be determined.

LEPTIN AS A SIGNAL FOR STARVATION

As discussed earlier, the ability to store energy in adipose tissue represents a major adaptation against the threat of starvation. Starvation triggers a complex array of neural, metabolic, and hormonal responses that maintain energy supply to the brain and vital organs. As glucose levels fall during prolonged fasting, there is a corresponding decrease in insulin and an increase in counterregulatory hormones (e.g., glucagon, epinephrine, and glucocorticoids), leading to a switch from carbohydrate- to fat-based metabolism. Triglyceride breakdown generates fatty acids to be used by muscles, kidneys, and various organs. Partial oxidation of fatty acids also generates ketones that can be utilized by the brain. Other responses to starvation include suppression of thyroid and gonadal hormones, inhibition of immune function, activation of the hypothalamic–pituitary–adrenal axis, decreased thermogenesis, and increased appetite. These changes are remarkably similar to the phenotype of leptin-deficient *ob/ob* mice, suggesting that the reduction in leptin mediates the metabolic and neuroendocrine response to starvation. We substantiated this hypothesis by showing that leptin administration blunted the expected rise in corticosterone and corticotropin and prevented the inhibition of thyroid hormone, growth hormone, and reproductive and immune function during fasting (102). An association between low plasma levels of leptin and obesity was reported in Pima Indians (109) and in mouse strains prone to diet-induced obesity (110). However, this finding has not been confirmed in other studies (111,112).

The role of leptin in mediating the response to fasting has been investigated in humans (113,114). In patients maintained at 10% weight reduction, chronic leptin treatment designed to prevent the fall in leptin blunted the typical reduction in energy expenditure and thyroid hormone associated with caloric deprivation (113). Another study showed that replacement of leptin within the physiologic range in fasted humans normalized the levels of thyrotropin, T3, gonadotropins, and testosterone (114). However, in contrast to rodents, leptin did not affect the pituitary–adrenal axis during fasting (114). The diurnal leptin rhythm as well as leptin pulses are attenuated in patients with hypothalamic amenorrhea; however, whether there is a causal relationship between weight reduction, low leptin level, and disruption of menstrual cycles remains to be determined (115).

Insulin and the Control of Glucose Uptake and Lipogenesis in the Adipocyte

Insulin is a regulator of virtually all aspects of adipocyte biology, and adipocytes are one of the most highly insulin-responsive cell types (116). Insulin promotes triglyceride stores in adipocytes by several mechanisms, including the fostering of the differentiation of preadipocytes to adipocytes and, in mature adipocytes, the stimulation of glucose transport and triglyceride synthesis (lipogenesis), and the inhibition of lipolysis. Insulin also increases the uptake of fatty acids derived from circulating lipoproteins by stimulating the activity of lipoprotein lipase in adipose tissue (117). The metabolic effects of insulin are mediated by a broad array of tissue-specific actions that involve both rapid changes in protein phosphorylation and function, as well as changes in gene expression. The fundamental biologic importance of these actions of insulin is evidenced by the fact that the insulin signaling cascade that initiates these events is largely conserved in evolution from *Caenorhabditis elegans* to humans (118).

The initial molecular signal for insulin action involves activation of the insulin receptor tyrosine kinase, which results in phosphorylation of insulin-responsive substrates (IRSs) on multiple tyrosine residues. These phosphotyrosine residues act as docking sites for many SH2 domain-containing proteins, including the p85 regulatory subunit of phosphoinositide 3-kinase (PI 3-kinase). Binding of the p110 catalytic subunit of PI 3-kinase to p85 activates the lipid kinase and this promotes glucose transport (119). Whereas activation of PI 3-kinase is necessary for full stimulation of glucose transport by insulin, emerging evidence suggests that it is not sufficient and another pathway may also be necessary (120–122). The signals downstream of PI 3-kinase are not known, and there is evidence of a role for the serine/threonine kinase, Akt (protein kinase B [PKB]) (123,124), and possibly protein kinase C (PKC) such as λ or ζ (125). Most likely, the pathways that mediate the metabolic effects of insulin diverge downstream of PI 3-kinase (122,124) and show differential sensitivity to varying levels of insulin. For example, the antilipolytic effect of insulin requires much lower insulin concentrations than does stimulation of glucose transport. Hence, even in insulin-resistant states when glucose transport is impaired, sensitivity to the antilipolytic effect of insulin is preserved, resulting in maintenance or expansion of adipose stores. Insulin also activates the ras–mitogen-activated protein kinase (MAPK) signaling cascade. This pathway appears to be important for the mitogenic effects of insulin, but most data do not implicate the MAPK pathway in the well-studied metabolic actions of insulin.

Insulin also regulates gene transcription in adipocytes. The transcription factor ADD-1/SREBP-1c may play a critical role in the actions of insulin to regulate adipocyte gene expression [(126–128) and references therein] by inducing genes involved in lipogenesis and repressing those involved in fatty acid oxidation. Transcription factors of the forkhead family also play a major role in transducing insulin signals to the nucleus (129). Foxol, for example, plays an important role in gluconeogenesis by interacting with PGC1α (130). The relative functions of the ADD-1/SREBP and forkhead pathways deserve further investigation.

For a more detailed review of the molecular mechanism of insulin action, the reader is referred to Chapter 9.

INSULIN RESISTANCE IN OBESITY AND TYPE 2 DIABETES

The term *insulin resistance* usually connotes resistance to the effects of insulin on glucose uptake, metabolism, or storage. Insulin resistance is one of the major pathogenic factors in type 2 diabetes and is often associated with other pathologic states, including hypertension, hyperlipidemia, atherosclerosis, and polycystic ovary disease (this combined set of complications has been termed the *metabolic syndrome*, or *syndrome X*) [discussed in references (131) and (132)]. However, whereas it is still not known precisely how obesity promotes insulin resistance, recent new discoveries have expanded our knowledge in this area. In addition, another new concept is that insulin resistance and hyperinsulinemia, in addition to being *caused by* obesity, may actually *contribute to* the development of obesity (116,133).

Insulin resistance in obesity and type 2 diabetes is manifest by decreased insulin-stimulated glucose transport and metabolism in adipocytes and skeletal muscle and by impaired suppression of hepatic glucose output (131). These functional defects may result, in part, from impaired insulin signaling in all three target tissues and, in adipocytes, also from downregulation of the major insulin-responsive glucose transporter, GLUT4. In both adipocytes and muscle, the cascade of insulin binding to its receptor, receptor phosphorylation and activation of tyrosine kinase activity, and phosphorylation of insulin-responsive substrate proteins are all reduced. There are also tissue-specific alterations. For example, in adipocytes from obese humans with type 2 diabetes, IRS-1 expression is reduced, resulting in decreased IRS-1–associated PI 3-kinase activity, and IRS-2 becomes the main docking protein for PI 3-kinase (134). In contrast, in the skeletal muscle of obese subjects with type 2 diabetes, levels of IRS-1 and IRS-2 protein are normal but PI 3-kinase activity associated with both IRS-1 and IRS-2 is impaired.

One mechanism for the signaling defects in adipocytes in the obese state may be the increased expression and activity of several protein tyrosine phosphatases (PTPs) that dephosphorylate and thus terminate signaling propagated through tyrosyl phosphorylation events. Some data indicate that the expression and/or activity of at least three PTPs, including PTP1B, leukocyte antigen–related phosphatase (LAR) and Src-homology-phosphatase 2 (SHP2), are increased in muscle and adipose tissue of obese humans, and PTP1B and LAR have been shown to dephosphorylate the insulin receptor and IRS1 *in vitro* in rodents (135,136). Overexpression of either PTB-1B or LAR in skeletal muscle impairs its insulin-signaling capability and causes systemic insulin resistance (136,137). Mice with a targeted deletion of the *PTP1B* gene display increased insulin sensitivity and resistance to diet-induced obesity (138) that is due, at least in part, to increased energy expenditure. By contrast, targeted disruption of LAR in mice has been reported to significantly disrupt glucose homeostasis (139). The increased insulin sensitivity in the PTP1B$^{-/-}$ mice is seen in muscle and liver but not in adipocytes. PTP1B also regulates leptic signaling directly at the step of JAK2 phosphorylation (140,141). Thus, PTP1B appears to regulate leptin and insulin signaling independently.

REDUCTION OF GLUCOSE DISPOSAL INTO ADIPOSE TISSUE IN OBESITY

The action of insulin to lower blood glucose levels results from suppression of hepatic production of glucose and an increase in the uptake of glucose into muscle and fat. Muscle has long been considered to be the major site of insulin-stimulated glucose uptake *in vivo*, with adipose tissue contributing relatively little to total body glucose disposal. Support for this conclusion comes from the finding that measurements of 2-deoxyglucose uptake *in vivo* show at least ten times more glucose per milligram of tissue going into muscle than into WAT (142). Because muscle mass is considerably greater than WAT mass, at least in lean rodents and humans, this observation has been taken to indicate the prominent contribution of muscle to glucose disposal. Glucose transport into BAT is higher than into many muscle groups, but the mass of BAT is small even in rodents, making this an unlikely site to account for large amounts of total body glucose uptake. Thus, it has been viewed as unlikely that diminished glucose uptake into fat could account for diminished whole-body glucose uptake. Transgenic studies, however, indicate a greater role for glucose uptake into fat in systemic glucose homeostasis than was previously believed. For example, genetic overexpression of GLUT4 selectively in fat was shown to enhance whole body insulin sensitivity and glucose tolerance (143) even in overtly diabetic mice (144). Furthermore, targeted gene disruption to "knockout" *GLUT4* selectively from fat results in a degree of insulin resistance similar to that seen with muscle-specific knockout of *GLUT4* (145). This insulin resistance is associated with acquired impairments in insulin signaling and metabolic activity in muscle and liver. Whether this insulin resistance results directly from the absence of glucose transport in adipose tissue or indirectly from possible effects of altered glucose uptake on the release of other molecules from adipocytes remains a key question. Likely candidates for indirect effects are FFA, leptin, tumor necrosis factor α (TNF-α), ACRP30 (also called adiponectin), and resistin (discussed below). However, at least in these rodent models with adipose-specific knockout of *GLUT4*, serum FFAs, leptin levels, adiponectin levels, and adipocyte expression of TNF-α are normal. Undoubtedly, there are other, as yet undiscovered, molecules secreted from fat that influence systemic metabolism.

IMPACT OF THE LOCATION OF BODY FAT ON INSULIN RESISTANCE

Large epidemiologic studies reveal that the risk for diabetes, and presumably insulin resistance, rises as body fat content (measured by body mass index [BMI]) increases from the very lean to the very obese, implying that the "dose" of body fat has an effect on insulin sensitivity across a broad range (146,147), with some ethnic differences noted (148). Although this relationship is seen with measures of general adiposity such as BMI, it is interesting that all sites of adiposity do not contribute equally to diabetes risk. Central (i.e., intraabdominal) fat depots are much more strongly linked than peripheral (gluteal/subcutaneous) fat depots to insulin resistance, type 2 diabetes, and cardiovascular disease (149). The reason for this is not known. It is possible that a common, unknown factor, either genetic or environmental, produces both insulin resistance and central adiposity. Alternatively, perhaps some biochemical feature of intraabdominal adipocytes directly influences systemic insulin sensitivity.

A leading hypothesis is that intraabdominal adipocytes are more lipolytically active. This is postulated to be due either to their complement of ARs or to postreceptor signaling that promotes increased basal lipolysis. The increased intraportal FFA levels and flux might inhibit insulin clearance and promote insulin resistance by mechanisms that are still uncertain and have been reviewed elsewhere (150). Hyperinsulinemia per se also can cause insulin resistance by downregulating insulin receptors and desensitizing postreceptor pathways. This concept is supported by experimental overexpression of insulin in the livers of otherwise normal transgenic mice. This insulin transgene resulted in an age-related reduction in the expression of insulin receptor, glucose intolerance, and hyperlipidemia without any primary genetic defect in insulin action or secretion (151). Another hypothesis is that intraabdominal adipocytes secrete a different mixture of factors (qualitatively or quantitatively) compared with adipocytes in other depots and that these factors are more likely to impair insulin action systemically. These issues deserve further investigation.

BOTH LIPOTOXICITY AND LIPOATROPHY AS CAUSES OF INSULIN RESISTANCE

The term *lipotoxicity* has been coined to describe some of the negative consequences of excess adipose stores in obesity. These include insulin resistance, lipid accumulation in nonadipose tissues, and other adverse effects (152). Paradoxically, the *absence* of adipose tissue, or lipoatrophy, may result in similar pathology. The expanded adipose depot in obesity results in elevated plasma FFA levels due to increased release from the expanded adipose mass and probably also to impaired hepatic metabolism. Elevated FFA levels impair the ability of insulin to suppress hepatic glucose output and to stimulate glucose uptake into skeletal muscle and inhibit insulin secretion from pancreatic β-cells. The defect in muscle may involve impaired activation of PI 3-kinase, possibly due to elevations in PKCθ (153). An acquired loss of PI 3-kinase activation in muscle also is seen as a result of a high-fat diet (154). In humans, the triglyceride content of muscle correlates directly with insulin resistance and the fatty acid composition of muscle phospholipids influences insulin sensitivity (155). The signaling pathways mediating the lipid accumulation in nonadipose tissues and the mechanisms by which such lipotoxic impairment of function occurs are not known. However, recent studies of β-cells suggest that long-chain fatty acids may exert adverse effects via their induction of the overproduction of ceramide (156). It will be important to determine if fatty acids alter gene expression through binding as ligands to transcription factors of the PPAR family.

Severe deficiency or absence of fat, known as lipodystrophy, also is associated with severe insulin resistance in humans and rodents. In mouse models of lipodystrophy, leptin treatment (157) or fat transplantation (158) reverses the insulin resistance and diabetes. Thus, deficiency of leptin, and quite possibly other secreted products from adipocytes, impairs insulin sensitivity in the mouse. This is further supported by the increased insulin sensitivity and the absence of triglyceride deposits in muscle and liver in mice with markedly reduced adipose tissue due to transgenic overexpression of leptin (159). Consistent with these preclinical studies in animal models, studies in patients with lipodystrophy treated with leptin (160–162) support the concept that leptin might serve a therapeutic role in normalizing triglyceride levels and improving glycemic control, perhaps through direct effects on lipid oxidation that have been reported in animal models (163).

Control of Mobilization of Triglyceride Stores in Adipocytes by Sympathetic Nervous System Activity

In times of caloric excess, energy is stored in adipocytes in the form of triglycerides. These can be formed from preexisting fatty acids in the circulation that become esterified to glycerol, or the acyl moieties can be generated de novo from the oxidation of glucose to acetyl-CoAs and their subsequent condensation [Charts 10.1 and 11.1 of reference (164)]. However, in times of net caloric deprivation, whether it occurs in response to extended food scarcity or fasting, sustained intense physical activity, or even during the later hours of sleep (overnight fasting), the drop in blood glucose triggers the sympathetic nervous system (SNS) to release the catecholamines epinephrine and norepinephrine. This occurs either as the release of norepinephrine from nerve terminals innervating adipose tissue or as the secretion of epinephrine into the circulation from the adrenals. Sympathetic innervation is more profuse in BAT than in WAT, indicating that neural-derived norepinephrine plays a greater role in the former, while catecholamines derived from the circulation play a greater role in WAT. Nevertheless, substantial noradrenergic stimulation can exist in the immediate vicinity of the nerve terminals present in WAT.

The ARs are the recipients of these catecholamine signals. They are members of the large family of G protein–coupled receptors that are integral membrane proteins of the plasma membrane. Of the two main families, α-AR and β-AR, the β-ARs mediate catecholamine-driven mobilization of stored triglycerides in adipose tissue. This is achieved by β-AR–initiated triggering of a classic signaling cascade: activation of adenylyl cyclase, synthesis of increased intracellular levels of cyclic adenosine monophosphate (cAMP), and activation of the cAMP-dependent PKA, all of which culminate in the phosphorylation of hormone-sensitive lipase (HSL), the rate-limiting enzyme that initiates cleavage of triglycerides into FFAs and glycerol. This activated state of HSL can also be reversibly dephosphorylated by the actions of insulin. Thus, a balance is maintained between the recruitment and storage of metabolic fuel through the catecholamine and insulin hormone systems, respectively. There are three subtypes of β-ARs (β_1-AR, β_2-AR, and β_3-AR), all expressed in adipocytes, and the relative proportions of these subtypes can vary by species and metabolic status [reviewed in reference (40)]. Extensive pharmacologic and physiologic studies have established (165–167), as reviewed in references (40,168), and molecular genetic manipulations confirm (169,170) that all three β-AR subtypes together control the response to the SNS.

The basic biochemical scheme for the stimulation of lipolysis is presented in Figure 13.7. Also included in this figure (see details in legend) is an expanded view of this process that reflects new developments in our understanding of the downstream signaling cascades triggered by β-AR activation in adipocytes [reviewed in reference (40)]. These include the activation of various MAP kinase cascades in addition to the well-established cAMP/PKA pathway. These include ERK1/2 MAPK and p38 MAPK. They are independent of each other and activated by different mechanisms in adipocytes in response to catecholamines. Activation of the ERK1/2 MAP kinases by β-adrenergic agonists occurs as a result of receptor coupling to G_i (171) and does not involve PKA (172), while p38 MAPK activation is downstream of β-agonist increases in cAMP levels and PKA activity (172,173). The ERK pathway appears to account for between 15% and 20% of total lipolysis (174,175). Pharmacologic analyses suggest that at low concentrations of catecholamine essentially all lipolysis is activated by PKA, while the ERK1/2 pathway may be most significant at higher concentrations of epinephrine and norepinephrine (175). By contrast, there is no apparent involvement of the p38 MAPK pathway in β-agonist–stimulated lipolysis (175). While we have yet to establish the functional consequences of p38 MAPK activation in white adipocytes, there is a very clear indication that in brown adipocytes the classic cAMP-dependent stimulation of the *UCP1* gene requires this pathway (77,174). These new findings require additional studies to establish the metabolic consequences of these simultaneous signaling cascades emanating from β-ARs, and there must be follow-up studies using samples of primary adipose tissue from humans to assess the importance of this ERK pathway in humans.

In addition to the β-adrenergic stimulation of lipolysis, catecholamines can also be antilipolytic themselves through their interaction with the α_2-ARs resulting in inhibition of cAMP production. The balance between the relative amounts of the β-AR and α_2-AR can thus also determine the relative efficacy of catecholamines for triglyceride hydrolysis. There is some evidence from experimental studies in animals and humans that a shift to a higher α_2/β ratio can contribute to obesity and a net lipid storage (176).

A variety of other metabolic enzymes and processes are also activated by β-adrenergic–stimulated phosphorylation, including glycogen synthase and phosphorylase kinase. Other evidence indicates that the adipocyte-derived hormone leptin is also regulated by the catecholamines. In animal models, as well as in humans, the secretion of leptin is decreased by β-agonists

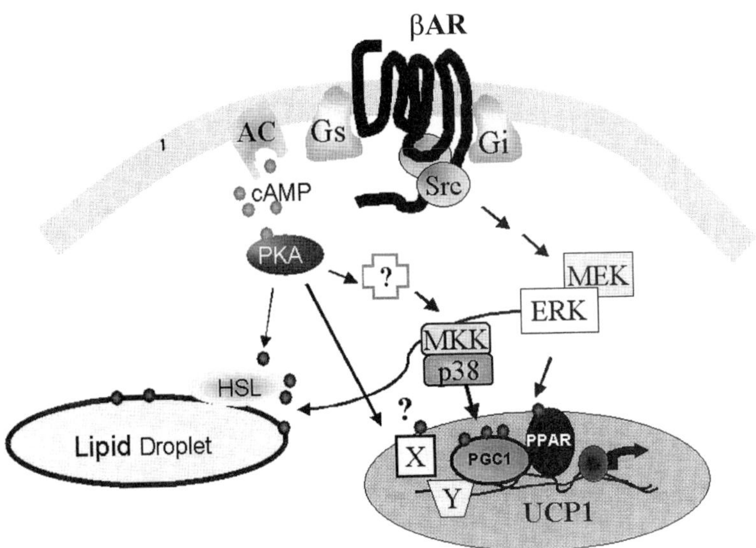

Figure 13.7. The β-adrenergic receptors (β-ARs) mediate the response of the catecholamines norepinephrine and epinephrine to stimulate lipolysis and thermogenesis in white and brown fat. Not shown is the fact that three β-AR subtypes are expressed together in adipocytes. Their signaling mechanism is classically defined as coupling to the stimulatory heterotrimeric G protein G_s, leading to activation of adenylyl cyclase (AC), increased in cyclic adenosine monophosphate (cAMP) production, and activation of the cAMP-dependent protein kinase (PKA). Downstream targets of PKA phosphorylation include hormone-sensitive lipase (HSL), perilipin, and various nuclear transcription factors for the modulation of gene expression. In brown adipocytes, expression of the uncoupling protein 1 (UCP1) is increased by this pathway. As illustrated in the figure, β_3AR couples interchangeably to both G_s and G_i to generate two distinct signaling events: the activation of PKA and ERK1/2. β-ARs also activate p38 MAP kinase (p38) downstream of PKA. The biochemical events linking PKA to MKK3/6 and p38 MAPK is currently unknown *(open cross),* but this pathway is required for transactivation of the *UCP1* gene. Some candidate factors that may be targets of these phosphorylation pathways are indicated, including PPAR-γ and its coactivator, PGC1. Other as-yet-undefined molecules could exist that are targets of these kinases (X and Y).

(177–179), but the mechanism(s) responsible for this suppression by β-ARs, including how leptin secretion is regulated, is not yet understood. Curiously, although it has been generally accepted that the increase in lipolysis during fasting is a direct consequence of catecholamine/β-adrenergic receptor-stimulated events, recent results from studies of mice that lack all three β-adrenergic receptor subtypes reveal that the lipolytic response to fasting is unimpaired (180). Additional work will be needed to establish whether this observation is peculiar to the animal model or also is relevant to humans.

When treated in the laboratory with β_3-AR–selective agonists, a variety of mammals exhibit a vigorous thermogenic response akin to cold exposure, supporting the notion that the β_3-AR plays a significant role in this thermogenic response (181–187). However, one of the most puzzling and immensely intriguing features observed is the de novo appearance of brown adipocytes within typical white adipose depots, suggesting a close interplay between these two adipocyte "species." The source of these brown adipocytes is unknown. They may arise from proliferation, but no supporting evidence has been found. There is currently discussion in the field that small pockets of "dedifferentiated" brown adipocytes from the neonatal period may be present in white adipose depots that express very low amounts of β_3-AR but that might be triggered to redifferentiate (9). However, as discussed below, while this response to catecholamines clearly has a predominant cAMP component, other evidence indicates that MAP kinase pathways may also modulate sympathetically driven brown adipocyte growth/survival.

Further support for a direct role of adipocytes in regulating systemic glucose homeostasis also comes from studies in which rodents or humans were treated with a β_3-adrenergic agonist (183,188,189). Since β_3-ARs are expressed almost exclusively in fat, effects of these agents would be expected to be initiated by alterations in fat. Treatment with the β_3-agonist results in enhanced sensitivity both of whole body glucose uptake and of suppression of hepatic glucose production (188). These effects are accompanied by increased glucose uptake in adipose tissue with no effect on muscle. Thus, increasing glucose uptake selectively in fat with β_3-AR agonists may improve whole body glucose uptake, with the effects in fat indirectly resulting in increased insulin sensitivity in liver. β_3-AR agonists may also work by changing the release of some adipocyte product that influences systemic insulin sensitivity. Quite apart from their effects in brown adipocytes, there is also newer evidence for white adipocytes to contribute to UCP1-independent thermogenesis in response to β_3-adrenergic agonists, and that white adipocyte mitochondria can, under certain conditions, exhibit high oxidative metabolic capacity (190,191).

Other Hormones and Cytokines Secreted by Adipose Tissue: Contribution to Insulin Resistance and Cardiovascular Dysfunction

Adipose tissue produces and secretes factors in addition to leptin that act in an autocrine, paracrine, or endocrine fashion to regulate adipogenesis and various systemic functions. In this section, we will discuss the potential involvement of adipose-derived steroids, proinflammatory cytokines, complement factors, and peptide hormones in adipogenesis, glucose homeostasis, and cardiovascular function.

SEX STEROIDS AND GLUCOCORTICOIDS

Adipose tissue does not synthesize steroid hormones de novo. However, adipose stromal cells are involved in steroid interconversion [reviewed in reference (192)]. 17-β-Hydroxysteroid oxidoreductase converts androstenedione to testosterone, and cytochrome P450–dependent aromatase mediates the conversion of estrone to estradiol. The levels of male and female sex steroids in various fat depots are thought to determine fat distribution (193,194). There is a strong association of androgens, central obesity, insulin resistance, and dyslipidemia with increased cardiovascular risk [reviewed in reference (195)]. It is possible that the rise in cardiovascular morbidity at menopause is determined in part by a relative increase in androgens and central adiposity.

The ratio of active to inactive glucocorticoids (cortisol vs. cortisone) in various fat depots is regulated by 11-β-hydroxysteroid dehydrogenase (type 1) (11-βHSD-1) [reviewed in reference (196)]. 11-β-HSD is regulated by insulin and in turn influences the local metabolism of glucocorticoids in adipose tissue. A link between local glucocorticoid metabolism, especially the expression or activity of 11-β-HSD, fat distribution, and glucose and lipid metabolism has been proposed by some investigators and supported by data from studies in transgenic mice (197, 198). Based on these observations and the well-known association between chronic hypercortisolism in Cushing syndrome and central obesity, insulin resistance, diabetes, hypertension, and cardiovascular morbidity, it has been tempting to speculate that excess local production of cortisol in adipose tissue could be a predisposing factor (199). Cortisol may also alter sex-steroid metabolism in adipose tissue by increasing aromatase activity. However, the pathophysiologic significance of this pathway is less clear.

Recent genetic studies in mice have provided important insights into the role of adipose-derived glucorticoids in metabolism and cardiovascular regulation (200,201). Mice with transgenic overexpression of 11βHSD-1 in adipocytes have normal circulating levels of corticosterone (the predominant glucocorticoid in rodents; however, local glucocorticoid concentration is increased in adipose tissue (201). As predicted, these mice develop visceral obesity and features of the metabolic syndrome, including insulin resistance, impairment of glucose tolerance, dyslipidemia, hypertension, and hepatic steatosis (200,201). Conversely, deletion of 11βHSD-1 in mice prevents diet-induced obesity and improves glucose tolerance, insulin sensitivy, and lipid levels (202).

TUMOR NECROSIS FACTOR-α AND OTHER PROINFLAMMATORY CYTOKINES

The role of TNF-α in the pathogenesis of septic shock, autoimmune disease, and cachexia associated with infection and cancer is well known. TNF-α is expressed as a 26-kDa transmembrane cell-surface protein and cleaved into the circulating biologically active 17-kDa form. TNF-α interacts with 55-kDa (p55) and 75-kDa (p75) membrane receptors. In addition to serving as the signal transmission mediator of TNF-α, alternatively processed forms of these receptors exist that are capable of being secreted into the circulation and consequently can alter TNF-α plasma concentrations and bioactivity. TNF-α reduces body weight by decreasing appetite, increasing lipolysis, and promoting adipocyte apoptosis (203). Systemic TNF-α infusion has been reported to blunt insulin-mediated glucose disposal and the ability of insulin to suppress hepatic glucose production (204). However, immunoneutralization of TNF-α improved insulin sensitivity in some rodents and humans, but not in others (205). Since these observations indicated that obesity and insulin resistance in rodents are associated with elevated adipose tissue–derived TNF-α (206), many studies have explored this connection in greater detail in an effort to determine the role of TNF-α in disturbing the process or maintenance of adipogenesis and lipid and glucose metabolism.

Potential mechanisms mediating TNF-α effects on insulin resistance include increased lipolysis and FFAs; inhibition of GLUT4, insulin receptor, and IRS-1 synthesis; inhibition of PPAR-γ function; and increased IRS-1 Ser/Thr phosphorylation or protein tyrosine phosphatase (PTPase) activity [reviewed in reference (207)]. TNF-α may act in a classical endocrine manner at distant target tissues (e.g., muscle, liver, and brain) to regulate glucose balance. On the other hand, TNF-α may stimulate lipolysis by a paracrine or autocrine mechanism and secondarily alter insulin sensitivity. Other proinflammatory cytokines produced by adipose tissue include interleukin (IL)-1 and IL-6 [see reference (208) and references therein]. The acute-phase C-reactive protein is stimulated by IL-6 and is positively correlated with insulin resistance, obesity, and endothelial dysfunction (209), but further study is required to determine whether IL-6 is a causative link between adipose tissue and the predilection to thromboembolism in obesity.

COAGULATION AND COMPLEMENT FACTORS

Proteins involved in the coagulation and fibrinolytic pathways [e.g., fibrinogen and plasminogen activator inhibitor-1 (PAI-1)] are increased in obesity. PAI-1 is produced mainly by the liver, but significant amounts are synthesized by adipose tissue (210). As with IL-6, there is a significant positive correlation between plasma PAI-1 levels, visceral adiposity, and cardiovascular risk, suggesting that PAI-1 might play a role in thromboembolic complications associated with obesity (211–213).

The link between nutritional deprivation and impaired immunity is well known (214,215). However, there is increasing evidence in support of an independent role of adipose tissue–derived factors in immune regulation. For example, an association between adipose tissue and the complement system was initially suggested by the occurrence of C3 deficiency in a patient with partial lipodystrophy (216). The complement system consists of ~20 proteins that mediate the response to infection and tissue injury. Complement activation via the classical pathway is triggered by antigen-antibody complexes, leading to activation of C1, C4, and C2 to form C4b2b. In the alternate pathway, C3 is hydrolyzed to a C3b-like factor, binds factor B, and is cleaved by factor D to form priming convertase C3bBb. The latter cleaves C3 into C3a and C3b, which interact with factors B and D to form amplification convertase C3bBb. Together the classical and alternate pathways activate the terminal complement factors C5–C9 to produce a membrane attack complex.

Differentiated 3T3-F442A adipocytes synthesize and secrete complement D (adipsin) (217), C3, and B and have been shown to activate the proximal alternate complement pathway in the absence of infection (218). Studies in animal models of obesity demonstrated severe reduction in the expression of adipsin from adipose tissue in genetic obesity (e.g., *ob/ob*, *db/db*), as well as acquired obesity (e.g., monosodium glutamate–treated mice and cafeteria-fed mice) in rodents (219). These findings, and the fact that human adipocytes also express and secrete adipsin (220), led to the notion that adipsin might be involved in obesity and related metabolic abnormalities. However, in humans, unlike rodents, blood concentrations of adipsin are increased in obese individuals and decreased with fasting or in conditions of lipoatrophy (221,222). This difference in the regulation of adipsin may be due in part to hypercortisolism, which is a prominent feature in the leptin-deficient, genetically obese rodents (223). Studies in nonmutant, diet-induced obese animals would be more instructive about whether there is a true species difference in these studies.

A role for the complement system in adipocyte biology was further suggested when a small protein (molecular weight 14,000 kDa) termed acylation-stimulating protein (ASP) was identified in human serum and shown to stimulate triglyceride synthesis in fibroblasts (224). The protein was subsequently found to be identical to C3a-*des*-Arg and derived from the cleavage of C3a by carboxypeptidase. The synthesis of C3a from C3 requires complement factors B and D (the latter being adipsin). Plasma concentrations of ASP are higher in obese than in lean individuals. Moreover, there is a sexual dimorphism of ASP such that the levels are higher in obese women than obese men, which may be the result of higher ASP production in subcutaneous adipose tissue; a depot that tends to be larger in women than in men. Consistent with a role of ASP as a mediator of lipogenesis, ASP deficiency in mice has been associated with increased postprandial levels of fatty acids and reduced triglyceride synthesis (225). As a result, it has been proposed that dysregulation of the ASP pathway may increase postprandial lipemia and alter lipoprotein profiles, thereby predisposing to the metabolic syndrome X and increased cardiovascular risk. However, since the genetic disruption of ASP expression also results in loss of complement factor C3 itself, additional definitive studies with nonpeptide analogues of ASP would provide important confirmation of the role of ASP.

ADIPONECTIN/ACRP30

Adiponectin, also known by other names, including adipocyte complement-related protein–30 kDa (ACRP30) (226), AdipoQ (227), gelatin-binding-protein-28 (228,229), and adipocyte-most-abundant protein (230), is synthesized and secreted exclusively by differentiated adipocytes. The protein has 247 amino acids and four main domains (231). The globular C-terminal domain shares sequence homology with the family of complement C1q-like proteins, including human type VII and X collagen, hibernation-regulated proteins, and precerebellin. The other domains consist of an NH_2-terminal signal sequence, nonhomologous sequence, and a collagenlike region. Although expression and plasma levels of ACRP30/adiponectin/AdipoQ originally were shown to be stimulated by insulin and decreased in obese mice, its functional role was unclear until recently [discussed in reference (232)].

Injection of purified adiponectin was reported to prevent the postprandial elevation of plasma fatty acid levels, in part by stimulating fatty acid oxidation in muscle (233). Moreover, adiponectin reduced body weight without affecting food intake, suggesting an effect on peripheral metabolism. Supporting this idea was the finding that adiponectin inhibited hepatic glucose production in rodents under clamp conditions (234). More recently, studies in rodents show that adiponectin activates AMP kinase in both muscle and liver (235). Furthermore, this report shows that dominant-negative adenovirus-delivered AMP kinase blocks the effects of adiponectin on phospho-*enol*-pyruvate carboxykinase (PEPCK) expression in liver and blunts the glucose-lowering effects of adiponectin in normal mice. Hence, AMP kinase is necessary for at least some of the metabolic effects of adiponectin, at least in the liver. Other work from this group also shows that targeted disruption of the adiponectin gene results in severe insulin resistance on a high-fat diet and increased susceptibility to atherosclerosis (236,237). In humans, plasma adiponectin levels are decreased in obesity, type 2 diabetes, and coronary artery disease (229,238–240). The ability of adiponectin to modulate coronary risk may occur by altering the expression of adhesion molecules (241–243). It is interesting that, as the search for the mechanisms underlying the insulin-sensitizing effects of thiazolidinediones continues, several reports have identified adiponectin as a target gene that is upregulated by thiazolidinediones. Insight into the type of receptor for adiponectin to search for has been unclear, since the primary sequence of the molecule did not suggest a structure.

However, an imaginative approach to this problem was the crystallization of adiponectin, wherein it was discovered that the structure of the globular head domain bore striking resemblance to that of another cytokine, TNF-α (Fig. 13.8), thus suggesting that a receptor of similar structural organization and signaling properties might exist for adiponectin (231). However, amidst debate about whether the functionally relevant moiety is the full-length protein or the globular head domain, or whether features of the molecule involved in signaling are distinct from other domains with separate functions, it was reported that adiponectin is modified post-translationally by hydroxylation and glycosylation and exists as low molecular weight (trimers) and higher molecular weight structures (244). These multiple forms are present in plasma in both rodents and humans and, importantly, the ratio of high molecular weight (HMW) to low molecular weight (LMW) adiponectin in circulation is a better predictor of glucose homeostasis than the absolute concentration (244). To understand adiponectin's ability to confer insulin-sensitizing properties requires understanding the receptor(s), their signaling cascade, and their regulation. Two reports of distinct receptor types for adiponectin have been described, the first being a pair of unusual molecules with a predicted architecture like an inverted G protein–coupled receptor (245) and the other as a member of the cadherin family (246). The tissue distributions and activation pathways of these receptors, and perhaps others yet to be described, will likely prove an exciting new direction for understanding how adipose tissue communicates with other metabolic tissues, and might someday yield new therapeutic strategies for metabolic disease.

ANGIOTENSINOGEN

Although angiotensinogen, the precursor of angiotensin II (Ang II), is produced mainly by the liver, adipose tissue also is considered an important source (247). In support of this view, proteins of the renin–angiotensin system (RAS) [e.g., renin, non-renin–angiotensin enzymes (chymase, cathepsins D and G, and tonin), angiotensin-converting enzyme, and Ang II receptors] are expressed by adipose tissue (248,249). The physiologic role of the RAS in adipose tissue is yet to be fully understood. Angiotensinogen mRNA and protein levels are regulated by nutritional status in rats, leading to a rapid decline with fasting and an increase when feeding is resumed (250). Expression of angiotensinogen mRNA is markedly increased during adipocyte differentiation (251,252). Ang II stimulates prostacyclin synthesis, adipocyte differentiation, and lipogenesis (253), suggesting that adipose-derived angiotensin may regulate adipocyte differentiation and growth, as is the case in other tissues. Targeted deletion of angiotensinogen in mice decreased adipose tissue mass and blood pressure, whereas transgenic overexpression of angiotensinogen in adipose tissue increased blood pressure and resulted in obesity (254,255). Furthermore, mice with transgenic overexpression of 11βHSD-1, leading to increased glucocorticoids in adipose tissue, develop hypertension in association with activation of the RAS, confirming a crucial involvement of adipose-derived RAS in the pathogenesis of cardiovascular complications of obesity (256).

RESISTIN

Thiazolidinediones (TZDs) are used as "insulin-sensitizing" agents for the treatment of type 2 diabetes. Although there is a strong correlation between the binding of TZD to the transcription factor PPAR-γ and the antidiabetic action of TZDs, the gene targets of PPAR-γ that mediate insulin sensitivity are not known. A screen for novel TZD-regulated genes resulted in the discovery of a protein that is induced during adipocyte differentiation and suppressed by TZDs (257). The protein, named resistin (257) or FIZZ3 (258), is encoded by a single mRNA transcript (750 residues) and is highly expressed in WAT and to a lesser degree in BAT. A low level of expression, potentially due to WAT, was detected in murine mammary tissue (257,259).

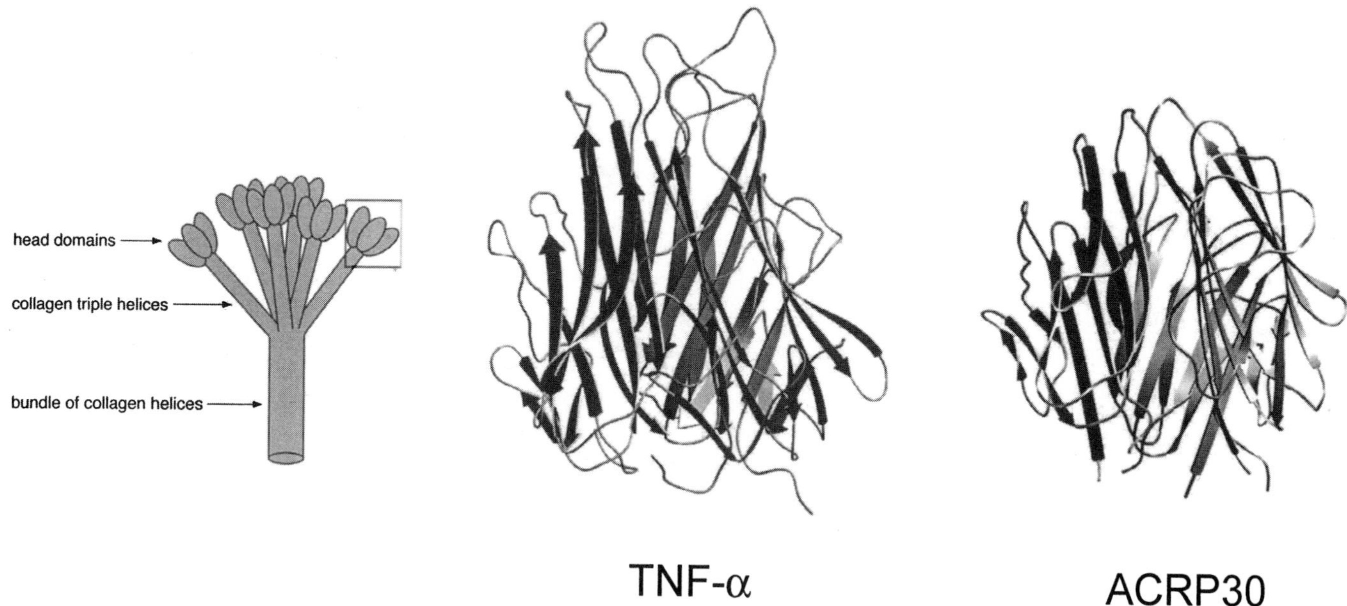

Figure 13.8. Crystal structure of the head domain of Acrp30 (adiponectin, AdipoQ) reveals tertiary structure homology with the cytokine TNF-α. (From Shapiro L, Scherer PE. The crystal structure of a complement-1q family protein suggests an evolutionary link to tumor necrosis factor. *Curr Biol* 1998;8:335–338, with permission. Copyright © 1998 Cell Press.)

Resistin protein was localized by immunostaining in the cytoplasm of white adipocytes. The deduced amino acid sequence includes an NH_2-terminal signal sequence and a unique pattern of cysteine residues. The latter is conserved among a family of resistinlike molecules (RELMs; also named FIZZ1) (258).

Resistin was shown to be secreted into the medium by transfected 293T cells and readily detected in mouse serum (257). More significantly, resistin mRNA and protein were regulated by nutrition and decreased with fasting and increased following refeeding (257). Resistin was found to be markedly elevated in genetically obese mice (*ob/ob* and *db/db*) and mice with diet-induced obesity. Neutralization of resistin with IgG-purified antiresistin serum decreased glucose levels in mice with diet-induced obesity. Moreover, antiresistin IgG improved insulin sensitivity. The function of recombinant resistin was analyzed *in vivo* and in differentiated adipocytes. Intraperitoneal administration of FLAG-tagged resistin improved glucose tolerance in mice and increased insulin-stimulated uptake of glucose in 3T3-L1 adipocytes.

The gene encoding rat resistin has recently been cloned (260). Unlike murine resistin, rat resistin encodes two mRNA transcripts and is highly induced by insulin (261). Human resistin-like molecules have been identified (262,263). As is the case with adiponectin, the crystal structures of resistin (Fig. 13.9) and RELM-β reveal complex trimeric and multimeric forms (264). Infusion of resistin or RELM-β into rodents, or transgenic overexpression of resistin, increases hepatic glucose production (264,265). Conversely, deletion of the resistin gene or attenuation of circulating resistin levels via specific antisense oligodeoxynucleotide to resistin mRNA decreases endogenous hepatic glucose production in mice, the latter effect being associated with suppression of AMP kinase (266,267). Both rat and mouse resistin are decreased by fasting, and stimulated by refeeding and specifically by insulin and glucose (261,268). In contrast to rodents, human resistin is expressed mainly by mononuclear cells in the stromavascular compartments of adipose tissue, instead of adipocytes (269). Moreover, the biology of resistin in humans is uncertain, in regard to its association with body fat, glucose, and insulin (270).

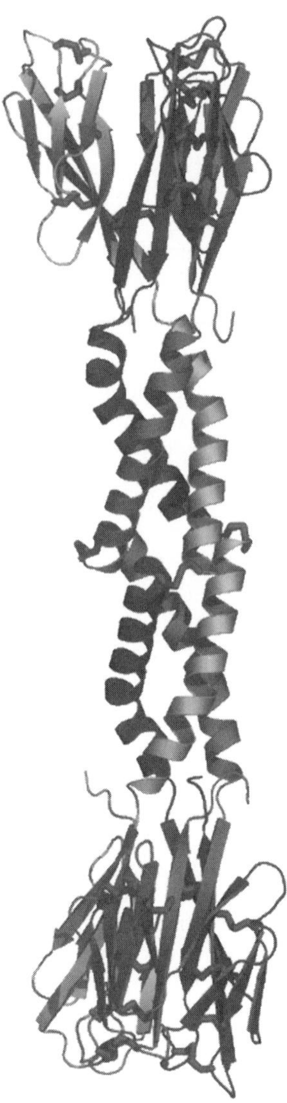

Figure 13.9. Ribbon diagram of resistin structure. A single resistin protomer, composed of a carboxy-terminal disulfide-rich globular domain and an amino-terminal α-helical region, assemble to form trimer-dimer hexamers. In both resistin and RELMβ (not shown) structures, each protomer from one trimer is disulfide linked to a protomer from the associated trimer. (Reprinted with permission from Patel SD, Rajala MW, Rossetti L, et al. Disulfide-dependent multimeric assembly of resistin family hormones. *Science* 2004;304:1154–1158. Copyright 2004 AAAS.)

SUMMARY

The biology of adipocytes has advanced from their being considered an inert storage depot for excess caloric energy and body cushioning and relegated to the "connective tissue" section of histology textbooks to having the status of a full-fledged member of the endocrine system that deserves a chapter of its own! The discovery of leptin and a host of other molecules that are secreted from adipose tissue, with important effects on glucose homeostasis and insulin sensitivity, marks a new era in which we are beginning to understand how organ systems communicate their energy demands and reserves. Many questions remain concerning the regulation of adipocyte development, the molecular mechanisms of leptin secretion and action, and the physiology of adiponectin and its target tissues. Similarly, even seemingly well-established mechanisms of biochemical events in adipocytes, such as catecholamine stimulation of lipolysis and thermogenesis, are undergoing revisions as more-elaborate signal transduction pathways are revealed and as new molecules are discovered that are critical to gene regulation and metabolic homeostasis. This inaugural chapter on the biology of adipocytes is an acknowledgment of how far this cell type has come as a player in our understanding of the pathogenesis of type 2 diabetes and the links between obesity, diabetes, and cardiovascular disease.

REFERENCES

1. Mokdad AH, Bowman BA, Ford ES, et al. The continuing epidemics of obesity and diabetes in the United States. *JAMA* 2001;286:1195–1200.
2. Reitman ML, Arioglu E, Gavrilova O, et al. Lipoatrophy revisited. *Trends Endocrinol Metab* 2000;11:410–416.
3. Zhang Y, Proenca R, Maffei M, et al. Positional cloning of the mouse obese gene and its human homologue. *Nature* 1994;372:425–432.
4. Ahima RS, Flier JS. Adipose tissue as an endocrine organ. *Trends Endocrinol Metab* 2000;11:327–332.
5. Hull D, Segall MM. Distinction of brown from white adipose tissue. *Nature* 1966;212:469–472.
6. Fawcett DW. A comparison of the histological organization and histochemical reactions of brown fat and ordinary fat. *J Morphol* 1952;90:363–372.
7. Giordano A, Morroni M, Santone G, et al. Tyrosine hydroxylase, neuropeptide Y, substance P, calcitonin gene–related peptide and vasoactive intestinal peptide in nerves of rat periovarian adipose tissue: an immunohistochemical and ultrastructural investigation. *J Neurocytol* 1996;25:125–136.
8. Bartness TJ, Bamshad M. Innervation of mammalian white adipose tissue: implications for the regulation of total body fat. *Am J Physiol* 1998;275: R1399–1411.
9. Cinti S. *The adipose organ.* Milan, Italy: Editrice Kurtis, 1999.

10. Cushman SW. Structure-function relationships in the adipose cell, I: ultrastructure of the isolated adipose cell. *J Cell Biol* 1970;46:326–341.
11. Cushman SW. Structure-function relationships in the adipose cell, II: pinocytosis and factors influencing its activity in the isolated adipose cell. *J Cell Biol* 1970;6:342–353.
12. Greenberg AS, Egan JJ, Wek SA, et al. Perilipin, a major hormonally regulated adipocyte-specific phosphoprotein associated with the periphery of lipid storage droplets. *J Biol Chem* 1990;11341–11346.
13. Bjorntorp P. The regulation of adipose tissue distribution in humans. *Int J Obes Relat Metab Disord* 1996;20:291–302.
14. Montague CT, O'Rahilly S. The perils of portliness: causes and consequences of visceral adiposity. *Diabetes* 2000;49:883–888.
15. Stern JS, Greenwood MR. A review of development of adipose cellularity in man and animals. *Fed Proc* 1974;33:1952–1955.
16. Bjorntorp P. Size, number and function of adipose tissue cells in human obesity. *Horm Metab Res* 1974[Suppl 4]:77–83.
17. Faust IM, Johnson PR, Stern JS, et al. Diet-induced adipocyte number increase in adult rats: a new model of obesity. *Am J Physiol* 1978;235:E279–E286.
18. Carpentier J, Perrelet A, Orci, L. Morphological changes of the adipose cell plasma membrane during lipolysis. *J Cell Biol* 1977;72:104–117.
19. Napolitano L, Gagne H. Lipid-depleted white adipose cells: an electron microscope study. *Anat Rec* 1963;147:273–278.
20. Belfrage E. Vasodilatation and modulation of vasoconstriction in canine subcutaneous adipose tissue caused by activation of beta-adrenoceptors. *Acta Physiol Scand* 1978;102:459–468.
21. Fukumura D, Ushiyama A, Duda DG, et al. Paracrine regulation of angiogenesis and adipocyte differentiation during in vivo adipogenesis. *Circ Res* 2003;93:88e–97.
22. Rupnick MA, Panigraphy D, Zhang CY, et al. Adipose tissue mass can be regulated through the vasculature. *Proc Natl Acad Sci U S A* 2002;99:10730–10735.
23. Brakenhielm E, Cao R, Gao B, et al. Angiogenesis inhibitor, TNP-470, prevents diet-induced and genetic obesity in mice. *Circ Res* 2004;94:1579–1588.
24. Miyazawa-Hoshimoto S, Takahashi K, Bujo H, et al. Elevated serum vascular endothelial growth factor is associated with visceral fat accumulation in human obese subjects. *Diabetologia* 2003;46:1483–1438.
25. Mick GJ, Wang X, McCormick K. White adipocyte vascular endothelial growth factor regulation by insulin. *Endocrinology* 2002;143:948–953.
26. Kolonin MG, Saha PK, Chan L, et al. Reversal of obesity by targeted ablation of adipose tissue. *Nat Med* 2004;10:625–632.
27. Wellen KE, Hotamisligil GS. Obesity-induced inflammatory changes in adipose tissue. *J Clin Invest* 2003;112:1785–1788.
28. Weisberg SP, McCann D, Desai M, et al. Obesity is associated with macrophage accumulation in adipose tissue. *J Clin Invest* 2003;112:1796–1808.
29. Xu H, Barnes GT, Yang Q, et al. Chronic inflammation in fat plays a crucial role in the development of obesity-related insulin resistance. *J Clin Invest* 2003;112:1821–1830.
30. Kim JK, Kim YJ, Fillmore JJ, et al. Prevention of fat-induced insulin resistance by salicylate. *J Clin Invest* 2001;108:437–446.
31. Lindberg O. *Brown adipose tissue.* New York: American Elsevier Publishing, 1970.
32. Smith R. Thermogenic activity of the hibernating gland in the cold-acclimated rat. *Physiologist* 1961;4:113.
33. Ball E, Jungas R. On the action of hormones which accelerate the rate of oxygen consumption and fatty acid release in rat adipose tissue *in vitro*. *Proc Natl Acad Sci U S A* 1961;47:932–941.
34. Bukowiecki L, Collet A, Follea N, et al. Brown adipose tissue hyperplasia: a fundamental mechanism of adaptation to a cold and hyperphagia. *Am J Physiol* 1982;242:E353–E359.
35. Géloën A, Collet AJ, Bukowiecki LJ. Role of sympathetic innervation in brown adipocyte proliferation. *Am J Physiol* 1992;263:R1176–R1181.
36. Girardier L. The regulation of the biological furnace of warm blooded animals. *Experientia* 1977;33:1121–1131.
37. Cannon, B, Hedin A, Nedergaard J. Exclusive occurrence of thermogenin antigen in brown adipose tissue. *FEBS Lett* 1982;150:129–132.
38. Ricquier D, Bouillaud F. Mitochondrial uncoupling proteins: from mitochondria to the regulation of energy balance. *J Physiol* 2000;529(Pt 1):3–10.
39. Merklin RJ. Growth and distribution of human fetal brown fat. *Anat Rec* 1974;178:637–645.
40. Collins S, Surwit RS. The β-adrenergic receptors and the control of adipose tissue metabolism and thermogenesis. In: Means AR, ed. *Recent progress in hormone research.* Bethesda, MD: Endocrine Society Press, 2001:309–328.
41. Lean ME, James WP, Jennings G, et al. Brown adipose tissue in patients with phaeochromocytoma. *Int J Obes* 1986;10:219–227.
42. Greenwood MR, Hirsch J. Postnatal development of adipocyte cellularity in the normal rat. *J Lipid Res* 1974;15:474–483.
43. Hausman GJ, Richardson RL. Cellular and vascular development in immature rat adipose tissue. *J Lipid Res* 1983;24:522–532.
44. Rosen ED, Walkey CJ, Puigserver P, et al. Transcriptional regulation of adipogenesis. *Genes Dev* 2000;14:1293–1307.
45. Surwit RS, Feinglos MN, Rodin J, et al. Differential effects of fat and sucrose on the development of obesity and diabetes in C57BL/6J and A/J mice. *Metabolism* 1995;44:645–651.
46. Imai T, Takakuwa R, Marchand S, et al. Peroxisome proliferator-activated receptor gamma is required in mature white and brown adipocytes for their survival in the mouse. *Proc Natl Acad Sci U S A* 2004;101:4543–4547.
47. Green H, Kehinde O. Sublines of mouse 3T3 cells that accumulate lipid. *Cell* 1974;1:113–116.
48. Morrison RF, Farmer SR. Insights into the transcriptional control of adipocyte differentiation. *J Cell Biochem* 1999[Suppl 32–33]:59–67.
49. Tontonoz P, Hu E, Spiegelman BM. Stimulation of adipogenesis in fibroblasts by PPAR gamma2, a lipid-activated factor. *Cell* 1994;79:1147–1156.
50. Wu Z, Rosen ED, Brun R, et al. Cross-regulation of C/EBPα and PPARγ controls the transcriptional pathway of adipogenesis and insulin sensitivity. *Mol Cell* 1999;3:151–158.
51. Hamm JK, el Jack AK, Pilch PF, et al. Role of PPAR gamma in regulating adipocyte differentiation and insulin-responsive glucose uptake. *Ann N Y Acad Sci* 1999;892:134–145.
52. Dixon TM, Daniel KW, Farmer SR, et al. CAATT/enhancer binding protein-α is required for transcription of the β_3AR gene during adipogenesis. *J Biol Chem* 2001;276:722–728.
53. Tontonoz P, Hu E, Graves RA, et al. mPPARγ2: tissue-specific regulator of an adipocyte enhancer. *Genes Dev* 1994;8:1224–1234.
54. Kliewer SA, Forman BM, Blumberg B, et al. Differential expression and activation of a family of murine peroxisome proliferator-activates receptors. *Proc Natl Acad Sci U S A* 1994;91:7355–7359.
55. Bernlohr DA, Angus CW, Lane MD, et al. Expression of specific mRNAs during adipose differentiation: identification of an mRNA encoding a homologue of myelin P2 protein. *Proc Natl Acad Sci U S A* 1984;81:5468–5472.
56. Graves RA, Tontonoz P, Ross SR, et al. Identification of a potent adipocyte-specific enhancer: involvement of an NF-1-like factor. *Genes Dev* 1991;5:428–437.
57. Graves RA, Tontonoz P, Spiegelman BM. Analysis of a tissue-specific enhancer: ARF6 regulates adipogenic gene expression. *Mol Cell Biol* 1992;12:1202–1208.
58. Rosen ED, Sarraf P, Troy AE, et al. PPAR gamma is required for the differentiation of adipose tissue in vivo and in vitro. *Mol Cell* 1999;4:611–617.
59. Zhang J, Fu M, Cui T, et al. Selective disruption of PPARgamma 2 impairs the development of adipose tissue and insulin sensitivity. *Proc Natl Acad Sci U S A* 2004;101:10703–10708.
60. Rosen ED, Hsu CH, Wang X, et al. C/EBPalpha induces adipogenesis through PPARgamma: a unified pathway. *Genes Dev* 2002;16:22–26.
61. Ren D, Collingwood TN, Rebar EJ, et al. PPARgamma knockdown by engineered transcription factors: exogenous PPARgamma2 but not PPARgamma1 reactivates adipogenesis. *Genes Dev* 2002;16:27–32.
62. Xu HE, Lambert MH, Montana VG, et al. Molecular recognition of fatty acids by peroxisome proliferator-activated receptors. *Mol Cell* 1999;3:397–403.
63. Lang M, Pelkonen O. Metabolism of xenobiotics and chemical carcinogenesis. *IARC Sci Publ*; 1999:13–22.
64. Linhart HG, Ishimura-Oka K, DeMayo F, et al. C/EBPalpha is required for differentiation of white, but not brown, adipose tissue. *Proc Natl Acad Sci U S A* 2001;98:12532–12537.
65. Kubota N, Terauchi Y, Miki H, et al. PPAR gamma mediates high-fat diet-induced adipocyte hypertrophy and insulin resistance. *Mol Cell* 1999;4:597–609.
66. Barak Y, Nelson MC, Ong ES, et al. PPAR gamma is required for placental, cardiac, and adipose tissue development. *Mol Cell* 1999;4:585–595.
67. He W, Barak Y, Hevener A, et al. Adipose-specific peroxisome proliferator-activated receptor gamma knockout causes insulin resistance in fat and liver but not in muscle. *Proc Natl Acad Sci U S A* 2003;100:15712–15717.
68. Kozak UC, Held W, Kreutter D, et al. Adrenergic regulation of the mitochondrial uncoupling protein gene in brown fat tumor cells. *Mol Endocrinol* 1992;6:763–772.
69. Kozak UC, Kozak LP. Norepinephrine-dependent selection of brown adipocyte cell lines. *Endocrinology* 1994;134:906–913.
70. Ross SR, Choy L, Graves RA, et al. Hibernoma formation in transgenic mice and isolation of a brown adipocyte cell line expressing the uncoupling protein gene. *Proc Natl Acad Sci U S A* 1992;89:7561–7565.
71. Irie Y, Asano A, Canas X, et al. Immortal brown adipocytes from p53-knockout mice: differentiation and expression of uncoupling proteins. *Biochem Biophys Res Commun* 1999;255:221–225.
72. Rohlfs EM, Daniel KW, Premont RT, et al. Regulation of the uncoupling protein gene (Ucp) by β_1, β_2, β_3-adrenergic subtypes in immortalized brown adipose cell lines. *J Biol Chem* 1995;270:10723–10732.
73. Vidal H. Gene expression in visceral and subcutaneous adipose tissues. *Ann Med* 2001;33:547–555.
74. Spiegelman BM, Frank M, Green H. Molecular cloning of mRNA from 3T3 adipocytes. Regulation of mRNA content for glycerophosphate dehydrogenase and other differentiation-dependent proteins during adipocyte development. *J Biol Chem* 1983;258:10083–10089.
75. Puigserver P, Wu Z, Park C, et al. A cold-inducible coactivator of nuclear receptors linked to adaptive thermogenesis. *Cell* 1998;92:829–839.
76. Wu Z, Puigserver P, Andersson U, et al. Mechanisms controlling mitochondrial biogenesis and respiration through the thermogenic coactivator PGC-1. *Cell* 1999;98:115–124.
77. Cao W, Daniel KW, Robidoux J, et al. p38 mitogen-activated protein kinase is the central regulator of cyclic AMP-dependent transcription of the brown fat uncoupling protein 1 gene. *Mol Cell Biol* 2004;24:3057–3067.
78. Kennedy GL. The role of depot fat in the hypothalamic control of food intake in the rat. *Proc R Soc Lond* 1953;140:579–592.
79. Friedman JM, Halaas JL. Leptin and the regulation of body weight in mammals. *Nature* 1998;395:763–770.
80. Coleman DL, Hummel KP. Effects of parabiosis of normal with genetically diabetic mice. *Am J Physiol* 1969;217:1298–1304.

81. Coleman DL. Effects of parabiosis of obese with diabetes and normal mice *Diabetologia* 1973;9:294–298.
82. Tartaglia LA, Dembski M, Weng X, et al. Identification and expression cloning of a leptin receptor, OB-R. *Cell* 1995;83:1263–1271.
83. Lee G-H, Proenca R, Montez JM, et al. Abnormal splicing of the leptin receptor in diabetic mice. *Nature* 1996;379:632–635.
84. Ahima RS, Flier JS. Leptin. *Annu Rev Physiol* 2000;62:413–437.
85. Mueller WM, Gregoire FM, Stanhope KL, et al. Evidence that glucose metabolism regulates leptin secretion from cultured rat adipocytes. *Endocrinology* 1998;139:551–558.
86. Wang J, Liu R, Hawkins M, et al. A nutrient-sensing pathway regulates leptin gene expression in muscle and fat. *Nature* 1998;393:684–688.
87. Bluher M, Michael MD, Peroni OK, et al. Adipose tissue selective insulin receptor protects against obesity and obesity-related glucose intolerance. *Dev Cell* 2002;3:25–38.
88. Pelleymounter MA, Cullen MJ, Baker MB, et al. Effects of the *obese* gene product on body weight regulation in *obob* mice. *Science* 1995;269:540–543.
89. Halaas JL, Gajiwala KS, Maffei M, et al. Weight-reducing effects of the plasma protein encoded by the *obese* gene. *Science* 1995;269:543–546.
90. Campfield LA, Smith FJ, Guisez Y, et al. Recombinant mouse OB protein: evidence for a peripheral signal linking adiposity and central neural networks. *Science* 1995;269:546–549.
91. Collins S, Kuhn CM, Petro AE, et al. Role of leptin in fat regulation. *Nature* 1996;380:677.
92. Sivitz WI, Fink BD, Morgan DA, et al. Sympathetic inhibition, leptin, and uncoupling protein subtype expression in normal fasting rats. *Am J Physiol* 1999;277:E668–677.
93. Elmquist JK, Elias CF, Saper CB. From lesions to leptin: hypothalamic control of food intake and body weight. *Neuron* 1999;22:221–232.
94. DeFalco J, Tomishima M, Liu H, et al. Virus-assisted mapping of neural inputs to a feeding center in the hypothalamus. *Science* 2001;291:2608–2613.
95. Schwartz MW. Brain pathways controlling food intake and body weight. *Exp Biol Med* (Maywood) 2001;226:978–981.
96. Tartaglia LA. The leptin receptor. *J Biol Chem* 1997;272:6093–6096.
97. Bjorbaek C, Elmquist JK, Frantz JD, et al. Identification of SOCS-3 as a potential mediator of central leptin resistance. *Mol Cell* 1998;1:619–625.
98. Elmquist JK. Hypothalamic pathways underlying the endocrine, autonomic, and behavioral effects of leptin. *Physiol Behav* 2001;74:703–708.
99. Niswender KD, Morton GJ, Stearns WH, et al. Intracellular signalling. Key enzyme in leptin-induced anorexia. *Nature* 2001;413:794–795.
100. Obici S, Zhang BB, Karkanias G, et al. Hypothalamic insulin signaling is required for inhibition of glucose production *Nat Med* 2002;8:1376–1382.
100a. Minokoshi Y, Kim YB, Peroni OD, et al. Leptin stimulates fatty-acid oxidation by activating AMP-activated protein kinase. *Nature* 2002;415:339–343.
100b. Andersson U, Filipsson K, Abbott CR, et al. AMP-activated protein kinase plays a role in the control of food intake. *J Biol Chem* 2004;279:12005–12008.
100c. Minokoshi Y, Alquier T, Furukawa N, et al. AMP-kinase regulates food intake by responding to hormonal and nutrient signals in the hypothalamus. *Nature* 2004;428:569–574.
101. Barsh GS, Farooqi IS, O'Rahilly S. Genetics of body-weight regulation. *Nature* 2000;404:644–651.
102. Ahima RS, Prabakaran D, Mantzoros C, et al. Role of leptin in the neuroendocrine response to fasting. *Nature* 1996;382:250–252.
103. Farooqi IS, Matarese G, Lord GM, et al. Beneficial effects of leptin on obesity, T cell hyporesponsiveness, and neuroendocrine dysfunction of human congenital leptin deficiency. *J Clin Invest* 2002;110:1093–2003.
104. Cohen P, Zhao C, Cai X, et al. Selective deletion of leptin receptor in neurons leads to obesity. *J Clin Invest* 2001;108:1113–1121.
104a. El-Haschimi K, Pierroz DD, Hileman SM, et al. Two defects contribute to hypothalamic leptin resistance in mice with diet-induced obesity. *J Clin Invest* 2000;105:1827–1832.
104b. Munzberg H, Flier JS, Bjorbaek C. Region-specific leptin resistance within the hypothalamus of diet-induced obese mice. *Endocrinology* 2004;Jul 22.
105. Bates SH, Stearns WH, Dundon TA, et al. STAT3 signalling is required for leptin regulation of energy balance but not reproduction. *Nature* 2003;421: 856–859.
106. Gao Q, Wolfgang MJ, Neschen S, et al. Disruption of neural signal transducer and activator of transcription 3 causes obesity, diabetes, infertility, and thermal dysregulation. *Proc Natl Acad Sci U S A* 2004;101:4661–4666.
107. Mori H, Hanada R, Hanada T, et al. Socs3 deficiency in the brain elevates leptin sensitivity and confers resistance to diet-induced obesity. *Nat Med* 2004; 10:739–743.
108. Howard JK, Cave BJ, Oksanen LJ, et al. Enhanced leptin sensitivity and attenuation of diet-induced obesity in mice with haploinsufficiency of Socs3. *Nat Med* 2004;10:734–738.
109. Ravussin E, Pratley RE, Maffei M, et al. Relatively low plasma leptin concentrations precede weight gain in Pima Indians. *Nat Med* 1997;3:238–240.
110. Surwit R, Petro A, Parekh P, et al. Low plasma leptin in response to dietary fat in diabetes- and obesity-prone mice. *Diabetes* 1997;46:1516–1520.
111. Fox CS, Esparza J, Nicolson M, et al. Is a low leptin concentration, a low resting metabolic rate, or both the expression of the "thrifty genotype"? Results from Mexican Pima Indians. *Am J Clin Nutr* 1998;68:1053–1057.
112. Surwit RS, Edwards CL, Murthy S, et al. Transient effects of long-term leptin supplementation in the prevention of diet-induced obesity in mice. *Diabetes* 2000;49:1203–1208.
113. Rosenbaum M, Murphy EM, Heymsfield SB, et al. Low dose leptin administration reverses effects of sustained weight-reduction on energy expenditure and circulating concentrations of thryoid hormoes. *J Clin Endocrinol Metab* 2002;87:2391–2394.
114. Chan JL, Heist K, DePaoli AM, et al. The role of falling leptin levels in the neuroendocrine and metabolic adaptation to short-term starvation in healthy men. *J Clin Invest* 2003;111:1409–1421.
115. Laughlin GA, Yen SS. Hypoleptinemia in women athletes: absence of a diurnal rhythm with amenorrhea. *J Clin Endocrinol Metab* 1997;82:318–321.
116. Kahn BB, Flier JS. Obesity and insulin resistance. *J Clin Invest* 2000;106: 473–481.
117. Fielding BA, Frayn KN. Lipoprotein lipase and the disposition of dietary fatty acids. *Br J Nutr* 1998;80:495–502.
118. Paradis S, Ruvkun G. Caenorhabditis elegans Akt/PKB transduces insulin receptor-like signals from AGE-1 PI3 kinase to the DAF-16 transcription factor. *Genes Dev* 1998;12:2488–2498.
119. White MF. The IRS-signaling system: a network of docking proteins that mediate insulin and cytokine action. *Recent Prog Horm Res* 1998;53:119–138.
120. Staubs PA, Nelson JG, Reichart DR, et al. Platelet-derived growth factor inhibits insulin stimulation of insulin receptor substrate-1-associated phosphatidylinositol 3-kinase in 3T3-L1 adipocytes without affecting glucose transport. *J Biol Chem* 1998;273:25139–25147.
121. Czech MP, Corvera S. Signaling mechanisms that regulate glucose transport. *J Biol Chem* 1999;274:1865–1868.
122. Wang Q, Somwar R, Bilan PJ, et al. Protein kinase B/Akt participates in GLUT4 translocation by insulin in L6 myoblasts. *Mol Cell Biol* 1999;19:4008–4018.
123. Kitamura T, Ogawa W, Sakaue H, et al. Requirement for activation of the serine-threonine kinase Akt (protein kinase B) in insulin stimulation of protein synthesis but not of glucose transport. *Mol Cell Biol* 1998;18:3708–3717.
124. Kotani K, Ogawa W, Matsumoto M, et al. Requirement of atypical protein kinase C lambda for insulin stimulation of glucose uptake but not for Akt activation in 3T3-L1 adipocytes. *Mol Cell Biol* 1998;18:6971–6982.
125. Kitamura T, Kitamura Y, Kuroda S, et al. Insulin-induced phosphorylation and activation of cyclic nucleotide phosphodiesterase 3B by the serine-threonine kinase Akt. *Mol Cell Biol* 1999;19:6286–6296.
126. Kim J, Sarraf P, Wright M, et al. Nutritional and insulin regulation of fatty acid synthetase and leptin gene expression through ADD1/SREBP1. *J Clin Invest* 1998;101:1–9.
127. Shimomura I, Bashmakov Y, Horton JD. Increased levels of nuclear SREBP-1c associated with fatty livers in two mouse models of diabetes mellitus. *J Biol Chem* 1999;274:30028–30032.
128. Foretz M, Guichard C, Ferre P, et al. Sterol regulatory element binding protein-1c is a major mediator of insulin action on the hepatic expression of glucokinase and lipogenesis-related genes. *Proc Natl Acad Sci U S A* 1999;96: 12737–12742.
129. Kops GJ, Burgering BM. Forkhead transcription factors: new insights into protein kinase B (c-Akt) signaling. *J Mol Med* 1999;77:656–665.
130. Puigserver P, Rhee J, Donovan J, et al. Insulin-regulated hepatic gluconeogenesis through FOXO1-PGC-1alpha interaction. *Nature* 2003;423:550–555.
131. Reaven GM. Pathophysiology of insulin resistance in human disease. *Physiol Rev* 1995;75:473–486.
132. Bergman RN, Van Citters GW, Mittelman SD, et al. Central role of the adipocyte in the metabolic syndrome. *J Invest Med* 2001;49:119–126.
133. Martin T, Collins S, Surwit RS. The C57BL/6J mouse as a model of insulin resistance and hypertension. In: Hansen BC, ed. *Lessons from animal diabetes*. Madras: Newgen Imaging Systems, 2002:73–86.
134. Rondinone CM, Wang LM, Lonnroth P, et al. Insulin receptor substrate (IRS) 1 is reduced and IRS-2 is the main docking protein for phosphatidylinositol 3-kinase in adipocytes from subjects with non-insulin-dependent diabetes mellitus. *Proc Natl Acad Sci U S A* 1997;94;4171–4175.
135. Goldstein B, Bittner-Kowalczyk J, White A, et al. Tyrosine dephosphorylation and deactivation of insulin receptor substrate-1 by protein-tyrosine phosphatase 1B: possible facilitation by the formation of a ternary complex with the Grb2 adaptor protein. *J Biol Chem* 2000;275:4283–4289.
136. Zabolotny JM, Kim YB, Peroni OD, et al. Overexpression of the LAR (leukocyte antigen-related) protein-tyrosine phosphatase in muscle causes insulin resistance. *Proc Natl Acad Sci U S A* 2001;98:5187–5192.
137. Zabolotny JM, Haj FG, Kim YB, et al. Transgenic overexpression of protein-tyrosine phosphatase 1B in muscle causes insulin resistance, but overexpression with leukocyte antigen-related phosphatase does not additively impair insulin action. *J Biol Chem* 2004;279:24844–24851.
138. Elchebly M, Payette P, Michaliszyn E, et al. Increased insulin sensitivity and obesity resistance in mice lacking the protein tyrosine phosphatase-1B gene. *Science* 1999;283:1544–1548.
139. Ren JM, Li PM, Zhang WR, et al. Transgenic mice deficient in the LAR protein-tyrosine phosphatase exhibit profound defects in glucose homeostasis. *Diabetes* 1998;47:493–497.
140. Cheng A, Uetani N, Simoncic PD, et al. Attenuation of leptin action and regulation of obesity by protein tyrosine phosphatase 1B. *Dev Cell* 2002;2:497–503.
141. Zabolotny JM, Bence-Hanulec JM, Stricker-Krongrad KK, et al. PTP1B regulates leptin signal transduction in vivo. *Dev Cell* 2002;2:489–495.
142. Kraegen EW, James DE, Jenkins AB, et al. Dose-response curves for in vivo insulin sensitivity in individual tissues in rats. *Am J Physiol* 1985;248:E353–362.
143. Shepherd PR, Gnudi L, Tozzi E, et al. Adipose tissue hyperplasia and enhanced glucose disposal in transgenic mice overexpressing GLUT4 selectively in adipose tissue. *J Biol Chem* 1993;268:22243–22246.
144. Tozzo E, Gnudi L, Kahn BB. Amelioration of insulin resistance in streptozocin diabetic mice by transgenic overexpression of GLUT4 driven by an adipose-specific promoter. *Endocrinology* 1997;138:1604–1611.

145. Abel ED, Peroni O, Kim JK, et al. Adipose-selective targeting of the GLUT4 gene impairs insulin action in muscle and liver. *Nature* 2001;409:729–733.
146. Colditz GA, Willett WC, Stampfer MJ, et al. Weight as a risk factor for clinical diabetes in women. *Am J Epidemiol* 1990;132:501–513.
147. Bjorntorp P. Body fat distribution, insulin resistance, and metabolic diseases. *Nutrition* 1997;13:795–803.
148. Okosun IS. Racial differences in rates of type 2 diabetes in American women: how much is due to differences in overall adiposity? *Ethn Health* 2001;6: 27–34.
149. Kissebah AH, Krakower GR. Regional adiposity and morbidity. *Physiol Rev* 1994;74:761–811.
150. Bergman RN, Ader M. Free fatty acids and pathogenesis of type 2 diabetes mellitus. *Trends Endocrinol Metab* 2000;11:351–356.
151. Patti M-E, Kahn CR. Lessons from transgenic and knockout animals about noninsulin-dependent diabetes mellitus. *Trends Endocrinol Metab* 1996;7: 311–319.
152. Unger RH. Lipotoxicity in the pathogenesis of obesity-dependent NIDDM. *Diabetes* 1995;44:863–870.
153. Griffin ME, Marcucci MJ, Cline GW, et al. Free fatty acid-induced insulin resistance is associated with activation of protein kinase C theta and alterations in the insulin signaling cascade. *Diabetes* 1999;48:1270–1274.
154. Zierath JR, Houseknecht KL, Gnudi L, et al. High-fat feeding impairs insulin-stimulated GLUT4 recruitment via an early insulin-signaling defect. *Diabetes* 1997;46:215–223.
155. Borkman M, Storlien LH, Pan DA, et al. The relation between insulin sensitivity and the fatty-acid composition of skeletal-muscle phospholipids. *N Engl J Med* 1993;328:238–244.
156. Shimabukuro M, Higa M, Zhou YT, et al. Lipoapoptosis in beta-cells of obese prediabetic fa/fa rats. Role of serine palmitoyltransferase overexpression. *J Biol Chem* 1998;273:32487–32490.
157. Shimomura I, Hammer RE, Ikemoto S, et al. Leptin reverses insulin resistance and diabetes mellitus in mice with congenital lipodystrophy. *Nature* 1999;401:73–76.
158. Gavrilova O, Marcus-Samuels B, Graham D, et al. Surgical implantation of adipose tissue reverses diabetes in lipoatrophic mice. *J Clin Invest* 2000;105:271–278.
159. Ogawa Y, Masuzaki H, Hosoda K, et al. Increased glucose metabolism and insulin sensitivity in transgenic skinny mice overexpressing leptin. *Diabetes* 1999;48:1822–1829.
160. Savage DB, O'Reilly S. Leptin: a novel therapeutic role in lipodystrophy. *J Clin Invest* 2002;109:1285–1286.
161. Petersen KF, Oral EA, Dufour S, et al. Leptin reverses insulin resistance and hepatic steatosis in patients with severe lipodystrophy. *J Clin Invest* 2002;109: 1345–1350.
162. Oral EA, Simha V, Ruiz E, et al. Leptin-replacement therapy for lipodystrophy. *N Engl J Med* 2002;346:570–578.
163. Minokoshi Y, Kim YB, Peroni OD, et al. Leptin stimulates fatty-acid oxidation by activating AMP-activated protein kinase. *Nature* 2002;415:339–343.
164. Salway J. *Metabolism at a glance*, 2nd ed. Blackwell Science: Oxford, 1999.
165. Galitzky J, Reverte M, Portill M, et al. Coexistence of beta 1-, beta 2-, and beta 3-adrenoceptors in dog fat cells and their differential activation by catecholamines. *Am J Physiol* 1993;264:E403–E412.
166. Collins S, Daniel KW, Rohlfs EM, et al. Impaired expression and functional activity of the beta 3- and beta 1-adrenergic receptors in adipose tissue of congenitally obese (C57BL/6J ob/ob) mice. *Mol Endocrinol* 1994;8:516–527.
167. Atgie C, D'Allaire F, Bukowiecki LJ. Role of beta1- and beta3-adrenoceptors in the regulation of lipolysis and thermogenesis in rat brown adipocytes. *Am J Physiol* 1997;273:C1136–C1142.
168. Rohrer DK. Physiological consequences of β-adrenergic receptor disruption. *J Mol Med* 1999;76:764–772.
169. Bachman ES, Dhillon H, Zhang CY, et al. BetaAR signaling is required for diet-induced thermogenesis and obesity resistance. *Science* 2002;297:843–845.
170. Jimenez M, Leger B, Canola K. et al. Beta(1)/beta(2)/beta(3)-adrenoceptor knockout mice are obese and cold-sensitive but have normal lipolytic responses to fasting. *FEBS Lett* 2002;530:37–40.
171. Soeder KS, Snedden SK, Cao W, et al. The β_3-adrenergic receptor activates mitogen-activated protein kinase in adipocytes through a Gi-dependent mechanism. *J Biol Chem* 1999;274:12017–12022.
172. Cao W, Medvedev AV, Daniel KW, et al. β-Adrenergic activation of p38 MAP kinase in adipocytes: cAMP induction of the uncoupling protein-1 (UCP1) gene requires p38 MAP kinase. *J Biol Chem* 2001;276:27077–27082.
173. Moule SK, Denton RM. The activation of p38 MAPK by the beta-adrenergic agonist isoproterenol in rat epididymal fat cells. *FEBS Lett* 1998;439:287–290.
174. Greenberg AS, Shen WJ, Muliro K, et al. Stimulation of lipolysis and hormone-sensitive lipase via the extracellular signal-regulated kinase pathway. *J Biol Chem* 2001;276:45456–45461.
175. Robidoux JR, Cao W, Cyr M, et al. Protein kinase A and ERK1/2 mitogen-activated protein kinases work in concert to mediate the β-adrenergic stimulation of lipolysis (submitted for publication).
176. Lafontan M, Berlan M. Fat cell α_2-adrenoceptors: the regulation of fat cell function and lipolysis. *Endocr Rev* 1995;16:716–738.
177. Gettys TW, Harkness PJ, Watson PM. The β_3-adrenergic receptor inhibits insulin-stimulated leptin secretion from isolated rat adipocytes. *Endocrinology* 1996;137:4054–4057.
178. Donahoo WT, Jensen DR, Yost TJ, et al. Isoproterenol and somatostatin decrease plasma leptin in humans: a novel mechanism regulating leptin secretion. *J Clin Endocrinol Metab* 1997;82:4139–4143.
179. Scriba D, Aprath-Husmann I, Blum WF, et al. Catecholamines suppress leptin release from in vitro differentiated subcutaneous human adipocytes in primary culture via beta1- and beta2-adrenergic receptors. *Eur J Endocrinol* 2000;143:439–445.
180. Jimenez M, Leger B, Canola K, et al. beta(1)/beta(2)/beta(3)-adrenergic receptor knockout mice are obese and cold-sensitive but have normal lipolytic responses to fasting. *FEBS Lett* 2002;530:37.
181. Champigny O, Ricquier D, Blondel O, et al. β_3-Adrenergic receptor stimulation restores message and expression of brown-fat mitochondrial uncoupling protein in adult dogs. *Proc Natl Acad Sci U S A* 1991;88:10774–10777.
182. Himms-Hagen J, Cui J, Danforth E Jr, et al. Effect of CL-316,243, a thermogenic β_3-agonist, on energy balance and brown and white adipose tissues in rats. *Am J Physiol* 1994;266:R1371–R1382.
183. Collins S, Daniel KW, Petro AE, et al. Strain-specific response to β_3-adrenergic receptor agonist treatment of diet-induced obesity in mice. *Endocrinology* 1997;138:405–413.
184. Ghorbani M, Himms-Hagen J. Appearance of brown adipocytes in white adipose tissue during CL 316,243-induced reversal of obesity and diabetes in Zucker fa/fa rats. *Int J Obes Relat Metab Disord* 1997;21:465–475.
185. Fisher MH, Amend AM, Bach TJ, et al. A selective human beta3 adrenergic receptor agonist increases metabolic rate in rhesus monkeys. *J Clin Invest* 1998;101:2387–2393.
186. Sasaki N, Uchida E, Niiyama M, et al. Anti-obesity effects of selective agonists to the β3-adrenergic receptor in dogs. II. Recruitment of thermogenic brown adipocytes and reduction of adiposity after chronic treatment with a β_3-adrenergic agonist. *J Vet Med Sci* 1998;60:465–469.
187. Ghorbani M, Claus TH, Himms-Hagen J. Hypertrophy of brown adipocytes in brown and white adipose tissues and reversal of diet-induced obesity in rats treated with a beta3-adrenoceptor agonist. *Biochem Pharmacol* 1997;54: 121–131.
188. de Souza CJ, Hirshman MF, Horton ES. CL-316,243, a beta3-specific adrenoceptor agonist, enhances insulin-stimulated glucose disposal in nonobese rats. *Diabetes* 1997;46:1257–1263.
189. Weyer C, Tataranni PA, Snitker S, et al. Increase in insulin action and fat oxidation after treatment with CL 316,243, a highly selective beta3-adrenoceptor agonist in humans. *Diabetes* 1998;47:1555–1561.
190. Granneman JG, Burnazi M, Zhu Z, et al. White adipose tissue contributes to UCP1-independent thermogenesis. *Am J Physiol Endocrinol Metab* 2003;285: E1230–1236.
191. Wilson-Fritch L, Burkart A, Bell G, et al. Mitochondrial biogenesis and remodeling during adipogenesis and in response to the insulin sensitizer rosiglitazone. *Mol Cell Biol* 2003;23:1085–1094.
192. Simpson ER, Zhao Y, Agarwal VR, et al. Aromatase expression in health and disease. *Recent Prog Horm Res* 1997;52:185–213.
193. Deslypere JP, Verdonck L, Vermeulen A. Fat tissue: a steroid reservoir and site of steroid metabolism. *J Clin Endocrinol Metab* 1985;61:564–570.
194. Jensen MD. Androgen effect on body composition and fat metabolism. *Mayo Clin Proc* 2000;75[Suppl]:S65–68.
195. Tchernof A, Despres JP. Sex steroid hormones, sex hormone-binding globulin, and obesity in men and women. *Horm Metab Res* 2000;32:526–536.
196. Seckl JR, Walker BR. Minireview: 11beta-hydroxysteroid dehydrogenase type 1—a tissue-specific amplifier of glucocorticoid action. *Endocrinology* 2001; 142:1371–1376.
197. Stewart PM. Cortisol, hypertension and obesity: the role of 11 beta-hydroxysteroid dehydrogenase. *J R Coll Physicians Lond* 1998;32:154–159.
198. Masuzaki H, Paterson J, Shinyama H, et al. A transgenic model of visceral obesity and the metabolic syndrome. *Science* 2001;294:2166–2170.
199. Bujalska IJ, Kumar S, Stewart PM. Does central obesity reflect "Cushing's disease of the omentum"? *Lancet* 1997;349:1210–1213.
200. Masuzaki H, Paterson J, Shinyama H, et al. A transgenic model of visceral obesity and the metabolic syndrome. *Science* 2001;294:2166–2170.
201. Morton NM, Paterson JM, Masuzaki H, et al. Novel adipose tissue-mediated resistance to diet-induced visceral obesity in 11β-hydroxysteroid dehydrogenase type 1-deficient mice. *Diabetes* 2004;53:931–938.
202. Morton NM, Holmes MC, Fievet C, et al. Improved lipid and lipoprotein profile, hepatic insulin sensitivity, and glucose tolerance in 11β-hydroxysteroid dehydrogenase type 1 null mice. *J Biol Chem* 2004;276:41293–41300.
203. Beutler B, Cerami A. The biology of cachectin/TNF—a primary mediator of the host response. *Annu Rev Immunol* 1989;7:625–655.
204. Lang CH, Dobrescu C, Bagby GJ. Tumor necrosis factor impairs insulin action on peripheral glucose disposal and hepatic glucose output. *Endocrinology* 1992;130:43–52.
205. Hotamisligil G, Shargill N, Spiegelman B. Adipose expression of tumor necrosis factor-alpha: direct role in obesity-linked insulin resistance. *Science* 1993;259:87–91.
206. Hotamisligil GS, Arner P, Caro JF, et al. Increased adipose tissue expression of tumor necrosis factor-α in human obesity and insulin resistance. *J Clin Invest* 1995;95:2409–2415.
207. Hotamisligil GS. The role of TNFalpha and TNF receptors in obesity and insulin resistance. *J Intern Med* 1999;245:621–625.
208. Fried SK, Bunkin DA, Greenberg AS. Omental and subcutaneous adipose tissues of obese subjects release interleukin-6: depot difference and regulation by glucocorticoid. *J Clin Endocrinol Metab* 1998;83:847–850.
209. Yudkin JS, Stehouwer CD, Emeis JJ, et al. C-reactive protein in healthy subjects: associations with obesity, insulin resistance, and endothelial dysfunction: a potential role for cytokines originating from adipose tissue? *Arterioscler Thromb Vasc Biol* 1999;19:972–978.

210. Shimomura I, Funahashi T, Takahashi M, et al. Enhanced expression of PAI-1 in visceral fat: possible contributor to vascular disease in obesity. *Nat Med* 1996;2:800–803.
211. Samad F, Loskutoff DJ. Hemostatic gene expression and vascular disease in obesity: insights from studies of genetically obese mice. *Thromb Haemost* 1999;82:742–747.
212. Funahashi T, Nakamura T, Shimomura I, et al. Role of adipocytokines on the pathogenesis of atherosclerosis in visceral obesity. *Intern Med* 1999;38: 202–206.
213. Loskutoff DJ, Fujisawa K, Samad F. The fat mouse. A powerful genetic model to study hemostatic gene expression in obesity/NIDDM. *Ann N Y Acad Sci* 2000;902:272–281.
214. Chandra RK. Nutrition and the immune system: an introduction. *Am J Clin Nutr* 1997;66:460S–463S.
215. Faggioni R, Feingold KR, Grunfeld C. Leptin regulation of the immune response and the immunodeficiency of malnutrition. *FASEB J* 2001;15: 2565–2571.
216. Sisson JG, West RJ, Fallow J, et al. The complement abnormalities of lipodystrophy. *N Engl J Med* 1976;294:461–465.
217. Cook KS, Min HY, Johnson D, et al. Adipsin: a circulating serine protease homolog secreted by adipose tissue and sciatic nerve. *Science* 1987;237: 402–405.
218. Choy LN, Rosen BS, Spiegelman BM. Adipsin and an endogenous pathway of complement from adipose cells. *J Biol Chem* 1992;267:12736–12741.
219. Flier JS, Cook KS, Usher P, et al. Severely impaired adipsin expression in genetic and acquired obesity. *Science* 1987;237:405–408.
220. White RT, Damm D, Hancock N, et al. Human adipsin is identical to complement factor D and is expressed at high levels in adipose tissue. *J Biol Chem* 1992;267:9210–9213.
221. Napolitano A, Lowell BB, Damm D, et al. Concentrations of adipsin in blood and rates of adipsin secretion by adipose tissue in humans with normal, elevated and diminished adipose tissue mass. *Int J Obes Relat Metab Disord* 1994; 18:213–218.
222. Esterbauer H, Krempler F, Oberkofler H, et al. The complement system: a pathway linking host defence and adipocyte biology. *Eur J Clin Invest* 1999; 29:653–656.
223. Coleman DL. Inherited obesity-diabetes syndromes in the mouse. In: *Mammalian genetics and cancer: the Jackson Laboratory Fiftieth Anniversary Symposium*. New York: Alan R Liss, 1979:145–158.
224. Baldo A, Sniderman AD, St-Luce S, et al. The adipsin-acylation stimulating protein system and regulation of intracellular triglyceride synthesis. *J Clin Invest* 1993;92:1543–1547.
225. Murray I, Sniderman AD, Havel PJ, et al. Acylation stimulating protein (ASP) deficiency alters postprandial and adipose tissue metabolism in male mice. *J Biol Chem* 1999;274:36219–36225.
226. Scherer P, Williams S, Fogliano M, et al. A novel serum protein similar to C1q, produced exclusively in adipocytes. *J Biol Chem* 1995;270:26746–26749.
227. Hu E, Liang P, Spiegelman BM. AdipoQ is a novel adipose-specific gene dysregulated in obesity. *J Biol Chem* 1996;271:10697–10703.
228. Nakano Y, Tobe T, Choi-Miura NH, et al. Isolation and characterization of GBP28, a novel gelatin-binding protein purified from human plasma. *J Biochem* (Tokyo) 1996;120:803–812.
229. Arita Y, Kihara S, Ouchi N, et al. Paradoxical decrease of an adipose-specific protein, adiponectin, in obesity. *Biochem Biophys Res Commun* 1999;257:79–83.
230. Maeda K, Okubo K, Shimomura I, et al. cDNA cloning and expression of a novel adipose specific collagen-like factor, apM1 (AdiPose most abundant gene transcript 1). *Biochem Biophys Res Commun* 1996;221:286–289.
231. Shapiro L, Scherer PE. The crystal structure of a complement-1q family protein suggests an evolutionary link to tumor necrosis factor. *Curr Biol* 1998;8:335–338.
232. Berg AH, Combs TP, Scherer PE. ACRP30/adiponectin: an adipokine regulating glucose and lipid metabolism. *Trends Endocrinol Metab* 2002;13:84–89.
233. Fruebis J, Tsao TS, Javorschi S, et al. Proteolytic cleavage product of 30-kDa adipocyte complement-related protein increases fatty acid oxidation in muscle and causes weight loss in mice. *Proc Natl Acad Sci U S A* 2001;98:2005–2010.
234. Combs TP, Berg AH, Obici S, et al. Endogenous glucose production is inhibited by the adipose-derived protein Acrp30. *J Clin Invest* 2001;108:1875–1881.
235. Yamauchi T, Kamon J, Minokoshi Y, et al. Adiponectin stimulates glucose utilization and fatty-acid oxidation by activating AMP-activated protein kinase. *Nat Med* 2002;8:1288–1295.
236. Kubota N, Terauchi Y, Yamauchi T, et al. Disruption of adiponectin causes insulin resistance and neointimal formation. *J Biol Chem* 2002;277:25863–25866.
237. Maeda N, Shimomura I, Kishida K, et al. Diet-induced insulin resistance in mice lacing adiponectin/ACRP30. *Nat Med* 2002;8:731–737.
238. Yang WS, Lee WJ, Funahashi T, et al. Weight reduction increases plasma levels of an adipose-derived anti-inflammatory protein, adiponectin. *J Clin Endocrinol Metab* 2001;86:3815–3819.
239. Weyer C, Funahashi T, Tanaka S, et al. Hypoadiponectinemia in obesity and type 2 diabetes: close association with insulin resistance and hyperinsulinemia. *J Clin Endocrinol Metab* 2001;86:1930–1935.
240. Hotta K, Funahashi T, Bodkin NL, et al. Circulating concentrations of the adipocyte protein adiponectin are decreased in parallel with reduced insulin sensitivity during the progression to type 2 diabetes in rhesus monkeys. *Diabetes* 2001;50:1126–1133.
241. Ouchi N, Kihara S, Arita Y, et al. Adipocyte-derived plasma protein, adiponectin, suppresses lipid accumulation and class A scavenger receptor expression in human monocyte-derived macrophages. *Circulation* 2001;103: 1057–1063.
242. Ouchi N, Kihara S, Arita Y, et al. Adiponectin, an adipocyte-derived plasma protein, inhibits endothelial NF-kappaB signaling through a cAMP-dependent pathway. *Circulation* 2000;102:1296–1301.
243. Hotta K, Funahashi T, Arita Y, et al. Plasma concentrations of a novel, adipose-specific protein, adiponectin, in type 2 diabetic patients. *Arterioscler Thromb Vasc Biol* 2000;20:1595–1599.
244. Pajvani UB, Hawkins M, Combs TP, et al. Complex distribution, not absolute amount of adiponectin, correlates with thiazolidinedione-mediated improvement in insulin sensitivity. *J Biol Chem* 2004;279:12152–12162.
245. Yamauchi T, Kamon J, Ito Y, et al. Cloning of adiponectin receptors that mediate antidiabetic metabolic effects. *Nature* 2003;423:762–769.
246. Hug C, Wang J, Ahmad NS, et al. T-cadherin is a receptor for hexameric and high-molecular-weight forms of Acrp30/adiponectin. *Proc Natl Acad Sci U S A* 2004;101:10308–10313.
247. Cassis LA, Saye J, Peach MJ. Location and regulation of rat angiotensinogen messenger RNA. *Hypertension* 1988;11:591–596.
248. Engeli S, Gorzelniak K, Kreutz R, et al. Co-expression of renin-angiotensin system genes in human adipose tissue. *J Hypertens* 1999;17:555–560.
249. Karlsson C, Lindell K, Ottosson M, et al. Human adipose tissue expresses angiotensinogen and enzymes required for its conversion to angiotensin. II. *J Clin Endocrinol Metab* 1998;83:3925–3929.
250. Frederich RC Jr, Kahn BB, Peach MJ, et al. Tissue-specific nutritional regulation of angiotensinogen in adipose tissue. *Hypertension* 1992;19:339–344.
251. Saye JA, Cassis LA, Sturgill TW, et al. Angiotensinogen gene expression in 3T3-L1 cells. *Am J Physiol* 1989;256:C448–451.
252. Saye J, Lynch KR, Peach MJ. Changes in angiotensinogen messenger RNA in differentiating 3T3-F442A adipocytes. *Hypertension* 1990;15:867–871.
253. Safonova I, Aubert J, Negrel R, et al. Regulation by fatty acids of angiotensinogen gene expression in preadipose cells. *Biochem J* 1997;322: 235–239.
254. Massiera F, Seydoux J, Geloen A, et al. Angiotensinogen-deficient mice exhibit impairment of diet-induced weight gain with alteration in adipose tissue development and increased locomotor activity. *Endocrinology* 2001;142:5220–5225.
255. Massiera F, Bloch-Faure M, Ceiler D, et al. Adipose angiotensinogen is involved in adipose tissue growth and blood pressure regulation. *FASEB J* 2001;15:2727–2729.
256. Masuzaki H, Yamamoto H, Kenyon CJ, et al. Transgenic amplification of glucocorticoid action in adipose tissue causes high blood pressure in lmice. *J Clin Invest* 2003;112:83–90.
257. Steppan CM, Bailey ST, Bhat S, et al. The hormone resistin links obesity to diabetes. *Nature* 2001;409:307–312.
258. Holcomb IN, Kabakoff RC, Chan B, et al. FIZZ1, a novel cysteine-rich secreted protein associated with pulmonary inflammation, defines a new gene family. *EMBO J* 2000;19:4046–4055.
259. Steppan CM, Brown EJ, Wright CM, et al. A family of tissue-specific resistin-like molecules. *Proc Natl Acad Sci U S A* 2001;98:502–506.
260. Kim KH, Lee K, Moon YS, et al. A cysteine-rich adipose tissue-specific secretory factor inhibits adipocyte differentiation. *J Biol Chem* 2001;276: 11252–11256.
261. Way JM, Gorgun CZ, Tong Q, et al. Adipose tissue resistin expression is severely suppressed in obesity and stimulated by peroxisome proliferator-activated receptor gamma agonists. *J Biol Chem* 2001;276:25651–25653.
262. McTernan PG, McTernan CL, Chetty R, et al. Increased resistin gene and protein expression in human abdominal adipose tissue. *J Clin Endocrinol Metab* 2002;87:2407–2410.
263. Savage DB, Sewter CP, Klenk ES, et al. Resistin/Fizz3 expression in relation to obesity and peroxisome proliferator-activated receptor-gamma action in humans. *Diabetes* 2001;50:2199–2202.
264. Patel SD, Rajala MW, Rossetti L, et al. Disulfide-dependent multimeric assembly of resistin family hormones. *Science* 2004;304:1154–1158.
265. Satoh H, Nguyen MT, Miles PD, et al. Adenovirus-mediated chronic "hyper-resistinemia" leads to in vivo insuln resistance in normal rats. *J Clin Invest* 2004;114:224–231.
266. Banerjee RR, Rangwala SM, Shapiro JS, et al. Regulation of fasted blood glucose by resistin. *Science* 2004;303:1195–1198.
267. Muse ED, Obici S, Bhanot S, et al. Role of resistin in diet-induced hepatic insulin resistance. *J Clin Invest* 2004;114:232–239.
268. Rajala MW, Qi Y, Patel HR, et al. Regulation of resistin expression and circulating levels in obesity, diabetes, and fasting. *Diabetes* 2004;53:1671–1679.
269. Savage DB, Sewter CP, Klenk ES, et al. Resistin/Fizz3 expression in relation to obesity and peroxisome proliferator-activated receptor-gamma action in humans. *Diabetes* 2001;50:2199–2202.
270. Steppan CM, Lazar MA. The current biology of resistin. *J Intern Med* 2004; 255:439–447.

CHAPTER 14
Biology of Skeletal Muscle

Alison C. Jozsi and Laurie J. Goodyear

ANATOMY

The human body contains more than 600 different skeletal muscles, collectively comprising the largest single organ of the body. The morphology of skeletal muscle at both the microscopic and macroscopic levels is intimately tied to its primary function, which is contractile activity. Each skeletal muscle in the body is covered by a dense connective tissue layer called the epimysium (Fig. 14.1). Extending inward from the epimysium is the perimysium, which surrounds small bundles of individual muscle fibers. Each individual muscle fiber within these bundles is surrounded by the endomysium, a thin layer of connective tissue. Within the endomysium is the cell membrane, which in muscle is called the sarcolemma. A dense capillary network extends throughout skeletal muscle, with several capillaries surrounding each muscle fiber. Individual cylindrical fibers do not always extend from one end of the muscle to the other; therefore, the connective tissue surrounding the muscle fiber bundles may be important for translating the mechanical forces of contraction throughout the length of the entire muscle group (1).

Muscle fibers contain dense networks of contractile proteins that are arranged precisely to achieve muscle contraction and body movement. Each muscle fiber is a single muscle cell. Fibers are roughly cylindrical, with the diameter of the fiber ranging between 10 and 100 μm (1). The length of fibers is variable, with some fibers extending the entire length of the muscle and to a length of 35 cm. The strength of a muscle fiber is directly proportional to its cross-sectional area, which can change dynamically commensurate with neuromuscular activity and muscle use.

Skeletal Muscle Organelles

Some of the organelles in the muscle fiber are similar to those in other eukaryotic cells but are named differently, such as the sarcolemma, the sarcoplasm, and the sarcoplasmic reticulum, which correspond to the plasma membrane, the cytoplasm, and the endoplasmic reticulum, respectively, of other eukaryotic cells. The sarcoplasm of the muscle fiber differs from the cytoplasm of most eukaryotic cells in that it contains a large quantity of stored glycogen. The sarcoplasmic reticulum is a longitudinal network of tubules within the muscle fiber that runs parallel to and surrounds the myofibrils (Fig. 14.2). The sarcoplasmic reticulum stores calcium, which is released during excitation of the muscle fiber. The transverse tubule system (T tubule) is a tubular network of membranous sacs that intertwines the myofibrils and facilitates the transmission of nerve impulses, as well as the transport of extracellular glucose, oxygen, and other electrolytes, to the individual myofibrils. The T tubules are formed by invaginations of the sarcolemma into and around the muscle fibers (1).

Although many of the organelles inside muscle fibers are common to most eukaryotic cells, muscle fibers are unique in many ways. For example, unlike most eukaryotic cells, which contain single, centrally located nuclei, muscle fibers are multinucleated, and these nuclei are located peripherally along the cell (Fig. 14.2). The nuclei likely act as local governing centers of cellular functions and adaptation to various stimuli and also function as integrated centers that communicate stimuli along the length of the muscle fiber to enable cohesive adaptation (2). The ratio of nuclei to cytoplasmic domain in a muscle fiber seems to be tightly regulated and dependent on the neuromuscular

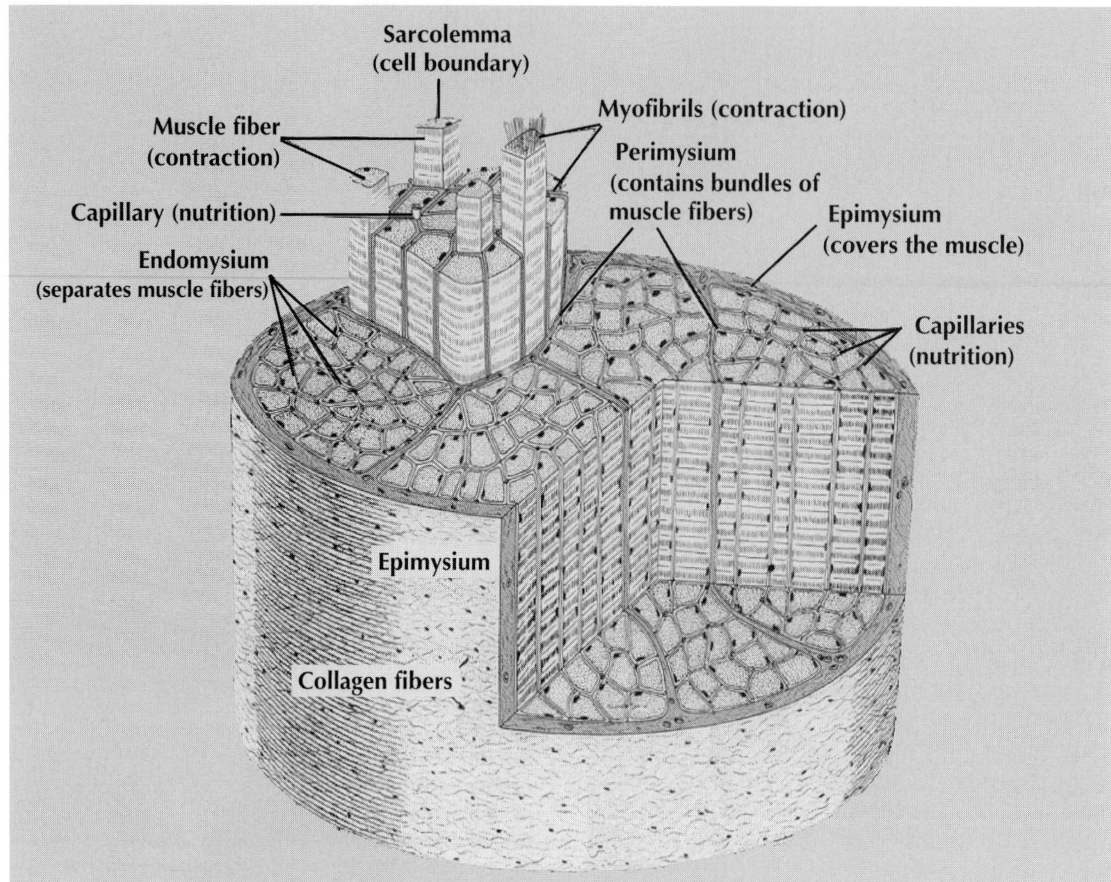

Figure 14.1. Skeletal muscle morphology. Each muscle cell (fiber) is composed of thousands of myofibrils. The membrane surrounding an entire skeletal muscle is called the epimysium. The epimysium invaginates into the muscle and surrounds clusters of individual muscle fibers. The sarcolemma surrounds individual muscle fibers. Each muscle fiber is surrounded by numerous capillaries, which provide oxygen and nutrients. (From Junqueira LC, Carneiro J, Kelley RO. *Basic histology*, 8th ed. Stamford, CT: Appleton & Lange, 1995, with permission.)

activity of the muscle fiber (2). Although mature muscle cells are postmitotic, skeletal muscle tissue has unique regenerative capacity afforded by quiescent myogenic cells called satellite cells that lie between the sarcolemma and the basal lamina of muscle fibers. The precise chemical and physical signals that activate satellite cells from their quiescent state to proliferate and differentiate into mature muscle fibers are still unclear.

Neuromuscular Junction

Muscle contraction occurs following the initiation and propagation of an action potential along a motor nerve to its endings on muscle fibers. The motor nerve enters the muscle and branches out between the muscle fascicles; these branches may then innervate a single muscle fiber or hundreds of muscle fibers. A motor unit is composed of a single nerve fiber and the cluster of muscle fibers that the nerve innervates. The site of neural innervation at the muscle cell surface is called the neuromuscular junction or the motor end plate (Fig. 14.3). The nerve axon terminus contains many mitochondria and synaptic vesicles containing the neurotransmitter acetylcholine. The space between the nerve axon terminus and the muscle fiber is called the synaptic cleft. To increase the surface area for acetylcholine receptors in the synaptic cleft, the sarcolemma is extensively folded in the region of the neuromuscular junction. There is a marked density of nuclei, mitochondria, ribosomes, and glycogen molecules in the sarcoplasm below the synaptic cleft (3).

Sarcomeric Structure

Each muscle fiber is composed of thousands of myofibrils, each of which is a cylindrical filament that runs parallel to the longitudinal axis of the muscle fiber (Fig. 14.4A). The myofibrils consist of a specialized arrangement of myosin and actin filaments, also called thick and thin filaments, respectively. These filaments interact to produce muscle contraction. Each actin filament is connected at one end to a protein structure called the Z line (or Z disc). The area containing actin and myosin filaments between two Z lines is called the sarcomere. Sarcomeres exist as repeating units along the full length of the myofibril and represent the functional (contraction-producing) unit of the muscle (4). The Z line is composed of two major proteins, α-actinin and desmin, which hold adjacent sarcomeres together. Titin is another very important myofibrillar protein that provides a lattice-like support structure that enables the side-by-side arrangement of myosin and actin. The actin filaments extend outward from the Z line into the sarcomere, and myosin filaments surround the actin filaments. The area on either side of the Z line

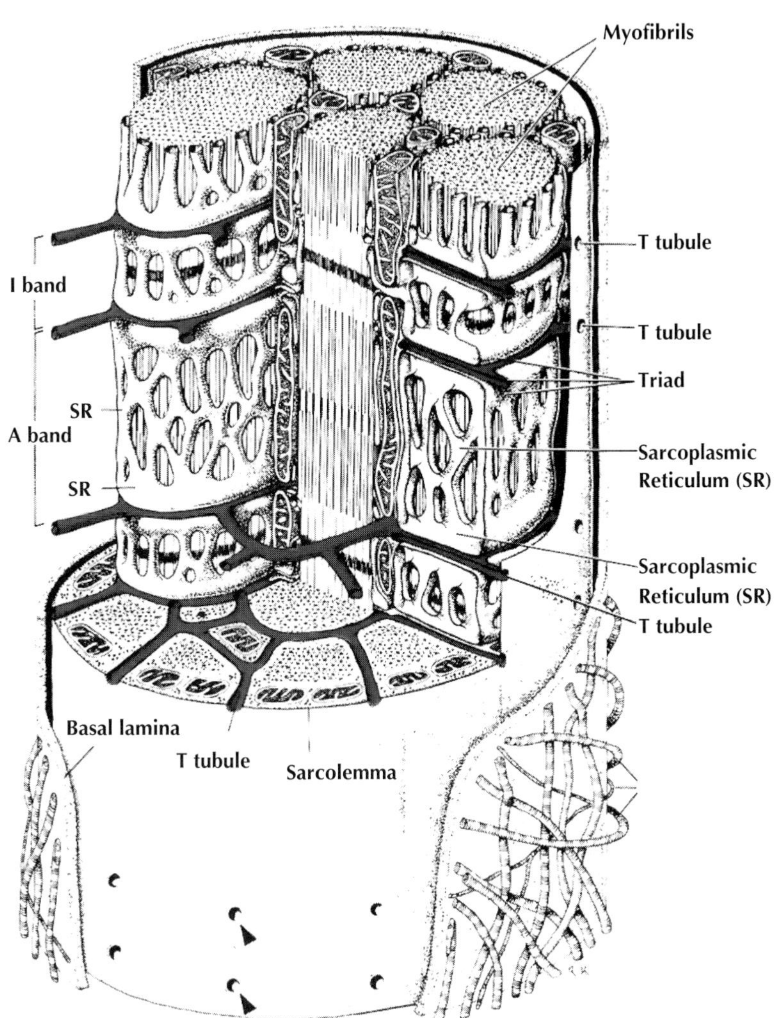

Figure 14.2. Intracellular architecture of the skeletal muscle fiber. The sarcolemma, the sarcoplasm, and the sarcoplasmic reticulum correspond to the plasma membrane, the cytoplasm, and the smooth endoplasmic reticulum, respectively, of other eukaryotic cells. The sarcolemma invaginates into the muscle fibers, creating the transverse tubule (T tubule) system, which facilitates the delivery of glucose, oxygen, and electrolytes to the myofibrils and the transmission of nerve impulses. (From Junqueira LC, Carneiro J, Kelley RO. *Basic histology*, 8th ed. Stamford, CT: Appleton & Lange, 1995, with permission.)

that is occupied only by actin filaments, with no overlap by myosin filaments, is the I band ("I" for isotropic; does not alter polarized light). The A band is the dark area in the middle of a sarcomere where the actin filaments are overlapped by myosin filaments ("A" for anisotropic; birefringent in polarized light) (1). When the muscle is not contracting, there is an area in the middle of the sarcomere occupied only by myosin filaments (H zone). When the muscle sarcomeres shorten, the actin filaments are pulled inward to completely overlap myosin filaments, and the H band disappears (4). The spatial arrangement of the thick myosin and thin actin filaments relative to one another, along with the other myofibrillar proteins that facilitate their interaction, yields a striated pattern observable under the light microscope (Fig. 14.4B).

A myosin filament consists of approximately 200 myosin molecules lined up end to end and side by side. Myosin has been studied extensively, and it is the diverse features of this protein that lead to the tremendous variation in contractile velocity and force production with different fiber types. Each myosin molecule is composed of two identical heavy chains and four light chains (Fig. 14.5A). The heavy chains are cylindrical proteins twisted around each other in a double-helical formation, each with a globular head at one end. The globular head portion of the myosin protein is able to bind both actin and adenosine triphosphate (ATP), as well as to hydrolyze ATP via intrinsic adenosine triphosphatase (ATPase) activity (5). Two myosin light chains are associated with each globular head region of the heavy chains and are thought to regulate the ATPase activity of the myosin head, thereby influencing the speed of muscle contractions. The three-dimensional structure of the myosin molecule is such that a portion of the cylindrical chain and the globular polypeptide head of the myosin molecule extend sideways from the helical body of the filament and form a cross-bridge to the actin filaments. Each cross-bridge is flexible at the place where the cylindrical arm begins to extend outward from the straight chain, as well as where the globular head meets this arm. These hinged regions enable both the extension of the globular myosin head away from the helical portion and movement of the myosin head when it is associated with the actin molecule, as is the case during contraction. The bundles of myosin filaments are twisted around each other so that each pair of myosin heads are separated by precisely 120 degrees, thereby ensuring that cross-bridges extend in all directions from the myosin filaments to interact with actin molecules (5).

The actin filament is composed of a double-helical arrangement of spherical actin monomers, each approximately 40 kilodaltons (kDa) (Fig. 14.5B). The actin monomers are called G-actin, and polymerized G-actin forms filamentous F-actin. Each G-actin monomer has one adenosine diphosphate (ADP) molecule bound to it; it is thought that this ADP molecule provides the binding site for the myosin cross-bridge. These active sites

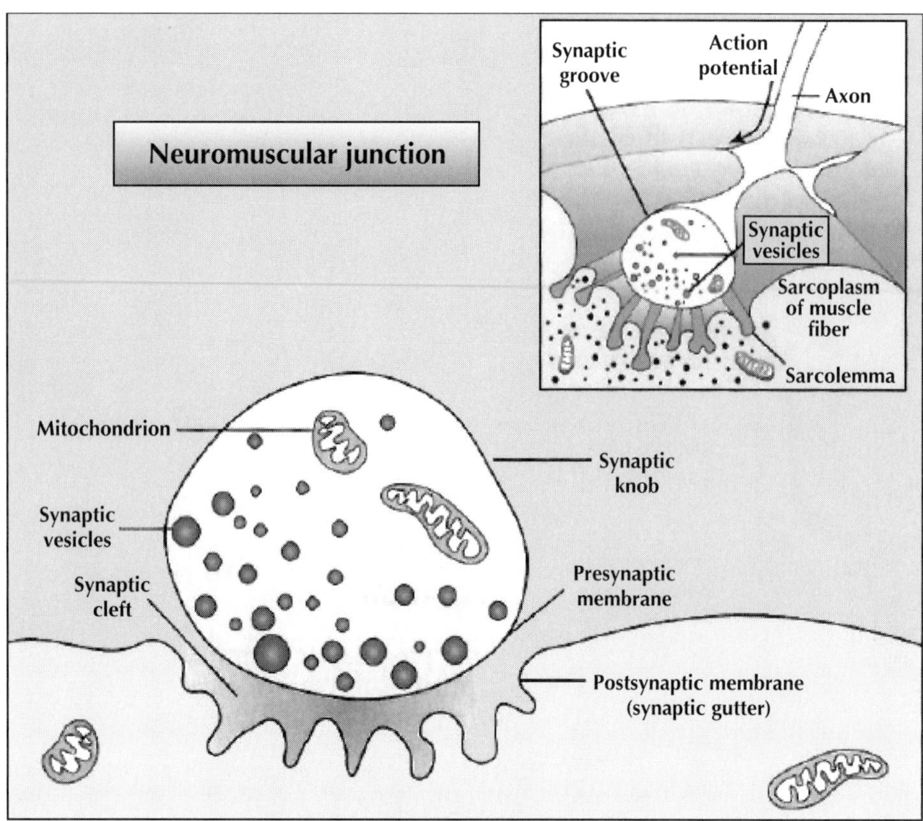

Figure 14.3. The motor end plate or neuromuscular junction. The inset shows the axon of a single motor neuron invaginating into the sarcolemma of a single muscle fiber. In the enlarged view, note that the nerve axon terminus contains many mitochondria and synaptic vesicles with the neurotransmitter acetylcholine. The space between the nerve axon terminus and the muscle fiber is called the synaptic cleft. Upon transmission of the nerve impulse to the axon terminus, acetylcholine is released from synaptic vessels into the cleft, thereby increasing the permeability of sarcolemmal and, subsequently, T tubule and sarcoplasmic reticulum (SR) membranes, resulting in calcium efflux from the SR for interaction with myofilaments and muscle contraction. (From Akert K. *Structures and functions of synapses.* New York: Raven Press, 1972, with permission.)

are also staggered for optimal interaction with the axially separated myosin cross-bridges. Two other proteins, tropomyosin and troponin, are associated with the actin filament. Troponin molecules bind approximately every seventh actin monomer along the filament. Troponin is composed of three subunits, Tn-I, Tn-C, and Tn-T (1). The Tn-T subunit binds troponin to tropomyosin and thereby attaches tropomyosin to the actin polymer. The troponin-tropomyosin complex blocks the active sites on actin for myosin cross-bridge formation when calcium is not present. The Tn-C subunit of troponin binds calcium during excitation of the muscle, which results in a conformational change that frees the active site and allows contraction to occur. The Tn-I subunit can inhibit tropomyosin when calcium is not present.

CONTRACTION OF SKELETAL MUSCLE

Skeletal muscle fibers shorten or contract when calcium is released into the sarcoplasm. Calcium release is coupled to depolarization of sarcolemmal and transverse tubule membranes. Taken together, this series of events has been defined as "excitation-contraction coupling." Membrane excitation occurs when the action potential reaches the nerve terminus, causing the synaptic vesicles in the nerve terminus to release acetylcholine into the synaptic cleft. The acetylcholine binds to acetylcholine-gated channels on the sarcolemma and increases the sarcolemmal permeability to sodium, resulting in membrane depolarization and the development of another action potential. The action potential and membrane depolarization is propagated across the entire sarcolemma and into the muscle fiber via the transverse tubule system and the sarcoplasmic reticulum (3). Translation of the action potential and subsequent depolarization of the sarcoplasmic reticulum culminates in the release of calcium into the sarcoplasm and the initiation of contraction.

Following release from the sarcoplasmic reticulum, the calcium ions bind the actin regulatory troponin-tropomyosin complex, thereby releasing the actin active sites so that actin-myosin cross-bridges may form. A basic description of muscle shortening or contraction can be provided by breaking the process into several steps (Fig. 14.6). The myosin ATPase enzyme in the globular myosin head cleaves a molecule of ATP to ADP + Pi (inorganic phosphate), the latter of which remains bound to the myosin head. The energy yielded from ATP hydrolysis causes a conformational change in the myosin head, during which the head extends perpendicular toward and attaches to the actin filament. When the myosin head attaches to the actin filament, the head moves inward toward the cylindrical arm of the myosin filament and pulls the actin filament in the same direction. The inward motion of the myosin head causes a conformational change that releases the bound ADP molecule, and a new ATP molecule binds. The binding of the new ATP molecule causes another structural change in the globular myosin head that releases the head from the actin active site. This cycle of ATP cleavage, myosin-actin attachment, and pulling actin forward repeats until the Z lines (to which the end of the actin filaments are attached) within each sarcomere have been pulled all the way in to the ends of the myosin filaments. This repeating process results in muscle contraction (5). With the cessation of the action potential, calcium is actively transported back into the sarcoplasmic reticulum, troponin can once again inhibit the actin-myosin binding site, and muscle relaxation begins.

Neuromuscular junction

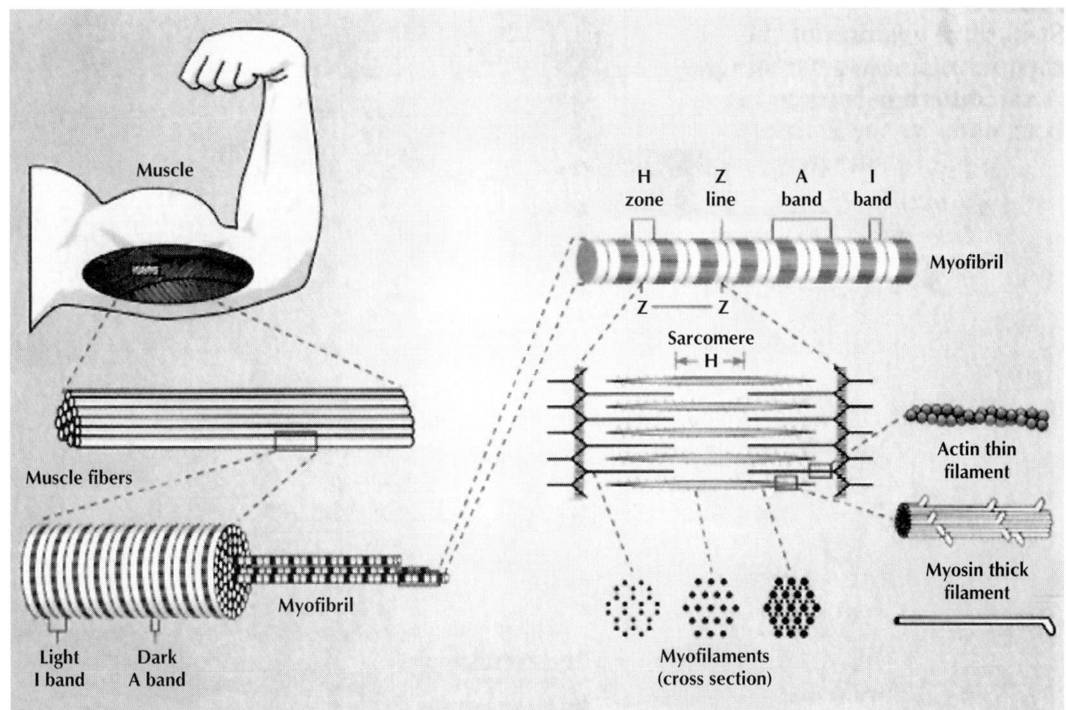

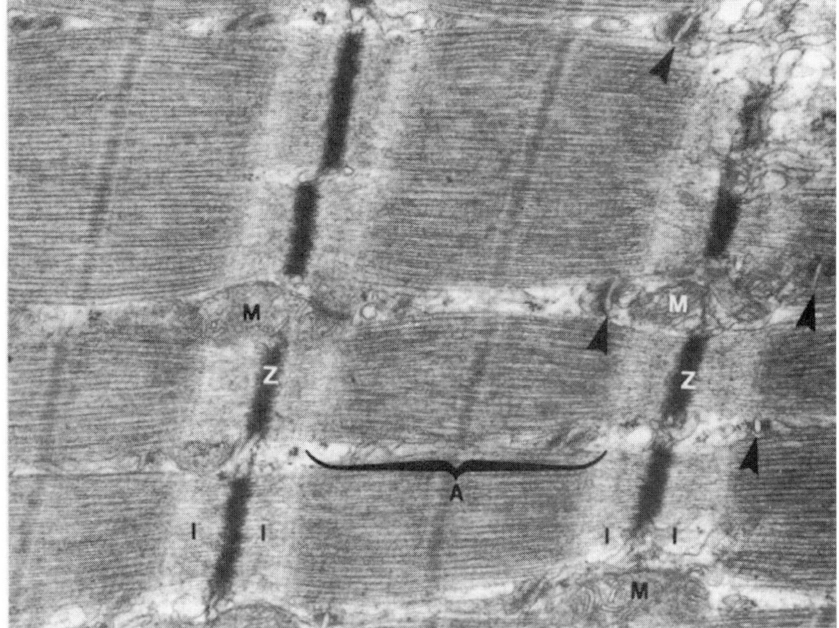

Figure 14.4. A: Diagram of the components of the skeletal muscle sarcomere. Each skeletal muscle is composed of numerous skeletal muscle fibers (*left*), which themselves are composed of thousands of myofilaments, consisting of two major proteins, actin and myosin. Actin filaments extend outward from a structure called the Z line (composed of two major proteins, α-actinin and desmin), and myosin filaments surround the actin filaments. This myofilament arrangement is repeated along the length of the fiber and produces a striated pattern, called the sarcomere, that is visible by light microscopy. The area on either side of the Z line that is occupied only by actin filaments, with no overlap by myosin filaments, is called the I band ("I" for isotropic; does not alter polarized light). The A band is the dark area in the middle of a sarcomere where the actin filaments are overlapped by myosin filaments ("A" for anisotropic; birefringent in polarized light). **B:** An electron micrograph of a longitudinal section of skeletal muscle. The Z lines (*Z*), I bands (*I*), and A band (*A*) of one sarcomere are clearly marked, and *M* indicates the presence of mitochondria between adjacent myofibrils. Arrows indicate triads. (**A** from Vander A. *Human physiology*, New York: McGraw-Hill, 1985, with permission; **B** from Junqueira LC, Carneiro J, Kelley RO. *Basic histology*, 8th ed. Stamford, CT: Appleton & Lange, 1995, with permission.)

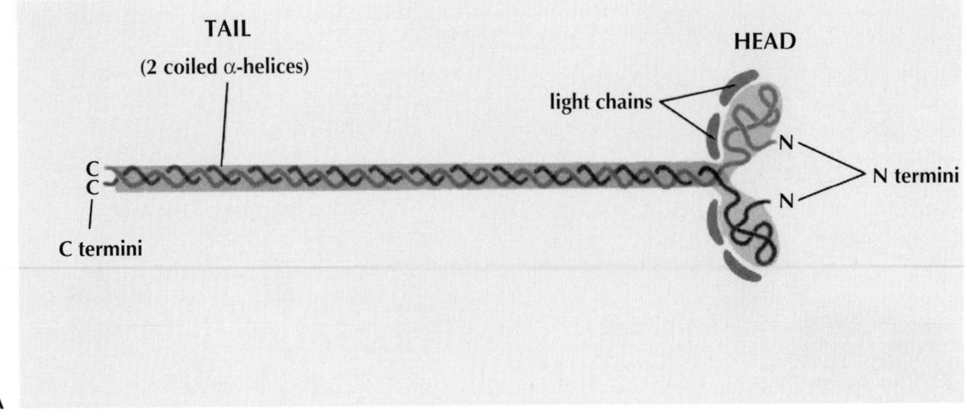

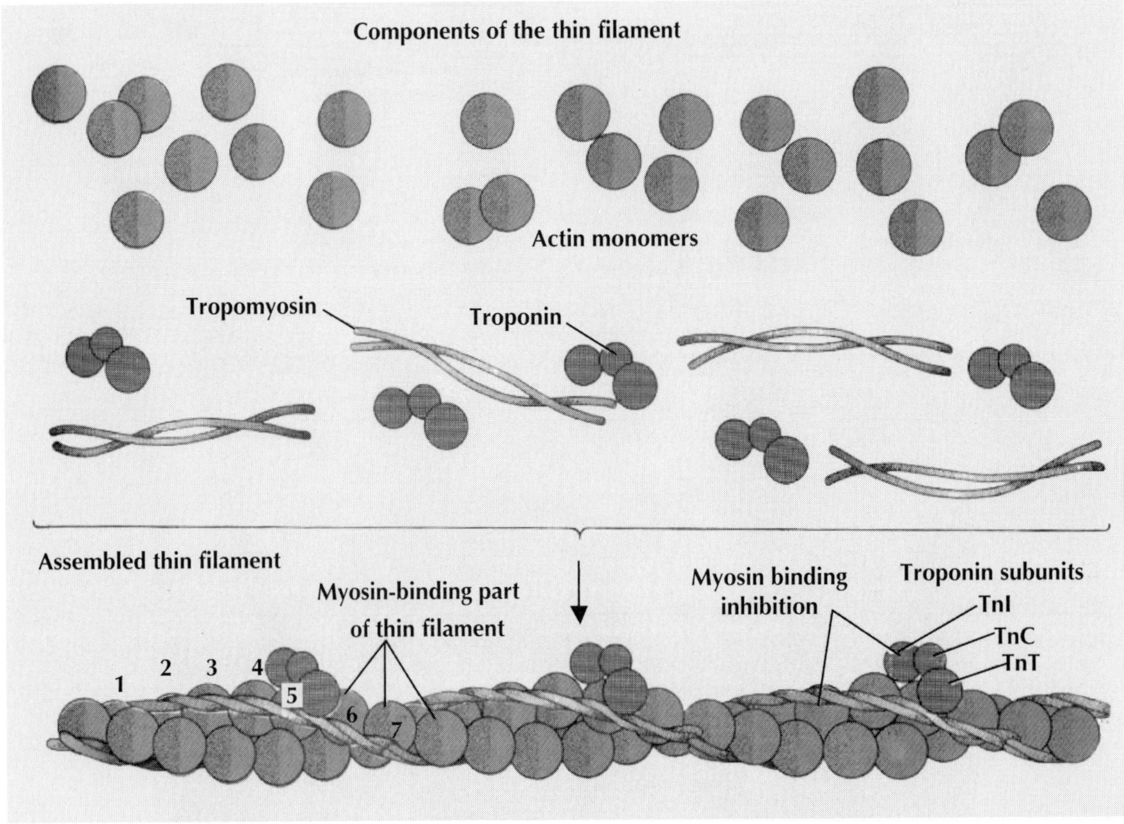

Figure 14.5. A: Diagram of a myosin filament, which is composed of two heavy chains and two light chains. On the C-termini, the heavy chains form a tail of two coiled α-helices, and at the N-termini, two opposing globular heads. The N-terminus or globular head region of the myosin molecule binds actin and has adenosine triphosphatase (ATPase) activity. Four light chains are associated with the globular head portion of the heavy chains, and these are thought to regulate the ATPase activity of the myosin head. **B:** Diagram of the actin filament, which is composed of three proteins: G-actin monomers polymerized to form the F-actin filament and two regulatory proteins, tropomyosin and troponin. Troponin is composed of three subunits, troponin-T, -I, and -C, which bind tropomyosin, inhibit tropomyosin, and bind calcium, respectively, during the cycle of muscle contraction and relaxation. (**A** from Alberts B, Bray D, Lewis J, et al. *Molecular biology of the cell.* New York: Garland Publishing, 1983, with permission; **B** from Junqueira LC, Carneiro J, Kelley RO. *Basic histology*, 8th ed. Stamford, CT: Appleton & Lange, 1995, with permission.)

When an action potential is propagated to all the nerve endings in a motor unit, all of the muscle fibers in the motor unit contract together. Therefore, motor units are modeled according to the intensity of the contraction required and the degree of motor control needed for various movements. In regions of the body where fine motor control is necessary, each nerve axon may innervate only one muscle fiber. Where coarser control is satisfactory but the development of great tension is desirable, as in moving a limb, larger motor units predominate, in which one motor nerve innervates clusters of muscle fibers (3).

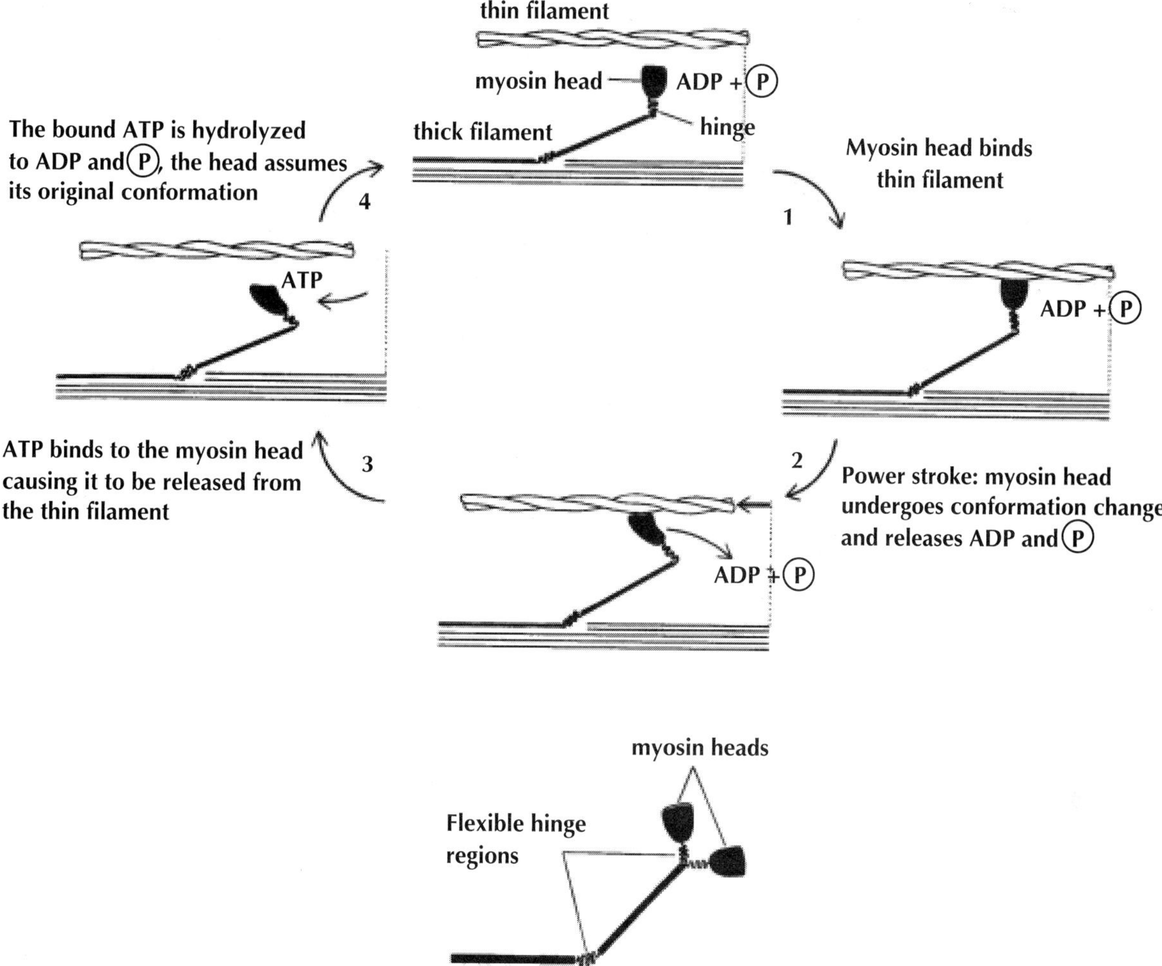

thin filament
myosin head
ADP + (P)
thick filament
hinge
The bound ATP is hydrolyzed to ADP and (P), the head assumes its original conformation
4
Myosin head binds thin filament
1
ATP
ADP + (P)
ATP binds to the myosin head causing it to be released from the thin filament
3
2
Power stroke: myosin head undergoes conformation change and releases ADP and (P)
ADP + (P)
myosin heads
Flexible hinge regions

Figure 14.6. Schematic of the interaction of myosin and actin filaments to produce muscle contraction. After cleaving a bound adenosine triphosphate (ATP) molecule, the myosin head undergoes a conformation change and extends upward toward and attaches to the actin filament. The head then moves inward toward the arm of the myosin filament and pulls the actin filament in the same direction. The inward motion of the myosin head releases the bound ADP molecule, and a new ATP molecule binds. The binding of the new ATP molecule causes another structural change in the globular myosin head that releases the head from the actin active site. This cycle results in muscle contraction. (From Alberts B, Bray D, Lewis J, et al. *Molecular biology of the cell.* New York: Garland Publishing, 1983, with permission.)

TYPES OF SKELETAL MUSCLE FIBERS

The muscle fibers differ tremendously morphologically, biochemically, and physiologically. Different muscle fiber types can be characterized by histologic methods according to myofibrillar ATPase activity or aerobic or anaerobic enzyme activity. For example, a reciprocal staining pattern occurs with acid or alkaline preincubation of muscle cross-sections, followed by myosin ATPase staining that reflects the spectrum of fiber types in the muscle. By this method, skeletal muscle was first divided into two major fiber types, type I and type II. Type I fibers are usually red, and type II fibers are white, proportional to the myoglobin content in the muscle. These fiber types are, as stated above, reciprocal in their metabolic enzymatic activities; slow-twitch type I fibers have low myosin ATPase activity and high aerobic oxidative enzyme activity, whereas fast-twitch type II fibers have high ATPase activity, low oxidative enzyme activity, and high anaerobic glycolytic enzyme activity. Investigations over the past 40 years have demonstrated that classifying fiber types by myosin ATPase is an oversimplification, and, in fact, muscle fibers commonly express several myosin isoforms at one time. Muscle fibers display a continuum of myosin isoforms, and a given fiber can alter its myosin ATPase, metabolic, and physiologic characteristics along either direction of this continuum, related to the stimuli received. For example, the human soleus muscle is a postural muscle and as such, contains primarily slow-twitch, oxidative type I fibers. However, under non–weight-bearing conditions, the soleus begins to express type IIa fibers, an intermediate fiber type that tends to be high in oxidative and glycolytic enzymes and in ATPase activity. With time, the soleus will progress further to a type IIb fiber phenotype, acquiring even more glycolytic and fast-contractile characteristics.

Skeletal muscle fibers display tremendous morphologic and biochemical plasticity in response to different stimuli, including altered energy status, gravity/mechanical load, neural stimulation, and intracellular calcium. It is clear that motor nerve activity influences muscle growth and fiber type by regulating muscle gene expression (6). The regulation of fiber type–specific gene expression likely occurs through both the pattern of electrical activity (and the resultant calcium release) and the trophic factors released at nerve termini. For example, it has been shown that reinnervation of muscles by motor neurons with a different firing pattern results in muscle fiber transformation. Similarly, remodeling of muscle fiber type distribution, myofibrillar proteins, mitochondria number, and metabolic enzymes has been observed following long-term electrical stimulation; a slow-to-fast fiber transformation is achieved with phasic high-frequency stimulation, and a fast-to-slow transition is achieved through chronic low-frequency stimulation. Chronic low-frequency stimulation decreases the surface area of the neuromuscular junctions and the postsynaptic folds. Many studies have documented an increase in type I slow-twitch fibers with endurance training, and the opposite fiber type transformation (an increase in type IIa fibers) has been shown following high-intensity, short-duration sprint training.

Calcineurin is a calcium/calmodulin-dependent phosphatase and is activated by sustained calcium elevation. Calcineurin is known to dephosphorylate the transcription factor nuclear activated T cells (NFAT), which enables NFAT to translocate into the nucleus and activate gene transcription in T cells. It has been proposed that calcineurin could regulate muscle-specific gene expression by transducing the different calcium signals transmitted through either tonic neural activity or intermittent bursts of neural activity. Calcium concentrations are relatively high in slow muscles and low in fast muscles. Activated calcineurin can upregulate slow fiber–specific gene promoters, and inhibiting calcineurin results in slow-to-fast fiber transformation (7). Further, the transcriptional activation of slow-fiber genes is mediated by the NFAT and MEF2 transcription factors.

CHANGES IN MUSCLE MORPHOLOGY AND FUNCTION IN DIABETES

In addition to the well-established metabolic changes in skeletal muscle associated with the progression of diabetes (see below and other chapters), there can be deleterious changes in muscle morphology associated with the advancement of this disease. It is often difficult to determine the evolution of such morphologic change because these types of alterations may precipitate from other end-organ complications, decreased activity, and/or increasing age. Some changes are observed only with long-term, uncontrolled type 1 diabetes.

A rare but severe complication of poorly controlled, long-duration type 1 diabetes is acute-onset diabetic muscle infarction (DMI). DMI is characterized by edema, tenderness, and muscle weakness and commonly presents in the vastus lateralis, thigh adductors, biceps femoris, and infrequently the triceps surae. Histologic assessments demonstrate edema; large areas of necrosis, fibrosis, regenerating fibers, and lymphocyte infiltration; and vascular thickening and thrombosis (8,9).

Characterizing the etiology and pathophysiology of type 1 diabetes through patient examination is limiting, as the physiology, genetics, and environment cannot be controlled. Several animal models of type 1 diabetes have been used to enable more comprehensive characterization and therapeutic and preventive strategies. One of the most commonly utilized models is administration of low-dose streptozotocin, which is toxic to β-cells, with diabetes ensuing after a few days (10). Animal models of diabetes have been used to study the time course of morphologic, neurologic, and vascular changes in skeletal muscle with diabetes. Diabetes progression can be associated with atrophy of skeletal muscle fibers, muscle weakness, diminished nerve activity, and decreased skeletal muscle blood flow (11–13). Diabetic neuropathies affect both sensory and motor nerves, as well as the autonomic nervous system. The physiologic derangements leading to neuropathies are not well defined, but it is hypothesized that hypoxia (precipitating from diabetic vasculitis) and hyperglycemia are primarily involved, as normalizing blood glucose is the most effective therapy (10). Hypoxia results in part from decreased capillary bed density and luminal diameter, resulting in diminished blood flow and oxygen delivery to the skeletal muscle (11). Alterations in the neuromuscular junction, muscle architecture, excitation-contraction coupling, and contractile properties have also been observed in streptozotocin-induced models of diabetes (12,14,15). A decrease in the number of synaptic vesicles and lower resting and end-plate potentials have been observed following induction of diabetes in mice. Further, streptozotocin-induced diabetes causes ultrastructural changes in the nerves and muscle fibers, including disrupted neurofilament and microfilament architecture and swollen and disrupted organelles (15). Similarly, a decrease in twitch tension and calcium mobilization in the sarcoplasmic reticulum has been observed in streptozotocin-treated mice (12,14). Together, these alterations may significantly decrease skeletal muscle contractile function.

SKELETAL MUSCLE METABOLISM

The metabolic rate in skeletal muscle is finely regulated by the acute energy requirements of the tissue and by hormonal mechanisms. In the resting condition, the major source of fuel for skeletal muscle is circulating nonesterified free fatty acids, providing approximately 85% to 90% of the required fuel (16). In the postprandial condition, when insulin is released from the pancreas, glucose uptake into muscle increases and the free glucose is rapidly phosphorylated by hexokinase to glucose-6-phosphate. If the muscle is not actively contracting, the majority of glucose-6-phosphate is shunted toward nonoxidative glucose disposal, resulting in increased muscle glycogen. The presence of high levels of glycogen in skeletal muscle is a unique feature of the sarcoplasm compared with the cytosol of other cell types.

Skeletal muscle is also unique among tissues because of its need to respond rapidly to large changes in cellular metabolism. There is only enough ATP stored within muscle fibers to sustain contractile activity for less than 1 or 2 seconds. The first source of energy used to restore ATP is phosphocreatine, which is stored within the muscle at levels that are approximately five times higher than those of ATP. When the chemical bond between creatine and phosphate is broken, the phosphate ion is transferred to ADP to form ATP by a reversible reaction catalyzed by creatine kinase. However, phosphocreatine as an energy source for ATP regeneration is also limited, capable of supporting only a few seconds of maximal muscle contractions. Energy is then provided for the resynthesis of ATP both by the anaerobic breakdown of glucose and glycogen to pyruvate and lactate and by the aerobic oxidation of carbohydrates, lipids, and proteins. The details of these metabolic pathways, along with a thorough discussion of their interactions, are described in other chapters in this text (Chapters 8, 16, 17, and 24).

Fatty Acid Metabolism

Of the various lipids in the body, fatty acids are the most important metabolic fuel for skeletal muscle. Sources of fatty acids can include triglycerides stored in the muscle or triglycerides stored in adipose cells within the muscle tissue (17). However, the majority of fatty acids are derived from the uptake of circulating fatty acids bound to albumin and circulating triglycerides present in the lipid core of very-low-density lipoproteins and chylomicrons. The enzyme lipoprotein lipase (LPL) is required to hydrolyze the fatty acids from circulating lipoprotein triglyceride before fatty acid transport across the vascular endothelium can occur (17). LPL activity is much higher in slow-twitch type I fibers than in more glycolytic type II fibers. Insulin downregulates LPL activity by decreasing LPL transcription and, therefore, its abundance.

The circulating fatty acids have to be transported into the mitochondria for oxidation, passing through the vascular endothelium, the interstitial space, the sarcolemma, and finally the outer and inner mitochondrial membranes. The transport of fatty acids across the vascular endothelium has not been clearly elucidated, but it is accepted that the fatty acids diffuse through the endothelium following release from albumin and are likely to rebind to interstitial albumin and to be brought to the sarcolemmal membrane. Transport across the sarcolemmal membrane is mediated by a transmembrane fatty acid transporter (FAT) found in a variety of tissues, including fat and muscle (17), although the mechanism and kinetics of this transporter are not fully understood. Once inside the sarcoplasm, fatty acids bind to fatty acid binding protein (FABP) and diffuse across the sarcoplasmic space to the mitochondrial membrane. The fate of fatty acids within skeletal muscle is either storage, in the form of triglyceride, or oxidation. After esterification to coenzyme A (CoA) by fatty acyl CoA synthetase, activated fatty acids can be transported into the mitochondria by carnitine to be oxidized (17). Carnitine acyl transferase I in the outer mitochondrial membrane converts fatty acyl CoA to acyl carnitine, which crosses the inner membrane via the carnitine–acyl carnitine translocase, in exchange for free carnitine. In the inner mitochondrial membrane, carnitine acyl transferase II catalyzes the exchange of the carnitine in the acyl carnitine for CoA, yielding intramitochondrial fatty acyl CoA, to be oxidized through the Krebs cycle.

Obesity and type 2 diabetes are associated with increased circulating levels of fatty acids and triglycerides and decreased muscle oxidation of fatty acids, leading to the accumulation of triglycerides in muscle (18). Lipid accumulation in muscle and liver is known to impair insulin signaling and metabolic enzyme activity and is strongly linked to the development of skeletal muscle insulin resistance and the multitude of diabetic metabolic complications (19). Indeed, it has been shown that interventions such as weight loss induced by dietary restriction and physical activity or treatment with peroxisome proliferator-activator receptor-γ agonists, the thiazolidinediones, can decrease muscle triglyceride content and improve insulin sensitivity (18,19). The precise mechanisms for the decrease in oxidation of fatty acids in skeletal muscle and the increase in lipid esterification in diabetes and obese states are unclear. However, proportional decreases in carnitine palmityl transferase 1 activity, the long-chain fatty acyl CoA mitochondrial translocase, and oxidative enzymes are consistent with a reduction in mitochondrial content or function or both (20).

Another mechanism by which altered intramuscular fatty acids have been proposed to induce insulin resistance in muscle is through the Randle glucose–fatty acid cycle. The Randle cycle suggests that glucose and fatty acids are oxidized reciprocally by skeletal muscle on the basis of their availability. An increase in fatty acid oxidation would lead to an increase in mitochondrial acetyl CoA, an inhibition of pyruvate dehydrogenase, and an increase in cellular citrate. The increase in citrate would lead to a downregulation of phosphofructokinase and, therefore, a decreased glycolytic rate. Decreased glycolytic flux would lead to an accumulation of glucose-6-phosphate and inhibition of hexokinase II, resulting in an increase in intracellular glucose and a decrease in glucose uptake (20). However, a series of investigations in which nuclear magnetic resonance (NMR) spectroscopy was employed to assess muscle glycogen and glucose-6-phosphate concentrations clearly demonstrated that fat-induced insulin resistance decreased glucose-6-phosphate concentrations and glycogen synthesis in muscle, likely due to a decrease in insulin-receptor signaling and glucose transport. As an alternative mechanism, it was proposed that the increase in by-products of fatty acid metabolism (fatty acyl CoA, diacylglycerol, and ceramides) activates serine/threonine kinases that phosphorylate insulin receptor substrate (IRS) proteins 1 and 2, thereby decreasing insulin signaling to phosphatidyl inositol 3-kinase (PI 3-kinase) and glucose transport (21).

Carbohydrate Metabolism

The maintenance of levels of skeletal muscle ATP through the oxidation of carbohydrate involves multiple steps. Of the three principal monosaccharides digested in the body, glucose is the major fuel source for oxidation, and under normal conditions, fructose and galactose are of minor importance. Once glucose is transported into skeletal muscle fibers, it is committed to cellular metabolism via phosphorylation by hexokinase to form glucose-6-phosphate. Glucose-6-phosphate then has one of three fates: (a) oxidation to pyruvate in the glycolytic pathway; (b) oxidation in the pentose phosphate pathway; or (c) synthesis to glycogen by glycogenolysis. The transport and metabolism of glucose are critical for cellular homeostasis in skeletal muscle, and under normal physiologic conditions, it is the transport process that is rate limiting for glucose utilization (22).

GLUCOSE TRANSPORT

The ability of skeletal muscle to remove glucose from the circulation in response both to food consumption and to physical exercise is a critical factor for the maintenance of euglycemia in humans. Glucose is transported into the muscle by a process of facilitated diffusion, utilizing glucose-transporter carrier proteins. Transport in muscle occurs through an increase in the maximal velocity of transport, without an appreciable change in the substrate concentration at which glucose transport is half maximal (23). Glucose transporters are a family of structurally related proteins that are expressed in a tissue-specific manner (24). In mouse, rat, and human skeletal muscle, GLUT4 is the major isoform present, whereas expression of the GLUT1 and GLUT5 isoforms is much lower (25,26). Studies of GLUT4 knockout mice reveal that this transporter is necessary for normal rates of basal, insulin-stimulated, and exercise-stimulated glucose transport (27,28).

Insulin and exercise increase glucose transport in skeletal muscle through the translocation of GLUT4 from an intracellular compartment to the sarcolemma and transverse tubules (29,30). The combination of exercise and insulin can have additive or partially additive effects on glucose transport, as well as an additive effect on GLUT4 recruitment to the cell surface, suggesting that there are different mechanisms leading to the stimulation of muscle glucose transport by exercise and insulin (29). GLUT4 translocation in skeletal muscle occurs by the exocytosis, trafficking, docking, and fusion of GLUT4-containing storage compartment or "vesicles" into the cell-surface membranes. Understanding of the composition, specificity, and trafficking of GLUT4 vesicles is still limited. Several of the so-called SNARE (soluble *N*-ethylmaleimide attachment protein receptor) proteins have been proposed to be involved in the regulation of the docking and fusion of GLUT4-containing vesicles. Following stimulation, the vesicle-associated SNARE proteins (v-SNARE), including vesicle-associated membrane protein-2 (VAMP-2), bind to the target-membrane SNARE proteins (t-SNARE), which include syntaxin 4 and SNAP23. This complex is thought to facilitate the fusion of GLUT4-containing vesicles into the cell-surface membrane. In studies with syntaxin 4 heterozygous knockout mice, syntaxin 4 has been shown to be a major molecule responsible for the regulation of insulin-stimulated GLUT4 redistribution and glucose transport in skeletal muscle (31). The roles of the SNARE proteins in exercise-stimulated GLUT4 translocation are less well understood, although VAMP2 has been shown to translocate to the cell surface in response to exercise (32).

There can be profound decreases in insulin action in people with type 2 diabetes, and impaired insulin-stimulated glucose transport at the level of skeletal muscle is a critical factor in the pathogenesis of this disease. The mechanism of the decreased insulin-stimulated glucose transport has not been fully elucidated, although, somewhat surprisingly, it is now well established that people with type 2 diabetes have normal levels of GLUT4 protein in their skeletal muscles (30). However, individuals with type 2 diabetes do have defective insulin-stimulated glucose uptake and GLUT4 translocation (33,34). Defects could include impaired ability of the GLUT4-containing vesicles to dock and fuse to the plasma membrane and/or T tubules or changes in specific activity of the glucose transporters on the membrane. Similar to the findings in humans, defects in GLUT4 translocation have been observed in animal models of type 2 diabetes and obesity (35,36). In contrast, exercise-stimulated glucose uptake and GLUT4 translocation in the Zucker rat (36–38) and in diabetic subjects (39) are normal. These studies reveal that the translocation machinery is intact in patients with type 2 diabetes but that there are likely to be defects in the insulin signal transduction system leading to GLUT4 translocation. The fact that the exercise stimulus functions via an independent mechanism that is able to bypass defects in insulin action, leading to normal glucose uptake into skeletal muscle, makes this mechanism a potential target for drug development.

GLYCOGEN METABOLISM

Glycogen is synthesized and stored within muscle fibers in response to feeding and in the period following exercise. The first step in glycogen synthesis is isomerization of glucose-6-phosphate to glucose-1-phosphate, which then is followed by conversion to uridine diphosphate (UDP)–glucose. UDP-glucose donates glucosyl residues to the priming protein glycogenin, which then passes linked glucosyl units to glycogen synthase and branching enzyme to assemble glycogen. The formation of α(1→4) oligosaccharides by glycogen synthase is considered to be the rate-limiting step in glycogen biosynthesis in skeletal muscle (40,41). Glycogen synthase is a multimeric protein consisting of four 85- to 90-kDa polypeptides. Catalytic activity of the enzyme is regulated by phosphorylation and dephosphorylation of up to nine serine residues. Net phosphorylation of glycogen synthase by various kinases leads to a reduction in catalytic activity, whereas dephosphorylation by phosphatases increases activity. Even when glycogen synthase is in the most highly phosphorylated form, maximal activity can be achieved by the allosteric effector glucose-6-phosphate. Therefore, net activity of glycogen synthase *in vivo* is controlled by a combination of allosteric regulation by glucose-6-phosphate and hierarchical phosphorylation and dephosphorylation of specific serine residues.

Glycogenolysis, the breakdown of glycogen, occurs in skeletal muscle in response to exercise and starvation. Muscle does not express glucose-6-phosphatase; therefore, glycogen breakdown in this tissue does not result in the release of glucose into the circulation. The rate-limiting enzyme for glycogenolysis is glycogen phosphorylase. Insulin inhibits the phosphorylation of the inactive form phosphorylase (b) to the active form (a). In contrast, the release of epinephrine results in glycogenolysis by a phosphorylation cascade that includes increasing levels of cytic adenosine monophosphate (cAMP) levels and cAMP-dependent protein kinase, leading to the phosphorylation and activation of phosphorylase b kinase.

Skeletal muscle of patients with type 2 diabetes is characterized by deficiencies in glycogen storage. NMR studies have indicated that persons with type 2 diabetes have a 60% reduction in muscle glycogen synthetic rate and that this reduction is not related to alterations in the glycogen synthase enzyme. Instead, this decrement in glycogen storage is due to alterations in glucose transport and hexokinase II activity that reduce the availability of glucose-6-phosphate (21,42). Patients with poorly controlled type 1 diabetes also have muscle insulin resistance, as evidenced by a decrease in the rate of glycogen synthesis (43). In this condition there is decreased glycogen turnover and glycogen phosphorylase (44), but these alterations are not due to primary defects in glycogen synthase activity (43).

Amino Acid Metabolism

There is a common misconception that the contribution of protein and amino acid metabolism to overall skeletal muscle metabolism is insignificant. However, as evidenced by dramatic changes in muscle size when the muscle is subjected to an increase (e.g., resistance exercise) or decrease (e.g., bed rest) in load, it is clear that the skeletal muscle has a tremendous capacity to alter rates of protein synthesis and degradation to adjust to changes in its fuel requirements. Understanding the regulation of protein synthesis and degradation in skeletal muscle has become an important research focus for the development of therapeutics to offset muscle wasting that occurs with trauma or in disease states such as diabetes, AIDS, cancer, or sepsis.

Because muscle is the largest source of protein in the body, the breakdown and synthesis of muscle proteins play a significant role in the maintenance of circulating levels of amino acids, acid–base balance, and, importantly, the generation of three-carbon intermediates for the Krebs cycle and gluconeogenesis. The interplay of muscle, hepatic, and renal protein turnover largely influences the pool of free amino acids, in addition to the rate of transport between the blood and tissues through transmembrane amino acid transporters. There is a dearth of knowledge about the specificity and kinetics of amino acid transporters, as compared with that about the glucose transporter. The transporters have generally been classified as system-A, for short-chain neutral amino acids, or system-L, for large neutral amino acids, for example (45). The translocation of amino acid transporters from endosomal sites, like glucose transporters, was not demonstrated until recently, when it was shown that insulin stimulates the exocytosis (although not the translocation or activity) of system-A transporters (SAT2) from a chloroquine-sensitive endosomal compartment in skeletal muscle (46). In general, alanine is a major muscle metabolite transported by system-A transporters, which are sodium dependent and insulin sensitive. System-L (insulin insensitive) transports branched chain amino acids (BCAA) and aromatic amino acids and is sodium independent and insulin insensitive. System-N (sodium dependent) transports glutamine, asparagine, histidine, and 3-methylhistidine across the sarcolemmal membrane. The activity of system-N is elevated following trauma or sepsis, for example, because glutamine is a major substrate for immune cells. The upregulation of both system-A and system-N appears to occur in response to changes in concentrations of the amino acid pool, resulting in transcriptional activation of genes encoding these transporters, whereas system-L appears to be regulated primarily by blood flow and the magnitude of the BCAA gradient across the muscle. BCAA cannot be degraded by the liver and therefore is taken up and degraded primarily by the muscle. Muscle breakdown of BCAA provides an abundant nitrogen source, which is used to synthesize alanine and glutamine and released by the muscle into the circulation (45).

Diabetes can be associated with skeletal muscle atrophy. Muscle atrophy results primarily from an increase in myofibrillar protein breakdown, which occurs through the activation of the ubiquitin proteasomal system (13,47). Streptozotocin-induced diabetes is associated with an increase in the mRNA levels of several proteasomal subunits and ubiquitin, the abundance of ubiquitin-protein conjugates/rate of conjugation, and the rate of ATP-dependent protein degradation, which is suppressed by proteasome inhibitors (48,49). These data suggest a role for the ubiquitin proteasomal system in mediating diabetic muscle atrophy.

SKELETAL MUSCLE SIGNALING

Biologic functions in mammalian cells involve the integration of highly regulated signaling cascades. A deviation from physiologic homeostasis is communicated to the inside of the cell by physical and biochemical interactions with the cell surface. In the case of skeletal muscle, signaling cascades can be grouped by the similarity of the events surrounding the initiation of the signal or the intracellular molecules and patterns of activation following signal initiation. This section will focus on insulin and exercise signaling mechanisms that have been implicated in the regulation of metabolic and transcriptional processes in skeletal muscle, because these have particular relevance for diabetes.

Insulin Signaling

In skeletal muscle, numerous biologic events require communication between the extracellular and intracellular compartments of the muscle fibers in response to insulin. Insulin signaling is initiated by the binding of insulin to the α-subunits of its cell-surface receptor, followed by phosphorylation of the insulin receptor on multiple tyrosine residues. Phosphotyrosine residues on the insulin receptor then interact with phosphotyrosine binding domains on several proteins, including the IRS proteins, of which IRS-1 and IRS-2 are expressed in skeletal muscle. Tyrosine-phosphorylated IRS can then act as docking proteins and interact with SH2 domains of other intracellular proteins, including the regulatory subunit of class I_A PI 3-kinases, resulting in the activation of the associated enzyme catalytic subunit (50,51). Activation of class I_A PI 3-kinases leads to the formation of specific phospholipids, including phosphatidyl inositol $(3,4,5)P_3$, which are critical for the recruitment of downstream molecules such as Akt to the membrane for phosphorylation by phosphoinositide-dependent protein kinase-1 (PDK-1). The activation of class I_A PI 3-kinases is critical for the actions of insulin, as nearly all physiologic responses of mammalian cells to insulin are prevented by pharmacologic inhibition or by overexpression of dominant-negative mutants of class I_A PI 3-kinase (52).

GLUCOSE TRANSPORT

The complete signaling mechanism leading to insulin-stimulated glucose transport remains elusive. It is now well established that PI 3-kinase is necessary, but not sufficient, for insulin-stimulated glucose uptake in skeletal muscle and other insulin-sensitive tissues. Some data support a role for the serine/threonine kinase Akt (also known as protein kinase B, PKB) downstream of PI 3-kinase in insulin-stimulated glucose transport. Overexpression of constitutively active forms of Akt in muscle cells mimics the actions of insulin on glucose transport (53,54), and mice deficient in the Akt2 isoform exhibit reduced insulin-stimulated glucose transport in isolated adult skeletal muscles (55).

GLYCOGEN SYNTHESIS

The dephosphorylation of serine residues on glycogen synthase that increases the catalytic activity of the enzyme could be due to the inhibition of a protein kinase that phosphorylates these regulatory sites or to the stimulation of a phosphatase that dephosphorylates them, or both. Several enzymes have been shown to exhibit specificity toward these sites *in vitro*. Signaling proteins that have been proposed to regulate glycogen synthase activity in muscle include protein phosphatase-1 ($PP1_G$) and glycogen synthase kinase-3 (GSK-3) (40,41). $PP1_G$ is a muscle-specific, type 1 serine/threonine phosphatase that is capable of dephosphorylating all nine regulatory sites of glycogen synthase (40,41). $PP1_G$ is a heterodimer consisting of a catalytic subunit and a regulatory subunit (R_{GL}) that targets the protein to glycogen and sarcoplasmic reticulum membranes (40,41). $PP1_G$ has been proposed to mediate insulin-stimulated glycogen synthesis in skeletal muscle (56). It has been hypothesized that insulin binding to its receptor would lead to 90-kDa ribosomal S6 kinase (RSK2)–induced phosphorylation of R_{GL}, which would then enable $PP1_G$ to dephosphorylate and activate glycogen synthase (56). However, it has since been demonstrated that mice deficient in R_{GL} display a normal activation of glycogen synthase in response to insulin treatment (57), strongly suggesting that $PP1_G$ is not necessary for insulin-stimulated glycogen metabolism. On the other hand, there is a great deal of evidence suggesting that insulin-stimulated glycogen synthase activation is mediated in part through a PI 3-kinase–dependent mechanism that leads to the inhibition of GSK-3 (40,41).

PROTEIN SYNTHESIS

The effect of insulin to increase muscle protein has been recognized for many years; however, whether the importance of insulin actions on protein metabolism is to increase the synthetic rate or to decrease protein degradation has not been resolved. It is known that the ability of insulin to stimulate protein synthesis is absent when the availability of amino acids is inadequate (58). Combining these two ideas, a recent investigation (59) demonstrated that combined administration of insulin and leucine elevated rates of protein synthesis by more than 50%. The mechanism of insulin action on protein synthesis appears to be through (a) the increased phosphorylation of the translational repressor, eukaryotic initiation factor (eIF) 4E binding protein-1 (4E-BP1), releasing its inhibitory effect on the formation of the eIF4G*eIF4E complex and the initiation of protein translation, and (b) increased phosphorylation and activation of the ribosomal protein S6 kinase (p70S6 kinase) (59).

GENE TRANSCRIPTION

Recent investigations have demonstrated that insulin signaling in skeletal muscle leads to an increase in metabolic gene expression (60–65). In regard to insulin signaling, insulin has been shown to mediate an increase in the gene expression of the p85α regulatory subunit of PI 3-kinase, whereas inhibition of the PI 3-kinase/Akt/p70S6 kinase pathway blocks this effect (61). Interestingly, insulin has been shown to increase GLUT4 and hexokinase II transcription, and this effect of insulin may also be mediated through the PI 3-kinase/p70S6 kinase pathway (62,63). The increased expression of glycogen phosphorylase in skeletal muscle in diabetic muscle also appears to be mediated by insulin signaling and may contribute to the glycogen storage deficiency observed with diabetes (65).

ALTERATIONS IN INSULIN SIGNALING WITH DIABETES

Skeletal muscle is the largest storage reservoir for glucose in the body, and defects in insulin action to promote glucose uptake by muscle can result in elevations in circulating concentrations of glucose and altered storage of glycogen by muscle. As discussed in a previous section, in insulin-resistant states such as obesity and type 2 diabetes, expression of GLUT4 protein is normal in skeletal muscle but translocation of GLUT4 is defective (66–68). These defects are thought to be a consequence of impaired intracellular signaling. In some conditions this may involve defective activation of PI 3-kinase, which results, at least in part, from decreased expression of the p85 regulatory subunit (69,70). Insulin-stimulated activation of PI 3-kinase is impaired in skeletal muscle in rodent models of genetic obesity and hyperinsulinemic diabetes (71,72), in rats rendered insulin resistant with high-fat feeding (73) or glucocorticoid treatment (74), and in humans with obesity (69) and type 2 diabetes (70).

Downstream of PI 3-kinase, defective insulin-stimulated Akt activation has been shown in nonobese humans with type 2 diabetes (75). In contrast, muscle biopsy samples obtained from obese and from obese diabetic subjects have demonstrated normal insulin-stimulated Akt1, Akt2, and Akt3 activation despite marked reductions in glucose disposal, IRS-1– and IRS-2–associated PI 3-kinase activity, and glycogen synthase activity (76). (GSK-3) a downstream target of Akt, has been reported to be altered in human subjects with type 2 diabetes. Muscle biopsy samples obtained from people with type 2 diabetes were shown to have 25% to 50% greater expression of GSK-3α and β protein and substantially elevated total GSK-3 activity (77). Significant inverse correlations also were observed between expression of GSK-3 protein and insulin-stimulated glycogen synthase activity and whole-body rates of glucose disposal, suggesting that GSK-3 may contribute to peripheral insulin resistance. In addition to Akt and GSK-3 being potential mediators of insulin resistance, there are reports of the atypical protein kinase (PKC) isoforms, λ/ζ, being downstream of PI 3-kinase in insulin signaling. Interestingly, insulin-stimulated PKC λ/ζ activity in skeletal muscle of individuals who are obese or obese with type 2 diabetes is reduced compared with the activity in lean control subjects, and this decrease in activation may be due to the reduced expression of PKC λ/ζ protein in the skeletal muscle of the patients (78). Thus, there is good evidence that insulin resistance in skeletal muscle may stem from impaired expression and/or function of multiple insulin signaling proteins that are likely critical for insulin action on glucose transport and glycogen synthesis. The mechanisms that lead to the downregulation of these skeletal muscle signaling proteins are not fully understood at this time.

Exercise Signaling

Multiple insulin-independent signaling pathways may lead to stimulation of glucose transport in skeletal muscle. Exercise is probably the most physiologically relevant of these stimuli; the intracellular signaling molecules leading to contraction-stimulated glucose transport are less well defined than those for insulin. In contrast to the effects of insulin, exercise does not increase tyrosine phosphorylation of the insulin receptor, IRS-1, IRS-2, or PI 3-kinase activity (79). Furthermore, wortmannin, a PI 3-kinase inhibitor, does not inhibit glucose transport in isolated rat muscle incubated and contracted *in vitro* (80–82). A study of genetically altered knockout mice that do not express insulin receptors in skeletal muscles has shown that exercise can normally increase glucose transport, whereas insulin-stimulated glucose transport in muscle is fully inhibited (83). Likewise, IRS-2 knockout mice have normal rates of exercise-stimulated glucose transport (84). Thus, although exercise and insulin both recruit GLUT4 to the plasma membrane and activate glucose transport, proximal insulin signaling events are not necessary for exercise to increase GLUT4 translocation or glucose transport in skeletal muscle.

Studies implicating the AMP-activated protein kinase (AMPK) as a critical signaling molecule for the regulation of multiple metabolic and growth processes in contracting skeletal muscle have provided exciting advances in the field of skeletal muscle biology. AMP kinase is a member of a metabolite-sensing protein kinase family that acts as a fuel gauge monitoring cellular energy levels and is the mammalian homologue of the SNF-1 protein kinase in *Saccharomyces cerevisiae*, which is critical for the adaptation of yeast to nutrient stress (85). When AMPK "senses" decreased energy storage, it acts to switch off ATP-consuming pathways and to switch on alternative pathways for ATP regeneration. AMPK is rapidly activated in skeletal muscle under numerous conditions, including contraction, hypoxia, uncoupling of oxidative phosphorylation, and osmotic shock (86). AMPK is activated by an increase in the AMP/ATP ratio by a mechanism that involves allosteric modification, phosphorylation by an AMPK kinase, and decreases in phosphatase activities.

Initial evidence in support of a role for AMPK in contraction-stimulated glucose transport came from studies using 5-aminoimidazole-4-carboxamide ribonucleoside (AICAR). AICAR is taken up into skeletal muscle and metabolized by adenosine kinase to form ZMP, the monophosphorylated derivative that mimics the effects of AMP on AMPK (87,88). AICAR can stimulate glucose transport in the absence of insulin, similar to the effects of exercise (88,89), and AICAR-stimulated transport is not inhibited by wortmannin, the pharmacologic inhibitor of PI 3-kinase. Furthermore, the increase in glucose transport with the combination of maximal AICAR plus maximal insulin treatments is partially additive, whereas there is no additive effect on glucose transport with the combination of AICAR plus contraction (88). Short-term infusion of rats with AICAR (and glucose to maintain euglycemia) also increases 2-deoxyglucose transport in multiple muscle types. Interestingly, patients with type 2 diabetes have normal activation of AMPK in skeletal muscle (90). The recent generation of a transgenic mouse expressing an inactive (dominant-negative) AMPK protein has suggested that AMPK may only be part of the mechanism leading to contraction-stimulated glucose transport (91). Elucidating additional mechanisms for contraction-stimulated glucose transport will be an important goal for skeletal muscle research in the next several years.

In addition to glucose transport, AMPK has been proposed to mediate the effects of muscle contractile activity on multiple other metabolic and transcriptional events in skeletal muscle. The initial studies showing AMPK activation in skeletal muscle provided the first evidence that AMPK plays an important role in the regulation of fatty acid oxidation during exercise (92–94). This occurs through AMPK phosphorylation of the β isoform of acetyl-CoA carboxylase (ACCβ), resulting in ACC inactivation, a decrease in malonyl-CoA content, and a subsequent increase in fatty acid oxidation after removing the inhibition of carnitine palmitoyl transferase I (92–94). Evidence for regulation of glycogen metabolism by AMPK in skeletal muscle is more controversial. *In vitro* AMPK can phosphorylate proteins involved in glycogen metabolism, including Ser^7 on glycogen synthase *in vitro* (95), which would be expected to inhibit glycogen synthesis (96), and phosphorylase kinase (95), the immediate upstream effector of glycogen phosphorylase. On the other hand, there is also compelling evidence that AMPK functions to increase glycogen synthesis, because chronic AICAR treatment for 5 to 28 days increases glycogen content in both type I and type II fibers (97,98). However, because chronic AICAR treatment causes numerous metabolic responses as well as increased GLUT4 content in skeletal muscle (97), the increased glycogen content may be due to the effects of AICAR on metabolism rather than direct regulation of glycogen synthase or glycogen phosphorylase.

Studies of SNF-1, the AMPK homologue in yeast, have provided evidence that AMPK plays an important role in the regulation of gene transcription (85). Studies of skeletal muscle support the concept that AMPK is involved in gene regulation, because chronic administration of AICAR via daily injections for 5 to 28 days significantly increases the expression of GLUT4 and hexokinase in multiple muscles composed of different fiber types, including epitrochlearis, gastrocnemius (99), and red and white quadriceps muscles (97). Furthermore, AICAR infusion resulted in significantly increased transcription of the genes encoding uncoupling protein 3 (UCP3), heme oxygenase-1 (HO-1), hexokinase II, and GLUT4 in rat gastrocnemius muscles (100). The mechanism by which AMPK modulates gene transcription remains unclear. However, these studies raise the possibility that AMPK is a key intermediary in the effects of a single bout of exercise in altering the induction of multiple genes. The accumulation of these individual effects of each exercise bout may lead to adaptations by muscle to chronic exercise training.

SUMMARY

The past 20 years have brought considerable advances in understanding the biochemistry underlying skeletal muscle contraction and metabolism. Of particular relevance to diabetes is the considerable enhancement of our understanding of the molecular mechanisms of insulin action as well as of the mechanism by which contractile activity enhances carbohydrate metabolism in skeletal muscle. With the continued development of novel methodologies for investigating signal transduction, metabolism, and transcriptional regulation in skeletal muscle, progress in this important area should continue in the near future.

REFERENCES

1. Junqueira LC, Carneiro J, Kelley RO, eds. Muscle tissue. In: *Basic histology*. Stanford, CT: Appleton & Lange, 1995:181–196.
2. Roy RR, Monke SR, Allen DL, et al. Modulation of myonuclear number in functionally overloaded and exercised rat plantaris fibers. *J Appl Physiol* 1999;87:634–642.
3. Guyton AC ed. *Excitation of skeletal muscle contraction: Neuromuscular transmission and excitation-contraction coupling*. Philadelphia: WB Saunders, 1991.
4. McArdle WD, Katch FI, Katch VL, eds. Skeletal muscle: structure and function. In: *Exercise physiology: energy, nutrition, and human performance*. Malvern, PA: Lea & Febiger, 1991:348–366.
5. Guyton AC, Hall JE. Contraction of skeletal muscle. In: *Textbook of medical physiology*, 10th ed. Philadelphia: WB Saunders, 2000:67–78
6. Schiaffino S, Murgia M, Serrano AL, et al. How is muscle phenotype controlled by nerve activity? *Ital J Neurol Sci* 1999;20:409–412.
7. Berchtold MW, Brinkmeier H, Muntener M. Calcium ion in skeletal muscle: its crucial role for muscle function, plasticity, and disease. *Physiol Rev* 2000;80:1215–1265.
8. Umpierrez GE, Stiles RG, Kleinbart J, et al. Diabetic muscle infarction. *Am J Med* 1996;101:245–250.
9. Lafforgue P, Janand-Delenne B, Lassman-Vague V, et al. Painful swelling of the thigh in a diabetic patient: diabetic muscle infarction. *Diabetes Metab* 1999;25:255–260.
10. Mordes JP, Greiner DL, Rossini AA. Animal models of autoimmune diabetes mellitus. In: LeRoith D, Taylor SI, Olefsky JM, eds. *Diabetes mellitus: a fundamental and clinical text*. Philadelphia: Lippincott Williams & Wilkins, 2000:435–436.
11. Kindig CA, Sexton WL, Fedde MR, et al. Skeletal muscle microcirculatory structure and hemodynamics in diabetes. *Respir Physiol* 1998;111:163–175.
12. Fahim MA, el Sabban F, Davidson N. Muscle contractility decrement and correlated morphology during the pathogenesis of streptozotocin-diabetic mice. *Anat Rec* 1998;251:240–244.
13. Furuno K, Goodman MN, Goldberg AL. Role of different proteolytic systems in the degradation of muscle proteins during denervation atrophy. *J Biol Chem* 1990;265:8550–8557.
14. Eibschutz B, Lopaschuk GD, McNeill JH, et al. Ca2+-transport in skeletal muscle sarcoplasmic reticulum of the chronically diabetic rat. *Res Commun Chem Pathol Pharmacol* 1984;45:301–304.
15. Fahim MA, Hasan MY, Alshuaib WB. Early morphological remodeling of neuromuscular junction in a murine model of diabetes. *J Appl Physiol* 2000;89:2235–2240.
16. Ahlborg G, Felig P, Hagenfeldt L, et al. Substrate turnover during prolonged exercise in man. Splanchnic and leg metabolism of glucose, free fatty acids, and amino acids. *J Clin Invest* 1974;53:1080–1090.
17. van der Vusse GJ, Reneman RS. Lipid metabolism in skeletal muscle. In: Rowell LB, Shepherd JT, eds. *Handbook of physiology*. New York: Oxford University Press, 1996:952.
18. Kelley DE, Goodpaster BH. Skeletal muscle triglyceride. An aspect of regional adiposity and insulin resistance. *Diabetes Care* 2001;24:933–941.
19. Kraegen EW, Cooney GJ, Ye JM, et al. The role of lipids in the pathogenesis of muscle insulin resistance and beta cell failure in type II diabetes and obesity. *Exp Clin Endocrinol Diabetes* 2001;109:S189–S201.
20. Kelley DE, Mandarino LJ. Fuel selection in human skeletal muscle in insulin resistance: a reexamination. *Diabetes* 2000;49:677–683.
21. Shulman GL. Perspective series: cellular mechanisms of insulin resistance. *J Clin Invest* 2000;106:171–176.
22. Kubo K, Foley JE. Rate-limiting steps for insulin-mediated glucose uptake into perfused rat hindlimb. *Am J Physiol* 1986;250:E100–E102.
23. Nesher R, Karl IE, Kipnis DM. Dissociation of effects of insulin and contraction on glucose transport in rat epitrochlearis muscle. *Am J Physiol* 1985;249: C226–C232.
24. Bell GI, Burant CF, Takeda J, et al. Structure and function of mammalian facilitative sugar transporters. *J Biol Chem* 1993;268:19161–19164.
25. Klip A, Paquet MR. Glucose transport and glucose transporters in muscle and their metabolic regulation. *Diabetes Care* 1990;13:228–242.
26. Kayano T, Burant CF, Fukumoto H, et al. Human facilitative glucose transporters. Isolation, functional characterization, and gene localization of cDNAs encoding an isoform (GLUT5) expressed in small intestine, kidney, muscle, and adipose tissue and an unusual glucose transporter pseudogene-like sequence (GLUT6). *J Biol Chem* 1990;265:13276–13282.
27. Zisman A, Peroni OD, Abel ED, et al. Targeted disruption of the glucose transporter 4 selectively in muscle causes insulin resistance and glucose intolerance. *Nat Med* 2000;6:924–928.
28. Katz EB, Stenbit AE, Hatton K, et al. Cardiac and adipose tissue abnormalities but not diabetes in mice deficient in GLUT4. *Nature* 1995;377: 151–155.
29. Hayashi T, Wojtaszewski JF, Goodyear LJ. Exercise regulation of glucose transport in skeletal muscle. *Am J Physiol* 1997;273:E1039–E1051.
30. Goodyear LJ, Kahn BB. Exercise, glucose transport, and insulin sensitivity. *Annu Rev Med* 1998;49:235–261.
31. Yang C, Coker KJ, Kim JK, et al. Syntaxin 4 heterozygous knockout mice develop muscle insulin resistance. *J Clin Invest* 2001;107:1311–1318.
32. Kristiansen S, Hargreaves M, Richter EA. Exercise-induced increase in glucose transport, GLUT-4, and VAMP-2 in plasma membrane from human muscle. *Am J Physiol* 1996;270:E197–E201.
33. Zierath JR, He L, Guma A, et al. Insulin action on glucose transport and plasma membrane GLUT4 content in skeletal muscle from patients with NIDDM. *Diabetologia* 1996;39:1180–1189.
34. Garvey WT, Maianu L, Zhu JH, et al. Evidence for defects in the trafficking and translocation of GLUT4 glucose transporters in skeletal muscle as a cause of human insulin resistance. *J Clin Invest* 1998;01:2377–2386.
35. King PA, Horton ED, Hirshman MF, et al. Insulin resistance in obese Zucker rat (fa/fa) skeletal muscle is associated with a failure of glucose transporter translocation. *J Clin Invest* 1992;90:1568–1575.

36. Brozinick JT Jr, Etgen GJ, Yaspelkis BB, et al. Glucose uptake and GLUT-4 protein distribution in skeletal muscle of obese Zucker rat. *Am J Physiol* 1994;267:R236–R243.
37. Brozinick JT Jr, Etgen GJ Jr, Yaspelkis BB, et al. Contraction-activated glucose uptake is normal in insulin-resistant muscle of the obese Zucker rat. *J Appl Physiol* 1992;73:382–387.
38. King PA, Betts JJ, Horton ED, et al. Exercise, unlike insulin, promotes glucose transporter translocation in obese Zucker rat muscle. *Am J Physiol* 1993;265: R447–R452.
39. Kennedy JW, Hirshman MF, Gervino EV, et al. Acute exercise induces GLUT4 translocation in skeletal muscle of normal human subjects and subjects with type 2 diabetes. *Diabetes* 1999;48:1192–1197.
40. Lawrence JC Jr, Roach PJ. New insights into the role and mechanism of glycogen synthase activation by insulin. *Diabetes* 1997;46:541–547.
41. Srivastava AK, Pandey SK. Potential mechanism(s) involved in the regulation of glycogen synthesis by insulin. *Mol Cell Biochem* 1998;182:135–141.
42. Shulman RG. Nuclear magnetic resonance studies of glucose metabolism in non-insulin-dependent diabetes mellitus subjects. *Mol Med* 1996;2:533–540.
43. Roden M, Shulman GI. Applications of NMR spectroscopy to study muscle glycogen metabolism in man. *Annu Rev Med* 1999;50:277–290.
44. Cline GW, Magnusson I, Rothman DL, et al. Mechanism of impaired insulin-stimulated muscle glucose metabolism in subjects with insulin-dependent diabetes mellitus. *J Clin Invest* 1997;99:2219–2224.
45. Rennie M. Influence of exercise on protein and amino acid metabolism. In: Rowell LB, Shepherd JT, eds. *Handbook of physiology*. New York: Oxford University Press, 1996:1035.
46. Hyde R, Peyrollier K, Hundal HS. Insulin promotes the cell surface recruitment of the sat2/ata2 system A amino acid transporter from an endosomal compartment in skeletal muscle cells. *J Biol Chem* 2002;277:13628–13634.
47. Solomon V, Goldberg AL. Importance of the ATP-ubiquitin-proteasome pathway in the degradation of soluble and myofibrillar proteins in rabbit muscle extracts. *J Biol Chem* 1996;271:26690–26697.
48. Merforth S, Osmers A, Dahlmann B. Alterations of proteasome activities in skeletal muscle tissue of diabetic rats. *Mol Biol Rep* 1999;26:83–87.
49. Lecker SH, Solomon V, Price SR, et al. Ubiquitin conjugation by the N-end rule pathway and mRNAs for its components increase in muscles of diabetic rats. *J Clin Invest* 1999;104:1411–1420.
50. Cheatham B, Vlahos CJ, Cheatham L, et al. Phosphatidylinositol 3-kinase activation is required for insulin stimulation of pp70 S6 kinase, DNA synthesis, and glucose transporter translocation. *Mol Cell Biol* 1994;4:4902–4911.
51. Clarke JF, Young PW, Yonezawa K, et al. Inhibition of the translocation of GLUT1 and GLUT4 in 3T3-L1 cells by the phosphatidylinositol 3-kinase inhibitor, wortmannin. *Biochem J* 1994;300:631–635.
52. Shepherd PR, Withers DJ, Siddle K. Phosphoinositide 3-kinase: the key switch mechanism in insulin signalling. *Biochem J* 1998;333:471–490.
53. Ueki K, Yamamoto-Honda R, Kaburagi Y, et al. Potential role of protein kinase B in insulin-induced glucose transport, glycogen synthesis, and protein synthesis. *J Biol Chem* 1998;273:5315–5322.
54. Hajduch E, Alessi DR, Hemmings BA, et al. Constitutive activation of protein kinase B alpha by membrane targeting promotes glucose and system A amino acid transport, protein synthesis, and inactivation of glycogen synthase kinase 3 in L6 muscle cells. *Diabetes* 1998;47:1006–1013.
55. Cho H, Mu J, Kim JK, et al. Insulin resistance and a diabetes mellitus-like syndrome in mice lacking the protein kinase Akt2 (PKB beta). *Science* 2001; 292:1728–1731.
56. Dent P, Lavoinne A, Nakielny S, et al. The molecular mechanism by which insulin stimulates glycogen synthesis in mammalian skeletal muscle. *Nature* 1990;348:302–308.
57. Suzuki Y, Lanner C, Kim JH, et al. Insulin control of glycogen metabolism in knockout mice lacking the muscle-specific protein phosphatase PP1G/RGL. *Mol Cell Biol* 2001;21:2683–2694.
58. Wolfe RR. Effects of insulin on muscle tissue. *Curr Opin Clin Nutr Metab Care* 2000;3:67–71.
59. Anthony JC, Reiter AK, Anthony TG, et al. Orally administered leucine enhances protein synthesis in skeletal muscle of diabetic rats in the absence of increases in 4E-BP1 or S6K1 phosphorylation. *Diabetes* 2002;51:928–936.
60. Xu GG, Rothenberg PL. Insulin receptor signaling in the beta-cell influences insulin gene expression and insulin content: evidence for autocrine beta-cell regulation. *Diabetes* 1998;47:1243–1252.
61. Roques M, Vidal H. A phosphatidylinositol 3-kinase/p70 ribosomal S6 protein kinase pathway is required for the regulation by insulin of the p85alpha regulatory subunit of phosphatidylinositol 3-kinase gene expression in human muscle cells. *J Biol Chem* 1999;274:34005–34010.
62. Jones JP, Dohm GL. Regulation of glucose transporter GLUT-4 and hexokinase II gene transcription by insulin and epinephrine. *Am J Physiol* 1997;273: E682–E687.
63. Osawa H, Sutherland C, Robey RB, et al. Analysis of the signaling pathway involved in the regulation of hexokinase II gene transcription by insulin. *J Biol Chem* 1996;271:16690–16694.
64. Antoine PJ, Bertrand F, Auclair M, et al. Insulin induction of protein kinase C alpha expression is independent of insulin receptor Tyr1162/1163 residues and involves mitogen-activated protein kinase kinase 1 and sustained activation of nuclear p44MAPK. *Endocrinology* 1998;139:3133–3142.
65. Kahn RC, Loeken MR. Expression of the gene encoding glycogen phosphorylase is elevated in diabetic rat skeletal muscle and is regulated by insulin and cyclic AMP. *Diabetologia* 1996;39:183–189.
66. Kahn BB. Facilitative glucose transporters. Regulatory mechanisms and dysregulation in diabetes. *J Clin Invest* 1992;89:1367–1374.
67. Pedersen O, Bak JF, Andersen PH, et al. Evidence against altered expression of GLUT1 or GLUT4 in skeletal muscle of patients with obesity or NIDDM. *Diabetes* 1990;39:865–870.
68. Handberg A, Vaag A, Damsbo P, et al. Expression of insulin regulatable glucose transporters in skeletal muscle from type 2 (non-insulin-dependent) diabetic patients. *Diabetologia* 1990;33:625–627.
69. Goodyear LJ, Giorgino F, Sherman LA, et al. Insulin receptor phosphorylation, insulin receptor substrate-1 phosphorylation, and phosphatidylinositol 3-kinase activity are decreased in intact skeletal muscle strips from obese subjects. *J Clin Invest* 1995;95:2195–2204.
70. Bjornholm M, Kawano Y, Lehtihet M, et al. Insulin receptor substrate-1 phosphorylation and phosphatidylinositol 3-kinase activity in skeletal muscle from NIDDM subjects after in vivo insulin stimulation. *Diabetes* 1997;46: 524–527.
71. Folli F, Saad MJA, Backer JM, et al. Regulation of phosphatidylinositol 3-kinase activity in liver and muscle of animal models of insulin-resistant and insulin-deficient diabetes mellitus. *J Clin Invest* 1993;92:1787–1794.
72. Heydrick SJ, Jullien D, Gautier N, et al. Defect in skeletal muscle phosphatidylinositol-3-kinase in obese insulin-resistant mice. *J Clin Invest* 1993; 91:1358–1366.
73. Zierath JR, Houseknecht KL, Gnudi L, et al. High-fat feeding impairs insulin-stimulated GLUT4 recruitment via an early insulin-signaling defect. *Diabetes* 1997;46:215–223.
74. Saad MJ, Folli F, Kahn JA, et al. Modulation of insulin receptor, insulin receptor substrate-1 and phosphatidylinositol 3-kinase in liver and muscle of dexamethasone-treated rats. *J Clin Invest* 1993;92:2065–2072.
75. Krook A, Roth RA, Jiang XJ, et al. Insulin-stimulated Akt kinase activity is reduced in skeletal muscle from NIDDM subjects. *Diabetes* 1998;47: 1281–1286.
76. Kim YB, Nikoulina SE, Ciaraldi TP, et al. Normal insulin-dependent activation of Akt/protein kinase B, with diminished activation of phosphoinositide 3-kinase, in muscle in type 2 diabetes. *J Clin Invest* 1999;104: 733–741.
77. Nikoulina SE, Ciaraldi TP, Mudaliar S, et al. Potential role of glycogen synthase kinase-3 in skeletal muscle insulin resistance of type 2 diabetes. *Diabetes* 2000;49:263–270.
78. Kim YB, Kotani K, Ciaraldi TP, et al. Insulin-stimulated PKC lamda zeta activity is impaired in muscle of insulin resistant subjects. *Diabetes* 2001;50:A62(abst).
79. Goodyear LJ, Giorgino F, Balon TW, et al. Effects of contractile activity on tyrosine phosphoproteins and phosphatidylinositol 3-kinase activity in rat skeletal muscle. *Am J Physiol* 1995;268:E987–E995.
80. Lee AD, Hansen PA, Holloszy JO. Wortmannin inhibits insulin-stimulated but not contraction-stimulated glucose transport activity in skeletal muscle. *FEBS Lett* 1995;361:51–54.
81. Yeh JI, Gulve EA, Rameh L, et al. The effects of wortmannin on rat skeletal muscle. Dissociation of signaling pathways for insulin- and contraction-activated hexose transport. *J Biol Chem* 1995;270:2107–2111.
82. Lund S, Holman GD, Schmitz O, et al. Contraction stimulates translocation of glucose transporter GLUT4 in skeletal muscle through a mechanism distinct from that of insulin. *Proc Natl Acad Sci U S A* 1995;92:5817–5821.
83. Wojtaszewski JF, Higaki Y, Hirshman MF, et al. Exercise modulates postreceptor insulin signaling and glucose transport in muscle-specific insulin receptor knockout mice. *J Clin Invest* 1999;104:1257–1264.
84. Higaki Y, Wojtaszewski JFP, Hirshman MF, et al. Insulin receptor substrate-2 is not necessary for insulin- and exercise-stimulated glucose transport in skeletal muscle. *J Biol Chem* 1999;274:20791–20795.
85. Hardie DG, Carling D, Carlson M. The AMP-activated/SNF1 protein kinase subfamily: metabolic sensors of the eukaryotic cell? *Annu Rev Biochem* 1998;67:821–855.
86. Hayashi T, Hirshman MF, Fujii N, et al. Metabolic stress and altered glucose transport: activation of AMP-activated protein kinase as a unifying coupling mechanism. *Diabetes* 2000;49:527–531.
87. Merrill GF, Kurth EJ, Hardie DG, et al. AICA riboside increases AMP-activated protein kinase, fatty acid oxidation, and glucose uptake in rat muscle. *Am J Physiol* 1997;273:E1107–E1112.
88. Hayashi T, Hirshman MF, Kurth EJ, et al. Evidence for 5' AMP-activated protein kinase mediation of the effect of muscle contraction on glucose transport. *Diabetes* 1998;47:1369–1373.
89. Bergeron R, Russell III RR, Young LH, et al. Effect of AMPK activation on muscle glucose metabolism in conscious rats. *Am J Physiol* 1999;276: E938–E944.
90. Musi N, Fujii N, Hirshman MF, et al. AMP-activated protein kinase (AMPK) is activated in muscle of subjects with type 2 diabetes during exercise. *Diabetes* 2001;50:921–927.
91. Mu J, Brozinick JT Jr, Valladares O, et al. A role for AMP-activated protein kinase in contraction- and hypoxia-regulated glucose transport in skeletal muscle. *Mol Cell* 2001;7:1085–1094.
92. Winder WW, Hardie DG. Inactivation of acetyl-CoA carboxylase and activation of AMP-activated protein kinase in muscle during exercise. *Am J Physiol* 1996;270:E299–E304.
93. Hutber CA, Hardie DG, Winder WW. Electrical stimulation inactivates muscle acetyl-CoA carboxylase and increases AMP-activated protein kinase. *Am J Physiol* 1997;272:E262–E266.

94. Vavvas D, Apazidis A, Saha AK, et al. Contraction-induced changes in acetyl-CoA carboxylase and 5′-AMP- activated kinase in skeletal muscle. *J Biol Chem* 1997;272:13255–13261.
95. Carling D, Hardie DG. The substrate and sequence specificity of the AMP-activated protein kinase. Phosphorylation of glycogen synthase and phosphorylase kinase. *Biochim Biophys Acta* 1989;1012:81–86.
96. Skurat AV, Wang Y, Roach PJ. Rabbit skeletal muscle glycogen synthase expressed in COS cells. Identification of regulatory phosphorylation sites. *J Biol Chem* 1994;269:25534–25542.
97. Winder WW, Holmes BF, Rubink DS, et al. Activation of AMP-activated protein kinase increases mitochondrial enzymes in skeletal muscle. *J Appl Physiol* 2000;88:2219–2226.
98. Buhl ES, Jessen N, Schmitz O, et al. Chronic treatment with 5-aminoimidazole-4-carboxamide-1-beta-D-ribofuranoside increases insulin-stimulated glucose uptake and GLUT4 translocation in rat skeletal muscles in a fiber type-specific manner. *Diabetes* 2001;50:12–17.
99. Holmes BF, Kurth-Kraczek EJ, Winder WW. Chronic activation of 5′-AMP-activated protein kinase increases GLUT-4, hexokinase, and glycogen in muscle. *J Appl Physiol* 1999;87:1990–1995.
100. Stoppani J, Hildebrandt AL, Neufer PD. Activation of AMP-activated protein kinase increases transcription of metabolic genes in rat gastrocnemius muscle. *FASEB J* 2001;15:A415(abst).

CHAPTER 15
Regulation of Hepatic Glucose Metabolism

Daryl K. Granner and Donald K. Scott

INTRODUCTION

Background

Glucose provides a major energy supply for mammalian cells; however, some tissues are much more dependent than others on this source. For example, glucose is the primary energy source for the brain and renal medulla and is essentially the sole provider for red blood cells and the retina. The total daily consumption of glucose in a 70-kg person is about 160 g. The brain uses about 120 g of this. Therefore, tissues that make up about 5% of the body weight consume more than 75% of the glucose metabolized each day. Some 10 to 15 g of glucose is available in the extracellular fluid (ECF), and ~300 g can be stored in the glycogen reservoirs. Thus, less than a 24-hour supply of glucose is directly available in circumstances when no exogenous supply is available. A constant supply of glucose must be available, as moderate hypoglycemia (<50 mg/dL) causes disabling symptoms and severe hypoglycemia (<20 mg/dL) can have devastating and irreversible effects on the central nervous system (CNS). By contrast, hyperglycemia must be avoided, as this causes its own set of deleterious consequences, albeit on a considerably longer time scale.

An intricate mechanism has evolved for maintaining ECF glucose within a relatively narrow range. In broad physiologic terms (Fig. 15.1), this involves the regulated production of glucose by the liver from glycogenolysis and gluconeogenesis and, to a lesser extent, from gluconeogenesis in the kidneys and small intestine. This is counterbalanced by the regulated peripheral clearance of glucose by tissues such as skeletal muscle, adipose tissue, and the splanchnic bed, including the liver. This chapter concerns the homeostatic role the liver plays in these processes by serving as a consumer, producer, and reservoir for glucose. Descriptions of the control processes involved in glucose homeostasis generally center on hormonal regulation (Fig. 15.1). A major thesis of this chapter is that glucose and/or glucose metabolism is a (the) central player in these events. This point will be made by first outlining the general steps in metabolic control, then by illustrating how these processes affect glucose metabolism, and vice versa.

Intracellular Symbols of Energy Charge, Glucose Homeostasis, and Carbon Balance

Multicellular organisms have elaborate mechanisms for sensing changes in the external environment and for generating signals that can then be transduced into an appropriate compensatory response (Table 15.1).

Glucose homeostasis is a case in point. Acute hypoglycemia results in the immediate release of glucagon, which binds to the hepatocyte plasma membrane and thereby promotes the generation of cyclic adenosine monophosphate (cAMP). cAMP is therefore an intracellular symbol of hypoglycemia (1). Hyperglycemia, through insulin release and the subsequent activation of phosphodiesterases that hydrolyze cAMP, reduces the concentration of this nucleotide. A low-molecular-weight activator

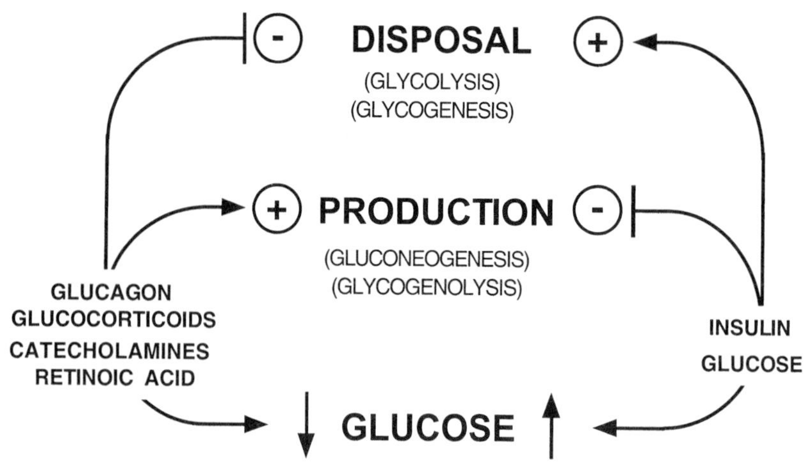

Figure 15.1. Overview of the hormonal regulation of glucose metabolism in the liver.

of phosphofructokinase-1 (PFK1) was found in the livers of rats given a glucose load and was absent in the livers of rats treated with glucagon (2,3). This molecule, fructose-2,6-bisphosphate (F-2,6-P_2), is thus a symbol of hyperglycemia. As discussed below, F-2,6-P_2 activates glycolysis and inhibits gluconeogenesis, as would be expected of a symbol of hyperglycemia, for which the maintenance of homeostasis requires that glucose utilization be promoted and its production inhibited. Glucose metabolism is a major source of adenosine triphosphate (ATP), which is synthesized by successive phosphorylation steps from AMP. The intracellular levels of AMP and ATP, or the AMP/ATP ratio, are thus a reflection of energy sufficiency or depletion, as the case may be, within the cell. Citrate, an early intermediate in the citric acid cycle, is a symbol of the carbon supply necessary for a variety of biosynthetic pathways. Alanine, synthesized in a single step from pyruvate, serves a similar purpose. Although probably not a complete list, cAMP, F-2,6-P_2, AMP/ATP, citrate, and alanine play key roles, by a variety of mechanisms that will be described below, in regulating hepatic glucose metabolism, which is a major source of energy and carbon for various biosynthetic reactions.

Metabolic Pathways

The elucidation of metabolic pathways, along with the principles that govern the regulation of these pathways, is one of the major achievements of 20th century biological research. The deciphering of how thousands of reactions are coordinated, as well as the purification and characterization of the enzymes involved, was accomplished using techniques that often were very primitive by contemporary standards. This set the stage for more recent developments that allow for the analysis of components of these pathways by overexpression of an enzyme in a tissue of interest, or the selective removal of an enzyme, by transgenic and gene knockout technologies. These, and other newer techniques, are providing supportive evidence for the fundamental importance of certain enzymatic steps and have led to the discovery of regulatory processes heretofore unappreciated. The regulation of glucose metabolism in the liver, the topic of this chapter, has been of central interest to investigators for more than 100 years. As will be discussed below, many of the principles of metabolic regulation were derived from these studies.

TABLE 15.1. Intracellular Symbols of Metabolic Balance

Change	Symbol
Hypoglycemia	cAMP
Hyperglycemia	Fructose-2,6-bisphosphate
Low energy charge	AMP; high AMP/ATP ratio
High energy charge	ATP; low AMP/ATP ratio
Carbon supply	Citrate, alanine

cAMP, cyclic adenosine monophosphate; ATP, adenosine triphosphate.

CONTROL MECHANISMS

A living cell is an intricate machine, and it generally has several ways of regulating critical processes, with redundant systems for backup support. Most disturbances of a cell, even quite severe ones, are tolerated because, under normal circumstances, homeostatic mechanisms restore the affected process (or processes) to, or near, the original state.

Simple Control Mechanisms

The simplest type of control is afforded by substrate availability. Flux through an enzyme step is directly related to the concentration of substrate and to the affinity of the enzyme for that substrate. For example, hexokinases catalyze the phosphorylation of glucose to form glucose-6-phosphate (G-6-P). The Michaelis-Menten constant (K_m) for the 100-kDa hexokinases (HK-I–III) is low (20–120 μM), so these enzymes are very efficient at low ECF glucose concentrations (4). Glucokinase, a 50-kDa hexokinase found in liver and pancreatic β-cells, has a K_m for glucose of 5 to 10 mM, so it is very active when glucose concentrations in the ECF are high, particularly in the portal circulation, as happens after a meal (5). These high glucose concentrations are well above the K_m of the 100-kDa hexokinases, which are relatively less influential under such circumstances. Glucokinase therefore plays an important role in hepatic glucose clearance during the postprandial period. Substrate availability provides a very rapid and simple control mechanism and is a major control mechanism in unicellular organisms. However, these organisms are relatively defenseless in the face of large changes of substrate availability, particularly when the substrate is not abundant.

Substrates and reaction products afford another type of direct regulation in which they affect their own concentration by influencing the activity or amount of an enzyme by positive or negative mechanisms. Positive control occurs when a downstream component activates a subsequent enzyme and promotes forward flux, or induces the synthesis of an enzyme that accomplishes the same purpose. Fructose-1,6-bisphosphate (F-1,6-P_2) activates a downstream enzyme, pyruvate kinase (PK), and thus promotes glycolytic flux (6); (Fig. 15.2). This provides a mechanism for ensuring that flux continues in the forward direction, but it generally does not afford fine-tuning of substrate concentration or flux because it is unidirectional. Negative feedback control, which is much more common than positive control, occurs when the product of a reaction is capable of feedback inhibition of upstream enzyme activity or synthesis. Negative feedback control can be exerted at many upstream reaction steps in a pathway and helps define the points at which metabolic-control strength is exerted. This mechanism, analogous to the function of a thermostat in temperature control, adjusts substrate concentration in a narrow range around a preset value. When the concentration of the reaction product falls, negative feedback inhibition is relieved and the reaction (or reactions) produces more of the regulatory molecule. High concentrations shut down the system, thus providing up-and-down fine-tuning. For example, physiologic levels of G-6-P, the product of the hexokinase reaction, provide feedback inhibition of the 100-kDa hexokinases but not of glucokinase (7). This provides for appropriately regulated levels of the branch-point substrate G-6-P in most tissues. Tissues or organs wherein glucokinase is the predominant hexokinase, such as liver and pancreatic β-cells, are able to continuously phosphorylate glucose owing to the lack of feedback inhibition by G-6-P, the reaction product. The liver is thus able to clear glucose in the postprandial state, and β-cells are able to employ glucokinase as a glucose sensor for regulated secretion of insulin (8). Substrate availability and feedback/feedforward control are prominent mechanisms in single-cell organisms.

Complex Control Mechanisms

Simple regulatory systems are advantageous in that they provide very rapid and quickly reversible control. The major disadvantages are that the unicellular organism is susceptible to major environmental changes of substrate availability and the regulation is provided by molecules that are themselves reaction

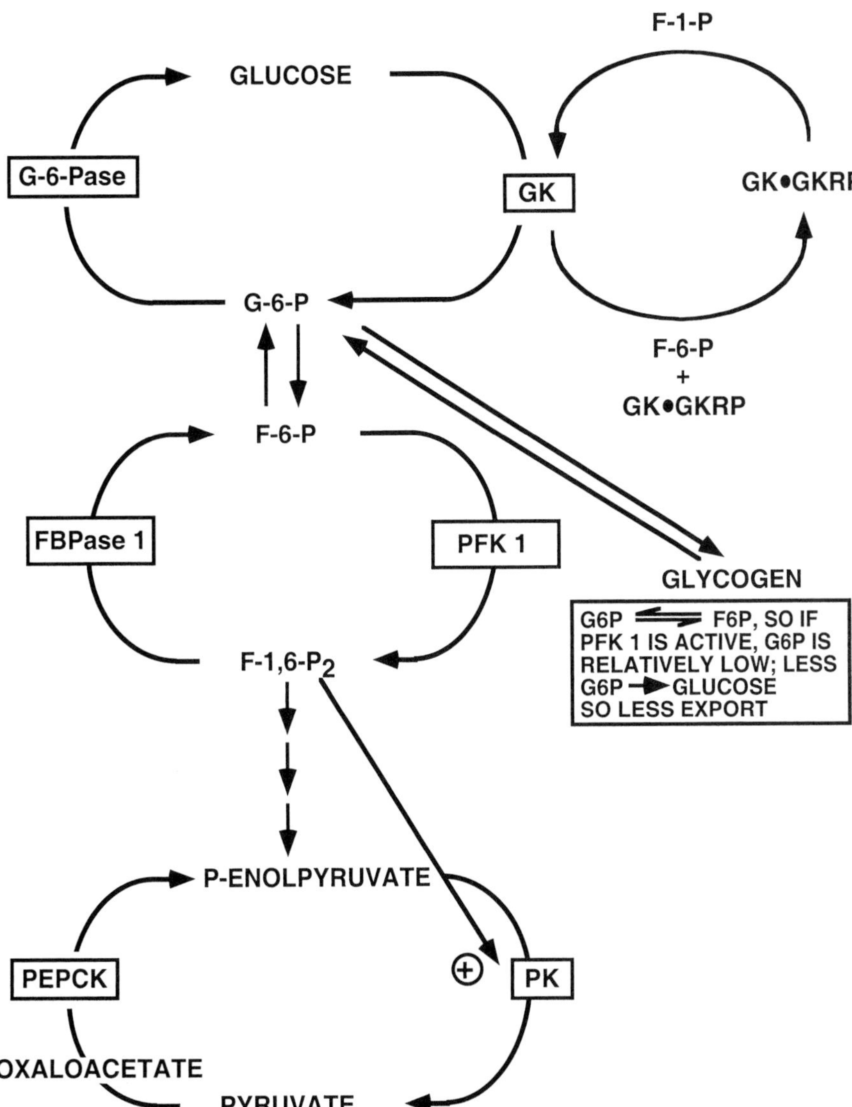

Figure 15.2. A simple control mechanism is provided by substrate availability, which influences the activity or amount of metabolic enzymes. G-6-P, glucose-6-phosphate; F-6-P, fructose-6-phosphate; F-1-P, fructose-1-phosphate; F-1,6-P_2, fructose-1,6-bisphosphate; GK, glucokinase; GKRP, glucokinase regulatory protein; G-6-Pase, glucose-6-phosphatase; FBPase, fructose-1,6-bisphosphatase; PFK 1, phosphofructokinase-1; PEPCK, phosphoenolpyruvate carboxykinase; PK, pyruvate kinase.

components. As noted, these mechanisms are frequently employed in glucose metabolism in multicellular organisms. However, the complexity of these organisms is such that certain environmental changes that are threats to survival are often perceived by one tissue or organ and the responses that allow for homeostasis are facilitated by one or more distant organs. Communication between the sensors of the environment and the organs or tissues that provide the appropriate response to recognized challenges is accomplished by the nervous and endocrine systems. For example, hypoglycemia is perceived by the CNS, which triggers the release of glucocorticoids, catecholamines, and glucagon and the inhibition of insulin secretion (Fig. 15.1). These hormones, the so-called first messengers, provide much of the cell-cell communication necessary for the coordinated response that restores the ECF glucose level to the normal range. A variety of intracellular molecules serve as so-called second messengers, including cAMP, cyclic guanosine monophosphate (cGMP), calcium ion, and various phosphatidylinositides. These molecules share several properties. They act as intracellular symbols of particular environmental changes, and more than one of these may be symbols of the same challenge, e.g., hypoglycemia. The concentration of these molecules is labile within the cell, as befits their regulatory potential. In contrast to the simple mechanisms of regulation described above, none of these molecules is a component (substrate or product) of a reaction pathway, nor are they structural analogues of such components. Finally, these regulatory molecules all initiate signal transduction cascades that result in the ultimate biologic response. Again, these cascades are not mutually exclusive, as different signals can activate the same, or complementary, steps in a given pathway. A wide variety of metabolic control mechanisms are affected by these signals, including allostery, posttranslational protein modification, protein translocation, protein-protein interaction, and changes in the amount of key proteins (Table 15.2).

ALLOSTERIC CONTROL

Some of the enzymes and proteins involved in glucose homeostasis are regulated by allosteric control mechanisms. Rather than exhibiting classical Michaelis-Menten kinetics, in which there is a hyperbolic association between substrate binding and enzyme activity, a plot of enzyme activity against substrate concentration shows a sigmoidal relationship. This occurs when substrate binding to one active site influences, in a cooperative fashion, binding to a second site in the same molecule. For example, the reaction velocity of PFK1 increases in a sigmoidal fashion as the concentration of the substrate, fructose-6-phosphate (F-6-P), increases (9–11) (Fig. 15.4B, center panel). Some molecules regulate activity of the allosteric enzyme by binding to regulatory sites distinct from substrate binding sites. The allosteric regulator F-2,6-P_2 significantly shifts the velocity of the PFK1 reaction for the substrate F-6-P to the left (12,13) (Fig. 15.4B, center panel).

POSTTRANSLATIONAL MODIFICATION OF PROTEINS

Several dozen different types of posttranslational modifications alter the activity of proteins, including many enzymes involved in glucose homeostasis. Modification of enzyme activity by phosphorylation of serine, threonine, or tyrosine residues is a particularly common mechanism. First described in the control of enzymes of glycogen metabolism, regulation by phosphorylation, and dephosphorylation, is employed in many different signal transduction pathways. For example, the binding of glucagon to its cell-surface receptor on the hepatocyte results in the activation of adenylyl cyclase and the production of cAMP from ATP. cAMP activates a kinase cascade that catalyzes the phosphorylation of phosphorylase b on the serine 14 residue of each monomer of this enzyme (14). This phosphorylation results in the conversion of the inactive phosphorylase b to the active phosphorylase a form and glycogen degradation by phosphorolysis.

PROTEIN TRANSLOCATION

The movement of proteins from one cellular compartment to another, with a subsequent change in activity or function of that protein, is an important control mechanism. One of the first examples of this control mechanism is the insulin-promoted movement of the glucose transporter 4 (GLUT4) from an intracellular reservoir to the plasma membrane in skeletal muscle and adipose cells (15,16). In the absence of insulin, there is a continuous movement of GLUT4 into and out of the plasma membrane. The interaction of insulin with its cell-surface receptor activates one or more signal transduction pathways that promote GLUT4 vesicle exocytosis in excess of transporter internalization. The role of phosphoinositide 3-kinase (PI 3-kinase), with possible involvement of downstream kinases such

TABLE 15.2. Control Mechanisms Employed in Hepatic Glucose Homeostasis

Process	Example
Substrate utilization	Glucokinase has a higher K_m for glucose than hexokinases I–III
Positive feedforward control	Fructose-1,6-bisphosphate stimulates pyruvate kinase activity
Negative feedback control	Glucose-6-phosphate inhibits hexokinases I–III
Allosteric control	Fructose-2,6-bisphosphate activates phosphofructokinase-1
Protein modification	cAMP promotes the phosphorylation of phosphorylase
Protein translocation	Glucokinase moves from nucleus to cytoplasm
Protein-protein interaction	Glucokinase regulatory protein associates with glucokinase
Regulation of protein amount	Insulin increases general mRNA translation
Regulation of gene transcription	Glucose inhibits phosphoenolpyruvate carboxykinase gene transcription

cAMP, cyclic adenosine monophosphate.

as protein kinase B (PKB) and protein kinase C (PKCζ/λ), is quite well established in this process (17,18). However, the activation of PI 3-kinase may not be totally sufficient. The role of various signal transduction pathways in moving the GLUT4 vesicle into and out of the plasma membrane remains to be established. Nonetheless, activation of the insulin signal transduction pathway (or pathways) results in a marked enhancement of glucose entry into skeletal muscle and adipose cells because of a protein translocation process.

PROTEIN–PROTEIN INTERACTION

Interactions with other proteins influence the activity of certain proteins. A complex array of protein-protein interactions is involved in regulating the transcription of genes that encode enzymes involved in glucose homeostasis, as will be described below. The interaction of glucokinase with the glucokinase regulatory protein (GKRP) is a pertinent example of a protein-protein interaction (19) and of how more than one mechanism is employed to facilitate a given process, in this case glucose phosphorylation. When glucokinase is bound to GKRP, a reaction facilitated by the allosteric binding of F-6-P to the GKRP (Fig. 15.3), glucokinase is inactive and located in the nucleus of hepatocytes. The exchange of F-6-P with fructose-1-phosphate (F-1-P) results in the dissociation of GKRP from glucokinase and the translocation of the latter to the cytosol, where it is an active enzyme. The regulation of glucokinase activity thus involves allosteric control, protein-protein interaction, and protein translocation, in addition to substrate control. The amount of the enzyme can also be influenced by the rate of transcription of the glucokinase gene.

REGULATION OF PROTEIN AMOUNT

The examples described above, in one way or another, regulate activity without changing the amount of enzymes or proteins. Several mechanisms also are employed to change the amount of a specific protein in a cell such as a hepatocyte. The concentration of a protein in the cell at any instant represents a balance between the relative rates of its synthesis and degradation. This balance is different for all proteins and is a regulatable process. The rate of synthesis of a protein (mRNA translation) is directly related to the amount of the encoding mRNA and the efficiency of translation of that specific mRNA. Translation is an exceedingly complex, multistep process, and it is extensively regulated. Insulin affects a critical step, the formation of the active translation factor eukaryotic initiation factor-4E (eIF-4E). Stimulation of cells by insulin and other growth factors results in activation of the mammalian target of rapamycin (mTOR) and mitogen-activated protein (MAP) kinase pathways and the phosphorylation of eIF-4E (20). This phosphoprotein associates with several other translation factors to form the eIF-4F complex, which binds to the mRNA cap and allows for translation initiation (20). This mechanism is thought to be responsible for the general anabolic effects of insulin, and it could come to play in enhancing the synthesis of specific proteins.

About 1% to 2% of total body proteins turn over each day in humans, and the liver is actively involved in this process. Hepatic proteins have markedly different turnover rates, measured as the half-life ($t_{1/2}$), the time required for a protein to be reduced to 50% of its initial value. This is an important concept, particularly in view of regulation, as the time required to move from one steady state to another, either up or down, is a function of the turnover time of the protein (or any other substance for that matter, e.g., mRNA, lipid, drug). Thus, one can calculate that about five turnover times are required to effect a change of steady state, e.g., 100→50→25→12.5→6.25→3.13, or vice versa. This has useful predictive value in considering how long it will take for an induced or repressed enzyme (or mRNA) to reach its new steady-state level. For example, the $t_{1/2}$ for phosphoenolpyruvate carboxykinase (PEPCK) mRNA and protein are ~0.6 and 2.0 hours, respectively (21). After the addition of glucocorticoids, a PEPCK gene inducer, the new steady states for the mRNA and protein are reached in ~3 and 10 hours, respectively, assuming there are no effects of the inducer on mRNA or protein turnover (and in this case and others there often are).

The $t_{1/2}$ for liver proteins varies from 30 minutes to more than 150 hours. In general, proteins that play a key role in metabolic regulation, such as PEPCK, tyrosine aminotransferase, and hydroxymethylglutaryl–coenzyme A (HMG-CoA) reductase, have short $t_{1/2}$ values in the range of 0.5 to 2 hours, and as

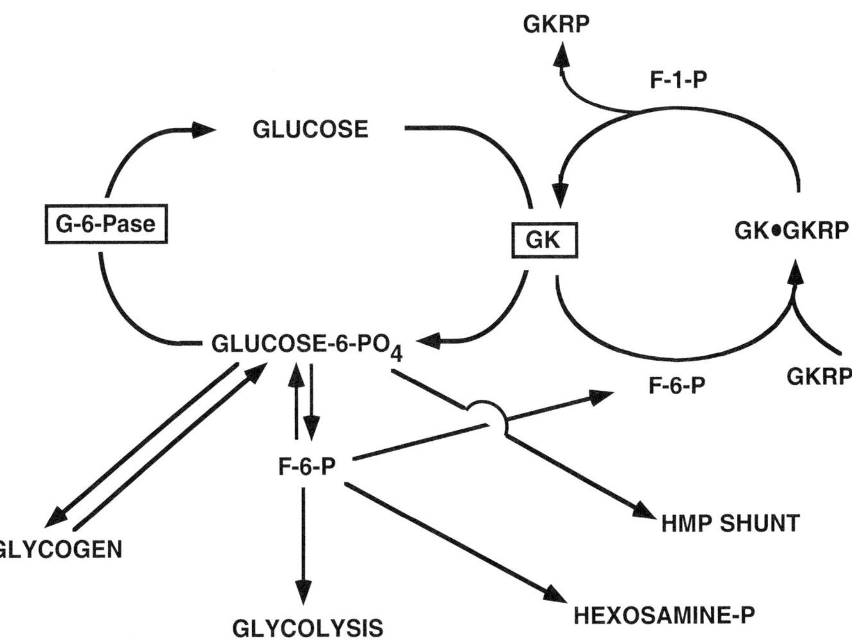

Figure 15.3. Regulation of the glucose/glucose-6-phosphate (G-6-P) cycle. G-6-P is a branch point for several metabolic pathways. G-6-Pase, glucose-6-phosphatase; GK, glucokinase; GKRP, glucokinase regulatory protein; F-6-P, fructose-6-phosphate; F-1-P, fructose-1-phosphate; Hmp-hexose monophosphate.

mentioned above, these rates can be decreased or increased in response to physiologic signals. Metabolic flux can thus be significantly influenced by the turnover of key enzymes. By contrast, other enzymes, such as aldolase or lactate dehydrogenase, have prolonged $t_{1/2}$ values in the range of more than 100 hours. Changes in the amount of such enzymes are not involved in acute adaptive processes.

REGULATION OF GENE TRANSCRIPTION

The rules of turnover are also applicable to a consideration of the concentration of a specific mRNA in the hepatocyte. The amount of a given mRNA represents the balance between its synthesis, from gene transcription, and its degradation. mRNAs, like proteins, have markedly different turnover times. In the liver, these range from a $t_{1/2}$ of 10 to 15 minutes to a $t_{1/2}$ of days for different individual mRNAs. In general, a specific mRNA turns over more rapidly than its cognate protein, and mRNAs that encode enzymes involved in acute metabolic regulation have shorter $t_{1/2}$ values than those that direct the synthesis of the so-called housekeeping proteins (21). In addition, hormones that regulate the rate of transcription of a gene also often affect the rate of turnover of the respective mRNA. Thus, glucocorticoids and cAMP increase the rate of transcription of the PEPCK gene, and they both prolong the $t_{1/2}$ of PEPCK mRNA (22,23). The net result of these two effects is to increase the amount of this mRNA in the hepatocyte and prolong its presence. This provides for more PEPCK synthesis and an extended influence of the enzyme on gluconeogenic flux.

Much more is understood about the regulation of mRNA synthesis than is known about its degradation. As will be described in detail below, complex arrays of protein-DNA and protein-protein interactions are involved in the regulation of the initiation phase of transcription of specific genes. These assemblies are controlled by a series of events that follow in sequence from the interaction of a hormone with the target cell. Regulation of the activity of PEPCK in the hepatocyte provides a case in point. This enzyme is not appreciably affected by feedforward, feedback, or allosteric control mechanisms, nor is its activity subject to change as a result of posttranslational modification of the protein, by protein-protein interactions, or by its location in the hepatocyte. Changes of PEPCK activity are attributable to alterations in the amount of the enzyme in the cell, which is directly related to the amount of PEPCK mRNA available for translation. This amount is principally determined by the rate of PEPCK mRNA synthesis, although degradation of the mRNA can also be important in certain circumstances (22,23). cAMP enhances PEPCK gene transcription by first promoting the phosphorylation of a protein, cAMP response element binding protein (CREB), that binds to the cAMP response element (CRE) in the PEPCK gene promoter (24,25). This phospho–CREB-CRE complex triggers the assembly of a set of protein-protein interactions that result in enhanced initiation of transcription through the PEPCK gene promoter (26). Glucocorticoids bind to the cytosolic glucocorticoid receptor (GR), which then dissociates from a chaperone protein and translocates into the hepatocyte nucleus to bind to the glucocorticoid response element (GRE). Occupation of the GRE by the GR triggers a different series of protein-DNA and protein-protein interactions that also result in an enhanced rate of PEPCK gene transcription and, in sequence, increased mRNA and protein synthesis and enzyme activity (27,28). Insulin, through its signal transduction cascade, inhibits PEPCK gene transcription and also slows the rate of PEPCK mRNA translation (27,29). Thus, the regulation of PEPCK activity, which has significant control strength in gluconeogenesis, is regulated by several mechanisms.

Metabolic Control Analysis

Until recently the guiding principle in metabolic control has been the idea that there is a single rate-controlling step in any metabolic pathway. Flux through such a pathway could thus be increased or decreased by changing the activity of that single rate-determining enzyme. The advent of recombinant DNA technology enabled investigators to rather easily change the expression of a given enzyme in a cell; yet this often does not result in the change of flux predicted by the rate-limiting enzyme hypothesis. These results were not surprising to students of metabolic control analysis, a concept first proposed by Kacser some 30 years ago (30). Metabolic control is assessed by measuring all enzyme activities, their kinetic properties, the substrates and products of each reaction, and the relevant regulatory molecules in a particular pathway. An analysis of the data allows one to assign a quantitative control strength value (C) to each step in this pathway. The sum of the C values for a pathway equals 1.0. High C values indicate high control strength. When appropriately analyzed, it is apparent that control strength can be distributed among the several steps in a pathway, and the C value for a given step can be changed by different metabolic circumstances. An examination of glucose metabolism in the isolated, beating heart provides a good example of these principles. In a heart preparation perfused with a physiologic concentration of glucose, control of the early steps of glucose metabolism is distributed between glucose transport (C value of 0.4) and glucose phosphorylation (C value of 0.6) (31). The addition of insulin results in a remarkable change in the distribution of control strength. Under these conditions the C value for glucose transport is now negligible (0.0002), whereas the C value for glucose phosphorylation increases to 0.97 (31). Phosphoglucoisomerase accounts for the other 0.02. Metabolic control analysis also allows one to assign relative importance to a set of reactions within a complex pathway. For instance, in the case cited, the distribution of control provided by transport/phosphorylation (0.58), glycolysis (0.25), and glycogen synthesis (0.17) was assessed.

At equilibrium, the supply of an end product by the series of enzymes and substrates equals the demand afforded by product utilization and degradation. Thus, the demand side can also influence metabolic control by providing a pull on the system. Two recent studies illustrate the importance of this concept. In studying tryptophan biosynthesis in yeast, investigators first showed that exogenous provision of excessive amounts of the first enzyme in the biosynthetic pathway did not increase flux to tryptophan. All of the enzymes in the pathway had to be overexpressed to increase flux (32). This illustrates the point made above about so-called rate-limiting steps. Of more interest was the observation that the biosynthetic enzymes ("supply side") accounted for only about 25% of the control strength. The other 75% was presumably provided by the "demand side," e.g., the use of tryptophan for protein synthesis. This is similar to the example cited above, in which, in the heart, glycolysis and glycogen synthesis exert control strength downstream from glucose transport/phosphorylation (31). That demand may also be an important control step as illustrated in another recent report. Glycolysis, as noted above, provides ATP from glucose. Yeasts engineered to have an excess of the ATP-degrading enzyme adenosine triphosphatase (ATPase) have a remarkable increase in glycolytic flux (33). This observation is pertinent to the topic of this chapter. The energy charge in these cells, as reflected in a low AMP/ATP ratio, resulted in increased glycolytic flux. As described in detail below, a low AMP/ATP ratio promotes flux through the critical glycolytic enzymes PFK1 and PK in hepatocytes. It thus is important to recognize that supply and demand are both significant, that control is distributed, and that this distribution is subject to change according to metabolic circumstances.

GLUCOSE AUTOREGULATION IN LIVER

Glucose Transport by Hepatocytes

Glucose enters all cells by facilitated diffusion (from a high to low concentration) through one of the members of the glucose transporter family of proteins (34). This is basically a unidirectional process in cells that cannot produce glucose, as one of the four hexokinase family members (HK-I–IV) rapidly converts glucose to G-6-P, which cannot be exported by the glucose transporter. The activity of these hexokinases keeps the intracellular free-glucose concentration low, so most cells have a net uptake of glucose due to inward, passive diffusion. The only regulation of this process is afforded by the extracellular glucose concentration (substrate control) and by G-6-P, which inhibits (by negative feedback) the 100-kDa hexokinases (isoforms I–III).

Hepatocytes, which can produce glucose from glycogenolysis and gluconeogenesis, can export and import glucose. The direction of glucose flux depends on the concentration gradient. Under certain metabolic conditions (e.g., fasting or hormonal conditions that favor glycogenolysis and/or gluconeogenesis), hepatocytes release glucose into the ECF. The ability of the hepatocyte to effect net glucose release is a function of its high K_m hepatic transporter coupled with a regulatable high K_m hexokinase (HK-IV, or glucokinase). When hormonal conditions favor glucose utilization (high insulin, low glucagon), glucokinase activity is high, intracellular glucose is rapidly phosphorylated, and glucose entry is facilitated along a downhill gradient. When conditions favor glycogenolysis or gluconeogenesis (low insulin, high glucagon), glucokinase activity is reduced, the low rate of glucose phosphorylation results in intracellular accumulation of glucose, and glucose is exported by facilitated diffusion. The hepatic GLUT2 transporter has a K_m for glucose of ~40 mM and generally functions with pseudo first-order kinetics with respect to the intracellular or extracellular glucose concentration (34). Because the portal vein glucose concentration normally does not exceed 10 mM, transport is not limiting for either hepatic glucose import or export. Because of this feature there is no need for regulation of the hepatic glucose transporter.

General Features of Hepatic Substrate Cycles

Hepatic glucose production and utilization involve the movement of substrates through three major cycles (2,35) (Fig. 15.2). Hepatic glucose production, by gluconeogenesis, is a biosynthetic pathway. Glucose utilization, by glycolysis, is a degradative pathway. Degradative and biosynthetic pathways are usually catalyzed by separate sets of enzymes. This affords unique, but flexible, control of each pathway. The latter is particularly important in this instance, as the production of a single molecule of glucose from gluconeogenesis requires the expenditure of six high-energy bonds [four ATP and two guanosine-triphosphate (GTP)], whereas glucose degradation to two pyruvate molecules results in the production of two ATP molecules. Futile cycling between the cycles involved in gluconeogenesis and glycolysis could thus be very wasteful in terms of energy consumption and heat production. In general, a negative free-energy charge (AMP, or a high AMP/ATP ratio) promotes glycolysis, and a high free-energy charge (ATP, or a low AMP/ATP ratio) favors the gluconeogenic pathway.

The direction and magnitude of substrate movement, along either the glycolytic or the gluconeogenic pathway, is controlled by six enzymes that catalyze essentially irreversible reactions and thus have high metabolic control strength (2). The three enzymes that catalyze the glycolytic reactions must be bypassed by three different enzymes that direct the gluconeogenic pathway and vice versa. The activity of these six enzymes is modulated by acute (seconds to minutes) and chronic (minutes to hours) regulatory mechanisms. The acute regulation of hepatic glucose metabolism occurs through hormone-mediated changes in enzymatic activity, principally the phosphorylation or dephosphorylation of two key enzymes, PK and phosphofructokinase-2/fructose-2,6-bisphosphatase (PFK2/FBPase2, the bifunctional enzyme), and the allosteric regulation of GK by GKRP and of PFK1 and FBPase1 by F-2,6-P_2 (2,3). Hormones also exert chronic effects on glucose metabolism by changing the rate of enzyme synthesis. These chronic effects are mediated through alterations of the rate of mRNA synthesis and, in some cases, by changes in the rate of degradation of specific mRNAs.

The net flux through the glucose/G-6-P, F-6-P/F-1,6-P_2, and phosphoenolpyruvate/pyruvate cycles depends on the relative activity of the enzymes illustrated in Figure 15.2. Conditions favoring gluconeogenesis (the combination of high plasma glucagon, catecholamine, and glucocorticoid levels with a low plasma insulin level, as occurs when animals are starved or fed a low-carbohydrate diet) result in increased activity of PEPCK, FBPase1, and glucose-6-phosphatase (G-6-Pase) and a coordinate decrease in the activity of GK, PFK1, and PK. Reciprocal changes in the activities of these enzymes occur when animals are fed a carbohydrate diet, particularly after a prolonged fast (2,3). In this situation, the plasma insulin concentration increases, levels of the counterregulatory hormones decrease, and glycolysis predominates. The F-6-P/F-1,6-P_2 substrate cycle is also regulated by a subcycle in which the amount of the regulatory molecule F-2,6-P_2 is controlled by the bifunctional enzyme (2,3). The relative activity of these seven enzymes, established by the interaction of several hormones, determines whether the hepatocyte is a consumer or producer of glucose. The activity of the enzymes involved in the cycles is controlled by all of the control mechanisms described above. Many other enzymes are also involved in these processes; however, they catalyze equilibrium reactions that are not rate determining.

Regulation of the Glucose/Glucose-6-phosphate Cycle

Upon entering the hepatocyte through the GLUT2 transporter, glucose is converted to G-6-P by the enzyme glucokinase (Fig. 15.3). Glucokinase is an unusual member of the hexokinase family. Its K_m for glucose is greater than 5 mM, whereas the K_m for HK-I–III (glucokinase is HK-IV) varies between 20 and 120 μM (4,5). This difference in K_m values gives the brain, muscle, and red blood cells, which have isoforms I–III, preference when the glucose supply is limited. Portal vein and liver sinusoidal glucose concentrations are high after a meal. Hepatocytes efficiently convert glucose to G-6-P because glucokinase (HK-IV) works most efficiently at this elevated glucose concentration (7). Also, unlike HK-I–III, glucokinase is not subject to feedback inhibition by physiologic concentrations of the reaction product, G-6-P (7). Because GLUT2 operates by facilitated diffusion, the activity of glucokinase, which keeps intracellular glucose concentrations very low, determines glucose clearance by hepatocytes.

This cycle is important because G-6-P is a branch-point substrate for, or a product of, the glycolytic, gluconeogenic, glycogen formation/degradation, hexosamine, and hexose monophosphate shunt pathways (Fig. 15.3). The balance of glucose phosphorylation and G-6-P hydrolysis, and thus the production or metabolism of glucose, as well as the avoidance of futile substrate cycling, requires the interplay of a number of control mechanisms.

Glucokinase activity is not altered by covalent modification, but its activity is regulated by an allosteric mechanism and by changes in the amount of the protein (2,19). Glucose phosphorylation, by glucokinase, results in increased intracellular levels of G-6-P. Although physiologic concentrations of G-6-P do not inhibit glucokinase, G-6-P is in near equilibrium with F-6-P through the action of the reversible enzyme phosphoglucoisomerase. F-6-P increases the affinity of binding of the nuclear GKRP to glucokinase (19). When bound to GKRP, glucokinase is found primarily in an inactive form in the nucleus of the hepatocyte (36–38). This complex is subject to allosteric regulation, as the inhibition of glucokinase by F-6-P is reversed by F-1-P, which competes with F-6-P for binding to the GKRP (19). F-1-P binding causes a conformational (allosteric) change of GKRP. This results in the dissociation of glucokinase, which can then translocate to the cytoplasm as an active enzyme (38). Thus fructose, which is converted to F-1-P by fructokinase, promotes hepatic glucose clearance by its indirect activation of glucokinase (38) (Fig. 15.3).

Glucokinase gene transcription, glucokinase mRNA, and glucokinase activity are decreased when plasma glucagon is high and plasma insulin is low (e.g., fasting or diabetes) (7,37,39–41). Refeeding a diet high in carbohydrate results in an increase of these parameters. A 20- to 30-fold increase in transcription occurs within 30 to 60 minutes after the injection of insulin into a diabetic rat or after the addition of insulin to primary cultures of hepatocytes (40–42). Glucokinase mRNA increases accordingly (40,41), and a significant increase of glucokinase activity and attendant flux from glucose to G-6-P ensues (43). The inhibitory effect of glucagon (or cAMP, its intracellular messenger) on glucokinase gene transcription is dominant over the stimulatory effect of insulin, because cAMP blocks the effects of insulin at all concentrations of insulin in cultured cell systems (44). These hormone effects are not dependent on the presence of glucose in the medium (41,44).

G-6-Pase is a multisubunit enzyme located on membranes of the endoplasmic reticulum. It has a K_m for G-6-P of about 2 mM, which generally exceeds the concentration of this substrate in the hepatocyte (34). Therefore, the enzyme is usually quite active, and glucose phosphorylation and G-6-P hydrolysis are controlled by substrate concentrations to a significant extent. G-6-Pase is not known to be regulated by allosteric or posttranslational modifications.

It has been known for some time that hepatic G-6-Pase activity is increased by starvation and in diabetic rats (45). These conditions favor glycogenolysis and gluconeogenesis, which, when coupled with elevated G-6-Pase levels and decreased GK activity (and decreased glycolysis), result in net carbon flux toward glucose and its export from the hepatocyte. It therefore is not surprising that insulin reduces, and cAMP increases, G-6-Pase gene transcription (46), just as occurs with the PEPCK gene, which encodes another gluconeogenic enzyme. Insulin inhibits transcription of the G-6-Pase gene in the absence of other hormones and exerts a dominant inhibitory effect over the actions of cAMP and glucocorticoids (46). This effect of insulin requires the PI 3-kinase signal transduction pathway and appears to be exerted, at least in part, through the TGGT-GTTTTG DNA element used in the PEPCK gene promoter (46).

How is glucose flux through this cycle regulated and how is futile cycling avoided? Net glucose output occurs during active glycogenolysis and gluconeogenesis. The G-6-P generated by these processes is readily hydrolyzed because its concentration is still well below the K_m of G-6-Pase (34). Futile cycling by phosphorylation of glucose is prevented by several mechanisms. First, the glucose readily exits the hepatocyte through the GLUT2 transporter and is diluted in the ECF. Second, the interconversion of G-6-P and F-6-P allows GKRP to bind and sequester glucokinase in an inactive form. Finally, the hormonal conditions that promote glucose production through glycogenolysis and gluconeogenesis (high glucagon/low insulin) combine to inhibit subsequent steps in the glycolytic pathway that would divert G-6-P from its hydrolysis to glucose (see below). Net glucose uptake and utilization, as occurs after a glucose load is presented to the liver, requires that the rate of glucose phosphorylation exceeds that of G-6-P hydrolysis. High intracellular levels of glucose increase flux through glucokinase simply because of substrate availability. The hormonal changes consequent to a glucose load (high insulin/low glucagon) activate glycogen synthesis and the downstream glycolytic enzymes (see below). These processes "pull" G-6-P toward utilization. One consequence of reduced G-6-P levels is a reduction of F-6-P and reduced binding of glucokinase to the inhibitory GKRP and thus continued glucose phosphorylation. Therefore, a series of regulatory steps combine to effect net glucose utilization.

Regulation of the Fructose-6-phosphate/ Fructose-1,6-bisphosphate Cycle

G-6-P can be directed along several metabolic pathways; thus the conversion of F-6-P to F-1,6-P_2 is the first committed step in glycolysis, and PFK1 is the most important enzyme in this process. The entire array of intracellular symbols of energy charge and glucose homeostasis operate through a number of mechanisms to provide complex regulation of the F-6-P/ F-1,6-P_2 substrate cycle (2,9) (Fig. 15.4A), which is a major determinant of glycolytic/gluconeogenic flux in liver. One objective of this regulation is to stimulate glycolysis when the energy charge is low and to provide a carbon supply for biosynthetic processes. By contrast, gluconeogenesis is stimulated when signals of glucose deficiency predominate and the energy charge is high.

F-1,6-P_2 affects substrate cycling at the pyruvate/phosphoenolpyruvate substrate cycle by feedforward activation of pyruvate kinase (47). F-1-6-P_2 levels are controlled by the activities of the gluconeogenic enzyme FBPase1 and by PFK1, the opposing glycolytic enzyme. The activity of these enzymes, and net flux through the F-6-P/F-1,6-P_2 cycle, are modulated by hormones that reflect the dietary status (48–51). For example, food deprivation results in the release of glucagon, which leads to the production of cAMP, an intracellular symbol of glucose deficiency. cAMP increases FBPase1 activity and gluconeogenesis, while inhibiting PFK1 activity and flux through glycolysis. By contrast, a glucose meal, with attendant insulin secretion and the consequent reduction of cAMP, results in the activation of PFK1 and the inhibition of FBPase1. This favors flux through glycolysis. Intracellular symbols of energy charge, AMP/ATP and citrate, are also involved in the regulation of these enzymes. High levels of ATP reduce the affinity of PFK1 for its substrate, F-6-P, by an allosteric mechanism (52) (see sigmoidal curve in Fig. 15.4B, left panel). Glycolysis also provides a carbon source for a variety of biosynthetic reactions. Citrate, as an early intermediate in the citric acid cycle, is a symbol of carbon sup-

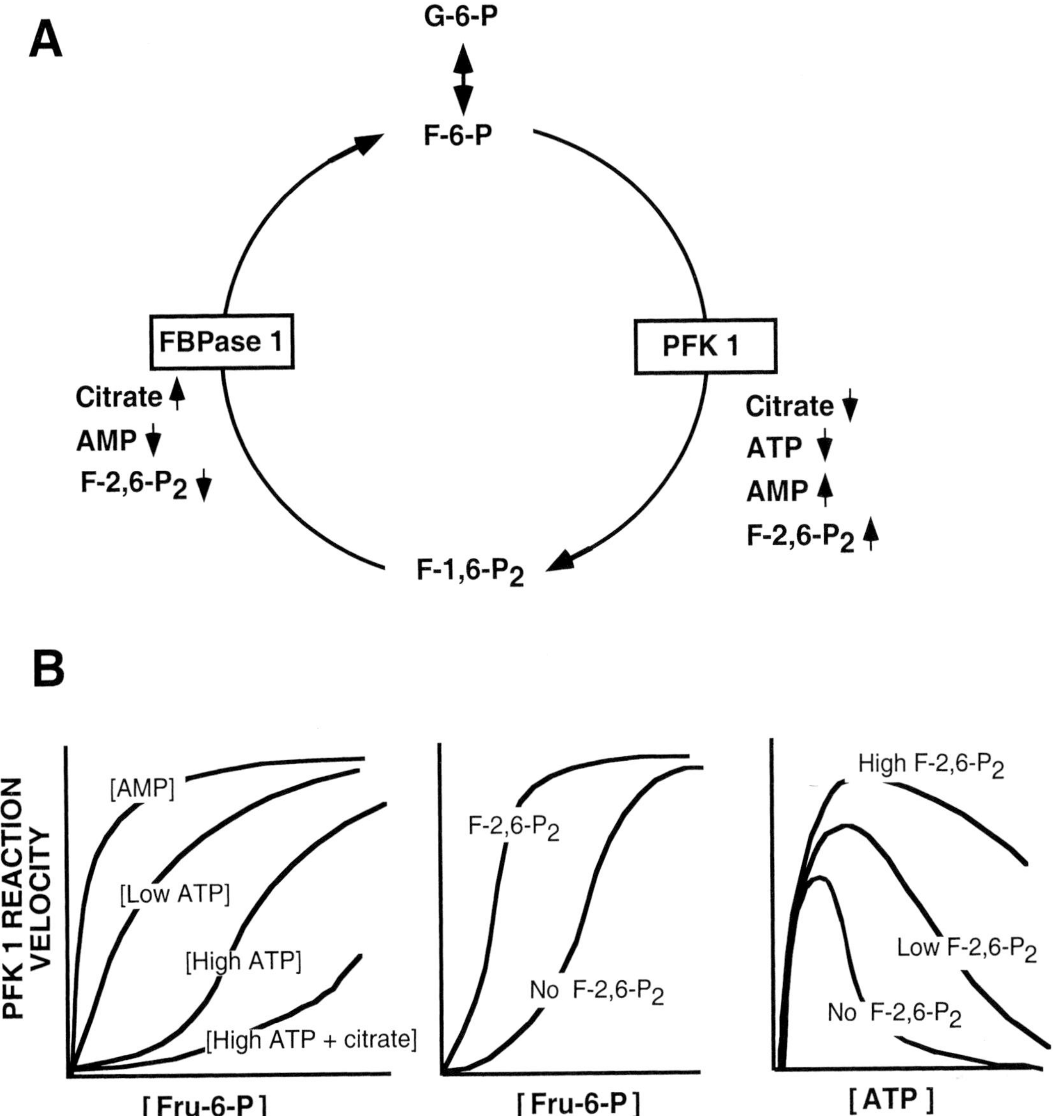

Figure 15.4. Regulation of the fructose-6-phosphate/fructose-1,6-bisphosphate (F-6-P/F-1,6-P_2) cycle. **A:** Glycolysis is stimulated when the energy charge of the cell is low, whereas gluconeogenesis is stimulated when glucose is deficient and the energy charge is high. **B:** Reaction velocities of phosphofructokinase-1 (PFK 1) are influenced by molecular symbols of carbon supply and energy charge. G-6-P, glucose-6-phosphate; ATP, adenosine triphosphate; AMP, adenosine monophosphate; FBPase, fructose-1,6-bisphosphatase; F-2,6-P_2, fructose-2,6-bisphosphate.

ply. Citrate provides feedback control of the PFK1 reaction by enhancing the inhibitory effect of ATP. This puts an additional brake on glucose degradation when the carbon supply is sufficient. Citrate also causes a reciprocal activation of FBPase1. The net effect of this is decreased glycolytic and increased gluconeogenic flux. AMP, a symbol of a low energy charge, counteracts the effect of ATP on PFK1 and is an inhibitor of FBPase1 (Fig. 15.4B, left panel). Thus, PFK1 activity is high when the energy charge is low and low when the energy charge is high.

For some time it was not clear how these effectors interacted to regulate the enzymes that drive this substrate cycle. Both enzymes are substrates for cAMP-dependent protein kinase, and it was first thought that this was the mechanism whereby these activities were altered [see reference (2) for review]. However, *in vitro* phosphorylation by cAMP-dependent protein kinase (PKA) had little effect on the activity of these enzymes (52,53). Furthermore, the inhibition of PFK1 activity seen in crude extracts of hepatocytes incubated with glucagon disappeared on partial purification of the enzyme (54). It was subsequently shown that a low-molecular-weight effector, F-2,6-P_2, is involved in the regulation of both PFK1 and FBPase1 by cAMP (2,3,55,56).

The synthesis of F-2,6-P_2 involves the PFK2 reaction (F-6-P + ATP $\rightarrow$ F-2,6-P_2 + ADP), whereas its degradation is catalyzed by a specific FBPase2 reaction (F-2,6-$P_2$$\rightarrow$F-6-P + P) (Fig. 15.5). A unique bifunctional enzyme, PFK2/FBPase2, catalyzes both of these reactions (57). Phosphorylation of this enzyme by PKA on serine 32 results in inhibition of the kinase and activation of the bisphosphatase and thus in low levels of F-2,6-P_2. Dephosphorylation results in opposite changes of the enzyme activities and increased levels of F-2,6-P_2 (58). These changes explain the rapid modulation of F-2,6-P_2 that occurs when β-adrenergic agonists and glucagon (high cAMP) or insulin (low cAMP) are added to isolated hepatocytes (59,60).

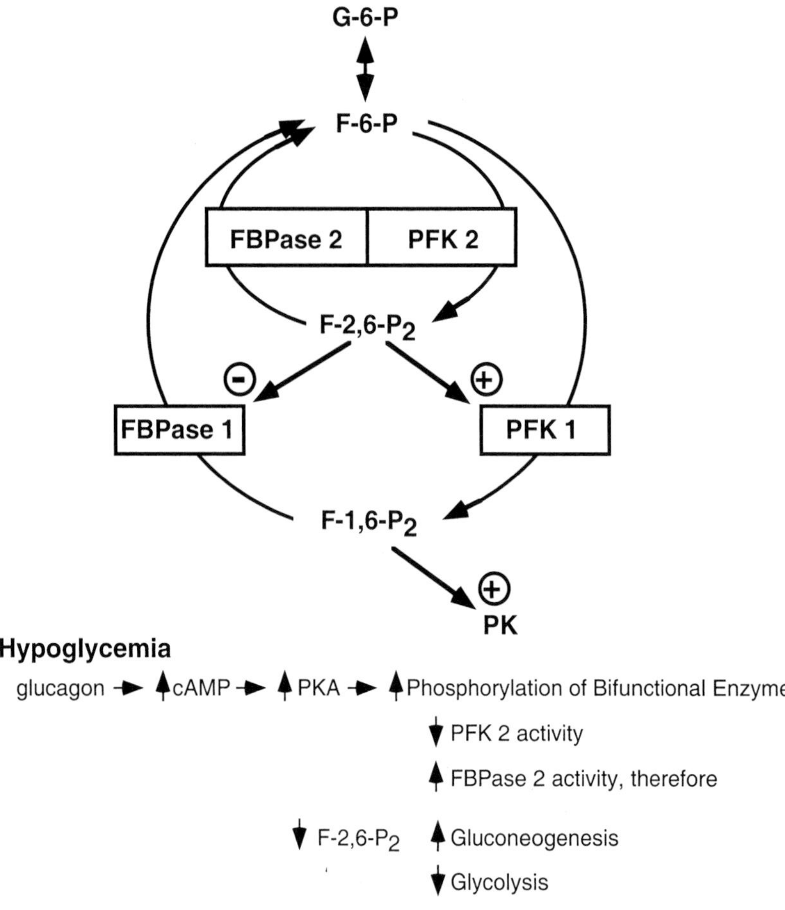

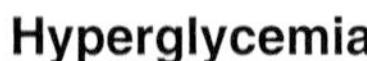

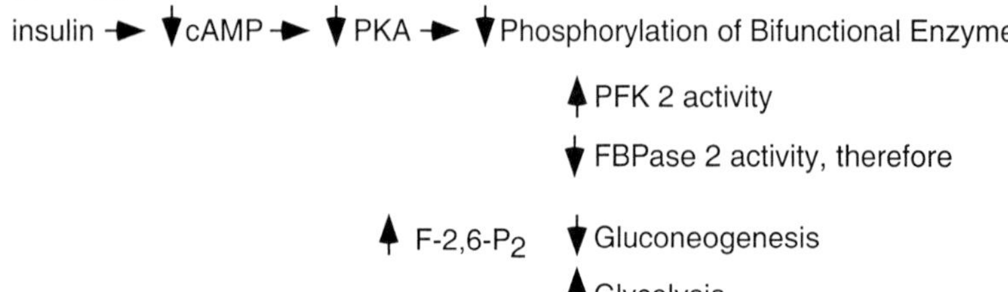

Figure 15.5. Regulation of the fructose-6-phosphate/fructose-2,6-bisphosphate (F-6-P/F-2,6-P_2) subcycle. F-2,6-P_2 is a powerful allosteric regulator of both phosphofructokinase-1 (PFK 1) and FBPase 1 and so determines whether glycolysis or gluconeogenesis prevails. G-6-P, glucose-6-phosphate; FBPase 2/PFK 2, fructose-2,6-bisphosphatase/phosphofructokinase-2 (the bifunctional enzyme); FBPase 1, fructose-1,6-bisphosphatase; PK, pyruvate kinase; cAMP, cyclic adenosine monophosphate; PKA, cAMP-dependent protein kinase.

F-2,6-P_2 increases the affinity of PFK1 for F-6-P (Fig. 15.4B, center panel) and thus is a potent activator of the enzyme. It is a competitive inhibitor of FBPase1 (2,9,12,55,56). Therefore, gluconeogenesis prevails when the glucagon/insulin ratio is elevated, as in starvation or diabetes, because cAMP levels are high and F-2,6-P_2 is low. The opposite situation occurs after refeeding or insulin administration. In this case, glycolysis, and the generation of three-carbon fragments for lipogenesis, prevails.

AMP and F-2,6-P_2, symbols of a low energy charge and hyperglycemia, respectively, interact synergistically to stimulate PFK1. In so doing, these agents override the inhibitory effects that citrate and ATP have on this enzyme. In a reciprocal action, AMP and F-2,6-P_2 inhibit the gluconeogenic enzyme FBPase1. The sensitivity of PFK1 to F-2,6-P_2 exceeds that of FBPase1. This partial inhibition allows for some cycling through the gluconeogenic part of this cycle, even in the fed state. This escape provides some relief from potential problems related to lactate accumulation (and acidosis) from excessive glycolysis (3).

Other features of the regulation of this cycle are noteworthy. F-6-P, the substrate of the PFK2 reaction, is a noncompetitive inhibitor of the FBPase2 reaction (61). Conditions that favor the increase of F-6-P, such as a glucose load or glycogenolysis mediated by α-adrenergic agonists, vasopressin and angiotensin, none of which act through cAMP (62), promote the formation of F-2,6-P_2 and stimulate glycolysis. However, the cAMP effect is dominant over that of glucose. PKA-mediated phosphorylation of the bifunctional enzyme results in reduced concentrations of F-2,6-P_2 even in the presence of glucose (3).

This cycle is functionally entwined with the cycles that precede and follow it. As mentioned above, F-6-P is in near equilibrium with G-6-P. F-6-P promotes flux down the glycolytic pathway by serving as a substrate for the formation of the allosteric regulator F-2,6-P_2. It also enhances the net formation of this important molecule by inhibiting FBPase2, the enzyme that degrades it. F-2,6-P_2 stimulates PFK1, which converts F-6-P to F-1,6-P_2. This reduces the level of F-6-P, which results in the release of GK inhibition by GKRP and hence in an increase in glucose flux through phosphorylation. The other product of this cycle, F-1,6-P_2 causes feedforward activation of pyruvate kinase, a key component of the downstream substrate cycle.

The primary regulation of this substrate cycle involves alterations of enzyme activity. Long-term regulation, by changes in the rate of synthesis of these proteins, also occurs (35). cAMP inhibits expression of the PFK1 and bifunctional enzyme genes. Glucocorticoids enhance the level of bifunctional enzyme mRNA. Insulin has opposite effects on these genes, but this effect requires glucose and is probably due more to this than to insulin. This is discussed in detail below. Glucocorticoids are potent inducers of bifunctional enzyme gene expression. These hormones increase the rate of transcription of the gene in livers of adrenalectomized rats, in primary hepatocytes, and in FTO-2B hepatoma cells. Like glucocorticoids, insulin causes a 10- to 20-fold increase of bifunctional enzyme mRNA in hepatoma cells. These effects require glucose (see below) and are completely blocked by the concomitant addition of cAMP. FBPase1 gene expression is increased severalfold in diabetic animals, and insulin reduces this to the baseline value. cAMP, by contrast, is reported to increase FBPase1 mRNA in cultured hepatocytes. These effects on the FBPase1 gene have been difficult to replicate and extend. The primary regulation of this component of the cycle appears to be accomplished through regulation of enzyme activity.

Regulation of the Pyruvate/ Phosphoenolpyruvate Cycle

This cycle is regulated by the glycolytic enzyme PK and the gluconeogenic enzyme PEPCK (Fig. 15.6). The PK reaction plays a critical role in the regulation of glycolysis and thus is an important site of nutrient and hormonal regulation. Glucagon (cAMP) strongly inhibits flux through PK, whereas epinephrine, which primarily exerts α-adrenergic, cAMP-independent effects in liver, is not very effective (63,64). Insulin, by decreasing cAMP levels, relieves the inhibition of PK activity caused by glucagon and increases flux through this enzyme (64–66).

The liver isozyme of PK (L-PK) is an allosteric enzyme. It exhibits sigmoidal kinetics for its substrate, phosphoenolpyruvate, and is activated by F-1,6-P_2 by a feedforward mechanism. This promotes glycolytic flux. L-PK is inhibited through allosteric mechanisms by alanine and ATP. The inhibitory effect of glucagon (cAMP) on L-PK is explained by the observation that the enzyme is phosphorylated by PKA (67). Phosphorylation increases the apparent K_m of the enzyme for phosphoenolpyruvate, and the phosphorylated enzyme is more readily inhibited by alanine and ATP than is the nonphosphorylated enzyme (Fig. 15.6). There are many subtle interplays between these regulatory systems, but the important point is that the inhibition of PK allows for the accumulation of PEP and its routing through the gluconeogenic pathway. It also prevents excessive production of lactate. These events are important during starvation, when gluconeogenesis is essential. Thus, in metabolic conditions that favor gluconeogenesis over glycolysis, cAMP as a symbol of glucose deficiency, alanine as a symbol of carbon supply, and ATP as a symbol of energy sufficiency combine to shut down flux through PK.

The activity of PEPCK, in contrast to that of PK, is not significantly affected by allosteric or posttranslation modifications, such as phosphorylation. There is thus no short-term or acute regulation of PEPCK. Rather, all changes of PEPCK activity are due to changes in the amount of the enzyme present in the hepatocyte. This is primarily controlled by the amount of PEPCK mRNA. A variety of effectors, including glucocorticoids, cAMP, thyroid hormones, and retinoic acid stimulate transcription of the PEPCK gene (27,68). These agents enhance gluconeogenic flux by this mechanism. Insulin and glucose act independently to exert dominant inhibition of PEPCK gene transcription and of gluconeogenesis, even in the presence of the inducers (27,69). A great deal has been learned about how these various hormones and metabolic signals converge to regulate the transcription of this gene. This is discussed in more detail below. Several of these agents also have effects on the stability of PEPCK mRNA. Glucocorticoids and cAMP enhance the rate of transcription of the gene, and both stabilize the mRNA against degradation (22,23,27). These combined effects result in a net increase of the mRNA and enhanced rates of translation of the protein.

PK is also subject to transcriptional control by many of these same effectors, but in a direction opposite to that exerted on the PEPCK gene. L-PK mRNA, decreased in starved or diabetic rats, is restored to normal levels by the refeeding of a carbohydrate diet or insulin. Both effects involve an increased rate of L-PK gene transcription; however, the insulin effect is delayed (compared with the rapid effect on the PEPCK gene) and is indirect. Further studies showed that glucose, or more exactly a metabolite of glucose, is the direct effector (70,71). Insulin, by promoting glucose phosphorylation through stimulating GK, supplies this glucose metabolite and is thus acting indirectly (35,70,71). Glucagon, acting through cAMP, inhibits transcription

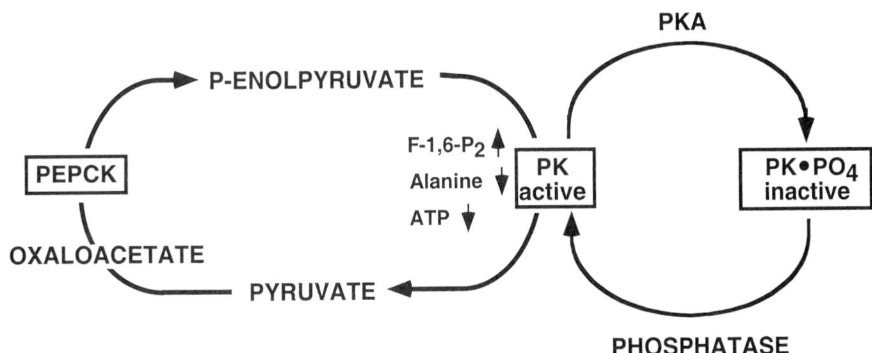

Figure 15.6. Regulation of the phosphoenolpyruvate (PEP)/pyruvate cycle. Pyruvate kinase (PK) is regulated by allostery, phosphorylation, and its biosynthesis, whereas phosphoenolpyruvate carboxykinase (PEPCK) is regulated primarily by control of its biosynthesis. F-1,6-P_2, fructose-1,6-bisphosphate; PKA, cAMP-dependent protein kinase; ATP, adenosine triphosphate.

of the L-PK gene. The cAMP effect is dominant over the effects of insulin/glucose (72). As with PEPCK, but in reverse, cAMP increases the rate of degradation of L-PK mRNA, and insulin/glucose stabilizes this mRNA (72).

In summary, cAMP, which causes a potent inhibition of PK by phosphorylation, also reduces the amount of the enzyme in the hepatocyte. Insulin reverses this phosphorylation effect by reducing the cAMP concentration in the cell but also works with glucose to promote an increase in the amount of the enzyme. cAMP, with glucocorticoids and retinoic acid, increases the amount of the gluconeogenic enzyme PEPCK in hepatocytes. Insulin and glucose, which inhibit gluconeogenesis, do so in part by reducing the amount of PEPCK in the cell. Thus, there is a multilevel, reciprocal regulation of the activity and the amount of the enzymes that drive the phosphoenolpyruvate/pyruvate substrate cycle.

Regulation of Glycogen Metabolism

After a meal enriched with carbohydrates, glucose in excess of that needed for immediate consumption is stored as glycogen, which is used as the body's primary reservoir of glucose during fasting. The regulation of the synthesis of glycogen (glycogenesis) or the breakdown of glycogen into glucose (glycogenolysis) is critically important for glucose homeostasis. Glycogenesis and glycogenolysis are controlled by a set of enzymes that are subject to a broad range of regulatory mechanisms, including phosphorylation, substrate availability, protein-protein interactions, allostery, and subcellular localization. In the fed state, glucose and insulin promote glycogenesis, whereas glucagon and its second messenger, cAMP, promote glycogenolysis in the fasted state. A familiar theme is that these agents often have reciprocal effects; i.e., they promote flux through one pathway while inhibiting flux through the other [for reviews see references (14) and (73–75)]. Another recurring theme is that glucose, or its metabolites, is a direct participant in the reactions that control its disposal into glycogen and its formation from glycogen.

The synthesis of glycogen in the liver begins with the influx of glucose through the GLUT2 transporter, whereupon it is phosphorylated to G-6-P by glucokinase (Fig. 15.7). G-6-P, converted to G-1-P by phosphoglucomutase, is then conjugated with uridine 5′-diphosphate by uridine diphosphate (UDP)–glucose pyrophosphorylase to form UDP-glucose. Two additional enzymes are required for glycogenesis: (a) glycogen synthase, which serially adds UDP-glucose subunits in a linear array through the formation of α-1,4-glycosidic bonds, and (b) branching enzyme, which causes a bifurcation of the growing glycogen chain through the formation of α-1,6-glycosidic bonds (14).

Glycogenolysis is mediated by the active form of the enzyme glycogen phosphorylase (phosphorylase a), which removes G-1-P residues from the glycogen polymer. G-1-P is converted to G-6-P by phosphoglucomutase and to glucose by G-6-ase (Fig. 15.7). Phosphorylase a is converted from the inactive form (phosphorylase b) by phosphorylase kinase, an enzyme that adds a phosphate group to serine 14 of phosphorylase b (14). Phosphorylase kinase, in turn, is activated by PKA (76). PKA is activated by an increase in the second messenger cAMP, which is an intracellular symbol of glucose deficiency, as described above. Thus, hypoglycemia results in the activation of phosphorylase a, which leads to the breakdown of glycogen and the production of glucose. This process is regulated by a phosphorylation cascade that amplifies the initial signal (glucagon) to promote a large biological response (glycogenolysis) (14,75) and by glucose (or G-6-P) itself.

Glycogenesis is regulated by glycogen synthase activity, whereas glycogenolysis is regulated by phosphorylase activity. The metabolic logic of the regulation of glycogen synthesis and degradation is evident in the observation that effectors that increase the activity of one enzyme decrease the activity

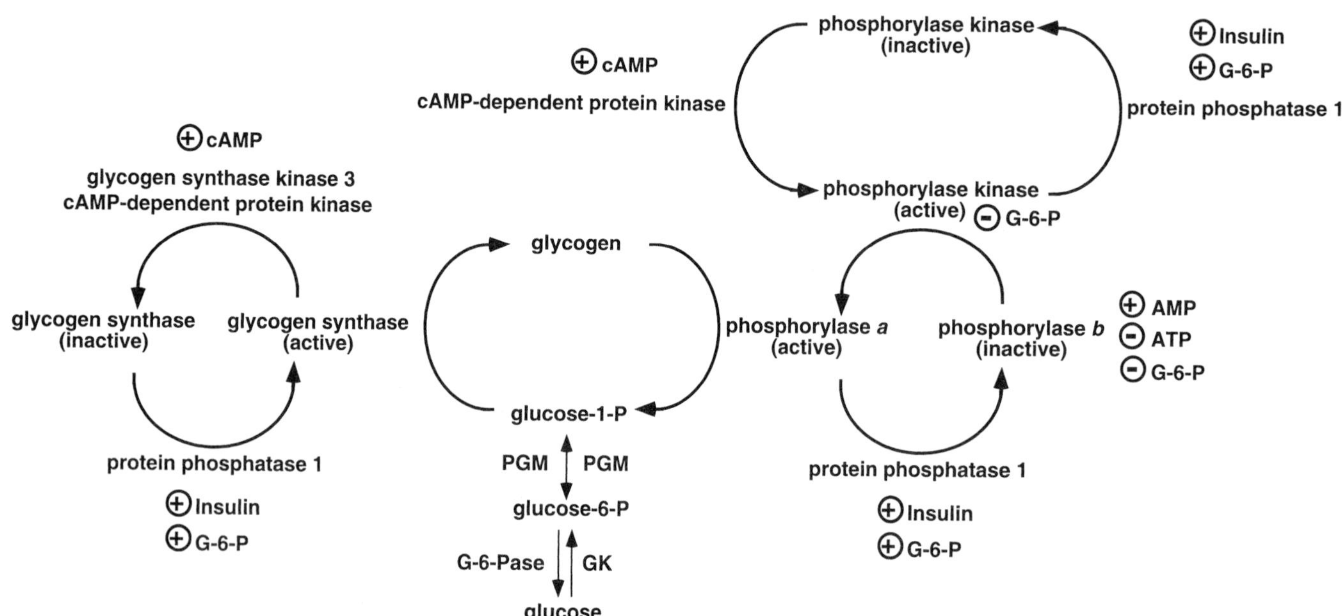

Figure 15.7. Regulation of glycogen metabolism. Glycogenesis and glycogenolysis are regulated in a reciprocal manner. Elevated cyclic adenosine monophosphate (cAMP) concentrations increase cAMP-dependent protein kinase and glycogen synthase kinase 3 activity, leading to decreased glycogenesis and increased glycogenolysis, whereas increased insulin and glucose-6-phosphate (G-6-P) levels increase protein phosphatase 1 activity, leading to increased glycogenesis and decreased glycogen degradation. G-1-P, glucose-1-phosphate; G-6-Pase, glucose-6-phosphatase; GK, glucokinase; PGM, phosphoglucomutase.

of the other. This reciprocity allows glycogen synthase and phosphorylase to act as molecular switches that rapidly change the liver from a glucose-producing to a glucose-storing organ, or vice versa, depending on the metabolic needs of the organism.

The activity of glycogen synthase, like that of phosphorylase, is regulated by the phosphorylation of several serine residues. Fasting [high glucagon (cAMP) and low insulin] results in phosphorylation and enzyme inactivation. After a carbohydrate-enriched meal, the concerted actions of insulin and glucose increase glycogen synthase activity by promoting the removal of the inhibitory phosphate residues. Insulin increases the activity of protein phosphatase 1 (PP1), the phosphatase that removes the inhibitory phosphates (77). In addition, insulin decreases the activity of the kinases that promote phosphorylation and enzyme inhibition, specifically PKA and glycogen synthase kinase 3 (78). The first product of glucose metabolism, G-6-P, binds to glycogen synthase and causes a conformational change that makes the enzyme a better substrate for PP1 (73). In addition, G-6-P promotes the proper intracellular localization of glycogen synthase (see below).

Whereas insulin and G-6-P activate glycogen synthase, thereby promoting glycogenesis, these two effectors reciprocally inhibit the activity of phosphorylase a, the active form of the enzyme that is primarily responsible for glycogenolysis (Fig. 15.7). G-6-P binds to the active site of phosphorylase a, and this has two consequences: (i) it is a competitive inhibitor with glycogen for binding to the active site of the enzyme, and (ii) the binding of G-6-P causes a conformational change in phosphorylase a that makes it a better substrate for PP1, thereby facilitating the conversion of the enzyme to its inactive form (phosphorylase b). Owing to the high transport capacity of GLUT2, and the high K_m of glucokinase, the concentration of G-6-P inside hepatocytes is proportional to the plasma glucose level. Therefore, phosphorylase a acts as a sensor of plasma glucose levels; the higher the glucose concentration, the more G-6-P is able to bind to the active site of phosphorylase a and inhibit glycogenolysis (14). Phosphorylase a is also inactivated by dephosphorylation, which is mediated by the insulin-dependent activation of PP1. In addition, PP1 dephosphorylates and inactivates phosphorylase kinase (Fig. 15.7). Furthermore, insulin decreases the intracellular concentration of cAMP by activating phosphodiesterases, the enzymes that degrade this effector molecule (78). Thus, insulin disrupts the entire cAMP-dependent kinase signaling cascade that activates phosphorylase b, while simultaneously acting to dephosphorylate and activate glycogen synthase. G-6-P also acts reciprocally on both rate-controlling enzymes, inactivating phosphorylase a and activating glycogen synthase, respectively (Fig. 15.7).

SPATIAL ORGANIZATION OF GLYCOGEN METABOLISM

The enzymes of glycogen metabolism exhibit a spatial organization that has profound effects on the regulation of glycogen synthesis and degradation. A family of proteins named glycogen targeting subunits (the liver-specific form is designated G_L) act as a scaffold for most of the enzymes involved in the regulation of glycogen metabolism. G_L is distributed in a gradient within the hepatocyte (75). The highest concentration is found near the plasma membrane, and the lowest concentration is near the center of the cell. Glycogen particles have the same subcellular distribution (73). G_L, which was originally studied as a subcellular targeting subunit of PP1, also has binding sites for glycogen, glycogen synthase, phosphorylase a, and phosphorylase kinase (75). Thus, all of the significant players in glycogen metabolism are localized on one scaffolding protein. This arrangement increases the local concentration of these enzymes and increases the efficiency of these sequential reactions. The differential localization of enzymes on G_L has other important regulatory implications. For example, the binding of phosphorylase a to G_L results in the allosteric inhibition of PP1, which results in reduced phosphorylation of glycogen synthase and thus in the activation of this enzyme. In addition, insulin and glucose promote the translocation of glycogen synthase from an intracellular site to the plasma membrane, presumably to G_L, although the mechanism of this translocation is not completely understood (75). Under some circumstances, the abundance of G_L is rate limiting for glycogen storage. Diabetic animals have decreased glycogen storage and decreased amounts of G_L. Glucose-intolerant animals injected with a recombinant adenovirus that expresses a G_L family member in the liver have increased hepatic glycogen content and normalized oral glucose tolerance (79).

In summary, glycogen metabolism is spatially restricted within hepatocytes and is controlled by a relatively small set of regulatory proteins. Glycogenesis is controlled by glycogen synthase, whose activity is increased by signals related to hyperglycemia and decreased by signals related to hypoglycemia. Glycogenolysis is controlled by glycogen phosphorylase, whose activity is increased by a phosphorylation cascade initiated by the fasting state and decreased by insulin during the fed state, which interferes with the former signaling cascade. G-6-P regulates its own abundance using a feedback control mechanism, inhibiting glycogenolysis by the repression of phosphorylase a activity and promoting glycogenesis by increasing glycogen synthase activity.

Regulation of Glucose Metabolism by Gene Transcription

Flux through metabolic pathways depends on the amount of critical enzymes present in the cell. An intricate set of mechanisms controls the rate of synthesis of the mRNAs that encode these enzymes. These control mechanisms are responsive to changes in the concentration of the hormones and effectors that provide overall metabolic control. As described above, hormones such as glucagon (acting through cAMP), glucocorticoids, retinoic acid, thyroid hormone, and insulin regulate the rate of transcription of genes that direct the synthesis of metabolic enzymes (Fig. 15.8). Glucose or, more likely, certain of its metabolic products are also directly involved in this process (see further on).

The paradigm that developed as a result of studies conducted about 25 years ago held that a ligand-receptor complex bound to a specific region of DNA in the promoter of target genes and that this interaction somehow resulted in a change in the frequency of transcription initiation. This valuable concept quickly led to the definition of specific, short DNA sequences that indeed could bind the ligand-receptor complex. This in turn led to the definition of discrete DNA sequences that could mediate the function of each hormone. These DNA sequences were called hormone response elements, or HREs. Often, but not always, this simple HRE could function in the context of a heterologous promoter/reporter system (Fig. 15.9A). It soon became apparent, however, that none of these hormone effectors employs an exclusive, or single, HRE that simply binds a ligand–hormone receptor complex to regulate transcription. It now appears that most, if not all, HREs function in necessary concert with accessory factors in the context of natural promoters. These multicomponent complexes include the receptor and accessory factor binding sites and are termed hormone response units (HRUs) or composite elements (80). Interestingly, some of the components of one HRU are components of another HRU and participate in the response to more than one

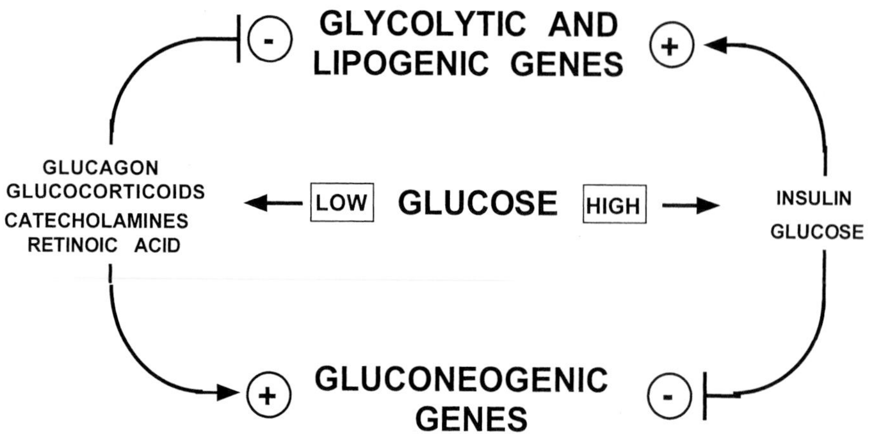

Figure 15.8. Regulation of glucose metabolism by gene transcription. An array of hormonal and nutritional signals regulate genes whose products catalyze reactions of glucose metabolism. The coordinated and reciprocal actions of these effectors contribute to glucose homeostasis.

hormone (81). In addition to this collection of protein-DNA interactions, a number of protein-protein interactions between the DNA-bound ligand-receptor and accessory factor complexes and one or more coregulatory proteins are required for the assembly of a functional transcription complex. This is illustrated schematically in Figure 15.9B.

This concept is well illustrated by the arrangement of the PEPCK gene promoter. The PEPCK gene promoter is divided into several HRUs, including the following: a cAMP response unit (CRU) that is assembled in response to glucagon, which acts by the cAMP signaling pathway; a glucocorticoid response unit (GRU) that is assembled in response to glucocorticoids; a retinoic acid response unit (RARU); and an insulin response unit (IRU) (24,81–84) (Fig. 15.10). Whereas the CRU, GRU, and RARU mediate increased expression of the PEPCK gene, the IRU is necessary for dominant repression by insulin.

Whereas a simple HRE may provide an "off-or-on" control, an HRU provides a more flexible and versatile regulation of gene transcription and may allow for a more precise control of gene expression. The assembly of multiple HRUs has been called a metabolic control domain (MCD) (26,80,85,86). As discussed above, different hormones recruit different sets of transcription factors and coactivators to the PEPCK gene promoter. Our current thinking is that this arrangement may explain the phenomena of additivity, synergism, and dominant repression observed in the presence of different combinations of hormones. The MCD may thus be an organizational structure that integrates the action of a variety of hormonal signals to provide a transcriptional response that is appropriate for a particular physiologic situation.

Although not as extensively characterized as the PEPCK MCD, several other genes that encode enzymes and proteins involved in metabolism appear to be regulated by a similar mechanism. Examples include the tyrosine aminotransferase, insulin-like growth factor binding protein-1 (IGFBP-1), G-6-Pase, PK, glucokinase, aldolase, and bifunctional enzyme genes (80).

Regulation of Hepatic Gene Expression by Glucose

An animal that ends a prolonged fast with a meal enriched in carbohydrates exhibits a characteristic pattern of gene expression

A. CONTROL BY A SIMPLE HORMONE RESPONSE ELEMENT

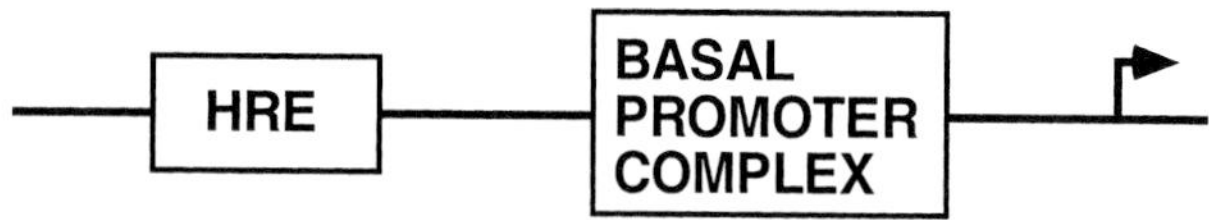

B. CONTROL BY A HORMONE RESPONSE UNIT

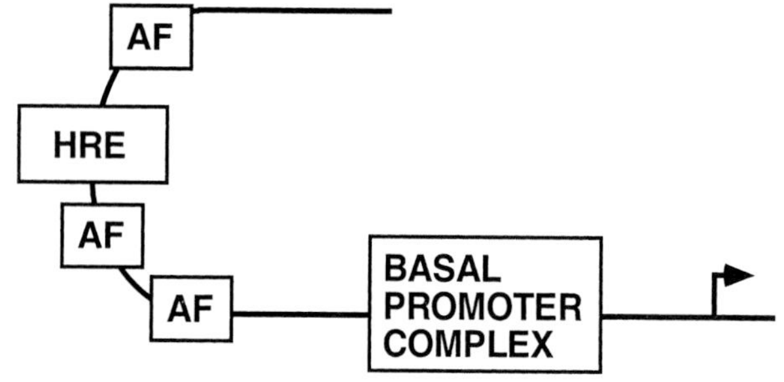

Figure 15.9. Hormonal regulation of gene transcription. The transcription of genes is regulated by either simple hormone response elements (**A,** HRE) or more commonly by hormone response units (**B,** HRU), which require the presence of additional DNA-binding proteins called accessory factors (AF).

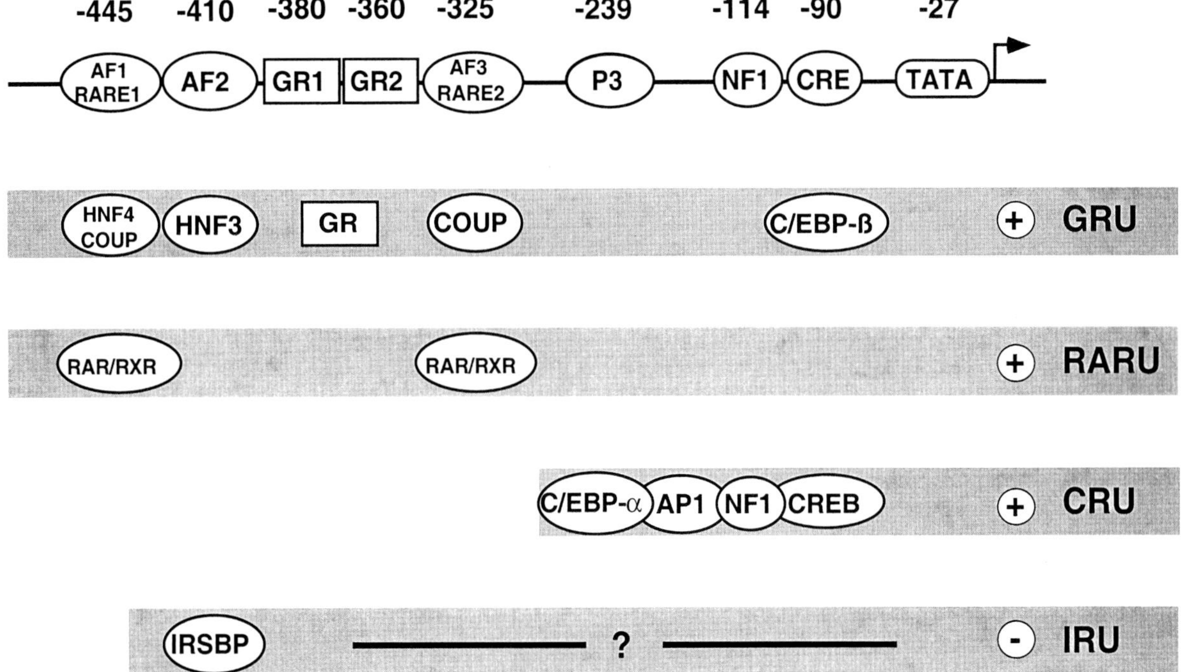

Figure 15.10. The metabolic control domain of the phosphoenolpyruvate carboxykinase (PEPCK) gene promoter. The metabolic control domain is composed of overlapping hormone response units. This arrangement allows for the integration of a variety of hormonal and environmental signals to provide an appropriate physiologic response. The numbers at the top of the figure represent the distance in base pairs from the transcription start site of individual elements characterized in the PEPCK promoter. The shaded portion contains the names of proteins that bind these elements and that are involved in the individual response units, shown on the right. GRU, glucocorticoid response unit; RARU, retinoic acid response unit; CRU, cAMP response unit; IRU, insulin response unit.

that contributes to the regulation of the plasma glucose level. These changes include an increase in the transcription of the genes that encode glycolytic and lipogenic enzymes and a decrease in the transcription of genes that encode gluconeogenic and ketogenic enzyme genes (87,88). Thus, hepatic glucose utilization is increased and glucose production is diminished, providing an impetus toward normal glucose levels. This programmatic change in gene expression, as discussed further on, requires the concerted actions of both insulin and glucose (Fig. 15.11).

Glucose exerts, through its metabolism, very strong effects on the transcription of genes that encode the enzymes that regulate its utilization and production. Because the glucose transporter, GLUT2, is not rate limiting in the liver, glucose clearance by hepatocytes is regulated primarily by the presence, abundance, and activity of glucokinase, as described above (5). Glucose flux through glucokinase acts as a sensor of the intrahepatic glucose concentration (5). Because glucokinase gene expression requires the presence of insulin and insulin decreases plasma glucose, it is very difficult to separate the effects of insulin and glucose *in vivo*. Cultures of isolated hepatocytes and hepatoma cells provide a system in which various environmental conditions can be carefully controlled. For example, in such systems insulin induces transcription of the glucokinase gene in the absence of glucose, but it has no effect on the PK gene (which appeared to be regulated by insulin *in vivo*). Reasoning that insulin induced glucokinase synthesis, and glucokinase initiated glucose metabolism, Kahn and coworkers tested whether glucokinase expression, in the absence of insulin, would stimulate PK gene transcription (89). Indeed, in hepatocytes treated with either retrovirus or adenovirus constructs that express glucokinase, glucose can stimulate transcription of the PK gene and repress the PEPCK gene in the absence of insulin (69,89).

How does glucose metabolism alter gene transcription? G-6-P, the product of the glucokinase reaction, can be directed through a number of metabolic pathways, including glycolytic, glycogenic, the hexose monophosphate shunt, or the glucosamine pathways (Fig. 15.12). In principle, any of these pathways could generate a metabolite that could act as a second messenger of glucose flux and therefore influence the transcription of genes encoding the enzymes of glucose utilization and production. Two candidate signaling metabolites, G-6-P and xylulose-5-P (xyl-5-P), have been identified. G-6-P is considered a candidate because its concentration rises and falls in a time course that precedes the comparable changes of mRNA levels of genes that are regulated by glucose (90). Xyl-5-P, a metabolite of the hexose monophosphate shunt, is also a candidate. Hepatocytes treated with xylitol, which is rapidly converted to xyl-5-P, show the same pattern of gene expression as cells treated with glucose (91). Furthermore, the xylitol effect occurs at very low concentrations, as would be expected for a signaling metabolite. What is particularly intriguing about the possibility of xyl-5-P as a signaling metabolite is that this molecule is known to stimulate the activity of protein phosphatase 2A (PP2A), which dephosphorylates PFK2, thereby increasing F-2,6-P_2 levels and increasing the activity of PFK1 and flux through glycolysis (92). In addition, as described below, the activation of PP2A increases the nuclear localization of a transcription factor that is involved in the stimulation of glucose-responsive genes (93).

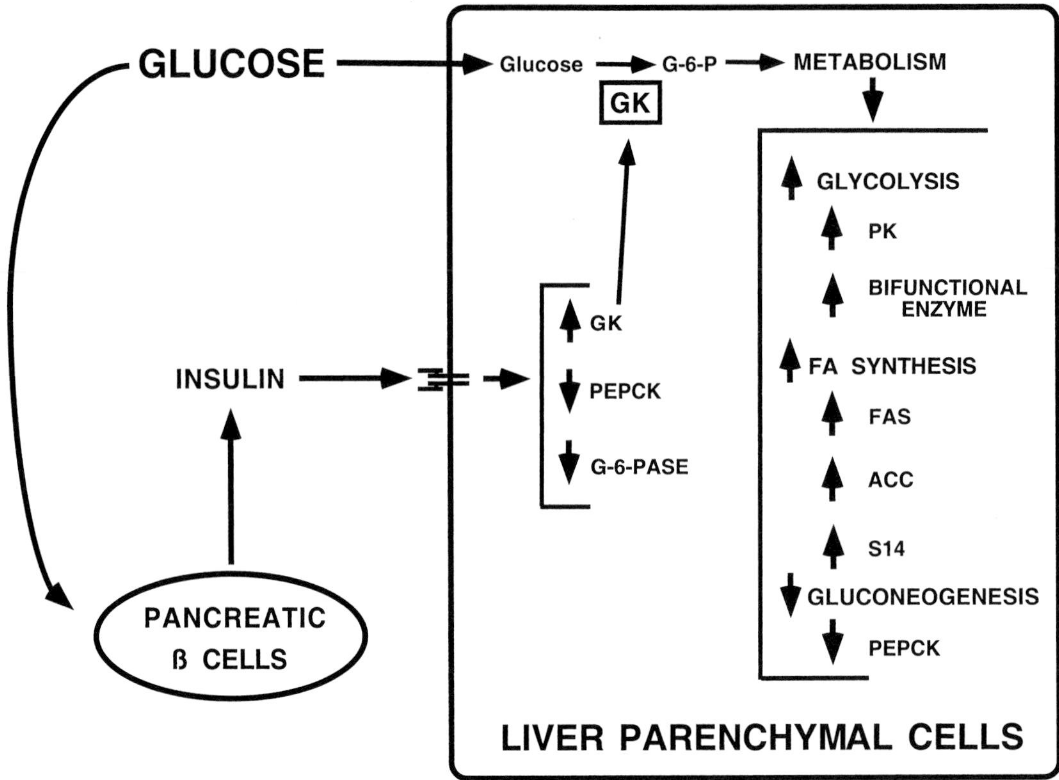

Figure 15.11. The concerted actions of insulin and glucose on metabolic enzyme gene expression. Insulin increases the expression of glucokinase (GK), allowing glucose signaling metabolites to alter the expression of metabolic genes in a coordinated fashion. G-6-P, glucose-6-phosphate; PEPCK, phosphoenolpyruvate carboxykinase; G-6-Pase, glucose-6-phosphatase; PK, pyruvate kinase; FA, fatty acid; FAS, fatty acid synthase; ACC, acetyl-CoA carboxylase; S14, spot 14 protein.

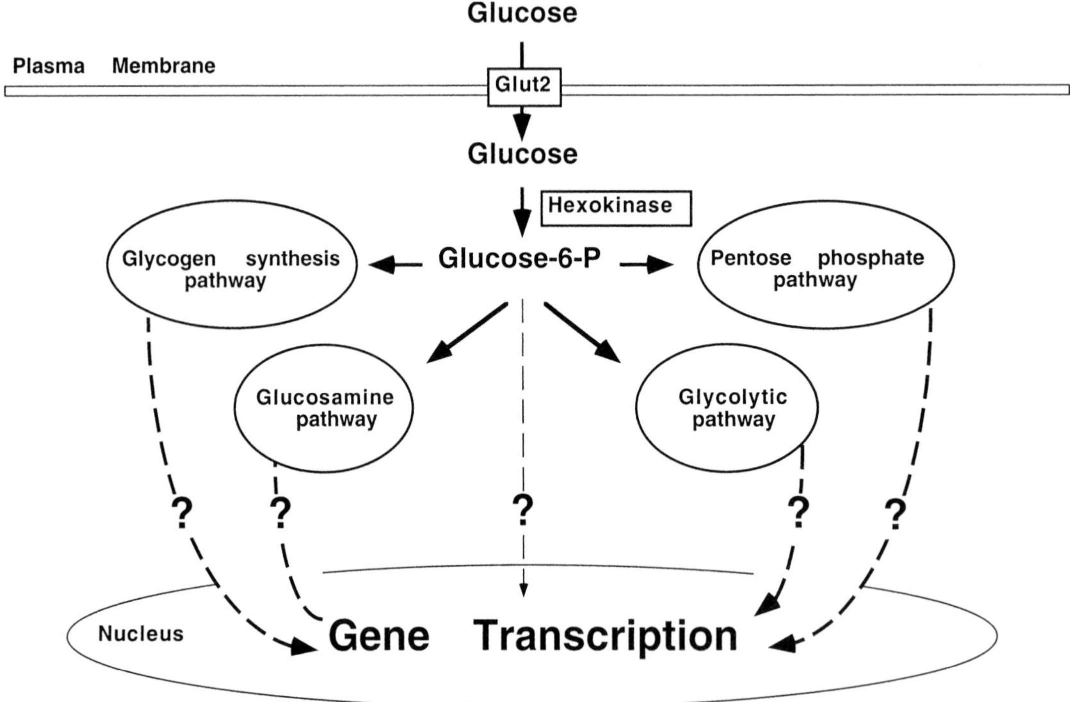

Figure 15.12. The metabolism of glucose provides a metabolic signal that alters gene transcription. The glucose signaling metabolite may be glucose-6-phoshate (G-6-P) or may originate from any metabolic pathway through which G-6-P is directed.

The glucose or carbohydrate response elements (ChoREs) of two genes, spot 14 (S14) and PK, have been studied in great detail. The function of the protein encoded by the S14 gene is incompletely understood, but it probably regulates lipid biosynthesis, a pathway that depends on the three-carbon molecules derived from glycolysis. The ChoREs of the PK and S14 genes are very similar; they each consist of two E-boxes separated by five base pairs (94). An E-box is a DNA element that binds to transcription factors having a basic helix-loop-helix (bHLH) DNA binding motif. Indeed, many bHLH transcription factors bind to the ChoREs, but it has been difficult to assign particular factors to the regulation of the glucose response. For example, upstream stimulating factor (USF) binds quite well to both the S14 and PK ChoREs *in vitro* (95,96). However, these elements can be mutated so that USF no longer binds but the element still conveys a glucose response (95). This observation made it clear that other factors are involved in the glucose response.

A transcription factor, termed the carbohydrate response element binding protein (ChREBP), has many of the characteristics expected of a protein that mediates the glucose response. ChREBP, isolated from the livers of fed animals, binds to the PK gene ChoRE more abundantly than when it is isolated from the livers of fasted animals. Furthermore, its binding activity is regulated by phosphorylation. ChREBP, when phosphorylated, is localized in the cytoplasm and is unable to bind DNA. Moreover, it is phosphorylated by PKA. Thus, when cAMP levels are high, as during a fast, ChREBP is prevented from activating the PK gene; the phosphorylation of one amino acid prevents nuclear localization, and the other restricts DNA binding (93). The termination of a fast with a meal enriched in carbohydrates results in increased glucose flux through glycolysis and the hexose monophosphate shunt, which activates PP2A, perhaps by increasing xyl-5-P. This results in the dephosphorylation and nuclear translocation of ChREBP, allowing this transcription factor to bind to the ChoREs of target genes. ChREBP is also regulated by fatty acids. Polyunsaturated fatty acids (PUFA) inhibit the effect glucose has on gene transcription. ChREBP is also phosphorylated by AMP kinase, an enzyme whose activity increases as the AMP/ATP ratio rises. Ingestion of PUFA increases AMP levels about 30-fold without changing ATP levels, and this increases AMP kinase activity about twofold. AMP levels rise as a consequence of fatty acid activation, a reaction that is required for fatty acid oxidation. The phosphorylation of ChREBP by AMP kinase, on an amino acid residue distinct from the PKA sites, prevents the factor from binding to DNA (97). Thus, ChREBP can be viewed as a nutrient sensor, balancing the requirements for glycolysis and lipogenesis by monitoring whether the available exogenous metabolic fuel is carbohydrate or fat.

However, this is not the complete story of glucose-regulated gene expression. It was noted above that glucose per se stimulates the coordinated expression of many glycolytic and lipogenic genes and represses the PEPCK gene in the absence of insulin, provided that glucokinase is present. However, the magnitude of the response of the PK, fatty acid synthase, and other genes is not as great with glucose alone as it is when both insulin and glucose are present, even with abundant glucokinase. Therefore, glucose and insulin may act together to elicit the carbohydrate response. Thus, for example, insulin is required for glucokinase activity (44). A transcription factor, sterol regulatory element binding protein-1c (SREBP-1c), is stimulated by insulin and can mimic the insulin-mediated induction of glucokinase in some systems (98). SREBP-1c overexpression in transgenic animals results in a pattern of expression of glycolytic and lipogenic enzymes consistent with the fed state—even when the mice are fasted. Furthermore, the carbohydrate response is reduced, but not completely blocked, in animals lacking SREBP-1c (99,100). A recent series of experiments led to a possible explanation of these observations. The fatty acid synthase gene promoter has two distinct DNA elements that are involved in the glucose/insulin response. One is a ChoRE and one is an SREBP binding site. The ChoRE binds to a ChREBP (or closely related transcription factor), and the SREBP binding site binds to SREBP-1c. If either site is mutated in the fatty acid synthase (FAS) gene promoter, only a very weak response to glucose remains. However, the binding of both factors, in the presence of insulin, allows a strong synergistic response to glucose—one that essentially matches the physiologic response (101). Thus, glucose and insulin act together to coordinately regulate enzymes involved in glucose and lipid homeostasis.

INTEGRATION AND VALIDATION OF THESE CONCEPTS BY CURRENT TECHNIQUES

The analysis of metabolic control has benefited greatly from experimental approaches developed in recent years. One can now perturb a cell by transfection of the corresponding cDNA to increase a specific mRNA or by the use of antisense or interfering RNA to decrease a specific mRNA. The consequent increase or reduction of the cognate protein allows one to test for the role of a specific enzyme in a particular metabolic process.

Another technique available for studies of the regulation of glucose metabolism is the use of nonreplicative recombinant adenoviruses. These viruses are constructed with vectors wherein an essential gene for the lytic cycle (E1A) is replaced with cDNAs that express genes of interest, such as metabolic enzyme genes. When driven by a strong promoter like the cytomegalovirus promoter, very high levels of expression can be achieved. Adenoviruses have the advantage of being highly infectious, with 70% to 100% of cultured cells positive for gene transfer. In addition, they have a wide host range, so that most cultured cells are transduced by adenoviruses very effectively. Furthermore, recombinant adenoviruses, unlike retroviruses, efficiently transfer genes to terminally differentiated primary cells because they do not require cell division for infection and subsequent gene expression (102).

It is also possible to manipulate the amount of specific gene products in the context of an intact animal. The expression of a particular protein can be enhanced by the pronuclear injection of a construct that consists of a promoter and a selected cDNA that has appropriate initiation and termination signals. If one employs a promoter from a gene that is ubiquitously expressed (e.g., the SV40 promoter), the protein will be expressed in all tissues. Tissue-specific expression can be achieved by using a promoter from a gene that is restricted to the tissue of interest (e.g., albumin for liver, myosin for muscle). Certain limitations to these experiments are imposed by the fact that copy number and insertion site cannot be controlled in these transgenic experiments.

Another powerful technique involves the so-called gene-knockout approach. Constructs are made in which a system known as Cre-loxP provides for the deletion of a DNA segment and subsequent genetic recombination. If an essential portion of the coding region of a gene is targeted by the Cre-loxP, the protein will be rendered functionless. Knockout mice are generated by introducing Cre recombinase sites (or loxP sites) on both sides of the gene to be removed, or knocked out, in embryonic stem cells. The embryonic stem cells are then introduced into blastocysts, which are placed into the uterus of pseudopregnant mice. The offspring and subsequent generations become transgenic mice containing loxP sites on either side of the gene to be knocked out. These mice can then be crossed with a transgenic strain that expresses the Cre recombinase, either in all cells or in specific tissues if the expression of Cre is driven by a tissue-specific promoter (103).

These approaches have been used to confirm ideas of how hepatic glucose metabolism is accomplished, to define alternative metabolic pathways, to illustrate new regulatory principles, and to explore how certain pathways might be involved in diabetes mellitus. A few vignettes, which summarize much larger stories, are used to illustrate these points.

1. *The role of PEPCK in gluconeogenesis.* The conversion of oxaloacetate to phosphoenolpyruvate, catalyzed by the enzyme PEPCK, is an important early step in gluconeogenesis. PEPCK is the most highly regulated of the gluconeogenic enzymes, which underscores the importance of this step (68). Unrestrained glucose production from gluconeogenesis is an important pathophysiologic feature in type 2 diabetes (104); hence abnormal regulation of PEPCK, particularly faulty suppression of the transcription of this gene by insulin, has been implicated in this disease. Bosch and colleagues generated transgenic mice in which excessive amounts of PEPCK mRNA were produced in the liver (105). These mice had hyperglycemia, abnormal responses to a glucose load, and a metabolic picture similar to that of type 2 diabetes.

   The treatment of fasted animals with 3-mercaptopicolinic acid, an inhibitor of PEPCK, causes hypoglycemia (106). Treatment of neonatal mice with this compound, when emerging gluconeogenesis is critical for glucose homeostasis, is lethal. PEPCK is thus an important gluconeogenic enzyme. However, it does not control the only route to gluconeogenesis. The cytosolic PEPCK gene was knocked out by the Cre-loxP method. Animals in which the gene was knocked out in all tissues died in the neonatal period, as did animals given 3-mercaptopicolinic acid (107). A different result was obtained when the gene was selectively eliminated in liver. These mice are viable and can maintain euglycemia even after a 24-hour fast (107). They thus have managed to maintain gluconeogenesis (perhaps from an alternative hepatic route or from kidney or small intestine) and thereby avoid the disastrous CNS consequences of hypoglycemia. There is a metabolic cost to the use of an alternative route that does not involve hepatic PEPCK, as these mice have steatosis, a fatty liver. Thus, these studies show that there are important alternative routes to gluconeogenesis, that the route through PEPCK is preferred, and that the unrestrained expression of PEPCK can result in the altered glucose homeostasis similar to that seen in type 2 diabetes.
2. *The role of glucokinase in hepatic glucose clearance and glycogen synthesis.* The effects of overexpression of a particular metabolic enzyme on the regulation of glucose metabolism have been studied using recombinant adenoviruses. An example is provided by the overexpression of glucokinase or HK-I in freshly isolated rat hepatocytes. Hepatocytes express two different hexokinases, glucokinase and HK-I. Glucokinase provides about 75% of the glucose-phosphorylating capacity of the cell, and the remainder is provided by HK-I (108). Recall that the low K_m HK-I is maximally active at fasting levels of glucose and is inhibited by physiologic concentrations of its reaction product, G-6-P. In contrast, glucokinase has a K_m for glucose of about 8 mM, well within the physiologic range (~4–12 mM), so that glucokinase activity increases with increasing concentrations of glucose (5), and glucokinase is not inhibited by physiologic concentrations of G-6-P. Primary hepatocytes were transduced with recombinant adenoviruses that express either glucokinase or HK-I at titers that provided an equivalent glucose-phosphorylating capacity to investigate the role these hexokinases play in the regulation of glycolysis and glycogen synthesis (108). As expected, overexpression of glucokinase dramatically increases both glucose flux through glycolysis and glycogen synthesis when cells are incubated in glucose at concentrations of 5 mM or greater. The increase in glycolytic flux is linear with respect to glucose concentration, whereas the increase in glycogen synthesis is sigmoidal, with the greatest increase occurring between 5 and 10 mM. Thus a threshold of G-6-P abundance must be reached before glycogen synthesis begins (108). In stark contrast, HK-I overexpression increased glucose flux through glycolysis (particularly at low glucose levels; at high glucose levels it is inhibited by G-6-P) but had no effect on glycogen synthesis. These results were observed despite the fact that, at 5-mM glucose, the concentration of intracellular G-6-P was identical when either glucokinase or HK-I was overexpressed (108).

   How is it that G-6-P produced from HK-I has different metabolic effects than G-6-P produced from glucokinase? One possible explanation lies in the different cellular compartments in which glucokinase and HK-I reside. HK-I is partitioned into two compartments. It is bound to the mitochondria, where the high local concentrations of ATP increase its activity, and it is diffusely distributed throughout the cytoplasm. The overexpression of HK-I does not alter the relative distribution of HK-I in the cell (108). By contrast, glucokinase is localized in the nucleus, bound to the GKRP, until glucose concentrations rise above 5 mM, at which time it migrates into the cytoplasmic compartment (109). Glycogen is synthesized in the cytoplasm, and the major regulatory enzymes, including glycogen synthase, are bound to the scaffolding protein, G_L (75). Glycogen synthase is activated by G-6-P. Thus, by virtue of its strategic cellular translocation, glucokinase produces G-6-P that is more efficiently funneled into glycogen than the relatively distantly located HK-I.

   In another experiment, a transgenic mouse strain with the glucokinase gene flanked by loxP sites ($GK^{lox/lox}$) was crossed with a transgenic strain with the liver-specific albumin promoter driving the expression of cre recombinase (Alb-cre). The result was a liver-specific glucokinase knockout transgenic mouse ($GK^{lox/lox}$ + Alb-cre), providing a model to study the metabolic perturbations caused by a lack of hepatic glucokinase in the whole animal (110). These animals appear to be normal, having only a slightly elevated plasma glucose level. However, when the animals were fasted or fed or infused with an appropriate amount of glucose to reach a predetermined hyperglycemic concentration (an experimentally induced glucose clamp), a number of metabolic effects were noted. Fasting $GK^{lox/lox}$ + Alb-cre mice have a 40% higher plasma glucose concentration than controls, and fed animals have twofold higher plasma insulin levels, suggesting the animals are insulin resistant. Under a hyperglycemic clamp, these animals showed a 90% reduction in the ability to synthesize glycogen, and several glucose-responsive genes were inappropriately regulated. In addition, the $GK^{lox/lox}$ + Alb-cre mice secreted 70% less insulin in response to the hyperglycemic clamp. These studies demonstrated that glucokinase plays an important role in glucose homeostasis by virtue of its requirement for glucose uptake and utilization in the liver and by indirect effects on pancreatic insulin secretion (110).

3. *The role of F-2,6-P_2 in the regulation of glucose metabolism.* Another study that used recombinant adenoviruses to test specific questions about glucose metabolism in the liver was performed using a double mutant of the bifunctional enzyme that ensures high kinase activity and low phosphatase activity (111). Recall that the bifunctional enzyme produces the allosteric effector, F-2,6-P_2, which activates PFK1 and inhibits FBPase1 (58). Lange and colleagues constructed a mutant of the bifunctional enzyme (Bif-DM) that contains an alanine substitution of serine 32, which prevents the phosphorylation and inactivation of the enzyme by cAMP (111). In addition, the Bif-DM has an alanine that replaces histidine 258, which decreases the phosphatase activity of the enzyme. This combination of mutations results in a very high kinase-to-phosphatase activity ratio, and its expression increases the abundance of F-2,6-P_2. The Bif-DM was introduced into recombinant adenoviruses, which were infused into the livers of normal mice or mice that had been treated with streptozotocin to destroy pancreatic β-cells, a model of type 1 diabetes. Overexpression of the Bif-DM in streptozotocin-treated diabetic mice resulted in near-normal plasma blood glucose, lactate, free fatty acid, and triglyceride levels and increased hepatic glycogen stores relative to levels in diabetic controls (111). These results are consistent with the idea that F-2,6-P_2 increases flux through glycolysis and glycogen synthesis and decreases flux through gluconeogenesis. The above study was essentially repeated in kk mice, animals that are a model of type 2 diabetes (112). In the latter studies, diabetic kk mice treated with the Bif-DM adenovirus had near-normal blood glucose levels along with a gene expression pattern of glycolytic, lipogenic, and gluconeogenic genes that reflects a fed rather than a diabetic state (112). These experiments demonstrate that F-2,6-P_2 is a powerful regulator of glucose metabolism *in vivo*.

CONCLUSION

The definition of the metabolic pathways and of the intricate mechanisms by which flux through these pathways is regulated represents one of the most important achievements of 20th century biological science. This understanding underpins the explanation of the metabolic consequences of hundreds of monogenic diseases. More complex genetic (and environmental) diseases, such as diabetes mellitus, will ultimately be understood on this basis as well. Although much has been learned, it is apparent that important control mechanisms are still being discovered and that known mechanisms are being refined and expanded upon.

The examples discussed in this chapter point to the fact that glucose is an important regulator of its own production, storage, and metabolism in the liver. A further understanding of this process will no doubt help reveal secrets about the role this organ plays in diabetes mellitus.

REFERENCES

1. Tomkins GM. The metabolic code. *Science* 1975;189:760–763.
2. Pilkis SJ, Granner DK. Molecular physiology of the regulation of hepatic gluconeogenesis and glycolysis. *Annu Rev Physiol* 1992;54:885–909.
3. Hue L. Regulation of gluconeogenesis in liver. In: *Handbook of physiology, the endocrine system.* New York: Oxford University Press, 2001:649–657.
4. Wilson JE. Hexokinases. *Rev Physiol Biochem Pharmacol* 1995;26:65–198.
5. Printz RL, Magnuson MA, Granner DK. Mammalian glucokinase. *Annu Rev Nutr* 1993;13:463–496.
6. Flory W, Peczon BD, Koeppe RE, et al. Kinetic properties of rat liver pyruvate kinase at cellular concentrations of enzyme, substrates and modifiers. *Biochem J* 1974;141:127–131.
7. Weinhouse S. Regulation of glucokinase in liver. *Curr Top Cell Regul* 1976; 11:1–50.
8. Matschinsky FM. Regulation of pancreatic beta-cell glucokinase: from basics to therapeutics. *Diabetes* 2002;51[Suppl 3]:S394–S404.
9. Hers HG, Hue L. Gluconeogenesis and related aspects of glycolysis. *Annu Rev Biochem* 1983;52:617–653.
10. Pilkis SJ, el-Maghrabi MR, Claus TH. Hormonal regulation of hepatic gluconeogenesis and glycolysis. *Annu Rev Biochem* 1988;57:755–783.
11. Uyeda K. Phosphofructokinase. *Adv Enzymol Relat Areas Mol Biol* 1979;48: 193–244.
12. Kemp RG, Marcus F. Effects of fructose-2,6-bisphosphate on 6-phosphofructo-1-kinase and fructose-1,6-bisphosphatase. In: *Fructose-2,6-bisphosphate.* Boca Raton, FL: CRC Press, 1990:17–37.
13. Liu R, Fromm HJ. The sites of interaction of fructose-2,6-bisphosphate and fructose-1,6-bisphosphate with their target enzymes: 6-phosphofructo-1-kinase and fructose-1,6-bisphosphatase. In: *Fructose-2,6-bisphosphate.* Boca Raton, FL: CRC Press, 1990:39–49.
14. Bollen M, Keppens S, Stalmans W. Specific features of glycogen metabolism in the liver. *Biochem J* 1998;336:19–31.
15. Suzuki K, Kono T. Evidence that insulin causes translocation of glucose transport activity to the plasma membrane from an intracellular storage site. *Proc Natl Acad Sci U S A* 1980;77:2542–2545.
16. Cushman SW, Wardzala LJ. Potential mechanism of insulin action on glucose transport in the isolated rat adipose cell. Apparent translocation of intracellular transport systems to the plasma membrane. *J Biol Chem* 1980;255:4758–4762.
17. Czech MP, Corvera S. Signaling mechanisms that regulate glucose transport. *J Biol Chem* 1999;274:1865–1868.
18. Pessin JE, Saltiel AR. Signaling pathways in insulin action: molecular targets of insulin resistance. *J Clin Invest* 2000;106:165–169.
19. Van Schaftingen E. A protein from rat liver confers to glucokinase the property of being antagonistically regulated by fructose 6-phosphate and fructose 1-phosphate. *Eur J Biochem* 1989;179:179–184.
20. Lawrence JC Jr, Brunn GJ. Insulin signaling and the control of PHAS–I phosphorylation. *Prog Mol Subcell Biol* 2001;6:1–31.
21. Hargrove JL, Schmidt FH. The role of mRNA and protein stability in gene expression. *FASEB J* 1989;3:2360–2370.
22. Petersen DD, Koch SR, Granner DK. 3′ Noncoding region of phosphoenolpyruvate carboxykinase mRNA contains a glucocorticoid-responsive mRNA-stabilizing element. *Proc Natl Acad Sci U S A* 1989;86:7800–7804.
23. Hod Y, Hanson RW. Cyclic AMP stabilizes the mRNA for phosphoenolpyruvate carboxykinase (GTP) against degradation. *J Biol Chem* 1988;263:7747–7752.
24. Quinn PG, Wong TW, Magnuson MM, et al. Identification of basal and cyclic AMP regulatory elements in the promoter of the phosphoenolpyruvate carboxykinase gene. *Mol Cell Biol* 1988;8:3467–3475.
25. Park EA, Roesler WJ, Liu J, et al. The role of the CCAAT/enhancer-binding protein in the transcriptional regulation of the gene for phosphoenolpyruvate carboxykinase (GTP). *Mol Cell Biol* 1990;10:6264–6272.
26. Waltner-Law M, Duong DT, Daniels MC, et al. Elements of the glucocorticoid and retinoic acid response units are involved in cAMP-mediated expression of the PEPCK Gene. *J Biol Chem* 2003;278:10427–10435.
27. Sasaki K, Cripe TP, Koch SR, et al. Multihormonal regulation of phosphoenolpyruvate carboxykinase gene transcription: dominant role of insulin. *J Biol Chem* 1984;259:15242–15251.
28. Duong DT, Waltner-Law ME, Sears R, et al. Insulin inhibits hepatocellular glucose production by utilizing liver-enriched transcriptional inhibitory protein to disrupt the association of CREB-binding protein and RNA polymerase II with the phosphoenolpyruvate carboxykinase gene promoter. *J Biol Chem* 2002;277:32234–32242.
29. Sasaki K, Granner DK. Regulation of phosphoenolpyruvate carboxykinase gene transcription by insulin and cAMP: reciprocal actions on initiation and elongation. *Proc Natl Acad Sci U S A* 1988;85:2954–2958.
30. Kacser H, Burns JA. The control of flux. *Symp Soc Exp Biol* 1973;27:65–104.
31. Kashiwaya Y, Sato K, Tsuchiya N, et al. Control of glucose utilization in working perfused rat heart. *J Biol Chem* 1994;269:25502–25514.
32. Niederberger P, Prasad R, Miozzari G, et al. A strategy for increasing an in vivo flux by genetic manipulations. The tryptophan system of yeast. *Biochem J* 1992;287:473–479.
33. Koebmann BJ, Westerhoff HV, Snoep JL, et al. The glycolytic flux in *Escherichia coli* is controlled by the demand for ATP. *J Bacteriol* 2002;184: 3909–3916.
34. Thomas HM, Brant AM, Colville CA, et al. Tissue-specific expression of facilitative glucose transporters: a rationale. *Biochem Soc Trans* 2002;20:538–542.
35. Granner D, Pilkis S. The genes of hepatic glucose metabolism. *J Biol Chem* 1990;265:10173–10176.
36. Brown KS, Kalinowski SS, Megill JR, et al. Glucokinase regulatory protein may interact with glucokinase in the hepatocyte nucleus. *Diabetes* 1997;46: 179–186.
37. Agius L, Peak M, Van Schaftingen E. The regulatory protein of glucokinase binds to the hepatocyte matrix, but, unlike glucokinase, does not translocate during substrate stimulation. *Biochem J* 1995;309:711–713.

38. de la Iglesia N, Veiga-da-Cunha M, Van Schaftingen E, et al. Glucokinase regulatory protein is essential for the proper subcellular localisation of liver glucokinase. *FEBS Lett* 1999;456:332–338.
39. Niemeyer H, Perez N, Rabajille E. Interrelation of actions of glucose, insulin, and glucagon on induction of adenosine triphosphate: D-hexose phosphotransferase in rat liver. *J Biol Chem* 1966;241:4055–4059.
40. Iynedjian PB, Ucla C, Mach B. Molecular cloning of glucokinase cDNA. Developmental and dietary regulation of glucokinase mRNA in rat liver. *J Biol Chem* 1987;262:6032–6038.
41. Magnuson MA, Andreone TL, Printz RL, et al. Rat glucokinase gene: structure and regulation by insulin. *Proc Natl Acad Sci U S A* 1989;86:4838–4842.
42. Sibrowski W, Seitz HJ. Rapid action of insulin and cyclic AMP in the regulation of functional messenger RNA coding for glucokinase in rat liver. *J Biol Chem* 1984;259:343–346.
43. Christ B, Probst I, Jungermann K. Antagonistic regulation of the glucose/glucose 6-phosphate cycle by insulin and glucagon in cultured hepatocytes. *Biochem J* 1986;238:185–191.
44. Iynedjian PB, Jotterand D, Nouspikel T, et al. Transcriptional induction of glucokinase gene by insulin in cultured liver cells and its repression by the glucagon-cAMP system. *J Biol Chem* 1989;264:21824–21829.
45. Nordlie RC, Arion WJ, Hanson TL, et al. Biological regulation of liver microsomal inorganic pyrophosphate-glucose phosphotransferase, glucose 6-phosphatase, and inorganic pyrophosphatase. Differential effects of fasting on synthetic and hydrolytic activities. *J Biol Chem* 1968;243:1140–1146.
46. O'Brien RM, Streeper RS, Ayala JE, et al. Insulin-regulated gene expression. *Biochem Soc Trans* 2001;29:552–558.
47. Claus TH, El-Maghrabi MR, Pilkis SJ. Modulation of the phosphorylation state of rat liver pyruvate kinase by allosteric effectors and insulin. *J Biol Chem* 1979;254:7855–7864.
48. Clark MG, Bloxham DP, Holland PC, et al. Estimation of the fructose 1,6-diphosphatase-phosphofructokinase substrate cycle and its relationship to gluconeogenesis in rat liver in vivo. *J Biol Chem* 1974;249:279–290.
49. Clark MG, Kneer NM, Bosch AL. et al. The fructose 1,6-diphosphatase-phosphofructokinase substrate cycle. A site of regulation of hepatic gluconeogenesis by glucagon. *J Biol Chem* 1974;249:5695–5703.
50. Van Schaftingen E, Hue L, Hers HG. Control of the fructose-6-phosphate/fructose 1,6-bisphosphate cycle in isolated hepatocytes by glucose and glucagon. Role of a low-molecular-weight stimulator of phosphofructokinase. *Biochem J* 1980;92:887–895.
51. Van Schaftingen E, Hue L, Hers HG. Study of the fructose 6-phosphate/fructose 1,6-biphosphate cycle in the liver in vivo. *Biochem J* 1980;92: 263–271.
52. Sakakibara R, Uyeda K. Differences in the allosteric properties of pure low and high phosphate forms of phosphofructokinase from rat liver. *J Biol Chem* 1983;258:8656–8662.
53. Pilkis SJE, El-Maghrai MR. Hormonal regulation of the Fru 6-P/Fru,1,6-P_2 substrate cycle. In: *Hormonal control of gluconeogenesis.* Boca Raton, FL: CRC Press, 1986:199–221.
54. Claus TH, Schlumpf JR, el-Maghrabi MR, et al. Mechanism of action of glucagon on hepatocyte phosphofructokinase activity. *Proc Natl Acad Sci U S A* 1980;77:6501–6505.
55. Claus TH, El-Maghrabi MR, Regen DM, et al. The role of fructose 2,6-bisphosphate in the regulation of carbohydrate metabolism. *Curr Top Cell Regul* 1984;23:57–86.
56. Hers HG, Van Schaftingen E. Fructose 2,6-bisphosphate 2 years after its discovery. *Biochem J* 1982;206:1–12.
57. Pilkis SJ, Chrisman T, Burgress B, et al. Rat hepatic 6-phosphofructo 2-kinase/fructose 2,6-bisphosphatase: a unique bifunctional enzyme. *Adv Enzyme Regul* 1983;21:147–173.
58. Pilkis SJ, Claus TH, Kurland IJ, et al. 6-Phosphofructo-2-kinase/fructose-2,6-bisphosphatase: a metabolic signaling enzyme. *Annu Rev Biochem* 1995;64: 799–835.
59. Garrison JC, Wagner JD. Glucagon and the Ca^{2+}-linked hormones angiotensin II, norepinephrine, and vasopressin stimulate the phosphorylation of distinct substrates in intact hepatocytes. *J Biol Chem* 1982;257:13135–13143.
60. Pilkis SJ, Chrisman TD, El-Maghrabi MR, et al. The action of insulin on hepatic fructose 2,6-bisphosphate metabolism. *J Biol Chem* 1983;258:1495–1503.
61. Van Schaftingen E. Fructose 2,6-bisphosphate. *Adv Enzymol Relat Areas Mol Biol* 1987;59:315–395.
62. Exton JH. Molecular mechanisms involved in alpha-adrenergic responses. *Mol Cell Endocrinol* 1981;23:233–264.
63. Feliu JE, Hue L, Hers HG. Hormonal control of pyruvate kinase activity and of gluconeogenesis in isolated hepatocytes. *Proc Natl Acad Sci U S A* 1976;73:2762–2766.
64. Blair JB, Cimbala MA, Foster JL, et al. Hepatic pyruvate kinase. Regulation by glucagon, cyclic adenosine 3′-5′-monophosphate, and insulin in the perfused rat liver. *J Biol Chem* 1976;251:3756–3762.
65. Pilkis SJ, Claus TH, Riou JP, et al. Possible role of pyruvate kinase in the hormonal control of dihydroxyacetone gluconeogenesis in isolated hepatocytes. *Metabolism* 1976;25:1355–1360.
66. Pilkis SJ, Riou JP, Claus TH. Hormonal control of glucose synthesis from [U-14C]dihydroxyacetone and glycerol in isolated rat hepatocytes. *J Biol Chem* 1976;251:7841–7852.
67. Engstrom D, Ekman P, Humble E, et al. Pyruvate kinase. *Enzymes* 1987; 18:47–75.
68. Hanson RW, Reshef L. Regulation of phosphoenolpyruvate carboxykinase (GTP) gene expression. *Annu Rev Biochem* 1997;66:581–611.
69. Scott DK, O'Doherty RM, Stafford JM, et al. The repression of hormone-activated PEPCK gene expression by glucose is insulin-independent but requires glucose metabolism. *J Biol Chem* 1998;273:24145–24151.
70. Vaulont S, Kahn A. Transcriptional control of metabolic regulation genes by carbohydrates. *FASEB J* 1994;8:28–35.
71. Towle HC. Metabolic regulation of gene transcription in mammals. *J Biol Chem* 1995;270:23235–23238.
72. Decaux JF, Antoine B, Kahn A. Regulation of the expression of the L-type pyruvate kinase gene in adult hepatocytes in primary culture. *J Biol Chem* 1989;264:11584–11590.
73. Guinovart JJ, Gomez-Foix AM, Seoane J, et al. Bridging the gap between glucose phosphorylation and glycogen synthesis in the liver. *Biochem Soc Trans* 1997;25:157–160.
74. Radziuk J, Pye S. Hepatic glucose uptake, gluconeogenesis and the regulation of glycogen synthesis. *Diabetes Metab Res Rev* 2001;17:250–272.
75. Newgard CB, Brady MJ, O'Doherty RM, et al. Organizing glucose disposal: emerging roles of the glycogen targeting subunits of protein phosphatase-1. *Diabetes* 2000;49:1967–1977.
76. Newgard CB, Hwang PK, Fletterick RJ. The family of glycogen phosphorylases: structure and function. *Crit Rev Biochem Mol Biol* 1989;24:69–99.
77. Dent P, Lavoinne A, Nakielny S, et al. The molecular mechanism by which insulin stimulates glycogen synthesis in mammalian skeletal muscle. *Nature* 1990;348:302–308.
78. Cross DA, Alessi DR, Cohen P, et al. Inhibition of glycogen synthase kinase-3 by insulin mediated by protein kinase B. *Nature* 1995;378:785–789.
79. Gasa R, Clark C, Yang R, et al. Reversal of diet-induced glucose intolerance by hepatic expression of a variant glycogen-targeting subunit of protein phosphatase-1. *J Biol Chem* 2002;277:1524–1530.
80. Lucas PC, Granner DK. Hormone response domains in gene transcription. *Annu Rev Biochem* 1992;61:1131–1173.
81. Sugiyama T, Scott DK, Wang JC, et al. Structural requirements of the glucocorticoid and retinoic acid response units in the phosphoenolpyruvate carboxykinase gene promoter. *Mol Endocrinol* 1998;12:1487–1498.
82. O'Brien RM, Lucas PC, Forest CD, et al. Identification of a sequence in the PEPCK gene that mediates a negative effect of insulin on transcription. *Science* 1990;249:533–537.
83. O'Brien RM, Lucas PC, Yamasaki T, et al. Potential convergence of insulin and cAMP signal transduction systems at the phosphoenolpyruvate carboxykinase (PEPCK) gene promoter through CCAAT/enhancer binding protein (C/EBP). *J Biol Chem* 1994;269:30419–30428.
84. Imai E, Stromstedt P, Quinn PG, et al. Characterization of a complex glucocorticoid response unit in the phosphoenolpyruvate carboxykinase gene. *Mol Cell Biol* 1990;10:4712–4719.
85. Hall RK, Scott DK, O'Brien RM, et al. From metabolic pathways to metabolic control domains: multiple factors bind the PEPCK AF1/retinoic acid response element. In: Mornex R, Jaffiol C, Lecler J, eds. *Progress in endocrinology. Proceedings of the Ninth International Congress on Endocrinology, Nice, 1992.* London: Parthenon Publishing, 1993;777–782.
86. Scott DK, Mitchell JA, Granner DK. The orphan receptor COUP-TF binds to a third glucocorticoid accessory factor element within the phosphoenolpyruvate carboxykinase gene promoter. *J Biol Chem* 1996;271:31909–31914.
87. Vaulont S, Vasseur-Cognet M, Kahn A. Glucose regulation of gene transcription. *J Biol Chem* 2000;275:31555–31558.
88. Towle HC, Kaytor EN, Shih H-M. Regulation of the expression of lipogenic enzyme genes by carbohydrate. *Annu Rev Nutr* 1997;17:405–433.
89. Doiron B, Cuif M-H, Kahn A, et al. Respective roles of glucose, fructose, and insulin in the regulation of the liver-specific pyruvate kinase gene promoter. *J Biol Chem* 1994;269:10213–10216.
90. Mourrieras F, Foufelle F, Foretz M, et al. Induction of fatty acid synthase and S14 gene expression by glucose, xylitol and dihydroxyacetone in cultured rat hepatocytes is closely correlated with glucose 6-phosphate concentrations. *Biochem J* 1997;326:345–349.
91. Doiron B, Cuif M-H, Chen R, et al. Transcriptional glucose signaling through the glucose response element is mediated by the pentose phosphate pathway. *J Biol Chem* 1996;271:5321–5324.
92. Nishimura M, Uyeda K. Purification and characterization of a novel xylulose 5-phosphate-activated protein phosphatase catalyzing dephosphorylation of fructose-6-phosphate,2-kinase:fructose-2,6-bisphosphatase. *J Biol Chem* 1995; 270:26341–26346.
93. Yamashita H, Takenoshita M, Sakurai M, et al. A glucose-responsive transcription factor that regulates carbohydrate metabolism in the liver. *Proc Natl Acad Sci U S A* 2001;98:9116–9121.
94. Shih H-M, Liu Z, Towle HC. Two CACGTG motifs with proper spacing dictate the carbohydrate regulation of hepatic gene transcription. *J Biol Chem* 1995;270:21991–21997.
95. Kaytor EN, Shih H, Towle HC. Carbohydrate regulation of hepatic gene expression. Evidence against a role for the upstream stimulatory factor. *J Biol Chem* 1997;272:7525–7531.
96. Kennedy HJ, Viollet B, Rafiq I, et al. Upstream stimulatory factor-2 (USF2) activity is required for glucose stimulation of L-pyruvate kinase promoter activity in single living islet beta-cells. *J Biol Chem* 1997;272:20636–20640.
97. Kawaguchi T, Osatomi K, Yamashita H, et al. Mechanism for fatty acid "sparing"; effect on glucose-induced transcription: regulation of carbohydrate-responsive element-binding protein by AMP-activated protein kinase. *J Biol Chem* 2002;277:3829–3835.
98. Foretz M, Guichard C, Ferre P, et al. Sterol regulatory element binding protein-1c is a major mediator of insulin action on the hepatic expression of

glucokinase and lipogenesis-related genes. *Proc Natl Acad Sci U S A* 1999;96: 12737–12742.

99. Shimomura I, Shimano H, Korn BS, et al. Nuclear sterol regulatory element-binding proteins activate genes responsible for the entire program of unsaturated fatty acid biosynthesis in transgenic mouse liver. *J Biol Chem* 1998;273:35299–35306.
100. Shimano, H. Yahagi, N, Amemiya-Kudo M, et al. Sterol regulatory element-binding protein-1 as a key transcription factor for nutritional induction of lipogenic enzyme genes. *J Biol Chem* 1999;274:35832–35839.
101. Koo SH, Dutcher AK, Towle HC. Glucose and insulin function through two distinct transcription factors to stimulate expression of lipogenic enzyme genes in liver. *J Biol Chem* 2001;276:9437–9445.
102. Becker TC, Noel RJ, Coats WS, et al. Use of recombinant adenovirus for metabolic engineering of mammalian cells. *Methods Cell Biol* 1994;43:161–189.
103. van der Weyden L, Adams DJ, Bradley A. Tools for targeted manipulation of the mouse genome. *Physiol Genomics* 2002;11:133–164.
104. Kahn C. Insulin action, diabetogenes, and the cause of type II diabetes. *Diabetes* 1994;43:1066–1084.
105. Valera A, Pujol A, Pelegrin M, et al. Transgenic mice overexpressing phosphoenolpyruvate carboxykinase develop non-insulin-dependent diabetes mellitus. *Proc Natl Acad Sci U S A* 1994;91:9151–9154.
106. DiTullio NW, Berkoff CE, Blank B, et al. 3-mercaptopicolinic acid, an inhibitor of gluconeogenesis. *Biochem J* 1974;138:387–394.
107. She P, Shiota M, Shelton KD, et al. Phosphoenolpyruvate carboxykinase is necessary for the integration of hepatic energy metabolism. *Mol Cell Biol* 1974;20:6508–6517.
108. O'Doherty RM, Lehman DL, Seoane J, et al. Differential metabolic effects of adenovirus-mediated glucokinase and hexokinase overexpression in rat primary hepatocytes. *J Biol Chem* 1996;271:20524–20530.
109. Agius L. The physiological role of glucokinase binding and translocation in hepatocytes. *Adv Enzyme Regul* 1996;38:303–331.
110. Postic C, Shiota M, Niswender KD, et al. Dual roles for glucokinase in glucose homeostasis as determined by liver and pancreatic beta cell-specific gene knock-outs using Cre recombinase. *J Biol Chem* 1996;274: 305–315.
111. Wu C, Okar DA, Newgard CB, et al. Overexpression of 6-phosphofructo-2-kinase/fructose-2,6-bisphosphatase in mouse liver lowers blood glucose by suppressing hepatic glucose production. *J Clin Invest* 2001;107: 91–98.
112. Wu C, Okar DA, Newgard CB, et al. Increasing fructose 2,6-bisphosphate overcomes hepatic insulin resistance of type 2 diabetes. *Am J Physiol Endocrinol Metab* 2002;282:E38–E45.

CHAPTER 16
Fat Metabolism in Diabetes

Ananda Basu and Michael D. Jensen

The pathophysiology of diabetes mellitus involves impairments in insulin secretion and insulin action. Whereas type 1 diabetes results from extreme impairment or absence of insulin secretion, an important causal factor in type 2 diabetes is resistance to insulin action, with impairment in insulin secretion progressing as the disease continues. In both type 1 and type 2 diabetes, major changes in fatty acid metabolism are concomitant with alterations in carbohydrate metabolism. As will be discussed, perturbations in the release of free fatty acids (FFAs) by adipose tissue result in an increase in plasma concentrations of FFAs. Abnormally high concentrations of FFAs can lead to defects in insulin action. In addition, recent evidence suggests high plasma concentrations of FFAs can affect the secretory capacity of pancreatic β-cells.

OVERVIEW OF FATTY ACID METABOLISM

In the postabsorptive state, muscle, heart, liver, and renal cortex use fatty acids as their primary fuel (1). In humans, in contrast to rodents, there is very little *de novo* synthesis of fatty acids (2), either in adipose tissue or in the liver. Hence, the proximate source of fatty acids in humans is dietary, with the fatty acids generally stored in adipose tissue or oxidized (3).

In the postprandial absorptive state, dietary fatty acids are packaged in the intestinal mucosa as chylomicrons and transported by the lymphatic system to the circulation. These triglyceride-rich particles are cleared rapidly under normal circumstances, with the majority of the lipid content stored in adipose tissue (3). The cholesterol-rich chylomicron remnant particles are cleared by the liver by binding to specific receptors (low-density lipoprotein receptor–related protein) on hepatocytes.

Plasma FFAs derive almost exclusively from lipolysis of adipose tissue triglycerides by hormone-sensitive lipase (HSL), which is so named because of its responsiveness to insulin and catecholamines. The one apparent exception is following the ingestion of a mixed meal, when some plasma FFAs arise from the rapid hydrolysis of plasma chylomicron triglycerides by lipoprotein lipase (LPL), an enzyme that acts primarily to allow tissue uptake of circulating triglycerides (4). In the postabsorptive state, lipolysis by adipose tissue HSL is likely the overwhelming, if not the only, source of FFAs (5).

The hydrolysis of circulating lipoprotein triglyceride is mediated by LPL at the capillary lumen (6). LPL activity is greatest in adipose tissue, where its regulation is reciprocal to that of HSL. During the postabsorptive state, HSL is activated, whereas LPL is inhibited; in the absorptive state, HSL is inhibited and LPL is activated. The regulation of LPL activity also is tissue specific, with LPL activity in adipose tissue stimulated by insulin, whereas LPL activity in skeletal muscle is unaffected by insulin (7,8).

After their release from adipose tissue, circulating FFAs are bound to albumin, which is a very effective solubilizer. FFAs are rapidly removed from the circulation by various tissues, with a half-life of less than 4 minutes (5), and they supply 25% to 50% of energy requirements postabsorptively in adults. FFAs not utilized for oxidative needs are reesterified, probably to a large extent in the liver, and exported as very-low-density lipoprotein (VLDL) triglyceride. The VLDL triglyceride is then re-stored primarily in adipose tissue. FFAs can thus be released in excess of energy needs without disastrous consequences because the cycle of FFA to VLDL triglyceride back to adipose tissue triglyceride is relatively efficient under most circumstances.

Plasma concentrations of FFAs reflect the balance between their release and uptake, but this relationship is not linear over the physiologic range (9,10). At low flux rates, a disproportionate decrease in plasma concentrations of FFAs occurs, whereas at very high flux rates, plasma levels of FFAs may increase to a greater degree than would be predicted if the relationship between flux and concentrations were linear. Basal FFA flux typically exceeds the fatty acid oxidation rate (measured by indirect calorimetry) by 50% to 100%; the excess FFAs are thought to be reesterified into triglycerides in the liver (11) and muscle (12–15). FFA clearance increases dramatically with exercise, such that at the onset of exercise plasma concentrations of FFAs may decrease even while rates of FFA release are increasing. Thus, although FFA concentrations are a reasonable indicator of FFA release, it is not possible to use concentration values to make quantitative estimates of release rates, and in some circumstances FFA concentrations can be misleading with respect to changes in lipolysis.

Many hormones regulate lipolysis in adipose tissue, thereby influencing the rate of FFA release. Given the profound disturbance of fat metabolism in diabetes mellitus and the fact that insulin administration to a large extent reverses the abnormalities, it is important to understand the role of insulin in the regulation of adipose tissue metabolism. Insulin is the major regulator of adipose tissue lipolysis through its inhibition of the activity of HSL, thereby reducing the release of FFAs and glycerol. Lipolysis is normally exquisitely sensitive to suppression by insulin, with a half-maximal effect occurring at concentrations of approximately 12 pmol/L. To put this in perspective, fasting concentrations of insulin typically may vary from approximately 6 to 60 pmol/L (16). Adipose tissue is much more sensitive than many other tissues to insulin in this regard. Lipolysis is more sensitive than glucose uptake and metabolism to changes in insulin concentrations (11,16). In addition to insulin, other important endogenous inhibitors of lipolysis include ketone bodies (which also stimulate insulin secretion), adenosine, and FFAs themselves (17–20).

Several hormones accelerate the release of FFAs from adipose tissue and therefore raise plasma concentrations of FFAs. Catecholamines (epinephrine and norepinephrine) are the most important stimulators of lipolysis, although growth hormone (GH) and, to a lesser degree, cortisol, also increase the release of FFAs. Catecholamines stimulate the activity of adenyl cyclase through their β-adrenergic effect, hence increasing the tissue availability of cyclic adenosine monophosphate (cAMP), which in turn stimulates the activity of HSL (2). Catecholamines reach adipose tissue through the circulation or via adrenergic nerve terminals, and the relative importance of their local neural versus systemic origin has not been fully established.

In contrast, glucocorticoids promote lipolysis via synthesis of new HSL protein through a cAMP-independent pathway (2). Cortisol may be an important promoter of lipolysis only in conditions of relative insulin deficiency and marked cortisol elevations, as in uncontrolled diabetes or stress states (21–24). This conclusion is based on experimental observations that cortisol does not stimulate lipolysis during cortisol infusion unless compensatory hyperinsulinemia is prevented by a pancreatic somatostatin clamp (21). There is evidence that the effect of GH on lipolysis depends on the synthesis of proteins involved in the formation of cAMP (2,22,25,26). However, the creation of acute GH deficiency results in a lower availability of FFAs within several hours (27), and pulsatile delivery of GH results in enhanced lipolysis within 60 to 90 minutes. These observations suggest that GH may have some direct stimulatory effects on lipolysis *in vivo*. Other weaker stimulators of lipolysis include thyroxine, tumor necrosis factor-α (TNF-α), and prostaglandin I_2 (28–30). Insulin antagonizes the effects of these lipolytic hormones. The antilipolytic effects of insulin and drugs such as nicotinic acid are accounted for by inhibition of adenyl cyclase activity (2).

ASSESSMENT OF FATTY ACID METABOLISM

Both *in vitro* and *in vivo* approaches have been used to study fatty acid metabolism. The *in vitro* approach permits the investigator to control a maximum number of variables during studies of lipolytic regulation. However, *in vivo* studies allow a more physiologic assessment and an understanding of the metabolic processes in the context of the whole organism.

In vivo methods for studying systemic lipolysis (10,31,32) include isotope-dilution techniques, selective catheterization of adipose tissue venous drainage, and adipose tissue microdialysis. Regional lipolytic rates can be measured with the arteriovenous catheterization (33–35) or microdialysis techniques (34). The combination of arteriovenous catheterization and isotope-dilution techniques allows investigators to collect information regarding regional fatty acid kinetics (uptake and release). This approach is perhaps one of the most useful techniques for gaining an understanding of regional FFA metabolism *in vivo*.

Systemic appearance and disappearance of FFAs can be accurately measured with isotope-dilution techniques under both steady-state and non–steady-state conditions. An intravenous tracer infusion coupled with arterialized venous or arterial blood sampling provides data that mirror the physiology of the release by adipocytes of FFAs into the venous circulation for delivery to tissues via the arterial circulation. Under conditions of stable FFA concentrations and flux (steady state), the rate of FFA appearance equals its rate of disappearance. FFA flux is calculated using the ratio of tracer infusion rate and the specific activity or enrichment of the tracer in plasma FFAs (32).

The choice of isotopic tracers is important in the assessment of FFA kinetics. Although there are slight regional differences in the metabolism of different fatty acids (36), the kinetics of the long-chain fatty acids are sufficiently similar to consider the rate of appearance of a single fatty acid such as palmitate or oleate representative of FFA turnover in humans. Differences in the kinetics of linoleate and stearate (the other major long-chain fatty acids) compared with the kinetics of FFAs as a whole are such that tracers of these FFAs are not used to measure FFA flux (36,37). Both stable isotopic tracers (^{13}C or ^{2}H) and radioactive tracers (^{14}C or ^{3}H) are used. The main disadvantage of ^{14}C or ^{3}H tracers relates to radiation exposure. They are unacceptable for use in pregnant women and in children, and some institutions and governments place severe restrictions on the administration of radioisotopes to humans for research purposes. The use of stable isotopic tracers of FFAs provides the advantage of avoiding radiation exposure; however, relatively large amounts of tracer (requiring substantial amounts of albumin) are needed for standard gas chromatography and mass spectroscopy analysis. Recent advances in stable isotope approaches appear to have overcome some of these limitations (38).

Isotopic tracers of glycerol have been used to measure systemic lipolysis. The rate of appearance of glycerol is considered to reflect whole-body adipose tissue lipolysis, because adipose tissue does not contain glycerol kinase, the enzyme needed for reuse of glycerol for esterification of fatty acids (39–44). Recent studies of glycerol metabolism have suggested that this assumption is unlikely to be rigorously correct (45); thus, the rate of glycerol appearance is not a totally reliable measure of total adipose-tissue lipolysis in humans.

Regional FFA kinetics can be estimated with arteriovenous catheterization techniques combined with isotopic-tracer approaches and measurement of plasma flow (46), as well as by microdialysis techniques (47–51). Regional rates of FFA release can be related to regional fat content to assess the lipolytic rates of different adipose tissue beds. Regional fat mass usually is assessed by imaging studies [computed tomography (CT) or

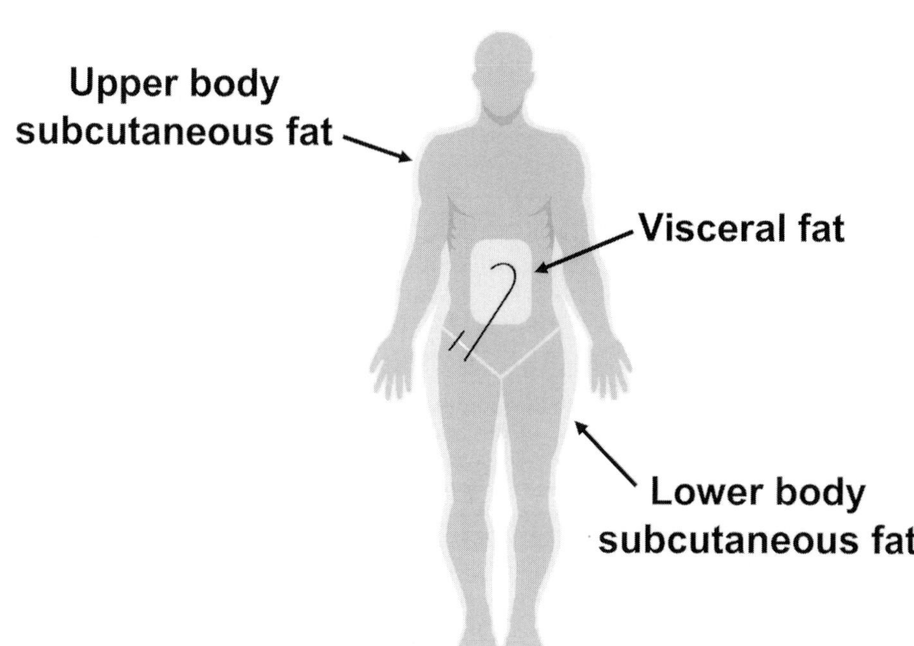

Figure 16.1. Approach to assessing regional adipose tissue release of free fatty acid (FFA) and regional uptake of FFA. A combination of vascular catheterization techniques (femoral artery, femoral vein, and hepatic vein catheters), FFA isotope-dilution studies, and measurement of regional plasma flow is used. Systemic release of FFAs can then be apportioned to leg, splanchnic, and nonsplanchnic upper body [total – (legs + splanchnic)] regions.

magnetic resonance imaging (MRI)] (52) and/or by dual-energy x-ray absorptiometry (53). For the most part, these approaches allow accurate measurement of systemic and regional (leg, splanchnic, and nonsplanchnic upper body) FFA kinetics. It should be noted that FFAs released into the portal circulation by omental and mesenteric adipose tissues are partially taken up by the liver before reaching the systemic circulation (5,15). Therefore, this portion of "hidden" or "unseen" visceral lipolysis cannot be accurately determined despite the use of tracer techniques and arteriovenous catheterization approaches. Nevertheless, it is possible to use the combination of regional catheterization and isotope-dilution techniques to determine the relative contribution of the splanchnic bed, leg, and nonsplanchnic upper-body adipose tissue to systemic lipolysis (Fig. 16.1).

Several agents have been used to manipulate FFA availability to determine the effects of FFA on tissue function. The agents most commonly used to lower plasma FFA concentrations are nicotinic acid (54) and acipimox (55–57). Etomoxir (57,58) (inhibits carnitine acyltransferase) has been used to inhibit FFA oxidation without lowering FFA concentrations. FFA plasma levels have been raised by intravenous infusion of a lipid emulsion to raise serum levels of triglycerides together with heparin to release LPL into the circulation (6,59), thereby generating FFA by the intravascular hydrolysis of triglycerides.

GLUCOSE–FATTY ACID INTERACTIONS

In 1963, Philip Randle and coworkers first described an interaction between glucose and fatty acid metabolism (60), which subsequently has been termed the *glucose–fatty acid cycle* or *Randle cycle*. Studying rat heart muscle and diaphragm, they observed that increasing fatty acid oxidation by these tissues impaired their oxidation of glucose. The mechanism they suggested involved increased mitochondrial ratios of [acetyl-CoA]/[CoA] and [NADH$^+$]/[NAD] as a result of increased fatty acid oxidation. They proposed that these changes inhibit pyruvate dehydrogenase and thus limit the entry of pyruvate derived from glycolysis into the mitochondria for participation in the citric acid cycle. In addition, increased acetyl coenzyme (acetyl-CoA) derived from β-oxidation leads to accumulation of citrate that in turn inhibits phosphofructokinase, one of the key regulators of glycolysis. This results in the accumulation of intracellular glucose-6-phosphate, which further inhibits hexokinase II, the glucose-phosphorylating enzyme present in muscle (57,60). Reduced activity of hexokinase II serves to reduce glucose transport into the muscle cells. Subsequently, this metabolic cycle was extended to involve inhibition of nonoxidative glucose metabolism by inhibition of glycogen synthase by elevated FFA levels (61–63).

Recognition of the glucose–fatty acid cycle as observed in studies of laboratory rats brought appropriate attention to the interactions between FFAs and glucose. Much subsequent work has shown that equally important glucose-FFA interactions occur in humans but that these result from quite different regulatory mechanisms (64,65). Human studies failed to show either reduced activity of glycogen synthase and pyruvate dehydrogenase enzymes in skeletal muscle biopsies as a consequence of FFA elevation (induced by lipid emulsion–heparin infusion) (66) or an elevation in citrate or carnitine palmitoyltransferase activity reflecting increased fatty acid oxidation (62). Intramuscular concentrations of glucose-6-phosphate were not increased in response to FFA concentrations as high as 0.5 mM during hyperinsulinemia (61), suggesting reduced glucose transport/phosphorylation as an alternative primary cause of reduced glucose uptake. Concordant findings have been reported using nuclear MRI to study human skeletal muscle during a euglycemic hyperinsulinemic clamp in the presence of elevated FFA levels (64,65). Reductions in insulin-receptor substrate-1–associated phosphatidylinositol 3-kinase activity were found, which could lead to inhibition of glucose transport into the myocytes. In addition, it was shown that non–insulin-mediated glucose uptake was not reduced as a result of elevated FFA concentrations in nondiabetic humans, suggesting that the effect of fatty acids on glucose transport is mediated through the insulin-responsive glucose transport system (67).

In recent years, a reverse "glucose–fatty acid" cycle has been proposed (68,69), through which hyperglycemia in the presence of elevated FFA concentrations reduces fat oxidation. This could result from a reduction in the entry of fatty acids into the mitochondria as a consequence of inhibition of carnitine acyltransferase activity (68), although increased reesterification of fatty acids in sensitive tissues represents another potential mechanism that has not been studied. In summary, although the glucose–fatty acid cycle involves a clear reciprocal relationship between glucose and fatty acid oxidation in muscle, the fundamental mechanism by which this occurs is likely different from that originally proposed on the basis of rat studies. Nevertheless, whatever the cellular mechanism of this vital metabolic cycle, elevated levels of FFAs impair the stimulation of glucose uptake by insulin in human skeletal muscle, and this represents a major site of altered glucose metabolism in individuals with type 2 diabetes.

Glucose uptake also occurs in the liver, especially during hyperglycemia. It is unclear whether the glucose–fatty acid cycle exists with respect to hepatic glucose uptake. *In vitro* studies of rat hepatocytes have shown a time- and dose-dependent reduction in activity of hepatic glucokinase with exposure to long-chain fatty acids (70). Because glucokinase activity, not glucose transport, is thought to be the rate-limiting step in hepatic glucose uptake (71–73), the elevated level of FFAs in type 2 diabetes could reduce hepatic uptake of glucose. This, in turn, could contribute to reduced rates of hepatic glycogen synthesis and aggravate postprandial hyperglycemia in diabetes.

FREE FATTY ACIDS AND THE LIVER

Early studies demonstrated that FFAs can stimulate gluconeogenesis from lactate and alanine in the perfused rat liver (74,75), and evidence for the stimulation of gluconeogenesis by FFAs *in vivo* was obtained subsequently (76,77). The proposed mechanisms include generation of acetyl-CoA from FFAs, activation of pyruvate carboxylase, and inhibition of pyruvate dehydrogenase enzymes. FFA oxidation also generates the reduced form of nicotinamide adenine dinucleotide phosphate (NADPH) and adenosine triphosphate (ATP). The former facilitates conversion of glycerol to glucose, and the latter favors the conversion of 1,3-phosphoglycerate to glyceraldehyde 3-phosphate. Further support for this hypothesis came from studies that found increased activity of the Cori cycle (a surrogate marker of gluconeogenesis) without any change in endogenous glucose production in the postabsorptive state subsequent to a lipid emulsion–heparin infusion (78). A more recent study showed that elevation of FFAs increased the relative contribution of gluconeogenesis to endogenous glucose production in the postabsorptive state, as measured by the deuterated water technique, although the absolute rate of endogenous glucose production did not increase (79).

The "single-gateway hypothesis" has recently been proposed as a mechanism that attributes a central role for FFAs in the determination of insulin effects on carbohydrate metabolism (80). According to this model, insulin traverses the endothelial cell boundaries in skeletal muscle and adipose tissue to stimulate glucose uptake and inhibit lipolysis, respectively. The declining FFA level in turn reduces endogenous glucose production primarily by reducing levels of the substrates necessary for gluconeogenesis. Direct support for this hypothesis has been provided by a number of investigators (81), and a positive correlation (82,83) between FFA concentrations and endogenous glucose production has been reported (84). Furthermore, acipimox (an inhibitor of lipolysis) allowed normal insulin-mediated suppression of endogenous glucose production by insulin in type 2 diabetes (85), whereas maintenance of elevated FFA concentrations with lipid emulsion–heparin reversed the effect of acipimox (80).

Whatever the mechanism, it appears clear that elevated FFA concentrations result in higher rates of gluconeogenesis and impairment of insulin suppression of endogenous glucose production.

FREE FATTY ACIDS AND INSULIN KINETICS

Data from a prospective study have shown a predictive value of elevated FFA concentrations for the future development of type 2 diabetes in Pima Indians (86). However, this correlation was not significant after adjusting for acute insulin response, suggesting that the relationship may relate to the inhibitory effects of FFAs on insulin secretion and not solely to their effect on glucose disposal. Both *in vivo* and *in vitro* experiments have implicated elevations in FFA concentrations in altered insulin secretion and insulin kinetics.

In one study, the infusion of a lipid emulsion for 48 hours to elevate FFA levels in healthy subjects was shown to increase glucose-stimulated insulin secretion (determined by C-peptide deconvolution techniques) during a hyperglycemic clamp (87). The increase in insulin secretion was not accompanied by a change in insulin clearance. In contrast, another study demonstrated a reduced acute insulin response to an intravenous glucose tolerance test after increasing FFA concentration with a 24-hour lipid-emulsion infusion, whereas a 6-hour lipid-emulsion infusion enhanced the acute insulin response to intravenous glucose (88). A third study showed greater glucose-stimulated insulin secretion during acute (90-minute) FFA elevation but unaltered glucose-stimulated insulin secretion after chronic (48-hour) FFA elevation (89). During both acute and chronic FFA elevations, the insulin sensitivity index (SI) obtained by application of the minimal model to the intravenous glucose tolerance test was impaired. Estimation of the "disposition index" (the product of SI and insulin secretion rate) revealed that during acute FFA elevation, higher insulin secretion compensated for reduced SI and normalized the disposition index. In contrast, during chronic FFA elevation, insulin secretion failed to compensate for the reduced SI, thereby resulting in a reduced disposition index. The insulin clearance rate also was reduced during chronic FFA elevation.

The mechanism of FFA effects on insulin secretion has been investigated through both *in vivo* and *in vitro* animal experiments. In female Wistar rats exposed to prolonged (48 hours) high FFA concentrations, basal insulin and C-peptide concentrations were shown to increase, whereas glucose-stimulated insulin secretion during a two-step hyperglycemic clamp was substantially reduced (90). A study in prediabetic Zucker fatty rats demonstrated a rise in plasma FFA concentrations coincident with decreases in glucose-stimulated insulin secretion and the GLUT2 glucose transporter content of β-cells (91). Reversal of elevated FFA levels by pair feeding with lean littermates corrected all of the observed β-cell abnormalities. *In vitro* studies of rat islets cultured for a week in medium containing 2 mM FFA demonstrated increased basal insulin secretion at 3 mM glucose, whereas the first-phase insulin response to glucose was reduced by 68%. Similar results were obtained in islets harvested from prediabetic animals (91). Others have reported that long-term (48-hour) exposure of rat islets to FFA (92) increased basal insulin secretion but resulted in a 30% to 50% decrease in proinsulin biosynthesis and insulin secretion induced by hyperglycemia. Results from other studies in rats have indicated that chronically elevated FFA levels reduce β-cell insulin content by increasing basal insulin secretion to an extent that is not compensated for by increased proinsulin biosynthesis (93). Levels of preproinsulin mRNA were elevated, suggesting that FFA may inhibit the translation of proinsulin mRNA. In the INS-1 clonal pancreatic cell line, long-chain fatty acids were shown to inhibit the expression of the acetyl-CoA carboxylase gene (94). This could increase fatty acid oxidation in the β-cell, thereby potentially causing glucose insensitivity. FFAs induce expression of the carnitine acyltransferase I gene in the INS-1 cell line, providing an additional mechanism for stimulation of fatty acid oxidation. FFA elevation also has been shown to reduce GLUT2 and glucokinase levels in rat pancreatic islets (95) and to open K^+-ATP channels, thereby inhibiting insulin secretion (96). In summary, there is substantial evidence for FFA effects on insulin secretory pathways, which may contribute to the altered physiology of type 2 diabetes.

Insulin clearance or degradation is thought to be a receptor-mediated process (97). Normally, approximately 50% of the insulin secreted by the pancreas is cleared via interactions with insulin receptors in liver parenchymal cells (97,98). Approximately 50% of insulin degradation takes place at the surface of the hepatocyte cell membrane (97). Internalization of the insulin-receptor complex by an endocytic mechanism then follows and is coupled to cleavage of the insulin molecule by various proteases. Of the insulin that is not cleared by hepatocytes, approximately 25% is removed by the kidney and the rest is removed by muscle, adipose tissue, and other tissues. Elevated circulating concentrations of FFAs have been shown to reduce hepatic clearance of insulin, hence contributing to peripheral hyperinsulinemia. Isolated rat hepatocytes show a dose-dependent decline in cell-surface insulin-receptor binding when exposed to palmitate, one of the major FFAs (99). This was attributed to a reduction in the number of insulin receptors as well to a reduction in the amount of internalized insulin within the hepatocytes. Similar effects of oleic acid have been described (100). On the basis of current evidence, it is reasonable to hypothesize that elevated FFA levels in individuals with type 2 diabetes have a significant role in decreasing hepatic clearance of insulin, thereby contributing to peripheral hyperinsulinemia.

INSULIN REGULATION OF LIPOLYSIS IN TYPE 2 DIABETES

Lean, nondiabetic humans are exquisitely sensitive to insulin-induced inhibition of lipolysis and, hence, to rates of FFA appearance (7,16). Persons with upper-body obesity and persons with type 2 diabetes have increased plasma concentrations of FFAs in the postabsorptive (101) and postprandial states (84,102), suggesting that dysregulation of FFA metabolism could play a role in the pathogenesis of hyperglycemia. Resistance to the inhibitory effects of insulin on lipolysis occurs in individuals with upper-body obesity and type 2 diabetes (7,101). Euglycemic stepwise insulin-clamp studies have shown reduced suppression of lipolysis by insulin in nonobese subjects with type 2 diabetes (11). Furthermore, rates of lipolysis during the postabsorptive stage have been shown to be higher in obese diabetic than in matched nondiabetic subjects (103). Experiments performed in our laboratory compared subjects with type 2 diabetes with equally obese healthy controls in the presence of comparable hyperglycemia (approximately 9 mM) and insulin levels (104). We found significantly increased rates of whole-body lipolysis in the diabetic individuals, resulting in modest elevations of FFA concentrations.

Because of evidence for regional heterogeneity in rates of FFA release by adipose tissue, it is important to understand the relative contribution of various adipose tissue beds to systemic FFAs. Therefore, in the above-mentioned study (104), regional splanchnic, leg, and nonsplanchnic upper-body release of FFAs was measured. Although FFA release from each adipose tissue bed was greater in diabetic than nondiabetic subjects, the relative contributions of the different regions to systemic lipolysis did not vary between the two groups. The major component of systemic lipolysis in both the diabetic and the nondiabetic subjects was the upper-body nonsplanchnic region, accounting for approximately 75% of FFA release (105). The importance of upper-body nonsplanchnic adipose tissue in delivering excess FFA to the systemic circulation was further demonstrated by a study of postprandial metabolism of FFA in upper-body obese and lower-body obese women (106). Postprandial release of FFA was 240% greater in the women with upper-body obesity despite higher insulin concentrations, and 73% of the excess FFA originated from the upper-body nonsplanchnic region (Fig. 16.2). It appears that although visceral fat is an excellent marker for abnormal FFA metabolism, it is not the major source of excess FFA.

Thus, type 2 diabetes is associated with higher fasting and postprandial FFA concentrations than occur in equally obese nondiabetic subjects. There still is some uncertainty, however, about how much of the resistance to insulin inhibition of lipolysis in persons with diabetes is a result of the metabolic state itself and how much is due to the associated features of upper-body or visceral obesity that frequently also are present.

TYPE 2 DIABETES AND BODY FAT DISTRIBUTION

Insulin resistance is one of the common links between type 2 diabetes, obesity, hypertension, dyslipidemia, hyperinsulinemia, and increased cardiovascular disease and mortality. This clustering of metabolic abnormalities has been termed the *metabolic syndrome, syndrome X*, or the *insulin resistance syndrome*, as proposed by Reaven (107). Vague (108) was the first to report that obesity-related adverse health and metabolic consequences occur predominantly in those with a masculine or upper-body fat distribution as opposed to a lower-body fat distribution. The relationships between the components of the metabolic syndrome inclusive of type 2 diabetes are stronger with upper-body obesity (as measured by waist-hip ratio) than with obesity per se (106,109,110). In particular, abdominal or visceral fat is most strongly associated with the presence of insulin resistance and the components of syndrome X (111–113). Visceral fat can be estimated using CT or MRI scans of the abdomen. Several large heritability studies [the HERITAGE family study (114) and the Quebec Family Study (115)] reported genetic and familial tendencies toward the development of visceral fat. Furthermore, the Nurses' Health Study (116) confirmed that being overweight increases the relative risk of type 2 diabetes and that the waist-hip ratio and waist circumference are powerful independent predictors of type 2 diabetes and coronary artery disease in U.S. women (117). Several investigators have confirmed a similar association of visceral adiposity with glucose intolerance and elevated plasma insulin, C-peptide, and triglyceride levels in men (112,118,119) and premenopausal women (120). Not all studies, however, support the conclusion that visceral fat is the best correlate of insulin resistance. Glucose disposal rates in middle-aged men with various degrees of adiposity were found to best relate to abdominal subcutaneous fat in one study (121). Body fat topography has also been shown to have different effects on glucose disposal rates in premenopausal women. Studies in nonobese women confirmed that total body fat mass appeared to be the primary determinant of insulin sensitivity, with abdominal visceral fat exerting a somewhat more significant effect in obese women (111).

In vitro studies have consistently shown that intraabdominal visceral fat (omental and mesenteric) has a high fractional lipolytic rate when compared with other fat depots in the body.

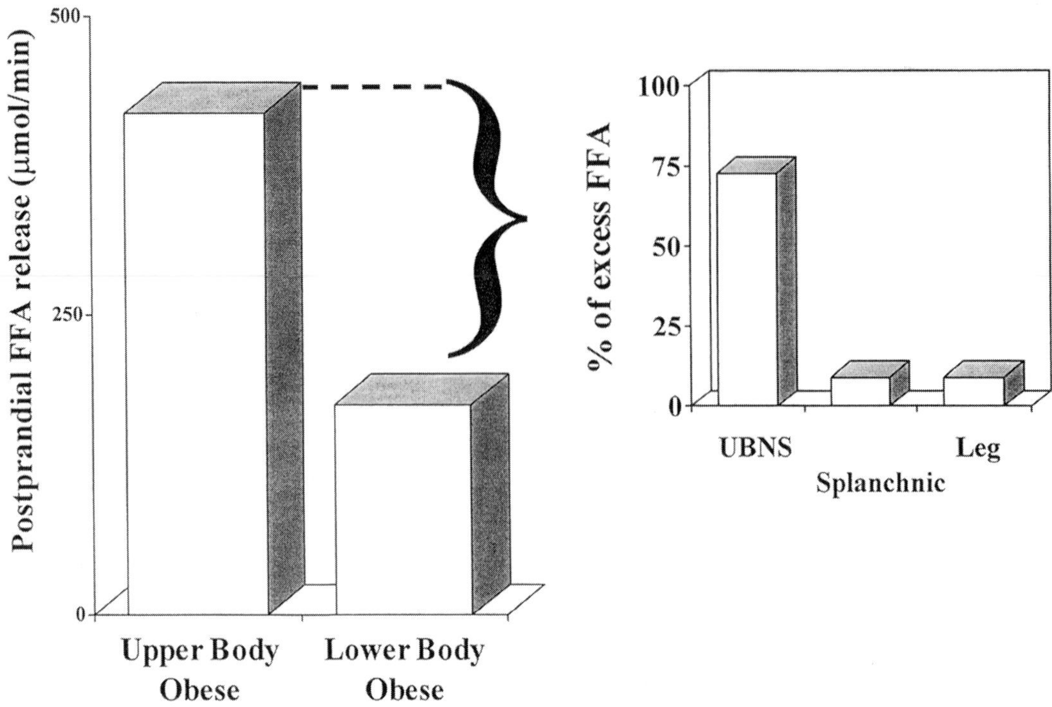

Figure 16.2. Left: Systemic release of free fatty acid (FFA) during ingestion of a meal in women who are upper-body obese and lower-body obese. **Right:** Relative amount of "excess" FFA release from the three different adipose tissue regions in the group with upper-body obesity. UBNS, upper-body nonsplanchnic. (Data are from Guo Z, Hensrud DD, Johnson CM, et al. Regional postprandial fatty acid metabolism in different obesity phenotypes. *Diabetes* 1999;48:1586–1592.)

As such, visceral fat could play a significant quantitative role (approximately 26% of upper-body release of FFA), which is out of proportion to its absolute mass (46). There is therefore a distinct possibility that in addition to the arterial delivery of FFAs to the liver, the delivery of FFAs through the portal route could have significant effects on the liver. This in turn could, by increasing the supply of gluconeogenic substrates, contribute to a reduction in insulin suppression of gluconeogenesis, resulting in an increase in endogenous glucose production. Furthermore, an increase in the availability of FFAs could also reduce insulin-stimulated peripheral glucose disposal (mainly in skeletal muscle, which is the most relevant site of insulin resistance). As discussed earlier, increased delivery of FFAs to the liver could potentially reduce hepatic insulin extraction (122,123), thereby contributing to peripheral hyperinsulinemia. This in turn, by suppressing subcutaneous adipose tissue lipolysis, potentially could magnify the ratio of visceral to systemic lipolysis (124).

The authors' laboratory conducted a series of experiments (125) to determine the effects of regional fat distribution on regional lipolysis in obesity (4,9,46). We found that rates of systemic lipolysis were greater in premenopausal women with upper-body obesity than in a matched group with lower-body obesity, especially during hyperinsulinemia. The majority of FFA release originated from the nonsplanchnic (subcutaneous) upper-body region. We found that the antilipolytic effect of a mixed meal was reduced in women with upper-body obesity compared with those with lower-body obesity or in nonobese women. A separate series of experiments also has revealed regional heterogeneity of insulin-regulated lipolysis, with the visceral adipose tissue being more resistant than leg adipose tissues to insulin-induced lipolysis. Further explorations on the regional postprandial FFA metabolism in different obesity phenotypes revealed a major contribution of nonsplanchnic upper-body tissues to total FFA flux in women with upper-body obesity, accounting for the greater postprandial FFA availability in these women. The nonvisceral upper-body source of postprandial release of FFA suggested that visceral fat might be a marker but not the source of excess postprandial FFA in obesity. Of interest, reduction of visceral fat by surgical removal (126) or by caloric restriction (127) in Sprague-Dawley rats has been shown to reverse hepatic insulin resistance. The finding that surgical removal of intraabdominal fat improves some aspects of insulin resistance suggests that there may be direct effects on hepatic metabolism unrelated to release of FFA by visceral adipose tissue. Other possible explanations for this observation include differences between rat and human physiology or indirect effects of intraabdominal fat on FFA release by subcutaneous adipose tissue.

There are a number of other hypotheses regarding the link between visceral adipose tissue and hepatic insulin resistance. These include potential roles of TNF-α, interleukin-6, and leptin (128). The presence of enlarged adipocytes in subcutaneous abdominal adipose tissue is predictive of adverse consequences of upper-body obesity (129), although this could be a result of resistance to insulin-mediated suppression of lipolysis (86,130). A large average fat-cell volume was found to be predictive of type 2 diabetes independent of age, gender, percent body fat, and body fat distribution in Pima Indians (131).

A recent study (132) has suggested a link between visceral adipose tissue and glucocorticoids. In this study, mice overexpressing the enzyme 11-β-hydroxysteroid dehydrogenase-1 (which converts the inactive form of glucocorticoids to the active form in mice and in humans) in adipose tissue developed visceral obesity, insulin-resistant diabetes, and hyperlipidemia that were exaggerated by a high-fat diet. Hence, it is possible that increased adipocyte expression of this enzyme

TABLE 16.1. Effect of Free Fatty Acids on Diabetes-related Physiologic Function

Physiologic function	Effects of FFAs
Glucose metabolism	
Insulin-mediated glucose uptake	Elevated FFAs inhibit insulin action
Insulin-mediated suppression of endogenous glucose production	Failure to suppress FFAs impairs effects of insulin
Glucose-mediated uptake of glucose	None
Glucose-mediated suppression of endogenous glucose production	Elevated FFAs impair suppression[140]
Insulin secretion	
Short-term	Stimulation of insulin secretion
Long-term	Inhibition of insulin secretion; possible islet toxicity
Insulin clearance	Reduced hepatic clearance of insulin
VLDL metabolism	Increased FFA associated with greater production of VLDL triglycerides

FFAs, free fatty acids; VLDL, very-low-density lipoprotein.

could potentially be a molecular etiology for visceral obesity and the metabolic syndrome. Another recent report (133) has shown increased 11-β-hydroxysteroid dehydrogenase-1 activity in adipose tissue of obese humans, lending further support to a link between visceral obesity and glucocorticoid metabolism.

Recent studies also have examined the relationship of subdivisions of subcutaneous abdominal adipose tissue to insulin resistance. Deep subcutaneous abdominal adipose tissue, separated from the superficial abdominal adipose tissue by a fascial plane, has been shown to have a strong negative correlation with insulin-stimulated glucose disposal (134). Misra et al. (135) have also reported that the deep subcutaneous adipose tissue located in the posterior as opposed to the anterior half of the abdomen is more closely correlated with insulin resistance.

TYPE 2 DIABETES AND METABOLISM OF VERY-LOW-DENSITY LIPOPROTEIN TRIGLYCERIDES

Type 2 diabetes has a well-known association with hypertriglyceridemia. In addition, fasting hypertriglyceridemia in subjects with type 2 diabetes has been linked to postprandial lipid and lipoprotein abnormalities. In 1976, Kissebah and colleagues (136) noted that FFA levels correlated with increased turnover of VLDL in subjects with type 2 diabetes, suggesting that increased hepatic production of VLDL may be driven by excess FFA. Although the patients with diabetes were hyperinsulinemic at the end of the study, no correlation was found between plasma insulin levels and the rate of VLDL turnover. A subsequent series of investigations clearly established that elevation of plasma FFA levels acutely stimulates VLDL production in nondiabetic individuals (137). These studies further showed that elevating plasma FFA levels in hyperinsulinemic subjects attenuates but does not completely abolish the suppressive effects of insulin on VLDL production. This suggested that in healthy individuals the acute inhibition of VLDL production by insulin is due only in part to suppression of FFA and may also be due to an FFA-independent process.

In considering the mechanism of FFA effects, it is relevant to note that degradation of the important VLDL protein apoB is inhibited by the FFA oleate (138,139). Thus, increased hepatic FFA delivery, as characteristically occurs in type 2 diabetes, may stimulate the assembly and secretion of apoB-containing VLDL by targeting apoB for secretion rather than intracellular degradation.

CONCLUDING COMMENTS

This chapter has provided a review of the causes and consequences of altered fat metabolism in diabetes mellitus. Although our knowledge of the intricate regulating interrelationships between FFA levels, insulin secretion and action, glucose metabolism, and triglyceride metabolism undoubtedly will undergo further advances, it is clear that FFA levels have a key role in contributing to the metabolic disturbances of diabetes (summarized in Table 16.1). Therapeutic approaches that lower FFA levels and restore FFA metabolism can be expected to have substantial beneficial effects in patients with diabetes. Lowered FFA levels in response to metformin and thiazolidinediones may contribute to the therapeutic efficacy of these agents, and the development of new agents that lower FFA levels in diabetes should be considered an important goal.

Acknowledgments

Preparation of this chapter was supported by grants DK 45343, DK 40484, DK 29953, DK 50456 (Minnesota Obesity Center) and by the Mayo Foundation.

REFERENCES

1. Hellerstein MK, Christiansen M, Kaempfer S, et al. Measurement of de novo hepatic lipogenesis in humans using stable isotopes. *J Clin Invest* 1991;87:1841–1852.
2. Mayes PA. Lipid transport and storage. In: Murray RK, Granner, DK, Mayes, PA, Rodwell VW. *Harper's biochemistry*, 24th ed. Norwalk, CT: Appleton & Lange, 1996:254–270.
3. Romanski SA, Nelson RM, Jensen MD. Meal fatty acid uptake in adipose tissue: gender effects in nonobese humans. *Am J Physiol Endocrinol Metab* 2000;279:E455–E462.
4. Roust LR, Jensen MD. Postprandial free fatty acid kinetics are abnormal in upper body obesity. *Diabetes* 1993;42:1567–1573.
5. Jensen MD. Assessment of free fatty acid metabolism. In: Draznin B, Rizza R, eds. *Clinical research in diabetes and obesity: methods, assessment and metabolic regulation.* Totowa, NJ: Humana Press, 1997:125–136.
6. Eckel RH. Lipoprotein lipase: a multifunctional enzyme relevant to common metabolic diseases. *N Engl J Med* 1989;320:1060–1068.
7. Coppack SW, Jensen MD, Miles JM. In vivo regulation of lipolysis in humans. *J Lipid Res* 1994;35:177–193.

8. Farese RV Jr, Yost TJ, Eckel RH. Tissue-specific regulation of lipoprotein lipase activity by insulin/glucose in normal-weight humans. *Metabolism* 1991;40:214–216.
9. Jensen MD, Haymond MW, Rizza RA, et al. Influence of body fat distribution on free fatty acid metabolism in obesity. *J Clin Invest* 1989;83:1168–1173.
10. Kanaley JA, Mottram CD, Scanlon PD, et al. Fatty acid kinetic responses to running above or below lactate threshold. *J Appl Physiol* 1995;79:439–447.
11. Groop LC, Bonadonna RC, DelPrato S, et al. Glucose and free fatty acid metabolism in non-insulin-dependent diabetes mellitus. Evidence for multiple sites of insulin resistance. *J Clin Invest* 1989;84:205–213.
12. Guo Z, Jensen MD. Intramuscular fatty acid metabolism evaluated with stable isotopic tracers. *J Appl Physiol* 1998;84:1674–1679.
13. Groop LC, Bonadonna RC, Shank M, et al. Role of free fatty acids and insulin in determining free fatty acid and lipid oxidation in man. *J Clin Invest* 1991;87:83–89.
14. Havel RJ, Kane JP, Balasse EO, et al. Splanchnic metabolism of free fatty acids and production of triglycerides of very low density lipoproteins in normotriglyceridemic and hypertriglyceridemic humans. *J Clin Invest* 1970;49:2017–2035.
15. Basso LV, Havel RJ. Hepatic metabolism of free fatty acids in normal and diabetic dogs. *J Clin Invest* 1970;49:537–547.
16. Jensen MD, Caruso M, Heiling V, et al. Insulin regulation of lipolysis in nondiabetic and IDDM subjects. *Diabetes* 1989;38:1595–1601.
17. Wahrenberg H, Lonnqvist F, Arner P: Mechanisms underlying regional differences in lipolysis in human adipose tissue. *J Clin Invest* 1989;84:458–467.
18. Burns TW, Langley PE, Terry BE, et al. The role of free fatty acids in the regulation of lipolysis by human adipose tissue cells. *Metabolism* 1978;27:1755–1762.
19. Leibel RL, Forse RA, Hirsch J. Effects of rapid glucose infusion on in vivo and in vitro free fatty acid re-esterification by adipose tissue of fasted obese subjects. *Int J Obes* 1989;13:661–671.
20. Coppack SW, Frayn KN, Humphreys SM, et al. Effects of insulin on human adipose tissue metabolism in vivo. *Clin Sci* 1989;77:663–670.
21. Divertie GD, Jensen MD, Miles JM. Stimulation of lipolysis in humans by physiological hypercortisolemia. *Diabetes* 1991;40:1228–1232.
22. Horber FF, Marsh HM, Haymond MW. Differential effects of prednisone and growth hormone on fuel metabolism and insulin antagonism in humans. *Diabetes* 1991;40:141–149.
23. Shamoon H, Hendler R, Sherwin RS. Altered responsiveness to cortisol, epinephrine, and glucagon in insulin-infused juvenile-onset diabetics. A mechanism for diabetic instability. *Diabetes* 1980;29:284–291.
24. Birkenhager JC, Timmermans HA, Lamberts SW. Depressed plasma FFA turnover rate in Cushing's syndrome. *J Clin Endocrinol Metab* 1976;42:28–32.
25. Goodman HM, Grichting G. Growth hormone and lipolysis: a reevaluation. *Endocrinology* 1983;113:1697–1702.
26. Boyle PJ, Avogaro A, Smith L, et al. Role of GH in regulating nocturnal rates of lipolysis and plasma mevalonate levels in normal and diabetic humans. *Am J Physiol* 1992;263:E168–E172.
27. Cersosimo E, Danou F, Persson M, et al. Effects of pulsatile delivery of basal growth hormone on lipolysis in humans. *Am J Physiol* 1996;271:E123–E126.
28. Saunders J, Hall SE, Sonksen PH. Glucose and free fatty acid turnover in thyrotoxicosis and hypothyroidism, before and after treatment. *Clin Endocrinol* 1980;13:33–44.
29. Starnes HF Jr, Warren RS, Jeevanandam M, et al. Tumor necrosis factor and the acute metabolic response to tissue injury in man. *J Clin Invest* 1988;82:1321–1325.
30. Axelrod L. Insulin, prostaglandins, and the pathogenesis of hypertension. *Diabetes* 1991;40:1223–1227.
31. Miles JM, Ellman MG, McLean KL, et al. Validation of a new method for determination of free fatty acid turnover. *Am J Physiol* 1987;252:E431–E438.
32. Jensen MD, Rogers PJ, Ellman MG, et al. Choice of infusion-sampling mode for tracer studies of free fatty acid metabolism. *Am J Physiol* 1988;254:E562–E565.
33. Butler PC, Home PD. The measurement of metabolite exchange across muscle beds. *Baillieres Clin Endocrinol Metab* 1987;1:863–878.
34. Frayn KN, Coppack SW, Humphreys SM, et al. Metabolic characteristics of human adipose tissue in vivo. *Clin Sci* 1989;76:509–516.
35. Meek SE, Nair KS, Jensen MD: Insulin regulation of regional free fatty acid metabolism. *Diabetes* 1999;48:10–14.
36. Hagenfeldt L, Wahren J, Pernow B, et al. Uptake of individual free fatty acids by skeletal muscle and liver in man. *J Clin Invest* 1972;51:2324–2330.
37. Spitzer JJ. Application of tracers in studying free fatty acid metabolism of various organs in vivo. *Fed Proc* 1975;34:2242–2245.
38. Guo Z, Nielsen S, Burguera B, et al. Free fatty acid turnover measured using ultralow doses of [U-13C] palmitate. *J Lipid Res* 1997;38:1888–1895.
39. Klein S, Coyle EF, Wolfe RR. Fat metabolism during low-intensity exercise in endurance-trained and untrained men. *Am J Physiol* 1994;267:E934–E940.
40. Romijn JA, Klein S, Coyle EF, et al. Strenuous endurance training increases lipolysis and triglyceride-fatty acid cycling at rest. *J Appl Physiol* 1993;75:108–113.
41. Wolfe RR, Klein S, Carraro F, et al. Role of triglyceride-fatty acid cycle in controlling fat metabolism in humans during and after exercise. *Am J Physiol* 1990;258:E382–E389.
42. Miyoshi H, Shulman GI, Peters EJ, et al. Hormonal control of substrate cycling in humans. *J Clin Invest* 1988;81:1545–1555.
43. Wolfe RR, Herndon DN, Jahoor F, et al. Effect of severe burn injury on substrate cycling by glucose and fatty acids. *N Engl J Med* 1987;317:403–408.
44. Boden G, Chen X, Desantis RA, et al. Effects of insulin on fatty acid reesterification in healthy subjects. *Diabetes* 1993;42:1588–1593.
45. Kurpad A, Khan K, Calder AG, et al. Effect of noradrenaline on glycerol turnover and lipolysis in the whole body and subcutaneous adipose tissue in humans in vivo. *Clin Sci* 1994;86:177–184.
46. Martin ML, Jensen MD. Effects of body fat distribution on regional lipolysis in obesity. *J Clin Invest* 1991;88:609–613.
47. Arner P, Kriegholm E, Engfeldt P. In situ studies of catecholamine-induced lipolysis in human adipose tissue using microdialysis. *J Pharmacol Exp Ther* 1990;254:284–288.
48. Arner P, Krieghold E, Engfeldt P, et al. Adrenergic regulation of lipolysis in situ at rest and during exercise. *J Clin Invest* 1990;85:893–898.
49. Arner P, Bolinder J, Eliasson A, et al. Microdialysis of adipose tissue and blood for in vivo lipolysis studies. *Am J Physiol* 1988;255:E737–E742.
50. Jansson PA, Smith U, Lonnroth P. Interstitial glycerol concentration measured by microdialysis in two subcutaneous regions in humans. *Am J Physiol* 1990;258:E918–E922.
51. Jansson PA, Smith U, Lonnroth P. Evidence for lactate production by human adipose tissue in vivo. *Diabetologia* 1990;33:253–256.
52. Jensen MD, Kanaley JA, Reed JE, et al. Measurement of abdominal and visceral fat with computed tomography and dual-energy x-ray absorptiometry. *Am J Clin Nutr* 1995;61:274–278.
53. Jensen MD, Kanaley JA, Roust LR, et al. Assessment of body composition with use of dual-energy x-ray absorptiometry: evaluation and comparison with other methods. *Mayo Clin Proc* 1993;68:867–873.
54. Canner PL, Berge KG, Wenger NK, et al: Fifteen year mortality in Coronary Drug Project patients: long-term benefit with niacin. *J Am Coll Cardiol* 1986;8:1245–1255.
55. Fulcher GR, Walker M, Catalano C, et al. Metabolic effects of suppression of nonesterified fatty acid levels with acipimox in obese NIDDM subjects. *Diabetes* 1992;4:1400–1408.
56. Vaag A, Skott P, Damsbo P, et al. Effect of the antilipolytic nicotinic acid analogue acipimox on whole-body and skeletal muscle glucose metabolism in patients with non-insulin-dependent diabetes mellitus. *J Clin Invest* 1991;88:1282–1290.
57. Randle PJ, Priestman DA, Mistry S, et al. Mechanisms modifying glucose oxidation in diabetes mellitus. *Diabetologia* 1994;37[Suppl 2]:S155–S161.
58. Bailey JW, Jensen MD, Miles JM. Effects of intravenous methyl palmoxirate on the turnover and oxidation of fatty acids in conscious dogs. *Metabolism* 1991;40:428–431.
59. Bensadoun A. Lipoprotein lipase. *Annu Rev Nutr* 1990;11:217–237.
60. Randle PJ, Hales CN, Garland PB, et al. The glucose fatty-acid cycle: its role in insulin sensitivity and the metabolic disturbances of diabetes mellitus. *Lancet* 1963;1:7285–7289.
61. Boden G, Chen X, Ruiz J, et al. Mechanisms of fatty acid-induced inhibition of glucose uptake. *J Clin Invest* 1994;93:2438–2446.
62. Boden G, Jadali F, White J, et al. Effects of fat on insulin-stimulated carbohydrate metabolism in normal men. *J Clin Invest* 1991;88:960–966.
63. Kelley DE, Mokan M, Simoneau JA, et al. Interaction between glucose and free fatty acid metabolism in human skeletal muscle. *J Clin Invest* 1993;92:91–98.
64. Dresner A, Laurent D, Marcucci M, et al. Effects of free fatty acids on glucose transport and IRS-1–associated phosphatidylinositol 3-kinase activity. *J Clin Invest* 1999;103:253–259.
65. Roden M, Price TB, Perseghin G, et al. Mechanism of free fatty acid-induced insulin resistance in humans. *J Clin Invest* 1996;97:2859–2865.
66. Saloranta C, Koivisto V, Widen E, et al. Contribution of muscle and liver to glucose-fatty acid cycle in humans. *Am J Physiol* 1993;264:E599–E605.
67. Baron AD, Brechtel G, Edelman SV: Effects of free fatty acids and ketone bodies on in vivo non-insulin-mediated glucose utilization and production in humans. *Metabolism* 1989;38:1056–1061.
68. Sidossis LS, Mittendorfer B, Chinkes D, et al. Effect of hyperglycemia-hyperinsulinemia on whole body and regional fatty acid metabolism. *Am J Physiol* 1999;276:E427–E434.
69. Sidossis LS, Wolfe RR. Glucose and insulin-induced inhibition of fatty acid oxidation: the glucose-fatty acid cycle reversed. *Am J Physiol* 1996;270:E733–E738.
70. Lea MA, Weber G. Role of enzymes in homeostasis. Inhibition of the activity of glycolytic enzymes by free fatty acids. *J Biol Chem* 1968;243:1096–1102.
71. Johnson JH, Newgard CB, Milburn JL, et al. The high K_m glucose transporter of islets of Langerhans is functionally similar to the low affinity transporter of liver and has an identical primary sequence. *J Biol Chem* 1990;265:6548–6551.
72. Mueckler M. Facilitative glucose transporters. *Eur J Biochem* 1994;219:713–725.
73. Gould GW, Holman GD. The glucose transporter family: structure, function and tissue-specific expression. *Biochem J* 1993;295:329–341.
74. Struck E, Ashmore J, Wieland O. Effects of glucagon and long chain fatty acids on glucose production by isolated perfused rat liver. *Adv Enzyme Regul* 1966;4:219–224.
75. Herrera MG, Kamm D, Ruderman NB, et al. Non-hormonal factors in the control of gluconeogenesis. *Adv Enzyme Regul* 1966;4:225–235.
76. Ferrannini E, Barrett EJ, Bevilacqua S, et al. Effect of fatty acids on glucose production and utilization in man. *J Clin Invest* 1983;72:1737–1747.

77. Boden G, Jadali F. Effects of lipid on basal carbohydrate metabolism in normal men. *Diabetes* 1991;40:686–692.
78. Clore JN, Glickman PS, Nestler JE, et al. In vivo evidence for hepatic autoregulation during FFA-stimulated gluconeogenesis in normal humans. *Am J Physiol* 1991;261:E425–E429.
79. Chen X, Iqbal N, Boden G. The effects of free fatty acids on gluconeogenesis and glycogenolysis in normal subjects. *J Clin Invest* 1999;103:365–372.
80. Bergman RN. New concepts in extracellular signaling for insulin action: the single gateway hypothesis. *Recent Prog Horm Res* 1997;52:359–385.
81. Rebrin K, Steil GM, Mittelman SD, et al. Causal linkage between insulin suppression of lipolysis and suppression of liver glucose output in dogs. *J Clin Invest* 1996;98:741–749.
82. Lewis GF, Vranic M, Giacca A. Role of free fatty acids and glucagon in the peripheral effect of insulin on glucose production in humans. *Am J Physiol* 1998;275:E177–E186.
83. Lewis GF, Zinman B, Groenewoud Y, et al. Hepatic glucose production is regulated both by direct hepatic and extrahepatic effects of insulin in humans. *Diabetes* 1996;45:454–462.
84. Groop LC, Saloranta C, Shank M, et al. The role of free fatty acid metabolism in the pathogenesis of insulin resistance in obesity and noninsulin-dependent diabetes mellitus. *J Clin Endocrinol Metab* 1991;72:96–107.
85. Saloranta C, Franssila-Kallunki A, Ekstrand A, et al. Modulation of hepatic glucose production by non-esterified fatty acids in type 2 (non-insulin-dependent) diabetes mellitus. *Diabetologia* 1991;34:409–415.
86. Paolisso G, Tataranni PA, Foley JE, et al. A high concentration of fasting plasma non-esterified fatty acids is a risk factor for the development of NIDDM. *Diabetologia* 1995;38:1213–1217.
87. Boden G, Chen X, Rosner J, et al. Effects of a 48-h fat infusion on insulin secretion and glucose utilization. *Diabetes* 1995;44:1239–1242.
88. Paolisso G, Gambardella A, Amato L, et al. Opposite effects of short- and long-term fatty acid infusion on insulin secretion in healthy subjects. *Diabetologia* 1995;38:1295–1299.
89. Carpentier A, Mittelman SD, Lamarche B, et al. Acute enhancement of insulin secretion by FFA in humans is lost with prolonged FFA elevation. *Am J Physiol* 1999;276:E1055–E1066.
90. Mason TM, Goh T, Tchipashvili V, et al. Prolonged elevation of plasma free fatty acids desensitizes the insulin secretory response to glucose in vivo in rats. *Diabetes* 1999;48:524–530.
91. Lee Y, Hirose H, Ohneda M, et al. Beta-cell lipotoxicity in the pathogenesis of non-insulin-dependent diabetes mellitus of obese rats: impairment in adipocyte-beta-cell relationships. *Proc Natl Acad Sci U S A* 1994;91:10878–10882.
92. Zhou YP, Grill VE. Long-term exposure of rat pancreatic islets to fatty acids inhibits glucose-induced insulin secretion and biosynthesis through a glucose fatty acid cycle. *J Clin Invest* 1994;93:870–876.
93. Bollheimer LC, Skelly RH, Chester MW, et al. Chronic exposure to free fatty acid reduces pancreatic beta cell insulin content by increasing basal insulin secretion that is not compensated for by a corresponding increase in proinsulin biosynthesis translation. *J Clin Invest* 1998;101:1094–1101.
94. Brun T, Assimacopoulos-Jeannet F, Corkey BE, et al. Long-chain fatty acids inhibit acetyl-CoA carboxylase gene expression in the pancreatic beta-cell line INS-1. *Diabetes* 1997;46:393–400.
95. Gremlich S, Bonny C, Waeber G, et al. Fatty acids decrease IDX-1 expression in rat pancreatic islets and reduce GLUT2, glucokinase, insulin, and somatostatin levels. *J Biol Chem* 1997;272:30261–30269.
96. Larsson O, Deeney JT, Branstrom R, et al. Activation of the ATP-sensitive K^+ channel by long chain acyl-CoA. A role in modulation of pancreatic beta-cell glucose sensitivity. *J Biol Chem* 1996;271:10623–10626.
97. Duckworth WC, Bennett RG, Hamel FG: Insulin degradation: progress and potential. *Endocr Rev* 1998;19:608–624.
98. Duckworth WC. Insulin degradation: mechanisms, products, and significance. *Endocr Rev* 1988;9:319–345.
99. Hennes MM, Shrago E, Kissebah AH. Receptor and postreceptor effects of free fatty acids (FFA) on hepatocyte insulin dynamics. *Int J Obes* 1990;14: 831–841.
100. Svedberg J, Bjorntorp P, Smith U, et al. Free-fatty acid inhibition of insulin binding, degradation, and action in isolated rat hepatocytes. *Diabetes* 1990; 39:570–574.
101. Skowronski R, Hollenbeck CB, Varasteh BB, et al. Regulation of non-esterified fatty acid and glycerol concentration by insulin in normal individuals and patients with type 2 diabetes. *Diabet Med* 1991;8:330–333.
102. Reaven GM, Hollenbeck C, Jeng CY, et al. Measurement of plasma glucose, free fatty acid, lactate, and insulin for 24 h in patients with NIDDM. *Diabetes* 1988;37:1020–1024.
103. Nurjhan N, Consoli A, Gerich J. Increased lipolysis and its consequences on gluconeogenesis in non-insulin-dependent diabetes mellitus. *J Clin Invest* 1992;89:169–175.
104. Basu A, Basu R, Shah P, et al. Effects of type 2 diabetes on the ability of insulin and glucose to regulate splanchnic and muscle glucose metabolism: evidence for a defect in hepatic glucokinase activity. *Diabetes* 2000;49:272–283.
105. Basu A, Basu R, Shah P, et al. Systemic and regional free fatty acid metabolism in type 2 diabetes. *Am J Physiol* 2001;280:E1000–E1006.
106. Despres JP, Allard C, Tremblay A, et al. Evidence for a regional component of body fatness in the association with serum lipids in men and women. *Metabolism* 1985;34:967–973.
107. Reaven GM: Syndrome X: 6 years later. *J Intern Med* 1994;736[Suppl]:13–22.
108. Vague J. The degree of masculine differentiation of obesities: a factor determining predisposition to diabetes, atherosclerosis, gout and uric calculous disease. *Am J Clin Nutr* 1956;4:20–34.
109. Anderson AJ, Sobocinski KA, Freedman DS, et al. Body fat distribution, plasma lipids, and lipoproteins. *Arteriosclerosis* 1988;8:88–94.
110. Thompson CJ, Ryu JE, Craven TE, et al. Central adipose distribution is related to coronary atherosclerosis. *Arterioscler Thromb* 1991;11:327–333.
111. Bonora E, Prato S, Bonadonna RC, et al. Total body fat content and fat topography are associated differently with in vivo glucose metabolism in nonobese and obese nondiabetic women. *Diabetes* 1992;41:1151–1159.
112. Pouliot MC, Despres JP, Nadeau A, et al. Visceral obesity in men. Associations with glucose tolerance, plasma insulin, and lipoprotein levels. *Diabetes* 1992;41:826–834.
113. Seidell JC, Bjorntorp P, Sjostrom L, et al. Visceral fat accumulation in men is positively associated with insulin, glucose, and C-peptide levels, but negatively with testosterone levels. *Metabolism* 1990;39:897–901.
114. Rice T, Despres JP, Daw EW, et al. Familial resemblance for abdominal visceral fat: the HERITAGE Family Study. *Int J Obes Relat Metab Disord* 1997;21: 1024–1031.
115. Perusse L, Despres JP, Lemieux S, et al. Familial aggregation of abdominal visceral fat level: results from the Quebec family study. *Metabolism* 1996;45: 378–382.
116. Carey VJ, Walters EE, Colditz GA, et al. Body fat distribution and risk of non-insulin-dependent diabetes mellitus in women. The Nurses' Health Study. *Am J Epidemiol* 1997;145:614–619.
117. Rexrode KM, Carey VJ, Hennekens CH, et al. Abdominal adiposity and coronary heart disease in women. *JAMA* 1998;280:1843–1848.
118. Sparrow D, Borkan GA, Gerzof SG, et al. Relationship of fat distribution to glucose tolerance. Results of computed tomography in male participants of the Normative Aging Study. *Diabetes* 1986;35:411–415.
119. Fujioka S, Matsuzawa Y, Tokunaga K, et al. Contribution of intra-abdominal fat accumulation to the impairment of glucose and lipid metabolism in human obesity. *Metabolism* 1987;36:54–59.
120. Despres JP, Moorjani S, Tremblay A, et al. Relation of high plasma triglyceride levels associated with obesity and regional adipose tissue distribution to plasma lipoprotein-lipid composition in premenopausal women. *Clin Invest Med* 1989;12:374–380.
121. Abate N, Garg A, Peshock RM, et al. Relationships of generalized and regional adiposity to insulin sensitivity in men. *J Clin Invest* 1995;96: 88–98.
122. Peiris AN, Mueller RA, Smith GA, et al. Splanchnic insulin metabolism in obesity. Influence of body fat distribution. *J Clin Invest* 1986;78:1648–1657.
123. Hennes MM, Dua A, Kissebah AH. Effects of free fatty acids and glucose on splanchnic insulin dynamics. *Diabetes* 1997;46:57–62.
124. Bjorntorp P. Metabolic implications of body fat distribution. *Diabetes Care* 1991;14:1132–1143.
125. Guo Z, Hensrud DD, Johnson CM, et al. Regional postprandial fatty acid metabolism in different obesity phenotypes. *Diabetes* 1999;48:1586–1592.
126. Barzilai N, She L, Liu BQ, et al. Surgical removal of visceral fat reverses hepatic insulin resistance. *Diabetes* 1999;48:94–98.
127. Barzilai N, Banerjee S, Hawkins M, et al. Caloric restriction reverses hepatic insulin resistance in aging rats by decreasing visceral fat. *J Clin Invest* 1998;101:1353–1361.
128. Barzilai N, She L, Liu L, et al. Decreased visceral adiposity accounts for leptin effect on hepatic but not peripheral insulin action. *Am J Physiol Endocrinol Metab* 1999;277:E291–E298.
129. Bjorntorp P, Gustafson A, Persson B. Adipose tissue fat cell size and number in relation to metabolism in endogenous hypertriglyceridemia. *Acta Med Scand* 1971;190:363–367.
130. Bjorntorp P, Bengtsson C, Blohme G, et al. Adipose tissue fat cell size and number in relation to metabolism in randomly selected middle-aged men and women. *Metabolism* 1971;20:927–935.
131. Reynisdottir S, Dauzats M, Thorne A, et al. Comparison of hormone-sensitive lipase activity in visceral and subcutaneous human adipose tissue. *J Clin Endocrinol Metab* 1977;82:4162–4166.
132. Masuzaki H, Paterson J, Shinyama H, et al: A transgenic model of visceral obesity and the metabolic syndrome. *Science* 2001;294:2166–2170.
133. Rask E, Olsson T, Soderberg S, et al: Tissue-specific dysregulation of cortisol metabolism in human obesity. *J Clin Endocrinol Metab* 2001;86:1418–1421.
134. Kelley DE, Thaete FL, Troost F, et al: Subdivisions of subcutaneous abdominal adipose tissue and insulin resistance. *Am J Physiol Endocrinol Metab* 2000;278:E941–E948.
135. Misra A, Garg A, Abate N, et al: Relationship of anterior and posterior subcutaneous abdominal fat to insulin sensitivity in nondiabetic men. *Obes Res* 1997;5:93–99.
136. Kissebah AH, Alfarsi S, Adams PW, et al: Role of insulin resistance in adipose tissue and liver in the pathogenesis of endogenous hypertriglyceridaemia in man. *Diabetologia* 1976;2:563–571.
137. Lewis GF, Uffelman KD, Szeto LW, et al. Interaction between free fatty acids and insulin in the acute control of very low density lipoprotein production in humans. *J Clin Invest* 1995;95:158–166.
138. Ginsberg HN. Diabetic dyslipidemia: basic mechanisms underlying the common hypertriglyceridemia and low HDL cholesterol levels. *Diabetes* 1996;45 [Suppl 3]:S27–S30.
139. Cummings MH, Watts GF, Umpleby AM, et al. Acute hyperinsulinemia decreases the hepatic secretion of very-low-density lipoprotein apolipoprotein B-100 in NIDDM. *Diabetes* 1995;44:1059–1065.
140. Rossetti L, Hawkins M, Shamoon H, et al. Scientific Sessions of the 60th Annual Meeting of the American Diabetes Association, San Antonio, TX, June 2000 (abst).

CHAPTER 17

Alterations in Protein Metabolism in Diabetes Mellitus

Craig S. Stump and K. Sreekumaran Nair

HISTORICAL PERSPECTIVE

Before insulin treatment became readily available, stunted growth, cachexia, and muscle wasting were well recognized in patients with type 1 diabetes mellitus (1,2). Indeed, this association has been known for millennia, as documented in ancient Sanskrit literature describing diabetes mellitus as "honey-urine-disease" (3). The Greek physician Aretaeus described diabetes as a condition with "melting of flesh into urine." Alternatively, the anticatabolic effect of insulin therapy has been well documented during the past 80 years (1,4,5). This anticatabolic effect is associated with normalization of urinary losses of nitrogen (4,6); increases in body cell mass, as indexed by total body potassium (7); and decreases in the concentrations of amino acids, especially of branched-chain amino acids (BCAA) (8,9). Intraarterial infusion of insulin during the postabsorptive state in subjects without diabetes decreases the net amino acid release from the forearm, indicating a net decrease in protein breakdown (10). Collectively, these observations demonstrate the important anabolic effects of insulin in humans. However, the mechanism by which insulin promotes the growth and maintenance of lean tissue continues to be debated, and the effects of insulin on the synthesis and breakdown of a variety of individual proteins remains an area of intense research.

This chapter reviews current knowledge of protein turnover in type 1 and type 2 diabetes mellitus. It describes the specific effects of insulin and other selected hormones on the components of protein turnover (i.e., protein breakdown and protein synthesis) and gives a general overview of the mechanisms by which insulin affects protein synthesis and breakdown within the cell. Although emphasizing human studies, it discusses important work from animal and *in vitro* studies and notes the discrepancies between different experimental approaches.

BALANCING PROTEIN SYNTHESIS AND BREAKDOWN

The balance between protein synthesis and breakdown determines the protein content of the whole body and individual tissues, as well as the concentrations of specific proteins. Consequently, protein turnover is not only important for increasing and maintaining cell size but also fundamental to tissue remodeling, adaptation, and repair. Specific proteins are synthesized and catabolized at variable rates in response to particular functional demands upon the cell. In considering the proteins involved in the regulation of processes such as differentiation, growth, energy production, or gene repair, it is important to recognize that small alterations in protein balance may have large effects on cell function. Changes in the content, function, and integrity of specific proteins involved with these types of cellular processes probably contribute to the chronic complications associated with diabetes mellitus. However, an understanding of the underlying mechanisms is complicated by the regulation of protein turnover by a number of hormones other than insulin, including cortisol, glucagon, growth hormone, insulin-like growth factors and other growth factors, thyroid hormones, and testosterone. Substrates such as amino acids, fatty acids, and ketones and different physiologic states such as fasting, exercise, pregnancy, aging, and chronic disease also influence protein turnover. Recent advances in molecular biology and isotopic tracer technology have enhanced the capacity to study human protein metabolism. The human genome project provides information that sets the stage for a new era of investigation that not only will help define the functions of proteins encoded by newly identified genes but also will provide insight into their regulation and turnover dynamics. This undoubtedly will expand our understanding of the influence of diseases such as diabetes mellitus on protein metabolism and the impact of altered protein dynamics on the course of diabetes.

EFFECTS OF INSULIN ON PROTEIN TURNOVER

Insulin has been shown to stimulate protein synthesis both *in vitro* and *in situ* (11–16). Studies in animals with low insulin levels, as occurs with fasting or β-cell destruction, have clearly shown that insulin replacement stimulates protein synthesis (12,17,18–21). Increased protein synthesis has been demonstrated in muscle tissue of nondiabetic animals after insulin administration in some (22,23) but not all (24) studies. The absence of an observed insulin effect in some reports may be related to the ages of animals studied and diminished insulin action in older animals (23–25). Studies on perfused or incubated rat diaphragm (26), skeletal muscle (12), and heart (17,21) have shown that insulin also decreases the breakdown of muscle protein.

The effects of insulin on protein metabolism in healthy human subjects without diabetes are less clear. In general, whole-body protein synthesis is not stimulated when insulin is infused during the postabsorptive state (fasting) (27–29). However, when insulin is infused under these conditions, circulating amino acids, especially BCAA, decrease in a dose-dependent manner (8,9,30). In contrast, when insulin is secreted in response to a meal under physiologic conditions, there is a simultaneous influx of dietary amino acids. Therefore, the lack of increase in protein synthesis observed in postabsorptive studies possibly relates to a decrease in the availability of amino acids. This concept is supported by studies that have examined the effects of infusing amino acids together with insulin in healthy subjects without diabetes (31–36). It generally has been observed that protein synthesis increases when insulin and amino acids are infused at rates sufficient to produce hyperinsulinemia and hyperaminoacidemia (32,36,37) but not with hyperinsulinemia and normal physiologic levels of amino acids (33). One study demonstrated that infusion of supraphysiologic doses of insulin together with amino acid supplementation can stimulate protein synthesis by more than 100% in forearm muscle of healthy subjects without diabetes (38). This protocol was designed to simulate, at the local muscle level, the high insulin concentrations used in many of the *in vitro* studies examining protein turnover. Therefore, the findings may help reconcile the observation of increased protein synthesis *in vitro* with the general absence of changes in protein synthesis *in vivo* in the presence of physiologic doses of insulin. In contrast to protein synthesis, the inhibitory effect of insulin on protein breakdown is readily demonstrated in subjects without diabetes even in the absence of infused amino acids (27,33,36,39,40). Similarly, several (27,28,39,41), but not all (42) studies measuring protein turnover in human limb muscle vascular beds have demonstrated decreased protein breakdown with insulin infusion. To summarize, findings in humans without diabetes concur with *in vitro* analyses and most animal studies in the demonstration of inhibitory effects of insulin on protein breakdown. By contrast, effects of insulin on protein synthesis in different experimental systems have not been consistent.

MECHANISMS OF INSULIN ACTION

Protein turnover in specific tissues and cell types is known to be affected differently in diabetes mellitus, depending on the degree of insulin deficiency, amino acid availability, and the level of glycemic control (40,43,44). It is likely that proteins in individual cellular subfractions (cytoplasm, mitochondria, nuclei, and contractile structures) respond differently to the effects of insulin and that these responses may be influenced by diabetes mellitus. The pathways by which insulin influences cellular processes such as gene transcription, messenger RNA (mRNA) stability, protein targeting for breakdown, and enzyme regulation undoubtedly are complex and exquisitely regulated. Knowledge of specific signaling pathways mediating insulin effects on protein synthesis and breakdown is advancing, and this new understanding will likely lead to practical new approaches to the management of the complications of diabetes mellitus.

Protein Synthesis

Although the role of insulin in regulating protein synthesis in humans remains uncertain, stimulation of protein synthesis by insulin in various *in vitro* models has been clearly shown (11–16). These somewhat divergent findings probably are related in part to methodologic issues. For example, it is difficult to show direct effects of insulin on gene expression and subsequent protein synthesis in intact animals because insulin deficiency and/or replacement results in concurrent changes in substrate concentrations and fluxes, changes in concentrations of counterregulatory hormones, and other factors. To circumvent this problem, investigators often attempt to maintain concentrations of glucose, amino acids, and various hormones by using clamp techniques. However, it is probably impossible to control all the known and still unknown factors that affect protein synthesis. For this reason, cell lines, primary cell cultures, tissue cultures, and *in situ* preparations represent useful systems for examining a more controlled cellular environment. These experimental models have the advantage of making it possible to evaluate insulin effects on gene expression in isolation or as a permissive or augmenting influence with other selected factors, but have the disadvantage of often uncertain physiologic relevance of the observed findings.

Insulin may influence protein synthesis through numerous sites of regulation (14,15), including effects on gene transcription (mRNA production), mRNA stability, ribosome biogenesis, initiation and elongation steps of mRNA translation, and the regulation of preexisting enzymes (Fig. 17.1). The effect of insulin

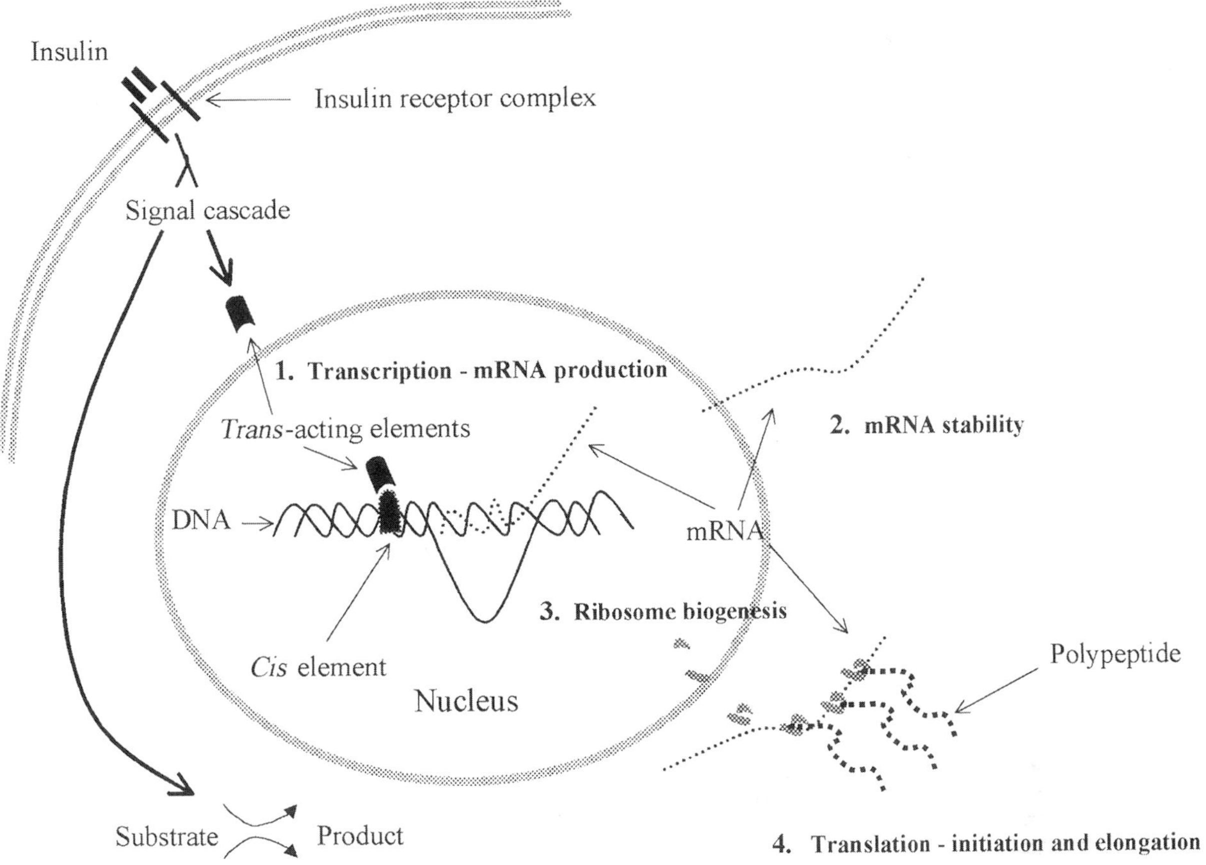

Figure 17.1. Sites of action of insulin in the regulation of protein synthesis. Insulin action depends on binding to the insulin receptor complex and initiation of a cascade of steps leading to its ultimate effect on protein synthesis. Insulin effects have been shown at various levels: (*1*) transcription of genetic message to mRNA; (*2*) contribution to mRNA stability; (*3*) biogenesis of ribosomes; and (*4*) translation—both at initiation and elongation. (See text for details of effects of each of these steps.)

on gene transcription is usually viewed in terms of the *cis/trans* hypothesis, in which intracellular *trans*-acting factors bind to *cis*-acting DNA sites in the nucleus. The specific gene sites affected by insulin are referred to as insulin response sequences or elements (IRSs/IREs), which are usually located in the gene promoter region. Positive or negative effects can be mediated through these *cis/trans* interactions. Reputed IREs for a variety of genes, including glyceraldehyde 3-phosphate dehydrogenase, pyruvate kinase, glucagon, phosphoenolpyruvate carboxykinase (PEPCK), and insulin-like growth factor binding protein 1, have been identified (15). The transmission of the insulin signal to these genes could presumably upregulate the encoded protein, in isolation or in addition to the effects of insulin on general cellular protein synthesis, by producing more mRNA for translation. Examples of mRNAs that are selectively increased by insulin include eukaryotic elongation factor 2 (eEF-2) (45), phosphorylated heat- and acid-stable protein (PHAS-I) (46), and myosin heavy chain α (47).

Insulin can also exert a selective influence on protein synthesis by stabilizing specific mRNA species. Degradation of mRNA can be measured by a decrease in radiolabel in an mRNA species prelabeled before the experiment, usually in the presence of transcription inhibitors. In these studies, stabilization of mRNA by insulin has been demonstrated for glycerol 3-phosphate dehydrogenase, glycogen phosphorylase, and glucose transporter 1 (GLUT1), among others (15,48). Conversely, insulin has been shown to destabilize some mRNAs, such as PEPCK (49,50) and GLUT4 (50). This leads to the interesting observation that insulin can stabilize some mRNA species and destabilize others within the same cell, further demonstrating the intricacy by which insulin regulates cell function. An example is the divergent effect of insulin on the stability of glycogen phosphorylase (48) and phosphoenolpyruvate carboxykinase mRNAs within hepatocytes (49). The specific mechanisms by which insulin influences mRNA stability are poorly understood at present.

Protein translation involves a complex set of reactions that decode the genetic information provided by mRNA into a polypeptide chain. Translation usually is divided into three phases: initiation, elongation, and termination. Protein-chain initiation involves binding of a methionyl-transfer RNA (tRNA) to a start codon in the mRNA, which in turn binds to 40S and 60S ribosomal subunits. The resulting mRNA-ribosome unit then adds tRNA-bound amino acid residues to the elongating peptide chain. Termination is the phase in which the completed polypeptide chain is released from the ribosome. Translational efficiency, particularly with regard to the initiation and elongation phases, has been a major focus of investigations of the effects of insulin on cellular protein synthesis. This is important because increases in translational efficiency have the potential to increase protein synthesis without necessarily changing the total RNA content. The mechanisms by which insulin affects translation have been the topic of a recent comprehensive review (51). In general, this occurs through a series of interactions of the mRNA, ribosomal subunits, and specific binding and initiation factors, often involving the phosphorylation of one or more of these factors (52–56). Initiation starts with the binding of methionyl-tRNA to the 40S ribosomal subunit mediated by eIF-2 (51,57). It is noteworthy that eIF-2 will bind methionyl-tRNA only when the eIF-2 is complexed with guanosine triphosphate (GTP). Another initiation factor, eIF-2B, controls the recycling of eIF-2 between its GTP-bound and guanosine diphosphate (GDP)–bound forms. Methionyl-tRNA recruitment to the 40S ribosomal subunit is followed by mRNA binding and subsequent joining to the 60S ribosomal subunit. The resulting 80S initiation complex is then competent to enter the elongation phase. Insulin regulates the initiation of translation in part by enhancing the binding of mRNA to the 40S ribosomal subunit. One important step in this process requires attachment of the eIF–4E (cap-binding protein) and the eIF-4E–binding proteins PHAS-1 (4E-BP1) and eIF-4G to the 7-methyl guanine cap structure at the 5′ end of eukaryotic mRNAs (13,58,53,54). Insulin and perhaps other hormones stimulate this process by enhancing the phosphorylation of PHAS-1, dissociating it from eIF-4E so that eIF-4E can complex with eIF-4G, which associates with the 40S ribosomal subunit (58). Insulin has also been shown to increase the activity of eIF-2B, which regenerates eIF-2 as noted above (54,59). Rats made insulin deficient by blocking insulin secretion with diazoxide show a large decrease in the binding of eIF-4E to eIF-4G and an increase in eIF-4E * 4E-BP1 complex formation (56).

Insulin may increase protein synthesis by selectively upregulating the initiation of translation of mRNAs containing a polypyrimidine tract at their 5′ transcriptional start site. These mRNAs encode important components of the translational apparatus, including ribosomal proteins and translational elongation factors that would likely increase the overall capacity of the cell for protein synthesis. Translation of such 5′-polypyrimidine mRNAs appears to be regulated in part via multisite phosphorylation of the 40S ribosomal protein S6 by p70 S6 kinase ($p70^{S6K}$) (60,61). An increase in S6 phosphorylation has been observed in a variety of cells in culture exposed to insulin [reviewed in references (14,62–64)], and S6 phosphorylation generally correlates with increased protein synthesis (63). Investigators have shown that expression of a dominant interfering mutant of $p70^{S6K}$, which prevents the activation of wild-type $p70^{S6K}$, blocks serum-activated translation of 5′-polypyrimidine tract mRNA in human kidney 293 cells (61).

The elongation phase of protein synthesis involves the progressive addition of amino acyl-tRNAs to the ribosomal mRNA complex, causing a lengthening of the peptide chain until termination. At least two elongation factors (eEF-1 and eEF-2) are important in facilitating this process. The eEF-1 factor is complexed with GTP in a fashion similar to that described above for eIF-2, and GTP-bound eEF-2 mediates the attachment of amino acyl-tRNA to the ribosome. Subsequently, eEF-2 is required for the movement of the ribosome relative to the mRNA and for migration of the amino acyl-tRNA from the acceptor site to the peptidyl site of the ribosome (65). Like eEF-1, eEF-2 is a phosphoprotein and is regulated by insulin. Phosphorylation of eEF-2 by way of eEF-2 kinase results in its complete inactivation (66). Insulin appears to increase the rate of elongation by the inactivation of eEF-2 kinase through a pathway sensitive to the antifungal agent rapamycin, which is discussed in greater detail below (67). Collectively, these studies indicate that insulin may enhance important steps in translation initiation and elongation. The significance of these steps in insulin-stimulated protein synthesis and the steps that are rate limiting remain to be determined.

The capacity of the cell to synthesize protein can be determined in part by the abundance of ribosomes. As noted above, ribosomes are essential components of the translational machinery, and their biogenesis involves the synthesis of approximately 80 ribosomal proteins and four rRNA species transcribed by RNA polymerases I (18S, 28S, 5.8S) or III (5S) (68,69). Production of ribosomal precursor molecules is dependent on the stage of cellular development, nutrient levels, growth factors, and hormones (69,70). Nucleoli contain the rRNA genes and are the sites of rRNA synthesis, processing, and assembly into ribosomes. To accommodate the demand for rapid production of large numbers of ribosomes, the rRNA transcription units are repeated in tandem up to 1,000 times in eukaryotic nucleolar sites (71). From the nucleolus, the components must be packaged and moved to the cytoplasm, where translation occurs. Insulin has been shown to increase the synthesis of ribosomal proteins fourfold in chick embryo fibroblasts (72) and to stimulate ribosomal protein synthesis in mouse myoblasts (73).

Although the mechanisms by which insulin increases the cellular content of functional ribosomal complexes are still largely unknown, there is evidence for a significant effect of insulin on posttranscriptional events (72,73). For example, the addition of insulin results in a selective increase in the fraction of ribosomal protein mRNAs associated with polysomes in mouse myoblasts (73), and the association of polysomes with the cellular cytoskeleton is increased in response to insulin when protein synthesis increases (74,75). The synthesis of rRNA species also is stimulated by insulin in a variety of cell types, including fibroblasts (72,76), myoblasts (73), and hepatocytes (77). Changes in rDNA transcription can involve changes in chromatin structure to permit the formation of initiation complex, alterations in RNA polymerase activity, or alterations in associated transcription factors. Insulin-stimulated increases in rRNA transcription in mouse fibroblasts and a rat hepatoma cell line are not associated with a change in the cellular content of RNA polymerase I (76). However, increases in upstream binding factor (UBF) and RNA polymerase I–associated factor 53 have been observed; both appear to aid in recruitment of RNA polymerase I to the rDNA promoter. It is interesting that overexpression of UBF in mouse fibroblasts was able to directly stimulate rDNA transcription (76). Finally, insulin may also diminish the rate of ribosome degradation (14,77,78).

The transmission of the insulin signal from outside the cell through the plasma membrane and cytoplasm and into the nucleus, where it can influence *trans*-acting factors, is an important component of insulin action. At least two general pathways by which insulin may affect gene transcription have been suggested. The first is the classical signal transduction in which formation of an insulin-receptor complex at the plasma membrane transmits a cascading signal through the cytoplasm into the nucleus via second-messenger molecules and protein phosphorylation/dephosphorylation reactions. The second, and less firmly established, pathway involves the effects of insulin on intracellular receptors (79). This hypothesis is supported by several reports of mediation of changes in transcription by internalized insulin (79–81) through nuclear insulin receptors (82,83). Whether direct insulin interactions with nuclear receptors and DNA IREs have important effects on protein synthesis is unknown.

Although direct nuclear actions may be significant, insulin is thought to exert most of its effects by changing the phosphorylation state of various regulatory proteins important to protein synthetic pathways via classical signal transduction (14). This pathway involves autophosphorylation of insulin receptors initiated by the binding of insulin, followed by increased tyrosine phosphorylation of intracellular proteins such as insulin-receptor substrates (IRS-1, IRS-2, IRS-3, and IRS-4) and the protein Shc. IRS-1 is the best characterized of the IRS family of proteins. Its phosphorylated tyrosine sites are thought to associate with high-affinity *src* homology 2 domain (SH2)–containing proteins such as on the 85-kDa regulatory subunit (p85) of phosphoinositide 3-kinase (PI 3-kinase). Of note, both the insulin receptor and IRS-1 appear to be required for the insulin-mediated stimulation of general and growth-related protein synthesis (84). PI 3-kinase is emerging as the only phosphotyrosine-activated effector downstream of IRS-1 that is essential for protein synthesis (84–87). LY 294002, a specific inhibitor of PI 3-kinase, completely prevents insulin-mediated stimulation of protein synthesis in rat skeletal muscle (86). A number of other effectors downstream of IRS-1 are also being investigated for their roles in insulin signaling to protein synthesis, including protein kinase C (59,88), ras (89), mitogen-activated protein (MAP) kinases (85), $p70^{S6K}$ (85), and PHAS-1 (13,55,86,90).

There appear to be essentially two mechanisms of insulin-stimulated protein synthesis, one controlled by PI 3-kinase and the other by the GTP-binding protein $p21^{ras}$ (87,88). The insulin-stimulated PI 3-kinase pathway appears to exert its effect primarily by way of the Ser/Thr protein kinase Akt and subsequent activation of $p70^{S6K}$ (91) and PHAS-1 (92). Akt and $p70^{S6K}$ can be activated directly by the products of PI 3-kinase, phosphatidylinositol 3,4-bisphosphate and phosphatidylinositol 3,4,5-trisphosphate (93). The use of the antifungal agent rapamycin helps in characterizing the pathway downstream of PI 3-kinase and Akt by acting at the level of TOR (target of rapamycin; mTOR in mammalian cells), a novel protein kinase, which appears to be on the pathway between Akt and both $p70^{S6K}$ and PHAS-1. Rapamycin inhibits activation of both of these factors (46,84,86,88,94) and attenuates insulin-stimulated protein synthesis (13,85,86). Alternatively, there appears to be a rapamycin-independent pathway involving an atypical protein kinase C isoform (PKCζ) downstream from PI 3-kinase involved in insulin-stimulated protein synthesis (88). It has been suggested that one pathway, through PKCζ, leads to general or "housekeeping" protein synthesis, whereas the other pathway, through Akt, stimulates growth-regulated protein synthesis (88).

Insulin stimulates Ras activity by two known mechanisms that involve binding the Grb/SOS complex by either Shc or IRS-1 (51,95) and subsequently leading to the formation of the active GTP-bound state of Ras. Ras then stimulates a cascade of protein serine/threonine kinase events that involve Raf, MEK, and the MAP kinases ERK1 and ERK2 (96,97). However, it is uncertain whether the activation of the MAP kinases contributes significantly to insulin-stimulated protein synthesis (13,84,98). Furthermore, it is important to note that the PI 3-kinase and $p21^{ras}$ branches are not completely separate and that there is evidence that PI 3-kinase may be upstream of ras under some conditions (87,99,100). Of interest is the finding that increases in IRS-1 tyrosine phosphorylation (101), PI 3-kinase activity (102), p85–PI 3-kinase mRNA expression (101), and Akt kinase activity (103) in response to insulin are diminished in skeletal muscle of patients with type 2 diabetes.

Protein Breakdown

A normal 70-kg adult synthesizes and degrades approximately 280 g of protein each day under standardized conditions (104). Most of this protein turnover occurs within cells. Intracellular protein turnover is continuous, albeit at vastly different rates (i.e., different protein half-lives), depending on the identity, function, and location of the protein, as well as on the physiologic state of the organism. Catabolic states such as acute starvation or untreated type 1 diabetes result in increased protein breakdown, particularly from skeletal muscle, which is an important reservoir of amino acids under these conditions. The resulting increase in circulating amino acids provides precursors for protein resynthesis and for gluconeogenesis in the liver, and the BCAA offer an additional energy source for the remaining muscle tissue. The amino acids from protein breakdown also are crucial for maintaining synthesis rates of essential proteins such as clotting factors produced by the liver. Fortunately, the regulation of cellular protein breakdown is highly specific and precise—often able to select less essential proteins for breakdown, to the overall benefit of the organism. The regulatory mechanisms responsible for this specificity in protein breakdown remain to be defined. Rapid or sustained breakdown of protein, as occurs in starvation, catabolic disease states, and other severe physiologic stresses, may result not only in losses in muscle mass but also in an overall disruption of homeostasis. Understanding the cellular mechanisms involved in protein breakdown is an essential step toward developing pharmacologic or other interventions that might reduce excessive losses of essential proteins during catabolic conditions.

It is important to emphasize that the influence of protein breakdown extends to the regulation of cell function under all physiologic conditions and not just to catabolic states. Generally, this essential regulatory process is observed as enzymes, transcription factors, receptors, and other signaling proteins undergo selective degradation. For example, the levels of gluconeogenic enzymes, such as PEPCK, increase in rat liver with fasting and promptly decrease after refeeding (105,106). Such rapid fluctuations in hepatic cell enzyme content require a significant change in the ratio of protein breakdown to protein synthesis. Another example of the mediation of metabolic change by protein breakdown is evident in the degradation of enzymes such as glutamine synthetase, ornithine decarboxylase, and 3-hydroxy-3-methylglutaryl coenzyme A (HMG-CoA) reductase in response to the accumulation of their reaction products (107). Alternatively, a decrease in the breakdown of a family of proteins known as heat-shock proteins (e.g., hsp70) occurs when cells are exposed to heat treatment (108). Heat-shock proteins appear to be cytoprotective during a variety of cellular insults, in part by facilitating the recovery of metabolic pathways that have been perturbed by cellular stress (109). It is interesting that hsp70 and cofactors known as DnaJ homologues are themselves essential in the preparation of certain abnormal proteins for breakdown in eukaryotic cells (110). In summary, protein breakdown is essential for cellular well-being through its roles in eliminating potentially lethal accumulations of abnormal, damaged, or foreign proteins; promoting normal tissue remodeling and repair; facilitating regulation of numerous metabolic pathways; and providing nutritive substrates in catabolic states. Defects in protein breakdown mechanisms clearly have the potential to cause abnormal tissue growth, whereas accelerated protein breakdown can result in tissue or organ wasting.

Our information on the control of protein breakdown is limited compared with that on insulin-mediated protein synthesis. Nevertheless, it is known that cellular protein breakdown can occur via several mechanisms, including (a) lysosomal pathways, (b) the adenosine triphosphate (ATP)–dependent ubiquitin-proteosome pathway, (c) Ca^{2+}-dependent proteases, and (d) ATP-independent pathways. Protein degradation within lysosomes involves several acid proteases called cathepsins and other hydrolases. Lysosomal pathways are responsible for degrading the long-lived protein pool ($t_{1/2}$ ~40 hours) in the liver, which includes the vast majority (>99%) of hepatic proteins (111).

Amino acid and/or insulin deprivation, glucagon, and β-agonists have been shown to induce lysosomal autophagy of this hepatic protein pool. A short-lived hepatic protein pool ($t_{1/2}$ ~10 minutes) is also present but does not appear to be regulated and probably is subject to nonlysosomal breakdown. In most tissues, lysosomal pathways are primarily those responsible for degrading extracellular, membrane, and organellar proteins. Examples include the downregulation of plasma membrane receptors or the breakdown of proteins identified by the immune system and presented on cell-surface major histocompatibility complex class II molecules. Lysosomal mechanisms can account for up to 10% to 20% of overall protein breakdown in skeletal muscle (112) but are quantitatively unimportant when considering protein breakdown during catabolic states.

The majority of proteins in mammalian cells are degraded by the ubiquitin-proteosome pathway, which is particularly important during catabolic conditions (113). This process involves the selective marking of proteins for breakdown by covalent conjugation to a small protein called ubiquitin (Fig. 17.2). The mechanism involves the formation by an E1 ubiquitin-conjugating enzyme of a high-energy thioester linkage with the COOH-terminal end of the peptide ubiquitin, a process that requires ATP. The activated ubiquitin is then transferred to carriers called E2 proteins, and the carboxyl group is coupled to the ε-amino groups of lysines on the target proteins by a ubiquitin-protein ligase known as E3. Multiple ubiquitin molecules are added in a chain, and the targeted protein then is recognized and degraded by an ATP-dependent complex known as the 26S proteosome (104). Ubiquitin conjugation appears to be the rate-limiting step of the pathway (114,115). The 26S proteosome consists of a 20S core proteosome and a 19S complex that recognizes ubiquitin-conjugated proteins (104). Nonspecific protein digestion is prevented in part by limiting proteolysis to unfolded proteins. This specificity is accomplished via the 19S complex, which catalyzes the unfolding of ubiquitin-targeted proteins and facilitates their transport into the central chamber of the 20S core proteosome for proteolytic cleavage (90,116–118). A variety of specific E2 carrier protein and E3 enzyme pairs impart another important level of selectivity through their capacity to catalyze the ubiquitization of certain targeted proteins or classes of proteins (119,115,120). One particular pair, $E2_{14k}$ and E3α, account for most of the ubiquitin conjugation that occurs in soluble extracts from skeletal muscle (121). Conjugation by this pathway has been termed the "N-end rule pathway" (122). This term originates from the fact that E3α recognizes proteins that contain basic and hydrophobic amino acids at the NH_2-terminus.

Studies of muscles removed from acidotic and septic animals have been used to assess the involvement of the ubiquitin-proteosome pathway in catabolic states. When these muscles are incubated in the presence of a specific proteosome inhibitor (MG132), protein breakdown decreases to levels similar to those in control muscles (123–125). Studies of atrophying muscles under similar conditions have demonstrated an increase in levels of mRNAs that encode for several components of the ubiquitin-proteosome pathway, including ubiquitin, E2, and certain proteosomal subunits (112,126–128). However, this increase has not necessarily resulted in increases in the corresponding encoded proteins (126).

There is evidence for the involvement of the ubiquitin-proteosome pathway in accelerated protein breakdown in animal models of diabetes mellitus. For example, increases in muscle protein in rats made acutely insulinopenic with injections of streptozotocin can be greatly blunted by inhibition of ATP synthesis (129). This does not occur with selective inhibitors of lysosomal function or calcium-dependent proteases. In another study, the ubiquitin-proteosome and calcium-dependent pathways, but not the lysosomal pathway, were shown to be activated in muscles from streptozotocin-treated rats (130). Further evidence for upregulation of the ubiquitin-proteosome system in muscle during insulinopenia are the increases in mRNAs for proteosome and ubiquitin subunits and in the transcription rate of the ubiquitin gene (129). An interesting finding is an increase in ubiquitin binding to endogenous muscle proteins in acutely diabetic rats (126). This increase in ubiquitization occurs primarily through the N-end rule pathway and appears to be rate limiting for protein

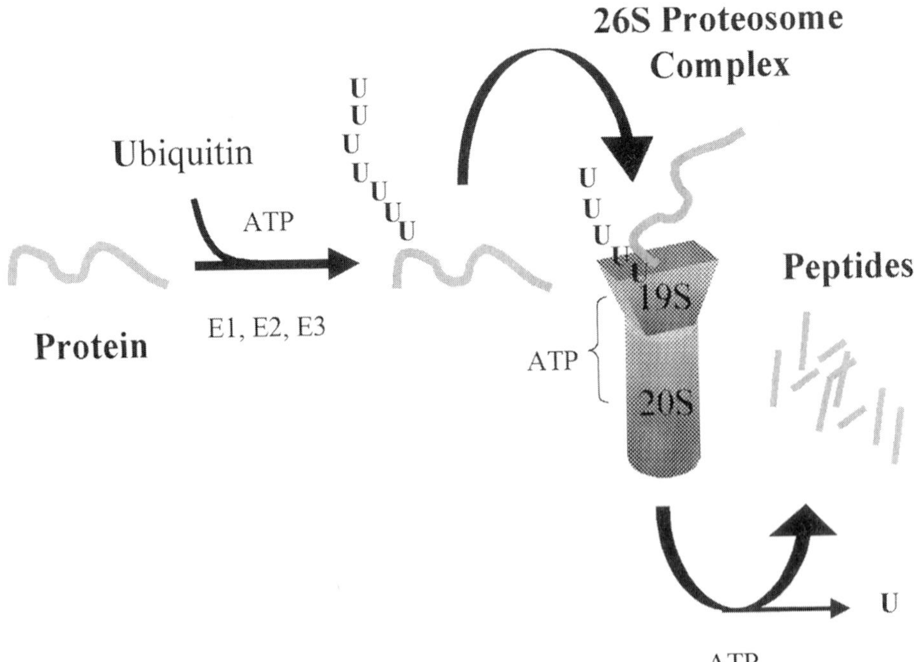

Figure 17.2. The ubiquitin-proteosome pathway for protein breakdown. Proteins are marked for degradation by covalent conjugation to multiple ubiquitin molecules (U) forming a chain. This process is mediated by E1, E2, and E3 proteins and is adenosine triphosphate (ATP) dependent. The targeted protein is degraded by the 26S proteosome complex, which consists of a 20S core proteosome and a 19S complex that recognizes ubiquitin-conjugated proteins. Proteins bind to the 19S subunit and are transferred to 20S proteosome, a process that releases the ubiquitin chain and requires ATP. Multiple proteolytic sites within the 20S proteosome degrade the protein (details are given in text).

breakdown. Treatment of diabetic rats with insulin for at least 24 hours reverses the breakdown of muscle protein and returns the mRNAs for the ubiquitin-proteosome pathway to control levels (131). The potential for interplay of insulin depletion with other hormone systems is illustrated by an apparent glucocorticoid requirement for pathway activation. This can be observed in the prevention of accelerated muscle protein breakdown in diabetic rats by adrenalectomy and the restoration of accelerated protein breakdown with subsequent administration of glucocorticoids (131). Increased cortisol levels are not universally observed in humans during insulin deprivation, and cortisol dependency of ubiquitin-proteosome–mediated protein breakdown under these conditions remains to be established. Collectively, these findings suggest that the ubiquitin-proteosome pathway is important in stimulating the breakdown of muscle protein during severe insulin deprivation and that insulin limits ubiquitin-proteosome activity under normal conditions. The molecular mechanisms that cause the inhibition of protein breakdown in response to physiologic as opposed to pathologic changes in circulating insulin levels remain to be established.

PROTEIN-TURNOVER METHODOLOGY

Whole-Body Study Methods

Most studies examining whole-body protein turnover in humans use a model based on the assumption that the entire protein pool exists as one compartment (Fig. 17.3). With this model, net protein turnover can be calculated as the difference between the degradation and synthesis of body protein. Net urinary nitrogen loss approximates net protein loss. The balance between protein breakdown, protein synthesis, amino acid oxidation, and exogenous amino acid input from dietary proteins determines the pool of free amino acids. A labeled (stable or radioactive isotope) essential amino acid (e.g., L-[1-^{13}C] or [1-^{14}C]leucine) can be used in tracer amounts in a primed continuous infusion to estimate whole-body protein synthesis, breakdown, and amino acid oxidation. The acquisition of a plateau steady state in the plasma, which is essential for the validity of these calculations, can be reached within 90 to 180 minutes of infusion. In the postabsorptive state, dietary protein can be effectively eliminated from the model so that free-leucine enrichment is diluted only by the appearance of leucine from protein breakdown. Consequently, protein breakdown can be estimated directly from leucine flux when leucine is labeled in the carboxyl moiety (1-C), which is not synthesized in the body. Because the only known fates of leucine are protein synthesis and oxidation, whole-body protein synthesis under steady-state conditions often is estimated by subtracting leucine oxidation from leucine flux. Leucine oxidation can be calculated from $^{13}CO_2$ production using ^{13}C enrichment of α-ketoisocaproate (KIC), which is the immediate transamination product of intracellular leucine (132–134). Similar measurements can be obtained using other isotopic amino acid tracers including [$^{2}H_3$]phenylalanine, [^{15}N]phenylalanine, and L-[1-^{13}C,^{15}N]leucine, albeit using somewhat different assumptions and having unique advantages for specific applications [reviewed in references (133) and (135)]. For example, L-[1-^{13}C,^{15}N]leucine can be used to determine nitrogen flux of leucine or transamination or both (136–138).

Methods for the Study of Regional Protein Metabolism

Measurement of whole-body protein dynamics represents the combined changes occurring in all the tissues of the body. Therefore, this method yields little information about the specific contributions of different tissues, organ beds, or proteins. It can be important to assess more localized protein dynamics,

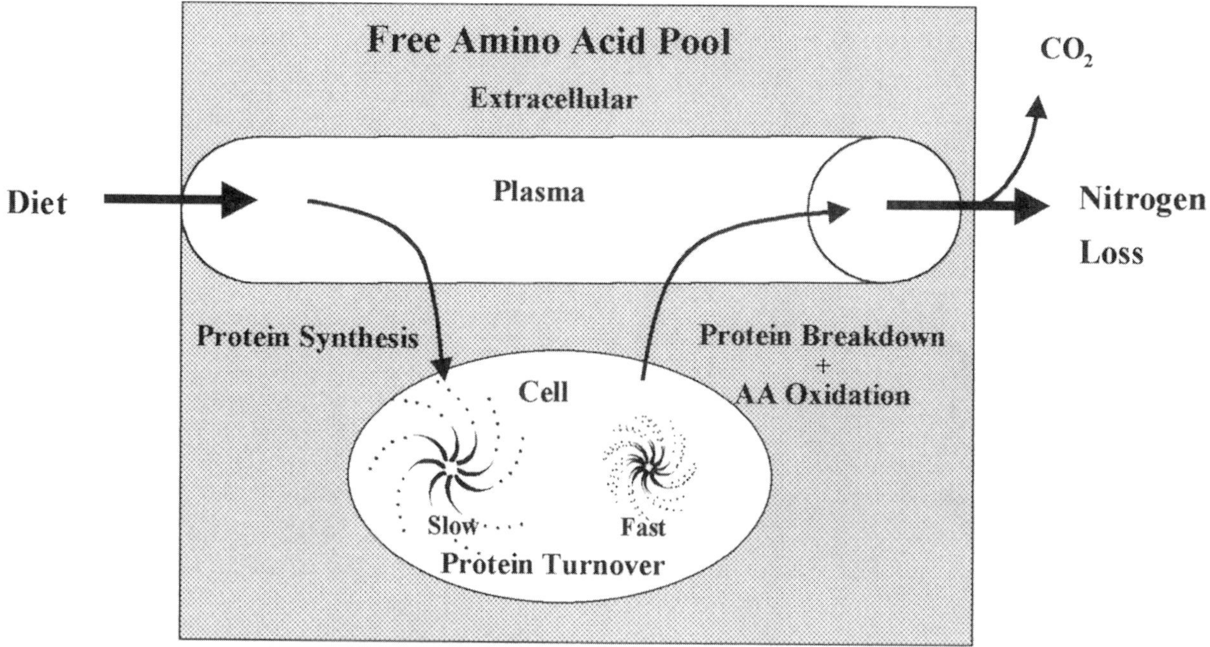

Figure 17.3. A model for *in vivo* protein turnover. The traditional way of determining protein balance is by measuring the net loss of nitrogen (nitrogen intake minus nitrogen output), which is determined by the balance between protein breakdown and protein synthesis. Although organs such as skeletal muscle constitute the major stores of body proteins, the pace of turnover (breakdown and synthesis) of proteins in muscle is much slower than that in other organs, such as gut and liver. As a result, the major contributors to the whole-body protein turnover are those organs with a fast rate of protein turnover. AA, amino acid.

because protein turnover occurs in individual tissues at distinct rates, and in the same tissue, specific proteins can be synthesized and degraded at different rates (139–142). For example, skeletal muscle constitutes greater than 60% of the cell mass in most individuals, while contributing less than 30% to the whole-body protein synthesis (44). This is the consequence of a much slower overall protein synthesis rate in skeletal muscle than in other tissues such as the liver (139). Some proteins in skeletal muscle are synthesized at slower rates [e.g., myosin heavy chain (143)] than others [e.g., mitochondrial proteins (144)]. Similarly, the rates of synthesis of some liver proteins, including apoB-100 and fibrinogen, are faster than the rate of synthesis of albumin (145). Individual proteins also are affected differently by factors regulating protein turnover, as indicated, for example, by the differential effect of insulin on the hepatic synthesis rates of albumin and fibrinogen (145,146). Although it is essential to measure the synthesis rates of individual proteins when considering mechanisms underlying abnormal protein levels, regional studies across tissue and organ beds also have great importance for understanding the interorgan transfer of amino acids that is essential for maintaining optimal whole-body function over a range of physiologic conditions. It is important to recognize that insulin is a key hormone regulating interorgan transfer of amino acids, as well as a regulator of the synthesis of specific proteins.

Many techniques are available for measuring protein turnover from individual tissue beds and synthesis rates of specific proteins. Some methods involve measuring the flux of labeled amino acids in the steady state and blood flow across a limb or tissue bed through arterial and venous sampling. For example, protein turnover in skeletal muscle can be measured by placing a venous catheter in the femoral vein or a deep forearm vein that drains primarily muscle tissue. An arterial catheter is also placed so that blood entering the muscle bed can be sampled. These techniques are helpful for estimating the relative contribution of skeletal muscle to whole-body protein turnover. However, their interpretation is complicated by the fact that in most cases multiple tissues constitute a given vascular bed. Although tissues such as bone, skin, and fat may be minor contributors in a limb, they ultimately cannot be discounted when protein synthesis and breakdown are considered. As an alternative method, the incorporation of labeled amino acids into mixed proteins or individual proteins from tissue biopsy samples (e.g., vastus lateralis muscle) can be measured to determine the effects of hormones, substrates, and altered physiologic states on rates of protein synthesis in specific tissue types (133). In this way the contributions to protein synthesis of minor tissues within a vascular bed can be eliminated. *In vivo* measurement of protein breakdown from a tissue bed or anatomic region remains limited to arteriovenous studies.

TYPE 1 DIABETES MELLITUS

Whole-Body Protein Turnover

Numerous studies have demonstrated increased protein breakdown and increased protein synthesis, indicated by a high leucine flux and nonoxidative leucine flux, respectively, in type 1 diabetes during insulin deprivation (31,35,36,138,147–151). An increase in amino acid oxidation with insulin deficiency has also been demonstrated in many studies by increases in leucine oxidation and urinary nitrogen excretion. Furthermore, leucine nitrogen flux resulting from leucine transamination is increased. A net catabolic effect occurs during insulin deprivation because the increase in protein breakdown is greater than the increase in protein synthesis. Insulin infusion can reduce both whole-body protein breakdown and synthesis, but the magnitude of the effect on breakdown exceeds that of synthesis, resulting in net protein anabolism (138,147–149,152). These responses have been confirmed in prepubertal children with type 1 diabetes (153). The effect of infusing amino acids with insulin has been studied in patients with type 1 diabetes, as described earlier in this chapter for subjects without diabetes. These investigations consistently demonstrate decreases in endogenous protein breakdown and increases in leucine oxidation (31,34,35). In addition, there is evidence for increased whole-body protein synthesis during insulin and amino acid infusion in two of the published studies (34,35) but not in a third study (31). Therefore, decreased availability of amino acid substrate may contribute to the reduction in protein synthesis observed in the studies that replace insulin without amino acid supplementation. In summary, insulin deprivation associated with type 1 diabetes results in greater increases in whole-body protein breakdown than protein synthesis, resulting in negative net protein balance. Reintroducing insulin appears to improve whole-body protein balance primarily by suppressing protein breakdown.

Regional Protein Turnover

Regional studies of protein turnover are important for determining amino acid traffic from one organ bed to another under various conditions (Fig. 17.4). Amino acid isotope labeling techniques combined with measurements of amino acid concentrations can be used to determine whether a change in protein synthesis and/or breakdown causes a net exchange of amino acids across an organ or tissue bed. With this approach, the skeletal muscle bed has been found to be a major donor of amino acids in the postabsorptive state (40). Muscle releases amino acids as a consequence of increased protein breakdown. The amino acids are taken up by the splanchnic bed (presumably by the liver) and used for synthesis of essential proteins such as clotting factors. During the postprandial state, amino acids absorbed from a meal are taken up in part by the liver and then released to the circulation. Skeletal muscle ultimately takes up a major portion of the circulating amino acids, thus resulting in a transition from net release to net uptake of amino acids. Circulating insulin levels decrease progressively in the postabsorptive state, facilitating protein breakdown, whereas increased circulating insulin and amino acids in the postprandial state not only decrease muscle protein breakdown but also increase the incorporation of amino acids into muscle proteins. It has been demonstrated that insulin deprivation in patients with type 1 diabetes leads to protein breakdown in the splanchnic bed and leg skeletal muscle, whereas protein synthesis increases almost exclusively in the splanchnic bed (138) (Fig. 17.5). Again, a net release of amino acids from muscle occurs during insulin deprivation because of an increase in protein breakdown (Fig. 17.6). By contrast, amino acid uptake increases in the splanchnic bed as a consequence of increased protein synthesis to an extent that exceeds a coincident increase in protein breakdown.

Skeletal Muscle

Skeletal muscle is an extremely important contributor to insulin effects on protein metabolism not only because it represents 50% of total body protein but also because it represents the majority of insulin-responsive tissue in the body. Studies of patients with type 1 diabetes during transient insulin deprivation have

A. Postabsorptive or Low Insulin State

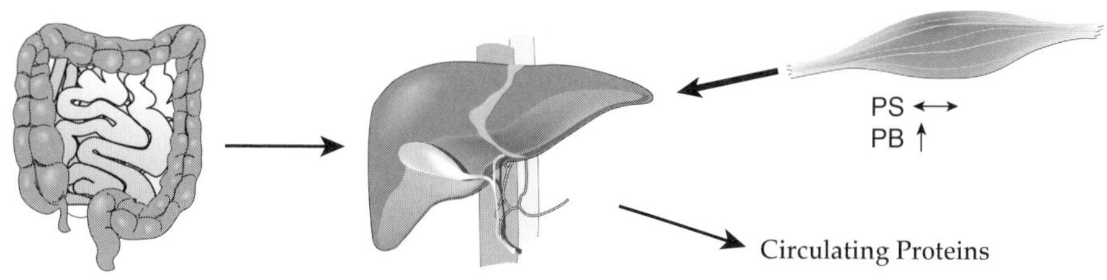

B. Postprandial or High Insulin State

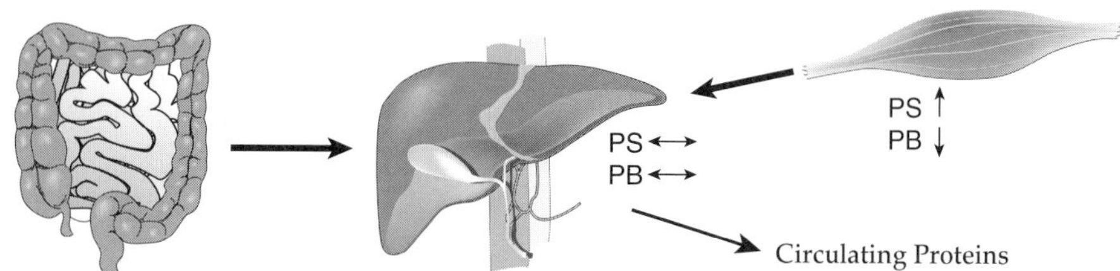

Figure 17.4. Amino acid exchanges across the major organs. The splanchnic bed (presumably reflecting predominantly liver) is a net receiver of amino acids during the postabsorptive state. Liver gets a continuous supply of amino acids so that the synthesis of various essential circulating proteins such as clotting factors can be maintained. There is a net release of amino acids from skeletal muscle [by increasing protein breakdown (PB)] during the postabsorptive state. In contrast, during the postprandial state, muscle is a net receiver of amino acids [by increased protein synthesis (PS) or reduced protein breakdown] and the splanchnic bed (presumably following the absorption of amino acids from the meal) is a net releaser of amino acids. Insulin is the key hormone involved in the regulation of amino acid release from muscle. Insulin inhibits muscle protein breakdown and facilitates the net uptake of amino acids in skeletal muscle in the postprandial state (131).

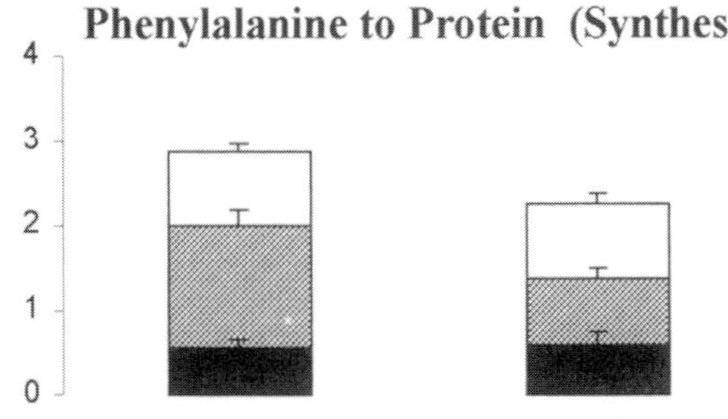

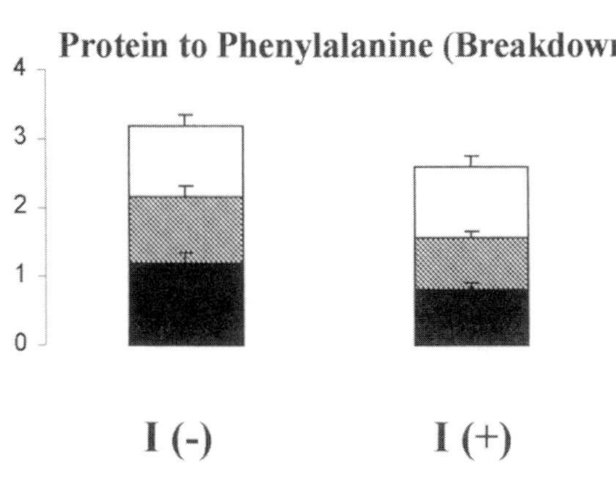

Figure 17.5. Regional protein dynamics in persons with type 1 diabetes during insulin deprivation [I(-)] and insulin treatment [I(+)]. Splanchnic protein turnover is represented by gray, skeletal muscle protein turnover by black, and turnover of other proteins by white. During insulin deprivation, protein breakdown was higher than protein synthesis in skeletal muscle, whereas in the splanchnic bed, protein synthesis was higher than protein breakdown. Insulin treatment decreased both protein breakdown and protein synthesis in the splanchnic bed, resulting in no net change in protein loss. In contrast, insulin treatment decreased only protein breakdown in skeletal muscle, thus resulting in a decrease in net protein loss. Consequently, the entire decrease in protein synthesis observed at the whole-body level during insulin replacement occurred in the splanchnic bed, and the entire protein conservation due to insulin treatment was caused by a decrease in muscle protein breakdown. (Adapted from Nair KS, Ford GC, Ekberg K, et al. Protein dynamics in whole body and in splanchnic and leg tissues in type 1 diabetic patients. *J Clin Invest* 1995;95:2926–2937.)

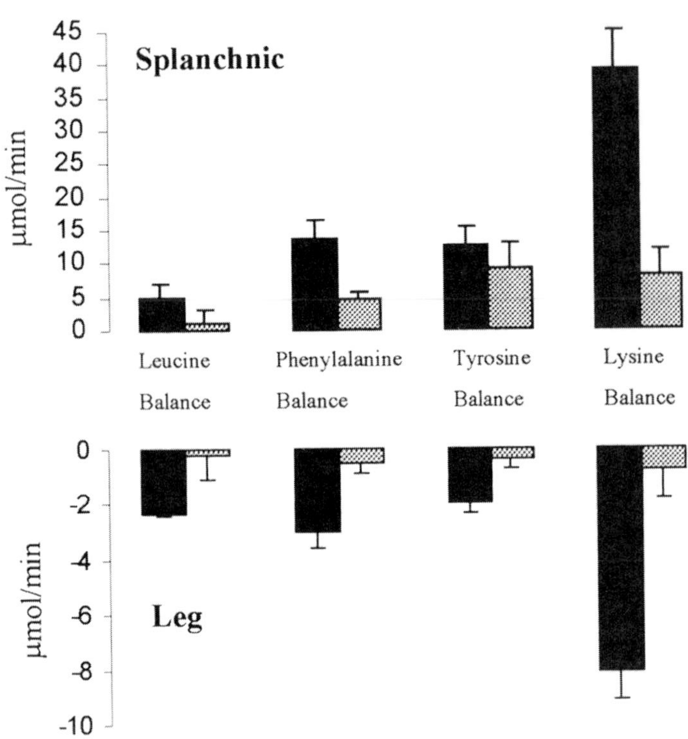

Figure 17.6. Splanchnic bed and leg amino acid balance in patients with type 1 diabetes during insulin deprivation (*black*) and replacement (*gray*). A net release of amino acids from the leg muscle bed and a net uptake of amino acids by the splanchnic bed occur during insulin deprivation. Leucine, phenylalanine, tyrosine, and lysine balance became less negative with insulin replacement in the leg, whereas they became less positive in the splanchnic bed. (Adapted from Nair KS, Ford GC, Ekberg K, et al. Protein dynamics in whole body and in splanchnic and leg tissues in type 1 diabetic patients. *J Clin Invest* 1995;95:2926–2937.)

consistently documented increases in the breakdown of muscle protein without an effect on the synthesis of muscle protein (28,31,132,138,152,154,155,164). These findings are consistent with *in vitro* and *in vivo* studies reporting increased protein breakdown in skeletal muscle from diabetic rats (19,78,129, 130,156–158). However, unlike in humans with type 1 diabetes, rates of synthesis of muscle protein in rats with alloxan- and streptozotocin-induced diabetes (20,158–162) and in eviscerated dogs (163) are consistently decreased compared with rates in control animals. In addition, a recent study demonstrated a significant decrease in protein synthesis in rat muscle during diazoxide-induced postprandial insulin deficiency (56). Collectively, these studies indicate that the loss in muscle protein associated with a deficiency in circulating insulin is caused by an increase in the breakdown of muscle protein, resulting in an increased release of amino acids. Despite the evidence that insulin is a promoter of protein synthesis, acute insulin withdrawal does not appear to decrease protein synthesis in human skeletal muscle.

In cross-limb arteriovenous studies of insulin infusion in patients with type 1 diabetes, most (138,154,155), but not all (152), have demonstrated decreases in protein breakdown, suggesting a direct effect on skeletal muscle. By contrast, protein synthesis measured across the limbs of patients with type 1 diabetes remains unchanged with insulin replacement (138,143, 154,155). Other investigations have used incorporation of amino acids with an isotopic label into protein to measure protein synthesis rates in muscle fractions. These studies also have shown that rates of synthesis of mixed muscle protein (132) and skeletal muscle myosin heavy-chain protein (143) remain unchanged in patients with type 1 diabetes when insulin is replaced (31,143, 154). Again, these findings differ from *in vitro*, *in situ*, and other animal models of insulin deprivation (11–14,16), which consistently have shown that the addition of insulin stimulates protein synthesis (12,15,17,18,20,21). The discrepancy between human and animal studies may represent species differences, the difference between growing rodents and mature humans, or the acute versus chronic nature of the insulin deficiency. Recent studies in a pig model (165) and in nondiabetic humans (166) demonstrated that insulin selectively stimulates the synthesis rate of muscle mitochondrial proteins with no significant effect on myosin heavy chain or sarcoplasmic proteins. These human studies, showing the effect of insulin on muscle mitochondrial protein synthesis, were performed while glucose and amino acids were infused to prevent the insulin-induced fall of these substrates.

Splanchnic Bed

Insulin replacement in patients with type 1 diabetes decreases protein turnover (synthesis and breakdown) in the splanchnic bed (138). The decrease in splanchnic protein synthesis appears to account completely for the decrease in whole-body protein synthesis observed under these conditions. Whether changes in splanchnic protein turnover occur in the liver or intestine or both is not clearly established. In one study (167), a decrease in the rate of protein synthesis was demonstrated in duodenal mucosa obtained endoscopically from insulin-deprived patients with type 1 diabetes. The decrement in mucosal protein synthesis was corrected with insulin treatment. This raises the possibility that diminished synthesis of intestinal mucosal protein may contribute to the development of gastrointestinal complications in patients with poorly controlled type 1 diabetes. Protein turnover and protein balance may be particularly important for gut mucosa remodeling because of the rapid turnover rate of this tissue. The observation that hepatic synthesis of plasma proteins such as fibrinogen is increased during insulin deprivation in patients with type 1 diabetes supports the hypothesis that liver also is a contributor to the increased rate of splanchnic protein synthesis under these conditions (146). Insulin and amino acids have been shown to suppress the breakdown of hepatic proteins in perfused rat liver (140, 168,169), and degradation of hepatic protein is more rapid in livers from diabetic rats than in normal rats (170). A recent human study demonstrated that although insulin has only a limited effect on splanchnic protein turnover, insulin-induced changes in circulating amino acids or increases in amino acids profoundly affect splanchnic protein breakdown (reduction) and protein synthesis (stimulation) (171).

Renal Hypertrophy

The kidney is another organ system that significantly contributes to whole-body protein balance (172), and alterations in protein turnover may contribute to renal complications in patients with diabetes (173). Hypertrophy of the kidney is a consistent finding in early type 1 diabetes in humans (174) and in animal models of diabetes (175–177). An early study attributed the net increase in rat kidney protein mass following streptozotocin induction of diabetes entirely to inhibition of protein breakdown (178). Alternatively, streptozotocin treatment of mice was shown to increase kidney protein breakdown, as determined by a double isotope pulse-chase valine labeling technique, despite the finding of renal hypertrophy (175). This increase in protein breakdown involved mitochondrial, nuclear, microsomal, and cytosolic fractions of the kidney. It therefore was hypothesized that both renal protein synthesis and breakdown are increased with insulin deficiency. However, the increase in protein breakdown during the early stages of diabetes is less than the increase in protein synthesis, resulting in renal hypertrophy. In agreement with this hypothesis are *in vitro* findings of studies of proximal-tubule suspensions from animal kidneys. One study reported higher rates of protein breakdown for incubated opossum proximal tubules in the absence of insulin (179). Another study demonstrated a nearly twofold increase in the incorporation of [^{3}H]valine into proteins obtained from streptozotocin-treated rat proximal tubules compared with that of controls (180). Alternatively, studies of proximal tubules isolated from rats with streptozotocin-induced diabetes have reported decreased protein breakdown rates *in vitro* (181,182). Thus, there is not complete agreement in the literature about the primary mechanism for renal hypertrophy seen in animal models of diabetes. Further studies on renal protein turnover in human diabetes also are needed.

TYPE 2 DIABETES MELLITUS

Whole-Body Protein Turnover

The effects of type 2 diabetes on protein metabolism are less well understood than the effects of type 1 diabetes. Unlike patients with type 1 diabetes, patients with type 2 diabetes are similar to obese individuals without diabetes in terms of protein stores (183). In addition, nitrogen balance studies have shown that lean body mass is preserved in patients with type 2 diabetes even in the setting of hyperglycemia and reduced dietary intake of protein (184). Most studies using isotope-labeled amino acid tracer techniques support the hypothesis that whole-body protein metabolism is affected modestly, if at all, in type 2 diabetes (185–188). For example, whole-body leucine carbon flux (^{13}C), leucine nitrogen flux (^{15}N), and leucine oxidation were not different in obese women without diabetes and obese women with type 2 diabetes (186). In addition, more rigorous insulin therapy that improved plasma glucose did not alter leucine kinetics. Welle and Nair (188) observed an absence of change in leucine kinetics following improved glucose control in obese women with type 2 diabetes after 2 weeks of treatment with an oral hypoglycemic agent (glyburide) and again after 2 weeks of insulin therapy. Luzi et al. (185) found no significant differences in decreased leucine flux, leucine oxidation, and nonoxidative leucine flux during euglycemic hyperinsulinemic clamps in the postabsorptive state in patients with type 2 diabetes and control subjects. When these subjects were given a combined insulin and amino acid infusion, plasma leucine concentration, leucine oxidation, and nonoxidative flux increased and leucine flux decreased as compared with basal values. However, the changes were similar for the subjects with and without diabetes. Alternatively, Denne et al. (189) reported findings consistent with increased whole-body protein breakdown in patients with type 2 diabetes. This study documented an increased rate of whole-body phenylalanine flux in obese subjects with type 2 diabetes during poor glycemic control as compared with obese control subjects without diabetes. Although the rate of protein breakdown was reduced during a hyperinsulinemic euglycemic clamp in the subjects with diabetes, the suppression was not different from that observed in the control subjects. Subsequent treatment of hyperglycemia with intensive insulin therapy did not alter the results in the basal or hyperinsulinemic condition.

Gougeon et al. (190–192) studied integrated feeding-fasting protein metabolism in patients with type 2 diabetes as compared with that in obese subjects without diabetes by a 60-hour oral [^{15}N]glycine method in which urine [^{15}N]urea enrichment is used to measure nitrogen flux and calculate protein synthesis and breakdown. The data suggested that whole-body nitrogen flux, protein synthesis, and protein breakdown are greater in hyperglycemic patients with type 2 diabetes on an isoenergetic diet than in obese control subjects without diabetes. In addition, patients with type 2 diabetes on a low-energy diet with preserved protein content did not completely equilibrate negative nitrogen balance over a 6-week period, in contrast to obese control subjects, despite restoring glycemia to near-normal levels (190). However, exogenous insulin (191) or oral hypoglycemic agents (192) in doses sufficient to improve hyperglycemia improved the altered protein metabolism in the patients with type 2 diabetes.

Collectively, these results suggest that there is a dissociation between the effects of insulin on protein and carbohydrate metabolism in type 2 diabetes. Most studies indicate that whole-body protein metabolism is essentially normal in the postabsorptive state. This suggests that the maximal effect of insulin on protein turnover may occur at basal levels of insulin and that further increases in circulating insulin necessary to achieve normal glucose levels may not have any additional effects. Alternatively, integrated fed-fasting whole-body protein metabolism in patients with type 2 diabetes may be altered during poor glycemic control. This condition requires further investigation.

Regional Protein Turnover

Reports documenting regional protein dynamics in patients with type 2 diabetes are limited. The effects of type 2 diabetes on 3-methylhistidine excretion, an index of myofibrillar protein breakdown, have been studied to a limited extent. In two studies, increases in urinary excretion of 3-methylhistidine were demonstrated in patients with poorly controlled type 2 diabetes as compared with healthy subjects (193) and obese subjects (192) without diabetes. In both studies, excretion of 3-methylhistidine decreased with improved glycemic control. However, patients with type 2 diabetes appear to be less sensitive than patients with type 1 diabetes to glycemic control (193). By contrast, one study using arteriovenous techniques across the leg showed a decrease in [$^{2}H_5$]phenylalanine flux in obese subjects with type 2 diabetes as compared with obese subjects without diabetes, suggesting a decrease in breakdown of skeletal muscle protein (189). Furthermore, euglycemic hyperinsulinemia reduced protein breakdown by 42% across the leg in the subjects without diabetes but did not inhibit breakdown in the subjects with diabetes. Of interest is the increase in BCAA concentrations in obese patients with type 2 diabetes (194,195). However, BCAA concentrations in nonobese subjects with type 2 diabetes and nonobese healthy subjects are comparable (185). Moreover, BCAA levels do not change with improved glycemic control in subjects with type 2 diabetes (186). Limited data are available examining splanchnic protein metabolism in type 2 diabetes. One study reported that postprandial splanchnic uptake of [^{14}C]phenylalanine from a standardized meal in nonobese subjects with type 2 diabetes is not different from that in normal control subjects (196).

ADDITIONAL FACTORS

Other Hormones

Insulin deprivation results in changes in a number of other hormones and substrates (Table 17.1). In many instances, these changes are dependent on the duration of insulin insufficiency. For example, increases in glucagon and growth hormone can occur in the short term, whereas catecholamines, cortisol, and insulin-like growth factor (IGF-1) remain relatively unchanged. An increase in IGF-binding proteins, however, may reduce the free IGF-1 levels (197). After a longer period of insulin deprivation, levels of cortisol, epinephrine, and norepinephrine may increase and the level of IGF-1 may decrease (198). Whole-body studies in humans have shown that elevated concentrations of glucagon during insulin deficiency cause substantial increases in leucine oxidation and resting metabolic rate and a slight increase in protein breakdown (199,200). When insulin is present at normal concentrations, the protein breakdown associated with hyperglucagonemia is normalized (201,202) but leucine oxidation is not (199,202). Furthermore, a somatostatin-induced decline in glucagon levels decreases leucine oxidation but not protein breakdown as indexed by leucine flux (199). These findings suggest that insulin deficiency increases protein breakdown but that hyperglucagonemia is primarily responsible for the increased leucine oxidation observed during insulin deprivation. Glucagon appears to exert its effects primarily on the liver with no apparent effect on skeletal muscle in humans (44).

The roles of the adrenal hormones cortisol and epinephrine in diabetes-induced protein turnover are largely unknown. High-dose glucocorticoids have been shown to increase protein breakdown (203,204) and oxidation (205). However, even though glucocorticoid-induced muscle wasting in humans is well described in Cushing syndrome and during administration of high doses in treatment of various diseases, the effects of these conditions on skeletal muscle protein dynamics remain uncertain (44). Whole-body measurements suggest that epinephrine infusion decreases protein breakdown in the short term (206,207), with no apparent effect after prolonged exposure (208). In skeletal muscle, epinephrine administration appears to decrease protein breakdown and synthesis initially, with improved net protein balance occurring after prolonged treatment, primarily due to a return to normal synthesis rates (209). The anabolic effect of catecholamines is further supported by the use of the potent β-agonist clenbuterol in livestock (210) and by some athletes (211) to increase muscle mass.

Infusion of growth hormone acutely decreases leucine oxidation and increases whole-body protein synthesis (212). Nonmuscle protein synthesis appears to be the greatest contributor to the increases in whole-body protein synthesis observed after administration of growth hormone. However, in studies that measure both protein synthesis and breakdown, positive net muscle protein balance is consistently demonstrated with systemic growth hormone replacement (44). Growth hormone also appears to blunt the decrease in muscle protein breakdown observed in the presence of insulin (213). The direct effects of growth hormone on protein turnover are difficult to distinguish from the effects mediated by IGF-1. One study found that local infusion of growth hormone increased muscle protein synthesis to a greater extent than systemic delivery of growth hormone (214). This suggests a direct action of growth hormone on muscle protein synthesis; however, actions through locally produced IGF-1 and/or IGF-binding proteins in this study cannot be excluded (215,216). Locally delivered IGF-1 has been shown to stimulate synthesis of muscle protein (44,217–219), whereas systemic infusion does not increase whole-body protein synthesis (220). In summary, during insulin deprivation the effects of the so-called counterregulatory hormones may be as important to the changes observed in protein metabolism as insulinopenia itself.

Substrates

Circulating levels of glucose, ketoacids, fatty acids, and amino acids all increase during insulin deprivation. BCAA, especially leucine, have been shown to inhibit whole-body protein breakdown and specifically decrease muscle protein breakdown, while increasing leucine oxidation (198,221). Therefore, increased levels of BCAA may play a pivotal role in preventing rapid depletion of body protein during insulin deficiency. As discussed above, amino acid supplementation to obtain hyperaminoacidemia during insulin infusion usually results

TABLE 17.1. Changes in Hormones and Substrates with Insulin Deprivation

Hormone	Change	Substrate	Change
Glucagon	++	Glucose	++
Cortisol	NC or +	Fatty acids	++
Epinephrine	NC or +	Ketones	+
Norepinephrine	NC or +	Amino acids	++
Growth hormone	+		
Insulin-like growth factor	NC or −		

++, marked increase; +, increase; −, decrease; NC, no change.
Adapted from Nair KS, Schwenk WF. Factors controlling muscle protein synthesis and degradation. *Curr Opin Neurol* 1994;7:471–474, with permission.

in an increase in protein synthesis. Glucose concentration per se has no apparent effect on protein turnover in humans (222). Increased levels of fatty acids are associated with decreases in protein breakdown and leucine oxidation, suggesting a general anabolic effect (203,223). There appears to be no effect of fatty acids on protein synthesis. Alternatively, infusion of β-hydroxybutyrate decreases urinary nitrogen loss and leucine oxidation, while increasing whole-body and muscle protein synthesis (224).

CONCLUSION

It is well established that protein turnover is greatly increased with a net negative nitrogen balance during short-term insulin deprivation in patients with type 1 diabetes. This increased protein loss is almost exclusively due to increased breakdown of muscle protein. Insulin has been shown to act at different levels of the protein synthetic process, although short-term insulin infusion in individuals without diabetes or short-term insulin deprivation in patients with type 1 diabetes has no apparent effect on mixed muscle protein synthesis. Alternatively, insulin seems to have distinct effects on different tissue protein pools and individual proteins. Changes in whole-body or regional protein turnover are much less apparent in type 2 diabetes than in type 1 diabetes. However, little is known about the effects of insulin-resistant conditions on protein turnover in subcellular compartments or on the synthesis of individual proteins. Changes in the turnover dynamics of proteins affecting key regulatory pathways, cellular structure, and/or energy production may be critical to the pathogenesis of diabetes or its associated complications. The subcellular pathways affecting protein synthesis and breakdown in diabetes mellitus are being defined. An exciting era of investigation has been introduced by the sequencing of the human genome and the subsequent development of genome-wide search strategies. Consequently, identifying the protein products of promising diabetes candidate genes will move forward, and protein characterization and an understanding of regulatory events, including turnover dynamics, will become critical. Challenges awaiting investigators include further definition of the contribution of various cell and tissue types to regional protein turnover (e.g., splanchnic bed). In addition, the effects of counterregulatory and other hormones on protein synthesis and breakdown in patients with diabetes need to be more clearly defined. The development of more sophisticated techniques that will aid in the measurement of protein synthesis and breakdown in individual cell compartments and specific proteins will be essential for understanding and ultimately modulating the underlying mechanisms.

Acknowledgments

This work was supported by NIH grants RO1 DK41973 and MO1 RR00585, David Murdock-Dole Professorship (K. S. Nair), and the Mayo Clinic Clinician Investigator Training Program (C. S. Stump).

REFERENCES

1. Geyelin HR, Harrop G, Murray MF, et al. The use of insulin in juvenile diabetes. *J Metab Res* 1922;11:767–791.
2. Osler W, ed. *Practice of medicine*. New York: D. Appleton, 1895;320–330.
3. Frank LL. Diabetes mellitus in the text book of old Hindu medicine. *Am J Gastroenterol* 1957;27:76–95.
4. Atchley DW, Loeb RF, Richards DW, et al. On diabetic acidosis: a detailed study of electrolyte balances following the withdrawal and reestablishment of insulin therapy. *J Clin Invest* 1933;12:297–326.
5. Nair KS, Copeland KC. Protein metabolism in type-I diabetic patients. In: *Protein metabolism in diabetes*. London: Smith-Gordon, 1992;233–242.
6. Solchey SS, Allan FN. The relationship of phosphates to carbohydrate metabolism: The time relationship of the changes in phosphate excretion caused by insulins. *Biochem J* 1924;18:1170–1184.
7. Walsh CH, Soler NG, James H, et al. Studies in whole body potassium and whole body nitrogen in newly diagnosed diabetics. *Q J Med* 1976;45:295–301.
8. Felig P, Wahren J, Sherwin R, et al. Amino acid and protein metabolism in diabetes mellitus. *Arch Intern Med* 1977;137:507–513.
9. Luck JM, Morrison G, Wilbur LF. The effect of insulin on the amino acid content of blood. *J Biol Chem* 1928;77:151–156.
10. Pozefsky T, Santis MR, Soeldner JS, et al. Insulin sensitivity of forearm tissues in prediabetic man. *J Clin Invest* 1973;22:1608–1615.
11. Jefferson LS, Koehler JO, Morgan HE. Effect of insulin on protein synthesis in skeletal muscle of an isolated perfused preparation of rat hemicorpus. *Proc Natl Acad Sci U S A* 1972;69:816–820.
12. Jefferson LS, Li JB, Rannels SR. Regulation by insulin of amino acid release and protein turnover in the perfused rat hemicorpus. *J Biol Chem* 1977;252: 1476–1483.
13. Kimball SR, Horetsky RL, Jefferson LS. Signal transduction pathways involved in the regulation of protein synthesis by insulin in L6 myoblasts. *Am J Physiol* 1998;274:C221–C228.
14. Kimball SR, Vary TC, Jefferson LS. Regulation of protein synthesis by insulin. *Annu Rev Physiol* 1994;56:321–348.
15. O'Brien RM, Granner DK. Regulation of gene expression by insulin. *Physiol Rev* 1996;76:1109–1161.
16. Stirewalt WS, Low RB. Effects of insulin in vitro on protein turnover in rat epitrochlearis muscle. *Biochem J* 1983;210:323–330.
17. Curfman GD, O'Hara DS, Hopkins BE, et al. Suppression of myocardial protein degradation in the rat during fasting. Effects of insulin, glucose, and leucine. *Circ Res* 1980;46:581–589.
18. Jefferson LS, Rannels DE, Munger BL, et al. Insulin in the regulation of protein turnover in heart and skeletal muscle. *Fed Proc* 1974;33:1098–1104.
19. Pain VM, Albertse EC, Garlick PJ. Protein metabolism in skeletal muscle, diaphragm, and heart of diabetic rats. *Am J Physiol* 1983;245:E604–E610.
20. Pain VM, Garlick PJ. Effect of streptozotocin diabetes and insulin treatment on the rate of protein synthesis in tissues of the rat in vivo. *J Biol Chem* 1974;249:4510–4514.
21. Rannels DE, Kao R, Morgan HE. Effect of insulin on protein turnover in heart muscle. *J Biol Chem* 1975;250:1694–1701.
22. Garlick PJ, Grant I. Amino acid infusion increases the sensitivity of muscle protein synthesis in vivo to insulin. Effect of branched-chain amino acids. *Biochem J* 1988;254:579–584.
23. Wray-Cahen D, Nguyen HV, Burrin DG, et al. Response of skeletal muscle protein synthesis to insulin in suckling pigs decreases with development. *Am J Physiol* 1998;275:E602–E609.
24. Mosoni L, Houlier ML, Mirand PP, et al. Effect of amino acids alone or with insulin on muscle and liver protein synthesis in adult and old rats. *Am J Physiol* 1993;264:E614–E620.
25. Baillie AG, Garlick PJ. Attenuated responses of muscle protein synthesis to fasting and insulin in adult female rats. *Am J Physiol* 1992;262:E1–E5.
26. Fulks RM, Li JB, Goldberg AL. Effects of insulin, glucose, and amino acids on protein turnover in rat diaphragm. *J Biol Chem* 1975;250:290–298.
27. Denne SC, Liechty EA, Liu YM, et al. Proteolysis in skeletal muscle and whole body in response to euglycemic hyperinsulinemia in normal adults. *Am J Physiol* 1991;261:E809–E814.
28. Gelfand RA, Barrett EJ. Effect of physiologic hyperinsulinemia on skeletal muscle protein synthesis and breakdown in man. *J Clin Invest* 1987;80:1–6.
29. McNurlan MA, Essen P, Thorell A, et al. Response of protein synthesis in human skeletal muscle to insulin: an investigation with L-[$^2H_5$]phenylalanine. *Am J Physiol* 1994;267:E102–E108.
30. Fukagawa NK, Minaker KL, Rowe JW, et al. Insulin-mediated reduction of whole body protein breakdown. Dose-response effects on leucine metabolism in postabsorptive men. *J Clin Invest* 1985;76:2306–2311.
31. Bennet WM, Connacher AA, Smith K, et al. Inability to stimulate skeletal muscle or whole body protein synthesis in type 1 (insulin-dependent) diabetic patients by insulin-plus-glucose during amino acid infusion: studies of incorporation and turnover of tracer L-[1-^{13}C]leucine. *Diabetologia* 1990;33: 43–51.
32. Castellino P, Luzi L, Simonson DC, et al. Effect of insulin and plasma amino acid concentrations on leucine metabolism in man. Role of substrate availability on estimates of whole body protein synthesis. *J Clin Invest* 1987;80: 1784–1793.
33. Flakoll PJ, Kulaylat M, Frexes-Steed M, et al. Amino acids augment insulin's suppression of whole body proteolysis. *Am J Physiol* 1989;257:E839–E847.
34. Inchiostro S, Biolo G, Bruttomesso D, et al. Effects of insulin and amino acid infusion on leucine and phenylalanine kinetics in type 1 diabetes. *Am J Physiol* 1992;262:E203–E210.
35. Luzi L, Castellino P, Simonson DC, et al. Leucine metabolism in IDDM. Role of insulin and substrate availability. *Diabetes* 1990;39:38–48.
36. Tessari P, Inchiostro S, Biolo G, et al. Differential effects of hyperinsulinemia and hyperaminoacidemia on leucine-carbon metabolism in vivo. Evidence for distinct mechanisms in regulation of net amino acid deposition. *J Clin Invest* 1987;79:1062–1069.

37. Giordano M, Castellino P, Ohno A, et al. Differential effects of amino acid and ketoacid on protein metabolism in humans. *Nutrition* 2000;16:15–21.
38. Hillier TA, Fryburg DA, Jahn LA, et al. Extreme hyperinsulinemia unmasks insulin's effect to stimulate protein synthesis in the human forearm. *Am J Physiol* 1998;274:E1067–E1074.
39. Heslin MJ, Newman E, Wolf RF, et al. Effect of hyperinsulinemia on whole body and skeletal muscle leucine carbon kinetics in humans. *Am J Physiol* 1992;262:E911–E918.
40. Meek SE, Persson M, Ford GC, et al. Differential regulation of amino acid exchange and protein dynamics across splanchnic and skeletal muscle beds by insulin in healthy human subjects. *Diabetes* 1998;47:1824–1835.
41. Moller-Loswick AC, Zachrisson H, Hyltander A, et al. Insulin selectively attenuates breakdown of nonmyofibrillar proteins in peripheral tissues of normal men. *Am J Physiol* 1994;266:E645–E652.
42. Biolo G, Declan Fleming RY, Wolfe RR. Physiologic hyperinsulinemia stimulates protein synthesis and enhances transport of selected amino acids in human skeletal muscle. *J Clin Invest* 1995;95:811–819.
43. Abu-Lebdeh HS, Nair KS. Protein metabolism in diabetes mellitus. *Baillieres Clin Endocrinol Metab* 1996;10:589–601.
44. Rooyackers OE, Nair KS. Hormonal regulation of human muscle protein metabolism. *Annu Rev Nutr* 1997;17:457–485.
45. Levenson RM, Nairn AC, Blackshear PJ. Insulin rapidly induces the biosynthesis of elongation factor 2. *J Biol Chem* 1989;264:11904–12011.
46. Lin TA, Kong X, Saltiel AR, et al. Control of PHAS-I by insulin in 3T3-L1 adipocytes. Synthesis, degradation, and phosphorylation by a rapamycin-sensitive and mitogen-activated protein kinase-independent pathway. *J Biol Chem* 1995;270:18531–18538.
47. Dillmann WH, Barrieux A, Shanker R. Influence of thyroid hormone on myosin heavy chain mRNA and other messenger RNAs in the rat heart. *Endocr Res* 1989;15:565–577.
48. Rao PV, Pugazhenthi S, Khandelwal RL. The effects of streptozotocin-induced diabetes and insulin supplementation on expression of the glycogen phosphorylase gene in rat liver. *J Biol Chem* 1995;270:24955–24960.
49. Christ B, Nath A. The glucagon-insulin antagonism in the regulation of cytosolic protein binding to the 3′ end of phosphoenolpyruvate carboxykinase mRNA in cultured rat hepatocytes. Possible involvement in the stabilization of the mRNA. *Eur J Biochem* 1993;215:541–547.
50. Flores-Riveros JR, McLenithan JC, Ezaki O, et al. Insulin down-regulates expression of the insulin-responsive glucose transporter (GLUT4) gene: effects on transcription and mRNA turnover. *Proc Natl Acad Sci U S A* 1993; 90:512–516.
51. Proud CG, Denton RM. Molecular mechanisms for the control of translation by insulin. *Biochem J* 1997;328(Pt 2):329–341.
52. Harmon CS, Proud CG, Pain VM. Effects of starvation, diabetes and acute insulin treatment on the regulation of polypeptide-chain initiation in rat skeletal muscle. *Biochem J* 1984;223:687–696.
53. Kimball SR, Jefferson LS, Fadden P, et al. Insulin and diabetes cause reciprocal changes in the association of eIF-4E and PHAS-I in rat skeletal muscle. *Am J Physiol* 1996;270:C705–C709.
54. Kimball SR, Jurasinski CV, Lawrence JC Jr, et al. Insulin stimulates protein synthesis in skeletal muscle by enhancing the association of eIF-4E and eIF-4G. *Am J Physiol* 1997;272:C754–C759.
55. Lin TA, Kong X, Haystead TA, et al. PHAS-I as a link between mitogen-activated protein kinase and translation initiation. *Science* 1994;266:653–656.
56. Sinaud S, Balage M, Bayle G, et al. Diazoxide-induced insulin deficiency greatly reduced muscle protein synthesis in rats: involvement of eIF4E. *Am J Physiol* 1999;276:E50–E61.
57. Merrick WC. Mechanism and regulation of eukaryotic protein synthesis. *Microbiol Rev* 1992;56:291–315.
58. Azpiazu I, Saltiel AR, DePaoli-Roach AA, et al. Regulation of both glycogen synthase and PHAS-I by insulin in rat skeletal muscle involves mitogen-activated protein kinase-independent and rapamycin-sensitive pathways. *J Biol Chem* 1996;271:5033.
59. Welsh GI, Proud CG. Evidence for a role for protein kinase C in the stimulation of protein synthesis by insulin in Swiss 3T3 fibroblasts. *FEBS Lett* 1993;316:241–246.
60. Dufner A, Thomas G. Ribosomal S6 kinase signaling and the control of translation. *Exp Cell Res* 1999;253:100–109.
61. Jefferies HB, Fumagalli S, Dennis PB, et al. Rapamycin suppresses 5′TOP mRNA translation through inhibition of p70s6k. *EMBO J* 1997;16:3693–3704.
62. Erikson RL. Structure, expression, and regulation of protein kinases involved in the phosphorylation of ribosomal protein S6. *J Biol Chem* 1991;266: 6007–6010.
63. Proud CG. Protein phosphorylation in translational control. *Curr Top Cell Regul* 1992;32:243–369.
64. Sturgill TW, Wu J. Recent progress in characterization of protein kinase cascades for phosphorylation of ribosomal protein S6. *Biochim Biophys Acta* 1991;1092:350–357.
65. Proud CG. Peptide-chain elongation in eukaryotes. *Mol Biol Rep* 1994;19: 161–170.
66. Redpath NT, Price NT, Severinov KV, et al. Regulation of elongation factor-2 by multisite phosphorylation. *Eur J Biochem* 1993;213:689–699.
67. Redpath NT, Foulstone EJ, Proud CG. Regulation of translation elongation factor-2 by insulin via a rapamycin-sensitive signalling pathway. *EMBO J* 1996;15:2291–2297.
68. Eichler DC, Craig N. Processing of eukaryotic ribosomal RNA. *Prog Nucleic Acid Res Mol Biol* 1994;49:197–239.
69. Larson DE, Zahradka P, Sells BH. Control points in eucaryotic ribosome biogenesis. *Biochem Cell Biol* 1991;69:5–22.
70. Zahradka P, Larson DE, Sells BH. Regulation of ribosome biogenesis in differentiated rat myotubes. *Mol Cell Biochem* 1991;104:189–194.
71. Long EO, Dawid IB. Repeated genes in eukaryotes. *Annu Rev Biochem* 1980;49:727–764.
72. DePhilip RM, Chadwick DE, Ignotz RA, et al. Rapid stimulation by insulin of ribosome synthesis in cultured chick embryo fibroblasts. *Biochemistry* 1979;18:4812–4817.
73. Hammond ML, Bowman LH. Insulin stimulates the translation of ribosomal proteins and the transcription of rDNA in mouse myoblasts. *J Biol Chem* 1988;263:17785–11791.
74. Hesketh JE, Pryme IF. Evidence that insulin increases the proportion of polysomes that are bound to the cytoskeleton in 3T3 fibroblasts. *FEBS Lett* 1988;231:62–66.
75. Vedeler A, Pryme IF, Hesketh JE. Insulin and step-up conditions cause a redistribution of polysomes among free, cytoskeletal-bound and membrane-bound fractions in Krebs II ascites cells. *Cell Biol Int Rep* 1990;14:211–218.
76. Hannan KM, Rothblum LI, Jefferson LS. Regulation of ribosomal DNA transcription by insulin. *Am J Physiol* 1998;275:C130–C138.
77. Antonetti DA, Kimball SR, Horetsky RL, et al. Regulation of rDNA transcription by insulin in primary cultures of rat hepatocytes. *J Biol Chem* 1993;268:25277–25284.
78. Ashford AJ, Pain VM. Effect of diabetes on the rates of synthesis and degradation of ribosomes in rat muscle and liver in vivo. *J Biol Chem* 1986;261: 4059–4065.
79. Harada S, Smith RM, Jarett L. Mechanisms of nuclear translocation of insulin. *Cell Biochem Biophys* 1999;31:307–319.
80. Jans DA. Nuclear signaling pathways for polypeptide ligands and their membrane receptors? *FASEB J* 1994;8:841–847.
81. Miller DS. Stimulation of RNA and protein synthesis by intracellular insulin. *Science* 1988;240:506–509.
82. Kim SJ, Kahn CR. Insulin induces rapid accumulation of insulin receptors and increases tyrosine kinase activity in the nucleus of cultured adipocytes. *J Cell Physiol* 1993;157:217–228.
83. Vigneri R, Pliam NB, Cohen DC, et al. In vivo regulation of cell surface and intracellular insulin binding sites by insulin. *J Biol Chem* 1978;253:8192–8197.
84. Mendez R, Myers MG Jr, White MF, et al. Stimulation of protein synthesis, eukaryotic translation initiation factor 4E phosphorylation, and PHAS-I phosphorylation by insulin requires insulin receptor substrate 1 and phosphatidylinositol 3-kinase. *Mol Cell Biol* 1996;16:2857–2864.
85. Dardevet D, Sornet C, Vary T, et al. Phosphatidylinositol 3-kinase and p70 s6 kinase participate in the regulation of protein turnover in skeletal muscle by insulin and insulin-like growth factor I. *Endocrinology* 1996;137:4087–4094.
86. Grzelkowska K, Dardevet D, Balage M, et al. Involvement of the rapamycin-sensitive pathway in the insulin regulation of muscle protein synthesis in streptozotocin-diabetic rats. *J Endocrinol* 1999;160:137–145.
87. Sharma PM, Egawa K, Huang Y, et al. Inhibition of phosphatidylinositol 3-kinase activity by adenovirus-mediated gene transfer and its effect on insulin action. *J Biol Chem* 1998;273:18528–18537.
88. Mendez R, Kollmorgen G, White MF, et al. Requirement of protein kinase C zeta for stimulation of protein synthesis by insulin. *Mol Cell Biol* 1997;17:5184–5192.
89. Egawa K, Sharma PM, Nakashima N, et al. Membrane-targeted phosphatidylinositol 3-kinase mimics insulin actions and induces a state of cellular insulin resistance. *J Biol Chem* 1999;274:14306–14314.
90. Lawrence JC Jr, Fadden P, Haystead TA, et al. PHAS proteins as mediators of the actions of insulin, growth factors and cAMP on protein synthesis and cell proliferation. *Adv Enzyme Regul* 1997;37:239–267.
91. Burgering BM, Coffer PJ. Protein kinase B (c-Akt) in phosphatidylinositol-3-OH kinase signal transduction. *Nature* 1995;376:599–602.
92. Scott PH, Brunn GJ, Kohn AD, et al. Evidence of insulin-stimulated phosphorylation and activation of the mammalian target of rapamycin mediated by a protein kinase B signaling pathway. *Proc Natl Acad Sci U S A* 1998;95: 7772–7777.
93. Franke TF, Yang SI, Chan TO, et al. The protein kinase encoded by the Akt proto-oncogene is a target of the PDGF-activated phosphatidylinositol 3-kinase. *Cell* 1995;81:727–736.
94. Brunn GJ, Williams J, Sabers C, et al. Direct inhibition of the signaling functions of the mammalian target of rapamycin by the phosphoinositide 3-kinase inhibitors, wortmannin and LY294002. *EMBO J* 1996;15:5256–5267.
95. Sasaoka T, Draznin B, Leitner JW, et al. Shc is the predominant signaling molecule coupling insulin receptors to activation of guanine nucleotide releasing factor and p21ras-GTP formation. *J Biol Chem* 1994;269:10734–10738.
96. Cheatham B, Kahn CR. Insulin action and the insulin signaling network. *Endocr Rev* 1995;16:117–142.
97. Jhun BH, Meinkoth JL, Leitner JW, et al. Insulin and insulin-like growth factor-I signal transduction requires p21ras. *J Biol Chem* 1994;269:5699–5704.
98. Sale EM, Atkinson PP, Arnott CH, et al. Role of ERK1/ERK2 and p70S6K pathway in insulin signalling of protein synthesis. *FEBS Lett* 1999;446: 122–126.
99. Sjolander A, Yamamoto K, Huber BE, et al. Association of p21ras with phosphatidylinositol 3-kinase. *Proc Natl Acad Sci U S A* 1991;88:7908–7912.

100. Yamauchi K, Holt K, Pessin JE. Phosphatidylinositol 3-kinase functions upstream of Ras and Raf in mediating insulin stimulation of c-fos transcription. *J Biol Chem* 1993;268:14597–14600.
101. Bjornholm M, Kawano Y, Lehtihet M, et al. Insulin receptor substrate-1 phosphorylation and phosphatidylinositol 3-kinase activity in skeletal muscle from NIDDM subjects after in vivo insulin stimulation. *Diabetes* 1997;46: 524–527.
102. Andreelli F, Laville M, Ducluzeau PH, et al. Defective regulation of phosphatidylinositol-3-kinase gene expression in skeletal muscle and adipose tissue of non-insulin-dependent diabetes mellitus patients. *Diabetologia* 1999; 42:358–364.
103. Krook A, Roth RA, Jiang XJ, et al. Insulin-stimulated Akt kinase activity is reduced in skeletal muscle from NIDDM subjects. *Diabetes* 1998;47:1281–1286.
104. Mitch WE, Goldberg AL. Mechanisms of muscle wasting. The role of the ubiquitin-proteasome pathway. *N Engl J Med* 1996;335:1897–1905.
105. Giffin BF, Drake RL, Morris RE, et al. Hepatic lobular patterns of phosphoenolpyruvate carboxykinase, glycogen synthase, and glycogen phosphorylase in fasted and fed rats. *J Histochem Cytochem* 1993;41:1849–1862.
106. Van Remmen H, Ward WF. Effect of age on induction of hepatic phosphoenolpyruvate carboxykinase by fasting. *Am J Physiol* 1994;267:G195–G200.
107. Kulka RG. Modulation of protein degradation in mammalian cells by ligands and stress. *Revis Biol Celular* 1989;21:321–345.
108. Mohsenzadeh S, Xu C, Fracella F, et al. Heat shock inhibits and activates different protein degradation pathways and proteinase activities in *Neurospora crassa*. *FEMS Microbiol Lett* 1994;124:215–224.
109. Welch WJ, Kang HS, Beckmann RP, et al. Response of mammalian cells to metabolic stress; changes in cell physiology and structure/function of stress proteins. *Curr Top Microbiol Immunol* 1991;167:31–55.
110. Sherman MY, Goldberg AL. Involvement of molecular chaperones in intracellular protein breakdown. *EXS* 1996;77:57–78.
111. Mortimore GE, Poso AR, Lardeux BR. Mechanism and regulation of protein degradation in liver. *Diabetes Metab Rev* 1989;5:49–70.
112. Wing SS, Goldberg AL. Glucocorticoids activate the ATP-ubiquitin-dependent proteolytic system in skeletal muscle during fasting. *Am J Physiol* 1993;264: E668–E676.
113. Ding X, Price SR, Bailey JL, et al. Cellular mechanisms controlling protein degradation in catabolic states. *Miner Electrolyte Metab* 1997;23:194–197.
114. Ciechanover A. The ubiquitin-proteasome proteolytic pathway. *Cell* 1994; 79:13–21.
115. Coux O, Tanaka K, Goldberg AL. Structure and functions of the 20S and 26S proteasomes. *Annu Rev Biochem* 1996;65:801–847.
116. Hershko A, Ciechanover A. The ubiquitin system for protein degradation. *Annu Rev Biochem* 1992;61:761–807.
117. Goldberg AL. Functions of the proteasome: the lysis at the end of the tunnel. *Science* 1995;268:522–523.
118. Lowe J, Stock D, Jap B, et al. Crystal structure of the 20S proteasome from the archaeon T. acidophilum at 3.4 A resolution. *Science* 1995;268:533–539.
119. Ciechanover A, Schwartz AL. The ubiquitin-mediated proteolytic pathway: mechanisms of recognition of the proteolytic substrate and involvement in the degradation of native cellular proteins. *FASEB J* 1994;8:182–191.
120. Scheffner M, Huibregtse JM, Vierstra RD, et al. The HPV-16 E6 and E6-AP complex functions as a ubiquitin-protein ligase in the ubiquitination of p53. *Cell* 1993;75:495–505.
121. Solomon V, Lecker SH, Goldberg AL. The N-end rule pathway catalyzes a major fraction of the protein degradation in skeletal muscle. *J Biol Chem* 1998;273:25216–25222.
122. Varshavsky A. The N-end rule: functions, mysteries, uses. *Proc Natl Acad Sci U S A* 1996;93:12142–12149.
123. Bailey JL, Wang X, England BK, et al. The acidosis of chronic renal failure activates muscle proteolysis in rats by augmenting transcription of genes encoding proteins of the ATP-dependent ubiquitin-proteasome pathway. *J Clin Invest* 1996;97:1447–1453.
124. Hobler SC, Tiao G, Fischer JE, et al. Sepsis-induced increase in muscle proteolysis is blocked by specific proteasome inhibitors. *Am J Physiol* 1998;274: R30–R37.
125. Tawa NE Jr, Odessey R, Goldberg AL. Inhibitors of the proteasome reduce the accelerated proteolysis in atrophying rat skeletal muscles. *J Clin Invest* 1997;100:197–203.
126. Lecker SH, Solomon V, Price SR, et al. Ubiquitin conjugation by the N-end rule pathway and mRNAs for its components increase in muscles of diabetic rats. *J Clin Invest* 1999;104:1411–1420.
127. Taillandier D, Aurousseau E, Meynial-Denis D, et al. Coordinate activation of lysosomal, Ca^{2+}-activated and ATP-ubiquitin-dependent proteinases in the unweighted rat soleus muscle. *Biochem J* 1996;316(Pt 1):65–72.
128. Temparis S, Asensi M, Taillandier D, et al. Increased ATP-ubiquitin-dependent proteolysis in skeletal muscles of tumor-bearing rats. *Cancer Res* 1994;54: 5568–5573.
129. Price SR, Bailey JL, Wang X, et al. Muscle wasting in insulinopenic rats results from activation of the ATP-dependent, ubiquitin-proteasome proteolytic pathway by a mechanism including gene transcription. *J Clin Invest* 1996;98:1703–1708.
130. Pepato MT, Migliorini RH, Goldberg AL, et al. Role of different proteolytic pathways in degradation of muscle protein from streptozotocin-diabetic rats. *Am J Physiol* 1996;271:E340–E347.
131. Mitch WE, Bailey JL, Wang X, et al. Evaluation of signals activating ubiquitin-proteasome proteolysis in a model of muscle wasting. *Am J Physiol* 1999;276: C1132–C1138.
132. Nair KS. *Energy and protein metabolism in diabetes and obesity* [dissertation]. London: Council of National Academic Awards, 1984.
133. Nair KS. Assessment of protein metabolism in diabetes. In: Draznin B, Rizza R, eds. *Clinical research in diabetes mellitus*. Totowa, NJ: Humana Press, 1996.
134. Wolfe RR, Goodenough RD, Wolfe MH, et al. Isotopic analysis of leucine and urea metabolism in exercising humans. *J Appl Physiol* 1982;52:458–466.
135. Wagenmakers AJ. Tracers to investigate protein and amino acid metabolism in human subjects. *Proc Nutr Soc* 1999;58:987–1000.
136. Matthews DE, Bier DM, Rennie MJ, et al. Regulation of leucine metabolism in man: a stable isotope study. *Science* 1981;214:1129–1131.
137. Matthews DE, Motil KJ, Rohrbaugh DK, et al. Measurement of leucine metabolism in man from a primed, continuous infusion of L-[1-^{3}C]leucine. *Am J Physiol* 1980;238:E473–E479.
138. Nair KS, Ford GC, Ekberg K, et al. Protein dynamics in whole body and in splanchnic and leg tissues in type 1 diabetic patients. *J Clin Invest* 1995;95:2926–2937.
139. Baumann PQ, Stirewalt WS, O'Rourke BD, et al. Precursor pools of protein synthesis: a stable isotope study in a swine model. *Am J Physiol* 1994;267:E203–E209.
140. Mortimore GE, Poso AR, Kadowaki M, et al. Multiphasic control of hepatic protein degradation by regulatory amino acids. General features and hormonal modulation. *J Biol Chem* 1987;262:16322–16327.
141. Nair KS. Muscle protein turnover: methodological issues and the effect of aging. *J Gerontol A Biol Sci Med Sci* 1995;50[Spec no.]:107–112.
142. Measurement of protein synthesis in cells and tissues. In: Stirewalt WS, Nair KS, eds. *Protein metabolism in diabetes mellitus*. London: Smith-Bordon, 1992: 27–33.
143. Charlton MR, Balagopal P, Nair KS. Skeletal muscle myosin heavy chain synthesis in type 1 diabetes. *Diabetes* 1997;46:1336–1340.
144. Rooyackers OE, Adey DB, Ades PA, et al. Effect of age on in vivo rates of mitochondrial protein synthesis in human skeletal muscle. *Proc Natl Acad Sci U S A* 1996;93:15364–15369.
145. De Feo P, Volpi E, Lucidi P, et al. Physiological increments in plasma insulin concentrations have selective and different effects on synthesis of hepatic proteins in normal humans. *Diabetes* 1993;42:995–1002.
146. De Feo P, Gaisano MG, Haymond MW. Differential effects of insulin deficiency on albumin and fibrinogen synthesis in humans. *J Clin Invest* 1991;88: 833–840.
147. Nair KS, Ford GC, Halliday D. Effect of intravenous insulin treatment on in vivo whole body leucine kinetics and oxygen consumption in insulin-deprived type 1 diabetic patients. *Metabolism* 1987;36:491–495.
148. Nair KS, Garrow JS, Ford C, et al. Effect of poor diabetic control and obesity on whole body protein metabolism in man. *Diabetologia* 1983;25:400–403.
149. Pacy PJ, Thompson GN, Halliday D. Measurement of whole-body protein turnover in insulin-dependent (type 1) diabetic patients during insulin withdrawal and infusion: comparison of. *Clin Sci* (Lond) 1991;80:345–352.
150. Robert JJ, Beaufrere B, Koziet J, et al. Whole body de novo amino acid synthesis in type 1 (insulin-dependent) diabetes studied with stable isotope-labeled leucine, alanine, and glycine. *Diabetes* 1985;34:67–73.
151. Umpleby AM, Boroujerdi MA, Brown PM, et al. The effect of metabolic control on leucine metabolism in type 1 (insulin-dependent) diabetic patients. *Diabetologia* 1986;29:131–141.
152. Tessari P, Biolo G, Inchiostro S, et al. Effects of insulin on whole body and forearm leucine and KIC metabolism in type 1 diabetes. *Am J Physiol* 1990;259:E96–E103.
153. Vogiatzi MG, Nair KS, Beckett PR, et al. Insulin does not stimulate protein synthesis acutely in prepubertal children with insulin-dependent diabetes mellitus. *J Clin Endocrinol Metab* 1997;82:4083–4087.
154. Bennet WM, Connacher AA, Jung RT, et al. Effects of insulin and amino acids on leg protein turnover in IDDM patients. *Diabetes* 1991;40:499–508.
155. Pacy PJ, Bannister PA, Halliday D. Influence of insulin on leucine kinetics in the whole body and across the forearm in post-absorptive insulin dependent diabetic (type 1) patients. *Diabetes Res* 1991;18:155–162.
156. Dice JF, Walker CD, Byrne B, et al. General characteristics of protein degradation in diabetes and starvation. *Proc Natl Acad Sci U S A* 1978;75:2093–2097.
157. Nakhooda AF, Wei CN, Marliss EB. Muscle protein catabolism in diabetes: 3-methylhistidine excretion in the spontaneously diabetic "BB" rat. *Metabolism* 1980;29:1272–1277.
158. Rodriguez T, Alvarez B, Busquets S, et al. The increased skeletal muscle protein turnover of the streptozotocin diabetic rat is associated with high concentrations of branched-chain amino acids. *Biochem Mol Med* 1997;61:87–94.
159. Ashford AJ, Pain VM. Insulin stimulation of growth in diabetic rats. Synthesis and degradation of ribosomes and total tissue protein in skeletal muscle and heart. *J Biol Chem* 1986;261:4066–4070.
160. Farrell PA, Fedele MJ, Hernandez J, et al. Hypertrophy of skeletal muscle in diabetic rats in response to chronic resistance exercise. *J Appl Physiol* 1999;87:1075–1082.
161. Fedele MJ, Hernandez JM, Lang CH, et al. Severe diabetes prohibits elevations in muscle protein synthesis after acute resistance exercise in rats. *J Appl Physiol* 2000;88:102–108.
162. Millward DJ, Garlick PJ, Nnanyelugo DO, et al. The relative importance of muscle protein synthesis and breakdown in the regulation of muscle mass. *Biochem J* 1976;156:185–188.

163. Forker LL, Chaikoff IL, Enteman C, et al. Formation of muscle protein in diabetic dogs studied with S^{35}-methionine. *J Biol Chem* 1951;188:37–48.
164. Pacy PJ, Nair KS, Ford C, et al. Failure of insulin infusion to stimulate fractional muscle protein synthesis in type 1 diabetic patients. Anabolic effect of insulin and decreased proteolysis. *Diabetes* 1989;38:618–624.
165. Boirie Y, Short KR, Ahlman B, et al. Tissue-specific regulation of mitochondrial and cytoplasmic protein synthesis rates by insulin. *Diabetes* 2001;50: 2652–2658.
166. Stump CS, Short KR, Bigelow ML, et al. Effect of insulin on human skeletal muscle mitochondrial ATP production, protein synthesis, and mRNA transcripts. *Proc Natl Acad Sci U S A* 2003;100:7996–8001.
167. Charlton M, Ahlman B, Nair KS. The effect of insulin on human small intestinal mucosal protein synthesis. *Gastroenterology* 2000;118:299–306.
168. Mortimore GE, Mondon CE. Inhibition by insulin of valine turnover in liver. Evidence for a general control of proteolysis. *J Biol Chem* 1970;245: 2375–2383.
169. Woodside KH, Mortimore GE. Suppression of protein turnover by amino acids in the perfused rat liver. *J Biol Chem* 1972;247:6474–6481.
170. Green M, Miller LL. Protein catabolism and protein synthesis in perfused livers of normal and alloxan-diabetic rats. *J Biol Chem* 1960;235:3202–3208.
171. Nygren J, Nair KS. Differential regulation of protein dynamics in splanchnic and skeletal muscle beds by insulin and amino acids in healthy human subjects. *Diabetes* 2003;52:1377–1385.
172. Garibotto G, Tessari P, Robaudo C, et al. Protein turnover in the kidney and the whole body in humans. *Miner Electrolyte Metab* 1997;23:185–188.
173. Liu S, Barac-Nieto M. Renal protein degradation in streptozotocin diabetic mice. *Diabetes Res Clin Pract* 1997;34:143–148.
174. Osterby R, Gundersen HJ. Fast accumulation of basement membrane material and the rate of morphological changes in acute experimental diabetic glomerular hypertrophy. *Diabetologia* 1980;18:493–500.
175. Garlick PJ, Albertse EC, McNurlan MA, et al. Protein turnover in tissues of diabetic rats. *Acta Biol Med Ger* 1981;40:1301–1307.
176. Heidland A, Ling H, Vamvakas S, et al. Impaired proteolytic activity as a potential cause of progressive renal disease. *Miner Electrolyte Metab* 1996;22:157–161.
177. Schwieger J, Fine LG. Renal hypertrophy, growth factors, and nephropathy in diabetes mellitus. *Semin Nephrol* 1990;10:242–253.
178. Seyer-Hansen K. Renal hypertrophy in experimental diabetes mellitus. *Kidney Int* 1983;23:643–646.
179. Tsao TC, Shi JD, Mortimore GE, et al. Modulation of kidney cell protein degradation by insulin. *J Lab Clin Med* 1990;116:369–376.
180. Barac-Nieto M, Liu SM, Spitzer A, et al. Renal protein synthesis in diabetes mellitus: effects of insulin and insulin-like growth factor I. *Am J Kidney Dis* 1991;17:658–660.
181. Rabkin R, Shechter P, Shi JD, et al. Protein turnover in the hypertrophying kidney. *Miner Electrolyte Metab* 1996;22:153–156.
182. Shechter P, Boner G, Rabkin R. Tubular cell protein degradation in early diabetic renal hypertrophy. *J Am Soc Nephrol* 1994;4:1582–1587.
183. Bogardus C, Taskinen MR, Zawadzki J, et al. Increased resting metabolic rates in obese subjects with non-insulin-dependent diabetes mellitus and the effect of sulfonylurea therapy. *Diabetes* 1986;35:1–5.
184. Henry RR, Wiest-Kent TA, Scheaffer L, et al. Metabolic consequences of very-low-calorie diet therapy in obese non-insulin-dependent diabetic and nondiabetic subjects. *Diabetes* 1986;35:155–164.
185. Luzi L, Petrides AS, De Fronzo RA. Different sensitivity of glucose and amino acid metabolism to insulin in NIDDM. *Diabetes* 1993;42:1868–1877.
186. Staten MA, Matthews DE, Bier DM. Leucine metabolism in type II diabetes mellitus. *Diabetes* 1986;35:1249–1253.
187. Umpleby AM, Scobie IN, Boroujerdi MA, et al. Diurnal variation in glucose and leucine metabolism in non-insulin-dependent diabetes. *Diabetes Res Clin Pract* 1990;9:89–96.
188. Welle S, Nair KS. Failure of glyburide and insulin treatment to decrease leucine flux in obese type II diabetic patients. *Int J Obes* 1990;14:701–710.
189. Denne SC, Brechtel G, Johnson A, et al. Skeletal muscle proteolysis is reduced in noninsulin-dependent diabetes mellitus and is unaltered by euglycemic hyperinsulinemia or intensive insulin therapy. *J Clin Endocrinol Metab* 1995;80:2371–2377.
190. Gougeon R, Pencharz PB, Marliss EB. Effect of NIDDM on the kinetics of whole-body protein metabolism. *Diabetes* 1994;43:318–328.
191. Gougeon R, Pencharz PB, Sigal RJ. Effect of glycemic control on the kinetics of whole-body protein metabolism in obese subjects with non-insulin-dependent diabetes mellitus during iso- and hypoenergetic feeding. *Am J Clin Nutr* 1997;65:861–870.
192. Gougeon R, Styhler K, Morais JA, et al. Effects of oral hypoglycemic agents and diet on protein metabolism in type 2 diabetes. *Diabetes Care* 2000;23:1–8.
193. Marchesini G, Forlani G, Zoli M, et al. Muscle protein breakdown in uncontrolled diabetes as assessed by urinary 3-methylhistidine excretion. *Diabetologia* 1982;23:456–468.
194. Caballero B, Wurtman RJ. Differential effects of insulin resistance on leucine and glucose kinetics in obesity. *Metab Clin Exp* 1991;40:51–58.
195. Petrides AS, Luzi L. Effect of insulin and amino acids on leucine kinetics in NIDDM. *Diabetes* 1987;36:29(abst).
196. Biolo G, Tessari P, Inchiostro S, et al. Fasting and postmeal phenylalanine metabolism in mild type 2 diabetes. *Am J Physiol* 1992;263:E877–E883.
197. Salgado LR, Semer M, Nery M, et al. Effect of glycemic control on growth hormone and IGFBP-1 secretion in patients with type 1 diabetes mellitus. *J Endocrinol Invest* 1996;19:433–440.
198. Nair KS, Schwenk WF. Factors controlling muscle protein synthesis and degradation. *Curr Opin Neurol* 1994;7:471–474.
199. Charlton MR, Nair KS. Role of hyperglucagonemia in catabolism associated with type 1 diabetes: effects on leucine metabolism and the resting metabolic rate. *Diabetes* 1998;47:1748–1756.
200. Nair KS, Halliday D, Matthews DE, et al. Hyperglucagonemia during insulin deficiency accelerates protein catabolism. *Am J Physiol* 1987;253: E208–E213.
201. Couet C, Fukagawa NK, Matthews DE, et al. Plasma amino acid kinetics during acute states of glucagon deficiency and excess in healthy adults. *Am J Physiol* 1990;258:E78–E85.
202. Hartl WH, Miyoshi H, Jahoor F, et al. Bradykinin attenuates glucagon-induced leucine oxidation in humans. *Am J Physiol* 1990;259:E239–E245.
203. Beaufrere B, Tessari P, Cattalini M, et al. Apparent decreased oxidation and turnover of leucine during infusion of medium-chain triglycerides. *Am J Physiol* 1985;249:E175–E182.
204. Darmaun D, Matthews DE, Bier DM. Physiological hypercortisolemia increases proteolysis, glutamine, and alanine production. *Am J Physiol* 1988;255:E366–E373.
205. Beaufrere B, Horber FF, Schwenk WF, et al. Glucocorticosteroids increase leucine oxidation and impair leucine balance in humans. *Am J Physiol* 1989;257:E712–E721.
206. Kraenzlin ME, Keller U, Keller A, et al. Elevation of plasma epinephrine concentrations inhibits proteolysis and leucine oxidation in man via beta-adrenergic mechanisms. *J Clin Invest* 1989;84:388–393.
207. Miles JM, Nissen SL, Gerich JE, et al. Effects of epinephrine infusion on leucine and alanine kinetics in humans. *Am J Physiol* 1984;247:E166–E172.
208. Matthews DE, Pesola G, Campbell RG. Effect of epinephrine on amino acid and energy metabolism in humans. *Am J Physiol* 1990;258:E948–E956.
209. Fryburg DA, Gelfand RA, Jahn LA, et al. Effects of epinephrine on human muscle glucose and protein metabolism. *Am J Physiol* 1995;268:E55–E59.
210. Mitchell GA, Dunnavan G. Illegal use of beta-adrenergic agonists in the United States. *J Anim Sci* 1998;76:208–211.
211. Prather ID, Brown DE, North P, et al. Clenbuterol: a substitute for anabolic steroids? *Med Sci Sports Exerc* 1995;27:1118–1121.
212. Copeland KC, Nair KS. Acute growth hormone effects on amino acid and lipid metabolism. *J Clin Endocrinol Metab* 1994;78:1040–1047.
213. Fryburg DA, Louard RJ, Gerow KE, et al. Growth hormone stimulates skeletal muscle protein synthesis and antagonizes insulin's antiproteolytic action in humans. *Diabetes* 1992;41:424–429.
214. Fryburg DA, Barrett EJ. Growth hormone acutely stimulates skeletal muscle but not whole-body protein synthesis in humans. *Metabolism* 1993;42:1223–1227.
215. Florini JR, Ewton DZ, Coolican SA. Growth hormone and the insulin-like growth factor system in myogenesis. *Endocr Rev* 1996;17:481–517.
216. Yarasheski KE. Growth hormone effects on metabolism, body composition, muscle mass, and strength. *Exerc Sport Sci Rev* 1994;22:285–312.
217. Fryburg DA. Insulin-like growth factor I exerts growth hormone- and insulin-like actions on human muscle protein metabolism. *Am J Physiol* 1994;267: E331–E336.
218. Fryburg DA. NG-monomethyl-L-arginine inhibits the blood flow but not the insulin-like response of forearm muscle to IGF-I: possible role of nitric oxide in muscle protein synthesis. *J Clin Invest* 1996;97:1319–1328.
219. Fryburg DA, Jahn LA, Hill SA, et al. Insulin and insulin-like growth factor-I enhance human skeletal muscle protein anabolism during hyperaminoacidemia by different mechanisms. *J Clin Invest* 1995;96:1722–1729.
220. Elahi D, McAloon-Dyke M, Fukagawa NK, et al. Effects of recombinant human IGF-I on glucose and leucine kinetics in men. *Am J Physiol* 1993; 265:E831–E838.
221. Louard RJ, Barrett EJ, Gelfand RA. Effect of infused branched-chain amino acids on muscle and whole-body amino acid metabolism in man. *Clin Sci* (Lond) 1990;79:457–466.
222. Heiling VJ, Campbell PJ, Gottesman IS, et al. Differential effects of hyperglycemia and hyperinsulinemia on leucine rate of appearance in normal humans. *J Clin Endocrinol Metab* 1993;76:203–206.
223. Tessari P, Nissen SL, Miles JM, et al. Inverse relationship of leucine flux and oxidation to free fatty acid availability in vivo. *J Clin Invest* 1986;77: 575–581.
224. Nair KS, Welle SL, Halliday D, et al. Effect of beta-hydroxybutyrate on whole-body leucine kinetics and fractional mixed skeletal muscle protein synthesis in humans. *J Clin Invest* 1988;82:198–205.

CHAPTER 18
Rodent Models for the Study of Diabetes

Clayton E. Mathews and Edward H. Leiter

Patients with diabetes share the clinical symptom of hyperglycemia accompanied by either insufficient circulating insulin or inadequate insulin action, but the genetic and environmental interactions leading to the metabolic disorder are complex because of etiopathologic heterogeneity. Because of the multifaceted nature of diabetes, etiologic dissection of diabetes in humans has been difficult. Much of the current understanding of diabetes etiopathogenesis has evolved from analysis of animal models in which either insulin-dependent or insulin-resistant forms of diabetes develop spontaneously. As early as the late 19th century, the importance of animals in the study of human disease was established when Oscar Minkowski (1a,1b) discovered the link between the pancreas and diabetes by pancreatectomizing dogs. The use of dogs and their pancreata by Banting and Best (1c,1d) in the 1920s in their discovery and isolation of insulin as a treatment for humans with insulin-dependent diabetes stands as a landmark in the history of medicine.

While animals have been used for physiologic and pharmacologic studies of diabetes for more than 100 years, animals with genetic syndromes that are models for various forms of diabetes in humans have been developed only during the last 50 years. Since the previous edition of this book, there has been an explosive increase in the number of new mouse models generated by gene-targeting technology wherein specific genes are disrupted (1e). Genetically engineered mutant mice used in diabetes research may or may not serve as good models for the natural course of the development of diabetes in humans but provide valuable tools for evaluating the role of a single gene in the maintenance of either metabolic or immunologic homeostasis (2). The focus of this chapter is rodent models of spontaneously occurring diabetes. We discuss information on targeted mutations of diabetogenic significance only to aid in understanding the spontaneous disease syndrome, especially autoimmune (type 1 or insulin-dependent) diabetes mellitus in the nonobese diabetic (NOD) mouse.

Research involving the available rodent models of both type 1 diabetes and type 2 diabetes (non–insulin-dependent) tends to be compartmentalized, with immunologists and immunogeneticists focusing on the NOD and BB (BioBreeding) rat models of type 1 diabetes. In turn, investigators interested in mechanisms of metabolic control and in obesity focus on the models of type 2 diabetes. This "division of interest" can obscure an important "lesson" taught by viewing the totality of rodent models available. Such a survey would suggest potential pathologic synergism among genomes selected for susceptibility to type 1 or type 2 diabetes. For instance, it is not difficult to envisage that combinations of genes contributing to impaired immune tolerance (a defect associated with type 1 diabetes) might interact deleteriously with genes contributing to impaired β-cell function or impaired glucose tolerance (IGT; both defects proposed to be central to the etiopathogenesis of certain types of type 2 diabetes). One such deleterious interaction was uncovered by mating type 1 diabetes–prone NOD mice to a wild-derived inbred strain carrying a predisposition to obesity (3,4). The biology of the pancreatic β-cell now provides a common meeting ground for researchers in both type 1 and type 2 diabetes. This chapter will describe a variety of relatively new inbred strains generated by sib matings of outbred Swiss (or CD-1) mice. The progenitor-outbred population is considered a model of an outbred human population segregating genetic susceptibility for type 1 and type 2 diabetes. Extensive inbreeding of pairs of mice from this family produced lean, glucose-tolerant strains (SWR, SJL, FVB), strains moderately obese and exhibiting IGT (NON, NSY), and strains developing overt type 2 diabetes with moderate (ALS) or more pronounced obesity (TallyHo) (Table 18.1). An interesting aspect to this family of mice is that it also contains the NOD strain, the most widely used animal model of type 1 diabetes. This chapter will discuss the available models of type 1 and type 2 diabetes in current use. The first portion of the chapter discusses in detail the mouse and rat models of type 1 diabetes. The remainder of the chapter will briefly cover several models of non–immune-mediated insulin-sensitive diabetes and then briefly describe each of the 15 rodent models of type 2 diabetes. The intent of

TABLE 18.1. Characteristics of ICR-Derived Strains

	NSY	NON	ALS	CTS	ALR	Tally Ho
Body size	?	+	+++	++++	+++	+++
Obesity	—	−/+	++	+	++	++++
IGT	++	++	++++	+++	—	++++
β-cell function	↓ with age	↓ with age	Normal	?	Normal	?
Islet changes	?	Normal	Hyperplasia	?	PVPD	?
Type 2 diabetes	Yes	No	Yes	No	No	Yes
ROS sensitivity	?	++	++++	?	Resistant	?

NSY, Nagoya-Shibata-Yasuda; NON, nonobese normal; ALS, alloxan-induced diabetes susceptible; CTS, cataract Shinogi; ALR, alloxan-induced diabetes resistant; ROS, reactive oxygen sensitivity; PVPD, perivascular/periductal insulitis; IGT, impaired glucose tolerance;?, not defined for the given strain.

this chapter is to provide a guide for the interested investigator so that careful selection and use of the appropriate systems can be made.

ANIMAL MODELS OF SPONTANEOUS TYPE 1 (INSULIN-DEPENDENT) DIABETES MELLITUS

Type 1 diabetes mellitus, or insulin-dependent diabetes mellitus (IDDM), is an endocrine disease in humans that, in most cases, results from an autoimmune destruction of the insulin-producing β-cells within the pancreatic islets of Langerhans (5). Clinical presentation of symptoms of type 1 diabetes (fasting hyperglycemia, glycosuria, and ketoacidosis) is usually abrupt in onset and is indicative of destruction of more than 90% of the β-cell population of the endocrine pancreas. The underlying autoimmune processes producing this level of extensive β-cell destruction, however, are believed to be chronic in nature. The two most intensively studied rodent models of autoimmune type 1 diabetes, the NOD mouse and the BB rat, clearly establish that T lymphocytes are both initiators and the final effectors of β-cell destruction (6). Certain clinical and immunopathologic differences distinguish these two models, indicating that the pathways leading to autoimmune type 1 diabetes in humans may be diverse. Because of the greater definition of the mouse genome, coupled with the ease of introducing transgenes and genetically targeted mutations ("knockouts") into this genome, the NOD mouse has surpassed the BB rat as the more commonly studied model of type 1 diabetes. Yet, given important genera differences between *Mus* and *Rattus* in the pathogenesis of type 1 diabetes, investigators considering a rodent model of type 1 diabetes for therapeutic intervention studies should look for efficacy in both the mouse and the rat models if the ultimate goal is to extrapolate such therapies to humans. The clinical heterogeneity of type 1 diabetes is illustrated by a dominant negative mutation in one of the two mouse insulin genes, creating an insulin-dependent syndrome in the absence of autoimmunity in the C57BL/6J-*Ins2^{Akita}* mouse, a new model to be described below (7). A final example of this clinical heterogeneity is an insulin-responsive diabetes superimposed upon a monogenic obesity syndrome represented in a C57BLKS/J stock congenic for the *fat* mutation at the carboxypeptidase E locus (*Cpe^{fat}*).

Nonobese Diabetic Mice

ORIGINS AND RELATED STRAINS

NOD is a descriptor string denoting the nonobese diabetic inbred strain developed by inbreeding of ICR (Swiss) mice in Japan (9). The strain is best referred to as NOD, since not all NOD mice will develop diabetes, although most mice of this strain develop insulitis. The discovery of these mice emphasizes the role of serendipity in science. The NOD and certain of the NOD-related inbred strains were developed from Jcl:ICR progenitors at the Shionogi Research Laboratories in Aburahi, Japan, by Dr. S. Makino (8–10). Selection for dominant cataract with microphthalmia was the initial objective of the breeding program in Makino's laboratory. This selective breeding program led to the development of the CTS (cataract Shionogi) strain, in which all mice develop cataracts, and of NCT, a cataract-free control strain. At the sixth generation of inbreeding (F6), Makino noticed that some mice that were free of cataracts exhibited high fasting blood glucose levels. By selective breeding of F6 sibs and their progeny that exhibited this phenotype, Makino hoped to develop a new inbred strain exhibiting spontaneous diabetes. At the same time, he recognized the need for a euglycemic control strain and simultaneously inbred F6 sibs and their progeny that exhibited normal fasting blood glucose levels. In 1974, at the 20th generation of inbreeding (F20), a female spontaneously developed overt type 1 diabetes associated with heavy leukocytic infiltrations within the pancreatic islets (insulitis). Paradoxically, this female was not found in the line being selected for fasting hyperglycemia. Instead, the female with spontaneous type 1 diabetes was found in the line being inbred as a diabetes-free euglycemic control line. The progeny of this diabetic female were the founders of the NOD strain. Since the line originally selected for high fasting glucose levels never progressed to overt diabetes at the time that type 1 diabetes appeared in the euglycemic control (the latter now the NOD) line, the former strain was designated NON, for nonobese normal, and more recently, redesignated as nonobese nondiabetic (8,11). It was serendipitous not only that Makino coselected a euglycemic "control" line but also that his screening of this line was sufficiently rigorous to permit the discovery of that the "exceptional" female and the selection of her progeny to produce the NOD strain. Another serendipitous happenstance was that the husbandry environment in Makino's vivarium was sufficiently free of murine pathogenic agents such that the diabetic phenotype could develop (see the section "Critical Role of Environment"). It should be noted that while subsequent inbreeding of ICR mice in Japan produced other inbred strains, including the ILI (ICR-L line-Ishibe), NSY (Nagoya-Shibata-Yasuda), ALS (alloxan-induced diabetes susceptible), and ALR (alloxan-induced diabetes resistant), none of the latter have developed spontaneous, autoimmune type 1 diabetes (although some that will be described in sections to follow have developed IGT, pre–type 2 diabetes, or overt type 2 diabetes) (12–14).

Distribution of NOD and its closely related strains was tightly restricted to Japan within the first 5 years of their development (15). However, NOD mice are now widely available from suppliers in Japan (NOD/Shi from Clea, Tokyo), the United States (NOD/LtJ from The Jackson Laboratory, Bar Harbor, ME; and NOD/MrkTac from Taconic, Germantown, NY), and Europe (NOD/HlBom, Bomholtgard, Ay, Denmark). Substrain differences have been reported, notably, the very low incidence of type 1 diabetes present in the NOD/Wehi substrain in Australia (16). To avoid substrain divergence resulting from accumulation of recessive mutations distinct from those being fixed in the source colony, new breeders from the source colony can be imported every 10 to 20 generations to maintain uniformity with the mice being studied by other investigators.

CRITICAL ROLE OF ENVIRONMENT

Investigators studying NOD mice must be aware of the critical role of a specific pathogen-free environment in allowing penetrance of the underlying genetic susceptibility (17). The investigator has to choose between two options: maintaining a NOD breeding colony on site or ordering the requisite number of mice necessary for specific studies. Whichever option is selected, the investigator must house the mice in a specific pathogen–free (SPF) vivarium maintained to high standards of cleanliness and good animal care practice to achieve the diabetes frequencies mentioned above [reviewed in reference (18)]. This is necessary because NOD mice are subject to protective immunomodulation when stimulated by a broad spectrum of extrinsic pathogens, including viruses, bacteria, or their products or when fed semipurified diets lacking diabetogenic catalysts (6).

CLINICAL COURSE OF TYPE 1 DIABETES

In marked contrast to the male gender–biased susceptibility observed in rodent models of type 2 diabetes to be discussed later, one of the mouse-specific characteristics of type 1 diabetes pathogenesis in NOD mice is that it is female gender–biased. This bias is presumably attributable to the development of larger lymphoid organs in females than in males and the stronger response of females to immunization. In high-incidence colonies of NOD mice, the incidence in females typically reaches 80% to 90% by 24 weeks of age, whereas the incidence in males is lower and much more variable, usually reaching more than 40% by 30 weeks of age in SPF colonies. In the author's (EHL) colony of NOD/Lt males at The Jackson Laboratory, the frequency of type 1 diabetes in males varies from year to year, with a recorded low of 40% by 30 weeks of age and a high of 70% by 24 weeks of age. One of the unusual characteristics of the development of type 1 diabetes in NOD mice is that insulin therapy is not obligatory to sustain life over the first 2 to 4 weeks following the first diagnosis of hyperglycemia or glycosuria. This, in part, represents the ability of diabetic NOD mice to resist development of severe ketoacidosis (19). Diabetic NOD/Lt mice in the author's colony must exhibit chronically high blood glucose levels (>500 mg/dL) before severe ketonemia can be demonstrated. For example, a diabetic NOD/Lt female with a glucose level of 337 mg/dL had a β-hydroxybutyrate level of only 0.5 mg/dL, a nondiabetic background level. A dipstick test of this mouse's urine was also negative for ketones (acetoacetic acid). Two chronically diabetic NOD/Lt females (glucose levels of 913 and 954 mg/dL) also were negative for urine ketones but did exhibit blood levels of β-hydroxybutyrate of 10 and 20 mg/dL. Ketone bodies in urine appear only after the establishment of pronounced ketonemia. It should be noted that ketone bodies in the blood of chronically diabetic mice are considerably lower than those in humans, probably because mice can metabolize blood ketones to lactate (20). As hyperglycemia and glycosuria become more severe, mice exhibit polyuria, dehydration, and weight loss. Complete protocols for monitoring the diabetic state have been published elsewhere (18). In vivaria where high levels of NOD intra-islet insulitis develop, but unknown environmental factors suppress the transition to clinical type 1 diabetes, the onset of disease in both males and females can be precipitated by treatment with cyclophosphamide (21). Commonly, 200 mg/kg of body weight is administered intraperitoneally initially, with a second injection given 2 weeks later if required. Cyclophosphamide-accelerated type 1 diabetes is a particularly useful tool for synchronizing activation of diabetogenic effectors in young (7- to 10-week-old) NOD/Lt males.

CONTROL OF BLOOD GLUCOSE LEVELS WITH INSULIN IN DIABETIC MICE

It is exceedingly difficult to maintain stable normoglycemia in a diabetic mouse (NOD or otherwise) by insulin injection, although life span can be extended. A protocol used by Dr. M. Hattori (Joslin Diabetes Center, Boston, MA) (22) entails twice-daily subcutaneous insulin (a 1:1 mixture of regular and NPH insulin administered at 7:30 a.m. and 4:00 p.m.). The dose of insulin (between 0.5 and 1.0 units) is adjusted according to the severity of matinal and evening glycosuria. Table 18.2 shows random glucose and glycosylated hemoglobin (HbA_1) measurements in diabetic animals with and without insulin treatment.

TABLE 18.2. Hemoglobin A_1 Levels in Diabetic Nonobese Diabetic Mice With and Without Insulin Treatment

Mice (n)	Age at HbA_1 assay (mo)	Duration of diabetes at HbA_1 assay (wk)	HbA_1 (%)	Blood glucose (mg/dL)
Diabetic NOD				
Insulin (9)	7.0 ± 0.9	6.0 ± 1.5	6.4 ± 0.5[a]	370 ± 2[a,b]
No insulin (6)	5.8 ± 0.7	4.7 ± 0.4	9.2 ± 0.5[a]	439 ± 26[a,b]
Nondiabetic NOD (6)	3.9 ± 0.7	—	3.3 ± 0.2	73 ± 4
C57BL/6 (4)	6–7	—	3.6 ± 0.1	120 ± 2

NOD, nonobese diabetic.
Values are mean ± SEM.
[a] $P < 0.002$ (Student's *t* test, two-tailed).
[b] Two of the six mice showed blood glucose levels of more than 500 mg/dL (the upper limit of the glucometer).
From Karasik A, Hattori M. Use of animal models in the study of diabetes. In: Kahn CR, Weir GC, eds. *Joslin's diabetes mellitus*, 13th ed. Philadelphia: Lea & Febiger; 1994:317–350. Copyright © 1994 by the Joslin Diabetes Center.

CONTROL STRAINS FOR NONOBESE DIABETIC MICE

An important issue for investigators studying genes and phenotypes in the NOD mouse is that of an appropriate control. The literature shows that C57BL/6J (B6) or BALB/c are commonly used as "standard" strains against which to compare NOD immunophenotypes or gene sequences. However, since neither strain was Swiss-derived, the differences observed could represent normal variation expected for independently derived mouse strains. Selection of a control strain depends on the nature of the experiment and the hypotheses being tested. A partial listing of possible control strains and their potential uses is provided in Table 18.3. For an investigator interested in associating a particular genetic polymorphism with a phenotype associated with NOD diabetes, it is logical to compare the NOD genotype/phenotype with that found in NOD-related but type 1 diabetes–resistant inbred strains. These include mice with a common Swiss origin but with differences in their major histocompatiblity complex (MHC) haplotype and/or other non-MHC genes (designated *Idd* loci) conferring various degrees of resistance to type 1 diabetes. Figure 18.1 provides an illustration wherein Swiss-derived strains were surveyed for the phenotype of high percentages of T lymphocytes in the peripheral blood and spleen, an NOD strain characteristic very possibly associated with the resistance of these T lymphocytes to apoptosis (23). This complex phenotype is not unique to NOD; it also is characteristic of the SJL/J strain. SJL/J (*H2s*) mice are highly susceptible to experimental allergic encephalomyelitis (EAE). A genetic contribution to the SJL strain susceptibility to EAE colocalizes to a 0.15-cM region on chromosome (Chr) 3 that also confers susceptibility to type 1 diabetes (*Idd3*) in outcrosses of NOD with certain type 1 diabetes–resistant strains (24,25). The logical candidate within this interval is the *Il2* gene, with NOD and SJL showing identity for an *Il2* gene polymorphism associated with a presumed hyperglycosylated interleukin-2 (IL-2) molecule (26,27). However, it is unknown whether the SJL trait of high numbers of peripheral T cells cosegregates with EAE susceptibility and the SJL *Il2* allele. Indeed, SWR/J, another Swiss-derived strain, also shares the *Il2* polymorphism with NOD but does not exhibit the T lymphoaccumulation phenotype (Fig. 18.1). This does not exclude the *Il2* polymorphism as a contributor to the phenotype but illustrates that genetic control of the trait is oligo- or multigenic. These examples also illustrate the value of comparing NOD to more than one control strain.

Because it is $H2^{g7}$-identical, but diabetes- and insulitis-resistant, NOR/Lt is an NOD-related strain frequently used to evaluate the effect of changes in non-MHC genes. This is a recombinant congenic strain arising from outcross of NOD with

TABLE 18.3. Control Strains and Stocks for Nonobese Diabetic (NOD) Mice

Strain/stock name	Characteristics and uses
A. Related inbred strains	
ALR/LtJ	Genome scan shows close relation to NOD/Lt, including very similar $H2^{gx}$ haplotype; strongly resistant to free radical–mediated stress; diabetes- and insulitis-free. Available from JAX.
NOR/LtJ	$H2^{g7}$-identical recombinant congenic strain (~87.5% NOD/LtJ genome, 12.5% C57BLKS/J genome). Resistant to intraislet insulitis and diabetes-free; useful for immunopathologic comparisons since periinsulitis develops. Available from JAX.
ILI/ShiJos	$H2^{g7}$-identical Swiss-derived strain; diabetes- and insulitis-free. Little additional information because strain still not distributed by Japanese investigators.
SWR/J	Common derivation from Swiss mice; immunocompetent; useful as control when studying immune defects in NOD/LtJ mice. $H2^{q}$ haplotype; available from JAX.
SJL/J	Common derivation from Swiss mice; like NOD, exhibit high % of $CD4^+$ and $CD8^+$ T lymphocytes in spleen (T-lymphoaccumulation phenotype). $H2^{S}$ haplotype; available from JAX.
NON/LtJ	Related to NOD/LtJ; IDDM-resistant MHC; males develop IGT, and NON mice become relatively $CD8^+$ T cell–deficient with age; useful for genetic analysis of diabetes susceptibility genes. $H2^{nbl}$ haplotype; available from JAX.
B. MHC congenics	
NOD.B10-$H2^{b}$ NOD.NON-$H2^{nbl}$ NOD.SWR-$H2^{q}$	Diabetes-resistant MHC on NOD genetic background; exhibit some but not all immune dysfunctions of NOD/LtJ mice; useful in dissecting the role of MHC vs. non-MHC gene in producing immunologic abnormalities. All available from JAX.
NON.NOD-$H2^{g7}$ B6.NOD-$H2^{g7}$	Diabetogenic NOD MHC on type 1 diabetes–resistant backgrounds; exhibit some but not all immune dysfunctions of NOD mice; useful in dissecting the role of MHC vs. non-MHC gene in producing immunologic abnormalities. Both available from JAX.
C. NOD congenics with mutations affecting immunocompetence	
NOD-$B2m^{null}$	MHC class I–deficient; CD8 T lymphocyte–deficient; diabetes-resistant; excellent source for insulitis-free, MHC class I–negative islets for transplantation studies. Available from JAX.
NOD-$Prkdc^{scid}$ NOD-$Ragl^{null}$	T and B lymphocyte–deficient; C5-deficient (Hc^0); low NK cells; insulitis and diabetes free; high incidence of thymomas later in life; useful as source for insulitis-free islets and as recipients in adoptive transfer studies for delineating the role of T-cell subsets in causing diabetes. Available from JAX.
NOD-*scid*.$B2m^{null}$	T and B lymphocyte–deficient, C5-deficient (Hc^0), low NK cells, class I–deficient; excellent source for insulitis-free, MHC class I–negative islets for transplantation studies. Available from JAX.
NOD-$Igh\text{-}6^{null}$	B lymphocyte–deficient; useful for studying the role of B lymphocytes as essential APC in autoimmune diabetes. Available from JAX.
NOD-$Ifng^{null}$ NOD-$IL4^{null}$ NOD-$IL10^{null}$	Deficient in interferon-γ, interleukin-4, or interleukin-10; useful for examining the role of T_H1 and T_H2 cytokines in development of type 1 diabetes. The NOD.$IL10^{tml}$ mouse develops colitis with rectal prolapse. Available from JAX.

JAX, The Jackson Laboratory; NOD, nonobese diabetic; IDDM, insulin-dependent diabetes mellitus; MHC, major histocompatibility complex; IGT, impaired glucose tolerance; APC, antigen-presenting cell.

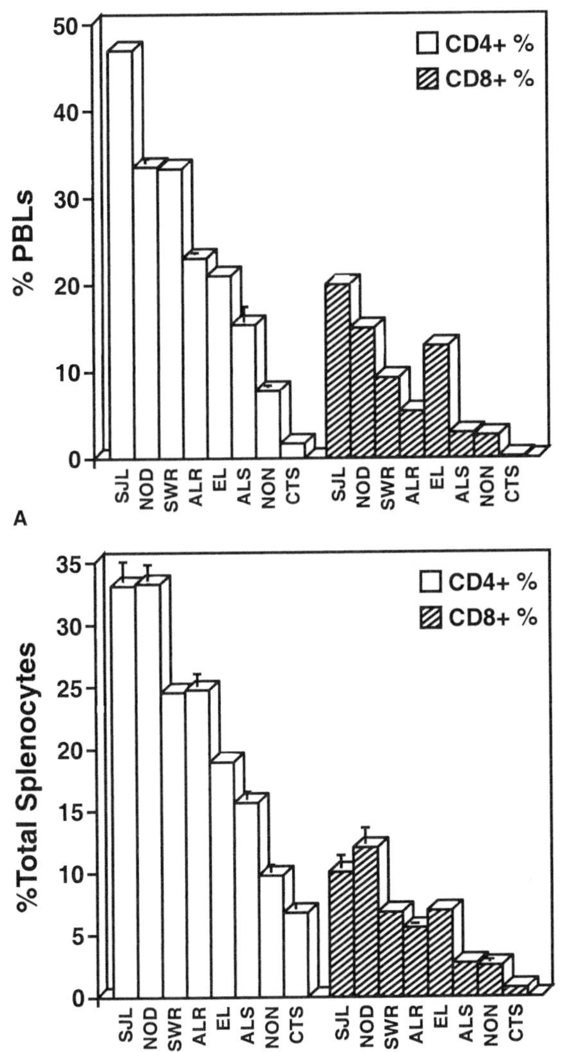

Figure 18.1. Variation in CD4⁺ and CD8⁺ T cell percentages of **(A)** peripheral blood leukocytes (PBLs) and **(B)** splenic leukocytes from the females of Swiss-derived inbred mouse strains.

C57BLKS/J (28). As discussed in detail below, the major genetic determinant of diabetes susceptibility in NOD mice is their $H2^{g7}$ MHC haplotype (K^d, A^{g7}, E^{null}, D^b). If an investigator is interested in analyzing the diabetogenic functions of the NOD $H2^{g7}$ MHC haplotype, stocks congenic for MHC haplotypes conferring resistance to type 1 diabetes are available for analysis of the selection of an autoimmune repertoire. Conversely, the diabetogenic NOD $H2^{g7}$ haplotype is available for study on the type 1 diabetes–resistant B6 background and in recombinant congenic strains (RCS) between CBA and NOD (29). During the initial period of NOD investigations in Japan, destruction of pancreatic β-cells was firmly established as a T lymphocyte–mediated process [reviewed in reference (10)]. For analysis of the diabetogenic potency of specific NOD T-cell clones or populations of immune effectors, NOD stocks congenic for immunodeficiency-producing mutations blocking development of functional T lymphocytes and/or B lymphocytes are available for adoptive-transfer studies. It has recently been demonstrated that B lymphocytes are essential antigen-presenting cells (APCs) for initiation of type 1 diabetes (B lymphocyte–deficient NOD mice congenic for the *Igμ* targeted mutation were protected from type 1 diabetes) (30). Therefore, T and B lymphocyte–deficient NOD mice congenic for either the $Prkdc^{scid}$ (severe combined immunodeficiency mutation; henceforth denoted as *scid*) or targeted mutations in the recombinase-activating gene (*Rag1*, *Rag2*) provide useful diabetes- and insulitis-free mice for adoptive-transfer studies without a requirement for prior irradiation (31–34). The NOD-*Rag1* and -*Rag2* congenics do not exhibit the DNA repair defects associated with the *scid* mutation and hence can tolerate sublethal irradiation. Moreover, thymic lymphomagenesis, a strain characteristic of NOD-*scid*, is slower to develop in NOD-*Rag* mice (32). Further, these stocks provide an excellent source of NOD pancreatic islets free of insulitic infiltrates. Not included in Table 18.3 is a listing of a growing battery of congenic stocks with defined chromosomal regions bearing non-MHC *Idd* loci affecting diabetes-related immunophenotypes (35). Certain of these will be discussed below in the section on genetic control of type 1 diabetes.

INSULITIS AND DEVELOPMENT OF TYPE 1 DIABETES

Insulitis, the disruption of islet structure and function by infiltrating leukocytes, is the major pathognomonic feature of the development of type 1 diabetes in NOD mice (8). In these mice, the development of insulitis is not abrupt; rather, the first stages are detectable in females around the time of weaning (4 weeks), at least 2 to 3 months before development of overt diabetes. Islets develop in the perivascular/periductular areas of the pancreas. Insulitis initiates as "periinsulitis," a pervasive leukocytic infiltrate emanating from the pancreatic vasculature and secretory ducts. Periinsulitis is not unique to NOD/Lt mice; for example, it can be detected in older mice of the related, but diabetes-resistant, NON/Lt strain, as well as in the diabetes-resistant NOR/Lt strain (36,37). However, what distinguishes the histologic appearance of insulitis in NOD mice from that observed either in the T-lymphopenic BBDR (BB diabetes-prone) rat or in humans is the unusually large numbers of leukocytes associated with all the pancreatic vascular spaces, including the lymphatics (lymphoaccumulation) (38). Lymphoaccumulation is not restricted to the pancreas; increased percentages of T lymphocytes are found in peripheral blood, in lymphoid organs, and in other endocrine tissues. Data in Figure 18.1 comparing NOD/Lt to other ICR (Swiss)-derived inbred strains illustrate this phenomenon. Perhaps reflective of this phenomenon, lymphoid tumors are common in aging NOD/Lt mice that remain free of type 1 diabetes (39). Accumulation of leukocytic infiltrates around the perivascular and periductular regions of the pancreas and subsequent development of progressively more severe insulitis (Fig. 18.2), usually initiates between 3 and 5 weeks in NOD females and several weeks later in males. These intrapancreatic lymphoaccumulations primarily, but not exclusively, comprise T lymphocytes (CD4⁺ >CD8⁺) (40–42). B lymphocytes and macrophage/dendritic cells also are found in the infiltrates (43). Although initially few in number, T lymphocytes capable of adoptively transferring type 1 diabetes into T and B lymphocyte–deficient NOD/LtSz-*scid* recipients can be isolated from islet donors as young as 3 weeks old (44).

Periinsular leukocytic aggregates around NOD islets usually initiate at one pole but eventually surround the entire islet perimeter (periinsulitis). After initiation of periinsulitis (usually in 3- to 5-week-old females and several weeks later in males), only a subset of islets observed in a microscopic field appears to be penetrated by leukocytes. However, as the mice transit through puberty, an increased prevalence of islet profiles showing intra-islet leukocytic infiltrates, coupled with erosion of between 25% and 90% of the insulin-stainable β-cell mass, is noted (18). The early insulitis, although leading to complete destruction of a percentage of islets in a given pancreas, appears

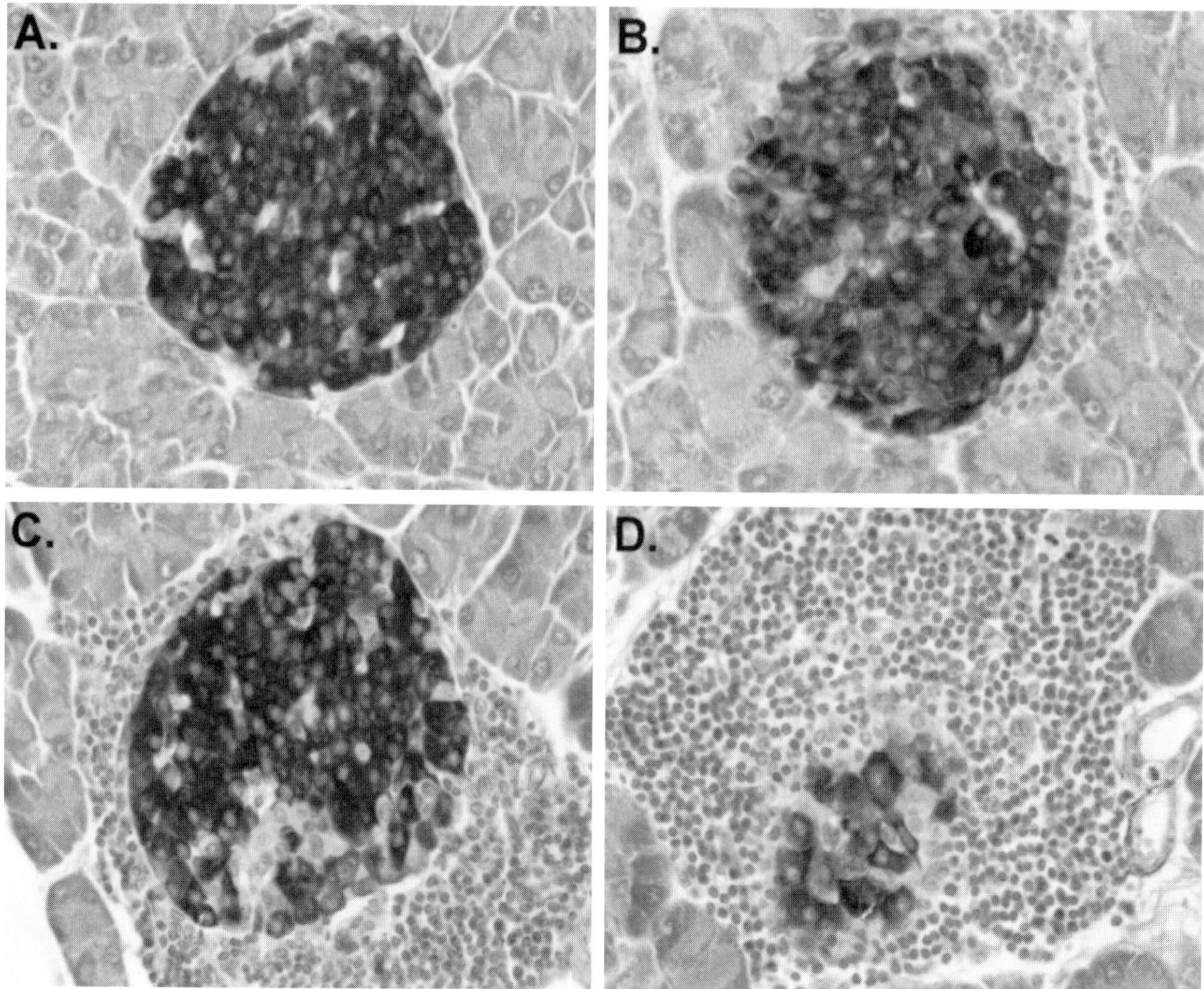

Figure 18.2. Illustration of the various stages of insulitis development in NOD/Lt mice. Islet profiles shown all were photographed in the same pancreas stained with aldehyde fuchsin to identify granulated β-cells. **A:** Unaffected islet at the level of section examined. **B:** Islet showing periinsulitis initiating at one pole. **C:** More extensive insulitis producing erosion of β-cell mass. **D:** Terminal stages of insulitis. Islet residua eventually comprise exclusively non-β endocrine cells.

to be partially compensated by a period of islet growth. During the period between 5 and 12 weeks, NOD/Lt islets are actually quite large in comparison to those of the closely related NON/Lt strain despite the heavy leukocytic aggregations surrounding or penetrating many of the islets in the former. Basal plasma insulin levels are significantly higher in NOD mice of both sexes between 4 and 6 weeks of age compared with levels in C57BL/6 (B6) mice bred in the same vivarium (45). Similarly, NOD fetal pancreas in organ culture secretes higher levels of insulin than does fetal BALB/c pancreas (46). Marked decreases in pancreatic insulin content are demonstrable in NOD/Lt females at around 12 weeks of age and several weeks later in males (47). At this time, increased numbers of atrophic "end-stage" islet profiles are detected. Immunocytochemical staining of these islet residua detects primarily non–β-islet endocrine cells. When more than 90% of the β-cell mass of the pancreas is destroyed, clinical symptoms of diabetes (hyperglycemia, glycosuria, polydipsia, and polyuria) appear abruptly (48). Although intra-islet insulitis initiates early after weaning, some immunoregulatory mechanism apparently keeps many of the infiltrating T lymphocytes in a resting state until a later activation event allows more widespread destruction of the β-cell mass (47,49).

CELLULAR AND MOLECULAR ANALYSIS OF THE INSULITIC PROCESS: "MACROPHAGE INSULITIS"

In considering the insulitis process, the reader should be reminded that important substrain and environmental differences distinguish extant colonies of NOD mice around the world (39). Hence, a longitudinal analysis of cellular and molecular events descriptive of insulitic progression in one colony may not exactly match an analysis of the same parameters in a separate colony. This is especially true for reverse transcriptase–polymerase chain reaction (RT-PCR) estimations of cytokine messenger RNAs (mRNAs) expressed in longitudinal studies.

Islet-associated macrophages may mediate cytopathic events indirectly (through secretion of lymphocyte chemoattractants and through the presentation of autoantigens to them) or directly (via secretion of toxic monokines, prostanoids, nitric oxide, and other reactive oxygen species). An immunocytochemical study of NOD mice from a colony in Paris detected ER-MP23$^+$ and MOMA-1$^+$ macrophages/dendritic-like cells as the first leukocytes to appear around swollen periinsular vessels in 3-week-old mice of both sexes (50); this was termed "macrophage insulitis." At 7 weeks, periinsular accumulations of leukocytes were reported that contained, in addition to the ER-MP23$^+$ and MOMA-1$^+$ cells, a BM8$^+$ cell described as a phagocytotic macrophage. A shift in location from the periinsular space to the islet interior of BM8$^+$ macrophages was associated with intra-islet insulitis and occurred earlier and at higher frequency in the pancreas of females than in the pancreas of males (50). In NOR/Lt mice, in which heavy periinsulitis develops with age, macrophages penetrate into the islet interior but T cells do not, possibly suggesting absence of a critical chemokine (36). Analysis by RT-PCR of spontaneously developing insulitis in NOD mice shows that, although individual islets within a single pancreas may exhibit a T-lymphocyte population expressing a relatively oligoclonal spectrum of T-cell receptor (TCR) genes, pooled islets exhibit a much more diverse spectrum of TCR clonotypes (51). The islet-reactive CD4$^+$ T-cell clones now available from NOD spleens or islets show a diverse array of TCR α- and β-chain rearrangements (52,53). Interestingly, among the H2-K^d-restricted CD8$^+$ islet-reactive clones isolated from NOD pancreatic islets, a more restricted TCR-α gene utilization has been noted, with up to 30% to 35% using an identical Vα17 to Jα42 TCR gene rearrangement (54,55).

As discussed in more detail below, CD4$^+$ T lymphocytes of NOD mice are strongly biased to secrete a T-helper 1 (T_H1) spectrum of proinflammatory lymphokines, especially interferon-γ (IFN-γ). IL-12 and IL-18 are two cytokines associated with the deviation of T lymphocytes toward a T_H1 cytokine profile. Both are expressed at high levels in NOD splenic and islet-infiltrating macrophages (56,57). In the cyclophosphamide (CY)-accelerated model of diabetogenesis in NOD mice, a T_H1-insulitis in NOD/Bom was correlated with upregulation of IL-12 and IL-18 mRNA levels in both spleen and pancreas (56,57). The importance of these monokines is indicated by the observation that onset of type 1 diabetes was retarded by a T_H2 deviation achieved by chronic treatment of prediabetic NOD/Lt females with an IL-12 antagonist (58). An elegant quantitative RT-PCR analysis found I-Aβ^{g7} and Igμ transcript levels to be elevated by 20-fold in islets from 20-day-old NOD/Jsd mice compared with nondiabetic control strains (59). However, these markers for intra-islet APCs encompassing both macrophages and B lymphocytes failed to distinguish NOD/Jsd females that transited to overt type 1 diabetes at a high frequency (80% to 85% by 30 weeks) from NOD/Jsd males that were quite resistant to type 1 diabetes (10% to 15% diabetic by 30 weeks). Fox and Danska (36) subsequently used their quantitative RT-PCR techniques to compare a variety of APC-specific and T lymphocyte–specific transcript levels in NOD/Jsd versus the *$H2^{g7}$* identical, but insulitis- and diabetes-resistant NORLt strain. They reported independent genetic regulation of the macrophage insulitis (found in NOD and NOR) from the more advanced phase involving T-lymphocyte penetration (found primarily in NOD) (36). These findings support the concept that clear "checkpoints" in the development of insulitis exist. The swollen periinsular vasculature prior to lymphocyte penetration of islets described above is associated with increased expression of MHC class II and addressin on vascular endothelium. These changes probably facilitate the NOD strain-characteristic T-lymphocyte accumulation in the pancreatic lymphatics and the subsequent extravasation of $\alpha_4\beta_7$-integrin—positive lymphocytes into the periinsular zones (60,61).

CELLULAR ANALYSIS OF THE INSULITIC PROCESS: THE ROLE OF T AND B LYMPHOCYTES

Small numbers of T lymphocytes (both CD4$^+$ and CD8$^+$), as well as B lymphocytes, are present in the early insulitic lesions (41,62). Studies of adoptive transfer into NODLtSz-*scid* mice confirmed previous reports that pathogenic contributions from both CD4$^+$ and CD8$^+$ subsets are required in the natural progression of the disease (63,64). CD4$^+$ splenic T lymphocytes preactivated *in situ* in overtly diabetic donors can adoptively transfer type 1 diabetes into NOD/LtSz-*scid* recipients in the absence of the CD8$^+$ subset. In contrast, both CD4$^+$ and CD8$^+$ subsets are required to transfer type 1 diabetes if isolated from young, prediabetic donors (63). In NOD/LtSz-*scid* mice, CD8$^+$ T lymphocytes adoptively transferred into NOD-*scid* recipients cannot home to islets in the absence of CD4$^+$ cells (63). The mutual dependency of CD4$^+$ and C8$^+$ T lymphocytes for initiation of disease in adoptive transfers into NOD-*scid* is elegantly illustrated by using NOD-*scid* recipients also homozygous for a targeted β-2 microglobulin (*B2m*) gene. The islets in these recipients do not express MHC class I cell surface molecules and thus do not serve as CD8$^+$ targets. When splenic T lymphocytes from NOD donors of various ages are transferred into this immunodeficient stock, only those from overtly diabetic donors transfer type 1 diabetes in the absence of class I–expressing islets (54, 65). Thus, the earliest initiation, and all but the final phases of autoimmune pancreatic β-cell destruction, require MHC class I–dependent T cells that are able to recognize cognate antigen on MHC class I–expressing β-cell targets. The contributions of CD4$^+$ T cell–secreted cytokines to the development of insulitis through various checkpoints are discussed in the next section.

Adoptive-transfer studies have focused attention on the pathogenic contributions of T lymphocytes, which, when derived from diabetic donors, are able to transfer disease into young recipients without recruitment of host B lymphocytes (66). However, B lymphocytes serving as APCs to amplify T-lymphocyte responses to β-cell autoantigens are essential diabetogenic catalysts in NOD mice. This was established by the discovery that NOD/Lt mice rendered B lymphocyte–deficient either by congenic transfer of a disrupted immunoglobulin heavy-chain gene (Igμ "knockout") or by treatment with antibody to μ chain rarely developed type 1 diabetes (67–69). The absence of B lymphocytes rather than the potential presence of any diabetes resistance genes inadvertently transferred with the genetically disrupted Igμ locus on Chr 12 was demonstrated by abrogation of resistance to type 1 diabetes following repopulation of these mice with B lymphocytes. Autoantibodies, most likely maternal in origin, are found on β-cells from islets of 2- to 3-week-old donors (41). However, such autoantibodies are apparently not required for pathogenesis, since passive transfer of purified serum immunoglobulins from diabetic NOD/Lt donors into these NOD/Lt.*$Ig\mu^{null}$* mice, in contrast to repopulation by B lymphocytes, failed to abrogate the resistance to type 1 diabetes of this stock. It is not known whether the B lymphocytes infiltrating the islet play essential roles in presentation to T lymphocytes of β-cell autoantigens released by T lymphocyte– and/or macrophage-catalyzed β-cell lysis.

MOLECULAR ANALYSIS OF THE INSULITIC PROCESS: THE CHANGING CYTOKINE PROFILE OF ISLET-INFILTRATING LYMPHOCYTES AND THE T_H1-T_H2 PARADIGM

One of the most unusual aspects of the diabetogenic process in NOD mice is that the autoimmune destruction of β-cells can be drastically retarded by so many different manipulations (70). In essence, the immune dysregulation of NOD mice that predisposes the strain to type 1 diabetes, particularly impaired APC function, can be partially corrected by immunostimulation (71). In some instances, the damage mediated by the insulitic process can be halted or reversed at quite a late stage in disease progression (72). In almost all cases in which the consequences of a protective manipulation have been investigated at the level of cytokine expression in the pancreas and, more germane, in the islet-infiltrating lymphocytes, a deviation in the spectrum of cytokine profiles expressed is indicated that suggests a $T_H1 \rightarrow T_H2$ shift has occurred (73,74). Whereas more than 140 manipulations can drastically retard the onset of hyperglycemia in NOD mice, a much smaller number (mostly entailing transgenic or gene targeting manipulations of genes associated with antigen presentation) are capable of completely suppressing the development of insulitis. This paradox of disease suppression, but not insulitis elimination, has given rise to the concept that a "benign" or "nondestructive" form of insulitis that is present in juvenile NOD mice (or NOD male mice in some colonies) can either be maintained or be elicited through maturity. It is widely held that T lymphocytes producing proinflammatory cytokines associated with the T_H1 phenotype, especially IFN-γ, are more likely to effect tissue damage in either spontaneous or experimentally induced T lymphocyte–mediated diseases in mice. Although IL-2 is sometimes used as a paradigm T_H1 cytokine, NOD/Lt T lymphocytes are low producers of IL-2 on a per-cell basis, and the NOD's IL-2 allele may prove to be the susceptibility gene at the *Idd3* locus (75). T_H2 functions [especially the production of IL-4, IL-10, and transforming growth factor-β (TGF-β)] are viewed as protective, or at least as neutral. The genomic makeup of NOD mice predisposes their $CD4^+$ T lymphocytes to respond to antigenic stimulation in a T_H1-biased fashion. As noted previously, NOD macrophages express high levels of IL-12 and IL-18 mRNA (56,57,76,77). This would perhaps partially explain why IFN-γ responses dominate over IL-4/IL-10 secretory responses in NOD mice.

A longitudinal analysis of cytokine gene expression in a colony of NOD/Jsd mice with a marked gender difference in the frequency of type 1 diabetes illustrates the changing cytokine profile that accompanies the progression of NOD mice toward frank hyperglycemia (59). Quantitative RT-PCR analysis showed that islet-infiltrating lymphocytes in males maintained a higher ratio of IL-4/IFN-γ transcripts through puberty than did females, with the increased likelihood of the development of type 1 diabetes in the latter associated with waning expression of T_H2 transcripts (59). These types of data reinforce the concept that insulitic destruction of β-cells in NOD mice is represented neither by a continuous linear regression line nor by an abrupt, late-activating process but rather by a gradual and chaotic progression wherein both regulatory events (including the changing endocrine milieu imposed by puberty and reproduction) and stochastic events (the particular subpopulation of $CD4^+$ and $CD8^+$ T lymphocytes "resident" in any given islet) determine the rate at which the diabetes threshold of more than 90% β-cell destruction is reached. The finding that many immunomodulatory interventions that retard type 1 diabetes development in this model produce a $T_H1 \rightarrow T_H2$ deviation is generally assumed to be evidence that the deviation itself was the basis for the retarded destruction of β-cells by islet-infiltrating effectors. However, recent analysis of NOD stocks congenic for disrupted genes encoding IFN-γ, IFN-γ receptor β chain, IL-4, and IL-10 has forced a reevaluation of this rather simplistic, but attractive concept.

NOD mice congenic for either a disrupted IFN-γ or IFN-γ receptor β gene (e.g., unresponsive to IFN-γ signaling while producing high levels of T_H2 cytokines) develop type 1 diabetes, while NOD stocks homozygous for disrupted IL-4 and IL-10 genes do not become diabetic at an accelerated rate (35,78,79). Although NOD mice congenic for a disrupted IFN-γ receptor α subunit have been reported to be resistant to type 1 diabetes, a subsequent report indicates that the resistance is not the result of the targeted allele on Chr 10 but rather a contribution of strain 129 genome in tight linkage (80,81). Treatment of standard prediabetic NOD mice with the nonspecific immunomodulator BCG (bacille Calmette-Guérin) induced resistance to type 1 diabetes resistance with a $T_H1 \rightarrow T_H2$ deviation. This treatment also protected NOD stocks congenic for disrupted IL-4 or IL-10 genes (35,82). Surprisingly, the IFN-γ–deficient stock is not protected by BCG (35). Collectively, these observations suggest that the $T_H1 \rightarrow T_H2$ deviation so commonly associated with protective immunomodulatory protocols are consequences, rather than causes, of the deviation. A number of studies have shown that NOD APCs, particularly macrophages, are not fully mature and hence fail to provide normal costimulatory signals such as IL-1, while producing high levels of prostaglandin E_2 (83,84). The resistance of NOD peripheral T lymphocytes to activation-induced cell death (AICD) may explain the T_H1 bias, since T_H1 cells normally are more prone to AICD than are T_H2 cells (85,86). Hence, if certain type 1 diabetes–preventative protocols differentially stimulate the AICD of β-cell autoreactive T lymphocytes in a way that preferentially spares those producing T_H2 cytokines, it would give the appearance of a $T_H1 \rightarrow T_H2$ cytokine shift (35).

MOLECULAR ANALYSIS OF THE INSULITIC PROCESS: THE ROLE OF THE β-CELL AND CANDIDATE β-CELL AUTOANTIGENS

A number of genetic and molecular genetic manipulations designed to limit the T-cell receptor repertoire available to $CD4^+$ and/or $CD8^+$ T cells in the NOD mouse generally fail to prevent type 1 diabetes (87). Hence, the NOD thymus is extremely flexible in its ability to generate a diabetogenic T-cell repertoire, even when rearranged TCR transgenes dictate a repertoire predominantly skewed to an "irrelevant" antigen [e.g., lymphocytic choriomeningitis virus (LCMV) peptide not expressed in NOD β-cells]. The broad spectrum of TCR clonotypes of both $CD4^+$ and $CD8^+$ T cell lines and clones reported to produce β-cytotoxicity effects in the NOD mouse reinforce the diversity of antigens recognized. An unresolved issue is whether a single β-cell autoantigen is targeted initially, followed by "downstream" immune reactivities as other antigens are processed and presented following the initial destruction of a few β-cells. The most commonly discussed candidate autoantigens in humans (based upon spontaneous autoantibody development) are insulin, glutamic acid decarboxylase (GAD), and IA-2, a putative tyrosine phosphatase localized in β-granules (88–91). Debate about NOD mice has focused on whether insulin or GAD represents the primary autoantigen. T-lymphocyte responses to GAD peptides appear earlier than to other candidate autoantigens, including carboxypeptidase E, peripherin, and heat-shock protein 60 (92). Administration of autoantigens in tolerogenic doses to prediabetic NOD mice can retard the development of type 1 diabetes (93,94). A rather controversial report that GAD67 is the primary autoantigen in NOD β-cells has not been replicated and is suspect because of the claims of easily detectable GAD67 protein in NOD β-cells by immunocytochemistry (95). Based on the plasticity of the T-cell repertoire capable of destroying NOD islets, the most conservative position regarding β-cell autoantigens in the NOD model is that a multiplicity must exist, each individually capable of serving as a target for autoimmune initiation. As noted above, $CD8^+$ T lymphocytes are essential for such initiation, suggesting that the initiating event entails recognition of autoantigenic peptide presented by the β-cell target or vascular endothelium near the β-cells.

Most studies examining the interaction between NOD T lymphocytes and their β-cell targets assume that if the appropriate autoantigen(s) is present and there are T lymphocytes in the periphery with the appropriate TCR clonotype(s), then type

1 diabetes will ensue. This is not necessarily true. Both rodent and human β-cells have very weak defenses against oxidative stress (96). NOD β-cells appear typical of most mouse strains in being quite sensitive to cell death mediated by combinations of monokines and IFN-γ. Analysis of β-cells from ALR/Lt mice, a strain closely related to NOD and selected for resistance to type 1 diabetes induced by a low dose of alloxan, has demonstrated that genes expressed at the β-cell level, and presumably associated with dissipation of reactive oxygen species, can protect against both toxic combinations of cytokines and monokines, as well as against islet-reactive cytotoxic T cells isolated from NOD islets and capable of recognizing antigens presented by ALR/Lt islets (13,97–99).

GENETICS OF TYPE 1 DIABETES

"Idd" loci: What and How Many?

A provisional nomenclature exists to describe murine chromosomal regions carrying genes capable of modulating susceptibility of type 1 diabetes. Such loci, designated *"Idd"* loci are uncovered either by out-crossing NOD mice to type 1 diabetes–resistant strains of mice and then doing segregation analysis or by genetically disrupting specific genes and analyzing the consequences on the development of type 1 diabetes (100). Segregation analysis has shown that many strains harbor potential *"Idd"* susceptibility contributions but that the NOD strain is unfortunate in terms of the large numbers randomly inbred into them during the generation of the strain. If the large numbers of genes shown by gene-targeting experiments to be essential for mediation of the diabetogenic process are excluded and only *"Idd"* loci identified by out-crossing NOD to type 1 diabetes-resistant strains are considered, linkage of more than 19 loci on 10 chromosomes have been reported [reviewed in references (39,87)]. Although originally given sequential numbers as they were reported in the literature, segments of chromosomes now carrying genes capable of modifying the frequency of type 1 diabetes are simply being described by molecular markers physically delimiting the region (generally simple sequence repeat–containing alleles). As noted above, certain of the susceptibility linkages derive from the genomes of type 1 diabetes–free outcross partner strains, and in one case, admixture of a wild-derived strain's genome produced a male gender–biased type 2 diabetes (3,4). To further complicate matters, a chromosomal segment identified initially through segregation analysis as containing a single *"Idd"* generally yields multiple loci when subcongenic analysis is conducted. Classical genetic segregation analysis greatly underestimates the actual number of genes required for the development of type 1 diabetes since transgenic and gene-targeting technologies being applied to analyze the genetic control of the development of type 1 diabetes in NOD mice are providing an ever-expanding panoply of contributory *"Idd"* loci, only a few of which will be discussed. Although most genomic manipulation by transgenic or gene "knockout" technology has focused on genes expressed in the immune system, it is now clear that genes expressed systemically and within the pancreatic β-cell can also be important modifiers of susceptibility (101). A discussion of the MHC-linked diabetogenic contributions (*"Idd1"*) will suffice to underscore the complexity of *"Idd"* loci and their interactions.

Paramount Role of Major Histocompatiblity Complex

The first genetic analysis of type 1 diabetes in the NOD mice reported a recessive susceptibility for clinical disease linked to MHC (102). Because the MHC complex contains genes essential for antigen processing and presentation, as well as for immune cell function, and given evidence indicative of broad-based immunotolerogenic defects in NOD mice, it is not surprising that $H2^{g7}$, encompassing both common class I alleles, a rare class II A^{g7} allele, and absence of class II E (the HLA-DR homologue), provides the major component of genetic susceptibility (103–105). Indeed, specific amino acid substitutions in the H2-Ab^{g7} chain reflect similar residues present in the human *HLA-DQ0302* allele linked to increased susceptibility to type 1 diabetes in whites. These include a histidine residue at position 56 and a serine residue at position 57 of the β chain. Recent radiographic crystallographic analysis helps to understand the diabetogenic properties of the I-A^{g7} molecule. The NOD I-A^{g7} molecule behaved very much like I-A^d, a MHC class II molecule that shares the same β chain with I-A^{g7} but contains proline and aspartic acid at residues 56–57 of the β chain and protects from diabetes. Binding affinities of a large collection of peptides are comparable for I-A^{g7} and I-A^d. Presence of negatively charged residues in the C-terminal region of the peptide increases binding affinity to I-A^{g7}. Exchange of the aspartic acid, as found in I-A^d, by a serine at position β57, increases the size of the P9 pocket of I-A^{g7} and exposes positively charged residues. As a consequence, the I-A^{g7} P9 pocket can bind negatively charged residues and residues with larger side chains than does I-A^d. These two features expand the peptide repertoire of I-A^{g7} by several-fold in comparison to I-A^d. Immunoprecipitation studies suggested that I-A^{g7}-peptide complexes are more unstable than similar MHC class II complexes from B6 (106). This might imply that I-A^{g7} bound more peptides, but with lower affinities such that cytopathic T-effectors are not centrally or peripherally deleted.

Molecular Dissection of "Idd1"

The diabetogenic relevance of the nested set of five nucleotide substitutions between position 248–252 converting a conserved proline residue at amino acid position 56 to histidine and aspartic acid 57 to serine was confirmed separately by production of transgenic stocks of NOD mice expressing Ab^{g7} alleles modified by site-specific mutagenesis to convert either the histidine 56 residue to proline or the serine 57 residue to aspartic acid (107–110). Further demonstration that *"Idd1"* comprised at least two linked, but separable susceptibility components was provided by the demonstration that the development of type 1 diabetes was also drastically suppressed or completely prevented in stocks of NOD mice expressing *H2-Ea*transgenes that restored H2-E expression on APC (107,109–111). It is not only the MHC class II region that contributes susceptibility in NOD mice but rather multiple loci in the extended haplotype. The requirement for MHC class I expression for cytopathic $CD8^+$ T-lymphocyte targeting of islet β-cells has been detailed above. It is noteworthy that extended haplotype analysis of human genes in linkage disequilibrium with *HLA-DR* and *-DQ* alleles conferring susceptibility to type 1 diabetes indicates additional susceptibility components toward the class I region (112). Analysis of NOD stocks congenic for recombinant haplotypes generated by crossover between $H2^{g7}$ and $H2^{209}$ provide evidence of additional *"Idd"* contributors centromeric to a *Lmp2* recombinatorial hotspot that both includes and extends proximal to the *H2-K* gene (113). One of these could represent *"Idd16,"* initially mapped in linkage disequilibrium to *Idd1* on Chr 17 (114). Because of this complexity, it is difficult to discuss whether the haplotype contributes susceptibility in a dominant or recessive fashion. Segregants heterozygous for $H2^{g7}$ may develop subclinical levels of insulitis (suggesting dominant $H2^{g7}$ contributions to this important diabetes subphenotype) and may even develop overt type 1 diabetes following cyclophosphamide treatment (115,116). However, type 1 diabetes rarely develops spontaneously in such heterozygotes, especially when an *Ea* product is expressed by the other H2 haplotype (116). In this regard, the NOD model diverges from the human situation, where certain HLA heterozygous haplotypes increase rather than suppress susceptibility to type 1 diabetes (117). In summary, "*Idd1*" is a collective descriptor for multiple disease-predisposing alleles within or linked to the MHC complex.

Diabetogenesis Entails Complex Major Histocompatibility Complex–Non-major–Histocompatibility Complex Interactions

Susceptibility to type 1 diabetes in segregating hybrids following outcross of NOD to other mouse strains is inherited as a polygenic threshold liability, requiring a complex interaction between the *H2*^{g7} haplotype and numerous other MHC-unlinked genes (118). None of the non-MHC genes present in the NOD genome contributes the same risk as the extended MHC haplotype, but homozygosity for *H2*^{g7} in the absence of a diverse collection of the NOD strain's collection of non-MHC susceptibility modifiers is insufficient to trigger type 1 diabetes (119). Unraveling the genetic basis for the development of type 1 diabetes in the NOD mouse is complicated by interactions between the NOD mouse's diabetogenic *H2*^{g7} and the welter of non-MHC "*Idd*" loci, none of which alone is sufficient to elicit type 1 diabetes. This can be demonstrated by developing B6 stocks congenic for long "*Idd*" susceptibility intervals from NOD (120). Although some level of periinsulitis can be seen, severe insulitis does not develop, even when bicongenic stocks are analyzed that carry both the non-MHC interval and the NOD "*Idd1*" genes on Chr 17 (121). Genetic analysis is further complicated by the finding that the set of non-MHC genes segregated are not constant but vary depending upon the type 1 diabetes–resistant partner strain used in the outcross. An "*Idd*" exerting a strong effect in one cross may not be detectable at all in another outcross combination. The situation is made even more complex by the knowledge that strong environmental influences, as well as intergenic interactions, affect gene penetrances and ultimate presentation of clinical disease. The interested reader is referred to a recent review of current knowledge of the locations and potential functions of the most intensively studied of the known non-MHC loci (87). Several examples are provided below to illustrate the nature and complexity of the intergenic "cross-talk" required for diabetogenesis.

Illustrations of Diabetogenic Epistasis

Segregation analysis between *H2*^{g7}-identical NOD/Lt and NOR/Lt mice permitted elucidation of a Chr 2/Chr 17 (MHC) interaction. Even though the MHC class I alleles of NOD and NOR mice (*H2K*^{d}, *H2D*^{b}) are commonly expressed in non–autoimmune-prone strains, they acquire diabetogenic function in NOD mice (122). A relatively long segment of NOR/Lt-derived genome on Chr 2 containing at least two resistance genes (collectively described as "*Idd13*") provided partial protection from type 1 diabetes in a NOD congenic stock (123). Included in this congenic interval was an NOR-derived *B2m*^{b} allele, replacing the equally common *B2m*^{a} allele expressed by NOD. This seemed an unlikely candidate gene for an "*Idd13*" component since these two MHC class I–binding proteins differed at only a single amino acid and did not alter total expression levels of MHC class I molecules. However, conformational analysis indeed showed that dimerization of NOD MHC class I K^{d} and D^{b} chains with the alternative β2m isoforms differentially altered their structural conformation (123). The type 1 diabetes–free NOD.*B2m*^{null} stock described above provided the means for a rigorous test of *B2m* candidacy by transgenic insertion directly into these zygotes of transgenes encoding either β2m isoform. A CD8^{+} T-cell repertoire was positively selected in both lines, but only the line with the reconstituted expression of the *B2m*^{a} (NOD-type) isoform developed type 1 diabetes (87). This represents the first empirical demonstration of the molecular nature of a non-MHC "*Idd*" candidate.

In addition to this Chr 2/Chr 17 (MHC) epistatic interaction, a recent genetic analysis of the markedly different course of insulitis progression in NOR versus NOD has suggested an epistatic interaction between the Chr 2 "*Idd13*" region containing the *B2m* candidate and Chr 1 ("*Idd5.2*" region) (124). Epistasis has also been reported among "*Idd*" loci on Chr 3, specifically the *Idd3* locus marked by the *Il2* allele and more distal loci denoted as "*Idd10/17/18*" (116).

Genetics of Mouse Type 1 Diabetes and the Identification of Human Type 1 Diabetes Genes

Although the *H2*^{g7} haplotype was originally thought to be unique to the NOD mouse, this haplotype is shared by the type 1 diabetes–free ILI strain (125). Several of its diabetogenic components (e.g., the class II alleles and the *H2-K*^{d} allele) also present in the related ALR and CTS strains (126,127). Since the ALR/Lt strain exhibits remarkable genetic resistance to autoimmune stress, it is clear that "diabetogenic" MHC alleles are not inherently diabetogenic but acquire diabetogenic potency only in the context of the non-MHC background (101). Moreover, not all of the susceptibility alleles will derive from the NOD genome, and some admixtures can produce type 2 rather than type 1 diabetes (4). What is the implication of this complexity for the inheritance of type 1 diabetes in humans? Will identification of mouse "*Idd*" loci identify possible homologous susceptibility regions in the human genome? There are a number of reasons why many of the known non-MHC mouse "*Idd*" loci are not matched by type 1 diabetes loci in the syntenic regions of the human genome. Important genus-specific differences distinguish mice from humans. The human *IDDM2* locus has been identified in both association and linkage studies and is defined by polymorphisms in a VNTR (variable number of tandem repeats) upstream of the human insulin (*INS*) gene (128). Although proinsulin/insulin represents a major type 1 diabetes autoantigen in both humans and NOD mice, an NOD homologue of the human *INS* gene (mouse *Ins2* on distal Chr 7) has not been detected in most segregation analyses (129,130). This lack of concordance might be expected because mice express two genes for insulin (the additional gene is *Ins1* on Chr 19). The "*Idd3*" (*Il2*) linkage is one of the strongest and most commonly identified non-MHC loci segregating in NOD outcrosses; the *IL2* gene in the homologous 4q26-q27 region in humans has not yet been implicated as a major type 1 diabetes–susceptibility locus (25). Of all the non-MHC loci identified in NOD outcrosses, the "*Idd5.1*" region containing the *Cd152* (*Ctla4*) locus may be reflected by the *IDDM12* linkage to the homologous region on human 2q33 (131,132). Despite the finding that non-MHC genes contributing to the development of type 1 diabetes in NOD mice often are not reflected by demonstration in humans of linkage to the syntenic region, the value of the mouse system is to elucidate specific immunologic or endocrinologic dysfunctions that are entrained when sufficient numbers of "*Idd*" genes are present. While the human *IL2* structural gene has not been implicated as a gene for type 1 diabetes, it is certainly possible that an unlinked gene, acting in *trans*, could confer a higher risk for type 1 diabetes by affecting IL-2 glycosylation state, as is implicated in the NOD mouse. Even if the controlling genes are not transposable from mice to humans in a one-to-one ratio, many of the phenotypes diagnostic of high susceptibility may be common. Further discussion of the similarities and differences between humans and mice in this regard is found in Chapter 21.

CELLULAR BASIS FOR GENETIC SUSCEPTIBILITY

Defective Antigen-Presenting Cell Functions

Although T lymphocytes often are the focus of studies describing immunotolerogenic defects in the NOD mouse, studies using bone marrow chimeras have demonstrated that the origin of many of the defects can be traced to APC dysfunction (macrophage, dendritic cells, and B lymphocytes). Diminished levels of antigen presentation by MHC molecules represent one likely mechanism whereby immune tolerance is not fully acquired. Both intrathymic and peripheral tolerance induction also requires costimulatory signals delivered to T lymphocytes by APC. Considerable evidence indicates that the APC of NOD mice maintained in SPF environments are deficient in ability to provide sufficiently high levels of costimulation. NOD macrophages maturing from bone marrow precursors do not become as functionally mature as macrophages from control strains (83,133,134). This blunted functional development is indicated by subnormal lipopolysaccharide (LPS)–stimulated IL-1 secretion and by reduced CD86 (B7-2) gene expression (83, 133,135). D-galactosamine–sensitized NOD mice are resistant to doses of LPS and TNF-α that produce lethal hepatocellular injury and apoptosis in B6 mice (136). These hypofunctions are negatively reinforced by constitutive expression of the normally inducible prostaglandin E_2 synthase gene (*Pgst2* on Chr 1) and hence secrete higher than normal levels of prostaglandin E_2 (84). Defects in both the high-affinity Fcγ1 receptor and Fcγ2 receptor have been reported (84,137). Both defects might be expected to affect the ability of macrophages to phagocytose monomeric IgG2c and IgG2b antibodies, respectively (the NOD mouse expresses the IgG2c and not the IgG2a isotype as is commonly assumed) (138). Glutathione levels are lower in NOD macrophages than in the NOR/Lt control strain, possibly contributing both to reduced capacity to process and present MHC class II–restricted antigens to $CD4^+$ T cells and to the T_H1 bias in response to antigen priming (139,140). Some anomalies in development of marrow-derived NOD dendritic cells have also been reported (141). Vitamin D metabolism is also disturbed in NOD macrophages (141a). The ability of many different microbial immunomodulators, such as CFA, BCG, and OK432, to upregulate APC function and to promote T-lymphocyte apoptosis links APC defects in costimulatory signaling to this major defect in the NOD T-lymphocyte compartment (e.g., their resistance to multiple forms of apoptosis) (35,142). Indeed, the high production of prostaglandin E_2 from NOD macrophages could contribute to T-lymphocyte apoptosis resistance by antagonizing TCR-coupled protein kinase C (PKC) second-messenger activities.

Thymocyte/T-lymphocyte Anomalies

The T-lymphocyte accumulation characteristic of NOD mice, reflected at its most extreme by the formation of what appear to be lymphoid follicles in the perivascular spaces of the pancreas and submandibular salivary glands, is a secondary reflection of resistance to AICD. Both NOD thymocytes and peripheral T lymphocytes are relatively resistant to AICD, as well as to apoptosis induced by dexamethasone, irradiation, or stress (143–148). A less severe resistance of male thymocytes to AICD may explain the reduced male susceptibility to type 1 diabetes (149). As discussed above, elevated prostaglandin E_2 levels may account for the association between poor proliferation in response to TCR cross-linking agents and reduced ability of thymocytes/T lymphocytes to activate TCR-coupled PKC second-messenger pathways (150). The earliest thymic immigrants, especially in females, may be enriched for effector T lymphocytes versus regulatory cells, because thymectomy at 3 weeks of age accelerates the onset of type 1 diabetes in females, but interestingly, not in NOD males (151).

IL-2 is now recognized not only as a growth factor for T lymphocytes but also as a required factor for AICD. The *Il2^b^* allele expressed by NOD is distinguished from the *Il2^a^* allele expressed by NON, BALB/c, and C57BL strains by presence of a T→C point mutation producing at residue 6 a Ser→Pro substitution, a four–amino-acid insertion at residue 8 (Ser-Ser-Pro-Thr), and a deletion of four glutamine residues within a polyglutamine stretch between residues 19 and 30 (152,153). *Il2* is an attractive candidate gene not only because IL-2 treatment of prediabetic NOD mice suppresses the development of type 1 diabetes but also because genetic disruption of the *Il2* gene produces severe lymphoproliferative disease with widespread tissue infiltrates, including pancreatitis and insulitis (71,154). Production by NOD splenic T lymphocytes of bioactive IL-2 on a "per-cell" basis was less than that from SWR/Bm, another Swiss-derived strain that shares the $Il2^b$ allotype (155,156). The NOD-produced molecule is associated with a higher glycosylation state, and this may affect either half-life or ability to induce AICD (157).

Numerous defects in T-regulatory cell functions have been reported in NOD mice (158). Among the presumed regulatory cells are natural killer T (NKT) cells. Representing a small population (<3%) of peripheral lymphoid cells, they are $CD3^+$, $CD8^-$, and either $CD4^-$ or $CD4^+$. Their selection entails recognition of glycolipid antigens presented by the nonclassical MHC class I–like CD1 molecule (159). Deficiencies in both number and immunoregulatory function of NOD NKT cells have been reported (160,161). These deficiencies include a low level of IL-4 secretion, a defect that can be corrected either by IL-7 treatment or by congenic transfer of B6 genes regulating natural killer (NK) and NKT function (including their NK1.1 phenotypic marker) in the "*Idd6*" type 1 diabetes–resistance region (162–164). Enriched populations of cells with an NKT phenotype can protect NOD mice from type 1 diabetes, leading to the suggestion that T_H2 cytokine secretion by these cells mediates the protection (162). However, NKT cells stimulated *in vitro* and *in vivo* actually produce more IFN-γ than IL-4 (165,166). Indeed, type 1 diabetes–resistant NOD.B6-"*Idd6*" mice produce more serum IFN-γ upon stimulation with α-galactosyl ceramide than do standard NOD mice (164). Hence, the molecular basis for NKT-mediated protection may be more complicated than a simple T_H1 to T_H2 deviation.

POLYGLANDULAR AUTOIMMUNITY

Salivary and Lacrimal/Harderian Glands

The multiplicity of immunodeficiencies characteristic of NOD mice leads to leukocytic infiltrations into endocrine organs in addition to pancreatic islets. Particularly notable are heavy infiltrations of the submandibular salivary gland (sialoadenitis) and the lacrimal and harderian gland of the eye (dacryoadenitis). Both sialoadenitis and dacryoadenitis in NOD mice develop after puberty, considerably later than insulitis. Splenic T lymphocytes from both overtly diabetic and young prediabetic NOD mice adoptively transfer these lesions into NOD/LtSz-*scid* mice (167). Although T lymphocytes are present, the infiltrates are not associated with a loss of glandular acinar cells as extensive as the progressive loss of β-cells in the pancreas (168,169). Since the sialoadenitis impairs salivary flow rates and protein content, and since NOD mice also develop leukocytic infiltrates in their lacrimal and harderian glands, NOD mice may serve as a model for Sjögren syndrome in humans (170). Although loss of salivary gland structural integrity is not as extensive as in Sjögren syndrome in humans, xerostomia ("dry mouth"), a clinical condition often associated with both Sjögren syndrome and type 1 diabetes in humans, is reflected in NOD mice (170). The dacryoadenitis develops at fourfold higher frequency in postpubertal males than females and can be suppressed by male castration, while tamoxifen treatment significantly increased frequency of this lesion in males (171). Its autoimmune nature was documented by upregulation of inflammatory T_H1 cytokine genes in the infiltrating T lymphocytes (171). As is the case for insulitis, salivary gland infiltrates are composed primarily of $CD4^+$ cells with smaller numbers of $CD8^+$ cells and with a diversity of TCR clonotypes represented (172). Insulin and insulin-like growth factors I and II are found at low concentrations in mouse saliva, as well as in parotid and submandibular glands, and hence may represent a potential target antigen (173). TNF-α is apparently involved in lesion development, since treatment of NOD mice with a soluble TNF-receptor p55 subunit inhibits infiltration in both submandibular and lacrimal glands (174). NOD strain–specific anomalies in the development of the submandibular gland were found in NOD/LtSz-*scid* mice lacking functional T and B lymphocytes (175). Hence, these developmental anomalies may trigger sialoadenitis when a functional immune system is present. An interesting aspect of the sialoadenitis in NOD mice is the potential role of autoantibodies. B lymphocyte–deficient NOD/Lt.$Ig\mu^{null}$ mice rarely develop type 1 diabetes, but they do develop sialoadenitis and dacryoadenitis in the absence of insulitis and type 1 diabetes (176). Passive transfer into these immunoglobulin-deficient mice of serum immunoglobulins either from standard NOD mice or from patients with primary Sjögren syndrome, but not from healthy controls, inhibited binding of ligands to muscarinic receptors on salivary membranes (176).

Thyroid Glands

Another common histopathologic lesion described in NOD mice is the presence of leukocytic infiltrates in the thyroid follicles (thyroiditis). This is of interest because autoimmune thyroid disease (Grave disease or Hashimoto thyroiditis) is frequently associated with type 1 diabetes in humans. However, the spontaneously developing lesions in NOD are not so severe that clinical manifestations of hypothyroidism appear. If goiters are induced and followed by iodine loading, severe lesions causing hypothyroidism are elicited (177,178).

Splenocytes from diabetic NOD/Lt donors also adoptively transferred thyroiditis into NOD/LtSz-*scid* recipients, albeit at a lower efficiency than insulitis (167). Spontaneous development of thyroiditis varies widely among different NOD colonies, with differences in environmental factors such as dietary iodine content representing possible explanations (179). Parathyroiditis has also been reported in one colony (180). Criteria for assessing thyroiditis may be partially responsible for the variability between colonies. A confounding factor in the diagnosis of both thyroiditis or parathyroiditis in NOD mice is the presence of a high frequency of thymic ectopies to the thyroid gland (181). Thymic ectopies are present at ~20% frequency in this author's (EHL) NOD/Lt colony, but significant leukocytic infiltration into thyroid interstitium or into follicles is relatively rare (~5% of mice sampled to 16 weeks of age). In a colony of NOD mice with a low incidence of diabetes accompanied by a high incidence (77%) of subclinical thyroiditis, as well as by antithyroid autoantibodies in older mice, thyroiditis was clearly independent from spontaneous development of type 1 diabetes (182). This was reinforced by the findings in a NOD colony in Paris with a high frequency of type 1 diabetes accompanied by a high incidence (20.5%) of thyroiditis in nondiabetic survivors (mostly males) aged to 90 weeks (183). When this incidence was compared with that of a diabetes-resistant NOD stock congenic for the $H2^k$ haplotype (associated with high susceptibility of the CBA/J inbred strain to experimentally induced thyroiditis), a significantly higher (30.3%) frequency of thyroiditis was noted (183). An age-associated increase in MHC class II expression on macrophages and thyroid epithelial cells has been noted (184). Clinically significant lesions comparable to Hashimoto thyroiditis can be induced in NOD mice by administration of a diet high in sodium iodide following induction of goiters using a diet low in iodine in combination with treatment with phenylthiourea (178). NOD/Mrk congenic for an intra-MHC recombinant haplotype ($H2^{h4}$) expressing $H2\text{-}K^k$ and $H2\text{-}A^k$ alleles will develop thyroiditis following exposure to sodium iodide alone (116).

AGING-ASSOCIATED PATHOLOGIES

Cancer

In addition to these polyendocrinopathies, leukocytic infiltrates of varying intensity can be found in liver (mild focal hepatitis), kidney (focal nephritis), and muscle (myositis) (185). If development of type 1 diabetes in NOD mice is prevented such that life span is extended, this strain exhibits a virtual "Pandora's box" of pathologies (185). A spectrum of tumors has been identified in the research colony at The Jackson Laboratory. Of these, lymphomas are those diagnosed most frequently. This propensity for lymphomagenesis in the absence of diabetes is starkly illustrated by the near 100% frequency of thymic lymphomas in NOD/LtSz-*scid* mice and B (follicle center) cell lymphomas in NOD/LtSz-Rag^{null} congenic mice (32,186). Osteosarcomas, a relatively rare tumor in mice, are also detected at a relatively high frequency in standard NOD/Lt mice in The Jackson Laboratory research colony (186).

Hearing Defects

NOD mice are severely hearing-impaired, developing a progressive hearing loss as assessed by auditory-evoked brain-stem responses (187,188). In most NOD mice, hearing loss progresses to complete deafness by 3 months. CBA/J mice have normal hearing. Three recombinant congenic stocks have been produced by outcross of NOD mice to CBA/LtJ, followed by a backcross to CBA and then inbreeding of first backcross progeny (29). Testing of auditory-evoked brain-stem response of these three recombinant congenic lines carrying mixtures of *NODLt* and *CBALtJ* genes indicates that this trait is under polygenic control, since one line hears as well as CBA and two lines have moderately impaired hearing. Because all three lines share the $H2^{g7}$ MHC haplotype with NOD, genes within this complex are excluded.

Hemolytic Anemia

Hemolytic anemia accompanied by development of Coombs-positive autoantibodies, reticulocytosis, splenomegaly, and jaundice, has been observed in aging (older than 200 days) mice of both the NOD/Wehi and NOD/Lt substrains maintained in Australia (189). In the low-diabetes-incidence NOD/Wehi substrain, 14 of 17 nondiabetic mice were affected by 550 days.

EXPERIMENTALLY INDUCED LESIONS

NOD mice are susceptible to a variety of experimentally induced organ-specific immune diseases, including drug-induced diabetes, lupus, colitis, encephalomyelitis, and thyroiditis. Not surprisingly, young NOD/Lt males, like outbred CD1 males, are susceptible to induction of type 1 diabetes by multiple low doses of the fungal antibiotic streptozotocin (190). This sensitivity is independent of autoimmune T-cell involvement, since NOD/LtSz-*scid* males are even more sensitive to low doses of this diabetogen (190). Injection of a single dose of 2.6 × 10^7 heat-killed *Mycobacterium tuberculosis* (BCG) intravenously into 8-week-old NOD mice prevented diabetes but precipitated a syndrome similar to systemic lupus erythematosus (191). Exposure of NOD/Lt mice to 3.5% dextran sodium sulfate in the drinking water for 5 days elicits a severe colitis (192). Experimental allergic encephalomyelitis can be induced in NOD mice using a peptide fragment (residues 56–70) in adjuvant from proteolipid protein (193). The NOD allele at the "*Idd3*" locus (in the region of the gene encoding IL-2) has been shown to be a component of this strain's high susceptibility to encephalitis induction (24). A similar demyelinating disease can be induced by injection of the MOG peptide (residues 35–55) in adjuvant; this model is prevented by treatment with anti–IL-12 antibody. A single intravenous injection of pertussin without adjuvant into NOD mice induced a T-cell–mediated encephalitis (194).

The BioBreeding Rat

INSULITIS AND DEVELOPMENT OF TYPE 1 DIABETES: COMPARISONS WITH NONOBESE DIABETIC

BioBreeding (BB) rats are a diabetes-prone strain derived from outbred Wistar rats from a commercial colony in Canada (195). The interested reader is referred to comprehensive recent reviews (196–200). Spontaneous type 1 diabetes was discovered in 1974, and selective breeding for that phenotype ensued. As with NOD mice, multiple substrains of BB rats exist, and lymphoid infiltrates are not limited to the pancreatic islets (201). The best-characterized BB colonies are those developed at the University of Massachusetts Medical School and now commercially distributed by Biomedical Research Models (Worcester, MA). A diabetes-resistant substrain (BBDR/Wor) has been selected, as have several diabetes-prone (BBDP/Wor) lines. These BB rats are fully inbred and characterized. In the Worcester virus-antibody-free (VAF) barrier colony, the frequency of type 1 diabetes in both sexes of DP rats exceeds 90%, whereas no spontaneous type 1 diabetes develops in VAF BBDR/Wor rats. A major genetic and phenotypic difference distinguishing the DR from the various DP strains is the presence in the DP line of a recessive mutation, lymphopenia (*Lyp*), on Chr 4 (202–204). Although DP rats develop a thymus of normal size and cellularity, recent thymic T lymphocyte emigrants to the periphery [phenotypically Thy-1^+ and not yet expressing a cell-surface adenosine diphosphate (ADP)–ribosyltransferase (formerly designated RT6 and now designated ART2)] are very short-lived (205,206). The consequence is a profound T-lymphopenia/lymphocytopenia. Hence, these rats are severely immunocompromised, as reflected by impaired T-lymphocyte function *in vitro*, impaired ability to reject foreign tissue grafts, increased susceptibility to B-lymphomagenesis, and requirement for special husbandry procedures to protect against infections by opportunistic pathogens. This obviously contrasts sharply with NOD mice, whose T lymphocytes are long-lived in the periphery, present in large numbers, and express a functional ortholog of rat RT6 (now designated as ART2 in both genera) (207). Whereas BBDP rats are strongly immunocompromised, as evidenced by difficulty in rejecting non-islet allografted tissues and being susceptible to infectious pathogens, NOD T cells are capable of rapidly rejecting allografted tissues, and NOD mice are remarkably pathogen-resistant. There are many additional distinctions between BB rats and NOD mice in the diabetes syndrome itself, reviewed elsewhere, and some are summarized in Table 18.4 (6,197,198).

GENETICS OF TYPE 1 DIABETES

Superficially, the genetic basis for the spontaneous development of type 1 diabetes in rat models appears less complex than that in the NOD mouse or in humans. However, this may relate to the level of study of the process, since initially the genetics of type 1 diabetes in NOD mice was also inferred to be less complex, and possibly only oligogenic (100,102). As in humans and mice, the detection of "*Idd*" loci in the rat genome has been facilitated by the development of polymorphic microsatellite markers that can now be scored by automated methods (201). Segregation analysis between BBDP crossed with other type 1 diabetes–resistant strains have established that the MHC class II alleles encoded by the *RT1^u* haplotype of the BB rat are essential for diabetogenesis (201,208–211). This MHC susceptibility, designated "*Iddm2*," is permissive for insulitis in the heterozygous state; however, most diabetic segregants are MHC homozygotes. Analyses of insulitis and development of type 1 diabetes following outcross of diabetes-prone BB/Wor rats of the "NB" subline to *RT1^u* congenic stocks of PVG rats carrying recombinants in the class I versus class II region have established the requirement for the RT1-D^u/B^u alleles at the two class II loci (homologues of human DQ and DR, respectively) (210). Unlike

TABLE 18.4. Comparison of Differences Between Three Rodent Models of Type 1 Diabetes

Phenotype/treatment	BBDP rat	BBDR rat[a]	NOD mouse
T-lymphopenic	Yes	No	No
Virus exposure	Not required	Kilham rat virus triggers type 1 diabetes	Virus exposure protects
High-dose poly I:C treatment	Accelerates type 1 diabetes	Accelerates type 1 diabetes in RT6 depletion model	Retards type 1 diabetes
Cyclophosphamide treatment	Inhibits type 1 diabetes	Induces type 1 diabetes	Induces type 1 diabetes
NK cell number and function	High	High	Virtually absent
NKT cell number and function	Low	Normal	Low
Hemolytic complement	Present	Present	Absent (C5)
Insulin required immediately after onset of type 1 diabetes	Yes	Yes	No
Ketoacidosis	Yes	Not diabetic	Very mild until late stages
Gender difference in susceptibility	F = M	F = M	F >> M

BBDP, BioBreeding diabetes-prone; BBDR, BioBreeding diabetes-resistant; NOD, nonobese diabetes; NK, natural killer; F, female; M, male.
[a]References are to unmanipulated, nondiabetic rats.

the nonexpression of H2-E molecules on APC of the NOD mouse, APC of the BB rat do express the DR homologue (RT1-D^u). Sequence analysis of the BB rat DQ homologue (RT1-B^u) showed it differed from both the high diabetes risk–conferring human HLA-DQβ alleles and the NOD H2-Ab^{g7} molecule. In contrast to NOD mice and humans, the BB rat allele contains an aspartic acid at residue 57 of the β chain instead of exhibiting "diabetogenic" non-Asp substitutions (212,213). All $RT1^u$-expressing rat strains carry the requisite class II "*Iddm2*" alleles. Class I alleles from non-$RT1^u$–positive rat strains apparently will substitute for the RT1-A^u, E^u, and C^u class I alleles. Interestingly, although insulitis and thyroiditis were suppressed in class II heterozygous segregants in one outcross/backcross analysis, thyroiditis (another characteristic immune pathology of the BBDP-NB subline used in the outcross) was not (210).

"*Iddm1*" was initially assigned to the recessive *Lyp* (lymphopenia) mutation in BBDP rats on Chr 4, in tight linkage to the neuropeptide Y (*Npy*) locus (202). The gene mutation that yields the lymphopenia phenotype has been positional cloned to the immune associated nucleotide 5 (*Ian5*) locus by two groups (213a,213b). Although most diabetic probands in segregation analyses between BBDP stocks and nonlymphopenic stocks, including BBDR, have been homozygous for this mutation, the traits (lymphopenia versus type 1 diabetes) have occasionally been separated, leading to the speculation that another locus in tight linkage with the *Lyp* mutation was contributing (204,214). Such a locus, designated "*Iddm4*" and proposed to be involved in insulitis initiation, has been discovered in outcross between BBDR and an inbred WF stock followed by backcross to WF (215). As noted above, BBDR rats express a wild-type allele at the *Lyp* locus and therefore, like WF rats, are not T-lymphopenic. However, unlike WF rats, BBDR rats can be turned diabetic by the anti-RT6.1 antibody plus treatment with poly I:C. Since the backcross was made to the type 1 diabetes–resistant (but $RT1^u$-identical) WF strain, type 1 diabetes in susceptible genotypes had to be induced by transient T-cell depletion using an anti-RT6.1 monoclonal antibody together with treatment with poly I:C. The poly I:C presumably activates T-effector cells surviving the depletion. An ortholog for "*Iddm4*" in the NOD mouse, if it existed, would be the "*Idd6*" segment on mouse Chr 6. Suggestive evidence for another diabetogenic locus on Chr 3, this time contributed by the WF parent and designated "*Iddm6*," also was noted, as was another locus on Chr X designated "*Iddm5*." The existence of "*Iddm3*" was originally inferred based on outcross of BBDP to Fisher 344 rats (202). This designation was subsequently used to describe suggestive evidence for a locus on Chr 18 contributing to development of spontaneous type 1 diabetes in outcross of BBDP/OK (a distinct line of BB rats in Germany) to the DA strain (216–219). Additional evidence for weak linkages following outcross to other nondiabetic strains was suggested in certain of these latter studies.

CELLULAR ANALYSIS OF THE INSULITIC PROCESS

In marked contrast to the periweaning onset of lymphoaccumulation and periinsulitis in NOD mice, the development of insulitis in BB rats does not occur around weaning, but rather focuses around and into the islets after the development of puberty and within 2 to 3 weeks of the (abrupt) onset of clinical symptoms. Indeed, the abrupt onset of hyperglycemia and the requirement for immediate insulin therapy are other factors distinguishing BB rats from NOD mice (Table 18.4); the latter often can survive for 3 to 4 weeks after first detection of hyperglycemia such that when diabetic splenocyte donors are used for adoptive transfer experiments these donors generally have not been maintained by daily insulin injections. As is true for NOD mice, most BBDP rats develop insulitis whether or not they develop diabetes and, as in NOD females, peak onset occurs after puberty, with more than 90% of diabetic animals identified between 8 and 16 weeks of age. Interestingly, this same time frame corresponds to the period of peak development of type 1 diabetes in NOD/Lt females. In common with NOD mice, the earliest phase of the insulitis process in BBDP rats also seems to be a phase in which both permeability changes in the pancreatic vascular endothelium and "macrophage insulitis" are noted (201).

Perhaps because of the paucity in BBDP rats of mature peripheral T lymphocytes, especially those expressing the $OX8^+/OX19^+$ T cytotoxic/suppressor phenotype, the $OX8^+/OX19^-$ asialoGM1$^+$ NK cell was initially implicated as a primary effector of β-cell destruction (200). Cells with this NK-like phenotype appeared to be the most prevalent of the islet-infiltrating leukocytes, but an NK cell–specific monoclonal antibody to the NKR-P1 receptor failed to reduce the frequency of diabetes in BBDP rats (220). Pathogenic roles for rat $CD4^+$ ($W3/25^+$) and $CD8^+$ ($OX8^+/OX19^+$) T lymphocytes were indicated by the finding that concanavalin A (con A)–activated splenocytes from acutely diabetic BBDP donors would adoptively transfer type 1 diabetes into young prediabetic BB or athymic nude recipients. Treatment of prediabetic BBDP rats with the nondepleting anti-CD4 monoclonal antibody, W3/25, reduced the frequency of type 1 diabetes, but not insulitis, whereas treatment with pan-T (OX19) monoclonal antibody completely prevented insulitis and type 1 diabetes without a reduction in the NK population (200). That both $CD4^+$ and $CD8^+$ T lymphocyte subsets synergistically contributed to insulitis was shown using manipulated T lymphocytes from the nonlymphopenic BBDR strain. Treatment of these nominally diabetes-resistant rats with a depleting monoclonal antibody to ART2/RT6 (the cell-surface ADP ribosyltransferase marking ~70% of mature peripheral T lymphocytes) could rapidly elicit insulitis and type 1 diabetes within a 2-week period if the rats were conventionally housed (see next section) (221). The availability of MHC-identical WAG-athymic nude rats allowed adoptive transfer experiments showing that transfer of both $CD4^+$ and $CD8^+$ subsets from BBDR donors treated with anti-RT6DR were required for rapid and efficient transfer of type 1 diabetes (222). Cotransfer of $RT6^+$ T lymphocytes from untreated BBDR donors with the RT6-depleted population blocked this pathogenesis, confirming the presence of a regulatory population of $RT6^+$ suppressor cells in the BBDR rat. Presumably, the absence of this regulatory population due to the T lymphopenia produced by the *Lyp* gene accounts for the high spontaneous incidence in the BBDP strain. It has since been shown that other inbred rat strains without spontaneous development of type 1 diabetes nevertheless contain potential diabetogenic T-cell clones in the periphery whose autoreactivities are suppressed by thymus-derived regulatory cells (223). It is interesting that the BBDP, but not the BBDR, rat, resembles the NOD mouse in exhibiting a deficiency in a NKP-R1$^+$ NKT subset (224). NKT cells from Wistar rats expressing RT6 conferred protection against recurrent pancreatic transplant rejection in BBDP recipients, suggesting that these cells were regulatory and capable of deviating autoaggressive cells to a T_H2 phenotype (225).

THE BB DIABETES-PRONE RAT AS A MODEL OF ENVIRONMENTALLY TRIGGERED TYPE 1 DIABETES

Environmental triggers may exist that are capable of unleashing autoreactive function in T lymphocytes that escape thymic deletion and are normally held under immunoregulatory control in the periphery. In the case of type 1 diabetes, human pathogenic viruses often are discussed as potential diabetogenic catalysts, but this has been exceedingly difficult to prove (226). Diabetogenesis in the BB/Wor rat was initially assumed to be relatively unaffected by its physical environment (227). However, this view has altered radically with the discovery that the rare sporadic breakout of type 1 diabetes in a nonbarrier colony of BBDR/Wor rats correlated with seropositivity to Kilham rat virus (KRV). Subsequent study showed that experimental infection of BBDR rats with this parvovirus rapidly led to insulitis and the development of type 1 diabetes (228). KRV infects lymphoid tissues, but not islet cells, so the catalytic effect on diabetogenesis was assumed to entail immunomodulation (229). Even rat strains not prone to diabetes that have the appropriate RT1 class I A^u and class II B/D^u restriction elements can be rendered diabetic by KRV exposure in combination with either anti-ART2/RT6 monoclonal antibody or administration of poly I:C (230). This effect is dependent on both $CD4^+$ and $CD8^+$ T lymphocytes, macrophages, and/or macrophage-secreted monokines and is virus-specific, because exposure of BBDP rats to LCMV virus reduces the incidence of type 1 diabetes (230,231). The ability of a virus to act as a diabetogenic trigger in rats makes this murine genus much more suitable for analysis of the role of viruses in type 1 diabetes than is the NOD mouse, in which viral exposure stimulates protective immunoregulatory mechanisms (Table 18.4).

MOLECULAR ANALYSIS OF THE INSULITIC PROCESS

Studies performed on the cytokine genes expressed by islet-infiltrating leukocytes in the BB rat are supportive of comparable studies done in NOD mice, indicating that pathogenesis is driven by a T_H1 cytokine spectrum. Consistent with the early "macrophage insulitis" described in the DP model, increased expression of IL-12p40 mRNA has been reported (232,233). Upregulated IFN-γ transcripts, with minimal or undetectable IL-4 and IL-10 transcripts, were found in islet-infiltrating leukocytes (233,234). The advantage of the RT6-depleted BBDR model is that insulitis development is rapid and synchronous, with macrophages and a few T lymphocytes present within 10 days of treatment and a progressively more florid insulitis developing between days 10 and 18 (235). A T_H1 cytokine profile similar to that developing in BBDP rats was observed in BBDR rats following $RT6^+$ T-cell depletion (233). Feeding BBDP rats a semipurified diet that reduces the incidence of type 1 diabetes is associated with reduced IFN-γ transcript levels and increased IL-10 and TGF-β transcript levels (236). Activation of macrophages by poly I:C correlates with induction of IFN-α/β gene transcription, translation, and secretion. Whereas poly I:C, which mimics a double-stranded RNA viral genome, like most viral infections, prevents type 1 diabetes in NOD mice, only a low dose can inhibit the development of type 1 diabetes in DP-BB rats (71,237). When administered at a dose of 10 μg per g of weight, poly I:C accelerates the development of type 1 diabetes in both DP and DR rats (238). Islets of unmanipulated DP, but not DR, rats showed increasing IFN-α transcript levels with age, and poly I:C-induced type 1 diabetes in DR rats was similarly correlated with induced expression of this cytokine (238). Unlike prediabetic NOD mice and BBDR/Wor rats in which cyclophosphamide treatment promotes a rapidly destructive insulitis, in BB rats this treatment inhibits the development of type 1 diabetes (239).

OTHER ENDOCRINOPATHIES: THYROIDITIS

The BBDP rat shares with the NOD mice the susceptibility to subclinical thyroiditis and sialitis development (196). The thyroiditis can be exacerbated by environmental manipulation to produce clinically significant lesions and hypothyroidism (177,178). Spontaneous lesions are more commonly encountered in diabetic (59%) versus nondiabetic (11%) BBDP/Wor rats (240). The University of Massachusetts, Worcester, developed six substrains of lymphopenic BB rats. Although the incidence of type 1 diabetes among these substrains was relatively constant, major differences (ranging between 4.9% and 100%) in incidences of spontaneous or excess iodine-elicited thyroiditis were observed (241). The immunoregulatory defects induced by the lymphopenia (*Lyp*) mutation are critical in this pathology, since it is rare in genetic segregation analysis between BB rats and nonlymphopenic strains to identify nonlymphopenic rats with thyroiditis (242). In a genetic analysis in which all diabetics were homozygous for $RT1.B^u$ class II genes, thyroiditis was distributed equally between $RT1.B^u$ homozygotes and heterozygotes (242). Thyroiditis can be transferred into athymic rats by the same population of con A–activated BB splenocytes that transfer type 1 diabetes (243). However, the antigens recognized between β-cells and thyrocytes are presumably not common, since insulin prophylactic therapy can retard insulitis but not the severity of thyroiditis (244).

AVAILABILITY

Information on the status of BB rat colonies can be obtained from the *International Index of Laboratory Animals* and the Institute for Laboratory Animal Research (ILAR) Web site (http://dels.nas.edu/ilar/). The major American supplier of BB rats is Biomedical Research Models (http://www.biomere.com); the major European vendor is M&B, A/S, Ry, Denmark (http://www.m-b.dk/).

Komeda Diabetes-Prone Rats

ORIGINS AND FREQUENCY OF TYPE 1 DIABETES

Spontaneous development of autoimmune type 1 diabetes with histopathologic characteristics (insulitis) very similar to those observed in BB rats was first reported in the Long-Evans-Tokushima lean (LETL) strain in 1991 (245). Although sharing the *RT1^u* MHC haplotype with BBDP rats, LETL rats were not T-lymphopenic or T-lymphocytopenic. Probably because these rats are not T-lymphopenic, the extent of insulitic infiltrates around islets appears more extensive than that observed in BBDP rats (246). As in the NOD and BB rat models, polyglandular infiltrates were observed in salivary and lacrimal glands (245). After 20 generations of inbreeding, the frequency of type 1 diabetes was 21.1% in males and 15% in females. Seven cycles of further selected breeding of diabetic versus nondiabetic parents from the original LETL strain by Komeda and colleagues (246) has led to the isolation of a nonlymphopenic diabetes-free control substrain (LETL-KND) and a nonlymphopenic line with a high incidence of type 1 diabetes (LETL-KDP). In the latter, type 1 diabetes was first detected at 60 days. A cumulative frequency of type 1 diabetes of ~70% for both sexes was attained by 120 days of age and one of 82% was obtained by 220 days, whereas KND rats remained free of type 1 diabetes. Onset of type 1 diabetes in KDP rats, as in BB rats, was abrupt, and diabetic rats exhibited reduced pancreatic insulin content (246). Severe insulitis was observed in all KDP rats by 220 days of age, yet only periinsulitis was observed in KND rats.

GENETICS

A search for genetic polymorphisms among 165 microsatellites tested found no differences among the KDP, KND, and the original LETL strains (246). Three mapping crosses have been reported wherein the LETL-KDP substrain has been out-crossed to the related LETO (Long-Evans Tokushima obese) strain, as well as to the Tester Moriyama (TM) strain and the unrelated

Brown Norway (BN/Sea) strain. LETO and TM strains were *RT1*^{u} identical with LETL-KDP, whereas BN rats express the *RT1*^{n} MHC haplotype. All F1 hybrids were type 1 diabetes-free, such that backcrosses to KDP were performed. All three backcrosses confirmed the presence of a diabetogenic recessive locus on Chr 11, designated *Iddm/kdp1* (247). In outcross to TM, weak evidence linked *Iddm/kdp1* to insulitis severity and overt type 1 diabetes development. Positional cloning has identified a C to T transition mutation in Casitas B-lineage lymphoma b (*Cblb*) as the major susceptibility gene in KDP rat diabetes (247a). In the mapping cross with BN, eight of nine backcross mice were homozygous for the *RT1*^{u} haplotype of LETL, indicating linkage to *Iddm2* (MHC).

AVAILABILITY

At the time of this writing, these strains have not been made available for distribution outside of Japan.

Single Gene Mutations Producing Insulin-Responsive Diabetes

C57BL/6NJCL-INSULIN2^{AKITA}

Strain Origin and Diabetic Phenotype

An autosomal dominant mutation producing juvenile-onset hyperglycemia in the absence of obesity was discovered in C57BL/6N mice in Akita, Japan (248). The mutation was initially named *Mody4* and mapped to distal Chr 7. The initial gene symbol assigned was *Mody* (for maturity-onset diabetes of the young). This choice was based on the autosomal dominant mode of inheritance and the findings that the β-cells in the pancreatic islets failed to develop a normal mass and that β-cell secretory responses to glucose were subnormal (248,249). Heterozygous males in the source colony developed severe hyperglycemia at weaning (4 weeks), whereas heterozygous mutant females developed a less severe hyperglycemia. Histologic analysis showed a dearth of islets; those detected were extremely atrophic and devoid of granulated β-cells. This histopathology was similar to that observed in mice rendered insulin-dependent diabetic by treatment with chemical diabetogens. Despite the juvenile onset of hyperglycemia, heterozygous diabetic males were both viable and fertile. In Japan, the mutation is maintained by breeding diabetic male heterozygotes to wild-type females. The C57BL/6NJcl-*Ins2*^{Akita} mouse has features observed in certain human *MODY* families. Indeed, the model was initially described as a model for early-onset type 2 diabetes. The initial linkage marker, *D7Mit189*, maps within 3 cM of *Ins2*, the ortholog of the human *INS* gene and one of the two insulin genes in the mouse (the other, *Ins1*, is on Chr 19). Sequencing of the *Ins2* gene in these mutant mice indeed confirmed the presence of a missense mutation at residue 96 that converted a cysteine (TGC) to a tyrosine (TAC) at amino acid residue 7 of the A chain (7). This is a critical substitution, since the A7 cysteine is required to form the interchain disulfide bond with the corresponding cysteine at the seventh amino acid residue on the B chain. In heterozygous *Ins2*$^+$*Ins2*^{Akita} mice, the conformational change leading to defective proinsulin chain folding of the mutant insulin triggers massive compensatory "quality-control" mechanisms in the endoplasmic reticulum (suggesting an influx of chaperonins). These responses are so massive that not only is proinsulin processing from the mutant allele blocked but folding and processing of *Ins1* gene products are also strongly inhibited. This disruption in normal processing in the regulated secretory pathway leads to the failure of β-cells to secrete normal levels of mature insulin and, hence, to early development of hyperinsulinemia. The failure of the islet β-cell mass to develop normally further suggests a role for insulin as an autonomous β-cell growth factor. The knowledge of the molecular basis for the syndrome led to the mutant symbol change from *Mody4* to *Ins2*^{Akita}.

The mutant stock was imported to The Jackson Laboratory in 1999, where the mutation has been maintained by backcrossing heterozygous males to normal C57BL/6J females. Comparison of the development of hyperglycemia and of survival of heterozygotes versus that of mutant homozygotes maintained on a 6% fat diet (PMI, NIH-31) showed that homozygotes rarely survived beyond 12 weeks of age. As was noted in Japan, heterozygous mutants remained viable for relatively long periods in the face of chronic hyperglycemia, with the development of hyperglycemia progressing more slowly in females than in males. Groups of four heterozygous males and females sampled for plasma glucose levels at 6 weeks of age exhibited comparable initial mean hyperglycemia (325 ± 57 mg/dL for males vs. 325 ± 57 mg/dL for females). The mean plasma glucose levels in the same mice at 12 and 18 weeks were 12 and 18 weeks, mean plasma glucose in males was 645 ± 109 (12 weeks) and ± 101 (18 weeks), whereas the averages in females were 341 ± 78 (12 weeks) and 398 ± 61 (18 weeks). Sensitivity of hyperglycemic *Ins2*^{Akita} mice to exogenously administered insulin had not previously been tested in Japan. A pair of hyperglycemic males tested at The Jackson Laboratory was insulin-responsive. This observation has important implications for the use of this model for testing insulin replacement therapies.

Potential Research Uses

Islets from *Ins2*^{Akita} mice are β-cell–depleted, and residual β-cells release very little mature insulin. This fact, coupled with the finding that the mutant mice respond to exogenously administered insulin, indicates that this model would serve as an excellent substitute for mice made insulin-dependent diabetic by treatment with diabetogens such as alloxan or streptozotocin. Chemically diabetic mice are widely used for the study of the effects of chronic hyperglycemia and diabetic complications. The difficulty has been that these chemical diabetogens may produce unwanted toxic side effects on multiple organ systems in addition to the pancreatic β-cells, thus complicating interpretations of damage produced by hyperglycemia versus direct toxin-induced damage. The observation that *Ins2*^{Akita} mice spontaneously develop an insulin-responsive hyperglycemia but will survive with chronic hyperglycemia without insulin therapy further suggests that they will be an excellent source of diabetic recipients for allogeneic or xenogeneic islets in studies designed to investigate induction of transplantation tolerance. Indeed, preliminary studies at The Jackson Laboratory indicate that intrarenal transplantation of 400 syngeneic C57BL/6 wild-type islets can correct the hyperglycemia.

Availability

C57BL/6J-*Ins2*^{Akita} mice are available as heterozygotes from The Jackson Laboratory (stock number 003548). Controls are B6-$^{+/+}$ segregants.

C57BL MICE CARRYING THE *FAT* MUTATION AT THE CARBOXYPEPTIDASE E LOCUS

Origin and Diabetic Phenotype

The autosomal recessive *fat* mutation arose spontaneously in 1972 in the HRS/J inbred strain (250). Obesity manifesting by 8 weeks of age was preceded by marked increases in immunologically detectable insulins (both proinsulins I and II and insulins I and II) in serum. Blood glucose levels were modestly elevated above normal such that insulin resistance was presumed. The phenotype elicited by the *fat* mutation proved to be heavily influenced by the inbred strain background. When the *fat* mutation was transferred from the HRS/J background to C57BLKS/J (BKS), a male gender–biased diabetes developed (250). Since hyperinsulinemia was accompanied by obesity, the model was originally considered to represent an insulin-resistant model of type 2 diabetes. However, on the BKS background, the diabetes syndrome produced by this mutation differs markedly from that produced by either the *Lep*^{ob} (leptin-deficient ob/ob) or *Lepr*^{db} (leptin receptor–deficient db/db) mutations on the same background. Unlike the latter two mutations, neither hypercorticism nor the glucocorticoid-induced shifts in hepatic sex steroid metabolism were elicited by the *fat* mutation (250). Another major distinction was the absence of hyperphagia in the BKS-*fat* homozygous mice (250). Finally, the hyperglycemic BKS-*fat* homozygotes were markedly sensitive to exogenously administered insulin, a finding that indicated that the molecular basis for the diabetes syndrome was a defect in proinsulin processing, a defect that could easily be explained by a defective carboxypeptidase E gene (250).

Genetics

The *fat* mutation had been mapped to Chr 8 within the vicinity of the carboxypeptidase E (*Cpe*) locus (251). CPE was initially identified as the carboxypeptidase involved with the biosynthesis of the enkephalins (252). Based on the broad neuroendocrine distribution and substrate specificity of CPE, this enzyme was thought to be involved with the processing of all neuroendocrine peptides that are produced from precursors by selective cleavage at sites containing basic amino acids (253). Following endopeptidase action, most peptides require removal of the C-terminal basic amino acids to generate the bioactive form of the peptide. In some cases, further processing to generate a C-terminal amide moiety also is required for bioactivity; this step is mediated by the enzyme peptidylglycine-α-amidating monooxygenase (254).

CPE is an important component of proinsulin processing in the β-cell. The unexpected discovery that *fat* mice were sensitive to exogenously administered insulin despite high serum levels of endogenous insulins, coupled with colocalization of the *Cpe* and *fat* genes to Chr 8, prompted an evaluation of the levels of CPE activity in *fat/fat* mice. Mutant mice were indeed found to have extremely low levels of CPE-like activity. Analysis of the *Cpe*^{fat} gene revealed a point mutation within the coding region, which substituted a proline for a serine (251). When the mutant form of CPE was expressed in a variety of cell culture systems, the resulting protein was inactive and was rapidly degraded within the cell prior to secretion, suggesting that the *Cpe*^{fat}is a null allele (281,255).

Potential Research Uses

The pleiotropic actions of the *Cpe*^{fat} mutation leading to obesity development are not resolved. The working hypothesis is that the defective CPE leads to loss of a peptide or peptides that function to control nutrient partitioning rather than caloric intake. Although the specific peptide or peptides has not been identified, a large number of peptides are detected with C-terminally extended basic residues in *Cpe*^{fat}/*Cpe*^{fat} mouse brain; none of these peptide precursors are found in control mouse brains, since CPE activity rapidly removes the C-terminal basic residues as soon as the endopeptidase has cleaved the precursor. Further studies are needed to determine the pleiotropic imbalances that underlie excess fat accumulation in *Cpe*^{fat}/*Cpe*^{fat} mice. The *Cpe*^{fat} mutation has led to discovery of several new members of the carboxypeptidase family and to novel neuroendocrine peptides. In the absence of CPE, the *Cpe*^{fat}/*Cpe*^{fat} mice presumably survive due to the ability of additional carboxypeptidases, such as carboxypeptidase D, to partially compensate in the processing of neuroendocrine peptides. The function of the other novel members of the carboxypeptidase family remains elusive, but it is unlikely that these other proteins participate in peptide processing. Further studies are needed to investigate the proposal that several of the novel members of the carboxypeptidase family function as binding proteins rather than active enzymes.

Availability

The BKS-*Cpe*^{fat} stock at N11 is available from The Jackson Laboratory. More recently, the mutation has been transferred onto the C57BL/6J inbred strain background, and this stock is available from The Jackson Laboratory. This latter congenic stock offers the advantages that the B6 background is free of the malocclusion and polycystic kidney lesions that are strain characteristic pathologies resident in the BKS inbred strain background. Homozygous mutants do not reproduce such that the stocks are maintained by heterozygous matings or by mating heterozygous males to females (e.g., NOD-*Prkdc*^{scid}) carrying ovarian transplants of mutant female ovaries.

ANIMAL MODELS OF TYPE 2 (NON–INSULIN-DEPENDENT) DIABETES MELLITUS

The onset of hyperglycemia, the hallmark symptom of all forms of diabetes, is the result of the breakdown either in insulin production or in insulin action or a combination of the two. Either can be primary and, if severe enough, either alone can be sufficient to produce hyperglycemia. In many cases, onset of type 2 (or non–insulin-dependent) diabetes occurs when compensatory mechanisms for insulin resistance drive β-cell failure. A host of errors, both genetic and environmental, is thought to be able to initiate insulin insufficiency and/or insulin resistance in humans. These phenotypes, which are checkpoints in the development of diabetes, also are present in rodents. A large array of rodent models exist for the study of type 2 diabetes, and although these models manifest hyperglycemia, the stresses needed for onset of diabetes, as well as the associated phenotypes, are, as in humans, drastically different.

Mouse Models of Type 2 Diabetes

SINGLE GENE MUTATIONS THAT PREDISPOSE MOUSE STRAINS TO TYPE 2 DIABETES

Spontaneous mutations in the mouse gene for leptin (*Lep*) and its receptor (*Lepr*), as well as "yellow" mutations at the agouti (*A*) locus, have been intensively studied because of their ability to produce diabetogenic obesity syndromes. The mutation formerly named *obese*, *ob*, is now designated *Lep*^{ob}; the mutation formerly named *diabetes*, *db*, is now designated *Lepr*^{db}. There is a plethora of reviews on the roles of mutations in these three genes (256–258); therefore, only a cursory review of the mutations and the phenotypes they elicit will appear in this chapter. The discovery that these monogenic obesity mutations are potentially diabetogenic, with their potential wholly dependent on genetic modifiers in the inbred strain background, provides major insight as to the complexity of type 2 diabetes etiopathogenesis in humans. Human morbid obesity syndromes elicited by mutations in the orthologous *LEP* and *LEPR* loci are rare and not reflective of the "garden variety" diet-influenced obesities contributing to the prevalent forms of human type 2 diabetes (259–261). Nevertheless, the diabetes syndromes elicited by interactions between a monogenic obesity mutation, background genetic modifiers, and environmental factors provide model systems for analysis of how an obesity-associated type 2 diabetes syndrome develops.

Mutations in Leptin (Lep^{ob})

The *ob* mutation (Lep^{ob}) was first described in 1950 and mapped to Chr 6 (262). In 1994 the *ob* mutation was found to be in the gene for leptin (263). Currently, there are two known obesity-producing mutations at the *Lep* locus; these have been designated Lep^{ob} (also known as $Lep^{ob\text{-}1J}$) and $Lep^{ob\text{-}2J}$. Mice carrying these mutations do not produce leptin, a hormone produced by adipose tissue that provides information on the level of fat stores to the hypothalamus and acts as a satiety factor, regulating appetite and energy expenditure in mammals. Hence, leptin-deficient *ob/ob* mice are always highly sensitive to the weight-reducing effects of leptin. Leptin decreases food intake and increases the basal metabolic rate (264–266). Lep^{ob} mice are also infertile, and administration of recombinant leptin to Lep^{ob} mutants restores reproductive function, indicating that leptin is involved in more than energy balance and food intake (267). Administration of leptin to these mice corrects most of the pleiotropic metabolic anomalies associated with this mutation (268).

B6-Lep^{ob} mice begin to develop obesity at weaning that becomes progressively more severe with age, and they exhibit hyperphagia throughout life. Insulin resistance is a key phenotype of the B6-Lep^{ob} mouse. It has been shown that, in both muscle and liver, multiple deleterious alterations in the insulin signaling contribute to the peripheral insulin insensitivity (269). Hyperinsulinemia is detectable at 15 days of age in Lep^{ob} mice and increases with age, reaching 10 to 50 times the level of age- and sex-matched, identical strain controls. Yet, hyperinsulinemic B6-Lep^{ob} mice develop only mild hyperglycemia (270,271). The highest plasma insulin levels are at ~7 months of age; afterwards, the levels decline but are highly variable (272). This increase in circulating insulin is witnessed in the pancreas as an increase in β-cell mass, with islet hypertrophy and hyperplasia. Islet volume of old B6-Lep^{ob} can be increased 10-fold compared with that of controls. Due to the increase in circulating insulin and a lower β-cell mass in young as compared with old B6-Lep^{ob} mice, younger mice have islets that are degranulated and stain poorly for insulin, whereas old mice have well-granulated islets (273).

As noted above, the diabetogenicity of the Lep^{ob} mutation is dependent on strain background. Whereas the B6 background can compensate for the diabetogenic effects of the mutation by sustained β-cell hypertrophy and hyperplasia, such compensation was not observed when the Lep^{ob2J} mutation occurred spontaneously on the SM/J background, with severe diabetes resulting (EHL, unpublished data, 1991). When transferred onto the closely related C57BLKS/J (BKS) by intercross followed by five cycles of backcross to BKS, the phenotype of BKS-Lep^{ob} homozygotes was similar in most respects to the chronic and severe diabetes syndrome produced by the $Lepr^{db}$ mutation on the same background. The major difference would be that the BKS-Lep^{ob} diabetes syndrome would be treatable with leptin, whereas the BKS-$Lepr^{db}$-induced syndrome would not (see below). B6 mice with the Lep^{ob} have been used for years for therapeutic interventions to prevent the obesity and mild hyperglycemia. The appropriate controls would be the +/+ littermate because heterozygous mice have been reported to have some intermediate phenotypes.

Mutations in the Leptin Receptor (db)

The recessive autosomal diabetes (*db*) mutation, which maps to Chr 4, spontaneously arose on the C57BLKS/J (BKS) stock at The Jackson Laboratory (274,275). The cloning of this mutation revealed that, as originally proposed based on parabiosis experiments between normal mice and *ob* and *db* mutants, the *db* mutation encoded a loss-of-function mutation at the leptin receptor (*Lepr*) locus. Including the $Lepr^{db}$, more than nine mutations in *Lepr* have been identified, including db^{2j}, db^{3j}, db^{5j}, db^{ad}, db^{pas1}, db^{pas2} db^{ad}, db^{dmpg}, and db^{rtnd} (256). For the purpose of this review, we will focus on BKS-$Lepr^{db}$. In this mutant stock, hyperinsulinemia is present as early as 10 days of age (274). As is the case with mice carrying the *ob* mutation, mice with the $Lepr^{db}$ weigh less than littermate controls before weaning, but the post-weaning phenotype is hyperphagia and a continued increase in adiposity. Hyperglycemia establishes between 4 and 8 weeks of age. By 12 weeks of age, insulin levels are elevated up to ten times that of the +/+ controls (274,276). Unlike the massive obesity in mice carrying the *ob* mutation, BKS-$Lepr^{db}$ only reach 60 g. When mice reach 4 to 6 months of age, the blood insulin levels diminish and the mice enter the phase of insulin insufficiency in the face of severe insulin resistance. Pancreatic morphology follows the demand for insulin. In young $Lepr^{db}$ mice, the islets are of normal size and well granulated. As the demand for insulin increases, so too does the β-cell mass. This stage is followed by β-cell failure, driven by necrosis and islet atrophy (277).

The demand for increased insulin production is due to insulin insensitivity at the level of the target organ in obese $Lepr^{db}$ mice. Hepatic production of glucose is hyperactive in mice with defective leptin receptors, adding to the hyperglycemic state. Treatment with exogenous insulin is not effective, and *in vitro* studies show a highly suppressed ability of muscle and adipose cell to transport glucose in response to insulin (278). While GLUT4 expression is not affected, cell-surface expression of insulin receptor is decreased and is inversely correlated with the insulin levels (279). Further, receptor kinase activity is also diminished when compared with that in controls (280).

Mice with mutations in the leptin receptor have been used for years for therapeutic interventions to prevent the obesity and mild hyperglycemia. The appropriate controls would be the +/+ littermates or mice from the identical strain.

"Yellow" Mutations at the Agouti Locus

Like the autosomal recessive mutations at the *Lep* and *Lepr* loci that are associated with diabesity (diabetes and obesity), dominant "yellow" mutations at the agouti (*A*) locus (Chr 2) produce obesity, with the development of hyperglycemia dependent on inbred strain background and gender. This obese phenotype is in direct correlation to the amount of yellow in the coat color [for reviews see references (281,282)]. The *A* gene product is a secreted paracrine factor that regulates pigment in hair-follicle melanocytes. The mutations at the *A* locus (A^{y}, A^{vy}, A^{iy}, A^{sy}, A^{hvy}, A^{iapy}) produce systemic expression of a protein of 131 amino acids that is normally only expressed at high levels in the dermal layer of the skin. Most of the cloned mutations at *A* are due to the insertion of an intracisternal A particle (IAP) retrotransposon upstream of the gene. This insertion disrupts the endogenous promoter's control of expression (283–287). The impact of these mutations is detected on both insulin secretion and action. Peripherally, agouti promotes lipogenesis by increasing fatty acid synthase (FAS) expression and activity in a Ca^{2+}-dependent manner (288,289). Insulin and agouti act in an additive manner to induce FAS expression and activity in adipocytes, as the FAS promoter contains both an insulin and agouti response element (288). Insulin treatment of mice that have agouti mutations increases adiposity. β-Cell phenotypes also are affected by the *A* gene product, as expression of the agouti protein in β-cells causes the hypersecretion of insulin (290–292).

The ectopic expression of agouti protein results in yellow fur, obesity, insulin resistance, hyperinsulinemia, and hyperglycemia. Further phenotypes include increased linear growth and skeletal mass, as well as increased susceptibility to tumors. The severity of these phenotypes varies among mouse strains. Mouse strains such as KK or ALS are very sensitive, with males and females affected and presenting hyperglycemia; strains such as ALR are almost completely resistant to the onset of hyperglycemia, while still manifesting the obesity syndrome (293). In mice with severe phenotypes, the onset of hyperinsulinemia begins at 6 weeks of age and insulin levels continue to increase with age (294,295). The increase in circulating insulin is proceeded by β-cell hyperplasia and hypertrophy (296). The type 2 diabetes syndrome that is driven by mutations the *A* locus is very complex, with important contributions from multiple endocrine glands. Removal of the adrenal glands prevents hyperglycemia and reduces obesity, and hypophysectomy ablates the diabetes and the hyperinsulinemia but has only a small effect on the level of obesity (297–300).

Appropriate controls for use in experiments with mice carrying mutations at the *A* locus would be mice of the identical strain that are *A/A* at the agouti locus. Mice carrying A^{y}, A^{vy}, A^{iy}, A^{sy}, A^{hvy}, A^{iapy} are available from The Jackson Laboratory.

ALLOXAN-SUSCEPTIBLE MICE: A MODEL OF NUTRITIONALLY EVOKED TYPE 2 DIABETES

Strain Origin and Diabetic Phenotype

ALS (alloxan-susceptible) mice were derived from outbred CD-1 mice by selection for sensitivity to alloxan-induced diabetes concomitant with selection for an alloxan-resistant line now designated ALR. Alloxan is a potent generator of free radicals. The basis for the differential alloxan sensitivity of the ALS/Lt and ALR/Lt strains was correlated with differential ability to dissipate free-radical stress (97). ALS mice respond to a relatively low concentration of alloxan (47 to 49 mg/kg) with development of insulin-dependent diabetes within 24 hours after administration. One of the unusual features of this chemically induced diabetes is the relationship between plasma insulin and glucose. In most strains, alloxan induces massive β-cell necrosis and release of insulin stores within hours after administration, producing an immediate hyperinsulinemia that, in turn, elicits an initial drop in blood glucose levels before hyperglycemia is detected. In alloxan-treated ALS/Lt mice, the expected immediate hyperinsulinemia is not accompanied by transient hypoglycemia, but rather by hyperglycemia. Indeed, unlike other strains rendered insulin dependent by alloxan treatment, ALS/Lt males made diabetic at 10 weeks of age by an alloxan dose of 52 mg/kg (intravenous) failed to respond to insulin therapy. This was suggestive of an underlying insulin resistance. Longitudinal measurements of plasma insulin and glucose levels in completely untreated ALS/Lt males maintained on a chow diet containing 4%, 6%, or 11% fat confirmed underlying defects in glucose homeostasis associated with a progressively more severe insulin resistance (301). Males exhibited marked glucose intolerance as early as 6 weeks of age. At this age, plasma insulin levels were moderately increased (4.7 ± 0.7 ng/mL) and increased progressively with age (14.5 ± 1.4 ng/mL by 12 weeks; 40 ± 15 ng/mL by 20 weeks). Mice of either sex are large and exhibit moderate obesity as they age [male ALS have 8.5% body fat as measured by dual energy x-ray absorptiometry (DEXA)]. Histologic examination of pancreatic sections of unmanipulated ALS males shows increased islet volume and islet-cell hypertrophy and hyperplasia. Females of this strain on a chow diet containing 6% fat are neither glucose-intolerant nor hyperinsulinemic. ALS/Lt females do exhibit increased islet numbers compared with closely related control strains, which include ALR/Lt, NON/Lt, and NOD/Lt.

Although ALS males present these pre–type 2 diabetes phenotypes, the incidence of overt hyperglycemia is sporadic and very low, even when mice are fed a diet containing 11% fat by weight. However, type 2 diabetes can be induced in 100% of ALS males if they are placed on a chow diet containing 11% fat and are singly housed. Under these conditions, these mice have a significantly increased plasma glucose level 2 weeks after the onset of the treatment and 100% will become hyperglycemic by 6 weeks after the onset of the stress. Plasma insulin levels under this stress attain exceedingly high levels, attaining an average of 212 ± 131 ng/mL after 8 weeks of stress (301). Histologic examination reveals severe degranulation of the pancreatic islets. The volume of islets of ALS/Lt males subjected to dietary stress is increased over that of the already large islets of ALS/Lt males, apparently due to an increase in the number of islet cells rather than to cell hypertrophy.

The ALS/Lt strain should prove especially valuable for analyzing the relationship between reactive oxygen species and the development of type 2 diabetes and its complications, because many of the pathologic changes associated with diabetic hyperglycemia entail increased production of reactive oxygen species. ALS/Lt males, when compared with ALR/Lt males, show significantly lower ratios of reduced-to-oxidized glutathione, as well as an increase in circulating lipid peroxides (97,98). These ratios decrease with age in ALS and correlate with onset of hyperinsulinemia and impaired glucose intolerance. That progressive free-radical damage is associated with dietary fat–induced development of type 2 diabetes in ALS/Lt males was shown by inclusion of the antioxidant lipoic acid in the diabetogenic diet. This manipulation markedly reduced hyperinsulinemia, led to improved glucose tolerance, and prevented the dietary induction of type 2 diabetes. These indications of a reduction in the ability of ALS mice to dissipate free-radical stress suggest that ALS males will serve as interesting models for the study the effects of oxidative stress on type 2 diabetes and its complications (301).

PHENOTYPES WITH MUTATIONS PREDISPOSING TO OBESITY OR TYPE 2 DIABETES

The yellow mutation (A^{y}) at the agouti locus on Chr 2 has been moved onto both the ALS and ALR backgrounds for comparison (293). The incidence of diabetes at 24 weeks of age in ALS males and females heterozygous for A^{y} was 100% and 60%, respectively. Only 50% of ALS.A^{y} males survived to 50 weeks. Pancreatic β-cell function in males was virtually abolished by 24 weeks, as evidenced by absence of circulating insulin. ALS.A^{y} females hypersecreted insulin as early as 16 weeks of age, even when fasting.

Potential Research Uses

The progressive development of pre–type 2 diabetes metabolic anomalies in the ALS male, coupled with the ability of dietary and behavioral stress to push the male across a threshold into clinical type 2 diabetes, provides investigators with an unusual opportunity to study the contributions of reactive oxygen species to the development of these phenotypes, and especially the progressively more severe peripheral insulin resistance. Since the genome of this strain is being characterized, it may also provide important new genetic insights into the genetics of type 2 diabetes.

Availability

ALS/Lt mice are available from The Jackson Laboratory. Control strains for research with the ALS include the co-selected ALR/Lt strain (systemically high free-radical dissipation and mild obesity without impaired glucose tolerance and hyperinsulinemia). ALS/Lt mice exhibit considerable genome sharing with the related NON/Lt strain, including *H2* haplotype ($H2^{nb1}$) and *Thy1* allele (Thy^{1a}). Although NON/Lt males share the phenotype of impaired glucose tolerance with ALS/Lt males, the former are differentiated by impaired insulin secretory responses (302). SWR/J, another Swiss-derived strain with normal glucose tolerance and plasma insulin levels, can be used as a lean control strain.

C57BL/6J MICE (A MODEL OF NUTRITIONALLY EVOKED TYPE 2 DIABETES)

Diabetic Phenotype

While used as a control strain for many studies of type 2 diabetes, the C57BL/6 (B6) male is a model for diet-induced type 2 diabetes. The studies and phenotypes described in this section may call into question the validity of the C57Bl/6J as a control strain for studies of type 2 diabetes. Males fed a diet high in fat and simple carbohydrate (58% fat by kcal) develop hyperglycemia, hyperinsulinemia, hyperlipidemia, and increased adiposity (303). The type 2 diabetes phenotypes are associated with insulin resistance and poor insulin secretion. Insulin secretory responses from islets isolated from B6 mice fed a high-fat/high-simple carbohydrate (HFHSC) diet were blunted compared with those in controls (304,305). Plasma levels of leptin in B6 mice remain significantly lower than those in controls. HFHSC feeding of B6 mice increased body weight in the absence of hyperphagia (306,307). This suggests that the B6 strain exhibits an increased feed efficiency when compared with that in the control nondiabetic A/J strain, and this was shown, as B6 mice gain more weight per calories consumed (306). This increase in feed efficiency drives the increase in adiposity via increased fat cell number (303). The increase in specific fat-pad size, particularly the mesenteric fat depot, is important for the onset of type 2 diabetes in this model. It is interesting that the BKS males, which are susceptible to severe diabetes induced by the Lep^{ob} and $Lepr^{db}$ mutations, are much more resistant to obesity induced by a HFHSC diet (308).

Complications

HFHSC feeding has been shown to cause diabetes-like symptoms during pregnancy (309).

Potential Research Uses

Since many humans with type 2 diabetes can control their diabetic conditions with dietary changes and exercise, the model of diet-induced type 2 diabetes is important for studying the diabetogenic changes induced by diet and the interventions that can reverse the phenotypes. This should be an excellent model of dietary, exercise, and pharmaceutical interventions. Gestational IGT can also be induced in this strain.

Availability

Young C57BL/6J males can be obtained from The Jackson Laboratory. See (310) for the control and diabetogenic diets. In addition to B6 males maintained on standard chow, the type 2 diabetes–resistant A/J male fed HFHSC diet has been used for metabolic comparison in most of the published work.

NAGOYA-SHIBATA-YASUDA MICE

Strain Origin and Diabetic Phenotype

The Nagoya-Shibata-Yasuda (NSY) mouse strain was inbred from outbred Jcl:ICR stock by selecting for impaired glucose tolerance (311). Impaired glucose tolerance was shown to be male-specific and to develop by 12 weeks of age (14). The cumulative incidence of IGT is 98% in males and 31% in females at 48 weeks of age, with increased adiposity and mild hyperinsulinemia. Fasting plasma insulin level was higher in male NSY mice than in male C3H/He control mice (545 ± 73 vs. 350 ± 40 pmol/L, $p < 0.05$, at 36 weeks, respectively). Decrease of glucose-stimulated insulin secretion *in vitro* can be detected by 12 weeks of age. Blunted insulin secretion in response to a glucose challenge was seen in all males by 24 weeks of age. The diminished β-cell function drives the impaired glucose tolerance. Pancreatic insulin content was higher in male NSY mice than in male C3H/He mice (76 ± 8 vs. 52 ± 5 ng/mg wet weight, $p < 0.05$, at 36 weeks of age). No abnormal morphologic findings exist such as hypertrophy or inflammatory changes in the pancreatic islets at any age tested.

Genetics

The cumulative incidence of impaired glucose tolerance and fatty liver in reciprocal F1 hybrid males was 100% (25 of 25) in (C3H × NSY) F1 and 97% (29 of 30) in (NSY × C3H) F1 at 48 weeks of age (312). Insulin resistance also was inherited dominantly but was more severe in F1 hybrid males in both directions than measured in parental NSY males, suggesting that the combined interaction of the C3H and NSY genomes produced a more severe pre–type 2 diabetes phenotype. Adiposity and impaired glucose-stimulated insulin secretion were both inherited in a recessive autosomal fashion, while body mass index was inherited as a codominant trait. Genetic dissection of the F2 generation using microsatellite markers throughout the genome mapped three major loci involved in IGT (313). $Nidd1^{nsy}$ (Chr 11) and $Nidd4^{nsy}$ (unmapped) influenced insulin secretion, and $Nidd2^{nsy}$ (Chr 14) and $Nidd3^{nsy}$ (Chr 6) appeared to affect insulin sensitivity. The $Nidd3^{nsy}$ locus also affected epididymal fat weight. Positional cloning of susceptibility genes for type 2 diabetes in NSY mice has not been completed. Currently, a candidate susceptibility gene for $Nidd1^{nsy}$ is *Tcf2* (encoding the HNF1β transcription factor) because NSY has a rare sequence variant in the DNA-binding domain (314).

Complications

The life span of NSY mice was found to be 618.7 ± 72.5 days (315), considerably shorter than that of C57BL/6 mice. Amyloid deposition was present in the tongue, esophagus, stomach, small intestine, large intestine, rectum, lung, heart, and adrenal glands and to a slight degree in the liver and the spleen. The most dominant amyloid deposition in NSY mice was seen in the glomerulus of the kidneys. NSY mice that lived for more than 400 days showed rising levels of blood urea nitrogen and large amounts of amyloid deposits in the glomerulus of the kidneys. NSY mice die of renal amyloidosis. Immunologic methods revealed evidence of $ApoA_{II}$ in the amyloid deposits of NSY mice (315). In NSY males glomerular basement membrane thickens with the progression of the type 2 diabetes and lesions can be inhibited by lysozyme treatment (316).

Potential Research Uses

The polygenic nature of type 2 diabetes in the NSY mouse coupled with its the kidney complications make this strain a unique and useful tool for gene discovery and evaluating new agents for the improvement of kidney function in diabetic patients (314).

Availability

Possible controls for the NSY are the closely related SWR/J (lean control), NON/LtK (IGT, impaired insulin secretion control), ALS/LtJ (IGT, hyperinsulinemic mildly obese control), or the ALR/LtJ (mild obesity, no impaired glucose tolerance). The NSY strain is available from Japan SLC, Shizuoka, Japan.

TALLYHO MICE

Strain Origin and Diabetic Phenotype

The TallyHo (TH) strain was derived from two male ancestors of an outbred Theiler Original colony that had late-onset (~26 weeks of age) polyuria and glucosuria. The TH strain has been selected based on breeding only hyperglycemic males from the original deviant stock. This strain is now maintained as inbred at The Jackson Laboratory. The progenitor population from which this strain was derived is unknown, but this albino strain appears to be of Swiss origin on the basis of its $H2^s$ MHC haplotype (shared with Swiss-derived SJL/J mice).

As with many mouse strains predisposed to type 2 diabetes, in the TH strain type 2 diabetes is sexually dimorphic, with only males of the strain exhibiting all phenotypes of type 2 diabetes. TH mice grow quickly, with males and females reaching 45 g by 26 weeks. At 26 weeks of age, TH males and females are obese [adiposity index, defined as weight of five fat pads (g)/body weight minus five fat pads = 0.18 ± 0.12 males; 0.39 ± 0.01 females], hyperlipidemic (TG = 652 ± 35 males; 349 ± 24 females) (total cholesterol = 213 ± 6 males; 132 ± 10 females) (FFA = 0.32 ± 0.02 males; 0.33 ± 0.03 females), hyperinsulinemic (16 ± 2.1 males; 7 ± 1.9 females), yet only males are hyperglycemic (544 ± 24 males; 162 ± 9 females). By 14 weeks of age, all males have nonfasting plasma glucose levels higher than 300 mg/dL and insulin levels higher than 3 ng/mL. Pancreatic islets of 20-week-old TH males are hypertrophied, and β-cells are degranulated (317).

Genetics

For the genetic dissection of the diabetes-associated traits from TH, outcrosses and first backcrosses to the nondiabetic and unrelated B6 and CAST/Ei (CAST) strains were used. Because of the male-specific susceptibility to diabetes, only males were used for both sets of genetic experiments. No F1 mice in either cross became diabetic. Quantitative-trait loci (QTL) mapping was performed for the phenotypes of plasma glucose (PG), BW, and fat pad weight. In the crosses with the B6 mice, two significant linkages were detected for PG. These were *Tanidd1* (Chr 19) and *Tanidd2* (Chr 13). The *Tanidd1* locus also was found to be associated with increased body weight. These QTL exhibited a recessive mode of inheritance. Further, for the traits of body weight and fat-pad weights alone, two separate QTL were discovered. Chr 7 was significantly linked to increased body weight. Unlike the loci for PG, this body weight–associated QTL showed that, even though the TH was the strain susceptible to obesity, the heterozygotes at this locus showed the greater body weights. A QTL controlling fat-pad weight only was located on Chr 4. Again, heterozygotes showed significantly higher values than the TH homozygotes.

Potential Research Uses

The TallyHo male provides a new model for the study of polygenic type 2 diabetes. Like the TSOD strain described below, complete disease penetrance in males makes this strain a unique and very useful tool for gene discovery and the evaluation of new antidiabetic agents.

Availability

TallyHo mice are available from The Jackson Laboratory. Although B6 has been used as a control strain for TallyHo, Swiss-derived strains such as the lean SJL/J or SWR/J strains with normal glucose tolerance and plasma insulin levels may provide a more closely related backgrounds for comparison.

TSUMURA, SUZUKI, OBESE DIABETES MICE

Strain Origin and Diabetic Phenotype

The Tsumura, Suzuki, obese diabetes (TSOD) inbred strain was established in 1992 following selective breeding of outbred Slc:ddY progenitors exhibiting high body weight and glycosuria in males (318). Type 2 diabetes in this strain is male gender–specific, with 100% exhibiting diabetes by 20 weeks of age. Hyperinsulinemia is demonstrable at 13 weeks of age and probably develops earlier. Male TSOD mice are hyperphagic throughout life and exhibit rapid weight gain during the peripubertal period (319). Blood lipid profiles of TSOD males are also abnormal, with cholesterol and triglycerides increasing with age. Histologic examination of the pancreas reveals hypertrophy of the pancreatic islets. Immunostaining of pancreatic sections for insulin and glucagon at 52 weeks of age demonstrates a significant decrease in insulin-positive staining of pancreatic islets, suggesting either partially or completely β-degranulated islets compared with insulin-positive control, nondiabetic TSNO (Tsumura, Suzuki, non-obesity) or to Slc:ddy males. Glucagon staining of islet α-cells is equivalent in TSOD and TSNO controls.

Genetics

Genetic outcrosses of TSOD with BALB/cA showed that the genetics of the development of type 2 diabetes in the TSOD parental males is recessive and under polygenic control, as no type 2 diabetes developed in either F1 or F2 males (319). A genome-wide screen for loci linked to glucose intolerance, insulin secretion, and body weight allowed mapping of three QTL controlling these diabetes-related phenotypes. The major genetic determinant of glucose intolerance was identified on Chr 11 and designated *Nidd4*. While *Nidd4* is located near the *Nidd3* locus reported in the NZO genome, the phenotypic effects and QTL peaks presumably distinguish these QTL (320). Two separate body-weight QTL were found on Chr 1 (*Nidd6*) and Chr 2 (*Nidd5*). *Nidd5* on Chr 2 also significantly affected insulin secretion in response to a glucose challenge. *Nidd5* is located in the region that contains Obesity QTL 3 (*Obq3*) (321).

Potential Research Uses

The polygenic nature of type 2 diabetes in the TSOD mouse coupled with complete disease penetrance in males make this strain a unique and very useful tool for gene discovery and for evaluating new antidiabetic agents (319).

Availability

The TSOD and the concomitantly derived TSNO control are not distributed.

NEW ZEALAND OBESE MICE

Strain Origin and Diabetic Phenotype

New Zealand Obese (NZO) is an inbred strain derived in New Zealand from outbred stock from the Imperial Cancer Research Fund Laboratories in London (322). Selection was initially for agouti coat color and later for polygenic obesity (both increased abdominal and subcutaneous adiposity) when this phenotype developed at F10. NZO neonates have high birth weights, and mice of both sexes are large and at weaning, have an elevated amount of carcass fat (323). The adiposity is more reflective of adipocyte hypertrophy than of hyperplasia (324). The related (but nonobese) New Zealand Chocolate (NZC) strain is sometimes used as a control strain for metabolic studies conducted using NZO/Wehi mice from the colony in Melbourne, Australia (325–327). NZO mice have not been as extensively studied as their well-studied sister strains, the autoimmune-prone New Zealand Black (NZB) and New Zealand White (NZW) strains, or the monogenic obesity mutants described above, because they are difficult to breed and, until recently, have not been available from commercial suppliers. Certain earlier studies in the literature describing the metabolic, endocrinologic, and pathophysiologic characteristics of NZO mice may not accurately describe the current generations of NZO substrains available for research [reviewed in reference (328)]. More recent generations of NZO/Wehi mice develop juvenile-onset obesity associated with hyperphagia, IGT, insulin resistance, and leptin resistance but do not develop overt diabetes under the current animal husbandry conditions at the Walter and Eliza Hall Institute in Melbourne (329). NZO/Hl is another currently studied substrain maintained for over 30 years by Dr. Lieselotte Herberg at the Diabetes Research Institute, Düsseldorf, and now distributed by Bomholtgard/Denmark. Approximately 40% to 50% of group-caged virgin NZO/Hl males, but not females, will transit from IGT into overt type 2 diabetes between 12 and 20 weeks of age when maintained on a chow diet containing 4.5% fat (320). This "cluster" comprised those males showing the greatest rate of body weight gain between 4 and 8 weeks of age. Genetic backcross analysis between NZO/Hl and either NON/Lt or SJL/J has confirmed that obesity-induced diabetes (diabesity) in this polygenic obesity model represents a complex threshold phenomenon whereby the rate of early adiposity development establishes a diabetogenic level of insulin and leptin resistance (330,331).

Hepatic insulin resistance and excessive glucose output have been documented as early abnormalities in NZO males (332), yet the mechanism of this hepatic resistance is quite different from the insulin resistance developing in the more intensively studied Lep^{ob} and $Lepr^{db}$ mice. In the latter, genes encoding glycolytic (glucokinase, pyruvate kinase) and gluconeogenic [phosphoenolpyruvate carboxykinase (PEPCK), glucose 6-phosphatase] enzymes that should be suppressed in chronically hyperinsulinemic mutant mice are not. In contrast, these same genes respond normally to insulin in NZO mice (325). This difference may relate to absence in NZO/Lt mice of the severe hypercorticism characteristic of Lep^{ob} and $Lepr^{db}$ mice (our unpublished observations). Hence, alternative mechanisms must be considered. Indeed, metabolic analysis of NZO mice suggests that hepatic insulin resistance is the consequence of increased lipid availability, particularly from glycerol gluconeogenesis, due to early postpartum increases in the hepatic activity of fructose 1,6-bisphosphatase (326,327). In the NZO/HlLt colony at The Jackson Laboratory, hepatic glycogen depletion and lipidosis is a consistent histopathologic feature and is particularly severe in those males crossing the threshold into overt type 2 diabetes. Although the unusually high body weights are evident by 2 weeks of age in NZO/HlLt males, plasma levels of insulin and leptin are not elevated until a later maturational stage (9 to 12 weeks of age). A drawback limiting widespread study is the difficulty in identifying an appropriate control, since obesity is polygenic in etiology. Obesity in NZO mice is characterized by widespread accumulation of subcutaneous as well as visceral fat. The obesity in these mice is accompanied by glucose intolerance in males associated with increased hepatic and peripheral insulin resistance (332). In marked contrast to genetically obese Lep^{ob} and $Lepr^{db}$ mice, in these mice the genes encoding certain gluconeogenic and glycolytic enzymes in the liver retain normal responsiveness to insulin, although evidence for an inappropriately active fructose 1,6-biphosphatase has been obtained (325).

Defects in glucose stimulated insulin secretion in the β-cells of NZO mice both *in vitro* and *in vivo* have been reported (332, 333). The defect appears to be in the early part of the glycolytic pathway between glucose transport and the triose isomerase step, since normal levels of insulin secretion are stimulated by glyceraldehyde but not by glucose (333). A defect in pancreatic polypeptide (PP) secretion has also been suggested, although numbers of PP cells immunocytochemically detectable in NZO/Hl and NZO/HlLt islets increase as the mice age [reference (334) and EHL, unpublished observation]. A previous report that transplantation of either allogeneic islets into NZO mice or treatment with avian or bovine PP reversed diabetes, hyperinsulinemia, and weight gain led to the proposal that a genetic deficiency in PP was responsible for the diabetes syndrome in NZO (335,336). However, this seems unlikely given more recent unpublished immunocytochemical evidence that PP is present in abundance in islets of NZO/Hl and NZO/HlLt mice.

With regard to the diabetogenic subphenotypes of plasma/serum glucose and insulin, data provided are from the author's (EHL) colony of NZO/HlLt mice maintained at The Jackson Laboratory on a low-fat (6%) chow diet. As noted above, obesity is juvenile-onset; mean body weight for a group of 10 weanling 4-week-old males was 25.8 g. By 8 weeks, mean weight had increased to 42.7 g. At this age, plasma insulin and leptin levels are not yet markedly increased above a normal range (2 to 3 ng/mL) and the mice are normoglycemic. By 16 weeks of age, when body weights are ≥50 g (total carcass fat = 20 g or higher by DEXA measurement), a range of plasma insulin levels between 4 and 16 ng/mL is observed. Those mice with the highest body weights and plasma insulin values at 16 weeks generally exhibit plasma glucose values higher than 250 mg/dL and develop a more pronounced hyperglycemia by 20 to 24 weeks (plasma glucose ranges increasing to between 300 and 400 mg/dL). Untreated diabetic males maintain chronic hyperglycemia at these levels for many months without loss of weight. Hence, hyperglycemia is late-onset and chronic once it is established.

Genetics

Genetic segregation analysis has confirmed that a large number of NZO-derived codominant polygenes capable of additive or epistatic interactions underlie the development of obesity (321, 330,337). QTL for both obesity and diabetes subphenotypes (plasma glucose and insulin) are distributed over a large number of chromosomes. When NZO is out-crossed to the unrelated Swiss-derived NON/Lt strain, which is a model for IGT, the two parental genomes "synergize" to produce a frequency of type 2 diabetes of 90% to 100% in F1 males (320). Among the numerous obesity QTL contributing to obesity ("*Obq*" or "*Nob*"), only a subset are required for the development of diabesity when NON/Lt is the outcross partner strain (330,337,338). Complex epistatic interactions between genotype and factors in the postparturition environment (e.g., in milk from obese dams) have been further shown to be important contributors to the early development of obesity in NZO × NON out-cross (330). In contrast, outcross of NZO to SJL, another unrelated Swiss-derived strain without IGT, prevents the development of type 2 diabetes in F1 males (338). Both NON/Lt and SJL/J outcross partners contribute a diabetogenic locus on Chr 4 near the leptin receptor locus that interacts synergistically with obesity contributions from NZO (320,331). NZO mice express the same leptin receptor variant ($Lepr^{A720T/T1044I}$) as the related NZB strain, which is neither hyperphagic nor markedly obese (339). This variant appears to signal normally following activation by ligand (338). However, the NZO allele at this locus or another gene in tight linkage enhances the weight-increasing effects of the NZO allele at *Nob1* (Chr 5) and the serum insulin-increasing effects of the NZO allele at *Nob2* (Chr 19) (338). One of the authors (EHL) has used NZO/HlLt as the donor strain and NON/Lt as the recipient background to produce recombinant congenic strains fixed for different combinations of NZO-derived "*Obq*"; certain of these combinations are capable of triggering diabesity spontaneously, while other combinations are diabetogenic if appropriate environmental stress (increased dietary fat) is applied.

Immunologic Anomalies

Since NZO mice originated from the same outbred stock that gave rise to the autoimmune-predisposed New Zealand Black (NZB) and New Zealand White (NZW) inbred strains, it is not surprising that NZO mice share with each of the latter two strains certain autoimmune proclivities. Indeed, the NZO is the only other inbred strain other than NZW known to express the recombinant $H2^z$ MHC haplotype associated with lupus development in (NZB × NZW) F1 mice. Other immune anomalies shared with (NZB × NZW) F1 mice include development of autoantibodies to both native and denatured single-strand DNA, as well as deposition of IgG antibodies on the glomerular basement membrane (340,341). The NZO strain has an additional immune peculiarity—development of autoantibodies to the insulin receptor (342). While these autoantibodies may contribute to insulin resistance, they are not predictive of hyperglycemia in males (EHL, unpublished observation). Histologic analysis of pancreata of aging NZO/Hl mice of both sexes reveal accumulations of leukocytes around pancreatic ducts and vasculature; since pancreatic islets also cluster around ducts and blood vessels, a periinsulitis forms around some of the islets. This periinsulitis differs from that observed in other strains of mice in that the content of $CD19^+$ B lymphocytes is high relative to that of $CD3^+$ T lymphocytes. Indeed, NZO/HlLt mice share with NZB and NZW mice the presence of elevated numbers of $CD5^+$ B lymphocytes in spleen (EHL, unpublished observations). These B1-B lymphocytes are thought to provide natural immunity and autoimmunity in contrast to the acquired immunity provided by B2-B lymphocytes (343). However, the humoral autoimmunity potentially generated in NZO mice by these cells against islet or other factors associated with glucose tolerance are likely to be secondary to and not causal for the diabetes syndrome, since levels of B1-B lymphocytes are higher in diabetes-resistant NZO/HlLt females when compared with diabetic or nondiabetic NZO/HlLt males (EHL, unpublished observations).

Complications. The principal complication described in NZO has been nephropathy characterized by an age-dependent increase in cellularity of glomerular tufts and mesangium, as well as mild thickening of the glomerular basement membrane due to the deposition of IgG (340,341). However, these changes probably are reflective of the generalized immune anomalies extant in NZO rather than to diabetes, since the changes are more pronounced in the diabetes-resistant females than in the more diabetes-prone males.

Potential research uses. Because type 2 diabetes in humans is polygenic in nature and associated with obesity in >80% of cases, the late-developing diabesity syndrome in NZO males makes this an excellent model for the human disease. Since the livers of NZO mice accumulate lipids as the mice age, this strain is exceptionally useful for screening insulin sensitizers, such as thiazolidinediones, for potential hepatotoxicity.

Husbandry Issues

NZO/Hl and NZO/HlLt mice are poor breeders and produce small litters when they do breed. Interestingly, hyperglycemia rarely develops in breeding males but frequently develops in group-caged virgin males, indicating an essential role for neuroendocrine factors in diabetogenesis. We have overcome the reproductive problems of NZO/HlLt mice by supplementing the NIH-31 (4% fat) diet with 0.001% CL316,243, a β_3-adrenergic receptor agonist known to suppress obesity development in genetically obese mice (344). NZO/HlLt mice of both sexes maintained on a CL-supplemented diet for only a month from weaning to retard the rate of weight gain and then placed on standard NIH-31 (4% fat) diet mate almost immediately.

Availability

NZO/HlLtJ mice are commercially available from The Jackson Laboratory (Bar Harbor, ME), and NZO/HlBom mice are available from Bomholtgard (Ry, Denmark). The recombinant congenic lines of NON/Lt mice carrying interval-specific segments of NZO genome producing various degrees of obesity and diabesity can be obtained from the author (EHL) at The Jackson Laboratory.

Rat Models of Type 2 Diabetes

BUREAU OF HOME ECONOMICS RATS

Strain Origin and Diabetic Phenotype

The Bureau of Home Economics (BHE/Cdb) is a subline of the parent BHE stock housed at the Genetic Resource Unit, National Center for Research Resources, National Institutes of Health. In 1975, the development of the BHE/Cdb strain began with selection criteria of hyperglycemia, hyperlipidemia, and the absence of obesity (345). After 36 generations, 75% of the rats showed fasting hyperglycemia and hyperlipidemia. Thereafter, all matings have been maintained along maternal lines and the diabetic phenotypes have strengthened to 95%. The IGT present in the BHE/Cdb is due primarily to a maternally inherited defect in glucose-stimulated insulin secretion (GSIS) (346–348). BHE/Cdb rats have an average life span of 600 to 700 days if fed the stock diet (Purina Chow), with renal disease as the primary cause of death. If the animals are fed a purified diet having a composition similar to that consumed by humans, the impaired glucose tolerance appears at 100 days of age, and in this setting, 100% of the animals are intolerant. Various hepatic abnormalities in metabolic control have been observed before the development of glucose intolerance. Among these are a 200% increase in *de novo* fatty acid and cholesterol synthesis, a 40% increase in gluconeogenesis, and a 20% reduction in the efficiency of ATP synthesis (349–351).

Feeding BHE/Cdb rats purified diets containing sucrose as the carbohydrate source and coconut oil as the fat source resulted in a further increase in fatty acid synthesis, an increase in gluconeogenesis, and a further disruption in the coupling of mitochondrial respiration (352,353). Thyroxin, which has been shown to increase the synthesis of a variety of proteins in oxidative phosphorylation, was administered to "rescue" respiration (354–356). An increase in shuttle activity and Mg-ATPase activity were observed, but no increase in coupling efficiency was recorded; in fact, deterioration in coupling efficiency was observed (353). With all substrates, the mitochondria respired normally but the energy generated by the respiratory chain was not fully captured in the high-energy bond of ATP, implying an error in the ATPase. The observation that the Mg-ATPase was increased with thyroxin treatment showed that the F_1 portion of the ATP synthase was functioning normally. As a result of these observations, it appeared that the uncoupling occurred because the F_o, although increased in amount, was not fully functional.

Normal diurnal rhythms are lost as humans progress toward type 2 diabetes (357–359). These changes in rhythm are associated with losses in the rhythms of blood glucose, insulin sensitivity, growth hormone, and fatty acids, suggesting that prediabetic humans adjust their metabolic patterns in an effort to retain some control of glucose homeostasis. This phenotype of altered circadian rhythm is exhibited by the BHE/Cdb rat with a noticeable change in diurnal pattern at 200 days. Dietary stress that accelerates the onset of diabetes will also accelerate the onset of the perturbed diurnal pattern (360). In all cases, the alteration of the diurnal rhythm precedes the onset of type 2 diabetes.

Genetics

In genetic crosses of the BHE/Cdb with nondiabetic Sprague Dawley (SD) rats, reciprocal F1 males and females have shown that the type 2 diabetes phenotypes of the BHE/Cdb are maternally inherited (346,347). Because of the error in F_0ATPase function, the mitochondrial genes for the subunits ATP synthase 6 and 8 were sequenced from BHE/Cdb and SD rats at 50 and 300 days of age (361). Four single-base differences were detected when comparing BHE/Cdb to SD rats. The base sequences in the SD rats were identical to the Genbank sequence (362). Of the four differences, only the mutation at base pair 8,204 altered the amino acid sequence. At this position, the SD codes for a guanine while the BHE/Cdb cell codes for adenine. This substitution replaces an aspartic acid with asparagine in a critical portion polar pocket of the F_0 molecule, through which the protons flow for the synthesis of ATP. This pocket spans the membrane and is surrounded by the membrane lipid. A polar amino acid instead of an acidic amino acid at this spot results in a reduction in the efficiency of ATP synthesis (363–365). When this occurs there is a reduction in the capture of the energy generated by the respiratory chain that is captured in the high-energy bond of the ATP. A reduction in the efficiency of ATP synthesis can be assessed indirectly through the determination of sensitivity to oligomycin. As has been shown in humans with a subunit 6 mutation somewhat similar to the one found in the BHE/Cdb rats, mitochondria from BHE/Cdb rats have a reduced sensitivity to oligomycin (366).

Potential Research Uses

The BHE/Cdb was the first animal model in which a defect in a mitochondrial gene was directly linked to a disease phenotype. This rat model not only has a diabetic phenotype but also shows heart defects and severe kidney disease. Therefore, this animal provides a unique opportunity for studying therapies for human mitochondrial diseases. As energy metabolism is an essential component in GSIS, the BHE also provides the opportunity to study therapies for increased mitochondrial function that would lead to improved insulin secretion. Because of the kidney disease, the BHE also serves as a model for the study of renal complications in the context of type 2 diabetes.

Availability

The BHE/Cdb is available without restriction from the NIH Animal Genetic Resource (Dr. Carl Hansen, Veterinary Resources Program, National Institutes of Health, Building 14F, Room 101, 14 Service Road South, MSC 5590, Bethesda, MD 20892-5590; Phone: (301) 402-3027: Fax: (301) 402-4258: E-mail: hansenc@ors.od.nih.gov). Control strains used in experiments with the BHE/Cdb have been the Wistar and SD rats.

E STILMANN SALGADO RATS

Strain Origin and Diabetic Phenotype

In 1978, spontaneous fasting hyperglycemia was detected in some males of a IIM albino rat line, resulting in the derivation by inbreeding of a diabetic line designated as the IIMe/Fm eSS (e Stilmann Salgado) (367). Type 2 diabetes in the eSS rat is characterized by early onset of IGT that worsens with age in the absence of obesity. Males are far more severely affected than females. While biochemical and histopathologic manifestations are more severe in males than in females, orchidectomization does not effect the diabetic evolution. Conversely, ovariectomy appears to be a worsening factor (368). Early in life, male eSS rats exhibit normal plasma glucose levels in the fasted state, while impaired glucose tolerance persists after glucose load (369). Despite their IGT, male rats of the eSS strain demonstrate fasting hyperglycemia and glycosuria (370). An improvement in the metabolic disturbances was registered in diabetic eSS males under long-term food deprivation (371).

Histopathologic examination of the pancreas reveals marked changes. The pancreatic islet structure is disrupted, and islets became smaller and more scattered with advancing age (371). The volume and density of β-cells decreases with age. The diabetic rats show disruption of the islet structure and fibrosis in the stroma. Defects in pancreatic histology begin as early as 6 months of age and progressively deteriorate. The volume density of endocrine tissue is diminished, as is β-cell volume density and percentage. This decrease in the endocrine pancreas is accompanied by a concomitant increase in the volume density of exocrine pancreatic tissue and not β-islet cells. Pancreatic β-cells showed an increase in the volume density of endoplasmic reticulum, immature secretory granules, and an apparent decrease in volume density of total secretory granules and microtubules of lysosomes (372,373).

eSS rats show diabetic lipid alterations at 5 months of age. Blood, liver, kidney, and testes all showed lipid alterations when compared with age- and sex-matched Wistar controls. Most noteworthy were the triglyceride and cholesterol profiles of the blood and liver (369,374). Feeding the eSS rats purified diets rich in lipids led to marked obesity and increased levels of circulating insulin, yet had no effect on the timing of onset of type 2 diabetes (370). A diet high in carbohydrates and fiber led to a leaner rat that was free of diabetes. High-protein diets appear to have the most detrimental effect on eSS rats. eSS rats fed this diet had the earliest onset of IGT; the highest levels of triglycerides, total cholesterol, and HDL-cholesterol; and the fewest islets of Langerhans at 23 months of age.

Complications

A diffuse glomerulosclerosis, interstitial lymphocyte infiltrates, and tubular nephrosis are present in kidneys (371). eSS rats as young as 6 months of age have increasing proteinuria and uremia as compared with Wistar controls (375). At 6 months of age, eSS rats exhibit areas of tubular dilatation with protein cylinders, and demonstrate increased capsular, glomerular, and Henle thin-loop diameters. At 18 months of age, glomeruli show diffuse hypertrophy of mesangial tissue and thickening of the basement membrane, with worsening proteinuria. Kidneys at this age are overtly damaged, with areas of markedly atrophic and dilated tubules containing acidophilic proteinaceous material.

Dietary manipulation of the eSS rat can markedly alter the onset of diabetic complications. While the feeding of a high-protein diet exacerbates the diabetic phenotype, this diet has extremely detrimental effects driving severe renal lesions and cataracts, which were total and bilateral in some cases. High-fat diets do not worsen the diabetic kidney abnormalities, but this diet does increase the incidence of cataracts.

Potential Research Uses

The eSS rat, while not genetically defined, could prove to be an exceptional model not only for the study of the pathogenesis of type 2 diabetes but also for the onset of complications. The slow progression through IGT toward overt hyperglycemia has produced a much more "human" model for the onset of type 2 diabetes. Much like the human with type 2 diabetes, the eSS rat loses β-cell function and mass with age, making this a nice tool for therapeutic interventions for the maintenance of the endocrine pancreas in the preclinical type 2 diabetes situation. While Wistar rats have been used in most of the studies with eSS rats, the lack of a genetic definition does not allow for the assumption of a more closely related nondiabetic control. Availability of dietary intervention to exacerbate or ameliorate the diabetic phenotype allows for either the more rapid progression of the diabetic phenotype or for a possible control. Because the female rats of this strain do not develop type 2 diabetes phenotypes, they could serve as controls. The possibilities of crosses between the eSS strain and rats of the spontaneously hypertensive SHR could lead to an excellent rat model for diabetic macrovascular complications.

Availability

The eSS rats are apparently not distributed.

GOTO-KAKIZAKI RATS

Strain Origin and Diabetic Phenotype

The Goto-Kakizaki (GK) inbred rat strain was derived from an outbred Wistar stock by selective breeding, with the highest blood glucose levels during an oral glucose tolerance test (376). Glucose intolerance was present in all rats after the sixth generation, and inbreeding was started at the ninth generation (377). The current stock of GK rats, available to the scientific community, is maintained at Charles River Japan and is in its 87th generation.

When compared with the control Wistar stock, GK rats of both sexes exhibit both mildly elevated blood glucose (GK: 154 ± 5 mg/dL female and 154 ± 4 male vs. Wistar: 120 ± 2 female and 122 ± 2 male) and plasma insulin (GK: 6.8 ± 0.3 ng/mL female and 6.3 ± 0.4 male vs. Wistar: 4.3 ± 0.4 female and 3.9 ± 0.2 male) levels at 8 weeks of age (378). While these pre–type 2 diabetes parameters are only mildly altered compared with those of the controls, as early as 4 days after birth, GK rats maintain a sharply reduced β-cell mass (35% of that of age-matched Wistar controls) and pancreatic insulin reserves that are only 31% of control values (379). By 4 months of age, the islets of GK rats maintain fewer β-cells, have a reduced islet insulin content, and exhibit abnormal islet morphology (380,381). A defect thought to be primary to the type 2 diabetes of the GK strain is decreased GSIS (rise in insulin levels of 42% in females and 17% in males of sex- and age-matched Wistar controls). Results from perifusion mirror the *in vivo* data, with first- and second-phase insulin secretion severely decreased. Study of the biochemical mechanisms behind the aberrant GSIS has shown that GK islets are impaired in many of the pathways important for insulin secretion. Decreased adenylate cyclase activity in GK islets has been reported, and an increase in the adenylate cyclase activity by forskolin restored GSIS (382). Defects in energy and shuttle metabolism leading to reduced K^+ ATP channel activity have been proposed as crucial to the type 2 diabetes of GK rats (383–386). SNAP-25 and syntaxin 1A, proteins essential for the process of membrane docking and fusion for exocytosis of insulin granules during insulin secretion, are reduced. Only the overexpression of SNAP-25 in GK islets restored GSIS to levels of control islets (387).

Genetics. GK rats have been extensively studied for the strain-specific genetic contributions to type 2 diabetes. Inheritance patterns of GK-derived type 2 diabetes phenotypes have been evaluated in crosses of the inbred GK strain with three nondiabetic control strains [Wistar, Fisher 344 (F344) and Brown Norway (BN).] GK × Wistar F1 hybrids were assessed for fasting blood glucose (oG), IGT, and GSIS. In all three instances, male and female reciprocal F1 showed intermediate phenotypes (388). This would suggest a polygenic inheritance of the type 2 diabetes phenotypes.

For a more detailed genetic comparison, both the BN and F344 rat strains have been used in GK outcrosses. Genetic analysis reported the results of reciprocal F2 crosses with the BN. These F2 rats were analyzed for oG and fasting insulin (oI), as well as IGT, GSIS, arginine-stimulated insulin secretion (ASIS), body weight (BW), and adiposity index (AI). Two significant and five suggestive genetic linkages were reported for crosses with the BN strain. The strongest linkage for IGT (*Nidd/gk1*) was detected on Chr 1, under a broad, 64-cM peak. Statistical analysis also revealed that this peak held suggestive significance for the phenotypes of AI, oG, and ASIS. Further, a suggestive linkage for IGT was detected on Chr 5 (*Nidd/gk4*). In both instances, the GK contributed recessive susceptibility for IGT. On Chr 7, a significant linkage for body weight was detected and named *bw/gk1*. Again, this peak was quite broad, and the GK genome contributed in a recessive fashion to increased body weight. The AI phenotype also segregated suggestively in this region of Chr 7. The four other loci all held suggestive status but controlled two or more phenotypes. *Nidd/gk2* (Chr 2) controlled oI and ASIS, *Nidd/gk3* (Chr 4) affected GSIS and ASIS, *Nidd/gk5* (Chr 8) had modest influence on GSIS and BW, and, last, *Nidd/gk6* (Chr 17) modulated oG and BW.

Concurrent to the GK × BN genetic analysis, was a report assessing the genetic susceptibility to type 2 diabetes of GK in F2 crosses to the nondiabetic inbred F344. Genetic responsibilities for the type 2 diabetes phenotypes of IGT, oI, GSIS, and BW were determined (389). In accord with the GK × BN genetic analysis, a recessive locus controlling IGT was detected on Chr 1. In this case, however, because of the use of an increased number of F2 rats, the peak for statistical significance was shortened to a confidence region only 20 cM in length. This locus, termed *Niddm1*, was inherited in a recessive manner and was not contributory to any other diabetes-related phenotype. Further, two significant loci for IGT also were detected on Chr 2 (*Niddm2*) and 10 (*Niddm3*). The inheritance patterns of *Niddm2* and *Niddm3* are consistent with the action of the GK alleles in a recessive or additive manner to perturb glucose tolerance.

The genetic contributions of *Niddm1* have been further analyzed by synthesizing F344 background recombinant congenic strains carrying Chr 1 segments from GK. Three RCS have been developed, a long congenic (*Niddm1a* carries a 52-cM region) and two smaller congenics that overlap *Niddm1b* (28 cM) and *Niddm1i* (22 cM), and assessed for IGT and GSIS (390). All three recombinant congenic strains are significantly less tolerant than the F344 parentals to glucose. Analysis of the subcongenic lines for GSIS differentiated these two chromosomal regions. Contained within the *Niddm1b* congenic interval are GK-derived genes that control increased oI, while rats of the *Niddm1i* recombinant congenic strain exhibit poor GSIS, yet maintain increased islet insulin reserves. Last, genetically delimiting the *Niddm1b* region has resulted in the mapping of this locus to a 1-cM interval. Testing of candidate genes in this region has led to the identification of a unique GK-derived allele for insulin-degrading enzyme (*Ide*), which maintains a single novel nucleotide difference (391). Analysis of this variant has shown that it maintains decreased insulin degradation activity, which is thought to contribute to the lack of insulin action on GK muscle cells.

Potential Research Uses

With alterations in multiple pathways essential for the maintenance of proper release of insulin by islets in response to glucose or other physiologic secretogogues, the GK rat provides a model for the study of islet growth and differentiation, of pharmacologic agents to improve insulin secretion, and of the genetic factors contributing to type 2 diabetes. Genetic analyses of loci *Niddm2-6* as well as of *Bw/gk1* are of clear research significance. Pharmacologic agents for improved insulin secretion are of value in patients with type 2 diabetes as well as those with type 1 diabetes. Studies aimed at increasing β-cell cAMP or increasing the activity of guanosine triphospate (GTP)–binding proteins have shown that pharmacologic agents can reverse the impaired insulin secretory responses of the GK rat, and this model would be an excellent choice for investigation of new compounds that increase insulin secretion. Study of gene expression in GK rats also has led to an increase in the understanding of insulin secretory vesicle docking and fusion mechanisms. Knowledge of how to regulate docking and fusion proteins could lead to therapies not only for insulin secretion but also for GLUT4 translocation in peripheral insulin targets. GK rats have also been used for both nutritional and therapeutic interventions.

Availability

While the GK rat is an excellent choice for an array of research questions, this rat strain is difficult to obtain and the research can be restrained by the supplier. Currently, the GK strain may not be bred or crossed, therefore eliminating the ability to perform *any* genetic experiments. Control strains for research with the GK would include the Wistar stock. Wistar is used because the GK was selected and inbred from an outbred Wistar population. Use of Wistar for a control in metabolic or gene-expression experiments is common. The F344 and BN strains are inbred strains that have been crossed to the GK strain for analysis of the genetic susceptibility loci for type 2 diabetes. The knowledge of the major genetic components and the production of congenic lines of F344 carrying GK-derived *Niddm* loci make the F344 an important control as well.

OTSUKA LONG-EVANS TOKUSHIMA FATTY RATS

Strain Origin and Diabetic Phenotype

The Otsuka Long-Evans Tokushima fatty (OLETF) rat strain was derived from an outbred Long-Evans colony at Charles River Canada (St. Constant, Quebec, Canada) that had shown polyuria, polydipsia, and mild obesity (392,393). To establish the OLETF inbred strain, selection was based on the phenotype of spontaneous hyperglycemia. Since 1989, the OLETF has been maintained as an inbred strain at the Tokushima Research Institute, Otsuka Pharmaceutical Company (Tokushima, Japan) (392). After the first 20 generations of inbreeding, the incidence of spontaneous hyperglycemia has been approximately 50% at 24 weeks of age and more than 90% by 65 weeks of age. Type 2 diabetes in OLETF rats is sexually dimorphic, with females exhibiting a greatly reduced incidence and a much later onset compared with males (394). Orchidectomy reduces the incidence of hyperglycemia to 20%, whereas ovariectomy increases the incidence of type 2 diabetes to 30%. Furthermore, treatment of castrated males with testosterone restores the incidence to 89%. At the time of the selection of the OLETF, the control LETO (Long-Evans Tokushima Otsuka) strain was coselected as a nondiabetic control.

Phenotypes associated with high risk for developing type 2 diabetes begin to appear in OLETF males at 24 weeks. At this age, males show elevated circulating levels of glucose and insulin and have IGT. These phenotypes deteriorate with age, and by 65 weeks of age the incidence of hyperglycemia and hypoinsulinemia in males is higher than 90% (392,393). In females, phenotypes associated with type 2 diabetes are not present at 55 weeks of age, but approximately one third have IGT 10 weeks later (395). When compared with the control LETO male and female, OLETF rats gain weight more rapidly with age and maintain an increased body weight (392). By 16 weeks of age, insulin-stimulated glucose transport is decreased in OLETF compared with that in LETO males, yet OLETF males have impaired GSIS throughout life. As early as 16 weeks of age, males hypersecrete insulin in response to glucose, but by 65 weeks the males fail to release insulin after a glucose challenge (392). These changes in the insulin secretory capacity are mirrored by the pancreatic islet morphology. There is an increase and deterioration in islet mass as the endocrine pancreas proceeds through three stages. The first or early stage (at less than 9 weeks of age) shows the presence of mild lymphocyte infiltration; at the second stage (10 to 40 weeks of age), β-cells become hyperplastic, with increasing fibrosis in or around islets; and finally after 40 weeks, islets atrophy (393). Diabetic changes are seen at the peripheral levels as well. Although there was no difference in GLUT4 expression or level of GLUT4 protein, there were clear differences in adipocyte GLUT4 translocation compared with that in LETO controls at 7 weeks of age (396). Translocation of GLUT4 in muscle also is reduced in OLETF compared with the LETO controls, yet this abnormality begins at 30 weeks of age (396,397). One clear finding from work with the OLETF is that the insulin resistance precedes impairment of pancreatic β-cell function. Experiments have also shown that obesity is necessary for the development of type 2 diabetes in OLETF males and that insulin resistance may be closely related to fat deposition in the abdominal cavity (398,399).

Genetics

For the determination of the genetic susceptibility determinants of the OLETF, outcrosses were performed with three nondiabetic control strains, F344, LETO, and the Brown Norway (BN). Male progeny from F1, F2, and first backcross generations have been used for genetic analysis. F1 hybrids resulting from the cross of OLETF of any of the three strains did not become diabetic, suggesting that the inheritance pattern of the OLETF susceptibility allele(s) was recessive. Studies in which OLETF was crossed with F344 included very few F2 males in the analysis, yet the incidence was drastically different in the reciprocal groups (400). In the 161 (OLETF × F344) F2 males used in the study, 5% progressed to type 2 diabetes, while an additional 7% had IGT. On the other hand, none of the 44 (F344 × OLETF) F2 males became diabetic. In the BC1 generation created by crossing (F344 × OLETF) females with OLETF males, the incidence of type 2 diabetes was 67%, with an additional 11% proceeding only to IGT. In the genetic segregation analysis, a highly significant linkage was observed for postprandial hyperglycemia near the *P-450ald* locus on Chr 1 and for the marker *D7Mit11* on Chr 7. These two markers were also statistically suggestive for the phenotypes of fasting glucose and body weight. Four other regions on Chr 1, 2, 5, and 17 were detected as influencing body weight, fasting glucose level, or postprandial hyperglycemia independently. This analysis, like that for type 2 diabetes of other murine models, suggests control by multiple genetic loci (401). A second group has repeated these studies with increased sample sizes for the F2 population, with very similar results (402).

Reciprocal F2 crosses of LETO with OLETF showed no difference, with an incidence of type 2 diabetes of approximately 12%. Of the BC1 [(OLETF × LETO) F1 × OLETF)], 44% of the males progressed to diabetes. The percentages of affected or diabetic animals, ~12% in an F2 and ~50% in a BC1, suggested that there was only a single locus controlling the type 2 diabetes phenotype of the OLETF when crossed with the LETO (400).

Genetic linkage analysis confirmed a single major diabetes locus on the Chr X that segregates with type 2 diabetes. This locus has been named *Odb1*.

The third set of crosses to identify diabetogenic genes involved in the development of spontaneous type 2 diabetes in the OLETF rat was performed in F2 (OLETF × BN) and BC1 [(OLETF × BN) F1 × OLETF] male offspring. In both the F2 and BC1 generations, diabetes was highly associated with the Hooded (*H*) coat color. The gene *H* is located on rat Chr 14 (403). In this cross, the marker that showed peak significance for the hyperglycemia phenotype was the gene for cholecystokinin type A receptor (*Cckar*). The maximum logarithm of the odds (LOD) score for this locus, designated *Odb2*, was 16.7 (404). Statistical tests have determined that the *Odb2* locus accounts for 55% of the total variance, or is responsible for ~50 of the type 2 diabetes in the OLETF rats (404). *Odb2* colocalizes with the gene encoding cholecystokinin A receptor (*Cckar*), which mediates the trophic effect of cholecystokinin on pancreas. *Cckar* is disrupted in the OLETF rat due to a 165-bp deletion in exon1 (405,406). Genetic segregation analysis has also showed that the *Obd1* and *Obd2* act in a synergistic fashion for type 2 diabetes in the OLETF rat (406). Both of these loci are required in homozygosity from OLETF to cause elevated plasma glucose levels.

Complications

While OLETF rats do weigh more than the nondiabetic control LETO rats for most of their life span, at 80 weeks of age, males generally lose weight and by 90 weeks of age they weigh less than the LETOs. This weight loss is most likely due to the diabetic condition. Levels of urinary protein of the OLETF begin to rise at 25 weeks of age and continue to do so for the remainder of life, reaching levels greater than 800 mg/dL late in life (396). Histologic changes are present and become worse with age. Fibrin caps are detected as early as 30 weeks. These deposits precede the thickening of the basement membrane, which thickens to the point of capillary occlusion (407). These lesions are called *capsular drop* and are present in human diabetic glomerulopathy (408). After the onset of diabetes, the OLETF rat displays hallmarks of macrovascular disease. Diabetic OLETF males are hypertensive, have thickening of artery walls, and show aberrant ventricular diastolic dynamics (409–412).

Potential Research Uses

Genetic predisposition for type 2 diabetes and obesity are major risk factors for the development of type 2 diabetes, and the interactions between these factors are likely to be important in the etiology of this disease. Further genetic dissection of *Odb1* is of clear research importance. The OLETF has been studied for dietary, exercise, and pharmaceutical interventions before and after the initiation of type 2 diabetes. As with many models of type 2 diabetes, caloric restriction can prevent type 2 diabetes and improve insulin sensitivity (413). This is most likely due to the key interactions of body fat or obesity and genetic susceptibility. Exercise training has also been shown to be effective in preventing the development of hyperglycemia (414–416). Exercise improved insulin sensitivity, yet there was no effect on islet morphology. The OLETF has also been used to test drug therapies for type 2 diabetes and the related complications. Troglitazone and metformin have both been successfully used to treat the type 2 diabetes phenotypes of OLETF. Troglitazone treatment reduced circulating glucose, insulin, cholesterol, and triglyceride levels to normal (417). Troglitazone treatment completely prevented or reversed histologic alterations such as fibrosis, fatty replacement, and inflammatory cell infiltration in the pancreas (417). Interestingly, sections of the liver from the untreated OLETF rats showed mild fatty changes in the central zone of the hepatic lobule, whereas those from the troglitazone-treated OLETF rats appeared normal, with no fat deposition in the hepatocytes. Further, no significant influences on serum levels of markers of liver dysfunction [aspartate aminotransferase (AST) and alanine aminotransferase (ALT)] were detected. Troglitazone, as well as metformin, significantly decreased systolic blood pressure (418).

Availability

Control strains for experimentation with the OLETF include the co-selected nondiabetic, nonobese LETO. Obese controls could include the obese Zucker (*fa/fa*) rat. For metabolic experiments, a control could be the outbred Long-Evans or Sprague Dawley, but a better candidate would be an inbred rat strain such as the Brown Norway (BN), the F344, or Wistar. OLETF males can be obtained from Otsuka America Pharmaceutical, Maryland Research Laboratories, 9900 Medical Center Drive, Rockville, MD 20850. However, the following restrictions apply: Otsuka America Pharmaceutical only provides 4- to 6-week-old male rats without charge, but the investigator has to pay for the transportation fees. They also require that the investigator submit a research protocol and a letter of undertaking (forms are available from the company). Any investigators who are interested in this model should contact the above address for details.

ZUCKER DIABETIC FATTY RATS

Strain Origin and Diabetic Phenotype

The derivation of the Zucker rat began almost 40 years ago (419). Most published studies on Zucker rats are on the non-inbred obese Zucker (ZF). The selection of the inbred Zucker diabetic fatty (ZDF) strain used Zucker (*fa/fa*) rats that had progressed to a diabetic phenotype. After two generations of brother–sister matings, a consistent reproducible diabetic phenotype was achieved in obese males fed Purina 5008 6% fat diet at Eli Lilly and Company (420). The characteristics listed in this chapter are for the commercially available ZDF/Gmi-*fa/fa* and are listed on the Genetic Models, Inc. (GMI) Web site (http://www.criver.com/products/genetic_models/index.html).

In obese males fed Purina 5008 6% fat diet, hyperglycemia begins to develop after 7 weeks of age. All obese males (*fa/fa*) are diabetic after 10 weeks, with serum glucose levels greater than 500 mg/dL. Hyperinsulinemia precedes hyperglycemia, but by 19 weeks of age, insulin levels drop. At 6 week of age, insulin-resistant ZDF and ZF rats are hyperinsulinemic compared with the Lean Zucker control (ZLC) (*fa*/+ or +/+) rat yet have normal plasma glucose levels (421). The diabetic state can be exacerbated with diets higher in fat or high in simple sugars. The development of diabetes between 7 and 12 weeks of age is associated with changes in islet morphology, and the islets of diabetic animals are markedly hypertrophic, with multiple irregular projections into the surrounding exocrine pancreas. In addition, multiple defects in the normal pattern of insulin secretion are present. The islets of prediabetic ZDF rats secrete significantly more insulin in response to glucose and show a left-ward shift in the dose-response curve relating glucose concentration to insulin secretion (422). Islets of prediabetic animals also demonstrate defects in the normal oscillatory pattern of insulin secretion, indicating an impairment of the normal feedback control between glucose and insulin secretion (422). The islets from diabetic animals show further impairment in the ability to respond to a glucose stimulus (422).

By 12 weeks of age, hypersecretion of insulin at 5.0 mmol/L glucose was observed in perifused islets from both obese groups relative to that in the ZLC rat (421). Islets from ZDF rats failed to increase insulin secretion in response to increased glucose concentration. Insulin secretion from ZF islets at 2.8 mmol/L glucose was two to four times greater than secretion from islets of lean ZDF littermate controls (ZLC) (423). Peak first- and second-phase insulin secretory responses of perifused ZDF islets to 20 mM glucose were also significantly greater (424–426). GLUT2, the high-K_m facilitative glucose transporter expressed by β-cells, is underexpressed in ZDF islets. Islets of diabetic rats exhibit a marked decrease in the volume of GLUT2-positive β-cells and a reduction in the number of GLUT2-immunoreactive sites per unit of β-cell plasma membrane. The deficiency of GLUT2 can neither be induced in ZDF β-cells by *in vivo* or *in vitro* exposure to high levels of glucose nor prevented in β-cells of prediabetic ZDF rats by elimination of hyperglycemia (427). ZDF islet glucokinase and hexokinase activity have been shown to be significantly increased compared with that of the ZLC (421). The glycolytic flux at 2.8 mmol/L glucose was significantly higher in ZDF islets versus ZLC islets and was suppressed by mannoheptulose inhibition of glycolysis. Inhibition of glycolysis or fatty acid oxidation also significantly inhibited basal insulin secretion in ZDF islets but not in ZLC islets. As in other animal models of type 2 diabetes, ZDF islets also show impairment in energy production pathways important for GSIS. The enzyme activities of mitochondrial glycerol phosphate dehydrogenase and pyruvate carboxylase were severely decreased compared with those of control Wistar rats and decreased with age and to a greater extent with diabetes onset (428).

In ZDF rats, severity of diabetes is highly correlated with increased GLUT2 in liver and decreased GLUT4 in adipose tissue, heart, and skeletal muscle (429). Further, an inverse correlation with hyperglycemia and proteins responsible for peripheral tissue GLUT4 vesicle mobilization and membrane docking and fusion has been documented. Cellubrevin, VAMP-2, and syntaxin-4 protein levels are elevated (2.8-, 3.7-, and 2.2-fold, respectively) in skeletal muscle from ZDF rats compared with lean controls. Restoration of normoglycemia and normoinsulinemia in ZDF rats with rosiglitazone (30 μmol/kg) normalizes cellubrevin, VAMP-2, and syntaxin 4 protein to levels approaching those observed in lean control animals.

The onset of type 2 diabetes in obese Zucker diabetic fatty (*fa/fa*) rats is preceded by a striking increase in the plasma levels of free fatty acids (FFAs) and by a sixfold rise in triglyceride content in the pancreatic islets. The latter finding provides clear evidence of elevated tissue levels of long-chain fatty acyl CoA, which can impair β-cell function (430). Overaccumulation of fat in pancreatic islets of obese ZDF rats and subsequent lipotoxicity are believed to cause β-cell failure and diabetes (431). ZDF pancreatic islets have an approximately 50-fold increase in fat, maintain an increased acetyl CoA carboxylase and fatty acid synthetase activities compared with ZLC, and lack a normal proinsulin mRNA response to FFAs (432). Furthermore, the FFA induces a fourfold greater rise in β-cytotoxic nitric oxide (NO), up-regulates mRNA of inducible nitric oxide synthase (iNOS), and reduces insulin output (433). Ceramide, a fatty acid–containing inducer of apoptosis, is significantly increased in ZDF islets (434,435). Pharmacologic therapy with triacsin C, an inhibitor of fatty acyl–CoA synthetase, and troglitazone, an enhancer of FFA oxidation in ZDF islets, both significantly limit β-cell death. These agents also reduce iNOS mRNA and NO production, which are involved in FFA-induced apoptosis (434).

Changes in gene expression are also evident in islets from prediabetic and diabetic ZDF rats compared with age-matched control animals. In prediabetic animals, there is no change in levels of insulin mRNA. However, there was a significant 30% to 70% reduction in the levels of a large number of other islet mRNAs, including glucokinase, mitochondrial glycerol-3-phosphate dehydrogenase, voltage-dependent Ca^{2+} and K^+ channels, Ca^{2+}-ATPase, and transcription factor islet-1 mRNA. In addition, there is a 40% to 50% increase in the levels of glucose-6-phosphatase and 12-lipoxygenase mRNA. Furthermore, changes in gene expression in the islets from diabetic ZDF rats include a decrease in levels of insulin mRNA that is associated with reduced islet insulin levels (422). Compared with control islets, expression of mRNA encoding C- and D-isoforms of α1-subunits of β-cell L-type voltage-dependent Ca^{2+} channels was significantly reduced in islets isolated from ZDF rats. Intracellular Ca^{2+} concentration responses in ZDF islets after glucose, KCl, or BAY K 8644 (a Ca^{2+} channel activator) stimulation are markedly attenuated, whereas responses evoked by carbachol (a Ca^{2+} channel blocker) were unimpaired, consistent with a specific decrease in intracellular Ca^{2+} in the diabetic islets. This reduction is accompanied by loss of pulsatile insulin secretion from ZDF islets treated with oscillatory increases of external glucose concentration (436).

Genetics

The fatty (*fa*) gene was mapped to rat Chr 5 in crosses between 13 M/Vc *fa*/+ and the genetically distant BN (437,438). This region of rat Chr 5 is syntenic to mouse Chr 4 and human Chr 1. All three of these genetic segments contain the leptin receptor (*Lepr*). Representing a rat ortholog to the $Lepr^{db}$ mutation in the mouse, the *fa* mutation is also a mutation in the leptin receptor. Sequencing of leptin receptor complemetary DNA (cDNA) yielded a single nucleotide mutation of A→C at position 880, causing an amino acid difference from a Q (glutamine) to a P (proline) (437,439,440). Mutations of the nucleotide sequence that lead to the substitution of proline for any other amino acid generally have devastating effects on the resulting protein structure. The *fa* mutation occurs in a conserved portion of the LEPR molecule and, unlike the *db* mutation, does not disrupt *Lepr* gene expression (440). The mutation is in the extracellular domain yet also has no effect on ligand binding (439). A major difference in the *Lepr-fa* is that this mutation imparts constitutive behavior to a heterologous intracellular signaling domain (441). This constitutive activation of the receptor-induced signaling cascade may induce a desensitization of the leptin signaling pathways.

The genetic factors that contribute to the susceptibility to type 2 diabetes of the ZDF rat have not been determined. One study has examined the phenotype of impaired β-cell function that characterizes both lean and obese ZDF rats. Although the analysis is incomplete, the authors have shown that the significantly decreased GSIS is a recessively inherited trait (442).

Complications

Animal models of diabetic complications are rare. The ZDF presents the opportunity to study important complications associated with diabetes: neuropathy and nerve damage. In studies in which ZDF rats are fed a diet high in cholesterol for 4 weeks, the rats experience decreases in velocity of peripheral nerve conduction and a diabetic neuropathy that presents, to some degree, morphologic changes resembling those of the human with type 2 diabetes (420).

Potential Research Uses

Historically, ZDF rats have been well utilized for research in many facets of diabetes, including nutritional interventions, gene expression, and drug development (443). As with many models of type 2 diabetes, caloric restriction is effective in limiting or preventing diabetes in the ZDF rat (444). The ZDF rat has been used extensively for therapeutic interventions. Efficacy of TZDs (thiazolidinediones), such as troglitazone and rosiglitazone, has been shown, as these drugs improve many of the type 2 diabetes phenotypes. Troglitazone prevents the development of diabetes, lowers serum triglycerides, improves β-cell function (GSIS), and insulin action, and significantly decreases levels of glycosylated hemoglobin (445–448). If administered before or if started early in the diabetes, rosiglitazone prevents the onset of hyperglycemia and proteinuria, but if started late (21 weeks of age), no effect is detected (449). ZDF rats have also been used for drug discovery in the attempt to determine new non-TZD high-affinity ligands for peroxisome proliferator-activator receptor-γ (PPARγ). Treatment with JTT-501 from the prediabetic stage controlled glycemia and lipidemia and prevented the development of diabetic complications (450). Chronic oral administration of GW1929 to ZDF rats resulted in dose-dependent decreases in circulating glucose, FFAs, and triglycerides compared with pretreatment values, as well as significant decreases in glycosylated hemoglobin (448). Furthermore, GW1929 treatment improved both first- and second-phase insulin secretion in response to glucose (448). Conjugated linoleic acid, which also activates PPARα, is able to normalize impaired glucose tolerance and improve hyperinsulinemia in the prediabetic ZDF rat (451).

ZDF rats can also be used for the study of diabetic complications and for testing therapeutic interventions. Zenarestat, an aldose reductase inhibitor, has been used in ZDF rats, and when compared with untreated ZDF controls, improved nerve dysfunction in peripheral neuropathy (452). Further crosses of the ZDF with rats from strains that have been selectively bred for disease phenotypes, such as the SHR (spontaneously hypertensive rat) or the SHHF (spontaneously hypertensive heart failure), could prove valuable in creating better models of diabetic complications. F1 hybrid rats from ZDF *fa*/+ outcrosses with the SHHF-*facp*/+ (SHHF/Mcc-*facp*/*facp* rats) have been made to determine renal function, renal morphology, hemodynamics, and metabolic status (453). The ZDF × SHHF F1 rats express insulin resistance, hypertension, obesity, and develop a more severe renal dysfunction than that seen in either parental stock homozygous for the respective *fatty* alleles

Availability

ZDF/Gmi rats can be obtained from Genetic Models (Indianapolis, IN). Control strains include the ZLC, as well as the obese Zucker (*fa*/*fa*) and lean Zucker (+/+ or *fa*/+). Wistar and Sprague Dawley rats have also been used as controls. Because of contractual obligations with the University of Indiana, certain restrictions apply to the ZDF rats purchased from GMI, including a no-breeding clause on all ZDF rats sold. This has severely limited studies into the genetic basis of the type 2 diabetes of ZDF rats.

Gerbil Models of Type 2 Diabetes

PSAMMOMYS OBESUS: A MODEL OF NUTRITIONALLY EVOKED TYPE 2 DIABETES

Strain Origin and Diabetic Phenotype

The *Psammomys obesus* (a member of the Gerbillinae family) also referred to inappropriately as the *sand rat*, is a model of nutritionally evoked type 2 diabetes. In the natural habitat (deserts of the Dead Sea and southern Algeria), *Psammomys* is not hyperglycemic but will transition into type 2 diabetes when fed *ad libitum* a calorie-dense laboratory feed. In the laboratory setting, the fertility of *Psammomys* can generally be maintained only when the animals are fed a mix of lab chow mixed with the native diet of salt bush (454). Like some rat models of type 2 diabetes, the *Psammomys* is an outbred model of type 2 diabetes, and research colonies differ in disease profile and most likely in genetic makeup. The phenotypes associated with type 2 diabetes in the *Psammomys* are obesity, impaired glucose tolerance, hyperinsulinemia, and finally hyperglycemia (455). A recent publication reported that *Psammomys* from the colony at the Hebrew University of Jerusalem, Israel, maintained on a diet that consisted of 70% starch, 17% protein, and 3% fat, had blood glucose values higher than 350 mg/dL and insulin levels of more than 15 ng/mL only 26 days after the onset of a high-calorie diet (456,457). Further, GSIS is defective in this gerbil, with blunted first- and second-phase insulin secretion (458). The defect that causes the type 2 diabetes is thought to be peripheral. Two reports (459,460) have shown that the hepatic insulin receptors bind insulin poorly. This is thought to abolish the control of insulin over gluconeogenesis, which is twice as high in *Psammomys* as in laboratory animals (459). Yet, fat and muscle cell insulin resistance is thought to be manifest through the overexpression of the PKCε, which highly correlates with the failure of the insulin receptor to signal (460). Due to the insulin resistance syndrome, the islets show enhanced insulin synthesis and β-cell hypertrophy in the effort to compensate. Ten percent of the *Psammomys* proceed to the point of β-cell failure. At this time, the phenotypes are hypoinsulinemia and ketosis (455).

Complications

Diabetic cataract formation is a long-term complication of diabetes in humans. The *Psammomys* offers the unique opportunity to study the initiation of cataractogenesis under the control of hyperglycemia. Bilateral cataracts form in the *Psammomys* fed a high-calorie diet, and treatments that lower the blood glucose levels prevent the cataracts (456).

Potential Research Uses

Like other animal models of nutritionally induced diabetes, *P. obesus* provides the opportunity to study the interactions of diet and the phenotypes of type 2 diabetes. At this time, *Psammomys* has not been used in studies with TZDs. Pharmaceutical interventions have been made with both vanadium salts and lipoic acid. The effects of lipoic acid in the treatment of type 2 diabetes are questionable, but lipoic acid is effective in preventing the development of cataracts (456). Vanadium salts decrease circulating glucose and insulin levels and improved the peripheral sensitivity to insulin (457). This gerbil would be an excellent candidate for the study of the effects of exercise on the development and persistence of type 2 diabetes. The onset of ketosis is very rare in animal models of diabetes. That a small proportion of *P. obesus* develops ketosis indicates that this model presents an opportunity to study the ketotic state driven by natural occurrences.

Availability

P. obesus are available from Harlan Laboratories, Ein Kerem, Jerusalem, 91120, POB 12085, Israel.

Acknowledgments

The writing of this chapter was supported by National Institutes of Health grants F32DK09865, DK36175, and DK27722 and grants from the Juvenile Diabetes Research Foundation International and the American Diabetes Association. We thank Drs. Arthur Like and John Mordes (University of Massachusetts, Worcester) for providing information on the BB/Wor rats.

REFERENCES

1a. Von Mering J, Minkowski O. Nach pancreas extirpation. *Arch Exp Pathol Pharmakol* 1890;26:371–381.

1b. Minkowski O. Weitere mittheilungen uber den diabetes mellitus nach exstirpatation des pankreas. *Berliner Klin Wochenschr* 29:90–94.

1c. Banting FG, Best CH, Doffin GM, Gilchrist JA. Quatitative parallelism of effect of insulin in man, dog, and rabbit (Abstract). *Am J Physiol* 1923;63:391.

1d. Banting FG, Best CH. The internal secretion of the pancreas. *J Lab Clin Invest* 1922;7:251–266.

1e. Mauvais-Jarvis F, Kahn CR. Understanding the pathogenesis and treatment of insulin resistance and type 2 diaetes mellitus: what can we learn from transgenic and knockout mice? *Diabetes Metab* 2000;26:433–448.

2. Accili D, Nakae J, Kim JJ, et al. Targeted gene mutations define the roles of insulin and IGF-I receptors in mouse embryonic development. *J Pediatr Endocrinol Metab* 1999;12:475–485.
3. Hattori M, Yamato E, Hirokawa KJ, et al. Male backcross mice of NOD with Mus spretus Spain predominantly develop diabetes regardless of MHC homozygosity and heterozygosity. *Diabetes* 1992;41:93A.
4. Hattori M, Yamato E, Matsumoto E, et al. Occurrence of pretype I diabetes (pre-IDDM) and type II diabetes (NIDDM) in BC1 [(NOD × *Mus spretus*)F1 × NOD] mice. In: Shafrir E, ed. *Lessons from animal diabetes, VI.* Boston: Birkhauser, 1996:83–95.
5. Mehta V, Palmer JP. The natural history of the IDDM disease process. In: Palmer JP, ed. *Prediction, prevention and genetic counseling in IDDM.* New York: John Wiley & Sons, 1996:3–16.
6. Serreze DV, Leiter EH. Insulin dependent diabetes mellitus (IDDM) in NOD mice and BB rats: origins in hematopoietic stem cell defects and implications for therapy. In: Shafrir E, ed. *Lessons from animal diabetes, V.* London: Smith-Gordon, 1995:59–73.
7. Wang J, Takeuchi T, Tanaka S, et al. A mutation in the insulin 2 gene induces diabetes with severe pancreatic beta-cell dysfunction in the Mody mouse. *J Clin Invest* 1999;103:27–37.
8. Makino S, Kunimoto K, Muraoka Y, et al. Breeding of a non-obese, diabetic strain of mice. *Exp Anim* 1980;29:1–8.
9. Makino S, Hayashi Y, Muraoka Y, et al. Establishment of the nonobese-diabetic (NOD) mouse. In: Sakamoto N, Min HK, Baba S, eds. *Current topics in clinical and experimental aspects of diabetes mellitus.* Amsterdam: Elsevier, 1985: 25–32.
10. Kikutani H, Makino S. The murine autoimmune diabetes model: NOD and related strains. In: Dixon FJ, ed. *Advances in immunology.* New York: Academic Press, 1992:285–322.
11. Makino S, Yamashita H, Kunimoto K, et al. Breeding of the NON mouse and its genetic characteristics. In: Sakamoto N, Hotta N, Uchida K, eds. *Current concepts of a new animal model: the NON mouse.* Tokyo: Elsevier Science Publishers, 1992:4–10.
12. Hattori M, Fukuda M, Ichikawa T, et al. A single recessive non-MHC diabetogenic gene determines the development of insulitis in the presence of an MHC-linked diabetogenic gene in NOD mice. *J Autoimmun* 1990;3:1–10.
13. Ino T, Kawamoto Y, Sato K, et al. Selection of mouse strains showing high and low incidences of alloxan-induced diabetes. *Jikken Dobutsu* 1991;40: 61–67.
14. Ueda H, Ikegami H, Yamato E, et al. The NSY mouse: a new animal model of spontaneous NIDDM with moderate obesity. *Diabetologia* 1995;39:503–508.
15. Leiter EH. NOD mice and related strains: origins, husbandry, and biology. In: Leiter EH, Atkinson MA, eds. *NOD mice and related strains: research applications in diabetes, AIDS, cancer, and other diseases.* Austin, TX: R.G. Landes, 1998:1–35.
16. Baxter AG, Adams MA, Mandel TE. Comparison of high- and low-diabetes incidence NOD mouse strains. *Diabetes* 1989;38:1296–1300.
17. Bowman MA, Leiter EH, Atkinson MA. Autoimmune diabetes in NOD mice: a genetic programme interruptible by environmental manipulation. *Immunol Today* 1994;15:115–120.
18. Leiter E. The NOD mouse: a model for insulin dependent diabetes mellitus. In: Coligan JE, Kruisbeek AM, Margulies DM, et al, eds. *Current protocols in immunology.* New York: John Wiley & Sons, 1997:15.9.1–15.9.23.
19. Harano Y, Nakano T, Kosugi K, et al. Evaluation of ketosis and a role of insulin-antagonistic hormones in NOD mouse. In: Tarui S, Tochino Y, Nonaka K, eds. *Insulitis and type 1 diabetes: lessons from the NOD mouse.* Tokyo: Academic Press, 1986:233–238.
20. Coleman DL. Acetone metabolism in mice: increased activity in mice heterozygous for obesity genes. *Proc Natl Acad Sci U S A* 1980;77:290–293.
21. Harada M, Makino S. Promotion of spontaneous diabetes in non-obese diabetes-prone mice with cyclophosphamide. *Diabetologia* 1984;27:604–606.
22. Karasik A, Hattori M. Use of animal models in the study of diabetes. In: Kahn CR, Weir GC, eds. *Joslin's diabetes mellitus,* 13th ed. Philadelphia: Lea & Febiger, 1994:317–350.
23. Colucci F, Bergman M-L, Penha-Gonclaves C, et al. Apoptosis resistance of nonobese diabetic peripheral lymphocytes linked to the *Idd5* diabetes susceptibility region. *Proc Natl Acad Sci U S A* 1997;94:8670–8674.
24. Encinas JA, Wicker LS, Peterson LB, et al. QTL influencing autoimmune diabetes and encephalomyelitis map to a 0.15-cM region containing Il2. *Nat Genet* 1999;21:158–160.
25. Lyons PA, Armitage N, Argentina F, et al. Congenic mapping of the type 1 diabetes locus, Idd3, to a 780-kb region of mouse chromosome 3: identification of a candidate segment of ancestral DNA by haplotype mapping. *Genome Res* 2000;10:446–453.
26. Chesnut K, She JX, Cheng I, et al. Characterizations of candidate genes for IDD susceptibility from the diabetes-prone NOD mouse strain. *Mamm Genome* 1993;4:549–554.
27. Podolin P, Wilusz M, Cubbon R, et al. Differential glycosylation of interleukin-2, the molecular basis for the NOD *Idd3* type 1 diabetes gene? *Cytokine* 2000;12:477–482.
28. Prochazka M, Serreze DV, Frankel WN, et al. NOR/Lt mice: MHC-matched diabetes-resistant control strain for NOD mice. *Diabetes* 1992;41:98–106.
29. Reifsnyder PC, Flynn JC, Gavin AL, et al. Genotypic and phenotypic characterization of 6 new recombinant congenic strains containing NOD/Shi and CBA/J genome. *Mamm Genome* 1998;10:161–167.
30. Serreze DV, Fleming SA, Chapman HD, et al. B-lymphocytes are critical antigen presenting cells for the initiation of T cell mediated autoimmune insulin dependent diabetes in NOD mice. *J Immunol* 1998;161:3912–3918.
31. Shultz LD, Schweitzer PA, Christianson SW, et al. Multiple defects in innate and adaptive immunological function in NOD/LtSz-*scid* mice. *J Immunol* 1995;154:180–191.
32. Shultz LD, Lang PA, Christianson SW, et al. NOD/LtSz-Rag1(null) mice: an immunodeficient and radioresistant model for engraftment of human hematolymphoid cells, HIV infection, and adoptive transfer of NOD mouse diabetogenic T cells. *J Immunol* 2000;164:2496–2507.
33. Soderstrom I, Bergman ML, Colucci F, et al. Establishment and characterization of RAG-2 deficient non-obese diabetic mice. *Scand J Immunol* 1996;43: 525–530.
34. Worthen SM, Leiter EH, Shultz LD. The NOD-scid mouse: a model system for T cell transfer of diabetes [abstract]. *Diabetes* 1990;39:68A.
35. Serreze DV, Chapman HD, Post CM, et al. T* to Th2 cytokine shifts in nonobese diabetic mice: sometimes an outcome rather than the cause of diabetes resistance elicited by immunostimulation. *J Immunol* 2001;166:1352–1359.
36. Fox CJ, Danska JS. Independent genetic regulation of T-cell and antigen-presenting cell participation in autoimmune islet inflammation. *Diabetes* 1998; 47:331–338.
37. McAleer M, Reifsnyder P, Palmer S, et al. Crosses of NOD mice with the related NON strain: a polygenic model for type I diabetes. *Diabetes* 1995; 44:1168–1195.
38. Atkinson MA, Leiter EH. The NOD mouse model of type 1 diabetes: as good as it gets? *Nat Med* 1999;5:601–604.
39. Leiter EH. Genetics and immunogenetics of NOD mice and related strains. In: Leiter EH, Atkinson MA, eds. *NOD mice and related strains: research applications in diabetes, AIDS, cancer, and other diseases.* Austin, TX: R.G. Landes, 1998:37–69.
40. Jarpe AJ, Winter WE, Peck AB. The changing profile of mononuclear cell populations infiltrating the islets of Langerhan during the progressive insulitis phase in prediabetic NOD mice. *Allerg Immunol* 1990;9:283–292.
41. Jarpe A, Hickman M, Anderson J, et al. A. Flow cytometric enumeration of mononuclear cell populations infiltrating the islets of Langerhan in prediabetic NOD mice: development of a model of autoimmune insulitis for type I diabetes. *Reg Immunol* 1991;3:305–317.
42. Miyazaki A, Hanafusa T, Yamada K, et al. Predominance of T lymphocytes in pancreatic islets and spleen of pre-diabetic non-obese diabetic (NOD) mice: a longitudinal study. *Clin Exp Immunol* 1985;60:622–630.
43. Faveeuw C, Gagnerault MC, Lepault F. Isolation of leukocytes infiltrating the islets of Langerhans of diabetes-prone mice for flow cytometric analysis. *J Immunol Methods* 1995;187:163–169.
44. Rohane PW, Shimada A, Kim DT, et al. Islet infiltrating lymphocytes from prediabetic NOD mice rapidly transfer diabetes to NOD-*scid/scid* mice. *Diabetes* 1995;44:550–554.
45. Amrani A, Durant S, Throsby M, et al. Glucose homeostasis in the nonobese diabetic mouse at the prediabetic stage. *Endocrinology* 1998;139:1115–1124.
46. Wilson SS, Deluca D. NOD fetal thymus organ-culture—an *in vitro* model for the development of T-cells involved in IDDM. *J Autoimmun* 1997;10:461–472.
47. Gaskins HR, Prochazka M, Hamaguchi K, et al. Beta cell expression of endogenous xenotropic retrovirus distinguishes diabetes susceptible NOD/Lt from resistant NON/Lt mice. *J Clin Invest* 1992;90:2220–2227.
48. Debussche X, Lormeau B, Boitard C, et al. Course of pancreatic beta cell destruction in prediabetic NOD mice a histomorphometric evaluation. *Diabete Metab* 1994;20:282–290.
49. Lafferty KJ. Immunobiology of autoimmune diabetes. *Res Immunol* 1997;148: 313–319.
50. Jansen A, Homo-Delarche F, Hooijkaas H, et al. Immunohistochemical characterization of monocytes-macrophages and dendritic cells involved in the initiation of the insulitis and β-cell destruction in NOD mice. *Diabetes* 1994; 43:667–675.
51. Sarukhan A, Gombert J-M, Olivi M, et al. Anchored polymerase chain reaction based analysis of the VB repertoire in the non-obese diabetic (NOD) mouse. *Eur J Immunol* 1994;24:1750.
52. Haskins K, Portas M, Bergman B, et al. Pancreatic islet-specific T-cell clones from nonobese diabetic mice. *Proc Natl Acad Sci U S A* 1989;86:8000–8004.
53. Verdaguer J, Schmidt D, Averill N, et al. Spontaneous autoimmune diabetes in monoclonal T-cell nonobese diabetic mice. *J Exp Med* 1997;186:1663–1676.
54. DiLorenzo TP, Graser RT, Chapman HD, et al. Major histocompatibility complex class I restricted T cells are required for all but the end stages of diabetes development in nonobese diabetic mice and use a prevalent T cell receptor alpha chain gene rearrangement. *Proc Natl Acad Sci U S A* 1998;95:2538–2543.

55. Santamaria P, Utsugi T, Park B-J, et al. Beta-cell-cytotoxic CD8+ T cells from nonobese diabetic mice use highly homologous T cell receptor a chain CDR3 sequences. *J Immunol* 1995;154:2494–2503.
56. Rothe H, Jenkins N, Copeland N, et al. Active stage of autoimmune diabetes is associated with the expression of a novel cytokine, IGIF, which is located near *Idd2*. *J Clin Invest* 1997;99:469–474.
57. Rothe H, Hibino T, Martin S, et al. Systemic production of interferon-gamma, inducing factor (IGIF) versus local IFN-gamma expression involved in the development of T* insulitis in NOD mice. *J Autoimmun* 1997;10:251–256.
58. Trembleau S, Penna G, Gregori S, et al. Deviation of pancreas-infiltrating cells to TH2 by interleukin-12 antagonist administration inhibits autoimmune diabetes. *Eur J Immunol* 1997;27:2330–2339.
59. Fox C, Danska J. IL-4 expression at the onset of islet inflammation predicts nondestructive insulitis in nonobese diabetic mice. *J Immunol* 1997;158: 2414–2424.
60. Faveeuw C, Gagnerault MC, Kraal G, et al. Homing of lymphocytes into islets of Langerhans in prediabetic non-obese diabetic mice is not restricted to autoreactive T cells. *Int Immunol* 1995;7:1905–1913.
61. Yang XD, Michie SA, Tisch R, et al. Cell adhesion molecules: a selective therapeutic target for alleviation of IDDM. *J Autoimmun* 1994;7:859–864.
62. Signore A, Pozzilli P, Gale EAM, et al. The natural history of lymphocyte subsets infiltrating the pancreas of NOD mice. *Diabetologia* 1989;32:282–289.
63. Christianson SW, Shultz LD, Leiter EH. Adoptive transfer of diabetes into immunodeficient NOD-*scid/scid* mice: relative contributions of CD4+ and CD8+ T lymphocytes from diabetic versus prediabetic NOD.NON-*Thy* 1^a donors. *Diabetes* 1993;42:44–55.
64. Miller BJ, Appel MC, O'Neil JJ, et al. Both the Lyt-2+ and L3T4+ T cell subsets are required for the transfer of diabetes in nonobese diabetic mice. *J Immunol* 1988;140:52–58.
65. Serreze DV, Chapman HD, Varnum DS, et al. Initiation of autoimmune diabetes in NOD/Lt mice is MHC class I-dependent. *J Immunol* 1997;158:3978–3986.
66. Bendelac A, Boitard C, Bedossa P, et al. Adoptive T cell transfer of autoimmune nonobese diabetic mouse diabetes does not require recruitment of host B lymphocytes. *J Immunol* 1988;141:2625–2628.
67. Akashi T, Nagafuchi S, Anzai K, et al. Direct evidence for the contribution of B cells to the progression of insulitis and the development of diabetes in nonobese diabetic mice. *Int Immunol* 1997;9:1159–1164.
68. Noorchashm H, Noorchashm N, Kern J, et al. B-cells are required for the initiation of insulitis and sialitis in nonobese diabetic mice. *Diabetes* 1997;46:941–946.
69. Serreze DV, Chapman HD, Varnum DS, et al. B lymphocytes are essential for the initiation of T cell mediated autoimmune diabetes: analysis of a new "speed congenic"stock of NOD.$Ig\mu^{null}$ mice. *J Exp Med* 1996;184:2049–2053.
70. Atkinson MA. NOD mice as a model for therapeutic interventions in human insulin dependent diabetes mellitus. In: Leiter EH, Atkinson MA, eds. *NOD mice and related strains: research applications in diabetes, AIDS, cancer, and other diseases*. Austin, TX: R. G. Landes, 1998:145–172.
71. Serreze DV, Hamaguchi K, Leiter EH. Immunostimulation circumvents diabetes in NOD/Lt mice. *J Autoimmun* 1989;2:759–776.
72. Bach J-F. Insulin-dependent diabetes mellitus as an autoimmune disease. *Endocr Rev* 1994;15:516–542.
73. Delovitch TL, Singh B. The nonobese diabetic mouse as a model of autoimmune diabetes: immune dysregulation gets the NOD. *Immunity* 1997;7:291–297.
74. Liblau RS, Singer SM, McDevitt HO. T* and Th2 CD4+ T cells in the pathogenesis of organ specific autoimmune diseases. *Immunol Today* 1995;16:34–38.
75. Denny P, Lord CJ, Hill NJ, Goy JV, et al. Mapping of the IDDM locus *Idd3* to a 0.35cM interval containing the *interleukin-2* gene. *Diabetes* 1997;46:695–700.
76. Rothe H, Hartmann B, Geerlings P, et al. Interleukin-12 gene-expression of macrophages is regulated by nitric-oxide. *Biochem Biophys Res Commun* 1996; 224:159–163.
77. Rothe H, Burkart V, Faust A, et al. Interleukin-12 gene expression mediates the accelerating effect of cyclophosphamide in autoimmune disease. *Ann N Y Acad Sci* 1996;795:397–399.
78. Hultgren B, Huang XJ, Dybdal N, et al. Genetic absence of gamma-interferon delays but does not prevent diabetes in NOD mice. *Diabetes* 1996;45:812–817.
79. Serreze DV, Post CM, Chapman HD, et al. Interferon-gamma receptor signaling is dispensable in the development of autoimmune type 1 diabetes in NOD mice. *Diabetes* 2000;49:2007–2011.
80. Kanagawa O, Xu G, Tevaarwerk A, et al. Protection of nonobese diabetic mice from diabetes by gene(s) closely linked to IFN-gamma receptor loci. *J Immunol* 2000;164:3919–3923.
81. Wang B, Andre I, Gonzalez A, et al. Interferon-gamma impacts at multiple points during the progression of autoimmune diabetes. *Proc Natl Acad Sci U S A* 1997;94:13844–13849.
82. Sadelain MWJ, Qin H-Y, Lauzon J, et al. Prevention of type 1 diabetes in NOD mice by adjuvant immunotherapy. *Diabetes* 1990;39:583–589.
83. Serreze DV, Gaedeke JW, Leiter EH. Hematopoietic stem cell defects underlying abnormal macrophage development and maturation in NOD/Lt mice: defective regulation of cytokine receptors and protein kinase C. *Proc Natl Acad Sci U S A* 1993;90:9625–9629.
84. Clare-Salzler M. The immunopathogenic roles of antigen presenting cells in the NOD mouse. In: Leiter EH, Atkinson MA, eds. *NOD mice and related strains: research applications in diabetes, AIDS, cancer, and other diseases*. Austin, TX: R. G. Landes; 1998:101–120.
85. Varadhachary AS, Perdow SN, Hu C, et al. Differential ability of T cell subsets to undergo activation-induced cell death. *Proc Natl Acad Sci U S A* 1997;94:5778–5783.
86. Zhang X, Brunner T, Carter L, et al. Unequal death in T helper (Th)1 and Th2 effectors: T*, but not Th2, effectors undergo rapid Fas/FasL-mediated apoptosis. *J Exp Med* 1997;185:1837–1849.
87. Serreze DV, Leiter EH. Genes and pathways underlying autoimmune diabetes in NOD mice. In: von Herrath M, ed. *Molecular pathology of insulin-dependent diabetes mellitus*. New York: Karger; 2001.
88. Baekkeskov S, Kanaani J, Jaume JC, et al. Does GAD have a unique role in triggering IDDM? *J Autoimmun* 2000;15:279–286.
89. Hawa MI, Fava D, Medici F, et al. Antibodies to IA-2 and GAD65 in type 1 and type 2 diabetes: isotype restriction and polyclonality. *Diabetes Care* 2000; 23:228–233.
90. Wegmann DR, Eisenbarth GS. It's insulin. *J Autoimmun* 2000;15:286–291.
91. Yoon JW, Sherwin RS, Kwon H, et al. Has GAD a central role in type 1 diabetes? *J Autoimmun* 2000;15:273–278.
92. Kaufman DL, Clare-Salzler M, et al. Spontaneous loss of T-cell tolerance to glutamic acid decarboxylase in murine insulin-dependent diabetes. *Nature* 1993;366:69–72.
93. Muir A, Schatz D, Maclaren N. Antigen-specific immunotherapy—oral tolerance and subcutaneous immunization in the treatment of insulin-dependent diabetes. *Diabetes Metab Rev* 1993;9:279–287.
94. Tisch R, Yang XD, Liblau RS, et al. Administering glutamic acid decarboxylase to NOD mice prevents diabetes. *J Autoimmun* 1994;7:845–850.
95. Yoon JW, Yoon CS, Lim Hw, et al. Control of autoimmune diabetes in NOD mice by GAD expression or suppression in β cells. *Science* 1999;284:1183–1186.
96. Eizirik DL, Hoorens A. β-cell dysfunction and death. *Adv Mol Cell Biol* 1999; 29:47–73.
97. Mathews C, Leiter E. Constitutive differences in anti-oxidant defense status distinguish alloxan aesistant (ALR/Lt) and alloxan susceptible (ALS/Lt) mice. *Free Radic Biol Med* 1999;27:499–455.
98. Mathews C, Leiter E. Resistance of ALR/Lt islets to free radical mediated diabetogenic stress is inherited as a dominant trait. *Diabetes* 1999;48: 2189–2196.
99. Mathews CE, Graser R, Savinov A, et al. The NOD/Lt-related ALR/Lt strain: unusual resistance of beta cells to autoimmune killing uncovers a role for beta-cell expressed resistance determinants. *Proc Natl Acad Sci U S A* 2001;98:235–240.
100. Prochazka M, Leiter EH, Serreze DV, et al. Three recessive loci required for insulin-dependent diabetes in NOD mice. *Science* 1987;237:286–289.
101. Mathews CE, Graser R, Savinov A, et al. The NOD/Lt-related ALR/Lt strain: unusual resistance of beta cells to autoimmune killing uncovers a role for beta-cell expressed resistance determinants. *Proc Natl Acad Sci U S A* 2001;98: 235–240.
102. Hattori M, Buse JB, Jackson RA, et al. The NOD mouse: recessive diabetogenic gene in the major histocompatibility complex. *Science* 1986;231: 733–735.
103. Markees TG, Serreze DV, Phillips NE, et al. NOD mice have a generalized defect in their response to transplantation tolerance induction. *Diabetes* 1999; 48:967–974.
104. Serreze DV. The identity and ontogenic origins of autoreactive T lymphocytes in NOD mice. In: Leiter EH, Atkinson MA, eds. *NOD mice and related strains: research applications in diabetes, aids, cancer, and other diseases*. Austin, TX: R. G. Landes; 1998:71–99.
105. Shimada A, Charlton B, Rohane P, et al. Immune regulation in type 1 diabetes. *J Autoimmun* 1996;9:263–269.
106. Carrasco-Marins E, Shimizu J, et al. The class II MHC I-A^{g7} molecules from nonobese diabetic mice are poor peptide binders. *J Immunol* 1996;156: 450–458.
107. Slattery RM, Kjer-Nielsen L, Allison J, et al. Prevention of diabetes in nonobese diabetic I-A^k transgenic mice. *Nature* 1990;345:724–726.
108. Acha-Orbea H, McDevitt HO. The first external domain of the nonobese diabetic mouse class II I-Aβ chain is unique. *Proc Natl Acad Sci U S A* 1987;84: 2435–2439.
109. Miyazaki T, Uno M, Uehira M, et al. Direct evidence for the contribution of the unique I-A^{nod} to the development of insulitis in non-obese diabetic mice. *Nature* 1990;345:722–724.
110. Lund T, O'Reilly L, Hutchings P, et al. Prevention of insulin-dependent diabetes mellitus in non-obese diabetic mice by transgenes encoding modified I-A β-chain or normal I-E α-chain. *Nature* 1990;345:727–729.
111. Hanson MS, Cetkovic-Cvrlje M, et al. Quantitative thresholds of MHC class II I-E expressed on hematopoietically derived APC in transgenic NOD/Lt mice determine level of diabetes resistance and indicate mechanism of protection. *J Immunol* 1996;157:1279–1287.
112. Lie BA, Sollid LM, Ascher H, et al. A gene telomeric of the HLA class I region is involved in predisposition to both type 1 diabetes and coeliac disease. *Tissue Antigens* 1999;54:162–168.
113. Hattori M, Yamato E, Itoh N, et al. Homologous recombination of the MHC class I K region defines new MHC-linked diabetogenic susceptibility gene(s) in nonobese diabetic mice. *J Immunol* 1999;163:1721–1724.
114. Ikegami H, Makino S, Yamato Y, et al. Identification of a new susceptibility locus for insulin-dependent diabetes mellitus by ancestral haplotype congenic mapping. *J Clin Invest* 1995;96:1936–1942.
115. Melanitou E, Joly F, Lathrop M, et al. Evidence for the presence of insulin-dependent diabetes-associated alleles on the distal part of mouse chromosome 6. *Genome Res* 1998;8:608–620.
116. Wicker LS, Todd JA, Peterson LB. Genetic control of autoimmune diabetes in the NOD mouse. *Annu Rev Immunol* 1995;13:179–200.

117. Friday RP, Trucco M, Pietropaolo M. Genetics of type 1 diabetes mellitus. *Diabetes Nutr Metab* 1999;12:3–26.
118. McAleer MA, Reifsnyder P, Palmer SM, et al. Crosses of NOD mice with the related NON strain: a polygenic model for type I diabetes. *Diabetes* 1995;44: 1186–1195.
119. Leiter EH. Lessons from the animal models: the NOD mouse. In: Palmer JP, ed. *Diabetes prediction, prevention, and genetic counselling*. London: John Wiley & Sons, 1996:201–226.
120. Yui MA, Muralidharan K, Moreno-Altamirano B, et al. Production of congenic mouse strains carrying NOD-derived diabetogenic genetic intervals: an approach for the genetic dissection of complex traits. *Mamm Genome* 1996; 7:331–334.
121. Yui MA, Muralidharan K, Moreno-Altamirano B, et al. Production of congenic mouse strains carrying NOD-derived diabetogenic genetic intervals: an approach for the genetic dissection of complex traits. *Mamm Genome* 1996; 7:331–334.
122. Serreze DV, Chapman HC, Gerling IC, et al. Initiation of autoimmune diabetes in NOD/Lt mice is MHC class I-dependent. *J Immunol* 1997;158: 3978–3986.
123. Serreze DV, Bridgett MB, Chapman HD, et al. Subcongenic analysis of the *Idd13* locus in NOD/Lt mice: evidence for several susceptibility genes including a possible diabetogenic role for β2-microglobulin. *J Immunol* 1998; 160:1472–1478.
124. Fox CJ, Paterson AD, Mortin-Toth SM, et al. Two genetic loci regulate T cell-dependent islet inflammation and drive autoimmune diabetes pathogenesis. *Am J Hum Genet* 2000;67:67–81.
125. Hattori M, Fukuda M, Ichikawa T, et al. A single recessive non-MHC diabetogenic gene determines the development of insulitis in the presence of an MHC-linked diabetogenic gene in NOD mice. *J Autoimmun* 1990;3:1–10.
126. Graser RT, Mathews CE, Leiter EH, et al. MHC characterization of ALR and ALS mice: respective similarities to the NOD and NON strains. *Immunogenetics* 1999;49:722–726.
127. Mathews CE, Graser RT, Serreze DV, et al. Re-evaluation of the major histocompatibility complex genes of the NOD progenitor CTS/Shi strain. *Diabetes* 2000;49:131–134.
128. Vafiadis P, Bennett S, Todd J, et al. Insulin expression in human thymus is modulated by *INS* VNTR alleles at the *IDDM2* locus. *Nat Gen* 1997;15: 289–292.
129. French M, Allison J, Dempseyc M, et al. Transgenic expression of mouse proinsulin-II prevents diabetes in nonobese diabetic mice. *Diabetes* 1997;46: 34–39.
130. Wong FS, Karttunen J, Dumont C, et al. Identification of an MHC class I-restricted autoantigen in type 1 diabetes by screening an organ-specific cDNA library. *Nat Med* 1999;5:1026–1031.
131. Hill NJ, Lyons PA, Armitage N, et al. The NOD *Idd5* locus controls insulitis and diabetes and overlaps the orthologous CTLA4/IDDM12 and NRAMP1 loci in humans. *Diabetes* 2000;49:1744–1747.
132. Marron M, Raffel L, Serranor M, et al. Insulin-dependent diabetes-mellitus (IDDM) is associated with CTLA4 polymorphisms in multiple ethnic-groups. *Hum Mol Gen* 1997;6:1275–1282.
133. Serreze DV, Gaskins HR, Leiter EH. Defects in the differentiation and function of antigen presenting cells in NOD/Lt mice. *J Immunol* 1993;150: 2534–2543.
134. Langmuir PB, Bridgett MM, Bothwell ALM, et al. Bone marrow abnormalities in the non-obese diabetic mouse. *Int Immunol* 1993;5:169–177.
135. Dahlen E, Hedlund G, Dawe K. Low CD86 expression in the nonobese diabetic mouse results in the impairment of both T cell activation and CTLA-4 up-regulation. *J Immunol* 2000;164:2444–2456.
136. Bahjat FR, Dharnidharka VR, Fukuzuka K, et al. Reduced susceptibility of nonobese diabetic mice to TNF-alpha and D-galactosamine-mediated hepatocellular apoptosis and lethality. *J Immunol* 2000;165:6559–6567.
137. Prins J-B, Todd J, Rodriques N, et al. Linkage on chromosome 3 of autoimmune diabetes and defective Fc receptor for IgG in NOD mice. *Science* 1993;260:695–698.
138. Martin R, Silva A, Lew A. The IgH-1 sequence of the nonobese diabetic (NOD) mouse assigns it to the IgG2C isotype. *Immunogenetics* 1997;46: 167–168.
139. Piganelli JD, Martin T, Haskins K. Splenic macrophages from the NOD mouse are defective in the ability to present antigen. *Diabetes* 1998;47: 1212–1218.
140. Peterson JD, Herzenberg LA, Vasquez K, et al. Glutathione levels in antigen-presenting cells modulate T* versus Th2 response patterns. *Proc Natl Acad Sci U S A* 1998;95:3071–3076.
141. Lee M, Kim AY, Kang Y. Defects in the differentiation and function of bone marrow-derived dendritic cells in non-obese diabetic mice. *J Korean Med Sci* 2000;15:217–223.
141a. Overbergh L, Decallonne B, Valckx D, et al. Identification and immune regulation of 25-hydroxyvitamin D-1-alpha-hydroxylase in murine macrophages. *Clin Exp Immunol* 2000;120:139–146.
142. Decallonne B, Overbergh L, Casteels KM, et al. Streptococcal wall component OK432 restores sensitivity of non-obese diabetic (NOD) thymocytes to apoptotic signals. *Diabetologia* 2000;43:1302–1308.
143. Leijon K, Hammarström B, Holmberg D. Non-obese diabetic (NOD) mice display enhanced immune responses and prolonged survival of lymphoid cells. *Int Immunol* 1994;6:339–345.
144. Penha-Goncalves C, Leijon K, et al. Type 1 diabetes and the control of dexamethazone-induced apoptosis in mice maps to the same region on chromosome 6. *Genomics* 1995;28:398–404.
145. Colucci F, Cilio CM, Lejon K, et al. Programmed cell death in the pathogenesis of murine IDDM: resistance to apoptosis induced in lymphocytes by cyclophosphamide. *J Autoimmun* 1996;9:271–276.
146. Lamhamedi Cherradi SE, Luan JJ, et al. Resistance of T-cells to apoptosis in autoimmune diabetic (NOD) mice is increased early in life and is associated with dysregulated expression of Bcl-x. *Diabetologia* 1998;41:178–184.
147. Martins TC, Aguas AP. NOD mice are resistant to depletion of thymic cells caused by acute stress or infection. *Autoimmunity* 1999;29:273–280.
148. Radosevic K, Casteels KM, Mathieu C, et al. Splenic dendritic cells from the non-obese diabetic mouse induce a prolonged proliferation of syngeneic T cells: a role for an impaired apoptosis of NOD T cells? *J Autoimmun* 1999;13: 373–382.
149. Casteels KM, Gysemans CA, Waer M, et al. Sex difference in resistance to dexamethasone-induced apoptosis in NOD mice: treatment with 1,25(OH)2D3 restores defect. *Diabetes* 1998;47:1033–1037.
150. Rapoport M, Lazarus A, Jaramillo A, et al. Thymic T cell anergy in autoimmune nonobese diabetic mice is mediated by deficient T cell receptor regulation of the pathway of $p21^{ras}$ activation. *J Exp Med* 1993;177:1221–1226.
151. Dardenne MF, Lepault A, Bendelac A, et al. Acceleration of the onset of diabetes in NOD mice by thymectomy at weaning. *Eur J Immunol* 1989;19: 889–895.
152. Ghosh S, Palmer SM, Rodrigues NR, et al. Polygenic control of autoimmune diabetes in nonobese diabetic mice. *Nat Genet* 1993;4:404–409.
153. Chesnut K, Shie J-X, Cheng I, et al. Characterization of candidate genes for IDD susceptibility from the diabetes-prone NOD mouse strain. *Mamm Genome* 1993;4:549–554.
154. Horak I, Lohler J, Ma A, et al. Interleukin-2 deficient mice: a new model to study autoimmunity and self-tolerance. *Immunol Rev* 1995;148:35–44.
155. Serreze DV, Leiter EH. Defective activation of T suppressor cell function in nonobese diabetic mice. Potential relation to cytokine deficiencies. *J Immunol* 1988;140:3801–3807.
156. Serreze DV, Leiter EH, Christianson GJ, et al. MHC class I deficient NOD-*B2m*^{null} mice are diabetes and insulitis resistant. *Diabetes* 1994;43:505–509.
157. Podolin PL, Wilusz MB, Cubbon RM, et al. Differential glycosylation of interleukin 2, the molecular basis for the NOD *Idd3* type 1 diabetes gene? *Cytokine* 2000;12:477–482.
158. Bach JF, Chatenou L, Carnaud C, et al. Autoimmune diabetes—how many steps for one disease. *Res Immunol* 1997;148:332–338.
159. Bendelac A, Rivera MN, Park SH, et al. Mouse CD1-specific NK1 T cells: development, specificity, and function. *Annu Rev Immunol* 1997;15:535–562.
160. Gombert J, Herbelin A, Tancrede E C, et al. Early defect of immunoregulatory T-cells in autoimmune diabetes. *C R Acad Sci III* 1996;319:125–129.
161. Baxter AG, Kinder SJ, Hammond KJL, et al. Association between alpha-beta-$TCR^{+}CD4^{-}CD8^{-}$ T-cell deficiency and IDDM in NOD/Lt mice. *Diabetes* 1997; 46:572–582.
162. Hammond KJL, Poulton LD, Palmisano PA, et al. aβ$(TCR)^{+}$ $CD4^{-}CD8^{-}$(NKT) thymocytes prevent insulin-dependent diabetes mellitus in non-obese diabetic (NOD/Lt) mice by the influence of interleukin (IL)-4 and/or IL-10. *J Exp Med* 1998;187:1285–1292.
163. Gombert JM, Tancredebohin E, Hameg A, et al. IL-7 reverses NK1(+) T cell-defective IL-4 production in the non-obese diabetic mouse. *Int Immunol* 1996; 8:1751–1758.
164. Carnaud C, Gombert JM, Donnars O, et al. Protection against diabetes and improved NK/NKT cell performance in NOD.NK1.1 mice congenic at the NK complex. *J Immunol* 2001;166:2404–2411.
165. Serizawa I, Koezuka Y, Amao H, et al. Functional natural killer T cells in experimental mouse stains, including NK1.1-strains. *Exp Anim* 2000;49: 171–180.
166. Arase H, Arase N, Saito T. Interferon gamma production by natural killer (NK) cells and $NK1.1^{+}$ T cells upon NKR-P1 cross-linking. *J Exp Med* 1996; 183:2391–2396.
167. Christianson SW, Shultz LD, Leiter EH. Adoptive transfer of diabetes into immunodeficient NOD-*scid/scid* mice: relative contributions of $CD4^{+}$ and $CD8^{+}$ T lymphocytes from diabetic versus prediabetic NOD.NON-Thy-1^{a} donors. *Diabetes* 1993;42:44–55.
168. Yanagi K, Haneji N, Hayashi Y, et al. Analysis of T-cell receptor V-beta usage in the autoimmune sialadenitis of nonobese diabetic (NOD) mice. *Clin Exp Immunol* 1997;110:440–446.
169. Papaccio G, Sellitti S, Salvatore G, et al. The Harderian gland in autoimmune diabetes of the nonobese diabetic mouse. *Microsc Res Tech* 1996;34: 156–165.
170. Hu Y, Nakagawa Y, Purushotham KR, et al. Functional changes in salivary glands of autoimmune disease-prone NOD mice. *Am J Physiol* 1992;263: E607–E614.
171. Takahashi M, Ishimaru N, Yanagi K, et al. High incidence of autoimmune dacryoadenitis in male non-obese diabetic (NOD) mice depending on sex steriod. *Clin Exp Immunol* 1997;109:555–561.
172. Skarstein K, Wahren M, Zaura E, et al. Characterization of T-cell receptor repertoire and anti-ro/ssa autoantibodies in relation to sialadenitis of NOD mice. *Autoimmunity* 1996;22:9–16.
173. Kerr M, Lee A, Wang P, Purushotham K, et al. Detection of insulin and insulin-like growth factors I and II in saliva and potential synthesis in the salivary glands of mice. *Biochem Pharmacol* 1995;49:1521–1531.
174. Hunger RE, Muller S, Laissue JA, et al. Inhibition of submandibular and

lacrimal gland infiltration in nonobese diabetic mice by transgenic expression of soluble TNF-receptor p55. *J Clin Invest* 1996;98:954–961.
175. Robinson CP, Yamamoto H, Peck AB, et al. Genetically programmed development of salivary gland abnormalities in the NOD (nonobese diabetic)-*scid* mouse in the absence of detectable lymphocytic infiltration: a potential trigger for sialoadenitis of NOD mice. *Clin Immunol Immunopathol* 1996;79:50–59.
176. Robinson CP, Brayer J, Yamachika S, et al. Transfer of human serum IgG to NOD.Igμ^{null} mice reveals a role for autoantibodies in the loss of secretory function of exocrine tissues in Sjoren's syndrome. *Proc Natl Acad Sci U S A* 1998;95:7538–7543.
177. Delemarr F, Simons P, Drexhage H. The BB rat as a model for autoimmune-thyroiditis—relevance for the pathogenesis of human disease. *Exp Clin Endocrinol Diabetes* 1996;104:10–12.
178. Many MC, Maniratunga S, Varis I, et al. Two-step development of Hashimoto-like thyroiditis in genetically autoimmune prone non-obese diabetic mice: effects of iodine-induced cell necrosis. *J Endocrinol* 1995;147:311–320.
179. Many MC, Maniratu S, Denef JF. The nonobese diabetic (NOD) mouse—an animal model for autoimmune thyroiditis. *Exp Clin Endocrinol Diabetes* 1996; 104:17–20.
180. Krug J, Williams AJK, Beales PE, et al. Parathyroiditis in the non-obese diabetic mouse—a new finding. *J Endocrinol* 1991;131:193–196.
181. Many M-C, Drexhage HA, Denef J-F. High frequency of thymic ectopy in thyroids from autoimmune prone nonobese diabetic female mice. *Lab Invest* 1993;69:364–367.
182. Bernard NF, Ertug F, Margolese H. High incidence of throiditis and anti-thyroid autoantibodies in NOD mice. *Diabetes* 1991;41:40–46.
183. Damotte D, Colomb E, Charreir J, et al. Analysis of susceptibility of NOD mice to spontaneous and experimentally-induced thyroiditis. *Eur J Immunol* 1997;27:2854–2882.
184. Margolese H, Okeefe C, Chung F, et al. Expression of major histocompatibility complex class II antigen in NOD mouse thyroid. *Autoimmunity* 1994;17: 1–11.
185. Leiter EH. The NOD mouse meets the "Nerup Hypothesis." Is diabetogenesis the result of a collection of common alleles present in unfavorable combinations? In: Vardi P, Shafrir E, eds. *Frontiers in diabetes research: lessons from animal diabetes, III*. London: Smith-Gordon, 1990:54–58.
186. Prochazka M, Gaskins HR, Shultz LD, et al. The NOD-*scid* mouse: a model for spontaneous thymomagenesis associated with immunodeficiency. *Proc Natl Acad Sci U S A* 1992;89:3290–3294.
187. Atkinson M, Gendreau P, Ellis T, et al. NOD mice as a model for inherited deafness. *Diabetologia* 1997;40:868.
188. Zheng QY, Johnson KR, Erway LC. Assessment of hearing in 80 inbred strains of mice by ABR threshold analyses. *Hear Res* 1999;130:94–107.
189. Baxter AG, Mandel TE. Hemolytic anemia in non-obese diabetic mice. *Eur J Immunol* 1991;21:2051–2055.
190. Gerling IC, Freidman H, Greiner DL, et al. Multiple low dose streptozotocin-induced diabetes in NOD-*scid/scid* mice in the absence of functional lymphocytes. *Diabetes* 1994;43:433–440.
191. Baxter AG, Horsfall AC, Healey D, et al. Mycobacteria precipitate an SLE-like syndrome in diabetes-prone NOD mice. *Immunology* 1994;83:227–231.
192. Mahler M, Leiter EH, Birkenmeier EH, et al. Differential susceptibility of inbred mouse strains to dextran sulfate sodium-induced colitis. *Am J Physiol* 1998;274:G544–G551.
193. Amor S, Baker D, Groome N, et al. Identification of major encephalitogenic epitope of proteolipid protein (residues 56-70) for the induction of experimental allergic encephalomyelitis in Biozzi AB/H and nonobese diabetic mice. *J Immunol* 1993;150:5666–5672.
194. Winer S, Astsaturov I, Cheung R, et al. Type I diabetes and multiple sclerosis patients target islet plus central nervous system autoantigens; nonimmunized nonobese diabetic mice can develop autoimmune encephalitis. *J Immunol* 2001;166:2831–2841.
195. Nakhooda AF, Like AA, Chappel CI, et al. The spontaneously diabetic Wistar rat metabolic and morphologic studies. *Diabetes* 1976;26:100–112.
196. Crisa L, Mordes J, Rossini A. Autoimmune diabetes in the BB rat. *Diabetes Metab Rev* 1992;8:4–37.
197. Rossini AA, Handler ES, Mordes JP, et al. Human autoimmune diabetes mellitus: lessons from BB rats and NOD mice—caveat emptor. *Clin Immunol Immunopathol* 1995;74:2–9.
198. Mordes JP, Groen H, Bortell R, et al. Autoimmune diabetes mellitus in the BB rat. In: Sima AAF, Shafrir E, eds. *Animal models of diabetes: a primer*. Amsterdam: Harwood Academic Publishers, 2001:1–41.
199. Mordes JP, Bortell R, Doukas J, et al. The BB/Wor rat and the balance hypothesis of autoimmunity. *Diabetes Metab Rev* 1996;12:103–109.
200. Like AA, Weringer EJ. Autoimmune diabetes in the biobreeding/Worcester rat. In: Lefèbvre PJ, Pipeleers DG, eds. *The pathology of the endocrine pancreas in diabetes*. Berlin, Heidelberg: Springer-Verlag, 1988:269–284.
201. Mordes JP, Desemone J, Rossini AA. The BB rat. *Diabetes Metab Rev* 1987;3: 725–750.
202. Jacob HJ, Pettersson A, Wilson D, et al. Genetic dissection of autoimmune type 1 diabetes in the BB rat. *Nat Genet* 1992;2:56–60.
203. Hornum L, Jackerott M, Markholst H. The rat T-cell lymphopenia resistance gene (*Lyp*) maps between D4Mit6 and Npy on RNO4. *Mamm Genome* 1995;6: 371–372.
204. Markholst H, Eastman S, Wilson D, et al. Diabetes segregates as a single locus in crosses between inbred BB rats prone or resistant to diabetes. *J Exp Med* 1991;174:297–300.
205. Iwakoshi NN, Goldschneider I, Tausche F, et al. High frequency apoptosis of recent thymic emigrants in the liver of lymphopenic diabetes-prone BioBreeding rats. *J Immunol* 1998;160:5838–5850.
206. Bortell R, Kanaitsuka T, Stevens LA, et al. The RT6 (Art2) family of ADP-ribosyltransferases in rat and mouse. *Mol Cell Biochem* 1999;193:61–68.
207. Koch-Nolte F, Duffy T, Nissen M, et al. New monoclonal antibody detects a developmentally regulated mouse ecto ADP ribosyltransferase on T cells: subset distribution, inbred strain variation, and modulation by T cell activation. *J Immunol* 1999;163:6014–6022.
208. Colle E, Guttman RD, Fuks A, et al. Genetics of the spontaneous diabetic syndrome: interaction of MHC and non-MHC associated factors. *Mol Biol Med* 1986;3:13–23.
209. Ellerman KE, Like AA. A major histocompatibility complex class II restriction for BioBreeding Worcester diabetes-inducing T cells. *J Exp Med* 1995;182: 923–930.
210. Awata T, Guberski DL, Like AA. Genetics of the BB rat: association of autoimmune disorders (diabetes, insulitis, and thyroiditis) with lymphopenia and major histocompatibility complex class II. *Endocrinology* 1995;136: 5731–5735.
211. Colle E. Genetic susceptibility to the development of spontaneous insulin-dependent diabetes mellitus in the rat. *Clin Immunol Immunopathol* 1990;57: 1–9.
212. Holowachuk EW, Greer MK. Unaltered class II histocompatibility antigens and pathogenesis of IDDM in BB rats. *Diabetes* 1989;38:267–271.
213. Chao NJ, Timmerman L, McDevitt HO, et al. Molecular characterization of MHC class II antigens (beta 1 domain) in the BB diabetes-prone and -resistant rat. *Immunogenetics* 1989;29:231–234.
213a. MacMurray AJ, Moralejo DH, Kwitek AE, et al. Lymphopenia in the BB rat model of type 1 diabetes is due to a mutation in a novel immune-associated nucleotide (Ian)-related gene. *Genome Res* 2002;12:1029–1039.
213b. Hornum L, Romer J, Markholst H. The diabetes-prone BB rat carries a frameshift mutation in Ian4, a positional candidate of Iddm1. *Diabetes* 2002; 51:1972–1979.
214. Like AA, Guberski DL, Butler L. Diabetic BioBreeding/Worcester (BB/Wor) rats need not be lymphopenic. *J Immunol* 1986;136:3254–3258.
215. Martin AM, Blankenhorn EP, Maxson MN, et al. Non-major histocompatibility complex-linked diabetes susceptibility loci on chromosomes 4 and 13 in a backcross of the DP-BB/Wor rat to the WF rat. *Diabetes* 1999;48:50–58.
216. Kloting I, Kovacs P. Genes of the immune system cosegregate with the age at onset of diabetes in the BB/OK rat. *Biochem Biophys Res Commun* 1998;242: 461–463.
217. Kloting I, Schmidt S, Kovacs P. Mapping of novel genes predisposing or protecting diabetes development in the BB/OK rat. *Biochem Biophys Res Commun* 1998;245:483–486.
218. Kloting I, Van Den Brande J, Kovacs P. Quantitative trait loci for blood glucose confirm diabetes predisposing and protective genes, IDDM4 and IDDM5, in the spontaneously diabetic BB/OK rat. *Int J Mol Med* 1998;2: 597–601.
219. Kloting I, Vogt L, Serikawa T. Locus on chromosome 18 cosegregates with diabetes in the BB/OK rat subline. *Diabete Metab* 1995;21:338–344.
220. Ellerman K, Wrobleski M, Rabinovitch A, et al. Natural killer cell depletion and diabetes mellitus in the BB/Wor rat (revisited). *Diabetologia* 1993;36: 596–601.
221. Greiner DL, Mordes JP, Handler ES, et al. Depletion of RT6.1[+] T lymphocytes induces diabetes in resistant Biobreeding/Worcester (BB/W) rats. *J Exp Med* 1987;166:461–475.
222. Whalen BJ, Greiner DL, Mordes JP, et al. Adoptive transfer of autoimmune diabetes mellitus to athymic rats: synergy of CD4(+) and CD8(+) T cells and prevention by RT6(+) T cells. *J Autoimmun* 1994;7:819–831.
223. Saoudi A, Seddon B, Fowell D, et al. The thymus contains a high-frequency of cells that prevent autoimmune diabetes on transfer into prediabetic recipents. *J Exp Med* 1996;184:2393–2398.
224. Iwakoshi NN, Greiner DL, Rossini AA, et al. Diabetes prone BB rats are severely deficient in natural killer T cells. *Autoimmunity* 1999;31:1–14.
225. Tori M, Ito T, Kitagawa-Sakakida S, et al. Importance of donor-derived lymphocytes in the protection of pancreaticoduodenal or islet grafts from recurrent autoimmunity: a role for RT6+NKR-P1+ T cells. *Transplantation* 2000;70: 32–38.
226. Trucco M, Laporte R. Exposure to superantigens as an immunogenetic explanation of type I diabetes mini-epidemics. *J Pediatr Endocrinol Metab* 1995; 8:3–10.
227. Rossini AA, Williams RM, Mordes JP, et al. Spontaneous diabetes in the gnotobiotic BB/W rat. *Diabetes* 1979;28:1031–1032.
228. Guberski D, Thomas V, Shek W, et al. Induction of type 1 diabetes by Kilham's rat virus in diabetes-resistant BB/Wor rats. *Science* 1991;254: 1010–1013.
229. Brown DW, Welsh RM, Like AA. Infection of peripancreatic lymph nodes but not islets precedes Kilham rat virus-induced diabetes in BB/Wor rats. *J Virol* 1993;67:5873–5878.
230. Ellerman KE, Richards CA, Guberski DL, et al. Kilham rat virus triggers T-cell-dependent autoimmune diabetes in multiple strains of rats. *Diabetes* 1996;45:557–562.
231. Chung YH, Jun HS, Kang Y, et al. Role of macrophages and macrophage-derived cytokines in the pathogenesis of Kilham rat virus-induced autoimmune diabetes in diabetes-resistant Biobreeding rats. *J Immunol* 1997;159: 466–471.

232. Kolb-Bachofen V, Schaermeyer U, Hoppe T, et al. Diabetes manifestation in BB rats is preceded by pan-pancreatic presence of activated inflammatory macrophages. *Pancreas* 1992;7:578–584.
233. Zipris D, Greiner DL, Malkani S, et al. Cytokine gene expression in islets and thyroids of BB rats. IFN-gamma and IL-12p40 mRNA increase with age in both diabetic and insulin-treated non-diabetic BB rats. *J Immunol* 1996;156: 1315–1321.
234. Rabinovitch A, Suarezpinzon W, Elsheikh A, et al. Cytokine gene expression in pancreatic islet-infiltrating leukocytes of BB rats: expression of T* cytokines correlates with beta-cell destructive insulitis and IDDM. *Diabetes* 1996;45:749–754.
235. Jiang Z, Handler ES, Rossini AA, et al. Immunopathology of diabetes in the RT6-depleted diabetes resistant BB/Wor rat. *Am J Pathol* 1990;137:767–777.
236. Scott FW, Cloutier HE, Kleemann R, et al. Potential mechanisms by which certain foods promote or inhibit the development of spontaneous diabetes in BB rats—dose, timing, early effect on islet area, and switch in infiltrate from T* to TH2 cells. *Diabetes*1997;46:589–598.
237. Sobel DO, Goyal D, Chung YH, et al. Low dose poly I-C prevents diabetes in the diabetes prone BB rat. *J Autoimmun* 1998;11:343–352.
238. Huang XJ, Hultgren B, Dybdal N, et al. Islet expression of interferon-alpha precedes diabetes in both the BB rat and streptozotocin-treated mice. *Immunity* 1994;1:469–478.
239. Sobel DO, Ahvazi B, Jun HS, et al. Cyclophosphamide inhibits the development of diabetes in the diabetes-prone BB rat. *Diabetologia* 2000;43: 986–994.
240. Sternthal E, Like AA, Sarantis K, et al. Lymphocytic thyroiditis and diabetes in the BB/W rat. A new model of autoimmune endocrinopathy. *Diabetes* 1981;30:1058–1061.
241. Rajatanavin R, Appel MC, Reinhardt W, et al. Variable prevalence of lymphocytic thyroiditis among diabetes-prone sublines BB/Wor rats. *Endocrinology* 1991;128:153–157.
242. Awata T, Kanazawa Y. Genetic-markers for insulin-dependent diabetes-mellitus in Japanese. *Diabet Res Clin Pract* 1994;24:S83–S87.
243. McKeever U, Mordes JP, Greiner DL, et al. Adoptive transfer of autoimmune diabetes and thyroiditis to athymic rats. *Proc Natl Acad Sci U S A* 1990;87: 7618–7622.
244. Gottlieb PA, Handler ES, Appel MC, et al. Insulin treatment prevents diabetes mellitus but not thyroiditis in RT6-depleted diabetes resistant BB/Wor rats. *Diabetologia* 1991;34:296–300.
245. Kawano K, Kirashima T, Mori S, et al. New inbred strain of Long-Evans Tokushima lean rats with IDDM without lymphopenia. *Diabetes* 1991;40: 1375–1381.
246. Komeda K, Noda M, Kanazawa M, et al. Establishment of 2 substrains, diabetes-prone and nondiabetic, from Long-Evans Tokushima-Lean (LETL) rats. *J Endocrinol* 1998;45:737–744.
247. Yokoi N, Kanazawa M, Kitada K, et al. A non-MHC locus essential for autoimmune type 1 diabetes in the Komeda diabetes-prone rat. *J Clin Invest* 1997;100:2015–2021.
247a. Yokoi N, Komeda K, Wang HY, et al. Cblb is a major susceptibility gene for rat type 1 diabetes mellitus. *Nat Genet* 2002;31:391–394.
248. Yoshioka M, Kayo T, Ikeda T, et al. A novel locus, Mody4, distal to D7Mit189 on chromosome 7 determines early-onset NIDDM in nonobese C57BL/6 (Akita) mutant mice. *Diabetes* 1997;46:887–894.
249. Kayo T, Koizumi A. Mapping of murine diabetogenic gene *mody* on chromosome 7 at D7Mit258 and its involvement in pancreatic islet and beta cell development during the perinatal period. *J Clin Invest* 1998;101:2112–2118.
250. Coleman DL, Eicher EM. Fat (*fat*) and tubby (*tub*), two autosomal recessive mutations causing obesity syndromes in the mouse. *J Hered* 1990;81:424–427.
251. Naggert JK, Fricker LD, Varlamov O, et al. Hyperproinsulinaemia in obese *fat/fat* mice associated with a carboxypeptidase E mutation which reduces enzyme activity. *Nat Genet* 1995;10:135–142.
252. Fricker LD, Snyder SH. Enkephalin convertase: purification and characterization of a specific enkephalin-synthesizing carboxypeptidase localized to adrenal chromaffin granules. *Proc Natl Acad Sci U S A* 1982;79:3886–3890.
253. Fricker LD. Carboxypeptidase E. *Annu Rev Physiol* 1988;50:309–321.
254. Eipper BA, Mains RE. Peptide alpha-amidation. *Annu Rev Physiol* 1988;50: 333–344.
255. Varlamov O, Leiter E, Fricker L. Induced and spontaneous mutations at Ser^{202} of carboxypeptidase E: effect on enzyme expression, activity, and intracellular routing. *J Biol Chem* 1996;271:13981–13986.
256. Leiter EH, Herberg L. The polygenetics of diabesity in mice. *Diabetes Rev* 1997;5:131–148.
257. Kim JH, Nishina PM, Naggert JK. Genetic models for non insulin dependent diabetes mellitus in rodents. *J Basic Clin Physiol Pharmacol* 1998;9:325–345.
258. Robinson SW, Dinulescu DM, Cone RD. Genetic models of obesity and energy balance in the mouse. *Annu Rev Genet 2000*;34:687–745.
259. Mammes O, Betoulle D, Aubert R, et al. Association of the G-2548A polymorphism in the 5′ region of the LEP gene with overweight. *Ann Hum Genet* 2000;64:391–394.
260. Ohshiro Y, Ueda K, Nishi M, et al. A polymorphic marker in the leptin gene associated with Japanese morbid obesity. *J Mol Med* 2000;78:516–520.
261. Roth H, Korn T, Rosenkranz K, et al. Transmission disequilibrium and sequence variants at the leptin receptor gene in extremely obese German children and adolescents. *Hum Genet* 1998;103:540–546.
262. Ingalls KA, Dickie MM, Snell GD. Obese, a new mutation in the mouse genome. *J Hered* 1950;41:317–318.
263. Zhang Y, Proenca R, Maffei M, et al. Positional cloning of the mouse *obese* gene and its human homologue. *Nature* 1994;372:425–432.
264. Campfield LA, Smith FJ, Guisez Y, et al. Recombinant mouse OB protein: evidence for a peripheral signal linking adiposity and central neural networks. *Science* 1995;269:546–549.
265. Halaas JL, Gajiwala KS, Maffei M, et al. Weight-reducing effects of the plasma protein encoded by the *obese* gene. *Science* 1995;269:543–546.
266. Pelleymounter MA, Cullen MJ, Baker MB, et al. Effects of the *obese* gene product on body weight regulation in *ob/ob* mice. *Science* 1995;269:540–543.
267. Chehab F, Lim M, Lu R. Correction of the sterility defect in homozygous obese female mice by treatment with the human recombinant leptin. *Nat Genet* 1996;12:318–320.
268. Friedman JM. Leptin, leptin receptors and the control of bodyweight. *Nutr Rev* 1998;56:S38–S46.
269. Kerouz NJ, Horsch D, Pons S, et al. Differential regulation of insulin receptor substrates-1 and -2 (IRS-1 and IRS-2) and phosphatidylinositol 3-kinase isoforms in liver and muscle of the obese diabetic (ob/ob) mouse. *J Clin Invest* 1997;100:3164–3172.
270. Frigeri LG, Wolff GL, Robel G. Impairment of glucose tolerance in yellow (Avy/A) (BALB/c X VY) F-1 hybrid mice by hyperglycemic peptide(s) from human pituitary glands. *Endocrinology* 1983;113:2097–2105.
271. Genuth SM, Przybylski RJ, Rosenberg DM. Insulin resistance in genetically obese, hyperglycemic mice. *Endocrinology* 1971;88:1230–1280.
272. Leiter E, Herberg L. The polygenetics of diabesity in mice. *Diabetes Rev* 1997; 5:131–148.
273. Herberg L, Coleman D. Laboratory animals exhibiting obesity and diabetes syndromes. *Metabolism* 1977;26:59–99.
274. Coleman DL, Hummel KP. Hyperinsulinemia in preweaning diabetes (*db*) mice. *Diabetologia* 1974;10:607–610.
275. Hummel KP, Dickie MM, Coleman DL. Diabetes, a new mutation in the mouse. *Science* 1966;153:1127–1128.
276. Coleman DL. Obese and diabetes: two mutant genes causing diabetes-obesity syndromes in mice. *Diabetologia* 1978;14:141–148.
277. Like AA, Chick WL. Studies in the diabetic mutant mouse, I: light microscopy and radioautography of pancreatic islets. *Diabetologia* 1970;6:207–215.
278. Chan TM, Dehaye JP. Hormone regulation of glucose metabolism in the genetically obese-diabetic mouse (db/db): glucose metabolism in the perfused hindquarters of lean and obese mice. *Diabetes* 1981;30:3211–3218.
279. Koranyi L, James D, Mueckler M, et al. Glucose transporter levels in spontaneously obese (*db/db*) insulin-resistant mice. *J Clin Invest* 1995;85:962–967.
280. Shargill NS, Tatoyan A, el-Refai MF, et al. Impaired insulin receptor phosphorylation in skeletal muscle membranes of db/db mice: the use of a novel skeletal muscle plasma membrane preparation to compare insulin binding and stimulation of receptor phosphorylation. *Biochem Biophys Res Commun* 1986;137:286–294.
281. Michaud EJ, Mynatt RL, Miltenberger RJ, et al. Role of the agouti gene in obesity. *J Endocrinol* 1997;155:207–209.
282. Miltenberger RJ, Mynatt RL, Wilkinson JE, et al. The role of the agouti gene in the yellow obese syndrome. *J Nutr* 1997;137:1902S–1907S.
283. Bultman S, Michaud E, Woychik R. Molecular characterization of the mouse agouti locus. *Cell* 1992;71:1195–1204.
284. Duhl DM, Stevens ME, Vrieling H, et al. Pleiotropic effects of the mouse lethal yellow (Ay) mutation explained by deletion of a maternally expressed gene and the simultaneous production of agouti fusion RNAs. *Development* 1994;120:1695–1708.
285. Michaud EJ, van Vugt MJ, Bultman SJ, et al. Differential expression of a new dominant agouti allele (A^{iapy}) is correlated with methylation state and is influenced by parental lineage. *Genes Dev* 1994;8:1463–1472.
286. Michaud EJ, Bultman SJ, Klebig ML, et al. A molecular model for the genetic and phenotypic characteristics of the mouse lethal yellow (Ay) mutation. *Proc Natl Acad Sci U S A* 1994;91:2562–2566.
287. Miller M, Duhl D, Vrieling H, Cordes S, et al. Cloning of the mouse agouti gene predicts a secreted protein ubiquitously expressed in mice carrying the lethal yellow mutation. *Genes Dev* 1993;7:454–467.
288. Claycombe KJ, Wang Y, Jones BH, et al. Transcriptional regulation of the adipocyte fatty acid synthase gene by agouti: interaction with insulin. *Physiol Genomics* 2000;3:157–162.
289. Claycombe KJ, Xue BZ, Mynatt RL, et al. Regulation of leptin by agouti. *Physiol Genomics* 2000;2:101–105.
290. Jones BH, Kim JH, Zemel MB, et al. Upregulation of adipocyte metabolism by agouti protein: possible paracrine actions in yellow mouse obesity. *Am J Physiol* 1996;270:E192–E196.
291. Zemel MB, Kim JH, Woychik RP, et al. Agouti regulation of intracellular calcium: role in the insulin resistance of viable yellow mice. *Proc Natl Acad Sci U S A* 1995;92:4733–4737.
292. Zemel MB. Insulin resistance vs. hyperinsulinemia in hypertension: insulin regulation of Ca^{2+} transport and Ca^{2+}-regulation of insulin sensitivity. *J Nutr* 1995;125:1738S–1743S.
293. Sekiguchi F, Ishibashi K, Kawamoto Y, et al. Diabetic peculiarity of the ALS-A^y and ALR-A^y strains. *Exp Anim* 1991;40:323–329.
294. Frigeri LG, Wolff GL, Robel G. Impairment of glucose tolerance in yellow (Avy/A) (BALB/c X VY) F-1 hybrid mice by hyperglycemic peptide(s) from human pituitary glands. *Endocrinology* 1983;113:2097–2105.
295. Gill AM, Yen TT. Effects of ciglitazone on endogenous plasma islet amyloid polypeptide and insulin sensitivity in obese-diabetic viable yellow mice. *Life Sci* 1991;48:703–710.

296. Warbritton A, Gill AM, Yen TT, et al. Pancreatic islet cells in preobese yellow Avy/- mice: relation to adult hyperinsulinemia and obesity. *Proc Soc Exp Biol Med* 1994;206:145–151.
297. Salem MA, Lewis UJ, Haro LS, et al. Effects of hypophysectomy and the insulin-like and anti-insulin pituitary peptides on carbohydrate metabolism in yellow Avy/A (BALB/c x VY)F1 hybrid mice. *Proc Soc Exp Biol Med* 1989; 191:408–419.
298. Salem MA, Wolff GL. Potentiation of response to insulin and anti-insulin action by two human pituitary peptides in lean agouti A/a, obese yellow Avy/A, and C57BL/6J-ob/ob mice. *Proc Soc Exp Biol Med* 1989;191:113–123.
299. Shimizu H, Shargill NS, Bray GA. Adrenalectomy and response to corticosterone and MSH in the genetically obese yellow mouse. *Am J Physiol* 1989;256:R494–R500.
300. Shimizu H, Shargill NS, Bray GA, et al. Effects of MSH on food intake, body weight and coat color of the yellow obese mouse. *Life Sci* 1989;45:543–552.
301. Mathews CE, Bagley RB, Caldwell JC, et al. NIDDM in a new mouse model elicited by low free radical scavenging potential combined with behavioral and dietary stress. *Diabetes* 2001;50:A517.
302. Hasegawa G, Hata M, Nakano K, et al. Diabetic syndrome in the NON mouse. In: Sakamoto N, Hotta N, Uchida K, eds. *Current concepts of a new animal model: the NON mouse.* Amsterdam: Elsevier Science Publishers, 1992: 41–50.
303. Rebuffe-Scrive M, Surwit R, Feinglos M, et al. Regional fat distribution and metabolism in a new mouse model (C57BL/6J) of non-insulin-dependent diabetes mellitus. *Metabolism* 1993;42:1405–1409.
304. Wencel HE, Smothers C, Opara EC, et al. Impaired second phase insulin response of diabetes-prone C57BL/6J mouse islets. *Physiol Behav* 1995;57: 1215–1220.
305. Lee SK, Opara EC, Surwit RS, et al. Defective glucose-stimulated insulin release from perifused islets of C57BL/6J mice. *Pancreas* 1995;11:206–211.
306. Surwit RS, Feinglos MN, Rodin J, et al. Differential effects of fat and sucrose on the development of obesity and diabetes in C57BL/6J and A/J mice. *Metabolism* 1995;44:645–651.
307. Surwit RS, Edwards CL, Murthy S, et al. Transient effects of long-term leptin supplementation in the prevention of diet-induced obesity in mice. *Diabetes* 2000;49:1203–1207.
308. Surwit R, Seldin M, Kuhn C, et al. Diet-induced obesity and diabetes in C57BL/6J and C57BL/KsJ mice. *Mouse Genome* 1994;92:523–525.
309. Livingston EG, Feinglos MN, Kuhn CM, et al. Hyperinsulinemia in the pregnant C57BL/6J mouse. *Horm Metab Res* 1994;26:307–308.
310. Parekh PI, Petro AE, Surwit RS, et al. Reversal of diet induced obesity and diabetes on C57BL/6J mice. *Metabolism* 1998;47:1089–1096.
311. Shibata M, Yasuda B. Spontaneously occurring diabetes in NSY mice. *Jikken Dobutsu* 1979;28:584–590.
312. Ueda H, Ikegami H, Kawaguchi Y, et al. Paternal-maternal effects on phenotypic characteristics in spontaneously diabetic Nagoya-Shibata-Yasuda mice. *Metabolism* 2000;49:561–656.
313. Ikegami H, Ueda H, Kawaguchi Y, et al. Positional cloning of susceptibility genes for non-insulin-dependent diabetes mellitus. *Nippon Ronen Igakkai Zasshi* 1998;35:290–293.
314. Ueda H, Ikegami H, Kawaguchi Y, et al. Genetic analysis of late-onset type 2 diabetes in a mouse model of human complex trait. *Diabetes* 1999;48: 1168–1174.
315. Shimizu K, Morita H, Niwa T, et al. Spontaneous amyloidosis in senile NSY mice. *Acta Pathol Jpn* 1993;43:215–221.
316. Shibata M, Kishi T, Yasuda B, et al. The inhibitory effect of lysozyme on the glomerular basement membrane thickening in spontaneous diabetic mice (NSY mice). *Tohoku J Exp Med* 1986;149:39–46.
317. Kim JH, Sen S, Avery CS, et al. Genetic analysis of a new mouse model for non-insulin dependent diabetes. *Genomics* 2001;74:273–286.
318. Suzuki W, Iizuka S, Tabuchi M, et al. A new mouse model of spontaneous diabetes derived from ddY strain. *Exp Anim* 1999;48:181–189.
319. Hirayama I, Yi Z, Izumi S, et al. Genetic analysis of obese diabetes in the TSOD mouse. *Diabetes* 1999;48:1183–1191.
320. Leiter EH, Reifsnyder PC, Flurkey K, et al. Non-insulin dependent diabetes genes in mice: deleterious synergism by both parental genomes contributes to diabetogenic thresholds. *Diabetes* 1998;47:1287–1295.
321. Taylor BA, Phillips SJ. Obesity QTLs on mouse chromosomes 2 and 17. *Genomics* 1997;43:249–257.
322. Bielschowsky M, Bielschowsky F. A new strain of mice with hereditary obesity. *Proc Univ Otago Med Sch* 1953;31:29–31.
323. Crofford OB, Davis CK. Growth characteristics, glucose tolerance, and insulin sensitivity of New Zealand obese mice. *Metabolism* 1965;14:271–280.
324. Herberg L. Insulin resistance in abdominal and subcutaneous obesity: comparison of C57BL/6J-ob/ob with New Zealand obese mice. In: Shafrir E, Renold A, eds. *Frontiers in diabetes research, II: lessons from animal diabetes.* London: John Libbey, 1988:367–373.
325. Andrikopoulos S, Rosella G, Gaskin E, et al. Impaired regulation of hepatic fructose-1, 6-bisphosphatase in the New Zealand obese mouse model of NIDDM. *Diabetes* 1993;42:1731–1736.
326. Andrikopoulos S, Proietto J. The biochemical basis of increased hepatic glucose production in a mouse model of type 2 (non-insulin-dependent) diabetes mellitus. *Diabetologia* 1995;38:1389–1396.
327. Andrikopoulos S, Rosella G, Kaczmarczyk SJ, et al. Impaired regulation of hepatic fructose-1,6-bisphosphatase in the New Zealand obese mouse: an acquired defect. *Metabolism* 1996;45:622–626.
328. Proietto J, Larkins RG. A perspective on the New Zealand obese mouse. In: Shafrir E, ed. *Lessons from animal models of diabetes, IV.* London: Smith-Gordon, 1993:65–73.
329. Thorburn AW, Holdsworth A, Proietto J, et al. Differential and genetically separable associations of leptin with obesity-related traits. *Int J Obes* 2000; 24:742–750.
330. Reifsnyder PC, Churchill G, Leiter EH. Maternal environment and genotype interact to establish diabesity in mice. *Genome Res* 2000;10:1568–1578.
331. Plum L, Kluge R, Giesen K, et al. Type 2 diabetes-like hyperglycemia in a backcross model of NZO and SJL mice: characterization of a susceptibility locus on chromosome 4 and its relation with obesity. *Diabetes* 2000;49:1590–1596.
332. Veroni M, Proietto J, Larkins R. Evolution of insulin resistance in New Zealand obese mice. *Diabetes* 1991;40:1480–1487.
333. Larkins R, Simeonova L, Veroni M. Glucose utilization in relation to insulin secretion in NZO and C57BL mouse islets. *Endocrinology* 1980;107:1634–1638.
334. Gates RJ, Lazarus NR. The ability of pancreatic polypeptides (APP and BPP) to return to normal the hyperglycemia, hyperinsulinaemia, and weight gain of New Zealand obese mice. *Horm Res* 1977;8:189–202.
335. Gates RJ, Smith R, Hunt MI, et al. Return to normal of blood-glucose, plasma-insulin, and weight gain in New Zealand obese mice after implantation of islets of Langerhans. *Lancet* 1972;7777:567–570.
336. Gates R, Hunt M, Lazarus N. Further studies on the amelioration of the characteristics of New Zealand Obese (NZO) mice following implantation of islets of Langerhans. *Diabetologia* 1974;10:401–406.
337. Taylor BA, Wnek C, Schroeder D, et al. Multiple obesity QTLs identified in an intercross between the NZO (New Zealand obese) and the SM (small) mouse strains. *Mamm Genome* 2001;12:95–103.
338. Kluge R, Giesen K, Bahrenberg G, et al. Quantitative trait loci for obesity and insulin resistance (Nob1, Nob2) and their interaction with the leptin receptor allele (LeprA720T/T1044I) in New Zealand obese mice. *Diabetologia* 2000;43: 1565–1572.
339. Igel M, Becker W, Herberg L, et al. Hyperleptinemia, leptin resistance, and polymorphic leptin receptor in the New Zealand obese mouse. *Endocrinology* 1997;138:4234–4239.
340. Melez KA, Harrison LC, Gilliam JN, et al. Diabetes is associated with autoimmunity in the New Zealand obese (NZO) mouse. *Diabetes* 1980;29:835–840.
341. Melez KA, Attallah AM, Harrison ET, et al. Immune abnormalities in the diabetic New Zealand obese (NZO) mouse: insulin treatment partially suppresses splenic hyperactivity measured by flow cytometric analysis. *Clin Immunol Immunopathol* 1985;36:110–119.
342. Harrison LC, Itin A. A possible mechanism for insulin resistance and hyperglycaemia in New Zealand obese mice. *Nature* 1979;279:334–336.
343. Hamano Y, Hirose S, Ida A, et al. Susceptibility alleles for aberrant B-1 cell proliferation involved in spontaneously occurring B-cell chronic lymphocytic leukemia in a model of New Zealand white mice. *Blood* 1998;92: 3772–3779.
344. Collins S, Daniel KW, Petro AE, et al. Strain-specific response to beta(3)-adrenergic receptor agonist treatment of diet-induced obesity in mice. *Endocrinology* 1997;138:405–413.
345. Berdanier CD. Non-insulin-dependent diabetes in the nonobese BHE/cdb rat. In: Shafrir E, ed. *Lessons from animal diabetes.* London: Smith-Gordon, 1994:231–246.
346. Mathews C, Everts H, Flatt W, et al. ATP production is reduced in rats having an ATPase 6 mutation. *Int J Diabetes* 2002 *(in press).*
347. Mathews CE, McGraw RA, Dean R, et al. Inheritance of a mitochondrial DNA defect and impaired glucose tolerance in BHE/Cdb rats. *Diabetologia* 1999;42:35–40.
348. Matschinsky FM. Banting Lecture 1995. A lesson in metabolic regulation inspired by the glucokinase glucose sensor paradigm. *Diabetes* 1996;45: 223–241.
349. Lakshmanan MR, Berdanier CD, Veech RL. Comparative studies on lipogenesis and cholesterogenesis in lipemic BHE rats and normal Wistar rats. *Arch Biochem Biophys* 1977;183:355–360.
350. Berdanier CD. Rat strain differences in gluconeogenesis by isolated hepatocytes. *Proc Soc Exp Biol Med* 1982;169:74–79.
351. Berdanier CD, Thomson AR. Comparative studies on mitochondrial respiration in four strains of rats rattus norvegicus. *Comp Biochem Physiol* 1986;85B: 531–535.
352. Deaver OE, Wander RC, McCusker RH, et al. Diet effects on membrane phospholipid fatty acids and mitochondrial function in BHE rats. *J Nutr* 1986; 116:1148–1155.
353. Kim MC, Berdanier CD. Glucose homeostasis in thyroxine-treated BHE/cdb rats fed corn oil or hydrogenated coconut oil. *J Nutr Biochem* 1993;4:10–19.
354. Hood DA, Simoneau J-A, Kelly AM, et al. Effect of thyroid status on the expression of metabolic enzymes during chronic stimulation. *Am J Physiol* 1992;263:C788–C793.
355. Soboll S. Thyroid hormone action on mitochondrial energy transfer. *Biochim Biophys Acta* 1993;1144:1–16.
356. Van Itallie CM. Thyroid hormone and dexamethasone increase the levels of a messenger ribonucleic acid for a mitochondrially encoded subunit but not for a nuclear-encoded subunit of cytochrome c oxidase. *Endocrinology* 1990;127:55–62.
357. Jarrett RJ, Keen H. Diurnal variation of oral glucose tolerance: a possible pointer to the evolution of diabetes mellitus. *BMJ* 1969;2:341–344.
358. Jarrett RJ, Keen H. Further observations on the diurnal variation of oral glucose tolerance. *BMJ* 1970;4:334–337.

359. Sassone-Corsi P. Molecular clocks: mastering time by gene regulation. *Nature* 1998;392:871–874.
360. Mathews CE, Wickwire K, Flatt W, et al. Attenuation of circadian rhythms of food intake and respiration in aging diabetes-prone BHE/Cdb rats. *Am J Physiol* 2000;279:R230–R238.
361. Mathews CE, McGraw R, Berdanier C. A point mutation in the mitochondrial DNA of diabetes-prone BHE/cdb rats. *FASEB J* 1995;9:1638–1642.
362. Gadaleta G, Pepe G, DeCandia G, et al. The complete nucleotide sequence of the *Rattus norvegicus* mitochondrial genome: cryptic signals revealed by comparative analysis between vertebrates. *J Mol Evol* 1989;28:497–516.
363. Brown GC, Lakin-Thomas PL, et al. Control of respiration and oxidative phosphorylation in isolated rat liver cells. *Eur J Biochem* 1990;192:355–362.
364. Brown GC. Control of respiration and ATP synthesis in mammalian mitochondria and cells. *Biochem J* 1992;284:1–13.
365. Hafner RP, Brown GC, Brand MD. Analysis of the control of respiration rate, phosphorylation rate, proton leak rate and protonmotive force in isolated mitochondria using the 'top-down' approach of metabolic control theory. *Eur J Biochem* 1990;188:313–319.
366. Kim S-B, Berdanier CD. Oligomycin sensitivity of mitochondrial F1Fo ATPase in diabetes prone BHE/cdb rats. *Am J Physiol* 1999;277:E702–E707.
367. Tarres MC, Martinez SM, Liborio MM, et al. Diabetes mellitus en una linea endocriada de ratas. *Mendeliana* 1981;5:39–48.
368. Tarres MC, Martinez SM, Montenegro SM, et al. Influence of gonadectomy in eSS diabetic rats. *Rev Esp Fisiol* 1997;53:211–216.
369. Tarres MC, Martinez SM, Montenegro SM, et al. Relationship of diet, biomass and expression of diabetes in eSS rats. *Medicina* (B Aires) 1990;50:235–243.
370. Martinez SM, Tarres MC, Montenegro S, et al. Intermittent dietary restriction in eSS diabetic rats. Effects on metabolic control and skin morphology. *Acta Diabetol Lat* 1990;27:329–336.
371. Martinez SM, Tarres MC, Montenegro S, et al. Spontaneous diabetes in eSS rats. *Acta Diabetol Lat* 1988;25:303–313.
372. Gomez Dumm CL, Semino MC, Gagliardino JJ. Quantitative morphological changes in endocrine pancreas of rats with spontaneous diabetes mellitus. *Virchows Arch B Cell Pathol Incl Mol Pathol* 1989;57:375–381.
373. Gomez Dumm CL, Semino MC, Gagliardino JJ. Sequential morphological changes in pancreatic islets of spontaneously diabetic rats. *Pancreas* 1990;5: 533–539.
374. de Gomez Dumm IN, Montenegro S, Tarres MC, et al. Early lipid alterations in spontaneously diabetic rats. *Acta Physiol Pharmacol Ther Latinoam* 1998;48: 228–234.
375. Daniele SM, Arriaga S, Martinez SM, et al. Onset and evolution of nephropathy in rats with spontaneous diabetes mellitus. *J Physiol Biochem* 2000;56:45–53.
376. Goto Y, Kakizaki M, Masaki N. Spontaneous diabetes produced by selective breeding of normal wistar rats. *Proc Jpn Acad* 1975;51:80–85.
377. Suzuki K-I, Goto Y, Toyata T. Spontaneously diabetic GK (Goto-Kakizaki) rats. In: Shafrir E, ed. *Lessons from animal diabetes*. London: Smith-Gordon, 1992:107–116.
378. Portha B, Serradas P, Bailbe D, et al. β-cell insensitivity to glucose in the GK rat, a spontaneous nonobese model for type II diabetes. *Diabetes* 1991;40:486–491.
379. Movassat J, Saulnier C, Serradas P, et al. Impaired development of pancreatic beta-cell mass is a primary event during the progression to diabetes in the GK rat. *Diabetologia* 1997;40:916–925.
380. Movassat J, Saulnier C, Portha B. Beta-cell mass depletion precedes the onset of hyperglycaemia in the GK rat, a genetic model of non-insulin-dependent diabetes mellitus. *Diabete Metab* 1995;21:365–370.
381. Portha B, Giroix MH, Serradas P, et al. Beta-cell function and viability in the spontaneously diabetic GK rat: information from the GK/Par colony. *Diabetes* 2001;50:S89–S93.
382. Salehi A, Henningsson R, Mosen H, et al. Dysfunction of the islet lysosomal system conveys impairment of glucose-induced insulin release in the diabetic GK rat. *Endocrinology* 1999;140:3045–3053.
383. Ostenson CG, Abdel-Halim SM, Rasschaert J, et al. Deficient activity of FAD-linked glycerophosphate dehydrogenase in islets of GK rats. *Diabetologia* 1993;36:722–726.
384. Ostenson CG, Khan A, Abdel-Halim SM, et al. Abnormal insulin secretion and glucose metabolism in pancreatic islets from the spontaneously diabetic GK rat. *Diabetologia* 1993;36:3–8.
385. Tsuura Y, Ishida H, Okamoto Y, et al. Glucose sensitivity of ATP-sensitive K+ channels is impaired in beta-cells of the GK rat: a new genetic model of NIDDM. *Diabetes* 1993;42:1446–1453.
386. Tsuura Y, Ishida H, Okamoto Y, et al. Reduced sensitivity of dihydroxyacetone on ATP-sensitive K+ channels of pancreatic beta cells in GK rats. *Diabetologia* 1994;37:1082–1087.
387. Nagamatsu S, Nakamichi Y, Yamamura C, et al. Decreased expression of t-SNARE, syntaxin 1, and SNAP-25 in pancreatic beta-cells is involved in impaired insulin secretion from diabetic GK rat islets: restoration of decreased t-SNARE proteins improves impaired insulin secretion. *Diabetes* 1999;48:2367–2373.
388. Abdel-Halim S, Guenifi A, Luthman H, et al. Impact of diabetic inheritance on glucose tolerance and insulin secretion in spontaneously diabetic GK-Wistar rats. *Diabetes* 1994;43:281–288.
389. Galli J, Li L-S, Glaser A, Östenson C-G, et al. Genetic analysis of non-insulin dependent diabetes mellitus in the GK rat. *Nat Genet* 1996;12:31–37.
390. Galli J, Fakhrai-Rad H, Kamel A, et al. Pathophysiological and genetic characterization of the major diabetes locus in GK rats. *Diabetes* 1999;48: 2463–2470.
391. Fakhrai-Rad H, Nikoshkov A, Kamel A, et al. Insulin-degrading enzyme identified as a candidate diabetes susceptibility gene in GK rats. *Hum Mol Genet* 2000;9:2149–2158.
392. Kawano K, Hirashima T, Saitoh Y, et al. Spontaneous long-term hyperglycemic rat with diabetic complications. Otkuka Long-Evans Tokushima fatty (OLETF) strain. *Diabetes* 1992;41:1422–1428.
393. Kawano K, T. H, Mori S, Natori T. OLEFT (Otsuka Long-Evans Tokushima fatty) rat: a new NIDDM rat strain. *Diabet Res Clin Pract* 1994;24:S317–S320.
394. Shi K, Mizuno A, Sano T, et al. Sexual difference in the incidence of diabetes mellitus in Otsuka-Long-Evans-Tokushima-fatty rats: effects of castration and sex hormone replacement on its incidence. *Metabolism* 1994;43: 1214–1220.
395. Kawano K, Hirashima T, Mori S, et al. Spontaneously diabetic rat "OLETF" as a model for NIDDM in humans. In: Shafrir E, ed. *Lessons in animal diabetes*. Boston: Birkhauser, 1996:225–236.
396. Toide K, Man ZW, Asahi Y, et al. Glucose transporter levels in a male spontaneous non-insulin-dependent diabetes mellitus rat of the Otsuka Long-Evans Tokushima Fatty strain. *Diabetes Res Clin Pract* 1997;38:151–160.
397. Sato T, Man ZW, Toide K, et al. Plasma membrane content of insulin-regulated glucose transporter in skeletal muscle of the male Otsuka Long-Evans Tokushima Fatty rat, a model of non-insulin-dependent diabetes mellitus. *FEBS Lett* 1997;407:329–332.
398. Ishida K, Mizuno A, Murakami T, et al. Obesity is necessary but not sufficient for the development of diabetes mellitus. *Metabolism* 1996;45:1288–1295.
399. Okauchi N, Mizuno A, Zhu M, et al. Effects of obesity and inheritance on the development of non-insulin-dependent diabetes mellitus in Otsuka-Long-Evans-Tokushima fatty rats. *Diabet Res Clin Pract* 1995;29:1–10.
400. Hirashima T, Kawano K, Mori S, et al. A diabetogenic gene (Odb-1) assigned to the X-chromosome in Oletf rats. *Diabet Res Clin Pract* 1995;27:91–96.
401. Nara V, Gao M, Sawamura M, et al. Genetic-analysis of non-insulin-dependent diabetes-mellitus in the Otsuka Long-Evans Tokushima fatty rat. *Biochem Biophys Res Commun* 1997;241:200–204.
402. Kanemoto N, Hishigaki H, Miyakita A, et al. Genetic dissection of "OLETF," a rat model for non-insulin-dependent diabetes mellitus. *Mamm Genome* 1998;9:419–425.
403. Hirashima T, Kawano K, Mori S, et al. A diabetogenic gene, ODB2, identified on chromosome 14 of the OLETF rat and its synergistic action with ODB1. *Biochem Biophys Res Commun* 1996;224:420–425.
404. Moralejo DH, Ogino T, Wei SW, et al. A major quantitative trait locus co-localizing with cholecystokinin type a receptor gene influences poor pancreatic proliferation in a spontaneously diabetogenic rat. *Mamm Genome* 1998;9: 794–798.
405. Takiguch S, Takata Y, Kataoka K, et al. Disrupted cholecystokinin type-a receptor (CCKAR) gene in OLETF rats. *Gene* 1997;197:169–175.
406. Takiguchi S, Takata Y, Takahash N, et al. A disrupted cholecystokinin-A receptor gene induces diabetes in obese rats synergistically with *Odb1* gene. *Am J Physiol* 1998;37:E265–E270.
407. Kawano K, Mori S, Hirashima T, et al. Examination of the pathogenesis of diabetic nephropathy in OLETF rats. *J Vet Med Sci* 1999;61:1219–1228.
408. Barrie HJ, Askanazy CL, Smith GW. More glomerular changes in diabetes. *Can Med Assoc J* 1952;66:428–435.
409. Kosegawa I, Katayama S, Kikuchi C, et al. Metformin decreases blood pressure and obesity in OLETF rats via improvement of insulin resistance. *Hypertens Res* 1996;19:37–41.
410. Mizushige K, Yao L, Noma T, et al. Alteration in left ventricular diastolic filling and accumulation of myocardial collagen at insulin-resistant prediabetic stage of a type II diabetic rat model. *Circulation* 2000;101:899–907.
411. Mizushige K, Noma T, Yao L, et al. Effects of troglitazone on collagen accumulation and distensibility of aortic wall in prestage of non-insulin-dependent diabetes mellitus of Otsuka Long-Evans Tokushima fatty rats. *J Cardiovasc Pharmacol* 2000;35:150–155.
412. Yao L, Mizushige K, Noma T, et al. Improvement of left ventricular diastolic dynamics in prediabetic stage of a type II diabetic rat model after troglitazone treatment. *Angiology* 2001;52:53–57.
413. Okauchi N, Mizuno A, Yoshimoto S, et al. Is caloric restriction effective in preventing diabetes mellitus in the Otsuka Long Evans Tokushima fatty rat, a model of spontaneous non-insulin-dependent diabetes mellitus? *Diabetes Res Clin Pract* 1995;27:97–106.
414. Shima K, Shi K, Sano T, et al. Is exercise training effective in preventing diabetes mellitus in the Otsuka-Long-Evans-Tokushima fatty rat, a model of spontaneous non-insulin-dependent diabetes mellitus? *Metabolism* 1993;42: 971–977.
415. Shima K, Shi K, Mizuno A, et al. Effects of difference in amount of exercise training on prevention of diabetes mellitus in the Otsuka-Long-Evans-Tokushima fatty rats, a model of spontaneous non-insulin-dependent diabetes mellitus. *Diabetes Res Clin Pract* 1994;23:147–154.
416. Shima K, Shi K, Mizuno A, et al. Exercise training has a long-lasting effect on prevention of non-insulin-dependent diabetes mellitus in Otsuka-Long-Evans-Tokushima fatty rats. *Metabolism* 1996;45:475–480.
417. Jia DM, Tabaru A, Akiyama T, et al. Troglitazone prevents fatty changes of the liver in obese diabetic rats. *J Gastroenterol Hepatol* 2000;15:1183–1191.
418. Kosegawa I, Chen S, Awata T, et al. Troglitazone and metformin, but not glibenclamide, decrease blood pressure in Otsuka Long Evans Tokushima fatty rats. *Clin Exp Hypertens* 1999;21:199–211.
419. Zucker LM, Zucker TF. Fatty, a new mutation in the rat. *J Hered* 1961;52: 275–278.

420. Peterson RG, Shaw WN, Neel M-A, et al. Zucker diabetic fatty rat as a model for non-insulin-dependent diabetes mellitus. *ILAR News* 1990;32:16–19.
421. Cockburn BN, Ostrega DM, Sturis J, et al. Changes in pancreatic islet glucokinase and hexokinase activities with increasing age, obesity, and the onset of diabetes. *Diabetes* 1997;46:1434–1439.
422. Tokuyama Y, Sturis J, Depaoli AM, et al. Evolution of beta-cell dysfunction in the male Zucker diabetic fatty rat. *Diabetes* 1995;44:1447–1457.
423. Zhou YP, Cockburn BN, Pugh W, et al. Basal insulin hypersecretion in insulin-resistant Zucker diabetic and Zucker fatty rats: role of enhanced fuel metabolism. *Metabolism* 1999;48:857–864.
424. Zawalich WS, Kelley GG. The pathogenesis of NIDDM: the role of the pancreatic beta cell. *Diabetologia* 1995;38:986–991.
425. Sturis J, Pugh WL, Tang J, et al. Alterations in pulsatile insulin secretion in the Zucker diabetic fatty rat. *Am J Physiol* 1994;267:E250–E259.
426. Sturis J, Pugh WL, Tang J, et al. Prevention of diabetes does not completely prevent insulin secretory defects in the ZDF rat. *Am J Physiol* 1995;269: E786–E792.
427. Orci L, Ravazzola M, Baetens D, et al. Evidence that down-regulation of beta-cell glucose transporters in non-insulin-dependent diabetes may be the cause of diabetic hyperglycemia. *Proc Natl Acad Sci U S A* 1990;87:9953–9957.
428. MacDonald MJ, Tang J, Polonsky KS. Low mitochondrial glycerol phosphate dehydrogenase and pyruvate carboxylase in pancreatic islets of Zucker diabetic fatty rats. *Diabetes* 1996;45:1626–1630.
429. Slieker LJ, Sundell KL, Heath WF, et al. Glucose transporter levels in tissues of spontaneously diabetic Zucker fa/fa rat (ZDF/drt) and viable yellow mouse (Avy/a). *Diabetes* 1992;41(2):187–193.
430. Lee Y, Hirose H, Zhou YT, et al. Increased lipogenic capacity of the islets of obese rats: a role in the pathogenesis of NIDDM. *Diabetes* 1997;46:408–413.
431. Lee Y, Hirose H, Ohneda M, et al. Beta-cell lipotoxicity in the pathogenesis of non-insulin-dependent diabetes mellitus of obese rats: impairment in adipocyte-beta-cell relationships. *Proc Natl Acad Sci U S A* 1994;91:10878–10882.
432. Zhou YT, Shimabukuro M, Lee Y, et al. Enhanced de novo lipogenesis in the leptin-unresponsive pancreatic islets of prediabetic Zucker diabetic fatty rats: role in the pathogenesis of lipotoxic diabetes. *Diabetes* 1998;47:1904–1908.
433. Shimabukuro M, Ohneda M, Lee Y, et al. Role of nitric oxide in obesity-induced beta cell disease. *J Clin Invest* 1997;100:290–295.
434. Shimabukuro M, Zhou YT, Levi M, et al. Fatty acid induced beta cell apoptosis: a link between obesity and diabetes. *Proc Natl Acad Sci U S A* 1998;95: 2498–2502.
435. Shimabukuro M, Higa M, Zhou YT, et al. Lipoapoptosis in beta-cells of obese prediabetic fa/fa rats. Role of serine palmitoyltransferase overexpression. *J Biol Chem* 1998;273:32487–32490.
436. Roe MW, Worley JF, Tokuyama Y, et al. NIDDM is associated with loss of pancreatic beta-cell L-type Ca^{2+} channel activity. *Am J Physiol* 1996;270: E133–E140.
437. Chua SCJ, Chung W, Wu-Peng X, et al. Phenotypes of mouse *diabetes* and rat *fatty* due to mutations in the OB (leptin) receptor. *Science* 1996;271:994–996.
438. Truett G, Bahary N, Friedman J, et al. Rat obesity gene fatty (*fa*) maps to chromosome 5: evidence for homology with the mouse gene diabetes (*db*). *Proc Natl Acad Sci U S A* 1991;88:7806–7809.
439. Chua SC Jr, White DW, Wu-Peng XS, et al. Phenotype of fatty due to Gln269Pro mutation in the leptin receptor (Lepr). *Diabetes* 1996;45:1141–1143.
440. Phillips M, Liu Q, Hammond H, et al. Leptin receptor missense mutation in the *fatty* Zucker rat. *Nat Genet* 1996;13:18–19.
441. White D, Wang Y, Chua S, et al. Constitutive and impaired signaling of leptin receptors containing the Gln→Pro extracellular domain fatty mutation. *Proc Natl Acad Sci U S A* 1997;94:10657–10662.
442. Griffen SC, Wang J, German MS. A genetic defect in beta-cell gene expression segregates independently from the fa locus in the ZDF rat. *Diabetes* 2001;50: 63–68.
443. Harmon JS, Gleason CE, Tanaka Y, et al. *In vivo* prevention of hyperglycemia also prevents glucotoxic effects on PDX-1 and insulin gene expression. *Diabetes* 1999;48:1995–2000.
444. Ohneda M, Inman LR, Unger RH. Caloric restriction in obese pre-diabetic rats prevents beta-cell depletion, loss of beta-cell GLUT 2 and glucose incompetence. *Diabetologia* 1995;38:173–179.
445. Sreenan S, Keck S, Fuller T, et al. Effects of troglitazone on substrate storage and utilization in insulin-resistant rats. *Am J Physiol* 1999;276:E1119–E1129.
446. Zhang B, Graziano MP, Doebber TW, et al. Down-regulation of the expression of the obese gene by an antidiabetic thiazolidinedione in zucker diabetic fatty rats and db/db mice. *J Biol Chem* 1996;271:9455–9459.
447. Shimabukuro M, Zhou YT, Lee Y, et al. Induction of uncoupling protein-2 mRNA by troglitazone in the pancreatic islets of Zucker diabetic fatty rats. *Biochem Biophys Res Commun* 1997;237:359–361.
448. Brown KK, Henke BR, Blanchard SG, et al. A novel *N*-aryl tyrosine activator of peroxisome proliferator-activated receptor-gamma reverses the diabetic phenotype of the Zucker diabetic fatty rat. *Diabetes* 1999;48:1415–1424.
449. Smith SA, Lister CA, Toseland CD, et al. Rosiglitazone prevents the onset of hyperglycaemia and proteinuria in the Zucker diabetic fatty rat. *Diabetes Obes Metab* 2000;2:363–372.
450. Shibata T, Takeuchi S, Yokota S, et al. Effects of peroxisome proliferator-activated receptor-alpha and -gamma agonist, JTT-501, on diabetic complications in Zucker diabetic fatty rats. *Br J Pharmacol* 2000;130:495–504.
451. Houseknecht KL, Vanden Heuvel JP, Moya-Camarena SY, et al. Dietary conjugated linoleic acid normalizes impaired glucose tolerance in the Zucker diabetic fatty fa/fa rat. *Biochem Biophys Res Commun* 1998;244:678–682.
452. Shimoshige Y, Ikuma K, Yamamoto T, et al. The effects of zenarestat, an aldose reductase inhibitor, on peripheral neuropathy in Zucker diabetic fatty rats. *Metabolism* 2000;49:1395–1399.
453. Tofovic SP, Kusaka H, Kost CK, et al. Renal function and structure in diabetic, hypertensive, obese ZDFxSHHF-hybrid rats. *Ren Fail* 2000;22:387–406.
454. Aharonson Z, Shani J, Sulman FG. Hypoglycaemic effect of the salt bush (*Atriplex halimus*)—a feeding source of the sand rat (*Psammomys obesus*). *Diabetologia* 1969;5:379–383.
455. Ziv E, Shafrir E. *Psammomys obesus*: nutritionally induced NIDDM-like syndrome on a "thrifty gene" background. In: Shafrir E, ed. *Lessons from animal diabetes*. London: Smith-Gordon, 1995:285–300.
456. Borenshtein D, Ofri R, Werman M, et al. Cataract development in diabetic sand rats treated with alpha-lipoic acid and its gamma-linolenic acid conjugate. *Diabetes Metab Res Rev* 2001;17:44–50.
457. Shafrir E, Spielman S, Nachliel I, et al. Treatment of diabetes with vanadium salts: general overview and amelioration of nutritionally induced diabetes in the *Psammomys obesus* gerbil. *Diabetes Metab Res Rev* 2001;17:55–66.
458. Hahn HJ, Gottschling HD, Schafer H. Apparent discrepancy between the insulin secretory responses *in vivo* and *in vitro* in carbohydrate-intolerant sand rats. *Diabetologia* 1979;17:367–369.
459. Kanety H, Moshe S, Shafrir E, et al. Hyperinsulinemia induces a reversible impairment in insulin receptor function leading to diabetes in the sand rat model of non-insulin-dependent diabetes mellitus. *Proc Natl Acad Sci U S A* 1994;91:1853–1857.
460. Ikeda Y, Olsen GS, Ziv E, et al. Cellular mechanism of nutritionally induced insulin resistance in *Psammomys obesus*: overexpression of protein kinase epsilon in skeletal muscle precedes the onset of hyperinsulinemia and hyperglycemia. *Diabetes* 2001;50:584–592.

SECTION III

Diabetes: Definition, Genetics, and Pathogenesis

CHAPTER 19

Definition, Diagnosis, and Classification of Diabetes Mellitus and Glucose Homeostasis

Peter H. Bennett and William C. Knowler

Diabetes mellitus is a heterogeneous group of metabolic disorders characterized by chronic hyperglycemia. Some forms of diabetes mellitus are characterized in terms of their specific etiology or pathogenesis, but the underlying etiology of the most common forms remains unclear. Regardless of the etiology, diabetes progresses through several clinical stages during its natural history. Persons developing the disease can be categorized according to clinical stages and other characteristics even in the absence of knowledge of the etiology.

DEFINITION OF DIABETES MELLITUS

Diabetes mellitus is characterized by chronic hyperglycemia with disturbances of carbohydrate, fat, and protein metabolism resulting from defects in insulin secretion, insulin action, or both. When fully expressed, diabetes is characterized by fasting hyperglycemia, but the disease can also be recognized during less overt stages, most usually by the presence of glucose intolerance. The effects of diabetes mellitus include long-term damage, dysfunction, and failure of various organs, especially the eyes, kidneys, heart, and blood vessels. Diabetes may present with characteristic symptoms such as thirst, polyuria, blurring of vision, weight loss, and polyphagia, and in its most severe forms, with ketoacidosis or nonketotic hyperosmolarity, which, in the absence of effective treatment, leads to stupor, coma, and death. Often symptoms are not severe or may even be absent. Hyperglycemia sufficient to cause pathologic functional changes may quite often be present for a long time before the diagnosis is made. Consequently, diabetes often is discovered because of abnormal results from a routine blood or urine glucose test or because of the presence of a complication. In some instances diabetes may be apparent only intermittently, as, for example, with glucose intolerance in pregnancy or gestational diabetes, which may remit after parturition. In some individuals the likelihood of developing diabetes may be recognized even before any abnormalities of glucose tolerance are apparent. During the evolution of type 1 diabetes, for example, immunologic disturbances such as islet cell or other antibodies are present, and these may precede clinically apparent disease by months or even years (1). In some families it is possible to recognize certain gene mutations that are strongly associated with certain forms of diabetes, such as variations in the glucokinase gene or hepatic nuclear factor genes that cause youth or early adult-onset diabetes (2). These genetic abnormalities are detectable at any time.

Although a number of specific causes of diabetes mellitus have been identified, the etiology and pathogenesis of the more common types are less clearly understood. The majority of cases of diabetes fall into two broad etiopathogenetic categories, now called type 1 and type 2 diabetes (3,4), but the extent of heterogeneity among these types remains uncertain. Because of the increasing number of forms of diabetes for which a specific etiology can be recognized, the current clinical classification, proposed by the American Diabetes Association (ADA) in 1997 (3) and adopted by the World Health Organization

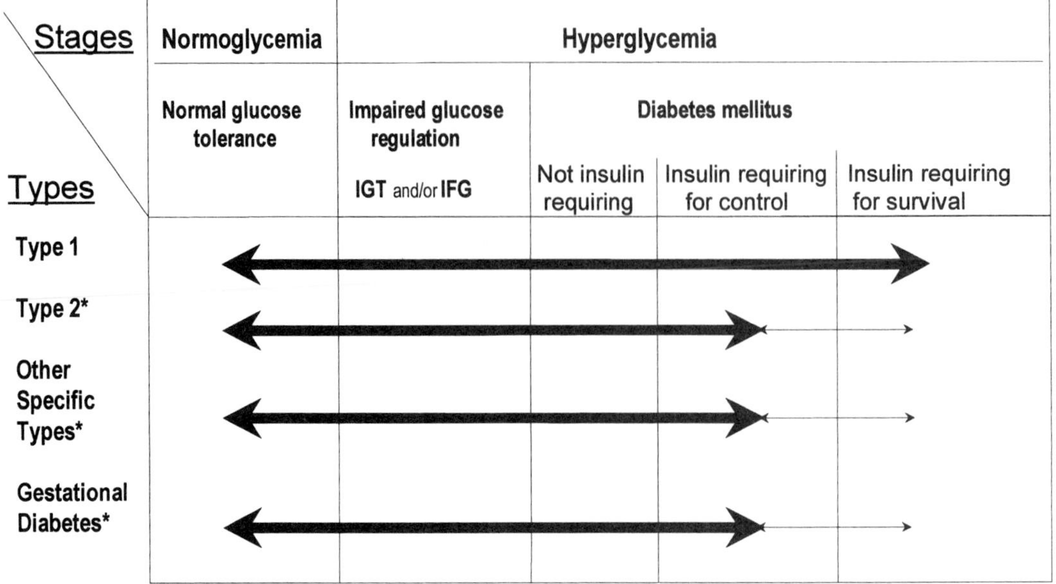

Figure 19.1. Clinical stages and etiologic types of diabetes.

(WHO) in 1999 (4) and that supersedes the previously internationally recognized 1985 WHO classification (5), now classifies diabetes according to both clinical stages and etiologic types (Fig. 19.1). The clinical staging reflects that diabetes progresses through several stages during its natural history and that individual subjects may move from one stage to another in either direction.

CLINICAL STAGES

Individuals who ultimately develop diabetes pass through several clinical stages during its development. Initially, glucose regulation is normal and no abnormality of glycemia can be identified even if these individuals undergo an oral glucose tolerance test (OGTT). This stage is followed by a period of variable duration in which glucose regulation is impaired. They may have some abnormality of the fasting glucose concentration, or if they receive an OGTT, they may demonstrate impaired glucose tolerance. Diabetes itself is characterized by either fasting glycemia or marked abnormalities of glucose tolerance, or both. Once diabetes develops, glycemia may be controlled by lifestyle changes such as diet and increased physical activity in some patients, whereas in others insulin or oral hypoglycemic agents are needed for its control or to prevent ketosis and ketoacidosis. If insulin is required to prevent ketosis, such patients are designated as "insulin requiring for survival." In all forms of diabetes, there may be remission in the extent of hyperglycemia. Patients may revert to having impaired glucose regulation or even normal glycemia, particularly if diabetes is of recent onset. This is seen most frequently in patients with recent-onset type 2 diabetes, in whom lifestyle intervention and/or early aggressive treatment of the glycemia may result in apparent reversal of the abnormality with reversion to impaired or normal glucose tolerance (6). This may also be seen in type 1 diabetes, in which after a short period of insulin treatment, there may be a variable period when insulin is no longer required for survival and glucose tolerance may improve—the so-called honeymoon period. Eventually such patients do need insulin treatment for survival (7). Gestational diabetes often is followed by improved glucose tolerance following parturition, and for a variable period, such women may be normoglycemic. With a subsequent pregnancy, gestational diabetes is likely to recur. Many women who have had gestational diabetes develop diabetes within a few years when they are not pregnant; thus, even in the face of normal glycemia, such women can be recognized as being at high risk of developing type 2 diabetes (8).

All subjects with diabetes can be classified according to clinical stage regardless of the underlying etiology of the diabetes. The stage of glycemia may change over time, depending on the extent of the underlying disease process. The disease process may be present but may not have progressed far enough to cause clinically identifiable abnormalities of glucose metabolism. For example, antibodies to islet cells, insulin, or glutamic acid decarboxylase (GAD) in a normoglycemic individual indicate a high likelihood for ultimate progression to type 1 diabetes (9). There are few sensitive or specific early indicators of the likelihood for development of type 2 diabetes, but the disease process may be identified before the development of overt diabetes.

Impaired glucose regulation refers to the metabolic stage intermediate between normal glucose homeostasis and diabetes that can be identified by impaired glucose tolerance (IGT) or impaired fasting glucose (glycemia) (IFG) (3,4). IFG and IGT are not synonymous and may represent different abnormalities of glucose regulation, although they may occur together. Individuals with either of these states of impaired glucose regulation have a high risk of progressing to diabetes (10–12). IGT can be assessed only if OGTTs are carried out, whereas IFG refers to fasting glucose concentrations that are lower than those required for the diagnosis of diabetes but higher than those usually found in subjects with normal glucose tolerance. Subjects with IGT or IFG usually have normal or slightly elevated levels of glycosylated hemoglobin (13). IGT is frequently associated with the

TABLE 19.1. Etiologic Classification of Disorders of Glycemia

Type 1 (β-cell destruction, usually leading to absolute insulin deficiency)
- A. Autoimmune
- B. Idiopathic

Type 2 (may range from predominantly insulin resistance with relative insulin deficiency to a predominantly secretory defect with or without insulin resistance)

Other specific types (see Table 19.2)
- Genetic defects of β-cell function
- Genetic defects in insulin action
- Diseases of the exocrine pancreas
- Endocrinopathies
- Drug- or chemical-induced
- Infections
- Uncommon forms of immune-mediated diabetes
- Other genetic syndromes sometimes associated with diabetes

Gestational diabetes

presence of other indicators of the metabolic or insulin resistance syndrome (14).

ETIOLOGIC TYPES

The etiologic classification of diabetes mellitus currently recommended by WHO and the ADA is presented in Table 19.1. This classification differs considerably from the previously recommended classification, which used the terms *insulin-dependent diabetes* and *non–insulin-dependent diabetes* (5). These terms, however, were frequently misused and at best classified patients based on treatment needs rather than on etiologic characteristics. The terms *type 1* and *type 2* diabetes (with Arabic numerals) have been adopted for the most common forms of diabetes mellitus.

TYPE 1 DIABETES MELLITUS

Type 1 diabetes is the form of the disease due primarily to β-cell destruction. This usually leads to a type of diabetes in which insulin is required for survival. Individuals with type 1 diabetes are metabolically normal before the disease is clinically manifest, but the process of β-cell destruction can be detected earlier by the presence of certain autoantibodies. Type 1 diabetes usually is characterized by the presence of anti-GAD, anti–islet cell, or anti-insulin antibodies, which reflects the autoimmune processes that have led to β-cell destruction. Individuals who have one of more of these antibodies can be subclassified as having type 1A, immune-mediated type 1 diabetes (3,4).

Particularly in nonwhites, type 1 diabetes can occur in the absence of autoimmune antibodies and without evidence of any autoimmune disorder. In this form of type 1 diabetes, the natural history also is one of progressive disease with marked hyperglycemia resulting in an insulin requirement for prevention of ketosis and survival. Such individuals are classified as having type 1B, or idiopathic, diabetes (15).

Type 1A diabetes shows strong associations with specific haplotypes or alleles at the DQ-A and DQ-B loci of the human leukocyte antigen (HLA) complex (16). The rate of β-cell destruction is quite variable, being rapid in some individuals, especially in infants and children, and slower in adults. Some have modest fasting hyperglycemia that can rapidly change to severe hyperglycemia or ketoacidosis, and others, particularly adults, may retain some residual β-cell function for many years and have sometimes been termed as having "latent autoimmune diabetes" (17,18). Such individuals may become dependent on insulin for survival only many years after the detection of diabetes. Individuals with type 1 diabetes have low or undetectable levels of insulin and plasma C-peptide. Patients with type 1A diabetes are also more likely to have other concomitant autoimmune disorders, such as Graves disease, Hashimoto thyroiditis, Addison disease, vitiligo, or pernicious anemia.

Type 1B, or idiopathic, diabetes is characterized by low insulin and C-peptide levels similar to those in type 1A. Such patients are prone to ketoacidosis, although they have no clinical evidence of autoimmune antibodies. Many of these patients are of African or Asian origin. They may suffer from episodic ketoacidosis, but the pathogenetic basis for their insulinopenia remains obscure.

TYPE 2 DIABETES MELLITUS

Type 2 diabetes is the most common form of diabetes. It is characterized by disorders of insulin action and insulin secretion, either of which may be the predominant feature. Usually, both are present at the time diabetes becomes clinically manifest. Although the specific etiology of this form of diabetes is not known, autoimmune destruction of the β-cells does not occur.

Patients with type 2 diabetes usually have insulin resistance and relative, rather than absolute, insulin deficiency. At the time of diagnosis of diabetes, and often throughout their lifetimes, these patients do not need insulin treatment to survive, although ultimately many require it for glycemic control. This form of diabetes is associated with progressive β-cell failure with increasing duration of diabetes (19). Ketoacidosis seldom occurs spontaneously but can arise with stress associated with another illness such as infection.

Most patients with type 2 diabetes are obese when they develop diabetes, and obesity aggravates the insulin resistance. Type 2 diabetes frequently goes undiagnosed for many years because the hyperglycemia develops gradually and in the earlier stages is not severe enough to produce the classic symptoms of diabetes; however, such patients are at increased risk of developing macrovascular and microvascular complications. Their circulating insulin levels may be normal or elevated yet insufficient to control blood glucose levels within the normal range because of their insulin resistance. Thus, they have relative, rather than absolute, insulinopenia. Insulin resistance may improve with weight reduction or pharmacologic treatment and results in normalization of their glycemia. Type 2 diabetes is seen frequently in women who have a previous history of gestational diabetes and in individuals with other characteristics of the insulin resistance syndrome, such as hypertension or dyslipidemia.

Patients who are not obese and who have relatives with type 1 diabetes, especially those of European origin, may present with a clinical picture consistent with type 2 diabetes but may have autoantibodies similar to those found in type 1 diabetes. Such patients have type 1A diabetes yet may appear to have type 2 diabetes unless antibody determinations are made.

The risk of developing type 2 diabetes increases with age, obesity, and physical inactivity. Type 2 diabetes shows strong familial aggregation, so that persons with a parent or sibling with the disease are at increased risk, as are individuals with obesity, hypertension, or dyslipidemia and women with a history of gestational diabetes. The frequency of type 2 diabetes varies considerably among different racial or ethnic subgroups. Persons of Native American, Polynesian or Micronesian, Asian-Indian,

Hispanic, or African-American descent are at higher risk than persons of European origin (20). Although the disease is most commonly seen in adults, the age of onset tends to be earlier in persons of non-European origin. The disease can occur at any age and is now seen in children and adolescents (21–24).

OTHER SPECIFIC TYPES OF DIABETES

Other specific types of diabetes are those in which the underlying defect or disease process can be identified in a relatively specific way or those that have other distinctive, distinguishing features. This category encompasses a variety of types of diabetes secondary to other specific conditions or associated with particular diseases or syndromes with a distinct etiology.

The categories and many of the causes of other specific types of diabetes are shown in Table 19.2. These include genetic defects of β-cell function, which encompass several types of diabetes that are associated with specific monogenic defects. Most of these are characterized by a dominant pattern of inheritance and the onset of hyperglycemia at an early age. They are often referred to as maturity-onset diabetes of the young (MODY). They are characterized by impaired insulin secretion with minimal or no defects in insulin action. They are inherited in an autosomal dominant pattern but are heterogeneous. A number of specific genetic defects have been identified, including variations in hepatic nuclear factor 4α (HNF4α) (MODY1), glucokinase (MODY2), HNF1α (MODY3), insulin-promoting factor 1 (IPF1) (MODY4), and HNF3β genes (MODY5) (2). There are also some forms of MODY for which the genetic defect remains to be identified. Another form of autosomal dominant diabetes is due to a mutation in the K_{ATP} channel subunit (SUR1) of the sulfonylurea receptor that gives rise to congenital hyperinsulimemia and loss of insulin secretory capacity in young adults, leading to impairment of glucose tolerance and diabetes in middle age (25).

Another genetic defect of β-cell function is due to a mutation in mitochondrial DNA. The mitochondrial DNA variant, Leu-Ala at position 3243, leads to diabetes mellitus associated with deafness (26). Because this form of diabetes is due to a mitochondrial defect, it may be suspected when there is evidence of maternal inheritance, particularly when associated with deafness. The same mitochondrial variant also is found in the MELAS syndrome (mitochondrial myopathy, encephalopathy, lactic acidosis, and stroke-like syndrome), although diabetes is not part of this syndrome (27).

Some forms of diabetes are associated with rare autosomal dominantly inherited genetic defects of insulin or insulin action (28). In one form affected individuals are unable to convert proinsulin to insulin. In general the glucose intolerance is mild. Structurally abnormal insulins, from specific mutations in the insulin gene, with resultant impaired receptor binding, have been identified in a few families. Affected individuals may have either mildly impaired or even normal glucose

TABLE 19.2. Other Specific Types of Diabetes Mellitus

Genetic defects of β-cell function	**Diseases of the exocrine pancreas**
Chromosome 20, HNF4α (MODY1)	Fibrocalculous pancreatopathy
Chromosome 7, glucokinase (MODY2)	Pancreatitis
Chromosome 12, HNF1α (MODY3)	Trauma/pancreatectomy
Chromosome 13, IPF1 (MODY4)	Neoplasia
Chromosome 17, HNF3β (MODY5)	Cystic fibrosis
Mitochondrial DNA, A3243G mutation	Hemochromatosis
Others	Wolcott-Rallison syndrome
Genetic defects in insulin action	Others
Type A insulin resistance	**Endocrinopathies**
Leprechaunism	Cushing syndrome
Rabson-Mendenhall syndrome	Acromegaly
Lipoatrophic diabetes	Pheochromocytoma
Others	Glucagonoma
Other genetic syndromes sometimes associated with diabetes	Hyperthyroidism
	Somatostatinoma
Down syndrome	Others
Friedreich ataxia	**Drug- or chemical-induced**
Huntington disease	Nicotinic acid
Klinefelter syndrome	Glucocorticoids
Laurence-Moon-Biedl syndrome	Thyroid hormone
Myotonic dystrophy	α-adrenergic agonists
Porphyria	β-adrenergic agonists
Prader-Willi syndrome	Thiazides
Turner syndrome	Phenytoin
Wolfram syndrome	Pentamidine
Others	Pyriminil (Vacor)
Uncommon forms of immune-mediated diabetes	Interferon-α
Insulin autoimmune syndrome (antibodies to insulin)	Others
	Infections
Anti–insulin receptor antibodies	Congenital rubella
"Stiff-man" syndrome	Cytomegalovirus
Others	Others

HNF4α, hepatic nuclear factor 4α; MODY, maturity-onset diabetes of the young; HNF1α, hepatic nuclear factor 1α; IPF1, insulin-promoting factor 1; HNF3β, hepatic nuclear factor 3β.

metabolism but have high circulating levels of insulin or C-peptide. A number of specific mutations of the insulin receptor gene have been identified that also result in impaired insulin action (29). Although these are rare causes of diabetes, they should be considered if circulating insulin levels are exceptionally high and if there are other clinical characteristics of insulin resistance syndromes such as acanthosis nigricans, ovarian dysfunction, hyperandrogenism, lipodystrophy, or extreme hypertriglyceridemia. The possibility of diabetes due to antibodies in the insulin receptor should be entertained if other autoimmune diseases such as systemic lupus erythematosus, Sjögren syndrome, or ataxia-telangiectasia are present. Defects of insulin action with a genetic basis are present in leprechaunism, the Rabson-Mendenhall syndrome, and lipoatrophic diabetes.

Diabetes mellitus may be secondary to a variety of diseases of the exocrine pancreas. Fibrocalculous pancreatopathy, which was considered one of the subtypes of "malnutrition-related" diabetes in the 1985 WHO classification, is now placed in that category. Diabetes may also result from pancreatitis, pancreatectomy, neoplastic disease of the pancreas, cystic fibrosis, and hemochromatosis. One specific form of exocrine pancreatic deficiency associated with a genetic abnormality of the PEK gene is the rare Wolcott-Rallison syndrome, which is associated with early-onset diabetes and multiple epiphyseal dysplasia (30).

Diabetes mellitus may result from several endocrinopathies. It may occur in association with Cushing syndrome, acromegaly, pheochromocytoma, glucagonoma, hyperthyroidism, and somatostatinoma.

A variety of drugs or chemicals have been associated with the development of diabetes. These include glucocorticoids, nicotinic acid, diazoxide, phenytoin, and pentamidine. When diabetes is associated with such agents, it is often uncertain whether or not the drug has been the direct cause of the diabetes or the diabetes has appeared coincidentally in association with administration of the drug (31).

A few specific infections may result in diabetes mellitus, including congenital rubella and cytomegalovirus infections (32). There are also a number of other relatively rare genetic syndromes sometimes associated with diabetes.

GESTATIONAL DIABETES MELLITUS

Gestational diabetes mellitus (GDM) is carbohydrate intolerance associated with hyperglycemia of variable severity with the onset or first recognition during pregnancy (3,4). It does not exclude the possibility that unrecognized glucose intolerance or diabetes may have antedated pregnancy. Women who become pregnant who are known to have diabetes that antedates pregnancy, however, do not have GDM.

In early pregnancy, fasting and postprandial glucose concentrations are normally lower than in nonpregnant women. Any elevation of fasting or postprandial glucose levels at this time may well reflect the presence of diabetes that antedates pregnancy, but specific criteria for designating abnormality at this time of pregnancy have not been established. Furthermore, normal glucose levels in early pregnancy do not establish that GDM will not develop later.

Individuals with a high risk of GDM include older women, those with a previous history of glucose intolerance, those with a history of babies large for gestational age, women from certain ethnic groups at high risk for type 2 diabetes, and any pregnant woman who has any elevation of fasting or casual blood glucose levels.

Gestational diabetes can have deleterious consequences for both the fetus and mother. Diabetes occurring before or recognized during pregnancy with elevated fasting glucose concentrations is associated with an increased risk of intrauterine fetal death during the last 4 to 8 weeks of gestation and other complications, including congenital abnormalities (33). GDM without severe fasting hyperglycemia has not been associated with increased perinatal mortality, but GDM of any severity increases the risk of fetal macrosomia (34). Neonatal hypoglycemia, jaundice, polycythemia, and hypocalcemia are other fetal complications of GDM. Offspring of women with GDM or with type 2 diabetes preceding pregnancy are at increased risk of obesity, glucose intolerance, and diabetes in adolescence or as young adults (35).

Women with high-risk characteristics for diabetes, such as marked obesity, a previous history of GDM, glycosuria, or a strong family history of diabetes, should undergo glucose testing as soon as feasible during pregnancy. Screening pregnant women from high-risk populations during the first trimester of pregnancy is appropriate to detect previously undiagnosed diabetes or glucose intolerance. Women who have a fasting plasma glucose level of 126 mg/dL or greater or a casual plasma glucose level of 200 mg/dL or greater at any time during pregnancy meet the thresholds for the diagnosis of diabetes. If confirmed, such levels preclude the need for any glucose challenge to establish the diagnosis of diabetes. Formal systematic testing for GDM usually is performed between 24 and 28 weeks of gestation.

Women with any of the following characteristics should receive formal testing for GDM between 24 and 28 weeks of gestation: those aged 25 and older, overweight women, women who are members of an ethnic group with a high prevalence of diabetes, women with first-degree relatives with diabetes, women with a history of abnormal glucose tolerance, or women with a poor obstetrical history (36). Following delivery, women who have GDM should be reclassified. Some women with GDM will have diabetes or impaired glucose regulation following parturition, but in the majority, glucose regulation will return to normal after delivery. Such women, however, carry a high risk of progressing to diabetes in subsequent years (8,37).

IMPAIRED GLUCOSE TOLERANCE

IGT is a stage of impaired glucose regulation that is present in individuals whose glucose tolerance is above the conventional normal range but lower than the level considered diagnostic of diabetes (3,4). IGT cannot be defined on the basis of fasting glucose concentrations; an OGTT is needed to categorize such individuals. Persons with IGT do have a high risk of developing diabetes, although not all do so (38). Some revert to normal glucose tolerance, and others continue to have IGT for many years. Persons with IGT have a greater risk than persons of similar age with normal glucose tolerance of developing arterial disease (39), but they rarely develop the more specific microvascular complications of diabetes, such as retinopathy or nephropathy, unless they develop diabetes (3,40).

IGT is more frequent in obese than in nonobese persons and often is associated with hyperinsulinemia and insulin resistance. IGT may be attributable to a wide variety of causes, including certain medications and many of the specific genetic syndromes or other conditions associated with diabetes (see Table 19.2). Nonetheless, in most subjects, IGT represents a transient stage between normal glucose tolerance and the development of type 2 diabetes.

Because persons with IGT have a high risk of progressing to type 2 diabetes, several randomized clinical trials have been conducted among such individuals. These trials have shown that the development of diabetes can be reduced or delayed by the use of lifestyle interventions such as dietary measures to reduce weight and increased physical activity (41–43). Several drugs, such as metformin (43), acarbose (44), and troglitazone (45), also reduce the incidence of type 2 diabetes in persons with IGT.

IMPAIRED FASTING GLUCOSE

IFG is also a stage of impaired glucose homeostasis. This category was introduced in the 1997 ADA and 1999 WHO classifications to include individuals whose fasting glucose levels were above normal but below those diagnostic for diabetes (3,4).

Individuals with fasting plasma glucose concentrations of 100 to 125 mg/dL (5.6 to <7.0 mmol/L) are now considered to have IFG (46). If an OGTT is performed, some of these individuals will have IGT and some may have diabetes (2 hours postload plasma glucose concentration ≥ 200 mg/dL, or ≥ 11.1 mmol/L) (Table 19.3). Consequently, it is prudent, and recommended by WHO, that such individuals, if possible, have an OGTT to exclude diabetes.

The category of IFG was introduced by the ADA in 1997 at the same time that the concentration of fasting plasma glucose for the diagnosis of diabetes was lowered to 126 mg/dL or greater (≥7.0 mmol/L). The range of fasting glucose concentrations for IFG was set originally at 110 to 125 mg/dL (6.1 to < 7.0 mmol) but was revised in 2003 to 100 to 125 mg/dL (5.6 to < 7.0 mmol/L). IFG and IGT identify substantially different subsets of the population (47). Although both categories contain individuals with a high risk of progressing to type 2 diabetes (10–12,48), the proportion with IFG in most populations is smaller than that with IGT (47,48). The modified cut-point recommended in the 2003 ADA report (46) is likely to be adopted by the WHO in the near future.

DIAGNOSTIC CRITERIA FOR DIABETES AND RELATED STAGES OF IMPAIRED GLUCOSE HOMEOSTASIS

If a patient has symptoms such as thirst, polyuria, unexplained weight loss, drowsiness or coma, and marked glucosuria, the diagnosis of diabetes can be established by demonstrating fasting hyperglycemia (3,4). If the fasting glucose concentration is in the diagnostic range for diabetes, an OGTT is not required for diagnosis. A confirmatory test should be performed because a diagnosis of diabetes carries considerable and lifelong consequences for the patient, and intraindividual variation or incomplete fasting may result in a spurious diagnosis. On the other hand, if the patient is asymptomatic or has only minimal symptoms and fasting blood or plasma concentrations are not diagnostic, an OGTT is required to confirm or exclude the diagnosis of diabetes (Table 19.4).

Normal glucose tolerance cannot be established on the basis of a fasting glucose determination alone. In healthy subjects, fasting glucose levels are less than 100 mg/dL (<5.5 mmol/L) in venous or capillary plasma and 90 mg/dL or less (≤ 5.0 mmol/L) in whole blood, but subjects with fasting levels below these limits may exhibit IGT (4). Subjects with fasting glucose levels above those characteristic for healthy subjects but below those diagnostic of diabetes also have a high likelihood of having either diabetes or IGT. Such levels represent a primary indication for an OGTT to confirm or exclude the diagnosis of diabetes or IGT.

ORAL GLUCOSE TOLERANCE TEST

The OGTT should be administered in the morning after the patient has had at least 3 days of unrestricted diet (>150 g of carbohydrate daily) and usual physical activity. The test should be preceded by an overnight fast of 10 to 16 hours, during which the patient may drink water. The patient may not smoke during the test. Factors that may influence interpretation of the results of the test should be recorded (e.g., medications, inactivity,

TABLE 19.3. Diagnostic Criteria for Diabetes Mellitus and Related Stages of Glycemia[a]

	Glucose concentration, mg/dL (mmol/L)	
	Capillary whole blood[b]	Venous plasma
Diabetes mellitus		
Fasting	≥110 (≥6.1)	≥126 (≥7.0)
or		
2-hour postglucose	≥200 (≥11.1)	≥200 (≥11.1)
Impaired glucose tolerance		
Fasting (if measured)	<110 (<6.1)	<126 (<7.0)
and		
2-hour postglucose	140–199 (7.8–11.0)	140–199 (7.8–11.0)
Impaired fasting glycemia		
Fasting	NA[c]	100–125 (5.6–6.9)[c]
and (if measured)		
2-hour postglucose	<140 (<7.8)[d] <200 (<11.1)[e]	<140 (<7.8)[d] <200 (<11.1)[e]

NA, not applicable.
[a]The 2-hour postglucose values are those measured after a 75-g oral glucose load.
[b]If glucose concentrations are measured on *venous whole blood*, the cut-off levels for postload values are different (4).
[c]According to 2003 ADA recommendations (46). No equivalent capillary whole blood values proposed.
[d]According to 1999 WHO recommendations (4).
[e]According to 1997 ADA recommendations (3).

TABLE 19.4. Categories of Hyperglycemia According to Venous Plasma Glucose Concentrations

	Fasting plasma glucose level			
	Normal[a]	Impaired[a]	Diabetes	
2-Hour postload plasma glucose level	<100 mg/dL (<5.5 mmol/L)	100–125 mg/dL (5.6–6.9 mol/L)	≥126 mg/dL (≥7.0 mmol/L)	Not done
<140 mg/dL (<7.8 mmol/L)	Normal[b]	IFG	Diabetes	"Normal"
140–199 mg/dL (7.8–11.0 mmol/L)	IGT[b]	IFG/IGT[c]	Diabetes	IGT
≥200 mg/dL (≥11.1 mmol/L)	Diabetes[b]	Diabetes[b]	Diabetes	Diabetes
Not done	"Normal"	IFG	Diabetes	Unknown

IFG, impaired fasting glucose; IGT, impaired glucose tolerance.
[a]The 1997 American Diabetes Association (ADA) and 1999 World Health Organization (WHO) recommendations for fasting plasma glucose values were as follows: normal, <110 mg/dL (6.1 mmol/L); impaired, 110–125 mg/dL (6.1–6.9 mmol/L). The values listed in the table reflect the most recent 2003 ADA Expert Committee recommendations (46).
[b]These categories are identifiable only if an oral glucose tolerance test is performed.
[c]This category is currently classified by the ADA recommendations as IFG and IGT and by the WHO as IGT. Because these subjects have approximately twice the risk of developing diabetes as those with IFG only or IGT only, it is preferable to state that they have both IFG and IGT.

infection). Such factors should be taken into account in interpreting the results of the test.

After the fasting blood sample is collected, the subject should drink 75 g of anhydrous glucose (or partial hydrolysates of starch with an equivalent carbohydrate content) in 150 to 300 mL of water over the course of 5 minutes. For children, the glucose load should be 1.75 g/kg of body weight, up to a total of 75 g of glucose. Blood samples are drawn before (fasting) and 2 hours after the test load.

Unless the glucose concentration is determined immediately, the blood sample should be collected in a tube containing sodium fluoride (6 mg/mL of whole blood) and centrifuged promptly to separate out the plasma. The plasma should be frozen until the glucose measurement is done.

The results of the OGTT should be interpreted according to the criteria given in Table 19.3 or Table 19.4. It is important to note that the diagnostic levels differ according to whether capillary or venous blood is collected and whether the glucose concentrations are reported as plasma or whole blood glucose concentrations.

DIAGNOSTIC CRITERIA FOR GESTATIONAL DIABETES

Testing for GDM is performed between the 24th and 28th week of pregnancy in women who are not known to have diabetes. Evaluation of GDM is done by one of two approaches. An OGTT may be performed using a 75-g oral glucose load, as is done in the nonpregnant state. An alternative method, widely used in the United States, is to screen in two stages, initially measuring plasma glucose concentrations 1 hour after a 50-g oral glucose load. For women whose venous plasma glucose values are 140 mg/dL or higher, either a 100-g or a 75-g OGTT is then performed on a subsequent day. Because of the widespread use of the 100-g OGTT among obstetricians in the United States, diagnostic values for GDM with either the 100-g or the 75-g oral glucose load have been recommended by the ADA (36) (Table 19.5). WHO recommends a single standard 75-g OGTT after an overnight fast, giving an oral load of 75 g of anhydrous glucose in 250 to 300 mL of water, with measurement of plasma glucose levels fasting and after 2 hours (4).

TABLE 19.5. Diagnostic Criteria (Venous Plasma Glucose Values) for Gestational Diabetes Mellitus According to ADA Clinical Practice and WHO Recommendations

	ADA clinical practice[a](36)		WHO(4)
	75-g Oral glucose load, mg/dL (mmol/L)	100-g Oral glucose load, mg/dL (mmol/L)	75-g Oral glucose load, mg/dL (mmol/L)
Fasting	95 (5.3)	95 (5.3)	≥126 (≥7.0)
1 Hour	180 (10.0)	180 (10.0)	or
2 Hour	155 (8.6)	155 (8.6)	
3 Hour	NA	140 (7.8)	≥140 (≥7.8)

ADA, American Diabetes Association; WHO, World Health Organization; NA, not applicable.
[a]Two or more of the venous plasma concentrations must be met or exceeded for a positive diagnosis. The test should be done in the morning after an overnight fast between 8 and 14 hours and after at least 3 days of unrestricted diet (≥150 g carbohydrate per day) and unlimited physical activity. The subject should remain seated and should not smoke throughout the test.

These tests identify different women as having high-risk pregnancies and different risks of adverse fetal outcome (49,50).

Use of the 75-g test has gained wide acceptance in many parts of the world, but less so in the United States. The WHO recommendation is that women with 2-hour venous plasma values of 140 mg/dL or higher (≥7.8 mmol/L), or fasting venous plasma values of 126 mg/dL or higher (≥7.0 mmol/L), or equivalent values if glucose is measured in whole blood, be considered to have GDM (Table 19.5).

THE IMPACT OF RECENT CHANGES IN CLASSIFICATION AND DIAGNOSTIC CRITERIA

As noted earlier, the currently recommended classification and criteria for diabetes differ from those recommended in earlier years (5). The major changes in classification have been to move toward an etiologically based classification because of increasing knowledge about some of the specific underlying causes of diabetes. This trend is likely to continue.

The terms *insulin-dependent* and *non–insulin-dependent* diabetes no longer appear in the classification. These terms were often misused, frequently reflecting the type of treatment that the patients were receiving rather than their actual type of diabetes. In addition, there is now greater certainty that type 1 diabetes is due primarily to pancreatic β-cell destruction, and this frequently can be documented by the presence of specific types of antibodies, as well as insulinopenia. The class of malnutrition-related diabetes is no longer recognized, as this was heterogenous, and one of its forms, fibrocalculous pancreatic diabetes, is clearly secondary to a specific form of pancreatic disease (4). The other form of diabetes formerly described as "malnutrition related" is now generally considered to be type 2 diabetes that occurs in malnourished persons.

Knowledge of specific forms of diabetes attributable to mutations in specific genes has expanded enormously, and such cases can now be classified very specifically if they are investigated in detail. Importantly, this information has led to circumstances in which susceptibility to the development of some types of diabetes can be identified before hyperglycemia is evident.

The introduction of clinical staging has been prompted by the recognition that all forms of diabetes pass through a number of stages associated with different degrees of metabolic dysfunction. Furthermore, it now has been established that progression from normal glucose tolerance to overt diabetes can be halted or delayed and that reversion to less severe states of dysglycemia is possible. On the other hand, hyperglycemia may be present, but specific information or knowledge enabling precise etiologic classification may not be available for many patients. Such individuals can be classified according to clinical stage in the absence of specific knowledge of causation.

The clinical stage of IFG has been introduced in the most recent classifications. This category was introduced because fasting blood or plasma glucose measurements represent the most common means used to screen or test for diabetes in clinical practice. Fasting glucose values considered diagnostic of diabetes have been lowered to be more equivalent to those found when the 2-hour plasma value after an oral glucose load is 200 mg/dL or greater (≥11.1 mmol/L) (3). This change increases the likelihood of a correct diagnosis of diabetes when only a fasting glucose concentration is determined, but the fasting level diagnostic of diabetes is well beyond the normal range in persons with normal glucose tolerance. Consequently, the stage of IFG was defined to accommodate and recognize individuals whose fasting glucose levels were above normal yet not diagnostic of diabetes.

Application of these revised criteria has shown that only a minority of persons with IGT have IFG, and vice versa. Yet persons with IFG only or IGT only are at considerable risk for the development of diabetes. In addition, there is some evidence that IFG is more likely than IGT to be associated with a reduction in insulin secretion, whereas IGT is associated with insulin resistance (48). This suggests that different mechanisms may be responsible for these two states. Whether or not these differences will ultimately have different implications for management and intervention to prevent progression to diabetes remains to be determined.

CONCLUSION

The recent classification system for diabetes and related states of hyperglycemia has focused on etiopathogenesis whenever possible. Although the underlying causes of the more common forms of diabetes are still unknown, their characteristics are sufficiently distinct for classification to be made with reasonable certainty in most instances. This, along with defined clinical stages, provides a clinically useful framework that can be modified as more precise information on the specific etiology of certain forms of diabetes becomes known. The classification and staging also provide a framework for further research into the etiology, treatment, and prevention of the many forms of diabetes.

REFERENCES

1. Rewers M, Norris JM, Eisenbarth GS, et al. Beta-cell autoantibodies in infants and toddlers without IDDM relatives: Diabetes Autoimmunity Study in the Young (DAISY). *J Autoimmun* 1996;9:405–410.
2. Almind K, Doria A, Kahn CR. Putting the genes for type II diabetes on the map. *Nat Med* 2001;7:277–279.
3. Gavin JR III, Alberti KGMM, Davidson MB, et al. Report of the Expert Committee on the Diagnosis and Classification of Diabetes Mellitus. *Diabetes Care* 1997;20:1183–1197.
4. WHO Consultation Group. *Definition, diagnosis and classification of diabetes mellitus and its complications*, 2nd ed. Part 1: Diagnosis and classification of diabetes mellitus WHO/NCD/NCS/99. Geneva: World Health Organisation, 1999:1–59.
5. WHO Study Group. *Diabetes mellitus*. Technical Report Series 727. Geneva: World Health Organization, 1985.
6. Savage PJ, Bennion LJ, Bennett PH. Normalization of insulin and glucagon secretion in ketosis-resistant diabetes mellitus with prolonged diet therapy. *J Clin Endocrinol Metab* 1979;49:830–833.
7. Agner T, Damm P, Binder C. Remission in IDDM: prospective study of basal C-peptide and insulin dose in 268 consecutive patients. *Diabetes Care* 1987;10:164–169.
8. O'Sullivan JB. Diabetes mellitus after GDM. *Diabetes* 1991;40[Suppl 2]: 131–135.
9. Bingley PJ, Christie MR, Bonifacio E, et al. Combined analysis of autoantibodies improves prediction of IDDM in islet cell antibody-positive relatives. *Diabetes* 1994;43:1304–1310.
10. Gabir MM, Hanson RL, Dabelea D, et al. The 1997 American Diabetes Association and 1999 World Health Organization criteria for hyperglycemia in the diagnosis and prediction of diabetes. *Diabetes Care* 2000;23:1108–1112.
11. Shaw JE, Zimmet PZ, de Courten M, et al. Impaired fasting glucose or impaired glucose tolerance. What best predicts future diabetes in Mauritius? *Diabetes Care* 1999;22:399–402.
12. de Vegt F, Dekker JM, Jager A, et al. Relation of impaired fasting and postload glucose with incident type 2 diabetes in a Dutch population: The Hoorn Study. *JAMA* 2001;285:2109–2113.
13. Harris MI, Flegal KM, Cowie CC, et al. Prevalence of diabetes, impaired fasting glucose, and impaired glucose tolerance in U.S. adults. The Third National Health and Nutrition Examination Survey, 1988–1994. *Diabetes Care* 1998;21: 518–524.
14. DeFronzo RA, Ferrannini E. Insulin resistance: a multifaceted syndrome responsible for NIDDM, obesity, hypertension, dyslipidemia and atherosclerotic cardiovascular disease. *Diabetes Care* 1991;14:173–194.
15. Tanaka S, Kobayashi T, Momotsu T. A novel subtype of type 1 diabetes mellitus. *N Engl J Med* 2000;342:1835–1837.

16. Greenbaum CJ, Cuthbertson D, Eisenbarth GS, et al. Islet cell antibody positive relatives with HLA-DQA1*0102, DQB1*0602: identification by the Diabetes Prevention Trial-1. *J Clin Endocrinol Metab* 2000;85:1255–1260.
17. Zimmet PZ, Tuomi T, Mackay IR, et al. Latent autoimmune diabetes mellitus in adults (LADA): the role of antibodies to glutamic acid decarboxylase in diagnosis and prediction of insulin dependency. *Diabet Med* 1994;11: 299–303.
18. Groop LC, Bottazzo GF, Doniach D. Islet cell antibodies identify latent type 1 diabetes in patients aged 35–75 years at diagnosis. *Diabetes* 1986;35: 237–241.
19. Turner RC, Cull CA, Frighi V, et al. Glycemic control with diet, sulfonylurea, metformin, or insulin in patients with type 2 diabetes mellitus: progressive requirement for multiple therapies (UKPDS 49). UK Prospective Diabetes Study (UKPDS) Group. *JAMA* 1999;281:2005–2012.
20. King H, Rewers M. Global estimates for prevalence of diabetes mellitus and impaired glucose tolerance in adults. WHO Ad Hoc Diabetes Reporting Group. *Diabetes Care* 1993;16:157–177.
21. Fagot-Campagna A, Pettitt DJ, Engelgau MM, et al. Type 2 diabetes among North American children and adolescents: an epidemiologic review and a public health perspective. *J Pediatr* 2000;136:664–672.
22. Dabelea D, Pettitt DJ, Jones KL, et al. Type 2 diabetes mellitus in minority children and adolescents. An emerging problem. *Endocrinol Metab Clin North Am* 1999;28:709–729.
23. Dabelea D, Hanson RL, Bennett PH, et al. Increasing prevalence of type II diabetes in American Indian children. *Diabetologia* 1998;41:904–910.
24. Kaufman FR. Type 2 diabetes mellitus in children and youth: a new epidemic. *J Pediatr Endocrinol Metab* 2002;15[Suppl 2]:737–744.
25. Huopio H, Otonkoski T, Vauhkonen I, et al. A new subtype of autosomal dominant diabetes attributable to a mutation in the gene for sulfonylurea receptor 1. *Lancet* 2003;361:301–307.
26. Maassen JA. Mitochondrial diabetes: pathophysiology, clinical presentation, and genetic analysis. *Am J Med Genet* 2002;115:66–70.
27. Moraes CT, Ricci E, Bonilla E, et al. The mitochondrial tRNA(Leu(UUR)) mutation in mitochondrial encephalomyopathy, lactic acidosis, and strokelike episodes (MELAS): genetic, biochemical, and morphological correlations in skeletal muscle. *Am J Hum Genet* 1992;50:934–949.
28. Steiner DF, Tager HS, Chan SJ, et al. Lessons learned from molecular biology of insulin-gene mutations. *Diabetes Care* 1990;13:600–609.
29. Taylor SI. Lilly Lecture: molecular mechanisms of insulin resistance. Lessons from patients with mutations in the insulin-receptor gene. *Diabetes* 1992;41:1473–1490.
30. Stoss H, Pesch HJ, Pontz B, et al. Wolcott-Rallison syndrome: diabetes mellitus and spondyloepiphyseal dysplasia. *Eur J Pediatr* 1982;138:120–129.
31. Ferner RE. Drug-induced diabetes. *Baillieres Clin Endocrinol Metab* 1992; 6:849–866.
32. Jaeckel E, Manns M, Von Herrath M. Viruses and diabetes. *Ann N Y Acad Sci* 2002;958:7–25.
33. Comess LJ, Bennett PH, Burch TA, et al. Congenital anomalies and diabetes in the Pima Indians of Arizona. *Diabetes* 1969;18:471–477.
34. Pettitt DJ, Knowler WC, Baird HR, et al. Gestational diabetes: infant and maternal complications of pregnancy in relation to third-trimester glucose tolerance in the Pima Indians. *Diabetes Care* 1980;3:458–464.
35. Pettitt DJ, Baird HR, Aleck KA, et al. Excessive obesity in offspring of Pima Indian women with diabetes during pregnancy. *N Engl J Med* 1983;308: 242–245.
36. American Diabetes Association. Gestational diabetes mellitus. *Diabetes Care* 2004;27[Suppl 1]:S88–S90.
37. Kjos SL, Peters RK, Xiang A, et al. Predicting future diabetes in Latino women with gestational diabetes. Utility of early postpartum glucose tolerance testing. *Diabetes* 1995;44:586–591.
38. Edelstein SL, Knowler WC, Bain RP, et al. Predictors of progression from impaired glucose tolerance to NIDDM: an analysis of six prospective studies. *Diabetes* 1997;46:701–710.
39. The DECODE study group. Glucose tolerance and mortality: comparison of WHO and American Diabetes Association diagnostic criteria. European Diabetes Epidemiology Group. Diabetes epidemiology: collaborative analysis of diagnostic criteria in Europe. *Lancet* 1999;354:617–621.
40. Gabir MM, Hanson RL, Dabelea D, et al. Plasma glucose and prediction of microvascular disease and mortality: evaluation of 1997 American Diabetes Association and 1999 World Health Organization criteria for diagnosis of diabetes. *Diabetes Care* 2000;23:1113–1118.
41. Pan XR, Li GW, Hu YH, et al. Effects of diet and exercise in preventing NIDDM in people with impaired glucose tolerance. The Da Qing IGT and Diabetes Study. *Diabetes Care* 1997;20:537–544.
42. Tuomilehto J, Lindstrom J, Eriksson JG, et al. Prevention of type 2 diabetes mellitus by changes in lifestyle among subjects with impaired glucose tolerance. *N Engl J Med* 2001;344:1343–1350.
43. The Diabetes Prevention Program Research Group: reduction in the incidence of type 2 diabetes with lifestyle intervention or metformin. *N Engl J Med* 2002;346:393–403.
44. Chiasson JL, Josse RG, Gomis R, et al. Acarbose for prevention of type 2 diabetes mellitus: the STOP-NIDDM randomised trial. *Lancet* 2002;359:2072–2077.
45. Buchanan TA, Xiang AH, Peters RK, et al. Preservation of pancreatic beta-cell function and prevention of type 2 diabetes by pharmacological treatment of insulin resistance in high-risk hispanic women. *Diabetes* 2002;51:2796–2803.
46. Genuth S, Alberti KG, Bennett P, et al. Follow-up report on the diagnosis of diabetes mellitus. *Diabetes Care* 2003;26:3160–3167.
47. The DECODE study group. Age- and sex-specific prevalences of diabetes and impaired glucose regulation in 13 European cohorts. *Diabetes Care* 2003; 26:61–69.
48. Unwin N, Shaw J, Zimmet P, et al. Impaired glucose tolerance and impaired fasting glycaemia: the current status on definition and intervention. *Diabet Med* 2002;19:708–723.
49. Pettit DJ, Bennett PH, Hanson RL, et al. Comparison of World Health Organization and National Diabetes Data Group procedures to detect abnormalities of glucose tolerance during pregnancy. *Diabetes Care* 1994;17:1264–1268.
50. De Sereday MS, Damiano MM, Gonzalez CD, et al. Diagnostic criteria for gestational diabetes in relation to pregnancy outcome. *J Diabetes Complications* 2003;17:115–119.

CHAPTER 20
Epidemiology of Diabetes Mellitus

James H. Warram and Andrzej S. Krolewski

In this chapter, we will review the descriptive epidemiology of type 1 and type 2 diabetes mellitus and discuss its relevance to the etiology of the disease (1). However, it is first necessary to define some of the indices used to estimate diabetes frequency in populations (2).

SOME USEFUL DEFINITIONS

Prevalence, Incidence Rate, and Cumulative Incidence

The number of persons in a particular place at a particular time who have diabetes (e.g., in Massachusetts on July 1, 2001) is a frequently cited statistic. Expressed as a proportion, this number is commonly called the prevalence rate or, preferably, *prevalence,* so it is not confused with the incidence rate, which is defined below. The prevalence in Massachusetts is the accumulation of persons who acquired diabetes before July 1, 2001, but the size of this collection depends on not only the frequency of new cases but also on how long these persons remain alive to be counted. For example, a marked increase in the prevalence of insulin-dependent diabetes followed the discovery of insulin, although we have no evidence that the number of new cases that developed each year increased.

To express diabetes frequency in a manner suitable for drawing conclusions regarding etiology of the disease, we use the *incidence rate*. The incidence rate is calculated by dividing the number of *new* cases of diabetes in Massachusetts residents during the 12 months of 2001, for example, by the number of nondiabetic individuals residing in Massachusetts during that year. Typically, the incidence rate is expressed as the number of new cases per 100,000 persons observed for a year (called *person-years*).

When an incidence rate is calculated according to a characteristic such as age, sex, or race, the results are referred to as a *specific rate*. The age-specific incidence rate of diabetes varies enormously across the normal life span, and populations typically have different age distributions. Meaningful comparisons among populations must therefore be based on a particular age-specific rate or, for simplicity, on a summary of age-specific rates determined by a technique that gives each population the same age distribution (2). This produces age-adjusted or age-standardized rates. Alternatively, one can compare populations that have different age structures by calculating the *cumulative incidence* of diabetes at specific ages in each population.

Cumulative incidence or *cumulative risk* of diabetes is calculated from the age-specific incidence rate by use of life-table methods (2). One begins with an arbitrary number of births (e.g., 1,000 births) and applies the age-specific incidence rate to the number of persons who remain unaffected after each successive year of age. By accumulating the cases from previous ages, one obtains the proportion of the original 1,000 children born who would be affected by each successive age in a population. By extending this process to the whole life span, one obtains the lifetime risk of diabetes. In a specific instance, the prevalence of diabetes at a certain age may be a reasonable estimate of cumulative incidence at that age. For example, type 2 diabetes–related mortality before the age of 55 years is negligible. Therefore, the prevalence of type 2 diabetes in the age group 45 through 54 years is a reasonable estimate of the cumulative incidence at age 50 years. However, at older ages, prevalence typically underestimates cumulative incidence of diabetes because persons with early onset of the disease may have died.

DIFFERENCES IN DISTRIBUTION OF TYPE 1 AND TYPE 2 DIABETES

The incidence rate is the most informative measure of the frequency of diabetes in a population for the study of etiologic factors. For the computation of the incidence rate, new cases of diabetes must be recognized and counted. Type 1 diabetes is easily recognized, and virtually all new cases are ascertained in a society with access to medical care. Recognition of new cases of type 2 diabetes, however, depends on the severity of symptoms, diagnostic activity of the medical-care system, and the choice of diagnostic criteria (3).

Data on the incidence rate of diabetes in Rochester, Minnesota, as ascertained through medical-care institutions, show how the incidence rate of type 1 diabetes varies according to age (Table 20.1) (4,5). Among the nondiabetic population of Rochester, type 1 diabetes developed in 7 to 27 individuals per 100,000 per year—depending on the age group being counted. The risk increases during the first and second decades of life, levels off during the third and fourth decades, and increases again thereafter, suggesting that there are two peaks of occurrence of type 1 diabetes, one centered in the second decade and the other in the sixth and seventh decades. The incidence rate of type 2 diabetes increases steadily with age (Table 20.1), with an almost 100-fold increase from early childhood to old age.

The sets of age-specific incidence rates can be summarized as cumulative incidence rates (i.e., the cumulative risk in a cohort of individuals followed from birth and exposed to the age-specific rates). For the age-specific rates in Table 20.1, the cumulative risk by age 70 years would be 1% for type 1 diabetes and 11% for type 2 diabetes.

EPIDEMIOLOGY OF TYPE 1 DIABETES

Any hypothesis put forward regarding the etiology of type 1 diabetes must account for the characteristics of its distribution in human populations that are discussed below. Most studies of type 1 diabetes have considered only the disease occurrence in children, typically under the age of 15 years. Therefore, this review is largely restricted to a consideration of the characteristics of diabetes occurring in the first two decades of life (the first peak in Table 20.1). Little is known about the determinants of type 1 diabetes occurring in adults (the second peak in Table 20.1).

TABLE 20.1. Age-Specific Incidence Rates of Type 1 and Type 2 Diabetes per 100,000 Person-Years in Rochester, 1960 through 1969

Age (y)	Type 1	Type 2
0–9	6.5	0.0
10–19	12.5	7.5
20–29	9.5	9.5
30–39	6.9	66.8
40–49	17.3	155.4
50–59	25.8	322.2
60–69	26.9	612.8
Cumulative incidence rate (%) by age 70	1.05	11.10

Adapted from Melton LJ III, Palumbo PJ, Chu C-P. Incidence of diabetes mellitus by clinical type. *Diabetes Care* 1983;6:75–86; Melton LJ, Palumbo PJ, Dwyer MS, et al. Impact of recent changes in diagnostic criteria on the apparent natural history of diabetes mellitus. *Am J Epidemiol* 1983;117:559–565; and Krolewski AS, Warram JH, Rand LI, et al. Epidemiologic approach to the etiology of type 1 diabetes mellitus and its complications. *N Engl J Med* 1987;317:1390–1398.

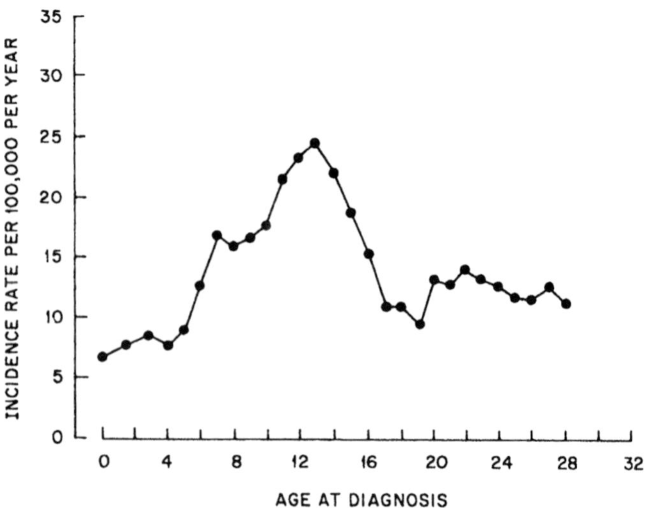

Figure 20.1. Incidence rate of type 1 diabetes according to individual years of age. (Adapted from Christau B, Kromann H, Christy M, et al. Incidence of insulin-dependent diabetes mellitus (0–29 years at onset) in Denmark. *Acta Med Scand Suppl* 1979;624:54–60.)

Variation in Incidence of Type 1 Diabetes with Age

Type 1 diabetes rarely occurs during the first year of life. Of nearly 10,000 incident cases included in the Finnish Childhood Diabetes Registry between 1965 and 1996, only 37 cases (0.4%) had onset before the first birthday (7). The incidence rises sharply until age 12 to 14 years, and then declines. The relationship with age is clearly seen in Figure 20.1, in which the incidence rate of type 1 diabetes in Denmark is presented according to age (8). A similar pattern is seen in most other countries, regardless of whether their overall incidence of type 1 diabetes is high or low.

Data on the incidence of type 1 diabetes with onset after the age of 30 years are scarce. In a population study of two counties in Denmark (9), the rate was 8.2 per 100,000 when very stringent diagnostic criteria for type 1 diabetes were used, and the age at onset resembled that for type 1 diabetes in Rochester, Minnesota (Table 20.1). When the criteria were relaxed to consider all patients treated with insulin from the onset of diabetes as having type 1 diabetes, the incidence rate rose to 35.8 per 100,000, with the difference being due to an increased magnitude of the peak in the oldest decades of age.

Variation in Incidence of Type 1 Diabetes among Races and Countries

Interest in the epidemiology of diabetes in the last two decades has resulted in the publication of a multitude of papers on the incidence rate in most areas of the world. A sample of these data illustrates the large magnitude of the geographic variation in the occurrence of type 1 diabetes (Fig. 20.2) (10). According to a recent compilation of data from 100 studies conducted in 50 countries, the lowest age-adjusted incidence rates for the population aged 0 to 14 years are in Asia, the Caribbean, and Latin America (ranging from 0.1 to 3.5 per 100,000 per year) and the highest are in Nordic countries, the United Kingdom, Canada, New Zealand, Portugal, and Sardinia (ranging from 21.2 to 36.8 per 100,000 per year) (11). The incidence rate of type 1 diabetes

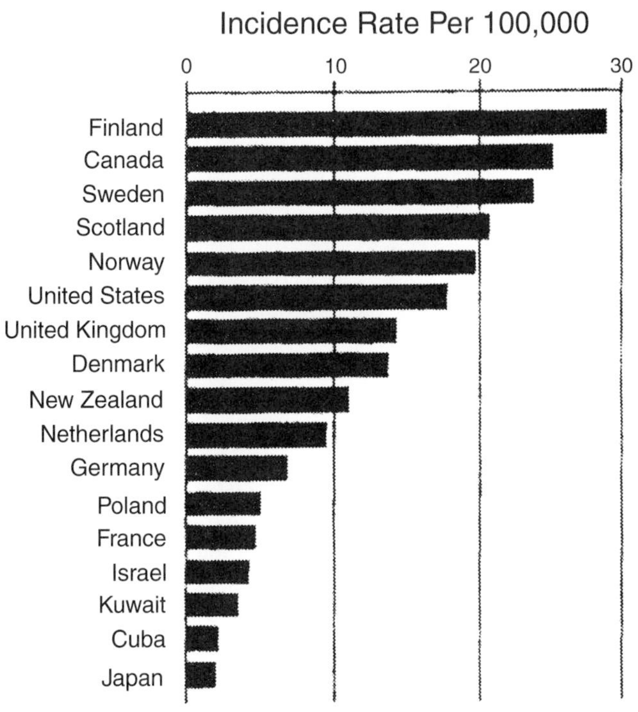

Incidence Rate Per 100,000

0 10 20 30

Finland
Canada
Sweden
Scotland
Norway
United States
United Kingdom
Denmark
New Zealand
Netherlands
Germany
Poland
France
Israel
Kuwait
Cuba
Japan

Figure 20.2. Incidence rate of type 1 diabetes in children less than 15 years old (per 100,000) in various populations. (From Patrick SL, Moy CS, LaPorte RE. The world of insulin-dependent diabetes mellitus: what international epidemiologic studies reveal about the etiology and natural history of IDDM. *Diabetes Metab Rev* 1989;5:571–578.)

in the white population in the United States, represented by three studies, ranges from 11.7 to 16.4 per 100,000 per year. This gives the United States a rank close to that for high-risk populations.

Data on the occurrence of type 1 diabetes according to race in the United States have been accumulating during the last two decades. In general, the reported incidence rate for nonwhites is lower than that for whites in the population aged 0 to 14 years. For example, in Allegheny County, Pennsylvania, the race-specific incidence rates during the 5-year period 1978 to 1983 were 16.2 and 11.8 per 100,000 for white and black children, respectively (11). During a similar calendar period in Jefferson County, Alabama, and in San Diego, California, the rates were much lower for blacks (4.4 and 3.3 per 100,000, respectively), although the rates for whites were similar in the three locales (12). Curiously, during a more recent period (1990 to 1994), the incidence rate in Allegheny County for blacks aged 10 to 14 years rose to equal that for whites and the rate for blacks aged 15 to 19 years exceeded that for whites (13). The reported rate among Hispanic children aged 0 to 14 years ranges from 9.7 per 100,000 in Colorado to 4.1 per 100,000 in California, while the incidence rate in Mexico is among the lowest in the world (12).

In summary, the accumulated data on the incidence of type 1 diabetes during the last 20 years demonstrate that type 1 diabetes occurs in most racial and ethnic groups but that the risk is highest among white populations (11). While genes may in part determine these differences among races, the range of variation within the white population is almost as great as the range among races. Therefore, an important question to be resolved is how much of the variation within and between racial groups is due to genetic differences and how much is due to exposure to different environmental factors.

Temporal Increase in Incidence of Type 1 Diabetes

The pattern of occurrence of type 1 diabetes over time can be important evidence in discriminating between alternative etiologic hypotheses. In particular, a lack of variability from generation to generation is a feature of many genetic traits. If, on the other hand, there is significant variability over time, nongenetic factors are presumably important. The particular pattern of variation may suggest specific environmental factors that can be investigated as components of the etiology of type 1 diabetes. Several types of variation over time have been described: long-term trends, a seasonal cycle, and episodic changes over a few years.

The few sources of data that contribute to an analysis of long-term trends in the incidence of type 1 diabetes in the United States are summarized in Figure 20.3 (6). During the first three decades of the 20th century, the incidence rate of type 1 diabetes in the white population younger than age 15 years was fairly constant. However, during the next three decades, the rate almost tripled. Data from several other countries are compatible with those from the United States. The incidence rate for children younger than age 15 years in Oslo, Norway, rose from 6.2 for the years 1925 through 1954 to 10.8 for the years 1956 through 1965 (14) and then to 20.5 for the years 1973 through 1982 (15), values quite close to those in the United States. In Finland, where the incidence of type 1 diabetes is higher than in the United States, a steady increase in the incidence rate for children aged 1 to 14 has been documented since 1965, reaching a value of 44.8 per 100,000 per year in 1996. The increase was greatest in the age group 1 to 4 years (Table 20.2) (16).

During the period 1989 to 1994, 44 centers representing most European countries collaborated in a study of the time trend in incidence rate of type 1 diabetes. The average annual increase in incidence was 3.4% overall, but it varied among centers and by age. As in the Finnish study, the increase was steepest for the age group 0 to 4 years (6.3% per year) and lowest for the age group 10 to 14 years (17). The reason for the secular increase in the incidence of type 1 diabetes in so many populations is unclear. In several regards, this long-term trend in the occurrence of type 1 diabetes resembles aspects of the emergence of poliomyelitis early in the 20th century. It has been speculated

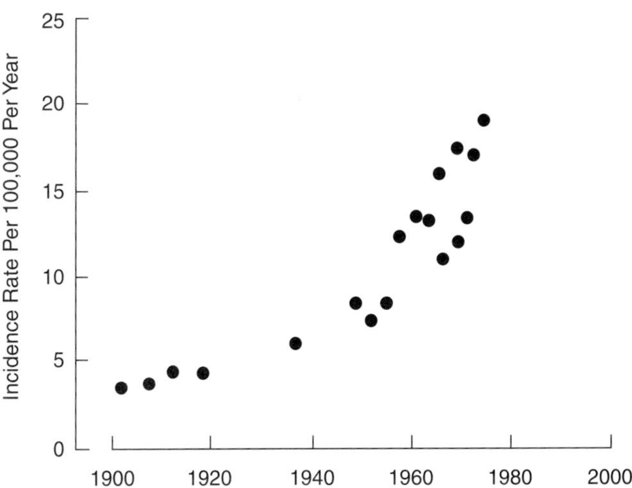

Figure 20.3. Incidence rate of type 1 diabetes in children in the white population of the United States from 1900 to 1976. (From Krolewski AS, Warram JH, Rand LI, et al. Epidemiologic approach to the etiology of type 1 diabetes mellitus and its complications. *N Engl J Med* 1987;317:1390–1398.)

TABLE 20.2. Increase in the Incidence Rate (Per 100,000 Person-Years) of Type 1 Diabetes in Children Younger Than 15 Years in Finland between 1965 and 1996

	Incidence rates in indicated calendar time period			Increase (%)
Age group (y)	1965–1974	1975–1984	1985–1996	1965–1996
1–4	15.8	22.0	33.2	110
5–9	24.9	33.7	40.8	64
10–14	32.7	41.4	45.2	38

Adapted from Tuomilehto J, Karvonen M, Pitkäniemi J, et al. Record-high incidence of type 1 (insulin-dependent) diabetes mellitus in Finnish children: the Finnish Childhood Type 1 Diabetes Registry Group. *Diabetologia* 1999;42:655–660.

that, by analogy, delayed exposure to a common virus may predispose to autoimmunity involving β-cells (6).

Seasonal variability in diagnoses of type 1 diabetes attracted much attention in the 1970s (18,19). It has since been established, however, that type 1 diabetes has a long subclinical period, so the seasonal pattern in diagnoses presumably results from the seasonal occurrence of factors that precipitate the appearance of symptoms in asymptomatic cases (such as common infections) or that result in closer observation of children (such as the return to school). The issue has been revisited recently with data provided by 16 centers representing 11 countries in Europe plus Israel (20). In most populations, a sinusoidal model with the peak incidence in a winter month was statistically significant. Interestingly, the exceptions were the two Scandinavian countries represented in the analysis (Norway and Finland). The pattern did not vary by gender or age group.

Recently, some attention has focused on short-term (year-to-year) variability in the incidence of type 1 diabetes. An apparent epidemic during 1982 through 1984 was described in midwestern Poland (21). The incidence rate in children under 18 years old in those years was double that between 1970 and 1981. Similar "epidemics" in the U.S. Virgin Islands and Jefferson County, Alabama, in 1984 have been described (22,23). The basis for these variations remains unresolved, but many attempts have been made to link them with epidemics of infectious diseases. However, because the subclinical period for type 1 diabetes typically lasts for several years, it is difficult to establish an etiologic link between a specific infection and the diabetes "epidemic," if such a link does exist.

Environmental Triggers of Type 1 Diabetes

The long-term trend in the occurrence of type 1 diabetes resembles aspects of the emergence of poliomyelitis early in the 20th century and has prompted speculation that, by analogy, delayed exposure to a common virus may predispose to destruction of the β-cells (6). Epidemiologic evidence supporting this hypotheses is the low risk of type 1 diabetes associated with markers of crowding or early social mixing, such as attendance at day care centers (24,25). Evidence of the role of enteroviral infections, particularly Coxsackie B, has recently been reviewed (26). Markers of recent infection have been associated in many different circumstances with type 1 diabetes: the presence of antibodies at the time of onset of type 1 diabetes, at the onset of islet autoimmunity, and even in maternal serum obtained during the gestation of children who subsequently developed diabetes. Although acute destruction of the β-cells by a virus, as originally supposed, is incompatible with the long subclinical period during which islet-cell antibodies are detectable, viral infection may play a role as initiator of autoimmunity, as promoter of progression of autoimmunity to type 1 diabetes, or both (26).

Concern about early exposure to cow's milk protein as a trigger of β-cell autoimmunity and the subsequent development of type 1 diabetes in susceptible individuals receives a lot of attention. The epidemiologic evidence suggesting this hypothesis came from a case-control study that found a decreased frequency/duration of breastfeeding in cases. The effect could be due to a lack of a protective effect of breastfeeding or to exposure to an initiator of autoimmunity in cow's milk. Subsequent studies have been inconsistent in replicating this finding, and the overall small magnitude of the effect can plausibly be attributed to recall bias (27). Preliminary results of follow-up studies that monitor the appearance of autoimmunity to β-cells in high-risk infants and small children have not found any association with early exposure to cow's milk (28).

Clustering of Type 1 Diabetes in Families

Studies of the pattern of disease occurrence in families are another approach to evaluating the relative contributions of genes and environment to disease etiology. The study of twins provides an appealing simple design. The premise is that monozygotic twins carry identical genotypes but that dizygotic twins are no more similar genotypically than nontwin siblings. A more frequent concordance for diabetes among monozygotic twins than among dizygotic twins, therefore, favors a greater role of genetic factors. Unfortunately, the simplicity of the study design is negated by the small size of the twin population and the rarity of type 1 diabetes. The chief problems are the small sample size if the twin sample is population-based and uncertainty about ascertainment biases if it is not. With these caveats in mind, the best estimate of the concordance rate for type 1 diabetes in monozygotic twins appears to be in the neighborhood of 45%, whereas that for dizygotic twins is about 25% (29). While this result argues for a role of genes, it also supports a major role of environment. The concordance rate for monozygotic twins is far below 100%, indicating that genes are not a sufficient cause. Moreover, the concordance rate for dizygotic twins is higher than for nontwin siblings, presumably due to the greater sharing of environmental exposures by twin siblings than by nontwin siblings (29).

A more useful measure of familial aggregation is the sibling recurrence-risk ratio, which is defined as the ratio of the risk of disease in the siblings of cases to the risk in the general population. A ratio greater than 1 indicates familial aggregation. Although such aggregation is not exclusively the result of genetic factors and may reflect environmental exposures that are also shared by family members, strong familial aggregation (ratio greater than 6) is unlikely to be due solely to environmental exposures (30).

Three studies, two conducted at the Joslin Diabetes Center in Boston and one conducted at the Steno Hospital in Copenhagen, permit computation of the cumulative risk of diabetes up to age 50 years for the siblings of type 1 diabetes probands. In all three studies, the probands (patients with type 1 diabetes that brought the families into the study) were diagnosed before age 21 years. In the earlier Joslin Diabetes Center study, 289 probands were diagnosed during the years 1928 through 1938 and their 589 siblings were followed to a median age of 49 years (31). In the later Joslin study, 168 probands were diagnosed in the years 1948 through 1960 and their 335 siblings were followed to a median age of 41 years (32). In the Danish study, 187 probands were diagnosed during the years 1918 through 1944 and their 375 siblings were followed to a median age of 52 years (33). The three studies yielded almost identical estimates of the cumulative risks by age 50 years (Fig. 20.4). For comparison, the cumulative risk at age 50 years in the general population was calculated to be 0.5% (Table 20.1). Thus, the risk to siblings by age 50 years seems to be approximately 10%, or 20 times the risk in the general population.

A sibling recurrence-risk ratio of this magnitude (20 times the population risk) is strong evidence of the role of genes in the etiology of type 1 diabetes (see Chapter 23). However, it is important to note that the major histocompatibility locus (also known as *IDDM1*) on chromosome 6 is responsible for only half of the familial clustering of type 1 diabetes (34). The rest is presumably due to other genetic factors or shared family environment. Possible evidence of the impact of environment is suggested in the results of these three studies of the sibling recurrence risk. Despite the close agreement regarding the cumulative risk at age 50 years, there are interesting and statistically significant differences in the cumulative incidence rates at younger ages.

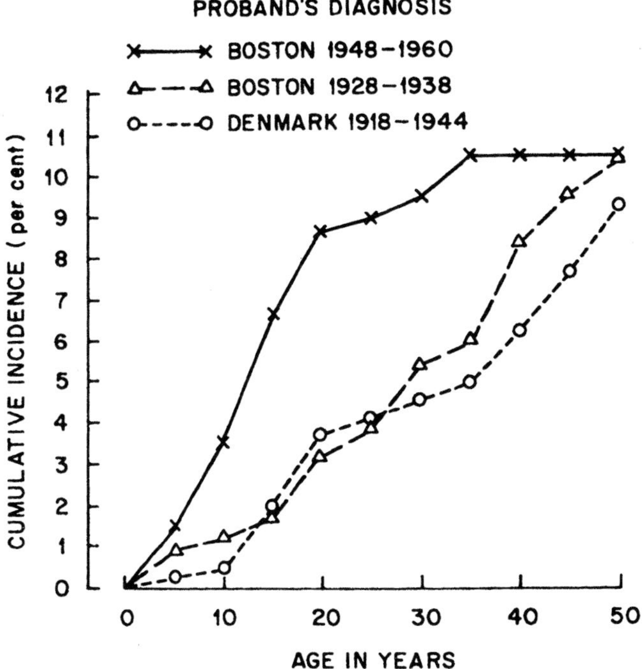

Figure 20.4. Cumulative incidence of type 1 diabetes in the siblings of probands with type 1 diabetes, as estimated in three different studies of families. (From Warram JH, Krolewski AS. Changing age-at-onset of diabetes in siblings of probands with insulin-dependent diabetes. *Am J Hum Gen* 1985;37[Suppl]:A208[abst].)

The cumulative risk of diabetes by age 15 years was 6.3% for the siblings of the 1950s cohort of the Joslin patients but only 1.7% and 1.9% for the siblings in the earlier Joslin and Danish studies, respectively. Results very similar to those of the recent Joslin study were reported for a study in Wisconsin of 194 probands with type 1 diabetes whose diagnosis was made before the age of 30 years during the years 1984 through 1987. The cumulative risk of type 1 diabetes was 10.5% by age 20 years in the sibling (35). This three- to fourfold increase in early-onset diabetes in the siblings of recently diagnosed probands suggests that there is a shift toward a younger age at clinical onset of type 1 diabetes in a population enriched with susceptible individuals. The previously discussed secular trend in the incidence rates of type 1 diabetes in the general population of children younger than age 15 years also might reflect a shift toward earlier manifestation of type 1 diabetes in susceptible individuals (36).

Evidence consistent with this hypothesized interaction between susceptibility and a changing environment has come from a recent collaborative study of sibling recurrence risk in 15 European countries plus Israel (37). The country-specific sibling recurrence risk was highly correlated with the risk of diabetes in that country (Spearman correlation 0.71). Because the sharing of genes among siblings is the same in all populations, this correlation must be due to variation in environmental factors that have similar effects on the siblings of index cases and the general population.

Parent–offspring pairs are another type of first-degree familial relationship that can be examined for familial aggregation of type 1 diabetes. A few follow-up studies of children of a parent with type 1 diabetes permit estimation of the cumulative risk of type 1 diabetes in the offspring up to the age of 20 years. As was found for siblings, the risk is much higher than for the general population, but surprisingly, there is a significant difference between the rate for offspring of diabetic fathers and the rate for offspring of diabetic mothers. For the offspring of diabetic fathers, the cumulative incidence of type 1 diabetes by age 20 years is 6%, or 20 times that for the general population (38,39). For the offspring of diabetic mothers, the corresponding cumulative incidence is approximately 2%, which is only seven times that in the general population (40). In two small studies of offspring born to women who did not develop type 1 diabetes until after the birth of the child (41,42), the children appeared to have a risk of type 1 diabetes similar to that of the children of fathers with type 1 diabetes. These data suggest that exposure to a diabetic environment in utero may have a protective effect on the offspring, perhaps by inducing immunologic tolerance to the antigen involved in the autoimmune destruction of the pancreatic β-cells (41).

Another factor that seems to modify the clustering of type 1 diabetes in families is the age of the proband at onset of type 1 diabetes (43). Regardless of the gender of the diabetic parent in the studies just described, the risk for offspring was approximately two times higher if type 1 diabetes in the parent was diagnosed before the age of 11 years rather than later (Fig. 20.5). Similar results were obtained in a Danish study of offspring of parents with type 1 diabetes (42). These findings suggest that environmental factors played a larger role in the etiology of diabetes when the age at onset is older rather than younger.

The risk for offspring of mothers with type 1 diabetes was lower than that for offspring of fathers with type 1 diabetes regardless of the parent's age at diagnosis, and the pattern was the same if the offspring of diabetic mothers were further strat-

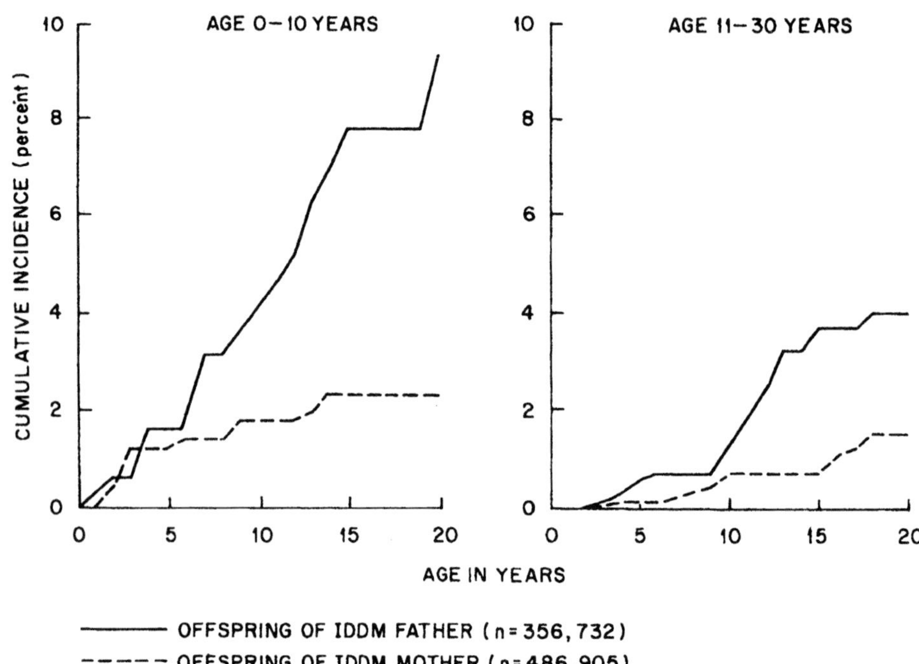

Figure 20.5. Cumulative incidence of type 1 diabetes in the offspring of a parent with type 1 diabetes according to gender and age at diagnosis of diabetes in the parent proband. (From El-Hashimy M, Angelico MC, Martin BC, et al. Factors modifying the risk of IDDM in offspring of an IDDM parent. *Diabetes* 1995;44: 295–299.)

ified by maternal age (data not shown). For simplicity, the cumulative-incidence curves in Figure 20.5 have been adjusted for maternal age by the direct method using the age distribution for the mothers of the total group of children (43). A similar age-dependence of the recurrence risk in relatives has been reported for twin (29) and nontwin siblings (35).

In summary, large variation in the occurrence of type 1 diabetes within and between racial/ethnic groups has been amply demonstrated by population-based studies. The rising incidence rate in many of these populations points to the major role of environmental determinants in the occurrence of diabetes in susceptible individuals. Advances in our knowledge of genes responsible for susceptibility will depend heavily on study designs based on families. At the same time, studies of the pattern of occurrence of diabetes within families have already yielded some clues as to the nature of the environmental determinants of disease manifestation in susceptible individuals. To characterize both the genetic and environments factors underlying the complex etiology of type 1 diabetes, future research should emphasize study designs based on families rather than on geographic populations.

EPIDEMIOLOGY OF TYPE 2 DIABETES

For epidemiologic studies, diabetes that develops in adults may be considered as type 2 diabetes. While this unquestionably results in some misclassification of the type of diabetes, cases of type 1 diabetes represent a very small proportion of new cases of diabetes developing in adults (Table 20.1). In this chapter, we discuss the descriptive epidemiology of type 2 diabetes together with its major risk factors. In contrast to type 1 diabetes, data on incidence rates of type 2 diabetes are sparse. Therefore, to describe the occurrence of type 2 diabetes in human populations, we have supplemented the available incidence data with prevalence data. Data obtained on the U.S. population are preferentially cited in this chapter.

Variation in Occurrence of Type 2 Diabetes According to Age

The development of type 2 diabetes is profoundly influenced by attained age. For example, in the 1960s in the white population of Rochester, Minnesota, the incidence of type 2 diabetes increased from 10 per 100,000 to 612 per 100,000 person-years, respectively, for individuals aged 20 to 29 and 60 to 69 years (Table 20.1). Similar findings were obtained in cohort studies conducted in other populations (44–46). The profound effect of age on risk of type 2 diabetes has also been demonstrated in many cross-sectional studies, although the prevalence of diabetes in the oldest groups in such studies usually underestimates the cumulative risk due to high mortality (see Chapter 47).

The best data on the prevalence of diabetes, diagnosed as well as undiagnosed, are available from the National Health and Nutrition Examination Survey III (NHANES III) conducted between 1988 and 1994 (47). NHANES III describes a probability sample of 18,825 U.S. adults aged 20 years and older who were interviewed to ascertain the history of physician-diagnosed diabetes. A subsample of 6,587 adults had fasting plasma glucose values determined and diabetes diagnosed according to the 1997 criteria of the American Diabetes Association (47,48).

The overall prevalence of diagnosed diabetes in the adult US population was 5.1%. The prevalence of undiagnosed diabetes was 2.7%. In adults, the prevalence of diabetes in non-Hispanic blacks and Mexican Americans was 1.6 and 1.9 times higher, respectively, than in non-Hispanic whites. In all races, men and women had a similar prevalence of diabetes. The prevalence of type 2 diabetes, both diagnosed and undiagnosed, in the U.S. population according to attained age and race is shown in Figure 20.6. In all three groups, the total prevalence of diabetes rose rapidly from a range of 1.4% to 3.0% for age category 20 to 39 years to a range of 17.3% to 29.3% in age category 60 to 74 years, being lowest in all age categories for non-Hispanic whites. The prevalence of type 2 diabetes in individuals 75 years or older did not increase further, most likely as a result of higher mor-

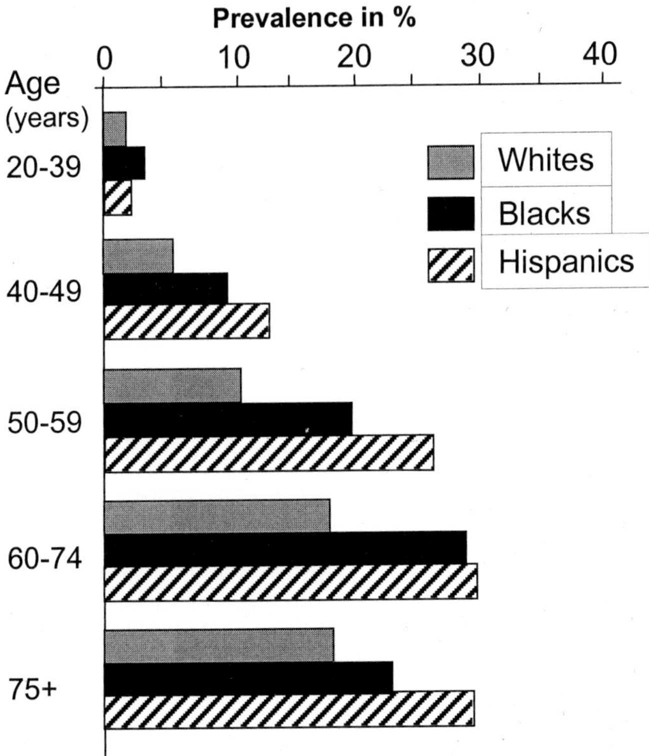

Figure 20.6. Prevalence of diagnosed and undiagnosed diabetes in U.S. adults by age and race or ethnic group based on data from the Third National Health and Nutrition Examination Survey, 1988–1994. (From Harris MI, Goldstein DE, Flegal KM, et al. Prevalence of diabetes, impaired fasting glucose, and impaired glucose tolerance in U.S. adults: the Third National Health and Nutritional Survey, 1988–1994. *Diabetes Care* 1998;21:518–524.)

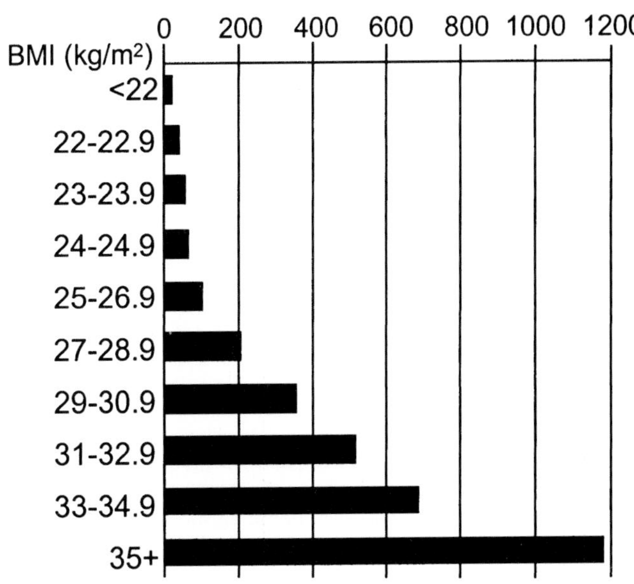

Figure 20.7. Incidence of type 2 diabetes according to body mass index (BMI) in a large cohort of US women followed up for 14 years. (From Colditz GA, Willett WC, Rotnitzky A, et al. Weight gain as a risk factor for clinical diabetes mellitus in women. *Ann Intern Med* 1995; 122: 481–486.)

tality in individuals with diabetes than in those without diabetes (see Chapter 47).

Variation in Incidence of Type 2 Diabetes According to Obesity

As early as 1921, Elliott P. Joslin published a report in which he showed that the risk of developing diabetes (type 2 according to our current criteria) was higher in obese than nonobese individuals (49). Similar findings were obtained in many subsequent case–control and cross-sectional studies, although the estimates of the effect varied due to problems associated with unreliable measurement of obesity, lack of distinction between type 1 and type 2 diabetes, and selection of unrepresentative study groups.

Over the last decade, excellent data on the risk of developing type 2 diabetes according to various indices of body weight have been obtained in several prospective studies. In the largest of these, the 14-year follow-up of the Nurses' Health Study, 2,204 new cases of type 2 diabetes were observed during 1.5 million person-years of observation (50). The age-adjusted incidence rates of type 2 diabetes increased continuously with increasing body weight (Fig. 20.7). An association of risk with increasing weight was evident even within the nonobese range. The incidence rate increased from 13 to 104 per 100,000 person-years comparing women whose body mass index (BMI) was in the range "less than 22" to those whose BMI was in the range "25 to 26.9." Although this was a steep gradient, the largest absolute increases in risk were found in the obese range. From the lowest BMI group in the obese range "27 to 28.9" to the highest "35+," the incidence rate rose from 200 to 1,190 per 100,000 person-years. The most extreme level of obesity (35+) represented only 3% of the population but contributed 26% of the incidence cases of type 2 diabetes. Both a high weight before age 18 years and a large weight gain during adulthood (after age 18 years) contributed significantly to the risk of subsequent type 2 diabetes. However, BMI at the baseline of the follow-up (age range, 30 to 55 years) had the most significant impact on the risk of type 2 diabetes (Fig. 20.7). Similar findings were obtained during follow-up for 5 years of a cohort of 51,529 U.S. male health professionals, 40 to 75 years of age at baseline (51), as well as in several other prospective studies (52–55).

Most studies used BMI as the measure of obesity. However, it has been postulated that fat mass, particularly visceral fat mass, is associated with insulin resistance and that indices of visceral fat such as waist–hip ratio or waist circumference might therefore be better predictors of risk of type 2 diabetes (56). These issues were examined specifically in one of the reports from the Nurses' Health Study (57). The total cohort was divided into quintiles of BMI, and each quintile was divided further according to classes of waist–hip ratio or waist circumference. In each quintile of BMI, the risk of type 2 diabetes increased steadily with higher class of waist–hip ratio or waist circumference. Interestingly, the latter was a much stronger predictor of the risk of type 2 diabetes than the former. When the data were adjusted for other covariates and controlled for BMI, the relative risk of type 2 diabetes for the 90th percentile of waist circumference (97 cm) versus the 10th percentile (67 cm) was 5.1 (95% confidence interval, 2.9 to 8.9). It is important to emphasize that, in models that included both BMI and waist circumference, BMI remained a strong predictor of risk of type 2 diabetes, although its effect was attenuated. Similar findings were reported in the follow-up study of the U.S. male health professionals (51). However, in this very large study of males, the effect of baseline BMI on the risk of type 2 diabetes was much stronger and the effect of waist circumference much weaker than in the Nurses' Health Study (57). Many other studies examined these issues and indicated a more significant role of visceral fat than BMI on the risk of type 2 diabetes. However, most of these studies did not have sufficient statistical power to dissect the independent effects of visceral fat as opposed to total fat reflected in BMI.

Variation in Incidence of Type 2 Diabetes According to Physical Activity

Although ecologic studies have suggested an inverse relationship between physical activity and the risk of type 2 diabetes, only recently has direct evidence of a protective effect of regular physical activity emerged from several large prospective studies. The earliest study was conducted in male alumni of the University of Pennsylvania and showed the beneficial effect of exercise primarily among those who were obese or had a family history of diabetes (52). In the Physicians' Health Study, which followed 21,271 male physicians for 5 years, a protective effect of exercise against type 2 diabetes also was demonstrated, and again the effect was mainly in obese physicians (58). Similar conclusions were drawn from a follow-up study among middle-aged Finnish men (59). In women, the protective effect of exercise against type 2 diabetes seems to be more universal. For example, the Nurses' Health Study showed that the protective effect of exercise against type 2 diabetes was similar in obese and nonobese individuals and in those with and without a family history of diabetes (60,61) (Fig. 20.8). Similar observations were made in a 12-year follow-up study of 34,257 women aged 55 to 69 years participating in the Iowa Women's Health Study Cohort (62).

The dose response between intensity of physical activity and risk of type 2 diabetes was estimated in most of the studies. In three studies in men (52,58,59), the risk of type 2 diabetes decreased with increasing amounts of exercise, whereas in the three other studies in women (60–62), the degree of protection against type 2 diabetes was the same in the subjects who exercised the most as it was in those who exercised only moderately. In summary, however, all studies showed that individuals with a modest level of exercise had a significantly lower risk of type 2 diabetes than did those who were completely sedentary. When adjusted for other risk factors, the relative risk of type 2 diabetes in individuals with a modest level of exercise ranged between 0.69 and 0.74 in comparison with the risk in individuals with a sedentary lifestyle.

Secular Trends in Occurrence of Type 2 Diabetes

The occurrence of type 2 diabetes has been increasing in the U.S. population over the last 50 years. The following review considers incidence and prevalence data separately. Whereas incidence measures directly the changes over time in the risk of diabetes, prevalence may reflect changes not only in risk over time but also in survival of individuals with diabetes.

The best incidence data on the occurrence of type 2 diabetes over the last 50 years were obtained in the population of Rochester, Minnesota (63). In that population, which is predominantly white and serves as a population laboratory for investigation of human diseases, all individuals older than 30 years and with newly diagnosed type 2 diabetes were identified during the period 1945 through 1989. The age-adjusted incidence rates for four periods within that interval are shown in Figure 20.9 accord-

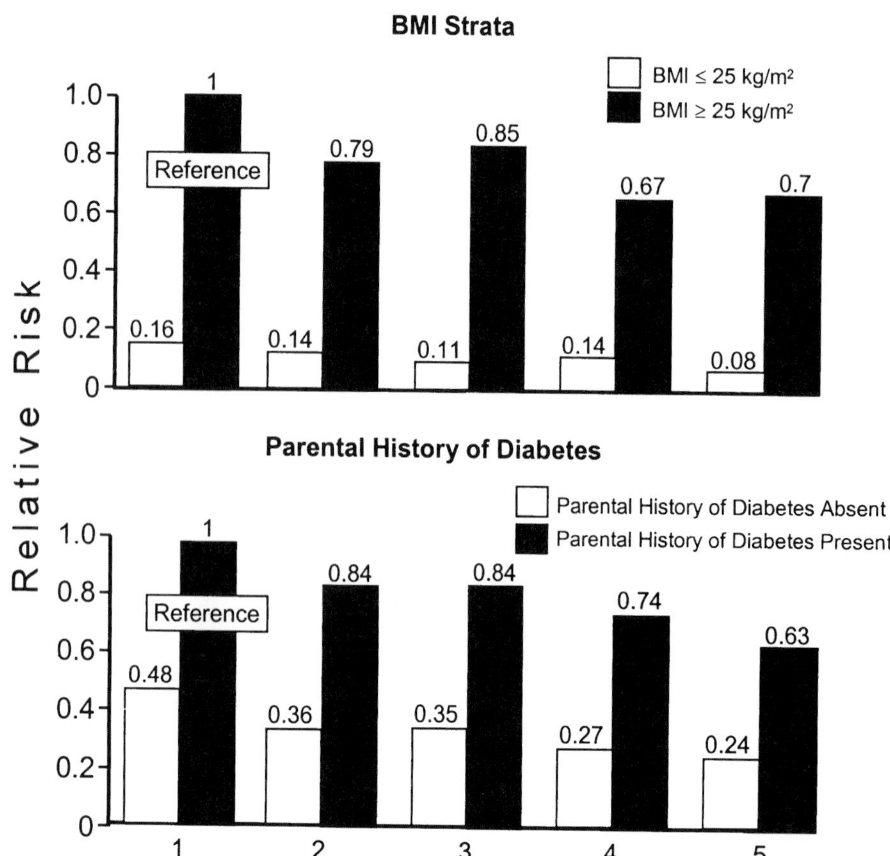

Figure 20.8. Relative risk of type 2 diabetes according to quintile of physical activity as measured by the metabolic equivalent task (MET) score, which is based on time spent per week on each of eight common physical activities, including walking. The results are stratified according to body mass index (BMI) and parental history of diabetes and were adjusted for other covariates. (From Hu FB, Sigal RJ, Rich-Edwards JW, et al. Walking compared with vigorous physical activity and risk of type 2 diabetes in women: a prospective study. *JAMA* 1999;282:1433–1439.)

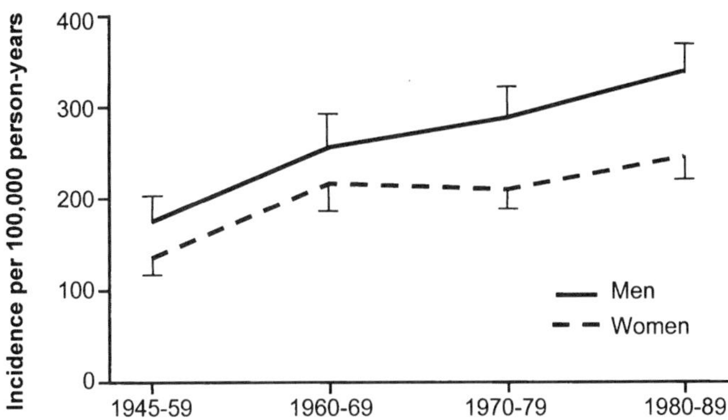

Figure 20.9. Age-adjusted, sex-specific incidence rates (95% confidence intervals represented by bars) for type 2 diabetes according to calendar time in adult residents of Rochester, Minnesota. (From Leibson CL, O'Brien PC, Atjinson E, et al. Relative contribution of incidence and survival to increasing prevalence of adult-onset diabetes mellitus: a population-based study. *Am J Epidemiol* 1997;146:12–22.)

ing to gender. The rates were higher in men than in women, and they increased between the periods 1945 through 1959 and 1980 through 1989: in men from 174 per 100,000 to 331 per 100,000 person-years and in women from 135 per 100,000 to 239 per 100,000 person-years. This represents an increase of 90% in men and 77% in women. Interestingly, similar methodology was used to analyze an additional period, 1990 through1994, and the incidence rates for type 2 diabetes had further increased significantly to 449 per 100,000 person-years in men and to 319 per 100,000 person-years in women (64). These increases could not be accounted for by more active screening for undiagnosed diabetes.

There are only a few other reports that examined the incidence of type 2 diabetes according to calendar time. Reported trends in diabetes incidence rates based on data from the National Health Interview Surveys during the period 1935 through 1968 are very similar to those observed in the Rochester population over the period 1945 through 1969. Subsequently, the rates rose in the Rochester population but in the National Health Interview Survey, data showed no change in the incidence of type 2 diabetes since 1968 (65). In contrast to the latter, a study by the Centers for Disease Control and Prevention (CDC) found a 48% increase in the incidence of self-reported diabetes between 1980 and 1994 in the U.S. population (66). A study in Cincinnati, Ohio, was conducted to determine the occurrence of type 2 diabetes in adolescents (67). The incidence of type 2 diabetes in adolescents increased in that area from 0.7 per 100,000 person-years in 1982 to 7.2 per 100,000 person-years in 1994. Recent results from the San Antonio Heart Study also showed a rapid increase in the incidence of type 2 diabetes in an adult population (68). During the period 1980 and 1987, the incidence rates of diagnosed and undiagnosed type 2 diabetes increased in Mexican Americans and non-Hispanic whites by 95% and 63%, respectively. After adjustment for other risk factors, including BMI, the increase in incidence according to calendar time was significant in Mexican Americans and borderline in non-Hispanic whites.

There have been many studies demonstrating an increasing prevalence of diabetes during the last century. Once again, the most reliable data on the prevalence of diagnosed diabetes according to calendar time were obtained for the population of Rochester, Minnesota (63). The age- and sex-adjusted prevalence of type 2 diabetes in the population aged 45 years in the census years 1970, 1980, and 1990 increased from 3.5% to 4.5% and then to 5.1%, respectively. Trends in the prevalence of self-reported diabetes were examined in telephone surveys conducted by CDC in random samples of adults in 50 states for the period 1990 to 1998 (69). Overall, the prevalence of diabetes rose from 4.9% to 6.5% during this period, and the increase was similar across sexes, races, and education levels. Table 20.3 shows the changes in diabetes prevalence according to age. The highest increase in prevalence of type 2 diabetes occurred in the age category 30 to 59 years. The interpretation of these data should be qualified, however, because only physician-diagnosed diabetes was considered. It is possible that the observed increase in prevalence was the results of improved ascertainment of patients with undiagnosed diabetes. However, this interpretation is not supported by the results on prevalence of type 2 diabetes obtained in NHANES II and NHANES III. With use of the recently adopted American Diabetes Association (ADA) criteria for a diagnosis of type 2 diabetes, the prevalence of diagnosed and undiagnosed diabetes in the U.S. population 40 to 74 years of age increased from 8.8% in 1976 through 1980 to 12.3% in 1988 through 1994 (47).

In summary, the prevalence of type 2 diabetes has been increasing in the U.S. population and this is accounted for in large part by an increased incidence of type 2 diabetes and not by increased survival of patients with diabetes (63). This increase seems to have accelerated during the last 20 years. Although there have not been direct studies, the increases in incidence and prevalence of type 2 diabetes seem to follow an increase in occurrence of obesity in the U.S. population (70).

TABLE 20.3. Changes in Prevalence of Diagnosed Diabetes in the U.S. Population from 1990 to 1998 According to Age

	Prevalence (%)			
Age group (y)	1990	1998	Difference	% Difference
18–29	1.5 (0.15)	1.6 (0.12)	0.1	9.1
30–39	2.1 (0.16)	3.7 (0.18)	1.6	69.9
40–49	3.6 (0.26)	5.1 (0.22)	1.5	39.8
50–59	7.5 (0.44)	9.8 (0.38)	2.3	30.9
60–69	10.9 (0.50)	12.8 (0.45)	1.9	17.1
70+	11.6 (0.50)	12.7 (0.39)	1.1	10.1

Values in parentheses are standard error.
From Mokdad AH, Ford ES, Bowman BA, et al. Diabetes trends in the U.S.: 1990–1998. *Diabetes Care* 2000;23:1278–1283.

Variation in Occurrence of Type 2 Diabetes among Races and Countries

Consideration of geographic and ethnic differences in the occurrence of type 2 diabetes can be used to evaluate environmental as well as genetic determinants of diabetes. Because the occurrence of type 2 diabetes is similar in men and women, we simplified this review by presenting the prevalence of type 2 diabetes for one sex (men) and for a specific age range (30 to 64 years). The latter can be considered a rough estimate of the cumulative incidence of diabetes by age 50 years. To the extent possible, we have used only previously published data from various population studies conducted in the late 1970s and in the 1980s that were age-standardized and included diagnosed and undiagnosed diabetes (71).

The prevalence of diagnosed and undiagnosed type 2 diabetes in various ethnic groups in the United States and around the world is summarized in Figure 20.10. The highest prevalence of type 2 diabetes is in the Pima and Papago Indians in Arizona. By age 50 years, almost one half of this Native-American population had diabetes. This is an extraordinary high prevalence of diabetes. Most likely, this results from the combination of the extremely high prevalence of obesity in that population together with a high frequency of genetic susceptibility to type 2 diabetes. Other populations of Native Americans also have a high prevalence of type 2 diabetes, although none so high as that in the Pima and Papago Indians (77). The next highest prevalence of type 2 diabetes in the United States is in Mexican Americans living in the states bordering Mexico. The prevalence in non-Hispanic whites is less than half that in Mexican Americans, while that for non-Hispanic blacks is intermediate between the two. Note that this ranking of the three racial groups according to the prevalence of type 2 diabetes (based on NHANES II in 1976 to 1980) persisted in the 1988 to 1994 NHANES III data (Fig. 20.6) despite the increasing prevalence of type 2 diabetes between the two surveys (47).

The prevalence of type 2 diabetes in European populations is similar or slightly lower than that in the non-Hispanic white U.S. population, indicating a similarity of environmental and genetic determinants in the two locations. On the other hand, the prevalence of type 2 diabetes is much lower in blacks in Africa than in non-Hispanic blacks in the United States. Although the explanation for these differences is unknown, a recent study showed that a large proportion of this variability could be accounted for by differences in BMI (78).

Significant differences in the prevalence of type 2 diabetes according to location were observed for three other racial/ethnic groups (Fig. 20.10). The prevalence of type 2 diabetes is very low in Chinese in Mainland China, intermediate in Chinese in Singapore, and very high in Chinese living on the island of Mauritius in the Indian Ocean. Prevalence data for Indians are somehow more complicated. The prevalence of diabetes is moderate in rural India, high in urban India, and high or very high in Indians in many other countries where the prevalence of type 2 diabetes in the aboriginal populations is very low (e.g., Tanzania or Fiji) (71). These data indicate that Indians as an eth-

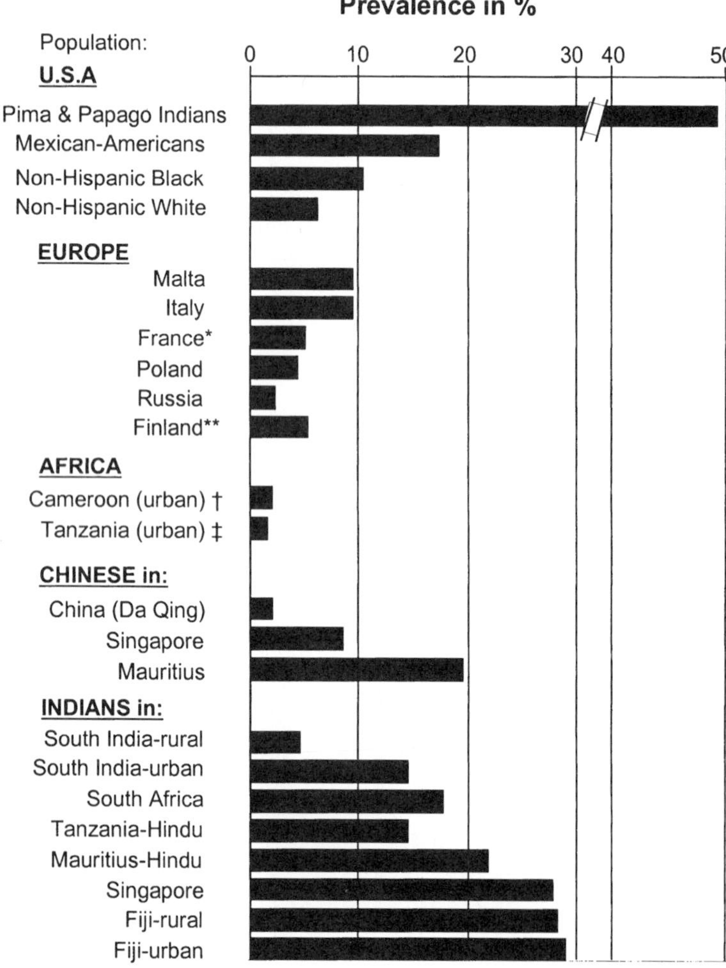

Figure 20.10. Prevalence of type 2 diabetes in men 30 to 64 years old in various populations screened for undiagnosed diabetes. (Adapted from King H, Rewers M, WHO Ad Hoc Diabetes Reporting Group. Global estimates for prevalence of diabetes mellitus and impaired glucose tolerance in adults. *Diabetes Care* 1993;16:157–177 * adapted from Charles MA, Balkau B, Vauzelle-Kervroedan F, et al. Revision of diagnostic criteria for diabetes. *Lancet* 1996;348:1657–1658, and Will new diagnostic criteria for diabetes mellitus change phenotype of patients with diabetes? Reanalysis of European epidemiologic data. DECODE Study Group on behalf of the European Diabetes Epidemiology Study Group. *BMJ* 1998;317:371–375; ** adapted from Charles MA, Balkau B, Vauzelle-Kervroedan F, et al. Revision of diagnostic criteria for diabetes. *Lancet* 1996;348:1657–1658; † adapted from Mbanya JCN, Ngogang J, Salah JN, et al. Prevalence of NIDDM and impaired glucose tolerance in a rural and an urban population in Cameroon. American Diabetes Association. *Diabetologia* 1997;40:824–829 and Levitt NS, Unwin NC, Bradshaw D, et al. Application of the new ADA criteria for the diagnosis of diabetes to population studies in sub-Sahara Africa. *Diabet Med* 2000;17:381–385; and ‡ adapted from McLarty DG, Swai ABM, Kitange HM, et al. Prevalence of diabetes and impaired glucose tolerance in rural Tanzania. *Lancet* 1989;1:871–875 and Levitt NS, Unwin NC, Bradshaw D, et al. Application of the new ADA criteria for the diagnosis of diabetes to population studies in sub-Sahara Africa. *Diabet Med* 2000;17:381–385.)

nic group have a high risk of type 2 diabetes, most likely due to genetic susceptibility.

In summary, there is large variability in the occurrence of type 2 diabetes according to racial/ethnic group. Large variability in the occurrence of type 2 diabetes within the same racial/ethnic group (e.g., the Chinese) according to geography may be accounted for by different frequencies of environmental factors, such as physical activity and obesity in each of these locations. On the other hand, the very high or high prevalence of type 2 diabetes in Native Americans and in Indians is most likely the result of interactions between a high population frequency of genetic susceptibility to type 2 diabetes and very high prevalence of environmental factors such obesity, physical inactivity, or other, as yet unknown, risk factors.

Clustering of Type 2 Diabetes in Families

As alluded to in the previous section, type 2 diabetes has a complex etiology involving both environmental exposures and genetic susceptibility. To select the most effective study designs for evaluating the role of genetic susceptibility and to devise strategies for identifying susceptibility genes for type 2 diabetes, one has to obtain specific information about the pattern of aggregation of diabetes in families of index cases with type 2 diabetes.

A widely used measure of familial aggregation is the sibling recurrence-risk ratio, designated λ_S, which is defined as the ratio of the risk of disease manifestation in siblings of cases compared with the disease risk in the general population (79,80). A ratio above unity suggests familial aggregation. Pincus and White (81), almost 70 years ago, were the first to use this kind of approach to describe aggregation of diabetes in families of index cases attending the Joslin Clinic. However, they and many subsequent researchers used various choices other than the general population risk for the reference risk; for example, the prevalence of diabetes in siblings of individuals without diabetes or in siblings of individuals with diabetes who had no parent with diabetes (82–88). These values underestimate the population risk and, therefore, overestimate familial aggregation.

As part of our efforts to identify informative families for mapping genes for type 2 diabetes diagnosed in middle age, we surveyed a random sample ($N = 563$) of such patients at the Joslin Clinic in Boston, Massachusetts, to obtain information about the occurrence of diabetes in their relatives. In the published report, we examined the λ_S for type 2 diabetes in these families according to parental history of diabetes and selected phenotypic characteristics of index cases (89).

Estimates of the sibling recurrence risk of type 2 diabetes obtained in our study and three other studies conducted in US white families are summarized in Table 20.4. The data in the three other studies were reanalyzed, and the results of all four studies were compared with the general population risk at comparable ages based on NHANES III (47). The first study was conducted in a population-based sample of patients with type 2 diabetes enrolled into the Wisconsin Epidemiologic Study of Diabetic Retinopathy (86). Index cases ($N = 923$) were aged 68 years (on average) at examination and were questioned about the history of diabetes in their families. The prevalence of diabetes in their 3,965 siblings was reported according to parental diabetes status. If neither parent had diabetes, the prevalence of diabetes in the siblings was 10.4%. If one parent was affected with diabetes, the prevalence of diabetes in siblings was 17.8%, and if both parents were affected, the prevalence of diabetes increased to 25.2% (Table 20.4). The second study, involving 9,164 index cases with type 2 diabetes and their 25,659 siblings, obtained results almost identical to those of the first study (87). In addition to the two studies of siblings of index cases, a recent report described the occurrence of diabetes in the offspring of the Framingham Heart Study population according to the parents' diabetes status (88). Diabetes in the offspring was ascertained by history and by examination during 20 years of follow-up. Unlike the other studies, parental diabetes was ascertained directly by examination of the parents during 40 years of follow-up rather than being based on the report of an offspring. The prevalence of diabetes in the offspring with no diabetic parent was 6.1%, 16.5% in offspring with one diabetic parent, and 26.2% in offspring of two diabetic parents. It is remarkable that the prevalence of diabetes in the offspring is so similar to the prevalence of diabetes in siblings in the two other studies. Our

TABLE 20.4. Estimates of the Diabetes Recurrence-Risk Ratio in Siblings (λ_S) or Offspring (λ_O) of Index Cases with Diabetes in Four US Studies According to Parental History of Diabetes

Authors (ref)	No. of siblings or offspring	Mean age, y[a]	Reference risk from NHANES III	λ (%) by parental history of diabetes: No diabetic parent	One diabetic parent	Two diabetic parents	Standardized estimate of λ_S[b]
Estimates based on prevalence							
Klein et al. (86)	3,965[c]	68	11.3	0.9 (10.4)	1.6 (17.8)	2.2 (25.2)	1.2
Karter et al. (87)	25,659[c]	59	9.5	0.8 (7.8)	1.8 (17.2)	2.8 (26.5)	1.2
Meigs et al. (88)[d]	2,527[e]	54	7.6	0.8 (6.1)	2.2 (16.5)	3.4 (26.2)	—
Estimates based on cumulative incidence							
Joslin study (89)	1,657[c]	65	11.3	1.2 (14.0)	2.6 (29.2)	3.7 (41.9)	1.8

NHANES III, National Health and Nutrition Examination III.
[a]For the studies of Klein et al. (86) and Karter et al. (87), the average age of siblings was assumed to be the same as that of index cases.
[b]Standardized by the direct method to the distribution of parental history of diabetes in the study by Klein et al. (86).
[c]Siblings.
[d]Estimates of λ_O are shown for the offspring according to the diabetes status in parents.
[e]Offspring.
Adapted from Weijnen CF, Rich SS, Meigs JB, et al. Risk of diabetes in siblings of index cases with type 2 diabetes: implication for genetic studies. *Diabet Med* 2002;19:41–50.

study is the fourth summarized in Table 20.4. The frequency of occurrence of diabetes in the siblings is presented as cumulative risk by age 65 years. The cumulative risks of diabetes in siblings of index cases with no diabetic parent, one diabetic parent, and two diabetic parents were 14.0%, 29.2%, and 41.9%, respectively.

Recurrence-risk ratios (sibling or offspring) according to parental history of diabetes (Table 20.4) were obtained by dividing the prevalence in each study by the corresponding age-specific prevalence of diagnosed diabetes in NHANES III (47). In all studies, siblings of index cases without a history of parental diabetes had a risk of diabetes similar to that in the general population, suggesting that the contribution of a genetic component was inconsequential in this subgroup. The λ_S was elevated only in families with one or two diabetic parents. The ratios are quite consistent across studies. For example, in families with one diabetic parent, it ranged from a low of 1.6 to a high of 2.6 for the estimate based on cumulative incidence. The distribution of index cases according to parental history of diabetes varied among the studies, with the proportion with a positive parental history being highest in the our study based on patients at the Joslin Clinic. An overall λ_S for comparisons among the studies of siblings was obtained by standardizing the rates specific to each type of parental history in each study to the distribution of parental histories of diabetes in the Wisconsin study, the only population-based sample of index cases. The adjusted λ_S for our study is lower than the unadjusted value because of the reduced weight given to families with affected parents. The overall estimates of λ_S from these three studies ranged from 1.2 to 1.8.

In our study we found that the λ_S of type 2 diabetes was particularly high (λ_S = 3.5) if a parent and grandparent reported diabetes. Moreover, if the family history of diabetes was an affected grandparent, aunt, or uncle *instead of a parent*, the risk was similar to that in families with no history of diabetes (13.2% ± 2.5%) and not different from the risk in the general population. Therefore, the risk of diabetes appeared to be transmitted primarily through affected rather than unaffected parents. This is consistent with the low (meaning similar to the general population) λ_S for type 2 diabetes in families with no affected parents. In the population-based Wisconsin Epidemiologic Study of Diabetic Retinopathy, 31% of the index cases with type 2 diabetes reported a parent with diabetes, whereas the proportion with a diabetic parent in our study was 50%.

To examine whether familial aggregation of type 2 diabetes varied with the age at diagnosis of diabetes, we partitioned the families at the mean age at diagnosis in the index case (47 years) (89). The cumulative incidence of diabetes by age 65 years in the siblings of index cases with a diagnosis of diabetes at young ages (28.4%) was significantly higher than that in the siblings of index cases with a diagnosis at an older age (19.9%). This difference largely vanished when the siblings were also stratified according to the number of affected parents. A young age at diagnosis of diabetes was itself associated with a history of diabetes in one or both parents: 62.3% of the index cases who were young at diagnosis reported an affected parent as compared with 46.7% of those who were older at diagnosis.

Obesity in the index case was associated with a reduced recurrent risk of type 2 diabetes in siblings. In families with no parental history of diabetes, the siblings of obese index cases had the same diabetes risk as obese individuals in the general population (λ_S = 0.9), whereas the risk in siblings of nonobese index cases was twice that in the nonobese general population (λ_S = 2.1) (89). If the nonobese index case had an affected parent, λ_S increased to 4.1. The significant clustering of diabetes in siblings of nonobese index cases points to an important role of genetic susceptibility to type 2 diabetes in the families of nonobese index cases and stands in contrast to the absence of evidence of a role of genetic susceptibility in the families of obese index cases. This conclusion is consistent with epidemiologic observations that obesity and a family history of diabetes are independent risk factors for the development of type 2 diabetes (90–93).

Overall, a family history of diabetes, particularly in parents, is a significant risk factor for the development of type 2 diabetes. However, it accounts for only a moderate proportion of cases with type 2 diabetes in the general population. At most, the proportion is 31%, which was the frequency of parental diabetes in the population-based Wisconsin study (86). The λ_S for type 2 diabetes is low (λ_S = 1.8). This is consistent with a hypothesis that type 2 diabetes is a complex disease caused by both environmental and genetic factors. With such a low λ_S, the identification of the genetic factors may be a challenging task. Based on the results discussed above, an optimal strategy for collecting families for linkage studies would be to select families through nonobese probands with type 2 diabetes or probands with a history of "vertical" transmission through an affected grandparent and a parent. Restriction of family ascertainment in this manner would reduce heterogeneity at both the phenotypic and genetic levels and therefore would make the task of findings the putative susceptibility genes for type 2 diabetes feasible.

REFERENCES

1. Krolewski AS, Warram JH. Epidemiology of diabetes mellitus. In: Marble A, Krall LP, Bradley RF, et al., eds. *Joslin's diabetes mellitus*, 12th ed. Philadelphia: Lea & Febiger, 1985:12–42.
2. Rothman KJ, Greenland S. Measures of disease frequency. In: Rothman KJ, Greenland S, eds. *Modern epidemiology*, 2nd ed. Philadelphia: Lippincott-Raven Publishers, 1998:29–46.
3. Harris MI, Eastman RC, Cowie CC, et al. Comparison of diabetes diagnostic categories in the U.S. population, according to 1997 American Diabetes Association and 1980–1985 World Health Organization diagnostic criteria. *Diabetes Care* 1997;20:1859–1862.
4. Melton LJ III, Palumbo PJ, Chu C-P. Incidence of diabetes mellitus by clinical type. *Diabetes Care* 1983;6:75–86.
5. Melton LJ, Palumbo PJ, Dwyer MS, et al. Impact of recent changes in diagnostic criteria on the apparent natural history of diabetes mellitus. *Am J Epidemiol* 1983;117:559–565.
6. Krolewski AS, Warram JH, Rand LI, et al. Epidemiologic approach to the etiology of type I diabetes mellitus and its complications. *N Engl J Med* 1987; 317:1390–1398.
7. Karvonen M, Pitkäniemi J, Tuomilehto J. The onset age of type 1 diabetes in Finnish children has become younger: the Finnish Childhood Diabetes Registry Group. *Diabetes Care* 1999;22:1066–1070.
8. Christau B, Kromann H, Christy M, et al. Incidence of insulin-dependent diabetes mellitus (0–29 years at onset) in Denmark. *Acta Med Scand Suppl* 1979; 624:54–60.
9. Mølbak AG, Christau B, Marner B, et al. Incidence of insulin-dependent diabetes mellitus in age groups over 30 years in Denmark. *Diabet Med* 1994;11: 650–655.
10. Patrick SL, Moy CS, LaPorte RE. The world of insulin-dependent diabetes mellitus: what international epidemiologic studies reveal about the etiology and natural history of IDDM. *Diabetes Metab Rev* 1989;5:571–578.
11. Karvonen M, Viik-Kajander M, Moltchanova E, et al. Incidence of childhood type 1 diabetes worldwide: Diabetes Mondiale (DiaMond) Project Group. *Diabetes Care* 2000;23:1516–1526.
12. Diabetes Epidemiology Research International Group. Geographic patterns of childhood insulin-dependent diabetes mellitus: *Diabetes* 1988;37:1113–1119.
13. Libman IM, LaPorte RE, Becker D, et al. Was there an epidemic of diabetes in nonwhite adolescents in Allegheny County, Pennsylvania? *Diabetes Care* 1998; 21:1278–1281.
14. Ustvedt HJ, Olsen E. Incidence of diabetes mellitus in Oslo, Norway 1956–65. *Br J Prev Soc Med* 1977;31:251–257.
15. Joner G, Søvik O. Incidence, age at onset and seasonal variation of diabetes mellitus in Norwegian children, 1973–1977. *Acta Paediatr Scand* 1981;70: 329–335.
16. Tuomilehto J, Karvonen M, Pitkäniemi J, et al. Record-high incidence of type 1 (insulin-dependent) diabetes mellitus in Finnish children: the Finnish Childhood Type I Diabetes Registry Group. *Diabetologia* 1999;42:655–660.

17. EURODIAB ACE Study Group. Variation and trends in incidence of childhood diabetes in Europe: *Lancet* 2000;355:873–876.
18. Gleason RE, Kahn CB, Funk IB, et al. Seasonal incidence of insulin-dependent diabetes (IDDM) in Massachusetts, 1964–1973. *Int J Epidemiol* 1982;11:39–45.
19. Gamble DR. The epidemiology of insulin-dependent diabetes, with particular reference to the relationship of virus infection to its etiology. *Epidemiol Rev* 1980;2:49–70.
20. Lévy-Marchal C, Patterson C, Green A. Variation by age group and seasonality at diagnosis of childhood IDDM in Europe: the EURODIAB ACE Study Group. *Diabetologia* 1995;38:823–830.
21. Rewers M, LaPorte RE, Walczak M, et al. Apparent epidemic of insulin-dependent diabetes mellitus in midwestern Poland. *Diabetes* 1987;36:106–113.
22. Tull ES, Roseman JM, Christian CLE. Epidemiology of childhood IDDM in U.S. Virgin Islands from 1979 to 1988: evidence of an epidemic in early 1980s and variation by degree of racial admixture. *Diabetes Care* 1991;14:558–564.
23. Wagenknecht LE, Roseman JM, Herman WH. Increased incidence of insulin-dependent diabetes mellitus following an epidemic of coxsackievirus B5. *Am J Epidemiol* 1991;133:1024–1031.
24. Patterson CC, Carson DJ, Hadden DR. Epidemiology of childhood IDDM in Northern Ireland 1989–1994: low incidence in areas with highest population density and most household crowding—Northern Ireland Diabetes Study Group. *Diabetologia* 1996;39:1063–1069.
25. McKinney PA, Okasha M, Parslow RC, et al. Early social mixing and childhood type 1 diabetes mellitus: a case-control study in Yorkshire, UK. *Diabet Med* 2000;17:236–242.
26. Graves PM, Norris JM, Pallansch MA, et al. The role of enteroviral infections in the development of IDDM: limitation of current approaches. *Diabetes* 1997; 46:161–168.
27. Norris JM, Scott FW. A meta-analysis of infant diet and insulin-dependent diabetes mellitus: do biases play a role? *Epidemiology* 1996;7:87–92.
28. Norris JM, Beaty B, Klingensmith G, et al. Lack of association between early exposure to cow's milk protein and beta-cell autoimmunity: Diabetes Autoimmunity Study in the Young (DAISY). *JAMA* 1996;276:609–614.
29. Kumar D, Gemayel N, Deapen D, et al. North-American twins with IDDM: genetic, etiological, and clinical significance of disease concordance according to age, zygosity, and the interval after diagnosis in the first twin. *Diabetes* 1993; 42:1351–1363.
30. Khoury MJ, Beaty TH, Liang KY. Can familial aggregation of disease be explained by aggregation of environmental risk factors? *Am J Epidemiol* 1988;127:674–683.
31. Gottlieb MS. Diabetes in offspring and siblings of juvenile- and maturity-onset-type diabetics. *J Chronic Dis* 1980;33:331–339.
32. Warram JH, Krolewski AS. Changing age-at-onset of diabetes in siblings of probands with insulin-dependent diabetes. *Am J Hum Genet* 1985;37[Suppl]: A208(abst).
33. Degnbol B, Green A. Diabetes mellitus among first- and second-degree relatives of early onset diabetics. *Ann Hum Genet* 1978;42:25–47.
34. Risch N. Assessing the role of HLA-linked and unlinked determinants of disease. *Am J Hum Genet* 1987;40:1–14.
35. Allen C, Palta M, D'Alessio DJ. Risk of diabetes in siblings and other relatives of IDDM subjects. *Diabetes* 1991;40:831–836.
36. Kurtz Z, Peckham CS, Ades AE. Changing prevalence of juvenile-onset diabetes mellitus. *Lancet* 1988;2:88–90.
37. The Eurodiab Ace Study Group and the Eurodiab Ace Substudy 2 Study Group. Familial risk of type 1 diabetes in European children: *Diabetologia* 1998;41:1151–1156.
38. Warram JH, Krolewski AS, Gottlieb MS, et al. Differences in risk of insulin-dependent diabetes in offspring of diabetic mothers and diabetic fathers. *N Engl J Med* 1984;311:149–152.
39. LaPorte RE, Fishbein HA, Drash AL, et al. The Pittsburgh insulin-dependent diabetes mellitus (IDDM) registry: the incidence of insulin-dependent diabetes mellitus in Allegheny County, Pennsylvania (1965–1976). *Diabetes* 1981; 30:279–284.
40. Warram JH, Krolewski AS, Kahn CR. Determinants of IDDM and perinatal mortality in children of diabetic mothers. *Diabetes* 1988;37:1328–1334.
41. Warram JH, Martin BC, Krolewski AS. Risk of IDDM in children of diabetic mothers decreases with increasing maternal age at pregnancy. *Diabetes* 1991; 40:1679–1684.
42. Lorenzen T, Pociot F, Stilgren L, et al. Predictors of IDDM recurrence risk in offspring of Danish IDDM patients: Danish IDDM Epidemiology and Genetics Group. *Diabetologia* 1998;41:666–673.
43. El-Hashimy M, Angelico MC, Martin BC, et al. Factors modifying the risk of IDDM in offspring of an IDDM parent. *Diabetes* 1995;44:295–299.
44. Vanderpump MP, Tunbridge WM, French JM, et al. The incidence of diabetes mellitus in an English community: a 20-year follow-up of the Whickham Survey. *Diabet Med* 1996;13:741–747.
45. Blanchard JF, Ludwig S, Wajda A et al. Incidence and prevalence of diabetes in Manitoba 1986–1991. *Diabetes Care* 1996;19:807–811.
46. Vilbergson S, Sigurdsson G, Sigvaldason H, et al. Prevalence and incidence of NIDDM in Iceland: evidence for stable incidence among males and females 1967–1991—the Reykjavik Study. *Diabet Med* 1997;14:491–498.
47. Harris MI, Goldstein DE, Flegal KM, et al. Prevalence of diabetes, impaired fasting glucose, and impaired glucose tolerance in U.S. adults: the Third National Health and Nutritional Survey, 1988–1994. *Diabetes Care* 1998;21:518–524.
48. Resnick HE, Harris MI, Brock DB, et al. American Diabetes Association diabetes diagnostic criteria, advancing age, and cardiovascular disease risk profiles: results from the Third National Health and Nutrition Examination Survey. *Diabetes Care* 2000;23:176–180.
49. Joslin EP. The prevention of diabetes mellitus. *JAMA* 1921;76:79–84.
50. Colditz GA, Willett WC, Rotnitzky A, et al. Weight gain as a risk factor for clinical diabetes mellitus in women. *Ann Intern Med* 1995; 122:481–486.
51. Chan JM, Rimm EB, Colditz GA, et al. Obesity, fat distribution, and weight gain as risk factors for clinical diabetes in men. *Diabetes Care* 1994; 17:961–969.
52. Helmrich SP, Ragland DR, Leung RW, et al. Physical activity and reduced occurrence of non-insulin-dependent diabetes mellitus. *N Engl J Med* 1991;325: 147–152.
53. Cassano PA, Rosner B, Vokonas PS, et al. Obesity and body fat distribution in relation to the incidence of non-insulin-dependent diabetes mellitus. *Am J Epidemiol* 1992;136:1474–1486.
54. Perry IJ, Wannamethee SG, Walker MK, et al. Prospective study of risk factors for development of non-insulin dependent diabetes in middle age British men. *BMJ* 1995;310:560–564.
55. Hanson RL, Narayan KMV, McCance DR, et al. Rate of weight gain, weight fluctuation, and incidence of NIDDM. *Diabetes* 1995; 43:261–266.
56. Kissebah AH, Vydelingum N, Murray R, et al. Relation of body fat distribution to metabolic complications of obesity. *J Clin Endocrinol Metab* 1982; 54: 254–260.
57. Carey VJ, Walters EE, Colditz GA, et al. Body fat distribution and risk of non-insulin-dependent diabetes mellitus in women: the Nurses' Health Study. *Am J Epidemiol* 1997;145:614–619.
58. Manson JE, Nathan DM, Krolewski AS, et al. A prospective study of exercise and incidence of diabetes among US male physicians. *JAMA* 1992;268:63–67.
59. Lynch J, Helmrich SP, Lakka TA, et al. Moderately intense physical activities and high levels of cardiorespiratory fitness reduce the risk of non-insulin-dependent diabetes mellitus in middle-aged men. *Arch Intern Med* 1996;156:1307–1314.
60. Manson JE, Rimm EB, Stampfer MJ, et al. Physical activity and incidence of non-insulin dependent diabetes mellitus in women. *Lancet* 1991; 338:774–778.
61. Hu FB, Sigal RJ, Rich-Edwards JW, et al. Walking compared with vigorous physical activity and risk of type 2 diabetes in women: a prospective study. *JAMA* 1999;282:1433–1439.
62. Folsom AR, Kushi LH, Hong CP. Physical activity and incident diabetes mellitus in postmenopausal women. *Am J Public Health* 2000;90:134–138.
63. Leibson CL, O'Brien PC, Atjinson E, et al. Relative contribution of incidence and survival to increasing prevalence of adult-onset diabetes mellitus: a population-based study. *Am J Epidemiol* 1997;146:12–22.
64. Burke J, Ransom J, O'Brien P, et al. An update of the incidence of diabetes in Rochester, Minnesota through 1994. *Diabetes* 2001;44[Suppl 1]:A202(abst).
65. Kenney SJ, Aubert RE, Geiss LS. Prevalence and incidence of non-insulin-dependent diabetes. In: National Diabetes Data Group, eds. *Diabetes in America*, 2nd ed. Bethesda, MD: National Institute of Diabetes and Digestive and Kidney Diseases, 1995:7–67; NIDDKD publication 95-1468.
66. Trends in the prevalence and incidence of self-reported diabetes mellitus—United States, 1980–1994. *MMWR Morbid Mortal Wkly Rep* 1997;46:1014–1018.
67. Pinhas-Hamiel O, Dolan LM, Daniels SR, et al. Increased incidence of non-insulin-dependent diabetes mellitus among adolescents. *J Pediatr* 1996;128: 608–615.
68. Burke JP, Williams K, Gaskill SP, et al. Rapid risk in the incidence of type 2 diabetes from 1987 to 1996: results from the San Antonio Heart Study. *Arch Intern Med* 1999;159:1450–1456.
69. Mokdad AH, Ford ES, Bowman BA, et al. Diabetes trends in the U.S.: 1990–1998. *Diabetes Care* 2000;23:1278–1283.
70. Kuczmarski RJ, Flegal KM, Campbell SM, et al. Increasing prevalence of overweight among US adults: The National Health and Nutrition Examination Surveys, 1960 to 1991. *JAMA* 1994;272:205–211.
71. King H, Rewers M, WHO Ad Hoc Diabetes Reporting Group. Global estimates for prevalence of diabetes mellitus and impaired glucose tolerance in adults. *Diabetes Care* 1993;16:157–177.
72. Charles MA, Balkau B, Vauzelle-Kervroedan F, et al. Revision of diagnostic criteria for diabetes. *Lancet* 1996;348:1657–1658.
73. DECODE Study Group on behalf of the European Diabetes Epidemiology Study Group. Will new diagnostic criteria for diabetes mellitus change phenotype of patients with diabetes? Reanalysis of European epidemiologic data. *BMJ* 1998;317:371–375.
74. Mbanya JCN, Ngogang J, Salah JN, et al. Prevalence of NIDDM and impaired glucose tolerance in a rural and an urban population in Cameroon: American Diabetes Association. *Diabetologia* 1997;40:824–829.
75. McLarty DG, Swai ABM, Kitange HM, et al. Prevalence of diabetes and impaired glucose tolerance in rural Tanzania. *Lancet* 1989;1:871–875.
76. Levitt NS, Unwin NC, Bradshaw D, et al. Application of the new ADA criteria for the diagnosis of diabetes to population studies in sub-Sahara Africa. *Diabet Med* 2000;17:381–385.
77. Burrows NR, Geiss LS, Engelgau MM, et al. Prevalence of diabetes among Native Americans and Alaska Natives, 1990–1997: an increasing burden. *Diabetes Care* 2000;23:1786–1790.
78. Cooper RS, Rotimi CN, Kaufman JS, et al. Prevalence of NIDDM among populations of the African diaspora. *Diabetes Care* 1997;20:343–348.
79. Penrose LS. The genetic background of common diseases. *Acta Genet* 1953; 4:257–265.
80. Risch N. Linkage strategies for genetically complex traits, I: multi-locus models. *Am J Hum Genet* 1990;46:222–228.
81. Pincus G, White P. On the inheritance of diabetes mellitus, II: further analysis of family histories. *Am J Med Sci* 1934;188:159–169.

82. Harris H. The familial distribution of diabetes: a study of the relatives of 1241 diabetic propositi. *Ann Eugenic* 1950;15:95–119.
83. Simpson N. Diabetes in the families of diabetics. *Can Med Assoc J* 1968; 98:427–432.
84. Kobberling J, Tillil H. Empirical risk figures for first degree relatives of non-insulin-dependent diabetics. In: Kobberling J, Tattersall R, eds. *The genetics of diabetes mellitus.* New York: Academic Press, 1982:201–209.
85. Gottlieb MS. Diabetes in offspring and siblings of juvenile and maturity-onset-type diabetics. *J Chronic Dis* 1980;33:331–339.
86. Klein BEK, Klein R, Moss SE, et al. Parental history of diabetes in a population based study. *Diabetes Care* 1996;8:827–830.
87. Karter AJ, Rowell SE, Ackerson LM, et al. Excess maternal transmission of type 2 diabetes: the Northern California Kaiser Permanente Diabetes Registry. *Diabetes Care* 1999; 22:938–943.
88. Meigs JB, Cupples LA, Wilson PWF. Parental transmission of type 2 diabetes mellitus: the Framingham Offspring Study. *Diabetes* 2000;49: 2201–2207.
89. Weijnen CF, Rich SS, Meigs JB, et al. Risk of diabetes in siblings of index cases with type 2 diabetes: implications for genetic studies. *Diabet Med* 2002;19:41–50.
90. Colditz GA, Willett WC, Stampfer MJ, et al. Weight as a risk factor for clinical diabetes in women. *Am J Epidemiol* 1990;132:501–513.
91. Chan JM, Rimm EB, Colditz GA, et al. Obesity, fat distribution, and weight gain as risk factors for clinical diabetes in men. *Diabetes Care* 1994;17:961–969.
92. Hanson RL, Pettitt DJ, Bennett PH, et al. Familial relationship between obesity and NIDDM. *Diabetes* 1995;44:418–422.
93. Morris RD, Rimm DL, Hartz AJ, et al. Obesity and heredity in the etiology of non-insulin-dependent diabetes mellitus in 32,662 adult white women. *Am J Epidemiol* 1989;130:112–121.

CHAPTER 21
Genetics of Type 1 Diabetes

Helena Reijonen and Patrick Concannon

It has long been recognized that certain forms of diabetes cluster within families. In families with type 1 diabetes, the risk of developing disease increases with genetic relatedness to a proband. Defining the underlying mechanisms of genetic susceptibility has been an important goal of research in type 1 diabetes for a number of reasons. Identification of genes that contribute to the risk of type 1 diabetes should provide new insights into the underlying mechanism of disease development and create new opportunities for therapeutic intervention. Definition of the genetic factors that predispose to type 1 diabetes should enhance the ability to predict who in the population may be at risk for type 1 diabetes, and such improved prediction may facilitate the development of novel preventive therapies. For example, the size of clinical trials could be reduced and the risks of therapies with potential side effects could be balanced by increased confidence that a highly specific "at-risk" population was being targeted.

Beginning in the early 1980s, the development of new tools and technologies for genetic-linkage analysis and positional cloning has resulted in the identification of genes underlying many genetic disorders. However, for type 1 diabetes, and indeed for most autoimmune disorders, progress toward identifying the underlying susceptibility genes has been slow. At the heart of this problem is the fact that these disorders share a common complicating factor for genetic studies—their mode of inheritance is unknown. The greatest single risk factor for type 1 diabetes is having an identical (monozygotic) twin with the disorder. However, the concordance rate for monozygotic twins is far less than 100%, with most studies placing the rate in the range of 25% to 50% (1). Concordance rates in monozygotic twins reflect the total familial contribution to risk, some of which will also be environmental, further lessening the expected role of genetic risk factors. This means that environmental factors, familial and nonfamilial, likely account for a significant fraction of the risk of developing type 1 diabetes.

Risk for type 1 diabetes declines as genetic relatedness to a proband in a family declines but remains elevated relative to the population risk in first-, second-, and even third-degree relatives of a proband. The risk to siblings of a proband is not significantly different from that to offspring, suggesting that the genetic variance in type 1 diabetes is additive. Under a strictly additive model, the relationship between genetic relatedness to a proband and risk of type 1 diabetes should be a linear function of the population prevalence. However, an examination of the risk of type 1 diabetes in second- and third-degree relatives suggests a nonlinear relationship. This argues against the possibility that a single locus with reduced penetrance accounts for type 1 diabetes risk and is most consistent with models in which multiple genes combine in an additive fashion to confer risk (2).

The combination of a substantial environmental component to risk and the presumed actions of an unspecified number of genes conspires to obscure the relationship between the genotype at any specific locus and the phenotype of type 1 diabetes. The weakness of this link between the disease phenotype and underlying genotype complicates efforts to define the underlying genetic elements responsible for susceptibility by genetic-linkage approaches. In a linkage-based approach, an investigator searches the genome in a systematic manner, typically by genotyping polymorphic markers spaced at defined intervals, in the hope of identifying markers that cosegregate with disease. Linkage approaches are very powerful and have resulted in the identification of genes responsible for many inherited disorders with known modes of inheritance. However, when applied to a genetically complex disorder, like type 1 diabetes, the inability of the investigator to specify a known mode of inheritance for the disorder can dramatically reduce the power of this approach. As a result, many investigators have turned to other approaches for mapping and identifying type 1 diabetes genes that, while less powerful, are relatively model-independent. The two general categories of approaches that have been used most extensively are those designed to detect allelic association and those that use identity-by-descent methods for the detection of linkage.

GENETIC APPROACHES TO IDENTIFICATION OF SUSCEPTIBILITY GENES IN COMPLEX DISORDERS

Linkage Mapping Approaches

Because of the difficulties in applying traditional parametric approaches for detecting linkage to complex disorders, many investigators have opted for less powerful, but more flexible, nonparametric approaches. As with traditional parametric approaches, a systematic scan of the entire genome using regularly spaced polymorphic markers is carried out. However, the individuals used in these analyses are affected relative pairs—most commonly affected sibling pairs (ASPs). The rationale is that relatives who share a disease phenotype are more likely to share whatever genetic elements act to increase familial aggregation for that phenotype. Thus, the investigator searches for regions of the genome that are more frequently shared among affected relative pairs than would be expected by chance. These approaches to mapping can be carried out with only the affected sibling (sib) pairs. However, substantially greater power to detect linkage can be achieved if parental genotypes are also available either by direct determination or by inference through the genotyping of additional relatives, so that alleles identical by descent can be identified in the affected offspring.

Equally as important as the methodology used for the mapping of susceptibility genes are the criteria used for assessing what constitutes significant evidence of genetic linkage. The strength of the evidence for linkage at a given site in a genome scan is typically reported in the form of a LOD (logarithm of the odds) score, a z score, or a p value. Although these different measures can all be interconverted, there are important distinctions between them. An LOD score is the log-likelihood ratio of the data under the hypothesis that the proportion of alleles shared has the observed value as compared with the hypothesis that there is no excess of allele sharing. Sometimes, this value is reported as a maximized LOD score (MLS), indicating that it has been maximized over a series of parameters. A z score represents the number of standard deviations by which the observed proportion of alleles shared between ASPs exceeds 0.50. The p value represents the chance of the observed deviation in allele sharing under independent assortment. In evaluating such significance measures, it is important to distinguish between locus-specific, or point-wise, significance and genome-wide significance. Point-wise significance refers to the evaluation of a single test of a hypothesis of linkage at one point in the genome. Genome-wide significance requires that results meet a much higher standard since it reflects the evaluation of multiple tests performed at markers spanning the genome (as in a genome scan) to find the most significant results.

Completing a genome-wide scan for linkage in a collection of nuclear families with reasonable power (3) (e.g., 100 to 200) requires a significant effort. Therefore, investigators are anxious to have some positive findings to report. This enthusiasm must, however, be balanced with the recognition that accumulating large numbers of reported linkages that do not reproduce in subsequent studies is counterproductive. Several investigators have suggested guidelines for evaluating the significance of findings in human genome scans that involve a series of thresholds corresponding to the likelihood of observing a given effect on allele sharing due to random chance (4,5). These classifications are as follows: (a) *suggestive linkage* is statistical evidence that would be expected to arise one time at random in a genome-wide scan and corresponds to a p value of 7.4×10^{-4} or, in ASPs, to an MLS or LOD of 2.2; (b) *significant linkage* is statistical evidence expected to arise 0.05 times in a genome-wide scan and corresponds to a p value of 2.2×10^{-5} or an LOD of 3.6; (b) *highly significant linkage* is statistical evidence expected to occur only 0.001 times in a genome-wide scan and corresponds to a p value of 3×10^{-7} or an LOD of 5.4. These guidelines are helpful in evaluating the relative strength of findings of linkage at different sites in the genome and will be used throughout this chapter with these meanings. However, it is important to remember that these are only guidelines; excessive adherence to fixed thresholds for significance may exclude important findings.

A convenient metric for quantitating the contributions of inheritance to risk in genetically complex disorders, such as type 1 diabetes, is the term λ (6), which is the ratio of the risk to an individual with a defined relation to an affected proband to the population risk for a given disorder. For example, for type 1 diabetes in the white population in the United States, the risk to a sibling of an affected proband is approximately 6%, whereas the population risk is approximately 0.4%, yielding a λs value (λ for affected sib pairs) of approximately 15. Higher λ values correspond to greater familial contributions to risk. Thus, complex disorders with higher λ values are more likely to be amenable to genetic-mapping approaches targeted at identifying the genes that contribute to susceptibility. λ can also be used to quantitate the contribution of individual loci by comparing the observed frequency of ASPs who share no parental alleles for a given marker to the expected frequency if inheritance at the locus is random (0.25). Locus-specific λ values, calculated in this way, can be used to rank the contributions of individual loci and, with some assumptions about the way in which different loci might interact, to estimate the contribution of individual loci to the overall λ for the disorder. In addition, λ values can be used as a tool to estimate the power of a study to detect linkage. The number of ASPs necessary to detect a locus of a given effect can be estimated prior to collecting data, and, conversely, the power to exclude linkage for a locus with a given λ value can be calculated for an existing data set.

Association Approaches

Association studies seek to identify alleles at polymorphic markers that are significantly over- or underrepresented among unrelated cases as compared with controls. In the ideal situation, such a result arises because the polymorphism under study is directly involved in disease predisposition. Consequently, association studies tend to focus on specific candidate genes where there is some a priori expectation that the polymorphism under study might affect gene function and that the gene might be involved in the development of type 1 diabetes. A given marker tested by such an approach also may detect association that does not reflect direct involvement of the tested polymorphism in the disease process. Again, in an idealized situation, this result can occur when alleles at the true disease-predisposing locus are either physically close to the marker under study or of recent origin. Such a condition arises when there has not been sufficient time for recombination to randomize the relationship between alleles at the two polymorphic sites. Alleles at such loci are said to be in linkage disequilibrium. The ability to indirectly sample the role of multiple polymorphic loci using a single marker via linkage disequilibrium is a potential advantage of the association approach but also necessitates careful follow-up studies in the event of a positive result to determine where the biologically relevant polymorphisms are located. Allelic association with disease also can arise for spurious reasons, the most common being that there is unrecognized structure in the population being studied such that marker allele frequencies differ between cases and controls at loci that are not linked to a disease-causing polymorphism.

Association studies often are done in a case–control format in which allele frequencies or population frequencies for a marker under study are compared between affected and unaffected populations. The case–control format is appealing because it is relatively easy to ascertain subjects for such a study and the overall number of genotypes required is generally less than for family studies. However, there are also some family-based approaches for detecting allelic association that reduce the risk of errors due to unrecognized structure in the case or control population. These approaches require information from additional unaffected relatives of the cases to establish parental genotypes for the marker under study. These family-based tests fall into two broad categories. One category is typified by the "haplotype relative risk" or HRR approach, in which allele frequencies are compared using the pools of parental alleles (7–9) transmitted or not transmitted to affected offspring as the case and control groups, respectively. The other category includes variants of the transmission/disequilibrium test (TDT), in which actual transmissions from heterozygous parents to affected offspring are tallied on a family-by-family basis (10). The TDT is, in reality, a test for both linkage and association and builds on the fact that, whereas linkage at a given marker can be detected in the absence of association, true association should not occur in the absence of linkage. Family-based methods for association testing are much more resistant to errors arising from population structure. Indeed, on theoretical grounds, the TDT is unaffected by such effects, making it the method of choice in populations in which structure cannot be ruled out (11).

Although a well-designed case–control study with carefully selected subjects should be relatively free from errors arising from population substructure, family-based approaches for detecting association still have definite advantages. In the case of type 1 diabetes, where the disease has a relatively early age at onset, the challenge in obtaining biologic samples from both parents and an affected child ("trios") is much reduced. Currently, the primary applications of association testing are in the evaluation of candidate genes and the narrowing of regions implicated in linkage studies as possibly containing type 1 diabetes susceptibility genes. However, genome-wide association testing is theoretically possible and may ultimately become the preferred approach for mapping genes in complex diseases such as type 1 diabetes (12). Implementation of such an approach is currently limited by the lack of an established method for evaluating the statistical evidence for association at specific sites in the face of the huge volume of tests that would need to be performed to extend such an approach across the genome. In addition, the density of markers required to carry out a comprehensive genome-wide scan for association is theoretically quite large and could potentially overwhelm the laboratory methods currently in use for genotyping (13). However, recent studies indicating that the human genome can be parsed into "haplotype blocks" of relatively modest diversity raise hopes that whole-genome association studies might be accomplished using a selected set of polymorphic markers that effectively tag these blocks (14–17). Such an approach will require the definition of haplotype blocks present in human populations—a haplotype map.

Positional Cloning and Gene Identification

Association-based and linkage-based approaches identify only the regions that may contain susceptibility genes; a significant effort is still required in any such region to determine unambiguously the identity of the gene or genes that contribute to susceptibility. Linkage approaches have some advantages over association studies as an initial screening tool for identifying candidate regions, because linkage can typically be detected over greater distances than can association. However, this strength of linkage-based approaches is a weakness at the next step of gene identification, because the regions that are identified in such studies often span tens of millions of nucleotides and encompass numerous genes. Since it is impossible in a genetically complex disorder to identify families that are truly linked to a particular susceptibility gene and separate them from those that share parental alleles by chance alone, observed recombination events cannot be used to define a more restricted region containing the gene of interest. Indeed, the standard approach to limiting such regions further has been to carry out association studies using markers within the region. In contrast to linkage-based approaches, association studies, if positive, implicate genes within a much narrower physical region, because linkage disequilibrium typically does not extend over large physical distances unless the study population is inbred and/or has passed through a population bottleneck in recent history (13). However, this means that most candidate markers or genes tested for association will return nonpositive results. Because association studies do not provide exclusionary data, they are difficult to apply systematically. Genome-wide linkage disequilibrium or haplotype maps, when available, should help to address this problem (14–17). Ultimately, regardless of the approach taken, genetic information alone will not identify susceptibility genes in a complex disorder such as type 1 diabetes. Biologic studies will usually be required to demonstrate that a given allele or group of alleles has an effect on the function of a gene or its product and that the gene or its product plays a role in the pathogenesis of type 1 diabetes.

THE SEARCH FOR TYPE 1 DIABETES SUSCEPTIBILITY GENES

A relatively large number of chromosomal regions have been implicated as harboring susceptibility genes for type 1 diabetes on the basis of results from genetic linkage or association studies. Two, the HLA and insulin gene regions, are generally accepted and have been designated *IDDM1* and *IDDM2*, respectively. Both *IDDM1* and *IDDM2* were initially identified by association testing in a case–control format (18,19) and subsequently confirmed by linkage studies and further family-based association testing (20–23). A comparison of observed-to-expected allele sharing in ASPs for markers within the HLA region suggests that a substantial fraction (on the order of 50%) of the familial risk for type 1 diabetes is contributed by the inheritance of genes within this region (24). The contribution of the insulin gene region is substantially less and is estimated to account for only 8% to 10% of the familial risk for type 1 diabetes (20). Additional putative type 1 diabetes susceptibility loci designated *IDDM3* to *IDDM15* and *IDDM18* have been defined on the basis of increased allele sharing in ASPs or from evidence of genetic association obtained by TDT analyses in similar collections of families. The *IDDM17* locus was defined on the basis of linkage studies in a single large pedigree (25). Finally, several additional chromosomal regions, Xp13–p11, 16q22–24, and 1q42, are reported to show suggestive to significant evidence of linkage to type 1 diabetes in genome scans but have not been assigned "IDDM" designations (26–28).

Five genome-wide scans for linkage to type 1 diabetes in ASPs have been reported. The studies of Davies et al. (24) and Hashimoto et al. (29) were the first such scans completed in any genetically complex disorder. Data analysis in these studies was performed by two-point evaluation of allele-sharing data at each marker. Larger subsequent genome scans completed by Mein et al. (26) and Concannon et al. (27) partially overlapped these earlier studies in the families used but used more informative multipoint approaches for assessing the evidence for linkage, as did a completely independent genome scan in Scandinavian families by Nerup et al. (30). The results from these genome-wide scans have been interpreted as suggesting the existence of numerous susceptibility loci for type 1 diabetes in humans. However, for many of these putative loci, the evidence for linkage in the initial reports did not attain a genome-wide significance level. Subsequent follow-up studies have, in some cases, been supportive of initial reports and, in other cases, negative. This inconsistency in the findings of different studies is a significant impediment to efforts to identify the relevant genes that contribute to susceptibility. Because fine mapping of such linked regions cannot proceed by analysis of observed recombination events, the currently accepted method of localizing susceptibility genes in such regions is to methodically test genetic markers spanning the region at high density in the hope of detecting evidence of allelic association with disease. The labor involved in performing such an analysis in even one suspected region is immense, especially because the confidence intervals for such regions are typically quite broad. Obviously, an investigator wants to apply such an approach only in those regions for which the supporting evidence is the strongest. This requires some prioritization of potential target regions based on the evidence for linkage. When independent genome-wide scans report largely nonoverlapping sets of putative linked loci, their utility for prioritizing these sites for further study is limited.

Two approaches to evaluating the significance of findings of linkage in complex diseases such as type 1 diabetes are to carry out either confirmation or extension studies. The first of these approaches, confirmation studies, relies on independent replication to strengthen the evidence for linkage. Since even when there is no linked disease susceptibility locus, a statistically significant finding will occur with a frequency of 5%, confirmation studies can play an important role by testing the reproducibility of such findings. Unlike the initial report of linkage, it may not be necessary to hold a confirmation study to the same level of statistical significance. Simulations indicate that to have sufficient power to attain replication at a genome-wide level of significance, a confirmation study might have to use impracticably large sample sizes (31). Therefore, a more appropriate standard may be to require a locus-specific significance level for a replication ($p = 0.01$). When an initial finding is only suggestive of linkage, then the second approach, extension studies, in which data from all studies are merged and jointly analyzed, is more appropriate until such a locus attains a genome-wide significance level (4).

Both confirmation and extension studies involve the joint analysis of data from multiple sources. A difficulty with both approaches is the challenge of making the analyses as inclusive as possible. Published data will tend to be selected for positive results. There is always a danger that negative results that might substantially affect the outcome of such analyses may not be incorporated simply because they are not reported. For extension studies, the ideal approach is to pool the raw data and carry out a single analysis. In the case of two-point analyses of allele sharing, it is possible to add reported results from different studies together in an extension study. In general, the same practice cannot be used with multipoint LOD scores except in the rare event that the independent studies that are to be merged all used the same markers, genetic maps, and methods for analysis. While two-point analyses of linkage data at specific markers allow relatively easy pooling across studies, multipoint analysis methods can extract substantially greater linkage information from a comparable collection of families. Therefore, caution is appropriate in considering significance levels reported from extension or replication studies that exclude data obtained by one method or the other.

The following sections summarize the evidence supporting the existence of reported "IDDM" loci in humans as well as some additional regions implicated by linkage studies but lacking such official designations. It is important to keep in mind that although these regions have been given locus designations, which may include the name of the most "interesting" candidate gene, in most cases what is being discussed is not a specific locus but a large chromosomal region that may contain hundreds of genes, any one or combination of which might contribute to disease susceptibility. The cytogenetic localizations provided for each of these regions are, therefore, just estimates and are taken from the relevant publications reporting the putative loci.

IDDM1 (6p21.3)

Identification of HLA Associations with Type 1 Diabetes

The first evidence of allelic association between the HLA complex and type 1 diabetes was reported for the HLA-B15 allele and was based on serology (32). In subsequent studies, a positive association of type 1 diabetes with HLA-B8 and a negative association with B7 were established (33,34). Higher risks were shown to be associated with HLA class II specificities, namely DR3 and DR4, whereas DR2 (now renamed DR15) was suggested to be involved in protection (35). DR3 is in linkage disequilibrium with B8, and DR4 is in disequilibrium with B15. More than 90% of white patients with type 1 diabetes have DR3 and/or DR4 as compared with 40% to 50% of controls (35). The greatest risk of type 1 diabetes is conferred by the simultaneous presence of DR3 and DR4, which are found together in 30% to 50% of patients (36,37) but in only 1% to 6% of controls. These associations with HLA antigens were defined initially by serologic or cellular typing methods. Restriction fragment length polymorphism (RFLP), allele-specific oligonucleotide typing, and direct nucleotide sequencing subsequently enabled the specific identification of genes associated with risk for type 1 diabetes. These molecular studies indicated that the primary susceptibility genes are situated in the HLA-DQ rather than the DR region (a schematic map of the HLA gene region is shown in Fig. 21.1). In most populations studied, the HLA alleles most strongly associated with type 1 diabetes are DQB1*0302 and/or DQB1*0201, which are in linkage disequilibrium with DRB1*0401 and DRB1*0301, respectively. (By convention, HLA alleles are named with a four-character alphanumeric code indicating the locus, followed by an asterisk and a four-digit number indicating the specific allele at that locus. For example DQB1*0302 refers to a specific polymorphic allele, 0302, at the DQB1 locus that encodes the β chain of the heterodimeric HLA-DQ molecule.)

HLA-DQ and HLA-DR as Predisposing Alleles for Type 1 Diabetes

Although numerous studies have emphasized the primary role of HLA-DQ in predisposition to type 1 diabetes (36,38), the involvement of HLA-DR loci cannot be excluded (39–52). The DR4-DQA1*0301-DQB1*0302 haplotype is associated with sus-

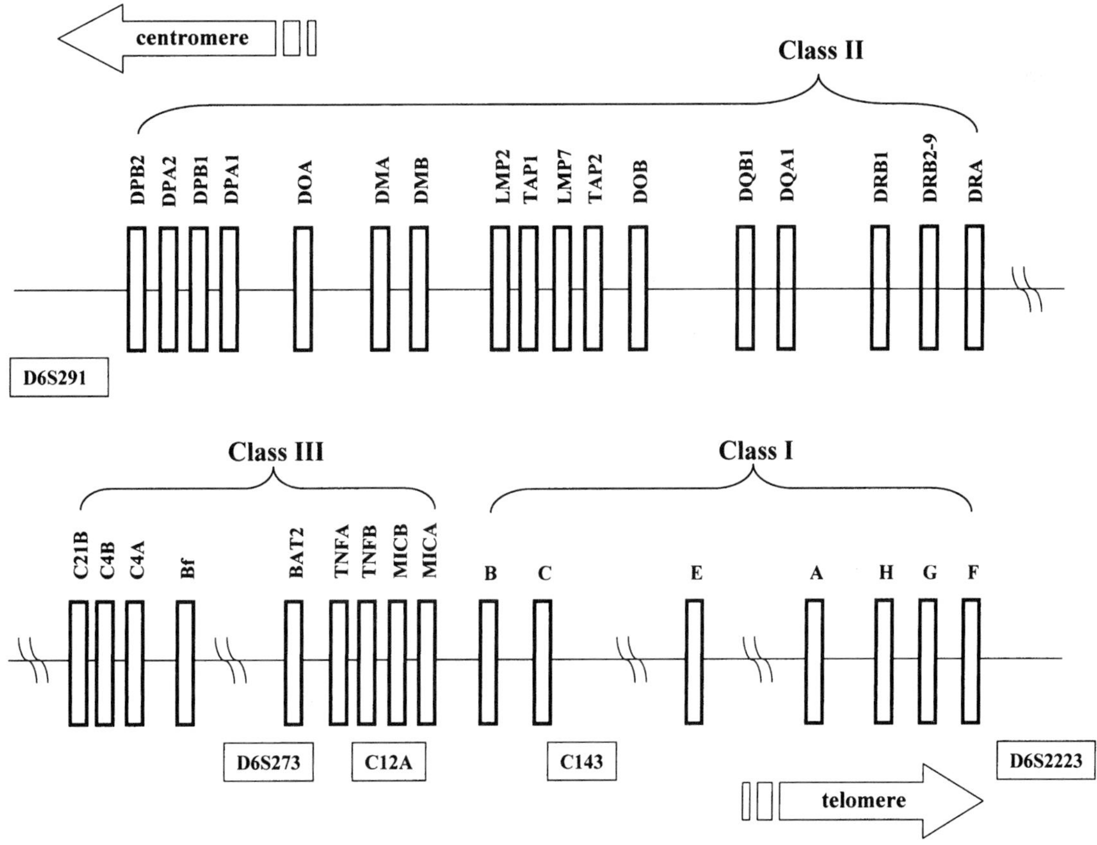

Figure 21.1. A map of the HLA region. The HLA region covers ~3,500 kilobase of chromosome 6p21.3. The HLA genes are divided into three groups. HLA class II genes encode α- and β-chains of the class II antigen-presenting molecules. HLA class I genes encode the α-polypeptide chain of the class I molecules, while the β-chain is encoded on chromosome 15 by the β-microglobulin gene. The genes in the HLA class III region encode complement proteins, some cytokines, and additional enzymes. The genes in the HLA class I and II regions are highly polymorphic, with the exception of *DRBA,* which is nonpolymorphic. Alleles of the genes are indicated by a four-digit number followed by an asterisk. The map shows only selected HLA genes among the ~150 genes mapped to the region. The distances between the loci are approximate. Microsatellite markers are shown as framed.

ceptibility to type 1 diabetes in most populations studied (36,41–43), but certain DR4 haplotypes are more prevalent among patients as compared with controls, suggesting a role for both DR and DQ molecules in the pathogenic process. Likewise, studies in the nonobese diabetic (NOD) mouse, a rodent model of type 1 diabetes, suggest that more than one gene in the major histocompatibility complex (the mouse equivalent of HLA) contributes to diabetes susceptibility (see Chapter 18 for detailed discussion of the NOD mouse model). DRB1*0401, 0402, and 0405 are positively associated with type 1 diabetes, whereas DRB1*0403 is not, even though these alleles all occur on haplotypes in conjunction with DQB1*0302 (39–42,44–47). In Scandinavian populations, the DRB1*0404-DQB1*0302 haplotype is decreased in frequency among patients (48–50). In the Oriental populations, the DRB1*0406-DQA1*0301-DQB1*0302 haplotype is negatively associated with type 1 diabetes (42,51–54). The role of all DR4 haplotypes cannot be jointly evaluated in a single population because the frequency of DR4 subtypes varies considerably in different ethnic groups and some haplotypes are very rare. For example, in Scandinavia, almost all DR4 haplotypes carry the DRB1*0401 or 0404 alleles, while DRB1*0406 is observed at high frequency only in the Oriental populations. Nevertheless, based on transracial association data, the DRB1*04 alleles can be ranked in the following order with respect to risk of type 1 diabetes: DRB1*0405 = 0402 = 401 > 404 > 403 ~ 0406 (48).

HLA-Encoded Protection

The DRB1*1501-DQA1*0102-DQB1*0602 haplotype is negatively associated with type 1 diabetes across multiple ethnic groups, whereas the DRB1*1301-DQA1*0103-DQB1*0603 haplotype is associated with reduced susceptibility (41,42,55). DQB1*0602 and 0603 differ only at amino acid position 30, whereas DQA1*0102 and DQA1*0103 differ only at amino acid positions 25 and 41 (56). The apparent protection from type 1 diabetes conferred by DQB1*0602 and 0603 appears to be dominant in nature (38,57–59). No patient with type 1 diabetes homozygous for DQB1*0602 or 0603 has been described so far. However, the protection conferred by these DQ alleles is not absolute, as patients positive for DQB1*0602 allele have been described (60–63). In these patients, the other DQB1 allele is typically one that is associated with high risk of disease. Another DQB1 allele that is also reduced in frequency among patients with type 1 diabetes in some populations is DQB1*0301 (36), although the protection observed with this allele is neither as global nor as significant as with DQB1*0602 and 0603. The negative association with DQB1*0301 is most prominent when it is present on DRB1*1101 haplotypes. However, it is also seen with those DR*04 haplotypes that confer susceptibility, suggesting that one protective DQ allele on a haplotype can neutralize any predisposing effect (46,47).

HLA Associations with Type 1 Diabetes in Different Ethnic Populations

The frequencies of HLA alleles and their haplotypic combinations differ greatly across various ethnic groups (41,64). There is also variance in the haplotypes associated with type 1 diabetes. For example, the DRB1*0405-DQA1*0301-DQB1*0302, DRB1*0405-DQA1*0301-DQB1*0401, and DRB1*0802-DQA1*0301-DQB1*0302 haplotypes are positively associated with type 1 diabetes in the Japanese population, whereas DRB1*0406-DQA1*0301-DQB1*0302 has a negative association (42,51,54). DR9 is positively associated with type 1 diabetes both in the Oriental populations and in populations of African descent, but these haplotypes differ in their DQB1 loci (42,53,65). In Orientals, DR9 haplotypes carry DQA1*0301-DQB1*0303 (as in white populations), whereas in Africans, DR9 is linked with DQA1 *301-DQB1*0201. DR7 is increased only in patients of African descent with type 1 diabetes (66). This particular haplotype carries the DQA1*0301 allele, which is positively associated with disease, whereas DR7 in whites is in linkage disequilibrium with the disease-neutral DQA1*0201 allele.

The strength of DRB1*0301 as a risk allele varies among populations; DR3-associated susceptibility is stronger in southern as compared with northern Europeans. In the latter group, DRB1*0301-DQB1*0201 haplotypes alone do not confer an increased risk for type 1 diabetes, and no excess of homozygotes for this haplotype is observed among patients (67). However, in Sardinia, the major susceptibility haplotype is DRB1*0301-DQA1*0501-DQB1*0201, and homozygosity for this haplotype is significantly increased among patients (68). In the Japanese population, the DRB1*0301-DQB1*0201 haplotype is rare (42,69). In the Chinese population, DR3/9 heterozygosity is strongly associated with type 1 diabetes (70,71). This is most likely due to the low frequency of risk-associated DR4 subtypes in this population. These differences in HLA haplotype frequencies in the general population may help explain the low disease incidence in these ethnic groups.

Synergistic Effects on Risk Associated with Heterozygous Combinations of HLA Alleles

The greatest HLA-encoded risk of type 1 diabetes is conferred by the simultaneous presence of DQA1*0301-DQB1*0302 and DQA1*0501-DQB1*0201 (40,67). This combination of haplotypes is found in ~40% of the patients, whereas the frequency in healthy controls is only 3%. The increased risk associated with heterozygosity for these two haplotypes is inconsistent with a simple additive effect. One proposed explanation is that this genotypic combination might facilitate the formation of heterodimers between the α- and β-chains that are encoded by alleles present on different parental chromosomes in *trans* (72–74). Because both the α- and β-chains of DQ molecules display allelic polymorphism, potentially four distinct DQ molecules can be formed in a heterozygous individual. While it has been demonstrated that these *trans*-dimers can be formed and are very stable, no T cells restricted by these molecules have been isolated from DQB1*0302/0201 heterozygous individuals with type 1 diabetes (75,76). The heterodimers encoded in *trans* in heterozygous individuals are DQA1*0301-DQB1*0201 and DQA1*0501-DQB1*0302. The former is encoded in *cis* on DR7 and DR9 haplotypes that are common among patients of African descent with type 1 diabetes (55,77). A second possible explanation for the increased risk associated with DQB1*0302/0201 heterozygosity is that it reflects the effects of additional genes beyond DQ. These might be other HLA class II genes known to have an effect on susceptibility, such as DR or DP, or even genes within the HLA complex that do not encode antigen-presenting molecules. As discussed below, such effects often are attributed to the HLA-DR3 haplotype that is associated with many different autoimmune disorders beyond type 1 diabetes.

Effects of Genes outside the HLA-DR-DQ Region and the Natural History of the Disease

As discussed above, other genes within the HLA region may make important contributions to susceptibility to type 1 diabetes by modifying the risk conferred by DR or DQ alleles or independently of their role. The tight linkage disequilibrium that exists between different polymorphic HLA genes complicates the identification of primary risk-conferring genes in association studies. Transracial studies and analysis of ancestral haplotypes have been valuable tools in mapping genes in the HLA region with potential roles in disease susceptibility. The recent use of microsatellite markers in linkage studies with well-matched patients and controls has suggested the existence of additional genes within the HLA region that may be involved in disease predisposition.

Several studies have reported associations between class I alleles and the natural history of type 1 diabetes [e.g., faster progression and earlier onset of the disease in patients who are positive for the HLA-A24 (78–80) or B18 haplotypes (81,82)]. A strong correlation between complete loss of residual β-cell function and the presence of HLA-A24 has been reported among Japanese patients (83). The B18-DR3-DQB1*0201 haplotype has been associated with a higher disease risk than the B8-DR3-DQB1*0201 haplotype (81,84). A30-B18-DR3-DQB1*0201 confers an independent association with type 1 diabetes, as homozygosity for it is enough to increase risk (68), whereas A1-B8-DR3-DQB1*0201 confers significant susceptibility only when it is present together with DR4-DQB1*0302. Analyzing DR3-B8 and DR3-B18 ancestral haplotypes, Degli-Esposti and colleagues (85) predicted that the region between HLA-B and the BAT2 loci could contain a gene or genes that contributed to risk for type 1 diabetes. A role of HLA-B alleles (or a gene in the region surrounding the HLA-B locus) also was suggested in a study in which HLA-B39 was shown to be increased in DRB1*0404-positive disease-associated haplotypes (49,50).

Recent studies on extended DR3 or DR4 haplotypes using dense sets of microsatellite markers suggested that at least two different genes in the HLA region beside the DQ and DR loci could be involved in disease susceptibility. A Belgian case–control study with DQB1*0302/0201-positive subjects tested for association with eight microsatellite markers spanning a region extending from 6-centiMorgan (cM) telomeric of HLA-F to 2-cM centromeric of HLA-DP. The study provided evidence for an association of one additional region with type 1 diabetes beside DQ. This region mapped near the microsatellite locus D6S273, just centromeric of tumor necrosis factor (86). This finding was confirmed in a northern white/British family study using a variant of the TDT called "homozygous parent TDT analysis." In this approach, transmissions of marker alleles from heterozygous parents are tallied only in families in which the parents are homozygous for known type 1 diabetes susceptibility alleles (DRB, DQA, and DQB) (87). An independent study of Finnish patients and controls stratified for DRB1*0401/301 or DRB1*0404/301 suggested that a genomic region near HLA-B contributes to diabetes susceptibility (88). The 240-kilobase (kb) region between C12A and C143 mapped in this study included the HLA-B, HLA-C, MICA, and MICB genes, as well as the less well-characterized P5-1 3.8-1.1 genes (89). The regions identified in these various microsatellite marker studies may well overlap, since the boundaries of the regions are not clearly defined with the markers utilized. Both sets of studies, when considered together with the previous data on ancestral haplotypes, suggest that there is an unrecognized diabetes susceptibility gene that maps to the centromeric end of the class I region near HLA-B.

A second region reported to display positive association with type 1 diabetes independent of the class II genes has been localized telomeric to the class I region (87). The allelic association in this region is detected with the microsatellite marker D6S2223, which is located 2.5-kb telomeric to HLA-F. This study also used the homozygous parent TDT in 225 selected families. The observed association was further confirmed in cases and controls matched for DR and DQ alleles. Presence of allele 3 at the D6S2223 loci appeared to decrease the risk conferred by the DR3-DQA1*0501-DQB1*0201 haplotype. This supports the notion that there is heterogeneity in DR3-positive haplotypes in their contribution to diabetes risk, as discussed above. It is interesting that the same microsatellite polymorphism also was found to display a similar association with celiac disease, another DR3-associated disorder (90). Further analyses will be required to determine if a gene or genes in this region contribute to diabetes susceptibility and whether it has a broader predisposing effect in autoimmunity.

The *TAP1* and *TAP2* genes in the class II region encode a heterodimeric molecule that is involved in the transport of peptides into the endoplasmic reticulum, where they are bound by class I molecules. The TAP protein is required for efficient loading and presentation of peptides in class I molecules and thus is an attractive candidate gene for diabetes susceptibility. Other candidate loci in the same region centromeric to DQ are LMP2/7 and DMA/B that encode proteins involved in antigen processing and the loading of peptides onto class II molecules, respectively. TAP1 and TAP2 polymorphisms have been extensively studied, and positive associations have been reported between TAP2 alleles and type 1 diabetes, but these associations appear to be secondary to DQ (91–96). An independent positive association of LMP2 and LMP7 with diabetes has been described in a case–control study in patients in the United States (97), while other reports have been negative (98,99). The association of LMP2 and/or LMP7 polymorphisms with type 1 diabetes also was studied using TDT analysis in Norwegian and British white families, but, once again, no independent association was observed (100,101). There is similar controversy with regard to the independent association of DMA and DMB with diabetes. No primary association between DMA or DMB and type 1 diabetes was found in a French case–control study (102). This was confirmed in an Italian study that analyzed transmission of DQA-DQB-TAP2-DMB haplotypes in affected individuals in type 1 diabetes families (103). In contrast, a German case–control study described a positive association of DMB*0101 and a negative association of DMA*0102 with diabetes (104). In this study, the patients and controls were stratified only for DQA1*0501. Therefore, association due to linkage to DQ could not be excluded.

Studies of HLA-DP alleles have provided evidence both for and against an independent role of DP in predisposition to type 1 diabetes. A positive association between DPB1*0301 and diabetes has been described in some white populations (105–107) and DPB1*0201 in the Japanese population (108). However, in other studies no significant difference in the distribution of DP alleles was observed between patients and controls (42,109,110).

Summary of the Role of Genes within the HLA Region in Susceptibility to Type 1 Diabetes

Allelic associations between type 1 diabetes and genes within the HLA complex were first observed more than 20 years ago, and these associations have been confirmed in numerous case–control and linkage studies since then. The strong linkage disequilibrium that exists between the polymorphic sites within the HLA complex has hampered the identification of the genes that are primarily involved in disease susceptibility or protection. However, most studies have shown that DQB1*0302 as a single allele confers a higher risk than DRB1*04, although a modifying effect of the *DRB1* gene is obvious in the haplotypes that represent different DRB1*04 subtypes. Positive association of the DRB1*03-DQA1*0501-DQB1*0201 haplotype with diabetes might be due to DRB1*03 or another, still unknown, gene linked to it. Since the presence of the DR3 haplotype predisposes to many autoimmune disorders, this association may not be specific for type 1 diabetes but could be related to a more general dysfunction in immune regulation. HLA-encoded protection is generally dominant over susceptibility. Protective effects of the alleles DQB1*0602 or 0603 and DRB1*403 or 406 can be seen across ethnic populations, whereas the frequency and strength of the most common risk-associated alleles, DQB1*0302 and 0201, vary in different populations. In most populations, ~75% to 90% of the patients are positive for DQB1*0302, which apparently is the predominant susceptibility allele, whereas the DR3-DQB1*0201 haplotype seems to be a more minor predisposing genetic factor. However, the presence of these two haplotypes together greatly amplifies the risk of type 1 diabetes.

IDDM2 (11p15.5)

Genetic association between type 1 diabetes and a polymorphic region located immediately 5′ of the insulin gene was first reported in a case–control study in 1984 (19). The marker used was a "variable number of tandem repeats" (VNTR) polymorphism consisting of many copies of a 14-nucleotide repeat. Initial studies classed these alleles into three groups—short (class I), intermediate (class II), and long (class III)—based on the size of the repeated region. The short class I alleles were observed to be associated with type 1 diabetes.

The finding of an association between class I alleles of the insulin VNTR polymorphism and type 1 diabetes suggested that a gene or genes in the region contributed to disease susceptibility. Because the VNTR did not obviously affect the coding region of any known gene, additional polymorphisms in and around the insulin gene and the flanking insulin-like growth factor and tyrosine hydroxylase genes were identified and tested for linkage and association with type 1 diabetes (111). These polymorphic sites all displayed similar degrees of association with type 1 diabetes in cases and controls (22). Stratification of cases by HLA type suggested higher relative risks associated with homozygosity at these insulin gene polymorphisms in patients who had the HLA-DR4 haplotype. Assays of transmissions of insulin alleles from heterozygous parents in multiplex families revealed an excess of transmission of alleles at two markers, the 5′ insulin VNTR and a *Pst*I RFLP, specifically to $DR4^+$ affected individuals. This effect was significant only for paternal transmissions, raising the possibility that imprinting, which is known to occur in this region of chromosome 11, might play a role in susceptibility to type 1 diabetes through an effect on *IDDM2*. These studies have been interpreted as mapping the *IDDM2* locus to a region of 4.1 kb surrounding the insulin gene, although alternative interpretations have been proposed (111,112).

The 4.1-kb region flanking the insulin gene contains four candidate polymorphisms that exist in near-complete linkage disequilibrium (22). Three of these polymorphisms are biallelic, whereas the fourth, the 5′ VNTR polymorphism, is characterized by variation both in the length of individual repeats and in their nucleotide sequences. Bennett et al. (20) carried out a detailed analysis of the association between marker haplotypes at *IDDM2* and type 1 diabetes. They identified specific marker haplotypes that were either predisposing or protective for type 1 diabetes and concluded, on the basis of a comparison of the alleles at various markers present on these haplotypes, that susceptibility to type 1 diabetes at the *IDDM2* locus mapped to the VNTR polymorphism itself. Similar results were reported by Owerbach and Gabbay (113). Subdivision of the pool of class I alleles at the VNTR revealed that, although the alleles in this size class were generally associated with susceptibility to type 1 diabetes, there were differences in the frequencies with which specific alleles were transmitted to affected offspring in multiplex families. Whether these differences reflect specific predisposing or protective effects of different allele sizes or random variation in the analyses due to small sample sizes remains unresolved (113–115).

The strong statistical evidence of association between type 1 diabetes and alleles of the insulin VNTR polymorphism suggests that variation at that site contributes to disease susceptibility; a biologic mechanism is then required to explain this effect. By examining the pancreatic expression of the insulin gene in individuals heterozygous for a polymorphism within the gene, Bennett et al. (20) demonstrated that, although expression was biallelic, the ratio of transcripts from each allele varied with the identity of the insulin VNTR alleles present. Kennedy et al. (116) further demonstrated that the VNTR region was active as a transcriptional regulator in pancreatic β-cells. However, the two studies reported discordant results as to which class of VNTR alleles was associated with increased transcription of the insulin gene in islets. Since insulin is a known β-cell autoantigen in type 1 diabetes, variation in expression level or in the tissue specificity of transcription could play a role in regulating induction of immunologic tolerance independent of expression in islet cells. Consistent with this possibility, two studies have reported transcription of the insulin gene in the thymus (117,118). In both cases, the protective class III VNTR alleles were associated with increased steady-state levels of insulin messenger RNA (mRNA) in the thymus. These studies suggest a model for the role of the insulin gene VNTR in type 1 diabetes susceptibility in which negative selection of insulin-specific autoreactive T cells depends on the overall expression level of insulin in the thymus.

IDDM3 (15q26)

Using the approach of linkage mapping in ASPs, Field et al. (119) defined the *IDDM3* locus on chromosome 15q26 on the basis of increased allele sharing at the microsatellite marker D15S107. In 250 families of Canadian ($N = 25$), British ($N = 100$), or American ($N = 125$) origin, the maximum two-point LOD score was 2.54. Most evidence for linkage at D15S107 appeared to derive from families in which affected sibs did not share HLA-DR alleles, suggesting the possibility of genetic heterogeneity.

Multiple follow-up studies have tested for linkage with type 1 diabetes at *IDDM3*. Two-point analyses of allele sharing at D15S107 failed to provide significant supporting evidence (120–122), although modestly increased allele sharing was observed in two of three studies. Summing the sharing data from individual nonoverlapping follow-up studies provides only modest supporting evidence for *IDDM3* ($p = 0.05$) (120). Multipoint analysis of linkage data from genome-wide scans in collections of American or British families overlapping with those used to originally define *IDDM3* similarly provides little supporting evidence (26,27). In one study, a locus with $\lambda s \geq 1.5$ could be excluded from the region with a LOD of −3.6 (27).

IDDM4 (11q13)

Three independent studies reported initial evidence for a type 1 diabetes susceptibility locus on chromosome 11q that was designated *IDDM4*. Davies et al. (24) reported evidence of increased allele sharing for a marker near the *FGF3* (fibroblast growth factor 3) gene from a genome-wide scan of 96 UK families with type 1 diabetes. Hashimoto et al. (29) reported similar evidence for the same marker in a collection of French and U.S. families. Both groups used a two-stage approach in which they carried out their genome-wide scan in a subset of their available families and then genotyped only markers displaying increased allele sharing in a second set of families. Field et al. (119) also reported evidence of linkage at *FGF3* in their report describing *IDDM3*. In none of these reports did the evidence for linkage attain a genome-wide significance level. Summing the raw allele-sharing data across these initial studies and excluding possible overlapping families, the evidence still attains only a p value of 0.01. All three initial studies further stratified the families studied by HLA sharing and by the presence of specific HLA-DR alleles but with conflicting results. In the first report, the evidence for linkage was contributed largely by those families sharing one or zero parental alleles (24), whereas in the second, the evidence for linkage came from those families sharing two parental alleles at HLA (29). The third report saw no significant effect from HLA stratification (119). These discordant results raise the question of whether such stratified analyses are actually helpful as a tool for initial identification of linked regions or are more appropriate as a method for further investigation of already confirmed findings. Repeated analyses under different models of gene–gene interaction will tend to increase the possibility of obtaining false-positive results.

Several confirmation studies have been performed in the *IDDM4* region. Luo et al. (120) summed the allele sharing across multiple studies, including their own, to obtain a MLS of 5.0 in the *IDDM4* region. Some caution in the interpretation of this value is warranted, however, because two of the sets of data included in this meta-analysis contain families from the same collection and may overlap. Also, these data are from two-point analyses that were summed despite their not having been performed with the same markers. Nevertheless, even if previously published data are eliminated and the analysis is confined to only those families genotyped by Luo et al., a significant MLS value of 3.9 is obtained.

Fine-mapping of the *IDDM4* region has provided some evidence for allelic association within the region with several markers. In an international study of 707 ASPs, an MLS of 2.7 was reported in the *IDDM4* region (123). Furthermore, there was evidence of decreased transmission of a specific haplotype of two markers in the region to affected offspring in families ($p = 4.3 \times 10^{-4}$). Additional evidence of association with alleles of a microsatellite marker in the region, D11S987, was reported by Eckenrode et al. (124), who also tested for, but failed to detect, allelic associations with polymorphisms within two candidate genes, Fas-associated death domain and galanin.

More recently, multipoint analyses of two large genome scans that together scanned more than 750 independent families failed to provide any significant evidence of linkage to *IDDM4* (MLS = 0.5 and MLS = 0.43) (26,27).

IDDM5 (6q25–q27)

IDDM5 was originally identified on the basis of modestly increased allele sharing at the marker ESR (MLS = 1.5) located on the long arm of chromosome 6 (24). Stratification by either HLA sharing or the presence of specific HLA-DR alleles did not increase the evidence for linkage. In an extension study, Davies et al. (125) genotyped additional markers in this region and performed multipoint analyses. The increased linkage information afforded by these two approaches strengthened the evidence for linkage (MLS = 2.42). However, further extension of these results through the addition of data from a second genome scan reduced the evidence of linkage to an MLS of 1.3 (26). One independent confirmation study provided significant two-point evidence of linkage at ESR (MLS = 4.5) (120). However, an independent genome scan that used multipoint analyses of genotyping data from a set of families overlapping with those used in this report did not find significant evidence of linkage in this region (MLS = 1.46) (27).

IDDM6 (18q21)

A potential susceptibility locus for type 1 diabetes on chromosome 18q12–q21 was originally suggested in 1981 on the basis of evidence of genetic linkage at the Kidd blood group locus (126). The original type 1 diabetes genome scan by Davies et al. (24) revealed modest but not significant evidence of linkage in this region (MLS = 1.1). A large-scale extension study using data from 1,457 families did not greatly strengthen the evidence for linkage (MLS = 1.6) (127). Nevertheless, a search for association with common alleles at various microsatellite markers in the region by TDT was carried out in the same set of families, providing nominally significant evidence of linkage disequilibrium after correction for multiple testing ($p = 0.036$). Addition of more families to this analysis (to a total of 1,708) and testing for association with specific marker haplotypes modestly increased the strength of the allelic association in this region ($p = 0.01$) (128). Neither of two large genome scans analyzed by multipoint methods yielded significant evidence of linkage at *IDDM6* (26,27).

IDDM7 (2q31–q33)

Like *IDDM6*, the *IDDM7* locus corresponds to a region where modest evidence of linkage to type 1 diabetes was observed in an early genome scan (24) and that was followed up by association testing using TDT. No study to date has reported significant or even suggestive evidence of linkage at *IDDM7*, with the highest reported MLS in any study being 1.53 (129). However, later studies of the chromosome 2q regions assigned two additional loci to this region, *IDDM12* and *IDDM13*. The relationship between these three loci that cluster within a 20- to 30-cM region is unclear. A joint multipoint analysis of linkage data from several genome scans in ASPs of U.S. and U.K. origin revealed a single peak on 2q with an MLS of 2.62 that may reflect the effects of one or more of these loci (130).

In the case of *IDDM7*, the primary evidence supporting its existence has come from association studies. In the initial description of *IDDM7*, there was evidence of allelic association with type 1 diabetes at the marker D2S152, but only in certain populations (e.g., patients from the United States but not from the United Kingdom) and only prior to correction for multiple testing. A subsequent focused test for association at just the implicated allele of D2S152 in 1,551 families provided nominally significant evidence of association ($p = 0.05$) (131). Studies by other groups have reported similarly modest results. Evidence of association was reported in Danish families ($p = 0.034$) (132). However, there was no evidence in independent studies of U.S. families (133) or of Basque families (134). Case–control studies of U.S. and of Chinese patients also failed to reveal evidence of association (133).

IDDM8 (6q25–q27)

In addition to the evidence of linkage at ESR (*IDDM5*), a second marker on chromosome 6q, D6S264, provided some modest evidence of linkage in the initial genome scan of Davies et al. (24) (MLS = 1.2). These data were extended by Luo et al. (121), who obtained an MLS of 2.0 at D6S264 and an MLS of 2.8 at a nearby marker, D6S281, in an independent set of families. When the two-point linkage data at D6S264 from these studies were added together, the MLS was suggestive of linkage (MLS = 3.4), and this region was designated *IDDM8*. A further extension study by Luo et al. (120) resulted in significant two-point evidence of linkage at D6S281 (MLS = 3.6). Neither of two subsequently reported genome scans analyzed by multipoint methods yielded even suggestive evidence of linkage at *IDDM8* (MLS = 1.9 and MLS = 1.14) (26,27). However, when data from these genome scans are merged and jointly analyzed, there is increased evidence for linkage in the *IDDM8* region in families in which both ASPs have early age at onset (130). In addition, a linkage disequilibrium study of the *IDDM8* region reported that several marker haplotypes in the region displayed preferential transmission to affected offspring by TDT (uncorrected $p = 0.01$) (135).

IDDM9 (3q22–q25)

IDDM9 was defined on the basis of increased allele sharing at the marker D3S1303 after stratification by HLA sharing in the initial genome scan in type 1 diabetes by Davies et al. (24). The highest reported MLS in the region in any study is 1.1, although HLA-stratified analyses have yielded LOD scores as high as 2.4 (26).

IDDM10 (10p11–q11)

In the genome scan of Davies et al. (24), an MLS of 1.3 was detected at the marker D10S193 at 10p11. An extension study incorporating data from 312 families and multipoint analysis increased the evidence for linkage in the region (MLS = 2.44) (136). TDT analyses with microsatellite markers in the region, or with a marker immediately flanking the *GAD65* gene (137), failed to reveal significant evidence of association after correction for multiple testing. A further extension study incorporating data from 356 families from the United Kingdom provided significant evidence of linkage in the *IDDM10* region (MLS = 4.7) (26). There was little evidence of linkage in a comparable study of U.S. families (MLS = 0.4) (27). However, when data from these latter two genome scans are merged and analyzed together, there is suggestive evidence of linkage in the *IDDM10* region (MLS = 2.8) (130).

IDDM11 (14q24.3–q31)

Significant two-point evidence of linkage was reported at the marker D14S67 in a study of 254 multiplex type 1 diabetes families (MLS = 4.02), defining the *IDDM11* locus (138). All of the evidence for linkage appeared to derive from the subset of families with 50% or fewer sharing of HLA alleles. No other study has reported significant evidence of linkage in this region, including two other genome scans that together incorporated 225 of the 254 families used in the initial report (26,27).

IDDM12 (2q33)

Studies in the NOD mouse model of type 1 diabetes have localized a putative susceptibility locus, *Idd5*, to proximal mouse chromosome 1, a region that is homologous with the long arm of human chromosome 2 (139,140). On the basis of this observation, Nistico et al. (141) tested for linkage or association between markers in the 2q33 region and type 1 diabetes. In a set of 48 Italian families, they observed suggestive evidence of linkage at the marker D2S72 (MLS = 3.39). However, in larger collections of families from the United Kingdom ($N = 284$), Sardinia ($N = 123$), and the United States ($N = 180$), there was no evidence of linkage at D2S72. D2S72 is located close to the *CTLA4* gene, an appealing candidate for a type 1 diabetes susceptibility gene due to its role in regulating cellular immune responses. A biallelic polymorphism (A/G, Thr/Ala) of unknown functional consequences located in the leader peptide of CTLA-4 was analyzed by TDT within type 1 diabetes families. Preferential transmission of the "G" allele of this marker to affected individuals was observed ($p = 0.002$).

No subsequent study has reported any significant evidence of linkage to type 1 diabetes in the 2q33 region. Numerous studies, both family-based and population-based, have, however, examined the evidence of association between polymorphism in the *CTLA4* gene and type 1 diabetes utilizing the A/G polymorphism in the leader peptide, a C/T polymorphism 318 nucleotides upstream from the transcription start site, or a dinucleotide repeat polymorphism in the 3′ untranslated region. There is some evidence that the A/G polymorphism may have effects on the expression or function of the CTLA-4 protein (142). Kristiansen et al. (143) jointly analyzed the reports of association between *CTLA4* alleles and type 1 diabetes. Across the 813 families genotyped in the studies they reviewed, there was persistent, although modest, evidence of preferential transmission of the "G" allele of the A/G polymorphism to affected offspring ($p = 0.002$). Case–control studies have also provided some sporadic evidence of an association of this allele with type 1 diabetes.

It is important to recall that *CTLA4* was originally investigated as a candidate gene, and follow-up studies have focused on only a narrow collection of polymorphisms. Association at the A/G polymorphism in *CTLA4* may reflect the effect of another nearby polymorphism with actual etiologic effects. For example, the *CD28* gene is located immediately adjacent to *CTLA4*, and, given its role in T-cell costimulatory events, it is also a potential candidate gene. Marron et al. (144) have begun to address this issue by testing multiple markers in the D2S72-CTLA4-D2S105 region for association with type 1 diabetes, both alone and in haplotypes. These studies reveal that the most significant evidence of association clusters immediately in and around the *CTLA4* gene, suggesting that further screening for new polymorphisms in this region may be warranted.

IDDM13 (2q34)

As in the report of *IDDM12*, other studies have searched for linkage between type 1 diabetes and markers on human chromosome 2q based on the localization of *Idd5* in the NOD mouse and the syntenic relationship between mouse chromosome 1 and human chromosome 2 (145). Suggestive evidence of linkage was observed slightly distal to *IDDM12*, with an MLS of 3.3 at the marker D2S164 (145). This evidence for linkage was enhanced when first-degree relatives positive for islet cell antibodies who had not progressed to frank diabetes were included in the analysis as affected, suggesting that the putative susceptibility gene in the region might be involved in the early stages of development of type 1 diabetes. This finding would be consistent with an orthologous relationship to the *Idd5* locus in the NOD mouse that controls the development of insulitis (139,140).

IDDM13 is one of three putative susceptibility loci for type 1 diabetes localized to a 20- to 30-cM region of chromosome 2q. It has proven difficult to confirm these reports of linkage or to determine if they represent distinct susceptibility loci. One subsequent large genome scan has provided suggestive evidence of linkage on 2q (MLS = 2.62), but the distribution of increased LOD scores that was observed in this region did not provide compelling evidence for multiple loci (130). A few markers in the region of *IDDM13* have been tested for association with type 1 diabetes, as have a few candidate genes such as insulin growth factor–binding proteins 2 and 5, but none have provided significant confirmatory evidence (146–148).

IDDM15 (6q21)

The HLA locus dominates the evidence of linkage to type 1 diabetes on chromosome 6. Delépine et al. (149) noted that evidence of linkage to HLA extended over a surprisingly large interval and hypothesized the existence of an additional susceptibility locus, independent of *IDDM1*, *IDDM5*, and *IDDM8*. They reported suggestive evidence for linkage at the marker D6S283 located 32 cM away from HLA ($p = 0.0002$ after correction for the effect of HLA). Additional suggestive evidence of linkage at D6S283 was reported in a separate genome scan (MLS = 1.71 to 2.27, dependent on mapping function used) (27). However, there is likely some overlap in the families used in these two studies. A completely independent genome scan of 424 families (464 ASPs) of Scandinavian origin revealed significant evidence of linkage at *IDDM15* (MLS = 4.8) (30).

IDDM17 (10q25)

IDDM17 is unique among IDDM loci in that it was defined by linkage studies in a single large Bedouin Arab pedigree rather than by the analysis of many small nuclear families (25). In this pedigree, autoimmune diabetes is reported to display oligogenic inheritance and is associated with two HLA-DR3 haplotypes. Studies of this pedigree provided the strongest evidence of linkage to markers in the chromosome 10q25 region. All affected individuals share a common haplotype of microsatellite markers in this region spanning approximately 8 cM. Whether the *IDDM17* locus plays a substantial role in predisposition to type 1 diabetes in the general population remains to be resolved. Genome scans have reported only modest evidence of linkage in this region. However, in one study, 10q25 was highlighted as one of only nine genomic regions in which LOD scores greater than 1.0 were observed (27).

IDDM18 (5q33–q34)

The *IDDM18* locus was defined based on a candidate gene study focusing on the *IL12B* gene (150). *IL12B* is an excellent candidate for a gene involved in the development of type 1 diabetes because it promotes the differentiation of the T_H1 subset of T cells, and cells of this phenotype are thought to play a critical role in the diabetogenic process. Linkage analysis with markers in the 5q33-q34 region, where the *IL12B* gene is localized, in a collection of British and Australian families with type 1 diabetes yielded suggestive evidence of linkage (MLS = 2.3) when the data were stratified by HLA status. A single nucleotide polymorphism in the 3′ untranslated region of the *IL12B* gene displayed a strong allelic association with type 1 diabetes in each of two independent sets of families tested by TDT (58.4% of 283 transmissions, $p = 0.0025$, in the first set and 64.7% of 156 transmissions, $p = 0.00014$, in the second set). The steady-state mRNA levels for *IL12B* were compared in two B-cell lines, each homozygous for different alleles at the polymorphism in the 3′ untranslated region. The cell line homozygous for the allele that had displayed an excess of transmissions in the TDT analyses expressed higher levels of *IL12B* mRNA.

Several follow-up studies have sought to confirm the reported evidence of linkage and association at the *IDDM18* locus as well as to examine the relationship between the specific polymorphism in the 3′ untranslated region and the expression of the *IL12B* gene. A study of American, British, Finnish, Romanian, and Sardinian families failed to detect evidence of linkage or association with type 1 diabetes at the *IDDM18* locus (151). In this same study, an examination of a panel of 19 B-cell lines revealed substantial variation in the level of *IL12B* mRNA and no clear correlation with the genotype of the polymorphism in the 3′ untranslated region. A second study of the same set of American families also failed to observe the reported association between the polymorphism in the 3′ untranslated region of the *IL12B* gene and type 1 diabetes but did observe 50% increased expression from the implicated allele in lymphocytes from three individuals (152). Additional studies of Norwegian families with type 1 diabetes and an Italian case–control population did not detect evidence of association at the *IDDM18* locus (153,154).

ADDITIONAL LOCI (Xp13–p11, 16q22–q24, 1q42)

Several additional linkages to type 1 diabetes have been reported in genome scans but have not been assigned "IDDM" designations. Cucca et al. (28) reported evidence for linkage at Xp13–p11. While overall evidence for linkage was weak, within the subset of patients who were DR3/X heterozygotes (where X was not DR4), an MLS of 3.5 was obtained. Recently, the *scurfin* gene, which, when mutated, results in a recessive neonatal autoimmune diabetes, was mapped to this region and is a potential candidate (155–157).

In a study of 356 type 1 diabetes families from the UK that extended the original genome scan of Davies et al., suggestive evidence of linkage was detected at chromosome 16q22–q24 (MLS = 3.4) (26). Subsequent merging of the data from this genome scan with that from several scans of U.S. families strengthened the evidence for linkage in this region (MLS = 4.13) (130).

Finally, suggestive evidence of linkage (MLS = 3.31) was reported at the marker D1S1617, on chromosome 1q42 in one study. This was the strongest evidence of linkage at any site other than HLA in a genome scan of 212 ASPs (27). Increasing the sample size and marker density for this region reduced the strength of the evidence for linkage (MLS = 2.46) but provided some evidence of allelic association with several closely spaced markers in the region.

The largest single genome scan completed in type 1 diabetes studied families from Denmark, Sweden, and Norway (30). Despite the use of a standardized ascertainment protocol and the greater homogeneity of genetic background in this population compared with others that had previously been studied by genome-wide scanning, only the *IDDM1* and *IDDM15* regions yielded significant evidence of linkage. However, three unique regions yielded LOD scores greater than 2.0, chromosome 2p (near the marker D2S113), chromosome 5 (near the marker D5S407), and chromosome 16p (in the interval between D16S407 and D16S287).

SUMMARY

Given the efforts of multiple investigators that have gone into mapping susceptibility loci for type 1 diabetes using genome-wide scans in ASPs, why have results, such as those summarized in the foregoing, appeared to be so inconsistent? There are a number of possible explanations. First, it needs to be recognized that failure to replicate a finding in an independent set of families does not imply that the initial report was incorrect. A series of studies, each reporting only modest evidence of linkage at a particular site, might well attain genome-wide significance in aggregate if the raw data were to be pooled and analyzed.

A second issue is that of power to detect linkage. The current set of genome scans for type 1 diabetes, although each an ambitious undertaking, have only good power to detect loci with very strong effects (e.g., $\lambda s > 2.0$). This is adequate to detect the effect of *IDDM1* in all studies but may not be adequate to allow consistent detection of other, non-HLA, loci that make more modest contributions to familial aggregation.

A third issue that may impact the ability to detect type 1 diabetes susceptibility genes by linkage studies is the possibility of heterogeneity in the patient population. Although the clinical diagnosis of type 1 diabetes can be made with confidence at the time β-cells have been largely ablated, there may be a variety of biochemical and immunologic pathways whereby patients reach this point. These different pathways may reflect the impact of polymorphism in different sets of genes. In such a situation, the extensive pooling of families required for genome scans may be counterproductive. It may be useful to consider incorporating additional phenotypic information into such studies. For example, the use of age at onset as a tool to identify a subset of patients whose disease is more strongly "genetic" has a long and successful history. Similar approaches in type 1 diabetes linkage studies that use not only age at onset but also other phenotypic manifestations to generate more homogeneous collections of families or patients for linkage or association studies may be warranted (130,158,159).

A fourth issue to consider regarding the variability in results between linkage studies in type 1 diabetes is the difficulty of accounting for the joint effects of multiple genes on susceptibility. Some of the reported type 1 diabetes linkages (e.g., *IDDM4*) attain statistical significance only when families to be analyzed are stratified on the basis of inheritance at other loci, usually *IDDM1* or *IDDM2*. It is a very reasonable hypothesis that there are statistically significant interactions between loci in type 1 diabetes. However, care must be exercised in testing multiple models of interaction as a means of searching for these loci. Repeated reanalysis of linkage data under different models, while a well-intentioned approach to uncover susceptibility loci, also increases the likelihood of false positive results. Carrying out analyses on various subsets of families requires that any findings meet a higher level of significance. When such a correction is applied, some reported linkages based on stratified analyses no longer attain statistical significance (160). Further development of statistical methods that can efficiently take into account the joint effects of multiple susceptibility genes might dramatically improve our ability to extract linkage information even from existing sets of data.

Finally, some of the reported loci may simply be false-positives. While it is not possible to rule out very small contributions to risk at any of these loci, it is worth noting that some are supported by only the most modest evidence, well below the thresholds cited earlier for even suggestive evidence and lacking convincing supporting evidence from association studies. Other loci are supported by suggestive or significant evidence of linkage in only a single study and are not supported by other studies. Finally, there is discordance between results obtained by two-point, as compared with multipoint analyses, for some loci, even in cases in which there is substantial overlap in the collection of families analyzed by the two different approaches.

FUTURE DIRECTIONS

To the famous fictional detective, Sherlock Holmes, even the absence of evidence could provide useful clues to solve a mystery.

> "Is there any point to which you would wish to draw my attention?"
> "To the curious incident of the dog in the night-time."
> "The dog did nothing in the night-time."
> "That was the curious incident,"
> remarked Sherlock Holmes. (161)

How can the mystery of the apparently discordant results for type 1 diabetes susceptibility loci be resolved? The "curious" behavior of the *IDDM2* locus in previously published genome scans may similarly provide an important clue. There is highly significant evidence from association studies that a gene or genes in the *IDDM2* region contribute to susceptibility to type 1 diabetes (20). Despite this, genome-wide scans completed to date have consistently failed to provide significant evidence of linkage at *IDDM2* (24,26,27,29,30,130). These genome-wide scans do provide strong exclusionary evidence for loci with effects comparable to and even somewhat less than *IDDM1* (e.g., loci with $\lambda s \geq 2.0$). However, the λ value for *IDDM2* is likely less than 1.3. If *IDDM2* is typical of the remaining susceptibility loci for type 1 diabetes, the sporadic nature of reports of linkage at other locations in the genome may simply represent a basic problem in sampling. In 1994, when Davies et al. (24) published the first genome-wide scan for linkage in type 1 diabetes, the collection of 96 families they used for their scan seemed quite large. However, if most type 1 diabetes susceptibility loci actually have λs values much lower than 1.5, significantly larger collections of ASPs will be necessary to have adequate power to detect their effects (3). It is clearly feasible to ascertain much larger collections of multiplex type 1 diabetes families than have been studied to date. However, in the near term, power could easily be increased by merging and jointly analyzing the raw genotyping data from already completed studies.

Some insight into the value of such an approach can be gained from the study of Cox et al. (130), who merged the primary data from what were currently the two largest published genome scans (26,27) and added new data from a further unpublished scan to obtain a data set that included 767 multiplex type 1 diabetes families. Within this collection, 667 of the families had been genome-scanned at a marker density of at least one marker for every 10 cM. The remaining 100 families had been used for targeted follow-up studies of regions where linkage had previously been reported. Multipoint analyses in this large set of data revealed three regions where the evidence for linkage was significant, *IDDM1* (LOD = 65.8), *IDDM2* (LOD = 4.28), and 16q22–q24 (LOD = 4.13). There was suggestive evidence of linkage at four more sites, *IDDM10*, *IDDM7*, *IDDM15*, and 1q42. Two points are of particular importance with regard to this study. First, addition of more families clearly increased the power to detect linkage. Of particular note was the magnitude of the evidence for linkage *IDDM2*, which was not anticipated based on the results in prior individual analyses of genome scans. This was not solely the result of genotyping markers, such as the insulin VNTR, that were known in advance to be located immediately at the *IDDM2* locus. If the data in this analysis for the 11p15 region are restricted to just the framework set of markers used in a typical genome scan, the evidence for linkage is still suggestive (LOD = 2.53). This brings up the second point that increasing marker density also increases power to detect linkage at an established site such as *IDDM2*.

These points, that increasing sample size and marker density can increase the power to detect linkage, are obvious to geneticists but merit emphasizing in the context of the genetics of type 1 diabetes. It may well be that to obtain unambiguous mapping of at least the most important type 1 diabetes susceptibility genes it will be necessary to study many more families at higher marker densities than has been done in the past. As a first step toward such a goal, investigators in the genetics of type 1 diabetes could help themselves by taking a consortium approach—merging all of the existing data from published studies and carrying out joint analyses. At the time of this writing, an effort to establish a type 1 diabetes genetics consortium to facilitate such an approach is under way. Such an effort should clarify some of the apparent conflicts in the current data regarding type 1 diabetes susceptibility loci and help prioritize those chromosomal regions most likely to contain susceptibility loci for the even harder work ahead of identifying the relevant genes.

REFERENCES

1. Barnett AH, Eff C, Leslie RDG, et al. Diabetes in identical twins: a study of 200 pairs. *Diabetologia* 1981;20:87–93.
2. Rich SS. Mapping genes in diabetes: genetic epidemiological perspective. *Diabetes* 1990;39:1315–1319.
3. Risch N. Linkage strategies for genetically complex traits, II: the power of affected relative pairs. *Am J Hum Genet* 1990;46:229–241.
4. Lander E, Kruglyak L. Genetic dissection of complex traits: guidelines for interpreting and reporting linkage results. *Nat Genet* 1995;11:241–247.
5. Thomson G. Identifying complex disease genes: progress and paradigms. *Nat Genet* 1994;8:108–110.
6. Risch N. Linkage strategies for genetically complex traits, I: multilocus models. *Am J Hum Genet* 1990;46:222–228.
7. Terwilliger JD, Ott J. A haplotype-based 'haplotype relative risk' approach to detecting allelic associations. *Hum Hered* 1992;42:337–346.
8. Falk CT, Rubinstein P. Haplotype relative risks: an easy reliable way to construct a proper control sample for risk calculations. *Ann Hum Genet* 1987;51(pt 3):227–233.
9. Thomson G. Mapping disease genes: family-based association studies. *Am J Hum Genet* 1995;57:487–498.
10. Spielman RS, McGinnis RE, Ewens WJ. Transmission test for linkage disequilibrium: the insulin gene region and insulin-dependent diabetes mellitus. *Am J Hum Genet* 1993;52:506–516.
11. Ewens WJ, Spielman RS. The transmission/disequilibrium test: history, subdivision, and admixture. *Am J Hum Genet* 1995;57:455–464.
12. Risch N, Merikangas K. The future of genetic studies of complex human diseases. *Science* 1996;273:1516–1517.
13. Kruglyak L. Prospects for whole-genome linkage disequilibrium mapping of common disease genes. *Nat Genet* 1999;22:139–144.
14. Daly MJ, Rioux JD, Schaffner SF, et al. High-resolution haplotype structure in the human genome. *Nat Genet* 2001;29:229–232.
15. Reich DE, Cargill M, Bolk S, et al. Linkage disequilibrium in the human genome. *Nature* 2001;411:199–204.
16. Gabriel SB, Schaffner SF, Nguyen H, et al. The structure of haplotype blocks in the human genome. *Science* 2002;296:2225–2229.
17. Dawson E, Abecasis GR, Bumpstead S, et al. A first-generation linkage disequilibrium map of human chromosome 22. *Nature* 2002;418:544–548.
18. Nerup J, Platz P, Andersen OO, et al. HL-A antigens and diabetes mellitus. *Lancet* 1974;2:864–866.
19. Bell GI, Horita S, Karam JH. A polymorphic locus near the human insulin gene is associated with insulin-dependent diabetes mellitus. *Diabetes* 1984;33: 176–183.
20. Bennett ST, Lucassen AM, Gough SC, et al. Susceptibility to human type 1 diabetes at IDDM2 is determined by tandem repeat variation at the insulin gene minisatellite locus. *Nat Genet* 1995;9:284–292.
21. Cox NJ, Baker L, Spielman RS. Insulin-gene sharing in sib pairs with insulin-dependent diabetes mellitus: no evidence for linkage. *Am J Hum Genet* 1988; 42:167–172.
22. Julier C, Lucassen A, Villedieu P, et al. Multiple DNA variant association analysis: application to the insulin gene region in type 1 diabetes. *Am J Hum Genet* 1994;55:1247–1254.
23. Bennett ST, Wilson AJ, Cucca F, et al. IDDM2-VNTR-encoded susceptibility to type 1 diabetes: dominant protection and parental transmission of alleles of the insulin gene-linked minisatellite locus. *J Autoimmun* 1996;9:415–421.
24. Davies JL, Kawaguchi Y, Bennett ST, et al. A genome-wide search for human type 1 diabetes susceptibility genes. *Nature* 1994;371:130–136.
25. Verge CF, Vardi P, Babu S, et al. Evidence for oligogenic inheritance of type 1 diabetes in a large Bedouin Arab family. *J Clin Invest* 1998;102:1569–1575.
26. Mein CA, Esposito L, Dunn MG, et al. A search for type 1 diabetes susceptibility genes in families from the United Kingdom. *Nat Genet* 1998;19:297–300.
27. Concannon P, Gogolin-Ewens KJ, Hinds D, et al. A second-generation screen of the human genome for susceptibility to insulin-dependent diabetes mellitus (IDDM). *Nat Genet* 1998;19:292–296.
28. Cucca F, Goy JV, Kawaguchi Y, et al. A male-female bias in type 1 diabetes and linkage to chromosome Xp in MHC HLA-DR3-positive patients. *Nat Genet* 1998;19:301–302.
29. Hashimoto L, Habita C, Beressi JP, et al. Genetic mapping of a susceptibility locus for insulin-dependent diabetes mellitus on chromosome 11q. *Nature* 1994;371:161–164.
30. Nerup J, Pociot F. A genomewide scan for type 1-diabetes susceptibility in Scandinavian families: identification of new loci with evidence of interactions. *Am J Hum Genet* 2001;69:1301–1313.
31. Suarez BK, Hampe CL, Van Eerdewegh P. Problems of replicating linkage claims in psychiatry. In: Gershon ES, Cloninger CR, eds. *Genetic approaches to mental disorders.* Washington, DC: American Psychiatric Press, 1994:23–46.
32. Singal DP, Blajchman MA. Histocompatibility (HLA) antigens, lymphocytotoxic antibodies and tissue antibodies in patients with diabetes mellitus. *Diabetes* 1973;22:429–432.
33. Nerup JO, Platz PO, Anderson OO, et al. HLA-antigens and diabetes mellitus. *Lancet* 1974;2:864–866.
34. Cudworth AG, Woodrow JC. HLA system and diabetes mellitus. *Diabetes* 1975;24:345–349.
35. Svejgaard A, Platz P, Ryder LP. HLA and disease 1982—a survey. *Immunol Rev* 1983;70:193–218.
36. Wassmuth R, Lernmark A. The genetics of susceptibility to diabetes [Review]. *Clin Immunol* 1989;53:358–399.
37. Deschamps I, Beressi JP, Khalil I, et al. The role of genetic predisposition to type I (insulin-dependent) diabetes mellitus. *Ann Med* 1991;23:427–435.
38. Thorsby E, Ronningen KS. Particular HLA-DQ molecules play a dominant role in determining susceptibility or resistance to type 1 (insulin-dependent) diabetes mellitus. *Diabetologia* 1993;36:371–377.
39. Sheehy MJ, Scharf SJ, Rowe JR, et al. A diabetes-susceptible HLA haplotype is best defined by a combination of HLA-DR and -DQ alleles. *J Clin Invest* 1989;83:830–835.
40. Caillat-Zucman S, Garchon H-J, Timsit J, et al. HLA genetic heterogeneity of insulin dependent diabetes mellitus: indication for an age dependent susceptibility gradient. *J Clin Invest* 1992;90:2242–2250.
41. Caillat-Zucman S, Djilali-Saiah I, Timsit J, et al. Insulin dependent diabetes mellitus (IDDM): 12th International Histocompatibility Workshop study. In: Charron D, ed. *Genetic diversity of HLA: functional and medical implications—proceedings of the 12th International Histocompatibility Workshop and Conference,* Vol 1. Paris: EDK, 1997:389–398.
42. Ronningen KS, Spurkland A, Tait BD, et al. HLA class II associations in insulin-dependent diabetes mellitus among blacks, caucasoids, and Japanese. In: Tsuji K, Aizawa M, Sasazuki T, eds. *HLA 1991.* Oxford: Oxford University Press, 1993:713–722.
43. Todd JA. Genetic control of autoimmunity in type I diabetes. *Immunol Today* 1990;11:122–129.
44. Erlich HA, Zeidler A, Chang J, et al. HLA class II alleles and susceptibility and resistance to insulin dependent diabetes mellitus in Mexican-American families. *Nat Genet* 1993;3:358–364.
45. Van der Auwera B, Van Waeyenberge C, Schuit F, et al. DRB1*0403 protects against IDDM in Caucasians with the high-risk heterozygous DQA1*0301-DQB*0302/DQA1*0501-DQB1*0201 genotype. *Diabetes* 1995;44:527–530.
46. Cucca F, Lampis R, Frau F, et al. The distribution of DR4 haplotypes in Sardinia suggests a primary association of type I diabetes with DRB1 and DQB1 loci. *Hum Immunol* 1995;43:301–308.
47. Donner H, Seidl C, Van der Auwera B, et al. HLA-DRB1*04 and susceptibility to type 1 diabetes mellitus in a German/Belgian family and German case-control study: the Belgian Diabetes Registry. *Tissue Antigens* 2000;55: 271–274.
48. Undlien DE, Friede T, Rammensee HG, et al. HLA-encoded genetic predisposition in IDDM: DR4 subtypes may be associated with different degrees of protection. *Diabetes* 1997;46:143–149.
49. Reijonen H, Nejentsev S, Tuokko J, et al. HLA-DR4 subtype and -B alleles in DQB1*0302-positive haplotypes associated with IDDM. *Eur J Immunogenet* 1997;24:357–363.
50. Nejentsev S, Reijonen H, Adojaan B, et al. The effect of HLA-B allele on the IDDM risk defined by DRB1*04 subtypes and DQB1*0302. *Diabetes* 1997;46: 1888–1892.
51. Awata T, Kanazawa Y. Genetic markers for insulin-dependent diabetes mellitus in Japanese. *Diabetes Res Clin Pract* 1994;24[Suppl]:S83–S87.
52. Huang HS, Peng JT, She JY, et al. HLA-encoded susceptibility to insulin-dependent diabetes mellitus is determined by DR and DQ genes as well as

their linkage disequilibria in a Chinese population. *Hum Immunol* 1995;44 210–219.
53. Park YS, Wang CY, Ko KW, et al. Combinations of HLA DR and DQ molecules determine the susceptibility to insulin-dependent diabetes mellitus in Koreans. *Hum Immunol* 1998;59:794–801.
54. Yasunaga S, Kimura A, Hamaguchi K, et al. Different contribution of HLA-DR and -DQ genes in susceptibility and resistance to insulin-dependent diabetes mellitus (IDDM). *Tissue Antigens* 1996;47:37–48.
55. Todd JA, Mijovic C, Fletcher J, et al. Identification of susceptibility loci for insulin-dependent diabetes mellitus by trans-racial gene mapping. *Nature* 1989;338:587–589.
56. Marsh SGE, Bodmer JG. HLA class II nucleotide sequences, 1992. *Tissue Antigens* 1992;40:229–243.
57. Pugliese A, Gianani R, Moromisato R, et al. HLA-DQB1*0602 is associated with dominant protection from diabetes even among islet cell antibody-positive first-degree relatives of patients with IDDM. *Diabetes* 1995;44:608–613.
58. Sanjeevi CB, Landin-Olsson I, Kockum I, et al. Effects of the second HLA-DQ haplotype on the association with childhood insulin-dependent diabetes mellitus. *Tissue Antigens* 1995;45:148–152.
59. Baisch JM, Weeks T, Giles T, et al. Analysis of HLA-DQ genotypes and susceptibility in insulin-dependent diabetes mellitus. *N Engl J Med* 1990;322: 1836–1841.
60. Erlich HA, Griffith RL, Bugawan TL, et al. Implication of specific DQB1 alleles in genetic susceptibility and resistance by identification of IDDM siblings with novel HLA-DQB1 allele and unusual DR2 and DR1 haplotypes. *Diabetes* 1991;40:478–481.
61. Zeliszewski D, Tiercy J-M, Boitard C, et al. Extensive study of DRB, DQA, and DQB gene polymorphisms in 23 DR2-positive insulin dependent diabetes mellitus patients. *Hum Immunol* 1992;33:140–147.
62. Reijonen H, Ilonen J, Akerblom HK, et al. Multi-locus analysis of HLA class II genes in DR2-positive IDDM haplotypes in Finland. *Tissue Antigens* 1994; 43:1–6.
63. Sanjeevi CB, Lybrand TP, Landin-Olsson M, et al. Analysis of DRB1, DRB5, DQA1 and DQB1 genes and molecular modeling of DR2 molecules in DR2 positive patients with type I diabetes. *Tissue Antigens* 1994;44:110–119.
64. Cambon TA. HLA population genetics. In: Levy-Marchal C, Czernichow P, eds. *Epidemiology and etiology of insulin-dependent diabetes mellitus in the young.* Vol 21. Basel: Pediatric Adolescence Endocrinology Karger, 1992:130–157.
65. Sugihara S, Sakamaki T, Konda S, et al. Association of HLA-DR, DQ genotype with different beta-cell functions at IDDM diagnosis in Japanese children. *Diabetes* 1997;46:1893–1897.
66. Mijovic CH, Jenkins D, Jacobs KH, et al. HLA-DQA1 and -DQB1 alleles associated with genetic susceptibility to IDDM in a black population. *Diabetes* 1991;40:748–753.
67. Ronningen KS, Spurkland A, Iwe T, et al. Distribution of HLA-DRB1, -DQA1 and -DQB1 alleles and DQA1-DQB1 genotypes among Norwegian patients with insulin-dependent diabetes mellitus. *Tissue Antigens* 1991;37:105–111.
68. Cucca F, Muntoni F, Lampis R, et al. Combinations of specific DRB1, DQA1, DQB1 haplotypes are associated with insulin-dependent diabetes mellitus in Sardinia. *Hum Immunol* 1993;37:85–94.
69. Awata T, Kuzuya T, Matsuda A, et al. Genetic analysis of HLA class-II alleles and susceptibility to type I (insulin-dependent) diabetes mellitus in Japanese subjects. *Diabetologia* 1992;35:419–424.
70. Hawkins BR, Lam KS, Ma JT, et al. Strong association of HLA-DR3/DRw9 heterozygosity with early-onset insulin-dependent diabetes mellitus in Chinese. *Diabetes* 1987;36:1297–1300.
71. Penny MA, Jenkins D, Mijovic CH, et al. Susceptibility to IDDM in a Chinese population—role of HLA class II alleles. *Diabetes* 1992;41:914–919.
72. Nepom BS, Schwarz D, Palmer JP, et al. Transcomplementation of HLA genes in IDDM. HLA-DQ alpha- and beta-chains produce hybrid molecules in DR3/4 heterozygotes. *Diabetes* 1987;36:114–117.
73. Charron DJ, Lotteau V, Turmel P. Hybrid HLA-DC antigens provide molecular evidence for gene transcomplementation. *Nature* 1984;312:157–159.
74. Gjertsen HA, Lundin KEA, Ronningen KS, et al. T cells recognizing an HLA-DQ αβ heterodimer encoded in cis by the DR4DQw4 haplotype and in trans by DR4DQw8/DRw8DQw4 heterozygous cells. *Hum Immunol* 1990;30: 226–232.
75. Kwok WW, Thurtle P, Nepom GT. A genetically controlled pairing anomaly between HLA-DQα and HLA-DQβ chains. *J Immunol* 1989;143:3598–3601.
76. Kwok WW, Kovats S, Thurtle P, et al. HLA-DQ allelic polymorphisms constrain patterns of class II heterodimer formation. *J Immunol* 1993;150: 2263–2272.
77. Jenkins D, Mijovic C, Fletcher J, et al. Identification of susceptibility loci for type 1 (insulin-dependent) diabetes by trans-racial gene mapping. *Diabetologia* 1990;33:387–395.
78. Honeyman MC, Harrison LC, Drummond B, et al. Analysis of families at risk for insulin-dependent diabetes mellitus reveals that HLA antigens influence progression to clinical disease. *Mol Med* 1995;1:576–582.
79. Kobayashi T, Tamemoto K, Nakanishi K, et al. Immunogenetic and clinical characterization of slowly progressive IDDM. *Diabetes Care* 1993;16:780–788.
80. Mizota M, Uchigata Y, Moriyama S, et al. Age-dependent association of HLA-A24 in Japanese IDDM patients. *Diabetologia* 1996;39:371–373.
81. Deschamps I, Marcelli-Barge A, Poirier JC, et al. Two distinct HLA-DR3 haplotypes are associated with age related heterogeneity in type I (insulin-dependent) diabetes. *Diabetologia* 1988;31:896–901.
82. Tait BD, Harrison LC, Drummond BP, et al. HLA antigens and age at diagnosis of insulin-dependent diabetes mellitus. *Hum Immunol* 1995;42:116–122.
83. Nakanishi K, Kobayashi T, Murase T, et al. Association of HLA-A24 with complete beta-cell destruction in IDDM. *Diabetes* 1993;42:1086–1093.
84. Vicario JL, Martinez-Laso J, Corell A, et al. Comparison between HLA-DRB and DQ DNA sequences and classic serological markers as type-1 (insulin-dependent) diabetes-mellitus predictive risk markers in the Spanish population. *Diabetologia* 1992;35:475–481.
85. Degli-Esposti MA, Leaver AL, Christiansen FT, et al. Ancestral haplotypes: conserved population MHC haplotypes. *Hum Immunol* 1992;34:242–252.
86. Hanafi Moghaddam PH, de Knijf P, Roep BO, et al. Genetic structure of IDDM1. Two separate regions in the major histocompatibility complex contribute to susceptibility or protection. Belgian Diabetes Registry. *Diabetes* 1998;47:263–269.
87. Lie BA, Todd JA, Pociot F, et al. The predisposition to type 1 diabetes linked to the human leukocyte antigen complex includes at least one non-class II gene. *Am J Hum Genet* 1999;64:793–800.
88. Nejentsev S, Gombos Z, Laine AP, et al. Non-class II HLA gene associated with type 1 diabetes maps to the 240-kb region near HLA-B. *Diabetes* 2000;49: 2217–2221.
89. The MHC Sequencing Consortium. Complete sequence and gene map of a human major histocompatibility complex. *Nature* 1999;401:921–923.
90. Lie BA, Sollid LM, Ascher H, et al. A gene telomeric of the HLA class I region is involved in predisposition to both type 1 diabetes and coeliac disease. *Tissue Antigens* 1999;54:162–168.
91. Caillat-Zucman S, Daniel S, Djilali-Saiah I, et al. Family study of linkage disequilibrium between TAP2 transporter and HLA class II genes. Absence of TAP2 contribution to association with insulin-dependent diabetes mellitus. *Hum Immunol* 1995;44:80–87.
92. Ronningen KS, Undlien DE, Ploski R, et al. Linkage disequilibrium between TAP2 variants and HLA class II alleles; no primary association between TAP2 variants and insulin-dependent diabetes mellitus. *Eur J Immunol* 1993;23: 1050–1056.
93. Nakanishi K, Kobayashi T, Murase T, et al. Lack of association of the transporter associated with antigen processing with Japanese insulin-dependent diabetes mellitus. *Metabolism* 1994;43:1013–1017.
94. Cucca F, Congia M, Trowsdale J, et al. Insulin-dependent diabetes mellitus and the major histocompatibility complex peptide transporters TAP1 and TAP2: no association in a population with a high disease incidence. *Tissue Antigens* 1994;44:234–240.
95. Esposito L, Lampasona V, Bosi E, et al. HLA DQA1-DQB1-TAP2 haplotypes in IDDM families: no evidence for an additional contribution to disease risk by the TAP2 locus. *Diabetologia* 1995;38:968–974.
96. Jackson DG, Capra JD. TAP2 association with insulin-dependent diabetes mellitus is secondary to HLA-DQB1. *Hum Immunol* 1995;43:57–65.
97. Deng GY, Muir A, Maclaren NK, et al. Association of LMP2 and LMP7 genes within the major histocompatibility complex with insulin-dependent diabetes mellitus: population and family studies. *Am J Hum Genet* 1995;56: 528–534.
98. van Endert PM, Liblau RS, Patel SD, et al. Major histocompatibility complex-encoded antigen processing gene polymorphism in IDDM. *Diabetes* 1994;43: 110–117.
99. Kawaguchi Y, Ikegami H, Fukuda M, et al. Absence of association of TAP and LMP genes with type 1 (insulin-dependent) diabetes mellitus. *Life Sci* 1994;54:2049–2053.
100. Undlien DE, Akselsen HE, Joner G, et al. No independent associations of LMP2 and LMP7 polymorphisms with susceptibility to develop IDDM. *Diabetes* 1997;46:307–312.
101. McTernan CL, Stewart LC, Mijovic CH, et al. Assessment of the non-HLA-DR-DQ contribution to IDDM1 in British Caucasian families: analysis of LMP7 polymorphisms. *Diabet Med* 2000;17:661–666.
102. Djilali-Saiah I, Benini V, Schmitz J, et al. Absence of primary association between DM gene polymorphism and insulin-dependent diabetes mellitus or celiac disease. *Hum Immunol* 1996;49:22–27.
103. Esposito L, Lampasona V, Bonifacio E, et al. Lack of association of DMB polymorphism with insulin-dependent diabetes. *J Autoimmun* 1997;10:395–400.
104. Siegmund T, Donner H, Braun J, et al. HLA-DMA and HLA-DMB alleles in German patients with type 1 diabetes mellitus. *Tissue Antigens* 1999;54: 291–294.
105. Baisch JM, Capra JD. Analysis of HLA genotypes and susceptibility to insulin-dependent diabetes mellitus: association maps telomeric to HLA-DP. *Scand J Immunol* 1992;36:331–340.
106. Tait BD, Harrison LC, Drummond BP, et al. HLA antigens and age at diagnosis of insulin-dependent diabetes mellitus. *Hum Immunol* 1995;42:116–122.
107. Noble JA, Valdes AM, Cook M, et al. The role of HLA class II genes in insulin-dependent diabetes mellitus: molecular analysis of 180 Caucasian, multiplex families. *Am J Hum Genet* 1996;59:1134–1148.
108. Nishimaki K, Kawamura T, Inada H, et al. HLA DPB1*0201 gene confers disease susceptibility in Japanese with childhood onset type I diabetes, independent of HLA-DR and DQ genotypes. *Diabetes Res Clin Pract* 2000;47: 49–55.
109. Balducci-Silano PL, Layrisse ZE. HLA-DP and susceptibility to insulin-dependent diabetes mellitus in an ethnically mixed population: associations with other HLA-alleles. *J Autoimmun* 1995;8:425–437.
110. Lie BA, Akselsen HE, Joner G, et al. HLA associations in insulin-dependent

diabetes mellitus: no independent association to particular DP genes. *Hum Immunol* 1997;55:170–175.
111. Lucassen AM, Julier C, Beressi JP, et al. Susceptibility to insulin dependent diabetes mellitus maps to a 4.1 kb segment of DNA spanning the insulin gene and associated VNTR. *Nat Genet* 1993;4:305–310.
112. Doria A, Lee J, Warram JH, et al. Diabetes susceptibility at IDDM2 cannot be positively mapped to the VNTR locus of the insulin gene. *Diabetologia* 1996; 39:594–599.
113. Owerbach D, Gabbay KH. Localization of a type I diabetes susceptibility locus to the variable tandem repeat region flanking the insulin gene. *Diabetes* 1993;42:1708–1714.
114. McGinnis RE, Spielman RS. Insulin expression: is VNTR allele 698 really anomalous? *Nat Genet* 1995;10:378–380.
115. McGinnis RE, Spielman RS. Insulin gene 5′ flanking polymorphism: length of class 1 alleles in number of repeat units. *Diabetes* 1995;44:1296–1302.
116. Kennedy GC, German MS, Rutter WJ. The minisatellite in the diabetes susceptibility locus IDDM2 regulates insulin transcription. *Nat Genet* 1995;9: 293–298.
117. Vafiadis P, Bennett ST, Todd JA, et al. Insulin expression in human thymus is modulated by INS VNTR alleles at the IDDM2 locus. *Nat Genet* 1997;15: 289–292.
118. Pugliese A, Zeller M, Fernandez A Jr, et al. The insulin gene is transcribed in the human thymus and transcription levels correlated with allelic variation at the INS VNTR-IDDM2 susceptibility locus for type 1 diabetes. *Nat Genet* 1997;15:293–297.
119. Field LL, Tobias R, Magnus T. A locus on chromosome 15q26 (IDDM3) produces susceptibility to insulin-dependent diabetes mellitus. *Nat Genet* 1994; 8:189–194.
120. Luo DF, Buzzetti R, Rotter JI, et al. Confirmation of three susceptibility genes to insulin-dependent diabetes mellitus: IDDM4, IDDM5 and IDDM8. *Hum Mol Genet* 1996;5:693–698.
121. Luo DF, Bui MM, Muir A, et al. Affected-sib-pair mapping of a novel susceptibility gene to insulin-dependent diabetes mellitus (IDDM8) on chromosome 6q25-q27. *Am J Hum Genet* 1995;57:911–919.
122. Zamani M, Pociot F, Raeymaekers P, et al. Linkage of type I diabetes to 15q26 (IDDM3) in the Danish population. *Hum Genet* 1996;98:491–496.
123. Nakagawa Y, Kawaguchi Y, Twells RC, et al. Fine mapping of the diabetes-susceptibility locus, IDDM4, on chromosome 11q13. *Am J Hum Genet* 1998;63: 547–556.
124. Eckenrode S, Marron MP, Nicholls R, et al. Fine-mapping of the type 1 diabetes locus (IDDM4) on chromosome 11q and evaluation of two candidate genes (FADD and GALN) by affected sibpair and linkage-disequilibrium analyses. *Hum Genet* 2000;106:14–18.
125. Davies JL, Cucca F, Goy JV, et al. Saturation multipoint linkage mapping of chromosome 6q in type 1 diabetes. *Hum Mol Genet* 1996;5:1071–1074.
126. Hodge SE, Anderson CE, Neiswanger K, et al. Close genetic linkage between diabetes mellitus and Kidd blood group. *Lancet* 1981;2:893–895.
127. Merriman T, Twells R, Merriman M, et al. Evidence by allelic association-dependent methods for a type 1 diabetes polygene (IDDM6) on chromosome 18q21. *Hum Mol Genet* 1997;6:1003–1010.
128. Merriman TR, Eaves IA, Twells RC, et al. Transmission of haplotypes of microsatellite markers rather than single marker alleles in the mapping of a putative type 1 diabetes susceptibility gene (IDDM6). *Hum Mol Genet* 1998;7: 517–524.
129. Copeman JB, Cucca F, Hearne CM, et al. Linkage disequilibrium mapping of a type 1 diabetes susceptibility gene (IDDM7) to chromosome 2q31-q33. *Nat Genet* 1995;9:80–85.
130. Cox NJ, Wapelhorst B, Morrison VA, et al. Seven regions of the genome show evidence of linkage to type 1 diabetes in a consensus analysis of 767 multiplex families. *Am J Hum Genet* 2001;69:820–830.
131. Esposito L, Hill NJ, Pritchard LE, et al. Genetic analysis of chromosome 2 in type 1 diabetes: analysis of putative loci IDDM7, IDDM12, and IDDM13 and candidate genes *NRAMP1* and *IA-2* and the interleukin-1 gene cluster: IMDIAB Group. *Diabetes* 1998;47:1797–1799.
132. Kristiansen OP, Pociot F, Bennett EP, et al. IDDM7 links to insulin-dependent diabetes mellitus in Danish multiplex families but linkage is not explained by novel polymorphisms in the candidate gene GALNT3: the Danish Study Group of Diabetes in Childhood and the Danish IDDM Epidemiology and Genetics Group. *Hum Mutat* 2000;15:295–296.
133. Luo DF, Maclaren NK, Huang HS, et al. Intrafamilial and case-control association analysis of D2S152 in insulin-dependent diabetes. *Autoimmunity* 1995;21:143–147.
134. Perez DN, Bilbao JR, Nistico L, et al. No evidence of association of chromosome 2q with type 1 diabetes in the Basque population. *Diabetologia* 1999; 42:119–120.
135. Owerbach D. Physical and genetic mapping of IDDM8 on chromosome 6q27. *Diabetes* 2000;49:508–512.
136. Reed P, Cucca F, Jenkins S, et al. Evidence for a type 1 diabetes susceptibility locus (IDDM10) on human chromosome 10p11-q11. *Hum Mol Genet* 1997; 6:1011–1016.
137. Wapelhorst B, Bell GI, Risch N, et al. Linkage and association studies in insulin-dependent diabetes with a new dinucleotide repeat polymorphism at the GAD_{65} locus. *Autoimmunity* 1995;21:127–130.
138. Field LL, Tobias R, Thomson G, et al. Susceptibility to insulin-dependent diabetes mellitus maps to a locus (IDDM11) on human chromosome 14q24.3-q31. *Genomics* 1996;33:1–8.
139. Cornall RJ, Prins JB, Todd JA, et al. Type 1 diabetes in mice is linked to the interleukin-1 receptor and Lsh/Ity/Bcg genes on chromosome 1. *Nature* 1991;353:262–265.
140. Hill NJ, Lyons PA, Armitage N, et al. NOD Idd5 locus controls insulitis and diabetes and overlaps the orthologous CTLA4/IDDM12 and NRAMP1 loci in humans. *Diabetes* 2000;49:1744–1747.
141. Nistico L, Buzzetti R, Pritchard LE, et al. The CTLA-4 gene region of chromosome 2q33 is linked to, and associated with, type 1 diabetes. *Hum Mol Genet* 1996;5:1075–1080.
142. Kouki T, Sawai Y, Gardine CA, et al. CTLA-4 gene polymorphism at position 49 in exon 1 reduces the inhibitory function of CTLA-4 and contributes to the pathogenesis of Graves' disease. *J Immunol* 2000;165:6606–6611.
143. Kristiansen OP, Larsen ZM, Pociot F. CTLA-4 in autoimmune diseases—a general susceptibility gene to autoimmunity? *Genes Immun* 2000;1:170–184.
144. Marron MP, Zeidler A, Raffel LJ, et al. Genetic and physical mapping of a type 1 diabetes susceptibility gene (IDDM12) to a 100-kb phagemid artificial chromosome clone containing D2S72-CTLA4-D2S105 on chromosome 2q33. *Diabetes* 2000;49:492–499.
145. Morahan G, Huang D, Tait BD, et al. Markers on distal chromosome 2q linked to insulin-dependent diabetes mellitus. *Science* 1996;272:1811–1813.
146. Larsen ZM, Kristiansen OP, Mato E, et al. IDDM12 (CTLA4) on 2q33 and IDDM13 on 2q34 in genetic susceptibility to type 1 diabetes (insulin-dependent). *Autoimmunity* 1999;31:35–42.
147. Fu J, Ikegami H, Kawaguchi Y, et al. Association of distal chromosome 2q with IDDM in Japanese subjects. *Diabetologia* 1998;41:228–232.
148. Owerbach D, Naya FJ, Tsai MJ, et al. Analysis of candidate genes for susceptibility to type 1 diabetes: a case-control and family association study of genes on chromosome 2q31-35. *Diabetes* 1997;46:1069–1074.
149. Delépine M, Pociot F, Habita C, et al. Evidence of a non-MHC susceptibility locus in type 1 diabetes linked to HLA on chromosome 6. *Am J Hum Genet* 1997;60:174–187.
150. Morahan G, Huang D, Ymer SI, et al. Linkage disequilibrium of a type 1 diabetes susceptibility locus with a regulatory IL12B allele. *Nat Genet* 2001;27: 218–221.
151. Dahlman I, Eaves IA, Kosoy R, et al. Parameters for reliable results in genetic association studies in common disease. *Nat Genet* 2002;30:149–150.
152. Davoodi-Semiromi A, Yang JJ, She JX. IL-12p40 is associated with type 1 diabetes in Caucasian-American families. *Diabetes* 2002;51:2334–2336.
153. Johansson S, Lie BA, Thorsby E, et al. The polymorphism in the 3′ untranslated region of IL12B has a negligible effect on the susceptibility to develop type 1 diabetes in Norway. *Immunogenetics* 2001;53:603–605.
154. Nistico L, Giorgi G, Giordano M, et al. IL12B polymorphism and type 1 diabetes in the Italian population: a case-control study. *Diabetes* 2002;51: 1649–1650.
155. Bennett CL, Christie J, Ramsdell F, et al. The immune dysregulation, polyendocrinopathy, enteropathy, X-linked syndrome (IPEX) is caused by mutations of FOXP3. *Nat Genet* 2001;27:20–21.
156. Ramsdell F, Peake J, Faravelli F, et al. X-linked neonatal diabetes mellitus, enteropathy and endocrinopathy syndrome is the human equivalent of mouse scurfy. *Nat Genet* 2001;27:18–20.
157. Chatila TA, Blaeser F, Ho N, et al. JM2, encoding a fork head-related protein, is mutated in X-linked autoimmunity-allergic dysregulation syndrome. *J Clin Invest* 2000;106:R75–R81.
158. Paterson AD, Petronis A. Age of diagnosis-based linkage analysis in type 1 diabetes. *Eur J Hum Genet* 2000;8:145–148.
159. Paterson AD, Petronis A. Age and sex based genetic locus heterogeneity in type 1 diabetes. *J Med Genet* 2000;37:186–191.
160. Lernmark A, Ott J. Sometimes it's hot, sometimes it's not. *Nat Genet* 1998;19: 213–214.
161. Doyle AC. Memoirs of Sherlock Holmes. In: *The complete Sherlock Holmes.* New York: Doubleday, 1960:335–350.

Color Plates

ADIPOSE TISSUE

A: White fat cells. The cytoplasm appears as a thin rim at the periphery of the cell. Stored fat is the predominant component of the cell. The nucleus is flattened in the cytoplasm, permitting maximum storage of fat globules. The fat cell lipid is in the form of a single droplet, and these cells are described as unilocular. **B:** Brown fat is an uncommon variety of fat found in specific locations in the body. Unlike the more common white fat, brown fat cells contain a number of small lipid droplets; hence the name multilocular fat. (From Bergman RA, Afifi AK, Heidger PM. *Atlas of Microscopic Anatomy,* 2nd ed. Philadelphia: WB Saunders, 1989, with permission.)

Plate I

FAT CELLS
Panniculus adiposus

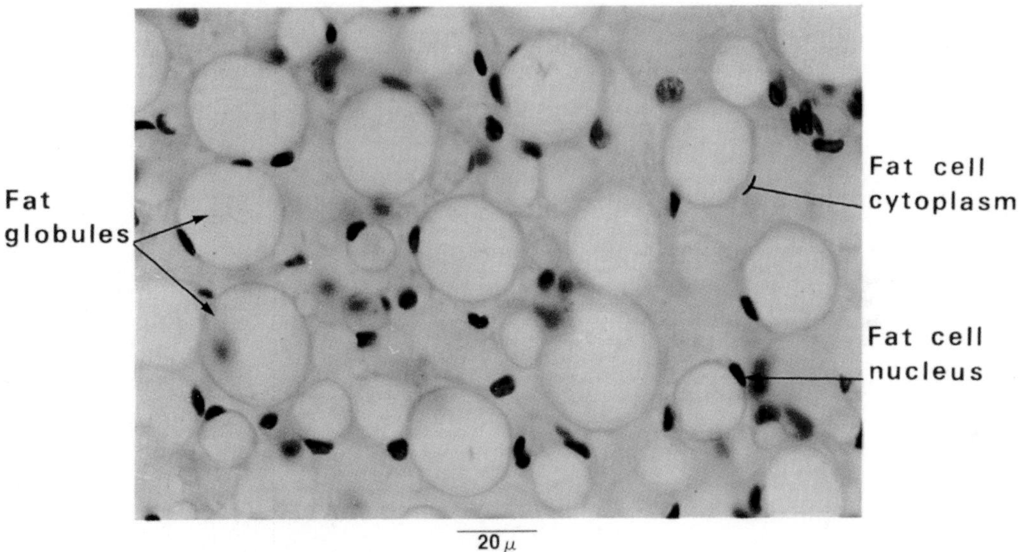

Human, 10 % Formalin, H. & E., 612 x.

A

BROWN FAT
Mediastinum

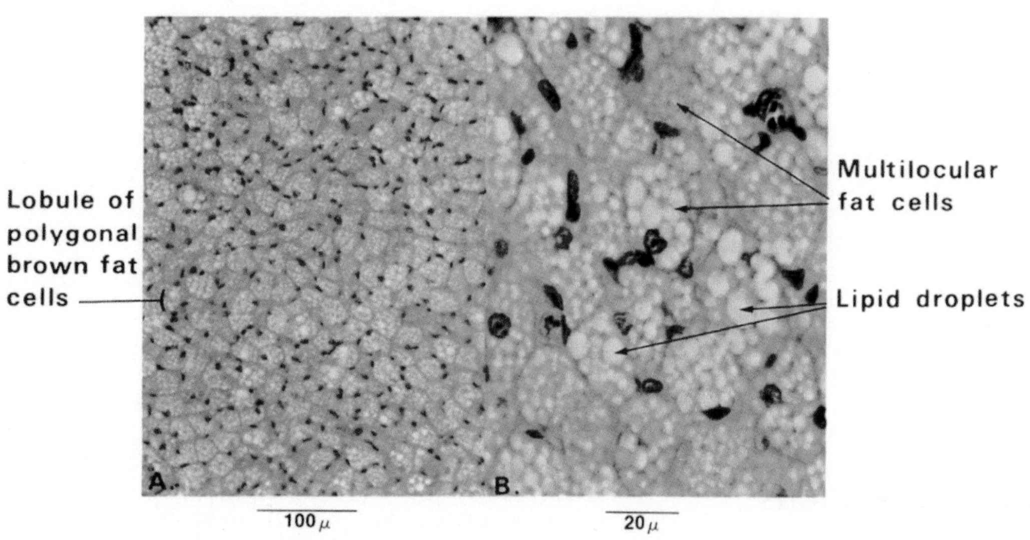

Rhesus monkey, Helly's fluid, H. & E., A. 162 x., B. 612 x.

B

SKIN MANIFESTATIONS

A: Acanthosis of the neck in a young woman with severe insulin resistance and obesity. **B:** Acute neuropathic ulcer in a 34-year-old man with diabetes who has had previous amputations for osteomyelitis secondary to ulceration. **C, D:** Necrobiosis lipoidica in a 24-year-old patient with type 1 diabetes. **E:** Disseminated granuloma annulare. **F:** Eruptive xanthomata of the abdomen in a 45-year-old patient with uncontrolled type 1 diabetes. **G, H:** Perforating folliculitis in a 50-year-old patient with diabetes with retinopathy and nephropathy.

Plate II

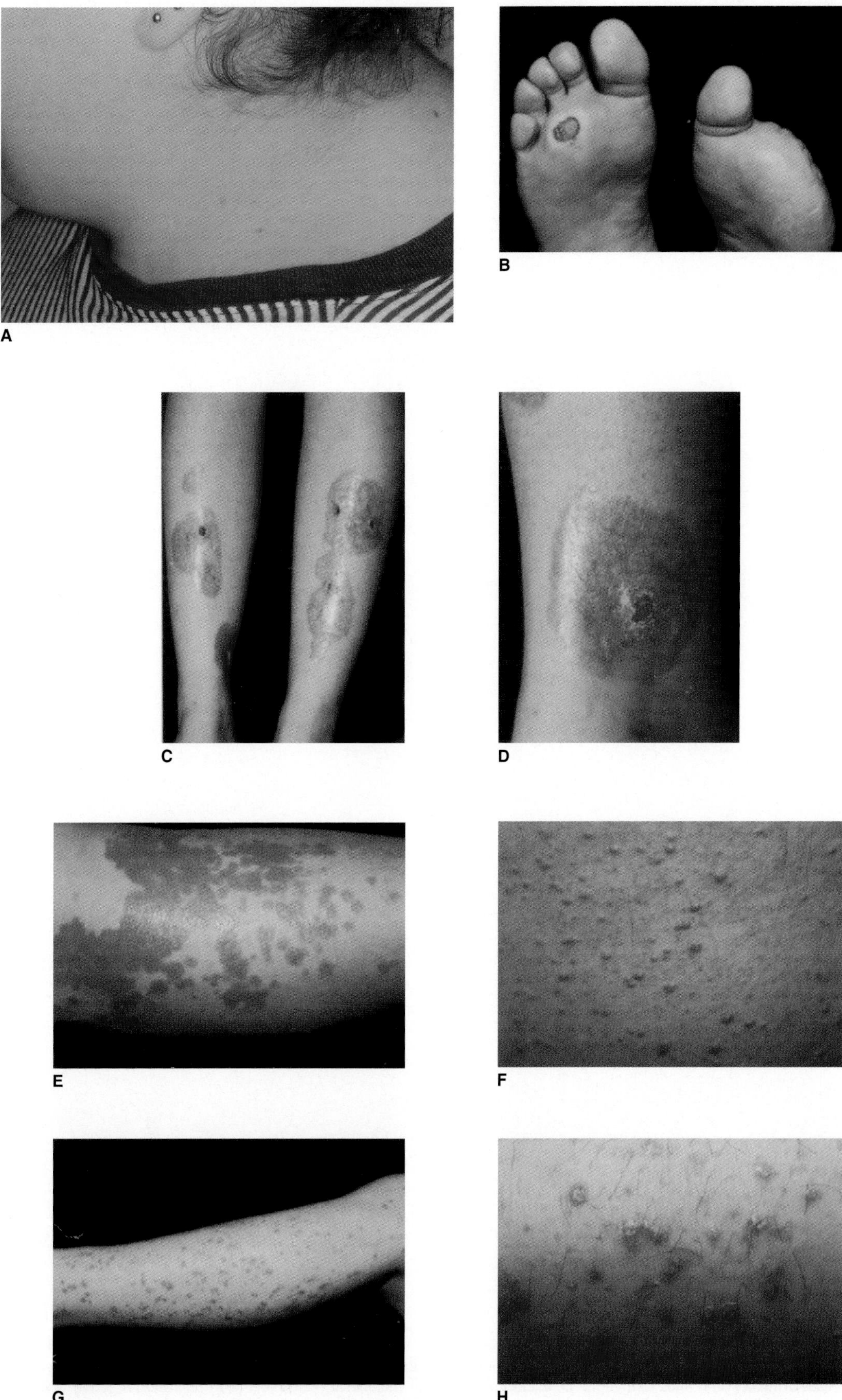

ULCERS

A: Early neuropathic ulcer over fifth metatarsal prominence. **B:** Chronic heel ulcer. **C:** Neuropathic forefoot ulcer over first metatarsal head with callus formation. **D, E:** Deceptively small metatarsal head ulcer with necrotic toe. Note true extent of ulcer, penetrating the foot to the dorsum.

Plate III

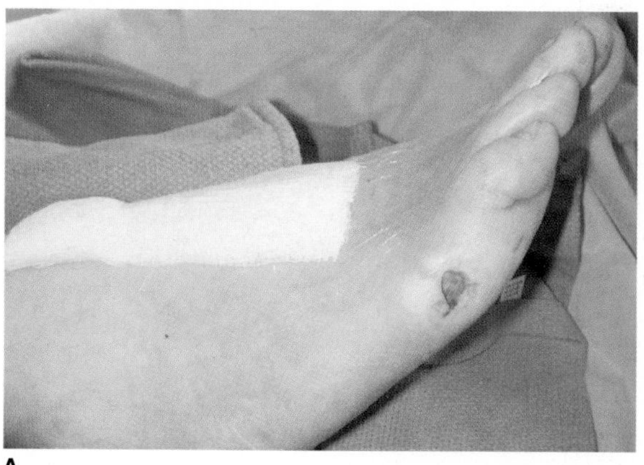
A

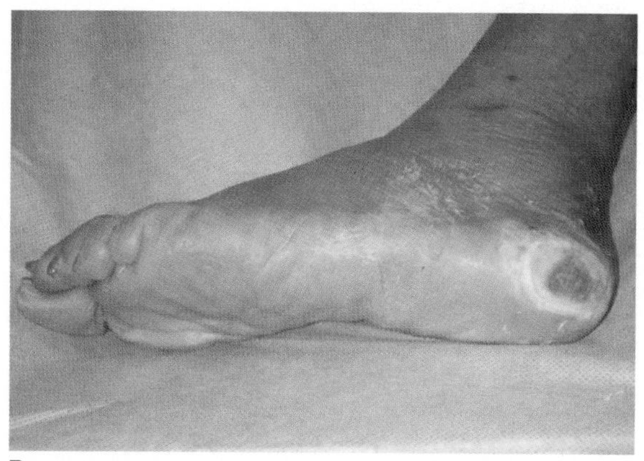
B

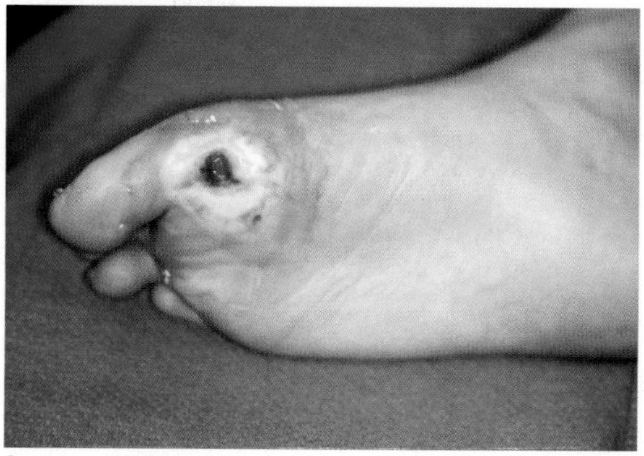

C

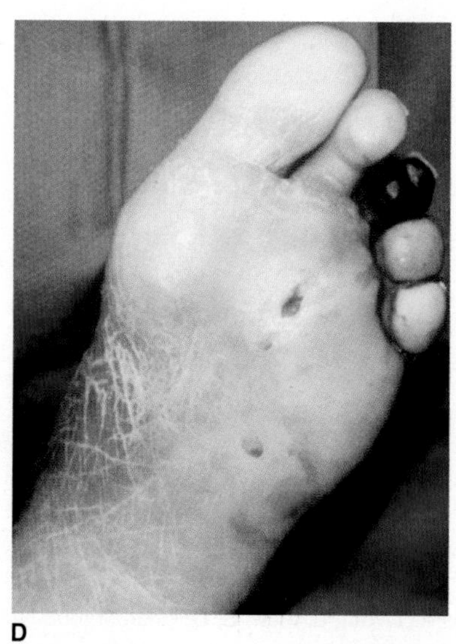
D

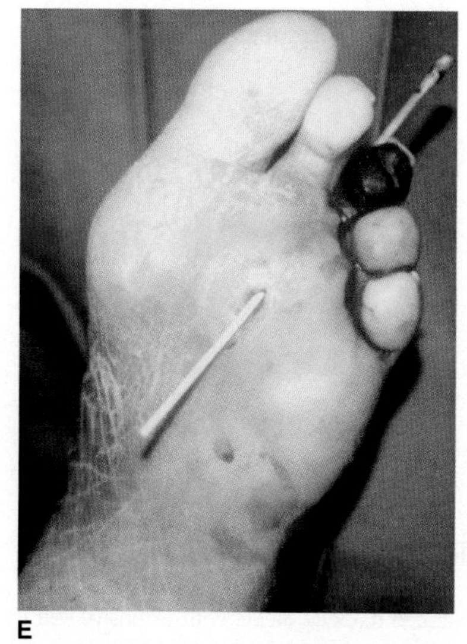
E

ULCERS AND CHARCOT FOOT

A, B: Advanced diabetic ulcers with extensive soft tissue and bone loss. Note clawing of toes. **C, D:** Charcot foot. Note ulcer forming over area of abnormally high pressure in this misshapen foot.

Plate IV

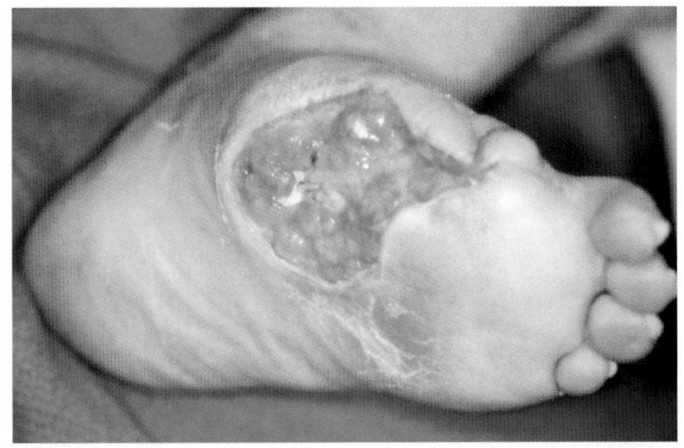

A

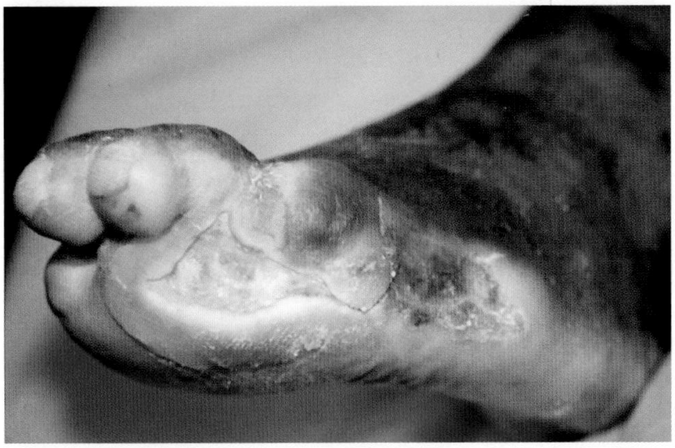

B

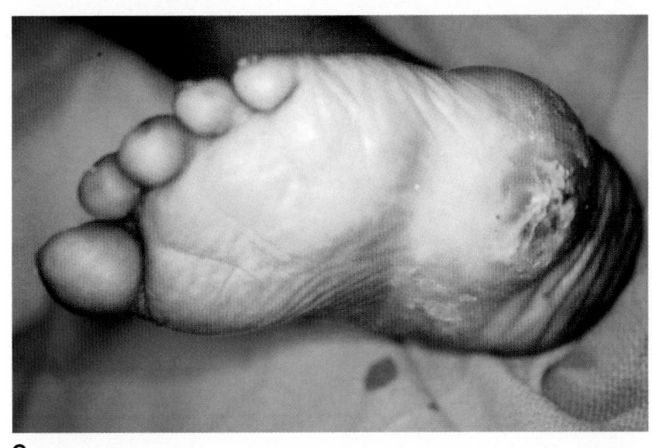

C

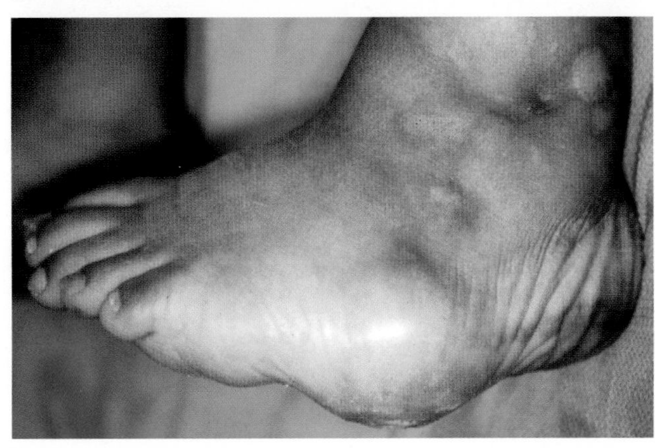

D

CHAPTER 22

Genetics of Type 2 Diabetes

Alessandro Doria

Type 2 diabetes, or non–insulin-dependent diabetes (NIDDM), is one of the most common metabolic disorders affecting humans. Approximately 14 million Americans have been diagnosed with this disease, and at least one third more are estimated to be affected without knowing it (1,2). Recent population surveys also indicate a striking increase in the prevalence of this disease in the United States, especially in younger people, with a 33% increase overall and a 70% increase in the 30- to 39-year age group during the 8-year period from 1990 to 1998 (2). Type 2 diabetes is now also a common diagnosis in the pediatric age group (3). The increasing number of affected people, together with the extensive list of long-term complications, including accelerated atherosclerosis, nephropathy, retinopathy, and neuropathy, makes type 2 diabetes a major health problem (4). The economic burden of diabetes is in excess of $100 billion annually in the United States alone. These factors have created a compelling need to understand the important role of genetic and environmental alterations in the etiology of this disease—to provide critical clues to the primary defects in this disorder, to allow tests that identify individuals at high risk of type 2 diabetes who may benefit from preventive programs, and to foster the development of new drugs to treat or prevent it.

GENES AND TYPE 2 DIABETES

Unlike type 1 diabetes, which is due to a single pathophysiologic defect (autoimmune destruction of β-cells resulting in a lack of endogenous insulin), most patients with type 2 diabetes exhibit two apparently different defects: (a) an impairment in the ability of muscle and fat to respond to insulin with increased glucose uptake and of liver to respond with decreased glucose output, i.e., insulin resistance; and (b) a failure of the β-cell to compensate for this insulin resistance by appropriately increasing insulin secretion (5) (Fig. 22.1). Although there are notable exceptions, in most longitudinal studies, insulin resistance can be demonstrated early in life before any evidence of glucose intolerance, whereas the β-cell failure develops somewhat later, in association with impaired glucose tolerance (5–8).

The contribution of genetic factors to the development of insulin resistance, impaired insulin secretion, and type 2 diabetes has been known for many years (9,10). Supporting evidence includes the familial clustering of these traits (9–11), the higher concordance rate of type 2 diabetes in monozygotic versus dizygotic twins (12–14), and the high prevalence of type 2 diabetes in certain ethnic groups (e.g., Pima Indians or Mexican Americans) (8,15) (see Chapter 20 for further discussion of this topic). On the other hand, environmental factors also appear to play a role, as indicated by the increasing incidence of type 2 diabetes during the past decade, the well-known links to diet and lifestyle, and the differences in risk of type 2 diabetes among genetically similar populations living in different areas (2,16). Thus, diabetes can be viewed as a complex disorder, with genetic factors conferring an increased *susceptibility* upon which environmental factors must act in order for hyperglycemia to develop (Fig. 22.2). This model is analogous to those proposed for other multifactorial disorders such as cancer and hypertension (17). It is estimated that between 25% and 70% of the occurrence of type 2 diabetes can be attributed to genetic factors (14).

Studies of the patterns of inheritance indicate that multiple genes probably are involved, although their number and relative contributions are uncertain (18,19). As schematically illustrated in Figure 22.3, different loci may contribute to the etiology of type 2 diabetes by interacting with each other within the same causal complex (*epistasis*). However, genes may also belong to different causal pathways, each being responsible for the development of diabetes in different subsets of indi-

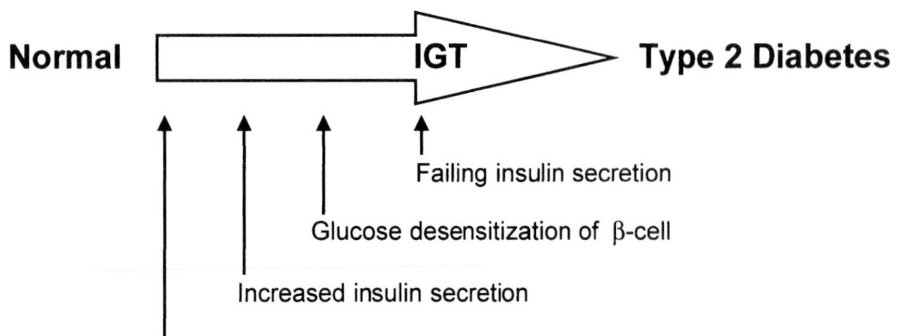
Normal
IGT
Type 2 Diabetes
Failing insulin secretion
Glucose desensitization of β-cell
Increased insulin secretion
Decreased insulin sensitivity

Figure 22.1. Model of the progressive pathogenesis of type 2 diabetes. In most individuals, there is a slow progression from normal or impaired glucose tolerance (IGT) to overt diabetes. This depends on interaction between genetic and environmental factors that regulate insulin sensitivity or the ability of β-cell to secrete insulin.

viduals (*genetic heterogeneity*). Some loci may be necessary but not sufficient (e.g., locus A in Fig. 22.3), whereas others may be neither necessary nor sufficient for the development of diabetes (e.g., loci B, C, and D). In this context, certain genes may predominate, their effects being more important than others (*major gene effects*). Some genetic characteristics may act only if patients are in the homozygous state (*recessive inheritance*), while for others the presence of only one allele may suffice (*dominant inheritance*). Furthermore, genetic susceptibility and environmental factors may interact in several different ways. For instance, environmental factors, such as excess caloric intake or sedentary lifestyle, may be responsible for the onset (initiation) of the metabolic abnormalities or β-cell damage, while genetic factors may be involved in regulating the rate of progression to overt diabetes. In other cases, genetic characteristics may be necessary from the very beginning for environmental factors to initiate the cascade of events leading to diabetes. Some of these genes may act at the level of insulin action while others may be involved in the regulation of insulin secretion.

This complexity makes the task of finding the genes for type 2 diabetes a formidable one. For instance, because of the important role played by environmental factors, cases of type 2 diabetes that are due entirely to nongenetic causes (so-called *phenocopies*) may be relatively frequent, especially in older populations. Conversely, diabetes may not develop in a substantial proportion of individuals carrying a susceptible genetic background because they have not been exposed to a diabetogenic environment or because they are not old enough (so-called *nonpenetrants*). Under these circumstances, research approaches that have been successful in identifying genes for mendelian disorders are difficult and of limited power. These problems, however, are counterbalanced by several major developments that have occurred during the past decade, namely the development of the polymerase chain reaction (20), the discovery of the class of DNA polymorphisms known as microsatellites and their systematic characterization as markers (21), the construction of genetic and physical maps of the human genome (22), the development of nonparametric methods of analysis of genetic data (23), and, finally, the completion of the Human Genome Project, which has provided the full human genome sequence and an initial catalogue of human genetic variation (24,25). The availability of these new tools carries with it the promise of finding the genes responsible for complex disorders, including type 2 diabetes.

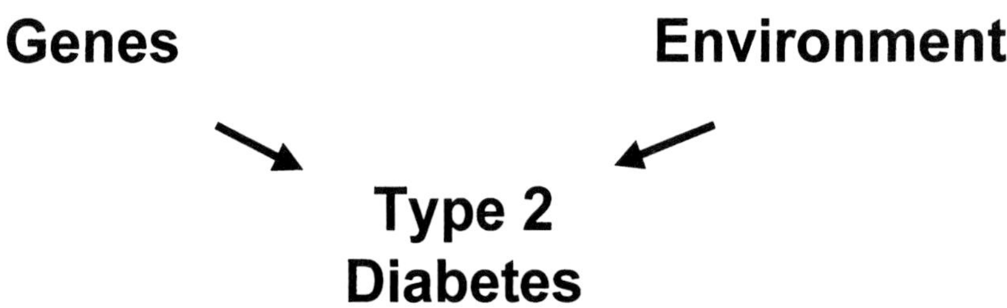
Genes
Environment
Type 2 Diabetes
• Higher concordance in monozygotic than dizygotic twins
• Clustering in families
• High prevalence in certain ethnic groups (e.g. Pima, Mexican-Americans).
• Links to life-style and diet
• Different incidence in genetically similar population living in different areas
• Type 2 diabetes secondary to other conditions

Figure 22.2. Contribution of genes and environment to the pathogenesis of type 2 diabetes. Available evidence supporting a role of genetic factors is listed on the left; the evidence for environmental factors is on the right.

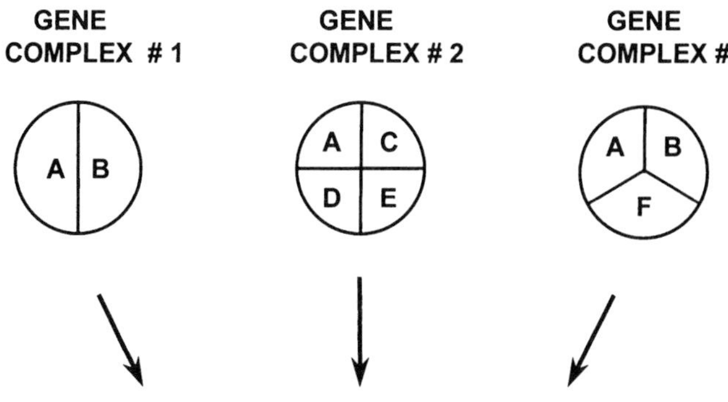

Figure 22.3. Illustration of the complex genetics of type 2 diabetes. Multiple type 2 diabetes genes (indicated by different letters of the alphabet) interact one with each other within different causal complexes that all lead to increased genetic susceptibility to the disease.

THE SEARCH FOR TYPE 2 DIABETES GENES

A powerful approach to the identification of genetic variants that predispose to type 2 diabetes is to investigate their association with the disease in human populations (26,27). In their simplest version, these studies compare the distribution of the alleles of a polymorphic locus between unrelated cases with type 2 diabetes and nondiabetic controls representative of the population from which cases have arisen (26). Any significant difference in allele distribution between cases and controls can be considered as evidence that this polymorphism or one associated (i.e., in *linkage disequilibrium*) with it contributes to the susceptibility to type 2 diabetes. Being case-control studies, association studies can be analyzed with the standard epidemiologic tools for evaluating disease risk according to various exposures, so that the presence of interaction between two loci or between a locus and environmental exposures can easily be tested. While straightforward in concept, association studies must be designed and analyzed according to established epidemiologic principles (26). False-positive results may arise due to unrecognized population differences between cases and controls (population stratification), while false-negative results can result from inappropriate study design such as inadequate sample size or inappropriate selection of cases and controls. The detection of small genetic effects may require several hundreds of cases and controls, especially if the linkage disequilibrium between the marker and the candidate susceptibility locus is weak (26,27). Despite these potential problems, association studies have nevertheless proved to be useful tools for detecting genetic contributions to human disorders, including diabetes. This is best exemplified by the case of HLA and type 1 diabetes (28).

It is estimated that about 11 million common variants (*polymorphisms*)—about 1 every 300 base pairs (bp)—are present along the human genome (29). Different combinations of these sequence differences account for heritable variation among individuals, including susceptibility to type 2 diabetes. Despite the remarkable progress in biotechnology, testing all 11 million variants for association with type 2 diabetes is not a feasible task at this time. To circumvent this problem, it has been proposed that the analysis be limited to a subset of polymorphisms that are spaced at regular intervals along the genome and serve as markers for intervening variants in linkage disequilibrium with these. The Human Genome Project has generated an extensive map of *single-nucleotide polymorphisms* (SNPs) that can be used for this task (25), but the number of markers needed to cover the whole genome may be disproportionally high [up to 500,000 according to one simulation (30)]. Another issue of concern is the stochastic variance of linkage disequilibrium throughout the genome, making the prospect of an effective whole-genome screen through this approach uncertain (31,32). Because of these constraints, association studies have thus far been focused on specific *candidate genes* selected according to two different strategies: (a) the study of genes that have been demonstrated to have a role in glucose homeostasis (*functional candidate genes*), and (b) the investigation of genes placed in chromosomal regions that are found to be inherited together (*linked*) with type 2 diabetes in whole-genome screens of families (*positional candidate genes*) (33). Such genome scans for linkage are not as sensitive as association studies, especially in the case of multifactorial disorders, but have the great advantage of not being limited to genes that are known to play a role in glucose metabolism (27). Both strategies have been widely used during the past decade and have led to the identification of many potential genes for type 2 diabetes (34). The most important of these loci, along with their positions along the genome, are reported in Figure 22.4.

MONOGENIC FORMS OF DIABETES

The search has been particularly successful for special types of familial diabetes that are transmitted with a mendelian mode of inheritance and share some clinical features with type 2 diabetes. While these syndromes are fairly rare, their study has provided insights into the etiology of more common forms of type 2 diabetes and has led to the identification of new classes of candidate genes. Three main categories of monogenic forms of diabetes have been identified to date: maturity-onset diabetes of the young (MODY), genetic syndromes of extreme insulin resistance, and mitochondrial diabetes.

Maturity-Onset Diabetes of the Young

The term MODY was first introduced by Tattersall and Fajans in 1975 to indicate type 2–like diabetes with early onset (before age 25) and an autosomal dominant mode of inheritance (35). It is now clear that forms of autosomal dominant diabetes can occur after age 25 and that the inheritance pattern is more important than age at onset for the diagnosis (36–38). Autosomal dominant diabetes probably accounts for 1% to 3% of all cases of diabetes, although precise estimates of its prevalence are not available. The presence of large families with multiple affected members, coupled with the simple pattern of inheritance, has facilitated genetic studies of this disorder. Six different forms of MODY have been identified to date, each involving a mutation in a different gene located on a different chromosome (Table 22.1).

The first MODY gene to be recognized was glucokinase (*GCK1*) (39–42), followed by hepatocyte nuclear factors (HNF) 1α and 4α (43,44). Glucokinase is the first enzyme involved in glucose metabolism in the β-cell (45), whereas HNF1α and HNF4α are transcription factors that regulate the expression of several genes in the liver and the β-cell (46,47). Glucokinase mutations are present in greater than 50% of French patients with MODY but are less frequent in other populations, repre-

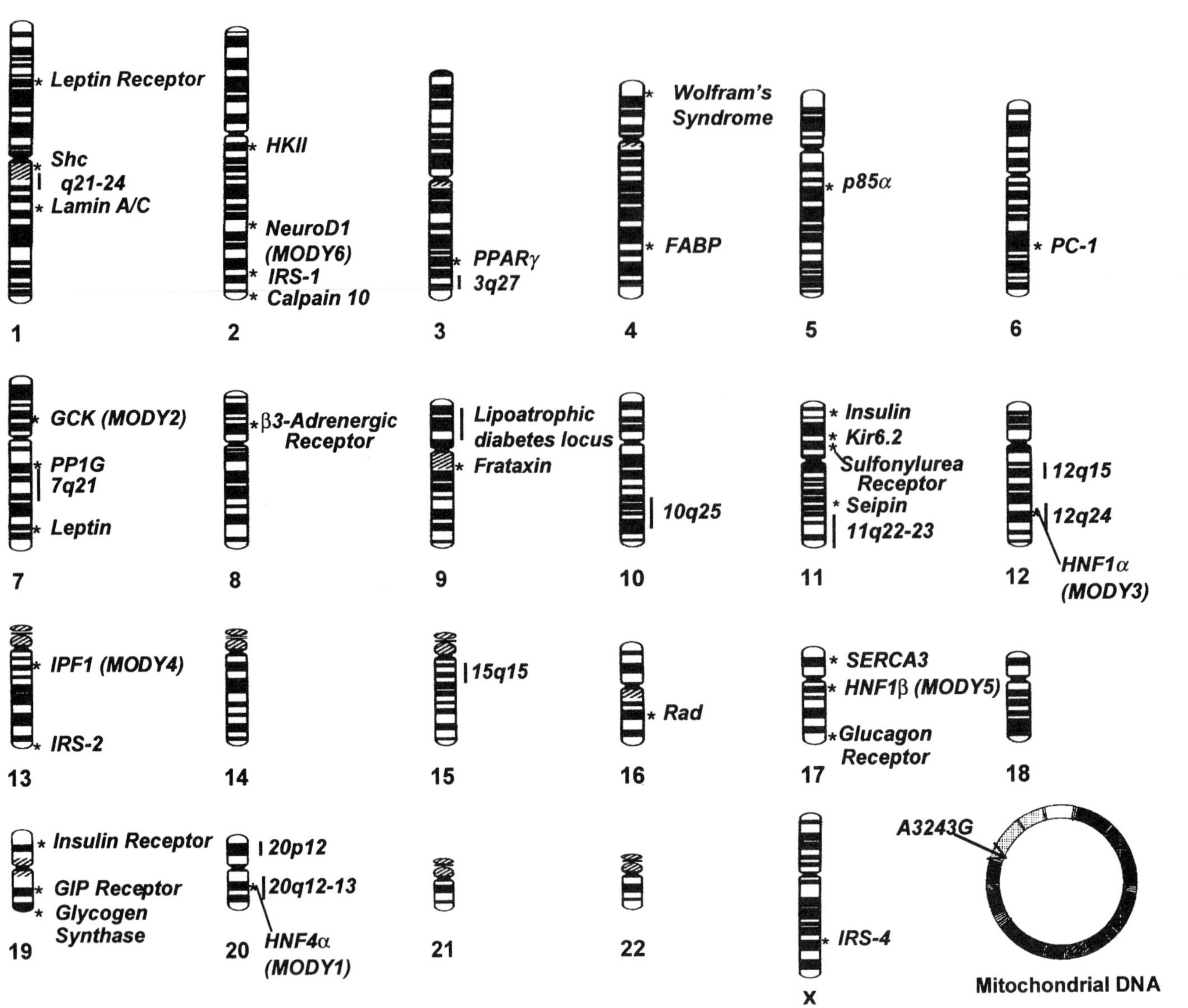

Figure 22.4. Location of potential type 2 diabetes genes in the human genome. (Modified from Almind K, Doria A, Kahn CR. Putting the genes for type II diabetes on the map. *Nat Med* 2001;7:277–279.)

TABLE 22.1. Genes Found to Be Mutated in Autosomal Dominant Diabetes or Maturity-Onset Diabetes of the Young

Gene	Chromosomal region	Clinical characteristics	Study
Glucokinase	7p15	Mild diabetes or impaired glucose tolerance, young age at diagnosis, rare microvascular complications	Vionnet et al. (41) Stoffel et al. (42)
HNF1α	12q24	Severe diabetes, young age at diagnosis, frequent need for insulin therapy, microvascular complications	Yamagata et al. (43)
HNF4α	20q12–q13	Mild to severe diabetes, young age at diagnosis, subtle liver abnormalities	Yamagata et al. (44)
IPF1/PDX1	13q12	Mild diabetes, variable age at diagnosis, pancreatic agenesis (homozygosis)	Stoffers et al. (37)
HNF1β	17q12–q21	Mild to severe diabetes, young age at diagnosis, nondiabetic kidney disease, genital malformations	Horikawa et al. (50) Lindner et al. (52)
neuroD1/BETA2	2q32	Mild to severe diabetes, variable age at diagnosis	Malecki et al. (38)

senting 10% to 25% of cases in the United States and the United Kingdom and only 1% of cases in Japan (48). Mutations in HNF1α and HNF4α account for approximately 70% of cases of MODY in the United States and the United Kingdom (48,49). Rarer forms of MODY have also been found associated with mutations in other three transcription factors expressed in the liver and the β-cell, namely insulin promoter factor 1 (IPF1, also known as *PDX1, IDX1,* or *STF1*), HNF1β, and neuroD1 (also known as BETA2) (37,38,50). MODY due to mutations in IPF1 has been described in a single family, in which the homozygous proband had pancreatic agenesis and the heterozygous parents had diabetes (51). Diabetes due to mutations in HNF1α is also very rare and often associated with kidney cystic disease, genital malformations, or both (52,53). Two mutations in neuroD1 have been described, one in a typical MODY pedigree, the other in a family with "typical" type 2 diabetes, but with an autosomal dominant mode of inheritance (38).

A prominent feature of all forms of MODY is a defect of insulin secretion (54,55). In the case of glucokinase mutations, this is due to an impairment of the β-cell glucose sensor caused by a decrease in the ability of glucokinase to phosphorylate glucose, resulting in inappropriately low fasting concentrations of insulin in relation to glycemic levels (45). For mutations in transcription factors, the cause of diabetes is less clear. One hypothesis is that a reduced activity of these transcription factors may impair the differentiation of islet cells during development, thereby reducing the number of functional β-cells in affected individuals (56–59). Another possibility is that these mutations directly affect the expression of genes required for glucose transport and metabolism in the β-cell (60). Also a direct effect on the expression of the insulin gene cannot be ruled out, especially for IPF1 and neuroD1, which are known regulators of insulin gene transcription (61,62). A clarification is expected from the postmortem analysis of islets from mutation carriers and from expression profile studies aimed at identifying the target genes of these transcription factors.

From a clinical standpoint, mutations in the glucokinase gene cause a rather mild form of diabetes (Table 22.1). Hyperglycemia is often diagnosed early in life, but fasting blood glucose values rarely exceed 130 mg/dL and the occurrence of diabetic complications is rare (54,63). Diabetes associated with mutations in HNF1α, HNF4α, and HNF1β is generally more severe (Table 22.1) (55). The insulin response to a glucose load is severely impaired, with insulin levels during an oral glucose tolerance test (OGTT) rarely exceeding 20 to 30 μU/mL (36,55). About 50% of diabetic carriers need insulin therapy, and diabetic complications are more common than in MODY due to glucokinase mutations (55,63). Diabetes due to IPF1 mutations is milder and is diagnosed at a slightly older age than is MODY due to HNF mutations (37). Of the two families thus far described as carrying neuroD1 mutations (38), one has a phenotype resembling that of MODY due to HNF1α mutations (young age at diagnosis, low prevalence of obesity, low insulin levels), while the phenotype in the other is more similar to that of common type 2 diabetes (older age at diagnosis, high prevalence of obesity, conserved insulin secretion).

While these are the general features of diabetes associated with different MODY genes, there is wide variability in the clinical presentation within the same MODY subtype. Some of this variability may be accounted for by the different nature of mutations segregating with diabetes in different families (*allelic heterogeneity*). However, large variation in the age at onset and severity of diabetes also is observed among carriers of identical mutations. This variability may be due to the presence of environmental or genetic factors that act as modifiers of the phenotype associated with each mutation. For instance, it has been hypothesized that co-inheritance of common type 2 diabetes susceptibility genes may determine a more severe presentation of MODY (64). Thus, MODY might not be the simple, monogenic disorder that has usually been considered, and further study of known MODY forms may lead to the discovery of new loci playing important roles in glucose homeostasis.

Finally, the six genes thus far identified do not account for all cases of autosomal dominant diabetes. In France and England, approximately 25% of MODY pedigrees do not show linkage with glucokinase, HNF1α, or HNF4α (48,65). The proportion of cases not accounted for by known genes appears to be even higher among families with an older age at diagnosis of diabetes (36). Available data suggest that some of these families are characterized by a pure insulin secretion defect, similar to that of HNF1α diabetes, whereas others are predominantly insulin-resistant, similar to common type 2 diabetes (36) (Fig. 22.5). Thus, a high degree of genetic heterogeneity is expected. Recent data from the laboratories of the Joslin Diabetes Center indicate that a locus accounting for diabetes in some of these families may be placed on chromosome 12q, 50 cM centromeric to HNF1α (66).

Genetic Syndromes of Extreme Insulin Resistance

Although rarer than MODY, syndromes of severe insulin resistance have been known for several years. Forms that have been described include leprechaunism, Rabson-Mendenhall syndrome, type A and type B syndromes, and lipodystrophies (67–71). Leprechaunism is a congenital syndrome characterized by severe insulin resistance of peripheral tissues, intrauterine and neonatal growth retardation, elfin facies, and early death (67). The Rabson-Mendenhall syndrome becomes evident during childhood, with severe insulin resistance, abnormal nails and dentition, accelerated growth, precocious pseudopuberty, and pineal hyperplasia (68). The type A syndrome of insulin resistance primarily affects young women, who present with severe hyperinsulinemia (>50 μU/mL in the fasting state), hyperandrogenism, polycystic ovary, and acanthosis nigricans (hyperpigmented and hyperkeratotic lesions in skinfold areas) (69). The type B syndrome has features similar to those of type A but affects older women and is often accompanied by autoimmune features (69). Finally, lipodystrophies are characterized by complete (lipoatrophic diabetes) or partial lack of adipose tissue, hepatosplenomegaly, hyperlipidemia, and severe insulin resistance, which can be present at birth or appear later in life (70,71).

Mutations in the insulin-receptor gene (*INSR*) impairing insulin action underlie all cases of leprechaunism and Rabson-Mendenhall syndrome described to date (72). Mutations in this gene are also responsible for a good proportion of cases of type A syndrome (72,73). Some of these sequence differences lead to a lower number of receptors because of decreased synthesis, increased degradation, or abnormal translocation from the endoplasm to the cell membrane (72). Other mutations are instead associated with decreased affinity of the receptor for insulin or impaired tyrosine kinase activity (72,73). In many instances, these forms are inherited in an autosomal recessive fashion, with some patients being homozygotes for a single mutation and others being compound heterozygotes who inherited two different mutant alleles, one from each parent. A few patients appear to have mutations in only one allele, suggesting an autosomal dominant pattern of inheritance, but the

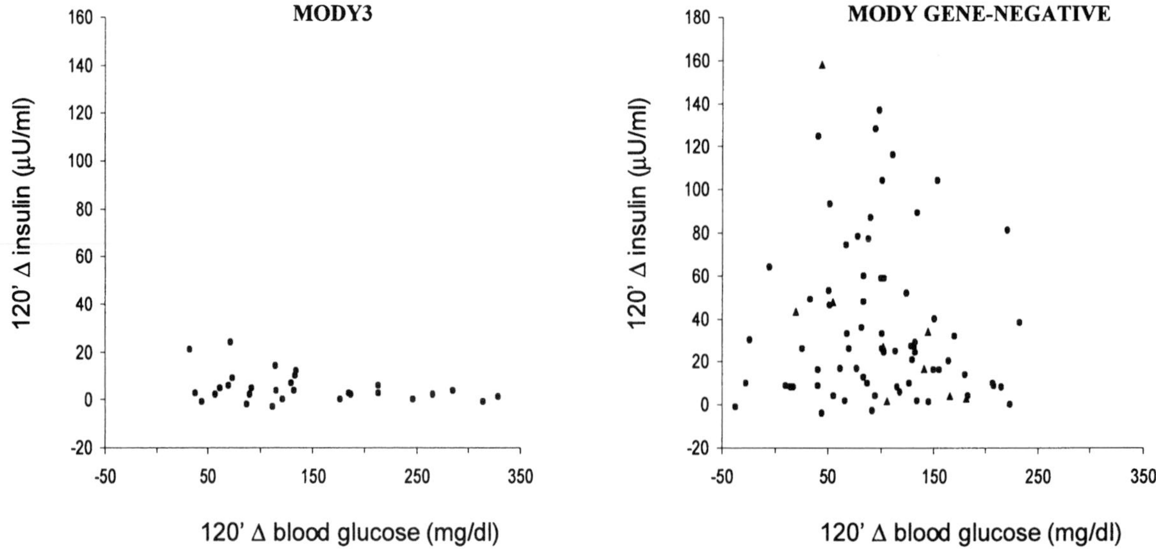

Figure 22.5. Relationship between increments in insulin secretion and blood glucose during oral glucose tolerance test (OGTT; 120′ Δ, change 2 hours after glucose ingestion) in maturity-onset diabetes of the young (MODY). Data are reported on the left for diabetic carriers of HNF1α mutations (MODY3) and on the right for diabetic members of families with early-onset, autosomal dominant type 2 diabetes not accounted for by known MODY genes (MODY gene–negative). Only individuals not treated with insulin were considered. MODY 3 subjects are characterized by a pure insulin secretion defect, while a more heterogeneous pattern is visible among MODY gene–negative subjects. (Copyright © 1999. From Doria A, Yang Y, Malecki M, et al. Phenotypic characteristics of early-onset autosomal-dominant type 2 diabetes unlinked to known maturity-onset diabetes of the young (MODY) genes. *Diabetes Care* 1999;22:253–261, with permission from the American Diabetes Association.)

presence of as yet unidentified mutations in the "healthy" allele cannot be excluded in these cases.

Autosomal dominant forms of partial lipodystrophy (Dunnigan-Kobberling type) have recently been found to be due to mutations in the lamin A/C gene (*LMNA*) on chromosome 1q21 (74,75). Lamins are the main components of the nuclear lamina, the proteinaceous layer that is apposed to the inner nuclear membrane (76). The *LMNA* gene codes for two of these proteins, lamin A and C, through alternative splicing. Most of the mutations associated with partial lipodystrophy cluster on a 15-bp region of exon 8 of the *LMNA* gene and affect the globular C-terminal domain of the lamin A/C proteins (74,75). Especially frequent are substitutions of a highly conserved arginine at position 482. Little is known, however, about the mechanisms linking these mutations to lipodystrophy, insulin resistance, and hyperlipoproteinemia. Lamins are expressed in all tissues, where they play a role in DNA replication, chromatin organization, nuclear-pore arrangement, and anchorage of nuclear envelope proteins (76). Of note, mutations in the *LMNA* gene have also been found to be associated with Emery-Dreyfuss muscular dystrophy and dilated cardiomyopathy and conduction-system disease (77,78). In contrast with partial lipodystrophy, mutations in these disorders are distributed across several exons. Thus, the region around residue 482 in the globular domain of lamins A/C may determine specific functions in the adipocyte, the impairment of which leads to lipodystrophy. Mutations in the *LMNA* gene, however, do not appear to be involved in the etiology of generalized lipodystrophy [lipoatrophic diabetes or Berardinelli-Seip syndrome (BSCL)] (79). A locus linked with some of these forms (*BSCL2*) has recently been mapped to chromosome 11q13 and shown to correspond to the human homologue of the murine guanine nucleotide-binding protein (G protein), γ3-linked gene (*GnG31g*) (80). *BSCL2* is most highly expressed in brain and testis and codes for a protein, called seipin, of unknown function. Another *BSCL* locus (*BSCL1*) has been mapped on 9q34 in *BSCL2*-negative families, but the identity of the gene that is involved is unknown (80).

Mitochondrial Diabetes

The mitochondrial genome consists of a circular 16,569-bp DNA molecule containing the genes for ribosomal and transfer RNAs and for some proteins of the respiratory chain. This DNA (mtDNA) has several unique features. First, it is transmitted only through the maternal side, since the sperm sheds its mitochondria during penetration into the ovum (81). Second, it exists in the cell in several copies—as many as a few thousand in cells with a high mitochondrial content. Finally, it is prone to a high degree of mutation and rearrangement, which, however, often affect only a fraction of the mtDNA, a phenomenon known as *heteroplasmy*. For each mutation, levels of heteroplasmy vary, being much higher in nondividing tissues such as muscle and brain than in rapidly dividing cells such as leukocytes.

A variety of syndromes associated with point mutations or deletions in the mtDNA have been described. Most of these concern tissues that have a high demand for energy, such as skeletal muscle and brain. The maternally inherited diabetes and neurosensory deafness (MIDD) syndrome is caused by a single nucleotide mutation (A3243G) in the mtDNA encoding the transfer RNA (tRNA) for leucine (82–85). Rare cases of MIDD have also been observed in association with mtDNA deletions or duplications (86). These mitochondrial defects are thought to result in altered oxidative metabolism in the β-cell, leading to an impairment in the production of ATP that is needed for glucose-stimulated release of insulin (87,88). A reduction in the oxidative metabolism of glucose in peripheral tissues may also contribute to the development of hyperglycemia, but its role is uncertain. The MIDD syndrome accounts for approximately 1% of individuals with diabetes.

Mitochondrial diabetes usually is characterized by an early onset of hyperglycemia (often before age 30), which is due to impaired insulin secretion and is followed by a rapid progression to insulin dependence (84,85). In some instances, MIDD can be misdiagnosed as type 1 diabetes (if insulin is required from the onset) or type 2 diabetes (if it can be managed with diet or oral medications), but patients are generally negative for islet-cell antibody and do not show increased prevalence of obesity (85). Impaired hearing, which can be so severe as to require the use of a hearing aid, is present in the majority of patients with MIDD and becomes manifest as a loss of high-frequency perception. The A3243G mutation also may lead to the so-called MELAS syndrome (mitochondrial myopathy, encephalopathy, lactic acidosis, and stroke-like episodes), which may or may not be associated with diabetes (89). Differences in phenotypic expression of the mitochondrial defects may be due to variations in the degree of heteroplasmy and to the tissue distribution of heteroplasmic mtDNA (85). The variable degree of heteroplasmy may also be responsible for difficulties in identifying the mitochondrial mutations responsible for the MIDD syndrome.

MULTIFACTORIAL FORMS OF TYPE 2 DIABETES

Because of the complex genetics, the search for genes involved in common, multifactorial type 2 diabetes has not been as successful. Many potential type 2 diabetes genes have been identified (Fig. 22.4), but findings have been difficult to replicate in most cases. Several factors contribute to these variable results. An important issue may be the presence of genetic heterogeneity, with different genes contributing to type 2 diabetes in different populations. Even within the same ethnic group, different subtypes of type 2 diabetes may be accounted for by different genes, making the results of association studies heavily dependent on how affected cases or families are selected. Discrepancies also can occur because of population differences in the linkage disequilibrium between markers and causal variants. Other important factors concern methodologic issues regarding the study design and the analysis of data. False-positive results can arise from multiple hypothesis testing or, in association studies, from unrecognized ethnic differences between cases and controls (so-called population stratification). Conversely, studies may fail to replicate true positive results because of inadequate statistical power or of failure to account for gene-gene or gene-environment interactions. All these factors must be carefully considered when weighing the evidence supporting or excluding the role of a certain locus. As discussed above, two main approaches have been followed to identify genes for multifactorial forms of type 2 diabetes: (a) studies of functional candidate genes and (b) whole-genome screens followed by the study of positional candidate genes.

Studies of Functional Candidate Genes

Selection of this class of candidate genes for type 2 diabetes has been based upon the biochemical function and expression pattern of the encoded proteins, which, if altered, might be implicated in the pathogenesis of the disease. Since both insulin resistance and a deficit of insulin production are involved in the etiology of type 2 diabetes (5), genes known to be involved in insulin action or β-cell function have been intensely investigated. Because of the strong links between obesity and type 2 diabetes, many studies have also considered genes involved in the regulation of the energy balance and in the development and metabolism of adipose tissue.

GENES INVOLVED IN INSULIN ACTION

Insulin action at the cellular level is the result of a complex network of signaling events (90) (Fig. 22.6). Binding of insulin to its

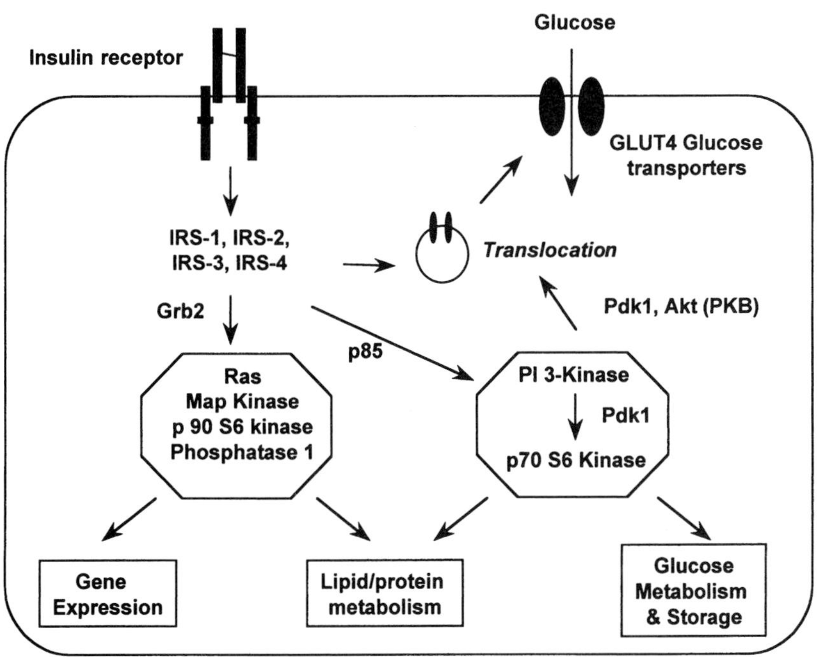

Figure 22.6. Schematic model of the cellular pathways involved in insulin signaling. IRS, insulin-receptor substrate; PDK, phosphoinositide-dependent protein kinase; PKB, protein kinase B; Grb, growth factor receptor–bound protein; p 90 S6 kinase and p 70 S6 kinase, 90 kDa and 70 kDa ribosomal kinase, respectively; PI, phosphatidylinositol.

receptor leads to activation of the insulin receptor tyrosine kinase, which results in phosphorylation of tyrosine residues on a family of insulin receptor substrates. These tyrosine-phosphorylated substrates then bind to and activate a number of intracellular proteins in the insulin signaling cascade, the most important of which for metabolic effects is phosphatidylinositol (PI) 3-kinase. Docking of these proteins in turn activates specific signal transduction pathways (for instance, the translocation of glucose transporters to the plasma membrane) mediating the cellular effects of insulin.

Insulin Receptor. Despite the relatively high frequency of insulin-receptor mutations in syndromes of severe insulin resistance, genetic variability in the insulin receptor gene does not appear to play a major role in common forms of type 2 diabetes. Initial studies demonstrated several polymorphisms in the coding regions, some affecting the amino acid sequence, but none of these were shown to be more frequent in subjects with type 2 diabetes as compared with controls (91,92). Results were similarly negative in populations with a high prevalence of insulin resistance such as Pima Indians and in linkage analyses of families (93–95). More recently, a significant association has been reported between type 2 diabetes and the Val985Met variant in two Dutch populations (96). This polymorphism appears to confer a twofold increase in the risk of type 2 diabetes but, being rather rare, can account for only a handful of cases of type 2 diabetes. Since the *INSR* gene is rather large, noncoding regions have not been extensively screened for variation. Thus, one cannot rule out the existence of variants in as-yet unscreened regulatory elements that increase susceptibility to diabetes by impairing insulin-receptor expression. Indeed, a decrease in the number of insulin receptors is observed in type 2 diabetes, although this is common to all hyperinsulinemic states and is thought to be due to downregulation of the receptor through increased degradation (97). An additional factor is the alternative splicing of the messenger RNA, which originates two forms of the receptor differing by 12 amino acids near the C-terminus of the α-subunit (98,99). These two receptor isoforms exhibit subtle differences in binding affinities, tyrosine kinase activities, and internalization kinetics (100–102). Differences in the expression of these two subtypes between patients with type 2 diabetes and nondiabetic controls have been reported in the literature, but the significance of this result is controversial because not all studies have found this difference and the functional differences between the two isoforms are rather small (103–105). Whether the alternative splicing is under the control of genetic variants is unknown at this time.

Insulin-Receptor Substrates. One of the best-characterized molecules in the intracellular insulin action cascade is insulin-receptor substrate-1 (IRS-1), a 131-kilodalton (kDa) cytosolic protein that is tyrosine phosphorylated by the insulin receptor (106,107). In animal models, heterozygous disruption of IRS-1 does not lead to frank hyperglycemia but acts epistatically to potentiate other genetic defects in the production of diabetes (108,109). A total of nine amino acid substitutions have been identified in this molecule to date in white and Japanese populations (110–122). The most prevalent of these is a glycine-to-arginine substitution placed at codon 972 between two potential tyrosine phosphorylation sites binding the p85 subunit of PI 3-kinase (110). This variant has been examined for association with type 2 diabetes in more than 14 populations (110–122). While initial studies suggested an association with type 2 diabetes (110), the carrier frequency varies considerably among different populations (from 0.01 to 0.19) and an association with type 2 diabetes has not been observed in all populations (Fig. 22.7). If all these studies are considered together in a meta-analysis, the relative risk of type 2 diabetes associated with the Gly972Arg variant is not significantly different from 1 [odds ratio (OR): 1.05, 95% confidence interval (CI) 0.83–1.33]. Results are similar if the meta-analysis is performed separately for whites and Asians.

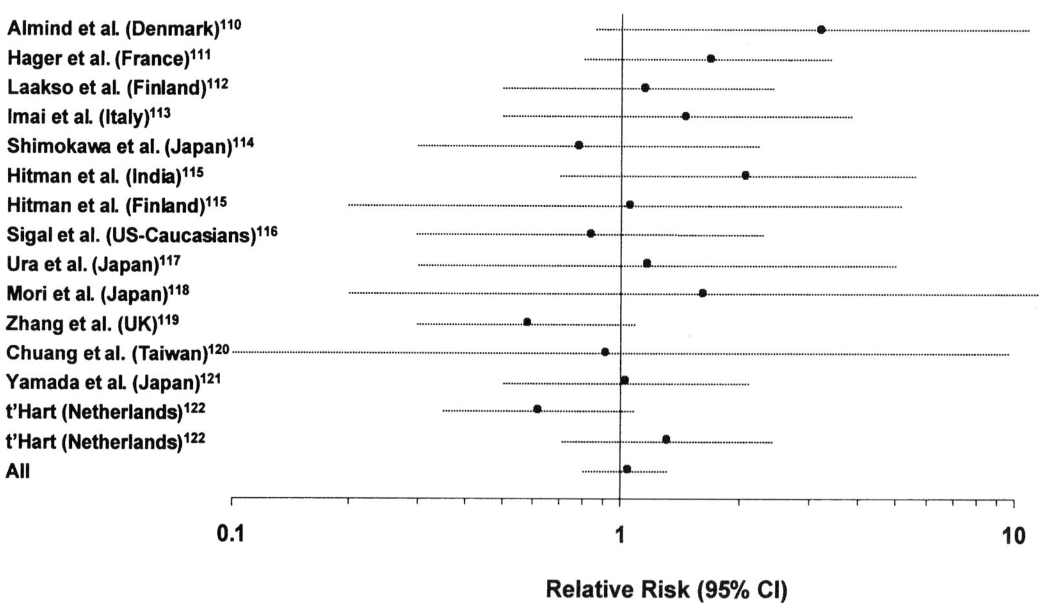

Figure 22.7. Estimated risk of type 2 diabetes associated with the IRS-1 Gly972Arg variant. For each study, the solid circles represent the odds ratio for 972Arg carriers and the dotted line indicates the 95% confidence interval. Odds ratios were not significantly different across studies ($p = 0.50$, Breslow-Day test). "All" indicates the Mantel-Haenszel estimate of the common relative risk based on all published studies (4,306 individuals).

Despite these negative results, IRS-1 cannot be easily dismissed as a possible type 2 diabetes gene. All the studies above considered cases of type 2 diabetes that were not selected on the basis of patients' insulin sensitivity or body weight. In contrast, it has been shown that the Gly972Arg is specifically associated with a subset of type 2 diabetes characterized by obesity and marked insulin resistance (115,123). Furthermore, functional data support a role for this variant in the etiology of insulin resistance. Transfection studies have consistently shown that the Arg^{972} allele is associated with a 40% decrease in IRS-1–associated PI 3-kinase activity and a 25% to 40% decrease in binding of the p85 subunit of PI 3-kinase to IRS-1 (124,125). It is interesting that expression of this variant in β-cells decreases both glucose and sulfonylurea-stimulated insulin secretion and that carriers of this allele have lower insulin-secretion rates during hyperglycemic clamp than do noncarriers (126,127). Thus, the Gly972Arg variant has the potential to contribute to both insulin resistance and the defective β-cell compensation characteristic of type 2 diabetes.

IRS-2 has been also at the center of intense investigation following the report that homozygous disruption of this gene in mice results in a phenotype similar to human type 2 diabetes (128). However, all three amino acid substitutions that have been identified in humans (Leu647Val, Gly879Ser, and Gly1057Asp) do not appear to be associated with type 2 diabetes, although nondiabetic Asp^{1057} homozygotes may have decreased insulin levels both in the fasting state and during OGTT (129–131). Variability in the coding region of the IRS-4 gene (placed on chromosome X) has also been excluded as a possible genetic determinant of type 2 diabetes (132). No information is available on the role of IRS-3, as the gene for this protein has been identified in mouse and rat but not in humans.

PI 3-Kinase. PI 3-kinase is the major protein that is bound and activated by phosphorylated IRSs (90). This molecule phosphorylates the inositol ring of phosphatidylinositol, producing phosphatidylinositol 4-phosphate (P), -4,5-P2, and 3,4,5-P3, which propagate the insulin signal to downstream pathways (133). A reduction in the insulin response of this enzymatic activity has been reported in muscle and adipose tissue from insulin-resistant subjects with type 2 diabetes (134). The enzyme consists of a catalytic subunit (p110) coupled to a regulatory subunit (p85) having two isoforms (α and β) encoded by different genes (135). A third regulatory subunit with lower molecular weight has also been isolated (p55γ) along with low-molecular-weight splice variants of p85α (136). A relatively common amino acid substitution (Met326Ile) has been identified in the p85α isoform (137). This residue is highly conserved across species and is placed in proximity to one of the two SH2 domains that interact with phosphorylated IRSs. While the Ile326 allele is not associated with type 2 diabetes, it was correlated with reductions in whole-body glucose effectiveness and intravenous glucose disappearance in healthy Danish subjects (137). In sharp contrast with these findings, the variant had an "antidiabetogenic" effect in Pima women, as indicated by a significantly higher acute insulin response during OGTT in Ile/Ile homozygotes (138). No effect was observed in Japanese patients (139). Results of *in vitro* experiments have failed to show significant difference in insulin-stimulated lipid kinase activity and phosphotyrosine recruitment between Met326 and Ile326 allele (140). Thus, if this polymorphism affects insulin action, its effect is probably minor. A rare variant of p85α (Arg409Gln) has been described in one subject with extreme insulin resistance and appears to be associated with lower insulin-stimulated PI 3-kinase activity (140). A screening of the p110 catalytic unit in Finnish subjects has identified two polymorphisms in the 5′ flanking region, but these are not associated with diabetes (141). The effect of genetic variability in the p85β and p55γ isoforms has not been investigated to date.

Genes Involved in Glucose Transport and Metabolism. While insulin has pleiotropic effects on cellular functions, the actions that have been specifically shown to be impaired in type 2 diabetes are those related to glucose uptake and incorporation into glycogen (5). In muscle and fat cells, insulin stimulates glucose uptake by inducing the translocation of glucose transporter 4 (GLUT4) from intracellular compartments to the cell surface and activates glycogen synthase by promoting its dephosphorylation (90). Both effects appear to involve the activation of the phosphoinositide-dependent protein kinase-1 (PDK1) and protein kinase B (PKB, also known as AKT) (Fig. 22.6), which have been both screened for amino acid variants in subjects with insulin resistance. However, only silent polymorphisms have been found (142). Likewise, variability in the GLUT4 gene (17p13) does not seem to contribute to type 2 diabetes. Sequence differences in GLUT4 promoter and coding sequence have been identified, but are either extremely rare or equally frequent in type 2 diabetic cases and nondiabetic controls (92,143–145).

The glycogen synthase gene (19q13) has been intensively investigated because of the finding of multiple defects in the activity of this enzyme in the skeletal muscle of patients with type 2 diabetes (146). An *Xba*I restriction fragment length polymorphism (RFLP) placed in intron 14 has been reported to be associated with type 2 diabetes, impaired nonoxidative glucose metabolism, and arterial hypertension in Finland (147). This finding has been replicated by the same authors in a different sample of unrelated Finnish individuals and in affected sib-pairs (148,149) but has not been confirmed in populations from France, Japan, and the United States (150,151, and A. S. Krolewski, personal communication). An association has been found in Pima Indians and Japanese but concerns a dinucleotide repeat rather than the *Xba*I polymorphism (152). A possible explanation is that both the *Xba*I polymorphism and the dinucleotide repeat are markers in linkage disequilibrium with as-yet-unidentified disease variants that are characteristic of specific populations. None of the amino acid polymorphisms identified to date appear to contribute to insulin-resistant phenotypes, although the very rare Pro442Ala variant has been shown to significantly decrease the ability of the enzyme to synthesize glycogen (153,154). A polymorphism in the regulatory G subunit of the glycogen synthase–activating protein phosphatase 1 (Asp905Tyr) may have a minor impact on insulin sensitivity in Danes, while a common variant in the 3′-untranslated region (UTR), causing a tenfold difference in reporter mRNA half-life, may contribute to insulin resistance in Pima Indians and aboriginal Canadians (155–157).

Inhibitors of Insulin Action. All the candidate genes described above have been selected based on the hypothesis that a genetically determined deficiency in elements of insulin action pathways leads to insulin resistance. An alternative concept is that insulin resistance may be due to a genetically determined excess in the expression or activity of inhibitors of insulin action. Several proteins that inhibit insulin signaling have been identified to date, and some of these have been investigated for a genetic contribution to type 2 diabetes (Fig. 22.8).

Rad is a member of a unique family of Ras-related guanosine triphosphatases that was identified by subtraction cloning between skeletal muscle of a type 2 diabetic individual and a nondiabetic subject (158). Rad expression is

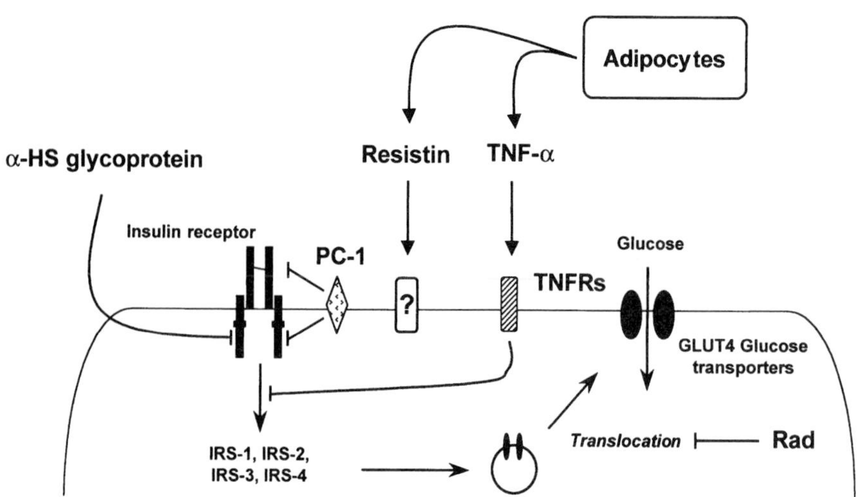

Figure 22.8. Natural inhibitors of insulin signaling and their action sites. TNF, tumor necrosis factor; TNFRs, TNF receptors; IRS, insulin-receptor substrate; PC, plasma cell membrane glycoprotein.

increased in about 20% of subjects with type 2 diabetes, its content being correlated to body weight and resting metabolic rate. The overexpression of this protein in cultured myocytes and adipocytes inhibits insulin-stimulated uptake of glucose through an effect on the intrinsic activity of GLUT4 molecules rather than on their translocation (159,160). The gene coding for Rad consists of 5 exons spanning about 3.7 kb on chromosome 16q (161). In a white population from the United States, a significant association was found between type 2 diabetes and the rare alleles of a composite trinucleotide repeat polymorphism placed in intron 2 (162). Carriers of these alleles had a threefold increase in the risk of diabetes as compared with noncarriers. This association, however, was not confirmed in Finns (163). By contrast, an association was detected in Japanese, but the alleles associated with type 2 diabetes are different from those found in whites in the United States (164). These discrepancies may reflect ethnic differences in the pattern of linkage disequilibrium between the trinucleotide repeat marker in exon 2 and a causal variant at the Rad locus or its vicinity.

Another potential inhibitor of insulin action is the plasma cell membrane glycoprotein-1 (PC-1), a transmembrane protein with phosphodiesterase and pyrophosphatase activity (165). When overexpressed in cultured cells, PC-1 inhibits insulin receptor tyrosine kinase activity by a direct interaction with the insulin receptor α-subunit (166). In nonobese, nondiabetic subjects, the PC-1 content of skeletal muscle is inversely correlated to both *in vivo* insulin action and *in vitro* stimulation of the insulin receptor tyrosine kinase activity (167). An amino acid variant identified in PC-1 (Lys121Gln) has been reported to contribute to insulin resistance in a nondiabetic population from Sicily, primarily by impairing insulin receptor kinase activity (168). Gln^{121} carriers have a threefold increase in the risk of being hyperinsulinemic and insulin resistant but have no increase in risk of developing type 2 diabetes (168). Fibroblasts from these subjects show an impairment of insulin-receptor autophosphorylation in the presence of normal PC-1 levels. Similar findings of association have been obtained in a family-based study from Sweden but not in a large population-based study from Denmark (169,170). In Mexican Americans, a major locus for fasting insulin concentrations and insulin-resistance traits has recently been mapped to the same region of the PC-1 gene on chromosome 6q22–q23 (171). Whether this locus corresponds to the PC-1 gene in this population awaits further investigation.

Other studies have considered circulating inhibitors of insulin action. pp63, also known as α-HS glycoprotein, was identified in extracts of rat liver (172). In both rodents and humans, this protein is present at relatively high levels in the circulation, where it might act on peripheral tissues involved in insulin action. pp63 has been shown to inhibit the insulin receptor tyrosine kinase and insulin-stimulated DNA synthesis (173). Thus far, however, there is no evidence for genetic alterations in expression, secretion, or action of this protein in type 2 diabetes. A circulating inhibitor that has been more intensively studied is tumor necrosis factor-α (TNF-α), a potent cytokine with a wide range of proinflammatory activities (174). TNF-α may contribute to the insulin resistance of infection or stress and also to type 2 diabetes, since TNF-α is hypersecreted by adipocytes in obesity (175). Exposure to TNF-α decreases glucose uptake *in vitro* and *in vivo*, and homozygous disruption of the TNF-α gene protects mice from obesity-induced insulin resistance (175,176). However, whether genetic variability in this cytokine contributes to the development of type 2 diabetes in humans remains unclear. The human TNF-α gene lies in the class III region of the major histocompatibility complex, centromeric to the HLA-B locus and telomeric to HLA-DR. The rare allele of a polymorphism in the promoter region (G/A at position -308) is associated with increased TNF-α expression and more severe disease in infections such as malaria and leishmaniasis (177,178). The same polymorphism was found to be associated with indices of insulin resistance in a Spanish population but not in studies from the United States, Germany, Denmark, United Kingdom, Japan, and Hong Kong (179–184). Another promoter variant (G/A at -238) was reported to be associated with impaired insulin sensitivity in the United Kingdom, but this was not confirmed in other populations (179–185). The role of variability in the two TNF-α receptor (TNFR1 and TNFR2) has been less investigated. Only one report has been published to date describing lower insulin sensitivity in carriers of an allele in the 3′ UTR of TNFR2 (186).

GENES INVOLVED IN INSULIN SECRETION

Pancreatic β-cells sense glucose and other nutrients and respond to this signal by synthesizing and secreting insulin to promote the utilization and storage of these substrates (45). The signal for insulin secretion is provided by the utilization of glucose in the β-cell (Fig. 22.9). After being transported into the cell by a high-capacity, Na^+-independent carrier (GLUT2),

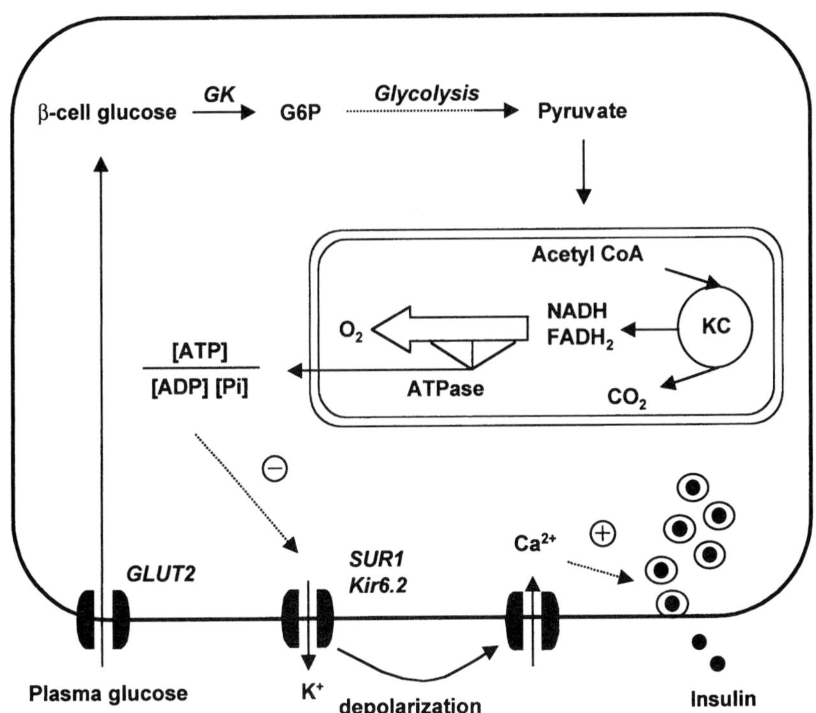

Figure 22.9. Schematic model of the β-cell glucose sensor and insulin secretion pathways. GK, glucokinase; G6p, glucose 6-phosphate; KC, Krebs cycle.

glucose is phosphorylated by the enzyme glucokinase and is metabolized in glycolysis and the Krebs cycle. The ensuing increase in energy production raises the intracellular ATP/ADP ratio, which in turn inhibits adenine nucleotide–sensitive potassium channels (45). The resulting depolarization opens voltage sensitive Ca^{2+} channels, leading to an increase in cytosolic Ca^{2+}, which ultimately induces the fusion of insulin granules with the plasma membrane and insulin release. β-Cells also respond to glucose by increasing preproinsulin biosynthesis in the endoplasmic reticulum, although the mechanisms by which glucose exerts transcriptional and translational control of preproinsulin mRNA are poorly understood. All genes whose products are placed in these pathways are obvious candidate genes for type 2 diabetes. Additional candidate genes are those that are involved in the development and turnover of β-cells (e.g., β-cell–specific transcription factors) or are part of hormonal systems regulating β-cell activity.

GLUT2 and Glucokinase. Because of their central role in glucose sensing, GLUT2 and glucokinase were among the first genes to be investigated for association or linkage with type 2 diabetes. An additional reason to study glucokinase was the finding that glucokinase mutations cause MODY (54). This raised the hypothesis that sequence differences resulting in a milder impairment of glucokinase activity may be responsible for forms of diabetes with a later onset. It is now clear that genetic variability at these two loci does not play a major role in common type 2 diabetes. An association between a *Taq*I RFLP in the GLUT2 gene and type 2 diabetes was reported in British individuals but has not been confirmed in other populations (187–190). A mutation (Val197Ile) abolishing GLUT2 activity, and possibly causing diabetes, has been described in a single patient with type 2 diabetes (191). Several other allelic variants have been detected in this gene, but none has shown association with overt type 2 diabetes or glucose intolerance (192). Results have been similarly negative for glucokinase. Initial studies reported an association between some microsatellite alleles and late-onset type 2 diabetes in African Americans, Mauritian Creoles, and Japanese, but mutations affecting glucokinase expression or structure were not found in these populations (193–197). More recently, a common variant in the islet-specific promoter of this gene (-30 G to A) has been reported to be associated with reduced insulin secretory responses to oral glucose, although results have not been consistent across populations (198–200). Attempts to demonstrate linkage between the glucokinase locus and type 2 diabetes have also been negative in family studies from France, England, and Utah (201–203).

Ion Channels. Adenine nucleotide–sensitive potassium channels (K_{ATP}) play a pivotal role in coupling glucose metabolism to insulin release. The K_{ATP} channels of β-cells consist of two subunits: the inward rectifier K^+ channel Kir6.2 and a regulatory subunit, which also serves as the sulfonylurea receptor (SUR1) (204). The genes coding for the two subunits are clustered at 11p15, with the Kir6.2 gene (also known as *KCNJ11*) placed immediately 3′ of *SUR1* (also known as *ABCC8*). Rare mutations in both subunits have been observed in persistent hyperinsulinemic hypoglycemia of infancy, a rare disorder characterized by unregulated insulin secretion despite severe hypoglycemia (205,206). However, the evidence for a contribution of these two loci to type 2 diabetes is controversial. Two polymorphisms in the *SUR1* gene have received particular attention. One corresponds to a C-to-T substitution placed in intron 15 at a short distance (3 bp) from the exon 16 acceptor side; the other is a synonymous polymorphism in exon 18 (a C-to-T substitution at codon 759). In the first report to be published, the allele "C" in intron 15 and the allele "T" in exon 18 were both significantly associated with type 2 diabetes in two different white populations (207) (Table 22.2). However, the association with the SNP in intron 15 was not unequivocally confirmed in subsequent reports (208–217). Among 10 studies, only three detected significant differences between cases and controls, and in one of these, the allele "T" rather than "C" was associated with diabetes (Table 22.2). Results are more convinc-

TABLE 22.2. Results of Association Studies Concerning the *SUR1* Gene in Type 2 Diabetes

		Intron 15 (−3C→T)					Exon 18 (C→T)				
		Type 2 diabetes		Controls			Type 2 diabetes		Controls		
Study	Country	*n*	C	*n*	C	*p*	*n*	T	*n*	T	*p*
Inoue et al. (207)	US (Utah)	134	.60	104	.49	.02	144	.059	107	.014	.01
Inoue et al. (207)	UK	187	.60	120	.43	<.0001	186	.073	129	.033	.02
Hani et al. (208)	France	168	.48	106	.50	NS	170	.038	115	.009	.03
Ohta et al. (209)	Japan	100	.46	67	.50	NS	—	—	—	—	—
Hansen et al. (210)	Denmark	419	.55	244	.56	NS	392	.052	249	.026	.03
Ishiyama-Shigemoto et al. (211)	Japan	236	.54	220	.53	NS	—	—	—	—	—
Ji et al. (212)	China	86	.68	148	.55	.007	—	—	—	—	—
Hart et al. (213)	Netherlands	388	.52	336	.59	.01	388	.069	313	.053	NS
van Tilburg et al. (214)	Netherlands	566	.59	150	.54	NS	—	—	—	—	—
Rissanen et al. (215)	Finland	40	.60	377	.43	.009	40	.050	377	.030	NS
Gloyn et al. (216)	UK	364	.47	328	.42	NS	356	.062	324	.060	NS
Meirhaeghe et al. (217)	France	122	.53	1250	.46	.04	—	—	—	—	—

NS, not significant.

ing for the SNP in exon 18. In this case, a significant or suggestive association with type 2 diabetes has been found in four of five replication studies, although the proportion of diabetes cases accounted for by this variant is probably small (208,210,213,215,216). A role of this variant in glucose homeostasis also is supported by studies among nondiabetic individuals showing lower C-peptide fasting levels and acute insulin response in nondiabetic carriers (210). Being a synonymous substitution, this SNP is probably a nonfunctional marker in linkage disequilibrium with an as-yet-unidentified causal variant. Variability in the Kir6.2 gene could also play a role in type 2 diabetes, but the evidence is controversial (218,219).

Preproinsulin Gene. Six extremely rare mutations have been identified to date in the insulin gene on 11p15 [reviewed by Steiner et al. (220)]. Three of these concern the primary sequence of the A- or B-chains: insulin Chicago (B Phe25Leu), insulin Wakayama (A Val3Leu), and insulin Los Angeles (B Phe24Ser). These mutations impair the binding of insulin to its receptor and are associated with high circulating levels of insulin, modest hyperglycemia, and an increase in the half-life of the hormone (because much of insulin clearance is due to receptor-mediated uptake). The other three mutations result in an impairment of the processing of proinsulin to insulin. Two of these are localized at the proinsulin-processing site (Arg65His and Arg65Leu) and prevent the recognition by the dibasic protease that cleaves the C-peptide from the proinsulin molecule. The other (a His-to-Asp substitution at position 10 of the B-chain) alters the processing of proinsulin by interfering with its binding to zinc and its crystallization in β-cell secretory granules. These three mutations have minor effects on glucose metabolism and are characterized by high circulating concentrations of proinsulin. Since these mutations are very rare, carriers are usually heterozygotes. It is unclear whether so few (pro)insulin variants have been reported because of the mild or nonexisting phenotype, because of the lack of screening, or because of a low mutation frequency at this site.

As mutations in the coding region of the preproinsulin gene have not been found to be involved in common forms of type 2 diabetes, it has been hypothesized that the observed deficit of insulin secretion in type 2 diabetes might be related to abnormalities in regulatory elements of the gene. In this regard, considerable interest has been drawn to a complex polymorphism located 5′ of the insulin gene in the proximity of promoter/enhancer sequences, which could affect, at least theoretically, expression of the insulin gene (221). The polymorphism consists of a variable number of tandem repeats (VNTR), which can be subdivided into three classes (I, II, and III) according to their length. While an association has consistently been found between homozygosity for class I alleles and type 1 diabetes, this does not seem to be the case for type 2 diabetes (222–224). A recent U.K. study using a family-based design (transmission disequilibrium test) has detected a preferential transmission of class III alleles from heterozygous fathers, but not mothers, to type 2 diabetic probands (225). This result, which would implicate imprinted genes in the pathogenesis of type 2 diabetes, has not yet been confirmed by any other group. Another study has described a rare 8-bp insertion/deletion in the insulin gene promoter among African Americans, but its contribution to type 2 diabetes seems to be small, if any (226).

The enzymes processing preproinsulin to mature insulin (prohormone convertases 1 and 2 and carboxypeptidase E) have also been investigated as possible type 2 diabetes loci. These studies were based on the hypothesis that the relative insulin-deficiency characteristic of type 2 diabetes may be due to the release of disproportionate amount of biologically inactive insulin precursors. Indeed, subjects with type 2 diabetes show a marked increase in the proportion of circulating proinsulin, and mice carrying mutations in carboxypeptidase E (*fat/fat* mice) develop obesity and diabetes (227,228). However, several studies have excluded a role of processing enzyme polymorphisms to the development of type 2 diabetes in humans (229,230). Mutations in prohormone convertase 1 have been identified but only in a rare genetic syndrome characterized by childhood obesity, gestational diabetes, and other endocrine disorders (231).

β-Cell Transcription Factors. The development of β-cells is regulated by a complex network of transcription factors organized in a hierarchical fashion (Fig. 22.10) (56,232). Some of these factors also control β-cell physiology in the adult life by modulating the expression of genes involved in glucose metabolism and the insulin gene itself (60–62). The discovery that rare mutations in these factors cause MODY has also implicated

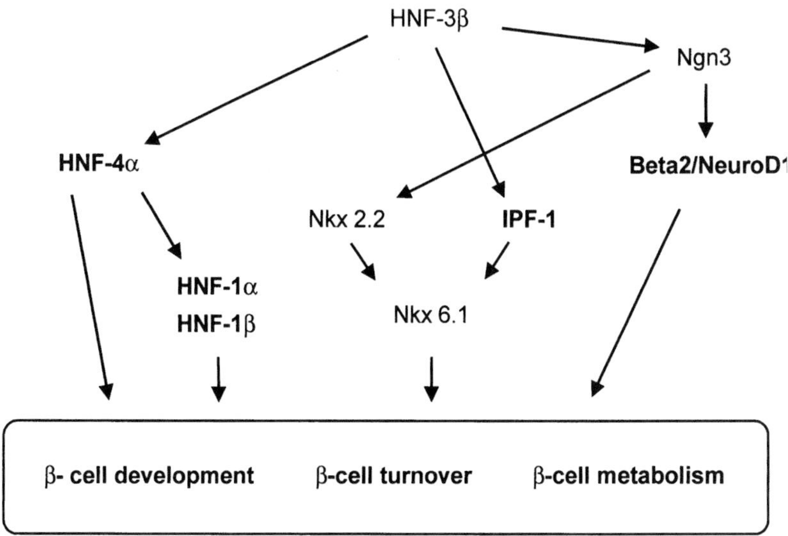

Figure 22.10. Transcriptional network in β-cells. Transcription factors that are mutated in maturity-onset diabetes of the young (MODY) are indicated in bold.

these genes in type 2 diabetes. In particular, it has been hypothesized that common variants, distinct from MODY mutations, may determine a slight impairment of β-cell function that may become evident only if there is an increased demand for insulin as in the presence of insulin resistance. Indeed, the chromosomal region of HNF1α (MODY3) on 12q24 has been found to be linked with type 2 diabetes among families with poor insulin response from Botnia (Finland), and in a single family from Australia (233,234). No mutations, however, were identified in the HNF1α coding region in these families, indicating that either the mutations are placed in as-yet unscreened regulatory regions or the gene responsible for these findings is a different one. Other studies have also suggested that polymorphisms in HNF1α do not play a major role in common type 2 diabetes, although these may be associated with slight abnormalities of insulin secretion (235–238). Linkage with type 2 diabetes has also been found in the HNF4α region on 20q in many studies, but genetic variability in this gene does not seem to be responsible for these findings (239–243). No association has been found between variants in neuroD1 and "garden variety" type 2 diabetes (38,244).

In contrast with these negative results, two recent papers have reported associations between IPF1 variants and type 2 diabetes. In England, Macfarlane et al. (245) have detected three missense mutations (C18R, D76N, and R197H) that are associated with decreased IPF1-binding activity and impaired activation of the insulin gene in response to hyperglycemia. These variants are rare overall (present in 1% of the population) but are associated with a threefold increase in the risk of type 2 diabetes. One of these mutations (D76N) has also been detected by researchers in France, where it is also significantly associated with type 2 diabetes (246). In the latter study, another variant was identified (InsCCG243) that was linked to type 2 diabetes in two families (246). Thus, it appears that genetic variability in IPF1 may indeed contribute to the development of type 2 diabetes, although this effect probably concerns a small proportion of cases and is not present in all populations (247). Several other transcription factors (HNF3β, HNF4γ, HNF6, neuroD4, PAX4) have been screened for sequence differences associated with type 2 diabetes with negative results (248–253). A weak association has been reported for a polymorphism in the neurogenin gene, but this has not been confirmed in other populations (251–253). New candidates in this class are expected to emerge from the expression profiling of β-cells.

Incretins. Another hypothesis is that the impairment in insulin secretion in type 2 diabetes is due to genetic alterations in extrapancreatic hormonal systems regulating β-cell function. GLP-1 (glucagon-like peptide-1) and GIP (glucose-dependent insulinotropic polypeptide) are gut hormones that act as incretins, activating specific receptors on the β-cell and augmenting insulin release after oral ingestion of carbohydrates, as compared with the intravenous intake (254–256). The effectiveness of GIP is generally diminished or lacking in patients with type 2 diabetes, whereas the efficacy of GLP-1 is maintained (257,258). One variant (Gly198Cys) in the GIP receptor identified in Japanese patients exhibits increased GIP-induced cAMP response in transfected CHO cells (259), and a common Glu354Gln variant is associated with decreased C-peptide levels during fasting and 30-minute post-OGTT in normal glucose-tolerant Danish white subjects (260). However, none of the identified amino acid variants showed associations with type 2 diabetes (259,260).

OBESITY GENES

Because obesity is closely correlated to the development of type 2 diabetes and has some degree of heritability (261), genes with a potential role in obesity have also been considered in the search for type 2 diabetes genes. Body weight is finely regulated by hypothalamic pathways controlling the balance between energy intake and expenditure (262). This control is achieved through effects on behavior, the autonomic nervous system and the neuroendocrine system, regulating feeding and physical activity, energy expenditure, and the utilization of metabolic substrates. Much progress has been made over the past decade in understanding the molecular mechanisms mediating these effects, in part through the cloning of genes responsible for animal models of obesity (261,262). These studies have generated a long list of potential candidate genes, many of which have been investigated for contributions to obesity and type 2 diabetes.

Central Nervous System Mediators. Effects promoting weight gain are mediated in the hypothalamus by orexigenic (feeding-inducing) neuropeptides, the best characterized of which are NPY and AgRP, whereas effects promoting weight loss involve anorexigenic neuromediators such as α-MSH and CART (the cocaine- and amphetamine-regulated transcript) (263). All these peptides propagate their signals by interacting with specific receptors (e.g., MC4R receptor for α-MSH and AgRP) expressed in downstream neurons (263). Mutations causing rare forms of morbid obesity have been found in the precursor of α-MSH [propiomelanocortin (POMC)] and in the enzyme involved in its processing (prohormone convertase 1) (231,264). However, because of the concomitant lack of adrenocorticotropic hormone (ACTH) activity, these mutations are associated with hypoglycemia rather than hyperglycemia. Mutations are more frequent in the MC4R receptor and may be responsible for up to 4% to 5% of cases of morbid obesity [body mass index (BMI) >40 kg/m^2], especially those showing an autosomal dominant mode of inheritance (265–268). However, no association with common, multifactorial forms of obesity or diabetes has been found to date for any of these genes (229,230,269–272).

Leptin and Leptin Receptor. A major breakthrough in obesity research was the discovery that adipose tissue regulates its own mass and metabolism through a feedback circuit involving the hormone leptin (273). Leptin is produced by the adipose tissue, crosses the blood–brain barrier, and interacts with specific receptors in the hypothalamus, where it inhibits the release of orexigenic mediators NPY and AgRP while inducing the anorexigenic peptides α-MSH and CART (274–276). Mutations in leptin or the leptin receptor cause severe obesity in mice (273,275,276). The importance of this pathway has also been demonstrated in humans by the discovery of three rare mutations: one that causes a truncated receptor and early-onset obesity, a second rare mutation associated with low serum leptin levels, and a rare frame-shift mutation causing a truncated form of leptin that is associated with severe early onset obesity (277–279). Nevertheless, several population studies indicate that such variants are rare and not a common cause of obesity or type 2 diabetes in humans (280,281).

β$_3$-Adrenergic Receptor and Uncoupling Proteins. The β$_3$-adrenergic receptor (β3AR) stimulates lipolysis and thermogenesis in adipocytes and has been intensively examined for potential implications in obesity and diabetes (282). Carriers of a Trp64Arg polymorphism have been suggested to have increased capacity to gain weight and accelerated onset of type 2 diabetes (283–285). These findings, however, have not been uniformly replicated (286,287). *In vivo* and *in vitro* investigations also have provided conflicting results. Two studies have shown a reduced agonist response associated with the Arg64 variant (288,289), whereas other studies demonstrate no functional effect (290–292). A recent meta-analysis of 31 published studies including more than 9,000 individuals indicates that the Arg64 alleles may indeed be associated with increased body weight, but this effect is quite small (0.3 kg/m^2 BMI difference between carriers and noncarriers) (293). A minor effect on the natural history of diabetes may also be present, with Arg64 carriers developing hyperglycemia about 2 years earlier than noncarriers (293).

Uncoupling proteins (UCPs), which promote the dissipation of energy as heat in the mitochondria of adipocytes and other tissues (294,295), have also been intensively investigated. Three UCP genes (UCP1, UCP2, UCP3) coding for proteins with different activities and patterns of expression have thus far been identified and searched for sequence differences (295). Results have been particularly interesting for a C/T polymorphism placed in the UCP3 promoter, 55 bp upstream of the transcription start (-55T/C) and in proximity of the putative TATA box (296–299). Subjects homozygous for the C allele have a significantly lower expression of UCP3 mRNA in skeletal muscle (296). The same allele also was associated with increased body weight in a study in the United Kingdom and with increased risk of type 2 diabetes in two populations from France (297–299). Other variants have been implicated in obesity or insulin-resistance phenotypes, but results have been less consistent.

Peroxisome Proliferator-Activated Receptor-γ (PPARγ). PPARγ is a transcription factor that plays a key role in regulation of adipocyte differentiation and is also the receptor for insulin-sensitizing drugs of the thiazolidenedione class (300). This factor has two isoforms (PPARγ1 and PPARγ2) that result from alternative splicing (301). Both have ligand-dependent and ligand-independent transcriptional activities. PPARγ2 has 28 additional amino acids at its amino-terminus that make its ligand-independent activity 5 to 10 times higher than that of PPARγ1. Two rare mutations (Pro467Leu and Val290Met) in this transcription factor have recently been found to be associated with severe insulin resistance and diabetes in addition to hypertension (302). Both of the identified variants are markedly transcriptionally impaired, and the mutated receptors are able to inhibit the action of coexpressed wild-type PPARγ, indicating a dominant negative effect (302). Another amino acid variant identified in a German population (Pro115Gln) was found exclusively in obese subjects (BMI >29 kg/m^2) (303). A functional study of the variant showed reduced phosphorylation of a nearby serine residue (Ser114) and accelerated differentiation of the cells into adipocytes (303). This variant has not been observed in other populations. A more frequent amino acid polymorphism, also affecting the transcriptional activity, has been described in PPARγ2 (Pro12Ala) (304,305). In one of the first reports, the Ala12 allele (frequency of 0.12) was significantly associated with lower BMI and improved insulin sensitivity, with Ala12 carriers having four times less risk of diabetes than carriers (304). Another report, published at the same time on a different journal, showed instead an association between Ala12 allele and *higher* BMI in a lean to moderately obese cohort and a cohort of very obese subjects from North America (305). These conflicting results were in part reconciled by a Danish study indicating that the variant might have divergent modulating effect on BMI, being associated with higher BMI in obese subjects and lower BMI in the control group (306). Although studies from other populations have not always been able to confirm these associations, most have shown a tendency to a lower risk of diabetes among Ala12 carriers (306–316) (Fig. 22.11). This has been confirmed by a recent report based on both family-based and population-based studies including a total of 3,000 individuals (310). However, the protection associated with the Ala12 allele appears to be modest (relative risk, 0.80, corresponding to a 1.25-fold risk of diabetes for the Pro12 allele). Similar risk estimates are obtained when all studies performed to date are considered in a meta-analysis (Fig. 22.11). The protection conferred by the Ala12 variant appears to be much more pronounced in Japanese (OR, 0.50; 95% CI, 0.4–0.65) than in whites (OR, 0.86; 95% CI, 0.76–0.98). The reasons for these racial differences are unclear, but a possible explanation is that the Ala12 variant must interact with other genetic or environmental factors to confer strong protection. Some of these may be characteristic of the Japanese population.

OTHER CANDIDATE GENES

Homozygous expansion of a GAA repeat in the frataxin gene has been linked to Friedreich ataxia. Thirty percent of patients suffering form the disease have abnormal glucose tolerance, with about 10% having overt diabetes (317). A study of populations in Germany and the United States have shown that intermediate expansions of the frataxin gene are associated with type 2 diabetes (318). This association, however, has not been observed in France, The Netherlands, Denmark, and United Kingdom (319–322). *In vitro* frataxin has been shown to play a role in mitochondrial oxidative metabolism (323).

An association between type 2 diabetes and a glucagon receptor variant at codon 40 was found in French and Sardinian

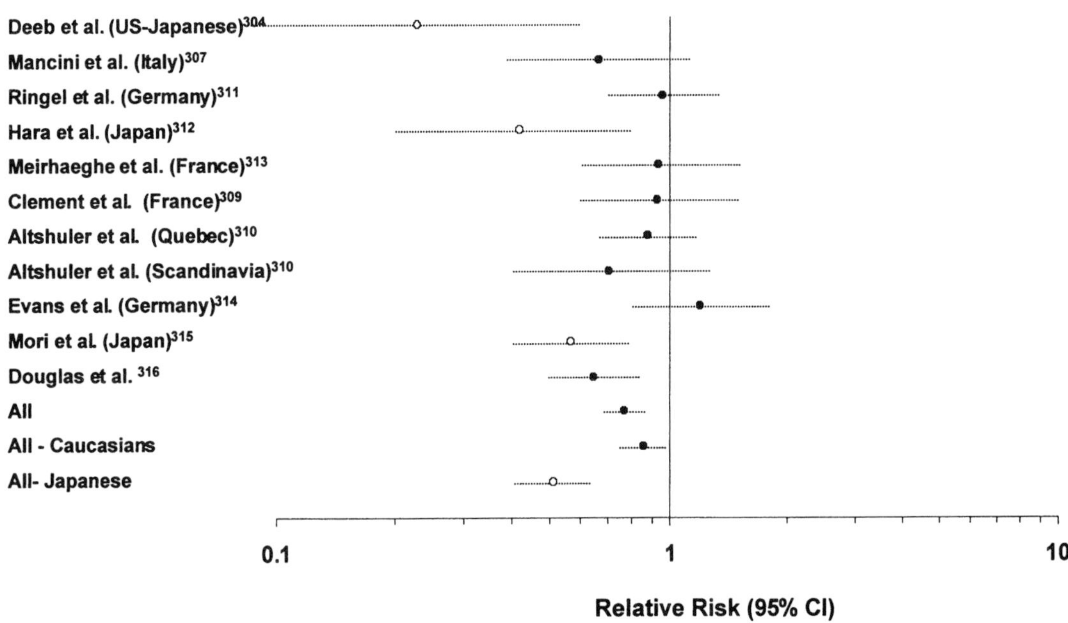

Figure 22.11. Estimated risk of type 2 diabetes associated with the peroxisome proliferator-activated receptor-γ (PPARγ) Pro12Ala variant. For each study, the solid circle represents the odds ratio for 12Ala carriers and the dotted line indicates the 95% confidence interval. For consistency with other reports, only population-based data from the study by Altshuler et al. (310) are included. Mantel-Haenszel estimates of the common relative risks are reported for all published studies (All, n = 10,227), for studies in caucasians (All-caucasians, n = 5,713), and for studies in Japanese only (All-Japanese, n = 4,514). The risk estimate in caucasians was significantly different from that in Japanese.

populations (324). This variant has been shown in transfection studies to confer a reduced sensitivity to glucagon (325), suggesting that an impairment in the insulinotropic effects of glucagon might be the link with diabetes. However, also in this case, the association has not been replicated in other populations (326,327).

Genome-Screen and Positional Candidate Genes

While functional candidate gene studies can be successful in some cases [a good example is the discovery of glucokinase as a MODY gene (39,40)], this approach is limited by two important factors. First, only a small proportion of the estimated 30,000 or more genes that exist in the human genome have known biologic function (24). Second, our knowledge of the cellular pathways involved in insulin action and secretion, and more generally in glucose homeostasis, is far from complete. These limitations can be overcome by an alternative approach based on the systematic screening of the whole genome for chromosomal regions that are linked, i.e., are transmitted together with the disease in families. Genes in these regions, which are defined as *positional* as opposed to functional candidate genes, can then be screened for sequence differences associated with type 2 diabetes. This strategy (positional cloning) has been extremely successful in identifying the genes for a variety of mendelian disorders (33,328,329). Many of these genes were not previously known, or if they were, they would not have been chosen as candidates because of their functions. A notable example is the identification of lamin A/C, coding for nuclear envelope proteins, as the gene responsible for partial lipodystrophy (74,75). The price to pay for extending the search to the whole genome is the lower sensitivity of linkage studies as compared with direct tests of associations (27).

Genome-wide screens for linkage are performed by genotyping members of affected families at many polymorphic loci that are spaced at regular intervals throughout the genome. This task has been greatly facilitated during the last decade by the construction of dense maps of highly polymorphic markers (microsatellites) that can be analyzed in an automated fashion (21,22). Most genome screens are based on 400 of such markers, corresponding to a 10 cM spacing. The marker information is used to test whether any of the chromosomal regions represented by each marker co-segregates (i.e., is linked) with the disease. For Mendelian disorders, this is accomplished by comparing the likelihood that a segregation pattern is due to linkage with the disease to the likelihood that it is due to chance. Results are expressed as LOD scores, i.e., the $\log_{10}$ of the ratio of the two likelihoods (330). A LOD of 3.0, corresponding to odds of 1,000:1 in favor of linkage, is usually taken as a significant result. This approach is quite powerful but requires the specification of parameters defining the mode of inheritance (hence the name of *parametric* analysis) and the availability of large, multigenerational families that can be analyzed individually.

These constraints limit the application of these analytic methods to multifactorial forms of type 2 diabetes. In many instances, the mode of inheritance is ambiguous, making the task of defining the parameters for linkage analysis extremely difficult. The late onset of the disease may also hamper the assembling of large families, because the parents of affected individuals are often deceased and the offspring are too young to develop hyperglycemia. Thus, genome screens for type 2 diabetes genes have usually relied on *nonparametric* methods of analysis. A common nonparametric approach consists of investigating whether affected sibling pairs share any chromosomal region more frequently than expected on the basis of chance (331). Because of the complexity and heterogeneity of type 2 diabetes, large numbers of sib-pairs must be studied to have enough power to detect significant genetic contributions. More elaborate and powerful study designs based on the same principle are possible using different kinds of affected-relative pairs from extended families (e.g., uncle-nephew) (332,333). In general, nonparametric studies are not as powerful as parametric approaches but are easier to assemble, do not need specification of a mode of inheritance, and, since only affected subjects are considered, avoid the problem of nonpenetrants. Nonparametric methods can also be used to evaluate linkage with quantitative traits relevant to type 2 diabetes (e.g., fasting or postchallenge glycemia or insulinemia, BMI) rather than with diabetes itself (334,335). This approach assumes that genes influencing variation in these traits among nondiabetic subjects may also be involved in regulating susceptibility to type 2 diabetes.

At least 12 genome screens for type 2 diabetes genes have been performed during the past 5 years using a combination of these techniques (233,336–346). Similar to functional candidate gene studies, these screens have produced conflicting results and their interpretation is often challenging. In addition to the issues discussed above (genetic heterogeneity, variable power of studies), there are other important factors contributing to these variability. One concerns the definition of significant linkage. Some studies have reported results based on the stringent criteria proposed by Lander and Kruglyak (347) to account for the multiple comparisons that are performed in a whole-genome screen. In other cases, results are reported according to less stringent criteria, increasing the chances of not missing significant gene effects but also inflating the false-positive rate. Results of different studies may also be difficult to compare because of differences in study designs (e.g., sib-pairs vs. extended families) or recruitment criteria (e.g., younger vs. older onset of diabetes). These differences may confer different power to studies of similar size. As clarified by the work of Risch in the early 1990s (348), the power of sib-pair studies is a function of the recurrence-risk in siblings, or λ_s, a measure of the genetic component of a disease that is defined as the ratio between the risk of the disease in siblings of affected cases and the risk in the general population. Several recent studies have estimated the overall λ_s for type 2 diabetes to be only 1.2, suggesting that environmental factors, as opposed to genetic factors, contribute to a large proportion of the disease in the general population (349–351). However, the λ_s is elevated to 1.6 to 2.2 in families with one diabetic parent and higher in families with two diabetic parents (349–351). In a study of the families of 600 patients of the Joslin Diabetes Center, the λ_s is even higher (3.5) in those families in which the affected parent also had an affected parent (J. Warram and A. Krolewski, personal communication). Thus, by focusing on families with vertical transmission through three generations, the likelihood of identifying susceptibility genes for type 2 diabetes is greatly increased, but results obtained with these families may be difficult to replicate in unselected collection of sib-pairs. Because of the frequent use of different marker maps and study design, it may also be difficult to judge whether the type 2 diabetes locus of one study corresponds to the locus found in another report. Nonetheless, despite these problems, several chromosomal regions have been identified that appear to be significantly linked to type 2 diabetes in different genome screens (Table 22.3), and efforts are in progress to identify the genes responsible for these findings through association studies.

CHROMOSOME 2q37 AND CALPAIN 10

The chromosomal region at 2q37 was the first locus to be identified as being significantly linked with type 2 diabetes in a whole-genome screen (336). This study included a total of 440 affected sib-pairs recruited in Star County, Texas, where 97% of the population is Mexican American. The reason to study this ethnic group was the high incidence of type 2 diabetes in this population (severalfold higher than in the general U.S. population) and the high a priori likelihood that a few major genes could account for diabetes. The genome screen was based on a map of 490 markers (8–9 cM spacing), through which four regions, placed on chromosomes 2, 15, 7, and 3, were identified as potentially linked with type 2 diabetes (336). The best evidence was found at 2q37, where marker *D2S125* showed a LOD score of 4.0, meeting the genome-wide criteria for significant evidence of linkage (LOD score >3.6). This locus, named *NIDDM1*, was subsequently found to interact with another locus on chromosome 15 near *CYP19*, with the combined analysis of the two loci raising the LOD scores from 4.0 to 7.3 at *NIDDM1* and from 1.3 to 4.0 at *CYP19* (Fig. 22.12) (352). No evidence for these two loci could be found in non-Hispanic whites of different origins and in Japanese, suggesting that these genes may be specific to the Mexican-American population (336,353). This hypothesis, however, is contradicted by the absence of linkage at this location in Mexican Americans from the San Antonio Family Diabetes Study and in Pima Indians, who share part of their genetic background with Mexican Americans (337,338).

Recent evidence from the same research group indicates that *NIDDM1* may correspond to the gene coding for the cysteine protease calpain 10 (354). In the original screen, the one-LOD support interval (the region in which the LOD score is within one unit from the peak score) spanned 7 cM, corresponding to a physical size of 1.7 Mb. Because none of the known genes placed in this interval was an obvious candidate for type 2 dia-

TABLE 22.3. Chromosomal Regions That Have Been Found to Be Linked with Type 2 Diabetes Mellitus

Population	Study design	Linked regions	Study
Mexican Americans (County Starr)	Affected sib-pairs	2q37, 15q21, 3p14	Hanis et al. (336)
Whites (Botnia)	Extended families	12q24	Mahtani et al. (233)
Pima Indians (Arizona)	Affected sib-pairs	1q21–q23, 11q23, 7q22–q31	Hanson et al. (337)
Mexican Americans (San Antonio)	Extended families	10q25, 6q22–q23	Duggirala et al. (171,338)
Whites (Utah)	Extended families	1q21–q23	Elbein et al. (339)
Whites (Amish)	Extended families	1q21–q23, 14q12	St. Jean et al. (340)
Whites, blacks, Mexican Americans	Affected sib-pairs	12q15, 5q12, Xq24–q26, 3p22–q24	Ehm et al. (341)
Whites (Finland)	Affected sib-pairs	20q11–q13, 20p12, 11q14, 2p24	Ghosh et al. (342)
Whites (France)	Affected sib-pairs	3q27–qter, 1q21–q23	Vionnet et al. (343)
Whites (Ashkenazi)	Affected sib-pairs	20q11–q12, 4q34	Permutt et al. (344)
Whites (Scandinavia)	Extended families	18p11	Parker et al. (346)
Whites (UK/Ireland)	Affected sib-pairs	1q21–q23	McCarthy et al. (345)

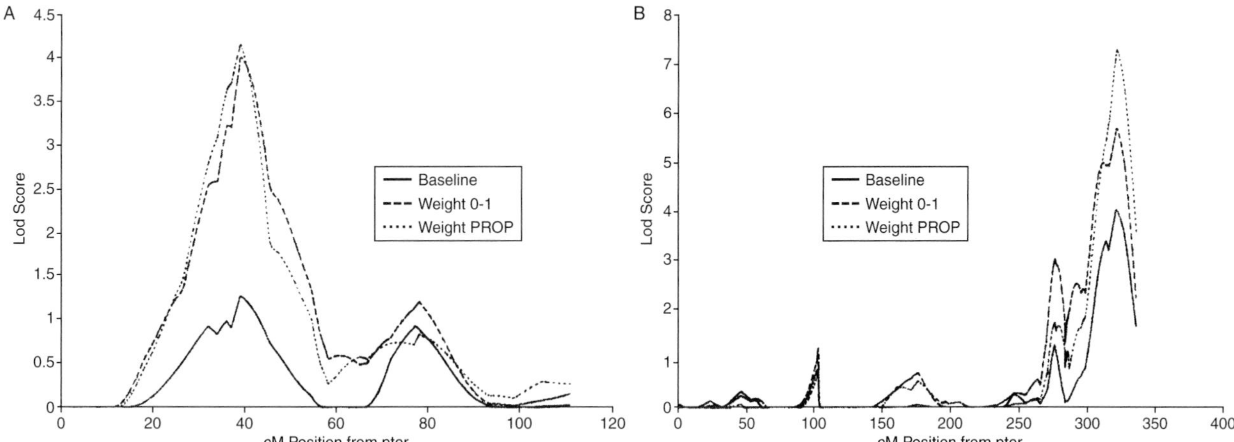

Figure 22.12. Interaction between *NIDDM1* and *CYP19* locus. **A:** Multipoint allele-sharing analysis of chromosome 15 weighted for linkage at *NIDDM1* on chromosome 2. **B:** Multipoint allele sharing analysis of chromosome 2 weighted by the evidence for linkage at *CYP19* on chromosome 15. The analysis was performed by assigning weight 0 to families with negative LOD score and 1 to families with positive LOD scores (Weight 0–1), or by assigning weights proportional to the evidence for linkage (Weight PROP). (Reprinted from Cox NJ, Frigge M, Nicolae DL, et al. Loci on chromosomes 2 (NIDDM1) and 15 interact to increase susceptibility to diabetes in Mexican Americans. *Nat Genet* 1999;21:213–215, with permission.)

betes, anonymous markers placed in this region were tested for association with type 2 diabetes. Results turned out positive for several SNPs placed in the region of the calpain 10 gene. The association with diabetes was particularly evident for a haplotype resulting from the combination of three SNPs (SNP-43 in intron 3, -19 in intron 6, and -63 in the 3′ region). Most important, this association could account for the linkage observed in the genome screen. The most common haplotype combination observed in Mexican Americans with type 2 diabetes was 112/121, which was associated with a threefold increase in the risk of diabetes as compared with the risk in carriers of other genotypes. A similar association was found in white populations from Finland and Germany, although this haplotype combination was rarer than in Mexican Americans. Variation at this locus is estimated to account for about 15% and 5% of type 2 diabetes in Mexican Americans and whites not of Mexican ethnicity, respectively (354).

While these results may represent the first example of positional cloning of a gene for a complex disorder, several issues must be addressed before calpain 10 can be unequivocally accepted as a type 2 diabetes gene. It is unclear, for instance, whether the three SNPs, which are all placed in noncoding regions, have biologic effects themselves or simply define a haplotype that is in linkage disequilibrium with the causal variant. SNP-43 has been shown to affect the binding of nuclear proteins from islet extract and to modulate gene expression *in vitro* in experiments with reporter genes (354). These data have been confirmed by *in vivo* experiments showing an association between SNP-43 and calpain-10 expression in skeletal muscle (355). Whether this is true for the other two SNPs and whether the combination of the three SNPs has a specific effect on expression of calpain 10 remains to be determined. It is also unclear why the association concerns 112/121 heterozygotes but not 112/112 or 121/121 homozygotes. A possible explanation is that two causal variants, one in linkage disequilibrium with haplotype 112 the other with 121, must interact to increase susceptibility to type 2 diabetes. However, none of the variants in the calpain 10 coding sequence are in tight linkage disequilibrium with the risk haplotypes, and the same appears to be true for all SNPs in the two flanking genes: *RNEPL1*, encoding for a protein homologous to aminopeptidase B; and *GPR35*, encoding for a G-protein–coupled receptor. Finally, there are uncertainties about whether these findings can completely account for the evidence of linkage at the *NIDDM1* locus. Since the initial screening for association was performed with a rather sparse SNP map (1 SNP every 80 kb, on average), one cannot exclude that another, perhaps more important, type 2 gene exists at this location and has been missed in this screen.

If the calpain 10 is really a type 2 diabetes gene, this implicates a completely new pathway in the regulation of glucose metabolism. Calpains (or calcium-activated neutral proteases) are a family of nonlysosomal cysteine proteases that are found in all human tissues (356). These enzymes modulate intracellular signaling and cellular differentiation and proliferation by cleaving specific substrates and causing activation or inactivation of protein functions (357). The presence of *CAPN10* mRNA in pancreatic islets, muscle, and liver suggests that calpain 10 may affect insulin secretion, insulin action, and hepatic glucose production. Indeed, carriers of the SNP-43 risk allele, who have lower calpain 10 expression in skeletal muscle, show decreased rates of fasting- and insulin-induced glucose turnover as a result of a decreased rate of glucose oxidation (355). If alterations of oxidative metabolism also occur in the pancreatic islets, variability at the calpain 10 locus might then explain both insulin resistance and the impairment of β-cell compensation observed in type 2 diabetes. Other calpain genes may be involved in the proportion of cases of type 2 diabetes that are not accounted for by calpain 10, and it is particularly interesting that one of these, *CAPN3*, is located in the region of chromosome 15 that interacts with *NIDDM1* (352).

CHROMOSOME 12q

At least two type 2 diabetes loci may exist on the long arm of chromosome 12. One (termed *NIDDM2*) corresponds to the same location of *MODY3* (*HNF1α*) at the telomeric end of 12q (233). Linkage at this locus was found in a genome screen of extended pedigrees from the Botnia district on the western coast of Finland, a region that was chosen for genetic studies because of the genetic homogeneity of its population and the availability of many large families. Analysis of the full collection of families (26 extended pedigrees) revealed no significant or even suggestive evidence for susceptibility loci predisposing to type 2 diabetes. However, significant linkage (LOD score = 3.65) was found in the *MODY3* region among the families in the lowest quartile of insulin levels during OGTT. The age at diabetes diagnosis in these families (58 years) was indistinguishable from that among the remaining families in the study, indicating that these findings were not due to misclassification of MODY as type 2 diabetes. Significant linkage at this location has subsequently been reported in a single, large family of Pacific Island origin (LOD score = 3.6), although this pedigree is characterized by insulin resistance and obesity rather than a defect in insulin secretion (234). Some evidence of linkage, although far from significant levels, has been found in white families by Bowden et al. and Ehm et al. (LOD scores = 1.4 and 1.45, respectively) (240,341) but not by other authors. The overlap between *NIDDM2* and *MODY3* initially suggested that these two loci may correspond to different alleles of the same gene, with severe mutations causing MODY and milder polymorphisms leading to later-onset type 2 diabetes. However, this hypothesis seems unlikely since no sequence differences associated with common type 2 diabetes have been identified in the *MODY3* gene *HNF1α* to date (235–238). No other obvious candidate gene is present at this site.

The second locus that has been identified on 12q is placed 50 cM centromeric to *NIDDM2/MODY3*. Suggestive linkage (LOD score = 3.1) was found at this location by Bektas et al. (66) in 26 white families with early-onset type 2 diabetes transmitted with an autosomal dominant mode of inheritance. Similar to the Botnia study, the evidence of linkage was particularly strong among families with poor insulin response to glucose (Fig. 22.13). The critical region defined by the recombinants spans 5 to 6 cM around marker *D12S1052* (358). A LOD score of 2.8 was found in the same region in the GENNID study, a large, multiethnic family collection sponsored by the American Diabetes Association (341). This finding, however, could not be replicated in a second GENNID population (so-called phase 2 families), and other genome screens have not detected linkage at this location. These discrepancies highlight the difficulties that are generally encountered in trying to replicate linkage results for multifactorial disorders. In the presence of genetic heterogeneity and epistasis, replication may require a much more powerful set than that needed for the original detection, since the fortuitous circumstances that led to detection of linkage in the first sample are unlikely to be replicated in the second sample unless a much larger number of families are examined.

CHROMOSOME 20

The long arm of chromosome 20 contains one of the most interesting regions that has been thus far identified in the search for type 2 diabetes genes. Attention initially was drawn to this chromosome by the mapping of *MODY1* on 20q13 (359). Testing the hypothesis that this locus, later identified as *HNF4α*, may also be involved in common forms of type 2 diabetes, several groups have performed linkage studies specifically targeted at this chromosome. While initial efforts failed to obtain positive results, three subsequent studies employing more informative markers and larger collections of families found suggestive linkage at this location. One study, conducted by Ji et al. in large white families with multiple affected members, showed evidence of linkage in a subset of families with age at diagnosis older than 47 years (239). The multipoint nonparametric LOD score reached 2.4 for two tightly linked markers (*D20S178* and *D20S197*) placed 8 cM telomeric to *HNF4α*. The addition of more markers and families subsequently raised the LOD score to 6.1 ($P = 1.8 \times 10^{-5}$) and refined the mapping to the 10 cM between markers *D20S119* and *D20S428* (Fig. 22.14) (360). It is interesting that the families showing evidence of linkage were characterized by insulin resistance rather than by poor insulin secretion, suggesting that this was a true type 2 diabetes locus rather than a MODY locus. The second study, also conducted in white pedigrees, suggested linkage in the very same region (LOD score = 1.5), despite the small number of sib-pairs that were used in this analysis (240). With slight differences in location, linkage at chromosome 20q13 also was observed in a study from France examining a total of 301 affected sib-pairs from 148

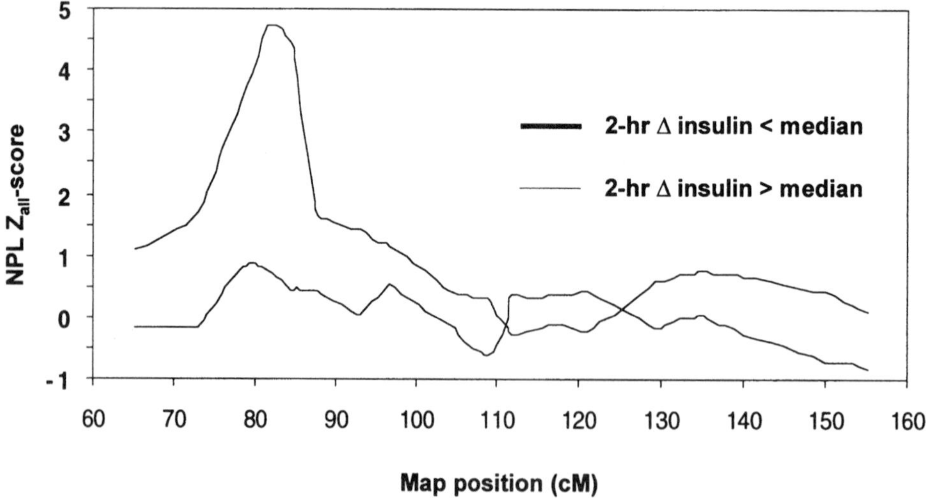

Figure 22.13. Type 2 diabetes locus on chromosome 12q15 in 32 families from the Joslin Diabetes Center with early-onset, autosomal dominant type 2 diabetes (66). Multipoint analysis was performed using GENEHUNTER (333) after families were subdivided into two groups based on the median within-family insulin increment during oral glucose tolerance testing (OGTT; 2-hr Δ, change after glucose ingestion). Evidence of linkage was present only among the families with insulin response below the median. NPL Z scores can be converted to LOD scores through the equation $LOD = Z^2/4.62$.

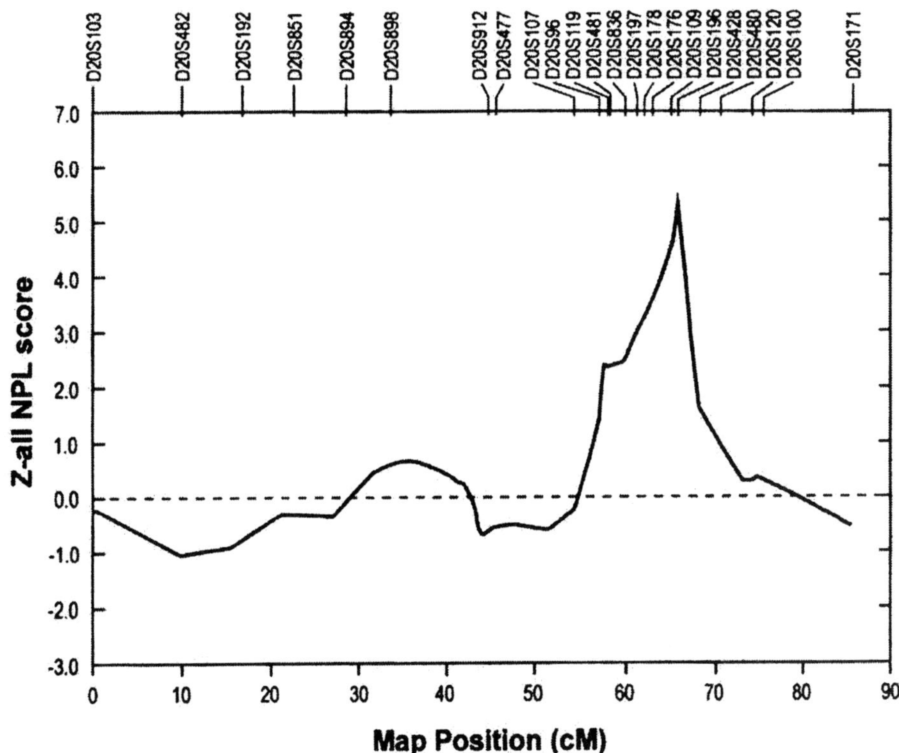

Figure 22.14. Evidence of a type 2 diabetes locus on chromosome 20q12–q13 in 43 Joslin families. Results were obtained by multipoint analysis using GENEHUNTER (332). The maximum score was obtained at marker D20S196 and corresponded to a p value of 1.8×10^{-5} in the entire set of families. (Copyright © American Diabetes Association. From Klupa T, Malecki MT, Pezzolesi M, et al. Further evidence for a susceptibility locus for type 2 diabetes on chromosome 20q13–q13.2. *Diabetes* 2000;49: 2212–2216, with permission from the American Diabetes Association.)

type 2 diabetes pedigrees (241). The evidence was particularly strong in a subset of families with age at diagnosis younger than 45 years, in which a linkage peak (LOD = 2.7) was found 10 cM telomeric to the locus reported in the other two studies. A smaller peak (LOD score = 1.8) was also observed 15 cM centromeric to this locus.

Confirmation of the existence of at least one type 2 diabetes locus on 20q13 has recently come from the results of the FUSION (Finland-United States Investigation of NIDDM Genetics) study, an international collaborative effort to map and positionally clone genes predisposing to type 2 diabetes in Finnish subjects (242). The Finnish population is believed to derive from a small group of founders with little subsequent immigration, a feature that minimizes the chances of genetic heterogeneity. The FUSION study includes 719 affected sib-pairs from 478 families. In a 10 cM genome screen, the strongest evidence of linkage was found on chromosome 20, where three peaks were identified, at 0 to 25 cM (LOD score = 1.99), 50 to 60 cM (LOD score = 2.04), and 63 to 72 cM (LOD score = 2.15) (242). The last two peaks, which might correspond to two separate loci or might be the expression of a single type 2 diabetes locus, are located in close proximity to the intervals linked with type 2 diabetes in previous studies. This locus or loci may interact with a putative locus on 2p, as suggested by a joint analysis of the two chromosomes increasing the 20q13 LOD score to 5.5 (342). Additional evidence for a type 2 diabetes locus on 20q has been provided by a genome screen in Ashkenazi Jews and studies of nondiabetic families demonstrating linkage with obesity, percent body fat, and fasting insulin levels (344,361,362).

Although other reports could not replicate these findings, the fact that six independent studies point to the same chromosomal region is highly indicative of the existence of a type 2 diabetes gene around 20q13. The identity of this gene or genes is unknown at this time. Extensive screening for mutations has failed to identify sequence differences associated with type 2 diabetes in the *HNF4α* gene (*MODY1*) (243). The finding of association between type 2 diabetes and a marker placed 8 cM telomeric of *HNF4α* also makes a role of this gene unlikely (360). Other good candidate genes in this region include protein tyrosine phosphatase-B, a regulator of insulin signaling that may influence insulin sensitivity, and CAAT/enhancer-binding-protein β, which is an inhibitor of insulin gene transcription (363,364). Collaborative efforts are under way to map this locus precisely and to positionally clone the gene or genes that are responsible for the linkage with type 2 diabetes. The sequence information and the SNP map generated by the Human Genome Project (24,25) are invaluable tools for this task.

CHROMOSOME 1q21–q23

Evidence for linkage at this location was first provided by a genome screen in Pima Indians, a Native-American population with an exceptionally high incidence of type 2 diabetes and obesity (365). This study included 551 affected sib-pairs with diabetes diagnosed before age 45 years, who were recruited from a longitudinal study of the Gila River Indian Community in central Arizona. While the best evidence for linkage was found at 11q in the overall population, a LOD score of 4.1 was observed at 1q21 near marker *D1S2127* (192 cM) in the subset of sib-pairs who were younger than 25 years old at diabetes diagnosis (Fig. 22.15) (337). Suggestive evidence of linkage near this location also was found in the overall group in an analysis comparing sib-pairs concordant for diabetes with discordant sib-pairs (LOD score = 2.5 at 171 cM). The presence of a type 2 diabetes locus at 1q21–q23 has subsequently been confirmed by genome screens in white populations. The first one, considering 42 extended families of northern European ancestry from Utah, detected a LOD score of 4.3 between *CRP* and *APOA2* (204 cM) under a recessive model of inheritance (339). Results were similarly positive in a nonparametric analysis, although they could not be confirmed in a replication set of 20 similarly ascertained but smaller families. The second study, considering 148 nuclear families from France, detected a LOD score of 3.0 at *APOA2* in

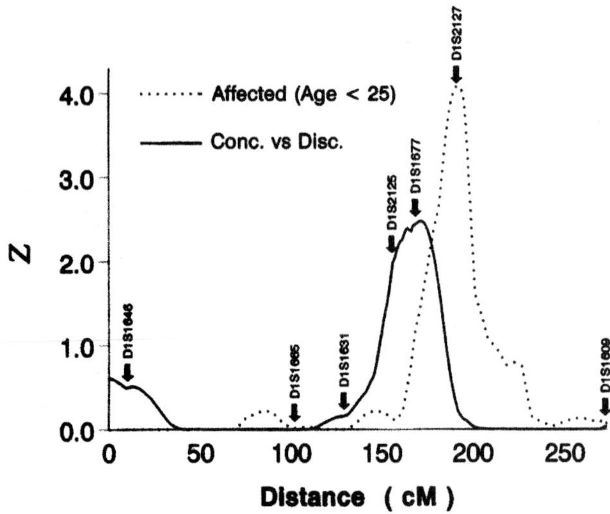

Figure 22.15. Multipoint results for linkage with type 2 diabetes at 1q21 in Pima Indians. In the analyses comparing concordant with discordant sib-pairs, the age at onset of diabetes was <45 years. (Reprinted from Hanson RL, Ehm MG, Pettitt DJ, et al. An autosomal genomic scan for loci linked to type II diabetes mellitus and body-mass index in Pima Indians. *Am J Hum Genet* 1998;63:1130–1138, with permission.)

a subset of 57 families with a lean phenotype (BMI <27 kg/m^2), suggesting that this may be a true diabetes locus rather than an obesity-susceptibility locus (343). Preliminary data from the British Diabetic Association Warren 2 consortium (812 affected sib-pairs) indicate that evidence of linkage at 1q21–q23 may also be present in that population (345). Similar to the original finding in Pima Indians, linkage seems to be stronger among families with early onset of diabetes (LOD score = 2.2). Furthermore, familial combined hyperlipidemia, which is characterized by insulin resistance and a propensity to glucose intolerance, has been also mapped to the same region of chromosome 1 in a study from Finland (366). By contrast, no evidence of linkage at this location has been found in the FUSION and GENNID studies or in Mexican Americans (338,341,342).

The 1-LOD support interval at 1q21–q23 spans 6–19 cM, depending on the study. This region is very rich in genes, many of which are plausible candidates for susceptibility to type 2 diabetes. An example is *KCNJ9,* a G-protein-coupled inwardly rectifying potassium channel, which might be involved in insulin secretion. A significant association has been found in Pima Indians between diabetes and several noncoding SNPs of this gene, but it does not account for the linkage observed at this location (367). Another interesting gene placed in this region is *LMNA*, which is mutated in autosomal dominant forms of partial lipodystrophy and insulin resistance (74,75). A silent polymorphism in intron 10 of the *LMNA* gene is associated with large adipocyte size in the abdominal subcutaneous tissue (a phenotype that predicts insulin resistance) but not with type 2 diabetes itself (368). No study has been published to date on apolipoprotein A2 (*APOA2*), which is placed in the middle of the linked interval and could play a role in the susceptibility to type 2 diabetes through an effect on free fatty acid metabolism.

OTHER CHROMOSOMAL REGIONS

Suggestive or significant linkage with type 2 diabetes has been found at several other chromosomal regions, although some of these results still await replication. In Mexican Americans from the San Antonio Family Diabetes Study, Duggirala et al. (338) have found significant evidence of a susceptibility locus on chromosome 10q influencing age at onset of diabetes (LOD score = 3.75) and linked with type 2 diabetes itself (LOD score = 2.9). This locus may account for up to 65% of the total variation in age at diagnosis of diabetes observed in this population. Another locus has been identified in the same population at 6q22–q23 that is linked with fasting insulin levels and other insulin resistance–related phenotypes such as BMI and triglycerides (171). Insulin-action inhibitor PC-1 is placed in this region, but whether variability in this gene accounts for the finding of linkage remains to be determined. A locus for type 2 diabetes (LOD score = 1.7) and BMI (LOD score = 3.6) has been identified at 11q23–q25 in Pima Indians (337). More recently, significant linkage has been demonstrated by Vionnet et al. (343) at 3q27 in French families with diabetes diagnosed before age 45 (LOD score = 4.7). Suggestive LOD scores have been found at the same location in Pima Indians for quantitative trait loci (QTL) controlling acute insulin response, insulin resistance, and waist-hip ratio (369). A locus may also be present on chromosome 18p11 conferring susceptibility to type 2 diabetes in association with obesity (346).

FUTURE DIRECTIONS

The magnitude of the search for genetic determinants of type 2 diabetes has increased exponentially during the past decade, evolving from a limited set of small association studies based on few RFLPs to whole-genome screens employing hundreds of polymorphisms genotyped in an automated way. In the process, our general understanding of the genetics of type 2 diabetes has become more mature. We now know that the existence of type 2 diabetes genes having effects as strong as that of HLA in type 1 diabetes is unlikely. We have also learned that type 2 diabetes may be much more genetically heterogeneous than expected, and new analytic methods have been developed to account for this heterogeneity as well as for gene-gene interactions (352). The crucial importance of finding replication has also been established, and it is now the rule to take positive results with extreme caution until these are confirmed in other populations.

Although major type 2 diabetes genes have yet to be identified (perhaps with the exception of calpain 10), several interesting leads have been produced that will be pursued during the next few years. The first task on the agenda is to identify the genes that are responsible for the linkage peaks detected by genome screens. Despite the imminent availability of the finished human genome sequence, finding these genes will not be an easy endeavor. In contrast with mendelian disorders, linkage peaks for complex diseases are rather large, being often defined on the basis of probabilities rather than firm recombination events. Hundreds of genes may be placed in a linked interval, and prioritizing the analysis of these genes may be misleading, as illustrated by the surprising role of lamins in some forms of lipoatrophic diabetes (74,75). Thus, there will be the need to narrow linked loci to diabetes-associated haplotypes by typing large numbers of cases and controls for hundreds of anonymous SNPs. The public SNP database that is being developed (25) will be a valuable tool for this task, but fine mapping through SNPs may prove difficult if there is allelic heterogeneity (different variants at the same locus contributing to diabetes in different people), as observed in MODY (43). If SNPs associated with diabetes are identified, extensive functional analysis at the molecular level will be necessary to distinguish the causal variants from all other SNPs that are in linkage disequilibrium.

Studies of functional candidate genes will be instrumental in identifying moderate gene effects that are below the detection threshold of linkage studies. Thus far, two important factors have been limiting functional candidate gene studies: the slow pace at which candidate genes have been identified by cellular physiology studies and the low throughput with which genes could be screened and typed for polymorphisms. So far, only a very small proportion of the genes involved in insulin action and secretion have been screened for association with type 2 diabetes. However, this scenario is rapidly changing. A large number of genes with putative roles in insulin action or secretion and the pathophysiology of diabetes are being identified by expression-profiling efforts making use of microarray technology. Many of these loci can be extensively screened for sequence variants by high-throughput technologies. Thus, the scope of association studies will quickly broaden to the analysis of hundreds of candidate genes in very large populations.

All these studies will require good physiologic phenotyping to identify more homogeneous disease subgroups together with a precise characterization of environmental exposures to analyze gene-environment interactions. Ultimately, however, it seems likely that over the next decade most cases of type 2 diabetes will be genetically classified and a new era of prediction and attempts at prevention may begin.

REFERENCES

1. Warram JH, Rich SS, Krolewski AS. Epidemiology and genetics of diabetes mellitus. In: Kahn CR, Weir G, eds. *Joslin's diabetes mellitus*, 13th ed. Philadelphia: Lea & Febiger, 1994:201–215.
2. Mokdad AH, Ford ES, Bowman BA, et al. Diabetes trends in the U.S.: 1990–1998. *Diabetes Care* 200;23:1278–1283.
3. Glaser NS. Non-insulin-dependent diabetes mellitus in childhood and adolescence. *Pediatr Clin North Am* 1997;44:307–337.
4. Diabetes Research Working group. *Conquering diabetes. A strategic plan for the 21st century.* Bethesda, MD: National Institutes of Health, 1999. NIH publication no. 99-4398.
5. Kahn CR. Insulin action, diabetogenes, and the cause of type II diabetes. *Diabetes* 1994;43:1066–1084.
6. Martin BC, Warram JH, Krolewski AS, et al. Role of glucose and insulin-resistance in the development of type II diabetes mellitus: results of a 25-years follow-up study. *Lancet* 1992;340:925–929.
7. Gulli G, Ferrannini E, Stern M, et al. The metabolic profile of NIDDM is fully established in glucose-tolerant offspring of two Mexican-American NIDDM parents. *Diabetes* 1992;41:1575–1586.
8. Knowler WC, Pettitt DJ, Saad MF, et al. Diabetes mellitus in Pima Indians: incidence, risk factors and pathogenesis. *Diabetes Metab Rev* 1990;6:1–27.
9. Pincus G, White P. On the inheritance of diabetes mellitus. II. Further analysis of family histories. *Am J Med Sci* 1034;188:159–169.
10. Harris H. The familial distribution of diabetes: a study of the relatives of 1241 diabetic propositi. *Ann Eugenet* 1950;15:95–119.
11. Gottlieb MS. Diabetes in offsprings and siblings of juvenile- and maturity-onset type diabetics. *J Chronic Dis* 1980;33:331–339.
12. Newman B, Selby JV, King M-C, et al. Concordance for type 2 (non-insulin-dependent) diabetes mellitus in male twins. *Diabetologia* 1987;30:763–768.
13. Medici F, Hawa M, Ianari A, et al. Concordance rate for type 2 diabetes mellitus in monozygotic twins: actuarial analysis. *Diabetologia* 1999;42:146–150.
14. Poulsen P, Kyvik KO, Vaag A, et al. Heritability of type 2 (non-insulin dependent) diabetes mellitus and abnormal glucose tolerance—a population-based twin study. *Diabetologia* 1999;42:125–127.
15. Flegal KM, Ezzati TM, Harris MI, et al. Prevalence of diabetes in Mexican-Americans, Cubans, and Puerto Ricans from the Hispanic Health and Nutrition Examination Survey, 1982–84. *Diabetes Care* 1991;14[Suppl 3]: 628–638.
16. Kawate R, Yamakido M, Nishimoto Y, et al. Diabetes mellitus and its vascular complications in Japanese migrants on the Island of Hawaii. *Diabetes Care* 1979;2:161–170.
17. Williams RR, Hunt SC, Hasstedt SJ, et al. Definition of genetic factors in hypertension. A search for major genes, polygenes and homogeneous subtypes. *J Cardiovasc Pharmacol* 1988;2[Suppl 3]:7–20.
18. Rich SS. Mapping genes in diabetes: genetic epidemiological perspective. *Diabetes* 1990;39:1315–1319.
19. Cook JT, Shields DC, Page RC, et al. Segregation analysis of NIDDM in Caucasian families. *Diabetologia* 1994;37:1231–1240.
20. Saiki RK, Scharf S, Faloona F, et al. Enzymatic amplification of beta-globin genomic sequences and restriction site analysis for diagnosis of sickle cell anemia. *Science* 1985;230:1350–1354.
21. Weber JL. Informativeness of human (dC-dA)n-(dG-dT)n polymorphisms. *Genomics* 1990;7:524–530.
22. Hudson TJ, Stein LD, Gerety SS, et al. An STS-based map of the human genome. *Science* 1995;270:1945–1954.
23. Lander ES, Schork NJ. Genetic dissection of complex traits. *Science* 1994; 265:2037–2048.
24. Lander ES, Linton LM, Birren B, et al. Initial sequencing and analysis of the human genome. *Nature* 2001;409:860–921.
25. Sachidanandam R, Weissman D, Schmidt SC, et al. A map of human genome sequence variation containing 1.42 million single nucleotide polymorphisms. *Nature* 2001;409:928–933.
26. Cox NJ, Bell GI. Disease associations: chance, artifacts, or susceptibility genes? *Diabetes* 1989;39:947–950.
27. Risch N, Merikangas K. The future of genetic studies of complex human diseases. *Science* 1996;273:1516–1517.
28. Svejgaard A, Ryder LP. HLA genotype distribution and genetic models of insulin-dependent diabetes mellitus. *Ann Hum Genet* 1981;45:293–298.
29. Kruglyak L, Nickerson DA. Variation is the spice of life. *Nat Genet* 2001; 27:234–236.
30. Kruglyak L. Prospects for whole-genome linkage disequilibrium mapping of common disease genes. *Nat Genet* 1999;22:139–144.
31. Roberts L. SNP mappers confront reality and find it daunting. *Science* 2000; 287:1898–1899.
32. Weiss KM, Terwilliger JD. How many diseases does it take to map a gene with SNPs? *Nat Genet* 2000;26:151–157.
33. Collins FS. Positional cloning moves from perditional to traditional. *Nature Genet* 1995;9:347–350.
34. Almind K, Doria A, Kahn CR. Putting the genes for type II diabetes on the map. *Nat Med* 2001;7:277–279.
35. Tattersall RB, Fajans SS. A difference between the inheritance of classical juvenile-onset and maturity-onset type diabetes of young people. *Diabetes* 1975;24:44–53.
36. Doria A, Yang Y, Malecki M, et al. Phenotypic characteristics of early-onset autosomal-dominant type 2 diabetes unlinked to known maturity-onset diabetes of the young (MODY) genes. *Diabetes Care* 1999;22:253–261.
37. Stoffers DA, Ferrer J, Clarke WL, et al. Early-onset type-II diabetes mellitus (MODY4) linked to IPF1. *Nat Genet* 1997;17:138–139.
38. Malecki MT, Jhala US, Antonellis A, et al. Mutations in NEUROD1 are associated with the development of type 2 diabetes mellitus. *Nat Genet* 1997;23:323–328.
39. Froguel P, Vaxillaire M, Sun F, et al. Close linkage of glucokinase locus on chromosome 7p to early-onset non-insulin-dependent diabetes mellitus. *Nature* 1992;356:162–164.
40. Hattersley AT, Turner RC, Permutt MA, et al. Linkage of type 2 diabetes to the glucokinase gene. *Lancet* 1992;339:1307–1310.
41. Vionnet N, Stoffel M, Takeda J, et al. Nonsense mutation in the glucokinase gene causes early-onset non-insulin-dependent diabetes mellitus. *Nature* 1992;356:721–722.
42. Stoffel M, Patel P, Lo YMD, et al. Missense glucokinase mutation in maturity-onset diabetes of the young and mutation screening in late-onset diabetes. *Nat Genet* 1992;2:153–156.
43. Yamagata K, Oda N, Kaisaki PJ, et al. Mutations in the hepatocyte nuclear factor-1alpha gene in maturity-onset diabetes of the young. *Nature* 1996;384:455–458.
44. Yamagata K, Furuta H, Oda N, et al. Mutations in the hepatocyte nuclear factor-4alpha gene in maturity-onset diabetes of the young. *Nature* 1996;384: 458–460.
45. Matschinky F, Liang Y, Kesavan P, et al. Glucokinase as pancreatic β-cell glucose sensor and diabetes gene. *J Clin Invest* 1993;92:2092–2098.
46. Tronche F, Bach I, Chouard T, et al. Hepatocyte nuclear factor 1 (HNF1) and liver gene expression. In: Tronche F, Yaniv M, eds. *Liver gene expression.* Austin, TX: Landes, 1994:155–181.
47. Sladek FM. Hepatocyte nuclear factor 4 (HNF 4). In: Tronche F, Yaniv M, eds. *Liver gene expression.* Austin, TX: Landes, 1994:207–230.
48. Frayling TM, Bulamn MP, Ellard S, et al. Mutations in the hepatocyte nuclear factor-1alpha gene are a common cause of maturity-onset diabetes of the young in the U.K. *Diabetes* 1997;46:720–725.
49. Glucksmann MA, Lehto M, Tayber O, et al. Novel mutations and a mutational hotspot in the MODY3 gene. *Diabetes* 1997;46:1081–1086.
50. Horikawa Y, Iwasaki N, Hara M, et al. Mutation in hepatocyte nuclear factor-1 beta gene (TCF2) associated with MODY. *Nat Genet* 1997;7:384–385.
51. Stoffers DA, Zinkin NT, Stanojevic V, et al. Pancreatic agenesis attributable to a single nucleotide deletion in the human IPF1 gene coding sequence. *Nat Genet* 1997;15:106–110.
52. Lindner TH, Njolstad PR, Horikawa Y, et al. A novel syndrome of diabetes mellitus, renal dysfunction and genital malformation associated with a partial deletion of the pseudo-POU domain of hepatocyte nuclear factor-1beta. *Hum Mol Genet* 1999;8:2001–2008.
53. Bingham C, Ellard S, Allen L, et al. Abnormal nephron development associated with a frameshift mutation in the transcription factor hepatocyte nuclear factor-1 beta. *Kidney Int* 2000;57:898–907.
54. Froguel P, Zouali H, Vionnet N, et al. Familial hyperglycemia due to mutations in glucokinase. Definition of a subtype of diabetes mellitus. *N Engl J Med* 1993;328:697–702.

55. Lehto M, Tuomi T, Mahtani MM, et al. Characterization of the MODY3 phenotype. Early-onset diabetes caused by an insulin secretion defect. *J Clin Invest* 1997;99:582–591.
56. Duncan SA, Navas MA, Dufort D, et al. Regulation of a transcription factor network required for differentiation and metabolism. *Science* 1998;281: 692–695.
57. Naya FJ, Huang HP, Qiu Y, et al. Diabetes, defective pancreatic morphogenesis, and abnormal enteroendocrine differentiation in BETA2/neuroD-deficient mice. *Genes Dev* 1997;11:2323–2334.
58. Jonsson J, Carlsson L, Edlund T, et al. Insulin-promoter-factor 1 is required for pancreas development in mice. *Nature* 1994;371:606–609.
59. Pontoglio M, Sreenan S, Roe M, et al. Defective insulin secretion in hepatocyte nuclear factor 1alpha-deficient mice. *J Clin Invest* 1998;101:2215–2222.
60. Stoffel M, Duncan SA. The maturity-onset diabetes of the young (MODY1) transcription factor HNF4alpha regulates expression of genes required for glucose transport and metabolism. *Proc Natl Acad Sci U S A* 1997;94: 13209–13214.
61. Naya FJ, Stellrecht CM, Tsai MJ. Tissue-specific regulation of the insulin gene by a novel basic helix-loop-helix transcription factor. *Genes Dev* 1995;9: 1009–1019.
62. Marshak S, Totary H, Cerasi E, et al. Purification of the beta-cell glucose-sensitive factor that transactivates the insulin gene differentially in normal and transformed islet cells. *Proc Natl Acad Sci U S A* 1996;93:15057–15062.
63. Velho G, Vaxillaire M, Boccio V, et al. Diabetes complications in NIDDM kindreds linked to the MODY3 locus on chromosome 12 q. *Diabetes Care* 1996; 19:915–919.
64. Tack CJ, Ellard S, Hattersley AT. A severe clinical phenotype results from the co-inheritance of type 2 susceptibility genes and a hepatocyte nuclear factor-1α mutation. *Diabetes Care* 2000;23:424–425.
65. Vaxillaire M, Boccio V, Philippi A, et al. A gene for maturity onset diabetes of the young maps to chromosome 12q. *Nat Genet* 1995;9:418–423.
66. Bektas A, Suprenant ME, Wogan LT, et al. Evidence of a novel type 2 diabetes locus 50 cM centromeric to NIDDM2 on chromosome 12q. *Diabetes* 1999; 48:2246–2251.
67. Donohue WL, Uchida IA. Leprechaunism: a euphemism for a rare familial disorder. *J Pediatr* 1954;45:505–519.
68. Rabson SM, Mendenhall EN. Familial hypertrophy of pineal body, hyperplasia of adrenal cortex and diabetes mellitus. *Am J Clin Pathol* 1956;26:283–290.
69. Kahn CR, Flier JS, Bar RS, et al. The syndromes of insulin resistance and acanthosis nigricans. Insulin-receptor disorders in man. *N Engl J Med* 1976;294: 739–745.
70. Berardinelli W. An undiagnosed endocrinometabolic syndrome: report of two cases. *J Clin Endocrinol* 1954;4:193–204.
71. Kobberling J, Dunnigan MG. Familial partial lipodystrophy: two types of an X linked dominant syndrome, lethal in the hemizygous state. *J Med Genet* 1986;3:120–127.
72. Taylor SI. Lilly Lecture: molecular mechanisms of insulin resistance. Lessons from patients with mutations in the insulin-receptor gene. *Diabetes* 1992;41: 1473–1490.
73. Flier JS. Lilly Lecture: syndromes of insulin resistance. From patient to gene and back again. *Diabetes* 1992;41:1207–1219.
74. Shackleton S, Lloyd DJ, Jackson SN, et al. LMNA, encoding lamin A/C, is mutated in partial lipodystrophy. *Nat Genet* 2000;24:153–156.
75. Cao H, Hegele RA. Nuclear lamin A/C R482Q mutation in Canadian kindreds with Dunnigan-type familial partial lipodystrophy. *Hum Mol Genet* 2000;9:109–112.
76. Stuurman N, Heins S, Aebi U. Nuclear lamins: their structure, assembly, and interactions. *J Struct Biol* 1998;22:42–66.
77. Bonne G, Di Barletta MR, Varnous S, et al. Mutations in the gene encoding lamin A/C cause autosomal dominant Emery-Dreifuss muscular dystrophy. *Nat Genet* 1999;21:285–288.
78. Fatkin D, MacRae C, Sasaki T, et al. Missense mutations in the rod domain of the lamin A/C gene as causes of dilated cardiomyopathy and conduction-system disease. *N Engl J Med* 1999;341:1715–1724.
79. Vigouroux C, Magre J, Vantyghem MC, et al. Lamin A/C gene: sex-determined expression of mutations in Dunnigan-type familial partial lipodystrophy and absence of coding mutations in congenital and acquired generalized lipoatrophy. *Diabetes* 2000;49:1958–1962.
80. Magre J, Delepine M, Khallouf E, et al. Identification of the gene altered in Berardinelli-Seip congenital lipodystrophy on chromosome 11q13. *Nat Genet* 2001;28:365–370.
81. Giles RE, Blanc H, Cann HM, et al. Maternal inheritance of human mitochondrial DNA. *Proc Natl Acad Sci U S A* 1980;77:6715–6719.
82. van den Ouweland JM, Lemkes HH, Ruitenbeek W, et al. Mutation in mitochondrial tRNA(Leu)(UUR) gene in a large pedigree with maternally transmitted type II diabetes mellitus and deafness. *Nat Genet* 1992;1:368–371.
83. Reardon W, Ross RJ, Sweeney MG, et al. Diabetes mellitus associated with a pathogenic point mutation in mitochondrial DNA. *Lancet* 1992;340: 1376–1379.
84. Kadowaki T, Kadowaki H, Mori Y, et al. A subtype of diabetes mellitus associated with a mutation of mitochondrial DNA. *N Engl J Med* 1994;330:962–968.
85. Maassen JA, Kadowaki T. Maternally inherited diabetes and deafness: a new diabetes subtype. *Diabetologia* 1996;39:375–382.
86. Ballinger SW, Shoffner JM, Hedaya EV, et al. Maternally transmitted diabetes and deafness associated with a 10.4 kb mitochondrial DNA deletion. *Nat Genet* 1992;1:11–15.
87. Soejima A, Inoue K, Takai D, et al. Mitochondrial DNA is required for regulation of glucose-stimulated insulin secretion in a mouse pancreatic beta cell line, MIN6. *J Biol Chem* 1996;271:26194–26199.
88. van den Ouweland JM, Maechler P, Wollheim CB, et al. Functional and morphological abnormalities of mitochondria harbouring the tRNA(Leu)(UUR) mutation in mitochondrial DNA derived from patients with maternally inherited diabetes and deafness (MIDD) and progressive kidney disease. *Diabetologia* 1999;42:485–492.
89. Goto Y, Nonaka I, Horai S. A mutation in the tRNA(Leu)(UUR) gene associated with the MELAS subgroup of mitochondrial encephalomyopathies. *Nature* 1990;348:651–653.
90. Kahn CR. Insulin signaling and the molecular mechanisms of insulin-resistance. In: Imura H, Kasuga M, Nakao K, eds. *Genetic and pathogenetic aspects of multifactorial diseases*. Uehara Memorial Foundation Symposium-1999. New York: Elsevier Science B.V., 1999:61–77.
91. O'Rahilly S, Choi WH, Patel P, et al. Detection of mutations in insulin-receptor gene in NIDDM patients by analysis of single-stranded conformation polymorphisms. *Diabetes* 1991;40:777–782.
92. Kusari J, Verma US, Buse JB, et al. Analysis of the gene sequences of the insulin receptor and the insulin-sensitive glucose transporter (GLUT-4) in patients with common-type non-insulin-dependent diabetes mellitus. *J Clin Invest* 1991;88:1323–1330.
93. Moller DE, Yokota A, Flier JS. Normal insulin-receptor cDNA sequence in Pima Indians with NIDDM. *Diabetes* 1989;38:1496–1500.
94. Cox NJ, Epstein PA, Spielman RS. Linkage studies on NIDDM and the insulin and insulin-receptor genes. *Diabetes* 1989;38:653–658.
95. Elbein SC, Sorensen LK, Taylor M. Linkage analysis of insulin-receptor gene in familial NIDDM. *Diabetes* 1992;41:648–656.
96. Hart LM, Stolk RP, Heine RJ, et al. Association of the insulin-receptor variant Met-985 with hyperglycemia and non-insulin-dependent diabetes mellitus in the Netherlands: a population-based study. *Am J Hum Genet* 1996;59: 1119–1125.
97. Roth J, Taylor SI. Receptors for peptide hormones: alterations in diseases of humans. *Annu Rev Physiol* 1982;44:639–651.
98. Seino S, Bell GI. Alternative splicing of human insulin receptor messenger RNA. *Biochem Biophys Res Commun* 1989;159:312–316.
99. Goldstein BJ, Dudley AL. Heterogeneity of messenger RNA that encodes the rat insulin-receptor is limited to the domain of exon 11. *Diabetes* 1992;41: 1293–1300.
100. Mosthaf L, Grako K, Dull TJ, et al. Functionally distinct insulin receptors generated by tissue-specific alternative splicing. *EMBO J* 1990;9:2409–2413.
101. McClain DA. Different ligand affinities of the two human insulin receptor splice variants are reflected in parallel changes in sensitivity for insulin action. *Mol Endocrinol* 1991;5:734–769.
102. Kellerer M, Lammers R, Ermel B, et al. Distinct alpha-subunit structures of human insulin receptor A and B variants determine differences in tyrosine kinase activities. *Biochemistry* 1992;31:4588–4596.
103. Mosthaf L, Vogt B, Haring HU, et al. Altered expression of insulin receptor types A and B in the skeletal muscle of non-insulin-dependent diabetes mellitus patients. *Proc Natl Acad Sci U S A* 1991;88:4728–4730.
104. Benecke H, Flier JS, Moller DE. Alternatively spliced variants of the insulin receptor protein. Expression in normal and diabetic human tissues. *J Clin Invest* 1992;89:2066–2070.
105. Norgren S, Zierath J, Galuska D, et al. Differences in the ratio of RNA encoding two isoforms of the insulin receptor between control and NIDDM patients. The RNA variant without Exon 11 predominates in both groups. *Diabetes* 1993;42:675–681.
106. Sun XJ, Rothenberg P, Kahn CR, et al. Structure of the insulin receptor substrate IRS-1 defines a unique signal transduction protein. *Nature* 1991;352: 73–77.
107. Araki E, Sun XJ, Haag BL, et al. Human skeletal muscle insulin receptor substrate-1. Characterization of the cDNA, gene, and chromosomal localization. *Diabetes* 1991;42:1041–1054.
108. Araki E, Lipes MA, Patti ME, et al. Alternative pathway of insulin signalling in mice with targeted disruption of the IRS-1 gene. *Nature* 1994;372:186–190.
109. Bruning JC, Winnay J, Bonner-Weir S, et al. Development of a novel polygenic model of NIDDM in mice heterozygous for IR and IRS-1 null alleles. *Cell* 1994;8:561–572.
110. Almind K, Biorbaek C, Vestergaard H, et al. Amino acid polymorphisms of insulin receptor substrate-1 in non-insulin-dependent diabetes mellitus. *Lancet* 1993;342:828–832.
111. Hager J, Zouali H, Velho G, et al. Insulin receptor substrate (IRS-1) gene polymorphism in French NIDDM families. *Lancet* 1993;342:1430.
112. Laakso M, Malkki M, Kekalainen P, et al. Insulin receptor substrate-1 variants in non-insulin-dependent diabetes. *J Clin Invest* 1994;94:1141–1146.
113. Imai Y, Fusco A, Suzuki Y, et al. Variant sequences of insulin receptor substrate-1 in patients with non-insulin-dependent diabetes mellitus. *J Clin Endocrinol Metab* 1994;79:1655–1658.
114. Shimokawa K, Kadowaki H, Sakura H, et al. Molecular scanning of the glycogen synthase and insulin receptor substrate-1 genes in Japanese subjects with non-insulin-dependent diabetes mellitus. *Biochem Biophys Res Commun* 1994;202:463–469.
115. Hitman GA, Hawrami K, McCarthy MI, et al. Insulin receptor substrate-1 gene mutations in NIDDM; implications for the study of polygenic disease. *Diabetologia* 1995;38:481–486.
116. Sigal RJ, Doria A, Warram JH, et al. Codon 972 polymorphism in the insulin

receptor substrate-1 gene, obesity, and risk of noninsulin-dependent diabetes mellitus. *J Clin Endocrinol Metab* 1996;81:1657–1659.
117. Ura S, Araki E, Kishikawa H, et al. Molecular scanning of the insulin receptor substrate-1 (IRS-1) gene in Japanese patients with NIDDM: identification of five novel polymorphisms. *Diabetologia* 1996;39:600–608.
118. Mori H, Hashiramoto M, Kishimoto M, et al. Amino acid polymorphisms of the insulin receptor substrate-1 in Japanese noninsulin-dependent diabetes mellitus. *J Clin Endocrinol Metab* 1995;80:2822–2826.
119. Zhang Y, Wat N, Stratton IM, et al. UKPDS 19: heterogeneity in NIDDM: separate contributions of IRS-1 and beta 3-adrenergic-receptor mutations to insulin resistance and obesity respectively with no evidence for glycogen synthase gene mutations. UK Prospective Diabetes Study. *Diabetologia* 1996;39:1505–1511.
120. Chuang LM, Lai CS, Yeh JI, et al. No association between the Gly971Arg variant of the insulin receptor substrate 1 gene and NIDDM in the Taiwanese population. *Diabetes Care* 1996;19:446-449.
121. Yamada K, Yuan X, Ishiyama S, et al. Codon 972 polymorphism of the insulin receptor substrate-1 gene in impaired glucose tolerance and late-onset NIDDM. *Diabetes Care* 1998;21:753–756.
122. Hart LM, Stolk RP, Dekker JM, et al. Prevalence of variants in candidate genes for type 2 diabetes mellitus in The Netherlands: the Rotterdam study and the Hoorn study. *J Clin Endocrinol Metab* 1999;84:1002–1006.
123. Clausen JO, Hansen T, Bjorbaek C, et al.. Insulin resistance: interactions between obesity and a common variant of insulin receptor substrate-1. *Lancet* 1995;346:397–402.
124. Almind K, Inoue G, Pedersen O, et al. A common amino acid polymorphism in insulin receptor substrate-1 causes impaired insulin signaling. Evidence from transfection studies. *J Clin Invest* 1996;97:2569–2575.
125. Yoshimura R, Araki E, Ura S, et al. Impact of natural IRS-1 mutations on insulin signals: mutations of IRS-1 in the PTB domain and near SH2 protein binding sites result in impaired function at different steps of IRS-1 signaling. *Diabetes* 1997;46:929–936.
126. Porzio O, Federici M, Hribal ML, et al. The Gly972Arg amino acid polymorphism in IRS-1 impairs insulin secretion in pancreatic beta cells. *J Clin Invest* 1999;104:357–364.
127. Stumvoll M, Fritsche A, Volk A, et al. The Gly972Arg polymorphism in the insulin receptor substrate-1 gene contributes to the variation in insulin secretion in normal glucose-tolerant humans. *Diabetes* 2001;50:882–885.
128. Withers DJ, Gutierrez JS, Towery H, et al. Disruption of IRS-2 causes type 2 diabetes in mice. *Nature* 1998;391:900–904.
129. Bernal D, Almind K, Yenush L, et al. Insulin receptor substrate-2 amino acid polymorphisms are not associated with random type 2 diabetes among caucasians. *Diabetes* 1998;47:976–979.
130. Kalidas K, Wasson J, Glaser B, et al. Mapping of the human insulin receptor substrate-2 gene, identification of a linked polymorphic marker and linkage analysis in families with type II diabetes: no evidence for a major susceptibility role. *Diabetologia* 1998;41:1389–1391.
131. Bektas A, Warram JH, White MF, et al. Exclusion of insulin receptor substrate 2 (IRS-2) as a major locus for early-onset autosomal dominant type 2 diabetes. *Diabetes* 1999;48:640–642.
132. Almind K, Frederiksen SK, Ahlgren MG, et al. Common amino acid substitutions in insulin receptor substrate-4 are not associated with type II diabetes mellitus or insulin resistance. *Diabetologia* 1998;41:969–974.
133. Carpenter CL, Cantley LC. Phosphoinositide kinases. *Curr Opin Cell Biol* 1996;8:153–158.
134. Bjornholm M, Kawano Y, Lehtihet M, et al. Insulin receptor substrate-1 phosphorylation and phosphatidylinositol 3-kinase activity in skeletal muscle from NIDDM subjects after in vivo insulin stimulation. *Diabetes* 1997;46: 524–527.
135. Otsu M, Hiles I, Gout I, Fry MJ, et al. Characterization of two 85 kd proteins that associate with receptor tyrosine kinases, middle-T/pp60c-src complexes, and PI3-kinase. *Cell* 1991;65:91–104.
136. Antonetti DA, Algenstaedt P, Kahn CR. Insulin receptor substrate 1 binds two novel splice variants of the regulatory subunit of phosphatidylinositol 3-kinase in muscle and brain. *Mol Cell Biol* 1996;6:2195–2203.
137. Hansen T, Andersen CB, Echwald SM, et al. Identification of a common amino acid polymorphism in the p85alpha regulatory subunit of phosphatidylinositol 3-kinase: effects on glucose disappearance constant, glucose effectiveness, and the insulin sensitivity index. *Diabetes* 1997;46:494–501.
138. Baier LJ, Wiedrich C, Hanson RL, et al. Variant in the regulatory subunit of phosphatidylinositol 3-kinase (p85alpha): preliminary evidence indicates a potential role of this variant in the acute insulin response and type 2 diabetes in Pima women. *Diabetes* 1998;47:973–975.
139. Kawanishi M, Tamori Y, Masugi J, et al. Prevalence of a polymorphism of the phosphatidylinositol 3-kinase p85 alpha regulatory subunit (codon 326 Met→Ile) in Japanese NIDDM patients. *Diabetes Care* 1997;20:1043.
140. Baynes KC, Beeton CA, Panayotou G, et al. Natural variants of human p85 alpha phosphoinositide 3-kinase in severe insulin resistance: a novel variant with impaired insulin-stimulated lipid kinase activity. *Diabetologia* 2000;43: 321–331.
141. Kossila M, Sinkovic M, Karkkainen P, et al. Gene encoding the catalytic subunit p110beta of human phosphatidylinositol 3-kinase: cloning, genomic structure, and screening for variants in patients with type 2 diabetes. *Diabetes* 2000;49:1740–1743.
142. Hansen L, Fjordvang H, Rasmussen SK, et al. Mutational analysis of the coding regions of the genes encoding protein kinase B-alpha and -beta, phosphoinositide-dependent protein kinase-1, phosphatase targeting to glycogen, protein phosphatase inhibitor-1, and glycogenin: lessons from a search for genetic variability of the insulin-stimulated glycogen synthesis pathway of skeletal muscle in NIDDM patients. *Diabetes* 1999;48:403–407.
143. Choi WH, O'Rahilly S, Buse JB, et al. Molecular scanning of insulin-responsive glucose transporter (GLUT4) gene in NIDDM subjects. *Diabetes* 1991;40:1712–1718.
144. Buse JB, Yasuda K, Lay TP, et al. Human GLUT4/muscle-fat glucose-transporter gene. Characterization and genetic variation. *Diabetes* 1992;41:1436–1444.
145. Bjorbaek C, Echwald SM, Hubricht P, et al. Genetic variants in promoters and coding regions of the muscle glycogen synthase and the insulin-responsive GLUT4 genes in NIDDM. *Diabetes* 1994;43:976–983.
146. Thorburn AW, Gumbiner B, Bulacan F, et al. Multiple defects in muscle glycogen synthase activity contribute to reduced glycogen synthesis in non-insulin dependent diabetes mellitus. *J Clin Invest* 1994;87:489–495.
147. Groop LC, Kankuri M, Schalin-Jantti C, et al. Association between polymorphism of the glycogen synthase gene and non-insulin-dependent diabetes mellitus. *N Engl J Med* 1993;328:10–14.
148. Orho-Melander M, Almgren P, Kanninen T, et al. A paired-sibling analysis of the XbaI polymorphism in the muscle glycogen synthase gene. *Diabetologia* 1999;42:1138–1145.
149. Schalin-Jantti C, Nikula-Ijas P, Huang X, et al. Polymorphism of the glycogen synthase gene in hypertensive and normotensive subjects. *Hypertension* 1996;27:67–71.
150. Zouali H, Velho G, Froguel P. Polymorphism of the glycogen synthase gene and non-insulin-dependent diabetes mellitus. *N Engl J Med* 1993;328:1568.
151. Kadowaki T, Kadowaki H, Yazaki Y. Polymorphism of the glycogen synthase gene and non-insulin-dependent diabetes mellitus. *N Engl J Med* 1993;328: 1568–1569.
152. Majer M, Mott DM, Mochizuki H, et al. Association of the glycogen synthase locus on 19q13 with NIDDM in Pima Indians. *Diabetologia* 1996;39:314–321.
153. Rissanen J, Pihlajamaki J, Heikkinen S, et al. New variants in the glycogen synthase gene (Gln71His, Met416Val) in patients with NIDDM from eastern Finland. *Diabetologia* 1997;40:1313–1419.
154. Orho-Melander M, Shimomura H, et al. Expression of naturally occurring variants in the muscle glycogen synthase gene. *Diabetes* 1999;8:918–920.
155. Hansen L, Reneland R, Berglund L, et al. Polymorphism in the glycogen-associated regulatory subunit of type 1 protein phosphatase (PPP1R3) gene and insulin sensitivity. *Diabetes* 2000;49:298–230.
156. Hegele RA, Harris SB, Zinman B, et al. Variation in the AU(AT)-rich element within the 3′-untranslated region of PPP1R3 is associated with variation in plasma glucose in aboriginal Canadians. *J Clin Endocrinol Metab* 1998;83: 3980–3983.
157. Xia J, Scherer SW, Cohen PT, et al. A common variant in PPP1R3 associated with insulin resistance and type 2 diabetes. *Diabetes* 1998;47:1519–1524.
158. Reynet C, Kahn CR. Rad: a member of the Ras family overexpressed in muscle of type II diabetic humans. *Science* 1993;262:1441–1444.
159. Zhu J, Reynet C, Caldwell JS, et al. Characterization of Rad, a new member of Ras/GTPase superfamily, and its regulation by a unique GTPase-activating protein (GAP)-like activity. *J Biol Chem* 1995;270:4805–4812.
160. Moyers JS, Bilan PJ, Reynet C, et al. Overexpression of Rad inhibits glucose uptake in cultured muscle and fat cells. *J Biol Chem* 1996;271:23111–23116.
161. Caldwell JS, Moyers JS, Doria A, et al. Molecular cloning of the human rad gene: gene structure and complete nucleotide sequence. *Biochim Biophys Acta* 1996;1316:145–148.
162. Doria A, Caldwell JS, Ji L, et al. Trinucleotide repeats at the rad locus. Allele distributions in NIDDM and mapping to a 3-cM region on chromosome 16q. *Diabetes* 1995;44:243–247.
163. Orho M, Carlsson M, Kanninen T, et al. Polymorphism at the rad gene is not associated with NIDDM in Finns. *Diabetes* 1996;45:429–433.
164. Yuan X, Yamada K, Ishiyama-Shigemoto S, et al. Analysis of trinucleotide-repeat combination polymorphism at the rad gene in patients with type 2 diabetes mellitus. *Metabolism* 1999;48:173–175.
165. Maddux BA, Sbraccia P, Kumakura S, et al. Membrane glycoprotein PC-1 and insulin resistance in non-insulin-dependent diabetes mellitus. *Nature* 1995; 373:448–451.
166. Maddux BA, Goldfine ID. Membrane glycoprotein PC-1 inhibition of insulin receptor function occurs via direct interaction with the receptor alpha-subunit. *Diabetes* 2000;49:13–19.
167. Frittitta L, Spampinato D, Solini A, et al. Elevated PC-1 content in cultured skin fibroblasts correlates with decreased in vivo and in vitro insulin action in nondiabetic subjects: evidence that PC-1 may be an intrinsic factor in impaired insulin receptor signaling. *Diabetes* 1998;47:1095–1100.
168. Pizzuti A, Frittitta L, Argiolas A, et al. A polymorphism (K121Q) of the human glycoprotein PC-1 gene coding region is strongly associated with insulin resistance. *Diabetes* 1999;48:1881–1884.
169. Gu HF, Almgren P, Lindholm E, et al. Association between the human glycoprotein PC-1 gene and elevated glucose and insulin levels in a paired-sibling analysis. *Diabetes* 2000;49:1601–1603.
170. Rasmussen SK, Urhammer SA, Pizzuti A. The K121Q variant of the human PC-1 gene is not associated with insulin resistance or type 2 diabetes among Danish Caucasians. *Diabetes* 2000;49:1608–1611.
171. Duggirala R, Blangero J, Almasy L, et al. A major locus for fasting insulin concentrations and insulin resistance on chromosome 6q with strong pleiotropic effects on obesity-related phenotypes in nondiabetic Mexican Americans. *Am J Hum Genet* 2001;68:1149–1164.

172. Colombo BM, Falquerho L, Manenti G, et al. Expression of the pp63 gene encoding the insulin receptor tyrosine kinase inhibitor in proliferating liver and in liver tumors. *Biochem Biophys Res Commun* 1991;180:967–971.
173. Srinivas PR, Wagner AS, Reddy LV, et al. Serum alpha 2-HS-glycoprotein is an inhibitor of the human insulin receptor at the tyrosine kinase level. *Mol Endocrinol* 1993;7:1445–1455.
174. Old LJ. Tumor necrosis factor (YNF). *Science* 1985;230:630–632.
175. Hotamisligil GS, Shargill NS, Spiegelman BM. Adipose expression of tumor necrosis factor-alpha: direct role in obesity-linked insulin resistance. *Science* 1993;259:87–91.
176. Uysal KT, Wiesbrock SM, Marino MW, et al. Protection from obesity-induced insulin resistance in mice lacking TNF-alpha function. *Nature* 1997;389: 610–614.
177. Wilson AG, Symons JA, McDowell TL, et al. Effects of a polymorphism in the human tumor necrosis factor alpha promoter on transcriptional activation. *Proc Natl Acad Sci U S A* 1997;94:3195-3199.
178. McGuire W, Hill AV, Allsopp CE, et al. Variation in the TNF-alpha promoter region associated with susceptibility to cerebral malaria. *Nature* 1994;371: 508–510.
179. Fernandez-Real JM, Gutierrez C, Ricart W, et al. The TNF-alpha gene Nco I polymorphism influences the relationship among insulin resistance, percent body fat, and increased serum leptin levels. *Diabetes* 1997;46:1468–1472.
180. Walston J, Seibert M, Yen CJ, et al. Tumor necrosis factor-alpha-238 and -308 polymorphisms do not associate with traits related to obesity and insulin resistance. *Diabetes* 1999;48:2096–2098.
181. Koch M, Rett K, Volk A, Maerker E, et al. The tumour necrosis factor alpha 238 G→A and -308 G→A promoter polymorphisms are not associated with insulin sensitivity and insulin secretion in young healthy relatives of type II diabetic patients. *Diabetologia* 2000;43:181–184.
182. Ishii T, Hirose H, Saito I, et al. Tumor necrosis factor alpha gene G-308A polymorphism, insulin resistance, and fasting plasma glucose in young, older, and diabetic Japanese men. *Metabolism* 2000;49:1616–1618.
183. Lee SC, Pu YB, Thomas GN, et al. Tumor necrosis factor alpha gene G-308A polymorphism in the metabolic syndrome. *Metabolism* 2000;49:1021–1024.
184. Rasmussen SK, Urhammer SA, Jensen JN, et al. The -238 and -308 G→A polymorphisms of the tumor necrosis factor alpha gene promoter are not associated with features of the insulin resistance syndrome or altered birth weight in Danish Caucasians. *J Clin Endocrinol Metab* 2000;85:1731–1734.
185. Day CP, Grove J, Daly AK, et al. Tumour necrosis factor-alpha gene promoter polymorphism and decreased insulin resistance. *Diabetologia* 1998;41: 430–434.
186. Fernandez-Real JM, Vendrell J, Ricart W, et al. Polymorphism of the tumor necrosis factor-alpha receptor 2 gene is associated with obesity, leptin levels, and insulin resistance in young subjects and diet-treated type 2 diabetic patients. *Diabetes Care* 2000;23:831–837.
187. Alcolado JC, Baroni MG, Li SR. Association between a restriction fragment length polymorphism at the liver/islet cell (GluT 2) glucose transporter and familial type 2 (non-insulin-dependent) diabetes mellitus. *Diabetologia* 1991; 34:734–736.
188. Matsutani A, Koranyi L, Cox N, et al. Polymorphisms of GLUT2 and GLUT4 genes. Use in evaluation of genetic susceptibility to NIDDM in blacks. *Diabetes* 1990;39:1534–1542.
189. Patel P, Bell GI, Cook JT, et al. Multiple restriction fragment length polymorphisms at the GLUT2 locus: GLUT2 haplotypes for genetic analysis of type 2 (non-insulin-dependent) diabetes mellitus. *Diabetologia* 1991;34:817–821.
190. Tanizawa Y, Riggs AC, Chiu KC, et al. Variability of the pancreatic islet beta cell/liver (GLUT 2) glucose transporter gene in NIDDM patients. *Diabetologia* 1994;37:420–427.
191. Mueckler M, Kruse M, Strube M, et al. A mutation in the Glut2 glucose transporter gene of a diabetic patient abolishes transport activity. *J Biol Chem* 1994; 269:17765–17767.
192. Moller AM, Jensen NM, Pildal J, et al. Studies of genetic variability of the glucose transporter 2 promoter in patients with type 2 diabetes mellitus. *J Clin Endocrinol Metab* 2001;86:2181–2186.
193. Chiu KC, Province MA, Permutt MA. Glucokinase gene is genetic marker for NIDDM in American blacks. *Diabetes* 1992;41:843–849.
194. Chiu KC, Province MA, Dowse GK, et al. A genetic marker at the glucokinase gene locus for type 2 (non-insulin-dependent) diabetes mellitus in Mauritian Creoles. *Diabetologia* 1992;35:632–638.
195. Noda K, Matsutani A, Tanizawa Y, et al. Polymorphic microsatellite repeat markers at the glucokinase gene locus are positively associated with NIDDM in Japanese. *Diabetes* 1993;42:1147–1152.
196. Chiu KC, Tanizawa Y, Permutt MA. Glucokinase gene variants in the common form of NIDDM. *Diabetes* 1993;42:579–582.
197. Eto K, Sakura H, Shimokawa K, et al. Sequence variations of the glucokinase gene in Japanese subjects with NIDDM. *Diabetes* 1993;42:1133–1137.
198. Stone LM, Kahn SE, Fujimoto WY, et al. A variation at position -30 of the beta-cell glucokinase gene promoter is associated with reduced beta-cell function in middle-aged Japanese-American men. *Diabetes* 1996;45:422–428.
199. Zaidi FK, Wareham NJ, McCarthy MI, et al. Homozygosity for a common polymorphism in the islet-specific promoter of the glucokinase gene is associated with a reduced early insulin response to oral glucose in pregnant women. *Diabet Med* 1997;14:228–234.
200. Rissanen J, Saarinen L, Heikkinen S, et al. Glucokinase gene islet promoter region variant (G→A) at nucleotide -30 is not associated with reduced insulin secretion in Finns. *Diabetes Care* 1998;21:1194–1197.
201. Zouali H, Vaxillaire M, Lesage S, et al. Linkage analysis and molecular scanning of glucokinase gene in NIDDM families. *Diabetes* 1993;42:1238–1245.
202. Elbein SC, Hoffman M, Chiu K, et al. Linkage analysis of the glucokinase locus in familial type 2 (non-insulin-dependent) diabetic pedigrees. *Diabetologia* 1993;36:141–145.
203. Cook JT, Hattersley AT, Christopher P, et al. Linkage analysis of glucokinase gene with NIDDM in Caucasian pedigrees. *Diabetes* 1992;41:1496–1500.
204. Ashcroft FM, Gribble FM. ATP-sensitive K+ channels and insulin secretion: their role in health and disease. *Diabetologia* 1999;42:903–919.
205. Thomas PM, Cote GJ, Wohllk N, et al. Mutations in the sulfonylurea receptor gene in familial persistent hyperinsulinemic hypoglycemia of infancy. *Science* 1995;268:426–429.
206. Thomas P, Ye Y, Lightner E. Mutation of the pancreatic islet inward rectifier Kir6.2 also leads to familial persistent hyperinsulinemic hypoglycemia of infancy. *Hum Mol Genet* 1996;5:1809–1812.
207. Inoue H, Ferrer J, Welling CM, et al. Sequence variants in the sulfonylurea receptor (SUR) gene are associated with NIDDM in Caucasians. *Diabetes* 1996;45:825–831.
208. Hani EH, Clement K, Velho G, et al. Genetic studies of the sulfonylurea receptor gene locus in NIDDM and in morbid obesity among French Caucasians. *Diabetes* 1997;46:688–694.
209. Ohta Y, Tanizawa Y, Inoue H, et al. Identification and functional analysis of sulfonylurea receptor 1 variants in Japanese patients with NIDDM. *Diabetes* 1998;47:476–481.
210. Hansen T, Echwald SM, Hansen L, et al. Decreased tolbutamide-stimulated insulin secretion in healthy subjects with sequence variants in the high-affinity sulfonylurea receptor gene. *Diabetes* 1998;47:598–605.
211. Ishiyama-Shigemoto S, Yamada K, Yuan X, et al. Clinical characterization of polymorphisms in the sulphonylurea receptor 1 gene in Japanese subjects with type 2 diabetes mellitus. *Diabet Med* 1998;15:826–829.
212. Ji L, Han X, Wang H. Sulfonylurea receptor gene polymorphism is associated with non-insulin dependent diabetes mellitus in Chinese population. *Zhonghua Yi Xue Za Zhi* 1998;78:774–775.
213. Hart LM, de Knijff P, Dekker JM, et al. Variants in the sulphonylurea receptor gene: association of the exon 16-3t variant with type II diabetes mellitus in Dutch Caucasians. *Diabetologia* 1999;42:617–620.
214. van Tilburg JH, Rozeman LB, van Someren H, et al. The exon 16-3t variant of the sulphonylurea receptor gene is not a risk factor for type II diabetes mellitus in the Dutch Breda cohort. *Diabetologia* 2000;43:681.
215. Rissanen J, Markkanen A, Karkkainen P, et al. Sulfonylurea receptor 1 gene variants are associated with gestational diabetes and type 2 diabetes but not with altered secretion of insulin. *Diabetes Care* 2000;23:70–73.
216. Gloyn AL, Hashim Y, Ashcroft SJ, et al. Association studies of variants in promoter and coding regions of beta-cell ATP-sensitive K-channel genes SUR1 and Kir6.2 with Type 2 diabetes mellitus (UKPDS 53). *Diabet Med* 2001;18: 206–212.
217. Meirhaeghe A, Helbecque N, Cottel D, et al. Impact of sulfonylurea receptor 1 genetic variability on non-insulin-dependent diabetes mellitus prevalence and treatment: a population study. *Am J Med Genet* 2001;101:4–8.
218. Inoue H, Ferrer J, Warren-Perry M, et al. Sequence variants in the pancreatic islet beta-cell inwardly rectifying K+ channel Kir6.2 (Bir) gene: identification and lack of role in Caucasian patients with NIDDM. *Diabetes* 1997;46: 502–507.
219. Hansen L, Echwald SM, Hansen T, et al. Amino acid polymorphisms in the ATP-regulatable inward rectifier Kir6.2 and their relationships to glucose- and tolbutamide-induced insulin secretion, the insulin sensitivity index, and NIDDM. *Diabetes* 1997;46:508–512.
220. Steiner DF, Tager HS, Chan SJ, et al. Lessons learned from molecular biology of insulin-gene mutations. *Diabetes Care* 1990;13:600–609.
221. Bell GI, Selby MJ, Rutter WJ. The highly polymorphic region near the human insulin gene is composed of simple tandemly repeating sequences. *Nature* 1982;295:31–35.
222. Bell GI, Horita S, Karam JH: A polymorphic locus near the human insulin gene is associated with insulin-dependent diabetes mellitus. *Diabetes* 1984;33: 176–183.
223. Julier C, Hyer RN, Davies J, Merlin F, et al. Insulin-IGF2 region on chromosome 11p encodes a gene implicated in HLA-DR4-dependent diabetes susceptibility. *Nature* 1991;354:155–159.
224. Elbein S, Rotwein P, Permutt MA, et al. Lack of association of the polymorphic locus in the 5′ flanking region of the human insulin gene and diabetes in American blacks. *Diabetes* 1985;34:433–439.
225. Huxtable SJ, Saker PJ, Haddad L, et al. Analysis of parent-offspring trios provides evidence for linkage and association between the insulin gene and type 2 diabetes mediated exclusively through paternally transmitted class III variable number tandem repeat alleles. *Diabetes* 2000;49:126–130.
226. Olansky L, Welling C, Giddings S, et al. A variant insulin promoter in non-insulin-dependent diabetes mellitus. *J Clin Invest* 1992;89:1596–1602.
227. Yoshioka N, Kuzuya T, Matsuda A, et al. Serum proinsulin levels at fasting and after oral glucose load in patients with type 2 (non-insulin-dependent) diabetes mellitus. *Diabetologia* 1988;31:355–360.
228. Naggert JK, Fricker LD, Varlamov O, et al. Hyperproinsulinaemia in obese fat/fat mice associated with a carboxypeptidase E mutation which reduces enzyme activity. *Nat Genet* 1995;10:135–142.
229. Utsunomiya N, Ohagi S, Sanke T, et al. Organization of the human carboxypeptidase E gene and molecular scanning for mutations in Japanese subjects with NIDDM or obesity. *Diabetologia* 1998;41:701–705.

230. Kalidas K, Dow E, Saker PJ, et al. Prohormone convertase 1 in obesity, gestational diabetes mellitus, and NIDDM: no evidence for a major susceptibility role. *Diabetes* 1998;47:287–289.
231. Jackson RS, Creemers JW, Ohagi S, et al. Obesity and impaired prohormone processing associated with mutations in the human prohormone convertase 1 gene. *Nat Genet* 1997;16:303–306.
232. Edlund H. Transcribing pancreas. *Diabetes* 1998;47:1817–1823.
233. Mahtani MM, Widen E, Lehto M, et al. Mapping of a gene for type 2 diabetes associated with an insulin secretion defect by a genome scan in Finnish families. *Nat Genet* 1996;14:90–96.
234. Shaw JT, Lovelock PK, Kesting JB, et al. Novel susceptibility gene for late-onset NIDDM is localized to human chromosome 12q. *Diabetes* 1998;47: 1793–1796.
235. Iwasaki N, Oda N, Ogata M, et al. Mutations in the hepatocyte nuclear factor-1alpha/MODY3 gene in Japanese subjects with early- and late-onset NIDDM. *Diabetes* 1997;46:1504–1508.
236. Urhammer SA, Rasmussen SK, Kaisaki PJ, et al. Genetic variation in the hepatocyte nuclear factor-1 alpha gene in Danish Caucasians with late-onset NIDDM. *Diabetologia* 1997;40:473–475.
237. Baier LJ, Permana PA, Traurig M, et al. Mutations in the genes for hepatocyte nuclear factor (HNF)-1alpha, -4alpha, -1beta, and -3beta; the dimerization cofactor of HNF-1; and insulin promoter factor 1 are not common causes of early-onset type 2 diabetes in Pima Indians. *Diabetes Care* 2000;23:302–304.
238. Urhammer SA, Fridberg M, Hansen T, et al. A prevalent amino acid polymorphism at codon 98 in the hepatocyte nuclear factor-1alpha gene is associated with reduced serum C-peptide and insulin responses to an oral glucose challenge. *Diabetes* 1997;46:912–916.
239. Ji L, Malecki M, Warram JH, et al. New susceptibility locus for NIDDM is localized to human chromosome 20q. *Diabetes* 1997;46:876–881.
240. Bowden DW, Sale M, Howard TD, et al. Linkage of genetic markers on human chromosomes 20 and 12 to NIDDM in caucasian sib pairs with a history of diabetic nephropathy. *Diabetes* 1997;46:882–886.
241. Zouali H, Hani EH, Philippi A, et al. A susceptibility locus for early-onset non-insulin dependent (type 2) diabetes mellitus maps to chromosome 20q, proximal to the phosphoenolpyruvate carboxykinase gene. *Hum Mol Genet* 1997;6:1401–1408.
242. Ghosh S, Watanabe RM, Hauser ER, et al. Type 2 diabetes: evidence for linkage on chromosome 20 in 716 Finnish affected sib pairs. *Proc Natl Acad Sci U S A* 1999;96:2198–2203.
243. Malecki MT, Antonellis A, Casey P, et al. Exclusion of the hepatocyte nuclear factor 4alpha as a candidate gene for late-onset NIDDM linked with chromosome 20q. *Diabetes* 1998;47:970–972.
244. Dupont S, Vionnet N, Chevre JC, et al. No evidence of linkage or diabetes-associated mutations in the transcription factors BETA2/NEUROD1 and PAX4 in type II diabetes in France. *Diabetologia* 1999;42:480–484.
245. Macfarlane WM, Frayling TM, Ellard S, et al. Missense mutations in the insulin promoter factor-1 gene predispose to type 2 diabetes. *J Clin Invest* 1999;104:R33–R39.
246. Hani EH, Stoffers DA, Chevre JC, et al. Defective mutations in the insulin promoter factor-1 (IPF-1) gene in late-onset type 2 diabetes mellitus. *J Clin Invest* 1999;104:R41–R48.
247. Hansen L, Urioste S, Petersen HV, et al. Missense mutations in the human insulin promoter factor-1 gene and their relation to maturity-onset diabetes of the young and late-onset type 2 diabetes mellitus in Caucasians. *J Clin Endocrinol Metab* 2000;85:1323–1326.
248. Plengvidhya N, Antonellis A, Wogan LT, et al. Hepatocyte nuclear factor-4gamma: cDNA sequence, gene organization, and mutation screening in early-onset autosomal-dominant type 2 diabetes. *Diabetes* 1999;48:2099–2102.
249. Horikawa Y, Horikawa Y, Cox NJ, et al. Beta-cell transcription factors and diabetes: no evidence for diabetes-associated mutations in the gene encoding the basic helix-loop-helix transcription factor neurogenic differentiation 4 (NEUROD4) in Japanese patients with MODY. *Diabetes* 2000;49:1955–1957.
250. Hinokio Y, Horikawa Y, Furuta H, et al. Beta-cell transcription factors and diabetes: no evidence for diabetes-associated mutations in the hepatocyte nuclear factor-3beta gene (HNF3B) in Japanese patients with maturity-onset diabetes of the young. *Diabetes* 2000;49:302–305.
251. Kim SH, Warram JH, Krolewski AS, et al. Mutation screening of the neurogenin-3 gene in autosomal dominant diabetes. *J Clin Endocrinol Metab* 2001; 86:2320–2322.
252. Jensen JN, Hansen L, Ekstrom CT, et al. Polymorphisms in the neurogenin 3 gene (NEUROG) and their relation to altered insulin secretion and diabetes in the Danish caucasian population. *Diabetologia* 2001;44:123–126.
253. Okada T, Tobe K, Hara K, et al. Variants of neurogenin 3 gene are not associated with type II diabetes in Japanese subjects. *Diabetologia* 2001;44:241–244.
254. Orskov C. Glucagon-like peptide-1, a new hormone of the entero-insular axis. *Diabetologia* 1992;35:701–711.
255. Ding WG, Gromada J. Protein kinase A-dependent stimulation of exocytosis in mouse pancreatic beta-cells by glucose-dependent insulinotropic polypeptide. *Diabetes* 1997;46:615–621.
256. Habener JF. The incretin notion and its relevance to diabetes. *Endocrinol Metab Clin North Am* 1993;22:775–794.
257. Nauck MA, Heimesaat MM, Orskov C, et al. Preserved incretin activity of glucagon-like peptide 1 [7-36 amide] but not of synthetic human gastric inhibitory polypeptide in patients with type-2 diabetes mellitus. *J Clin Invest* 1993;91:301–307.
258. Elahi D, McAloon-Dyke M, Fukagawa NK, et al. The insulinotropic actions of glucose-dependent insulinotropic polypeptide (GIP) and glucagon-like peptide-1 (7-37) in normal and diabetic subjects. *Regul Pept* 1994;51:63–74.
259. Kubota A, Yamada Y, Hayami T, et al. Identification of two missense mutations in the GIP receptor gene: a functional study and association analysis with NIDDM: no evidence of association with Japanese NIDDM subjects. *Diabetes* 1996;45:1701–1705.
260. Almind K, Ambye L, Urhammer SA, et al. Discovery of amino acid variants in the human glucose-dependent insulinotropic polypeptide (GIP) receptor: the impact on the pancreatic beta cell responses and functional expression studies in Chinese hamster fibroblast cells. *Diabetologia* 1998;41:1194–1198.
261. Barsh GS, Farooqi IS, O'Rahilly S. Genetics of body-weight regulation. *Nature* 2000;404:644–651.
262. Spiegelman BM, Flier JS. Obesity and the regulation of energy balance. *Cell* 2001;104:531–543.
263. Schwartz MW, Woods SC, Porte D Jr, et al. Central nervous system control of food intake. *Nature* 2000;404:661–671.
264. Krude H, Biebermann H, Luck W, et al. Severe early-onset obesity, adrenal insufficiency and red hair pigmentation caused by POMC mutations in humans. *Nat Genet* 1998;19:155–157.
265. Yeo GS, Farooqi IS, Aminian S, et al. A frameshift mutation in MC4R associated with dominantly inherited human obesity. *Nat Genet* 1998;20:111–112.
266. Vaisse C, Clement K, Guy-Grand B, et al. A frameshift mutation in human MC4R is associated with a dominant form of obesity. *Nat Genet* 1998;20: 113–114.
267. Hinney A, Schmidt A, Nottebom K, et al. Several mutations in the melanocortin-4 receptor gene including a nonsense and a frameshift mutation associated with dominantly inherited obesity in humans. *J Clin Endocrinol Metab* 1999;84:1483–1486.
268. Vaisse C, Clement K, Durand E, et al. Melanocortin-4 receptor mutations are a frequent and heterogeneous cause of morbid obesity. *J Clin Invest* 2000;106:253–262.
269. Echwald SM, Sorensen TI, Andersen T, et al. Mutational analysis of the proopiomelanocortin gene in Caucasians with early onset obesity. *Int J Obes Relat Metab Disord* 1999;3:293–298.
270. Challis BG, Yeo GS, Farooqi IS, et al. The CART gene and human obesity: mutational analysis and population genetics. *Diabetes* 2000;49:872–875.
271. Norman RA, Permana P, Tanizawa Y, et al. Absence of genetic variation in some obesity candidate genes (GLP1R, ASIP, MC4R, MC5R) among Pima Indians. *Int J Obes Relat Metab Disord* 1999;23:163–165.
272. Roche C, Boutin P, Dina C, et al. Genetic studies of neuropeptide Y and neuropeptide Y receptors Y1 and Y5 regions in morbid obesity. *Diabetologia* 1997; 40:671–675.
273. Zhang Y, Proenca R, Maffei M, et al. Positional cloning of the mouse obese gene and its human homologue. *Nature* 1994;372:425–432.
274. Tartaglia LA, Dembski M, Weng X, et al. Identification and expression cloning of a leptin receptor, OB-R. *Cell* 1995;83:1263–1271.
275. Chua SC Jr, Chung WK, Wu-Peng XS, Z et al. Phenotypes of mouse diabetes and rat fatty due to mutations in the OB (leptin) receptor. *Science* 1996;271: 994–996.
276. Chen H, Charlat O, Tartaglia LA, et al. Evidence that the diabetes gene encodes the leptin receptor: identification of a mutation in the leptin receptor gene in db/db mice. *Cell* 1996;84:491–495.
277. Clement K, Vaisse C, Lahlou N, et al. A mutation in the human leptin receptor gene causes obesity and pituitary dysfunction. *Nature* 1998;392:398–401.
278. Strobel A, Issad T, Camoin L, Ozata M, et al. A leptin missense mutation associated with hypogonadism and morbid obesity. *Nat Genet* 1998;18:213–215.
279. Montague CT, Farooqi IS, Whitehead JP, et al. Congenital leptin deficiency is associated with severe early-onset obesity in humans. *Nature* 1997;387: 903–908.
280. Maffei M, Stoffel M, Barone M, et al. Absence of mutations in the human OB gene in obese/diabetic subjects. *Diabetes* 1996;45:679–682.
281. Silver K, Walston J, Chung WK, et al. The Gln223Arg and Lys656Asn polymorphisms in the human leptin receptor do not associate with traits related to obesity. *Diabetes* 1997;46:1898–1900.
282. Lowell BB, Flier JS. Brown adipose tissue, beta 3-adrenergic receptors, and obesity. *Annu Rev Med* 1997;48:307–316.
283. Walston J, Silver K, Bogardus C, et al. Time of onset of non-insulin-dependent diabetes mellitus and genetic variation in the beta 3-adrenergic-receptor gene. *N Engl J Med* 1995;333:343–347.
284. Widen E, Lehto M, Kanninen T, et al. Association of a polymorphism in the beta 3-adrenergic-receptor gene with features of the insulin resistance syndrome in Finns. *N Engl J Med* 1995;333:348–351.
285. Clement K, Vaisse C, Manning BS, et al. Genetic variation in the beta 3-adrenergic receptor and an increased capacity to gain weight in patients with morbid obesity. *N Engl J Med* 1995;333:352–354.
286. Buettner R, Schaffler A, Arndt H, et al. The Trp64Arg polymorphism of the beta 3-adrenergic receptor gene is not associated with obesity or type 2 diabetes mellitus in a large population-based Caucasian cohort. *J Clin Endocrinol Metab* 1998;83:2892–2897.
287. Gagnon J, Mauriege P, Roy S, et al. The Trp64Arg mutation of the beta3 adrenergic receptor gene has no effect on obesity phenotypes in the Quebec Family Study and Swedish Obese Subjects cohorts. *J Clin Invest* 1996;98: 2086–2093.
288. Pietri-Rouxel F, St John Manning B, et al. The biochemical effect of the naturally occurring Trp64→Arg mutation on human beta3-adrenoceptor activity. *Eur J Biochem* 1997;247:1174–1179.

289. Hoffstedt J, Poirier O, Thorne A, et al. Polymorphism of the human beta3-adrenoceptor gene forms a well-conserved haplotype that is associated with moderate obesity and altered receptor function. *Diabetes* 1999;48:203–205.
290. Candelore MR, Deng L, Tota LM, et al. Pharmacological characterization of a recently described human beta 3-adrenergic receptor mutant. *Endocrinology* 1996;137:2638–2641.
291. Li LS, Lonnqvist F, Luthman H, et al. Phenotypic characterization of the Trp64Arg polymorphism in the beta 3-adrenergic receptor gene in normal weight and obese subjects. *Diabetologia* 1996;39:857–860.
292. Snitker S, Odeleye OE, Hellmer J, et al. No effect of the Trp64Arg beta 3-adrenoceptor variant on in vivo lipolysis in subcutaneous adipose tissue. *Diabetologia* 1997;40:838–842.
293. Fujisawa T, Ikegami H, Kawaguchi Y, et al. Meta-analysis of the association of Trp64Arg polymorphism of beta 3-adrenergic receptor gene with body mass index. *J Clin Endocrinol Metab* 1998;83:2441–2444.
294. Kozak LP, Harper ME. Mitochondrial uncoupling proteins in energy expenditure. *Annu Rev Nutr* 2000;20:339–363.
295. Ricquier D, Bouillaud F. Mitochondrial uncoupling proteins: from mitochondria to the regulation of energy balance. *J Physiol* 2000;529:3–10.
296. Schrauwen P, Xia J, Walder K, et al. A novel polymorphism in the proximal UCP3 promoter region: effect on skeletal muscle UCP3 mRNA expression and obesity in male non-diabetic Pima Indians. *Int J Obes Relat Metab Disord* 1999;23:1242–1245.
297. Halsall D, Luan J, Saker P, et al. Uncoupling protein 3 genetic variants in human obesity: the c-55t promoter polymorphism is negatively correlated with body mass index in a UK Caucasian population. *Int J Obes Relat Metab Disord* 2001;25:472–477.
298. Otabe S, Clement K, Dina C, et al. A genetic variation in the 5′ flanking region of the UCP3 gene is associated with body mass index in humans in interaction with physical activity. *Diabetologia* 2000;43:245–249.
299. Meirhaeghe A, Amouyel P, Helbecque N, et al. An uncoupling protein 3 gene polymorphism associated with a lower risk of developing type II diabetes and with atherogenic lipid profile in a French cohort. *Diabetologia* 2000;43:1424–1428.
300. Tontonoz P, Hu E, Spiegelman BM. Stimulation of adipogenesis in fibroblasts by PPAR gamma 2, a lipid-activated transcription factor. *Cell* 1994;79:1147–1156.
301. Fajas L, Auboeuf D, Raspe E, et al. The organization, promoter analysis, and expression of the human PPARgamma gene. *J Biol Chem* 1997;272:18779–18789.
302. Barroso I, Gurnell M, Crowley VE, et al. Dominant negative mutations in human PPARgamma associated with severe insulin resistance, diabetes mellitus and hypertension. *Nature* 1999;402:880–883.
303. Ristow M, Muller-Wieland D, Pfeiffer A, et al. Obesity associated with a mutation in a genetic regulator of adipocyte differentiation. *N Engl J Med* 1998;339:953–959.
304. Deeb SS, Fajas L, Nemoto M, et al. A Pro12Ala substitution in PPARgamma2 associated with decreased receptor activity, lower body mass index and improved insulin sensitivity. *Nat Genet* 1998;20:284–287.
305. Beamer BA, Yen CJ, Andersen RE, et al. Association of the Pro12Ala variant in the peroxisome proliferator-activated receptor-gamma2 gene with obesity in two Caucasian populations. *Diabetes* 1998;47:1806–1808.
306. Ek J, Urhammer SA, Sorensen TI, et al. Homozygosity of the Pro12Ala variant of the peroxisome proliferation-activated receptor-gamma2 (PPAR-gamma2): divergent modulating effects on body mass index in obese and lean Caucasian men. *Diabetologia* 1999;42:892–895.
307. Mancini FP, Vaccaro O, Sabatino L, et al. Pro12Ala substitution in the peroxisome proliferator-activated receptor-gamma2 is not associated with type 2 diabetes. *Diabetes* 1999;48:1466–1468.
308. Hamann A, Munzberg H, Buttron P, et al. Missense variants in the human peroxisome proliferator-activated receptor-gamma2 gene in lean and obese subjects. *Eur J Endocrinol* 1999;141:90–92.
309. Clement K, Hercberg S, Passinge B, et al. The Pro115Gln and Pro12Ala PPAR gamma gene mutations in obesity and type 2 diabetes. *Int J Obes Relat Metab Disord* 2000;24:391–393.
310. Altshuler D, Hirschhorn JN, Klannemark M, et al. The common PPARgamma Pro12Ala polymorphism is associated with decreased risk of type 2 diabetes. *Nat Genet* 2000;26:76–80.
311. Ringel J, Engeli S, Distler A, et al. Pro12Ala missense mutation of the peroxisome proliferator activated receptor gamma and diabetes mellitus. *Biochem Biophys Res Commun* 1999;254:450–453.
312. Hara K, Okada T, Tobe K, Yasuda K, et al. The Pro12Ala polymorphism in PPAR gamma2 may confer resistance to type 2 diabetes. *Biochem Biophys Res Commun* 2000;271:212–216.
313. Meirhaeghe A, Fajas L, Helbecque N, et al. Impact of the peroxisome proliferator activated receptor gamma2 Pro12Ala polymorphism on adiposity, lipids and non-insulin-dependent diabetes mellitus. *Int J Obes Relat Metab Disord* 2000;24:195–199.
314. Evans D, de Heer J, Hagemann C, et al. Association between the P12A and c1431t polymorphisms in the peroxisome proliferator activated receptor gamma (PPAR gamma) gene and type 2 diabetes. *Exp Clin Endocrinol Diabetes* 2001;109:151–154.
315. Mori H, Ikegami H, Kawaguchi Y, et al. The Pro12→Ala substitution in PPAR-gamma is associated with resistance to development of diabetes in the general population: possible involvement in impairment of insulin secretion in individuals with type 2 diabetes. *Diabetes* 2001;50:891–894.
316. Douglas JA, Erdos MR, Watanabe RM, et al. The peroxisome proliferator-activated receptor-gamma2 Pro12A1a variant: association with type 2 diabetes and trait differences. *Diabetes* 2001;50:886–890.
317. Durr A, Cossee M, Agid Y, et al. Clinical and genetic abnormalities in patients with Friedreich's ataxia. *N Engl J Med* 1996;335:1169–1175.
318. Ristow M, Giannakidou E, Hebinck J, et al. An association between NIDDM and a GAA trinucleotide repeat polymorphism in the X25/frataxin (Friedreich's ataxia) gene. *Diabetes* 1998;47:851–854.
319. Dupont S, Dubois D, Vionnet N, et al. No association between the Friedreich's ataxia gene and NIDDM in the French population. *Diabetes* 1998;47:1654–1656.
320. Hart LM, Ruige JB, Dekker JM, et al. Altered beta-cell characteristics in impaired glucose tolerant carriers of a GAA trinucleotide repeat polymorphism in the frataxin gene. *Diabetes* 1999;48:924–926.
321. Dalgaard LT, Hansen T, Urhammer SA, et al. Intermediate expansions of a GAA repeat in the frataxin gene are not associated with type 2 diabetes or altered glucose-induced beta-cell function in Danish Caucasians. *Diabetes* 1999;48:914–917.
322. Lynn S, Hattersley AT, McCarthy MI, et al. Intermediate expansions of a X25/frataxin gene GAA repeat and type II diabetes: assessment using parent-offspring trios. *Diabetologia* 2000;43:384–385.
323. Ristow M, Pfister MF, Yee AJ, et al. Frataxin activates mitochondrial energy conversion and oxidative phosphorylation. *Proc Natl Acad Sci U S A* 2000;97:12239–12243.
324. Hager J, Hansen L, Vaisse C, et al. A missense mutation in the glucagon receptor gene is associated with non-insulin-dependent diabetes mellitus. *Nat Genet* 1995;9:299–304.
325. Hansen LH, Abrahamsen N, Hager J, et al. The Gly40Ser mutation in the human glucagon receptor gene associated with NIDDM results in a receptor with reduced sensitivity to glucagon. *Diabetes* 1996;45:725–730.
326. Huang X, Orho M, Lehto M, et al. Lack of association between the Gly40Ser polymorphism in the glucagon receptor gene and NIDDM in Finland. *Diabetologia* 1995;38:1246–1248.
327. Ambrosch A, Lobmann R, Dierkes J, et al. Analysis of the Gly40Ser polymorphism in the glucagon receptor gene in a German non-insulin-dependent diabetes mellitus population. *Clin Chem Lab Med* 1999;37:719–721.
328. Gusella JF, Wexler NS, Conneally PM, et al. A polymorphic DNA marker genetically linked to Huntington's disease. *Nature* 1983;306:234–238.
329. Wooster R, Bignell G, Lancaster J, et al. Identification of the breast cancer susceptibility gene BRCA2. *Nature* 1995;378:789–792.
330. Morton NE. Sequential tests for the detection of linkage. *Am J Hum Genet* 1955;7:277–318.
331. Goldgar DE. Sib pair analysis. In: Haines JL, Peiricak-Vance MA, eds. *Approaches to gene mapping in complex human diseases*. New York: Wiley-Liss, 1998:273–303.
332. Weeks DE, Lange K. The affected-pedigree-member method of linkage analysis. *Am J Hum Genet* 1988;42:315–326.
333. Kruglyak L, Daly MJ, Reeve-Daly MP, et al. Parametric and nonparametric linkage analysis: a unified multipoint approach. *Am J Hum Genet* 1996;58:1347–1363.
334. Haseman JK, Elston RC. The investigation of linkage between a quantitative trait and a marker locus. *Behav Genet* 1972;2:3–19.
335. Almasy L, Blangero J. Multipoint quantitative-trait linkage analysis in general pedigrees. *Am J Hum Genet* 1998;62:1198–1211.
336. Hanis CL, Boerwinkle E, Chakraborty R, E et al. A genome-wide search for human non-insulin-dependent (type 2) diabetes genes reveals a major susceptibility locus on chromosome 2. *Nat Genet* 1996;13:161–166.
337. Hanson RL, Ehm MG, Pettitt DJ, et al. An autosomal genomic scan for loci linked to type II diabetes mellitus and body-mass index in Pima Indians. *Am J Hum Genet* 1998;63:1130–1138.
338. Duggirala R, Blangero J, Almasy L, et al. Linkage of type 2 diabetes mellitus and of age at onset to a genetic location on chromosome 10q in Mexican Americans. *Am J Hum Genet* 1999;64:1127–1140.
339. Elbein SC, Hoffman MD, Teng K, et al. A genome-wide search for type 2 diabetes susceptibility genes in Utah Caucasians. *Diabetes* 1999;48:1175–1182.
340. St. Jean PL, Mitchell BD, Hsueh WC, et al. Type 2 diabetes loci in the Old Order Amish. *Diabetes* 1999;48[Suppl 1]:A46.
341. Ehm MG, Karnoub MC, Sakul H, et al. Genomewide search for type 2 diabetes susceptibility genes in four American populations. *Am J Hum Genet* 2000;66:1871–1881.
342. Ghosh S, Watanabe RM, Valle TT, et al. The Finland-United States investigation of non-insulin-dependent diabetes mellitus genetics (FUSION) study. I. An autosomal genome scan for genes that predispose to type 2 diabetes. *Am J Hum Genet* 2000;67:1174–1185.
343. Vionnet N, Hani El-H, Dupont S, et al. Genomewide search for type 2 diabetes-susceptibility genes in French whites: evidence for a novel susceptibility locus for early-onset diabetes on chromosome 3q27-qter and independent replication of a type 2-diabetes locus on chromosome 1q21-q24. *Am J Hum Genet* 2000;67:1470–1480.
344. Permutt MA, Wasson JC, Suarez BK, et al. A genome scan for type 2 diabetes susceptibility loci in a genetically isolated population. *Diabetes* 2001;50:681–685.
345. McCarthy MI, Hattersley AT, Walker M, et al. Genome scan linkage data from a large European family collection support localization of a type 2 diabetes susceptibility gene to chromosome 1q21-23. *Diabetes* 2001;50[Suppl 1]:A27.

346. Parker A, Meyer J, Lewitzky S, et al. A gene conferring susceptibility to type 2 diabetes in conjunction with obesity is located on chromosome 18p11. *Diabetes* 2001;50:675–680.
347. Lander E, Kruglyak L. Genetic dissection of complex traits: guidelines for interpreting and reporting linkage results. *Nat Genet* 1995;11:241–247.
348. Risch N. Linkage strategies for genetically complex traits. II. The power of affected relative pairs. *Am J Hum Genet* 1990;46:229–241.
349. Klein BEK, Klein R, Moss SE, et al. Parental history of diabetes in a population-based study. *Diabetes Care* 1996;8:827–830.
350. Karter AJ, Rowell SE, Ackerson LM, et al. Excess maternal transmission of type 2 diabetes. The Northern California Kaiser Permanente Diabetes Registry. *Diabetes Care* 1999;22:938–943.
351. Meigs JB, Cupples LA, Wilson PWF. Parental transmission of type 2 diabetes mellitus: The Framingham Heart Study. *Diabetes* 2000;49:2201–2207.
352. Cox NJ, Frigge M, Nicolae DL, et al. Loci on chromosomes 2 (NIDDM1) and 15 interact to increase susceptibility to diabetes in Mexican Americans. *Nat Genet* 1999;21:213–215.
353. Ghosh S, Hauser ER, Magnuson VL, et al. A large sample of Finnish diabetic sib-pairs reveals no evidence for a non-insulin-dependent diabetes mellitus susceptibility locus at 2qter. *J Clin Invest* 1998;102:704–709.
354. Horikawa Y, Oda N, Cox NJ, et al. Genetic variation in the gene encoding calpain-10 is associated with type 2 diabetes mellitus. *Nat Genet* 2000;26: 163–175.
355. Baier LJ, Permana PA, Yang X, et al. A calpain-10 gene polymorphism is associated with reduced muscle mRNA levels and insulin resistance. *J Clin Invest* 2000;106:R69–R73.
356. Saido TC, Sorimachi H, Suzuki K. Calpain: new perspectives in molecular diversity and physiological-pathological involvement. *FASEB J* 1994;8: 814–822.
357. Carafoli E, Molinari M. Calpain: a protease in search of a function? *Biochem Biophys Res Commun* 1998;247:193–203.
358. Bektas A, Hughes JN, Warram JH, et al. Type 2 diabetes locus on 12q15. Further mapping and mutation screening of two candidate genes. *Diabetes* 2001; 50:204–208.
359. Bell GI, Xiang KS, Newman MV, et al. Gene for non-insulin-dependent diabetes mellitus (maturity-onset diabetes of the young subtype) is linked to DNA polymorphism on human chromosome 20q. *Proc Natl Acad Sci U S A* 1991;88:1484–1488.
360. Klupa T, Malecki MT, Pezzolesi M, et al. Further evidence for a susceptibility locus for type 2 diabetes on chromosome 20q13.1-q13.2. *Diabetes* 2000;49: 2212–2216.
361. Lembertas AV, Perusse L, Chagnon YC, et al. Identification of an obesity quantitative trait locus on mouse chromosome 2 and evidence of linkage to body fat and insulin on the human homologous region 20q. *J Clin Invest* 1997; 100:1240–1247.
362. Lee JH, Reed DR, Li WD, et al. Genome scan for human obesity and linkage to markers in 20q13. *Am J Hum Genet* 1999;64:196–209.
363. Elchebly M, Payette P, Michaliszyn E, et al. Increased insulin sensitivity and obesity resistance in mice lacking the protein tyrosine phosphatase-1B gene. *Science* 1999;283:1544–1548.
364. Wang L, Shao J, Muhlenkamp P, et al. Increased insulin receptor substrate-1 and enhanced skeletal muscle insulin sensitivity in mice lacking CCAAT/enhancer-binding protein beta. *J Biol Chem* 2000;275:14173–14181.
365. Knowler WC, Bennett PH, Hamman RF, et al. Diabetes incidence and prevalence in Pima Indians: a 19-fold greater incidence than in Rochester, Minnesota. *Am J Epidemiol* 1978;108:497–505.
366. Pajukanta P, Nuotio I, Terwilliger JD, et al. Linkage of familial combined hyperlipidaemia to chromosome 1q21-q23. *Nat Genet* 1998;18:369–373.
367. Wolford JK, Hanson RL, Kobes S, et al. Linkage disequilibrium between polymorphisms in the KCNJ9 gene with type 2 diabetes mellitus in Pima Indians. *Mol Genet Metab* 2001;73:97–103.
368. Weyer C, Wolford JK, Hanson RL, et al. Subcutaneous abdominal adipocyte size, a predictor of type 2 diabetes, is linked to chromosome 1q21-q23 and is associated with a common polymorphism in LMNA in Pima Indians. *Mol Genet Metab* 2001;72:231–238.
369. Pratley RE, Thompson DB, Prochazka M, et al. An autosomal genomic scan for loci linked to prediabetic phenotypes in Pima Indians. *J Clin Invest* 1998; 101:1757–1764.

CHAPTER 23
Type 1 Diabetes Mellitus

George S. Eisenbarth

FORMS OF TYPE 1 DIABETES

During the past two decades, an accumulating body of information has led to the recognition that the predominant form of insulin-dependent diabetes mellitus (IDDM) is of immune etiology, that the disease can present at any age, and that individuals are not insulin-dependent early in the course of disease (1–6). Given this body of information, an expert committee of the American Diabetes Association has divided the "idiopathic" (e.g., not pancreatitis, mitochondrial DNA mutations) forms of diabetes resulting from β-cell loss and/or severe insulin secretory deficiency into type 1A and type 1B (1). Type 1A is the immune-mediated form and is best characterized by the presence of islet autoantibodies (see below) and insulitis (7,8), with selective destruction of islet β-cells (e.g., glucagon-producing cells are spared). In addition, type 1A diabetes is strongly associated with specific human leukocyte antigen (HLA) alleles (4,9,10) and almost always progresses to severe insulin deficiency (11). The term type 1B diabetes is reserved for forms of diabetes with severe insulin deficiency without evidence of β-cell autoimmunity (1). An interesting form of potential type 1B diabetes was reported in Japan (12). The patients had lymphocytic infiltration of the exocrine pancreas (with increased serum amylase levels) and an acute development of diabetes such that, at the time of diabetes onset, levels of glycosylated hemoglobin (HbA_{1c}) were normal despite marked hyperglycemia. Japan has one of the lowest incidences of type 1A diabetes in the world, and thus type 1B forms of diabetes are likely to represent a larger proportion of their cases of childhood type 1 diabetes than that seen in other countries. In Europe and the United States, fewer than 10% of non-Hispanic white children presenting with diabetes do not have type 1A diabetes. In contrast, among African-American children and Hispanic-American children, almost one half do not have type 1A diabetes, with the majority believed to have early onset type 2 diabetes and relatively few having type 1B diabetes. In particular, a subset of African-American children can present with ketoacidosis but do not express islet autoantibodies, lack HLA alleles associated with type 1A diabetes, and often can be treated with oral hypoglycemic medications after resolution of their acute illness (13–15).

The present "etiologic" classification of diabetes is not completely satisfactory, since specific diagnostic markers are lacking for many forms of "idiopathic" diabetes (type 2 and type 1B), and some individuals with type 1A diabetes may even lack islet autoantibodies if they are tested only once at diagnosis. In addition, no combination of HLA alleles is completely diagnostic for type 1A diabetes. Only 20% to 50% of the patients with type 1A diabetes have the highest-risk HLA genotype (DR 3/4 DQ2/DQ8 heterozygous) compared with the 2.4% of individuals without diabetes who have this genotype (16). Approximately 1% of children with type 1A diabetes have highly "protective" HLA alleles (e.g., DQB1*0602) compared with 20% of the general public with these alleles. Given "biochemical" assays for islet autoantibodies with specificity set at greater than the 99th percentile, the terms *autoantibody-positive* and *antibody-negative* diabetes are perhaps more precise descriptors. Caveats for such designations include the loss of islet autoantibodies prior to the development of overt diabetes that occurs in a subset of children and the observation that individuals can have both type 1 and type 2 diabetes (17,18). Figure 23.1 illustrates first-phase insulin secretion (1+3 minute insulin on intravenous glucose tolerance testing) for a markedly obese teenager who progressed to overt diabetes. At the time of diagnosis of diabetes, the fasting insulin level was approximately 25 μU/mL, and although the sum of insulin at 1+3 minutes (50 μU/mL) was above the first percentile (of 48 μU/mL), there was essentially no glucose-stimulated insulin secretion. This child with islet autoantibodies and progressive loss of first-phase insulin secretion has both type 1A diabetes and evidence of insulin resistance (marked by high fasting levels of insulin and obesity).

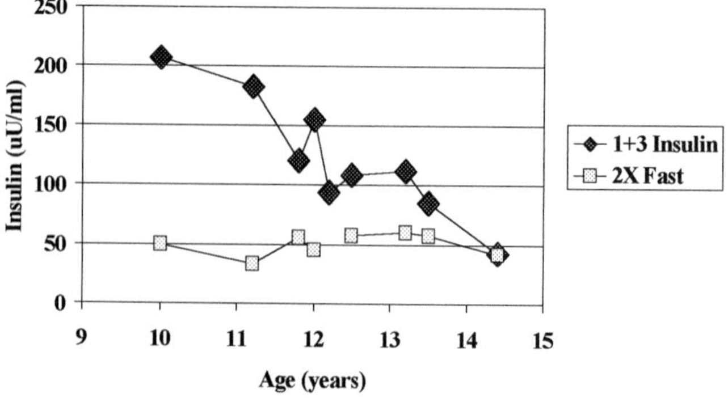

Figure 23.1. Progression to diabetes of an overweight teenager (BMI 30–35) with evidence of both type 1 and insulin resistance. Fasting insulin ranged between 17 μU/mL and 36 μU/mL during the prodrome to diabetes (normal children fasting insulin usually <5 μU/mL), suggesting insulin resistance. At time of diagnosis of diabetes, fasting insulin decreased to 21 μU/mL, and twice the fasting insulin was equivalent to the 1+3 minute insulin post-glucose, indicating no first-phase insulin response to glucose.

The category of diabetes that will expand with increased knowledge is that of "other specific forms of diabetes," which will include the subset of "immune-mediated diabetes." At present the best example of a defined form of type 1A diabetes is that in patients with diabetes as part of the autoimmune polyendocrine syndrome type 1 caused by a mutation of the *AIRE* (autoimmune regulator) gene on chromosome 21 (19) (see below).

Does the classification of diabetes matter? Most children presenting with diabetes have type 1A diabetes, and most adults have type 2 diabetes. We believe it does matter when providing prognostic information (20), information concerning likely associated disorders [e.g., autoimmune disorders for type 1A diabetes (21) and manifestations of insulin resistance for type 2 diabetes], for assessing genetic risk for relatives (22), and in providing some guidance concerning therapy [insulin versus oral medications (e.g., insulin secretagogues and insulin sensitizers)] (23). Patients with islet autoantibodies and who have diabetes are probably best treated with insulin even if they are not currently "insulin dependent (24)." Oral agents rapidly lose their efficacy in adults with type 1A diabetes.

CLINICAL RAMIFICATIONS OF AN AUTOIMMUNE DIATHESIS

In that type 1A diabetes is of immune etiology, it marks an inherited failure in the maintenance of self-tolerance. It is thus not surprising that individuals with diabetes and their relatives are at increased risk for a series of autoimmune disorders (25–28). The presence of type 1A diabetes is also a "marker" for the presence of specific HLA alleles that are associated with many immunologic disorders. The associated disorders are so prevalent among patients with type 1A diabetes, and some are so devastating when not diagnosed early, both a high index of suspicion and screening for asymptomatic disease are warranted. Four important disorders are Addison's disease (28), celiac disease (29–36), thyroid autoimmunity (37–40), and pernicious anemia (41–43). In addition, two major autoimmune polyendocrine syndromes are recognized, termed autoimmune polyendocrine syndrome type-I (APS-I) and APS-II (44).

Addison's Disease

When Addison's disease develops in a patient with type 1 diabetes, insulin requirements often decrease, with accompanying hypoglycemia. Such a decrease in insulin requirements can occur in the absence of the characteristic hyperpigmentation associated with Addison's disease. Excellent radioassays for 21-hydroxylase autoantibodies associated with Addison's disease now exist that have a sensitivity greater than 95% and a specificity exceeding 99% (28,45). Figure 23.2 illustrates the expression of 21-hydroxylase autoantibodies in patients with type 1A diabetes. We have screened more than 2,000 patients for 21-hydroxylase autoantibodies, and approximately 1 (1.5%) of 60 are positive for autoantibody. Among 30 with 21-hydroxylase autoantibodies, five had Addison's disease at initial testing. For three of the patients, the diagnosis of Addison's disease could have been made on the basis of symptoms and signs, including a severe hypotensive crisis in one (46). For one patient with apparent Addison's disease, the diagnosis was made only at age 17, but the child had missed a year of school at age 10 because of fatigue. Although the diagnosis for this child pre-

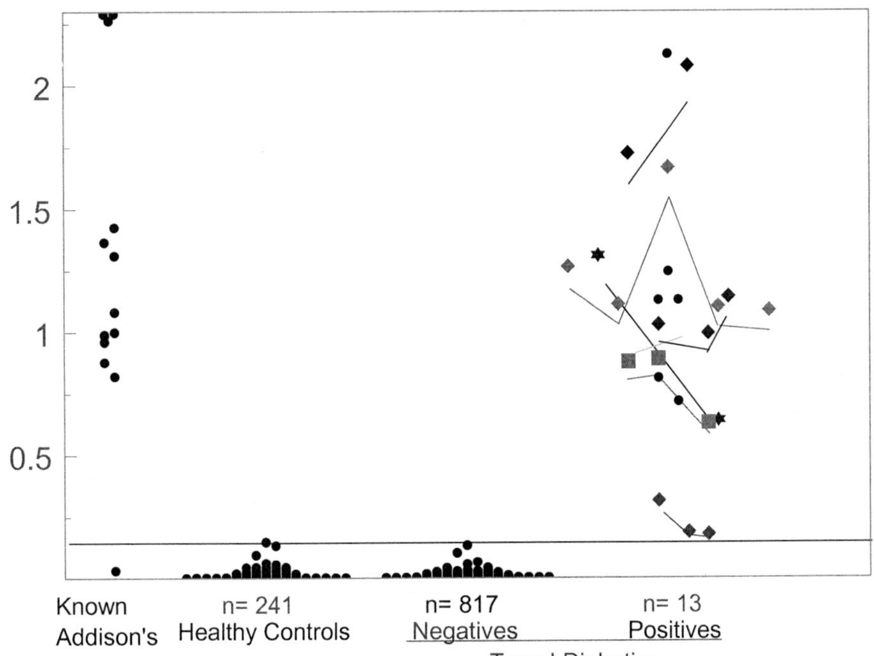

Figure 23.2. 21-Hydroxylase autoantibodies among patients with type 1A diabetes. Connected lines represent sequential measurements in the same patient. Positivity set at an index greater than all 241 healthy controls. A total of 957 patients with type 1 diabetes were included in the analysis, 15 of whom were positive. (Reprinted from Yu L, Brewer KW, Gates S, et al. DRB1*04 and DQ alleles: expression of 21-hydroxylase autoantibodies and risk of progression to Addison's disease. *J Clin Endocrinol Metab* 1999;84:328–335, with permission. Copyright 1999, The Endocrine Society.)

sumably could have been made before detection of 21-hydroxylase autoantibodies on screening, it was not. The typical clinical history for patients with Addison's disease includes years of symptoms before diagnosis.

For the remaining 25 non-Addison's patients with 21-hydroxylase autoantibodies, we annually measure adrenocorticotropic hormone and cortisol after Cortrosyn. Determined in part by their HLA alleles (highest risk with HLA genotype DR3 and DR4 with DRB1*0404, lower risk with DRB1*0401), some patients with autoantibodies are unlikely to progress to overt disease (28). Studies using immunofluorescent assays for adrenal autoantibodies (47) indicate that approximately one third to one half of those who are positive for this autoantibody are likely to progress to Addison's disease and that the risk of Addison's disease among patients with type 1 diabetes will exceed 1 per 200, in contrast to a risk in the general population of 1 per 10,000 (Table 23.1).

Celiac Disease

Celiac disease, both in the general population and in patients with type 1A diabetes, is usually asymptomatic (29,31,48). In the United States, it is likely that celiac disease is not diagnosed in more than 90% of the patients with the disease. Similar to Addison's disease and type 1 diabetes, celiac disease is associated with HLA alleles DR3 and DR4 (the DQ allele DQ2 in particular). As for Addison's disease, there now exist excellent assays for autoantibodies associated with celiac disease. The endomysial autoantigen has now been cloned and found to be the molecule tissue transglutaminase (49). Approximately one third of patients with type 1 diabetes who are DQ2 homozygous are positive for transglutaminase autoantibodies (30). Twelve percent of patients with type 1A diabetes express transglutaminase autoantibodies, and one half of these have high levels of the autoantibody.

Approximately one-half of patients with type 1 diabetes who express transglutaminase autoantibodies have celiac disease, as determined by biopsy. A higher level of transglutaminase autoantibodies correlates with findings indicative of celiac disease on an intestinal biopsy. In the general population, 0.5% of the population have celiac disease (screening for transglutaminase autoantibodies followed by intestinal biopsy). Asymptomatic patients with transglutaminase autoantibodies show evidence of metabolic abnormalities, particularly decreased growth. Osteoporosis and gastrointestinal malignancy (50) are associated with untreated symptomatic disease.

Celiac disease is a remarkable immune-mediated disorder in that an inducing environmental factor is known, namely the wheat protein gliadin (51–53). Removal of wheat from the diet results in the loss of transglutaminase autoantibodies and resolution of the intestinal lesions (54). A gluten-free diet also reduces the development of intestinal malignancies (55). There is evidence that oats need not be proscribed for patients with celiac disease (54). A wheat-restricted diet, combined with the

TABLE 23.1. Patients with Type 1 Diabetes Mellitus Screened for Autoantibodies: Examples of Associated Autoimmune Disorders in a Population of Patients with Type 1A Diabetes Mellitus

Disease	% Autoantibody-positive	% Developing disease
Addison's disease	21-Hydroxylase (1.5%) (28)	0.5% (28)
Celiac disease	Transglutaminase (12%) (30)	6% (30)
Autoimmune thyroid	Peroxidase or thyroglobulin (25%)	4%
Pernicious anemia	Parietal cell antibodies (21%)	2% (56)

dietary restrictions associated with type 1 diabetes, is a considerable burden. Nevertheless, given the high prevalence of celiac disease among patients with type 1A diabetes, we recommend screening with measurement of transglutaminase autoantibodies. Following the diagnosis of celiac disease, lifetime avoidance of wheat and other gliadin-containing proteins is recommended.

Thyroid Autoimmunity

Thyroid autoimmunity is very common among patients with type 1A diabetes. Approximately one fourth of patients with type 1A diabetes express thyroid autoantibodies. Only a subset of individuals with thyroid autoantibodies progress to overt thyroid disease (Hashimoto thyroiditis resulting in hypothyroidism or Graves disease). Thus, rather than assaying for thyroid autoantibodies, we routinely measure thyrotropin levels (approximately every 2 years with sensitive assays), allowing diagnosis of both early thyroid failure and Graves disease.

Other Autoimmune Disorders

In addition to their risk for Addison's disease, thyroid autoimmunity, and celiac disease, patients or their relatives with type 1A diabetes are at risk for a series of other autoimmune disorders. With specific autoimmune diseases (e.g., myasthenia gravis, Addison's disease, celiac disease, Graves disease), there is a reciprocal increased risk of type 1A diabetes. Anecdotal reports indicate that it is more frequent to observe type 1A diabetes in siblings of patients with multiple sclerosis than in the patients themselves. The high-risk haplotype for multiple sclerosis, DRB1*1501 and DQB1*0602, is one of the most important haplotypes protective against type 1A diabetes. Juvenile rheumatoid arthritis is a "non-organ"–specific disorder apparently also associated with type 1A diabetes. Disorders such as lupus erythematosus that are treated with glucocorticoids that induce insulin-resistant diabetes are difficult to assess for association with diabetes. Pernicious anemia occurs at an earlier average age in patients with endocrine autoimmunity, but even among patients with diabetes, pernicious anemia usually occurs in adults. A detailed study using the Belgian Diabetes Registry found pernicious anemia in approximately 10% of patients with parietal cell antibodies (38,42).

Autoimmune Polyendocrine Syndromes

Two important autoimmune syndromes are autoimmune polyendocrine syndrome type I (APS-I) (56) and autoimmune polyendocrine syndrome type II (APS-II) (27). Although APS-I is extremely rare, it is one autoimmune syndrome for which a mutation causing the disease has been defined (19,57)—a mutation of a gene termed *autoimmune regulator*, on the long arm of chromosome 21. APS-I characteristically develops in early infancy with mucocutaneous candidiasis, Addison's disease, and hypoparathyroidism. An individual may have one or all three disorders, and his or her affected siblings may have different disorders of the syndrome. These patients are also at risk for autoimmune hepatitis. Approximately 18% of patients with APS-I develop type 1 diabetes (56). It appears that more patients have anti–glutamic acid decarboxylase (GAD) autoantibodies than progress to overt diabetes, but similar to patients with standard type 1A diabetes, those with multiple autoantibodies (insulin and islet cell antibody [ICA] 512 in addition to GAD) are at high risk of progression (20).

The APS-II syndrome is characterized by two or more organ-specific autoimmune disorders, including Addison's disease, Graves disease, type 1A diabetes, and thyroiditis (27). This syndrome is strongly influenced by HLA alleles, and the majority of patients with Addison's disease have high-risk alleles DR3 and DR4 (DQ2 and DQ8), similar to patients with type 1A diabetes (21). In comparison to patients with type 1A diabetes, patients with APS-II syndrome have an excess of DRB1*0404 alleles, while most patients with type 1A diabetes have DRB1*0401, 0402, and 0405 alleles. There is a tendency for patients with APS-II syndrome with Addison's disease to develop type 1A diabetes later in life, and prediction of disease again relies on the presence of multiple islet autoantibodies. There is also a tendency for more patients with type 1A diabetes in the setting of APS-II to have "protective" or non–high-risk HLA alleles compared with the usual patient with only type 1A diabetes. At present, the genes outside of the HLA region that underlie risk of APS-II have not been identified, although some studies of type IA diabetes have reported an association of Addison's disease and Graves disease with polymorphisms of the genes *CTLA-4* (58–61) and *MIC-A* (62,63).

The XPID syndrome (*X*-linked syndrome of *p*olyendocrinopathy, *i*mmune dysfunction and *d*iarrhea) (64–67) was mapped to the X chromosome and results from mutations of the Foxp3 gene. This rare syndrome with overwhelming immunologic abnormalities results in type 1 diabetes, enteropathy with villous atrophy, chronic dermatitis, variable immunodeficiency, and death in infancy. The diabetes often presents in neonates. Mice with the *scurfy* mutation develop lymphoproliferative disease, increased cytokine release, and wasting potentially associated with high levels of tumor necrosis factor-α. Similar to the etiologic gene *AIRE* for the APS-I syndrome, the *scurfy* gene is thought to be a transcription factor. The specific genes whose abnormal regulation results in this spectrum of illnesses are unknown, but it is now known that the Foxp3 gene is essential for the generation of CD4+ CD25+ regulatory T cells.

STAGES IN THE DEVELOPMENT OF TYPE 1A DIABETES MELLITUS

Type 1A diabetes can develop at any age. For example, Cilio and colleagues have described a child with fulminant autoimmunity and diabetes presenting at birth and we have followed the mother of a child with diabetes who developed type 1A diabetes at age 69 (67). Given this wide spectrum of age at diagnosis, long-term prospective studies are necessary to define the course of the disease. Such studies have benefited from the discovery of islet autoantibodies (68) and from the realization that type 1A diabetes is a chronic autoimmune disorder (69). We divide the development of type 1A diabetes into a series of stages beginning with genetic susceptibility (Fig. 23.3) and ending with complete or nearly complete β-cell destruction associated with a lack of C-peptide secretion. Studies of monozygotic twins illustrate many of the stages associated with type 1A diabetes. In that monozygotic twins are identical for all germline–encoded polymorphisms and mutations, if diabetes develops in one twin of a pair, the other twin is at high risk of developing diabetes (70,71). However, because diabetes does not develop in all such twins or activate autoimmunity (as evidenced by a lack of islet autoantibodies) (72), a subset of genetically susceptible individuals do not progress beyond stage I.

Factors that induce the expression of islet autoantibodies are currently poorly defined. The great majority of individuals expressing islet autoantibodies that react with multiple islet antigens progress to loss of first-phase insulin secretion on intravenous glucose tolerance testing and eventually to overt diabetes (73,74). Islet autoantibodies can appear during the first year of life but also can first develop in adults. Figure 23.4 illus-

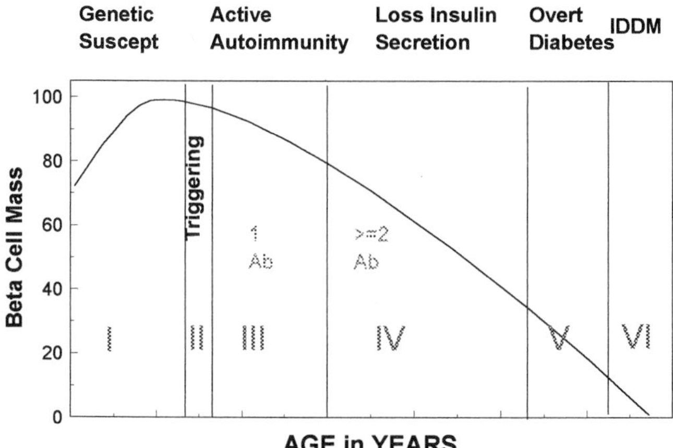

Figure 23.3. Stages in the development of type 1A diabetes. (Modified from Eisenbarth GS. Type I diabetes mellitus. A chronic autoimmune disease. *N Engl J Med* 1986;314:1360–1368, with permission. Copyright © 1986, Massachusetts Medical Society. All rights reserved.)

trates the course of an identical twin whose islet autoantibodies were first detected at age 42 at the time of diagnosis of diabetes, even though his twin mate developed diabetes at age 12. A subset of individuals who express islet autoantibodies are found not to progress to diabetes with long-term follow-up. These individuals usually express a single islet autoantibody, such as antibodies that react only with the molecule GAD (75,76). Progressive loss of first-phase insulin secretion characteristically precedes the development of hyperglycemia (77–79).

The detection of progressive loss of first-phase insulin secretion in the presence of islet autoantibodies led to the hypothesis that type 1A diabetes is a "chronic" autoimmune disorder (69). In that data concerning the prediabetic pancreas are limited, chronic progressive islet destruction remains a hypothesis. An alternative hypothesis is that chronic loss of first-phase insulin secretion results from functional inhibition of insulin secretion by the immune system and that the actual destruction of pancreatic β-cells is acute and follows a long latency period during which islet autoantibodies are expressed (80,81). We believe this is unlikely, given the available histologic data and the observation that loss of β-cell mass correlates with loss of first-phase insulin secretion (82). In particular, the pancreases of identical twins of patients with type 1A diabetes, when biopsied (on the occasion of living related donor transplantation), appear normal (83). Pancreases from individuals who have died at the

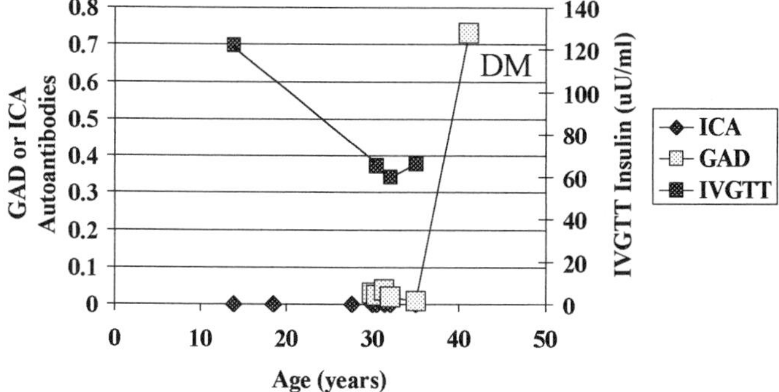

Figure 23.4. Late appearance of anti-islet autoantibodies in an initially discordant monozygotic twin of a patient with type 1A diabetes. IVGTT, intravenous glucose tolerance test; ICA, islet cytoplasmic antibodies; GAD, antibodies to glutamic acid decarboxylase.

onset of diabetes often have lost most β-cells but still have a significant mass of islet β-cells remaining (84). Several years after the onset of diabetes, as reflected by loss of C-peptide secretion, this remaining β-cell mass is lost. It thus appears that the chronic destruction that precedes type 1A diabetes continues after the development of hyperglycemia.

The histology of the pancreas in individuals at the onset of diabetes shows a diversity of islet lesions. Within islets, β-cells are selectively destroyed (84). This specificity of β-cell destruction is very dramatic, and for islets containing no β-cells, there is no insulitis. Thus, the same section of the pancreas may contain normal islets, islets with β-cells and insulitis, and islets lacking all β-cells and without insulitis (pseudoatrophic islets). This spotty process is conceptually similar to vitiligo, with destruction of patches of melanocytes. This destruction of β-cells of individual islets probably underlies the chronic progression to type 1A diabetes.

GENETICS OF TYPE 1A DIABETES MELLITUS

Familial Aggregation

The great majority of individuals in whom type 1A diabetes develops do not have a first-degree relative with the disorder (85% to 90%). If one has a first-degree relative with type 1A diabetes, the risk of diabetes is, however, much greater than that for the general population. In the United States, type 1A diabetes develops in approximately 1 in 300 individuals, compared with 1 in 20 first-degree relatives (85). The risk of diabetes in relatives can be stratified according to their relationship to the proband and by laboratory testing (e.g., HLA typing and determination of autoantibody expression).

Monozygotic twins of a patient with type 1A diabetes have an overall risk of developing type 1A diabetes of approximately 50% (72,86–89). This overall concordance for monozygotic twins is likely to be a composite of a number of different genetic syndromes resulting in type 1A diabetes, each syndrome potentially with a different concordance. In that only some of the genes contributing to the development of type 1A diabetes are currently known, concordance rates for specific genetic syndromes cannot be calculated accurately.

We have analyzed the development of diabetes in two large series of monozygotic twins, one from the United States (72) and the other from Great Britain (90). All twins in the study were selected to be discordant at the time of initial study. Both diabetes concordance and expression of islet autoantibodies were studied. Over time, diabetes develops in more twins. There is no duration of discordance at which the risk of diabetes disappears. Approximately 20% of those twins who became concordant did so after 15 years of discordance (91). With statistical methods to correct for pairs of twins who were both concordant at initial study and for discordant twins still being observed, the overall concordance is 50%. There is a marked difference in the hazard rate of progression to diabetes related to the age of the proband at diabetes onset (92). If the index twin (first diabetic twin) developed type 1A diabetes after age 20, concordance was less than 5%, compared with a concordance greater than 50% if the index twin developed diabetes before age 20. If the first twin developed type 1A diabetes before the age of 10, almost 5% of discordant twins per year developed diabetes in the first years of discordance, and the rate decreased to 1% per year only by 20 years of follow-up. In contrast, if diabetes developed in the first twin after age 20, the initial hazard rate was low and remained at approximately 1% per year for the duration of follow-up. These differences in concordance and hazard rates may reflect differences in genetic forms of type 1A diabetes for groups of twins subdivided by the age of the proband twin at diagnosis of diabetes.

Discordant dizygotic twins have a diabetes risk that is similar to that of non-twin siblings of patients with diabetes: approximately 6% (72). The difference between monozygotic and dizygotic twins most likely represents a difference in the inherited genes shared with the proband (100% for monozygotic twins; mean of 50% for dizygotic twins). There is one report that dizygotic twins have a very high prevalence of islet autoantibodies (87), but with reanalysis and exchange of sera, the high prevalence of islet autoantibodies was not confirmed. Dizygotic twins do not have increased expression of islet autoantibodies compared with that in their siblings (72), and when monozygotic twins express islet autoantibodies, they usually progress to overt diabetes (72,92).

Offspring of a father and siblings of patients with type 1A diabetes have a similar risk of type 1A diabetes, while offspring of a mother with type 1A diabetes have a somewhat decreased risk (93). The difference in risk between offspring of mothers versus fathers with type 1A diabetes has not yet been explained. Preliminary data from the Diabetes Autoimmunity Study in the Young (DAISY) (94) suggest that offspring of fathers with type 1 diabetes more often are DQ8/DQ2 heterozygous than are offspring of mothers with type 1 diabetes. This may contribute to a slightly higher diabetes risk (Table 23.2).

As will be discussed, the ratio of the overall risk of diabetes of a sibling of a patient with type 1 diabetes is 6% and the general population risk is 0.4%, giving a sibling familial aggregation ratio, λ–s of 15 (6/0.4) (10). This number provides some estimate of the influence of being a sibling in terms of familial (shared genetic and sibling environmental background) risk of developing type 1A diabetes. For genetic disorders, a λ–s of 15 is a moderate association. The most important locus for type 1A diabetes is the HLA region of chromosome 6. Polymorphisms 5′ of the insulin gene also contribute to the familial aggregation. A major portion of the genetic risk of type 1 diabetes cannot currently be assigned to specific genes (10,95,96).

The Major Histocompatibility Complex

The most important determinants of type 1A diabetes are genes within the major histocompatibility complex (MHC) on chromosome 6p21 (33,97). The MHC is approximately 4 million base pairs long with more than 200 known or predicted transcripts (5). The region is divided into class I [containing the classical histocompatibility antigens HLA (human leukocyte antigens) A, B, and C], class II (containing immune response genes, HLA-DP, -DQ, and -DR), and the class III region with genes of the complement cascade, as well as other genes influencing immune function. There are also other genes within this complex not related to immune function, such as the gene for 21-hydroxylase, an enzyme of adrenal steroidogenesis, and the gene determining hemochromatosis telomeric to the MHC.

HLA-DQ, -DR, -A, -B, and -C molecules are extremely polymorphic, with hundreds of different alleles (e.g., as of January 2000, 241 alleles for DRB1 had been identified) (98). An individual inherits one allele of each gene from each parent. The series of alleles on a given chromosome inherited from a parent are termed a haplotype. By typing alleles of multiple family members, one can determine the four haplotypes of a nuclear family (two haplotypes for each parent). Alleles of different genes in a population are often not randomly associated with each other on the same chromosome; it is then stated that the alleles are in linkage dysequilibrium. For example, the class I HLA alleles A1 and B8 and the class II alleles DR3 and DQ2 (DQ2=DQA1*0501, DQB1*0201) are commonly associated with each other on chromosomes (99–101). The term *linkage dysequilibrium* implies that not enough evolutionary time has elapsed for these allelic associations to be randomized by crossing-over events between alleles. This "DR3" haplotype that encodes a high risk for diabetes has been termed an ancestral or extended haplotype (102, 103). Because all of these alleles, as well as alleles of other genes within this extended haplotype, are inherited as a unit, the specific combination of alleles determining diabetes risk is difficult to pinpoint. Other HLA haplotypes do not show as extensive linkage dysequilibrium, and the primary importance of DQ and DR alleles to diabetes risk is apparent.

The nomenclature for HLA alleles has changed almost with each modern edition of the Joslin text but is unlikely to change again because it is now based on variants of nucleotide sequence of the HLA genes rather than serologic typing (98). For DQ molecules, both the α and β chain of the molecule are polymorphic; thus to specify a DQ molecule, one must specify both chains (e.g., DQA1*0501, DQB1*0201). In contrast, for DR molecules, the DR α chain is not polymorphic and only the DR β chain is specified (DRB1*0301). If a chain has a "silent" nucleotide polymorphism (amino acid sequence not changed), a fifth digit is added (e.g., DRB1*03011). The nucleotide sequences are typically determined with direct sequencing and computer analysis. With automated sequencers and polymerase chain reaction amplification of DNA, direct sequencing is relatively simple. The direct sequencing of two alleles (one for each chromosome) of an individual can result in a small amount of ambiguity for certain combinations of alleles. This is usually not a problem, and the sequences provide

TABLE 23.2. Approximate Frequency of Islet Autoantibodies (Ab+) and Development of Diabetes Mellitus for Initially Nondiabetic Relatives

Relationship	% DM	% Ab+ (GAD, 512, or insulin)	Comment
Monozygotic twin	50%	50%	Almost all Ab+ progress to DM
Dizygotic twin	6%	10%	Risk similar to sibling
Sibling	3.2%[a]	7.4%	—
Offspring father	4.6%	6.5%	Diabetes risk greater than offspring of diabetic mother
Offspring mother	3%	5%	Lower risk relative to offspring of diabetic father
Parent	1%	4.1%	Many parents with single Ab+
DR3/4,DQ8 sibling	>25%	>50%	Highest risk for non-twin relative

[a]Lifetime diabetes risk is approximately 6% for siblings followed from birth. The difference in the percentage of dizygotic twins and siblings with diabetes mellitus is within the error of the estimates.

TABLE 23.3. Risk of Type 1A Diabetes Mellitus Associated with DR and DQ Haplotypes

Risk	DRB1	DQA1	DQB1
High	0401, 0402, 0405	0301	0302 (DQ8)
	0301	0501	0201 (DQ2)
Moderate	0801	0401	0402
	0404	0301	0302 (DQ8)
	0101	0101	0501
	0901	0301	0303
Weak or moderate protection	0401	0301	0301
	0403	0301	0302 (DQ8)
	0701	0201	0201
	1101	0501	0301
Strong protection	1501	0102	0602 (DQ6)
	1401	0101	0503
	0701	0201	0303

much more information concerning exact alleles compared with that obtained with older methods of typing for HLA alleles.

One can define HLA disease associations with individual alleles of single genes (e.g., alleles of DQB or DRB), with haplotypes (e.g., alleles of HLA-A, -B, -DQ, -DR on a single chromosome), and with genotypes (alleles of both chromosome 6 haplotypes possessed by an individual). In a physiologic sense, genotypes contribute to diabetes risk (104–108). With so many different alleles, and different haplotypes, there are millions of theoretical genotypes. In practice, the genotypes associated with type 1A diabetes risk or protection are relatively limited, and specifying genotypes for DQ (DQA and DQB) and DRB alleles provides the great bulk of relevant information (Table 23.3). The disease associations of genotypes can be complex. For instance, DQA chains coded for by one haplotype can combine with DQB chains of the other haplotype and influence diabetes risk. DQB1*0301 is in linkage dysequilibrium with DR4 but is not a high-risk allele (and is relatively protective). Thus, most white patients with type 1A diabetes have the DQB1*0302 allele on their DR4 haplotypes and not DQB1*0301 (109). The DQB1*0301 appears to be protective primarily in patients who also have a DR3 haplotype (with DQA1*0501, DQB1*0201) on their other chromosome. However, in combination with other haplotypes, such as the DR1(DQA1*0101, DQB1*0501), DQB1*0301 increases diabetes risk (110–112).

The prevalence of given genotypes (and haplotypes) varies among populations, but given the same DQ and DR genotypes, the influence of HLA on type 1A diabetes is similar for populations throughout the world (113). Thus, even in populations with a very low incidence of type 1A diabetes (e.g., Korea and Japan), when similar genotypes are present, they confer increased or decreased risk of diabetes. Investigators have attempted to encapsulate the HLA-DQ risk by reference to several specific amino acids. The most common rule is that aspartic acid at position 57 of the DQB is protective and that arginine at DQA 52 is associated with increased diabetes risk, but there are many exceptions (114). Figure 23.5 illustrates the transmission of a series of DQB alleles from parents to children with type 1A diabetes (115). The transmission test corrects for differences in the prevalence of alleles in the population, as transmissions are counted only from parents heterozygous for the specific allele (115,116). If DQ alleles did not influence diabetes risk, all alleles would be transmitted 50% of the time to children with diabetes. As is apparent from the figure, there is a tremendous spectrum of transmission frequencies for different alleles, and a similar spectrum is documented by studies of large populations (117). The rules concerning aspartic acid at position 57 provide little predictive power. For instance DQB1*0402 is one of the alleles with the highest transmission frequency, DQB1*0301 is intermediate, and DQB1*0602 is one of the most protective alleles. All have aspartic acid at position 57 of their DQB chain. Since we currently can define all of the polymorphisms of these chains, knowledge of the complete sequence rather than of single amino acid polymorphism is preferred for assessing diabetes risk.

HLA-associated protection from type 1A diabetes is dominant relative to susceptibility (108,118). The three most protective molecules are DQA1*0102 with DQB1*0602, DQA1*0201 with DQB1*0303, and DRB1*1401. The latter two molecules are relatively rare, whereas in most populations, more than 20% of individuals have DQA1*0102, DQB1*0602 and fewer than 2% of children with type 1A diabetes have this allele. Note that both DQ and DR alleles can protect against the development of type 1A diabetes; this observation is similar to findings in animal models, in which alleles of the equivalent genes (I-A, DQ; and I-E, DR) both can provide protection (119,120). Transmission of haplotypes from parents to affected offspring was analyzed for the Norwegian NODIAB study (116) and the HBDI (Human Biologic Disease Interchange) repository (121). This allowed analysis of rare "recombinant" haplotypes such as DRB1*0101 or 1404 with DQA1*0101, DQB1*0503 in comparison to the usual DRB1*1401, DQA1*0101, DQB1*0503 haplotype (Table

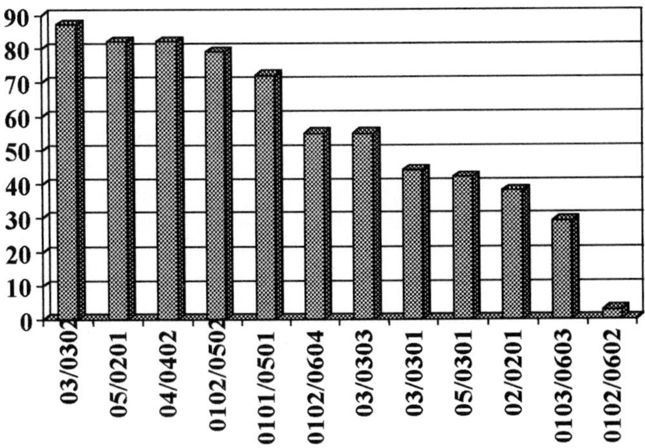

Figure 23.5. Percent transmission of DQA1/B1 alleles from parents heterozygous for the indicated allele to affected children. The first number refers to DQα and the second to DQβ. (Copyright © 1998 American Diabetes Association. From Kawasaki E, Noble J, Erlich H, et al. Transmission of DQ haplotypes to patients with type 1 diabetes. *Diabetes* 1998; 47:1971–1973. Reprinted with permission from the American Diabetes Association.)

TABLE 23.4. Evidence that DQB1*0602 and DRB1*1401 Haplotypes Are Protective (Transmission of Haplotypes from Parent to Affected Child)

Parental haplotype	DRB1*1501/*DQB1*0602*	DRB1***X**/*DQB1*0602*	DRB1*1501/DQB1***X**
Transmission to diabetic child	2/313 (0.6%)	0/6 (0%)	5/11 (46%)
Parental haplotype	*DRB1*1401*/DQB1*0503	DRB1***Y**/DQB1*0503	*DRB1* 1401*/DQB1***Y**
Transmission to diabetic child	0/40 (0.0%)	2/4 (50%)	No parents with such a haplotype

X, allele not DQB1*0602 or DRB1*1501; **Y**, allele not DRB1*1401 or DQB1*0503.

23.4). The DRB1*1401 allele was transmitted to none of 40 diabetic offspring, whereas DQB1*0503 without DRB1*1401 was transmitted to 2 of 4 diabetic offspring. In this case, DRB1*1401 apparently determines protection. DQB1*0602 was transmitted to 0 of 6 diabetic offspring for haplotypes without DRB1*1501; transmission of DQB1*0602 with DRB1*1501 was also rare (2 of 313). In contrast, DRB1*1501 without DQB1*0602 was transmitted to 5 of 11 diabetic offspring. For this haplotype, DQB1*0602 apparently provides protection (Table 23.4).

To date we have found 13 (1.5%) of 877 individuals with type 1A diabetes (as evidenced by positivity for islet autoantibody and the presence of diabetes) with DQB1*0602. Their DQB sequence did not differ from the standard sequence (97,118). One patient had the APS-I syndrome, although overall it is likely that, in patients with APS-1, DQB1*0602 is also protective for diabetes but not for Addison's disease (26,56). Another child had high levels of 21-hydroxylase autoantibodies, often associated with polyendocrine autoimmunity. Thus, we suspect that some individuals with DQB1*0602 and type 1A diabetes are likely to have variant genetic forms of type 1A diabetes. Among the patients with DQB1*0602, the other allele is usually a high-risk HLA allele [10 (77%) of 13 DQ8 or DQ2]. Two of the three patients lacking DQ8 and DQ2 had DQB1*0402 (n = 2). Analysis of islet autoantibody–positive relatives of Diabetes Prevention Trial Type-1, for which the presence of DQB1*0602 is an exclusion criteria, indicates that 7% of cytoplasmic islet cell antibody (ICA)–positive relatives are positive for DQB1*0602 (122). There was an increased prevalence of DQB1*0602 among African-American ICA-positive relatives, again suggesting genetic heterogeneity (122).

The highest risk genotype for type 1A diabetes consists of DRB1*0301/DQA1*0501, DQB1*0201 (DQ2) with DRB1*0401 (or 0402, or 0405)/DQA1*0301, DQB1*0302 (DQ8) (9). This genotype occurs in approximately 2.4% of newborns in Denver, Colorado, and in approximately 40% of children with type 1A diabetes (16). A newborn with this genotype without a relative with type 1A diabetes is estimated to have a risk of diabetes of approximately 6%. In contrast, a sibling of a patient with type 1A diabetes with the same genotype has a risk of developing diabetes that is greater than 25%. We believe the greatly enhanced risk for a relative relates both to non-MHC genes inherited by such relatives and to other HLA alleles associated with increased diabetes risk. A number of other HLA genotypes are associated with high to moderate risk for type 1A diabetes, including DR 4/4, DQ 8/8 (DQ8 = DQA1*0301, DQB1*0302); DR 3/3, DQ 2/2 (DQ2 = DQA1*0501, DQB1*0201); DR 1/4, DQ 1/8; DR 1/4, DQ 1/7 (DQ7 = DQA1*0301, DQB1*0301). The DRB1 allele DRB1*0403 modifies the risk of diabetes associated with DQA1*0301, DQB1*0302 (DQ8) such that the haplotype DRB1*0403, DQA1*0301, DQB1*0302 is slightly protective (105, 123).

Genotypes consisting of both DR and DQ alleles appear to underlie the bulk of MHC-associated susceptibility. Nevertheless, there are likely to be alleles of other genes within the MHC contributing to susceptibility to diabetes. Class I alleles that present peptides to cytotoxic CD8 T lymphocytes are likely to influence disease risk or the age of development of type 1A diabetes. The allele A24 is reported to be associated with a younger age of onset of type 1A diabetes, and there is evidence that HLA-A2 influences diabetes risk (124). Alleles of the nontypical HLA allele, termed MIC-A, have been reported to be associated both with type 1A diabetes and with Addison's disease (63). Alleles of several microsatellite markers (repeat elements) that simply mark chromosomal regions are reported to be associated with diabetes risk and subdivide haplotypes with fixed DR and DQ alleles. Such analyses are particularly difficult because of the extensive linkage dysequilibrium of alleles of genes within the MHC and the importance of class II alleles (DR and DQ, as well as influence of DP) (125,126).

The Insulin Gene

Another locus clearly associated with risk for type 1A diabetes is the insulin gene locus (127–129). Alleles of a variable nucleotide tandem repeat 5′ of the insulin gene influence the risk of type 1A diabetes. This tandem repeat has been divided into three major sizes, and the longest tandem repeats are associated with decreased risk of type 1A diabetes. The longer tandem-repeat group is also associated with increased expression of insulin messenger RNA within the thymus (130,131). In animal models, expression of minute amounts of insulin message within the thymus correlates with protection from diabetes and insulitis (132,133). An attractive hypothesis is that insulin is a key molecular target and that greater thymic expression of insulin leads to tolerance and thus decreased risk of diabetes.

Oligogenic versus Polygenic Inheritance

Genes within the MHC and the insulin locus account for approximately 50% of the familial aggregation of type 1A diabetes. The remaining familial aggregation is probably due to additional inherited polymorphisms/mutations, and the lack of 100% concordance of identical twins could be due to somatic mutation, random rearrangement of genes (e.g., rearrangements in the T-cell receptor), differences in environmental exposures, or stochastic events. We believe that non-MHC genetic loci are of major importance. For one of the best animal models of type 1A diabetes, the NOD mouse, the inheritance is polygenic, with more than 15 different genetic loci influencing susceptibility to diabetes (134–136).

Diabetes in the NOD mouse is a potential example of a single form of human type 1A diabetes. This is not strictly accurate, in that NOD mice are brother-sister mated for more than 20 generations (inbred) and thus have no genetic variability. NOD mice are not diallelic at any locus. Humans have different alleles at more than 100,000 loci, many within coding regions of

TABLE 23.5. Confirmed and Putative Loci Associated with Type 1A Diabetes Mellitus

Locus	Chromosome	Marker	Comment
IDDM1	6p21.31	HLA	50% of the familial aggregation
IDDM2	11p15.5	5′ Insulin	Influence on thymic insulin expression
IDDM3	15q26	D15S107	—
IDDM4	11q13	FGF3	—
IDDM5	6q25	ESR	—
IDDM6	18q21	D18S64	—
IDDM7	2q31–31	D2S152	—
IDDM8	6q27	D6S1590	—
IDDM9	3q21	D3S1303	—
IDDM10	10p11–q11	D10S193	—
IDDM11	14q4.3–14q31	—	—
IDDM12	2q33	CTLA-4	CTLA-4 candidate
IDDM13	2q34	D2S164	—
IDDM14	6q21	—	"Confirmed" locus besides IDDM1 and IDDM2
IDDM15	10q25.1	D10S1681	Oligogenic inheritance

genes. The inbred nature of the NOD mouse may relate to the ease with which multiple small genetic changes, as well as therapeutic interventions, prevent diabetes (135). Such ease of prevention is less likely in humans. Other animal models do not show a polygenic form of inheritance but show an "oligogenic" inheritance, with a few major loci (including the histocompatibility complex) determining diabetes risk (137,138).

Whether human type 1A diabetes is polygenic or oligogenic is currently debated. Practical ramifications of the mode of inheritance are likely to relate to the ease of defining genes underlying susceptibility, identifying at-risk individuals, and discovering pathways for prevention of diabetes. We favor the hypothesis that type 1A diabetes is oligogenic but heterogeneous (139). Namely, in most families, one to three loci determine diabetes susceptibility but different families have different major "diabetogenes." The bulk of the effort to define diabetogenic loci has involved the study of hundreds of families with two siblings (sib pairs) with type 1A diabetes. These studies have implicated more than 15 loci associated with diabetes risk but have been difficult to replicate (96). For example, several studies have suggested that a polymorphism of CTLA-4 may contribute to diabetes risk in certain populations but not in others (Table 23.5) (140–145). A missense mutation of the LYP gene (PTPN22; lymphocyte tyrosine phosphatase) is a major "autoimmune" allele (Arg620Trp) and has an odds ratio of approximately 1.7 for type 1 diabetes (145a).

If type 1A diabetes is heterogeneous and if no specific genetic syndrome accounts for more than 20% of cases of type 1A diabetes, one may need to define relevant genes by studying specific families before application to mixed populations. We have studied a Bedouin Arab family from Israel that has 21 members with type 1A diabetes. In this family, diabetes is associated with typical HLA alleles and with a locus on chromosome 10, currently termed IDDM17 (139). Individuals homozygous for related 10q25.1 haplotypes and with DR3 have a 40% risk of developing type 1A diabetes. In contrast, relatives lacking DR3 or who are not homozygous have a risk of type 1A diabetes lower than 2%. This suggests that a major diabetogene on chromosome 10 is segregating with diabetes and that diabetes develops from a combination of this locus and high-risk HLA alleles.

None of the putative non-MHC loci except for LYP and the insulin gene contribute to the assessment of risk for type 1A diabetes, and it is likely that genes, rather than loci, will need to be defined before such studies will be of major influence. The Genome Project should greatly facilitate studies to identify these genes, and it is now possible to create detailed maps of any region of the human genome and, thus, to analyze transmission and linkage dys-equilibrium for specific haplotypes.

ENVIRONMENTAL FACTORS

A number of potential environmental causes of type 1 diabetes have been reported, but few have been established beyond doubt. However, there are examples of autoimmune diseases that not only are caused by environmental factors but also can be prevented or treated through avoidance of these factors (e.g., celiac disease). These diseases occur only through a strong interaction between environmental factors and specific alleles of mainly HLA genes, suggesting the futility of defining "genetic" versus "environmental" etiology.

Celiac disease, discussed earlier in this chapter, is induced by ingestion of wheat protein gliadin (146–148) in a person with DQ2 or DQ8 haplotypes. Removal of wheat from the diet results in the loss of transglutaminase autoantibodies and resolution of the intestinal lesions (149). There is some evidence that the delayed introduction of wheat into infant feeding in recent years has prevented a substantial number of symptomatic cases, although some of such prevented cases may manifest with milder symptoms later in life. Rheumatic fever, another autoimmune disease, is induced by streptococcal infection of a host with an HLA-DR4 genetic background. It has been nearly eradicated in many countries with the introduction of antibiotics and guidelines for diagnosis and treatment of streptococcal infections.

Diabetes in patients with congenital rubella syndrome is perhaps the only form of type 1A diabetes proven to be caused by a viral infection (150–152). Non-congenital rubella infection does not appear to be associated with diabetes risk. At present it is not clear whether congenital rubella is associated with endocrine autoimmunity caused by direct infection of target tissues, the triggering of autoimmunity (153), or the induction of changes in the immune system that lead to autoimmunity (154). Although only a small proportion of cases of type 1A diabetes have been found to be caused by congenital rubella infection, this is the only type of autoimmune diabetes that we currently can prevent (using live attenuated rubella vaccine, a component of the MMR vaccine).

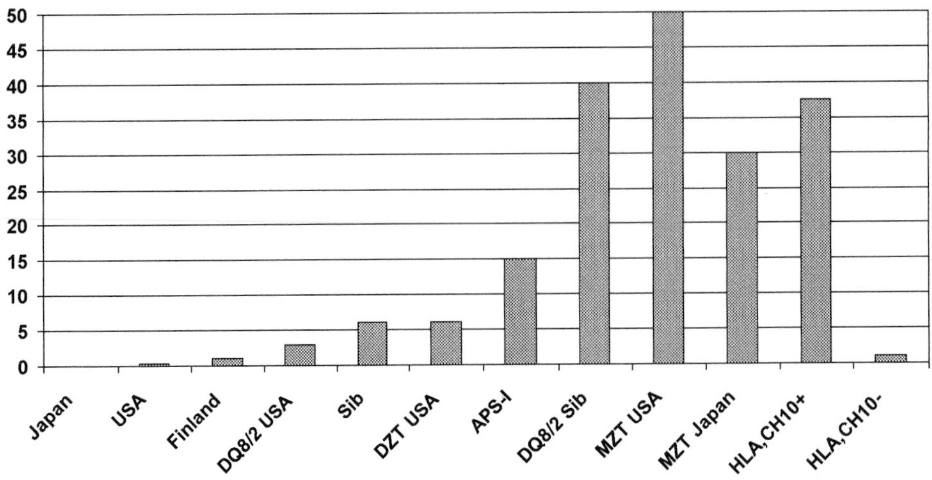

Figure 23.6. Prevalence of type 1A diabetes: geographic and genetic variation. DZT, dizygotic twin; MZT, monozygotic twin; HLA,Ch10+, patient from a Bedouin Arab family with HLA DR3 and homozygous for IDDM17 diabetes-associated haplotypes (Japan, 0.02%; USA, 0.3%; Finland, 1%).

Figure 23.6 contrasts prevalence of type 1A diabetes for a series of countries with dramatic differences in its incidence and compares such diabetes prevalence to diabetes risk, taking into account genetic information. The incidence of type 1A diabetes varies geographically by more than 45-fold (e.g., in Japan the approximate incidence is 1 in 100,000 compared with Finland, where it is 45 in 100,000) (155–159). Nevertheless, even the highest-risk Scandinavian countries have a prevalence of type 1A diabetes less than 3%, while an identical twin of a patient with type 1A diabetes from Japan has a diabetes concordance of approximately 30% (88).

A sibling or offspring of a patient with type 1A diabetes with HLA DQ8/DQ2 has a diabetes risk of approximately 20% to 40% (17,160), and an individual with this genotype from the general U.S. population has a risk of approximately 6%. In addition, a dizygotic twin of a patient with type 1A diabetes has a risk of diabetes very similar to that of a sibling (72). This suggests that, if there are environmental factors triggering the development of type 1A diabetes, they account for a relatively small amount of the familial aggregation of the disease. This may explain the difficulty finding such environmental factors. One exception previously discussed is the rare congenital rubella syndrome that is strongly associated with the development of thyroiditis and type 1A diabetes (161–163) and recent reports from two studies that introduction of cereal before 3 months of age increases risk (160a,160b).

TRIGGERING OF AUTOIMMUNITY

The most prominent proposed environmental triggers for type 1A diabetes are infections (particularly viruses), vaccination, and dietary factors (163). There is lack of clear consensus concerning the etiologic role of any of these factors. For both the NOD mouse and the BB rat, the development of diabetes is enhanced when animals are raised in a germ-free environment (164). This suggests that, for both of these animal models, infections are not necessary for the development of diabetes. In fact, when either animal becomes infected with relatively common viruses, the development of diabetes decreases. The BB rat has a severe T-cell lymphopenia inherited in an autosomal recessive manner (165–169). For strains of BB rats termed DR (diabetes resistant) that lack the T-cell lymphopenia locus, diabetes can be induced with a number of immunostimulatory maneuvers, including infection with the rat Kilham virus or with induction of the expression of interferon-α with injection of poly-IC (polyinosinic-polycytidylic acid, a synthetic double-stranded RNA) (170). Of note, administration of poly-IC induces diabetes and insulitis or just insulitis in a broad range of rat strains with "HLA" class II U alleles (diabetes and insulitis strains: lew1.WR1, PVG.RT1^u, PVG.R8, WF, and WAG; only insulitis-LOU strain). In animal models, several forms of "vaccination" prevent diabetes (e.g., BCG vaccination for NOD mice), and dietary modification, usually with removal of complex proteins from the diet, decreases the development of diabetes (171–173). Thus, such manipulations are potential triggers of autoimmunity or may provide therapies (e.g., removal of triggering factors) of relevance to diabetes prevention.

HUMAN DIABETES

Viruses

Viral infections may initiate autoimmunity or precipitate diabetes in subjects with autoimmunity. Cytoplasmic ICA or insulin autoantibodies have been detected after mumps (174), rubella, measles, chickenpox (175), Coxsackie virus (176), and ECHO-4 virus (177) infections, but most reported studies have used assays of questionable specificity—not the current fluid-phase GAD65 and ICA512 (IA-2) autoantibody assays. Fetuses and newborns may be particularly at risk because of their propensity to develop persistent infection, as shown by the example of congenital rubella infection (162).

Congenital rubella infection is clearly associated with the development of type 1A diabetes and is associated with the development of a series of autoimmune disorders (especially autoimmune thyroid disease). Diabetes occurs in individuals with high-risk HLA alleles and occurs years after the rubella infection (178). Other congenital infections, particularly enteroviral infections (179), have been reported to be associated with type 1A diabetes.

Both β-cell autoimmunity (180) and diabetes (181) may be caused by enteroviral infections, perhaps acquired in utero (180,182). A molecular mimicry between the P2-C protein of Coxsackie virus and the GAD protein (183) could have a role.

Presence of antibodies to enteroviruses in persons with autoimmunity does not, however, prove a causal relationship. People with autoimmunity may be more prone to enteroviral infection, may have a stronger humoral response to infection because of their particular HLA genotypes, or may be in a nonspecific hyperimmune state marked by elevation in levels of antibody to a variety of exogenous antigens (184). However, if the enteroviral infections are indeed associated with triggering of both autoimmunity *and* diabetes, one of the following mechanisms could operate: (a) enteroviral infections may act in a manner similar to poly-IC (mimic of double-stranded RNA) that induces diabetes in MHC-susceptible rat strains (170); (b) several distinct infections may be necessary, the first, early in ontogenesis, leads to a low-grade persistent infection while the subsequent infections with a similar virus initiate and sustain autoimmunity until the final "hit" results in β-cell loss sufficient to cause diabetes (185,186); (c) enteroviral infection does not trigger autoimmunity, but recurrent acute lytic infections of β-cells promote β-cell loss and diabetes in persons with autoimmunity; (d) persistent enteroviral infection of β-cells impairs insulin secretion without cell lysis and promotes diabetes in persons with autoimmunity; or (e) an acute or chronic enteroviral infection of peri-insular tissue leads to β-cell destruction from abundance of free radicals—the "innocent bystander theory." These hypotheses are based on extensive studies in animal models [reviewed in reference (187)] but have been extremely difficult to test in human populations because of the need to follow prospectively large groups of young children at risk for type 1 diabetes (188). Most early studies have attempted to correlate evidence (either antibodies or enteroviral RNA) with diabetes at onset. With current knowledge of the long prodromal phase that precedes type 1A diabetes, evidence that β-cell function is severely compromised years prior to diabetes, and the current ability to predict diabetes, it is unlikely that infections at the onset of diabetes have a primary pathogenic role. Thus, infections at onset may simply represent one of a number of stresses that either bring a patient to medical attention or increase the need for insulin and is thus associated with development of overt hyperglycemia. A recent prospective study of development of islet autoantibodies failed to find an association between enteroviral infections during pregnancy and the development of islet autoantibodies in offspring (2 mothers [10%] with infection of 21 children developing autoantibodies versus 17 mothers [16%] with infection of 104 control children). In contrast, the same study reported that 26% (33 of 125) of the prospectively observed children in whom islet autoantibodies developed and 18% (103 of 567) control children had evidence of enteroviral infection and that enteroviral infection and RNA were more often present during the 6-month interval before the development of islet autoantibodies. A very similar study from the United States addressing the same question failed to find an association of enteroviral infection with development or appearance of islet autoantibodies (189). The lack of confirmatory studies and small differences in enteroviral infections even in "positive" studies suggests that, if enteroviral infections do have a role, it is minor. It is certainly possible that only some strains of enteroviruses induce type 1A diabetes, but to date identification of specific strains in prospective studies, such as those from Finland, are negative, with a wide variety of enteroviral infections documented in young children developing islet autoimmunity.

In that type 1A diabetes is thought to be a T cell–mediated disease rather than autoantibody-mediated, studies of T-cell responses to enteroviruses are of interest. Hyoty and coworkers recently reported that children with recent-onset diabetes less often had T-cell responses to Coxsackie B4 virus than did control children and children with long-standing diabetes (190). They interpret this as suggesting that enterovirus-specific T cells are within the islets. The alternative hypothesis that enterovirus-specific T cells are unrelated to diabetes onset is perhaps as probable.

If infections are related to the development of type 1A diabetes, it is likely that the environmental factor is relatively ubiquitous, in that diabetes develops in the majority of individuals with high genetic susceptibility (e.g., monozygotic twins and DQ8/DQ2 siblings of patients). Honeyman and coworkers, following up evidence that a peptide of rotavirus is similar to GAD and IA-2 (ICA512), reported that rotavirus infection, a common cause of childhood gastroenteritis, was associated with an increase in levels of islet autoantibodies, although rotaviral infections were equally frequent for controls and cases (191). On many occasions, islet autoantibodies appeared without rotavirus infection, and the small change in autoantibodies used to correlate with rotavirus infections makes it essential that the reported findings be confirmed in other studies.

Vaccination

The NOD mouse model of type 1A diabetes is finely balanced in terms of the development of diabetes, and as recently reviewed, more than 100 different therapies can prevent the development of disease in this model. Thus, it is not too surprising that a number of vaccines administered to NOD mice prevent the development of diabetes. It was initially observed that complete Freund adjuvant administered to mice prevented diabetes, and follow-up studies indicated that the related vaccine, BCG, also prevented disease. This has led to trials in humans, in which BCG administration was found to have no influence on the loss of C-peptide secretion after diagnosis of diabetes (192,193).

A more important consideration is whether standard vaccines or the schedule of vaccination increases or decreases the development of childhood diabetes. A recent editorial in the *Journal of Epidemiology and Community Health* discussed the propensity in "postmodern medicine" to focus on risks of vaccination, with most reported adverse events falling in categories of "no data" or "data inadequate to assess causality" (194). This perhaps appropriately encapsulates claims that standard childhood vaccination is related to development of type 1A diabetes. Studies such as the DAISY study in Denver with prospective evaluation of children for the first appearance of islet autoantibodies and then progression to diabetes provide no evidence for changes in vaccination timing or regimen as related to islet autoimmunity (189).

Dietary Factors

For both the NOD mouse and the BB rat, modification of diet can modify the development of diabetes. In particular, diets that lack complex proteins (amino acids rather than proteins) are associated with decreased development of diabetes. In the NOD mouse model, a diet with gluten restriction (the dietary factor in celiac disease) decreases development of diabetes. The area of greatest interest has related to milk proteins; particularly bovine albumin given to young children.

In humans, a proposed protective effect of breast feeding on the incidence of type 1 diabetes (195) has attracted enormous interest. The association between cow's milk and autoimmunity and diabetes remains controversial (196–198). If this association is real, it could be due to a molecular mimicry between bovine serum albumin (BSA) and pancreatic autoantigen ICA69 (196,197) or to the effect of β-casein immunostimulating hexapeptide present in enzymatic hydrolysate of milk from *Bos taurus* cows but not from *Bos indicus* cows (R. B Elliott and N. J. Bibby, unpublished data). Subsequent human studies have given a variety of results: (a) diabetic children were significantly less likely than nondiabetic children to have been breast-fed (199–201); (b) there was no significant difference between the frequency of breast feeding in diabetic and nondiabetic children (202–211); or (c) diabetic children were significantly more likely than nondiabetic children to have been breast-fed (212). Certain studies suggested that the longer children had been breast-fed, the lower their risk for developing diabetes (200,201,213,214), whereas other studies did not show that protection increased with a longer duration of breast feeding (208,210,212,215). A meta-analysis of selected studies suggested that children with diabetes are 60% more likely than nondiabetic children to have had an early exposure to cow's milk (216). A major limitation of most of the aforementioned studies is that the data on infant diet were based on long-term maternal recall, which is subject to error (217). In fact, studies using prospectively collected records to assess infant diet (208,210,218) did not find the associations between type 1 diabetes and infant diet exposures that were found in studies that relied on recalled data. This suggests that there may be bias in the retrospective assessment of infant diet. The DAISY study has found no association between early exposure to cow's milk and β-cell autoimmunity in young siblings and offspring of patients with diabetes (219); this lack of association was also seen when the analyses were restricted to the highest-risk HLA genotypes: DR3/4,DQB1*0302, DR3/3 or DRx/4,DQB1*0302. Groups propose to gather definitive data concerning avoidance of cow's milk through a trial in newborn relatives with high-risk HLA genotypes (220,221). In a pilot study, type 1 diabetes developed in one child in the intervention group ($n = 10$) at the age of 14 months despite compliance with the intervention (breastfeeding or casein hydrolysate until the age of 9 months) and prevention of the development of antibody to BSA (222). This raises questions of whether BSA exposure is not relevant or whether it should be avoided for a period longer than 9 months, perhaps for life, similar to the elimination of gluten in celiac disease.

There are many other potential dietary factors, including vitamins, that may influence the development of diabetes. Toxic doses of nitrosamine compounds can cause diabetes (223–225) because of the generation of free radicals. The effect of dietary exposure to nitrate, nitrite, or nitrosamine on risk for human type 1 diabetes is less clear (226–228). Breast milk and vitamin supplements are important sources of antioxidants and theoretically may reduce the concentration of free radicals and thus the risk of β-cell damage. A number of additional environmental toxins have been implicated in the etiology of type 1 diabetes (225,229) but have never been fully explored in a cohort study. Multiple exposures to dietary β-cell toxins may render genetically resistant individuals susceptible to diabetogenic viruses, leading to type 1 diabetes (230).

In that the incidence of type 1A diabetes has increased dramatically in many countries during the past four decades, it is likely that some factors in the environment are changing. At present, these factors are unknown. An alternative explanation could be the explanation proposed for the recent increase in childhood asthma (231), that is, that the prevalence of suppressive environmental factors is decreasing. A candidate for such suppressive factors, in analogy to animal models, is the possibility that many childhood infections decrease, rather than increase, such risk. Evidence for such a protective effect in humans is not available. Measles immunization, but not polio immunization, has been reported to be associated with lower risk of type 1 diabetes (232); however, the effects of current mass immunization programs against potentially diabetogenic viruses are virtually unknown.

HUMORAL AUTOIMMUNITY

During the past 15 years, remarkable progress has been made in defining target autoantigens recognized by islet autoantibodies (233–235). The earliest test for islet autoantibodies was the cytoplasmic islet cell antibody (ICA) assay (68). This test uses frozen sections of human pancreas. The binding of immunoglobulin from patients to islets, as contrasted to binding with acinar pancreas, forms the basis for the test. Studies of cytoplasmic islet cell autoantibodies greatly aided studies of pathophysiology and facilitated the prediction of type 1A diabetes (236–238). The cytoplasmic ICA assay detects autoantibodies reacting with the ICA512 (IA-2), GAD, a ganglioside, and additional islet antigens (239–242). When cytoplasmic ICA autoantibodies react only with GAD, the antibodies react with human pancreas but fail to react with mouse pancreas; and on rat pancreas, the antibodies react specifically with islet β-cells. These antibodies are called "restricted" or "selective" and are usually associated with a relatively low progression to diabetes. The pattern of reactivity relates to the almost complete absence of GAD from mouse islets, β-cell specificity of GAD expression in rat islets, and the presence of GAD in all islet cells (e.g., α, β, γ, and δ) of human islets. Restricted ICA staining can be totally absorbed by incubating sera with GAD while standard ICA staining is not absorbed with GAD.

Quantitative assays are now available for autoantibodies reacting with three major islet autoantigens: insulin, GAD65, and ICA512 (IA-2) (20). Determination of autoantibodies reacting with these three molecules has supplanted, to a great extent, the determination of ICA, although there are ICA autoantibodies that are not GAD- or ICA512-reactive. Nevertheless, the detection of ICA in the absence of the previous three autoantibodies is associated with a very low risk of progression to diabetes (74,243,244), and the ICA test suffers from difficulty in standardization (20) and, in a number of laboratories, in reproducibility. Thus, we presently do not use the ICA test but measure insulin, GAD, and ICA512 (IA-2) autoantibodies.

INSULIN

Insulin was the first islet autoantigen to be characterized. Insulin autoantibodies were found to be present in children at the onset of type 1 diabetes before the administration of exogenous insulin (245). Insulin antibodies develop in essentially everyone treated with subcutaneous insulin (including human insulin) after several weeks to months of therapy. Thus, positivity for insulin autoantibodies/antibodies of insulin-treated patients provides no information relative to the diagnosis of type 1A diabetes.

Insulin is the smallest of the defined protein islet autoantigens (51 amino acids), consisting of disulfide-linked A and B chains. Insulin autoantibodies react with a conformational determinant of insulin, requiring residues of both the A and B chains. Perhaps related to the small size of the insulin molecule, almost all of the autoantibodies react with a similar determinant, centered at a pocket with the A13 leucine residue at its base (246). In that this pocket is relatively invariant for most species of insulin, insulin autoantibodies react well with human, bovine, porcine, and even rat insulin. In contrast, guinea pig insulin is nonreactive, and changing a single amino acid, A13 leucine, to tryptophan decreases binding of insulin autoantibodies by more than 100-fold. There are reports that proinsulin autoantibodies, distinct from insulin autoantibodies, are associated with type 1 diabetes (247). Most studies indicate that proinsulin autoantibodies can be absorbed by insulin, and the measurement of proinsulin autoantibodies does not increase the sensitivity of detecting autoantibodies (246).

Insulin autoantibodies are of high apparent affinity and very low capacity (10^{-12} M), and this may relate to the poor performance of the enzyme-linked immunosorbent assay (ELISA) for insulin autoantibodies (246). At the time of the initial discovery of insulin autoantibodies, there was debate about whether fluid-phase radioassays or assays with insulin bound to plastic (ELISAs) should be used. ELISAs are the standard assay format for many immunologic assays. It rapidly became apparent that ELISAs for insulin autoantibodies did not detect disease-relevant autoantibodies (248), although such assays readily detected the insulin antibodies generated after subcutaneous insulin therapy.

Until recently, the fluid-phase radioassays essential for detection of insulin autoantibodies were cumbersome and required a large volume of serum (20). Williams and coworkers modified the standard insulin autoantibody assays that used polyethylene glycol precipitation of antibodies to an assay that used protein A bound to Sepharose beads (249,250). Serum volumes were dramatically decreased with such an assay. Perhaps more important, several situations in which the polyethylene glycol–based assays artifactually indicated the presence of autoantibodies do not give false-positive results with protein A–based assays (250). Polyethylene glycol precipitation depends on decreasing the solubility of proteins in sera and is thus not specific for antibodies. In contrast, Sepharose–protein A precipitation is antibody-specific. Both cord blood and hemolyzed sera produce false-positive signals for insulin antibodies with polyethylene glycol precipitation (250–252).

The protein A–Sepharose-based assay for insulin autoantibodies has been modified to allow high throughput (253). In particular, we use assays with 96-well membrane filtration to separate autoantibody-bound from free ^{125}I-insulin. Scintillation fluid is added directly to the 96-well plates; these assays are, in many respects, as convenient as ELISA-based assays, but require working with low levels of radioactivity. With such an assay, not only are prediabetic humans found to produce insulin autoantibodies but similar antibodies are found in prediabetic NOD mice (Fig. 23.7) (253).

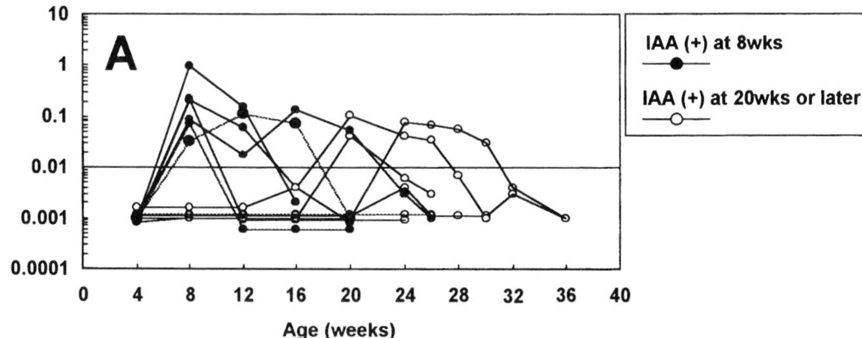

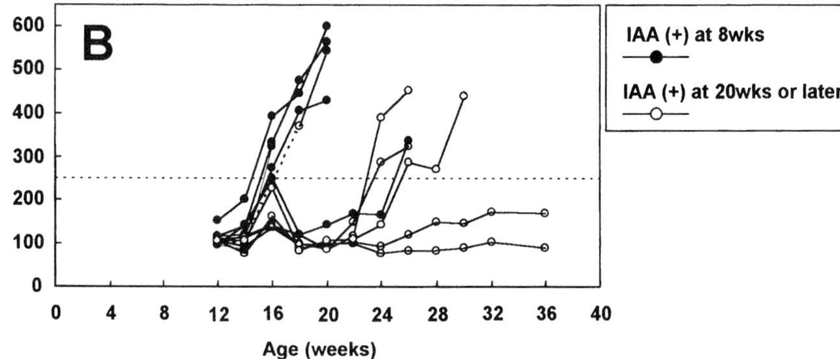

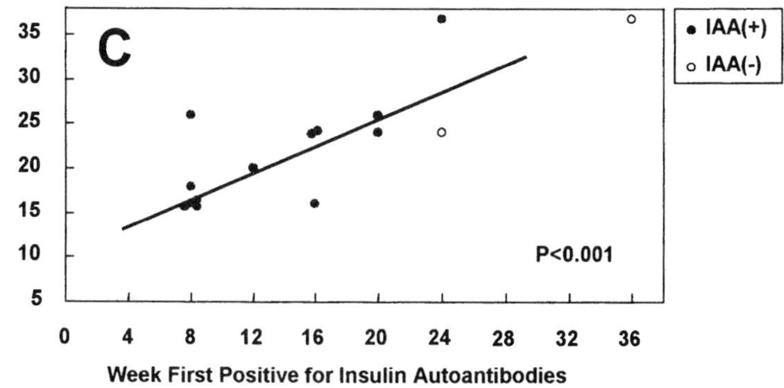

Figure 23.7. Insulin autoantibodies (IAA) of NOD mice. Mice developing insulin autoantibodies at 8 weeks of age develop diabetes earlier. **A:** Time course of insulin autoantibodies. **B:** Time course of glucose (open symbols: mice with late development of insulin autoantibodies). **C:** Correlation of first appearance of insulin autoantibodies and age of diabetes onset. (Reprinted from Yu L, Robles DT, Abiru N, et al. Early expression of anti-insulin autoantibodies of man and the NOD mouse: evidence for early determination of subsequent diabetes. *Proc Natl Acad Sci U S A* 2000;97:1701–1706, with permission. Copyright 2000 National Academy of Sciences, U.S.A.)

TABLE 23.6. Caveats of Autoantibody Determination

Caveat	Suggestion
Assays vary dramatically in sensitivity/specificity and ability to standardize (20,354)	Do not use cytoplasmic ICA assay. Use "biochemical autoantibody" assays with documented proficiency testing and specificity ≥99% (i.e., <.01 normal controls positive)
Insulin antibodies appear after insulin therapy	Do not measure insulin antibodies several weeks after insulin treatment
Specific autoantibodies expressed vary, with insulin autoantibodies most common in young children and GAD autoantibodies, in adults (24,253)	Measure multiple "biochemical" autoantibodies
Single autoantibodies, such as restricted ICA that is only GAD antibodies, confer low risk (76,355)	Measure multiple "biochemical" autoantibodies. If GAD or ICA is only antibody, test absorption of ICA with GAD
Subset of patients who are apparently type 1A express no known autoantibody	HLA typing, insulin secretion, and clinical history (e.g., autoimmunity) may aid diagnosis
Autoantibodies can appear at any age and often develop sequentially (253,281)	Measurement over time is important
Antibodies reacting with a single islet autoantigen do not always indicate β-cell autoimmunity (73,74)	Antibodies reacting with multiple epitopes of a single molecule or multiple islet antigens are more likely to be disease associated
Autoantibodies can disappear, and "mistakes" in handling sera can approach true positive rate in low-risk populations (294)	Do not rely on determination of autoantibodies in single serum sample

Insulin is the only identified β-cell–specific islet autoantigen. The autoantibodies reacting with insulin are also unique in that there is a remarkable inverse relationship between the age at which diabetes develops and the levels of insulin autoantibodies (254–256). Essentially all children in whom type 1A diabetes develops before the age of 5 years express insulin autoantibodies, while approximately one half of individuals in whom type 1A diabetes develops after the age of 15 years lack insulin autoantibodies. We believe this relationship is the result of an association between higher levels of insulin autoantibodies and a more rapid course of β-cell destruction and thus a more rapid progression to diabetes (257). An important exception to this correlation is that progression of diabetes is limited in individuals who have only insulin autoantibodies (e.g., no ICA512 or GAD65 autoantibodies) (243).

For children younger than 2 years of age, insulin autoantibodies are usually the first autoantibodies to appear and, characteristically, their appearance is followed by the development of GAD65 autoantibodies and then of ICA512 autoantibodies (17,252,253,257–259). For many children in whom type 1A diabetes develops during the first few years of life, multiple autoantibodies appear over several months to 1 year, with the first autoantibody often present by the time they are 6 months old. Transplacental insulin antibodies usually disappear by 6 months of age but, as with other autoantibodies (particularly GAD autoantibodies), they can be present in some infants for up to 1 year. It is well recognized that infants of mothers with diabetes frequently have transplacental islet autoantibodies. Such transplacental antibodies may be present even when the mother does not have diabetes, in that a nondiabetic mother may express islet autoantibodies that are then detectable in her children (Table 23.6).

GLUTAMIC ACID DECARBOXYLASE

The discovery that the 64-kDa islet autoantigen was GAD provided one of the most important assays for islet autoantibodies (260). Patients with the rare neurologic disorder stiff man syndrome were found to express autoantibodies reacting with Purkinje cells, and these antibodies reacted with GAD (261). Although stiff man syndrome is rare, the expression of GAD autoantibodies is relatively common for patients with type 1A diabetes and their relatives and is rarely associated with stiff man syndrome. Mapping of the epitopes recognized by GAD65 autoantibodies indicates that essentially the entire surface of the molecule is a target for GAD autoantibodies (262). This suggests that the native folded GAD65 is the immunogen during β-cell destruction. Most autoantibodies react with conformational epitopes of GAD65, and few react with GAD67. With extremely high titer GAD autoantibodies (e.g., patients with stiff man syndrome or restricted ICA), GAD67-reactive antibodies also are present. Both GAD65 and GAD67 are present in cytoplasmic microvesicles of neurons and in multiple different endocrine cells. Within human islets, GAD65 is expressed in all islet cells (α, β, γ, PP), even though only β-cells are destroyed.

ICA512 (IA-2)/IA-2β (PHOGRIN)

The molecule ICA512 was originally identified as an islet autoantigen with the screening of an islet expression library with sera from patients with diabetes (263,264). The initial sequencing of the ICA512 clone had several errors in base calling that resulted in an altered predicted reading frame, and thus initial ELISAs for ICA512 autoantibodies used a C-terminus–shortened clone (265). Even with the shorter clone and the use of the ELISA methodology, the presence of ICA512 autoantibodies in patients developing type 1A diabetes was apparent. The ICA512 molecule also was identified in studies of insulinoma cells and was given the designation IA-2 (266). Several investigators independently discovered a related molecule termed IA-2β (267), or phogrin (268,269). The importance of autoantibodies to this family of molecules for prediction of the development of diabetes was demonstrated before the sequences of ICA512 and IA-2β were defined. Patients' sera precipitated enzymatic digests of metabolically labeled islet molecules (270,271).

ICA512 and IA-2β are structurally related, and both have sequence homology to tyrosine phosphatase–like molecules, although no enzyme activity has been demonstrated for either molecule (272). ICA512 and IA-2β are widely distributed in neuronal and endocrine tissues, and the molecules are associated with islet secretory granules. The autoantibodies react with the portion of the molecule that remains intra-cytoplasmic when secretory granules fuse with the plasma membrane. Most of the autoantibodies react with the ICA512 molecule and may cross-react with IA-2β. Relatively few individuals developing diabetes have IA-2β autoantibodies without ICA512 autoantibodies, whereas approximately 10% of patients developing diabetes have ICA512 autoantibodies in the absence of IA-2β autoantibodies (272–277). In addition, almost all anti–IA-2β reactivity can be adsorbed with the ICA512 molecule.

Similar to their producing autoantibodies that react with the GAD65 molecule, individuals developing type 1A diabetes produce autoantibodies reacting with a large number of epitopes of ICA512 (273,276). Included among the epitopes is an alternatively spliced form of ICA512 that lacks the transmembrane exon (exon 13). This ICA512 clone [termed ICA512bdc (bdc = Barbara Davis Center)] was found with the screening of an islet expression library with patient sera, similar to the original studies by Rabin and coworkers (278, 279). A subset of patients has autoantibodies reacting with full-length ICA512 but not ICA512bdc, and vice versa, with approximately 10% of sera specifically reacting with only one of the two molecules. Recent studies indicate that expression of messenger RNA for the two forms differs between thymus and islets, with islets expressing both forms and the thymus expressing only the ICA512bdc form (280).

ICA512 autoantibodies are probably the most specific of the "biochemical" autoantibodies identified to date. When ICA512 autoantibodies are detected, individuals usually already express antibodies reacting with insulin or GAD65 (281). Nevertheless, a significant number of individuals with new-onset diabetes express only ICA512 autoantibodies. For a few individuals, ICA512 autoantibodies may be the only autoantibody detected in the prediabetic phase of the disease. With so many epitopes of ICA512 recognized by autoantibodies, it is relatively easy to construct autoantibody assays that use portions of the molecule. Mennuni and colleagues utilized a phage display library to define a number of ICA512 epitopes (282); they cloned non-overlapping fragments of ICA512 and developed autoantibody radioassays. Disease-associated autoantibodies react with multiple ICA512 epitopes, while the rare control individual expressing ICA512 antibodies appears to have antibodies reacting with only a single epitope. We believe it is likely that many such antibodies in controls are not related to islet β-cell destruction but may simply represent cross-reactivity of a given serum antibody (among millions) with a portion of the sequence of ICA512.

T-CELL AUTOIMMUNITY

A large series of diabetogenic T-cell clones have been derived from the NOD mouse model of type 1 diabetes. These T-cell clones are able to transfer diabetes to young or immunodeficient recipients, indicating that T cells are sufficient to transfer diabetes. These clones are both CD8 (cytotoxic) and CD4 "helper" (Th1, Th2, Th0) and recognize a series of different islet autoantigens (283–289). The Th1 (T-helper 1) CD4 clones can produce diabetes without CD8 T cells, probably through the cytokines that they produce. Th2 clones are complex, with some producing diabetes and others protecting from diabetes. The target antigen of many of the clones is unknown. An interesting series of clones react with peptides of insulin—particularly insulin B-chain peptide amino acids B:9–23—and others with a beta cell–specific molecule termed IGRP (islet-specific glucose-6-phosphatase catalytic subunit–related protein) (289a). Many of these clones were developed by isolating T cells directly from islets of NOD mice.

In contrast to T-cell clones of the NOD mouse, the production of T-cell clones and the assessment of the T-cell reactivity of patients with type 1A diabetes have been limited. For humans, T lymphocytes are obtained from peripheral blood, rather than from islets or lymphoid organs. It has been difficult to measure T-cell autoreactivity reliably in a way that would distinguish a patient with diabetes from a normal control. In an international T-cell workshop, with "blinded" peptides sent to multiple laboratories, none of the laboratories were able to distinguish T cells of controls versus those of patients with new-onset type 1 A diabetes. It is likely that more sensitive and specific assays will need to be developed to allow accurate T-cell determination. Newer techniques are being applied, including MHC+peptide avidin conjugates ("tetramers") reacting with T-cell receptors, assays that measure cytokine secretion of specific cells (ELISPOT), and assays dependent on separation of T-cell subsets. The potential importance of T-cell assays is illustrated by studies in which monitoring of islet transplants detected T-cell autoreactivity and alloreactivity (290).

NATURAL HISTORY OF TYPE 1A DIABETES

Childhood Onset

A number of recent studies have reported on children followed from birth for the expression of autoantibodies and the development of type 1A diabetes (252,253,257,291,292). Three of the largest of these studies are the DAISY study from Denver, Colorado (16), the BabyDiab study from Germany (253), and a series of studies from Finland [e.g., DIPP (Diabetes Prediction and Prevention) and TRIGR (Trial in Genetically at Risk)] (258,292). The DAISY and studies from Finland have evaluated both first-degree relatives of patients with type 1A diabetes and individuals from the general population following HLA typing. The BabyDiab study has evaluated primarily the offspring of mothers with type 1 diabetes. In general, results of the evaluation of these different populations appear concordant, despite wide geographic differences and some differences in autoantibody methodology (e.g., reliance or lack of reliance on the cytoplasmic ICA assay). Transplacental autoantibodies disappear relatively slowly, with a small percentage of infants having antibodies persisting until 1 year of age. Islet autoantibodies can be present during the first several months of life but often develop by 9 months of age (252,253,257,258,293). An increasing percentage of children develop autoantibodies between the ages of 9 months and 3 years. The first autoantibodies in infants are usually insulin autoantibodies—usually at very high levels. A subset of these infants lose antibody expression as they progress to overt diabetes, while most progressors express multiple islet autoantibodies until the onset of diabetes (20,75,294). The autoantibodies are usually persistent, although a few individuals lose antibody expression without progressing to diabetes (294). Very few children who express autoantibodies that react with more than a single islet antigen have only transient expression of autoantibodies.

Persistent, but not transient, autoantibodies are strongly related to genetic risk factors of type 1A diabetes (294). In the

TABLE 23.7. Caveats of Intravenous Glucose Tolerance Testing

Caveat	Suggestion
In young children, a "first"-test lack of response is not infrequent (356)	Never rely on a single test
Lack of carbohydrate intake may blunt first-phase insulin secretion	Dietary preparation similar to oral glucose tolerance testing
Type 1A diabetes mellitus and severe insulin resistance may coexist in the same individual	Subtracting 2× the fasting insulin from the 1+3 minute insulin may reveal lack of glucose-stimulated insulin secretion
When below the first percentile, first-phase insulin secretion may remain low for a number of years before onset of diabetes (357)	Long-term follow up is recommended
A subset of normal individuals has, by definition, first-phase secretion at the first percentile (78)	In the absence of islet autoantibodies, especially in athletes, low first-phase insulin secretion may not be significant
First-phase insulin secretion varies considerably and increases at puberty	Never rely on a single test and interpret small changes in first-phase secretion with caution

DAISY study, none of the children with transient islet autoantibodies had the highest-risk HLA genotype, DR3/4, DQ2/8. Transient islet autoantibodies occur in less than 2% of both first-degree relatives and individuals from the general population, and the incidence of transient antibodies was not increased in relatives of patients with diabetes. In contrast, persistent islet autoantibodies are greatly increased among first-degree relatives and especially relatives with the genotype DQ8/2. Siblings of patients with type 1A diabetes with the genotype DQ8/2 have more than a 50% risk of developing islet autoantibodies by age 3 years. The risk in offspring with DQ8/2 is also very high, but approximately one-half that of siblings. In contrast, DQ8/2 individuals from the general population have a risk of less than 5%. Given the presence of islet autoantibodies in such young children, most go on to express multiple islet autoantibodies, and life-table analysis suggests a high rate of progression to overt diabetes.

Loss of first-phase insulin secretion precedes the development of type 1A diabetes, and severe abnormalities of insulin secretion (below the first percentile) are a risk factor in children for rapid progression to diabetes (77,79,238,295–299). The Australian family study has confirmed earlier reports of progressive loss of first-phase insulin secretion before overt diabetes (79). At present, most groups assess first-phase insulin secretion with the ICARUS protocol, measuring fasting insulin, and insulin 1 and 3 minutes after a bolus of intravenous glucose (300). Caveats concerning first-phase insulin testing are listed in Table 23.7.

It has long been recognized that many individuals have type 2 diabetes and are not aware of their illness. In a similar manner, with glucose tolerance testing (GTT), "silent type 1A diabetes" is found to be present in high-risk populations (e.g., islet autoantibody–positive relatives), even among children (122). Such children typically have normal fasting glucose levels, but glucose levels exceed 200 mg/dL at 2 hours with oral GTT. Almost all such individuals we have followed have progressed to overt diabetes, and given the classification of the American Diabetes Association Expert Committee, with an oral GTT diagnosis of diabetes, we institute insulin therapy (298). A subset of these individuals may be treated with relatively low doses of long-acting insulin for several years. In contrast to this recommendation, some diabetes experts treat only those individuals with fasting hyperglycemia.

Latent Autoimmune Diabetes of Adults

It is now clear that type 1A diabetes can occur at any age. The oldest individual we have followed to the development of diabetes was 69 years old, the mother of a patient with type 1A diabetes. She expressed multiple islet autoantibodies, with first-phase insulin secretion below the first percentile for more than a year before the onset of diabetes. Multiple studies indicate that between 5% and 30% of patients initially thought to have type 2 diabetes have type 1A diabetes (24,104,301). If type 1A diabetes develops in an adult, usually, but not always, the disease course is very slow. Such patients are best identified by the expression of islet autoantibodies, and of GAD65 autoantibodies in particular. Given the presence of islet autoantibodies, such individuals as a group "rapidly" (usually within 3 years) progress and require insulin therapy (24). Their HLA alleles more closely resemble those of patients with type 1A diabetes, although the frequency of DQ8/DQ2 is lower (104). Given the large number of patients with a diagnosis of type 2 diabetes (estimated to be ten times more than the number with type 1A diabetes), patients with latent autoimmune diabetes of adults (LADA) probably comprise almost one half of all patients with type 1A diabetes. In some countries, such as Japan, it is hypothesized that the majority of cases of type 1A diabetes develop in adults (302).

At present it has not been proven that patients with LADA should be treated with insulin at the onset of diabetes. Although oral hypoglycemic therapy will rapidly be ineffective in these patients and they are at increased risk for ketoacidosis, they are often treated with oral agents and observed for failure to maintain adequate glucose control. One small study from Japan suggested that immediate insulin therapy, in comparison to therapy with oral hypoglycemic agents, was associated with longer preservation of C-peptide secretion (303). In general, we treat autoantibody-positive adult patients with insulin, often with relatively low doses of long-acting insulin, early in their disease course.

PREDICTION OF DIABETES

Given current knowledge of the "natural" history of type 1A diabetes, the disorder can be predicted, such that trials for diabetes prevention have been instituted. The closer an individual is to the development of overt diabetes, the more accurate the prediction. Large-scale prediction of type 1A diabetes will likely not be essential until there is a proven preventive therapy. At present, most prediction of type 1A diabetes is coupled to trials for the prevention of diabetes. There are isolated individuals for whom disease screening is warranted. The clearest such indication relates to relatives of patients with type 1A diabetes who will donate either a kidney or a portion of their pancreas. It is generally felt that such individuals expressing islet autoantibodies or with abnormal metabolic function (e.g., oral and intravenous GTT) are not good candidates as living-related donors.

Approximately 1 of 200 children with diabetes have been reported to die at the onset of type 1A diabetes (304,305). The clinical histories for most of these children are similar, with symptoms of diabetes overlooked by the first health care professionals who evaluate the child. The child then presents with ketoacidosis and develops cerebral edema. This can occur even when a family member has type 1 diabetes. It is believed that slow correction of hyperosmolarity helps to prevent cerebral edema, but this catastrophic complication is not predictable. With improved critical care facilities and early mannitol therapy, a number of children are now surviving cerebral edema, although many with stroke-like complications. In a family in which a high risk of diabetes for a child has been identified, most children are diagnosed before severe metabolic decompensation and then treated at onset of hyperglycemia as outpatients (305a). Given these risks, individual families request screening for diabetes risk.

During stress, a significant number of children develop hyperglycemia that is transient (306,307). The majority of these individuals do not progress to overt diabetes and appear to not be at increased risk for type 1A diabetes. Transient hyperglycemia is more common in children without a family history of type 1A diabetes and in children in whom hyperglycemia develops in the setting of severe stress (e.g., infection, steroid therapy). Type 1A diabetes develops in approximately 5% to 10% of children with transient hyperglycemia. These children usually express islet autoantibodies and have a severe loss of first-phase insulin secretion. Overt type 1A diabetes usually develops within months to several years.

Type 1A diabetes develops in approximately 5% of women with gestational diabetes (308). In contrast to the majority of women with gestational diabetes, those with type 1A diabetes usually express islet autoantibodies. Monitoring of such women is warranted, with institution of therapy (usually insulin) at the first indication of metabolic decompensation.

The current mainstays of diabetes prediction can be divided into three categories, genetic, autoantibody, and metabolic. At present, the only known environmental factor that increases the risk of type 1A diabetes is congenital rubella infection.

Genetic

A family history of type 1A diabetes increases risk of diabetes, as do specific HLA genotypes (309). Table 23.2 subdivides risk by relationship to proband with diabetes and HLA genotypes. High risk indicates individuals heterozygous for HLA DR3/4, DQ2/8. Moderate-risk genotypes include DR4/4 and DR1/4. Low-risk genotypes include most other genotypes not indicated as high-risk, moderate-risk, or protective. Protective genotypes include those with DQA1*0102, DQB1*0602, DQA1*201, DQB1*0303, or DRB1*1401 (71) (Table 23.8).

Autoantibody

The best current predictor for the development of type 1A diabetes is the expression of two or more biochemically assayed islet autoantibodies (insulin, GAD65, and ICA512 specifically set at ≥99th percentile) (74,242,244). Approximately 80% of individuals developing type 1A diabetes express two or more of these autoantibodies. With assays for the autoantibodies set at the 99th percentile of normal controls, on a single serum sample, approximately 3% of normal individuals express one or more antibodies, while fewer than 1 in 300 express two or more of these autoantibodies. In that the expression of multiple islet autoantibodies is approaching the prevalence of type 1A diabetes in the general population, it is likely that prediction of type 1A diabetes is now feasible for both relatives and the general population. Limited experience suggests that the positive predictive value of multiple autoantibodies for the development of diabetes will be as good (or within a factor of two) as prediction among relatives (75,253,310–312).

TABLE 23.8. Approximate Genetic Risk of Type 1A Diabetes Mellitus

	Identical twin	Sibling	Offspring	General population
Unknown HLA	50%	6%	4%	0.3%
High-risk HLA	70%	40%	20%	6%
Protective HLA	Unknown	Unknown	Unknown	0.03%

A large number of studies have confirmed the utility of what has been termed "combinatorial" autoantibody prediction (20, 313). Figure 23.8 illustrates the progression to diabetes of first-degree relatives of patients with type 1A diabetes subdivided by expression of zero, one, two, or three autoantibodies reacting with insulin, GAD65, or ICA512). We do not include determination of cytoplasmic ICA in the counting of autoantibodies expressed, in that cytoplasmic ICA may represent GAD65 or ICA512 autoantibodies and not a distinctive specificity. A number of studies have indicated that the presence of both cytoplasmic ICA and GAD65 autoantibodies increases risk of diabetes relative to the presence of either autoantibody alone. This is likely related to using the ICA assay and its correlation with the presence of ICA512 autoantibodies or the presence of higher titer GAD65 autoantibodies (73,75).

At present, not enough information is available to define the prognosis of individuals with multiple islet autoantibodies with DQB1*0602 (106,118,121,122,314). Many such individuals with DQB1*0602 express only a single autoantibody. Some DQB1*0602 relatives expressing multiple islet autoantibodies have been followed to the development of diabetes.

Metabolic

Progressive metabolic deterioration precedes type 1A diabetes and, similar to type 2 diabetes, asymptomatic hyperglycemia is present in a significant number of individuals. Oral GTT is the "gold" standard for the diagnosis of diabetes but is unnecessary if fasting hyperglycemia is present (fasting glucose ≥126 mg/dL). Before hyperglycemia develops, individuals progressing to diabetes lose insulin secretion following intravenous administration of glucose. Almost all individuals who become hyperglycemic secondary to type 1A diabetes have first-phase insulin secretion below the first percentile of normal months to years before diabetes develops.

Dual-Parameter Model

Different patients with type 1A diabetes progress to diabetes at very different rates. The presence of multiple islet autoantibod-

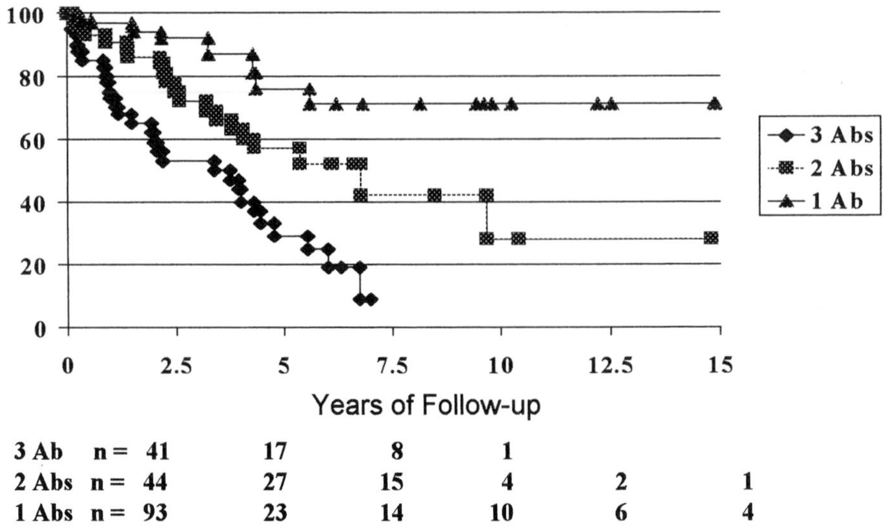

Figure 23.8. Progression of diabetes of relatives subdivided by number of autoantibodies (Abs) (GAD, ICA512, insulin) recognizing different autoantigens. (Copyright © 1996 American Diabetes Association. From Verge CF, Giannani R, Kawasaki E, et al. Prediction of type I diabetes in first-degree relatives using a combination of insulin, GAD, and ICA512 bdc/IA-2 autoantibodies. *Diabetes* 1996;45:926–933. Reprinted with permission from the American Diabetes Association.)

ies indicates a high risk of progression. A combination of loss of first-phase insulin secretion and the presence of higher levels of insulin autoantibodies aids in predicting approximate time to onset of diabetes, accounting for approximately one half of the variance in time to the development of overt diabetes (256).

PREVENTION OF DIABETES

Rationale for Maintenance of C-Peptide

At the diagnosis of type 1A diabetes, most patients have significant insulin secretory capacity. The amount of islet β-cells remaining probably ranges between 10% and 50% of normal islet mass. When a patient presents with overt diabetes, and especially with ketoacidosis, there is little insulin secretion, probably as a consequence of the toxic effects of hyperglycemia on insulin secretion. Following insulin therapy and normalization of glucose levels, many patients develop a "honeymoon" phase of their diabetes, with normalization of glucose, increased insulin secretion, and a need for relatively low doses of insulin. C-peptide, the connecting peptide of proinsulin, is secreted in equimolar concentrations with insulin and is a measure of insulin secretion for patients who are receiving exogenous insulin. With time (ranging from months to years) after the diagnosis of diabetes, additional β-cells are killed and C-peptide secretion decreases progressively. By 3 to 5 years of type 1A diabetes, most children produce no C-peptide [in the Diabetes Care and Complications Trial (DCCT), at 5 years of diabetes, 8% of adults, but 3% of adolescents, had a meal-stimulated C-peptide level greater than 0.2 nmol/L]. This loss of C-peptide correlates with increasing insulin needs; metabolic deterioration, including risk of severe hypoglycemia with exclusive dependence on exogenous insulin therapy; and a marked increase in variation in blood glucose levels. Studies from the DCCT indicate that even minimal residual preservation of C-peptide correlates with improved diabetes control (315). Given this information, preservation of C-peptide is a major outcome measure in trials to prevent β-cell destruction after the onset of diabetes (315a).

Prevention of further β-cell destruction after diabetes onset is an important clinical goal. Studies of cyclosporin A demonstrated that this potent immunosuppressive agent is sufficient to prevent C-peptide loss for as long as it is administered (316–319). It does not, however, prevent recurrence of hyperglycemia when it is administered after onset of diabetes, but it does moderate the metabolic dysfunction. Recurrent hyperglycemia in the patients treated with cyclosporin A at diagnosis of diabetes reflects increasing insulin resistance in the setting of limited β-cell mass. In addition, once cyclosporin A is discontinued, C-peptide secretion is lost and insulin dependence rapidly ensues. Risks of cyclosporin A include the risks of immunosuppression and, of importance, nephrotoxicity. These risks make it a poor choice for preventing further β-cell destruction. Trials of less toxic therapies, such as azathioprine (320, 321), methotrexate (322), BCG vaccination (323), nicotinamide (324–326), anti-thymocyte globulin (327), and oral insulin (328, 329), have had minimal, if any, positive benefits. Trials of newer modalities [e.g., "non-activating" anti-CD3 monoclonal antibodies (330) and mycophenolate mofetil] are under way with promising data for initial anti-CD3 trial (329a). From studies of pancreas and islet transplantation, it is clear that there are drug regimens that can halt immune-mediated β-cell destruction, and it is likely that safe modalities to preserve β-cell mass will be developed.

Primary/Secondary/Tertiary Prevention

Given the stages in the development of type 1A diabetes illustrated in Figure 23.3 and the ability to identify individuals in these stages, one can envision prevention trials for each of the stages. We have already discussed prevention after diabetes onset. As one goes backwards in the natural history of type 1A diabetes, prediction of diabetes becomes less secure, and thus analysis of the risk-to-benefit ratio requires modalities with minimal to "no" toxicity. One can envision primary prevention trials, aimed at preventing the development of islet autoimmunity; secondary prevention trials, aimed at preventing β-cell destruction after the activation of islet autoimmunity (currently usually marked by the presence of multiple islet autoantibodies); and tertiary prevention trials after the onset of diabetes or following islet transplantation. It is not clear that modalities effective earlier in the course of the disease will be effective later in disease. In animal models, there is one example of a therapy that is effective at the onset of diabetes but not earlier (331). In addition to these considerations, trials for prevention before the presence of autoimmunity or the development of diabetes require relatively large screening programs to identify individuals at risk. With the many agents that prevent diabetes in animal models, it is likely that initial trials will be carried out in patients with new-onset disease. Therapies effective and safe at that stage would be applied to autoantibody-positive, high-risk relatives of patients with diabetes, and depending on the agent, potentially to genetically at-risk individuals. As discussed, islet autoimmunity develops in approximately 40% of siblings of patients with type 1A diabetes with DR3/4; thus, trials can also be designed for this group. If a safe and effective therapy is identified, it should be possible, with current technology, to identify individuals at risk for diabetes, both for relatives and for the general population among whom the bulk of type 1A diabetes develops (156).

Current Prevention Trials

The two largest current prevention trials were a nicotinamide trial (ENDIT), primarily in Europe, and a trial of oral or parenteral insulin therapy [Diabetes Prevention Trial-1 (DPT-1)] carried out by the National Institutes of Health in the United States and Canada. Both trials were based initially on animal data, followed by pilot trials in humans (324,332,333). One small negative nicotinamide trial has been reported since the start of the large ENDIT trial (334). Trials of oral insulin after diabetes onset have not shown preservation of C-peptide (328,329). The ENDIT trial has closed enrollment, and there was no influence of nicotinamide or progression to diabetes.

The DPT-1 consists of two separate trials, one of oral insulin (to induce oral tolerance) and the other of parenteral insulin with daily subcutaneous low-dose insulin and annual intravenous insulin. More than 90,000 first-degree relatives have been screened for expression of islet autoantibodies; of those with autoantibodies, relatives either with loss of first-phase insulin secretion (parenteral trial) or with insulin autoantibodies and normal first-phase insulin secretion (oral trial) are eligible for trial participation. A manuscript describing the oral trial is awaited, while the parenteral trial showed no prevention of diabetes. (334a)

Finland is the country with the highest incidence of type 1 diabetes. The childhood incidence is now approximately 50 in 100,000, which is twice the current approximate incidence in the state of Colorado and more than 50 times that in Japan. Given this high incidence, two major prevention trials are under way. The DIPP (Diabetes Prediction and Prevention) trial is evaluating mucosal administration (nasal) of insulin for individuals expressing islet autoantibodies (335). The trial initially screens newborns with HLA typing to identify those with high-risk HLA alleles. The TRIGR (Trial in Genetically at Risk) is targeting high-risk infants with diet modification (removal of cow's milk), with a hypothesis that exposure to bovine albumin before 9 months of age induces diabetes (220).

Future Prevention Trials

A remarkable number of new agents for immunotherapy are being introduced into clinical research and practice. Many of these agents are potentially applicable to the autoimmunity of type 1A diabetes. With the current knowledge of the genetics and natural history of type 1A diabetes, these agents are likely to be studied for prevention of autoimmune β-cell destruction.

It is very likely that potent immunosuppressive agents can prevent β-cell destruction similar to that achieved with cyclosporin A. The drug rapamycin, part of a protocol for successful islet transplantation (336), will probably be evaluated in the near future if its toxicity profile does not change with wider use in transplantation. Mycophenolate mofetil is an inhibitor of de novo purine biosynthesis. It is more potent than azathioprine and has replaced azathioprine in pancreas transplant regimens, thereby allowing a decrease in the use of glucocorticoids. Trials to prevent progressive β-cell destruction with mycophenolate mofetil in patients with new-onset type 1A diabetes are about to be initiated.

A number of monoclonal antibodies targeting T lymphocytes are being studied or are likely to be studied in patients with new-onset diabetes. CD3 autoantibodies have been used for more than a decade in organ transplantation, but the standard antibody activates a cytokine "storm." Newer monoclonal antibodies, altered such that they do not bind complement, have been used to induce long-lasting disease remission in NOD mice and are now being studied in patients with new-onset type 1A diabetes (329a,330,331,337). Similar concepts apply to monoclonal antibodies to the interleukin-2 (IL-2) receptor, one of which was used for islet transplantation in combination with rapamycin and low-dose FK506.

Perhaps the most exciting group of reagents entering clinical trials for diabetes prevention go under the rubric of "immunologic vaccination." In animal models, a series of autoantigens can be administered to prevent disease. Both an altered peptide ligand of insulin peptide B:9–23 (338) and a heat-shock peptide (p277) (339) are now in clinical trials. Following phase I trials, initial trials will evaluate patients with recent-onset diabetes. In that the tools for monitoring the relevant immune response to such therapies are in their infancy, the success of such trials are far from assured.

UNUSUAL DIABETES-RELATED AUTOIMMUNITY

Insulin Autoimmune Syndrome (Hirata Syndrome)

High levels of insulin autoantibodies are associated with hypoglycemia (340). It is thought that the hypoglycemia is the result of nonregulated release of insulin from bound autoantibody. Such high levels of insulin autoantibodies can be the result of the production of monoclonal antibodies by plasmacytomas. This is even less common than the rare Hirata syndrome (340,341), in which patients spontaneously produce polyclonal insulin autoantibodies. This latter syndrome is strongly HLA-restricted, with more than 90% of patients having DRB1*0406 (342). Most patients with the syndrome are Asian, and disease induction is associated with sulfhydryl-containing drugs and methimazole, in particular (343). Therapy usually consists of discontinuing the inducing medication.

Autoantibodies to Insulin Receptor

Autoantibodies reacting with the insulin receptor also can produce hypoglycemia (344). In addition, some patients present with insulin resistance and hyperglycemia, and individuals with the syndrome can have both hypoglycemia and hyperglycemia. This suggests that autoantibodies reacting with the insulin receptor can act as both agonists and antagonists (344). Patients with this syndrome often have non–organ-specific autoimmunity (e.g., DNA autoantibodies) (345). Therapy has included plasma exchange, immunosuppression, and one report of treatment with insulin-like growth factor-1 (346).

Insulin "Allergy/Hypersensitivity"

Lipohypertrophy and lipoatrophy of the site of injection, painful inflammation following insulin injection, and systemic reactions to insulin are all potential reactions to insulin (347). Delayed hypersensitivity and allergic reactions, uncommon even with animal insulin, appear to be even less common with human insulin (348). In the past when such reactions occurred, individuals were switched from one species of insulin to another (e.g., bovine, porcine, human) or to one form of insulin to another (NPH versus lente insulin). With current use of human insulin, the formulation of insulin is still of importance (regular, NPH, lente), and there exists the possibility of utilizing genetically altered insulin such as lispro (349) insulin, and there is one report of successful pancreatic transplantation (350). Although lispro insulin represents a modified insulin, it does not appear to be more immunogenic than regular human insulin, perhaps because of its more rapid absorption (IgE-mediated allergic reactions even to lispro insulin are reported) (351).

IgE-mediated allergy to insulin, if mild, usually is treated with an antihistamine such as cetirizine (351) and, if severe, usually is treated with insulin desensitization. Desensitization to both protamine and insulin has been reported. Patients with local delayed hypersensitivity reactions to insulin may also be treated by the addition of small amounts of dexamethasone injected directly with the insulin (352). There is one report of pancreatic transplantation to treat intractable insulin allergy (350).

Islet/Pancreas Transplantation

Islet and pancreas transplantation for type 1A diabetes faces two immunologic barriers, recurrent autoimmunity and transplant alloimmunity (353). The importance of autoimmunity was demonstrated by transplantation of the tail of the pancreas between identical twins (83). The twins receiving the pancreas developed diabetes years before transplantation, whereas the donor twins were normal (83). Although the transplants initially restored euglycemia, they were rapidly destroyed. Such transplants, even though they are between identical twins, are now performed only with immunosuppression of the recipient.

Until recently, although pancreas transplantation with immunosuppression was successful, islet transplants almost universally failed. Investigators in Edmonton have recently reported sequential successful islet transplants using a new immunosuppressive protocol (336). Their protocol uses anti-IL-2R antibodies and a combination of rapamycin and low-dose FK506. Among the transplant recipients, insulin antibodies were suppressed while GAD autoantibodies were unchanged, with as yet a limited duration of follow up (<1 year). These studies suggest that the very aggressive destruction of islet transplants can now be overcome with immunosuppression. The Edmonton regimen also prevents the development of increased levels of islet autoantibodies that have been associated with the failure of transplants with other regimens. Clinical experience with rapamycin is, however, relatively limited, and further study and clinical experience will be needed to assess risks and benefits of this therapy.

CONCLUSION

Type 1A diabetes results from immune-mediated destruction of islet β-cells. The disorder, with a long chronic progressive phase, is now predictable for the great majority of individuals. Trials of potential preventive therapies are presently under way, but no therapy has demonstrated safety and efficacy. With excellent animal models and extensive studies in humans, we believe it is only a matter of time before insulitis, like hepatitis, becomes a treatable disorder. Once treatments are available, depending on the stage of disease for optimal intervention, it is likely that type 1A diabetes will become one of the first autoimmune disorders for which there is screening on a public-health scale. It is important to recognize the autoimmune disorders that are frequently associated with type 1 diabetes and to institute therapies before the development of irreversible morbidity. In the future, it is hoped that the family of organ-specific autoimmune diseases will be addressed as preventable public-health menaces.

Acknowledgments

We thank Marian Rewers for reviewing this chapter and offering his suggestions concerning environmental factors.

REFERENCES

1. American Diabetes Association. Report of the Expert Committee on the Diagnosis and Classification of Diabetes Mellitus. *Diabetes Care* 1997;20:1183-1197.
2. Bellgrau D, Eisenbarth GS. Immunobiology of autoimmunity. In: Eisenbarth GS, ed. *Endocrine and organ specific autoimmunity.* Austin, TX: RG Landes, 1999:1–18.
3. Bach JF. Etiology and pathogenesis of human insulin-dependent diabetes mellitus. In: Volpe R, ed. *Autoimmune endocrinopathies.* Totowa, NJ: Humana Press, 1999:293–307.
4. Nepom GT, Kwok WW. Perspectives in diabetes: molecular basis for HLA-DQ associations with IDDM. *Diabetes* 1998;47:1177–1184.
5. Thorsby E. Invited anniversary review: HLA associated diseases. *Hum Immunol* 1997;53:1–11.
6. Mordes JP, Greiner DL, Rossini AA. Animal models of autoimmune diabetes mellitus. In: LeRoith D, Taylor SI, Olefsky JM, eds. *Diabetes mellitus: a fundamental and clinical text.* Philadelphia: Lippincott-Raven, 1996:349–360.
7. Foulis AK, Clark A. Pathology of the pancreas in diabetes mellitus. In: Kahn CR, Weir GC, eds. *Joslin's diabetes mellitus,* 13th ed. Philadelphia: Lea & Febiger, 1994:265–281.
8. Foulis AK, McGill M, Farquharson MA. Insulitis in type 1 (insulin-dependent) diabetes mellitus in man—macrophages, lymphocytes, and interferon-gamma containing cells. *J Pathol* 1991;165:97–103.
9. Noble JA, Valdes AM, Cook M, et al. The role of HLA class II genes in insulin-dependent diabetes mellitus: molecular analysis of 180 Caucasian, multiplex families. *Am J Hum Genet* 1996;59:1134–1148.
10. Todd JA. From genome to aetiology in a multifactorial disease, type 1 diabetes. *Bioassays* 1999;21:164–174.
11. Anonymous. Epidemiology of severe hypoglycemia in the diabetes control and complications trial. The DCCT Research Group. *Am J Med* 1991;90: 450–459.
12. Imagawa A, Hanafusa T, Miyagawa J. A novel subtype of type 1 diabetes mellitus characterized by a rapid onset and an absence of diabetes-related antibodies. Osaka IDDM Study Group. *N Engl J Med* 2000;342:301-307.
13. Winter WE, Maclaren NK, Riley WJ, et al. Maturity-onset diabetes of youth in black Americans. *N Engl J Med* 1987;316:285–291.
14. Pinhas-Hamiel O, Dolan LM, Daniels SR, et al. Increased incidence of non-insulin-dependent diabetes mellitus among adolescents. *J Pediatr* 1996;128: 608–615.
15. Pinhas-Hamiel O, Dolan LM, Zeitler PS. Diabetic ketoacidosis among obese African-American adolescents with NIDDM. *Diabetes Care* 1997;20:484–486.
16. Rewers M, Bugawan TL, Norris JM, et al. Newborn screening for HLA markers associated with IDDM: diabetes autoimmunity study in the young (DAISY). *Diabetologia* 1996;39:807–812.
17. Schenker M, Hummel M, Ferber K, et al. Early expression and high prevalence of islet autoantibodies for DR3/4 heterozygous and DR4/4 homozygous offspring of parents with type I diabetes: the German BABYDIAB study. *Diabetologia* 1999;42:671–677.
18. Rosenbloom AL, Joe JR, Young RS, et al. Emerging epidemic of type 2 diabetes in youth. *Diabetes Care* 1999;22:345–354.
19. Aaltonen J, Björses P, Perheentupa J, et al. An autoimmune disease, APECED,

caused by mutations in a novel gene featuring two PHD-type zinc-finger domains. *Nat Genet* 1997;17:399–403.
20. Verge CF, Stenger D, Bonifacio E, et al. Combined use of autoantibodies (IA-2 autoantibody, GAD autoantibody, insulin autoantibody, cytoplasmic islet cell antibody) in type 1 diabetes: combinatorial islet autoantibody workshop. *Diabetes* 1998;47:1857–1866.
21. Redondo MJ, Eisenbarth GS. Autoimmune polyendocrine syndrome type II. In: Eisenbarth GS, ed. *Endocrine and organ specific immunity.* Austin, TX: RG Landes, 1999:41–61.
22. Pugliese A. Genetic protection from insulin-dependent diabetes mellitus. *Diab Nutr Metab* 1997;10(4):169–179.
23. Abiru N, Takino H, Yano M, et al. Clinical evaluation of non-insulin-dependent diabetes mellitus patients with autoantibodies to glutamic acid decarboxylase. *J Autoimmun* 1996;9:683–688.
24. Turner R, Stratton I, Horton V, et al. UKPDS 25: autoantibodies to islet-cell cytoplasm and glutamic acid decarboxylase for prediction of insulin requirement in type 2 diabetes. UK Prospective Diabetes Study Group. *Lancet* 1997; 350:1288–1293.
25. Balducci-Silano PL, Connor E, Maclaren NK. Association between insulin-dependent diabetes mellitus and other autoimmune diseases. In: LeRoith D, Taylor SI, Olefsky JM, eds. *Diabetes mellitus: a fundamental and clinical text.* Philadelphia: Lippincott-Raven, 1996:333–339.
26. Neufeld M, Maclaren NK, Blizzard RM. Two types of autoimmune Addison's disease associated with different polyglandular autoimmune (PGA) syndromes. *Medicine* (Baltimore) 1981;60:355–362.
27. Verge CF, Eisenbarth GS. Immunoendocrinopathy syndromes. In: Wilson JD, Foster DW, eds. *Williams textbook of endocrinology.* Philadelphia: WB Saunders, 1998:1651–1662.
28. Yu L, Brewer KW, Gates S, et al. DRB1*04 and DQ alleles: expression of 21-hydroxylase autoantibodies and risk of progression to Addison's disease. *J Clin Endocrinol Metab* 1999;84:328–335.
29. Bao F, Rewers M, Scott F, et al. Celiac disease. In: Eisenbarth GS, ed. *Endocrine and organ specific autoimmunity.* Austin, TX: RG Landes, 1999:85–96.
30. Bao F, Yu L, Babu S, et al. One third of HLA DQ2 homozygous patients with type 1 diabetes express celiac disease associated transglutaminase autoantibodies. *J Autoimmun* 1999;13:143–148.
31. Hoffenberg EJ, Bao F, Eisenbarth GS, et al. G.S. Silent celiac disease in American children at genetic risk. *J Pediatr Gastroenterol Nutr* 2000;31:S65(abstr).
32. Savilahti E, Ormala T, Saukkonen T, et al. Jejuna of patients with insulin-dependent diabetes mellitus (IDDM) show signs of immune activation. *Clin Exp Immunol* 1999;116:70–77.
33. Vitoria JC, Castano L, Rica I, et al. Association of insulin-dependent diabetes mellitus and celiac disease: a study based on serologic markers. *J Pediatr Gastroenterol Nutr* 1998;27:47–52.
34. Acerini CL, Ahmed ML, Ross KM, et al. Coeliac disease in children and adolescents with IDDM: Clinical characteristics and response to gluten-free diet. *Diabet Med* 1997;15:38–44.
35. Lorini R, Scotta MS, Cortona L, et al. Celiac disease and type I (insulin-dependent) diabetes mellitus in childhood: follow-up study. *J Diabetes Complications* 1996;10:154–159.
36. Saukkonen T, Savilahti E, Reijonen H, et al, and Childhood Diabetes in Finland Study Group. Coeliac disease: frequent occurrence after clinical onset of insulin-dependent diabetes mellitus. *Diabet Med* 1995;13:464–470.
37. Fernández-Castañer M, Molina A, López-Jiménez L, et al. Clinical presentation and early course of type 1 diabetes in patients with and without thyroid autoimmunity. *Diabetes Care* 1999;22:377–381.
38. Holl RW, Bohm B, Loos U, et al. Thyroid autoimmunity in children and adolescents with type 1 diabetes mellitus. Effect of age, gender and HLA type. *Horm Res* 1999;52:113–118.
39. Lorini R, d'Annunzio G, Vitali L, et al. IDDM and autoimmune thyroid disease in the pediatric age group. *J Pediatr Endocrinol Metab* 1996;9:89–94.
40. Gerstein HC. Incidence of postpartum thyroid dysfunction in patients with type I diabetes mellitus. *Ann Intern Med* 1993;118:419–423.
41. Davis RE, McCann VJ, Stanton KG. Type 1 diabetes and latent pernicious anaemia. *Med J Aust* 1992;156:160–162.
42. De Block CE, De Leeuw I, Van Gaal LF. High prevalence of manifestations of gastric autoimmunity in parietal cell antibody positive type 1 (insulin-dependent) diabetic patients: the Belgian Diabetes Registry. *J Clin Endocrinol Metab* 1999;84:4062–4067.
43. Snow CF. Laboratory diagnosis of vitamin B12 and folate deficiency: a guide for the primary care physician. *Arch Intern Med* 1999;159:1289–1298.
44. Eisenbarth GS, Gottlieb P. Immunoendocrinopathy syndromes. In: Larsen PR, Kronenberg H, Melmed S, et al. *Williams textbook of endocrinology*, 10th ed. Philadelphia: WB Saunders, 2003.
45. Betterle C, Volpato M, Pedini B, et al. Adrenal-cortex autoantibodies and steroid-producing cells autoantibodies in patients with Addison's disease: comparison of immunofluorescence and immunoprecipitation assays. *J Clin Endocrinol Metab* 1999;84:618–622.
46. Brewer KW, Parziale VS, Eisenbarth GS. Screening patients with insulin-dependent diabetes mellitus for adrenal insufficiency. *N Engl J Med* 1997;337: 202.
47. Furmaniak J, Sanders J, Rees Smith B. Autoantigens in the autoimmune endocrinopathies. In: Volpe R, ed. *Autoimmune endocrinopathies.* Totowa, NJ: Humana Press, 1999:183–216.
48. Not T, Horvath K, Hill ID, et al. Celiac disease risk in the USA: high prevalence of antiendomysium antibodies in healthy blood donors. *Scand J Gastroenterol* 1998;33:494–498.
49. Dietrich W, Ehnis T, Bauer M, et al. Identification of tissue transglutaminase as the autoantigen of celiac disease. *Nat Med* 1997;3:797–801.
50. O'Connor TM, Cronin CC, Loane JF, et al. Type 1 diabetes mellitus, coeliac disease, and lymphoma: a report of four cases. *Diabet Med* 1999;16:614–617.
51. Arentz-Hansen H, Korner R, Molberg O, et al. The intestinal T cell response to alpha-gliadin in adult celiac disease is focused on a single deamidated glutamine targeted by tissue transglutaminase. *J Exp Med* 2000;191:603–612.
52. van de Wal Y, Kooy YMC, van Veelen PA, et al. Small intestinal T cells of celiac disease patients recognize a natural pepsin fragment of gliadin. *Proc Natl Acad Sci U S A* 1998;95:10050–10054.
53. Sjöström H, Lundin KEA, Molberg O, et al. Identification of a gliadin T-cell epitope in coeliac disease: general importance of gliadin deamidation for intestinal T-cell recognition. *Scand J Immunol* 1998;48:111–115.
54. Hoffenberg EJ, Haas J, Drescher A, et al. A trial of oats in newly diagnosed celiac disease. *J Pediatr* 2000;137:361–366.
55. Holmes GKT, Prior P, Lane MR, et al. Malignancy in coeliac disease—effect of a gluten free diet. *Gut* 1989;30:333–338.
56. Perheentupa J, Miettinen A. Autoimmune polyendocrinopathy-candidiasis-ectodermal dystrophy. In: Eisenbarth GS, ed. *Endocrine and organ specific autoimmunity.* Austin, TX: RG Landes, 1999.
57. Scott HS, Heino M, Peterson P, et al. Common mutations in autoimmune polyendocrinopathy-candidiasis-ectodermal dystrophy patients of different origins. *Mol Endocrinol* 1998;2:1112–1119.
58. Vaidya B, Imrie H, Geatch DR, et al. Association analysis of the cytotoxic T lymphocyte antigen-4 (CTLA-4) and autoimmune regulator-1 (AIRE-1) genes in sporadic autoimmune Addison's disease. *J Clin Endocrinol Metab* 2000;85:688–691.
59. Kemp EH, Ajjan RA, Husebye ES. A cytotoxic T lymphocyte antigen-4 (CTLA-4) gene polymorphism is associated with autoimmune Addison's disease in English patients. *Clin Endocrinol* 1998;49:609–613.
60. Heward JM, Allahabadia A, Armitage M, et al. The development of Graves' disease and the CTLA-4 gene on chromosome 2q33. *J Clin Endocrinol Metab* 1999;84:2398–2401.
61. van der Auwera BJ, Vandewalle CL, Schuit FC, et al. CTLA-4 gene polymorphism confers susceptibility to insulin-dependent diabetes mellitus (IDDM) independently from age and from other genetic or immune disease markers. The Belgian Diabetes Registry. *Clin Exp Immunol* 1997;10:98–103.
62. Gambelunghe G, Falorni A, Ghaderi M, et al. Microsatellite polymorphism of the MHC class I chain-related (MIC-A and MIC-B) genes marks the risk for autoimmune Addison's disease. *J Clin Endocrinol Metab* 1999;84:3701–3707.
63. Gambelunghe G, Ghaderi M, Cosentino A, et al. Association of MHC Class I chain-related A (MIC-A) gene polymorphism with type 1 diabetes. *Diabetologia* 2000;43:507–514.
64. Powell BR, Buist NR, Stenzel V. An X-linked syndrome of diarrhea, polyendocrinopathy, and fatal infection in infancy. *J Pediatr* 1982;100:731–737.
65. Bennett CL, Yoshioka R, Kiyosawa H, et al. X-Linked syndrome of polyendocrinopathy, immune dysfunction, and diarrhea maps to Xp11.23-Xq13.3. *Am J Hum Genet* 2000;66:461–468.
66. Ferguson PJ, Blanton SH, Saulsbury FT, et al. Manifestations and linkage analysis in X-linked autoimmunity-immunodeficiency syndrome. *Am J Med Genet* 2000;90:390–397.
67. Cilio CM, Bosco A, Moretti C, et al. Congenital autoimmune diabetes mellitus [Letter]. *N Engl J Med* 2000;342:1529–1531.
68. Bottazzo GF, Florin-Christensen A, Doniach D. Islet-cell antibodies in diabetes mellitus with autoimmune polyendocrine deficiencies. *Lancet* 1974;2: 1279–1283.
69. Eisenbarth GS. Type I diabetes mellitus. A chronic autoimmune disease. *N Engl J Med* 1986;314:1360–1368.
70. Redondo MJ, Yu L, Hawa M, et al. Late progression to type 1 diabetes of discordant twins of patients with type 1 diabetes: combined analysis of two twin series (United States and United Kingdom). *Diabetes* 1999;48:780(abst).
71. Johnston C, Millward BA, Hoskins P, et al. Islet-cell antibodies as predictors of the later development of type I (insulin-dependent) diabetes. *Diabetologia* 1989;32:382–386.
72. Redondo MJ, Rewers M, Yu L, et al. Genetic determination of islet cell autoimmunity in monozygotic twin, dizygotic twin, and non-twin siblings of patients with type 1 diabetes: prospective twin study. *BMJ* 1999;318:698–702.
73. Bingley PJ, Christie MR, Bonifacio E, et al. Combined analysis of autoantibodies improves prediction of IDDM in islet cell antibody-positive relatives. *Diabetes* 1994;43:1304–1310.
74. Verge CF, Gianani R, Kawasaki L, et al. Prediction of type I diabetes in first-degree relatives using a combination of insulin, GAD, and ICA512bdc/IA-2 autoantibodies. *Diabetes* 1996;45:926–933.
75. Bingley PJ, Bonifacio E, Williams AJK, et al. Prediction of IDDM in the general population: strategies based on combinations of autoantibody markers. *Diabetes* 1997;46:1701–1710.
76. Wagner R, McNally JM, Bonifacio E, et al. Lack of immunohistological changes in the islets of nondiabetic, autoimmune, polyendocrine patients with β-selective GAD-specific islet cell antibodies. *Diabetes* 1994;43:851–856.
77. Srikanta S, Ganda OP, Jackson RA, et al. Type I diabetes mellitus in monozygotic twins: chronic progressive beta cell dysfunction. *Ann Intern Med* 1983; 99:320–326.
78. Srikanta S, Ganda OP, Rabizadeh A, et al. First-degree relatives of patients with type I diabetes mellitus. Islet cell antibodies and abnormal insulin secretion. *N Engl J Med* 1985;313:461–464.
79. Colman PG, McNair P, Steele C, et al. Linear decline in insulin production prior to development of type 1 diabetes—a reality. *Diabetes* 2000;49:A36(abst).

80. Gazda LS, Charlton B, Lafferty KJ. Diabetes results from a late change in the autoimmune response of NOD mice. *J Autoimmun* 1997;10:261–270.
81. Shimada A, Charlton B, Taylor-Edwards C, et al. β-cell destruction may be a late consequence of the autoimmune process in nonobese diabetic mice. *Diabetes* 1996;45:1063–1067.
82. McCulloch DK, Raghu PK, Johnston C, et al. Defects in beta-cell function and insulin sensitivity in normoglycemic streptozotocin-treated baboons: a model of preclinical insulin-dependent diabetes. *J Clin Endocrinol Metab* 1988; 67:785–792.
83. Sutherland DE, Sibley R, Xu XA, et al. Twin-to-twin pancreas transplantation: reversal and reenactment of the pathogenesis of type I diabetes. *Trans Assoc Am Physicians* 1984;97:80–87.
84. Foulis AK, Liddle CN, Farquharson MA, et al. The histopathology of the pancreas in type I diabetes (insulin dependent) mellitus: a 25-year review of deaths in patients under 20 years of age in the United Kingdom. *Diabetologia* 1986;29:267–274.
85. Eisenbarth GS. Genetic basis of autoimmune diabetes. In: Williams G, Habener JF, eds. *Metabolic basis of common inherited diseases*. Philadelphia: Harcourt Health Sciences/WB Saunders, 2003.
86. Hawkes CH. Twin studies in diabetes mellitus. *Diabet Med* 1997;17:347–352.
87. Petersen JS, Kyvik KO, Bingley PJ, et al. Population based study of prevalence of islet cell autoantibodies in monozygotic and dizygotic Danish twin pairs with insulin dependent diabetes mellitus. *BMJ* 1997;314:1575–1579.
88. Ikegami H, Ogihara T. Genetics of insulin-dependent diabetes mellitus. *Endocrinol J* 1996;43:605–613.
89. Kyvik KO, Green A, Beck-Nielsen H. Concordance rates of insulin dependent diabetes mellitus: a population based study of young Danish twins. *BMJ* 1995;311:913–917.
90. Fava D, Gardner S, Pyke D, et al. Evidence that the age at diagnosis of IDDM is genetically determined. *Diabetes Care* 1998;21:925–929.
91. Redondo MJ, Yu L, Hawa M, et al. Heterogeneity of type 1 diabetes: analysis of monozygotic twins in Great Britain and the United States. *Diabetologia*, 2001;44:354–362.
92. Hawa M, Rowe R, Lan MS, et al. Value of antibodies to islet protein tyrosine phosphatase-like molecule in predicting type 1 diabetes. *Diabetes* 1997;46: 1270–1275.
93. El-Hashimy M, Angelico MC, Martin BC, et al. Factors modifying the risk of IDDM in offspring of an IDDM parent. *Diabetes* 1995;44:295–299.
94. Rewers M, Ziegler A. Primary prevention of type 1 diabetes. Presented at the Fourth Congress of the Immunology of Diabetes Society, November 10–15, 1999.
95. Pugliese A. Unraveling the genetics of insulin-dependent type 1A diabetes: the search must go on. *Diabetes Rev* 1999;7:39–54.
96. Lernmark Å, Ott J. Sometimes it's hot, sometimes it's not. *Nat Genet* 1998;19: 213–214.
97. Pugliese A, Eisenbarth GS, Type 1 diabetes mellitus of man: genetic susceptibility and resistance. In: Eisenbarth GS, ed. *Type 1 diabetes: molecular, cellular, and clinical immunology*. New York: Oxford University Press, 1996:134–152.
98. Bodmer JG, Marsh SG, Albert ED, et al. Nomenclature for factors of the HLA system, 1996. *Hum Immunol* 1997;53:98–128.
99. Raum D, Awdeh Z, Yunis EJ, et al. Extended major histocompatibility complex haplotypes in type I diabetes mellitus. *J Clin Invest* 1996;4:449–454.
100. Valdes AM, Thomson G. Detecting disease-predisposing variants: the haplotype method. *Am J Hum Genet* 1997;60:703–716.
101. Price P, Witt C, Allcock R, et al. The genetic basis for the association of the 8.1 ancestral haplotype (A1,B8,DR3) with multiple immunopathological diseases. *Immunol Rev* 1999;167:257–274.
102. Lau HT, Yu M, Fontana A, et al. Prevention of islet allograft rejection with engineered myoblasts expressing FasL in mice. *Science* 1996;273:109–112.
103. Dawkins RL, Martin E, Saueracker G, et al. Supratypes and ancestral haplotypes in IDDM: potential importance of central non-HLA MHC genes. *J Autoimmun* 1990;3:63–68.
104. Horton V, Stratton I, Bottazzo GF, et al. Genetic heterogeneity of autoimmune diabetes: age of presentation in adults is influenced by HLA DRB1 and DQB1 genotypes (UKPDS 43). UK Prospective Diabetes Study (UKPDS) Group. *Diabetologia* 1999;42:608–616.
105. Van der Auwera B, Van Waeyenberge C, Schuit F, et al, and Belgian Diabetes Registry. DRB1*0403 protects against IDDM in Caucasians with the high-risk heterozygous DQA1*0301-DQB1*0302/DQA1*501-DQB1*0201 genotype. *Diabetes* 1995;44:527–530.
106. Huang W, She J-X, Muir A, et al. High risk HLA-DR/DQ genotypes for IDD confer susceptibility to autoantibodies but DQB1*0602 does not prevent them. *J Autoimmun* 1994;7:889–897.
107. Ronningen KS, Spurkland A, Iwe T, et al. Distribution of HLA-DRB1, -DQA1 and -DQB1 alleles and DQA1-DQB1 genotypes among Norwegian patients with insulin-dependent diabetes mellitus. *Tissue Antigens* 1991;37:105–111.
108. Baisch JM, Weeks T, Giles R, et al. Analysis of HLA-DQ genotypes and susceptibility in insulin-dependent diabetes mellitus. *N Engl J Med* 1990;22: 1836–1841.
109. Kockum I, Sanjeevi CB, Eastman S, et al. Population analysis of protection by HLA-DR and DQ genes from insulin-dependent diabetes mellitus in Swedish children with insulin-dependent diabetes and controls. *Eur J Immunogenet* 1995;22:443–465.
110. Tait BD, Mraz G, Harrison LC. Association of HLA-DQw3 (TA10-) with type 1 diabetes occurs with DR3/4 but not DR1/4 patients. *Diabetes* 1987;37: 926–929.
111. Awata T, Kuzuya T, Matsuda A, et al. Genetic analysis of HLA class II alleles and susceptibility to type I (insulin-dependent) diabetes mellitus in Japanese subjects. *Diabetologia* 1992;35:419–424.
112. Rich SS, Reusch J, Panter S, et al. Is there a genetic connection between IDDM and NIDDM? *Diabetes* 1986;35:95.
113. Park Y, Erlich H, Noble J, et al. Identical transmission pattern of HLA DRB1/DQB1 haplotypes to patients with type 1A diabetes among Koreans and Caucasians. *Diabetes* 1998;7:27A(abst).
114. Khalil I, D'Auriol L, Gobet M, et al. A combination of HLA-DQ beta Asp 57-negative and HLA-DQ alpha Arg 52 confers susceptibility to insulin-dependent diabetes mellitus. *J Clin Invest* 1990;85:1315–1319.
115. Kawasaki E, Noble J, Erlich H, et al. Transmission of DQ haplotypes to patients with type 1 diabetes. *Diabetes* 1998;47:1971–1973.
116. Lie BA, Ronningen KS, Akselsen HE, et al. Application and interpretation of transmission/disequilibrium tests: transmission of HLA-DQ haplotypes to unaffected siblings in 526 families with type 1 diabetes. *Am J Hum Genet* 2000; 66:740–743.
117. Undlien DE, Kockum I, Ronningen KS, et al. HLA associations in type 1 diabetes among patients not carrying high-risk DR3-DQ2 or DR4-DQ8 haplotypes. *Tissue Antigens* 1999;54:543–551.
118. Pugliese A, Kawasaki E, Zeller M, et al. Sequence analysis of the diabetes-protective human leukocyte antigen-DQB1*0602 allele in unaffected, islet cell antibody-positive first degree relatives and in rare patients with type 1 diabetes. *J Clin Endocrinol Metab* 1999;84:1722–1728.
119. Hattori M, Buse JB, Jackson RA, et al. The NOD mouse: recessive diabetogenic gene within the major histocompatibility complex. *Science* 1986;231: 733–735.
120. Acha-Orbea H, McDevitt HO. The first external domain of the nonobese diabetic mouse class II I-A chain is unique. *Proc Natl Acad Sci U S A* 1987;84: 2435–2439.
121. Redondo MJ, Kawasaki E, Mulgrew CL, et al. DR and DQ associated protection from type 1 diabetes: comparison of DRB1*1401 and DQA1*0102-DQB1*0602. *J Clin Endocrinol Metab* 2000;85:3793–3797.
122. Greenbaum CJ, Cuthbertson D, Eisenbarth GS, et al. Islet cell antibody positive relatives with HLA-DQA1*0102, DQB1*0602: identification by the Diabetes Prevention Trial-1. *J Clin Endocrinol Metab* 2000;85:1255–1260.
123. Sheehy MJ, Scharf SJ, Rowe JR, et al. A diabetes-susceptible HLA haplotype is best defined by a combination of HLA-DR and -DQ alleles. *J Clin Invest* 1989;83:830–835.
124. Nakanishi K, Kobayashi T, Murase T, et al. Human leukocyte antigen-A24 and -DQA1*0301 in Japanese insulin-dependent diabetes mellitus: independent contributions to susceptibility to the disease and additive contributions to acceleration of beta-cell destruction. *J Clin Endocrinol Metab* 1999;84:3721–3725.
125. Noble JA, Valdes AM, Thomson G, et al. The HLA class II locus DPB1 can influence susceptibility to type 1 diabetes. *Diabetes* 2000;49:121–125.
126. Lie BA, Akselsen HE, Jones G, et al. HLA association in insulin-dependent diabetes mellitus: no independent association to particular DP genes. *Hum Immunol* 1997;55:170–175.
127. Bell GI, Horita S, Karam JH. A polymorphic locus near the human insulin gene is associated with insulin-dependent diabetes mellitus. *Diabetes* 1984;33: 176–183.
128. Bennett ST, Lucassen AM, Gough SCL, et al. Susceptibility to human type I diabetes at IDDM2 is determined by tandem repeat variation at the insulin gene minisatellite locus. *Nat Genet* 1995;9:284–292.
129. Bennett ST, Wilson AJ, Cucca F, et al. IDDM2-VNTR-encoded susceptibility to type 1 diabetes: dominant protection and parental transmission of alleles of the insulin gene-linked minisatellite locus. *J Autoimmun* 1996;9:415–421.
130. Vafiadis P, Bennett ST, Todd JA, et al. Insulin expression in human thymus is modulated by INS VNTR alleles at the IDDM2 locus. *Nat Genet* 1997;15: 289–292.
131. Pugliese A, Zeller M, Fernandez A, et al. The insulin gene is transcribed in the human thymus and transcription levels correlate with allelic variation at the INS VNTR-IDDM2 susceptibility locus for type I diabetes. *Nat Genet* 1997;15:293–297.
132. Hanahan D. Peripheral-antigen-expressing cells in thymic medulla: factors in self-tolerance and autoimmunity. *Curr Opin Immunol* 1998;10:656–662.
133. Smith KM, Olson DC, Hirose R, et al. Pancreatic gene expression in rare cells of thymic medulla: evidence for functional contribution to T cell tolerance. *Int Immunol* 1997;9:1355–1365.
134. Leiter EH. Lessons from the animal models: the NOD mouse. In: Palmer JP, ed. *Prediction, prevention, and genetic counseling in IDDM*. Chichester, England: Wiley, 1996:201–227.
135. Atkinson MA, Leiter EH. The NOD mouse model of type 1 diabetes: as good as it gets? *Nat Med* 1999;5:601–604.
136. Wicker LS, Todd JA, Peterson LB. Genetic control of autoimmune diabetes in the NOD mouse. *Annu Rev Immunol* 1995;13:179–200.
137. Martin AM, Maxson MN, Leif J, et al. Diabetes-prone and diabetes-resistant BB rats share a common major diabetes susceptibility locus, iddm4: additional evidence for a "universal autoimmunity locus" on rat chromosome 4. *Diabetes* 1999;48:2138–2144.
138. Kawano K, Hirashima T, Moris S, et al. New inbred strain of Long-Evans Tokushima lean rats with IDDM without lymphopenia. *Diabetes* 1991;40: 1375–1381.
139. Verge CF, Vardi P, Babu S, et al. Evidence for oligogenic inheritance of type 1A diabetes in a large Bedouin Arab family. *J Clin Invest* 1998;102:1569–1575.
140. Larsen ZM, Kristiansen OP, Mato E, et al. IDDM12 (CTLA4) on 2q33 and IDDM13 on 2q34 in genetic susceptibility to type 1 diabetes (insulin-dependent). *Autoimmunity* 1999;31:35–42.

141. Donner H, Rau H, Walfish PG, et al. CTLA4 alanine-17 confers genetic susceptibility to Graves' disease and to type-1 diabetes mellitus. *J Clin Endocrinol Metab* 1997;82:143–146.
142. Marron MP, Raffel LJ, Garchon HJ, et al. Insulin-dependent diabetes mellitus (IDDM) is associated with CTLA4 polymorphisms in multiple ethnic groups. *Hum Mol Genet* 1997;6:1275–1282.
143. Todd JA, Farrall M. Panning for gold: genome-wide scanning for linkage in type I diabetes. *Hum Mol Genet* 1996;5:1443–1448.
144. She J-X, Marron MP. Genetic susceptibility factors in type 1 diabetes: linkage disequilibrium and functional analyses. *Curr Opin Immunol* 1998;10:682–689.
145. Concannon P, Gogolin-Ewens KJ, Hinds DA, et al. A second-generation screen of the human genome for susceptibility to insulin-dependent diabetes mellitus. *Nat Genet* 1998;19:292–296.
145a. Bottini N, Muscumeci L, Alonso A, et al. A functional variant of lymphoid tyrosine phosphatase is associated with type 1 diabetes. *Nat Genet* 2004;36: 337–338.
146. Copeman JB, Cucca F, Hearne CM, et al. Linkage disequilibrium mapping of type 1 diabetes susceptibility gene (IDDM7) to chromosome 2q31-q33. *Nat Genet* 1995;9:80–85.
147. Luo D-F, Bui MM, Muir A, et al. Affected-sib-pair mapping of a novel susceptibility gene to insulin-dependent diabetes mellitus (IDDM8) on chromosome 6q25-q27. *Am J Hum Genet* 1995;57:911–919.
148. Field LL, Tobias R, Thomson G, et al. Susceptibility to insulin-dependent diabetes mellitus maps to a locus (IDDM11) on human chromosome 14q24.3-q31. *Genomics* 1996;33:1–8.
149. Morahan G, Huang D, Tait BD, et al. Markers on distal chromosome 2q linked to insulin-dependent diabetes mellitus. *Science* 1996;272:1811–1813.
150. Atkinson MA, Maclaren NK, Luchetta R. Insulitis and diabetes in NOD mice reduced by prophylactic insulin therapy. *Diabetes* 1990;39:933–937.
151. Daniel D, Wegmann DR. Protection of nonobese diabetic mice from diabetes by intranasal or subcutaneous administration of insulin peptide B-(9-23). *Proc Natl Acad Sci U S A* 1996;93:956–960.
152. Hamman RF, Cook M, Keefer S, et al. Medical care patterns at the onset of insulin-dependent diabetes mellitus: association with severity and subsequent complications. *Diabetes Care* 1985;8:94–100.
153. Karjalajnen S, Salema P, Ilonen J. A comparison of childhood and adult type 1 diabetes mellitus. *N Engl J Med* 1989;320:881–886.
154. Levy-Marchal C, Papoz L, de Beaufort C, et al. Clinical and laboratory features of type I diabetic children at time of diagnosis. *Diabet Med* 1992;9: 279–284.
155. Karvonen M, Tuomilehto J, Libman I, et al, and WHO DIAMOND Project Group. A review of the recent epidemiological data on the worldwide incidence of type 1 (insulin-dependent) diabetes mellitus. *Diabetologia* 1993;36: 883–892.
156. Rewers M, Norris JM. Epidemiology of type I diabetes. In: Eisenbarth GS, Lafferty KJ, eds. *Type I diabetes: molecular, cellular, and clinical immunology*. New York: Oxford University Press, 1996:172–208.
157. Karvonen M, Pitkaniemi J, Tuomilehtov J. The onset age of type 1 diabetes in Finnish children has become younger. The Finnish Childhood Diabetes Registry Group. *Diabetes Care* 1999;22:1066–1070.
158. Muntoni S. New insights into the epidemiology of type 1 diabetes in Mediterranean countries. *Diabetes Metab Res Rev* 1999;15:133–140.
159. Dorman JS, McCarthy B, McCanlies E, et al, and the WHO DiaMond Molecular Epidemiology Sub-Project Group. Molecular IDDM epidemiology: international studies. *Diabetes Res Clin Pract* 1996;34:S17–S23.
160. Eisenbarth GS, Elsey C, Yu L, et al. Infantile anti-islet autoimmunity: DAISY study. *Diabetes* 1998;45[Suppl 1]:A219(abstr).
160a. Norris JM, Barriga K, Klingensmith G, et al. Timing of cereal exposure in infancy and risk of islet autoimmunity. The Diabetes Autoimmunity Study in the Young (DAISY). *JAMA* 2003;290:1713–1720.
160b. Ziegler AG, Schmid S, Huber D, et al. Early infant feeding and risk of developing type 1 diabetes-associated autoantibodies. *JAMA* 2003;290: 1721–1728.
161. Ou D, Jonsen LA, Metzger DL, et al. CD4+ and CD8+ T-cell clones from congenital rubella syndrome patients with IDDM recognize overlapping GAD65 protein epitopes. Implications for HLA class I and II allelic linkage to disease susceptibility. *Hum Immunol* 1999;60:652–664.
162. Shaver KA, Boughman JA, Nance WE. Congenital rubella syndrome and diabetes: a review of epidemiologic, genetic, and immunologic factors. *Am Ann Deaf* 1985;130:526–532.
163. Ginsberg-Fellner F, Witt ME, Yagihashi S, et al. Congenital rubella syndrome as a model for type I (insulin-dependent) diabetes mellitus: increased prevalence of islet cell surface antibodies. *Diabetologia* 1984;27[Suppl]:87–89.
164. Rossini AA, Greiner DL, Friedman HP, et al. Immunopathogenesis of diabetes mellitus. *Diabetes Rev* 1993;1:43–75.
165. Jackson R, Rassi N, Crump A, et al. The BB diabetic rat. Profound T-cell lymphocytopenia. *Diabetes* 1981;30:887–889.
166. Jackson RA, Buse JB, Rifai R, et al. Two genes required for diabetes in BB rats. Evidence from cyclical intercrosses and backcrosses. *J Exp Med* 1984;159:1629–1636.
167. Markholst H, Eastman S, Wilson D, et al. Diabetes segregates as a single locus in crosses between inbred BB rats prone or resistant to diabetes. *J Exp Med* 1991;174:297–300.
168. Awata T, Guberski DL, Like AA. Genetics of the BB rat: association of autoimmune disorders (diabetes, insulitis, and thyroiditis) with lymphopenia and major histocompatibility complex class II. *Endocrinology* 1995;136: 5731–5735.
169. Jacob HJ, Pettersson A, Wilson D, et al. Genetic dissection of autoimmune type I diabetes in the BB rat. *Nat Genet* 1992;2:56–60.
170. Ellerman KE, Like AA. Susceptibility to diabetes is widely distributed in normal class IIu haplotype rats. *Diabetologia* 2000;43:890–898.
171. Daneman D, Fishman L, Clarson C, et al. Dietary triggers of insulin-dependent diabetes in the BB rat. *Diabetes Res* 1987;5:93–97.
172. Reddy S, Bibby NJ, Wu D, et al. A combined casein-free-nicotinamide diet prevents diabetes in the NOD mouse with minimum insulitis. *Diabetes Res Clin Pract* 1995;29:83–92.
173. Scott FW, Sarwar G, Cloutier HE. Diabetogenicity of various protein sources in the diet of the diabetes-prone BB rat. *Adv Exp Med Biol* 1988;246:277–285.
174. Helmke K, Otten A, Willems WR, et al. Islet cell antibodies and the development of diabetes mellitus in relation to mumps infection and mumps vaccination. *Diabetologia* 1986;29:30–33.
175. Bodansky HJ, Grant PJ, Dean BM, et al. Islet-cell antibodies and insulin autoantibodies in association with common viral infections. *Lancet* 1986;2: 1351–1353.
176. Champsaur H, Bottazzo GF, Bertrams J, et al. Virologic, immunologic and genetic factors in insulin-dependent diabetes mellitus. *J Pediatr* 1982;100: 15–20.
177. Uriarte A, Cabrera E, Ventura R, et al. Islet cell antibodies and ECHO-4 virus infection. *Diabetologia* 1987;30:590A(abst).
178. Rubinstein P, Walker ME, Fedun B, et al. The HLA system in congenital rubella patients with and without diabetes. *Diabetes* 1982;31:1088–1091.
179. Dahlquist G, Källén B. Early neonatal events and the disease incidence in nonobese diabetic mice. *Pediatr Res* 1997;42:489–491.
180. Hyöty H, Hiltunen M, Knip M, et al, and The Childhood Diabetes in Finland (DiMe) Study Group. A prospective study of the role of coxsackie B and other enterovirus infections in the pathogenesis of IDDM. *Diabetes* 1995;44:652–657.
181. Clements GB, Galbraith DN, Taylor KW. Coxsackie B virus infection and onset of childhood diabetes. *Lancet* 1995;346:221–223.
182. Dahlquist GG, Ivarsson S, Lindberg B, et al. Maternal enteroviral infection during pregnancy as a risk factor for childhood IDDM. A population-based case-control study. *Diabetes* 1995;44:408–413.
183. Kaufman DL, Erlander MG, Clare-Salzler M, et al. Autoimmunity to two forms of glutamate decarboxylase in insulin-dependent diabetes mellitus. *J Clin Invest* 1992;89:283–292.
184. Graves PM, Rewers M. The role of enteroviral infections in the development of IDDM: limitations of current approaches. *Diabetes* 1997;46:161–168.
185. Oldstone MB, Nerenberg M, Southern P, et al. Virus infection triggers insulin-dependent diabetes mellitus in a transgenic model: role of anti-self (virus) immune response. *Cell* 1991;65:319–331.
186. Ohashi P, Oehen SH, Buerki K, et al. Ablation of "tolerance" and induction of diabetes by virus infection in viral antigen transgenic mice. *Cell* 1991;65: 305–317.
187. Rewers M, Atkinson M. The possible role of enteroviruses in diabetes mellitus. In: Rotbart HA, ed. *Human enterovirus infections*. Washington, DC: American Society for Microbiology, 1996:353–385.
188. Dahlquist G. Environmental risk factors in human type 1 diabetes—an epidemiological perspective. *Diabetes Metab Rev* 1998;11:37–46.
189. Graves PM, Barriga KJ, Norris JM, et al. Lack of association between early childhood immunizations and beta-cell autoimmunity. *Diabetes Care* 1999;22: 1694–1697.
190. Juhela S, Hyoty H, Roivainen M, et al. T-cell responses to enterovirus antigens in children with type 1 diabetes. *Diabetes* 2000;49:1308–1313.
191. Honeyman MC, Coulson BS, Stone NL, et al. Association between rotavirus infection and pancreatic islet autoimmunity in children at risk of developing type 1 diabetes. *Diabetes* 2000;49:1319–1324.
192. Allen HF, Klingensmith GJ, Jensen P, et al. Effect of BCG vaccination on new-onset insulin-dependent diabetes mellitus: a randomized clinical study. *Diabetes Care* 1998;22:1703–1707.
193. Pozzilli P. BCG vaccine in insulin-dependent diabetes mellitus. IMDIAB Group. *Lancet* 1997;349:1520–1521.
194. Jefferson T. Real or perceived adverse effects of vaccines and the media—a tale of our times [Editorial]. *J Epidemiol Community Health* 2000;54:402–403.
195. Borch-Johnsen K, Joner G, Mandrup-Poulsen J, et al. Relation between breast-feeding and incidence rates of insulin-dependent diabetes mellitus. A hypothesis. *Lancet* 1984;2:1083–1086.
196. Martin JM, Trink B, Daneman D, et al. Milk proteins in the etiology of insulin-dependent diabetes mellitus (IDDM). *Ann Med* 1991;23:447–452.
197. Karjalainen J, Martin JM, Knip M, et al. A bovine albumin peptide as a possible trigger of insulin-dependent diabetes mellitus. *N Engl J Med* 1992;327:302–307.
198. Atkinson MA, Bowman MA, Kao K, et al. Lack of immune responsiveness to bovine serum albumin in insulin-dependent diabetes. *N Engl J Med* 1993;329: 1853–1858.
199. Glatthaar C, Whittall DE, Welborn TA, et al. Diabetes in Western Australian children: descriptive epidemiology. *Med J Aust* 1988;148:117–123.
200. Metcalfe MA, Baum JD. Family characteristics and insulin dependent diabetes. *Arch Dis Child* 1992;67:731–736.
201. Mayer ES, Hamman RF, Gay EC, et al. Reduced risk of IDDM among breast-fed children: The Colorado IDDM Registry. *Diabetes* 1988;37:1625–1632.
202. Kostraba JN, Dorman JS, LaPorte RE, et al. Early infant diet and risk of IDDM in blacks and whites. A matched case-control study. *Diabetes Care* 1992;15: 626–631.
203. Kostraba JN, Cruickshanks KJ, Lawler-Heavner J, et al. Early exposure to cow's milk and solid foods in infancy, genetic predisposition and risk of IDDM. *Diabetes* 1993;42:288–295.

204. Patterson CC, Carson DJ, Hadden DR, et al. A case-control investigation of perinatal risk factors for childhood IDDM in Northern Ireland and Scotland. *Diabetes Care* 1994;17:376–381.
205. Blom L, Dahlquist G, Nystrom L, et al. The Swedish childhood diabetes study—social and perinatal determinants for diabetes in childhood. *Diabetologia* 1989;32:7–13.
206. Fort P, Lanes R, Dahlem S, et al. Breast feeding and insulin-dependent diabetes mellitus in children. *J Am Coll Nutr* 1986;5:439–441.
207. Siemiatycki J, Colle E, Campbell S, et al. Case-control study of IDDM. *Diabetes Care* 1989;12:209–216.
208. Kyvik KO, Green A, Svendsen A, et al. Breast feeding and the development of type 1 diabetes mellitus. *Diabet Med* 1991;9:233–235.
209. Bodington MJ, McNally PG, Burden AC. Cow's milk and type I childhood diabetes: no increase in risk. *Diabet Med* 1994;11:663–665.
210. Samuelsson U, Johansson C, Ludvigsson J. Breast-feeding seems to play a marginal role in the prevention of insulin-dependent diabetes mellitus. *Diabetes Res Clin Pract* 1993;19:203–210.
211. Soltesz G, Jeges S, Dahlquist G. Non-genetic risk determinants for type 1 (insulin-dependent) diabetes mellitus in childhood. Hungarian Childhood Diabetes Epidemiology Study Group. *Acta Paediatr* 1994;83:730–735.
212. Nigro G, Campea L, De Novellis A, et al. Breast-feeding and insulin-dependent diabetes mellitus [Letter]. *Lancet* 1985;1:467.
213. Virtanen SM, Rasanen L, Aro A, et al. Infant feeding in Finnish children less than 7 yr of age with newly diagnosed IDDM. Childhood Diabetes in Finland Study Group. *Diabetes Care* 1991;14:415–417.
214. Virtanen SM, Rasanen L, Aro A, et al. Feeding in infancy and the risk of type 1 diabetes mellitus in Finnish children. The Childhood Diabetes in Finland Study Group. *Diabet Med* 1992;9:815–819.
215. Verge CF, Howard NJ, Irwig L, et al. Environmental factors in childhood IDDM. A population-based, case-control study. *Diabetes Care* 1994;17:1381–1389.
216. Gerstein HC. Cow's milk exposure and type I diabetes mellitus—a critical overview of the clinical literature. *Diabetes Care* 1994;17:13–19.
217. Vobecky JS, Vobecky J, Froda S. The reliability of the maternal memory in a retrospective assessment of nutritional status. *J Clin Epidemiol* 1988;41: 261–265.
218. Golding J, Haslum M. Breast-feeding and diabetes [Letter]. *Med Sci Res* 1987; 15:1135.
219. Norris JM, Beaty B, Klingensmith G, et al. Lack of association between early exposure to cow's milk protein and β-cell autoimmunity: Diabetes Autoimmunity Study in the Young (DAISY). *JAMA* 1996;276:609–614.
220. Akerblom HK, Savilahti E, Saukkonen TT, et al. The case for elimination of cow's milk in early infancy in the prevention of type 1 diabetes: the Finnish experience. *Diabetes Metab Rev* 1993;9:269–278.
221. Gerstein HC, Simpson JR, Atkinson S, et al. Feasibility and acceptability of a proposed infant feeding intervention trial for the prevention of type I diabetes. *Diabetes Care* 1995;18:940–942.
222. Martikainen A, Saukkonen T, Kulmala PK, et al. Disease-associated antibodies in offspring of mothers with IDDM. *Diabetes* 1996;45:1706–1710.
223. Schein PS, Alberti KG, Williamson DH. Effects of streptozotocin on carbohydrate and lipid metabolism in the rat. *Endocrinology* 1971;89:827–834.
224. Banerjee S. Effect of certain substances of the prevention of diabetogenic action of alloxan. *Science* 1947;128–130.
225. Pont A, Rubino JM, Bishop D, et al. Diabetes mellitus and neuropathy following Vacor ingestion in man. *Arch Intern Med* 1979;139:185–187.
226. Virtanen SM, Jaakkola L, Rasanen L, et al, and The Childhood Diabetes in Finland Study Group. Nitrate and nitrite intake and the risk for type I diabetes in Finnish children. *Diabet Med* 1994;11:656–662.
227. Kostraba JN, Gay EC, Rewers M, et al. Nitrate levels in community drinking waters and risk of IDDM. *Diabetes Care* 1992;15:1505–1508.
228. Dahlquist GG, Blom LG, Persson LA, et al. Dietary factors and the risk of developing insulin dependent diabetes in childhood. *BMJ* 1990;300: 1302–1306.
229. Elias D, Prigozin H, Polak N, et al. Autoimmune diabetes induced by the beta-cell toxin STZ. Immunity to the 60-kDa heat shock protein and to insulin. *Diabetes* 1994;43:992–998.
230. Toniolo A, Onodera T, Yoon JW, et al. Induction of diabetes by cumulative environmental insults from viruses and chemicals. *Nature* 1980;288:383–385.
231. Douek IF, Leech NJ, Gillmor HA, et al. Children with type-1 diabetes and their unaffected siblings have fewer symptoms of asthma. *Lancet* 1999;353: 1850.
232. Blom L, Nystrom L, Dahlquist G. The Swedish childhood diabetes study. Vaccinations and infections as risk determinants for diabetes in childhood. *Diabetologia* 1991;34:176–181.
233. Abiru N, Eisenbarth GS. Autoantibodies and autoantigens in type 1 diabetes: role in pathogenesis, prediction and prevention. *Can J Diabetes Care* 1999;23: 59–65.
234. Bonifacio E. Humoral immune markers: islet cell antibodies. In: Palmer JP, ed. *Prediction, prevention, and genetic counseling in IDDM.* Chichester, England: Wiley, 1996:43–62.
235. Christie MR. Humoral immune markers: antibodies to glutamic acid decarboxylase. In: Palmer JP, ed. *Prediction, prevention, and genetic counseling in IDDM.* Chichester, England: Wiley, 1996:77–96.
236. Gorsuch AN, Spencer KM, Lister J, et al. Can future type I diabetes be predicted? A study in families of affected children. *Diabetes* 1982;31:862–866.
237. Gorsuch AN, Spencer KM, Lister J, et al. Evidence for a long prediabetic period in type I (insulin-dependent) diabetes mellitus. *Lancet* 1981;2: 1363–1365.
238. Srikanta S, Ganda OP, Eisenbarth GS, et al. Islet cell antibodies and beta cell function in monozygotic triplets and twins initially discordant for type I diabetes mellitus. *N Engl J Med* 1983;308:322–325.
239. Dotta F, Gianani R, Previti M, et al. Autoimmunity to the GM2-1 islet ganglioside before and at the onset of type I diabetes. *Diabetes* 1996;45:1193–1196.
240. Yu L, Gianani R. GAD autoantibody levels in ICA positive relatives with restricted ICA. *Diabetes* 1993;42:65A(abst).
241. Seissler J, de Sonnaville JJ, Morgenthaler NG, et al. Immunological heterogeneity in type I diabetes: presence of distinct autoantibody patterns in patients with acute onset and slowly progressive disease. *Diabetologia* 1998;41:891–897.
242. Maclaren N, Lan M, Coutant R, et al. Only multiple autoantibodies to islet cells (ICA), insulin, GAD65, IA-2 and IA-2beta predict immune-mediated (type 1) diabetes in relatives. *J Autoimmun* 1999;12:279–287.
243. Verge CF, Gianani R, Kawasaki E, et al. Number of autoantibodies (against insulin, GAD or ICA512/IA2) rather than particular autoantibody specificities determines risk of type I diabetes. *J Autoimmun* 1996;9:379–383.
244. Bonifacio E, Genovese S, Braghi S, et al. Islet autoantibody markers in IDDM: risk assessment strategies yielding high sensitivity. *Diabetologia* 1995;38: 816–822.
245. Palmer JP, Asplin CM, Clemons P, et al. Insulin antibodies in insulin-dependent diabetics before insulin treatment. *Science* 1983;222:1337–1339.
246. Castano L, Ziegler AG, Ziegler R, et al. Characterization of insulin autoantibodies in relatives of patients with type 1 diabetes. *Diabetes* 1993;42: 1202–1209.
247. Bohmer K, Keilacker H, Kuglin B, et al. Proinsulin autoantibodies are more closely associated with type 1 (insulin-dependent) diabetes mellitus than insulin autoantibodies. *Diabetologia* 1991;34:830–834.
248. Greenbaum C, Palmer JP, Kuglin B, et al, and Participating Laboratories. Insulin autoantibodies measured by radioimmunoassay methodology are more related to insulin-dependent diabetes mellitus than those measured by enzyme-linked immunosorbent assay: results of the Fourth International Workshop on the Standardization of Insulin Autoantibody Measurement. *J Clin Endocrinol Metab* 1992;74:1040–1044.
249. Williams AJK, Bingley PJ, Bonifacio E, et al. A novel micro-assay for insulin autoantibodies. *J Autoimmun* 1997;10:473–478.
250. Naserke HE, Dozio N, Ziegler A-G, et al. Comparison of a novel micro-assay for insulin autoantibodies with the conventional radiobinding assay. *Diabetologia* 1998;41:681–683.
251. Bilbao JR, Calvo B, Urrutia I, et al. Anti-insulin activity in normal newborn cord-blood serum: absence of IgG-mediated insulin binding. *Diabetes* 1997; 46:713–716.
252. Naserke HE, Bonifacio E, Ziegler A-G. Immunoglobulin G insulin autoantibodies in BABYDIAB offspring appear postnatally: sensitive early detection using a protein A/G-based radiobinding assay. *J Clin Endocrinol Metab* 1999; 84:1239–1243.
253. Yu L, Robles DT, Abiru N, et al. Early expression of anti-insulin autoantibodies of man and the NOD mouse: evidence for early determination of subsequent diabetes. *Proc Natl Acad Sci U S A* 2000;97:1701–1706.
254. Arslanian SL, Becker DJ, Rabin B, et al. Correlates of insulin antibodies in newly diagnosed children with insulin-dependent diabetes before insulin therapy. *Diabetes* 1985;34:926–930.
255. Vardi P, Ziegler AG, Matthews JH, et al. Concentration of insulin autoantibodies at onset of type I diabetes. Inverse log-linear correlation with age. *Diabetes Care* 1988;11:736–739.
256. Eisenbarth GS, Gianani R, Yu L, et al. Dual parameter model for prediction of type 1 diabetes mellitus. *Proc Assoc Am Physicians* 1998;110:126–135.
257. Bonifacio E, Scirpoli M, Kredel K, et al. Early autoantibody responses in prediabetes are IgG1 dominated and suggest antigen-specific regulation. *J Immunol* 1999;163:525–532.
258. Kimpimaki T, Kulmala P, Savola K, et al. Disease-associated autoantibodies as surrogate markers of type 1 diabetes in young children at increased genetic risk. Childhood Diabetes in Finland Study Group. *J Clin Endocrinol Metab* 2000;85:1126–1132.
259. Colman PG, McNair P, Margetts H, et al. The Melbourne Pre-Diabetes Study: prediction of type 1 diabetes mellitus using antibody and metabolic testing. *Med J Aust* 1998;169:81–84.
260. Baekkeskov S, Aanstoot H-J, Christgau S, et al. Identification of the 64K autoantigen in insulin-dependent diabetes as the GABA-synthesizing enzyme glutamic acid decarboxylase [published erratum appears in *Nature* 1990;347:782]. *Nature* 1990;347:151–156.
261. Solimena M, DeCamilli P. Autoimmunity to glutamic acid decarboxylase (GAD) in stiff-man syndrome and insulin-dependent diabetes mellitus. *Trends Neurosci* 1991;14:452–457.
262. Schwartz HL, Chandonia JM, Kash SF, et al. High-resolution autoreactive epitope mapping and structural modeling of the 65 kDa form of human glutamic acid decarboxylase. *J Mol Biol* 1999;287:983–999.
263. Rabin DU, Pleasic SM, Palmer-Crocker R, et al. Cloning and expression of IDDM-specific human autoantigens. *Diabetes* 1992;41:183–186.
264. Rabin DU, Pleasic SM, Shapiro JA, et al. Islet cell antigen 512 is a diabetes-specific islet autoantigen related to protein tyrosine phosphatases. *J Immunol* 1994;152:3183–3188.
265. Kawasaki E, Yu L, Gianani R, et al. Evaluation of islet cell antigen (ICA) 512/IA-2 autoantibody radioassays using overlapping ICA512/IA-2 constructs. *J Clin Endocrinol Metab* 1997;82:375–380.
266. Lan MS, Lu J, Goto Y, Notkins AL. Molecular cloning and identification of a receptor-type protein tyrosine phosphatase, IA-2, from human insulinoma. *DNA Cell Biol* 1994;13:505–514.

267. Lu J, Li Q, Xie H, et al. Identification of a second transmembrane protein tyrosine phosphatase, IA-2 β, as an autoantigen in insulin-dependent diabetes mellitus: precursor of the 37-kDa tryptic fragment. *Proc Natl Acad Sci U S A* 1996;93:2307–2311.
268. Wasmeier C, Hutton JC. Molecular cloning of phogrin, a protein-tyrosine phosphatase homologue localized to insulin secretory granule membranes. *J Biol Chem* 1996;271:18161–18170.
269. Kawasaki E, Hutton JC, Eisenbarth GS. Molecular cloning and characterization of the human transmembrane protein tyrosine phosphatase homologue, phogrin, an autoantigen of type 1 diabetes. *Biochem Biophys Res Commun* 1996;227:440–447.
270. Christie MR, Vohra G, Champagne P, et al. Distinct antibody specificities to a 64-kD islet cell antigen in type 1 diabetes as revealed by trypsin treatment. *J Exp Med* 1990;172:789–794.
271. Payton MA, Hawkes CJ, Christie MR. Relationship of the 37,000- and 40,000-Mr tryptic fragments of islet antigens in insulin-dependent diabetes to the protein tyrosine phosphatase-like molecule IA-2 (ICA512). *J Clin Invest* 1995; 96:1506–1511.
272. Kawasaki E, Eisenbarth GS, Wasmeier C, et al. Autoantibodies to protein tyrosine phosphatase-like proteins in type I diabetes: overlapping specificities to phogrin and ICA512/IA-2. *Diabetes* 1996;45:1344–1349.
273. Kawasaki E, Yu L, Rewers MJ, et al. Definition of multiple ICA512/phogrin autoantibody epitopes and detection of intramolecular epitope spreading in relatives of patients with type 1 diabetes. *Diabetes* 1998;47:733–742.
274. Leslie RD, Atkinson MA, Notkins AL. Autoantigens IA-2 and GAD in type I (insulin-dependent) diabetes. *Diabetologia* 1999;42:3–14.
275. Medici F, Hawa MI, Giorgini A, et al. Antibodies to GAD65 and a tyrosine phosphatase-like molecule IA-2ic in Filipino type 1 diabetic patients. *Diabetes Care* 1999;22:1458–1461.
276. Naserke HE, Ziegler AG, Lampasona V, et al. Early development and spreading of autoantibodies to epitopes of IA-2 and their association with progression to type 1 diabetes. *J Immunol* 1998;161:6963–6969.
277. Savola K, Bonifacio E, Sabbah E, et al, and the Childhood Diabetes in Finland Study Group. IA-2 antibodies—a sensitive marker of IDDM with clinical onset in childhood and adolescence. *Diabetologia* 1998;41:424–429.
278. Gianani R, Rabin DU, Verge CF, et al. ICA512 autoantibody radioassay. *Diabetes* 1995;44:1340–1344.
279. Park Y, Kawasaki E, Yu L, et al. Humoral autoreactivity to an alternatively spliced variant of ICA512/IA2 in type 1 diabetes. *Diabetologia* 2000;43: 1293–1301.
280. Diez J, Zeller M, Park Y, et al. Differential splicing of the IA-2/ICA512 gene in pancreas and lymphoid organs as a permissive genetic mechanism for autoimmunity against the IA-1/ICA512 type 1 diabetes autoantigen. *Diabetes* 2001;50:895–900.
281. Yu L, Rewers M, Gianani R, et al. Anti-islet autoantibodies develop sequentially rather than simultaneously. *J Clin Endocrinol Metab* 1996;81:4264–4267.
282. Mennuni C, Santini C, Lazzaro D, et al. Identification of a novel type 1 diabetes-specific epitope by screening phage libraries with sera from pre-diabetic patients. *J Mol Biol* 1997;268:599–606.
283. Wong FS, Janeway CAJ. The role of CD4 vs. CD8 T cells in IDDM. *J Autoimmun* 1999;13:290–295.
284. Peterson JD, Haskins K. Transfer of diabetes in the NOD-scid mouse by CD4 T-cell clones. Differential requirement for CD8 T-cells. *Diabetes* 1996;45: 328–336.
285. Abiru N, Wegmann D, Kawasaki E, et al. Dual overlapping peptides recognized by insulin peptide B:9-23 reactive T cell receptor AV13S3 T cell clones of the NOD mouse. *J Autoimmun* 2000;14:231–237.
286. Wegmann DR, Norbury-Glaser M, Daniel D. Insulin-specific T cells are a predominant component of islet infiltrates in pre-diabetic NOD mice. *Eur J Immunol* 1994;24:1853–1857.
287. Anderson B, Park BJ, Verdaguer J, et al. Prevalent CD8+ T cell response against one peptide/MHC complex in autoimmune diabetes. *Proc Natl Acad Sci U S A* 1999;96:9311–9316.
288. Santamaria P, Utsugi T, Park B-J, et al. Beta-cell-cytotoxic CD8+ T cells from nonobese diabetic mice use highly homologous T cell receptor β-chain CDR3 sequences. *J Immunol* 1995;154:2494–2503.
289. DiLorenzo TP, Graser RT, Ono T, et al. Major histocompatibility complex class I-restricted T cells are required for all but the end stages of diabetes development in nonobese diabetic mice and use a prevalent T cell receptor alpha chain gene rearrangement. *Proc Natl Acad Sci U S A* 1998;95: 12538–12543.
289a. Lieberman SM, Evans AM, Han B, et al. Identification of the β cell antigen targeted by a prevalent population of pathogenic CD8+ T cells in autoimmune diabetes. *Proc Natl Acad Sci U S A* 2003;100:8384–8388.
290. Roep BO, Stobbe I, Duinkerken G, et al. Auto- and alloimmune reactivity to human islet allografts transplanted into type 1 diabetic patients. *Diabetes* 1999;48:484–490.
291. Colman PG, Steele C, Couper JJ, et al. Islet autoimmunity in infants with a type I diabetic relative is common but is frequently restricted to one autoantibody. *Diabetologia* 2000;43:203–209.
292. Kulmala P, Savola K, Reijonen H, et al. Genetic markers, humoral autoimmunity, and prediction of type 1 diabetes in siblings of affected children. Childhood Diabetes in Finland Study Group. *Diabetes* 2000;49:48–58.
293. Ziegler A-G, Hummel M, Schenker M, et al. Autoantibody appearance and risk for development of childhood diabetes in offspring of parents with type 1 diabetes. The 2-year analysis of the German BABYDIAB study. *Diabetes* 1999;48:460–468.
294. Yu J, Yu L, Bugawan TL, et al. Transient anti-islet autoantibodies: infrequent occurrence and lack of association with genetic risk factors. *J Clin Endocrinol Metab* 2000;85:2421–2428.
295. Tuomi T, Björses P, Falorni A, et al. Antibodies to glutamic acid decarboxylase and insulin-dependent diabetes in patients with autoimmune polyendocrine syndrome type I. *J Clin Endocrinol Metab* 1996;81:1488–1494.
296. Böhmer KP, Kolb H, Kuglin B, et al. Linear loss of insulin secretory capacity during the last six months preceding IDDM. *Diabetes Care* 1994;17:138–141.
297. Wagner R, Genovese S, Bosi E, et al. Slow metabolic deterioration towards diabetes in islet cell antibody positive patients with autoimmune polyendocrine disease. *Diabetologia* 1994;37:365–371.
298. Bleich D, Jackson RA, Soeldner JS, et al. Analysis of metabolic progression to type I diabetes in ICA+ relatives of patients with type I diabetes. *Diabetes Care* 1990;13:111–118.
299. Srikanta S, Ganda OP, Gleason RE, et al. Pre-type I diabetes. Linear loss of beta cell response to intravenous glucose. *Diabetes* 1984;33:717–720.
300. Bingley P. Interactions of age, islet cell antibodies, insulin autoantibodies, and first-phase insulin response in predicting risk of progression to IDDM in ICA+ relatives: the ICARUS data set. *Diabetes* 1996;45:1720–1728.
301. Carlsson A, Sundkvist G, Groop L, et al. Insulin and glucagon secretion in patients with slowly progressing autoimmune diabetes (LADA). *J Clin Endocrinol Metab* 2000;85:76–80.
302. Kobayashi T, Sugimoto T, Itoh T, et al. The prevalence of islet cell antibodies in Japanese insulin-dependent and non-insulin-dependent diabetic patients studies by indirect immunofluorescence and by a new method. *Diabetes* 1986;35:335–340.
303. Kobayashi T, Nakanishi K, Murase T, et al. Small doses of subcutaneous insulin as a strategy for preventing slowly progressive β-cell failure in islet cell antibody-positive patients with clinical features of NIDDM. *Diabetes* 1996;45:622–626.
304. Dorman JS, LaPorte RE, Kuller LH, et al. The Pittsburgh insulin-dependent diabetes mellitus (IDDM) morbidity and mortality study: mortality results. *Diabetes* 1984;33:271–276.
305. Scibilia J, Finegold D, Dorman J, et al. Why do children with diabetes die? *Acta Endocrinol Suppl (Copenh)* 1986;279:326–333.
305a. Barker JM, Goehrig SH, Barriga K, et al. Clinical characteristics of children diagnosed with type 1 diabetes through intensive screening and follow-up. *Diabetes Care* 2004;27:1399–1404.
306. Herskowitz-Dumont R, Wolfsdorf JI, Jackson RA, et al. Distinction between transient hyperglycemia and early insulin-dependent diabetes mellitus in childhood: a prospective study of incidence and prognostic factors. *J Pediatr* 1993;123:347–354.
307. Ricker AT, Herskowitz R, Wolfsdorf JI, et al. Prognostic factors in children and young adults presenting with transient hyperglycemia or impaired glucose tolerance. *Diabetes* 1986;35[Suppl 1]:93A(abst).
308. Füchtenbusch M, Ferber K, Standl E, et al. Prediction of type I diabetes postpartum in patients with gestational diabetes mellitus by combined islet cell autoantibody screening: a prospective multicenter study. *Diabetes* 1997;46: 1459–1467.
309. Kobberling J, Tillil H. Risk to family members of becoming diabetic: a study on the genetics of type I diabetes. *Pediatr Adolesc Endocrinol* 1986;15:26–38.
310. Krischer JP, Schatz DA, Silverstein JH, et al. Islet cell antibodies (ICA) predict the development of IDD in the school age general population as effectively as in unaffected relatives. *Autoimmunity* 1993;15[Suppl]:74(abst).
311. Bosi EP, Garancini MP, Poggiali F, et al. Low prevalence of islet autoimmunity in adult diabetes and low predictive value of islet autoantibodies in the general adult population of northern Italy. *Diabetologia* 1999;42:840–844.
312. Strebelow M, Schlosser M, Ziegler B, et al. Karlsburg type I diabetes risk study of a general population: frequencies and interactions of the four major type I diabetes-associated autoantibodies studied in 9419 schoolchildren. *Diabetologia* 1999;42:661–670.
313. Eisenbarth GS. Combinatorial autoantibody screening for prediction of type I diabetes. *Clin Res* 1993;41:154A(abst).
314. Pugliese A, Gianani R, Moromisato R, et al. HLA-DQB1*0602 is associated with dominant protection from diabetes even among islet cell antibody-positive first-degree relatives of patients with IDDM. *Diabetes* 1995;44:608–613.
315. Anonymous. Effect of intensive therapy on residual beta-cell function in patients with type 1 diabetes in the diabetes control and complications trial. A randomized, controlled trial. The Diabetes Control and Complications Trial Research Group. *Ann Intern Med* 1998;128:517–523.
315a. Palmer JP, Fleming GA, Greenbaum CJ, et al. C-peptide is the appropriate outcome measure for type 1 diabetes clinical trials to preserve beta-cell function: Report of an ADA workshop, 21–22 October 2001. *Diabetes* 2004;53:250–264.
316. Hramiak IM, Dupre J, Finegood DT. Determinants of clinical remission in recent-onset IDDM. *Diabetes Care* 1993;16:125–132.
317. Martin S, Schernthaner G, Nerup J, et al. Follow-up of cyclosporin A treatment in type I (insulin-dependent) diabetes mellitus: lack of long-term effects. *Diabetologia* 1991;34:429–434.
318. Assan R, Feutren G, Debray-Sachs M, et al. Metabolic and immunological effects of cyclosporine in recently type I diabetes mellitus. *Lancet* 1985;1:67–71.
319. Carel J-C, Boitard C, Eisenbarth G, et al. Cyclosporine delays but does not prevent clinical onset in glucose intolerant pre-type 1 diabetic children. *J Autoimmun* 1996;9:739–745.
320. Harrison LC, Colman PG, Dean B, et al. Increase in remission rate in newly diagnosed type I diabetic subjects treated with azathioprine. *Diabetes* 1985; 34:1306–1308.

321. Silverstein J, Maclaren N, Riley W, et al. Immunosuppression with azathioprine and prednisone in recent-onset insulin-dependent diabetes mellitus. *N Engl J Med* 1988;319:599–604.
322. Buckingham BA, Sandborg CI. A randomized trial of methotrexate in newly diagnosed patients with type 1 diabetes mellitus. *Clin Immunol* 2000;96:86–90.
323. Klingensmith G, Allen H, Hayward A, et al. Vaccination with BCG at diagnosis does not alter the course of IDDM. *Diabetes* 1997;46:193A(abst).
324. Chase HP, Butler-Simon N, Garg S, et al. A trial of nicotinamide in newly diagnosed patients with type 1 (insulin-dependent) diabetes mellitus. *Diabetologia* 1990;33:444–446.
325. Pozzilli P, Visalli N, Ghirlanda G, et al. Nicotinamide increases C-peptide secretion in patients with recent onset type 1 diabetes. *Diabet Med* 1989;6: 568–572.
326. Elliott RB, Chase HP, Pilcher CC, et al. Effect of nicotinamide in preventing diabetes (IDDM) in children. *J Autoimmun* 1990;3:61A(abst).
327. Eisenbarth GS, Srikanta S, Jackson R, et al. Anti-thymocyte globulin and prednisone immunotherapy of recent onset type I diabetes mellitus. *Diabetes Res* 2:271–276.
328. Chaillous L, Lefevre H, Thivolet C, et al. Oral insulin administration and residual beta-cell function in recent-onset type 1 diabetes: a multicentre randomised controlled trial. *Lancet* 2000;356:545–549.
329. Pozzilli P, Pitocco D, Visalli N, et al. No effect of oral insulin on residual beta-cell function in recent-onset type I diabetes (the IMDIAB VII). IMDIAB Group. *Diabetologia* 2000;43:1000–1004.
329a. Herold KC, Hagopian W, Auger JA, et al. Anti-CD3 monoclonal antibody in new-onset type 1 diabetes mellitus. *N Engl J Med* 2002;346:1692–1698.
330. Herold KC, Bluestone JA, Montag AG, et al. Prevention of autoimmune diabetes with nonactivating anti-CD3 monoclonal antibody. *Diabetes* 1992;41: 385–391.
331. Chatenoud L, Primo J, Bach JF. CD3 antibody-induced dominant self tolerance in overtly diabetic NOD mice. *J Immunol* 1997;158:2947–2954.
332. Keller RJ, Jackson RA, Eisenbarth GS. Preservation of beta cell function in islet cell antibody (ICA) positive first degree relatives treated with insulin. *Diabetes* 1992;41[Suppl 1]:50A(abst).
333. Füchtenbusch M, Rabl W, Grassl B, et al. Delay of type 1 diabetes in high risk, first degree relatives by parenteral antigen administration: the Schwabing Insulin Prophylaxis Pilot Trial. *Diabetologia* 1998;41:536–541.
334. Lampeter EF, Klinghammer A, Scherbaum WA, et al. The Deutsche Nicotinamide Intervention Study: an attempt to prevent type 1 diabetes. DENIS Group. *Diabetes* 1998;47:980–984.
334a. Effects of insulin in relatives with type 1 diabetes mellitus. *N Engl J Med* 2002;346:1685–1691.
335. Lonnrot M, Korpela K, Knip M, et al. Enterovirus infection as a risk factor for beta-cell autoimmunity in a prospectively observed birth cohort: the Finnish Diabetes Prediction and Prevention Study. *Diabetes* 2000;49: 1314–1318.
336. Shapiro AM, Lakey JR, Ryan EA, et al. Islet transplantation in seven patients with type 1 diabetes mellitus using a glucocorticoid-free immunosuppressive regimen. *N Engl J Med* 2000;343:230–238.
337. Chatenoud L, Thervet E, Primo J, et al. Anti-CD3 antibody induces long-term remission of overt autoimmunity in nonobese diabetic mice. *Proc Natl Acad Sci U S A* 1994;91:123–127.
338. Wegmann DR, Eisenbarth GS. It's insulin. *J Autoimmun* 2000;15:286–291.
339. Ablamunits V, Elias D, Reshef T, et al. Islet T cells secreting IFN-gamma in NOD mouse diabetes: arrest by p277 peptide treatment. *J Autoimmun* 1998;11: 73–81.
340. Uchigata Y, Hirata Y. Insulin autoimmune syndrome (IAS, Hirata disease). In: Eisenbarth G, ed. *Endocrine and organ specific autoimmunity*. Austin, TX: RG Landes, 1999:133–148.
341. Hirata Y, Ishizu H, Ouchi N, et al. Insulin autoimmunity in a case with spontaneous hypoglycaemia. *Jpn J Diabetes* 1970;13:312–319.
342. Uchigata Y, Kuwata S, Tokunaga K, et al. Strong association of insulin autoimmune syndrome with HLA-DR4. *Lancet* 1992;339:393–394.
343. Hirata Y. Methimazole and insulin autoimmune syndrome with hypoglycemia. *Lancet* 1983;2:1037–1038.
344. Rodriguez O, Collier E, Arakaki R, et al. Characterization of purified autoantibodies to the insulin receptor from six patients with type B insulin resistance. *Metabolism* 1992;41:325–331.
345. Taylor SI, Barbetti F, Accili D, et al. Syndromes of autoimmunity and hypoglycemia. Autoantibodies directed against insulin and its receptor. *Endocrinol Metab Clin North Am* 1989;18:123–143.
346. Yamamoto T, Sato T, Mori T, et al. Clinical efficacy of insulin-like growth factor-1 in a patient with autoantibodies to insulin receptors: a case report. *Diabetes Res Clin Pract* 2000;49:65–69.
347. Lebovitz HE. Insulin allergy and insulin resistance. *Curr Ther Endocrinol Metab* 1997;6:500–504.
348. Schernthaner G. Immunogenicity and allergenic potential of animal and human insulins. *Diabetes Care* 1993;16:155–165.
349. Panczel P, Hosszufalusi N, Horvath MM. Advantage of insulin lispro in suspected insulin allergy. *Allergy* 2000;55:409–410.
350. Oh HK, Provenzano R, Hendrix J, et al. Insulin allergy resolution following pancreas transplantation alone. *Clin Transplant* 1998;12:593–595.
351. Gonzalo MA, De Argila D, Revenga F, et al. Cutaneous allergy to human (recombinant DNA) insulin. *Allergy* 1998;53:106–107.
352. Loeb JA, Herold KC, Barton KP, et al. Systematic approach to diagnosis and management of biphasic insulin allergy with local anti-inflammatory agents. *Diabetes Care* 1989;12:421–423.
353. Stegall MD, Lafferty KJ, Kam I, et al. Evidence of recurrent autoimmunity in human allogeneic islet transplantation. *Transplantation* 1996;61:1272–1274.
354. Boitard C, Bonifacio G, Bottazzo GF, et al. Immunology and Diabetes Workshop: report on the Third International (Stage 3) Workshop on the Standardisation of Cytoplasmic Islet Cell Antibodies. Held in New York, NY, October 1987. *Diabetologia* 1988;31:451–452.
355. Gianani R, Pugliese A, Bonner-Weir S, et al. Prognostically significant heterogeneity of cytoplasmic islet cell antibodies in relatives of patients with type I diabetes. *Diabetes* 1992;41:347–353.
356. Allen HF, Jeffers BW, Klingensmith GJ, et al. First-phase insulin release in normal children. *J Pediatr* 1993;123:733–738.
357. Vardi P, Crisa L, Jackson RA, et al. Predictive value of intravenous glucose tolerance test insulin secretion less than or greater than the first percentile in islet cell antibody positive relatives of type I (insulin-dependent) diabetic patients. *Diabetologia* 1991;34:93–102.

CHAPTER 24

Insulin Resistance and Its Role in the Pathogenesis of Type 2 Diabetes

Meredith Hawkins and Luciano Rossetti

The term *insulin resistance* generally refers to resistance to the metabolic effects of insulin, including the suppressive effects of insulin on endogenous glucose production, the stimulatory effects of insulin on peripheral (predominantly skeletal muscle) glucose uptake and glycogen synthesis, and the inhibitory effects of insulin on adipose tissue lipolysis.

Following its discovery by Banting and Best in 1921, insulin rapidly entered the clinical arena and dramatically extended the life spans of individuals with type 1 diabetes mellitus. Chronic treatment with exogenous insulin permitted the recognition of individuals with very high insulin requirements, indicating resistance to the hormone (1). Many such individuals had secondary causes for insulin resistance, including high titers of antibodies to insulin after chronic treatment with insulin from animal sources (2), as well as rare genetic defects in insulin signaling (3). However, the thriving of patients with type 1 diabetes into their later years and the treatment of individuals with type 2 diabetes with insulin revealed the phenomenon of insulin resistance secondary to obesity and aging, which was widely recognized by the 1970s (3). Many of the considerable advances of the past three decades in understanding the pathogenesis of insulin resistance will be reviewed below.

CLINICAL FEATURES AND SIGNIFICANCE OF INSULIN RESISTANCE

The clinical importance of insulin resistance cannot be overstated, given the mortality and morbidity associated with the many disorders that are likely a consequence of this condition. Indeed, there is considerable epidemiologic evidence linking insulin resistance with glucose intolerance and type 2 diabetes, hypertension, dyslipidemia, atherosclerosis, and many cancers (4–8). It is generally accepted that insulin resistance plays a major role in the development of type 2 diabetes (9). Because currently an estimated 170 million people worldwide have type 2 diabetes (10), this is clearly an important association. Indeed, prospective studies have revealed that insulin resistance predates the onset of type 2 diabetes by 10 to 20 years and is the best clinical predictor of subsequent development of type 2 diabetes (11,12). Furthermore, insulin resistance is a consistent finding in patients with type 2 diabetes (3,13–15). However, the development of frank diabetes mellitus appears to require an additional defect in insulin secretion (11). In the absence of a defect in β-cell function, individuals can compensate indefinitely for insulin resistance with appropriate hyperinsulinemia (11). Hence, many individuals with marked insulin resistance may never progress to type 2 diabetes. However, the risk of atherosclerosis is apparently comparable in nondiabetic, insulin-resistant individuals and in those with type 2 diabetes (16).

Metabolic Syndrome

Reaven formally recognized the clinically significant association between insulin resistance and cardiovascular risk factors in his description of the *syndrome of insulin resistance* in 1988 (17). The most recent definition of the metabolic syndrome was established as a consensus by the National Cholesterol Education Program (NCEP) Adult Treatment Panel III (ATPIII) in 2001 (18). Based on the panel's guidelines, diagnosis of the metabolic syndrome requires the presence of at least three of the following five criteria: elevated fasting plasma glucose levels (>110 mg/dL), visceral obesity (waist circumference >35 inches in women and 40 inches in men), hypertension (>130/85 mm Hg), hypertriglyceridemia (>150 mg/dL), and low high-density lipoprotein (HDL) cholesterol (<40 mg/dL in men and <50 mg/dL in women). By this definition, the estimated prevalence of the metabolic syndrome in the United States is currently greater than 20% among all adults older than 20 years of age, and greater than 40% among the population older than 50 (19).

Other recognized components of the syndrome include systemic inflammation, a prothrombotic state, and increased oxidant stress (20). The increased circulating levels of tumor necrosis factor-α (TNF-α), interleukin-6 (IL-6), and other proinflammatory cytokines may contribute to some of the metabolic features of the metabolic syndrome, whereas the increased levels of plasminogen activator inhibitor-1 (PAI-1) appear to heighten the risk of atherothrombosis (21). Indeed, an increased risk of atherosclerotic disease mortality and morbidity is conferred by the metabolic syndrome. Other associated clinical disorders include polycystic ovarian syndrome, nonalcoholic fatty liver disease, and sleep apnea (14).

Contributions of Tissue-Specific Insulin Resistance

Defects in the ability of insulin to stimulate skeletal muscle glucose uptake and to suppress hepatic glucose production and adipose tissue lipolysis all tend to coexist in insulin-resistant individuals with established type 2 diabetes (22). It has been speculated that the onset of insulin resistance in some tissues may precede the onset in others. Although it has been proposed that insulin resistance develops later in the liver than in skeletal muscle, hepatic glucose production is inappropriately unsuppressed in the presence of hyperinsulinemia during the development of insulin resistance (23). Additionally, marked hepatic insulin resistance precedes the onset of peripheral insulin resistance secondary to moderate fat feeding (24). Various experimental models have been developed to define organ-specific contributions of insulin resistance to hyperglycemia and other metabolic abnormalities.

SKELETAL MUSCLE

A universally recognized feature of type 2 diabetes is skeletal muscle insulin resistance, secondary to either genetic or metabolic factors (25). Insulin clamp studies have permitted the measurement of peripheral and hepatic glucose fluxes in the presence of fixed glucose and insulin levels by means of continuous intravenous infusions and frequent measurement of plasma glucose levels (26,27). These sophisticated physiologic measures have revealed that skeletal muscle is quantitatively the most important tissue involved in systemic glucose homeostasis, because it accounts for ~80% of glucose disposal following glucose infusion or ingestion (11). Thus, decreased ability of insulin to stimulate glucose disposal by this tissue is of considerable importance to whole-body glucose homeostasis.

Indeed, impaired insulin-dependent glucose uptake and phosphorylation have been documented at early stages in the development of type 2 diabetes (28). Several transgenic mouse models have examined the impact of isolated defects in skeletal muscle insulin action on whole-body glucose intolerance. Conditional inactivation of the insulin receptor in skeletal muscle by Cre-mediated recombination gave rise to a model of the metabolic syndrome, with increased fat stores and hypertriglyceridemia (29). Despite the changes in fat metabolism, these muscle-specific insulin receptor knockout (MIRKO) mice did not develop hyperinsulinemia and diabetes, suggesting that there was adequate shunting of glucose utilization from muscle to adipose tissue to prevent excursions in blood glucose (30). Another model of severe skeletal muscle insulin resistance was generated by crossing mice heterozygous for a systemic insulin receptor knockout with mice bearing a dominant-negative insulin receptor transgene in muscle. Despite a greater than 90% decrease in insulin receptor kinase activity and reduced insulin-stimulated glucose uptake, these mice still did not develop diabetes (31).

The findings stand in sharp contrast to studies showing that ablation of the insulin-dependent glucose transporter GLUT4 in skeletal muscle can cause diabetes (32). There are several explanations for this apparent contradiction. In mice lacking the insulin receptor in muscle, both the contraction-activated pathway (33,34) and the insulin-like growth factor I (IGF-I) signaling pathway (35) can compensate for the ablation of insulin signaling. The former, which activates adenosine monophosphate (AMP)–activated protein kinase and thereby stimulates translocation of glucose transporters (36), remains intact in MIRKO mice. The importance of the IGF-I signaling system in muscle metabolism is highlighted by a mouse model of combined ablation of insulin and IGF-I receptor function in skeletal muscle (37). Unlike mice with isolated ablation of the insulin receptor in skeletal muscle, these mice develop frank diabetes and other metabolic features characteristic of insulin resistance. Together, these models confirm the central role of skeletal muscle as a site of insulin action, yet indicate that there are alternate pathways leading to glucose uptake and GLUT4 translocation in skeletal muscle that can compensate in mice lacking the insulin receptor.

Insulin-stimulated 3-*O*-methylglucose transport into isolated skeletal muscle from patients with type 2 diabetes is substantially lower than in normal controls, demonstrating that decreased skeletal muscle uptake contributes to impaired peripheral glucose uptake (36,38). A uniform finding in both obesity and type 2 diabetes is decreased insulin receptor substrate-1 (IRS-1)–associated tyrosine phosphorylation and 1-phosphatidylinositol 3-kinase (PI 3-kinase) activity in skeletal muscle (39–41). Of note, insulin action on glucose transport is normalized in isolated muscle strips from patients with type 2 diabetes after a 2-hour *in vitro* incubation in the presence of 5 mM glucose (42). Similarly, a more recent report provided evidence that proximal insulin signaling parameters elicit a normal response in cultured myotubes prepared from muscle biopsies from insulin-resistant nondiabetic subjects (43). These findings support the hypothesis that insulin resistance of skeletal muscle in individuals with type 2 diabetes is at least in part secondary to an altered metabolic milieu, as will be explored further under "Environmental" Factors Contributing to Insulin Resistance.

In addition to this downregulation of proximal insulin signaling, several negative regulators of insulin signaling are upregulated in insulin resistance. Plasma-cell differentiation factor-1 (PC-1) is a membrane glycoprotein with ectonucleotide pyrophosphatase activity that seems to act as an intrinsic inhibitor of insulin receptor tyrosine kinase activity (44,45). In healthy subjects with no clinically significant defects in glucose metabolism, PC-1 expression in muscle is negatively correlated with insulin sensitivity and *in vitro* stimulation of muscle insulin receptor tyrosine kinase activity (46,47). It has been suggested that increased expression of PC-1 in skeletal muscle of obese subjects is more strongly associated with downregulation of insulin receptor tyrosine phosphorylation than with decreased insulin receptor expression, but this requires further investigation (48).

Phosphotyrosine phosphatases (PTPases) are enzymes that dephosphorylate the insulin receptor and its substrates, thereby turning off the insulin signal. Total membrane-bound tyrosine phosphatase activity is increased in skeletal muscle of patients with type 2 diabetes (49), particularly protein-tyrosine phosphatase-1B (PTP-1B) (50), which negatively regulates phosphorylation of the insulin receptor and IRS-1 (51). Mice with ablation of the *PTP1B* gene demonstrate increased insulin sensitivity and enhanced insulin-stimulated phosphorylation of the insulin receptor in both skeletal muscle and liver (52). These mice are also resistant to weight gain on a high-fat diet, demonstrating the potential importance of this enzyme in mediating the central effects of insulin on appetite, discussed under Brain. Selective reduction of PTP1B protein and messenger RNA (mRNA) in liver and fat normalized plasma glucose levels, reduced hyperinsulinemia, and reduced expression of gluconeogenic enzymes in genetically obese and diabetic mice (53). These promising *in vivo* rodent data have prompted a highly motivated search for pharmacologic inhibitors of this enzyme (54).

ADIPOSE TISSUE

Insulin resistance in adipose tissue is characterized by decreased suppression of adipose tissue lipolysis by insulin, resulting in elevated circulating levels of free fatty acids (FFAs). Indeed, the suppressive effect of insulin on FFA levels is impaired in obese insulin-resistant individuals (55,56) and in type 2 diabetes (57). The presence of the same defect in glucose-tolerant first-degree relatives of patients with type 2 diabetes (58,59) suggests that abnormal insulin-mediated suppression of plasma FFA is an early defect in those with a genetic predisposition to insulin resistance. Although it has been suggested that increased FFA levels in obese individuals are due primarily to expansion of body-fat depots (60,61), the suppressive effect of insulin on FFA levels is also reduced in nonobese insulin-resistant individuals (62).

Transgenic models of adipocyte-specific disruption of insulin signaling have been generated to address the impact of decreased adipocyte insulin action on systemic fat and glucose metabolism. Conditional ablation of the insulin receptor in white and brown adipocytes with an adipose-specific fatty acid binding protein aP2 promoter (63) caused a marked decrease in gonadal fat mass and whole-body triglyceride content. Moreover, these fat-specific insulin receptor knockout (FIRKO) mice are resistant to weight gain with aging or hypothalamic insult and are protected against hyperphagia-induced glucose intolerance. Since the aP2 promoter would also target macrophages, these mice may also have been spared the adverse metabolic effects of systemic inflammation, discussed below. Thus, although insulin signaling is required for triglyceride storage in adipocytes, it may not be essential for normal glucose metabolism.

By contrast, knockout of the insulin-dependent glucose transporter GLUT4 in fat induced hepatic and skeletal muscle insulin resistance and glucose intolerance (64). However, fasting serum FFA levels were suppressed appropriately in response to insulin in these knockout mice, suggesting that the insulin resistance was relatively selective for glucose uptake. Furthermore, these mice displayed normal muscle triglyceride content and normal levels of leptin and TNF-α. Thus, the insulin resistance observed in these mice may be secondary to chronic hyperinsulinemia or to altered secretion of adipocyte-derived molecules that mediate insulin action in other tissues (see below).

Ob/ob mice that lack the adipose tissue fatty acid binding protein aP2 have reduced adipose tissue lipolysis and increased adipose tissue mass, together with a paradoxical reduction in plasma lipids and an improvement in insulin sensitivity and insulin secretion (65). This suggests that enlargement of adipose tissue mass may have protective effects against insulin resistance. This concept of adipose tissue providing a "sink" to protect other tissues from the toxic effects of excessive fatty acids is supported by the observation that overexpression of GLUT4 in adipose tissue of transgenic mice causes both an increase in adipose tissue mass and an improvement in whole-body insulin sensitivity (66,67). Further evidence for beneficial effects of adipose tissue will be provided in the subsequent discussion of lipodystrophy and fatless mice and the reversal of insulin resistance with adipose tissue transplantation in those transgenic models.

LIVER

There has been considerable controversy about whether hepatic glucose production is directly regulated by insulin or is mediated via extrahepatic metabolic effects. In particular, it has been proposed that insulin suppresses glucose production by reducing flux of amino acids and FFA from muscle and adipose tissue to the liver, thereby also reducing gluconeogenesis (68–72). Normal inhibitory action of insulin on hepatic glucose production appears to require normal insulin responsiveness at the level of adipose tissue. Indeed, the ability of peripheral insulin to regulate glucose production appears to be at least in part due to its ability to suppress circulating FFA levels (73,74).

Evidence for a direct effect of insulin on hepatic glucose production is provided by a mouse model in which the insulin receptor is ablated in muscle and adipose tissue, with normal insulin signaling in the liver (75). These mice maintain normal hepatic insulin sensitivity and do not progress to diabetes despite impaired glucose tolerance, suggesting that hepatic insulin resistance is required for the onset of overt diabetes. This model may also suggest that insulin resistance in the liver is an intrinsic abnormality of insulin signaling in the hepatocyte. Indeed, mice with conditional, liver-specific knockout of the insulin receptor (LIRKO) exhibit marked insulin resistance, glucose intolerance, and an inability of insulin to suppress hepatic glucose production and regulate hepatic gene expression (76,77). Furthermore, the liver might actually affect peripheral insulin action. Some evidence for an association between hepatic fat accumulation and peripheral insulin resistance is presented below in the discussion of the metabolic effects of intrahepatocellular triglyceride.

BRAIN

Hypothalamic resistance to the central appetite-suppressing and metabolic effects of insulin may play seminal roles in the development of insulin resistance. The insulin receptor is widely expressed in several brain areas (78) and has been implicated in the regulation of satiety (79). Although glucose disposal in the majority of neurons occurs in an insulin-independent manner, neurons in the hypothalamus and other discrete brain areas express the insulin-responsive glucose transporter GLUT4 (80). The potential role of brain insulin signaling has been studied by

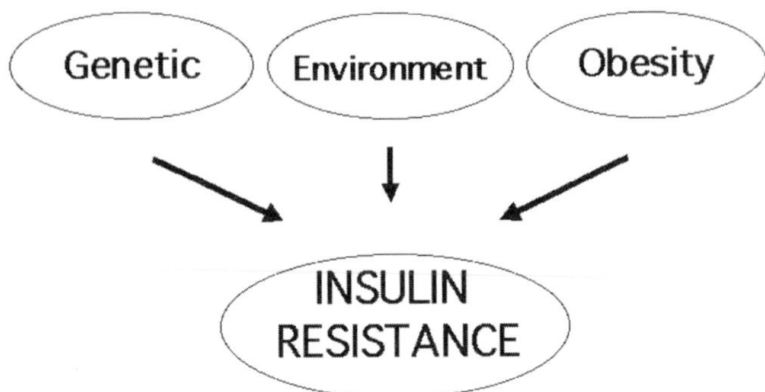

Figure 24.1. Pathogenesis of insulin resistance: contributions of genes, obesity, and environment. "Environment" refers to a variety of factors, including hormones, increased nutrient availability, and age.

generating a neuron-specific insulin receptor knockout (NIRKO), resulting in increased food intake and moderate diet-dependent obesity (81).

The metabolic effects of insulin action in the brain have recently been examined using intracerebroventricular injections of antisense oligonucleotides and blocking antibodies to the insulin receptor (82). These manipulations caused a targeted impairment in hypothalamic insulin receptor function in rats, with a rapid onset of hyperphagia and a significant increase in fat mass after only 7 days, similar to the NIRKO mouse. Of particular note, this central inhibition of insulin action also dramatically reduced the ability of exogenously infused insulin to blunt hepatic glucose output, demonstrating an important role for the hypothalamic insulin receptor in the regulation of hepatic glucose metabolism (83).

An Integrated Model of Insulin Resistance

As shown in Figure 24.1, it is likely that several factors contribute to impaired insulin action in most individuals with insulin resistance. The following sections will discuss the interrelationship between genetic inheritance, obesity, and environmental factors in the pathogenesis of insulin resistance.

GENETIC CAUSES OF INSULIN RESISTANCE

Defects in both insulin action and insulin secretion are present in type 2 diabetes, and both are believed to be genetically predetermined (84). A strong genetic basis for insulin resistance is suggested by the high prevalence in certain populations, particularly the Nauru Islanders of the Pacific (85), the Pima Indians in Arizona (86), and the urban Wanigela people in Papua New Guinea (87). Although the current epidemic levels of insulin resistance and type 2 diabetes in these populations have followed the introduction of a "Westernized" lifestyle characterized by high caloric intake and physical inactivity, their prevalence is much higher in these populations than in populations of other ethnic groups with the same lifestyle. Furthermore, there is a nearly 100% concordance in diagnosis of type 2 diabetes between monozygotic twins but only a 20% concordance between dizygotic twins (88). To date, documented monogenic inheritance of insulin resistance has been limited to a few families with extreme forms of the disorder, as described in the next section.

Extreme Insulin Resistance

To date, several rare mutations in genes associated with insulin action have been linked to extreme insulin resistance (Fig. 24.2). Although these are all rare conditions, their study has been helpful in elucidating issues pertinent to more general pathophysiology of insulin resistance. All of the following genetic conditions are associated with typical clinical manifestations: hyperinsulinemia, dyslipidemia, hypertension, and impaired glucose tolerance or insulin-resistant diabetes (89). Acanthosis nigricans is a characteristic skin lesion in insulin resistance, consisting of velvety and papillomatous pigmented hyperkeratosis of the flexures and neck (90). In women, extreme insulin resistance is also associated with hyperandrogenism, hirsutism, menstrual abnormalities, and polycystic ovarian disease.

INSULIN RECEPTOR MUTATIONS

Severe insulin resistance has been reported in conjunction with more than 100 naturally occurring mutations in the insulin receptor gene (91,92), as well as in the complete absence of insulin receptors (93). The varying severity and diversity of their phenotypes have resulted in the description of several clinical syndromes of severe insulin resistance (94).

Leprechaunism is the most extreme form of these syndromes, characterized by intrauterine growth retardation and characteristic dysmorphic features including prominent eyes, thick lips, upturned nostrils, low-set posteriorly rotated ears, and thick skin with lack of subcutaneous fat (95). Life expectancy is extremely short, with death usually before 1 year of age. Milder syndromes of insulin resistance have been reported in patients whose insulin receptor mutations do not lead to a complete loss of insulin receptor function (96). Children with the somewhat milder *Rabson-Mendenhall* syndrome have life expectancies of up to 15 years and display different dysmorphic features, with premature or dysplastic teeth and gingival hyperplasia, as well as growth retardation. Despite postprandial hyperglycemia, affected children with either syndrome demonstrate fasting hypoglycemia due to inappropriately elevated fasting insulin levels. *Type A insulin resistance* is the mildest syndrome of insulin receptor gene mutations and is characterized by a classic triad of insulin resistance, acanthosis nigricans, and hyperandrogenism (in females) (97). Most patients with type A insulin resistance are heterozygous for a single mutant allele, most frequently a mutation in the tyrosine kinase domain of the receptor (98), and most such patients do not develop diabetes. However, patients with two mutant alleles tend to develop overt diabetes in childhood or adolescence (99).

The pronounced mitogenic features and fasting hypoglycemia in individuals with the above syndromes, despite the marked resistance to the metabolic effects of insulin, suggest that the high circulating insulin levels may be mediating these mitogenic effects through the homologous IGF-I receptor (100). Indeed, this receptor homology has been exploited therapeutically in the treatment of diabetes in these patients. Daily injections of IGF-I were effective in lowering both fasting and postprandial plasma glucose concentrations for up to 16 months in 11 patients with extreme insulin resistance (101). Even more dramatically, a recent report demonstrated that treatment of a patient with leprechaunism from infancy until 7 years of age with recombinant human IGF-I maintained her growth rate and hemoglobin A_{1C} level nearly within the normal range (102).

INSULIN-MEDIATED PSEUDOACROMEGALY

A syndrome of severe insulin resistance has been described in which patients develop pathologic tissue growth similar in appearance to that of acromegaly but without elevated levels of growth hormone or IGF-I (103). Although neither insulin nor IGF-I can activate PI 3-kinase or stimulate glucose uptake in cultured skin fibroblasts from these individuals, mitogen-activated protein kinase (MAPK) phosphorylation and downstream mitogenic signaling by both hormones are intact. No defects have

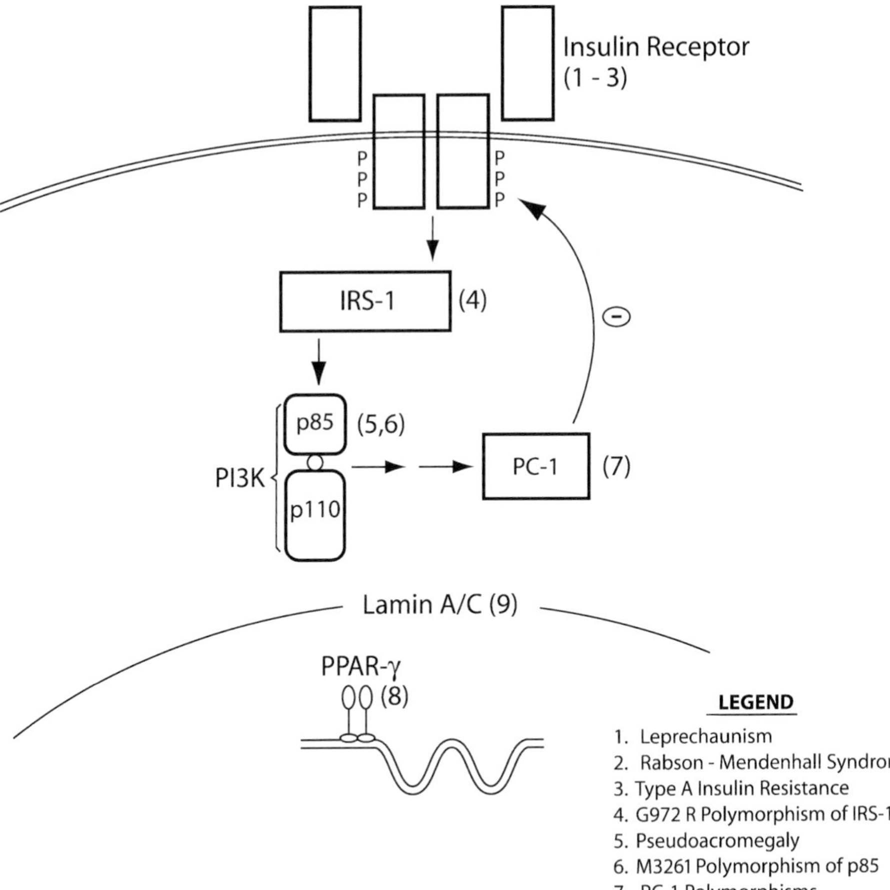

Figure 24.2. Genetic causes of insulin resistance identified in humans. This schematic representation depicts the cellular localization of proteins in which mutations or polymorphisms have been identified in association with extreme insulin resistance. In the case of the insulin receptor, multiple mutations have been identified that contribute to the syndromes indicated. Numerically, the mutations/polymorphisms/syndromes are as follows: *(1)* leprechaunism; *(2)* Rabson-Mendenhall syndrome; *(3)* type A insulin resistance; *(4)* G972R polymorphism of insulin receptor substrate-1 (IRS-1); *(5)* pseudoacromegaly; *(6)* M3261 polymorphism of p85; *(7)* Plasma-cell differentiation factor-1 (PC-1) polymorphisms; *(8)* P115Q mutation of peroxisome proliferator-activated receptor γ (PPARγ); *(9)* familial partial lipodystrophy (lamin A/C mutations). PI3K, 1-phosphatidylinositol 3-kinase.

been documented in the structure, expression, or activation of the insulin receptor, IRS-1, or p85α, suggesting a selective defect of postreceptor insulin signaling to metabolic pathways. The acromegaloid tissue growth is likely due to activation of the intact mitogenic signaling pathways by the severe hyperinsulinemia (104).

MUTATIONS IN THE PEROXISOME PROLIFERATOR-ACTIVATED RECEPTOR γ

The nuclear receptor peroxisome proliferator-activated receptor γ (PPARγ) appears to play a vital role in both adipocyte differentiation and insulin action, underscoring the important interactions between these two phenomena (105–107). A direct link between insulin sensitivity and PPARγ action in humans was strongly suggested by the discovery of a small number of individuals with heterozygous loss-of-function mutations within the ligand-binding domain of the PPARγ receptor (108–110). These dominant-negative and other mutations result in the clinical features of severe insulin resistance described above and partial lipodystrophy of the limbs and buttocks, sparing the face and central abdominal adipose depots (111). The associated lipodystrophy appears to result from the inability of subcutaneous abdominal adipose tissue to trap and store FFA postprandially (112). Although thiazolidinediones are of limited benefit in this syndrome, the tyrosine-based receptor agonist farglitazar corrected defects in ligand binding and restored transcriptional function in cells from affected individuals and may offer a therapeutic approach to improving insulin action in these patients.

By contrast, a missense mutation at codon 115 (Pro115Gln) was associated with severe obesity in four unrelated German subjects (113). Overexpression of the mutant receptor in murine fibroblasts led to accelerated differentiation of the cells into adipocytes and greater cellular accumulation of triglyceride when compared with the wild-type receptor. Although it might be expected that this constitutively active form of PPARγ might cause heightened insulin sensitivity, interpretation of the lower insulin levels in these subjects relative to obese controls was complicated by the fact that three of the four subjects had type 2 diabetes.

Of potentially more general relevance to type 2 diabetes, a common polymorphism in the *PPARγ* gene may confer protection from type 2 diabetes (114,115). A Pro12Ala polymorphism in the *PPARγ* gene was associated with improved insulin sensitivity among more than 1,000 middle-aged and elderly Finns (114). This mutation occurs in the region of the *PPARγ* gene that encodes a protein segment unique to the PPARγ2 isoform and is within the domain of PPARγ that enhances ligand-independent activation (116). Subsequently, an analysis of more than 3,000 Scandinavian individuals in a study using a multilayered design revealed that this common polymorphism was associated with a small but significant reduction in risk of type 2 diabetes (relative risk 0.78) relative to the prevalent proline form (115). In contrast with an earlier report (114), a recent meta-analysis demonstrated an increase in body mass index (BMI) among obese (but not lean) Ala12 homozygotes (117). The disparate effects of the *PPARγ* gene Pro12Ala polymorphism on BMI in obese and lean individuals suggest that the impact of this genetic variant can be modified by other environmental and/or genetic factors. In general, PPARγ expression is increased in the adipose tissue of obese subjects, but a low-calorie diet can downregulate its expression (118). It has been shown that when the dietary ratio of polyunsaturated fat to saturated fat is low, the BMI in Ala12 carriers is greater than that in Pro12 homozygotes, but when the ratio is high, the opposite is seen (119). This gene-nutrient interaction may explain, in part, the disparate effects of the Ala12 variant on BMI in obese and lean subjects.

LIPODYSTROPHY

This diverse group of disorders is characterized by severe insulin resistance and partial or complete absence of adipose tissue. The study of these rare genetic variants is important in gaining understanding of the relationship between body-fat distribution and insulin resistance. Following earlier descriptions of affected individuals, Dunnigan (120) first described a family with the syndrome of *familial partial lipodystrophy* (FPLD) in 1974. Patients with FPLD appear normal at birth but lose subcutaneous fat from their extremities and the gluteal region after puberty. This results in prominent, well-defined musculature in these areas, while fat deposition within the face and neck, axillae, back, labia majora, and abdominal cavity is markedly increased (121). Magnetic resonance imaging studies of these individuals have revealed a complete lack of subcutaneous fat in affected areas, with preservation of intermuscular, intraabdominal, intrathoracic, and bone-marrow fat and excessive accumulation of intramuscular fat (122). Recent genetic studies in families with FPLD have identified several mutations in the *LMNA* gene, which encodes lamin A and C (123,124). These proteins perform important structural functions in the nuclear membranes of adipocytes and myocytes and participate in DNA replication in these terminally differentiated cells (125). The reason for the regional distribution of the lipodystrophy remains to be determined.

By contrast, *congenital generalized lipodystrophy* is characterized by a total lack of adipose tissue and by insulin resistance from birth or infancy. The clinical features of insulin resistance (described above) are accompanied by an anabolic syndrome with muscular hypertrophy, hepatomegaly, and hypertrophic cardiomyopathy, the last being frequently lethal by early adulthood (126). This striking clinical syndrome is associated with mutations of two distinct genes on different chromosomes: the gene (*AGPAT2*) encoding 1-acylglycerol-3-phosphate-*O*-acyltransferase and a gene homologous to the murine guanine nucleotide-binding protein (G protein), *BSCL2*. Because the AGPAT2 enzyme catalyzes the acylation of lysophosphatidic acid to form phosphatidic acid, a key intermediate in the biosynthesis of triacylglycerol and glycerophospholipids, mutations in *AGPAT2* probably cause congenital generalized lipodystrophy by inhibiting triacylglycerol synthesis and storage in adipocytes (127). The gene *BSCL2* is most highly expressed in brain and testis and encodes a protein (seipin) of unknown function. Most of the variants are null mutations and probably result in a severe disruption of the protein (128). Potential mechanisms whereby lipodystrophy may cause insulin resistance are discussed below.

The various *monogenic* syndromes of insulin resistance described above reveal that there is considerable heterogeneity of phenotype among those affected with the identified mutations. Because this heterogeneity does not necessarily appear to be explained by gene penetrance or degree of defect in insulin signaling, it suggests that other factors (genetic or environmental or both) may be important in determining phenotype, even in these extreme genetic variants.

Commonly Occurring Polymorphisms

In addition to the extreme forms of insulin resistance associated with the rare genetic mutations described above, analysis of more commonly occurring polymorphisms of genes with relevance to insulin action has revealed the association of several such polymorphisms with increased incidence of type 2 diabetes.

INSULIN-SIGNALING PATHWAY

In a Caucasian population, individuals homozygous for a common codon 326Met>Ile variant of the p85 subunit of PI 3-kinase demonstrated reduced insulin sensitivity, although no increased incidence of type 2 diabetes (129). Several IRS-1 polymorphisms are more common among individuals with type 2 diabetes than among nondiabetic controls and have been studied extensively in many populations (130). Obese carriers of the G972R polymorphism in a Caucasian population demonstrated decreased insulin sensitivity and increased prevalence of metabolic cardiovascular risk factors (130). Transfection of this common IRS-1 variant into myeloid progenitor cells stably overexpressing the insulin receptor resulted in decreased binding of the p85 regulatory subunit of PI 3-kinase to IRS-1 and decreased IRS-1–associated PI 3-kinase activity (131). In a Japanese population, the combined prevalence of several IRS-1 polymorphisms was threefold greater among patients with type 2 diabetes, and both diabetic and nondiabetic carriers of the various polymorphisms demonstrated reduced insulin sensitivity (132).

Several genetic studies have examined whether polymorphisms in the locus for *adiponectin*, 3q27, could affect the circulating levels of adiponectin and whether these polymorphisms were associated with increased risk for the development of type 2 diabetes. Evidence for the effects of this adipose-specific circulating protein on insulin action will be discussed below. The results of one study showed evidence of linkage with the metabolic syndrome (133), whereas another showed evidence of a type 2 diabetes susceptibility locus at 3q27 in a French population with early-onset diabetes (134). Polymorphisms within the adiponectin locus were also linked with increased risk for type 2 diabetes in a Japanese cohort (135).

DIGENIC

There are a few examples of potential interactions between separate genes in conferring increased risk of insulin resistance (136). The combined effect of PC-1 (K121Q) and PPARγ2 (P12A) polymorphisms results in significant increases in BMI and insulin levels and impairments in both insulin sensitivity and insulin secretion. Additionally, a family has been described in which five individuals with severe insulin resistance (but no unaffected family members) were doubly heterozygous for frameshift/premature stop mutations in two unlinked genes, *PPARG* and *PPP1R3A*. These genes encode PPARγ and protein phosphatase 1 regulatory subunit 3, the muscle-specific regulatory subunit of protein phosphatase 1.

TRANSGENIC MOUSE MODELS OF HUMAN POLYGENIC BASIS OF DIABETES INHERITANCE

Given the complex genetic interactions that likely contribute to human diabetes, insulin receptor (Ir) heterozygous mutants have been used to mimic genetic interactions leading to type 2 diabetes. A first step in this direction was the development of a polygenic model of insulin-resistant diabetes by generating mice with combined heterozygous Ir and Irs1 mutations. Whereas Irs1 heterozygotes are normal and only ~5% of $Ir^{+/-}$ heterozygotes develop diabetes, mice doubly heterozygous for both Ir- and Irs1-null alleles ($Ir/Irs1^{+/-}$) develop severe hyperinsulinemia and hyperplasia of pancreatic β-cells. Nearly half of these mice ultimately become frankly hyperglycemic (137), similar to the increased risk of diabetes in first-degree relatives of patients with type 2 diabetes (138). These characteristics of the Ir/Irs1$^{+/-}$ mouse are consistent with an oligogenic mode of inheritance of type 2 diabetes, in which two subclinical defects of gene function could account for virtually the entire genetic susceptibility to the disease. Even further increases in the incidence of diabetes occurred when these mice were crossed with mice doubly heterozygous for Ir and IRS-2 (Ir/Irs2$^{+/-}$). Diabetes developed in 40% of the triple heterozygotes (139), providing a useful experimental model for the complex genetic interactions that are likely to contribute to the inheritance of type 2 diabetes. Thus, even such a major predisposing allele as the null insulin receptor mutation has a modest effect alone but can contribute importantly to a predisposing background. This is confirmed by the widely variable prevalence of diabetes (<2% to 85%) observed when the double-heterozygous knockout mice are bred onto different genetic backgrounds (140).

"THRIFTY GENOTYPE" VERSUS "THRIFTY PHENOTYPE"

These concepts highlight interesting aspects of gene-environment interactions. The high prevalence of insulin resistance and type 2 diabetes in certain population groups is consistent with effects of nutrient availability on gene selection over a long time. Because food supply was neither predictable nor consistent throughout most of the history of *Homo sapiens*, it is likely that ancestral hunter-gatherers experienced alternating cycles of feast and famine (141). It is postulated that the evolutionary pressures in the late Paleolithic era favored the selection of "thrifty genes" for efficient intake and utilization of fuel stores (142), thereby promoting storage of fuel for periods of impending famine. It does not appear that the genome has changed appreciably over the past 10,000 years, and certainly not with the explosion in the prevalence of type 2 diabetes during the past 40 to 100 years (143). Indeed, genes that favored survival in the late Paleolithic era would be maladaptive in the face of the current combination of continuous food abundance and physical inactivity. The complexity of gene-gene and gene-environment interactions discussed above suggests that the thrifty genotype is polygenic and includes genes that would impact an individual's response to environmental factors.

There is also considerable epidemiologic evidence suggesting that nutrient availability may condition the patterns of an individual's gene expression at early developmental stages. Indeed, intrauterine growth retardation is strongly linked with subsequent development of obesity or insulin resistance or both in later life (144). Many animal models have been generated to explore possible mechanisms for this association (145). In particular, maternal protein restriction has been shown to be associated with many metabolic defects in adult offspring, including resistance to the effects of insulin on peripheral glucose uptake (146) and hepatic glucose production (147), as well as defective insulin signaling in adipocytes (148) and hypertension (149). As opposed to the evolutionary pressures described above, the effects of fetal deprivation have been termed the "thrifty phenotype" (150). This suggests that the metabolism of the liver, muscle, and adipose tissue may be programmed by maternal nutrition during gestation and lactation and that an individual programmed to survive on minimal nutrients in utero may suffer adverse consequences in adult life in response to plentiful nutrition. Early growth restriction combined with subsequent supranormal nutrition in these experimental models results in the clinical features of the insulin resistance syndrome.

IMPACT OF OBESITY ON INSULIN ACTION

The quantity of body fat varies widely in mammals, ranging from 2% to 50% of body mass (151). This large variation in fat mass is apparently determined both by an individual's genetic background (152) and by environmental factors, including diet and physical activity (153). Excess body fat, or obesity, is an important factor in the pathogenesis of insulin resistance and substantially increases the risk of type 2 diabetes.

The Obesity Epidemic

In the United States of America, successive cross-sectional nationally representative surveys such as the National Health and Nutrition Examination Surveys (NHANES I: 1971–1974; NHANES II: 1976–1980; NHANES III: 1988–1994) permit the study of trends in weight over time. Disturbingly, the prevalence of obesity (BMI ≥ 30.0) showed a large increase from NHANES II to NHANES III: NHANES I, 14.1%; NHANES II, 14.5%; and NHANES III, 22.5% (154). In NHANES III, the crude prevalence of overweight and obesity (BMI > 25.0) among adults was 59.4% for men, 50.7% for women, and 54.9% overall. During this time of rising prevalence in obesity, the levels of physical activity have decreased and important shifts in diet have occurred (155), including increased consumption of sugars and energy-dense foods (156). Average daily caloric intake by people in the United States aged 2 years and older increased by 194 kcal/day from 1977 to 1996, with the largest increases in caloric intake among adolescents and young adults (157).

This highly disturbing trend is not limited to the United States or even to developed countries (158). Analyses of economic and food availability data for 1962 through 1994 have revealed a major shift in the structure of the global diet, with an uncoupling of the classic relationship between incomes and fat intakes (159). Global availability of cheap vegetable oils and fats has resulted in greatly increased fat consumption among people in low-income nations, including many countries in Asia, Latin America, North Africa, the Middle East and the urban areas of sub-Saharan Africa. Consequently, obesity is becoming a significant health issue even in countries with lower levels of gross national product and is aggravated by high urbanization rates (160). As expected, dramatic increases in the consumption of low-cost fat and simple carbohydrate calories have resulted in steep increases in incidence of overweight and obesity even among the poorest individuals in these countries (161).

The following section will highlight the metabolic effects of obesity and putative mechanisms whereby obesity contributes to insulin resistance. The impact of increased nutrients will be examined separately below, in light of substantial evidence that both factors impact insulin action.

Adipose Tissue as an Endocrine Organ

Besides being the body's principal site for energy storage, white adipose tissue influences whole-body insulin action both through release of FFAs and by secretion of adipose-derived proteins. The latter include both proinflammatory peptides, discussed below, and several newly identified hormones that appear to have dramatic effects on glucose metabolism and insulin action (162,163).

ADIPONECTIN

Adiponectin (also known as Acrp30, AdipoQ, and GBP28) is a 30-kDa adipose-specific secretory protein that appears to enhance insulin sensitivity (164,165). Decreased circulating levels of this hormone accompany obesity and insulin resistance in both humans and animal models (166–168). Indeed, adiponectin levels were negatively correlated with hyperinsulinemia and degree of insulin resistance in both Pima Indian and Japanese groups (168,169). As described above, genetic polymorphisms of the adiponectin gene are associated with increased incidence of insulin resistance and diabetes. Although there do not appear to be acute effects of nutrient excess or deprivation on adiponectin levels, chronic caloric restriction (which enhances insulin action) increases adiponectin levels (170,171). Furthermore, high baseline plasma levels of adiponectin are associated with a substantially reduced risk of development of type 2 diabetes (172). The experimental models discussed below suggest that low plasma levels of adiponectin contribute to the pathogenesis of insulin resistance and type 2 diabetes.

Pharmacologic treatment with adiponectin in rodents increases hepatic insulin sensitivity, with decreased glucose production. It was first noted that a single injection of purified recombinant adiponectin caused a transient decrease in basal glucose levels in various mouse models, with temporary correction of hyperglycemia without affecting insulin levels in ob/ob, nonobese diabetic, and streptozotocin-treated mice (173). Additionally, adiponectin increased the ability of subphysiologic levels of insulin to suppress glucose production in isolated hepatocytes (173). Infusion of adiponectin in conscious mice resulted in improved hepatic insulin action measured during euglycemic hyperinsulinemic clamp studies, with enhanced suppression of glucose production (174). Adiponectin stimulated phosphorylation and activation of the 5′AMP-activated protein kinase (AMPK) in skeletal muscle and in liver, together with stimulation of fatty acid oxidation and glucose uptake in myocytes, reduced gluconeogenesis in the liver, and reduction of glucose levels *in vivo* (175). Blocking AMPK activation inhibited all of these effects, suggesting that stimulation of glucose utilization and fatty acid oxidation by adiponectin occurs through activation of AMPK.

The phenotypes of adiponectin-deficient and transgenic adiponectin-overproducing animal models further substantiate an important role for adiponectin in mediating insulin action. Using a dominant mutation in the collagenous domain of adiponectin to generate a transgenic mouse, Combs et al (176). demonstrated that approximately threefold elevations in circulating adiponectin levels were associated with enhanced insulin-mediated suppression of endogenous glucose production and increased phosphorylation of AMPK in liver. Conversely, mouse models with a disruption of the adiponectin locus display moderate insulin resistance and impaired FFA clearance on a normal chow diet and an earlier onset of diet-induced insulin resistance (177,178).

It has recently been reported that adiponectin circulates in two discrete forms: as a relatively low-molecular-weight (LMW) hexamer and as a high-molecular-weight (HMW) multimeric structure (179). The ratio of these two oligomeric forms (HMW/LMW) has recently been shown to correlate more tightly with insulin action than do total circulating adiponectin levels (180). Furthermore, although pharmacologic activation of PPARγ with thiazolidinediones increases adiponectin levels, the most striking effect is a selective proportional increase in the HMW form with close association with improved hepatic insulin action (180). This suggests that the HMW form is the active circulating form of adiponectin, and that its favorable effects on glucose metabolism are predominantly at the level of the liver.

LEPTIN

Leptin is a 16-kDa protein secreted from adipose tissue, the product of the defective obesity gene identified by positional cloning in the obese, hyperinsulinemic *ob/ob* mouse (181). Circulating leptin concentrations in humans correlate closely with fasting insulin concentrations and the percentage of body fat, making leptin a marker of obesity and the insulin resistance syndrome. Leptin infusion acutely increases glucose uptake under euglycemic, hyperinsulinemic conditions in rats (182). Indeed, acute leptin administration enhances the ability of insulin to inhibit hepatic glucose production but does not affect peripheral insulin action (183). By contrast, chronic leptin administration induces metabolically favorable changes in body composition that include decreased visceral adiposity and reduced muscle accumulation of triglyceride (184). These leptin-induced changes in body composition are associated with improved sensitivity to the metabolic effects of insulin on skeletal muscle (184).

Recent findings suggest that these favorable effects on body composition and lipid storage may be due to leptin-induced stimulation of β-oxidation via activation of AMPK in muscle and liver (185,186). When activated, AMPK decreases adenosine triphosphate (ATP)–consuming anabolic pathways such as glucose-regulated transcription, protein synthesis, cholesterol synthesis, and fatty acid and triglyceride synthesis and increases ATP-producing catabolic pathways such as increased glucose transport, β-oxidation, glycolysis, and mitochondrial biogenesis. Other potential mechanisms whereby leptin could influence insulin action include its regulation of immune function and hormone secretion (187). Profound leptin deficiency in ob/ob mice is accompanied by impaired T-cell immunity (188). Furthermore, the immunosuppression associated with acute starvation is reversed when exogenous leptin is administered (189). Leptin also alters the regulation of hormones in the hypothalamus-pituitary-adrenal axis and affects growth hormone, prolactin, and a number of other anterior pituitary hormones (190), many of whose effects on insulin action are discussed above. A discussion of mechanisms whereby leptin deficiency contributes to hyperinsulinemia and insulin resistance in lipodystrophy is provided below. Thus, defective leptin action may contribute to insulin resistance in the metabolic syndrome.

It has been postulated that leptin resistance can develop in the face of high circulating levels of the hormone. This is supported by the fact that leptin levels are increased in most mouse models of insulin resistance associated with obesity. Furthermore, diet-induced obese mice are resistant to the effects of leptin administration (191). Indeed, resistance to the central anorectic effects of leptin develops rapidly in the face of nutrient excess (192). However, leptin was effective in increasing energy expenditure in obese individuals after a sustained weight reduction of ~10% of their previous body weight (193). This suggests that it may be possible to regain leptin sensitivity with weight loss and/or nutrient restriction, which may also have favorable implications for insulin action.

RESISTIN

Resistin is a 10-kDa adipose tissue–specific hormone recently identified in a screen for transcripts upregulated during adipogenesis and downregulated by treatment with a PPARγ agonist (194). Whereas injection of resistin into wild-type mice impaired glucose tolerance and insulin action, neutralizing antibodies improved insulin action in obese diabetic mice (194). When resistin was infused at near-physiologic levels in normal rats, lower rates of glucose infusion were necessary to maintain basal glucose levels during a hyperinsulinemic clamp study (195). The insulin resistance caused by resistin infusion was wholly accounted for by an increase in the rate of glucose production, suggesting that resistin has rapid inhibitory effects on hepatic rather than peripheral insulin sensitivity.

Despite this compelling evidence for acute effects of resistin on *in vivo* insulin action, there remains considerable uncertainty about the significance of resistin to the long-term regulation of insulin action in animals and humans. Indeed, resistin mRNA appears to be downregulated in most mouse models of insulin resistance (196). Additionally, resistin expression was very low in isolated adipocytes from human adipose tissue explants (197) and was actually higher in monocytes (198) and other non-adipocyte cells of adipose tissue (199) than in adipocytes. Furthermore, although some studies suggest a link between resistin levels and BMI or insulin sensitivity in humans (200–202), others have failed to reveal such a connection (203–205). However, it is possible that serum levels do not correlate with tissue mRNA or protein levels, a phenomenon observed for other adipokines under certain conditions (206). Given the challenges of reliably measuring plasma levels of resistin, most published papers on this topic report only tissue resistin transcript levels, and therefore more studies will be necessary to determine the clinical relevance of resistin in obesity and in the development of insulin resistance.

Obesity and Inflammation

There is growing evidence that the relationship between inflammation and insulin resistance is not merely correlative but actually causative (207). Epidemiologic data from several large studies have demonstrated a link between insulin resistance and systemic inflammation in both type 2 diabetes and nondiabetic populations (208–210). Adipose tissue produces many proinflammatory molecules, including TNF-α, IL-6, transforming growth factor-β, C-reactive protein, and monocyte chemotactic (chemoattractant) protein-1 (MCP-1), and circulating levels of these "adipokines" are increased in obesity (211–216).

Adipose-derived proinflammatory molecules are believed to induce systemic insulin resistance and to contribute to the pathogenesis of many metabolic complications of obesity, including type 2 diabetes and atherosclerosis (210). Although definitive human evidence is still accumulating, substantial experimental evidence links proinflammatory molecules with insulin resistance. The proinflammatory cytokine TNF-α has been demonstrated to mediate insulin resistance as a result of obesity in several rodent models (217). Expression of TNF-α was increased in white adipose tissue from different rodent models of obesity and diabetes (217), with elevations in TNF-α protein both locally and systemically. Neutralization of TNF-α in insulin-resistant rats caused a significant increase in the peripheral uptake of glucose in response to insulin (217,218). Furthermore, mice lacking either the TNF-α ligand or one of its receptors were partially protected from obesity-induced insulin resistance (219,220). TNF-α directly decreases insulin sensitivity and increases lipolysis in adipocytes (221,222). Expression of TNF-α is increased in white adipose tissue in obese and insulin-resistant states (223). Multiple mechanisms have been suggested to account for these metabolic effects of TNF-α, including direct effects on insulin signaling, downregulation of genes that are required for normal insulin action, induction of elevated FFA levels via stimulation of lipolysis, and negative regulation of PPARα (224).

Although neutralizing TNF-α with circulating antibodies did not cause metabolic improvement in humans with type 2 diabetes (225), this does not exclude the possibility of important paracrine effects of this cytokine on fat tissue. Despite the protean studies demonstrating a link between TNF-α and insulin resistance, there is no evidence that TNF-α directly causes insulin resistance in skeletal muscle. Indeed, TNF-α activates NF-B, a transcription factor that regulates the expression of many inflammatory molecules (226). It is therefore possible that the predominant effects of TNF-α are to stimulate the production of other cytokines, some of which ultimately exert direct effects on muscle. In addition to TNF-α, other cytokines are known to have metabolic effects. IL-6 also increases lipolysis and has been implicated in the hypertriglyceridemia and increased serum FFA levels associated with obesity (227). Additionally, IL-6 induces cellular insulin resistance in hepatocytes (228). Recently, the chemokine MCP-1 also was shown to impair adipocyte insulin sensitivity (229).

Historically, it has been known that high doses of salicylates are able to lower blood glucose concentrations (230). Indeed, TNF-α activates NF-B by stimulating IB kinase complex (IKK) activity, and salicylate has been demonstrated to inhibit TNF-α–induced stimulation of IKK activity (231). It was recently shown that reduced signaling through the IKKβ pathway, a key pathway in tissue inflammation, either by salicylate-based inhibitors or decreased IKKβ expression, is accompanied by improved insulin sensitivity *in vivo* (232,233). Ultimately, aspirin treatment inhibits serine phosphorylation of IRS-1 in TNF-α–treated cells through targeting multiple serine kinases (234). High-dose aspirin treatment for 2 weeks resulted in significant reductions in fasting plasma glucose in nine patients with type 2 diabetes, with reduced basal rates of hepatic glucose production and improved insulin-stimulated peripheral glucose uptake (235).

Independent studies have recently indicated that obesity in rodents and humans is associated with increased infiltration of macrophages into adipose tissue (236–238). These findings suggest an intriguing mechanism for the increased production of proinflammatory peptides by adipose tissue in obesity. With the onset of obesity, secretion of low levels of TNF-α by adipocytes is believed to stimulate preadipocytes to produce MCP-1, a chemoattractant specific for monocytes and macrophages (237). Increased secretion of leptin by adipocytes may also contribute to macrophage accumulation by stimulating transport of macrophages to adipose tissue (239) and promoting adhesion of macrophages to endothelial cells, respectively (240). Adipocytes also produce colony-stimulating factor-1 (CSF-1), the primary regulator of macrophage differentiation and survival (241). Therefore, increasing adiposity may result in adipose-derived signals such as MCP-1, causing increased monocyte influx. The production of CSF-1 by adipocytes may then create a permissive microenvironment for these monocytes to differentiate and survive as mature adipose tissue macrophages. Once activated macrophages are present in sufficient numbers within adipose tissue, it is likely that they cooperate with adipocytes and other cell types to perpetuate a vicious circle of macrophage recruitment and production of inflammatory cytokines, ultimately causing systemic insulin resistance.

Adipocyte cell size is highly correlated with indicators of systemic insulin resistance, dyslipidemia, and risk for developing type 2 diabetes (242–245). Potential mechanisms whereby adipocyte hypertrophy may perturb adipocyte function and thereby influence systemic glucose and lipid metabolism (246) include induction of sterol regulatory element binding protein-2 (SREBP-2) and its target genes (247) and secretion of increased quantities of secreted products such as leptin (248) or TNF-α (249). The data for humans and mice show that adipocyte size is a strong predictor of the percentage of macrophages in adipose tissue (237). The close relationship between adipocyte size and the abundance of macrophages in adipose tissue suggests that the influence of adipocyte size on adipocyte function may be conveyed through a paracrine pathway involving adipose tissue macrophages (237).

Visceral fat mass, which includes both mesenteric and omental intraabdominal fat depots, is more closely correlated with obesity-associated pathology than is overall adiposity (250–252). Proposed mechanisms for the negative metabolic effects of visceral fat include unrestrained lipolysis with increased circulating FFA levels, a specific increase in portal delivery of FFA, and unfavorable secretion profiles of adipose-derived proteins. Relative to subcutaneous fat cells, visceral fat cells are more sensitive to the lipolytic effect of catecholamines and less sensitive to the antilipolytic effect of insulin (253). Furthermore, the venous effluent of visceral fat depots leads directly into the portal vein, resulting in greater FFA flux to the liver in viscerally obese individuals (254). Increased hepatic delivery of fatty acids results in hepatic insulin resistance and in decreased insulin clearance, with secondary effects of peripheral insulin resistance (254).

Additionally, visceral versus subcutaneous fat might display different secretion profiles of proteins with systemic metabolic roles. Comparisons of the relative expression of metabolically relevant genes have revealed a few depot-specific expression patterns that may be consistent with a metabolically adverse role of visceral adipose tissue. These include increased expression of resistin in visceral fat, versus increased expression of leptin and IRS-1 in subcutaneous fat (255). Possible explanations for hormonal contributions to visceral adiposity include the observed increase in gene expression of receptors for glucocorticoids and androgens in this depot (255). However, there are some noteworthy limitations to these comparisons, including the observation that the insulin-sensitizing protein adiponectin is expressed at higher levels by visceral adipocytes (256). The example of adiponectin may provide important insights into the secretion patterns of these adipose depots, because plasma adiponectin levels fall markedly with visceral adiposity (257), in concert with decreased adiponectin expression in visceral fat with obesity (258). This suggests that adipocyte size and/or degree of lipid engorgement affects its secretion profile and that visceral adipose tissue may display altered secretion of proteins with expansion of this depot.

The relative contribution of the above factors to the metabolic effects of visceral fat has recently been examined in elegant studies with several rodent models of insulin resistance. Surgical removal of epididymal and perinephric fat pads dramatically lowered insulin levels and improved insulin action in both diet-induced and genetically obese rodent models without altering portal or peripheral FFA levels (259,260). Intriguingly, removal of the visceral fat pads also resulted in marked decreases in the gene expression of TNF-α and leptin in subcutaneous fat. This suggests that there may be "cross-talk" between adipose depots, and indicates an important role for the secretory products of visceral fat both in the biology of subcutaneous fat and in the induction of insulin resistance.

Abnormalities of Fat Deposition

LIPODYSTROPHY

In apparent contradiction to the above models of obesity-induced insulin resistance, similar metabolic features are paradoxically observed in the presence of decreased body fat, including insulin resistance, hyperlipidemia, and diabetes (121). The severity of the metabolic abnormalities varies widely and correlates roughly with the degree of fat deficiency.

Lipodystrophies can be subdivided into two major types: familial and acquired. The main subtypes of familial lipodystrophies (congenital generalized lipodystrophy and FPLD) have been described above. Whereas patients with acquired generalized lipodystrophy (Lawrence syndrome) have generalized loss of subcutaneous fat, those with acquired partial lipodystrophy (Barraquer-Simons syndrome) have fat loss limited to the face, trunk, and upper extremities (261–263). These acquired lipodystrophy syndromes occur approximately three times more frequently in women, begin during childhood, and are associated with underlying autoimmune disorders such as dermatomyositis and scleroderma.

Lipodystrophy is also encountered frequently in patients infected with human immunodeficiency virus (HIV), particularly among those receiving HIV-1 protease inhibitors (264,265). This HIV-associated lipodystrophy is characterized by loss of subcutaneous fat from the extremities and face but excess fat deposition in the neck and trunk. Among the proposed mechanisms for this finding is the possibility that HIV protease inhibitors impair adipocyte differentiation, because they have been shown to block preadipocyte differentiation *in vitro* (266). However, lipodystrophy has also been observed in HIV-infected patients treated with other antiretroviral agents who have never received protease inhibitors (267). This opens the possibility that HIV-associated lipodystrophy may not be caused by a specific drug regimen but may instead be a consequence of HIV infection per se in effectively treated patients (267). Other causes of acquired localized lipodystrophies include drugs, pressure, injection of insulin or growth hormone, and panniculitis (268).

Several fatless transgenic mouse models may be helpful in elucidating the mechanism (or mechanisms) whereby lipodystrophy causes insulin resistance. In the models described below, selected genes were selectively expressed in adipose tissue by means of the promoter/enhancer of the *Ap2* (adipocyte fatty acid binding protein) gene. With Ap2-targeted expression of an attenuated diphtheria toxin, mice displayed progressive adipose tissue atrophy and necrosis, with a 90% reduction in fat-pad weight by 10 months of age (269). Adipose-selective expression of a dominant-negative protein called A-ZIP/F inactivates several transcription factors implicated in adipocyte growth and differentiation, resulting in complete absence of visible white adipose tissue at all times during development (270). Unexpectedly, white adipose tissue–deficient mice were also generated by adipose-specific expression of a constitutively active form of the transcription factor SREBP-1c, which stimulates transcription of genes regulating fatty acid biosynthesis (271).

These rodent models are all severely insulin resistant and have a phenotype similar to that of patients with severe lipodystrophy, including increased accumulation of triglyceride in muscle and liver. Indeed, the lack of white adipose tissue causes leptin deficiency, which probably contributes to the insulin resistance and tissue triglyceride accumulation (272,273). However, although leptin normalized glucose levels and nearly normalized insulin levels in the aP2–SREBP-1c mice (274) and in humans with lipodystrophy (275), it had a more modest effect on glucose and insulin levels in A-ZIP/F-1 mice (276). Although it is possible that higher doses and/or more prolonged treatment with leptin would be more effective in the latter model, this may underscore the loss of other important functions or factors provided by adipose tissue. The lack of white adipose tissue to take up and store fat leads to increased blood levels of FFA and triglycerides and to tissue triglyceride accumulation. Increased circulating FFAs and increased tissue triglyceride deposition have also been proposed as a cause of insulin resistance, through purported mechanisms discussed below. Probably more important, there is an accumulation of intracellular fatty acid metabolites (fatty acyl-CoAs [coenzyme A], diacylglycerol, and ceramides, among others) in these insulin-responsive tissues, which leads to acquired defects in insulin signaling and insulin resistance. Another important factor contributing to hyperinsulinemia in fatless mice may be the reduced plasma leptin levels, because leptin has been shown to negatively regulate insulin secretion (277,278).

As further evidence for multiple metabolic effects of fat tissue, the severe metabolic defects in these rodent lipodystrophy models are reversed in a dose-dependent manner by surgical transplantation of wild-type adipose tissue (279–283). However, it is intriguing to note that transplantation of adipose tissue lacking leptin is unable to reverse the metabolic abnormalities associated with lipoatrophy (284). The modest effects of leptin alone in the same model (280) suggest the potential importance of other secreted proteins from leptin-primed adipose tissue.

By contrast to the above models, fatless Irs1/Irs3 double knockout mice do not have increased triglyceride levels in liver or muscle yet manifest metabolic characteristics similar to those in lipodystrophic patients and in other transgenic mouse models (285,286). The fact that tissue triglyceride accumulation is not an essential component of lipodystrophic insulin resistance raises important questions about whether abnormal muscle and liver fat causes insulin resistance, as discussed below. Of note, the hyperglycemia and hyperinsulinemia of the Irs1/Irs3 double knockout mice are reversed by adenovirus-mediated expression of leptin in the liver.

Thus, both too little and too much fat can cause insulin resistance. Perhaps obesity and lipodystrophy have more similarities than may initially be apparent. In both cases, a storage defect within adipocytes (due either to massive engorgement with lipid or to a paucity of differentiated adipocytes) leads to excess accumulation of triglyceride in nonadipose tissues (discussed below) and decreased secretion of certain adipokines with favorable metabolic effects. In the case of obesity, the greater overall fat mass in obese individuals will result in an elevation of fatty acid flux to nonadipose tissues, even in the absence of a qualitative abnormality in adipose tissue metabolism (287). Also, increased adiposity may result in proportionally greater secretion of hormones and other adipokines that negatively impact insulin action and in decreased secretion of those with favorable effects. Notable examples would include the decrease in adiponectin and increase in inflammatory mediators with obesity.

INTRAMYOCELLULAR TRIGLYCERIDE ACCUMULATION

Intramuscular triglyceride accumulation is associated with muscle insulin resistance in lean and obese, nondiabetic, and type 2 diabetic humans (288–290). Sophisticated nuclear magnetic resonance (NMR) spectroscopy imaging of muscle lipid accumulation permits the clear distinction of intramyocellular triglyceride (IMTG) deposition from intercellular striation (291,292) and has demonstrated that IMTG is strongly associated with insulin resistance (293). Despite a considerable amount of interest in this area, it remains to be determined whether muscle accumulation of triglyceride is merely a marker of other metabolic abnormalities or plays a causative role in the development of insulin resistance.

A central question in the etiology of IMTG accumulation in insulin-resistant individuals is whether triglycerides accumulate as a result of increased total FFA flux to muscle or of a primary defect in fatty acid oxidation (254). Muscle from obese, insulin-resistant individuals appears to have a reduced capacity for uptake and oxidation of circulating FFAs (294,295), which might be attributable to defects of fatty acid oxidation at the levels of carnitine palmitoyltransferase-1 (CPT-1) or at a subsequent step or both (296). The CPT-1 enzyme controls the entry of long-chain fatty acyl-CoA (LCFA-CoA) into the mitochondria and is the initial and rate-limiting step in the oxidation of fatty acids. Of note, prolonged pharmacologic inhibition of muscle CPT-1 in rats causes the accumulation of IMTG and the development of insulin resistance (297). Additionally, plasma delivery of FFA itself, as well as glucose delivery and plasma insulin levels, may determine the rate of muscle fatty acid oxidation (298–300) through tissue accumulation of malonyl-CoA. There is increased availability of circulating FFAs in insulin-resistant individuals (254). McGarry et al. (301) first identified malonyl-CoA as a biochemical sensor implicated in the switch from fatty acid to glucose oxidation, because malonyl-CoA is a potent allosteric inhibitor of CPT-1 (302). In the presence of high circulating levels of glucose, insulin, and FFA, the accumulation of malonyl-CoA inhibits CPT-1 and reduces fatty acid oxidation, favoring lipid storage into triglycerides. Experimental evidence suggests that excessive FFA delivery to muscle from the circulation can be a source of triglyceride accumulation in muscle (303,304). An extramuscular defect of fatty acid metabolism could contribute to the intramyocellular triglyceride accumulation and the skeletal muscle lipotoxic effects seen in obesity and type 2 diabetes (254). Together, these findings suggest that impaired muscle fatty acid oxidation and increased FFA delivery have synergistic effects on IMTG accumulation and muscle insulin resistance in patients with obesity and insulin resistance (305).

In studies of the relationship between IMTG and insulin action, many apparent clinical and experimental paradoxes suggest that IMTG may be a marker for other metabolic defects. Triglycerides accumulate in the muscle tissue of highly physically trained athletes (306), who demonstrate enhanced insulin sensitivity. A woman found to be homozygous for a missense mutation in the carnitine palmitoyltransferase II gene had decreased muscle fat oxidation and markedly impaired insulin-stimulated glucose uptake yet normal IMTG (307). Thus, it has been suggested that muscle triglyceride may not have adverse metabolic consequences in muscle that has the capacity for efficient lipid utilization (307). The onset of type 2 diabetes is associated with a marked increased accumulation of intramyocellular lipid (IMCL) despite no further worsening in insulin action. Additionally, although there was an initial correlation between IMCL and insulin resistance in individuals with type 2 diabetes, near-normalization of plasma glucose with insulin infusion for ~3 days increased IMCL without changing insulin action, such that postinsulin levels of IMCL were actually positively correlated with insulin sensitivity (308). Furthermore, in several cultured cell models, the accumulation of intracellular triglyceride actually appeared to be protective against toxic cellular effects of fatty acids (309). Whereas oleic acid supplementation promoted triglyceride accumulation and was associated with normal cell viability, excess palmitic acid was poorly incorporated into triglyceride and induced apoptosis. Moreover, in cells lacking the enzyme that catalyzes the final step in mammalian triglyceride synthesis, oleate induced cellular lipotoxicity. Although these studies exonerated intracellular triglyceride from proapoptotic effects of lipid accumulation, they did not specifically examine insulin action or identify a putative effector (or effectors) of lipotoxicity.

Indeed, a more consistent relationship has been demonstrated between insulin stimulation of glucose uptake and suppression of LCFA-CoA in skeletal muscle (310). Whereas improved insulin action and reduced LCFA-CoA resulted from both a bout of exercise and short-term caloric restriction, decreased muscle triglyceride was observed only with caloric restriction. There are several potential mechanisms whereby increased LCFA-CoA could inhibit muscle glucose metabolism (310). Increased LCFA-CoA could lead secondarily to increases in the concentration of diacylglycerol, phosphatidic acid, and triglycerides and activation of one or more protein kinase C (PKC) isoforms, which would downregulate insulin signaling. Other proposed mechanisms whereby increases in LCFA-CoA could cause insulin resistance include alterations in membrane fluidity (311,312), direct inhibition of enzymes such as glycogen synthase (313), and acylation of proteins involved in GLUT4 translocation (314). LCFA-CoAs would be expected to accumulate in the cytosol under conditions of increased FFA availability and decreased fatty acid oxidation, as was described above in the context of insulin resistance. States of energy excess, glucose, insulin, and citrate result in increased malonyl-CoA, which is paralleled by a rise in cytosolic LCFA-CoA.

INTRAHEPATOCELLULAR TRIGLYCERIDE ACCUMULATION

Nonalcoholic hepatic steatosis (fat infiltration) is frequently observed in obese subjects (315,316) and can range from mild hepatic steatosis to steatohepatitis, fibrosis, and cirrhosis (317,318). Although liver biopsy is considered the "gold standard" for quantification of liver triglyceride accumulation, localized ^{1}H magnetic resonance spectroscopy provides a noninvasive and highly specific estimation of hepatic fat *in vivo* (319,320). As with the relationship between IMCL and insulin action, it remains to be determined whether hepatic steatosis causes or develops as a consequence of hepatic and/or peripheral insulin resistance (321). Several recent observations demonstrating correlations between intrahepatocellular triglyceride (IHTG) and both hepatic and peripheral insulin action will be presented here along with proposed theories for how IHTG might impact insulin action.

Hepatic steatosis is associated with decreased requirements for glucose infusion during hyperinsulinemic clamp studies, indicating insulin resistance that could be either hepatic or peripheral (322). Likewise, percent hepatic fat was the obesity-associated parameter best correlated with daily insulin dose in subjects with stable type 2 diabetes (323). Nonobese, nondiabetic subjects with biopsy-proven nonalcoholic fatty liver disease demonstrated both reduced insulin-mediated suppression of hepatic glucose production (approximately a twofold increase relative to nonsteatotic controls) and reduced insulin-stimulated glucose disposal (by ~ 50%) and insulin resistance comparable to that of individuals with type 2 diabetes (324). Likewise, stratification of healthy nondiabetic men by IHTG revealed impaired suppression of glucose production by insulin in the men with higher hepatic fat content (325). A small decrease in insulin-stimulated glucose disposal in the higher IHTG group was not significant; however, these subjects were less insulin resistant than those in the previous study. Among individuals with type 2 diabetes, the presence of hepatic steatosis as detected by computed tomography (CT) scanning was associated with reduced insulin-stimulated glucose uptake, whereas only the male subjects demonstrated impaired suppression of glucose production by insulin (326). In a group of healthy nondiabetic subjects, IHTG demonstrated a stronger inverse correlation than IMCL with insulin sensitivity, and this relationship remained significant when corrected for visceral fat content (327).

These intriguing associations between IHTG and peripheral insulin action are consistent with a transgenic mouse model in which decreasing IHTG improved muscle insulin action (328). Liver-specific enhancement of fatty acid oxidation was associated with increased insulin-stimulated peripheral glucose uptake, even though IMCL was actually increased in some muscles (328). Although there is currently no definitive explanation for these observations, it has been proposed that an as yet unidentified liver factor increases glucose uptake into skeletal muscle, because raw liver extracts increased the glucose uptake in isolated rat hindquarter (329). It is conceivable that increased hepatic fat accumulation might interfere with the production or release of this factor, resulting in impaired peripheral insulin action.

"ENVIRONMENTAL" FACTORS CONTRIBUTING TO INSULIN RESISTANCE

Medical Conditions That Result in Insulin Resistance

Insulin resistance has been reported to result from many medical conditions. A discussion of the impaired insulin action that results from many endocrinopathies follows in the next section, and the association of insulin resistance with lipodystrophies is discussed elsewhere in this chapter. One of the first medical causes of insulin resistance to be identified was the presence of antibodies to insulin receptor (type B insulin resistance) (330,331). Although frequently encountered when animal insulin was in wide usage, clinically significant levels of antibodies to insulin receptor have also been described in the presence of various autoimmune disorders, including systemic lupus erythematosus (332). Insulin resistance is also a characteristic feature of renal failure and uremia and improves with dialysis (333,334). The cause of the insulin resistance in renal failure is likely to be multifactorial. Loss of muscle mass and decreased physical fitness, accumulation of uremic toxins, raised levels of growth hormone and glucagon, metabolic acidosis, and dyslipidemia have all been proposed as potential mechanisms (335).

Hepatic cirrhosis is frequently associated with glucose intolerance and insulin resistance (336,337). Although the mechanism (or mechanisms) underlying the insulin insensitivity are unknown, they may include elevation in circulating FFAs and insulin levels, both shown below to inhibit insulin action. Studies of glucose tolerance demonstrated defects in insulin secretion and insulin action, both of which were related to the degree of hepatic iron deposition, in a large kindred with familial hemochromatosis (338). Indeed, iron overload appears to impair both hepatic and peripheral insulin action early in the course of hereditary hemochromatosis (prior to overt hepatic cirrhosis), and phlebotomy may improve insulin action in affected individuals (339,340). In addition, transfusion-induced iron overload in thalassemia major was shown to be associated with insulin resistance, apparently proportional to the degree of liver disease (341).

Insulin resistance has been recognized in patients with any of several types of cancer, particularly malignancies of the gastrointestinal tract and pancreas (342,343). It has been proposed that inflammatory mediators contribute to this insulin resistance, particularly TNF-α and IL-6 (344–346). Potential mechanisms whereby these cytokines inhibit insulin action are discussed below.

Hormonal Mediators of Insulin Action

Insulin resistance has been documented in the presence of many syndromes of abnormal hormone levels, particularly states of hormone excess. These endocrinopathies will be described in some detail, as these disease states shed light on the role of hormones in the pathogenesis of insulin resistance (Fig. 24.3).

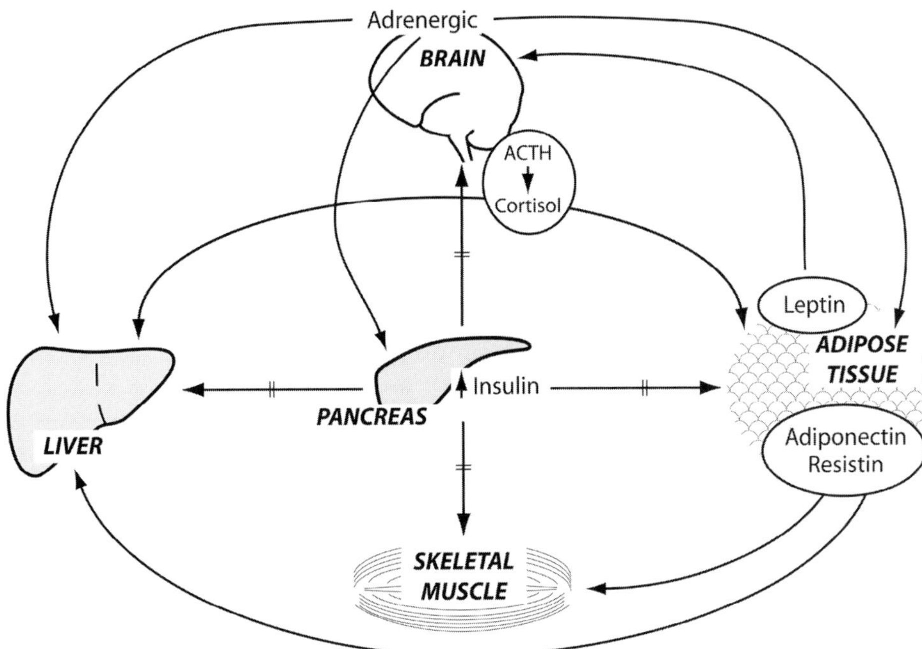

Figure 24.3. The contribution of hormonal hypersecretion to insulin resistance. The diagram identifies hormones whose circulating levels are increased in the metabolic syndrome and shows the tissue-specific effects of hormonal hypersecretion on insulin action, including the effects of hyperinsulinemia per se. ACTH, adrenocorticotropic hormone.

Hyperinsulinemia is the classic indicator of insulin resistance and may itself contribute to the insulin resistance in type 2 diabetes and obesity. Indeed, elevating plasma insulin levels for 7 days in normal rats results in impaired insulin-mediated glucose uptake (347). Additionally, euglycemic, hyperinsulinemic clamp studies have revealed decreased peripheral glucose uptake in patients with insulinoma (348). Moreover, insulin receptor levels are normal or only mildly impaired in type 1 diabetes (349) and are generally increased in animal models of hypoinsulinemic diabetes (350). Amelioration of hyperinsulinemia by streptozotocin treatment in two obese-animal models corrected the decreased levels of insulin receptor expression (351). These data suggest that hyperinsulinemia causes downregulation of the insulin receptor due to increased internalization and degradation after insulin binds to its receptor, leading to secondary insulin resistance (352). Thus chronic hyperinsulinemia in the metabolic syndrome, likely secondary to nutrient excess and insufficient caloric expenditure, in turn contributes to insulin resistance.

Counterregulatory hormones (cortisol, epinephrine, norepinephrine, glucagon, and growth hormone) play significant roles in antagonizing insulin action after hypoglycemia (353). Of note, 24-hour infusions of cortisol impaired insulin-induced suppression of glucose production and stimulation of glucose utilization in normal volunteers (354). Peripheral glucose uptake is also markedly reduced in individuals with Cushing syndrome, even as compared with obese individuals (355). It has been proposed that the metabolic syndrome is associated with hyperactivity of the hypothalamic-pituitary-adrenal axis and that the enhanced cortisol secretion contributes to insulin resistance (356).

It is not clear whether increased sympathetic nervous system activity, which may occur in the metabolic syndrome (357), contributes to decreased insulin signaling. However, in white adipocytes (358), stimulation of the β-adrenergic receptor decreases insulin-stimulated PI 3-kinase activity. Desensitization of β-adrenergic receptors by isoproterenol increases insulin-stimulated glucose uptake in white adipocytes (359). A naturally occurring mutation of the β_3-adrenergic receptor (W64R) has been associated with increased abdominal obesity and early-onset type 2 diabetes (360), although this remains controversial. In isolated human omental adipocytes, the W64R variant shows decreased β-agonist–induced lipolysis (361), providing a potential mechanism whereby omental adipocity may be increased in patients with this variant. Pheochromocytoma-associated decreases in peripheral insulin action corrected rapidly following surgical resection, suggesting that the insulin resistance was secondary to the pheochromocytoma (362). Among the postulated mechanisms for this insulin resistance are increased levels of norepinephrine (363) or epinephrine or both (364,365).

Growth hormone acts at several levels to block insulin actions, including the inhibition of phosphorylation of the insulin receptor and one of its principal signaling molecules, IRS-1, in response to insulin administration. This leads to reduced sensitivity to insulin both in stimulating peripheral glucose uptake and in suppressing glucose production (366). Furthermore, an excess of growth hormone leads to mobilization of FFAs, which inhibit insulin-stimulated glucose oxidation by acting as a competitive energy source, thus leading to further worsening of insulin resistance. Most patients with acromegaly have some degree of insulin resistance (367). These abnormalities have been reversed by surgical resection of growth hormone–secreting tumors (368) and by administering agents that block growth hormone action (369). Although one study reported that long-term octreotide therapy decreased the secretion of growth hormone, the decrease did not correct the insulin resistance (370). In contrast to growth hormone, IGF-I appears to enhance insulin action and may partially counteract the insulin-opposing effects of growth hormone.

Systemic Effects of Nutrient Excess on Insulin Action

Along with the dramatic lifestyle changes described above, with unprecedented increases in nutrient intake, it is likely that biochemical adaptations that evolved to deal with famine now predispose to nutrient-induced insulin resistance. Teleologically,

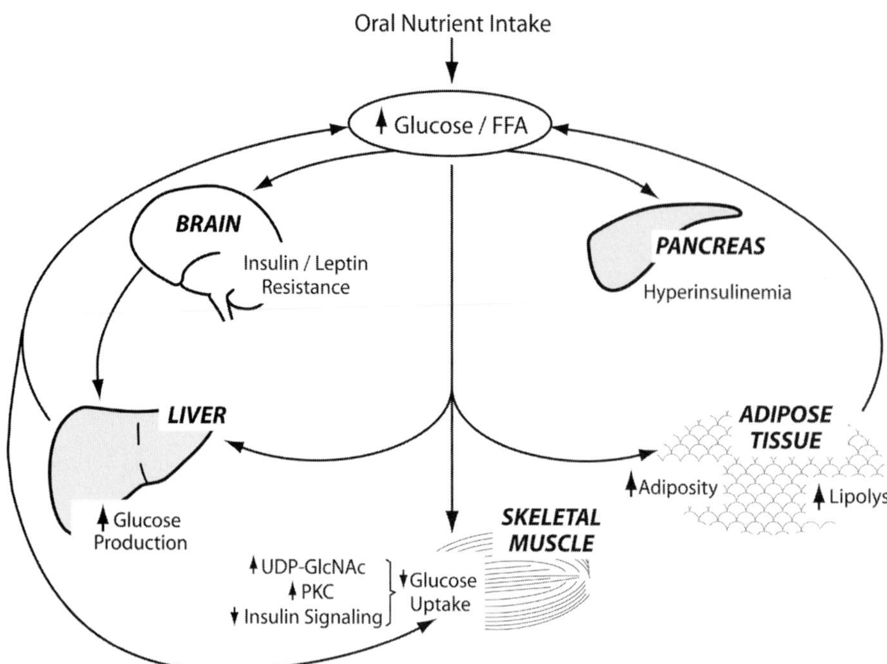

Figure 24.4. Systemic impact of nutrient excess. The diagram shows tissue sources and effects of increased availability of glucose and free fatty acids. FFA, free fatty acids; UDP-GlcNAc, uridine diphosphate-*N*-acetylglucosamine; PKC, protein kinase C.

downregulation of insulin action may have protected cells from potentially toxic effects of further influx of glucose and other nutrients (371). This concept is predicated upon the ability of the cell to "sense" nutrient availability via various mechanisms, which need to be tightly coupled to insulin signaling or glucose transport or both. This review will focus on the effects of increased availability of glucose and FFAs on potential nutrient-sensing pathways and ultimately on insulin action (Fig. 24.4).

GLUCOSE

Glucose toxicity refers to the inhibitory effects of chronic hyperglycemia on insulin secretion and action (372). Hyperglycemia-induced insulin resistance includes downregulation of the glucose transport system by hyperglycemia and a defect in insulin-stimulated glycogen synthesis. Initial clinical evidence of this phenomenon came from the observation that patients with poorly controlled type 1 diabetes are insulin resistant and that this insulin resistance can be ameliorated by tight glycemic control (373,374). Normalization of blood glucose levels with phlorizin treatment completely corrected insulin-mediated glucose metabolism in diabetic rats (375) and restored insulin-mediated glucose transport in adipose cells without restoring glucose transporter gene expression (376). Furthermore, in diabetic GK rats, an animal model of lean type 2 diabetes, normalization of glycemia by phlorizin treatment improves glucose tolerance, insulin signaling, and glucose transport in skeletal muscle (377,378).

Following the serendipitous observation that the amino acid glutamine was required for the desensitization by high levels of glucose to insulin in primary cultures of adipocytes, Marshall et al. (379) demonstrated with a series of elegant studies that the flux of glucose through the hexosamine biosynthetic pathway (HBP) is required for glucose-induced insulin resistance. He determined that glucose-induced desensitization of the glucose transport system could be prevented by glutamine analogues that inhibit glutamine:fructose-6-phosphate amidotransferase (GFAT), the initial and rate-limiting enzyme in hexosamine biosynthesis (380,381) (Fig. 24.5). After transport and phosphorylation of glucose to glucose 6-phosphate, the latter is used primarily in the synthesis of glycogen and in glycolysis. A small fraction (1% to 3%) of incoming glucose, after its conversion to fructose 6-phosphate, enters the HBP. The final step in the HBP is the formation of uridine diphosphate (UDP)-*N*-acetylglucosamine (GlcNAc), which is a main substrate for protein glycosylation and whose intracellular levels are nutritionally regulated (382–385). The activities of many cytoplasmic and nuclear proteins appear to be regulated by glycosylation on their serine and/or threonine residues, including important enzymes and transcriptional factors (386,387). The HBP could be considered a prime example of a biochemical mechanism of nutrient sensing, in that it becomes activated by increased glucose fluxes (388).

Administration of glucosamine, which enters the HBP at a point distal to enzymatic amidation by GFAT, induced cellular insulin resistance to a degree comparable to that of hyperglycemia, even in the presence of normal glucose levels (389). Glucose-induced insulin resistance is blunted by inhibiting GFAT activity and expression (390), suggesting that the deleterious effects of hyperglycemia are mediated by activation of HBP. *In vivo*, infusion of glucosamine into conscious rats induced a pattern of impaired insulin-stimulated glucose uptake and glycogen synthesis that was similar to the glucose toxicity model described above (381). Furthermore, the effects of glucosamine infusion and chronic hyperglycemia were not additive in diabetic rats, indicating that it is likely that increased flux through the hexosamine pathway could account for the insulin resistance observed with hyperglycemia. The link between insulin resistance and HBP has been validated in transgenic models in which the overexpression of GFAT in muscle and fat leads to peripheral insulin resistance (391,392). HBP induces insulin resistance by inhibiting multiple sites in the insulin-signaling cascade, particularly activation of PI 3-kinase by insulin (393). Several groups have shown that insulin-dependent glucose uptake, as well as glycogen synthesis, is downregulated by HBP activation (394,395).

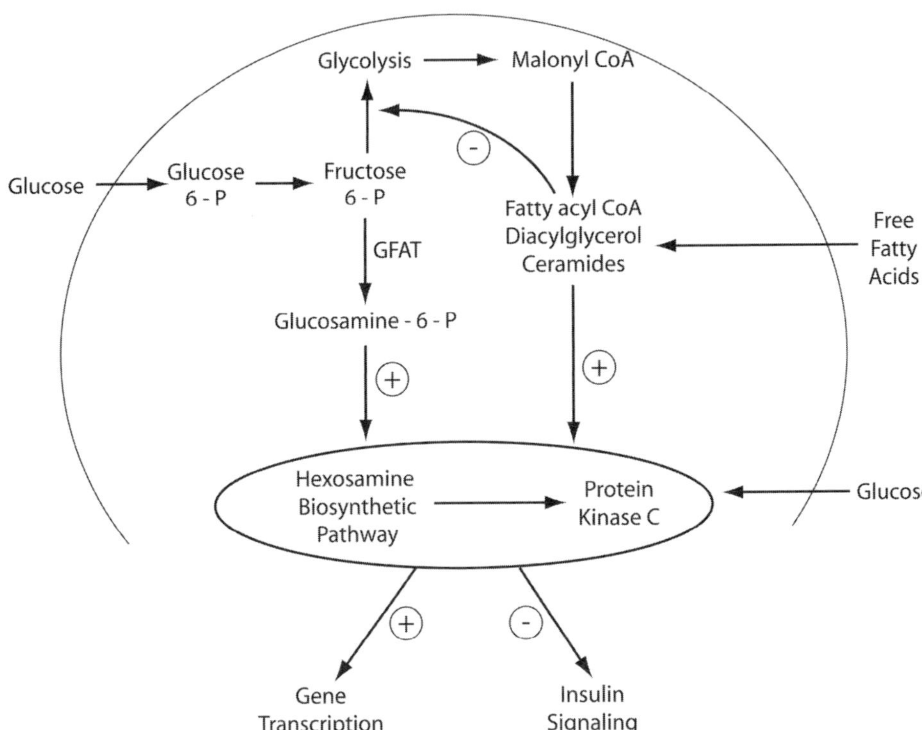

Figure 24.5. The role of nutrient-sensing pathways in the induction of nutrient-mediated insulin resistance. In the presence of increased glucose and insulin, intracellular generation of malonyl-CoA results in increased fatty acyl-CoA. Both the hexosamine biosynthetic pathway and protein kinase C (PKC) are activated by increased glucose and fatty acyl-CoA, and both probably contribute to insulin resistance by impacting gene transcription and insulin signaling. Increased flux through the hexosamine pathway has been shown to activate PKC. GFAT, glutamine:fructose-6-phosphate amidotransferase; P, phosphate.

Another potential mechanism for glucose-induced downregulation of insulin action is activation of the serine kinase PKC, described above. PKC is activated by the intracellular metabolite diacylglycerol, whose intracellular concentration increases in a glucose-dependent manner during exposure of isolated muscles to hyperinsulinemia (396). In NIH3T3 cells overexpressing the insulin receptor, PKC inhibitors blocked insulin desensitization by glucose (397). An intriguing potential link between glucose-induced activation of the HBP and PKC was provided by the recent observation that both hyperglycemia and glucosamine activate PKCβ and PKCδ (398). Indeed, cotransfection of dominant-negative versions of these PKC isoforms prevented the activation of PAI-1 promoter transcription by both sugars, because PAI-1 gene expression is known to be regulated by the HBP via glycosylation of the transcription factor Sp-1 (399). The potential collaborative role of these pathways in mediating insulin resistance is schematically outlined in Fig. 24.5.

INCREASED LEVELS OF CIRCULATING FREE FATTY ACIDS

Chronic elevations in circulating FFA levels are a classic feature of insulin resistance and type 2 diabetes (269,400). Their impact on insulin action in both skeletal muscle and liver will be discussed separately below.

Skeletal Muscle. Inadequate suppression of fatty acid oxidation by insulin is a common feature of various forms of insulin resistance in humans (401), and a strong, inverse correlation between glucose and lipid oxidation has been observed in obese subjects with type 2 diabetes (402). Randle et al. (403) first recognized this relationship between carbohydrate and lipid metabolism in heart and diaphragm muscle. The ensuing hypothesis was that a glucose–fatty acid cycle operates by decreasing the rate of oxidation of the alternate substrate in the presence of increased availability of the other (404). As initially proposed by Randle, an increase in fatty acid availability results in an elevation of the intramitochondrial acetyl CoA/CoA and NADH/NAD^+ (reduced form of nicotinamide adenine dinucleotide/oxidized form of nicotinamide adenine dinucleotide) ratios, with subsequent inactivation of pyruvate dehydrogenase. This in turn causes an increase in citrate concentrations, leading to inhibition of phosphofructokinase. Subsequent increases in intracellular concentrations of glucose-6-phosphate were predicted to inhibit hexokinase II activity, resulting in an increase in intracellular glucose concentration and a decrease in muscle glucose uptake.

Many *in vivo* studies in both humans and animals have emphasized that, although an increase in circulating FFA levels during insulin-clamp studies promptly decreased the rate of carbohydrate oxidation, defective glucose uptake could be detected only after 3 to 4 hours of lipid infusion (405–408). Recent observations have led to a proposed mechanism whereby increased FFA levels lead to downregulation of insulin signaling in human skeletal muscle (409). Increased FFA levels have been shown to enhance phosphorylation of serine/threonine sites on insulin receptor substrates (IRS-1 and IRS-2), in turn reducing the ability of the insulin receptor substrates to activate PI 3-kinase and glucose transport (410). Moreover, an acute elevation of plasma fatty acids for 5 hours resulted in activation of the serine kinase PKCθ in skeletal muscle, which was associated with decreased tyrosine phosphorylation of IRS-1 (411). Chalkley et al. (412) have reported that lipid infusion for a comparable duration increased muscle levels of triglyceride and LCFA-CoA, which would be expected to cause an increase in diacylglycerol, a known potent activator of PKCθ (413). Activation of other PKC isoforms has recently been shown to be altered in skeletal muscle in FFA-induced insulin resistance. Increasing FFA levels for 2 hours in nondiabetic humans increased membrane-associated PKCβ2 and PKCθ (414). Additionally, fatty acid infusion reduced insulin-stimulated activation of PKCλ/ζ, an atypical PKC isoform required for insulin stimulation of glucose uptake and GLUT4 translocation, in muscle of normal rats (415).

Increased FFA levels may also promote inflammation. It has recently been hypothesized that FFAs may cause skeletal muscle insulin resistance by activating the serine kinase IKK-β, which subsequently leads to increased serine phosphorylation of IRS-1 (416). High-dose salicylate therapy, long known to be effective in lowering blood sugar levels in type 2 diabetes (417), has many antiinflammatory actions, including inhibition of IKK-β. Both high-dose salicylate therapy and targeted disruption of IKK-β prevented fat-induced insulin resistance and inactivation of IRS-1–associated PI 3-kinase in skeletal muscle (416).

The HBP, whose role in glucose-induced insulin resistance was discussed above, may provide a unifying mechanism for the metabolic effects of both glucose and FFAs (418). FFAs can inhibit the entry of fructose-6-phosphate into the glycolytic pathway, thereby causing a shunt of fructose-6-phosphate toward the formation of glucosamine-6-phosphate (419). Increased concentration of acetyl-CoA, derived in the mitochondria from the oxidation of fatty acids, decreases the rate of pyruvate oxidation via inhibition of pyruvate dehydrogenase (420). Furthermore, the entry of fructose-6-phosphate into the glycolytic pathway is also limited by the inhibition of phosphofructokinase, mediated by an increased concentration of citrate (403) or a decreased concentration of xylulose-5-phosphate or both (421). Indeed, sustained elevations in FFA levels in normal rats induced defects in insulin action and accumulation of skeletal muscle UDP-GlcNAc comparable to those observed in the presence of hyperglycemia and glucosamine infusion (382), suggesting that the increased intracellular fructose-6-phosphate provides substrate for the hexosamine pathway. Incubation of human myotubes with the saturated fatty acids palmitate and stearate resulted in a threefold to fourfold increase in expression of the mRNA of GFAT, the rate-limiting enzyme of the hexosamine pathway (422).

Liver. Increased circulating FFA levels also impair the suppressive effects of insulin on hepatic glucose production. Various mechanisms appear to contribute to this phenomenon. FFAs have been shown to stimulate gluconeogenesis *in vitro* (423), probably due to both increased production of ATP and NADH (424) and increased gluconeogenic gene expression (425). Additionally, chronic high-fat feeding in rats is associated with an increase in the activity ratio of hepatic glucose-6-phosphatase/glucokinase, thus favoring increased hepatic glucose output (426). Although this model also demonstrated hyperinsulinemia and other metabolic abnormalities, it has recently been shown that increased FFA levels per se acutely induce the expression of hepatic glucose-6-phosphatase in normal rats (427). Transcriptional regulation of hepatic genes by lipids could potentially be mediated via the PPARs (428). Combined elevations of malonyl-CoA and cytosolic long-chain CoA may contribute to increased hepatic glucose production in obesity and type 2 diabetes (254). Conversely, hyperinsulinemia promotes conditions favoring FFA biosynthesis, thus further aggravating the metabolic conditions. High levels of malonyl-CoA, by suppressing CPT-1, induce a preferential flux away from FFA oxidation and toward esterification, with increased production of triglycerides and very-low-density lipopolysaccharides and an exacerbation of the hyperlipidemia and insulin resistance (254).

Oxidative Stress

Inducing conditions of oxidative stress in *in vitro* models results in reduced responsiveness to insulin (429) and impaired insulin signaling (430). Furthermore, the antioxidant lipoic acid prevents the induction of insulin resistance in the presence of oxidative stress (431). It has been proposed that activation of common stress-activated signaling pathways such as nuclear factor-KB, p38 MAPK, and NH_2-terminal Jun kinases/stress-activated protein kinases by glucose and possibly FFAs leads to both insulin resistance and impaired insulin secretion (432,433). Increased oxidative stress has recently been proposed as a potential unifying mechanism among many nutrient-activated pathways (434). Indeed, increased nutrient availability increases the production of reactive oxygen species and thereby results in activation of PKC isoforms, increased formation of glucose-derived advanced glycation end-products, and increased glucose flux through the aldose reductase pathway (434). Although this relationship has been well established in endothelial cell models of diabetic complications, the role of oxidative stress in nutrient-mediated activation of PKC will likely also prove relevant in the pathogenesis of insulin resistance.

Aging

The final "environmental" factor that appears to contribute to insulin resistance is advancing age. An increased incidence of insulin resistance and type 2 diabetes has frequently been observed with both natural aging and progeria syndromes (435,436). Various characteristic features of aging that could predispose to insulin resistance include increased fat mass and particularly increased visceral adiposity (437,438), increased circulating levels of inflammatory proteins, and increased cellular accumulation of triglycerides (439). A consistent observation in multiple experimental models of aging is that chronic restriction of caloric intake markedly improves survival and prevents the onset of insulin resistance (440). It has been hypothesized that the beneficial effects of caloric restriction on the metabolic alterations of aging are largely accounted for by its prevention of visceral fat accumulation (441). Potential support for this theory is provided by the recent obervation that removal of visceral fat prevented insulin resistance and glucose intolerance in aging rat models of obesity and insulin resistance without altering plasma levels of FFAs (442).

It has recently been proposed that an age-associated decline in mitochondrial functions contributes to insulin resistance in the elderly (439). Indeed, mitochondrial oxidative and phosphorylation function as assessed by *in vivo* $^{13}C/^{31}P$ NMR spectroscopy was reduced by ~40% in association with increased intramyocellular and intrahepatocellular lipid content and decreased insulin-stimulated glucose uptake. Finally, it has been proposed that aging-induced resistance to the effects of leptin on fat distribution and insulin action contributes to the increased tissue lipid accumulation and insulin resistance (443). Of note, this aging-associated leptin resistance appears to be independent of fat mass, because long-term caloric restriction induced reductions in fat mass yet no improvement in sensitivity to leptin (444).

CONCLUSIONS

Obesity and type 2 diabetes are currently at epidemic levels both in the United States and around the world. Even more sobering is the prediction that, at current growth rates, the global prevalence of type 2 diabetes can be expected to essentially double within the next 20 years. Because the mortality and morbidity currently attributable to type 2 diabetes are already very high, the anticipated increase in the prevalence of type 2 diabetes is likely to bring an enormous healthcare burden. Although accompanying defects in insulin secretion are required for the development of frank diabetes, the significant contribution of insulin resistance to the pathogenesis of both type 2 diabetes and atherosclerotic disease underscores the clinical significance of this defect in hormone action.

As reviewed above, insulin resistance develops from the complex interplay of genes, obesity, and "environment," with the latter including nutritional and hormonal factors, as well as advancing age. Given the stable nature of the human genome, the burgeoning prevalence of insulin resistance is likely due to a rapid and dramatic lifestyle progression from hunting and gathering to farming to sedentary overeating. Indeed, genes that were selected over many millennia to favor energy efficiency and storage now appear to be highly maladaptive in the face of nutrient excess. There are complex and additive mechanisms whereby nutrient excess leads to insulin resistance, including the hormonal and proinflammatory effects of increased fat mass, as well as direct effects of nutrients on insulin action via nutrient-sensing pathways. To prevent toxic accumulation of nutrients in insulin-sensitive tissues such as skeletal muscle, activation of nutrient-sensing pathways such as the HBP and PKC may be interconnecting mechanisms to detect nutrient excess and inhibit further insulin-mediated glucose uptake.

Averting a global health crisis will require a reckoning of the toxic effects of current lifestyle trends and a radical adjustment in the ratio of calories consumed to calories expended.

REFERENCES

1. Rabinowitz D. Some endocrine and metabolic aspects of obesity. *Annu Rev Med* 1970;21:241–258.
2. Soeldner JS, Steinke J. Insulin resistance. *Med Clin North Am* 1965;49: 939–946.
3. Roth J, Kahn CR, Lesniak MA, et al. Receptors for insulin, NSILA-s, and growth hormone: applications to disease states in man. *Recent Prog Horm Res* 1975;31:95–139.
4. Folsom AR, Kushi LH, Anderson KE, et al. Associations of general and abdominal obesity with multiple health outcomes in older women: the Iowa Women's Health Study. *Arch Intern Med* 2000;160:2117–2128.
5. Chow W-H, Gridley G, Fraumeni JF, et al. Obesity, hypertension, and the risk of kidney cancer in men. *N Engl J Med* 2000;343:1305–1311.
6. Calle EE, Thun JM, Petrelli JM, et al. 1999. Body-mass index and mortality in a prospective cohort. *N Engl J Med* 1999;341:1097–1002.
7. DeFronzo RA. Insulin resistance: a multifaceted syndrome responsible for NIDDM, obesity, hypertension, dyslipidaemia and atherosclerosis. *Neth J Med* 1997;50:191–197.
8. Barrett-Connor EL. Obesity, atherosclerosis, and coronary artery disease. *Ann Intern Med* 1985;103:1010–1019.
9. O'Rahilly S. Science, medicine, and the future. Non-insulin dependent diabetes mellitus: the gathering storm. *BMJ* 1997;314:955–959.
10. Global Burden of Disease Estimate of 176,525,312 Individuals with Diabetes Mellitus in 2000. Data generated by World Health Organization and available at http://www.who.int/ncd/dia/databases4.htm
11. Warram JH, Martin BC, Krolewski AS, et al. Slow glucose removal rate and hyperinsulinemia precede the development of type II diabetes in the offspring of diabetic patients. *Ann Intern Med* 1990;113:909–915.
12. Lillioja S, Mott DM, Howard BV, et al. Impaired glucose tolerance as a disorder of insulin action. Longitudinal and cross-sectional studies in Pima Indians. *N Engl J Med* 1988;318:1217–1225.
13. Haffner SM, Stern MP, Dunn J, et al. Diminished insulin sensitivity and increased insulin response in nonobese, nondiabetic Mexican Americans. *Metabolism* 1990;39:842–847.
14. Reaven GM, Bernstein R, Davis B, et al. Nonketotic diabetes mellitus: insulin deficiency or insulin resistance? *Am J Med* 1976;60:80–88.
15. DeFronzo RA. The triumvirate: beta-cell, muscle, liver: a collusion responsible for NIDDM. *Diabetes* 1988;37:667–687.
16. Despres JP, Lamarche B, Mauriege P, et al. Hyperinsulinemia as an independent risk factor for ischemic heart disease. *N Engl J Med* 1996;334: 952–957.
17. Reaven GM. Banting Lecture. Role of insulin resistance in human disease. *Diabetes* 1988;37:1595–1607.
18. Expert Panel on Detection, Evaluation, and Treatment of High Blood Cholesterol in Adults. Executive Summary of the Third Report of the National Cholesterol Education Program (NCEP) Expert Panel on Detection, Evaluation, and Treatment of High Blood Cholesterol in Adults (Adult Treatment Panel III). *JAMA* 2001;285:2486–2497.
19. Ford ES, Giles WH, Dietz WH. Prevalence of the metabolic syndrome among US adults: findings from the Third National Health and Nutrition Examination Survey. *JAMA* 2002; 16;287:356–359.
20. Kereiakes DJ, Willerson JT. Metabolic syndrome epidemic. *Circulation* 2003;108:1552–1553.
21. Sakkinen PA, Wahl P, Cushman M, et al. Clustering of procoagulation, inflammation, and fibrinolysis variables with metabolic factors in insulin resistance syndrome. *Am J Epidemiol* 2000;152:897–907.
22. Groop LC, Bonadonna RC, DelPrato S, et al. Glucose and free fatty acid metabolism in non-insulin-dependent diabetes mellitus. Evidence for multiple sites of insulin resistance. *J Clin Invest* 1989;84:205–213.
23. DeFronzo RA, Ferrannini E, Simonson DC. Fasting hyperglycemia in non-insulin-dependent diabetes mellitus: contributions of excessive hepatic glucose production and impaired tissue glucose uptake. *Metabolism* 1989;38: 387–395.
24. Kim SP, Ellmerer M, Van Citters GW, et al. Primacy of hepatic insulin resistance in the development of the metabolic syndrome induced by an isocaloric moderate-fat diet in the dog. *Diabetes* 2003;52:2453–2460.
25. Ferrannini E, Galvan AQ, Gastaldelli A, et al. Insulin: new roles for an ancient hormone. *Eur J Clin Invest* 1999;29:842–852.
26. DeFronzo RA, Tobin JD, Andres R. Glucose clamp technique: a method for quantifying insulin secretion and resistance. *Am J Physiol* 1979;237:E214–E223.
27. Bergman RN, Steil GM, Bradley DC, et al. Modeling of insulin action in vivo. *Annu Rev Physiol* 1992;54:861–883.
28. Cline GW, Petersen KF, Krssak M, et al. Impaired glucose transport as a cause of decreased insulin-stimulated muscle glycogen synthesis in type 2 diabetes. *N Engl J Med* 1999;341:240–246.
29. Bruning JC, Michael MD, Winnay JN, et al. A muscle-specific insulin receptor knockout exhibits features of the metabolic syndrome of NIDDM without altering glucose tolerance. *Mol Cell* 1998;2:559–569.
30. Kim JK, Michael MD, Previs SF, et al. Redistribution of substrates to adipose tissue promotes obesity in mice with selective insulin resistance in muscle. *J Clin Invest* 2000;105:1791–1797.
31. Okamoto H, Accili D. In vivo mutagenesis of the insulin receptor. *J Biol Chem* 2003;278:28359–28362.
32. Zisman A, Peroni OD, Abel ED, et al. Targeted disruption of the glucose transporter 4 selectively in muscle causes insulin resistance and glucose intolerance. *Nat Med* 2000;6:924–928.
33. Wojtaszewski JF, Higaki Y, Hirshman MF, et al. Exercise modulates postreceptor insulin signaling and glucose transport in muscle-specific insulin receptor knockout mice *J Clin Invest* 1999;104:1257–1264.
34. Mu J, Brozinick JT Jr, Valladares O, et al. A role for AMP-activated protein kinase in contraction- and hypoxia-regulated glucose transport in skeletal muscle. *Mol Cell* 2001;7:1085–1094.
35. Shefi-Friedman L, Wertheimer E, Shen S, et al. Increased IGFR activity and glucose transport in cultured skeletal muscle from insulin receptor null mice. *Am J Physiol Endocrinol Metab* 2001;281:E16–E24.
36. Zierath JR, He L, Guma A, et al. Insulin action on glucose transport and plasma membrane GLUT4 content in skeletal muscle from patients with NIDDM. *Diabetologia* 1996;39:1180–1189.
37. Fernandez A, Kim J, Yakar S, et al. Functional inactivation of the IGF-I and insulin receptors in skeletal muscle causes type 2 diabetes. *Genes Dev* 2001;15: 1926–1934.
38. Zierath JR, Wallberg-Henriksson H. From receptor to effector: insulin signal transduction in skeletal muscle from type II diabetic patients. *Ann N Y Acad Sci* 2002;967:120–134.
39. Goodyear LJ, Giorgino F, Sherman LA, et al. Insulin receptor phosphorylation, insulin receptor substrate-1 phosphorylation, and phosphatidylinositol 3-kinase activity are decreased in intact skeletal muscle strips from obese subjects. *J Clin Invest* 1995;95:2195–2204.
40. Bjornholm M, Kawano Y, Lehtihet M, et al. Insulin receptor substrate-1 phosphorylation and phosphatidylinositol 3-kinase activity in skeletal muscle from NIDDM subjects after *in vivo* insulin stimulation. *Diabetes* 1997;46: 524–527.
41. Zierath JR, Krook A, Wallberg-Henriksson H. Insulin action in skeletal muscle from patients with NIDDM. *Mol Cell Biochem* 1998;182:153–160.
42. Zierath JR, Galuska D, Nolte LA, et al. Effects of glycemia on glucose transport in isolated skeletal muscle from patients with NIDDM: *in vitro* reversal of muscular insulin resistance. *Diabetologia* 1994;37:270–277.
43. Krutzfeldt J, Kausch C, Volk A, et al. Insulin signaling and action in cultured skeletal muscle cells from lean healthy humans with high and low insulin sensitivity. *Diabetes* 2000;49:992–998.
44. Maddux BA, Sbraccia P, Kumakura S, et al. Membrane glycoprotein PC-1 in the insulin resistance of non-insulin dependent diabetes mellitus. *Nature* 1995;373:448–451.
45. Goldfine ID, Maddux BA, Youngren JF, et al. Membrane glycoprotein PC-1 and insulin resistance. *Mol Cell Biochem* 1998;182:177–184.
46. Frittitta L, Spampinato D, Solini A, et al. Elevated PC-1 content in cultured skin fibroblasts correlates with decreased *in vivo* and *in vitro* insulin action in nondiabetic subjects: Evidence that PC-1 may be an intrinsic factor in impaired insulin receptor signaling. *Diabetes* 1998;47:1095–1100.
47. Kumakura S, Maddux BA, Sung CK. Overexpression of membrane glycoprotein PC-1 can influence insulin action at a post-receptor site. *J Cell Biochem* 1998;3:366–377.
48. Youngren JF, Maddux BA, Sasson S, et al. Skeletal muscle content of membrane glycoprotein pc-1 in obesity: relationship to muscle glucose transport. *Diabetes* 1996;10:1324–1328.
49. Urano T, Emkey R, Feig LA. Ral-GTPases mediate a distinct downstream signaling pathway from Ras that facilitates cellular transformation. *EMBO J* 1996;15:810–816.

50. Ahmad F, Azevedo J, Cortright R, et al. Alterations in skeletal muscle protein-tyrosine phosphatase activity and expression in insulin-resistant human obesity and diabetes. *J Clin Invest* 1997;100:449–458.
51. Goldstein BJ, Ahmad F, Ding W, et al. Regulation of the insulin signalling pathway by cellular protein-tyrosine phosphatases. *Mol Cell Biochem* 1998; 182:91–99.
52. Elchebly M, Payette P, Michaliszyn E, et al. Increased insulin sensitivity and obesity resistance in mice lacking the protein tyrosine phosphatase-1b gene. *Science* 1999;283:1544–1548.
53. Zinker BA, Rondinone CM, Trevillyan JM, et al. PTP1B antisense oligonucleotide lowers PTP1B protein, normalizes blood glucose, and improves insulin sensitivity in diabetic mice. *Proc Natl Acad Sci U S A* 2002;99: 11357–11362.
54. Wagner JA. Early clinical development of pharmaceuticals for type 2 diabetes mellitus: from preclinical models to human investigation. *J Clin Endocrinol Metab* 2002;87:5362–5366.
55. Campbell PJ, Carlson MG, Nurjhan N. Fat metabolism in human obesity. *Am J Physiol* 1994;266:E600–E605.
56. Jensen MD, Haymond MW, Rizza RA, et al. Influence of body fat distribution on free fatty acid metabolism in obesity. *J Clin Invest* 1989;83:1168–1173.
57. Groop LC, Saloranta C, Shank M, et al. The role of free fatty acid metabolism in the pathogenesis of insulin resistance in obesity and noninsulin-dependent diabetes mellitus. *J Clin Endocrinol Metab* 1991;72:96–107.
58. Eriksson JW, Smith U, Waagstein F, et al. Glucose turnover and adipose tissue lipolysis are insulin-resistant in healthy relatives of type 2 diabetes patients: is cellular insulin resistance a secondary phenomenon? *Diabetes* 1999; 48:1572–1578.
59. Gelding SV, Coldham N, Niththyananthan R, et al. Insulin resistance with respect to lipolysis in non-diabetic relatives of European patients with type 2 diabetes. *Diabet Med* 1995;12:66–73.
60. Groop LC, Bonadonna RC, Simonson DC, et al. Effect of insulin on oxidative and nonoxidative pathways of free fatty acid metabolism in human obesity. *Am J Physiol* 1992;263:E79–E84.
61. Bjorntorp P, Bergman H, Varnauskas E. Plasma free fatty acid turnover rate in obesity. *Acta Med Scand* 1969;185:351–356.
62. Abbasi F, McLaughlin T, Lamendola C, et al. Insulin regulation of plasma free fatty acid concentrations is abnormal in healthy subjects with muscle insulin resistance. *Metabolism* 2000;49:151–154.
63. Bluher M, Michael MD, Peroni OD, et al. Adipose tissue selective insulin receptor knockout protects against obesity and obesity-related glucose intolerance. *Dev Cell* 2002;3:25–38.
64. Abel ED, Peroni O, Kim JK, et al. Adipose-selective targeting of the GLUT4 gene impairs insulin action in muscle and liver. *Nature* 2001;409:729–733.
65. Uysal KT, Scheja L, Wiesbrock SM, et al. Improved glucose and lipid metabolism in genetically obese mice lacking aP2. *Endocrinology* 2000;141: 3388–3396.
66. Shepherd PR, Gnudi L, Tozzo E, et al. 1 Adipose cell hyperplasia and enhanced glucose disposal in transgenic mice overexpressing GLUT4 selectively in adipose tissue. *J Biol Chem* 1993;268:22243–22246.
67. Tozzo E, Gnudi L, Kahn BB. Amelioration of insulin resistance in streptozotocin diabetic mice by transgenic overexpression of GLUT4 driven by an adipose-specific promoter. *Endocrinology* 1997;138:1604–1611.
68. Cherrington AD. Banting Lecture 1997. Control of glucose uptake and release by the liver in vivo. *Diabetes* 1999;48:1198–1214.
69. Ader M, Bergman RN. Peripheral effects of insulin dominate suppression of fasting hepatic glucose production. *Am J Physiol* 1990;245:E1020–E1032.
70. Giacca A, Fisher SJ, Shi ZO, et al. Importance of peripheral insulin levels for insulin-induced suppression of glucose production in depancreatized dogs. *J Clin Invest* 1992;90:1769–1777.
71. Mittelman SD, Fu YY, Rebrin K, et al. Indirect effect of insulin to suppress endogenous glucose production is dominant, even with hyperglucagonemia. *J Clin Invest* 1997;100:3121–3130.
72. Sindelar DK, Balcom JH, Chu CA, et al. A comparison of the effects of selective increases in peripheral or portal insulin on hepatic glucose production in the conscious dog. *Diabetes* 1996;45:1594–1605.
73. Sindelar DK, Chu CA, Rohlie M, et al. The role of fatty acids in mediating the effects of peripheral insulin on hepatic glucose production in the conscious dog. *Diabetes* 1997;46:187–196.
74. Saloranta C, Taskinen M, Widen E, et al. Metabolic consequences of sustained suppression of free fatty acids by acipimox in patients with NIDDM. *Diabetes* 1993;42:1559–1566.
75. Lauro D, Kido Y, Castle AL, et al. Impaired glucose tolerance in mice with a targeted impairment of insulin action in muscle and adipose tissue. *Nat Genet* 1998;20:294–298.
76. Michael MD, Kulkarni RN, Postic C, et al. Loss of insulin signaling in hepatocytes leads to severe insulin resistance and progressive hepatic dysfunction. *Mol Cell* 2000;6:87–97.
77. Fisher SJ, Kahn CR. Insulin signaling is required for insulin's direct and indirect action on hepatic glucose production. *J Clin Invest* 2003;111:463–468.
78. Havrankova J, Roth J, Brownstein M. Insulin receptors are widely distributed in the central nervous system of the rat. *Nature* 1978;272:827–829.
79. Porte D Jr, Seeley RJ, Woods SC, et al. Obesity, diabetes and the central nervous system. *Diabetologia* 1998;41:863–881.
80. Leloup C, Arluison M, Kassis N, et al. Discrete brain areas express the insulin-responsive glucose transporter GLUT4. *Brain Res Mol Brain Res* 1996;38:45–53.
81. Bruning JC, Gautam D, Burks DJ, et al. Role of brain insulin receptor in control of body weight and reproduction. *Science* 2000;289:2122–2155.
82. Obici S, Feng Z, Karkanias G, et al. Decreasing hypothalamic insulin receptors causes hyperphagia and insulin resistance in rats. *Nat Neurosci* 2002; 5:566–572.
83. Obici S, Zhang BB, Karkanias G, et al. Hypothalamic insulin signaling is required for inhibition of glucose production. *Nat Med* 2002;8:1376–1382.
84. LeRoith D. Beta-cell dysfunction and insulin resistance in type 2 diabetes: role of metabolic and genetic abnormalities. *Am J Med* 2002;113[Suppl 6A]:3S–11S.
85. Rubinstein H, Zimmet P. *Phosphate, wealth, and health in Nauru: a study of lifestyle change*. Brolga: Gundaroo, 1993.
86. Knowler W, Pettitt D, Saad M, et al. Diabetes mellitus in the Pima Indians: incidence, risk factors and pathogenesis. *Diabetes Metab Rev* 1990;6:1–27.
87. Diamond J. The double puzzle of diabetes. *Nature* 2003;423:599–602.
88. Hales C, Barker D. Type 2 (non-insulin-dependent) diabetes mellitus: the thrifty phenotype hypothesis. *Diabetologia* 1992;35:595–601.
89. O'Rahilly S, Farooqi IS, Yeo GS, et al. Minireview: human obesity-lessons from monogenic disorders [review]. *Endocrinology* 2003;144:3757–3764.
90. Torley D, Bellus GA, Munro CS. Genes, growth factors and acanthosis nigricans. *Br J Dermatol* 2002;147:1096–1101.
91. Taylor SI. Insulin action, insulin resistance, and type 2 diabetes mellitus. In: Scriver CR, Beaudet AL, Sly WS, et al, eds. *The metabolic and molecular bases of inherited disease,* 8th ed. New York; McGraw-Hill, 2000:1433–1470.
92. Virkamaki A, Ueki K, Kahn CR. Protein-protein interaction in insulin signaling and the molecular mechanisms of insulin resistance. *J Clin Invest* 1999; 103:931–943.
93. Krook A, Brueton L, O'Rahilly S. Homozygous nonsense mutation in the insulin receptor gene in infant with leprechaunism. *Lancet* 1993;342: 277–278.
94. Taylor SI, Accili D, Cama A, et al. Mutations in the insulin receptor gene in patients with genetic syndromes of insulin resistance. *Adv Exp Med Biol* 1991;293:197–213.
95. Donohue LW, Uchida I. Leprechaunism. A euphemism for a rare familial disorder. *J Pediatr* 1954;45:505–519.
96. Longo N, Wang Y, Smith SA, et al. Genotype-phenotype correlation in inherited severe insulin resistance. *Hum Mol Genet* 2002;11:1465–1475.
97. Moller DE, Yakota A, White MF, et al. A naturally occurring mutation of insulin receptor alanine 1134 impairs tyrosine kinase function and is associated with dominantly inherited insulin resistance. *J Biol Chem* 1990;265: 14979–14985.
98. Taylor SI, Accili D, Haft CR, et al. Mechanisms of hormone resistance: lessons from insulin-resistant patients. *Acta Paediatr Suppl* 1994;399:95–104.
99. Kadowaki T, Kadowaki H, Rechler MM, et al. Five mutant alleles of the insulin receptor gene in patients with genetic forms of insulin resistance. *J Clin Invest* 1990;86:254–264.
100. Fradkin JE, Eastman RC, Lesniak MA, et al. Specificity spillover at the hormone receptor—exploring its role in human disease. *N Engl J Med* 1989; 320:640–645.
101. Kuzuya H, Matsuura N, Sakamoto M, et al. Trial of insulin-like growth factor 1 therapy for patients with extreme insulin resistance syndromes. *Diabetes* 1993;42:696–705.
102. Nakae J, Kato M, Murashita M, et al. Long-term effect of recombinant human insulin-like growth factor I on metabolic and growth control in a patient with leprechaunism. *J Clin Endocrinol Metab* 1998;83:542–549.
103. Flier JS, Moller DE, Moses AC, et al. Insulin-mediated pseudoacromegaly: clinical and biochemical characterization of a syndrome of selective insulin resistance. *J Clin Endocrinol Metab* 1993;76:1533–1541.
104. Dib K, Whitehead JP, Humphreys PJ, et al. Impaired activation of phosphoinositide 3-kinase by insulin in fibroblasts from patients with severe insulin resistance and pseudoacromegaly. A disorder characterized by selective postreceptor insulin resistance. *J Clin Invest* 1998;101:1111–1120.
105. Tontonoz P, Hu E, Spiegelman BM. Stimulation of adipogenesis in fibroblasts by PPAR2, a lipid-activated transcription factor. *Cell* 1994;79:1147–1156.
106. Day C. Thiazolidinediones: a new class of antidiabetic drugs. *Diabet Med* 1999;16:179–192.
107. Maeda N, Takahashi M, Funahashi T, et al. PPAR ligands increase expression and plasma concentrations of adiponectin, an adipose-derived protein. *Diabetes* 2001;50:2094–2099.
108. Barroso I, Gurnell M, Crowley VEF, et al. Dominant negative mutations in human PPAR are associated with severe insulin resistance, diabetes mellitus and hypertension. *Nature* 1999;402:880–883.
109. Agarwal AK, Garg A. A novel heterozygous mutation in peroxisome proliferator-activated receptor-gene in a patient with familial partial lipodystrophy. *J Clin Endocrinol Metab* 2002;87:408–411.
110. Hegele RA, Henian C, Frankowski C, et al. PPARG F388L, a transactivation-deficient mutant, in familial partial lipodystrophy. *Diabetes* 2002;51: 3586–3590.
111. Gurnell M. PPARgamma and metabolism: insights from the study of human genetic variants. *Clin Endocrinol* 2003;59:267–277.
112. Savage DB, Tan GD, Acerini CL, et al. The human metabolic syndrome resulting from dominant-negative mutations in the nuclear receptors and PPAR. *Diabetes* 2003;52:910–917.
113. Ristow M, Muller-Wieland D, Pfeiffer A, et al. Obesity associated with a mutation in a genetic regulator of adipocyte differentiation. *N Engl J Med* 1998;339:953–959.

114. Deeb SS, Fajas L, Nemoto M, et al. A Pro12Ala substitution in PPAR2 associated with decreased receptor activity, lower body mass index and improved insulin sensitivity. *Nat Genet* 1998;20:284–287.
115. Altshuler D, Hirschhorn JN, Klannemark M, et al. The common PPAR Pro12Ala polymorphism is associated with decreased risk of type 2 diabetes. *Nat Gen* 2000;26:76–80.
116. Werman A, Hollenberg A, Solanes G, et al. Ligand-independent activation domain in the N terminus of peroxisome proliferator-activated receptor gamma (PPARgamma). Differential activity of PPARgamma1 and -2 isoforms and influence of insulin. *J Biol Chem* 1997;272:20230–20235.
117. Masud S, Ye S; SAS Group. Effect of the peroxisome proliferator activated receptor-gamma gene Pro12Ala variant on body mass index: a meta-analysis. *J Med Genet* 2003;40:773–780.
118. Vidal-Puig AJ, Considine RV, Jimenez-Linan M, et al. Peroxisome proliferator-activated receptor gene expression in human tissues. Effects of obesity, weight loss, and regulation by insulin and glucocorticoids. *J Clin Invest* 1997;99:2416–2422.
119. Luan J, Browne PO, Harding AH, et al. Evidence for gene-nutrient interaction at the PPARgamma locus. *Diabetes* 2001;50:686–689.
120. Dunnigan MG, Cochrane MA, Kelly A, et al., Familial lipoatrophic diabetes with dominant transmission: a new syndrome. *Q J Med* 1974;43:33–48.
121. Garg A, Peshock RM, Fleckenstein JL, et al. Adipose tissue distribution pattern in patients with familial partial lipodystrophy (Dunnigan variety). *J Clin Endocrinol Metab* 1999;84:170–174.
122. Szczepaniak LS, Babcock EE, Schick F, et al. Measurement of intracellular triglyceride stores by H spectroscopy: validation in vivo. *Am J Physiol* 1999; 276(5 Pt 1):E977–E989.
123. Cao H, Hegele RA. Nuclear lamin A/C R482Q mutation in Canadian kindreds with Dunnigan-type familial partial lipodystrophy. *Hum Mol Genet* 2000;9:109–112.
124. Shackleton S Lloyd DJ, Jackson SN, et al. LMNA, encoding lamin A/C, is mutated in partial lipodystrophy. *Nat Genet* 2000;24:153–156.
125. Hegele RA. Molecular basis of partial lipodystrophy and prospects for therapy. *Trends Mol Med* 2001;7:121–126.
126. Seip M, Trygstad O. Generalized lipodystrophy, congenital and acquired (lipoatrophy). *Acta Paediatr Suppl* 1996;413:2–28.
127. Agarwal AK, Arioglu E, De Almeida S, et al. AGPAT2 is mutated in congenital generalized lipodystrophy linked to chromosome 9q34. *Nat Genet* 2002; 31:21–32.
128. Magre J, Delepine M, Khallouf E, et al. Identification of the gene altered in Berardinelli-Seip congenital lipodystrophy on chromosome 11q13. *Nat Genet* 2001;28:365–370.
129. Hansen T, Andersen CB, Echwald SM, et al. Identification of a common amino acid polymorphism in the p85alpha regulatory subunit of phosphatidylinositol 3-kinase: effects on glucose disappearance constant, glucose effectiveness, and the insulin sensitivity index. *Diabetes* 1997;46: 494–501.
130. Clausen JO, Hansen T, Bjorbaek C, et al. Insulin resistance: interactions between obesity and a common variant of insulin receptor substrate-1. *Lancet* 1995;346:397–402.
131. Almind K, Inoue G, Pedersen O, et al. A common amino acid polymorphism in insulin receptor substrate-1 causes impaired insulin signaling. Evidence from transfection studies. *J Clin Invest* 1996;97:2569–2575.
132. Ura S, Araki E, Kishikawa H, et al. Molecular scanning of the insulin receptor substrate-1 (IRS-1) gene in Japanese patients with NIDDM: identification of five novel polymorphisms. *Diabetologia* 1996;39:600–608.
133. Kissebah AH, Sonnenberg G, Myklebust J, et al. Quantitative trait loci on chromosomes 3 and 17 influence phenotypes of the metabolic syndrome. *Proc Natl Acad Sci U S A* 2000;97:14478–14483.
134. Vionnet N, Hani El H, Dupont S, et al. Genomewide search for type 2 diabetes–susceptibility genes in French whites: evidence for a novel susceptibility locus for early-onset diabetes on chromosome 3q27-qter and independent replication of a type 2-diabetes locus on chromosome 1q21–q24. *Am J Hum Genet* 2000;67:1470–1480.
135. Takahashi M, Arita Y, Yamagata K, et al. Genomic structure and mutations in adipose-specific gene, adiponectin. *Int J Obes Relat Metab Disord* 2000;24: 861–868.
136. Savage DB, Agostini M, Barroso I, et al. Digenic inheritance of severe insulin resistance in a human pedigree. *Nat Genet* 2002;31:379–384.
137. Bruning JC, Winnay J, Bonner-Weir S, et al. Development of a novel polygenic model of NIDDM in mice heterozygous for IR and IRS-1 null alleles. *Cell* 1997;88:561–572.
138. Ghosh S, Collins FS. The geneticist's approach to complex disease. *Annu Rev Med* 1996;47:333–353.
139. Kido Y, Burks DJ, Withers D, et al. Tissue-specific insulin resistance in mice with mutations in the insulin receptor, IRS-1, and IRS-2. *J Clin Invest* 2000;105:199–205.
140. Kido Y, Philippe N, Schaffer AA, et al. Genetic modifiers of the insulin resistance phenotype in mice. *Diabetes* 2000;49:589–596.
141. Eaton SB, Konner M, Shostak M. Stone agers in the fast lane: chronic degenerative diseases in evolutionary perspective. *Am J Med* 1988;84:739–749.
142. Neel JV. Diabetes mellitus a "thrifty" genotype rendered detrimental by "progress"? *Am J Hum Genet* 1962;14:352–353.
143. Chakravarthy M, Booth FW. Eating, exercise, and "thrifty" genotypes: connecting the dots toward an evolutionary understanding of modern chronic diseases. *J Appl Physiol* 2004;96:3–10.
144. Desai M, Crowther NJ, Ozanne SE, et al. Adult glucose and lipid metabolism may be programmed during fetal life [review]. *Biochem Soc Trans* 1995;23: 331–335.
145. Ozanne SE. Metabolic programming in animals. *BMJ* 2001;60:143–152.
146. Ozanne SE, Wang CL, Coleman N, et al. Altered muscle insulin sensitivity in the male offspring of protein-malnourished rats. *Am J Physiol* 1996;271(6 Pt 1): E1128–E1134.
147. Ozanne SE, Smith GD, Tikerpae J, et al. Altered regulation of hepatic glucose output in the male offspring of protein-malnourished rat dams. *Am J Physiol* 1996;270(4 Pt 1):E559–E564.
148. Ozanne SE, Nave BT, Wang CL, et al. Poor fetal nutrition causes long-term changes in expression of insulin signaling components in adipocytes. *Am J Physiol* 1997;273(1 Pt 1):E46–E51.
149. Ozanne SE, Hales CN. The long-term consequences of intra-uterine protein malnutrition for glucose metabolism. *Proc Nutr Soc* 1999;58:615–619.
150. Hales CN, Desai M, Ozanne SE. The thrifty phenotype hypothesis: how does it look after 5 years? *Diabet Med* 1997;14:189–195.
151. Reitman ML, Arioglu E, Gavrilova O, et al. Lipoatrophy revisited. *Trends Endocrinol Metab* 2000;11:410–416.
152. Comuzzie AG, Allison DB. The search for human obesity genes. *Science* 1998;280:1374–1377.
153. Hill JO, Peters JC. Environmental contributions to the obesity epidemic. *Science* 1998;280:1371–1374.
154. Flegal KM, Carroll MD, Kuczmarski RJ, et al. Overweight and obesity in the United States: prevalence and trends, 1960–1994. *Int J Obes Relat Metab Disord* 1998;22:39–47.
155. McCrory MA, Fuss PJ, Hays NP, et al. Overeating in America. Association between restaurant food consumption and body fatness in healthy adult men and women ages 19 to 80. *Obes Res* 1999;7:564–571.
156. Popkin BM, Nielsen SJ. The sweetening of the world's diet. *Obes Res* 2003;11:1325–1332.
157. Nielsen SJ, Siega-Riz AM, Popkin BM. Trends in energy intake in U.S. between 1977 and 1996: similar shifts seen across age groups. *Obes Res* 2002;10:370–378.
158. Popkin BM. The nutrition transition and obesity in the developing world. *J Nutr* 2001;131:871S–873S.
159. Drewnowski A, Popkin BM. The nutrition transition: new trends in the global diet. *Nutr Rev* 1997;55:31–43.
160. Popkin BM. Urbanization, lifestyle changes and the nutrition transition. *World Dev* 1999;27:1905–1916.
161. Monteiro CA, D'A Benicio MH, Conde WL, et al. Shifting obesity trends in Brazil. *Eur J Clin Nutr* 2000;54:342–346.
162. Havel PJ. Control of energy homeostasis and insulin action by adipocyte hormones: leptin, acylation stimulating protein, and adiponectin. *Curr Opin Lipidol* 2002;13:51–59.
163. Rajala MW, Scherer PE. Minireview: the adipocyte: at the crossroads of energy homeostasis, inflammation, and atherosclerosis. *Endocrinology* 2003;144:3765–3773.
164. Scherer PE, Williams S, Fogliano M, et al. A novel serum protein similar to C1q, produced exclusively in adipocytes. *J Biol Chem* 1995;270:26746–26749.
165. Pajvani UB, Scherer PE. Adiponectin: systemic contributor to insulin sensitivity. *Curr Diab Rep* 2003;3:207–213.
166. Hotta K, Funahashi T, Arita Y, et al. Plasma concentrations of a novel, adipose-specific protein, adiponectin, in type 2 diabetic patients. *Arterioscler Thromb Vasc Biol* 2000;20:1595–1599.
167. Hotta K, Funahashi T, Bodkin NL, et al. Circulating concentrations of the adipocyte protein adiponectin are decreased in parallel with reduced insulin sensitivity during the progression to type 2 diabetes in rhesus monkeys. *Diabetes* 2001;50:1126–1133.
168. Weyer C, Funahashi T, Tanaka S, et al. Hypoadiponectinemia in obesity and type 2 diabetes: close association with insulin resistance and hyperinsulinemia. *J Clin Endocrinol Metab* 2001;86:1930–1935.
169. Arita Y, Kihara S, Ouchi N, et al. Paradoxical decrease of an adipose-specific protein, adiponectin, in obesity. *Biochem Biophys Res Commun* 1999;257: 79–83.
170. Combs TP, Berg AH, Rajala MW, et al. Sexual differentiation, pregnancy, calorie restriction, and aging affect the adipocyte-specific secretory protein adiponectin. *Diabetes* 2003;52:268–276.
171. Yang WS, Lee WJ, Funahashi T, et al. Weight reduction increases plasma levels of an adipose-derived anti-inflammatory protein, adiponectin. *J Clin Endocrinol Metab* 2001;86:3815–3819.
172. Spranger J, Kroke A, Mohlig M, et al. Adiponectin and protection against type 2 diabetes mellitus. *Lancet* 2003;361:226–228.
173. Berg AH, Combs T, Du X, et al. The adipocyte-secreted protein Acrp30 enhances hepatic insulin action. *Nat Med* 2001;7:947–953.
174. Combs TP, Berg AH, Obici S, et al. Endogenous glucose production is inhibited by the adipose-derived protein Acrp30. *J Clin Invest* 2001;108:1875–1881.
175. Yamauchi T, Kamon J, Minokoshi Y, et al. Adiponectin stimulates glucose utilization and fatty-acid oxidation by activating AMP-activated protein kinase. *Nat Med* 20028:1288–1295.
176. Combs TP, Pajvani UB, Berg AH, et al. A transgenic mouse with a deletion in the collagenous domain of adiponectin displays elevated circulating adiponectin and improved insulin sensitivity. *Endocrinology* 2004;145: 367–383.
177. Maeda N, Shimomura I, Kishida K, et al. Diet-induced insulin resistance in mice lacking adiponectin/ACRP30. *Nat Med* 2002;8:731–737.

178. Kubota N, Terauchi Y, Yamauchi T, et al. Disruption of adiponectin causes insulin resistance and neointimal formation. *J Biol Chem* 2002;277: 25863–25866.
179. Pajvani UB, Du X, Combs TP, et al. Structure-function studies of the adipocyte-secreted hormone Acrp30/adiponectin: implications for metabolic regulation and bioactivity. *J Biol Chem* 2003;278:9073–9085.
180. Pajvani UB, Hawkins M, Combs TP, et al. Complex distribution, not absolute amount of adiponectin, correlates with thiazolidinedione-mediated improvement in insulin sensitivity. *J Biol Chem*. 2004;279:12152–12162.
181. Zhang Y, Proenca R, Maffei M, et al. Positional cloning of the mouse obese gene and its human homologue. *Nature* 1994;372:425–432.
182. Sivitz WI, Walsh SA, Morgan DA, et al. Effects of leptin on insulin sensitivity in normal rats. *Endocrinology* 1997;138:3395–3401.
183. Rossetti L, Massillon D, Barzilai N, et al. Short term effects of leptin on hepatic gluconeogenesis and in vivo insulin action. *J Biol Chem* 1997;272:27758–27763.
184. Barzilai N, Wang J, Massilon D, et al. Leptin selectively decreases visceral adiposity and enhances insulin action. *J Clin Invest* 1997;100:3105–3110.
185. Minokoshi Y, Kim YB, Peroni OD, et al. Leptin stimulates fatty-acid oxidation by activating AMP-activated protein kinase. *Nature* 2002;415:339–343.
186. Minokoshi Y, Kahn BB. Role of AMP-activated protein kinase in leptin-induced fatty acid oxidation in muscle. *Biochem Soc Trans* 2003;31:196–201.
187. Huang L, Li C. Leptin: a multifunctional hormone. *Cell Res* 2000;10:81–92.
188. Lord GM, Matarese G, Howard JK, et al. Leptin modulates the T-cell immune response and reverses starvation-induced immunosuppression. *Nature* 1998;394:897–901.
189. Farooqi IS, Matarese G, Lord GM, et al. Beneficial effects of leptin on obesity, T cell hyporesponsiveness, and neuroendocrine/metabolic dysfunction of human congenital leptin deficiency. *J Clin Invest* 2002;110:1093–1103.
190. Popovic V, Damjanovic S, Dieguez C, et al. Leptin and the pituitary. *Pituitary* 2001;4:7–14.
191. Hukshorn CJ, van Dielen FM, Buurman WA, et al. The effect of pegylated recombinant human leptin (PEG-OB) on weight loss and inflammatory status in obese subjects. *Int J Obes Relat Metab Disord* 2002;26:504–509.
192. Wang J, Obici S, Morgan K, et al. Overfeeding rapidly induces leptin and insulin resistance. *Diabetes* 2001;50:2786–2791.
193. Rosenbaum M, Murphy EM, Heymsfield SB, et al. Low dose leptin administration reverses effects of sustained weight-reduction on energy expenditure and circulating concentrations of thyroid hormones. *J Clin Endocrinol Metab* 2002;87:2391–2394.
194. Steppan CM, Bailey ST, Bhat S, et al. The hormone resistin links obesity to diabetes. *Nature* 2001;409:307–312.
195. Rajala MW, Obici S, Scherer PE, et al. Adipose-derived resistin and gut-derived resistin-like molecule-β selectively impair insulin action on glucose production. *J Clin Invest* 2003;111:225–230.
196. Way JM, Gorgun CZ, Tong Q, et al. Adipose tissue resistin expression is severely suppressed in obesity and stimulated by peroxisome proliferator-activated receptor agonists. *J Biol Chem* 2001;276:25651–25653.
197. Janke J, Engeli S, Gorzelniak K, et al. Resistin gene expression in human adipocytes is not related to insulin resistance. *Obes Res* 2002;10:1–5.
198. Patel L, Buckels AC, Kinghorn IJ, et al. Resistin is expressed in human macrophages and directly regulated by PPAR activators. *Biochem Biophys Res Commun* 2003 300:472–476.
199. Fain JN, Cheema PS, Bahouth SW, et al. Resistin release by human adipose tissue explants in primary culture. *Biochem Biophys Res Commun* 2003;300: 674–678.
200. McTernan CL, McTernan PG, Harte AL, et al. Resistin, central obesity, and type 2 diabetes. *Lancet* 2002;359:46–47.
201. McTernan PG, McTernan CL, Chetty R, et al. Increased resistin gene and protein expression in human abdominal adipose tissue. *J Clin Endocrinol Metab* 2002;87:2407.
202. Degawa-Yamauchi M, Bovenkerk JE, Juliar BE., et al. Serum resistin (FIZZ3) protein is increased in obese humans. *J Clin Endocrinol Metab* 2003;88: 5452–5455.
203. Lee JH, Chan JL, Yiannakouris N, et al. Circulating resistin levels are not associated with obesity or insulin resistance in humans and are not regulated by fasting or leptin administration: cross-sectional and interventional studies in normal, insulin-resistant, and diabetic subjects. *J Clin Endocrinol Metab* 2003;88:4848–4856.
204. Lee H, Chan JL, Yiannakouris N, et al. Circulating resistin levels are not associated with obesity or insulin resistance in humans and are not regulated by fasting or leptin administration: cross-sectional and interventional studies in normal, insulin-resistant, and diabetic subjects. *J Clin Endocrinol Metab* 2003;88:4848–4856.
205. Savage DB, Sewter CP, Klenk ES, et al. Resistin/Fizz3 expression in relation to obesity and peroxisome proliferator-activated receptor-gamma action in humans. *Diabetes* 2001;50:2199–2202.
206. Combs TP, Berg AH, Rajala MW, et al. Sexual differentiation, pregnancy, calorie restriction and aging affect the adipocyte-specific secretory protein Acrp30/adiponectin. *Diabetes* 2003;52:268–276.
207. Pickup JC, Crook MA. Is type II diabetes mellitus a disease of the innate immune system? *Diabetologia* 1998;41:1241–1248.
208. Grimble RF. Inflammatory status and insulin resistance. *Curr Opin Clin Nutr Metab Care* 2002;5:551–559.
209. Pickup JC, Mattock MB, Chusney GD, et al. NIDDM as a disease of the innate immune system: association of acute-phase reactants and interleukin-6 with metabolic syndrome X. *Diabetologia* 1997;40:1286–1292.
210. Festa A, D'Agostino R Jr, Howard G, et al. Chronic subclinical inflammation as part of the insulin resistance syndrome: the Insulin Resistance Atherosclerosis Study (IRAS). *Circulation* 2000;102:42–47.
211. Hotamisligil GS, Shargill NS, Spiegelman BM. Adipose expression of tumor necrosis factor-alpha: direct role in obesity-linked insulin resistance. *Science* 1993;259:87–91.
212. Vgontzas AN, Papanicolaou DA, Bixler EO, et al. Elevation of plasma cytokines in disorders of excessive daytime sleepiness: role of sleep disturbance and obesity. *J Clin Endocrinol Metab* 1997;82:1313–1316.
213. Samad F, Yamamoto K, Pandey M, et al. Elevated expression of transforming growth factor-beta in adipose tissue from obese mice. *Mol Med* 1997;3:37–48.
214. Visser M, Bouter LM, McQuillan GM, et al. Elevated C-reactive protein levels in overweight and obese adults. *JAMA* 1999;282:2131–2135.
215. Weyer C, Yudkin JS, Stehouwer CD, et al. Humoral markers of inflammation and endothelial dysfunction in relation to adiposity and in vivo insulin action in Pima Indians. *Atherosclerosis* 2002;161:233–242.
216. Sartipy P, Loskutoff DJ. Monocyte chemoattractant protein 1 in obesity and insulin resistance. *Proc Natl Acad Sci U S A* 2003;100:7265–7270.
217. Hotamisligil GS, Shargill NS, Spiegelman BM. Adipose expression of tumor necrosis factor-alpha: direct role in obesity-linked insulin resistance. *Science* 1993;259:87–91.
218. Borst SE, Bagby GJ. Neutralization of tumor necrosis factor reverses age-induced impairment of insulin responsiveness in skeletal muscle of Sprague-Dawley rats. *Metabolism* 2002;51:1061–1064.
219. Uysal KT, Wiesbrock SM, Marino MW, et al. Protection from obesity-induced insulin resistance in mice lacking TNF-alpha function. *Nature* 1997;389: 610–614.
220. Uysal KT, Wiesbrock SM, Hotamisligil GS. Functional analysis of tumor necrosis factor (TNF) receptors in TNF-alpha-mediated insulin resistance in genetic obesity. *Endocrinology* 1998;139:4832–4838.
221. Hotamisligil GS, Murray DL, Choy LN, et al. Tumor necrosis factor alpha inhibits signaling from the insulin receptor. *Proc Natl Acad Sci U S A* 1994;91: 4854–4858.
222. Zhang HH, Halbleib M, Ahmad F, et al. Tumor necrosis factor-alpha stimulates lipolysis in differentiated human adipocytes through activation of extracellular signal-related kinase and elevation of intracellular cAMP. *Diabetes* 2002;51:2929–2935.
223. Uysal KT, Wiesbrock SM, Hotamisligil GS. Functional analysis of tumor necrosis factor (TNF) receptors in TNF-alpha-mediated insulin resistance in genetic obesity. *Endocrinology* 1998;139:4832–4838.
224. Moller DE. Potential role of TNF-alpha in the pathogenesis of insulin resistance and type 2 diabetes. *Trends Endocrinol Metab* 2000;11:212–217.
225. Ofei F, Hurel S, Newkirk J, et al. Effects of an engineered human anti-TNF-alpha antibody (CDP571) on insulin sensitivity and glycemic control in patients with NIDDM. *Diabetes* 1996;45:881–885.
226. Zandi E, Rothward DM, Delhase M, et al. The IB kinase complex (IKK) contains two kinase subunits, IKK and IKKβ, necessary for IB phosphorylation and NF-B activation. *Cell* 1997;91:243–252.
227. Nonogaki K, Fuller GM, Furetes NL, et al. Interleukin-6 stimulates hepatic triglyceride secretion in rats. *Endocrinology* 1995;136:2143–2149.
228. Senn JJ, Klover PJ, Nowak IA, et al. Interleukin-6 induces cellular insulin resistance in hepatocytes. *Diabetes* 2002;51:3391–3399.
229. Sartipy P, Loskutoff DJ. Monocyte chemoattractant protein 1 in obesity and insulin resistance. *Proc Natl Acad Sci U S A* 2003;100:7265–7270.
230. Baron SH. Salicylates as hypoglycemic agents. *Diabetes Care* 1982;5:64–71.
231. Yin M-J, Yamamoto Y, Gaynor RB. The anti-inflammatory agents aspirin and salicylate inhibit the activity of IB kinase-β. *Nature* 1998;396:77–80.
232. Yuan M, Konstantopoulos N, Lee J, et al. Reversal of obesity- and diet-induced insulin resistance with salicylates or targeted disruption of Ikkbeta. *Science* 2001;293:1673–1677.
233. Hundal RS. Petersen KF, Mayerson AB, et al. Mechanism by which high-dose aspirin improves glucose metabolism in type 2 diabetes. *J Clin Invest* 2002;109:1321–1326.
234. Gao Z, Zuberi A, Quon MJ, et al. Aspirin inhibits serine phosphorylation of insulin receptor substrate 1 in tumor necrosis factor-treated cells through targeting multiple serine kinases. *J Biol Chem* 2003;278:24944–24950.
235. Hundal RS, Petersen KF, Mayerson AB, et al. Mechanism by which high-dose aspirin improves glucose metabolism in type 2 diabetes. *J Clin Invest* 2002;109:1321–1326.
236. Xu H, Barnes GT, Yang O, et al. Chronic inflammation in fat plays a crucial role in the development of obesity-related insulin resistance. *J Clin Invest* 2003;112:1821–1830.
237. Weisberg SP, McCann D, Desai M, et al. Obesity is associated with macrophage accumulation in adipose tissue. *J Clin Invest* 2003;112: 1796–1808.
238. Moraes RC, Blondet A, Birkenkamp-Demtroeder K, et al. Study of the alteration of gene expression in adipose tissue of diet-induced obese mice by microarray and reverse transcription-polymerase chain reaction analyses. *Endocrinology* 2003;144:4773–4782.
239. Sierra-Honigmann MR, Nath AK, Murakami C, et al. Biological action of leptin as an angiogenic factor. *Science* 1998;281:1683–1686.
240. Maeda N, Shimomura I, Kishida K, et al. Diet-induced insulin resistance in mice lacking adiponectin/ACRP30. *Nat Med* 2002;8:731–737.
241. Levine JA, Jensen MD, Eberhardt NL, et al. Adipocyte macrophage colony-stimulating factor is a mediator of adipose tissue growth. *J Clin Invest* 1998;101:1557–1564.

242. Schneider BS, Faust IM, Hemmes R, et al. Effects of altered adipose tissue morphology on plasma insulin levels in the rat. *Am J Physiol* 1981;240:E358–E362.
243. Weyer C, Wolford JK, Hansen RL, et al. Subcutaneous abdominal adipocyte size, a predictor of type 2 diabetes, is linked to chromosome 1q21–q23 and is associated with a common polymorphism in LMNA in Pima Indians. *Mol Genet Metab* 2001;72:231–238.
244. Weyer C, Foley JE, Bogardus C, et al. Enlarged subcutaneous abdominal adipocyte size, but not obesity itself, predicts type II diabetes independent of insulin resistance. *Diabetologia* 2000;43:1498–1506.
245. Stern JS, Batchelor BR, Hollander N, et al. Adipose-cell size and immunoreactive insulin levels in obese and normal-weight adults. *Lancet* 1972;2: 948–951.
246. Hissin PJ, Foley JE, Wardzala LJ, et al. Mechanism of insulin-resistant glucose transport activity in the enlarged adipose cell of the aged, obese rat. *J Clin Invest* 1982;70:780–790.
247. Le Lay S, Kried S, Farnier C, et al. Cholesterol, a cell size-dependent signal that regulates glucose metabolism and gene expression in adipocytes. *J Biol Chem* 2001;276:16904–16910.
248. Friedman JM. Obesity in the new millennium. *Nature* 2000;404:632–634.
249. Hotamisligil GS, Shargill NS, Spiegelman BM. Adipose expression of tumor necrosis factor-alpha: direct role in obesity-linked insulin resistance. *Science* 1993;259:87–91.
250. Stolk RP, Meijer R, Mali WP, et al. Ultrasound measurements of intraabdominal fat estimate the metabolic syndrome better than do measurements of waist circumference. *Am J Clin Nutr* 2003;77:857–860.
251. DiPietro L, Katz LD, Nadel ER. Excess abdominal adiposity remains correlated with altered lipid concentrations in healthy older women. *Int J Obes Relat Metab Disord* 1999;23:432–436.
252. Abate N, Garg A, Peshock RM, et al. Relationship of generalized and regional adiposity to insulin sensitivity in men with NIDDM. *Diabetes* 1996;45:1684–1693.
253. Kahn BB, Flier JS. Obesity and insulin resistance. *J Clin Invest* 2000;106: 473–481.
254. Lewis GF, Carpentier A, Adeli K, et al. Disordered fat storage and mobilization in the pathogenesis of insulin resistance and type 2 diabetes. *Endocr Rev* 2002;23:201–229.
255. Montague CT, O'Rahilly S. The perils of portliness: causes and consequences of visceral adiposity. *Diabetes* 2000;49:883–888.
256. Motoshima H, Wu X, Sinha MK, et al. Differential regulation of adiponectin secretion from cultured human omental and subcutaneous adipocytes: effects of insulin. and rosiglitazone. *J Clin Endocrinol Metab* 2002;87:5662–5667.
257. Staiger H, Tschritter O, Machann J, et al. Relationship of serum adiponectin and leptin concentrations with body fat distribution in humans. *Obes Res* 2003;11:368–372.
258. Milan G, Granzotto M, Scarda A, et al. Resistin and adiponectin expression in visceral fat of obese rats: effect of weight loss. *Obes Res* 2002;10:1095–1103.
259. Barzilai N, She L, Liu BQ, et al. Surgical removal of visceral fat reverses hepatic insulin resistance. *Diabetes* 1999;48:94–98.
260. Gabriely I, Ma XH, Yang XM, et al. Removal of visceral fat prevents insulin resistance and glucose intolerance of aging: an adipokine-mediated process? *Diabetes* 2002;51:2951–2958.
261. Lawrence RD. Lipodystrophy and hepatomegaly with diabetes, lipaemia, and other metabolic disturbances: a case throwing new light on the action of insulin. *Lancet* 1946;724–731, 773–775.
262. Hubler A, Abendroth K, Keiner T, et al. Dysregulation of insulin-like growth factors in a case of generalized acquired lipoatrophic diabetes mellitus (Lawrence syndrome) connected with autoantibodies against adipocyte membranes. *Exp Clin Endocrinol Diabetes* 1998;106:79–84.
263. Spranger A, Spranger M, Tasman AJ, et al. Barraquer-Simons syndrome (with sensorineural deafness): a contribution to the differential diagnosis of lipodystrophy syndromes. *Am J Med Genet* 1997;71:397–400.
264. Barbaro G. HIV-associated lipodystrophy: pathogenesis and clinical features. *Adv Cardiol* 2003;40:97–104.
265. Kino T, Mirani M, Alesci S, et al. AIDS-related lipodystrophy/insulin resistance syndrome. *Horm Metab Res* 2003;35:129–136.
266. Zhang B, MacNaul K, Szalkowski D, et al. Inhibition of adipocyte differentiation by HIV protease inhibitors. *J. Clin Endocrinol Metab* 1999;84:4274–4277.
267. Madge S, Kinloch-de-Loes S, Mercey D, et al. Lipodystrophy in patients naive to HIV protease inhibitors. *AIDS* 1999;13:735–737.
268. Garg A. Lipodystrophies. *Am J Med* 2000;108:143–152.
269. Burant CF, Sreenan S, Hirano K, et al. Troglitazone action is independent of adipose tissue. *J Clin Invest* 1997;100:2900–2908.
270. Moitra J, Mason MM, Olive M, et al. Life without white fat: a transgenic mouse. *Genes Dev* 1998;12:3168–3181.
271. Shimomura I, Hammer RE, Richardson JA, et al. Insulin resistance and diabetes mellitus in transgenic mice expressing nuclear SREBP-1c in adipose tissue: model for congenital generalized lipodystrophy. *Genes Dev* 1998;12: 3182–3194.
272. Friedman JM, Halaas JL. Leptin and the regulation of body weight in mammals. *Nature* 1998;395:763–770.
273. Shimabukuro M, Koyama K, Chen G, et al. Direct antidiabetic effect of leptin through triglyceride depletion of tissues. *Proc Natl Acad Sci U S A* 1997;94: 4637–4641.
274. Shimomura I, Hammer RE, Ikemoto S, et al. Leptin reverses insulin resistance and diabetes mellitus in mice with congenital lipodystrophy. *Nature* 1999;401:73–76.
275. Oral EA, Simha V, Ruiz E, et al. Leptin-replacement therapy for lipodystrophy. *N Engl J Med* 2002;346:570–578.
276. Gavrilova O, Marcus-Samuels B, Leon LR, et al. Leptin and diabetes in lipoatrophic mice. *Nature* 2000;403:850.
277. Kulkarni RN, Wang ZL, Wang RM, et al. Leptin rapidly suppresses insulin release from insulinoma cells, rat and human islets and, in vivo, in mice. *J Clin Invest* 1997;100:2729–2736.
278. Kieffer TJ, Habener JF. The adipoinsular axis: Effects of leptin on pancreatic β-cells. *Am J Physiol Endocrinol Metab* 2000;278:E1–E14.
279. Gavrilova O, Marcus-Samuels B, Graham D, et al. Surgical implantation of adipose tissue reverses diabetes in lipoatrophic mice. *J Clin Invest* 2000;105: 271–278.
280. Kim JK, Gavrilova O, Chen Y, et al. Mechanism of insulin resistance in A-ZIP/F-1 fatless mice. *J Biol Chem* 2000;275:8456–8460.
281. Shimomura I, Hammer RE, Ikemoto S, et al. Leptin reverses insulin resistance and diabetes mellitus in mice with congenital lipodystrophy. *Nature* 1999;401:73–76.
282. Gavrilova O, Marcus-Samuels B, Leon L.R, et al. Leptin and diabetes in lipoatrophic mice. *Nature* 2000;403:850–851.
283. Ebihara K, Ogawa Y, Masuzaki H, et al. Transgenic overexpression of leptin rescues insulin resistance and diabetes in a mouse model of lipoatrophic diabetes. *Diabetes* 2001;50:1440–1448.
284. Colombo C, Cutson JJ, Yamauchi T, et al. Transplantation of adipose tissue lacking leptin is unable to reverse the metabolic abnormalities associated with lipoatrophy. *Diabetes* 2002;51:2727–2733.
285. Laustsen PG, Michael MD, Crute BE, et al. Lipoatrophic diabetes in Irs1(-/-)/ Irs3(-/-) double knockout mice. *Genes Dev* 2002;16:3213–3222.
286. Reitman ML, Arioglu E, Gavrilova O, et al. Lipoatrophy revisited. *Trends Endocrinol Metab* 2000;11:410–416.
287. Robinson C, Tamborlane WV, Maggs DG, et al. Effect of insulin on glycerol production in obese adolescents. *Am J Physiol* 1998;274:E737–E743.
288. Phillips DI, Caddy S, Ilic V, et al. Intramuscular triglyceride and muscle insulin sensitivity: evidence for a relationship in nondiabetic subjects. *Metabolism* 1996;45:947–950.
289. Goodpaster BH, Thaete FL, Simoneau JA, et al. Subcutaneous abdominal fat and thigh muscle composition predict insulin sensitivity independently of visceral fat. *Diabetes* 1997;46:1579–1585.
290. Pan DA, Lillioja S, Kriketos AD, et al. Skeletal muscle triglyceride levels are inversely related to insulin action. *Diabetes* 1997;46:983–988.
291. Schick F, Machann J, Brechtel K, et al. MRI of muscular fat. *Magn Reson Med* 2002;47:720–727.
292. Szczepaniak LS, Babcock EE, Schick F, et al. Measurement of intracellular triglyceride stores by H spectroscopy: validation in vivo. *Am J Physiol* 1999; 276:E977–E989.
293. Sinha R, Dufour S, Petersen KF, et al. Assessment of skeletal muscle triglyceride content by (1)H nuclear magnetic resonance spectroscopy in lean and obese adolescents: relationships to insulin sensitivity, total body fat, and central adiposity. *Diabetes* 2002;51:1022–1027.
294. Kelley DE, Goodpaster B, Wing RR, et al. Skeletal muscle fatty acid metabolism in association with insulin resistance, obesity, and weight loss. *Am J Physiol* 1999;277:E1130–E1141.
295. Simoneau JA, Veerkamp JH, Turcotte LP, et al. Markers of capacity to utilize fatty acids in human skeletal muscle: relation to insulin resistance and obesity and effects of weight loss. *FASEB J* 1999;13:2051–2060.
296. Kim JY, Hickner RC, Cortright RL, et al. Lipid oxidation is reduced in obese human skeletal muscle. *Am J Physiol Endocrinol Metab* 2000;279:E1039–E1044.
297. Dobbins RL, Szczepaniak LS, Bentley B, et al. Prolonged inhibition of muscle carnitine palmitoyltransferase-1 promotes intramyocellular lipid accumulation and insulin resistance in rats. *Diabetes* 2001;50:123–130.
298. Sidossis LS, Mittendorfer B, Chinkes D, et al. Effect of hyperglycemia-hyperinsulinemia on whole body and regional fatty acid metabolism. *Am J Physiol* 276:E427–E434.
299. Sidossis LS, Stuart CA, Shulman GI, et al. Glucose plus insulin regulate fat oxidation by controlling the rate of fatty acid entry into the mitochondria. *J Clin Invest* 1999;98:2244–2250.
300. Sidossis LS, Wolfe RR. Glucose and insulin-induced inhibition of fatty acid oxidation: the glucose-fatty acid cycle reversed. *Am J Physiol* 1996;270:E733–E738.
301. McGarry JD, Mannaerts GP, Foster DW. A possible role for malonyl-CoA in the regulation of hepatic fatty acid oxidation and ketogenesis. *J Clin Invest* 1977;60:265–270.
302. Saha AK, Kurowski TG, Ruderman NB. A malonyl-CoA fuel-sensing mechanism in muscle: effects of insulin, glucose, and denervation. *Am J Physiol* 1995;269:E283–E289.
303. Boden G, Lebed B, Schatz M, et al. Effects of acute changes of plasma free fatty acids on intramyocellular fat content and insulin resistance in healthy subjects. *Diabetes* 2001;50:1612–1617.
304. Oakes ND, Bell KS, Furler SM, et al. Diet-induced muscle insulin resistance in rats is ameliorated by acute dietary lipid withdrawal or a single bout of exercise: parallel relationship between insulin stimulation of glucose uptake and suppression of long-chain fatty acyl-CoA. *Diabetes* 1997;46:2022–2028.
305. Kelley DE, Goodpaster BH. Skeletal muscle triglyceride. An aspect of regional adiposity and insulin resistance. *Diabetes Care* 2001;24:933–941.

306. Hoppeler H, Billeter R, Horvath PJ, et al. Muscle structure with low- and high-fat diets in well-trained male runners. *Int J Sports Med* 1999;20:522–526.
307. Haap M, Thamer C, Machann J, et al. Metabolic characterization of a woman homozygous for the ser113leu missense mutation in carnitine palmitoyl transferase II. *J Clin Endocrinol Metab* 2002;87:2139–2143.
308. Anderwald C, Bernroider E, Krssak M, et al. Effects of insulin treatment in type 2 diabetic patients on intracellular lipid content in liver and skeletal muscle. *Diabetes* 2002;51:3025–3032.
309. Listenberger LL, Han X, Lewis SE, et al. Triglyceride accumulation protects against fatty acid-induced lipotoxicity. *Proc Natl Acad Sci U S A* 2003;100: 3077–3082.
310. Ruderman NB, Saha AK, Vavvas D, et al. Malonyl-coA, fuel sensing, and insulin resistance. *Am J Physiol Endocrinol Metab* 1999;276:E1–E18.
311. Prentki M, Corkey BE. Are the beta-cell signaling molecules malonyl-CoA and cystolic long-chain acyl-CoA implicated in multiple tissue defects of obesity and NIDDM? *Diabetes* 1996;45:273–283.
312. Ruderman NB, Saha AK, Vavvas DJ, et al. Lipid abnormalities in muscle of insulin-resistant rodents. The malonyl CoA hypothesis. *Ann N Y Acad Sci* 1997;827:221–230.
313. Wititsuwannakul D, Kim K-H. Mechanism of palmityl coenzyme A inhibition of liver glycogen synthase. *J Biol Chem* 1977;252:7812–7817.
314. Sleeman MW, Donegan NP, Heller-Harrison R, et al. Association of acyl-CoA synthetase-1 with GLUT4-containing vesicles. *J Biol Chem* 1998;273:3132–3135.
315. Marceau P, Biron S, Hould FS, et al. Liver pathology and the metabolic syndrome X in severe obesity. *J Clin Endocrinol Metab* 1999;84:1513–1517.
316. Ludwig J, Viggiano TR, McGill DB, et al. Nonalcoholic steatohepatitis: Mayo Clinic experiences with a hitherto unnamed disease. *Mayo Clin Proc* 1980; 55:434–438.
317. Dixon JB, Bhathal PS, O'Brien PE. Nonalcoholic fatty liver disease: predictors of nonalcoholic steatohepatitis and liver fibrosis in the severely obese. *Gastroenterology* 2001;121:91–100.
318. Matteoni CA, Younossi ZM, Gramlich T, et al. Nonalcoholic fatty liver disease: a spectrum of clinical and pathological severity. *Gastroenterology* 1999;116: 1413–1419.
319. Thomsen C, Becker U, Winkler K, et al. Quantification of liver fat using magnetic resonance spectroscopy. *Magn Reson Imaging* 1994;12:487–495.
320. Longo R, Ricci C, Masutti F, et al. Fatty infiltration of the liver. Quantification by 1H localized magnetic resonance spectroscopy and comparison with computed tomography. *Invest Radiol* 1993;28:297–302.
321. Garg A, Misra A. Hepatic steatosis, insulin resistance, and adipose tissue disorders. *J Clin Endocrinol Metab* 2002;87:3019–3022.
322. Sanyal AJ, Campbell-Sargent C, Mirshahi F, et al. Nonalcoholic steatohepatitis: association of insulin resistance and mitochondrial abnormalities. *Gastroenterology* 2001;120:1183–1192.
323. Ryysy L, Hakkinen AM, Goto T, et al. Hepatic fat content and insulin action on free fatty acids and glucose metabolism rather than insulin absorption are associated with insulin requirements during insulin therapy in type 2 diabetic patients. *Diabetes* 2000;49:749–758.
324. Marchesini G, Brizi M, Bianchi G, et al. Nonalcoholic fatty liver disease: a feature of the metabolic syndrome. *Diabetes* 2001;50:1844–1850.
325. Seppälä-Lindroos A, Vehkavaara S, Häkkinen A-M, et al. Fat accumulation in the liver is associated with defects in insulin suppression of glucose production and serum free fatty acids independent of obesity in normal men. *J Clin Endocrinol Metab* 2002;87:3023–3028.
326. Kelley DE, McKolanis TM, Hegazi RAF, et al. Fatty liver in type 2 diabetes mellitus: relation to regional adiposity, fatty acids, and insulin resistance. *Am J Physiol Endocrinol Metab* 2003;285: E906–E916.
327. Hwang JH, Hawkins M, Stein D, et al. Simultaneous measurement of intrahepatic, intramyocellular and visceral fat content by in vivo magnetic resonance methods: relation to insulin sensitivity. In: *Proceedings of the International Society of Magnetic Resonance in Medicine*, 2004;11:P503.
328. An J, Shiota M, Newgard C. Amelioration of muscle insulin resistance by activation of fat oxidation in liver. *Diabetes* 2003;52[Suppl 1]:296.
329. Petersen KF, Tygstrup N. A liver factor increasing glucose uptake in rat hindquarters. *J Hepatol* 1994;20:461–465.
330. Flier JS, Kahn CR, Jarrett DB, et al. The immunology of the insulin receptor. *Immunol Commun* 1976;5:361–373.
331. Flier JS. Lilly Lecture: syndromes of insulin resistance. From patient to gene and back again. *Diabetes* 1992;41:1207–1219.
332. Taylor SI, Accili D, Haft CR, et al. Mechanisms of hormone resistance: lessons from insulin-resistant patients. *Acta Paediatr Suppl* 1994;399:95–104.
333. Alvestrand A. Carbohydrate and insulin metabolism in renal failure. *Kidney Int Suppl* 1997;62:S48–S52.
334. Mak RH, DeFronzo RA. Glucose and insulin metabolism in uremia. *Nephron* 1992;61:377–382.
335. Schmitz O, Orskov L, Lund S, et al. Glucose metabolism in chronic renal failure with reference to GH treatment of uremic children. *J Pediatr Endocrinol* 1993;6:53–59.
336. Farrer M, Fulcher GR, Johnson AJ, et al. Effect of acute inhibition of lipolysis on operation of the glucose-fatty acid cycle in hepatic cirrhosis. *Metabolism* 1992;41:465–470.
337. Taylor R, Heine RJ, Collins J, et al. Insulin action in cirrhosis. *Hepatology* 1985; 5:64–71.
338. Rowe JW, Wands JR, Mezey E, et al. Familial hemochromatosis: characteristics of the precirrhotic stage in a large kindred. *Medicine* (Baltimore) 1977; 56:197–211.
339. Hramiak IM, Finegood DT, Adams PC. Factors affecting glucose tolerance in hereditary hemochromatosis. *Clin Invest Med* 1997;20:110–118.
340. Fernandez-Real JM, Penarroja G, Castro A, et al. Blood letting in high-ferritin type 2 diabetes: effects on insulin sensitivity and beta-cell function. *Diabetes* 2002;51:1000–1004.
341. Pappas S, Donohue SM, Denver AE, et al. Glucose intolerance in thalassemia major is related to insulin resistance and hepatic dysfunction. *Metabolism* 1996;45:652–657.
342. Copeland GP, Leinster SJ, Davis JC, et al. Insulin resistance in patients with colorectal cancer. *Br J Surg* 1987;74:1031–1035.
343. Isaksson B, Strommer L, Friess H, et al. Impaired insulin action on phosphatidylinositol 3-kinase activity and glucose transport in skeletal muscle of pancreatic cancer patients. *Pancreas* 2003;26:173–177.
344. McCall JL, Tuckey JA, Parry BR. Serum tumour necrosis factor alpha and insulin resistance in gastrointestinal cancer. *Br J Surg* 1992;79:1361–1363.
345. Makino T, Noguchi Y, Yoshikawa T, et al. Circulating interleukin 6 concentrations and insulin resistance in patients with cancer. *Br J Surg* 1998;85: 1658–1662.
346. Noguchi Y, Yoshikawa T, Marat D, et al. Insulin resistance in cancer patients is associated with enhanced tumor necrosis factor-alpha expression in skeletal muscle. *Biochem Biophys Res Commun* 1998;253:887–892.
347. Koopmans SJ, Ohman L, Haywood JR, et al. Seven days of euglycemic hyperinsulinemia induces insulin resistance for glucose metabolism but not hypertension, elevated catecholamine levels, or increased sodium retention in conscious normal rats. *Diabetes* 1997;46:1572–1578.
348. Del Prato S, Riccio A, Vigili de Kreutzenberg S, et al. Mechanisms of fasting hypoglycemia and concomitant insulin resistance in insulinoma patients. *Metabolism* 1993;42:24–29.
349. Hjollund E, Pedersen O, Richelsen B, et al. Glucose transport and metabolism in adipocytes from newly diagnosed untreated insulin-dependent diabetics. Severely impaired basal and postinsulin binding activities. *J Clin Invest* 1985;76:2091–2096.
350. Pedersen O, Hjollund E. Insulin receptor binding to fat and blood cells and insulin action in fat cells from insulin-dependent diabetics. *Diabetes* 1982; 31:706–715.
351. Hurrell DG, Pedersen O, Kahn CR. Alterations in the hepatic insulin receptor kinase in genetic and acquired obesity in rats. *Endocrinology* 1989; 125:2454–2462.
352. Freidenberg GR, Reichart DR, Olefsky JM, et al. Reversibility of defective adipocyte insulin receptor kinase activity in non-insulin-dependent diabetes mellitus. Effect of weight loss. *J Clin Invest* 1988;82:1398–1406.
353. Gerich JE. Lilly Lecture 1988. Glucose counterregulation and its impact on diabetes mellitus. *Diabetes* 1988;37:1608–1617.
354. Rizza RA, Mandarino LJ, Gerich JE. Cortisol-induced insulin resistance in man: impaired suppression of glucose production and stimulation of glucose utilization due to a postreceptor detect of insulin action. *J Clin Endocrinol Metab* 1982;54:131–138.
355. Karnieli E, Cohen P, Barzilai N, et al. Insulin resistance in Cushing's syndrome. *Horm Metab Res* 1985;17:518–521.
356. Bjorntorp P, Rosmond R. The metabolic syndrome—a neuroendocrine disorder? *Br J Nutr* 2000;83[Suppl 1]:S49–S57.
357. Reaven GM, Lithell H, Landsberg L. Hypertension and associated metabolic abnormalities—the role of insulin resistance and the sympathoadrenal system. *N Engl J Med* 1996;334:374–381.
358. Ohsaka Y, Tokumitsu Y, Nomura Y. Suppression of insulin-stimulated phosphatidylinositol 3-kinase activity by the β_3-adrenoceptor agonist CL316243 in rat adipocytes. *Growth Regul* 1997;402:246–250.
359. Green A, Carroll RM, Dobias SB. Desensitization of β-adrenergic receptors in adipocytes causes increased insulin sensitivity of glucose transport. *Am J Physiol* 1996;271:E271–E276.
360. Widen E, Lehto M, Kanninen T, et al. Association of a polymorphism in the β_3-adrenergic-receptor gene with features of the insulin resistance syndrome in Finns. *N Engl J Med* 1995;333:348–351.
361. Umekawa T, Yoshida T, Sakane N, et al. Trp64Arg mutation of β_3-adrenoceptor gene deteriorates lipolysis induced by β_3-adrenoceptor agonist in human omental adipocytes. *Diabetes* 1999;48:117–120.
362. Wiesner TD, Bluher M, Windgassen M, et al. Improvement of insulin sensitivity after adrenalectomy in patients with pheochromocytoma. *J Clin Endocrinol Metab* 2003;88:3632–3636.
363. Luo S, Luo J, Cincotta AH. Chronic ventromedial hypothalamic infusion of norepinephrine and serotonin promotes insulin resistance and glucose intolerance. *Neuroendocrinology* 1999;70:460–465.
364. Niklasson M, Holmang A, Lonnroth P. Induction of rat muscle insulin resistance by epinephrine is accompanied by increased interstitial glucose and lactate concentrations. *Diabetologia* 1998;41:1467–1473.
365. Bessey PQ, Brooks DC, Black PR, et al. Epinephrine acutely mediates skeletal muscle insulin resistance. *Surgery* 1983;94:172–179.
366. Hansen I, Tsalikian E, Beaufrere B, et al. Insulin resistance in acromegaly: defects in both hepatic and extrahepatic insulin *Am J Physiol* 1986;250(3 Pt 1): E269–E273.
367. Clemmons DR. Roles of insulin-like growth factor-I and growth hormone in mediating insulin resistance in acromegaly [review]. *Pituitary* 2002;5: 181–183.
368. Wasada T, Aoki K, Sato A, et al. Assessment of insulin resistance in acromegaly associated with diabetes mellitus before and after transsphenoidal adenomectomy. *Endocr J* 1997;44:617–620.

369. Rose DR, Clemmons DR. Growth hormone receptor antagonist improves insulin resistance in acromegaly. *Growth Horm IGF Res* 2002;12:418–424.
370. Breidert M, Pinzer T, Wildbrett J, et al. Long-term effect of octreotide in acromegaly on insulin resistance. *Horm Metab Res* 1995;27:226–230.
371. Obici S, Rossetti L. Minireview: nutrient sensing and the regulation of insulin action and energy balance. *Endocrinology* 2003;144:5172–5178.
372. Rossetti L, Giaccari A, DeFronzo RA. Glucose toxicity [review]. *Diabetes Care* 1990;13:610–630.
373. Leslie RD, Taylor R, Pozzilli P. The role of insulin resistance in the natural history of type 1 diabetes. *Diabet Med* 1997;14:327–331.
374. Yki-Jarvinen H. Glucose toxicity. *Endocr Rev* 1992;13:415–431.
375. Rossetti L, Smith D, Shulman GI, et al. Correction of hyperglycemia with phlorizin normalizes tissue sensitivity to insulin in diabetic rats. *J Clin Invest* 1987;79:1510–1515.
376. Kahn BB, Shulman GI, DeFronzo RA, et al. Normalization of blood glucose in diabetic rats with phlorizin treatment reverses insulin-resistant glucose transport in adipose cells without restoring glucose transporter gene expression. *J Clin Invest* 1991;87:561–570.
377. Krook A, Kawano Y, Song XM, et al. Improved glucose tolerance restores insulin-stimulated AKT kinase activity and glucose transport in skeletal muscle from diabetic Goto-Kakizaki (GK) rats. *Diabetes* 1997;46:2110–2114.
378. Song XM, Kawano Y, Krook A, et al. Muscle fiber-type specific defects in insulin signal transduction to glucose transport in diabetic Goto-Kakizaki rats. *Diabetes* 1999;48:664–670.
379. Marshall S, Bacote V, Traxinger RR. Discovery of a metabolic pathway mediating glucose-induced desensitization of the glucose transport system. Role of hexosamine biosynthesis in the induction of insulin resistance. *J Biol Chem* 1991;266:4706–4712.
380. Nelson BA, Robinson KA, Buse MG. High glucose and glucosamine induce insulin resistance via different mechanisms in 3T3-L1 adipocytes. *Diabetes* 2000;9:981–991.
381. Rossetti L, Hawkins M, Chen W, et al. In vivo glucosamine infusion induces insulin resistance in normoglycemic but not in hyperglycemic conscious rats. *J Clin Invest* 1995;96:132–140.
382. Hawkins M, Barzilai N, Liu R, et al. Role of the glucosamine pathway in fat-induced insulin resistance. *J Clin Invest* 1997;99:2173–2182.
383. Hawkins M, Angelov I, Liu R, et al. The tissue concentration of UDP-N-acetylglucosamine modulates the stimulatory effect of insulin on skeletal muscle glucose uptake. *J Biol Chem* 1997;272:4889–4895.
384. Gazdag AC, Wetter TJ, Davidson RT, et al. Lower calorie intake enhances muscle insulin action and reduces hexosamine levels. *Am J Physiol Regul Integr Comp Physiol* 2000;278:R504–R512.
385. Wang J, Obici S, Morgan K, et al. Overfeeding rapidly induces leptin and insulin resistance. *Diabetes* 2001;50:2786–2791.
386. Wells L, Vosseller K, Hart GW. Glycosylation of nucleocytoplasmic proteins: signal transduction and O-GlcNAc. *Science* 2001;291:2376–2378.
387. Hart GW. Dynamic *O*-linked glycosylation of nuclear and cytoskeletal proteins. *Annu Rev Biochem* 1997;66:315–335.
388. Obici S, Rossetti L. Minireview: nutrient sensing and the regulation of insulin action and energy balance. *Endocrinology* 2003;144:5172–5178.
389. Marshall S, Bacote V, Traxinger RR. Discovery of a metabolic pathway mediating desensitization of the glucose transport system: role of hexosamine biosynthesis in the induction of insulin resistance. *J Biol Chem* 1991;266:4706–4712.
390. Marshall S, Bacote V, Traxinger RR. Complete inhibition of glucose-induced desensitization of the glucose transport system by inhibitors of mRNA synthesis. Evidence for rapid turnover of glutamine:fructose-6-phosphate amidotransferase. *J Biol Chem* 1991;266:10155–10161.
391. Cooksey RC, McClain DA. Transgenic mice overexpressing the rate-limiting enzyme for hexosamine synthesis in skeletal muscle or adipose tissue exhibit total body insulin resistance. *Ann N Y Acad Sci* 2002;967:102–111.
392. Cooksey RC, Hebert LF Jr, Zhu JH, et al. Mechanism of hexosamine-induced insulin resistance in transgenic mice overexpressing glutamine:fructose-6-phosphate amidotransferase: decreased glucose transporter GLUT4 translocation and reversal by treatment with thiazolidinedione. *Endocrinology* 1999;140:1151–1157.
393. Hawkins M, Hu M, Yu J, et al. Discordant effects of glucosamine on insulin-stimulated glucose metabolism and phosphatidylinositol 3-kinase activity. *J Biol Chem* 1999;274:31312–31319.
394. Wells L, Vosseller K, Hart GW. A role for N-acetylglucosamine as a nutrient sensor and mediator of insulin resistance. *Cell Mol Life Sci* 2003;60:222–228.
395. Parker GJ, Lund KC, Taylor RP, et al. Insulin resistance of glycogen synthase mediated by o-linked N-acetylglucosamine. *J Biol Chem* 2003;278:10022–10027.
396. Chen KS, Heydrick SJ, Brown ML, et al. Insulin increases a biochemically distinct pool of diacylglycerol in the rat soleus muscle. *Am J Physiol* 1994;266: E479–E485.
397. Haring HU, Tippner S, Kellner M, et al. Modulation of insulin receptor signaling. Potential mechanisms of a cross talk between bradykinin and the insulin receptor [review]. *Diabetes* 1996;45[Suppl 1]:S115–S119.
398. Goldberg HJ, Whiteside CI, Fantus IG. The hexosamine pathway regulates the plasminogen activator inhibitor-1 gene promoter and Sp1 transcriptional activation through protein kinase C-beta I and -delta. *J Biol Chem* 2002;277: 33833–33841.
399. Du XL, Edelstein D, Rossetti L, et al. Hyperglycemia-induced mitochondrial superoxide overproduction activates the hexosamine pathway and induces plasminogen activator inhibitor-1 expression by increasing Sp1 glycosylation. *Proc Natl Acad Sci U S A* 2000;97:12222–12226.
400. Reaven GM, Hollenbeck C, Jeng C-Y, et al. Measurement of plasma glucose, free fatty acid, lactate, and insulin for 24h in patients with NIDDM. *Diabetes* 1988;37:1020–1024.
401. Arslanian SA, Kahlan SC. Correlations between fatty acid and glucose metabolism. *Diabetes* 1994;43:908–914.
402. Felber JP, Ferrannini E, Golay A. Role of lipid oxidation in pathogenesis of insulin resistance of obesity and type II diabetes. *Diabetes* 1987;36:1341–1350.
403. Randle PJ, Garland PB, Hales CN, et al. The glucose fatty acid cycle: its role in insulin sensitivity and the metabolic disturbances of diabetes mellitus. *Lancet* 1963;1:785–789.
404. Randle PJ, Garland PB, Newsholme EA, et al. The glucose fatty acid cycle in obesity and maturity onset diabetes mellitus. *Ann N Y Acad Sci* 1965;131: 324–333.
405. Boden G, Jadali F, White J, et al. Effects of fat on insulin-stimulated carbohydrate metabolism in normal men. *J Clin Invest* 1991;88:960–966.
406. Boden G, Chen X, Ruiz J, et al. Mechanisms of fatty acid-induced inhibition of glucose uptake. *J Clin Invest* 1994;93:2438–2446.
407. Kelley D, Mokan M, Simoneau J-A, et al. Interaction between glucose and free fatty acid metabolism in human skeletal muscle. *J Clin Invest* 1993;92: 91–98.
408. Roden M, Price T, Perseghin G, et al. Mechanism of free fatty acid-induced insulin resistance in humans. *J Clin Invest* 1996;97:2859–2865.
409. Shulman GI. Cellular mechanisms of insulin resistance. *J Clin Invest* 2000;106: 171–176.
410. Yu C, Chen Y, Cline GW, et al. Mechanism by which fatty acids inhibit insulin activation of insulin receptor substrate-1 (IRS-1)-associated phosphatidylinositol 3-kinase activity in muscle. *J Biol Chem* 2002;277:50230–50236.
411. Griffin ME, Marcucci MJ, Cline GW, et al. Free fatty acid-induced insulin resistance is associated with activation of protein kinase C and alterations in the insulin signaling cascade. *Diabetes* 1999;48:1270–1274.
412. Chalkley SM, Hettiarachchi M, Chisholm DJ, et al. Five-hour fatty acid elevation increases muscle lipids and impairs glycogen synthesis in the rat. *Metabolism* 1998;47:1121–1126.
413. Schmitz-Peiffer C, Browne CL, Oakes ND, et al. Alterations in the expression and cellular localization of protein kinase C isozymes epsilon and theta are associated with insulin resistance in skeletal muscle of the high-fat-fed rats. *Diabetes* 1997;46:169–178.
414. Itani SI, Ruderman NB, Schmieder F, et al. Lipid-induced insulin resistance in human muscle is associated with changes in diacylglycerol, protein kinase C, and I kappa B-alpha. *Diabetes* 2002;51:2005–2011.
415. Kim YB, Shulman GI, Kahn BB. Fatty acid infusion selectively impairs insulin action on Akt1 and protein kinase C lambda/zeta but not on glycogen synthase kinase-3. *J Biol Chem* 2002;277:32915–32922.
416. Kim JK, Kim YJ, Fillmore JJ, et al. Prevention of fat-induced insulin resistance by salicylate. *J Clin Invest* 2001;108:437–446.
417. Williamson RT, Lond MD. On the treatment of glycosuria and diabetes mellitus with sodium salicylate. *BMJ* 1901;1:760–762.
418. Hawkins M, Barzilai N, Liu R, et al. Role of the glucosamine pathway in fat-induced insulin resistance. *J Clin Invest* 1997;99:2173–2182.
419. Patti ME. Nutrient modulation of cellular insulin action. *Ann N Y Acad Sci* 1999;892:187–203.
420. Randle PJ, Kerbey AL, Espinal J. Mechanisms decreasing glucose oxidation in diabetes and starvation: role of lipid fuels and hormones. *Diabetes Metab Rev* 1988;4:623–638.
421. Liu Y, Uyeda K. A mechanism for fatty acid inhibition of glucose utilization in liver. Role of xylulose-5-P. *J Biol Chem* 1996;271:8824–8830.
422. Weigert C, Klopfer K, Kausch C. Palmitate-induced activation of the hexosamine pathway in human myotubes: increased expression of glutamine: fructose-6-phosphate aminotransferase. *Diabetes* 2003;52:650–656.
423. Williamson JR, Kreisberg RA, Felts PW. Mechanism for the stimulation of gluconeogenesis by fatty acids in perfused rat liver. *Proc Natl Acad Sci U S A* 1966;6:247–254.
424. Williamson J, Browning E, Scholz R. Control mechanisms of gluconeogenesis and ketogenesis. *J Biol Chem* 1969;250:4607–4616.
425. Antras-Ferry J, Le Bigot G, Robin P, et al. Stimulation of phosphoenolpyruvate carboxykinase gene expression by fatty acids. *Biochem Biophys Res Commun* 1994;203:385–391.
426. Oakes ND, Cooney GJ, Camilleri S, et al. Mechanisms of liver and muscle insulin resistance induced by chronic high-fat feeding. *Diabetes* 1997;46: 1768–1774.
427. Massillon D, Barzilai N, Hawkins M, et al. Induction of hepatic glucose-6-phosphatase gene expression by lipid infusion. *Diabetes* 1997;46:153–157.
428. Rodriguez JC, Gil-Gomez G, Hegardt FG, et al. Peroxisome proliferator-activator receptor mediates induction of the mitochondrial 3-hydroxy-3-methyl-glutaryl-CoA synthase gene by fatty acids. *J Biol Chem* 1994;269: 18767–18772.
429. Rudich A, Kozlovsky N, Potashnik R, et al. Oxidant stress reduces insulin responsiveness in 3T3-L1 adipocytes. *Am J Physiol* 1997;272(5 Pt 1): E935–E940.
430. Tirosh A, Rudich A, Potashnik R, et al. Oxidative stress impairs insulin but not platelet-derived growth factor signalling in 3T3-L1 adipocytes. *Biochem J* 2001;355(Pt 3):757–763.

431. Rudich A, Tirosh A, Potashnik R, et al. Lipoic acid protects against oxidative stress induced impairment in insulin stimulation of protein kinase B and glucose transport in 3T3-L1 adipocytes. *Diabetologia* 1999;42:949–957.
432. Evans JL, Goldfine ID, Maddux BA, et al. Oxidative stress and stress-activated signaling pathways: a unifying hypothesis of type 2 diabetes. *Endocr Rev* 2002;23:599–622.
433. Talior I, Yarkoni M, Bashan N, et al. Increased glucose uptake promotes oxidative stress and PKC-delta activation in adipocytes of obese, insulin-resistant mice. *Am J Physiol Endocrinol Metab* 2003;285:E295–E302.
434. Nishikawa T, Edelstein D, Du XL, et al. Normalizing mitochondrial superoxide production blocks three pathways of hyperglycaemic damage. *Nature* 2000;404:787–790.
435. Ferrannini E, Natali A, Capaldo B, et al. Insulin resistance, hyperinsulinemia, and blood pressure: role of age and obesity: European Group for the Study of Insulin Resistance (EGIR). *Hypertension* 1997;30:1144–1149.
436. Rosenbloom AL, Kappy MS, DeBusk FL, et al. Progeria: insulin resistance and hyperglycemia. *J Pediatr* 1983;102:400–402.
437. Cefalu WT, Wang ZQ, Werbel S, et al. Contribution of visceral fat mass to the insulin resistance of aging. *Metabolism* 1995;44:954–959.
438. Shimokata H, Tobin JD, Muller DC, et al. Studies in the distribution of body fat. I. Effects of age, sex, and obesity. *J Gerontol* 1989;44:M66–M73.
439. Petersen KF, Befroy D, Dufour S, et al. Mitochondrial dysfunction in the elderly: possible role in insulin resistance. *Science* 2003;300:1140–1142.
440. Heilbronn LK, Ravussin E. Calorie restriction and aging: review of the literature and implications for studies in humans. *Am J Clin Nutr* 2003;78:361–369.
441. Barzilai N, Banerjee S, Hawkins M, et al. Caloric restriction reverses hepatic insulin resistance in aging rats by decreasing visceral fat. *J Clin Invest* 1998;101:1353–1361.
442. Gabriely I, Ma XH, Yang XM, et al. Removal of visceral fat prevents insulin resistance and glucose intolerance of aging: an adipokine-mediated process? *Diabetes* 2002;51:2951–2958.
443. Ma XH, Muzumdar R, Yang XM, et al. Aging is associated with resistance to effects of leptin on fat distribution and insulin action. *J Gerontol A Biol Sci Med Sci* 2002;57:B225–B231.
444. Gabriely I, Ma XH, Yang XM, et al. Leptin resistance during aging is independent of fat mass. *Diabetes* 2002;51:1016–1021.

CHAPTER 25
β-Cell Dysfunction in Type 2 Diabetes Mellitus

Jack L. Leahy

Type 2 diabetes mellitus is a worldwide health crisis; the World Health Organization predicts an incidence of 300 million by 2025 (1). The past decade has seen great progress in our understanding of the pathogenesis of type 2 diabetes (Fig. 25.1). The initial event is a genetic predisposition for glucose intolerance. Although specific polymorphisms or mutated genes are not yet known, many that affect the liver, skeletal muscle, adipose, β-cells, or brain physiology will undoubtedly be uncovered. Lifestyle and environmental factors also determine whether glucose intolerance develops (2). An observation from many cross-sectional and longitudinal studies is the presence of insulin resistance (from obesity, a high-fat diet, inactivity, aging, or a genetic basis) early in the course, even predating the hyperglycemia (3–7). This observation is so well known that type 2 diabetes is understood by most students and practicing physicians to be a disease of insulin resistance. However, several lines of investigation, summarized below, have established a crucial role for β-cell dysfunction.

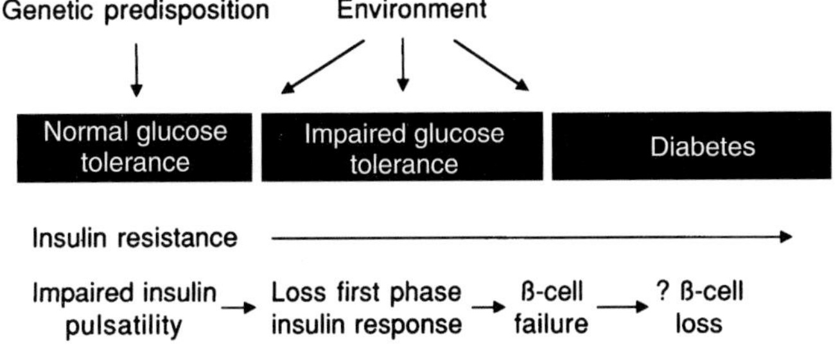

Figure 25.1. Proposed schema for the pathogenesis of type 2 diabetes. Predicted time points for the onset of various aspects of the β-cell dysfunction in this disease that are shown are based on the available literature, as reviewed in the chapter.

- β-Cell dysfunction is always found in type 2 diabetes. Furthermore, it occurs early and likely predates the hyperglycemia (8–10).
- Insulin resistance changes little during the progression from impaired glucose tolerance (IGT) to diabetes. In contrast, β-cell function undergoes substantial change. Cross-sectional and longitudinal studies have shown an increase in fasting insulin level and in insulin response to oral glucose in the early phases of the disease that keep glycemia normal despite the presence of insulin resistance, followed by a decrease when fasting glycemia surpasses 140 mg/dL (11,12). This inverted U-shaped curve of insulin levels (Fig. 25.2) was initially used to support the importance of insulin resistance in the early stages of the disease, as reflected in the increasing insulin output. However, more recent interest has focused on the decline—the so-called *β-cell failure*—as it coincides with, and is thought to cause, the progression from IGT to overt diabetes (9,10,13–15). Further, prospective study of persons with normal glucose tolerance (16) or IGT (17) showed that those with the lowest insulin response to a meal or to an oral glucose challenge (*low insulin responders*) carry the highest risk for developing type 2 diabetes later in life. These experimental observations highlight the importance of β-cell function in determining the glycemic status of at-risk persons.

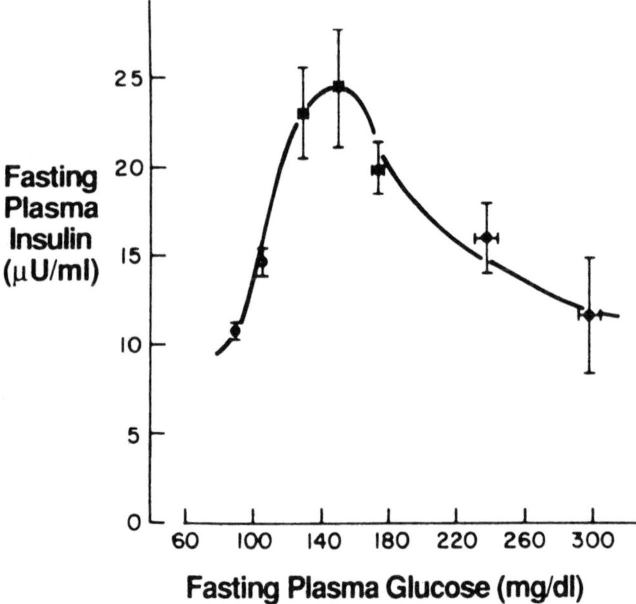

Figure 25.2. Fasting immunoreactive plasma insulin levels in nonobese subjects stratified by the level of glycemia. (From DeFronzo RA, Ferrannini E, Simonson DC. Fasting hyperglycemia in noninsulin-dependent diabetes mellitus: contributions of excessive hepatic glucose production and impaired tissue glucose uptake. *Metabolism* 1989;38:387–395, with permission.)

- Following the onset of diabetes, the β-cell dysfunction is reversible to a large degree by intensive glycemic control (18–20). In one of these studies (20), insulin pumps were used for 21 days in persons with type 2 diabetes. Improvement was observed not only in β-cell function but also in insulin-mediated suppression of hepatic glucose production and in some lessening of insulin resistance. These findings established the concept that part of the diabetes phenotype is acquired from metabolic derangements in the prediabetes/IGT phase of the disease through glucotoxicity (21,22), β-cell exhaustion (23), or less well defined mechanisms. Dysmetabolism-induced acquired tissue dysfunction explains why type 2 diabetes presents a relatively uniform clinical syndrome in different ethnic groups and populations despite presumed diverse genetic causes.
- Over time, type 2 diabetes becomes less responsive to oral hypoglycemic therapy in tandem with worsening β-cell function (24,25). The working assumption is that pathogenic elements that lead to a loss in β-cell mass become operative.
- There is little information from human studies regarding the biochemical and molecular basis for the β-cell dysfunction in type 2 diabetes because of the unavailability of pancreatic biopsy. Instead, animals—both rodents and larger animals—have been the major venue of investigation, as their β-cell (dys)function with diabetes closely resembles that of humans. Animal studies have identified a panoply of β-cell abnormalities with diabetes. We do not yet know which mechanisms operate in humans, but it seems certain that the β-cell dysfunction will be multifaceted and will entail multiple mechanisms.

To summarize, there is now general acceptance that β-cell dysfunction plays a crucial and necessary role in type 2 diabetes. Indeed, most investigators in the field consider defective insulin secretion and tissue insulin resistance of equal importance in the development of this disease; in the vast majority of affected persons, both must be present for the diabetes syndrome to occur (26). Whether defective insulin secretion and tissue resistance to insulin represent pleiotropic tissue effects of a single defect or multiple abnormalities is unknown. Another understanding is that type 2 diabetes is a progressive disease. Loss of β-cell function, and possibly of β-cell mass, is believed to underlie this progression, highlighting the pivotal role of the β-cell in determining the natural history of this disease. Many excellent reviews on β-cell dysfunction in type 2 diabetes are available (27–32).

NORMAL β-CELL FUNCTION

Pancreatic β-cells regulate the storage and metabolism of cellular fuels through their secretion of insulin. This crucial function is accomplished through a feedback loop whereby glycemia upregulates β-cell function—insulin secretion, proinsulin biosynthesis, processing of proinsulin to insulin, and β-cell replication rate—and the secreted insulin in turn lowers glycemia by inhibiting hepatic and renal glucose production and increasing glucose uptake into target organs, primarily skeletal muscle. Glucose regulation of insulin secretion occurs directly (*glucose-induced insulin secretion*) and also through modulation of the insulin response to insulinotropic hormones, nutrients, and neurotransmitters (*glucose potentiation of nonglucose secretagogues*; Fig. 25.3). These dual aspects of glucose-regulated insulin secretion are a potent modulatory system that ensures that the tissues' needs for insulin are exactly met in the fasting and post-

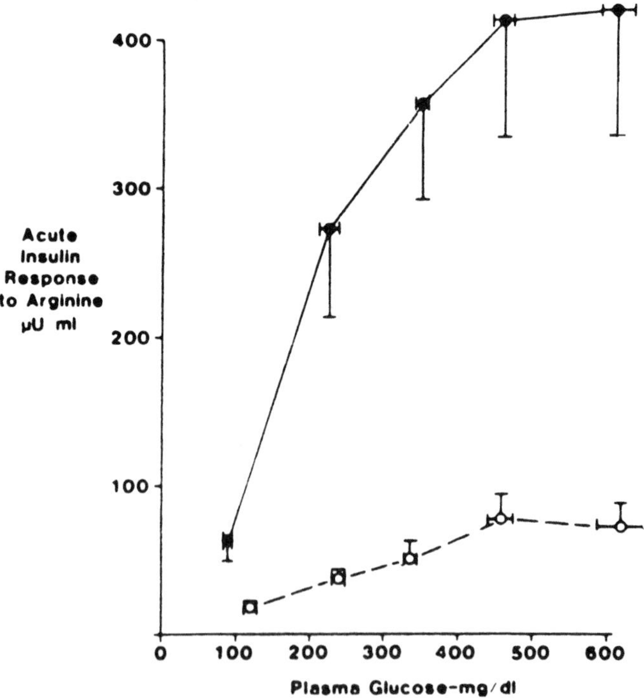

Figure 25.3. Acute insulin responses to 5 g of intravenous arginine at five different glucose levels in eight subjects with type 2 diabetes (*open circles*) and eight control subjects (*closed circles*). Insulin responses at all of the glucose levels are markedly attenuated in the subjects with type 2 diabetes. (From Ward WK, Bolgiano DC, McKnight B, et al. Diminished B cell secretory capacity in patients with noninsulin-dependent diabetes mellitus. *J Clin Invest* 1984;74:1318–1328, with permission from the American Society for Clinical Investigation.)

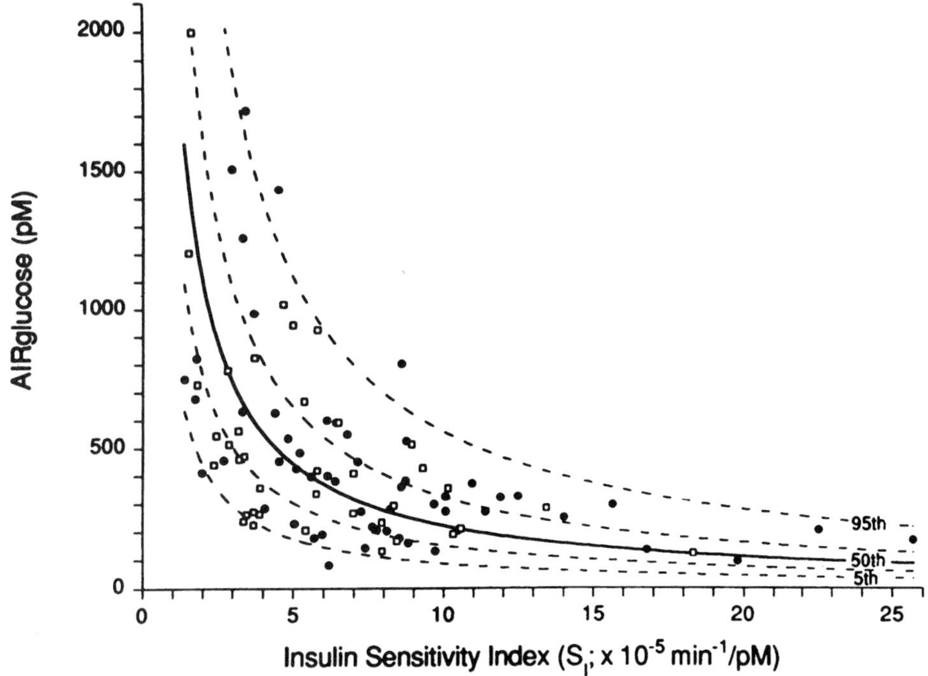

Figure 25.4. Curvilinear relationship between insulin sensitivity (S_I) and the first-phase insulin response (AIRglucose) in 93 normoglycemic subjects: 55 men (*closed circles*) and 38 women (*open squares*). Lines depicting the 5th, 25th, 50th, 75th, and 95th percentiles are shown. (Copyright © 1993 from the American Diabetes Association. From Kahn SE, Prigeon RL, McCulloch DK, et al. Quantification of the relationship between insulin sensitivity and β-cell function in human subjects: evidence for a hyperbolic function. *Diabetes* 1993;42:1663–1672, with permission from the American Diabetes Association.)

prandial states. The need for insulin is for the most part determined by the sensitivity of tissue to insulin—a curvilinear relationship exists with insulin secretion (Fig. 25.4) (33). Thus, even wide variations in insulin sensitivity such as the insulin resistance of puberty (34), pregnancy (35), and aging (36) do not normally affect glycemia. Also, dysfunction of the system can be determined by graphing insulin sensitivity and secretion from the experimental population to see if these values fall on the curvilinear curve (10,37,38). Another *in vivo* approach to testing the glucose-sensing character of β-cells uses a graded glucose infusion to produce a progressive increase in glycemia (39).

It is not only the amount of insulin released that is important. An acute increase in glycemia that can be approximated experimentally with intravenous glucose elicits a large burst of insulin secretion that lasts 5 to 7 minutes (*first phase*) followed by sustained insulin secretion that lasts for the duration of the hyperglycemia (*second phase*). Meals also induce a biphasic pattern of insulin secretion, although the phases are less distinct, with the early phase ascribed to the first 30 minutes and the later phase to the remaining postprandial hyperinsulinemia (1 to 2 hours normally). The biphasic pattern is necessary for normal mealtime glucose tolerance, with the concept being that the first phase primes the insulin-sensitive tissues for the coming food. Supporting this notion are studies that experimentally disrupted the early insulin response to a meal in otherwise healthy, normoglycemic subjects, causing impaired insulin-mediated tissue glucose disposal and excessive postprandial glycemia (40,41).

Insulin secretion occurs as oscillatory pulsations with a periodicity of 11 to 14 minutes, thought to be necessary to fully regulate hepatic glucose production (42,43). Also, large bursts of insulin release (*ultradian oscillations*) occur several times a day, particularly with meals (44), increasing the efficiency of nutrient clearance following meals (45).

Thus, the β-cell functions in a highly complex fashion that regulates the timing and overall insulin response to a meal to preserve normoglycemia. Quantitative insulin release and the pulsatile patterns can be tested *in vivo* by means of frequent insulin measurements to an appropriate stimulus. Also, the glucose-sensing and pulsatile-secretion characteristics can be jointly tested with an oscillatory glucose infusion that causes small increases and decreases in plasma glucose levels. Insulin secretion normally attains an oscillatory pattern termed *entrainment* (46,47). Failure of entrainment has been identified as an early defect in insulin secretion that precedes abnormal responses to more traditional tests. *In vivo* testing has been aided by several technical advances over the last few years. Insulin-specific assays are now widely available that have eliminated the cross-reactivity with proinsulin and its conversion intermediates (which are biologically inactive) that affected earlier assays. Also, insulin is secreted into the portal vein and undergoes a substantial first-pass clearance by the liver (approximately 50%). Thus, insulin levels in the peripheral circulation only approximate insulin secretion. Many investigators now analyze C-peptide values—the portion of proinsulin that is removed as it is converted to insulin. C-peptide is secreted with insulin in an equimolar ratio but undergoes minimal hepatic degradation and thus can be used for calculating true rates of insulin secretion (48,49).

β-CELL DYSFUNCTION IN TYPE 2 DIABETES

β-Cell Unresponsiveness to Glucose

The distinctive β-cell defect in type 2 diabetes is the loss of the first phase of glucose-induced insulin secretion (Fig. 25.5). This observation was first made in the late 1960s, when persons with

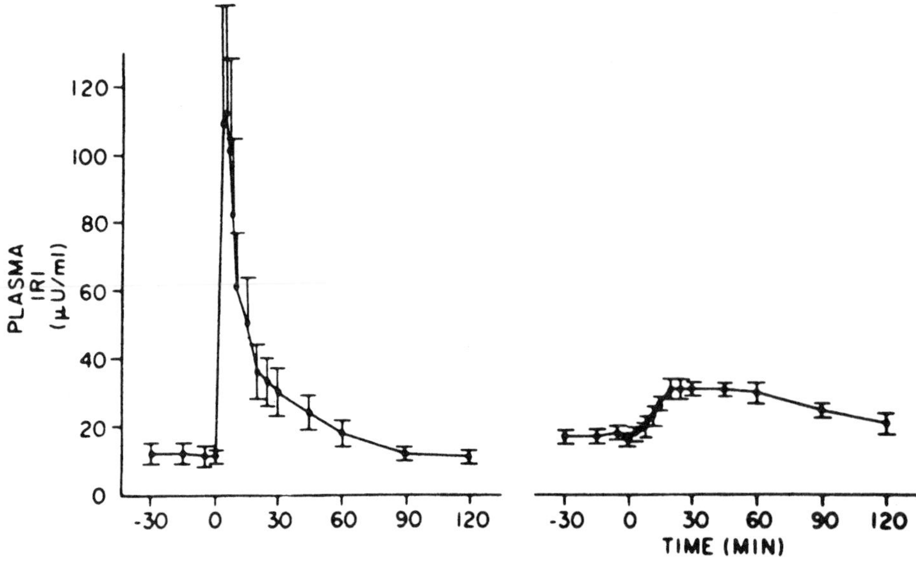

Figure 25.5. Plasma immunoreactive insulin response to 20-g bolus of intravenous glucose in nine subjects with type 2 diabetes (*right*) and nine normoglycemic control subjects (*left*). The first-phase insulin response (from 0 to 10 minutes) is totally lacking in the subjects with type 2 diabetes. In contrast, the second phase (from 10 minutes continuing for the duration of hyperglycemia) is intact in the subjects with diabetes and is greater than in the controls because of the persistent hyperglycemia in the subjects with diabetes following the glucose administration. (Reprinted from Pfeifer MA, Halter JB, Porte D Jr. Insulin secretion in diabetes mellitus. *Am J Med* 1981;70:579–588, with permission from Elsevier Science.)

type 2 diabetes were noted to have a delayed insulin response to intravenous glucose, and later was recognized as loss of the first phase. The second phase is also impaired but to a lesser degree (50,51). Subsequent investigation showed that this defect was fully established by the time the fasting glucose level reached 115 mg/dL (52), clearly predating overt diabetes, but was not present in persons with truly normal glucose levels in whom type 2 diabetes developed later (3,6). Thus, it first appears in the prediabetes state, termed IGT, which is clinically manifest as excess postprandial excursions of glycemia. Given the importance of the first-phase insulin response for normal prandial glucose tolerance (40,41), it follows that this defect is an important cause of the IGT state. Attesting to this idea is a study that simulated a burst of insulin with a short-term insulin infusion at the beginning of a meal in persons with type 2 diabetes, which resulted in a marked improvement in postprandial glycemia (53).

A major advance in our understanding occurred with the demonstration that intensive glycemic control restored the first-phase insulin response in subjects with type 2 diabetes (19). At about the same time, glucose-induced insulin secretion was shown to be impaired in diabetic animals (discussed subsequently). An important observation, made in diabetic rats, is that phloridzin reverses the defect (54). Phloridzin promotes glycosuria; it is used experimentally in diabetic animals to restore normoglycemia without changing insulinemia, thus helping to identify pathogenic effects of hyperglycemia. The understanding that has evolved from these findings is that the defect in glucose-induced insulin secretion occurs when β-cells are exposed to a "toxic" environment of an abnormally high level of glycemia (so-called *glucose toxicity*).

Insulin responses to nonglucose secretagogues are less impaired than those to glucose. When the defective glucose-induced insulin secretion was first investigated, nonglucose agents were thought to be unaffected, a finding that led to the idea that the glucose response was uniquely deranged (*selective glucose unresponsiveness*). However, later studies that were more carefully controlled for glycemia in the subjects with and without diabetes made it clear that responses to nonglucose secretogogues also were impaired, although less so than those to glucose. This challenged the concept that glucose unresponsiveness is the prototypical β-cell abnormality in type 2 diabetes; however, subsequent investigation (55) showed that the basis for the defective nonglucose-mediated secretion was impaired glucose potentiation (Fig. 25.3). The time of onset for the glucose potentiation defect is not as well defined as that for glucose-induced insulin secretion, and it is not clear if these dual abnormal effects of glucose on insulin secretion represent a single defect or separate biochemical/molecular defects in glucose sensing by the β-cell. Viewed together, type 2 diabetes entails defective glucose regulation of insulin secretion through both pathways—glucose-induced insulin secretion (in particular the first phase) and glucose potentiation—emphasizing why fasting and postprandial hyperglycemia are defining characteristics of this disease.

For many years there was confusion about how β-cell dysfunction could be present in the prediabetes/IGT state, in particular the loss of the first-phase response, when countless studies had showed hyperinsulinemia (both fasting and after a glucose challenge or a meal) at that time (Fig. 25.2). Insight into this seeming paradox came with the understanding of the importance of the early insulin response for control of postprandial glycemia (40,41); loss of this early response results in an excessive meal-induced rise in glycemia, and this hyperglycemia causes the late insulin response to exceed that seen normally. Previous studies had generally looked at insulin levels 2 hours after a meal or oral glucose challenge and thus had missed the defect in early insulin secretion. This concept is shown in Figure 25.6, which shows the 30-minute and 2-hour insulin values after oral glucose challenge across a wide range of glycemia (29). Note the disparity as the early insulin response decreases with increasing glycemia at a time when later insulin release is increasing.

Thus, a characteristic feature of type 2 diabetes is loss of the first-phase insulin response to a meal. It occurs early in the

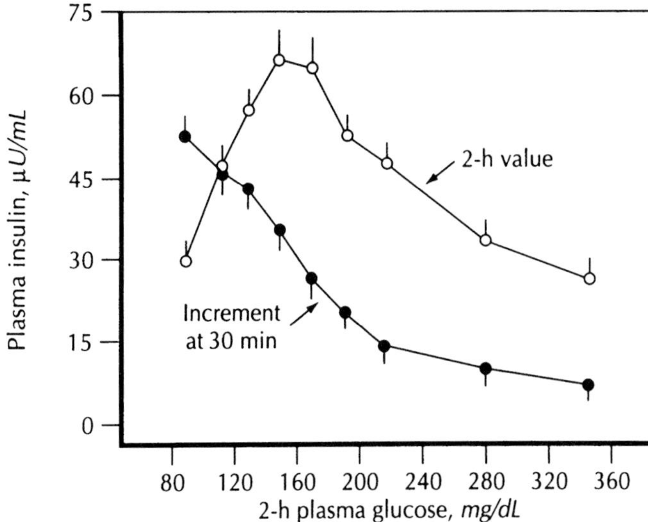

Figure 25.6. Comparison of 30-minute and 2-hour plasma insulin responses during oral glucose tolerance tests as a function of 2-hour plasma glucose values in 294 subjects. (From Gerich J, Van Haeften T. Insulin resistance versus impaired insulin secretion as the genetic basis for type 2 diabetes. *Curr Opin Endocrinol Diabetes* 1998;5:144–148, with permission.)

course of type 2 diabetes, predating fasting hyperglycemia, and is a major cause of the postprandial hyperglycemia that characterizes IGT and overt diabetes. This concept underlies the recent use of drugs for type 2 diabetes (meglitinides and phenylalanine derivatives) that are taken at meals to induce a rapid, short-lived insulin response.

Abnormal Pulsatile Secretion of Insulin

The pattern of orderly oscillations of insulin secretion with an 11- to 14-minute periodicity is lost in type 2 diabetes (56). Relatives of persons with type 2 diabetes show this defect when their glucose tolerance is normal (57,58), showing that it occurs early in the course of the disease. This might imply a genetic etiology. Countering that idea is a recent study showing recovery of oscillations in persons with type 2 diabetes after an overnight infusion of somatostatin, which pharmacologically blocks insulin release—interpreted by the authors as indicating that depletion of a readily releasable pool of insulin granules underlies the oscillation defect (59).

It is now generally accepted that the abnormal insulin pulsatility impairs normal regulatory control of insulin over hepatic glucose production. However, this understanding is relatively recent. The importance of the pulsatility defect was uncertain when first observed, as the magnitude of the pulsations in the normoglycemic control subjects was quite small (56): It was difficult to appreciate that such a minor effect would have any physiologic importance. Those studies used blood from the peripheral circulation. Insulin is secreted into the portal vein and undergoes substantial hepatic extraction. The breakthrough came with the understanding that the pulses are in fact large and are damped by hepatic extraction so that only a small fraction escapes the liver (42,60). Thus, the abnormal peripheral pulsations in type 2 diabetes represent very distorted insulin delivery to the liver, fitting with the idea of major dysregulation to the insulin-hepatic system. Future treatments might target this abnormality. For example, glucagon-like peptide-1 (GLP-1), which is under investigation as a hypoglycemic therapy for type 2 diabetes, increases pulsatile insulin secretion (61).

The ultradian oscillations—the large bursts of insulin that occur every 1 to 2 hours and more frequently with meals—also are disrupted in type 2 diabetes (62,63). This fact is well established, but the impact on glucose homeostasis is not totally clear. Regardless, pulsatile delivery of insulin holds a physiologic advantage, as evidenced by studies that have shown a greater hypoglycemic effect of pulsed versus continuously infused exogenous insulin (64). As such, loss of the pulsatile pattern of insulin secretion in type 2 diabetes disrupts this aspect of the glucose homeostasis system.

Increased Proinsulin-to-Insulin Ratio

The blood levels of insulin precursors (proinsulin and its conversion intermediates, which have only weak biologic activity) are disproportionately increased relative to insulin in type 2 diabetes (65,66). The same observation has been made in patients with diabetes caused by cystic fibrosis (67), a finding that raises the possibility that this disproportionate increase is another manifestation of hyperglycemia-induced β-cell dysfunction. However, the relationship of this increased ratio to hyperglycemia has been confused by seemingly inconsistent data. Most cross-sectional data show that the increased proinsulin/insulin ratio in type 2 diabetes occurs after the onset of hyperglycemia (68,69), with the ratio increasing as glycemia worsens (69,70). In disagreement are reports of an increased proinsulin/insulin ratio in the absence of glucose intolerance in populations at high risk for type 2 diabetes (71,72). Treatment studies to determine how reversal of hyperglycemia affects the proinsulin/insulin ratio also have not clarified its dependence on abnormal glycemia, because both improvement (73) and no effect (74) have been reported. Insight into this conundrum has come from the previously mentioned study that administered an overnight infusion of somatostatin to persons with type 2 diabetes; the proinsulin/insulin ratio was normalized by this pharmacologic inhibition of insulin secretion (59). This observation suggests that excessive insulin secretion, as opposed to hyperglycemia per se, underlies the raised proinsulin/insulin ratio. Another study of type 2 diabetes (75) and a study in diabetic sand rats (76) made a similar conclusion.

Our laboratory has studied diabetic rats in an effort to gain insight into the mechanistic basis for the raised proinsulin/insulin ratio (77–79). We first studied rats that had 90% of their pancreas removed (90% pancreatectomy) and observed an increased abundance of proinsulin-like peptides relative to insulin in pancreatic extracts, suggesting that the underlying defect was the storage, and subsequent secretion, of material enriched in proinsulin (77). We made the same observation in normal rats that received 48-hour infusions of glucose (78). That study showed the increased ratio resulted from a decreased insulin content, not from an increased proinsulin content (Fig. 25.7). Also, co-infusion of diazoxide to inhibit insulin secretion blocked the increase in the proinsulin/insulin ratio, results analogous to those seen in humans infused with somatostatin (59). These findings are in accord with the previously stated concept that an ongoing hypersecretion of insulin leading to depletion of the releasable insulin stores is the cause of the enhancement in proinsulin secretion, likely through secretion of immature, proinsulin-enriched granules. Confirmatory evidence was obtained by infusing normal rats for 3 days with large amounts of the insulin secretagogue tolbutamide (plus glucose to keep them euglycemic) and observing a raised percentage of proinsulin in pancreatic extracts (78). Furthermore, this concept implies that there is no biochemical or molecular defect in the proinsulin-processing pathway in diabetes, which we demonstrated to be the case in glucose-infused rats (79).

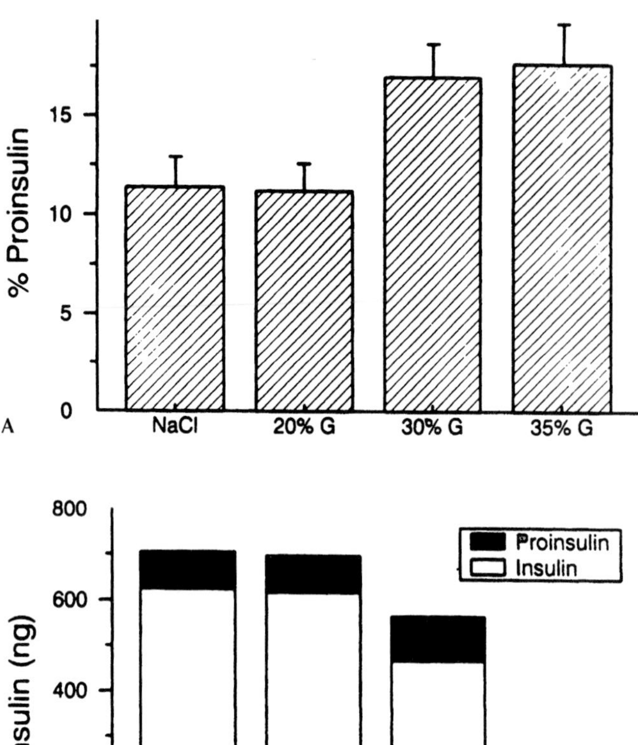

Figure 25.7. Relative proportion of proinsulin in pancreatic extracts from rats that received a 48-hour infusion with glucose. Pancreases underwent extraction, insulin/proinsulin precipitation, and separation of the insulins and proinsulins by high-performance liquid chromatography. Immunoreactive insulin and proinsulin were determined as the areas under the curve of the different peaks measured by insulin radioimmunoassay. **A:** % proinsulin = plasma immunoreactive insulin response (IRI) proinsulin/(IRI insulin + IRI proinsulin). **B:** IRI insulin and proinsulin in chromatography samples. Note that an increase in % proinsulin resulted from a decrease in insulin content not from an increase in proinsulin content. (Copyright © 1993, American Diabetes Association. From Leahy JL. Increased proinsulin/insulin ratio in pancreas extracts of hyperglycemic rats. *Diabetes* 1993;42:22–27. Reprinted with permission from the American Diabetes Association.)

Thus, the increased proportion of stored and circulating proinsulin in the diabetic rats appears to be secondary to a hypermobilization of granules, which leads to a rapid transit time and thus to incomplete processing to fully mature insulin. This hypersecretion scenario fits perfectly with the findings in patients with type 2 diabetes (59,75). However, enhanced insulin secretion per se is not enough to raise the proinsulin/insulin ratio, as is apparent from studies of nondiabetic obese subjects who are hyperinsulinemic but who have normal to lowered proinsulin/insulin ratios (68,80). Instead, some underlying element of β-cell dysfunction must be present as well.

β-CELL MASS AND STRUCTURE IN TYPE 2 DIABETES

The preceding discussion was of abnormalities that affect β-cell function. A second topic is whether the mass of β cells is lowered in type 2 diabetes and if so why? Relatively little is known about this subject, as investigation has been hampered by the inability to obtain pancreatic biopsy samples from free-living humans. Further, there is no noninvasive way to assess β-cell mass, although interest in the development of techniques that will allow that goal to be reached is growing. We are thus dependent on autopsy studies that have quantified pancreatic β-cell mass. However, these studies are few and are open to interpretation because of incomplete physiologic/clinical information about the subjects or of inexact matching with controls. Finally, the technical challenge of measuring β-cell mass in humans is substantial, which means that none of the available studies (81–83) are large. As such, they usually are viewed collectively, leading to the conclusion that the β-cell mass is modestly lowered in type 2 diabetes. Illustrating that conclusion is the study by Klöppel et al. (83), which is noteworthy not only because it is one of the largest but also because it controlled for obesity. They observed a doubling of β-cell mass in the obese versus nonobese control subjects (showing why weight matching of subjects is so important for this kind of study) and a 50% reduction in β-cell mass in the obese and nonobese diabetic subjects compared with their weight-matched controls (83).

That β-cell mass is decreased in type 2 diabetes is generally well accepted, but it is not known when it occurs or how it is temporally related to the β-cell failure that leads to the development of hyperglycemia. This early stage of diabetes is characterized by considerable recovery of β-cell function following intensive glycemic control (18–20), which has led some to conclude that abnormalities in β-cell function, not mass, are foremost. In contrast, the United Kingdom Prospective Diabetes Study (UKPDS), a study of intensive treatment in new-onset type 2 diabetes, reported increases in glycemia over time, in tandem with worsening of β-cell function, whether diet, sulfonylurea, metformin, or insulin therapy was used (24,25). This observation has led to speculation that the waning β-cell function in longstanding diabetes stems from a declining β-cell mass. The cause of that effect is not known. It is clearly not immune-mediated and is thus distinct from type 1 diabetes: morphologically, the islets appear relatively normal (except for amyloid infiltration, which is discussed below), and insulitis is never present (84). Also missing is evidence for the hyperactivity that might be expected in response to the hyperglycemia, with few mitotic figures found (84) and only modest degranulation seen (85). A recent finding in some diabetic animals is increased β-cell apoptosis (86–89), although its relevance for human type 2 diabetes is unknown.

Islet Amyloid

The best-studied mechanism that might lead to accelerated β-cell death in type 2 diabetes is the development of islet amyloid (90–93). Islet amyloid deposits were first described nearly 100 years ago by Opie (94). Although these deposits were found commonly in type 2 diabetes, they were thought to hold little significance until the seminal study of Howard that correlated islet morphology with the clinical and metabolic status of *Macaca nigra* monkeys as they went from nondiabetes to diabetes (95). Howard reported that the appearance of islet amyloid coincided with, or immediately preceded, hyperglycemia and concluded that amyloid-induced destruction of islet β-cells caused metabolic progression to diabetes. This relationship, which also was observed in cats (96), spurred substantial interest in islet amyloid.

A breakthrough in this field occurred with the identification and cloning, simultaneously by two groups, of the peptide that makes up the amyloid deposits. This peptide was termed *amylin*; the more common term today is *islet amyloid polypeptide* (IAPP) (97,98). IAPP is a 37-amino-acid peptide normally produced in β-cells that is copackaged with insulin in secretory granules. The 25- to 28-amino acid sequence is conserved in humans, monkeys, and cats [Ala-Ile-Leu-Ser], all of which develop islet amyloid in tandem with diabetes. This amino acid sequence is necessary for the formation of amyloid fibrils, as shown by the lack of fibril formation *in vitro* or *in vivo* of IAPP from animals that lack this sequence (rats, guinea pigs, and mice). This dichotomy has proven useful for studies in transgenic mice that have overexpressed human IAPP in β-cells, as there is no risk of amyloid formation from the mouse's own IAPP (99,100). The normal function of IAPP remains controversial. It slows gastric emptying—whether this effect is physiologic or pharmacologic is debated—and clinical trials are in progress of the ability of an analogue of IAPP to decrease postprandial glucose excursions in persons with diabetes (101).

The effects of IAPP on β-cells have been studied extensively *in vitro* and *in vivo*. When placed in solution, IAPP forms fibrils, and these aggregates have been shown to be cytotoxic to islets *in vitro* (102,103). However, the relevance of this observation *in vivo* is debated. Studies in transgenic mice that have overexpressed human IAPP have resulted in amyloid deposition and diabetes (99,100). However, a concern is that this requires very high levels of IAPP expression (99) or an accompanying insult, such as insulin resistance from growth hormone or dexamethasone treatment (104), or a high-fat diet (100). Whether this corequirement shows that IAPP is nonpathologic under normal conditions or that physiologically nonrelevant circumstances are required to induce pathogenic outcomes is still not clear.

Crucial questions must be answered before confirmation of a pathogenic role for IAPP and the amyloid deposits. There is no doubt that islets with amyloid deposits have a small β-cell mass with cellular distortion and destruction. The crucial question is which came first? Is the deposition of amyloid an early event that precedes hyperglycemia or does it occur only after mild hyperglycemia (and thus the β-cell functional failure) has developed? Do IAPP aggregates then induce functional and/or β-cell structural damage? Alternatively, is type 2 diabetes associated with β-cell death through an effect that is unrelated to IAPP such that the cellular stores of IAPP are released and form amyloid extracellularly among the cellular debris? Currently, there are no answers to these questions. However, studies of pancreas specimens that have been collected at autopsy from subjects who span the full range from nondiabetes to severe diabetes are in progress. The key information obtained from these studies should help determine the role of islet amyloid in this disease.

MECHANISMS OF β-CELL DYSFUNCTION

Glucose Toxicity

The hypothesis has been advanced that chronic hyperglycemia causes alterations in β-cell function, termed *glucose toxicity*. The idea started with the observation of substantial recovery of β-cell function in type 2 diabetes following treatments that restored normoglycemia (18–20). Also influential was the observation that diabetic animals have β-cell dysfunction similar to that in humans with type 2 diabetes (discussed below), supporting a causative effect of the metabolic environment. Subsequent biochemical and molecular studies of β-cell lines and islet tissue have uncovered plausible mechanisms for hyperglycemia-induced β-cell dysfunction. The term *glucose toxicity* was coined to represent tissue dysfunction from a hyperglycemic environment. Our own usage of the term is focused on the idea of a direct impairment effect of the raised glycemia on β-cell function as opposed to *exhaustion*, which is an indirect effect of hyperglycemia acting through a nonsustainable hypersecretion of insulin (23). The difference may seem subtle but becomes clear when reversal studies are performed with inhibitors of insulin secretion, as will be discussed subsequently. Generally, terminology that holds no exact mechanistic meaning is not advised. Regardless, the literature on type 2 diabetes and β-cell dysfunction is replete with these terms, and readers need to be familiar with their meanings.

Multiple rat models of experimental hyperglycemia have been studied for β-cell function, including the administration of streptozotocin during the neonatal period (105–107), partial pancreatectomy (108,109), and *in vivo* glucose infusions (110,111). Studies have also been carried out in a variety of rodents with spontaneous hyperglycemia, including GK rats (112), Zucker diabetic fatty (ZDF) rats (113), Otsuka Long-Evans Tokushima fatty (OLETF) rats (114), and many others. A universal finding is that secretion in response to glucose is impaired as opposed to secretion in response to nonglucose secretagogues such as arginine, glucagon, or tolbutamide, which are relatively unaffected (Fig. 25.8). This pattern of selective unresponsiveness to glucose closely resembles the pattern in human type 2 diabetes, as described. Just as important in terms of the concept of glucose toxicity is the complete absence of β-cell unresponsiveness to glucose with normoglycemia, as determined in studies of animals without a genetic predisposition to diabetes or before the onset of hyperglycemia in animals that later go on to develop diabetes (113,114). This concept is further supported by the finding that glucose-induced insulin secretion *in vitro* or *in vivo* is recovered with therapies that reverse the hyperglycemia (115–117). The most influential of these studies in terms of identifying hyperglycemia as the causative factor was a study of phloridzin. As previously discussed, phloridzin promotes glycosuria and restores normoglycemia without changing plasma insulin or other metabolic factors and thus identifies tissue dysfunction related to hyperglycemia. Rossetti et al. (54) reported correction of the β-cell dysfunction in 90% pancreatectomized diabetic rats after phloridzin treatment.

Many biochemical and molecular mechanisms for the induction of β-cell dysfunction by hyperglycemia have been proposed based on studies of islet tissue from diabetic animals or the use of superphysiologic glucose concentrations *in vitro*. The proposed mechanisms include excess glycogen storage (118), impaired glucose transport into the β-cell (119), impaired activity of key signaling pathways such as the glycerol phosphate shuttle (120,121) or pyruvate carboxylase (121,122), defective ATP-sensitive channel activity (123–125), reduced expression of voltage-dependent calcium channels (126,127), defective hydrolysis of membrane inositol phospholipids (128), cycling of glucose-6-phosphate back to glucose through increased glucose-6-phosphatase activity (129–131), altered Na^+-K^+-ATPase activity coupled with reduced myoinositol uptake (132), and loss of β-cell differentiation (133). That there are so many possible mechanisms clearly demonstrates how "toxic" a hyperglycemic environment is for β-cells. Stated another way, it is almost certain that the β-cell dysfunction in human type 2 diabetes will stem from multiple biochemical/molecular defects.

β-Cell Exhaustion

A related concept is *β-cell exhaustion* or *overwork*, which we (23,134) and others (59) view as β-cell dysfunction from a nonsustainable hyperstimulation of insulin secretion. In that case, hyperglycemia is the stimulus for the β-cell dysfunction but is not the operative mechanism. This subtlety is revealed when reversal strategies are undertaken that use inhibitors of insulin

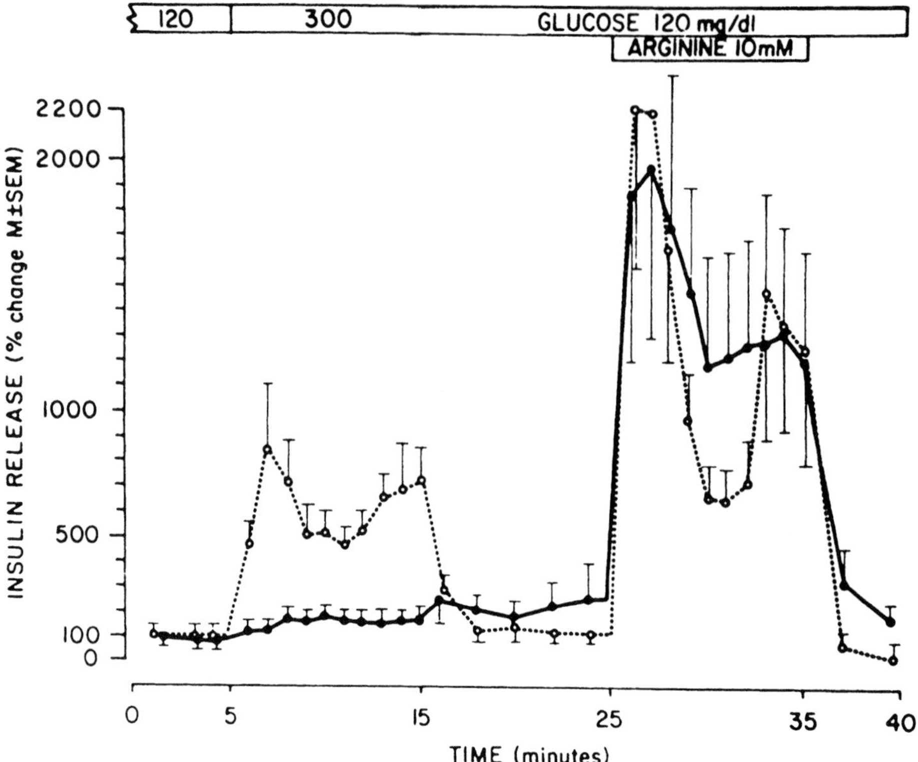

Figure 25.8. Insulin secretory responses to glucose and arginine in the perfused pancreatic remnant of 90% pancreatectomized diabetic rats (*solid line*) and normoglycemic control rats (*dotted line*). Studies were performed 8 to 11 weeks after pancreatectomy or sham surgery. Note the pattern of selective glucose unresponsiveness in the diabetic rats, as reflected in the brisk insulin response to arginine but the absence of response to a high level of glucose. (From Bonner-Weir S, Trent DF, Weir GC. Partial pancreatectomy in the rat and subsequent defect in glucose-induced insulin release. *J Clin Invest* 1983;71:1544–1553, with permission from the American Society for Clinical Investigation.)

secretion. The most studied inhibitor is diazoxide, although somatostatin has also been used. Glycemia is unchanged in these studies, or sometimes worsens, so that detrimental tissue effects of hyperglycemia versus hyperstimulated insulin secretion can be identified separately.

Support for the concept of β-cell exhaustion began with Sako and Grill (135), who reported that diazoxide prevented β-cell dysfunction in normal rats that were made hyperglycemic by a 48-hour glucose infusion *in vivo*. These investigators also showed a protective effect of diazoxide during long-term *in vitro* incubation of islets with high glucose and made the additional observation that the diazoxide effect resulted from preventing the insulin content of β-cells from declining below a critical level (136). Glucose-infused rats are markedly hyperinsulinemic, and the hyperglycemia is by necessity short term, so the applicability of the Sako and Grill study to the more usual situation of normal to subnormal plasma insulin levels with long-term diabetes was unclear. We treated rats that were diabetic from a 90% pancreatectomy with diazoxide for 5 days: Glucose-potentiated insulin secretion in response to arginine (a commonly used nonglucose secretagogue) normalized (Fig. 25.9). In contrast, the direct effect of glucose on insulin secretion improved minimally. The recovery of glucose potentiation occurred in tandem with normalization of the insulin content for the β-cell mass (137). A second mode for lowering insulin secretion, a 40-hour fast, produced similar results—a marked improvement in glucose potentiation but no change in glucose-induced insulin secretion—this time using GLP-1^{7-37} as the nonglucose secretagogue (138). GLP-1^{7-37} is a member of the incretin family of gut-released peptides that potentiate meal-induced insulin secretion (139,140). Both of these studies noted a linear correlation between the insulin content of the pancreas and glucose-potentiated secretion of insulin before and after treatments, findings that agree with those of Grill's laboratory concerning the crucial role of insulin content in the exhaustion concept (136). To further test the exhaustion hypothesis, we investigated the prediction that upregulation of insulin secretion in nondiabetic rats sufficient to lower the insulin content should impair glucose-potentiated secretion of insulin. Normal rats received a 48-hour infusion of high-dose tolbutamide (insulin secretagogue) plus enough glucose to maintain normoglycemia: The insulin content of the pancreas declined 50%, and as predicted, glucose-potentiated insulin secretion in response to arginine declined exactly in parallel (141).

These findings support a causative role for excessive insulin release in the defective glucose-potentiated secretion of insulin with chronic hyperglycemia. The concept is that a substrate, cofactor, cellular fuel, or other required substance is depleted, resulting in a lowered insulin response to meals. Our studies have focused on the potential role of the releasable pool of insulin stores as that factor. As already discussed, the same pathogenic mechanism has been linked to the increased proinsulin to insulin ratio and the abnormal pulsatile insulin secretion in type 2 diabetes (59). It is important to note that results supporting the exhaustion concept have been obtained in studies of human type 2 diabetes. Diazoxide therapy (142), a 4-day fast (143), and overnight infusion of somatostatin (59) all improved insulin secretion as opposed to their normal

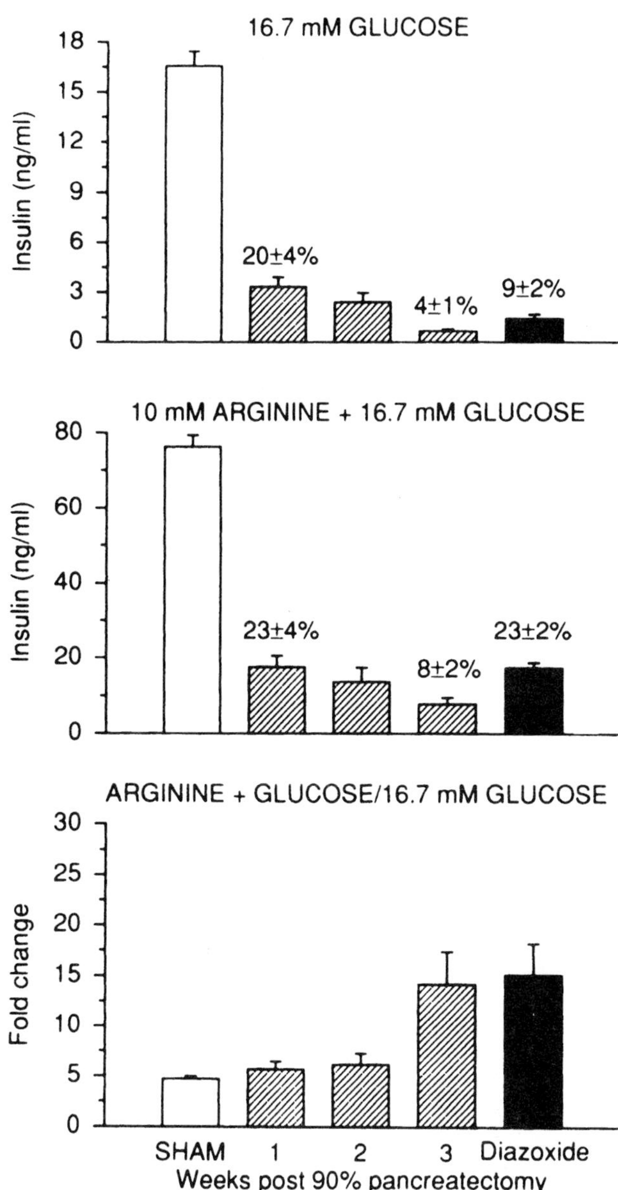

Figure 25.9. Increased insulin secretion with diazoxide therapy in rats made diabetic by 90% pancreatectomy. Insulin secretion in response to 16.7 mM glucose and 16.7 mM glucose/10 mM arginine was assessed with the *in vitro* perfused pancreas at weekly intervals after a 90% pancreatectomy. The percentage values above the bars are fractional output calculated from the results for the sham-operated control rats (*open bars*). Note the decrease in both insulin responses at 3 weeks after surgery, showing the onset of defective glucose responsiveness and glucose potentiation. A 5-day treatment period with diazoxide partially blocked the decrease in glucose-induced insulin secretion and normalized that to glucose/arginine (*solid bars*). (Data from Leahy JL, Bumbalo LM, Chen C. Diazoxide causes recovery of β-cell glucose responsiveness in 90% pancreatectomized diabetic rats. *Diabetes* 1994;43:173–179; and Leahy JL, Bumbalo LM, Chen C. Beta-cell hypersensitivity for glucose precedes loss of glucose-induced insulin secretion in 90% pancreatectomized rats. *Diabetologia* 1993;36:1238–1244.)

inhibitory effect, replicating the results in studies of diabetic rats (137,138).

Impaired Proinsulin Biosynthesis

It has been suggested that transcriptional control of proinsulin biosynthesis is impaired by chronic hyperglycemia and that this is a cause of the lowered insulin secretion in type 2 diabetes (144,145). This idea stems from extensive *in vitro* studies of β-cell lines and isolated islets that established that several factors related to a high glucose environment cause defective activation of proinsulin transcription; these factors include lowered expression/binding of the activators PDX-1 (pancreatic duodenum homeobox factor-1; also termed somatostatin transcription factor-1 and islet duodenum homeobox-1) (146) and rat insulin promoter element 3b1-activator (147) and increased expression of the inhibitor C/EBPβ (148). Additional support has come from studies in diabetic rats. Zangen et al. (149) reported impaired proinsulin transcription that paralleled lowered expression of PDX-1 in 90% pancreatectomized diabetic rats. Seufert et al. (150) reported similar results in ZDF rats in association with upregulation of C/EBPβ expression (150). Harmon et al. (151) prevented hyperglycemia in ZDF rats with troglitazone, thereby eliminating the lowered gene expression of proinsulin, in association with recovery of PDX-1 expression/binding. A recent cross-sectional study of diabetic rats with various levels of hyperglycemia suggested that inhibition of gene expression of proinsulin requires severe hyperglycemia (133). We speculate that this effect plays a role in the β-cell dysfunction of markedly hyperglycemic type 2 diabetes but not in the β-cell failure of new-onset diabetes, in which hyperglycemia is typically mild for most patients.

Lipotoxicity

Other metabolic disruptions beside hyperglycemia make up the diabetic environment, including hypertriglyceridemia and elevated circulating and tissue levels of free fatty acids. A hypothesis about the pathogenesis of β-cell dysfunction secondary to these factors, called *lipotoxicity*, has evolved based on several experimental findings (152–155). Islets cultured with elevated levels of fatty acids develop β-cell dysfunction reminiscent of that in type 2 diabetes, namely lowered glucose-induced insulin release, impaired proinsulin synthesis, and accelerated β-cell apoptosis (156,157). Plausible biochemical and molecular mechanisms for the β-cell dysfunction were identified soon afterward. Fatty acids were shown to lower expression of IDX-1 (also called PDX-1), which is a key transcription factor for β-cell development, glucose metabolism, and proinsulin synthesis (158). Also, the well-known effect of fatty acids to impair glucose oxidation through lowered activation of pyruvate dehydrogenase, the so-called *Randle cycle* (159,160), was shown to be operative in fatty acid-cultured islets and was implicated in the lowered glucose-induced secretion of insulin (161). The most influential studies have been the extensive studies of ZDF rats by the Unger laboratory (155,162,163). These rats are obese and hyperlipidemic, and the males have large stores of triglyceride in islets in tandem with the spontaneous development of diabetes. These investigators have identified a well-characterized biochemical sequence of altered islet triglyceride metabolism that was shown to correlate with β-cell dysfunction and apoptosis. Unclear, however, is whether the findings from these studies of ZDF rats can be applied to other hyperlipidemic states, since the genetic abnormality in ZDF rats is a mutated leptin receptor that blocks leptin action and a leptin deficiency plays a central role in their identified pathogenic sequence (164,165).

Despite these findings, there remains uncertainty about the lipotoxicity concept. Of concern are the observations from several studies that used long-term lipid infusions in nondiabetic humans; most found minimal to no detrimental effect on insulin secretion (166–169). This is not surprising, as nondiabetic insulin-resistant states entail supernormal β-cell function/insulin secretion (33) despite the common occurrence of hypertriglyceridemia (170). Also, reexamination of the biochemical defects that were purported to cause the fatty acid–induced β-cell dysfunction has led to questioning of some of the original findings. We (171) and others (172) observed no Randle cycle–induced impairment of glucose oxidation in fatty acid–cultured islets or β-cells. Also, the reported inhibitory effect of fatty acids on proinsulin biosynthesis (156) was not confirmed by an in-depth analysis (173). Finally, hyperlipidemia or raised islet triglyceride stores are clearly not mandatory for β-cell dysfunction in diabetic rats (174). None of these negative data eliminate the possibility of lipid-induced β-cell dysfunction. However, the concept needs to be investigated further to determine the role of lipid-induced dysfunction (if any) in type 2 diabetes.

SUMMARY

Debate about the importance of β-cell dysfunction in the pathogenesis of type 2 diabetes is over. Prospective studies of the progression to type 2 diabetes have highlighted the crucial role played by β-cell dysfunction. A notable example is the study from Weyer et al. that monitored insulin action, insulin secretion, and endogenous glucose output in 17 Pima Indians as they progressed from normal glucose tolerance to diabetes, compared with 31 Pima Indians who retained normal glucose tolerance over the same time (10). In those in whom diabetes developed, defects in both insulin secretion and insulin action were present when they were normoglycemic, but it was the lowering of the insulin response to intravenous glucose that best correlated with the progression from normoglycemia to diabetes. In addition, there is now a clear understanding that β-cell dysfunction continues to exert a major influence once diabetes develops, with a particular focus on the progression from oral monotherapy, to therapy with a combination of oral agents, to insulin therapy likely reflecting deteriorating β-cell function (24,25).

The past decade has seen considerable progress in our understanding of potential pathogenic mechanisms, and we are optimistic that we are on the threshold of identifying prevention and/or therapeutic strategies that will preserve β-cell function in this disease. However, major challenges remain, the foremost being the determination of the molecular, biochemical, and genetic bases for the β-cell dysfunction. Animal models have been the major investigative tools until now, but their relevance to human disease is still uncertain. Ways must be found to identify the defects that occur in humans and to design experimental systems that reproduce the human pathogenic condition. We must clarify the role of β-cell dysfunction versus loss of β-cell mass in the disease. The identification of ways of imaging β-cells noninvasively for both function and mass is a key requirement. Biochemical and molecular investigation into normal β-cell function and development must continue. Some of the most important recent advances are based on defining how β-cells work normally, for example, how β-cells grow and develop (175,176) and the role of islet neogenesis (177) are important topics of active investigation. Also, a functional role for "the insulin signaling cascade" within β-cells was identified just a few years ago (178–180). It is plausible that future breakthroughs will take advantage of signaling pathways or other aspects of β-cell physiology that are not yet known to exist.

It is almost certain that in the next decade our treatment of type 2 diabetes will change to take advantage of the incredible, and ongoing, scientific advances. Much attention will be focused on prevention. A reasonable prediction is that β-cell–directed therapies will play a crucial role in both endeavors.

REFERENCES

1. King H, Rewers M, WHO Ad Hoc Diabetes Reporting Group. Global estimates for prevalence of diabetes mellitus and impaired glucose tolerance in adults. *Diabetes Care* 1993;16:157–177.
2. Hamman R. Genetic and environmental determinants of non-insulin-dependent diabetes mellitus (NIDDM). *Diabetes Metab Rev* 1992;8:287–338.
3. Lillioja S, Mott DM, Howard B, et al. Impaired glucose tolerance as a disorder of insulin action: longitudinal and cross-sectional studies in Pima Indians. *N Engl J Med* 1988;318:1217–1225.
4. Lillioja S, Mott DM, Spraul M, et al. Insulin resistance and insulin secretory dysfunction as precursors of non-insulin-dependent diabetes mellitus. Prospective studies of Pima Indians. *N Engl J Med* 1993;329:1988–1992.
5. Eriksson J, Franssila-Kallunki A, Ekstrand A, et al. Early metabolic defects in persons at increased risk for non-insulin-dependent diabetes mellitus. *N Engl J Med* 1989;321:337–343.
6. Warram JH, Martin BC, Krolewski AS, et al. Slow glucose removal rate and hyperinsulinemia precede the development of type II diabetes in the offspring of diabetic parents. *Ann Intern Med* 1990;113:909–915.
7. Martin BC, Warram JH, Krolewski AS, et al. Role of glucose and insulin resistance in development of type 2 diabetes mellitus: results of a 25-year follow-up study. *Lancet* 1992;340:925–929.
8. Leahy JL. Natural history of beta-cell dysfunction in NIDDM. *Diabetes Care* 1990;13:992–1010.
9. Mitrakou A, Kelley D, Mokan M, et al. Role of reduced suppression of glucose production and diminished early insulin release in impaired glucose tolerance. *N Engl J Med* 1992;326:22–29.
10. Weyer C, Bogardus C, Mott DM, et al. The natural history of insulin secretory dysfunction and insulin resistance in the pathogenesis of type 2 diabetes mellitus. *J Clin Invest* 1999;104:787–794.
11. DeFronzo RA, Ferrannini E, Simonson DC. Fasting hyperglycemia in non-insulin-dependent diabetes mellitus: contributions of excessive hepatic glucose production and impaired tissue glucose uptake. *Metabolism* 1989;38: 387–395.
12. Saad MF, Knowler WC, Pettitt DJ, et al. Sequential changes in serum insulin concentration during development of noninsulin-dependent diabetes. *Lancet* 1989;1:1356–1359.
13. Saad MF, Knowler WC, Pettitt DJ, et al. A two-step model for development of non-insulin-dependent diabetes. *Am J Med* 1991;90:229–235.
14. Beck-Nielsen H, Groop LC. Metabolic and genetic characterization of prediabetic states. Sequence of events leading to non-insulin-dependent diabetes mellitus. *J Clin Invest* 1994;94:1714–1721.
15. Swinburn BA, Gianchandani R, Saad MF, et al. In vivo beta-cell function at the transition to early non-insulin-dependent diabetes mellitus. *Metabolism* 1995;44:757–764.
16. Efendic S, Grill V, Luft R, et al. Low insulin response: a marker of prediabetes. *Adv Exp Med Biol* 1988;246:167–174.
17. Kadowaki T, Miyake Y, Hagura R, et al. Risk factors for worsening to diabetes in subjects with impaired glucose tolerance. *Diabetologia* 1984;26:44–49.
18. Kosaka K, Kuzuya T, Akanuma Y, et al. Increase in insulin response after treatment of overt maturity-onset diabetes is independent of the mode of treatment. *Diabetologia* 1980;18:23–28.
19. Vague P, Moulin J-P. The defective glucose sensitivity of the β-cell in noninsulin dependent diabetes: improvement after twenty hours of normoglycemia. *Metabolism* 1982;31:139–142.
20. Garvey WT, Olefsky JM, Griffin J, et al. The effect of insulin treatment on insulin secretion and insulin action in type II diabetes mellitus. *Diabetes* 1985; 34:222–234.
21. Rossetti L, Giaccari A, DeFronzo RA. Glucose toxicity. *Diabetes Care* 1990;13: 610–630.
22. Yki-Järvinen H. Toxicity of hyperglycaemia in type 2 diabetes. *Diabetes Metab Rev* 1998;14 [Suppl 1]:S45–S50.
23. Leahy JL. β-cell dysfunction with chronic hyperglycemia: the "overworked β-cell" hypothesis. *Diabetes Rev* 1996;4:298–319.
24. U.K. Prospective Diabetes Study Group. U.K. prospective diabetes study 16. Overview of 6 years' therapy of type II diabetes: a progressive disease. *Diabetes* 1995;44:1249–1258.
25. Turner RC, Cull CA, Frighi V, et al. Glycemic control with diet, sulfonylurea, metformin, or insulin in patients with type 2 diabetes mellitus: progressive requirement for multiple therapies (UKPDS 49). *JAMA* 1999;281:2005–2012.
26. Weir GC. Which comes first in non-insulin-dependent diabetes mellitus: insulin resistance or beta-cell failure? Both come first. *JAMA* 1995;273: 1878–1879.
27. Polonsky KS, Sturis J, Bell GI. Seminars in Medicine of the Beth Israel Hospital, Boston. Non-insulin-dependent diabetes mellitus—a genetically programmed failure of the beta cell to compensate for insulin resistance. *N Engl J Med* 1996;334:777–783.
28. Ferrannini E. Insulin resistance versus insulin deficiency in non-insulin-dependent diabetes mellitus: problems and prospects. *Endocr Rev* 1998;19: 477–490.
29. Gerich J, Van Haeften T. Insulin resistance versus impaired insulin secretion as the genetic basis for type 2 diabetes. *Curr Opin Endocrinol Diabetes* 1998;5: 144–148.
30. Kjos SL, Buchanan TA. Gestational diabetes mellitus. *N Engl J Med* 1999;341: 1749–1756.

31. Kahn SE. The importance of the beta-cell in the pathogenesis of type 2 diabetes mellitus. *Am J Med* 2000;108[Suppl 6a]:2S–8S.
32. Weir GC, Bonner-Weir S. Insulin secretion in type 2 diabetes mellitus. In: LeRoith D, Taylor SI, Olefsky JM, eds. *Diabetes mellitus: a fundamental and clinical text*, 2nd ed. Philadelphia: Lippincott Williams & Wilkins, 2000: 595–603.
33. Kahn SE, Prigeon RL, McCulloch DK, et al. Quantification of the relationship between insulin sensitivity and β-cell function in human subjects: evidence for a hyperbolic function. *Diabetes* 1993;42:1663–1672.
34. Amiel SA, Sherwin RS, Simonson DC, et al. Impaired insulin action in puberty. A contributing factor to poor glycemic control in adolescents with diabetes. *N Engl J Med* 1986;315:215–219.
35. Boden G. Fuel metabolism in pregnancy and in gestational diabetes mellitus. *Obstet Gynecol Clin North Am* 1996;23:1–10.
36. Boden G, Chen X, DeSantis RA, et al. Effects of age and body fat on insulin resistance in healthy men. *Diabetes Care* 1993;16:728–733.
37. Roder ME, Schwartz RS, Prigeon RL, et al. Reduced pancreatic β cell compensation to the insulin resistance of aging: impact on proinsulin and insulin levels. *J Clin Endocrinol Metab* 2000;85:2275–2280.
38. Elbein SC, Wegner K, Kahn SE. Reduced beta-cell compensation to the insulin resistance associated with obesity in members of caucasian familial type 2 diabetic kindreds. *Diabetes Care* 2000;23:221–227.
39. Byrne MM, Sturis J, Polonsky KS. Insulin secretion and clearance during low-dose graded glucose infusion. *Am J Physiol* 1995;268:E21–E27.
40. Calles-Escandon J, Robbins DC. Loss of early phase of insulin release in humans impairs glucose tolerance and blunts thermic effect of glucose. *Diabetes* 1987;36:1167–1172.
41. Luzi L, DeFronzo RA. Effect of loss of first-phase insulin secretion on hepatic glucose production and tissue glucose disposal in humans. *Am J Physiol* 1989; 257:E241–E246.
42. Porksen N, Nyholm B, Veldhuis JD, et al. In humans at least 75% of insulin secretion arises from punctuated insulin secretory bursts. *Am J Physiol* 1997; 273:E908–E914.
43. Butler P. Pulsatile insulin secretion. *Novartis Found Symp* 2000;227:190–205.
44. Polonsky KS, Sturis J, Van Cauter E. Temporal profiles and clinical significance of pulsatile insulin secretion. *Horm Res* 1998;49:178–184.
45. Sturis J, Scheen AJ, Leproult R, et al. 24-hour glucose profiles during continuous or oscillatory insulin infusion. Demonstration of the functional significance of ultradian insulin oscillations. *J Clin Invest* 1995;95:1464–1471.
46. Sturis J, Van Cauter E, Blackman JD, et al. Entrainment of pulsatile insulin secretion by oscillatory glucose infusion. *J Clin Invest* 1991;87:439–445.
47. Porksen N, Juhl C, Hollingdal M, et al. Concordant induction of rapid in vivo pulsatile insulin secretion by recurrent punctuated glucose infusions. *Am J Physiol* 2000;278:E162–E170.
48. Shapiro ET, Tillil H, Miller MA, et al. Insulin secretion and clearance. Comparison after oral and intravenous glucose. *Diabetes* 1987;36:1365–1371.
49. Van Cauter E, Mestrez F, Sturis J, et al. Estimation of insulin secretion rates from C-peptide levels. Comparison of individual and standard kinetic parameters for C-peptide clearance. *Diabetes* 1992;41:368–377.
50. Perley MJ, Kipnis DM. Plasma insulin responses to oral and intravenous glucose: studies in normal and diabetic subjects. *J Clin Invest* 1967;46:1954–1962.
51. Cerasi E, Luft R. The plasma insulin response to glucose infusion in healthy subjects and in diabetes mellitus. *Acta Endocrinol (Copenh)* 1967;55:278–304.
52. Brunzell JD, Robertson RP, Lerner RL, et al. Relationships between fasting plasma glucose levels and insulin secretion during intravenous glucose tolerance tests. *J Clin Endocrinol Metab* 1976;42:222–229.
53. Bruce DG, Chisholm DJ, Storlien LH, et al. Physiological importance of deficiency in early prandial insulin secretion in non-insulin-dependent diabetes. *Diabetes* 1988;37:736–744.
54. Rossetti L, Shulman GI, Zawalich W, et al. Effect of chronic hyperglycemia on in vivo insulin secretion in partially pancreatectomized rats. *J Clin Invest* 1987;80:1037–1044.
55. Ward WK, Bolgiano DC, McKnight B, et al. Diminished β cell secretory capacity in patients with noninsulin-dependent diabetes mellitus. *J Clin Invest* 1984;74:1318–1328.
56. Lang DA, Matthews DR, Burnett M, et al. Brief, irregular oscillations of basal plasma insulin and glucose concentrations in diabetic man. *Diabetes* 1981;30: 435–439.
57. O'Rahilly S, Turner RC, Matthews DR. Impaired pulsatile secretion of insulin in relatives of patients with non-insulin-dependent diabetes. *N Engl J Med* 1988;318:1225–1230.
58. Schmitz O, Porksen N, Nyholm B, et al. Disorderly and nonstationary insulin secretion in relatives of patients with NIDDM. *Am J Physiol* 1997;272: E218–E226.
59. Laedtke T, Kjems L, Porksen N, et al. Overnight inhibition of insulin secretion restores pulsatility and proinsulin/insulin ratio in type 2 diabetes. *Am J Physiol* 2000;279:E520–528.
60. Porksen N, Munn S, Steers J, et al. Effects of glucose ingestion versus infusion on pulsatile insulin secretion. The incretin effect is achieved by amplification of insulin secretory burst mass. *Diabetes* 1996;45:1317–1323.
61. Juhl CB, Schmitz O, Pincus S, et al. Short-term treatment with GLP-1 increases pulsatile insulin secretion in type II diabetes with no effect on orderliness. *Diabetologia* 2000;43:583–588.
62. Polonsky KS, Given BD, Hirsch LJ, et al. Abnormal patterns of insulin secretion in non-insulin-dependent diabetes mellitus. *N Engl J Med* 1988;318: 1231–1239.
63. Sturis J, Polonsky KS, Shapiro ET, et al. Abnormalities in the ultradian oscillations of insulin secretion and glucose levels in type 2 (non-insulin-dependent) diabetic patients. *Diabetologia* 1992;35:681–689.
64. Matthews DR, Naylor BA, Jones RG, et al. Pulsatile insulin has greater hypoglycemic effect than continuous delivery. *Diabetes* 1983;32:617–621.
65. Mako ME, Starr JI, Rubenstein AH. Circulating proinsulin in patients with maturity onset diabetes. *Am J Med* 1977;63:865–869.
66. Temple RC, Carrington CA, Luzio SD, et al. Insulin deficiency in non-insulin-dependent diabetes. *Lancet* 1989;1:293–295.
67. Hartling SG, Garne S, Binder C, et al. Proinsulin, insulin, and C-peptide in cystic fibrosis after an oral glucose tolerance test. *Diabetes Res* 1988;7: 165–169.
68. Saad MF, Kahn SE, Nelson RG, et al. Disproportionately elevated proinsulin in Pima Indians with noninsulin-dependent diabetes mellitus. *J Clin Endocrinol Metab* 1990;70:1247–1253.
69. Yoshioka N, Kuzuya T, Matsuda A, et al. Serum proinsulin levels at fasting and after oral glucose load in patients with type 2 (non-insulin-dependent) diabetes mellitus. *Diabetologia* 1988;31:355–360.
70. Kahn SE, Leonetti DL, Prigeon RL, et al. Relationship of proinsulin and insulin with noninsulin-dependent diabetes mellitus and coronary heart disease in Japanese-American men: impact of obesity. *J Clin Endocrinol Metab* 1995;80:1399–1406.
71. Kahn SE, Leonetti DL, Prigeon RL, et al. Proinsulin as a marker for the development of NIDDM in Japanese-American men. *Diabetes* 1995;44:173–179.
72. Haffner SM, Stern MP, Miettinen H, et al. Higher proinsulin and specific insulin are both associated with a parental history of diabetes in nondiabetic Mexican-American subjects. *Diabetes* 1995;44:1156–1160.
73. Yoshioka N, Kuzuya T, Matsuda A, Iwamoto Y. Effects of dietary treatment on serum insulin and proinsulin response in newly diagnosed NIDDM. *Diabetes* 1989;38:262–266.
74. Prigeon RL, Jacobson RK, Porte D Jr, et al. Effect of sulfonylurea withdrawal on proinsulin levels, β cell function, and glucose disposal in subjects with noninsulin-dependent diabetes mellitus. *J Clin Endocrinol Metab* 1996;81: 3295–3298.
75. Kahn SE, Halban PA. Release of incompletely processed proinsulin is the cause of the disproportionate proinsulinemia of NIDDM. *Diabetes* 1997;46: 1725–1732.
76. Gadot M, Ariav Y, Cerasi E, et al. Hyperproinsulinemia in the diabetic *Psammomys obesus* is a result of increased secretory demand on the beta-cell. *Endocrinology* 1995;136:4218–4223.
77. Leahy JL, Halban PA, Weir GC. Relative hypersecretion of proinsulin in rat model of NIDDM. *Diabetes* 1991;40:985–989.
78. Leahy JL. Increased proinsulin/insulin ratio in pancreas extracts of hyperglycemic rats. *Diabetes* 1993;42:22–27.
79. Alarcon C, Leahy JL, Schuppin GT, et al. Increased secretory demand rather than a defect in the proinsulin conversion mechanism causes hyperproinsulinemia in a glucose-infusion rat model of non-insulin-dependent diabetes mellitus. *J Clin Invest* 1995;95:1032–1039.
80. Koivisto VA, Yki-Jarvinen H, Hartling SV, et al. The effect of exogenous hyperinsulinemia on proinsulin secretion in normal man, obese subjects, and patients with insulinoma. *J Clin Endocrinol Metab* 1986;63:1117–1120.
81. Maclean N, Ogilvie RF. Quantitative estimation of the pancreatic islet tissue in diabetic subjects. *Diabetes* 1955;4:367–376.
82. Saito K, Yaginuma N, Takahashi T. Differential volumetry of A, B, and D cells in the pancreatic islets of diabetic and nondiabetic subjects. *Tohoku J Exp Med* 1979;129:273–283.
83. Klöppel G, Löhr M, Habich K, et al. Islet pathology and the pathogenesis of type 1 and type 2 diabetes mellitus revisited. *Surv Synth Pathol Res* 1985;4: 110–125.
84. Gepts W, Lecompte PM. The pancreatic islets in diabetes. *Am J Med* 1981;70: 105–115.
85. Bell ET. The incidence and significance of degranulation of the beta cells in the islets of Langerhans in diabetes mellitus. *Diabetes* 1953;2:125–129.
86. Shimabukuro M, Zhou YT, Levi M, et al. Fatty acid-induced beta cell apoptosis: a link between obesity and diabetes. *Proc Natl Acad Sci U S A* 1998;95: 2498–2502.
87. Pick A, Clark J, Kubstrup C, et al. Role of apoptosis in failure of beta-cell mass compensation for insulin resistance and beta-cell defects in the male Zucker diabetic fatty rat. *Diabetes* 1998;47:358–364.
88. Koyama M, Wada R, Sakuraba H, et al. Accelerated loss of islet beta cells in sucrose-fed Goto-Kakizaki rats, a genetic model of non-insulin-dependent diabetes mellitus. *Am J Pathol* 1998;153:537–545.
89. Donath MY, Gross DJ, Cerasi E, et al. Hyperglycemia-induced beta-cell apoptosis in pancreatic islets of *Psammomys obesus* during development of diabetes. *Diabetes* 1999;48:738–744.
90. Clark A, Charge SB, Badman MK, et al. Islet amyloid polypeptide: actions and role in the pathogenesis of diabetes. *Biochem Soc Trans* 1996;24:594–599.
91. Westermark P. Islet pathology of non-insulin-dependent diabetes mellitus (NIDDM). *Diabet Med* 1996;13[Suppl 6]:S46–S48.
92. Kahn SE, Andrikopoulos S, Verchere CB. Islet amyloid: a long-recognized but underappreciated pathological feature of type 2 diabetes. *Diabetes* 1999;48: 241–253.
93. Butler PC: Islet amyloid and its potential role in the pathogenesis of type 2 diabetes mellitus. In: LeRoith D, Taylor SI, Olefsky JM, eds. *Diabetes mellitus: a fundamental and clinical text,* 2nd ed. Philadelphia: Lippincott Williams & Wilkins, 2000:141–146.

94. Opie EL. The relation of diabetes mellitus to lesions of the pancreas: hyaline degeneration of the islands of Langerhans. *J Exp Med* 1900-1901;5:527–540.
95. Howard CF Jr. Longitudinal studies on the development of diabetes in individual *Macaca nigra*. *Diabetologia* 1986;29:301–306.
96. Johnson KH, O'Brien TD, Jordan K, et al. Impaired glucose tolerance is associated with increased islet amyloid polypeptide (IAPP) immunoreactivity in pancreatic beta cells. *Am J Pathol* 1989;135:245–250.
97. Westermark P, Wernstedt C, Wilander E, et al. Amyloid fibrils in human insulinoma and islets of Langerhans of the diabetic cat are derived from a neuropeptide-like protein also present in normal islet cells. *Proc Natl Acad Sci U S A* 1987;84:3881–3885.
98. Cooper GJS, Willis AC, Clark A, et al. Purification and characterization of a peptide from amyloid-rich pancreases of type 2 diabetic patients. *Proc Natl Acad Sci U S A* 1987;84:8628–8632.
99. Janson J, Soeller WC, Roche PC, et al. Spontaneous diabetes mellitus in transgenic mice expressing human islet amyloid polypeptide. *Proc Natl Acad Sci U S A* 1996;93:7283–7288.
100. Verchere CB, D'Alessio DA, Palmiter RD, et al. Islet amyloid formation associated with hyperglycemia in transgenic mice with pancreatic beta cell expression of human islet amyloid polypeptide. *Proc Natl Acad Sci U S A* 1996;93:3492–3496.
101. Kong MF, Stubbs TA, King P, et al. The effect of single doses of pramlintide on gastric emptying of two meals in men with IDDM. *Diabetologia* 1998;41:577–583.
102. Lorenzo A, Razzaboni B, Weir GC, et al. Pancreatic islet cell toxicity of amylin associated with type-2 diabetes mellitus. *Nature* 1994;368:756–760.
103. Janson J, Ashley RH, Harrison D, et al. The mechanism of islet amyloid polypeptide toxicity is membrane disruption by intermediate-sized toxic amyloid particles. *Diabetes* 1999;48:491–498.
104. Couce M, Kane LA, O'Brien TD, et al. Treatment with growth hormone and dexamethasone in mice transgenic for human islet amyloid polypeptide causes islet amyloidosis and beta-cell dysfunction. *Diabetes* 1996;45: 1094–1101.
105. Bonner-Weir S, Trent DF, Honey RN, et al. Responses of neonatal rat islets to streptozotocin: limited β-cell regeneration and hyperglycemia. *Diabetes* 1981;30:64–69.
106. Weir GC, Clore ET, Zmachinski CJ, et al. Islet secretion in a new experimental model for non-insulin-dependent diabetes. *Diabetes* 1981;30:590–595.
107. Giroix MH, Portha B, Kergoat M, et al. Glucose insensitivity and amino acid hypersensitivity of insulin release in rats with non-insulin-dependent diabetes: a study with the perfused pancreas. *Diabetes* 1983;32:445–451.
108. Bonner-Weir S, Trent DF, Weir GC. Partial pancreatectomy in the rat and subsequent defect in glucose-induced insulin release. *J Clin Invest* 1983;71:1544–1553.
109. Leahy JL, Bonner-Weir S, Weir GC. Minimal chronic hyperglycemia is a critical determinant of impaired insulin secretion after an incomplete pancreatectomy. *J Clin Invest* 1988;81:1407–1414.
110. Leahy JL, Cooper HE, Deal DA, et al. Chronic hyperglycemia is associated with impaired glucose influence on insulin secretion: a study in normal rats using chronic in vivo glucose infusions. *J Clin Invest* 1986;77:908–915.
111. Leahy JL, Cooper HE, Weir GC. Impaired insulin secretion associated with near normoglycemia: study in normal rats with 96-h in vivo glucose infusions. *Diabetes* 1987;36:459–464.
112. Portha B, Serradas P, Bailbé D, et al. β-Cell insensitivity to glucose in the GK rat a spontaneous nonobese model for type II diabetes. *Diabetes* 1991;40: 486–491.
113. Tokuyama Y, Sturis J, DePaoli AM, et al. Evolution of beta-cell dysfunction in the male Zucker diabetic fatty rat. *Diabetes* 1995;44:1447–1457.
114. Kanazawa M, Tanaka A, Nomoto S, et al. Alterations of insulin and glucagon secretion from the perfused pancreas before, at the onset and after the development of diabetes in male Otsuka Long-Evans Tokushima fatty (OLETF) rats. *Diabetes Res Clin Pract* 1997;38:161–167.
115. Grill V, Westberg M, Ostenson CG. β Cell insensitivity in a rat model of non-insulin-dependent diabetes. Evidence for a rapidly reversible effect of previous hyperglycemia. *J Clin Invest* 1987;80:664–669.
116. Leahy JL, Weir GC. Beta-cell dysfunction in hyperglycaemic rat models: recovery of glucose-induced insulin secretion with lowering of the ambient glucose level. *Diabetologia* 1991;34:640–647.
117. Kergoat M, Bailbe D, Portha B. Insulin treatment improves glucose-induced insulin release in rats with NIDDM induced by streptozocin. *Diabetes* 1987; 36:971–977.
118. Marynissen G, Leclercg-Meyer V, et al. Perturbation of pancreatic islet function in glucose-infused rats. *Metabolism* 1990;39:87–95.
119. Thorens B, Weir GC, Leahy JL, et al. Reduced expression of the liver/beta-cell glucose transporter isoform in glucose-insensitive pancreatic beta cells of diabetic rats. *Proc Natl Acad Sci U S A* 1990;87:6492–6496.
120. Giroix M-H, Rasschaert J, Bailbe D, et al. Impairment of glycerol phosphate shuttle in islets from rats with diabetes induced by neonatal streptozocin. *Diabetes* 1991;40:227–232.
121. MacDonald MJ, Tang J, Polonsky KS. Low mitochondrial glycerol phosphate dehydrogenase and pyruvate carboxylase in pancreatic islets of Zucker diabetic fatty rats. *Diabetes* 1996;45:1626–1630.
122. MacDonald MJ, Efendic S, Ostenson CG. Normalization by insulin treatment of low mitochondrial glycerol phosphate dehydrogenase and pyruvate carboxylase in pancreatic islets of the GK rat. *Diabetes* 1996;45:886–890.
123. Purrello F, Vetri M, Vinci C, et al. Chronic exposure to high glucose and impairment of K+-channel function in perifused rat pancreatic islets. *Diabetes* 1990;39:397–402.
124. Tsuura Y, Ishida H, Okamota Y, et al. Impaired glucose sensitivity of ATP-sensitive K+ channels in pancreatic beta-cells in streptozotocin-induced NIDDM rats. *Diabetes* 1992;41:861–865.
125. Tsuura Y, Ishida H, Okamoto Y, et al. Glucose sensitivity of ATP-sensitive K^+ channels is impaired in beta-cells of the GK rat. A new genetic model of NIDDM. *Diabetes* 1993;42:1446–1453.
126. Iwashima Y, Pugh W, Depaoli AM, et al. Expression of calcium channel mRNAs in rat pancreatic islets and down-regulation following glucose infusion. *Diabetes* 1993;42:948–953.
127. Roe MW, Worley JF 3rd, Tokuyama Y, et al. NIDDM is associated with loss of pancreatic beta-cell L-type Ca^{2+} channel activity. *Am J Physiol* 1996;270: E133–E140.
128. Zawalich WS, Zawalich KC, Shulman GI, et al. Chronic in vivo hyperglycemia impairs phosphoinositide hydrolysis and insulin release in isolated perifused rat islets. *Endocrinology* 1990;126:253–260.
129. Kahn A, Chandramouli V, Ostenson C-G, et al. Evidence for the presence of glucose cycling in pancreatic islets of the ob/ob mouse. *J Biol Chem* 1989;264:9732–9733.
130. Kahn A, Chandramouli V, Ostenson C-G, et al. Glucose cycling in islets from healthy and diabetic rats. *Diabetes* 1990;39:456–459.
131. Khan A, Chandramouli V, Ostenson CG, et al. Glucose cycling is markedly enhanced in pancreatic islets of obese hyperglycemic mice. *Endocrinology* 1990;126:2413–2416.
132. Xia M, Laychock SG. Insulin secretion, myo-inositol transport, and Na(+)-K(+)-ATPase in glucose-desensitized rat islets. *Diabetes* 1993;42:1392–1400.
133. Jonas JC, Sharma A, Hasenkamp W, et al. Chronic hyperglycemia triggers loss of pancreatic beta cell differentiation in an animal model of diabetes. *J Biol Chem* 1999;274:14112–14121.
134. Leahy JL. Detrimental effects of chronic hyperglycemia in the pancreatic β-cell. In: LeRoith D, Taylor SI, Olefsky JM, eds. *Diabetes mellitus: a fundamental and clinical text*, 2nd ed. Philadelphia: Lippincott Williams & Wilkins, 2000:115–125.
135. Sako Y, Grill VE. Coupling of β-cell desensitization by hyperglycemia to excessive stimulation and circulating insulin in glucose-infused rats. *Diabetes* 1990;39:1580–1583.
136. Bjorklund A, Grill V. β-Cell insensitivity in vitro: reversal by diazoxide entails more than one event in stimulus-secretion coupling. *Endocrinology* 1993;132:1319–1328.
137. Leahy JL, Bumbalo LM, Chen C. Diazoxide causes recovery of β-cell glucose responsiveness in 90% pancreatectomized diabetic rats. *Diabetes* 1994;43: 173–179.
138. Hosokawa YA, Hosokawa H, Chen C, et al. Mechanism of impaired glucose-potentiated insulin secretion in diabetic 90% pancreatectomy rats: study using GLP-1 (7-37). *J Clin Invest* 1996;97:180–186.
139. Fehmann HC, Goke R, Goke B. Cell and molecular biology of the incretin hormones glucagon-like peptide-I and glucose-dependent insulin releasing polypeptide. *Endocr Rev* 1995;16:390–410.
140. Drucker DJ. Glucagon-like peptides. *Diabetes* 1998;47:159–169.
141. Hosokawa YA, Leahy JL. Parallel reduction of pancreas insulin content and insulin secretion in 48-h tolbutamide-infused normoglycemic rats. *Diabetes* 1997;46:808–813.
142. Greenwood RH, Mahler RF, Hales CN. Improvement in insulin secretion in diabetes after diazoxide. *Lancet* 1976;1:444–447.
143. Féry F, Balasse EO. Glucose metabolism during the starved-to-fed transition in obese patients with NIDDM. *Diabetes* 1994;43:1418–1425.
144. Robertson RP, Harmon J, Tanaka Y, et al. Glucose toxicity of the β-cell. In: LeRoith D, Taylor SI, Olefsky JM, eds. *Diabetes mellitus: a fundamental and clinical text*, 2nd ed. Philadelphia: Lippincott Williams & Wilkins, 2000:125–132.
145. Briaud I, Rouault C, Reach G, et al. Long-term exposure of isolated rat islets of Langerhans to supraphysiologic glucose concentrations decreases insulin mRNA levels. *Metabolism* 1999;48:319–323.
146. Olson LK, Sharma A, Peshavaria M, et al. Reduction of insulin gene transcription in HIT-T15 β-cells chronically exposed to high glucose concentration is associated with loss of STF-1 transcription factor expression. *Proc Natl Acad Sci U S A* 1995;92:9127–9131.
147. Sharma A, Olson LK, Robertson RP, et al. The reduction of insulin gene transcription in HIT-T15 β-cells chronically exposed to high glucose concentrations is associated with the loss of RIPE3b1 and STF-1 transcription factor expression. *Mol Endocrinol* 1995;9:1127–1134.
148. Lu M, Seufert J, Habener JF. Pancreatic β-cell-specific repression of insulin gene transcription by CCAAT/enhancer-binding protein β. Inhibitory interactions with basic helix-loop-helix transcription factor E47. *J Biol Chem* 1997; 272:28349–28359.
149. Zangen DH, Bonner-Weir S, Lee CH, et al. Reduced insulin, GLUT2, and IDX-1 in β-cells after partial pancreatectomy. *Diabetes* 1996;46:258–264.
150. Seufert J, Weir GC, Habener JF. Differential expression of the insulin gene transcriptional repressor CCAAT/enhancer-binding protein beta and transactivator islet duodenum homeobox-1 in rat pancreatic β-cells during the development of diabetes mellitus. *J Clin Invest* 1998;101:2528–2539.
151. Harmon JS, Oseid EA, Gleason CE, et al. Prevention of hyperglycemia and glucotoxic effects on insulin gene expression by troglitazone in ZDF rats. *Diabetes* 1999;48:1995–2000.
152. Unger RH. Lipotoxicity in the pathogenesis of obesity-dependent NIDDM. Genetic and clinical implications. *Diabetes* 1995;44:863–870.
153. Prentki M, Corkey BE. Are the beta-cell signaling molecules malonyl-CoA

and cystolic long-chain acyl-CoA implicated in multiple tissue defects of obesity and NIDDM? *Diabetes* 1996;45:273–283.
154. McGarry JD, Dobbins RL. Fatty acids, lipotoxicity and insulin secretion. *Diabetologia* 1999;42:128–138.
155. Unger RH, Yan-Ting Z, Orci L. Lipotoxicity. In: LeRoith D, Taylor SI, Olefsky JM, eds. *Diabetes mellitus: a fundamental and clinical text*, 2nd ed. Philadelphia: Lippincott Williams & Wilkins, 2000:132–141.
156. Zhou YP, Grill VE. Long-term exposure of rat pancreatic islets to fatty acids inhibits glucose-induced insulin secretion and biosynthesis through a glucose fatty acid cycle. *J Clin Invest* 1994;93:870–876.
157. Milburn JL Jr, Hirose H, Lee YH, et al. Pancreatic beta-cells in obesity. Evidence for induction of functional, morphologic, and metabolic abnormalities by increased long chain fatty acids. *J Biol Chem* 1995;270:1295–1299.
158. Gremlich S, Bonny C, Waeber G, et al. Fatty acids decrease IDX-1 expression in rat pancreatic islets and reduce GLUT2, glucokinase, insulin, and somatostatin levels. *J Biol Chem* 1997;272:30261–30269.
159. Randle PJ, Priestman DA, Mistry S, et al. Mechanisms modifying glucose oxidation in diabetes mellitus. *Diabetologia* 1994;37[Suppl 2]:S155–S161.
160. Randle PJ. Regulatory interactions between lipids and carbohydrates: the glucose fatty acid cycle after 35 years. *Diabetes Metab Rev* 1998;14:263–283.
161. Zhou YP, Grill VE. Palmitate-induced beta-cell insensitivity to glucose is coupled to decreased pyruvate dehydrogenase activity and enhanced kinase activity in rat pancreatic islets. *Diabetes* 1995;44:394–399.
162. Shimabukuro M, Zhou YT, Levi M, et al. Fatty acid-induced beta cell apoptosis: a link between obesity and diabetes. *Proc Natl Acad Sci U S A* 1998;95: 2498–2502.
163. Shimabukuro M, Higa M, Zhou YT, et al. Lipoapoptosis in beta-cells of obese prediabetic fa/fa rats. Role of serine palmitoyltransferase overexpression. *J Biol Chem* 1998;273:32487–32490.
164. Zhou YT, Shimabukuro M, Lee Y, et al. Enhanced de novo lipogenesis in the leptin-unresponsive pancreatic islets of prediabetic Zucker diabetic fatty rats: role in the pathogenesis of lipotoxic diabetes. *Diabetes* 1998;47: 1904–1908.
165. Unger RH, Zhou YT, Orci L. Regulation of fatty acid homeostasis in cells: novel role of leptin. *Proc Natl Acad Sci U S A* 1999;96:2327–2332.
166. Paolisso G, Gambardella A, Amato L, et al. Opposite effects of short- and long-term fatty acid infusion on insulin secretion in healthy subjects. *Diabetologia* 1995;38:1295–1299.
167. Boden G, Chen X, Rosner J, et al. Effects of a 48-h fat infusion on insulin secretion and glucose utilization. *Diabetes* 1995;44:1239–1242.
168. Carpentier A, Mittelman SD, Lamarche B, et al. Acute enhancement of insulin secretion by FFA in humans is lost with prolonged FFA elevation. *Am J Physiol* 1999;276:E1055–E1066.
169. Carpentier A, Mittelman SD, Bergman RN, et al. Prolonged elevation of plasma free fatty acids impairs pancreatic beta-cell function in obese nondiabetic humans but not in individuals with type 2 diabetes. *Diabetes* 2000; 49:399–408.
170. Golay A, Swislocki AL, Chen YD, et al. Effect of obesity on ambient plasma glucose, free fatty acid, insulin, growth hormone, and glucagon concentrations. *J Clin Endocrinol Metab* 1986;63:481–484.
171. Liu YQ, Tornheim K, Leahy JL. Glucose-fatty acid cycle to inhibit glucose utilization and oxidation is not operative in fatty acid-cultured islets. *Diabetes* 1999;48:1747–1753.
172. Segall L, Lameloise N, Assimacopoulos-Jeannet F, et al. Lipid rather than glucose metabolism is implicated in altered insulin secretion caused by oleate in INS-1 cells. *Am J Physiol* 1999;277:E521–E528.
173. Bollheimer LC, Skelly RH, Chester MW, et al. Chronic exposure to free fatty acid reduces pancreatic beta cell insulin content by increasing basal insulin secretion that is not compensated for by a corresponding increase in proinsulin biosynthesis translation. *J Clin Invest* 1998;101:1094–1101.
174. de Souza CJ, Capotorto JV, Cornell-Kennon S, et al. Beta-cell dysfunction in 48-hour glucose-infused rats is not a consequence of elevated plasma lipid or islet triglyceride levels. *Metabolism* 2000;49:755–759.
175. Nielsen JH, Svensson C, Galsgaard ED, et al. Beta cell proliferation and growth factors. *J Mol Med* 1999;77:62–66.
176. Bonner-Weir S. Perspective: postnatal pancreatic beta cell growth. *Endocrinology* 2000;141:1926–1929.
177. Wilkin TJ. Neogenesis of islet cells. *Diabetes Metab Rev* 1998;14:331–333.
178. Withers DJ, Gutierrez JS, Towery H, et al. Disruption of IRS-2 causes type 2 diabetes in mice. *Nature* 1998;391:900–904.
179. Withers DJ, Burks DJ, Towery HH, et al. Irs-2 coordinates Igf-1 receptor-mediated beta-cell development and peripheral insulin signalling. *Nat Genet* 1999;23:32–40.
180. Aspinwall CA, Qian WJ, Roper MG, et al. Roles of insulin receptor substrate-1, phosphatidylinositol 3-kinase, and release of intracellular Ca^{2+} stores in insulin-stimulated insulin secretion in beta-cells. *J Biol Chem* 2000;275: 22331–22338.

CHAPTER 26

Maturity-Onset Diabetes of the Young

Andrew T. Hattersley

The early clinical descriptions recognized that maturity-onset diabetes of the young (MODY) was a monogenic form of diabetes with a single gene mutation causing diabetes within a family. Our understanding of MODY has been transformed by defining the genes involved in this condition. MODY initially was defined solely by clinical criteria, but now a genetic subclassification is possible based on the description of six genes in which mutations have been described. With the description of the etiologic genes, there have been new clinical insights, and with each gene resulting in the description of discrete clinical and physiologic entities for mutation. The definition of the underlying molecular genetics frequently helps determine the likely clinical course, prognosis, and best treatment options. Recent classifications of diabetes by the American Diabetes

Association (ADA) and the World Health Organization (WHO) (1) have recognized this by classifying MODY now as discrete subtypes of diabetes arising from mutations in specific β-cell genes. MODY is probably the first area of diabetes in which molecular genetics has played a clear clinical as well as research role.

EARLY DESCRIPTIONS OF MATURITY-ONSET DIABETES OF THE YOUNG

In the pre-insulin era, it was recognized that some patients with diabetes did not die and that these patients typically had a parent with diabetes. Cammidge noted in 1928 that "a dominant inheritance is almost invariably associated with a good prognosis" (2). It is likely that this is the first recognition of a clinical subgroup that was later known as MODY.

Strongly inherited young-onset familial diabetes subsequently was recognized and studied by Fajans in the 1960s and 1970s (3,4). In 1974, Tattersall recognized that an autosomal dominant inheritance was a feature of this condition (5). The term *MODY* was coined in 1975, although initially this stood for maturity-onset type diabetes of young people (6). Subsequently, a large number of families with variable phenotypes were described throughout the world. Although some of the phenotypic variation resulted in the use of different definitions, it became apparent that there was clinical heterogeneity in MODY, even if only white families with an age of onset of 25 years were considered (4,7). This clinical heterogeneity is now explicable in terms of genetic heterogeneity (8).

CLINICAL DEFINITION OF MATURITY-ONSET DIABETES OF THE YOUNG

In the vast majority of patients, it is now possible to define MODY as diabetes associated with β-cell dysfunction resulting from a specific mutation in a MODY-related gene. However, it is clearly not feasible to perform genetic studies on all subjects, and hence clinical criteria still are necessary to identify those patients in whom a mutation is likely. In addition, some subjects have MODY but the etiologic genes have not yet been defined. Criteria we propose are those used in genetic studies in the United Kingdom and France (8).

Early Onset Non–Insulin-Dependent Diabetes

By definition, a family is considered to have early onset diabetes if at least one and ideally two members of the family are diagnosed with diabetes before the age of 25 years, although it is recognized that other family members, particularly in older generations, may be diagnosed later.

Patients are considered non–insulin-dependent if 5 years after diagnosis they either are not receiving insulin treatment or are insulin treated but have significant levels of circulating C-peptide. Family members are considered to be affected either if they had diabetes by WHO criteria or, particularly in the case of glucokinase mutations, if they had fasting hyperglycemia (>6 mmol/L or >108 mg/dL) (9,10).

Autosomal Dominant Inheritance

The minimal criterion for autosomal dominant inheritance is the occurrence of diabetes in two generations, although most MODY families have at least three or more generations affected. In an autosomal dominant condition, only one of the two parents of an affected child should be affected. Therefore, considerable caution should be taken before defining a family in which both parents have diabetes as a MODY family, especially because children who inherit a "double gene dose" of type 2 diabetes from both parents also may have an earlier onset of diabetes (11).

Other Features

While early-onset, non–insulin-dependent diabetes and an autosomal dominant inheritance have typically been used for the definition of MODY, other features can help in identifying whether a particular family has MODY. The most important features follow:

- *β-cell dysfunction:* β-cell dysfunction rather than insulin resistance is a characteristic of MODY. A young subject with acanthosis nigricans, the cutaneous marker of marked insulin resistance, is very unlikely to have MODY.
- *Lean-body habitus*: Subjects with MODY mutations do not need to be obese to develop diabetes, in marked contrast to most subjects with childhood or early onset type 2 diabetes (12). However, MODY cannot be excluded if a subject is obese, as most series suggest that obesity is similar to that seen in the normal population. However, it is unlikely to be a consistent feature of diabetes throughout a family.

DEFINITION OF THE GENETIC BASIS OF MATURITY-ONSET DIABETES OF THE YOUNG

The development of modern genetic techniques centered on the use of the polymerase chain reaction in the early 1990s has considerably helped in defining the genes in MODY. The definition of genes in monogenic MODY families was always likely to be considerably easier than defining genes in polygenic type 1 and type 2 diabetes, in which there are multiple genes and a large environmental component. The early onset favored the collection of large, multigeneration pedigrees that greatly facilitated analysis and gave a single family sufficient power to define a new locus or gene (9,13,14). Candidate genes were also relatively easy to define, as all families had a β-cell defect.

The breakthroughs in defining the genetic etiology came through the use of linkage methods. A candidate-gene approach was used in defining the role of the glucokinase gene in French and English MODY pedigrees (9,10). The major breakthrough, however, was the use of linkage to localize etiologic genes with a positional mapping approach that identified susceptibility loci on chromosome 20q (MODY1) and 12q (MODY3) (13,15). The MODY gene on 12q was defined as being hepatic nuclear factor (HNF) 1α (16). This was a seminal finding that led to the rapid recognition that HNF4α was the MODY1 gene (17). It also clearly indicated that HNF1β (MODY5), which forms heterodimers with HNF1α, was also an excellent candidate gene. The role of the HNF in β-cell function had previously been unsuspected. The description of insulin-promoter factor (IPF) 1 (also known as PDX1) as the MODY4 gene arose from observations in a family initially investigated because the proband had pancreatic agenesis, a condition seen in the IPF1 knockout mouse (14,18). It was shown that heterogeneity for a severe mutation caused MODY, while homozygosity for this mutation caused pancreatic agenesis.

A variety of approaches have therefore led to the identification of the genes involved in MODY. These observations opened new areas of understanding and research on β-cell physiology, pathophysiology, and genetics.

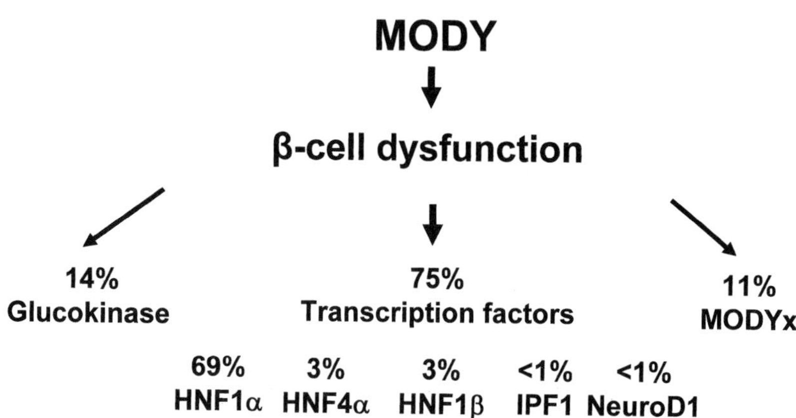

Figure 26.1. Distribution of MODY in the United Kingdom MODY collection. (Data from 131 families from Frayling TM, Evans JC, Bulman MP, et al. Beta-cell genes and diabetes: molecular and clinical characterization of mutations in transcription factors. *Diabetes* 2001;50[Suppl 1]: S94–S100; and A. T. Hattersley and S. Ellard, unpublished.)

RELATIVE PREVALENCE OF THE DIFFERENT SUBGROUPS OF MATURITY-ONSET DIABETES OF THE YOUNG

Large national collections, particularly in the United Kingdom and France, allow assessment of the relative prevalence of the different subgroups of MODY. Figure 26.1 shows the relative contribution of the six known genes in United Kingdom pedigrees that have been collected principally from adult hospital clinics (19).

Although the prevalence of the mutations varies, HNF1α (MODY3) is the commonest cause in most MODY series. This depends on the strictness of the criteria for MODY used when recruiting families, the predominant method of recruiting families, and racial origin. In two large collections from France and Italy, glucokinase (MODY2) is the most prevalent subtype (20,21). This probably represents the detection of asymptomatic, mild fasting hyperglycemia in children based on recruitment from pediatric clinics or by screening young children in family studies (22). In contrast, the majority of other MODY series are recruited from adult diabetes clinics, where the majority of patients have symptomatic diabetes, so MODY3, with more marked hyperglycemia, is more common. It does appear that, even allowing for differences in diagnostic criteria and ascertainment, the prevalence of the known MODY genes is considerably lower in Japanese and Chinese series than in series of European whites.

As the different genetic subgroups of MODY have clear differences in clinical and physiologic phenotypes, they are discussed separately below and summarized in Table 26.1. A genetic classification is clinically useful, as the phenotypic differences between MODY2 and MODY3 are as marked as the differences between type 2 diabetes and either MODY2 or MODY3.

TABLE 26.1. Comparison of the Different Subtypes of Maturity-Onset Diabetes of the Young

Characteristic	HNF4α (MODY1)	Glucokinase (MODY2)	HNF1α (MODY3)	IPF1 (MODY4)	HNF1β (MODY5)	MODYx
Chromosomal location	20q	7p	12q	13q	17q	Unknown
Frequency in U.K.	3%	14%	69%	<1%	4%	12%
Mutations	No evidence of a common mutation	No evidence of a common mutation	C insertion in the exon 4 C tract (codon 291) in 10%–15% of families with mutations	D76N found in many populations but type 2 not MODY	No evidence of a common mutation	Not known
Penetrance of mutations at age 40 y	>90%	45% (>90% FPG >6 mmol/L)	>95%	?>80%	>95%	Not known
Onset of hyperglycemia	Adolescence Early adulthood	Early childhood (from birth)	Adolescence Early adulthood	?Early adulthood	?Similar to HNF1α	Uncertain
Severity of hyperglycemia	Progressive May become severe	Mild with minor deterioration with age	Progressive May be severe	Limited data: ?less penetrant than HNF1α	May be severe	Variable
Microvascular complications	Frequent	Rare	Frequent	Limited data	Frequent	Variable
Pathophysiology	β-cell dysfunction	β-cell dysfunction Glucose sensing disorder	β-cell dysfunction	β-cell dysfunction	β-cell dysfunction and insulin resistance	β-cell dysfunction
Non–diabetes-related features	Low plasma triglycerides	Reduced birth weight	Low renal threshold for glucose	Pancreatic agenesis in homozygotes	Renal cysts Renal failure	

HNF4α MUTATIONS (MATURITY-ONSET DIABETES OF THE YOUNG-1)

Molecular Genetics

MODY1 was the first genetic locus to be defined in MODY (13). The localization of the gene to the long arm of chromosome 20 by Bell et al. (13) was possible because of the collection of DNA samples and careful longitudinal study of the extensive RW pedigree by Fajans (23). Fine mapping of this gene was difficult, as linkage to MODY1 was rare (10). The major breakthrough in defining the MODY1 gene was the identification of the MODY3 gene as HNF1α (16). This led to the rapid recognition that HNF4α was the MODY1 gene and to the identification of a nonsense mutation Q268X that co-segregated with MODY in the RX pedigree (17) (see below).

Mutations in HNF4α are considerably less common than mutations in HNF1α, with fewer than 20 mutations being described during the first 5 years following the description of the gene [reviewed in reference (24)]. These mutations are distributed throughout the gene and consist of nonsense, frameshift, and missense mutations. Recently, it has been shown that the main HNF4α isomer in the β-cell uses a far-upstream promoter and alternative exon 1 (25). This P2 promoter has HNF1 and IPF1 binding sites. The critical regulatory role of these binding sites in the β-cell has been established by studies in HNF1α knockout animals and the finding of a mutation that causes MODY in the IPF1 binding site (25,26).

Phenotype of Patients with HNF4α Mutations

CLINICAL CHARACTERISTICS

The clinical phenotype of HNF4α mutations is far more similar to the phenotype seen with HNF1α mutations than the phenotype seen with the glucokinase mutations (Table 26.1). Children younger than 10 years of age who have HNF4α mutations usually have normal glucose tolerance and develop diabetes in adolescence or early adulthood. In some families, the age at diagnosis is older than that in HNF1α families, but this is not a consistent finding (27). Patients show worsening glycemia with increasing age as the result of progressive β-cell dysfunction.

HNF4α is expressed in a wide range of cell types and tissues. Secretion of both glucagon from the α-cells and the pancreatic polypeptide (PP) cells is also reduced in patients with MODY1 (28).

PENETRANCE OF MUTATIONS

HNF4α generally has a high penetrance, with the majority of subjects with a diagnosis of diabetes by the age of 25 years. Teenagers and young adults who have carried the mutation but who had not developed diabetes on repeated glucose tolerance testing have been described. In some families, the older age of diagnosis probably reflects reduced penetrance of specific mutations (27,29).

TREATMENT

As in patients with HNF1α mutations, those with HNF4α mutations show a progressive deterioration in glycemia and frequently require oral agents and insulin. Some patients have been successfully maintained for decades on sulfonylureas (30) and, like patients with MODY3, may be sensitive to the hypoglycemic effects of sulfonylurea therapy.

COMPLICATIONS

Both microvascular and macrovascular complications are frequent. The frequency is thought to be similar to that in subjects with type 1 or type 2 diabetes (4).

EXTRAPANCREATIC FEATURES

The main extrapancreatic manifestations described result from reduced transcription of hepatic target genes of HNF4α. Reduced concentrations of the apolipoproteins $apoA_{II}$, $apoC_{III}$, and possibly apoB are found in patients with MODY1 but not in patients with type 2 diabetes (31,32). Triglyceride levels are decreased in patients with MODY1 in contrast to patients with type 2 diabetes, in whom levels are usually increased. This elevation probably reflects decreased lipoprotein lipase activity resulting from the reduction in apolipoproteins (31). In contrast to patients with mutations in HNF1α, low renal threshold for glucose has not been reported in patients with MODY1.

PATHOPHYSIOLOGY

Patients with HNF4α mutations have progressive β-cell dysfunction. This β-cell dysfunction is characterized by an inability to increase insulin secretion when blood glucose levels are high (33). In contrast to HNF1α, prolonged hyperglycemia (18 hours) does not prime the β-cell in nondiabetic individuals (33).

CLASSIFICATION

The separation of patients with HNF4α mutations from patients with mutations in other transcription factors would normally require molecular genetic diagnosis. The ADA classification proposes that an etiologic diagnosis be used, for example, genetic defect in β-cell function; chromosome 20 HNF4α.

PREVALENCE

Mutations in HNF4α are far less common than mutations in HNF1α. In the United Kingdom, families with HNF4α mutations represent 2% to 4% of MODY families (Fig. 26.1).

Disease Mechanisms in Maturity-Onset Diabetes of the Young-1

FUNCTIONAL CHARACTERISTICS OF MATURITY-ONSET DIABETES OF THE YOUNG-1 MUTATIONS

The functional characteristics of HNF4α mutations associated with MODY1 have been studied extensively [reviewed in reference (24)]. The principal mutation mechanism is haploinsufficiency, with the majority of mutations showing a considerable reduction of transcription activity *in vitro*: They are not "dominant-negative" mutations, because they do not significantly interfere with the activity of wild-type HNF4α. The HNF4α mutation associated with later-onset type 2 diabetes shows intermediate activity *in vitro* between wild-type and the mutations causing MODY (27).

Mechanisms Involved in Development of Diabetes in Maturity-Onset Diabetes of the Young

The mechanisms resulting in heterozygous mutations in the HNF4α gene that cause β-cell dysfunction are not fully established. Studies by Stoffel and Duncan (34) using embryonic stem cells have established that HNF4α regulates the expression of genes encoding components of the glucose-dependent insulin-secretion pathway, including glucose transporter 2; the glycolytic enzymes aldolase B and glyceraldehyde 3-phosphate dehydrogenase; and liver pyruvate kinase. The progressive loss of β-cell function is hard to explain purely by altered levels of glucose transport and metabolism and may reflect a progressive reduction in β-cell mass due to altered β-cell turnover.

GLUCOKINASE MUTATIONS (MATURITY-ONSET DIABETES OF THE YOUNG-2)

Molecular Genetics

GLUCOKINASE AS A CANDIDATE GENE FOR MATURITY-ONSET DIABETES OF THE YOUNG

Glucokinase was the first MODY gene identified. The role of glucokinase in insulin secretion made it an ideal candidate gene for MODY. Glucokinase is one of four isoforms of hexokinase, enzymes that catalyze the first step in the metabolism of glucose: its phosphorylation to glucose-6-phosphate. Glucokinase is expressed principally in pancreatic β-cells and in hepatocytes. In β-cells, glucose phosphorylation is closely linked with the initiation of insulin secretion (35,36). Unlike the other hexokinases, glucokinase has a low affinity for glucose (K_m of 5.5 mmol/L or 99 mg/dL plasma glucose concentration) and is not inhibited by its product. These features allow β-cells and hepatocytes to change rates of glucose phosphorylation at physiologic glucose concentrations (4–15 mmol/L or 72–270 mg/dL). Glucokinase had consequently been termed the *pancreatic glucose sensor* (36).

MUTATIONS OF THE GLUCOKINASE GENE CAUSE MATURITY-ONSET DIABETES OF THE YOUNG

The characteristic of glucokinase strongly suggested that this might be an important candidate gene in type 2 diabetes. Tanizawa and colleagues in Permutt's laboratory at Washington University in St. Louis cloned the human gene and showed that it had a structure similar to that of the rat gene, with 12 exons and discrete pancreatic and hepatic promoters (37). The identification of two microsatellite polymorphisms flanking the glucokinase gene led to the description in early 1992 of linkage in French and English MODY pedigrees (9,10).

MOLECULAR GENETICS OF THE GLUCOKINASE GENE

The demonstration of linkage between MODY and the glucokinase gene was quickly followed by the characterization of the human gene and the detection of mutations (38–40). The first mutation was reported in 1992 (38), and more than 100 mutations of the glucokinase gene have now been described in many populations, with the majority found in France and Italy (20,21, 38–43). All these mutations have been associated with mild to moderate hyperglycemia.

It is interesting that one mutation is associated with the opposite phenotype, that is, hypoglycemia associated with hyperinsulinemia (44). This is due to a gain-of-function mutation that results in overproduction of insulin. Homozygous loss-of-function mutations in the glucokinase gene have recently been shown to result in permanent neonatal diabetes that is severe and requires insulin treatment from birth (45).

Mutations associated with hyperglycemia are distributed throughout the gene, and different mutation mechanisms, with nonsense, missense, frameshift, and splice-site mutations, having all been described. The mutations associated with MODY2 have been shown to have reduced activity when expressed *in vitro*. Many mutations alter the maximal activity of the enzyme for glucose phosphorylation or alter its affinity for glucose (46). Other mutations, distant from the glucose binding cleft of the enzyme (encoded by exons 5, 6, 7, and 8), either can alter the structure by a major alteration in protein structure as a result of nonconservative changes in amino acid or can alter adenosine triphosphate phosphorylation (47,48).

Phenotype of Patients with Glucokinase Mutations

CLINICAL CHARACTERISTICS

Despite the wide variety of mutations (49), alterations in the glucokinase gene result in a discrete phenotype, summarized in Table 26.1. An increased fasting blood glucose is a consistent feature, and the majority of patients have blood glucose values within a tight range of 6 to 8 mmol/L or 108 to 144 mg/dL (Fig. 26.2). A fasting glucose level below 5.5 mmol/L is extremely rare in MODY2 patients, and no patients with mutations have had fasting glucose values consistently below 5.5 mmol/L (50). There is a mild deterioration in fasting blood glucose levels with age, but blood glucose levels in patients in their eighth and ninth decades still rarely exceeded 9 mmol/L (50–52). This mild hyperglycemia is present very early in life, and patients have been described who have hyperglycemia in the first weeks of life (53). Recent observations showing altered birth weight and fetal growth support the concept that these changes in the β-cell function are present before birth (43).

Patients with glucokinase mutations are usually asymptomatic throughout their life and rarely have symptoms of hyperglycemia. The vast majority will be detected by screening either for routine medical examinations, during pregnancy, or family screening when MODY is suspected (9,54). In most patients, the age of diagnosis is the age at which they are first tested. While being diagnosed young is supportive of a glucokinase mutation, the fact that a patient is diagnosed only in old age should not be used to exclude the diagnosis. More than in any other type of diabetes, MODY2 may be diagnosed decades after the age of onset.

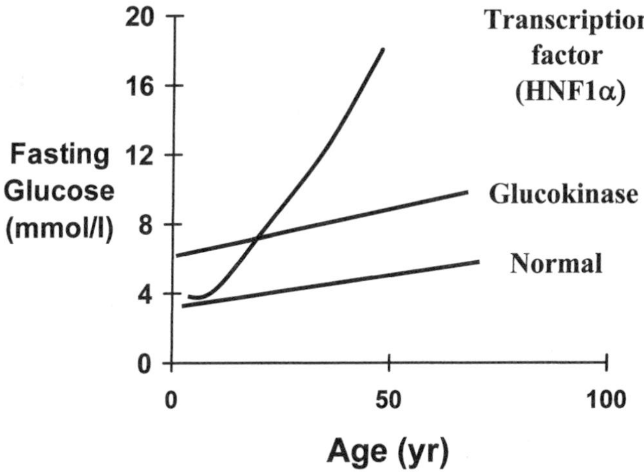

Figure 26.2. Diagrammatic representation of the change in fasting glucose with age in untreated patients with HNF1α and glucokinase mutations. (Based on data from Hattersley AT. Maturity-onset diabetes of the young: clinical heterogeneity explained by genetic heterogeneity. *Diabet Med* 1998;15:15–24; Stride A, Vaxillaire M, Tuomi T, et al. The genetic abnormality in the beta cell determines the response to an oral glucose load. *Diabetologia* 2002;45:427–435; and Pearson ER, Velho G, Clark P, et al. Beta-cell genes and diabetes: quantitative and qualitative differences in the pathophysiology of hepatic nuclear factor-1alpha and glucokinase mutations. *Diabetes* 2001;50[Suppl 1]:S101–S107.)

TREATMENT

Patients with glucokinase mutations rarely need any pharmacologic treatment (51,52). The majority of patients with glucokinase mutations (>85%) are treated with diet alone. Avoiding unrefined carbohydrate may not be as important as in patients with type 2 diabetes, because most patients with glucokinase mutations show little increment in their blood glucose on receiving 75 g of glucose in an oral glucose tolerance test (50,52,55). Another interesting observation is that body mass index makes little difference to the level of glycemia in patients with glucokinase mutations (50,51). This is in marked contrast to patients with type 2 diabetes, in whom weight loss can very effectively reduce glycemia. In patients with glucokinase mutations, this is probably because the fasting hyperglycemia is due to a defect in glucose sensing; thus, as in the healthy subject, increased insulin resistance as a result of obesity results in compensatory hyperinsulinemia rather than hyperglycemia. The only time that patients with glucokinase mutations are likely to consistently receive treatment is during pregnancy (see below).

COMPLICATIONS

Patients with MODY2 rarely suffer from microvascular complications (42,51), probably because their hyperglycemia is mild. The rare cases of proliferative retinopathy and diabetic retinopathy reported in the French series may represent coincidental conventional type 2 diabetes in patients who also have a glucokinase mutation. It is hard to assess whether patients with MODY2 have significant macrovascular complications, because only 500 patients have been described in the literature. An increased risk of macrovascular disease is seen in patients with impaired glucose tolerance, so an increased risk might be expected in subjects with glucokinase mutations (56). However, in contrast to patients with impaired glucose tolerance, patients with glucokinase mutations have normal fasting lipid concentrations (51), are not significantly insulin resistant (9), and have less postprandial hyperglycemia (50,52,55). These factors are all likely to reduce the macrovascular risk in patients with glucokinase mutations.

PATHOPHYSIOLOGY

In keeping with our understanding of the biochemistry of glucokinase, patients with glucokinase mutations have been shown to have β-cell dysfunction characterized as a defect in glucose sensing (9,51,57,58). First-phase insulin response to an intravenous glucose bolus is well preserved (57).

Patients with glucokinase mutations do not show the features of insulin resistance seen in type 2 diabetes. Insulin concentrations and plasma lipids are normal, and in most series there is no increase in insulin resistance (9,51). In a large series of French patients, a small but statistically significant increase in insulin resistance was found in patients with glucokinase mutations with diabetes compared both with patients with glucokinase mutations who have only fasting hyperglycemia and with normal controls (59). There are many possible explanations of this result: severe glucokinase mutations may affect both β-cell function and insulin sensitivity, the insulin resistance was secondary to glucose toxicity, or these patients had other genetic or environmental influences that predispose to type 2 diabetes resulting in their reduced glucose tolerance and insulin resistance. It has clearly been demonstrated that patients with glucokinase mutations do have reduced hepatic glycogen synthesis, confirming that glucokinase is a rate-determining step in the liver as well as in the pancreatic β-cell (60).

CLASSIFICATION

The same glucokinase mutation has been identified in patients who were defined as having MODY, type 2 diabetes, or gestational diabetes (40,61), depending on when the diagnosis was made. There was no evidence of a different phenotype in these three groups (62). This shows the difficulties of a clinical classification for which the time of diagnosis determines the classification of the type of diabetes. Patients with a glucokinase mutation appeared to have a discrete phenotype, and hence a classification based on etiology had been proposed (62,63) and supported by the ADA as "genetic defects of β-cell function; chromosome 7, glucokinase" (64).

PREVALENCE

The prevalence of glucokinase mutations is difficult to assess, because the mild hyperglycemia and absence of symptoms means patients frequently do not receive a diagnosis. No large-scale population studies to assess the prevalence of glucokinase mutations have been done. In the white population, approximately 2% of the population will be diagnosed as having gestational diabetes, and of these, approximately 2% to 5% (65) will have a glucokinase mutation. This would suggest a population prevalence of 0.04% to 0.1%.

The prevalence of patients with MODY who have glucokinase mutations ranges from as high as 56% in France (20), to 12.5% in the United Kingdom (43), and to less than 1% in Japan (66). This probably reflects differences in ascertainment (see previous section), as well as a genuinely lower prevalence in Japan than in Europe.

Glucokinase Mutations and Pregnancy

DIAGNOSIS OF GLUCOKINASE MUTATIONS AS GESTATIONAL DIABETES

Patients with glucokinase mutations are frequently diagnosed during screening in pregnancy. In the series of European whites, the prevalence of glucokinase mutations ranged from 0% to 6% (65). The recognition of subjects with glucokinase mutations is important, because they have a different clinical course both within and outside pregnancy compared with most other subjects with gestational diabetes. Patients' clinical characteristics can be used to detect those who are most likely to have a glucokinase mutation. Specific criteria favoring a diagnosis of a glucokinase mutation have been shown to be persistent fasting hyperglycemia, a small increment on the oral glucose tolerance test (<3 mmol/L or <54 mg/dL), and a family history of mild hyperglycemia (65).

FETAL GROWTH IN PREGNANCIES OF WOMEN WITH GLUCOKINASE MUTATIONS

Fetal growth in pregnant patients with MODY2 has been shown to be dependent on whether the fetus has inherited the mutation from its mother (43). Fetal insulin secretion is a key determinant of fetal growth, acting mainly during the third trimester when the weight of the fetus increases markedly. Macrosomic children born to mothers with diabetes in pregnancy have increased fetal insulin secretion in response to fetal pancreatic sensing of maternal hyperglycemia. Factors that alter fetal insulin secretion will therefore alter intrauterine growth by altering fetal insulin-mediated growth.

A glucokinase mutation in a pregnant mother will result in maternal hyperglycemia, hence increasing fetal insulin secretion and fetal growth. Inheritance of the mutation by the fetus will result in reduced sensing of the maternal glucose by the fetal pancreas and hence reduced fetal insulin secretion and

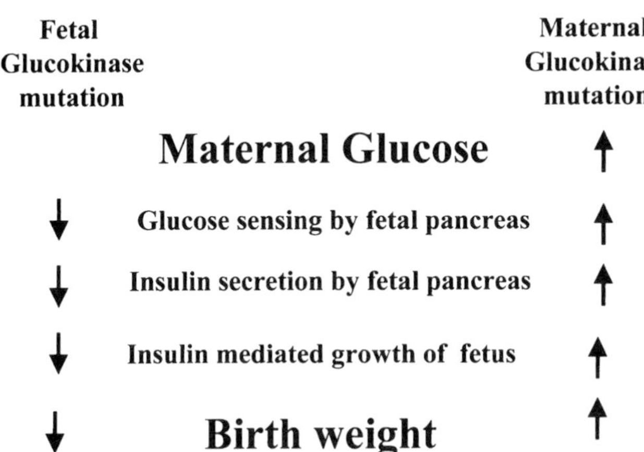

Figure 26.3. The contradictory effects of a fetal and maternal glucokinase mutation on birth weight are mediated by the fetal mutation resulting in reduced fetal insulin secretion and a maternal glucokinase mutation resulting in maternal hyperglycemia and hence in increased fetal insulin secretion.

reduced intrauterine growth. The two contradictory effects of glucokinase mutations are shown in Figure 26.3. The effects of inheriting a glucokinase mutation by either mother or fetus are considerable. Children born to mothers with a glucokinase mutation were 601 g heavier at birth than children born to mothers without a glucokinase mutation, and children who inherited a glucokinase mutation weighed 521 g less than children without a glucokinase mutation. Figure 26.4 shows the effects of fetal and maternal mutations on mean birth weight centiles, showing that the two effects are additive. When both mother and fetus had the glucokinase mutation, two opposing effects canceled out and the baby was of normal weight.

These observations have important theoretical implications. They establish that glucokinase plays a key role in the sensing of glucose by the fetus in utero. It also led to a more wide-ranging hypothesis described as the "fetal insulin hypothesis" (67). This proposes that genetic defects that alter either fetal insulin secretion or fetal insulin action could, by reducing insulin-mediated growth, reduce birth weight. This therefore provides a potential explanation of the association seen between low birth weight and diabetes in adult life. This association had previously been attributed to intrauterine programming as the result of intrauterine malnutrition. The relative importance of these two factors may vary between populations and requires further study. It is likely that both the intrauterine environment and fetal genetics are important in explaining the association.

MANAGEMENT OF PREGNANCIES INVOLVING GLUCOKINASE MUTATIONS

The observations of the impact of glucokinase mutations on fetal growth are important for the management of the pregnancies of mothers who have glucokinase mutations. These mothers will have fasting hyperglycemia that will not respond to dietary measures. Most modern recommendations suggest that such patients are treated with insulin, achieving normoglycemia, and many subjects with glucokinase mutations therefore are treated with insulin during pregnancy. However, recent observations have suggested that the fetal genotype is a far greater determinant of pregnancy outcome than is treatment of the mother with insulin. In addition, it is debatable whether the achievement of maternal euglycemia is desirable if the baby has a mutation, because this may result in a small baby (68). The baby is small if the fetus inherits a mutation from the father and is born in a normal mother (67,69). Treatment decisions in glucokinase gestational diabetes should therefore be related to fetal growth as shown by scans rather than to maternal glycemia levels alone, as has been proposed in other types of gestational diabetes. Fetal hypoglycemia is not seen when the fetus has inherited the mutation, and the newborn child will have mild fasting hyperglycemia that is unlikely to progress [reference (53); and G. Spyer and A. T. Hattersley, unpublished data].

The recognition that a patient has a glucokinase mutation is also important for the subsequent treatment of the mother. It is likely that, even if she has been receiving very large doses of insulin, she will not require pharmacologic therapy after the pregnancy. In contrast, in subjects with gestational diabetes that is not due to a glucokinase mutation, deterioration to type 2 diabetes over the following 10 years is unlikely.

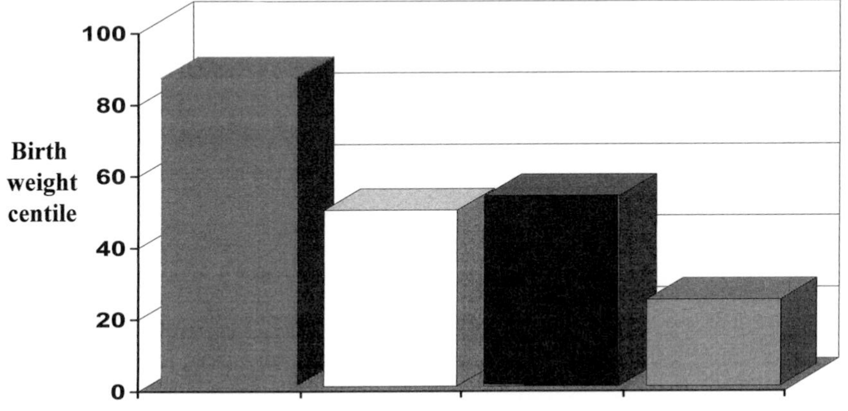

Figure 26.4. Birth weight centile according to maternal and fetal mutation status in families with glucokinase mutations. (Data from Hattersley AT, Beards F, Ballantyne E, et al. Mutations in the glucokinase gene of the fetus result in reduced birth weight. *Nat Genet* 1998;19:268–270.)

HNF1α MUTATIONS (MATURITY-ONSET DIABETES OF THE YOUNG-3)

Molecular Genetics

Graeme Bell's group in Chicago and collaborators from France, the United Kingdom, Japan, Denmark, and the United States were first to show that the transcription factor HNF1α encoded the MODY3 gene (16). Studies of MODY pedigrees in United Kingdom (70), Germany (71), France (72), Denmark (73), Italy (74), Finland (75), North America (75), and Japan (76) confirmed that HNF1α mutations are the most common known cause of MODY. Although many different mutations occur, approximately 15% of the families with an HNF1α mutation have an insertion of an extra nucleotide (C) in the C tract in exon 4, leading to a frameshift (mutation P291fsinsC). This common mutation is thought to result from a hotspot for spontaneous mutations rather than representing a single distantly related family (71,75,77). More than 100 other mutations have been found scattered throughout the gene and consist of frameshift, missense, nonsense, and splice-site mutations.

Phenotype of Patients with HNF1α Mutations

CLINICAL CHARACTERISTICS

The phenotype associated with HNF1α mutations is markedly different from that found in patients with glucokinase mutations (Table 26.1 and Fig. 26.2). Most subjects under the age of 10 years have a normal fasting blood glucose level and normal glucose tolerance. In adolescence and early adulthood, subjects with HNF1α mutations may show no, or only minimal, elevation of fasting blood glucose level but are frequently diabetic on the 2-hour value in an oral glucose tolerance test (50). The mean age for the clinical diagnosis of diabetes is 23 years. Most subjects present with symptoms related to hyperglycemia (54). Glycosuria is an early marker as a result of the reduced renal threshold in these patients (78,79).

PENETRANCE OF MUTATIONS

HNF1α mutations have a high penetrance, with the majority of subjects having diabetes by the age of 25 years (52,70). However, diabetes was not diagnosed until middle or old age in some subjects found to carry HNF1α mutations; it is difficult to determine whether this is due to a delayed diagnosis, a later onset of diabetes, or both. Frequently, the subjects with HNF1α mutations who do not have diabetes on testing are young and diabetes is likely to develop later in life (70). Some individuals reach early middle age without having diabetes, and these unusual cases probably represent reduced penetrance of the gene mutation (80). These subjects may compensate for their β-cell defect by being sensitive to the insulin or may have a less severe β-cell defect.

TREATMENT

In contrast to the relatively stable mild hyperglycemia seen in patients with glucokinase mutations, once diabetes develops in patients with HNF1α mutations, they show progressive deterioration in their glucose tolerance (Fig. 26.2). Their treatment requirements are also likely to increase as they get older. Approximately one third of subjects with diabetes who have HNF1α mutations are treated by diet; one third, with oral agents; and one third, with insulin. The patients receiving insulin tend to be older and more obese than those treated with diet or oral agents. Some patients are misdiagnosed as having type 1 diabetes because they present with osmotic symptoms in their late teens or early twenties with a random blood glucose in the region of 15 to 20 mmol/L and are started immediately on insulin treatment. Such patients may be recognized by their autosomal dominant family history, the absence of typical type 1 diabetes human leukocyte antigen markers, excellent glycemic control despite relatively low doses of insulin (usually <0.5 U/kg), and an absence of ketoacidosis even when insulin is omitted.

Patients with HNF1α mutations may show marked sensitivity to the hypoglycemic action of sulfonylureas (81,82). This is particularly marked at diagnosis and during the first 10 years of disease. This may result in marked symptomatic hypoglycemia while starting therapy. In patients with type 2 diabetes, metformin and sulfonylureas are equally effective in reducing hyperglycemia, but in patients with HNF1α mutations, there have been reports of marked deterioration in glycemic control on transferring from sulfonylureas to metformin, with a subsequent decrease in glycosylated hemoglobin A_{1c} (HbA_{1c}) of 4% to 5% when they return to sulfonylureas (82). Therefore, low-dose sulfonylureas are the appropriate first-line medication for patients with HNF1α mutations, although they must be introduced with caution. This is an example of pharmacogenetics and is a clear reason for establishing the cause of early onset non–insulin-dependent diabetes.

COMPLICATIONS

Microvascular complications, particularly retinopathy, can develop, especially if treatment of hyperglycemia is inadequate (60,83). This means that it is important to strive for excellent glycemic control. The pattern of complications and also of vascular dysfunction is similar to that seen in type 1 diabetes (84). In both of these subgroups of diabetes, the primary pathophysiology is in the β-cell, with insulin resistance and dyslipidemia less frequently seen than in type 2 diabetes.

PATHOPHYSIOLOGY

The pathophysiology in patients with HNF1α mutations is a progressive β-cell defect (8,52,85). Physiologic experiments have shown that the patients who have inherited the HNF1α mutation but are not yet diabetic show adequate insulin when fasting but are unable to increase their insulin secretion as glucose levels rise. Once patients have established diabetes, insulin secretion is reduced at all glucose values (85). Prolonged hyperglycemia (18 hours) primes the β-cell in nondiabetic but not in diabetic mutation carriers (85). Increased sensitivity to insulin is seen in mutation carriers, and the mechanism for this is unknown (52)

CLASSIFICATION

Most subjects with HNF1α mutations present with symptomatic diabetes and have hyperglycemia in the diabetic range by adolescence or early adulthood. The recent ADA classification now suggests an etiologic diagnosis be used, for example, genetic defect in β-cell function; chromosome 12 HNF1α.

PREVALENCE

Mutations in HNF1α are the commonest cause of diabetes in European white patients with MODY. If strict criteria are used, then a prevalence of this form of MODY among patients with MODY is 50% to 90%, but the prevalence is lower when less stringent criteria are used. We estimate that these patients account for approximately 1% to 2% of white patients in a diabetes clinic, although many of these cases may not be formally recognized as MODY (86). This would result in a population frequency of approximately 0.02% to 0.04%.

Extrapancreatic Manifestations: Low Renal Threshold for Glucose

The early descriptions of MODY described a discrete subgroup of MODY families who had a low renal threshold before diabetes develops (5,87). It has now been shown that these patients had a mutation in HNF1α (65) and that a low renal threshold is a feature of other patients with MODY3 (78,79). This is probably due to reduced expression of the high-capacity/low-affinity sodium-glucose transporter-2 (SGLT-2), reducing glucose reabsorption in the proximal tubule (88).

Disease Mechanisms with HNF1α Mutations

The disease mechanisms that result in HNF1α mutations causing β-cell dysfunction are complex. There is evidence that dominant-negative mutations in cell lines reduce many critical components of carbohydrate metabolism, resulting in reduced GLUT2 transporter expression and mitochondrial dysfunction (89–91). In addition, there is evidence of increased apoptosis and reduced β-cell proliferation (91–94).

One fascinating feature is that mutations in the different transcription factors result in a very similar pattern of β-cell dysfunction even though there is considerable variation in the extrapancreatic features (see previous section). This would suggest a common mechanism or common pathway resulting in β-cell dysfunction. There is increasing evidence that the MODY transcription factors show considerable interaction and form a regulatory network that maintains β-cell function and hence normal glucose homeostasis (95) (Fig. 26.5). It has recently been established that much of the interaction occurs at the β-cell alternative upstream (P2) promoter in HNF4α (25,26). Through binding sites in this alternative promoter, HNF1α, HNF1β, and IPF1 can increase HNF4α expression and, conversely, HNF4α can increase expression of HNFα through a binding site in the HNF1α promoter. This would suggest not only that HNF4α regulates HNF1α expression but that HNF1α regulates HNF4α expression in β-cells. The critical role of this network is shown, as both mutations in the HNF4α P2 promoter and the HNF1α promoter are sufficient to result in MODY (25,74).

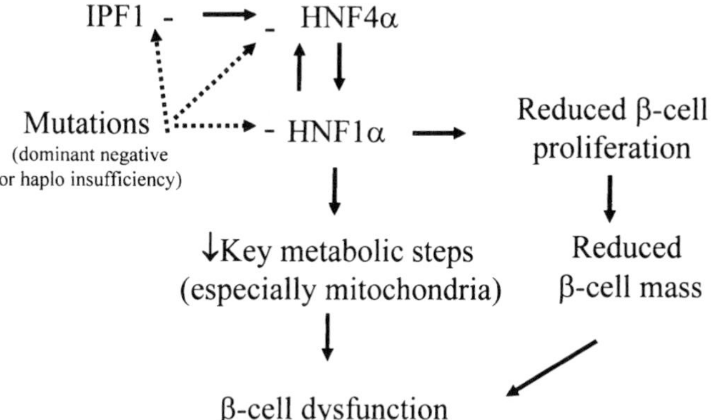

Figure 26.5. Possible mechanisms by which transcription factor mutations in MODY result in cell dysfunction. Note that IPF1, HNF4α, and HNF1α form a regulatory network and may result in β-cell dysfunction by common pathways.

INSULIN PROMOTER FACTOR 1 MUTATIONS (MATURITY-ONSET DIABETES OF THE YOUNG-4)

Molecular Genetics

Elegant clinical science led to the identification of the IPF1, also known as PDX1, as a cause of MODY. The key role of IPF1 in the development of the pancreas was illustrated by the presence of pancreatic agenesis in mice with a homozygous knockout of IPF1. Stoffers and colleagues (18) studied a child with pancreatic agenesis and found a homozygous frameshift mutation that had dominant-negative characteristics *in vitro* (96). They noticed that there were multiple generations with diabetes on both sides of the family and went on to show that the heterozygous frameshift mutation co-segregated with non–insulin-dependent diabetes in both parents' families, with a significant total LOD (logarithm of the odds) score of 3.43 (14). No other IPF1 mutations causing MODY have been described.

Phenotype of Patients with Mutations in Insulin Promoter Factor 1

CLINICAL PHENOTYPE

Defining the clinical phenotype is difficult, because there is only one published family to date. This family met standard criteria for MODY, but there is evidence that this gene was less penetrant than a typical HNF1α mutation (14). Two individuals who inherited the mutation had apparently had normal glucose levels at 22 and 23 years, and the mean age at diagnosis was 35 years (range, 17–68), which is considerably older than the 23 years seen with HNF1α mutations.

PREVALENCE

In France, Japan (97), and the United Kingdom (98), no IPF1 mutations that cause MODY have been found. However, in French families, perfect co-segregation with early onset type 2 diabetes has been shown with moderately severe missense mutations, suggesting IPF1 mutations can result in a monogenic form of type 2 diabetes. Other milder missense mutations were shown to predispose but not to cause early onset type 2 diabetes in the United Kingdom, French, and Swedish pedigrees (98–100).

PHYSIOLOGY

Physiologic studies have shown that carriers of IPF1 mutations that cause MODY have severe β-cell dysfunction, particularly in response to glucose, but, like patients with MODY3, are insulin sensitive (101). Less severe mutations that predispose to type 2 diabetes also resulted in reduced insulin secretion, particularly first-phase insulin secretion (99). It is likely that variation of the severity of the mutation seen *in vitro* explains the variation in phenotype. The less severe missense IPF1 mutations are likely to be part of a polygenic predisposition to type 2 diabetes rather than to a simple monogenic etiology seen in MODY, and hence the pathophysiology is less clear-cut.

HNF1β MUTATIONS (MATURITY-ONSET DIABETES OF THE YOUNG-5)

Molecular Genetics

HNF1β forms heterodimers with HNF1α and was therefore a clear candidate gene for MODY. The first description of an

HNF1β mutation was in a Japanese subject with MODY (102). HNF1β mutations are rare causes of MODY both in Japan and the United Kingdom (102,103). With the recognition that these patients usually present with nondiabetic renal disease before diabetes, many more families have been identified from renal clinics. The majority of the 15 HNF1β mutations described to date have presented with kidney disease in children or young adults (104) and are nonsense or frameshift mutations in early exons [reviewed in reference (24)].

Phenotype of Patients with HNF1β Mutations

The striking feature of MODY5 has been that these subjects, in addition to having early onset diabetes, have all had nondiabetic renal disease. We therefore recently proposed the term *renal cysts and diabetes* (RCAD) for the clinical syndrome associated with HNF1β mutations (105).

DIABETES PHENOTYPE

HNF1β mutations result in early onset non–insulin-dependent diabetes of a severity similar to that in patients with mutations in HNF1α. Children and young adults have been described who have normal or impaired glucose tolerance, suggesting that there is a progressive deterioration in β-cell function. The mean age at diagnosis is the early 20s. Physiologic studies in a single subject showed a clear β-cell defect (106), and it is likely that this is the pathophysiology in all subjects, although, in contrast to HNF1α, preliminary studies suggest that subjects with HNF1β mutations are insulin resistant (E. R. Pearson, C. Bingham, and A. T. Hattersley, unpublished observations).

COMPLICATIONS

Subjects have been described who have proliferative retinopathy, suggesting that these patients, like carriers of HNF1α mutation, are at risk of microvascular complications (102).

RENAL PHENOTYPE

In the initial description of HNF1β mutations, patients with mutations had end-stage renal failure and proteinuria (102). Subsequent study of these patients (107) and other publications have shown that these features represent a non–diabetes-related renal phenotype of HNF1β mutations. In a second Japanese family, all members of a family who had an HNF1β mutation had at least one renal manifestation (108). These included cysts in the kidney on ultrasound, end-stage renal failure, and proteinuria. These renal manifestations were seen in young children with mutations at a time when they were not diabetic (108). Nondiabetic renal disease has been a consistent feature of all families with HNF1β mutations [for a review, see reference (104)].

The renal manifestations of MODY5 are the result of abnormal development of the kidney, and abnormal renal morphology may be observed on scans as early as 17 weeks of pregnancy (106,108). The renal disease varies, with three discrete renal histologic manifestations having been described: oligomeganephronia (109), cystic dysplasia (106), and familial hypoplastic glomerulocystic kidney disease (105). It is uncertain what determines the morphology of the renal defect, but it probably reflects the functional characteristics of the mutation (24). Additional families will be needed to establish if there is a reproducible association between the phenotypes and the functional characteristics of the mutation.

Renal cysts have been seen in some members of all families with HNF1β mutations. Equally, there is considerable variation in the severity of renal dysfunction associated with a single mutation. End-stage renal disease will develop in approximately 50% of subjects before the age of 45 years. Other developmental disorders have been seen in association with HNF1β mutations, including uterine abnormalities (104,109), a lantern jaw, and pyloric stenosis (106). The salient clinical features of the RCAD syndrome in patients with MODY5 are summarized in Table 26.2.

TABLE 26.2. Features of Patients with HNF1β Mutations Causing Renal Cysts and Diabetes (RCAD)

Clinical feature	Percent of subjects with HNF1β mutations and details
Renal cysts	70%
Renal impairment	73%
Renal histology (includes)	Glomerulocystic kidney disease
	Renal dysplasia
	Oligomeganephronia
Diabetes	66%
	Mean age at diagnosis 23.6 y (range, 10–61 y)
	Most nondiabetic subjects are <20 y
Other features	
Short stature	20% <2 SD below mean height
Hyperuricemia and gout	20% (clinical gout)
Uterine abnormalities	17%
Hypospadias	17%
Joint laxity	Rare
Hearing loss	Rare
Prognathism	Rare
Pyloric stenosis	Rare
Learning difficulties	Rare

Pathophysiology of HNF1β Mutations

The common feature of all the renal lesions is that they likely result from abnormal development of the kidney, and the vast majority result from abnormal development of the nephron. HNF1β has been shown to be expressed in very early stages of embryologic development of the kidney. A critical role in the development of the kidney was not apparent from transgenic mice, as the HNF1β heterozygous mouse has no phenotype and HNF1β homozygosity is lethal to the embryo. It is uncertain if the pancreatic β-cell lesion that results in diabetes in later life is the result of abnormal pancreatic development.

NEUROD1 AND ISLET-BRAIN-1 MUTATIONS (MATURITY-ONSET DIABETES OF THE YOUNG-6)

Mutations in NeuroD1 (110) and Islet-Brain-1 (111) have been described in early onset familial type 2 diabetes. One NeuroD1 family met the clinical criteria for MODY, although in this family there was not perfect co-segregation with diabetes (110). NeuroD1 mutations were not detected in United Kingdom, French, or Japanese MODY series. However, recently a missense mutation was described in a MODY family from Iceland that showed complete co-segregation with diabetes, strengthening the case that NeuroD1 should be considered MODY6. No detailed descriptions of clinical characteristics or pathophysiology are available for the NeuroD1 MODY families.

NO GENE DEFINED MATURITY-ONSET DIABETES OF THE YOUNG-X

The genes are still undefined for a significant proportion of MODY families. In the United Kingdom and France, this accounts for approximately 15% of MODY cases, but the proportion is considerably higher in Japan.

One interesting subgroup of MODY for which the underlying molecular genetics have not be defined is a subgroup of youth-onset diabetes in black patients termed atypical diabetes mellitus (ADM) (112,113). ADM represent 10% of youth-onset diabetes in blacks. These young people present acutely with weight loss and frequently with ketoacidosis, but months to years after diagnosis, atypical diabetes mellitus reverts to a non–insulin-requiring course similar to MODY in whites. ADM was found in at least two generations in 75% of the families; there was no evidence of pancreatic autoimmunity, and insulin secretion was intermediate between secretion in nondiabetic controls and patients with classic type 1 diabetes (112).

In the absence of an underlying genetic defect, it is difficult to make precise statements on the phenotype of MODYx. Some families who do not have a mutation in the known MODY genes have been defined by less rigorous criteria. In such families, diabetes may result from a high concentration of polygenic influences rather than a single gene. In those families in which there is likely to be a single gene mutation segregating, there still appears to be some heterogeneity. In the French and United Kingdom series, the phenotype in MODYx families was intermediate between the phenotypes in MODY2 and MODY3. Genetic analysis using a combination of reverse genetics and candidate gene studies will help define these families further. Key candidate genes are likely to be involved in gene transcription, development, or glucose sensing in the pancreatic islet.

USING MOLECULAR GENETIC INFORMATION IN THE MANAGEMENT OF PATIENTS WITH MATURITY-ONSET DIABETES OF THE YOUNG

We have reached a level of scientific understanding such that molecular genetic information can help in the clinical management of patients. The potential advantages and disadvantages of diagnostic and predictive genetic testing are outlined in Table 26.3. For patients with diabetes, a molecular genetic diagnosis will allow a definitive diagnosis of MODY to be made and the subtype to be classified and hence will help with treatment and prediction of the likely prognosis and clinical course. A young child with a slightly increased fasting glucose level can be predicted to have a very different clinical course and treatment if he or she has a glucokinase mutation, a mutation in HNF1α, or neither of these and a high level of islet cell antibodies. For this reason, the United Kingdom, France, and other European countries have introduced diagnostic molecular genetic testing. Details of diagnostic testing for patients and their physicians are available on the website: www.diabetesgene.org. An area of uncertainty is the degree of medical supervision necessary for patients with glucokinase gene mutations. Certainly, close follow-up of children who have only mildly increased fasting glucose levels is not warranted, and repeated contact with a diabetes clinic dealing predominantly with type 1 diabetes may be detrimental. We cannot assume that older patients will not have diabetic complications, particularly as there is no evidence that these patients are

TABLE 26.3. Advantages and Disadvantages of Diagnostic and Predictive Testing in MODY

Possible advantages	Possible disadvantages
Diagnostic testing	
Confirm diagnosis of MODY: Not type 1 or type 2 Diagnosis in other family members Identification of subtype: Extrapancreatic features Specific treatment Pregnancy outcome Clinical care: Targeted follow-up Advice re: clinical course Complication screening	Implications for family: Awareness of 50% risk to child Cost implications: Full sequencing of gene required as only 15% have common mutation—expensive
Predictive testing	
Possible advantages	**Possible disadvantages**
Reduced uncertainty Positive result: Adaptation Reduced delay in diagnosis of diabetes Misdiagnosis of type 1 or type 2 diabetes unlikely Negative result: No screening required	Relationships and emotions: Effect on family relationships Feelings of guilt and blame Positive result: Uncertainty of when diabetes will develop Confirms 50% risk to each child Insurance implications

protected from developing polygenic type 2 diabetes. Annual follow-up of adults, including measurement of HbA_{1c}, is probably all that is required. Only the few patients with an elevated HbA_{1c} will require more careful follow-up or treatment.

Mutation-based genetic testing can predict, with a high degree of accuracy, whether MODY is likely to develop in an unaffected first-degree relative. Full genetic counseling should be provided for individuals who seek predictive genetic testing. The child of a patient with MODY may find it helpful to know whether or not they have inherited a mutation, especially if they reach the age of 25 and are apparently unaffected. If they do not have the mutation, then the risk of diabetes would be the same as that of the population and hence screening on an annual basis would no longer be necessary. Testing of young children may also be beneficial, but this is considerably more controversial (114,115). This area of clinical practice needs to be studied carefully before its widespread introduction into clinical use.

CONCLUSION

The definition of the underlying genes in MODY has developed from the early clinical description. Mutations in six discrete genes have been shown to cause MODY: glucokinase, hepatocyte nuclear factor 1α (HNF1α), hepatocyte nuclear factor 4α (HNF4α), hepatocyte nuclear factor 1β (HNF1β), insulin-promoter factor 1 (IPF1), and NeuroD1. The description of these genes has allowed us to understand much of the clinical and physiologic heterogeneity seen in MODY. Molecular genetic testing provides new possibilities for the classification of MODY and possibly for the prediction and eventually the prevention of diabetes within these families.

Acknowledgments

I am very grateful to Diabetes UK, the Wellcome Trust, the European Union, the Medical Research Council, Northcott Devon Medical Foundation, DIRECT, PPP Healthcare Trust, The Darlington Trust, The Royal Devon and Exeter NHS Trust, Perkin Elmer Biosystems, and the University of Exeter for supporting our work on MODY.

Many outstanding colleagues in Exeter, Birmingham, and Oxford and our collaborators throughout the world have contributed to the ideas in this chapter and are gratefully acknowledged.

REFERENCES

1. WHO Study Group, Report of a WHO Consultation. *Part 1: Diagnosis and classification of diabetes mellitus.* Geneva: World Health Organisation, 1999.
2. Cammidge PJ. Diabetes mellitus and heredity. *BMJ* 1928;2:738–741.
3. Tattersall R. Maturity-onset diabetes of the young: a clinical history. *Diabet Med* 1998;15:11–14.
4. Fajans SS. Scope and heterogeneous nature of MODY [Review]. *Diabetes Care* 1990;13:49–64.
5. Tattersall RB. Mild familial diabetes with dominant inheritance. *Q J Med* 1974;3:339–357.
6. Tattersall RB, Fajans SS. A difference between the inheritance of classical juvenile-onset and maturity-onset type diabetes of young people. *Diabetes* 1975;24:44–53.
7. Tattersall RB, Mansell PI. Maturity onset-type diabetes of the young (MODY): one condition or many? [Review]. *Diabet Med* 1991;8:402–410.
8. Hattersley AT, Maturity-onset diabetes of the young: clinical heterogeneity explained by genetic heterogeneity. *Diabet Med* 1998;15:15–24.
9. Hattersley AT, Turner RC, Permutt MA, et al. Linkage of type 2 diabetes to the glucokinase gene. *Lancet* 1992;339:1307–1310.
10. Froguel P, Vaxillaire M, Sun F, et al. Close linkage of glucokinase locus on chromosome 7p to early-onset non-insulin-dependent diabetes mellitus. *Nature* 1992;356:162–164.
11. O'Rahilly S, Spivey RS, Holman RR, et al. Type II diabetes of early onset: a distinct clinical and genetic syndrome? *BMJ* 1987;294:923–928.
12. Fagot-Campagna A, Pettitt D, Engelgau M, et al. Type 2 diabetes among North American children and adolescents: an epidemiologic review and a public health perspective. *J Pediatr* 2000;136:664–672.
13. Bell GI, Xiang KS, Newman MV. Gene for non-insulin dependent diabetes mellitus (maturity-onset diabetes of the young subtype) is linked to DNA polymorphism on human chromosome 20q. *Proc Natl Acad Sci U S A* 1991; 1484–1488.
14. Stoffers DA, Ferrer J, Clarke WL, et al. Early-onset type-II diabetes mellitus (MODY4) linked to IPF1. *Nat Genet* 1997;17:138–139.
15. Vaxillaire M, Boccio V, Philippi A, et al. A gene for maturity onset diabetes of the young (MODY) maps to chromosome 12q. *Nat Genet* 1995;9:418–423.
16. Yamagata K, Oda N, Kaisaki PJ, et al. Mutations in the hepatic nuclear factor 1 alpha gene in maturity-onset diabetes of the young (MODY3). *Nature* 1996; 384:455–458.
17. Yamagata K, Furuta H, Oda N, et al. Mutations in the hepatocyte nuclear factor 4 alpha gene in maturity-onset diabetes of the young (MODY1). *Nature* 1996;384:458–460.
18. Stoffers DA, Zinkin NT, Stanojevic V, et al. Pancreatic agenesis attributable to a single ncleotide deletion in the human IPF1 gene coding sequence. *Nat Genet* 1997;15:106–110.
19. Frayling TM, Evans JC, Bulman MP, et al. Beta-cell genes and diabetes: molecular and clinical characterization of mutations in transcription factors. *Diabetes* 2001;50[Suppl 1]:S94–S100.
20. Froguel P, Zouali H, Vionnet N, et al. Familial hyperglycemia due to mutations in glucokinase. Definition of a subtype of diabetes mellitus. *N Engl J Med* 1993;328:697–702.
21. Massa O, Meschi F, Cuesta-Munoz A, et al. High prevalence of glucokinase mutations in Italian children with MODY. Influence on glucose tolerance, first-phase insulin response, insulin sensitivity and BMI. Diabetes Study Group of the Italian Society of Paediatric Endocrinology and Diabetes (SIEDP). *Diabetologia* 2001;44:898–905.
22. Froguel P, Velho G, Cohen D, et al. Strategies for the collection of sibling-pair data for genetic studies in type 2 (non-insulin-dependent) diabetes mellitus [letter]. *Diabetologia* 1991;34:685.
23. Cox NJ, Xiang KS, Fajans SS, et al. Mapping diabetes-susceptibility genes. Lessons learned from search for DNA marker for maturity-onset diabetes of the young [review]. *Diabetes* 1992;41:401–407.
24. Ryffel GU. Mutations in the human genes encoding the transcription factors of the hepatocyte nuclear factor (HNF)1 and HNF4 families: functional and pathological consequences. *J Mol Endocrinol* 2001;27:11–29.
25. Thomas H, Jaschkowitz K, Bulman M, et al. A distant upstream promoter of the HNF-4alpha gene connects the transcription factors involved in maturity-onset diabetes of the young. *Hum Mol Genet* 2001;10:2089–2097.
26. Boj SF, Parrizas M, Maestro MA, et al. A transcription factor regulatory circuit in differentiated pancreatic cells. *Proc Natl Acad Sci U S A* 2001;98: 14481–14486.
27. Hani EH, Suaud L, Boutin P, et al. A missense mutation in hepatocyte nuclear factor-4 alpha, resulting in a reduced transactivation activity, in human late-onset non-insulin-dependent diabetes mellitus. *J Clin Invest* 1998;101: 521–526.
28. Ilag LL, Tabaei BP, Herman WH, et al. Reduced pancreatic polypeptide response to hypoglycemia and amylin response to arginine in subjects with a mutation in the HNF-4alpha/MODY1 gene. *Diabetes* 2000;49:961–968.
29. Bulman M, Dronsfield MJ, Frayling T, et al. A missense mutation in the hepatocyte nuclear factor 4 alpha gene in a UK pedigree with maturity-onset diabetes of the young. *Diabetologia* 1997;40:859–863.
30. Fajans SS, Brown MB. Administration of sulfonylureas can increase glucose-induced insulin secretion for decades in patients with maturity-onset diabetes of the young. *Diabetes Care* 1993;16:1254–1261.
31. Lehto M, Bitzen PO, Isomaa B, et al. Mutation in the HNF-4 alpha gene affects insulin secretion and triglyceride metabolism. *Diabetes* 1999;48:423–425.
32. Shih DQ, Dansky HM, Fleisher M, et al. Genotype/phenotype relationships in HNF-4 alpha/MODY1: haploinsufficiency is associated with reduced apolipoprotein (AII), apolipoprotein (CIII), lipoprotein(a), and triglyceride levels. *Diabetes* 2000;49:832–837.
33. Byrne MM, Sturis J, Fajans S, et al. Altered insulin secretory responses to glucose in subjects with a mutation in the MODY1 gene on chromosome 20. *Diabetes* 1995;44:699–704.
34. Stoffel M, Duncan SA. Identification of target genes of hepatocyte nuclear factor 4a (HNF-4a). *Diabetes* 1997;46[Suppl 1]):51A(abst).
35. Meglasson MD, Matschinsky FM. Pancreatic islet glucose metabolism and regulation of insulin secretion. *Diabetes Metab Rev* 1986;2:163–214.
36. Matschinsky FM. Glucokinase as glucose sensor and metabolic signal generator in pancreatic b-cell and hepatocytes. *Diabetes* 1990;30:647–752.
37. Tanizawa Y, Matsutani A, Chiu KC, et al. Human glucokinase gene: isolation, structural characterization, and identification of a microsatellite repeat polymorphism. *Mol Endocrinol* 1992;6:1070–1081.
38. Vionnet N, Stoffel M, Takeda J, et al. Nonsense mutation in the glucokinase gene causes early-onset non-insulin-dependent diabetes mellitus. *Nature* 1992; 356:721–722.
39. Stoffel M, Froguel P, Takeda J, et al. Human glucokinase gene: isolation, characterization, and identification of two missense mutations linked to early-onset non-insulin-dependent. *Proc Natl Acad Sci U S A* 1992;89:698–702.
40. Stoffel M, Patel P, Lo YM, et al. Missense glucokinase mutation in maturity-

onset diabetes of the young and mutation screening in late-onset diabetes. *Nat Genet* 1992;2:153–156.
41. Eto K, Sakura H, Shimokawa K, et al. Sequence variations of the glucokinase gene in Japanese subjects with NIDDM. *Diabetes* 1993;42:1133–1137.
42. Velho G, Blanche H, Vaxillaire M, et al. Identification of 14 new glucokinase mutations and description of the clinical profile of 42 MODY-2 families. *Diabetologia* 1997;40:217–224.
43. Hattersley AT, Beards F, Ballantyne E, et al. Mutations in the glucokinase gene of the fetus result in reduced birth weight. *Nat Genet* 1998;19:268–270.
44. Glaser B, Kesavan P, Haymen M, et al. Familial hyperinsulinism caused by an activating glucokinase mutation. *N Engl J Med* 1998;338:226–230.
45. Njolstad P, Sovik O, Cuesta-Munoz A, et al. Permanent neonatal diabetes mellitus due to glucokinase deficiency: an inborn error of the glucose/insulin signaling pathway. *N Engl J Med* 2001;344:1588–1592.
46. Gidh-Jain M, Takeda J, Xu LZ. Glucokinase mutations associated with non-insulin dependent (type 2) diabetes mellitus have decreased enzymatic activity: implications for structure/function relationships. *Proc Natl Acad Sci U S A* 1993;90:1932–1936.
47. Burke CV, Buettger CW, Davis EA, et al. Cell-biological assessment of human glucokinase mutants causing maturity-onset diabetes of the young type 2 (MODY-2) or glucokinase-linked hyperinsulinaemia (GK-HI). *Biochem J* 1999; 342(Pt 2):345–352.
48. Liang Y, Kesavan P, Wang LQ, et al. Variable effects of maturity-onset-diabetes-of-youth (MODY)-associated glucokinase mutations on substrate interactions and stability of the enzyme. *Biochem J* 1995;309(pt 1):167–173.
49. Hattersley AT. Glucokinase mutations and type 2 diabetes. In: Lightman S, ed. *Horizons in medicine*. Bristol: Blackwell Science, 1996:440–449.
50. Stride A, Vaxillaire M, Tuomi T, et al. The genetic abnormality in the beta cell determines the response to an oral glucose load. *Diabetologia* 2002;45:427–435.
51. Page RC, Hattersley AT, Levy JC, et al. Clinical characteristics of subjects with a missense mutation in glucokinase. *Diabet Med* 1995;12:209–217.
52. Pearson ER, Velho G, Clark P, et al. Beta-cell genes and diabetes: quantitative and qualitative differences in the pathophysiology of hepatic nuclear factor-1alpha and glucokinase mutations. *Diabetes* 2001;50[Suppl 1]:S101–S107.
53. Prisco F, Iafusco D, Franzese A, et al. MODY 2 presenting as neonatal hyperglycaemia: a need to reshape the definition of "neonatal diabetes"? *Diabetologia* 2000;43:1331–1332.
54. Appleton M, Ellard S, Bulman M, et al. Clinical characteristics of the HNF1a (MODY3) and glucokinase mutations. *Diabetologia* 1997;40:A161(abst).
55. O'Rahilly S, Hattersley A, Vaag A, et al. Insulin resistance as the major cause of impaired glucose tolerance: a self-fulfilling prophesy? *Lancet* 1994;344: 585–589.
56. Jarrett RJ, McCartney P, Keen H. The Bedford Survey: ten year mortality rates in newly diagnosed diabetics, borderline diabetics and normoglycaemic controls and risk indices for coronary heart disease in borderline diabetics. *Diabetologia* 1982;22:79–84.
57. Velho G, Froguel P, Clement K, et al. Primary pancreatic beta-cell secretory defect caused by mutations in glucokinase gene in kindreds of maturity onset diabetes of the young. *Lancet* 1992;340:444–448.
58. Byrne MM, Sturis J, Clement K, et al. Insulin secretory abnormalities in subjects with hyperglycemia due to glucokinase mutations. *J Clin Invest* 1994;93: 1120–1130.
59. Clement K, Pueyo ME, Vaxillaire M, et al. Assessment of insulin sensitivity in glucokinase-deficient subjects. *Diabetologia* 1996;39:82–90.
60. Velho G, Petersen KF, Pereseghin G, et al. Impaired hepatic glycogen-synthesis in glucokinase-deficient (MODY2) subjects. *J Clin Invest* 1996;98:1755–1761.
61. Saker PJ, Hattersley AT, Barrow B, et al. High prevalence of a missense mutation of the glucokinase gene in gestational diabetic patients due to a founder-effect in a local population. *Diabetologia* 1996;39:1325–1328.
62. Hattersley AT, Turner RC. Mutations of the glucokinase gene and type 2 diabetes [review]. *Q J Med* 1993;86:227–232.
63. Chiu KC, Tanizawa Y, Permutt MA. Glucokinase gene variants in the common form of NIDDM. *Diabetes* 1993;42:579–582.
64. Report of the Expert Committee on the Diagnosis and Classification of Diabetes Mellitus. *Diabetes Care* 1997;20:1183–1197.
65. Ellard S, Beards F, Allen LIS, et al. A high prevalence of glucokinase mutations in gestational diabetic subjects selected by clinical criteria. *Diabetologia* 2000;43:250–253.
66. Katagiri H, Asano T, Ishihara H, et al. Nonsense mutation of glucokinase gene in late-onset non-insulin-dependent diabetes mellitus. *Lancet* 1992;340: 1316–1317.
67. Hattersley AT, Tooke JE. The fetal insulin hypothesis: an alternative explanation of the association of low birthweight with diabetes and vascular disease. *Lancet* 1999;353:1789–1792.
68. Spyer G, Hattersley AT, Sykes JE, et al. Influence of maternal and fetal glucokinase mutations in gestational diabetes. *Am J Obstet Gynecol* 2001;185:240–241.
69. Velho G, Hattersley AT, Froguel P. Maternal diabetes alters birth weight in glucokinase-deficient (MODY2) kindred but has no influence on adult weight, height, insulin secretion or insulin sensitivity. *Diabetologia* 2000;43:1060–1063.
70. Frayling T, Bulman MP, Ellard S, et al. Mutations in the hepatocyte nuclear factor 1 alpha gene are a common cause of maturity-onset diabetes of the young in the United Kingdom. *Diabetes* 1997;46:720–725.
71. Kaisaki PJ, Menzel S, Lindner T, et al. Mutations in the hepatocyte nuclear factor 1 a gene in MODY and early-onset NIDDM: evidence for a mutational hotspot in exon 4. *Diabetes* 1997;45:528–535.
72. Vaxillaire M, Rouard M, Yamagata K, et al. Identification of nine novel mutations in the hepatocyte nuclear factor 1 alpha gene associated with maturity-onset diabetes of the young (MODY3). *Hum Mol Genet* 1997;6:583–586.
73. Hansen T, Eiberg H, Rouard M, et al. Novel MODY3 mutations in the hepatic nuclear factor-1a gene: evidence for a hyperexcitability of pancreatic B-cells to intravenous secretagogues in a glucose tolerant carrier of a P447L mutation. *Diabetes* 1997;46:726–730.
74. Gragnoli C, Lindner T, Cockburn BN, et al. Maturity-onset diabetes of the young due to a mutation in the hepatocyte nuclear factor-4 alpha binding site in the promoter of the hepatocyte nuclear factor-1 alpha gene. *Diabetes* 1997; 46:1648–1651.
75. Glucksmann MA, Lehto M, Tayber O, et al. Novel mutations and a mutational hotspot in the MODY3 gene. *Diabetes* 1997;46:1081–1086.
76. Iwasaki N, Oda N, Ogata M, et al. Mutations in the hepatocyte nuclear factor-1a/MODY3 gene in Japanese subjects with early- and late-onset NIDDM. *Diabetes* 1997;46:1504–1508.
77. Frayling TM, Bulman MP, Appleton M, et al. A rapid screening method for hepatocyte nuclear factor 1 alpha; prevalence in maturity-onset diabetes of the young and late-onset non-insulin dependent diabetes. *Hum Genet* 1997; 101:351–354.
78. Menzel R, Kaisaki PJ, Rjasanowski I, et al. A low renal threshold for glucose in diabetic patients with a mutation in the hepatocyte nuclear factor-1alpha (HNF-1alpha) gene. *Diabet Med* 1998;15:816–820.
79. Bingham C, Ellard S, Nicholls AJ, et al. The generalized aminoaciduria seen in patients with hepatocyte nuclear factor-1alpha mutations is a feature of all patients with diabetes and is associated with glucosuria. *Diabetes* 2001;50: 2047–2052.
80. Lehto M, Tuomi T, Mahtani MM, et al. Characterization of the MODY3 phenotype. Early-onset diabetes caused by an insulin secretion defect. *J Clin Invest* 1997;99:582–591.
81. Sovik O, Njolstad P, Folling I, et al. Hyperexcitability to sulphonylurea in MODY3. *Diabetologia* 1998;41:607–608.
82. Pearson ER, Liddell WG, Shepherd M, et al. Sensitivity to sulphonylureas in patients with hepatocyte nuclear factor 1 alpha gene mutations: evidence for pharmacogenetics in diabetes. *Diabet Med* 2000;17:543–545.
83. Isomaa B, Henricsson M, Lehto M, et al. Chronic diabetic complications in patients with MODY3 diabetes. *Diabetologia* 1998;41:467–473.
84. Lee BC, Appleton M, Shore AC, et al. Impaired maximum microvascular hyperaemia in patients with MODY 3 (hepatocyte nuclear factor-1alpha gene mutations). *Diabet Med* 1999;16:731–735.
85. Byrne MM, Sturis J, Menzel S, et al. Altered insulin secretory responses to glucose in diabetic and nondiabetic subjects with mutations in the diabetes susceptibility gene MODY3 on chromosome 12. *Diabetes* 1996;45:1503–1510.
86. Appleton M, Hattersley AT. Maturity onset diabetes of the young: a missed diagnosis. *Diabet Med* 1996[Suppl 2]:AP3.
87. Tattersall RB. The present status of maturity-onset type diabetes of young people (MODY). In: Kobberling R, Tattersal J, eds. *The genetics of diabetes mellitus*. London: Academic Press, 1982:261–270.
88. Pontoglio M, Prie D, Cheret C, et al. HNF1 alpha controls renal glucose reabsorption in mouse and man. *EMBO Rep* 2000;1:359–365.
89. Wang H, Maechler P, Hagenfeldt KA, et al. Dominant-negative suppression of HNF-1alpha function results in defective insulin gene transcription and impaired metabolism-secretion coupling in a pancreatic beta-cell line. *EMBO J* 1998;17:6701–6713.
90. Wang H, Antinozzi PA, Hagenfeldt KA, et al. Molecular targets of a human HNF1 alpha mutation responsible for pancreatic beta-cell dysfunction. *EMBO J* 2000;19:4257–4264.
91. Shih DQ, Screenan S, Munoz KN, et al. Loss of HNF-1alpha function in mice leads to abnormal expression of genes involved in pancreatic islet development and metabolism. *Diabetes* 2001;50:2472–2480.
92. Wobser H, Dussmann H, Kogel D, et al. Dominant-negative suppression of HNF-1 alpha results in mitochondrial dysfunction, INS-1 cell apoptosis, and increased sensitivity to ceramide-, but not to high glucose-induced cell death. *J Biol Chem* 2002;277:6413–6421.
93. Hagenfeldt-Johansson KA, Herrera PL, Wang H, et al. Beta-cell-targeted expression of a dominant-negative hepatocyte nuclear factor-1 alpha induces a maturity-onset diabetes of the young (MODY)3-like phenotype in transgenic mice. *Endocrinology* 2001;142:5311–5320.
94. Yamagata K, Nammo T, Moriwaki M, et al. Overexpression of dominant-negative mutant hepatocyte nuclear fctor-1 alpha in pancreatic beta-cells causes abnormal islet architecture with decreased expression of E-cadherin, reduced beta-cell proliferation, and diabetes. *Diabetes* 2002;51:114–123.
95. Shih DQ, Stoffel M. Dissecting the transcriptional network of pancreatic islets during development and differentiation. *Proc Natl Acad Sci U S A* 2001;98: 14189–14191.
96. Stoffers DA, Stanojevic V, Habener JF. Insulin promoter factor-1 gene mutation linked to early-onset type 2 diabetes mellitus directs expression of a dominant negative isoprotein. *J Clin Invest* 1998;102:232–241.
97. Hara M, Lindner TH, Paz VP, et al. Mutations in the coding region of the insulin promoter factor 1 gene are not a common cause of maturity-onset diabetes of the young in Japanese subjects. *Diabetes* 1998;47:845–846.
98. Macfarlane W, Frayling T, Ellard S, et al. Missense mutations in the insulin promoter factor 1 (IPF-1) gene predispose to type 2 diabetes. *J Clin Invest* 1999;104:R33–R39.
99. Hani EH, Stoffers DA, Chevre JC, et al. Defective mutations in the insulin promoter factor-1 (IPF-1) gene in late-onset type 2 diabetes mellitus. *J Clin Invest* 1999;104:R41–8.

100. Weng J, MacFarlane W, Lehto M, et al. Functional consequences of mutations in the MODY4 gene (IPF-1) and co-existence with MODY3 mutation. *Diabetologia* 2001;44:249–258.
101. Clocquet AR, Egan JM, Stoffers DA, et al. Impaired insulin secretion and increased insulin sensitivity in familial maturity-onset diabetes of the young 4 (insulin promoter factor 1 gene). *Diabetes* 2000;49:1856–1864.
102. Horikawa Y, Iwasaki N, Hara M, et al. Mutation in hepatocyte nuclear factor-1b gene (TCF2) associated with MODY. *Nat Genet* 1997;17:384–385.
103. Beards F, Frayling T, Bulman M, et al. Mutations in hepatocyte nuclear factor 1 beta are not a common cause of maturity-onset diabetes of the young in the U.K. *Diabetes* 1998;47:1152–1154.
104. Bingham C, Ellard S, Cole TR, et al. Solitary functioning kidney and diverse genital tract malformations associated with hepatocyte nuclear factor-1beta mutations. *Kidney Int* 2002;61:1243–1251.
105. Bingham C, Bulman M, Ellard S, et al. Mutations in the HNF1-beta gene are associated with familial hypoplastic glomerulocystic kidney disease. *Am J Hum Genet* 2001;68:219–224.
106. Bingham C, Ellard S, Allen L, et al. Abnormal nephron development associated with a frameshift mutation in the transcription factor hepatocyte nuclear factor-1 beta. *Kidney Int* 2000;57:898–907.
107. Iwasaki N, Ogata M, Tomonaga O, et al. Liver and kidney function in Japanese patients with maturity-onset diabetes of the young. *Diabetes Care* 1998;21:2144–2148.
108. Nishigori H, Yamada S, Kohama T, et al. Frameshift mutation, A263fsinsGG, in the hepatocyte nuclear factor-1 beta gene associated with diabetes and renal dysfunction. *Diabetes* 1998;47:1354–1355.
109. Lindner TH, Njolstad PR, Horikawa Y, et al. A novel syndrome of diabetes mellitus, renal dysfunction and genital malformation associated with a partial deletion of the pseudo-POU domain of hepatocyte nuclear factor-1beta. *Hum Mol Genet* 1999;8:2001–2008.
110. Malecki MT, Jhala US, Antonellis A, et al. Mutations in NEUROD1 are associated with the development of type 2 diabetes mellitus. *Nat Genet* 1999;23: 323–328.
111. Waeber G, Delplanque J, Bonny C, et al. The gene MAPK8IP1, encoding islet-brain-1, is a candidate for type 2 diabetes. *Nat Genet* 2000;24:291–295.
112. Winter WE, MacLaren NK, Riley WJ, et al. Maturity onset diabetes of youth in black Americans. *N Engl J Med* 1987;316:285–291.
113. Winter WE, Nakamura M, House DV, Monogenic diabetes mellitus in youth. The MODY syndromes. *Endocrinol Metab Clin North Am* 1999;28:765–785.
114. Shepherd M, Ellis I, Ahmad AM, et al. Predictive genetic testing in maturity-onset diabetes of the young (MODY). *Diabet Med* 2001;18:417–421.
115. Shepherd M, Hattersley AT, Sparkes AC. Predictive genetic testing in diabetes: a case study of multiple perspectives. *Qual Health Res* 2000;10:242–259.

CHAPTER 27

Secondary Forms of Diabetes

Om P. Ganda

The term *secondary diabetes* generally refers to diabetes or glucose intolerance that develops in association with disorders (or factors) other than those currently defined as type 1 or type 2 diabetes mellitus or gestational diabetes mellitus. According to the classification system developed by the Expert Committee on the Diagnosis and Classification of Diabetes Mellitus (1), the subclass "secondary diabetes" contains a variety of types of diabetes, in some of which the etiologic relationship is known (e.g., diabetes secondary to pancreatic disease, endocrine disease, or administration of certain drugs). In others, an etiologic relationship is suspected because of a higher frequency of association of diabetes with a syndrome or condition (e.g., a number of genetic syndromes). The extent of glucose intolerance in patients with secondary forms of diabetes varies widely, presenting as insulin-requiring or non–insulin-requiring overt diabetes, simulating type 1 (insulin-dependent diabetes mellitus) or type 2 diabetes (non–insulin-dependent diabetes mellitus) or as milder forms such as impaired fasting glucose (IFG), impaired glucose tolerance (IGT), or minimally abnormal glucose tolerance, considered nondiagnostic. Another complexity in the evolution of secondary diabetes is that an underlying coexisting predisposition to primary diabetes might be unmasked, a not uncommon occurrence, considering the prevalence of diabetes and the presumed genetic underpinnings of diabetes in the population.

Table 27.1 presents a classification of various forms of secondary diabetes. When diabetes is secondary to pancreatic disorders, particularly when β-cell mass is greatly reduced, e.g., by malignancy or pancreatectomy, or when diabetes is due to chemical agents toxic to the β-cell, e.g., pentamidine or pyriminil (Vacor), overt diabetes with or without ketoacidosis often will result, depending on the extent of β-cell loss. On the other hand, when diabetes is secondary to endocrinopathies leading to counterregulatory hormone production (e.g., acromegaly, Cushing syndrome, hyperthyroidism), overt diabetes, or ketoacidosis are unusual, thanks to the capacity of the β-cell reserve (2,3). Thus, the net metabolic outcome in patients with secondary diabetes depends on the direct or indirect impact of the underlying disorders on (a) insulin secretion, i.e., inhibition or compensatory hyperinsulinemia; (b) insulin sensitivity, i.e., glucose utilization; and (c) hepatic glucose output.

TABLE 27.1. A Classification of Secondary Forms of Diabetes or Impaired Glucose Tolerance

A. Pancreatic disorders
  a. Pancreatectomy
  b. Pancreatitis
  c. Cystic fibrosis
  d. Pancreatic cancer
  e. Hemochromatosis
B. Endocrinopathies
  a. Disorders of growth hormone secretion
    1. Acromegaly
    2. Growth hormone deficiency states
  b. Hyperprolactinemic states
  c. Glucocorticoid excess (Cushing syndrome)
  d. Catecholamine excess (pheochromocytoma)
  e. Primary hyperaldosteronism
  f. Hyperthyroidism
  g. Disorders of calcium and phosphorus metabolism
  h. Tumors of endocrine pancreas or gut (see Chapter 70)
    1. Glucagonoma
    2. Somatostatinoma
    3. Pancreatic cholera syndrome
    4. Carcinoid syndrome
    5. Multiple endocrine neoplasia (MEN) syndromes
  i. Polyglandular deficiency syndromes (see Chapter 69)
  j. Polyneuropathy, organomegaly, endocrinopathy, monoclonal gammopathy, skin changes (POEMS) syndrome
C. Drugs, chemical agents, and toxins
  a. Diuretics and antihypertensive agents: Thiazides; chlorthalidone; loop diuretics (furosemide, ethacrynic acid, metolazone); diazoxide; clonidine; β-adrenergic antagonists
  b. Hormones: Glucocorticoids, adrenocorticotropic hormone, α-adrenergic agonists, growth hormone, glucagon, oral contraceptives, progestational agents
  c. Psychoactive agents: Lithium, opiates, ethanol, phenothiazines, atypical antipsychotics
  d. Anticonvulsants: Diphenylhydantoins (Dilantin)
  e. Antineoplastic agents: Streptozotocin, L-asparaginase, mithramycin
  f. Antiprotozoal agents: Pentamidine
  g. Rodenticides: Pyriminil (Vacor)
  h. Miscellaneous: Nicotinic acid, immunosuppressants, *N*-nitrosamines, theophylline, protease inhibitors
D. Genetic syndromes
  a. Pancreatic deficiencies
    1. Congenital absence of pancreatic islets
    2. Cystic fibrosis
    3. Hereditary relapsing pancreatitis
  b. Inborn errors of metabolism
    1. Glycogen storage disease
    2. Acute intermittent porphyria
  c. Severe to extreme insulin resistance syndromes (see Chapter 28)
    1. Type A syndrome: Classic and variants
    2. Type B syndrome: Associated with autoantibodies to insulin receptor
    3. Leprechaunism
    4. Lipodystrophic syndromes
    5. Rabson-Mendenhall syndrome (precocious puberty, dental dysplasia, dystrophic nails)
    6. Ataxia-telangiectasia
    7. Alstrom syndrome (obesity, retinitis pigmentosa, deafness)
    8. Myotonic dystrophy
  d. Obesity-associated insulin resistance
    1. Laurence-Moon-Biedl syndrome
    2. Bardet-Biedl syndrome
    3. Prader-Willi syndrome
    4. Achondroplasia
  e. Progeroid syndromes
    1. Werner syndrome
    2. Cockayne syndrome (microcephaly, dwarfism, deafness, nephropathy)
  f. Chromosomal defects
    1. Down syndrome (trisomy 21)
    2. Klinefelter syndrome (47,XXY)
    3. Turner syndrome (45,XO)
  g. Hereditary neuromuscular disorders
    1. Muscular dystrophy
    2. Huntington chorea
    3. Friedreich ataxia (spinocerebellar ataxia)
    4. Machado disease (ataxia, dysarthria, nystagmus)
    5. Herrmann syndrome (photomyoclonus, dementia, deafness, nephropathy)
    6. Stiff-man syndrome
    7. DIDMOAD syndrome (diabetes insipidus, diabetes mellitus, optic atrophy, deafness), or Wolfram syndrome, and variants
    8. Mitochondrial DNA disorders (maternally inherited diabetes and deafness, MIDD)

PANCREATIC DIABETES

Pancreatectomy

Diabetes that results from pancreatectomy is, in a mechanistic sense, the prototype of insulin-deficient secondary diabetes. The amount of human pancreas that must be surgically removed or pathologically destroyed before the development of fasting hyperglycemia is a matter of some debate. Of interest, elegant studies in baboons revealed that after induction of diabetes with streptozotocin, the animals developed fasting hyperglycemia and a reduction in β-cell function *in vivo* when 40% to 50% of the β-cell mass was still detectable by islet morphometric assessment (4). Furthermore, of 28 healthy human donors who underwent 50% pancreatectomy, 7 (25%) developed glucose intolerance and a deterioration in insulin secretion after 8 to 15 months (5) (Fig. 27.1). However, none of these individuals developed overt diabetes during this time. It has been suggested that development of diabetes in partially pancreatectomized humans depends on several additional factors, such as rate of regeneration of β-cells, changes in nutritional status caused by weight loss and concomitant exocrine insufficiency, and the glucagon deficiency resulting from loss of α-cells (6).

Subtotal or total pancreatectomy theoretically provides a model for diabetes with "pure" insulin deficiency, because glucagon also should be absent (7). However, there are many reports of normal or elevated levels of immunoreactive glucagon (IRG) originating from extrapancreatic sources (gastrointestinal) in such patients (8–10). In most studies, the majority of this IRG comprised larger-molecular-weight material, which does not have biologic activity, but small quantities of 3500-kDa pancreatic glucagon may also be detectable (8). The biologic significance of extrapancreatic glucagon in these patients is not known, and their levels of IRG do not respond to arginine administration, although paradoxical stimulation in response to oral glucose or mixed meals has been reported (8,10).

The clinical presentation of diabetes in pancreatectomized humans differs from that of type 1 diabetes in several respects:

- Because of coexisting exocrine deficiency, pancreatectomized individuals present a nutritional challenge. They tend to be leaner than patients with type 1 diabetes and present with various degrees of malabsorption despite treatment with pancreatic enzyme supplements. Consequently, their insulin requirements are lower than those of weight-matched patients with type 1 diabetes (11).
- Pancreatectomized patients are more prone to hypoglycemia and may have a more sluggish and delayed recovery from hypoglycemia. The reasons for these differences are multiple. Glucose turnover and gluconeogenesis are considerably diminished, and levels of gluconeogenic precursors (alanine, lactate, pyruvate) are markedly increased owing to lack of glucagon (12,13); these changes are reversible by physiologic replacement of glucagon. Furthermore, epinephrine release in response to hypoglycemia may be markedly blunted (14), possibly due to recurrent episodes

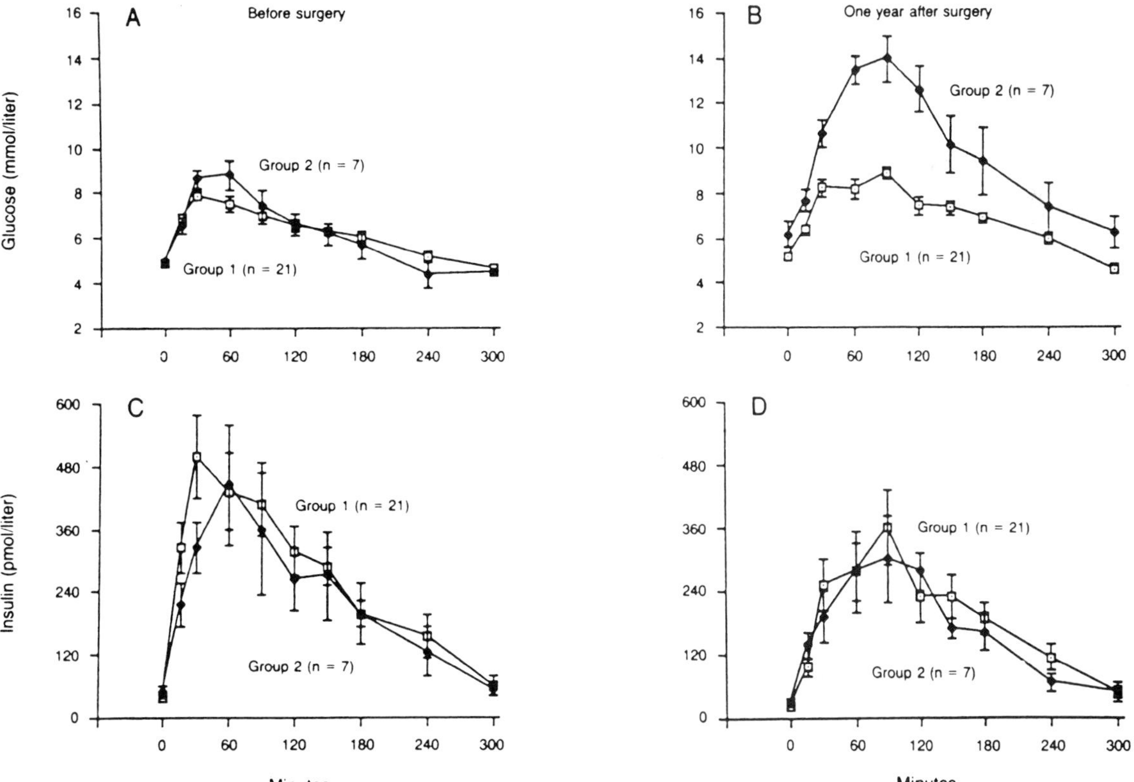

Figure 27.1. Mean (± SEM) serum glucose levels **(A, B)** and serum insulin levels **(C, D)**, measured before and 1 year after hemipancreatectomy during 5-hour oral glucose tolerance tests in 21 transplant donors with normal glucose tolerance at 1 year (*group 1; open squares*) and 7 donors with abnormal glucose tolerance at 1 year (*group 2; closed circles*). (From Kendall DM, Sutherland DER, Najarian JS, et al. Effects of hemipancreatectomy on insulin secretion and glucose tolerance in healthy humans. *N Engl J Med* 1990;322:898–903, with permission. Copyright © 1990 Massachusetts Medical Society. All rights reserved.)

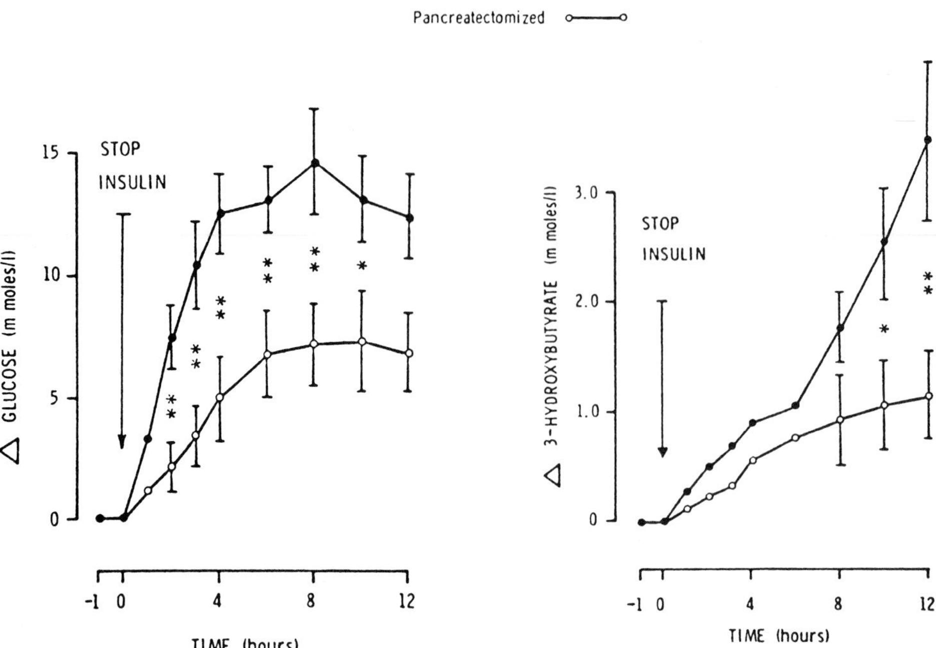

Figure 27.2. Changes in blood concentrations (mean ± SEM) of glucose and 3-hydroxybutyrate in patients with type 1 diabetes (n = 6) and pancreatectomized subjects (n = 4) after withdrawal of insulin. $^{*}P < 0.05$; $^{**}P < 0.02$. (From Barnes AJ, Bloom SR, Alberti KGMM, et al. Ketoacidosis in pancreatectomized man. *N Engl J Med* 1977;296:1250–1253, with permission. Copyright © 1977 Massachusetts Medical Society. All rights reserved.)

of hypoglycemia. Thus, combined defects in glucagon and epinephrine may underlie prolonged and delayed recovery from hypoglycemia in such patients.

- Ketonemia and ketoacidosis are less severe in pancreatectomized patients despite comparable stimulation of lipolysis. As shown in Figure 27.2, withdrawal of insulin for 12 hours from totally pancreatectomized subjects (n = 4) and age- and weight-matched patients with type 1 diabetes (n = 6) resulted in about a 50% reduction in the magnitude of hyperglycemia and hyperketonemia in the former (15). There were no significant differences in levels of free fatty acids and glycerol. Glucagon was undetectable before and after insulin withdrawal in pancreatectomized subjects (7,15). These studies strongly support the important role of glucagon in the promotion of ketogenesis but also argue against a primary role of glucagon in the induction of ketoacidosis.
- The issue of insulin sensitivity and peripheral glucose utilization following pancreatectomy is controversial. Although some investigators reported increased cellular insulin binding and enhanced hepatic and extrahepatic insulin sensitivity (16), others observed a state of peripheral insulin resistance (17) that was further impaired by glucagon replacement (18). Some of these discrepancies may be explained by differences in patient characteristics and alcohol intake and by the lack of consistent control for the induction of insulin resistance by antecedent hyperglycemia per se.

Pancreatitis

Diabetes secondary to pancreatitis accounts for fewer than 1% of cases of diabetes in the United States and other Western countries. However, in many parts of the world (especially tropical countries), the proportion is much higher.

Transient hyperglycemia may be seen in up to 50% of patients with acute pancreatitis in the absence of further attacks, but persistent diabetes develops—presumably as a result of ongoing chronic, painless pancreatitis—in fewer than 5% of such individuals during long-term follow-up in the absence of further attacks (19). On the other hand, in patients with chronic, relapsing pancreatitis, the incidence of diabetes increases over the years, being present in about 40% to 50% of patients after 20 years, with an additional 25% to 30% having IGT (19,20). Among patients with fibrocalcific pancreatitis, up to 80% to 90% have overt diabetes or IGT (19,20). In Western societies, the etiology of chronic pancreatitis is largely alcohol related in both patients with and without biliary disease. The precise mechanisms by which chronic pancreatic inflammation leads to glucose intolerance are not established, but compromised blood flow to islets from fibrotic scarring of exocrine pancreas may play a role. Insulin and C-peptide secretory responses to various secretagogues, including orally and intravenously administered glucose, sulfonylureas, glucagon, and amino acids, are impaired, and these abnormalities are correlated with the magnitude of exocrine pancreatic dysfunction (19,21,22). Glucagon levels are markedly increased in acute pancreatitis, both in the basal state and following stimulation with alanine. This increase may contribute to the transient hyperglycemia frequently seen in this situation (23). In chronic pancreatitis, the basal glucagon levels are normal or elevated, but the responses to amino acids (9,23) or to insulin-induced hypoglycemia (24,25) usually are found to be blunted. In some studies, however, levels of glucagon-like immunoreactivity were increased after stimulation (20,26), perhaps due to glucagon derived from extrapancreatic sources, but the significance of this observation is uncertain. Finally, in a small series of patients with chronic pancreatitis, a partial hepatic insulin resistance was shown in the presence of pancreatic polypeptide (PP) deficiency, which was reversible by PP infusion (27).

Patients with diabetes secondary to chronic pancreatitis may show a delayed recovery from hypoglycemia, a situation similar to that seen in pancreatectomized subjects. However, the incidence and severity of hypoglycemia in these patients are influenced by a number of other factors, e.g., alcohol intake, nutritional status, and state of malabsorption.

Subtle abnormalities of pancreatic exocrine function may sometimes be seen in patients with type 1 or type 2 diabetes (28,29), a finding that suggests the loss of a trophic effect of islet cell secretion on acinar cell function. These abnormalities, usually asymptomatic, may occasionally be difficult to differentiate from chronic, painless pancreatitis and may make additional diagnostic workup necessary.

Cystic Fibrosis

Cystic fibrosis (CF), one of the most common autosomal recessive disorders in the white population, leads to chronic progressive pulmonary disease and pancreatic insufficiency. With the increasing life expectancy of patients with CF, the incidence of diabetes due to CF has been increasing as a comorbidity. IGT or diabetes has been reported in up to 50% of adult patients with CF (30–32). Progressive insulin deficiency develops because of fibrotic destruction of islets and a marked decrease in β-cell mass (31). In addition, islet amyloid deposition was detected in 69% of 41 diabetic cases in one series (33). The extent of glucose intolerance depends also on additional factors, e.g., malnutrition, infections, and liver dysfunction. Recently, an increased prevalence of mutations in the cystic fibrosis transmembrane conductance regulator (CFTR) gene was reported in patients with "idiopathic" chronic pancreatitis as well as "alcoholic" chronic pancreatitis in the absence of any diagnostic features of CF (34,35). In most of these patients, one abnormal allele was detected. Thus, heterozygosity for CFTR mutation might be an underlying defect in many adult patients presenting with chronic pancreatitis.

Pancreatic Cancer

Pancreatic malignancy, leading to loss of β-cell mass, is a well-known cause of diabetes. However, whether diabetes is a risk factor for pancreatic malignancy remains controversial. In some case-control studies, diabetes could not be shown to be a risk factor, after excluding patients with recent onset (<3 years) of hyperglycemia (36). However, in a large meta-analysis of 20 case-control or cohort studies, a twofold relative risk of pancreatic cancer was found, even after excluding those with diabetes of up to 5 years of duration (37). Furthermore, in a large, prospective cohort study, with a 25-year duration of follow-up, a progressive increase in the risk of pancreatic cancer was seen with increasing glucose levels following a glucose load at baseline (38). Whether hyperglycemia itself or the associated metabolic abnormalities, e.g., hyperinsulinemia or abnormalities in the insulin-like growth factor (IGF) axis, are involved in pancreatic carcinogenesis is unclear. In a series of patients with pancreatic cancer, with or without diabetes, levels of islet amyloid polypeptide (IAPP) were more than twice as high in those with diabetes compared with those with normal glucose tolerance (39).

HEMOCHROMATOSIS

Prevalence and Clinical Features

Hemochromatosis is the most common autosomal recessive disorder; the gene frequency is 7% to 10% among white populations, and the disease prevalence is 2 to 4 per 1,000 population (40–44). The disease is expressed three to five times more frequently in men than in women, since about 60% to 80% of homozygous women do not accumulate iron significantly because of menstrual blood loss and pregnancies.

The hemochromatosis gene (HFE) has been localized to chromosome 6, and two missense point mutations, C282Y and H63D, account for 65% to 100% of all patients of European descent (41,44). H63D is not deleterious by itself but probably acts synergistically in persons who are also heterozygotes for C282Y. In large series of participants, gene frequencies for C282Y and H63D mutations were 5% to 6% and 13% to 15%, respectively, whereas about 2% were compound heterozygotes. However, only about 50% of homozygotes for C282Y express clinical features of hemochromatosis, more commonly men than women (45,46).

Iron deposition occurs primarily in parenchymal cells of liver, pancreas, adrenals, anterior pituitary, myocardium, and skeletal muscle. The classic triad of hepatomegaly, diabetes, and skin pigmentation ("bronze diabetes"), once considered common, is in fact not a frequent association, considering the changing clinical presentation associated with early diagnosis and earlier treatment (41,45). Some of the common presenting symptoms are hepatomegaly with or without abdominal pain, arthralgias, fatigue, and impotence. Presence of symptoms usually correlates with the severity of iron accumulation as documented by liver biopsy and with the presence of cirrhosis. Cirrhosis was present at diagnosis in about 70% of patients prior to the availability of genetic tests (47). Hepatocellular carcinoma develops in about 15% to 30% of patients, depending on patients' longevity, despite the successful removal of iron.

Hemochromatosis may have a number of secondary causes, including sideroblastic anemias (chiefly thalassemia major), chronic hemolytic anemias, multiple blood transfusions, porphyria cutanea tarda, and dietary or medical iron overload, e.g., consumption of iron-rich beer among the Bantus (40,41). None of these conditions is linked with HFE gene mutations (41). The severity of total-body iron load produced by these states is variable but is usually less than the loads of 30 g or more seen in primary (idiopathic) hemochromatosis. Alcohol promotes iron absorption but does not, by itself, result in hemochromatosis.

Diabetes in Hemochromatosis

Abnormal glucose tolerance occurs in up to 75% to 80% of patients with hemochromatosis; of these, 50% to 60% have overt diabetes (45,47,48). Similarly, glucose intolerance was present in about 50% of patients with thalassemia major following chronic transfusion therapy (49,50). In a large series of patients with hemochromatosis, 25% had first-degree relatives with diabetes (48).

Conversely, hemochromatosis was diagnosed in 1.3% of 894 patients with diabetes by the old criteria in Italy, where the gene frequency is lower (51). The prevalence in age- and sex-matched controls was 0.2%. The pathogenesis of glucose intolerance in iron-overload states remains controversial, because multiple factors, including cirrhosis, pancreatic iron deposition, and underlying primary diabetes, can be involved. However, the severity of cirrhosis and iron load is correlated with the degree of glucose intolerance, and the control of diabetes improves in 35% to 45% of all patients following iron depletion (40,47).

Studies of β-cell and α-cell function in the presence of iron overload have revealed several interesting features. Patients who develop overt diabetes usually have impaired β-cell function (48,49), and about 40% to 50% of them require insulin therapy. However, in patients studied in a precirrhotic stage and in those who have not developed overt diabetes, significant hyperinsulinemia was observed in response to oral glucose (52,53) and during a hyperglycemic clamp (53). Furthermore, rates of insulin-mediated glucose disposal were impaired in patients with transfusion-induced iron overload in the latter study (53). These observations suggest that insulin resistance secondary to hepatic or extrahepatic (muscle?) iron deposition precedes the β-cell dysfunction and overt diabetes that eventually develop. However, the mechanism of insulin resistance produced by iron overload remains unknown. In histopathologic studies, an increase in β-cell mass was demonstrated in a small number of nondiabetic or mildly diabetic patients with iron overload (54). However, whether iron infiltration of pancreatic islets explains the later β-cell dysfunction remains controversial. In patients with hemochromatosis, glucagon secretion was augmented by arginine and was not suppressed by oral glucose (55,56), responses similar to those seen in primary diabetes. In this respect, the α-cell responses seem to differ from those seen in patients with chronic pancreatitis (21,22) and are in keeping with the observation that iron deposition in islets, albeit variable, is restricted to β-cells (54).

In making the diagnosis of hemochromatosis, it should be noted that biochemical tests of iron metabolism, i.e., determinations of serum iron, transferrin saturation, and ferritin levels, are helpful but are not as specific for the diagnosis as is the hepatic histology (41). The availability of genetic tests helps diagnosis in relatives at early stages (45). Recently, attention was drawn to the presence of hyperferritinemia in 10% to 30% of unselected patients with type 2 diabetes (57). In most cases, the hyperferritinemia in such patients resolved spontaneously or proved to be due to other causes when follow-up studies were done (58). An underlying chronic inflammatory state also may result in a nonspecific increase in iron stores in patients with insulin resistance; the relevance of this to development of diabetes and its complications needs further study (59). Such studies underscore the need for confirmation of results, particularly when patients with diabetes are being screened for hemochromatosis.

Management and Prognosis

Regular phlebotomy treatment, often lifelong, remains the treatment of choice for hemochromatosis. Successful iron depletion, initiated early in the course of disease, clearly reduces the incidence and progression of cirrhosis, improves diabetes control, and frequently reduces damage to other target organs and overall morbidity and mortality (41,47). In a large prospective study of 163 patients, with a mean follow-up period of 10.5 ± 5.6 years, the major determinants of reduced survival included the presence of cirrhosis, diabetes, and failure of iron depletion (47) (Fig. 27.3). Mortality ratios (observed/expected) for liver cancer, cardiomyopathy, cirrhosis, and diabetes were 219, 306, 13, and 7, respectively, for patients with hematochromatosis as compared with those for the general population in this study. Successful iron depletion, however, did not protect from the development of liver cancer.

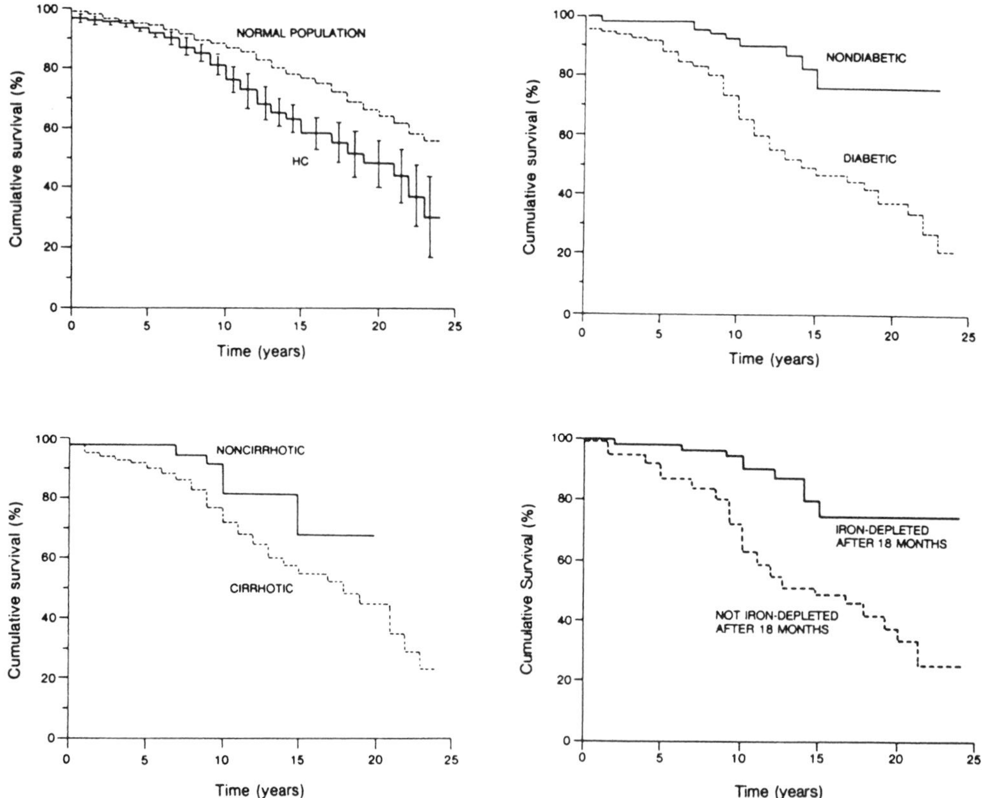

Figure 27.3. Cumulative survival in 163 patients with hemochromatosis compared with normal population and in the same patients with ($n = 112$) or without ($n = 51$) cirrhosis; with ($n = 89$) or without ($n = 74$) diabetes; and depleted ($n = 77$) or not depleted ($n = 75$) of iron during the first 18 months of venesection (see text for details). All differences were statistically significant ($P < 0.05$ to < 0.002 by log-rank test). (From Niederau C, Fischer R, Sonnenberg A, et al. Survival and causes of death in cirrhotic and noncirrhotic patients with primary hemochromatosis. *N Engl J Med* 1985;313:1256–1262, with permission. Copyright © 1985 Massachusetts Medical Society. All rights reserved.)

TABLE 27.2. Sites of Actions of Major Diabetogenic Hormones in Humans

	Liver			Muscle		Adipose tissue	
Hormone	β-cell secretion	Glycogen[a]	Gluconeogenesis	Glucose	Amino acid release	Glucose uptake	Lipolysis
Growth hormone	+	+	+	−	?	−	+
Glucocorticoids	+	+	+	−	+	−	+
Catecholamines	−	−	+	−	−	?	+
Glucagon	+	−	+	0	?	0	?
Thyroid hormones	+	−	+	0	0	?	+

+, stimulation; −, inhibition; 0, no effect; ?, uncertain.
[a]Net effect on glycogen content via glycogen synthesis or glycogenolysis.

In patients unable to undergo phlebotomy, such as those with thalassemia or other forms of anemia, chelation therapy with deferoxamine is an alternative for which the outcome is often successful (41,60,61), although the effects of this regimen on diabetes control have not been studied.

ENDOCRINOPATHIES

The major sites of action of various counterregulatory hormones on target organs and the principal mechanisms of their diabetogenic effects are listed in Table 27.2.

Disorders of Growth Hormone Secretion

Classic experiments, using crude pituitary extracts, performed more than 60 years ago demonstrated a relationship between the anterior pituitary and diabetes (62). In rat pancreatic monolayer cultures derived from an islet tumor cell line (63) or neonatal pancreas (64), growth hormone (GH) stimulated β-cell replication, an effect that was claimed to be independent of GH-induced insulin-like growth factors (64). However, chronic administration of GH in experimental animals over prolonged periods has been shown to result in hypersecretion of insulin followed by eventual loss of β-cells and permanent diabetes (65).

SECRETION AND METABOLIC EFFECTS OF GROWTH HORMONE

The physiology of GH secretion and its diverse metabolic effects on carbohydrate, protein, and lipid metabolism in humans have been studied extensively (66–68). In healthy subjects, GH release is stimulated by hypoglycemia, sleep, exercise, stress, and amino acids and is inhibited by hyperglycemia. Recently, a 28-amino-acid gastric hormone, ghrelin, has been identified as a potent ligand for GH secretagogue receptor (GHS-R), probably mediating GH secretion in response to various stimuli via neurons in the hypothalamus secreting growth hormone–releasing hormone (GHRH) (69). Infusions of GH in healthy subjects that produce increments in plasma GH levels within the supraphysiologic range (up to 30 to 50 ng/mL) initially result in acute but transient (2 to 4 hours) insulin-like effects, i.e., suppression of hepatic glucose production and enhancement of peripheral glucose clearance (69–72). In fact, insulin levels increase over this period, offering an explanation for some portion of these effects. Subsequently, over a 2- to 12-hour period, similar increments or increments closer to the physiologic range (73) are associated with the "delayed" insulin-antagonistic effects. The primary site of GH-induced insulin resistance resides at the level of peripheral tissues (72,73), as first suggested by the elegant studies of forearm perfusion by Zierler and Rabinowitz (74). Although an effect of GH on inhibition of peripheral glucose uptake is well established, the lipolytic effect has not always been confirmed (67,75).

The understanding of the cellular site of insulin resistance induced by GH is complicated; multiple coexisting factors are involved, including GH concentrations, GH-binding proteins, presence or absence of hyperinsulinemia, and glucose intolerance. In most studies of healthy subjects given GH infusions or of patients with acromegaly, binding of insulin to receptors on circulating monocytes or hepatocytes was found to be little affected as a result of reciprocal effects on receptor number and affinity (72,73,66,76). However, in acromegalic patients with fasting hyperglycemia, the compensatory increase in receptor affinity that occurs in such patients with normoglycemia may fail to occur, a factor contributing to glucose intolerance (77). In cultured adipocytes, GH was shown to inhibit the expression of the gene for the glucose transporter GLUT1 but not that for the transporter GLUT4 (78). Thus, probably both postreceptor and receptor defects in insulin action underlie the diabetogenic effects of GH excess, although the precise nature of these defects remains unknown.

DIABETES IN ACROMEGALY

Anterior pituitary adenomas that hypersecrete GH account for more than 90% of cases of acromegaly (79). Other causes include ectopic (nonpituitary) sources of GH or GHRH, e.g., pancreatic islet cell tumors, carcinoid tumors, and hypothalamic hamartomas.

Glucose intolerance is prevalent in patients with acromegaly, affecting about 60% to 70%. However, overt diabetes requiring treatment occurs in only 10% to 30% of patients (80–83). Even more frequent than glucose intolerance is evidence for insulin resistance, which is manifested by a striking hyperinsulinemia in response to orally or intravenously administered glucose and other secretagogues, as well as markedly attenuated responses to exogenous insulin (67,68,84). Defects in both hepatic action and peripheral glucose disposal have been described in studies using insulin clamp techniques (70,73). Overall, GH levels in individual patients correlate poorly with both hyperinsulinemia and the severity of glucose intolerance. A better correlation of disease activity and glucose intolerance is found with serum levels of insulin-like growth factor 1 (IGF-1) (67,68) or

IGF-binding protein 3 (IGFBP-3) (85). In contrast to patients with acromegaly with normal or impaired glucose tolerance, insulin secretion is quite blunted by the time overt diabetes develops, with or without ketosis (68,84), a finding reminiscent of that in animal models of metasomatotrophic diabetes (65). However, coexistent primary diabetes (type 1 or type 2) may also be present, particularly if diabetes persists after successful treatment of acromegaly in such patients. Considerable evidence exists from studies of somatostatin infusion that lipolytic and ketogenic effects of GH supervene only after significant insulinopenia (71,86). Successful treatment of acromegaly, with normalization of GH and IGF-1, is usually accompanied by striking improvements in glucose tolerance and a reversal of hyperinsulinemia, as well as by normalization of insulin sensitivity (68,82–84). However, the results are unpredictable in those with overt, symptomatic diabetes (84,87). Lack of a complete remission in many patients may be due to incomplete cure of acromegaly, defined as suppression of GH to less than 2.5 ng/mL or to less than 1 ng/mL after oral glucose, using newer, ultrasensitive assays (88). Some have argued that this cut-off should be even lower, i.e., less than 0.5 ng/mL (89). The increase in mortality rate in acromegaly may persist unless GH levels are suppressed to the near-normal range (90,91). Moreover, glucose intolerance and hypertension are independent determinants of acromegalic cardiomyopathy (92).

The long-acting somatostatin analogue octreotide has been shown to be a useful adjunct in the treatment of acromegaly. In large, multicenter trials lasting up to 30 months of 58 and 103 patients, most of whom had previously been treated with surgery or radiotherapy (93,94), treatment with octreotide for 6 months or more resulted in substantial improvement in about 65% of patients. However, biochemical cure, defined by GH less than 5 ng/mL and normal IGF-1, occurred in about 50% of patients, and only approximately 2% to 40% of patients fulfilled the more stringent criterion of GH suppression to less than 2 ng/mL in both of these large series of patients (93,94).

Regarding the effects of octreotide therapy on glucose tolerance, the results from various reports indicate a mixed outcome, depending on the baseline metabolic status (68). On the one hand, in patients with overt diabetes or IGT, significant improvement in glucose tolerance or normalization of diabetes may result after several weeks of treatment. Impressive decreases in insulin requirements among the diabetic subjects within the largest randomized multicenter trial were observed (94). Normalization of GH and IGF-1 was associated with improvements in insulin sensitivity and greater suppression of hepatic glucose output as determined by the euglycemic-hyperinsulinemic clamp technique, whereas peripheral glucose disposal was not affected (95). On the other hand, in patients with normal or minimally impaired glucose tolerance, treatment with octreotide resulted in slight improvement, no change, or even a worsening of glucose tolerance, despite improvements in GH and IGF-1 levels (68,93,96). Thus, an adverse outcome in glucose homeostasis may be seen in some nondiabetic acromegalic patients following treatment with octreotide, depending on baseline characteristics such as β-cell reserve and degree of insulin resistance. Finally, long-term octreotide therapy may result in other side effects, the most important of which is the 40% to 50% incidence of cholelithiasis and/or biliary sludge (94).

Recently, results with longer-acting somatostatin analogues (octreotide LAR and lanreotide) have shown comparable decreases in GH and IGF-1 levels, but the long-term effects on glucose homeostasis with these agents are awaited. Similarly, impressive data on short-term clinical outcome with the growth hormone receptor antagonist, pegvisomant, in a large series of patients with acromegaly were reported recently (97). A 50% decrease in the insulin levels with a modest decrease in glucose levels was reported in that study after 12 to 18 months of follow-up. The long-term effects of this novel approach on glucose intolerance will be of interest.

DIABETES ASSOCIATED WITH ISOLATED GROWTH HORMONE DEFICIENCY

The presence of diabetes in GH-deficient dwarfs presents an interesting paradox. However, it has been known for a number of years that exogenous administration of GH to both normal and hypopituitary subjects augments the insulin response to a variety of secretagogues before a significant change in blood glucose occurs (98). Martin and Gagliardino (99) showed a β-cytotropic effect of GH on isolated pancreatic islets of rats *in vitro*. Similarly, some workers have shown direct effects of GH on islet β-cell replication in neonatal rat-islet monolayer cultures (63,65).

The majority of adult sexual ateliotic dwarfs with monotropic GH deficiency, studied by Merimee and coworkers (100), showed evidence of a mild to moderately severe glucose intolerance and insulin deficiency. It is interesting that after 10 years of follow-up, there was no evidence of diabetic microangiopathy in these dwarfs, despite worsening of glucose intolerance (101). On the one hand, these observations support the concept of a permissive role of GH in the pathogenesis of diabetic vascular disease. On the other hand, the incidence and severity of microangiopathy in patients with acromegaly with a striking increase of ambient GH concentrations do not appear to be increased and may indeed be significantly lower than in patients with genetic diabetes. Further studies on groups of patients well matched for the degree and duration of hyperglycemia are required to settle this question.

A number of long-term follow-up studies in adult patients with hypopituitarism have suggested an increased cardiovascular mortality even after replacement of other hormones (102). This has been ascribed partly to an atherogenic lipid profile, visceral adiposity, and insulin resistance in such patients. Administration of GH in such patients may restore, although not normalize, the cardiovascular risk profile (103). On the other hand, short-term studies with GH therapy over 12 to 30 months also have reported adverse effects on glucose tolerance and insulin sensitivity in hypopituitary adults (104,105). Retinal changes, mimicking diabetic retinopathy, were reported in two nondiabetic patients after 14 to 17 months of treatment with GH (106). However, only 12 cases of overt diabetes were reported among 8,136 GH-treated children (107).

GH is currently being proposed by some as a therapeutic agent for several indications e.g., preservation of lean body mass during aging, human immunodeficiency virus (HIV)–related disorders, prolonged illness, osteoporosis, enhancing tissue repair following surgery or trauma, and stimulation of muscle mass in athletes. Besides its potential for diabetogenic effects, other long-term risks of GH therapy need to be studied before specific recommendations can be made (108).

Hyperprolactinemia

The human prolactin molecule shares considerable homology with the human GH molecule, and an even greater homology exists between their respective mRNAs (79), similarities that suggest a common evolutionary origin. The precise role of prolactin in human physiology is poorly understood (109). A diabetogenic effect of prolactin has been suggested but has not been established in humans. Hyperprolactinemic states are sometimes associated with mild glucose intolerance; however, the difference is of only marginal statistical significance when levels are compared with those for controls (110,111). In one study of 26 patients with prolactinomas, basal levels of glucose and insulin were comparable to those for controls, despite the presence of chronic endogenous hyperprolactinemia in these patients (110). However, oral glucose tolerance was significantly impaired and associated with insulin insensitivity, as reflected by hyperinsulinemia. It is interesting that both glucose intolerance and hyperinsulinism improved after treatment with bromocriptine, which reduced levels of prolactin. Similarly, in a group of nine patients with hyperprolactinemia and the amenorrhea-galactorrhea syndrome, four of whom had pituitary tumors, mild impairment in glucose tolerance associated with elevated basal levels and postglucose insulin levels was found in comparisons with matched controls (111). These changes were similar in some ways to those normally seen in late pregnancy. Whether prolactin causes insulin resistance leading to hyperinsulinemia or exerts direct effects on the β-cell, or both, is not known.

Cushing Syndrome

METABOLIC EFFECTS OF GLUCOCORTICOIDS

Glucocorticoids, like GH, are the principal insulin-antagonistic hormones. They have diverse metabolic effects on liver, adipose tissue, and muscle (112,113). In the liver, glucocorticoids serve as the key promoters of gluconeogenesis by accelerating the biochemical events at every rate-limiting step. Specifically, glucocorticoids stimulate (a) hepatic uptake of amino acids; (b) activation of pyruvate carboxylase in generating pyruvate from amino acids; and (c) activation of phosphoenolpyruvate carboxykinase (PEPCK), the unidirectional rate-limiting enzyme in the initiation of the cascade of gluconeogenesis from pyruvate. Insulin antagonizes the response of PEPCK gene transcription to glucocorticoids and cyclic adenosine monophosphate (cAMP) (114). Paradoxically, glucocorticoids enhance glycogen deposition, an insulin-like effect. It has been proposed that glycogenesis in response to glucocorticoids may be mediated by insulin (112). However, this effect may well be a direct consequence of activation of glycogen synthase by glucocorticoids (113).

At the level of adipose tissue and muscle, glucocorticoids antagonize insulin-mediated uptake and utilization of glucose (115,116). This effect is mediated at the cellular level by multiple mechanisms, including a decrease in insulin receptor affinity (76,117) and defects in insulin receptor signaling (115–117). Dexamethasone was shown to inhibit glucose transport by causing translocation of glucose transporters from the plasma membrane, an effect reversible by insulin (116). Glucocorticoids also exert a permissive effect on lipolysis by promoting the activation of cAMP-dependent hormone-sensitive lipase, a key enzyme inhibited by insulin (112). The net clinical effect of glucocorticoid excess in humans is a relocation of fat depots, which results in the typical truncal obesity of Cushing syndrome. The precise mechanism by which this unique pattern of fat redistribution develops remains unexplained. However, adipose tissues from various sites do show metabolic differences. Lipoprotein lipase activity is increased and lipolytic activity is decreased in abdominal adipose tissue in comparison to that in femoral adipose tissue in patients with Cushing syndrome (118). Glucocorticoids also augment proteolysis in skeletal muscle (112,113), and the relative distribution of types of muscle fibers may be altered (118). Finally, glucocorticoids may have a direct inhibitory effect on insulin release at the level of Ca^{2+}-induced exocytosis (119).

GLUCOCORTICOID-INDUCED DIABETES

In healthy humans, short-term increments in plasma cortisol levels within the range seen in moderate stress situations (~40 μg/dL) result in a slight increase in levels of glucose, which is mediated by both hepatic and extrahepatic effects (120,121), as well as in a significant increase in levels of ketones and branched-chain amino acids (121). However, the effects of chronic administration of moderate doses of glucocorticoids to healthy humans are usually compensated for by increased insulin release, which results in minimal changes in glucose levels. Thus, the spectrum of glucose intolerance in patients with Cushing syndrome or exogenous steroid use depends in large part on endogenous β-cell reserve, a situation similar to that in acromegaly. Glucose intolerance occurs in 75% to 80% of patients with Cushing syndrome, but only 10% to 15% of patients develop overt diabetes (122,123). Almost all patients, however, manifest basal and stimulated hyperinsulinemia and insulin resistance.

A contributory diabetogenic effect of glucocorticoid excess is stimulation of glucagon secretion. Glucocorticoid administration over 3 to 4 days in healthy subjects induced an augmented α-cell responsiveness both during the basal state and following protein ingestion or amino acid infusion (124,125). This effect may be mediated by hyperaminoacidemia brought about by augmented proteolysis and perhaps by decreased glucose utilization by α-cells or some other direct effect of corticosteroids on α-cells.

Pheochromocytoma

METABOLIC EFFECTS OF CATECHOLAMINES

Catecholamines influence insulin secretion directly and produce anti-insulin effects at several loci in intermediary metabolism (126,127). In the human, basal insulin secretion is inhibited by α_2-adrenergic and augmented by β_2-adrenergic stimulation (127,128). The net effect on insulin secretion is governed by the relative local concentrations of epinephrine, norepinephrine, and various other secretagogues. However, the inhibitory effects on the α-receptor generally predominate over the stimulatory effects on the β-receptor. Stimulation of the α-receptor also may promote glucagon secretion. The role of catecholamines in the physiologic regulation of insulin secretion is still uncertain. A 29-amino-acid polypeptide, galanin, was shown to be contained in sympathetic nerve endings in the islets and is proposed to be an additional mediator of insulin inhibition by sympathetic activation (129). In patients with preexisting glucose intolerance, the acute effects of physiologic increments in epinephrine levels on β-cell inhibition are exaggerated, producing greater hyperglycemia than in controls (130).

Catecholamines stimulate hepatic glucose output by promoting glycogenolysis and gluconeogenesis, the former being the predominant immediate effect (127). Glycogenolysis results from the β-adrenergic stimulation of adenyl cyclase, which leads to the release of cAMP. In addition, epinephrine also stimulates hepatic glycogenolysis via a cAMP-independent, Ca^{2+}-dependent pathway involving the α-adrenergic pathway (131). The effects of catecholamines (mainly epinephrine) on adipose tissue (lipolysis) and muscle (glycogenolysis) are mediated primarily via β-adrenergic receptors. In response to β-adrenergic agonists, proteolysis is inhibited (132), but oxidation of branched-chain amino acids is enhanced (133). However, the significance of these effects of catecholamines on muscle nitrogen balance requires further elucidation.

DIABETES IN PHEOCHROMOCYTOMA

Glucose intolerance occurs in about 30% of patients with pheochromocytoma (126,127,134). Multiple mechanisms may contribute to this intolerance, including (a) the α_2-adrenergic inhibition of insulin secretion, (b) β-adrenergic stimulation of hepatic glycogenolysis and gluconeogenesis, and (c) enhanced lipolysis. Overt diabetes and ketoacidosis are distinctly unusual. Administration of α-adrenergic blocking agents, e.g., phentolamine or phenoxybenzamine, characteristically improves insulin secretion and glucose tolerance (126,135,136). Glucagon levels were surprisingly normal in the basal state (135,136) and markedly suppressed in response to arginine (137) or hypoglycemia (138), findings suggesting normal regulation by hyperglycemia despite an enormous increase in circulating catecholamine levels. However, others have reported a normal increase with arginine (126). Surgical removal of the tumor usually restores or improves glucose tolerance within several weeks (134,137); however, in some cases, it may take up to several months.

Primary Hyperaldosteronism

The triad of hypertension, hypokalemia, and glucose intolerance (Conn syndrome) was described in 1955 (139). Contrary to previous estimates, this syndrome accounts for no more than 2% of cases of hypertension (140,141). Glucose intolerance, previously thought to be present in about 50% of patients with Conn syndrome, is somewhat less common and is usually mild. It probably is the result, to a variable degree, of K^+ depletion, which may be responsible for blunted insulin secretion (139,142) and perhaps for increased glycogenolysis. In healthy men, K^+ depletion of 200 to 500 mEq (110% of total body K^+) during 5- to 14-day periods was shown to result in mild glucose intolerance, whereas insulin sensitivity remained essentially unchanged (143). However, it is not certain if the glucose intolerance seen in Conn syndrome is completely explained by K^+ depletion (144).

Hyperthyroidism

Hyperthyroidism is associated with significant aberrations of carbohydrate, lipid, and protein metabolism (145). This state is characterized by increased oxygen consumption, rapid gastric emptying, enhanced gluconeogenesis and glycogenolysis, increased lipolysis and ketogenesis, and increased proteolysis. Many of these effects are reproducible in experimental hyperthyroidism induced in nondiabetic (146) or diabetic (147) individuals. The insulin clearance rate was found to be increased by about 40% (148). The data on peripheral glucose disposal and insulin sensitivity are controversial, perhaps because of differences in the methods used. Some studies reported a decreased peripheral insulin sensitivity (149), whereas most others found it to be normal (148) or increased (146,150) compared with that in controls, primarily because of enhanced rates of glucose oxidation as determined by indirect calorimetry.

An increased incidence of glucose intolerance, usually of mild-to-moderate severity, was documented in 30% to 50% of patients with hyperthyroidism (145,151). Increased sympathetic sensitivity mediated via a β-adrenergic mechanism (126) probably contributes to the increased propensity to lipolysis and ketogenesis in such patients (146,152). Elevated levels of free fatty acids might also contribute to glucose intolerance. In patients with preexisting diabetes, the metabolic consequences of untreated hyperthyroidism on hepatic glucose production, lipolysis, and insulin clearance would facilitate the deterioration of glycemic control and even the development of recurrent ketoacidosis (153). In previously nondiabetic individuals, glucose intolerance persisted in 32% (7 of 22) of patients with hyperthyroidism after 12 years of posttreatment follow-up (151). This may be explained, at least in part, on the basis of common autoimmune mechanisms underlying Graves disease and type 1 diabetes.

Disorders of Calcium and Phosphorus Metabolism

Disorders of calcium and phosphorus metabolism may occasionally be associated with significant changes in insulin secretion or sensitivity or both. Hyperinsulinemia in primary hyperparathyroidism has been reported (154,155) and found to correlate with calcium levels (155), whereas glucose tolerance was preserved. Glucose intolerance has been reported in up to 40% of patients with primary hyperparathyroidism (156), suggesting a state of insulin insensitivity due to raised levels of intracellular calcium. On the other hand, experimental hypophosphatemia was shown to produce insulin insensitivity in dogs (157) and humans (158) and may thus be a possible mediator of insulin resistance in primary hyperparathyroidism. In secondary hyperparathyroidism induced by diet in dogs (157) or in patients with renal insufficiency who had undergone parathyroidectomy (159), no evidence was noted of any direct effects of parathyroid hormone itself on glucose disposal or insulin secretion. However, some patients with diabetes who underwent parathyroidectomy for primary hyperparathyroidism showed an increased sensitivity to endogenous and exogenous insulin postoperatively (156). The α-cell responses to arginine, to a protein meal, and to glucose were found to be normal before and after removal of the parathyroid adenoma (156). For discussions of tumors of the endocrine pancreas or gut and of polyglandular deficiency syndromes see Chapters 69 and 70.

POEMS Syndrome (Polyneuropathy, Organomegaly, Endocrinopathy, Monoclonal Gammopathy, Skin Changes)

POEMS syndrome is a rare form of plasma cell disorder associated with an osteosclerotic type of myeloma and several systemic features. About 100 cases have been reported (160,161). Other eponyms of this entity include Takatsuki syndrome and Crow-Fukase syndrome. In most cases (>90%), the M-component is of the γ-light-chain type. A relationship of this syndrome to multicentric angiofollicular lymph node hyperplasia (Castleman disease) has also been suggested (162). The etiology of these entities is obscure, but they appear to be secondary to a defect in immunoglobulin synthesis.

Glucose intolerance has been reported in 30% to 50% of cases (140,141). Other endocrine features include hypogonadism, hypothyroidism, hyperprolactinemia, and adrenal insufficiency.

DRUGS, CHEMICAL AGENTS, AND TOXINS

Administration of a variety of drugs or chemical agents (Table 27.1) is known to induce glucose intolerance or diabetes in previously nondiabetic subjects or to exacerbate hyperglycemia in patients with previously diagnosed diabetes. The diabetogenic effects may be brought about by effects on islet cell function, either directly or indirectly, or on insulin action at hepatic or extrahepatic sites or may be due to variable combinations of these factors. Table 27.3 presents the principal mechanisms of effects of certain therapeutic agents more commonly associated with glucose intolerance or diabetes.

Diuretics and β-Adrenergic Antagonists

The diabetogenic effects of diuretics, particularly high-dose thiazides and chlorthalidone, and β-adrenergic antagonists have been well recognized in clinical practice (163). A 12-year follow-up epidemiologic study revealed that the risk of developing diabetes over the risk in controls was increased 3- to 4-fold in subjects receiving thiazides, 5- to 6-fold in those receiving β-adrenergic blockers, and 11-fold in subjects receiving both drugs (164). Other large surveys have reported a 40% to 80% increased risk for initiation of treatment for diabetes with

TABLE 27.3. Sites of Action of Drugs or Agents More Commonly Associated with Diabetes or Glucose Intolerance

	Impaired insulin secretion	Impaired insulin action	Comments
Diuretics			
Thiazide	+	±	Effects primarily mediated by K^+ depletion
Loop diuretics	+	0	
Diphenylhydantoin	+	0	Direct β-cell effects
Pentamidine	+	0	Structurally similar to streptozotocin and alloxan
Pyriminil (Vacor)	+	±	
Glucocorticoids	0	+	Also cause hyperglucagonemia
Oral contraceptives	0	+	Effects less prominent than effects of glucocorticoids
Nicotinic acid	0	+	Minimal effects in healthy subjects
β-Adrenergic antagonists	+	+	Effects more common with nonselective agents
Diazoxide	+	+	A nondiuretic thiazide
Cyclosporine	+	+	Often used in combination with glucocorticoids
Opiates	+	±	Also stimulate glucagon secretion
Protease inhibitors	0	+	Associated with lipodystrophy

thiazides and with use of multiple antihypertensive agents with or without thiazides (165). For thiazides, most studies have indicated that the mechanism involved in this increased risk is an insulin secretory defect caused by hypokalemia and that the defect can be corrected by K^+ replacement (144,166). Diazoxide, a nondiuretic thiazide, has pronounced inhibitory effects on the β-cell as well as peripheral effects (167).

For β-blockers, an inhibitory effect on β-cell secretion would be anticipated. Indeed, in some cases, drugs such as propranolol precipitated hyperglycemic, hyperosmolar, non-ketotic coma (168). Moreover, evidence of peripheral effects of propranolol resulting in insulin resistance has also been reported (163).

In a large prospective study of subjects with hypertension, β-blocker use over 3 to 6 years was associated with a 28% increased risk for developing diabetes after adjustment of other risk factors (169). However, the relationship with the type of β-blocker was not studied. The diabetogenic effects of β-blockers should not negate the proven benefits of these agents in reducing mortality in patients with known coronary heart disease.

Diphenylhydantoins

Phenytoin (Dilantin) has direct inhibitory effects on β-cell secretion (170). This effect appears to be dose related, and hyperglycemic, nonketotic coma precipitated by phenytoin toxicity has been reported (163,170).

Glucocorticoids

Glucocorticoid-induced glucose intolerance is characterized by insulin resistance and hyperinsulinemia. As discussed earlier, as in patients with Cushing syndrome, chronic administration of glucocorticoids induces distinct effects on hepatic and extrahepatic sites.

Pentamidine and Pyriminil

Pentamidine, an antiprotozoal agent, and pyriminil (Vacor), a nitrosourea-derived rodenticide, resemble streptozotocin and alloxan chemically. Pentamidine is used in prophylaxis and treatment of *Pneumocystis carinii* infection in patients with acquired immunodeficiency syndrome (AIDS), and an increase in the incidence of insulin-dependent diabetes following its use has been reported (171,172). Use of aerosolized pentamidine, the currently preferred route, has minimized the effects of this agent on carbohydrate metabolism. Similarly, accidental or intentional ingestion of pyriminil may result in the development of insulin-dependent diabetes with or without ketoacidosis as a result of β-cell destruction (173,174). The sequence of events leading to diabetes following use of these agents is similar to that seen with streptozotocin and initially involves a release of insulin from lysed β-cells that lasts for hours and frequently is associated with hypoglycemia and a delayed persistent hyperglycemia caused by β-cell loss after days to weeks (172–174).

Nicotinic Acid

Nicotinic acid in higher dosage causes glucose intolerance by inducing peripheral insulin insensitivity (175). In healthy individuals this is accompanied by minimal changes in glucose tolerance because of adaptive hyperinsulinemia. However, significant hyperglycemia or deterioration in glucose tolerance may result in some patients with a limited β-cell reserve or preexisting diabetes (176,177).

Immunosuppressants

An increased incidence of diabetes in transplant recipients receiving cyclosporine has been reported (163,178). This increase is probably independent of the concomitant diabetogenic effects of corticosteroids in these patients (178,179). Direct inhibitory effects of cyclosporine on β-cells, as well as peripheral effects on glucose transport, have been implicated (163,178). The diabetogenic effects may be more pronounced in African Americans (180). Tacrolimus (FK-506) has also been reported to be associated with an increased incidence of diabetes or worsening of preexisting glucose intolerance (179,181).

Opiates

A hyperglycemic effect of morphine and other opiates has been recognized. Human islets produce β-endorphins and enkephalins. In healthy and diabetic subjects, infusions of β-endorphin resulted in hyperglycemia accompanied by hyperglucagonemia (182). These results are in keeping with the observation of impaired β-cell responsiveness to glucose in subjects addicted to narcotics (183).

Alcohol

Light-to-moderate consumption of alcohol (one to three drinks daily) has been associated with enhanced insulin sensitivity, compared with that in nondrinkers (184). In an epidemiologic survey of a more than 12,000 participants followed up over a period of 3 to 6 years, an intake of more than three drinks of alcohol per day was associated with a 50% increased risk of diabetes in men, whereas no increase in men or women was seen with more moderate intake (185).

Protease Inhibitors

Several recent studies have reported an association between the use of highly active antiretroviral therapy, particularly protease inhibitors, in patients with HIV-related illness and a dysmetabolic syndrome characterized by lipodystrophy, insulin resistance, dyslipidemia, and hyperglycemia (186–188). Many such patients have IGT with variable rates of progression to overt diabetes. In a 5-year study of 221 HIV-infected patients, 5% developed hyperglycemia after the initiation of protease inhibitors (187). IGT was reported in 16% in another series (186). Drugs known to improve insulin sensitivity, e.g., metformin and thiazolidinediones, are undergoing trials in this syndrome and appear to be reasonable choices; long-term results are awaited (189,190).

Atypical Antipsychotics

A number of anecdotal reports have recently pointed to a potential diabetogenic effect of atypical antipsychotic agents, particularly clozapine and olanzapine (191–194). In one series of 82 patients treated with clozapine over a period of 5 years, 30% were diagnosed with diabetes, most requiring treatment (192). Although some of the adverse effects of these agents may be secondary to the weight gain seen with these agents, other mechanisms, including their direct effects on insulin action and islet cell function, need to be explored (194,194a). Severe mental illness and its associated lifestyle changes, by themselves, are known to be associated with increased risk for obesity and diabetes. Therefore, controlled trials with these agents are needed, as outlined by several national organizations (194a).

GENETIC SYNDROMES

More than 50 distinct rare genetic syndromes are associated with glucose intolerance (195). Some of these represent chromosomal defects such as Down syndrome (trisomy 21), Klinefelter syndrome, and Turner syndrome, whereas many others are single-gene defects (Table 27.1). In addition to congenital pancreatic disorders and certain inborn errors of metabolism, a variety of disorders characterized by severe or extreme insulin resistance caused by structural or functional abnormalities of the insulin receptor may produce glucose intolerance or non–insulin-dependent diabetes (see Chapter 28). Examples of genetic disorders linked to obesity-associated insulin resistance include Prader-Willi syndrome (196), Laurence-Moon-Biedl syndrome, and its variant, Bardet-Biedl syndrome (BBS) (197). About 45% of patients with the BBS are glucose intolerant. This disorder, previously thought to be a single-gene recessive disease, has recently been proposed to be a more complex genetic disorder requiring three mutant alleles (198).

In some of the genetic syndromes, a striking incidence of insulin-dependent diabetes, simulating typical autoimmune type 1 diabetes, is an integral feature. Examples include stiff-man syndrome, an autoimmune disorder (see Chapter 23), and several other hereditary neurologic disorders, including Friedreich ataxia (199); DIDMOAD (diabetes insipidus, diabetes mellitus, optic atrophy, sensorineural deafness), also known as Wolfram syndrome, and its variants (200); and maternally inherited diabetes and deafness due to mitochondrial gene mutations (201). In Friedreich ataxia, up to 20% of patients have diabetes, although some may be non–insulin-dependent for variable periods. In contrast, in Wolfram syndrome, autopsy studies have shown a selective loss of islet β-cells (202), a finding explaining the onset of diabetes in early childhood and the absolute insulin requirement in these patients. Urinary tract abnormalities and renal failure, in the absence of diabetic nephropathy, are very common in Wolfram syndrome, and 60% mortality by age 35 was reported in a series of 68 patients (203).

The maternally inherited diabetes and deafness (MIDD) syndrome is due to an A-to-G point mutation at position 3243 of mitochondrial DNA, encoding leucine transfer RNA. Mitochondrial gene mutations are characterized by oxidative phosphorylation defects leading to a variety of clinical syndromes, including a group of myopathies, such as Kearns-Sayre syndrome, Leber hereditary optic neuropathy, myoclonic epilepsy with ragged red fibers (MERRF), and a syndrome of myopathy, encephalopathy, lactic acidosis, and stroke-like episodes (MELAS) (204). In a series of 54 patients from France, MIDD was characterized by lack of obesity and by mild diabetes at onset but progressing to insulin dependency in about 50% of patients by 10 years (201). Myopathy, including cardiomyopathy and neuropsychiatric features, was commonly observed, and a specific retinal lesion, macular-pattern dystrophy, was much more common than diabetic retinopathy. Neurosensory deafness was present in virtually all patients.

CHRONIC COMPLICATIONS IN SECONDARY FORMS OF DIABETES

Whether chronic complications of diabetes (microangiopathy, neuropathy, and macroangiopathy) are a consequence of long-term hyperglycemia per se or require additional metabolic, hormonal, or genetic factors is a controversial issue. If hyperglycemia per se is the most important factor, one would expect an equivalent incidence and prevalence of these complications in secondary forms of diabetes. However, in practical terms, such comparisons of complications in primary versus secondary diabetes are difficult in view of (a) the milder severity of hyperglycemia in most patients with secondary diabetes, (b) the relatively shorter durations of follow-up in patients with secondary diabetes either because of poor prognosis of underlying disease or because of adequate treatment of the disorder with amelioration of hyperglycemia, and (c) lack of genetic markers for the detection of primary diabetes in association with secondary diabetes.

Despite these limitations, there is evidence that diabetic microvascular disease and neuropathy are mainly a function of severity and duration of hyperglycemia, and this view is strengthened by the demonstration of microangiopathic lesions in animal models of diabetes induced by alloxan or streptozotocin and of amelioration of these lesions by insulin treatment. In diabetes secondary to chronic pancreatitis or pancreatectomy, careful comparisons with patients with type 1 diabetes matched for age, sex, and duration and treatment of diabetes revealed a similar prevalence of retinopathy in the two groups (205,206). In another human model, that of pyriminil-induced insulin-dependent diabetes (173,174), a striking

TABLE 27.4. Pyriminil (Vacor)-induced Diabetes and Microangiopathy

Group	n	Age (yr)	Duration (yr)	HbA_1 (%)	QCBM (A)	DR (%)	Proteinuria (%)
Type 1 diabetes	16	27 ± 2	6.2 ± 0.3	11.9	2287 ± 144[a]	25	6
Pyriminil	18	28 ± 2	4.7 ± 1.5	12.1	2320 ± 149[a]	44	28
Control	20	28 ± 2	—	—	1781 ± 46	0	0

DR, diabetic retinopathy; QCBM, quadriceps capillary basement membrane width.
[a] $P < 0.001$ vs. controls.
Data are from Feingold KR, Lee TH, Chung MY, et al. Muscle capillary basement membrane within patients with Vacor-induced diabetes mellitus. *J Clin Invest* 1986;78:102–107.

prevalence of diabetic retinopathy, overt proteinuria, and thickened muscle capillary basement membranes was observed that was equal to or even greater than that in matched patients with type 1 diabetes (207) (Table 27.4). This form of diabetes is akin to chemically induced diabetes in animals and excludes the potentially confounding variable of a genetic factor or factors.

In one respect, however, the type of retinopathy in secondary forms of diabetes differs from that in genetic diabetes—i.e., severe or proliferative retinopathy is rare or quite infrequent. This difference may be due in part to a lack of the concomitant increase in GH or related growth factors that may be involved in the progression of proliferative retinopathy in patients with genetic diabetes (208,209). GH at physiologic concentrations was shown to enhance proliferation of human retinal microvascular endothelial cells in cultures (210). Dwarfs with isolated growth hormone deficiency and glucose intolerance do not develop retinopathy (or macrovascular disease) (211), and pituitary ablation was shown to arrest or retard the progression of proliferative retinopathy (212). Similarly, in patients with hemochromatosis, a blunted GH responsiveness was associated with only a mild background retinopathy (213). On the other hand, background retinopathy was reported in the absence of GH in a patient with diabetes following pancreatectomy (214). However, no proliferative retinopathy was observed in this patient despite 24 years of diabetes and the presence of severe nephropathy and neuropathy. Proliferative retinopathy is also rare in patients with acromegaly, despite their having marked elevations in levels of GH for many years. Overall, the available evidence supports the concept that GH is involved in the progression, but not in the initiation, of at least some of the long-term diabetic vascular complications.

REFERENCES

1. Report of the Expert Committee on the Diagnosis and Classification of Diabetes Mellitus. *Diabetes Care* 1997;20:1183–1197.
2. Seldin DW, Tarail R. Effect of hypertonic solutions on metabolism and excretion of electrolytes. *Am J Physiol* 1949;159:160–174.
3. Seltzer HS, Harris VL. Exhaustion of insulogenic reserve in maturity-onset diabetic patients during prolonged and continuous hyperglycemic stress. *Diabetes* 1964;13:6–13.
4. McCulloch DK, Koerker DJ, Kahn SE, et al. Correlations of in vivo β-cell function tests with β-cell mass and pancreatic insulin content in streptozocin-administered baboons. *Diabetes* 1991;40:673–679.
5. Kendall DM, Sutherland DER, Najarian JS, et al. Effects of hemipancreatectomy on insulin secretion and glucose tolerance in healthy humans. *N Engl J Med* 1990;322:898–903.
6. Weir GC, Bonner-Weir S, Leahy JL. Islet mass and function in diabetes and transplantation. *Diabetes* 1990;39:401–405.
7. Barnes AJ, Bloom SR. Pancreatectomised man: a model for diabetes without glucagon. *Lancet* 1976;1:219–221.
8. Boden G. Extrapancreatic glucagon in human subjects. In: Unger RH, Orci L, eds. *Glucagon: physiology, pathophysiology, and morphology of the pancreatic A-cells.* New York: Elsevier, 1981:349–357.
9. Tiengo A, Bessioud M, Valverde I, et al. Absence of islet alpha cell function in pancreatectomized patients. *Diabetologia* 1982;22:25–32.
10. Holst JJ, Pedersen JH, Baldissera F, et al. Circulating glucagon after total pancreatectomy in man. *Diabetologia* 1983;25:396–399.
11. Del Prato S, Tiengo A, Baccaglini U, et al. Effect of insulin replacement on intermediary metabolism in diabetes secondary to pancreatectomy. *Diabetologia* 1983;25:252–259.
12. Bajorunas DR, Fortner JG, Jaspan J, et al. Total pancreatectomy increases the metabolic response to glucagon in humans. *J Clin Endocrinol Metab* 1986;63:439–346.
13. de Kreutzenberg SV, Maifreni L, LiSato G, et al. Glucose turnover and recycling in diabetes secondary to total pancreatectomy: effect of glucagon infusion. *J Clin Endocrinol Metab* 1990;70:1023–1029.
14. Polonsky KS, Herold KC, Gilden JL, et al. Glucose counterregulation in patients after pancreatectomy: comparison with other clinical forms of diabetes. *Diabetes* 1984;33:1112–1119.
15. Barnes AJ, Bloom SR, Alberti KGMM, et al. Ketoacidosis in pancreatectomized man. *N Engl J Med* 1977;296:1250–1253.
16. Nosadini R, Del Prato S, Tiengo A, et al. Insulin sensitivity, binding, and kinetics in pancreatogenic and type I diabetes. *Diabetes* 1982;31:346–355.
17. Yki-Järvinen H, Kiviluoto T, Taskinen M-R. Insulin resistance is a prominent feature of patients with pancreatogenic diabetes. *Metabolism* 1986;35:718–727.
18. Bajorunas DR, Dresler CM, Horowitz GD, et al. Basal glucagon replacement in chronic glucagon deficiency increases insulin resistance. *Diabetes* 1986;35:556–562.
19. Bank S. Chronic pancreatitis: clinical features and medical management. *Am J Gastroenterol* 1986;81:153–167.
20. Sjoberg, RJ, Kidd GS. Pancreatic diabetes mellitus. *Diabetes Care* 1989; 12:715–724.
21. Kalk WJ, Vinik AI, Jackson WPU, et al. Insulin secretion and pancreatic exocrine function in patients with chronic pancreatitis. *Diabetologia* 1979;16:355–358.
22. Andersen BN, Krarup T, Pedersen NT, et al. B cell function in patients with chronic pancreatitis and its relation to exocrine pancreatic function. *Diabetologia* 1982;23:86–89.
23. Donowitz M, Hendler R, Spiro HM, et al. Glucagon secretion in acute and chronic pancreatitis. *Ann Intern Med* 1975;83:778–781.
24. Persson I, Gyntelberg F, Heding LG, et al. Pancreatic-glucagon-like immunoreactivity after intravenous insulin in normals and chronic-pancreatitis patients. *Acta Endocrinol* 1971;67:401–404.
25. Larsen S, Hilsted J, Philipsen EK, et al. Glucose counter-regulation in diabetes secondary to chronic pancreatitis. *Metabolism* 1990;39:138–143.
26. Kalk WJ, Vinik AI, Paul M, et al. Immunoreactive glucagon responses to intravenous tolbutamide in chronic pancreatitis. *Diabetes* 1975;24:851–855.
27. Brunicardi FC, Chaiken RL, Ryan AS, et al. Pancreatic polypeptide administration improves abnormal glucose metabolism in patients with chronic pancreatitis. *J Clin Endocrinol Metab* 1996;81:3566–3572.
28. Williams JA, Goldfine ID. The insulin-pancreatic acinar axis. *Diabetes* 1985;34:980–986.
29. Baron JH, Nabarro JDN. Pancreatic exocrine function in maturity-onset diabetes mellitus. *BMJ* 1973;4:25–27.
30. Allen HF, Gay EC, Klingensmith GJ, et al. Identification and treatment of cystic fibrosis-related diabetes. A survey of current medical practice in the U.S. *Diabetes Care* 1998;21:943–948.
31. Moran A, Hardin D, Rodman D, et al. Diagnosis, screening and management of cystic fibrosis related diabetes mellitus: a consensus conference report. *Diabetes Res Clin Pract* 1999;45:61–73.
32. Moran A, Phillips J, Milla C. Insulin and glucose excursion following premeal insulin lispro or repaglinide in cystic fibrosis-related diabetes. *Diabetes Care* 2001;24:1706–1710.
33. Couce M, O'Brien TD, Moran A, et al. Diabetes mellitus in cystic fibrosis is characterized by islet amyloidosis. *J Clin Endocrinol Metab* 1996;81:1267–1272.
34. Cohn JA, Jowell PS. Are mutations in the cystic fibrosis gene important in chronic pancreatitis? *Surg Clin North Am* 1999;79:723–731.
35. Sharer N, Schwarz M, Malone G, et al. Mutations of the cystic fibrosis gene in patients with chronic pancreatitis. *N Engl J Med* 1998;339:645–652.

36. Gullo L, Pezzilli R, Morselli-Labate AM. Diabetes and the risk of pancreatic cancer. Italian Pancreatic Cancer Study Group. *N Engl J Med* 1994;331: 81–84.
37. Everhart J, Wright D. Diabetes mellitus as a risk factor for pancreatic cancer. A meta-analysis. *JAMA* 1995;273:1605–1609.
38. Gapstur SM, Gann PH, Lowe W, et al. Abnormal glucose metabolism and pancreatic cancer mortality. *JAMA* 2000:283:2552–2558.
39. Permert J, Larsson J, Westermark GT, et al. Islet amyloid polypeptide in patients with pancreatic cancer and diabetes. *N Engl J Med* 1994;330: 313–318.
40. Crosby WH. Hemochromatosis: current concepts and management. *Hosp Pract* 1987;22:173–192.
41. Andrews NC. Disorders of iron metabolism. *N Engl J Med* 1999;341:1986–1995.
42. Beutler E, Felitti V, Gelbart T, et al. The effect of HFE genotypes on measurements of iron overload in patients attending a health appraisal clinic. *Ann Intern Med* 2000;133:329–337.
43. Sanchez AM, Schreiber GB, Bethel J, et al. Prevalence, donation practices, and risk assessment of blood donors with hemochromatosis. *JAMA* 2001;286:1475–1481.
44. Steinberg KK, Cogswell ME, Chang JC, et al. Prevalence of C282Y and H63D mutations in the hemochromatosis (HFE) gene in the United States. *JAMA* 2001;285:2216–2222.
45. Bulaj ZJ, Ajioka RS, Phillips JD, et al. Disease-related conditions in relatives of patients with hemochromatosis. *N Engl J Med* 2000;343:1529–1535.
46. Olynyk JK, Cullen DJ, Aquilia S, et al. A population-based study of the clinical expression of the hemochromatosis gene. *N Engl J Med* 1999;341:718–724.
47. Niederau C, Fischer R, Sonnenberg A, et al. Survival and causes of death in cirrhotic and in noncirrhotic patients with primary hemochromatosis. *N Engl J Med* 1985;313:1256–1262.
48. Dymock IW, Cassar J, Pyke DA, et al. Observations on the pathogenesis, complications, and treatment of diabetes in 115 cases of haemochromatosis. *Am J Med* 1972;52:203–210.
49. Lassman MN, Genel M, Wise JK, et al. Carbohydrate homeostasis and pancreatic islet cell function in thalassemia. *Ann Intern Med* 1974;80:65–69.
50. Saudek CD, Hemm RM, Peterson CM. Abnormal glucose tolerance in β-thalassemia major. *Metabolism* 1977;26:43–52.
51. Conte D, Manachino D, Colli A, et al. Prevalence of genetic hemochromatosis in a cohort of Italian patients with diabetes mellitus. *Ann Intern Med* 1998;128:370–373.
52. Niederau C, Berger M, Stremmel W, et al. Hyperinsulinaemia in non-cirrhotic haemochromatosis: impaired hepatic insulin degradation? *Diabetologia* 1984;26:441–444.
53. Merkel PA, Simonson DC, Amiel SA, et al. Insulin resistance and hyperinsulinemia in patients with thalassemia major treated by hypertransfusion. *N Engl J Med* 1988;318:809–814.
54. Rahier JR, Loozen S, Goebbels RM, et al. The hemochromatotic human pancreas: a quantitative immunohistochemical and ultrastructural study. *Diabetologia* 1987;30:5–12.
55. Passa P, Luyckx AS, Carpentier JL, et al. Glucagon secretion in diabetic patients with idiopathic haemochromatosis. *Diabetologia* 1977;13:509–513.
56. Nelson RL, Baldus WD, Rubenstein AH, et al. Pancreatic α-cell function in diabetic hemochromatotic subjects. *J Clin Endocrinol Metab* 1979;49:412–416.
57. Ford ES, Cogswell ME. Diabetes and serum ferritin concentration among U.S. adults. *Diabetes Care* 1999:22:1978–1983.
58. O'Brien T, Bassett B, Burray DM, et al. Usefulness of biochemical screening of diabetic patients for hemochromatosis. *Diabetes Care* 1990;13:532–534.
59. Fernández-Real JM, Lopez-Bermejo A, Ricard W. Cross-talk between iron metabolism and diabetes. *Diabetes* 2002;51:2348–2354.
60. Schafer AI, Rabinowe S, LeBoff MS, et al. Long-term efficacy of deferoxamine iron chelation therapy in adults with acquired transfusional iron overload. *Arch Intern Med* 1985;145:1217–1221.
61. Bronspiegel-Weintrob N, Olivieri NF, Tyler B, et al. Effect of age at the start of iron chelation therapy on gonadal function in β-thalassemia major. *N Engl J Med* 1990;323:713–719.
62. Young FG. The relation of the anterior pituitary gland to carbohydrate metabolism. *BMJ* 1939;2:393–396.
63. Fong HKW, Chick WL, Sato GH. Hormones and factors that stimulate growth of a rat islet tumor cell line in serum-free medium. *Diabetes* 1981;30:1022–1028.
64. Rabinovitch A, Quigley C, Rechler MW. Growth hormone stimulates islet B-cell replication in neonatal rat pancreatic monolayer cultures. *Diabetes* 1983;32:307–312.
65. Pierluissi J, Campbell J. Metasomatotrophic diabetes and its induction: basal insulin secretion and insulin release responses to glucose, glucagon, arginine and meals. *Diabetologia* 1980;18:223–228.
66. Daughaday WH. Growth hormone: normal synthesis, secretion, control and mechanisms of action. In: DeGroot LJ, Besser GM, Cahill GF Jr, et al, eds. *Endocrinology*, Vol 1, 2nd ed. Philadelphia: WB Saunders, 1989:318–329.
67. Press M. Growth hormone and metabolism. *Diabetes Metab Rev* 1988;4: 391–414.
68. Ganda OP, Simonson DS, Growth hormone, acromegaly and diabetes. *Diabetes Rev* 1993;1:2886–3000.
69. Arvat E, Maccario M, Di Vito L, et al. Endocrine activities of ghrelin, a natural growth hormone secretagogue (GHS), in humans: comparison and interactions with hexarelin, a nonnatural peptidyl GHS, and GH-releasing hormone. *J Clin Endocrinol Metab* 2001:86:1169–1174.
70. Hansen I, Taslikian E, Beaufrere B, et al. Insulin resistance in acromegaly: defects in both hepatic and extrahepatic insulin action. *Am J Physiol* 1986;250: E269–E273.
71. Metcalfe P, Johnston DG, Nosadini R, et al. Metabolic effects of acute and prolonged growth hormone excess in normal and insulin-deficient man. *Diabetologia* 1981;20:123–128.
72. Bratusch-Marrian PR, Smith D, DeFronzo RA. The effect of growth hormone on glucose metabolism and insulin secretion in man. *J Clin Endocrinol Metab* 1982;55:973–982.
73. Rizza RA, Mandarino LJ, Gerich JE. Effects of growth hormone on insulin action in man: mechanisms of insulin resistance, impaired suppression of glucose production, and impaired stimulation of glucose utilization. *Diabetes* 1982;31:663–669.
74. Zierler KL, Rabinowitz D. Roles of insulin and growth hormone, based on studies of forearm metabolism in man. *Medicine* (Baltimore) 1963;42: 385–402.
75. Fineberg SE, Merimee TJ. Acute metabolic effects of human growth hormone. *Diabetes* 1974;23:499–504.
76. Kahn CR, Goldfine ID, Neville DM Jr, et al. Alterations in insulin binding induced by changes in vivo in the levels of glucocorticoids and growth hormone. *Endocrinology* 1978;103:1054–1066.
77. Muggeo M, Saviolakis GA, Businaro V, et al. Insulin receptor on monocytes from patients with acromegaly and fasting hyperglycemia. *J Clin Endocrinol Metab* 1983;56:733–738.
78. Tai PK, Liao J-F, Chen EH, et al. Differential regulation of two glucose transporters by chronic growth hormone treatment of cultured 3T3-F442A adipose cells. *J Biol Chem* 1990;265:21828–21834.
79. Melmed S, Braunstein GD, Chang RJ, et al. Pituitary tumors secreting growth hormone and prolactin. *Ann Intern Med* 1986;105:238–253.
80. Jadresic A, Banks LM, Child DF, et al. The acromegaly syndrome: relation between clinical features, growth hormone values, and radiologic characteristics. *Q J Med* 1982;202:189–204.
81. Nabarro JD. Acromegaly. *Clin Endocrinol* (Oxf) 1987:26:481–512.
82. Molitch ME. Clinical manifestations of acromegaly. *Endocrinol Metab Clin North Am* 1992:21:597–614.
83. Ezzat S, Forster MJ, Berchtold P, et al. Acromegaly. Clinical and biochemical features in 500 patients. *Medicine* (Baltimore) 1994;73:233–240.
84. Sönksen PH, Greenwood FC, Ellis JP, et al. Changes of carbohydrate tolerance in acromegaly with progress of the disease and in response to treatment. *J Clin Endocrinol Metab* 1967;27:1418–1430.
85. Grinspoon S, Clemmons D, Swearingen B, et al. Serum insulin-like growth factor-binding protein-3 levels in the diagnosis of acromegaly. *J Clin Endocrinol Metab* 1995;80:927–932.
86. Gerich JE, Lorenzi M, Bier DM, et al. Effects of physiologic levels of glucagon and growth hormone on human carbohydrate and lipid metabolism: studies involving administration of exogenous hormone during suppression of endogenous hormone secretion with somatostatin. *J Clin Invest* 1976:57: 875–884.
87. Moller N, Schmitz O, Joorgensen JO, et al. Basal- and insulin-stimulated substrate metabolism in patients with active acromegaly before and after adenomectomy. *J Clin Endocrinol Metab* 1992;74:1012–1019.
88. Giustina A, Barkan A, Casanueva FF, et al. Criteria for cure of acromegaly: a consensus statement. *J Clin Endocrinol Metab* 2000;85:526–529.
89. Trainer PJ. Acromegaly—consensus, what consensus? *J Clin Endocrinol Metab* 2002;87:3534–3536.
90. Bates AS, Van't Hoff W, Jones JM, et al. An audit of outcome of treatment in acromegaly. *Q J Med* 1993;86:293–299.
91. Rajasoorya C, Holdaway IM, Wrightson P, et al. Determinants of clinical outcome and survival in acromegaly. *Clin Endocrinol* (Oxf) 1994;41:95–102.
92. Colao A, Baldelli R, Marzullo P, et al. Systemic hypertension and impaired glucose tolerance are independently correlated to the severity of the acromegalic cardiomyopathy. *J Clin Endocrinol Metab* 2000;85:193–199.
93. Sassolas G, Harris AG, James-Deidier A. Long term effect of incremental doses of the somatostatin analog SMS 201-995 in 58 acromegalic patients. French SMS 201-995 approximately equal to Acromegaly Study Group. *J Clin Endocrinol Metab* 1990;71:391–397.
94. Newman CB, Melmed S, Snyder PJ, et al. Safety and efficacy of long-term octreotide therapy of acromegaly: results of a multicenter trial in 103 patients—a clinical research center study. *J Clin Endocrinol Metab* 1995;80: 2768–2775.
95. Ho KK, Jenkins AB, Furler SM, et al. Impact of octreotide, a long-acting somatostatin analogue, on glucose tolerance and insulin sensitivity in acromegaly. *Clin Endocrinol* (Oxf) 1992;36:271–279.
96. Breidert M, Pinzer T, Wildbrett J, et al. Long-term effect of octreotide in acromegaly on insulin resistance. *Horm Metab Res* 1995;27:226–230.
97. Van der Lely AJ, Hutson RK, Trainer PJ, et al. Long-term treatment of acromegaly with pegvisomant, a growth-hormone receptor antagonist. *Lancet* 2001;358:1754–1759.
98. Daughaday WH, Kipnis DM. The growth-promoting and anti-insulin actions of somatotropin. *Recent Prog Horm Res* 1966;22:49–99.
99. Martin JM, Gagliardino JJ. Effect of growth hormone on the isolated pancreatic islets of rat in vitro. *Nature* 1967;213:630–631.
100. Merimee TJ, Fineberg SE, McKusick VA, et al. Diabetes mellitus and sexual ateliotic dwarfism: a comparative study. *J Clin Invest* 1970;49:1096–1102.
101. Merimee TJ. A follow-up study of vascular disease in growth-hormone-deficient dwarfs with diabetes. *N Engl J Med* 1978;298:1217–1222.

102. Thomas AM, Berglund L. Growth hormone and cardiovascular disease: an area in rapid growth. *J Clin Endocrinol Metab* 2001;86:1871–1873.
103. Colao A, Di Somma C, Cuocolo A, et al. Improved cardiovascular risk factors and cardiac performance after 12 months of growth hormone (GH) replacement in young adult patients with GH deficiency. *J Clin Endocrinol Metab* 2001;86:1874–1881.
104. Beshyah SA, Henderson A, Niththyananthan R, et al. The effects of short and long-term growth hormone replacement therapy in hypopituitary adults on lipid metabolism and carbohydrate tolerance. *J Clin Endocrinol Metab* 1995;80:356–363.
105. Rosenfalck AM, Maghsoudi S, Fisker S, et al. The effect of 30 months of low-dose replacement therapy with recombinant human growth hormone (rhGH) on insulin and C-peptide kinetics, insulin secretion, insulin sensitivity, glucose effectiveness, and body composition in GH-deficient adults. *J Clin Endocrinol Metab* 2000;85:4173–4181.
106. Koller EA, Green L, Gertner JM, et al. Retinal changes mimicking diabetic retinopathy in two nondiabetic, growth hormone-treated patients. *J Clin Endocrinol Metab* 1998;83:2380–2383.
107. Czernichow P, Albertsson-Wikland K, et al. Growth hormone treatment and diabetes: survey of the Kabi Pharmacia International Growth Study. *Acta Paediatr Scand Suppl* 1991;379:104–107.
108. Thornes MO. Critical evaluation of the safety of recombinant growth hormone administration: statement from the Growth Hormone Research Society. *J Clin Endocrinol Metab* 2001;86:1868–1870.
109. Katznelson L, Klibanski A. Prolactin and its disorders. In: Becker KL, ed. *Principles and practice of endocrinology and metabolism,* 3rd ed. New York: Lippincott Williams & Wilkins, 2001:145–153.
110. Landgraf R, Landgraf-Leurs MMC, Weissmann A, et al. Prolactin: a diabetogenic hormone. *Diabetologia* 1977;13:99–104.
111. Gustafson AB, Banasiak MF, Kalkhoff RK, et al. Correlation of hyperprolactinemia with altered plasma insulin and glucagon: similarity to effects of late human pregnancy. *J Clin Endocrinol Metab* 1980;51:242–246.
112. Cahill GF Jr. Action of adrenal cortical steroids on carbohydrate metabolism. In: Christy NP, ed. *The human adrenal cortex.* New York: Harper and Row, 1971:205–238.
113. Exton JH, Miller TB Jr, Harper SC, et al. Carbohydrate metabolism in perfused livers of adrenalectomized and steroid-replaced rats. *Am J Physiol* 1976;230:163–170.
114. O'Brien RM, Lucas PC, Forest CD, et al. Identification of a sequence in the PEPCK gene that mediates a negative effect of insulin on transcription. *Science* 1990;249:533–537.
115. Olefsky JM. Effect of dexamethasone on insulin binding, glucose transport and glucose oxidation of isolated rat adipocytes. *J Clin Invest* 1975;56: 1499–1508.
116. Horner HC, Munck A, Lienhard GE. Dexamethasone causes translocation of glucose transporters from the plasma membrane to an intracellular site in human fibroblasts. *J Biol Chem* 1987;262:17696–17702.
117. Yasuda K, Hines E III, Kitabchi AE. Hypercortisolism and insulin resistance: comparative effects of prednisone, hydrocortisone, and dexamethasone on insulin binding of human erythrocytes. *J Clin Endocrinol Metab* 1982;55: 910–915.
118. Rebuffé-Scrive M, Krotkiewski M, et al. Muscle and adipose tissue morphology and metabolism in Cushing's syndrome. *J Clin Endocrinol Metab* 1988;67: 1122–1128.
119. Lambillotte C, Gilon P, Henquin JC. Direct glucocorticoid inhibition of insulin secretion. An in vitro study of dexamethasone effects in mouse islets. *J Clin Invest* 1997;99:414–423.
120. Rizza RA, Mandarino LJ, Gerich JE. Cortisol-induced insulin resistance in man: impaired suppression of glucose production and stimulation of glucose utilization due to a postreceptor defect of insulin action. *J Clin Endocrinol Metab* 1982;54:131–138.
121. Shamoon H, Soman V, Sherwin RS. The influence of acute physiological increments of cortisol on fuel metabolism and insulin binding to monocytes in normal humans. *J Clin Endocrinol Metab* 1980;50:495–501.
122. Pupo AA, Wajchenberg BL, Schnaider J. Carbohydrate metabolism in hyperadrenocorticism. *Diabetes* 1966;15:24–29.
123. Boyle DJ. Cushing's disease, glucocorticoid excess, glucocorticoid deficiency, and diabetes. *Diabetes Rev* 1993;1:301–308.
124. Marco J, Calle C, Roman D, et al. Hyperglucagonism induced by glucocorticoid treatment in man. *N Engl J Med* 1973;288:128–131.
125. Wise JK, Hendler R, Felig P. Influence of glucocorticoids on glucagon secretion and plasma amino acid concentrations in man. *J Clin Invest* 1973;52: 2774–2782.
126. Cryer PE. Catecholamines, pheochromocytoma, and diabetes. *Diabetes Rev* 1993;1:309–317.
127. Landsberg L, Young JB. Catecholamines and the adrenal medulla. In: Wilson JD, Foster DW, eds. *Williams textbook of endocrinology,* 7th ed. Philadelphia: WB Saunders, 1985:891–965.
128. Robertson RP, Halter JB, Porte D Jr. A role for alpha-adrenergic receptors in abnormal insulin secretion in diabetes mellitus. *J Clin Invest* 1976;57:791–795.
129. Dunning BE, Taborsky GJ Jr. Galanin—sympathetic neurotransmitter in endocrine pancreas? *Diabetes* 1988;37:1157–1162.
130. Ortiz-Alonso FJ, Herman WH, Zobel DL, et al. Effect of epinephrine on pancreatic β-cell and α-cell function in patients with NIDDM. *Diabetes* 1991;40: 1194–1202.
131. Strickland WG, Blackmore PF, Exton JH. The role of calcium in alpha-adrenergic inactivation of glycogen synthase in rat hepatocytes and its inhibition by insulin. *Diabetes* 1980;29:617–622.
132. Garber AJ, Karl IE, Kipnis DM. Alanine and glutamine synthesis and release from skeletal muscle. IV. β-Adrenergic inhibition of amino acid release. *J Biol Chem* 1976;251:851–857.
133. Shamoon H, Jacob R, Sherwin RS. Epinephrine-induced hypoaminoacidemia in normal and diabetic human subjects: effect of beta blockade. *Diabetes* 1980; 29:875–881.
134. Stenström G, Sjöström L, Smith U. Diabetes mellitus in phaeochromocytoma: fasting blood glucose levels before and after surgery in 60 patients with phaeochromocytoma. *Acta Endocrinol* 1984;106:511–515.
135. Vance JE, Buchanan KD, O'Hara D, et al. Insulin and glucagon responses in subjects with pheochromocytoma: effect of alpha adrenergic blockade. *J Clin Endocrinol Metab* 1969;29:911–916.
136. Turnbull DM, Johnston DG, Alberti KGMM, et al. Hormonal and metabolic studies in a patient with a pheochromocytoma. *J Clin Endocrinol Metab* 1980; 51:930–933.
137. Hamaji M. Pancreatic α- and β-cell function in pheochromocytoma. *J Clin Endocrinol Metab* 1979;49:322–325.
138. Bolli G, DeFeo P, Massi-Benedetti M, et al. Circulating catecholamine and glucagon responses to insulin-induced blood glucose decrement in a patient with pheochromocytoma. *J Clin Endocrinol Metab* 1982;54:447–449.
139. Conn JW. Hypertension, the potassium ion and impaired carbohydrate tolerance. *N Engl J Med* 1965;273:1135–1143.
140. Kotchen TA, Guthrie GP Jr. Renin-angiotensin-aldosterone and hypertension. *Endocrinol Rev* 1980;1:78–99.
141. Young WF Jr, Hogan MJ, Klee GG, et al. Primary aldosteronism: diagnosis and treatment. *Mayo Clin Proc* 1990;65:96–110.
142. Podolsky S, Melby JC. Improvement of growth-hormone response to stimulation in primary aldosteronism with correction of potassium deficiency. *Metabolism* 1976;25:1027–1032.
143. Sagild U, Andersen V, Andreasen PB. Glucose tolerance and insulin responsiveness in experimental potassium depletion. *Acta Med Scand* 1961;169:243–251.
144. Gorden P. Glucose intolerance with hypokalemia: failure of short-term potassium depletion in normal subjects to reproduce the glucose and insulin abnormalities of clinical hypokalemia. *Diabetes* 1973;22:544–551.
145. Loeb JN. Metabolic changes in thyrotoxicosis. In: Braverman LE, Utiger RD, Ingbar SH, Werner SC, eds. *Werner and Ingbar's the thyroid: a fundamental and clinical text,* 7th ed. Philadelphia: Lippincott Williams & Wilkins, 1996: 687–693.
146. Sandler MP, Robinson RP, Rabin D, et al. The effect of thyroid hormones on gluconeogenesis and forearm metabolism in man. *J Clin Endocrinol Metab* 1983;56:479–485.
147. Bratusch-Marrain PR, Komjati M, Waldhäusl WK. Glucose metabolism in noninsulin-dependent diabetic patients with experimental hyperthyroidism. *J Clin Endocrinol Metab* 1985;60:1063–1068.
148. Randin J-P, Tappy L, Scazziga B, et al. Insulin sensitivity and exogenous insulin clearance in Graves' disease: measurement by the glucose clamp technique and continuous indirect calorimetry. *Diabetes* 1986;35:178–181.
149. Shen D-C, Davidson MB, Kuo S-W, et al. Peripheral and hepatic insulin antagonism in hyperthyroidism. *J Clin Endocrinol Metab* 1988;66:565–569.
150. Foss MC, Paccola GMGF, Saad MJA, et al. Peripheral glucose metabolism in human hyperthyroidism. *J Clin Endocrinol Metab* 1990;70:1167–1172.
151. Maxon HR, Kreines KW, Goldsmith RE, et al. Long-term observations of glucose tolerance in thyrotoxic patients. *Arch Intern Med* 1975;135:1477–1480.
152. Beylot M, Riou JP, Bienvenu F, et al. Increased ketonaemia in hyperthyroidism: evidence for a β-adrenergic mechanism. *Diabetologia* 1980;19: 505–510.
153. Cooppan R, Kozak GP. Hyperthyroidism and diabetes mellitus: an analysis of 70 patients. *Arch Intern Med* 1980;140:370–373.
154. Kim H, Kalkhoff RK, Costrini NV, et al. Plasma insulin disturbances in primary hyperparathyroidism. *J Clin Invest* 1971;50:2596–2605.
155. Yasuda K, Hurukawa Y, Okuyama M, et al. Glucose tolerance and insulin secretion in patients with parathyroid disorders: effect of serum calcium on insulin release. *N Engl J Med* 1975;292:501–504.
156. Taylor WH, Khaleeli AA. Coincident diabetes mellitus and primary hyperparathyroidism. *Diabetes Metab Res Rev* 2001;17:175–180.
157. Harter HR, Santiago JV, Rutherford WE, et al. The relative roles of calcium, phosphorus, and parathyroid hormone in glucose- and tolbutamide-mediated insulin release. *J Clin Invest* 1976;58:359–367.
158. DeFronzo RA, Lang R. Hypophosphatemia and glucose intolerance: evidence for tissue insensitivity to insulin. *N Engl J Med* 1980;303:1259–1263.
159. Amend WJC Jr, Steinberg SM, Lowrie EG, et al. The influence of serum calcium and parathyroid hormone upon glucose metabolism in uremia. *J Lab Clin Med* 1975;86:435–444.
160. Miralles GD, O'Fallon JR, Talley NJ. Plasma-cell dyscrasia with polyneuropathy. The spectrum of POEMS syndrome. *N Engl J Med* 1992;327:1919–1923.
161. Soubrier MJ, Dubost JJ, Sauvezie BJ. POEMS syndrome: a study of 25 cases and a review of the literature. French Study Group on POEMS Syndrome. *Am J Med* 1994;97:543–553.
162. Feigert JM, Sweet DL, Coleman M, et al. Multicentric angiofollicular lymph node hyperplasia with peripheral neuropathy, pseudotumor cerebri, IgA dysproteinemia, and thrombocytosis in women: a distinct syndrome. *Ann Intern Med* 1990;113:362–367.
163. Pandit MK, Burke J, Gustafson AB, et al. Drug-induced disorders of glucose tolerance. *Ann Intern Med* 1993;118:529–539.
164. Bengtsson C, Blohmé G, Lapidus L, et al. Do antihypertensive drugs precipitate diabetes? *BMJ* 1984;289:1495–1497.
165. Gurwitz JH, Bohn RL, Glynn RJ, et al. Antihypertensive drug therapy and the initiation of treatment for diabetes mellitus. *Ann Intern Med* 1993;118:273–278.

166. Grunfeld C, Chappell DA. Hypokalemia and diabetes mellitus [Editorial]. *Am J Med* 1983;75:553–554.
167. Trube G, Rorsman P, Ohno-Shosaku T. Opposite effects of tolbutamide and diazoxide on the ATP-dependent K^+ channel in mouse pancreatic beta-cells. *Pflugers Arch* 1986;407:493–499.
168. Podolsky S, Pattavina CG. Hyperosmolar nonketotic diabetic coma: a complication of propranolol therapy. *Metabolism* 1973;22:685–693.
169. Burris JF. Beta-blockers, dyslipidemia, and coronary artery disease. A reassessment. *Arch Intern Med* 1993;153:2085–2092.
170. Pace CS, Livingston E. Ionic basis of phenytoin sodium inhibition of insulin secretion in pancreatic islets. *Diabetes* 1979;28:1077–1082.
171. Bouchard P, Sai P, Reach G, et al. Diabetes mellitus following pentamidine-induced hypoglycemia in humans. *Diabetes* 1982;31:40–45.
172. Assan R, Perronne C, Assan D, et al. Pentamidine-induced derangements of glucose homeostasis. Determinant roles of renal failure and drug accumulation. A study of 128 patients. *Diabetes Care* 1995;18:47–55.
173. LeWitt PA. The neurotoxicity of the rat poison Vacor: a clinical study of 12 cases. *N Engl J Med* 1980;302:73–77.
174. Karam JH, Lewitt PA, Young CW, et al. Insulinopenic diabetes after rodenticide (Vacor) ingestion: a unique model of acquired diabetes in man. *Diabetes* 1980;29:971–978.
175. Kahn SE, Beard JC, Schwartz MW, et al. Increased β-cell secretory capacity as mechanism for islet adaptation to nicotinic acid-induced insulin resistance. *Diabetes* 1989;38:562–568.
176. Garg A, Grundy SM. Nicotinic acid as therapy for dyslipidemia in non-insulin-dependent diabetes. *JAMA* 1990;264:723–726.
177. Elam MB, Hunninghake DB, Davis KB, et al. Effect of niacin on lipid and lipoprotein levels and glycemic control in patients with diabetes and peripheral arterial disease: the ADMIT study: a randomized trial. Arterial Disease Multiple Intervention Trial. *JAMA* 2000;284:1263–1270.
178. Teuscher AU, Seaquist ER, Robertson RP. Diminished insulin secretory reserve in diabetic pancreas transplant and nondiabetic kidney transplant recipients. *Diabetes* 1994;43:593–598.
179. Montori VM, Basu A, Erwin PJ, et al. Posttransplantation diabetes. A systematic review of the literature. *Diabetes Care* 2002;25:583–592.
180. Sumrani NB, Delaney V, Daskalakis P, et al. Retrospective analysis of post-transplantation diabetes mellitus in black renal allograft recipients. *Diabetes Care* 1991;14:760–762.
181. Kawai T, Shimada A, Kasuga A. FK506-induced autoimmune diabetes. *Ann Intern Med* 2000;132:511.
182. Feldman M, Kiser RS, Unger RH, et al. Beta-endorphin and the endocrine pancreas: studies in healthy and diabetic human beings. *N Engl J Med* 1983;308:349–353.
183. Giugliano D. Morphine, opioid peptides, and pancreatic islet function. *Diabetes Care* 1984;7:92–98.
184. Facchini F, Chen YD, Reaven GM. Light-to-moderate alcohol intake is associated with enhanced insulin sensitivity. *Diabetes Care* 1994;17:115–119.
185. Kao WH, Puddey IB, Boland LL, et al. Alcohol consumption and the risk of type 2 diabetes mellitus: atherosclerosis in communities study. *Am J Epidemiol* 2001;154:748–775.
186. Carr A, Samaras K, Thorisdottir A, et al. Diagnosis, prediction, and natural course of HIV-1 protease-inhibitor-associated lipodystrophy, hyperlipidaemia, and diabetes mellitus: a cohort study. *Lancet* 1999;353:2093–2099.
187. Tsiodras S, Mantzoros C, Hammer S, et al. Effects of protease inhibitors on hyperglycemia, hyperlipidemia, and lipodystrophy: a 5-year cohort study. *Arch Intern Med* 2000;160:2050–2056.
188. Martinez E, Mocroft A, Garcia-Viejo MA, et al. Risk of lipodystrophy in HIV-1-infected patients treated with protease inhibitors: a prospective cohort study. *Lancet* 2001;357:592–598.
189. Hadigan C, Corcoran C, Basgoz N, et al. Metformin in the treatment of HIV lipodystrophy syndrome: a randomized controlled trial. *JAMA* 2000;284: 472–477.
190. Walli R, Michl GM, Muhlbayer D, et al. Effects of troglitazone on insulin sensitivity in HIV-infected patients with protease inhibitor-associated diabetes mellitus. *Res Exp Med* (Berl) 2000;199:253–262.
191. Henderson DC. Clozapine: diabetes mellitus, weight gain, and lipid abnormalities. *J Clin Psychiatry* 2001:62[Suppl 23]:39–44.
192. Goldstein LE, Henderson DC. Atypical antipsychotic agents and diabetes mellitus. *Pry Psych* 2001;7:65–68.
193. Koro CE, Fedder DO, L'Italian GJ, et al. Assessing of independent effect of olanzapine and risperidone on risk of diabetes among patients with schizophrenia: population based nested case-control study. *BMJ* 2002;325: 243–247.
194. Lean MEJ, Pajonk FG. Patients on atypical antipsychotic drugs. Another high-risk group for type 2 diabetes. *Diabetes Care* 2003;26:1597–1605.
194a. ADA, APA, AACE, NAASD. Consensus development conference on antipsychotic drugs and obesity and diabetes. *Diabetes Care* 2004;27:596–601.
195. Rotter JI, Vadheim CM, Rimoin DL. Genetics of diabetes mellitus. In: Rifkin H, Porte H, eds. *Diabetes mellitus: theory and practice*. New York: Elsevier, 1990: 378–413.
196. Bray GA, Dahms WT, Swerdloff, RS, et al. The Prader-Willi syndrome: a study of 40 patients and a review of the literature. *Medicine* (Baltimore) 1983; 62:59–80.
197. Green JS, Parfrey PS, Harnett JD, et al. The cardinal manifestations of Bardet-Biedl syndrome, a form of Laurence-Moon-Biedl syndrome. *N Engl J Med* 1989;321:1002–1009.
198. Katsanis N, Ansley SJ, Badano JL, et al. Triallelic inheritance in Bardet-Biedl syndrome, a Mendelian recessive disorder. *Science* 2001:293:2256–2259.
199. Schoenle EJ, Boltshauser EJ, Baekkeskov S, et al. Preclinical and manifest diabetes mellitus in young patients with Friedreich's ataxia: no evidence of immune process behind the islet cell destruction. *Diabetologia* 1989;32: 378–381.
200. Barrett TG, Bundey SE, Macleod AF. Neurodegeneration and diabetes: UK nationwide study of Wolfram (DIDMOAD) syndrome. *Lancet* 1995;346: 1458–1463.
201. Guillausseau PJ, Massin P, Dubois-LaForgue D, et al. Maternally inherited diabetes and deafness: a multicenter study. *Ann Intern Med* 2001;134 (9 Pt 1):721–728.
202. Karasik A, O'Hara C, Srikanta S, et al. Genetically programmed selective islet β-cell loss in diabetic subjects with Wolfram's syndrome. *Diabetes Care* 1989;12:135–138.
203. Kinsley BT, Swift M, Dumont RH, et al. Morbidity and mortality in the Wolfram syndrome. *Diabetes Care* 1995;18:1566–1570.
204. Leonard JV, Schapira AH. Mitochondrial respiratory chain disorders II: neurodegenerative disorders and nuclear gene defects. *Lancet* 2000;355: 389–394.
205. Tiengo A, Segato T, Briani C, et al. The presence of retinopathy in patients with secondary diabetes following pancreatectomy or chronic pancreatitis. *Diabetes Care* 1983;6:570–574.
206. Couet C, Genton P, Pointel JP, et al. The prevalence of retinopathy is similar in diabetes mellitus secondary to chronic pancreatitis with or without pancreatectomy and in idiopathic diabetes mellitus. *Diabetes Care* 1985;8: 323–328.
207. Feingold KR, Lee TH, Chung MY, et al. Muscle capillary basement membrane within patients with Vacor-induced diabetes mellitus. *J Clin Invest* 1986;78:102–107.
208. Passa P, Gauville C, Canivet J. Influence of muscular exercise on plasma levels of growth hormone in diabetics with and without retinopathy. *Lancet* 1974;2:72–74.
209. Merimee TJ, Zapf J, Froesch ER. Insulin-like growth factors: studies in diabetes with or without retinopathy. *N Engl J Med* 1983;309:527–530.
210. Rymaszewski Z, Cohen RM, Chomczynski P. Human growth hormone stimulates proliferation of human retinal microvascular endothelial cells in vitro. *Proc Natl Acad Sci U S A* 1991;88:617–621.
211. Merimee TJ. A follow-up study of vascular disease in growth-hormone-deficient dwarfs with diabetes. *N Engl J Med* 1978;298:1217–1222.
212. Sharp PS, Fallon TJ, Brazier OJ, et al. Long-term follow-up of patients who underwent yttrium-90 pituitary implantation for treatment of proliferative diabetic retinopathy. *Diabetologia* 1987;30:199–207.
213. Passa P, Rousselie F, Gauville C, et al. Retinopathy and plasma growth hormone levels in idiopathic hemochromatosis with diabetes. *Diabetes* 1977;26:113–120.
214. Rabin D, Bloomgarden ZT, Feman SS, et al. Development of diabetic complications despite the absence of growth hormone in a patient with post-pancreatectomy diabetes. *N Engl J Med* 1984;310:837–839.

CHAPTER 28

Syndromes of Extreme Insulin Resistance

Allison B. Goldfine and Alan C. Moses

Glucose homeostasis depends on a balance between the production of glucose predominantly by the liver and the utilization of glucose by insulin-dependent tissues (muscle and fat) and insulin-independent tissues (brain and kidney). Insulin controls glucose homeostasis primarily through the suppression of hepatic glucose production and stimulation of peripheral (and to a lesser degree, splanchnic) glucose uptake. Insulin resistance occurs when the ability of endogenous or exogenous insulin to promote glucose clearance is impaired (1). Several pathophysiologic conditions are associated with insulin resistance of varying severity (Table 28.1). Medical treatment of patients with these conditions may be difficult but often leads to improved insulin action.

Syndromes of extreme insulin resistance represent the far end of the spectrum of insulin resistance. In general, the syndromes of extreme insulin resistance are caused by genetic defects in the insulin action pathway or in pathways that intersect with the insulin action pathway, or by the presence of autoantibodies to the insulin receptor that affect receptor function, or by autoantibodies to insulin itself (Table 28.2).

DEFINITION OF SEVERE INSULIN RESISTANCE

Patients with severe insulin resistance may be euglycemic if their β-cells are able to produce sufficient insulin to compensate for the defect in signaling, or they may have only impaired postprandial glucose tolerance, or they may have overt diabetes. Thus, the characterization of these patients differs, depending on the level of glycemia. For individuals with normal glucose levels, serum insulin levels are a good index of the severity of insulin resistance, because the ability of the β-cell to produce insulin, together with the magnitude of the peripheral insulin resistance, will determine the overall degree of hyperinsulinemia. Although there is no established value above which a fasting insulin level reflects severe insulin resistance, in the absence of obesity a fasting insulin value greater than 30 to 50 μU/mL and/or a postprandial insulin level or an insulin level following glucose challenge that is greater than 200 μU/mL should warrant further evaluation. However, identifiable genetic defects are less likely to be found when stimulated insulin levels are less than 1,000 μU/mL.

As patients progress to impaired glucose tolerance or overt hyperglycemia, the β-cell defect may progress and insulin levels may decline. For patients receiving insulin therapy, insulin resistance may be defined according to the insulin dose required to achieve glucose control. Because the normal adult secretes an average of 25 to 40 units of insulin daily (0.3 to 0.5 U/kg per day) and about 70% of exogenous insulin is bioavailable, any patient requiring more than 60 to 100 units of insulin every 24 hours has some degree of insulin resistance. However, for clinical purposes, the requirement of more than 1.5 to 2.0 U/kg body weight suggests more severe insulin resistance and the need for further evaluation. Behavioral problems or improper diabetes management

TABLE 28.1. Conditions Frequently Associated with Clinical Insulin Resistance

Obesity
Hypertension
Hypercholesterolemia
Type 2 diabetes mellitus
Physiologic states (puberty, pregnancy)
Severe stress (sepsis, burns)
Metabolic abnormalities (acidosis, uremia, hyperglycemia, hyponatremia)
Endocrine (acromegaly, Cushing's syndrome or disease, pheochromocytoma)

should be rigorously excluded as the cause of "insulin resistance." The exclusion of these causes may require careful evaluation of the patient's dietary and drug history and understanding of insulin therapy. Often hospitalization may be necessary to reveal a behavioral problem.

CLINICAL FINDINGS ASSOCIATED WITH EXTREME INSULIN RESISTANCE

The most common clinical features associated with severe insulin resistance include acanthosis nigricans, ovarian dysfunction with hyperandrogenism and hirsutism, and lipoatrophy.

Acanthosis Nigricans

Acanthosis nigricans is characterized by a velvety rash with papillomatosis, hyperkeratosis, and hyperpigmentation in the epidermis (Fig. 28.1). Lesions are commonly found at the neck and axillae and occasionally in the antecubital fossae and other areas. When severe, acanthosis nigricans can involve the entire face and much of the truncal skin. Acanthosis nigricans has been observed in a variety of clinical settings, including several endocrinopathies and internal malignancies, particularly gastrointestinal cancer (2). However, when present, acanthosis nigricans typically indicates at least a moderate degree of underlying insulin resistance.

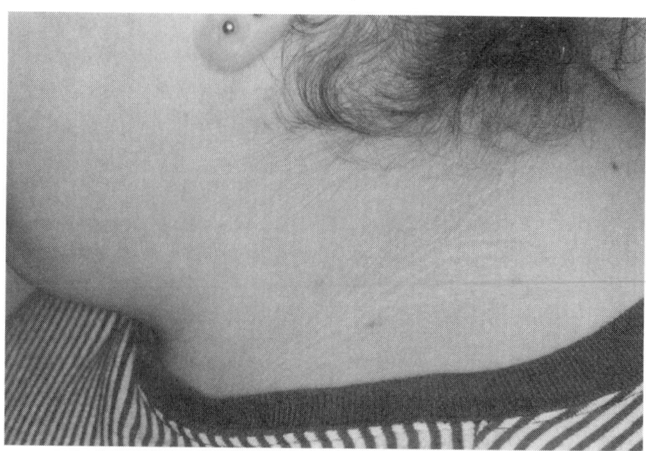

Figure 28.1. Acanthosis of the neck in a young woman with severe insulin resistance and obesity.

When specifically searched for, the frequency of acanthosis nigricans may be higher than previously thought. In an unselected population of 1,412 schoolchildren in Texas, acanthosis nigricans was present equally among boys and girls, with a prevalence of 7.1% (3). The acanthosis nigricans was more frequently noted in obese children, and its severity was correlated with the fasting plasma insulin level. Acanthosis nigricans is even more common in selected groups of patients and was shown to affect up to 29% of women with hyperandrogenism referred to a subspecialty clinic and up to 50% of obese women with polycystic ovarian disease (4). Many of these patients have variants of the type A syndrome with moderate insulin resistance that at least partially reverts with weight loss (see below).

TABLE 28.2. Classification of Syndromes of Severe Insulin Resistance

Genetic defects in insulin receptor
Type A syndrome
Rabson-Mendenhall syndrome
Leprechaunism
Immunologic, autoimmune
Antibodies to the insulin receptor
Type B syndrome
Ataxia-telangiectasia
Antibodies to insulin
Disorders of unknown etiology
Lipotrophic diabetes
Congenital
Dominant inheritance (Köbberling-Dunnigan syndrome)
Autosomal recessive inheritance (Seip syndrome)
Acquired
Generalized (Lawrence syndrome)
Partial lipoatrophy

Pseudoacromegaly

Pseudoacromegaly, including frontal bossing, prominence of the jaw and malocclusion of the teeth, macroglossia, increased hand and foot size, skin tags, increased skin thickness, and median nerve entrapment at the carpal tunnel, has been described in some patients with severe insulin resistance (Fig. 28.2). The development of either acanthosis nigricans or an acromegalic appearance has been attributed to direct effects of hyperinsulinemia on skin tissue that result in epidermal hypertrophy. The presence of marked hyperinsulinemia in some patients is sufficient to bind to and activate the insulin-like growth factor 1 (IGF-1) receptor. IGF-1 receptors have a substantially lower affinity for insulin than do insulin receptors themselves, but when the ambient concentration of insulin is sufficiently high, IGF-1 receptors may become activated by a mechanism that has been called "specificity spillover" (5,6). Thus, increased stimulation of the IGF-1 receptor by hyperinsulinemia may be an important mechanism for the stimulation of epidermal growth in acanthosis nigricans. In addition, these mechanisms also may play an important role in the increased production of ovarian androgens in insulin-resistant states. In some patients, it is likely that insulin resistance is limited to insulin-receptor pathways involved in acute metabolic effects such as glucose transport or amino acid uptake and that "growth" effects of insulin are unrestrained and, in fact, accentuated by the hyperinsulinemia.

Hyperandrogenism-Ovarian Dysfunction

Hyperandrogenism-ovarian dysfunction, presenting with primary or secondary amenorrhea or irregular menstrual cycles, is very common in female patients with syndromes of severe insulin resistance, with amenorrhea being more common in those with more severe resistance (7). The menstrual irregularity is associated with an increased production of ovarian androgens, leading to moderately elevated serum testosterone levels and various degrees of hirsutism and virilization (8). Moreover, free or bioavailable testosterone levels may be increased disproportionately in these patients owing to a decrease in sex hormone–binding globulin. The ovaries are typically polycystic and hyperthecotic. Although the exact pathophysiology of such ovarian dysfunction is not known, insulin may cause ovarian hyperstimulation via its own receptor or by cross-reacting with the receptors for IGF-1, which also are present in the ovary. Luteinizing hormone has also been shown to act synergistically with insulin to promote the production of androgen by the ovaries (9).

HIRSUTISM AND VIRILIZATION

Hirsutism, the development of excessive androgen-stimulated terminal hair in a female, may occur with severe insulin resistance. Virilization, including defeminizing signs such as loss of the female body contour or frank masculinization with clitoromegaly and deepening of the voice, increased muscle mass, temporal balding, and increased libido, is less common.

Lipoatrophy or Lipodystrophy

Lipoatrophy or lipodystrophy, a marked reduction in subcutaneous adipose tissue that occurs in a segmental or generalized distribution (Fig. 28.3), is an additional clinical sign associated with the insulin resistance syndromes of leprechaunism and lipoatrophic diabetes. Lipoatrophy can be classified as focal or generalized and congenital or acquired. If lipoatrophy is localized to sites of insulin injection, it can be the result of a form of insulin allergy in individuals without marked insulin resistance. Descriptions of various forms of lipodystrophy are provided later in this chapter.

CHARACTERIZATION OF INSULIN RESISTANCE

Patients suspected of having a syndrome of severe insulin resistance and who are not receiving exogenous insulin may be characterized by fasting and postprandial or post–glucose challenge serum insulin levels. The standard oral glucose tolerance test with both insulin and glucose levels is a rapid and reliable initial diagnostic evaluation. The more markedly elevated these levels, the more severe the resistance and the more likely that the evaluation will reveal an identifiable underlying defect, such as when the fasting insulin level is above 50 mIU/L and the postprandial levels are above 200 to 500 mIU/L, although in some affected patients they may exceed 1,000 mIU/L (with normal values between 2 and 20 mIU/L). The hyperinsulinemia commonly observed in these patients develops by two complementary mechanisms. One is an increase in insulin secretion by the pancreatic β-cell in response to persistent elevations in fasting or postprandial glucose levels, and the other results from defects in the peripheral action of insulin associated with a striking reduction in the metabolic clearance of circulating insulin (10).

Several additional procedures are used clinically to evaluate the severity of insulin resistance. These tests vary in their complexity both in performance and in interpretation. They share the common element of administering exogenous insulin to rule out the unlikely possibility of an abnormal endogenous insulin molecule (insulin mutation) as the cause of hyperinsulinemia. The *insulin tolerance test* (ITT) assesses the glucose-lowering effect of an intravenous insulin bolus (6). After an overnight fast, in a normal individual, an intravenous bolus injection of a dose of regular insulin of 0.1 U/kg of body weight will reduce the blood glucose level to a value 50% or less of the initial value or may provoke frank hypoglycemia. A patient with peripheral insulin resistance will require a higher dose of injected insulin (≥0.2 U/kg) to produce this reduction in the fasting glucose level. If the patient requires an insulin bolus of 0.3 U/kg or more to induce hypoglycemia, the diagnosis of extreme insulin resistance is certain. Given the importance of the diagnosis, a serum insulin level should be obtained 10 minutes after insulin injection to confirm that insulin entered the vascular compartment.

In the *steady-state plasma glucose test* (SSPG), also known as the triple-infusion test, somatostatin is infused to suppress endogenous insulin production, and fixed doses of insulin and glucose are co-infused. At steady state, the higher the glucose level for a given insulin dose administered, the more insulin resistant the subject. The *frequently sampled intravenous glucose tolerance test* (FSIVGTT) provides a standardized method to assess both the pancreatic β-cell secretory capacity and periph-

A

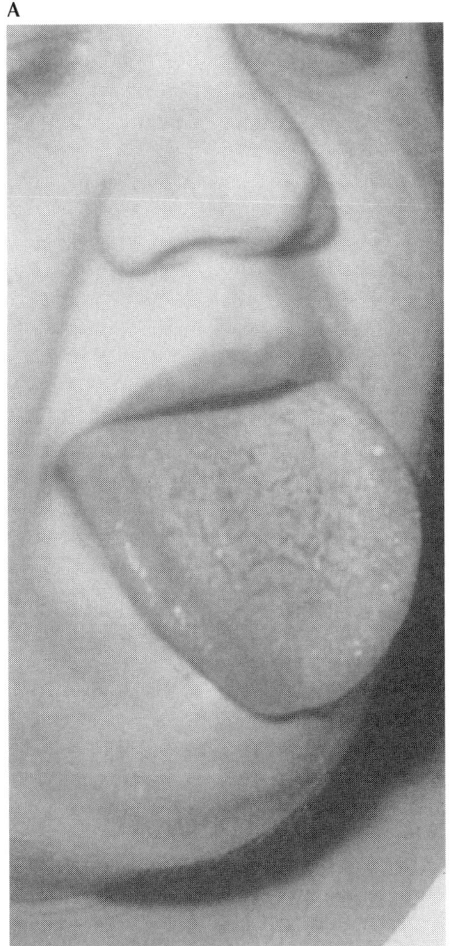

Figure 28.2. A: Tongue enlargement seen in the insulin-resistant patient with pseudoacromegaly.

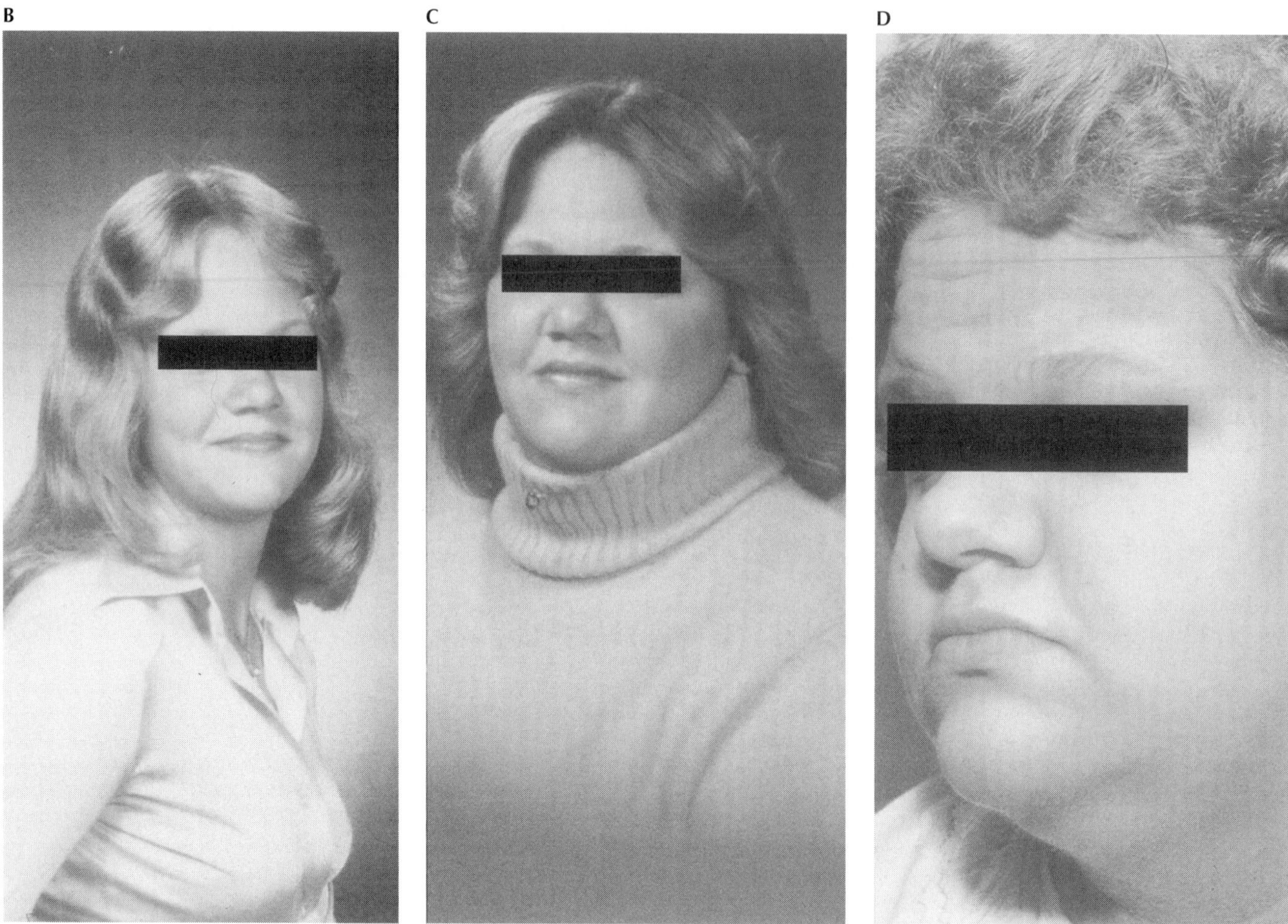

Figure 28.2. (*continued*) **B–D:** Progressive pseudoacromegaly in a young woman with severe insulin resistance. Note the progressive coarsening of facial features. (**A, B** from Flier JS, Moller DE, Moses AC, et al. Insulin-mediated pseudoacromegaly: clinical and biochemical characterization of a syndrome of selective insulin resistance. *J Clin Endocrinol Metab* 1993;76:1533–1541, with permission. Copyright 1993. The Endocrine Society.)

eral glucose uptake in response to a bolus intravenous administration of glucose (0.3 g/kg). Additional information on insulin sensitivity is gained by the administration of insulin (0.03 to 0.05 U/kg) 20 minutes after the glucose load. *Euglycemic-hyperinsulinemic clamp* studies are considered the gold standard for measurement of insulin action but are more difficult to perform. A dose-response curve to exogenous insulin is generated by measuring the variable infusion rate of glucose required to maintain euglycemia. The steady-state rate of peripheral glucose utilization (M value) is measured as milligrams of glucose used per kilogram of body weight per minute. Studies have demonstrated total-body glucose clearance to be reduced by 35% to 40% in subjects with type 2 diabetes as compared with that of age- and weight-matched healthy controls, with similar or more modest reduction in insulin sensitivity in persons with obesity, hypertension, and hyperlipidemia (1). More severe reductions are seen in persons with syndromes of extreme insulin resistance. In type 2 diabetes, the primary site of reduced insulin-mediated glucose uptake appears to be located in the peripheral (muscle) tissue (11), and both oxidative and nonoxidative (glycogen storage) components of glucose metabolism may be impaired (12).

INSULIN RESISTANCE DUE TO MUTATIONS IN THE INSULIN-RECEPTOR GENE

Although more than 60 naturally occurring mutations in the insulin-receptor gene have been characterized, three distinct clinical syndromes are associated with mutations in this receptor. All share the clinical features of acanthosis nigricans and hyperandrogenism.

Leprechaunism

Leprechaunism (also known as Donohue syndrome), the most severe of the conditions associated with mutations in the insulin-receptor gene, is characterized additionally by intrauterine growth retardation, a characteristic bird-like facies, fasting hypoglycemia, and glucose intolerance despite insulin levels that may be more than 100 times the normal values (Fig. 28.4). Most patients die within the first year of life. The condition is associated with homozygous mutations in either the coding sequence or the regulatory domains of both alleles of the insulin-receptor gene. Rare patients have two null alleles and totally lack functional insulin receptors.

A

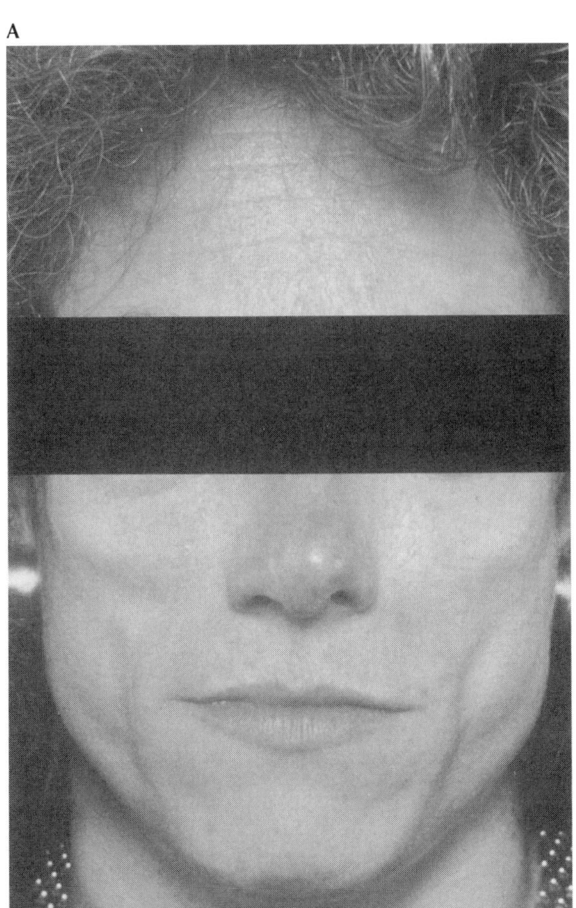

B

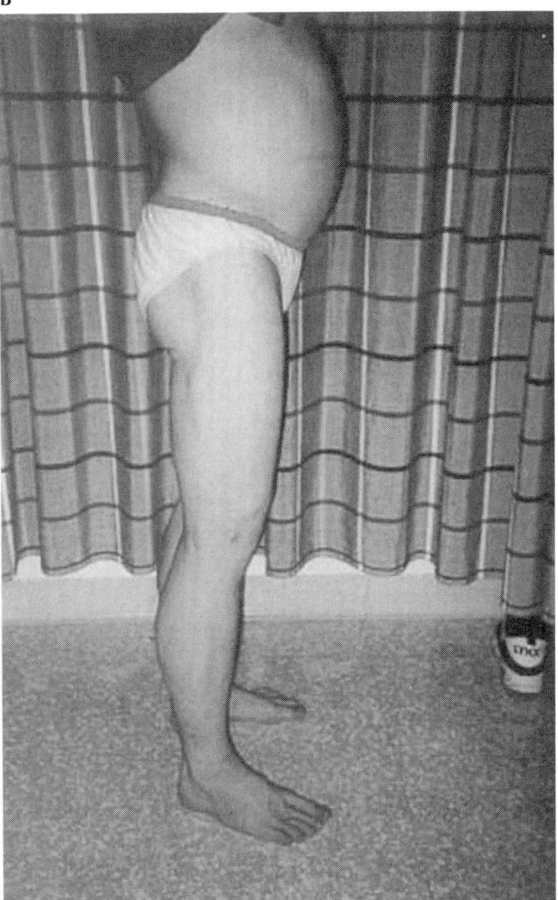

C

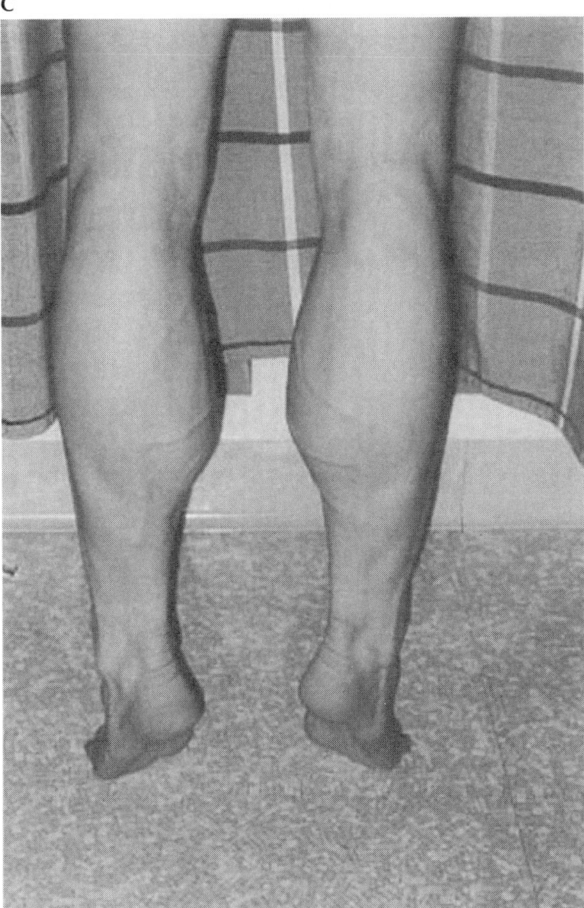

Figure 28.3. A: Lipoatrophy affecting the face in a patient with partial lipoatrophy. **B, C:** Lipoatrophy affecting the body and legs. Note the protuberant abdomen caused by marked hepatomegaly and the apparent muscular hypertrophy of the calves.

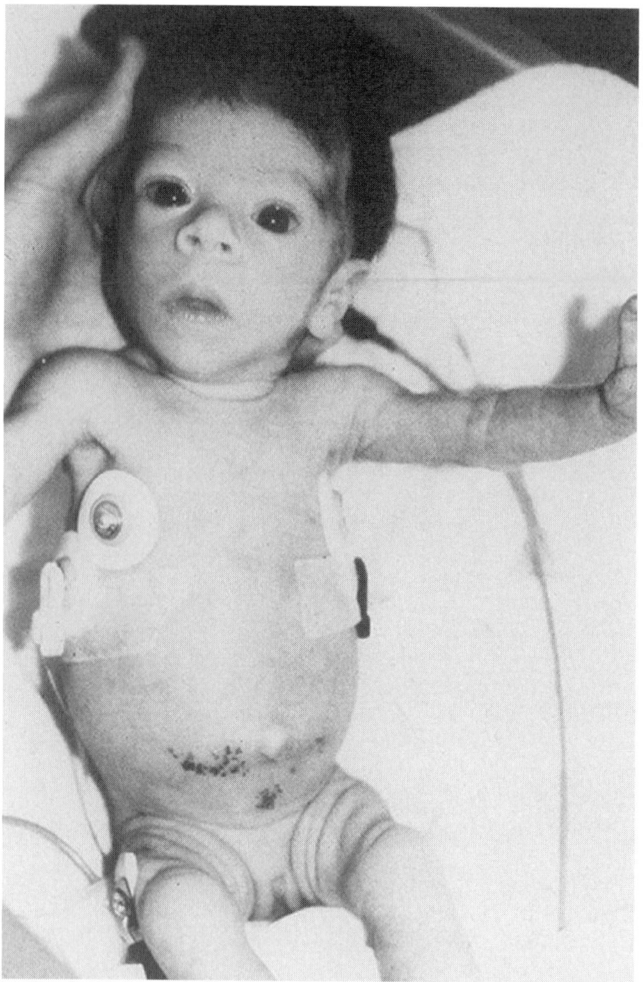

Figure 28.4. Infant affected with Donohue syndrome (leprechaunism). (From Kahn CR, Goldstein BJ, Reddy SSK. Hereditary and acquired syndromes of insulin resistance. In: Pickup J, Williams G, eds. *Textbook of diabetes*. Oxford: Blackwell Scientific Publications, 1991:276–285, with permission.)

Rabson-Mendenhall Syndrome

Patients with Rabson-Mendenhall syndrome demonstrate abnormalities in the teeth and nails and pineal gland hyperplasia. These patients may survive until adolescence, and many have compound heterozygous mutations in the insulin receptor, producing severe impairment of receptor function.

Type A Syndrome

The type A syndrome of insulin resistance is the least severe of the receptor mutation disorders. Affected females generally also demonstrate significant hyperandrogenism. Patients are neither obese nor lipoatrophic. Although many use the term type A syndrome to identify patients with mutations in one allele of the insulin receptor, many use the term to describe patients who demonstrate the triad of hyperandrogenism, insulin resistance, and acanthosis nigricans (HAIR-AN). Because only a minority of the patients who manifest this triad have heterozygous mutations in the insulin receptor, it is likely that mutations exist in postreceptor insulin-signaling transduction proteins. Likewise, when this triad is seen in the setting of obesity, it is less likely to be associated with a mutation in the insulin receptor than with additional polygenic factors rendering the patient susceptible to the clinical syndrome.

Mutations of the insulin receptor have been described in the insulin-binding domain, the transmembrane domain, and at or near phosphotyrosine sites; not all of these defects are associated with severe insulin resistance and the acromegaloid and hyperandrogenic features. In addition, specific mutations in the insulin receptor are found in only a minority of patients with a severe insulin resistance syndrome.

Insulin action at the cellular level is complex (reviewed in Chapter 6). Postreceptor insulin signaling proteins have been assessed carefully in patients with severe insulin resistance in whom no receptor defect could be identified. There is a small increase in frequency in variations in the insulin-receptor substrate 1 (IRS-1) sequence in subjects with type 2 diabetes as compared with controls (~15% vs. 5%, respectively), and some studies suggest that these may have some functional significance (13,14). IRS-1 variants may be more common among patients with severe insulin resistance; however, as these variants are also present in unaffected persons, they are not likely to account fully for the severe insulin resistance (15,16). Phosphatidylinositol 3-kinase (PI 3-kinase) is central in insulin-mediated glucose disposal and consists of a regulatory domain splice variants p85α and p85β and a catalytic domain p110. Variants of p85α, Met^{326}Ile, have been described in humans and do not appear to be associated with decreased activity; however, an Arg^{409}Gln mutation has been identified in a patient with severe insulin resistance and is associated with lower activity *in vitro* and higher fasting glucose levels in the carriers within the proband's family (17). In addition, impaired insulin activation of PI 3-kinase has been demonstrated in fibroblasts from severely insulin-resistant patients (18,19) . Expression levels of genes for other proteins appear altered in some patients with type 2 diabetes, such as the gene belonging to the Ras–guanosine triphosphate superfamily, RAD (ras-associated with diabetes), which has been found to be overexpressed in muscle tissue of patients with type 2 diabetes (20), although the clinical significance of this finding remains uncertain and has not been demonstrated in conditions of extreme resistance.

The role of peroxisome proliferator-activated receptors (PPARs) in modulating insulin sensitivity has only recently been appreciated with the discovery of the thiazolidinedione class of drugs. These agents have been demonstrated to be potent insulin sensitizers, although the molecular mechanisms of action are only partially understood (see Chapter 41). The drugs bind to and activate an orphan nuclear receptor PPARγ and regulate the transcription of a number of insulin-responsive genes, including glucose transporters, critical for the control of glucose metabolism. PPARs exist as heterodimers with another nuclear receptor, RXR, and effects are dependent on the presence of separate insulin-regulated transcription factors. Two dominant negative heterozygote mutations in the ligand-binding domain of the PPARγ receptor have been identified in severely insulin-resistant, hypertensive patients with overt diabetes (21).

At the molecular level, multiple alterations in the insulin action cascade have been shown to be present and to contribute to the insulin resistance of type 2 diabetes and the insulin resistance syndromes; however, the relative importance of these alterations remains controversial. These changes are regulatory and include downregulation of the insulin receptor, decreased receptor kinase activity, decreased phosphorylation of receptor substrates, and defects in glucose transporter translocation (22–26) . In addition to these signaling defects, several inhibitors of insulin action, such as cytokines, may be involved in the pathophysiology of diabetes. For example, tumor necrosis factor-α (TNF-α), which is expressed by adipose tissue and increased in human obesity, inhibits insulin-receptor kinase activity, and neutralization of TNF-α improves muscle insulin sensitivity in insulin-resistant rats (27). Similarly, the transmembrane glycoprotein PC-1, a threonine-specific protein kinase, nonspecifically inhibits the activity of insulin-receptor tyrosine kinase and has been isolated from fibroblasts of a patient with severe insulin resistance (28), although a primary role for this kinase in the etiology of insulin resistance remains unproven. Although such regulatory involvement may be present in or contribute to syndromes of severe insulin resistance, none has been clearly demonstrated to date.

LIPOATROPHIC DIABETES

Lipoatrophic diabetes encompasses a genetically heterogeneous group of rare syndromes characterized by insulin-resistant diabetes associated with a regional or complete absence of subcutaneous adipose tissue and presence of hypertriglyceridemia. Several forms of this condition have been reported according to mode of inheritance and extent and regional distribution of the lipoatrophy (29). These include congenital types of generalized lipoatrophic diabetes, which may exhibit either dominant inheritance (Köbberling-Dunnigan syndrome) or recessive inheritance (Berardinelli-Seip syndrome). In addition, syndromes of acquired total lipoatrophy (Lawrence syndrome) and various types of acquired partial lipoatrophy have been described.

Congenital Lipoatrophy

DOMINANT INHERITANCE (KÖBBERLING-DUNNIGAN VARIETY)

By studying pedigrees of congenital lipoatrophy with dominant inheritance in Scotland and Germany, Köbberling and Dunnigan delineated two clinical subtypes with characteristic distributions of subcutaneous fat that appear to be consistent within each pedigree (30–32). In type 1 familial lipodystrophy, the loss of subcutaneous fat is confined to the limbs, with sparing of the face and trunk, and intracavity fat deposits. In type 2 congenital lipoatrophy syndrome, the trunk, with the exception of the vulva, also is affected, giving the impression of labial hypertrophy. Associated clinical features variably expressed in the pedigrees include severe hyperlipidemia, acanthosis nigricans, hepatosplenomegaly, tuberoeruptive xanthomata, elevated basal metabolic rate, and insulin-resistant diabetes without ketoacidosis. Genetic characterization of at least 10 kindreds with this condition demonstrates linkage to chromosome 1q, with evidence of a common founder haplotype (33,34). At least five different missense mutations have been identified in the *LMNA* gene associated with this condition. The protein product of the gene is lamin A/C, a component of the nuclear envelope. Lamins A and C are two alternatively transcribed products of the *LMNA* gene and are members of the intermediate filament family of proteins that form components of the nuclear lamina, a protein-rich fibrous area below the inner nuclear membrane. The defects in nuclear lamin A/C have been confirmed in additional affected kindreds, but not all patients with the phenotypic characteristics of the syndrome manifest mutations in this gene (35). The lipoatrophic disorder may be caused by a gene tightly linked to this site; however, evidence supports a direct involvement of the *LMNA* mutation in the disease, and there may be a series of genetic mutations responsible for the phenotype. Heterozygous mutations in *LMNA*, which are more extensive and involve several exons, have been associated with an autosomal dominant form of muscular dystrophy, the Emery-Dreifuss variant (36), characterized by muscle contractures and a cardiac conduction defect and with an age-related dilated cardiomyopathy and conduction system disease, CMD1A (37). Rodent models with a targeted deletion of this gene develop postnatal cardiac and skeletal muscle dystrophy and a loss of white adipose tissue (38). *LMNA* is expressed ubiquitously in cells; thus, the site-specific amino acid substitutions associated with these three distinct clinical syndromes reveal distinct functional domains of the lamin A/C protein to the different cell types. Further studies may reveal the role of lamin A/C in adipocyte function and insulin action.

RECESSIVE INHERITANCE (BERARDINELLI-SEIP SYNDROME)

The autosomal recessive form of congenital generalized lipoatrophy has been reported to occur more widely (39) than the dominant variety (40). Parental consanguinity is frequent, and cases are equally distributed among males and females. The absence of subcutaneous fat and muscular hypertrophy is noted in early infancy, although the diabetes typically appears during or after puberty. Imaging studies and autopsy demonstrate a near-complete absence of metabolically active adipose tissue from the subcutaneous area, from the intraabdominal, retroperitoneal, and epicardial regions, as well as from the bone marrow. Unlike with the dominantly inherited Köbberling-Dunnigan syndromes, both facial fat and buccal fat are affected. In contrast, mammary fat tissue may be spared, and mechanical adipose tissue is present in the palms, soles, scalp, and perineal areas. Loss of subcutaneous adipose tissue causes the thyroid, peripheral veins, and skeletal muscles to appear more prominent, and actual muscular hypertrophy may occur.

Growth and maturation of bone during the first 4 to 5 years of life are frequently accelerated. Acromegalic facies, along with thick skin and large hands and feet, may be present. Acanthosis nigricans is often a later development. Umbilical herniation is common. Hepatomegaly, resulting from increased stores of lipid and glycogen, is frequently observed and can be massive. Hypertriglyceridemia with eruptive xanthomas, lipemia retinalis, and episodic pancreatitis also may occur. Polycystic ovaries and menstrual irregularity are common in affected females. Mental retardation, psychiatric disturbances, and intracerebral disorders localized to the region of the third ventricle have also been associated with congenital lipoatrophy.

Laboratory studies of patients with recessive, congenital lipoatrophic diabetes have demonstrated a striking elevation of the basal metabolic rate with normal thyroid function. Despite the acromegaloid appearance, circulating levels of growth hormone are normal. A striking type IV or type V hyperlipoproteinemia typically is present and appears to be due to increased synthesis and decreased clearance of lipoproteins (41). When diabetes has been present for years, long-term diabetic complications have been described, including nephropathy with proteinuria and hypertension, peripheral neuropathy, and diabetic retinopathy. The hepatomegaly often leads to portal hypertension and irreversible cirrhosis, which is commonly the cause of death in patients with this disorder.

Previous studies of candidate genes involved in insulin action and lipid metabolism have not identified the molecular basis of this form of lipodystrophy; however, two chromosomal loci have been identified in association with this disorder. Genetic characterization of 17 carefully ascertained patients with the syndrome demonstrated linkage with the chromosomal locus 9q34. Initially termed BSL1, the gene responsible was revealed to encode

1-acylglycerol-3-phosphate *O*-acyltransferase 2 (AGPAT2) (42). AGPAT2 is abundantly expressed in adipose tissue and catalyzes the acylation of lysophosphatidic acid to form phosphatidic acid, an intermediate in the biosynthesis of triacylglycerol and glycerophospholipids; mutations in this gene thereby inhibit triacylglycerol synthesis and storage in adipocytes. The second locus, identified as BSCL2 and located on chromosome 11q13, is found in cohorts from Norway and Lebanon (43a). The defect has been identified within the gene that encodes a protein termed *seipin*, of unknown function and with little homology to known proteins. Seipin is widely expressed, with particularly high levels in the brain. Several variants of this locus are found with the syndrome; most are null mutations and probably result in a severe disruption of the protein. As subsets of patients do not have mutations in either of these genes, additional loci will likely be identified (43b). Other candidate genes include a series of proteins involved in adipocyte differentiation. Transgenic mice with altered expression of the transcription factors sterol responsive element binding protein 1 (SREBP1c) (44) and CCAAT/enhancer binding protein (C/EBP) (45) demonstrate features similar to those of congenital generalized lipodystrophy and support a role for transcription factor involvement in the syndrome. Although no mutations in PPARγ have been identified to date in patients with Berardinelli-Seip lipoatrophic syndromes (46,47), evidence is beginning to suggest a role for these nuclear regulatory proteins in the disease, and a heterozygous mutation in the PPARγ coding region in exon 6 at a highly conserved residue in one patient with a familial partial lipodystrophy (48) suggests a role for this gene in some forms of the disorder.

Acquired Lipoatrophy

GENERALIZED FORM

Acquired, generalized lipoatrophy was first described by Lawrence in 1946 (49). Affected patients exhibit a generalized absence of body fat, insulin-resistant nonketotic diabetes mellitus, an elevated basal metabolic rate with hyperhidrosis, and hyperlipidemia with hepatosplenomegaly. The occurrence of this condition is sporadic, without familial inheritance. In many cases, a viral illness precedes the development of lipoatrophy, but a direct viral etiology has not been demonstrated. The onset is usually in childhood or shortly after puberty, and this condition has a 2:1 preponderance in females. Clinical diabetes typically follows the onset of lipoatrophy by an average of 4 years. In the Lawrence syndrome, as in the congenital form of lipoatrophic diabetes, hepatomegaly can lead to cirrhosis, which may be the ultimate cause of death. Accelerated atherosclerosis also may occur and contribute to premature coronary artery disease.

PARTIAL LIPOATROPHY

Several forms of acquired, partial loss of subcutaneous adipose tissue have been described (50). In partial lipoatrophy, the most common pattern is loss of fat from the face and trunk with normal or actually increased fat deposition below the waist. Occasionally, only the lower half of the body is affected or lipodystrophy is segmental in a dermatomal distribution.

Familial occurrence of partial lipoatrophy has also been described, although the mode of inheritance is not clearly Mendelian. Acquired partial lipoatrophy may represent a less severe variant of the generalized disorder (Lawrence syndrome), and families have been described in which both forms of the disease occur. In rare cases, the partial form may develop into generalized total lipoatrophy. Like acquired generalized lipoatrophy, females are affected predominantly, the onset of partial lipoatrophy usually occurs in childhood, and in some cases onset has been preceded by an infectious illness.

Patients with partial lipoatrophy frequently have hypocomplementemia, which also has been associated with membranoproliferative (mesangiocapillary) glomerulonephritis in some individuals (51,52). These alterations have not been observed in the congenital lipoatrophic disorders. The reduction in levels of serum complement is due to the presence of an IgG autoantibody that binds to and stabilizes the C3 convertase enzyme. The result of this antibody action is an increase in the splitting of complement factor C3 and the activation of the alternative pathway of complement. This autoantibody is indistinguishable from the C3 nephritic factor observed in patients with membranoproliferative glomerulonephritis who do not have partial lipodystrophy, and the relationship between the complement system defect and the clinical lipodystrophy remains obscure.

Pathogenesis

As described above, multiple molecular and genetic mechanisms underlie the lipoatrophic syndromes. A direct role for the insulin receptor has not been demonstrated in these disorders. Studies on several siblings in a pedigree with recessive congenital lipodystrophy revealed heterogeneity in the function and expression of the insulin receptor in cultured cells, as well as a variant sequence of the insulin-receptor gene in the family members (53). The abnormalities were not fully linked to the clinical expression of the lipodystrophy, a finding that supports a complex nature of the genetic and metabolic defects in this syndrome that may lead to secondary effects on the insulin receptor. No circulating insulin inhibitors or antibodies directed at insulin or the insulin receptor have been found that account for the insulin resistance in patients with lipoatrophic diabetes. However, one case of total acquired lipodystrophy with diabetes but normal circulating insulin levels was associated with increased clearance of circulating insulin or accelerated degradation of insulin at target tissues (54).

Direct examination of cultured fibroblasts from several patients with generalized lipodystrophy has suggested that the severe insulin resistance in this syndrome may actually be due to a postbinding defect in insulin action that affects primarily glucose uptake or glucose metabolism (55). Furthermore, both insulin and IGF-1 receptors from these fibroblasts were found to have defects in their tyrosine kinase activity, suggesting that a signaling abnormality common to these related receptors may play a role in the pathogenesis of the insulin resistance (56).

Other mechanisms have been suggested to play a role in the development of lipoatrophic syndromes but have not been clearly established. A potential association between the immune system and disorders of adiposity and energy balance may ultimately be found in a serum protein named *adipsin*, which is secreted by adipocytes into the bloodstream. Adipsin has been shown to have serine protease activity identical to that of complement factor D, a process that is the initial step in the activation of the alternative pathway (57). It is interesting that both factor D activity and levels of adipsin mRNA are dramatically reduced in several models of genetic obesity in mice, a finding suggesting a possible role for adipsin in the energy balance of certain states of obesity (58). Some years ago the presence of a circulating lipid-mobilizing factor was thought to be causally associated with lipoatrophic diabetes, but this component remains poorly characterized. This factor was initially isolated from the urine of lipoatrophic patients and, when injected into animals, produced insulin resistance and lipolysis of fat stores (59). The factor was not specific for this syndrome, because it was later found in the urine of diabetic patients with proteinuria (60). However, clinical data on both of these mechanisms remain inconclusive.

The presence of elevated metabolic rate, hyperlipidemia, and insulin resistance suggests hyperactivity of the sympathetic nervous system, but plasma and urinary levels of catecholamine have not been consistently elevated in the patients studied (61,62) . However, segmental dysfunction of the adrenergic nervous system or regional differences in the response of adipose tissue to circulating hormones may be etiologic factors in the unique distribution of affected adipose tissue in partial lipodystrophy (63,64).

The association of increased hypothalamic releasing factors in the circulation of lipoatrophic patients has raised the possibility of a hypothalamic role in the etiology of these conditions. Because an accumulation of dopamine within the hypothalamus might lead to accelerated release of hypothalamic hormones, drugs that affect dopamine synthesis or action were tested in lipoatrophic patients. The neuroleptic agent pimozide, which reduces levels of hypothalamic dopamine, was initially described as producing dramatic clinical improvement in several prepubertal or peripubertal patients with lipoatrophy (65). However, subsequent reports demonstrated no clinical benefit from pimozide and diminish the practical therapeutic value of this drug (66,67). Fenfluramine, a dopamine-blocking agent that also lowers serotonin levels, has also been used in a few patients with lipoatrophic diabetes. This agent was initially found to increase the sensitivity of a few patients to exogenous insulin and to improve the hyperhidrosis and hyperlipidemia; however, no consistent long-term beneficial effect has been observed in other studies (68), and the agent is no longer available in the United States (69,70).

The possibility that a hypothalamic lesion might play a role in these disorders is suggested by the frequent occurrence of tumors of the third ventricle in patients with congenital lipoatrophic diabetes (71). It is of interest that, in the diencephalic syndrome of infancy, anterior hypothalamic tumors have also been found to occur in association with diminished body fat, elevated metabolic rate, and accelerated growth. A boy with acquired lipoatrophic diabetes associated with stenosis of the aqueduct of Sylvius demonstrated dramatic clinical improvement after placement of a ventriculocisternal shunt, providing further evidence that hypothalamic dysfunction may contribute to the perturbed metabolic state (67).

Management

Because the etiology of insulin-resistant diabetes in the lipoatrophic syndromes is enigmatic, therapy has consisted of attempts at maintaining the blood glucose level within a reasonable range. Caloric restriction may improve the hyperlipemia and carbohydrate tolerance in patients with lipoatrophic diabetes (70,72). Good control of blood glucose levels may be difficult to achieve in patients with lipodystrophy because of the fixed nature of the underlying abnormalities in peripheral insulin action or glucose uptake found in many of these patients. Some benefit has been demonstrated with the insulin-sensitizing agents, including the biguanide agent metformin and the thiazolidinedione compound troglitazone. In addition to the improvements in insulin sensitivity, thiazolidinedione compounds have been associated with increased adipocyte development (73) and thus seem particularly suited to treat this condition. In a cohort of 13 patients treated over 6 months, troglitazone substantially lowered levels of glycosylated hemoglobin, fasting triglycerides, and free fatty acids and lowered the respiratory quotient, suggesting increased oxidation of fat, while body fat increased (74). However, this agent has been associated with impaired liver function, the rate of which may be increased in patients with the underlying fatty liver seen in severe insulin resistance, and has been removed from the market. A few patients currently are being treated with other thiazolidinedione compounds, but it is too early to identify any as a superior product for this condition.

The adipocyte hormone leptin is important in regulating energy balance, and lipoatrophic patients are deficient in leptin. Genetically engineered rodent models of lipoatrophic diabetes demonstrate that the metabolic abnormalities improve with surgical fat transplantation (75), and leptin replacement can reverse insulin resistance and diabetes (76). Treatment with recombinant leptin for 4 months has been studied in a small cohort of humans with lipoatrophic conditions (77), demonstrating improved glycosylated hemoglobin, decreased triglycerides and liver volume, and reduced need for other antidiabetic agents.

Attempts at dietary therapy for lipoatrophic diabetes with omega-3 fatty acids resulted in a reduction in serum triglyceride levels and an amelioration of pancreatitis in at least one patient but at the expense of more severe glucose intolerance caused by an inhibition of insulin secretion (78). Limited studies have been conducted using recombinant human IGF-1 in insulin-resistant and lipoatrophic patients, with some suggestion of metabolic improvement (79). As described above, neuroleptic agents have been used in the treatment of lipoatrophic diabetes, with transient or no improvement noted in most cases.

Medical or dietary therapy has not accomplished a reversal of the lipoatrophy with the reappearance of subcutaneous fat tissue. In a case of acquired partial lipodystrophy, however, transplantation of autologous adipose tissue to the face was recently reported to provide a favorable cosmetic improvement (80).

IMMUNOLOGIC INSULIN RESISTANCE

In several syndromes of extreme insulin resistance, the insulin action pathway in target cells is intact but the effectiveness of circulating insulin is blocked by the presence of antibodies that react with the insulin receptor or the insulin molecule itself.

Antibodies to Insulin

Antibodies to insulin are less common today than previously as treatment has shifted from relatively impure preparations of animal insulins to more purified human insulin of recombinant origin. Intermittent exposure is more likely to generate an immune response than is continuous treatment. Insulin resistance due to high-titer immunoglobulin G (IgG) antibodies is extremely uncommon and occurs in well under 0.01% of insulin-treated patients with diabetes. In rare situations the high circulating levels of antibodies to insulin can serve as a reservoir for insulin and contribute to episodes of spontaneous or fasting severe or prolonged hypoglycemia. Most patients receiving insulin therapy, including the human insulins, develop measurable antibodies to insulin; thus, a quantitative measurement of competitive protein binding is necessary to confirm that these antibodies are clinically relevant to the resistance. In insulin-resistant patients, the concentration of antibody measured by binding capacity usually exceeds 5 units of insulin per liter of plasma. In rare cases, switching to an insulin analogue may be an effective form of treatment. Immunosuppression or plasmapheresis also may be effective. Rarely, endogenous high-titer antibodies to insulin appear in the absence of insulin therapy and are associated with autoimmune disease.

Type B Syndrome of Insulin Resistance: Autoantibodies to Insulin Receptor

The type B syndrome of severe insulin resistance is an autoimmune syndrome of circulating antibodies directed at the insulin receptor (81–83) that causes both target-cell insulin resistance and endogenous hyperinsulinemia and most often presents in the fourth to sixth decade of life. Like other autoimmune disorders, this condition has a female preponderance (female-to-male ratio, 2:1) and is often associated with other autoimmune phenomena, such as an increased erythrocyte sedimentation rate, elevated levels of γ-globulins, and autoantibodies to nuclear antigens or DNA. In fact, up to one third of the patients satisfy criteria for the diagnosis of systemic lupus erythematosus or Sjögren syndrome (84). Some of the clinical features of this disorder, such as the severity of the acanthosis nigricans, tend to follow the severity of the underlying insulin resistance.

PATHOGENESIS

Laboratory studies of antibodies to the insulin receptor isolated from patients with type B insulin resistance have demonstrated that these polyclonal antibodies can affect any of several vital aspects of the insulin action pathway. Most often, the antibodies to the insulin receptor cause a decrease in the affinity of the insulin receptor for insulin and lead to peripheral insulin resistance by acting as competitive antagonists of insulin binding. Other receptor antibodies that do not affect hormone binding can interfere with signal transduction by the insulin receptor, accelerate turnover of the insulin receptor, or lead to postreceptor desensitization of the insulin action pathway. Because the antibodies are typically polyclonal, several types of biochemical effects may be elicited by different classes of antibodies to the receptor even in an individual patient (85).

Further clinical heterogeneity of the type B syndrome has been observed in several patients who have developed or have presented with fasting hypoglycemia in association with the presence of circulating antibodies to the insulin receptor (86). In contrast to the patients with severe insulin resistance, these patients exhibit antibodies to the insulin receptor that can interact with the insulin-binding domain of the receptor in a positive manner and actually mimic the actions of insulin. In these individuals, the insulin-like activity of the antibodies is clinically manifest as an erratic hypoglycemic syndrome that may be confused with an islet cell tumor.

As with other autoimmune disorders, the symptoms may wax and wane over time, with the clinical severity dependent on both variation in titer and properties of the circulating autoantibodies. Remarkable clinical heterogeneity has been observed in some patients with type B syndrome, whose condition has actually evolved from one of severe insulin resistance to a hypoglycemic state. This development may occur because of changes in the abundance or activity of free autoantibodies in the circulation, which can have variable effects on insulin action in target tissues. These combined effects obviously can complicate the precise management of blood glucose control in these patients. A fraction of patients experience spontaneous remission of the disorder over a 2- to 3-year period.

In laboratory studies, the chronicity of exposure also has been shown to play an important role in the cellular effects of particular antibodies to the receptor (87). Thus, acute exposure of cultured cells to receptor antibodies may have insulinomimetic effects, whereas exposure for several hours may result in insulin resistance as a consequence of accelerated internalization and degradation of the receptors in the target cells (88). As in other autoimmune disorders, the type B syndrome arises from a defect in the regulation of the immune system rather than from an abnormality of the tissue insulin receptors. This conclusion is supported by the observation that insulin sensitivity appears to be normal in patients with the type B syndrome during periods of antibody remission. Furthermore, normal function of insulin receptors has been demonstrated in cultured cells from patients with type B syndrome, and insulin resistance can be mimicked by incubating the patient's cells with serum containing the receptor antibodies.

Several methods are used by specialized clinical laboratories to detect the presence of antibodies to the insulin receptor, which are typically polyclonal and of the IgG class (89,90). These include the binding-inhibition assay, the immunoprecipitation assay, and an assay of insulin-like activity in the γ-globulin fraction of the patient's serum (Table 28.3). The first method, which depends on the ability of the antibody to inhibit the binding of insulin to its receptor on cultured human lymphoblastoid cells, is the method most commonly used. However, the specificity of this technique may be affected by the presence of nonspecific inhibitors of insulin binding that may be found in the plasma of individuals without receptor antibodies.

The immunoprecipitation assay is performed by incubating the patient's serum with affinity-labeled insulin receptors and isolating the immune complexes that result in a positive test (90). This assay is somewhat more difficult to perform but is more sensitive than the binding-inhibition assay and can detect antibodies directed at sites other than the insulin-binding domain of the receptor. Flow cytometry has also been used to demonstrate the presence of antibodies to insulin receptor in the serum of patients with the type B syndrome (91). Assays based on the insulin-like activity of the antibodies are sensitive but are not specific for antibodies to insulin receptor and may give a positive response to other factors in the patient's circulation.

It is interesting that, in addition to immunosuppressive and plasmapheresis approaches, administration of recombinant human IGF-1 has improved both insulin sensitivity and glycemic control in some patients (92).

Ataxia-telangiectasia

Low-molecular-weight IgM antibodies to insulin receptors have been described in several patients with ataxia-telangiectasia (93). Ataxia-telangiectasia is a rare recessive syndrome characterized by progressive cerebellar ataxia, oculocutaneous telangiectasia, recurrent upper and lower respiratory tract infections,

TABLE 28.3. Evaluation of Pathogenetic Mechanism in Patients with Extreme Insulin Resistance

- Patient with associated autoimmune features: suspect type B syndrome
  - Measurement of antibodies to insulin receptor
    - Insulin receptor binding-inhibition assay
    - Insulin receptor immunoprecipitation assay
  - Assay of serum insulin-like activity
    - Flow cytometry
- Patient with suspected antibodies to insulin
  - Quantitative measurement of antibodies to insulin by competitive protein-binding assay
- Patient with clinical features of type A syndrome or leprechaunism
  - Biochemical studies of insulin-receptor function
  - Molecular analysis of insulin-receptor gene
  - Assay of postreceptor defect in cultured cells

and a variety of immunologic abnormalities. About 60% of patients with this syndrome have glucose intolerance, hyperinsulinemia, and a decreased sensitivity to exogenous insulin. As in the typical type B syndrome, the insulin receptors on cultured fibroblasts are normal, indicating that there is no underlying defect in the insulin receptor itself.

Acknowledgment

The authors gratefully acknowledge the work of Barry J. Goldstein, MD, who authored this chapter in the 13th edition, portions of which have been carried forward into the current text.

REFERENCES

1. Chen L, Komiya I, Inman L, et al. Molecular and cellular responses of islets during perturbations of glucose homeostasis determined by in situ hybridization histochemistry. *Proc Natl Acad Sci U S A* 1989;86:1367–1371.
2. Brown J, Winkelmann RK. Acanthosis nigricans: a study of 90 cases. *Medicine* (Baltimore) 1968;47:33–51.
3. Stuart CA, Pate CJ, Peters EJ. Prevalence of acanthosis nigricans in an unselected population. *Am J Med* 1989;87:269–272.
4. Dunaif A, Graf M, Mandeli J, et al. Characterization of groups of hyperandrogenic women with acanthosis nigricans, impaired glucose tolerance, and/or hyperinsulinemia. *J Clin Endocrinol Metab* 1987;65:499–507.
5. Fradkin JE, Eastman RC, Lesniak MA, et al. Specificity spillover at the hormone receptor—exploring its role in human disease. *N Engl J Med* 1989; 320:640–645.
6. Taylor SI. Receptor defects in patients with extreme insulin resistance. *Diabetes Metab Rev* 1985;1:171–202.
7. Flier JS, Kahn CR, Roth J. Receptors, antireceptor antibodies and the mechanism of insulin resistance. *N Engl J Med* 1979;300:413–419.
8. DeClue TJ, Shah SC, Marchese M, et al. Insulin resistance and hyperinsulinemia induce hyperandrogenism in a young type B insulin-resistant female. *J Clin Endocrinol Metab* 1991;72:1308–1311.
9. Poretsky L, Kalin MF. The gonadotropic function of insulin. *Endocr Rev* 1987;8:132–141.
10. Flier JS, Minaker KL, Landsberg L, et al. Impaired in vivo insulin clearance in patients with severe target-cell resistance to insulin. *Diabetes* 1982;31:132–135.
11. DeFronzo RA, Gunnarson R, Biorkman O, et al. Effects of insulin on peripheral and splanchnic glucose metabolism in non-insulin dependent (type II) diabetes mellitus. *J Clin Invest* 1985;76:149–155.
12. Felber JP, Ferrannini E, Golay A, et al. Role of lipid oxidation in the pathogenesis of insulin resistance in obesity and type II diabetes. *Diabetes* 1987;36:1341–1350.
13. Almind K, Bjorbaek C, Vestergaard H, et al. Amino acid polymorphisms of insulin receptor substrate-1 in non-insulin-dependent diabetes mellitus. *Lancet* 1993;342:828–832.
14. Yoshimura R, Araki E, Ura S, et al. Impact of natural IRS-1 mutations of insulin signals: mutations of IRS-1 in the PTB domain and near SH2 protein binding sites result in impaired function at different steps of IRS-1 signaling. *Diabetes* 1997;46:929–936.
15. Panz VR, Raal FJ, O'Rahilly S, et al. Insulin receptor substrate-1 gene variants in lipoatrophic diabetes mellitus and non-insulin-dependent diabetes mellitus: a study of South African black and white subjects. *Hum Genet* 1997;101: 118–119.
16. Whitehead JP, Humphreys P, Krook A, et al. Molecular scanning of the insulin receptor substrate 1 gene in subjects with severe insulin resistance: detection and functional analysis of a naturally occurring mutation in a YMXM motif. *Diabetes* 1998;47:837–839.
17. Baynes KC, Beeton CA, Panayotou G, et al. Natural variants of human p85 alpha phosphoinositide 3-kinase in severe insulin resistance: a novel variant with impaired insulin-stimulated lipid kinase activity. *Diabetologia* 2000;43: 321–331.
18. Dib K, Whitehead JP, Humphreys PJ, et al. Impaired activation of phosphoinositide 3-kinase by insulin in fibroblasts from patients with severe insulin resistance and pseudoacromegaly. A disorder characterized by selective postreceptor insulin resistance. *J Clin Invest* 1998;101:1111–1120.
19. Kausch C, Bergemann C, Hamann A, et al. Insulin-mediated pseudoacromegaly in a patient with severe insulin resistance: association of defective insulin-stimulated glucose transport with impaired phosphatidylinositol 3-kinase activity in fibroblasts. *Exp Clin Endocrinol Diabetes* 1999;107:148–154.
20. Doria A, Caldwell JS, Ji L, et al. Trinucleotide repeats at the *rad* locus: allele distributions in NIDDM and mapping to a 3-cM region on chromosome 16q. *Diabetes* 1995;44:243–247.
21. Barroso I, Gurnell M, Crowley VE, et al. Dominant negative mutations in human PPARgamma associated with severe insulin resistance, diabetes mellitus and hypertension. *Nature* 1999;402:880–883.
22. Caro JF, Sinha MK, Raju SM, et al. Insulin receptor kinase in human skeletal muscle from obese subjects with and without non-insulin-dependent diabetes. *J Clin Invest* 1987;79:1330–1337.
23. Reaven GM. Banting lecture 1988. Role of insulin resistance in human disease. *Diabetes* 1988;37:1595–1607.
24. Kahn CR. Insulin action, diabetogenes, and the cause of type II diabetes (Banting Lecture). *Diabetes* 1994;43:1066–1084.
25. Olefsky JM, Nolan JJ. Insulin resistance and non-insulin-dependent diabetes mellitus: cellular and molecular mechanisms. *Am J Clin Nutr* 1995;61:980S–986S.
26. Kerouz NJ, Horsch D, Pons S, et al. Differential regulation of insulin receptor substrates-1 and -2 (IRS-1 and IRS-2) and phosphatidylinositol 3-kinase isoforms in liver and muscle of the obese diabetic (ob/ob) mouse. *J Clin Invest* 1997;100:3164–3172.
27. Hotamisligil GS, Shargill NS, Spiegelman BM. Adipose expression of tumor necrosis factor-alpha: direct role in obesity-linked insulin resistance. *Science* 1993;259:87–91.
28. Sbraccia P, Goodman PA, Maddux BA, et al. Production of inhibitor of insulin-receptor tyrosine kinase in fibroblasts from patient with insulin resistance and NIDDM. *Diabetes* 1991;40:295–299.
29. Podolsky S. Lipoatrophic diabetes and leprechaunism. In: Podolsky S, Viswanathan M, eds. *Secondary Diabetes*. New York: Raven Press, 1980;335–352.
30. Dunnigan MG, Cochrane MA, Kelly A, et al. Familial lipoatrophic diabetes with dominant transmission. A new syndrome. *Q J Med* 1974;43:33–48.
31. Kobberling J, Willms B, Kattermann R, et al. Lipodystrophy of the extremities. A dominantly inherited syndrome associated with lipatrophic diabetes. *Humangenetik* 1975;29:111–120.
32. Kobberling J, Dunnigan MG. Familial partial lipodystrophy: two types of an X linked dominant syndrome, lethal in the hemizygous state. *J Med Genet* 1986;23:120–127.
33. Jackson SN, Pinkney J, Bargiotta A, et al. A defect in the regional deposition of adipose tissue (partial lipodystrophy) is encoded by a gene at chromosome 1q. *Am J Hum Genet* 1998;63:534–540.
34. Shackleton S, Lloyd DJ, Jackson SN, et al. LMNA, encoding lamin A/C, is mutated in partial lipodystrophy. *Nat Genet* 2000;24:153–156.
35. Speckman RA, Garg A, Du F, et al. Mutational and haplotype analyses of families with familial partial lipodystrophy (Dunnigan variety) reveal recurrent missense mutations in the globular C-terminal domain of lamin A/C. *Am J Hum Genet* 2000;66:1192–1198.
36. Bonne G, Di Barletta MR, Varnous S, et al. Mutations in the gene encoding lamin A/C cause autosomal dominant Emery-Dreifuss muscular dystrophy. *Nat Genet* 1999;21:285–288.
37. Fatkin D, MacRae C, Sasaki T, et al. Missense mutations in the rod domain of the lamin A/C gene as causes of dilated cardiomyopathy and conduction-system disease. *N Engl J Med* 1999;341:1715–1724.
38. Sullivan T, Escalante-Alcalde D, Bhatt H, et al. Loss of A-type lamin expression compromises nuclear envelope integrity leading to muscular dystrophy. *J Cell Biol* 1999;147:913–920.
39. Seip M, Trygstad O. Generalized lipodystrophy. *Arch Dis Child* 1963;38: 447–453.
40. Berardinelli W. A undiagnosed endocrino-metabolic syndrome: report of two cases. *J Clin Endocrinol Metab* 1954;14:193–204.
41. Enzi G, Digito M, Baldo-Enzi, G et al. Lipid metabolism in lipoatrophic diabetes. *Horm Metab Res* 1988;20:587–591.
42. Agarwal AK, Arioglu E, De Almeida S, et al. AGPAT2 is mutated in congenital generalized lipodystrophy linked to chromosome 9q34. *Nat Genet* 2002;31: 21–23.

43a. Magre J, Delepine M, Khallouf E, et al. Identification of the gene altered in Berardinelli-Seip congenital lipodystrophy on chromosome 11q13. *Nat Genet* 2001;28:365–370.

43b. Agarwal AK, Simha V, Oral EA, et al. Phenotypic and genetic heterogeneity in congenital generalized lipodystrophy. *J Clin Endocrinol Metab* 2003;88: 4840–4847.

44. Cole PA, Grace MR, Phillips RS, et al. The role of the catalytic base in the protein tyrosine kinase Csk. *J Biol Chem* 1995;270:22105–22108.
45. Moitra J, Mason MM, Olive M, et al. Life without white fat: a transgenic mouse. *Genes Dev* 1988;12:3168–3181.
46. Okazawa H, Mori H, Tamori Y, et al. No coding mutations are detected in the peroxisome proliferator-activated receptor-gamma gene in Japanese patients with lipoatrophic diabetes. *Diabetes* 1997;46:1904–1906.
47. Vigouroux C, Fajas L, Khallouf E, et al. Human peroxisome proliferator-activated receptor-gamma2: genetic mapping, identification of a variant in the coding sequence, and exclusion as the gene responsible for lipoatrophic diabetes. *Diabetes* 1998;47:490–492.
48. Agarwal AK, Garg A. A novel heterozygous mutation in peroxisome proliferator-activated receptor-gamma gene in a patient with familial partial lipodystrophy. *J Clin Endocrinol Metab* 2002;87:408–411.
49. Lawrence RD. Lipodystrophy and hepatomegaly with diabetes, lipaemia, and other metabolic disturbances: a case throwing new light on the action of insulin. *Lancet* 1946;1:724–731.
50. Senior B, Gellis SS. The syndromes of total lipodystrophy and of partial lipodystrophy. *Pediatrics* 1964;330:593–612.
51. Ipp MM, Minta JO, Gelfand EW. Disorders of the complement system in lipodystrophy. *Clin Immunol Immunopathol* 1977;7:281–287.
52. Sissons JG, West RJ, Fallows J, et al. The complement abnormalities of lipodystrophy. *N Engl J Med* 1976;294:461–465.

53. Kriauciunas KM, Kahn CR, Muller-Wieland D, et al. Altered expression and function of the insulin receptor in a family with lipoatrophic diabetes. *J Clin Endocrinol Metab* 1988;67:1284–1293.
54. Golden MP, Charles MA, Arquilla ER, et al. Insulin resistance in total lipodystrophy: evidence for a pre-receptor defect in insulin action. *Metabolism* 1985;34:421–428.
55. Magré J, Reynet C, Capeau J, et al. In vitro studies of insulin resistance in patients with lipoatrophic diabetes. Evidence for heterogeneous postbinding defects. *Diabetes* 1988;37:421–428.
56. Magré J, Grigorescu F, Reynet C, et al. Tyrosine-kinase defect of the insulin receptor in cultured fibroblasts from patients with lipoatropic diabetes. *J Clin Endocrinol Metab* 1989;69:142–150.
57. Rosen BS, Cook KS, Yaglom J, et al. Adipsin and complement factor D activity: an immune-related defect in obesity. *Science* 1987;237:405–408.
58. Flier JS, Cook KS, Usher P, et al. Severely impaired adipsin expression in genetic and acquired obesity. *Science* 1987;237:405–408.
59. Foss I, Trygstad O. Lipoatrophy produced in mice and rabbits by a fraction prepared from the urine from patients with congenital generalized lipodystrophy. *Acta Endocrinol* (Copenh) 1975;80:398–416.
60. Louis LH, Conn JW. A urinary diabetogenic peptide in proteinuric diabetic patients. *Metabolism* 1969;18:556–563.
61. Jensen MD. Adrenergic regulation of lipolysis in a patient with lipoatrophy of the upper body. *Mayo Clin Proc* 1991;66:704–710.
62. Huseman C, Johanson A, Varma M, et al. Congenital lipodystrophy: an endocrine study in three siblings. I. Disorders of carbohydrate metabolism. *J Pediatr* 1978;93:221–226.
63. Steinberg T, Gwinup G. Lipodystrophy, a variant of lipoatrophic diabetes. *Diabetes* 1967;16:715–721.
64. Davidson MB, Young RT. Metabolic studies in partial lipodystrophy of the lower trunked extremities. *Diabetologia* 1975;11:561–568.
65. Corbin A, Upton GV, Mabry CC, et al. Diencephalic involvement in generalized lipodystrophy: rationale and treatment with the neuroleptic agent, pimozide. *Acta Endocrinol* (Copenh) 1974;77:209–220.
66. Rossini AA, Self J, Aki TT, et al. Metabolic and endocrine studies in a case of lipoatrophic diabetes. *Metabolism* 1977;26:637–560.
67. Hager A, Heding LG, Larsson Y, et al. Pancreatic B-cell function and abnormal urinary peptides in a boy with lipoatrophic diabetes and stenosis of the aqueduct of Sylvius. *Acta Paediatr Scand* 1980;69:537–545.
68. Trygstad O, Foss I. Congenital generalized lipodystrophy and experimental lipoatrophic diabetes in rabbits treated successfully with fenfluramine. *Acta Endocrinol* (Copenh) 1977;85:436–448.
69. Trygstad O, Seip M, Oseid S. Lipodystrophic diabetes treated with fenfluramine. *Int J Obes* 1977;1:287–292.
70. Wilson TA, Melton T, Clarke WL. The effect of fenfluramine and caloric restriction on carbohydrate homeostasis in patients with lipodystrophy. *Diabetes Care* 1985;6:160–165.
71. Krolewski AS, Warram JH. Epidemiology of diabetes mellitus. In: Marble A, Krall LP, Bradley RF, et al, eds. *Joslin's diabetes mellitus*, 12th ed. Philadelphia: Lea & Febiger, 1985;12–42.
72. Schwartz R. Generalized lipoatrophy, hepatic cirrhosis, disturbed carbohydrate metabolism and accelerated growth (lipoatrophic diabetes): longitudinal observations and metabolic studies. *Am J Med* 1960;28:973–985.
73. Tontonoz P, Hu E, Spiegelman BM. Stimulation of adipogenesis in fibroblasts by PPAR gamma 2, a lipid-activated transcription factor [published erratum appears in *Cell* 1995;80:following 957]. *Cell* 1994;79:1147–1156.
74. Arioglu E, Duncan-Morin J, Sebring N, et al. Efficacy and safety of troglitazone in the treatment of lipodystrophy syndromes. *Ann Intern Med* 2000;133:263–274.
75. Gavrilova O, Marcus-Samuels B, Graham D, et al. Surgical implantation of adipose tissue reverses diabetes in lipoatrophic mice. *J Clin Invest* 2000;105:271–278.
76. Shimomura I, Hammer RE, Ikemoto S, et al. Leptin reverses insulin resistance and diabetes mellitus in mice with congenital lipodystrophy. *Nature* 1999;401:73–76.
77. Oral EA, Simha V, Ruiz E, et al. Leptin-replacement therapy for lipodystrophy. *N Engl J Med* 2002;346:570–578.
78. Stacpoole PW, Alig J, Kilgore LL, et al. Lipodystrophic diabetes mellitus. Investigations of lipoprotein metabolism and the effects of omega-3 fatty acid administration in two patients. *Metabolism* 1988;37:944–951.
79. Moses AC, Morrow LA, O'Brien M, et al. Insulin-like growth factor I (rhIGF-I) as a therapeutic agent for hyperinsulinemic insulin-resistant diabetes mellitus. *Diabetes Res Clin Pract* 1995;28[Suppl]:S185–S194.
80. Hurwitz PJ, Sarel R. Facial reconstruction in partial lipodystrophy. *Ann Plast Surg* 1982;8:253–257.
81. Reddy SSK, Kahn CR. Insulin resistance: a look at the role of insulin receptor kinase. *Diabet Med* 1988;5:621–629.
82. Kahn CR, Flier JS, Muggeo M, et al. Autoantibodies to the insulin receptor in insulin diabetes. In: Irvine WJ, ed. *Immunology of diabetes mellitus*. Edinburgh: Teviot Sci Publishing, 1980;205–218.
83. Taylor SI, Barbetti F, Accili D, et al. Syndromes of autoimmunity and hypoglycemia. Autoantibodies directed against insulin and its receptor. *Endocrinol Metab Clin North Am* 1989;18:123–143.
84. Tsokos GC, Gorden P, Antonovych T, et al. Lupus nephritis and other autoimmune features in patients with diabetes mellitus due to autoantibody to insulin receptors. *Ann Intern Med* 1985;102:176–181.
85. DePirro R, Roth R, Rossetti L, et al. Characterization of the serum from a patient with insulin resistance and hypoglycemia. *Diabetes* 1984;33:301–304.
86. Taylor SI, Grunberger G, Marcus-Samuels B, et al. Hypoglycemia associated with antibodies to the insulin receptor. *N Engl J Med* 1982;307:1422–1426.
87. Grunfeld C, Van Obberghen E, Karlsson FA, et al. Antibody-induced desensitization of the insulin receptor: studies of the mechanism of desensitization in 3T3-L1 fatty fibroblasts. *J Clin Invest* 1980;66:1124–1134.
88. Taylor SI, Marcus-Samuels B. Anti-receptor antibodies mimic the effect of insulin to down-regulate insulin receptors in cultured human lymphoblastoid (IM-9) cells. *J Clin Endocrinol Metab* 1984;58:182–186.
89. Flier JS, Kahn CR, Jarrett DB, et al. Characterization of antibodies to the insulin receptor: a cause of insulin resistant diabetes in man. *J Clin Invest* 1976;58:1442–1449.
90. Taylor SI, Underhill LH, Marcus-Samuels B. Assay of antibodies directed against cell surface receptors. *Methods Enzymol* 1985;109:656–667.
91. Maron R, Jackson RA, Jacobs S, et al. Analysis of the insulin receptor by anti-receptor antibodies and flow cytometry. *Proc Natl Acad Sci U S A* 1984;81:7446–7450.
92. Gabbay RA, O'Brien M, Moses AC. Rh-IGF-1 improves insulin sensitivity and glycemic control in some patients with the type B syndrome of severe insulin resistance. *Diabetes* 1999;48:A93(abst).
93. Bar RS, Levis WR, Rechler MM, et al. Extreme insulin resistance in ataxia telangiectasia: defect in affinity of insulin receptors. *N Engl J Med* 1978;298:1164–1171.

CHAPTER 29

Diabetes in Minorities in the United States

A. Enrique Caballero

As human beings, we all share innumerable biologic, psychological, spiritual, and social elements. At the same time, we are each different enough in some or all these elements to make us unique. An evident and closer share of genetically transmitted physical characteristics, history, nationality, religion, language, traditions, and cultural heritage provides the basis to our integration into races or ethnic groups. Race is defined primarily by genetically transmitted physical characteristics, whereas ethnicity is a broader concept that refers to the sharing of a common and distinctive racial, national, religious, linguistic, or cultural heritage. Whites account for three fourths of the population in the United States. However, an increasing number of other racial and ethnic groups in the country contribute to the wide heterogeneity of the current population. In quantitative terms, these groups are known as the "minorities." In the United States, the largest minority groups are Hispanics or Latinos, African Americans, Native Americans, Alaska natives, and Asian and Pacific Islanders.

Significant information on the health status of these groups has become available (1). Whereas the reported prevalence and incidence rates of type 1 diabetes in these groups are lower than those in whites, those reported for type 2 diabetes and its complications are higher in these groups (1).

Type 2 diabetes is a heterogeneous disease that results from a combination of genetic and environmental factors. Many studies have shown that these minority groups have a strong genetic predisposition for the development of type 2 diabetes. The "thrifty gene" hypothesis has emerged as a possible explanation for this genetic tendency to the development of diabetes. This hypothesis, first proposed in 1962, suggests that populations of indigenous people who experienced alternating periods of feast and famine gradually developed adaptations that increased the efficiency of their storage of fat during periods of plenty to better survive famine. However, now that food supplies have become more constant and abundant, this genetic adaptation has become detrimental, leading to an increased prevalence of obesity and type 2 diabetes in some populations (2,3). Much research has been devoted to identifying the precise nature of the "thrifty gene or genes." Unfortunately, no uniform genes across ethnic groups have been identified to fully support this hypothesis.

Environmental factors have undoubtedly contributed to the increase in risk for obesity and diabetes in these populations. The best data to support this concept come from the multiple studies that have found that the rates of type 2 diabetes and obesity are significantly higher in some minority groups in the United States than in the same racial and ethnic groups in their country of origin (4–13). Studies comparing their rates of diabetes in urban and rural areas also support this notion (14,15). The common elements of "Westernization" that increase the risk for obesity, diabetes, and related diseases include a diet higher in total calories and fat but lower in fiber and a decreased expenditure of energy because of labor-saving devices. In addition, particular aspects of preferred foods and lifestyle practices in each of these groups certainly play a role in the development of diabetes and its management. We now have a better understanding of how obesity, insulin resistance, diabetes, and cardiovascular disease are interrelated (16,17).

The high rates of diabetes in these populations represent a serious burden to the healthcare system in the United States. The burden comes not only from the high rates of diabetes and complications that they exhibit but also from the lack of widely available culturally and linguistically appropriate programs that demonstrate basic understanding of the needs and characteristics of each of the minority groups. Differences in cultural background do not impose a barrier for diabetes care per se. These differences do impose a barrier to the medical system and health professionals only when we lack the cultural competence to provide adequate care. A general call for action in developing research and clinical programs for minority populations has been posed by the U.S. government. New information being generated can increase our understanding of the challenges and opportunities in these groups. The goal of this chapter is to contribute to this effort by presenting information on various aspects of diabetes in the largest minority groups in the United States. For each group, general information is included on the population, diabetes epidemiology and pathophysiology, categories at risk for diabetes, microvascular and macrovascular complications, cultural and lifestyle factors related to diabetes, and prevention strategies.

DIABETES IN HISPANICS/LATINOS

The Hispanic/Latino Population

DEFINITION

Hispanic or *Latino* refers to a person of Cuban, Mexican, Puerto Rican, South or Central American, or other Spanish culture or origin regardless of race (18). Historically, Spaniards, blacks, and Native Americans have contributed, to one degree or another, to the contemporary Hispanic populations. An example of these contributions is presented in Figure 29.1.

DEMOGRAPHICS

According to the 2000 U.S. census, there are approximately 35 million Hispanics in the United States, representing 12.5% of the population. For the first time, Hispanics represent the country's largest minority group (18) (Table 29.1). It is certainly the fastest growing group, and it is estimated that, by the year 2050, Hispanics will number 97 million and will constitute 25% of the U.S. population (19). The largest Hispanic groups in the country are Mexican Americans (66%), Central/South Americans (15%), Puerto Ricans (9%), and Cuban Americans (4%). The majority of Hispanics live in the South Central and Southwestern United States, but their numbers are increasing rapidly in many states in the North and Northeast. The mean age of Hispanics is 36.7 years, whereas it is 43.8 years in whites. Approximately one third of the Hispanic population is younger than 18 years old; thus, Hispanics are considered to be the youngest population in the United States (18).

Diabetes Epidemiology

PREVALENCE AND INCIDENCE OF DIABETES

Type 1 Diabetes. Overall, the rates of type 1 diabetes are lower among Hispanics than among the white population, as shown in a study of Mexican-American and white children in Colorado (20). A study in Philadelphia found a similar incidence of type 1 diabetes in Puerto Rican children and their white counterparts (21). Because genetic, immunologic, and environmental factors are involved in the development of type 1 diabetes, differences

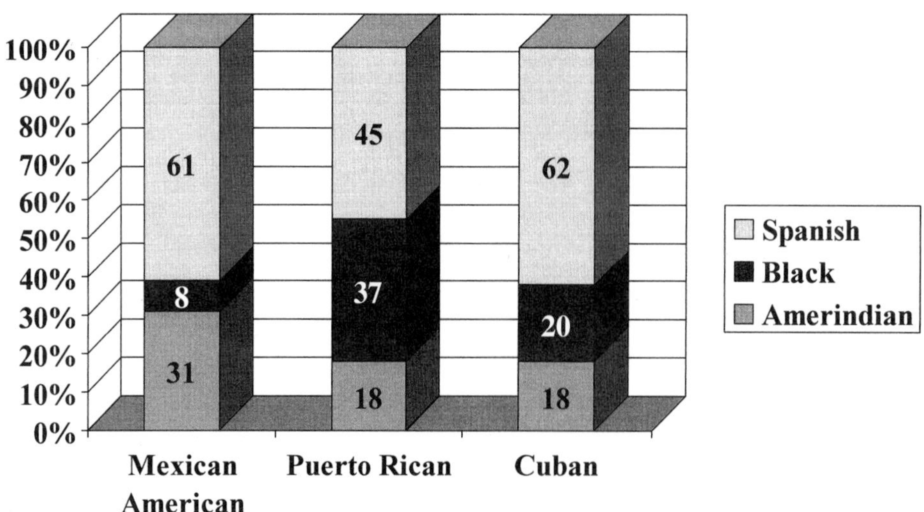

Figure 29.1. Genetic origins of major Hispanic groups based on distribution of polymorphic markers and trihybrid model of ancestry. (From Hanis CL, Hewett-Emmett D, Betrin TK, et al. Origins of U.S. Hispanics. Implications for diabetes. *Diabetes Care* 1991;14:618–627.)

TABLE 29.1. Distribution of U.S. Population by Race/Ethnicity in the 2000 U.S. Census

Race/ethnicity	Number[a]	Total population (%)[a]
Total population	281,421,906	
White/Caucasian	211,460,626	75.1
Hispanic/Latino	35,305,818	12.5
Black/African American	34,658,190	12.3
Asian	10,242,998	3.6
Native American and Alaska Native	2,475,956	0.9
Native Hawaiian and other Pacific Islander	398,835	0.1
Others	15,359,073	5.5

[a]Numbers and percentages do not add up to 100% because of the way data were collected.
From US Bureau of Census. Table DP-1. Profile of Characteristics for the United States 2000.

in these factors may account for distinct prevalence rates among Hispanic subgroups.

Type 2 Diabetes. The most recent prevalence data in the United States are from the National Health and Nutrition Examination Survey III (NHANES III), conducted from 1988 to 1994 by the National Center for Health Statistics of the Centers for Disease Control and Prevention (22,23). This study included a representative sample of the U.S. civilian noninstitutionalized population to assess the prevalence of total, diagnosed, and undiagnosed diabetes, as well as categories at risk for type 2 diabetes, such as impaired fasting glucose (IFG) and impaired glucose tolerance (IGT) (24), in the general population as a whole and in non-Hispanic whites, non-Hispanic blacks, and Hispanics (25). The Hispanic population in this survey was represented by Mexican Americans, who constitute the largest Hispanic group in the United States. Overall, the prevalence of diabetes in Hispanic Americans was 1.9 times higher that in non-Hispanic whites. Figure 29.2 shows the prevalence rates, according to age and gender, of diagnosed and undiagnosed diabetes and IFG in adults older than 20 years of age in these various populations. The prevalence rates of diagnosed diabetes, undiagnosed diabetes, total diabetes, and IFG were significantly higher in Hispanic Americans than in non-Hispanic whites and similar or higher than in non-Hispanic blacks. When considering only those between the age of 40 and 74 years of age, the prevalence of diabetes (diagnosed and undiagnosed) was 11.2% for non-Hispanic whites and 20.3% for Mexican Americans. The prevalence of IGT, according to the 1980–1985 World Health Organization (WHO) (26,27) criteria, was 20.2% for Mexican Americans, and 15.3% for non-Hispanic whites. Similarly, other studies have reported higher prevalence and incidence rates of diabetes in Hispanics than in whites (28–32).

Subgroup Analysis. *Age.* In practically every age group, the prevalence of diabetes is higher in Mexican Americans than in non-Hispanic whites. The proportion of the Mexican-American population with diabetes increases from less than 1% among those younger than 39 years old to as high as approximately 25% among those 60 to 74 years old (25) (Fig. 29.3). These rates incorporate only diagnosed cases; thus, overall rates of diabetes are higher in all age groups. This is also applicable to young Hispanic adults, adolescents, and children, who have been found to have high prevalence of obesity and type 2 diabetes (33,34).

Gender. The NHANES III study showed a higher prevalence of diagnosed diabetes among Mexican-American women older than 20 years of age than among Mexican-American men (10.9% vs. 7.7%) (25). On the other hand, the prevalence of undiagnosed diabetes in the same population was 5.4% in men and 3.6% in women. Therefore, the overall rate of diabetes is similar in men and women (13.1% and 14.5%, respectively). In addition, although the prevalence of IFG was higher in men (11.6%) than in women (6.3%), that of IGT, which was evaluated only in those between 40 and 74 years of age, was higher in women (22.3%) than in men (18.2%) (25).

Hispanic subgroups. The Hispanic Health and Nutrition Examination Survey (HHANES) was conducted in 1982 to 1984

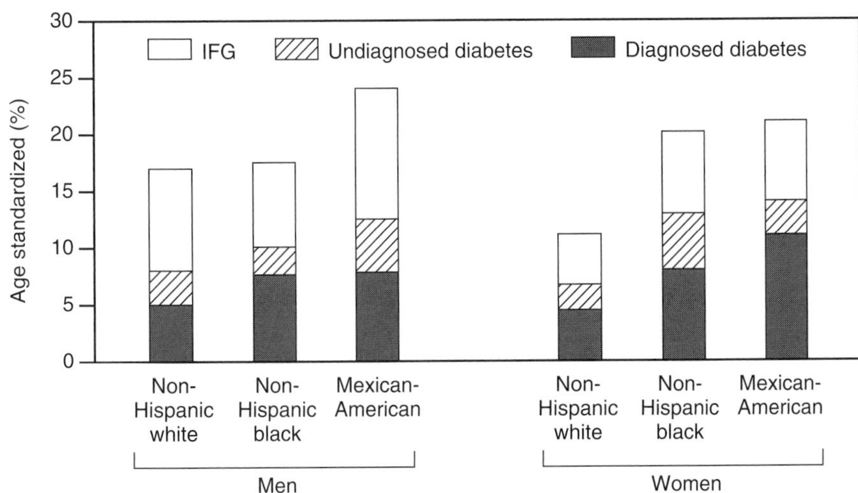

Figure 29.2. Prevalence of diagnosed and undiagnosed diabetes and impaired fasting glucose in the U.S. population greater than 20 years old, by sex and racial/ethnic group. (From Harris MI, Flegal KM, Cowie CC, et al. Prevalence of diabetes, impaired fasting glucose, and impaired glucose tolerance in U.S. adults: The Third National Health and Nutrition Examination Survey (NHANES), 1988–94. *Diabetes Care* 1998;21:518–524.)

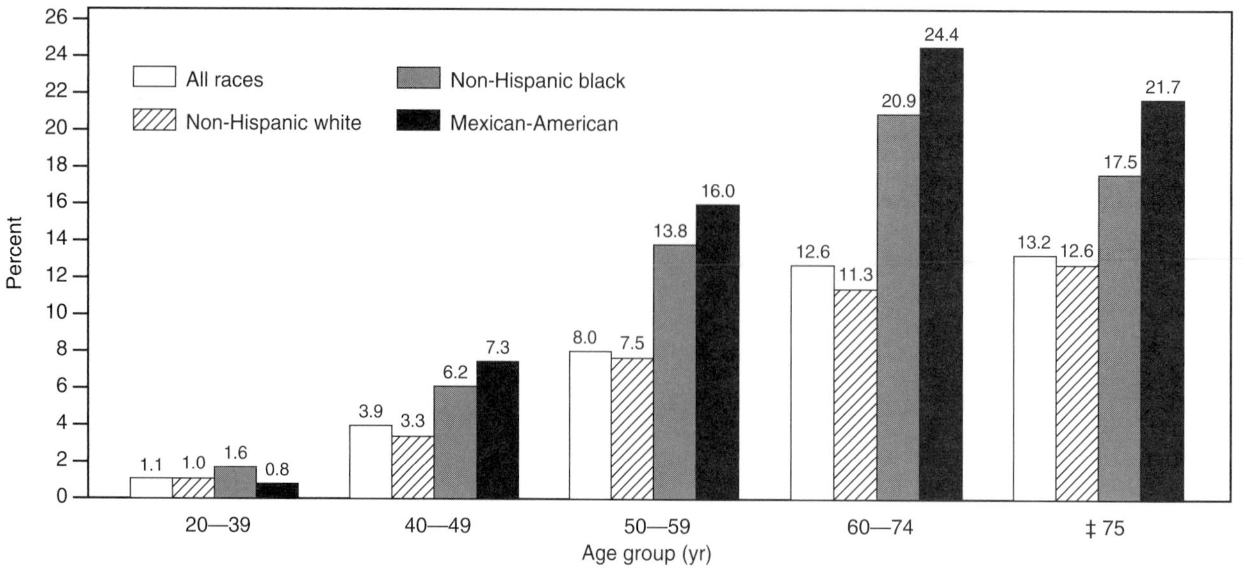

Figure 29.3. Percentage of U.S. population with diagnosed diabetes by age and race/ethnicity. Percentage is based on medical history interview in subject asked about previous diagnosis by a physician. (From Harris MI, Flegal KM, Cowie CC, et al. Prevalence of diabetes, impaired fasting glucose, and impaired glucose tolerance in U.S. adults: The Third National Health and Nutrition Examination Survey (NHANES), 1988–94. *Diabetes Care* 1998;21:518–524.)

to address the prevalence of diabetes in three Hispanic populations: Mexican Americans in the Southwestern United States; Cuban Americans in Miami, Florida; and Puerto Ricans in the New York city area (35). In this survey, the total rate for diabetes (diagnosed and undiagnosed) in adults between 20 and 74 years of age was 27.7% in Mexican Americans, 30.2% in Puerto Ricans, and 18.2% in Cuban Americans (the corresponding rates for non-Hispanic whites and non-Hispanic blacks in this survey were 13.6% and 22.6%) (Fig. 29.4). This lower rate of diabetes in Cuban Americans may be due to a lower proportion of Native American and African genes and a higher socioeconomic level. There are no available data for other Hispanic subgroups in the United States.

MORTALITY

Few studies address diabetes-specific mortality rates in the Hispanic population in the United States. The Starr County Diabetes Study found that Mexican Americans with diabetes, particularly those with chronic complications, such as proliferative retinopathy (36), experience premature and excessive mortality as compared with the general population. In addition, a study conducted in New Mexico showed that diabetes mortality rates

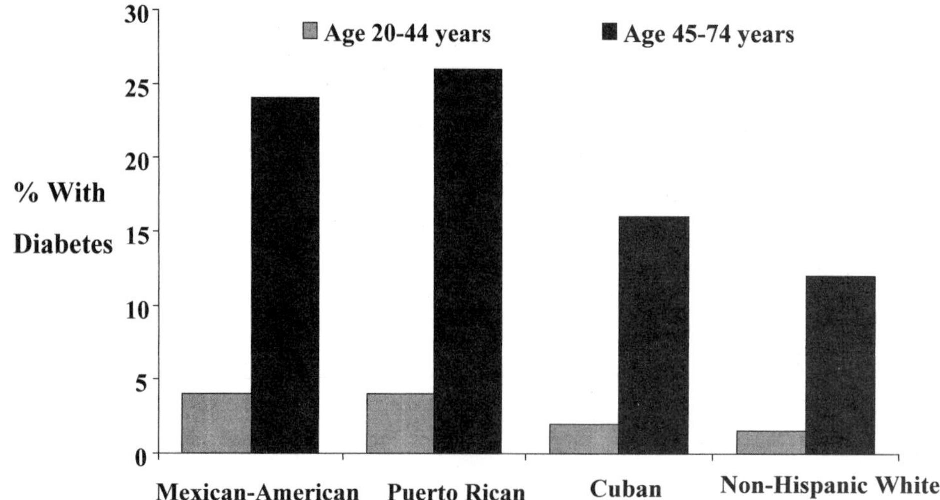

Figure 29.4. Prevalence of type 2 diabetes in some Hispanic subgroups and in whites: from HHANES data. (From Flegal KM, Ezzati TM, Harris MI, et al. Prevalence of diabetes in Mexican Americans, Cubans, and Puerto Ricans from the Hispanic Health and Examination Survey (HHANES), 1982–84. *Diabetes Care* 1991;14[Suppl 3]:628–638.)

among Hispanics in that area gradually increased between 1958 and 1994 and that these rates are higher than those in whites (37).

Pathophysiology of Type 2 Diabetes

GENETIC PREDISPOSITION

The three primary ancestors of Hispanics are Spaniards, native Indians, and Africans. Clearly, the rates of diabetes are higher in both the native Indian and African groups. The differences in rates of diabetes in the various Hispanic subgroups have been explained by the various degrees of genetic influence from these main groups (Fig. 29.1). Thus, a group such as the Puerto Ricans, who have a significant genetic contribution by Africans and native Indians, have shown a high rate of diabetes, whereas Cuban Americans, for whom the genetic contribution of these two groups is lower, have a lower rate of diabetes (35). Yet, even among Cuban Americans, whose reported rate of diabetes is the lowest among Hispanics, the rate of diabetes is higher than that among non-Hispanic whites (35) (Fig. 29.4). The prevalence rate for diabetes in Spain is higher than that in the non-Hispanic white population in the United States, suggesting that even Spanish admixture may be an important factor in explaining the higher rates of diabetes in Hispanics (38).

The nature of the precise genes that increase the risk for diabetes in this population is still unknown, although interesting information about potential genetic factors is now becoming available (39,40). Whatever the predisposing genes, it is evident that people with a family history of type 2 diabetes have an increased risk of the disease. The San Antonio Heart Study showed that the prevalence of diabetes among Mexican Americans who have first-degree relatives (e.g., parents) with diabetes is twice that of those with no family history of diabetes (41). In addition, the full metabolic profile of insulin resistance is fully established in the offspring of people with type 2 diabetes in this population (42). Strictly speaking, besides sharing a genetic background, first-degree relatives of persons with diabetes usually share environmental factors that may also participate in increasing the overall risk.

INSULIN RESISTANCE

Among people without diabetes in the NHANES III survey, insulin levels were higher in Mexican Americans than in non-Hispanic whites, a finding that suggests more insulin resistance in this population and, therefore, their greater predisposition for type 2 diabetes. Several other studies also have shown higher rates of hyperinsulinemia in Hispanics than in non-Hispanic whites, even after adjusting for obesity and body-fat distribution (43,44). In a more detailed evaluation of insulin resistance, the Insulin Resistance and Atherosclerosis Study found that nondiabetic Hispanics have significantly higher insulin resistance and a higher acute insulin response than do nondiabetic whites, although this difference disappears after adjustments are made for obesity and body-fat distribution (45). Therefore, although there is enough evidence to support a high prevalence of insulin resistance in Hispanics, the extent of its dependence on the degree and distribution of adiposity is not known.

INSULIN SECRETION

Acute insulin secretion has been reported to be higher in Hispanic Americans than in the non-Hispanic white population (45). This may represent a compensatory response of β-cell function to the degree of insulin resistance in this population. However, insufficient insulin secretion relative to the degree of insulin resistance is considered a crucial independent factor in the development of type 2 diabetes in this population (46).

OBESITY

Obesity is a major risk factor for type 2 diabetes in any population. Recent U.S. data show that the age-adjusted prevalence of combined overweight and obesity [body mass index (BMI) >25] in Mexican-American women older than age 20 years is 65.9%. The corresponding proportion in Mexican-American men is 63.9% (47). These rates are higher than in white women and white men, who have rates of 49.2% and 61%, respectively (47). Figure 29.5 shows the combined overweight and obesity (BMI >25) rates by gender in the Hispanic, non-Hispanic black, and non-Hispanic white population according to the NHANES III study (47). Other studies previously showed that Mexican-American adults and children, particularly women, have substantially higher rates of obesity than do non-Hispanic white Americans (48,49). The rate for diabetes has also been described to increase with each higher level of percent desirable weight in Mexican Americans, Puerto Ricans, and Cuban Americans (50). The localization of adipose tissue in the Mexican-American population has also been addressed, with upper body obesity being an important contributing factor for the development of type 2 diabetes (51,52). Low income level has also been reported to correlate with obesity. Among Mexican-American women age 20 to 74 years, the age-adjusted prevalence of overweight is 46% for women living below the poverty line as compared with 40% for those living above the poverty line (53). In an interesting finding, now applicable to many populations, low birthweight

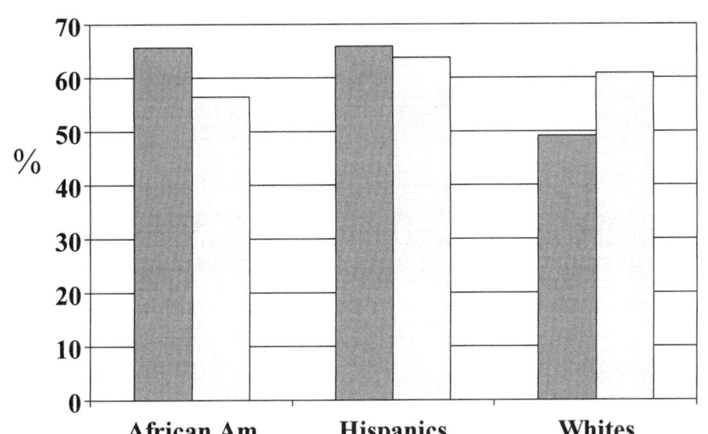

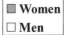

Figure 29.5. Age-adjusted prevalence of combined overweight and obesity rates (body mass index >25) in Hispanic, African-American, and white adults in the United States. (From Flegal KM, Carroll MD, Kuczmarski RJ, et al. Overweight and obesity in the United States: prevalence and trends, 1960–1994. *Int J Obes Relat Disord* 1998;22:39–47.)

is associated with the development of type 2 diabetes in Hispanics (54).

Categories at Risk for Diabetes

IMPAIRED FASTING GLUCOSE AND IMPAIRED GLUCOSE TOLERANCE

Rates of IFG and IGT are higher in Hispanics than in non-Hispanic whites. The age- and sex-standardized rate of IFG in people older than 20 years of age in the NHANES III survey was 8.9% in Hispanics, 7% in blacks, and 6.8% in whites (25). Rates of IGT among adults age 40 to 74 years in the same study were also higher for Mexican Americans (20.2%) than for non-Hispanic white Americans (15.3%) and blacks (14%) (25).

GESTATIONAL DIABETES

The prevalence of gestational diabetes in Hispanics is two to three times higher than that in the general population (55). The risk of type 2 diabetes among Hispanic women who had gestational diabetes has been explored in a study of Mexican-American women in Southern California. This study showed that 12% of women with gestational diabetes progress to type 2 diabetes each year. This figure is about four times higher than that in the white population (56). Hispanic women with gestational diabetes represent an important group considered for diabetes prevention programs.

Microvascular Complications

RETINOPATHY

In the San Antonio Heart Study, the rate of diabetic retinopathy was 2.3 times higher among Mexican Americans than among non-Hispanic white Americans, even after controlling for duration of diabetes, severity of hyperglycemia, age, and systolic blood pressure (57). In concordance with these findings, the NHANES III study also found that the prevalence of diabetic retinopathy was twice as high in Mexican Americans as in whites and that this difference was not explained by duration of diabetes, glycemic control, or mode of diabetes treatment (58). In contrast, the San Luis Valley Diabetes Study found lower rates of retinopathy in Hispanics than in non-Hispanic whites (59,60). These opposite findings are not well understood but may reflect differences in some characteristics of the Hispanic groups included in these studies. The results of all three studies coincided in that severity and duration of diabetes was significantly associated with diabetic retinopathy.

The risk for microvascular complications is closely related to glycemic control. The NHANES III study found that 40.8% of Mexican Americans had glycosylated hemoglobin A_{1c} (HbA_{1c}) values greater than 8% as compared with 35.7% of non-Hispanic whites (61). In a subgroup analysis by gender, 44.5% of Mexican-American men had HbA_{1c} values greater than 8%. In this study, education, income, health insurance coverage, and number of physician visits per year were not associated with poor glycemic control and did not seem to explain the differences observed by ethnicity. Another study suggested that lack of outpatient health insurance is associated with a higher rate of microvascular complications in Mexican Americans (62).

NEPHROPATHY

All stages of diabetic nephropathy are more frequent in Hispanics than in non-Hispanic whites. The San Antonio Heart Study showed that the prevalence of clinical nephropathy, defined by the presence of proteinuria, was 2.8 times higher and that the prevalence of microalbuminuria was 3.5 times higher in Mexican Americans than in non-Hispanic whites with diabetes. These differences remained statistically significant after adjusting for age and duration of diabetes (63). The NHANES III data also showed a higher prevalence of clinical proteinuria in Mexican Americans than in whites (11% vs. 5%) (50). However, the San Luis Valley Diabetes Study showed no difference in the incidence of diabetic nephropathy in Hispanics and non-Hispanic whites (59). Some clinical differences among these groups may explain these discrepant results.

The risk of end-stage renal disease (ESRD) due to diabetes, mostly type 2, has been reported to be six times higher in Mexican Americans than in whites (64,65). This increased risk does not seem to be completely explained by a higher prevalence of diabetes. Survival among Hispanics receiving hemodialysis appears to be better than among whites, perhaps because of a lower cardiovascular risk (66).

NEUROPATHY

The San Luis Valley Diabetes Study found no significant difference in the prevalence of diabetic neuropathy in Hispanics and non-Hispanic whites (59). In this study, symptoms and a physical examination, including vibration threshold, were taken into consideration to define diabetic neuropathy. In contrast, in the 1989 National Health Interview Survey, symptoms of sensory neuropathy were reported more frequently by Mexican Americans than by whites or African Americans (67).

Macrovascular Complications

CARDIOVASCULAR DISEASE

In the general population, no significant differences exist in the prevalence of nonfatal coronary heart disease (CHD), defined by electrocardiogram, among whites, blacks, and Hispanics (68). With regard to the diabetic population, studies in Texas and Colorado found lower rates of myocardial infarction in Mexican Americans than in non-Hispanic whites. Mexican Americans, men in particular, also exhibit a decreased prevalence of fatal myocardial infarction as compared with non-Hispanic whites (69,70). More studies are needed to determine whether this finding is consistent and applicable to other Hispanic subgroups.

Associated Cardiovascular Risk Factors. Findings from NHANES III indicate that the age-adjusted prevalence rate of metabolic syndrome was higher in Hispanics (Mexican Americans) than in the white population (31.9% vs. 23.7%). The age-adjusted individual metabolic abnormalities considered to define the metabolic syndrome were all higher in Hispanics than in whites: abdominal obesity, 45.7% vs 37.2%; hypertriglyceridemia, 37.7% vs 31.1%; low high-density lipoprotein (HDL) cholesterol, 39.6% vs. 37.9%; high blood pressure, 36.6% vs. 32.8%; and diabetes or IFG, 20% vs. 11.9% (71). With regard to hypertension, not all studies have shown a higher prevalence rate in Hispanics than in whites (72). In fact, the NHANES III study showed that, in the population with type 2 diabetes, the frequency of hypertension was significantly lower in Mexican Americans than in non-Hispanic whites (54% vs. 66%) (73). The prevalence rate of dyslipidemia was also lower in Hispanics than in non-Hispanic whites (51% vs. 65%) (73). Dyslipidemia in Hispanics is clearly associated with the degree of insulin resistance (74).

PERIPHERAL VASCULAR DISEASE AND AMPUTATIONS

Lavery et al. (75) found a higher incidence of diabetes-related lower-extremity amputations among Hispanics than among whites in Texas and California. In the San Antonio Heart Study, the rate of peripheral vascular disease also was higher in Mexican Americans with type 2 diabetes than among non-Hispanic whites, although in this case, this increased incidence was not statistically significant after adjusting for the prevalence of diabetes (76). Of interest are the lower in-hospital mortality rates due to amputations among Hispanics than among whites. It is not known whether this difference is related to a lower cardiovascular risk in Hispanics (77). Certainly, preventing amputations is an important task in people with diabetes in diverse populations (78).

CEREBROVASCULAR DISEASE

In a multicenter evaluation of nondiabetic subjects, the Insulin Resistance and Atherosclerosis Study found that common carotid artery intimal-medial thickness was significantly lower in Hispanics than in non-Hispanic whites, suggesting a lower degree of atherosclerosis (79). This difference remained even after adjusting for major cardiovascular risk factors and insulin sensitivity. This measure of atherosclerosis exhibited a clear relationship with the degree of insulin resistance in the study groups. No difference between Hispanics and whites was seen regarding the internal carotid artery measures (79). However, the degree of thickness of internal carotid artery plaque was lower in Hispanics than in blacks and whites in the Northern Manhattan Stroke Study (80).

Lifestyle and Cultural Factors

As previously mentioned, the prevalence of obesity is higher in the Hispanic population. An interesting cultural aspect about obesity is that the desire to lose weight may not be as strong among some Hispanics as among people of some other cultures. It is well known that in some societies women equate thinness with beauty; however, some Hispanic women, particularly older women, may equate physical robustness with physical health. As a result, being overweight may be considered normal and in some instances preferable to being slimmer (81,82). Food preferences are shared but are not necessarily the same for all Hispanic subgroups. There are differences in traditional foods among people from the many countries in Central and South America. The diet of Mexican Americans has been found to be slightly more atherogenic than the diet of whites (83). However, this concept cannot be generalized to all Hispanic subgroups. Even more, some traditional foods may have some beneficial effects in diabetes (84,85).

With regard to physical activity, the HHANES showed that the prevalence of diabetes was lower among Hispanic men with high levels of work-related physical activity than among those who had less physically demanding work (35). Unfortunately, The NHANES III survey found that 65% of Mexican-American men and 74% of Mexican-American women reported little or no leisure-time physical activity (86). Exercise was found to be inversely predictive of the incidence of type 2 diabetes among Mexican-American men but not among Mexican-American women (87).

The process of acculturation of Hispanics, and perhaps of other groups, to mainstream U.S. society has been described in terms of having two limbs: an ascending limb at which people adopt unhealthy food choices and become more sedentary, and a potential descending limb, at which people become progressively more affluent and try to adopt a healthier lifestyle (88). This latter stage, reflecting a higher level of acculturation, has been correlated with reduced prevalence of type 2 diabetes among Mexican Americans (89). For some other social aspects, lower socioeconomic status and education level is linked to a higher prevalence of diabetes (90,91).

Another important cultural aspect of diabetes care is language. A significant proportion of Hispanics do not speak English, and the healthcare system does not always provide services in Spanish. This issue has represented a limitation for healthcare access (92, 93). A study conducted in a group of Hispanic patients with diabetes showed that recall of the disease process and treatment information was higher in patients who were seen by bilingual physicians than in patients who were seen by physicians who spoke only English (94).

Like any ethnic group, the Hispanic culture is rich in beliefs, traditions, practices, and attitudes. Among Hispanics, family and religion play a crucial role in day-to-day life. All these aspects offer an opportunity to develop culturally and linguistically appropriate services and educational programs for Hispanics (95).

DIABETES IN AFRICAN AMERICANS

The African-American Population

DEFINITION

Black or *African American* refers to people who have origins in any of the black racial groups of Africa (18).

DEMOGRAPHICS

According to the 2000 U.S. census, there are 34.7 million African-American people in the country, representing 12.3% of the total U.S. population (18). The median age of this population is 30 years. Approximately 33% are younger than 18 years of age and 8% are older than 65 years of age. The majority of African Americans live in the South (54%), and 16% live in the Midwest, 18% in the Northeast, and 10% in the West. The ten states with the largest black populations are New York, California, Texas, Florida, Georgia, Illinois, North Carolina, Maryland, Michigan, and Louisiana. Between 1990 and 2000, the rate of increase in the black population was greater than that of the total population (15.6% vs. 13.2%) (18).

Diabetes Epidemiology

PREVALENCE AND INCIDENCE OF DIABETES

Type 1 Diabetes. Rates of type 1 diabetes appear to be lower in African-American children than in white American children (96). Incidence rates have been reported at around 5 to 8 per 100,000 per year in the African-American population, as compared with 14 to 17 per 100,000 per year in the white population. The distinct incidence rates reported in black populations may be due to the different proportions of racial admixture, particularly with the white population (97). It is known that genetic factors play a significant role in the development of type 1 diabetes. The major histocompatibility genes (HLA) most frequently associated with type 1 diabetes are infrequent in this population (98).

Type 2 Diabetes. The prevalence of type 2 diabetes in African Americans is higher than in the non-Hispanic white population and similar to that in Hispanic-Americans. Figure 29.2 shows the most recent national data according to the NHANES III survey conducted from 1988 to 1994. The prevalence rate of diagnosed diabetes in African Americans older than 20 years of age is 8.2%, as compared with 4.8% in whites. Among those age 40 to 74 years in this survey, the prevalence rate was 18.2% for blacks and 11.2% for whites. Therefore, the prevalence of type 2 diabetes in African Americans is approximately 1.6 times higher than in whites (25). Over the past 35 years, the number of people diagnosed with diabetes in this population has significantly increased. The total diabetes prevalence in African Americans

40 to 74 years old has increased from 8.9% in 1976 to 1980 to 18.2% in 1988 to 1994. Other studies have also reported a higher prevalence of diabetes in blacks than in whites (99). The incidence of type 2 diabetes has also been reported to be distinctly higher in the black population than in the white population (100,101).

The rates for undiagnosed diabetes and IFG are also higher in African Americans than in whites (Fig. 29.2). It is estimated that among blacks there is one case of undiagnosed type 2 diabetes for every two diagnosed cases. This is similar to the proportion for other racial/ethnic groups in the United States. Identifying patients with diabetes is a major task in this group, as it is in the general population.

Subgroup Analysis. *Age.* The proportion of the African-American population with diabetes increases with age, increasing from less than 2% for people younger than 39 years old to as high as 21% for those 60 to 74 years old (25) (Fig. 29.3). These rates are based only on diagnosed cases of diabetes; therefore, the rates for total diabetes, which include undiagnosed cases, would be higher. Type 2 diabetes frequently develops in children and adolescents from this population (33).

Gender. The NHANES III survey found that the prevalence of diabetes in the African-American population is higher in women than in men at all ages (25). Among those age 20 years or older, the prevalence rate of diagnosed diabetes was 9.1% for women and 7.3% for men. The prevalence of undiagnosed diabetes in this study was 4.5% in women and 2.7% in men. However, the prevalence of IFG was 6.4% in women and 7.7% in men, whereas the prevalence of IGT was 13% in women and 15% in men.

MORTALITY

Diabetes is the seventh leading cause of death in the general African-American population and the fifth leading cause of death in people 45 years of age or older (102). In all age groups, the diabetes-related mortality rate is higher in African Americans than in whites (103). The overall mortality rate is 20% higher for black men and 40% higher for black women as compared with the rates in whites. These increased mortality rates have also been found in high-income areas (104).

Pathophysiology of Type 2 Diabetes

GENETIC PREDISPOSITION

As postulated in the "thrifty gene hypothesis," some populations, such as Africans, developed a genetic adaptation to "feast and famine" cycles to use food energy more efficiently. It is believed that this protective change has now become an unfavorable situation that increases the risk of type 2 diabetes (2,3). Unfortunately, the precise genes that increase the risk for diabetes in the African-American population have not been clearly identified. However, these genes are very likely involved in increasing insulin resistance, decreasing insulin production, or both.

INSULIN RESISTANCE

African Americans have been found to have a higher degree of insulin resistance than their white counterparts. The NHANES III survey found that insulin levels were higher in African Americans without diabetes than in whites without diabetes (50). Hyperinsulinemia is a compensatory mechanism for overcoming peripheral insulin resistance and is thus an indirect measure of insulin resistance. This finding was particularly evident in African-American women and is consistent with the high rates of obesity and diabetes reported in black women. The Insulin Resistance and Atherosclerosis Study found significantly higher levels of insulin resistance and acute insulin response in nondiabetic African Americans than in nondiabetic whites, even after adjusting for obesity and body fat distribution (45).

In an alarming fashion, the full-blown syndrome of insulin resistance and type 2 diabetes are now frequently noted in African-American children and adolescents (33). African-American children have been found to have higher acute insulin responses and lower insulin sensitivity than white children, even after adjusting for body composition, social-class background, and dietary patterns (105).

INSULIN SECRETION

Deficient insulin secretion has been considered an important pathophysiologic element in the development of type 2 diabetes in African Americans. It has been identified not only in people with type 2 diabetes but even in those with impaired glucose tolerance (106).

Some interesting atypical forms of diabetes have been described in this population. A form of diabetes that presents with features of type 1 diabetes, with an evident insulin-secretion deficiency but without the usual HLA associations, has been reported (107). An interesting form of diabetes, called "Flatbush diabetes," has also been described (108). These individuals present with ketoacidosis and a subsequent clinical course of type 2 diabetes. They are negative for antibody to glutamic acid decarboxylase and have an increased frequency of HLA-DR3 and -DR4 antigens (108). In addition, a ketosis-resistant diabetic syndrome associated with malnutrition has been reported in Jamaica. This form is associated with impaired insulin function and phasic insulin dependence (109). Some transient remission due to recovery of β-cell function after intensive glycemic control has also been reported in some African Americans (110).

OBESITY

Consistent with the higher rates of diabetes and insulin resistance, the prevalence of obesity is higher in African-American adults than in whites. Recent U.S. data show that the age-adjusted prevalence of combined overweight and obesity (BMI >25) in black women older than 20 years of age is 65.8%. The rate in black men is 56.5% (47). The corresponding rates in white women and white men are 49.2% and 61%, respectively (47) (Fig. 29.5). The difference between blacks and whites is noted only among women. In addition, the rates of central obesity, which is related to an increase in visceral fat that is clearly associated with the risk of diabetes, hypertension, and dyslipidemia, are also higher in the black population than in the white population.

It is tempting to believe that the higher rate of diabetes among African Americans is merely related to higher rates of obesity. However, the prevalence of diabetes is still higher in this population than in whites after adjusting for the presence of obesity and its degree and type (50,69). The extent to which obesity per se contributes to the higher rate of diabetes in blacks is uncertain; however, as in all populations, obesity is clearly a factor that increases the risk of diabetes and its associated metabolic abnormalities.

Categories at Risk for Type 2 Diabetes

IMPAIRED FASTING GLUCOSE AND IMPAIRED GLUCOSE TOLERANCE

According to the NHANES III study (25), the prevalence rate of IFG, standardized for sex and age, among adults older than

20 years of age was 7% for non-Hispanic blacks, 6.8% for whites, and 8.9% for Hispanics (Fig. 29.2). Application of the WHO diagnostic criteria for fasting and postchallenge plasma glucose to the NHANES III data gives a prevalence of IGT in people between 40 and 74 years of age of 14% for non-Hispanic blacks, 15.3% for non-Hispanic whites, and 20.2% for Hispanics (25).

GESTATIONAL DIABETES

Gestational diabetes develops in approximately 2% to 5% of all pregnant women. The likelihood of developing gestational diabetes is higher among those who generally have risk factors for type 2 diabetes, usually due to a combination of genetic predisposition and acquired factors such as obesity, unhealthy dietary patterns, and physical inactivity. African-American women have a high risk of type 2 diabetes and gestational diabetes develops 50% to 80% more frequently than in white women (111).

Microvascular Complications

RETINOPATHY

According to the NHANES III data, the prevalence of diabetic retinopathy is 40% to 50% higher in African Americans than in white Americans (58). African-American women have been found to have worse glycemic control than white women (61). The NHANES III study found that 45.7% of non-Hispanic blacks had HbA_{1c} values greater than 8% as compared with 35.7% of non-Hispanic whites. In a subgroup analysis by gender, 50% of non-Hispanic black women had HbA_{1c} values >8%. In this study, education, income, health insurance coverage, and number of physician visits per year were not associated with poor glycemic control (61). This factor may provide a partial explanation for the higher frequency of retinopathy. In addition, the high rates of hypertension in blacks also seem to play a role (112). However, in a 4-year follow-up study of middle-aged subjects with type 2 diabetes, the rate of development of retinopathy was higher (50% vs. 19%) in blacks than in whites. This result could not be explained by differences between the groups with respect to HbA_{1c} or blood pressure levels, type of diabetes treatment, or gender distribution (113). These findings suggest that African Americans may have an underlying predisposition for the development of retinopathy and perhaps for other diabetes-induced microvascular complications. Further research is needed to clarify this aspect.

NEPHROPATHY

All stages of diabetic nephropathy are more prevalent among African Americans than among whites. Several studies have demonstrated that the rates of microalbuminuria and clinical nephropathy (macroalbuminuria) are very high in the African-American population (114–116). In addition, ESRD due to diabetes is about four times more common in African Americans than in whites. After adjustment for the underlying increased prevalence of diabetes, this number is reduced to 2.6 (115). The high frequency of ESRD in African Americans seems to be influenced by the high rates of hypertension in this population. However, a study that adjusted for systolic blood pressure found that blacks still had a 63% higher risk of developing ESRD (117). As reported for the Hispanic population, African Americans have better survival rates after they develop kidney failure than do white Americans (118,119). The reason for this is unclear. It may be that blacks receive transplants less frequently, and therefore more patients who are eligible for transplants are placed on dialysis (119). In addition, the rates of voluntary withdrawal from dialysis are lower among African Americans than among whites. (120).

NEUROPATHY

Neuropathy is a very common complication in diabetes. Its prevalence depends on the diagnostic criteria. No particular difference in neuropathy rates has been reported in the African-American population as compared with whites or Hispanics (121).

Macrovascular Complications

CARDIOVASCULAR DISEASE

Although no significant differences in the prevalence of nonfatal myocardial infarction have been found among whites, blacks, and Hispanics in the general population (68), African Americans have the highest overall mortality rate due to CHD and the highest out-of-hospital coronary death rates, particularly at younger ages, of any ethnic group in the United States (122).

Associated Cardiovascular Risk Factors. A high incidence of hypertension has been reported in the African-American population. This increased rate seems to be related in part to the high prevalence of obesity and insulin resistance. However, there also seems to be a specific predisposition for the development of hypertension independent of the insulin resistance syndrome (123). Hypertension and left ventricular hypertrophy are more prevalent in African Americans, develop at younger ages, and are associated with mortality rates three to five times higher than the rates in whites (124).

Most population-based surveys indicate that total serum cholesterol levels are lower and the prevalence of hypercholesterolemia is similar or lower in African Americans than in whites (125). Levels of HDL cholesterol are approximately 20% higher in African-American men than in their white counterparts (126). Triglyceride levels in black men and women are generally lower than those in whites in both individuals with and without CHD (127). Levels of lipoprotein(a) are two to three times higher in African Americans than in whites, although they have not been independently associated with an increased cardiovascular risk (128–130). In the nondiabetic population, African Americans may exhibit the typical dyslipidemia associated with insulin resistance, consistent of high triglycerides, low HDL-cholesterol, and small LDL-cholesterol particles (73). Plasminogen activator inhibitor 1 activity has been found to be lower in African Americans than in whites, although this difference may be attributable to distinct dietary patterns (131).

PERIPHERAL VASCULAR DISEASE AND AMPUTATIONS

Among people with diabetes, the likelihood of an African American undergoing an amputation of a lower-extremity amputation is twofold higher than that in whites (75,76). An important contributing factor is the high prevalence of peripheral vascular disease in African Americans (132). In addition, rates of in-hospital amputation-related mortality are twice as high in African Americans as in whites (76).

CEREBROVASCULAR DISEASE

The Insulin Resistance and Atherosclerosis Study included the measurement of common carotid artery intimal-medial thickness in a white, black, and Hispanic nondiabetic population. African Americans had more atherosclerosis than did whites, even after adjusting for traditional cardiovascular risk factors and insulin sensitivity. Within the African-American population, this measurement was not significantly related to the degree of insulin resistance, perhaps because of an absence of wide variation in the degree of insulin resistance in this group (79). A high rate of carotid atherosclerosis in blacks has also been reported in another multiethnic population (80). In the general population, rates of cerebral vascular disease have also been reported to be higher among blacks than among whites, but no information about people with diabetes is available (133).

Lifestyle and Cultural Factors

Obesity contributes to the development of diabetes and plays a major role in establishing the course of the disease. Therefore, there has been strong interest in assessing how particular lifestyle factors may promote obesity in this population. There is wide variability in lifestyle patterns among people within each ethnic group. However, many individuals share preferences and attitudes. It has been found that black people consume more fat and sodium and less fiber than do white people (134). This may be a factor that increases the risk to diabetes, although no study has shown a clear cause-and-effect relationship. Another important factor in the natural history of diabetes is physical activity. The NHANES III survey found that 50% of black men and 67% of black women reported little or no leisure-time physical activity (86). These numbers are slightly higher than in the white population. Lifestyle factors are believed to play a major role in the development of type 2 diabetes in this population (135).

Not only are dietary factors and limited physical activity probable contributors to the high rate of obesity in this population, but also some women may not be very willing to lose weight. A study suggests that some African-American women consider obesity and robustness as indicators of good health (136).

Socioeconomic factors certainly influence the development of diabetes and its course. In the African-American population, low-income status and low educational level have been linked to the development of type 2 diabetes (137).

Common beliefs, attitudes, and traditions are part of the African-American culture, as in other cultures. All these factors in combination with social and economic elements need to be taken into account when establishing programs for African Americans with diabetes and at risk for the disease (138,139).

DIABETES IN NATIVE AMERICANS AND ALASKA NATIVES

The Native American and Alaska Native Population

DEFINITION

Native American and *Alaska Natives* refer to people having origins in any of the original peoples of North, Central, and South America and who maintain tribal affiliation or community attachment (18).

DEMOGRAPHICS

There are 2.5 million Native Americans and Alaska Natives in the United States, representing 0.9% of the total population in the country (18). The median age of this group is 28 years, whereas it is 38 years for whites. Approximately 44% of members of these groups are younger than 18 years of age, and 6.3% are older than 65 years of age. More of the nation's Native Americans, Eskimos, and Aleuts live in Oklahoma than in any other state (13%). Arizona, California, New Mexico, and Alaska are the next most popular states of residence. The subgroups with more people are Cherokee, Navajo, Sioux 1, Chippewa, Choctaw, Pueblo 2, and Apache. Pima Indians, a well-known subgroup with high diabetes prevalence rates, represent 0.8% of the Native American group. Since 1990, the Native American population has grown by 12%, while the non-Hispanic white population has increased by 3%. The projected growth of this group is 40% over the next 20 years.

Diabetes Epidemiology

PREVALENCE AND INCIDENCE OF DIABETES

Type 1 Diabetes. Type 1 diabetes is relatively rare in Native Americans and Alaska Natives. Some of the reported cases may in fact correspond to people who have some additional European white genetic background (140).

Type 2 Diabetes. On average, Native Americans and Alaska Natives are 2.8 times more likely than non-Hispanic whites of a similar age to have diagnosed diabetes (140). The diabetes rates in these populations are increasing rapidly. The Centers for Disease Control and Prevention reported an increase in the prevalence of diabetes from 5.2% to 8.5% among Native Americans and Alaska Natives between 1990 and 1998, an increase of 65% in 8 years (141). The Indian Health Service reported an increase in the age-adjusted prevalence rate of diabetes in these groups from 6.2% to 8% between 1990 and 1997, an increase of 29% in 7 years (142). However, these rates do not seem to accurately reflect the actual diabetes epidemic in some of these populations. Among adults older than 20 years old in the Navajo community, the reported age-adjusted prevalence rate of diabetes is 22.9% (143). Another screening study that included three Native American populations found that 40% to 70% of adults 45 to 74 years old have diabetes (144). Among Pima Indians, the most widely studied Native American group, the prevalence of type 2 diabetes is approximately 50% among individuals 30 to 64 years old and is considered to be the highest in the world (145). There are many other studies showing high rates of diabetes in Native Americans and Alaska Natives (146–157). It is interesting that the prevalence of diabetes is slightly lower among Alaskan Eskimos and Inuits than among non-Hispanic whites (140).

Subgroup Analysis. *Age.* In both men and women in every age group, the prevalence of type 2 diabetes is higher in Native Americans and Alaska Natives than in non-Hispanic whites (142) (Fig. 29.6). Native American children and adolescents frequently manifest type 2 diabetes (33). Among Pima Indian children, the prevalence of type 2 diabetes in girls 10 to 14 years old increased from 0.72% in the period 1967 to 1976 to 2.88% in the period 1987 to 1996 (158).

Gender. Among Native Americans and Alaska Natives, more women than men have diabetes (142) (Fig. 29.6). However, between 1990 and 1997, the prevalence increased at a greater rate among men than among women (37% vs. 25%) (141).

Native American and Alaska Native subgroups. The prevalence rates of diabetes among the many Native American and Alaska Native groups appear to be different. The recent survey from the Indian Health Service has reported various diabetes prevalence rates by the main geographic regions where these groups are found. The prevalence rates vary from around 3% in the Alaska region to 17.4% in the Atlantic region (142) (Fig. 29.7).

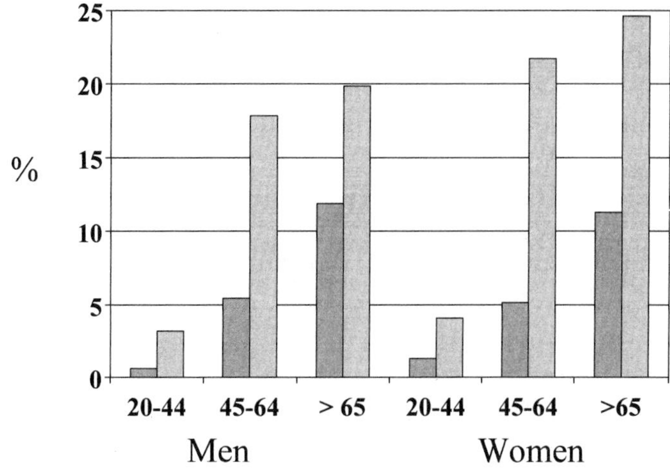

Figure 29.6. Prevalence of type 2 diabetes in Native Americans (*NA*) and Alaska Natives (*AN*) as compared with non-Hispanic (*NH*) whites by age group and gender. (From Rios Burrows N, Geiss LS, Engelgau MM, et al. Prevalence of diabetes among Native Americans and Alaska Natives, 1990–1997. *Diabetes Care* 2000;23: 1786–1790.)

MORTALITY

Diabetes was considered to be the sixth leading cause of death among Native Americans and Alaska Natives in the United States between 1984 and 1986. The adjusted mortality rate for diabetes in Native Americans was 4.3 times the rate in non-Hispanic whites between 1986 and 1988. Diabetes-related mortality rates are very similar in Aleuts, Eskimos, and Native Americans. In New Mexico, diabetes-related mortality increased by 564% and 1,110% for Native American men and women, respectively, from 1958 to 1994 (159,160). Several factors are thought to play an important role in increasing diabetes-related mortality among Native Americans and Alaska Natives, such as diabetes duration, the presence of cardiovascular risk factors, and proteinuria (140,161–167).

Pathophysiology of Type 2 Diabetes

GENETIC PREDISPOSITION

The nature of the primary genes responsible for increasing the risk of obesity and diabetes in Native Americans and Alaska Natives is still not well defined. In has been proposed that some genetic adaptation has occurred in many minority groups to survive the lack of constant food supplies in ancient times (2,3,168). One certain aspect is that individuals among the Native American population with the least genetic admixture with other groups have a higher risk of developing diabetes, which suggests an evident genetic predisposition for the disease (140).

Although members from the same family tend to share environmental factors that could increase the risk for diabetes, the high occurrence of diabetes among descendants of individuals with type 2 diabetes also suggests an important genetic influence (161,169). The high rates of diabetes in some subgroups such as Pima Indians has been seen as an excellent opportunity to conduct diabetes-related genetic studies (170). Some interesting information is now available from these studies in Pima Indians and other groups about genes that could explain some of the metabolic abnormalities that lead to diabetes in these groups (171–175).

INSULIN RESISTANCE

The high prevalence of diabetes in Pima Indians has allowed investigators to establish important prospective studies to aid in understanding the natural history of type 2 diabetes. These studies have contributed to the concept of a dual defect that leads to the development of diabetes: insulin secretory dysfunction and insulin resistance (176,177). Recent elegant studies have shown that both phenomena deteriorate progressively as

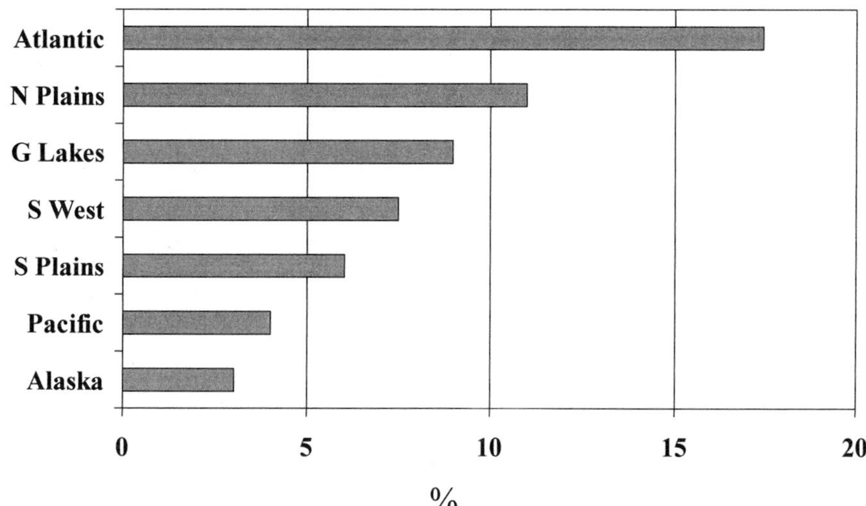

Figure 29.7. Age-adjusted prevalence of diagnosed diabetes by region among Native Americans and Alaska Natives from 1990 through 1997. (From Rios Burrows N, Geiss LS, Engelgau MM, et al. Prevalence of diabetes among Native Americans and Alaska Natives, 1990–1997. *Diabetes Care* 2000;23:1786–1790.)

individuals make the transition from normal glucose tolerance to impaired glucose tolerance to diabetes (178). In fact, both insulin resistance and insulin secretory dysfunction are independent risk predictors of worsening glucose tolerance during each stage of type 2 diabetes (179) (Fig. 29.8). Insulin resistance antedates the development of type 2 diabetes by many years and has been identified in young nondiabetic Pima Indians (180). The high rate of insulin resistance in this population is the result of lifestyle factors in addition to genetic predisposition. Some specific genetic abnormalities have been postulated to play a role in the development of insulin resistance (171–175).

INSULIN SECRETION

As already discussed, impaired insulin secretion is an important, independent factor in the progression to type 2 diabetes. Studies of Pima Indians have shown that insulin secretory dysfunction plays a significant independent role in the progression from normal glucose tolerance to IGT and to type 2 diabetes (178,179).

OBESITY

Obesity is an extremely common problem in Native American and Alaska Native communities (181). Approximately 95% of Pima Indians with type 2 diabetes are also overweight (182). Obesity increases the risk of developing type 2 diabetes in any population. Obesity is also an important factor among Pima Indians, and the duration of obesity has also been related to the development of type 2 diabetes (183,184). A more important role of central obesity over general adiposity as a predictor of type 2 diabetes has also been identified in Native American groups (185). Pima Indians have been identified as having a low metabolic rate that may contribute to the high rate of obesity in this group (140). In many populations, low birthweight has been associated with an increased risk for type 2 diabetes as adults. This association has also been found in Native Americans (186,187).

Categories at Risk for Type 2 Diabetes

IMPAIRED FASTING GLUCOSE AND IMPAIRED GLUCOSE TOLERANCE

In concordance with the high rate of obesity and type 2 diabetes among Native Americans and Alaska Natives, it is not surprising that a significant proportion of people in these groups have IFG and IGT (144,161). These are categories that indicate a considerable risk of developing type 2 diabetes.

GESTATIONAL DIABETES

The frequency of gestational diabetes has been reported for several Native American groups. In all of them, the rates are higher than in the general population (188–190). The rate for gestational diabetes varies among subgroups; for example, the rate of gestational diabetes is 14.5% among Zuni women, 5.8% among Yupik Eskimo women, and 3.4% among Navajo women. In all cases, the frequency of gestational diabetes is higher than in the white population, which is around 2%. Women with gestational diabetes have a high risk of type 2 diabetes. Type 2 diabetes develops during the first 10 years after pregnancy in approximately one third of Pima and Zuni Indian women who have had gestational diabetes (188).

Adult offspring of Pima Indian women who had gestational diabetes have a significantly higher risk of type 2 diabetes than do the offspring of women who did not have gestational diabetes (191–193). Therefore, exposure to diabetes in utero is a strong risk factor for diabetes in Pima Indians.

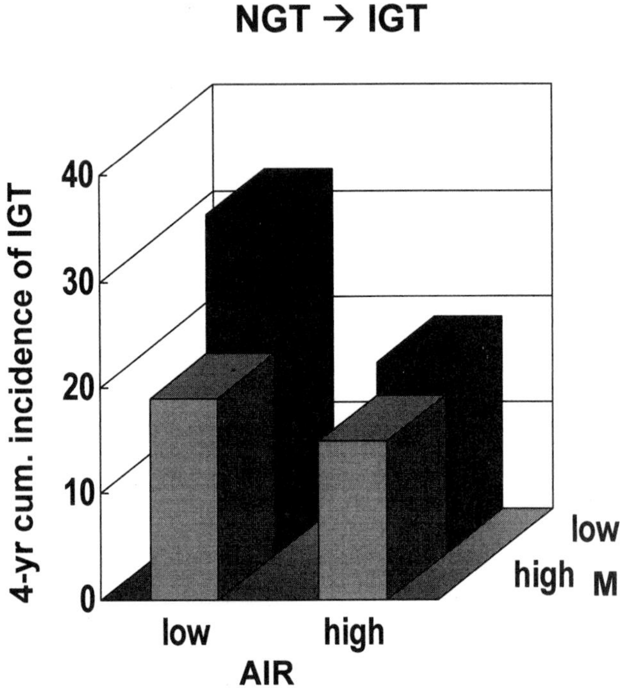

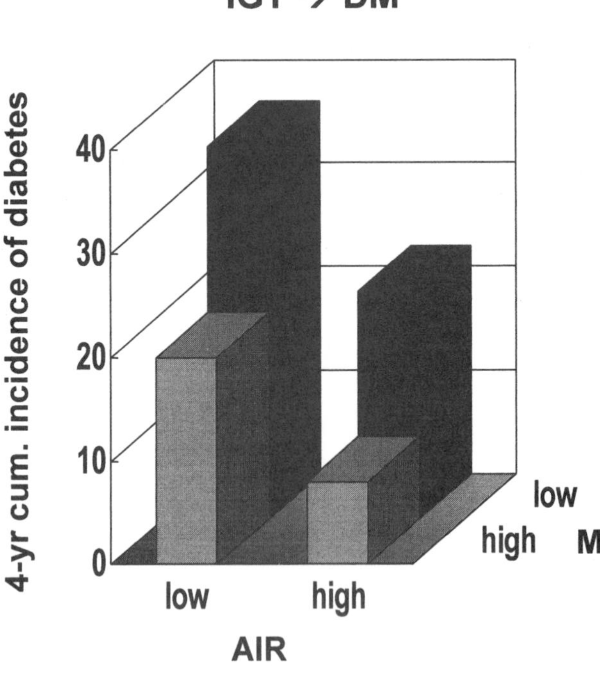

Figure 29.8. Progression from normal glucose tolerance (*NGT*) to impaired glucose tolerance (*IGT*) to diabetes mellitus (*DM*) in Pima Indians: independent effects of insulin action (*M*) and acute insulin secretory response (*AIR*). (From Weyer C, Tataranni PA, Bogardus C. Insulin resistance and insulin secretory dysfunction are independent predictors of worsening of glucose tolerance during each stage of type 2 diabetes development. *Diabetes Care* 2000;24:89–94.)

Microvascular Complications

RETINOPATHY

Diabetic retinopathy seems to be more prevalent among Native Americans and Alaska Natives than among the white population. The prevalence of diabetic retinopathy depends on the subgroup studied, duration of diabetes, presence of hypertension, and glycemic control, among others factors. Some studies of Pima and Oklahoma Indians show the high frequency of diabetic retinopathy (194–196).

NEPHROPATHY

As discussed for other minority groups, the rates of nephropathy at all stages are very high in Native Americans and Alaska Natives. High rates of microalbuminuria and clinical nephropathy have been reported (197–200). ESRD is the leading cause of death in Pima Indians (199). The rate of development of ESRD is six times higher in Native Americans with diabetes than among non-Hispanic whites with diabetes (201). An interesting finding among Alaska Natives is that ESRD is more likely to develop in women than men, and women are more likely to die of renal failure. Studies from other populations confirm this finding (202–204). The reason for these high rates of nephropathy among Native Americans and Alaska Natives is not well understood. However, there also seems to be a genetic predisposition for renal disease (205).

NEUROPATHY

Neuropathy can develop in Native Americans and Alaska Natives as a consequence of diabetes. No different rates of neuropathy have been reported in these groups in comparison to the rates in other populations (206,207).

Macrovascular Complications

CARDIOVASCULAR DISEASE

Cardiovascular disease is the leading cause of death among Native Americans with diabetes, particularly those with nephropathy (208,209). Cardiovascular mortality is higher in Native Americans than in non-Hispanic whites in the United States (210). However, the prevalence of coronary artery disease (CAD) in Pima Indians is not as high as expected for individuals with such a high rate of diabetes and hypertension (211).

The Strong Heart Study recently reported that prevalence of CAD was twofold to threefold lower among the communities in Arizona than among those in Oklahoma, South Dakota, and North Dakota. The lower prevalence of CAD among Native Americans in Arizona may be related to a low prevalence of smoking and a more favorable lipid profile, manifested by low concentrations of total and low-density lipoprotein cholesterol (212).

Associated Cardiovascular Risk Factors. Before 1950, the prevalence of hypertension in Native Americans was 8% to 10%, as compared with the national average of about 25% (213). However, in the past few years, hypertension has been reported to be higher in Native Americans than in the general population. This increasing rate may be due to changes in lifestyle (214). Similarly, cholesterol levels, which have traditionally been reported as lower in Native Americans than in the general population, have gradually increased over time (215).

PERIPHERAL VASCULAR DISEASE AND AMPUTATIONS

In general, rates of lower extremity amputation are high in some Native Americans but may vary by tribe. The rate of amputation is 3.7 times higher among Pima Indians than overall rates compiled previously for six states (216). Most studies suggest that amputations represent a major health problem in Native Americans (217,218). When data are analyzed by gender, several studies indicate a higher amputation rate among men than among women.

CEREBROVASCULAR DISEASE

Few data are available on stroke prevalence and incidence rates among Native Americans. The incidence of stroke in Alaska Natives was greatest among Eskimos, followed by Aleuts, and Indians. The overall incidence of stroke in Eskimo women was higher than in any other group studied (140).

Lifestyle and Cultural Factors

Native Americans and Alaska Natives have gone through an obvious process of lifestyle changes over many years. They have gradually incorporated a diet with more fat and less complex carbohydrates and have become more sedentary. These changes in the setting of the already discussed genetic predisposition for the development of obesity and diabetes have had a tremendously unfavorable impact on their rates of obesity and type 2 diabetes (219). An interesting study in Pima Indians showed that physical activity is associated with insulin sensitivity independent of its effect on body composition (220). There is a natural example of the severe impact that the adoption of an unhealthy diet and a more sedentary lifestyle can have on the development of type 2 diabetes. Pima Indians living in Mexico who consume a more traditional diet (less animal fat and more complex carbohydrates) and who are more physically active have a lower prevalence of type 2 diabetes than do Pima Indians living in Arizona (221).

It is well known that Native Americans have a genetic tendency for the development of obesity and, therefore, of type 2 diabetes (222). Culturally oriented programs to improve lifestyle in Native Americans with diabetes have been very successful in improving glycemic control and additional cardiovascular risk factors in this population (223–225). Native Americans and Alaska Natives have a rich culture with a vast array of traditions, beliefs, and behaviors. Understanding and respecting their culture has been a crucial element in establishing successful obesity and diabetes research and clinical care programs among these groups (226–228).

DIABETES IN ASIANS AND PACIFIC ISLANDERS

The Asian and Pacific Islander Population

DEFINITION

Asian refers to people having origins in any of the original peoples of the Far East, Southeast Asia, or the Indian subcontinent. *Pacific Islander* refers to people having origins in any of the original peoples of Hawaii, Guam, Samoa, or other Pacific Islands (18).

DEMOGRAPHICS

According to the recent 2000 U.S. census, there are 10.2 million Asians and Pacific Islanders in the country, representing 3.6% of the total population (18). Approximately 29% of them are younger than 18 years of age, and only 6.2% are older than 65 years of age, in contrast to the non-Hispanic white population, among whom the proportions are 24% and 14%, respectively. Since 1990, the Asian and Pacific Islander population has grown at a rate of about 4.5% per year. The Immigration Act of 1965 and the arrival of many Southeast Asian refugees under the

Refugee Resettlement Program after 1975 contributed to the increase in population observed in the past two decades. Six of every 10 Asians and Pacific Islanders reside in metropolitan areas in the western region, and approximately 73% are located within seven states: California, Hawaii, Illinois, New Jersey, New York, Texas, and Washington. The major subgroups are Chinese, Filipino, Asian Indian, Korean, Vietnamese, and Japanese. Some of the Asian subgroups, such as the Chinese and Japanese, have been in the United States for several generations. Others, such as the Hmong, Vietnamese, Laotians, and Cambodians, are comparatively recent immigrants. The major Pacific Islander subgroups are Hawaiian, Guamanian or Chamorro, and Samoan. Relatively few of the Pacific Islanders are foreign born.

Diabetes Epidemiology

PREVALENCE AND INCIDENCE OF DIABETES

Type 1 Diabetes. Type 1 diabetes among Asian children is relatively rare. The rate of type 1 of diabetes is significantly lower than among non-Hispanic whites. Both genetic and environmental factors are thought to be involved in the etiology of type 1 diabetes in any racial group. A good example of the influence of environmental factors is that the rates for type 1 diabetes in Japanese children in Hawaii have been reported to be higher than the rates for Japanese children in Tokyo (6).

Type 2 Diabetes. Few studies have addressed the prevalence of type 2 diabetes in Asian and Pacific Islander Americans in the United States. A study of Native Hawaiians showed that approximately 22% of persons older than age 30 years have type 2 diabetes. Among people between the ages of 60 and 64 years, about 40% of them have type 2 diabetes (229). This is considerably higher than the rate of type 2 diabetes in whites. In the Japanese population in the United States, approximately 37% of people between the ages of 45 and 74 years have diabetes (230–232). The prevalence of diabetes is lower in other subgroups, such as Polynesians (1.1% for men and 7.2% for women) (6). A distinct gender lifestyle pattern may explain this observed wide difference in diabetes prevalence. Similarly, in Western Samoa, a difference in diabetes prevalence in a rural and an urban community (3.4% vs 7.8%) has been found (6). Lifestyle factors, dietary habits, and level of physical activity play a major role in these differences.

Subgroup Analysis. *Age and gender*. The incidence of type 2 diabetes is increasing in young people, particularly members of minority groups (33). The rate of type 2 diabetes is also increasing gradually among Asians and Pacific Islanders, as it has been shown for Japanese children and adolescents (6). With regard to gender differences, there are no solid data to suggest that the prevalence of diabetes differs by gender per se. The study of Polynesians that shows a sevenfold higher rate of diabetes in women than in men seems to be explained by their clear differences in physical activity (6).

Asian and Pacific Islander subgroups. Filipinos have the highest prevalence of diabetes among the four largest ethnic Asian groups in Hawaii (Chinese, Filipino, Japanese, and Korean). However, the prevalence is higher in all groups than among whites (233).

MORTALITY

Diabetes is the fifth cause of death among Asians and Pacific Islanders, whereas it is the seventh leading cause of death in whites (6). However, a comparison of adjusted diabetes-related mortality rates in Asian and Pacific Islander Americans with those of other ethnic groups indicates that these rates are very close to the rate in whites (approximately 12 to 14 per 100,000) but two to three times lower than the rates reported for African Americans, Native Americans and Alaska Natives, and Hispanic Americans (6).

Pathophysiology of Type 2 Diabetes

GENETIC PREDISPOSITION

Among Asian and Pacific Islanders, like other minority groups in the United States, the rates of diabetes are higher than those in the white population. It is believed that genetic factors play a significant role in increasing the risk of developing type 2 diabetes in these groups. No data on specific genetic abnormalities that could explain this increased risk have emerged. However, as mentioned for other ethnic groups, whatever genetic factors are responsible for this predisposition may have been the result of an adaptation to conditions prevalent many years ago (2,3).

INSULIN RESISTANCE

Studies in Japanese-American and Japanese men with type 2 diabetes have provided interesting information. Insulin levels, an indirect measure of insulin resistance, have been evaluated in these two groups. Both groups exhibit hyperinsulinemia, consistent with the presence of insulin resistance. Insulin levels, measured during an oral glucose tolerance test, are higher in Japanese-American men than in Japanese men, suggesting a higher degree of insulin resistance. Japanese-American men are usually more obese than Japanese men. However, insulin levels in Japanese Americans continue to be higher than those in Japanese men even after adjusting for BMI. Therefore, factors other than obesity contribute to insulin resistance (234). As in all studied populations, insulin resistance is usually the result of a combination of genetic and environmental factors.

INSULIN SECRETION

A defect in insulin secretion is now considered an important element in the development of type 2 diabetes. It can be identified before the appearance of abnormalities in glucose tolerance. Studies of Japanese Americans have identified an early defect in insulin secretion before the development of type 2 diabetes (235). Once type 2 diabetes appears, this defect continues to have crucial importance in the progression of the disease.

OBESITY

Obesity, particular from visceral adiposity, was found to be a strong predictor of type 2 diabetes in a prospective study in Japanese-American men (236). Neither BMI, a measure of general adiposity (234), nor waist circumference (237) has been considered to be a good predictor of type 2 diabetes among Japanese Americans. Some specific measurements, such as increased leptin levels, are associated with an increased risk of type 2 diabetes in men, although not in women (238). Obesity in Asian-Americans and Pacific Islanders has become a significant problem, in part due to the adoption of a "Westernized" diet and a more sedentary lifestyle. This is reflected by data showing that Japanese people who have emigrated to Hawaii or the continental United States have twice the rates of obesity and diabetes of Japanese people in Japan (6).

Categories at Risk for Type 2 Diabetes

IMPAIRED FASTING GLUCOSE AND IMPAIRED GLUCOSE TOLERANCE

Studies of two different Asian and Pacific Islander subgroups have assessed categories at risk for type 2 diabetes. A study in

Native Hawaiians showed a prevalence rate of IGT of 15.6% in the adult population. Studies in Japanese Americans have also shown a higher rate of IGT than in the general U.S. population (231,239). A recent report suggests that Japanese Americans with IGT based on the 2-hour plasma glucose level have significant metabolic abnormalities despite having a normal fasting plasma glucose level (240). Therefore, classification of Japanese Americans by fasting plasma glucose levels does not allow the identification of all people with unfavorable cardiovascular risk profiles.

GESTATIONAL DIABETES

Little information is available on the prevalence of gestational diabetes among Asian American and Pacific Islander women. Those that have been reported are similar to those of non-Hispanic white women in the United States (approximately 2% to 3% of pregnancies) (6).

Microvascular Complications

NEPHROPATHY

Asian Americans and Pacific Islanders have a higher rate of ESRD than do whites. However, the prevalence of ESRD is lower than in other minority groups, such as African Americans, Hispanics, and Native Americans (241). No data on the incidence of retinopathy or neuropathy are available for Asians and Pacific Islanders.

Macrovascular Complications

CARDIOVASCULAR DISEASE AND CARDIOVASCULAR RISK FACTORS

CHD is one of the leading causes of death for both diabetic and nondiabetic Asians and Pacific Islander men and women (6).

Japanese Americans with impaired glucose tolerance and diabetes have an increased risk of CHD (242). Visceral adiposity, blood pressure, and plasma glucose levels are independent risk factors for incident CHD in diabetic and nondiabetic Japanese Americans (243). Obesity in this population is also associated with CHD (242). The typical dyslipidemia of the insulin-resistance syndrome, including high triglycerides, low HDL cholesterol, and small dense low-density lipoprotein particles, has been detected in this population. Dyslipidemia is associated with visceral adiposity and fasting insulin levels in nondiabetic Japanese Americans (244).

There are no published reports on the rate of amputations, peripheral vascular disease, or cerebral vascular disease in this population.

Lifestyle and Cultural Factors

Asians and Pacific Islanders have also suffered from the "westernization" effect of some particular diets and the lack of physical activity. Japanese Americans consume more calories, protein, fat, and carbohydrates than do Japanese individuals living in Japan. For example, the mean daily intake of fat in Japanese-American men is approximately 32.4 g while that of Japanese men in Japan is about 16.7 g. The diet of the latter group is based more on fish and plants (6).

Data also suggest that Japanese Americans are more sedentary than Japanese living in Japan (6). Therefore, the combination of a more unhealthy diet and less physical activity on the presence of some genetic factors has contributed to the fourfold increased rate of obesity and type 2 diabetes in some Asian groups in the United States compared with the same groups in their country of origin (245). Figure 29.9 compares the rate of diabetes in Japanese Americans in Seattle with the rate in Japanese individuals in Tokyo (234). People who come to the United States who preserve their original lifestyle, including a more balanced diet and more physical activity, seem to have a lower rate of diabetes than do those who adopt a more unhealthy lifestyle (246).

Other important cultural and lifestyle factors that influence the development of type 2 diabetes are income and educational level. A low level of either of these has been associated with an increased risk for type 2 diabetes among Japanese Americans (247). Another important element that influences access to and success in the healthcare system is language. Speaking a language different from that of healthcare providers has been found to be a barrier to diabetes care in the Asian population (248). Culturally and linguistically oriented programs are crucial to improving diabetes care in this population.

PREVENTION OF DIABETES IN MINORITY GROUPS

As stated throughout this chapter, people from minority groups have a significant risk of type 2 diabetes and its complications. Once diabetes develops, it is extremely difficult to achieve good metabolic control in any population. In some minority groups, such as Hispanics and African Americans, glycemic control tends to be even worse than that in whites.

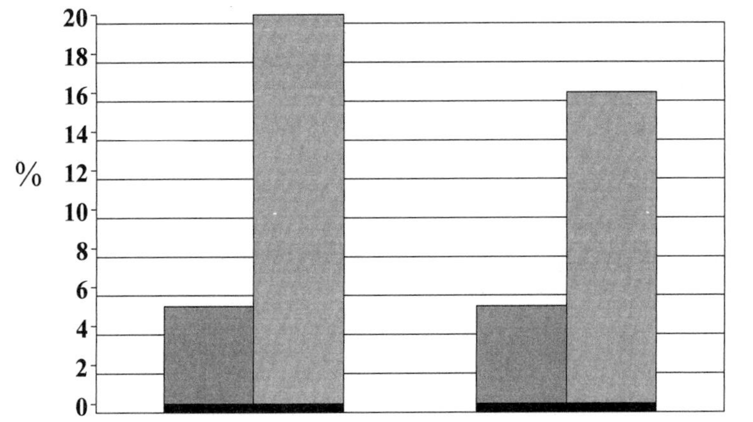

Figure 29.9. Prevalence of type 2 diabetes in Tokyo and Seattle among men and women greater than 40 years of age (1981 to 1988). (From Fujimoto W. The importance of insulin resistance in the pathogenesis of type 2 diabetes mellitus. *Am J Med* 2000;108[6A]:9S–14S.)

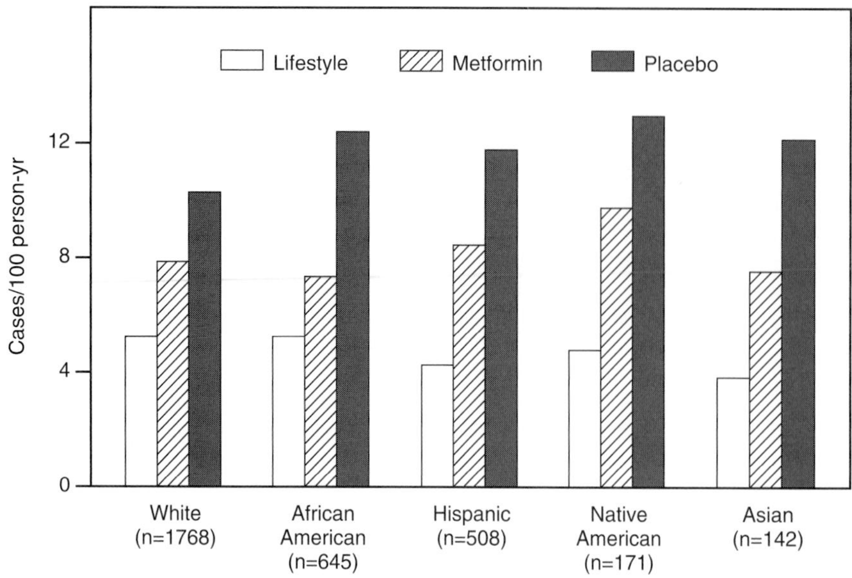

Figure 29.10. Percentage developing diabetes by race/ethnicity in the Diabetes Prevention Program. (From Knowler WC, Barrett-Connor E, Fowler SE, et al. Reduction in the incidence of type 2 diabetes with lifestyle intervention or metformin. *N Engl J Med* 2002;346:393–403.)

Because it is possible to identify individuals at risk for type 2 diabetes, the National Institutes of Health sponsored the recently completed Diabetes Prevention Program (249,250). This research project had the goal of preventing or delaying the progression to type 2 diabetes in individuals with IGT by having them participate in an intensive lifestyle modification program, taking metformin, or taking placebo. A total of 3,234 individuals were followed for an average of 2.8 years. Forty-five percent of the people in the study were from minority groups: African Americans, Hispanics, Native Americans, and Asians and Pacific Islanders. People in the intensive lifestyle modification group achieved a mean weight loss of 5% of their initial body weight by following a healthier meal plan and increasing their exercise level. The incidence of diabetes was 11 cases per 100 person-years in the placebo group, whereas the corresponding numbers for the group taking metformin and the group in the intensive lifestyle modification were 7.8 and 4.8, respectively. Therefore, the lifestyle intervention reduced the progression to diabetes by 58% and metformin treatment reduced it by 31%. These beneficial effects were observed in all ethnic groups (251) (Fig. 29.10). The Diabetes Prevention Program will continue to observe this population for a few more years.

SUMMARY

Type 2 diabetes represents a serious health problem among minority groups in the United States. The prevalence and incidence rates for obesity, diabetes, and its vascular complications are usually higher in these groups than in the white population. In all these groups, genetic factors that have not yet been well identified increase the risk of development of type 2 diabetes. In addition, acquired factors such as a diet rich in saturated fat and carbohydrates combined with a sedentary lifestyle have increased the prevalence of obesity and type 2 diabetes to epidemic proportions in minority groups. All minority groups have a unique culture, with particular beliefs, attitudes, and traditions. Understanding and respecting these aspects of their lives are necessary elements in the development and implementation of culturally and linguistically appropriate diabetes care programs. Diabetes prevention programs represent an excellent opportunity to reduce the burden of diabetes and its complications in minority groups in the United States.

REFERENCES

1. *Chronic diseases in minority populations.* Atlanta, GA: US Department of Health and Human Services, 1994.
2. Neel JV. The thrifty genotype revisited. In: Kobberling J, Tattersall R, eds. *The genetics of diabetes mellitus.* New York: Academic Press, 1982:283–293.
3. Neel JV. Diabetes mellitus: a thrifty genotype rendered detrimental by progress? *Am J Hum Genet* 1962;14:353–362.
4. Taylor R, Zimmet P. Migrant studies in diabetes epidemiology. In: Mann JI, Pyorala K, Teuscher A, eds. *Diabetes in epidemiological perspective.* New York: Churchill Livingstone, 1983:58–77.
5. Kawate R, Yamakido M, Nishimoto Y. Migrant studies among the Japanese in Hiroshima and Hawaii. In: Waldhausi WK, ed. Diabetes 1979. *Proceedings of the 10th Congress of the International Diabetes Federation*, Vienna, Austria, September 9–14, 1979. Princeton: Excerpta Medica, 1980:526–531.
6. Fujimoto WF. Diabetes in Asians and Pacific Islander Americans. In: National Diabetes Data Group. *Diabetes in America*, 2nd ed. Bethesda, MD. National Institute of Diabetes and Digestive and Kidney Diseases, 1995:661–681. NIDDKD publication 95-1468.
7. Kim EJ, Kims KS, Lee TH, Kim DY. The incidence of diabetes mellitus in urban and rural populations in Korea. In: Baba S, Goto Y, Fukui I, eds. *Diabetes mellitus in Asia: ecological aspects of epidemiology, complications and treatment.* New York: Excerpta Medica, 1976:41–44.
8. Tai TY, Yang CL, Chang CJ, et al. Epidemiology of diabetes mellitus in Taiwan, ROC—comparison between urban and rural areas. In: Vannasaeng S, Nitiyanant W, Chandraprasert S, eds. *Epidemiology of diabetes mellitus: Proceedings of the International Symposium on Epidemiology of Diabetes Mellitus. Bangkok, Thailand*: Crystal House PR, 1987:49–53.
9. Fernando RE. The status of diabetes mellitus in the Philippines. In: Baba JS, Goto Y, Fukui I, eds. *Diabetes mellitus in Asia: ecological aspects of epidemiology, complications and treatment.* New York: Excerpta Medica, 1976:123–127.
10. Kuzuya T, Ito C, Sasaki A, et al. Prevalence and incidence of diabetes in Japanese people compiled from the literature. A report of the Epidemiology Data Committee, The Japan Diabetes Society 1992;35:173–194.
11. Kitazawa Y, Murakami K, Goto Y, et al. Prevalence of diabetes mellitus detected by 75 g GTT in Tokyo, Thoku. *J Exp Med* 1983;141[Suppl]:229–234.
12. Haddock L, de Conty IT. Prevalence rates for diabetes mellitus in Puerto Rico. *Diabetes Care* 1991;14:676–684.
13. Stern MP, Gonzalez C, Mitchell BD, et al. Genetic and environmental determinants of type II diabetes in Mexico City and San Antonio. *Diabetes* 1992;41: 484–492.
14. Zimmet P, Faaiuso S, Ainuu J, et al. The prevalence of diabetes in the rural and urban Polynesian population of Western Samoa. *Diabetes* 1981;30: 45–51.
15. Marine N, Vinik AI, Edelstein I, et al. Diabetes, hyperglycemia and glycosuria among Indians, Malays and Africans (Bantu) in Cape Town, South Africa. *Diabetes* 1969;18:840–857.
16. Caballero AE. Endothelial dysfunction in obesity and insulin resistance: a road to diabetes and heart disease. *Obes Res* 2003;11:1278–1289.

17. Caballero AE. Endothelial dysfunction, inflammation, and insulin resistance: a focus on subjects at risk for type 2 diabetes. *Curr Diabetes Rep* 2004;46:237–246.
18. US Bureau of Census. United States Department of Commerce. Washington, DC: US Government Printing Office, 2000.
19. US Bureau of Census. *Population projections of the United States by age, sex, race and Hispanic Origin: 1995 to 2050*. Current population reports no. P25-1130. Washington, DC: US Government Printing Office, 1996.
20. Kostraba J, Gay EC, Cai Y, et al. Incidence of insulin-dependent diabetes mellitus in Colorado. *Am J Epidemiol* 1992;3:232–238.
21. Lipman TH. The epidemiology of type 1 diabetes in children 0–14 yr of age in Philadelphia. *Diabetes Care* 1993;16:922–925.
22. National Center for Health Statistics. *Plan and operation of the Third National Health and Nutrition Examination Survey, 1988–1994*. Hyattsville, MD: National Center for Health Statistics, 1994. Vital and Health Statistics ser. 1, no. 32.
23. National Center for Health Statistics. *Third National Health and Nutrition Examination Survey, 1988–1994, Reference manuals and reports: manual for medical technicians and laboratory procedures used for NHANES III* (CD-ROM). Hyattsville, MD; Centers for Disease Control and Prevention, 1996 (available from National Technical Information Service, Springfield VA, in Acrobat.PDF format with Acrobat Reader 2.0 access software, Adobe Systems).
24. American Diabetes Association. Report of the Expert Committee on the Diagnosis and Classification of Diabetes Mellitus. *Diabetes Care* 1997;20:1183–1197.
25. Harris MI, Flegal KM, Cowie CC, et al. Prevalence of diabetes, impaired fasting glucose, and impaired glucose tolerance in U.S. adults: The Third National Health and Nutrition Examination Survey (NHANES), 1988–94. *Diabetes Care* 1998;21:518–524.
26. World Health Organization. WHO Expert Committee on Diabetes Mellitus: Second Report. *World Health Organ Tech Rep Ser* 1980;646.
27. World Health Organization: Diabetes Mellitus: Report of a WHO Study Group. Geneva, *World Health Organ Tech Rep Ser* 1985;727.
28. Stern MP, Gaskill SP, Allen CR Jr, et al. Cardiovascular risk factors in Mexican Americans in Laredo, Texas: II. Prevalence and control of hypertension. *Am J Epidemiol* 1981;113:556–562.
29. Samet JM, Coultas DB, Howard CA, et al. Diabetes, gallbladder disease, obesity and hypertension among Hispanics in New Mexico. *Am J Epidemiol* 1988; 128:1302–1311.
30. Gardner LI Jr, Stern MP, Haffner SM, et al. Prevalence of diabetes in Mexican Americans. Relationship to percent of gene pool derived from Native Americans sources. *Diabetes* 1984;33:86–92.
31. Hanis CL, Ferrell RE, Barton SA, et al. Diabetes among Mexican Americans in Starr County, Texas. *Am J Epidemiol* 1983;118:659–672.
32. Haffner SM, Hazuda HP, Mitchell BD, et al. Increased incidence of type II diabetes mellitus in Mexican-Americans. *Diabetes Care* 1991;14:102–108.
33. Rosenbloom AL, Joe JR, Young RS, et al. Emerging epidemic of type 2 diabetes in youth. *Diabetes Care* 1999;22:345–354.
34. Neufeld ND, Raffel LJ, Landon C, et al. Early presentation of type 2 diabetes in Mexican-American youth. *Diabetes Care* 1998;21:80–86.
35. Flegal KM, Ezzati TM, Harris MI, et al. Prevalence of diabetes in Mexican Americans, Cubans, and Puerto Ricans from the Hispanic Health and Examination Survey (HHANES), 1982–84. *Diabetes Care* 1991;14[Suppl 3]: 628–638.
36. Hanis CL, Chu HH, Lawson K, et al. Mortality of Mexican Americans with NIDDM. Retinopathy and other predictors in Starr County, Texas. *Diabetes Care* 1993;16:82–89.
37. Gilliland FD, Owen C, Gilliland SS, et al. Temporal trends in diabetes mortality among American Indians and Hispanics in New Mexico: birth cohort and period effects. *Am J Epidemiol* 1997;145:422–431.
38. Lorenzo C, Serrano-Rios M, Martinez-Larrad MT, et al. Was the historic contribution of Spain to the Mexican gene pool partially responsible for the higher prevalence of type 2 diabetes in Mexican-origin populations? The Spanish Insulin Resistance Study Group, the San Antonio Heart Study, and the Mexico City Diabetes Study. *Diabetes Care* 2001;24:2059–2064.
39. Hanis CL, Hewett-Emmett D, Betrin TK, et al. Origins of U.S. Hispanics. Implications for diabetes. *Diabetes Care* 1991;14:618–627.
40. Mitchell BD, Kammerer CM, O'Connell P, et al. Evidence for linkage of postchallenge insulin levels with intestinal fatty-acid binding protein ($FABP_2$) in Mexican Americans. *Diabetes* 1995;44:1046–1053.
41. Mitchell BD, Valdez R, Hazuda HP, et al. Differences in the prevalence of diabetes and impaired glucose tolerance according to maternal or paternal history of diabetes. *Diabetes Care* 1993;16:1262–1267.
42. Gulli G, Ferranini E, Stern M, et al. The metabolic profile of NIDDM is fully established in glucose-tolerant offspring of two Mexican-American NIDDM parents. *Diabetes* 1992;41:1575–1586.
43. Boyko EJ, Keane EM, Marshall JA, et al. Higher insulin and C-peptide concentrations in Hispanic population at high risk for NIDDM. *Diabetes* 1991;40: 509–515.
44. Haffner SM, Bowsher R, Mykkanen L, et al. Proinsulin and specific insulin concentration in high and low risk populations for non-insulin dependent diabetes mellitus. *Diabetes* 1994;43:1490–1493.
45. Haffner SM, D'Agostino R, Saad MF, et al. Increased insulin resistance and insulin secretion in nondiabetic African-Americans and Hispanics compared with non-Hispanic whites. The Insulin Resistance Atherosclerosis Study. *Diabetes* 1996;45:742–748.
46. Haffner SM, Mietinen H, Gaskill SP, et al. Decreased insulin secretion and increased insulin resistance are independently related to the 7-year risk of non-insulin dependent diabetes mellitus in Mexican Americans. *Diabetes* 1995;44:1386–1391.
47. Flegal KM, Carroll MD, Kuczmarski RJ, et al. Overweight and obesity in the United States: prevalence and trends, 1960–1994. *Int J Obes Relat Disord* 1998; 22:39–47.
48. Kuzmarski RJ, Flegal KM, Campbell SM, et al. Increasing prevalence of overweight among U.S. adults. The National Health and Nutrition Examination Surveys (NHANES), 1960 to 1991. *JAMA* 1994;272:205–211.
49. Troiano RP, Flegal KM, Kuczmarski RJ, et al. Overweight prevalence and trends for children and adolescents. *Arch Pediatr Adolesc Med* 1995;149: 1085–1091.
50. Harris MI. Epidemiological correlates of NIDDM in Hispanics, whites and blacks in the US population. *Diabetes Care* 1991;14[Suppl 3]:639–648.
51. Joos SK, Mueller WH, Hanis CL, et al. Diabetes alert study: weight history and upper body obesity in diabetic and non-diabetic Mexican American adults. *Ann Hum Biol* 1984;11:167–171.
52. Haffner SM, Stern MP, Hazuda HP, et al. Upper body and centralized adiposity in Mexican Americans and non-Hispanic whites: relationship to body mass index and other behavioral and demographic variables. *Int J Obes* 1986;10:493–502.
53. US Interagency Committee on Nutrition Monitoring. US Public Health Service and US Department of Agriculture. *Nutrition monitoring in the United States: the directory of federal nutrition monitoring activities.* Hyattsville, MD: Department of Health and Human Service, 1989. DHHS publication no. (PHS) 89-1255.
54. Valdez R, Athens MA, Thompson GH, et al. Birth-weight and adult health outcomes in a biethnic population in the USA. *Diabetologia* 1994;37:624–631.
55. Hollingsworth DR, Vaucher Y, Yamamoto TR. Diabetes in pregnancy in Mexican Americans. *Diabetes Care* 1991;14:695–705.
56. Peters RK, Kjos SL, Xiang A, et al. Long-term diabetogenic effect of single pregnancy in women with previous gestational diabetes. *Lancet* 1996;347: 227–230.
57. Haffner SM, Fong D, Stern MP, et al. Diabetic retinopathy in Mexican Americans and non-Hispanic whites. *Diabetes* 1988;37:878–884.
58. Harris MI, Klein R, Cowie, CC, et al. Is the risk of diabetic retinopathy greater in non-Hispanic blacks and Mexican Americans than in non-Hispanic whites with type 2 diabetes? A U.S. population study. *Diabetes Care* 1998;21: 1230–1235.
59. Hamman RF, Franklin GA, Mayer E, et al. Microvascular complications of NIDDM in Hispanics and non-Hispanic whites. San Luis Valley Diabetes Study. *Diabetes Care* 1991;14:655–664.
60. Hamman RF, Marshall JA, Baxter J, et al. Methods and prevalence of non-insulin-dependent diabetes mellitus in a biethnic Colorado population: The San Luis Valley Diabetes Study. *Am J Epidemiol* 1989;129:295–311.
61. Harris MI, Eastman RC, Cowie CC, et al. Racial and ethnic differences in glycemic control of adults with type 2 diabetes. *Diabetes Care* 1999;22:403–408.
62. Pugh JA, Tuley MR, Hazuda HP, et al. The influence of outpatient insurance coverage on the microvascular complications of non-insulin-dependent diabetes in Mexican Americans. *J Diabetes Comp* 1992;6:236–241.
63. Haffner SM, Mitchell BD, Pugh JA, et al. Proteinuria in Mexican Americans and non-Hispanic whites with NIDDM. *Diabetes Care* 1989;12:530–536.
64. Pugh JA, Medina RA, Cornell JC, et al. NIDDM is the major cause of diabetic end-stage renal disease. More evidence from a tri-ethnic community. *Diabetes* 1995;44:1375–1380.
65. Pugh JA, Stern MP, Haffner SM, et al. Excess incidence of treatment of end-stage renal disease in Mexican Americans. *Am J Epidemiol* 1988;127:135–144.
66. Pugh JA, Tuley MR, Basu S. Survival among Mexican-Americans, non-Hispanic whites and African-Americans with end-stage renal disease: the emergence of a minority pattern of increased incidence and prolonged survival. *Am J Kidney Dis* 1994;23:803–807.
67. Harris MI, Cowie CC, Eastman RC. Symptoms of sensory neuropathy in adults with diabetes in the U.S. population. *Diabetes Care* 1993;16:1446–1452.
68. Ford ES, Giles WH, Croft JB. Prevalence of nonfatal coronary heart disease among American adults. *Am Heart J* 2000;139:371–377.
69. Carter JS, Pugh JA, Monterrosa A. Non-insulin dependent diabetes mellitus in minorities in the United States. *Ann Intern Med* 1996;125:221–232.
70. Lemon-Garber I, Villa RA, Caballero AE. Diabetes and cardiovascular disease. Is there a true Hispanic paradox? *Rev. Invest Clinica* 2004;56:282–296.
71. Ford ES, Giles WH, Dietz WH. Prevalence of the metabolic syndrome among US adults. Findings from the Third National Health and Nutrition Survey. *JAMA* 2002;287:356–359.
72. Hafner SM, Morales PA, Hazuda HP, et al. Level of control of hypertension in Mexican Americans and non-Hispanic whites. *Hypertension* 1993;21:83–88.
73. Harris MI. Racial and ethnic differences in health care access and health outcomes for adults with type 2 diabetes. *Diabetes Care* 2001;24:454–459.
74. Howard BV, Mayer-Davis EJ, Goff D, et al. Relationships between insulin resistance and lipoproteins in nondiabetic African Americans, Hispanics, and non-Hispanic whites: the Insulin Resistance Atherosclerosis Study. *Metabolism* 1998;47:1174–1179.
75. Lavery LA, van Houtum WH, Ashry HR, et al. Diabetes-related lower-extremity amputations disproportionately affect blacks and Mexican Americans. *South Med J* 1999;92:593–599.
76. Haffner SM, Mitchell BD, Stern MP, et al. Macrovascular complications in Mexican Americans with type II diabetes. *Diabetes Care* 1991;14:665–671.
77. Lavery L, Ashry H, Harkless L. Mortality associated with lower extremity amputations in minorities with diabetes. *Diabetes* 1994:43:29(abst).

78. Caballero AE, Habershaw SM, Pinzor MS. Preventing amputations in patients with diabetes. Caring for diverse populations. *Patient Care* 2000;5:113–133.
79. D'Agostino RB, Burke G, O'Leary D, et al. Ethnic differences in carotid wall thickness. The Insulin Resistance and Atherosclerosis Study. *Stroke* 1996;27: 1744–1749.
80. Sacco RL, Roberts K, Boden Albala B, et al. Race-ethnicity and determinants of carotid atherosclerosis in a multiethnic population. *Stroke* 1997;28:929–935.
81. Stern MP, Pugh JA, Gaskill SP, et al. Knowledge, attitudes, and behavior related to obesity and dieting in Mexican Americans and Anglos: the San Antonio Heart Study. *Am J Epidemiol* 1982;115:917–928.
82. Kimanyika S. Special issues regarding obesity in minority populations. *Ann Intern Med* 1993;119:650–654.
83. Haffner SM, Knapp JA, Hazuda HP, et al. Dietary intakes of macronutrients among Mexican Americans and Anglo Americans. The San Antonio Heart Study. *Am J Clin Nutr* 1985;42:1266–1275.
84. Frati-Munari A, Fernandez-Harp JA, de la Riva H, et al. Effects of nopal (Opuntia sp) on serum lipids, glycemia, and body weight. *Arch Invest Med* (Mex) 1983;14:117–125.
85. Frati AC, Gordillo BE, Altamriano P, et al. Acute hypoglycemic effect of Opuntia Streptacantha lemaire in NIDDM [Letter]. *Diabetes Care* 1990;13:455–456.
86. Crespo CJ, Keteyian SJ, Heath GW, et al. Leisure-time physical activity among U.S. adults. *Arch Intern Med* 1996;156:93–98.
87. Monterrosa AE, Haffner SM, Stern MP, et al. Sex difference in lifestyle factors predictive of diabetes in Mexican Americans. *Diabetes Care* 1995;18:448–456.
88. Stern MP, Knapp JA, Hazuda HP, et al. Genetic and environmental determinants of type II diabetes in Mexican Americans. Is there a descending limb to the modernization/diabetes relationship? *Diabetes Care* 1991;14:649–654.
89. Hazuda HP, Haffner SM, Stern MP, et al. Effects of acculturation and socioeconomic status on obesity and diabetes in Mexican Americans. The San Antonio Heart Study. *Am J Epidemiol* 1988;128:1289–1301.
90. Marshall JA, Hamman RF, Baxter J, et al. Ethnic differences in risk factors associated with the prevalence of non-insulin-dependent diabetes mellitus. The San Luis Valley Diabetes Study. *Am J Epidemiol* 1993;137:706–718.
91. Hazuda HP, Monterrosa A. Social class predicts 8-year incidence of diabetes in Mexican Americans and non-Hispanic whites. *Diabetes* 1992;41:179(abst).
92. Stein JA, Fox SA. Language preference as an indicator of mammography use among Hispanic women. *J Natl Cancer Inst* 1990;82:1715–1716.
93. Solis JM, Marks G, Garcia M, et al. Acculturation, access to care and use of preventive services by Hispanics: findings from HHANES 1982–1984. *Am J Public Health* 1990;80[Suppl]:11–19.
94. Seijo R, Gomez H, Freidenberg J. Language as a communication barrier in medical care Hispanic patients. *Hisp J Behav Sci* 1991;13:363–376.
95. Caballero AE, Monzillo L, Yohai F, et al. The short and long term effect of a non-traditional culturally oriented diabetes education program on the metabolic control of Hispanic patients with type 2 diabetes. *Diabetes* 2002;51 [Suppl 2]:A313.
96. Lorenzi M, Cogliero E, Schmidt NJ. Racial differences in the incidence of juvenile-onset type 1 diabetes: epidemiologic studies in southern California. *Diabetologia* 1985;28:734–738.
97. Tull ES, Makame MH, DERI Group. Evaluation of type 1 diabetes in black African-heritage populations: no time for further neglect. *Diab Med* 1992; 513–521.
98. Serjeanstson SW, Easteal S. Cross-ethnic group comparisons of HLA class II alleles and insulin dependent diabetes mellitus. *Baillieres Clin Endocrinol Metab* 1991;5:299–320.
99. O'Brien TR, Flanders WD, Decoufle P, et al. Are racial differences in the prevalence of diabetes in adults explained by differences in obesity? *JAMA* 1989;262:1485–1488.
100. Lipton RB, Liao Y, Cao G, et al. Determinants of incident non-insulin dependent diabetes mellitus among blacks and whites in a national sample. The NHANES I Epidemiologic Follow-up Study. *Am J Epidemiol* 1993;138: 826–839.
101. Watterhall SF, Olson DR, DeStefano F, et al. Trends in diabetes and diabetes complications, 1980–1987. *Diabetes Care* 1992;15:960–967.
102. Geiss LS, ed. *Diabetes surveillance*, 1997. Centers for Disease Control and Prevention, Atlanta, GA, 1997.
103. Gu K, Cowie CC, Harris MI. Mortality in adults with and without diabetes in a national cohort of the US population, 1971–93. *Diabetes Care* 1998;21: 1138–1145.
104. Poledknak AP. Mortality from diabetes mellitus, ischemic heart disease and cerebrovascular disease among blacks in a higher income area. *Public Health Rep* 1990;105:393–399.
105. Lindquist CH, Gower BA, Goran MI. Role of dietary factors in ethnic differences in early risk of cardiovascular disease and type 2 diabetes. *Am J Clin Nutr* 2000;71:725–732.
106. Osei K, Gaillard T, Schuster DP. Pathogenetic mechanisms of impaired glucose tolerance and type II diabetes in African-Americans. *Diabetes Care* 1997; 20:396–404.
107. Winter WE, Maclaren NK, Riley WJ, et al. Maturity-onset diabetes of youth in black Americans. *N Engl J Med* 1987;316:285–291.
108. Banerji MA, Chaiken RL, Huey H, et al. GAD antibody negative NIDDM in adult male black subjects with diabetic ketoacidosis and increased frequency of human leukocyte antigen DR3 and DR4. Flatbush diabetes. *Diabetes* 1994; 43:741–745.
109. Morrison EY, Ragoobirsingh D. J Type diabetes revisited. *J Natl Med Assoc* 1992;84:603–608.
110. McFarlane SL, Chaiken RL, Hirsch S, et al. Near-normoglycemic remission in African-Americans with type 2 diabetes mellitus is associated with recovery of beta cell function. *Diabet Med* 2001;18:10–16.
111. Dooley SL, Metzger BE, Cho NH. Gestational diabetes mellitus. Influence of race on disease prevalence and perinatal outcome in a U.S. population. *Diabetes* 1991;40[Suppl 2]:25–29.
112. Harris EL, Feldman S, Robinson CR, et al. Racial differences in the relationship between blood pressure and risk for retinopathy among individuals with NIDDM. *Diabetes Care* 1993;16:748–754.
113. Harris EL, Sherman SH, Georgopolous A. Black-white differences in risk of developing retinopathy among individuals with type 2 diabetes. *Diabetes Care* 1999;22:779–783.
114. Dasmahapatra A, Bale A, Raghuwanshi MP, et al. Incipient and overt diabetic nephropathy in African Americans with NIDDM. *Diabetes Care* 1994;17: 297–304.
115. Wingard DL, Barrett-Connor EL, Scheidt-Nave C, et al. Prevalence of cardiovascular and renal complications in older adults with normal or impaired glucose tolerance or NIDDM. A population based study. *Diabetes Care* 1993; 16:1022–1025.
116. Goldschmid MG, Domin WS, Ziemer DC, et al. Diabetes in urban African Americans. II. High prevalence of microalbuminuria and nephropathy in African Americans with diabetes. *Diabetes Care* 1995;18:955–961.
117. Brancatti FL, Kag MJ, Whelton PK, et al. End-stage renal disease in black and white diabetic men. A prospective cohort study. *Diabetes* 1994;43:26(abst).
118. Cowie CC, Port FK, Wolfe RA, et al. Disparities in incidence of diabetic end-stage renal disease by race and type of diabetes. *N Engl J Med* 1989;321: 1074–1079.
119. Cowie CC, Port FK, Rust KF, et al. Differences in survival between black and white patients with diabetic end-stage renal disease. *Diabetes Care* 1994; 17:681–687.
120. Port FK, Wolfe RA, Hawthorne VM, et al. Discontinuation of dialysis therapy as a cause of death. *Am J Nephrol* 1989;9:145–149.
121. Harris MI, Eastman R, Cowie C. Symptoms of sensory neuropathy in adults with NIDDM in the U.S. population. *Diabetes Care* 1993;16:1446–1452.
122. Gillium RF, Mussolino ME, Madans JH. Coronary heart disease incidence and survival in African-American women and men: the NHANES I epidemiologic follow-up study. *Ann Intern Med* 1997;127:111–118.
123. Harris MI. Noninsulin-dependent diabetes mellitus in black and white Americans. *Diabetes Metab Rev* 1990;6:71–90.
124. Clark LT. Primary prevention of cardiovascular disease in high-risk patients: physiologic and demographic risk factor differences between African American and white American populations. *Am J Med* 1999;107:22S–24S.
125. Hutchinson RG, Watson RL, Vavis CE, et al. Racial differences in risk factors for atherosclerosis: the ARIC study. *Angiology* 1997;48:279–290.
126. Freedman DS, Strogatz DS, Eaker E, et al. Differences between blacks and white men in correlates of high density lipoprotein cholesterol. *Am J Epidemiol* 1990;132:656–669.
127. Harris-Hooker S, Sanford GL. Lipids, lipoproteins and coronary heart disease in minority populations. *Atherosclerosis* 1994;108[Suppl]:S83–S104.
128. Howard BV, Le NA, Belcher JD, et al. Concentrations of Lp(a) in black and white young adults: relations to risk factors for cardiovascular disease. *Ann Epidemiol* 1994;4:341–350.
129. Sorrentino MJ, Vielhauer C, Eisenhart JD, et al. Plasma lipoprotein (a) protein concentration and coronary artery disease in black patients compared with white patients. *Am J Med* 1992;93:658–662.
130. Moliterno DJ, Jokinen EV, Miserz AR, et al. No association between plasma lipoprotein (a) concentrations and the presence or absence of coronary atherosclerosis in African-Americans. *Arterioscler Thromb Vasc Biol* 1995;15: 850–855.
131. Jerling JC, Vorster HH, Oosthuizen W, et al. Differences in plasminogen activator inhibitor 1 activity between blacks and whites may be diet related. *Haemostasis* 1994;24:364–368.
132. Wetterhall SF, Olson DR, DeStefano F, et al. Trends in diabetes and diabetic complications, 1980–1987. *Diabetes Care* 1992;15:960–967.
133. Aronow WS, Schoenfel MR. Prevalence of atherothrombotic brain infarction and extracranial carotid arterial disease, and their association in elderly blacks, Hispanics and whites. *Am J Cardiol* 1993;71:999–1000.
134. Kumanyika SK, Ewart CK. Theoretical and baseline considerations for diet and weight control of diabetes among blacks. *Diabetes Care* 1990;13: 1154–1162.
135. Lipton RB, Liao Y, Cao G, et al. Determinants of incident non-insulin dependent diabetes mellitus among blacks and whites in a national sample. The NHANES I Epidemiologic Follow-up Study. *Am J Epidemiol* 1993;138: 826–839.
136. Kumanyika S, Wilson JF, Guiford-Davenport M. Weight-related attitudes and behaviors of black women. *J Am Diet Assoc* 1993;93:416–422.
137. Auslander WF, Haire-Joshu D, Hosuton CA, et al. Community organization to reduce the risk of non-insulin-dependent diabetes among low-income African American women. *Ethn Dis* 1992;2:176–184.
138. Osei K. Diabetes prevention and intervention programs for African Americans: a single center experience. *Diabetes Spectrum* 1998;11:175–180.
139. McNabb WL, Quinn MT, Rosing L. Weight loss programs for inner-city black women with non-insulin dependent diabetes mellitus. PATHWAYS. *J Am Diet Assoc* 1993;93:75–77.
140. Gohdes D. Diabetes in North American Indians and Alaska Natives. In: National Diabetes Data Group. *Diabetes in America,* 2nd ed. Bethesda, MD.

National Institute of Diabetes and Digestive and Kidney Diseases, 1995: 683–701. NIDDKD publication 95-1468.
141. Mokdad AH, Bowman BA, Engelgau MM, et al. Diabetes trends among American Indians and Alaska Natives. *Diabetes Care* 2001;24:1508–1509.
142. Rios Burrows N, Geiss LS, Engelgau MM, et al. Prevalence of diabetes among Native Americans and Alaska Natives, 1990–1997. *Diabetes Care* 2000;23: 1786–1790.
143. Will JC, Strauss KF, Mendlein JM, et al. Diabetes mellitus among Navajo Indians: Findings from the Navajo Health and Nutrition Survey. *J Nutr* 1997; 127[Suppl 10]:2106S–2113S.
144. Lee ET, Howard BV, Savage PJ, et al. Diabetes and impaired glucose tolerance in three American Indian populations aged 45–74 years. *Diabetes Care* 1995;18:599–610.
145. Knowler WC, Bennett PH, Hamman RF, et al. Diabetes incidence and prevalence in Pima Indians: a 19-fold greater incidence than in Rochester, Minnesota. *Am J Epidemiol* 1978;108:497–505.
146. Murphy NJ, Schraer CD, Bulkow LR, et al. Diabetes mellitus in Alaskan Yup'ik Eskimos and Athabascan Indians after 25 yr. *Diabetes Care* 1992;15: 1390–1392.
147. Muneta B, Newman J, Wetterall S, et al. Diabetes and associated risk factors among Native Americans. *Diabetes Care* 1993;16:1619–1620.
148. Schraer CD, Lanier AP, Boyko EJ, et al. Prevalence of diabetes mellitus in Alaskan Eskimos, Indians, and Aleuts. *Diabetes Care* 1988;11:693–700.
149. Sugarman J, Percy C. Prevalence of diabetes in a Navajo Indian community. *Am J Public Health* 1989;79:511–513.
150. Martinez CB, Strauss K. Diabetes in St Regis Mohawk Indians. *Diabetes Care* 1993;16:260–262.
151. Freeman WL, Hosey GM, Diehr P, et al. Diabetes in American Indians of Washington, Oregon and Idaho. *Diabetes Care* 1989;12:282–288.
152. Acton K, Rogers B, Campbell G, et al. Prevalence of diagnosed diabetes and selected related conditions of six reservations in Montana and Wyoming. *Diabetes Care* 1993;16:263–265.
153. Rith-Najarian SJ, Valway SE, Gohdes DM. Diabetes in a northern Minnesota Chippewa tribe. Prevalence and incidence of diabetes and incidence of major complications, 1986–1988. *Diabetes Care* 1993;16:266–270.
154. Farrell MA, Quiggins PA, Owle PA, et al. Prevalence of diabetes and its complications in the Eastern Band of Cherokee Indians. *Diabetes Care* 1993;16: 253–256.
155. Carter J, Horowitz R, Wilson R, et al. Tribal differences in diabetes: prevalence among American Indians in New Mexico. *Public Health Rep* 1989; 104:665–669.
156. Johnson LG, Strauss K. Diabetes in Mississippi Choctaw Indians. *Diabetes Care* 1993;16:250–252.
157. Stahn RM, Gohdes D, Valway SE. Diabetes and its complications among selected tribes in North Dakota, South Dakota, and Nebraska. *Diabetes Care* 1993;16:244–247.
158. Dabelea D, Hanson RL, Bennett PH, et al. Increasing prevalence of type II diabetes in American Indian children. *Diabetologia* 1998;41:904–910.
159. Carter JS, Wiggins CL, Becker TM, et al. Diabetes mortality among New Mexico's American Indian, Hispanic, and non-Hispanic white populations, 1958–1987. *Diabetes Care* 1993;16:306–309.
160. Gilliland FD, Owen C, Gilliland SS, et al. Temporal trends in diabetes mortality among American Indians and Hispanics in New Mexico: birth cohort and period effects. *Am J Epidemiol* 1997;145:422–431.
161. Gohdes D, Kaufman S, Valway S. Diabetes in American Indians. *Diabetes Care* 1993;16[Suppl 1]:239–243.
162. Pettitt DJ, Lisse JR, Knowler WC, et al. Mortality as a function of obesity and diabetes mellitus. *Am J Epidemiol* 1982;115:359–366.
163. Sugarman JR, Hickey M, Hall T, et al. The changing epidemiology of diabetes mellitus among Navajo Indians. *West J Med* 1990;153:140–145.
164. Newman JM, DeStefano F, Valway SE, et al. Diabetes-associated mortality in Native Americans. *Diabetes Care* 1993;16:297–299.
165. Nelson RG, Bennett PH. Diabetic renal disease in Pima Indians. *Transplant Proc* 1989;21:3913–3915.
166. Knowler WC, Pettitt DJ, Saad MF, et al. Diabetes mellitus in the Pima Indians: incidence, risk factors and pathogenesis. *Diabetes Metab Rev* 1990;6:1–27.
167. Schraer CD, Adler AI, Mayer AM, et al. Diabetes complications and mortality among Alaska Natives: 8 years of observation. *Diabetes Care* 1997;20:314–316.
168. Williams RC, Steinberg AG, Gershowitz H, et al. GM allotypes in Native Americans: evidence for three distinct migrations across the Bering land bridge. *Am Phys Anthropol* 1985;66:1–19.
169. Lee ET, Anderson PS Jr, Bryan J, et al. Diabetes, parental diabetes, and obesity in Oklahoma Indians. *Diabetes Care* 1985;8:107–113.
170. Bogardus C, Lillioja S. Pima Indians as a model to study the genetics of NIDDM. *J Cell Biochem* 1992;48:337–343.
171. Baier LJ, Sacchettini JC, Knowler WC, et al. An amino acid substitution in the human intestinal fatty acid binding protein is associated with increased fatty acid binding, increased fat oxidation and insulin resistance. *J Clin Invest* 1995; 95:1281–1287.
172. Xia J, Scherer SW, Cohen PTW, et al. A common variant in PPP1R3 associated with insulin resistance and type 2 diabetes. *Diabetes* 1998;47:1519–1524.
173. Prochazca M, Thompson B, Scherer SW, et al. Linkage and association of insulin resistance and NIDDM with markers at 7q21.3-q22.1 in the Pima Indians. *Diabetes* 1995;44:42(abst).
174. Knowler WC, Williams RC, Pettit DJ, et al. Gm3,5, 13,14 and type 2 diabetes mellitus: an association in American Indians with genetic admixture. *Am J Hum Genet* 1988;43:520–526.
175. Silver K, Walston J, Cell FS, et al. A missense mutation in the B_3-adrenergic receptor gene in Pima Indians and its relationship to obesity and NIDDM. *Diabetes* 1995;44:42(abst).
176. Saad MF, Knowler WC, Pettit DJ, et al. A two-step model for development of non-insulin dependent diabetes. *Am J Med* 1991;90:229–235.
177. Lillioja S, Mott DM, Spraul M, et al. Insulin resistance and insulin secretory dysfunction as precursors of non-insulin dependent diabetes mellitus: prospective studies of Pima Indians. *N Engl J Med* 1993;329:1988–1992.
178. Weyer C, Bogardus C, Mott DM. The natural history of insulin secretory dysfunction and insulin resistance in the pathogenesis of type 2 diabetes. *J Clin Invest* 1999;104:787–794.
179. Weyer C, Tataranni PA, Bogardus C. Insulin resistance and insulin secretory dysfunction are independent predictors of worsening of glucose tolerance during each stage of type 2 diabetes development. *Diabetes Care* 2000;24: 89–94.
180. Lillioja S, Mott DM, Zawadski JK, et al. In vivo insulin action is familial characteristic in nondiabetic Pima Indians. *Diabetes* 1987;36:1329–1335.
181. Broussard BA, Johnson A, Himes JH, et al. Prevalence of obesity in American Indians and Alaska Natives. *Am J Clin Nutr* 1991;53[6 Suppl]:1535S–1542S.
182. Knowler WC, Pettitt DJ, Saad MF, et al. Obesity in the Pima Indians: its magnitude and relationship with diabetes. *Am J Clin Nutr* 1991;53[6 Suppl]: 1543S–1551S.
183. Knowler WC, Pettit DJ, Savage PJ, et al. Diabetes incidence in Pima Indians: contributions of obesity and parental diabetes. *Am J Epidemiol* 1981;113: 144–156.
184. Everhart JE, Pettitt DJ, Bennett PH, et al. Duration of obesity increases the incidence of NIDDM. *Diabetes* 1992;41:235–240.
185. Zsathmary EJ, Holt N. Hyperglycemia in Dogrib Indians of the Northwest territories, Canada: association with age and centripetal distribution of body fat. *Hum Biol* 1983;55:493–515.
186. McCance DR, Pettitt DJ, Hanson RL, et al. Birth weight and non-insulin dependent diabetes: thrifty genotype, thrifty phenotype, or surviving small baby genotype? *BMJ* 1994;308:942–945.
187. Knowler WC, Saad MF, Pettit DJ, et al. Determinants of diabetes mellitus in the Pima Indians. *Diabetes Care* 1993;16:216–227.
188. Benjamin E, Winteres D, Mayfield J, et al. Diabetes in pregnancy in Zuni Indian women. Prevalence and subsequent development of clinical diabetes after gestational diabetes. *Diabetes Care* 1993;16:1231–1235.
189. Livingston RC, Bachaman-Carter K, Frank C, et al. Diabetes mellitus in Tohon O'odham pregnancies. *Diabetes Care* 1993;16:318–321.
190. Sugarman JR. Prevalence of gestational diabetes in a Navajo Indian community. *West J Med* 1989;150:548–551.
191. Pettitt DJ, Aleck KA, Baird RH, et al. Congenital susceptibility to NIDDM: role of intrauterine environment. *Diabetes* 1988;37:622–628.
192. Pettit DJ, Knowler WC, Baird HR, et al. Gestational diabetes: infant and maternal complications of pregnancy in relation to third-trimester glucose tolerance in the Pima Indians. *Diabetes Care* 1980;3:458–644.
193. Pettitt DJ, Baird HR, Aleck KA, et al. Excessive obesity in offspring of Pima Indian women with diabetes during pregnancy. *N Engl J Med* 1983;308: 242–245.
194. Lee ET, Vee VS, Kinglsey RM, et al. Diabetic retinopathy in Oklahoma Indians with NIDDM. Incidence and risk factors. *Diabetes Care* 1992;15:1620–1627.
195. Lee ET, Lee VS, Lu M, Russell D. Development of proliferative retinopathy in NIDDM. A follow-up study of American Indians in Oklahoma. *Diabetes* 1992; 41:359–367.
196. Nelson RG, Wolfe JA, Horton MB, et al. Proliferative retinopathy in NIDDM. Incidence and risk factors in Pima Indians. *Diabetes* 1989;38:435–440.
197. Kunzelman CL, Knowler WC, Pettitt DJ, et al. Incidence of proteinuria in type 2 diabetes mellitus in the Pima Indians. *Kidney Int* 1989;35:681–687.
198. Lee ET, Lee VS, Lu M, et al. Incidence of renal failure in NIDDM. The Oklahoma Indian Diabetes Study. *Diabetes* 1994;43:572–579.
199. Nelson RG, Bennett PH. Diabetic renal disease in Pima Indians. *Transplant Proc* 1989;21:3913–3915.
200. Nelson RG, Kunzelman CL, Pettitt DJ, et al. Albuminuria in type 2 (non-insulin dependent) diabetes mellitus and impaired glucose tolerance in Pima Indians. *Diabetologia* 1989;32:870–876.
201. Agoda LY, Eggers PW. Renal replacement therapy in the United States: data from the Unites States Renal Data System. *Am J Kidney Dis* 1995;25:119–133.
202. Megill DM, Hoy WE, Woodruff SD. Rates and causes of end stage renal disease in Navajo Indians. 1971–1985. *West J Med* 1988;149:178–182.
203. Stahn RM, Gohdes D, Valway SE. Diabetes and its complications among selected tribes in North Dakota, South Dakota, and Nebraska. *Diabetes Care* 1993;16:244–247.
204. Quiggins PA, Farrell MA. Renal disease among the Eastern Band of Cherokee Indians. *Diabetes Care* 1993;16:342–345.
205. Pettit DJ, Saad MF, Bennett PH, et al. Familial predisposition to renal disease in two generations of Pima Indians with type 2 (non-insulin dependent) diabetes mellitus. *Diabetologia* 1990;33:438–443.
206. Rith-Najarian SJ, Stolusky T, Gohdes DM. Identifying diabetic patients at high risk for lower-extremity amputation in a primary health care setting. A prospective evaluation of simple screening criteria. *Diabetes Care* 1992;15: 1386–1389.
207. Rate RG, Knowler WC, Morse HG, et al. Diabetes mellitus in Hopi and Navajo Indians. Prevalence of microvascular complications. *Diabetes* 1983;32: 894–899.

208. Welty TK, Lee ET, Yeh J, et al. Cardiovascular disease risk factors among American Indians: The Strong Heart Study. *Am J Epidemiol* 1995;142: 269–287.
209. Lee ET, Russell D, Jorge N, et al. A follow-up study of diabetic Oklahoma Indians. Mortality and causes of death. *Diabetes Care* 1993;16:300–305.
210. Lee ET, Cowan LD, Welty TK, et al. All-cause mortality and cardiovascular disease mortality in three American Indian populations, aged 45–74, 1984–1988. *Am J Epidemiol* 1998;147:995–1008.
211. Nelson RG, Sievers ML, Knowler WC, et al. Low incidence of fatal coronary heart disease in Pima Indians despite high prevalence of non-insulin dependent diabetes. *Circulation* 1990;81:987–995.
212. Howard BV, Lee ET, Cowan LD, et al. Coronary heart disease prevalence and its relation to risk factors in American Indians. The Strong Heart Study. *Am J Epidemiol* 1995;142:254–268.
213. Hoy W, Light A, Megill D. Blood pressure in Navajo Indians and its association with type 2 diabetes and renal and cardiovascular disease. *Am J Hypertens* 1994;7:321–328.
214. Robbins DC, Knowler WC, Lee ET, et al. Regional differences in albuminuria among American Indians: an epidemic of renal disease. *Kidney Int* 1996; 49:557–563.
215. Powers DR, Wallin JD. End-stage renal disease in specific ethnic and racial groups. Risk factors and benefits of antihypertensive therapy. *Arch Intern Med* 1998;158:793–800.
216. Nelson RG, Gohdes DM, Everhart JE, et al. Lower-extremity amputation in NIDDM. 12-yr follow-up study in Pima Indians. *Diabetes Care* 1988;11:8–16.
217. Valway SE, Linkins RW, Gohdes DM. Epidemiology of lower-extremity amputations in the Indian Health Service, 1982–1987. *Diabetes Care* 1993;16: 349–353.
218. Wirth RB, Marfin AA, Grau DW, et al. Prevalence and risk factors for diabetes and diabetes-related amputation in American Indians in Southern Arizona. *Diabetes Care* 1993;16:354–356.
219. Reid JM, Fullmer SD, Pettigrew KD, et al. Nutrient intake of Pima Indian women: relationships to diabetes mellitus and gallbladder disease. *Am J Clin Nutr* 1971;24:1281–1289.
220. Kriska AM, Pereria MA, Hanson RL, et al. Association of physical activity and serum insulin concentrations in two populations at high risk for type 2 diabetes but differing by BMI. *Diabetes Care* 2001;24:1175–1180.
221. Ravussin E, Valencia ME, Esparaza J, et al. Effects of a traditional lifestyle on obesity in Pima Indians. *Diabetes Care* 1994;17:1067–1074.
222. Ravussin E, Lilloja S, Knowler WE, et al. Reduced rate of energy expenditure as a risk factor for body-weight gain. *N Engl J Med* 1988;318:467–472.
223. Leonard B, Leonard C, Wilson R. Zuni Diabetes Project. *Public Health Rep* 1986;101:282–288.
224. Narayan KM, Hoskin M, Kozak D, et al. Randomized clinical trial of lifestyle interventions in Pima Indians; a pilot study. *Diabet Med* 1998;15:66–72.
225. Gilliland SS, Azen SP, Perez GE. Strong in body and spirit. Lifestyle intervention for Native American adults with diabetes in New Mexico. *Diabetes Care* 2002;25:78–83.
226. Acton K, Valway S, Helgerson S, et al. Improving diabetes care for American Indians. *Diabetes Care* 1994;16:372–375.
227. Broussard BA, Bass MA, Jackson MY. Reasons for diabetic diet noncompliance among Cherokee Indians. *J Nutr Educ* 1982;14:56–57.
228. Smith CJ, Schakel SF, Nelson RG. Selected traditional and contemporary foods currently used by the Pima Indians. *J Am Diet Assoc* 1991;91:338–341.
229. Grandinetti A, Chang HK, Mau MK, et al. Prevalence of glucose intolerance among Native Hawaiians in two rural communities. *Diabetes Care* 1998; 21:549–554.
230. Fujimoto WY, Leonetti DL, Kinyoun JL, et al. Prevalence of diabetes mellitus and impaired glucose tolerance among second-generation Japanese-American men. *Diabetes* 1987;36:721–729.
231. Fujimoto WY, Leonetti DL, Bergstrom RW, et al. Glucose intolerance and diabetic complications among Japanese American women. *J Diab Res Clin Pract* 1991;13:113–129.
232. Burchfiel CM, Curb DJ, Rodriguez BL, et al. Incidence and predictors of diabetes in Japanese-American men. The Honolulu Heart Program. *Ann Epidemiol* 1995;5:33–43.
233. Sloan NR. Ethnic distribution of diabetes mellitus in Hawaii. *JAMA* 1963; 183:419–424.
234. Fujimoto W. The importance of insulin resistance in the pathogenesis of type 2 diabetes mellitus. *Am J Med* 2000;108[6A]:9S–14S.
235. Chen KW, Boyko EJ, Bergstrom RW, et al. Earlier appearance of impaired insulin secretion than of visceral adiposity in the pathogenesis of NIDDM: 5-year follow-up of initially non-diabetic Japanese American men. *Diabetes Care* 1995;18:747–753.
236. Boyko EJ, Fujimoto WY, Leonetti DL, et al. Visceral adiposity and risk of type 2 diabetes: a prospective study among Japanese Americans. *Diabetes Care* 2000;23:465–471.
237. McNeely MJ, Boyko EJ, Shofer JB. Standard definitions of overweight and central adiposity for determining diabetes risk in Japanese Americans. *Am J Clin Nutr* 2001;74:101–107.
238. McNeely MJ, Boyko EJ, Seigle DS, et al. Association between baseline plasma leptin levels and subsequent development of diabetes in Japanese Americans. *Diabetes Care* 1999;22:65–70.
239. Fujimoto WY, Bergstrom RW, Boyko EJ, et al. Diabetes and diabetes risk factors in second and third-generation Japanese Americans in Seattle, Washington. *Diabetes Res Clin Pract* 1994;24[Suppl]:S43–S52.
240. Liao D, Shofer JB, Boyko EJ, et al. Abnormal glucose tolerance and increased risk for cardiovascular disease in Japanese-Americans with normal fasting glucose. *Diabetes Care* 2001;24:39–44.
241. Incidence and causes of treated ESRD: USRDS, 1993 Annual Report. *Am J Kidney Dis* 1993;22[4 Suppl 2]:30–37.
242. Fujimoto WY, Bergstrom RW, Boyko EJ, et al. Coronary heart disease and NIDDM in Japanese-Americans. *Diabetes* 1996;54[Suppl 3]:S17–S18.
243. Fujimoto WY, Bergstrom RW, Boyko EJ, et al. Visceral adiposity and incident coronary heart disease in Japanese American men. The 10-year-follow-up results of the Seattle Japanese-American Community Diabetes Study. *Diabetes Care* 1999;22:1808–1812.
244. Boyko EJ, Leonetti DL, Bergstrom RW, et al. Visceral adiposity, fasting plasma insulin, and lipid and lipoprotein levels in Japanese Americans. *Int J Obes Relat Metab Disord* 1996;20:801–808.
245. Fujimoto WY, Bergstrom RW, Boyko EJ, et al. Type 2 diabetes and the metabolic syndrome in Japanese Americans. *Diabetes Res Clin Pract* 2000;50[Suppl 2]:S73–S76.
246. Huang B, Rodriguez BL, Burchfiel CM, et al. Acculturation and prevalence of diabetes among Japanese American men in Hawaii. *Am J Epidemiol* 1996; 144:674–681.
247. Leonetti DL, Tsunehara CH, Wahl PW, et al. Educational attainment and the risk of non-insulin-dependent diabetes or coronary heart disease in Japanese-American men. *Ethn Dis* 1992;2:326–336.
248. Uba L. Cultural barriers to health care for Southeast Asian refugees. *Public Health Rep* 1992;107:544–548.
249. Knowler WC, Barrett-Connor E, Fowler SE, et al. Designs and methods for a clinical trial in the prevention of type 2 diabetes. *Diabetes Care* 1999;22:623–634.
250. The Diabetes Prevention Program Research Group. The diabetes prevention program: baseline characteristics of the randomized cohort. *Diabetes Care* 2000;23:1619–1629.
251. Knowler WC, Barrett-Connor E, Fowler SE, et al. Reduction in the incidence of type 2 diabetes with lifestyle intervention or metformin. *N Engl J Med* 2002; 346:393–403.

CHAPTER 30

Diabetes—A Worldwide Problem

Paul Zimmet and Jonathan Shaw

In recent years, the global community has been preoccupied with the threat of a resurgence of infectious diseases, old ones such as tuberculosis and newer ones such as human immunodeficiency virus–acquired immunodeficiency syndrome (HIV-AIDS) and the Ebola virus. However, diabetes is a growing public health problem throughout the world. Currently, approximately 171 to 194 million people in the world have diabetes, the majority of the cases being type 2 (1,2). This number is expected to increase to more than 330 million by the year 2025—a doubling within a single generation. This spectacular increase in the frequency of type 2 diabetes is being paralleled by a similarly alarming increase in obesity (3), which is one of the major risk factors for type 2 diabetes (4). Because of the close linkage between these two conditions, Ziv and Shafrir have suggested the term "diabesity" to describe this association (5).

This dual epidemic, which was largely ignored by the public health community until recently, has come as a great surprise. In addition, the public health community, both national and international, has been very slow to recognize the huge socioeconomic and public health threat from diabetes and its devastating complications such as retinopathy, nephropathy, neuropathy, and, most importantly, cardiovascular disease (CVD) (6,7). However, diabetes and its huge personal and socioeconomic costs are increasingly being recognized as a major global health and societal problem, particularly by the World Health Organization (8) and the World Bank (9). Diabetes is now among the five leading causes of death due to disease in most countries (10). The costs are enormous economically, as well as in terms of health. By the most recent estimates, for example, diabetes costs the United States approximately $132 billion annually (11).

WORLDWIDE PREVALENCE OF DIABETES

Epidemiologic studies have provided overwhelming evidence that the prevalence of diabetes, particularly type 2 diabetes, is increasing rapidly in many nations (12). Between 1976 and 1988, the prevalence of diabetes (among people age 40 to 74 years) rose from 11.4% to 14.3% in the United States (13). In China (14), a prevalence of 3.1% in 1994 (in those older than 25 years), although relatively low by international standards, was almost two and a half times higher than a figure from the Chinese province of Da Qing 8 years earlier. Two cross-sectional studies in an urban south Indian population showed that the prevalence in persons older than age 20 years had increased from 8.3% in 1989 to 11.6% in 1995 (15). In Denmark, a 38% increase in diabetes prevalence has been reported over 22 years (16). Our data on the national prevalence in Australia reveal a prevalence of diabetes of 7.4% (16), whereas 20 years ago, the best estimate was 3.4% (17). Overall, the highest rates are seen in Native Americans and Pacific Islanders, followed by Hispanics or Mexican Americans, people originating from the Indian subcontinent, Southeast Asians, and African Americans. The prevalence in Europeans is somewhat lower, and diabetes remains rare only among indigenous peoples living a traditional lifestyle.

We recently published global diabetes estimates for 2003 and projections for the year 2025 (2) in order to raise the profile of diabetes in a global perspective. Furthermore, we hoped to encourage governments to initiate or improve local diabetes monitoring and prevention strategies. We estimated that 194 million people were likely to have diabetes globally in 2003 i.e., about 5.1% of the world population. By the year 2025, the total number of people with diabetes is projected to reach 330 million worldwide (Fig. 30.1). The region most likely to experience the main brunt of the epidemic is Asia. Here, diabetes could become two to three times more common than it is at present. Over the next 25 years, India alone is expected to see an increase from 36 to 73 million people with diabetes, and China will see a rise from 24 to 46 million.

THE EPIDEMIOLOGIC TRANSITION

Paradoxically, for many countries, type 2 diabetes has evolved as a major health problem in part because of increasing longevity (4). During the past century, improved nutrition, better hygiene, and the control of many communicable diseases have dramatically improved longevity, but these benefits have unmasked many age-related noncommunicable diseases,

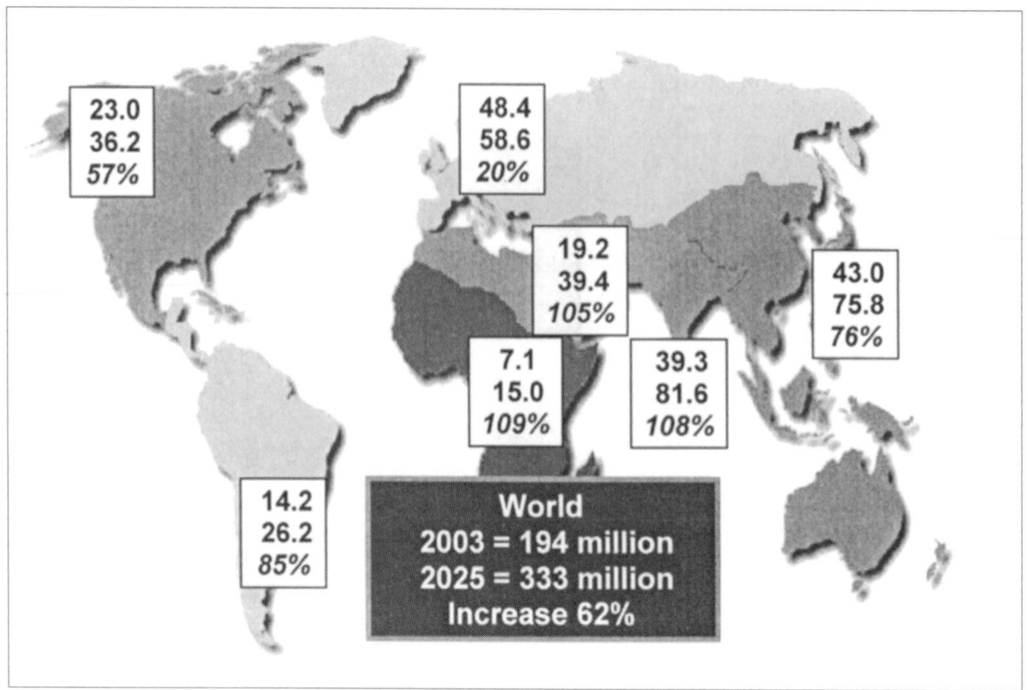

Figure 30.1. Numbers of people with diabetes by region for 2003 and 2025. Data shown are numbers (in millions) for 2003 (top number) and 2025 (middle number) and the percentage increase. (Data from Sicree R, Shaw JE, Zimmet PZ. The global burden of diabetes. In: Gan D, ed. *Diabetes atlas,* 2nd ed. Brussels: International Diabetes Federation, 2003:15–71.)

including type 2 diabetes and CVD (7,18). These formerly uncommon noncommunicable diseases have replaced many communicable diseases and are now major contributors to ill health and death.

This phenomenon of shifting disease patterns, termed *epidemiologic transition* by Orman (19), has occurred in developed countries over the past 50 years but is now affecting many developing countries. The transition has catapulted type 2 diabetes from its position as a rare disease at the beginning of the 20th century to its current position as a major global contributor to disability and death and one of the major health challenges of the 21st century (7).

Although changes in lifestyle and disease patterns are seen around the world, it is in the developing nations, where traditional lifestyles have been lost, that these events are played out most dramatically. The use of the term *traditional lifestyle* has at least two dimensions that should be clearly delineated (20). *Traditional* in the context of the history of indigenous people can mean the time before contact with the European settlers (precontact), i.e., historical dimension. Alternatively, it can denote a lifestyle according to behavioral traditions, which have an impact on patterns of physical activity, composition of the diet, amount of food, and other factors of daily living, that is, the behavioral dimension. It is within this context that we use it here, particularly in relation to the diabetes epidemic in the Pacific and in the indigenous population of Australia.

In his book *The Call Girls* (21), the late Arthur Koestler suggested the term "Coca-colonization" as a means to describe the impact of Western societies on traditional sociocultural habits and way of life in developing countries. The devastating results of Western intrusion into the lives of traditional-living indigenous communities can be seen from the Eskimos in the Arctic Circle to the Maori (Polynesians) in New Zealand and into the remote and idyllic islands and atolls of the Pacific Ocean (7). During the 19th century, European explorers and voyagers brought many communicable diseases, such as measles, whooping cough, tuberculosis, influenza and venereal diseases, to the Pacific Island communities. In that century, nearly all of the islands suffered a drastic decline in population as a result of these imported diseases. In the mid-18th century, there were about 250,000 Maori in New Zealand. The intrusion of European ways, weapons, and diseases soon decimated their numbers to 90,000, so that by the early 20th century the Maori in that country seemed to be a dying race (7,22). The same scenario was repeated in Australia, with devastating effect on the Aboriginal population (6).

From a historical and teleological perspective, the main causes of morbidity and mortality in all countries of the world were epidemics of communicable diseases, including typhoid, cholera, smallpox, diphtheria, and influenza, until the latter part of the 19th century (18). While some of these diseases remain epidemic in many Third World countries, industrialization and progressive modernization of societies have seen major improvements in housing, sanitation, water supply, and nutrition. Accompanied by the development of antibiotics and immunization programs, this scenario has radically changed the profile of diseases—initially in developed countries and later in many developing countries.

THE EPIDEMIC IN PROGRESS—WHAT ARE THE MAJOR FACTORS?

At the same time that the threat of communicable diseases has decreased, rapid socioeconomic development and "Coca-colonization" have resulted in a change in the way of life from traditional to modern (21). In virtually all populations, higher-fat diets and decreased physical activity have accompanied the benefits of modernization. Exercise has been engineered out of our daily lives, both in the workplace and at leisure (23). These lifestyle changes have been well documented in Canadian (24) and Native-American communities, Pacific and Indian Ocean island populations (25), and Australian Aboriginal communities (26). When combined with increasing longevity, these changes form the basis of the dynamic type 2 diabetes epidemic we are witnessing today.

The explosion of type 2 diabetes in Native-American and Pacific Island populations (with rates of up to 40% in communities where diabetes was virtually unknown 50 years previously) points the finger squarely at environmental causes, albeit in populations with a high genetic susceptibility to type 2 diabetes (4). The increase has occurred far too quickly to be the result of altered gene frequencies. However, the magnitude of the differences between ethnic groups when exposed to similar environments also implicates a significant genetic contribution. Jared Diamond, the noted American biologist and author, has suggested that the lifestyle-related diabetes epidemic in Native Americans and Pacific Islanders probably results from the collision of our old hunter-gatherer genes with the new 20th century way of life (27). The Western lifestyle must have unmasked the effects of preexisting genes, because the consistent result has been diabetes within a few decades.

In these communities, the former dependency on hunting and gathering, and later on subsistence agriculture, was replaced with a modern pattern characterized by a sedentary way of life and a diet of energy-dense processed foods, high in saturated fat, and usually exported from neighboring and perhaps well-meaning developed nations (7). For example, Australia and New Zealand export large quantities of consumable products rich in animal fats (e.g., canned meats and fatty joints) to the Pacific Islanders, foods that their own populations would be loathe to eat. Neel's thrifty-genotype hypothesis proposes that the genes selected over previous millennia to allow survival in times of famine by efficiently storing all available energy during times of feast are the very genes that lead to obesity under conditions of a constant high-energy diet (28,29).

Furthermore, Drewnowski and Popkin have proposed the concept of nutrition transition—the impact of globalization on the human diet (30). Analysis of economic and food availability data for 1962 through 1994 reveals a major shift in composition of the global diet marked by an uncoupling of the classic relationship between income and fat intake. The increasing availability of cheap vegetable oils and fats has resulted in greatly increased fat consumption in low-income nations. This trend means that the nutrition transition occurs at a lower level of gross national product and is further accelerated by high rates of urbanization. They conclude that, while economic development has led to improvements in food security and better health in some instances, the nutrition transition has had adverse effects such as increased rates of childhood obesity. To this, one would add the burden of type 2 diabetes and cardiovascular diseases, each of which may be preceded or aggravated by obesity.

DEVELOPMENT OF TYPE 2 DIABETES AT A YOUNGER AGE —"NINTENDO-NIZATION"

As the prevalence of type 2 diabetes increases, the disease is encroaching on younger and younger adults. Traditionally, type 2 diabetes is thought of as a disease of the middle aged and elderly, with typical onset after 50 years. Although it remains true that this group maintains its high relative risk (in relation to the risk in younger adults), the signs from high-risk populations have been that onset in the group 20 to 30 years of age is increasing (12). Even children are now becoming caught up in the "diabesity" epidemic. Among children in Japan, type 2 diabetes is already far more common than type 1 diabetes, accounting for 80% of cases of diabetes in childhood. Type 2 diabetes has been reported in children in a number of other populations (31,32), primarily those already known to have a high prevalence of diabetes in the adult population. Until recent times, autoimmune type 1 diabetes was the major form of diabetes among children and adolescents. Less than 3% of diabetic children had type 2 diabetes or other rare forms of diabetes (33). The situation has changed dramatically in recent years, with reports indicating that up to 45% of children with newly diagnosed diabetes have what appears to be typical (i.e., not maturity onset diabetes of the young) type 2 diabetes (33).

The increase in the prevalence of type 2 diabetes in this age group is due primarily to the increase in participation in sedentary activities such as television and computer usage, either for games or school work, with consequent reduction in sports activities. Add to this the increasing availability of energy-dense foods high in saturated fats and we have a "witches brew" to promote obesity and type 2 diabetes. We can now add "Nintendo-nization" to the collection of terms such as "Coca-colonization" and "Westernization." The socioeconomic and public-health impact of this downward shift in disease onset on society will be considerable through effects on the work force and premature morbidity and mortality—not to ignore the negative impact on fertility and reproduction.

This decline in the age of onset of type 2 diabetes is an important factor influencing the future burden of the disease, since onset in childhood heralds many years of disease and an accumulation of the full gamut of complications. Type 2 diabetes in children and adolescents has now become a major new challenge in diabetes. The American Diabetes Association has recently issued a consensus statement on the problem (33), and a number of pharmaceutical companies have embarked on clinical trials of oral agents in this age group. Affected children face up to 40 to 50 years of therapy, raising the issues of compliance with diet and with oral and insulin therapies, as well as the risk of complications, both microvascular and macrovascular, at a relatively young age.

TYPE 2 DIABETES AND THE EPIDEMIC OF CARDIOVASCULAR DISEASE

Type 2 diabetes is a multifactorial disease and shows heterogeneity in numerous respects (34,35). Our understanding of type 2 diabetes and related disorders such as impaired glucose tolerance (IGT) and impaired fasting glucose (IFG) is undergoing a radical change, particularly as there are data suggesting that the risk of complications, at least from macrovascular disease, commences many years before the onset of clinical diabetes (10). Previously, type 2 diabetes was regarded as a relatively distinct disease entity, but in reality, it is a descriptive term and a manifestation of a much broader underlying disorder (36). The manifestations include the metabolic syndrome (Fig. 30.2) (12), a cluster of CVD risk factors, which apart from glucose intolerance include hyperinsulinemia, dyslipidemia, hypertension, visceral obesity, hypercoagulability, and microalbuminuria. This combination of risk factors is partly responsible for the increased risk of CVD in people with diabetes. Attention has recently been drawn to the CVD epidemic now being seen in many developing nations (10). It should be noted that while IGT is predictive of future diabetes, it also carries a substantial risk of both current and subsequent CVD. IGT not only is predictive of future diabetes but also carries a substantial risk of both current and subsequent CVD (37–39). A similar risk probably is associated with IFG, but this is presently not as well substantiated (40).

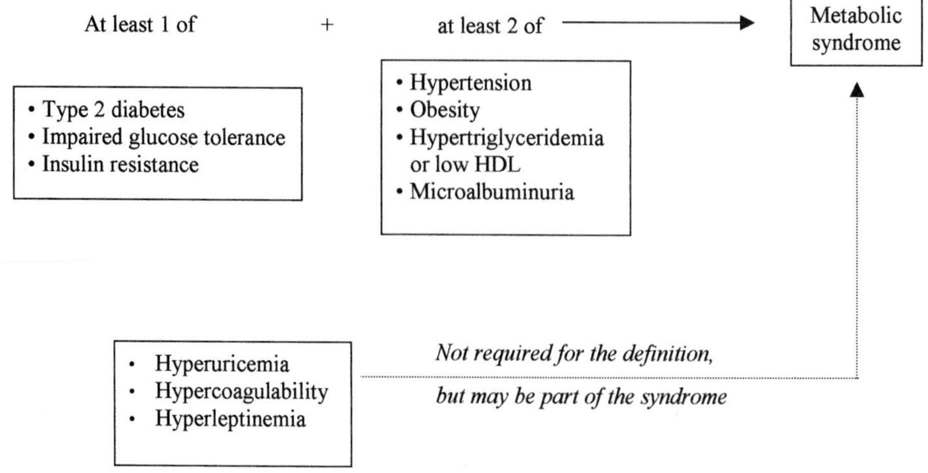

Figure 30.2. Metabolic syndrome as defined by the World Health Organization (34). Insulin resistance is defined as being within the highest quartile for the relevant population. Hypertension: BP ≥140/90. Obesity: body mass index ≥30 kg/m^2 or waist-to-hip ratio >0.90 for males and >0.85 for females. Hypertriglyceridema: triglycerides ≥1.7 mmol/L. Low high-density lipoproteins: <0.9 mmol/L for men and <1.0 mmol/L for women. Microalbuminuria: urinary albumin excretion rate ≥20 μg/min or albumin creatinine ratio ≥30 mg/min.

OTHER CATEGORIES OF GLUCOSE INTOLERANCE—ADDING TO THE EPIDEMIC

We believe that at least 300 million people worldwide have IGT (2). The prevalence of IGT varies widely, being 3% to 10% in European populations (41). It is much higher in some newly industrialized nations and groups with high prevalence of type 2 diabetes, such as Asian Indians, Native Americans, Pacific Islanders, and indigenous Australians. Recent data now suggest increasing rates in Europeans, with the recent national Australian diabetes study noting a prevalence of IGT of 10.6% (17).

IGT represents a key stage in the natural history of type 2 diabetes, as these persons are at higher future risk for diabetes than are the general population (42). Approximately 5% of those with IGT progress to diabetes annually, but some revert to normal glucose tolerance and others continue to have IGT. Therefore, predicting which persons with IGT at baseline in whom type 2 diabetes will develop presents a challenge. Evidence suggests that those with IGT who have one or more components of the metabolic syndrome are more likely to progress to diabetes (43).

The recently defined category of IFG recognizes the fact that elevated but nondiabetic fasting levels of glucose also carry an elevated risk of future diabetes and probably of CVD as well (40, 42). It is now clear that significant differences between IFG and IGT exist, even though they represent, in a broad sense, disorders with similar implications. Although the risk of an individual's progressing to diabetes is similar for IGT and IFG, many more progressors can be identified by IGT (42). The majority of people with either IGT or IFG do not have the other condition; indeed, approximately 20% of people with a fasting glucose level in the IFG range already have diabetes according to the 2-hour glucose criterion (42). Finally, and perhaps of greatest importance, the 2-hour postchallenge glucose level appears to be a better predictor of CVD and mortality than does the fasting glucose level (38).

In a study in Mauritius, we showed a definite gender difference in prevalence of IFG and IGT. IGT was more common in women and IFG was more common in men, and only a small but equal proportion of men and women had coexisting IFG and IGT (44). Other recent epidemiologic studies have reported similar sex differences in the prevalence of IFG and IGT (Table 30.1). The observation that IFG is more prevalent in males and IGT is usually more prevalent in females raises important questions about the underlying etiology of IFG and IGT and the ability of current glucose thresholds to identify high-risk categories equally among men and women.

Although the new category of IFG may broaden and improve our description of intermediate abnormal states in glucose metabolism, it should be seen as complementary to impaired glucose tolerance rather than as a replacement (42). Data from other populations have confirmed these findings; thus screening programs aimed at identifying people at risk of developing diabetes chance missing a considerable amount of information by relying solely on fasting plasma glucose levels.

Recent studies have highlighted the potential for lifestyle interventions focusing on dietary modification, physical activity, and weight loss in subjects with IGT to reduce progression to type 2 diabetes (45, 46). The American Diabetes Prevention Program and the Finnish Diabetes Prevention Study both

TABLE 30.1. Prevalence of Impaired Fasting Glucose and Impaired Glucose Tolerance in Males and Females from Different Populations

Glucose category	Country	Males (%)	Females (%)	Reference
IFG	Australia	8.1	3.4	17
	Mauritius	6.2	2.9	49
	USA	8.8	5.0	13
	Scandinavia	12.8	7.5	50
	Taiwan	24.3	18.3	51
IGT	Australia	9.2	11.9	17
	Mauritius	11.2	16.2	49
	USA	15.2	16.4	13
	Scandinavia	13.5	15.9	50
	Japan	12.0	16.5	52
	Singapore	14.9	15.2	53
	South Africa	7.6	4.4	54
	India	6.3	9.8	55

showed that the incidence of diabetes could be reduced by 58% with intensive lifestyle interventions. The reduction in the incidence of diabetes was directly associated with changes in lifestyle. The U.S. study also found that among these overweight subjects with IGT, metformin led to a 31% reduction in diabetes incidence. Buchanan and coworkers (47) have demonstrated a substantial reduction in the risk of developing type 2 diabetes with the use of troglitazone, and the Heart Outcomes Prevention Evaluation (HOPE) study suggests the possibility that angiotensin-converting enzyme (ACE) inhibitors may have a similar effect (48).

CONCLUSIONS

The international diabetes and public health communities need to adopt a more pragmatic view of the epidemic of diabesity. The current scenario is symptomatic of globalization with respect to its social, cultural, economic, and political significance. Type 2 diabetes will not be prevented by traditional medical approaches. What is required are major and dramatic changes in the socioeconomic and cultural status of people in developing countries and the disadvantaged minority groups in developed nations.

REFERENCES

1. Wild S, Roglic G, Green A, et al. Global prevalence of diabetes: estimates for the year 2000 and projections for 2030. *Diabetes Care* 2004;27:1047–1053.
2. Sicree R, Shaw JE, Zimmet PZ. The global burden of diabetes. In: Gan D, ed. *Diabetes atlas,* 2nd ed. Brussels: International Diabetes Federation, 2003:15–71.
3. Cameron AJ, Welborn TA, Zimmet PZ, et al. Overweight and obesity in Australia: the 1999–2000 Australian Diabetes Obesity and Lifestyle Study (AusDiab). *Med J Aust* 2003;178:427–432.
4. de Courten, M., Bennett PH, Tuomilehto J, Zimmet P. Epidemiology of NIDDM in non-Europids. In: Alberti K, DeFronzo RA, Keen H, eds. *International textbook of diabetes mellitus*, 2nd ed. New York: John Wiley & Sons, 1997:143–170.
5. Ziv E, Shafrir E. *Psammomys obesus*: nutritionally induced NIDDM-like syndrome on a "thrifty gene" background. In: Shafrir E, ed. *Lessons from animal diabetes.* London: Smith-Gordon, 1995:285–300.
6. Zimmet P, Lefebvre P. The global NIDDM epidemic: treating the disease and ignoring the symptom. *Diabetologia* 1996;39:1247–1248.
7. Zimmet P. Globalization, coca-colonization and the chronic disease epidemic: can the doomsday scenario be averted? *J Intern Med* 2000;247:301–310.
8. World Health Organisation. *The World Health Report 1997*. Geneva: WHO, 1997.
9. World Bank. *World Development Report 1993: Investing in health. World development indicators.* Oxford: Oxford University Press, 1993.
10. Zimmet P, Alberti K. The changing face of macrovascular disease in non-insulin dependent diabetes mellitus in different cultures: an epidemic in progress. *Lancet* 1997;350:S1–S4
11. Hogan P, Dall T, Nikolov P. Economic costs of diabetes in the US in 2002. *Diabetes Care* 2003;26:917–932.
12. Zimmet P. Diabetes epidemiology as a trigger to diabetes research. *Diabetologia* 1999;42:499–518.
13. Harris M, Flegal K, Cowie C, et al. Prevalence of diabetes, impaired fasting glucose, and impaired glucose tolerance in U.S. adults. The Third National Health and Nutrition Examination 1988–1994. *Diabetes Care* 1998;21:518–524.
14. Pan XR, Yang WY, Li GW, et al. Prevalence of diabetes and its risk factors in China, National Diabetes Prevention and Control Cooperative group. 1994. *Diabetes Care* 1997;20:664–1669.
15. Ramachandran A, Snehalatha C, Latha F, et al. Rising prevalence of NIDDM in an urban population in India. *Diabetologia* 1997;40:232–237.
16. Drivsholm T, Ibsen H, Schroll M, et al. Increasing prevalence of diabetes mellitus and impaired glucose tolerance among 60-year-old Danes. *Diabet Med* 2001;18:126–132.
17. Dunstan DW, Zimmet PZ, Welborn TA, et al. The rising prevalence of diabetes and impaired glucose tolerance: the Australian Diabetes, Obesity and Lifestyle Study. *Diabetes Care* 2002;25:829–834.
18. Hennekens G, Buring J. *Epidemiology in medicine.* Boston: Little, Brown and Company, 1987.
19. Orman A. The epidemiologic transition: a theory of the epidemiology of population change. *Milbank Q* 1971;49:509–538.
20. McMichael AJ, Beaglehole R. The changing global context of public health. *Lancet* 2000;356:495–499.
21. Koestler A. *The Call Girls.* London and Sydney: Pan Books, 1976.
22. Zimmet P, Dowse G, Finch C, et al. The epidemiology and natural history of NIDDM—lessons from the South Pacific. *Diabetes Metab Rev* 1990;6:91–124.
23. Pereira M, Kriska AM, Collins VR, et al. Occupational status and cardiovascular disease risk factors in a rapidly developing high-risk population of Mauritius. *Am J Epidemiol* 1998;148:148–159.
24. Harris S, Gittelsohn J, Hanley A, et al. The prevalence of NIDDM and associated risk factors in native Canadians. *Diabetes Care* 1997;20:185–187.
25. Zimmet P. Kelly West Lecture 1991. Challenges in diabetes epidemiology—from West to the rest. *Diabetes Care* 1992;15:232–252.
26. O'Dea K. Westernisation, insulin resistance and diabetes in Australian Aborigines. *Med J Aust* 1991;155:258–264.
27. Diamond J. Diabetes running wild. *Nature* 1992;357:362–363.
28. Neel J. Diabetes mellitus: a thrifty genotype rendered detrimental by "progress"? *Am J Hum Genet* 1962;14:353–362.
29. Dowse G, Zimmet P. The thrifty genotype in non-insulin-dependent diabetes: the hypothesis survives. *BMJ* 1993;306:532–533.
30. Drewnowski A, Popkin B. The nutrition transition: new trends in the global diet. *Nutr Rev* 1997;55:31–43.
31. Ehtisham S, Barrett T, Shaw N. Type 2 diabetes mellitus in UK children—an emerging problem. *Diabet Med* 2000;17:867–871.
32. Fagot-Campagna A, Narayan K. Type 2 diabetes in children. *BMJ* 2001;322: 377–387.
33. American Diabetes Association. Type 2 diabetes in children and adolescents. *Diabetes Care* 2000;23:381–389.
34. Alberti KGGM, Zimmet PZ. Definition, diagnosis and classification of diabetes mellitus and its complications. Part 1: diagnosis and classification of diabetes mellitus provisional report of a WHO consultation. *Diabet Med* 1998;15:539–553.
35. Zimmet P, Turner R, McCarty D, et al. Crucial points at diagnosis—type 2 diabetes or slow type 1 diabetes. *Diabetes Care* 1999;22:B59–B64.
36. Zimmet P. Hyperinsulinaemia—how innocent a bystander. *Diabetes Care* 1993; 16:56–70.
37. Harris M, Zimmet P. Classification of diabetes mellitus and other categories of glucose intolerance. In: Alberti K, DeFronzo RA, Keen H, eds. *International textbook of diabetes mellitus*, 2nd ed. Chichester, UK: John Wiley and Sons, 1997:9–23.
38. Shaw JE, Hodge AM, De Courten M, et al. Isolated post-challenge hyperglycaemia confirmed as a risk factor for mortality. *Diabetologia* 1999;42:1050–1054.
39. World Health Organization. *Prevention of diabetes mellitus.* Geneva: Technical Report Series no. 844. WHO, 1994.
40. DECODE Study Group. Glucose tolerance and mortality: comparison of WHO and American Diabetes Association diagnostic criteria. The DECODE Study Group. European Diabetes Epidemiology Group. Diabetes Epidemiology: Collaborative analysis of diagnostic criteia in Europe. *Lancet* 1999;354:617–621.
41. King H, Rewers M. Global estimates for prevalence of diabetes mellitus and impaired glucose tolerance in adults. *Diabetes Care* 1993;16:617–621.
42. Shaw JE, Zimmet PZ, De Courten M, et al. Impaired fasting glucose or impaired glucose tolerance. What best predicts future diabetes in Mauritius? *Diabetes Care* 1999;22:399–402.
43. Boyko EJ, de Courten M, Zimmet PZ, et al. Features of the metabolic syndrome predict higher risk of diabetes and impaired glucose tolerance: a prospective study in Mauritius. *Diabet Med* 2003;20:915–920.
44. Williams JW, Zimmet PZ, Shaw JE, et al. Gender differences in the prevalence of impaired fasting glycaemia and impaired glucose tolerance in Mauritius. Does sex matter? *Diabet Med* 2003;20:915–920.
45. Tuomilehto J, Lindstrom J, Eriksson JG, et al. Prevention of type 2 diabetes mellitus by changes in lifestyle among subjects with impaired glucose tolerance. *N Engl J Med* 2001;344:1343–1350.
46. Knowler WC, Barrett-Connor E, Fowler SE, et al. Reduction in the incidence of type 2 diabetes with lifestyle intervention or metformin. *N Engl J Med* 2002;346:393–403.
47. Buchanan TA, Xiang Ah, Peters RK, et al. Preservation of pancreatic beta-cell function and prevention of type 2 diabetes by pharmacological treatment of insulin resistance in high-risk hispanic women. *Diabetes* 2002;51:2796–2803.
48. Heart Outcomes Prevention Evaluation (HOPE) Study. Effects of ramipril on cardiovascular and microvascular outcomes in people with diabetes mellitus: results of the HOPE study and MICRO-HOPE substudy. *Lancet* 2000;355: 253–259.
49. Söderberg S, Zimmet P. Tuomilehto J, et al. Increasing prevalence of type 2 diabetes mellitus in all ethnic groups in Mauritius. *Diabet Med (in press).*
50. Tripathy D, Carlsson M, Almgren P, et al. Insulin secretion and insulin sensitivity in relation to glucose tolerance: lessons from the Botnia Study. *Diabetes* 2000;49:975–980.
51. Chen KT, Chen CJ, Gregg EW, et al. High prevalence of impaired fasting glucose and type 2 diabetes mellitus in Penghu Islets, Taiwan: evidence of a rapidly emerging epidemic? *Diabetes Res Clin Pract* 1999;44:59–69.
52. Sekikawa A, Eguchi H, Tominaga M, et al. Prevalence of type 2 diabetes mellitus and impaired glucose tolerance in a rural area of Japan. The Funagata diabetes study. *J Diabetes Complications* 2000;14:78–83.
53. Health Mo: National Health Survey 1998 Singapore. 1999.
54. Omar MA, Seedat MA, Dyer RB, et al. South African Indians show a high prevalence of NIDDM and bimodality in plasma glucose distribution patterns. *Diabetes Care* 1994;17:70–73.
55. Zargar AH, Khan AK, Masoodi SR, et al. Prevalence of type 2 diabetes mellitus and impaired glucose tolerance in the Kashmir Valley of the Indian subcontinent. *Diabetes Res Clin Pract* 2000;47:135–146.

SECTION

IV

Obesity and Lipoprotein Disorders

CHAPTER 31
Obesity

Eleftheria Maratos-Flier and Jeffrey S. Flier

Adipose tissue has three primary functions. Two are well recognized and defined: to serve as the site for storage of energy-rich fatty acids in the form of triglyceride and to effect the controlled release of the constituent fatty acids and glycerol in response to neural, endocrine, and local signals for metabolism at distant sites. A third and increasingly important role of adipose tissue is its function as an endocrine organ, releasing a variety of factors that regulate metabolism. Obesity is defined as a state of excessive adipose tissue mass and is best viewed as a syndrome or group of diseases rather than as a single disease entity. The importance of this state derives from its high prevalence in our society and its association with serious morbidity, not the least of which is a marked increase in the prevalence of type 2 diabetes. Specific syndromes of obesity, both in animal models and in humans, are associated with identified neural, endocrine, or genetic causes. However, the pathogenesis of obesity in the vast majority of humans is unknown and remains an unexplained chronic excess in caloric intake relative to energy needs. An understanding of obesity and its consequences requires the investigation of the many factors that control energy intake and energy expenditure, the two interrelated components of the energy-balance equation. As with our understanding of pathogenesis, our understanding of the molecular connection between obesity and its most important complications is limited, and our approach to therapy, as defined by clinical success rate, is extremely poor. In this chapter, we will review the current understanding of the pathogenesis, complications, and treatment of obesity.

DEFINITION AND INDICES OF OBESITY

The distribution of body weight in the population is a continuous function without a clear separation between lean and obese. The most medically relevant criterion relates to the identification of a weight that confers morbidity. The selection of a specific threshold is somewhat arbitrary, and a number of different criteria have been used. Initially, the approach was through the use of life insurance data (Metropolitan Life) that assess mortality as a function of body weight per height, adjusted for frame size, with obesity defined on purely statistical grounds as a weight that is 20% or more above the average weight per height (1). Over the past decade, calculation of body mass index (BMI) has evolved as a more standard measurement used to correlate weight with morbidity and mortality. BMI is calculated by determining weight in kilograms and dividing by the height in meters squared. This measurement has been used to define four classes of body weight. A BMI of less than 18.5 is considered *underweight* and carries a modestly increased risk of morbidity and mortality. A BMI between 18.5 and 24.9 is considered normal. A BMI of more than 25.0 but less than 29.9 is considered *overweight* or *preobese* and, statistically, carries a slightly increased risk of comorbidities such as diabetes and cardiovascular disease compared with the risk in normal-weight individuals. A BMI of more than 30 is considered in the *obese* category, which is further subdivided into class I (BMI, 30 to 39.9), class II (BMI, 40 to 49.9), and class III (BMI, >50). These categories of obesity carry respective risks of comorbidities that are moderate, severe, and very severe, respectively (2). A second approach to defining the obese state involves quantitation of adipose tissue, either directly or indirectly. Values are obtained for a reference group viewed as normal, and obesity is defined as levels of adiposity exceeding that seen in the reference group.

The definition of obesity can be refined on the basis of the realization that the accumulation of adipose tissue in different depots has distinct consequences. Thus, many of the most important complications of obesity, including insulin resistance, diabetes, hypertension, and hyperlipidemia, are linked to the amount of intraabdominal fat, rather than to lower-body fat (i.e., buttocks and leg) or subcutaneous abdominal fat (3,4). Abdominal fat, typically evident on physical examination, can be estimated by determining the waist-to-hip circumference ratio (with a ratio >0.72 considered abnormal), or more accurately quantified by dual-energy x-ray absorptiometry (DEXA) scanning or computed tomography.

PREVALENCE OF OBESITY

It is obvious from casual inspection of the population that obesity is prevalent in the United States, although the precise prevalence figures vary to some degree, depending on the nature of the population surveyed. In the United States, the prevalence of *overweight* or *preobesity*, i.e., a BMI of 25 to 29.9, has remained fairly constant at 40% for men and 24% for women over roughly a 30-year period (1960 to 1994). However, in the same period, the prevalence of a BMI higher than 30 has risen significantly, especially over the past decade. In 2001 more than 20% of all adults had a BMI greater than 30, compared with 12% of all adults in 1991. Obesity among adults aged 18 to 29 doubled from 7% in 1991 to 14% in 2001. Among people aged 50 to 59, more than 25% have a BMI greater than 30. When analyzed by race and ethnicity (Fig. 31.1A), a BMI greater than 30 was most prevalent among black, non-Hispanic people. Interestingly, rates of obesity correlate inversely with educational level and are almost twice as high in adults who have not completed high school as in adults who have finished college or graduate school (Fig. 31.1B). This indicates that environmental and cultural factors can act as inhibitors to weight gain. At present 60% of the male population and 50% of the female population have a BMI greater than 25, which is associated with increased risk of morbidity and mortality.

As noted above, an important predictor of the morbidity and mortality associated with obesity is the quantity of visceral fat. A rough index of the relative amounts of visceral and abdominal fat is the waist-to-hip ratio. The alternative patterns of body-fat distribution have been described as pear shaped (low waist-to-hip ratio) and apple shaped (higher waist-to-hip ratio). When the waist-to-hip ratio is less than 0.8, the relative risk of morbidities associated with obesity is lower than when the waist-to-hip ratio is greater than 1.0. Hence, the metabolic syndrome, which is a clustering of obesity and other cardiovascular risk factors, is more likely to be associated with visceral obesity (5).

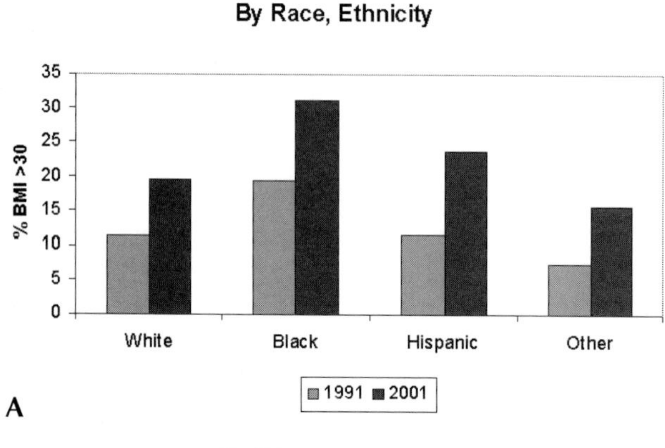

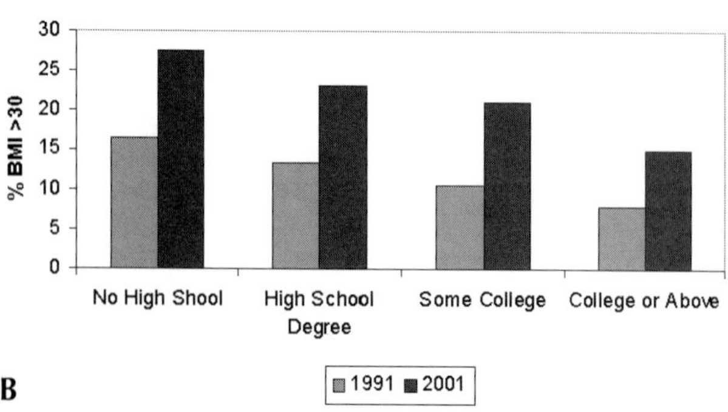

Figure 31.1. Prevalence rates of normal weight, overweight, and obesity in the adult U.S. population in 1991 and 2001. **A:** Rate of obesity by race, ethnicity. **B:** Rate of obesity by educational level. (Adapted from data from the Centers for Disease Control and Prevention.)

PATHOLOGIC CONSEQUENCES OF OBESITY

Obesity results in morbidity and mortality largely because of its association with other diseases, including diabetes, cardiovascular disease, hypertension, sleep apnea, endometrial cancer, colon cancer, and gallbladder disease. Overall, in the United States, the excess mortality of obesity accounts for 300,000 deaths per year. It was estimated that the total spent for both weight reduction and treatment of the consequences of obesity was $100 billion in the United States in 2001. This represents 5.5% to 7.0% of all medical expenses (3).

Diabetes

The increased risk for type 2 diabetes in individuals with obesity is considerable. In persons aged 20 to 44, obesity is associated with a fourfold increase in the relative risk of diabetes (4). In a study of a cohort of more than 50,000 U.S. male health professionals, the risk of diabetes correlated strongly with BMI. In men with a BMI of 35 or higher, the multivariate relative risk of diabetes was 42.1 compared with the risk in men with a BMI of less than 23. BMI appears to be the dominant risk factor for type 2 diabetes. Even men with average relative weight had a significant increase in risk when compared with men in lower weight groups. A similar increased risk exists for women. Among 43,581 women enrolled in the Nurses' Health Study, the relative risk for type 2 diabetes at the 90th percentile of BMI was 11.2 (6). Weight was the single most important predictor of diabetes. After adjustment for BMI, lack of exercise and a poor diet (i.e., foods with a high glycemic index and high in trans fat) were also associated with increased risk of diabetes (7). Another study examined new diagnoses of diabetes in a population between 18 and 44 years of age (8) and found an inverse correlation with age and BMI. Adults developing diabetes before age 44 had an average BMI of 39, whereas adults developing diabetes at 45 or older had an average BMI of 33. Among all adults, the odds ratio for developing diabetes is 6.38 for those with a BMI greater than 40 (9). The results of these and other studies lend support to the concept that the vast majority of cases of type 2 diabetes could be prevented by the adoption of therapies and lifestyle characteristics that decrease obesity.

Although the precise mechanism by which obesity contributes to insulin resistance and type 2 diabetes has not yet been defined, it is likely related to the production of various factors derived from the adipocyte that act on fat, liver, or muscle to impair insulin action. Obesity is itself associated with hyperinsulinemia, and insulin may induce insulin resistance through downregulation of the insulin receptor. Potential candidate substances produced by fat that may cause insulin resistance include tumor necrosis factor and other cytokines, such as interleukin-6, and resistin and adiponectin. Increased levels of free fatty acids are also capable of inhibiting insulin action. It is intriguing that a recent report found that treatment with high-dose salicylate markedly improved insulin resistance, suggesting that obesity may induce an inflammatory state that contributes to insulin resistance (10).

Cardiovascular Disease

Obesity is an independent risk factor for cardiovascular disease (11), including coronary artery disease and congestive heart failure, in both men and women. Waist-to-hip ratio is the best predictor, and it is noteworthy that increased waist-to-hip ratio has an effect in women even at the relatively low BMI of 25. Visceral obesity is associated with increased occurrence of hypertension and an atherogenic lipid profile (12,13), both of which contribute to the development of cardiovascular disease. In addition, in the obese state, there is a need for perfusion of a greater mass of tissue, resulting in an increase in cardiac work. Blood volume, stroke volume, and cardiac output are all increased and result in increased ventricular mass, which is reversible with weight loss (14,15).

Pulmonary Disease

Abnormalities in pulmonary function may be seen in obese patients (16–18). These range from quantitative abnormalities in pulmonary function tests that have no established clinical significance to major dysfunction replete with symptoms and morbid consequences. The increased metabolic rate in obese subjects increases O_2 consumption and CO_2 production, and these changes result in increased minute ventilation. In subjects with marked obesity, the compliance of the chest wall is reduced, the work of breathing is increased, and the respiratory reserve volume and vital capacity are reduced; a resultant mismatch between ventilation and perfusion may result in hypoxemia. Severe obesity may cause hypoventilation, defined by the development of CO_2 retention. The full designation of the obesity-hypoventilation, or pickwickian, syndrome includes somnolence, lethargy, and respiratory acidosis and typically also includes sleep apnea. Such patients may have reduced ventilatory drive to hypoxia and hypercapnia, as well as obstructive or mechanical causes of hypoventilation, and sleep studies may be necessary to distinguish among these.

Gallstones

Obesity is associated with enhanced biliary secretion of cholesterol. This results in supersaturation of bile and a higher incidence of gallstones—particularly cholesterol gallstones (19). Fasting, as opposed to more limited caloric restriction, increases the saturation of bile by reducing the phospholipid component, and cholecystitis induced by fasting is a well-recognized problem in obese individuals.

Cancer

Excess weight has been associated with increased rates of cancer. A recent study examining data for more than a million patients enrolled in the Cancer Prevention Study demonstrates convincingly that obese individuals are at increased risk for a number of cancers (20). The most dramatic increase in risk is seen for liver cancer. The relative risk of liver cancer was almost 2-fold higher in men with a BMI of 30.0 to 34.9 than in normal-weight individuals, and it was 4.5-fold higher in men with a BMI greater than 35. In men with a BMI higher than 35, the risk of stomach cancer was increased 1.94-fold, that of kidney cancer was increased 1.7-fold, and that of esophageal cancer was increased 1.6-fold over the risk in normal-weight individuals. The effect of obesity on cancers of the gastrointestinal tract was not as great in women, but the increase in relative risk in women was the same as that in men for kidney cancer. In women with a BMI greater than 35, the relative risk of cancer of the uterus was 2.8, of cancer of the cervix was 3.8, and of breast cancer was 1.7.

ENDOCRINE CONSEQUENCES OF OBESITY

Many alterations in endocrine function are seen in patients with established obesity. These changes can be induced by overeating, and normal function resumes after weight loss. Therefore, these changes are viewed as being secondary to the obese state. A possible causal link has been sought between some of these abnormalities and the pathogenesis of obesity, and thus they have undergone considerable scrutiny.

Endocrine Pancreas

As discussed earlier, hyperinsulinemia is a pervasive concomitant of obesity. Hyperinsulinemia results from an increased rate of insulin secretion (21), although patients with intraabdominal obesity may have decreased hepatic clearance of insulin (22). Hyperinsulinemia follows weight gain and reverses with weight loss and is most likely a consequence of insulin resistance that accompanies the obese state. Given the fact that, in the animal model of ventromedial hypothalamic lesions, hyperinsulinism driven by the vagus nerve may precede obesity (23), the possibility that a defect in central control of insulin secretion exists in a subset of persons with obesity should be considered. Studies of glucagon, somatostatin, pancreatic polypeptide, and amylin secretion in obesity have not been particularly revealing. However, more recent studies suggest that neuropeptides such as neuropeptide Y and melanocyte-stimulating hormone may have direct effects on the islet (24,25).

Thyroid

Given the known effect of thyroid hormone on basal metabolic rate, it is reasonable to speculate that defects in this axis might be a factor in obesity. In general, studies of obese individuals have revealed normal levels of thyroxine (T_4) and thyroid-stimulating hormone (TSH) but increased levels of triiodothyronine (T_3) in a minority of subjects. The increased T_3 levels are probably secondary to increased carbohydrate intake, and they decrease, as do values in nonobese subjects, in response to caloric restriction (26).

Gonadal Function

Marked obesity in men is associated with changes in both testosterone and estrogen metabolism, although these are usually without clinical consequences. Rates of estrogen production, primarily from androgen precursors, are increased, as are levels of estradiol (27). Decreased total testosterone levels are commonly observed and appear to be secondary to diminished levels of sex hormone–binding globulin (SHBG), with a preservation of normal levels of free testosterone. Levels of free testosterone may, however, be reduced in men with massive obesity (28). These changes may result in gynecomastia.

In women, marked obesity is associated with increased androgen production, increased peripheral conversion of androgen to estrogen, an increased rate of estrogen production, and decreased levels of SHBG. This constellation may be a major cause of the amenorrhea not infrequently seen in morbidly obese women. Upper-body obesity is associated with increased testosterone production, decreased SHBG, and increased levels of free testosterone in comparison to levels in obese women with lower-body or gynoid obesity (29–31). The fact that upper-body obesity also is associated with hyperinsulinemia has led to the hypothesis that insulin may be a factor that contributes to hyperandrogenism through actions on the ovary, as seems to be the case in syndromes of extreme insulin resistance. The increased peripheral production of estrogen from androstenedione, which occurs to a greater degree in women with lower-body obesity, may contribute to the increased incidence of uterine cancer in obese postmenopausal women (32).

Adrenal Function

The relationship between obesity and altered adrenal function can be addressed from a number of perspectives. The first relates to the clinical issue of whether a given patient with obesity, particularly one with hypertension and glucose intolerance, has Cushing syndrome. In 90% of obese individuals, the overnight cortisol response to 1 mg of dexamethasone given at midnight is normal, a finding sufficient to rule out Cushing syndrome. The 10% of individuals who fail to suppress cortisol production adequately on this test will suppress cortisol production normally in the formal 2-day low-dose dexamethasone test (33).

Obesity, however, is commonly associated with abnormalities of the cortisol axis, with increases in the rates of cortisol production and levels of urinary 17-hydroxysteroids frequently observed. Despite these findings, serum cortisol levels—including their diurnal variation—appear to be normal, and no clear defects in adrenocorticotropic hormone (ACTH) secretion have been observed (34). Thus, the precise basis for the increased cortisol production is unclear. One reason for interest in this area is the finding that cortisol is overproduced in a number of animal models of obesity, such as the *ob/ob* mouse and the *fa/fa* rat, and that removal of the adrenal gland markedly ameliorates many of the phenotypic and biochemical findings in these animals (35,36). The role, if any, of increased cortisol production in human obesity has not been established.

Pituitary Function

Obesity is clearly associated with defects in growth hormone secretion (37,38). Levels of growth hormone in response to many stimuli, including insulin-induced hypoglycemia, arginine, levodopa, exercise, sleep, and the physiologic regulator growth hormone–releasing hormone, are reduced in obese individuals. Treatment with cholinergic antagonists may reverse this defect (39). Because administration of growth hormone will reduce the percentage of body fat (40), these observations raise the obvious question of whether functional growth hormone deficiency is present in obesity. On the basis of levels of insulin-like growth factor-1, this would appear not to be the case. Many investigations of pituitary adrenal function in obesity have been carried out, in part because of the persistent interest in whether subtle hypothalamic dysfunction might be present in this disorder. A variety of findings with no obvious clinical relevance have been made (37).

ETIOLOGY OF OBESITY

Maintenance of a normal body weight requires a match of food intake to energy expenditure. Chronic positive energy balance leads to storage of calories in fat, mostly as fat but also as increased lean body mass (41), whereas negative balance leads to utilization of stores, including energy stored as glycogen, fat, and lean body mass. Both nutrient intake and energy expenditure are regulated by a complex interaction between the periphery and the central nervous system. Although not all aspects of central-peripheral interactions involved in energy balance are understood, key factors have been identified. For example, leptin from the adipocyte, ghrelin from the stomach, peptide YY from the gut, and insulin from the pancreas are all involved in the central regulation of energy balance. In the brain, more than a dozen peptides have been implicated in appetite and satiety. Among these peptides, neuropeptide Y, melanocyte-stimulating hormone, and agouti-related peptide in the arcuate nucleus, as well as melanin-concentrating hormone in the lateral hypothalamus, have emerged as important regulators (Fig. 31.2).

It is clear that in mammals the energy-balance equation tips readily toward the overconsumption of calories. The relative threat of starvation to survival apparently has exerted greater evolutionary influence than the long-term consequences of obesity. Indeed, in the wild, the most common cause of death among mice is starvation, as these animals cannot sustain themselves for longer than 3 to 4 days without food. In humans, one excess pound of fat will provide 3,500 calories, which represents adequate fuel for 2 to 3 days in the absence of any food intake.

Role of the Adipocyte in the Regulation of Food Intake

The adipocyte plays an important role in energy homeostasis. To compensate for fluctuations in the availability of food, mammals consume more calories than immediately required for metabolic needs and store excess calories. Calories may be stored as glycogen in the liver, triglycerides in adipocytes (particularly white adipose tissue), and protein in muscle. Adipocyte physiology is regulated by a number of signals, including nutrient availability, hormones, and neuronal input. For example, during a fast, levels of glucose and insulin fall, whereas those of glucocorticoids and growth hormone rise; in consequence, adipocyte triglycerides are metabolized to fatty acids and released into the circulation.

Although this role of the adipocyte in metabolic homeostasis has long been known, its role as an endocrine cell has only recently been recognized. Data suggesting that the adipocyte functions as more than a passive, externally regulated site for the storage of energy date back 10 to 15 years to the description of secretory products such as adipsin and angiotensinogen. Adipsin, a serine protease, is secreted by adipocytes and was found to be markedly decreased in some obese models such as the *ob/ob* mouse (42). Nutritionally regulated angiotensinogen secretion also was reported (43). However, the role of the adipocyte as a secretory cell was not fully appreciated until the discovery of leptin, a 16-kDa protein of the cytokine gene family, through genetic analysis of the *ob/ob* mouse (44). Since the discovery of the *ob* gene, adipocytes have been recognized to synthesize other factors that may contribute to energy balance.

LEPTIN

A spontaneous mutation in the leptin gene is associated with morbid obesity, hyperphagia, insulin resistance, and infertility in mice. Intriguing studies involving parabiotic mouse pairs had suggested that the syndrome involved the absence of a circulating factor (45,46). Identification of leptin confirmed that absence of a hormone, made in adipocytes and secreted into the circulation, caused the obesity syndrome and that replacement of this factor led to correction of the phenotype (47). Subsequent studies demonstrated an important action of leptin in the hypothalamus (48). The critical importance of leptin in humans was confirmed in studies of morbidly obese children lacking functional leptin alleles. These children, unable to make leptin (49), demonstrate continuous hyperphagia and respond to exogenously administered leptin with a resolution of hyperphagia and significant reductions in body weight (50).

Although the complete absence of leptin is associated with morbid obesity in rare examples of rodent and human obesity, most obese mammals, including humans, have high levels of circulating leptin. Circulating leptin levels correlate well with available fat stores (51), and administration of leptin in most obese states does not lead to decreases in appetite. These findings suggest that the dominant physiologic role of leptin is that of a "starvation signal," which is important in switching between fed and fasted states rather than in serving as an antiobesity hormone (37,52). In rodents, decreased leptin during fasting is associated with a series of metabolic changes that result in the suppression of reproductive hormones, growth hormone, and thyroid hormones and in the activation of the hypothalamic-pituitary axis with a resultant rise in corticosterone level. These changes can be mitigated by the administration of leptin during the fast. Furthermore, in mice, fasting is associated with a disruption of the estrous cycle, an effect that lasts for many days after the re-introduction of food. Administration of leptin during the fast attenuates this disruption. The physiologic dose response to leptin may be viewed as biphasic. Between absent and normal leptin levels, leptin is effective in signaling adequacy of fat stores, and leptin levels correlate with fat stores. However, when leptin concentrations rise above those associated with adequate adipose stores, leptin has little effect in limiting food intake and a state of "leptin resistance" develops.

ADIPONECTIN

Adiponectin (Acrp30) is a protein exclusively and abundantly expressed in adipose tissue. In mice, a single injection of adiponectin leads to a decrease in glucose levels, and in *ob/ob* mice, adiponectin abolishes hyperglycemia. In addition, treatment with adiponectin leads to an acute increase in fatty acid oxidation in muscle (53). In isolated hepatocytes, adiponectin leads to a reduction in the amount of insulin needed to suppress gluconeogenesis (54). In various forms of obesity, in both humans and mice, levels of adiponectin messenger RNA (mRNA) are decreased. At least one study has reported an increase in adiponectin after surgery for obesity (55). A recent study indicates that levels are genetically determined and may be associated with obesity (56). These data indicate that adiponectin is important in energy homeostasis and insulin sensitivity.

11-β HYDROXYSTEROID DEHYDROGENASE TYPE 1

The enzyme 11-β hydroxysteroid dehydrogenase type 1 (11-β HSD-1) plays an important role in determining intracellular glucocorticoid concentrations by regenerating active glucocorticoids from inactive cortisone. Activity of this enzyme is relatively increased in visceral fat as opposed to subcutaneous fat (57). Overexpression of the enzyme with a fat-specific transgene leads to a syndrome of visceral obesity that is associated with hyperphagia, insulin resistance, and hypertension (58). The activity of 11-β HSD-1 may be increased in humans with obesity.

Role of the Central Nervous System in the Regulation of Appetite

Although defects intrinsic to the adipocyte can lead to obesity, the establishment of excess adiposity requires the chronic

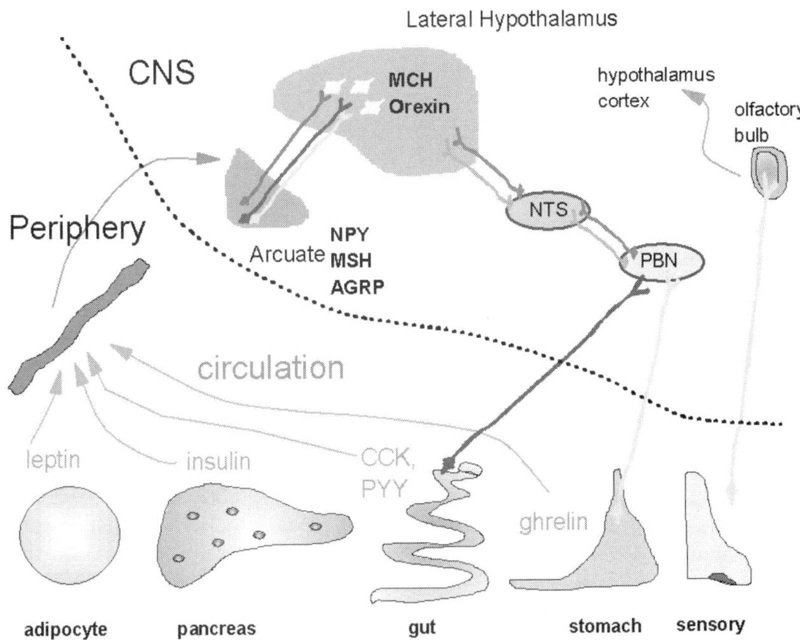

Figure 31.2. Factors in the periphery that impact energy homeostasis are from a variety of tissues and act in the central nervous system (CNS). Peptides known to be important for energy homeostasis include melanocyte-stimulating hormone (MSH), melanocyte-concentrating hormone (MCH), neuropeptide Y (NPY), agouti-related peptide (AGRP). and cocaine-amphetamine–related transcript (CART). Many other central peptides may also play a role in energy balance (orexin, corticotropin-releasing factor, urocortin, galanin, and neurotensin, among others); however, their roles are less well understood. Somatosensory inputs such as smell are also known to be important. CCK, cholecystokinin; PYY, peptide YY.

excessive ingestion of calories. The precise mechanisms by which appetite is regulated are still unknown; however, insights from animal models and from human beings with single-gene defects leading to obesity have made it clear that appetite and feeding are regulated processes. The initial observations that animals could be made lean or obese through hypothalamic lesions date back to studies performed in the 1930s and 1940s. Studies in rats and cats showed that electrical stimulation of the medial hypothalamus decreased eating, whereas surgically made ablative lesions led to hyperphagia and obesity. This led to the definition of the medial hypothalamus as a "satiety center." In contrast, electrical stimulation of the lateral hypothalamus led to increased feeding, whereas lesions of the lateral hypothalamus led to a syndrome of adipsia and aphagia. Hence, the lateral hypothalamus was identified as a feeding center. Despite these early findings, progress in understanding the role of the hypothalamus in obesity was slow. Indeed, for years obesity was viewed not as a medical process but as a moral fault. This view of obesity was partially modified when a series of studies in humans led to the observation that different individuals fed isocaloric diets normalized for weight might maintain, lose, or gain weight. However, the gradual change in the categorization of obesity from moral fault to a physiologic failure came with discoveries over the past decade that have defined a number of molecular mechanisms leading to leanness or obesity in both mice and humans. These discoveries also redefined the role of the adipocyte as a passive caloric storage depot to an endocrine cell.

The brain, particularly the hypothalamus, is key in the integration of signals that regulate appetite and feeding. The hypothalamus receives input from the periphery via neural afferents, hormones, and metabolites. Inputs from the vagus through the hindbrain provide information from the viscera, such as gut distention. Peripheral hormonal signals include leptin, insulin, cortisol, ghrelin, and cholecystokinin. Metabolites also may influence appetite, as it is known that hypoglycemia induces hyperphagia; however, the role of metabolites is less clear. A series of neuronal connections within the hypothalamus are involved in processing these signals.

Within the hypothalamus, the arcuate nucleus plays an important role in responding to signals from the periphery. A subset of neurons in this region of the hypothalamus express the long form of the leptin receptor and respond directly to the adipocyte hormone leptin. Leptin acts on one set of neurons that synthesize the two orexigenic peptides neuropeptide Y (NPY) and agouti-related peptide (AgRP) and a second population of neurons that synthesize the anorectic peptides melanocyte-stimulating hormone (α-MSH) and cocaine-amphetamine–related transcript (CART). Leptin acts to hyperpolarize the NPY/AgRP neurons, whereas it activates the α-MSH/CART neurons (59). A peptide in the lateral hypothalamus, melanin-concentrating hormone (MCH), also contributes to hunger, but it does not appear to be a direct target of leptin regulation.

The essential role of leptin in regulating these neurons is dramatically demonstrated in *db/db* mice, which lack the long form of the leptin receptor, and similarly in some human families that do not express the long form of the receptor. In both animals and humans (60), circulating levels of leptin are significantly elevated. However, because the hormone cannot signal the hypothalamus, affected individuals are hyperphagic and obese with a phenotype similar to that seen in animals lacking leptin.

THE MELANOCORTIN SYSTEM AND OBESITY

Thus far, the most extensively analyzed central system involved in the regulation of energy homeostasis is the melanocortin pathway. Disruption of this pathway along any of several steps leads to obesity in both mice and humans.

Insight into this pathway originally derived from examination of the obese, yellow mice known as agouti and expressing the mutated gene A^y (61). Normally, the peptide agouti is expressed only in skin, where it serves as a regulator of type I melanocortin 1 receptors (MC1-R) (62). Activation of these receptors by α-MSH leads to a conversion of yellow melanin to black melanin; agouti acts on the same receptor to prevent its activation by α-MSH. This system is responsible for coloration in mammals, as the relative signals from MSH and agouti lead to a mix of yellow and black melanin, which is perceived as brownish gray. The A^y gene has a mutation in the promoter that leads to constitutive expression of agouti in an unregulated fashion in all organs. In the skin, high levels of agouti block MSH signaling of MC1-R and yellow melanin is not converted to black melanin. Further analysis of the obese phenotype of these mice led to a recognition that ectopically expressed agouti blocked the action of MSH in the brain through the brain melanocortin receptors MC4-R and MC3-R (63).

Although the function of α-MSH as a neuropeptide that inhibits food intake had been described (64), the importance of this neuropeptide in energy homeostasis was not appreciated until analysis of the A^y mouse. This finding was confirmed by the generation of genetically engineered mice lacking either MC4-R or MC3-R. The phenotype of the MC4-R–ablated mouse closely mimics the obesity phenotype of the agouti mouse, although coat color is normal (65). Interestingly, the heterozygote animals also demonstrate weights intermediate between those of the homozygote and normal wild-type mice. The MC3-R knockout mouse also has abnormal energy expenditure.

Findings in the A^y mouse led to the search for an endogenous agouti-like factor that might regulate brain melanocortin receptors. An analogue of agouti, AgRP (66), with expression limited to arcuate neurons in the hypothalamus, was thus discovered. This neuropeptide plays an important role in energy homeostasis. Mice overexpressing AgRP mimic the phenotype of agouti mice, and AgRP is negatively regulated by leptin.

The melanocortin system has been shown to be important in humans. Screening of morbidly obese individuals with a history of early childhood obesity has revealed a prevalence of MC4-R mutations in up to 5% (67,68). Depending on the precise nature of the mutation, humans with a single mutated allele may be obese. A small number of individuals without functional genes for pre-opiomelanocortin (POMC), which is the gene encoding melanocortin, have a phenotype of early-onset obesity, red hair, and adrenal insufficiency (69). This demonstrates the importance of the POMC gene in regulating both body weight and pigmentation and adrenal function in humans.

AN ADIPO-HYPOTHALAMIC AXIS AND ENERGY BALANCE

On the basis of currently available knowledge, at least one pathway regulating energy balance can be defined (Fig. 31.3). Leptin, made in the adipocyte, is released into the circulation. It crosses the blood–brain barrier and acts on leptin receptors on neurons that make either NPY/AgRP or POMC/CART in the arcuate nucleus. Leptin suppresses NPY neurons and activates the POMC neurons. Activation of the POMC neurons leads to the production of MSH, which acts on the MC4-R in the brain and leads to a reduction in feeding. Mutations in leptin, leptin receptor, POMC, and MC4-R lead to obesity in both mice and humans. Furthermore, mutations of prohormone-converting enzyme-1 (PC-1) in humans (70) and certain converting enzymes in rodents that prevent the processing of POMC also lead to obesity (71).

OTHER NEUROPEPTIDES

A second hypothalamic system involved in the regulation of appetite and, potentially, in energy homeostasis is MCH and its receptors (MCH1-R and MCH2-R). MCH is a nonadecapeptide with expression limited to the lateral hypothalamic area of all mammals thus far studied. The peptide sequence is identical in rodents, humans, and sheep. As a pharmacologic agent injected into the brain, MCH rapidly increases appetite (72). Mice genetically altered to lack MCH are lean and have both slight hypophagia and a slight increase in energy expenditure (73). Mice overexpressing MCH have mild obesity and insulin resistance. MCH neurons project throughout the brain, including the cortex and the hindbrain. Rodents express only one receptor, MCHR-1, whereas humans and dogs express MCHR-1 and a second receptor with limited homology to MCHR-1, designated MCHR-2. The potential importance of the MCH system in humans has not yet been evaluated.

NPY is another peptide expressed in the brain that induces rapid and significant increases in feeding when it is injected into rodents (16). Chronic infusions in rodents lead to sustained hyperphagia, obesity, and insulin resistance (74). However, the precise role of NPY in the regulation of appetite remains elusive, because mice deficient in NPY have normal energy homeostasis (75) except for impaired refeeding after starvation (76). Mice lacking two of the NPY receptors believed to mediate the appetite effects of NPY have mild obesity. It is interesting that, when mice lacking NPY are bred to mice without leptin, the offspring show an attenuation of the obesity seen in the leptin-deficient mice and partial restoration of fertility (77). In addition, chronic infusion of NPY has recently been shown to lead to hypogonadism. These data suggest that excess NPY expression seen in hypoleptinemic states may be involved in mediating the infertility seen during starvation as well as in *ob/ob* mice and aleptinemic humans.

PERIPHERAL SIGNALS

A number of peptides originating from peripheral sources other than the adipocyte may be important in regulating body weight (78). These include but are not limited to ghrelin, cholecystokinin (CCK), glucagon-like peptide, and insulin. Such afferent signals may be responsible for short-term regulation of appetite and meal size.

CCK was the first afferent signal inhibiting appetite to be described (in 1975) (79,80). Injection of CCK stops feeding and has been shown to induce satiety in both rats and rhesus monkeys. More recent data indicate that CCK can act synergistically with leptin to induce greater reductions in feeding than those seen with leptin alone (81). Thus far, no deficits of CCK in human obesity have been defined, although CCK receptors remain a potential drug target.

Ghrelin, a peptide localized to the stomach and brain, is the endogenous ligand of the growth hormone secretagogue receptor. Ghrelin acts to stimulate appetite, and its secretion is decreased in both rodents and humans by the ingestion of nutrients (82,83) and increases before the initiation of a meal. In rats, chronic infusion of ghrelin, either systemically or into the cerebral ventricles, leads to hyperphagia and obesity, suggesting that it may play a role in long-term food intake (84). Recent findings indicate that ghrelin acts on NPY and AgRP neurons in the

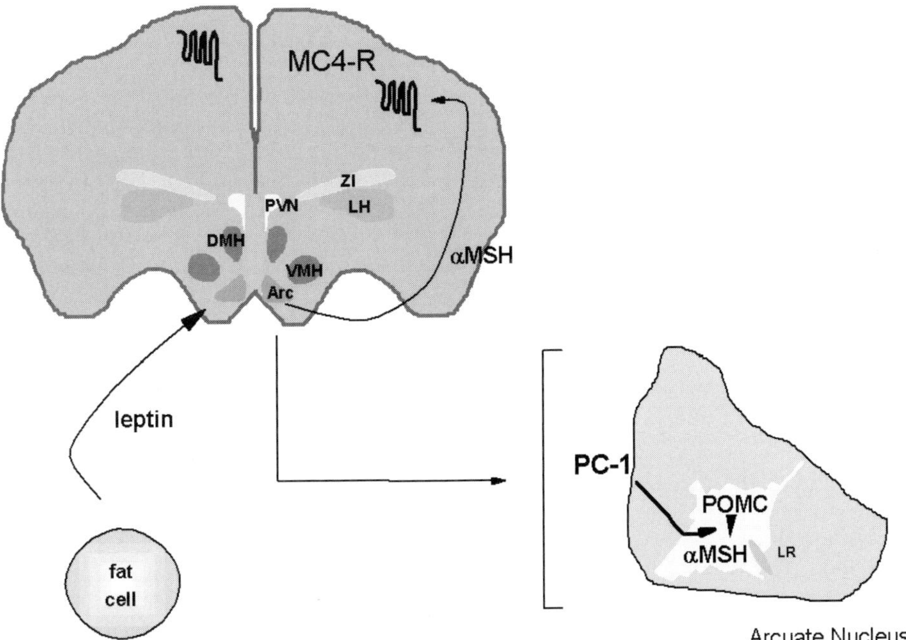

Figure 31.3. One pathway that is important in energy balance has been defined. Leptin, made in the adipocyte, is secreted into the blood. It crosses the blood–brain barrier and acts on cells in the arcuate nucleus (Arc), where it activates cells making the melanocyte-stimulating hormone (MSH) precursor pro-opiomelanocortin (POMC). POMC is converted to MSH (by prohormone-converting enzyme-1 [PC-1] in humans) and acts on one of the central melanocortin receptors, MC4-R. Disturbance of this pathway in rodents or humans leads to obesity, as documented by identification of mutations in leptin, leptin receptor, PC-1, POMC, and MC4-R. Other neuroanatomic areas involved in feeding that may participate in regulation of appetite and satiety include the lateral hypothalamus (LH) (melanin-concentrating hormone, cocaine-amphetamine–related peptide, orexin), the paraventricular nucleus (PVN) (corticotropin-releasing factor, urocortin), the zona incerta (ZI) (melanin-concentrating hormone), the ventromedial hypothalamus (VMH), and the dorsomedial hypothalamus (DMH).

arcuate nucleus (17). Interestingly, levels of circulating ghrelin are lower in obese than in normal-weight humans. Furthermore, weight loss in the obese leads to an increase in ghrelin levels toward normal levels. Thus, the decrease in ghrelin in obese subjects may reflect a failed attempt to decrease food consumption in the context of increased adiposity. When the subjects diet and go into negative caloric balance, ghrelin levels increase as the body attempts to regain lost calories. A recent study examined ghrelin regulation after gastric bypass surgery, one of the few procedures known to result in long-term weight loss. In this group, ghrelin levels decreased markedly after bypass surgery, suggesting that exclusion of the fundus of the stomach leads to alterations in the regulation of ghrelin (18). However, much remains to be done to define the precise physiology of this peptide. At least one report indicates that human obesity is associated with decreased circulating levels of ghrelin (85).

Glucagon-like peptide-1 (GLP-1), which is synthesized in the gut, acts to inhibit appetite. Injection of GLP-1 inhibits food intake in the rat, and repeated injections lead to weight loss. In contrast, treatment of animals with the GLP-1 antagonist exendin leads to increased food intake and an increase in body weight (86). A long-acting GLP-1 derivative, NN2211, reduces food intake and leads to weight loss in both normal rats and rats with diet-induced obesity. After a 7-day treatment period, animals manifested decreased energy expenditure, typically associated with weight loss (87). However, ablation of GLP-1 in mice is not associated with altered energy balance.

Peptide YY (PYY) is another peptide synthesized in the gut that appears to inhibit food intake in both rodents and humans (88). This contrasts with its action when administered directly into the central nervous system, which is to increase feeding. Further study will be required to establish the role of PYY in human obesity.

Insulin enters the brain from the peripheral circulation and also may play a role in reducing food intake through central nervous system mechanisms. Insulin entry into the brain occurs via a saturable system (89), and chronic insulin infusion is associated with weight loss (90). A mouse model of selective ablation of the insulin receptor from the brain is characterized by mild obesity and increased sensitivity to diet-induced obesity (91). Analyzing the role of insulin is extremely complex, as obesity is associated with hyperinsulinemia, suggesting that in obesity either insulin transport into the brain or insulin signaling within the brain may be impaired.

Abnormal Regulation of Energy Expenditure

Energy expenditure is an important determinant of body weight. Energy expenditure can be divided into several components: the resting, or basal, metabolic rate (RMR); the cost of metabolizing and storing food (thermic effect of food [TEF]); exercise-induced thermogenesis; and adaptive thermogenesis. Adaptive thermogenesis includes regulated responses to diet and environmental temperature. These changes act both to provide protection from the environment and to regulate energy homeostasis in relation to energy intake (92,93).

The RMR normally accounts for between 65% and 75% of the total daily energy expenditure. RMR measures the energy expended for maintenance of normal body functions at rest and is obtained by taking measurements several hours remote from food intake or exercise. The rate is determined in large part by fat-free mass but also is influenced by sex, age, physical conditioning, and genetic factors. RMR in absolute terms is almost always increased in obese individuals; however, when RMR is expressed in terms of fat-free mass, it is typically normal (36,94,95). These two expressions of RMR have different applications. RMR expressed in absolute terms is most relevant to the question of total energy expenditure in obese individuals (and by inference, if weight is stable, to food intake). RMR expressed per lean body mass is most relevant to the question of possible biochemical differences between lean and obese individuals that might predispose to efficient energy metabolism and weight gain. It is possible that some obese individuals in the so-called preobese state or after weight reduction have a reduction in RMR per unit of lean body mass. The molecular or physiologic basis for such a potential defect is not clear, but abnormalities of futile cycling (34) and energy-expensive processes such as ion pumping (35,44) have been proposed. It has been calculated that a low RMR by itself, i.e., in the absence of hyperphagia, would contribute only modestly to the tendency to gain weight, because the increased total RMR consequent to weight gain would counter any preceding reduction in RMR. In the absence of hyperphagia, an increased RMR would result in equilibration at a new, modestly increased weight. Thus, for major obesity to develop, dysregulation of food intake must coexist with any possible thermogenic defect.

TEF may account for as much 10% of energy ingested. It consists of the energy costs of absorbing and processing food and of thermogenesis in response to diet. Feeding acutely increases energy expenditure by as much as 25% to 40% in both rodents (38) and humans (39). The possibility that decreased TEF contributes to the development of obesity is controversial, and studies demonstrate both decreased and normal energy expenditure after meals (40,96).

Diet has significant effects on thermogenesis. During starvation, RMR can be reduced significantly, and a diet that diminishes body weight by 10% is associated with decreased energy expenditure (97). Nutrients in the diet also influence thermogenesis. For example, ingestion of low-protein diets increases overall total food consumption to meet protein demand. In this situation excess calories are not stored, but rather dissipated as heat (98). Interestingly, overfeeding is associated with increased energy expenditure, a process that may provide partial protection against the development of obesity and may be genetically determined (99). Environmental temperature also has significant effects on thermogenesis, as increased heat production is necessary to maintain body temperature with cold exposure. In rodents, exposure to a temperature of 4°C leads to significant increases in oxygen consumption. Acutely, part of this response is due to shivering. More chronically increased heat production comes from increased adaptive thermogenesis in brown adipose tissue. In humans, these effects are less marked, at least in part because of the ability of humans to vary the amount of clothing.

Adaptive thermogenesis in response to food intake and temperature change is regulated by the brain and is mediated by activation of the sympathetic nervous system, the hypothalamic-pituitary-thyroid axis, and various neuropeptides that have dual effects on appetite and energy expenditure (such as leptin, NPY, and MSH). These systems target uncoupling proteins, particularly in brown adipose tissue in rodents (100) and skeletal muscle in both rodents and humans (101). The significance of defects in adaptive thermogenesis in human obesity remains unclear.

The thermic effect of exercise is the most variable component of energy expenditure, and a possible causative role for this component in obesity has been studied. As with studies of food intake, progress has been limited by methodologic issues. Recent data derived from population studies indicate that obese persons spend fewer hours per week physically active than do people whose BMIs are lower. There also is an inverse association between socioeconomic status and physical activity. However, the potential impact of physical activity on weight loss may be limited for any given individual. For example, expenditure of 220 calories requires approximately 25 minutes of rapid walking (i.e., 17 minutes per mile). A person engaged in a regular exercise program three times per week might expend an additional 700 calories, which represents about 20% of a pound of fat. Hence, although lifestyle changes are important for weight loss and contribute significantly to cardiovascular health, their overall impact on energy balance is small. Nonexercise activity also contributes to thermogenesis in humans. This activity is associated with fidgeting, maintenance of posture, and other physical activities of daily life. In some humans, overfeeding is associated with an induction of nonexercise activity, which serves to dissipate energy and reduce weight gain, whereas other individuals may fail to increase nonexercise activity and have increased fat storage (102). One study examined nonexercise activity, such as fidgeting, activities of daily living, and posture maintenance, and found a correlation of "spontaneous physical activities" with overall habitual physical activity (103). This suggests that activity levels may be either genetically or culturally determined in individuals and raises the possibility that a predisposition toward physical activity can decrease the predisposition to obesity.

In summary, although thermogenesis is important in maintaining energy balance, there are few data to suggest that most patients with established obesity have decreased rates of total energy expenditure. Indeed, as RMR increases with body weight, most obese patients have total increased thermogenesis, implying that their total energy intake is also increased in absolute terms. Some evidence supports the claim, frequently encountered in clinical practice, that individuals destined to become obese but who are not yet obese may have modest reductions in energy expenditure that would permit the development of obesity despite a low energy intake. However, even if such a defect is present, its basis is unknown, and it is unlikely, on the basis of current knowledge, that efficient energy metabolism on its own plays a major role in the generation or maintenance of the obese state. In contrast, after weight reduction, there is an overall decrease in thermogenesis (104), which makes maintenance of weight loss difficult.

Endocrine Factors

There is no established endocrine cause for most cases of obesity. However, endocrinologists frequently are consulted because of concern that a patient may have Cushing syndrome or hypothyroidism. Endocrine syndromes that may be associated with obesity are listed in Table 31.1. Although obese patients may have central obesity, hypertension, and glucose tolerance, they are free of most other stigmata of Cushing syndrome, and for the most part this can be ruled out as a cause of obesity by the use of dexamethasone suppression testing (37,52). Some individuals with hypothyroidism become obese. This probably results from the decrease in metabolic rate and lower rate of lipolysis brought about by hypothyroidism. However, much of the weight gain in hypothyroidism is due to fluid accumulation with myxedema. Standard tests of thyroid function rule out the diagnosis in most obese patients. Other endocrine disorders that may be associated with obesity include insulinoma, male hypogonadism, growth hormone deficiency, and Turner syndrome.

Table 31.1. Endocrine Syndromes Associated with Obesity

1. Cushing syndrome
2. Hypothyroidism
3. Insulinoma
4. Craniopharyngioma
5. Turner syndrome
6. Male hypogonadism

TREATMENT OF OBESITY

Successful treatment of obesity, defined as treatment that results in sustained attainment of normal body weight and composition without producing unacceptable treatment-induced morbidity, is rarely achievable in clinical practice (96). Many therapeutic approaches can bring about short-term weight loss, but long-term success is infrequent regardless of the approach. Nevertheless, billions of dollars are spent annually in the United States in pursuit of this goal. Although many individuals diet solely in pursuit of cosmetic goals unrelated to any medically relevant definition of obesity, the need is great for effective and safe therapies for those individuals in whom obesity represents a major health risk.

Given the limitations, discomforts, and potential risks of available therapy, it is necessary to consider the risks of obesity-related morbidity in any individual. It is clear that the morbidity of obesity increases with BMI and that, for any BMI, greater waist-to-hip ratios confer greater risk. Moderate risk begins at a BMI of 30 and doubles with a BMI between 30 and 40 (5). In addition to the risk conferred by an increased BMI, diabetes, hypertension, and an atherogenic lipid profile, when present, each increases the impact of obesity on health. Through evaluation of these factors and assessment of the likelihood that an individual patient will respond to a particular therapeutic regimen, an individualized long-term treatment plan must be developed.

Diet

Reduction of caloric intake is the cornerstone of any therapy for obesity and is discussed extensively in Chapter 32. The fundamental goal is the reduction of energy intake to a level substantially below that of energy expenditure. This simple prescription is difficult to accomplish despite a wide variety of specific dietary approaches. A number of factors complicate the ability to predict the results with any given diet (105–107). Because energy expenditure increases with increasing obesity at any level of caloric intake, individuals who are more obese will lose weight more rapidly than those who are less obese. The rate of weight loss at any level of energy intake also is influenced by factors that increase energy expenditure, such as exercise and thyroid function, and by gender and age, because women and persons of advanced age have lower metabolic rates for any body weight. As discussed below, there are claims that specific features of a diet, i.e., level of carbohydrates or proteins, may influence its efficacy. Importantly, many obese individuals believe that they are resistant to weight loss despite severe caloric restriction. The issues related to energy expenditure in obesity and the possibility that some individuals have a metabolic predisposition to efficient metabolism was discussed earlier. Whatever the answer to that question, it must be emphasized that there are no reliable demonstrations of failure of weight loss among obese individuals placed on diets of 1,200 kilocalories (kcal) or less while under strict observation. On the other hand, diets that produce weight loss for inpatients are frequently unsuccessful when applied to outpatients, indicating problems with compliance with dietary regimens.

Apart from the initial weight loss consequent to natriuresis and fluid shifts, a deficit of 7,500 kcal is predicted to produce a weight loss of 1 kg (107). Therefore, a reduction in food intake by as little as 100 kcal per day should bring about a 5-kg weight loss over 1 year. It is clear from common experience, however, that attempts at dieting that rely on such small reductions in food intake are rarely successful. Thus, more severe reductions in energy intake are typically prescribed. Three general categories of calorie-restricted diets have been used (105).

Total starvation will produce the most rapid weight loss, although a greater fraction of the lost weight is from fluid losses than is found with other approaches. The extreme nature of the therapy, the need for close inpatient supervision, the excessive loss of lean body mass, and the occurrence of complications such as gout, renal stones, and hypotension have led to the virtual disappearance of this approach.

So-called very-low-calorie diets of 200 to 600 kcal were initially designed to supplement fasting, primarily with protein, with the goal being the prevention of loss of lean body mass (108). During the 1970s, formula supplements that contained low-quality protein derived largely from collagen and were deficient in essential amino acids led to excessive cardiovascular deaths (109). Contemporary versions of such diets use high-quality protein derived from soy, casein, egg, or lean fish or fowl and adequate quantities of other nutrients, including unsaturated fatty acids, potassium, magnesium, vitamins, and minerals. Whether or not carbohydrate should be a component of such diets, with the goal of minimizing ketosis and reducing the decrease in triiodothyronine but with the possible side effect of reducing conservation of lean body mass, is a subject of debate and is discussed more fully in Chapter 32. Recent application of such diets under medical supervision has not been associated with unexpected deaths (110,111). Indeed, institution of such therapy virtually always has beneficial effects: a prompt reduction in blood pressure in hypertensive patients and in blood glucose levels in diabetic patients, typically allowing medication to be discontinued, at least for the duration of the diet. The average weight loss is 1.5 kg per week, although, for several reasons, including the decline in metabolic rate that follows loss of lean body mass, the rate diminishes as weight is lost (112,113). Because regaining weight after cessation of dieting is extremely common, such diets make sense only as part of an overall plan to modify food intake chronically.

Many different diets that provide 800 to 1,000 kcal per day are in common use, and with adequate compliance by the patient, these diets should result in weight loss. Balanced low-calorie diets, as well as those that feature low amounts of carbohydrate or protein, have been advocated by different authorities. There are also many programs that recommend specific food combinations or unusual sequences for eating, but none of these approaches has any proven merit. However, dietary composition may play a role in long-term success in weight loss and weight maintenance. For example, a study comparing a moderate-fat diet consisting of 35% energy from fat and a low-fat diet in which 20% of energy was derived from fat demonstrated enhanced weight loss assessed by total weight loss, BMI change, and decrease in waist circumference in the group on the moderate-fat diet. Retention in the diet study was greater among those enrolled in the moderate-fat group, as 54% of patients continued actively participating in the weight loss program in this group compared with 20% in the low-fat diet group (114).

Recently, increased interest has focused on the possibility that diet content may affect appetite. For example, diets with a low glycemic index may be useful in preventing the development of obesity; subjects given test meals with different glycemic indexes and then allowed free access to food ate less after eating meals with a low glycemic index. Some data suggest that diets with a high glycemic index predispose to increased postprandial hunger, whereas diets focused on glycemic index and information regarding portion control lead to higher rates of success in weight loss, at least among adolescent populations (115). Low-carbohydrate diets such as the Atkins diet appear to be associated with significant weight loss. However, this diet has not been systematically studied, nor has long-term maintenance of weight loss.

A key aspect yet missing from diet therapy is education regarding diet aimed at preventing initial weight gain. Among the population, general information on caloric content is quite poor. It is also a noteworthy paradox that over the past 30 years, the U.S. population has gained weight while focusing on reducing saturated fat in the diet. Indeed, total fat content in the diet is lower today than at any time in the past several decades, yet obesity has achieved epidemic proportions. One possibility is that the focus on "low fat" deflected attention from a focus on portion control. Between 1970 and 1994, total daily per capita calorie consumption increased by 500 calories (Fig. 31.4). Approximately 80% of this increase derived from higher daily carbohydrate consumption, which increased by 100 g. In comparison, protein consumption increased minimally and fat consumption remained constant. During the same interval, yearly per capita meat consumption increased by 13 pounds, whereas cereal consumption increased by 65 pounds (Fig. 31.5). Although consumption of all food groups increased, the disproportionate increase of carbohydrates and cereals suggests that the focus on low-fat foods, which are necessarily high in carbohydrates, may be contributing to the obesity epidemic. This could occur because individuals either are more likely to discount calories derived from carbohydrates and hence consume more of these calories or experience increased hunger as a consequence of carbohydrate intake and respond with an overall increase in calorie consumption.

Exercise

It is appropriate to consider the therapeutic use of exercise for any patient with obesity. Because exercise increases energy expenditure, the most obvious purpose of exercise in obesity is to shift the energy balance equation toward a net negative. Unfortunately, long-term compliance with exercise programs is limited. This and the relatively small impact of moderate exercise on net energy balance combine to support the view that exercise is at best a small aid to weight loss in clinical practice (116). For example, a 150-pound person engaging in moderate exercise such as walking uphill at a grade of 4% at a pace of 3 miles per hour for 30 minutes will expend only 150 calories. Nevertheless, given the potential benefit of exercise on blood pressure, lipids, cardiovascular fitness, insulin sensitivity, and sense of well-being, attempts should be made to incorporate an exercise program into the therapeutic approach. In addition, exercise has positive effects on weight maintenance and thus may help to avoid regain of weight.

Drugs

At present, few drugs are available for the treatment of obesity, and the available agents lead to successful weight loss in only a limited number of patients. Orlistat (Xenical) is a synthetic fat that impairs absorption of ingested fat by inhibiting intestinal lipase. Expected weight loss is on the order of 5 to 15 kg. However, in some patients this relatively small degree of loss may be sufficient to improve comorbidity. In patients

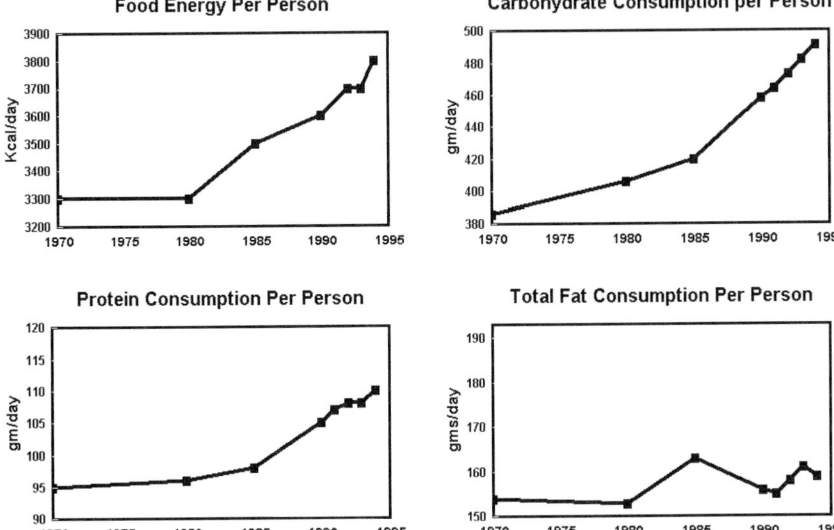

Figure 31.4. Daily per capita energy consumption. These panels show the source of calories. Overall daily energy consumption has increased by 500 calories over 15 years. Most of these increased calories derive from carbohydrate, as can be seen by comparing the increases in carbohydrate, protein, and fat consumption. (Adapted from data from the U.S. Department of Agriculture.)

with a recorded history of increasing weight gain over time, even the stabilization of body weight may be a desirable endpoint. Orlistat is not absorbed and has few systemic side effects, although supplementation with fat-soluble vitamins is recommended. Loose, fatty stools in some patients are a significant problem, leading to the termination of therapy. As with most other obesity treatments, it is unusual to sustain weight loss for more than 2 or 3 years after therapy.

A second available agent is sibutramine (Meridia), which inhibits reuptake of both serotonin and catecholamines at nerve intervals and acts both to decrease appetite and to increase thermogenesis (117). Expected weight loss is similar to that seen with orlistat. However, hypertension and tachycardia occur as relatively common side effects. This tends to limit the treatable population. Phentermine is still available and may be useful in some patients.

As seen with diet, long-term results after cessation of pharmacologic treatment are discouraging, with fewer than 10% of patients who achieved successful weight loss showing sustained long-term weight loss.

Surgery

Patients with massive obesity who are refractory to therapy are subject to major morbidity from their disease. A number of surgical procedures have been used to treat morbid obesity. Malabsorptive procedures such as jejunoileal bypass and biliopancreatic diversion lead to weight loss without changes in eating habits. These procedures have generally been abandoned because of their association with high rates of complications. Jejunoileal bypass may lead to hepatic failure, cirrhosis, protein malnutrition, vitamin deficiency, and metabolic bone disease.

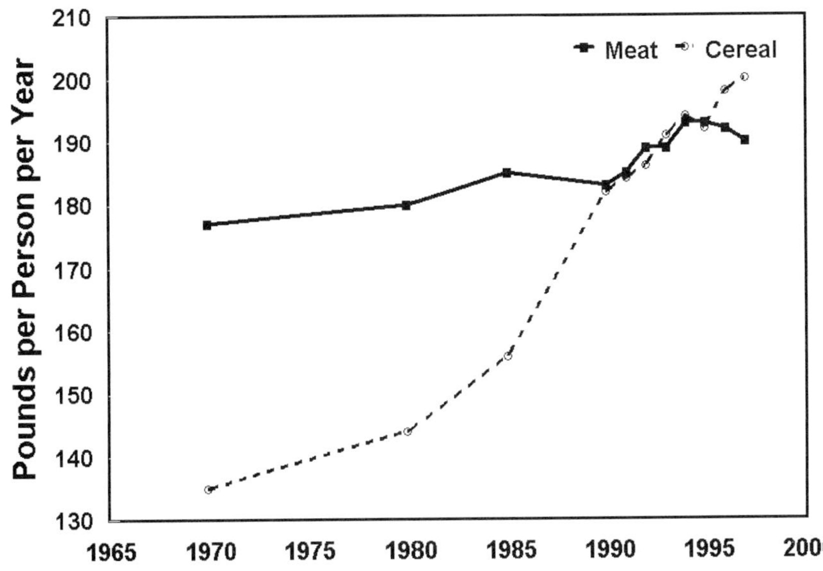

Figure 31.5. Yearly per capita meat and cereal consumption. (Adapted from data from the U.S. Department of Agriculture.)

Biliopancreatic diversion is associated with protein malnutrition, metabolic bone disease, and vitamin deficiency.

These malabsorptive procedures have been supplanted by procedures in which the major element is restriction of stomach capacity, including gastroplasty, gastric banding, and gastric bypass surgery (118). Gastroplasty involves stapling the stomach to exclude the fundus. In gastric banding, a prosthetic band encircles the proximal stomach and may be placed laparoscopically. Gastric bypass partitions the stomach into a small proximal pouch and a distal bypassed fundus; a gastrojejunostomy is used to drain the pouch. This configuration can lead to a "dumping syndrome" when a carbohydrate-rich meal is ingested; the potential for experiencing symptoms of dumping, including lightheadedness, nausea, palpitations, and diaphoresis, may contribute a behavioral component to weight loss. The success of gastroplasty appears to be relatively low, as fewer than 40% of patients maintain 50% excess weight loss at 3 years (119). Gastric banding is associated with variable success.

At present the Roux-en-Y gastric bypass procedure is recommended in patients with a BMI higher than 40 or in those with a BMI higher than 35 and a comorbidity such as diabetes, hypertension, or arthritis. When this procedure is performed in appropriately prescreened patients, 80% lose significant amounts of weight, and weight loss can be sustained indefinitely. Patients need to be evaluated by a nutritionist and must fully understand the consequences of the surgical procedure. All programs also require a psychological assessment. Severe depression and a history of bulimia or anorexia would disqualify a patient. The surgical procedure appears to be well tolerated. Following surgery, approximately 95% of patients with diabetes will experience a significant improvement in their glucose tolerance, ranging from an ability to maintain euglycemia without any medication to a marked reduction in dose and number of antidiabetic drugs. Hypercholesterolemia and hypertension almost always improve.

CONCLUSION

Overweight and obesity are major health problems associated with increased risk of diabetes and numerous other illnesses. Although increasingly prevalent, the available pharmacologic treatments are poor. Surgery, particularly Roux-en-Y bypass, is an established and useful therapy; however, this is applicable only for patients with significant obesity.

Successful treatment of most overweight and obese individuals will depend upon the future development of new therapies. It also requires a paradigm shift in viewing obesity as a disease that requires treatment, rather than deferring treatment until the complications develop.

REFERENCES

1. Build study, 1979. Chicago: Society of Actuaries and Association of Life Insurance Medical Directors of America, 1980.
2. James WP. What are the health risks? The medical consequences of obesity and its health risks. *Exp Clin Endocrinol Diabetes* 1998;106[Suppl 2]:1–6.
3. Thompson D, Wolf AM. The medical-care cost burden of obesity. *Obes Rev* 2001;2:189–197.
4. Vanitallie TB. Body weight, morbidity, and longevity. In: Bjorntorp P, Brodoff BN, eds. *Obesity*. Philadelphia: JB Lippincott Co, 1992.
5. Montague CT, O'Rahilly S. The perils of portliness: causes and consequences of visceral adiposity. *Diabetes* 2000;49:883–888.
6. Carry VJ, Walters EE, Colditz GA, et al. Body fat distribution and risk of non-insulin-dependent diabetes mellitus in woman. The Nurses' Health Study. *Am J Epidemiol* 1997;145:614–519.
7. Chan JM, Rimm EB, Colditz GA, et al. Obesity, fat distribution, and weight gain as risk factors for clinical diabetes in men. *Diabetes Care* 1994;9:961–969.
8. Hillier TA, Pedula KL. Characteristics of an adult population with newly diagnosed type 2 diabetes: the relationship of obesity and age of onset. *Diabetes Care* 2001;24:1522–1527.
9. Mokdad AH, Ford ES, Bowman BA, et al. Prevalence of obesity, diabetes and obesity-related health risk factors, 2001. *JAMA* 2003;289:76–79.
10. Lyon CJ, Law RE, Hsueh WA. Minireview: adiposity, inflammation and atherogenesis. *Endocrinology* 2003;144:2195–2200.
11. Hubert HB, Feinleib M, McNamara PM, et al. Obesity as an independent risk factor for cardiovascular disease: a 26-year follow-up of participants in the Framingham Heart Study. *Circulation* 1983;67:968–977.
12. Peeples LH, Carpenter JW, Israel RG, et al. Alterations in low-density lipoproteins in subjects with abdominal adiposity. *Metabolism* 1989;38:1029–1036.
13. Ostlund RE Jr, Staten M, Kohrt WM, et al. The ratio of waist-to-hip circumference, plasma insulin level, and glucose intolerance as independent predictors of the HDL_2 cholesterol level in older adults. *N Engl J Med* 1990;322:229–234.
14. Vaughan RW, Conahan TJ III. Part I: Cardiopulmonary consequences of morbid obesity. *Life Sci* 1980;26:2119–2127.
15. MacMahon SW, Wilcken DEL, MacDonald GJ. The effect of weight reduction on left ventricular mass: a randomized controlled trial in young, overweight hypertensive patients. *N Engl J Med* 1986;314:334–339.
16. Billington CJ, Brigg JE, Grace M, et al. Effects of intracerebroventricular injection of neuropeptide Y on energy metabolism. *Am J Physiol* 1991;260: R321–R327.
17. Cowley MA, Smith RG, Diano S, et al. The distribution and mechanism of action of ghrelin in the CNS demonstrates a novel hypothalamic circuit regulating energy homeostasis. *Neuron* 2003;37:649–661.
18. Cummings DE, Weigle DS, Frayo RS, et al. Plasma ghrelin levels after diet-induced weight loss or gastric bypass surgery. *N Engl J Med* 2002;346: 1623–1630.
19. Grundy SM. Mechanism of cholesterol gallstones formation. *Semin Liver Dis* 1983;3:97–111.
20. Calle EE, Rodriguez C, Walker-Thurmond K, et al. Overweight, obesity and mortality from cancer in a prospectively studied cohort of US adults. *N Engl J Med* 2003;348:1625–1635.
21. Polonsky KS, Given BD, Hirsch L, et al. Quantitative study of insulin secretion and clearance in normal and obese subjects. *J Clin Invest* 1988;81: 435–441.
22. Peiris AN, Mueller RA, Smith GA, et al. Splanchnic insulin metabolism in obesity: influence of body-fat distribution. *J Clin Invest* 1986;78:1648–1657.
23. Bray GA, York DA. Hypothalamic and genetic obesity in experimental animals: an autonomic and endocrine hypothesis. *Physiol Rev* 1979;59:719–809.
24. Wang ZL, Bennet WM, Wang RM, et al. Evidence of a paracrine role of neuropeptide-Y in the regulation of insulin release from pancreatic islets of normal and dexamethasone treated rats. *Endocrinology* 1994;135:200–206.
25. Fan W, Dinulescu DM, Butler AA, et al. The central melanocortin system can directly regulate serum insulin levels. *Endocrinology* 2000;141:3072–3079.
26. Danforth E Jr, Horton ES, O'Connell M, et al. Dietary-induced alterations in thyroid hormone metabolism during overnutrition. *J Clin Invest* 1979;64: 1336–1347.
27. Glass AR. Endocrine aspects of obesity. *Med Clin North Am* 1989;73:139–160.
28. Stanik S, Dornfeld LP, Maxwell MH, et al. The effect of weight loss on reproductive hormones in obese men. *J Clin Endocrinol Metab* 1981;53:828–832.
29. Kirschner MA, Samojlik E, Drejka M, et al. Androgen-estrogen metabolism in women with upper body versus lower body obesity. *J Clin Endocrinol Metab* 1990;70:473–479.
30. Glass AR, Dahms WT, Abraham G, et al. Secondary amenorrhea in obesity: etiologic role of weight-related androgen excess. *Fertil Steril* 1978;30:243–244.
31. Poretsky L. On the paradox of insulin-induced hyperandrogenism in insulin-resistant states. *Endocr Rev* 1991;12:3–13.
32. Kay TJ, Allen NE, Verkasalo PK, et al. Energy balance and cancer: the role of sex hormones. *Proc Nutr Soc* 2001;60:81–89.
33. Crapo L. Cushing's syndrome: a review of diagnostic tests. *Metabolism* 1979;28:955–977.
34. Glass AR. Endocrine aspects of obesity. *Med Clin North Am* 1989;73:139–160.
35. Arch JRS, Ainsworth AT, Cawthorne MA, et al. Atypical β-adrenoceptor on brown adipocytes as target for antiobesity drugs. *Nature* 1984;309:163–165.
36. James WPT, Davies HL, Bailes J, et al. Elevated metabolic rates in obesity. *Lancet* 1978;1:1122–1125.
37. Ahima RS, Prabakaran D, Mantzoros C, et al. Role of leptin in the neuroendocrine response to fasting. *Nature* 1996;382:250–252.
38. Berne C, Fagius J, Niklasson F. Sympathetic response to oral carbohydrate administration: evidence from microelectrode nerve recordings. *J Clin Invest* 1989;84:1403–1409.
39. Sims EA, Danforth E. Expenditure and storage of energy in man. *J Clin Invest* 1987;79:1019–1025.
40. Jéquier E, Schutz Y. Energy expenditure in obesity and diabetes. *Diabetes Metab Rev* 1988;4:583–593.
41. Forbes GB, Welle SL. Lean body mass in obesity. *Int J Obes* 1983;7:99–107.
42. Flier JS, Cook KS, Usher P, et al. Severely impaired adipsin expression in genetic and acquired obesity. *Science* 1987;237:405–408.
43. Frederich RC Jr, Kahn BB, Peach MJ, et al. Tissue-specific nutritional regulation of angiotensinogen in adipose tissue. *Hypertension* 1992;4:339–344.
44. Zhang Y, Proenca R, Maffei M, et al. Positional cloning of the mouse obese gene and its human homologue. *Nature* 1994;372:425–432.
45. Coleman DL. Effects of parabiosis of obese with diabetes and normal mice. *Diabetologia* 1973;9:294–298.
46. Coleman Dl, Hummel KP. Effects of parabiosis of normal with genetically diabetic mice. *Am J Physiol* 1969;217:1298–1304.
47. Halaas JL, Gajiwala KS, Maffei M, et al. Weight reducing effects of the plasma protein encoded by the obese gene. *Science* 1995;269:543–546.

48. Baskin D, Breininger J, Schwartz M. Leptin receptor mRNA identifies a subpopulation of neuropeptide Y neurons activated by fasting in the rat hypothalamus. *Diabetes* 1999;48:828–833.
49. Montague CT, Farooqui IS, Whitehead JP, et al. Congenital leptin deficiency is associated with severe early onset obesity in humans. *Nature* 1997;387:903–908.
50. Farooqui IS, Jebb SA, Langmack G, et al. Effect of recombinant leptin therapy in a child with congenital leptin deficiency. *N Engl J Med* 1999;341:879–894.
51. Considine RV, Sinha MK, Heiman ML, et al. Serum immunoreactive-leptin concentrations in normal-weight and obese humans. *N Engl J Med* 1996;334: 292–295.
52. Flier JS. What's in a name? In search of leptin's physiologic role. *J Clin Endocrinol Metab* 1998;83:1407–1413.
53. Fruebis J, Tsao TS, Javorschi S, et al. Proteolytic cleavage product of 30-kDa adipocyte complement-related protein increases fatty acid oxidation in muscle and causes weight loss in mice. *Proc Natl Acad Sci U S A* 2001;98:2005–2010.
54. Berg AH, Cobs TP, Du X, et al. The adipocyte-secreted protein Acrp30 enhances hepatic insulin action. *Nat Med* 2001;8:947–953.
55. Yang WS, Lee WJ, Funahashi T, et al. Weight reduction increases plasma levels of an adipose-derived anti-inflammatory protein, adiponectin. *J Clin Endocrinol Metab* 2001;86:3815–3819.
56. Comuzzi AG, Funahashi T, Sonnenberg G, et al. The genetic basis of plasma variation in adiponectin, a global endophenotype for obesity and the metabolic syndrome. *J Clin Endocrinol Metab* 2001;86:4321–4325.
57. Bujalska IJ, Kumar S, Stewart PM. Does central obesity reflect "Cushing's disease on the omentum"? *Lancet* 1997;349:1210–1213.
58. Masuzaki H, Paterson J, Shinyama H, et al. A transgenic model of visceral obesity and the metabolic syndrome. *Science* 2001;294:2166–2170.
59. Elmquist JK. Hypothalamic pathways underlying the endocrine, autonomic, and behavioral effects of leptin. *Physiol Behav* 2001;74:703–708.
60. Clement K, Vaisse C, Lahlou N, et al. A mutation in the human leptin receptor gene causes obesity and pituitary dysfunction. *Nature* 1997;392:398–401.
61. Yen TT, Gill AM, Frigeri LG, et al. Obesity, diabetes and neoplasia in the yellow Avy/-mice: ectopic expression of the agouti gene. *FASEB J* 1994;8:481–488.
62. Mountjoy KG, Robbins LS, Mortrud MT, et al. The cloning of a family of genes that encode the melanocortin receptors. *Science* 1992;387:903–908.
63. Lu D, Willard D, Patel IR, et al. Agouti protein is the antagonist of the melanocyte-stimulating hormone receptor. *Nature* 1994;371:799–802.
64. Tsujii S, Bray GA. Acetylation alters the feeding response to MSH and beta-endorphin. *Brain Res Bull* 1989;23:165–169.
65. Huszar D, Lynch C, Fairchild-Huntress V, et al. Targeted disruption of the melanocortin-4 receptor results in obesity in mice. *Cell* 1997;88:131–141.
66. Shutter JR, Graham M, Kinsey AC, et al. Hypothalamic expression of ART, a novel gene related to agouti, is up-regulated in obese and diabetic mutant mice. *Genes Dev* 1997;11:593–602.
67. Vaisse C, Clement K, Guy-Grand B, et al. A frameshift mutation in human MC4R is associated with a dominant form of obesity. *Nat Genet* 1998;20: 113–114.
68. Yeo GS, Farooqui IS, Aminian S, et al. A frameshift mutation in MC4R associated with dominantly inherited human obesity. *Nat Genet* 1998;20:111–112.
69. Krude H, Biebermann H, Luck W, et al. Severe early-onset obesity, adrenal insufficiency and red hair pigmentation caused by POMC mutations in humans. *Nat Genet* 1998;9:155–157.
70. Whitehead JP, Humphreys PJ, Dib K, et al. Expression of the putative inhibitor of the insulin receptor tyrosine kinase PC-1 in dermal fibroblasts from patients with syndromes of severe insulin resistance. *Clin Endocrinol* (Oxf) 1997;47:65–70.
71. Berman Y, Mzhavia N, Polonskaia A, et al. Impaired prohormone convertase in Cpe (fat)/CpE(fat) mice. *J Biol Chem* 2001;276:1466–1473.
72. Qu D, Ludwig DS, Gammeltoft S, et al. A role for melanin concentrating hormone in the central regulation of feeding behavior. *Nature* 1996; 380:243–246.
73. Shimada M, Tritos NA, Lowell BB, et al. Mice lacking melanin concentrating hormone are hypophagic and lean. *Nature* 1998;396:670–674.
74. Zarjevski N, Cusin I, Vetter R, et al. Chronic intracerebroventricular neuropeptide-Y administration to normal rats mimics hormonal and metabolic changes of obesity. *Endocrinology* 1993;133:753–1758.
75. Erickson JC, Clegg KE, Palmiter RD. Sensitivity to leptin and susceptibility to seizures of mice lacking neuropeptide Y. *Nature* 1996;381:415–421.
76. Segal-Lieberman G, Trombly DJ, Juthani V, et al. NPY ablation in C57BL/6 mice leads to mild obesity and to an impaired refeeding response to fasting. *Am J Physiol Endocrinol Metab* 2003;284:E1131–E1139.
77. Erickson JC, Hollopeter G, Palmiter RD. Attenuation of the obesity syndrome of ob/ob mice by the loss of neuropeptide Y. *Science* 1996;274:1704–1707.
78. Bray GA. Afferent signals regulating food intake. *Proc Nutr Soc* 2000;59: 373–384.
79. Antin J, Gibbs J, Holt J, et al. Cholecystokinin elicits the complete behavioral sequence of satiety in rats. *J Comp Physiol Psychol* 1975;89:784–790.
80. Smith GP, Gibbs J. Cholecystokinin: a putative satiety signal. *Pharmacol Biochem Behav* 1975;3:135–138.
81. Matson CA, Wiater MF, Kujiper JL, et al. Synergy between leptin and cholecystokinin (CCK) to control daily caloric intake. *Peptides* 1997;18:1275–1278.
82. Ariyasu H, Tkaya K, Tagami Y, et al. Stomach is a major source of circulating ghrelin and feeding state determines plasma ghrelin-like immunoreactivity levels in humans. *J Clin Endocrinol Metab* 2001;86:4753–4578.
83. Tschop M, Wawarta R, Riepl RL, et al. Post-prandial decrease of circulating human ghrelin levels. *J Endocrinol Invest* 2001;24:RC19–RC21.
84. Wren AM, Small CJ, Abbott CR, et al. Ghrelin causes hyperphagia and obesity in rats. *Diabetes* 2001;50:2540–2547.
85. Tschop M, Weyer C, Tataranni PA, et al. Circulating ghrelin levels are decreased in human obesity. *Diabetes* 2001;50:707–709.
86. Meeran K, O'Shea D, Edwards CM, et al. Repeated intracerebroventricular administration of glucagon-like peptide-1-(7-36) amide or exendin-(9-39) alters body weight in the rat. *Endocrinology* 1999;140:244–250.
87. Larsen PJ, Fledelius C, Knudsen LB, et al. Systemic administration of the long-acting GLP-1 derivative NN2211 induces lasting and reversible weight loss in both normal and obese rats. *Diabetes* 2001;50:2530–2539.
88. Batterham RL, Cowley MA, Small CJ, et al. Gut hormone PYY(3-36) physiologically inhibits food intake. *Nature* 2002;418:595–597.
89. Baura G, Foster DM, Porte D Jr, et al. Saturable transport of insulin from plasma into the central nervous system of dogs in vivo: a mechanism for regulated delivery to the brain. *J Clin Invest* 1993;92:1824–1830.
90. Woods S, Lotter E, McKay L, et al. Chronic intracerebroventricular infusion of insulin reduces food intake and body weight of baboons. *Nature* 1979;282: 503–505.
91. Bruning JC, Gautham D, Burks DJ, et al. Role of brain insulin receptor in control of body weight and reproduction. *Science* 2000;289:2066–2067.
92. Lowell BB, Spiegleman BM. Towards a molecular understanding of adaptive thermogenesis. *Nature* 2000;404:652–660.
93. Ricquier D, Buillaud F. Mitochondrial uncoupling proteins: from mitochondria to the regulation of energy balance. *J Physiol* 2000;529:3–10.
94. James WPT, Trayhurn P. Thermogenesis and obesity. *BMJ* 1981;37:43–48.
95. Blaza S, Garrow JS. Thermogenic response to temperature, exercise and food stimuli in lean and obese women, studied by 24 h direct calorimetry. *Br J Nutr* 1983;49:171–180.
96. Tappy L, Felber JP, Jéquier E. Energy and substrate metabolism in obesity and postobese state. *Diabetes Care* 1991;14:1180–1188.
97. Leibel RL, Rosenbaum M, Hirsch J. Changes in energy expenditure resulting from altered body weight. *N Engl J Med* 1995;332:621–628.
98. Rothwell NJ, Stock MJ. Effect of environmental temperature on energy balance and thermogenesis in rats fed normal or low protein diets. *J Nutr* 1987;117:833–847.
99. Bouchard C, Tremblay A, Despres JD, et al. The response to long-term overfeeding in identical twins. *N Engl J Med* 1990;322:1477–1482.
100. Nicholls DG, Locke RM. Thermogenic mechanisms in brown fat. *Physiol Rev* 1984;64:1–64.
101. Simonsen L, Bulow J, Madsen J, et al. Thermogenic response to epinephrine in the forearm and abdominal subcutaneous adipose tissue. *Am J Physiol* 1992;263:E850–E855.
102. Levine JA, Eberhard NL, Jensen MD. Role of nonexercise activity in resistance to fat gain in humans. *Science* 1999;283:212–214.
103. Snitker S, Tararanni PA, Ravussin E. Spontaneous physical activity in a respiratory chamber is correlated to habitual physical activity. *Int J Obes Relat Metab Disord* 2001;25:1481–1486.
104. Leibel RL, Hirsch J. Diminished energy requirements in reduced-obese patients. *Metabolism* 1984;33:164–170.
105. Bray GA, Gray DS. Treatment of obesity: an overview. *Diabetes Metab Rev* 1988;4:653–679.
106. Yang M-U, Van Itallie TB. Composition of weight lost during short-term weight reduction: metabolic responses of obese subjects to starvation and low-calorie ketogenic and nonketogenic diets. *J Clin Invest* 1976;58: 722–730.
107. Passmore R, Strong JA, Ritchie FJ. The chemical composition of the tissue lost by obese patients on a reducing regimen. *Br J Nutr* 1958;12:113–122.
108. Howard AN. The historical development, efficacy and safety of very-low-calorie diets. *Int J Obes* 1981;5:195–208.
109. Sours HE, Frattali VP, Brand CD, et al. Sudden death associated with very low calorie weight reduction regimens. *Am J Clin Nutr* 1981;34:453–461.
110. Vertes V, Genuth SM, Hazelton IM. Supplemented fasting as a large scale outpatient program. *JAMA* 1977;238:2151–2153.
111. Amatruda JM, Richeson JF, Welle SL, et al. The safety and efficacy of a controlled low energy (very-low-calorie) diet in the treatment of non-insulin dependent diabetes and obesity. *Arch Intern Med* 1988;148:873–877.
112. Miller DS, Parsonage S. Resistance to slimming: adaptation or illusion? *Lancet* 1975;1:773–775.
113. Wadden TA, Foster GD, Letizia KA, et al. Long-term effects of dieting on resting metabolic rate in obese outpatients. *JAMA* 1990;264:707–711.
114. McManus K, Antinoro L, Sacks F. A randomized controlled trial of a moderate-fat, low-energy diet compared with a low fat, low-energy diet for weight loss in overweight adults. *Int J Obes Relat Metab Disord* 2001;25: 1503–1511.
115. Spieth LE, Harnish JD, Lenders CM, et al. A low glycemic index diet in the treatment of pediatric obesity. *Arch Pediatr Adolesc Med* 2000;154:947–951.
116. Segal KR, Pi-Sunyer FX. Exercise and obesity. *Med Clin North Am* 1989;73:217–236.
117. Seagle HM, Bessesen D, Hill JO. Effects of sibutramine on resting metabolic rate and weight loss in overweight women. *Obes Res* 1998;68:1180–1186.
118. Mun E, Blackburn G, Matthews J. Current status of medical and surgical therapy for obesity. *Gastroenterology* 2001;120:669–681.
119. Nightengale ML, Sarr MG, Kelly KA, et al. Prospective valuation of vertical banded gastro-plasty as the primary operation for morbid obesity. *Mayo Clin Proc* 119;66:773–782.

CHAPTER 32

Treatment of Obesity

Xavier Pi-Sunyer

The recommendation for treating obesity is based on two premises. The first is that weight can be lost and that, once lost, the lower weight can be maintained. The second is that this improves health. The evidence suggests that both of these are true (1,2). A loss of 10% of baseline weight can be achieved and maintained (2). But losing weight and particularly maintaining weight loss is very difficult and often discouraging, and the failure rate is high. Given our still-limited knowledge of the etiology of obesity, the primary emphasis must be on self-control, and the primary agent for change is the patient, not the physician. Motivation and commitment from the patient are required, but the support, understanding, and knowledge of the physician are also extremely helpful.

Because physicians are accustomed to pharmacologic solutions for most of the diseases they treat, they are not well attuned to the tedious task of slow, difficult weight loss, with its plateaus, relapses, and disappointing statistics. As a result, other health professionals have become involved in treatment. Dietitians, exercise physiologists, psychologists, social workers, and nurses advise and treat patients who want to lose weight. While these other professionals can be very helpful and often are more effective, a physician should monitor the weight-loss program and treat any other associated risk factors and health problems that are present or may develop.

The assessment of obesity can be rapid and easy. A physician usually requires nothing more than a visual inspection to determine the need for weight loss. However, for a more quantitative assessment, there are simple techniques for categorizing and following a patient. The body mass index (BMI) is a useful guideline. It is calculated by dividing the weight in kilograms by the height in meters squared (kg/m^2) (3). It can also be found from a table relating height and weight to BMI (Table 32.1). There is a fairly good correlation between BMI and body fat (4). However, this correlation is far from perfect, and very athletic persons can be misclassified due to their increased muscularity, although there are very few such disparities. Normal, overweight, and obese categories of BMI are shown in Table 32.2. The upper limit of the recommended BMI range is set at 25 because the mortality curve begins to increase at higher BMI values (5). There has been some argument that the BMI threshold should be set higher in some groups (women, older persons) and lower in others, such as Asians. However, the BMI of 25 is a reasonable and useful compromise (6), alerting individuals and populations to increased health risk.

Obesity aggravates or precipitates a number of other risk factors and diseases, including insulin resistance, impaired glucose tolerance, diabetes mellitus, hypertension, dyslipidemia, coronary heart disease, congestive heart failure, thromboembolic disease, restrictive lung disease, sleep apnea, gout, degenerative arthritis, gallbladder disease, and infertility (7,8) (Table 32.3). In cases in which one or more of these conditions are present, more stringent standards of weight seem appropriate (9). Although the loss of weight is likely to ameliorate any associated conditions, therapy targeted specifically for these disorders is also often necessary.

The physician also needs to assess body-fat distribution. An excessive amount of fat in the trunk (central fat, upper-body fat) carries more health risk than does fat on the lower body (peripheral fat, lower-body fat). Central fat is independently associated with risk factors such as insulin resistance, hypertension, and dyslipidemia (10,11) and is an independent predictor of coronary heart disease and diabetes (12–15). A simple assessment can be done by measuring waist circumference (Table 32.2). Measuring waist circumference is described in Figure 32.1.

Weight gain develops because energy intake exceeds energy expenditure. Once obesity supervenes, however, there may be a new weight stability, with caloric intake becoming equivalent once again to caloric expenditure. For a person to lose weight, energy intake must be decreased and/or energy expenditure increased to disequilibrate the energy balance equation and create a caloric deficit.

TABLE 32.1. Body Mass Index Chart[a]

	Body mass index																
	19	20	21	22	23	24	25	26	27	28	29	30	31	32	33	34	35
	Body weight (pounds)																
Height (inches)																	
58	91	96	100	105	110	115	119	124	129	134	138	143	148	153	158	162	167
59	94	99	104	109	114	119	124	128	133	138	143	148	153	158	163	168	173
60	97	102	107	112	118	123	128	133	138	143	148	153	158	163	168	174	179
61	100	106	111	116	122	127	132	137	143	148	153	158	164	169	174	180	185
62	104	109	115	120	126	131	136	142	147	153	158	164	169	175	180	186	191
63	107	113	118	124	130	135	141	146	152	158	163	169	175	180	186	191	197
64	110	116	122	128	134	140	145	151	157	163	169	174	180	186	192	197	204
65	114	120	126	132	138	144	150	156	162	168	174	180	186	192	198	204	210
66	118	124	130	136	142	148	155	161	167	173	179	186	192	198	204	210	216
67	121	127	134	140	146	153	159	166	172	178	185	191	198	204	211	217	223
68	125	131	138	144	151	158	164	171	177	184	190	197	203	210	216	223	230
69	128	135	142	149	155	162	169	176	182	189	196	203	209	216	223	230	236
70	132	139	146	153	160	167	174	181	188	195	202	209	216	222	229	236	243
71	136	143	150	157	165	172	179	186	193	200	208	215	222	229	236	243	250
72	140	147	154	162	169	177	184	191	199	206	213	221	228	235	242	250	258
73	144	151	159	166	174	182	189	197	204	212	219	227	235	242	250	257	265
74	148	155	163	171	179	186	194	202	210	218	225	233	241	249	256	264	272
75	152	160	168	176	184	192	200	208	216	224	232	240	248	256	264	272	279
76	156	164	172	180	189	197	205	213	221	230	238	246	254	263	271	279	287

[a]To use the table, find the appropriate height in the left-hand column. Move across to a given weight. The number at the top of the column is the BMI at that height and weight. Pounds have been rounded off. From National Heart, Lung and Blood Institute. Clinical guidelines on the identification, evaluation, and treatment of overweight and obesity in adults—the evidence report. *Obes Res* 1998;6[Suppl 2]:51S–210S, with permission.

TABLE 32.2. Classification of Overweight and Obesity by Body-Mass Index, Waist Circumference, and Associated Disease Risk

Classification	BMI (kg/m^2)	Obesity class	Disease risk[a] relative to normal weight and waist circumference: M <102 cm (≤40 in) W <88 cm (≤35 in)	Disease risk[a] relative to normal weight and waist circumference: M >102 cm (>40 in) W >88 cm (>35 in)
Underweight	≤18.5		—	—
Normal[b]	18.5–24.9		—	—
Overweight	25.0–29.9		Increased	High
Obese	30.0–34.9	I	High	Very high
	35.0–39.9	II	Very high	Very high
Extremely obese	≥40	III	Extremely high	Extremely high

BMI, body mass index; M, men; W, women.
[a]Disease risk for type 2 diabetes mellitus, hypertension, and cardiovascular disease.
[b]Increased waist circumference can also be a marker for increased risk even in persons of normal weight.
From the National Heart, Lung and Blood Institute. Clinical guidelines on the identification, evaluation, and treatment of overweight and obesity in adults—the evidence report. *Obes Res* 1998;6[Suppl 2]:51S–210S, with permission.

TABLE 32.3. Diseases Associated with Obesity

Diabetes mellitus
Hypertension
Coronary heart disease
Thromboembolic disease
Restrictive lung disease
Sleep apnea
Degenerative arthritis
Gallbladder disease
Dyslipidemia
Cancer: endometrial, breast, prostate, colon

Body mass index																		
36	37	38	39	40	41	42	43	44	45	46	47	48	49	50	51	52	53	54
Body weight (pounds)																		
172	177	181	186	191	196	201	205	210	215	220	224	229	234	239	244	248	253	258
178	183	188	193	198	203	208	212	217	222	227	232	237	242	247	252	257	262	267
184	189	194	199	204	209	215	220	225	230	235	240	245	250	255	261	266	271	276
190	195	201	206	211	217	222	227	232	238	243	248	254	259	264	269	275	280	285
196	202	207	213	218	224	229	235	240	246	251	256	262	267	273	278	284	289	295
203	208	214	220	225	231	237	242	248	254	259	265	270	278	282	287	293	299	304
209	215	221	227	232	238	244	250	256	262	267	273	279	285	291	296	302	308	314
216	222	228	234	240	246	252	258	264	270	276	282	288	294	300	306	312	318	324
223	229	235	241	247	253	260	266	272	278	284	291	297	303	309	315	322	328	334
230	236	242	249	255	261	268	274	280	287	293	299	306	312	319	325	331	338	344
236	243	249	256	262	269	276	282	289	295	302	308	315	322	328	335	341	348	354
243	250	257	263	270	277	284	291	297	304	311	318	324	331	338	345	351	358	365
250	257	264	271	278	285	292	299	306	313	320	327	334	341	348	355	362	369	376
257	265	272	279	286	293	301	308	315	322	329	338	343	351	358	365	372	379	386
265	272	279	287	294	302	309	316	324	331	338	346	353	361	368	375	383	390	397
272	280	288	295	302	310	318	325	333	340	348	355	363	371	378	386	393	401	408
280	287	295	303	311	319	326	334	342	350	358	365	373	381	389	396	404	412	420
287	295	303	311	319	327	335	343	351	359	367	375	383	391	399	407	415	423	431
295	304	312	320	328	336	344	353	361	369	377	385	394	402	410	418	426	435	443

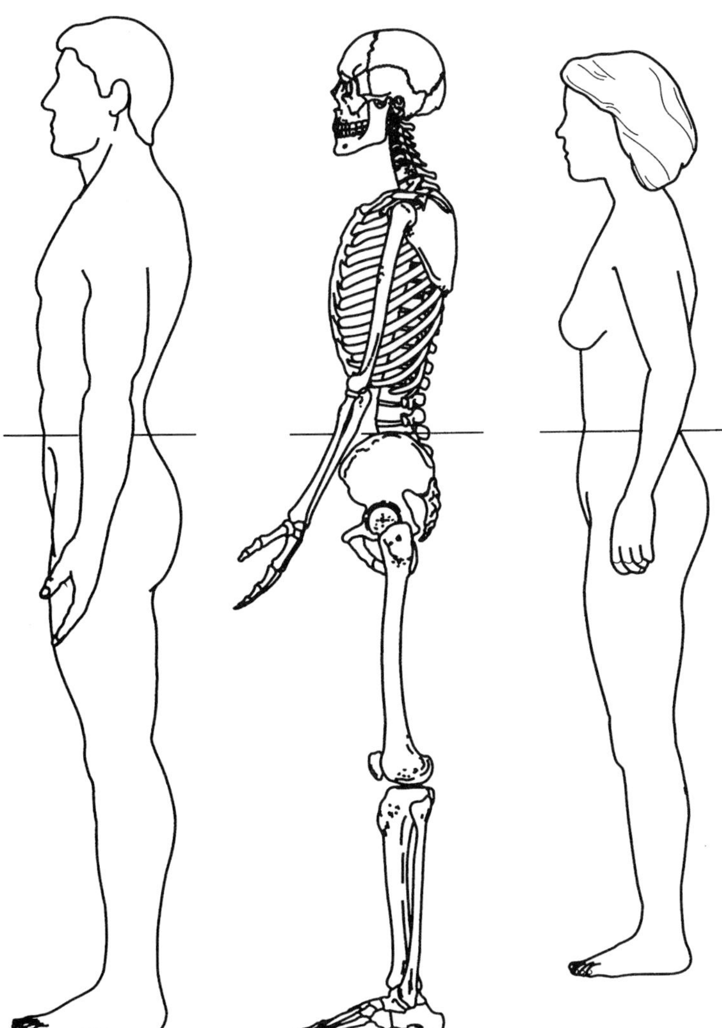

Figure 32.1. Measuring tape position for waist (abdominal) circumference. To define the level at which waist circumference is measured, a bony landmark is first located. The subject stands and the examiner, positioned at the right of the subject, palpates the upper hip bone to locate the right iliac crest. Just above the uppermost lateral border of the right iliac crest, a horizontal mark is drawn, then crossed with a vertical mark on the midaxillary line. The measuring tape is placed in a horizontal plane around the abdomen at the level of this marked point on the right side of the trunk. The plane of the tape is parallel to the floor and the tape is snug, but does not compress the skin. The measurement is made at a normal minimal respiration. (From National Heart, Lung, and Blood Institute. Clinical guidelines on the identification, evaluation, and treatment of overweight and obesity in adults—the evidence report. *Obes Res* 1998;6[Suppl]51S–210S, with permission.)

WEIGHT LOSS CAN IMPROVE HEALTH

Intentional weight loss in obese persons has been shown to improve health in both epidemiologic and clinical intervention studies. Williamson et al. (16) have shown that intentional weight loss decreases both cardiovascular and overall mortality. Weight loss also decreases morbidity (17).

Short-term studies have demonstrated that weight loss resulting from low-calorie diets, very-low-calorie diets, anorectic drugs, or bypass surgery is associated with increased insulin sensitivity, improved insulin secretion by islet cells, decreased hepatic glucose production, and improved glucose disposal (1,18–23). Wing et al. (24) conducted a long-term study in which diabetic patients lost an average of 5.6 ± 4.0 kg during the active intervention phase and maintained a weight loss of 4.5 ± 7.5 kg at 1 year. Those who were most successful in losing weight had significant improvements in fasting blood glucose and glycosylated hemoglobin values at 1 year even though they remained 20% above ideal body weight at the end of the study. Reductions in insulin dose or oral hypoglycemic medication were made for 100% of patients who lost 6.9 to 13.6 kg, 46% of those who lost 2.4% to 6.8 kg, and 40% of those who lost 0 to 2.3 kg. In the United Kingdom Prospective Diabetes Study (UKPDS) study (25), the response to diet was studied in 3,044 patients with newly diagnosed type 2 diabetes. Their mean fasting plasma glucose level was 12.1 ± 3.7 mmol/L. The investigators determined that the weight loss needed to achieve normalization was 16% of ideal body weight in patients with initial fasting plasma glucose levels of 6 to 8 mmol/L, 21% in those with levels of 8 to 10 mmol/L, 28% in those with levels of 10 to 12 mmol/L, 35% in those with levels of 12 to 14 mmol/L, and 41% in those with levels greater than 14.0 mmol/L. At the 15-month assessment, 482 patients maintained normal fasting plasma glucose levels. On average, they had slightly lower fasting plasma glucose levels at study entry and had lost more weight than did other patients (25). After 3 months, 742 patients achieved normal fasting plasma glucose levels. However, it is important to remember that there will be nonresponders, and obese individuals who remain hyperglycemic after a weight loss of 2.3 to 9.1 kg are unlikely to improve with further weight loss and should be considered for treatment with hypoglycemic agents (26).

Weight loss through diet and exercise can reduce the risk of the conversion of impaired glucose tolerance to frank diabetes. This has been shown in studies in China (27), Finland (28), and the United States (29). In the Diabetes Prevention Program in the United States, which studied more than 4,000 patients over 5 years, the progression to diabetes was decreased by 58% (29).

Ross and Rissanen (30) have shown effects of diet and exercise on insulin sensitivity, preferential loss of visceral fat, and blood pressure. The effect of weight loss on hypertension has now been documented in a number of randomized clinical trials. Long-term studies have confirmed the effectiveness of weight reduction in lowering blood pressure and enabling some patients to become normotensive without the use of antihypertensive drugs and for others to reduce the dosage of required drugs or the number of drugs taken (31–42). The marked improvement found in many unmedicated hypertensive patients suggests that weight reduction should be the initial treatment for an obese person with hypertension. In patients for whom elimination of antihypertensive drugs is not a realistic goal, weight loss can potentiate the effects of drug therapy (40,41,43).

The dyslipidemia of obesity is characterized by high triglycerides, reduced high-density lipoprotein (HDL) cholesterol, and small dense low-density lipoprotein (LDL) particles (44,45). With weight loss, triglycerides fall, HDL cholesterol rises, and small dense LDL particles become larger and less atherogenic (45). Short-term studies have confirmed the value of behavioral, low-calorie diet, and very-low-calorie diet interventions in decreasing total and LDL cholesterol levels and the HDL/LDL ratio and lowering triglyceride levels (46–50). Additional long-term studies, of greater than 1 year, have also been done and have shown a sustained improvement in the lipid profile of overweight and obese patients (33,36,51–54). Although some of these lipid changes are relatively small, they should not serve as a disincentive to embarking on a weight-loss program, because even modest improvements in lipid levels are associated with a decreased risk of cardiovascular disease (1,17,55).

Few trials have explicitly addressed the relationship between weight loss and cardiovascular disease per se. A 10-year study of 2,500 patients from the Framingham Study cohort conducted by Higgins et al. (36) found a positive association between weight loss and cardiovascular disease, although this finding almost certainly results from the fact that the study does not distinguish disease-related involuntary weight loss from voluntary weight reduction.

Respiratory function is often impaired in obese individuals because of reduced lung volume, altered respiratory patterns, and decreased respiratory system compliance (7). Obesity-hyperventilation syndrome and sleep apnea are the most common respiratory disorders associated with severe obesity (8). Short-term studies of sleep apnea have indicated that weight loss resulting from low-calorie diets or gastric bypass surgery is associated with a marked reduction in apneic episodes and night awakenings and with a general improvement in sleep patterns (56–61).

Obesity is often associated with an increased risk of gout (62), as is increased central fat distribution (63). When persons lose weight, their uric acid levels may initially increase (1,64), but precipitation of gout by weight-loss therapy in asymptomatic patients is uncommon (65). Uric acid levels rarely become high enough to necessitate medical treatment (66). Occasionally, large amounts of uricosuria and a predisposition to renal uric acid stone formation occur. When the appropriate diagnosis is made, urine alkalinization is the treatment of choice.

Cross-sectional studies have repeatedly found an association between increasing weight and increased prevalence of osteoarthritis of the knee (67–69) and, to a much lesser extent, of the hip (70). There have been just a few studies that have related weight reduction to the reduction of the onset of arthritis (71) or to the improvement of arthritic symptoms (72).

Obese persons are at a greater risk for developing gallstones than are persons of normal weight, probably because their bile is more highly saturated with cholesterol, their gallbladders are larger and less contractile, and their triglyceride levels tend to be higher (7). An association between loss of large amounts of weight and gallstone formation has been reported, although this finding has not been observed consistently (73–76). However, once individuals lose weight, their risk of gallstone formation and of cholecystitis decreases because the risk factors previously cited improve.

Available data suggest that obese persons may have a greater tendency to depression than do lean persons, but there are no data to suggest that obese persons are more prone to psychosis (77,78). The depression generally improves with weight loss (79).

GOALS OF THERAPY

Obesity is associated with increased health risk, and this is especially so in patients with diabetes (80). The goals of therapy are to improve health risk. There are two ways to approach the risk—one is to modify weight and the other is to focus on and try to modify other health-related variables (81). Focusing on other health-related variables can be done with individuals for whom the initiation of a weight-loss program seems impossible or impracticable.

It is common for patients who are beginning a weight-loss program to have faulty and unrealistic beliefs about how much and how rapidly they can lose weight. It is important to counsel them in this regard to prevent disappointment and attrition.

Most obese persons wish to lose all of their excess weight and return to normal weight (82). While this may be realistic for someone whose BMI is close to normal (26 to 30), it is not realistic for individuals whose BMIs are higher. For these persons, a weight loss goal should be set for a reduction of 10% to 15% from their present baseline weight (2) for a number of reasons. First, it is very difficult for most persons to lose more than this, and it is consequently damaging for their self-image, sense of success, and satisfaction when they set goals that are unreasonable and generally unattainable. Second, if a patient is pushed to lose more, such as can occur with very-low-calorie (300 to 500 kcal) diets, experience has shown that, while persons can lose weight quickly, they will generally regain it almost as quickly (83).

BEHAVIORAL THERAPY

The traditional technique of handing a patient a printed description of a 1,200- or a 1,500-kcal diet, complete with specific menus and specific portion sizes, and telling him or her to increase exercise without further instruction, has generally been unsuccessful. With inadequate education and support, patients quickly abandon such programs and never increase their activity.

In an effort to prevent such failure, the use of behavioral therapy has increased. Approaches to changing behavior began with Ferster et al. (84) and were greatly popularized by Stuart (85). The goal of such therapy was to modify maladaptive eating by improving environmental control. The aim was to change eating behavior (86). This approach was found to be too narrow, and more recent adaptations have recognized obesity as much more complex than just maladaptive eating, with influences from genetic, physiologic, psychological, and social factors (87). The newer approaches have targeted not only eating but also physical activity. In the 1970s, cognitive-behavioral techniques were initiated (88–90). A number of psychologists have written about these treatment techniques (91–95).

Table 32.4 summarizes weight losses in randomized clinical trials that combined behavior modification with moderate caloric restriction (96). It can be seen that there has been an improvement in weight loss over time, but generally because treatment programs are running longer, not because there is an increase in weight loss per week. On average, weight loss is close to 10% from baseline. It is depressing, however, that the baseline weight of the individuals being treated has increased dramatically, demonstrating how serious the problem of obesity is in the United States. The maintenance of the weight loss is difficult. While the majority are able to maintain their weight loss for at least a year, many regain most of their weight over the next 3 to 5 years (96,97). This seems to occur even when specific maintenance strategies are used in the program (98,99). It is interesting to note that some of the most successful results of behavioral programs have been reported in childhood obesity (100–102). Whether this is related to less fixed lifestyle habits at that age is not clear.

Behavioral change in a patient is attempted in small, possible, and reasonable steps with the help of a physician or other health professional. Behavioral change requires knowledge of nutrition, physical activity, and self. Nutritional knowledge means becoming familiar with the caloric content and energy density of foods, portion sizes, and less calorically dense cooking techniques. Knowledge about physical activity means learning about one's own capabilities and physical weaknesses and how to increase the time and the intensity of activity progressively and safely. Self-knowledge is crucial for dealing with individual maladaptive eating and activity behavior (103).

The first step in self-knowledge is to describe for oneself one's eating and activity behavior. Patients need to self-monitor so they will become aware of the amount, time, and circumstances of their eating and of their activity (or inactivity) patterns. This increased awareness is required so that corrective measures can be attempted. Once specific problems are identified, the next step is to begin to effect changes. Typical stimuli that lead to maladaptive eating behavior would be contact with persons or situations that increase stress, anxiety, or hostility. The particular stimuli should be identified, and patients need to make an effort to distance themselves from them. A further behavioral step is to develop techniques to control the act of eating and what is eaten. The most important of these is the technique of paying close attention to the act of eating. Others include becoming aware of the places where the person eats, the speed of eating, the portion sizes, and the frequency of eating. Some therapists have suggested that prompt reinforcement of behaviors that delay or control eating is very helpful. This would mean setting up some reward system (e.g., money, entertainment, and praise) as positive reinforcement for improved behavior (103).

TABLE 32.4. Summary Analysis of Selected Studies from 1974 to 1990 Providing Treatment by Behavior Therapy and Conventional Reducing Diet

Parameter	1974	1978	1984	1985–1987	1988–1990
Number of studies included	15	17	15	13	5
Sample size	53.1	54.0	71.3	71.6	21.2
Initial weight (kg)	73.4	87.3	88.7	87.2	91.9
Initial % overweight	49.4	48.6	48.1	56.2	59.8
Duration of treatment (wk)	8.4	10.5	13.2	15.6	21.3
Weight loss (kg)	3.8	4.2	6.9	8.4	8.5
Loss per week (kg)	0.5	0.4	0.5	0.5	0.4
Attrition (%)	11.4	12.9	10.6	13.8	21.8
Duration of follow-up (wk)	15.5	30.3	58.4	48.3	53.0
Loss at follow-up	4.0	4.1	4.4	5.3	5.6

Adapted from Wadden TA, Bartlett S. Very low calorie diets: an overview and appraisal. In: Wadden TA, Van Itallie TB, ed. *Treatment of the severely obese patient.* New York: Guilford Press, 1992:44–79, with permission.

There has been an effort in recent years to incorporate relapse-prevention strategies into the treatment effort (92, 104–106). While it is not clear that this has been very successful, it points to the need to maintain an effort even though there may well be missteps along the way.

The program needs to be adapted to each patient's goals and skills rather than to a physician's idea of how a patient should behave. This individualization of treatment is crucial for enhancing the chances of success in a motivated person.

The advantage of a behavioral approach is that both the patient and the therapist (which may include the group) focus on specific variables that seem to govern a particular person's behavior. Central to a behavioral analysis is the search by a patient and therapist for solutions to soluble, concrete problems. They may be relatively modest. This simplifies and focuses therapy. It has been the experience in our weight-control program that conducting behavioral therapy in a group setting is highly efficacious. The group setting leads to focused inquiry, mutual support, and group encouragement that are conducive to success. Many physicians have embraced group therapy as a way of reaching more patients effectively at lower cost.

Another advantage of a behavioral approach is that it gives patients the major responsibility for the weight-loss strategy so that, with success, they can attribute increased power to themselves. The treatment is reinforced when patients believe that positive results are attributable to their own efforts, and they gain increased confidence and a desire to continue.

The most important advantage of a behavioral approach is that it allows patients to change habits under the natural social and environmental conditions that they live in day to day. Thus, the new habits learned during weight loss can be continued during the very difficult period of weight maintenance, which is lifelong. This may be more difficult in programs in which the patient is taken off natural foods for a time and placed on a liquid diet and then is suddenly confronted with a return to regular food and the need to modify behavior. The learning may come too little and too late and may lead to failure and weight regain. Appropriate safeguards must be called on to prevent this, such as early start of nutrition education and physical activity, with self-monitoring occurring as solid food is re-introduced. It must be remembered that a behavioral program produces the slowest initial weight loss because calorie reduction is not radical and patients are encouraged to eat a balanced and sensible diet. This helps the patient to develop a long-term view and strategy. For continuing success, a patient needs to remain in treatment not just until goal weight is achieved but also well into the weight-maintenance period.

WEIGHT GOALS

Years ago, the goal in weight loss was to return the patient to a normal weight, but this is no longer the case. The reason has been the inability of individuals to lower their weight to this level and then to maintain it. As a result, the aim has changed to that of attaining a "healthy weight," that is, a weight that lowers health risk. Thus, the National Heart, Lung and Blood Institute (NHLBI) Evidence Report (2) states that there is evidence that one can lose and maintain a loss of 10% from baseline weight. Blackburn (107) has championed this approach, suggesting aiming at a 10% weight loss. This is also the approach in the report by the Institute of Medicine (108).

Thus, the evidence suggests that it is better to aim for a slow, attainable, and sustainable weight loss. One kilogram of lost weight, which will be part fat and part lean body mass, is equivalent to about 7,000 kcal. A caloric deficit of 700 kcal per day results in a 1-kg weight loss in 10 days; if the deficit is 1,000 kcal, it will take 7 days to lose 1 kg; if the daily deficit is 500 kcal, 14 days. Initial weight loss may be a bit faster because a water diuresis can occur. A nutritional and exercise regimen of diet and exercise that creates a deficit of 500 to 1,000 kcal per day is reasonable (2,29). Thus, a man weighing 100 kg whose calorie intake to maintain weight is 2,800 kcal needs to reduce intake to between 1,800 and 2,300 kcal. Such a diet should enable him to lose between 0.5 and 1 kg per week, assuming that there is no change in physical activity. If his ideal body weight is 70 kg, it would take him between 30 and 60 weeks to reach this weight. A clear realization of the need for the sustained effort over time required to reach the goal that is set is important for keeping a patient motivated and positively reinforced. Also, as mentioned, the goal should not be set at ideal weight but at a percentage from initial baseline weight that is known to improve comorbid conditions and that can realistically be maintained long term (1,17). For the previous case example, the goal should be set at 85 to 90 kg.

NUTRITION

Nutritional change is the most important component of a weight-loss program. To lose weight successfully, obese persons must lower caloric intake and maintain a reduced intake indefinitely. The nutritional change must be within the framework of a patient's current cultural food habits and preferences. While this is sometimes impossible when dietary habits are so poor that a radical restructuring is required, in most patients compliance is better when familiar foods are suggested. Factors such as available cooking facilities, ethnic background, family requirements, and economic background should not be ignored. Documentation of food intake (e.g., diet records) is an invaluable method of tracking dietary pitfalls, patterns, and progress, but physicians must be aware of perfect records unaccompanied by weight loss. These should serve as a signal that a patient may not be ready to work seriously on weight loss.

Energy expenditure should be estimated since resting metabolic rates (RMR) are not usually available to the average physician because obtaining them is too difficult and too expensive. A formula such as the Harris-Benedict equation for calculating basal metabolic rate can be helpful in estimating energy requirement (Table 32.5) (109). Multiplying the value thus obtained for RMR by 1.4 gives a reasonable approximation of 24-hour energy expenditure for a typical sedentary obese individual in our society. It is important to stress, however, that this will only give an approximation and will need to be adapted for each individual patient (110). An appropriate caloric deficit should be discussed with the patient. For example, a 120-kg male with a calculated 24-hour expenditure of 3,000 kcal may choose to lose 1 kg per week on 2,500 kcal per day rather than 1.5 kg per

TABLE 32.5. Harris-Benedict Equation (Energy Requirements)

Men: $BEE = [66 + (6.2 \times W) + (12.7 \times H) - (6.8 \times A)]$
Women: $BEE = [655 + (4.3 \times W) + (14.3 \times H) - (4.7 \times A)]$

BEE, basal energy expenditure; W, weight in kg; H, height in cm; A, age in years. For weight gain of approximately 1 kg/week, an additional 100 kcal/day should be provided. From Johnson MM, Chin R Jr, Haponik EF. Nutrition, respiratory function, and disease. In: Shils M, Olson J, Shike M, et al., eds. *Modern nutrition in health and disease,* 9th ed. Baltimore: Williams & Wilkins, 1999:1473–1490, with permission.

week on 2,000 kcal per day because for him the quantity of food eaten per day takes priority over the rate of weight loss. Such decisions should be made jointly by the patient and physician to help promote long-term compliance. A diet should be adequate nutritionally because it will be continued indefinitely, and this is possible without vitamin and mineral supplements only for diets of 1,100 to 1,200 kcal per day or more. To achieve this, patients must be instructed in the need for micronutrient-rich foods that they may not be used to eating regularly. With very hypocaloric diets, the nutrients most likely to be in deficit are iron, folacin, vitamin B_6, and zinc. If levels of calories fall below 1,200, vitamin and mineral supplements are necessary and should be prescribed: A multivitamin/multimineral tablet once a day is enough. Calcium should be supplemented at 1,000 mg per day and vitamin D at 400 IU per day to prevent bone mineral loss (111). Other extra macrominerals (sodium, potassium, magnesium) are usually not necessary unless patients go on very-low-calorie diets (300 to 500 kcal).

During weight loss, the goal should be reduction of adipose, rather than lean, tissue. While there is always some obligate loss of lean body mass (112), it should be kept to a minimum. Lean body mass can generally be spared during weight loss with a protein intake of 1.0 to 1.5 g per kg ideal body weight (calculated from Table 32.1 using a BMI of 25). The dietary sources of protein should be of high biologic value (e.g., egg whites, fish, poultry, lean beef, and low-fat dairy products). A vegetarian diet is acceptable, but the concept of protein complementation to assure adequate intake of essential amino acids must be explained to the patient and encouraged (113). The remainder of calories should come from carbohydrate (preferably high-fiber foods) and fat. Although the macronutrient ratio of fat to carbohydrate can vary according to the patient's preferences, it is important to obtain the antiketogenic, micronutrient, high-fiber benefits of carbohydrate, which occur with at least 100 g per day, and to get adequate amounts of fat-soluble vitamins and essential fatty acids from dietary fat.

In weight reduction, the emphasis therefore should be on micronutrient-dense food choices and away from "empty-calorie" selections. A brief discussion of basic nutrition will help alert the patient to appropriate food choices for maximizing the caloric restriction. A patient must learn that alcohol and sweets do not carry essential micronutrients. These should be avoided because they provide little more than excess calories. It should be made clear that although some fats are less atherogenic than others, all fats are high-energy, low-micronutrient foods and should be restricted to less than 30% of the total daily calories. Gram for gram, pure fat has more than double the caloric concentration of carbohydrate or protein (9 kcal/g vs. 4 kcal/g). Because carbohydrate often absorbs water during cooking, the actual caloric density of hydrated carbohydrate on the plate may be as low as 1 to 2 kcal/g. Decreasing fat foods in the diet will provide a substantial caloric decrease. In general, high-fat spreads, condiments, sauces, and gravies are far more detrimental in a weight-reduction program than are bread, potatoes, pasta, or rice, although a patient, if not properly instructed, can substitute carbohydrates totally for any fat restriction and end up eating as many calories as previously.

Many of the more popular media-touted diets have little scientific basis and simply play upon vulnerable persons' desperation to lose weight. These diets often ignore the concept of balanced nutrition by totally eliminating or providing insufficient amounts of a particular macronutrient (e.g., protein, carbohydrate, or fat). In time, this can result in a concurrent micronutrient imbalance. Such diets are unsound, and if they are followed for any significant time period, as any serious weight-control diet must be, untoward health consequences such as electrolyte imbalances, deficiency syndromes, or protein-malnutrition can ensue (114).

Very-low-calorie liquid diets (300 to 500 kcal/day) are generally counterproductive if carried out for a long period (83). Although weight loss can be large on such diets, the results are usually short-lived (114). A return to pre-diet weight after solid foods are resumed is the rule. Unless such diets are undertaken in the context of a complete medically supervised, stepwise program in which the very-low-calorie diet is replaced after a few weeks by a higher-calorie balanced diet and an intensive behavior-modification program, they accomplish little except for periodic loss of water and electrolytes. Such diets need to provide adequate high-quality protein to prevent protein malnutrition and possible cardiac morbidity (115). It is better to recommend diets that are no lower than 800 kcal. These have been found to be as efficacious and are safer (116).

An understanding of the U.S. Department of Agriculture food pyramid (Fig. 32.2) (117) may help the patient to adhere to a diet balanced in micronutrients and vitamins. By selecting judiciously from the grain, fruit, and vegetable groups (1–3), cutting down on the number of servings of the meat, milk, and fat groups (4–6), the patient can obtain adequate nutrients with a hypocaloric diet. Group 1 provides carbohydrate, protein, thiamine, niacin, vitamin E, iron, phosphorus, magnesium, zinc, and copper; group 2 and 3 provide carbohydrate, vitamins A and C, iron and magnesium; group 5 provides protein, fat, vitamins A and D, magnesium, calcium, phosphorus, and zinc; and group 6 provides essential fatty acids.

Patients are encouraged to select a wide variety of foods within these six food groups to alleviate boredom and monotony and thereby enhance compliance. The number of servings per day from each group will vary according to the individual's caloric restriction and macronutrient breakdown. Since portion sizes are crucial, they should be explained in terms of common household measures (e.g., spoonfuls, cups, ounces) and with the aid of food models. A patient should not lose more than 1% of body weight per week (114).

A common mistake made by patients is that they think that once they lose weight they can liberalize their diet. This is not true; as energy expenditure decreases with weight loss, an individual will need to continue to limit calorie intake if he or she does not want to regain the weight. Thus, the dietary plan that has been created should be continued. Patients generally plateau with regard to weight loss at about 6 months into their treatment program (118). At that point, the increased exercise and the decreased calorie intake come into a new equilibrium and no more weight is lost. To lose further at that time requires a stricter diet, greater exercise activity, or both.

EXERCISE

Because physical activity expends calories, increasing it is logical for any weight-loss program. Obese persons are generally very inactive. Many of them, particularly the heavier ones, have trouble walking even short distances and climbing steps and tend to avoid such situations. By staying so sedentary, they are close to their resting metabolic rate for most of the day. Increased physical activity has a strong impact on insulin sensitivity and improving glucose tolerance (119). Kelly and Goodpaster reviewed eight randomized studies (119) and found an improvement in insulin action. Exercise training can elicit improvement in insulin action in obesity within 1 week of intervention. In a study that compared the effect of aerobic to resistance exercise, they were found to be equally effective (120). Higher-intensity exercise is more effective (121). There is strong epidemiologic evidence that phys-

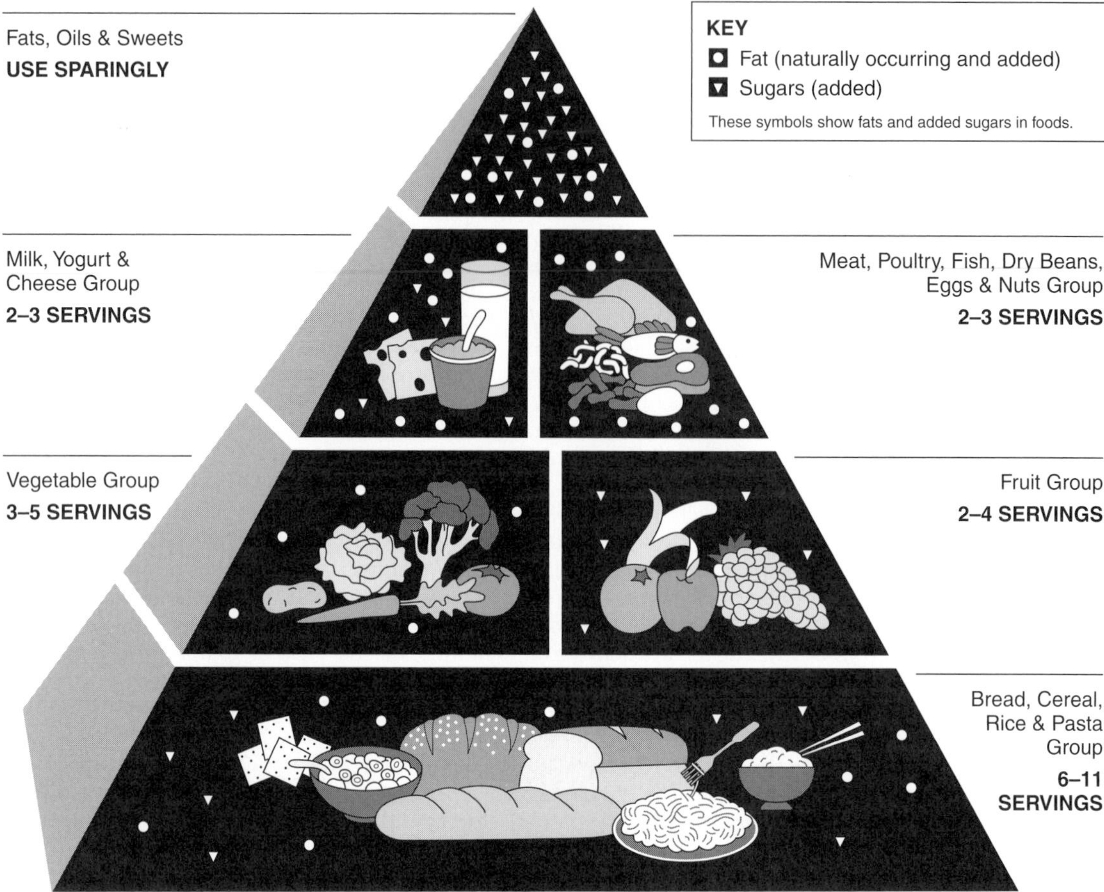

Figure 32.2. The US Department of Agriculture food pyramid. (From Center for Nutrition Policy. *The food guide pyramid.* Washington, DC: Department of Agriculture,1996. Report number: Home and Garden Bulletin 252.)

ical activity can reduce the risk of type 2 diabetes (120,122–127). Aerobic exercise also reduces blood pressure independent of change in weight. The blood-pressure effect depends on the initial blood pressure but not on initial BMI or age (128).

The importance of exercise in weight control programs has been widely debated. The NHLBI Expert Panel (2) reported that, in 10 of 12 studies that met their review criteria, subjects in the exercise study arm had larger weight losses than did the no-exercise controls. In a meta-analysis of studies, Garrow and Summerbell (129) came to the same conclusion. Table 32.6 shows the results of ten randomized clinical trials showing that exercise produces greater weight loss than the no-treatment control (130). One can then ask if exercise in combination with diet produces greater weight loss than diet alone. The NHLBI panel (2) found that 12 of 15 randomized clinical trials showed a greater weight loss (1.9 kg) and greater reduction in BMI (0.3 to 0.5 unit) in the group with combined diet and exercise than in the group with diet only. Reviewing 13 of these studies, Wing (130) found, however, that only 2 of the 13 showed a statistically significant difference in the weight loss between the group with diet alone and the group with diet plus exercise (Table 32.6). In four of the studies that had a diet plus resistance exercise training condition, there was again no statistically significant difference.

Another question is whether exercise in combination with diet can produce better maintenance of weight loss than diet alone. The NHLBI panel (2) found a 1.5- to 3-kg greater weight loss in the combined diet and exercise condition. Miller et al. (140) did a meta-analysis in which they found a nonsignificant difference of 6.6 kg vs. 8.6 kg in the diet vs. diet/exercise groups. Wing (130), in her review of six studies, found that two showed a significantly greater weight loss at 1 year for the diet/exercise group but that four others did not.

It may be that many of the persons on diet alone studied above started to exercise and the persons on exercise stopped, because these studies have all been analyzed by intent-to-treat criteria. There are data suggesting that those persons who exercise tend to maintain their weight better (141–143). To date, few have studied the effect of weight-resistance studies as opposed to aerobic exercise on weight loss and maintenance. Also, time requirements and intensity of exercise need to be better studied. Schoeller et al. (144) reported a requirement of 47 kilojoules per kilogram of body weight per day for weight maintenance after weight loss. Klem et al. (145), using data from the Weight Control Registry, reported that successful weight losers expend at least 2,800 kcal per week in physical activity, a number very similar to that found by Schoeller et al.

Obese persons must first be taught to walk, then to walk faster, and then, if possible, to run or bicycle or do aerobic dance or swim. An exercise program, however, should start slowly. An obese person who is pushed too rapidly can experience discomfort and subsequent avoidance. Careful observation for treatment of skin intertrigo, dependent edema, and foot or joint injuries is mandatory, particularly in obese diabetic patients who may have neuropathy and peripheral vascular disease.

The patient must learn how many calories are spent in various exercise activities. Table 32.7 lists some of these activities

TABLE 32.6. Weight Loss in Exercise-Alone Versus No-Treatment Control Group

Study	Duration	Exercise alone		Control		Significance[a]
		N	Weight loss	*N*	Weight loss	
Anderssen 1995 (131)	1 yr	49 M/F	−0.9 kg	43 M/F	+1.1 kg	S
Hammer 1989 (132)	4 mo	8 F	−6.7 kg	4 F	−5.8 kg	S
Helenius 1993 (133)	6 mo	39 M	−0.3 BMI	39 M	+0.3 BMI	S
Katzel[b] 1995 (134)	9 mo	49 M	−1%	18 M	+0.5%	NS
King[c] 1991 (135)	1 yr	29–35 F	−0.6 to +0.4 BMI	34 F	0 BMI	NS
		40–45 M	−0.9 to −0.2 BMI	41 M	+0.1 BMI	NS
Rönnemaa 1988 (136)	4 mo	13 M/F	−2.0 kg	12 M/F	+0.5 kg	S
Stefanick 1988 (137)	1 yr	43 F	−0.4 kg	45 F	+0.8 kg	NS
		47 M	−0.6 kg	46 M	+0.5 kg	NS
Verity 1989 (138)	4 mo	5 F	−2.1 kg	5 F	−2.9 kg	NS
Wood 1983 (139)	1 yr	48 M	−1.9 kg	33 M	+0.6 kg	S
Wood 1988 (52)	1 yr	47 M	−4.0 kg	42 M	+0.6 kg	S

S, significant; NS, not significant; BMI, body mass index.
[a]Significance of difference in weight loss for exercise vs control.
[b]Data interpreted from graph.
[c]This study included three exercise conditions: high-intensity group-based; high-intensity home-based; and low-intensity home-based. None differed in weight loss from controls.

TABLE 32.7. Approximate Energy Expenditure in Selected Activities for People of Different Weights

Activity	Energy expenditure (kcal/30 min) for indicated weight					
	110 lb	130 lb	150 lb	170 lb	190 lb	210 lb
Aerobic dancing						
Walking pace	99	114	132	150	168	186
Jogging pace	159	186	213	243	270	300
Running pace	204	240	276	315	351	387
Basketball	207	243	282	318	357	396
Canoeing—leisure	66	78	90	102	114	126
Canoeing—racing	156	183	210	237	267	294
Carpentry	78	93	105	120	135	147
Cycling—5.5 mph	96	114	132	147	165	183
Cycling—9.4 mph	150	17	204	231	258	285
Dancing—ballroom	78	90	105	117	132	144
Dancing—disco	156	183	210	237	267	294
Gardening	150	177	204	231	258	285
Golf	129	150	174	195	219	243
Judo	294	345	399	450	504	558
Lying or sitting down	33	39	45	51	57	63
Mopping floor	96	105	120	138	153	171
Running						
11.5 min/mi	204	240	276	315	351	387
9 min/mi	291	342	393	447	498	552
7 min/mi	366	417	468	522	573	624
5.5 min/mi	435	513	591	669	747	828
Skiing, cross-country	216	252	291	330	369	408
Standing quietly	39	45	51	57	66	72
Swimming						
Backstroke	255	300	345	390	435	486
Crawl	192	228	261	297	330	366
Table tennis	102	120	138	156	174	195
Tennis	165	192	222	252	282	312
Walking						
3 mph	102	114	126	138	153	165
4 mph	120	141	162	186	207	228

Adapted from Gutin B, Kessler G. *The high energy factor.* New York: Random House, 1983, with permission.

(146). However, most tables (including the one here) depicting caloric expenditure levels and type of activity have been compiled to reflect total caloric expenditure, not the amount above the resting metabolic rate. The actual caloric contribution of exercise is the difference between the calories expended per minute during exercise and the calories that a person would have expended just sitting or standing. It is instructive and often disappointing for patients to discover just how much exercise they must do to expend a significant number of calories. For instance, if an overweight woman's basal metabolic rate is 1,400 kcal per day, lying down awake she expends 1.1 kcal per minute; sitting, about 1.2 kcal per minute; walking slowly, about 1.9 kcal per minute; and walking on a treadmill at 4.0 miles per hour, 7.2 kcal per minute (147). Thus, the difference in caloric expenditure between sitting quietly and walking fast on a treadmill (at 4.0 miles per hour) is 6.0 kcal per minute. In an hour, the energy expended by walking 4 miles is only 360 calories higher than the subject would have expended just quietly sitting. A very significant and persistent commitment to exercise must be present for exercise to have any substantial effect on caloric balance and weight loss.

As a person loses weight, the energy expenditure required to carry his or her weight around decreases (147–149). As a result, for a given amount of time exercising, particularly if a person is carrying his or her weight, doing the same activity at the same intensity, less calories are lost. As a result, just to maintain energy expenditure at the same 24-hour level as before weight loss, more physical activity is required, either by increasing the amount of time or the intensity of the activity (148). This is a crucial point that must be explained to the patient; decreasing weight requires increasing activity because only maintaining activity similar to that before the weight loss results in a decreased energy expenditure.

FITNESS

It is known that unfit men have a higher cardiovascular mortality and all-cause mortality than do fit men, whether they are lean or obese (150–152). Decreased physical activity has been associated with an increased risk for diabetes, coronary heart disease, and stroke (122,153,154). At whatever level the BMI is in overweight individuals, it is important to advise increased physical activity. Exercise has been shown to improve lipid profiles (155), blood pressure (128), and insulin sensitivity (119).

PHARMACOTHERAPY

The combination of intense attempts at weight loss and of frustration at the difficulty of losing weight and maintaining it has led to a great interest in pharmacotherapy by patients and physicians. The renewed interest in pharmacotherapy is also an outgrowth of the recognition in recent years that obesity is a chronic disease with genetic underpinnings (156–158). Thus, the new thinking stresses the fact that a chronic disease cannot be cured but can be treated and that treatment is a life-long affair and may require medication for life rather than medication for a short period. The models for obesity then are diseases such as diabetes and hypertension, where chronic medication is an accepted modality of treatment for metabolic control and a cure is not the anticipated effect.

While drugs have a definite role in weight-loss programs, they are never primary but always adjunctive. Under no circumstances should they be used as the sole therapy, because the armamentarium is small and the efficacy quite low. Because obesity is a chronic and persistent condition, drug therapy should be started with the aim of continued use. As a result, safety aspects of the drugs are critically important.

Sibutramine and Orlistat

Only two drugs have been approved for long-term use in the United States: sibutramine (Meridia) and orlistat (Xenical). Their mechanisms of action differ. Sibutramine is both a norepinephrine and a serotonin re-uptake inhibitor working in the central nervous system at neural synapses. The re-uptake inhibition enhances the total time that these neurotransmitters remain in the neural synapse, increase their concentration in the synapse, and enhance neurotransmission. Weight reduction with sibutramine can be maintained for a year or longer at a significantly greater level than with placebo (159). The drug in randomized clinical trials produces at 6 months a 5% to 8% weight loss in comparison to a 1% to 4% weight loss for placebo (160–162). Because sibutramine enhances norepinephrine neurotransmission, it has an effect on blood pressure and heart rate. In randomized controlled trials, sibutramine did not lower blood pressure as much as did a similar amount of weight loss with placebo (161). There is also generally some elevation in heart rate (161). Careful monitoring is required when this drug is used, and it is not wise to use it in patients with more severe hypertension. Dosage begins with 10 mg a day and can go to 15 mg a day, in one morning dose. The drug has not been implicated in heart-valve abnormalities (163,164). Other adverse effects include dry mouth, headache, insomnia, and constipation (164). The drug improves lipid profile and uric acid levels, as well as glycemic control and insulin levels, as expected for the amount of weight loss (159,160,162,165,166).

Orlistat binds to gastrointestinal lipases. This inhibits the hydrolysis of ingested fat in the intestine and partially prevents its absorption. It effectively blocks absorption of about one-third of the fat ingested (167). Therefore, the more fat that is eaten the greater the steatorrhea. Randomized clinical trials have been carried out for up to 2 years (168,169). Weight loss at 1 year with orlistat was 10.2% in comparison to a loss of 6.1% with placebo (168). At 2 years, the orlistat group maintained a weight loss of 7.6% from baseline while placebo was 4.5% from baseline (168). To avoid excess steatorrhea, fat intake should not exceed 100 g or 35% of total calories. Levels of fat-soluble vitamins fall, even though they stay within the normal range (170). A multiple vitamin tablet should be taken daily to ensure maintenance of optimal levels of fat-soluble vitamins. Levels of cholesterol and triglycerides drop more than would be expected from the weight loss effect alone, no doubt related to its inhibition of fat absorption (171). Because the drug blocks the action of pancreatic lipase that is released when fat is ingested, it should be taken as the meal begins (120 mg three times a day). Side effects of the drug include flatulence with discharge, fecal urgency, fecal incontinence, steatorrhea, oily spotting, and increased frequency of defecation. The effects are generally not too severe, tend to get better with time, and certainly get better if fat intake is decreased.

Phentermine

Other anorectic drugs are available that have been approved for short-term use (3 months) in the United States. They act on the central nervous system, affecting either adrenergic or serotoninergic neurotransmission, or both. One such drug is phentermine, which is being widely used throughout the world for long-term therapy. There are two published long-term randomized clinical trials. The first was carried out for 24 weeks, with phentermine given continuously or intermittently every other week (172). Weight loss was about 20.5% vs. 6% with placebo, as good as or better than the weight loss in the sibutramine and orlistat trials. The second was carried out for 6 months, with a weight loss of 12.6% as compared with 9.2% in the placebo group (173). While phentermine was part of the phen-fen (phentermine-fenfluramine) therapy that caused heart-valve abnormalities (174) and was therefore banned by the U.S. Food and Drug Administration (FDA), the onus was placed on fenfluramine and not phentermine (175). To date, long-term use of phentermine has not evoked any known toxicity, though no further formal randomized control trials have been done. Because the treatment of obesity needs to be long-term, the fact that no real efficacy or safety studies have been done long-term with this drug is a problem. No studies are available on the risk/benefit of long-term therapy. If this drug is used long-term, it would be wise for a physician to obtain a signed informed consent form from the patients.

Other Drugs

The U.S. pharmacopeia includes a number of noradrenergic drugs in addition to phentermine. These include diethylpropion, phendimetrazine, benzphetamine, and the amphetamines. These drugs are approved by the FDA only for short-term use (no more than 12 weeks) and have significant abuse potential. The amphetamines are Drug Enforcement Agency (DEA) schedule II and are no longer used. The others are DEA schedule III. There have been no long-term studies of efficacy or safety of these drugs, and so they should not be used for longer than 12 weeks.

A number of drugs that have been approved for other uses have subsequently been found to have a weight-loss effect. Bupropion, an atypical antidepressant, is a weak reuptake inhibitor of norepinephrine, serotonin, and dopamine. Small weight losses have been reported, and most recently an 8-week clinical trial showed a 4.9% weight loss from baseline for drug in comparison to a 1.3% weight loss of placebo (176).

Topiramate is an anti-epileptic agent that has also been found to cause weight loss. It is presently in clinical trials of safety and efficacy. Adverse effects of the drug include renal stones and dizziness, fatigue, cognitive dysfunction, and somnolence (177).

Metformin, a widely used drug for glucose control in patients with type 2 diabetes, has been used for many years in Europe and has a good safety record. In the UKPDS study, metformin limited weight gain in patients with type 2 diabetes as compared with the weight gain induced with other drugs, such as sulfonylureas or insulin (178). Because metformin can cause lactic acidosis, particularly in patients with renal insufficiency, congestive heart failure, pulmonary or liver disease, it should not be used in such patients.

Herbal Preparations and Dietary Supplements

There have been 6-month trials in Europe of the combination of ephedrine and caffeine for weight loss (165,179,180) as well as of the combination of ephedrine, caffeine, and aspirin (181). These have all been found to be more effective than placebo.

Although some herbal products have active ingredients that could have plausible mechanisms of action, few have been tested for efficacy and safety in long-term trials. Boozer et al. (182) has done a 6-month randomized clinical trial comparing herbal ephedra/caffeine with a placebo, with a significantly greater weight loss with the active substance. However, blood pressure did not drop as much in the drug group as in the placebo group for a given level of weight loss. At the moment, the data are insufficient to permit recommendation of any of these preparations (183).

Thyroid preparations, digitalis, and diuretics should not be used for weight loss. Inhibitors of carbohydrate absorption (α-amylase, α-glucosidase, and sucrase inhibitors) do not work as weight reduction agents. While interest in possible thermogenic agents is growing, no satisfactory one is available.

It is important to emphasize that drugs for weight loss should always be used as an adjunct to diet and exercise modification (2). Addition of lifestyle modification to drug therapy results in a significantly greater weight loss, as has been clearly shown in a randomized trial of 1 year's duration (184).

There have been few studies of the combination of the two FDA-approved drugs. Wadden et al. (185) added orlistat after 1 year of sibutramine treatment and found no enhanced effect.

WEIGHT MAINTENANCE

Maintaining reduced weight following the achievement of weight loss has been extremely difficult. The reasons for this phenomenon are not clear. Weight loss results not only in loss of fat but also in loss of lean body mass. The average loss of weight in obese persons comprises about 75% fat to 25% lean (186). For reasons that are not clear, the heavier the individual, the more protected they are against loss of lean body mass as weight loss progresses (112).

While the mechanisms for the powerful drive to regain weight are not totally clear, a number of forces are relevant to the cause of this regain of weight.

First, persons on hypocaloric diets decrease their basal metabolic rate and therefore require fewer calories (187). Thus, as the weight loss proceeds, the caloric deficit becomes less than it was originally. At the end of the weight-loss phase, a patient will have a lower metabolic rate than previously. This happens because, as the patient loses weight, he or she will also lose lean body mass and the metabolic rate is directly related to the lean body mass (188). Thus, the patient will require fewer calories at the end of a weight loss period than he or she required before starting to lose weight (189).

Second, as people lose weight, they become more efficient. That is, they require less energy to do the same physical task (190). Thus, when a person who after a weight-loss phase returns to the total physical activity done previously, she or he will be in positive caloric balance because fewer calories are required to accomplish the same physical task. It is incumbent on every patient who has lost weight to increase his or her physical activity, and to increase it markedly (to some an extra 500 to 700 kcal per day).

Third, levels of lipoprotein lipase (LPL), an enzyme that breaks down circulating lipoprotein triglycerides and thus facilitates the entry of free fatty acids into cells, are increased in persons who are obese (11). With weight reduction, the responsiveness of adipose tissue LPL to meals is increased (11,191), suggesting a better ability to dispose of the triglyceride. This physiologic avidity, then, of the adipose cells for the triglyceride makes the post–weight-loss period a particularly difficult one in terms of regain.

Finally, there seems to be a heightened sensitivity to palatable foods (192). While this has not been adequately studied, there seems to be an enhanced taste threshold and an increased natural intake after a period of deprivation (193).

A common psychological change is actually overconfidence: the feeling that the weight can be lost and that the individual can deal with maintenance without help. This is clearly not the case. Studies have repeatedly shown that the longer the relationship between patient and the therapeutic team is continued, the greater the likelihood of success (194). As a result, caloric intake should be liberalized very carefully and slowly after goal weight has been reached, with daily weight monitoring. A permanent reduction in caloric intake is required because a patient's total energy expenditure will drop after weight loss. All the lifestyle changes learned during the weight-loss period must be continued, including the increased physical activity. If weight-loss drugs have been successful and without adverse effects, their chronic utilization can be recommended, with careful tracking for potential adverse effects.

A National Weight Control Registry (NWCR) has recruited persons who have lost significant amounts of weight and have kept at least 30 lb off for 1 year or longer (195). Participants lost an average of 66 lb (30 kg), and 14% lost more than 100 lb (45.4 kg); 89% modified food intake and maintained relatively high levels of physical activity (2,800 kcal weekly on average) to achieve weight loss. The diet strategy of nearly 90% of participants restricted the intake of certain types and/or amounts of foods; 43% counted calories and lipid intake, and 25% restricted grams of lipid. More than 44% ate the same foods they normally ate, but in reduced amounts.

The importance of physical activity for the NWCR members is great. Nearly all exercised as part of weight-maintenance strategy. Many walked briskly for 1 hour a day; 92% exercised at home; and approximately one third exercised regularly with friends. Women tended primarily to walk and do aerobic dancing and men to engage in competitive sports and resistance training.

SURGERY

Surgery is being used increasingly in patients who are severely obese (BMI >40) and who have tried all other forms of therapy and have failed to lose weight (196). Because of the significant rates of morbidity and even mortality from surgery, however, it is indicated only in patients in whom the obesity itself or an associated condition is severe. Patients with a BMI of ≥40 without associated health problems or with a BMI ≥35 and above with comorbid conditions can be considered for surgery (196). Obesity surgery should be performed only in centers with adequate support from anesthesia, pulmonary, cardiac, and metabolic divisions. The surgeon must be interested in the life-long follow-up of the patient. The surgery must be considered experimental, because no wholly adequate operation has yet been developed.

Various surgical procedures are being done for obesity. Vertical banded gastroplasty (VBG) is the most commonly done procedure. It consists of stapling the stomach vertically and creating a small opening 1 cm in diameter and a reservoir of 35 to 50 mL (Fig. 32.3B). Gastric banding is generally done laparoscopically and creates a configuration similar to VBG. Gastric bypass is a more complex operation in which a small 35- to 50-mL reservoir is created at the upper end of the stomach and a loop of small intestine is brought up and anastomosed to the opening of this reservoir in a Roux-en-Y procedure (Fig. 32.3A). The gastric bypass is the most effective procedure being done today, producing the greatest weight loss. In the Swedish Obesity Surgery (SOS) trial, a loss of 23% ± 10% of excess weight occurred over a period of 2 years with vertical gastroplasty and of 33% ± 10% with gastric bypass (197). Some surgeons are doing obesity surgery laparoscopically, using bands that are placed around the upper part of the stomach. Data available on gastric banding from the SOS show that the weight loss is even less than with the VBG (197). Side effects are less common and less serious than in the gastric bypass, and this operation is technically easier. The weight loss in all procedures can continue for up to 18 months and then levels off. Normal weight is not reached. The greater weight loss with the gastric bypass is traded off by greater surgical complications and mortality. Biliopancreatic diversion is not done in this country. The adverse effects are severe diarrhea and liver disease (198). Liposuction is a cosmetic plastic procedure for removing subcutaneous fat and cannot remove enough fat to affect health risk. Success rates of

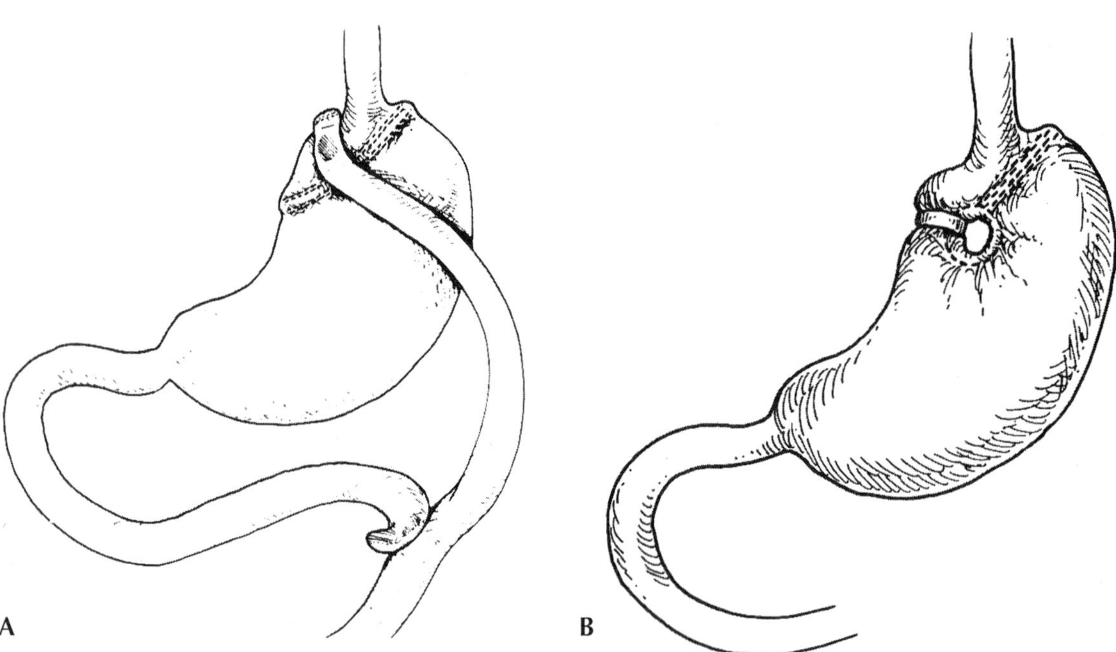

Figure 32.3. Surgical procedures for obesity. **A:** Roux-en-Y gastric bypass. **B:** Vertical banded gastroplasty.

surgical procedures vary, and there have been quite a few failures. These are generally related to poor operative technique or to a patient's eating around the procedure by frequent ingestion of small meals that include high-calorie liquids.

A long-term study of the risk-benefit ratio of obesity surgery as compared with medical treatment is presently being carried out in Sweden (199). Most recently, the 8-year report (200) has shown that, while lipids and diabetes have continued to improve, blood pressure has returned to its preoperative levels (201). Diabetes prevalence has been essentially stable at 10.8% in the operated group, whereas it has increased from 7.8% to 24.9% at 8 years of follow-up in the medically treated group (201). Thus, the results so far are quite positive.

CONCLUSION

The approach to the treatment of the obese patient is a difficult one. It requires significant input of time from the physician and, it is hoped, from other health professionals, such as dietitians and exercise physiologists. Weight loss is extremely difficult to attain, and the maintenance of the weight loss is even more difficult. Lifestyle change is crucial and must be sustained. Obesity is only contained; it is never really cured. Persistent efforts by the patient and the physician are crucial. It is important to stress prevention early in the progression of overweight because weight loss at that point is easier and more sustainable.

REFERENCES

1. Pi-Sunyer FX. Short-term medical benefits and adverse effects of weight loss. *Ann Intern Med* 1993;119:722–726.
2. National Heart, Lung, and Blood Institute. Clinical guidelines on the identification, evaluation, and treatment of overweight and obesity in adults—the evidence report. *Obes Res* 1998;6[Suppl 2]:51S–210S.
3. Lee IM, Paffenbarger RS. Quetelet's index and risk of colon cancer in college alumni. *J Natl Cancer Inst* 1992;84:1326–1331.
4. Zumoff B, Strain G, Miller L. Plasma free and non-sex-hormone-binding-globulin-testosterone are decreased in obese men in proportion to their degree of obesity. *J Clin Endocrinol Metab* 1990;70:929–931.
5. Troiano RP, Frongillo EA Jr, Sobal J, et al. The relationship between body weight and mortality: a quantitative analysis of combined information from existing studies. *Int J Obes Metab Relat Disord* 1996;20:63–75.
6. Bray G. In defense of a body mass index of 25 as the cut-off point for defining overweight. *Obes Res* 1998;6:461–462.
7. Pi-Sunyer FX. Medical hazards of obesity. *Ann Intern Med* 1993;119:655–660.
8. Pi-Sunyer FX. Health implications of obesity. *Am J Clin Nutr* 1991;53:1595S–1603S.
9. Pi-Sunyer FX. Weight and non-insulin dependent diabetes. *Am J Clin Nutr* 1996;63:426S–429S.
10. Kissebah A, Peiris AN, Evans D. Mechanisms associating body fat distribution to glucose intolerance and diabetes mellitus: window with a view. *Acta Med Scand Suppl* 1988;723:79–89.
11. Després JP. Lipoprotein metabolism in visceral obesity. *Int J Obes Metab Relat Disord* 1991;15[Suppl 2]:45–52.
12. Ohlson LO, Larsson B, Svärdsudd K, et al. The influence of body fat distribution on the incidence of diabetes mellitus: 13.5 years of follow up of the participants in the study of men born in 1913. *Diabetes* 1985;34:1055–1058.
13. Lapidus L, Bengtsson C, Larsson B, et al. Distribution of adipose tissue and risk of cardiovascular disease and death: a 12 year follow up of participants in the population study of women in Gothenburg, Sweden. *BMJ* 1984;289:1257–1261.
14. Larsson B, Svärdsudd K, Wilhelmsen L, et al. Abdominal adipose tissue distribution, obesity and risk of cardiovascular disease and death: 13-year follow up of participants in the study of men born in 1913. *BMJ* 1984;288:1401–1404.
15. Haffner SM, Mitchell BD, Hazuda HP, et al. Greater influence of central distribution of adipose tissue on incidence of non-insulin-dependent diabetes in women than men. *Am J Clin Nutr* 1991;53:1312–1317.
16. Williamson DF, Pamuk E, Thun M, et al. Prospective study of intentional weight loss and mortality in never-smoking overweight US white women aged 40–64 years. *Am J Epidemiol* 1995;141:1128–1141.
17. Pi-Sunyer FX. A review of long-term studies evaluating the efficacy of weight loss in ameliorating disorders associated with obesity. *Clin Ther* 1996;18:1006–1035.
18. Hughes T, Gwynne J, Switzer B, et al. Effects of caloric restriction and weight loss on glycemic control, insulin release and resistance, and atherosclerotic risk in obese patients with type II diabetes mellitus. *Am J Med* 1984;77:7–17.
19. Bitzen P-O, Melander A, Schersten B, et al. Efficacy of dietary regulation in primary health care patients with hyperglycaemia detected by screening. *Diabet Med* 1988;5:640–647.
20. Carpenter M, Bodansky H. Drug treatment of obesity in type 2 diabetes mellitus. *Diabet Med* 1990;7:99–104.
21. Henry R, Wiest-Kent T, Scheaffer L, et al. Metabolic consequences of very-low-calorie diet therapy in obese non-insulin-dependent diabetic and non-diabetic subjects. *Diabetes* 1986;35:155–164.
22. Henry R, Wallace P, Olefsky JM. Effects of weight loss on mechanisms of hyperglycemia in obese non-insulin-dependent diabetes mellitus. *Diabetes* 1986;35:990–998.
23. Henry R, Gumbiner B. Benefits and limitations of very-low-calorie diet therapy in obese NIDDM. *Diabetes Care* 1991;14:802–823.
24. Wing RR, Koeske R, E, et al. Long-term effects of modest weight loss in type II diabetic patients. *Arch Intern Med* 1987;147:1749–1753.
25. UK Prospective Diabetes Study 7: Response of fasting plasma glucose to diet therapy in newly presenting type II diabetic patients. UKPDS Group. *Metabolism* 1990;39:901–912.
26. Watt N, Spanheimer R, DiGirolamo M, et al. Prediction of glucose response to weight loss in patients with non-insulin-dependent diabetes mellitus. *Arch Intern Med* 1990;150:803–806.
27. Pan XR, Li GW, Hu YH, et al. Effects of diet and exercise in preventing NIDDM in people with impaired glucose tolerance. The Da Qing IGT and Diabetes Study. *Diabetes Care* 1997;20:537–544.
28. Tuomilehto J, Lindstrom J, Eriksson JG, et al. Prevention of type 2 diabetes mellitus by changes in lifestyle among subjects with impaired glucose tolerance. *N Engl J Med* 2001;344:1343–1350.
29. Diabetes Prevention Program Research Group. Reduction in the incidence of type 2 diabetes with lifestyle intervention or metformin. *N Engl J Med* 2002;346:393–403.
30. Ross R, Rissanen J. Mobilization of visceral and subcutaneous adipose tissue in response to energy restriction and exercise. *Am J Clin Nutr* 2002;60:695–703.
31. Scotte DE, Stunkard AJ. The effect of weight reduction on blood pressure in 301 obese patients. *Arch Intern Med* 1990;150:1701–1704.
32. Kanders B, Blackburn GL, Lavin P, et al. Weight loss outcome and health benefits associated with the Optifast program in the treatment of obesity. *Int J Obes Metab Relat Disord* 1998;13[Suppl 2]:131–134.
33. Mancini M, Di Biase G, Contaldo F, et al. Medical complication of severe obesity: importance of treatment by very-low-calorie diets: intermediate and long-term effects. *Int J Obes Metab Relat Disord* 1981;5:341–352.
34. Foley E, Benotti P, Borlase B, et al. Impact of gastric restrictive surgery on hypertension in the morbidly obese. *Am J Surg* 1992;163:294–297.
35. Bagdade J, Bierman EL, Porte D. The significance of basal insulin levels in the evaluation of the insulin response to glucose in diabetic and nondiabetic subjects. *J Clin Invest* 1967;46:1549–1557.
36. Higgins M, D'Agostino RB, Kannel W, et al. Benefits and adverse effects of weight loss: observations from the Framingham Study. *Ann Intern Med* 1993;119:758–763.
37. Langford HG, Blaufox M, Oberman A, et al. Dietary therapy slows the return of hypertension after stopping prolonged medication. *JAMA* 1985;253:657–664.
38. Stamler R, Stamler J, Grimm RH Jr, et al. Nutritional therapy for high blood pressure: final report of a four-year randomized clinical trial—the Hypertension Control Program. *JAMA* 1987;257:1484–1491.
39. Stevens V, Corrigan S, Obarzanek E, et al. Weight loss intervention in phase 1 of the trials of hypertension prevention. *Arch Intern Med* 1993;153:849–858.
40. Ramsay LE, Ramsay MH, Hettiarachchi J, et al. Weight reduction in a blood pressure clinic. *BMJ* 1978;2:244–245.
41. Heyden S, Borhani NO, Tyroler HA, et al. The relationship of weight change to changes in blood pressure, serum uric acid, cholesterol and glucose in the treatment of hypertension. *J Chronic Dis* 1985;38:281–288.
42. Davis BR, Blaufox M, Oberman A, et al. Reduction in long-term antihypertensive medication requirements: effects of weight reduction by dietary intervention in overweight persons with mild hypertension. *Arch Intern Med* 1993;153:1773–1782.
43. Wassertheil-Smoller S, Blaufox M, Oberman A, et al. The Trial of Antihypertensive Interventions and Management (TAIM) study. *Arch Intern Med* 1992;152:131–136.
44. Després JP, Moorjani S, Lupien PJ, et al. Regional distribution of body fat, plasma lipoproteins, and cardiovascular disease. *Arteriosclerosis* 1990;10:497–511.
45. Krauss RM. Triglycerides and atherogenic lipoproteins: rationale for lipid management. *Am J Med* 1998;105[Suppl]:58S–62S.
46. Follick M, Abrams D, Smith T, et al. Contrasting short- and long-term effects of weight loss on lipoprotein levels. *Arch Intern Med* 1984;144:1571–1574.
47. Carmena R, Ascaso J, Tebar J, et al. Changes in plasma high-density lipoproteins after body weight reduction in obese women. *Int J Obes Metab Relat Disord* 1984;8:135–140.
48. Fachnie J, Foreback C. Effects of weight reduction, exercise and diet modification on lipids and apolipoproteins A-1 and B in severely obese persons. *Henry Ford Hosp Med J* 1987;35:216–220.
49. Schieffer B, Moore D, Funke E, et al. Reduction of atherogenic risk factors by short-term weight reduction. *Klin Wochenschr* 1991;69:163–167.
50. Wylie-Rosett J, Swencionis C, Peters M, et al. A weight reduction intervention that optimizes use of practitioner's time, lowers glucose level, and raises HDL cholesterol level in older adults. *J Am Diet Assoc* 1994;94:37–42.

51. Hall Y, Stamler J, Cohen D, et al. Effectiveness of a low saturated fat, low cholesterol, weight-reducing diet for the control of hypertriglyceridemia. *Atherosclerosis* 1972;16:389–403.
52. Wood PD, Stefanick ML, Dreon D, et al. Changes in plasma lipids and lipoproteins in overweight men during weight loss through dieting as compared with exercise. *N Engl J Med* 1988;319:1173–1179.
53. Brolin R, Kenler H, Wilson A, et al. Serum lipids after gastric bypass surgery for morbid obesity. *Int J Obes Metab Relat Disord* 1990;14:939–950.
54. Weintraub M, Sundaresan P, Schuster B. Long-term weight control study VII (weeks 0–210). *Clin Pharmacol Ther* 1992;51:634–641.
55. Goldstein DJ. Beneficial health effects of modest weight loss. *Int J Obes* 1992; 16:397–415.
56. Peiser J, Lavie P, Ovnat A, et al. Sleep apnea syndrome in the morbidly obese as an indication for weight reduction surgery. *Ann Surg* 1984;199:112–115.
57. Charuzi I, Ovnat A, Peiser J, et al. The effects of surgical weight reduction on sleep quality in obesity-related sleep apnea syndrome. *Surgery* 1985;97:535–538.
58. Pons J-B and Montanari A. Eficacia de la perdida de peso en el tratamiento del sindrome de apneas obstructivas durante el sueño. Experiencia en 135 pacientes. *Med Clin (Barc)* 1992;98:45–48.
59. Aubert G. Alternative therapeutic approaches in sleep apnea syndrome. *Sleep* 1992;15:S69–S72.
60. Pasquali R, Colella P, Cirignotta F, et al. Treatment of obese patients with obstructive sleep apnea syndrome (OSAS): effect of weight loss and interference of otorhinolaringioatric pathology. *Int J Obes Metab Relat Disord* 1990;14: 207–217.
61. Rajala R, Partinen M, Sane T, et al. Obstructive sleep apnoea syndrome in morbidly obese patients. *J Intern Med* 1991;230:125–129.
62. Rimm AA, Werner LH, Yserloo BV, et al. Relationship of obesity and disease in 73,532 weight-conscious women. *Public Health Rep* 1975;90:44–54.
63. Seidell JC, Bakx JC, De Bower E, et al. Fat distribution of overweight persons in relation to morbidity and subjective health. *Int J Obes* 1985;9:363–374.
64. Anderson J, Hamilton C, Brinkman-Kaplan V. Benefits and risks of an intensive very-low-calorie-diet program for severe obesity. *Am J Gastroenterol* 1992; 87:6–15.
65. Atkinson R. Medical evaluation and monitoring of patients treated by severe caloric restriction. In: Wadden TA, Van Itallie TB, ed. *Treatment of the seriously ill patient.* New York: Guilford Press, 1992:273–289.
66. Atkinson RL, Kaiser DL. Effects of calorie restriction and weight loss on glucose and insulin levels in obese humans. *J Am Coll Nutr* 1985;4:411–419.
67. Felson DT, Zhang Y, Hannan M, et al. Risk factors for incident radiographic knee osteoarthritis in the elderly: the Framingham Study. *Arthritis Rheum* 1997;40:728–733.
68. Manninen P, Rihmaki H, Heliovaara M, et al. Overweight, gender and knee osteoarthritis. *Int J Obes Relat Metab Disord* 1996;20:595–597.
69. Anderson JJ, Felson DT. Factors associated with osteoarthritis of the knee in the first National Health and Nutrition Examination Survey (HANES I): evidence for an association with overweight, race, and physical demands of work. *Am J Epidemiol* 1988;128:178–189.
70. Hartz AJ, Fischer ME, Bril G, et al. The association of obesity with joint pain and osteoarthritis in the HANES data. *J Chronic Dis* 1986;39:311–319.
71. Felson DT, Zhang Y, Anthony M, et al. Weight loss reduces the risk for symptomatic knee ostearthritis in women. *Ann Intern Med* 1992;116:535–539.
72. Bradley M, Golden E. Powdered meal replacements—can they benefit overweight patients with concomitant conditions exacerbated by obesity? *Curr Ther Res* 1990;47:429–436.
73. Schlierf G, Schellenberg B, Stiehl A, et al. Biliary cholesterol saturation and weight reduction—effects of fasting and low-calorie diet. *Digestion* 1981;21: 44–49.
74. Reuben A, Quershi Y, Murphy G, et al. Effect of obesity and weight reduction on biliary cholesterol saturation and the response to chenodeoxycholic acid. *Eur J Clin Invest* 1985;16:133–142.
75. Heshka S, Spitz A, Nunez C, et al. Obesity and risk of gallstone development on a 1200 kcal/d (5025 Lk/d) regular food diet. *Int J Obes Relat Metab Disord* 1996;20:450–454.
76. Maclure KM, Hayes KC, Colditz GA, et al. Weight, diet, and the risk of symptomatic gallstones in middle-aged women. *N Engl J Med* 1989;321:563–569.
77. O'Neil PM, Jarrell MP. Psychological aspects of obesity in dieting. In: Wadden TA, Van Itallie TB, eds. *Treatment of the seriously obese patient.* New York: Guilford Press; 1992.
78. Stunkard AJ, Wadden TA. Psychological aspects of severe obesity. *Am J Clin Nutr* 1992:524S–532S.
79. Wilson GT. Relation of dieting and voluntary weight loss to psychological functioning and binge eating. *Ann Intern Med* 1993;119:727–730.
80. Maggio C, Pi-Sunyer FX. The prevention and treatment of obesity. *Diabetes Care* 1997;20:1744–1766.
81. Faith MS, Fontaine K, Cheskin L, et al. Behavioral approaches to the problems of obesity. *Behav Modif* 2000;24:459–493.
82. Foster GD, Wadden TA, Vogt RA, et al. What is a reasonable weight loss? Patients' expectations and evaluations of obesity treatment outcomes. *J Consult Clin Psychol* 1997;65:79–85.
83. Pi-Sunyer FX. The role of very-low-calorie diets in obesity. *Am J Clin Nutr* 1992;56:240S–243S.
84. Ferster C, Nurnberger J, Levitt E. The control of eating. *J Math* 1962;87–109.
85. Stuart R. Behavioral control of overeating. *Behav Res Ther* 1967;5:357–365.
86. Stunkard AJ, Berthold H. What is behavior therapy? A very short description of behavioral weight control. *Am J Clin Nutr* 1985;41:821–823.
87. Brownell KD, Wadden TA. Etiology and treatment of obesity: understanding a serious, prevalent, and refractory disorder. *J Consult Clin Psychol* 1992;60: 505–517.
88. Mahoney M. *Cognition and behavior modification.* Cambridge, MA: Ballinger, 1974.
89. Mahoney M, Mahoney K. *Permanent weight control.* New York: Norton, 1976.
90. Meichenbaum D. *Cognitive behavior modification.* New York: Plenum, 1977.
91. Brownell KD, Marlatt G, Lichtenstein E, et al. Understanding and preventing relapse. *Am Psychol* 1986;41:765–782.
92. Brownell KD, Rodin J. *The weight maintenance survival guide.* Dallas, TX: American Health, 1990.
93. Foreyt J, Goodrick G. Attributes of successful approaches to weight loss and control. *Appl Prevent Psychol* 1994;3:209–215.
94. Stunkard AJ. An overview of current treatments for obesity. In: Wadden TA, Van Itallie TB, ed. *Treatment of the severely obese patient.* New York: Guilford Press, 1992:33–43.
95. Wadden TA, Foster GD. Behavioral assessment and treatment of markedly obese patients. In: Wadden TA, Van Itallie TB, ed. *Treatment of the severely obese patient.* New York: Guilford Press, 1992:290–330.
96. Wadden TA, Bartlett S. Very low calorie diets: an overview and appraisal. In: Wadden TA, Van Itallie TB, ed. *Treatment of the severely obese patient.* New York: Guilford Press, 1992:44–79.
97. Wadden TA, Sternberg J, Letizia KA, et al. 5-Year perspective. *Int J Obes Metab Relat Disord* 1989[Suppl 2];13:39–46.
98. Cogan J, Rothblum E. Outcomes of weight-loss programs. *Genet Soc Gen Psychol Monogr* 1993;118:387–415.
99. Wilson GT. Behavioral treatment of obesity. *Adv Behav Res Ther* 1994;16:31–75.
100. Epstein LH, Valoski A, Kalarchian M, et al. Do children lose and maintain weight easier than adults? A comparison of child and parent weight changes from 6 months to 10 years. *Obes Res* 1995;3:411–417.
101. Epstein LH, Valoski A, Wing RR, et al. Ten-year follow-up of behavioral family-based treatment for obese children. *JAMA* 1990;264:2519–2523.
102. Epstein LH, Valoski A, Wing RR, et al. Ten-year outcomes of behavioral family-based treatment of childhood obesity. *Health Psychol* 1994;13:573–583.
103. Jeffery RW, Wing RR. Long-term effects of interventions for weight loss using food provision and monetary incentives. *J Consult Clin Psychol* 1995;63:793–796.
104. Brownell KD. Relapse and the treatment of obesity. In: Wadden TA, Van Itallie TB, ed. *Treatment of the severely obese patient.* New York: Guilford Press, 1992:437–455.
105. Prochaska J, DiClemente C. Common processes in change in smoking, weight control, and psychological distress. In: Shiffman S, Wills T, ed. *Coping and substance abuse.* New York: Academic Press, 1985:345–364.
106. Perri M. Improving maintenance of weight loss following treatment by diet and lifestyle modification. In: Wadden TA, Van Itallie TB, ed. *Treatment of the severely obese patient.* New York: Guilford Press, 1992:456–477.
107. Blackburn GL. Effect of degree of weight loss on health benefits. *Obes Res* 1995;3[Suppl 2]:211s–216s.
108. Committee to Develop Criteria for Evaluating the Outcomes of Approaches to Prevent and Treat Obesity. Institute of Medicine. *Weighing the options: criteria for evaluating weight-management programs.* Washington, DC: National Academy Press, 1995.
109. Johnson MM, Chin R Jr, Haponik EF. Nutrition, respiratory function, and disease. In: Shils M, Olson J, Shike M, et al, ed. *Modern nutrition in health and disease,* 9th ed. Baltimore: William & Wilkins, 1999:1473–1490.
110. Frankenfield DC, Muth ER, Rowe WA. The Harris-Benedict studies of human basal metabolism: history and limitations. *J Am Diet Assoc* 1998;98: 439–445.
111. US Department of Agriculture and US Department of Health and Human Services. *Dietary guidelines for Americans.* Washington, DC: US Government Publishing Office, 1995. Report no. Home and Garden Bulletin 232.
112. Van Itallie T, Yang MU. Current concepts in nutrition. Diet and weight loss. *N Engl J Med* 1977;297:1158–1161.
113. Johnston PK. Vegetarian nutrition. Proceedings of a symposium. *Am J Clin Nutr* 1994;59[Suppl]:1097S–1262S.
114. Nonas CA, Pi-Sunyer FX. Obesity. In: Morrison G, Hark L, ed. *Medical nutrition and disease,* 2nd ed. Cambridge, MA: Blackwell Science, 1999.
115. Lantigua RA, Amatruda JM, Biddle TL, et al. Cardiac arrhythmias associated with a liquid protein diet for the treatment of obesity. *N Engl J Med* 1980; 303:735–738.
116. Foster GD, Wadden TA, Peterson FJ, et al. A controlled comparison of three very-low-calorie diets: effects on weight, body composition, and symptoms. *Am J Clin Nutr* 1992;55:811–817.
117. Center for Nutrition Policy. *The food guide pyramid.* Washington, DC: Department of Agriculture, 1996. Report number: Home and Garden Bulletin 252.
118. Bray G, Greenway F. Current and potential drugs for treatment of obesity. *Endocr Rev* 1999;20:805–875.
119. Kelley DE, Goodpaster BH. Effects of physical activity on insulin action and glucose tolerance in obesity. *Med Sci Sports Exerc* 1999;31[November Suppl]: S619–S623.
120. Smutok M, Reece C, Kokkinos P, et al. Effects of exercise training modality on glucose tolerance in men with abnormal glucose regulation. *Int J Sports Med* 1994;15:283–289.
121. Kang J, Robertson R, Hagberg J, et al. Effect of exercise intensity on glucose and insulin metabolism in obese individuals and obese NIDDM patients. *Diabetes Care* 1996;19:341–349.
122. Helmrich S, Ragland D, Leung R, et al. Physical activity and reduced occur-

rence of non-insulin-dependent diabetes mellitus. *N Engl J Med* 1991;325: 147–152.
123. James S, Jamjoum L, Raghunathan T, et al. Physical activity and NIDDM in African-Americans: the Pitt County Study. *Diabetes Care* 1998;21:555–562.
124. Manson JE, Nathan DM, Krowleski A, et al. A prospective study of exercise and incidence of diabetes among U.S. male physicians. *JAMA* 1992;268:63–67.
125. Manson JE, Rimm EB, Stampfer MJ, et al. Physical activity and incidence of non-insulin dependent diabetes mellitus in women. *Lancet* 1991;338:774–778.
126. Pan D, Lillioja S, Kriketos A, et al. Skeletal muscle triglyceride levels are inversely related to insulin action. *Diabetes* 1997;46:983–988.
127. Perry I, Wannamethee S, Walker M, et al. Prospective study of risk factors for development of non-insulin dependent diabetes in middle aged British men. *BMJ* 1995;310:560–564.
128. Fagard R. Physical activity in the prevention and treatment of hypertension in the obese. *Med Sci Sports Exerc* 1999;31[November Suppl]:S624–S630.
129. Garrow J, Summerbell C. Meta-analysis: effect of exercise, with or without dieting, on the body composition of overweight subjects. *Eur J Clin Nutr* 1995;49:1–10.
130. Wing RR. Physical activity in the treatment of the adulthood overweight and obesity: current evidence and research issues. *Med Sci Sports Exerc* 1999;31 [November Suppl]:S547–S552.
131. Anderssen S, Holme I, Urdal P, et al. Diet and exercise intervention have favourable effects on blood pressure in mild hypertensives: the Oslo Diet and Exercise Study (ODES). *Blood Press* 1995;4:343–349.
132. Hammer RL, Barrier CA, Roundy ES, et al. Calorie-restricted low-fat diet and exercise in obese women. *Am J Clin Nutr* 1989;49:77–85.
133. Hellenius ML, de Faire U, Berglund B, et al. Diet and exercise are equally effective in reducing risk for cardiovascular disease. Results of a randomized controlled study in men with slightly to moderately raised cardiovascular risk factors. *Atherosclerosis* 1993;103:81–91.
134. Katzel LI, Bleecker ER, Colman EG, et al. Effects of weight loss vs aerobic exercise training on risk factors for coronary disease in healthy, obese, middle-aged and older men. A randomized controlled trial. *JAMA* 1995;274:1915–1921.
135. King AC, Haskell WL, Taylor CB, et al. Group- vs home-based exercise training in healthy older men and women. A community-based clinical trial. *JAMA* 1991;266:1532–1542.
136. Ronnemaa T, Marniemi J, Puukka P, et al. Effects of long-term physical exercise on serum lipids, lipoproteins and lipid metabolizing enzymes in type 2 (non-insulin-dependent) diabetic patients. *Diabetes Res* 1988;7:79–84.
137. Stefanick ML, Mackey S, Sheehan M, et al. Effects of diet and exercise in men and postmenopausal women with low levels of HDL cholesterol and high levels of LDL cholesterol. *N Engl J Med* 1998;339:12–20.
138. Verity LS, Ismail AH. Effects of exercise on cardiovascular disease risk in women with NIDDM. *Diabetes Res Clin Pract* 1989;6:27–35.
139. Wood PD, Haskell WL, Blair SN, et al. Increased exercise level and plasma lipoprotein concentrations: a one-year, randomized, controlled study in sedentary, middle-aged men. *Metabolism* 1983;32:31–39.
140. Miller W, Koceja D, Hamilton E. A meta-analysis of the past 25 years of weight loss research using diet, exercise or diet plus exercise intervention. *Int J Obes* 1997;21:941–947.
141. Wadden TA, Vogt R, Andersen R, et al. Exercise in the treatment of obesity: effects of four interventions on body composition, resting energy expenditure, and mood. *J Consult Clin Psychol* 1997;65:269–277.
142. Pronk N, Wing RR. Physical activity and long-term maintenance of weight loss. *Obes Res* 1994;2:587–599.
143. Wing RR. Physical activity in the treatment of the adulthood overweight and obesity: current evidence and research issues. *Med Sci Sports Exerc* 1999;31:S547–S552.
144. Schoeller D, Shay K, Kushner RF. How much physical activity is needed to minimize weight gain in previously obese women? *Am J Clin Nutr* 1997;66: 551–556.
145. Klem M, Wing RR, McGuire M, et al. A descriptive study of individuals successful at long-term maintenance of substantial weight loss. *Am J Clin Nutr* 1997;66:239–246.
146. Gutin B, Kessler G. *The high energy factor.* New York: Random House, 1983.
147. Woo R, Garrow JS, Pi-Sunyer FX. Effect of exercise on spontaneous calorie intake in obesity. *Am J Clin Nutr* 2002;36:470–477.
148. Woo R, Pi-Sunyer FX. Effect of increased physical activity on voluntary intake in lean women. *Metab Clin Exp* 1985;34:836–841.
149. Weigle DS, Brunzell JD. Assessment of energy expenditure in ambulatory reduced-obese subjects by the techniques of weight stabilization and exogenous weight replacement. *Int J Obes* 1990;14:69–77.
150. Barlow C, Kohl H III, Gibbons L, et al. Physical fitness, mortality and obesity. *Int J Obes Relat Metab Disord* 1995;19:S41–S44.
151. Lee C, Blair S, Jackson A. Cardiorespiratory fitness, body composition, and all-cause and cardiovascular disease mortality in men. *Am J Clin Nutr* 1999; 69:373–380.
152. Lee C, Jackson A, Blair S. US weight guidelines: is it also important to consider cardiorespiratory fitness? *Int J Obes Relat Metab Disord* 1998;22:S2–S7.
153. Haapanen N, Millunpalo I, Vuori P, et al. Association of leisure time physical activity with the risk of CHD. *Int J Epidemiol* 1997;26:739–747.
154. Hsieh S, Yoshinaga H, Muto T, et al. Regular physical activity and coronary risk factors in Japanese men. *Circulation* 1998;97:661–665.
155. Stefanick ML, Mackey S, Sheehan M, et al. Effects on diet and exercise in men and postmenopausal women with low levels of HDL cholesterol and high levels of low density lipoprotein (LDL) cholesterol. *N Engl J Med* 1998;339:12–20.
156. Bouchard C, Perusse L, Leblanc C, et al. Inheritance of the amount and distribution of human body fat. *Int J Obes* 1988;12:205–215.
157. Bouchard C, Tremblay A, Després JP, et al. The response to long-term overfeeding in identical twins. *N Engl J Med* 1990;24:1477–1482.
158. Stunkard AJ, Sorensen TI, Hanis C, et al. An adoption study of human obesity. *N Engl J Med* 1986;314:193–198.
159. McMahon F, Fujioka K, Singh B, et al. Efficacy and safety of sibutramine in obese white and African American patients with hypertension: a 1-year double-blind, placebo-controlled, multicenter trial. *Arch Intern Med* 2000;160: 2185–2191.
160. Fanghanel G, Cortinas L, Sanchez-Reyes L, et al. A clinical trial of the use of sibutramine for the treatment of patients suffering essential obesity. *Int J Obes Relat Metab Disord* 2000;24:144–150.
161. Bray GA, Blackburn GL, Ferguson JM, et al. Sibutramine produces dose-related weight loss. *Obes Res* 1999;7:189–198.
162. Fujioka K, Seaton TB, Rowe E, et al. Weight loss with sibutramine improves glycaemic control and other metabolic parameters in obese patients with type 2 diabetes mellitus. Sibutramine/Diabetes Clinical Study Group. *Diabetes Obes Metab* 2000;2:175–187.
163. Bach D, Rissanen A, Mendel CM, et al. Absence of cardiac valve dysfunction in obese patients treated with sibutramine. *Obes Res* 2002;7:363–369.
164. Anonymous. Sibutramine for obesity. *Med Lett Drugs Ther* 1998;40:32.
165. James WPT, Astrup A, Finer N, et al. Effect of sibutramine on weight maintenance after weight loss: a randomised trial. STORM Study Group. Sibutramine trial of obesity reduction and maintenance. *Lancet* 2000;356:2119–2125.
166. Finer N, Bloom S, Frost G, et al. Sibutramine is effective for weight loss and diabetic control in obesity with type 2 diabetes: a randomised, double blind, placebo-controlled study. *Diabetes Obes Metab* 200;2:105–112.
167. Heck A, Yanovski J, Calis J. Orlistat, a new lipase inhibitor for the management of obesity. *Pharmacotherapy* 2000;20:270–279.
168. Davidson MH, Hauptman J, DiGirolamo M, et al. Weight control and risk factor reduction in obese subjects treated for 2 years with orlistat: a randomized controlled trial. *JAMA* 1999;281:235–242.
169. Sjöström L, Rissanen A, Andersen T, et al. Randomised placebo-controlled trial of orlistat for weight loss and prevention of weight regain in obese patients. European Multicentre Orlistat Study Group. *Lancet* 1998;352:167–172.
170. Anonymous. *Physicians' desk reference*. 55th ed. Montvale, NJ: Medical Economics, 2001.
171. Mittendorfer B, Ostlund RE Jr, Patterson BW, et al. Orlistat inhibits dietary cholesterol absorption. *Obes Res* 2001;9:599–604.
172. Munro J, MacCuish A, Wilson E, et al. Comparison of continuous and intermittent anorectic therapy in obesity. *BMJ* 1968;1:352–362.
173. Willims RA, Foulsham BM. Weight reduction in osteoarthritis using phentermine. *Practitioner* 1981;225:231–232.
174. Connolly HM, Crary JL, McGoon MD, et al. Valvular heart disease associated with fenfluramine-phentermine. *N Engl J Med* 1997;28:581–598.
175. Connolly H, McGoon M. Obesity drugs and the heart. *Curr Probl Cardiol* 1999;24:745–792.
176. Gadde K, Krishnan K, Drezner M. Bupropion SR shows promise as an effective obesity treatment. *Obes Res* 1999;7:51S(abst).
177. Glauser T. Topiramate. *Epilepsia* 1999;40[Suppl 5]:S71–S80.
178. Effect of intensive blood-glucose control with metformin on complications in overweight patients with type 2 diabetes. UK Prospective Diabetes Study (UKPDS) Group. *Lancet* 1998;352:854–865.
179. Astrup A, Breum L, Toubro S, et al. The effect and safety of an ephedrine/caffeine compound compared to ephedrine, caffeine and placebo in obese subjects on an energy restricted diet. A double blind trial. *Int J Obes Relat Metab Disord* 1992;16:269–277.
180. Toubro S, Astrup A, Breum L, et al. Safety and efficacy of long-term treatment with ephedrine, caffeine and an ephedrine/caffeine mixture. *Int J Obes Relat Metab Disord* 1993;17[Suppl 1]:S69–S72.
181. Daly P, Krieger D, Dulloo A, et al. Ephedrine, caffeine and aspirin: safety and efficacy for treatment of human obesity. *Int J Obes Relat Metab Disord* 1993;17[Suppl 1]:S73–S78.
182. Boozer CN, Nasser J, Heymsfield SB, et al. Efficacy of an herbal mixture of ma huang and guarana for weight loss. *Int J Obes Rel Metab Disord* 2001;25:316–324.
183. Allison DB, Fontaine K, Heshka S, et al. Alternative treatments for weight loss: a critical review. *Crit Rev Food Sci Nutr* 2001;41:1–28.
184. Wadden TA, Berkowitz R, Sarwer D, et al. Benefits of lifestyle modification in the pharmacologic treatment of obesity: a randomized trial. *Arch Intern Med* 2001;161:218–227.
185. Wadden TA, Berkowitz RI, Womble LG, et al. Effects of sibutramine plus orlistat in obese women following 1 year of treatment by sibutramine alone: a placebo-controlled trial. *Obes Res* 2000;8:431–437.
186. Yang MU, Barbosa-Saldivar JL, Pi-Sunyer FX, et al. Metabolic effects of substituting carbohydrate for protein in a low-calorie diet: a prolonged study in obese patients. *Int J Obes* 1981;5:231–236.
187. Bray GA. Effect of caloric restriction on energy expenditure in obese patients. *Lancet* 1969;2:397–398.
188. Nelson KM, Weinsier RL, Long CL, et al. Prediction of resting energy expenditure from fat-free mass and fat mass. *Am J Clin Nutr* 1992;56:848–856.
189. Heshka S, Yang MU, Wang J, et al. Weight loss and change in resting metabolic rate. *Am J Clin Nutr* 1990;52:981–986.
190. Weigle DS, Sande KJ, Iverius PH, et al. Weight loss leads to a marked decrease in nonresting energy expenditure in ambulatory human subjects. *Metab Clin Exp* 2002;37:930–936.

191. Ong JM, Simsolo RB, Saghizadeh M, et al. Effects of exercise training and feeding on lipoprotein lipase gene expression in adipose tissue, heart, and skeletal muscle of the rat. *Metab Clin Exp* 1995;44:1596–1605.
192. Rodin J, Schank D, Striegel-Moore R. Psychological features of obesity. *Med Clin North Am* 1989;73:47–66.
193. Van Itallie TB, Kissileff HR. Physiology of energy intake: an inventory control model. *Am J Clin Nutr* 1985;42:914–923.
194. Perri MG, Nezu AM, Patti ET, et al. Effect of length of treatment on weight loss. *J Consult Clin Psychol* 1989;57:450–452.
195. McGuire MT, Wing RR, Klem ML, et al. What predicts weight regain in a group of successful weight losers? *J Consult Clin Psychol* 1999;67:177–185.
196. Gastrointestinal surgery for severe obesity: National Institutes of Health Consensus Development Conference Statement. *Am J Clin Nutr* 1992;55:615S–619S.
197. Sjöström CD, Lissner L, Wedel H, et al. Reduction in incidence of diabetes, hypertension and lipid disturbances after intentional weight loss induced by bariatric surgery: the SOS intervention study. *Obes Res* 1999;7:477–484.
198. Scopinaro N, Gianetta E, Adami GF, et al. Biliopancreatic diversion for obesity at eighteen years. *Surgery* 1996;119:261–268.
199. Sjöström L, Larsson B, Backman L, et al. Swedish Obese Subjects (SOS). Recruitment for an intervention study and a selected description of the obese state. *Int J Obes* 1992;16:465–479.
200. Sjöström CD, Peltonen M, Wedel H, et al. Differentiated long-term effects of intentional weight loss on diabetes and hypertension. *Hypertension* 2000;36:20–25.
201. Sjöström CD, Peltonen M, Sjöström L. Blood pressure and pulse pressure during long-term weight loss in the obese: the Swedish Obese Subjects (SOS) Intervention Study. *Obes Res* 2001;9:188–195.

CHAPTER 33
Pathophysiology and Treatment of Lipid Disorders in Diabetes

Barbara V. Howard and Wm. James Howard

An understanding of lipoprotein metabolism and how it influences diabetes is of particular importance because of the association of lipoproteins with cardiovascular disease, the leading cause of death among people with diabetes (1). Abnormalities in lipoproteins are very common in both type 1 and type 2 diabetes. Although alterations in lipoproteins appear to be an intrinsic part of these disorders, such alterations also are induced by diabetes-associated complications such as obesity and renal disease and are sometimes exacerbated by therapeutic regimens associated with the management of diabetic patients. The National Cholesterol Education Program (2) and the American Diabetes Association (ADA) (3) have focused attention on the necessity of managing lipid disorders. In diagnosing and treating lipid abnormalities in diabetes, particular consideration must be given to diabetes-specific targets, the relationship between glycemic control and lipoproteins, and the potential for a different response to lipid-lowering agents by individuals with diabetes. This chapter will review the basics of lipoprotein composition and metabolism, the alterations in lipoprotein composition and metabolism in diabetes, and therapeutic approaches to the management of lipid disorders in patients with diabetes.

LIPOPROTEIN METABOLISM

Structure and Classification

Lipoproteins are microemulsions composed of lipids (cholesterol, cholesteryl ester, triglyceride, and phospholipid) and proteins (apoproteins). Their function is to transport non–water-soluble cholesterol and triglycerides in plasma. Lipoproteins are spherical particles containing a central core of nonpolar lipids (primarily triglycerides and cholesteryl ester) and a surface monolayer of phospholipids and apoproteins. Free cholesterol is present primarily in the surface monolayer. [For a detailed review of lipoprotein structure and metabolism, the reader is referred to references (4) through (16)].

TABLE 33.1. Human Plasma Lipoproteins

Lipoprotein	Density (g/mL)	Electrophoretic mobility	Diameter (nm)	Chol/CE (%)	Triglyceride (%)[a]	Protein (%)
Chylomicrons	0.95	Origin	75–1200	5	86	2
VLDL	<1.006	Pre-β	30–80	15	55	10
IDL	1.006–1.019	Pre-β	25–35	38	23	19
LDL	1.019–1.063	β	18–25	50	5	22
Lp(a)	1.040–1.063	β	25–35	50	5	36
HDL	1.063–1.210	α	5–12	19	3	48

VLDL, very-low-density lipoprotein; IDL, intermediate-density lipoprotein; LDL, low-density lipoprotein; Lp(a), lipoprotein a; HDL, high-density lipoprotein; Chol, cholesterol; CE, cholesteryl ester.
[a]Approximate value.

Lipoproteins have been classified on the basis of their densities during ultracentrifugation (Table 33.1). Chylomicrons, particles that are primarily triglyceride bearing, are produced by the intestine after exogenous fat undergoes digestion. Very-low-density lipoproteins (VLDLs), also triglyceride-bearing lipoproteins, are secreted by the liver and carry endogenously produced triglyceride. Intermediate-density lipoproteins (IDLs) represent remnants of the metabolism of triglyceride-rich lipoproteins and also can be intermediates in the conversion of VLDLs to low-density lipoproteins (LDLs) (8,13,14–16). LDLs are the major cholesterol-bearing lipoproteins and are those most strongly related to the occurrence of cardiovascular disease. Lp(a) is a subclass of the LDL fraction that consists of LDL complexed to a large glycoprotein resembling plasminogen; this complex has also been associated with atherosclerosis (17). High-density lipoproteins (HDLs) are the smallest and densest of the lipoproteins. Although HDLs also transport substantial amounts of cholesterol, they are negatively associated with cardiovascular disease.

The metabolism and production of all lipoproteins are controlled by the apoproteins contained within the complex, by enzymes and proteins that moderate lipoprotein metabolism, and by specific cellular receptors that direct their interaction with cells. All known apoproteins (Table 33.2) have been sequenced and their genes localized (18,19). Most are hydrophobic proteins and serve as ligands for specific receptors involved in the metabolism of the various lipoproteins and as cofactors for enzymatic activities involved in lipoprotein metabolism. Several other proteins and enzymes play key roles in plasma lipoprotein transport, including lipoprotein lipase (8,9,16,20,21) and hepatic lipase (12,22), which catalyze the delipidation of triglyceride-rich particles; lecithin-cholesterol acyltransferase (LCAT) (23), which is responsible for the synthesis of virtually all cholesteryl esters in plasma lipoproteins; and cholesteryl ester transfer protein (CETP) (24,25), which facilitates the transfer of cholesteryl ester and triglycerides between lipoproteins during their metabolism. A number of cell receptors (Table 33.3) govern lipoprotein binding and uptake and lipid flux; they are described in the following sections on metabolism.

Formation and Metabolism of Chylomicrons

Chylomicrons are responsible for the transport of dietary triglycerides and cholesterol. Dietary triglycerides are hydrolyzed in the gut, releasing monoglycerides and fatty acids that are then reesterified to form triglycerides in the intestinal mucosal cell (Fig. 33.1) (5,7,8,10,11,16). These triglycerides are assembled with newly absorbed cholesterol, apoprotein (apo) B_{48}, and the A apoproteins. Upon secretion from the enterocyte, these assembled particles enter the lymphatic circulation and then the bloodstream, where they acquire C apoproteins and apoE by transfer from HDL. As chylomicrons enter the plasma, the triglycerides are rapidly hydrolyzed by the enzyme lipoprotein lipase (LPL), which resides on the surface of capillary endothelial cells. LPL is synthesized primarily in adipose tissue and striated muscle (8,10,16,20,21). It is secreted and transported to the endothelial surface, where it acts on triglyceride-rich particles. Its action requires the presence of apoC_{II} on the

TABLE 33.2. Major Apoproteins Associated with Plasma Lipoproteins

Apoprotein	Association						Function
	Chylomicrons	VLDL	IDL	LDL	HDL	Lp(a)	
ApoA_I	x	—	—	—	x	—	Cell cholesterol efflux Binds to HDL receptor
ApoA_{II}	—	—	—	—	x	—	Binds to HDL receptor
ApoA_{IV}	x	—	—	—	x	—	Cell cholesterol efflux
ApoB_{48}	x	—	—	—	—	—	Structure/clearance of chylomicrons
ApoB_{100}	—	x	x	x	—	x	Binds to B/E receptor
ApoC_{II}	x	x	x	—	x	—	Activates LPL
ApoC_{III}	x	x	x	—	x	—	Inhibits LPL
ApoE	x	x	x	—	x	—	Binds to B/E and remnant receptors
Apo(a)	—	—	—	—	—	x	Plasminogen antagonist

VLDL, very-low-density lipoprotein; IDL, intermediate-density lipoprotein; LDL, low-density lipoprotein; HDL, high-density lipoprotein; Lp(a), lipoprotein a; LPL, lipoprotein lipase.

TABLE 33.3. Cell Receptors Involved in Lipoprotein Metabolism

Receptor	Cell	Ligand	Function
B/E (LDL_R)	Liver	LDL	Clearance of LDL from plasma
	Peripheral cells	—	Cellular cholesterol uptake for membrane synthesis or biliary excretion
		VLDL remnants	Clearance of VLDL
			Conversion to LDL
LRP	Liver	Chylomicron remnants	Triglyceride and remnant clearance
SRA	Peripheral cells[a]	Oxidized LDL	Cholesterol accumulation—foam cell formation
SRB_1 (CLA_1)	Liver	HDL	Selective HDL cholesterol uptake
	Peripheral cells[a]	HDL	Selective HDL cholesterol efflux
		Modified LDL	Cholesterol accumulation—foam cell formation
CD-36	Peripheral cells[a]	Modified LDL	Cholesterol accumulation—foam cell formation
ABC_1	Peripheral cells[a]	HDL	Efflux of cellular cholesterol
HDL_R	Kidney	HDL	HDL excretion
			Steroid biosynthesis

B/E, apo B/E receptor; LDL, low-density lipoprotein; LDL_R, LDL receptor; LRP, LDL receptor-like protein; SRA, scavenger receptor class A; SRB_1, scavenger receptor class B, type 1; CLA_1, term for human receptor; CD-36, conjugated diene lipid hydroperoxide 36; ABC_1, ATP binding cassette 1; HDL, high-density lipoprotein; HDL_R, HDL receptor; VLDL, very-low-density lipoprotein.
[a]Especially macrophages in vessel wall.

surface of the lipoprotein, whereas $apoC_{III}$ inhibits LPL. LPL is induced in adipose tissue by insulin (26). The liberated free fatty acids are available for oxidative needs of peripheral cells, and excess free fatty acids are stored primarily in triglycerides in adipose tissue to serve as a future source of free fatty acids.

As triglyceride is depleted from the chylomicrons, phospholipids and A and C apoproteins are transferred to HDL. The residual chylomicron particle, which has lost 80% to 90% of its triglyceride and is now relatively cholesterol-enriched, is called a chylomicron remnant. These remnants are believed to be cleared by the liver via LDL receptor–like protein (LRP), a protein that resembles the apo B/E receptor but probably recognizes $apoB_{48}$ (27). The remnants thus enter lysosomes in the liver, from which cholesterol can enter metabolic pathways in the hepatocytes, including excretion into the bile. The remaining triglyceride enters the hepatic triglyceride stores.

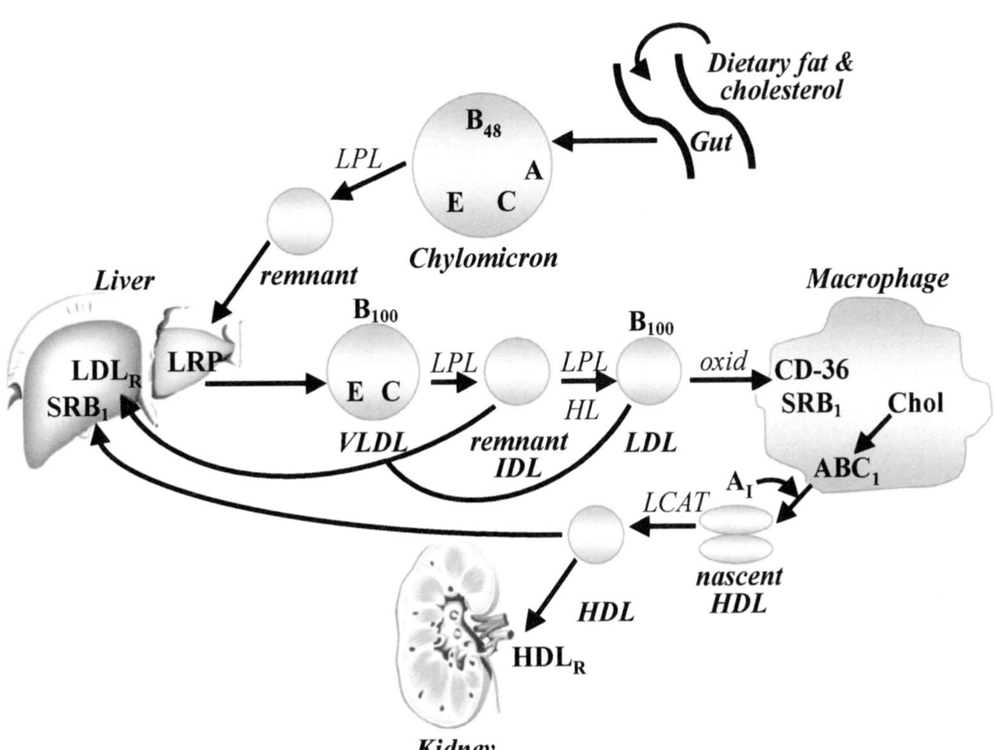

Figure 33.1. Schematic of lipoprotein metabolism. LDL_R, low-density lipoprotein receptor; SRB_1, scavenger receptor class B, type 1; LRP, LDL receptor-like protein; LPL, lipoprotein lipase; VLDL, very-low-density lipoproteins; IDL, intermediate-density lipoprotein; LDL, low-density lipoprotein; HL, hepatic lipase; oxid, oxidation; CD-36, conjugated diene lipid hydroperoxide; Chol, cholesterol; ABC_I, ATP binding cassette 1; LCAT, lecithin-cholesterol acyltransferase; HDL_R, HDL receptor; B_{48}, E, C_{II}, B_{100}, A_I, apoproteins (apo).

Very-Low-Density Lipoproteins

VLDLs are synthesized in the endoplasmic reticulum of hepatocytes and are composed of endogenous triglyceride derived from plasma free fatty acids, from chylomicron remnants, and from *de novo* lipogenesis (Fig. 33.1) (5,7,8,11,14,15). Post-translational regulation of VLDL assembly by glucose, fatty acids, and insulin is the major determinant of secretion (28). The concentration of circulating free fatty acids governs the rate of triglyceride esterification in the liver, and glucose—especially when glycogen synthesis is impeded—may stimulate *de novo* production of free fatty acids and thus triglycerides. Triglyceride transfer protein in the hepatocyte regulates the transport and assembly of triglyceride with apoB (28,29). Insulin is required for VLDL production, both for apoprotein synthesis and for its role in regulating several enzymes involved in lipogenesis (30). On the other hand, increases in insulin have been shown to inhibit VLDL secretion in hepatocytes by phosphorylating apoB, which impedes the assembly of apoB with lipids (28,31), and increases in insulin have been shown to inhibit VLDL production *in vivo* in human studies (32).

Nascent VLDLs, as secreted into the circulation, contain apoB$_{100}$ and small amounts of apoC and apoE. After VLDLs enter the circulation, they are metabolized in the same manner as chylomicrons by the enzyme LPL, with the fatty acids that are liberated following the same fate as those liberated from chylomicrons. After secretion, VLDLs acquire more C and E apoproteins by transfer from HDL. In addition, free cholesterol is progressively exchanged to HDL, where it is esterified and the cholesteryl ester is returned to VLDL. As VLDLs become progressively depleted of triglyceride, a portion of the surface, including cholesterol, apolipoproteins C and E, and phospholipids, is removed and contributes to nascent HDL particles (33). The enzyme hepatic lipase also plays a role in the metabolism of smaller VLDL particles during the latter stages of the VLDL catabolic cascade (22). The smaller remnants of VLDL are triglyceride-depleted, cholesterol-rich particles, some of which are isolated in the IDL compartment, although some remain in the VLDL compartment. These remnant particles are cleared from the circulation primarily by receptors in the liver. These receptors include both the B/E receptor (see below) and possibly LRP (27), which acts on chylomicron remnants. A portion of VLDL remnants is further metabolized, possibly within the intracellular spaces of the liver, by a process involving hepatic lipase, to form LDL. During this process, the remainder of apoproteins other than apoE is lost.

The mechanisms that determine which and how many VLDL particles are converted to LDL are not clearly understood. VLDL particles are believed to be secreted in a spectrum of sizes with various degrees of triglyceride enrichment. The larger VLDL particles appear to be more rapidly cleared and less likely to be converted to LDL (34). On the other hand, smaller VLDL particles that are richer in cholesterol may be preferentially converted to LDL. When apoE is missing or defective (as in type III hyperlipidemia) (14), clearance of chylomicron remnants and VLDL remnants is much slower than normal. These remnants accumulate in plasma and are not readily converted to LDL.

Low-Density Lipoproteins

As indicated above, LDLs are products of the metabolism of VLDL (Fig. 33.1) (4,5,7,8). The only apolipoprotein in LDL is apoB, and only one molecule of apoB is present per particle of LDL. Clearance of LDL is mediated by a specific receptor (the B/E receptor) present on the surface of both liver and peripheral cells (4). Once it is bound to the receptor, the lipoprotein is internalized by an endocytotic process (Fig. 33.2). The vesicle then fuses with a lysosome, where enzymes degrade the apoB and hydrolyze the cholesteryl ester to free cholesterol. Triglycerides and phospholipids may also be hydrolyzed. The influx of free cholesterol from LDL sets into motion a cascade of regulatory events aimed at controlling the cholesterol content of the cell. Esterification of cholesterol is stimulated by activation of acyl CoA cholesterol acyltransferase (ACAT). Simultaneously, *de novo* cholesterol production is inhibited by the inhibition of 3-hydroxy-3-methyl-glutaryl (HMG)-CoA reductase, the rate-limiting enzyme in cholesterol biosynthesis. Finally, accumulation of intracellular cholesterol limits the further uptake of cholesterol-rich lipoproteins by inhibiting synthesis of the B/E receptor.

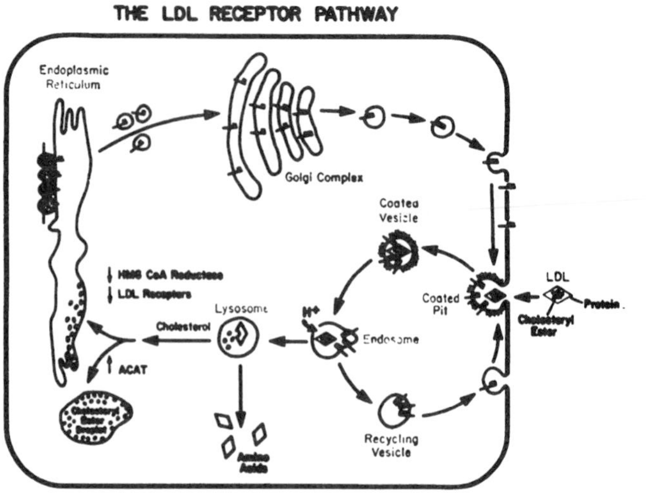

Figure 33.2. Binding and cellular metabolism of low-density lipoprotein (LDL). HMG, 3-hydroxy-3-methyl-glutaryl; ACAT, acyl CoA cholesterol acyltransferase. (From Brown MS, Goldstein JL. The LDL receptor and HMG-CoA reductase—two membrane molecules that regulate cholesterol homeostasis. *Curr Top Cell Regul* 1985;26:3–15, with permission.)

LDL may also be removed by clearance mechanisms mediated not by the B/E receptor but by phagocytic cells; such mechanisms include uptake by both nonspecific endocytosis and via the scavenger receptors—classes A (SRA) and B type 1 (SRB$_1$, known as CLA$_1$ in humans), and conjugated diene lipid hydroperoxide 36 (CD-36) receptors, which recognize altered (oxidized or glycated) LDL (35–39). This process is thought to be responsible for cholesterol deposition in macrophages of the vessel wall.

LDLs represent a spectrum of particles varying in density from larger cholesterol-rich particles (phenotype A) to smaller cholesterol-poor particles (phenotype B) (40,41). The latter usually occur when levels of triglyceride-rich lipoproteins are elevated as a result of CETP-mediated exchange between triglyceride and the cholesteryl ester from LDL followed by lipolysis of LDL triglyceride (42). These smaller, denser LDL particles are more susceptible to modification by oxidation (and glycation, see below), after which they are recognized and taken up by macrophages.

High-Density Lipoproteins

HDLs also are represented by a spectrum of particles of various sizes and densities (5,7,13). HDLs are secreted by the hepatocyte as small, cholesterol-poor/protein-rich particles that contain the A apoproteins as well as apoE. Small (nascent) HDLs also are produced by the intestine (Fig. 33.1). Some HDL particles contain both apoA$_I$ and apoA$_{II}$, whereas others contain only apoA$_I$. In the plasma, surface components of triglyceride-rich lipoproteins are transferred to HDL during lipolysis. In addi-

TABLE 33.4. Important Plasma Regulators of Lipoprotein Metabolism

Plasma regulator	Major source	Function
Lipoprotein lipase (LPL)	Adipose tissue Muscle Heart	Hydrolyzes triglycerides and phospholipids in chylomicrons and large VLDL
Hepatic lipase (HL)	Liver	Hydrolyzes triglycerides and phospholipids in small VLDL and HDL
Lecithin-cholesterol acyltransferase (LCAT)	Liver	Esterifies free cholesterol
Cholesteryl ester transfer protein (CETP)	Liver	Transfers cholesteryl ester and cholesterol between lipoproteins and cells

VLDL, very low-density lipoprotein; HDL, high-density lipoprotein.

tion, HDL particles are the sites of synthesis of cholesteryl ester from free cholesterol and lecithin through the enzyme LCAT, which circulates in association with HDL particles. HDLs participate in the catabolism of triglyceride-rich lipoproteins, serving as a source for cholesteryl esters and the C and E apoproteins and ultimately as the receptacle for surface components. During the lipolytic process, the size of the HDL particle increases. Larger particles are referred to as HDL_2 and the smaller HDL precursors are known as HDL_3.

HDLs, along with LCAT and CETP (Table 33.4), are important in the flux of cholesterol from cells to plasma lipoproteins and the liver (13,24,25,43,44). The ATP binding cassette 1 (ABC_1) receptor, which is present on macrophages and other peripheral cells, facilitates the transfer of cellular cholesterol to $apoA_1$, which is free in plasma or on nascent HDL particles. After conversion to cholesteryl ester by LCAT, the cholesteryl ester becomes trapped within the nonpolar center of HDL; this cholesteryl ester may circulate in HDL or be transferred to triglyceride-rich particles. The SRB_1 receptor may also mediate the removal of cholesterol and cholesteryl ester from peripheral cells or macrophages to HDL through a process of selective lipid transfer. This receptor mediates the transfer of cholesterol and cholesteryl ester from cells to HDL and from larger HDLs to the liver. This process represents a pathway for "reverse cholesterol transport," by which cholesterol from peripheral cells can be removed and transported to the liver for excretion in bile.

The mechanisms that control clearance of HDL are not well understood. Hepatic lipase may hydrolyze HDL phospholipids, which in turn may promote net transfer of cholesterol from the surface of HDL to the liver. A specific HDL receptor (HDL_R) on the kidney catalyzes specific uptake and degradation of HDL particles (45). This receptor also provides cholesterol to adrenal cells for steroidogenesis.

LIPOPROTEIN ALTERATIONS IN TYPE 2 DIABETES

The following summarizes commonly observed lipoprotein changes and their possible metabolic determinants in individuals with type 2 diabetes (Table 33.5) (for additional details, see references 30,46–55).

Triglycerides and Very-Low-Density Lipoproteins

The most common alteration of lipoproteins in type 2 diabetes is hypertriglyceridemia caused by an elevation in VLDL concentrations. In clinical descriptions of diabetic hypertriglyceridemia, an emphasis is often placed on individuals with extremely high levels of plasma and VLDL triglycerides. It is clear, however, from population-based studies (53,56) that type 2 diabetes generally is associated with only a 50% to 100% elevation in the plasma levels of total and VLDL triglycerides. Thus, it is likely that subjects with type 2 diabetes who have concentrations of total triglycerides greater than 350 to 400 mg/dL also have genetic defects in lipoprotein metabolism, the expression of which may be exacerbated by hyperglycemia (57) (see below).

Metabolic Determinants

One of the determinants of diabetic hypertriglyceridemia is the overproduction of VLDL triglyceride (58–60), which is most likely due to the increased flow of substrates, particularly glucose and free fatty acids, to the liver. In addition, individuals with type 2 diabetes appear to have a defect in clearance of VLDL triglyceride that parallels the degree of hyperglycemia (58–61). Studies to date suggest that LPL activity is decreased in individuals with type 2 diabetes, especially those with moderate to severe hyperglycemia who exhibit both insulin deficiency and insulin resistance (62). However, *in vivo* clearance defects have not consistently been observed in patients with type 2 diabetes, especially in those with greatly elevated triglyceride levels.

The metabolism of VLDL apoB may also be altered in type 2 diabetes. Subjects with type 2 diabetes have a decreased fractional catabolic rate for VLDL apoB similar to that for VLDL triglyceride (60). Overproduction of VLDL apoB also occurs in

TABLE 33.5. Lipoprotein Alterations in Type 2 Diabetes

Lipoprotein	Alterations
VLDL ↑	Increased production of triglyceride and apoB Decreased clearance of triglyceride and apoB Abnormal composition
LDL ↑→	Increased production of LDL apoB Decreased receptor-mediated clearance Triglyceride enrichment Smaller (more dense) particle distribution Glycation Oxidation
HDL ↓	Increased clearance of apoA Decreased proportion of large HDL Triglyceride enrichment Glycation Diminished reverse cholesterol transport
Chylomicron	Delayed clearance; remnant accumulation

VLDL, very-low density lipoprotein; LDL, low-density lipoprotein; HDL, high-density lipoprotein; apo, apoprotein.

type 2 diabetes, and it has been suggested that this overproduction is further increased by obesity (60). Although obese diabetic subjects have a higher VLDL-B production than do lean individuals, VLDL-B production may already be maximally stimulated in obese nondiabetic individuals (60). Thus, the extent of overproduction of VLDL triglyceride may be greater than that of apoB in type 2 diabetes, a situation that results in the production of larger triglyceride-rich VLDL particles.

The alterations in VLDL metabolism in type 2 diabetes are related in part to insulin resistance. Several studies have shown correlations between VLDL concentrations and measures of insulin resistance (30,52). Hyperinsulinemia and the central obesity that typically accompanies insulin resistance also are thought to lead to overproduction and impaired catabolism of VLDL. Metabolic alterations in insulin resistance that lead to VLDL overproduction include (a) increased free fatty acid and glucose levels, which regulate VLDL output from the liver, and (b) elevated triglyceride levels in the liver, which inhibit apoB degradation and result in increased assembly and secretion of VLDL. In addition, LPL levels are reduced in insulin resistance, which interferes with the normal lipoprotein metabolic cascade and results in decreased clearance of VLDL.

Triglyceride elevations in type 2 diabetes may also be due to delayed clearance of postprandial particles (63). Mechanisms of delayed clearance of chylomicrons are similar to those discussed for VLDL clearance.

Very-Low-Density Lipoprotein Composition

In addition to increases in the amount of VLDL, changes in VLDL composition in type 2 diabetes may reflect or be the cause of alterations in VLDL metabolism. Several studies suggest that individuals with diabetes, especially those with severe hyperglycemia, may have larger triglyceride-rich VLDL (60,64). This increased ratio of triglyceride to apoB may be a reflection of a disproportionate influence of type 2 diabetes on VLDL triglyceride production (see above). Subfractions of VLDL have been found to be enriched in the proportion of cholesterol-rich particles (65). These compositional changes may have implications for the increased propensity for atherosclerosis among individuals with type 2 diabetes, because cholesterol-enriched VLDL may be atherogenic. Changes in the distribution of apoE would have important implications for VLDL metabolism in type 2 diabetes because apoE influences the affinity of binding to receptors. An increased proportion of apoE in the VLDL of type 2 diabetes has been reported (66). Although differences in distribution of apoE phenotypes in diabetes have not been demonstrated, apoE sialation has been reported to be higher in diabetic than nondiabetic individuals, a change that may impair binding to the B/E receptor (67).

Additional evidence for abnormal VLDL in type 2 diabetes is that VLDLs from persons with type 2 diabetes have altered metabolic properties *in vitro*. VLDL isolated from normotriglyceridemic patients with type 2 diabetes produced a greater cellular accumulation of lipids in mouse peritoneal macrophages than did VLDL isolated from either normotriglyceridemic or hypertriglyceridemic nondiabetic control subjects (68). Thus, altered VLDL composition may contribute to metabolic abnormalities as well as to the atherosclerotic propensity of the VLDL particles.

Remnant particles from delayed chylomicron clearance may also be present in the VLDL fraction; they are subject to the same compositional alterations discussed for VLDL.

Low-Density Lipoprotein Cholesterol

Studies examining plasma concentrations of total and LDL cholesterol in type 2 diabetes vary by population, with some showing higher and some showing lower levels in type 2 diabetes than in control subjects. Data from the National Health and Nutrition Examination Survey (NHANES II) indicate that levels of LDL cholesterol in whites with diabetes are higher than for blacks with diabetes, after adjustment for relevant covariates (56). Lower LDL concentrations are also seen in American Indians with diabetes (53). It should be pointed out that in most population studies, the density ranges chosen for quantitation of LDL (1.006 to 1.063) result in the inclusion of the IDL fraction. It is possible that the increase in LDL in type 2 diabetes is the result of an increase in this IDL fraction.

METABOLISM

In individuals with type 2 diabetes and relatively severe hyperglycemia, the clearance rate for LDL apoB is reduced (60,69). Mildly hyperglycemic individuals with type 2 diabetes may have increased LDL production as well (69). Because LDL binding is stimulated by insulin (70), defects in LDL clearance in type 2 diabetes may be due to insulin resistance or relative insulin deficiency. This possibility is supported by the observation that clearance of LDL in type 2 diabetes is positively related to plasma insulin levels and to the insulin response from oral glucose challenge (69). Direct removal of VLDL apoB is also increased in individuals with type 2 diabetes and large, triglyceride-rich VLDL (60). Thus, the concentrations of LDL in type 2 diabetes may be influenced by two opposing phenomena. On one hand, decreased clearance in type 2 diabetes may lead to increased LDL; on the other hand, increased direct removal tends to lower production. The resultant concentration may thus be dependent on the relative magnitude of these two processes. Nevertheless, these alterations in the flux of both VLDL remnants and LDL particles, coupled with the changes in LDL composition, indicate that LDL in individuals with type 2 diabetes has significant atherogenic potential.

COMPOSITION

The composition of LDL in type 2 diabetes is altered, and these changes also may contribute significantly to abnormal metabolism and atherosclerosis. An increase in the proportion of small, dense, triglyceride-enriched LDL has consistently been observed (64,71–73). LDL particles from individuals with diabetes have a decreased ability to bind to receptors, and this decrease in binding is inversely related to the size and ratio of triglyceride to protein in LDL (74). LDL in diabetic individuals has been shown to be more rapidly oxidized (75). This may be in part because of the increased oxidative susceptibility of small, dense LDL particles, which are prevalent in diabetic individuals. Oxidized LDL particles are believed to play a major role in stimulating the atherosclerotic process because of their recognition by macrophage receptors (Table 33.3).

Increased plasma triglyceride levels, low HDL levels, and small, dense LDLs usually occur together in a lipoprotein pattern often referred to as atherogenic dyslipidemia (76). This abnormal pattern occurs in insulin resistance, is exacerbated in diabetes (52,77), and is derived in part from alterations in apoB metabolism because triglyceride-rich VLDLs are the precursors of denser LDL particles (78). Small, dense LDLs are slowly catabolized because they do not bind well to the B/E receptor.

Nonenzymatic glycation (or glycosylation) of apoB also may influence LDL metabolism in diabetes. Small, dense LDLs are more rapidly glycated. The extent of glycation of LDL in individuals with type 2 diabetes who have moderate hyperglycemia is approximately 2% to 5% (79), and this degree of glycation of lysine residues has been shown to decrease LDL catabolism *in vivo* by 5% to 25% (80). Glycated LDLs also appear to exhibit altered interactions with endothelial cells, stimulate cytokine production, and enhance cholesteryl ester synthesis in human macrophages (81). Moreover, glycated LDLs are more readily oxidized. Thus, the glycation of LDL may represent an important mechanism by which atherogenesis is increased in type 2 diabetes. Together, glycation and oxidation render LDLs more immunogenic; the formation of antibody-antigen complexes stimulates macrophage accumulation and further foam cell formation (82).

Finally, a pattern of abnormal cholesterol transport and transfer in the plasma has been shown in patients with type 2 diabetes. The transfer of LCAT-synthesized cholesteryl esters to VLDL and LDL is inhibited, with a concomitant increase in their transfer to HDL; this abnormal metabolic pattern is reversed by insulin therapy (83). The block in cholesteryl ester transfer activity in patients with type 2 diabetes is correlated with an increase in free cholesterol content of both LDL and VLDL. Therefore, in type 2 diabetes, this abnormal cholesteryl ester transfer may be related to an increased risk for atherosclerosis.

High-Density Lipoprotein Cholesterol

Almost as common as the observation of increased VLDL concentrations in type 2 diabetes is the finding of decreased concentrations of HDL cholesterol in individuals with type 2 diabetes.

METABOLISM

Individuals with type 2 diabetes have an increased rate of HDL clearance, as measured by $apoA_I$ and $apoA_{II}$ kinetics (84–86). Significant correlations have been found between HDL clearance and plasma concentrations of HDL cholesterol and $apoA_I$, and the increase in HDL clearance was directly related to plasma glucose levels. The finding of increased HDL clearance is consistent with lower VLDL clearance and lower LPL activity. Because HDL concentrations, especially of larger HDLs, increase during the lipolytic process, the decreases in LPL activity and impaired VLDL catabolism have been shown to be correlated with decreases in HDL concentrations in patients with type 2 diabetes. Elevated hepatic lipase activity also may contribute to the decrease in HDL concentrations in type 2 diabetes, because this enzyme also plays a key role in the metabolism of HDL. The changes in lipoprotein and hepatic lipases may act in concert to decrease HDL levels in type 2 diabetes.

COMPOSITION

There are several indications that the composition of HDLs in type 2 diabetes may be altered (52). These differences may be in part a reflection of alterations in the delipidation cascade. Decreased HDL concentrations in type 2 diabetes are reflected mostly in decreases in larger particles. As with LDL, in type 2 diabetes an increased proportion of triglyceride in HDL has been observed. These compositional changes appear to be related to the activity of adipose tissue LPL, because LPL deficiency may be a factor responsible for the altered distribution of HDL particles in untreated type 2 diabetes. Nonenzymatic glycation of HDL appears to interfere with HDL receptor binding (87). Thus, glycation of HDL may also play a role in the lower levels of HDL observed in diabetes. Finally, abnormalities in HDL composition have been noted even in individuals with optimal glycemic control (88). All of these alterations in HDL composition may impair the role of HDL in reverse cholesterol transport.

As stated above, the decreases in HDL concentration and changes in HDL composition are part of the dyslipidemia of insulin resistance. Changes in HDL metabolism in insulin resistance include (a) impaired VLDL lipolysis, which depletes HDL by impeding the transfer of apoproteins and cholesterol ester from triglyceride-rich lipoproteins to the HDL compartment; (b) increased activity of hepatic lipase, which facilitates HDL clearance; and (c) alterations in hepatic function, which inhibit production of $apoA_I$ (the main apoprotein of HDL) and/or hepatic secretion of nascent HDL (52).

Significant negative relationships between plasma concentrations of insulin and HDL have been observed in subjects with type 2 diabetes as well as a negative relationship between insulin resistance and HDL cholesterol that is independent of VLDL concentrations (53,63). These observations indicate that insulin or insulin resistance influences the concentration or composition of HDL in some way.

LIPOPROTEINS IN TYPE 1 DIABETES

The consideration of lipoprotein metabolism in type 1 diabetes is influenced by the requirement for insulin therapy. Thus, a spectrum of situations is possible, from the insulin-deficient ketoacidotic state with greatly elevated glucose, free fatty acids, ketones, and lipolytic hormones such as glucagon and epinephrine, to that seen when continuous insulin therapy is administered, in which an excess of insulin in peripheral plasma is found and glucose and fatty acid levels are close to normal (Fig. 33.3) (47–52). In the following sections, an attempt will be made to differentiate between these various degrees of control.

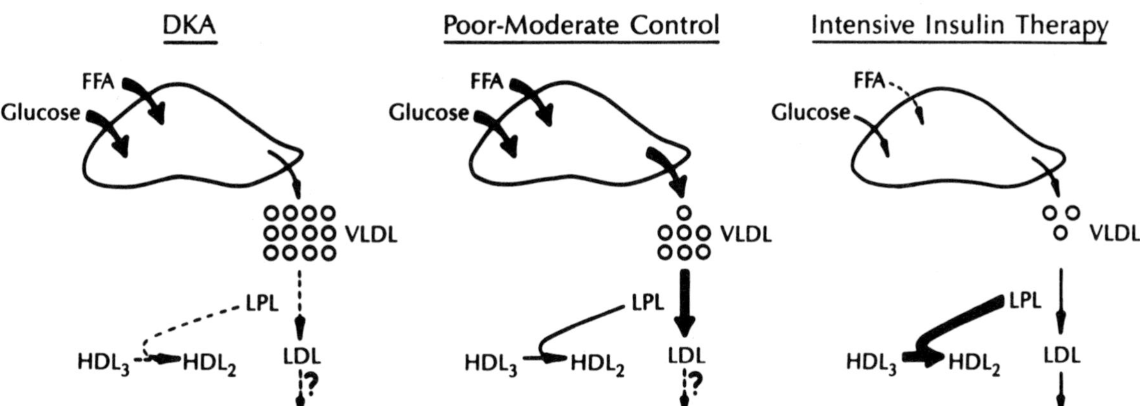

Figure 33.3. Spectrum of lipoprotein changes in type 1 diabetes with various degrees of control. DKA, diabetic ketoacidosis. See legend to Figure 33.1 for other abbreviations. (From Howard BV. Lipoprotein metabolism in diabetes mellitus. *J Lipid Res* 1987;28:613–628, with permission.)

Very-Low-Density Lipoproteins

Extreme elevations in VLDL levels have been recognized as being a common occurrence in diabetic ketoacidosis, the stage at which insulin concentrations are minimal (89). On the other hand, VLDL levels may not be elevated in individuals with type 1 diabetes who are receiving adequate therapy. It is now well established that elevations in VLDL triglycerides in type 1 diabetes are often correlated with the degree of diabetic control (90,91).

METABOLISM

In people with untreated type 1 diabetes, the fractional catabolic rate for endogenous triglyceride is decreased (92), as is the clearance rate for exogenous triglyceride (93). Thus, when insulin deficiency is extreme, clearance is impaired because the activity of LPL is dependent on insulin. In the early stages of insulin deficiency, production of VLDL is increased, probably because of the increase in mobilization of free fatty acids. This enhanced hepatic secretion of VLDL falls off in the later stages of ketoacidosis because of the decrease in hepatic protein synthesis secondary to the insulin deficiency. In poorly controlled but nonketotic patients with type 1 diabetes, both overproduction and decreased clearance are observed (94). Kinetic studies of VLDL triglyceride in subjects with type 1 diabetes with adequate conventional insulin therapy showed that production and fractional catabolic rates of VLDL triglycerides were normal when compared with rates in weight- and age-matched controls (95). Continuous subcutaneous insulin infusion produced a significant decline in VLDL triglyceride production to levels below those observed in nondiabetic subjects. There was no change in the mean fractional catabolic rate for VLDL triglyceride after insulin infusion. A similar decrease in plasma VLDL triglyceride production in type 1 diabetes was observed after treatment with the artificial β-cell (96). These latter studies indicate that rigorous insulin therapy can decrease rates of VLDL production and produce even subnormal levels of VLDL triglyceride.

During severe ketoacidosis when there is a marked insulin deficiency, hypertriglyceridemia is caused primarily by a deficiency in LPL activity, and overproduction of triglycerides may not occur despite elevated levels of free fatty acids. As insulin therapy is instituted, the situation changes. With moderate control (i.e., when insulin administration is suboptimal) there is both an overproduction of VLDL because of an increase in the level of free fatty acids and some deficiency in VLDL clearance because of the continued limitation in LPL. As stringent control is achieved with the administration of large amounts of peripheral insulin, VLDL clearance normalizes. VLDL production rates may fall to subnormal levels because excess insulin may suppress hepatic VLDL formation. Individuals with type 1 diabetes in this situation will have normal or even low-normal levels of circulating VLDL triglycerides.

Low-Density Lipoproteins

LDL concentration appears to vary directly with the extent of hyperglycemia. LDL levels are increased in poorly controlled type 1 diabetes. However, in many individuals with type 1 diabetes, LDL concentrations are not different from those of age- and weight-matched controls, and some type 1 diabetic subjects receiving insulin by means of a pump exhibit LDL concentrations considerably below those of controls.

METABOLISM

Fractional catabolic rates for LDL in subjects receiving conventional therapy or who have received 3 weeks of continuous subcutaneous insulin infusion are similar to those for nondiabetic controls. Improvement in glycemic control decreases LDL apoB production to levels below those of nondiabetic subjects. In uncontrolled type 1 diabetes, LDL fractional clearance is probably decreased because insulin appears to potentiate LDL binding to its receptor. With increased control, LDL metabolism may return to normal (97). Further, insulin deficiency may lead to overproduction of LDL in response to an increased influx of VLDL or its precursor or to impaired removal of VLDL remnants by the liver. Abnormalities in the VLDL particle also may influence conversion to LDL.

COMPOSITION

Individuals with type 1 diabetes may also have a preponderance of small, dense particles for the same reasons as those described for type 2 diabetes. LDLs isolated from patients with poorly controlled type 1 diabetes are taken up and degraded by fibroblasts at a lower rate than LDLs isolated from healthy subjects; when glucose concentrations are lowered by insulin therapy, the binding properties of LDLs return to normal (98). Glycated LDL and defects in cholesteryl ester transfer may be found in type 1, as well as in type 2, diabetes, although no studies on glycation in type 1 diabetes have yet been performed. Exposure of cells to lipoprotein-deficient serum obtained from patients with poorly controlled type 1 diabetes enhances the efficiency of LDL binding (99). It has been postulated that in type 1 diabetes, membrane changes may be induced that alter LDL binding.

High-Density Lipoproteins

It has been suggested that concentrations of HDL may be low in patients with untreated, insulin-deficient diabetes. Response of HDL to insulin therapy is slower than that of VLDL, but HDL increases with the degree of glycemic control. In several studies, HDL concentrations are similar or higher in patients with type 1 diabetes than in age-, sex-, and weight-matched controls. HDL levels may also be higher in those who are receiving insulin-pump therapy (91–97).

METABOLISM

One factor responsible for the decrease in HDL in patients with poorly controlled type 1 diabetes is low LPL activity. The reduced activity impairs lipolysis of VLDL and subsequently slows formation of HDL particles (62). Levels of both HDL cholesterol and phospholipids in type 1 diabetes have been shown to correlate positively with LPL activity; thus, greatly increased catabolism of triglyceride-rich lipoproteins in the presence of excess insulin might augment the HDL compartment. An inverse correlation has been observed between HDL and hepatic lipase activity in the plasma of type 1 diabetic subjects. Hepatic lipase activity may be lower in well-controlled type 1 diabetes and associated with a high ratio of HDL_2 to HDL_3; thus, the role of this enzyme in regulating HDL levels and the possible influence of insulin on this process are similar to those postulated for type 2 diabetes (100).

COMPOSITION

HDL elevations in well-controlled type 1 diabetes are generally due to an increase in larger particles. These observations confirm the hypothesis that the action of insulin, whether it occurs through the activity of LPL or via some other process, hastens the transfer of material to the HDL_2 compartment. Data indicate that alterations in HDL composition may be found in type 1 diabetes much as they are in type 2 diabetes. Lower concentrations of HDL are associated with HDL particles that are smaller and richer in triglycerides. Abnormalities in both triglyceride and $apoA_I$ content have been observed in the HDL of individuals with type 1 diabetes (101), and apoA$_I$ and apoA$_{II}$ content may also be decreased. ApoA has also been reported to be glycated in patients with type 1 diabetes (102).

RATIONALE FOR THERAPY FOR LIPID ABNORMALITIES IN DIABETES

Atherosclerotic macrovascular disease is the leading cause of morbidity and mortality in patients with diabetes mellitus. Both men and women with diabetes have a significantly increased risk of myocardial infarction (MI) (103–105), stroke, and peripheral gangrene (104,105). The risk for developing coronary heart disease (CHD) begins prior to the development of type 2 diabetes. By the time the diagnosis of type 2 diabetes is made, more than half of all diabetic individuals already have clinical CHD (106). Haffner et al. (107) compared this phenomenon to a clock that begins ticking with the onset of insulin resistance and accelerates with the development of hyperglycemia. In a Finnish cohort of patients with type 2 diabetes, Haffner and colleagues (108) demonstrated that diabetic patients without previous MI have as high a risk for a first MI as do nondiabetic patients with a history of MI for having a second infarction. In addition, patients with diabetes have an increased rate of MI-associated prehospital mortality (105,109), as well as increased morbidity and mortality during and after hospitalization (110–112). This is particularly true for women with diabetes (53,113) These data provide a strong rationale for treating cardiovascular risk factors in diabetic patients as aggressively as in nondiabetic patients with clinical CHD. Thus, diabetes confers a risk that is equivalent to that of known CHD. The ADA and the American Heart Association consider type 2 diabetes a CHD equivalent (104,114).

The evidence is unequivocal that an abnormal lipid profile is a significant risk factor for atherosclerotic macrovascular disease in patients with diabetes (115,116). Modification of lipid and other risk factors has clearly been shown to lower mortality due to cardiovascular disease (CVD) in the general population (117–127). This has underscored the need for management of CVD risk factors (in addition to control of hyperglycemia) in individuals with diabetes (114,128–130). The United Kingdom Prospective Diabetes Study (UKPDS) demonstrates that controlling lipids and blood pressure may be significantly more effective in preventing CVD than is controlling hyperglycemia (122,131). Thus, in individuals with diabetes, the management of lipid disorders, as well as total risk-factor management, is of paramount importance.

DIABETIC DYSLIPIDEMIA

The dyslipidemia associated with type 2 diabetes and insulin resistance typically consists of elevated triglycerides and decreased HDL cholesterol level (132). In such individuals, LDL cholesterol levels are generally not significantly abnormal, although they may be somewhat elevated in whites (133) and lower in other racial/ethnic groups. The frequently mild abnormality in LDL cholesterol concentration associated with diabetes belies a qualitative abnormality in the LDL structure, i.e., decreased size and increased density of the LDL particle (134). The metabolic processes responsible for these abnormalities have been discussed previously.

Although triglyceride levels are usually mildly elevated, diabetic and insulin-resistant patients are subject to known, nonhyperglycemic factors that induce hyperlipidemia. For example, diabetes may occur in the presence of a familial syndrome of abnormal triglyceride or LDL metabolism and secondary causes of hyperlipidemia (135–141). Pharmacologic agents or alcohol abuse also may increase triglyceride and LDL cholesterol levels or further decrease HDL cholesterol concentrations (142–144). Coincident hypothyroidism and renal and liver disease also increase lipid levels (145).

Even when LDL cholesterol is normal or within a range that might be considered low in nondiabetic individuals, LDL appears to be a very potent contributor to the development of CHD (146). Recent data from the Strong Heart Study illustrated that, in American Indians, LDL cholesterol level was the most significant predictor of increased CHD, despite an average LDL cholesterol level of approximately 115 mg/dL (146). In this study, LDL was a strong predictor of CHD at levels as low as 70 mg/dL (146).

Multiple studies in the general population now conclusively demonstrate that LDL cholesterol lowering is very effective in both primary and secondary CVD prevention (147). Three large clinical trials—the Scandinavian Simvastatin Survival Study (4S) (129), the Cholesterol and Recurrent Events (CARE) trial (148), and the Long-term Intervention with Pravastatin in Ischaemic Disease (LIPID) Trial (125)—have all shown that the use of a statin drug to lower LDL cholesterol over a wide range of LDL levels in patients with preexisting CHD is very effective in preventing all-cause mortality, death due to atherosclerotic events, nonfatal atherosclerotic events, and the need for revascularization. Unexpectedly, these studies also showed a reduced incidence of stroke with statin therapy in patients with preexisting CHD. Several diabetes substudies (129, 153) have demonstrated significant improvement with regard to CVD mitigation and prevention (123–127, 149–152). Two additional trials in individuals without preexisting CHD, the Air Force/Texas Coronary Atherosclerosis Prevention Study (AFCAPS/TexCAPS) (126) and West of Scotland Coronary Prevention Study (WOSCOPS), have shown similar results.

The 4S trial, which initially studied 202 patients with type 2 diabetes, showed that cholesterol lowering effected a 55% reduction in risk of major CHD events, bringing the risk close to that for nondiabetic individuals (129). A later analysis of the 4S cohort using the new diagnostic criteria for diabetes of the Expert Committee on the Diagnosis and Classification of Diabetes Mellitus (154) (i.e., a fasting plasma glucose cutpoint of 7.0 instead of 7.8 mmol/L) increased the size of the diabetic cohort in 4S from 202 to 483 (155), with similar results with regard to the efficacy of lipid lowering in preventing CVD.

The CARE study included a large number of participants with type 2 diabetes as well as individuals with impaired glucose tolerance and insulin resistance (130). In this study, aggressive lipid lowering reduced CVD risk in diabetic individuals to that in their nondiabetic counterparts. A similar observation was made in the LIPID trial (125), although the percentage of diabetic participants was small. The AFCAPS/TexCAPS trial demonstrated that CHD could be prevented in diabetic patients who had no prior history of CHD (126). The therapeutic effect of statin therapy in these trials was a significant lowering of LDL cholesterol levels. At least one subsequent analysis indicates that reduction in CVD risk is proportional to the degree of reduction in LDL cholesterol (156,157). Further, statins have been shown to lower triglyceride and raise HDL cholesterol levels (158).

The Veterans Affairs High-Density Lipoprotein Cholesterol Intervention Trial (VA-HIT) examined the effects of gemfibrozil in patients with average to low LDL levels, moderately elevated triglyceride levels, and significantly decreased HDL cholesterol (159). In this study, gemfibrozil therapy increased HDL cholesterol concentrations by 6% and lowered triglyceride levels by

31%. These changes in lipid levels resulted in a 24% decrease in relative risk of CVD. Results in the subcohort of 627 patients with diabetes were identical (159). Finally, the Post Coronary Artery Bypass Trial showed similar angiographic improvement between diabetic and nondiabetic subjects with aggressive therapy with lovastatin and low-dose warfarin (160).

Although none of the previously described trials was designed primarily for patients with diabetes, they strongly indicate that controlling lipid abnormalities in patients with diabetes is effective in preventing or ameliorating CVD. The first trial designed to study a diabetic population, the Diabetes Atherosclerosis Intervention Study (DAIS), examined the effects of fenofibrate therapy in patients with type 2 diabetes (161,162). This trial was also a secondary prevention trial, with its primary outcome an improved coronary angiogram with fenofibrate therapy. At the end of the 3-year study, in a cohort of 418 patients, repeated angiograms showed a significant 40% reduction in focal atherosclerotic lesions with a similar (although not statistically significant) reduction in diffuse atherosclerotic disease (163,164). Although the trial was not powered to observe clinical outcomes, fenofibrate also reduced the combined endpoints of MI, revascularization, and death by approximately 23%. The most impressive study of lipid reduction in patients with diabetes is the Heart Protection Study (164a). In this trial 20,536 adults were randomized to either simvastatin, 40 mg, or antioxidant vitamins. Of the participants in this trial, 5,963 were known prospectively to have diabetes mellitus. Of this group, 1,981 had existing CHD and 3,982 were without prior CHD. Simvastatin therapy resulted in a significant 20.2% reduction of CHD events. Antioxidant vitamins were ineffective in preventing CHD. Additional trials in patients with diabetes are in progress and will be reported in the near future. It is hoped that these trials will provide final conclusive evidence concerning the management of lipid disorders in patients with type 2 diabetes.

At present, there are no interventional studies of lipid lowering in patients with type 1 diabetes, whose lipid abnormalities differ significantly from those of patients with type 2 diabetes. Patients with type 1 diabetes are reported to have accelerated CVD, and their lipid abnormalities are very responsive to glucose control. (90,91,95–97,115) Severe hypertriglyceridemia secondary to hyperchylomicronemia and an increased concentration of VLDL may occur in patients with type 1 diabetes when acute glucose metabolism is significantly abnormal. Patients with moderately controlled type 1 diabetes have less severe abnormalities of all lipid subfractions. There have been reports of elevated Lp(a) in uncontrolled type 1 diabetes, but the studies are not consistent (165).

In view of the observed increase in CVD in type 1 diabetes (166–168) and the increased prevalence of lipid abnormalities in those patients (116), a trial of lipid lowering is needed. Because the lipid abnormalities of type 1 diabetes often respond to glucose control, the results of the Diabetes Control and Complications Trial (DCCT) are germane (169). Although therapy with hypolipidemic drugs was not used in the DCCT, microvascular and neurologic complications of type 1 diabetes were mitigated in patients who received intensive insulin therapy, with a nonsignificant reduction in macrovascular disease (170). This trend toward reduced macrovascular disease is of double importance because of the concern that intensive insulin therapy per se might be atherogenic.

GOALS OF THERAPY

The Adult Treatment Panel III (ATPIII) of the National Cholesterol Education Program (NCEP) has established the goal of an LDL cholesterol level less than100 mg/dL for patients with pre-existing CHD or CHD risk equivalents (171). In this subset of patients, the NCEP has also determined that an HDL cholesterol level less than 40 mg/dL and a triglyceride level higher than 150 mg/dL are major CHD risk factors (172). In a recent addendum to the ATPIII report, an optional goal of achieving an LDL-C of less than 70 mg/dL was proposed for very-high-risk individuals such as patients with diabetes and known CHD (172a).

Because of the significant increase in cardiovascular risk conferred by diabetes and insulin resistance, the ADA has convened a series of consensus panels to discuss the goals for therapy in patients with diabetes (172). Because CVD risk in individuals with diabetes is equal to that of nondiabetic individuals who have pre-existing coronary disease, the ADA recommends that a similar LDL cholesterol goal of 100 mg/dL be set for all patients with type 2 diabetes. The categories of risk for type 2 diabetes as determined by lipid levels are summarized in Table 33.6.

In patients with diabetes, lipid abnormalities other than elevated LDL cholesterol are also potentially atherogenic. Hypertriglyceridemia has been implicated as an important contributor to atherosclerotic CVD (ASCVD) in patients with diabetes (173). Both the World Health Organization Multi-National Trial (174) and the Paris Prospective Study (175) have shown that hypertriglyceridemia is a significant predictor of subsequent cardiovascular mortality in persons with diabetes. In the Stockholm Ischaemic Heart Disease Secondary Prevention Study (176), lowering triglyceride levels was the most important factor in decreasing total and cardiovascular mortality. As discussed previously, abnormalities in VLDL composition and delayed clearance of chylomicron remnants may contribute to the accelerated ASCVD in patients with diabetes. In addition, individuals with diabetes are known to accumulate IDL and remnants of VLDL, which are definitely known to be atherogenic (177). The presence of small, dense LDL is also correlated with hypertriglyceridemia (173,178); this more atherogenic form of LDL begins to accumulate when triglyceride levels exceed 100 to 150 mg/dL (178).

TABLE 33.6. Degree of Risk of Coronary Heart Disease by Lipoprotein Level (mg/dL) in Type 2 Diabetes

Risk	LDL	HDL Men	HDL Women	Triglyceride
High	≥130	<35	<45	≥400
Borderline	100–129	35–45	45–55	200–399
Low	<100	>45	>55	<200

HDL, high-density lipoprotein; LDL, low-density lipoprotein.
Data from American Diabetes Association. Management of dyslipidemia in adults with diabetes. *Diabetes Care* 2000;23[Suppl 1]:S57–S60.

Epidemiologic studies have shown an inverse relationship between HDL concentration and CHD (179). As stated previously, the VA-HIT (159) and Stockholm (176) studies demonstrated a significant effect of a therapeutically induced increase in HDL in the prevention of CHD. Further, the Cholesterol Lowering Atherosclerosis Study (CLAS) (180) and Familial Atherosclerosis Treatment Study (FATS) (181) suggest that increases in HDL play a role in slowing the progression of CHD. Raising HDL levels in patients with type 2 diabetes can be extremely difficult, although the VA-HIT study suggests that pharmacologic therapy can be effective and desirable (182).

Recent studies suggest that non-HDL cholesterol is a better predictor of CHD risk than is LDL cholesterol alone (183,184). Non-HDL is determined by subtracting HDL cholesterol from total cholesterol and reflects the remaining amount of LDL and VLDL. Because the latter lipid classes also are differentiated by the presence of $apoB_{100}$, non-HDL cholesterol is highly correlated with total apoB. In AFCAPS/TexCAPS, total apoB was the best predictor of cardiovascular risk; non-HDL cholesterol provided an acceptable and readily available surrogate for total apoB (126). This is particularly applicable to the dyslipidemia that accompanies insulin resistance and type 2 diabetes, when HDL cholesterol is often low and triglyceride levels are high because of accumulation of atherogenic remnant triglyceride-rich lipoproteins: remnant VLDL and chylomicrons. The therapeutic goals for patients with type 2 diabetes are shown in Table 33.7.

The lack of interventional data in patients with type 1 diabetes makes it difficult to set specific goals for lipid therapy. The recommendation of the most recent ADA consensus panel, however, represents the best available advice of a panel of experts (3). One significant difference between type 1 and type 2 diabetes is that the intensive insulin therapy in type 1 usually normalizes and often increases HDL levels and improves other lipid abnormalities (115).

TREATMENT OF HYPERGLYCEMIA IN PATIENTS WITH DIABETES

Nonpharmacologic Therapy

A great deal of epidemiologic evidence indicates that patients with even mild hyperglycemia are at increased risk for macrovascular disease (185). Although there is little evidence from interventional studies that control of hyperglycemia in patients with type 2 diabetes will prevent macrovascular disease, the UKPDS (186) and other clinical trials (187,188) demonstrated a reduction in microvascular disease in individuals with either type 1 (189) or type 2 (186,190) diabetes. Therefore, glycemic control should be a high priority in both patients with type 1 diabetes and those with type 2 diabetes. Recent evidence indicates that there is therapeutic value in immediate control of blood glucose in individuals with type 2 diabetes who are experiencing an acute MI. The Diabetes Mellitus, Insulin Glucose Infusion in Acute Myocardial Infarction (DIGAMI) study demonstrated an 11% reduction in mortality during the first year among diabetic patients who received an insulin/glucose infusion within 24 hours after acute MI (191). The benefits of such aggressive therapy persisted for 3.5 years.

TABLE 33.7. Proposed Therapeutic Goals for Men and Women with Type 2 Diabetes

Lipid fractions	Ideal goal (mg/dL)
Total cholesterol	≤170
LDL cholesterol	<100[a]
HDL cholesterol	≥45 for men ≥55 for women
Triglycerides	≥200
Non-HDL cholesterol	<130

LDL, low-density lipoprotein; HDL, high-density lipoprotein.
[a] Optional goal for very-high-risk individual: <70.
Adapted from American Diabetes Association. Management of dyslipidemia in adults with type 2 diabetes. *Diabetes Care* 2000;23[Suppl 1]:S57–S60.

Hyperglycemia in both forms of diabetes accentuates the typical lipid abnormalities seen in each diabetic syndrome. Controlling glucose has been shown to decrease triglyceride levels and to increase HDL cholesterol levels in both type 1 and type 2 diabetes, as stated previously. The nonpharmacologic and pharmacologic therapies for hyperglycemia have been discussed previously and will not be repeated here. However, it is worth noting that several of the hypoglycemic agents used to treat patients with diabetes have primary effects on lipid levels in addition to their effects on hyperglycemia. Metformin has been shown to lower triglyceride levels in individuals with type 2 diabetes (192), and several of the thiazolidinediones also may lower triglycerides and raise HDL (193). Thiazolidinediones must be used with caution, however, because their use is often associated with increased levels of LDL cholesterol (194,195). Data from several small studies suggest that this increase in LDL concentration may be the result of conversion of small, dense LDL to a more buoyant form (196). This claim requires further investigation, especially because of the lack of conclusive evidence from prospective interventional trials that such a change in LDL size will be beneficial.

Nonpharmacologic treatments for hyperglycemia should be vigorously applied to patients with diabetes, because these therapies can retard the progression of and improve the lipid abnormalities associated with the disease (197). In addition to its effects on hyperglycemia (197) and lipids (198), exercise has positive benefits on cardiac physiology (199). Because of recent controversy concerning the appropriate diet for patients with diabetes and lipids abnormalities, nutritional therapy will be discussed in more detail in the following section.

EXERCISE

Although exercise programs have not been shown to consistently improve glycemic control in patients with type 1 diabetes, exercise has long been advocated for these patients for its other beneficial effects (200). A position statement from the Council on Exercise of the ADA advocates exercise for patients with type 1 diabetes because of its potential to improve cardiovascular fitness (199). Several studies have shown that exercise in patients with type 1 diabetes decreases triglyceride levels and increases HDL cholesterol levels (199,200). The ADA Council on Exercise also has pointed out possible risks of exercise for individuals with type 1 diabetes: hyperglycemia, hypoglycemia, ketosis, cardiovascular ischemia and arrhythmias, exacerbation of proliferative retinopathy, and injury to the lower extremities (199).

In patients with type 2 diabetes, exercise may be even more important than in those with type 1 diabetes for the management of both hyperglycemia and dyslipidemia (199,200). Several prospective epidemiologic studies have shown that individuals who are less physically active have higher risk of developing type 2 diabetes (201–205), and a randomized trial showed that increased physical activity decreased the incidence of diabetes in individuals with impaired glucose tolerance (197). In considering the appropriate role of exercise in patients with type 2 diabetes, the ADA Council on Exercise emphasized the reduction of

ASCVD risk factors in its position statement (199) and recommended that moderate levels of physical activity be incorporated into daily living (206,207). Improvements in blood glucose, insulin resistance, and lipoprotein profile are thought to be realized by the cumulative effect of frequent, smaller bouts of activity (207). Again, however, the Council on Exercise points out risks of exercise in patients with type 2 diabetes, which are the same as those outlined for patients with type 1 diabetes (199). The Council strongly recommended that before individuals with type 2 diabetes begin an exercise program, they should undergo an evaluation specifically designed to diagnose previously unknown hypertension, nephropathy, retinopathy, neuropathy, and silent ischemic heart disease, which would include an exercise stress cardiogram for all patients older than 35 years.

In addition to direct effects on lipoproteins, exercise has several indirect benefits for lipoproteins in patients with type 2 diabetes (200,206). First, there is some evidence that weight-loss programs that incorporate exercise will be more successful than those focused on diet alone in maintaining weight reduction, with a resulting beneficial effect on lipid levels, as described below. In addition, there are direct effects of exercise training on reducing insulin resistance, a factor that may contribute to dyslipidemia, as discussed above. Exercise has also been shown to increase HDL cholesterol levels and lower triglycerides in individuals with type 2 diabetes.

DIET

Weight Loss

Weight loss is the conservative form of therapy for type 2 diabetes and has been discussed in Chapter 32. As stated previously, weight reduction in patients with type 2 diabetes has multiple benefits. A decrease in insulin resistance and hyperinsulinemia would be expected to have beneficial effects on hyperglycemia and dyslipidemia. Weight reduction in type 2 diabetes has been shown to lower triglyceride concentrations, increase HDL levels, and, in some studies, to lower LDL cholesterol levels (208,209). Even when hypoglycemic drug therapy is necessary, an appropriate diet will minimize the dose of drug required to control glucose levels.

Diet Composition

The dietary management of diabetes is discussed further in Chapter 36. The diet for patients with diabetes that is recommended by both the ADA (3,210) and the NCEP Expert Panel (2) (Table 33.8) stresses reducing the amount of saturated fat to less than 10% of total calories. This is the most important dietary strategy to lower LDL cholesterol. Cholesterol intake should be reduced to less than 300 mg per day. A maximum of 30% of total fat is recommended for most individuals, although there is flexibility depending on triglyceride levels (3,210). The rest of the diet should consist of 15% to 20% of calories from protein, five to eight servings of fruits and vegetables, and at least six servings of whole-grain products per day. Complex carbohydrates may account for 50% to 60% of total calories consumed. It is emphasized that this increase in the amount of complex carbohydrates in the diet should be accompanied by a concomitant increase in fiber intake (2,210–212). This is important because soluble fiber has an independent effect on cholesterol lowering (213). The NCEP has a second level of dietary recommendations for those with more severe hyperlipidemia (2), which include reducing saturated fat to less than 7% of calories and cholesterol to less than 200 mg per day.

There has been controversy concerning the desirable carbohydrate content of the diet in diabetes (211,214–217). For many years, it was believed that dietary carbohydrate should be restricted to prevent the complications of diabetes. In addition, studies in nondiabetics (218) and some studies in diabetics (216,217) have suggested that diets high in carbohydrate, especially those containing a large amount of simple sugars and low fiber, lead to increases in triglyceride levels and decreases in HDL levels, both of which will exaggerate the pattern of dyslipidemia already present in diabetes. There was also concern that metabolic control might deteriorate with increased consumption of carbohydrates, although this has not been borne out in clinical studies comparing high-carbohydrate and low-carbohydrate diets (219–221).

Most studies in diabetes (both types) have shown that replacing foods high in saturated fat with foods containing predominantly complex carbohydrate lowers both total and LDL cholesterol levels (212,215,222–224); this response has been noted in both lean and obese diabetic subjects. Decreases in HDL cholesterol concentrations have been observed in some (216,217) but not other studies in which complex carbohydrate replaced saturated fat (222). Decreases in HDL concentrations appear to be less pronounced in subjects with diabetes who have lower initial HDL concentrations. Significant increases in fasting triglyceride concentrations have been seen in some studies of subjects with type 2 diabetes on various solid-food, high-carbohydrate diets, usually when there is no additional increase

TABLE 33.8. Dietary Guidelines of the American Diabetes Association and the National Cholesterol Education Program

Nutrient	Step 1 diet	Step 2 diet
Total fat	<30% of total calories	<30% of total calories
Saturated fat	<10% of total calories	<7% of total calories
Polyunsaturated fat	≤10% of total calories	≤10% of total calories
Monounsaturated fat	10%–15% of total calories	10%–15% of total calories
Carbohydrates	50%–60% of total calories	50%–60% of total calories
Protein	10%–20% of total calories	10%–20% of total calories
Cholesterol	<300 mg/d	<200 mg/d
Total calories	To achieve and maintain desirable body weight	

Data from Management of dyslipidemia in adults with diabetes. Diabetes Association: Clinical Practice Recommendations 1998. *Diabetes Care* 1998;[Suppl 1]:S36–S39; and The Expert Panel. National Cholesterol Education Program. National Heart, Lung, and Blood Institute: report of the National Cholesterol Education Program Expert Panel on detection, evaluation, and treatment of high blood cholesterol in adults. *Arch Intern Med* 1998;148:36–69.

in the amount of fiber (222,223). An additional advantage of diets that are higher in carbohydrate and diets lower in fat is that they are lower in calories for comparable portion sizes and thus may promote weight reduction.

An alternative dietary approach that appears promising for the treatment of dyslipidemia in patients with type 2 diabetes who cannot or will not follow a high-carbohydrate diet is a diet high in monounsaturated fatty acids (184,216). Such diets reduce triglyceride and LDL concentrations and sometimes produce less lowering of HDL concentrations than do high-carbohydrate diets.

An additional dietary consideration for diabetic patients concerns intake of omega (ω)-3 polyunsaturated fatty acids. These fatty acids, which are found predominantly in fish oils, have a hypotriglyceridemic action in nondiabetic persons (225). Epidemiologic studies and clinical trials (226,227) provide evidence that diets high in fatty fish may help prevent CVD, and this effect has been attributed to the presence of ω-3 polyunsaturated fatty acids (228). Fish-oil supplements have been shown to reduce serum triglyceride levels in studies of patients with type 2 diabetes (229,230). However, increases in LDL cholesterol and apoB concentrations may occur in hypertriglyceridemic subjects given fish oil, a situation often observed in subjects with diabetes (231,232). Clinical trials have established that fish-oil supplementation does not have an adverse effect on glycemic control (232,233). Thus, diabetic patients should be encouraged to eat fish, and ω-3 supplements should be considered in those with cardiovascular disease.

Because of the role that oxidative processes play in acceleration of atherosclerosis, it has been widely suggested that antioxidant supplements (vitamins E and C) be prescribed to individuals with diabetes. Although there have been no randomized trials in patients with diabetes, two recent trials have shown that vitamin E supplementation does not lower risk for cardiovascular disease (234,235), raising the possibility that other micronutrients present in vitamin E– and C–containing foods may be protective. Thus, dietary guidelines stress increased intake of vegetables, fruits, and grains so that micronutrients may be derived from whole foods rather than from vitamin supplements.

In summary, on the basis of the NCEP and ADA recommendations, several changes in typical American diets should be made to lower LDL and prevent diabetic dyslipidemia, including decreasing saturated fat and cholesterol and increasing fruits, vegetables, grains, and dietary fiber. When followed consistently, these recommendations can often reduce or even eliminate the need for hypolipidemic medications.

Pharmacologic Therapy for Type 1 Diabetes and Its Relation to Dyslipidemia

Secondary causes of dyslipidemia should always be investigated before initiating pharmacologic therapy. As stated previously, the usual secondary pathologic and pharmacologic causes of lipid abnormalities are more frequently detected in patients with diabetes (135,136,141), and their effects on lipid metabolism are often more pronounced in conjunction with the diabetic syndrome. The presence of known CHD mandates aggressive therapy for lipid abnormalities in all patients with diabetes. The ADA consensus panel recommends aggressive lipid-lowering therapy regardless of whether CHD is present or absent (3,145).

In diabetic patients with known CHD and LDL cholesterol higher than 100 mg/dL, immediate pharmacologic therapy to correct diabetic dyslipidemia should be instituted. Combined diet, exercise, and hypolipidemic drug therapy should be instituted for all diabetic patients with CHD immediately upon confirmation of myocardial ischemia or infarction. A strong case can be made for initiating hypolipidemic drugs in the hospital when a patient is admitted for an acute coronary event or ischemia. Discharging patients on lipid-lowering therapy gives them and their referring physicians an important, strong message concerning the necessity for control of lipid risk factors. Early initiation of lipid-lowering therapy was shown to improve patient compliance (236) and maintain target lipid levels at 6-month follow-up (237). In addition to the importance of lowering LDL cholesterol levels, results of the VA-HIT and DAIS studies suggest that therapy to correct triglycerides (238) and HDL cholesterol (239) abnormalities may be of extreme importance in patients at high risk for coronary events (164). When triglycerides and/or HDL cholesterol are the targets for therapy, lowering of non-HDL cholesterol levels should be considered as a potential therapeutic goal (183).

Diet and exercise should always be an adjunct to pharmacologic therapy because these modalities will often be synergistic in the control of lipid abnormalities. Because LDL cholesterol is often spuriously lowered following an acute ischemic event, lipid levels should continue to be monitored after hospital discharge and the dose of hypolipidemic drugs titrated to maintain lipids at target levels. Patients who adopt intensive lifestyle changes (i.e., begin dieting and exercising) may be able to discontinue pharmacologic therapy (240).

The same lipid-lowering drugs are used in patients with and without diabetes. Table 33.9 shows the principal classes of lipid-

TABLE 33.9. Effect of Hypolipidemic Drugs on Lipid Fractions

	Lipoprotein fractions (% change)			
	Cholesterol			
Drug class	Total	LDL	HDL	Triglycerides
HMG CoA reductase inhibitors (statins)	↓ 25–30	↓ 30–60	↑ 5–15	↓ 20–45
Fibric acid derivatives	↓ 10–25	↓ 5–25[a]	↑ 10–35	↓ 20–50
Bile acid sequestrants	↓ 10–25	↓ 15–30	↑ 0–5	↑ 0–15[b]
Nicotinic acid preparations	↓ 10–25	↓ 20–30	↑ 10–35	↓ 30–50
Ezetemibe	↓ 15	↓ 20	↑ 5	↓ 5–10

LDL, low-density lipoprotein; HDL, high-density lipoprotein; HMG CoA, 3-hydroxy-3-methyl-glutaryl CoA.
[a]LDL levels may increase significantly in patients with hypertriglyceridemia who are taking gemfibrozil.
[b]Triglyceride levels may increase by ≥100% in patients with preexisting hypertriglyceridemia.

TABLE 33.10. Hypocholesterolemic Drugs

Drug class	Generic name	Trade name	Usual effective daily dose	Maximal daily dose
HMG CoA reductase inhibitors	Simvastatin	Zocor	10 mg	80 mg
	Lovastatin	Mevacor	20 mg	80 mg
	Atorvastatin	Lipitor	10 mg	80 mg
	Fluvastatin	Lescol	20 mg	40 mg
	Pravastatin	Pravachol	20 mg	80 mg
	Rosuvastatin	Crestor	5 mg	40 mg
Fibric acid derivatives	Gemfibrozil	Lopid	1,200 mg	1,200 mg
		Generic gemfibrozil		
	Fenofibrate	Tricor	160 mg	160 mg
	Clofibrate	Atromid S	2 g	2 g
Bile acid sequestrants	Cholestyramine	Questran		
		Questran Light	8–12 g	24 g
		Generic cholestyramine		
	Colestipol	Colestid	10–15 g	30 g
	Colesevelam hydrochloride	WelChol	3.75 g	4.375 g
Nicotinic acid preparations[a]	Niacin	Crystalline niacin	1,000–3,000 mg	9 g
		Niacor		
		Niaspan	500 mg	2,000 mg
Intestinal absorption inhibitor	Ezetemibe	Zetia	10 mg	10 mg

HMG CoA, 3-hydroxy-3-methyl-glutaryl CoA.
[a]With all the niacin agents, concomitant use of one aspirin daily may be indicated to prevent flushing.

lowering drugs and their effect on each lipid fraction, and Table 33.10 illustrates the various drugs available in each of these hypolipidemic classes, the usual effective dose, and the maximal daily dose for each medication.

HMG CoA REDUCTASE INHIBITORS (STATINS)

As shown in at least five large clinical trials (123–127), the statin drugs are the most effective pharmacologic agents for the prevention of CHD in both diabetic and nondiabetic patients and should be considered as the first line of therapy in patients with diabetic dyslipidemia. Although the primary effect of statins is to reduce LDL cholesterol levels, they are also effective in lowering triglyceride levels and have variable effects on HDL cholesterol. Statins competitively inhibit the rate-controlling enzyme of endogenous cholesterol biosynthesis, 3-hydroxy-3-methylglutaryl coenzyme A (HMG CoA) reductase, thus reducing cellular cholesterol production (241). The resultant decrease in levels of intracellular free cholesterol increases the activity of LDL receptor–mediated catabolism of LDL cholesterol (127,132,238).

The effect of the statin drugs on triglyceride levels is proportional to both baseline triglyceride levels and the degree of LDL lowering. Statins have little effect at triglyceride levels less than 150 mg/dL, a moderate effect at triglyceride levels in the 150- to 250-mg/dL range, and significant, dose-dependent reductions (22% to 45%) at triglyceride levels higher than 250 mg/dL (242). There also is evidence that statins may have clinically significant effects on HDL metabolism (158,243). Several of the previously mentioned large clinical trials demonstrated the ability of the naturally occurring statins—simvastatin, pravastatin, and lovastatin—to raise HDL levels. Questions recently have been raised about the effects of the more potent synthetic statins on HDL levels, and it has been suggested that higher doses of these statins may actually lower HDL cholesterol concentrations (158,243,244). In patients with diabetes, statins should be initiated at recommended doses and titrated at approximately 6-week intervals to achieve desired goal levels for LDL cholesterol. As in the general population, liver function tests should be administered at approximately 3-month intervals for the first year.

Six statins are now available (Table 33.10); they differ primarily in their effectiveness in lowering LDL at their maximum dose. The appropriate drug should be chosen to achieve the degree of LDL reduction that is desirable to reach the goal level. One potential significant difference between the drugs is their metabolism by hepatic cytochrome P450 enzymes (245,246). Pravastatin has a pattern of metabolism different from that of the other four agents: simvastatin, lovastatin, atorvastatin, and fluvastatin. Pravastatin is not metabolized by any of the P450 enzymes. Therefore, if prolonged use of a concomitant medication that inhibits P450 enzymes is required, the use of pravastatin should be considered. Typical examples of drugs that inhibit the P450 enzyme system are erythromycin and other macrolide antibiotics, oral antifungal agents, and protease inhibitors. Myositis has sometimes been observed when these medications have been used with one of the statins that requires metabolism by these hepatic enzymes (247). Even grapefruit juice is known to have effects on statin metabolism (248,249), and patients taking statins should be counseled to avoid grapefruit juice or to consume it in moderation (250). Although myositis and rhabdomyolysis have been reported side effects of statin–fibrate combinations in the past, 21 clinical trials conducted in the past decade have shown this combination to be effective and safe, with low incidences of complications (251).

Statin drugs are more effective if they are taken at night, particularly at bedtime, with the exception of atorvastatin, which is longer acting than the other statin drugs. In the event that a patient develops side effects such as liver function abnormalities or myositis with one of the statins, that agent should be discontinued. After the abnormality has resolved, one of the other statins can be tried cautiously with careful monitoring of liver function and creatine phosphokinase (CPK) levels. In the previously-cited five large clinical trials, which included more than 30,000 patients over an approximately 5-year period, the statin drugs effectively lowered LDL cholesterol levels and were also extremely well tolerated, with no significant differences in other causes of morbidity or mortality between the placebo and intervention groups (123–127). In addition to decreased total mortality, no increases in cancer, violent deaths, or suicidal deaths occurred in these trials; these had been observed in previous lipid-lowering studies prior to the use of statins (252).

The mechanism by which these agents prevent atherosclerotic events is very interesting. Although early trials that used coronary arteriography showed decreased angiographic progression in most patients and small degrees of regression in a minority of patients, the more significant effects on clinical endpoints suggested new mechanisms of action. It now appears that stabilization of small, lipid-rich plaques (253) and restoration of normal endothelial function (254) may well be the predominant modes of action of statin drugs in preventing atherosclerotic events. Because these beneficial effects occur relatively quickly (prevention of ischemic events can be observed as soon as 1 month after commencement of therapy) (255), lipid-lowering therapy with a statin drug should be instituted promptly, particularly in patients with pre-existing CHD.

A variety of pleiotropic effects have been associated with statin therapy, including reduction in thrombogenicity, inhibition of cellular proliferation, anti-inflammation, and changes in oxidative potential. The weight of the evidence, however, indicates that the reduction in coronary events is a class effect of the statins that is most closely related to the reduction in levels of LDL cholesterol (141,157,247,256).

FIBRIC ACID DERIVATIVES

The two recommended fibrates now available in the United States, gemfibrozil and fenofibrate, are described in Table 33.10. Although clofibrate can still be prescribed, it is not recommended because of the significant side effects observed in previous clinical trials (257,258). The predominant effects of fibrates are to significantly lower triglyceride levels and raise HDL cholesterol levels; however, fibrates differ in their effect on LDL cholesterol. Gemfibrozil has been prescribed widely for a number of years and was the drug used in the Helsinki Heart Study. In this trial, patients with the dyslipidemia typical of diabetes (i.e., hypertriglyceridemia and low HDL levels with or without elevation in LDL) were most responsive to the protective effects of gemfibrozil (259). One of the concerns with gemfibrozil, however, has been the association of an increase in LDL with a lowering of triglycerides (159,260). Fenofibrate, which has recently become available in the United States, has the advantage of lowering LDL levels, along with having effects similar to gemfibrozil on triglyceride and HDL concentrations (261).

As discussed previously, in addition to the Helsinki Heart Study, the more recent VA-HIT study has shown that gemfibrozil raises HDL levels, thus reducing the risk of macrovascular disease, including stroke (182). The DAIS trial has shown a similar effect for fenofibrate on angiographic outcomes and effects similar to gemfibrozil on clinical endpoints (164).

In patients with particularly high triglyceride levels and lower levels of LDL cholesterol, fibrates should be considered as initial therapy. Doses of fibrate should be instituted as indicated in Table 33.10, and serum triglycerides should be monitored. Effects of fibrate drugs on triglycerides may be observed within several weeks because of the rapid turnover of VLDL, as discussed previously.

Although it has been debated whether triglycerides are a risk factor for CHD, as discussed previously, recent data from a number of clinical trials indicate that even a moderate degree of hypertriglyceridemia in patients with diabetes increases the risk for a coronary event (262). A recent meta-analysis has shown a significant effect of triglyceride as a cardiovascular risk factor (263) and follow-up in the Prospective Cardiovascular Muenster (PROCAM) study has had similar results (264). It is interesting that extreme hypertriglyceridemia is not associated with the same degree of CHD risk (265), probably because the triglyceride-rich lipoproteins seen in patients with insulin resistance and type 2 diabetes are generally of the remnant variety and those seen in patients with higher levels of triglycerides exist in a larger, more buoyant, less atherogenic form. Extreme hypertriglyceridemia, particularly in type 1 diabetes, confers a significantly increased risk of pancreatitis (265) and should be lowered to the range that will reduce the risk of CHD without harming the pancreas (171).

BILE ACID SEQUESTRANTS

Cholestyramine and colestipol were among the earliest hypolipidemic drugs studied. Cholestyramine alone was shown to reduce CHD risk in the Lipid Research Clinics Coronary Primary Prevention Trial (LRC-CPPT) (119), the National Heart, Lung, and Blood Institute (NHLBI) Type II Intervention Trial (266), and in a secondary prevention trial conducted by the NHBLI that examined angiographic endpoints (267). Cholestyramine combined with a statin also was effective in reducing CHD risk (268–271). Low doses of a bile acid resin can further lower LDL cholesterol levels when combined with statins, fibric acid derivatives, or nicotinic acid. When used in the presence of preexisting hypertriglyceridemia, bile acid sequestrants may significantly raise triglyceride levels (141) and increase the risk of pancreatitis (136,141,272). In addition, patients with diabetes often have gastroparesis and other gastrointestinal syndromes that may be worsened by the use of bile acid sequestrants. Therefore, small doses of bile acid sequestrants can be used, after triglyceride levels are controlled, as adjunctive therapy to achieve additional LDL lowering and avoid the potential gastrointestinal side effects associated with higher doses of these agents. The new bile acid sequestrant, colesevelam hydrochloride, will eliminate or diminish such side effects (273).

INTESTINAL ABSORPTION INHIBITOR

Ezetemibe represents the first agent in a new class of lipid-lowering drugs, the intestinal cholesterol absorption inhibitors. This drug inhibits a sterol transferase located in the brush border of the small intestine, thereby reducing the absorption of intestinal intraluminal cholesterol. Dietary cholesterol contributes only 25% of the intraluminal cholesterol available to this transferase, with the remaining 75% coming from the liver. By inhibiting cholesterol absorption, chylomicron cholesterol, and chylomicron remnant cholesterol concentrations are reduced, with a significant decrease in the absorbed cholesterol delivered to the liver. A resulting upregulation of hepatic LOL receptors leads to a 18% to 20% reduction in LDL cholesterol concentration. In addition, triglycerides are reduced and HDL-C is slightly increased.

NICOTINIC ACIDS

Nicotinic acid, or niacin, is a cofactor in intermediary metabolism at physiologic doses less than 20 mg/dL (137). However, doses of 1,000 mg or more per day have significant positive effects on all lipid abnormalities. Niacin was the first agent to be shown to prevent CHD in the Coronary Drug Project (274) and was shown to lower all-cause mortality at 15-year follow-up (275). Niacin is the most effective drug in raising HDL levels, even at doses as low as 1,000 mg per day (136,141). Higher doses are usually required to alter triglyceride or LDL metabolism (276). The principal problem in using niacin is that it increases insulin resistance (137,140,141). Therefore, in individuals with type 2 diabetes, niacin should be used very sparingly and only in patients with severe hypertriglyceridemia that does not adequately respond to other forms of therapy such as a fibric acid derivative or fish-oil capsules (277). As mentioned above, small doses (1,000 mg per day) may be used to raise HDL cholesterol levels, but glucose metabolism should be followed very carefully. Because the undesirable effects are predominately on insulin resistance, there is no significant contraindication to the use of niacin in individuals with type 1 diabetes. However, this is seldom necessary because the triglyceride abnormalities in patients with type 1 diabetes usually respond to glucose control (115).

Niacin also has a number of other significant side effects, of which the most common are flushing and various dermatologic manifestations such as pruritus and rash (278). Niacin may be very hepatotoxic (279), particularly in some of the over-the-counter, long-acting forms. In addition, niacin is known to exacerbate inflammatory bowel disease, ulcers, and asthma.

COMBINATION THERAPY

Patients with severe diabetes-associated dyslipidemia often may require more than one drug to maximize control of all lipid fractions. Ezetemibe or bile acid sequestrants can be added to a statin to further decrease LDL-C levels without significant drug-drug interactions. In the case of the bile acid sequestrants, triglyceride levels should be reduced before this class of drugs is used in combination with a statin. When patients treated with gemfibrozil to control hypertriglyceridemia are noted to have an increase in LDL cholesterol level or when the LDL reduction induced by fenofibrate or gemfibrozil does not reach goal levels, a bile acid sequestrant can be added to the treatment regimen after triglyceride levels are under control (141). The combination of gemfibrozil or fenofibrate with a bile acid sequestrant and the combination of nicotinic acid with a bile acid sequestrant have both been shown to be effective in treating combined hyperlipidemia (141,280–282). Although the risk of using either niacin or a fibric acid derivative with a statin drug increases the risk of myositis, as discussed previously, the combination may be indicated in carefully selected patients with high-risk lipid profiles (251). Because both niacin and fibric acids may be hepatotoxic, the presence of abnormal liver function at baseline is a contradiction to combination therapy, and liver function should be carefully monitored during therapy. Niacin-induced hepatoxicity increases the risk of myositis from the resultant abnormality of drug metabolism associated with hepatic dysfunction (141). A fibrate/statin combination can be very effective in patients with the mixed dyslipidemia characteristic of type 2 diabetes and therefore may be necessary if control cannot be achieved by a single agent. Recent pharmacokinetic studies have indicated that gemfibrozil significantly increases the serum concentration of all statins secondary to the inhibition of the glucuronidation step in statin metabolism. For this reason, only fenofibrate should be used as combination therapy with any statin. In cases of mixed dyslipidemia, the statin dose should be maintained at the starting dose and the patient should be warned about the potential side effects of the fibrate/statin combination. CPK levels do not need to be monitored unless the patient develops signs or symptoms of myositis, in which case the statin should be immediately discontinued and CPK levels measured. A CPK level more than ten-times normal mandates immediate discontinuation of the combination therapy to prevent the more severe complication of rhabdomyolysis. There are no apparent differences among the statins and fibrate drugs in terms of the development of myositis. Any combination may be used, and all patients receiving them should be monitored closely. The previously discussed medications that are known to inhibit the metabolism of statin drugs (e.g., macrolide antibiotics, oral antifungal agents, and protease inhibitors) should not be used concomitantly because they will increase the risks associated with the statin/fibrate combination. Triple-drug therapy with nicotinic acid, a bile acid sequestrant, and a statin has been used in patients with severe hyperlipidemia (283). This triple-drug regimen is capable of lowering LDL cholesterol levels by 70% to 80% and can thereby normalize LDL levels even in patients with heterozygous familial forms of hypercholesterolemia or mixed hyperlipidemia.

OTHER CONSIDERATIONS

The Elderly Patient with Diabetes

Because the incidence of type 2 diabetes and of hypercholesterolemia increases with age, diabetic dyslipidemia is a frequent finding in older individuals. Although most of the major clinical trials have not studied elderly patients, the available data from a few studies and from epidemiologic studies such as the Framingham Study indicate that lipid disorders continue to be of concern in the geriatric age group (284–286). Because type 2 diabetes frequently has its onset when individuals are older than 60 years of age and because glucose intolerance increases the atherogenic potential of dyslipidemia and augments the natural tendency of cholesterol levels to increase with age, elderly people with diabetes are of special concern to the clinician (287). Studies from Framingham have suggested that CHD risk is significantly increased in elderly individuals with diabetes; therefore, it seems appropriate to reduce cholesterol levels in this group (286). Nonpharmacologic therapy should be effectively used before therapy with hypolipidemic drugs is considered. When drug therapy is necessary, both fibric acid derivatives and the statin drugs are effective hypolipidemic agents and seem to have no age-related side effects. However, as with all drug therapy for the elderly, special consideration should be given to the changes in metabolism that occur with aging, and doses should be carefully titrated for older individuals. The major clinical trials of statin therapy described previously (4S, LIPID, CARE, WOSCOPS, AFCAPS/TexCAPS, and HPS) (123–127) have all included patients over 60 years of age. Substudies of this older cohort have shown effectiveness of statin treatment equal to that in younger patients, with no evidence of increased toxicity.

Diabetic Nephropathy

Diabetic nephropathy is a frequent complication of both type 1 and type 2 diabetes. Diabetic renal disease usually presents with microalbuminuria and hypertension and then progresses to nephrotic syndrome and/or chronic renal insufficiency (288,299). A number of lipid abnormalities have been observed in patients with diabetic nephropathy, with hypertriglyceridemia and low levels of HDL cholesterol being the most common. However, combined hyperlipidemia and isolated elevations in LDL cholesterol levels also are seen in patients with diabetic renal disease (290). Bile acid resins have been administered to patients with nephrotic syndrome secondary to diabetes, and because these agents are not absorbed through the gastrointestinal tract, they do not appear to increase side effects in patients with renal disease. However, because of their limited capacity to lower LDL cholesterol levels and their propensity to elevate triglyceride levels, these agents are often not effective in controlling the lipid disorders of diabetic renal disease (290).

Statins used in patients with nephrotic syndrome appear to be effective in lowering LDL cholesterol levels and are well tolerated in patients with no deterioration of renal function (291). Because they are metabolized primarily by the liver, statins should also be safe for patients with mild renal insufficiency. However, because statins have not been studied in patients with more severe forms of diabetic nephropathy, they cannot be recommended for patients with significant deterioration of renal function. Atorvastatin has been used in patients with moderate renal insufficiency without side effects and with significant efficacy in reducing LDL cholesterol levels (292).

For patients whose primary lipid problem secondary to diabetic nephropathy is hypertriglyceridemia, fibric acid derivatives are of potential therapeutic benefit (293). Early studies with clofibrate in patients with renal insufficiency or nephrotic syndrome identified a significant problem with myositis, which in some cases was severe enough to produce rhabdomyolysis and worsening of renal failure (247,288,289,294). Although some studies have indicated that gemfibrozil and fenofibrate are beneficial in patients with nephrotic syndrome, fibric acid derivatives should be used with caution in patients with diabetic nephropathy because the predominant route of metabolism of these agents is renal excretion (290).

CONCLUSION

Macrovascular disease is the number one cause of morbidity and mortality in type 2 diabetes and is becoming increasingly important in type 1 diabetes. Although there has been an impressive decrease in CVD-related mortality in the general US population over the past 30 years, patients with diabetes have not experienced the same degree of decrease (295). Not only is diabetes an independent risk factor for arteriosclerosis, it also is frequently associated with insulin resistance and the accompanying risk factors of obesity, hypertension, and dyslipidemia. Hence, total risk factor management is mandatory in patients with diabetes, an approach strongly supported by the UKPDS and DAIS studies (131,164). Subgroup analyses of the participants in the major prospective statin trials also support aggressive management of LDL cholesterol levels (123–130). In addition, the therapeutic approach to any single risk factor must be designed so that it does not introduce or worsen other cardiovascular risk factors.

There is growing evidence not only that dyslipidemia is one of the most important contributors to arteriosclerosis but also that other risk factors for CHD may be lipid-dependent (296). Hence, an understanding of the pathophysiology and treatment of diabetic dyslipidemia is essential for the successful management of patients with diabetes.

It seems particularly appropriate to end this discussion with an often-quoted statement made by Dr. Elliot Joslin (297) in 1927.

> I believe the chief cause of premature development of arteriosclerosis in diabetes, save for advancing age, is an excess of fat, an excess of fat in the body (obesity), an excess of fat in the diet, and an excess of fat in the blood. With an excess of fat diabetes begins and from an excess of fat diabetics die, formerly of coma, recently of arteriosclerosis.

REFERENCES

1. Wingard DL, Barrett-Connor E. Heart disease and diabetes. In: *Diabetes in America,* 2nd ed. Washington, DC: National Institutes of Health, National Institute of Diabetes and Digestive and Kidney Diseases, 1995;19:429–448: NIH publication no. 95–1468.
2. The Expert Panel. National Cholesterol Education Program. National Heart, Lung, and Blood Institute: report of the National Cholesterol Education Program Expert Panel on detection, evaluation, and treatment of high blood cholesterol in adults. *Arch Intern Med* 1988;148:36–69.
3. Management of dyslipidemia in adults with diabetes. Diabetes Association: Clinical Practice Recommendations 1998. *Diabetes Care* 1998;21[Suppl 1]: S36–S39.
4. Brown MS, Goldstein JL. The LDL receptor and HMG-CoA reductase—two membrane molecules that regulate cholesterol homeostasis. *Curr Top Cell Regul* 1985;26:3–15.
5. Gotto AM Jr, Pownall HJ, Havel RJ. Introduction to the plasma lipoproteins. *Methods Enzymol* 1986;128:3–4.
6. Shepherd J. Lipoprotein metabolism: an overview. *Drugs* 1994;47[Suppl 2]: 1–10.
7. Havel RJ, Kane JP. Introduction: structure and metabolism of plasma lipoproteins. In: Scriver CR, Beaudet AL, Sly WS, Valle D, eds. *The metabolic and molecular basis of inherited disease,* 7th ed. New York: McGraw-Hill, 1995.
8. Kane JP, Havel RJ. Disorders of the biogenesis and secretion of lipoproteins containing the B apolipoproteins. In: Scriver CR, Beaudet AL, Sly WS, Valle D, eds. *The metabolic and molecular basis of inherited disease,* 7th ed. New York: McGraw-Hill, 1995.
9. Olivecrona T, Hultin M, Bergo M, et al. Lipoprotein lipase: regulation and role in lipoprotein metabolism. *Proc Nutr Soc* 1997;56:723–729.
10. Ginsberg HN. Lipoprotein physiology. *Endocrinol Metab Clin North Am* 1998; 27:503–519.
11. Hugh P, Barrett R. Kinetics of triglyceride rich lipoproteins: chylomicrons and very low density lipoproteins. *Atherosclerosis* 1998;141[Suppl 1]:S35–S40.
12. Santamarina-Fojo S, Haudenschild C, Amar M. The role of hepatic lipase in lipoprotein metabolism and atherosclerosis. *Curr Opin Lipidol* 1998;9:211–219.
13. Williams DL, Connelly MA, Temel RE, et al. Scavenger receptor BI and cholesterol trafficking. *Curr Opin Lipidol* 1999;10:329–339.
14. Brewer HB Jr. Hypertriglyceridemia: changes in the plasma lipoproteins associated with an increased risk of cardiovascular disease. *Am J Cardiol* 1999; 83:3F–12F.
15. Jong MC, Hofker MH, Havekes LM. Role of apoCs in lipoprotein metabolism: functional differences between apoC1, apoC2, and apoC3. *Arterioscler Thromb Vasc Biol* 1999;19:472–484.
16. Mahley RW, Ji ZS. Remnant lipoprotein metabolism: key pathways involving cell-surface heparan sulfate proteoglycans and apolipoprotein E. *J Lipid Res* 1999;40:1–16.
17. Scanu AM, Fless GM. Lipoprotein (a): heterogeneity and biological relevance. *J Clin Invest* 1990;85:1709–1715.
18. Brewer HB Jr, Santamarina-Fojo S, Hoeg JM. Molecular biology of lipoproteins, their receptors, and lipoprotein lipase: primary hyperlipidemias. Vol 3. In: Jeffers D, ed. *Primary hyperlipidemias.* New York: McGraw Hill, 1991:43–74.
19. Cole SA, Hixson JE. PCR methodology applied to genetic studies of lipoprotein metabolism and atherosclerosis. *Methods Mol Biol* 1998;110:1–34.
20. Garfinkel AS, Schotz MC. Lipoprotein lipase. In: Gotto AM, ed. *Plasma lipoproteins.* Amsterdam: Elsevier, 1987:335.
21. Jansen H, Breedveld B, Schoonderwoerd K. Role of lipoprotein lipases in postprandial lipid metabolism. *Atherosclerosis* 1998;141[Suppl 1]:S31–S34.
22. Connelly PW. The role of hepatic lipase in lipoprotein metabolism. *Clin Chim Acta* 1999;286:243–255.
23. Santamarina-Fojo S, Lambert G, Hoeg JM, et a. Lecithin-cholesterol acyltransferase: role in lipoprotein metabolism, reverse cholesterol transport and atherosclerosis. *Curr Opin Lipidol* 2000;11:267–275.
24. Yamashita S, Sakai N, Hirano K, et al. Molecular genetics of plasma cholesteryl ester transfer protein. *Curr Opin Lipidol* 1997;8:101–110.
25. Tall AR. Plasma cholesteryl ester transfer protein and high-density lipoproteins: new insights from molecular genetic studies. *J Intern Med* 1995;237:5–12.
26. Yki-Jarvinen H, Taskinen M-R, Koivisto VA, et al. Response of adipose tissue lipoprotein lipase activity and serum lipoproteins to acute hyperinsulinemia in man. *Diabetologia* 1984;27:364–369.
27. Beisiegel U, Weber W, Ihrke G, et al. The LDL-receptor-related-protein, LRP, is an apolipoprotein E-binding protein. *Nature* 1989;341:162–164.
28. Ginsberg HN. Role of lipid synthesis, chaperone proteins and proteasomes in the assembly and secretion of apoprotein B-containing lipoproteins from cultured liver cells. *Clin Exp Pharmacol Physiol* 1997;24:A29–A32.
29. Gordon DA. Recent advances in elucidating the role of the microsomal triglyceride transfer protein in apolipoprotein B lipoprotein assembly. *Curr Opin Lipidol* 1997;8:131–137.
30. Howard BV. Insulin resistance and lipid metabolism. *Am J Cardiol* 1999;84 [Suppl]:28J–32J.
31. Sparks CE, Sparks JD, Bolognino M, et al. Insulin effects on apolipoprotein B lipoprotein synthesis and secretion by primary cultures of rat hepatocytes. *Metabolism* 1986;35:1128–1136.
32. Lewis GF, Uffelman KD, Szeto LW, et al. Effect of acute hyperinsulinemia on VLDL triglyceride and VLDL apoB production in normal weight and obese individuals. *Diabetes* 1993;42:833–842.
33. Eisenberg S. High density lipoprotein metabolism. *J Lipid Res* 1984;25: 1017–1058.
34. Packard CJ, Munro A, Lorimer AR, et al. Metabolism of apolipoprotein B in large triglyceride-rich very low density lipoproteins of normal and hypertriglyceridemic subjects. *J Clin Invest* 1984;74:2178–2192.
35. Steinberg D, Parthasarathy S, Carew TE, et al. Beyond cholesterol: modifications of low-density lipoprotein that increase its atherogenicity. *N Engl J Med* 1989;320:915–924.
36. Stangl H, Hyatt M, Hobbs HH. Transport of lipids from high and low density lipoproteins via scavenger receptor-BI. *J Biol Chem* 1999;274:32692–32698.
37. de Villiers WJ, Smart EJ. Macrophage scavenger receptors and foam cell formation. *J Leukocyte Biol* 1999;66:740–746.
38. Nakata A, Nakagawa Y, Nishida M, et al. D36, a novel receptor for oxidized low-density lipoproteins, is highly expressed on lipid-laden macrophages in human atherosclerotic aorta. *Arterioscler Thromb Vasc Biol* 1999;19:1333–1339.

39. Calvo D, Gomez-Coronado D, Suarez Y, et al. Human CD36 in a high affinity receptor for the native lipoproteins HDL, LDL, and VLDL. *J Lipid Res* 1998;39:777–788.
40. Krauss RM, Burke DJ. Identification of multiple subclasses of plasma low density lipoproteins in normal humans. *J Lipid Res* 1982;23:97–104.
41. Austin MA, King MC, Vranizan KM, et al. Atherogenic lipoprotein phenotype: a proposed genetic marker for coronary heart disease risk. *Circulation* 1990;82:495–506.
42. Deckelbaum RJ, Galeano NF. Small dense low density lipoprotein: formation and potential mechanisms for atherogenicity. *Isr J Med Sci* 1996;32:464–468.
43. Gwynne JT. High-density lipoprotein cholesterol levels as a marker of reverse cholesterol transport. *Am J Cardiol* 1989;64:10G–17G.
44. Hill SA, McQuinn MJ. Reverse cholesterol transport: a review of the process and its clinical implications. *Clin Biochem* 1997;30:517–525.
45. Graham DL, Oram JF. Identification and characterization of a high density lipoprotein-binding protein in cell membranes by ligand blotting. *J Biol Chem* 1987;262:7439–7442.
46. Taskinen MR, Lahdenpera S, Syvanne M. New insights into lipid metabolism in non-insulin-dependent diabetes mellitus. *Ann Med* 1996;28:335–340.
47. Brunzell JD, Chait A, Bierman EL. Plasma lipoproteins in human diabetes mellitus. In: Alberti KGMM, Krall LD, eds. *The diabetes annual*. Amsterdam: Elsevier, 1985:463–479.
48. Reaven GM. Non-insulin-dependent diabetes mellitus, abnormal lipoprotein metabolism, and atherosclerosis. *Metabolism* 1987;36[Suppl 1]:1–8.
49. Dunn FL. Treatment of lipid disorders in diabetes mellitus. *Med Clin North Am* 1988;72:1379–1398.
50. Ginsberg HN. Relationship between diabetes mellitus and coronary artery disease. *Clin Diabetes* 1988;6[Suppl 4]:73–94.
51. Howard BV, Howard WJ. Dyslipidemia in non-insulin-dependent diabetes mellitus. *Endocr Rev* 1994;15:263–274.
52. Howard BV. Insulin actions in vivo: insulin and lipoprotein metabolism. In: Alberti KGMM, Zimmet P, DeFronzo RA, et al., eds. *International textbook of diabetes mellitus*, 2nd ed. Vol. 1. New York: John Wiley and Sons, 1997:531–539.
53. Howard BV, Cowan LD, Go O, et al. Adverse effects of diabetes on multiple cardiovascular disease risk factors in women. The Strong Heart Study. *Diabetes* 1998;21:1258–1265.
54. Georgopoulos A. Postprandial triglyceride metabolism in diabetes mellitus. *Clin Cardiol* 1999;22[6 Suppl]:II28–II33.
55. Evans M, Khan N, Rees A. Diabetic dyslipidaemia and coronary heart disease: new perspectives. *Curr Opin Lipidol* 1999;10:387–391.
56. Cowie CC, Howard BV, Harris MI. Serum lipoproteins in African Americans and whites with non-insulin-dependent diabetes in the US population. *Circulation* 1994;90:1185–1193.
57. Brunzell JD, Hazzard WR, Motulsky AG, et al. Evidence for diabetes mellitus and genetic forms of hypertriglyceridemia as independent entities. *Metabolism* 1975;24:1115–1121.
58. Abrams JJ, Ginsberg H, Grundy SM. Metabolism of cholesterol and plasma triglycerides in nonketotic diabetes mellitus. *Diabetes* 1982;31:903–910.
59. Dunn FL, Raskin P, Bilheimer DW, et al. The effect of diabetic control on very low-density lipoprotein-triglyceride metabolism in patients with type II diabetes mellitus and marked hypertriglyceridemia. *Metabolism* 1984;33:117–123.
60. Howard BV, Abbott WGH, Beltz WF, et al. Integrated study of low density lipoprotein metabolism and very low density lipoprotein metabolism in non-insulin-dependent diabetes. *Metabolism* 1987;36:870–877.
61. Malmstrom R, Packard CJ, Caslake M, et al. Defective regulation of triglyceride metabolism by insulin in the liver in NIDDM. *Diabetologia* 1997;40:454–462.
62. Taskinen MR. Lipoprotein lipase in diabetes. *Diabetes Metab Rev* 1987;3:551–570.
63. Mero N, Syvanne M, Taskinen MR. Postprandial lipid metabolism in diabetes. *Atherosclerosis* 1998;141[Suppl 1]:S53–S55.
64. Schonfeld G, Birge C, Miller JP, et al. Apolipoprotein B levels and altered lipoprotein composition in diabetes. *Diabetes* 1974;23:827–834.
65. Patti L, Swinburn B, Riccardi G, et al. Alterations in very-low-density lipoprotein subfractions in normotriglyceridemic non-insulin-dependent diabetics. *Atherosclerosis* 1991;91:15–23.
66. Fielding CJ, Castro GR, Donner C, et al. Distribution of apolipoprotein E in the plasma of insulin-dependent and non-insulin-dependent diabetics and its relation to cholesterol net transport. *J Lipid Res* 1986;27:1052–1061.
67. Eto M, Watanabe K, Iwashima Y, et al. Apolipoprotein E polymorphism and hyperlipemia in type II diabetics. *Diabetes* 1986;35:1374–1382.
68. Klein RL, Lyons TJ, Lopes-Virella MF. Metabolism of very low- and low-density lipoproteins isolated from normolipidaemic type 2 (non-insulin-dependent) diabetic patients by human monocyte-derived macrophages. *Diabetologia* 1990;33:299–305.
69. Kissebah AH, Alfarsi S, Evans DJ, et al. Plasma low density lipoprotein transport kinetics in noninsulin-dependent diabetes mellitus. *J Clin Invest* 1983;71:655–667.
70. Chait A, Bierman EL, Albers JJ. Low-density lipoprotein receptor activity in cultured human skin fibroblasts—mechanism of insulin-induced stimulation. *J Clin Invest* 1979;64:1309–1319.
71. Haffner SM, Mykkanen L, Stern MP, et al. Greater effect of diabetes on LDL size in women than in men. *Diabetes Care* 1994;17:1164–1171.
72. Gray RS, Robbins DC, Wang W, et al. Relation of LDL size to the insulin resistance syndrome and coronary heart disease in American Indians: the Strong Heart Study. *Arterioscler Thromb Vasc Biol* 1997;17:2713–2720.
73. Tan KC, Ai VH, Chow WS, et al. Influence of low density lipoprotein (LDL) subfraction profile and LDL oxidation on endothelium-dependent and independent vasodilation in patients with type 2 diabetes. *J Clin Endocrinol Metab* 1999;84:3212–3216.
74. Hiramatsu K, Bierman EL, Chait A. Metabolism of low-density lipoprotein from patients with diabetic hypertriglyceridemia by cultured human skin fibroblasts. *Diabetes* 1985;34:8–14.
75. Moro E, Alessandrini P, Zambon C, et al. Is glycation of low density lipoproteins in patients with type 2 diabetes mellitus a LDL pre-oxidative condition? *Diabet Med* 1999;16:663–669.
76. Grundy SM. Atherogenic dyslipidemia: lipoprotein abnormalities and implications for therapy. *Am J Cardiol* 1995;75:45B–52B.
77. Hseuh WA, Law RE. Cardiovascular risk continuum: implications of insulin resistance and diabetes. *Am J Med* 1998;105[1A]:4S–14S.
78. Demant T, Packard C. In vivo studies of VLDL metabolism and LDL heterogeneity. *Eur Heart J* 1998;19[Suppl H]:H7–H10.
79. Kim HJ, Kurup IV. Nonenzymatic glycosylation of human plasma low density lipoprotein: evidence for in vitro and in vivo glucosylation. *Metabolism* 1982;31:348–353.
80. Steinbrecher UP, Witztum JL. Glucosylation of low-density lipoproteins to an extent comparable to that seen in diabetes slows their catabolism. *Diabetes* 1984;33:130–134.
81. Lorenzi M, Cagliero E, Markey B, et al. Interaction of human endothelial cells with elevated glucose concentrations and native and glycosylated low density lipoproteins. *Diabetologia* 1984;26:218–222.
82. Lopez-Virella MF, Virella G. Immune mechanisms of atherosclerosis in diabetes mellitus. *Diabetes* 1992;41[Suppl 2]:86–91.
83. Fielding CJ, Reaven GM, Fielding PE. Human noninsulin-dependent diabetes: identification of a defect in plasma cholesterol transport normalized *in vivo* by insulin and *in vitro* by selective immunoadsorption of apolipoprotein E. *Proc Natl Acad Sci U S A* 1982;79:6365–6369.
84. Golay A, Zech L, Shi M-Z, et al. High density lipoprotein (HDL) metabolism in noninsulin-dependent diabetes mellitus: measurement of HDL turnover using tritiated HDL. *J Clin Endocrinol Metab* 1987;65:512–518.
85. Brinton EA, Eisenberg S, Breslow JL. Human HDL cholesterol levels are determined by apoA-I fractional catabolic rate, which correlates inversely with estimates of HDL particle size: effects of gender, hepatic and lipoprotein lipases, triglyceride and insulin levels, and body fat distribution. *Arterioscler Thromb* 1994;14:707–720.
86. Taskinen MR, Kahri J, Koivisto V, et al. Metabolism of HDL apolipoprotein A-I and A-II in type 1 (insulin dependent) diabetes mellitus. *Diabetologia* 1992;35;4:347–356.
87. Duell PB, Oram JF, Bierman EL. Nonenzymatic glycosylation of HDL and impaired HDL-receptor-mediated cholesterol efflux. *Diabetes* 1991;40:377–384.
88. Bagdade JD, Buchanan WE, Kuusi T, et al. Persistent abnormalities in lipoprotein composition in noninsulin-dependent diabetes after intensive insulin therapy. *Arteriosclerosis* 1990;10:232–239.
89. Bagdade JD, Porte D Jr, Bierman EL. Diabetic lipemia: a form of acquired fat-induced lipemia. *N Engl J Med* 1967;276:427–433.
90. Gonen B, White N, Schonfeld G, et al. Plasma levels of apoprotein B in patients with diabetes mellitus: the effect of glycemic control. *Metabolism* 1985;34:675–679.
91. Lopes-Virella MF, Wohltmann HJ, Loadholt CB, et al. Plasma lipids and lipoproteins in young insulin-dependent diabetic patients: relationship with control. *Diabetologia* 1981;21:216–223.
92. Nikkila EA, Kekki M. Plasma triglyceride transport kinetics in diabetes mellitus. *Metabolism* 1973;22:1–22.
93. Lewis B, Mancini M, Mattock M, et al. Plasma triglyceride and fatty acid metabolism in diabetes mellitus. *Eur J Clin Invest* 1972;2:445–453.
94. Ginsberg H, Mok H, Grundy S, et al. Increased production of very low density lipoprotein-triglyceride (VLDL-TG) in insulin-deficient diabetics. *Diabetes* 1977;26[Suppl 1]:399(abst).
95. Pietri AO, Dunn FL, Grundy SM, et al. The effect of continuous subcutaneous insulin infusion on very-low-density lipoprotein triglyceride metabolism in type I diabetes mellitus. *Diabetes* 1983;32:75–81.
96. Dunn FL, Carroll P, Vlachokosta F, et al. Effect of treatment with the artificial beta-cell on triglyceride metabolism in type I diabetes mellitus. *Diabetes* 1985;34[Suppl 1]:86A(abst).
97. Rosenstock J, Vega G-L, Raskin P. Improved diabetic control decreases LDL apoB synthesis in type I diabetes mellitus. *Arteriosclerosis* 1985;5:513A(abst).
98. Lopes-Virella MF, Sherer GK, Lees AM, et al. Surface binding, internalization and degradation by cultured human fibroblasts of low density lipoproteins isolated from type I (insulin-dependent) diabetic patients: changes with metabolic control. *Diabetologia* 1982;22:430–436.
99. Lopes-Virella MF, Sherer G, Wohltmann H, et al. Diabetic lipoprotein deficient serum: its effect in low density lipoprotein (LDL) uptake and degradation by fibroblasts. *Metabolism* 1985;34:1079–1085.
100. Nikkila EA, Kuusi T, Taskinen MR. Role of lipoprotein lipase and hepatic endothelial lipase in the metabolism of high density lipoproteins: a novel concept on cholesterol transport in HDL cycle. In: Carlson LA, Personow B, eds. *Metabolic risk factors in ischemic cardiovascular disease*. New York: Raven Press, 1982:205–215.
101. Eckel RH, Albers JJ, Cheung MD, et al. High density lipoprotein composition in insulin dependent diabetes mellitus. *Diabetes* 1981;30:132–138.
102. Curtiss LK, Witztum JL. Plasma apolipoproteins AI, AII, B, CI, and E are glucosylated in hyperglycemic diabetic subjects. *Diabetes* 1985;34:452–461.

103. Kannel WB, McGee DL. Diabetes and cardiovascular disease: the Framingham Study. *JAMA* 1979;241:2035–2038.
104. Anonymous. Diabetes mellitus: a major risk factor for cardiovascular disease—a joint editorial statement by the American Diabetes Association, the National Heart, Lung, and Blood Institute, the Juvenile Diabetes Foundation International, the National Institute of Diabetes and Digestive and Kidney Diseases, and the American Heart Association [Editorial; comment]. *Circulation* 1999;100:1132–1133.
105. Grundy SM, Benjamin IJ, Burke GL, et al. Diabetes and cardiovascular disease: a statement for healthcare professionals from the American Heart Association [see comments] [Review]. *Circulation* 1999;100:1134–1146.
106. Bahia L, Gomes MB, da Cruz P di M, et al. Coronary artery disease, microalbuminuria and lipid profile in patients with non-insulin dependent diabetes mellitus. *Arq Bras Cardiol* 1999;73:11–22.
107. Haffner SM, Stern MP, Hazuda HP, et al. Cardiovascular risk factors in confirmed prediabetic individuals. Does the clock for coronary heart disease start ticking before the onset of clinical diabetes? *JAMA* 1990;263:2893–2898.
108. Haffner SM, Lehto S, Ronnemaa T, et al. Mortality from coronary heart disease in subjects with type 2 diabetes and in nondiabetic subjects with and without prior myocardial infarction. *N Engl J Med* 1998;339:229–234.
109. Henry P, Richard P, Beverelli F, et al. [Diabetic coronary disease and risk of myocardial infarction] [French]. *Arch Mal Coeur Vaiss* 1999;92:219–223.
110. Orlander PR, Goff DC, Morrissey M, et al. The relation of diabetes to the severity of acute myocardial infarction and post-myocardial infarction survival in Mexican-Americans and non-Hispanic whites: the Corpus Christi Heart Project. *Diabetes* 1994;43:897–902.
111. Sprafka JM, Burke GL, Folsom AR, et al. Trends in prevalence of diabetes mellitus in patients with myocardial infarction and effect of diabetes on survival: the Minnesota Heart Survey. *Diabetes Care* 1991;14:537–543.
112. Miettinen H, Lehto S, Salomaa V, et al. Impact of diabetes on mortality after the first myocardial infarction. *Diabetes Care* 1998;21:69–75.
113. Galcera-Tomas J, Melgarejo-Moreno A, Garcia-Alberola A, et al. Prognostic significance of diabetes in acute myocardial infarction. Are the differences linked to female gender? *Int J Cardiol* 1999;69:289–298.
114. Grundy SM, Bazzarre T, Cleeman J, et al. Prevention Conference V: beyond secondary prevention: identifying the high-risk patient for primary prevention—medical office assessment. *Circulation* 2000;101:E3–E11.
115. O'Brien T, Nguyen TT, Zimmerman BR. Hyperlipidemia and diabetes mellitus. *Mayo Clin Proc* 1998;73:969–976.
116. Howard BV, Robbins DC, Sievers ML, et al. LDL cholesterol as a strong predictor of coronary heart disease in diabetic individuals with insulin resistance and low LDL: the Strong Heart Study. *Arterioscler Thromb Vasc Biol* 2000;20:830–835.
117. Canner PL, Berge KG, Wenger NK, et al. for the Coronary Drug Project Research Group. Fifteen year mortality in coronary drug project patients: long-term benefit with niacin. *J Am Coll Cardiol* 1986;8:1245–1255.
118. Lipid Research Clinics Program. The Lipid Research Clinics coronary primary prevention trial results, I: reduction in incidence of coronary heart disease. *JAMA* 1984;251:351–364.
119. Rifkind BM. Lipid Research Clinics Coronary Primary Prevention Trial: results and implications. *Am J Cardiol* 1984;54:30C–34C.
120. Frick MH, Elo O, Haapa K, et al. Helsinki Heart Study: primary-prevention trial with gemfibrozil in middle-aged men with dyslipidemia: safety of treatment, changes in risk factors, and incidence of coronary heart disease. *N Engl J Med* 1987;317:1237–1245.
121. Koskinen P, Manttari M, Manninen V, et al. Coronary heart disease incidence in NIDDM patients in the Helsinki Heart Study. *Diabetes Care* 1992;15:820–825.
122. Adler AI, Stratton IM, Neil HAW, et al. Association of systolic blood pressure with macrovascular and microvascular complications of type 2 diabetes (UKPDS 35): prospective observational study. *BMJ* 2000;321:412–419.
123. Randomised trial of cholesterol lowering in 4444 patients with coronary heart disease: the Scandinavian Simvastatin Survival Study (4S). *Lancet* 1994;344:1383–1389.
124. Sacks FM, Pfeffer MA, Moye LA, et al. The effect of pravastatin on coronary events after myocardial infarction in patients with average cholesterol levels. *N Engl J Med* 1996;335:1001–1009.
125. Anonymous. Prevention of cardiovascular events and death with pravastatin in patients with coronary heart disease and a broad range of initial cholesterol levels: the Long-Term Intervention with Pravastatin in Ischaemic Disease (LIPID) Study Group [see comments]. *N Engl J Med* 1998;339:1349–1357.
126. Downs JR, Clearfield M, Weis S, et al. Primary prevention of acute coronary events with lovastatin in men and women with average cholesterol levels: results of AFCAPS/TexCAPS. *JAMA* 1998;279:1615–1622.
127. Shepherd J, Cobbe SM, Ford I, et al. for the West of Scotland Coronary Prevention Study Group. Prevention of coronary heart disease with pravastatin in men with hypercholesterolemia. *N Engl J Med* 1995;333:1301–1307.
128. Haffner SM. Patients with type 2 diabetes: the case for primary prevention. *Am J Med* 1999;107:43S–45S.
129. Pyorala K, Pedersen TR, Kjekshus J, et al. Cholesterol lowering with simvastatin improves prognosis of diabetic patients with coronary heart disease: a subgroup analysis of the Scandinavian Simvastatin Survival Study (4S). *Diabetes Care* 1997;20:614–620.
130. Goldberg RB, Mellies MJ, Sacks FM, et al. Cardiovascular events and their reduction with pravastatin in diabetic and glucose-intolerant myocardial infarction survivors with average cholesterol levels: subgroup analyses in the cholesterol and recurrent events (CARE) trial: the CARE investigators. *Circulation* 1998;98:2513–2519.
131. Stratton IM, Adler AI, Neil HAW, et al. Association of glycemia with macrovascular and microvascular complications of type 2 diabetes (UKPDS 35): prospective observational study. *BMJ* 2000;321:405–412.
132. Howard BV. Pathogenesis of diabetic dyslipidemia. *Diabetes Rev* 1995;3: 423–432.
133. Harris MI. Hypercholesterolemia in diabetes and glucose intolerance in the U.S. population. *Diabetes Care* 1991;14:366–374.
134. Siegel RD, Cupples A, Schaefer EJ, et al. Lipoproteins, apolipoproteins, and low-density lipoprotein size among diabetics in the Framingham offspring study. *Metabolism* 1996;45:1267–1272.
135. Christlieb AR. Treatment selection considerations for the hypertensive diabetic patient. *Arch Intern Med* 1990;150:1167–1174.
136. Brown WV, Howard WJ. Treatment of lipoprotein disorders. *Cardiovasc Clin* 1990;20:157–176.
137. Brown WV, Field L, Howard WJ. Nicotinic acid and its derivatives. In: Rifkind B, ed. *Drug treatment of hyperlipidemia.* New York: Marcel Dekker, 1991.
138. Alderman JD, Pasternak RC, Sacks FM, et al. Effect of a modified, well-tolerated niacin regimen on serum total cholesterol, high density lipoprotein cholesterol and the cholesterol to high density lipoprotein ratio. *Am J Cardiol* 1989;64:725–729.
139. Henkin Y, Johnson KC, Segrest JP. Rechallenge with crystalline niacin after drug-induced hepatitis from sustained-release niacin. *JAMA* 1990;264:241–243.
140. Garg A, Grundy SM. Nicotinic acid as therapy for dyslipidemia in non-insulin-dependent diabetes mellitus. *JAMA* 1990;264:723–726.
141. Howard WJ, Brown WV. Pharmacologic therapy of hypercholesterolemia. *Curr Opin Cardiol* 1989;3:525–541.
142. Donahoo WT, Kosmiski LA, Eckel RH. Drugs causing dyslipoproteinemia. *Endocrinol Metab Clin North Am* 1998;27:677–697.
143. Lindner J, Seitz W, Hellich R. [Correlation between lipids, especially HDL-cholesterol, and increasing alcohol consumption] [German]. *Zeitschr Gesamte Innere Med Ihre Grenzgebiete* 1981;36:979–981.
144. Donahoo WT, Kosmiski LA, Eckel RH. Drugs causing dyslipoproteinemia. *Endocrinol Metab Clin North Am* 1998;27:677–697.
145. Liebson PR, Amsterdam EA. Prevention of coronary heart disease, I: primary prevention [Review]. *Disease-A-Month* 1999;45:497–571.
146. Howard BV, Robbins DC, Sievers ML, et al. LDL cholesterol as a strong predictor of coronary heart disease in diabetic individuals with insulin resistance and low LDL: the Strong Heart Study. *Arterioscler Thromb Vasc Biol* 2000;20:830–835.
147. Sacks FM, Ridker PM. Lipid lowering and beyond: results from the CARE study on lipoproteins and inflammation: cholesterol and recurrent events [Review]. *Herz* 1999;24:51–56.
148. Flaker GC, Warnica JW, Sacks FM, et al. Pravastatin prevents clinical events in revascularized patients with average cholesterol concentrations: cholesterol and recurrent events. CARE investigators. *J Am Coll Cardiol* 1999;34:106–112.
149. Vaughan CJ, Delanty N. Neuroprotective properties of statins in cerebral ischemia and stroke. *Stroke* 1999;30:1969–1973.
150. Bucher HC, Griffith LE, Guyatt GH. Effect of HMG coA reductase inhibitors on stroke: a meta-analysis of randomized, controlled trials. *Ann Intern Med* 1998;128:89–95.
151. MacMahon S, Sharpe N, Gamble G, et al. Effects of lowering average or below-average cholesterol levels on the progression of carotid atherosclerosis: results of the LIPID Atherosclerosis Substudy. *Circulation* 1998;97:1784–1790.
152. White HD, Simes J, Anderson NE, et al. Pravastatin therapy and the risk of stroke. *N Engl J Med* 2000;343:317–326.
153. Goldberg RB, Mellies MJ, Sacks FM, et al. Cardiovascular events and their reduction with pravastatin in diabetic and glucose-intolerant myocardial infarction survivors with average cholesterol levels: subgroup analyses in the cholesterol and recurrent events (CARE) trial: the CARE Investigators. *Circulation* 1998;98:2513–2519.
154. The Expert Committee on the Diagnosis and Classification of Diabetes Mellitus: Report of the Expert Committee on the Diagnosis and Classification of Diabetes Mellitus. *Diabetes Care* 1997;20:1–15.
155. Haffner SM, Alexander CM, Cook TJ, et al. Reduced coronary events in simvastatin-treated patients with coronary heart disease and diabetes or impaired fasting glucose levels: subgroup analyses in the Scandinavian Simvastatin Survival Study [see comments]. *Arch Intern Med* 1999;159:2661–2667.
156. LaRosa JC, He J, Vupputuri S. Effect of statins on risk of coronary disease: a meta-analysis of randomized controlled trials. *JAMA* 1999;282:2340–2346.
157. Kastelein JJ. The future of best practice [Review]. *Atherosclerosis* 1999;143 [Suppl 1]:S17–S21.
158. Crouse JR 3rd, Frohlich J, Ose L, et al. Effects of high doses of simvastatin and atorvastatin on high-density lipoprotein cholesterol and apolipoprotein A-I. *Am J Cardiol* 1999;83:1476–1477(abst 7).
159. Rubins HB, Robins SJ, Collins D, et al. Gemfibrozil for the secondary prevention of coronary heart disease in men with low levels of high-density lipoprotein cholesterol. Veterans Affairs High-Density Lipoprotein Cholesterol Intervention Trial Study Group. *N Engl J Med* 1999;341:410–418.
160. Hoogwerf BJ, Waness A, Cressman M, et al. Effects of aggressive cholesterol lowering and low-dose anticoagulation on clinical and angiographic outcomes in patients with diabetes: the Post Coronary Artery Bypass Graft Trial. *Diabetes* 1999;48:1289–1294.
161. Steiner G, Stewart D, Hosking JD. Baseline characteristics of the study population in the Diabetes Atherosclerosis Intervention Study (DAIS): World

Health Organization Collaborating Centre for the Study of Atherosclerosis in Diabetes. *Am J Cardiol* 1999;84:1004–1010.
162. Steiner G. The Diabetes Atherosclerosis Intervention Study (DAIS): a study conducted in cooperation with the World Health Organization—the DAIS Project Group. *Diabetologia* 1996;39:1655–1661.
163. Diabetes Atherosclerosis Intervention Study. *Endocrinology Update* July 10, 2000:1.
164. Fenofibrate retards atherosclerosis in diabetics—DAIS results. *Heartwire* June 27, 2000. Available at: http://www.theheart.org/documents/docs13500/13806. Accessed June 27, 2000.
164a. MRC/BHF Heart Protection Study of cholesterol lowering with simvastatin in 20,536 high-risk individuals: a randomized placebo-controlled trial. *Lancet* 2002;360:7–22.
165. Robbins DC, Howard BV. Lipoprotein(a) and diabetes [Editorial; comment]. *Diabetes Care* 1991;14:347–349.
166. Gotto AM Jr, LaRosa JC, Hunninghake D, et al. The cholesterol facts: a summary of the evidence relating dietary fats, serum cholesterol, and coronary heart disease: a joint statement by the American Heart Association and the National Heart, Lung, and Blood Institute. *Circulation* 1988;81:1721–1733.
167. Steiner G. From an excess of fat, diabetics die [Editorial]. *JAMA* 1989;262:398–399.
168. Sytkowski PA, Kannel WB, D'Agostino RB. Changes in risk factors and the decline in mortality from cardiovascular disease. The Framingham Heart Study. *N Engl J Med* 1990;322:1635–1641.
169. Anonymous. The effect of intensive treatment of diabetes on the development and progression of long-term complications in insulin-dependent diabetes mellitus: the Diabetes Control and Complications Trial Research Group. *N Engl J Med* 1993;329:977–986.
170. Zinman B. Glucose control in type 1 diabetes: from conventional to intensive therapy. *Clinical Cornerstone* 1998;1:29–38.
171. Expert Panel on Detection, Evaluation, and Treatment of High Blood Cholesterol in Adults. Executive Summary of the Third Report of the National Cholesterol Education Program (NCEP) Expert Panel on Detection, Evaluation, and Treatment of High Blood Cholesterol in Adults (Adult Treatment Panel III). *JAMA* 2001;285:2486–2497.
172. American Diabetes Association. Standards of medical care for patients with diabetes mellitus. *Diabetes Care* 2000;23[Suppl 1]:S57–S60.
172a. Grundy SM, Cleeman JI, Merz CN, et al. Implications of recent clinical trials for the National Cholesterol Education Program Adult Treatment Panel III guidelines. *Circulation* 2004;110:227–239.
173. Assmann G, Schulte H, Funke H, et al. The emergence of triglycerides as a significant independent risk factor in coronary artery disease. *Eur Heart J* 1998;19[Suppl M]:M8–M14.
174. West KM, Ahuja MMS, Bennett PH, et al. The role of circulating glucose and triglyceride concentrations and their interactions with other "risk factors" as determinants of arterial disease in nine diabetic population samples from the WHO multinational study. *Diabetes Care* 1983;6:361–369.
175. Fontbonne A, Eschwege E, Cambien F, et al. Hypertriglyceridaemia as a risk factor of coronary heart disease mortality in subjects with impaired glucose tolerance or diabetes: results from the 11-year follow-up of the Paris Prospective Study. *Diabetologia* 1989;32:300–304.
176. Carlson LA, Rosenhamer G. Reduction of mortality in the Stockholm Ischaemic Heart Disease Secondary Prevention Study by combined treatment with clofibrate and nicotinic acid. *Acta Med Scand* 1988;223:405–418.
177. Verges BL. Dyslipidaemia in diabetes mellitus: review of the main lipoprotein abnormalities and their consequences on the development of atherogenesis. *Diabetes Metab* 1999;25[Suppl 3]:32–40.
178. Krauss RM. Triglycerides and atherogenic lipoproteins: rationale for lipid management. *Am J Med* 1998;105:58S–62S.
179. American Diabetes Association. Role of cardiovascular risk factors in prevention and treatment of macrovascular disease in diabetes. *Diabetes Care* 1989;12:573–579.
180. Blankenhorn DH, Nessim SA, Johnson RL, et al. Beneficial effects of combined colestipol-niacin therapy on coronary atherosclerosis and coronary venous bypass grafts. *JAMA* 1987;257:3233–3240.
181. Brown BG, Zambon A, Poulin D, et al. Use of niacin, statins, and resins in patients with combined hyperlipidemia. *Am J Cardiol* 1998;81:52B–59B.
182. Scheen AJ. [Clinical study of the month. Usefulness of increasing HDL cholesterol in secondary prevention of coronary heart disease: results of the VA-HIT study] [French]. *Rev Med Liege* 1999;54:773–775.
183. Frost PH, Havel RJ. Rationale for use of non-high-density lipoprotein cholesterol rather than low-density lipoprotein cholesterol as a tool for lipoprotein cholesterol screening and assessment of risk and therapy. *Am J Cardiol* 1998;81:26B–31B.
184. Garg A, Grundy SM. Management of dyslipidemia in NIDDM. *Diabetes Care* 1990;13:153–169.
185. Sievers ML, Bennett PH, Nelson RG. Effect of glycemia on mortality in Pima Indians with type 2 diabetes. *Diabetes* 1999;48:896–902.
186. Anonymous. Intensive blood-glucose control with sulphonylureas or insulin compared with conventional treatment and risk of complications in patients with type 2 diabetes (UKPDS 33). UK Prospective Diabetes Study (UKPDS) Group. *Lancet* 1998;352:837–853.
187. Gaster B, Hirsch IB. The effects of improved glycemic control on complications in type 2 diabetes [Review]. *Arch Intern Med* 1998;158:134–140.
188. Gaster B. The effects of improved glycemic control on complications in type 2 diabetes. *Arch Intern Med* 1998;158:134–140.
189. Roshan B, Tofler GH, Weinrauch LA, et al. Improved glycemic control and platelet function abnormalities in diabetic patients with microvascular disease. *Metabolism* 2000;49:88–91.
190. Ohkubo Y, Kishikawa H, Araki E, et al. Intensive insulin therapy prevents the progression of diabetic microvascular complications in Japanese patients with non-insulin-dependent diabetes mellitus: a randomized prospective 6-year study [see comments]. *Diabetes Res Clin Pract* 1995;28:103–117.
191. Malmberg K. Prospective randomised study of intensive insulin treatment on long term survival after acute myocardial infarction in patients with diabetes mellitus: DIGAMI (Diabetes Mellitus, Insulin Glucose Infusion in Acute Myocardial Infarction) Study Group [see comments]. *BMJ* 1997;314:1512–1515.
192. DeFronzo RA, Goodman AM. Efficacy of metformin in patients with non-insulin-dependent diabetes mellitus: the Multicenter Metformin Study Group. *N Engl J Med* 1995;333:541–549.
193. Ghazzi MN, Perez JE, Antonucci TK, et al. Cardiac and glycemic benefits of troglitazone treatment in NIDDM: the Troglitazone Study Group. *Diabetes* 1997;46:433–439.
194. Wolffenbuttel BH, Gomis R, Squatrito S, et al. Addition of low-dose rosiglitazone to sulphonylurea therapy improves glycaemic control in type 2 diabetic patients. *Diabet Med* 2000;17:40–47.
195. Kumar S, Boulton AJ, Beck-Nielsen H, et al. Troglitazone, an insulin action enhancer, improves metabolic control in NIDDM patients: Troglitazone Study Group. *Diabetologia* 1996;39:701–709.
196. Howard BV, Howard WJ. LDL cholesterol and troglitazone therapy [Letter; comment]. *Diabetes Care* 1998;21:2201–2203.
197. Pan XR, Li GW, Hu YH, et al. Effects of diet and exercise in preventing NIDDM in people with impaired glucose tolerance: the Da Qing IGT and Diabetes Study. *Diabetes Care* 1997;20:537–544.
198. Rigla M, Sanchez-Quesada JL, Ordonez-Llanos J, et al. Effect of physical exercise on lipoprotein(a) and low-density lipoprotein modifications in type 1 and type 2 diabetic patients. *Metabolism* 2000;49:640–647.
199. American Diabetes Association. Position statement: diabetes mellitus and exercise. *Diabetes Care* 2000;23[Suppl 1]:S50–S54.
200. American Diabetes Association. Diabetes and exercise: the risk-benefit profile. In: Devlin JT, Ruderman N, eds. *The health professional's guide to diabetes and exercise*. Alexandria, VA, American Diabetes Association, 1995:3–4.
201. Frisch RE, Wyshak G, Albright TE, et al. Lower prevalence of diabetes in female former college athletes compared with nonathletes. *Diabetes* 1986;35:1101–1105.
202. Manson JE, Rimm EB, Stampfer MJ, et al. Physical activity and incidence of non-insulin-dependent diabetes mellitus in women. *Lancet* 1991;338:774–778.
203. Helmrich SP, Ragland DR, Leung RW, et al. Physical activity and reduced occurrence of non-insulin-dependent diabetes mellitus. *N Engl J Med* 1991;325:147–152.
204. Manson JE, Nathan DM, Krolewski AS, et al. A prospective study of exercise and incidence of diabetes among US male physicians. *JAMA* 1992;268:63–67.
205. Burchfiel CM, Sharp DS, Curb JD, et al. Physical activity and incidence of diabetes: the Honolulu Heart Program. *Am J Epidemiol* 1995;141:360–368.
206. Pate RR, Pratt M, Blair SN, Haskell WL, et al. Physical activity and public health: a recommendation from the Centers for Disease Control and Prevention and the American College of Sports Medicine. *JAMA* 1995;273:402–407.
207. Kriska A, ed. Physical activity and the prevention of type II (non-insulin dependent) diabetes. *Research Digest of the President's Council on Physical Fitness and Sports* 1997;series 2(10).
208. Pascale RW, Wing RR, Butler BA, et al. Effects of a behavioral weight loss program stressing calorie restriction versus calorie plus fat restriction in obese individuals with NIDDM of a family history of diabetes. *Diabetes Care* 1995;18:1241–1318.
209. Wing RR, Shoemaker M, Marcus MD, et al. Variables associated with weight loss and improvements in glycemic control in type II diabetic patients in behavioral weight control programs. *Int J Obes* 1990;14;6:495–503.
210. American Diabetes Association. Nutritional recommendations and principles for individuals with diabetes mellitus. *Diabetes Care* 2000;23[Suppl 1]:S1–S46.
211. Rivellese AA, Giacco R, Genovese S, et al. Effects of changing amount of carbohydrate in diet on plasma lipoproteins and apolipoproteins in type II diabetic patients. *Diabetes Care* 1990;13:446–448.
212. Riccardi G, Rivellese AA. Effects of dietary fiber and carbohydrate on glucose and lipoprotein metabolism in diabetic patients. *Diabetes Care* 1991;14;12:1115–1125.
213. Van Horn L. Fiber, lipids, and coronary heart disease. A statement for healthcare professionals from the Nutrition Committee, American Heart Association. *Circulation* 1997;95:2701–2704.
214. Coulston AM, Hollenbeck CB, Swislocki ALM, et al. Persistence of hypertriglyceridemic effect of low-fat high-carbohydrate diets in NIDDM patients. *Diabetes Care* 1989;12:94–101.
215. Abbott WGH, Swinburn B, Ruotolo G, et al. Effect of a high-carbohydrate, low-saturated-fat diet on apolipoprotein B and triglyceride metabolism in Pima Indians. *J Clin Invest* 1990;86:642–650.
216. Garg A. High-monounsaturated-fat diets for patients with diabetes mellitus: a meta-analysis. *Am J Clin Nutr* 1998;67[3 Suppl]:577S–582S.
217. Garg A, Bantle JP, Henry RR, et al. Effects of varying carbohydrate content of diet in patients with non-insulin-dependent diabetes mellitus. *JAMA* 1994;271:1421–1428.
218. NIH Consensus Development Conference Summary. Treatment of hypertriglyceridemia. *Arteriosclerosis* 1984;4:296–301.

219. Bantle JP, Laine CW, Thomas JW. Metabolic effects of dietary fructose and sucrose in types I and II diabetic subjects. *JAMA* 1986;256:3241–3246.
220. Bantle JP, Swanson JE, Thomas W, et al. Metabolic effects of dietary sucrose in type II diabetic subjects. *Diabetes Care* 1993;16:1301–1305.
221. Wise JE, Keim KS, Huisinga JL, et al. Effects of sucrose-containing snacks on blood glucose contol. *Diabetes Care* 1989;12:423–426.
222. Abbott WGH, Boyce VL, Grundy SM, et al. Effects of replacing saturated fat with complex carbohydrate in diets of subjects with NIDDM. *Diabetes Care* 1989;12:102–107.
223. Anderson JW, Zeigler JA, Deakins DA, et al. Metabolic effects of high-carbohydrate, high-fiber diets for insulin-dependent diabetic individuals. *Am J Clin Nutr* 1991;54:936–943.
224. Ginsberg HN, Kris-Etherton P, Dennis B, et al. Effects of reducing dietary saturated fatty acids on plasma lipids and lipoproteins in healthy subjects: the DELTA Study, protocol 1. *Arterioscler Thromb Vasc Biol* 1998;18:441–449.
225. Simons LA, Ruys J, Chang S, et al. Maintenance of plasma triglyceride-lowering through use of low-dose fish oils in the diet. *Artery* 1987;14:127–136.
226. Albert CM, Hennekens CH, O'Donnell CJ, et al. Fish consumption and risk of sudden cardiac death. *JAMA* 1998;279:23–28.
227. Siscovick DS, Raghunathan TE, King I, et al. Dietary intake and cell membrane levels of long-chain n-3 polyunsaturated fatty acids and the risk of primary cardiac arrest. *JAMA* 1995;274:1363–1367.
228. Leaf A, Weber PC. Cardiovascular effects of n-3 fatty acids. *N Engl J Med* 1988;318:549–557.
229. Hendra TJ, Britton ME, Roper DR, et al. Effects of fish oil supplements in NIDDM subjects: controlled study. *Diabetes Care* 1990;13:821–829.
230. Friday KE, Childs MT, Tsunehara CH, et al. Elevated plasma glucose and lowered triglyceride levels from omega-3 fatty acid supplementation in type II diabetes. *Diabetes Care* 1989;12:276–281.
231. Kasim S. Is there a role for fish oils in diabetes treatment? *Clin Diabetes* 1989;7: 93–100.
232. Mori TA, Vandongen R, Masarei JRL. Fish oil-induced changes in apolipoproteins in IDDM subjects. *Diabetes Care* 1990;13:725–732.
233. Sorisky A, Robbins DC. Fish oil and diabetes: the net effect [Editorial]. *Diabetes Care* 1989;12:302–304.
234. Ascherio A, Rimm EB, Hernan MA, et al. Relation of consumption of vitamin E, vitamin C, and carotenoids to risk for stroke among men in the United States [see comments]. *Ann Intern Med* 1999;130:963–970.
235. Yusuf S, Dagenais G, Pogue J, et al. Vitamin E supplementation and cardiovascular events in high-risk patients: the Heart Outcomes Prevention Evaluation Study Investigators. *N Engl J Med* 2000;342:154–160.
236. Fonarow GC, Gawlinski A. Rationale and design of the cardiac hospitalization atherosclerosis management program at the University of California Los Angeles. *Am J Cardiol* 2000;85:10A–17A.
237. Baller D, Notohamiprodjo G, Gleichmann U, et al. Improvement in coronary flow reserve determined by positron emission tomography after 6 months of cholesterol-lowering therapy in patients with early stages of coronary atherosclerosis. *Circulation* 1999;99:2871–2875.
238. Mooney A. Treating patients with hypertriglyceridaemia saves lives: triglyceride revisited. *Curr Med Res Opin* 1999;15:65–77.
239. Scheen AJ. [Clinical study of the month. Usefulness of increasing HDL cholesterol in secondary prevention of coronary heart disease: results of the VA-HIT study] [French]. *Rev Med Liege* 1999;54:773–775.
240. Ornish D, Brown SE, Scherwitz LW, et al. Can lifestyle changes reverse coronary heart disease? The Lifestyle Heart Trial. *Lancet* 1990;336:129–133.
241. Grundy SM. HMG-CoA reductase inhibitors for treatment of hypercholesterolemia. *N Engl J Med* 1988;319:24–33.
242. Stein EA, Lane M, Laskarzewski P. Comparison of statins in hypertriglyceridemia. *Am J Cardiol* 1998;81:66B–69B.
243. Kastelein JJP, Isaacsohn JL, Ose L, et al. Comparison of effects of simvastatin versus atorvastatin on high-density lipoprotein cholesterol and apolipoprotein A-I levels. *Am J Cardiol* 2000;86:221–223.
244. Jones P, Kafonek S, Laurora I, et al. Comparative dose efficacy study of atorvastatin versus simvastatin, pravastatin, lovastatin, and fluvastatin in patients with hypercholesterolemia (the CURVES study). *Am J Cardiol* 1998; 81:582–587.
245. Michalets EL. Update: clinically significant cytochrome P-450 drug interactions [see comments] [Review]. *Pharmacotherapy* 1998;18:84–112.
246. Rudy E. Using cytochrome P450 tables to predict drug interactions: caveats and cautions. *Drug Therapy Topics* (University of Washington Medical Center/Harborview Medical Center) 1998;28:1–42.
247. Knopp RH. Drug therapy: drug treatment of lipid disorders. *N Engl J Med* 1999;341:498–511.
248. Bailey DG, Malcolm J, Arnold O, et al. Grapefruit juice–drug interactions. *Br J Clin Pharmacol* 1998;46:101–110.
249. Kane GC, Laisky JJ. Drug–grapefruit juice interactions. *Mayo Clin Proc* 2000; 75:933–942.
250. Anonymous. Grapefruit juice influences certain cholesterol drugs [news]. *Mayo Clin Health Lett* 2000;18:4.
251. Shviro I, Leitersdorf E. The patient at risk: who should we be treating? *Br J Clin Pract* 1996;77A[Suppl]:24–27.
252. Wysowski DK, Gross TP. Deaths due to accidents and violence in two recent trials of cholesterol-lowering drugs. *Arch Intern Med* 1990;150:2169–2172.
253. Fuster V. Human lesion studies. *Ann N Y Acad Sci* 1997;811:207–224.
254. Cannon RO III. Cardiovascular benefit of cholesterol-lowering therapy: does improved endothelial vasodilator function matter? *Circulation* 2000;102: 820–822.
255. Vaughan CJ, Gotto AM Jr, Basson CT. The evolving role of statins in the management of atherosclerosis. *J Am Coll Cardiol* 2000;35:1–10.
256. Ansell BJ, Watson KE, Fogelman AM. An evidence-based assessment of the NCEP Adult Treatment Panel II Guidelines. *JAMA* 1999;282:2051–2057.
257. The Coronary Drug Project Research Group. Clofibrate and niacin in coronary heart disease. *JAMA* 1975;231:360–381.
258. Report of the Committee of Principal Investigators. WHO cooperative trial on primary prevention of ischaemic heart disease using clofibrate to lower serum cholesterol: mortality follow-up. *Lancet* 1980;2:379–385.
259. Tenkanen L, Manttari M, Manninen V. Some coronary risk factors related to the insulin resistance syndrome and treatment with gemfibrozil: experience from the Helsinki Heart Study. *Circulation* 1995;92:1779–1785.
260. Avogaro A, Piliego T, Catapano A, et al, for the Gemfibrozil Study Group. The effect of gemfibrozil on lipid profile and glucose metabolism in hypertriglyceridaemic well-controlled non-insulin-dependent diabetic patients. *Acta Diabet* 1999;36:27–33.
261. Anonymous. Choice of lipid-lowering drugs. *Med Lett Drugs Ther* 1998;40: 117–122.
262. Gotto AM Jr. Triglyceride as a risk factor for coronary artery disease. *Am J Cardiol* 1998;82:22Q–25Q.
263. Austin MA. Epidemiology of hypertriglyceridemia and cardiovascular disease. *Am J Cardiol* 1999;83:13F–16F.
264. Assmann G, Schulte H, Funke H, et al. The emergence of triglycerides as a significant independent risk factor in coronary artery disease. *Eur Heart J* 1998;19[Suppl M]:M8–M14.
265. Stalenhoef AF. [Serum triglycerides as a risk factor for atherosclerosis] [Dutch]. *Ned Tijdschr Geneeskd* 1999;143:284–287.
266. Brensike JF, Levy RI, Kelsey SF, et al. Effects of therapy with cholestyramine on progression of coronary arteriosclerosis: results of the NHLBI Type II Coronary Intervention Study. *Circulation* 1984;69:313–324.
267. Detre KM, Levy RI, Kelsey SF, et al. Secondary prevention and lipid lowering: results and implications. *Am Heart J* 1985;110:1123–1127.
268. Illingworth DR, Bacon S. Treatment of heterozygous familial hypercholesterolemia with lipid-lowering drugs. *Arteriosclerosis* 1989;9[1 Suppl]:I121–I134.
269. Brocard JJ, Keller U, Oberhansli A, et al. Effects and side effects of a 1-year treatment of primary hypercholesterolemia with simvastatin. *Schweiz Med Wochenschr* 1991;121:977–983.
270. Blankenhorn DH, Nessim SA, Johnson RL, et al. Beneficial effects of combined colestipol-niacin therapy on coronary atherosclerosis and coronary venous bypass grafts. *JAMA* 1987;257:3233–3240.
271. Brown G, Albers JJ, Fisher LD, et al. Regression of coronary artery disease as a result of intensive lipid-lowering therapy in men with high levels of apolipoprotein B. *N Engl J Med* 1990;323:1289–1298.
272. Denke MA, Grundy SM. Hypertriglyceridemia: a relative contraindication to the use of bile acid-binding resins? *Hepatology* 1988;8:974–975.
273. Davidson MH, Dillon MA, Gordon B, et al. Colesevelam hydrochloride (cholestagel): a new, potent bile acid sequestrant associated with a low incidence of gastrointestinal side effects. *Arch Intern Med* 1999;159:1893–1900.
274. Berge KG, Canner PL. Coronary drug project: experience with niacin: Coronary Drug Project Research Group. *Eur J Clin Pharmacol* 1991;40[Suppl 1]:S49–S51.
275. Canner PL, Berge KG, Wenger NK, et al. Fifteen year mortality in Coronary Drug Project patients: long-term benefit with niacin. *J Am Coll Cardiol* 1986; 8:1245–1255.
276. Crouse JR III. New developments in the use of niacin for treatment of hyperlipidemia: new considerations in the use of an old drug. *Coron Artery Dis* 1996;7:321–326.
277. Montori VM, Farmer A, Wollan PC, et al. Fish oil supplementation in type 2 diabetes: a quantitative systematic review. *Diabetes Care* 2000;23: 1407–1415.
278. Goldberg AC. Clinical trial experience with extended-release niacin (Niaspan): dose-escalation study. *Am J Cardiol* 1998;82:35U–38U; discussion 39U–41U.
279. Schwartz ML. Severe reversible hyperglycemia as a consequence of niacin therapy. *Arch Intern Med* 1993;153:2050–2052.
280. Illingworth DR. Lipid-lowering drugs: an overview of indications and optimum therapeutic use. *Drugs* 1987;33:259–279.
281. Crouse JR III. Hypertriglyceridemia: a contraindication to the use of bile acid binding resins. *Am J Med* 1987;83:243–248.
282. Witztum JL. Intensive drug therapy of hypercholesterolemia. *Am Heart J* 1987;113:603–609.
283. Malloy MJ, Kane JP, Kunitake ST, et al. Complementarity of colestipol, niacin and lovastatin in treatment of severe familial hyper-cholesterolemia. *Ann Intern Med* 1987;107:616–622.
284. Denke MA, Grundy SM. Hypercholesterolemia in elderly persons: resolving the treatment dilemma. *Ann Intern Med* 1990;112:780–792.
285. Kafonek SD, Kwiterovich PO. Treatment of hypercholesterolemia in the elderly [Editorial]. *Ann Intern Med* 1990;112:723–725.
286. Castelli WP, Wilson PWF, Levy D, et al. Cardiovascular risk factors in the elderly. *Am J Cardiol* 1989;63:12H–19H.
287. Stout RW. Diabetes and atheroma: 20-yr perspective. *Diabetes Care* 1990;13: 631–654.
288. Reddi AS, Camerini-Davalos RA. Diabetic nephropathy: an update. *Arch Intern Med* 1990;150:31–43.
289. Selby JV, FitzSimmons SC, Newman JM, et al. The natural history of epidemiology of diabetic nephropathy: implications for prevention and control. *JAMA* 1990;263:1954–1960.
290. Grundy SM. Management of hyperlipidemia of kidney disease [Editorial review]. *Kidney Int* 1990;37:847–853.

291. Vega GL, Grundy SM. Lovastatin therapy in nephrotic hyperlipidemia: effects on lipoprotein metabolism. *Kidney Int* 1988;33:1160–1168.
292. Hufnagel G, Michel C, Vrtovsnik F, et al. Effects of atorvastatin on dyslipidaemia in uraemic patients on peritoneal dialysis. *Nephrol Dial Transplantation* 2000;15:684–688.
293. Groggel GC, Cheung AK, Ellis-Benigni K, et al. Treatment of nephrotic hyperlipoproteinemia with gemfibrozil. *Kidney Int* 1989;36:266–271.
294. Appel GB, Appel AS. Lipid-lowering agents in proteinuric diseases. *Am J Nephrol* 1990;10[Suppl 1]:110–115.
295. Gu K, Cowie CC, Harris MI. Diabetes and decline in heart disease mortality in US adults. *JAMA* 1999;281:1291–1297.
296. Roberts WA. Atherosclerotic risk factors—are there ten or is there only one [Editorial]? *Am J Cardiol* 1989;64:552–554.
297. Joslin EP. Arteriosclerosis and diabetes. *Ann Clin Med* 1927;5:1061.

SECTION

V

Treatment of Diabetes Mellitus

CHAPTER 34
General Approach to the Treatment of Diabetes Mellitus

Ramachandiran Cooppan

Since the last edition of this textbook, major scientific advances have increased our understanding of the pathophysiology underlying both type 1 and type 2 diabetes and have fueled new approaches to therapy. New insights into the mechanism of insulin action and insulin resistance, greater understanding of the mechanisms of controlling insulin secretion, and advances in genetics and in immunology have contributed to this explosion of knowledge. Furthermore, a number of randomized prospective studies demonstrating the benefits of tight glycemic control and the availability of new oral therapies and insulin formulations provide a compelling rationale for improving the overall level of diabetes care.

The results of the Diabetes Control and Complications Trial (1), the Kumamoto Trial (2), and the United Kingdom Prospective Diabetes Study (3) have provided conclusive evidence that tight glycemic control will prevent the onset, as well as delay the progression, of the long-term microvascular complications of type 1 and type 2 diabetes. A more recent follow-up of the Kumamoto study (4) noted that the optimal degree of glycemic control to prevent or delay complications is a glycosylated hemoglobin (HbA_{1c}) level of less than 6.5%, a fasting glucose level of less than 110 mg/dL, and a 2-hour postprandial blood glucose level of less than 180 mg/dL.

DIABETES AS A WORLDWIDE HEALTHCARE PROBLEM

Diabetes mellitus has become an international healthcare crisis that requires new approaches to prevention and treatment. During the last 20 years, the prevalence of diabetes has increased dramatically in many parts of the world. Although genetic factors play a role in the etiology, especially of type 2 diabetes, the growing problem of obesity that parallels improved economic status in some developing countries is a major environmental factor in this epidemic of diabetes. On the other hand, in many parts of the developing world, low birth weight and maternal malnutrition during pregnancy may be a major factor underlying the insulin resistance syndrome and thus in an increased risk of diabetes in later life.

At least 120 million people throughout the world suffer from type 2 diabetes, and it is projected that the number will increase to 220 million by the year 2010. This disease is now a worldwide public health issue that not only costs many nations millions of dollars for healthcare but also robs many developing economies of their most precious resource, their workers. Data almost a decade old gave an estimated prevalence of type 2 diabetes in the United States of 14 million persons that caused an estimated 300,000 deaths and resulted in healthcare expenditures of $100 billion (5).

Some of the world's most highly indebted and poorest nations do not have sufficient resources to pay back their debt and to also provide care for patients with diabetes, adding to the problem. In these areas, a lack of adequate insulin supplies is a major problem for young children with type 1 diabetes, and many do not survive more than 1 year after onset of disease. Solutions to this problem must be forthcoming, because treatment for patients with type 1 diabetes exists and should be widely distributed (6).

CHANGING DIAGNOSTIC CRITERIA FOR DIABETES

In 1997, the American Diabetes Association (ADA) changed the diagnostic criteria for diabetes mellitus and recommended that the use of Roman numerals for the two major forms of diabetes mellitus be discontinued and that Arabic numerals 1 and 2 be used instead. The earlier change in the classification from insulin-dependent diabetes mellitus (IDDM) and non–insulin-dependent diabetes mellitus (NIDDM) to type 1 or type 2 was an attempt to move away from a treatment-based classification to one based on underlying pathophysiology. This new system removed the confusion that emerged when patients classified as having NIDDM under the old nomenclature were treated with insulin because of disease progression. Would these patients now be classified as having IDDM or were they merely patients with NIDDM who now required insulin therapy? The pathophysiologic approach allows for the spectrum of changes in the underlying disease process that develop with time and provides a rationale for treatment changes based on this progression.

In making these changes, the ADA also revised the diagnostic criteria for diabetes and introduced a new category, impaired fasting glucose (IFG). The old criteria required a fasting plasma glucose level of 140 mg/dL or higher or a glucose level of 200 mg/dL or higher 2 hours after a 75-g glucose challenge to establish a diagnosis of diabetes. These older criteria also were in line with the recommendations of the World Health Organization. The new criteria were developed to allow earlier diagnosis of diabetes that would, in turn, lead to early treatment and, it is hoped, to a reduction in diabetes-related complications (7). Studies in Egypt and the United States demonstrated a correlation between the development of retinopathy and a fasting glucose level of more than 108 to 116 mg/dL (8,9). Not all groups are enthusiastic about these changes in the diagnostic criteria. Some are concerned that undo emphasis on the fasting glucose concentrations will reduce the use of the oral glucose tolerance test that may be necessary to identify individuals with impaired glucose tolerance (IGT), which is associated with greater rate of progression to clinical diabetes and is a risk factor for cardiovascular disease (10,11). Furthermore, there is concern that the new criteria may increase the prevalence of diabetes in many parts of the world and strain already limited healthcare resources (12,13), although, of course, the new criteria do not increase the actual prevalence of diabetes but only that of diagnosed diabetes.

Advances in molecular biology and genetics have helped to elucidate the mechanism of insulin action and to identify specific gene mutations [e.g., glucokinase gene in maturity-onset diabetes of the young-2 (MODY 2)] that can lead to diabetes. In addition, outcome data clearly support the benefits of strict glycemic control in retarding both the development and progression of the long-term microvascular complications in both type 1 and type 2 diabetes mellitus. These studies on glucose control have been complemented by studies on macrovascular disease that demonstrate the major benefits derived from aggressive treatment of hypercholesterolemia and elevated blood pressure in patients with diabetes.

The increase in the number of oral medications for treating type 2 diabetes has now made it possible for providers not only to choose therapies based on the underlying pathophysiology of diabetes but also to use drugs that work synergistically by addressing different pathophysiologic abnormalities. The benefits of this approach, which often allows the use of submaximal doses of different agents, are improved glycemic control and a reduction of the adverse effects of the medications used. The challenge in type 2 diabetes is to start treatment early and to use combination therapies that address both the insulin resistance and insulin secretory defects of the disease. The introduction of rapid-acting human insulin, as well as the new long-acting insulin analogues, has made it possible to approximate normal insulin secretion through the use of basal and premeal (bolus) insulin regimens.

The "cure" for diabetes still eludes us. However, the progress made in the development of new approaches to growing and transplanting β-cells and in immunosuppressive therapy lends hope to the possibility that transplanted β-cells, even those not rendered immunoneutral, will survive for the long term and render patients with type 1 diabetes insulin-independent (14).

The approach to a chronic disease such as diabetes requires treatment goals that include both the maintenance of the well-being of the affected individual and the prevention of the long-term complications associated with the disease. The relationship of glucose control to the microvascular complications has been validated; the challenge is to make practical use of this information by improving the delivery of appropriate care. This requires close collaboration among all members of the healthcare team involved in the care of patients with diabetes. Despite the dramatic results of the Diabetes Control and Complications Trial (DCCT), for most patients, there has been no major shift in the care of type 1 diabetes that will provide the benefits noted in the intensive therapy trials.. It is gratifying that those patients who were in the intensive treatment arm of DCCT and are now part of the Epidemiology of Diabetes Interventions and Complications (EDIC) trial have continued to benefit from participation in the intensive treatment arm for as long as 4 years after the trial's end. Unfortunately, this group has experienced some deterioration in overall glycemic control outside the environment of a rigorously controlled clinical trial (15). The cost-effectiveness of intensive treatment also has been examined and found to be worthwhile compared with the cost of treating the complications when they occur. To achieve aggressive goals of glycemic control, self-monitoring of blood glucose (SMBG) must be a standard for all patients. Moreover, patients should have access to the appropriate monitoring equipment, independent of the type of diabetes, and with the frequency of testing determined by the medical professionals and the patient.

Many variations of practice guidelines for diabetes are now available; however, adherence to these guidelines has not been optimal in many instances (16). There are many reasons for this, and these must be assessed carefully if progress is to be made in this area. Current treatment guidelines are based on outcomes data derived from controlled clinical trials and extensive physician experience. A mechanism is now needed to translate these guidelines into a format that will be both practical and realistic in clinical practice. The care of patients with a chronic disease such as diabetes, while benefiting from the modern revolution in information technology, still has as its basis the caring, compassionate, and understanding relationships between the patient and members of the healthcare team. Unfortunately, current reimbursement systems do not support the establishment or maintenance of these relationships and thus work against efforts to provide optimal care to patients with diabetes.

The major clinical issue in patients with type 2 diabetes, in addition to that of achieving symptomatic control of hyperglycemia, is the enormous risk of cardiovascular disease and the problems arising from microvascular complications. An appreciation of the interrelationships of the various risk factors that lead to coronary heart disease and the benefits of treating these vigorously is growing rapidly. Multiple studies on cholesterol lowering [Scandinavian Simvastatin Survival Study (4S) and Cholesterol and Recurrent Events trial (CARE)] (17,18); blood pressure control [United Kingdom Prospective Diabetes Study (UKPDS) and Hypertension Optimal Treatment (HOT) study] (19,20); and the use of aspirin (21), inhibitors of angiotensin-converting enzyme [Heart Outcomes Prevention Evaluation trial (HOPE)] (22), and β-blockers reveal significant benefits in patients with diabetes. While these randomized controlled clinical trials have been conducted primarily in subjects without diabetes, the subgroups with diabetes also had significant reductions in major cardiovascular events and death. The recent data from the Atherosclerosis Risk in Communities (ARIC) Study showed that the risk for diabetes in patients with hypertension is increased by two and a half. The study also noted that the risk of development of diabetes was not increased by thiazide diuretics but was increased by β-blockers. However, the benefits of the use of β-blockers following myocardial infarction have been validated in the literature, so the risk of developing diabetes should be considered of secondary importance in this group of patients (23).

The treatment plan for patients with diabetes also will be affected by the prevalence of the disease in the population. The prevalence of type 2 diabetes is higher in certain ethnic groups, such as Native Americans (especially the Pima Indians) (24), Hispanic Americans, African Americans, and Asian Americans (25–27). For many of these groups, access to good medical care is affected by factors such as socioeconomic status, insurance coverage, cultural background, language barriers, individual and group health beliefs, educational level, and peer behavior. These factors present special problems that will have to be addressed if these patients are to achieve optimal outcomes.

Diabetes in the older population also is a special issue because of the increase in the prevalence of diabetes with aging, the multiple other conditions being treated in the elderly population, and the risks associated with polypharmacy. There is an urgent need to approach the treatment of diabetes in these patients with enthusiasm and to set appropriate goals for therapy. Treatment must be individualized, and the relationship of risks to benefits must always be carefully evaluated, but age, per se, is not a reason to alter the target goals for glycemic control. Although most elderly patients with diabetes have type 2 disease, many of them have type 1 (insulin-dependent diabetes) disease—not only because type 1 diabetes can present for the first time in the elderly but also because many patients with type 1 diabetes are living long enough to be included in the elderly group. The elderly do not always present with the classical symptoms and signs of hyperglycemia, so the physician must consider this diagnosis, especially in those with neuropathy, nonhealing ulcers, and recurrent infections (28).

Although this chapter will focus on the general approach to the treatment of the patient with diabetes in the outpatient setting, the principles also apply to inpatients. The material presented here is intended as a general overview of the treatment of diabetes; other chapters in this text are devoted to specific issues.

AN INITIAL APPROACH

Once the diagnosis of diabetes has been established, the question of initiating therapy must be addressed. Those patients who present with diabetic ketoacidosis or who are markedly hyperglycemic and symptomatic should be admitted to the hospital for urgent treatment. The need for hospitalization at diagnosis applies primarily to patients with type 1 diabetes, especially children.

At this initial stage, the physician or healthcare professional who is seeing the patient should obtain a detailed history and perform a complete examination with appropriate laboratory testing. The future progression of the patient's care will be affected by a number of factors, including the physician's treatment philosophy, the patient's healthcare beliefs and competence at self-care, and the availability of a team consisting of a dietitian, diabetes educator, exercise physiologist, and, when needed, social workers and psychologists. Unfortunately, not all components of this team may be available in the general office practice; however, most communities do have these resources, and patients should be referred to them, as appropriate, to achieve optimal glucose control.

The approach must consider the "whole person" with diabetes, not just the levels of glycemic control to be achieved or the therapy to be used to accomplish this (i.e., insulin or oral antidiabetic therapies). To this end, a strong, integrated team approach is the one most likely to succeed. Although, as noted above, the complete team may not exist in most cases, the physician and the patient can make considerable progress together, with other components of the team, especially the diabetes educator and dietitian, coming from the community.

The Patient History

A detailed history is the foundation of good diabetes care. Knowledge about the age of the patient and the clinical presentation often help the physician determine whether the patient has type 1 or type 2 diabetes. This is not a laboratory-validated diagnosis but a clinical assessment to assist in choosing the initial treatment. The clinician bases the classification on aspects of the patient's history such as age, body weight, family history, duration of symptoms, and the results of the blood glucose and the HbA_{1c} determinations. Considerable heterogeneity exists, especially in type 2 diabetes, in the clinical presentation as well as in the underlying pathophysiology. Some patients actually may have a slowly progressive form of autoimmune diabetes. These tend to be younger adults and generally require insulin therapy relatively soon. These patients can be diagnosed by measuring certain autoimmune markers in the blood, such as antibodies to insulin and glutamic acid decarboxylase (GAD). The increasing prevalence of type 2 diabetes in adolescents makes it necessary to differentiate type 1 from type 2 diabetes in this group of patients. Another problem is the difficulty in assigning a definite date for the onset of diabetes, particularly for type 2 diabetes, which can be asymptomatic for many years, a determination that has implications concerning the risk for diabetes complications. At the Joslin Clinic, both patients with new-onset diabetes and those seeking consultation for existing disease are mailed a detailed metabolic questionnaire about symptoms, current therapy, family history, exercise patterns, and other medical problems and therapies. Particular attention must be paid to histories of coronary artery disease, peripheral vascular disease, hypertension, and renal disease in the patient and the family. Patients also are asked to keep a record on a dietary assessment sheet or in a food diary for 2 or 3 days, including the times of their meals and the types and quantities of foods eaten. This information helps the dietitian design an appropriate meal plan based on the patient's food preferences and lifestyle. With new information-technology systems, patients can access these questionnaires electronically and enter the information from home. This will avoid mail delays, help get the information in a timely manner, and enhance the patient's visit with the physician.

Physical Examination

The physical examination is a fundamental part of the initial evaluation. Special attention should be paid to the height and weight, body mass index (BMI), blood pressure (lying down and standing up), and vascular status. A careful examination of peripheral pulses and auscultation of carotid and femoral vessels for bruits is extremely important in obtaining a baseline for the future. The neurologic examination must include a careful search for evidence of neuropathy. Not only are muscle strength and reflexes tested, vibration, position sense, and appreciation of application of a 10-g monofilament to the feet must also be assessed. While these clinical methods lack the precision of a detailed laboratory neurologic evaluation, they still permit the clinician to obtain a baseline picture and to obtain further investigations in appropriate patients.

In a study of 189 patients with diabetes and 88 control subjects, Thivolet et al. (29) used a graduated tuning fork to measure the sensitivity of the feet to vibratory sensations and noted that 51% of patients with clinical symptoms of neuropathy in the extremities, 70% of those with absent tendon reflexes, and 75% of those with abnormal nerve-conduction velocities had limited vibration sensation. On the other hand, the study by Dyck et al. (30) revealed the problems present in assessing the epidemiologic data on diabetic neuropathy. Part of the problem is the variety of clinical types of neuropathy and the characterization of neurologic dysfunction. With multiple clinical entities and variable presentation, the best the clinician can do is to look for and document the presence of neuropathy. In a recent study, Perkins et al. (31) reported on the usefulness of four simple tests: 10-g Semmes–Weinstein monofilament examination, superficial pain sensation, vibration testing by the on–off method, and vibration testing by the timed method. They found excellent sensitivity and specificity for each of the tests from the reported operating characteristics. The timed-vibration method took longer to perform than the others, but each of the other tests took less than 10 seconds and should therefore be part of the annual examination for neuropathy. If the history and physical examination are atypical for diabetes, an additional workup should be undertaken and a referral to a neurologist considered.

The physician also should pay special attention to the patient's feet, carefully palpating the dorsalis pedis and posterior tibial, popliteal, and femoral pulses. Skeletal deformities such as hallux valgus, bunions, callouses, and hammertoes must be carefully documented. The combination of vascular disease and neuropathy is the major cause of foot infection and nontraumatic amputation in patients with diabetes.

Finally, a careful funduscopic examination is done, although this should not substitute for an evaluation by an ophthalmologist with experience in diabetic eye disease. Some new methodologies using nonmydriatic digital retinal imaging serve as an excellent screening technique to prioritize the need for formal ophthalmologic evaluation.

Laboratory Studies

The choice of laboratory tests performed is in part determined by the clinical presentation of the patient. If the patient is in a state of diabetic ketoacidosis or is symptomatic from marked hyperglycemia, the degree of hyperglycemia, the acid–base status, electrolytes, and the presence of acetone are urgently assessed. For the nonacute situation, at the patient's first visit, the minimum tests required are a complete urinalysis and determinations of blood glucose and HbA_{1c}. It is now usual to add to these a chemistry panel that includes measurements of lipids, liver and kidney function, and electrolytes and a complete blood count. If possible, the lipid measurements should be done on the patient in the fasting state to obtain an accurate determination of the triglyceride level. It may be necessary for the patient to make a separate visit to the office or laboratory for these tests. In most cases, lipids also are evaluated on the first visit. Total cholesterol, triglycerides, high-density cholesterol, and low-density cholesterol are determined. Lipid studies are an important aspect of diabetes assessment because of the high risk of macrovascular disease, especially in the patient with type 2 diabetes (32).

A test for microalbuminuria also is recommended, since the presence of microproteinuria heralds the future development of renal disease (33,34) and is an independent risk factor for cardiovascular disease. Many different methods are available for determining the presence and degree of albumin excretion, including an albumin-to-creatinine ratio in a spot urine, timed urine collection, and 24-hour urine collection. The latter test also allows the determination of creatinine clearance. The test for albumin-to-creatinine ratio is now widely available and can easily be performed in the office, with the caveat that moderate to intense physical activity may result in a false increase in albumin excretion. It is usually not necessary in clinical practice to measure islet cell antibodies, insulin autoantibodies, or anti-GAD antibodies in patients at the clinical onset of the disease. The presence of anti-GAD antibodies may identify a subgroup of patients with adult-onset diabetes who actually have a slowly evolving form of autoimmune type diabetes [latent autoimmune diabetes of adults (LADA)]. These tests, together with the intravenous glucose tolerance test, are used in research settings to determine which patients are at high risk for developing diabetes (35,36). The routine measurement of insulin levels or C-peptide is not recommended as a routine test in clinical practice. In selected instances, these measurements may indicate the more appropriate selection of therapy. In the older patient or in patients with high blood pressure or a family history of cardiac disease, a baseline electrocardiogram should be performed. If additional cardiovascular risk factors are present or if the patient is planning to begin an exercise program, consideration should be given to performing a cardiac stress test. The physician can order a chest x-ray film and other studies as needed. Patients with type 1 diabetes should also have a thyrotropin level measured on the first visit because of the frequent coexistence of immune-mediated thyroid disease.

EDUCATION

For the patient with a chronic disease, education is a lifelong process and an opportunity to improve self-care techniques and to recognize the onset of complications. Access to printed educational materials and to the services of skilled diabetes nurse educators will help facilitate this process. Access to diabetes educational materials on the Internet is increasing, and providing advice about the most reliable sites for information can be an important part of the educational process. Care must be taken not to overwhelm the patient with a surfeit of information. The onset of diabetes, either type 1 or type 2, is a difficult time emotionally for the patient, and the physician must be a source of encouragement as well as a provider of treatment. The family should participate in the educational process as much as possible. In adults with diabetes, involving the spouse in the educational process can be very rewarding; however, the patient must be encouraged to accept responsibility unless there are mitigating conditions. The initial goals of education are to help the family understand the basic pathophysiology of diabetes and the differences between the insulin-dependent and non–insulin-dependent forms.

Patients with type 1 diabetes and their families learn basic skills necessary for the patient's survival. Such necessary skills include (a) insulin administration; (b) SMBG and testing for urine glucose and ketones; (c) adjusting insulin dosage and food intake for exercise; and (d) sick-day care and prevention of ketoacidosis and treatment of hypoglycemia.

Patients with type 2 diabetes are taught similar skills, although the emphasis is very much on the nutritional program and weight control. It is important for patients to realize that the loss of even small amounts of weight (10 to 20 lb) can be very beneficial for overall glucose control. The ability to self-monitor blood glucose also is important in these patients. Exercise helps obese patients lose weight, and if they request more than a simple exercise prescription, it is appropriate for the physician to refer them to an exercise physiologist. Care should be taken in prescribing vigorous exercise programs to older patients, especially those with diabetic complications such as neuropathy or retinopathy. There is also the issue of coronary disease and silent ischemia. If a question arises about the presence of coronary artery disease and whether exercise can be undertaken with safety, the patient should be referred to a cardiologist for appropriate testing. A study in 1999 by Janand-Delenne et al. (37) of 203 patients with type 1 or type 2 diabetes noted that 20.9% of male patients with type 2 diabetes had silent myocardial ischemia with significant lesions on cardiac catheterization. The authors thus recommended routine screening for men with type 2 diabetes of more than 10 years' duration or even less for those with more than one cardiovascular risk factor. Once the patient is cleared for an exercise program, he or she should exercise three to four times a week for at least 30 minutes for the program to be of any benefit.

Those patients who will be receiving oral hypoglycemic therapy must become knowledgeable about the action of these medications and their adverse effects. They also must understand that many patients will fail to respond to these agents with time and will need insulin therapy. When medication is prescribed, it is essential not only to instruct patients on how to take the pills but also to counsel them on when to stop taking them to avoid potentially serious adverse side effects. This is very important, because the number of new medications for diabetes has increased rapidly and, for many of them, we do not know the long-term effects.

At the initial visit it also is appropriate to discuss briefly the rationale for glucose control and the potential for complications. At this time, the physician's interpretation and understanding of the current literature on the relationship between the control of diabetes and complications and familiarity with the standards of care set by the ADA will be extremely important. If the physician is vague and noncommittal in presenting this issue, the patient may assume that tight control is not necessary. By individualizing therapy and building on a solid foundation of basic skills acquired by the patient, the physician is in a unique position to guide the patient toward improved control.

CLINICAL GOALS

It is evident from the earlier discussion that the type of diabetes influences the form of therapy chosen. In the patient with new-onset diabetes who has acutely decompensated type 1 diabetes or in the patient with previous diagnosed diabetes who is in poor control, the goals will include (a) elimination of ketosis; (b) elimination of symptoms of hyperglycemia such as polydipsia, polyuria, vaginitis, fatigue, and visual blurring; (c) restoration of normal blood chemistry values; (d) regaining of lost weight; and (e) restoration of sense of well-being. At this time, the emphasis for patients with previously diagnosed diabetes is on restoring those behaviors that will improve diabetes control and that will allow them to once again fully participate in their care. Glucose control at this time is directed toward getting patients to monitor their blood glucose, to improve adherence to prescribed medications, to become more confident at administering insulin, and to gather data on the patterns of glucose testing. This information becomes very important when one is working with the patient to plan the changes in insulin dosage and timing that will ensure that the glycemic goals set will be achieved.

Once the initial goals have been met, one can proceed to work on the plan necessary for long-term success. The general aim is the maintenance of health and well-being through control of the disease. It is important not to foster a lifestyle that is completely dominated by diabetes. Patients should control their diabetes and follow their desired lifestyle as much as possible. This is not always easy to accomplish, especially in patients with very unstable or "brittle" type 1 disease. A minority of patients are severely incapacitated, and care must be taken to set realistic goals and promote behavior that is not self-deprecating. For many patients and parents of young children, working with a counselor, psychologist, or psychiatrist can help alleviate feelings of guilt and depression.

As discussed in Chapter 42, for young children the goals are the maintenance of normal growth and development. Again, the lifestyle should be as close to normal as possible, without diabetes becoming the focal point of the family's existence. Ideally, children should be comfortable at school, participate in sports, and socialize with their peers without being made to feel different.

Marrying and having a family is important for young adults with diabetes. Helping women who wish to have children achieve a successful pregnancy is a very important aspect of diabetes care. Unless the physician has considerable experience in this area, it is preferable for the patient to be referred to a multidisciplinary team skilled in managing these high-risk pregnancies. However, all physicians should educate young women with diabetes on appropriate birth control methods and the importance of good glycemic control before conception.

Underlying all these goals is the desire to control the diabetes optimally so that long-term microvascular and macrovascular complications can be minimized. Since there currently is no way to predict who will develop long-term complications, it seems prudent to set a goal of optimal glycemic control, within the limits of safety, for all patients.

Before proceeding with therapy, it is useful for the physician to discuss with patients the different levels of success that may be achieved in the treatment of diabetes. In general, the goals of therapy can be referred to as minimal, average, and intensive. The goals as defined by the ADA (38) follow.

Minimal goals

1. HbA_{1c}, 11% to 13%; or total glycosylated hemoglobin (HbA_1), 13.0% to 15.0%
2. Many SMBG values of higher than 300 mg/dL
3. Tests for urinary glucose almost always positive
4. Intermittent, spontaneous ketonuria

Average goals

1. HbA_{1c}, 8% to 9.0%; or HbA_1, 10% to 11.0%
2. Premeal SMBG of 160 to 200 mg/dL
3. Tests for urinary glucose intermittently positive
4. Rare ketonuria

Intensive goals

1. HBA_{1c}, 6.0% to 7.0%; or HbA_1, 7% to 9%
2. Premeal SMBG of 70 to 120 mg/dL and postmeal SMBG of less than 180 mg/dL
3. Tests for urinary glucose essentially never positive
4. No ketonuria

In the most recent standards of glycemic control (38a), the ADA recommends an HbA_{1c} of less than 7%, a preprandial plasma glucose level of 90 to 130 mg/dL, and a postprandial plasma glucose level of less than 180 mg/dL.

Assessment of the level of diabetes control is best accomplished by measuring biochemical parameters. Clinical indexes such as body weight, frequency of polyuria, polydipsia, number of hypoglycemic reactions, fatigue, and sense of well-being are important clinical parameters but can be misleading about the overall level of control. It is true that patients with very poor control often can be identified easily by their symptoms; however, patients whose fasting glucose levels are 140 to 180 mg/dL and postprandial glucose levels are 180 to 240 mg/dL can feel quite well and present a false clinical picture of satisfactory diabetes control. In the past, daily urinary glucose measurements and random office glucose tests were relied on. However, the accuracy of urine testing can suffer in the presence of a high renal threshold, renal disease, or bladder neuropathy, and these limitations are not eliminated by the use of a double-voided urine specimen. Testing for the presence of ketones is still best accomplished with a urine sample.

During the last two decades, general availability of two innovations has revolutionized our approach to therapy. The first of these was SMBG (39), and the second was the development of reliable assays for glycosylated hemoglobin.

Self-Monitoring of Blood Glucose

Since its development, SMBG has developed into a sophisticated monitoring system. A variety of glucose-monitoring devices are now available that give a digital readout of the blood glucose concentration. The devices continue to be improved, and the time required for the test to be completed is now as short as 5 seconds. In addition, the size of the blood samples required has decreased, and many meters use a direct activation system. Some of the newest meters allow blood sampling both from the finger and from the forearm, thereby reducing the overuse and callousing of the fingers. These devices appear accurate enough for routine use by patients. For convenience, mechanical lancet devices are available for obtaining blood. Some of the newer glucose monitors include computerized memory to record the blood glucose levels, and some can be used in conjunction with more elaborate personal computers. Special machines are available for visually impaired patients. One concern about SMBG is the accuracy of the recordings as compared with those obtained in the laboratories of large clinics or research settings that use more sophisticated instruments. The patient may encounter many problems with SMBG in everyday use, even after receiving careful instruction on the technique by a diabetes nurse educator. One such difficulty involves the patient's ability to obtain a drop of blood, place it accurately on the reagent strip, and time the monitor carefully. Newer monitors that do not require wiping or timing and that allow the use of very small amounts of blood can help minimize these errors. A study performed by Jovanovic-Peterson et al. (40), in which four meter systems were compared, demonstrated the least variance from the control system (a glucose autoanalyzer) with a "no-wipe" system. Use of this system, which eliminated the need for blood removal and timing, greatly decreased the variability in test results.

For SMBG to be effective, its use must be accompanied by an educational program that helps the patient understand the factors affecting any particular blood glucose level and that provides appropriate options for corrections or adjustments. This knowledge is particularly necessary for patients involved in intensive insulin treatment programs.

There has been some discussion about the value of routine SMBG in patients with type 2 diabetes who are using diet or oral agents for control (41). Although these patients rarely will make treatment changes on the basis of information from SMBG, it can reinforce dietary principles and reveal the benefits of exercise and medication. Patients with type 2 diabetes who are receiving insulin should definitely use SMBG. Hypoglycemia occurs both in patients being treated with sulfonylurea drugs and those receiving insulin; in this setting SMBG can confirm a low glucose level and may help the healthcare provider adjust therapy on a more timely basis. The frequency of monitoring can easily be adjusted to the individual patient's needs and circumstances. SMBG is therefore an extremely valuable tool for daily diabetes management. The recent introduction of a subcutaneous continuous glucose-sensing monitor that can obtain a 3-day profile of blood glucose levels (240 readings) can be a very useful tool in selected patients. Such data can be very important in assessing the dose of preprandial insulin, in identifying unrecognized hypoglycemia, and in revealing the dawn effect. Rapid advances in new glucose monitoring systems are expected over the next few years.

Glycosylated Hemoglobin Assays

In the last decade a number of studies on glucose control and diabetic complications have been completed, and all use HbA_{1c} as a surrogate marker for risk. The standards of care of the ADA were revised based on the fasting blood glucose level as well as on the HbA_{1c} from these studies. Currently, laboratories can measure either the total glycosylated hemoglobin or the A_{1c} fraction. The latter is the test used in the large outcome studies. However, the assays have not been standardized, and because commercial laboratories use different methods, the reference ranges vary, making it difficult for the clinician to use the results if they vary constantly. Clinicians should use the same laboratory to measure A_{1c} in the same patient over time.

In normoglycemic subjects, a carbohydrate moiety is attached to a small proportion of hemoglobin A, thus creating what is called *glycosylated* or *glycated* hemoglobin (42). The glycosylated hemoglobin can be separated into three distinct fractions, which are designated A_{1a}, A_{1b}, and A_{1c}. Because of electrophoretic behavior of these minor hemoglobins, they are referred to as *fast hemoglobin*. The A_{1c} fraction is the most reactive site of the *N*-valine terminal of the B-chain, which accounts for 60% of the bound glucose.

In conditions of sustained hyperglycemia, such as in diabetes mellitus, the proportion of hemoglobin that is glycosylated increases substantially (43). This glycosylation is the result of posttranslational modification of hemoglobin A molecules; the binding of glucose is a nonenzymatic process that occurs continuously during the life of the red blood cell. Thus, the amount of glycosylated hemoglobin reflects the glycemic control of a patient during the 6- to 8-week period before the blood sample was obtained, given the average life span of a red blood cell of 120 days (44). The amount of glycosylated hemoglobin correlates well with fasting and postprandial blood glucose levels. Currently, the glycosylated hemoglobin can be measured by ion-exchange high-performance liquid chromatography (HPLC), affinity chromatography, and immunologic methods. In the DCCT study, an ion-exchange HPLC method was used, and data from this study have been adopted as the reference standard for assessing glucose control.

A recent study by Schnedl et al. (45) noted that there are more than 700 known variants of hemoglobin that may affect the currently used assays for glycosylated hemoglobin. They evaluated the effect of the following hemoglobin variants: Hb Graz, Hb Sherwood Forest, Hb O Padova, Hb D, and Hb S. They noted that the HPLC boronate affinity assay lacked the resolution necessary to separate out the variants and that the immunoassays resulted in falsely low levels of Hb Graz. It is therefore recommended that laboratories establish and validate assays for the local population to make allowances for any hemoglobin variants. The glycosylated hemoglobin assay is presently one of the most widely applied tests in the management of diabetes. It is useful for the assessment of glycemic control in patients with type 1 diabetes and in patients with type 2 diabetes.

Glycosylated hemoglobin values must be assessed with caution in patients with unstable diabetes. Levels of blood sugar in these patients fluctuate from very low to very high on an almost daily basis, a situation that can lead to unwanted symptoms of hyperglycemia and dangerous episodes of hypoglycemia (38). A study by Brewer et al. (46) suggested that using a pie-shaped graph of SMBG data with defined target-range parameters can aid patients and their families attain the desired HbA_{1c} goals. The authors set the target range for SMBG values for different times of the day and then determined the number of values that needed to be within or above that range to achieve the desired HbA_{1c}. For young adults 17 to 35 years of age using a target range of 70 to 150 mg/dl, at least 38% of the values needed to be in the target range and no more than 48% above the range to achieve an HbA_{1c} of less than 8%. The assay of glycosylated hemoglobin should be done every 3 to 4 months, with the goal of adjusting therapy to obtain the lowest value that does not place patients at undue risk for hypoglycemic reactions. In patients who have reached a goal and are very stable, the test can be done every 6 months. However, it is important that the information obtained from the test be communicated to the patient to use to improve adherence to the prescribed treatment plan. At present the HbA_{1c} is the best surrogate marker we have for setting goals of treatment. Efforts are under way to standardize the procedure for measuring glycosylated hemoglobin. Ultimately, this would result in a certification process for manufacturers and thus ensure standardization of the results used by the healthcare professional in setting glucose control goals for their patients.

INITIATION OF THERAPY

For most adult patients, initiation of treatment is safely accomplished in the outpatient setting. Very young children and patients with diabetic ketoacidosis or severe, uncontrolled diabetes usually require hospitalization. Although the decision to use insulin usually is made by the physician, it is extremely important to explain the rationale to patients and to include them in the decision process. Many have an understandable fear of injections and often regard this therapy as an indication of the presence of a more severe form of the disease. Insulin therapy needs to be presented as any other treatment option, and patients should be made to understand that one, two, or three injections per day may be needed, depending on their response. The physician also should review the issue of control and complications and develop initial goals with the patient.

At the Joslin Clinic, the decision to start insulin therapy is followed by a referral to a diabetes nurse educator, who will instruct the patient or a family member on the techniques that will be required. Patients will administer their first injection at this time under supervision. This also provides an opportunity to teach patients about the types of insulin available and their characteristic peaks and durations of activity and to review strategies for dealing with hypoglycemia and hyperglycemia. The present availability of very-fast-acting human insulin analogues, as well as a nonpeaking basal human insulin analogue, has increased the need to emphasize to patients the importance of coordinating the timing of meals and insulin injection according to the type of insulin used. The techniques for mixing regular with intermediate-acting insulins may be reviewed if the physician believes that these are appropriate insulin formulations for a specific patient. Premixed insulin [70% neutral protamine Hagedorn (NPH) and 30% crystalline zinc insulin or 75% neutral protamine lispro (NPL) and 25% lispro] can be used initially in patients who may not be able to master the mixing of insulins. This simplifies the treatment program, especially when patients have problems understanding and performing the mixing maneuvers. Furthermore, these premixed insulins are now available in prefilled syringes with a simple dose-dialing mechanism. In many cases, limitations in mixing insulins are due to problems such as cataracts, degenerative joint disease, previous cerebrovascular accidents, or severe neuropathy.

Most new patients who require insulin will receive human insulin of recombinant DNA origin. Allergy and lipoatrophy are uncommon with human insulins. Beef insulin and mixed beef–pork insulin should be avoided unless there are specific indications for their use or if human insulin is not available. These latter insulins are now being phased out in the United States. Patients also are instructed on SMBG at this time and are asked to maintain close contact with the nurse educator, who in turn reviews adjustments in insulin therapy and the patient's progress with the physician. In most patients, the blood glucose levels can be expected to be brought under control over a 4- to 6-week period. The patient often is seen several times within this interval so that the physician can monitor progress, modify therapy, and review any interim problems or concerns.

Most patients are not started on an intensive management program at this time, as it is necessary to allow the patient to adjust to the emotional and lifestyle changes that follow a diagnosis of diabetes. Intensive therapy with multiple daily injections or continuous subcutaneous insulin infusion is used for women who plan a pregnancy, patients who cannot control their glucose levels by conventional therapies, or patients whose lifestyles or complications, especially hypoglycemic unawareness, demand the greater flexibility and control that intensive programs offer (47).

Patients with known diabetes in poor control or with complications of diabetes will undergo a similar evaluation and physical examination. Attention is focused here on the patient's general approach to the disease, with a particular focus on the patient's acceptance of the disease and its treatment requirements. The Joslin Clinic offers an outpatient program called "DO IT," in which patients are seen by a team over a period of three and a half days. This program allows a comprehensive review of the patient's problems and for these problems to be addressed on an individual basis. This program has become necessary because, with the changing healthcare-insurance environment, the old inpatient education programs are no longer available in many institutions. Many patients have an overwhelming fear of hypoglycemia. Some will deliberately avoid using rapid-acting insulin or will omit their evening injections, which predictably results in hyperglycemia. Others will overcompensate and treat any symptoms as a sign of potential hypoglycemia and some will start to monitor glucose levels with excessive frequency in an effort to discover lower values in the hope of avoiding severe hypoglycemic reactions. It is important to review the nutritional programs, exercise habits, alcohol intake, and psychosocial status of these patients. Even some patients with diabetes of long duration do not appropriately time their insulin injection to their ingestion of calories. Also, some patients make the mistake of regularly injecting insulin at hypertrophied sites, with resultant unpredictability of insulin absorption. In general, no acute changes in the insulin program are made at an initial visit, but the patient frequently is asked to monitor blood glucose three to four times a day for the next month, with the focus being on the nutritional program. Changes of insulin therapy are made by telephone or at future visits. Patients with major psychological problems are referred to a psychologist or psychiatrist. Unless these issues are addressed, diabetes control will continue to be a problem.

Some patients will require hospitalization. At the hospital, the focus of the treatment will be education and close monitoring to identify potential problems such as nocturnal hypoglycemia with rebound hyperglycemia, hypoglycemic unawareness, or inherently unstable diabetes. Even though the present economic climate is making it more difficult to hospitalize these patients, there is no way of satisfactorily addressing some of these problems in the outpatient setting. If the patient is hospitalized, it is important to attempt to reproduce the patient's normal lifestyle as closely as possible, including the timing and content of meals and exercise. Complicated diabetes requires individualized therapy that is both complex and time-consuming. For appropriate individualized care to be provided for patients, specific issues that may interfere with optimal control must be identified and addressed carefully and sympathetically. Solutions that offer the patient the greatest opportunity for a successful outcome should be sought in consultation with the patient and the patient's family. Very often individuals with unstable glucose control will need to have their glycemic goals changed to avoid dangerous hypoglycemia, despite earlier encouragement to maintain "tight control."

Patients with type 2 diabetes may require insulin when they are first seen, particularly if they are very symptomatic and have lost weight. In some instances, insulin can be discontinued when control is achieved and adherence to diet has taken effect (48). However, many patients will require insulin indefinitely; this becomes obvious when they become ketonuric and hyperglycemic with a reduction in insulin dose.

The basis of therapy in type 2 diabetes is to promote lifestyle changes with a nutritional program designed to reduce calories and encourage weight loss. An exercise program is an essential part of any effort to lose weight. Glycemic control can often be improved by caloric restriction alone, even before significant weight loss occurs. At the same time, it is also important to pay close attention to the risk factors for macrovascular disease. This means controlling lipids and hypertension and counseling on smoking cessation and the value of glucose control. Patients with type 2 diabetes also are taught SMBG, and the frequency of testing is individualized. SMBG is always the preferred method of glucose monitoring, with urine testing being used only in special situations.

The decision to use oral antidiabetic therapies is generally made after a trial of nutritional therapy unless the initial random glucose level is higher than 350 mg/dL. In general, a 4- to 12-week trial period of diet and lifestyle modification is reasonable, and if the fasting glucose concentration remains higher than 140 mg/dL or postprandial values are higher than 200 mg/dL, treatment with oral pharmacologic agents is initiated. Much has changed in this area since the last edition of this textbook. The last 5 years have seen the introduction not only of new sulfonylureas but also of new nonsulfonylurea insulin secretagogues. The latter drugs are often more rapid acting than the sulfonylureas and may be very well suited in treating postprandial hyperglycemia. The biguanide metformin, which has been available in many parts of the world for decades, was introduced into the United States relatively recently. The α-glucosidase inhibitors offer another option for controlling blood glucose levels, especially after meals. A totally new class of oral medication, the thiozolidinediones, also is available. Drugs in this class are novel insulin-sensitizing agents that work through specific nuclear receptors.

The physician now is presented with a number of choices and tries clinically to match the presumed underlying abnormality in the individual patient to a particular pharmacologic approach. Because type 2 diabetes involves a dual defect, the early use of combination therapy may be very advantageous. Customarily, the patient will start with a sulfonylurea or an insulin sensitizer. It is very important for the healthcare provider to be aware of the contraindications to the use of each drug as well the monitoring requirements to avoid serious adverse reactions. Failure of control with a single drug will result in the use of a combination regimen that can take advantage of the different mechanisms of action. Substitution of drugs from one class to another is rarely successful; however, the addition of a drug from another class often improves glucose control.

The recently completed UKPDS demonstrated that many of the oral monotherapies will fail to control the blood glucose levels for longer than 5 years (3). Much of the failure is due to the progression of the β-cell defect, with continued reduction in insulin production. Some patients who fail to obtain control with the maximal dose of oral medication may benefit from the combined use of insulin and oral medication. Usually a bedtime dose of intermediate-acting insulin or a basal insulin analogue (48a) is given, with the oral drug being continued (49). If the patient has high blood glucose levels following supper, a mixture of a short-acting and an intermediate-acting insulin can be given before supper. It is often useful to use a premixed insulin (70/30 human insulin mixture or 75/25 lispro mixture) in patients who have difficulty with mixing or adjusting insulin dose. Several studies of combination therapy have been completed. Generally, patients who have residual endogenous insulin secretion respond best, although patients' responses vary greatly and treatments must be individualized (48).

For every patient, diabetes management must include a careful nutritional assessment and the implementation of a *realistic* dietary program. The goal of nutritional therapy in type 2 diabetes is the control of blood glucose levels, normalization of lipid levels, and maintenance of ideal body weight. For young children with diabetes, the goal should be the maintenance of normal growth and development, as well as of a reasonable body weight.

In general, the dietitian will prescribe a meal plan based on the individual patient's type of diabetes and mode of treatment. Patients receiving exogenous insulin must pay particular attention to the timing of meals and snacks to prevent undue fluctuation of the blood glucose levels. The meal plan is individualized with respect to weight goals, personal food preferences, and exercise habits. Many obese patients with diabetes may require special weight-loss programs and behavior modification therapy to maintain weight loss. Unfortunately, most patients do not succeed in their efforts to lose weight and to maintain weight loss for prolonged periods.

Diet therapy often is referred to as the cornerstone of treatment, particularly in type 2 diabetes. For the patient to benefit maximally from this aspect of patient management, a team approach, which includes the services of a skilled registered dietitian, is recommended. Although these skills are not always available in physician's offices, they are offered in local community hospitals and by some dietitians in private practice. A detailed discussion on this component of treatment is presented in Chapter 36 on nutritional therapy.

Exercise plays an important role in diabetes management. For patients with type 1 diabetes, exercise should not be thought of as the major way of improving glucose control but rather as part of the overall approach to maintaining a healthy lifestyle. Physical activity can benefit the patient by lowering the blood glucose level if overall control is good. However, care must be taken to instruct the patient on the possibility of physical exercise provoking hypoglycemic reactions or worsening control when undertaken in the presence of higher blood glucose levels and ketonuria. Furthermore, patients with the complications of retinopathy and neuropathy can place themselves in jeopardy with excessive exercise.

In general, patients who are free of complications can engage in any type of exercise. Certain activities, such as scuba diving, have to be assessed in light of the certification requirements issued by appropriate organizations. Patients often may benefit from a consultation with an exercise physiologist. In patients with type 2 diabetes, an individualized exercise program should be part of the overall treatment plan. Exercise helps promote weight loss, optimize glycemic control, and reduce cardiovascular risk. These patients need to be screened for early neuropathy or peripheral vascular disease before they start an exercise program. Silent ischemia is more common in patients with diabetes than in the general population, and appropriate patients should have a stress test before starting the exercise program. Routine screening of men with type 2 diabetes of longer than 10 years' duration or less if they have more than one cardiovascular risk factor is recommended because of the high prevalence of myocardial ischemia with significant lesions among men with type 2 diabetes (37). The program should be done three to four times a week to be effective, with appropriate warm-ups, setting target exercise levels with monitoring of pulse rate and cooling-down time. A further discussion of this important area appears in the editorial by Nesto (50) in the issue of *Diabetes Care* that published the above study [reference (37)].

FOLLOW-UP

A critical part of diabetes management is regular follow-up of patients. This is based on the goals established with the patient in the initial management plan. At each visit thereafter, the patient's progress is reviewed and ongoing problems are addressed. The frequency of visits depends on the individual patient, type of diabetes, goals of control, and other medical conditions. Patients starting insulin therapy need to be seen frequently initially, but once their condition has stabilized, they can be seen three to four times a year. In addition, patients are encouraged to maintain telephone contact with the other team members. Some patients with type 2 diabetes need to be seen only every 6 months.

As part of this follow-up process, an interim history is obtained, results of glucose monitoring are reviewed, and new problems or illnesses that affect diabetes control are addressed.

A comprehensive physical examination is done annually. At interim visits, previously abnormal findings are reevaluated and height, weight, and blood pressure are determined. For younger patients, an assessment of sexual maturation should be done. A complete, dilated eye examination by an ophthalmologist should be performed annually in all patients older than 30 years and in patients 12 to 30 years old who have had diabetes for more than 5 years.

A test for glycosylated hemoglobin should be done at least quarterly in patients with type 1 diabetes and semiannually in those with type 2 diabetes. The patient with adult-onset diabetes also may benefit from having either a fasting or postprandial glucose level checked as a means of judging overall glycemic control. A determination of fasting levels of triglycerides, cholesterol, and high-density lipoprotein (HDL) cholesterol should be performed annually and more often in patients with dyslipidemia. Urinalysis done at least yearly is useful. After 5 years of diabetes, patients should be tested for microalbuminuria yearly. If proteinuria is present, the patient's creatinine and blood urea nitrogen levels should be closely monitored; in addition, aggressive antihypertensive therapy and protein restriction should be considered.

At each visit the overall management plan, including the nutritional program and the exercise plan, is reviewed and modified as required. In addition, the overall emotional status of the patient is reviewed. This type of comprehensive care is extremely important for patients with a chronic, life-long disease such as diabetes. This chapter has reviewed the general principles of management of diabetes. Many of the details will be found in other chapters in this textbook. Since the last edition there have been many important advances in the understanding of the pathophysiology and treatment of diabetes. New diagnostic criteria have been developed, and new goals of treatment have been defined. Many studies demonstrating the value not only of glucose control but also of risk factor reduction and cardiovascular disease have been published and incorporated into the routine approach to diabetes management. In addition, therapeutic choices have increased greatly, and therapy can now be based on the underlying pathophysiologic mechanisms of disease. The primary goal in treating patients with diabetes is to help them avoid short-term problems and long-term complications. A recent study of adults with type 1 or type 2 diabetes investigated cognitive representations of illness, self-regulation of diabetes, quality-of-life, and behavioral factors. The authors found that individuals' understanding of diabetes and their perceptions of control over the disease were the most important predictors of outcome (51). This reinforces the need to continue to provide ongoing self-education for patients and to provide them with the evidence, now available, that control of diabetes is possible and that complications can be avoided.

To the practicing physician, diabetes offers the challenge of providing optimal patient care at every visit. It allows the physician the opportunity and privilege to practice not only the science but also the art of medicine.

REFERENCES

1. The effect of intensive treatment of diabetes on the development and progression of long-term complications in insulin dependent diabetes mellitus. Diabetes Control and Complications Trial Research Group. *N Engl J Med* 1993;329:977–986.
2. Ohkubo Y, Kishikawa H, Arak E, et al. Intensive insulin therapy prevents the progression of diabetic microvascular complications in Japanese patients with non insulin dependent diabetes mellitus: a randomized prospective 6-year study. *Diabetes Res Clin Pract* 1995;28:103–117.
3. Intensive blood glucose control with sulfonylureas or insulin compared with conventional treatment and the risk of complications in patients with type 2 diabetes (UKPDS 33): UK Prospective Diabetes Study (UKPDS) Group. *Lancet* 1998;352:837–853.
4. Shichiri M, Ohkubo Y, Kishikawa H, et al. Long term results of the Kumamoto study in optimal diabetes control in type 2 diabetic patients. *Diabetes Care* 2000;23[Suppl 2]:B21–B29.
5. Javitt JC, Chiang Y. Economic impact of diabetes. In: National Diabetes Data Group, eds. *Diabetes in America*. Bethesda, MD: National Institute of Diabetes and Kidney Diseases, 1995:601–611; NIH publication 95-1468.
6. Yudkin JS. Insulin for the world's poorest nations. *Lancet* 2000;355:919–921.
7. American Diabetes Association. Report of the Expert Committee of the Diagnosis and Classification of Diabetes Mellitus. *Diabetes Care* 2000;23[Suppl 1]: S4–S19.
8. McCance DR, Hanson RL, Charles MA, et al. Comparison of tests for glycated hemoglobin and fasting and two hour plasma glucose concentrations as diagnostic methods for diabetes. *BMJ* 1994;308:1323–1328.
9. Engelgau MM, Thompson TJ, Herman WH, et al. Comparison of fasting and 2-hour glucose and HbA_{1c} levels for diagnosing diabetes: diagnostic criteria and performance revisited. *Diabetes Care* 1997;20:785–791.
10. Alberti KGGM. The clinical implications of impaired glucose tolerance. *Diabet Med* 1996;13:927–937.
11. Glucose tolerance and mortality: comparison of WHO and American Diabetes Association diagnostic criteria. The Decode Study group. European Diabetes Epidemiology Group. Diabetes Epidemiology: collaborative analysis of diabetes criteria in Europe. *Lancet* 1999;354:617–621.
12. Levitt NS, Unwin NC, Bradshaw D, et al. Application of the new ADA criteria for the diagnosis of diabetes to populations studies in sub-Saharan Africa. *Diabet Med* 2000;17:381–385.
13. Shaw JE, Zimmet PZ, McCarty D, et al. Type 2 diabetes worldwide according to the new classification and criteria. *Diabetes Care* 2000;23[Suppl 2]:B5–B10.

14. Shapiro JAM, Lakey JRT, Ryan EA, et al. Islet transplantation in seven patients with type 1 diabetes mellitus using a glucocorticoid-free immunosuppressive regimen. *N Engl J Med* 2000;343:230–238.
15. Epidemiology of Diabetes Interventions and Complications (EDIC). Design, implementation, and preliminary results of a long-term follow-up of the Diabetes Control and Complications Trial cohort. *Diabetes Care* 1999;22:99–111.
16. American Diabetes Association. Standards of medical care for patients with diabetes mellitus. *Diabetes Care* 2000;23[Suppl 1]:S32–S42.
17. Randomised trial of cholesterol lowering in 4444 patients with coronary heart disease: the Scandinavian Survival Study (4S). *Lancet* 1994;344:1383–1389.
18. Sacks FM, Pfeffer MA, Lemuel A. The effect of pravastatin on coronary events after myocardial infarction in patients with average cholesterol levels. *N Engl J Med* 1996;335:1001–1009.
19. Tight blood pressure control and the risk of macrovascular and microvascular complications in type 2 diabetes (UKPDS 35): UK Prospective Diabetes Study Group. *BMJ* 1998;317:703–713.
20. Hansson L, Zanchetti A, Carruthers SG, et al. Effects of intensive blood pressure lowering and low-dose aspirin in patients with hypertension: principal results of the Hypertension Optimal Treatment (HOT) randomized trial: HOT Study Group. *Lancet* 1998;351:1755–1762.
21. Collaborative overview of randomised trials of antiplatelet therapy-1: prevention of death, myocardial infarction, and stroke by prolonged antiplatelet therapy in various categories of patients. Antiplatelet Trialists' Collaboration. *BMJ* 1994;308:81–106.
22. Effects of ramipril on cardiovascular and microvascular outcomes in people with diabetes mellitus: results of the HOPE Study and MICR-HOPE Substudy: Heart Outcomes Prevention Evaluation Study Investigators. *Lancet* 2000;355:253–259.
23. Gress TW, Nieto FJ, Shahar E, et al. Hypertension and antihypertensive therapy as risk factors for type 2 diabetes mellitus. *N Engl J Med* 2000;342:905–912.
24. Knowler WC, Pettitt DJ, Savage PJ, et al. Diabetes incidence in Pima Indians: contribution of obesity and paternal diabetes. *Am J Epidemiol* 1981;113:114–156.
25. Diehl AK, Stern MP. Special health problems of Mexican-Americans: obesity, gall bladder disease, diabetes mellitus and cardiovascular disease. *Adv Intern Med* 1989;34:13–56.
26. Fujimoto WF. Background and recruitment data for the US Diabetes Prevention Program. *Diabetes Care* 2000;23[Suppl 2]:B11–B13.
27. Kenny SJ, Aubert RE, Geiss LS. Prevalence and incidence of non-insulin-dependent diabetes. In: Harris MI, Cowie CC, Stern MJ, eds. *Diabetes in America,* 2nd ed. Bethesda, MD: National Institute of Diabetes and Kidney Diseases, 1995: 47–67; NIH publication 95-1468.
28. Minaker KL. What diabetologists should know about elderly patients. *Diabetes Care* 1990;13[Suppl 2]:34–46.
29. Thivolet C, el Farkh J, Petiot A, et al. Measuring vibration sensations with a graduated tuning fork: a simple and reliable means to detect diabetic patients at risk for neuropathic foot ulceration. *Diabetes Care* 1990;13:1077–1080.
30. Dyck PJ, Melton LJ 3rd, O'Brien PC, et al. Approaches to improve epidemiological studies of diabetic neuropathy: insights form the Rochester Diabetic Neuropathy Study. *Diabetes* 1997;46[Suppl 2]:S5–S8.
31. Perkins BA, Olaleye D, Zinman B, et al. Simple screening tests for peripheral neuropathy in the diabetes clinic. *Diabetes Care* 2001;24:250–256.
32. Haffner SM, Lehto S, Ronnemaa T, et al. Mortality from coronary heart disease in subjects with type 2 diabetes and in non-diabetic subjects with and without prior myocardial infarction. *N Engl J Med* 1998;339:229–234.
33. Mogensen CE. Prediction of clinical diabetic nephropathy in IDDM patients: alternatives to microalbuminuria? *Diabetes* 1990;39:761–767.
34. Mogensen CE. Microalbuminuria predicts clinical proteinuria and early mortality in maturity-onset diabetes. *N Engl J Med* 1984;310:356–360.
35. Ziegler AG, Ziegler R, Vardi P, et al. Life-table analysis of progression to diabetes of anti-insulin autoantibody-positive relatives of individuals with type I diabetes. *Diabetes* 1989;38:1320–1325.
36. Krischer JP, Schatz D, Riley WJ, et al. Insulin and islet cell autoantibodies as time-dependent covariates in the development of insulin dependent diabetes. *J Clin Endocrinol Metab* 1993;77:743–479.
37. Janand-Delenne B, Savin B, Habib G, Bory M, et al. Silent myocardial ischemia in patients with diabetes: who to screen. *Diabetes Care* 1999;22: 1396–1400.
38. *Physician's guide to insulin-dependent (type 1) diabetes: diagnosis and treatment.* Alexandria, VA: American Diabetes Association, 1988:18.
38a. American Diabetes Association. Standards of medical care in diabetes. *Diabetes Care* 2004;[Suppl 1]:S19.
39. American Diabetes Association. Tests of glycemia in diabetes. *Diabetes Care* 2000; 23[Suppl 1]:560–582.
40. Jovanovic-Peterson L, Peterson CM, Dudley JD, et al. Identifying sources of error in self monitoring blood glucose. *Diabetes Care* 1988;11:791–794.
41. Allen BT, Delong ER, Feusser JR. Impact of glucose self monitoring on non insulin treated patients with type II diabetes mellitus: randomized controlled trial comparing blood and urine testing. *Diabetes Care* 1990;13:1044–1050.
42. Bunn HF, Haney DN, Gabbay KH, et al. Further identification of the nature and linkage of the carbohydrate in hemoglobin A_{1c}. *Biochem Biophys Res Comm* 1975;67:103–109.
43. Rahbar S. An abnormal hemoglobin in red cells of diabetics. *Clin Chim Acta* 1968;22: 296–298.
44. Koenig RJ, Peterson CM, Jones RL. Correlation of glucose regulation and hemoglobin A_{1c} in diabetes mellitus. *N Engl J Med* 1976;295:417–420.
45. Schnedl WJ, Krause R, Halwach-Baumann G, et al. Evaluation of HbA_{1c} determination methods in patients with hemoglobinopathies. *Diabetes Care* 2000;23:339–344.
46. Brewer W, Chase HP, Owen S, et al. Slicing the pie. Correlating HbA_{1c} values with average glucose values in a pie-chart form. *Diabetes Care* 1998;21:209–212.
47. American Diabetes Association. Continuous subcutaneous insulin infusion. *Diabetes Care* 2000;23[Suppl 1]:S90.
48. Genuth S. Insulin use in NIDDM. *Diabetes Care* 1990;13:1240–1264.
48a. Riddle MC, Rosenstock J, Gerich J, on behalf of the insulin glargine 2002 study investigators. Randomized addition of glargine or human NPH insulin to oral therapy of type 2 diabetic patients. *Diabetes Care* 2003;26:3080–3086.
49. Riddle MC. Evening insulin. *Diabetes Care* 1991;13:676–686.
50. Nesto RW. Screening for asymptomatic coronary disease in diabetes. *Diabetes Care* 1999;22:1393–1395.
51. Watkins K, Connell CM, Fitzgerald JT, et al. Effect of adults' self-regulation of diabetes on quality-of-life outcomes. *Diabetes Care* 2000;23:1511–1515.

CHAPTER 35
Education in the Treatment of Diabetes

Richard S. Beaser, Katie Weinger, and Lisa M. Bolduc-Bissell

> This building given by thousands of patients and their friends provides an opportunity for many to control their diabetes by methods of teaching hitherto available to the privileged few.

Chiseled in stone on the front of the Joslin Clinic Building, erected in 1955, the above inscription reflected Elliott P. Joslin's conviction that education was not just a part of diabetes treatment, it was the treatment. Dr. Joslin's concern about educating both patients with diabetes and their families began more than 100 years ago, when such instruction was considered by many to be a luxury. Over the last two decades, the importance of education has become more widely recognized. As the World Health Organization commented in 1980, "Education is a cornerstone of diabetic therapy and vital to the integration of the diabetic into society" (1).

This growing recognition of the vital role of education in the treatment of diabetes led to the development and periodic updating of the National Standards for Diabetes Education by the National Diabetes Advisory Board in 1983 (2–4). This was followed by the development of a recognition program for diabetes education by the American Diabetes Association (ADA) (5) and of a certification program for diabetes educators by the American Association of Diabetes Educators (6) now administered by a separate organization, the National Certification Board for Diabetes Educators.

Progress in making educational programs available to everyone with diabetes has been slowed by the reluctance of third-party payers to reimburse for educational services in the United States (7). This is now changing. In 2001, the Center for Medicare and Medicaid Services (CMS) began paying for Medicare patients to attend group diabetes education programs and for medical nutrition therapy visits. Many private insurers followed suit. However, diabetes education programs are still at risk, with many closing their doors because of poor reimbursement. One nationwide study found that more than 60% of people with diabetes have received little or no diabetes education (8,9). Unfortunately, little evidence suggests that this is changing. Despite the obstacles, however, healthcare professionals who treat people with diabetes continue their commitment to patient education through the development of new programs and research into more effective methods of teaching the principles and practice of diabetes self-care.

WHY IS SELF-MANAGEMENT EDUCATION IMPORTANT IN THE TREATMENT OF DIABETES?

The importance of improved glycemic control in delaying the onset and progression of serious microvascular complications is now clear (10,11). Treatment of diabetes leading to improved control is a 24-hour-a-day activity and often includes important changes in lifestyle, most of which persons with diabetes must provide for themselves on a daily basis. These efforts require careful balancing of various lifestyle functions and activities that are integral parts of the daily routine. Thus, the goal of diabetes self-management education is not simply to increase knowledge about diabetes, but rather to support individuals with diabetes and their families in their efforts to incorporate diabetes treatment into their lifestyles. Of course, the more that people with diabetes understand how to make these required changes and what the rationale is behind them, the more successful they will be in their diabetes self-management.

Diabetes self-management education provides many benefits. Education allows people with diabetes to take control of their condition, integrating the daily routines of self-monitoring and discipline into their lifestyle rather than permitting this condition to overwhelm them and control their lives. Education in diabetes self-management trains people to take the necessary actions to improve their metabolic control, which helps maintain health and well-being and reduces the risk of diabetic complications. The well-educated person with diabetes may also decrease the costs related to the condition—both the direct cost of medical care and the indirect costs related to lost income or productivity (12).

Diabetes education is both an art and a fledging science. Only within these past 20 years has research begun to examine the role and effectiveness of education in diabetes self-management, and future research is needed to further evaluate and clarify optimal methods for this educational process (4). In addition, in this litigious age, as the value of education gains credence, the provision of proper education to people with diabetes by a healthcare provider may help reduce the risk of malpractice suits.

The evolution of the scientific component of diabetes education has traveled a long and somewhat bumpy road. Initial studies examining diabetes education were difficult to design, perform, and evaluate, and when they were completed, their validity was often the subject of controversy among healthcare professionals. One reason for this disagreement was the assumption by researchers studying diabetes education that it was an integral component of care. Thus, the usual study design contrasted intensive education with less-intensive education rather than with no education or a "placebo" form of education.

Some small studies comparing these two forms of education showed no differences in glycemic control between groups. For example, a trial comparing minimal versus intensive education showed similar improvement in the two groups (13). Good control was related to the duration of school education, absence of anxiety, and quality of control and degree of self-confidence upon entry into the study. A similar study, with admitted socioeconomic bias affecting some of these factors, showed that education led to improvements in knowledge and behavior but not in improvements in metabolic control (14). However, during the last two decades, many randomized clinical trials and smaller studies have examined the efficacy of diabetes education (4), and several well-done meta-analyses (15–19) that evaluated the quality of education summarized the results of research in diabetes education. These meta-analyses, along with more recent trials (20–24), provide convincing evidence that diabetes education is effective in supporting patients' efforts to improve and/or maintain physiologic and quality-of-life outcomes.

Currently, research in diabetes education has moved beyond the question of whether it is important and is beginning to focus on the science of education, addressing questions that clarify educational outcomes, determine which groups of patients respond best to which form of education, and evaluate which are the most efficient and cost-effective methods of providing education (25–28). Diabetes education already encompasses the family and social support; researchers are now beginning to consider public-health aspects of diabetes education at the community and possibly the national level (29).

Education Improves Well-Being and Quality of Life

People with diabetes must make what some perceive as being overwhelming lifestyle changes, yet their failure to accept these changes may result in inadequate diabetes control. Emotions related to the psychological burden of diabetes, such as anxiety, depression, and poor self-confidence, have been shown to be associated with poor control (13, 30–33). Thus, a properly designed education program not only should present facts but also should address the emotional responses to diabetes.

Education improves self-care practices (16,17,22,34) but a mere increase in knowledge and skills does not guarantee an improvement in metabolic parameters (14). Several psychological factors, having been implicated as barriers to improved glycemic control, play an important role in translation of knowledge and skills into the desired metabolic results. These factors include emotion-based coping styles (35,36), diabetes-related emotional distress (33), and lack of readiness to change (37). For individuals to be willing and able to make all the necessary lifestyle changes, they must have knowledge and skills *plus* a positive emotional outlook about their diabetes, believing that the changes they make will lead to better health.

An educational program that demonstrably improves parameters of emotional well-being in addition to addressing self-care practices has been shown to lead to improved metabolic control that was sustained over 6 months (38,39). The authors of these studies suggested that emotional well-being itself may contribute to improved self-care (38). Others contend that, for many patients, education about diabetes and self-care alone enhances emotional well-being (40–42), which further boosts self-care ability. In the first randomized controlled trial to demonstrate an additive effect of psychological intervention on glycemic control, Grey and her colleagues (43,44) demonstrated that adolescents who received training in coping skills along with methods of intensive diabetes treatment improved glycemic control and self-care behaviors more than did adolescents who received only intensive treatment instruction. However, whether emotional well-being leads to improvement in self-care or vice versa has not been clearly determined. More research is needed to clarify the associations among education, improved self-care, and improved emotional outlook.

Education Improves Self-Care Management

Even after one accepts that emotional well-being is a crucial component of the educational intervention, the complexity of the diabetes treatment regimen itself often leads to confusion and misunderstanding that interferes with the ability to manage one's diabetes. Diabetes education can play an important role in clarifying the treatment regimen, reinforcing the skills necessary to successfully manage diabetes, and supporting efforts to integrate self-management behaviors into one's life. Several meta-analyses and clinical trials examining the effects of diabetes education found that education leads to improved self-care behaviors as well as to improved knowledge, and metabolic and psychological outcomes (15–17,19,22,34,38,45). Rubin and his colleagues (45) noted a differential effect among self-care behaviors: behaviors requiring changes in lifestyle such as in diet and exercise were more difficult to maintain over time than were less-demanding behaviors such as self-monitoring of blood glucose (SMBG).

Education Improves Metabolic Control

The Diabetes Control and Complications Trial (DCCT) and the United Kingdom Prospective Diabetes Study (UKPDS) established the principle that improvement in glycemic control is beneficial and that maintaining glucose levels as near to normal as possible results in reduction in the risk of development and progression of serious microvascular complications. The importance of education to the training of patients with diabetes about their treatment and to supporting their self-management efforts to improve their glycemic control became apparent early during the 9-year course of the DCCT (46,47). Moreover, the importance of a multidisciplinary team consisting of at least one healthcare practitioner/educator such as a registered nurse or nutritionist was definitively documented (46–48). The roles of other team members, such as the podiatrist, psychologist, ophthalmologist, pharmacist, exercise physiologist, among others, are now being recognized as well (12,20–22,38,39,49–51).

Although initial studies attempting to demonstrate that education improves diabetes control produced variable results, again it was through meta-analyses that examined the cumulative evidence that the conclusion can be drawn that diabetes education can result in a moderate to large effect on improving glycemic control (15–19). For glycemic control, the magnitude of this effect was particularly evident in studies that were completed after measurements of glycosylated hemoglobin (HbA_{1c}) came into widespread use (15). Traditional diabetes education also resulted in improved knowledge and self-care behaviors with a small effect on psychological outcomes (17). Padgett and coworkers (16) found that diet instruction had the largest effect size while relaxation training had the weakest.

Other studies also have underscored the importance of selecting the right outcome criteria for measurement. If the wrong outcomes are measured, education may not appear to be responsible for the desired improvements, both when looked at in relation to various outcomes other than metabolic control (52) and when examined over extended periods (34,53). For example, the Diabetes Education Study reported minimal differences between the education and control groups in measurements of their knowledge but found numerous, significant differences in their skills and self-care behaviors. Such studies suggest that adult learning theory holds true: Individuals tend to learn what is important to them and what they can relate to their own life experience (54). Not surprisingly, discrepancies may exist between what healthcare providers teach and what individuals with diabetes perceive as important. These studies also point out the difficulties of measuring the effects of education after a single educational intervention that focuses primarily on facts about diabetes rather than on behaviors and that does not include ongoing follow-up (55) or that measures outcomes in terms of selected metabolic parameters only. Such limited studies often fail to detect all the potential long-term benefits of an ongoing educational experience (56). Others have made the important point that improved glycemic control may not be apparent unless other treatment factors, such as the treatment regimen and individual metabolism, are taken into account (57).

Although the studies cited suggest that education does improve metabolic control, most studies do not examine education in isolation. In an extensive review of the diabetes education literature, Clement (58) emphasized that negative studies did not examine diabetes education that was integrated into medical treatment. Therefore, one must conclude that education alone does not improve metabolic control. This point was nicely demonstrated in a randomized controlled study of nurse case management that included a 12-hour education program. After 1 year, the combined medical/education case management approach led to a greater improvement in glycemic control as measured by HbA_{1c} of 1.1% as compared with the control group receiving the usual care (21). These data and the emphasis that the DCCT placed on education to help patients reach glycemic targets (46,48,59–61) support the suggestion that the maximal benefit of diabetes education is realized when education is integrated into diabetes care.

Education Enhances the Prevention and Early Detection of Complications

Evidence is now emerging that diabetes education plays an important role in the prevention and early detection of diabetes complications. In fact, the Revised National Standards for Diabetes Self-Management Education have included prevention, detection, and treatment of both acute and chronic complications among the ten content areas for diabetes education (4).

A case–control study of 886 subjects with long-term diabetic complications and 1,888 control subjects without complications found that, in addition to being male, older, and having type 1 or insulin-treated type 2 diabetes, patients who did not receive any kind of educational intervention were at increased risk of developing complications. Furthermore, self-management of insulin, a skill that is usually dependent on receiving diabetes education, had a protective effect on the risk of complications (62).

In a randomized control trial of 352 patients and four healthcare provider practice teams, Litzelman and her colleagues (23) found that patients with type 2 diabetes who were assigned to an educational intervention with patient, healthcare provider, and educational systems were less likely to have serious foot lesions and more likely to report appropriate self-care behaviors than were patients assigned to usual care. In addition, healthcare providers who received practice guidelines, informational flow sheets on foot-related risk factors, and who had reminder notices placed on their patients charts were more likely to examine patients' feet and to refer patients for podiatry appointments.

Education Decreases Costs of Care

> While it is generally agreed that education can be a major factor in decreasing costs of hospitalization, not until this fact can be proven conclusively regarding diabetic patients will ample money be made available for the needed education.

This statement by Joslin's Dr. Leo Krall (63) opened the section in earlier editions of this text that discussed how education could decrease the cost of diabetes care. Finally, in this edition, the evidence is beginning to accrue that, indeed, Dr. Krall's wish for data may be coming true. However, the path to this conclusion has followed a difficult and convoluted route, and the conclusion has been slow to gain acceptance among many, particularly those responsible for paying the bills. In addition, as Krall pointed out at the Joslin symposium held at the 2000 International Diabetes Federation meetings, from a worldwide perspective, economic environments vary—not all of them resembling that of the United States.

Yet, spurred by the managed-care movement, cost-effectiveness and the impact on quality of life are now being measured, and slowly the recognition that diabetes education is a reasonable expense is beginning to gain acceptance. This trend is seeing a confluence of endpoints. Medical professionals are looking to improve parameters such as HbA_{1c} values or complication rates, assuming that the good stemming from improvements in these numbers is justification in and of itself. However, the people who pay the bills—the managed-care executives initially and, ultimately, the consumers of healthcare services—view parameters such as dollars and cents and, in particular, impact on quality of life for dollar spent to ensure that the benefits reaped by an intervention such as education warrant the expense.

Demonstrating that education is a cost worth bearing has been promulgated over the last few decades. However, during the 1990s, enough momentum seemed to have gathered for people to finally begin to accept this principle. Prior to that, a traditional endpoint was a reduction in hospitalizations, which may not necessarily reflect the entire picture in this new millennium in which outpatient medicine and pharmaceutical costs are a focus of the cost-conscious healthcare insurance executives. Nevertheless, hospitalizations are still costly and serve as a reasonable yardstick.

To get a sense of the battle that has been waged, we should look back to 1981, at the dawn of the era of "intensive insulin therapy" heralded by the availability of SMBG and HbA_{1c} measurements. This quiet revolution in diabetes management gave us the tools to target normoglycemia more realistically and to monitor glucose patterns in a normal setting without the need for hospitalization, yet increasing the importance of self-care skills if these new tools were to be used to their optimal efficacy.

At that time, educational deficits were clearly a cause for increased costs of medical interventions. In 1981, Geller and Butler (64) judged that 27% of the hospital admissions for diabetes complications over a 1-year period were the result of educational deficits and that an additional 20% were due to a combination of educational, psychological, and socioeconomic deficits. In a 1985 edition of this textbook, Krall (63) recounted the classic, but not scientifically controlled, report of 100 patients surveyed who were admitted to the Joslin Diabetes Center with foot infections. Only 38% of these patients had received any diabetes education. The same year, Scott et al. (65) from New Zealand suggested that education lowers admission rates among patients with diabetes. Of a group of 902 insulin-using patients, 79 required hospitalization, of whom 11% had received education previously and 89% had not.

In a 1983 report from Maine (66), based on its experiences as one of the few states that at that time provided some reimbursement for diabetes education, 38.5% fewer people were hospitalized and 28.3% fewer hospitalizations were necessary among patients who had participated in an educational program. The experience in Rhode Island reported in 1985 by Fishbein (67) also demonstrated a reduction in the number of admissions after attendance in an outpatient education program.

However, these and other studies that have appeared over the years had seemingly not provided convincing proof that education does save money. Criticisms of various studies, exemplified by a review by Kaplan and Davis (68), typified the dilemma. Reviewing studies used by the ADA to support third-party payment for outpatient education and nutritional counseling (69), these authors identified various defects in study design such as deficiencies in the use of control groups, in patient randomization, in cost accounting, and in clearly demonstrating actual savings. They also pointed out that duration of hospital stay and rate of hospital admission can be affected by multiple factors influencing hospitalization practices that are unrelated to diabetes education or even to actual medical conditions.

The crux of the argument at that time was expressed succinctly by Anderson (70) in a reply to the Kaplan and Davis report (68), pointing out that patients appear to need education to follow their daily routine of diabetes self-care. As with the impact on medical parameters cited earlier, asking that an educational program *alone* results in reduction in cost without considering the other variables that affect such outcome measures is ascribing more power to educational intervention than is warranted.

However, during the 1990s we passed a significant milestone, as those who view healthcare in the aggregate, rather than one patient at a time, began to recognize that patient education was an important component of the multifactorial effort to achieve improvements in diabetes control and reductions in complications and thus achieve better outcomes. Studies such as the DCCT and UKPDS provided enough momentum to establish the economic value, albeit indirect, of patient education. Although the DCCT had already proven that intensive therapy reduces microvascular and neuropathic complications (7,71), the cost-effectiveness of intensive therapy itself was subsequently demonstrated (72). Implicitly, patient education is central to establishing a successful intensive therapy program, and thus patient education contributes to a cost-effective outcome.

Concurrently, other studies examined the costs of care for patients with diabetes in the managed-care environment. In a health maintenance organization (HMO) in which 3.6% of the patients had diabetes, these patients accounted for more than three times their allotment of costs, or 11.9% of total healthcare delivery costs, attributable in significant part to long-term and short-term complications (73). This study suggests that reducing the occurrence of complications would generate savings, accomplished through disease management, which includes to a considerable degree, of course, patient education. Other studies further underscore these economic benefits of improving diabetes control and preventing complications (74–76), as well as the benefit of adding quality time to a person's life (77).

The ADA has participated in this argument for many years, strongly advocating proper support for patient education. Even before the DCCT results became available, the ADA stated that every patient has a right to accessible and affordable patient-education services (78) and has issued a policy statement that "supports and encourages reimbursement for outpatient education and nutrition counseling that meet acceptable standards for persons with diabetes" (69). Again, in 1990, the ADA issued a policy statement (79) that noted "the omission of outpatient education as a benefit in many insurance and healthcare financing plans constitutes a major barrier to the availability and accessibility of these services" and supported "adequate reimbursement and payment for outpatient diabetes education services that meet accepted standards." Such lack of coverage may be the result of either the failure of insurance companies to include coverage in their policies or a choice made by employers not to include such coverage in the insurance benefits they offer their employees when arranging insurance benefits.

More recently, the ADA stated (80) that "self-management education is a critical part of the medical plan for people with diabetes, such that medical treatment of diabetes without systematic self-management education can be regarded as substandard and unethical care." The ADA suggests that such education will ultimately reduce costs.

Throughout this period, economic factors as well as technologic advances have exerted an increasing influence on the setting for and scope of diabetes patient education. The ability to perform SMBG has eliminated the need to hospitalize a person just to monitor multiple glucose levels throughout the day. Inpatient education programs are now restricted to people with medical conditions that cannot be adequately addressed in an outpatient setting and thus justify hospitalization; the shorter hospital stays now mandated limit the extent of material that can be taught (81). Thus, diabetes education must increasingly be delivered through outpatient programs (82).

Ironically, however, the evolution from inpatient to outpatient education has been negatively influenced by economic factors as well. Inpatient education frequently was provided as part of the "overhead" service covered by the cost of hospitalization. However, because education is often inadequately covered by insurance in many states, the cost of outpatient education is often borne directly by the patient. Thus, because inpatient education is restricted and outpatient education is unaffordable, all education may be unavailable for most patients.

Outpatient education does, however, have advantages over inpatient education. There is flexibility of timing of the sessions, extension of the educational experience over weeks or months, ability to educate in a normal life setting rather than in an artificial inpatient environment, and the opportunity for follow-up sessions. The trends of recognition of both the quality and the importance of outpatient education hopefully will continue, but until all people with diabetes can have some access to insurance-supported outpatient education, the full potential cannot be met.

In summary, we are finally reaching the point at which most people accept that patient education can improve diabetes control and decrease the risk of acute and chronic complications and thus is a significant component of an overall management plan. These results, in turn, can lead to reduced costs and improved quality of life. Patient education *alone* does not accomplish this, but patient education as part of a comprehensive management program does. Thus, the cost of educational services and the supplies that must accompany them, such as test strips and meters, are slowly being included in many coverage plans—not universally, but it is happening.

The following was written in the last edition of this text: "We hope that in the next edition of this textbook the report on the financing of diabetes education will be quite different!"

Well, it is! Maybe it should not be termed "quite" different, but it is different enough and definitely evolving enough in the right direction to be most encouraging!

Malpractice Protection

Sensitivity to the potential for malpractice lawsuits for alleged negligence has become part of the practice of medicine. This concern also extends to the act of conveying information about diabetes. Legal precedents in United States law exist that require healthcare providers to be sure their patients receive adequate education and that outline the potential liability for either not educating or poorly educating their patients (83).

In light of the progress during the last decades in demonstrating that improved control and avoidance of complications can be accomplished through education, the risk of potential lawsuits stemming from inadequate or improper education is theoretically significant. Although economic motivation pushes healthcare organizations to recognize the need to support patient education, the humanistic approach of the healthcare providers that leads to the recommendation for such education (with, we hope, some crossover motivation in the best of all worlds!), both groups may be further encouraged by the potential for liability of not doing so.

Therefore, it is prudent for healthcare professionals to ensure that their patients receive education of proper quality. Unless a program is known to meet established standards, programs recognized by the ADA or educators certified by the National Certification Board for Diabetes Educators are the most reliable sources of proper education. Healthcare professionals should encourage patients to attend such programs and document in the patient's record that they did so.

THE DIABETES EDUCATION PROGRAM

Diabetes self-management education is the process of providing people with diabetes with experiences that favorably influence their understandings, attitudes, and practices related to living well with diabetes (84). At its best, an educational program empowers those with diabetes to achieve optimal self-management of their condition (85). A successful educational program does not occur by accident; it is carefully planned by the healthcare team and then executed by that team with the individual with diabetes as an integral part of the team. The most successful diabetes self-management education is individualized (37,61,86,87), is integrated into medical treatment, and addresses psychosocial and behavioral components of care (88,89).

The goal of any educational program is to help patients with diabetes gain the knowledge and skills that enable them to care for themselves and to develop the attitudes that will enable them to make behavioral changes. A national task force representing organizations interested in diabetes (ADA, Veterans Administration, Centers for Disease Control, Indian Health Service, American Dietetic Association, American Association of Diabetes Educators, Diabetes Research and Training Centers) has recently revised the National Standards for Diabetes Education (4) (Table 35.1). These standards provide guidelines for the format of diabetes education and a clear outline of the content areas that should be addressed (4). The ADA provides an education recognition program that evaluates diabetes education according to the National Standards and certifies those programs that meet or exceed the standards.

The Educators

In the years after the discovery of insulin, Dr. Joslin was among the first to recognize that the responsibility of patient care lay mainly with the patients themselves. "The patient is his own nurse, doctor's assistant and chemist," he wrote in the first comprehensive guide to self-care, *A Diabetic Manual for the Mutual Use of Doctor and Patient*, in 1924 (90), shortly after the discovery of insulin. Recognizing the need for patient education, Joslin showed his nurses how to give insulin, calculate the diet, and balance insulin requirements with that diet. These nurses then visited patients in their homes throughout New England, sometimes staying with families for weeks, to teach patients and families to plan menus, prepare food, and administer several injections daily.

The role of the "teaching nurse" has since evolved and expanded and now includes other healthcare providers with special diabetes-related skills. Diabetes educators, as they are now called, include nurses, nutritionists, social workers, exercise physiologists, psychologists, pharmacists, and physicians. Their expertise in diabetes care and education may qualify them to take an examination to become Certified Diabetes Educators (CDEs) or Board-Certified Advanced Diabetes Managers (BC-ADM).

These diabetes educators form the basis of the team approach to diabetes education (91). Working together in both inpatient and outpatient settings, each member of the team provides the patient with specialized expert services. For example, nurses help patients master the skills necessary to inject insulin and monitor blood glucose levels and adapt these skills to their lifestyle, nutritionists work with patients to develop realistic meal plans, and psychologists and social workers focus on coping mechanisms. The person with diabetes and key family members are now recognized as important players in the team who must be involved in the educational program (92–94). This multifaceted team effort, which includes the patient and the physician, provides the most complete approach to diabetes education and care (12,20,22,39,50).

The Setting for Education

Education for diabetes care may be provided in a variety of settings, such as clinics, hospitals, education centers, a physician's office, or the patient's home (95). The program can be formalized and presented in a classroom setting or provided in a one-to-one fashion. It may be presented in a carefully planned educational session or may arise spontaneously from responses to questions asked during a routine office visit (96).

In educational sessions, the size of the groups may vary and the forms of interaction used may include, but not be limited to, discussion, lecture, and interactive learning activities (97–99). Innovative educational techniques, such as programs incorpo-

TABLE 35.1. National Standards for Diabetes Self-Management Education (DSME)

Standard 1. The DSME entity will have documentation of its organizational structure, mission statement, and goals and will recognize and support quality DSME as an integral component of diabetes care.
Standard 2. The DSME will determine its target population, assess educational needs, and identify the resources necessary to meet the self-management needs of the target population(s).
Standard 3. An established system (committee, governing board, advisory body) involving professional staff and other stake holders will participate annually in a planning and review process that includes data analysis and outcome measurements and addresses community concerns.
Standard 4. The DSME entity will designate a coordinator with academic and/or experiential preparation in program management and the care of individuals with chronic diseases. The coordinator will oversee the planning, implementation, and evaluation of the DSME entity.
Standard 5. DSME will involve the interaction of the individuals with diabetes with a multifaceted educational instructional team, which may include a behaviorist, exercise physiologist, ophthalmologist, optometrist, pharmacist, physician, podiatrist, registered dietitian, registered nurse, other health care professionals, and paraprofessionals. DSME instructors are collectively qualified to teach the content areas. The instructional team must consist of at least a registered dietitian and a registered nurse. Instructional staff must be certified diabetes educators or have recent didactic and experiential preparation in education and diabetes management.
Standard 6. The DSME instructors will obtain regular continuing education in the areas of diabetes management, behavioral interventions, teaching and learning skills, and consulting skills.
Standard 7. A written curriculum, with criteria for successful learning outcomes, shall be available. Assessed needs of the individual will determine which content areas listed below are delivered.

- Describing the diabetes disease process and treatment options
- Incorporating appropriate nutritional management
- Incorporating physical activity into lifestyle
- Using medications (if applicable) for therapeutic effectiveness
- Monitoring blood glucose and urine ketones (when appropriate), and using the results to improve control
- Preventing, detecting, and treating complications
- Preventing (through risk-reduction behavior), detecting, and treating chronic complications
- Goal setting to promote health and problem solving for daily living
- Integrating psychosocial adjustment to daily life
- Promoting preconception care, management during pregnancy, and gestational diabetes management (if applicable)

Standard 8. An individualized assessment, development of an educational plan, and periodic reassessment between participant and instructor(s) will direct the selection of appropriate educational materials and interventions.
Standard 9. There shall be documenting of the individual's assessment, educational plan, intervention, education, and follow-up in the permanent confidential education record. Documentation also will provide evidence of collaboration among instructional staff, providers, and referral sources.
Standard 10. The DSME entity will use a continuous quality improvement process to evaluate the effectiveness of the education experience provided and determine opportunities for improvement.

rating computers, the Internet, and other audiovisual media, can enhance the educational program (99–102).

Availability of staff, the needs of patients, the subject matter, and economic factors often dictate the choice of setting. For example, general information about the various kinds of insulin and their respective activity patterns might be presented in a group setting. However, the teaching of specific skills such as drawing insulin into the syringe is best carried out on an individual basis or in small groups that are no larger than six people. This small size provides the healthcare professional with the opportunity to help each patient individually learn the techniques necessary for carrying out these essential activities. Similarly, general information about monitoring glucose levels might be presented in a group setting, but the actual learning of the skill should take place in a setting in which every patient can benefit from the individual attention of the healthcare professional. However, we must also keep in mind that reimbursement guidelines often dictate the details of such education sessions and their structure.

In addition, as with many other "school" settings, the educational experience is not limited to formalized instructional sessions; much of diabetes education occurs through the interactions among patients that take place in diabetes treatment units and camp-type settings (103,104). Information and understanding gained through the sharing of personal experiences can help patients improve both self-management and coping skills in ways not possible with more formalized instruction.

An example of such a program is the Diabetes Outpatient Intensive Treatment (DO IT) program at Joslin Diabetes Center (Table 35.2). This behavior modification program has evolved from the historic Diabetes Treatment Unit, an inpatient program originally intended for diabetes education and treatment. Because of current reimbursement for this education, the DO IT program permits the same medical management, with accompanying education and group cohesiveness but on an outpatient basis. During this 3.5-day program, patients are evaluated by a physician, nurse, dietitian, exercise physiologist, and mental health professional. After the initial assessment, the remaining 3 days consist of medical care and education. Free time is also available for social interaction among patients. Follow-up shortly after completion of the program is recommended, both via telephone and office visits, to ensure that patients are able to apply what they have learned during the program to their everyday lives.

Since 1992, the Joslin's DO IT program has been a recognized education program as per ADA standards. One criterion necessary to achieve this recognition is to prove the effectiveness of the program as it relates both to clinical aspects of diabetes care and to the quality of life of these persons with diabetes. These outcomes data have shown an average decrease in HbA_{1c} of levels of 1.5% over a 3- to 6-month period following the participation in the DO IT program. Attendees whose HbA_{1c} levels were greater than 10% were shown to reduce the level by an average of 2.5% during the same time period. In a clinical survey conducted after the program, participants of the program reported a 38% improvement in their perception of their diabetes-related problems. In addition, program evaluation has shown a decrease in emergency department visits, hospitalizations, and lost time from work or school for patients after their participation in the DO IT program.

TABLE 35.2. Schedule for 3-Day Program of the Diabetes Outpatient Intensive Treatment (DO-IT) Program of the Joslin Clinic

Activity	Times	Tuesday	Wednesday	Thursday
Lab	7:30–8:00 a.m.	X	X	X
Breakfast and self-instructional computer modules	8:00–9:15 a.m.	Check-in Choose from breakfast buffet Computer time	Check-in Choose from breakfast buffet Computer time	Check-in Choose from breakfast buffet Computer time
Class 1	9:15–10:00 a.m.	Diabetes Know-how	Exercise: Moving Toward Better Control	Blood Glucose Interpretation
Class 2	10:00–10:45 a.m.	Food for Thought	Responding to High Blood Glucose Levels	Understanding Fats
Break	10:45–11:00 a.m.			
Class 3	11:00–12:00 p.m.	Understanding Your Diabetes Medications	Healthy Food Choices	Staying on Top: Investing in Your Health
Lab	12:00–12:15 p.m.	X	X	X
Lunch	12:15–1:00 p.m.	Choose from lunch buffet	Choose from lunch buffet	Choose from lunch buffet
Exercise	1:00–2:00 p.m.	Exercise class	Exercise Class/family support group	Bringing It all Together
Class 4	2:00–2:45 p.m.	Skills Training (as needed) Check-out with case manager	Skills Training (as needed) Check-out with case manager	Final check-out with case manager

Who Should Be Educated

The National Standards for Diabetes Education recognizes that diabetes education is an integral component of diabetes care (4), and the ADA recommends education for all people with diabetes at the time of diagnosis and at regular intervals throughout their lifetime (5). These standards recognize the right of each person to understand the nature of his or her condition, to be given the tools to manage and control the condition, and to have this information updated routinely. Unfortunately, we are far short of that goal. However, in a survey of 2,318 persons with diabetes, 59% of those with type 1 diabetes, 49% of those with insulin-treated type 2 diabetes, and 24% of those with type 2 diabetes not treated with insulin had attended a class or program about diabetes at some time during the course of their illness (8). The challenge for the team is to gain access to the patient at regular intervals and to meet the needs of each patient through assessment, implementation, and evaluation.

Patient Assessment

Assessment of the patient's and family's readiness to learn is the first step in the educational process (37,105). Concurrent illnesses, new diagnosis of diabetes, or psychosocial problems may affect a patient's willingness or ability to learn. A patient who has just received a diagnosis of pancreatic carcinoma may not be ready to discuss insulin administration. Similarly, a patient recovering from surgery may be more interested in starting on solid food than learning self-monitoring techniques. The key to assessment is communication with the patient. If education starts when the patient is emotionally and experientially ready, there is a better chance of engaging him or her in the entire educational process (106).

The emotional response to diabetes can have an impact on the patient's ability to hear and absorb information. Denial may be the patient's first reaction to the diagnosis of diabetes and can impair his or her ability to learn (107). The healthcare provider can assist the patient by recognizing this response as denial, acknowledging that it may be a stage in the long process of adapting to a chronic illness, and supporting the patient's effort to cope with the disease. Involvement in support groups and individual therapy may help the patient move from denial to successful adaptation.

Assessment of knowledge, skills, and attitudes about diabetes is an ongoing process that starts with the initial chart review and interview. Many patients do not recall medical advice and some report never having received specific self-care recommendations (108–110). Assessment of the person's knowledge of his or her actual treatment prescription is as important for those with diabetes of long duration as for those with newly diagnosed diabetes. Use of a conversational style, rather than a question-and-answer session, helps to establish rapport and to give the healthcare professional some idea of the patient's lifestyle (111). The healthcare professional should learn to listen to the patient, to be sympathetic and understanding, and to accept that the patient's priorities may not be the same as those of the healthcare team. It is important to remember that diabetes is an intrusion into daily life, that most people will still have significant gaps in their knowledge about diabetes even after having the condition for 20 years, and that it is ultimately the patient who makes the final decisions about how he or she will approach the disease (94,112). Recognizing and accepting these realities will allow the healthcare professional to set reasonable, achievable, and mutually acceptable goals. The initial assessment should be clearly documented in the chart and updated on a regular basis (4,113–115).

Because the backgrounds of the team members may be very different, many different assessments take place. A registered dietitian, for example, may assess the current eating habits of someone newly diagnosed with diabetes and provide that person with a meal plan as close to this as possible. An exercise physiologist may teach a person with diabetes how to correctly adjust his or her insulin dose to prevent hypoglycemia during exercise. A nurse educator may assess a patient's skills and general diabetes knowledge and provide him or her with the necessary information. In some institutions, CDEs are seen as just that: diabetes educators.

Using this rationale, any CDE can meet the diabetes education needs of a patient to a certain extent. For example, if a patient needs to learn how to self-administer insulin and no nurse educator is available to do this, as a CDE, a registered dietitian or exercise physiologist could teach this skill. Then, at a later date, the patient may follow up with a nurse educator to review technique as well as acquire other necessary information related to insulin. Patients starting exercise programs can review general insulin or food adjustment with a nurse educator and then schedule to see an exercise physiologist for more detailed adjustments.

At the Joslin Clinic in Boston, educators use a team approach to patient assessment and education. A "new patient" to the clinic will see an educator solely for an educational assessment (i.e., to determine the patient's current level of diabetes knowledge and skills and to schedule appointments with "appropriate" educators based on this assessment). This serves two purposes: It enables the patient to recognize diabetes educators as a part of his or her healthcare team and allows an effective and efficient way to recognize and address the needs of the patient. The primary goal is to identify and focus on the educational needs of the patient.

The assessment process provides an opportunity for the patient and family to express their healthcare beliefs and their agenda for that visit and to express particular needs or goals (116). The information gained not only provides the healthcare team with data about educational needs but also guides the team in management issues. The team has the opportunity to answer questions, provide positive feedback, and encourage proper self-care behaviors.

In addition to assessing the patient's readiness to learn (37) and stage of adaptation to diabetes (117), the healthcare professional must obtain information on the patient's ethnic or cultural background, occupation, socioeconomic status, support systems, personality type, and health beliefs before looking at the patient's knowledge of diabetes (118). Other factors that may have an impact on learning include age, gender, literacy level, and level of education (119). This information is invaluable in getting a sense of the patient and the approach to education and treatment that would be most helpful and reasonable for that patient.

An evaluation of functional ability helps the healthcare provider plan how to teach skills such as SMBG and insulin administration (120). The patient's dexterity may be affected by arthritis or neuropathy. Vision changes due to retinopathy may be evident at a relatively young age. Some patients have a difficult time admitting to their vision deficit, so it is important to assess the patient's skill in these areas at the initial visit and again at regular intervals. Relatives or close friends should definitely be included in this part of the assessment process to determine whether they are willing and able to assume some responsibility for care of the patient.

Reported educational level appears to be a poor predictor of reading ability, because a person's actual reading level may be significantly lower. Nevertheless, it may be helpful to ask about educational experience (121). In this context, a question concerning how the person learns best will provide some guidelines for deciding whether to use audio, video, or written materials or a one-on-one or classroom setting. Recent research suggests that health literacy, the ability to understand instruction and health information, may impact how well individuals manage their diabetes (122).

What Is Taught

The educational plan is developed by the team—addressing educational needs and treatment goals identified by both the patient and the team. Education begins with "survival" knowledge (i.e., the information absolutely necessary for a person with diabetes to have to function independently and safely at home). For some, this may be as simple as identifying when to call the healthcare provider. For others, SMBG and use of insulin and glucagon may be survival skills. Everyone with diabetes must also have some general knowledge about diabetes to understand when it is necessary to call the healthcare provider for help.

The educational assessments done by various diabetes educators provide the basis for the individualization of teaching. Having determined the patient's knowledge about diabetes, psychosocial history, attitudes about diabetes, and eating and exercise habits, the educator can then formulate an educational plan that reflects the patient's specific needs.

As outlined by the National Standards for Diabetes Self-Management Education (Table 35.1) (4), the actual content of the diabetes education program is based on assessed needs of the individual or individuals. Diabetes education programs do not need to be structured in the model of a medical or nursing course on diabetes (89) but instead should be structured in a way that provides maximal benefits for patients in terms of health outcomes. Many education programs begin with areas identified by the patient as priorities. Addressing the patient's pressing issues then allows the patient to be more attentive to the issues the provider has identified as important (89).

The National Standards recommend that the curriculum include an explanation of diabetes disease process and treatment options to help individuals make informed treatment choices and facilitate self-directed behavior. An explanation of treatment modalities, including the use of insulin, insulin delivery systems, oral antidiabetes medications, the meal plan, and exercise, are important aspects of the curriculum. Other key components of a well-rounded educational program are methods for incorporating nutritional management and physical activity into one's lifestyle. The goals of monitoring; the types, descriptions, and limitations of monitoring devices; and instruction in the use and interpretation of SMBG results are also necessary parts of initial and ongoing education.

Patients also need information about the recognition, treatment, and prevention of acute complications such as hyperglycemia, hypoglycemia, and ketoacidosis and the prevention of chronic complications through risk-reduction behaviors (foot inspection and care). The effects of illness on diabetes and sick-day rules are a critical part of any diabetes education. Guidelines for monitoring blood glucose and urine ketones, for modifying food intake, and when to call the healthcare team are essential skills for the patient. Equally important components of care include helping patients set realistic, achievable goals for their diabetes care and discussion of the psychosocial adjustment to diabetes. Finally, patients may need specialty education during specific times such as preconception or pregnancy, the onset of complications, or the initiation of new treatments.

The section on prevention, treatment, and rehabilitation of chronic complications should include strategies for coping with the physical changes and losses that complications may bring. It is extremely important to stress the benefits that blood glucose control can have for both the short- and long-term. Focusing on the prevention of complications through risk reduction is a vital part of this section. A discussion of personal adaptation to life with a chronic disease and the impact of diabetes on the family will also help patients understand some of their feelings.

Care of the skin, teeth, and feet is part of the hygiene segment of a diabetes education program. Self-care measures that help prevent complications, address the need for regular checkups, and outline the effects of smoking, alcohol, and drug use are addressed in this section. The class on the benefits and responsibilities of care explores the patient–professional partnership in planning care and helps the patient develop short- and long-term goals. Exploration of the use of healthcare systems and community resources can help the patient find support and services in the community.

Educational Methods

Diabetes education has benefited from principles of adult learning (54) and instructional design (123). The use of basic educational principles as guides can increase the success of a diabetes education program, regardless of its setting. However, continued evaluation of the applicability and usefulness of principles borrowed from educational theory is important for the continued improvement of educational programs in diabetes (119). For example, the active involvement of the patient in all aspects of the educational endeavor, including decisions about the treatment program, is one such principle that is not universally recognized as being important for successful diabetes education.

Unfortunately, many diabetes education programs frequently foster too passive a role for the patient (124). Many educators have suggested that when patients participate in decisions about their care (86), improvements are seen in measures of both clinical condition and attitudes about health-related quality of life. In a controlled study, Greenfield and associates (125) met with patients before a scheduled office visit with their physicians to review past medical concerns and to focus and improve patients' information-seeking skills. Patients rehearsed negotiation skills, addressing obstacles, such as feelings of embarrassment or intimidation, that stood in the way of their gaining information from the physician. Patients so coached were twice as effective as those in the control group at eliciting information from the physician. Improvements in levels of HbA_1 were significantly greater in these individuals, as were reductions in factors such as days lost from work as a result of illness.

Others also have emphasized the relationship between treatment adherence and the ways in which the physician and the patient reach treatment decisions (126–129). Commenting on some of these studies, Sims and Sims (130) concluded that patients will adhere to their treatment plans more consistently if they feel a sense of ownership of the plans. Today, emphasis is placed on the influence of patient priorities on that person's ability to manage the self-care tasks required for their diabetes treatment. Each individual's priorities and life issues must be considered when the diabetes team, including the patient, sets goals and targets (112,131). The self-care goals that are set should be concrete, realistic, and measurable (132,133).

A study of adolescents (134) in a summer-school program for young people with diabetes demonstrated another important principle: Education and learning are more effective when people have an opportunity to actively address the questions and problems that actually affect them. One group of participants was randomly assigned to a social learning intervention approach to identify situations in which social pressures made it difficult for them to maintain their treatment regimen, and they rehearsed appropriate responses to these situations. The second group of adolescents underwent a more didactic, fact-oriented diabetes education program. Subsequent HbA_1 values were significantly lower among the adolescents in the social skills intervention group. Variables significantly correlated with good metabolic control included self-reported adherence with a diabetes regimen and attitudes toward self-care.

Of course, providing complete didactic information that is personally connected is also important and is associated with higher patient satisfaction. Ley et al. (135) provided patients with additional physician visits that were designed to assess previous patient education and understanding and to clarify areas of misunderstanding. These patients showed significantly more satisfaction with their care than did the control group. In a review of this subject, Tabak (136) concurred that patients' satisfaction is clearly related to the amount of information available that contributes to their understanding of their condition and that they can use in caring for themselves. It is also important that the provision and acquisition of information span a reasonable time period if patients are to remember and use it. For example, a study of a diet education program given over either 3 days or 11 weeks showed that the longer program was associated with significantly greater improvements in dietary behaviors (137). The need to pace both the provision and use of information has been demonstrated by others as well (109).

Reinforcement and repetition are also important components of an educational program (108). Often, this is accomplished through the preparation of written materials for patients. Unfortunately, there is frequently a mismatch between a patient's reading skills and the level of comprehension required to understand the materials (138,139).

In one study (140), only 28% of the patients had reading skills at or above the ninth-grade level: 59% read at the fifth- to eighth-grade level and 13% had reading skills below the fifth-grade level. By contrast, an evaluation of the educational materials used with these patients showed that 87% were written at the ninth-grade level or above, 13% at the fifth- to eighth-grade level, and none below the fifth-grade level. This means that 87% of the materials were comprehensible to only 28% of the patients, 13% were understood by 87%, and none were readable by 13%!

Formulas have been developed to determine the reading level of educational materials (141–145). Typically, recommendations for readability suggest that educational materials be geared toward the sixth-grade reading level. However, materials should be selected based on assessments of the reading levels of the targeted populations. Helpful strategies are available for developing health education materials for low-literacy groups (146). Most word-processing programs have readability statistics functions such as the Flesch–Kincaid grade level that will determine reading level. Education materials should also be available in the primary language of the targeted population. The National Institute of Diabetes and Digestive and Kidney Diseases of the National Institutes of Health maintains an up-to-date Web site (www.niddkk.nih.gov/health/diabetes/diabetes.htm) that provides diabetes health information, as well as reviews of diabetes information publications, in easy-to-read formats. These reviews are available in both English and Spanish. Joslin's Web site (www.joslin.org) is another source of useful diabetes information.

Finally, a successful education program provides patients with an opportunity to explore their attitudes toward the material being taught and to understand its implications for day-to-day living. Factors such as the patient's familial, social, and cultural environments; socioeconomic status; other health problems; and overall psychological and emotional well-being provide frames of reference from which patients approach diabetes care and their participation in it (149). The goals for diabetes education developed by the ADA acknowledge the importance of these factors (92). Anderson et al. (147) suggest a means of adapting an educational program to the patient's frame of reference through activities that stimulate an exploration of the meaning of diabetes to the patient and of the psychological adaptations required for the patient to cope with his or her concept of the disease.

Clearly, the implementation of the educational principles discussed above is most effective when the healthcare professional has received training in teaching skills (124,148–152).

Unfortunately, many health professionals involved in diabetes education are not adequately trained in these skills. Such training is strongly encouraged.

When Education Should Take Place

Education for diabetes care is an ongoing, life-long undertaking. However, there are identifiable stages in the progression of diabetes when educational interactions are particularly recommended. The ADA identified diabetes education goals for individuals and their families at diagnosis and throughout their life (92,96).

DIAGNOSIS STAGE

Upon receiving a diagnosis of diabetes, many people are overwhelmed both by the condition itself and by the idea of all the information they think they must absorb. Therefore, people with newly diagnosed diabetes should start by learning the minimum basic skills required for survival. They should learn to maintain reasonably satisfactory management of their diabetes while carrying out essential daily activities. They should become familiar with the medical nutritional principles that they will be following and be able to choose foods in the correct amounts to follow their meal plan. Patients should be taught SMBG, and some need to learn how to inject insulin. This initial education provided at or around the time of diagnosis can occur over several days, particularly if the person is hospitalized, or in small increments over several days or weeks for those who are outpatients.

ONGOING STAGE

Once patients have mastered the essential "survival skills" of diabetes management, they should progress to a more in-depth program of ongoing diabetes education to help them become even more sufficient at self-care and therefore at preventing complications. The challenge for patients in this stage is to learn and follow a complex and demanding regimen when the benefit of preventing complications is distant (117). Key issues concern adapting diabetes self-management to work, school, social, and family settings while coping with more typical life issues and crises. Self-management education programs are available in many education centers, clinics, hospitals, and community public-health programs. These programs, such as the DO IT program at the Joslin Clinic described earlier, not only provide information, knowledge, and skills but also support patient efforts to incorporate self-care tasks into everyday life (Table 35.2).

Periodic educational updates are extremely important after patients complete the initial in-depth training to enable them to meet changing needs at different times of their lives. People can learn new ways of managing diabetes, develop skills that enable them to adapt their management program to changing needs, and familiarize themselves with new resources and advances available for diabetes care.

ONSET OF COMPLICATIONS AND OTHER MAJOR POINTS OF CHANGE

Times of major life and health changes can signal the need for revisions in diabetes management and often make supplementary educational exposure necessary. Throughout the course of a pregnancy, for example, nutritional needs will change and insulin treatment programs may become more intensified, and pregnant women must learn to make these changes properly.

Another milestone at which supplementary education is necessary is at the appearance of early symptoms or signs of a major complication. This is typically a time when patients undergo enormous anxiety and fear and often seek diabetes education to help improve their glycemic control (117). Because improved control can slow the progression of major complications (7), diabetes education programs focus on helping individuals make lifestyle changes to integrate more successful self-management practices. For example, patients can learn to make changes in their routine that, if instituted early enough, may slow down the progression of kidney dysfunction. However, even for motivated patients, lifestyle changes can be difficult and frustrating.

MAXIMIZING THE EFFICACY OF EDUCATION

As pointed out previously, knowledge does not equal adherence to the self-care recommendations of the treatment plan. Nonadherence is not unique to diabetes nor is it a new problem. In fact, there are low rates of adherence with recommended treatment in a variety of chronic conditions. Older studies show that only 50% of patients are compliant with long-term medication and that only 25% are compliant when the condition is asymptomatic (153). In studies specific for diabetes, 80% of those studied administered insulin in an unacceptable manner, 58% gave the wrong dose, and 75% did not follow dietary recommendations (83). Other recent studies reflect similar results (154–156).

Difficulty with following the therapeutic recommendations presents a substantial obstacle to the achievement of medical treatment goals, diminishes the potential benefits of the treatment regimen, and makes evaluation of treatment efficacy inaccurate (157). There is no common profile of a nonadherent patient. Age, sex, education, income, or personality type cannot predict a patient's ability to successfully self-manage diabetes. Also, patients may be nonadherent in one area and not in others (158).

The patient's ability to manage diabetes is affected by a number of factors. The first is the individual's knowledge of the self-management recommendations. With a thorough assessment of the patient's knowledge of diabetes and of self-management recommendations, diabetes education can address this barrier by correcting misconceptions, determining patient priorities, and encouraging changes in behavior by helping patients set achievable and measurable goals. Acknowledgment of the imperfections and frustrations of the treatment plan helps to prepare the patient for the inevitable setbacks (159).

The second factor that impacts self-management behaviors is the patient's beliefs about healthcare. The health-belief model looks at whether the patient believes that he or she has diabetes, that it is serious, that the treatment is beneficial, and that the barriers to care are outweighed by its benefits (160–164). Health beliefs can be complicated and interrelated; thus, modification of some health beliefs alone may not result in improved physiologic outcomes of diabetes care (163,165,166). For example, health beliefs about the seriousness of diabetes of 79 participants were not related to clinic attendance, dietary intake, weight loss, or fasting glucose levels but did predict reductions in body mass index after 1 year (166). In addition, the realities of a person's life and the priorities the individual holds may differ from those of the healthcare provider. For example, a mother may put more emphasis on child-care duties or family requirements than on her own healthcare requirements. This type of barrier is difficult to overcome. In some cases, therapeutic goals and recommendations may require restructuring so that they better fit the patient's priorities and achieve at least some improvement in glycemia. Other approaches may involve the help of social services and of mental health professionals.

The characteristic coping styles of a patient may also be factors that determine adherence. Those patients who typically use a problem-focused coping style may be better able to self-manage their diabetes than those who employ a more emotion-focused approach (35,36). Denial of diabetes will not allow the patient to enter into an aggressive treatment regimen. On the other hand, those patients who tend to be obsessive/compulsive may need to be given permission to do less rather than encouraged to do more.

Another important factor is the treatment regimen itself. The greater the complexity and duration of the regimen, the more negative is its impact on treatment adherence (158). The more we ask patients to do and the longer we ask them to do it, the less likely they will be able to sustain compliance. In a study of patients with type 2 diabetes treated with oral medication, Paes et al. (156) found that patients taking one pill per day were adherent to the medication prescription on 79% of days, however, those taking two or three pills per day took medications as prescribed on only 66% and 38% of days, respectively.

The healthcare team can help modify this adherence barrier. A simplified and tailored regimen designed to meet individual lifestyle needs is more likely to be implemented successfully than is one that focuses on metabolic control alone. Clear, specific, simple, and concrete information and instructions in a diabetes education program will go far toward reducing the perceived complexity of treatment and improving the rate of adherence (108,167).

A final critical factor in the patient's ability to self-manage their diabetes is the healthcare provider. He or she can listen to the patient and modify the treatment regimen and/or alter his or her relationship with the patient as needed. In fact, the healthcare provider may be one of the most important factors influencing adherence.

The relationship between the healthcare provider and patient itself can have a positive or negative effect on compliance. Impersonality, inability to listen, and lack of warmth in the relationship between the healthcare provider and the patient can adversely affect patients' adherence to treatment (168). On the other hand, the healthcare provider's use of self-disclosure and positive nonverbal communication, such as smile, touch, and eye contact, can have a positive impact on compliance. Although time for providers is a precious commodity in today's stringent healthcare environment, taking a few minutes to check whether patients understand their self-management tasks, to address anticipated difficulties with the treatment regimen, or to answer additional questions can be quite beneficial to both the patient's self-management behaviors and to the healthcare provider/patient relationship.

In addition to working on a positive relationship with the patient, the healthcare provider can simplify the form of treatment and support the patient's efforts to manage his or her care.

ASSESSING OUTCOMES

"Outcome" refers to the hoped-for effect of an educational effort on diabetes management and overall quality of life for people with diabetes. Assessments of educational outcome have traditionally focused on physiologic improvements, which are the changes most easily measured. Today, these assessments attempt to determine how changes in knowledge and skills contribute to better self-care behavior and improvements in blood glucose levels, decreased complications, reduced use of healthcare services, and improved quality of life (20,24,55,147,169,170). However, as suggested earlier, healthcare professionals are recognizing that assessing outcomes by examining only the knowledge acquired and the skills learned as the sole factors involved in effecting beneficial self-care practices and metabolic control is too narrow a focus (57,70). There are many steps between an educational encounter and a medically or economically valuable outcome, with multiple factors influencing the process along the way. Knowledge and skills are only two factors that influence self-care behavior, and self-care behavior, although crucial for success, is only one component of a favorable outcome.

For example, improvements in self-care practices are unlikely to occur unless the patient is also helped to actively integrate his or her therapeutic regimen into the many facets of daily life. If the patient is expected to assume only a passive role in determining the regimen or in performing tasks and if his or her personal values and needs are ignored, no true progress is likely (78).

The ultimate purpose of assessing outcomes of educational efforts is to justify the cost and to ensure that the desired goal of improved health is reached. However, measuring the efficacy of education has been limited by the difficulty or impracticality of demonstrating a direct link between educational interaction and desired outcome while controlling for the other variables. Therefore, before beneficial outcomes can be measured, educational programs must be designed to address the multiple factors that encourage active patient participation in self-care that ultimately bring about an associated improvement in metabolic control, overall health, and quality of life (89). For example, one program made an effort to help patients develop a more accepting and positive personal response to having diabetes and to its treatment (147). Another program successfully affected self-care patterns, levels of HbA_1, and emotional well-being by specifically addressing these issues (38). Joslin's DO IT program also demonstrated improvements both in the glucose control parameters and in quality-of-life measurements. Currently, therefore, assessments of outcome look beyond knowledge and skills and focus on behaviors. Identification of about three specific, desired behavioral changes during the educational encounter permits subsequent evaluation based on whether these changes have occurred.

The challenge remains to design outcome assessments that trace the further progression from educational intervention, through behavioral changes, to desired outcome in terms of measurable medical parameters, improvements in quality of life, or economic parameters. To determine the exact effect of education, however, one must control for the other variables that affect the outcome, a challenge that remains formidable. Finally, assessment of all aspects of the process of education is as important as assessing outcomes (4,171).

CONCLUSION

Diabetes education programs that are evolving as part of multifaceted diabetes management efforts provided by skilled healthcare teams can help patients reach higher levels of adherence, metabolic control, and satisfaction by leading to their even more active participation in self-care. With such models of excellence and the growing recognition of the cost-effectiveness of educational intervention, these educational programs should be recognized as the bargain they are rather than as an additional financial burden on society. Diabetes patient education services must become accessible to all people with diabetes as an important component of the effort to extend quality medical care to all. To continue Dr. Krall's pattern of looking forward, we trust that by the *next* edition of this textbook, the hoped-for universal availability of patient education will be closer to a reality.

REFERENCES

1. WHO Expert Committee on Diabetes Mellitus. Education. Second report. Technical report series 646. Geneva: World Health Organization, 1980:58.
2. National standards for diabetes patient education programs. From the National Diabetes Advisory Board. *Diabetes Educ* 1984;9:11–14.
3. Funnell MM, Haas LB. National Standards for Diaetes Self-Management Education Programs. *Diabetes Care* 1995;18:100–116.
4. Mensing C, Boucher J, Cypress M, et al. National standards for diabetes self-management education. *Diabetes Care* 2000;23:682–689.
5. Quality recognition for diabetes patient education programs. Review criteria for national standards from the American Diabetes Association. *Diabetes Care* 1986;9:XXXVI–XL.
6. Paduano DJ, Anderson BJ, Ingram S, et al. Certification: progress and prospects for diabetes educators. National Certification Board for Diabetes Educators. *Diabetes Educ* 1987;13:206–208.
7. Sinnock P, Bauer DW. Reimbursement issues in diabetes. *Diabetes Care* 1984;7: 291–296.
8. Conrood BA, Betschart J, Harris MI. Frequency and determinants of diabetes patient education among adults in the U.S. population. *Diabetes Care* 1994;17: 852–858.
9. Cowie CC, Hanes MI. Ambulatory medical care for non-Hispanic whites, African-Americans, and Mexican-Americans with NIDDM in the U.S. *Diabetes Care* 1997;20:142–147.
10. Diabetes Control and Complications Trial Research Group. The effect of intensive treatment of diabetes on the development and progression of long-term complications in insulin-dependent diabetes mellitus. *N Engl J Med* 1993;329: 977–986.
11. UK Prospective Diabetes Study Group. Intensive blood-glucose control with sulphonylureas or insulin compared with conventional treatment and risk of complications in patients with type 2 diabetes mellitus (UKPDS 33). *Lancet* 1998;352:837–853.
12. Levetan CS, Salas JR, Wilets IF, et al. Impact of endocrine and diabetes team consultation on hospital length of stay for patients with diabetes. *Am J Med* 1995;99:22–28.
13. Korhonen T, Huttunen JK, Aro A, et al. A controlled trial on the effects of patient education in the treatment of insulin-dependent diabetes. *Diabetes Care* 1983;6:256–261.
14. Bloomgarden ZT, Karmally W, Metzger MJ, et al. Randomized controlled trial of diabetic patient education: improved knowledge without improved metabolic status. *Diabetes Care* 1987;10:263–272.
15. Brown SA. Effects of educational interventions in diabetes care: a meta-analysis of findings. *Nurs Res* 1988;37:223–230.
16. Padgett D, Mumford E, Hynes M, et al. Meta-analysis of the effects of educational and psychosocial interventions on the management of diabetes mellitus. *J Clin Epidemiol* 1988;41:1007–1030.
17. Brown SA. Studies of educational interventions and outcomes in diabetic adults: a meta-analysis revisited. *Patient Educ Couns* 1990;16:189–215.
18. Brown SA. Meta-analysis of diabetes education research: variations in intervention effects across studies. *Res Nurs Health* 1992;15:409–419.
19. Norris SL, Lau J, Smith SJ, et al. Self-management education for adults with type 2 diabetes: a meta-analysis of the effect on glycemic control. *Diabetes Care* 2002;25:1159–1171.
20. Abourizk NN, O'Connor PJ, Crabtree BF, et al. An outpatient model of integrated diabetes treatment and education: functional, metabolic, and knowledge outcomes. *Diabetes Educ* 1994;20:416–421.
21. Aubert RE, Herman WH, Waters J, et al. Nurse case management to improve glycemic control in diabetic patients in a health maintenance organization. *Ann Intern Med* 1998;129:605–612.
22. Glasgow RE, Toobert DJ, Hampson SE, et al. Improving self-care among older patients with type II diabetes: the "sixty-something..." study. *Patient Educ Couns* 1992;19:61–74.
23. Litzelman DK, Slemanda CW, Langefeld CD, et al. Reduction of lower extremity clinical abnormalities in patients with non-insulin-dependent diabetes mellitus: a randomized control trial. *Ann Intern Med* 1993;119:36–41.
24. Peyrot M, Rubin RR. Modeling the effect of diabetes education on glycemic control. *Diabetes Educ* 1994;20:143–148.
25. Peyrot M. Behavior change in diabetes education. *Diabetes Educ* 1999;25 [Suppl 6]:62–73.
26. Rickheim PL, Weaver TW, Flader JL, Kendall DM. Assessment of group versus individual diabetes education: a randomized study. *Diabetes Care* 2002;25:269–274.
27. Report of the AADE Diabetes Educational and Behavioral Research Summit. *Diabetes Educ* 1999 25[Suppl]26–35.
28. Report of the AADE Diabetes Educational and Behavioral Research Summit. *Diabetes Educ* 2001;27:899–907.
29. Glasgow RE. Outcomes of and for diabetes education research. *Diabetes Educ* 1999;25[Suppl 6]:74–88.
30. Jacobson AM, Weinger K. Treating depression in diabetic patients: is there an alternative to medications? *Ann Intern Med* 1998;129:656–657.
31. Kovacs M, Mukerji P, Iyengar S, et al. Psychiatric disorders and metabolic control among youths with IDDM: a longitudinal study. *Diabetes Care* 1996; 19:318–323.
32. Lustman P, Griffith LS, Clouse RE. Depression in adults with diabetes. *Semin Clin Neuropsychiatry* 1997;2:15–23.
33. Weinger K, Jacobson AM. Psychosocial and quality of life correlates of glycemic control during intensive treatment of type 1 diabetes. *Patient Educ Couns* 2001;42:123–131.
34. Mazzuca SA, Moorman NH, Wheeler ML, et al. The diabetes education study: a controlled trial of the effects of diabetes patient education. *Diabetes Care* 1986;9:1–10.
35. Peyrot MF, McMurray JF Jr. Stress buffering and glycemic control: the role of coping styles. *Diabetes Care* 1992;15:842–846.
36. Peyrot M, McMurry JF Jr, Kruger DF. A biopsychosocial model of glycemic control in diabetes: stress, coping and regimen adherence. *J Health Soc Behav* 1999;40:141–158.
37. Ruggerio L, Prochaska JO. Readiness for change: Introduction. *Diabetes Spectrum* 1993;6:22–24.
38. Rubin RR, Peyrot M, Saudek CD. Effect of diabetes education on self-care, metabolic control, and emotional well-being. *Diabetes Care* 1989;12:673–679.
39. Rubin RR, Peyrot M, Saudek CD. The effect of a diabetes education program incorporating coping skills training on emotional well-being and diabetes self-efficacy. *Diabetes Educ* 1993;19:210–214.
40. Wilson W, Ary DV, Biglan A, et al. Psychosocial predictors of self-care behaviors (compliance) and glycemic control in non-insulin-dependent diabetes mellitus. *Diabetes Care* 1986;9:614–622.
41. Jacobson AM, Hauser ST, Wolfsdorf JI. Psychological predictors of compliance in children with insulin-dependent diabetes. *Diabetes* 1986;35[Suppl 1]: 79A(abst).
42. Crabtree MK. Performance of diabetic self-care predicted by self-efficacy. *Diabetes* 1987;36[Suppl 1]:32A(abst).
43. Grey M, Boland EA, Davidson M, et al. Coping skills training for youths with diabetes on intensive therapy. *Appl Nurs Res* 1999;12:3–12.
44. Grey M, Boland EA, Davidson M, et al. Short-term effects of coping skills training as adjunct to intensive therapy in adolescents. *Diabetes Care* 1998;21:902–908.
45. Rubin RR, Peyrot M, Saudek CD. Differential effects of diabetes education on self-regulation and lifestyle behaviors. *Diabetes Care* 1991;14:335–338.
46. Implementation of treatment protocols in the Diabetes Control and Complications Trial. *Diabetes Care* 1995;18:361–376.
47. Delahanty L, Simkins SW, Camelon K. Expanded role of the dietitian in the Diabetes Control and Complications Trial: implications for clinical practice. The DCCT Research Group. *J Am Diet Assoc* 1993;93:768–772.
48. Franz MJ, Callahan T, Castle G. Changing roles: educators and clinicians. *Clin Diabetes* 1994;12:53–54.
49. Gilden JL, Hendryx M, Casia C, et al. The effectiveness of diabetes education programs for older patients and their spouses. *J Am Geriatr Soc* 1989;37: 1023–1030.
50. Koproski J, Pretto Z, Poretsky L. Effects of an intervention by a diabetes team in hospitalized patients with diabetes. *Diabetes Care* 1997;20:1553–1555.
51. Coast-Senior EA, Kroner BA, et al. Management of patients with type 2 diabetes by pharmacists in primary care clinics. *Ann Pharmacother* 1998;32:636–641.
52. Rettig BA, Shrauger DG, Recker RR, et al. A randomized study of the effects of a home diabetes education program. *Diabetes Care* 1986;9:173–178.
53. Mazzuca SA, Cohen SJ, Clark CM Jr, et al. The diabetes education study: two-year follow-up. *Diabetes* 1984;3[Suppl 1]:7A(abst).
54. Knowles M. *The adult learner: a neglected species*. Houston: Gulf Publishing Company, 1978.
55. Whitehouse FW, Whitehouse IJ, Smith J, et al. Teaching the person with diabetes: experience with a follow-up session. *Diabetes Care* 1979;2:35–38.
56. Anderson RM. Defining and evaluating diabetes patient education [Letter]. *Diabetes Care* 1983;6:619–620.
57. Glasgow RE, McCaul KD, Shafer LC. Self-care behaviors and glycemic control in type I diabetes. *J Chronic Dis* 1987;40:399–412.
58. Clement S. Diabetes self-management education. *Diabetes Care* 1995;18: 1204–1214.
59. Ahem JA, Kruger DF, Gatcomb PM, et al. Diabetes Control and Complications Trial (DCCT): the trial coordinator perspective—report of the DCCT Research Group. *Diabetes Educ* 1989;15:236–241.
60. Ahem J, Grove N, Strand T, et al. The impact of the trial coordinator in the Diabetes Control and Complications Trial (DCCT): the DCCT Research Group. *Diabetes Educ* 1993;19:509–512.
61. Lorenz RA, Bubb J, Davis D, et al. Changing behavior: practical lessons from the Diabetes Control and Complications Trial. *Diabetes Care* 1996;19:648–652.
62. Nicolucci A, Cavaliere D, Scorpiglione N, et al. A comprehensive assessment of the avoidability of long-term complications of diabetes. *Diabetes Care* 1996; 19:927–933.
63. Krall LP. Education: a treatment for diabetes. In: Marble A, Krall LP, Bradley RF, et al. *Joslin's diabetes mellitus*, 12th ed. Philadelphia: Lea & Febiger, 1985:465–484.
64. Geller J, Butler K. Study of educational deficits as the cause of hospital admission for diabetes mellitus in a community hospital. *Diabetes Care* 1981; 4:487–489.
65. Scott RS, Brown LJ, Clifford P. Use of health services by diabetic persons, II: hospital admissions. *Diabetes Care* 1985;8:43–47.
66. Zaremba MM, Willhoite B, Ra K. Self-reported data: reliability and role in determining program effectiveness. *Diabetes Care* 1985;8:486–490.
67. Fishbein HA. Precipitants of hospitalization in insulin-dependent diabetes mellitus (IDDM): a statewide perspective. *Diabetes Care* 1985;8[Suppl 1]:61–64.
68. Kaplan RM, Davis WK. Evaluating the costs and benefits of outpatient diabetes education and nutrition counseling. *Diabetes Care* 1986;9:81–86.
69. Third-party reimbursement for outpatient education and nutrition counseling. American Diabetes Association. *Diabetes Care* 1984;7:505–506.

70. Anderson RM. Assessing value of diabetes patient education [Letter]. *Diabetes Care* 1986;9:553.
71. Resource utilization and costs of care in the Diabetes Control and Complications Trial. *Diabetes Care* 1995;18:1468–1478.
72. Herman WH, Eastman RC. The effects of treatment on the direct costs of diabetes. *Diabetes Care* 1998;21[Suppl 3]:C19–C24.
73. Selby JV, Ray GT, Zhang D, Colby CJ. Excess costs of medical care for patients with diabetes in a managed care population. *Diabetes Care* 1997;20:1396–1402.
74. Gilmer TP, O'Connor PJ, Manning WG, et al. The cost to health plans of poor glycemic control. *Diabetes Care* 1997;20:1847–1853.
75. Rubin RJ, Dietrich KA, Hawk AK. Clinical and economic impact of implementing a comprehensive diabetes management program in managed care. *J Clin Endocrinol Metab* 1998;83:2635–2642.
76. Javor KA, Katsanos JG, McDonald RC, et al. Diabetic ketoacidosis changes relative to medical charges of adult patients with type 1 diabetes. *Diabetes Care* 1997;20:349–354.
77. Eastman RC, Javitt JC, Harman WH, et al. Model of complications of NIDDM. *Diabetes Care* 1997;20:735–744.
78. American Diabetes Association. ADA patient bill of rights. *Diabetes Forecast* 1983;36.
79. Third-party reimbursement for outpatient diabetes education and counseling. American Diabetes Association. *Diabetes Care* 1990;13[Suppl 1]:36.
80. Third-party reimbursement for diabetes care, self-management education, and supplies. American Diabetes Association. *Diabetes Care* 2000;23[Suppl 1]: S111–S112.
81. Martinez NC, Deane DM. Impact of prospective payment on the role of the diabetes educator. *Diabetes Educ* 1989;15:503–509.
82. Hiss RG, Frey ML, Davis WK. Diabetes patient education in the office setting. *Diabetes Educ* 1986;12:281–285.
83. McCaughrin WC. Legal precedents in American law for patient education. *Patient Counsel Health Educ* 1979;1:135–141.
84. Read DA, Greene WH. *Creative teaching in health*. New York: Macmillan, 1971:5.
85. Valentine V. Empowering patients for change. *Practical Diabetol* 1990;9:13.
86. Duchin SP, Brown SA. Patients should participate in designing diabetes educational content. *Patient Educ Couns* 1990;16:255–267.
87. Assal J, Jacquement S, Morel Y. The added value of therapy in diabetes: the education of patients for self-management of their disease. *Metabolism* 1997; 46[Suppl 1]:61–64.
88. Brown SA. Interventions to promote diabetes self-management: state of the science. *Diabetes Educ* 1999;25[Suppl 6]:52–61.
89. Funnell MM, Anderson RM. Putting Humpty Dumpty back together again: reintegrating the clinical and behavioral components in diabetes care and education. *Diabetes Spectrum* 1999;12:19–23.
90. Joslin EP. *A diabetic manual for the mutual use of doctor and patient*, 3rd ed. Philadelphia: Lea & Febiger, 1924:21.
91. Satterfield DW, Davidson JK. The team approach to evaluation, education, and treatment. In: Davidson JK, ed. *Clinical diabetes mellitus: a problem-oriented approach*. New York: Thieme, 1986:128–141.
92. Franz M, et al. *Goals for diabetes education. American Diabetes Association Task Group on Goals for Diabetes Education*. Alexandria, VA: American Diabetes Association. 1986.
93. Anderson RM, Funnell MM, Butler PM, et al. Patient empowerment: results of a randomized controlled trial. *Diabetes Care* 1995;18:943–949.
94. Williams GC, Freedman ZR, Deci EL. Supporting autonomy to motivate patients with diabetes for glucose control. *Diabetes Care* 1998;21:1644–1651.
95. Urban AD, Rearson MA, Murphy K. The diabetes center home care nurse: an integral part of the diabetes team. *Diabetes Educ* 1998;24:608–611.
96. Brink S, Simineria L, Hinnen-Hentzen D, et al. *Diabetes education goals*. Alexandria: VA: American Diabetes Association, 1995.
97. Pieber TR, Brunner GA, Schnedl WJ, et al. Evaluation of a structured outpatient group education program for intensive insulin treatment. *Diabetes Care* 1995;18:625–630.
98. Heller SR, Clarke P, Daly H, et al. Group education for obese patients with type 2 diabetes: greater success at less cost. *Diab Med* 1988;5:552–556.
99. Glasgow RE, Toobert DJ, Hampson SE, et al. A brief office-based intervention to facilitate diabetes dietary self-management. *Health Educ Res* 1995;10:467–478.
100. Glasgow RE, Toobert DJ, Hampson SE. Effects of a brief office-based intervention to facilitate diabetes dietary self-management. *Diabetes Care* 1996;19: 835–842.
101. Lewis D. The Internet as a resource for healthcare information. *Diabetes Educ* 1998;24:627–630, 632.
102. Lewis D. Computer-based patient education: use by diabetes educators. *Diabetes Educ* 1996;22:140–145.
103. Management of diabetes at diabetes camps. American Diabetes Association. *Diabetes Care* 1999;22:167–169.
104. Misuraca A, Di Gennaro M, Lioniello M, et al. Summer camps for diabetic children: an experience in Campania, Italy. *Diabetes Res Clin Pract* 1996;32:91–96.
105. Ruggerio L. Helping people with diabetes change behavior: from theory to practice. *Diabetes Spectrum* 2000;13:125–132.
106. Redman BK. *The process of patient education*, 6th ed. St. Louis: Mosby, 1988: 21–48.
107. Hamburg BA, Inoff GE. Coping with predictable crises of diabetes. *Diabetes Care* 1983;6:409–416.
108. Ley P. Satisfaction, compliance, and communication. *Br J Clin Psych* 1982;21: 241–254.
109. Page P, Verstraete DG, Robb JR, et al. Patient recall of self-care recommendations in diabetes. *Diabetes Care* 1981;4:96–98.
110. Ruggiero L, Glasgow R, Dryfoos JM, et al. Diabetes self-management. Self-reported recommendations and patterns in a large population. *Diabetes Care* 1997;20:568–576.
111. McLeod B. *Program development for diabetes*. Toronto: Canadian Diabetes Association, 1988.
112. Glasgow RE, Anderson RM. In diabetes care, moving from compliance to adherence is not enough. Something entirely different is needed. *Diabetes Care* 1999;22:2090–2092.
113. Liesenfeld B, Heekeren H, Schade G, et al. Quality of documentation in medical reports of diabetic patients. *Int J Qual Healthcare* 1996;8:537–542.
114. Midwest Medical Insurance Company Risk Management Committee. Medical record documentation—is yours a help or a hindrance in a lawsuit? *S Dakota J Med* 1998;51:51–52.
115. Grebe SK, Smith RB. Clinical audit and standardised follow up improve quality of documentation in diabetes care. *N Z Med J* 1995;108:339–342.
116. Resler MM. Teaching strategies that promote adherence. *Nurs Clin North Am* 1983;18:799–811.
117. Jacobson AM, Weinger K. Psychosocial complications in diabetes. In: Leahy J, Clark NG, Cefalu WT, eds. *Medical management of diabetes*. New York: Marcel Dekker, 2000:559–572.
118. Rosenstock IM. Understanding and enhancing patient compliance with diabetic regimens. *Diabetes Care* 1985;8:610–616.
119. Walker EA. Characteristics of the adult learner. *Diabetes Educ* 1999;25[Suppl 6]:16–24.
120 Alogna M. Assessment of patient knowledge and performance. In: Steiner G, Lawrence PA, eds. *Educating diabetic patients*. New York: Springer, 1981:146–153.
121. Barr P, Hess G, Frey ML. Relationship between reading levels and effective patient education. *Diabetes* 1986;35[Suppl 1]:48A(abst).
122. Schillinger D, Grumbach K, Piette J, et al. Association of health literacy with diabetes outcomes. *JAMA* 2002;288:475–482.
123. Gagné RM, Briggs LJ, Wager WW. *Principles of instructional design*. Fort Worth: Harcourt Brace Jovanovich College Publishers, 1992.
124. Lorenz RA. Teaching skills of health professionals. *Diabetes Educ* 1989;15: 149–152.
125. Greenfield S, Kaplan SH, Ware JE Jr. Patients' participation in medical care: effects on blood sugar control and quality of life in diabetes. *J Gen Intern Med* 1988;3:448–457.
126. Rost K. The influence of patient participation on satisfaction and compliance. *Diabetes Educ* 1989;15:139–143.
127. Roter DL. Patient participation in the patient-provider interaction: the effects of patient question asking on the quality of interaction, satisfaction and compliance. *Health Educ Monogr* 1977;5:281–315.
128. Rothert ML, Talarczyk GJ. Patient compliance and the decision-making process of clinicians and patients. *J Compliance Healthcare* 1987;2:55–71.
129. Stewart MA. What is a successful doctor-patient interview? A study of interactions and outcomes. *Soc Sci Med* 1984;19:167–175.
130. Sims DF, Sims EAH. Commentary. *Diabetes Spectrum* 1990;3:227–228.
131. Lutfey KE, Wishner WJ. Beyond 'compliance' is 'adherence.' Improving the prospect of diabetes care. *Diabetes Care* 1999;22:635–639.
132. Davis M, Eschelman ER, Mckay M. *The relaxation and stress reduction workbook*. Oakland, CA: New Harbinger Publications, 1988.
133. Strecher VJ, Seijts GH, Kok GJ, et al. Goal setting as a strategy for health behavior change. *Health Educ Q* 1995;22:190–200.
134. Kaplan RM, Chadwick MW, Schimmel LE. Social learning intervention to promote metabolic control in type I diabetes mellitus: pilot experiment results. *Diabetes Care* 1985;8:152–155.
135. Ley P, Bradshaw PW, Kincey JA, et al. Increasing patients' satisfaction with communications. *Br J Soc Clin Psychol* 1976;15:403–413.
136. Tabak ER. The relationship of information exchange during medical visits to patient satisfaction: a review. *Diabetes Educ* 1987;13:36–40.
137. Campbell LV, Barth R, Bosper JK, et al. Impact of intensive educational approach to dietary change in NIDDM. *Diabetes Care* 1990;13:841–847.
138. Hosey GM, Freeman WL, Stracqualursi F, et al. Designing and evaluating diabetes education material for American Indians. *Diabetes Educ* 1990;16: 407–414.
139. Overland JE, Hoskins PL, McGill MJ, et al. Low literacy: a problem in diabetes education. *Diabet Med* 1993;10:847–850.
140. McNeal B, Salisbury Z, Baumgardner P, et al. Comprehension assessment of diabetes education program participants. *Diabetes Care* 1984;7:232–235.
141. Dale E, Chall JS. *A formula for predicting readability*. Columbus: Ohio State University Press, 1948.
142. Flesch RF. A new readability yardstick. *J Appl Psychol* 1948;32:221–233.
143. Fry E. A readability formula that saves time. *J Reading* 1958;11:513–578.
144. McLaughlin GH. SMOG grading—a new readability formula. *J Reading* 1969; 12:639–646.
145. Doak CC, Doak LG, Root JH. *Teaching patients with low literacy skills*. Philadelphia: JB Lippincott Co, 1985.
146. Plimpton S, Root J. Materials and strategies that work in low literacy health communication. *Public Health Rep* 1994;109:86–92.
147. Anderson RM, Nowacek G, Richards F. Influencing the personal meaning of diabetes: research and practice. *Diabetes Educ* 1988;14:297–302.
148. Boulton C, Garth RY. *Students in learning groups: active learning through conversation*. San Francisco: Jossey-Bass, 1983:73–81.

149. Finkel DL, Monk GS. *Teachers and learning groups: dissolution of the atlas complex*. San Francisco: Jossey-Bass, 1983:83–97.
150. Istre SM. The art and science of successful teaching continuing education credit. *Diabetes Educ* 1989;15:67–76.
151. Lorenz RA. Training health professionals to improve the effectiveness of patient education programs. *Diabetes Educ* 1986[Suppl];12:204–209.
152. Sanson-Fisher RW, Campbell EM, Redman S, et al. Patient-provider interactions and patient outcomes. *Diabetes Educ* 1989;15:134–138.
153. Sackett DL. The magnitude of compliance and non-compliance. In: Sackett DL, Haynes RB, eds. *Compliance with therapeutic regimens.* Baltimore: The Johns Hopkins University Press, 1976:9–25.
154. Haynes RB, McKibbon KA, Kanani R. Systematic review of randomized trials of interventions to assist patients to follow prescriptions for medications. *Lancet* 1996;348:383–386.
155. Haynes RB, McKibbon KA, Kanani R. Systematic review of randomized trials of interventions to assist patients to follow prescriptions for medications. *Lancet* 1996;348:383–386.
156. Paes AHP, Bakker A, Soe-Agnie CJ. Impact of dosage frequency on patient compliance. *Diabetes Care* 1997;20:1512–1517.
157. Speers MA, Turk DC. Diabetes self care: knowledge, beliefs, motivation and action. *Patient Couns Health Educ* 1982;3:144–149.
158. Eraker SK, Becker MH. Improving compliance for the patient with diabetes. *Practical Diabetol* 1984;3:6–11.
159. Westberg J, Jason H. Building a helpful relationship: the foundation of effective patient education. *Diabetes Educ* 1986;12:374–378.
160. Becker MH. Theoretical models of adherence and strategies for improving adherence. In: Shumaker S, et al, eds. *The handbook of health behavior change.* New York: Springer, 1990.
161. Bradley C. Health beliefs and knowledge of patients and doctors in clinical practice and research. *Patient Educ Couns* 1995;26:99–106.
162. Bradley C. Measures of perceived control of diabetes. In: Bradley C, ed. *Handbook of psychology and diabetes.* Great Britain: Harwood Academic Publishing, 1994:291–331.
163. Wooldridge KL, Wallston KA, Graber AL, et al. The relationship between health beliefs, adherence, and metabolic control of diabetes. *Diabetes Educ* 1992;18:495–500.
164. Maiman LA, Becker MH. The clinician's role in patient compliance. *Trends Pharmacol Sci* 1980;1:457–459.
165. Coates VE, Boore JR. The influence of psychological factors on the self-management of insulin-dependent diabetes mellitus. *J Adv Nurs* 1998;27:528–537.
166. Polley BA, Jakicic JM, Venditti EM, et al. The effects of health beliefs on weight loss in individuals at high risk for NIDDM. *Diabetes Care* 1997;20:1533–1538.
167. Strowig S. Patient education: a model for autonomous decision-making and deliberate action in diabetes self-management. *Med Clin North Am* 1982;66:1293–1307.
168. Harris G. Filling the gaps between patients and professionals. *Diabetes Educ* 1987;13:133–136.
169. Tilly KF, Belton AB, McLachlan JFC. Continuous monitoring of health status outcomes: experience with diabetes education program. *Diabetes Educ* 1995;21:413–419.
170. Tildesley HD, Mair K, Sharpe J, et al. Diabetes teaching—outcome analysis. *Patient Educ Couns* 1996;29:59–65.
171. O'Connor PJ, Rush WA, Peterson J, et al. Continuous quality improvement can improve glycemic control for HMO patients with diabetes. *Arch Fam Med* 1996;5:502–506.

CHAPTER 36

Medical Nutrition Therapy

Karen Hanson Chalmers

A BRIEF HISTORY OF NUTRITION AND DIABETES

More than 50 years ago, Elliott Joslin stated:

> The diet in health is made up chiefly of carbohydrate; the diet in diabetes before the discovery of insulin was made up chiefly of fat. Insulin has changed all this. The task of the modern diabetic is not so much to learn how to live comfortably upon less carbohydrate and more fat, but rather to balance the carbohydrate in his diet with insulin so that he can utilize it and thus keep his urine sugar-free. (1)

Little did Dr. Joslin realize that his guidelines would still hold true at the beginning of the 21st century.

Patients have identified "diet" as one of the most challenging aspects of their diabetes regimen. However, countless events have resulted in positive changes in nutrition science as it relates to diabetes. From the rigidly controlled, semistarvation diets in ancient times to the present "all-foods-can-fit," we have arrived at nutrition science as we know it today—medical nutrition therapy.

One of the earliest references to a so-called diabetic diet was noted in a medical writing as far back as 1550 B.C., although for the first 3,500 years of diabetes history, no clear distinction was made between type 1 and type 2 diabetes. The writings recommended a diet high in carbohydrates, which included fruit, wheat grain, and sweet beer to stop the passing of too much urine. Aretaeus, a follower of Hippocrates, first used the name *diabetes* in the first century A.D. to describe the "melting down of flesh and limbs into the urine" (2). He concluded that diabetes was a disease of the stomach and should be treated with milk, gruel, cereals, fruits, and sweet wines. Milk, water, wine, and beer were used as the main fluids to relieve excessive thirst until the second century A.D., when diabetes was thought to be a disease of the kidneys. At this time, restriction of fluids was recommended. By the sixth century, diabetes was thought to be directly caused by overeating and thought to be a disease of "sweet urine" (3).

Little information about diabetes and food is mentioned again until the late 1600s, when the suggested diabetic diet returned to foods higher in carbohydrates, such as milk, bread, and barley water. Also, at this time, opium was introduced as a staple of the diet to decrease appetite, as physicians recognized that those people with diabetes who ate the least food lived the longest.

In the late 1700s, a French physician began prescribing undernutrition or semistarvation diets, interspersed with frequent periods of fasting, for those with diabetes. Finally, a physician from England related carbohydrates to high glucose levels and excessive urination. Again, the diet reverted back to low carbohydrates and included more fat and protein in the form of milk, butter, suet, and rancid meats. Low-carbohydrate vegetables were added only when the urine became completely sugar free. Although fat in the diabetic diet was further liberalized to add enough calories for survival, most people with diabetes could not adhere to the extremely limited quantity of food. Those people with diabetes who were "thin" did not survive, whereas those people with diabetes who were "fat" improved.

In the early 1900s, Dr. Frederick M. Allen, in the United States, developed his starvation diet and was one of the first to tailor foods in diets to his patients' preferences while still providing only 1,000 calories a day. Although many of his patients were malnourished, he is credited with helping many survive before the introduction of insulin therapy in 1921 (3).

The starvation diet disappeared with the discovery of insulin. The prescribed diabetic diet was still 4% carbohydrate, 21% protein, and 75% fat—all measured and weighed to exact amounts. Although no consistent food lists were available at the time, the carbohydrate foods were categorized according to the amount of carbohydrate each food contained, e.g., 5%, 10%, and 20% vegetables. Vegetables were cooked three times, the water changed each time to remove as much carbohydrate as possible. Even after insulin was initiated, Dr. Elliott P. Joslin continued to use a high-fat, carbohydrate-restricted diet for his "severe diabetics" and noted in his first preinsulin *Diabetic Manual* that "olive oil forms an excellent lunch for a diabetic" (1). Dr. Joslin gradually increased his diet for "mild diabetics" to 23% carbohydrate, 15% protein, and 62% fat.

In the 1940s, it became evident that there was a great need to develop consistent and standardized food values and to design a simple method for planning the diabetic diet. The American Dietetic Association, the American Diabetes Association, and the diabetes branch of the U.S. Public Health Service developed a method that became what we know today as the exchange system. Six "convenient" sample meal plans were developed that detailed the grams of carbohydrate, protein, and fat for various calorie amounts. These plans were developed to be used by the health professional, who would modify the plan to suit the particular needs of the patient. Although the meal plans were not meant to be distributed to patients, they soon became widely available.

In the early 1970s, the sample meal plans were being used extensively. These preplanned diets did not focus on nutrition education or on follow-up by a registered dietitian. Patients quickly lost their motivation to adhere to these diets, and their interest in nutrition quickly diminished. A 1973 publication by Kelly West, *Diet Therapy of Diabetes: An Analysis of Failure*, examined deterrents to successful diet therapy, which included lack of physician support in promoting adequate nutrition care and of third-party reimbursement for dietary instruction for outpatients (4).

In the 1970s, the high-carbohydrate diet was rediscovered (5,6), and the officially recommended diet was higher in complex carbohydrate and lower in fat and protein than most of the earlier diets. The attitude toward sucrose and other sugars became more liberal. The American Diabetes Association began emphasizing the need for nutrition education about the exchange system. This eventually led to the publication in 1971 of the Association's *Principles of Nutrition and Dietary Recommendations* (7). The exchange lists for meal planning were revised in 1976, 1986, and again in 1995; each revision placed an increasing emphasis on carbohydrates. These changes reflect a move from the main focus on the lethal effects of short-term complications (ketoacidosis and hypoglycemia) to a new focus: concern about long-term complications.

The exchange system continued to be taught and used and was perceived as the diabetic diet until the 1980s. However, surveys from dietitians who provided nutrition education for patients with diabetes identified a need for a variety of meal-planning methods to be used in addition to the exchange system. In 1987, the Diabetes Care and Education Practice Group of the American Dietetic Association promoted the concept of the individualization of the meal planning approach to diabetes nutritional care with new nutrition resources for diabetes meal planning (8). More and more people with diabetes were seeking a dietitian's care and counseling for updating their methods of meal planning.

Current medical nutrition therapy recommendations for overall health of persons with diabetes are the same as those for all healthy Americans, as seen in the *U.S. Dietary Guidelines* 2000 (9). These guidelines include the following:

- Aim for a healthy weight
- Choose a variety of grains daily, especially whole grains
- Choose a variety of fruits and vegetables daily
- Choose a diet that is low in saturated fat and cholesterol and moderate in total fat
- Choose beverages and foods to moderate your intake of sugars
- Choose and prepare food with less salt
- If you drink alcoholic beverages, do so in moderation.

The volume of research on issues of nutrition and diabetes and the number of changes in nutrition recommendations over recent years are now greater than ever. The evolution of new knowledge is rapidly affecting the management of diet for the patient with diabetes. Therefore, the 2000 Dietary Guidelines, which are published every 5 years by the Department of Health and Human Services (HHS) and the Department of Agriculture (USDA), are currently in the process of review in light of recent scientific evidence to determine if revision is needed in the 2005 sixth edition. The USDA's Food Guide Pyramid, which was introduced in 1992, is also under review. Prominent experts in nutrition and health are now proposing a revised food guide pyramid that clearly emphasizes the benefits of healthy fats, daily exercise, and avoidance of excessive intake of calories. Recommendations promote high fiber, healthy and unprocessed carbohydrates, as well as adequate consumption of fresh fruits and vegetables. Healthy sources of protein are encouraged, such as nuts, legumes, fish, poultry, and eggs, whereas red meat, butter, refined grains, potatoes, and sugar are minimized.

The availability of a greater variety in the types of oral antidiabetes agents and insulins, together with the availability of technology from self-monitoring of blood glucose to continuous blood glucose sensors and insulin pump therapy, has allowed increased flexibility in meal planning. A continued research focus on the glycemic response of the nutrients—carbohydrate, protein, and fat—is gradually changing how we think about diet in diabetes.

The dietary management of type 2 diabetes is now recognized to be quite different from that of type 1 diabetes. Our knowledge about the treatment of obesity in diabetes also has increased. In addition, attention is being given to the special considerations required among different subgroups of people with diabetes, specifically the needs of ethnic minority groups, pregnant women, growing children and adolescents, and the elderly. Emphasis is placed on providing individualized, flexible meal plans that people are willing and able to follow. Dramatic changes in our methods of diabetes education have also been instituted in recent years. New strategies, knowledge, and techniques for teaching and improving the overall management of diabetes, as well as dietary management, were clearly demonstrated in the 1993 published results of the Diabetes Control and Complications Trial (DCCT) for those with type 1 diabetes (10) and the smaller Stockholm Diabetes Intervention Study (11) of similar design. These studies recognized the importance of a coordinated team approach to the achievement of nutrition goals. The diabetes team used in the DCCT consisted of the patient and family as the primary participants, a diabetes nurse educator, a registered dietitian, a behaviorist, and the diabetologist. Today, exercise physiologists also have been included as important members of the diabetes team. The DCCT also provided specific information about important nutrition intervention strategies, based firmly on scientific evidence. In 1994, shortly after publication of the DCCT clinical findings, the American Diabetes Association published a revised set of nutrition guidelines, refocusing on an "individualized approach to nutrition self-management that is appropriate for the personal life-style and diabetes management goals of the individual with diabetes" (12).

The results of another 20-year landmark study, the United Kingdom Prospective Diabetes Study (UKPDS) (13), for those with type 2 diabetes, were published in 1998 and further confirmed that the intensive use of pharmacologic therapy, together with diet and exercise, would have clinical benefits. In 1996, recruitment began for a more recent randomized clinical trial, The Diabetes Prevention Program (DPP) (14). The DPP was designed to test strategies to prevent or delay glucose concentrations and impaired glucose tolerance (IGT). This major clinical trial compared intensive lifestyle intervention (diet and exercise) with metformin treatment in 3,234 people with impaired glucose tolerance. Lifestyle intervention worked as well in men and women and in all ethnic groups, reducing the risk of getting type 2 diabetes by 58%. It also worked well in people age 60 and older, reducing their development of diabetes by 71%. Metformin was also effective in men and women and in all ethnic groups, reducing their risk of getting type 2 diabetes by 31%, but not as effective in the older volunteers and in those who were less overweight. The trial ended a year early because the data had clearly answered the main research questions. This is the first major trial to show that diet and exercise can prevent or delay diabetes in a diverse American population of overweight people with IGT and a major step toward reversing the epidemic of type 2 diabetes in the United States. A recently launched trial, the Look AHEAD (Action for Health in Diabetes) study, will examine how diet and exercise affect heart attack, stroke, and cardiovascular-disease–related death in people with type 2 diabetes.

Diet still remains the cornerstone of diabetes self-management, but additional research is needed to improve the contribution that diet can make for effective diabetes self-management.

GOALS OF MEDICAL NUTRITION THERAPY

Today, there is no one "diabetic diet." The current nutrition recommendations can be defined simply as "a nutrition prescription based on assessment and treatment goals and outcomes" (15). The 1994 American Diabetes Association nutrition recommendations redistributed the calories provided from the various macronutrients (12), and these recommendations still hold true today. Table 36.1 gives a historical perspective of nutrition recommendations. The American Diabetes Association recommends that the distribution of calories from carbohydrate and fat be based on nutritional assessment and on blood glucose, weight, and lipid goals, with continued emphasis on a diet with fewer than 10% of calories from saturated fats and with 10% to 20% of calories from protein (lean).

TABLE 36.1. Historical Perspective of Nutrition Recommendations for People with Diabetes

	Distribution of calories (%)		
Year	**Carbohydrate**	**Protein**	**Fat**
Before 1921	—	Starvation diets	—
1921	20	10	70
1950	40	20	70
1971	45	20	35
1986	<60	12–20	<30
1994	Based on nutritional assessment and treatment goals	10–20	Based on nutritional assessment and treatment goals; <10% of calories from saturated fats

TABLE 36.2. Goals of Medical Nutrition Therapy

1. Attain and maintain optimal metabolic outcomes, including
   - Blood glucose levels as near normal as possible to safely prevent or reduce the risk for complications of diabetes
   - Optimal serum lipid profile to reduce the risk for macrovascular disease
   - Blood pressure levels that decrease the risk for macrovascular disease
2. Prevent and treat chronic complications of diabetes by
   - Modification of nutrient intake and lifestyle for prevention and treatment of obesity, dyslipidemia, cardiovascular disease, hypertension, and nephropathy
3. Improve health through healthy food choices and physical activity
4. Address individual needs, such as
   - Personal and cultural preferences and lifestyle while respecting the individual's wishes and willingness to change

The goals of medical nutrition therapy are summarized in Table 36.2, which outlines the most recent recommendations of the American Diabetes Association (15) and are discussed in more detail below.

Goals in Type 1 Diabetes

The primary goals of therapy for persons with type 1 diabetes are as follows:

- Provision of an individualized meal plan based on usual food intake and lifestyle. This plan is used as the basis for integrating insulin therapy into the usual eating and exercise patterns.
- Consistency of carbohydrate intake to allow the synchronization of mealtimes with times of insulin action for persons receiving *fixed insulin regimens.*
- Determination of premeal insulin dose and postprandial blood glucose response by monitoring of blood glucose levels and adjusting insulin doses for the amount of total carbohydrate consumed for persons receiving *intensive insulin therapy.*
- Prevention of weight gain is desirable, with attention therefore paid to total caloric intake from carbohydrate, protein, and fat, for persons with improved glycemic control.
- Adjustment of rapid- or short-acting insulin for deviations from usual eating and exercise habits is the preferred choice for prevention of hypoglycemia. Additional carbohydrate may be needed for unplanned exercise.

Goals in Type 2 Diabetes

The primary goals of therapy for persons with type 2 diabetes depend on body weight and level of glucose control.

- Emphasis on lifestyle changes that result in reduced caloric intake and increased energy expenditure through physical activity for those who are overweight and insulin resistant
- Achievement and maintenance of glucose, lipid, and blood pressure goals by reduction in dietary intake of carbohydrate, saturated fat, cholesterol, and sodium when necessary
- Maintenance of moderate caloric restriction and a nutritionally adequate meal plan with a reduction of carbohydrate and total fat—especially saturated fat—together with an increase in exercise for those with excessive weight
- Increase of activity and exercise to improve glycemia, decrease insulin resistance, and reduce cardiovascular risk factors

CALORIES

> The diet of the diabetic patient should contain the minimum number of calories which the normal individual would require under similar conditions. If the patient is allowed more than the minimum amount of food there is far more likelihood that a portion will be lost, unassimilated, and appear as sugar in the urine. (1)

Prescribing enough calories (kilocalories, or kcals) to achieve and maintain a desirable weight should be carefully considered. Caloric requirements for persons with diabetes are not different from those for persons without diabetes, assuming the person with diabetes is not losing calories through glycosuria. Caloric needs vary with a patient's weight, age, gender, activity level, and genetic background. The recommended calorie level is based on the weight that the patient and his or her healthcare provider acknowledge as one that can be achieved and maintained, for both the short term and the long term. This may not be the same as ideal body weight.

Persons with type 1 diabetes are often thin when the diagnosis is first made, and the diet should include enough calories to ensure normal growth and development and to sustain the usual level of physical activity. For infants, children, and adolescents, caloric intake should maintain consistent growth curves based on energy needs during periods of growth and

TABLE 36.3. Estimating Caloric Intake and Desirable Body Weight for Adults

Estimating caloric intake	
Basal calories: 10 kcal/lb desirable body weight	
Add calories for activity	
If sedentary, add 10% of estimated base calories	
If moderately active, add 20% of estimated base calories	
If strenuously active, add 40% of estimated base calories	
Adjustments[a]	
Estimating desirable body weights from frame size	
Women	100 lb for first 5 ft plus 5 lb for each additional inch
Men	106 lb for first 5 ft plus 6 lb for each additional inch
Small frame	Subtract 10%
Large frame	Add 10%

[a]Adjustments are approximate; weight changes should be monitored and compared with caloric intake.
Adapted from Vinik A, Wing RR. Nutritional management of the person with diabetes. In: Rifkin H, Porte D Jr, eds. *Diabetes mellitus*, 4th ed. New York: Elsevier, 1990.

sexual maturation. The prescribed calories must be adjusted on a regular basis. If diabetes is not properly controlled, growth may be retarded and the height potential may not be reached. Any abnormal or unexplained deviation in growth and weight demands an assessment of diabetes control, eating patterns, and caloric intake, as well as insulin dosage.

Persons with type 2 diabetes are often overweight when the diagnosis is first made. A moderate weight loss (5 to 9 kg), irrespective of the patient's starting weight, is perhaps the most important aspect of medical nutrition therapy and is associated with an improvement in lipids, blood glucose, and blood pressure (15–19). Weight loss leads to a reduction in insulin resistance and has long-term effects on the maintenance of reduced blood glucose levels. Overweight and obese patients with type 2 diabetes should be encouraged to attain a reasonable weight rather than attempting to achieve the traditionally defined desirable or ideal body weight. Setting intermediate weight goals may be useful when a patient becomes overwhelmed by the magnitude of his or her necessary weight loss. Weight management also should include behavioral modification to encourage healthy eating behaviors, together with increased physical activity. A moderate reduction in calories of approximately 250 to 500 kcal per day less than the average daily intake (calculated from a food history) can result in losses of 2 to 4 kg per month, a rate that is considered excellent.

Several different means of estimating desirable body weight and caloric needs are included in Table 36.3. The recommended calorie level need not be absolutely precise but should be considered a starting point for fine-tuning during follow-up until a level has been established that will help the patient achieve his or her goals for weight and blood glucose levels.

There is evidence to support the use of body mass index (BMI) (Table 36.4) in risk assessment for the diagnosis of diabetes or response to weight loss. The BMI provides a more accurate

TABLE 36.4. Body Mass Index Table

	19	20	21	22	23	24	25	26	27	28	29	30	31	32	33	34	35
Height (in.)								**Body weight (pounds)**									
58	91	96	100	105	110	115	119	124	129	134	138	143	148	153	158	162	167
59	94	99	104	109	114	119	124	128	133	138	143	148	153	158	163	168	173
60	97	102	107	112	118	123	128	133	138	143	148	153	158	163	168	174	179
61	100	106	111	116	122	127	132	137	143	148	153	158	164	169	174	180	185
62	104	109	115	120	126	131	136	142	147	153	158	164	169	175	180	186	191
63	107	113	118	124	130	135	141	146	152	158	163	169	175	180	186	191	197
64	110	116	122	128	134	140	145	151	157	163	169	174	180	186	192	197	204
65	114	120	126	132	138	144	150	156	162	168	174	180	186	192	198	204	210
66	118	124	130	136	142	148	155	161	167	173	179	186	192	198	204	210	216
67	121	127	134	140	146	153	159	166	172	178	185	191	198	204	211	217	223
68	125	131	138	144	151	158	164	171	177	184	190	197	203	210	216	223	230
69	128	135	142	149	155	162	169	176	182	189	196	203	209	216	223	230	236
70	132	139	146	153	160	167	174	181	188	195	202	209	216	222	229	236	243
71	136	143	150	157	165	172	179	186	193	200	208	215	222	229	236	243	250
72	140	147	154	162	169	177	184	191	199	206	213	221	228	235	242	250	258
73	144	151	159	166	174	182	189	197	204	212	219	227	235	242	250	257	265
74	148	155	163	171	179	186	194	202	210	218	225	233	241	249	256	264	272
75	152	160	168	176	184	192	200	208	216	224	232	240	248	256	264	272	279
76	156	164	172	180	189	197	205	213	221	230	238	246	254	263	271	279	287

	36	37	38	39	40	41	42	43	44	45	46	47	48	49	50	51	52	53	54
Height (in.)									**Body weight (pounds)**										
58	172	177	181	186	191	196	201	205	210	215	220	224	229	234	239	244	248	253	258
59	178	183	188	193	198	203	208	212	217	222	227	232	237	242	247	252	257	262	267
60	184	189	194	199	204	209	215	220	225	230	235	240	245	250	255	261	266	271	276
61	190	195	201	206	211	217	222	227	232	238	243	248	254	259	264	269	275	280	285
62	196	202	207	213	218	224	229	235	240	246	251	256	262	267	273	278	284	289	295
63	203	208	214	220	225	231	237	242	248	254	259	265	270	278	282	287	293	299	304
64	209	215	221	227	232	238	244	250	256	262	267	273	279	285	291	296	302	308	314
65	216	222	228	234	240	246	252	258	264	270	276	282	288	294	300	306	312	318	324
66	223	229	235	241	247	253	260	266	272	278	284	291	297	303	309	315	322	328	334
67	230	236	242	249	255	261	268	274	280	287	293	299	306	312	319	325	331	338	344
68	236	243	249	256	262	269	276	282	289	295	302	308	315	322	328	335	341	348	354
69	243	250	257	263	270	277	284	291	297	304	311	318	324	331	338	345	351	358	365
70	250	257	264	271	278	285	292	299	306	313	320	327	334	341	348	355	362	369	376
71	257	265	272	279	286	293	301	308	315	322	329	338	343	351	358	365	372	379	386
72	265	272	279	287	294	302	309	316	324	331	338	346	353	361	368	375	383	390	397
73	272	280	288	295	302	310	318	325	333	340	348	355	363	371	378	386	393	401	408
74	280	287	295	303	311	319	326	334	342	350	358	365	373	381	389	396	404	412	420
75	287	295	303	311	319	327	335	343	351	359	367	375	383	391	399	407	415	423	431
76	295	304	312	320	328	336	344	353	361	369	377	385	394	402	410	418	426	435	443

To use the table, find the appropriate height in the left-hand column. Move across to a given weight. The number at the top of the column is the BMI at that height and weight.
From National Institute of Health, National Heart, Lung, and Blood Institute, North American Association for the Study of Obesity. The practical guide: identification, evaluation, and treatment of overweight and obesity in adults. NIH publication no. 00-4084, October 2000.

TABLE 36.5. Classification of Overweight and Obesity by Body Mass Index, Waist Circumference, and Associated Disease Risk

	BMI (kg/m²)	Obesity class	Disease risk[a] relative to normal weight and waist circumference: M<102 cm (≤40 in.) W<88 cm (≤35 in.)	M>102 cm (>40 in.) W>88 cm (>35 in.)
Underweight	≤18.5		—	—
Normal[b]	18.5–24.9		—	—
Overweight	25.0–29.9		Increased	High
Obese	30.0–34.9	I	High	Very high
	35.0–39.9	II	Very high	Very high
Extremely obese	≥40	III	Extremely high	Extremely high

M, men; W, women.
[a]Disease risk for type 2 diabetes, hypertension, and cardiovascular disease.
[b]Increased waist circumference can also be a marker for increased risk even in persons of normal weight.
From National Institutes of Health, National Heart, Lung, and Blood Institute, North American Association for the Study of Obesity. The practical guide: identification, evaluation, and treatment of overweight and obesity in adults. NIH publication no. 00-4084, October 2000.

measure of total body fat than does assessment of body weight alone. Measurement of waist circumference (20) is particularly helpful when patients are categorized as normal or overweight. Men whose waist circumference is greater than 40 inches and women whose waist circumference is greater than 35 inches are at high risk of diabetes, dyslipidemia, hypertension, and cardiovascular disease because of excess abdominal fat. The relationship between BMI and waist circumference for defining risk is shown in Table 36.5.

CARBOHYDRATE

> The diet of the normal and diabetic individuals differs very little these days, chiefly because of the discovery of insulin. At one time my hospital patients did not have over 30 grams of carbohydrates per day, or the equivalent of about one ounce or two tablespoons of sugar. Today no patient has less than 150 grams of carbohydrate or the equivalent of 10 tablespoonfuls of sugar or 10 slices of bread. (1)

Calories from carbohydrate are variable and should be individualized on the basis of nutritional assessment, diabetes treatment goals, other medical issues, and the patient's eating habits and response of blood glucose to carbohydrate intake.

If protein contributes 10% to 20% of calories, carbohydrate and fat can be distributed between the remaining 80% and 90% of calories, after the blood glucose and lipid levels are taken into account (21). Although carbohydrate foods vary in the ability to promote good health, the total amount of carbohydrate consumed is more important than the source or the type of carbohydrate. Even sucrose-containing foods may be substituted for other carbohydrate grams and are acceptable as long as these foods are within the context of a healthy meal plan and metabolic control and desirable body weight are maintained.

A nutrition prescription (based on nutritional assessment and treatment goals) may result in a reduction in carbohydrate and dietary fat—particularly saturated fat—which in turn reduces cardiovascular risk. Although there are supportive studies indicating that high-carbohydrate meal plans improve glucose tolerance and insulin sensitivity (21–24), there is still some disagreement about what constitutes the optimal percentage of carbohydrate for persons with diabetes (25,26). Although some researchers are concerned about high-carbohydrate diets and their potential for influencing glucose and lipid metabolism and blood pressure (27–32), others have demonstrated that the limited elevation in lipids can be prevented if carbohydrate and fiber in the diet are increased in parallel (33–35). Joslin Diabetes Center has recently updated nutrition recommendations for people with type 2 diabetes who are overweight and obese. Although additional research will be required to define the maximum nutrients that promote both blood glucose control and weight loss success, we currently assess each patient individually to determine an appropriate meal plan composition based on reducing calories to achieve a negative caloric balance and using the guidelines below:

Carbohydrates. No more than 40% of total daily calorie intake should come from carbohydrates, which should be mainly low-glycemic-index foods such as vegetables, fruits, and whole and minimally processed grains. Refined carbohydrates or processed grains and starchy food such as pasta, bread, cereal, and white potatoes should be avoided or consumed in limited quantities.

Protein. To maintain muscle mass and energy expenditure, 30% of total daily calorie intake should come from protein. Preferable protein sources include fish, particularly cold water fish such as salmon, tuna, or sardines, and chicken, turkey, and other poultry and soy, rather than red or processed meat. Furthermore, data suggest that protein aids in the sensation of fullness and that low-protein meal plans are associated with increased hunger. Thus, protein may serve to reduce appetite and assist one in achieving and maintaining the desired lower calorie level.

Fat. Of total daily calorie intake 30% should come from fat, which should be mainly derived from monounsaturated and polyunsaturated fat (e.g., nuts, olive oil, canola oil) and fish, particularly those high in omega-3 fatty acids. Meats high in saturated fat, including beef, pork, lamb, and high-fat dairy products, should be consumed only in small amounts. Similarly, foods high in trans-fatty acids should be avoided.

The above distribution of nutrients for overweight and obese people with type 2 diabetes will

- Promote long-term weight loss in those with type 2 diabetes. The combination of restricting calories while increasing the intake of protein and low-glycemic-index foods may diminish the sensation of hunger.
- Improve blood glucose control because of the relatively lower carbohydrate content and the lower glycemic index of those carbohydrates that are consumed.

- Improve the body's response to insulin (insulin sensitivity), whether or not weight loss is achieved.
- Improve blood lipid profile, particularly triglycerides and high-density lipoprotein (HDL) cholesterol, whether or not weight loss is achieved.
- Reduce the stress on the insulin-producing cells in the pancreas by reducing the need for as much insulin.

It is also important to recognize that a meal plan prescription alone is not sufficient to maximize significant and sustained weight loss. Physical activity, behavior modification, and good support systems are extremely important adjuncts to the dietary prescription described above.

Glycemic Index

All complex carbohydrates and all simple carbohydrates (or sugars) traditionally were thought to generate different blood glucose responses based on molecular structure. However, an inconsistent relationship of glucose response demonstrated from so-called simple and complex carbohydrates suggests this terminology may be misleading and restrictive in meal planning. The position of the American Diabetes Association is that priority should be given to the total amount rather than the source of carbohydrate. Controversy is ongoing about whether the ingestion of similar amounts of carbohydrate foods produces different blood glucose and insulin responses and whether this information will have useful clinical applications.

In 1981, Jenkins et al. (36) suggested that the blood glucose and insulin response to a food could be expressed as a glycemic index, which quantifies the postprandial glucose response to a particular food in comparison to the response to a standard amount of glucose, or an attempt to classify foods by the extent to which they raise the blood glucose level. Glucose alone produces the largest increase in blood glucose level and is assigned a glycemic index of 100. Fiber-rich foods, acidic foods, and high-fat foods often have low glycemic indexes. The glycemic index of sucrose, a disaccharide made up of glucose and fructose, is lower than that of some starches, such as potatoes, because sucrose contains less pure glucose.

Those in favor of replacing foods having a high glycemic index with foods having a low glycemic index refer to studies demonstrating the value of the glycemic index in the dietary management of diabetes (37–46). However, others find that the study results are not consistent or predictable and not clinically useful (47–50). Another controversy exists over the impact of meals with a high glycemic index versus meals with a low glycemic index on weight loss and satiety. Ludwig (41) suggests that the ingestion of low-glycemic-index foods typically induces higher satiety than does the ingestion of high-glycemic-index foods and is followed by the intake of fewer calories at subsequent meals. It is theorized that slower rates of digestion and absorption of low-glycemic-index foods stimulate nutrient receptors in the gastrointestinal tract for a longer period, resulting in a longer period of feedback to the satiety center in the brain. Brand-Miller et al. (42) suggest that high-glycemic-index meals dictate differences in satiety and caloric intake because of the faster digestion and absorption and high insulin responses, and that they expand fat stores. Pi-Sunyer (49) takes the position that the data are not yet sufficient and that most of the data relating high-glycemic-index meals to increased food intake were collected in single-meal experimental designs. Although the weight-loss benefit of a low-glycemic-index diet compared with a high-glycemic-index diet is still only a hypothesis, it may be helpful to use the glycemic index as an additional weight-loss tool. A low-glycemic-index diet consisting of vegetables, fruits, and legumes, a moderate amount of protein and unsaturated fats, and fewer refined carbohydrate foods—along with overall decreased calorie intake and increased physical activity—will assist patients in their weight-loss efforts (40). As more long-term research trials on glycemic response to single foods and complete meals are conducted, the usefulness of this concept as a teaching tool is increasing (Table 36.6). However, the glycemic response to food depends not only on the amount and type of carbohydrate but also on other variables (Table 36.7), which could impact the glycemic effect of the carbohydrate food eaten. To further determine the impact of carbohydrate foods on blood glucose levels, researchers have come up with a way to describe the extent to which the blood glucose rises (GI) and remains high. This is called the glycemic load (GL). The GL provides a measure of the level of glucose in the blood, but also

TABLE 36.6. Glycemic Index of Common Carbohydrate Foods, Using Glucose as Standard

Greater than 70%	55%–70%	Less than 55%
French baguette, 1 oz	Pita bread, 2 oz	Pumpernickel, whole grain, 1 oz
Black bread, 1.7 oz	White bread, 1 oz	Sourdough bread, 1.5 oz (acid)
Corn flakes, 1 cup	Cheerios, 1 cup	All-bran with extra fiber, $\frac{1}{2}$ cup
Rice Chex, 1	Shredded wheat, $\frac{2}{3}$ cup	Frosted flakes, $\frac{3}{4}$ cup
Rice cakes, 3 plain	Stoned Wheat Thins, 3	Social Tea biscuits, 4
Vanilla wafers, 7	Shortbread cookies, 4	Twix chocolate cookie, 2 oz
Dates, 5	Pineapple, 2 slices	Cherries, 10 large
Watermelon, 1 cup	Raisins, $\frac{1}{4}$ cup	Banana, 1 medium
Tofu frozen dessert, $\frac{1}{2}$ cup	Ice cream, $\frac{1}{2}$ cup	Ice milk, $\frac{1}{2}$ cup
Angel food cake, 1 oz	Blueberry muffin, 2 oz	Pound cake, 3 oz
Jelly beans, 10 large	Coca-Cola, 1 can	Chocolate bar, 1.5 oz
Life Savers, 6	Honey, 1 tbsp	M & M chocolate peanuts, 1.7 oz
Baked potato without fat	White boiled potato	Sweet potato
Rice, instant, 1 cup	Basmati white rice, 1 cup	Brown rice, 1 cup
Millet, $\frac{1}{2}$ cup	Couscous, $\frac{1}{2}$ cup	Barley, $\frac{1}{2}$ cup
Bagel, 1 small	Macaroni and cheese, 1 cup	Spaghetti, white, 1 cup

Adapted from Brand-Miller J, Wolever TM, Colgiuri S, et al. *The glucose revolution: the authoritative guide to the glycemic index.* New York: Marlowe & Company, 1999.

TABLE 36.7. Factors Affecting Glycemic Response

Food factors	Human factors
Structure of the food	Variable rates of digestion and absorption
Food storage procedures	Stimulation of gut peptides
Presence of fat	Concomitant diseases
Protein/starch interrelationships	Body mass/weight
Cooking/processing method (particle size, blending, grinding)	Preprandial blood glucose level
Ripeness or maturity	Composition of previous meal
Presence and type of fiber	Exercise/activity
Resistant starch	Time of day
Soluble nonstarch polysaccharides	Gender and age
Resilience of cell structure	Ethnicity and race

the insulin demand produced by a normal serving of the food. The GL considers a food's GI as well as the amount of carbohydrate per serving and gives a more detailed picture.

- The GI determines how rapidly a particular carbohydrate food may raise blood glucose.
- The GL determines how much impact a carbohydrate food may have on blood glucose levels, depending on the number of grams of carbohydrate in a serving.

GI *divided* by 100 (glucose is set to equal 100) *multiplied* by the carbohydrate grams/serving = GL (51)

For example, it may be recommended that carrots be eliminated entirely owing to their very high GI value of 92. Common sense, however, tells us that carrots are a vegetable and provide fiber and healthy nutrients. For example:

1/2 cup carrots **GI** 92/100 × 4 g carb = **GL** of 3.7 = **Low GL**

2 cups carrots **GI** 92/100 × 16 g carb = **GL** of 15 = **Medium GL**

In general, the GI is highest if high GI foods are eaten in large quantities. Low GI foods usually have a low GL, but medium to high GI foods can range from low to high GL. Therefore, you can reduce the GL by limiting foods that have both a high GI and a high carbohydrate content.

Most agree that the ability of a person to adhere to a dietary regimen is inversely related to the complexity of the regimen. Calculating the glycemic index at each meal may be burdensome for some individuals. Because the exact effect of food on a person's blood glucose level is an individual response to specific foods and meals, patients are encouraged to identify their own glycemic index for certain foods by using self-management of blood glucose. Therefore, we may propose the use of the glycemic index as an adjunct to the dietary management tools already in use by our patients.

Information about glycemic index may be reviewed with patients who (a) track their carbohydrate intake and keep blood glucose and food records; (b) monitor their blood glucose levels at least two or three times per day and are willing to evaluate blood glucose levels following meals; (c) follow up with a registered dietitian to evaluate out-of-range blood glucose values that may be due to consumption of particular types of carbohydrate foods; (d) express an interest in making additional modifications in their eating plan to fine-tune glycemic control; and (e) express an interest in using information about glycemic index for helping to guide food choices for weight control.

The primary goal is for patients to achieve both glycemic and weight control while eating a variety of nutritionally balanced foods. It is not necessary to completely avoid foods with a high glycemic index, because many are healthy, nutritious foods that can be eaten in moderation. However, patients should be encouraged to include more unprocessed, high-fiber foods, for which a lower glycemic response has been generated. Examples of high-fiber foods include lentils, beans, legumes, raw and unpeeled fruits and vegetables, or foods that have been minimally cooked (52).

Because knowledge of food composition and physiology is not sufficient to permit a consistent prediction of glycemic responses, the principle that food choices can be refined to obtain maximal control of blood glucose remains a possibility for motivated individuals who closely monitor their blood glucose levels. Awareness of differences in glycemic response to food has played an important role in expanding our thinking about how to improve dietary management and our understanding of what occurs in the daily management of individuals with diabetes.

Sucrose

The inclusion of sucrose in the total carbohydrate content of the diet has not been found to impair blood glucose control in individuals with either type 1 or type 2 diabetes (15). Consumption of modest amounts of sucrose by persons with diabetes is acceptable as long as both metabolic control and weight are maintained. For instance, several investigators found no significant difference between the blood glucose responses of persons with diabetes when they consumed sucrose and when they consumed only starch (53–56).

In a recent study (57), nine children with type 1 diabetes were studied in a controlled setting to compare glycemic responses of isocaloric mixed meals that contained 2% sucrose (sucrose-free diet) and 17% sucrose (sucrose-containing diet). Insulin infusion was started the night before the beginning of the study period so that all of the children had fasting euglycemia. Diets were carefully matched for nutrient and energy content, with only small differences noted for fiber. The glycemic response was lower with the 17% sucrose diet than with the 2% sucrose diet over the 4-hour study period. The peak blood glucose response was earlier and lower with the 17% sucrose diet. The results suggest that moderate amounts of sucrose isocalorically exchanged for starch lowered the glycemic response between breakfast and lunch in children who were euglycemic before breakfast.

Other investigators have studied the blood glucose response in adults with type 1 and type 2 diabetes and found no significant difference between the blood glucose responses to their consumption of sucrose and the responses to their consumption of only starch (55,58).

The crossover study of Bantle et al. (55) with 12 patients with type 2 diabetes involved two study diets—a high-sucrose diet (19% kilocalories from sucrose) and a high-starch diet (<3% kilocalories from sucrose) for 28 days. The sucrose and starch diets provided about 55% kilocalories from carbohydrate, 15% kilocalories from protein, and 30% kilocalories from fat. The two diets contained almost identical amounts of dietary fiber, cholesterol, polyunsaturated fat, monounsaturated fat, and saturated fat. No significant differences were noted between the study diet with 19% of kilocalories from sucrose relative to a diet deriving its energy from starch on the mean plasma and urinary glucose, fasting serum cholesterol, HDL cholesterol, low-density lipoprotein (LDL) cholesterol, and triglycerides levels.

Available studies have allowed children and adults with diabetes to feel less constrained by allowing them a diet more consistent with the sucrose-containing diet of their peers. Realistic guidelines for including sucrose-containing foods in the diet also improves patient adherence to overall dietary management. However, sucrose does encourage the development of dental caries, and sucrose-containing foods may contain a significant number of calories, especially when combined with fat in dessert foods such as baked goods, ice cream, and chocolate bars. This may contribute to elevated serum lipid levels and weight gain in some people if they are not carefully monitored. These findings are indications of how glycemic indexing is making us reconsider strongly held doctrines and permitting us to develop improved dietary recommendations.

Fiber

The population with diabetes in the United States consumes, on average, only 16 g of fiber per day (59), which is below the recommended intake of 20 to 35 g/day for those with or without diabetes. Previous studies on fiber in diabetes have had somewhat inconsistent results, probably as a consequence of previously unrecognized differences in the amounts, types, and properties of fiber. The benefits of fiber in improving serum cholesterol levels and colonic function are well established (60), and the American Diabetes Association currently recommends the consumption of 20 to 35 g of fiber daily on the basis of these benefits. However, the effects of fiber on glycemia have been considered to be minimal (15).

Several studies have demonstrated that diets particularly high in fiber (especially soluble fiber) are associated with lower blood glucose and serum lipid levels. Water-soluble fibers, such as the pectins, gums, storage polysaccharides, and a few hemicelluloses found in fruits, legumes, lentils, roots, tubers, oats, and oat bran, have little influence on fecal bulk but may reduce serum levels of glucose and insulin (61–65). Wolever (66) reported that the amount of soluble fiber in whole foods is not closely related to glucose response but discerned a weak, but significant, correlation between the total dietary fiber and the glycemic response to a food. He postulated that the cell walls of foods that elicited a low glycemic response were sturdy and high in cellulose and hemicellulose. However, the differences in fiber components of foods did not explain all the variation in glycemic response. Water-insoluble fibers, such as cellulose, lignin, and most hemicelluloses found in whole-grain breads, cereals, and wheat bran, affect gastrointestinal transit time and fecal bulk but have little impact on plasma glucose, insulin, or cholesterol levels.

New evidence that high dietary fiber intake is beneficial in type 2 diabetes confirms previously published research (67–69). In a recent crossover study, Chandalia et al. (70) demonstrated that intake of dietary fiber, particularly soluble fiber, above the amounts recommended by the American Diabetes Association improves glycemic control and decreases hyperinsulinemia in patients with type 2 diabetes, in addition to the expected decrease in plasma lipid concentrations. Thirteen patients with type 2 diabetes followed two diets, each for 6 weeks. Both diets consisted of unfortified fiber foods, 15% protein, 55% carbohydrate, and 30% fat. The high-fiber study diet provided 50 g of total fiber daily, with soluble and insoluble fiber providing 25 g each. The American Diabetes Association study diet contained 24 g of total fiber per day, with soluble fiber contributing 8 g and insoluble fiber contributing 16 g. Daily plasma glucose levels were 10% lower with the high-fiber diet than with the American Diabetes Association diet. Rendell (71) stated that this study clearly pointed out the importance of dietary intervention in patients with diabetes and that the "decrease in the degree of hyperglycemia achieved in the study by Chandalia et al. by increasing patients' fiber intake is similar to that typically obtained by the addition of another oral hypoglycemic drug to the therapeutic regimen." As expected, the high-fiber diet resulted in lower fasting plasma total cholesterol, triglyceride, and very-low-density lipopolysaccharide (VLDL) concentrations than did the American Diabetes Association diet.

Although it is unclear if improved glycemic control associated with high fiber intake is due to an increase in soluble fiber, insoluble fiber, or both, the total amount of fiber from unfortified whole foods has now been better defined. A practical way of proceeding is to determine the current level of fiber in a patient's diet and to increase the amount of fiber *gradually* to a maximum of 50 g/day. The gradual introduction of the fiber minimizes gastrointestinal problems such as osmotic diarrhea and flatulence. Increased fiber intake should be accompanied by an increase of fluid intake and careful attention to self-monitoring of blood glucose levels. Intake of large quantities of fiber can delay or reduce peak glucose responses to carbohydrate and perhaps predispose an individual receiving antidiabetes medication to hypoglycemia if the dosage of the medication is not adjusted to compensate for this effect.

PROTEIN

> The quantity of protein required by diabetic patients varies with age, weight and activity of the case as well as with the condition of the kidneys. It is a safe rule at the beginning of treatment to increase the protein gradually up to the same quantity as that required by a normal individual. This is approximately 1 to 1.5 grams per kilogram body weight for adults but for children it may reach 3 grams. (1)

In a typical Western diet, the estimated protein intake is 1.1 to 1.4 g/kg of body weight for a 70-kg person ingesting 2,000 kcal/day, an amount considerably greater than the minimum recommended by the National Academy of Sciences (72). The 1989 Recommended Dietary Allowance (RDA) for protein continues to stand at 0.8 g/kg of body weight for adults. This translates to about 10% to 20% of total daily calories from protein from both animal and vegetable sources. There is no evidence to support a higher- or lower-than-average protein intake for those with diabetes.

Individuals whose diabetes is under good control appear to have the same protein requirements as individuals without diabetes. Thus, when insulin levels are normal, protein is conserved in the body and the use of amino acids for glucose synthesis is limited (73). However, severe insulin deficiency increases the loss of body protein, and those with poorly controlled diabetes may have increased needs for protein because their liver may use protein to synthesize glucose. A study by Nair et al. (74)

demonstrated that withdrawal of insulin resulted in a 97% increase in protein loss in subjects with type 1 diabetes.

Although there is no evidence that restricting protein will prevent or delay the onset of nephropathy (75), several small studies have suggested that patients with overt nephropathy would benefit from a prescribed protein restriction of 0.6 g/kg per day. Limiting protein consumption to 0.6 g/kg per day (although study participants achieved a restriction of only 0.7 g/kg per day) suggested a modest lowering of the rate of decline in the glomerular filtration rate. However, the Modified Diet in Renal Disease Study (only 3% of participants had type 2 diabetes and none had type 1 diabetes) did not indicate any clear benefit of protein restriction (76). The general consensus is to prescribe a protein intake of 0.8 g/kg per day in those patients with overt nephropathy, with a possible lowering to 0.6 g/kg per day once the glomerular filtration rate begins to decline and careful monitoring for possible protein deficiency and muscle weakness (15).

Because past dietary recommendations for persons with diabetes sometimes emphasized protein and because the average American eats more protein than is necessary to maintain health (15% to 20% of calories), current recommendations suggest that people with diabetes consume amounts similar to those consumed by people without diabetes. Evidence suggests that this amount of protein is not harmful.

Protein and Glucose Concentration

As early as 1915, Janney reported that 3.5 g of glucose could be produced as the result of a beef-protein meal for every gram of nitrogen excreted in the urine. If beef protein is 16% nitrogen, 56% of beef protein can be converted to glucose (77). However, several studies completed *after* Janney's calculation that focused on the effect of protein on glucose response suggested that protein ingestion by patients with and without diabetes did not elevate blood glucose levels. These important findings were "lost," and Janney's theoretical calculation prevailed. In recent years, several studies conducted by Nuttall et al. (78–80) continue to support that glucose concentration did not increase after protein ingestion in people with or without diabetes. In 1999, Gannon et al. (81) reported that the ingestion of 50 g of lean beef protein by participants with type 2 diabetes resulted in the appearance of only about 2.0 g as glucose in the circulation more than 8 hours later. This result was compared with that for patients who consumed only water. Although the ingestion of beef increased glucose concentration by 0.1 mmol/L at 1 hour, the concentration then decreased similarly to that of participants who consumed only water. Further questions arose when the plasma insulin level remained steady in the water group but the insulin level increased threefold and the plasma glucagon increased 50% in the protein group. If gluconeogenesis from protein is found, researchers can only theorize why glucose does not appear in the general circulation. Several theories, noted in a review of available research by Franz (77), suggest the following:

- The glucose converted from protein is much less than the theorized 50% to 60%, and the smaller amount of glucose from protein that actually enters the general circulation is offset by a corresponding increase in glucose use, as long as enough insulin is available.
- The conversion of glucose from protein is in fact 50% to 60%, but this glucose does not actually enter the general circulation. Gluconeogenesis from protein may occur slowly over 24 hours, and the glucose is disposed of over this long period.
- Increased insulin secretion caused by dietary protein results in rapid storage of the glucose as glycogen in the liver and skeletal muscles. This glycogen can be broken down to glucose when needed; however, the body does not identify the glucose entering the general circulation as a product from protein or carbohydrate.

Current studies of protein and its effects on blood glucose concentration have possible clinical implications for both type 1 and type 2 diabetes. For those with type 1 diabetes, possible increases in the protein content of the diet, which seems to have a minimal impact on glucose concentrations, while decreasing the carbohydrate content, may improve and stabilize blood glucose excursions. For those with type 2 diabetes, the ingestion of more protein along with less carbohydrate may increase the concentration of circulating insulin. These possibilities demonstrate the importance of examining the beneficial or potentially harmful effects of ingesting higher amounts of protein for those with diabetes.

FAT

> The discovery of insulin has lowered the fat in the diabetic's diet, because he can take more carbohydrate. Indirectly, . . . this may retard the development of hardening of the arteries. How much fat should a diabetic patient eat? The safest answer would be: as little as possibly above the normal quantity in order to maintain normal body weight. (1)

People with type 1 diabetes who maintain good control of blood glucose with insulin have plasma lipid levels similar to those of the general population of the same age and gender. However, the prevalence of hyperlipidemia and coronary heart disease (CHD) among patients with type 2 diabetes is twofold to fourfold higher than in the general population. Frequent lipid abnormalities are hypertriglyceridemia and decreased high-density lipoprotein cholesterol (HDL-C), although concentrations of low-density lipoprotein cholesterol (LDL-C) are often not significantly different from those in control populations. However, patients with type 2 diabetes are twice as likely as control populations to accumulate smaller, denser LDL particles, which may increase the risk of CHD even if LDL-C levels are not significantly increased (82,83).

According to recent research, different types and sources of fat have beneficial or detrimental effects on lipid levels.

- *Monounsaturated fats* are liquid at room temperature and derived primarily from oleic acid. Major dietary sources are olive, canola, and peanut oils; avocados; nuts; and olives. These nonessential fatty acids (NEFAs) help lower LDL-C levels and possibly raise HDL-C levels. Generally, about 10% to 15% of total calories may come from monounsaturated fats.
- *Polyunsaturated fats* are liquid at room temperature and derived from linoleic, linolenic, and arachidonic acids. Major dietary sources are corn, safflower, sesame, and soybean oils. These essential fatty acids (EFAs) are known to lower both LDL-C and plasma cholesterol levels. Omega-3 fatty acids, a type of polyunsaturated fat, lower plasma triglyceride and very-low-density lipopolysaccaride cholesterol (VLDL-C) levels. Major dietary sources are fatty fish, flaxseed and other vegetable oils, shortenings, and liquid or partially hydrogenated margarines.
- *Saturated fats* are mostly solid at room temperature and synthesized in the body from acetate. Major dietary sources are animal products such as butter, meat, lard, poultry skin, whole milk, cheese, sour cream, cream cheese, and tropical oils such

as coconut, cocoa butter, palm oil, and palm kernel oil. These NEFAs increase total serum cholesterol and LDL-C levels.

- *Trans-fats* are semisolid at room temperature. The chemical process of hydrogenation causes unsaturated fatty acids to become more saturated and alters the position of hydrogen atoms around the double bond (on opposite sides, or *trans*). This process increases the shelf life of foods. Major dietary sources are polyunsaturated vegetable oils in solid margarines, salad dressings, shortening, and many baked goods. Trans-fats increase LDL-C and decrease HDL-C and are associated with an increased risk of CHD.

Guidelines of the National Cholesterol Education Program: Adult Treatment Panel III

Research advances in the prevention and management of high cholesterol in adults led the National Cholesterol Education Program (NCEP) Expert Panel on Detection, Evaluation, and Treatment of High Blood Cholesterol in Adults (Adult Treatment Panel III, ATP III) to issue major new clinical practice guidelines in 2001 (84). In 1985, this program began to promote greater awareness by physicians and patients of CHD risk status by blood cholesterol level and to provide recommendations for dietary treatment and educational programs. Earlier guidelines were issued in 1988 and 1993.

The 2001 ATP III guidelines recommend a new set of therapeutic lifestyle changes (TLCs) that intensify the use of nutrition, physical activity, and weight control in the treatment of elevated blood cholesterol (Table 36.8). These guidelines reflect changes in the eating habits of Americans, including a decrease in the consumption of saturated fats and cholesterol. The present recommendations allow up to 35% of daily calories from total fat, provided mostly from unsaturated fat, which does not raise cholesterol levels. Abnormalities in lipid and carbohydrate metabolism in those with diabetes must be carefully assessed because of the potential risk of promoting higher triglyceride levels with a high-carbohydrate diet while attempting to decrease total and saturated fats to lower LDL-C (85). Some patients with high triglyceride or low HDL levels or both may need to eat more unsaturated fats to keep their triglyceride or HDL levels from worsening.

ATP III also encourages use of foods that contain plant stanols and sterols or are rich in soluble fiber to boost the LDL-lowering power of the diet. Plant stanols and sterols are included in certain margarines and salad dressings. Foods high in soluble fiber include cereal grains, beans, peas, legumes, and many fruits and vegetables. Additional guidelines stress the importance of weight control, which enhances the lowering of LDL levels and increases HDL levels; and physical activity, which improves HDL values and, for some, LDL values (86).

The recommendations for dietary fat intake for those with diabetes depends on treatment goals for existing hyperlipidemia and risk of CHD, as well as goals for blood glucose and weight. If the recommendations for dietary protein are for about 15% of total calories per day, the remaining 85% to 90% of calories may be distributed through fats and carbohydrates. The first line of defense is to get fewer than 7% of the allotted calories from saturated fat, with dietary cholesterol limited to less than 200 mg/day. Up to 10% of total calories should be from polyunsaturated fats, and up to 20% of total calories should be from monounsaturated fats. However, consumption of omega-3 polyunsaturated fats found in seafood does not need to be decreased in people with diabetes. The remaining calories can then be derived from complex carbohydrates, including whole grains, fruits, and vegetables.

Fat Replacers

The medical need to decrease fat in the diets of those with type 2 diabetes has increased the demand for palatable, lower-fat foods and has led to the creation of fat replacers. Fat replacers are used in many fat-free, nonfat, reduced-calorie, and low-fat foods in an attempt to lower fat and calorie intake. At present, most fat replacers are carbohydrate-based, but some are protein- or fat-based. One fat-based replacer, olestra, was approved by the Food and Drug Administration (FDA) in 1996 for use in snack foods and crackers. Studies of this synthetic oil indicated that it has the potential to lower total cholesterol and LDL-C in persons consuming either a high- or a low-cholesterol diet (87).

Although fat replacers have the potential to reduce total and saturated fat in the diet, patients must be educated to use them wisely within the context of an overall food plan. Unfortunately,

TABLE 36.8. Therapeutic Lifestyle Changes: Nutrient Composition of Therapeutic Lifestyle Changes Diet

Nutrient	Recommended intake
Saturated fat[a]	Less than 7% of total calories
Polyunsaturated fat	Up to 10% of total calories
Monounsaturated fat	Up to 20% of total calories
Total fat	25%–35% of total calories
Carbohydrate[b]	50–60% of total calories
Fiber	20–39 g/day
Protein	Approximately 15% of total calories
Cholesterol	Less than 200 mg/day
Total calories (energy)[c]	Balance energy intake and expenditure to maintain desirable weight and prevent weight gain

[a]Trans-fatty acids are another LDL-raising fat that should be limited in the diet.
[b]Carbohydrate should be derived predominantly from foods rich in complex carbohydrates, including grains, especially whole grains; fruits; and vegetables.
[c]Daily energy expenditure should include at least moderate physical activity (contributing ~200 kcal/day).
From the National Cholesterol Education Program Expert Panel on Detection, Evaluation, and Treatment of High Blood Cholesterol in Adults (Adult Treatment Panel III). *JAMA* 2001;285:19, with permission.

many patients with type 2 diabetes are not aware of the potential high-calorie content of fat-free foods made with fat replacers. These foods are created by using mixtures of carbohydrates or proteins to simulate the properties of fat and cannot be eaten liberally without affecting caloric intake, glycemia, and weight.

Plant Stanol Esters

A new dietary approach to helping manage serum cholesterol levels is now being used in the United States. Plant stanol esters (PSEs) occur naturally in plant products, especially oils, and are the saturated derivative of sitosterol known as sitostanol. PSEs are structurally similar to cholesterol and are virtually unabsorbed by the body. PSEs are found in soy and olive oils, corn, rye, rice, wheat, and wood. More than 20 published studies support the cholesterol-lowering effects of stanol esters. A landmark 15-month study by Miettinen et al. (88) in Finland focused attention on the cholesterol-lowering benefits of PSE in the form of margarine with and without sitostanol. After 1 year, total cholesterol was reduced by up to 10% and LDL-C by up to 14%; HDL-C and triglycerides were unaffected. A U.S. multicenter study (89) conducted in 1999 demonstrated the efficacy and safety of PSE spreads. At 2 weeks, significant reductions in total cholesterol and LDL-C were reported in all groups. At 12 weeks, an average reduction in LDL-C of 12% versus baseline was achieved. Researchers have concluded that PSE may be useful in the dietary approach to cholesterol lowering and suggest a benefit by adding PSE to NCEP III nutrition recommendations. The trade names of current plant PSE spreads on the market include Benecol® and Take Control®.

Soluble Fiber and Cholesterol

Chandalia et al. (70) also reaffirmed the results of previous reports of the cholesterol-reducing effects of soluble but not insoluble fiber. Thirteen patients with type 2 diabetes followed two diets, each for 6 weeks. The effects of the American Diabetes Association diet (total fiber, 24 g: 8 g of soluble fiber and 16 g of insoluble fiber) were compared with a high-fiber diet (total fiber, 50 g: 25 g of soluble fiber and 25 g of insoluble fiber). The high-fiber diet reduced total plasma cholesterol concentrations by 6.7%, reduced triglyceride concentrations by 10.2%, and reduced VLDL-C by 12.5%. The LDL-C was 6.3% lower with the high-fiber diet. There were no significant differences in HDL-C. This study demonstrated the positive effects of a high-fiber diet, particularly soluble fiber, on lowering plasma lipid concentrations.

Educating Patients about Fat Intake

A primary strategy for patients with hypercholesterolemia, before they use cholesterol-lowering medications, is nutrition education. Key education points for patients with diabetes should include the following:

- Understanding the difference between dietary and blood lipids and how to change and decrease the dietary fats to lower blood lipid levels.
- Reducing total fat intake to 25% to 35% of calories based on nutrition assessment, with fewer than 7% of calories from saturated fat while meeting needs for essential fatty acids (seafood).
- Shifting the emphasis from animal to vegetable sources of fat.
- Encouraging the use of liquid, unsaturated oils, plant stanols, and tub or liquid margarines and reducing the use of foods with partially hydrogenated oils.
- Emphasizing an increase in fiber by the inclusion of more whole grains, vegetables, and fruits.
- Recognizing that fat provides a concentrated source of calories in the diet and in body stores for those who want to lose weight loss or are obese.
- Reducing or eliminating alcohol intake for those with dyslipidemia, especially those with elevated triglyceride levels.

ALTERNATIVE SWEETENERS

Nutritive Sweeteners

In the past, the use of sucrose and glucose alone or in foods high in these sugars (corn syrup, fruit juice, honey, molasses, dextrose, and maltose) was restricted for those with diabetes. This dietary approach was a means of limiting excursions of blood glucose and limiting calories in the overweight person with diabetes. This approach gave rise to the development of alternative sweeteners—both caloric and noncaloric. For years, these alternative sweeteners have played a dominant role in providing persons with diabetes with sweetness in their diet, much as they do for those without diabetes. Some patients with diabetes may feel that sweeteners help them adhere to their "diet," contribute to better diabetes control, and are beneficial for weight reduction. Unfortunately, little scientific evidence supports these beliefs. The American Diabetes Association notes that "there is no evidence that foods sweetened with these sweeteners have any significant advantage or disadvantage over foods sweetened with sucrose in decreasing total calories or carbohydrate content of the diet or in improving overall diabetes control" (15).

Although fructose has previously been promoted as producing a smaller increase in blood glucose than equal amounts of sucrose and most starches, evidence suggests potential negative effects of large amounts of fructose (twice the amount usually consumed, or 20% of daily calories) on serum cholesterol and LDL-C (90). However, no recommendations have been made to avoid foods with naturally occurring fructose, such as fruits and vegetables, or even modest amounts of fructose-sweetened foods.

Sugar alcohols (polyols) such as sorbitol, mannitol, xylitol, isomalt, lactitol, maltitol, and hydrogenated starch hydrolysate are less sweet than sugar but do add bulk to foods. They are manufactured from monosaccharides, disaccharides, or polysaccharides for use in foods. Of note, sorbitol does not contribute to the sorbitol pathway that has been implicated in neuropathy and retinal changes. Once sorbitol has been metabolized in the liver, it is no longer available to the body (91). Polyols may elicit less of a glycemic response because they are absorbed more slowly and provide only 2.4 to 3.5 kcal/g as compared with 4 calories/g from other carbohydrates. The incomplete absorption of sugar alcohols, producing osmotic diarrhea when ingested in large amounts (50 g/day for sorbitol, 20 g/day for mannitol), constitutes the main drawback to their use (21). Sorbitol and mannitol must have warning labels affixed that state, "Excess consumption may have a laxative effect."

There is no concrete evidence that sugar alcohols reduce total calories or the total daily carbohydrate intake of those with diabetes. However, it is important that those with diabetes have a good understanding of the potential of nutritive sweeteners to affect blood glucose levels and to account for these effects.

Nonnutritive Sweeteners

Acesulfame K, aspartame, saccharin, and sucralose are the common noncaloric intense sweeteners used at present in the

United States. All have been approved by the FDA. An acceptable daily intake (ADI) is determined for these intense sweeteners, as for all food additives. ADI is defined as the amount of a food additive that can be safely consumed on a daily basis over a person's lifetime without having any adverse effects. The ADI also includes a 100-fold safety factor.

ACESULFAME K

Acesulfame K (acesulfame potassium) is a white, odorless, crystalline sweetener. It has no caloric value and is 200 times sweeter than sucrose. It is described as having a clean, fresh taste that does not linger, but some perceive that it has a bitter taste when used in large amounts (92). Acesulfame K is a derivative of acetoacetic acid with a structure somewhat similar to that of saccharin. Approved for use by the FDA in 1988, it is marketed in the United States under the brand name Sunette® when used as an ingredient in foods and as Sweet One® when sold as a table-top sweetener. Its advantages are its remarkable stability both in liquids and during baking or cooking. Acesulfame K is not metabolized by the body and is eliminated unchanged in the urine. It is heat stable and blends well with other sweeteners. The amount of potassium in this sweetener is minimal (only 10 mg of potassium per packet). No safety concerns have been raised about acesulfame K, and it is reported to be safe for all individuals. The ADI for both adults and children is 15 mg/kg per day (one packet contains about 0.4 g) (93).

ASPARTAME

Aspartame is a protein sweetener. It is the methyl ester of L-phenylalanine and L-aspartic acid. Intestinal esterases hydrolyze aspartame to aspartic acid, methanol, and phenylalanine. Medical nutrition therapy controls the use of aspartame products in persons with phenylketonuria, a homozygous, recessive inborn error of metabolism that makes them unable to metabolize the amino acid phenylalanine.

Aspartame is 160 to 220 times sweeter than sucrose. Aspartame contains 4 kcal/g but because of its intense sweetening ability provides negligible calories. It was first approved for use in 1981 and is marketed as NutraSweet® both in food products and as a table-top sweetener. Aspartame does not alter glycemic control in individuals with diabetes (94). It is metabolized in the gastrointestinal tract and at recommended intakes does not accumulate. Aspartame may decompose with long exposure to high temperatures and is not heat stable. The ADI for adults and children is 50 mg/kg body weight (37 mg in one packet, 200 mg in a 12-oz diet soda).

The FDA has addressed many concerns related to ingestion of aspartame for individuals with and without diabetes. A variety of safety concerns have been raised, i.e., that mild, nonspecific symptoms such as headaches, dizziness, and menstrual irregularities are associated with its ingestion and that the by-products of metabolism (methanol or its by-product formate) are toxic. This prompted the Centers for Disease Control and Prevention (CDC) to further evaluate aspartame. The CDC reported that data "do not provide for the existence of serious widespread, adverse health consequences" (95). Aspartame has repeatedly been determined to be safe for both the general public and people with diabetes.

SACCHARIN

Saccharin is a heat-stable, synthetic sweetener that is 200 to 700 times sweeter than sucrose. Saccharin is without caloric value because it is not metabolized and is excreted unchanged. Concern about the carcinogenic potential of saccharin has lingered for years, although a review of the literature has not yielded evidence that can justify governmental restriction (96–98). Although saccharin is synthetic and not a food additive, the Joint Expert Committee of Food Additions of the World Health Organization has set an ADI of 5 mg/kg body weight per day. The FDA has stated that saccharin poses no health hazard.

SUCRALOSE

Sucralose is the most recent noncaloric sweetener to be approved by the FDA (in 1998), and its use has been confirmed by many regulatory agencies throughout the world. It is 600 times sweeter than sugar and marketed under the name of Splenda®. Sucralose is made from sucrose through a chemical process that alters the sucrose molecule by replacing three hydrogen/oxygen groups with three chlorine atoms. Sucralose is not recognized by the body as either a sugar or a carbohydrate. It does not affect carbohydrate metabolism and is eliminated unchanged by the body (93,99).

Sucralose is heat stable and may be used in cooking and baking. The FDA states that no adverse or carcinogenic effects are associated with consumption of sucralose. The ADI for adults and children is 15 mg/kg body weight per day (93).

SODIUM

> Salt is of great service to the diabetic patient. The percentage of salt (sodium chloride) in the ocean and in the human blood is alike and the body tends to keep it constant. The first essential for a low sodium diet is to omit all salt either in the preparation of food or at the table. (1)

The recommended sodium intake for people with diabetes is the same as that for people without diabetes, with the main goal being not to exceed 3,000 mg/day. Some health professionals do, however, recommend no more than 2,400 mg/day, which is equivalent to 1 teaspoon of salt. Because the recommendations are the same as those for the general population, guidelines should be directed toward the entire family. Severe sodium restriction, however, may be harmful for persons whose diabetes is poorly controlled or who have postural hypotension or fluid imbalance.

Persons with diabetes have not been found to be more sensitive to sodium than persons without diabetes or to be at greater risk of developing hypertension associated with high sodium intake. Concern about sodium intake is directed primarily at individuals with congestive heart failure, nephropathy, and hypertension or who are at risk for the development of these complications. Routine monitoring of blood pressure will help identify those who may benefit from a reduction in sodium intake. The recommended intake of sodium is less than 2,400 mg/day for those with mild-to-moderate hypertension and less than 2,000 mg/day for those with hypertension and nephropathy.

Patients should always be cautioned about the use of salt substitutes, which often contain potassium rather than sodium. When consumed in excess, salt substitutes can be harmful, especially for people with kidney problems. As an alternative to salt substitutes, salt-free seasoning blends are readily available.

ALCOHOL

Adults with diabetes do not have to abstain from alcohol. Indeed, the guidelines for alcohol use in individuals with diabetes mirror those for the general population. However, restrictions on or abstinence from alcohol may be necessary for those with hypoglycemic unawareness, neuropathy, poor control of blood glucose or blood lipids, pancreatitis, obesity, or a history of alcohol abuse, or for those who are pregnant.

Some issues regarding the use of alcohol require attention. First, alcohol adds calories without nutritional benefit and has been shown to supplement rather than displace other calories (100). Suter et al. (101) and Flatt (102) demonstrated that, whereas carbohydrate and protein oxidation was mostly unaffected by the ingestion and metabolism of alcohol, fat oxidation was decreased by about 50%. Therefore, restriction of calories provided by ethanol is a dietary strategy that is positively related to success with weight loss. Second, excessive alcohol consumption by a person who is fasting or skipping meals can lead to hypoglycemia via inhibition of gluconeogenesis. This may pose a serious risk for those taking insulin or oral agents to control hyperglycemia. Even blood alcohol levels that do not exceed mild intoxication can result in hypoglycemia (21). Third, intoxication can impair a person's ability to follow a prescribed management plan or to recognize symptoms of hypoglycemia and obtain treatment if needed. Fourth, ingestion of alcohol increases the synthesis of lipoproteins, especially VLDL. Because some persons with diabetes are susceptible to hypertriglyceridemia, and because alcohol has the potential to raise triglyceride levels, alcohol ingestion should be discouraged. Recent studies, however, indicate that moderate amounts of alcohol have been associated with a decrease in CHD attributed to an increase in less dense HDL-C subfractions (15,103–106).

Alcohol Guidelines

- Alcohol use and abuse should be discussed as part of the education process for all persons with diabetes so that they know the facts about the effects of alcohol on glycemia.
- Excessive alcohol consumption may lead to erratic behavior, loss of consciousness, or seizures, particularly if food is not consumed with the alcohol. Alcohol should only be consumed with food or after the meal.
- For those with type 1 diabetes, alcohol should be taken in addition to their regular meal without omitting any food. Metabolism of alcohol does not require insulin.
- For those with type 2 diabetes, alcohol is best substituted for fat calories: One alcohol equivalent equals two fat exchanges (10 of fat).
- Glucagon is not effective in the treatment of alcohol-induced hypoglycemia because alcohol depletes glycogen stores.
- Alcohol should be used only when diabetes is under good control and in moderate amounts. Alcohol should be strictly avoided when driving.
- General recommendations for alcohol intake are no more than two alcohol equivalents per day for men and no more than one alcohol equivalent per day for women. An alcohol equivalent, which contains about 1 oz (15 g) of alcohol, is defined as 12 oz of beer, 5 oz of wine, or 1.5 oz of 80-proof distilled spirits (15).
- A person who ingests alcohol should always be encouraged to monitor blood glucose levels.
- Wearing identification is extremely important for individuals who choose to drink, because intoxication and symptoms of hypoglycemia can often be confused. Drinking alone should always be discouraged.

THE MICRONUTRIENTS: VITAMINS AND MINERALS

Intake of vitamins and minerals should meet recommended levels for good health. If dietary intake is balanced and adequate, there is usually no need for additional vitamin and mineral supplements for the majority of people with or without diabetes. Supplementation of vitamins and minerals should not be used in place of a varied, balanced diet to ensure adequate nutrients. However, those who may be at risk for micronutrient deficiencies and are likely to respond positively to multivitamin supplementation include (a) those who are on a very-low-calorie diet for weight reduction; (b) those who are taking medications that may alter certain micronutrients; (c) those who have documented micronutrient deficiencies such as anemia or osteoporosis; (d) those who are strict vegetarians; (e) pregnant or lactating women; (f) those who are elderly and confined or unable to eat; (g) children and teenagers who severely limit foods or whole food groups; and (h) those who have uncontrolled hyperglycemia with glycosuria, which can result in excess excretion of water-soluble vitamins.

Vitamins and minerals involved in carbohydrate and glucose metabolism that are topics of current research will be discussed briefly.

Chromium

Fortunately, most people with diabetes are not chromium deficient, and chromium supplementation is not recommended unless a deficiency is clearly documented. This trace mineral is needed to potentiate insulin action by the production of glucose tolerance factor. Chromium deficiency in both animal and human studies is associated with elevated blood glucose and lipid levels. Populations at risk for chromium deficiency include the elderly and those on long-term total parenteral alimentation. A study in China reported in 1997 (107) suggested a possible role for chromium supplementation. Individuals with type 2 diabetes were given either a 1,000-μg or 200-μg chromium picolinate supplement or a placebo. Both fasting blood glucose and glycosylated hemoglobin A_{1c} levels were decreased in all three groups, but those taking the 1,000-μg supplement had much larger decreases in fasting and 2-hour insulin concentrations and in total cholesterol. Although the study of Anderson et al. (108) in rats showed a lack of toxicity of chromium chloride and chromium picolinate at concentrations at extremely high limits of what is estimated to be safe, other studies have demonstrated that very large amounts of chromium picolinate caused severe chromosomal damage in animals (109). Until new research can clearly demonstrate the benefits and safety of chromium supplementation, the American Diabetes Association maintains that chromium supplementation is of no known benefit except for those with chromium deficiency (15).

Magnesium

The magnesium link to diabetes involves the transport of glucose across membranes and the oxidation of glucose. Magnesium deficiency has been associated with insulin resistance, carbohydrate intolerance, cardiac arrhythmias, congestive heart failure, retinopathy, and hypertension. Probably the most common cause of magnesium deficiency among those with diabetes is loss of magnesium through chronic glycosuria or diuretic use. A deficiency may lead to increased insulin resistance or may be a result of insulin resistance (110). Several small studies have found that supplementation with magnesium can improve glucose control and insulin sensitivity (111,112). The American Diabetes Association does not recommend routine evaluation of magnesium status in healthy individuals with diabetes but recommends routine evaluations for those people at high risk for magnesium losses, such as those with poor glycemic control (diabetic ketoacidosis and prolonged glycosuria), those receiving diuretics, those with intestinal malabsorption, those with calcium or potassium deficiencies, and pregnant women.

Antioxidants

Antioxidants have received wide attention in the past decade because of their ability to neutralize reactive free electrons and prevent toxic cellular damage. Although there are many antioxidants, including vitamins, minerals, and even plant substances, the emphasis has been on their role in reduction of cancer and cardiovascular risk. Vitamin E is receiving closer attention in people with diabetes. Vitamin E has been related to a decreased risk of cardiovascular disease. α-Tocopherol is considered the major antioxidant for LDL-C and has been reported to increase the oxidative resistance of LDL and improve nonoxidative glucose metabolism in people with type 2 diabetes (113,114). Recent research by Bursell et al. (115) demonstrated that vitamin E may reduce the risk of the development of nephropathy and eye disease. An 8-month trial evaluated 36 patients with type 1 diabetes of short duration. Patients were randomly assigned to either 1,800 IU vitamin E per day or placebo for 4 months and followed up and, after treatment crossover, were followed up for another 4 months. Oral vitamin E treatment appeared to effectively normalize retinal hemodynamic abnormalities and improve renal function without inducing a significant change in glycemic control.

Recommended dosages of vitamin E for people with cardiovascular disease should be in amounts no greater than 400 IU/day. Higher doses may increase the risk of stroke in people with high blood pressure and of bleeding for those patients receiving anticoagulants.

DESIGNING THE MEAL PLAN

> Treatment rests in the hands of the patient. It is by diet and exercise as well as by insulin, and the patients with the will to win and those who know the most, conditions being equal, can live the longest. There is no disease in which an understanding by the patient of the methods of treatment avails as much. Brains count. (1)

One of the primary reasons people with diabetes have such difficulty understanding "nutrition issues" is a lack of nutrition education and counseling by qualified professionals (e.g., registered dietitians). Instead, patients may simply be told to restrict "sugar" or "cut down on calories" or may be given a "sample menu" to follow without an adequate educational foundation. The DCCT provided important insight into the role of nutrition intervention in intensive diabetes treatment and stated that registered dietitians are best qualified to match appropriate meal-planning approaches to the needs of the patient (10).

The time required by the educator and person with diabetes depends on multiple factors, such as emotional status, extended support system, preconceived ideas about the "diabetic diet," and the person's social and cultural attitudes. The consideration and involvement of the person with diabetes are considered critical to devising a successful meal plan that the person is willing and able to follow to promote positive outcomes.

A qualified registered dietitian is an important member of the diabetes team, helping patients understand the relationships among nutrition, exercise, and medication. A dietitian can gather a detailed nutrition history that includes a person's usual intake, the frequency with which he or she eats outside the home, ethnic influences on food choices, food preferences, weight history, diets followed in the past, and food allergies. Caloric needs may then be estimated and developed into a workable meal plan. Meal plans also are based on an individual's lifestyle, sociocultural and economic characteristics, activity level, food preferences, type of diabetes, medications, and other dietary restrictions. The dietitian can instruct and counsel the patient about all of the aspects of nutrition care as it relates to sick-day food management, restaurant eating, carbohydrate counting for intensive insulin therapy, exercise, snacks, and how to incorporate "treats" into the meal plan within the context of overall healthy eating.

Nutrition information is usually presented in small, sequential stages. Initially, basic "survival skills" can be taught and individualized with only general guidelines provided, such as consistency with timing, amount and types of foods, and the relationships among food, activity, and medication. This visit should lay the groundwork in nutrition basics and serve to develop a sound and trusting relationship with the patient.

In later stages, more detailed information can be provided to extend and reinforce existing knowledge and help the patients make positive improvements in nutrition behavior through continuous reviews of food and blood glucose records, laboratory values, and weight status. In recent years, the importance of tailoring nutrition programs to the individual's cultural framework to include traditional foods has been emphasized. Educators must use educational techniques appropriate to the literacy of the individual. The need for tools and techniques suitable for various ethnic groups or learning styles has led to the development of a wide variety of teaching tools, educational materials, and meal-planning approaches.

Meal-Planning Approaches

A *meal-planning approach* simply means the educational resource used by the dietitian to teach the patient how to plan meals (116). Several meal-planning alternatives are available for persons with diabetes.

CARBOHYDRATE COUNTING

Basic carbohydrate (carb) counting may be used for those receiving conventional therapy, with or without insulin. This approach assumes that one carbohydrate choice is based on the amount of food that contains 15 g of carbohydrate (Table 36.9). Patients may simply be given a "carb allowance" to aim for at each meal, while enabling them to spend their allowance based on healthy choices, weight, blood glucose levels, or lipid abnormalities. Advanced carbohydrate counting may be used for those who want to achieve near-normal glucose levels with multiple daily injections of insulin or continuous subcutaneous insulin infusion. This approach coordinates food intake (carbohydrate) by matching the peak activity of insulin with the peak levels of glucose resulting from the digestion and absorption of food. This method allows more precise adjustment of premeal rapid- or short-acting insulin using an insulin/carbohydrate ratio. The ratio is based on the assumption that carbohydrate intake is the main consideration in determining meal-related insulin requirements, together with values from self-monitoring of blood glucose and premeal blood glucose targets set by the physician and the patient. A good understanding of how carbohydrate affects blood glucose, what food groups contain carbohydrate, and which reference books provide carbohydrate content of specific foods is necessary for this approach to be effective.

THE EXCHANGE SYSTEM

This meal-planning approach is based on three main food groups: the carbohydrate group (starch, fruit, milk, vegetables, and other carbohydrates), the meat and meat-substitute group

TABLE 36.9. Food Choices

Carbohydrate
Starch *15 gms carb, 3 gms pro*

Breads, Cereals, & Grains	Beans	Starchy Vegetables	Crackers/Snacks
1 slice (1 oz) bread	$\frac{1}{2}$ C beans, peas (garbanzo, pinto, kidney, white, black-eyed peas)	$\frac{1}{2}$ C corn/peas	3 C air-popped popcorn
$\frac{1}{4}$ (1 oz) large bagel		$\frac{1}{3}$ C baked beans	20 mini pretzels
6 inch tortilla or pita bread		1 C winter squash	6 whole grain crackers
$\frac{1}{2}$ English muffin		3 oz baked, boiled potato	3 graham crackers, $2\frac{1}{2}$″ sq
$\frac{1}{2}$ C cooked cereal		2 oz baked sweet potato	2 rice cakes, 4″ across
$\frac{3}{4}$ C dry cereal		$\frac{1}{2}$ C mashed potato	
2 rice cakes		$\frac{1}{2}$ C sweet potato	
2 slices low-calorie bread			
$\frac{1}{3}$ C cooked rice/pasta			

Fruit *15 gms carb*	Milk *15 gms carb, 8 gms pro*	Non-Starchy Vegetables *15 gms carb*	Other Carbs *15 gms carb*
1 sm (4 oz) fresh fruit, banana	**Fat-Free/Low-Fat (<3 gms fat)**	3 C raw vegetables (lettuce, mushrooms cauliflower, celery, cucumber, peppers, radishes)	1 oz angel food cake
$\frac{1}{2}$ C cnd fruit, juice	1 C fat-free/skim/1% milk		2″ sq unfrosted cake*
$\frac{1}{4}$ C dried fruit	6 oz fat-free, low fat, lite yogurt		2″ sq brownie*
$1\frac{1}{4}$ C watermelon	$\frac{1}{2}$ C evaporated skim milk		2 sm cookies*
$1\frac{1}{4}$ C strawberries	$\frac{1}{3}$ C dry fat-free milk		$\frac{1}{2}$ C ice cream*
1 C melon, raspberries	**Reduced-Fat (3–5 gms fat)**	$1\frac{1}{2}$ C cooked vegetables (asparagus, carrots, beets, broccoli, brussels sprouts, cabbage, green beans, spinach)	$\frac{1}{2}$ C sorbet
$\frac{3}{4}$ C black/blueberries	1 C 2%-milk yogurt		1 Tblsp. jam/jelly
$\frac{1}{2}$ grapefruit	1 C 2% soy/rice milk		1 Tblsp. honey/sugar
$\frac{1}{2}$ C ($5\frac{1}{2}$ oz) mango	6 oz reduced fat yogurt		
17 grapes		1 C vegetable juice	
2 Tblsp. raisins			

Protein—Meat and Meat Substitutes
0 gms carb, 7 gms pro

Very Lean (0–1 gms fat)	Lean (3 gms fat)	Medium-Fat (5 gms fat)	High-Fat (8 gms fat)
1 oz chicken/turkey (white, no skin)	1 oz chicken (dark, no skin)	1 oz beef (most products)	1 oz reg cheese (Swiss, American, cheddar)
1 oz cheese (<1 gm fat)	1 oz lean beef/pork (ham)	1 oz chicken (dark, with skin)	1 Tblsp. natural peanut butter
$\frac{1}{4}$ C egg substitute	1 oz cheese (1–3 gm fat)	1 oz feta/mozzarella cheese	1 oz pork
1 oz fish (haddock, flounder, shellfish)	1 oz turkey (dark meat, no skin)	1 egg	
	1 oz fish (salmon, swordfish)	4 oz tofu	
		1 oz veal	

Fat
0 gms carb, 5 gms fat

Monounsaturated (Heart Healthy)	Polyunsaturated (Heart Healthy)	Saturated (NOT Heart Healthy)
1 tsp. canola/olive/peanut oil	1 tsp. reg (1 Tblsp. lite) margarine	1 tsp. stick (2 tsp. whipped) butter
$\frac{1}{2}$ Tblsp. peanut butter	1 tsp. reg (1 Tblsp. lite) mayonnaise	2 Tblsp. reg (3 Tblsp. lite) sour cream
6 almonds/cashews	1 tsp. corn/safflower/soybean oil	2 Tblsp. half & half
10 peanuts	1 Tblsp. sunflower seeds	
	1 Tblsp. reg salad dressing	

Free Food
A free food has no more than 5 gms carb and 20 calories/serving. Limit to 3 servings per day.

1 C raw vegetables	1 Tblsp. fat-free cream cheese/nondairy creamer/mayonnaise/salad dressing/sour cream	
$\frac{1}{2}$ cooked vegetables	4 Tblsp. fat-free (1 tsp. lite) margarine	1 hard, sugar-free candy
$\frac{1}{4}$ C salsa	2 Tblsp. lite/fat-free whipped topping	Sugar-free gelatin dessert
Bouillon or broth	2 tsp. lite jam/jelly	Sugar-free gum
Coffee/tea	1 Tblsp. sugar-free syrup	Sugar-free soft drinks

Fast Food/Combination Food

Meat pizza, thin crust ($\frac{1}{4}$ of 10 inch pie)	$2\frac{1}{2}$ carbs/1 med-fat meat/3 fats
Cheese pizza, thin crust ($\frac{1}{4}$ of 10 inch pie)	2 carbs/2 med-fat meat/1 fat
Casserole/hot dish (1 c)	2 carb, 2 meat/pro

* Starred items also have additional fat that is not heart healthy.
Center for Innovation in Diabetes Education. Winter 2003.

TABLE 36.10. Nutrient Content of Exchanges

Group/list	Carbohydrate (g)	Protein (g)	Fat (g)	Calories
Carbohydrate				
Starch	15	3	1 or less	80
Fruit	15	—	—	60
Milk				
Skim	12	8	0–3	90
Reduced-fat	12	8	5	120
Whole	12	8	8	150
Other carbohydrates	15	Varies	Varies	Varies
Vegetables	5	2	—	25
Meat and meat substitutes				
Very lean	—	7	0–1	35
Lean	—	7	3	55
Medium-fat	—	7	5	75
High-fat	—	7	8	100
Fat	—	—	5	45

From *Exchange lists for meal planning*, with permission of the American Diabetes Association and the American Dietetic Association, © 1995.

(protein), and the fat group (Table 36.10). Examples of the specific amounts of carbohydrate, protein, fat, or combination of these nutrients in each food group are found in Table 36.9. Foods with similar nutrient values are listed together and may be exchanged or traded for any other food on the same list (117). Portion sizes for each food are listed and are measured after cooking. Exchange lists are used to achieve consistent timing and intake of nutrients and to provide some variety when planning meals. Initially, exchange lists and a meal plan can be a starting point for those patients on conventional therapy or intensive insulin management and can help them learn the carbohydrate content of foods.

GUIDELINE APPROACHES

Another simplified guideline approach, Healthy Food Choices, was successfully used in the DCCT (10). This approach provides an introduction to diabetes meal planning and is most often used in the first stage of nutrition education. It provides guidelines for making healthy food choices with an abbreviated, simplified exchange list.

MENU APPROACHES

This simplified approach is the basis of all meal-planning approaches and illustrates how meals can be designed to accommodate the patient's food preferences and lifestyle while maintaining a healthy dietary intake. Menus may be specific or offer several choices. This method involves the patient in the concept of portion size.

COUNTING APPROACHES

Calorie or fat-gram counting may be appropriate for the obese patient with type 2 diabetes. These self-monitoring methods engage the patient in recording daily food intake and will assist the patient and the dietitian to individualize nutrition goals and achieve weight loss by the patient. These methods also provide some structure in the form of a number of calories or fat grams to strive for on a daily basis while allowing flexibility and variety in meal planning.

In summary, any of these methods can be appropriate for any given individual, but development of an individual meal plan requires that the patient be educated in both the principles of good nutrition and their effective implementation.

MEDICAL NUTRITION THERAPY FOR THE ELDERLY

The healthcare provider who takes into consideration the changes that come with age can vastly improve the nutritional status of and care given to the elderly patient. In general, the elderly have a higher percentage of body fat, a lower lean body mass, and a lower caloric requirement. The extent of the decrease in caloric needs depends on health status and activity levels.

Eating patterns in the elderly can be significantly influenced by many physical, mental, and emotional factors, such as impaired vision, smell, hearing, and/or taste; decreased dexterity and memory; loneliness and depression; dental problems; illness and multiple medications; limited financial resources; and problems of mobility and transportation. Poor teeth and gums or ill-fitting dentures are widespread problems in the elderly and commonly lead to their consumption of softer foods high in sugar and fat. Foods containing greater amounts of fiber, such as fresh fruits, vegetables, or whole-grain cereals or breads, can be more difficult to chew. Depression and physical limitations can limit their access to food or ability to prepare it.

All of these factors contribute to the increased difficulties that the elderly person has in coping with the many demands imposed by diabetes. The important first step in nutritional management for the elderly patient is a complete assessment of all factors that affect nutrition. Obtaining necessary information from some elderly persons may be difficult because of a short attention span, poor short-term memory, or a severe deficit in mental capacity. Older persons may not be able to recall their diet clearly enough to provide the educator with the information necessary for making appropriate dietary recommendations. If possible, family or caregivers or both should be present during education sessions.

In general, it is probably best to keep the meal-planning regimen of the elderly simple. Nutritional goals should aim at the provision of simple, balanced, consistent meals that fit long-standing eating habits and the physical and psychological needs of the individual. Trying to change long-standing food habits by imposing new, rigid, and/or complicated meal plans may not be successful. On the other hand, many elderly have the time and interest to get highly involved in their diabetes management and will eagerly follow instructions when given the necessary support and information.

Last, financial difficulties and social isolation of the elderly and the dietary problems they create cannot be neglected. The dietitian must be sensitive to these needs and be prepared with useful suggestions. Many communities have a variety of support services for elderly citizens, and all health professionals should be familiar with the resources and services available.

MEDICAL NUTRITION THERAPY AND PREGNANCY

Optimal medical and nutritional care must begin before conception to ensure a healthy pregnancy and a positive outcome. In general, the nutritional requirements of a pregnant person with diabetes are essentially the same as those of a pregnant person without diabetes. However, pregnancy magnifies the importance of adherence to nutrition management principles for those with diabetes, the rigid control of glucose levels throughout the course of pregnancy, and the avoidance of ketonuria.

Nutrition management during pregnancy should begin at the earliest possible time. Caloric intake should be evaluated as soon as possible in the first trimester and at the start of each trimester thereafter to ensure adequate intake. During the first trimester of pregnancy, daily caloric levels may vary between 30 and 38 kcal/kg of ideal prepregnancy weight. During the second and third trimesters, this level is increased to 36 to 38 kcal/kg of ideal prepregnancy weight (118). These additional calories during the second and third trimesters are needed for increases in maternal blood volume and increases in breast, uterus, and adipose tissue; placental growth; fetal growth; and amniotic fluids (15). However, individualized caloric targets, blood glucose levels, and weight goals may be recommended. In addition, pregnant women need adequate protein (0.75 g/kg per day plus an additional 10 g per day) (15). For those with preexisting diabetes in pregnancy, three meals and three snacks should be spaced no less than 2 hours apart and no more than 4 hours apart. Distribution of calories is as follows: carbohydrate, 40% to 50% of total calories; protein, 20% to 25% of total calories; and fat, 30% to 40% of total calories.

Caloric requirements are based on pregravid weight, height, age, activity level, and usual intake. Weight gain must also be measured during pregnancy. Both actual weight and BMI may be used for weight assessment. The Joslin Diabetes Center's recommendations for weight gain during pregnancy are listed in Table 36.11. Pregnant women should gain only 2 to 5 pounds during the first trimester. Thereafter, a steady gain of about 1 pound per week is recommended. However, underweight women should gain 1.1 pounds per week, and overweight women should gain only 0.7 pound per week (116). In addition, special emphasis should be placed on the following:

- Meal planning to include appropriate calcium, folic acid, and other vitamins
- Modification of the meal plan to address nausea, vomiting, heartburn, and constipation
- Risk assessment and prevention of fasting hypoglycemia
- Adequate carbohydrate, protein, and fat intake at bedtime to prevent nocturnal hypoglycemia or ketones
- Current intake of sweeteners and caffeine
- Adjustment of calories for gestational age
- Weight-gain goals during pregnancy based on pregravid weight and clinical assessment.

MEDICAL NUTRITION THERAPY FOR CHILDREN AND ADOLESCENTS

Food and feeding issues are very important in the physical and psychological growth of children. Diet education must be approached differently and be responsive to each child, his or her developmental state, and family dynamics. The child with diabetes is adding the complexities of balancing food, insulin, and activity to the already demanding needs of physical maturation and psychological, social, and cultural development. Adolescents with diabetes face unique challenges. At a time when they are attempting to separate from and become independent of parents and authority, they must follow management routines frequently in conflict with this need as well as with their need to attain peer uniformity. Special attention must be paid to these needs to achieve the young person's maximal cooperation with dietary management.

It is now possible to provide a more positive approach to what could be a potentially negative topic for children and teens: nutrition management and diabetes. Healthcare providers on the diabetes team must not lose sight of the ability of food to provide more than nutrients, especially for this group. Changes in eating should not be viewed as restrictions and losses but as a healthful way for the whole family to eat. Every attempt should be made to design a meal plan that reflects the child's food preferences and the family's social and cultural attitudes. Flexibility and graduated goal setting are important keys to success, increasing the chances of the child's achieving optimal diabetes management and decreasing the development of complications. In the attempt to maintain the "pleasures of the table," it is essential that the nutrition guidelines promote "normal" healthy eating and prevent isolating and dividing the child and family in their food choices.

For the child with diabetes, frequent assessment of diet and careful monitoring of growth are necessary. Nutritional assessment should include the regular plotting of height and weight measurement on standard growth charts in an effort to detect any

TABLE 36.11. Recommended Weight Gain During Pregnancy

Description	% of ideal body weight	Body mass index (kg/m²)	Recommended weight gain during pregnancy (lb)
Underweight	<90	<19.8	25–40
Normal weight	90–120	19.8–26.0	25–35
Overweight	120–135	26.0–29.0	15–25
Obese	>135	>29.0	At least 15

From Beaser RC, and Staff of Joslin Diabetes Center. *Joslin's diabetes deskbook—a guide for primary care providers.* Copyright © 2001 by Joslin Diabetes Center. Reprinted with permission.

shift in growth. Meal plans will need to be adjusted on a regular basis to account for changes in growth rate and activity. There can be wide seasonal variations in caloric needs as children change activity patterns from school to home, on weekends or vacations, and from periods of sports activity to lulls between seasons. General guidelines to help develop a positive working relationship with the child or adolescent and their caretakers are as follows:

- Include children and teens in the interview to allow them to be part of the decision-making process.
- Do not refer to or label a child as a "diabetic"; these are children who happen to have diabetes.
- Interview prepubertal children separately and together with family to stimulate self-management.
- Provide reassurance that most of the child's usual foods can be included in his or her meal plan.
- Describe the meal plan as a "road map" for healthy eating, rather than a rigid diet.
- Stress healthy eating practices for the entire family rather than focusing on just the child with diabetes.
- Avoid negative words when counseling, such as cannot, do not, never, bad, restrict, and especially the word diet. In a child's mind, diet connotes deprivation, as well as a short-term process rather than an ongoing one.
- Ask about favorite foods and avoid eliminating these foods. Instead, stress balance, moderation, and variety.
- Review the reality of special treats for special occasions and relate treat foods to extra exercise and active days.
- Advise caregivers that omitting foods because of a single high blood glucose reading is not advisable.

Continued nutritional follow-up and education are required every 6 months to 1 year as the child grows and develops and as the family works to gain expertise in the nutritional management of diabetes.

SUMMARY

Nutrition management for the person with diabetes is one of the most important factors in the attainment and maintenance of good metabolic control. Devising meal plans that provide flexibility while conforming to guidelines based on current research is a constant challenge to the registered dietitian. To translate meal plans into an action plan for patients with diabetes, a registered dietitian must have a thorough understanding of all the components of diabetes management and help each person adapt diabetes to his or her lifestyle instead of adapting lifestyle to his or her diabetes. Although a great deal of information that improves our ability to manage diabetes continues to be generated, we do not yet have the final answers about what constitutes the "ultimate" dietary maneuvers. Therefore, it is important for the clinician to stay abreast of new research and knowledge and be willing to try new approaches to nutritional management of diabetes.

REFERENCES

1. Joslin EP. *Diabetic manual for doctor and patient,* 9th ed. Philadelphia: Lea & Febiger, 1953.
2. Wood FC Jr, Bierman EL. New concepts in diabetic dietetics. *Nutr Today* 1972;7:4–12.
3. Rafkin M. Diabetes and diet—partners with a past. *Diabetes Forecast* 1990; 43:50–51.
4. West KM. Diet therapy of diabetes: an analysis of failure. *Ann Intern Med* 1973;79:425–434.
5. Brunzell JD, Lerner RL, Hazzard WR, et al. Improved glucose tolerance with high carbohydrate feeding in mild diabetes. *N Engl J Med* 1971;284: 521–524.
6. Anderson JW, Herman RH, Sakim D. Effect of high glucose and high sucrose diets on glucose tolerance of normal men. *Am J Clin Nutr* 1973;26: 600–607.
7. American Diabetes Association Committee on Food and Nutrition. Special report: principles of nutrition and dietary recommendations for patients with diabetes mellitus. *Diabetes* 1971;20:633–634.
8. Green JA, Holler HJ, eds. *Meal planning approaches in the nutrition management of the person with diabetes.* Chicago: American Dietetic Association, 1987.
9. US Department of Agriculture, US Department of Health and Human Services. *U.S. dietary guidelines,* 5th ed. Hyattsville, MD: USDA Human Nutrition Information Service, Home and Garden Bulletin 232, 2000:30.
10. Diabetes Control and Complications Trial Research Group. The effect of intensive treatment of diabetes on the development and progression of long-term complications in insulin-treated diabetes mellitus. *N Engl J Med* 1993; 329:977–986.
11. Reichard P, Nillson BY, Rosenqvist V. The effect of long-term intensified insulin treatment of the development of microvascular complications of diabetes mellitus. *N Engl J Med* 1993;329:304–309.
12. American Diabetes Association. Nutritional recommendations and principles for individuals with diabetes mellitus: 1994. *Diabetes Care* 1994;17: 490–518.
13. UK Prospective Diabetes Study Group. Intensive blood-glucose control with sulphonylureas or insulin compared with conventional treatment and risk of complications in patients with type 2 diabetes (UKPDS 33). *Lancet* 1998;352: 837–853.
14. The Diabetes Prevention Program. Design and methods for a clinical trial in the prevention of type 2 diabetes. *Diabetes Care* 1999;22:623–634.
15. American Diabetes Association. Evidence-based nutrition principles and recommendations for the treatment and prevention of diabetes and related complications (position statement). *Diabetes Care* 2003;26[Suppl 1]:S51–S61.
16. Wing RR, Shoemaker M, Marcus MD, et al. Variables associated with weight loss and improvement in glycemic control in type II diabetic patients in behavioral weight control programs. *Int J Obes* 1990;14:495–503.
17. Reaven GM: Beneficial effect of moderate weight loss in older patients with non-insulin-dependent diabetes mellitus poorly controlled with insulin. *J Am Geriatr Soc* 1985;33:93–95.
18. Watts NG, Spanheimer RG, DiGirolamo M, et al. Prediction of glucose response to weight loss in patients with non-insulin-dependent diabetes mellitus. *Arch Intern Med* 1990;150:803–806.
19. Markovic TP, Jenkins AB, Campbell LV, et al. The determinants of glycemic responses to diet restriction and weight loss in obesity and NIDDM. *Diabetes Care* 1998;21:687–694.
20. National Institutes of Health, National Heart, Lung, and Blood Institute, North American Association for the Study of Obesity. The practical guide: identification, evaluation, and treatment of overweight and obesity in adults. NIH publication no. 00-4084, October 2000.
21. American Diabetes Association. Position statement: evidence-based nutrition principles and recommendations for the treatment and prevention of diabetes and related complications. *Diabetes Care* 2002;25:148–197.
22. Brunzell JD, Lerner RL, Hazzard WR, et al. Improved glucose tolerance with high carbohydrate feeding in mild diabetes. *N Engl J Med* 1971;284: 521–524.
23. Brunzell JD, Lerner RL, Porte D Jr, et al. Effect of a fat free, high carbohydrate diet on diabetic subjects with fasting hyperglycemia. *Diabetes* 1974;23: 138–142.
24. American Diabetes Association. Nutritional recommendations and principles for individuals with diabetes mellitus. *Diabetes Care* 1986;10:126–132.
25. Thompson RG, Hayford JT, Danney MM. Glucose and insulin responses to diet: effect of variations in source and amount of carbohydrate. *Diabetes* 1974;27:1020–1026.
26. Reaven GM. How high the carbohydrate [Editorial]. *Diabetologia* 1980;18: 409–413.
27. Jarrett RJ. More about carbohydrates [Letter]. *Diabetologia* 1981;21: 427–428.
28. Garg A, Bantle JP, Henry RR, et al. Effects of varying carbohydrate content of diet in patients with non-insulin-dependent diabetes mellitus. *JAMA* 1994;271:1421–1428.
29. Rasmussen OW, Thomsen C, Hansen KW, et al. Effects on blood pressure, glucose, and lipid levels of a high-monounsaturated fat diet compared with a high carbohydrate diet in NIDDM subjects. *Diabetes Care* 1993;16:1565–1570.
30. Rivellese AA, Giacco R, Genovese S, et al. Effects of changing amount of carbohydrate in diet on plasma lipoproteins and apolipoproteins in type II diabetic patients. *Diabetes Care* 1990;13:446–448.
31. Chen Y-DI, Swami S, Skowronski R, et al. Effect of variations in dietary fat and carbohydrate intake on postprandial lipemia in patients with non-insulin-dependent diabetes mellitus. *J Clin Endocrinol Metab* 1993;76:347–351.
32. Chen YD, Coulston AM, Zhou MY, et al. Why do low-fat high-carbohydrate diets accentuate postprandial lipemia in patients with NIDDM? *Diabetes Care* 1995;18:10–15.
33. Parillo M, Rivellese AA, Ciardullo AV, et al. A high-monounsaturated-fat/low-carbohydrate diet improves peripheral insulin sensitivity in non-insulin-dependent diabetic patients. *Metabolism* 1992;41:1373–1378.
34. Garg A, Grundy SM, Unger RH. Comparison of effects of high and low carbohydrate diets on plasma lipoproteins and insulin sensitivity in patients with mild NIDDM. *Diabetes* 1992;41:1278–1285.

35. O'Dea K, Traianedes K, Ireland P, et al. The effects of diet differing in fat, carbohydrate, and fiber on carbohydrate and lipid metabolism in type II diabetes. *J Am Diet Assoc* 1989;89:1076–1086.
36. Jenkins DJA, Wolever TM, Taylor RH, et al. Glycemic index of foods: a physiological basis for carbohydrate exchange. *Am J Clin Nutr* 1981;34:362–366.
37. Wolever TM, Nguyen PM, Chiasson JL, et al. Determinants of diet glycemic index calculated retrospectively from diet records of 342 individuals with non-insulin dependent diabetes mellitus. *Am J Clin Nutr* 1994;9:1265–1269.
38. Wolever TMS. The glycemic index: flogging a dead horse? *Diabetes Care* 1997;20:452–456.
39. Jarvi AE, Karlstrom BE, Granfeldt YE, et al. Improved glycemic control and lipid profile and normalized fibrinolytic activity on a low-glycemic index diet in type 2 diabetes patients. *Diabetes Care* 1999;22:10–18.
40. Giacco R, Parillo M, Rivellese AA, et al. Long-term dietary treatment with increased amounts of fiber-rich low-glycemic index natural foods improves blood glucose control and reduces the number of hypoglycemic events in type 1 diabetic patients. *Diabetes Care* 2000;10:1461–1466.
41. Ludwig DS. Dietary glycemic index and obesity. *J Nutr* 2000;130[2SSuppl]: 280S–283S.
42. Brand-Miller JC, Holt SH, Pawlak DB, et al Glycemic index and obesity. *Am J Clin Nutr* 2002;76:281S–285S.
43. Ludwig DS. The glycemic index: physiological mechanisms relating to obesity, diabetes, and cardiovascular disease. *JAMA* 2002;287:2414–2423.
44. Foster-Powell K, Holt SHA, Brand-Miller JC. International table of glycemic index and glycemic load values. *Am J Clin Nutr* 2002;76:5–56.
45. Jenkins DJA, Kendall CW, Augustin LS, et al. Glycemic index: overview of implications in health and disease. *Am J Clin Nutr* 2002;76:266S–273S.
46. Willett W, Manson J, Liu S. Glycemic index, glycemic load, and risk of type 2 diabetes. *Am J Clin Nutr* 2002;76:274S–280S.
47. Franz MJ, Horton ES, Bantle JP, et al. Nutrition principles for the management of diabetes and related complications [Technical Review]. *Diabetes Care* 1994;17:490–518.
48. Coulston AM, Reaven GM. Much ado about (almost) nothing. *Diabetes Care* 1997;20:241–243.
49. Pi-Sunyer FX. Glycemic index and disease. *Am J Clin Nutr* 2002;76: 2905–2908.
50. Franz MJ. Carbohydrate and diabetes: is the source or the amount of more importance? *Curr Diabetes Rep* 2001;1:177–186.
51. Brand-Miller J, Foster-Powell K, Holt S. *The new glucose revolution complete guide to glycemic index values.* New York: Marlowe & Company, 2003:5–8.
52. Wolever TM. Relationship between dietary fiber content and composition in foods and the glycemic index. *Am J Clin Nutr* 1990;51:72–75.
53. Hollenbeck CM, Coulston A, Donner C, et al. The effects of variations in percent of naturally occurring complex and simple carbohydrates on plasma glucose and insulin responses in individuals with non-insulin-dependent diabetes mellitus. *Diabetes* 1985;34:151–155.
54. Loghmani E, Rickard K, Washburne L, et al. Glycemic responses to sucrose-containing mixed meals in diets of children with insulin-dependent diabetes mellitus. *J Pediatr* 1991;119:531–537.
55. Bantle JP, Swanson JE, Thomas W, et al. Metabolic effects of dietary sucrose in type II diabetic subjects. *Diabetes Care* 1993;16:1301–1305.
56. Peterson DB, Lambert J, Gerrig S, et al. Sucrose in the diet of diabetic patients—just another carbohydrate? *Diabetologia* 1986;29:216–220.
57. Rickard KA, Loghmani E, Cleveland JL, et al. Lower glycemic response to sucrose in the diets of children with type 1 diabetes. *J Pediatr* 1998;133: 429–432.
58. Peters AL, Davidson MB, Eisenberg K. Effect of isocaloric substitution of chocolate cake for potato in type I diabetic patients. *Diabetes Care* 1990;13: 888–892.
59. National Health and Nutrition Examination Survey III (NHANES) 1988–94. NCHS CD-ROM series 11, no. 2A. ASCII version. Hyattsville, MD: National Center for Health Statistics, April 1998.
60. Bruce B, Spiller GA, Klevay LM, et al. A diet high in whole and unrefined foods favorably alters lipids, antioxidant defenses, and colonic function. *J Am Coll Nutr* 2000;19:61–67.
61. Kiehm TG, Anderson JAW, Ward K. Beneficial effects of a high carbohydrate, high fiber diet on hyperglycemic diabetic men. *Am J Clin Nutr* 1976;29: 895–899.
62. Simpson HCR, Simpson RW, Lousley S, et al. A high carbohydrate leguminous fiber diet improves all aspects of diabetic control. *Lancet* 1981;1:1–5.
63. Rivellese A, Riccardi G, Giacco A, et al. Effect of dietary fiber on glucose control and serum lipoproteins in diabetic patients. *Lancet* 1980;2:447–450.
64. Riccardi G, Rivellese A, Pacioni D, et al. Separate influence of dietary carbohydrate and fiber on the metabolic control in diabetes. *Diabetologia* 1984;26: 116–121.
65. Nuttall FQ. Dietary fiber in the management of diabetes. *Diabetes* 1993;42: 503–508.
66. Wolever TMS. Relationship between dietary fiber content and composition in foods and the glycemic index. *Am J Clin Nutr* 1990;51:72–75.
67. McMurry JF Jr, Baumgardner B. A high-wheat bran diet in insulin treated diabetes mellitus: assessment with the artificial pancreas. *Diabetes Care* 1984;7:211–214.
68. Hall SHE, Bolton TM, Hetenyi G Jr. The effect of bran on glucose kinetics and plasma insulin in non-insulin-dependent diabetes mellitus. *Diabetes Care* 1980;3:520–525.
69. Wursch P, Pi-Sunyer FX. The role of viscous soluble fiber in the metabolic control of diabetes: a review with special emphasis on cereals rich in beta-glucan. *Diabetes Care* 1997;20:1774–1780.
70. Chandalia M, Garg A, Lutjohann D, et al. Beneficial effects of high dietary fiber intake in patients with type 2 diabetes mellitus. *N Engl J Med* 2000;342: 1392–1398.
71. Rendell M. Dietary treatment of diabetes mellitus [Editorial]. *N Engl J Med* 2000;342:1440–1441.
72. Protein and amino acids. In: *Recommended dietary allowances*, 10th ed. Washington, DC: National Academy Press, 1989:52–77.
73. Cahill GF Jr. Starvation in man. *N Engl J Med* 1970;282:668–675.
74. Nair KS, Garrow JS, Ford C, et al. Effect of poor diabetic control and obesity on whole body protein metabolism in man. *Diabetologia* 1983;25:400–403.
75. Nyberg G, Norden G, Attman PO, et al. Diabetic nephropathy: is dietary protein harmful? *J Diabet Complications* 1987;1:37–40.
76. Levey AS, Adler S, Caggiula AWE, et al. Effects of dietary protein restriction on the progression of advanced renal disease in the Modification of Diet in Renal Disease Study. *Am J Kidney Dis* 1996;27:652–663.
77. Franz MJ. Protein controversies in diabetes. *Diabetes Spectrum* 2000;13: 132–141.
78. Nuttall FQ, Gannon MC: Plasma glucose and insulin response to macronutrients in nondiabetic and NIDDM subjects. *Diabetes Care* 1991;14: 824–838.
79. Westphal SA, Gannon MC, Nuttal RQ. The metabolic response to glucose ingested with various amounts of protein. *Am J Clin Nutr* 1990;52:267–272.
80. Khan MA, Gannon MC, Nuttal FQ. Glucose appearance rate following protein ingestion in normal subjects. *J Am Coll Nutr* 1992;11:701–706.
81. Gannon MC, Damberg G, Gupta V, et al. Ingested protein has little effect on glucose concentration or rate of glucose appearance in people with type 2 diabetes. *J Am Coll Nutr* 1999;18:546(abst 97).
82. Feingold KR, Grunfeld C, Pang M, et al. LDL subclass phenotypes and triglyceride metabolism in non-insulin dependent diabetes. *Arteriosclerosis* 1992;12:1496–1502.
83. American Diabetes Association. Management of dyslipidemia in adults with diabetes. *Diabetes Care* 2003;26[Suppl 1];S83–S86.
84. Executive Summary of The Third Report of the NCEP Expert Panel on Detection, Evaluation, and Treatment of High Blood Cholesterol in Adults (Adult Treatment Panel III). *JAMA* 2001;285:2486–2499.
85. Coulston AM, Hollenbeck CM, Swislocki ALM, et al. Persistence of hypertriglyceridemic effect of low fat, high carbohydrate diets in NIDDM patients. *Diabetes Care* 1989;12:94–101.
86. Executive Summary of the Third Report of the National Cholesterol Education Program (NCEP III), National Institutes of Health, NIH News Release, May 2001.
87. Warshaw HS, Franz MJ, Powers MA, et al. Fat replacers: their use in foods and role in diabetes medical nutrition therapy [Technical Review]. *Diabetes Care* 1996;19:1294–1301.
88. Miettinen TA, Puska P, Gylling H, et al. Reduction of serum cholesterol with sitostanol-ester margarine in a mildly hypercholesterolemic population. *N Engl J Med* 1995;333:1308–1312.
89. Nguyen TT, Croghan IT, Dale LC. Mayo Clinic and Foundation, Rochester, MN: European Atherosclerosis Society, 1998 (abst).
90. Bantle JP, Swanson JR, Thomas W, et al. Metabolic effects of dietary fructose in diabetic subjects. *Diabetes Care* 1992;15:1468–1476.
91. Geil PM: Complex and simple carbohydrates in diabetes therapy. In: Powers MA, ed. *Handbook of diabetes medical nutrition therapy*. Gaithersburg, MD: Aspen, 1996:303–319.
92. Lipinski GWV. The new intense sweetener acesulfame-K. *Food Chemistry* 1985;16:259–269.
93. American Dietetic Association. Use of nutritive and nonnutritive sweeteners (position statement). *J Am Diet Assoc* 1998;98:580–587.
94. Nehrling JK, Kobe P, McLane MP, et al. Aspartame use by persons with diabetes. *Diabetes Care* 1985;8:415–417.
95. Council on Scientific Affairs. Aspartame. Review of safety issues. *JAMA* 1985;254:400–402.
96. Morrison AS, Buring JE. Artificial sweeteners and cancer of the lower urinary tract. *N Engl J Med* 1980;302:537–541.
97. Morgan R, Wong O. A review of epidemiological studies on artificial sweeteners and bladder cancer. *Food Chem Toxicol* 1985;23:529–533.
98. Council on Scientific Affairs. Saccharin—review of safety issues. *JAMA* 1985;254:2622.
99. Mezitis N, Koch P, Maggio C, et al. Glycemic response to sucralose, a novel sweetener, in subjects with diabetes mellitus. *Diabetes Care* 1996;19:1004–1005.
100. DeCastro JM, Orozco S. Moderate alcohol intake and spontaneous eating patterns of humans: evidence of unregulated supplementation. *Am J Clin Nutr* 1990;52:246–253.
101. Suter PM, Schutz Y, Jequier E. The effect of ethanol on fat storage in healthy subjects. *N Engl J Med* 1992;326:983–987.
102. Flatt JP. Body weight, fat storage, and alcohol metabolism. *Nutr Rev* 1992;50:267–270.
103. Burr ML, Fehily AM, Butland BK, et al. Alcohol and high density lipoprotein cholesterol: a randomized controlled trial. *Br J Nutr* 1986;56: 81–86.
104. Steinberg D, Pearson TA, Kuller LH. Alcohol and atherosclerosis. *Ann Intern Med* 1991;114:967–976.
105. Suh I, Shaten BJ, Cutler JA, et al. Alcohol use and mortality from coronary heart disease: the role of high-density lipoprotein cholesterol. *Ann Intern Med* 1992;116:881–887.
106. Gaziano Jm, Buring JE, Breslow JL, et al. Moderate alcohol intake, increased levels of high density lipoprotein and its subfractions, and decreased risk of myocardial infarction. *N Engl J Med* 1993;329:1829–1834.

107. Anderson RA, Cheng N, Bryden NA, et al. Elevated intakes of supplemental chromium improve glucose and insulin variables in individuals with type 2 diabetes. *Diabetes* 1997;46:1786–1791.
108. Anderson RA, Bryden NA, Polansky MM. Lack of toxicity of chromium chloride and chromium picolinate. *J Am Coll Nutr* 1997;16: 273–279.
109. Stearns DM, Wise JP, Patierno SR, et al. Chromium (III) picolinate produces chromosome damage in Chinese hamster ovary cells. *FASEB J* 1995;17: 1643–1648.
110. Alzaid A, Dinneen S, Moyer T, et al. Effects of insulin on plasma magnesium in non-insulin dependent diabetes mellitus: evidence for insulin resistance. *J Clin Endocrinol Metab* 1995;80:1376–1381.
111. Lima JDL, Cruz T, Pousada JC, et al. The effect of magnesium supplementation in increasing doses on the control of type 2 diabetes. *Diabetes Care* 1998;21:682–686.
112. Paolisso G, Sgambato S, Cambardella A, et al. Daily magnesium supplements improve glucose handling in elderly subjects. *Am J Clin Nutr* 1992; 55: 1161–1167.
113. Ceriello A, Giugliano D, Quatraro A, et al. Vitamin E reduction of protein glycosylation in diabetes: new prospect for prevention of diabetic complications? *Diabetes Care* 1991;14:68–72.
114. Reaven PD, Herold DA, Barnett J, et al. Effects of vitamin E on susceptibility of low-density lipoprotein and low density lipoprotein subfractions to oxidation and on protein glycation in NIDDM. *Diabetes Care* 1995;18: 807–816.
115. Bursell SE, Clermont AC, Aiello LP, et al. High-dose vitamin E supplementation normalizes retinal blood flow and creatinine clearance in patients with type 1 diabetes. *Diabetes Care* 1999;22:1245–1251.
116. Diabetes Care and Education Dietetic Practice Group of the ADA. *Meal planning approaches for diabetes management*, 2nd ed. Alexandria, VA: American Dietetic Association, 1994.
117. American Diabetes Association and the American Dietetic Association. *Exchange lists for meal planning*. New York: American Diabetes Association, 1995.
118. Beaser RS, et al. *Joslin's diabetes deskbook—a guide for primary care providers*. Boston: Joslin Diabetes Center, 2001.

CHAPTER 37

Behavioral Research and Psychological Issues in Diabetes: Progress and Prospects

Barbara J. Anderson, Ann E. Goebel-Fabbri, and Alan M. Jacobson

Over the past half-century, there has been an explosion of research and clinical work focused on the central role of behavioral and psychological issues in the lives and care of persons living with chronic illness, particularly diabetes. Clinicians and researchers alike acknowledge that behavior (i.e., self-management behavior) is the most fundamental source of both the treatment and prevention of diabetes. Moreover, behavioral scientists play an important role in research focused on the prevention and cure of type 1 and type 2 diabetes. As described by Glasgow and colleagues (1), "The most compelling evidence of the complementarity of behavioral science and biology is the observation that clinical advances, such as intensive therapy, islet transplantation, or genetic testing and 'engineering,' raise rather than eliminate behavioral and psychological questions and needs." In the past decade, behavioral scientists and mental health clinicians have formed the Council of Psychology and Behavioral Medicine within the American Diabetes Association. Behavioral-science research has addressed broad-ranging issues about living with diabetes such as the impact of tight blood sugar control on the cognitive functioning and quality of life of the person with diabetes, how family members can help the person with diabetes live a healthy lifestyle, and what constitutes the most effective treatment for the person with diabetes who also has major depression. Research studies on behavioral and psychological aspects of diabetes are now published in medical journals as well as psychological journals. Most important, this attention to behavioral and psychological issues in the treatment of diabetes has refocused the field on health promotion in living with diabetes and on prevention of the disease itself. The "behavior specialist" is now a recognized member of the multidisciplinary diabetes care team.

We are writing this chapter for clinicians who work with persons living with diabetes. We have attempted to provide an up-to-date review of research progress focused on behavioral and psychological aspects of diabetes that are relevant to the professionals who care for persons with diabetes. We have divided this review into four sections. First we discuss psychosocial issues that are salient at each stage of development across the life cycle. Second, we discuss research on factors that affect adaptation to chronic illness: stress, coping, social and family environments, adherence, and "diabetes burnout." In the third major section, we focus on new paradigms of the patient-provider relationship. In the format of an "intervention table," we provide an overview of research on intervention strategies and techniques relevant to practicing clinicians. In our final section, we address special psychological problems that arise in the care of persons with diabetes, such as eating disorders, sexual functioning, and depression. To conclude, we review progress in and suggest prospects for future research on behavioral issues in diabetes.

DIABETES AND THE LIFE CYCLE

At each stage in the life cycle, the individual is confronted with a series of "developmental tasks" or goals in physical, psychological, and social domains. Within this context, diabetes presents people with unique additional demands at particular developmental stages. Persons with diabetes face the challenge of adapting to each normative developmental stage while balancing the influence of each new stage on the complex tasks of diabetes self-care and management.

The demands of diabetes self-care may exacerbate the pressures of normal development. At each stage of development, family members of persons with diabetes are confronted with the task of being sensitive to the importance of establishing a developmentally appropriate balance between the patient's need for independence and his or her need for family support and involvement in self-care tasks. This dilemma raises unique issues at different stages of child and adult development for families of patients with diabetes. The struggle to balance independence and dependence in the relationships between the person with diabetes and family members presents major coping tasks for all members of the family.

Childhood

It is well documented that the complex daily regimen of diabetes care can affect every aspect of family life and child and adolescent development (2–4).

Although diabetes is relatively rare among infants and toddlers, when it is diagnosed in this age group, the parents or caregivers are the real "patients" (5). Parents are faced initially with the challenge posed by their grief over the loss of a "healthy," "perfect" child. While still in the midst of this acute adjustment phase, parents must also learn the fundamentals of diabetes care and accommodate their family lives to include the daily tasks of disease management. Many parents, during this first phase of the disease, report increased marital conflict and feelings of depression; however, over time and with greater opportunities for diabetes education, parents report greater confidence and more flexibility in the diabetes regimen (6).

Diabetes in toddlers and children of preschool age presents parents and healthcare providers with the challenge of adapting diabetes care to the toddler's normal developmental struggle for independence. Children's natural drive toward autonomy is often reflected in refusals to cooperate when receiving injections or blood glucose monitoring and in conflicts about food. In this way, diabetes can fuel parent–child conflicts that typify this developmental stage. Parents can help foster their child's sense of independence without compromising diabetes care by allowing children to choose between two snacks, between injection sites, and which fingers to use for blood glucose monitoring. In addition, for children who are finicky eaters, administering Humalog injections after meals may help eliminate parent–child power struggles at mealtimes. Temper tantrums are common in children at this age, but they may also be indicative of hypoglycemia. Many parents identify difficulties in differentiating diabetes-related mood changes from age-appropriate behavior (6). Once hypoglycemia has been ruled out, parents need to set as firm limits as they would for their child if he or she did not have diabetes.

The transition to school is a particularly difficult time for parents of young children with diabetes. Parents struggle with anxiety about their child's safety and supervision. Parents should be encouraged to take an active role in educating daycare workers, nannies, babysitters, and teachers about signs and symptoms of high and low blood glucose levels, appropriate treatment of hypoglycemia, and the mechanics of blood glucose monitoring and insulin administration.

There is a growing body of evidence that mild cognitive deficits may result from recurrent, severe episodes of hypoglycemia in young children. Researchers using neuropsychological assessments have found significant differences in verbal intelligence, visual-motor coordination, and visuospatial abilities in comparing youths with diabetes to age-matched controls (7–10). Rovet and colleagues found that children diagnosed with diabetes before the age of 4 years had more frequent hypoglycemic seizures than did children diagnosed later in childhood, suggesting that severe hypoglycemia during the period of brain development may impair later cognitive functioning (10). In light of these findings, clinicians and caregivers of very young children with diabetes must actively avoid the trend toward intensive glycemic control advocated by the Diabetes Control and Complications Trial (11,12). Age-specific blood glucose ranges, aimed at preventing severe hypoglycemia, should be the standard of care for these young patients (13).

Because peer relationships are so important once children start school, it is important to be aware of the impact of diabetes on social functioning. Diabetes during the school-age years can affect the child's self-esteem. In fact, many studies link low self-esteem in children to poorly controlled diabetes (14,15). For this reason, children with diabetes should be encouraged to participate fully in school-based activities, sports, and clubs that can serve as sources of support for the development of positive self-esteem. For this to be accomplished, children may require individualized care plans in school (16) with changes in lunch schedules and extra time for snacks to prevent hypoglycemia. Parents may need to advocate for their child so that these safety precautions can be put in place to allow for full integration of children with diabetes into the regular school routine. Parents should be encouraged to work with school personnel to ensure that their child misses as little classroom time as possible. The overall goal of diabetes treatment during the school years should include the minimal disruption of successful experiences in school.

Adolescence

Research has consistently shown a decline in metabolic control of diabetes during adolescence—influenced partly by physiologic hormonal changes during puberty and partly by a decline in diabetes self-care during this time (17–19). The role of the peer group has been implicated in the decrease in self-care exhibited by adolescents with diabetes. Jacobson and colleagues (20) report that more than one-half of adolescents with newly diagnosed diabetes do not disclose their diabetes to their close friends and that 35% of these teens report that they believe their friends would like them more if they did not have diabetes. Other research has indicated that adolescents will skip needed insulin injections in an attempt to fit in with their peers or out of fear that diabetes self-care will draw negative attention to themselves (21,22). On the positive side, however, research on benefits of peer support for adolescents with diabetes shows that peer and family support in combination is directly associated with the integration of diabetes self-care behavior into daily adolescent routines (23,24).

A final area of diabetes management that poses a particular challenge across child development is the gradual transition of diabetes responsibilities from parent to child. The consensus is growing across research studies that children and adolescents given greater responsibility for diabetes management make a greater number of mistakes in self-care, are less consistent in adhering to their treatment plan, and have poorer metabolic control than those children whose parents remain involved in diabetes management (25–30). Results of these studies have led many clinicians to advocate a diabetes treatment approach whereby parents and teens share responsibility for the tasks of diabetes care. This involves open communication between parent and child to reduce diabetes-related conflicts about out-of-range blood sugars and to encourage a more matter-of-fact, problem-solving approach to blood sugar control. Each family needs to be encouraged to develop its own pattern of parent-adolescent teamwork so that the child with diabetes can continue to feel support for the daily burden of diabetes care and be less at risk for the development of diabetes adherence problems.

Early to Middle Adult Years

In contrast to the extensive empiric literature on child and adolescent development within the context of diabetes, relatively little research has been carried out on adaptation to diabetes during early adulthood. One area of interest has focused on examining the process of transitioning from pediatric management of diabetes to management in the adult healthcare system. In a survey of patients making this transition, Pacaud and colleagues (31) report that up to 50% of the patients surveyed reported delays or loss of regular medical follow-up during this transition period. One way of understanding the barrier to transitions in healthcare providers is implicated by findings reported by Wysocki and colleagues (32) that difficulties in adjusting to diabetes during adolescence persist into adulthood. Studies of this transition period, while rare, argue for the importance of interventions aimed at smoothing the transition of care from adolescence to adulthood. This is especially important for "high-risk" patients who have already been struggling with their diabetes management during childhood and adolescence.

The developmental tasks of middle adulthood are complex and take time to master. These tasks include household and lifestyle management, childrearing, and career management. During the middle adult years, each of these tasks involves acceptance of the inevitable processes of aging, as well as an investment in external social systems. According to Newman and Newman, "The tasks of middle adulthood demand an expanded conceptual analysis of social systems and a capacity to balance individual needs with system goals. The adult not only learns how to function effectively within larger groups, s/he comes to invest energy in those groups with which s/he can most readily identify" (33).

Diabetes imposes conflicts between an adult's responsibilities for maintaining his or her own health and blood sugar levels and responsibilities for meeting the needs of other family members (34). Few studies have been done on the impact of diabetes in a parent on the family environment of children (35). Interest has centered primarily on understanding the influence of spouse support. Ahlfield et al. (36) studied the impact of diabetes on marriage and quality of daily life. They report that adults with diabetes perceived that the disease interfered with family activities and finances more than did their spouses, who did not have diabetes. Significantly more men than women with diabetes felt that the disease was a source of friction in their marriage.

Shenkel and colleagues (37) reported that the importance of the diabetes treatment regimen to the spouse who did not have diabetes was directly related to level of adherence to the treatment plan in the spouse who had diabetes. Pieper et al. (38) reported that, in a sample of patients 40 years or older who had type 2 diabetes, the higher the rating that nondiabetic spouses gave to the benefits of diet the lower they perceived their ability to help the partner with diabetes. Dietary changes were most frequently rated as the most difficult part of the diabetic treatment regimen. Pieper et al. (38) concluded, "For the married person diagnosed as having diabetes in middle age or later life, lifestyle changes, especially in regard to diet and medications, may impact on marital adjustment. A lack of understanding of the impact of diabetes on the marital relationship may allow a couple to use diabetes to negatively influence their marriage and disease control."

Pregnancy

The experience of pregnancy for a woman with diabetes is shaped by a number of forces: the development of her self-concept, sexuality, and body image during childhood and adolescence; information she has received about diabetes as it relates to her ability to become pregnant and have a "normal, healthy" baby; the quality of her diabetes control before pregnancy; the presence of any diabetes complications before pregnancy; her access to highly specialized high-risk prenatal care; her resources for coping with the physical demands of diabetes self-management during pregnancy and with the emotional stress related to uncertain health outcomes for herself and the baby; and, finally, the availability of involvement and support from a partner and from her extended family and friends before, during, and immediately after the pregnancy.

Recent research documents the ability of women with diabetes to give birth to "normal, healthy" infants if they have tight blood glucose control at conception and can maintain it throughout pregnancy. More information is now available on the impact of pregnancy on the health of women with diabetes. Women with more advanced ocular, vascular, and renal complications are frequently advised not to become pregnant because of the potential for pregnancy to accelerate these physical complications and cause severe physical disability or even death of the mother. For these reasons, the decision about whether and when to become pregnant is a complex one for the woman with diabetes. Involvement and support from the partner are critical during this stressful decision-making period, especially if there are contraindications for pregnancy.

Medical management of diabetes is especially intense during pregnancy in terms of the frequency of contact with specialists and the daily diabetes self-care that is recommended. Insulin needs often decrease during the first trimester of pregnancy but increase during the second and third trimesters. Throughout the pregnancy, most women must increase the frequency of blood sugar monitoring to at least four times a day because the stabilization of blood-sugar levels is more difficult during pregnancy and because hypoglycemia and hyperglycemia present risks to the developing fetus.

Given the health risks of poorly controlled diabetes during pregnancy, it is surprising that the majority of women with diabetes do not have access to pre-pregnancy counseling. In fact, as few as 34% of women with diabetes receive conception guidance before they get pregnant (39), and fewer than half of pregnancies in women with diabetes are planned (40). Holing and colleagues (40) found that women who had unplanned pregnancies reported that their doctors had discouraged them from getting pregnant, whereas women with planned pregnancies reported that their doctors had reassured them of their ability to have a healthy baby despite their diabetes. Such research underscores the importance of positive prepregnancy education and supportive patient-doctor interactions that allow women with diabetes who are of childbearing age to feel that they can engage in family planning and work with their healthcare team to support a healthy pregnancy.

Despite the research advances and the increased likelihood of the delivery of a "healthy, normal" baby, a great deal of apprehension accompanies a pregnancy in the context of diabetes. In addition to the normal concerns that all pregnant women experience, the pregnant woman with diabetes must cope with concerns about the impact of her diabetes on the health of her baby and the reciprocal impact of pregnancy on her own health. Research by Langer and Langer (41) found that pregnant women with diabetes were significantly more anxious throughout their pregnancies than were women without diabetes. This increased anxiety may be fueled by the multiple physiologic tests that women with diabetes must undergo in order to assess the health and condition of the developing fetus throughout their pregnancy. The increased work involved in managing a pregnancy in conjunction with the intense emotional experience of the pregnancy make support from the husband or partner an extremely important factor in the outcome of pregnancy in diabetes. Support from extended family and friends also is critical in helping the pregnant woman maintain the discipline and emotional stability needed for the duration of the pregnancy.

Late Adulthood

In the later adult years, the primary developmental tasks concern the redirection of energy to new roles and activities, the acceptance of one's life and the physical and cognitive changes associated with aging, and the development of a point of view about death. Retirement requires many persons to find new outlets for their intellectual capacities and social supports. Little has been written about diabetes in the later adult years. Empiric data on coping issues facing the elderly patient with diabetes are not available. Retirement can place financial constraints on patients with diabetes, who may no longer have the same access to healthcare reimbursements through private employee-based health insurance.

Compared with their functioning in middle adulthood, later adulthood is a period when the normal physical deterioration of the aging process in combination with the onset and progression of diabetes complications realistically limit the functioning of many elderly patients. Moreover, elderly patients with diabetes frequently cope with multiple medical conditions and multiple complex medication schedules simultaneously. Thus, it may be difficult for family members and elderly patients to distinguish the deterioration related to the normal aging process from the progression of diabetes complications. Worry, frustration, and alienation may result from the decline in level of functioning. Moreover, depression is a serious and underrecognized problem among the elderly. In the patient with diabetes, depression can decrease their motivation and energy for diabetes-related self-care.

Healthcare professionals caring for elderly patients with diabetes must be alert to the need to assess issues of functional status. As such, they are encouraged to assess the patient's level of manual dexterity, quality of vision and hearing, and ability to be physically active. The functional status of each patient influences his or her ability to carry out the complex tasks of diabetes management; including administering medication doses accurately, monitoring blood glucose regularly, inspecting their feet, remembering medical recommendations and appointments, preparing meals, and engaging in exercise. If self-care abilities decline, flexible arrangements need to be made for greater family or professional involvement in diabetes treatment and decision-making. Younger family members find that they must become educated in diabetes and make decisions concerning living arrangements for an elderly parent with diabetes who is no longer able to inject insulin independently, to take medications at appropriate times, or to eat reliably.

In summary, across the life span—from infancy to the later adult years—the struggle to balance independence and dependence in the relationships between the person with diabetes and family members, especially with respect to self-care, presents unique coping challenges for patients with diabetes and their families.

ADAPTATION TO CHRONIC ILLNESS

One of the most significant outcomes of the growth of the fields of health psychology and behavioral medicine has been publication of scientific evidence of the contribution of psychological and social factors to human health, particularly to adaptation to chronic health problems, such as cancer, heart disease, stroke, and diabetes (42). This has led to a wide acceptance of the interplay between psychosocial factors and biologic outcomes in both type 1 and type 2 diabetes. Three broad psychosocial factors that impact a person's adaptation to chronic illness are stress, coping ability, and the social and family environment. Although these factors interact, each will be considered separately for purposes of review.

Stress

Numerous reports have examined the influence of emotionally stressful experiences on health status. For example, Rahe et al. (43), using scaled measures of life events, found that acute medical illnesses tend to occur at times of change. Other studies suggest that stressful experiences can be important etiologic factors in the pathophysiology of disabling chronic conditions, such as coronary vessel disease (44). The course of a chronic illness such as diabetes can also be affected by stressful experiences (45). Studies often emphasize the additive effects of multiple stressful life events. In addition to the number and intensity of these life events, their particular meaning to the individual also contributes to their ultimate influence on health status (45–47).

STRESS AND DIABETES ONSET

Interest in examining the role of psychological or environmental stressors in diabetes has a long history. Early reports (48) suggested that the onset of type 1 diabetes may be triggered by psychological stress in a physiologically susceptible individual. Stein and Charles (48), using retrospective documentation, found a higher prevalence of disturbances in infant feeding patterns in a small group of diabetic children than in their siblings. Since psychological stress can alter activity in the sympathetic nervous and adrenomedullary systems, elevate plasma cortisol levels, possibly enhance the secretion of glucagon and growth hormone (49), and affect immune functions (50), a theoretically relevant set of biologic pathways are present that could mediate a relationship between psychosocial stressors and diabetes onset. Indeed, some animal studies using the BB rat as a model of type 2 diabetes have indicated that an increase in environmental stress shortens the time to onset of overt diabetes mellitus (51).

Although stress, both psychological and physical, has been shown to have major effects on metabolic activity and has long been suspected of playing a role in the onset of type 1 diabetes (52), there is no solid evidence base for this connection between stress and diabetes onset. However, recent research in genetics, immunology, and endocrinology has identified a multicomponent model of the pathogenesis of type 1 diabetes that links autoimmune destruction of insulin-producing pancreatic β-cells with genetic and environmental factors. Existing studies of the role of stress in the development of type 1 diabetes have been limited by methodologic problems, including small subject samples and a reliance on retrospective accounts of major life stressors (52,53). Despite methodologic limitations, existing studies suggest that individuals with type 1 diabetes are more likely to report a major life stressor or family loss prior to the onset of symptoms of diabetes (48). A provocative recent paper by Thernlund and associates (54) reported that stressful life events during the first two years of life distinguished children who developed diabetes from matched healthy controls. The hypothesis is that major stressors, including illnesses, occurring early in the life of a genetically susceptible individual could impair immune function during this critical developmental period, which over time triggers the onset of type 1 diabetes.

Another recent line of research has examined the role of stress as a trigger for type 2 diabetes. Surwit and colleagues (56) noted the "mounting experimental evidence of altered sympathetic nervous system activity in type 2 diabetes" identified from several animal models. They have demonstrated that *ob/ob* mice differ from their lean littermates in having exaggerated blood glucose responses to environmental stressors and to the exogenous administration of epinephrine (55,56). Other research suggests that *ob/ob* mice may have enhanced adrenergic responses to environmental stress (57).

Research on obese but otherwise healthy men (58) shows that they exhibit an alteration in autonomic nervous system functioning—specifically a decrease in sympathetic and parasympathetic activity—associated with an increase in body fat. This finding indicates that a disordered homeostatic mechanism may exist that could promote excessive storage of energy by decreasing sympathetic activity but at the same time defend against weight gain by decreasing parasympathetic activity.

It is not clear whether these and other changes in neuroendocrine activity are causative, are related to the onset of hyperglycemia and/or hyperinsulinemia, or are simply chance findings without significance for the problem of type 2 diabetes. However, this is an area in which further research may elaborate the role of stress and central nervous system control in the onset and course of type 2 diabetes. There is consensus that type 2 diabetes is strongly genetically determined and most likely is polygenic and heterogeneous. Genes involved in some subtypes of type 2 diabetes have recently been identified (59): "There has been clear demonstration that obesity, physical inactivity, and other lifestyle factors are important environmental risk factors for the development of type 2 diabetes in the genetically-susceptible individual." Further research is needed to clarify the interplay between genetic factors, lifestyle factors, obesity, and stress in the onset of type 2 diabetes.

STRESS AND THE COURSE OF DIABETES

Stress has both direct and indirect effects on outcomes in chronic illness (60). It has been postulated that stress may affect the course of diabetes either directly through the stress hormones affecting blood glucose levels and insulin metabolism, or indirectly, through stress producing changes in self-care behavior (61). Stress, both psychological and physical, has been shown to have direct effects on metabolic activity (62). Physical stressors, such as illness or trauma, have been shown to cause hyperglycemia and eventual ketoacidosis in persons diagnosed with type 1 diabetes (63). Among children with type 1 diabetes, epinephrine infusion produced more elevated blood glucose levels and more rapid ketone release than among children without diabetes (64). Recent work examining negative life events among individuals with type 1 diabetes has suggested that these types of stressors have an adverse effect on glucose control (63,65). In contrast, studies of the effects of laboratory-induced stress on glycemic functioning of individuals with type 1 diabetes have been more equivocal (66). Possibly, differences across studies in the types of laboratory stressors investigated (e.g., noise, mental arithmetic) may have contributed to the contradictory findings, as not all subjects may find these experiences to be stressful. Indeed, studies examining the effects of stress hormones on glucose control have produced more consistent findings (62). Some research has suggested that there may be "stress-reactive" subgroups of individuals with diabetes for whom stress mainly affects metabolic control through direct physiological mechanisms (67,68).

In addition to a direct effect of stress on metabolic activity, stress has an indirect effect on metabolism by influencing the self-care behaviors of the person with diabetes, which in turn have an impact on metabolic control. Stressful events distract the person with diabetes from usual patterns of self-care. Stress causes disruptions in routines and decreases in resources and supports that are likely to result in less stable patterns of self-care behavior for patients with diabetes and their families. Thus, to the extent that the person's self-care behaviors are influencing metabolic control, by disrupting self-care behavior, stress indirectly influences metabolic control.

In summary, there are intriguing suggestions from initial studies of animal models of diabetes that psychological and physical stress may play a role in the onset of diabetes, especially type 1 diabetes. Definitive conclusions linking stress with the onset of either type 1 or type 2 diabetes await further multidisciplinary research. The evidence is stronger that stress affects the course of diabetes, both through a direct neuroendocrine effect and an indirect behavioral effect on the metabolic control of the person with diabetes.

STRESS AS A CONSEQUENCE OF DIABETES OR DIABETES-SPECIFIC DISTRESS

Health psychologists have recognized that in addition to the possible effects of stress on the onset or course of various chronic physical illnesses, "the chronic illness itself and its required treatment also constitute stressors that the individual must confront" (60). Polonsky and colleagues at the Joslin Diabetes Center (69) led one of the first scientific efforts to identify these diabetes-specific stressors. Moreover, this group has developed and validated a measure of diabetes-specific distress—PAID (*P*roblem *A*reas *i*n *D*iabetes). Because of the innovative and important perspective that understanding diabetes-specific distress can have for healthcare providers, in this section we list the 20 sources of diabetes-specific distress that affect patients that were identified by Polonsky and associates and measured in the PAID measure (69–71).

1. Not having clear and concrete goals for diabetes care
2. Feeling discouraged with the diabetes treatment plan
3. Feeling scared when thinking about living with diabetes
4. Uncomfortable social situations related to diabetes care (e.g., people nagging about what to eat)
5. Feelings of deprivation regarding food and meals
6. Feeling depressed when thinking about living with diabetes
7. Not knowing if moods or feelings are related to diabetes
8. Feeling overwhelmed by diabetes
9. Worrying about low blood sugar reactions
10. Feeling angry when thinking about living with diabetes
11. Feeling constantly concerned about food and eating
12. Worrying about the future and the possibility of serious complications
13. Feelings of guilt or anxiety when off track with respect to diabetes management
14. Not "accepting" diabetes
15. Feeling unsatisfied with the diabetes physician
16. Feeling that diabetes is taking up too much mental and physical energy every day

17. Feeling alone with diabetes
18. Feeling that friends and family are not supportive of diabetes management efforts
19. Coping with complications of diabetes
20. Feeling "burned out" by the constant effort needed to manage diabetes

Weinger and Jacobson (72) have demonstrated that higher levels of diabetes-specific distress in adults with type 1 diabetes relate to poorer metabolic control as well as to lower self-reported quality of life. Future research is needed to identify strategies for preventing diabetes-related distress and for intervening with patients overwhelmed by the stresses of living with diabetes. We now address the wide variation seen in how persons handle these diabetes-specific stressors as well as the stress of chronic illness.

Coping Ability

Coping is a broad construct that generally refers to "the strategies that people use to manage and master stressful circumstances and to minimize the negative impact of life stressors on psychological well-being" (73). The concept of coping introduces the concept of "person" or "individual difference" factors that influence an individual's adaptation to the stresses of chronic illness. From a biopsychosocial model, these individual factors (such as self-esteem, health beliefs, personal models, ego strength, and personality) affect and are affected by other factors in the model (social environment, disease itself, healthcare system).

Differences in coping styles and personality types influence the appraisal of stress (74) and therefore can affect the individual's experience of what constitutes a stressful life situation. Such individual differences may affect not only the emotional and behavioral consequences of stress, as noted earlier, but also the hormonal components of the stress response in cardiovascular illness (75) and perhaps in diabetes (76). Similarly, Wolff et al. (77) found that variations in personal coping styles are associated with variations in corticosteroid levels of individuals under stress.

Clearly, individual differences color the meaning and experience of being ill as well as the specific problems posed by that illness. These differences influence the management of a complex chronic illness such as diabetes. Understanding such individual differences can contribute to the thoughtful design of treatment plans.

Studies of a pattern of individual differences in response to the diagnosis of diabetes failed to identify a "diabetic personality" and proved unproductive overall (78). This led to study of the "cognitive and behavioral" strategies patients use to manage diabetes and their emotional responses (79). First, we need to consider the major set of coping tasks that face the person diagnosed with a chronic physical illness such as diabetes. Moos and Tsu (80) identified seven fundamental "adaptive tasks" with which the person with any chronic illness must cope:

1. Dealing with pain and incapacitation
2. Dealing with the hospital environment and special treatment procedures
3. Developing adequate relationships with professional staff
4. Preserving a reasonable emotional balance
5. Preserving a satisfactory self-image
6. Preserving relationships with family and friends
7. Preparing for an uncertain future

Coping skills is the term used to describe those individual differences in the ways in which persons face and handle stressful tasks such as those above.

Lazarus and Folkman (81) suggested that the coping process begins when a person appraises or evaluates the stressful situation and that the person evaluates both the stressful aspects of the situation as well as his or her ability to deal effectively with these stressors. Within this theory, individuals cope with stress in one of two major ways: by attempting to change the nature of the stressful situation (problem-focused coping) or by managing their emotional reactions to the stressful situation (emotion-focused coping) (74). *Emotion-focused coping* is described as directing energy away from the source of stress, by avoidance, denial, or distraction. *Problem-focused coping* refers to efforts to resolve the problem, to focus energy and resources on solving the problem or reducing stress. Studies with adolescents with type 1 diabetes give conflicting results about the relationship between these two types of coping skills and level of metabolic control (82,83). However, in studies with adolescents, consistent associations have been reported between self-care behavior and type of coping skill, with emotion-focused coping associated with poorer levels of self-care behavior (84,85).

COPING AND THE COURSE OF DIABETES

An increasing number of systematic studies point to the influence of individual characteristics on the course of diabetes, with respect to management (adherence), metabolic control, and overall adjustment (86,87). Self-esteem is one of the aspects of personality important in adaptation to diabetes. High or robust self-esteem may serve as a protective factor in a patient's adjustment to the vicissitudes of this complicated illness and to the potentially confusing, and at times inadvertently hurtful, responses of significant others such as family members, close friends, schoolmates, and colleagues. Along these lines, Jacobson et al. (88) have found that preadolescents and adolescents with low self-esteem had lower levels of adherence at the time of diagnosis and over time than did those with higher self-esteem.

Several studies have found that other aspects of patient adjustment and coping ability are linked to adherence and glycemic control (88,89). For example, a number of investigators have considered how the patient's level of socioemotional (ego) development may bear upon his or her experience of and response to type 1 diabetes. Ego development reflects the individual's maturation along the lines of impulse control, moral development, cognitive complexity, and interpersonal relationships (90). Barglow and colleagues (91) found that ego development was the best predictor of an adolescent's responsiveness to a brief intervention designed to enhance adherence and glycemic control. In contrast, psychopathology was not associated with the response to the educative intervention. These findings and theoretical considerations suggest that the level of ego development a patient has achieved can affect the benefits of educational and medical interventions designed to improve metabolic control, adherence, or coping strategies. Researchers have suggested that a higher level of ego development may provide an individual with the cognitive and emotional maturity needed to deal effectively with the demands of having a chronic illness (92). Further research is needed to develop interventions that are either tailored to individual differences in psychosocial functioning or designed to alleviate problems in psychosocial functioning that impede adherence among patients with diabetes.

COPING WITH THE DIABETES REGIMEN: REALISTIC EXPECTATIONS AND READINESS TO CHANGE

It is well documented that most people living with diabetes find it difficult to adhere to the daily demands of the diabetes medical regimen. According to Rubin (93), coping problems are common among people with type 1 and type 2 diabetes "largely because the demands of diabetes management are so substantial and unremitting. Specifically, the regimen is demanding and unpleasant, factors outside the patient's control often affect glycemic control, and the avoidance of diabetes-related complications cannot be guaranteed." It is paradoxical that although it is widely recognized that the treatment demands placed on the person with diabetes are complex and burdensome, many clinicians, family members, and patients themselves expect "perfect" adherence to this regimen. This expectation of "perfectionism" has been documented as one of the primary causes of "noncompliance" (94) and "diabetes burnout" (95). Clearly, having realistic expectations for the patient's self-management behavior is an important aspect of the coping process.

It has recently been recognized that the patient's "readiness to change" influences the process of coping with the demands of diabetes (96). Prochaska and DiClemente (97) suggest that patients can be identified as being in one of six stages of change—from "precontemplation," in which individuals are not currently engaged in behavioral change and do not intend to change, all the way to the "maintenance" stage at which individuals have made a healthy behavioral change and have maintained it for 6 months or longer. Future studies of the link between coping style and diabetes self-care must include these dimensions of realistic expectations for self-management behavior and of patients' "readiness to change."

The Social and Family Environments

The social/family environment is the third major psychosocial mediator of adaptation to chronic illness and maintenance of health. In recent years, increased attention has been given to the role of interpersonal or social support variables in the process of adaptation to chronic illness (73). Social support is thought to have a "buffering," "mediating," or "moderating" effect on the stress of living with a chronic illness. While most of this attention has focused on support from within families, there has been some investigation of the benefits of social support outside the family for the chronic diseases of cancer, acquired immunodeficiency syndrome (AIDS), Alzheimer's disease, and cardiovascular disease (73). However, very few empiric studies have examined the social environment outside the family for adults with diabetes (98). Social support such as "worksite, neighborhood, and community factors" in adults with diabetes have received almost no examination (1).

La Greca and colleagues (99,100) have conducted research on social supports outside the family for adolescents with diabetes and reported that peers and friends serve support functions for the adolescent with diabetes specifically different from those provided by the adolescents' family. Whereas families provided more support for daily management tasks (insulin, blood glucose monitoring), friends provided more support for the "lifestyle" aspects of diabetes management (i.e., providing companionship during exercise or when eating meals away from home). Moreover, peers represented a significant source of emotional support for adolescents living with diabetes. In summary, aside from the empiric research with adolescents (23,101), there has been little investigation of social support outside the family for individuals with diabetes.

THE FAMILY AS THE PRIMARY SOCIAL ENVIRONMENT FOR LIVING WITH DIABETES

Diabetes, like several other chronic physical diseases, places demands on the patient for self-care and for clinical decision-making responsibilities that require major adjustments in lifestyle (102). Moreover, these lifestyle adjustments affect many components of family life—food, activity, finances, and time (34). This section focuses on how characteristics of the family environment influence self-management behavior and health outcomes in the person with diabetes. First, it is critical to point out that the relationship between family characteristics and the patient's behavior and health is a bidirectional relationship. In other words, just as family stress has been reported to produce poor diabetes control, similarly, poor control may trigger stress among family members.

CHILDREN AND ADOLESCENTS WITH DIABETES

Empiric research has documented that successful management of a child's diabetes makes it necessary for families to redistribute responsibilities, reorganize their daily routines, and renegotiate family roles (17). When a very young child is diagnosed with diabetes, the parents are, in reality, the patient (4). Golden and colleagues (103) reported that the parents of children who are diagnosed with diabetes before the age of 5 years who receive training in intensive diabetes management and are provided multidisciplinary supports report less family stress, fewer hospitalizations, and fewer episodes of severe hypoglycemia in their very young children with diabetes as compared with families receiving standard diabetes care. With respect to school-aged children with diabetes, there is consensus from empiric studies that the following family characteristics are linked to both good metabolic control and adherence to the treatment regimen: parental warmth and caring; positive parental involvement with diabetes-related tasks; low levels of family conflict; family rules that are followed by all family members; and agreement between both parents about diabetes goals (13).

Longitudinal research by Jacobson and colleagues (88,104) revealed that the child's perception of family conflict at diagnosis was the strongest predictor of poor adherence over a 4-year follow-up period. In a study by Miller-Johnson and colleagues (105), parent–child conflict was related to both adherence and glycemic control. Multivariate analyses indicated that family conflict might interfere with glycemic control by disrupting adherence to treatment (105). The most significant family characteristic of school-aged children who have the best glycemic control and who are the most adherent to the diabetes treatment regimen is the sharing of responsibility for the tasks of the treatment regimen between parent and child (25,106,107).

Certain demographic characteristics of families have also been linked to metabolic outcomes in children with diabetes. Children with diabetes from single-parent families or from ethnic minority or lower socioeconomic backgrounds have been reported to be at increased risk for problems with adherence and diabetes control (108,109).

For adolescents with diabetes, family support has consistently been linked to optimal self-care behavior. However, family support does not consistently relate directly to metabolic outcomes (61). It has been suggested that family conflict has both a direct and an indirect effect on adherence by its impact on family interactions. In a comprehensive review of the literature on adolescents with diabetes, Skinner and colleagues (61) reported that a developmentally appropriate level of parent involvement in the tasks of diabetes management is the single most important predictor of positive adolescent health and self-care behavior outcomes.

ADULTS WITH DIABETES

In contrast to the broad range of studies of family factors and diabetes outcomes in children and adolescents, literature on the families of adults with diabetes is quite limited. The few early studies of adults with diabetes focused exclusively on the relationship of spouse support to adherence and metabolic control in the adult with diabetes. Schafer and colleagues (110) developed an objective questionnaire for assessing the frequency with which family members engage in behaviors defined as "supportive." For adults with type 1 diabetes, greater perceived negative spouse interactions were associated with poorer adherence. However, for adults with type 2 diabetes, no relationship was found between negative spouse interactions and adherence.

Recent work by Fisher and colleagues (111) has provided both a theoretical framework and empiric data on family characteristics of adults with type 2 diabetes from Hispanic and European-American ethnic backgrounds (98,111). Fisher et al. (98) identified four areas of family life that related to health outcomes for adults with type 2 diabetes (98): 1) family structure and organization; 2) family values and beliefs about the world; 3) family expression and management of emotions; 4) family problem solving. Using objective scales with excellent psychometric properties to measure the first three areas of family functioning, Fisher et al. (111) reported significant differences between characteristics of the family and disease management outcomes for Hispanic as compared with European-American families. The family's worldview and management of emotions was linked to disease management among European-American patients, whereas family structure/organization was linked to disease management among Hispanic patients. In general, optimal disease management is reported in families that are well organized, have clear and traditional gender roles, have an optimistic belief about life, and in which spouses are able to resolve differences of opinion about diabetes care.

In summary, there is a close connection between the disease-related coping and stress levels of the person with diabetes and his or her social environment. Especially for social influences within the family, levels of support and conflict have a significant impact on adherence and health outcomes in diabetes.

Adherence and Burnout

The Diabetes Control and Complications Trial (DCCT) proved that intensive insulin management of diabetes, aimed at achieving "near-normal" glycemia, significantly reduces the risk of medical complications of the disease (11,12). For most people with diabetes, achieving near-normal blood glucose levels means treatment with multiple daily injections of insulin, frequent blood glucose monitoring, or the use of a subcutaneous insulin infusion pump. While adherence to the diabetes self-care regimen is believed to be the most essential ingredient in diabetes management, patients commonly have difficulty with sustaining the burden of self-care over time. This was true in the era before dissemination of the DCCT findings, but with the hopeful news for medical outcomes from the DCCT, the number of daily diabetes self-care tasks (and therefore the daily burden of the disease) has increased for most people living with diabetes.

To complicate the matter, evidence shows that adherence is not a univariate phenomenon. One patient's adherence to a meal plan, for example, may be unrelated to adherence to a prescribed regimen of blood glucose monitoring. In general, few significant correlations have been found between the different components of adherence to the self-care regimen (112–115). Therefore, healthcare providers should not assume that a patient's difficulty with adherence to one component of the regimen indicates a global disavowal of the regimen. Initial assessment must include a careful examination of patients' adherence to each aspect of the regimen.

When people become overwhelmed by the complexity of their diabetes regimen, they may feel that nothing they do or how hard they try will have a positive impact on their disease course. This is what diabetes treatment teams are now referring to as the problem of "diabetes burnout," which Polonsky (95) has defined succinctly: "Burnout is what happens when you feel overwhelmed by diabetes and by the frustrating burden of diabetes self-care. People who have burned out realize that good diabetes care is important for their health, but they just don't have the motivation to do it. At a fundamental level, they are at war with their diabetes—and they are losing." When burnout is affecting the patient (or the diabetologist), it can be helpful to remember the words of Joan Hoover, an early diabetes advocate who was appointed to the first Congressional Advisory Committee on Diabetes in the 1970s: "Diabetes is not a do it yourself disease" (94). Diabetes management is burdensome and support of the patient is necessary. This support can include family members, friends, co-workers, and a multidisciplinary diabetes treatment team. Such a support system can help the patient set small, realistically attainable goals to help move gradually out of the struggle with burnout and toward improved diabetes management (116).

THE PATIENT–PROVIDER RELATIONSHIP

Over the last decade, empiric research has increasingly documented the importance of the patient–provider relationship to the adherence of patients with chronic disease to a particular treatment regimen and to health outcomes. The multicenter national Medical Outcomes Study demonstrated that a "collaborative relationship between patient and provider" and a "participatory decision-making style of physicians" (117) improved adherence and health outcomes in patients with chronic illnesses such as cancer, arthritis, and diabetes (118). DiMatteo and colleagues (119) reported that patient satisfaction with the interpersonal communication with their provider is related to adherence to the diabetes treatment regimen. More recently, Ciechanowski and colleagues (120) demonstrated that adherence to the diabetes regimen is associated with the type of attachment the adult patient displays in the context of the patient's perception of the quality of communication with the diabetes provider. Clearly, the behavior of the provider and the quality of the patient–provider relationship are now recognized as critical variables affecting adherence of patients with diabetes to the complex treatment regimen. Over the last decade a new paradigm of the patient-provider relationship has been described in diabetes: "patient empowerment" (121).

Patient Empowerment

As framed by R. Anderson, M. Funnell, and colleagues at the University of Michigan (122), the empowerment approach is based on three key principles: (a) More than 98% of diabetes care is provided by the patient; therefore, the patient is the locus of control and decision-making in the daily treatment of diabetes; (b) the primary goal of the healthcare team is to provide ongoing diabetes expertise, education, and psychosocial support so that patients can make informed decisions about their daily diabetes self-care; and (c) adult patients are much more likely to make and maintain behavior changes if those changes are personally meaningful and freely chosen. Perhaps the most defining characteristic of the empowerment approach is the philosophy that "the patient and the healthcare providers are equals" (123). Diabetes healthcare has benefited because the developers of the empowerment model have translated their philosophy into practical interventions and have provided empiric evidence for its effectiveness. In a randomized con-

TABLE 37.1. Office-based Interventions

Intervention	Description	Primary source
Blood Glucose Awareness Training (BGAT)	BGAT is a psychoeducational intervention designed for patients with type 1 diabetes. Its current version, BGAT-III, is a structured 8-week program, conducted in groups or individually, that provides patients with a systematic approach to enhance anticipation, prevention, awareness, and response to extreme fluctuations in blood glucose levels. The patients most likely to benefit from BGAT are those with poor ability to recognize/predict blood glucose extremes, on intensive insulin therapy, with reduced hypoglycemia awareness, with a history of recurrent severe hypoglycemia, with fear of hypoglycemia, with recurrent diabetic ketoacidosis, and/or with poor metabolic control.	Cox et al. (130) Gonder-Frederick et al. (131,132)
Motivational Interviewing (MI)	MI is a counseling strategy focused on persons reluctant or ambivalent about changing their behavior. Initially formulated for changing addictive behaviors, MI has recently been applied to behavior change in patients with diabetes and other health issues. It differs from a traditional, nondirective therapeutic approach in that the counselor offers advice and helps the patient explore and resolve ambivalence to enhance motivation for change.	Miller et al. (133) Smith et al. (134)
Stage of Change Counseling	Appropriate for use by healthcare providers not just by "counselors," this model of working with patients integrates the empowerment model and MI techniques with the transtheoretical model (Stages of Change Theory). It is a patient-centered approach that helps identify a person's readiness to change behavior and to then identify and prioritize self-management goals in diabetes. As such, it provides the healthcare provider with a framework that breaks down the process of change into a series of stages.	Doherty et al. (96) Prochaska et al. (97,135)
Pediatric office-based interventions	Several pediatric office-based interventions have recently reported encouraging, although preliminary, results. The impact of a "care-ambassador" intervention, a trained assistant to support parents of pediatric patients in making appointments regularly, resolving insurance and billing questions, and helping schedule specialty appointments has been shown to improve medical-visit follow-up and reduce costly adverse outcomes such as diabetes-related hospitalizations and emergency department visits.	Laffel et al. (136)
	A low-cost, family-based psychoeducational intervention aimed at sustaining parental involvement in diabetes-management tasks and reducing diabetes-related family conflict that has been used with adolescents and recently diagnosed pediatric patients. This eight-module intervention is implemented by a trained assistant at the time of the medical office visit. Preliminary results indicate that this intervention helps improve adherence, parent–child teamwork in diabetes management, and glycemic control.	Anderson et al. (137)
Cognitive Behavioral Therapy (CBT)	CBT aims at changing patients' thoughts about diabetes and diabetes self-care tasks that interfere with diabetes management as well as actual diabetes self-care behaviors. CBT involves consciously identifying and challenging maladaptive beliefs. Behavior change in this model is achieved by working gradually toward small, achievable goals. CBT can be implemented in individualized treatment or in a group format.	Weinger et al. (72) Van Der Ven et al. (138)
Coping Skills Training	This group-based treatment technique is aimed at helping adolescents and/or adults cope better with diabetes-related stressors and improving their treatment adherence. It has been shown to be effective when taught by a healthcare professional or a "counselor" with diabetes expertise. Coping Skills Training teaches positive coping skills to patients with diabetes through the use of role playing and active problem solving.	Grey et al. (139) Rubin et al. (140)
Support groups	Heterogeneous support groups for patients or loved ones of patients with diabetes can include people with either type 1 or type 2 diabetes. Another support group model involves a homogeneous group in which people with the same type of diabetes are group members.	Tattersall et al. (141)
	Internet-based discussion groups are being used to provide diabetes support and education for persons unable to access support groups in-person.	Zrebiec et al. (142)
Telephone-based telemedicine technologies	Telephone care is the most widely used technology as a supplement to office-based diabetes education. Telephone care has recently been extended to include "automated telephone disease management" (ATDM). ATDM involves assessment of both health and self-care problems that arose between outpatient visits, as well as education in the form of "health tips" or interactive dietary education modules. Two randomized studies showed that for patients with type 2 diabetes, ATDM as an adjunct to usual care improved glycemic outcomes, frequency of blood glucose monitoring, satisfaction with care, and self-efficacy to perform self-care activities. ATDM enhanced diabetes care for patients living at a remote distance from their diabetes provider and for non-English-speaking and illiterate patients.	Piette et al. (143,144)
Computer- and Internet-based telemedicine technologies	One of the first computer-based interventions in diabetes was pioneered by Glasgow and colleagues. This early intervention involved a 15-min touch-screen computer assessment to help patients identify personal dietary goals and barriers to achieving these goals. Responses were immediately scored and provided to patient and physician. The patient then met with a health educator to collaboratively develop an action plan that took into account the individual's barriers to adherence. This intervention was documented to be cost-effective and patients maintained improvements in diet and serum cholesterol over a 12-mo follow-up period. This work also demonstrated that older patients without previous Internet experiences effectively participated in Internet-based self-management support programs.	Feil et al. (145) Glasgow et al. (146,147)
	A computerized system to assess patients, code and analyze data, and provide feedback to both the patient and healthcare team has also been designed. The Diabetes Psychosocial Management Aid (DPMA) has been used successfully in an inner-city hospital with patients with low literacy and computer skills.	Welch et al. (148)
	Diabetes information has recently become available for education and support over the Internet from several Web-based sites.	www.jdrf.org; www.diabetes.org; www.childrenwithdiabetes.com; www.diabetes123.com; and www.joslin.harvard.edu

trolled trial, Anderson and colleagues (124) demonstrated that a 6-week empowerment intervention program, developed by Feste (125), significantly improved diabetes self-efficacy, diabetes attitudes, and glycemic control. The empowerment model has been described by Anderson and colleagues (122) as follows: "When appropriate changes in roles are made, both the health-care provider and the patient can find themselves part of a satisfying partnership that results in improved glycemic control for the patient and an enhanced sense of self-efficacy and level of satisfaction with care for both parties." Finally, the empowerment model is directed toward physicians, nutritionists, diabetes educators, and behavioral clinicians, all the members of the multidisciplinary team that has become the recommended standard for the care of patients with diabetes.

The Multidisciplinary Team in Diabetes Care

It has long been recognized that because diabetes is such a complex disease, patients need a multidisciplinary team of health professionals for optimal care (126). The current Standards of Medical Care for Patients with Diabetes Mellitus of the American Diabetes Association (127) recommend that "people with diabetes should receive their treatment and care from a physician-coordinated team. Such teams include, but are not limited to, physicians, nurses, dietitians, and mental health professionals with expertise and a special interest in diabetes." In reality, however, most patients with diabetes do not have access to a multidisciplinary team and receive their diabetes care in the office of an internist or family practice physician (128). Appropriately, behavioral scientists have recently focused on translating interventions to improve diabetes self-care behavior and quality of life (129) for office practices that do not have a multidisciplinary team as a resource for patients with diabetes. Table 37.1 presents an overview of the most recent and empirically tested of these interventions, with information about how to access more complete information for the clinician who would like to learn more about these intervention strategies.

SPECIAL PROBLEMS IN DIABETES

Psychiatric Disorders in Diabetes

The literature examining the relationship of diabetes to psychiatric disorders continues to grow. These studies focus primarily on the relationship of diabetes to depression, anxiety disorders, and eating disorders.

With regard to the incidence and prevalence of these disorders, it now appears that patients with type 1 diabetes are at particular risk for the development of depressive disorders. The development of depressive disorders, while increasing with the duration of diabetes and the development of complications also occurs relatively early in the course of illness before the onset of complications (149–151). While there is less research on anxiety disorders, a similar trend is emerging from these studies, especially among patients with type 1 diabetes (152,153). The causal links between psychiatric disorders and diabetes are not well understood, but growing evidence from research suggests the connection described in Fig. 37.1.

Most studies looking at the relationship of diabetes to psychiatric disorders are cross-sectional in design. Directionality and causality in these relationships has yet to be fully determined. A few longitudinal studies do suggest that patients with depressive disorders and or eating disorders appear to develop worse glycemic control and greater risk for retinopathy over time (154,155). Thus, as shown in Fig. 37.1, at least in patients with type 1 diabetes, it is reasonable to assume that diabetes itself may increase the risk of developing some specific psychiatric disorders and, when present, that diabetes outcomes are influenced negatively by their presence.

Studies of type 2 diabetes are less clear with regard to the development of psychiatric disorders, as has been pointed out by Talbot and Nouwen (156). The increased rates of depression in patients with type 2 diabetes appear to occur before the onset of illness, thereby raising an entirely different hypothesis about the etiologic relationship (i.e., that depressive disorders themselves may place patients at risk for developing diabetes). Sup-

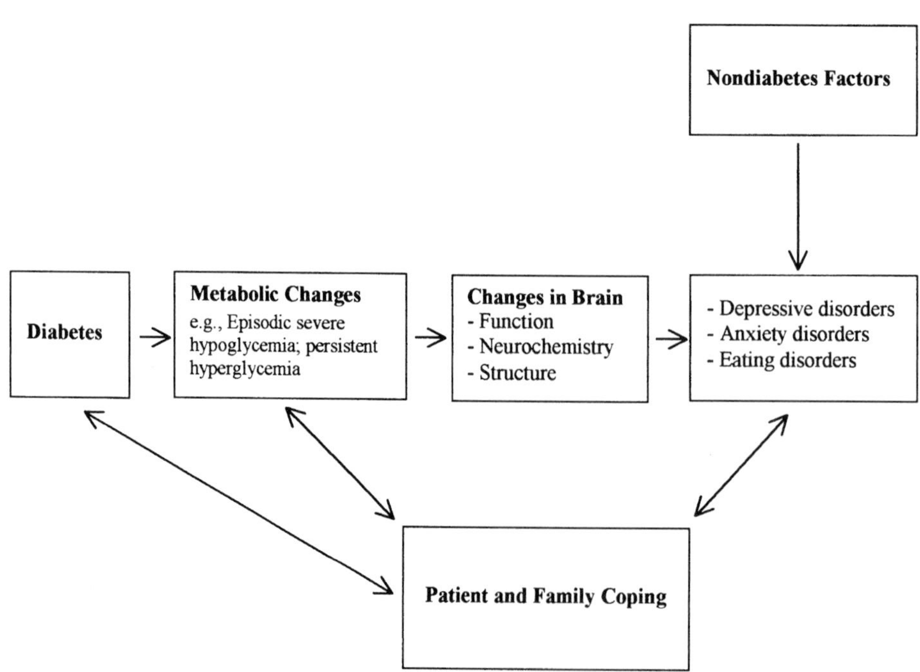

Figure 37.1. Hypothesized model of the relationship of diabetes and psychiatric disorders.

port for this hypothesis derives from the fact that patients with depression have alterations in the hypothalamic-pituitary axis, which lead to increased rates of cortisol production (157–159). Depressed patients also decrease physical activity and increase cardiovascular risk factors by smoking and eating high caloric and fatty foods, suggesting that individuals who are depressed may, because of their changes in lifestyle, develop type 2 diabetes (160–164).

Some investigators also have suggested that the metabolic problems of diabetes (increased rates of hypoglycemia and/or hyperglycemia) could themselves play a role in the development of depression. There is increasing evidence that diabetes leads to changes in the white matter of the brain (162) and that these abnormalities in the white matter, if present in the frontal lobe, may play a role in the development of depression (165). Changes in frontal white matter have been found in studies of depression in patients without medical illness and could lead to changes in the frontal–striatal tracks that regulate affect, thereby increasing risk for affect regulatory problems and consequently of depression (161,166–174). Whatever the direction of causality of the relationship, it does appear that successful treatment of depression and anxiety can lead to improved glycemic control in patients with diabetes (155).

In summary, the frequency of common psychiatric problems such as depression and anxiety disorders appears to be increased among patients with type 1 diabetes and there is now evidence that improved treatment can lead to better outcomes in terms of glycemic control. The combination of high prevalence of common psychiatric illnesses such as depression and anxiety disorders in patients with diabetes and other medical conditions and the treatability of some of these conditions means that it is critical to identify patients with these conditions early in their onset and to implement treatment strategies that are widely recognized to be successful with these patients. Based on a small number of studies, the efficacy of treatment of depression, including cognitive behavior therapy and antidepressant therapy, in patients with diabetes appears to be equivalent to the efficacy in patients without co-occurring chronic disease (175,176). Thus, attention to assessment of depression should be maintained when treating patients who are having problems adapting to diabetes, showing difficulties maintaining metabolic control, and/or other problems with adaptation and stress. These patients may well have an underlying treatable psychiatric condition. Screening measures such as the Symptom Checklist 90R (177) may be useful in identifying patients with diabetes and affective disorders. Moreover, diabetes-specific measures of quality of life, such as the Problem Areas in Diabetes Scale (PAID) (71,178) and the Diabetes Quality of Life Measure (DQOL) (179,180), may also be useful in screening patients who are at risk for these conditions.

Eating Disorders

There has been considerable interest in examining the impact of type 1 diabetes on the development of eating disorders. Although research results in this area are somewhat contradictory, the most recent controlled studies suggest an increased risk of eating disorders among female patients with type 1 diabetes. For example, Jones and colleagues (181) report that the risk of developing an eating disorder was 2.4 times higher in young women with type 1 diabetes than in age-matched women without diabetes. Some researchers have argued that diabetes-specific treatment issues, like the need to carefully monitor diet, exercise, and blood glucose may contribute to the development of eating disorder symptoms among women with diabetes (182). Researchers and clinicians have argued that the attention to food portions, blood sugars, and weight that is part of routine diabetes management parallels the rigid thinking about food and body image characteristic of women with eating disorders. Additionally, intensive insulin management of diabetes has been shown to be associated with weight gain (183).

Researchers who do not report higher rates of eating disorders in female patients with type 1 diabetes often do not include underdosing or omission of insulin as a purging symptom. Fairburn and colleagues (184) compared 56 women with type 1 diabetes to 67 age-matched women without diabetes using a structured diagnostic interview for eating disorders, the Eating Disorder Examination (EDE). They found that the difference in the rates of eating disorders between these groups was not statistically significant; however, they also highlighted the importance of thorough assessments of disordered eating and insulin misuse in this population—especially as a potential cause of poor glycemic control. These authors found widespread insulin misuse among women with diabetes and emphasize that this behavior is not limited to women who meet formal diagnostic criteria for eating disorders. In an 8-year follow-up of this same cohort of patients with diabetes, the authors note that had they included insulin misuse in their eating disorder group, 39% of the women would have been included in the eating disorder group (185). Another study examining disordered eating among adolescents with diabetes also reported no significance between-group differences in rates of eating disorders (186). However, the teens in this study were quite young, and only one half of them administered insulin without parental supervision. It may be that insulin manipulation or omission becomes a more significant problem in older adolescents, as parental supervision of insulin administration decreases.

When symptoms of disordered eating do not meet the level of severity to warrant a formal diagnosis of an eating disorder, intermittent insulin omission and dose reduction for weight loss purposes has been found to be a common practice among women with type 1 diabetes. For example, Polonsky and colleagues (187) found that 31% of a group of 341 women with type 1 diabetes between the ages of 13 and 60 years reported intentional insulin omission. Rates of omission peaked in late adolescence and early adulthood, with 40% of women between ages of 15 and 30 years reporting intentional omission. Insulin use and tighter blood sugar management caused significant psychological distress for these women; with 42.5% reporting fears that keeping their blood glucose in good control would cause weight gain, 44.3% reporting beliefs that taking insulin would cause weight gain, and 35.9% believing that good control would cause them to become fat (187). In addition, studies show that this behavior places women at heightened risk for medical complications of diabetes. Women reporting intentional insulin misuse had higher levels of glycosylated hemoglobin A_{1c} (HbA_{1c}), higher rates of hospital and emergency room visits, and higher rates of neuropathy and retinopathy than did women who did not report insulin omission (187). A report by Rydall and colleagues (154) lends further support to the link between insulin misuse and medical complications of diabetes. They found that disordered eating at baseline was associated with microvascular complications of diabetes 4 years later, with 86% of young women with serious eating disorders presenting with retinopathy compared with 43% of women with moderate eating disorders and 24% of women with no reported eating disturbance.

Women with type 1 diabetes may use insulin manipulation (i.e., administering reduced insulin doses or omitting necessary doses altogether) as a means of caloric purging. Intentionally induced glycosuria is a powerful weight-loss behavior unique to patients with type 1 diabetes. As mentioned above, it is also very dangerous, and places women at greater risk for developing infections, potentially fatal diabetic ketoacidosis (DKA), and long-term medical complications of diabetes. Once established as a long-standing behavior pattern, the problem of frequent insulin omission may be particularly difficult to treat. For this reason, early detection and intervention appears to be crucial. Open-ended questions such as, "Do you ever change your insulin dose or skip insulin doses to influence your weight?" can be helpful in screening for insulin omission, especially when patients have elevated HbA_{1c} values or unexplained DKA. Disordered eating behaviors are often well hidden, but patients should be encouraged to bring up and discuss issues such as their current level of satisfaction with their weight, their weight goals, and—if willing—their experiences with binge eating.

Neuropsychological Aspects of Diabetes

The number of studies of the potential for patients with type 1 and type 2 diabetes to develop problems in cognition and other signs of altered brain function has been growing. These studies have focused on three measures of the brain: cognitive ability; cortical evoked potentials; and magnetic resonance imaging (MRI)–based assessments of brain structure. This research suggests that patients with either type 1 or type 2 diabetes may be at increased risk for changes in brain structure, including white matter lesions and atrophy (162). Decrements in cognitive function, especially in areas of memory and psychomotor speed, have been found. Changes in cortical evoked potentials indicate the possibility of the risk for development of a central neuropathy. Older patients with type 2 diabetes appear to develop cognitive declines at earlier ages and higher rates than age-matched controls without medical illness. Children with onset of type 1 diabetes before the age of 6 years who were studied during adolescence and young adulthood also appear to demonstrate subtle cognitive performance problems (188–190). It is not clear whether these cognitive differences represent developmental delays or problems that persist into adulthood. In children especially, severe hypoglycemia causing seizure, coma, and unconsciousness has been considered as an important causative factor in the development of cognitive problems (188,189,191–197). A small body of research also suggests that persistent hyperglycemia also may play a role in declines in cognitive functioning (190,198). Finally, in older individuals, the development of cerebral vascular illness has been suggested to play an important role in cognitive decline (190).

Two large clinical trials carefully evaluated the impact of intensive diabetes treatment and severe hypoglycemia on the development of cognitive problems in patients with type 1 diabetes diagnosed when they were either adolescents or adults. These studies, the DCCT and the Stockholm Diabetes Intervention Study (SDIS), did not show an effect of intensive treatment or severe hypoglycemia on the development of cognitive problems (199,200). However, both studies had relatively short follow-up periods. Moreover, because of the nature of these trials, the number of severe hypoglycemic episodes was limited. Thus, these studies may understate the problem (201,202). A few other studies of adults do suggest the possibility that severe hypoglycemia in type 1 diabetes could play a role in the development of cognitive problems (201–203). The role of severe hypoglycemia in the development of cognitive problems remains highly controversial. Recently, there have been suggestions that the demonstrated problems in cognition, brain structure, and function may also be associated with the increased incidence of depression in patients with type 1 diabetes (204). To date, no studies have explicitly examined this hypothesis.

Sexual Functioning

It is well established that men commonly develop erectile dysfunction (ED) secondary to diabetes. The prevalence of ED in men with diabetes has been estimated at 35% to 70% (205). ED has been identified as contributing significantly to decreased quality of life in men with diabetes (206).

Longer duration of diabetes, poor glycemic control, and presence of diabetes complications such as diabetic neuropathy, vascular disease, retinopathy, and nephropathy are strongly correlated with the presence of ED in men with diabetes (207,208). In addition, the reported risk of ED is greater among men who smoke cigarettes and self-report symptoms of depression, anxiety, and treatment for hypertension (208). Since the medical treatments for depression, anxiety, and hypertension can also have side effects on sexual functioning, medical interventions for men with longer-term diabetes should be recommended after these risks are taken into account.

Although the organic component in ED has been widely recognized, psychosocial factors also may contribute to the development of ED in a significant subset of men with diabetes. Indeed, some research suggests that in as many as 20% of diabetic men with reported impotence, the dysfunction may have a primarily psychogenic origin (209,210). Any evaluation of ED must therefore be sensitive both to primary psychological factors and to secondary factors that may influence sexual functioning. For example, anxiety about performance may further exacerbate a partially dysfunctional episode in organically impaired individuals. Ignorance also may contribute to such problems. Many couples do not realize and are not informed that diabetes can promote ED and may misinterpret the source of the problem, believing that it is due to loss of love or to an extramarital interest. Most frequently, organic and psychological factors coexist, so that behavioral and psychological interventions may be valuable in facilitating adjustment to the limitations posed by the organic impairment.

Little research has focused on the impact of diabetes on the sexual functioning of women. In fact, since 1971, only 16 such studies have been published (211). These studies present conflicting evidence on the existence of diabetes-associated sexual problems in women. In their comprehensive review of the literature, Enzlin and colleagues (211) attempted to draw consensus between conflicting evidence from these studies. Thus far, it appears that women with diabetes may experience diminished libido and more pain during intercourse as compared with women without diabetes. However, women with diabetes appear to be at especially high risk for decreased or slowed sexual arousal. Researchers postulate that this may relate to inadequate vaginal lubrication, which occurs in 30% of women with diabetes (twice that of the population without diabetes). There is a lack of consistent evidence that diabetes causes problems with achieving orgasm in women.

Whereas there is growing consensus that sexual problems in men with diabetes are influenced by autonomic neuropathic damage, the etiology of sexual arousal problems in women with diabetes remains unclear at this time. Further study of the impact of diabetes and the complex interplay between psychological and physical factors on female sexuality is clearly needed.

CONCLUSION

In summary, we have provided an update of the significant progress made by behavioral scientists and clinicians focused on persons living with diabetes, their families, and their healthcare teams. During the last decade, the role of psychology in diabetes care has moved from a traditionally psychiatric or medical model to a biopsychosocial model, in which behavioral interventions in the form of telemedicine technology or behavioral strategies for optimizing self-management have been shown to improve biologic, psychological, and behavioral outcomes for persons with diabetes.

Now at the beginning of the 21st century, behavioral scientists focused on diabetes are prepared to apply their skills to an even broader spectrum of factors having an impact on the quality of life for persons living with diabetes (1). Increasingly, behavioral issues are seen as critical in basic research toward finding a cure for and preventing type 1 diabetes and identifying genetic and environmental risk factors that could be modified to prevent type 2 diabetes. With the advent of new efficacious treatments and innovative technologies, basic scientists and diabetes clinicians are seeking the contributions of behavioral scientists as they collaborate on the complex biopsychosocial dilemmas in curing, preventing, and treating diabetes.

REFERENCES

1. Glasgow RE, Fisher EB, Anderson BJ, et al. Behavioral science in diabetes. Contributions and opportunities. *Diabetes Care* 1999;22:832–843.
2. Faulkner MS, Clark FS. Quality of life for parents of children and adolescents with type 1 diabetes. *Diabetes Educ* 1998;24:721–727.
3. Silverstein JH, Johnson S. Psychosocial challenge of diabetes and the development of a continuum of care. *Pediatr Ann* 1994;23:300–305.
4. Wolfsdorf JI, Anderson BA, Pasquarello C. Treatment of the child with diabetes. In: Kahn CR, Weir G, eds. *Joslin's diabetes mellitus,* 13th ed. Philadelphia, Lea & Febiger, 1994:430–451.
5. Kushion W, Salisbury PJ, Seitz KW, et al. Issues in the care of infants and toddlers with insulin-dependent diabetes mellitus. *Diabetes Educ* 1991;17: 107–110.
6. Hatton DL, Canam C, Thorne S, et al. Parents' perceptions of caring for an infant or toddler with diabetes. *J Adv Nurs* 1995;22:569–577.
7. Ryan C, Longstreet C, Morrow L. The effects of diabetes mellitus on the school attendance and school achievement of adolescents. *Child Care Health Dev* 1985;11:229–240.
8. Ryan C, Vega A, Longstreet C, et al. Neuropsychological changes in adolescents with insulin-dependent diabetes. *J Consult Clin Psychol* 1984;52:335–342.
9. Ryan C, Vega A, Drash A. Cognitive deficits in adolescents who developed diabetes early in life. *Pediatrics* 1985;75:921–927.
10. Rovet JF, Ehrlich RM, Hoppe M. Intellectual deficits associated with early onset of insulin-dependent diabetes mellitus in children. *Diabetes Care* 1987; 10:510–515.
11. The effect of intensive treatment of diabetes on the development and progression of long-term complications in insulin-dependent diabetes mellitus: the Diabetes Control and Complications Trial Research Group. *N Engl J Med* 1993;329:977–986.
12. Effect of intensive diabetes treatment on the development and progression of long-term complications in adolescents with insulin-dependent diabetes mellitus: Diabetes Control and Complications Trial: the Diabetes Control and Complications Trial Research Group. *J Pediatr* 1994;125:177–188.
13. Anderson BJ, Brackett J. Diabetes during childhood. In: Snoek FJ, Skinner FJ, eds. *Psychology in diabetes care.* New York: Wiley, 2000:1–23.
14. Johnson SB. Psychosocial factors in juvenile diabetes: a review. *J Behav Med* 1980;3:95–116.
15. Ryden O, Nevander L, Johnsson P, et al. Family therapy in poorly controlled juvenile IDDM: effects on diabetic control, self-evaluation and behavioural symptoms. *Acta Paediatr* 1994;83:285–291.
16. Clark WL. Advocating for the child with diabetes. *Diabetes Spectrum* 1999;12: 230–236.
17. Jacobson AM, Hauser ST, Lavori P, et al. Family environment and glycemic control: a four-year prospective study of children and adolescents with insulin-dependent diabetes mellitus. *Psychosom Med* 1994;56:401–409.
18. Hoey H, Mortensen H, McGee H, et al. Is metabolic control related to quality of life? A study of 2103 children and adolescents with IDDM from 17 countries. *Diabet Res Clin Pract Suppl* 1994;44:S3.
19. Mortensen HB, Villumsen J, Volund A, et al. Relationship between insulin injection regimen and metabolic control in young Danish type 1 diabetic patients: comparison to non-diabetic children: the Danish Study Group of Diabetes in Childhood. *Diabet Med* 1992;9:834–839.
20. Jacobson AM, Hauser ST, Wertlieb D, et al. Psychological adjustment of children with recently diagnosed diabetes mellitus. *Diabetes Care* 1986;9:323–329.
21. Dunning PL. Young-adult perspectives of insulin-dependent diabetes. *Diabetes Educ* 1995;21:58–65.
22. Meldman LS. Diabetes as experienced by adolescents. *Adolescence* 1987;22: 433–444.
23. La Greca AM, Auslander WF, Greco P, et al. I get by with a little help from my family and friends: adolescents' support for diabetes care. *J Pediatr Psychol* 1995;20:449–476.
24. Wallander JL, Varni JW. Social support and adjustment in chronically ill and handicapped children. *Am J Community Psychol* 1989;17:185–201.
25. Anderson BJ, Auslander WF, Jung KC, et al. Assessing family sharing of diabetes responsibilities. *J Pediatr Psychol* 1990;15:477–492.
26. Anderson B, Ho J, Brackett J, et al. Parental involvement in diabetes management tasks: relationships to blood glucose monitoring adherence and metabolic control in young adolescents with insulin-dependent diabetes mellitus. *J Pediatr* 1997;130:257–265.
27. Burns KL, Green P, Chase HP. Psychosocial correlates of glycemic control as a function of age in youth with insulin-dependent diabetes. *J Adolesc Healthcare* 1986;7:311–319.
28. Ingersoll GM, Orr DP, Herrold AJ, et al. Cognitive maturity and self-management among adolescents with insulin-dependent diabetes mellitus. *J Pediatr* 1986;108:620–623.
29. Weissberg-Benchell J, Glasgow AM, Tynan WD, et al. Adolescent diabetes management and mismanagement. *Diabetes Care* 1995;18:77–82.
30. Wysocki T, Taylor A, Hough BS, et al. Deviation from developmentally appropriate self-care autonomy. Association with diabetes outcomes. *Diabetes Care* 1996;19:119–125.
31. Pacaud D, McConnell B, Huot C, et al. Transition from pediatric care to adult care for insulin-dependent diabetes patients. *Can J Diabetes Care* 1996;20: 14–20.
32. Wysocki T, Hough BS, Ward KM, et al. Diabetes mellitus in the transition to adulthood: adjustment, self-care, and health status. *J Dev Behav Pediatr* 1992; 13:194–201.
33. Newman BM, Newman PR. Development through life: a psychosocial approach. Homewood, IL: Dorsey Press, 1975.
34. Anderson BJ. Diabetes and adaptations in family systems. In: Holmes CS, ed. Neuropsychological and behavioral aspects of diabetes. New York: Springer-Verlag, 1990:85–101.
35. Anderson BJ, Kornblum HK. The family environment of children with a diabetic parent: issues for research. *Fam Syst Med* 1984;2:17–27.
36. Ahlfield JE, Soler NG, Marcus SD. The young adult with diabetes: impact of the disease on marriage and having children. *Diabetes Care* 1985;8:52–56.
37. Shenkel RJ, Rogers JP, Perfetto G, et al. Importance of "significant others" in predicting cooperation with diabetic regimen. *Int J Psychiatry Med* 1985;15: 149–155.
38. Pieper BA, Kushion W, Gaida S. The relationship between a couple's marital adjustment and beliefs about diabetes mellitus. *Diabetes Educ* 1990;16: 108–112.
39. Willhoite MB, Bennert HW Jr., Palomaki GE, et al. The impact of preconception counseling on pregnancy outcomes. The experience of the Maine Diabetes in Pregnancy Program. *Diabetes Care* 1993;16:450–455.
40. Holing EV, Beyer CS, Brown ZA, et al. Why don't women with diabetes plan their pregnancies? *Diabetes Care* 1998;21:889–895.
41. Langer N, Langer O. Pre-existing diabetics: relationship between glycemic control and emotional status in pregnancy. *J Matern Fetal Med* 1998;7:257–263.
42. Nicassio PM, Smith TW. Managing chronic illness: a biopsychosocial perspective. Washington, DC: American Psychological Association, 1995.
43. Rahe R, Meyer M, Smith M, et al. Social stress and illness onset. *J Psychosom Res* 1964;8:35–44.
44. Goldband S, Katkin E, Morell M. Personality and cardiovascular disorder: steps toward demystification. In: Sarason IG, Spielberger CD, eds. *Stress and anxiety*. New York: Wiley, 1979:351–370.
45. Johnson JH, Sarason IG. Moderator variables in life stress research. In: Sarason IG, Spielberger CD, eds. *Stress and anxiety*. New York: Wiley, 1979: 159–168.
46. Bibring GL. Psychiatry and medical practice in a general hospital. *N Engl J Med* 1956;254:366–372.
47. Klerman GL, Izen JE. The effects of bereavement and grief on physical health and general well-being. *Adv Psychosom Med* 1977;9:63–104.
48. Stein SP, Charles ES. Emotional factors in juvenile diabetes mellitus: a study of the early life experiences of eight diabetic children. *Psychosom Med* 1975;37: 237–244.
49. Kemmer FW, Bisping R, Steingruber HJ, et al. Psychological stress and metabolic control in patients with type I diabetes mellitus. *N Engl J Med* 1986;314: 1078–1084.
50. Kiecolt-Glaser JK, Fisher LD, et al. Marital quality, marital disruption, and immune function. *Psychosom Med* 1987;49:13–34.
51. Carter WR, Herrman J, Stokes K, et al. Promotion of diabetes onset by stress in the BB rat. *Diabetologia* 1987;30:674–675.
52. Surwit RS, McCubbin JA, Kuhn CM, et al. Alprazolam reduces stress hyperglycemia in ob/ob mice. *Psychosom Med* 1986;48:278–282.
53. Surwit RS, Feinglos MN, Livingston EG, et al. Behavioral manipulation of the diabetic phenotype in ob/ob mice. *Diabetes* 1984;33:616–618.
54. Thernlund GM, Dahlquist G, Hansson K, et al. Psychological stress and the onset of IDDM in children. *Diabetes Care* 1995;18:1323–1329.
55. Surwit RS, Feinglos MN, Scovern AW. Diabetes and behavior. A paradigm for health psychology. *Am Psychol* 1983;38:255–262.
56. Surwit RS, McCubbin JA, Livingston EG, et al. Classically conditioned hyperglycemia in the obese mouse. *Psychosom Med* 1985;47:565–568.

57. Kuhn CM, Cochrane C, Feinglos MN, et al. Exaggerated peripheral responses to catecholamines contributes to stress-induced hyperglycemia in the ob/ob mouse. *Pharmacol Biochem Behav* 1987;26:491–495.
58. Peterson HR, Rothschild M, Weinberg CR, et al. Body fat and the activity of the autonomic nervous system. *N Engl J Med* 1988;318:1077–1083.
59. Kahn CR. *Conquering diabetes: a strategic plan for the 21st century. 1999.* Report of the Diabetes Research Working Group. Bethesda, MD: National Institutes of Health, 1999. NIH publication 99-4398.
60. Feuerstein M, Labbe EE, Kuczmierczyk AR. *Health psychology: a psychobiological perspective.* New York: Plenum Press, 1986.
61. Skinner TC, Channon S, Howells L, et al. Diabetes during adolescence. In: Snoek FJ, Skinner TC, eds. *Psychology in diabetes care.* New York: Wiley, 2000: 25–59.
62. Taborsky GJ, Havel PJ, Porte D. Stress-induced activation of the neuroendocrine system and its effects on carbohydrate metabolism. In: Porte D, Sherwin RS, eds. *Ellenberg and Rifkin's diabetes mellitus,* 5th ed. Stamford, CT: Appleton & Lange, 1997:141–168.
63. Chase HP, Jackson GG. Stress and sugar control in children with insulin-dependent diabetes mellitus. *J Pediatr* 1981;98:1011–1013.
64. Baker L, Barcai A, Kaye R, et al. Beta adrenergic blockade and juvenile diabetes: acute studies and long-term therapeutic trial. Evidence for the role of catecholamines in mediating diabetic decompensation following emotional arousal. *J Pediatr* 1969;75:19–29.
65. Brand AH, Johnson JH, Johnson SB. Life stress and diabetic control in children and adolescents with insulin-dependent diabetes. *J Pediatr Psychol* 1986; 1:481–495.
66. Carter WR, Gonder-Frederick LA, Cox DJ, et al. Effect of stress on blood glucose in IDDM. *Diabetes Care* 1985;8:411–412.
67. Aiken LS, Wallender JL, Bell DSH, et al. A nomothetic-idiographic study of daily psychological stress and blood glucose in women with type 1 diabetes mellitus. *J Behav Med* 1994;17:535–548.
68. Hanson SL, Pichert JW. Perceived stress and diabetes control in adolescents. *Health Psychol* 1986;5:439–452.
69. Polonsky WH, Anderson BJ, Lohrer PA, et al. Assessment of diabetes-related distress. *Diabetes Care* 1995;18:754–760.
70. Polonsky WH, Welch GW. Listening to our patients' concerns: understanding and addressing diabetes-specific emotional distress. *Diabetes Spectrum* 1996;9: 8–10.
71. Welch GW, Jacobson AM, Polonsky WH. The Problem Areas in Diabetes Scale: an evaluation of its clinical utility. *Diabetes Care* 1997;20:760–766.
72. Weinger K, Jacobson AM. Psychosocial and quality of life correlates of glycemic control during intensive treatment of type 1 diabetes. *Patient Educ Couns* 2001;42:123–131.
73. Lyons RF, Sullivan MJ, Ritvo PG, et al. *Relationships in chronic illness and disability.* Thousand Oaks, CA: Sage Publications, 1995.
74. Lazarus RS. Psychological stress and coping in adaptation and illness. *Int J Psychiatry Med* 1974;5:321–333.
75. Cohen F. Personality, stress, and the development of physical illness. In: Stone GC, Cohen F, Adler NE, eds. *Health psychology: a handbook: theories, applications and challenges of a psychological approach to the healthcare system.* San Francisco: Jossey-Bass, 1979:77–112.
76. Stabler B, Surwit RS, Lane JD, et al. Type A behavior pattern and blood glucose control in diabetic children. *Psychosom Med* 1987;49:313–316.
77. Wolff CT, Friedman SB, Hofer MA, et al. Relationship between psychological defenses and mean urinary 17-hydroxycorticosteroid excretion rates. 1. A predictive study of parents of fatally ill children. *Psychosom Med* 1964;26: 576–591.
78. Dunn SM, Turtle JR. The myth of the diabetic personality. *Diabetes Care* 1981; 4:640–646.
79. Welch G, Dunn SM, Beeney LJ. The ATT39: a measure of psychological adjustment to diabetes. In: Bradley C, ed. *Handbook of psychology and diabetes: a guide to psychological measurement in diabetes research and management.* Chur, Switzerland: Harwood Academic Publishers, 1994:223–245.
80. Moos RH, Tsu VD. The crisis of psychological illness: an overview. In: Moos RH, ed. *Coping with physical illness.* New York: Plenum, 1977:3–21.
81. Lazarus RS, Folkman S. *Stress, appraisal and coping.* New York: Springer, 1984.
82. Delamater AM, Kurtz SM, Bubb J, et al. Stress and coping in relation to metabolic control of adolescents with type 1 diabetes. *J Dev Behav Pediatr* 1987;8: 136–140.
83. Grey M, Cameron ME, Thurber FW: Coping and adaptation in children with diabetes. *Nurs Res* 1991;40:144–149.
84. Band EB, Weisz JR. Developmental differences in primary and secondary control of coping and adjustment to juvenile diabetes. *J Clin Child Psychol* 19: 150–158.
85. Hanson CL, Henggeler SW, Harris MA, et al. Family system variables and the health status of adolescents with insulin-dependent diabetes mellitus. *Health Psychol* 1989;8:239–253.
86. Helz JW, Templeton B. Evidence of the role of psychosocial factors in diabetes mellitus: a review. *Am J Psychiatry* 1990;147:1275–1282.
87. Wertlieb D, Jacobson AM, Hauser ST. The child with diabetes: a developmental stress and coping perspective. In: Costa PY Jr, Vanden Bos GR, eds. *Psychological aspects of serious illness: chronic conditions, fatal diseases, and clinical care.* Washington, DC: American Psychological Association, 1990.
88. Jacobson AM, Hauser ST, Lavori P, et al. Adherence among children and adolescents with insulin-dependent diabetes mellitus over a four-year longitudinal follow-up, I: the influence of patient coping and adjustment. *J Pediatr Psychol* 1990;15:511–526.
89. Jacobson AM, Hauser ST, Wolfsdorf JI, et al. Psychological predictors of compliance in children with recent onset of diabetes mellitus. *J Pediatr* 1987;110: 805–811.
90. Hauser ST, Jacobson AM, Noam G, et al. Ego development and self-image complexity in early adolescence. Longitudinal studies of psychiatric and diabetic patients. *Arch Gen Psychiatry* 1983;40:325–332.
91. Barglow P, Edidin DV, Budlong-Springer AS, et al. Diabetic control in children and adolescents: psychosocial factors and therapeutic efficacy. *J Youth Adolesc* 1983;12:77–94.
92. Silver EJ, Bauman LJ, Coupey SM, et al. Ego development and chronic illness in adolescents. *J Pers Soc Psychol* 1990:305–310.
93. Rubin RR. Psychotherapy and counselling in diabetes mellitus. In: Snoek FJ, Skinner TJ, eds. *Psychology in diabetes care.* New York: Wiley, 2000:235–263.
94. Hoover JW. Patient 'burnout' can explain non-compliance. In: Krall LP, ed. *World book of diabetes in practice.* Vol 3. New York: Elsevier, 1988.
95. Polonsky WH: Diabetes burnout. Alexandria, VA: American Diabetes Association, 1999.
96. Doherty Y, James P, Roberts S. Stage of Change counselling. In: Snoek FJ, Skinner TJ, eds. *Psychology in diabetes care.* New York: Wiley, 2000:99–139.
97. Prochaska JO, DiClemente CC. Towards a comprehensive model of change. In: Miller WR, Heather N, eds. *Treating addictive behaviours: process of change.* NY: Plenum, 1986:1007–1030.
98. Fisher L, Chesla CA, Bartz RJ, et al. The family and type 2 diabetes: a framework for intervention. *Diabetes Educ* 1998;24:599–607.
99. La Greca AM. Social consequences of pediatric conditions: fertile area for future investigation and intervention. *J Pediatr Psychol* 1990;15:285–307.
100. La Greca AM. Peer influences in pediatric chronic illness: an update. *J Pediatr Psychol* 1992;17:775–784.
101. Kyngas H, Hentinen M, Barlow JH. Adolescents' perceptions of physicians, nurses, parents and friends: help or hindrance in compliance with diabetes self-care? *J Adv Nurs* 1998;27:760–769.
102. Drah AL, Becker D. Diabetes mellitus in the child: course, special problems, and related disorders. In: Katzen H, Mahler R, eds. *Diabetes, obesity, and vascular disease: advances in modern nutrition.* Vol 2. New York: Wiley, 1978: 615–643.
103. Golden MP, Russell BP, Ingersoll GM, et al. Management of diabetes mellitus in children younger than 5 years of age. *Am J Dis Child* 1985;139:448–452.
104. Hauser ST, Jacobson AM, Lavori P, et al. Adherence among children and adolescents with insulin-dependent diabetes mellitus over a four-year longitudinal follow-up, II: immediate and long-term linkages with the family milieu. *J Pediatr Psychol* 1990;15:527–542.
105. Miller-Johnson S, Emery RE, et al. Parent-child relationships and the management of insulin-dependent diabetes mellitus. *J Consult Clin Psychol* 1994;62:603–610.
106. Allen DA, Tennen H, McGrade BJ, et al. Parent and child perceptions of the management of juvenile diabetes. *J Pediatr Psychol* 1983;8:129–141.
107. La Greca AM. Children with diabetes and their families: coping and disease management. In: Field T, McCabe P, Schneiderman N, eds. *Stress and coping across development.* Hillsdale, NJ: Erlbaum, 1988:139–159.
108. Auslander WF, Anderson BJ, Bubb J, et al. Risk factors to health in diabetic children: a prospective study from diagnosis. *Health Soc Work* 1990;5: 133–142.
109. Kovacs M, Ho V, Pollock MH. Criterion and predictive validity of the diagnosis of adjustment disorder: a prospective study of youths with new-onset insulin-dependent diabetes mellitus. *Am J Psychiatry* 1995;152:523–528.
110. Schafer LC, McCaul KD, Glasgow RE. Supportive and nonsupportive family behaviors: relationships to adherence and metabolic control in persons with type I diabetes. *Diabetes Care* 1986;9:179–185.
111. Fisher L, Chesla CA, Skaff MM, et al. The family and disease management in Hispanic and European-American patients with type 2 diabetes. *Diabetes Care* 2000;23:267–272.
112. Glasgow RE, McCaul KD, Schafer LC. Barriers to regimen adherence among persons with insulin-dependent diabetes. *J Behav Med* 1986;9:65–77.
113. Glasgow RE, McCaul KD, Schafer LC. Self-care behaviors and glycemic control in type I diabetes. *J Chronic Dis* 1987;40:399–412.
114. Glasgow RE, Wilson W, McCaul KD. Regimen adherence: a problematic construct in diabetes research. *Diabetes Care* 1985;8:300–301.
115. Johnson SB, Silverstein J, Rosenbloom A, et al. Assessing daily management in childhood diabetes. *Health Psychol* 1986;5:545–564.
116. Wolpert HA, Anderson BJ. Metabolic control matters: why is the message lost in the translation? *Diabetes Care* 2001;24:1302–1303.
117. Kaplan SH, Gandek B, Rogers W, et al. Patients and visit characteristics related to physicians' participatory decision-making style. Results from the Medical Outcomes Study. *Med Care* 1995;33:1176–1187.
118. Kaplan SH, Greenfield S, Ware JE Jr. Assessing the effects of physician-patient interactions on the outcomes of chronic disease. *Med Care* 1989;27 [Suppl]:S110–S127.
119. DiMatteo MR, Sherbourne CD, Hays RD, et al. Physicians' characteristics influence patients' adherence to medical treatment: results from the Medical Outcomes Study. *Health Psychol* 1993;12:93–102.
120. Ciechanowski PS, Katon WJ, Russo JE, et al. The patient-provider relationship: attachment theory and adherence to treatment in diabetes. *Am J Psychiatry* 2001;158:29–35.

121. Anderson RM, Funnell MM. *The art of empowerment.* Alexandria, VA: American Diabetes Association, 2000.
122. Anderson RM, Funnell MM, Arnold MS. Using the empowerment approach to help patients change behavior. In: Anderson BJ, Rubin RR, eds. *Practical psychology for diabetes clinicians.* Alexandria, VA: American Diabetes Association, 1996:163–172.
123. Anderson R, Funnell M, Carlson A, et al. Facilitating self-care through empowerment. In: Snoek FJ, Skinner TC, eds. *Psychology in diabetes care.* New York: Wiley, 2001:69–97.
124. Anderson RM, Funnell MM, Butler PM, et al. Patient empowerment: results of a randomized controlled trial. *Diabetes Care* 1995;18:943–949.
125. Feste CC. *Empowerment: facilitating a path to personal self-care.* Elkhart, IN: Miles Diagnostic Division, 1991.
126. Drash AL. *Role of the family networks of social support, and the therapeutic team.* Bethesda, MD: National Diabetes Information Clearinghouse, 1980. NIH publication 80-1993.
127. American Diabetes Association. Clinical practice recommendations: 2001. *Diabetes Care* 2001;24[Suppl]:S33.
128. Glasgow RE, Eakin EG. Medical office-based interventions. In: Snoek FJ, Skinner TC, eds. *Psychology in diabetes care.* New York: Wiley, 2000:141–168.
129. Glasgow RE, Eakin EG. Dealing with diabetes self-management. In: Anderson BJ, Rubin RR, eds. *Practical psychology for diabetes clinicians.* Alexandria, VA: American Diabetes Association, 1996:53–62.
130. Cox D, Gonder-Frederick L, Polonsky W, et al. A multi-center evaluation of blood glucose awareness training-II. *Diabetes Care* 1995;18:523–528.
131. Gonder-Frederick LA, Cox DJ, Driesen NR, et al. Individual differences in neurobehavioral disruption during mild and moderate hypoglycemia in adults with IDDM. *Diabetes* 1994;43:1407–1412.
132. Gonder-Frederick L, Cox D, Clarke W, et al. Blood glucose awareness training. In: Snoek FJ, Skinner TC, eds. *Psychology in diabetes care.* New York: Wiley, 2000:169–205.
133. Miller WR, Rollnick S. *Motivational interviewing: preparing people to change addictive behavior.* New York: Guilford, 1991.
134. Smith DE, Heckemeyer CM, Kratt PP, et al. Motivational interviewing to improve adherence to a behavioral weigh-control program for older obese women with NIDDM: a pilot study. *Diabetes Care* 1997;20:52–54.
135. Prochaska JO, Norcross JC, DiClemente CC. *Changing for good.* New York: William Morrow, 1994.
136. Laffel LMB, Brackett J, Ho J, et al. Changing the process of diabetes care improves metabolic outcomes and reduces hospitalizations. *Qual Manage Healthcare* 1999;7:53–62.
137. Anderson BJ, Brackett J, Ho J, et al. An office-based intervention to maintain parent-adolescent teamwork in diabetes management. *Diabetes Care* 1999;22: 713–721.
138. Van Der Ven NCW, Chatrou M, Cnoek FJ. Cognitive behavioral group training. In: Snoek FJ, Skinner TC, eds. *Psychology in diabetes care.* New York: Wiley and Sons, 2000:207–234.
139. Grey M, Boland EA, Davidson M, et al. Short-term effects of coping skills training as adjunct to intensive therapy in adolescents. *Diabetes Care* 1998;21: 902–907.
140. Rubin RR, Peyrot M, Saudek CS. The effect of a diabetes education program incorporating coping skills training on emotional well-being and diabetes self-efficacy. *Diabetes Educ* 1993;19:210–214.
141. Tattersall RB, McCulloch DK, Aveline M. Group therapy in the treatment of diabetics. *Diabetes Care* 1985;8:180–188.
142. Zrebiec JF, Jacobson AM. What attracts patients with diabetes to an Internet support group: a 21-month longitudinal Website study. *Diabet Med* 2001;18:154–158.
143. Piette JD, McPhee A, Weinberger M, et al. Use of automated telephone disease management calls in an ethnically diverse sample of low-income patients with diabetes. *Diabetes Care* 1999;22:1302–1309.
144. Piette JD, Weinberger M, McPhee SJ, et al. Can automated calls with nurse follow-up improve self-care and glycemic control among vulnerable patients with diabetes: a randomized controlled trial. *Am J Med* 2000;108:20–27.
145. Feil EG, Glasgow RE, Boles S, et al. Who participates in Internet-based self-management programs? A study among novice computer users in a primary care setting. *Diabetes Educ* 2000;26:806–811.
146. Glasgow RE, Toobert DJ, Hampson SE. Effects of a brief office-based intervention to facilitate diabetes dietary self-management. *Diabetes Care* 1996;19: 835–842.
147. Glasgow RE, La Chance P, Toobert DJ, et al. Long-term effects and costs of brief behavioral dietary intervention for patients with diabetes delivered from the medical office. *Patient Educ Counsel* 1997;32:175–184.
148. Welch GW, De Groot M, Buckland GT, et al. Patient satisfaction with a computerized diabetes psychosocial assessment tool in a low literacy, inner-city hospital setting. *Diabetes* 1999;48[Suppl 1]:1408A(abst).
149. Samson JA, de Groot M, Jacobson AM. Comorbid psychiatric diagnoses in men and women with type 1 and type 2 diabetes mellitus. 2001. Unpublished work cited with permission.
150. Mayou R, Peveler R, Davies B, et al. Psychiatric morbidity in young adults with insulin-dependent diabetes mellitus. *Psychol Med* 1991;21:639–645.
151. Kovacs M, Obrosky DS, Goldston D, et al. Major depressive disorder in youths with IDDM: a controlled prospective study of course and outcome. *Diabetes Care* 1997;20:45–51.
152. Wells KB, Golding JM, Burnam MA. Chronic medical conditions in a sample of general population with anxiety, affective, and substance use disorders. *Am J Psychiatry* 1989;146:1440–1446.
153. Wells KB, Bolding JM, Burnam MA. Affective, substance use, and anxiety disorders in persons with arthritis, diabetes, heart disease, high blood pressure, or chronic lung conditions. *Gen Hosp Psychiatry* 1989;11:320–327.
154. Rydall AC, Rodin GM, Olmsted MP, et al. Disordered eating behavior and microvascular complications in young women with insulin-dependent diabetes mellitus. *N Engl J Med* 1997;336:1849–1854.
155. Lustman PJ, Anderson RJ, Freedland KE, et al. Depression and poor glycemic control: a meta-analytic review of the literature. *Diabetes Care* 2000;23: 934–942.
156. Talbot F, Nouwen A. A review of the relationship between depression and diabetes in adults: is there a link? *Diabetes Care* 2000;23:1556–1562.
157. Geringer ED. Affective disorders and diabetes mellitus. *Neuropsychol Behav Aspects Diabetes* 1990;239–272.
158. Cameron O, Kronfol Z, Greden J, et al. Hypothalamic-pituitary-adrenocortical activity in patients with diabetes mellitus. *Arch Gen Psychiatry* 1984;41: 1090–1095.
159. Hudson J, Hudson M, Rothschild A, et al. Abnormal results of dexamethasone suppression test in non-depressed patients with diabetes mellitus. *Arch Gen Psychiatry* 1984;41:1086–1089.
160. Araki Y, Nomura M, Tanaka H, et al. MRI of the brain in diabetes mellitus. *Neuroradiology* 1994;36:101–103.
161. Lyoo IK, Lee HK, Jung JH, et al. White matter hyperintensities on brain MRI in children with psychiatric disorders. 2001. Unpublished work cited with permission.
162. Dejgaard A, Gade A, Larsson H, et al. Evidence for diabetic encephalopathy. *Diabetic Med* 1991;8:162–167.
163. Schurhoff F, Bellivier F, Jouvent R, et al. Early and late onset bipolar disorders: two different forms of manic-depressive illness. *J Affect Disord* 2000;58: 215–221.
164. Woods BT, Yurgelun-Todd D, Mikulis D, et al. Age-related MRI abnormalities in bipolar illness: a clinical study. *Biol Psychiatry* 1995;38:846–847.
165. Jacobson AM, Weinger K, Jimerson D, et al. Factors related to the development of MRI abnormalities in type 1 diabetic patients. 2001. Unpublished work cited with permission.
166. Coffey CE, Figiel GS, Djang WT, et al. Subcortical hyperintensity on magnetic resonance imaging: a comparison of normal and depressed elderly subjects. *Am J Psychiatry* 1990;147:187–189.
167. Krishnan KR, McDonald WM, Escalona PR, et al. Magnetic resonance imaging of the caudate nuclei in depression: preliminary observations. *Arch Gen Psychiatry* 1992;49:553–557.
168. Brown FW, Lewine RJ, Hudgins PA, et al. White matter hyperintensity signals in psychiatric and nonpsychiatric subjects. *Am J Psychiatry* 1992;149: 620–625.
169. Buchsbaum MS, Wu J, DeLisi LE, et al. Frontal cortex and basal ganglia metabolic rates assessed by positron emission tomography with [18F]2-deoxyglucose in affective illness. *J Affect Disord* 1986;10:137–152.
170. Coffey CE, Figiel GS, Djang WT, et al. Leukoencephalopathy in elderly depressed patients referred for ECT. *Biol Psychiatry* 1988;24:143–161.
171. Coffey CE, Figiel GS, Djang WT, et al. Subcortical white matter hyperintensity on magnetic resonance imaging: Clinical and neuroanatomic correlates in the depressed. *J Neuropsychiatry* 1989;1:135–144.
172. Coffey CE, Wilkinson WE, Weiner RD, et al. Quantitative cerebral anatomy in depression: a controlled magnetic resonance imaging study. *Arch Gen Psychiatry* 1993;50:7–16.
173. Dolan RJ, Calloway SP, Thacker PF, et al. The cerebral cortical appearance in depressed subjects. *Psychol Med* 1986;16:775–779.
174. Figiel GS, Krishnan KR, Doraiswamy PM, et al. Subcortical hyperintensities on brain magnetic resonance imaging: a comparison of normal and bipolar subjects. *J Neuropsychiatry Clin Neurosci* 1991;3:18–22.
175. Jacobson AM, Weinger K. Treating depression in diabetic patients: is there an alternative to medications? *Ann Intern Med* 1998;129:656–657.
176. Lustman PJ, Griffith LS, Freedland KE, et al. Cognitive behavior therapy for depression in type 2 diabetes mellitus: a randomized, controlled trial. *Ann Intern Med* 1998;129:613–621.
177. Derogatis LR. SCL-90-R administration, scoring, and procedures manual, II. Towson, MD: Clinical Psychometric Research, 1983.
178. Polonsky W, Anderson BJ, Welch G, et al. Assessment of diabetes specific distress. *Diabetes Care* 1995;18:754–760.
179. Jacobson AM, Samson JA. The evaluation of two measures of quality of life in patients with type I and type II diabetes mellitus. *Diabetes Care* 1994;17: 267–274.
180. Jacobson AM. Psychological care of patients with insulin-dependent diabetes mellitus. *N Engl J Med* 1996;334:1249–1253.
181. Jones JM, Lawson ML, Daneman D, et al. Eating disorders in adolescent females with and without type 1 diabetes: cross sectional study. *BMJ* 2000;20:1563–1566.
182. Levine MD, Marcus MD. Women, diabetes, and disordered eating. *Diabetes Spectrum* 1997;10:191–195.
183. Carlson MG, Campbell PJ. Intensive insulin therapy and weight gain in IDDM. *Diabetes* 1993;42:1700–1707.
184. Fairburn CG, Peveler RC, Davies B, et al. Eating disorders in young adults with insulin dependent diabetes mellitus: a controlled study. *BMJ* 1991;303: 17–20.

185. Bryden KS, Neil A, Mayou RA, et al. Eating habits, body weight, and insulin misuse. A longitudinal study of teenagers and young adults with type 1 diabetes. *Diabetes Care* 1999;22:1956–1960.
186. Striegel-Moore RH, Nicholson TJ, et al. Prevalence of eating disorder symptoms in preadolescent and adolescent girls with IDDM. *Diabetes Care* 1992;15:1361–1368.
187. Polonsky WH, Anderson BJ, Lohrer PA. Disordered eating and regimen manipulation in women with diabetes: relationships to glycemic control. *Diabetes* 1992;40[Suppl 1]:540A(abst).
188. Ryan CM. Effects of diabetes mellitus on neuropsychological functioning: a lifespan perspective. *Sem Clin Neuropsychiatry* 1997;2:4–14.
189. Ryan C, Vega A, Drash A. Cognitive deficits in adolescents who developed diabetes early in life. *Pediatrics* 1985;75:921–927.
190. Ryan CM, Greckle M. Why is learning and memory dysfunction in type 2 diabetes limited to older adults. *Diabetes Metab Res Rev* 2000;16:308–315.
191. Bjorgaas M, Gimse R, Vik T, et al. Cognitive function in type 1 diabetic children with and without episodes of hypoglycaemia. *Acta Paediatr* 1997;86:148–153.
192. Hershey T, Bhargava N, Sadler M, et al. Conventional vs. intensive diabetes therapy in children with type 1 diabetes: effects on memory and motor speed. *Diabetes Care* 1999;22:1318–1324.
193. Rovet JF, Ehrlich RM. The effect of hypoglycemic seizures on cognitive function in children with diabetes: a 7-year prospective study. *J Pediatr* 1999;134:503–506.
194. Rovet J, Alverez M. Attentional functioning in children and adolescents with IDDM. *Diabetes Care* 1997;20:803–810.
195. Holmes CS, Richman LC. Cognitive profiles of children with insulin-dependent diabetes. *J Dev Behav Pediatr* 1985;6:323–326.
196. Rovet JF, Ehrlich RM, Czuchta D. Intellectual characteristics of diabetic children at diagnosis and one year later. *J Pediatr Psychol* 1990;15:775–788.
197. Rovet JF, Ehrlich RM, Czuchta D, Akler M. Psychoeducational characteristics of children and adolescents with insulin-dependent diabetes mellitus. *J Learn Disabil* 1993;26:7–22.
198. Leibson CL, Rocca WA, Hanson VA, et al. Risk of dementia among persons with diabetes mellitus: a population-based cohort study. *Am J Epidemiol* 1997;145:301–308.
199. Effects of intensive diabetes therapy on neuropsychological function in adults in the Diabetes Control and Complications Trial. *Ann Intern Med* 1996;124:379–388.
200. Reichard P, Pihl M, Rosenqvist U, et al. Complications in IDDM are caused by elevated blood glucose level: the Stockholm Diabetes Intervention Study (SDIS) at 10-year follow up. *Diabetologia* 1996;39:1483–1488.
201. Deary I, Crawford J, Hepburn DA, et al. Severe hypoglycemia and intelligence in adult patients with insulin-treated diabetes. *Diabetes* 1993;42:341–344.
202. Deary IJ, Frier BM. Severe hypoglycaemia and cognitive impairment in diabetes: link not proven. *BMJ* 1996;313:767–768.
203. Perros P, Deary IJ, Sellar RJ, et al. Brain abnormalities demonstrated by magnetic resonance imaging in adult IDDM patients with and without a history of recurrent severe hypoglycemia. *Diabetes Care* 1997;20:1013–1018.
204. Jacobson AM, Weinger K, Hill TC, et al. Brain functioning, cognition, and psychiatric disorders in patients with type 1 diabetes. *Diabetes* 2000;50[Suppl 1]:A132(abst).
205. Meisler AW, Carey MP, Lantinga LJ, et al. Erectile dysfunction in diabetes mellitus: a biopsychosocial approach to etiology and assessment. *Ann Behav Med* 1989;11:18–27.
206. NIH Consensus Conference. Impotence: NIH Consensus Development Panel on Impotence. *JAMA* 1993;270:83–90.
207. Klein R, Klein BE, Lee KE, et al. Prevalence of self-reported erectile dysfunction in people with long-term IDDM. *Diabetes Care* 1996;9:135–141.
208. Fedele D, Bortolotti A, Coscelli C, et al., on behalf of Gruppo Italiano Studio Deficit Erettile nei Diabetici. Erectile dysfunction in type 1 and type 2 diabetics in Italy. *Int J Epidemiol* 2000;29:524–531.
209. Karacan I, Salis PJ, Ware JC, et al. Nocturnal penile tumescence and diagnosis in diabetic impotence. *Am J Psychiatry* 1978;35:191–197.
210. Lehman TP, Jacobs JA. Etiology of diabetic impotence. *J Urol* 1983;129:291–294.
211. Enzlin P, Mathieu C, Vanderschueren D, et al. Diabetes mellitus and female sexuality: a review of 25 years' research. *Diabet Med* 1998;15:809–815.

CHAPTER 38
Exercise in Patients with Diabetes Mellitus

Jeanne H. Steppel and Edward S. Horton

Exercise has long been recognized as an important factor in the treatment of diabetes mellitus. Before the discovery of insulin, patients with diabetes, particular those with type 1 diabetes, were very limited in their ability to exercise, because it was almost impossible for them to avoid ketosis and dehydration. After insulin therapy was established as a mainstay treatment, exercise was no longer an elusive activity. With their ability to exercise, it became evident that hypoglycemia frequently developed both in the immediate postexercise period and during the 24 hours after exercise. It also was recognized that ketosis could be induced by exercise in patients with poor glucose control and that even patients with excellent control would sometimes develop hyperglycemia after vigorous exercise. As our understanding of exercise in the patient with type 1 diabetes has increased, the goal has been to manage glucose homeostasis and fuel metabolism so that patients can participate fully in all forms of exercise.

Exercise also plays a critical role in patients with type 2 diabetes. It can help improve insulin sensitivity and assist with reduction and maintenance of body weight in obese patients. Exercise, together with diet and pharmacologic therapies, is important as part of the overall approach to improving glycemic control and reducing cardiovascular risk factors. Indeed, exercise often is "prescribed" as a therapy for type 2 diabetes. The many benefits of exercise in these patients include improved long-term glycemic control as a result of the decrease in insulin resistance and of the cumulative blood glucose–lowering effects of individual bouts of exercise. In addition, regular exercise has been shown to improve lipid abnormalities and lower blood pressure (1–3). Finally, exercise also may be an important component of weight-loss regimens for these patients. When used in combination with dietary changes (especially calorie restriction), exercise promotes loss of adipose tissue with preservation of lean body mass (4,5). In addition, exercise may promote a beneficial redistribution of body fat. Abdominal adiposity appears to have a greater impact on insulin resistance than does fat deposition at other sites, and exercise has recently been shown to decrease abdominal fat in postmenopausal women (6). Unfortunately, there are some significant risks of exercise in the patient with type 2 diabetes, including symptomatic hypoglycemia, which can occur up to 24 hours after exercise; exacerbation of known or previously unknown cardiac disease; worsening of symptoms secondary to degenerative joint disease; and possible damage to joints in the setting of neuropathy. It is particularly important to screen patients with type 2 diabetes for existing cardiovascular disease before prescribing an exercise regimen.

There are several universal risks of exercise in patients with type 1 or type 2 diabetes. Most important, vigorous exercise can cause retinal hemorrhage or vitreous bleeding in patients with proliferative retinopathy. Maneuvers such as the Valsalva maneuver that increase intraabdominal pressure should be avoided, as should jarring head motions that might induce retinal detachment. In addition, patients with sensory neuropathy should refrain from high-impact exercise to reduce the risk of soft tissue and joint injury. The presence of autonomic neuropathy often makes performance of high-intensity exercise difficult because of decreased aerobic capacity and postural hypotension. Proteinuria tends to increase with exercise in patients with nephropathy. However, this is thought to merely be a result of a transient change in renal blood flow, as opposed to worsening of renal disease. Angiotensin-converting enzyme inhibitors have been shown to decrease this effect (7–9).

PHYSIOLOGY OF EXERCISE IN HEALTHY INDIVIDUALS

To understand metabolic regulation in patients with diabetes, it is helpful first to discuss the physiology of exercise in healthy individuals without diabetes. Several hormonal, cardiovascular, and neurologic responses that occur during exercise enable the body to respond to the increased energy demand.

In the resting fasted state, before exercise, blood glucose levels are maintained by a balance of the production of glucose by the liver and the uptake of glucose by body tissues (50% by the brain; 15% to 20% by skeletal muscle; and the remainder by kidney, splanchnic bed, blood cells, and other tissues). Glucose production by the liver early in fasting occurs predominantly via glycogenolysis, with only about 25% contributed by gluconeogenesis (Fig. 38.1). In patients with type 1 diabetes, up to 45% of glucose production during the nonexercising state derives from gluconeogenesis, even early in fasting.

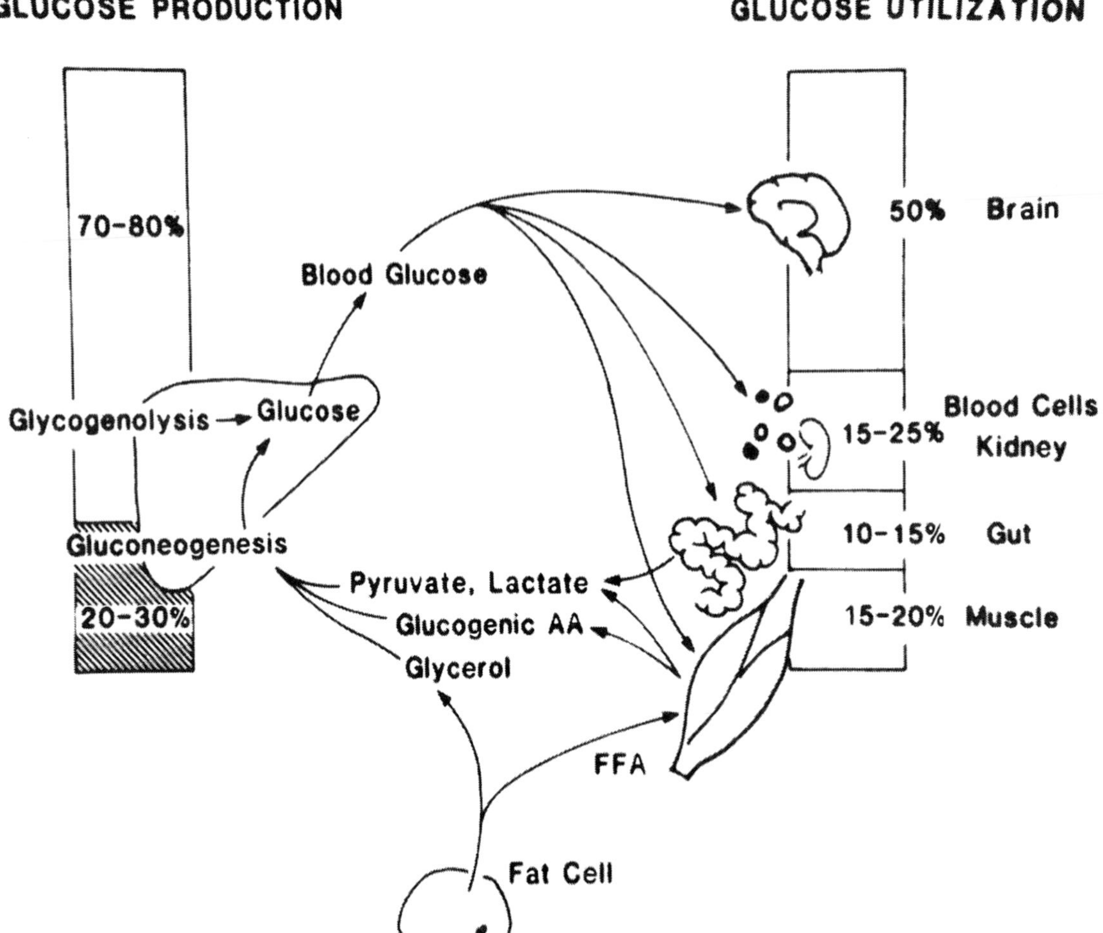

Figure 38.1. Glucose production and utilization in the resting, fasted state in normal man. AA, amino acids; FFA, free fatty acids. (Modified from Bjorkman O, Wahren J. In: Horton E, Terjung R, eds. *Exercise, nutrition, and energy metabolism.* New York: Macmillan Publishing, 1988;100–115, with permission.)

The sources of energy used by skeletal muscle vary markedly between times of rest and exercise. At rest, only 10% of the energy produced in skeletal muscle is from glucose oxidation, whereas 85% to 90% is from fatty acids and 1% to 2% is from amino acids (10). Carbohydrate metabolism increases significantly with the onset of exercise as the breakdown of glycogen in muscle increases. This is associated with the rapid generation of lactate, which enters the bloodstream. Within minutes of the onset of exercise, anaerobic metabolism switches to aerobic metabolism, and uptake of glucose and oxygen into muscle increases as the blood flow to muscle increases. The circulating glucose concentration is kept essentially constant as a result of a regulated matching of the hepatic production of glucose to the rate of glucose uptake by the muscle from the circulation. In addition to the shift in glucose metabolism during exercise, breakdown of triglycerides in adipose tissue releases fatty acids into the circulation as an alternative metabolic fuel. Glycerol released from the triglyceride backbone is taken up by the liver and used as a precursor for gluconeogenesis along with the release of amino acids from the skeletal muscle.

Once exercise stops, the increase in glucose uptake continues for a time to rebuild glycogen stores in the muscle. The rate of repletion of glycogen stores can vary dramatically, depending on intake of food. This occurs quite slowly in the fasted state; in the fed state, glycogen generally is replenished within 12 hours. Glycogen stores in skeletal muscle are repleted more rapidly than are those in the liver.

Multiple complex neurologic and hormonal responses play important roles in fuel homeostasis during exercise. These include activation of the sympathetic nervous system and a change in the ratios of insulin and the counterregulatory hormones. The shifts in the balance of these hormones, plus increased sympathetic tone, alter the metabolism of glucose, free fatty acids, and amino acids and change the body's ability to utilize oxygen and to maintain fluid status.

At the onset of exercise, the sympathetic nervous system is activated, with a resultant increase in heart rate and constriction of the blood vessels supplying the splanchnic bed, the kidneys, and muscles not involved directly in the exercise. This causes an increase in blood flow to the tissues most in need—the exercising muscles. In addition, epinephrine and norepinephrine play vital roles in stimulating breakdown of adipose tissue [β-adrenergic stimulation (11)] and suppressing insulin secretion (α-adrenergic stimulation). Catecholamines are also important in stimulating glycogenolysis during exercise.

Adjustments in insulin secretion are critical for the regulation of fuel metabolism during exercise. As mentioned above, the sympathetic nervous system suppresses secretion of insulin at the onset of exercise. Because insulin normally inhibits hepatic glucose production, the decrease in insulin allows the liver to increase glucose output. Insulin also suppresses lipolysis, and thus the decrease in insulin levels promotes the breakdown of adipose tissue triglycerides. As will be discussed later, the molecular mechanisms of glucose uptake during exercise are independent of insulin, so the decrease in serum insulin concentration does not affect the ability of the muscle to take up glucose from the circulation (12).

Glucagon is important in the regulation of glucose levels during vigorous or prolonged exercise but plays a smaller role in mild-to-moderate exercise. As the plasma glucose concentration begins to fall, glucagon acts as a counterregulatory hormone, contributing to the activation of glycogenolysis and to the increase in gluconeogenesis through accelerated uptake of amino acids by the liver (13). The role played by glucagon is generally larger in people who have not undergone physical training than in those who are trained athletes. Cortisol and growth hormone also act as counterregulatory hormones that help to block the effects of insulin during exercise. They may be especially important in antagonizing the effects of insulin in tissues that are not directly involved in exercise, thus increasing the amount of glucose available for the actively exercising muscles.

Several factors can alter fuel utilization and the extent of influence of the hormonal and neurologic regulators. These include physical training, intensity of exercise, duration of exercise, and the diet that precedes exercise. Physical training lowers the percentage of the maximum aerobic capacity ($VO_{2\,max}$) that is reached when doing an equivalent amount of work. Trained individuals depend more heavily on utilization of free fatty acids than of glucose for fuel. This appears to be important in developing endurance, because muscle glycogen stores in trained individuals do not become depleted as quickly as those in untrained individuals.

The intensity of exercise, defined as a percentage of $VO_{2\,max}$, also influences fuel metabolism. As the intensity rises, the role of glucose in providing fuel to the exercising muscles keeps increasing (Fig. 38.2), with the importance of lipolysis decreasing. The use of amino acids remains roughly the same. Once the $VO_{2\,max}$ is greater than 75%, carbohydrate becomes the main fuel consumed by muscle and the rate of glycogenolysis is increased.

The duration of exercise affects fuel metabolism as a consequence of a time-dependent shift from the utilization of carbohydrates to the utilization of free fatty acids. Glycogen stores become depleted after several hours of moderate continuous exercise, and lipolysis becomes the main source of fuel for exercising muscle. After depletion of glycogen stores, hepatic glucose production via gluconeogenesis is essential for maintenance of blood glucose concentrations. Sometimes in prolonged exercise such as marathon running, glycogen stores are depleted, the liver is unable to keep up with glucose requirements through gluconeogenesis, and hypoglycemia develops.

The composition of the diet preceding exercise can affect fuel metabolism during activity. A diet high in carbohydrates is associated with a greater rate of glucose oxidation and increased muscle glycogen stores. This may contribute to generally greater endurance in individuals who have had a carbohydrate-rich diet than in those with a carbohydrate-restricted diet. Some athletes therefore use a technique called "carbohydrate loading" before exercise to improve endurance.

Skeletal muscle is able to take up glucose from the circulation predominantly via the GLUT4 transporter protein (14).

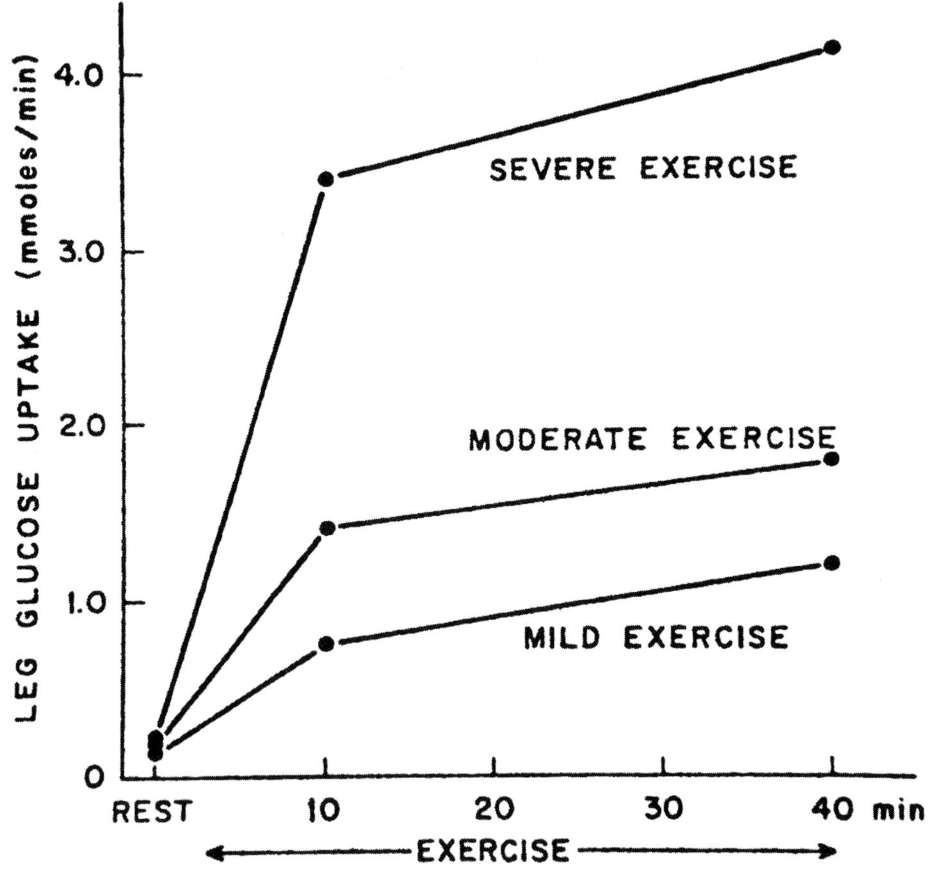

Figure 38.2. Leg uptake of glucose during bicycle ergometer exercise. Mild exercise is 25% to 30% of maximal capacity, moderate exercise is 50% to 60% of maximal capacity, and severe exercise is 75% to 90% of maximal capacity. (From Felig P, Warren J. Fuel homeostasis in exercise. *N Engl J Med* 1975; 293:1078–1084, with permission. Copyright © 1975 Massachusetts Medical Society.)

During exercise, GLUT4 is translocated from an intracellular location to the plasma membrane, similar to what occurs with insulin stimulation. There is now abundant evidence to indicate that the insulin-mediated and contraction-mediated mechanisms are distinct (15). Insulin-mediated signaling involves binding of insulin to the insulin receptor and causing its autophosphorylation and a cascade of reactions, including activation of insulin receptor substrate protein-1 (IRS-1) and phosphatidylinositol 3-kinase. Exercise-induced glucose transport does not involve either IRS-1 or phosphatidylinositol 3-kinase, although there may be activation of the signaling serine kinase Akt, which is located farther down in the insulin signaling pathway.

Numerous hypotheses have been proposed to explain the mechanism of exercise-induced glucose transport. Calcium flux in the muscle cell has been implicated, because glucose transport decreases when calcium release is blocked pharmacologically (15). Calcium is also thought to play an important role in the activation of enzymes such as protein kinase C, which are thought to be upstream of the mobilization of GLUT4. Another theory implicates nitric oxide as a potential mediator of contraction-induced glucose transport, because generation of nitric oxide increases during exercise (16). Although the uptake of glucose by muscle after contraction is not affected by inhibition of nitric oxide synthase, basal rates of glucose transport in muscle appear to be decreased (17). It is possible that nitric oxide modulates a unique pathway that affects glucose transport independent of either the insulin or the exercise pathway.

Evidence also has implicated mitogen-activated protein (MAP) kinase in the process of exercise-induced glucose transport. The MAP kinase signaling pathway contains several enzyme cascades that are activated with exercise. This appears to include both the ERK1/2 and JNK MAP kinases (18). In addition to potential effects on glucose uptake, the MAP kinase pathways likely regulate gene-transcription events that are involved in muscle growth and repair.

There currently is strong interest in the hypothesis that 5′-adenosine monophosphate–activated protein (AMP) kinase serves as a metabolic "fuel gauge" and key regulator of glucose uptake during exercise. AMP kinase activity increases markedly with exercise. Studies with activators and inhibitors of AMP kinase indicate that this is causally linked to the translocation of GLUT4 transporters (19,20). Fatty acid oxidation and insulin sensitivity may also be affected by exercise via this pathway. Several excellent review articles have covered the signaling pathways implicated in exercise-induced glucose transport (15,21,22).

EXERCISE AND GLUCOSE METABOLISM IN PATIENTS WITH TYPE 1 DIABETES

Physical exercise increases insulin sensitivity in individuals with diabetes (Fig. 38.3). This increased insulin sensitivity is thought to be caused by the increase in glucose uptake via GLUT4 resulting from the effect of exercise on the expression and translocation of the transporter to the skeletal muscle plasma membrane (23). This state of altered sensitivity can last for several hours (24). Highly trained athletes have better glucose tolerance, β-cell efficiency, and glucose utilization than do untrained individuals (25). In addition, athletes may exhibit a greater glycemic response to oral glucose secondary to adaptations in glucose absorption (26). The adaptations associated with training reverse rapidly once athletes stop their exercise programs (27).

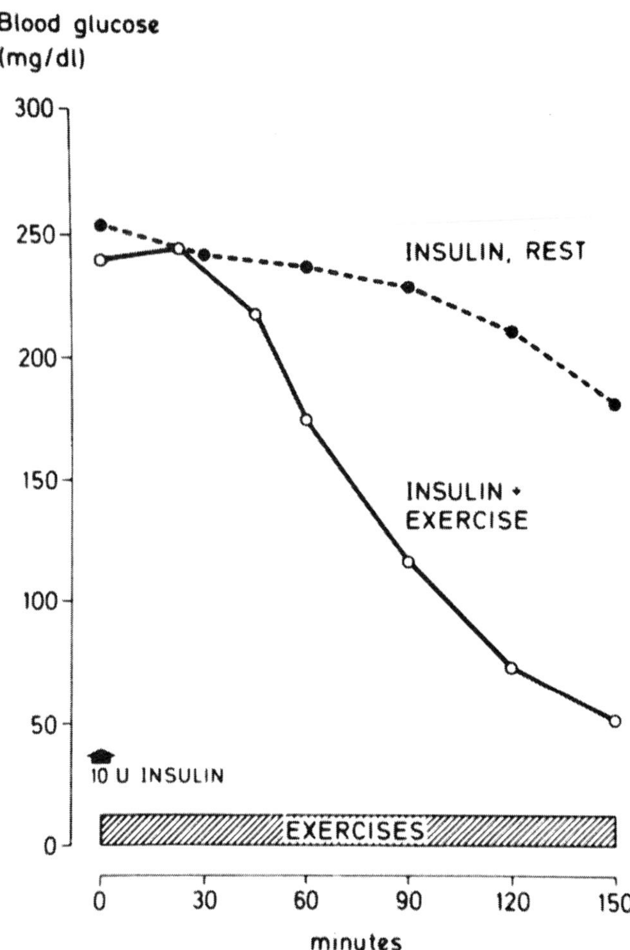

Figure 38.3. The effect of insulin on blood glucose at rest and with exercise in type 1 diabetes. (From Lawrence RD. *BMJ* 1926;1:648–650.)

In individuals with type 1 diabetes, unlike those without diabetes, regulatory events in the pancreatic islets induced by exercise cannot decrease insulin secretion, because insulin is derived by injection. Because insulin levels are sustained, the suppressive effect of insulin on the liver continues and hepatic production of glucose remains low at the same time that utilization of glucose by muscle rises. This results in a substantial risk of hypoglycemia. The risk of hypoglycemia in patients with diabetes is even greater if they have injected insulin into a subcutaneous site in an exercising limb, because increased blood flow can accelerate insulin absorption (28). This can be particularly problematic when very-short-acting insulin, such as lispro or aspart, is used (29). Because of the increased risk of hypoglycemia secondary to rapid absorption of recently administered insulin, it is recommended that vigorous exercise be avoided for 1 to 1.5 hours after injection. The site of insulin administration is also important and should be chosen with regard to the particular activity so as to avoid injecting insulin into an actively exercising area.

Because, as described above, insulin levels do not decline in response to activity in patients with type 1 diabetes, the normal upregulation of glycogenolysis and gluconeogenesis does not occur, the rate of muscle glucose uptake may not be matched, and hypoglycemia is likely to develop. This can cause problems particularly in patients who have tight glucose control, because they may have greater hypoglycemia unawareness and reduced counterregulatory responses (30). The presence of autonomic neuropathy may further contribute to a decreased counterregulatory response, as well as to a diminished ability to sense hypoglycemia.

As an approach to decreasing the risk of hypoglycemia during exercise, patients with type 1 diabetes often benefit from lowering their dose of short-acting insulin before exercise and ingesting carbohydrates before or during exercise. It often is effective to decrease the insulin dose by 25% to 50% before exercise and to avoid exercise for at least an hour after taking insulin. Patients should check their blood glucose levels before they exercise and consider a supplementary carbohydrate snack when their blood glucose level is below 100 mg/dL. The response of blood glucose to exercise may vary significantly among patients with diabetes, and thus precise adjustments in insulin and carbohydrate intake need to be individualized.

In some patients with type 1 diabetes, improved insulin sensitivity may persist for several hours after they stop exercising (Fig. 38.4), and these effects can last for up to 24 hours (31). The mechanism is not fully understood, but the increased sensitivity is thought to be due to a relatively high rate of glucose uptake by the exercised muscles and lower hepatic production of glucose as the glycogen stores are repleted (24). This may result in the development of hypoglycemia several hours after exercise. Therefore, it is often advisable to decrease doses of short- and intermediate-acting insulin before exercise (as noted above), and carbohydrate intake should be increased after exercise. As stated earlier, the treatment regimen needs to be tailored to each patient on the basis of his or her response to exercise.

It is important to recognize that different types of exercise can have distinct effects on blood glucose levels. Whereas moderate, sustained activity may lower plasma glucose concentrations and result in hypoglycemia in patients with type 1 diabetes, short bursts of high-intensity exertion can actually increase glucose levels and cause hyperglycemia (32) (Fig. 38.5). The glucose level in individuals without diabetes tends to rise modestly during brief intensive exercise, with a peak level occurring up to 15 minutes after cessation of activity. The glucose level then gradually drops during the next hour. The rise in glucose concentration is attributed to an increase in hepatic production of glucose that exceeds the rate of glucose uptake by exercising muscle. This likely reflects the dramatic stimulation of

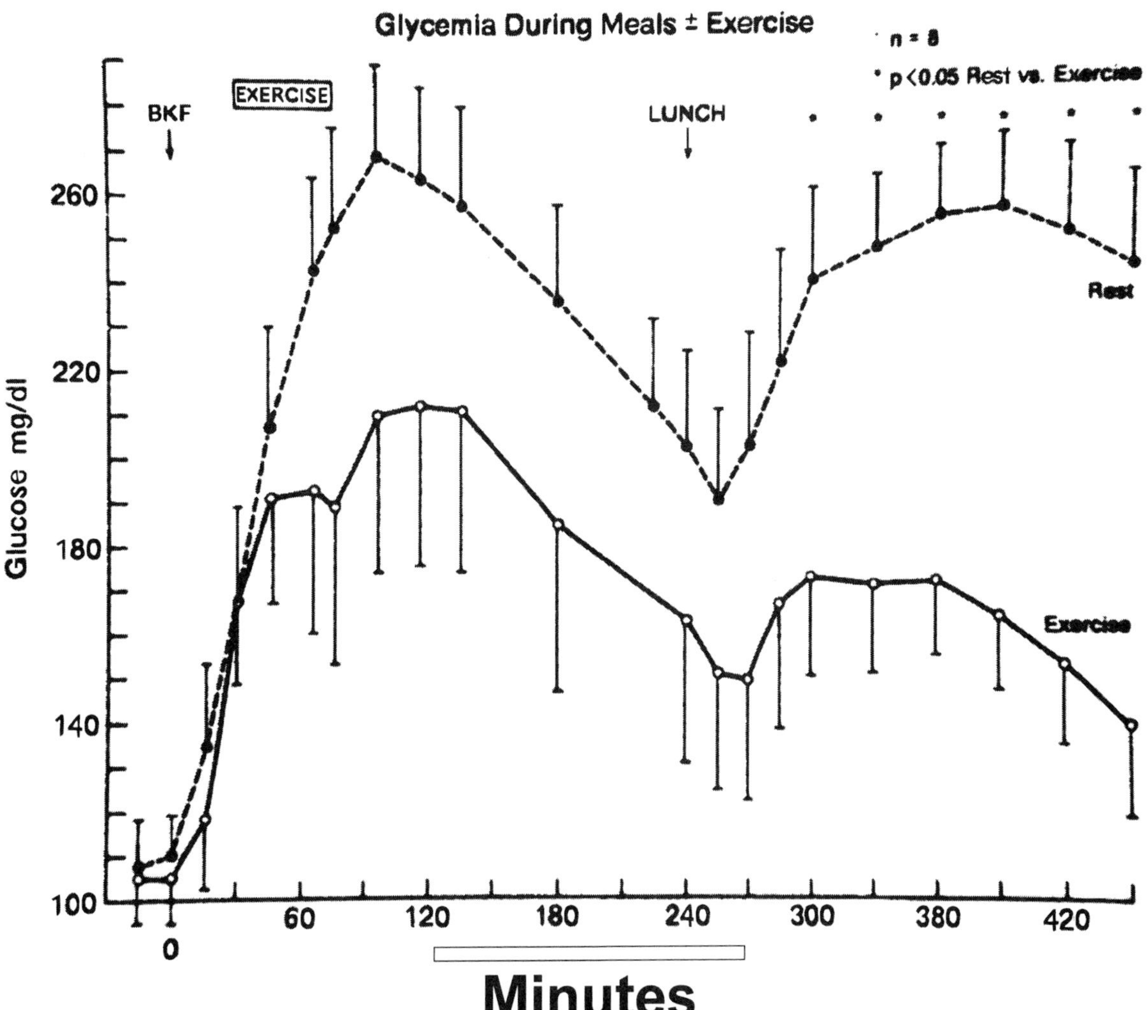

Figure 38.4. Glucose levels during breakfast (BKF) and lunch with rest and with 45 minutes of moderate exercise starting 30 minutes after breakfast in patients with type 1 diabetes. (Copyright © American Diabetes Association. From Caron D, Poussier P, Marliss EB, et al. The effect of postprandial exercise on meal-related glucose intolerance in insulin-dependent diabetic individuals. *Diabetes Care* 1982;5:364–369. Reprinted with permission from the American Diabetes Association.)

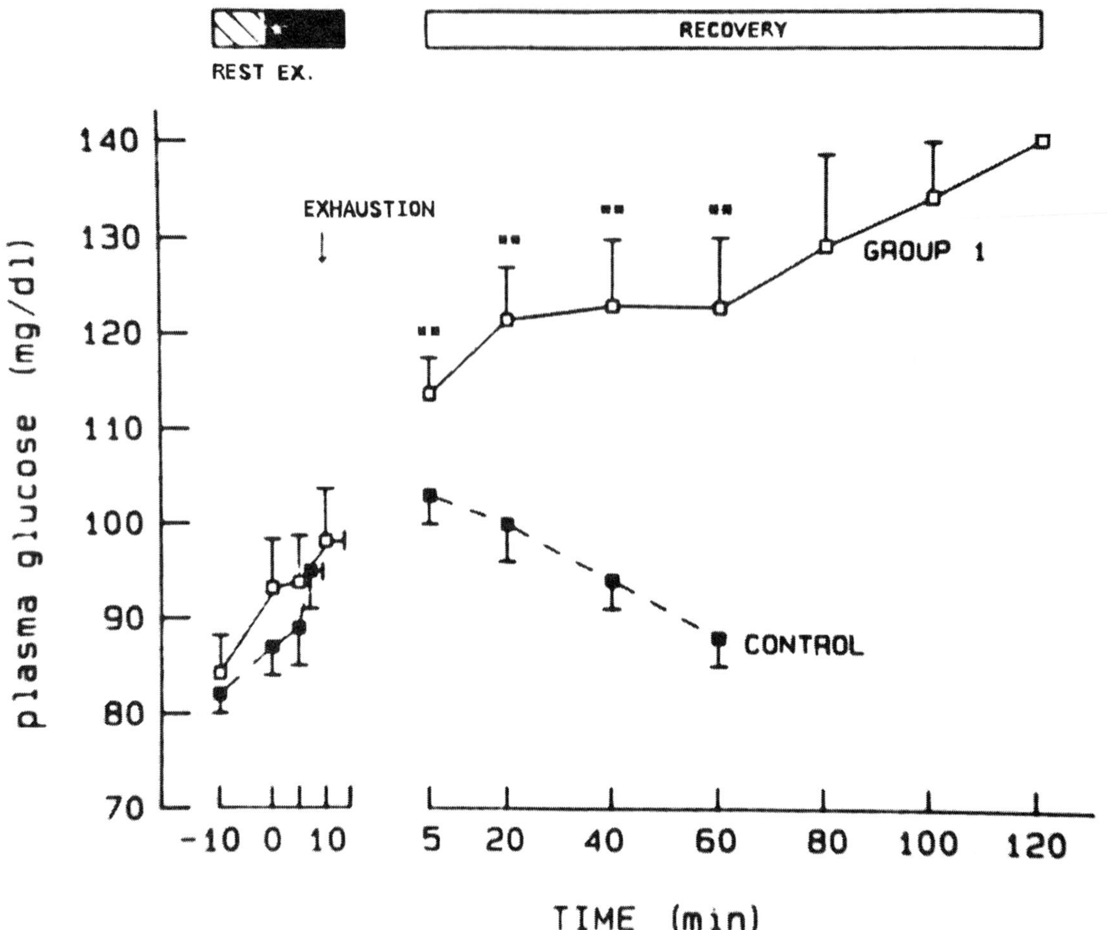

Figure 38.5. Glucose concentrations in control and diabetic subjects 10 minutes before intense exercise, then an exercise period at 80% $VO_{2\ max}$, then 2 hours of recovery. Group 1 consists of the diabetic subjects, all of whom had plasma glucose values of 70 to 120 mg/dL before the exercise test. (Copyright © American Diabetes Association. From Mitchell TH, Abraham G, Schiffrin A, et al. Hyperglycemia after intense exercise in IDDM subjects during continuous insulin infusion. *Diabetes Care* 1988;11:311–317. Reprinted with permission from the American Diabetes Association.)

the counterregulatory hormone secretion during intense exercise, which suppresses insulin release. Once exercise is completed, there is a compensatory increase in insulin secretion.

The rise in blood glucose with intensive exercise may last longer in individuals with type 1 diabetes than in those without diabetes. One study found that the postexercise hyperglycemia reached higher levels and lasted for a full 2-hour observation period in patients with type 1 diabetes after they exercised at 80% VO_{2max} (32). The higher glucose levels and prolonged hyperglycemia in patients with type 1 diabetes are likely due to increased hepatic production of glucose in the setting of counterregulatory hormone release. This is followed by an inability to increase insulin release after completion of exercise in response to the elevated blood glucose levels. Of note, the catecholamine response in patients with diabetes appears to be normal (33).

Although hyperglycemia can occur after intense exercise in diabetic patients with excellent glycemic control, patients with poor control who exercise often experience an even more marked increase in blood glucose levels, which can be accompanied by ketosis (Fig. 38.6). In the setting of insulin deficiency, fatty acid oxidation and glucose production by the liver are stimulated, contributing to increased ketogenesis and hyperglycemia (34). There also appears to be decreased clearance of ketones in patients with poorly controlled diabetes, because this is an insulin-stimulated response (35). It is recommended that patients with type 1 diabetes check both their blood glucose level and their urine or serum for ketones before exercising. If their serum glucose concentration is 250 mg/dL or higher and ketones are present, they should postpone exercise and administer insulin. If no ketones are present, it is generally safe for them to exercise. Indeed, moderate exercise may be helpful in improving the serum glucose level.

Recommendations for patients with type 1 diabetes should always be individualized, but there are some universal principles (Table 38.1). First, patients should always check blood glucose levels before exercise. If their glucose level is less than 100 mg/dL, they should take supplemental carbohydrate before initiating exercise. They also should exercise about 1 to 3 hours after a meal. If they take short-acting insulin with meals, they should plan to lower their dose of insulin at the meal before initiating activity. A general rule is to lower the short-acting insulin by at least 50%. If they take only intermediate-acting insulin, they may wish to lower the dose by 30% to 35% on the morning of the planned exercise. If patients are involved in high-intensity exercise with a $VO_{2\ max}$ greater than 80%, they may need supplemental insulin after exercise to counter postexercise hyperglycemia. For patients

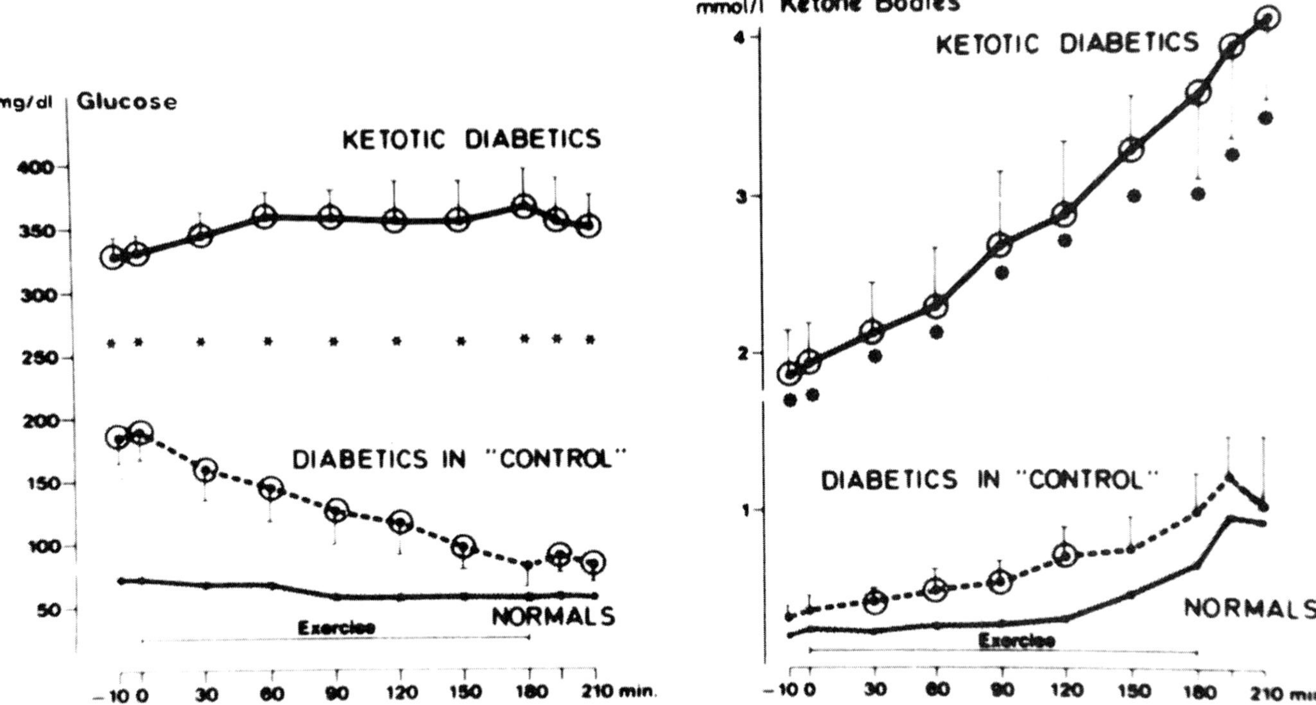

Figure 38.6. Glucose and ketone levels during exercise in patients with diabetes with good versus poor blood glucose control. (From Berger M, Berchtold P, Cuppers HJ, et al. Metabolic and hormonal effects of muscular exercise in juvenile type diabetes. *Diabetologia* 1977;13:355–365, with permission. Copyright 1977 by Springer-Verlag.)

on an insulin pump, the basal rate should be lowered and the premeal bolus decreased to avoid hypoglycemia. In addition, patients may need to take supplemental carbohydrates before exercising and at intervals during and after exercise. It is important to consider each patient's personal experience when developing an appropriate regimen and making adjustments.

EXERCISE IN PATIENTS WITH TYPE 2 DIABETES

There are many health benefits of exercise for patients with type 2 diabetes, including improvement in the circulating lipid profile and blood pressure. In addition to the benefits of acute exercise, prolonged physical training can improve insulin sensitivity and both fasting and postprandial glucose levels (36,37). It is thought that the greater insulin sensitivity from physical conditioning reflects an increase in glucose uptake by skeletal muscle rather than a decrease in hepatic glucose production. This may be linked to augmented translocation of GLUT4 glucose transporters to the plasma membrane, thus improving peripheral glucose uptake (38). Unfortunately, much of this effect disappears once exercise training is discontinued, often within days (39,40). In a recent meta-analysis of studies focusing on the effects of exercise training on glycemic control, the hemoglobin A_{1c} level was significantly lower in the exercise group than in the control group (41), indicating that exercise is beneficial to long-term glycemic control.

TABLE 38.1. Insulin Regimen for Exercise

- Multiple daily injections
  - Decrease short-acting insulin dose by 30–50% before exercise
  - Adjust postexercise doses based on glucose monitoring and experience with postexercise hypoglycemia
- Insulin pump therapy
  - Decrease basal infusion rate
  - Decrease or omit premeal boluses before exercise
  - Adjust postexercise basal rate and boluses based on glucose

Numerous studies have evaluated the effectiveness of exercise in the prevention of type 2 diabetes. Because insulin resistance plays an important role in the progression to type 2 diabetes, techniques to improve insulin sensitivity should theoretically delay or reverse this process. One study showed that Japanese persons living in Hawaii were much more likely than those living in Japan to develop diabetes. This was thought to be associated with decreased physical exercise and changes in diet in individuals who had immigrated to Hawaii as compared with those who lived in Japan (42). Subsequently, multiple studies confirmed that physical activity has a protective effect against the development of diabetes (43–46). Several important findings have emerged from these studies. First, the beneficial effect of physical activity appears to be independent of corrections in the risk factors for diabetes. In one study, the incidence of diabetes was reduced by 24% from the highest to the lowest activity group in men at high risk for developing diabetes [based on obesity, high blood pressure, and family history (44)]. In another study, women who participated in physical activity were found to have a decreased occurrence of diabetes, independent of other risk factors (45).

More recently, three important clinical trials evaluated the effects of exercise and lifestyle modification on the prevention of type 2 diabetes. The first study (the Da Qing Study) looked at 577 Chinese patients with impaired glucose tolerance. The subjects were divided into four groups according to the clinic they attended: a control group, a group treated with diet alone, a group treated with exercise alone, and a group treated with both diet and exercise. Patients received an oral glucose tolerance test every 2 years for a total of 6 years of follow-up. All of the treatment groups had a significant drop in the incidence of diabetes compared with the control group. Interestingly, the group with only exercise as an intervention had the highest overall reduction in diabetes incidence after adjustment for baseline blood glucose and body mass index (47).

A second study (the Finnish Diabetes Prevention Study) evaluated patients with impaired glucose tolerance. The subjects were randomly divided into two groups: a treatment group offered intensive lifestyle changes, including diet and exercise, and a nontreatment group. At the end of the study (after an average of 3.2 years of follow-up), the incidence of diabetes in the treatment group was reduced by 58%. The risk reduction was most significant in those patients who exercised for more than 4 hours per week and in those who had the largest weight loss (48).

Finally, the Diabetes Prevention Program, a large multicenter clinical trial, examined the incidence of diabetes in patients with impaired glucose tolerance who were randomized to placebo, lifestyle intervention, and metformin treatment groups. The lifestyle treatment group had a 58% reduction in the incidence of type 2 diabetes compared with controls. This was significantly better than the 31% reduction achieved with metformin.

In all of these studies, it is clear that prevention or reduction of obesity plays an important role in the prevention of type 2 diabetes. Exercise must be combined with calorie restriction in order to tip the energy balance in the direction of energy expenditure.

There are several universal recommendations that should be given to patients with type 2 diabetes before they begin an exercise regimen. Individuals older than 35 should be given an exercise test to screen for potential underlying asymptomatic coronary artery disease (49). Patients should undergo an ophthalmologic evaluation to ensure that proliferative retinopathy is addressed before they start to exercise. In addition, tests for microalbuminuria and peripheral and autonomic neuropathy should be performed. Exercise regimens should then be individualized. Ideally, aerobic activity should be of a level that can be sustained for at least 30 minutes, and the maximum heart rate should not be higher than 60% to 70% above the resting heart rate. It is important to allot time for warm-up and cool-down stretching exercises to avoid muscle injuries.

For patients to achieve the health benefits of exercise, it is suggested that they partake in physical activity at least 3 days per week, and they should be encouraged to increase the frequency to 5 to 7 days per week, if possible. If patients are receiving oral hypoglycemic agents or insulin, they should be aware of the potential for developing hypoglycemia during or after exercise. They may need to ingest additional carbohydrate to prevent low blood glucose levels, and adjustments to their medications may become necessary.

CONCLUSION

It has long been known that exercise has beneficial effects for people with diabetes. In the past, it was often difficult to avoid the hazards of exercise, particularly in patients with type 1 diabetes. More recently, a greater understanding of energy metabolism and fuel homeostasis has made it possible to include exercise as a realistic goal for almost all patients with diabetes. Improvements in glucose-monitoring technology have further contributed to the feasibility of active physical exercise programs for people with diabetes. In particular, personal blood glucose monitors have allowed patients to follow their blood glucose levels closely and thus readily develop individualized exercise regimens. This has made it much easier for individuals with diabetes to participate in competitive sports or endurance activities such as marathon running. It is important to address strategies for avoiding hypoglycemia (both during and after exercise), as well as hyperglycemia and ketosis, with all patients before they embark on routine exercise.

Patients with type 2 diabetes clearly benefit from frequent exercise. Physical activity plays an important part in the treatment strategy in these patients, as it decreases obesity and lowers blood pressure while improving insulin sensitivity, long-term glycemic control, and blood lipid profiles. Because of the risk of exercise unmasking ischemia as well as causing soft tissue and joint injury or retinal hemorrhage, it is critical that all patients have a complete history and physical examination before they engage in moderate or vigorous activity.

For all patients with diabetes, physician-patient interaction is key to establishing a successful exercise program. A team approach that involves coordination among exercise physiologists, nutritionists, diabetes educators, the physician, and the patient is usually the most effective way to create an individualized exercise regimen that provides benefits to the patient while avoiding potential harm.

REFERENCES

1. Kiens B, Lithell H. Lipoprotein metabolism influenced by training induced changes in human skeletal muscle. *J Clin Invest* 1989;83:558–564.
2. Haskell WL. The influence of exercise training on plasma lipids and lipoproteins in health and disease. *Acta Med Scand Suppl* 1986;711:25–37.
3. Whelton S, Chin A, Xin X, et al. Effect of aerobic exercise on blood pressure: a meta-analysis of randomized, controlled trials. *Ann Intern Med* 2002;136: 493–503.
4. Krotkiewski M, Mandroukas K, Sjostrom L, et al. Effects of long-term physical training on body fat, metabolism and blood pressure in obesity. *Metabolism* 1979;28:650–658.
5. Hill JO, Sparling PB, Shields TW, et al. Effects of exercise and food restriction on body composition and metabolic rate in obese women. *Am J Clin Nutr* 1987;46:622–630.
6. Irwin M, Yasui Y, Ulrich C, et al. Effect of exercise on total and intra-abdominal body fat in postmenopausal women—a randomized controlled trial. *JAMA* 2003;289:323–330.
7. Mogensen CE, Vittinghus E. Urinary albumin excretion during exercise in juvenile diabetes. A provocation test for early abnormalities. *Scand J Clin Lab Invest* 1975;35:295–300.
8. Viberti GC, Jarrett RJ, McCartney M, et al. Increased glomerular permeability to albumin induced by exercise in diabetic subjects. *Diabetologia* 1978;14: 293–300.
9. Poulsen PL, Ebbehoj E, Mogensen, CE. Lisinopril reduces albuminuria during exercise in low grade microalbuminuric type 1 diabetic patients: a double blind randomized study. *J Intern Med* 2001;249:433–440.
10. Ahlborg G, Felig P, Hagenfeldt L, et al. Substrate turnover during prolonged exercise. *J Clin Invest* 1974;53:1080–1090.
11. Stallknecht B, Lorentsen J, Enevoldsen LH, et al. Role of the sympathoadrenergic system in adipose tissue metabolism during exercise in humans. *J Physiol* 2001;536:283–294.
12. Richter EA, Ploug T, Galbo H. Increased muscle glucose uptake following exercise: no need for insulin during exercise. *Diabetes* 1985;34:1041–1048.
13. Wasserman DH, Lickley HLA, Vranic M. Interactions between glucagon and other counterregulatory hormones during normoglycemic and hypoglycemic exercise in dogs. *J Clin Invest* 1984;74:1401–1413.
14. Kennedy JW, Hirshman MF, Gervino EV, et al. Acute exercise induces GLUT-4 translocation in skeletal muscle of normal human subjects and subjects with type 2 diabetes. *Diabetes* 1999;48:1192–1197.
15. Hayashi T, Jorgen FPW, Goodyear LJ. Exercise regulation of glucose transport in skeletal muscle. *Am J Physiol* 1997;273:E1039–E1051.
16. Roberts CK, Barnard RJ, Jasman A, et al. Acute exercise increases nitric oxide synthase activity in skeletal muscle. *Am J Physiol Endocrinol Metab* 1999;277: E390–E394.
17. Higaki Y, Hirshman M, Fujii N, et al. Nitric oxide increases glucose uptake through a mechanism that is distinct from the insulin and contraction pathways in rat skeletal muscle. *Diabetes* 2001;50:241–247.
18. Aronson D, Violan MA, Dufresne SD, et al. Exercise stimulates the mitogen-activated protein kinase pathway in human skeletal muscle. *J Clin Invest* 1997;99:1251–1257.
19. Hayashi T, Hirshman MF, Kurth EJ, et al. Evidence for 5′AMP-activated protein kinase mediation of the effect of muscle contraction on glucose transport. *Diabetes* 1998;47:1369–1373.

20. Kurth-Kraczed EJ, Hirshman MF, Goodyear LJ, et al. 5′AMP-activated protein kinase activation causes GLUT4 translocation in skeletal muscle. *Diabetes* 1999;48:1667–1671.
21. Ryder JW, Chibalin AV, Zierath JR. Intracellular mechanisms underlying increases in glucose uptake in response to insulin or exercise in skeletal muscle. *Acta Physiol Scand* 2001;171:249–257.
22. Sakamoto K, Goodyear LJ. Intracellular signaling in contracting skeletal muscle. Review. *J Appl Physiol* 2002;93:369–383.
23. Goodyear LJ, Hirshman MF, Valyou PM, et al. Glucose transporter number, function and subcellular distribution in rat skeletal muscle after exercise training. *Diabetes* 1992;41:1091–1099.
24 Bogardus C, Thuillez P, Ravussin E, et al. Effect of muscle glycogen depletion in vivo in insulin action in man. *J Clin Invest* 1983;72:1605–1610.
25. Ryan AS, Muller DC, Elahi D. Sequential hyperglycemic-euglycemic clamp to assess β-cell and peripheral tissue: studies in female athletes. *J Appl Physiol* 2001;91:872–881.
26. Rose A, Howlett K, King D, et al. Effect of prior exercise on glucose metabolism in trained men. *Am J Physiol Endocrinol Metab* 2001; 281:E766–E767.
27. Lipman RL, Raskin P, Love T, et al. Glucose intolerance during decreased physical activity in man. *Diabetes* 1972;21:101–107.
28. Koivisto VA, Felig P. Effects of leg exercise on insulin absorption in diabetic patients. *N Engl J Med* 1978;298:77–83.
29. Yamakita T, Tomofusa I, Yamagami K, et al. Glycemic response during exercise after administration of insulin lispro compared with that after administration of regular human insulin. *Diabetes Res Clin Pract* 2002;57:17–22.
30. Amiel SA, Tamborlane WV, Simonson DC, et al. Defective glucose counterregulation after strict control of insulin-dependent diabetes mellitus. *N Engl J Med* 1987;316:1376–1383.
31. MacDonald MJ. Postexercise late-onset hypoglycemia in insulin-dependent diabetic patients. *Diabetes Care* 1987;10:584–588.
32. Mitchell TH, Abraham G, Schiffrin A, et al. Hyperglycemia after intense exercise in IDDM subjects during continuous subcutaneous insulin infusion. *Diabetes Care* 1988;11:311–317.
33. Purdon C, Brousson M, Nyveen SL, et al. The roles of insulin and catecholamines in the glucoregulatory response during intense exercise and early recovery in insulin-dependent diabetic and control subjects. *J Clin Endocrinol Metab* 1993;76:566–573.
34. Berger M, Berchtold P, Cuppers HJ, et al. Metabolic and hormonal effects of muscular exercise in juvenile type diabetics. *Diabetologia* 1977;13:355–365.
35. Fery F, de Maertalaer V, Balasse EO. Mechanism of the hyperketonaemic effect of prolonged exercise in insulin-deprived type I (insulin-dependent) diabetic patients. *Diabetologia* 1987;30:298–304.
36. Bjorntorp P, de Jounge K, Sjostrom L, et al. The effect of physical training on insulin production in obesity. *Metabolism* 1970;19:631–638.
37. Maiorana A, O'Driscoll G, Goodman C, et al. Combined aerobic and resistance exercise improves glycemic control and fitness in type 2 diabetes. *Diabetes Res Clin Pract* 2002;56:115–123.
38. Kennedy JW, Hirshman MF, Gervino EV, et al. Acute exercise induces GLUT4 translocation in skeletal muscle of normal human subjects and subjects with type 2 diabetes. *Diabetes* 1999;48:1192–1197.
39. Burstein R, Polychronakos C, Toews CJ, et al. Acute reversal of the enhanced insulin action in trained athletes. *Diabetes* 1985;34:756–760.
40. Mikines KJ, Sonne B, Farrell PA, et al. Effect of physical exercise on sensitivity and responsiveness to insulin in humans. *Am J Physiol* 1988;254:E248–E259.
41. Boule NG, Haddad E, Kenny GP, et al. Effects of exercise on glycemic control and body mass in type 2 diabetes mellitus: a meta-analysis of controlled clinical trials. *JAMA* 2001;286:1218–1227.
42. Kawate R, Yamakido M, Nishimoto Y, et al. Diabetes mellitus and its vascular complications in Japanese migrants on the island of Hawaii. *Diabetes Care* 1979;2:161–170.
43. Frisch RE, Wyshak G, Albright TE, et al. Lower prevalence of diabetes in female former college athletes compared with nonathletes. *Diabetes* 1986;35: 1101–1105.
44. Helmrich SP, Ragland DR, Leung RW, et al. Physical activity and reduced occurrence of non-insulin-dependent diabetes mellitus. *N Engl J Med* 1991;325: 147–152.
45. Manson JE, Rimm EB, Stampfer MJ, et al. Physical activity and incidence of non-insulin dependent diabetes mellitus in women. *Lancet* 1991;338:774–778.
46. Manson JE, Nathan DM, Krolewski AS, et al. A prospective study of exercise and incidence of diabetes among U.S. male physicians. *JAMA* 1992;268:63–67.
47. Pan XR, Li GW, Hu YH, et al. Effects of diet and exercise in preventing NIDDM in people with impaired glucose tolerance: the Da Qing IGT and Diabetes Study. *Diabetes Care* 1997;20:537–544.
48. Tuomilehto J, Lindstrom J, Eriksson J, et al. Prevention of type 2 diabetes mellitus by changes in lifestyle among subjects with impaired glucose tolerance. *N Engl J Med* 2001;344:1343–1350.
49. American College of Sports Medicine. *Guidelines for exercise testing and prescription*, 6th ed. Philadelphia: Lippincott Williams & Wilkins, 2000.

CHAPTER 39
Principles of Insulin Therapy

Alice Y. Y. Cheng and Bernard Zinman

HISTORICAL BACKGROUND

The isolation of insulin from dog pancreas and demonstration of its biologic effectiveness by Banting, Best, Collip, and MacLeod in 1921 at the University of Toronto represents one of the greatest medical discoveries of modern medicine (1). This antidiabetic substance, initially called isletin by Banting and Best and later named insulin by MacLeod, was purified sufficiently by Collip, the biochemist member of the team, so that it could be injected into humans (2). The first injection was given to a patient with diabetes, Leonard Thompson, on January 11, 1922, at the Toronto General Hospital (3). Improvements in insulin extraction and purification followed, facilitating the widespread use of insulin for patients with diabetes.

In 1936, Hagedorn discovered that the addition of fish protamine kept insulin in suspension so that it was absorbed slowly from subcutaneous sites, thus prolonging the effect of insulin (4). Scott and Fisher (5) discovered that zinc could further extend the action of protamine insulin, leading to the development of protamine zinc insulin. In 1946, NPH insulin (neutral protamine Hagedorn), a more stable form of protamine insulin, was introduced and remains in use today (6).

For the first 60 years of the insulin era, insulin was available only in bovine or porcine preparations. In the 1980s, human insulin was introduced (7), making animal insulin essentially obsolete. In the 1990s, insulin analogues with pharmacokinetics that were more appropriate for bolus (premeal) therapy were introduced and facilitated the improvement of subcutaneous insulin regimens (8). Over the last 80 years, great strides have been made to improve the treatment of diabetes with improved insulin formulations, increased ease of self-monitoring of blood glucose, and a better understanding of physiologic insulin requirements. Unfortunately, although we are much closer to the goal of physiologic insulin replacement, this goal remains elusive owing to the inherent limitations of administering insulin at a nonphysiologic site (subcutaneous tissue) (9).

TYPES OF INSULIN

The laboratory production of human insulin in the early 1980s has gradually resulted in the replacement of animal insulins as a viable therapeutic choice for patients with diabetes. Human insulins and newer insulin analogues produced by recombinant

TABLE 39.1. Approximate Pharmacokinetic Characteristics of Human Insulin and Insulin Analogues Following Subcutaneous Injection

Insulin	Onset of action	Peak of action	Duration of action	Blood glucose targets
Mealtime insulins				
Lispro	10–15 min	1–1.5 h	4–5 h	Postprandial
Aspart[a]	10–15 min	1–2 h	4–6 h	Postprandial
Regular	15–60 min	2–4 h	5–8 h	Postprandial Prior to next meal
Basal insulins				
NPH	2.5–3 h	5–7 h	13–16 h	Midafternoon (for morning NPH) Fasting glucose next morning (for bedtime NPH)
Lente	2.5–3 h	7–12 h	Up to 18 h	Similar to NPH
Glargine[b]	2–3 h	No peak	Up to 30 h	Similar to NPH
Ultralente	3–4 h	8–10 h	Up to 20 h	Similar to NPH
Detemir[c]	2–3 h	No peak	Up to 24 h	Similar to NPH

NPH, Neutral Protamine Hagedorn.
[a]Data from Mudaliar SR, Lindberg FA, Joyce M, et al. Insulin aspart: a fast acting analog of human insulin—absorption kinetics and action profile compared with regular human insulin in healthy non-diabetic subjects. *Diabetes Care* 1999;22:1501–1506.
[b]Data from Heinemann L, Linkeschova R, Rave K, et al. Time-action profile of the long-acting insulin analog insulin glargine (HOE 901) in comparison with those of NPH insulin and placebo. *Diabetes Care* 2000;23:644–649.
[c]Data from Heinemann L, Sinha K, Weyer C, et al. Time-action profile of the soluble, fatty acid acylated, long-acting insulin analogue NN304. *Diabet Med* 1999;16:332–338
Adapted from Heineman L, Richter B. Clinical pharmacology of human insulin. *Diabetes Care* 1993;16[Suppl S3]:90–101.

DNA technology are becoming the main insulins used in the current treatment of diabetes in most countries. Insulins for clinical use can be characterized according to their pharmacokinetic profiles. They are available in rapid-acting, short-acting, intermediate-acting, and long-acting preparations (10). Table 39.1 shows the onset, peak, and duration of action after subcutaneous injections of the insulins used commonly in therapy. The different time–action profiles make it feasible to pursue the goal of simulating physiologic insulin secretion, as shown in Figure 39.1; however, this goal remains difficult to achieve with the current formulations. Insulin replacement should be thought of in terms of mealtime (bolus) and basal insulins. The mealtime insulins are the rapid-acting analogues or short-acting regular human insulin. These insulins have been used to attempt to simulate the high levels of insulin seen in individuals without diabetes after ingestion of a meal. The basal insulins are the intermediate- and long-acting human insulins and analogue. They simulate the basal level of insulin occurring between meals, through the night, and with fasting. Insulin is commercially available in concentrations of 100 or 500 units/mL, designated U-100 or U-500. The U-500 concentration, which is available only in short-acting formulations, is used only in rare cases of insulin resistance when the patient requires extremely large doses of insulin.

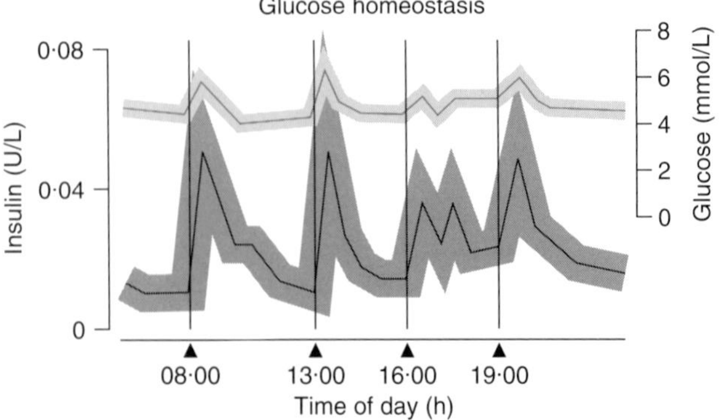

Figure 39.1 Normal insulin secretion in relation to meals and the overnight fasting state. (Redrawn from Owens DR, Zinman B, Bolli GB: Insulins today and beyond. *Lancet 2001*;358:739.)

Mealtime Insulins

RAPID-ACTING INSULIN ANALOGUES: LISPRO AND ASPART

The time–action profile of regular human insulin is unable to adequately mimic physiologic insulin secretion. Insulin in solution self-associates and forms larger aggregates called hexamers. These large aggregates need to dissociate after subcutaneous injection before diffusion of insulin into the circulation is possible (11). Therefore, analogues of human insulin have been developed that can dissociate rapidly from hexamers to monomers or that remain less associated in solution, thus allowing faster absorption and onset of action (10,11). The first rapidly acting insulin analogue approved for human administration was insulin lispro, in which the terminal proline and lysine residues of the B chain of insulin are inverted, resulting in decreased self-association properties of the insulin (8,12). Lispro insulin is absorbed much more rapidly than regular insulin. Lispro begins acting within 15 minutes, reaches peak biologic effects in 60 to 90 minutes, and continues to act for 4 to 5 hours. In comparison to regular insulin, lispro peaks more rapidly, achieves higher blood insulin concentrations more rapidly, and has been shown to lower postprandial glucose levels and decrease rates of hypoglycemia (13–17). The impact of lispro compared with regular insulin on levels of glycosylated hemoglobin (HbA_{1c}) has been variable (18–23). However, lispro provides more flexibility for patients at mealtimes because it does not need to be administered 30 minutes before a meal and the dose can readily be adjusted for changes in the carbohydrate content of the meal. Randomized controlled prospective trials have demonstrated that lispro is one of the preferred insulins for insulin pump therapy with continuous subcutaneous insulin infusion (CSII) and results in lower HbA_{1c} levels and less hypoglycemia (24–26). Lispro must be used with caution in patients with gastroparesis because of its rapid onset of action and the potential for early postprandial hypoglycemia. Patients with gastroparesis can delay the meal insulin injection until after they have consumed the meal to reduce the risk of hypoglycemia.

Insulin aspart is another very-rapid-acting insulin analogue. Similar to lispro, it is absorbed very rapidly after subcutaneous injection, resulting in higher peak concentrations compared with those achieved with regular insulin (27). Trials comparing insulin aspart and regular insulin in patients with type 1 diabetes show significantly reduced HbA_{1c} levels with no difference in the frequency of hypoglycemia (28–30). In type 2 diabetes, insulin aspart is comparable to regular insulin, with no significant difference in HbA_{1c} levels or frequency of hypoglycemia (31). Both insulin lispro and insulin aspart appear to be associated with a lower incidence of nocturnal hypoglycemia than regular human insulin. For these reasons, lispro and aspart are the insulins of choice for use before meals in most treatment regimens and particularly in multiple daily injection therapy (13–17,19–21,23, 28–30). The safety and efficacy of the use of aspart in CSII have also been demonstrated (31a).

SHORT-ACTING HUMAN INSULIN: REGULAR

As mentioned earlier, subcutaneously injected regular insulin, because of its relatively slow rate of absorption, is unable to mimic physiologic insulin secretion following a meal. Regular insulin has an onset of action 15 to 60 minutes after injection, a peak effect 2 to 4 hours after injection, and a duration of action ranging from 5 to 8 hours (11). Given the "short-acting" nature of regular insulin, it is used primarily as a mealtime insulin. Therefore, regular insulin should be administered approximately 30 to 45 minutes before a meal in order to match the kinetics of insulin absorption with the peak of carbohydrate absorption after the meal (11).

Basal Insulins

INTERMEDIATE-ACTING HUMAN INSULINS: NPH AND LENTE

Both NPH and lente insulins are modified into a suspension form to delay their absorption from subcutaneous sites, thereby prolonging their action. NPH insulin, first developed in 1946, has a longer duration of action than regular insulin (12). Its onset of action is within 2.5 to 3 hours of injection, with a peak action 5 to 7 hours after injection and a duration of action between 13 and 16 hours (12). Lente insulin, the other intermediate-acting insulin, was first introduced in the 1950s. Its onset of action is similar to that of NPH at 2.5 hours, its peak action is 7 to 12 hours after injection, and its duration of action is up to 18 hours (12). Given the more prolonged action of NPH and lente insulins, they are not ideal for controlling postprandial serum glucose levels. When given at appropriate times, these insulins are reasonably effective in lowering fasting plasma glucose and predinner plasma glucose levels (11). These insulins are used as the basal insulins and are necessary for adequate glycemic control in type 1 and type 2 diabetes. Currently, NPH insulin is the only intermediate-acting insulin available for the pen delivery system.

LONG-ACTING HUMAN INSULIN: ULTRALENTE

The role of long-acting insulin is to achieve basal insulin coverage with a relatively small or no pharmacologic/biologic peak action. Its onset of action is 4 hours after injection, its peak action is at 8 to 10 hours, and its duration of action is up to 20 hours (12). In clinical practice, its biologic action appears to be similar to that of intermediate-acting insulin. NPH and ultralente provide similar glycemic control when used as the basal insulin in a multiple daily injection regimen with lispro as the mealtime insulin (32). Most patients (75%) require only one injection of basal insulin per day given at bedtime (32). However, NPH seems to provide a slightly better daily glycemic profile than ultralente in those requiring two injections of basal insulin per day (32).

LONG-ACTING INSULIN ANALOGUE: GLARGINE

Glargine is a long-acting insulin analogue that was developed in an attempt to provide a more constant level of insulin than that achieved with the human intermediate- and long-acting insulin preparations (10,33–38). Glargine has a higher isoelectric point than human insulin and precipitates in the neutral environment of subcutaneous tissue, giving it its prolonged duration of action (10,33–36). Glargine is absorbed more slowly than the human long-acting insulin preparations, with no pronounced insulin peaks, decreasing the risk of nocturnal hypoglycemia (33,34,36–38). Insulin glargine has a greater affinity than human insulin for insulin-like growth factor 1 (IGF-1) receptors, and it has been suggested that this may lead to increased mitogenic potential in cell lines rich with IGF-1 receptors (39). However, the clinical significance of this hypothesis is still unknown (39).

Detemir is another long-acting insulin analogue that was developed using a different approach—binding to albumin. An aliphatic fatty acid has been acylated to the B29 amino acid, and the B30 amino acid has been removed (39a). This results in reversible binding between albumin and the fatty acid acylated to the insulin. After injection, 98% of the insulin is bound to albumin. The gradual release of the bound fraction from albumin allows for the sustained, prolonged action of detemir (39b). The time-action profile of insulin detemir is characterized by a peak activity at 6 to 8 hours after injection and prolonged 24-hour duration of action (39b). Detemir has been approved for release in Europe and has received preliminary approval from the FDA in the United States. Studies to date have shown less hypoglycemia and less variation in blood glucose levels with detemir as basal insulin in intensive regimens compared with NPH (39c–e).

Premixed Insulin

Premixed preparations of short- and intermediate-acting insulins are available in a wide range of ratios (90/10 to 50/50) (11). The most commonly used premixed insulin is 70/30, which contains 30% short-acting and 70% intermediate-acting insulin. A premixed insulin of 75% NPL (neutral protamine lispro) and 25% lispro, Humalog Mix 75/25, also is available (40). Humalog Mix 75/25 provides a relatively rapid peak in insulin activity, similar to lispro alone, and the NPL provides basal coverage similar to that of NPH (40). This allows improved postprandial glycemic control compared with that offered by 70/30 insulin (41,42). A premixed insulin of 30% aspart and 70% protaminated insulin aspart (NovoLog Mix 70/30) is also available. Like Humalog Mix 75/25, NovoLog Mix 70/30 provides improved postprandial glucose control and less hypoglycemia than 70/30 insulin (42a,b).

Use of premixed insulin avoids the potential problems of self-mixing and reduces the number of steps before injection, thereby reducing the number of possible errors. The premixed insulins are preferred by elderly patients and those with visual or fine-motor impairment (43). However, premixed insulins do not permit easy adjustment of mealtime and basal insulin doses and are inappropriate for patients with type 1 diabetes. They are valuable and frequently used in the treatment of type 2 diabetes.

TABLE 39.2. Goals of Insulin Therapy

1. Eliminate symptoms of hyperglycemia
2. Prevent diabetic ketoacidosis
3. Arrest severe catabolic state and regain lean body mass
4. Reduce frequent infections
5. Decrease fetal and maternal morbidity in pregnancy
6. Prevent and delay microvascular and macrovascular complications

GOALS OF THERAPY

Type 1 Diabetes

Insulin deficiency is the hallmark of type 1 diabetes. Insulin replacement is essential for life in people with type 1 diabetes to avoid a progressive catabolic state and ketosis. When used properly, insulin can eliminate clinical symptoms of hyperglycemia, prevent diabetic ketoacidosis, restore lean body mass and exercise capacity, decrease the incidence of certain infections, and improve the patient's sense of well-being. In addition, the use of insulin in intensive treatment regimens, with the goal of achieving near-normal plasma glucose concentrations, delays the onset and slows the progression of microvascular complications in patients with type 1 diabetes (44,45). Table 39.2 itemizes some of the principal goals of insulin therapy. The Diabetes Control and Complications Trial (DCCT) was a multicenter, randomized controlled trial comparing multiple daily injection therapy or continuous subcutaneous insulin infusion (intensive therapy) to therapy with one to two injections per day (conventional therapy) in 1,441 patients with type 1 diabetes, followed for a mean of 6.5 years (44). The intensive-therapy group, who achieved significantly lower HbA_{1c} levels than patients in the conventional-therapy groups, had a relative risk reduction of 76% for developing retinopathy and a 54% relative risk reduction for progression of retinopathy (44). The intensive-therapy groups had a 39% relative risk reduction for developing microalbuminuria and a 54% relative risk reduction for progressing to albuminuria (44). The intensive-therapy group also had a 64% relative risk reduction for developing neuropathy or experiencing progression of diagnosed neuropathy (46). Thus, intensive insulin therapy, which resulted in a lower HbA_{1c} level, was associated with a statistically and clinically significant reduction in microvascular complications in the intensive-therapy group. A follow-up study of the DCCT group, the Epidemiology of Diabetes Intervention and Complications (EDIC) study, showed that the risk reduction in microvascular complications from intensive therapy persists for at least 4 years despite increasing hyperglycemia (47). However, the benefit related to macrovascular complications is less clear (48). The DCCT showed a nonstatistically significant 41% relative risk reduction for macrovascular complications with intensive therapy; however, the study was not powered to detect a difference in macrovascular events, and the number of these events in the trial was low (49). There was also a relative risk reduction of 40% for developing elevated low-density lipoprotein (LDL) cholesterol levels in the intensive-therapy group (49). A recent meta-analysis of intensive therapy in type 1 diabetes showed that intensive therapy decreased the total number of macrovascular events but showed no significant effect on the number of patients affected or on mortality due to macrovascular disease (48). The need for insulin in type 1 diabetes for survival is apparent. However, the appropriate use of insulin with the goal of achieving near-normal serum glucose concentrations has benefits beyond those of mere survival and symptom relief.

The degree of glucose lowering to be sought depends on many factors and should be individualized for each patient. In the DCCT, the mean HbA_{1c} level achieved by the intensive-therapy group was approximately 7.2% compared with a mean of 9.0% in the conventional-therapy group (44). Therefore, the most recent clinical practice recommendations from the American Diabetes Association state that the primary treatment goal in type 1 diabetes should be blood glucose control approximating the median value achieved in the intensive-therapy group (50). Table 39.3 outlines the glycemic goals from the American Diabetes Association. In fact, any improvement in blood glucose control will slow the development and progression of microvascular complications. However, one must consider the risks of hypoglycemia when aiming for a low HbA_{1c} level. The intensive-treatment group in the DCCT had a threefold greater risk of severe hypoglycemia compared with the conventional-therapy group, but the rate of hypoglycemia decreased with time (44). Therefore, very tight control should not be attempted in patients unwilling or unable to participate actively in their glucose management. Patients with hypoglycemia unawareness or those susceptible to permanent injury from hypoglycemia, such as children or the elderly, can be managed with intensive therapy with multiple daily injections (MDI) or CSII but should have higher glycemic targets to avoid hypoglycemia (51–53). Appropriate diabetes education and self-monitoring of blood glucose are invaluable components of reducing hypoglycemia (51,53,54). Clinical judgment and common sense are required to determine the target premeal, postprandial, and

TABLE 39.3. Target Glycemic Control for Nonpregnant Adults with Diabetes

	Glucose level, mg/dL (mmol/L)		
Measurement	**Normal**	**Goal**	**Additional action suggested**
Whole blood (capillary blood glucose)			
Average preprandial glucose	<100 (<5.6)	80–120 (4.4–6.7)	<80 or >140 (<4.4 or >7.8)
Average bedtime glucose	<110 (<6.1)	100–140 (5.6–7.8)	<100 or >160 (<5.6 or >8.9)
Plasma			
Preprandial glucose	<110 (<6.1)	90–130 (5.0–7.2)	<90 or >150 (<5.0 or >8.3)
Postprandial glucose (1–2 h after beginning of meal)	<120 (<6.7)	<180 (<10.0)	<110 or >180 (<6.1 or >10.0)
HbA_{1c}	<6%	<7.0%	<8%

HbA_{1c}, glycosylated hemoglobin.

bedtime glucose levels for individual patients without placing them at undue risk for hypoglycemia (50,51,53,54).

Type 2 Diabetes

The initial treatment for type 2 diabetes generally does not include insulin. Diet, exercise, weight loss, and oral hypoglycemic agents are initially adequate therapies for achieving glycemic control. However, insulin is indicated for patients who are unable to achieve good glycemic control with a combination of oral agents, diet, and exercise (55). The goals of insulin therapy in type 2 diabetes are similar to those for type 1 diabetes. The elimination of clinical symptoms of hyperglycemia is an important goal. In addition, maintaining good glycemic control reduces the risk of microvascular and macrovascular complications. The United Kingdom Prospective Diabetes Study (UKPDS) was a multicenter, randomized, controlled study designed to establish whether intensive blood glucose control reduced the risk of macrovascular and microvascular complications in patients with type 2 diabetes (56) and to compare the relative effectiveness and safety of different pharmacologic approaches to therapy. The UKPDS studied 5,102 patients with type 2 diabetes and followed them for an average of 10 years (56). There was a 12% reduction in diabetes-related endpoints and a 25% risk reduction in microvascular endpoints for the intensive-therapy group (56). There was no significant difference within the intensive-therapy group (i.e., no difference between insulin and sulfonylureas). A smaller Japanese study also showed significant reductions in microvascular complications with improved HbA_{1c} levels (57). Although the original analysis of the UKPDS data showed a nonstatistically significant 16% risk reduction ($p = 0.052$) in macrovascular complications with intensive therapy (56), a recent analysis showed a significant relationship between macrovascular complications and hyperglycemia, as measured by the updated mean HbA_{1c} (58,59). For every 1% reduction in updated mean HbA_{1c}, there was a 14% risk reduction for myocardial infarction ($p < 0.0001$), a 12% risk reduction for stroke ($p = 0.035$), and a 43% risk reduction for amputation or death from peripheral vascular disease ($p < 0.0001$) (58).

In the UKPDS, the intensive-therapy group achieved a median HbA_{1c} value of 7.0%, compared with 7.9% in the conventional-therapy group (56). This suggests that the primary treatment goal for patients with type 2 diabetes should be similar to that for patients with type 1 diabetes. The target HbA_{1c} should also be as close to normal as possible without placing the patient at undue risk for severe hypoglycemia (60). There is a continuous relationship between the risks of microvascular complications and glycemia, such that for any decrease in HbA_{1c}, there is a corresponding reduction in the risk of complications (58,60).

Although the UKPDS provided suggestive data to support the claim that aggressive glycemic control reduces macrovascular complications, a landmark study from Denmark provided the best evidence, thus far, that aggressive glycemic control, in the context of a multifactorial approach, can reduce cardiovascular outcomes (60a). One hundred and sixty patients with type 2 diabetes and microalbuminuria were randomized to receive intensive multifactorial treatment or conventional diabetes care by their family physician or specialist. The target HbA_{1c} level in the intensive group was less than 6.5%. In addition to intensive glycemic control, blood pressure and cholesterol levels were aggressively treated. After a mean follow-up of 7.8 years, the intensively treated group experienced a 53% relative risk reduction ($p = 0.007$) in the composite primary outcome of cardiovascular death, myocardial infarction, stroke, revascularization, and amputation. Microvascular complications, including nephropathy, retinopathy, and autonomic neuropathy, were also significantly reduced. This study provided further support to the recommendation for aggressive glycemic control among patients with diabetes.

Aggressive therapy with insulin in patients with type 2 diabetes appears to be particularly indicated following myocardial infarction. The Diabetes Mellitus, Insulin Glucose Infusion in Acute Myocardial Infarction (DIGAMI) trial showed that intensive insulin therapy following an acute myocardial infarction decreases patient mortality (61,62). The use of an insulin–glucose infusion for at least 24 hours after an acute myocardial infarction followed by intensive insulin therapy reduced in-hospital all-cause mortality by 58% ($p < 0.05$) and 1-year all-cause mortality by 52% ($p < 0.02$) (61). The benefit persisted for several years after the event (62). Of interest, the most profound effect was seen in patients with the lowest apparent risk at the time of presentation (61).

TREATMENT STRATEGIES

The appropriate insulin regimen for an individual patient should take into account the patient's lifestyle, age, motivation, general health, self-management skills, and goals of treatment (18,63). Prior to initiating insulin therapy, the patient should receive appropriate education and support regarding the care and use of insulin, the recognition and treatment of hypoglycemia, and the management of sick days (18,63).

Type 1 Diabetes

As prescribed by diabetologists and endocrinologists, the commonly used insulin protocols for individuals with type 1 diabetes are MDI and CSII. The DCCT clearly shows that intensive therapy with MDI or CSII coupled with the appropriate education and frequent self-monitoring of blood glucose (SMBG) achieves a significant lowering of HbA_{1c} levels and reduction in the risk of microvascular complications compared with that achieved with less frequent injections (44). Unfortunately, even in the intensively treated cohort of the DCCT, after the completion of the clinical trial, glycemic control deteriorated, pointing out the necessity of continuing education and close clinical surveillance (48). Therefore, MDI or CSII, along with appropriate education, counseling, and support, is the preferred therapy for patients with type 1 diabetes.

MULTIPLE DAILY INJECTIONS

It is best to think about insulin therapy according to the pharmacokinetics of the available insulin preparations and the physiologic secretion of insulin in individuals without diabetes. Thus, we tend to think of basal insulin administration for the overnight and postabsorptive states and bolus insulin administration for mealtimes as an attempt to reproduce acute β-cell insulin release. This mealtime-basal routine usually requires at least four injections per day. A rapid-acting mealtime insulin analogue (lispro or insulin aspart) is the preferred insulin before each meal. As described earlier, the rapid onset of action of lispro or insulin aspart produces less postprandial hypoglycemia and less nocturnal hypoglycemia compared with regular insulin, which makes them ideal for an MDI regimen. NPH, ultralente, or glargine can be used as the basal insulin, classically at bedtime; however, different regimens are being used (32,37,43). It is likely that glargine (and perhaps detemir) will become the basal insulin of choice for MDI therapy because of their pharmacokinetic properties.

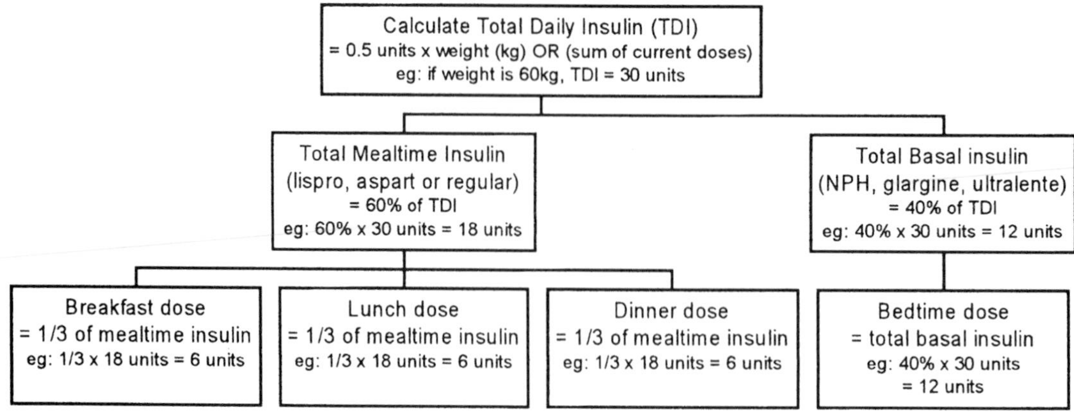

Figure 39. 2 Initiation of multiple daily injection insulin therapy (four injections per day). (From Cheng AY, Zinman B. Insulin for treating type 1 and type 2 diabetes. In: Gerstein HC, Haynes RB, eds. *Evidence-based diabetes care.* Hamilton, Ontario: BC Decker, 2001.)

Glargine, as the basal insulin in a MDI regimen, has been associated with improved fasting blood glucose levels and less hypoglycemia (36,37). The administration of a rapid-acting insulin analogue (lispro or insulin aspart) prior to each meal controls postprandial serum glucose concentrations, and the intermediate- or long-acting insulin controls fasting serum glucose concentrations. As shown in the DCCT, the risk of hypoglycemia is greater with MDI than with less frequent injections, primarily because of the tighter glycemic targets and improved control achieved (44). Therefore, patient education, self-monitoring, and a self-directed management approach are fundamental to achieving success with this therapy. Both clinician and patient have to be prepared to make adjustments to the regimen as necessary, including adjustment of glycemic targets to avoid severe hypoglycemia. Since lispro and insulin aspart are such rapidly acting insulins, a second injection of NPH or ultralente before breakfast may be required to provide basal insulin over the day and better control of predinner serum glucose concentrations. However, a controlled clinical trial (32) demonstrated that most patients (75%) required only one injection of intermediate-acting insulin. The actual doses of insulin used must be adjusted on an individual basis. However, the following is an empirical guide for choosing initial insulin doses for MDI (Fig. 39.2). The approximate total daily insulin (TDI) requirements for an individual not previously receiving insulin are 0.5 units/kg. If the patient is already receiving insulin, the TDI is the sum of all the current insulin doses. Approximately 60% should be rapid-acting mealtime insulin (lispro or insulin aspart) given before each meal. The breakfast meal usually requires a disproportionately higher dose of insulin than other meals for the calories consumed. The remaining 40% of the estimated TDI should be given as the basal insulin (NPH, ultralente, or glargine) at bedtime. Close self-monitoring of blood glucose and frequent adjustments are necessary to optimize glycemic control with the fewest episodes of hypoglycemia.

Many different MDI regimens, some outlined in Table 39.4, have been used by various individuals. However, all MDI regimens follow the same basic principles. Mealtime insulins (lispro, insulin aspart, or regular) are used in combinations with basal insulin (NPH, ultralente, or glargine) in an attempt to simulate physiologic insulin secretion.

TWICE-DAILY DOSING

Twice-daily (BID) injections are not recommended for patients with type 1 diabetes. Such a regimen provides neither optimal glycemic control nor sufficient flexibility for adjustments of insulin dose. It is important to note that NPH given before dinner increases the risk of hypoglycemia during the night; thus bedtime NPH insulin is more appropriate both to control fasting blood glucose levels and to reduce the risk of nocturnal hypoglycemia (11).

ADJUSTMENTS TO INSULIN FOR EXERCISE

Exercise is encouraged for patients with type 1 diabetes and should be prescribed on the basis of the patient's functional status and presence of complications. Patients receiving insulin may experience hypoglycemia during, immediately after, or many hours after exercise. This can be avoided by adjusting insulin therapy and nutritional intake to accommodate exercise. It is essential for the patient to collect self-monitored blood glucose data to determine his or her response to exercise. The glycemic level at the start of exercise, previously measured response to exercise, and intensity and duration of planned exercise need to be considered to make appropriate changes in insulin dose or to increase food intake as necessary (64).

Type 2 Diabetes

Insulin is indicated when adequate glycemic control cannot be achieved with diet, exercise, and multiple oral agents in patients with type 2 diabetes (55,65). Insulin can be used in conjunction with oral hypoglycemic agents or alone. Oral hypoglycemic agents include biguanides, sulfonylureas, α-glucosidase inhibitors, thiazolidinediones, and meglitinides. Studies have shown that regimens of insulin plus an oral agent are equivalent to or better than insulin-only regimens in some circumstances (55,66–70). In fact, adding metformin to insulin for

TABLE 39.4. Various Multiple Daily Injection Regimens

Before breakfast	Before lunch	Before dinner	Bedtime
MI	MI	MI	BI
MI + BI	MI	MI	BI
MI + BI	None	MI	BI
MI + BI	MI + BI	MI + BI	None

MI, mealtime insulin (lispro, aspart, regular); BI, basal insulin [Neutral Protamine Hagedorn (NPH), ultralente, glargine].

patients with poorly controlled type 2 diabetes lowers glucose and lipid levels more effectively than increasing the insulin dose alone (67). Different combinations of insulin and oral agents have been used to treat type 2 diabetes. A commonly used regimen is bedtime NPH insulin in combination with metformin with breakfast and dinner. This combination provides improved glycemic control, less hypoglycemia, and less weight gain compared with some other bedtime insulin regimens (55,66). Insulin glargine can be used in place of NPH insulin at bedtime in combination with oral agents (38). In fact, bedtime glargine causes less nocturnal hypoglycemia and provides better postdinner glucose control compared with bedtime NPH (38). Another commonly used combination regimen is BID dosing with intermediate-acting insulin given in the morning and at bedtime in combination with metformin. The thiazolidinediones also have been studied for patients with type 2 diabetes, and agents from this class of drugs are currently being used as monotherapy or in combination therapy (68–72). These drugs often are referred to as insulin sensitizers and act through the peroxisome proliferator-activated receptor-γ (PPARγ), a nuclear receptor that regulates the expression of several genes involved in glucose and lipid metabolism (71,72). They stimulate adipogenesis, reduce plasma triglyceride and free fatty acid concentrations, and improve insulin sensitivity (71,72). In insulin-treated patients with type 2 diabetes, the addition of thiazolidinediones significantly improved glycemic control and allowed for a significant reduction of daily insulin requirements (68–70).

Insulin-only regimens can also be used in type 2 diabetes in a manner similar to that used for type 1 diabetes. It is important to note that insulin deficiency in type 2 diabetes is progressive, and the likelihood that a patient will require insulin continues to increase over time. BID dosing regimens can be used in type 2 diabetes. Frequently, premixed 70/30 insulin (consisting of 70% NPH insulin and 30% regular human insulin) is given in the morning and before dinner. This regimen is suboptimal because NPH insulin given before dinner can lead to hypoglycemia during the night. However, this regimen is simple and may be the best option for patients who have difficulty mixing insulin. Usually two thirds of the total daily insulin is administered in the morning and the remaining one third is given in the evening for BID dosing regimens. The premixed insulin analogues (Humalog Mix 75/25 or Novolog 70/30) can be used in the same fashion, but it is injected immediately before a meal, allowing a little more flexibility (41,42). This premixed insulin provides similar overall glycemic control with improved postprandial glucose control and less nocturnal hypoglycemia compared with BID dosing with 70/30 insulin (41,42). The role of insulin glargine for providing basal replacement with less nocturnal hypoglycemia has been established in type 2 diabetes (38).

COMMON DELIVERY SYSTEMS

Several insulin delivery systems are commonly used, and choices should be made on the basis of personal preferences and needs. Particular attention should be paid to individuals who have impaired vision, problems with manual dexterity, or difficulty mixing various formulations of insulin.

Syringe and Needle

The traditional insulin delivery system is the syringe and needle. This delivery system is flexible, allows dosages to be adjusted readily, and allows some of the insulin formulations to be mixed for fewer injections per day. The limitations to this delivery system are the requirement for good eyesight and fine-motor skills to ensure that appropriate doses of insulin are drawn and administered. The vial, syringe, and needles need to be available whenever insulin administration might be required, and some individuals may find the apparatus cumbersome.

Pen Devices

Pen-cartridge devices are becoming more popular than the syringe-and-needle system. Replaceable insulin cartridges containing 150 to 300 units of regular, aspart, lispro, NPH, or premixed insulin are used in the pen devices. The dose is dialed into the device, and needles with a very fine gauge are used to minimize the discomfort of injection. This method of insulin administration is convenient, unobtrusive, easy to carry, and very useful for MDI regimens. However, insulins cannot be mixed, so two injections are necessary when both rapid-acting and intermediate-acting insulins are required unless premixed insulins are used (73).

Continuous Subcutaneous Insulin Infusion

External insulin infusion pumps first became available in the early 1980s and have evolved rapidly since then. Lispro or regular insulin is stored in a reservoir of the pump and is infused through a catheter into a transcutaneous catheter placed subcutaneously (73). A preprogrammed basal rate of insulin is delivered continuously. The patient can program the pump to provide more than one basal rate over a 24-hour period to best mimic the needs of the individual. There is complete flexibility in the timing of meals because the basal rate maintains glycemic control and boluses of insulin are delivered before the meal. The amount of mealtime insulin given can also be adjusted according to the preprandial blood value. As in all intensive treatment regimens, careful and frequent self-monitoring of blood glucose levels is essential. Adequate support must be provided for the patient with CSII. Although either lispro, aspart, or regular insulin can be used for CSII, there is evidence that lispro and aspart are superior to regular insulin in terms of glycemic control, postprandial blood glucose levels, and risk of hypoglycemia (24–26,31a). Therefore, lispro or aspart is the preferred insulin for CSII.

There are several advantages of the insulin pump over MDI. Patients are spared the burden of administering MDI. Also, the pump provides great flexibility with respect to meal timing and exercise programs. Insulin-pump therapy currently is the most physiologic way of replacing basal insulin, because rates of basal infusion can be changed to match different physiologic requirements.

CSII carries some patient risks and disadvantages that are not encountered with MDI. Since only short-acting insulins are used, any interruption of insulin delivery by pump malfunction, catheter blockage, or displacement of the subcutaneous catheter can result in a rapid deterioration in control and the development of ketoacidosis. However, the newer pumps with safety alarms indicating interrupted flow have dramatically decreased the incidence of this complication (73). Some studies have shown that interruption of CSII using lispro is associated with an earlier and greater metabolic deterioration than that with regular insulin (74,75). However, other studies have not shown a significant difference (76). The correction of any metabolic deterioration appears to be faster with lispro than with regular insulin (74–76). Special attention to self-care is essential to avoid subcutaneous infections. The subcutaneous catheter should be changed every 2 days. Some patients find the external pump cumbersome. Currently, the main barrier to CSII use is the substantial cost of equipment and supplies. CSII used by a well-trained patient can be an effective method of providing more physiologic insulin replacement.

PRACTICAL ASPECTS OF INSULIN USE

Storage

Insulin preparations are stable at room temperature. Insulin in use may be kept at room temperature for 30 days; however, there may be a slight loss in potency if the same vial is used for more than 30 days (77). If patients experience unexplained deterioration of their glycemic control, they should be instructed to inspect their insulin and possibly to change vials in an attempt to improve control. Vials of insulin not in use should be refrigerated. Extreme temperatures and excess agitation should be avoided. The insulin should be visually inspected before each use for changes such as clumping, frosting, precipitation, or a change in clarity or color.

Mixing Insulin

Many insulin regimens require a mixture of different insulin formulations administered at the same time. These insulin formulations either can be administered as two separate subcutaneous injections or can be mixed for a single injection. Commercially available premixed insulins may be appropriate for patients with type 2 diabetes if the insulin ratio matches the patient's insulin requirements. Pen devices do not allow for mixing insulins, so two injections are necessary. However, conventional insulin administration with syringe and needle does allow for mixing. NPH and regular insulin when mixed may be used immediately or stored for future use. Similarly, rapid-acting insulin analogues may be mixed with NPH or ultralente insulin and used without fear of significantly changing the pharmacokinetics of each component (77). Mixing regular insulin with lente or ultralente is not recommended except for patients whose glucose levels are already well controlled with such a mixture (77). The zinc present in the lente insulins can bind with the regular insulin, thereby delaying its onset of action in an unpredictable fashion (77). NPH insulin should not be mixed with lente insulins because zinc phosphate may precipitate. Insulin glargine cannot be mixed with other insulins because it is in solution at an acidic pH and will precipitate if mixed with pH-buffered insulin.

Insulin Injection Technique

The following description applies to the conventional syringe-and-needle administration of insulin. The top of the insulin vial should be cleaned with an alcohol swab. If the insulin is in suspension, the vial should be gently rolled between the hands to ensure that the suspension is uniform before the syringe is loaded. Before the insulin is drawn into the syringe, an amount of air equal to the dose of insulin should be injected into the vial to avoid creating a vacuum. The proper amount of insulin is then drawn into the syringe, and the air bubbles are expelled. If two insulin types are to be mixed, air should be injected into both bottles and the clear rapid- or short-acting insulin should be drawn first.

Insulin should be injected into the subcutaneous tissue. The skin should be gently pinched between the thumb and forefinger and injected at a perpendicular angle. The plunger should be pushed down, the skin released, and the needle then withdrawn. In thin people or children, the needle may need to be inserted at a 45-degree angle to avoid an intramuscular injection. Painful injections may be minimized by injecting the insulin at room temperature, making sure there are no air bubbles in the syringe before injection, keeping muscles in the injection area relaxed, penetrating skin quickly, and not reusing dull needles.

Insulin can be injected into sites with the most subcutaneous fat, which include the abdomen, anterior and lateral thigh, buttocks, and dorsal area of the arm. Within the abdomen, a circle with a 5.08-cm (2 in.) radius around the navel should be avoided. Injection into areas with little subcutaneous fat may result in intramuscular administration, which is painful and may result in faster insulin absorption (78). Insulin is absorbed more rapidly and consistently from the abdomen than from the arms, thighs, or buttocks (79) and from an extremity that is subsequently exercised, probably by increasing blood flow to the skin and perhaps by local muscle contraction (77). Massage of a local area that has been injected can increase the rate of insulin absorption, as can increased local skin temperature. Rotation of injection site is important to prevent lipohypertrophy or lipoatrophy (77). Rotation within one area is recommended as opposed to rotating to different areas within the body (77).

Blood Glucose Monitoring

All insulin-using patients should be encouraged to perform SMBG. With SMBG, patients can evaluate their goals of therapy and adjust their insulin regimens accordingly. A written or electronic record of the daily blood glucose levels is an invaluable tool for the physician and patient for guiding adjustment of the insulin regimen to accommodate fluctuations in insulin requirements. Many of the currently available glucose meters have memory, which simplifies record keeping. The frequency of monitoring depends on the insulin regimen used. The use of MDI of insulin requires multiple daily glucose monitoring, specifically before every meal and at bedtime. Specific situations, such as pregnancy and illness, may make more frequent monitoring necessary.

Implementation

One of the most critical components for successful implementation of any insulin regimen is education and support. This is especially true for implementing MDI or CSII therapy (44,50,51). All patients must be educated about the basics of insulin therapy, including all the previously discussed practical topics and about the complications and how to manage them. In addition, patients receiving MDI or CSII should learn how to self-manage their insulin therapy. They should learn about meal planning and carbohydrate counting, how to identify blood glucose patterns, potential hypoglycemic situations, and the principles of insulin dose adjustments and how to make appropriate adjustments for exercise, sick days, and travel. They should learn how to develop and adjust their own variable insulin dose scales (VIDS). These steps will empower patients and allow them to actively participate with their diabetes care team in their therapy. Education and support on a continuous basis not only improve overall glycemic control they also can decrease hypoglycemia and other adverse events (48,50,51,80).

COMPLICATIONS OF INSULIN THERAPY

Hypoglycemia

Hypoglycemia is the most frequent and feared complication of insulin treatment, with potentially serious sequelae (52,81). Poor timing of meals, exercise, and insulin treatment can lead to hypoglycemia (82). Previous episodes of repeated severe hypoglycemia requiring assistance or hypoglycemic unawareness are risk factors for severe hypoglycemia (80,82). In the DCCT, the frequency of severe hypoglycemia was increased threefold in the intensive-therapy group (82). The risk of severe hypoglycemia was inversely related to HbA_{1c} levels (44,52,82). When severe hypoglycemia occurs, one should investigate the specific circumstances of that episode, potentially raise glycemic targets, and improve education to avoid future episodes (51,53,54,80). Also, a period of meticulous prevention of hypoglycemia may reverse some hypoglycemia unawareness (51). The rates of hypoglycemia in type 2 diabetes are much lower than those in type 1 diabetes (56,57,83). In the UKPDS, the frequency of major hypoglycemic episodes was 1.8% per year in the insulin-treated group (56). In the study by Okhubo et al. (57), no major hypoglycemic episodes occurred with insulin-mediated intensive control over 7 years of follow-up. However, the same general principle applies in type 2 diabetes; namely, the risk of hypoglycemia is inversely related to the HbA_{1c} (84). Most patients experience symptoms when their plasma glucose levels decrease to 60 mg/dL (3.3 mmol/L). As plasma glucose levels decline further, more severe symptoms, specifically neurologic symptoms, appear (85). A complete discussion of hypoglycemia can be found in Chapter 40.

Weight Gain

Weight gain is another potential adverse effect of insulin use. In the DCCT, the incidence of becoming overweight during the median 6.5 years of follow-up was 41.5% in the intensive-therapy groups compared with only 26.9% in the conventional-therapy group ($p < 0.001$) (82). The risk of weight gain with insulin use in type 2 diabetes also has been well documented (56,57,82,86). In the UKPDS, the insulin group gained 4.0 kg (8.89 lb) more than the conventional-therapy group ($p < 0.001$) (56).

Several mechanisms have been proposed to explain the weight gain associated with insulin use. Improved glycemic control decreases glycosuria, thereby decreasing the loss of calories through the urine (87). The direct lipogenic effects of insulin on adipose tissue contribute to weight gain (87). Also, increasing insulin doses may cause recurrent mild hypoglycemia that only manifests itself as hunger. This may result in intake of excess calories. Therefore, diet therapy and weight-loss programs in conjunction with appropriate glycemic targets are extremely important in the management of diabetes.

The result of weight gain in insulin-treated patients is further insulin resistance, leading to the need for more insulin and a potentially greater weight gain. Obesity is associated with decreased responsiveness to insulin in muscle, liver, and fat (88) (discussed in detail in Chapter 31).

Lipoatrophy/Lipohypertrophy

Injection of less-purified insulin into subcutaneous fat can sometimes lead to localized loss of the fat. With the current more-purified insulins, this problem is uncommon. If insulin is injected into the area surrounding the affected sites, the subcutaneous fat will be restored over several months to years.

The opposite of lipoatrophy, lipohypertrophy, may occur at sites of insulin injection. Localized areas of increased swelling of subcutaneous fat can develop with repeated injection. The sensitivity to pain may decrease in these areas, and masses of fibrous tissue may develop. Insulin absorption from sites of lipohypertrophy may be erratic and unreliable. Rotating injection sites can prevent the development of lipohypertrophy. The excess tissue will regress gradually with time.

Atherosclerosis

For a number of years, there has been a concern that insulin promotes and accelerates atherosclerosis. Some studies have shown an association between high insulin levels and macrovascular disease (89–95). Others have shown that hyperinsulinemia is not an independent risk factor for macrovascular disease (96–100). It has been suggested that hyperinsulinemia merely reflects insulin resistance, which is closely associated with other risk factors for macrovascular disease (91,92,96–100). Therefore, insulin probably does not directly promote atherosclerosis. There is clearly no evidence that exogenous insulin use is associated with macrovascular disease, and its appropriate administration should not be discouraged (60). The UKPDS showed no increase in cardiovascular events or death in either the insulin or sulfonylurea group than in the conventionally treated patients, despite higher plasma insulin levels (56). As a consequence, one can safely conclude that exogenous insulin is not a risk factor for atherosclerosis.

Alternative Routes of Insulin Delivery

The benefits of achieving tight glycemic control are well established, and the insulin analogues play an important role in meeting appropriate bolus and basal insulin requirements. However, for this goal to be achieved, MDI of insulin or CSII are required. Despite the widespread use of insulin pen devices that are less painful and use smaller gauge needles, injection-related anxiety remains a common problem (101). Since the 1920s, there have been many attempts to find alternative routes of insulin delivery, including oral, rectal, transdermal, nasal, and pulmonary routes.

Attempts to develop an effective oral insulin began in 1923 (102). To date, these attempts have been largely unsuccessful because of the extensive enzymatic and chemical degradation that occurs in the gastrointestinal tract and the variable transit time of the gastrointestinal tract (103). Researchers have tried enclosing insulin within microspheres and concurrent administration of proteolytic enzyme inhibitors, with minimal success (104). Rectal insulin has been investigated but its variable poor bioavailability and lack of patient acceptance make this route of delivery impractical (105).

Transdermal delivery of insulin is an attractive option given the easy accessibility of skin; however, success has been limited because of the relative impermeability of the skin. Methods used to try to improve the permeability of skin include iontophoresis, low-frequency ultrasound, coupling with transferomes, and the application of photomechanical waves (103,106,107). The initial observations in animals and humans have been encouraging; however, further clinical studies are required.

Intranasal administration of aerosolized insulin seemed like another attractive option. However, the disadvantages are that the surface area of the nasal mucosa is relatively small, at approximately 150 cm^2, and absorption must occur quickly or the drug will be removed to the back of the nasopharynx by the mucociliary clearance mechanisms and swallowed (108). Clinical studies demonstrate poor bioavailability and a rapid but short-lived hypoglycemic effect (108). Large doses are required, despite the addition of enhancers, and patients experience irritation to the nose and nasal congestion (108). For these reasons, intranasal administration does not appear to be a viable route for delivering aerosolized insulin.

Beginning as early as 1925, investigators have tried to develop an effective means of intrapulmonary delivery of insulin (108). The surface area of the alveolar region of the lung is very large (75 to 100 m^2) and is highly permeable (0.1 μm) (103,108). It is well vascularized and has minimal mucociliary clearance. All these features favor the lung as an effective and efficient means of delivering insulin. However, effective delivery of aerosolized insulin to the alveolar region of the lung requires appropriate aerosol particle size, aerosol velocity, and inspiratory flow rate (103). Current delivery systems include dry-powder inhalation systems and aqueous insulin aerosol devices.

The dry-powder insulin inhalation system uses a holding chamber to capture the insulin cloud and allow for slow deep inhalations. Comparison with subcutaneous regular human insulin demonstrated faster onset of action and time to peak effect. The duration of action was between that of lispro and regular insulin (109,110). An open-label, proof-of-concept study in 73 patients with type 1 diabetes, comparing preprandial inhaled insulin plus bedtime subcutaneous ultralente insulin and usual MDI of subcutaneous insulin, demonstrated no difference in HbA_{1c}, fasting or postprandial blood glucose levels, and frequency or severity of hypoglycemia after 3 months (111). An open-label, noncontrolled study of 26 patients with type 2 diabetes using preprandial inhaled insulin plus bedtime ultralente insulin demonstrated decreased HbA_{1c} after 3 months (112). Inhaled insulin was well tolerated in both studies, and there was no change in pulmonary function.

The aqueous insulin aerosol device is breath-activated and releases insulin when inspiratory flow rate and volume are optimal. A clear dose–response curve and a rapid onset of action as compared with that of subcutaneous regular human insulin have also been demonstrated (113,114). Both insulin formulations have relatively poor bioavailability as compared with that of subcutaneous insulin. Enhancers have been incorporated to try to improve bioavailability, and early results have been promising (115).

Improved aerosol and delivery technology, ease of use, and patient satisfaction make intrapulmonary insulin the most promising alternative route of insulin delivery at this time. Adequate patient education to ensure proper technique is critical to the success of inhaled insulin. It is important to note that clinical studies to date have been performed in patients with normal pulmonary function tests. Data are unavailable for patients with abnormal pulmonary function. In addition, smokers are known to have more rapid absorption of intrapulmonary substances, and this may affect its clinical use in this population (108). There is also concern about the potential of high concentrations of insulin in the lungs to cause pulmonary vascular disease or other effects (116). No major adverse effects have been demonstrated to date, but long-term safety and efficacy studies are required before inhaled insulin delivery systems can be routinely incorporated into clinical practice.

CONCLUSIONS

The discovery of insulin by Banting, Best, Collip, and MacLeod in 1921 represents one of the greatest medical discoveries of modern medicine. Insulin and insulin analogues remain a fundamental component of diabetes management. Insulins are now available in a wide range of time–action profiles, and a number of different delivery systems are available. MDI or CSII is considered the standard of care for type 1 diabetes. For type 2 diabetes, a number of different insulins plus an oral agent or insulin-only options may be used. Regardless of the regimen chosen, proper education and support are critical and the goal should always be to achieve the best glycemic control with the fewest adverse events. When used properly, insulin therapy effectively reduces morbidity and mortality in patents with diabetes. The challenge for the future is to continue to improve insulin replacement and to achieve the elusive goal of physiologic replacement of insulin.

REFERENCES

1. Banting FM, Best CH. The internal secretion of the pancreas. *J Lab Clin Med* 1922;7:256–271.
2. Bliss M. *The discovery of insulin.* Chicago: McClelland & Stewart, 1996.
3. Best CH. The first clinical use of insulin. *Diabetes* 1956;5:65–67.
4. Hagedorn HC, Jensen BN, Krarup NB, et al. Protamine insulinate. *JAMA* 1936;106:177–180.
5. Scott D, Fisher A. Studies on insulin with protamine. *J Pharmacol Exp Ther* 1936;58:78–92.
6. Krayenbuhl C, Rosenberg T. Crystalline protamine insulin. *Rep Steno Mem Hosp* 1946;1:60–73.
7. Riggs AD. Bacterial production of human insulin. *Diabetes Care*, 1984;4:64–68.
8. Howey DC, Bowsher RR, Brunelle R, et al. [Lys (B28), Pro (B29)]—human insulin: a rapidly absorbed analogue of human insulin. *Diabetes* 1994;43: 396–402.
9. Zinman, B. The physiological replacement of insulin—an elusive goal. *N Engl J Med* 1989;321:363–370.
10. Lee WL, Zinman B. From insulin to insulin analogs: progress in the treatment of type 1 diabetes. *Diabetes Rev* 1998;6:73–88.
11. Burge MR, Schade DS. Insulins. *Endocrinol Metab Clin North Am* 1997;26: 575–598.
12. Heinemann L, Richter B. Clinical pharmacology of human insulin. *Diabetes Care* 1993;16[Suppl S3]:90–101.
13. Brunelle RL, Llewelyn J, Anderson JH, et al. Meta-analysis of the effect of insulin lispro on severe hypoglycemia in patients with type 1 diabetes. *Diabetes Care* 1998;21:1726–1731.
14. Anderson JH Jr, Brunelle RL, Koivisto VA, et al. Reduction of postprandial hyperglycemia and frequency of hypoglycemia in IDDM patients on insulin analog treatment: Multicenter Insulin Lispro Study Group. *Diabetes* 1997;46; 265–270.
15. Anderson JH Jr, Brunelle RL, Keohane P, et al. Mealtime treatment with insulin analogue improves postprandial hyperglycemia and hypoglycemia in NIDDM patients. *Arch Intern Med* 1997;157:1249–1255.
16. Pfutzner A, Kustner E, Forst T, et al. Intensive insulin therapy with insulin lispro in patients with type 1 diabetes reduces the frequency of hypoglycemic episodes. *Exp Clin Endocrinol* 1996;104:25–30.
17. Holleman F, Schmitt H, Rottiers R, et al. Reduced frequency of severe hypoglycemia and coma in well-controlled IDDM patients treated with insulin lispro. *Diabetes Care* 1997;20:1827–1832.
18. Meltzer S, Leiter L, Daneman D, et al. 1998 clinical practice guidelines for the management of diabetes in Canada. *Can Med Assoc J* 1998;159[Suppl 8]: S1–S29.
19. Ciofetta M, Lalli C, Del Sindaco P, et al. Contribution of postprandial versus interprandial blood glucose to Hb A1c in type 1 diabetes on physiologic intensive therapy with lispro insulin at mealtime. *Diabetes Care* 1999;22: 795–800.
20. Colombel A, Murat A, Krempf M, et al. Improvement of blood glucose control in type 1 diabetic patients treated with lispro and multiple NPH injections. *Diabet Med* 1999;16:319–324.
21. Mohn A, Matyka KA, Harris DA, et al. Lispro or regular insulin for multiple injection therapy in adolescence—differences in free insulin and glucose levels overnight. *Diabetes Care* 1999;22:27–32.
22. Ebeling P, Jansson P, Smith U, et al. Strategies toward improved control during insulin lispro therapy IDDM. *Diabetes Care* 1997;20:1287–1289.
23. Lalli C, Ciofetta M, Del Sindaco P, et al. Long-term intensive treatment of type 1 diabetes with the short-acting insulin analog lispro in variable combination with NPH insulin at mealtime. *Diabetes Care* 1999;22:468–477.
24. Zinman B, Tildesley H, Chiasson JL, et al. Insulin lispro in CSII: results of a double-blind crossover study. *Diabetes* 1996;104:25–30.
25. Melki V, Renard E, Lassmann-Vague V, et al. Improvement of HbA_{1c} and blood glucose stability in IDDM patients treated with lispro insulin analog in external pumps. *Diabetes Care* 1998;21:977–981.
26. Renner R, Pfutzner A, Trautmann M, et al. Use of insulin lispro in continuous subcutaneous insulin infusion treatment. *Diabetes Care* 1999;22: 784–788.
27. Mudaliar SR, Lindberg FA, Joyce M, et al. Insulin aspart: a fast acting analog of human insulin—absorption kinetics and action profile compared with reg-

ular human insulin in healthy non-diabetic subjects. *Diabetes Care* 1999;22: 1501–1506.
28. Home PD, Lindhom A, Riis AP, et al. Improved long-term blood glucose control with insulin aspart versus human insulin in people with type 1 diabetes. *Diabetes* 1999;48 [Suppl 1]:A358(abst).
29. Uwe B, Ebrahim S, Hirshberger S, et al. Effect of the rapid acting insulin analogue insulin aspart on quality of life and treatment satisfaction in type 1 diabetic patients. *Diabetes* 1999;48[Suppl 1]:A112(abst).
30. Raskin P, Guthrie RA, Leiter L, et al. Use of insulin aspart, a fast-acting insulin analog, as the mealtime insulin in the management of patients with type 1 diabetes. *Diabetes Care* 2000;23:583–588.
31. Raskin P, McGill J, Kilo C, et al. Human insulin analog (insulin aspart) is comparable to human insulin in type 2 diabetes. *Diabetes* 1999;48[Suppl 1]: A355(abst).
31a. Bode BW, Strange P. Efficacy, safety, and pump compatibility of insulin aspart used in continuous subcutaneous insulin infusion therapy in patients with type 1 diabetes. *Diabetes Care* 2001;24:69–72.
32. Zinman B, Ross S, Campos RV, et al. Effectiveness of human ultralente versus NPH insulin in providing basal insulin replacement for an insulin lispro multiple daily injection regimen: a double-blind randomized prospective trial. *Diabetes Care* 1999;22:603–608.
33. Rosskamp RH, Park G. Long-acting insulin analogs. *Diabetes Care* 1999; 22[Suppl 2]:B109–B113.
34. Luzio SD, Owens D, Evans M, et al. Comparison of the sc absorption of HOE 901 and NPH human insulin type 2 diabetic subjects. *Diabetes* 1999;48[Suppl 1]:A111(abst).
35. Heinemann L, Linkeschova R, Rave K, et al. Time-action profile of the long-acting insulin analog insulin glargine (HOE901) in comparison with those of NPH insulin and placebo. *Diabetes Care* 2000;23:644–649.
36. Ratner RE, Hirsch IB, Neifing JL, et al. Less hypoglycemia with insulin glargine in intensive insulin therapy for type 1 diabetes. *Diabetes Care* 2000; 23:639–643.
37. Rosenstock J, Park G, Zimmerman J, et al. Basal insulin glargine (HOE 901) versus NPH insulin in patients with type 1 diabetes on multiple daily insulin regimens. *Diabetes Care* 2000;23:1137–1142.
38. Yki-Jarvinen H, Dressler A, Ziemen M, et al. Less nocturnal hypoglycemia and better post-dinner glucose control with bedtime insulin glargine compared with bedtime NPH insulin during insulin combination therapy in type 2 diabetes. *Diabetes Care* 2000;23:1130–1136.
39. Bolli GB, Owens DR. Insulin glargine. *Lancet* 2000;356:443–445.
39a. Markussen J, Havelund S, Kurtzhals P, et al. Soluble, fatty acid acylated insulins bind to albumin and show protracted action in pigs. *Diabetologia* 1996;39:281-288.
39b. Heinemann L, Sinha K, Weyer C, et al. Time-action profile of the soluble, fatty acid acylated, long-acting insulin analogue NN304. *Diabet Med* 1999;16:332–338.
39c. Barnett AH. A review of basal insulins. *Diabet Med* 2003;20:873–885.
39d. Home P, Bartley P, Russell-Jones D, et al. Insulin detemir offers improved glycemic control compared with NPH insulin in people with type 1 diabetes: a randomized clinical trial. *Diabetes Care* 2004;27(5):1081–1087.
39e. Vague P, Selam JL, Skeie S, et al. Insulin detemir is associated with more predictable glycemic control and reduced risk of hypoglycemia than NPH insulin in patients with type 1 diabetes on a basal-bolus regimen with premeal insulin aspart. *Diabetes Care* 2003;26:590–596.
40. Heise T, Weyer C, Serwas A, et al. Time-action profiles of novel premixed preparations of insulin lispro and NPL insulin. *Diabetes Care* 1998;21: 800–803.
41. Kovisto VA, Tuominen JA, Ebeling P. Lispro mix25 insulin as premeal therapy in type 2 diabetic patients. *Diabetes Care* 1999;22:459–462.
42. Roach P, Yue L, Arora V. Improved postprandial glycemic control during treatment with Humalog Mix25, a novel protamine-based insulin lispro formulation. *Diabetes Care* 1999;22:1258–1261.
42a. Kapitza C, Rave K, Ostrowski K, et al. Reduced postprandial glycaemic excursion with biphasic insulin Aspart 30 injected immediately before a meal. *Diabet Med* 2004;21:500–501.
42b. Christiansen JS, Vaz JA, Metelko Z, et al. Twice daily biphasic insulin aspart improves postprandial glycaemic control more effectively than twice daily NPH insulin, with low risk of hypoglycaemia, in patients with type 2 diabetes. *Diabetes Obes Metab* 2003;5:446–454.
43. Coscelli C, Clabrese G, Fedele D, et al. Use of premixed insulin among the elderly. *Diabetes Care* 1992;15:1628–1630.
44. The Diabetes Control and Complication Trial Research Group. The effect of intensive treatment of diabetes on the development and progression of long-term complication in insulin-dependent diabetes mellitus. *N Engl J Med* 1993;329:977–986.
45. Reichard P, Britz A, Carlsson P, et al. Metabolic control and complications over 3 years in patients with insulin dependent diabetes (IDDM): the Stockholm Diabetes Intervention Study (SDIS). *J Intern Med* 1990;228:511–517.
46. The Diabetes Control and Complications Trial Research Group. The effect of intensive diabetes therapy on the development and progression of neuropathy. *Ann Intern Med* 1995;122:561–568.
47. The Diabetes Control and Complications Trial/Epidemiology of Diabetes Intervention and Complications Research Group. Retinopathy and nephropathy in patients with type 1 diabetes four years after a trial of intensive therapy. *N Engl J Med* 2000;342:381–389.
48. Lawson ML, Gerstein HC, Tsui E, Zinman B. Effect of intensive therapy on early macrovascular disease in young individuals with type 1 diabetes. *Diabetes Care* 1999;22[Suppl 2]:B35–B39.
49. The Diabetes Control and Complications Trial Research Group. Effect of intensive diabetes management on macrovascular events and risk factor in the Diabetes Control and Complications Trial. *Am J Cardiol* 1995;75:894–903.
50. American Diabetes Association. Implications of the diabetes control and complications trial: clinical practice recommendations 2001. *Diabetes Care* 2001;24[Suppl 1]:S25–S27.
51. Bolli GB. How to ameliorate the problem of hypoglycemia in intensive as well as nonintensive treatment of type 1 diabetes. *Diabetes Care* 1999;22[Suppl 2]:B43–B52.
52. The Diabetes Control and Complications Trial Research Group. Hypoglycemia in the diabetes control and complications trial. *Diabetes* 1997;46: 271–286.
53. Pampanelli S, Fanelli C, Lalli C, et al. Long-term intensive insulin therapy in IDDM: effects on HbA_{1c}, risk for severe and mild hypoglycemia, status of counterregulation and awareness of hypoglycemia. *Diabetologia* 1996;39: 677–686.
54. Schiel R, Muller UA, Ulbrich S. Long-term efficacy of a 5-day structured teaching and treatment programme for intensified conventional insulin therapy and risk for severe hypoglycemia. *Diabetes Res Clin Pract* 1997;35:41–48.
55. Yki-Jarvinen H, Kauppila M, Kujansuu E, et al. Comparison of insulin regimens in patients with non-insulin-dependent diabetes mellitus. *N Engl J Med* 1992;327:1426–1433.
56. UK Prospective Diabetes Study (UKPDS) Group. Intensive blood-glucose control with sulphonylureas of insulin compared with conventional treatment and risk of complications in patients with type 2 diabetes (UKPDS 33). *Lancet* 1998;352:837–853.
57. Okhubo Y, Kishikawa H, Araki E, et al. Intensive insulin therapy prevents the progression of diabetic microvascular complications in Japanese patients with non-insulin-dependent diabetes mellitus: a randomized prospective 6-year study. *Diabetes Res Clin Pract* 1995;28:103–117.
58. Stratton IM, Adler AI, Neil HAW, et al. Association of glycaemia with macrovascular and microvascular complications of type 2 diabetes (UKPDS 35): prospective observational study. *BMJ* 2000;321:405–412.
59. Adler AI, Stratton IM, Neil HAW, et al. Association of systolic blood pressure with macrovascular and microvascular complications of type 2 diabetes (UKPDS 36): prospective observational study. *BMJ* 2000;321:412–419.
60. American Diabetes Association. Implications of the United Kingdom Prospective Diabetes Study: Clinical practice recommendations 2001. *Diabetes Care* 2001;24[Suppl 1]: S28–S32.
60a. Gæde P, Pernille V, Larsen N, et al. Multifactorial intervention and cardiovascular disease in patients with type 2 diabetes. *N Engl J Med* 2003;348: 383–393.
61. Malmberg K, Ryden L, Hamsten A, et al. Effects of insulin treatment on cause-specific one-year mortality and morbidity in diabetic patients with acute myocardial infarction—DIGAMI Study Group (Diabetes Insulin-Glucose in Acute Myocardial Infarction). *Eur Heart J* 1996;17:1298–1301.
62. Malmberg K. Prospective randomised study of intensive insulin treatment on long term survival after acute myocardial infarction in patients with diabetes mellitus (DIGAMI). *BMJ* 1997;314:1512–1515.
63. American Diabetes Association. Standards of medical care for patients with diabetes mellitus. *Diabetes Care* 2004;27[Suppl 1]:S15–S35.
64. American Diabetes Association. Physical activity/exercise and diabetes. *Diabetes Care* 2004;27[Suppl 1]:S58–S62.
65. Wolfenbuttel BH, Sels JJ, Rondas-Colbers GJ, et al. Comparison of different insulin regimens in elderly patients with NIDDM. *Diabetes Care* 1996;19: 1326–1332.
66. Yki-Jarvinen H, Ryysy L, Nikkila K, et al. Comparison of bedtime insulin regimens in patients with type 2 diabetes mellitus. *Ann Intern Med* 1999;130: 389–396.
67. Relimpio F, Pumar A, Losada F, et al. Adding metformin versus insulin dose increase in insulin-treated but poorly controlled type 2 diabetes mellitus: an open-label randomized trial. *Diabet Med* 1998;15:997–1002.
68. Buse JB, Bumbiner B, Mathias NP, et al. Troglitazone use in insulin-treated type 2 diabetic patients. *Diabetes Care* 1998;21:1455–1461.
69. Schwartz S, Raskin P, Fonsec V, et al. Effect of troglitazone in insulin-treated patients with type II diabetes mellitus. *N Engl J Med* 1998;338:861–866.
70. Fonseca V, Graveline J, Nissel J. Long term experience with troglitazone in combination with insulin in type 2 diabetes mellitus. *Diabetes* 1998;47[Suppl 1]:A90(abst).
71. Scheen AJ, Lefebvre PJ. Troglitazone: antihyperglycemic activity and potential role in the treatment of type 2 diabetes. *Diabetes Care* 1999;22:1568–1577.
72. Schoonjans K, Auwerx J. Thiazolidinediones: an update. *Lancet* 2000;355: 1008–1010.
73. Saudek CD. Novel forms of insulin delivery. *Endocrinol Metab Clin North Am* 1997;26:599–610.
74. Guerci B, Meyer L, Salle A, et al. Comparison of metabolic deterioration between insulin analog and regular insulin after a 5-hour interruption of a continuous subcutaneous insulin infusion in type 1 diabetic patients. *J Clin Endocrinol Metab* 1999;84:2673–2678.
75. Reichel A, Rietzsch H, Kohler HJ, et al. Cessation of insulin infusion at night-time during CSII-therapy: comparison of regular human insulin and insulin lispro. *Exp Clin Endocrinol Diabetes* 1998;106:168–172.
76. Attia N, Jones TW, Holcombe J, et al. Comparison of human regular and lispro insulins after interruption of continuous subcutaneous insulin infusion and in the treatment of acutely decompensated IDDM. *Diabetes Care* 1998; 21:817–821.
77. American Diabetes Association. Insulin administration: clinical practice recommendations 2000. *Diabetes Care* 2001;24[Suppl 1]:S94–S97.

78. Vaag A, Handberg A, Lauritzen M, et al. Variation in absorption of NPH insulin due to intramuscular injection. *Diabetes Care* 1990;13:74–76.
79. Skyler JS. Insulin pharmacology. *Med Clin North Am* 1988;72:1337–1354.
80. Bott S, Bott U, Berger M, et al. Intensified insulin therapy and risk of severe hypoglycaemia. *Diabetologia* 1997;40:326–932.
81. McCrimmon RJ, Frier BM. Hypoglycemia, the most feared complication of insulin therapy. *Diabet Metab* 1994;20:503–512.
82. The Diabetes Control and Complications Research Group. Adverse events and their association with treatment regimens in the Diabetes Control and Complications Trial. *Diabetes Care* 1995;18:1415–1427.
83. Gerstein HC, Capes S. Advantages and perceived disadvantages of insulin therapy for patients with type 2 diabetes. *Can J Diab Care* 1999;23[Suppl 2]: 91–94.
84. Gaster B, Hirsch IB. The effects of improved glycemic control on complications in type 2 diabetes. *Arch Intern Med* 1998;158:134–140.
85. Gerich JE, Campbell PJ. Overview of counterregulation and its abnormalities in diabetes mellitus and other conditions. *Diabetes Metab Rev* 1988;4:93–111.
86. Trischitta V, Italia S, Mazzarino S. Comparison of combined therapies in treatment of secondary failure to glyburide. *Diabetes Care* 1992;15:539–543.
87. Torbay N, Bracco E, Geliebter A, et al. Insulin increases body fat despite control of food intake and physical activity. *Am J Physiol* 1985;258:R2120–R2144.
88. Field JB. Chronic insulin resistance. *Acta Diabetol Lat* 1970;7:220–242.
89. Welborn TA, Wearne K. Coronary heart disease incidence and cardiovascular mortality in Busselton with reference to glucose and insulin concentrations. *Diabetes Care* 1979;2:154–160.
90. Pyorala K, Savolainen E, Kaukola S, et al. Plasma insulin as a coronary heart disease risk factors: relationship to other risk factors and predictive value over 9.5 year follow up of the Helsinki Policemen Study population. *Acta Med Scand* 1985;701:7–14.
91. Fontbonne A, Charles MA, Thibult N, et al. Hyperinsulinaemia as a predictor of coronary heart disease mortality in a healthy population: the Paris Prospective Study, 15-year follow-up. *Diabetologia* 1991;34:356–361.
92. Fontbonne AM, Eschwege EM. Insulin and cardiovascular disease: Paris prospective study. *Diabetes Care* 1991;14:431–469.
93. Nishimoto Y, Miyazaki Y, Toki Y, et al. Enhanced secretion of insulin plays a role in the development of atherosclerosis and restenosis of coronary arteries: elective percutaneous transluminal coronary angioplasty in patients with effort angina. *J Am Coll Cardiol* 1998;32:1642–1649.
94. Fujiwara R, Kursumi Y, Hayashi T, et al. Relation of angiographically defined coronary artery disease and plasma concentrations of insulin, lipid, and apolipoprotein in normolipidemic subjects with varying degrees of glucose tolerance. *Am J Cardiol* 1995;75:122–126.
95. Kuusisto J, Mykkanen L, Pyorala K, et al. Hyperinsulinemic microalbuminuria: a new risk indicator for coronary heart disease. *Circulation* 1995;91: 831–837.
96. Yudkin JS, Denver AE, Mohamed-Ali V, et al. The relationship of concentrations of insulin and proinsulin-like molecules with coronary heart disease prevalence and incidence. *Diabetes Care* 1997;20:1093–1100.
97. Folsom AR, Szklo M, Stevens J, et al. A prospective study of coronary heart disease in relation to fasting insulin, glucose, and diabetes. *Diabetes Care* 1997; 20:935–942.
98. Mykkanen L, Laakso M, Pyorala K. High plasma insulin level associated with coronary heart disease in the elderly. *Am J Epidemiol* 1993;137:1190–1202.
99. Katz RJ, Ratner RE, Cohen RM, et al. Are insulin and proinsulin independent risk markers for premature coronary artery disease? *Diabetes* 1996;45: 736–741.
100. Hauhan A, Foote J, Petch MC, et al. Hyperinsulinemia, coronary artery disease and syndrome X. *J Am Coll Cardiol* 1994;23:364–368.
101. Zambanini A, Newson RB, Maisey M, et al. Injection related anxiety in insulin-treated diabetes. *Diabetes Res Clin Pract* 1999;46:239–246.
102. Winter LB. On the absorption of insulin from the stomach. *J Physiol* 1923;58: 18–21.
103. Cefalu WT. Novel routes of insulin delivery for patients with type 1 or type 2 diabetes. *Ann Med* 2001;33:579–586.
104. Modi P, Mihic M. Replacement of sc injections with Oralin in treatment of diabetes. *Diabetes Care* 2001;50:179.
105. Yamasaki Y, Shichiri M, Kawamori R, et al. The effectiveness of rectal administration of insulin suppository on normal and diabetic subjects. *Diabetes Care* 1981;4:454–458.
106. Lee S, McAuliffe DJ, Mulholland SE, et al. Photomechanical transdermal delivery of insulin in vivo. *Lasers Surg Med* 2001;28:282–285.
107. Kanikkannan N, Singh J, Ramarao P. Transdermal iontophoretic delivery of bovine insulin and monomeric human insulin analogue. *J Control Release* 1999;59:99–105.
108. Laube BL. Treating diabetes with aerosolized insulin. *Chest* 2001;120: 99S–106S.
109. Heinemann L, Traut T, Heise T. Time-action profile of inhaled insulin. *Diabet Med* 1997;14:63–72.
110. Laube BL, Benedict GW, Dobs AS. Time to peak insulin level, relative bioavailability, and effect of site of deposition of nebulized insulin in patients with noninsulin-dependent diabetes mellitus. *J Aerosol Med* 1998;11:153–173.
111. Skyler JS, Cefalu WT, Kourides IA, et al. Efficacy of inhaled human insulin in type 1 diabetes mellitus: a randomized proof-of-concept study. *Lancet* 2001; 357:331–533.
112. Cefalu WT, Skyler JS, Kourides IA, et al. Inhaled human insulin treatment in patients with type 2 diabetes mellitus. *Ann Intern Med* 2001;134:795.
113. Brunner GA, Balent B, Ellmerer M, et al. Dose-response relation of liquid aerosol inhaled insulin in type 1 diabetic patients. *Diabetologia* 2001;44: 305–308.
114. Farr SJ, McElduff A, Mather LE, et al. Pulmonary insulin administration using the AERx system: physiological and physicochemical factors influencing insulin effectiveness in healthy fasting subjects. *Diabetes Technol Ther* 2000;2:185–197.
115. Steiner S, Pfutzner A, Wilson BR, et al. Technosphere/Insulin—proof of concept study with a new insulin formulation for pulmonary delivery. *Exp Clin Endocrinol Diabetes* 2002;110:17–21.
116. Chan NN, Baldewag S, Tan TMN, et al. Inhaled insulin in type 2 diabetes [Letter]. *Lancet* 2001;357:1979.

CHAPTER 40

Iatrogenic Hypoglycemia

Stephanie Anne Amiel

No definition of good glycemic control in diabetes is complete unless it includes a statement about absence of hypoglycemia. Patients with diabetes and their families are well aware of this, and healthcare professionals responsible for patients with diabetes need to be equally well informed.

Hypoglycemia—literally, a low blood glucose concentration—is rarely encountered in healthy individuals. Glucose is normally the major metabolic fuel for the brain. Because the brain stores only trivial amounts of glucose as glycogen, the brain is dependent for normal function on an adequate supply of glucose from its circulation. Both the entry of glucose into the circulation and its removal therefrom vary widely with fasting and feeding and with rest and exertion. Elaborate and sensitive mechanisms exist to maintain glucose concentrations in the plasma within narrow limits—too high a concentration upsets the water balance in tissues, causes glycosuria, and accelerates tissue glycosylation, whereas too low a concentration results in cerebral dysfunction and ultimately coma and death. In health, hypoglycemia sufficient to cause clinically significant cognitive dysfunction does not occur because of the efficiency of the endogenous mechanisms of glucose homeostasis. Once these mechanisms are upset by diabetes *and its treatment*, clinically problematic hypoglycemia can occur.

Hypoglycemia can be defined in biochemical terms as a plasma glucose concentration below the normal range. It should be noted that glucose concentrations in plasma are approximately 10% higher than those in whole blood because red cells contain relatively low concentrations of glucose; arterial glucose levels are higher than venous levels, and capillary levels are between the arterial and venous levels. Research studies of hypoglycemia in human subjects often use arterialized venous glucose concentrations because they approximate those of the arterial system (and therefore the glucose supply to a tissue) and make arterial sampling unnecessary (1).

Fasting plasma glucose concentrations are considered normal if they are less than 6 mmol/L, although levels higher than 5.5 mmol/L are rarely seen in healthy individuals (2). The lower limit of normality is more equivocal. Healthy people rarely have a plasma glucose concentration lower than 4 mmol/L after an overnight fast, but levels of 2.8 mmol/L have been recorded in healthy people after prolonged fasting (3). Spontaneous, pathologic hypoglycemia, such as may occur in the presence of

TABLE 40.1. A Modification of Whipple's Triad for Diagnosis of Hypoglycemia in Diabetes Therapy

Presence of symptoms and/or signs compatible with a low plasma glucose concentration
Demonstrably low plasma glucose concentration (<3.5 mmol/L)
Rapid resolution with restoration of plasma glucose concentration

insulin- or insulin-like growth factor (IGF)–secreting tumors, requires for diagnosis the demonstration of plasma glucose levels of less than 2.8 mmol/L or even, according to some authorities, levels less than 2.2 mmol/L in women (4). However, detailed physiologic studies show a detectable impairment of higher cerebral function at plasma glucose levels of 3 mmol/L (arterialized venous plasma) (5), and there is evidence that recurrent plasma glucose levels of 3 mmol/L damage the endogenous protective mechanisms against more severe hypoglycemia (6). Nonpancreatic counterregulatory responses to hypoglycemia start at 3.5 to 3.6 mmol/L (see below). Thus, *in the context of the treatment of diabetes mellitus,* hypoglycemia is defined as a plasma glucose concentration of 3.5 mmol/L or less.

In diabetes, hypoglycemia is also often defined by its clinical presentation. Acute hypoglycemia is symptomatic, and Whipple's triad, although defined by a surgeon interested in insulinomas, remains a useful guide for defining episodes. The triad requires (a) symptoms attributable to a low plasma glucose concentration, (b) a measurably low plasma glucose concentration (less than 3.5 mmol/L in diabetes), and (c) rapid resolution of the symptoms after correction of the biochemical abnormality (7). However, as will be described later, patients with diabetes (and indeed those with insulinomas) can lose their ability to generate and detect the symptoms of early hypoglycemia (see Hypoglycemia Unawareness), and Whipple's original triad is best modified by the inclusion of the term "and signs" in the first criterion (Table 40.1).

Perhaps the most important clinical definition of acute hypoglycemia in diabetes therapy is the division into mild and severe. Many authorities also recognize an intermediate category of moderate. Mild hypoglycemia is defined as that which is recognized and treated by the patient, and severe hypoglycemia is defined as that which the patient is unable to self-treat because of cognitive impairment. Some authorities restrict the term "severe hypoglycemia" to episodes requiring parenteral therapy (intramuscular glucagon or intravenous glucose) and/or those resulting in coma or seizure. The classification "moderate hypoglycemia" usually refers to episodes that the patient could self-treat but resulted in significant life disruption. The lack of clarity in this definition has led to its disuse. The terms "mild" and "severe" hypoglycemia are not appropriately applied to degrees of *biochemical* hypoglycemia (Table 40.2).

TABLE 40.2. Clinical Classification of Acute Hypoglycemia

Mild	Symptomatic, self-treated, no major lifestyle disruption
Moderate	Symptomatic, self-treated, but with significant lifestyle disruption
Severe	Often (but not always) asymptomatic, but patient unable to self-treat because of cognitive impairment 1. Third-party help but not parenteral therapy 2. Parenteral therapy required (intramuscular glucagon or intravenous glucose) 3. Associated with coma or seizure

Commonly, the qualification concerning lifestyle disruption is omitted, leaving only "mild" and "severe" categories.

FREQUENCY OF HYPOGLYCEMIA

Formal studies of the frequency of hypoglycemic events must be compared carefully because of differences in definitions. This difficulty not withstanding, it is important to document the frequencies of hypoglycemic episodes in order to compare the effects of different therapeutic regimens and to determine clinical characteristics that put patients at risk.

Mild hypoglycemia, although often unpleasant, tends to be accepted as an inevitable consequence of glucose-lowering therapies. However, mild hypoglycemia should not be ignored, as it has the potential to increase the risk of severe episodes. In the Diabetes Control and Complications Trial (DCCT), which was conducted in patients with type 1 diabetes, the rate of severe hypoglycemia increased from approximately 20 episodes per 100 patient-years during conventional therapy to 60 per patient-year during intensified therapy (8). In contrast, the Dusseldorf group, using internally consistent definitions but different from those used in the DCCT, reported a decline in rates of severe hypoglycemia with intensified therapy from rates of 28 to 17 episodes per 100 patient-years (9).

COUNTERREGULATION: THE DAMAGED DEFENSES AGAINST SEVERE HYPOGLYCEMIA IN DIABETES

As the plasma glucose concentration begins to decrease, an orchestrated neurohumoral response acts to prevent hypoglycemia. The first component of this counterregulation is local to the pancreatic islets, with cessation of insulin secretion and stimulation of glucagon release by the pancreas. These responses promote hepatic production of glucose, which, in health, represents the most important mechanism for preventing hypoglycemia between meals. In people with diabetes, the insulin levels do not decrease as glucose levels fall, either because of persistent absorption of exogenous insulin or because of non–glucose-dependent elevation of insulin secretion by sulfonylureas. The lack of decline in plasma insulin concentration as glucose levels decrease then results in iatrogenic hypoglycemia.

In addition to their inability to modulate insulin levels as the plasma level of glucose decreases, patients with type 1 diabetes lose the ability to enhance glucagon production by pancreatic α-cells in response to hypoglycemia. Basal glucagon production and glucagon responses to other secretagogues are maintained, but the response to hypoglycemia is abrogated. This happens within 5 years of the onset of type 1 diabetes (10) and may be secondary to decreased β-cell activity. Glucagon responses are also lost late in the evolution of type 2 diabetes, and the glucagon response to hypoglycemia is reduced under experimental conditions in which β-cell activity is maintained by sulfonylureas (11,12).

In experimental studies, counterregulation (the spontaneous correction of a decreasing plasma glucose level) occurs even if the insulin and glucagon responses are inhibited (13), a consequence of secondary defense mechanisms involving the autonomic nervous system and adrenal medulla. Released epinephrine and norepinephrine stimulate endogenous glucose production and also inhibit glucose consumption by peripheral tissues. These actions occur through elevation of substrates for gluconeogenesis, including nonesterified fatty acids, which also inhibit peripheral glucose oxidation (14). Glucose is generated initially by hepatic glycogenolysis and subsequently by hepatic (and renal) gluconeogenesis (15,16). The activation of the sympathetic nervous system can be demonstrated not only by determining adrenal catecholamine secretion as blood glucose concentrations fall but also by determining sympathetic activity in muscle (17), recording perspiration (18), or measuring norepinephrine assumed to have "spilled over" from sympathetic nerve terminals.

A significant and probably growing number of patients with type 1 diabetes develop defects in the adrenal and autonomic responses to hypoglycemia. These occur independently of classical autonomic neuropathy, to which they are not mechanistically related (19) and represent an important risk factor for susceptibility to severe hypoglycemia. The defects are associated with a failure to generate the typical symptoms of autonomic activation. Affected patients, described as having *hypoglycemia unawareness,* are at greatly increased risk for severe hypoglycemia (20,21).

Growth hormone and cortisol are additional hormones with important roles in glucose homeostasis, and their absence can be associated with clinical hypoglycemia. Their roles in the response to acute hypoglycemia are less clear, and they certainly cannot compensate for defects in epinephrine secretion and autonomic responsiveness.

SYMPTOMS OF ACUTE HYPOGLYCEMIA

Early experts in diabetes, America's Elliot P. Joslin and Britain's R. D. Lawrence (22,23), divided the symptoms of acute hypoglycemia on physiologic principles into autonomic (attributable to activation of the autonomic nervous system and adrenal medulla) and neuroglycopenic categories (related to impaired glucose supply to the cerebral cortex). More recently, complex statistical packages have been used to group the symptoms reported by patients (or symptoms and signs reported by parents of children with diabetes) into related "families," with very similar results (Tables 40.3 and 40.4) (24,25). Clinically, the specific symptoms experienced are not important as long as the patient becomes aware of them at a glucose level when cognitive function is adequate to enable an effective response (i.e., ingestion of some rapidly absorbed carbohydrate). Many patients with type 1 diabetes report a greater dependence on neuroglycopenic symptoms than on autonomic symptoms over time.

The etiology of hunger, which represents a frequent symptom of hypoglycemia and most directly encourages resuscitative food intake, has not been clearly delineated. The satiety centers lateral to the hypothalamus may be involved. Leptin does not respond acutely in hypoglycemia, and the role of orexin is uncertain (26,27).

TABLE 40.3. Classification of Acute Hypoglycemia by Factor Analysis in Adults

Adrenergic	Neuroglycopenic	Other
Tremor	Dizziness	Hunger
Sweating	Confusion	Weakness
Anxiety	Tiredness	Blurred vision
Nausea	Difficulty speaking	—
Warmness	Inability to concentrate	—
Palpitations	Drowsiness	—
Shivering	—	—

From Deary IJ, Hepburn DA, MacLeod KM, et al. Partitioning the symptoms of hypoglycaemia using multi-sample confirmatory factor analysis. *Diabetologia* 1993;36:771–777, with permission. Copyright 1993 by Springer Verlag.

TABLE 40.4. Classification of Acute Hypoglycemia by Factor Analysis in Children

Neuroglycopenic and autonomic	Behavioral
Weakness	Headache
Trembling	Argumentative
Dizziness	Aggression
Poor concentration	Irritability
Hunger	Naughtiness
Sweating	Nausea
Confusion	Nightmares
Blurred/double vision	—
Slurred speech	—

From McCrimmon RJ, Gold AE, Deary IJ, et al. Symptoms of hypoglycemia in children with IDDM. *Diabetes Care* 1995;18:858–861.

INVESTIGATION OF RESPONSES TO ACUTE HYPOGLYCEMIA

The categorization of the symptoms of acute hypoglycemia discussed above was based on data collected from the description of symptoms and signs by patients and their family members. More detailed studies on the relationships between symptoms of acute hypoglycemia and the effect of diabetes and its therapy often have involved experimentally induced hypoglycemia. Insulin injection (i.e., the insulin tolerance test) is a high-risk procedure that results in an uncontrolled, rapid, variable, and often profound hypoglycemic challenge that will miss all but the most extreme variations in the counterregulatory response. A slow decline in plasma glucose level induced by a low-dose infusion can be useful for examining an individual's overall counterregulatory capacity (i.e., the ability to arrest or reverse a drop in glucose level) (28). However, the comparison of responses between individuals or groups of individuals may be complicated by the failure to achieve equal levels of hypoglycemia. As an alternative, controlled hypoglycemia can be induced with a modification of the euglycemic insulin clamp technique (29). In the slow-fall clamp, plasma glucose is controlled during a high-dose insulin infusion by means of an adjustable intravenous glucose infusion (Fig. 40.1). For patients with diabetes, plasma glucose often is regulated during the night preceding the study by an intravenous insulin infusion. This ensures that all subjects in a given study, with or without diabetes, are exposed to the same hypoglycemic challenge (i.e., similar initial glucose level, final glucose level, and rate of decline) (29). In some experimental protocols, the plasma glucose concentration is lowered in a series of steps, so that the glucose level associated with the onset of any one response can be determined for that individual or group of individuals. This technique first was used to determine the effect of the rate of glucose decline on the magnitude of the counterregulatory responses to a given moderate hypoglycemic challenge (29) and later to investigate the effects of intensified diabetes treatment on counterregulatory hormone responses (30). It is important to realize that the clamp technique does *not* exam-

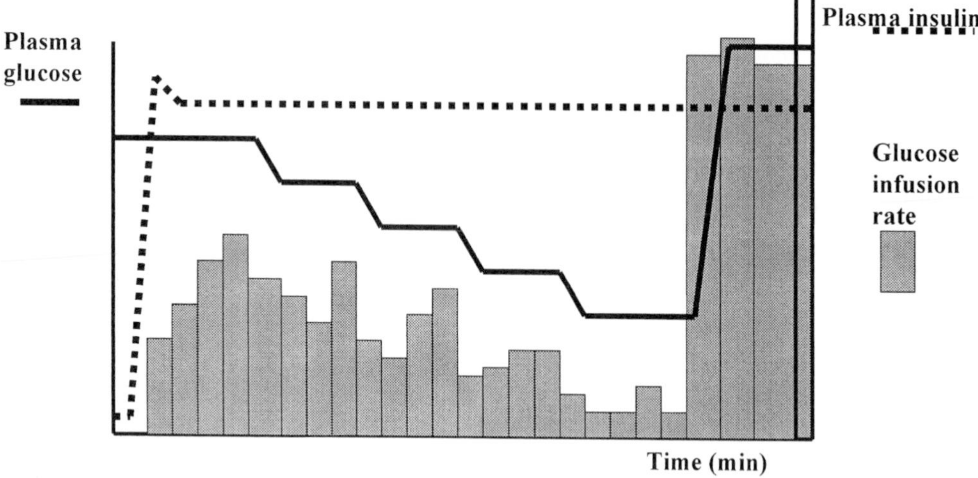

Figure 40.1. The stepped hypoglycemic clamp: a means of applying a controlled reproducible hypoglycemic challenge. A primed-continuous intravenous insulin infusion is started at time = 0 minutes, creating a predictable rapid square wave rise in circulating insulin levels (*black dotted line*). The subsequent hypoglycemia is controlled by a variable-rate glucose infusion (*bars*) adjusted according to the plasma glucose measurement made at the bedside every 5 minutes. (From Amiel SA, Simonson DC, Tamborlane WV, et al. Rate of glucose fall does not affect counterregulatory hormone responses to hypoglycemia in normal and diabetic humans. *Diabetes* 1987;36:518–522.)

ine counterregulation per se, because the glucose level is always under the control of the investigator.

Such studies show that acute hypoglycemia results in a hierarchy of responses. In healthy volunteers, epinephrine secretion begins at arterialized plasma glucose levels of 3.0 to 3.4 mmol/L, adrenergic symptoms at 3.2 mmol/L, and minor but detectable cognitive impairment (first shown as a slowing of complex reaction times) at 3.0 mmol/L (Fig. 40.2) (5,29–33). More extensive cognitive impairment has been shown at lower glucose levels (32). The hormonal and symptomatic responses occur at higher glucose levels in patients with poorly controlled diabetes (31,34). The initiation of hormonal responses, and especially of symptoms, before the onset of significant cognitive impairment during a progressive glucose decline is critical to a patient's ability to prevent severe hypoglycemia, giving a window of opportunity for recognition of the situation and for self-treatment (35).

The delineation of cognitive impairment during acute hypoglycemia is less clear. The brain is not a homogeneous organ, and specific brain functions use various brain regions that have different susceptibilities to hypoglycemia. The detection of hypoglycemia by glucose-sensing neurons and the initiation of the autonomic responses normally occur at or before the onset of cognitive changes (typically at arterialized plasma glucose levels of 3.4 mmol/L). For example, the slowing of choice reaction time occurs at glucose levels of 3 mmol/L, and the slowing of a simple motor activity such as finger tapping occurs at 2.4 mmol/L (Fig. 40.3).

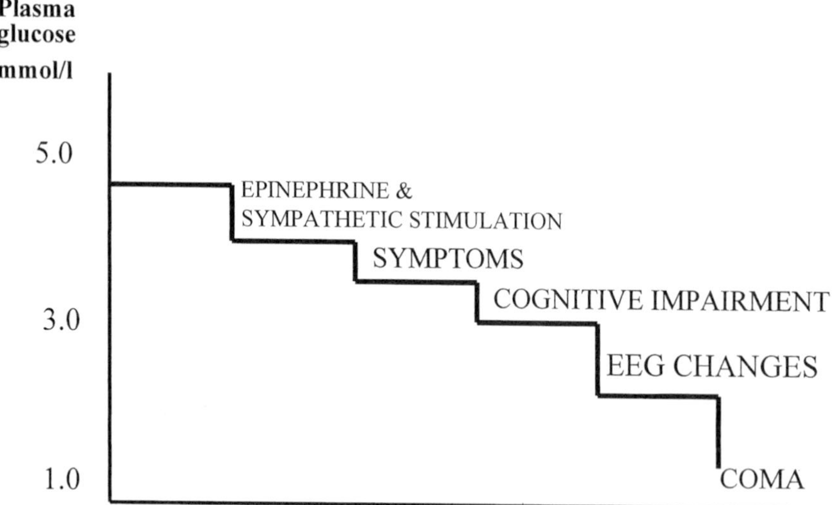

Figure 40.2. Normal hierarchy of responses to acute hypoglycemia. As plasma glucose level falls, the autonomic and symptomatic responses precede the onset of even mild cognitive impairment.

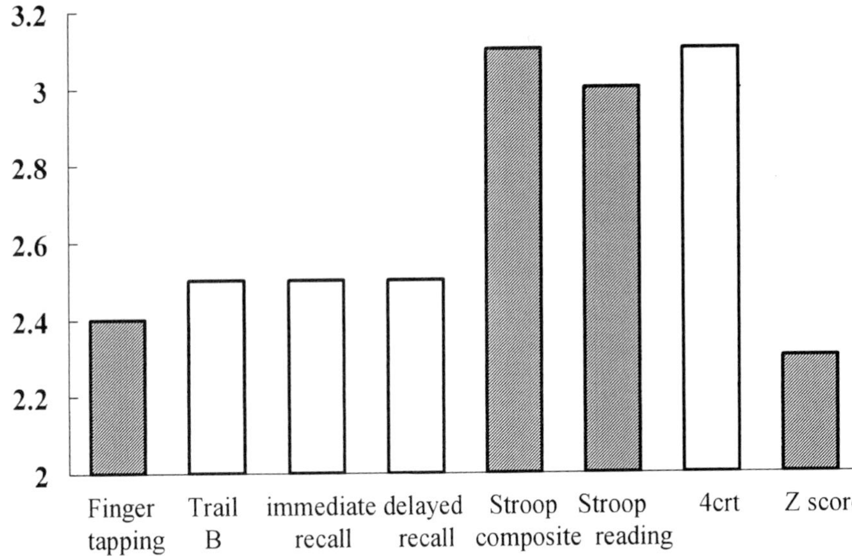

Figure 40.3. Glucose thresholds for onset of cognitive impairment in healthy volunteers. The data are acquired from clamp studies in which the rate of glucose decline is precisely controlled. It is important to note that different cognitive functions have different susceptibilities to hypoglycemia. Data for the two memory tests (immediate and delayed recall) and the composite Stroop score are from Cryer PE, Scott A, Segal MD, et al. Blood brain glucose transport is not increased following hypoglycemia. *Diabetes* 2000;39[Suppl 1]; the *z* scores are from Fanelli CG, Epifano L, Rambotti AM, et al. Meticulous prevention of hypoglycemia normalizes the glycemic thresholds and magnitude of most of neuroendocrine responses to, symptoms of, and cognitive function during hypoglycemia in intensively treated patients with short-term IDDM. *Diabetes* 1993;42:1683–1689; and the finger tapping, trail B, Stroop reading, and 4-choice reaction time (4crt) are from Hopkins DFC, Evans M, Lomas J, et al. Effects of antecedent control on cognitive function and symptoms during hypoglycaemia in type 1 diabetes. *Diabet Med* 1998;15[Suppl]:S4. The shaded bars represent cognitive functions that have been shown to manifest a degree of resistance to hypoglycemia in patients with hypoglycemia unawareness.

HYPOGLYCEMIA UNAWARENESS

The best defense a patient with diabetes has against severe hypoglycemia is subjective awareness of an early fall in plasma glucose concentrations and the immediate ingestion of a rapidly available carbohydrate. Loss of the ability to generate and/or perceive such symptoms—the syndrome of hypoglycemia unawareness—is a serious clinical problem, increasing the risk of severe hypoglycemia by about 10-fold (20,21). Such unawareness places the patient in danger, as he or she may experience blood glucose levels low enough to impair basic cognitive processes such as reaction times (5), making common tasks such as driving or operating heavy machinery potentially lethal. Less dramatic, but equally devastating, is the sudden inability to sustain logical thought or the sudden onset of uncharacteristic aggression, which can have serious professional and social consequences for the individual. Because, by definition, a patient with hypoglycemia unawareness cannot recognize his or her state, a full assessment of a patient's experience of hypoglycemia can be completed only by interviewing the people close to the patient in everyday life: the partner, other family members, or close friends (36).

An impaired ability to decrease insulin levels in response to hypoglycemia is integral to treatment with insulin or a sulfonylurea. Failure of the glucagon response in type 1 diabetes (and late insulin-deficient type 2) is apparently universal, and early studies also showed a marked diminution of the epinephrine response to hypoglycemia in patients with long-standing (10 years or more) type 1 diabetes (10). However, most patients with long-standing type 1 diabetes do retain an ability to recognize early hypoglycemia and defend against severe episodes, at least most of the time. Loss of awareness of hypoglycemia is certainly more common in long-duration type 1 diabetes than in diabetes of shorter duration (it has not been well described in type 2 diabetes), with 25% of patients in one general diabetes clinic with a duration of diabetes of more than 15 years reporting this problem. Such patients are at much higher risk of severe hypoglycemia (20,21). Similarly, more than a decade ago, patients with a history of recurrent severe hypoglycemia were found to have defective counterregulation, with impaired hormonal responses and an inability to arrest a glucose fall during low dose insulin infusion independent of diabetic neuropathy (19).

Interest in the problems of hypoglycemia awareness increased with the recognition that both asymptomatic (37) and severe symptomatic (8) hypoglycemia were more common in patients with type 1 diabetes randomized to receive intensified insulin therapy in the large trials of prevention of chronic complications (38). Investigation showed that patients receiving intensified therapy were less able than those receiving standard therapy to produce a counterregulatory response in the face of insulin infusion (as were previously studied patients with recurrent hypoglycemia) (39). The defect was found to be a lowering of the plasma glucose level needed to initiate the adrenergic and symptomatic responses (30), closing, if not obliterating, the gap between the onset of symptomatic protective responses and of cognitive impairment (Figs. 40.3 and 40.4).

There is little doubt that the detection of hypoglycemia and the initiation of the autonomic and adrenergic responses are centrally mediated. Animal studies show that maintenance of glucose supplies in a brain region around the ventromedial hypothalamus during systemic hypoglycemia prevents the counterregulatory response (40) and, conversely, that localized intracellular glucose deprivation (by deoxyglucose) in that brain region alone can induce a peripheral hyperglycemic "counterregulatory" hormonal response in euglycemic animals (41). Neurons from these and related brain areas can be excited by changes in glucose supply (42). In an experiment of nature, a patient with a sarcoid lesion in the same region showed abnormalities of glucose homeostasis and counterregulation until his lesion regressed with therapy (43). Glucose-sensing neurons also are present in the hepatic portal tract, as shown by animal experiments in which portal perfusion with glucose ameliorates the autonomic and adrenergic responses to systemic hypoglycemia (44,45), but their role in maintaining glucose supplies to the brain glucose is unclear. One hypothesis is that these neurons monitor glucose input from the gastrointestinal tract and may be able to moderate a centrally mediated counterregulatory response to systemic hypoglycemia once eating starts (46).

There is good circumstantial evidence that the trigger for autonomic and adrenergic counterregulation is a slowing of metabolic rate in the glucose-sensing neurons. Supplying the nonglucose substrates lactate or 3-hydroxybutyrate to support metabolism during experimentally induced hypoglycemia delays (i.e., shifts to lower glucose levels) the onset and magnitude of the epinephrine response, adrenergic symptoms, and cognitive impairment of acute hypoglycemia in volunteers (47–49). One popular current theory to explain the change in hypoglycemia sensitivity of the glucose-sensing mechanism is that an upregulation of glucose transporters and of glucose uptake by the brain occurs as a result of prior exposure to hypoglycemia (50–52). A study in patients with diabetes and healthy volunteers that calculated glucose consumption by the brain from measurements of cerebral blood flow and arteriovenous differences in glucose concentrations across the brain showed no effect of hypoglycemia in diabetic patients with a history of hypoglycemia unawareness, whereas hypoglycemia was associated with a decline in glucose uptake by the brain in symptomatic diabetic and nondiabetic subjects (53). A similar apparent adaptation in the handling of glucose by the brain also was induced in healthy volunteers by exposure to 56 hours of induced moderate hypoglycemia (54). The concept that the human brain can adapt to antecedent hypoglycemia by upregulating its ability to extract glucose and thus fails to trigger counterregulation because metabolism in the cerebral glucose sensor is better maintained is an attractive one. However, recent data obtained with positron emission tomography, measuring uptake in the brain of glucose labeled with a positron emitter, have been unable to confirm the data from the studies of arteriovenous difference (55,56). The discrepancies remain to be explained. One possibility is that adaptational changes are regional—all the described studies have measured only global glucose uptake by the brain. Regional differences in sensitivity to hypoglycemia itself have already been mentioned, and regional differences within the metabolic capacity of the brain and even of just the cerebral cortex have been suggested by further studies of nonglucose metabolic substrates in acute hypoglycemia (57).

The altered sensitivity of the brain's hypoglycemia sensing mechanisms in the hypoglycemia unawareness syndrome is well documented. There is debate about the extent to which this effect occurs in the cerebral cortex. The discrepancies in the literature are almost certainly due to differences in the cognitive function tests used to assess cortical function during acute hypoglycemia—some of which adapt (i.e., do not show evidence of deterioration until a more profound hypoglycemia has been reached) and some of which do not. It is clear that, in people with counterregulatory failure and hypoglycemia unawareness, the glucose level required to initiate the symptomatic counterregulatory responses is reduced below normal to a greater extent than any change in glucose level associated with detectable cognitive malfunction, narrowing or even closing the window of opportunity between subjective awareness and confusion.

It is not known how antecedent hypoglycemia alters the response to subsequent episodes. As explained above, in connection with the mechanisms of hypoglycemia unawareness, a possible mechanism is upregulation of glucose transporters in

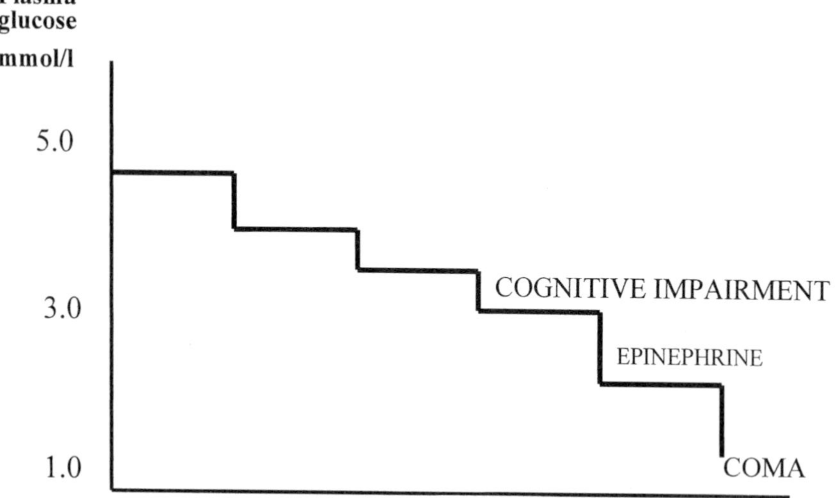

Figure 40.4. Disturbed hierarchy of responses to acute hypoglycemia after a preceding period of hypoglycemia. Counterregulatory failure is manifest as a lowering of the glucose level that induces an adrenergic counterregulatory response toward, or even below, that associated with the onset of cognitive impairment.

response to the initial hypoglycemic episodes; another is hypoglycemia-associated apoptosis of glucose-sensing cells (58). A suggested factor may be the adrenocorticotropic hormone or cortisol response to the initial insult (59,60), although how this might be involved in long-term hypoglycemia unawareness is unclear.

Whatever the mechanism, the link between the defective counterregulatory responses of hypoglycemia unawareness and hypoglycemia itself is strong. A series of research studies have demonstrated induction of counterregulatory failure and diminished symptomatic responses to experimentally induced hypoglycemia in both healthy volunteers and diabetic patients as a consequence of exposure to hypoglycemia during the day or night before the test stimulus (61–65). Such transient defects in the neuroendocrine response to hypoglycemia are very similar to those first demonstrated in intensively controlled diabetic patients with hypoglycemia unawareness: a lowering of the glucose level required to initiate the symptomatic and hormonal responses (particularly the epinephrine response) and a diminution of the hormonal response at any given glucose level. The relevance to the clinical syndrome of hypoglycemia unawareness in diabetic patients is confirmed by the demonstration that both the unawareness and the neurohumoral failure are either partially (66) or completely (67) reversible by scrupulous avoidance of hypoglycemia in daily living. It is important to note that the induction of temporary counterregulatory failure in experimental studies can be generated by modest prior decreases in plasma glucose concentrations (Table 40.5) and that reversibility in patients with diabetes can be achieved by successful avoidance of blood glucose concentrations lower than 3 mmol/L on home monitoring. This illustrates the danger of using definitions of hypoglycemia coined for the diagnosis of pathologic spontaneous hypoglycemia in the context of diabetes therapies.

It is important not to assume that counterregulatory defects induced by exposure to hypoglycemia itself are restricted to intensified insulin therapy regimens and tight glycemic control. The study by Cranston et al. (67) included six patients with poorly controlled diabetes receiving conventional therapy who, despite high levels of glycosylated hemoglobin and generally high plasma glucose concentrations, nevertheless experienced intermittent severe hypoglycemia with no warning. These patients also recovered symptomatic neurohumoral responses to induced hypoglycemia after a period of hypoglycemia avoidance, suggesting that the etiology of their counterregulatory failure was the same as that in patients receiving intensive therapy.

The failure to generate an adequate neurohumoral response to induced hypoglycemia in diabetic patients with hypoglycemia unawareness is probably enhanced by a diminished sensitivity to adrenergic stimulation. Reduced cardiovascular responses to infused β-agonists have been demonstrated in patients with diabetes prone to recurrent episodes of severe hypoglycemia (68,69), and perhaps loss of both epinephrine secretion and its effects are required to create the full syndrome of hypoglycemia unawareness and high risk of severe hypoglycemia. The reduced sensitivity to adrenergic stimulation may be reversible; one study that attempted to correct counterregulatory failure by hypoglycemia avoidance demonstrated restoration of adrenergic symptoms but not of epinephrine responses to induced hypoglycemia (70).

Variation in adrenergic sensitivity also may explain differences in the susceptibility of patients with classical diabetic autonomic neuropathy to hypoglycemia unawareness. These patients have diminished counterregulatory hormone responses to hypoglycemia (71) and increased risk of severe hypoglycemia (72), but there is no direct link between clinical autonomic neuropathy and counterregulatory failure (19). Patients with autonomic neuropathy may be more sensitive to any adrenergic stimulation that they can achieve (73). The failure of subjective awareness of hypoglycemia in these patients can also be partially restored by avoidance of hypoglycemia (74), which does not correct the neuropathy itself.

Recent data suggest genotypic variation may contribute to the risk of severe hypoglycemia. In particular, variants of the ACE gene have been demonstrated in some populations to be excessively represented in patients with severe hypoglycemia (75).

TABLE 40.5. The Hypoglycemic Stimuli Associated with Subsequent Counterregulatory Defects

Healthy volunteers
3.9 mmol/L for 2 h
3.3 mmol/L for 2 h
3 mmol/L for 2 h
2.9 mmol/L for 2 h (residual effect at 3 d)
Patients with diabetes
2.8 mmol/L for 2 h
2.8 mmol/L for 2 h twice a week
2.7 mmol/L for 3 h at night

Data from Davis SN, Shavers C, Mosqueda-Garcia R, et al. Effects of differing antecedent hypoglycemia on subsequent counterregulation in normal humans. *Diabetes* 1997;46:1328–1335; George E, Harris N, Bedford C, et al. Prolonged but partial impairment of the hypoglycaemic physiological response for following short-term hypoglycaemia in normal subjects. *Diabetologia* 1995;38:1183–1190; Hvidberg A, Fanelli CG, Hershey T, et al. Impact of recent antecedent hypoglycemia on hypoglycemic cognitive dysfunction on nondiabetic humans. *Diabetes* 1996;45:1030–1036; George E, Marques JL, Harris ND, et al. Preservation of physiological responses to hypoglycemia 2 days after antecedent hypoglycemia in patients with IDDM. *Diabetes Care* 1997;20:1293–1298; Ovalle F, Fanelli CG, Paramore DS, et al. Brief twice-weekly episodes of hypoglycemia reduce detection of clinical hypoglycemia in type 1 diabetes mellitus. *Diabetes* 1998;47:1472–1479; and Fanelli CG, Paramore DS, Hershey D, et al. Impact of nocturnal hypoglycemia on hypoglycemic cognitive dysfunction in type 1 diabetes. *Diabetes* 1998;47:1920–1927.

CLINICAL CAUSES OF HYPOGLYCEMIA AND APPROACHES TO MINIMIZING RISKS

It is important to recognize that acute hypoglycemia in diabetes, whether or not complicated by hypoglycemia unawareness, is caused by excessive insulin action. There are many important differences between therapeutic exogenous insulin and endogenous insulin: exogenous insulin is delivered peripherally not portally, has variable and nonphysiologic pharmacodynamics, and is unresponsive to changes in blood glucose concentrations.

Meal-Related Insulin and Hypoglycemia

Rapid-acting (regular) insulin, designed for prandial use, has too low a peak and too long a duration of action to mimic the short, sharp, prandial burst of insulin produced by the healthy pancreas in response to eating. Thus, if enough insulin is taken to prevent an excessive increase in glucose level with a meal, too much insulin may remain in the circulation 2 to 4 hours later. The problem may be compounded if an intermediate-acting insulin is administered with the preprandial regular insulin in an effort to cover the subsequent two meals (e.g., the use of a prebreakfast mixture of regular and intermediate-acting insulin to cover breakfast and lunch). Patients trying to gain control of immediate postprandial glycemia almost invariably need between-meal snacks to prevent hypoglycemia before the next meal (76). This represents one of the most troublesome aspects of such diabetes treatment regimens. The use of ultra–short-acting insulin analogues may reduce the dependence on snacks between meals (77,78), as may the use of twice-daily intermediate-acting insulin to provide basal insulin coverage and reduce the dependence on a meal-related regular insulin bolus to provide enough insulin to last from one meal to the next (9,79).

Basal Insulin Replacement and Nocturnal Hypoglycemia

Basal insulin coverage overnight often represents an even more significant problem in diabetes management. It has long been known that approximately 50% of insulin-treated patients experience nocturnal hypoglycemia (80), and this has recently been confirmed in studies in children (81–83). In one of these studies, the median glucose nadir was 1.9 mmol/L (range, 1.1 to 3.3 mmol/L) and the median duration was 270 minutes (range, 30 to 630 minutes) (82). Nocturnal hypoglycemia is often asymptomatic, possibly because it produces a much less vigorous counterregulatory hormone response during sleep than during wakefulness (84,85). This lack of a vigorous sympathetic response may explain the prolonged duration of episodes of nocturnal hypoglycemia episodes observed in children (82) and why nocturnal hypoglycemia can be profound enough to cause convulsions and seizures. It has been surprisingly difficult to demonstrate deleterious effects of nocturnal hypoglycemia on cognitive function the next day (82,86), except for the finding of a significant decline in feelings of well-being and mood. However, nocturnal hypoglycemia is capable of inducing defective counterregulation the following day (32) and should be avoided for this reason alone.

Significant difficulties result from the use of conventional intermediate-acting insulins for overnight insulin replacement in patients with type 1 diabetes. All have a marked peak-and-trough effect that does not match the physiologic pattern of nonprandial insulin secretion from the healthy pancreas. The predicted peak action is 4 to 8 hours after injection, with the subsequent decreased levels likely to leave the patient with insulin deficiency and hyperglycemia the next morning. Within the range of isophane and lente insulins, there are subtle differences in pharmacodynamics that sometimes can be exploited but the differences are not great (87). Less pure and animal insulins may last longer than the equivalent human insulins, with one study showing the lowest fasting glucose levels, dose-for-dose, with bovine insulin (87); however, a recent study specifically of nocturnal glycemic control with equivalent human and porcine insulins showed no difference in glycemic control or in the frequency of episodes of nocturnal hypoglycemia (88).

Delaying the administration of evening intermediate-acting insulin to defer the peak action into the time of the dawn phenomenon can often be useful (89), and one study showed reduced rates of hypoglycemia when nocturnal insulin replacement was by single-rate continuous subcutaneous insulin infusion (90). There is also a suggestion that the risk of nocturnal hypoglycemia may be diminished when basal insulin replacement is provided by twice-daily intermediate-acting insulins rather than by one evening dose (9,79). The new insulin analogues, glargine and detemir, which are designed to have a flatter, more prolonged, insulin action than conventional isophane and lente insulins, have been associated with reduced nocturnal hypoglycemia (91,92), although the first clinical trials have not shown a major impact on hypoglycemia in general (93).

The regular insulin given before the evening meal can be a significant contributor to nocturnal hypoglycemia. This has been shown by studies suggesting that the blood glucose test before the bedtime snack may be a good predictor of nocturnal hypoglycemia (94,95), although this is not a universal finding (81). Converting to an ultra–short-acting insulin analogue for meals reduces the risk of nocturnal hypoglycemia (96), although this results in significant hyperglycemia during the early part of the night (97,98). Adjusting bedtime snacking procedures may prevent such hyperglycemia, but this has not been confirmed in controlled studies.

Bedtime snacking is a long-established component of diabetes treatment regimens that is widely accepted as an approach to preventing nocturnal hypoglycemia. It most often is used to offset the late action of the regular insulin taken before the evening meal—as food intake is not likely to have a significant effect on blood glucose levels after 3 or 4 hours. Inclusion of uncooked cornstarch in the bedtime snack has been shown to reduce rates of nocturnal hypoglycemia, but the mechanism is uncertain (99). Because the amount of cornstarch ingested is very small, it is unlikely to function as a source of carbohydrate slowly absorbed over many hours. The suggested inclusion of substrates for gluconeogenesis in the bedtime snack has a logical appeal but has not been formally tested (100). The use of β-agonists at bedtime, effective in a research setting, demonstrated no effect in a clinical trial (101).

POSTHYPOGLYCEMIC HYPERGLYCEMIA AND HYPOGLYCEMIA

Belief in the Somogyi phenomenon, literally the occurrence of ketonuria the morning after a nighttime hypoglycemic episode, as an explanation for diabetic instability and fasting hyperglycemia, has a cyclic popularity (102). As discussed previously, it is likely that morning hyperglycemia results from a waning of the insulin effect from the previous day, with the earlier peak action of that same insulin causing the prior hypoglycemia (103). Early morning ketonuria is likely to arise from the same insulin deficiency, although ketosis also is undoubtedly augmented by elevations in stress hormones. Despite the frequent importance of insulin deficiency, posthypoglycemic hyperglycemia does occur and may explain why successful resolution of recurrent hypoglycemic episodes often is associated with lowering of glycosylated hemoglobin values and improved blood glucose control overall.

The mechanisms of posthypoglycemic hyperglycemia include a tendency to overtreat the hypoglycemic episode and the generation of insulin resistance as a result of hypoglycemia counterregulation. Contrary to traditional teaching, the effect of a single episode of hypoglycemia may be manifest as postprandial hyperglycemia the next day rather than as fasting hyperglycemia (104). The insulin resistance due to the catecholamine response is transient (105,106); a more prolonged effect appears to be attributable to growth hormone (107). This effect may be particularly pronounced in children, whose counterregulatory hormone response to hypoglycemia is greater than that in adults (108), especially when glycemic control is generally poor. The problem is compounded in adolescents, who, in addition to having a vigorous counterregulatory response, are also relatively insulin-resistant (109). No therapeutic compensation can be made for this—avoidance of the hypoglycemia is the essential therapeutic maneuver.

Paradoxically, the other change in blood glucose levels that should be anticipated following a hypoglycemic event is another hypoglycemic episode. This applies to more severe episodes of hypoglycemia and is presumably related to a counterregulatory deficit induced by the index episode (110). Patients receiving insulin should be aware of the risk of a second occurrence of hypoglycemia within 24 hours of a single severe episode.

HYPOGLYCEMIA IN TYPE 2 DIABETES MELLITUS

Compared with the information available about hypoglycemia in type 1 diabetes, knowledge about hypoglycemia in type 2 diabetes is limited. Severe hypoglycemia is much less common in type 2 diabetes, in which insulin resistance and residual pancreatic function presumably confer some protection. However, with progression of the disease process to an insulin-requiring state, the patient with type 2 diabetes may assume risks of hypoglycemia similar to those in patients with type 1 diabetes. The analysis of the effects of blood glucose control in type 2 diabetes in the United Kingdom Prospective Diabetes Study (UKPDS) clearly demonstrated an increased risk of severe hypoglycemia with intensification of control and the introduction of insulin (Fig. 40.5) (111).

Patients with type 2 diabetes whose therapy is limited to diet and exercise do not experience significant hypoglycemia, and it is extremely rare in those receiving metformin or thiazolidenediones, because these drugs act as an insulin sensitizer and thus do not prevent a decrease in the patient's endogenous insulin or an increase in glucagon as levels of plasma glucose decline. With insulin secretagogues, hypoglycemia can occur and can often be severe enough to produce neuroglycopenic symptoms (112–114). The long-acting sulfonylureas are particularly problematic, and the occurrence of confusion in elderly patients receiving sulfonylureas must always raise suspicion of hypoglycemia. Shorter-acting sulfonylureas and the metiglinides carry a lower risk of hypoglycemia (Fig. 40.6) (114,115).

Hypoglycemia induced by sulfonylureas can be prolonged and can recur after emergency treatment as a consequence of persistent drug action. Patients presenting with severe hypoglycemia secondary to sulfonylurea treatment should be hospitalized for observation; they often require parenteral glucose therapy.

There is controversy concerning the differences between the counterregulatory responses to hypoglycemia in type 1 and type 2 diabetes. Patients with type 2 diabetes are generally older than patients with type 1 diabetes, and normal aging has been associated with reduced counterregulatory hormone responses to induced hypoglycemia (116–118). Symptom generation and cognitive impairment in hypoglycemia occur more closely together in healthy older individuals, and this might be expected to increase the risk of severe hypoglycemia in older patients with type 2 diabetes (119,120).

There is good evidence that counterregulatory responses in patients with poorly controlled type 2 diabetes are initiated at high glucose levels, with a decrease in the levels of glucose that are associated with hormonal responses and subjective awareness as control is improved, at least with insulin (Fig. 40.7) (121). Preliminary evidence suggests that thresholds for at least some cognitive dysfunctions are not similarly mobile (121). Symptoms of hypoglycemia in patients with type 2 diabetes receiving insulin differ little from those of patients with type 1 diabetes (122), although elderly patients more readily present with neurologic symptoms such as incoordination, blurred vision, or slurred speech (122).

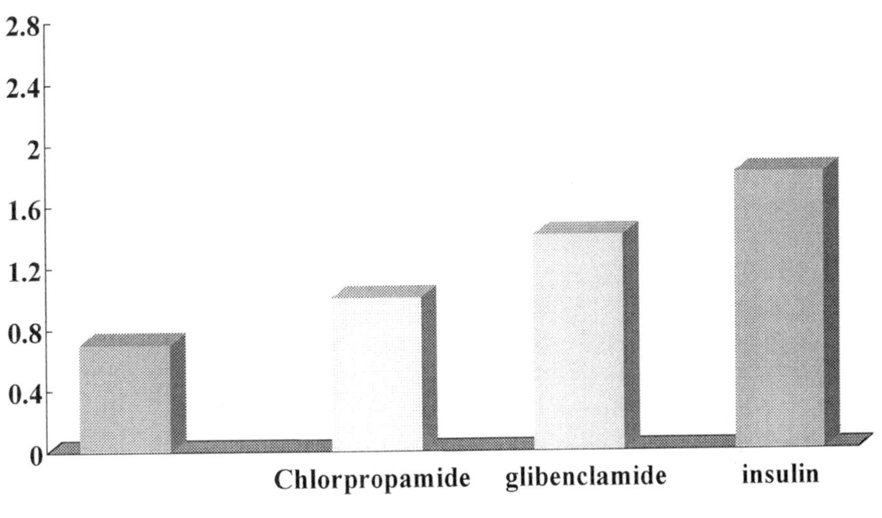

Figure 40.5. Incidence of severe hypoglycemia in the United Kingdom Prospective Diabetes Study. (From UK Prospective Diabetes Study Group. Intensive blood glucose control with sulphonylureas or insulin compared with conventional therapy and risk of complications in patients with type 2 diabetes mellitus: UKPDS 33. *Lancet* 1998;352:837–853.)

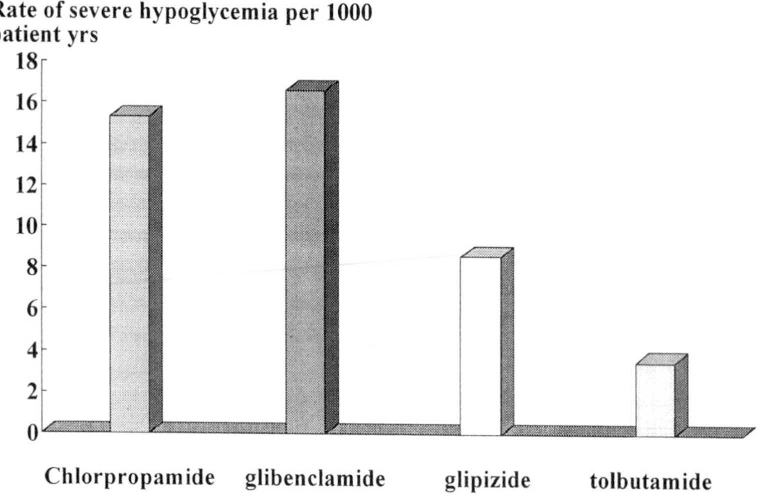

Figure 40.6. Incidence of severe hypoglycemia on different oral hypoglycemic agents. (From Shorr RI, Ray WA, Daugherty JR, et al. Antihypertensives and the risk of serious hypoglycemia in older persons using insulin or sulfonylureas. *JAMA* 1997;278:40–43.)

EXERCISE AND HYPOGLYCEMIA

Exercise is an important contributor to episodic hypoglycemia. The effects of exercise on blood glucose are immediate (as exercising muscle uses glucose), intermediate (lasting for 18 to 24 hours if the exercise is vigorous or prolonged), and chronic (in the sense that muscle is more sensitive than adipose tissue to insulin and that a fit body is more insulin-sensitive than an untrained body) (123–125).

The immediate hypoglycemic effect of exercise can be accommodated by reducing the dose of insulin that will be active at the time of planned exercise. Alternatively, rapidly available carbohydrate (fruit juice or glucose) can be taken during and after the exercise. Judicious use of home blood glucose monitoring helps the patient assess his or her own requirements for given intensities of exercise.

Vigorous or prolonged exertion will deplete liver and muscle glycogen, and the demand for glucose to restore these pools lasts at least 24 hours. People who exercise intermittently, either very vigorously or over prolonged periods, are likely to require significantly less insulin through the following night and possibly even the next day. Insulin requirements, including basal requirements, during sporting holidays (e.g., skiing) can fall by 30% to 50% (126). For a more detailed discussion of exercise in diabetes, see Chapter 38.

ALCOHOL AND HYPOGLYCEMIA

Alcoholic beverages often contain glucose, and the immediate response to alcohol ingestion, especially of beer and cider, is often hyperglycemia. The hyperglycemic effect of wine is very small. Alcohol is also an insulin sensitizer (127). It suppresses gluconeogenesis, an effect that can cause delayed hypoglycemia, as the body normally activates gluconeogenesis after several hours of fasting. This can, for example, cause significant hypoglycemia the morning after evening drinking. The effect is dose-dependent, and one or two drinks are therefore unlikely to have a major effect. However, individuals in tight glycemic control (and their friends and relatives) need to be aware of the risk. The likelihood of hypoglycemia is greatest in young people who combine alcohol intake (not necessarily excessive) with exercise—typically at overnight parties involving dancing. Young people have died as a result of this combination. Advising reduction in overnight insulin after evening or all-night parties where alcohol and/or exercise have been involved and warning relatives or friends of the risk next day should be advised.

Acutely, alcohol has been shown to diminish appreciation of hypoglycemic symptoms (128) and counterregulatory hormone responses (129) and can therefore be a contributor to severe hypoglycemia without warning signs.

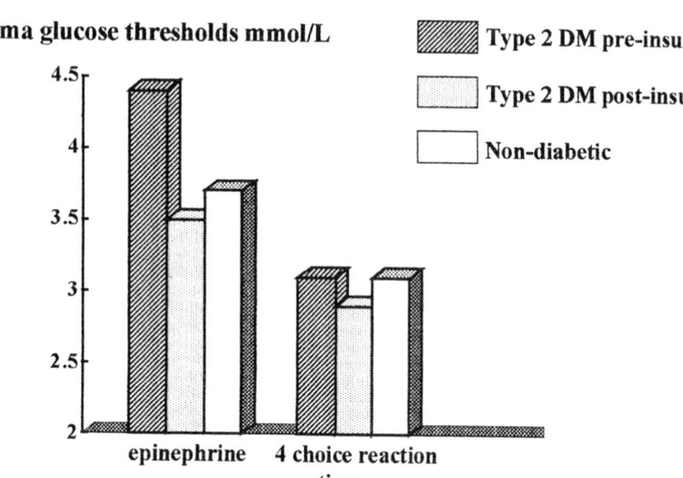

Figure 40.7. Arterialized plasma glucose thresholds for epinephrine release and slowing of 4-choice reaction time (a very sensitive measure of psychomotor coordination in hypoglycemia) during acute induced hypoglycemia in poorly controlled type 2 diabetes mellitus and after improving glycemic control with insulin on the right. (Data from Korzon-Burakowska A, Hopkins D, Matyka K, et al. Effects of glycemic control on protective responses against hypoglycemia on type 2 diabetes mellitus. *Diabetes Care* 1998;21:282–291.)

DRUGS AND HYPOGLYCEMIA

The risk that β-blockers may diminish appreciation of symptoms of hypoglycemia has not been substantiated in experimental studies indicating that exaggerated sweating enhanced subjective awareness of hypoglycemia (130). The use of β-blockers in diabetic patients with cardiovascular disease should not be avoided on the basis of the risk of hypoglycemia, although it makes sense to use cardioselective agents where appropriate.

Considerable discussion about there being a significantly increased risk of hypoglycemia with the use of angiotensin-converting enzyme (ACE) inhibitors (131) was followed by evidence (in a mixed group of patients with type 1 and type 2 diabetes) that the association was with antihypertensive therapy per se (132). ACE inhibitors do appear to enhance insulin sensitivity, but the effect is small. There were suggestions that the relationship was indirect—either through comorbidity for the conditions for which the ACE inhibitors were being used or as a consequence of modern diabetes management with intensified insulin therapy and vigorous use of ACE inhibitors. A report of an association between enalapril and risk of hypoglycemia specifically in patients receiving a sulfonylurea (133) was followed by a failure to observe increased hypoglycemia rates in users of ramipril in the HOPE (Heart Outcomes Prevention Evaluation) trial (again a mixture of patients with type 1 and type diabetes) (134). The possibility that hypoglycemic effects of ACE inhibitors are drug-specific rather than class-specific has not been excluded by available studies. At present, caution is advised when introducing or increasing the dose of an ACE inhibitor in a patient with tightly controlled diabetes, with advice given to increase home glucose monitoring until the dose is established. This is good practice when making any adjustment in medication for a patient with diabetes. The data do not in any way support the avoidance of ACE inhibitors in patients with diabetes.

Thyrotoxic patients have accelerated hepatic degradation of insulin. Treatment with hypothyroid drugs may then increase the risk of hypoglycemia, especially if the patient becomes significantly hypothyroid (135).

Finally, it has been suggested that changes in the nature, and particularly the species, of exogenous insulin used by a patient with diabetes can be associated with increased risk of hypoglycemia. In particular, concerns have been raised that synthetic human insulins may carry greater risk than older animal insulins of problematic hypoglycemia. A recent systematic review of available published studies found no evidence to support this claim, although it was noted that any study may fail to pick up an idiosyncratic effect with relevance to some individuals (136). There is no evidence that various insulin species have different effects on responses to hypoglycemia (e.g., differentially disposing to hypoglycemia unawareness), but it is good practice to use an insulin species with which the patient feels most confident.

MANAGEMENT OF HYPOGLYCEMIA

The Acute Event

Acute hypoglycemia is most safely treated with 15 to 20 g of oral glucose—ideally as glucose tablets; jelly, or glucose-containing drinks such as 150 to 200 mL of fresh fruit juice, nondiet lemonade, nondiet cola, or a slightly lesser amount of Lucozade (100 to 130 mL). Chocolate is best avoided because the fat content tends to retard glucose absorption. If no meal is planned within the hour after a hypoglycemic episode, additional complex carbohydrate (10 to 20 g) should also be ingested. The parenteral route should not be used if the patient is conscious and able to swallow.

It is useful if the patient can confirm the blood glucose concentration prior to treatment, since it will help subsequent management to know the level at which the patient experiences symptoms of hypoglycemia. Treatment of nonhypoglycemic, apparently symptomatic, episodes (blood glucose higher than 3.5 mmol/L) should be avoided unless the patient needs to be sure the glucose level is not falling further or is about to drive.

If the patient is too confused to swallow safely, corrective therapy must be administered parenterally. Absorption of honey or glucose gel through the buccal mucosa can sometimes be tried if the situation is not too extreme. Intramuscular glucagon (1 mg) can be administered by trained nonprofessionals and should be effective within 10 minutes (137). The action has been said to be as rapid as intravenous glucose, although anecdotally, intravenous glucose has been reported to be faster. Administration of glucagon should be followed by oral administration of 20 g of glucose after the patient is alert enough to swallow and thereafter of 40 g of a starchy carbohydrate to maintain recovery. The action of glucagon depends on stimulation of glycogenolysis, and it therefore may not be effective after prolonged fasting or in alcohol-induced hypoglycemia.

Intravenous glucose solutions should be given with care. The old regimen of 50 mL of 50% glucose provides too much glucose in a form that is very toxic to tissues. What matters is the total quantity of glucose given, and 75 to 100 mL of a 20% solution or even 150 to 200 mL of a 10% solution of glucose is much safer. There is a report of tissue necrosis requiring amputation of a hand as a consequence of extravasation of a 50% solution of glucose administered intravenously (138).

Prevention

Aspects of hypoglycemia prevention have been discussed in the section on minimization of risk, but it is important to note the need to review the therapeutic regimen in patients with problematic hypoglycemia. This includes episodes of hypoglycemia without patient awareness; episodes that a third party had to help treat; episodes when the patient lost self-control, resulting in embarrassment, underperformance at work, or accidents with or without physical damage to the patient or another person; and episodes when the patient lost consciousness or had a seizure.

Comorbidities that might increase hypoglycemia risk (deficiencies of cortisol, growth hormone, thyroid hormone and causes of malabsorption such as coelic disease, anorexia, or gastroparesis) should be excluded. However, the principal cause of hypoglycemia is excess insulin, and adjustment of the insulin regimen or changes in insulin secretagogues must be considered in any such patient. This should be coupled with education on proper management of other risk factors, such as the timing and content of meals and snacks, management of exercise, and the effects of alcohol. Adjustment of diabetes regimens to eliminate blood glucose values of less than 3 mmol/L may help a hypoglycemia-unaware patient regain hypoglycemia warnings and can frequently be accomplished without worsening the average glucose control. Examination of a patient's "typical" day in terms of meal times and exercise patterns often can reveal easily remediable risk factors. It is often worth comparing the patient's insulin distribution with the norm and, if there is a big discrepancy, trying to redistribute the total dose in line with textbook descriptions of requirements (e.g., in multiple daily insulin regimens, 40% to 60% of a total dose should be administered as basal insulin, with the remainder divided between meals—most for breakfast, least for lunch). A schema for altering therapy to reverse problematic hypoglycemia is

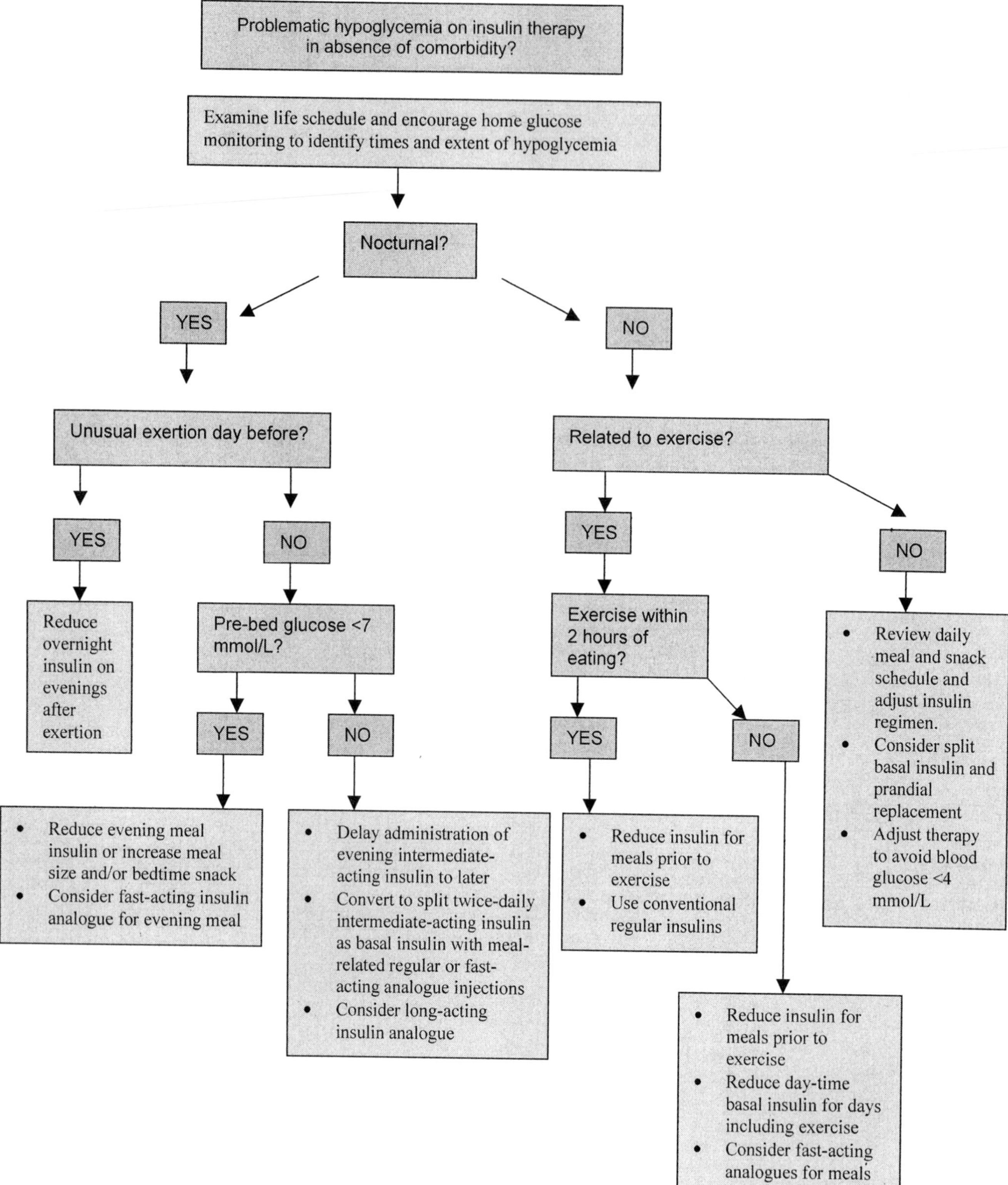

Figure 40.8. A proposed plan for the management of patients with problematic hypoglycemia.

illustrated in Figure 40.8. For patients with type 2 diabetes who are receiving sulfonylureas, reduced doses, administration of other hypoglycemic agents, and conversion to shorter-acting agents should all be considered. Ultimately, judicious use of continuous subcutaneous insulin therapy (insulin pump therapy) is effective (139,140). Islet transplantation remains a research procedure which can be effective in reducing hypoglycemia burden in insulin-sensitive type 1 patients when all else has failed (141).

Driving and Hypoglycemia

There is no clear evidence that patients with diabetes have an overall higher risk of automobile collisions than do other individuals. However, hypoglycemia is implicated as a cause of accidents (142), and it is possible that drivers with diabetes follow particularly safe driving practices to compensate. Much of the evidence on the incidence of automobile collisions was collected before the widespread introduction of intensified insulin therapy, and new studies therefore are needed (143). Ultimately, decisions about the fitness of patients with diabetes to drive must be made on an individual basis.

Patients with recurrent severe hypoglycemia and those who do not recognize hypoglycemia should not be permitted to drive. If these circumstances can be reversed by improving the mechanism of subjective hypoglycemia recognition, it is reasonable to consider the resumption of driving. It is a good strategy for such patients to verify their blood glucose level before driving and at 90-minute intervals during a long drive. The driver with diabetes should always carry glucose for rapid management of hypoglycemia should it occur. If a hypoglycemic episode develops, the patient should stop the car without delay, treat with glucose, wait 20 minutes, and recheck the blood glucose before resuming driving. This is important, because cognitive recovery from acute hypoglycemia may be delayed (144).

LONG-TERM EFFECTS OF ACUTE HYPOGLYCEMIA

Recovery from severe hypoglycemia with cognitive impairment, including coma or seizure, is generally complete. Rarely, patients suffer permanent brain damage, obvious at the time of recovery of consciousness, with slow improvement that can continue for weeks afterward. Permanent neurologic sequelae have most often been reported after massive deliberate or malicious overdosage and delayed restoration of blood glucose levels (145).

Hypoglycemic hemiplegia is an uncommon condition in which the patient wakes up after nocturnal hypoglycemia with a hemiparesis that resolves after minutes or hours. Patients may present with recurrent episodes. Although sometimes thought to indicate underlying circulatory defects, in one survey of 56 reported cases in adults, most of which involved a right-sided hemiparesis, only three of 16 who were investigated showed evidence of internal carotid artery stenosis (146). There are no data to suggest a poor prognosis. In children, there is no record of a preference for right- or left-sided neurologic signs, and one series of 44 children included 14 who underwent computed tomographic scans, which were normal in all but one (147).

Cumulative Damage from Recurrent Severe Hypoglycemia

The concern that recurrent severe hypoglycemia, *from which an apparently full recovery is made at the time,* might cause cumulative cortical damage and impaired cognitive function remains unresolved (148). In adults, there are data to suggest a greater decline in IQ scores over time and impaired decision times on formal testing in diabetic patients with a history of recurrent severe hypoglycemia (149). These are suggestive data, but the decrement in IQ was calculated, in a rather complicated manner, as the difference between the National Adult Reading Test score (which is said to be resistant to organic brain disease) and the Wechsler Adult Intelligence Scale (revised) score, adjusted to account for the difference in the way the two tests are performed. The increased loss was approximately a doubling of the normal reduction in IQ score with age. Another study found decreased performance in a word-recall test in diabetic patients with a history of severe hypoglycemia; ultimately it was unclear whether this was associated with diabetes per se rather than with hypoglycemia (150). Similarly, diabetes was found to be associated with prolongation of the evoked potential the P300 wave on electroencephalography, with no further effect of a history of severe hypoglycemia (151). However, another study concluded that there was decreased psychomotor performance only in diabetic patients with severe hypoglycemia and neuropathy, supporting the possibility of a diabetic central neuropathy or encephalopathy (152). In evaluating the possibility of hypoglycemia-induced damage of the central nervous system, it is important to recognize that factors other than subclinical organic brain damage may affect results of formal cognitive function testing. In particular, depression can have a very major effect and is rarely factored out of the cross-sectional studies. This may explain why an early study found equally decreased cognitive performance in patients from a diabetes clinic and patients from a gastroenterology clinic (153).

Neuroimaging has not produced definitive answers. Studies have generally been small and cross-sectional. One study found leukoaraiosis in two each of 11 diabetic patients with and without hypoglycemia but found imaging evidence of cortical atrophy in 5 of the 11 with recurrent hypoglycemia only (154). It is possible that both chronic hyper- and recurrent hypoglycemia have detrimental effects on cortical function, as evidenced by delayed reaction times in both very tightly controlled (and by implication more commonly hypoglycemic) and very poorly controlled diabetes (155).

None of the changes described amount to clinical dementia, but some patients, perhaps particularly those whose habits and situations require high cognitive input and fast reaction times, may be disadvantaged. Frank dementia has been documented in five patients with severe hypoglycemia, but advanced macrovascular disease may have been of etiologic significance (156).

There is clear evidence that intensified insulin therapy, despite its association with increased prevalence of severe hypoglycemia, does not cause cognitive impairment prospectively over time (157). This does not exonerate recurrent severe hypoglycemia, because conventionally treated patients also develop hypoglycemia and not all intensively treated diabetic patients experience problematic hypoglycemia, but it provides reassurance. An exhaustive breakdown of the DCCT data, collected prospectively, showed no evidence for diminished psychomotor performance in patients with more than five episodes of severe hypoglycemia as compared with those with fewer episodes (158).

The situation is slightly clearer regarding the effects of recurrent hypoglycemia on the developing brain. In children younger than 7 years, there is evidence of impaired intellectual performance at later times if diabetes develops very early (before the age of 7 years) and if there has been recurrent hypoglycemia *with seizures* (159). In such young children, one major aim of diabetes therapy must be the avoidance of hypoglycemia. Good blood glucose control is important for the optimization of growth and for the prevention of long-term complications of diabetes. However, it is at least as important to avoid severe hypoglycemia in young children, and slightly higher glycemic targets than those appropriate for adults and older children may be indicated.

SUDDEN DEATH AND HYPOGLYCEMIA

Death from acute hypoglycemia occurs but is very rare (160,161). Hypoglycemia has been implicated in occasional unexplained deaths in young people with diabetes (162). The diagnosis cannot be made retrospectively, as it is not possible to obtain firm postmortem evidence of hypoglycemia. Typically, the patient is found in an undisturbed bed with no evidence of preceding ketoacidosis (prodromal illness, evidence of vomiting) or a hypoglycemic seizure. Recent studies have shown that acute hypoglycemia is associated with lengthening of the QT interval on the electrocardiogram, which may predispose to serious arrhythmias (163,164). It has been suggested that the combination of a catecholamine surge and a drop in potassium level associated with hypoglycemia may precipitate a fatal cardiac arrhythmia in these, fortunately rare, cases. It is not known if an "at-risk" population can be identified, as the problem is so infrequent, but the potential catastrophic complication adds to concerns about avoiding problematic hypoglycemia in the course of insulin therapy.

REFERENCES

1. Liu D, Moberg E, Kollind K, et al. Arterial, arterialized venous, venous and capillary blood glucose measurements in normal man during hyperinsulinaemic euglycaemia and hypoglycaemia. *Diabetologia* 1992;35:287–290.
2. Alberti KG, Zimmet PZ. Definition, diagnosis and classification of diabetes mellitus and its complications, I: diagnosis and classification of diabetes mellitus provisional report of a WHO consultation. *Diabet Med* 1998;15:539–543.
3. Merimee TJ, Tyson JE. Stabilization of plasma glucose during fasting: normal variation in two separate studies. *N Engl J Med* 1974;291:1275–1278.
4. Marks V. The measurement of blood glucose and the definition of hypoglycemia. *Horm Metab Res* 1986[Suppl 6]:1–6.
5. Maran A, Lomas J, MacDonald IA, et al. Lack of preservation of higher brain function during hypoglycaemia in patients with intensively treated insulin dependent diabetes mellitus. *Diabetologia* 1995;38:1412–1418.
6. Heller SR, Cryer PE. Reduced neuroendocrine and symptomatic responses to subsequent hypoglycemia in non-diabetic humans. *Diabetes* 1991;40:223–226.
7. Whipple AO. Hyperinsulinism in relation to pancreatic tumour. *Surgery* 1944;16:289–298.
8. Epidemiology of severe hypoglycemia in the Diabetes Control and Complications Trial: the DCCT Research Group. *Am J Med* 1991;90:450–459.
9. Muller UA, Femerling M, Reinauer KM, et al. Intensified treatment and education of type 1 diabetes as clinical routine: a nationwide quality-circle experience in Germany—ASD (the Working Group on Structured Diabetes Therapy of the German Diabetes Association). *Diabetes Care* 1999;22[Suppl 2]:B29–B34.
10. Bolli G, DeFeo P, Campugnucci P, et al. Abnormal glucose counterregulation in insulin-dependent diabetes mellitus: interaction of anti-insulin antibodies and impaired glucagon secretion. *Diabetes* 1983;32:134–141.
11. Peacey SR, Rostami-Hodjegan A, George E, et al. The use of tolbutamide-induced hypoglycemia to examine the intraislet role of insulin in mediating glucagon release in normal humans. *J Clin Endocrinol Metab* 1997;82:1458–1461.
12. Landstedt-Hallin L, Adamson U, Lins PE. Oral glibenclamide suppresses glucagon secretion during insulin-induced hypoglycemia in patients with type 2 diabetes. *J Clin Endocrinol Metab* 1999;84:3140–3145.
13. Rizza RA, Cryer PE, Gerich JE. Role of glucagon, catecholamines, and growth hormone in human glucose counterregulation: effects of somatostatin and combined alpha- and beta-blockade on plasma glucose recovery and glucose flux rates following insulin induced hypoglycemia. *J Clin Invest* 1979;64:62–71.
14. Lee KU, Park JY, Kim CH, et al. Effect of decreasing plasma free fatty acids by acipimox on hepatic glucose metabolism in normal rats. *Metabolism* 1996;45:1408–1414.
15. Cersosimo E, Garlick P, Ferretti J. Renal substrate metabolism and gluconeogenesis during hypoglycemia in humans. *Diabetes* 2000;49:1186–1193.
16. Joseph SE, Heaton N, Potter D, et al. Renal glucose production compensates for the liver during the anhepatic phase of liver transplantation. *Diabetes* 2000;49:450–456.
17. Berne C, Fagius J. Metabolic regulation of sympathetic nervous system activity: lessons from intraneural nerve recordings. *Int J Obes Relat Metab Disord* 1993;17[Suppl 3]:S2–S6.
18. Peacey SR, George E, Rostami-Hodjegan A, et al. Similar physiological and symptomatic responses to sulphonylurea and insulin induced hypoglycaemia in normal subjects. *Diabet Med* 1996;13:634–641.
19. Ryder RE, Owens DR, Hayes DM, et al. Unawareness of hypoglycaemia and inadequate counterregulation: no causal relationship to diabetic autonomic neuropathy. *BMJ* 1990;301:783–787.
20. Gold AE, MacLeod KM, Frier BM. Frequency of severe hypoglycemia in patients with type I diabetes with impaired awareness of hypoglycemia. *Diabetes Care* 1994;17:697–703.
21. MacLeod KM, Hepburn DA, Frier BM. Frequency and morbidity of severe hypoglycaemia in insulin-treated diabetic patients. *Diabet Med* 1993;10:238–245.
22. Joslin EP. *Joslin's diabetes mellitus*. Philadelphia: Lea & Febiger, 1916.
23. Lawrence RD. Insulin hypoglycaemia: changes in nervous manifestations. *Lancet* 1941;2:602–604.
24. Deary IJ, Hepburn DA, MacLeod KM, et al. Partitioning the symptoms of hypoglycaemia using multi-sample confirmatory factor analysis. *Diabetologia* 1993;36:771–777.
25. McCrimmon RJ, Gold AE, Deary IJ, et al. Symptoms of hypoglycemia in children with IDDM. *Diabetes Care* 1995;18:858–861.
26. Wellhoener P, Fruehwald-Schultes B, Kern W, et al. Glucose metabolism rather than insulin is a main determinant of leptin secretion in humans. *J Clin Endocrinol Metab* 2000;85:1267–1271.
27. Cai XJ, Widdowson PS, Harrold J, et al. Hypothalamic orexin expression: modulation by blood glucose and feeding. *Diabetes* 1999;48:2132–2137.
28. White NH, Skor DA, Cryer PE, et al. Identification of type I diabetic patients at increased risk for hypoglycemia during intensive therapy. *N Engl J Med* 1983;308:485–491.
29. Amiel SA, Simonson DC, Tamborlane WV, et al. Rate of glucose fall does not affect counterregulatory hormone responses to hypoglycemia in normal and diabetic humans. *Diabetes* 1987;36:518–522.
30. Amiel SA, Sherwin RS, Simonson DC, et al. Effect of intensive insulin therapy on glycemic thresholds for counterregulatory hormone release. *Diabetes* 1988;37:901–907.
31. Boyle PJ, Schwartz NS, Shah SD, et al. Plasma glucose concentrations at the onset of hypoglycemic symptoms in patients with poorly controlled diabetes and in nondiabetics. *N Engl J Med* 1988;318:1487–1492.
32. Fanelli CG, Paramore DS, Hershey T, et al. Impact of nocturnal hypoglycemia on hypoglycemic cognitive dysfunction in type 1 diabetes. *Diabetes* 1998;47:1920–1927.
33. Mitrakou A, Ryan C, Veneman T, et al. Hierarchy of glycemic thresholds for counterregulatory hormone secretion, symptoms, and cerebral dysfunction. *Am J Physiol* 1991;260:E67–E74.
34. Korzon-Burakowska A, Hopkins D, Matyka K, et al. Effects of glycemic control on protective responses against hypoglycemia in type 2 diabetes mellitus. *Diabetes Care* 1998;21:282–291.
35. Amiel SA. Cognitive function testing in studies of acute hypoglycaemia: rights and wrongs? *Diabetologia* 1998;41:713–719.
36. Heller S, Chapman J, McCloud J, et al. Unreliability of reports of hypoglycaemia by diabetic patients. *BMJ* 1995;310:440.
37. Lager I, Attvall S, Blohme G, et al. Altered recognition of hypoglycaemic symptoms in type I diabetes during intensified control with continuous subcutaneous insulin infusion. *Diabet Med* 1986;3:322–325.
38. Egger M, Davey Smith G, Stettler C, et al. Risk of adverse effects of intensified treatment in insulin-dependent diabetes mellitus: a meta-analysis. *Diabet Med* 1997;14:919–928.
39. Amiel SA, Tamborlane WV, Simonson DC, et al. Defective glucose counterregulation after strict glycemic control of insulin-dependent diabetes mellitus. *N Engl J Med* 1987;316:1376–1383.
40. Borg MA, Sherwin RS, Borg WP, et al. Local ventromedial hypothalamus glucose perfusion blocks counterregulation during systemic hypoglycemia in awake rats. *J Clin Invest* 1997;99:361–365.
41. Borg WP, Sherwin RS, During MJ, et al. Local ventromedial hypothalamus glucopenia triggers counterregulatory hormone release. *Diabetes* 1995;44:180–184.
42. Silver IA, Erecinska M. Glucose-induced intracellular ion changes in sugar-sensitive hypothalamic neurons. *J Neurophysiol* 1998;79:1733–1745.
43. Fery F, Plat L, van de Borne P, et al. Impaired counterregulation of glucose in a patient with hypothalamic sarcoidosis. *N Engl J Med* 1999;340:852–856.
44. Hevener AL, Bergman RN, Donovan CM. Novel glucosensor for hypoglycemic detection localized to the portal vein. *Diabetes* 1997;46:1521–1525.
45. Hevener AL, Bergman RN, Donovan CM. Portal vein afferents are critical for the sympathoadrenal response to hypoglycemia. *Diabetes* 2000;49:8–12.
46. Smith D, Pernet A, Reid H, et al. The role of hepatic portal vein glucose sensing in modulating responses to hypoglycaemia. *Diabetologia* 2002;45:1416–1424.
47. Amiel SA, Archibald HR, Chusney G, et al. Ketone infusion lowers hormonal responses to hypoglycaemia: evidence for acute cerebral utilization of a non-glucose fuel. *Clin Sci* 1991;81:189–194.
48. Maran A, Cranston I, Lomas J, et al. Protection by lactate of cerebral function during hypoglycaemia. *Lancet* 1994;343:16–20.
49. Veneman T, Mitrakou A, Mokan M, et al. Effect of hyperketonemia and hyperlacticacidemia on symptoms, cognitive dysfunction and counterregu-

latory hormone responses during hypoglycemia in normal humans. *Diabetes* 1994;43:1311–1317.
50. Kumagai AK, Kang YS, Boado RJ, et al. Upregulation of blood-brain barrier GLUT1 glucose transporter protein and mRNA in experimental chronic hypoglycemia. *Diabetes* 1995;44:1399–1404.
51. Duelli R, Staudt R, Duembgen L, Kuschinsky W. Increase in glucose transporter densities of Glut3 and decrease of glucose utilization in rat brain after one week of hypoglycemia. *Brain Res* 1999;831:254–262.
52. McCall AL, Fixman LB, Fleming N, et al. Chronic hypoglycemia increases brain glucose transport. *Am J Physiol* 1986;251:E442–447.
53. Boyle PJ, Kempers SF, O'Connor AM, et al. Brain glucose uptake and unawareness of hypoglycemia in patients with insulin dependent diabetes mellitus. *N Engl J Med* 1995;333:1726–1731.
54. Boyle PJ, Nagy RJ, O'Connor AM, et al. Adaptation in brain glucose uptake following recurrent hypoglycemia. *Proc Natl Acad Sci U S A* 1994;91: 9352–9356.
55. Cryer PE, Scott A, Segal MD, et al. Blood brain glucose transport is not increased following hypoglycemia. *Diabetes* 2000;39[Suppl 1].
56. Cranston IC, Reed LJ, Marsden PK, Amiel SA. Changes in the regional brain ^{18}F-Fluorodeoxyglucose uptake at hypoglycemia in type 1 diabetic men associated with hypogylcemia unawareness and counter regulatory failures. *Diabetes* 2001;50:2329-2336.
57. Evans M, Amiel SA. Carbohydrates as a cerebral metabolic fuel. *J Paediatr Endocrinol Metab* 1998:11[Suppl 1]:99–102.
58. Tkacs NC, Dunn-Meynell AA, Levin BE Presumed apoptosis and reduced arcuate nucleus neuropeptide Y and pro-opiomelanocortin mRNA in non-coma hypoglycemia. *Diabetes* 2000;49:820–826.
59. Davis SN, Shavers C, Costa F, et al. Role of cortisol in the pathogenesis of deficient counterregulation after antecedent hypoglycemia in normal humans. *J Clin Invest* 1996;98:680–689.
60. Davis SN, Shavers C, Davis B, et al. Prevention of an increase in plasma cortisol during hypoglycemia preserves subsequent counterregulatory responses. *J Clin Invest* 1997;100:429–438.
61. Davis SN, Shavers C, Mosqueda-Garcia R, et al. Effects of differing antecedent hypoglycemia on subsequent counterregulation in normal humans. *Diabetes* 1997;46:1328–1335.
62. George E, Harris N, Bedford C, et al. Prolonged but partial impairment of the hypoglycaemic physiological response following short-term hypoglycaemia in normal subjects. *Diabetologia* 1995;38:1183–1190.
63. Hvidberg A, Fanelli CG, Hershey T, et al. Impact of recent antecedent hypoglycemia on hypoglycemic cognitive dysfunction in nondiabetic humans. *Diabetes* 1996;45:1030–1036.
64. Ovalle F, Fanelli CG, Paramore DS, et al. Brief twice-weekly episodes of hypoglycemia reduce detection of clinical hypoglycemia in type 1 diabetes mellitus. *Diabetes* 1998;47:1472–1479.
65. Fanelli CG, Paramore DS, Hershey T, et al. Impact of nocturnal hypoglycemia on hypoglycemic cognitive dysfunction in type 1 diabetes. *Diabetes* 1998;47:1920–1927.
66. Fanelli CG, Epifano L, Rambotti AM, et al. Meticulous prevention of hypoglycemia normalizes the glycemic thresholds and magnitude of most of neuroendocrine responses to, symptoms of, and cognitive function during hypoglycemia in intensively treated patients with short-term IDDM. *Diabetes* 1993;42:1683–1689.
67. Cranston I, Lomas J, Maran A, et al. Restoration of hypoglycaemia awareness in patients with long-duration insulin-dependent diabetes. *Lancet* 1994; 344:283–287.
68. Berlin I, Grimaldi A, Landault C, et al. Lack of hypoglycemic symptoms and decreased beta-adrenergic sensitivity in insulin-dependent diabetic patients. *J Clin Endocrinol Metab* 1988;66:273–278.
69. Fritsche A, Stumvoll M, Grub M, et al. Effect of hypoglycemia on beta-adrenergic sensitivity in normal and type 1 diabetic subjects. *Diabetes Care* 1998;21:1505–1510.
70. Dagogo-Jack S, Rattarasarn C, Cryer PE. Reversal of hypoglycemia unawareness, but not defective glucose counterregulation, in IDDM. *Diabetes* 1994;43:1426–1434.
71. Meyer C, Grossmann R, Mitrakou A, et al. Effects of autonomic neuropathy on counterregulation and awareness of hypoglycemia in type 1 diabetic patients. *Diabetes Care* 1998;21:1960–1966.
72. Stephenson JM, Kempler P, Perin PC, et al. Is autonomic neuropathy a risk factor for severe hypoglycaemia? The EURODIAB IDDM Complications Study. *Diabetologia* 1996;39:1372–1376.
73. Dejgaard A, Andersen P, Hvidberg A, et al. Increased cardiovascular, metabolic, and hormonal responses to noradrenaline in diabetic patients with autonomic neuropathy. *Diabet Med* 1996;13:983–989.
74. Fanelli C, Pampanelli S, Lalli C, et al. Long-term intensive therapy of IDDM patients with clinically overt autonomic neuropathy: effects on hypoglycemia awareness and counterregulation. *Diabetes* 1997;46:1172–1181.
75. Pedersen-Bjergaard U, Agerholm-Larsen B, Pramming S, et al. Prediction of severe hypoglycemia by angiotensin-converting enzyme activity and genotype in type 1 diabetes. *Diabetologia* 2003;46:89–96.
76. Orre-Pettersson AC, Lindstrom T, Bergmark V, et al. The snack is critical for the blood glucose profile during treatment with regular insulin preprandially. *J Intern Med* 1999;245:41–45.
77. Kong N, Ryder RE. What is the role of between meal snacks with intensive basal bolus regimens using preprandial lispro? *Diabet Med* 1999;16:325–331.
78. Ronnemaa T, Viikari J Reducing snacks when switching from conventional soluble to lispro insulin treatment: effects on glycaemic control and hypoglycaemia. *Diabet Med* 1998;15:601–607.
79. The DAFNE study group. A randomized control trial of training and intensive insulin management to enable dietary freedom in people with type 1 diabetes: The DAFNE (Dose Adjustment for Non Eating) trial. *BMJ* 2002;13:197–204.
80. Gale EA, Tattersall RB. Unrecognised nocturnal hypoglycaemia in insulin-treated diabetics. *Lancet* 1979;19:1049–1052.
81. Porter PA, Keating B, Byrne G, et al. Incidence and predictive criteria of nocturnal hypoglycemia in young children with insulin-dependent diabetes mellitus. *J Pediatr* 1997;130:366–372.
82. Matyka KA, Wigg L, Pramming S, et al. Cognitive function and mood after profound nocturnal hypoglycaemia in prepubertal children with conventional insulin treatment for diabetes. *Arch Dis Child* 1999;81:138–142.
83. Porter PA, Byrne G, Stick S, et al. Nocturnal hypoglycaemia and sleep disturbances in young teenagers with insulin dependent diabetes mellitus. *Arch Dis Child* 1996;75:120–123.
84. Jones TW, Porter P, Sherwin RS, et al. Decreased epinephrine responses to hypoglycemia during sleep. *N Engl J Med* 1998;338:1657–1662.
85. Matyka KA, Crowne EC, Havel PJ, et al. Counterregulation during spontaneous nocturnal hypoglycemia in prepubertal children with type 1 diabetes. *Diabetes Care* 1999;22:1144–1150.
86. Bendtson I, Gade J, Theilgaard A, et al. Cognitive function in type 1 (insulin-dependent) diabetic patients after nocturnal hypoglycaemia. *Diabetologia* 1992;35:898–903.
87. Tunbridge FK, Newens A, Home PD, et al. Double-blind crossover trial of isophane (NPH)- and lente-based insulin regimens. *Diabetes Care* 1989;12: 115–119.
88. George E, Bedford C, Peacey SR, et al. Further evidence for a high incidence of nocturnal hypoglycaemia in IDDM: no effect of dose for dose transfer between human and porcine insulins. *Diabet Med* 1997;14:442–448.
89. Fanelli CP, Pamparelli F, Porcellati F, et al. Administration of Nutral, Protamine Hagedorn insulin at bedtime versus with dinner in type 1 diabetes mellitus to avoid nocturnal hypoglycemia and improve control; a randomized clinical trial. *Ann Intern Med* 2002:136:504–514.
90. Kanc K, Janssen MM, Keulen ET, et al. Substitution of night-time continuous subcutaneous insulin infusion therapy for bedtime NPH insulin in a multiple injection regimen improves counterregulatory hormonal responses and warning symptoms of hypoglycaemia in IDDM. *Diabetologia* 1998;41:322–329.
91. Ratner RE, Hirsch IB, Neifing JL, et al. Less hypoglycemia with insulin glargine in intensive insulin therapy for type 1 diabetes: U.S. Study Group of Insulin Glargine in Type 1 Diabetes. *Diabetes Care* 2000;23:639–643.
92. Russell-Jones D, Simpson R, Hylleberg B, et al. Effects of QD insulin detemir or neutral protamine Hagedorn on blood glucose control in patients with type I diabetes mellitus using a basal-bolus regimen. *Clin Ther* 2004;26: 724–736.
93. Pieber TR, Eugene-Jolchine I, et al. Efficacy and safety of HOE 901 versus NPH insulin in patients with type 1 diabetes: the European Study Group of HOE 901 in Type 1 Diabetes. *Diabetes Care* 2000;23:157–162.
94. Shalwitz RA, Farkas-Hirsch R, et al. Prevalence and consequences of nocturnal hypoglycemia among conventionally treated children with diabetes mellitus. *J Pediatr* 1990;116:685–689.
95. Beregszaszi M, Tubiana-Rufi N, Benali K, et al. Nocturnal hypoglycemia in children and adolescents with insulin-dependent diabetes mellitus: prevalence and risk factors. *J Pediatr* 1997;131:27–33.
96. Heller SR, Amiel SA, Mansell P. Effect of the fast-acting insulin analog lispro on the risk of nocturnal hypoglycemia during intensified insulin therapy: U.K. Lispro Study Group. *Diabetes Care* 1999;22:1607–1611.
97. Ahmed AB, Home PD. The effect of the insulin analog lispro on nighttime blood glucose control in type 1 diabetic patients. *Diabetes Care* 1998;21:32–37.
98. Mohn A, Matyka KA, Harris DA, et al. Lispro or regular insulin for multiple injection therapy in adolescence: differences in free insulin and glucose levels overnight. *Diabetes Care* 1999;22:27–32.
99. Kaufman FR, Halvorson M, Kaufman ND. A randomized, blinded trial of uncooked cornstarch to diminish nocturnal hypoglycemia at diabetes camp. *Diabetes Res Clin Pract* 1995;30:205–209.
100. Saleh TY, Cryer PE. Alanine and terbutaline in the prevention of nocturnal hypoglycemia in IDDM. *Diabetes Care* 1997;20:1231–1236.
101. Hvidberg A, Rosenfalck A, Christensen NJ, et al. Long-term administration of theophylline and glucose recovery after hypoglycaemia in patients with type 1 diabetes mellitus. *Diabet Med* 1998;15:608–614.
102. Gale EA, Kurtz AB, Tattersall RB. In search of the Somogyi effect. *Lancet* 1980;2:279–282.
103. Bolli GB, Gottesman IS, Campbell PJ, et al. Glucose counterregulation and waning of insulin in the Somogyi phenomenon (posthypoglycemic hyperglycemia). *N Engl J Med* 1984;311:1214–1219.
104. Fowelin J, Attvall S, von Schenck H, et al. Postprandial hyperglycaemia following a morning hypoglycaemia in type 1 diabetes mellitus. *Diabet Med* 1990;7:156–161.
105. Attvall S, Ericksson BM, Fowelin J, et al. Early post-hypoglycemic insulin resistance in man is mainly an effect of β adrenergic stimulation. *J Clin Invest* 1987;80:437–442.
106. Fanelli CG, De Feo P, Porcellati F, et al. Adrenergic mechanisms contribute to the late phase of hypoglycemic glucose counterregulation in humans by stimulating lipolysis. *J Clin Invest* 1992;89:2005–2013.

107. Fowelin J, Attvall S, von Schenck H, et al. Characterization of the insulin-antagonistic effect of growth hormone in insulin-dependent diabetes mellitus. *Diabet Med* 1995;12:990–996.
108. Amiel SA, Simonson DC, Sherwin RS, et al. Exaggerated epinephrine responses to hypoglycemia in normal and insulin dependent diabetic children. *J Pediatr* 1987;110:832–837.
109. Amiel SA, Tamborlane WV, Simonson DC, et al. Impaired insulin action in puberty: a contributing factor to poor glycemic control in adolescents with diabetes. *N Engl J Med* 1986;315:215–219.
110. Cox D, Gonder-Frederick L, Schlundt D, et al. Recent hypoglycemia influences probability of subsequent hypoglycemia in type 1 patients. *Diabetes* 1993;42[Suppl 1]:126A.
111. UK Prospective Diabetes Study Group. Intensive blood glucose control with sulphonylureas or insulin compared with conventional therapy and risk of complications in patients with type 2 diabetes mellitus: UKPDS 33. *Lancet* 1998;352:837–853.
112. Chan TY Lee KK, Chan AW, et al. Utilization of antidiabetic drugs in Hong Kong: relation to the common occurrence of antidiabetic drug induced hypoglycemia amongst acute medical admissions and the relative prevalence of NIDDM. *Int J Clin Pharmacol Ther* 1996;34:43–46.
113. Tessier D, Dawson K, Tervault JP, et al. Glibenclamide vs gliclazide in type 2 diabetes of the elderly. *Diabet Med* 1994;11:974–980.
114. Shorr RI, Ray WA, Daugherty JR, et al. Individual sulfonylureas and serious hypoglycemia in older people. *J Am Geriatr Soc* 1996;44:751–755.
115. Wolffenbuttel BH, Landgraf R. A 1-year multicenter randomized double-blind comparison of repaglinide and glyburide for the treatment of type 2 diabetes: Dutch and German Repaglinide Study Group. *Diabetes Care* 1999;22:463–467.
116. Marker JC, Cryer PE, Clutter WE. Attenuated glucose recovery from hypoglycemia in the elderly. *Diabetes* 1993;41:671–678.
117. Meneilly GC, Cheung E, Tuokko H. Altered responses to hypoglycemia of healthy elderly people. *J Clin Endocrinol Metab* 1994;78:1341–1348.
118. Ortiz-Alonso FJ, Gaelecki A, Herman WH, et al. Hypoglycemia counterregulation in elderly humans: relationship to blood glucose levels. *Am J Physiol* 1994;267:E497–E506.
119. Brierley EJ, Broughton DL, James OFW, et al. Reduced awareness of hypoglycaemia in the elderly despite an intact counterregulatory response. *Q J Med* 1995;88:439–445.
120. Matyka K, Evans M, Lomas J, et al. Altered hierarchy of protective responses against severe hypoglycemia in normal aging in healthy men. *Diabetes Care* 1997;20:135–141.
121. Korzon-Burakowska A, Hopkins D, Matyka K, et al. Effects of glycemic control on protective responses against hypoglycemia in type 2 diabetes mellitus. *Diabetes Care* 1998;21:282–291.
122. Jaap AJ, Jones GC, McCrimmon RJ, et al. Perceived symptoms of hypoglycaemia in elderly type 2 diabetic patients treated with insulin. *Diabet Med* 1998;15:398–401.
123. Casey A, Mann R, Banister K, et al. Effect of carbohydrate ingestion on glycogen resynthesis in human liver and skeletal muscle, measured by (13)C MRS. *Am J Physiol Endocrinol Metab* 2000;278:E65–E75.
124. Krssak M, Petersen KF, Bergeron R, et al. Intramuscular glycogen and intramyocellular lipid utilization during prolonged exercise and recovery in man: a 13C and 1H nuclear magnetic resonance spectroscopy study. *J Clin Endocrinol Metab* 2000;85:748–754.
125. Koivisto VA, Sane T, Fyhrquist F, et al. Fuel and fluid homeostasis during long-term exercise in healthy subjects and type I diabetic patients. *Diabetes Care* 1992;15:1736–1741.
126. Sane T, Helve E, Pelkonen R, et al. The adjustment of diet and insulin dose during long-term endurance exercise in type 1 (insulin-dependent) diabetic men. *Diabetologia* 1988;31:35–40.
127. Lazarus R, Sparrow D, Weiss ST. Alcohol intake and insulin levels: the Normative Aging Study. *Am J Epidemiol* 1997;145:909–916.
128. Kerr D, MacDonald IA, Heller SR, et al. Alcohol causes hypoglycaemic unawareness in healthy volunteers and patients with type 1 (insulin-dependent) diabetes. *Diabetologia* 1990;33:216–221.
129. Flanagan D, Wood P, Sherwin R, et al. Gin and tonic and reactive hypoglycemia: what is important—the gin, the tonic, or both? *J Clin Endocrinol Metab* 1998;83:796–800.
130. Kerr D, MacDonald IA, Heller SR, et al. Beta-adrenoceptor blockade and hypoglycaemia: a randomised, double-blind, placebo controlled comparison of metoprolol CR, atenolol and propranolol LA in normal subjects. *Br J Clin Pharmacol* 1990;29:685–693.
131. Herings RM, de Boer A, Stricker BH, et al. Hypoglycaemia associated with use of inhibitors of angiotensin converting enzyme. *Lancet* 1995;345: 1195–1198.
132. Thamer M, Ray NF, Taylor T. Association between antihypertensive drug use and hypoglycemia: a case-control study of diabetic users of insulin or sulfonylureas. *Clin Ther* 1999;21:1387–1400.
133. Shorr RI, Ray WA, Daugherty JR, et al. Antihypertensives and the risk of serious hypoglycemia in older persons using insulin or sulfonylureas. *JAMA* 1997;278:40–43.
134. Effects of ramipril on cardiovascular and microvascular outcomes in people with diabetes mellitus: results of the HOPE study and MICRO-HOPE substudy: Heart Outcomes Prevention Evaluation Study Investigators. *Lancet* 2000;355:253–259.
135. Dimitriadis G, Baker B, Marsh H, et al. Effect of thyroid hormone excess on action, secretion, and metabolism of insulin in humans. *Am J Physiol* 1985; 248:E593–601.
136. Airey CM, Williams DR, Martin PG, et al. Hypoglycaemia induced by exogenous insulin—'human' and animal insulin compared. *Diabet Med* 2000;17: 416–432.
137. Collier A, Steedman DJ, Patrick AW, et al. Comparison of intravenous glucagon and dextrose in the treatment of severe hypoglycemia in the accident and emergency department. *Diabetes Care* 1987;10:712–715.
138. Koren I, Shalitin S, Vardi P. Hazardous outcome of treating hypoglycemia with 50% IV infusion. *Diabetologia* 2000;43[Suppl 1]:A195.
139. Bode BW, Steed RD, David PC. Reduction in severe hypoglycemia with long term subcutaneous insulin infusion in type 1 diabetes. *Diabetes Care* 1996; 19:324–327.
140. Rodrigues IAS, Reed HA, Ismail K, Amiel SA. Indications and efficacy of continuous subcutaneous insulin infusion (CSII) therapy in type 1 diabetes mellitus: in clinical warded. *Diabet Med* 2004 (in press).
141. Ryan EA, Shandro T, Green K, et al. Assessment of the severity of hypoglycemia and glycemic lability in type 1 diabetic subjects undergoing islet transplantation. *Diabetes* 2004;53:955–962.
142. Eadington DW, Frier BM. Accident risk of the diabetic driver. *Diabetes Care* 1989;12:597.
143. MacLeod KM. Diabetes and driving: towards equitable, evidence-based decision-making. *Diabet Med* 1999;16:282–290.
144. Evans ML, Pernet A, Lomas J, et al. Delay in onset of awareness of acute hypoglycemia and of restoration of cognitive performance during recovery. *Diabetes Care* 2000;23:893–897.
145. Cooper AJ. Attempted suicide using insulin by a non-diabetic: a case study demonstrating the acute and chronic consequences of profound hypoglycemia. *Can J Psychol* 1994;39:103–107.
146. Shintani S, Tsuruoka S, Shiigai T. Hypoglycaemic hemiplegia: a repeat SPECT study. *J Neurol Neurosurg Psychol* 1993;56:700–701.
147. Pococco M, Ronfani L. Transient focal neurological deficits associated with hypoglycemia in children with insulin dependent diabetes mellitus. *Acta Paediatr* 1998;87:542–544.
148. Deary IJ, Crawford JR, Hepburn DA, et al. Severe hypoglycemia and intelligence in adult patients with insulin-treated diabetes. *Diabetes* 1993;42: 341–344.
149. Langan SJ, Deary IJ, Hepburn DA, et al. Cumulative cognitive impairment following recurrent severe hypoglycaemia in adult patients with insulin-treated diabetes mellitus. *Diabetologia* 1991;34:337–344.
150. Sachon C, Grimaldi A, Digy JP, et al. Cognitive function, insulin-dependent diabetes and hypoglycaemia. *J Intern Med* 1992;231:471–475.
151. Kramer L, Fasching P, Madl C. Previous episodes of hypoglycemic coma are not associated with permanent cognitive brain dysfunction in IDDM patients on intensive insulin treatment. *Diabetes* 1998;47:1909–1914.
152. Ryan CM, Williams TM, Finegold DN, et al. Cognitive dysfunction in adults with type 1 (insulin-dependent) diabetes mellitus of long duration: effects of recurrent hypoglycaemia and other chronic complications. *Diabetologia* 1993;36:329–334.
153. Skenazy J, Bigler ED. Neuropsychological findings in diabetes mellitus. *J Clin Psychol* 1984;40:246–258.
154. Perros P, Deary IJ, Sellar RJ, et al. Brain abnormalities demonstrated by magnetic resonance imaging in adult IDDM patients with and without a history of recurrent severe hypoglycemia. *Diabetes Care* 1997;20:1013–1018.
155. Holmes CS, Tsalikian E, Yamada T. Blood glucose control and visual and auditory attention in men with insulin dependent diabetes. *Diabet Med* 1988;5:634–639.
156. Gold AE, Deary IJ, Jones RW, et al. Severe deterioration in cognitive function and personality in five patients with long-standing diabetes: a complication of diabetes or a consequence of treatment? *Diabet Med* 1994;11:499–505.
157. Effects of intensive diabetes therapy on neuropsychological function in adults in the Diabetes Control and Complications Trial. *Ann Intern Med* 1996;124:379–388.
158. Austin EJ, Deary IJ. Effects of repeated hypoglycemia on cognitive function: a psychometrically validated reanalysis of the Diabetes Control and Complications Trial data. *Diabetes Care* 1999;22:1273–1277.
159. Rovet J, Alvarez M. Attentional functioning in children and adolescents with IDDM. *Diabetes Care* 1997;20:803–810.
160. Edge JA, Ford-Adams ME, Dunger DB. Causes of death in children with insulin dependent diabetes 1990–96. *Arch Dis Child* 1999;81:318–323.
161. Laing SP, Swerdlow AJ, Slater SD, et al. The British Diabetic Association Cohort Study, I: all-cause mortality in patients with insulin-treated diabetes mellitus. *Diabet Med* 1999;16:459–465.
162. Tattersall RB, Gill GV. Unexplained deaths of type 1 diabetic patients. *Diabet Med* 1991;8:49–58.
163. Marques JL, George E, Peacey SR, et al. Altered ventricular repolarization during hypoglycaemia in patients with diabetes. *Diabet Med* 1997;14:648–654.
164. Landstedt-Hallin L, Englund A, Adamson U, et al. Increased QT dispersion during hypoglycaemia in patients with type 2 diabetes mellitus. *J Intern Med* 1999;246:299–307.

CHAPTER 41

Management of Hyperglycemia with Oral Antihyperglycemic Agents in Type 2 Diabetes

Harold E. Lebovitz

The management of hyperglycemia in patients with diabetes has changed significantly during the past several years as a result of numerous advances in our knowledge about the disorder and the application of this knowledge to the development of new strategies and treatments.

The quantitative relationship between glycemic control and the chronic microvascular, neuropathic, and macrovascular complications of diabetes have been defined by large long-term clinical studies in individuals with type 1 and type 2 diabetes (1–3). A clearer understanding of the physiologic mechanisms involved in regulating glucose metabolism has provided the basis for a more detailed analysis of the different pathophysiologic processes causing hyperglycemia (4–7). Methods for regulating fasting glycemia can be differentiated from methods for regulating postprandial hyperglycemia (8,9). New classes of antihyperglycemic agents are available that provide the means for selectively ameliorating the different mechanisms that cause hyperglycemia (10,11). Long-term follow-up data are sufficient to demonstrate that type 2 diabetes is a progressive disease and that therapy must change with disease progression (12). Combinations of oral antihyperglycemic agents or of oral antihyperglycemic agents and insulin are frequently necessary to achieve appropriate glycemic goals (13, 14). The impacts of the various classes of antihyperglycemic agents on cardiovascular risk factors have been established and are an important consideration in deciding which agents to use in a particular patient (15,16).

Effective management of hyperglycemia requires utilization of all of this new information. Initial evaluation of a patient requires establishment of the goals of therapy for that patient. Diabetes education reinforces those goals and helps the patient learn techniques and behavior that can help achieve those goals. The evaluation must include an assessment of whether the patient has the metabolic syndrome and, if so, which components of the syndrome. The selection of initial pharmacologic therapy is determined by these initial evaluations. Long-term management requires intermittent re-evaluation of the progression of the disease process and modification of the therapy to adjust to this changing pathophysiology. Effective use of current therapeutic agents and techniques can result in near normoglycemic control in most patients with type 2 diabetes.

GLYCEMIC GOALS OF THERAPY

A variety of approaches are used to define the goals for glycemic control in patients with diabetes. The levels achieved and shown to decrease chronic complications in intervention studies such as the Diabetes Control and Complications Trial (DCCT) in patients with type 1 diabetes or the United Kingdom Prospective Diabetes Study (UKPDS) in patients with type 2 diabetes can define the goals (1–3). In those studies, the intensively treated patients achieved mean or median hemoglobin A_{1c} (HbA_{1c}) levels approaching 7.0%. These levels were attainable in a large cohort of patients and significantly reduced, but did not prevent, chronic complications.

Another approach in defining the goal is to determine if there is a threshold of glycemic control only above which chronic complications occur. An analysis of the relationship between the mean HbA_{1c} and the development of retinopathy, nephropathy, or neuropathy in the entire DCCT cohort showed that there was no glycemic threshold short of normal glycemia throughout the entire range of HbA_{1c} (17). The data for sustained progression of retinopathy (Fig. 41.1) showed a constant 39% reduction in risk for each 10% reduction in absolute HbA_{1c}

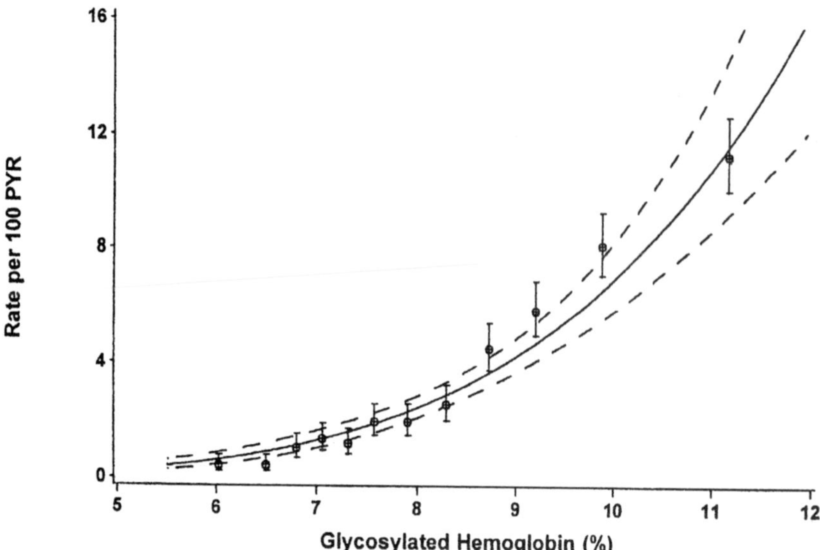

FIG. 41.1. Outcome data from the Diabetes Control and Complications Trial (DCCT) on the relationship between the risk of sustained progression of retinopathy and the mean HbA_{1c}. There is no glycemic threshold for retinopathy development and progression. Retinopathy progression decreased 39% for every 10% reduction in mean HbA_{1c} percentage. (Copyright © 1996 American Diabetes Association. From DCCT Research Group: The absence of a glycemic threshold for the development of long-term complications: the perspective of the Diabetes Control and Complications Trial. *Diabetes* 1996;45:1289–1298. Reprinted with permission from the American Diabetes Association.)

values (17). The epidemiologic data from the entire UKPDS similarly showed no glycemic threshold for either microvascular or macrovascular complications (Fig. 41.2) (18).

The lack of a glycemic threshold short of normal glycemia indicates that any level of increased glycemia, as well as the duration of the increase, can result in chronic complications. These data suggest that the goal for glycemic control in patients with diabetes should be levels as close to normal as possible, provided that they can be achieved without causing unacceptable side effects. For the standard HbA_{1c} assay, normoglycemia is considered to be less than 6.0%. Obviously, other clinical factors need to be considered in determining the glycemic goal for a particular individual. The age of the individual and life expectancy are important, because the benefits of glycemic control are greatest in those who live long enough to benefit from reduced complications. The achievement of very good glycemic control requires a motivated, educated, and cooperative patient.

Although identification of the ideal glycemic goal is near-normal glycemia, it is equally important to recognize that any improvement in glycemic control decreases complication rates. Because the complication rate increases nonlinearly with the HbA_{1c}, a 10% reduction in HbA_{1c} from 11% to 9.9% results in a reduction in risk of progression of retinopathy of 6.57 cases per 100 patient years (17). In contrast, a decrease from 8.0% to 7.2% reduces the risk by 0.95 cases per 100 patient years (17). Table 41.1 highlights the 9-year cumulative incidence of development of retinopathy progression or microalbuminuria in patients with type 1 diabetes at mean HbA_{1c} levels ranging from 6% to 8% (17).

In summary, the glycemic goal that can be readily achieved with an acceptable level of side effects is an HbA_{1c} of 7.0%. However, in young patients and in those who are not limited by side effects, a goal of 6.0% would appear to be more acceptable. While any improvement in HbA_{1c} is worthwhile, a level in the range of 7.0% or lower should be sought.

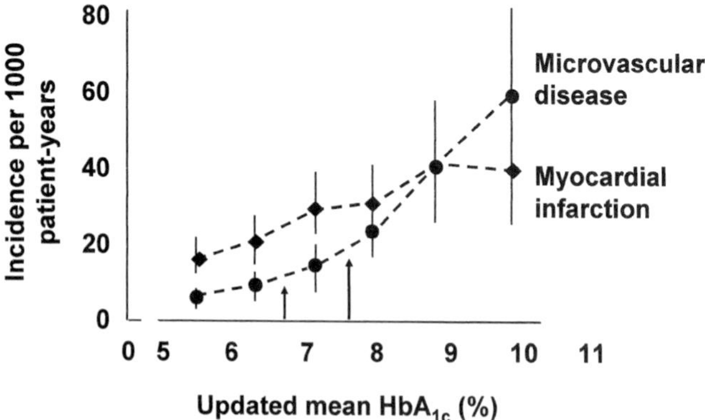

FIG. 41.2. Epidemiologic analyses of the relationships between mean HbA_{1c} over 11 years and the incidence of microvascular and macrovascular complications in the United Kingdom Prospective Diabetes Study (UKPDS). There was no glycemic threshold for either macrovascular or microvascular complications. (From Stratton IM, Adler AI, Neil HA, et al. Association of glycemia with macrovascular and microvascular complications of type 2 diabetes (UKPDS 35): prospective observational study. *BMJ* 2000;321:405–412, with permission.)

TABLE 41.1. Cumulative Incidence Rates Among Patients in the Diabetes Control and Complications Trial of Developing Complications over a 9-year Period as a Function of Mean HbA_{1c} Values

Mean HbA_{1c} value (%)	Cumulative incidence of retinopathy progression (%)	Cumulative incidence of risk of microalbuminuria (%)
8.0	20.0	26.0
7.0	11.0	19.0
6.0	5.5	13.0

Data from The absence of a glycemic threshold for the development of long-term complications: the perspective of the Diabetes Control and Complications Trial. *Diabetes* 1996;45:1289–1298.

FASTING VERSUS POSTPRANDIAL HYPERGLYCEMIA

Fasting plasma glucose (FPG) levels are determined primarily by hepatic and, to a lesser degree, by renal glucose production (4, 19,20). As the plasma glucose levels decrease during fasting, plasma insulin levels decrease proportionately. The decrease in plasma insulin causes an increase in adipose tissue lipolysis and skeletal muscle proteolysis and a decrease in uptake of glucose by peripheral tissue (21). At the level of the liver, the carbon skeleton from amino acids from muscle proteolysis serves as substrate and the free fatty acids from adipose tissue serve as energy source for the production of glucose. Glucose from glycogenolysis and gluconeogenesis provides the energy source for the nervous system, which has an insulin-independent requirement for glucose. Peripheral tissues use free fatty acids and ketones as their energy source. The plasma glucose level is determined by the rate of glucose production from the liver and kidney, because the rate of glucose utilization by the peripheral insulin-independent tissues is fixed. Normally, the plasma insulin level stabilizes at a level in which glucose production equals non–insulin-dependent uptake of glucose. Fasting hyperglycemia occurs when glucose production exceeds glucose utilization, as occurs with absolute or relative insulin deficiency at the level of the liver.

Postprandial plasma levels of glucose are determined in the initial phase by meal-mediated suppression of hepatic production of glucose and throughout the postprandial period by hepatic and muscle uptake of glucose (19,22). Glucose uptake requires higher plasma levels of insulin (such as those normally generated by meals) than does suppression of hepatic production of glucose. The regulation of postprandial plasma glucose therefore is highly dependent on the qualitative and quantitative aspects of meal-mediated insulin secretion, as well as by the sensitivity of muscle to insulin action (8). These phenomena account for the differential regulation of fasting and postprandial glucose that occurs in diabetes in general and in type 2 diabetes in particular.

There are many potential consequences of the differential regulation of fasting and postprandial plasma glucose levels. Postprandial hyperglycemia occurs several years before fasting hyperglycemia and is the initial phase of glucose intolerance. Contributions of postprandial hyperglycemia to the overall glycemic control, as estimated by the HbA_{1c}, will vary with the individual and the stage of glucose intolerance (23). Some data suggest that spikes in glucose excursion may have different quantitative effects on the metabolic mechanisms involved in the pathogenesis of chronic complications (24,25). Pharmacologic agents may differentially affect fasting and postprandial hyperglycemia (10,26,27). Near-normal glycemia cannot be achieved unless both fasting and postprandial hyperglycemia are controlled.

STAGES OF TYPE 2 DIABETES

Type 2 diabetes is the end stage of a process that involves progressive loss of pancreatic β-cell function (Fig. 41.3) (12). The initial phase of this process in the majority of patients is the development of insulin resistance (28,29). Studies of low-birth-weight infants indicate that insulin resistance can be recognized in children as young as 8 years of age (30). The normal compensatory response to insulin resistance is increased insulin secretion and compensatory hyperinsulinemia. As long as the compensatory hyperinsulinemia is sufficient to overcome the insulin resistance, fasting and postprandial plasma glucose levels remain normal. If the individual with insulin resistance has the genetic predisposition to develop type 2 diabetes, the abnormalities in the pancreatic β-cell will cause a progressive loss of insulin secretory function and a loss of first-phase insulin release (31,32). This results initially in impaired glucose tolerance (IGT) and subsequently in type 2 diabetes with only postprandial hyperglycemia (23). As pancreatic β-cell function continues to deteriorate, not only does postprandial insulin secretion become inadequate, so does basal insulin secretion, and fasting hyper-

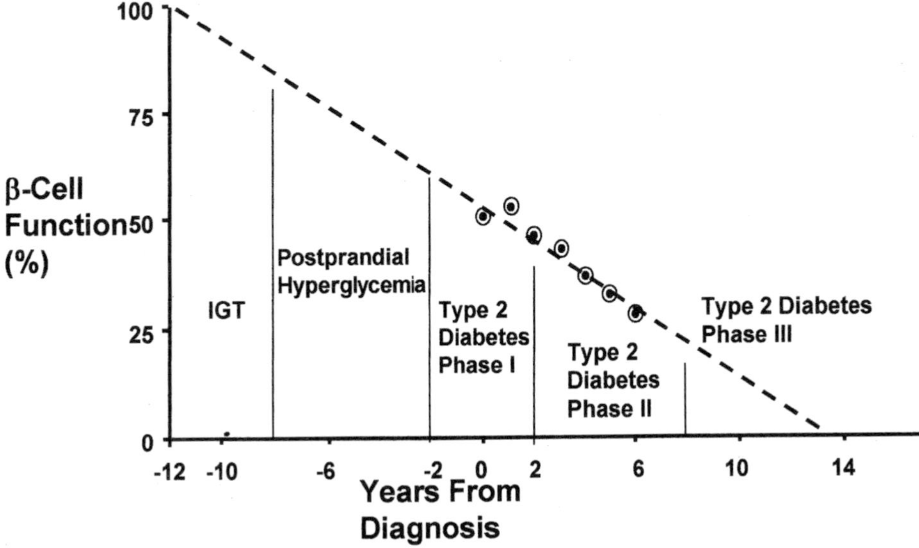

FIG. 41.3. Schematic representation of the stages of glucose intolerance as a function of pancreatic-cell insulin secretory capacity. The data points are taken from the HOMA (Homeostasis Model Assessment) calculation of percent normal-cell insulin secretory capacity as a function of time in a subset of the UKPDS population. The data are extrapolated both backward before the onset of clinical disease and forward into longer duration of disease. (Copyright © 1999 American Diabetes Association. From Lebovitz HE. Insulin secretogogues: old and new. *Diabetes Rev* 1999;7:139–153. Reprinted with permission from the American Diabetes Association.)

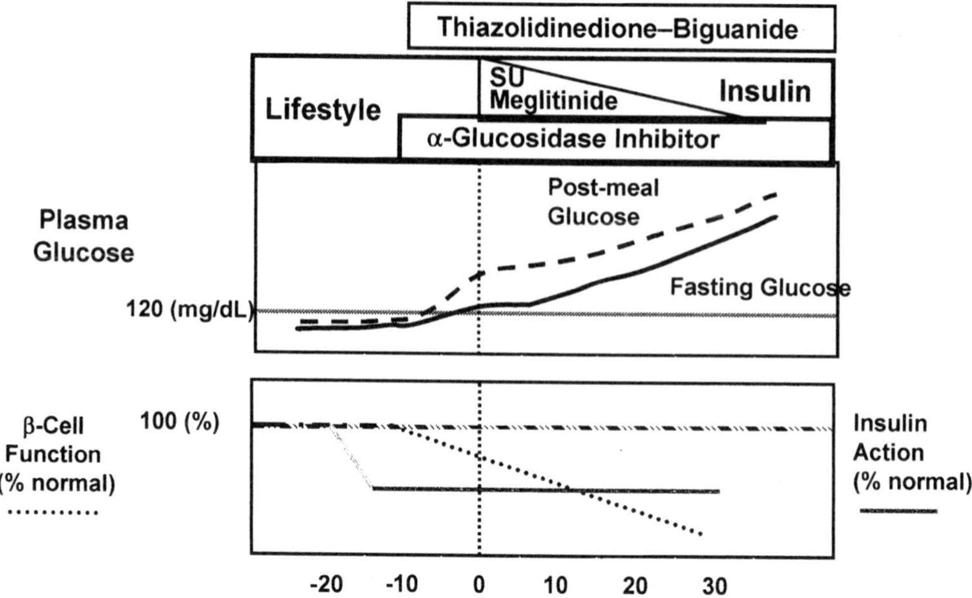

FIG. 41.4. Schematic representation of the natural history of the evolution of insulin-resistant type 2 diabetes and the matching of pathophysiology with the pharmacology of available treatments. SU, sulfonylureas.

glycemia ensues. During the clinical course of type 2 diabetes, insulin secretory function continues to decrease, and finally, after a number of years of clinical diabetes, many patients become severely insulin deficient and will require insulin-replacement therapy. Treatment of the abnormal glucose metabolism is determined by the stage of the disorder (Fig. 41.4).

INSULIN RESISTANCE AND ASSOCIATED ABNORMALITIES

In the report of the American Diabetes Association Expert Committee on the Diagnosis and Classification of Diabetes Mellitus, type 2 diabetes is characterized as ranging from predominately insulin resistance with relative insulin deficiency to predominately an insulin secretory defect with insulin resistance (33). In practical terms, about 85% of patients with type 2 diabetes have significant insulin resistance, which precedes the development of type 2 diabetes by many years, as noted previously. Insulin resistance is a separate entity from type 2 diabetes. Many individuals have insulin resistance and never develop type 2 diabetes because they do not have the pancreatic β-cell abnormalities (34,35).

Insulin resistance is associated with a cluster of metabolic abnormalities, and this is referred to as the *insulin resistance syndrome* or the *metabolic syndrome* (5,36,37). All of the components of the metabolic syndrome (Table 41.2) are cardiovascular risk factors. Because macrovascular disease is responsible for a large component of morbidity and mortality in patients with type 2 diabetes, their therapy must be directed at cardiovascular risk factors as well as hyperglycemia. An important issue in any antihyperglycemic treatment regimen is the effect that regimen might have on the components of the insulin resistance syndrome that are present.

TABLE 41.2. Components of the Metabolic Syndrome

Insulin resistance
Hyperinsulinemia
Central obesity
Increased systolic and diastolic blood pressure
Dyslipidemia
Increase in plasma triglycerides
Decrease in plasma HDL cholesterol
An LDL-particle pattern shifted to small, dense particles (type B pattern)
Procoagulant state
Increase in plasma fibrinogen
Increase in plasminogen activator inhibitor 1
Vascular abnormalities
Increase in urinary albumin excretion
Endothelial dysfunction
Hyperuricemia
Non-infectious inflammation

HDL, high-density lipoprotein; LDL, low-density lipoprotein.
From Lebovitz HE. *Clinician's manual on insulin resistance.* London: Science Press; 2002, with permission.

PHARMACOLOGY AND USE OF CURRENTLY APPROVED ORAL ANTIHYPERGLYCEMIC AGENTS AS MONOTHERAPY

The different major classes of oral antihyperglycemic agents in current use can be divided into those that increase insulin secretion, those that decrease insulin resistance, and those that modify the rate of glucose entry from the gastrointestinal tract (Fig. 41.5). Even within these classes there are striking differences among agents. Current data on the effectiveness of newer agents on glycemic control generally are derived from the large multicenter randomized placebo-controlled phase III studies presented to regulatory agencies for approval (13,14). These studies are heavily weighted with patients who had previously received an active agent that was discontinued. In those instances, the patients randomized to placebo have a very significant deterioration of glycemic control, while the patients in the actively treated group either maintain or show improved

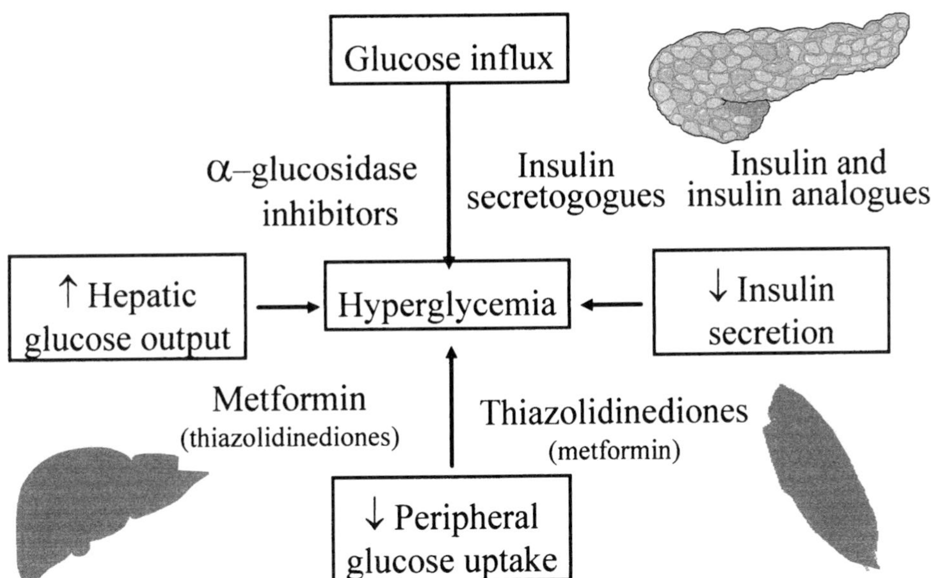

FIG. 41.5. Available pharmacologic agents ameliorate the hyperglycemia of type 2 diabetes by many different mechanisms. The antihyperglycemic effect of agents with different modes of action are additive. See Table 41.9.

glycemic control. Results are reported either as treatment effect, which is the difference between active treatment and placebo treatment, or as change from baseline, which is the difference in glycemic control at the end of the treatment period compared with that before the treatment period. The difference between treatment effect and decrease from baseline is significantly less in drug-naive patients with type 2 diabetes. Recent studies with antihyperglycemic drugs have shown that the decreases in HbA_{1c} with any treatment are directly proportional to the baseline HbA_{1c} levels (13). In drug-naive patients with type 2 diabetes in the rosiglitazone clinical trials (Fig. 41.6), it was apparent that the same dose of the same drug resulted in a 2.2%

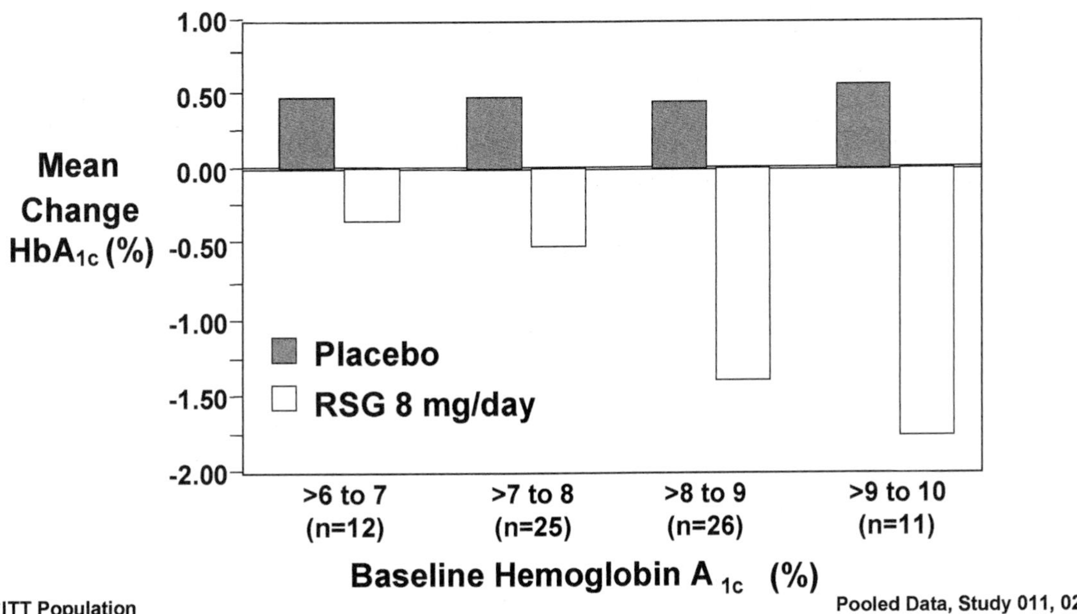

FIG. 41.6. The magnitude of glycemic response to every antihyperglycemic agent is inversely related to the baseline HbA_{1c}. The data here are from a cohort of drug-naive patients with type 2 diabetes treated in a double-blind placebo-controlled fashion with rosiglitazone at 8 mg/day. The placebo-treated patients had the same increase in HbA_{1c} regardless of their baseline HbA_{1c}.

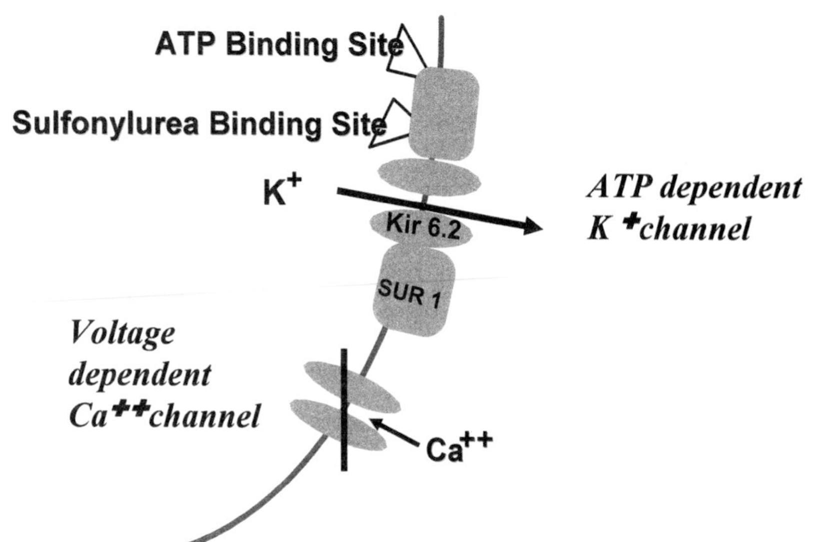

FIG. 41.7. The pancreatic β-cell K_{ATP} channel is open and extruding potassium ions when the plasma glucose level is low. The adjacent voltage-dependent calcium channel is closed. The K_{ATP} channel consists of two types of subunits: the Kir-6.2 subunit, which makes up the rectifier; and the SUR-1 subunit, which regulates opening and closing of the channel.

decrease in HbA_{1c} compared with placebo treatment at a baseline of 10.0% but in only a 0.8% decrease at a baseline of 7.0%. These effects of the nature of the populations studied and the baseline HbA_{1c} levels on glycemic responses are relevant because they show that it is not possible to compare the efficacy of different agents on glycemic control unless the comparison is derived from data generated from the same randomized double-blinded study.

Insulin Secretogogues

MECHANISM OF ACTION

The insulin secretogogues currently available stimulate the secretion of insulin by causing closure of the adenosine triphosphate (ATP)-dependent potassium channel (K_{ATP}) in the plasma membrane of the β-cell (38–40). The K_{ATP} channel is composed of two different types of subunits and is assembled from four subunits of each type (Fig. 41.7). The Kir-6.2 subunits make up the inward rectifier through which K^+ is transported from the intracellular compartment to the extracellular compartment. The SUR-1 subunit is attached to the Kir-6.2 subunit and regulates whether the K_{ATP} channel is open or closed. The SUR-1 subunit contains a binding site for sulfonylurea and related molecules, as well as binding sites for ATP and adenosine diphosphate (ADP). When the ATP:ADP ratio increases, as occurs when the plasma glucose level is elevated or when sulfonylureas or the newer insulin secretogogues bind to the SUR-1 subunit, the K_{ATP} channel closes (Fig. 41.8). When the K_{ATP} channel closes, K^+ accumulates at the plasma membrane and causes depolarization of the membrane adjacent to the closed channels. Depolarization of the membrane causes voltage-dependent L-type calcium channels in the microenvironment to open and for Ca^{2+} to enter the intracellular compartment from the extracellular compartment and increase the cytosolic Ca^{2+} concentration in the β-cell. The increase in Ca^{2+} stimulates the migration and exocytosis of the insulin granule.

All of the sulfonylureas and the newer non-sulfonylurea insulin secretogogues, repaglinide and nateglinide, act by binding to the SUR-1 subunits of the K_{ATP} channels, causing them to

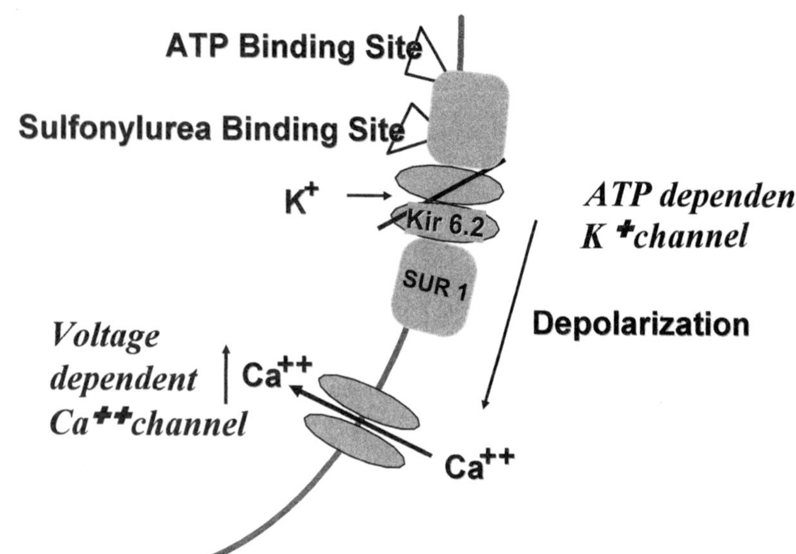

FIG. 41.8. When the plasma glucose level increases, the ATP:ADP ratio increases, causing the K_{ATP} channel to close. That initiates local depolarization of the plasma membrane, resulting in the opening of the L-type voltage-dependent calcium channels. Calcium ions enter the cell, and the rise in cytosolic calcium ion concentration stimulates insulin secretion.

TABLE 41.3. Factors Influencing the Clinical Effects of Insulin Secretogogues

Bioavailability following oral administration
Time to reach maximal concentration
Affinity for and kinetic interaction with SUR-1 subunit of the pancreatic β-cell K_{ATP} channel
Plasma half-life
Mechanism of metabolism and activity of metabolic products
Route of excretion
Interaction with other K_{ATP} channels
Side effects

close (41–43). Differences in the insulin secretory characteristics of the various insulin secretogogues are dependent on their pharmacokinetic properties and the affinity and kinetics of their binding to the SUR-1 subunit (41–43).

PHARMACOLOGY

The normal regulation of insulin secretion is tightly coupled to the plasma glucose level (44,45). Increasing plasma glucose levels, such as those that occur following ingestion of food, result in an almost immediate increase in insulin secretion. Decreasing plasma glucose levels are associated with a rapid decline in the secretion and plasma levels of insulin. Fasting is accompanied by reductions in insulin secretion sufficient to increase hepatic production of glucose to maintain glucose homeostasis. The ideal insulin secretogogue, therefore, would be one that restores to normal the defective early meal-mediated insulin secretion of type 2 diabetes, increases insulin secretion to adequately overcome the insulin resistance, stimulates insulin release only in response to elevated plasma glucose levels, and has little or no lag time in its insulin secretory response to rapidly changing plasma glucose levels. None of the available insulin secretogogues fulfills all of these properties.

Early postprandial hyperglycemia in the individual with diabetes is a consequence of delayed and inadequate early secretion of insulin (44–46). Late postprandial hypoglycemia in these subjects with type 2 diabetes results from an increase in drug-mediated late insulin secretion that is further accentuated if there is an early exaggerated postprandial hyperglycemia. Fasting or nocturnal hypoglycemia is more likely to occur in patients with type 2 diabetes administered insulin secretogogues that have long half-lives and stimulate insulin secretion in the presence of low glucose levels (45).

The factors determining the clinical effects of the available insulin secretogogues are listed in Table 41.3 and tabulated for each secretogogue in Table 41.4 (13,47). The major factors to consider in prescribing an insulin secretogogue are the rate of onset of its action, the duration of its action, the degree to which its action is dependent on the plasma glucose level, and its spectrum of side effects, including interaction with K_{ATP} channels in other tissues. The major complications of therapy with insulin secretogogues are hypoglycemia and weight gain, both of which are manifestations of the inability of these agents to simulate normal physiologic insulin secretion (47–50). The closer a particular insulin secretogogue can restore insulin secretory physiology to normal in the patient with type 2 diabetes, the less these two complications will occur. The effectiveness of all insulin secretogogues in stimulating insulin secretion and in reducing hyperglycemia is dependent of the presence of functioning β-cells. Insulin secretogogues are ineffective in patients with type 1 diabetes, in patients with latent autoimmune diabetes of adults (LADA), and in the later stages of type 2 diabetes when pancreatic β-cell function is markedly deficient.

K_{ATP} channels are present in many other tissues, including brain, myocardium, and vascular smooth muscle cells (38–40,51). The SUR subunit of the brain K_{ATP} channel is the same as that of the pancreatic β-cell (SUR-1), while the isoforms in myocardium and vascular smooth muscle cell are different (SUR-2A and SUR-2B). The abilities of various insulin secretogogues to interact with the different isoforms of the SUR subunit are not the same. This results in pharmacologic differences and has been postulated to produce clinical differences in side-effect profiles.

TABLE 41.4. Characteristics of Specific Insulin Secretogogues

Drug	Dose range (mg/day)	Peak level (hr)	Half-life (h)	Metabolites	Excretion
Sulfonylurea					
Tolbutamide	500–3,000	3–4	4.5–6.5	Inactive	Kidney
Chlorpropamide	100–500	2.4	36	Active or unchanged	Kidney
Tolazamide	100–1,000	3–4	7	Inactive	Kidney
Glipizide	2.5–25[a]	1–3	2–4	Inactive	Kidney 80%, bile 20%
Glipizide-GITS	5–20	Constant after several days of dosing	—	Inactive	Kidney 80%, bile 20%
Glyburide	1.25–20	~4	10	Inactive and weakly active	Kidney 50%, bile 50%
Glyburide, micronized formulation	1.5–12	2–3	~4	Inactive and weakly active	Kidney 50%, bile 50%
Glimeperide	1–8	2–3	9	Inactive and weakly active	Kidney 60%, bile 40%
Meglitinide					
Repaglinide	1.5–12[b]	0.75	1	Inactive	Bile
D-phenylalanine					
Nateglinide	180–360[b]	0.5–1.9	1.25		Urine

[a]Usual maximum effective dose.
[b]Divided into three doses each given before the meal.
Data from Lebovitz HE. Insulin secretogogues: old and new. *Diabetes Rev* 1999;7:139–153; and Lebovitz HE, Melander A. Sulfonylureas: basic aspects and clinical use. In: Alberti KGMM, Zimmet P, DeFronzo RA, Keen H, eds. *International textbook of diabetes,* 2nd ed. Chichester, UK: John Wiley & Sons, 1997:817.

SPECIFIC CLASSES OF INSULIN SECRETOGOGUES

Sulfonylureas

Sulfonylurea drugs have been used in the treatment of type 2 diabetes since the early 1950s. Extensive literature, including many review articles, is available (13,45,47). The major new information concerning the use of sulfonylureas in the treatment of type 2 diabetes has come from the UKPDS (12,52–54), the development programs of the newer sulfonylureas such as glimepiride (55), and recent studies investigating the effects of sulfonylureas on myocardial and vascular responses to ischemia (56–59).

The sulfonylurea drugs do not appear to correct the defect in early insulin secretion characteristic of type 2 diabetes (60,61). Their primary action is to increase the late stage of insulin secretion. This increases the likelihood of late postprandial and fasting hypoglycemia. The sulfonylurea drugs do not increase insulin biosynthesis and, indeed, seem to inhibit proinsulin biosynthesis *in vitro*. There is no evidence that they are either β-cytotropic or that they facilitate β-cell exhaustion (12,47). In the UKPDS, patients treated with sulfonylureas showed an increase in β-cell function for the first year but thereafter showed the same rate of loss of β-cell function as the conventionally treated group (12). Questions have been raised concerning the possibility that sulfonylureas, because of their prolonged effects on the pancreatic β-cell K_{ATP} channels, could lead to desensitization, with diminution of their pharmacologic effects. Several clinical studies showing that higher doses of sulfonylureas may be less effective than modest doses in lowering hyperglycemia provide some support for this hypothesis (62,63). Continuous *in vitro* incubation of β-cells with glyburide has been shown to lead to an increase in functionally deficient K_{ATP} channels (64).

Previous studies have shown that sulfonylureas can exert a variety of extrapancreatic actions in laboratory models *in vivo* and *in vitro* (47). It has been difficult to demonstrate conclusively any of these effects in humans. Some *in vivo* studies in humans have shown that sulfonylureas can lower plasma glucose levels under conditions in which the peripheral plasma insulin levels are unchanged. These studies have not excluded small changes in the portal vein insulin concentrations, which influence the liver but are not measurable in peripheral blood. Two effects of sulfonylureas that occur in humans that may result in extrapancreatic effects are interactions with K_{ATP} channels in other tissues (39) and direct effects on calcium ion–mediated exocytosis (65).

K_{ATP} channels in cardiac myocytes and vascular smooth muscle cells have SUR regulatory subunits, which differ somewhat from the SUR-1 subunit in β-cells (38–40). These different subunits change their binding characteristics such that they may have less affinity for some ligands that cause insulin secretion than for others. Brain-cell plasma membranes contain K_{ATP} channels that have the same regulatory subunit as pancreatic β-cells. It is therefore possible that some sulfonylureas might interact with K_{ATP} channels in tissues other than β-cells and cause extrapancreatic effects. Another mechanism by which specific sulfonylureas might cause extrapancreatic effects is through direct enhancement of calcium-mediated exocytosis of other hormones that are stored in secretory granules. Presently, there is little evidence that sulfonylureas exert any clinically significant extrapancreatic effects in humans. The only exception may be effects on the myocardial and vascular smooth muscle responses to ischemia and hypoxia.

Chlorpropamide. Chlorpropamide is a first-generation sulfonylurea that has been prescribed extensively worldwide for almost 40 years. At dosages ranging from 100 to 500 mg once a day, it is highly effective in reducing hyperglycemia, but because of its very long plasma half-life, it has been associated with a significant incidence of severe and protracted hypoglycemia, particularly in the elderly (47,66). Other significant side effects are water retention with hyponatremia and alcohol-induced facial flushing (45). Chlorpropamide is unique among sulfonylureas in that it stimulates secretion of antidiuretic hormones and potentiates an antidiuretic hormone effect in the renal tubules. The effect on water balance is thought to explain the observation in the UKPDS of an increase in systolic and diastolic blood pressure as well as a greater need for antihypertensive therapy in the 619 patients treated with chlorpropamide than in patients treated with insulin, glyburide, or conventional therapy (2). In the UKPDS, chlorpropamide treatment reduced HbA_{1c} significantly more than did glyburide or insulin; however, this was not accompanied by any greater reduction in risk for progression of retinopathy (2). Many previous studies have noted that hypoglycemia is a major risk of chlorpropamide treatment. Major hypoglycemic events occurred less frequently in the UKPDS in the chlorpropamide-treated cohort than in the glyburide-treated cohort (2).

Glyburide. Glyburide (glibenclamide) is currently the most widely prescribed sulfonylurea—but not because it is more effective or safer than other sulfonylureas. It is marketed as a formulation with poor and variable bioavailability (dosage 1.25–20 mg daily) and as a micronized formulation with relatively good and consistent bioavailability (dosage 1.5–12 mg daily) (45,47,67). Its efficacy in reducing hyperglycemia appears to be equal to that of other sulfonylureas, but it is associated with a high rate of serious side effects, including its long duration of action, with a rate of serious and fatal hypoglycemia that is significantly higher than that with other sulfonylureas, modest weight gain, and a relative lack of specificity on the different K_{ATP} channels (67–69). Careful evaluation of the 615 patients with type 2 diabetes treated with glyburide for a mean of 11 years in the UKPDS has clearly defined the characteristics of chronic glyburide therapy (2). It is most effective in controlling hyperglycemia in patients with newly diagnosed type 2 diabetes for the first year or 2 and then begins to lose effectiveness progressively with time (secondary failure or sulfonylurea ineffectiveness) (52–54). Glyburide treatment alone was relatively ineffective in controlling hyperglycemia after 4 or 5 years (54). The median decrease in HbA_{1c} in patients treated with glyburide as compared with patients receiving conventional (diet) treatment over 10 years was 0.7% (7.2% vs. 7.9%) (2). Weight gain occurred primarily in the first 3 or 4 years of treatment and was maintained throughout the study, so that at 10 years the glyburide-treated patients had gained 1.7 kg more than the conventionally treated patients (2). Serious hypoglycemia occurred primarily during the first few years of glyburide therapy, when it had been most effective in reducing hyperglycemia. Major hypoglycemic events were noted in approximately 1.4% of patients in year 1, 1.3% in year 2, and 0.4% in year 3 (2). These rates of serious hypoglycemic events are comparable to those reported in other large series and are greater than those with other sulfonylureas (Table 41.5) (68, 70–72).

Glipizide. Glipizide is a sulfonylurea that is available in both a short-acting formulation and in an extended-release formulation (glipizide-*g*astro*i*ntestinal *t*herapeutic *s*ystem, or glipizide-*GITS*) (45). The short-acting form is rapidly absorbed and is completely bioavailable. It is metabolized by oxidative hydroxylation and is eliminated with a half-life of 2 to 4 hours

TABLE 41.5. Serious Hypoglycemia Reported in Large Retrospective Studies

Study	Sulfonylurea	Rates of serious hypoglycemia[a] (per 100 person-years)
Tennessee Medicaid (13,963 patients; 20,715 person-years) (71)	All sulfonylureas	1.23
	Glyburide	1.66
	Glipizide	0.88
	Tolbutamide	0.35
VAMP-Research Data Base (33,243 patients) (72)	All sulfonylureas	1.77

[a]Serious hypoglycemia was defined in the Tennessee Medicaid Study as admission to the hospital emergency department or death, with a measured blood glucose level of <2.8 mmol/L; and in the VAMP Data Base, as a condition requiring the assistance of another person.

(45). Its elimination is not affected by mild to moderate renal insufficiency (creatinine clearance ≥30 mL/min) (45). Glipizide is administered once or twice a day. Its efficacy is equal to that of glyburide in controlling hyperglycemia, but because of its metabolism and more rapid elimination, therapy with glipizide is associated with less hypoglycemia (45). The official maximum dosage of glipizide in the United States is 40 mg per day, although available clinical studies show little or no benefit in giving more than 15 or 20 mg per day. Glipizide should be administered before meals, as its absorption may be mildly delayed by food ingestion.

The extended-release formulation of glipizide provides once-a-day dosage of 5 to 20 mg (73,74). Plasma levels of glipizide 24 hours after doses of 5 mg and 20 mg of glipizide-GITS (Glucotrol XL) are 54 ng/mL and 310 ng/mL, respectively. The decreases in HbA_{1c} in clinical trials with glipizide-GITS were 1.50% and 1.84% compared with placebo treatment. The decrease in HbA_{1c} was maximal at 5 mg per day. FPG level was reduced 57 mg/dL to 74 mg/dL compared with placebo treatment. The extended-release form appears to have glucose-lowering effects similar to those of immediate-release glipizide, as measured by the improvement in HbA_{1c}. In a study comparing glipizide-GITS to immediate-acting glipizide, the authors concluded that the glipizide-GITS formulation at dosages of 5 mg and 20 mg have an improved metabolic profile compared with that of immediate-acting glipizide; however, the design of the study makes such a conclusion tenuous. No increase in hypoglycemia was noted with the extended-acting form.

Glimepiride. Glimepiride is the newest of the sulfonylureas to be approved for use. It is said to be more selective for the β-cell K_{ATP} channel than for the cardiovascular tissue K_{ATP} channel (75). It appears to bind to a slightly different part of the sulfonylurea-binding site than does glyburide, although the two sulfonylureas displace each other from their respective binding sites. Glimepiride associates 2.5- to 3.0-fold faster and dissociates 8.0- to 9.0-fold faster than glyburide from its β-cell K_{ATP}-binding site (75,76). Insulin release is therefore more rapid and of shorter duration than that with glyburide. Hyperglycemic and euglycemic-hyperinsulinemic clamp studies in patients with type 2 diabetes demonstrated that glimepiride does not restore first-phase insulin secretion and that it increases second-phase insulin secretion, whole-body glucose uptake, and increases insulin sensitivity (61). Some studies have suggested that glimepiride reduces hyperglycemia with less insulin secretion than that required by other sulfonylureas, and this has led to the claim that glimepiride has an insulin-sparing action (57,77–80). The data are marginally significant, and additional studies are required to substantiate this claim. For glimepiride, as for all other sulfonylureas, there are claims that it has extrapancreatic effects. Some of the effects described are an increase in glucose uptake and utilization by an increase in the translocation of the GLUT4 transporter protein in adipose and muscle cells, an effect on the regulation of the intracellular routing of the insulin receptor complexes toward degradative pathways, and an increased association of the insulin receptor with protein kinase C isozymes (76,79). These extrapancreatic effects have been demonstrated in *in vitro* systems, and their relevance to glimepiride effects in humans is debatable.

Glimepiride is administered once daily at dosages ranging from 1 to 8 mg. The recommended starting dosage is 1 to 2 mg daily, and the average maintenance dosage is 1 mg to 4 mg daily (57,77–80). Glimepiride is absorbed quickly and achieves maximal blood glucose lowering within 2 to 3 hours, but its blood-glucose-lowering effect is still evident at 24 hours. Like most sulfonylureas, glimepiride is metabolized by the liver and its metabolites are excreted via the kidney. In a 1-year comparative clinical trial, glimepiride and glyburide were equivalent in controlling glycemia; however, fasting plasma insulin and C-peptide values were statistically significantly lower in patients treated with glimepiride than in patients treated with glyburide (77). Glimepiride reduced HbA_{1c} 1.2% to 1.9% and mean FPG 54 mg/dL to 76 mg/dL compared with placebo treatment in studies of monotherapy (57,78).

Glimepiride treatment is associated with lower rates of documented hypoglycemia than is glyburide treatment (1.7% vs. 2.4%) and with rates that are equivalent to those with glipizide (0.9% vs. 1.2%) (57,79,80).

Repaglinide

Repaglinide is a non-sulfonylurea insulin secretogogue. It is a member of the meglitinide family (Fig. 41.9) (81–83). The mechanism of action of insulin release for repaglinide is slightly different from that of sulfonylureas (44). Repaglinide interacts with a specific binding site on the SUR-1 subunit that is distinct from the glyburide sulfonylurea-binding site but still causes closure of the K_{ATP} channel. Repaglinide, unlike sulfonylureas, does not directly stimulate exocytosis of insulin granules (65). Repaglinide is rapidly absorbed orally, with the C_{max} occurring 45 to 50 minutes after ingestion and plasma levels returning to baseline in 3 to 4 hours (47,83). The pharmacokinetic and K_{ATP} channel interactive properties of repaglinide result in the more rapid release of insulin and for a shorter duration than with sulfonylureas. The insulin-releasing action of repaglinide commences within 30 minutes and facilitates early meal-related secretion of insulin. Its major insulin secretory effect subsides in approximately 4 hours. Because repaglinide is a short-acting

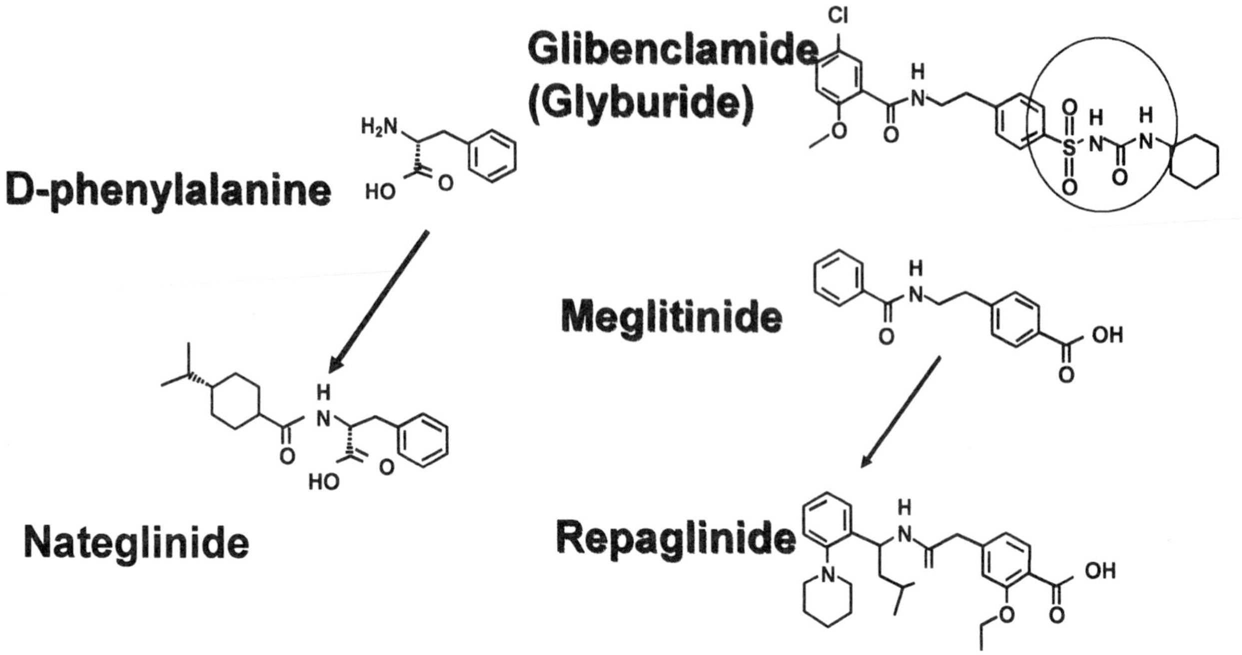

FIG. 41.9. Structure of the new rapid insulin secretogogues compared with a sulfonylurea such as glyburide.

insulin secretogogue, it must be taken within 30 minutes of each meal. When a meal is skipped or delayed, the administration of repaglinide should be altered similarly (84). The ability to alter the time and dose of repaglinide administration to match meal ingestion more closely reduces the likelihood of postprandial or fasting hypoglycemia. This is an advantage over traditional sulfonylurea treatment, although multiple doses of repaglinide per day are necessary. Repaglinide is administered as 0.5 mg to 4.0 mg before each meal, and the dose can be adjusted on the basis of the estimated calories and content of the meal (83,85).

Monotherapy with repaglinide in patients with type 2 diabetes was found to reduce mean HbA_{1c} by 1.7% and mean FPG by 62 mg/dL as compared with placebo treatment. One-year trials showed that the antihyperglycemic effects of repaglinide and glyburide are equivalent (86). Although repaglinide-treated patients experience hypoglycemia and weight gain, the magnitude is significantly less than with glyburide.

Repaglinide is metabolized by the liver, and 90% of the dose is excreted in the bile. Therefore, repaglinide is not contraindicated in patients with type 2 diabetes who have impaired renal function. The dose of repaglinide should be reduced in patients with clinically significant liver disease.

Nateglinide

Nateglinide is a D-phenylalanine derivative (Fig. 41.9) that does not contain a sulfonylurea moiety, is rapidly absorbed, and binds to the SUR-1 subunit of the K_{ATP} channel with binding characteristics quite different from those of sulfonylureas (43). When nateglinide is administered 10 minutes before the meal, its peak plasma level is achieved at a mean time of 0.92 hours and its mean half-time disappearance rate in plasma is 2.14 hours (10,87). Oral bioavailability is estimated to be 72%. The drug is metabolized by the mixed-function oxidase system of the liver (CYP3A4 and CYP2C9) before excretion (87). The drug and its metabolites are eliminated rapidly and completely. If nateglinide is taken after the meal, its rate of absorption is decreased, resulting in a 22% increase in the time to maximal plasma levels.

Binding and displacement studies with nateglinide and the β-cell K_{ATP} channel indicate that it dissociates very rapidly. Inhibition of the K_{ATP} channel current by the patch-clamp technique and its reversal confirm the rapid and short duration of nateglinide action on the channel. Nateglinide selectively binds to the K_{ATP} channel of the β-cell and binds relatively little to the K_{ATP} channel of vascular smooth muscle (relative binding, 45- to 311-fold relative selectivity) (51). It has a 1.6-fold selectivity for inhibition of the β-cell K_{ATP} channel current as compared with the cardiac K_{ATP} channel current. These properties of nateglinide are predictive of a rapid and short duration of stimulation of insulin secretion with little or no potential for effects on cardiac or vascular tissues.

Clinical data are consistent with what would be predicted from the pharmacologic properties. Administration of nateglinide to fasted patients with type 2 diabetes caused a small increase in plasma insulin levels (4–5 μU/mL), which peaked within an hour and caused a small decrease in plasma glucose over the 4-hour period following dosing (10,88,89). In contrast, when nateglinide was given to the same individuals 10 minutes before a meal, the plasma insulin levels increased by 30 minutes, peaked at 2 hours, and declined at 3 hours to those levels seen following treatment with placebo (88). Nateglinide increased meal-mediated plasma insulin levels in a dose-dependent manner, with a maximum effective dose of 120 mg.

When administered as monotherapy for 12 weeks to patients with type 2 diabetes whose glucose levels were inadequately controlled by diet and exercise (mean HbA_{1c} 8.4%; mean FPG 182 mg/dL), a dose of 120 mg administered 10 minutes before meals resulted in a decrease in HbA_{1c} of 0.55% and in a reduction in FPG of 21 mg/dL (10). A large randomized double-blind study in patients with type 2 diabetes, with washout of their previous treatment for 4 weeks, compared 24 weeks of treatment with 120 mg of nateglinide before each meal to 500 mg of metformin three times a day and to a combination of metformin and nateglinide (89). Placebo treatment resulted in a 0.5% increase in HbA_{1c}, whereas metformin treatment resulted in a 0.8% decrease and nateglinide treatment resulted in a 0.5% decrease. Combination nateglinide-metformin therapy resulted in greater improvement in glycemic control (1.4% decrease in HbA_{1c} and 40 mg/dL decrease in FPG) than did either drug alone. The major benefit of nateglinide treatment is a reduction in the postprandial glucose excursions.

The potential side effect of nateglinide is hypoglycemia. In the clinical studies completed to date, hypoglycemia appeared to be relatively uncommon and mild.

INSULIN SECRETOGOGUES AND CARDIOVASCULAR EFFECTS

Starting with the report of the results of University Group Diabetes Program in 1970, there has been an ongoing concern about whether sulfonylureas have a detrimental effect on the cardiovascular system (90). In that study, the authors noted that chronic treatment of patients with type 2 diabetes with tolbutamide for 8 years was associated with a statistically significant 75% increase in cardiovascular mortality as compared with the mortality in the placebo-treated controls. The design and results of that study were extensively criticized throughout the 1970s, and several subsequent studies failed to confirm their findings.

In the 1980s, K_{ATP} channels were found to be present in the plasma membranes of myocardial and vascular smooth muscle cells and in pancreatic β-cells, and ischemic preconditioning was discovered (91,92). Ischemic preconditioning is the phenomenon whereby a short period of ischemia followed by reperfusion transiently protects the myocardium from a subsequent more severe and prolonged ischemia and reduces the area of infarction in the ischemic region by as much as 75% to 80%. Information has accumulated that indicates that the mechanism responsible for ischemic preconditioning involves an opening of the myocardial and coronary artery K_{ATP} channels by the metabolic consequences of ischemia (93). The effects are an increase in K^+ efflux and a reduction in Ca^{2+} influx into the cells. The consequences are a shortening of the duration of the myocardial action potential, a reduction in contractility, energy conservation by the myocardium, and vasodilatation by the coronary artery. Another consequence of the K^+ changes, however, is a possible increase in ventricular arrhythmias.

When it was recognized that the primary action of sulfonylureas is to close the K_{ATP} channels in the pancreatic β-cells, the question arose as to the possible effects of sulfonylureas on cardiovascular K_{ATP} channels and whether sulfonylurea treatment might interfere with the protective effects afforded by the opening of K_{ATP} channels by ischemia in cardiovascular tissues (94). A series of studies were carried out, first in animal models and subsequently in humans, that have demonstrated that doses of glyburide in the range of the maximal prescribed doses can block ischemic preconditioning, presumably by closing the K_{ATP} channel (95,96).

The clinical significance of these observations is not clear. A retrospective study from the Mayo Clinic reported that patients with diabetes undergoing angioplasty for acute myocardial infarction had a risk of early mortality 2.77 times greater than patients receiving no therapy or receiving insulin (97). The Bypass Angioplasty Revascularization Investigation reported that patients with diabetes had greater long-term mortality following angioplasty than did patients without diabetes, but the two groups had similar mortality following bypass surgery. The sulfonylurea-treated patients in particular had greater mortality 4 to 7 years after the angioplasty (98). In contrast, Klamann et al. (99) have reported no increase in mortality or infarct size in a cohort of 245 patients with type 2 diabetes taking glyburide who were admitted with an acute myocardial infarction and followed for a mean of 6.5 years as compared with those not taking a sulfonylurea. Some investigators have indicated that patients with diabetes treated with glyburide may have a lower rate of ventricular arrhythmias.

All of the clinical and animal studies showing effects of the sulfonylureas on ischemic preconditioning have used glyburide as the sulfonylurea. The binding affinities of glyburide for the K_{ATP} channels in cardiovascular tissues and for those of the β-cell are almost equal (51). Tolbutamide has virtually no binding activity to the SUR-2 subunits (those in K_{ATP} channels in cardiovascular tissues). Glimepiride had no effect on blocking ischemic preconditioning in human studies in which glyburide abolished it (77). The non-sulfonylurea insulin secretogogues have very little binding affinity for the SUR-2 subunits and have a very high specificity for the SUR-1 (β-cell subunit) (51). Summarizing the data, one can make the following conclusions: (a) it is likely that insulin secretogogues with relatively equal specificity for the SUR-1 and SUR-2 subunits could affect cardiovascular responses under specific conditions; (b) the only condition under which a drug that closes the K_{ATP} channel might interfere with normal cardiovascular responses is one in which there is transient ischemia followed shortly thereafter by more prolonged ischemia; (c) the effects would be manifest as a greater area of infarction; (d) maximum doses of glyburide are most likely to interfere with the cardiovascular responses to ischemia; and (e) the new non-sulfonylurea insulin secretogogues are much less or not at all likely to produce those effects. Despite all of the studies, the question of whether sulfonylurea treatment has detrimental cardiovascular effects in humans remains controversial. There are currently no clinical data that unequivocally demonstrate an adverse effect of glyburide on outcomes related to cardiovascular events.

Insulin Sensitizers

The majority of patients with type 2 diabetes have insulin resistance and the metabolic disease syndrome as a component of their disorder. The normal compensatory response to insulin resistance is a sufficient increase in insulin secretion to overcome the insulin resistance and maintain normal glucose metabolism. Glucose intolerance is an indication that the individual's β-cells are not secreting enough insulin to overcome the insulin resistance adequately. The evolution of glucose intolerance in these individuals progresses from normal glucose tolerance with insulin resistance and compensatory hyperinsulinemia, to IGT with insulin resistance and decreasing compensatory hyperinsulinemia, to type 2 diabetes with insulin resistance and frankly inadequate secretion of insulin. A reduction in insulin resistance at each and every stage of the evolution of type 2 diabetes in such individuals will improve glucose metabolism by allowing their endogenous insulin to be more effective (77,100).

Additional benefits to be accrued from reducing insulin resistance are amelioration of some components of the metabolic syndrome (insulin resistance syndrome). These components increase macrovascular disease risk, and reduction of the components of the metabolic syndrome are as important to the health of the individual with type 2 diabetes as is the treatment of the hyperglycemia (101–103). Treatment of insulin resistance at the stage of IGT with metformin can slow the progression to type 2 diabetes by 31% over 3 years, although this effect is not as great as that with intensive lifestyle modification, which slows progression by 58% over 3 years (104). Thiazolidinedione treatment may also be highly effective in delaying or preventing the development of type 2 diabetes in insulin-resistant individuals, as troglitazone treatment of women with previous gestational diabetes decreased the development of diabetes by 56% over 30 months (TRIPOD study) (100). It has been postulated that treatment of insulin resistance itself in the absence of glucose intolerance may slow the development of atherosclerosis and macrovascular disease (36,101,103). Clinical trials to evaluate this possibility are under way.

The high prevalence of insulin resistance worldwide and its impact as a contributor to the development of so many diseases has made the discovery of drugs for the treatment of insulin resistance a very high priority for the pharmaceutical industry. Currently, two classes of oral agents, the biguanides and thiazolidinediones, are available to treat insulin resistance, and both are important agents for the treatment of type 2 diabetes. Metformin is the only widely available biguanide. Rosiglitazone and pioglitazone are the currently available thiazolidinediones. Troglitazone, which was the first thiazolidinedione to be marketed, was withdrawn from the market because its treatment was associated with rare cases of idiosyncratic liver toxicity with liver failure and death.

METFORMIN

Mechanism of Action

Metformin, a biguanide, has been used in the treatment of type 2 diabetes since the 1960s. Its mechanism of action has been studied extensively, and although many metabolic effects have been described in *in vitro* systems and animal models, the molecular and biochemical sites of action have eluded discovery (105–107). Metformin exerts several physiologic effects that contribute to its ability to decrease hyperglycemia in patients with type 2 diabetes. Patients taking metformin frequently complain of a metallic taste and often have some degree of anorexia (108). Treatment of patients with type 2 diabetes is usually associated with a mean weight loss of 2 to 3 kg, which is due primarily to a decrease in adipose tissue (52,109). This effect has been obscured in some studies by confounding weight gain associated with improved glycemic control and a reduction in glycosuria. Though not well documented, the weight loss usually is associated with a decrease in appetite. Recent studies show that the percent reduction in the visceral adipose tissue depot is significantly greater than that in the subcutaneous or total adipose tissue pool (110). The ability of metformin to increase insulin-mediated glucose disposal in skeletal muscle appears to be at best quite modest. Studies in the 1980s using the euglycemic hyperinsulinemic-clamp technique demonstrated that metformin significantly increased insulin-mediated glucose uptake by muscle. Those studies, however, did not control for weight loss or reduction in glucose toxicity resulting from improved glycemic control. Several subsequent studies in which weight loss was not a factor failed to show a significant effect of metformin on insulin-mediated glucose uptake in peripheral tissues. Two more recent studies, which were specifically designed to eliminate changes in weight and differences in glycemic control, found no effect and a small increase in insulin-mediated peripheral glucose uptake, respectively (9, 111). In contrast, all well-designed studies have shown marked effects of metformin in decreasing the elevated hepatic glucose production that is associated with fasting hyperglycemia (20, 109,112). The decrease in hepatic glucose production by metformin appears to be due primarily to a decrease in gluconeogenesis, although there is some contribution from a decrease in glycogenolysis (112). Administration of metformin has been shown to lower plasma levels of free fatty acids and to increase lipid oxidation in some, but not all, studies. The effects on lipid metabolism are modest and not likely to play a major role in decreasing hepatic glucose production (20,109,112,113). Metformin has no direct effects on pancreatic β-cells and does not influence insulin secretion directly but only through its influences on changing plasma glucose levels.

Pharmacokinetics and Metabolism

Metformin is incompletely and slowly absorbed from the small intestine, with a bioavailability of 50% to 60% from a 500-mg tablet taken in the fasting state (114). Absorption decreases with increasing dose, and administration with food decreases the extent of and slightly delays absorption. Peak plasma concentrations reach 1 μg/mL to 2 μg/mL 1 to 2 hours after an oral dose of 500 mg to 1,000 mg. Metformin is not bound to plasma proteins, has a plasma half-life of 1.5 to 4.9 hours, is not metabolized, and is rapidly cleared by the kidney (90% within 12 hours). These properties of metformin are quite important, since the drug does not accumulate in the body, and excessive plasma levels are unlikely to occur in the presence of normal renal function. These properties are in contrast to those of phenformin, a biguanide that is no longer available in most countries because of its occasional association with the development of lactic acidosis. Dose-response studies of the effect of metformin on glycemic control in patients with type 2 diabetes indicate that maximal effects occur at dosages of 1,750 to 2,000 mg per day (115). Metformin is administered twice or three times a day with meals, because that minimizes the gastrointestinal side effects.

Metformin is now also marketed as a long-acting preparation (metformin hydrochloride extended-release tablets). The peak plasma level following oral administration of this preparation occurs at 4 to 8 hours and is 20% lower than that following a comparable dose of the regular formulation of metformin (114). The extended-release formulation is administered at dosages of 500 to 2,000 mg given once daily with the evening meal. The peak plasma level attained with 1,000 and 2,000 mg were 1.1 μg/mL and 1.8 μg/mL, respectively.

Clinical Use

Administration of metformin to patients with type 2 diabetes results in a decrease in hepatic insulin resistance. The consequence is an increase in the effectiveness of endogenous portal vein insulin and a resultant decrease in hepatic glucose production and fasting hyperglycemia (9,109,112). Fasting plasma insulin levels are either unchanged or modestly reduced. A reduction in insulin resistance of muscle is a less consistent and relatively minor effect of metformin. Metformin treatment generally reduces hyperglycemia by approximately the same magnitude as sulfonylurea treatment, even though their mechanisms of action are entirely different (52,116).

While many clinical studies measuring the effects of metformin treatment in patients with type 2 diabetes have been published, relatively few have been randomized, been placebo-controlled, included large numbers of subjects, had treatment periods extending for more than a few months, and had adequate assessments of glycemic control. The registration studies done for metformin approval in the United States (116) and the UKPDS provide the best data relative to the clinical effectiveness of metformin (3). In the registration studies, metformin monotherapy in obese subjects with type 2 diabetes (mean baseline HbA_{1c} and FPG 8.3% and 240 mg/dL, respectively) for 29 weeks lowered mean HbA_{1c} 1.8% and mean FPG 58 mg/dL compared with placebo-treated controls. The glucose-lowering effect was greatest in subjects with the highest HbA_{1c} and FPG values and the least in those with the lowest HbA_{1c} and FPG values. The effect of metformin on glycemic control was due primarily to a decrease in FPG, as there was no significant reduction in the postprandial glucose excursions. Fasting plasma insulin and C-peptide levels were unchanged. Body weight did not change significantly. Metformin treatment resulted in small decreases in serum total cholesterol, low-density lipoprotein (LDL) cholesterol, and triglycerides.

In the UKPDS, 342 obese patients with newly diagnosed type 2 diabetes were randomized to metformin treatment and followed for a median duration of 10.7 years. The median HbA_{1c} for the first 5 years of metformin treatment was 6.7%. For the same time interval, the conventional control group had a value of 7.5%. For the second and third 5-year periods, the median HbA_{1c} for the metformin-treated group was 7.9% and 8.3%, respectively. Throughout the study, the median difference between the metformin and conventionally treated groups was 0.6%. Metformin treatment was associated with no weight gain, with a decrease in fasting plasma insulin levels, and with no significant incidence of hypoglycemia.

Studies comparing the effects of metformin and sulfonylureas on glycemic control in patients with type 2 diabetes consistently show equivalence, even though their modes of action are entirely different. The practical consequence of this finding is that replacement of sulfonylurea treatment by metformin or metformin by sulfonylureas does not improve glycemic control (116). There are, however, differences in effects on body weight and the incidence of hypoglycemia. In a 1-year study in which patients of normal weight were randomized to metformin or chlorpropamide, glycemic control in the two groups was remarkably the same, but the chlorpropamide-treated patients gained a mean of 4.6 kg while the metformin-treated patients lost a mean of 1.5 kg (117). Hypoglycemia does not occur with metformin monotherapy (105–107). Combining the two oral agents, however, is additive because they lower glycemia equally but by different mechanisms.

Metformin treatment has beneficial effects on many aspects of the insulin resistance syndrome (metabolic disease syndrome): it decreases obesity and particularly central obesity; has a small beneficial effect on decreasing serum triglycerides and LDL cholesterol; improves fibrinolysis by decreasing plasminogen activator inhibitor 1 (PAI 1); and frequently decreases plasma insulin levels (105,109,113). The metabolic disease syndrome is associated with an increase in clinical macrovascular disease. A drug that improves some or all of the components of the metabolic disease syndrome would be expected to decrease macrovascular disease. One of the major findings of the UKPDS was that treatment of the overweight patients with type 2 diabetes with metformin reduced the risk of myocardial infarction by 39% and of diabetes-related deaths by 42% (3). Those were highly significant reductions when compared with conventional treatment, but not when compared with the other intensive treatments, which were associated with small but statistically insignificant reductions even though they reduced HbA_{1c} to a degree equivalent to that with metformin.

While the data from the metformin primary prevention arm of the UKPDS appear valid, a substudy in the UKPDS comparing the effect of adding metformin to the regimen of patients poorly controlled with sulfonylureas showed a statistically significant increase in cardiovascular mortality when compared with those randomized to added placebo (3). A further analysis of the data compared with the results of the entire study suggested that the results were due to an unexplained decrease in mortality in the sulfonylurea-plus-placebo group rather than an increase in mortality in the sulfonylurea-plus-metformin group. Two recent retrospective studies have reported that diabetic patients treated with sulfonylureas plus metformin have a higher mortality than those treated with diet or sulfonylureas alone. A study of 2,275 patients with diabetes and coronary disease in Israel who were followed for a mean of 7.7 years found an increase in mortality in patients who received metformin in combination with glyburide compared with those on dietary or glyburide management alone (118). A Swedish study reported an increase in mortality in 169 patients taking sulfonylureas in combination with metformin as compared with 741 patients taking sulfonylureas alone (119). The major flaws in these studies are the lack of randomized cohorts, which means the groups are not comparable, and the retrospective analysis, which implies dissimilar care during the follow-up period. The substudy and two retrospective studies suggest that a definitive long-term study of the safety and efficacy of combination sulfonylurea and metformin therapy would be useful.

Side Effects

The major complications associated with metformin treatment are gastrointestinal symptoms (105,106,116). In general, the symptoms are dose-related and transient. They have been reported to occur in 5% to 20% of patients. The most common gastrointestinal symptoms are metallic taste, anorexia, nausea, abdominal pain, and diarrhea. Gastrointestinal symptoms can be minimized by starting therapy with low doses of metformin (500 mg) and increasing the dose slowly. Taking the drug with meals decreases the symptoms, and it is useful to initiate drug therapy with the evening meal.

Lactic acidosis is the most frequently discussed complication, although it is extremely rare and almost always occurs in clinical situations in which metformin is contraindicated (105,106,120). The reported incidence of lactic acidosis in patients receiving metformin is 3 per 100,000 patient years; the fatality rate is 50%. Almost all cases of lactic acidosis during metformin therapy have occurred in patients with impaired renal function or those who have illnesses that predispose to impaired renal function. Metformin is contraindicated in those patients (Table 41.6).

TABLE 41.6. Contraindications for Metformin Treatment

Decreased renal function: plasma creatinine ≥1.5 mg/dL for men and ≥1.4 mg/dL for women or a creatinine clearance <60 mL/min
Patients with congestive heart failure requiring pharmacologic management
Patients ≥80 years of age unless a creatinine clearance demonstrates adequate renal function
Liver disease
Chronic alcohol abuse
Sepsis or other acute illness with decreased tissue perfusion
During intravenous radiographic contrast administration

From Glucophage; Glucophage XR prescribing information. Bristol-Myers Squibb Co. Revised October 2000, with permission.

Vitamin B_{12} malabsorption was found in 30% of patients with diabetes during long-term treatment with metformin. In the large U.S. registration studies, serum vitamin B_{12} levels were decreased 29% during metformin treatment. Megaloblastic anemia during metformin treatment is very rare and can be treated by administering vitamin B_{12}. The mechanism of the malabsorption is unknown.

THIAZOLIDINEDIONES

Mechanism of Action

The thiazolidinediones were discovered in the late 1970s during screening for lipid-lowering agents. Ciglitazone, which was the original compound, was noted to reduce hyperglycemia, hyperinsulinemia, and hypertriglyceridemia in rodent models of insulin-resistant diabetes. During the 1980s, many derivatives containing the glitazone structure were synthesized and evaluated. The three thiazolidinediones eventually approved for clinical use were troglitazone, rosiglitazone, and pioglitazone (Fig. 41.10). Troglitazone was the first to be marketed and had reasonable efficacy in reducing insulin resistance and improving hyperglycemia in type 2 diabetes (121). Its use, however, was associated with the rare development of idiosyncratic liver toxicity, which could progress to hepatic failure and death, and troglitazone was removed from the market in March 2000 (122, 123). Rosiglitazone and pioglitazone have been approved for the treatment of type 2 diabetes since mid-1999. No evidence of significant liver toxicity has been found with either rosiglitazone or pioglitazone after almost 2 years of use and the treatment of more than 2 million patients (124).

The mechanism of action of the thiazolidinediones was discovered after their clinical effectiveness had been established. The thiazolidinediones were found to be ligands for an orphan receptor known as the peroxisome proliferator–activated receptor (PPAR) (125–127). This receptor is a member of the nuclear receptor superfamily of ligand-activated transcription factors. It is a heterodimer consisting of two subunits: one that binds thiazolidinediones and one that binds retinoids (Fig. 41.11). There are three subtypes of PPARs: PPAR-α, PPAR-δ, and PPAR-γ. The three subtypes have distinct actions. All three bind to specific response elements of genes that have central roles in the storage and catabolism of fatty acids. PPAR-α is present at high concentrations in the liver and is activated by fibrates, which are pharmacologic ligands for the receptor. PPAR-δ is ubiquitous, and its activation by specific pharmacologic ligands has a profound influence on lipoprotein metabolism. PPAR-γ is the receptor to which thiazolidinediones bind. The natural ligands for each of the PPARs are unknown, and the physiology of each is being studied actively. The three-dimensional structures of the PPAR class of receptors, as well as the sites involved that characterize each of the subtypes, have been defined, and it is now possible to design molecules that activate a single specific subtype or several subtypes simultaneously.

When thiazolidinediones bind to the PPAR-γ heterodimer, the heterodimer becomes activated and attaches to the PPAR-γ response elements of genes that contain such an element (Fig. 41.11). Binding to the response element is followed by incorporation of activator and inhibitor molecules, and gene transcription is either activated or inhibited. The specific genes that are PPARγ responsive are numerous (e.g., lipoprotein lipase, fatty acid–binding proteins, PEPCK) and involve the regulation of lipid metabolism, insulin action, and adipose tissue differentiation.

The major pharmacologic actions of thiazolidinediones *in vivo* are to increase insulin-mediated glucose uptake (decrease in insulin resistance) in muscle and to increase adipogenesis (37,128–131). Considerable controversy exists concerning the mechanism of both of these actions. PPARγ receptors are

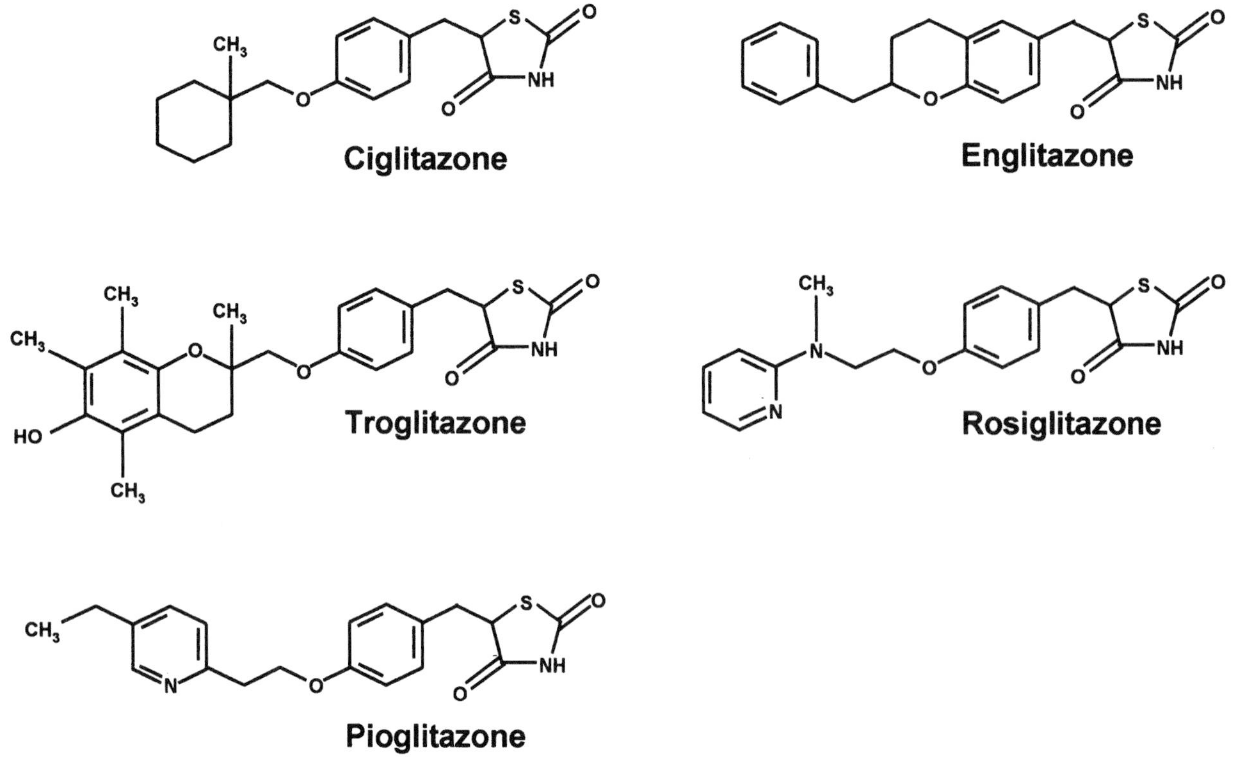

FIG. 41.10. Structure of commonly studied and currently available glitazones.

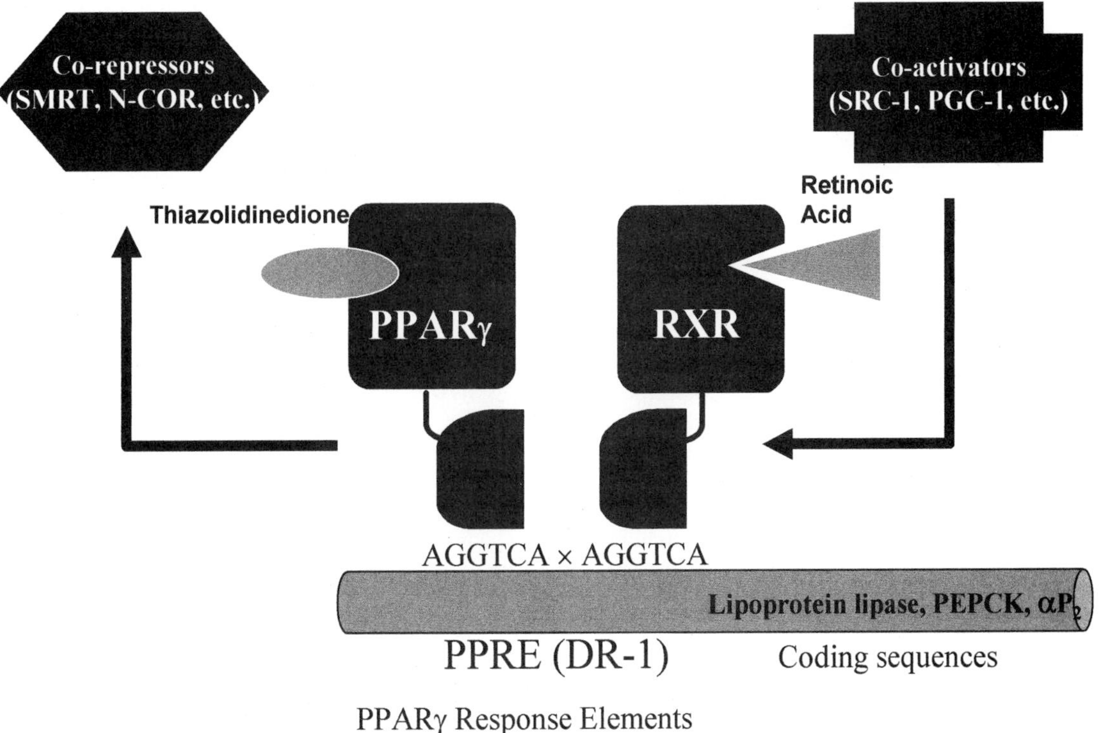

FIG. 41.11. Mechanism of action of thiazolidinediones. Thiazolidinediones bind to the PPARγ receptor of a heterodimeric intranuclear transcription factor. The activated transcription factor binds to genes with a PPARγ response element and, after interactions with appropriate coactivators and coinhibitors, either activates or inhibits transcription of the genes. (Adapted from Forman BM, Tontonoz P, Chen J, et al. 15-Deoxy-delta 12,14 prostaglandin J2 is a ligand for the adipocyte determination factor PPARγ. *Cell* 1995; 83:803–812.)

expressed primarily in adipose tissue (>10-fold higher than in muscle), yet the major quantitative effect in improving total body insulin sensitivity occurs in muscle. One strain of genetically engineered mice that lack adipose tissue (A-ZIP/F-1 phenotype) fail to respond to troglitazone or rosiglitazone therapy by a reduction in insulin resistance and hyperglycemia (132). In contrast, another genetically altered mouse (aP2/DTA) that has little or no white or brown adipose tissue responds to troglitazone with the expected improvement in insulin resistance and hyperglycemia (133). The latter data plus muscle cell culture studies showing that troglitazone increases glucose uptake suggest the possibility that the small number of PPAR-γ receptors in muscle and liver might mediate the insulin-sensitizing effects of thiazolidinediones. Recent studies, however, have emphasized that products released from adipose tissue such as free fatty acids and their metabolic derivatives rather than adipose tissue itself mediate the insulin resistance in muscle (7,134), and these products are elevated in the mice without peripheral adipose tissue (132). Other studies show that thiazolidinediones act on adipose tissue to decrease not only the circulating levels of free fatty acids but also protein factors such as tumor necrosis factor-α, resistin, and leptin that are released from adipose tissue and that can cause insulin resistance in muscle (135,136). Thiazolidinediones also stimulate the release of an adipose tissue hormone, adiponectin, which is associated with increased hepatic insulin sensitivity (137). Thus, whether the improvement in insulin action is secondary to a primary action on adipose tissue, is a specific effect on free fatty acid metabolism, or is a direct effect on muscle has not yet been resolved (125–127, 129). The second major unresolved issue is how a drug that increases the quantity of adipose tissue can decrease insulin resistance. In rodents, thiazolidinediones increase the number of small adipocytes and decrease the number of large adipocytes (138). The smaller cells are more sensitive to insulin and have a lower rate of lipolysis. In humans, thiazolidinediones increase adipogenesis in subcutaneous adipose tissue but have no effect on visceral adipose tissue (139,140). Thus, thiazolidinediones appear to facilitate adipogenesis but in a way that improves insulin sensitivity.

PPAR-γ receptors are present in moderate concentrations in macrophages, colonic epithelium, and endothelial and vascular smooth muscle cells. Their functions in these tissues are being investigated actively, as is the therapeutic potential of these drugs for the treatment of inflammatory bowel disease and the early lesions of atherosclerosis.

Pharmacokinetics and Metabolism

Rosiglitazone and pioglitazone are rapidly and well absorbed orally (141,142). Both are extensively metabolized in the liver by the CYP450 isoenzymes—rosiglitazone by CYP2C8 and CYP2C9 and pioglitazone by CYP2C8, CYP3A4, and several other CYP isoenzymes. Approximately two thirds of the rosiglitazone dose is excreted in the urine and approximately one third in the bile, whereas two thirds of the pioglitazone dose is excreted in the feces and one third in the urine. The plasma half-life of rosiglitazone is 3 to 4 hours and that of pioglitazone and its active metabolites is 16 to 24 hours. Both drugs can be administered safely to individuals with impaired renal function.

Clinical Use

Rosiglitazone is administered in doses of 4 to 8 mg given once or twice daily (130,141). Pioglitazone is given in doses of 15 to

45 mg administered once daily (131,142). These differences in effective doses reflect to some degree the differences in binding affinities of these two drugs for the human PPAR-γ receptor. When administered to patients with type 2 diabetes who are inadequately controlled with diet and increased physical activity, rosiglitazone at 4 and 8 mg daily decreased HbA_{1c} and FPG 1.2% and 58 mg/dL and 1.5% and 76 mg/dL, respectively. Pioglitazone at 15 and 45 mg daily decreased HbA_{1c} and FPG 1.0% and 39 mg/dL and 1.6% and 65 mg/dL, respectively. These data reflect comparisons to placebo treatment in the same studies. Of the patients treated with rosiglitazone at 4 mg twice a day, 59% achieved a HbA_{1c} level of less than 8% and 30% achieved a level less than 7%. The data on glycemic control with monotherapy indicate that the two thiazolidinediones are similar in efficacy. Because the patient populations studied had somewhat different clinical characteristics (patients treated with pioglitazone had poorer baseline glycemic control, were more obese, and were hypertriglyceridemic than those treated with rosiglitazone), any subtle differences noted in the responses to the two drugs may have been due to differences in the responsiveness of the different populations rather than any true differences of the effects of the drugs. Any presumed differences need to be substantiated by a comparison of comparably effective doses of the two drugs in the same randomized controlled study.

In addition to improving glycemic control, both pioglitazone and rosiglitazone improve many of the components of the insulin resistance syndrome (29,127–129). Both improve insulin sensitivity and decrease plasma insulin levels. Both improve the dyslipidemia characteristic of insulin resistance, that is, they both consistently increase plasma HDL cholesterol and have some effects on lowering plasma triglycerides. Differences in the effects of pioglitazone and rosiglitazone on dyslipidemia have been reported (143). Rosiglitazone produced a small increase in plasma concentrations of LDL cholesterol and reduced plasma triglycerides only if they were elevated. Preliminary data indicate that these changes may be due to a shift in the characteristics of the LDL particles from small, dense, very atherogenic particles to large, buoyant, less atherogenic ones and not to an increase in the number of particles. Pioglitazone treatment has been associated with a general reduction in plasma triglycerides and no increase in plasma levels of LDL cholesterol. As noted previously, a comparison of the effects of the two drugs on dyslipidemia in the same randomized study is necessary to clarify whether these drugs do indeed have somewhat different effects on serum lipids and lipoproteins.

The thiazolidinediones decrease plasma levels of PAI-1, which reduces the inhibition of fibrinolysis that is characteristic of insulin resistance (144). One of the more striking effects of treatment of patients with type 2 diabetes with thiazolidinediones is a 20% to 25% reduction in plasma levels of free fatty acids (130). Several studies have shown that thiazolidinediones reduce rates of urinary excretion of albumin independent of their effects on improving glycemia (145). The thiazolidinediones cause an increase in subcutaneous adipose tissue (~5%–8%) but either have no effect or slightly reduce visceral adipose tissue (128,146). Preliminary data indicate that thiazolidinediones improve the endothelial dysfunction that is characteristic of insulin resistance (16).

The decline in β-cell function characteristic of type 2 diabetes has been postulated to be related in part to detrimental effects of insulin resistance (147). Insulin resistance increases β-cell secretory function and as such increases the metabolic activity of the β-cell and also increases the secretion of amylin. Increased secretion of amylin can result in increased amyloid deposits within the islets and in destruction of β-cells. Increased metabolic activity of genetically programmed β-cells could lead to increased rates of apoptosis. It has been postulated that thiazolidinediones, by reducing insulin resistance, might decrease the rate of β-cell loss in patients with type 2 diabetes. Controlled studies comparing glyburide treatment with rosiglitazone for 1 year show better preservation of glucose control with rosiglitazone. One-year studies are inadequate to prove β-cell preservation and need to be followed up by 3- to 5-year studies. Studies in two rodent models of insulin-resistant diabetes have shown that rosiglitazone treatment does preserve β-cells in that setting (148). Recently reported studies (TRIPOD study) have shown that the administration of troglitazone to women who had previously had gestational diabetes decreases the rate of β-cell loss and can prevent the development or progression of type 2 diabetes (100). This effect is likely due to its reduction in insulin resistance, an effect shared by the two available thiazolidinediones, rosiglitazone and pioglitazone.

Side Effects

The major side effects observed with rosiglitazone and pioglitazone have been fluid retention with peripheral edema and, in unusual circumstances, congestive heart failure, and weight gain (37,128,141,142). Idiosyncratic liver toxicity with liver failure developed in a few people treated with troglitazone who then died. The clinical trials with troglitazone showed some changes in liver function that in retrospect were probably signals of potential hepatotoxicity (130). Serum alanine aminotransferase (ALT) levels greater than three times the upper limit of the reference range (ULRR) were recorded in 1.9% of the patients with type 2 diabetes treated with troglitazone compared with 0.6% of those who received placebo (Fig. 41.12). As many as 0.68% of the troglitazone-treated patients had serum ALT values 10 times or greater than the ULRR, and jaundice developed in two patients that reversed on drug withdrawal. In contrast, neither rosiglitazone nor pioglitazone showed any signal of hepatotoxicity during their clinical trials, and after approximately 2 years on the market, no significant severe hepatotoxicity has been associated with either drug.

A small increase in plasma volume appears to be related to activation of the PPAR-γ receptor, as judged by a small decrease in hemoglobin and hematocrit values (0.6 g/dL and 2.8%, respectively) (130,131). This change was not accompanied by any alteration in red blood cell mass in any patients with diabetes treated with any of the thiazolidinediones. Mild-to-moderate peripheral edema is observed in 3% to 5% of patients treated with a thiazolidinedione as monotherapy (37,128,130, 131). This increases to approximately 15% in patients treated with the combination of pioglitazone and insulin (128). The mechanism for the development of edema is presently unknown. The edema responds poorly to loop diuretics and inhibitors of angiotensin-converting enzymes. Rarely, severe edema can develop that is reversed with discontinuation of the drug. It is unclear to what extent thiazolidinedione treatment might precipitate heart failure in a susceptible patient, as there are no controlled data. It might be anticipated that an individual in borderline congestive heart failure would develop clinical failure if the plasma volume were expanded significantly. There is no evidence in 1- and 2-year studies of cardiovascular function that the thiazolidinediones have any detrimental effect on myocardial function (149).

The weight gain associated with thiazolidinedione treatment is due to a combination of fluid retention and an increase in adipose tissue. A primary action of thiazolidinediones is the differentiation of stem cells into adipocytes (126,127). In humans, PPAR-γ agonists differentiate subcutaneous adipose tissue stem cells into small adipocytes but appear to have no effect on the

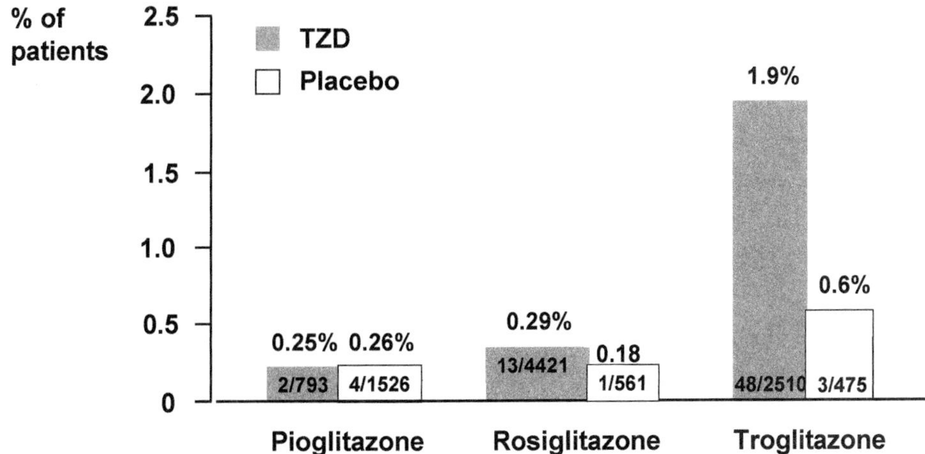

FIG. 41.12. The results of monitoring alanine aminotransferase (ALT) levels in the phase three clinical trials of troglitazone, rosiglitazone, and pioglitazone. The percentage of subjects with any ALT that is greater than three times the upper limit of the reference range (ULRR) is reported. Troglitazone treatment was associated with a significantly higher rate of abnormal values than was the placebo control. Neither rosiglitazone nor pioglitazone treatment showed any differences in abnormal values from their placebo controls.

differentiation of visceral adipose tissue stem cells (140). Several studies have examined the effect of either troglitazone or rosiglitazone on weight gain and adipose tissue distribution. All studies show a significant increase in total body fat and subcutaneous adipose tissue mass. Mass of visceral adipose tissue is usually not changed (128,146,150).

The effects on expansion of plasma volume usually are seen in the first 12 weeks of treatment and probably stabilize by 6 months. The few long-term studies on weight gain show increases that tend to slow down and stabilize after 12 months of treatment. Careful long-term studies of both edema and weight gain are needed to clarify these issues.

Potential Cardiovascular Benefits

Thiazolidinediones ameliorate many of the components of the insulin resistance syndrome, and one might anticipate that such actions would decrease the cardiovascular complications of type 2 diabetes (128,151). At the present time, clinical outcome studies are limited to a few preliminary observations that thiazolidinedione treatment preserves the patency of coronary artery stents by slowing the proliferation of the cells of the intima and media. There are many observations of improvement of endothelial function *in vivo*. The improvement of the dyslipidemia by increasing plasma high-density lipoprotein cholesterol, lowering elevated plasma triglycerides, and shifting LDL particles from small-dense to large-buoyant particles are significant and consistent effects of thiazolidinediones, as is the improvement in the procoagulant state. Although the current data are insufficient to recommend thiazolidinediones as primary treatment for improving macrovascular outcomes in patients with type 2 diabetes, one needs to be aware of the potential of these agents. Outcome studies are under way to determine the effects of these agents on clinical cardiovascular events.

α-GLUCOSIDASE INHIBITORS

The recognition of the importance of controlling postprandial hyperglycemia began when pharmacologic agents specifically targeted at postprandial plasma glucose levels became available. The first group of these agents were oral agents specifically designed to delay postprandial carbohydrate digestion and lower postprandial plasma glucose excursions. The α-glucosidase inhibitor acarbose is a pseudotetrasaccharide of microbial origin that was isolated and purified in the late 1970s and approved for the treatment of type 2 diabetes in the early 1990s (152). It acts exclusively on the gastrointestinal tract and specifically lowers postprandial glucose excursions.

Mechanism of Action

The digestion of complex carbohydrates involves initial cleavage by amylases in the small intestine into oligosaccharides (11, 153). Oligosaccharides are poorly absorbed and have to be cleaved into monosaccharides before absorption through the intestinal mucosa. The cleavage of oligosaccharides into monosaccharides occurs in the brush border of the enterocytes and is carried out by a variety of α-glucosidase enzymes (glucoamylase, sucrase, maltase, dextrinase, and isomaltase). The monosaccharides generated are absorbed rapidly. The digestion of complex carbohydrates normally occurs in the distal duodenum and proximal jejunum.

The cleavage of the oligosaccharides by the α-glucosidase enzyme involves binding of the oligosaccharides to a binding site on the enzyme, followed by hydrolytic cleavage. The α-glucosidase inhibitors compete with the oligosaccharides for the binding site. They bind to the site but cannot be hydrolyzed. They are classic competitive inhibitors. The mechanisms of action of the different α-glucosidase inhibitors are similar though not identical. Acarbose binds to glucoamylase, maltase, sucrase, and dextrinase. It binds to intestinal sucrase with a binding affinity 10^4 to 10^5 greater than that to sucrose. Acarbose has minimal effects on isomaltase and no effect on lactase, which is a β-glucosidase enzyme. Acarbose is also an inhibitor of pancreatic amylase. Voglibose inhibits most α-glucosidase enzymes but is weaker than acarbose at inhibiting sucrase and has little effect on pancreatic amylase. Neither acarbose nor voglibose interferes with glucose absorption through the intestinal sodium-dependent glucose transporter. Miglitol is an effective α-glucosidase inhibitor and has greater activity than acarbose on isomaltase. Miglitol has no effect on pancreatic amylase but does mildly interfere with glucose absorption by interacting with the intestinal sodium-dependent glucose transporter.

The consequence of administering an α-glucosidase inhibitor with the meal is that oligosaccharide cleavage is only partially accomplished in the upper small intestine. The rest of the oligosaccharides go into the middle and distal small intestine, where they are cleaved if the enterocytes contain sufficient enzyme. If enzyme is insufficient, the oligosaccharides go into the large intestine, where the bacteria ferment the carbohydrate and produce short-chain fatty acids, hydrogen gas, methane, and carbon dioxide.

Since carbohydrate digestion and absorption normally are complete in the upper jejunum, the amount of α-glucosidase enzyme in the middle and distal small intestine is low and insufficient to digest the carbohydrate load presented to it during the initiation of α-glucosidase treatment unless the therapy is initiated with a very low dose and the dose is increased very slowly over time.

Pharmacokinetics and Metabolism

Three α-glucosidase inhibitors are available: acarbose, voglibose, and miglitol (Fig. 41.13). Acarbose is a pseudotetrasaccharide that contains a nitrogen in place of an oxygen. Voglibose is a valiolamine derivative, and miglitol is a synthetic deoxynojirimycin analogue (11). The primary site of action of both acarbose and voglibose is at the enterocytes, since neither is significantly absorbed (acarbose <2%; voglibose 3%–5%). Miglitol is absorbed rapidly and excreted unchanged by the kidney. Although acarbose is not absorbed, it is metabolized in the colon by bacteria to several intermediates and 4-methylpyrogallol, which are absorbed, conjugated, and excreted as sulfates or glucuronidates. Because the α-glucosidase inhibitors are competitive inhibitors of the binding of oligosaccharides, they must be administered at the start of each meal.

Clinical Use

α-Glucosidase inhibitors must be given at the start of each meal. They are effective only if the diet contains at least 40% and preferably 50% carbohydrate. As noted previously, therapy must be initiated with very low doses and the doses titrated up quite slowly. For acarbose and miglitol, therapy should be started with 25 mg with the evening meal (153). After 2 weeks or so the dose can be increased to 25 mg with the start of breakfast and 25 mg with the start of the evening meal. After another several weeks, the dose can be increased to 25 mg at the start of each of the three major meals. Increasing the dose to 50 mg with each meal should also be done in incremental steps. If at any stage, gastrointestinal side effects become a significant problem, the dose should be reduced for several weeks and then the titration continued. Most patients will initially obtain a maximal effect on glycemia at 50 mg with each meal. Some, however, may need to have the dose increased slowly to 100 mg with each meal. The primary clinical effect of the α-glucosidase inhibitors is to decrease the postprandial glucose excursion in patients with either type 1 or type 2 diabetes. The mean decrease in the peak postprandial rise in plasma glucose level during acarbose monotherapy in diet-treated patients with type 2 diabetes is approximately 54 mg/dL and is associated with a

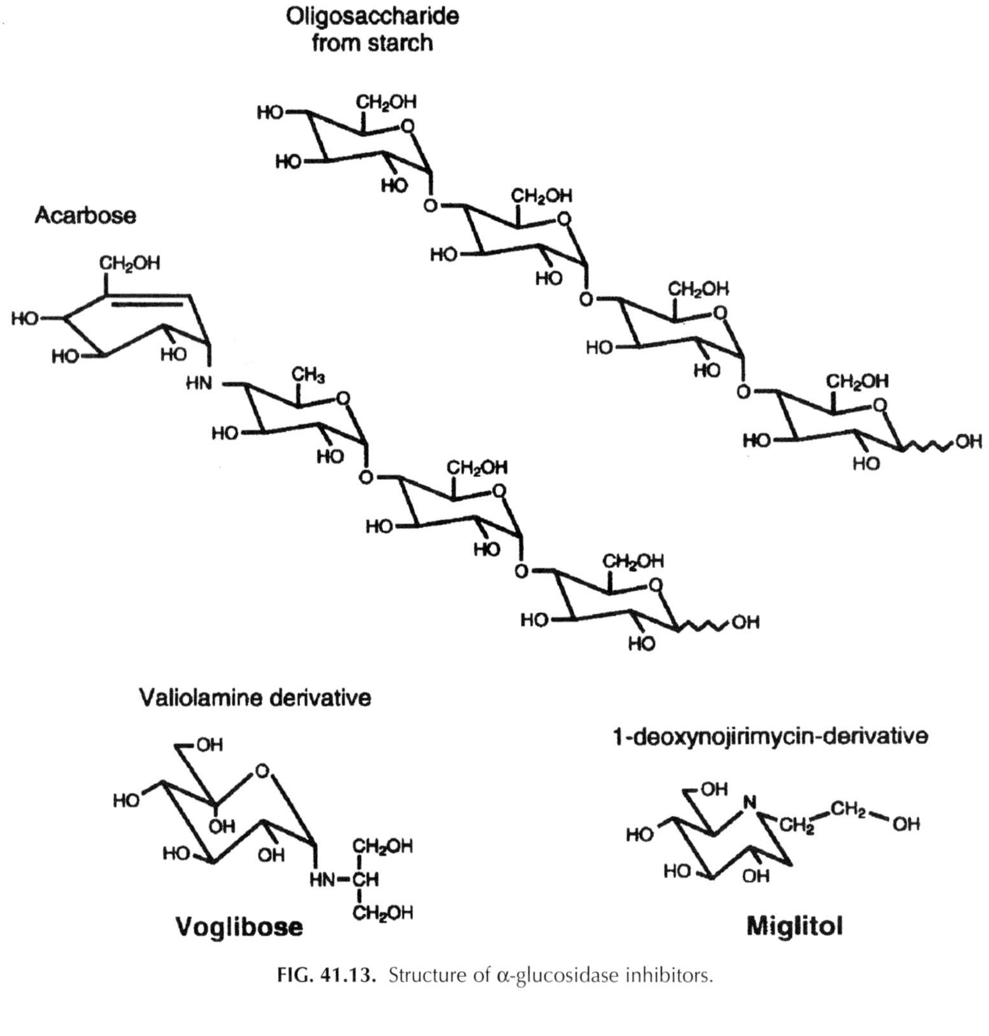

FIG. 41.13. Structure of α-glucosidase inhibitors.

mean decrease in HbA_{1c} of 0.9% (11,154). The mean decrease in FPG is approximately 24 mg/dL, and that is probably due to a reduction in glucose toxicity as a result of improved postprandial hyperglycemia. Voglibose is given at a dose of 0.1 to 0.2 mg with each major meal. There are no comparative data for voglibose and acarbose, but the few reported studies suggest that voglibose lowers mean HbA_{1c} between 0.3% and 0.7%

α-Glucosidase inhibitors are extremely effective for the treatment of severe hypoglycemia following gastrointestinal surgery and other forms of reactive hypoglycemia. Several studies have shown that α-glucosidase inhibitors given with the evening meal can reduce the incidence and severity of nocturnal hypoglycemia in patients with insulin-treated type 1 diabetes.

Other effects of α-glucosidase inhibitors are a slight reduction in mean weight (<1.0 kg), a decrease in postprandial plasma insulin levels, a small decrease in postprandial plasma triglycerides, and a modest increase in plasma levels of glucagon-like peptide-1 (11).

Side Effects

The major side effects of α-glucosidase inhibitor therapy are gastrointestinal and include abdominal discomfort, flatus, and diarrhea, which are due to an excessive amount of carbohydrate reaching the colon and undergoing fermentation (11,155). Rare cases of jaundice with cholestasis have been reported in patients in Japan treated with acarbose and voglibose. However, studies of acarbose administration to individuals with liver disease have not shown any significant worsening of the hepatic problems.

Hypoglycemia does not occur with monotherapy with these agents. The addition of an α-glucosidase inhibitor to a sulfonylurea, another insulin secretogogue, or insulin, may improve glycemic control such that hypoglycemia may occur. In such cases, the hypoglycemia must be treated with glucose because the digestion of sucrose and complex carbohydrates will be delayed.

COMBINATION THERAPY WITH ORAL AGENTS AND ORAL AGENTS AND INSULIN

Although all of the oral antidiabetic agents are reasonably effective as monotherapy in improving glycemic control and reducing HbA_{1c}, they are rarely able to restore glycemia to near normal and HbA_{1c} levels to less than 6.5% in patients with type 2 diabetes who present with fasting hyperglycemia and HbA_{1c} levels of 7% or greater (13). This is probably because the hyperglycemia is caused by the combination of metabolic defects that have caused the diabetes and the marked deficiency of β-cell function that has occurred by the time an individual has developed symptomatic hyperglycemia (12). Oral medications such as sulfonylureas and metformin that predominately lower FPG will decrease HbA_{1c} values 2.0% to 3.0% in patients with type 2 diabetes who have HbA_{1c} values 10% or greater by a combination of their specific pharmacologic actions and the resultant decrease in glucose toxicity (13,14,128). The same agents will lower HbA_{1c} only 0.5% to 1.0% when the baseline HbA_{1c} is between 6.0% and 8.0%. The same types of results are obtained with oral agents that lower both fasting and postprandial plasma glucoses, such as repaglinide and thiazolidinediones. Oral agents that primarily decrease postprandial plasma glucose levels will have a lesser absolute effect on HbA_{1c} levels (decrease of 0.5%–1.0% at a baseline HbA_{1c} of 8.0%–9.0%), but again their effects decrease as the baseline HbA_{1c} level decreases (13).

It appears that there is a limited benefit to improving glycemic control by ameliorating any one specific mechanism that accounts for the hyperglycemia in patients with type 2 diabetes. Generally, replacing an oral agent with one mechanism of action by another with a different mechanism of action does not result in better glycemic control (116,156). Combining agents with different modes of action, as depicted in Figure 41.5, produces additive effects on glycemic control; allows the use of submaximal doses of the agents, thereby decreasing unwanted side effects; and provides for complementary benefits on cardiovascular risk factors (13,14). Tables 41.7 and 41.8, which are from one of the author's recent reviews, illustrate these advantages (13). Table 41.9 summarizes the results of most of the published U.S. Food and Drug Administration registration studies that have examined the effects of combination oral antihyperglycemic agent therapy on glycemic control in patients with type 2 diabetes (13).

The main principles that underlie combination therapy (Table 41.10) start with the assessment of a patient's specific pathophysiology at the time of initiation of therapy. The assessment should determine (a) the presence or absence of significant insulin resistance; (b) the components, if any, of the insulin resistance syndrome that are present; (c) the stage of

TABLE 41.7. Direct Effects of Oral Antihyperglycemic Agents on Cardiovascular Risk Factors in Patients with Type 2 Diabetes

Cardiovascular risk factor	Sulfonylurea	Rapid-acting insulin secretogogues	Metformin	Thiazolidinediones	α-Glucosidase inhibitors
Insulin resistance	0	0	↓↓	↓↓↓	0
Hyperinsulinemia	0	0	↓↓	↓↓↓	↓↓↓
LDL cholesterol levels	0	0	↓	↑ or 0	0
LDL particle pattern	0	0	?	Large buoyant	0
HDL cholesterol levels	0	0	0	↑↑↑	0
Triglycerides	0	0	↓	↓↓	0
Lp(a)	0	0	↓↓	↑	0
PAI-1	0	0	↓↓	↓↓	0
Endothelial function	0	0	↑	↑↑↑	0
Body weight	↑↑	↑↑	↓↓	↑↑	0
Visceral adiposity	↑	?	↓↓	0 or ↓	

HDL, high-density lipoprotein; LDL, low-density lipoprotein; Lp(a), lipoprotein little A antigen; PAI, plasminogen activator inhibitor-1.
↑↑↑, marked increase; ↑↑, moderate increase; ↑, small increase; 0, no increase.
↓↓↓, marked decrease; ↓↓, moderate decrease; ↓, small decrease.
Modified from Lebovitz HE. Oral therapies for diabetic hyperglycemia. *Endocrinol Metab Clin North Am* 2001;30:909–933.

TABLE 41.8. Side Effects of Oral Antihyperglycemic Agents

Drug	Hypoglycemia	Weight gain	Edema	GI effects	Lactic acidosis	Liver toxicity
Glipizide-GITS	1+	1+	0	±	0	±
Gliburide	4+	2+	0	±	0	±
Glimepiride	2+	1+	0	±	0	±
Repaglinide	1+	1+	0	0	0	0
Nateglinide	1+	?	0	0	0	0
Metformin	0	↓	0	2+	1+	0
Acarbose	0	0	0	3+	0	±
Miglitol	0	0	0	3+	0	0
Rosiglitazone	0	3+	2+	0	0	0[a]
Pioglitazone	0	3+	2+	0	0	0[a]

0, none; ±, very infrequent; 1+, infrequent problem; 2+, occasional problem; 3+, moderate problem; 4+, significant problem; ↓, decrease.
[a]No evidence of liver toxicity but monitoring of liver function every 2 months for the first year of treatment still recommended.
Data from Lebovitz HE. Oral therapies for diabetic hyperglycemia. *Endocrinol Metab Clin North Am* 2001;30:909–933.

TABLE 41.9. Effect of Combination Therapy with Oral Antihyperglycemic Agents on Glycemic Control in Registration Studies

Drug	Dosage (mg/day)	Baseline mean HbA_{1c} (%)	Additional decrease in HbA_{1c} (%)[a]	Percentage attaining $HbA_{1c} \leq 7\%$
Metformin ≥2,000 mg/d +				
Glyburide	20	8.8	1.3 (1.7)	NA
Repaglinide	12	8.3	1.1 (1.4)	~60
Nateglinide	120	8.4	0.7 (1.9)	NA
Acarbose	600	7.8	0.8	NA
Rosiglitazone	8	8.9	1.2 (0.8)	28
Pioglitazone	30	9.9	0.8 (0.64)	NA
Rosiglitazone 8 mg/d +				
Repaglinide	12	9.2	1.15 (1.45)	NA
Sulfonylurea			1.4 (1.4)	NA
Pioglitazone 30 mg/d +				
Repaglinide	12	9.6	2.2 (1.9)	NA
Sulfonylurea		10.0	1.3 (1.2)	NA
Insulin[b] +				
Metformin	2,000	9.0	0.54 (2.1)	NA
Sulfonylurea		8.9	1.0 (1.8)	NA
Rosiglitazone	8	9.0	1.3 (1.2)	NA
Pioglitazone	30	9.9	1.0 (1.3)	NA

NA, not available.
[a]Difference from placebo treatment (difference from baseline).
[b]Insulin dose is usually decreased 15% to 25% when oral agents are added to an insulin treatment program in patients with type 2 diabetes.
Data from Lebovitz HE. Oral therapies for diabetic hyperglycemia. *Endocrinol Clin North Am* 2001;30:909–933.

TABLE 41.10. Guidelines for Developing Combination Therapy Strategy for Patients with Type 2 Diabetes

Assess patient's specific pathophysiology
- Is insulin resistance present?
- Are there any components of the insulin resistance syndrome?
- What is the stage of β-cell function?
- How abnormal are the fasting plasma glucose levels?
- What is the magnitude of postprandial hyperglycemia?
- Evaluate the patient for subclinical or clinical diabetic complications
- Estimate the patient's life expectancy

Define the goals of treatment
Select the appropriate insulin sensitizers
Select a method of increasing insulin availability
- Insulin secretogogue
- Insulin preparation

Decide if an α-glucosidase inhibitor has any advantage
In patients in whom glycemic control has been elusive, consider 48- to 72-hr continuous blood glucose monitoring or pattern testing with home glucose monitoring
Monitor HbA_{1c} every 3 mo

β-cell dysfunction; (d) the magnitude of both fasting and postprandial hyperglycemia; (e) the presence of subclinical and/or clinical complications of diabetes; and (f) the likely life expectancy of the patient. After the assessment, the goals for the planned therapeutic intervention should be defined. The choice of an insulin sensitizer needs to be made. Metformin and the thiazolidinediones have major differences in their effects. Rather than regarding them as competing agents, one might consider them as complementary agents. Frequently, there is a rationale for prescribing them in combination. The next choice is to decide whether β-cell function is sufficient to warrant the use of an insulin secretogogue or whether insulin or an insulin analogue should be used. If an insulin secretogogue is chosen, it is necessary to decide which one to use. Sulfonylureas are inexpensive and can be given once a day. Rapid-acting insulin secretogogues are expensive and must be administered with each meal. Weight gain and hypoglycemia are less with the rapid-acting insulin secretogogues. They also partially restore early postprandial insulin secretion and provide a much more flexible lifestyle. If insulin is elected, a choice of a basal, bedtime, or meal-related insulin or a combination of them must be made (see Chapter 39). If postprandial hyperglycemia is the major unresolved issue, the use of an α-glucosidase inhibitor as part of the therapeutic program might be desirable. Combinations of two and sometimes three oral antihyperglycemic agents may be necessary to reach the target glycemic goal.

The availability of devices that allow for continuous blood glucose monitoring for 48 to 72 hours has revolutionized our understanding of the individual variability that occurs in glucose regulation in patients with diabetes. These devices may assist in planning and modifying combination therapy in patients who are not achieving target goals with their current regimen, although the advantage of these devices over traditional home blood glucose monitoring four to seven times a day has not been determined.

Among the unanswered questions concerning combination therapy is whether it should be started at the time of clinical diagnosis or only after a trial of monotherapy has failed to achieve the target glycemic goal. The recent clinical trial comparing the efficacy of glyburide alone, metformin alone, and a combination of submaximal doses of glyburide and metformin on glycemic control in patients with type 2 diabetes inadequately controlled by diet and exercise showed better glycemic control with initial combination therapy than with monotherapy with either agent alone (157). It was unclear from that study whether the improved benefit resulted from some potentiating of effects or from a limitation of the dose of the monotherapy because of side effects.

The combination of one or more insulin sensitizers with an insulin secretogogue will result in target glycemic goals only if there is sufficient β-cell function remaining to allow endogenous insulin secretion in the presence of improved insulin sensitivity to regulate glucose and lipid metabolism appropriately. In many instances, and particularly after several years of clinical diabetes, β-cell function is so reduced that insulin secretogogues either need to be replaced by or supplemented with exogenous insulin preparations. An effective strategy is to administer either intermediate-acting insulin or glargine at 10:00 p.m. to regulate overnight hepatic glucose production, resulting in an FPG less than 110 mg/dL, or either an oral insulin sensitizer or a short-acting insulin secretogogue, or a combination of both, to regulate prandial glucose control (158,159). This type of program will decrease HbA_{1c} between 1.8% and 2.5% when the baseline HbA_{1c} with two oral agents is approximately 9.5% (Table 41.11). In the instances where β-cell insufficiency is so advanced that the patient with type 2 diabetes requires full insulin replacement therapy, it is also important to treat the insulin resistance (either effective lifestyle modification or insulin sensitizers), as it will decrease the quantity of insulin (160–162) that has to be administered and will improve the components of the insulin resistance syndrome, most of which are known cardiovascular risk factors (3,128,147, 163).

Therapy for type 2 diabetes with oral medications has become more complicated because of the availability of several new classes of drugs, particularly the insulin sensitizers. These drugs appear to be increasing the number of patients who can achieve target glucose values with oral therapy. In addition, these new drugs, used singly or in combination, may prolong the responses of improved glycemic control by improving β-cell function directly or indirectly. The long-term results of these combinations on clinical diabetes outcomes remain to be established by long-term intervention trials.

TABLE 41.11. Effects of Bedtime NPH Insulin and Daytime Oral Agents or Morning NPH Insulin on Glycemic Control in Patients with Type 2 Diabetes with Previous Poor Control with Oral Agents (Treatment Duration 1 yr)

Parameter	Glyburide	Metformin	Glyburide + metformin	Morning NPH insulin
Number of patients	22	19	23	24
ΔHbA_{1c} (%)	−1.9[a]	−2.5	−2.1[a]	−1.9[a]
Δ Body weight (lb)	+8.6[a]	+2.0	+7.9[a]	+10.1[b]
Δ Triglyceride (% change)	−30	−29	−17	−35
Insulin dose (U/day)				
Bedtime	24[b]	36	20[b]	24[b]
Morning				29
Hypoglycemia (%)	2.2[b]	1.1	1.8[a]	1.2

Hypoglycemia defined as fasting blood glucose level <63 mg/dL (3.5 mmol/L).
[a]$P < .05$ compared with bedtime NPH insulin + metformin.
[b]$P < .01$ compared with bedtime NPH insulin + metformin.
Data from Yki-Jarvinen H, Ryysy L, Nikkila K, et al. Comparison of bedtime insulin regimens in patients with type 2 diabetes mellitus: a randomized, controlled trial. *Ann Intern Med* 1999;130:389–396.

REFERENCES

1. Diabetes Control and Complications Trial Research Group. The effect of intensive treatment of diabetes on the development and progression of long-term complications in insulin-dependent diabetes mellitus. *N Engl J Med* 1993;329:977–986.
2. Intensive blood-glucose control with sulphonylureas or insulin compared with conventional treatment and risk of complications in patients with type 2 diabetes (UKPDS 33). UK Prospective Diabetes Study (UKPDS) Group. *Lancet* 1998;352:837–853.
3. Effect of intensive blood glucose control with metformin on complications in overweight patients with type 2 diabetes (UKPDS 34). UK Prospective Diabetes Study (UKPDS) Group. *Lancet* 1998;352:854–865.
4. Dostou J, Gerich J. Pathogenesis of type 2 diabetes mellitus. *Exp Clin Endocrinol Diabetes* 2001;109[Suppl 2]:S149–S156.
5. Reaven GM. Banting Lecture 1988. Role of insulin resistance in human disease. *Diabetes* 1998;37:1595–1607.
6. Ferrannini E. Insulin resistance versus insulin deficiency in non-insulin-dependent diabetes mellitus: problems and prospects. *Endocr Rev* 1998;19: 477–490.
7. Shulman GI. Cellular mechanisms of insulin resistance. *J Clin Invest* 2000;106: 171–176.
8. van Haeften TW, Pimenta W, Mitrakou A, et al. Relative contributions of beta-cell function and tissue insulin sensitivity to fasting and postglucose-load glycemia. *Metabolism* 2000;49:1318–1325.
9. Inzucchi SE, Maggs DG, Spollett GR, et al. Efficacy and metabolic effects of metformin and troglitazone in type 2 diabetes mellitus. *N Engl J Med* 1998; 338:867–872.
10. Hanefeld M, Dickinson S, Bouter KP, et al. Rapid and short-acting mealtime insulin secretion with nateglinide controls both prandial and mean glycemia. *Diabetes Care* 2000;23:202–207.
11. Lebovitz HE. Alpha-glucosidase inhibitors as agents in the treatment of diabetes. *Diabetes Rev* 1998;6:132–145.
12. UK Prospective Diabetes Study 16. Overview of 6 years' therapy of type II diabetes: a progressive disease. UK Prospective Diabetes Study Group. *Diabetes* 1995;44:1249–1258.
13. Lebovitz HE. Oral therapies for diabetic hyperglycemia. *Endocrinol Metab Clin North Am* 2001;30:909–933.
14. Inzucchi SE. Oral antihyperglycemic therapy for type 2 diabetes. Scientific review. *JAMA* 2002;287:360–372.
15. Lebovitz HE. Effects of oral antidiabetic agents in modifying macrovascular risk factors in type 2 diabetes. *Diabetes Care* 1999;22[Suppl 3]:C41–C44.
16. Parulkar AA, Pendergrass ML, Granda-Ayala R, et al. Nonhypoglycemic effects of thiazolidinediones. *Ann Intern Med* 2001;134:61–71.
17. The absence of a glycemic threshold for the development of long-term complications: the perspective of the Diabetes Control and Complications Trial. *Diabetes* 1996;45:1289–1298.
18. Stratton IM, Adler AI, Neil HA, et al. Association of glycemia with macrovascular and microvascular complications of type 2 diabetes (UKPDS 35): prospective observational study. *BMJ* 2000;321:405–412.
19. Mitrakou A, Kelley D, Mokan M, et al. Role of reduced suppression of glucose production and diminished early insulin release in impaired glucose tolerance. *N Engl J Med* 1992;326:22–29.
20. Roden M, Petersen KF, Shulman GI. Nuclear magnetic resonance studies of hepatic glucose metabolism in humans. *Recent Prog Horm Res* 2001;56: 219–237.
21. Newsholme EA, Dimitriadis G. Integration of biochemical and physiologic effects of insulin on glucose metabolism. *Exp Clin Endocrinol Diabetes* 2001; 109[Suppl 2]:S122–S134.
22. Gavin JR. Pathophysiologic mechanisms of postprandial hyperglycemia. *Am J Cardiol* 2001;88[Suppl]:4H–8H.
23. Harris MI, Klein R, Welborn TA, et al. Onset of NIDDM occurs at least 4–7 yr before clinical diagnosis. *Diabetes Care* 1992;15:815–819.
24. Haller H. The clinical importance of postprandial glucose. *Diabetes Res Clin Pract* 1998;40[Suppl]:S43–S49.
25. Ceriello A, Lizzio S, Bortolotti N, et al. Meal-generated oxidative stress in type 2 diabetic patients. *Diabetes Care* 1998;21:1529–1533.
26. Ratner RE. Controlling postprandial hyperglycemia. *Am J Cardiol* 2001;88 [Suppl]:26H–31H.
27. Bastyr EJ 3rd, Stuart CA, Brodows RG, et al. Therapy focused on lowering postprandial glucose, not fasting glucose, may be superior for lowering HbA1c. *Diabetes Care* 2000;23:1236–1241.
28. Stern MP, Morales PA, Valdez RA, et al. Predicting diabetes. Moving beyond impaired glucose tolerance. *Diabetes* 1993;42:706–714.
29. Lebovitz HE. Insulin resistance: definition and consequences. *Exp Clin Endocrinol Diabetes* 2001;109[Suppl 2]:S135–S148.
30. Bavdekar A, Chittaranjan S, Yajnik S, et al. Insulin resistance syndrome in 8-year-old Indian children. *Diabetes* 1999;48:2422–2429.
31. Gerich JE. The genetic basis of type 2 diabetes mellitus: Impaired insulin secretion versus impaired insulin sensitivity. *Endocr Rev* 1998;19:491–503.
32. Brunzell JD, Robertson RP, Lerner RL, et al. Relationships between fasting glucose levels and insulin secretion during intravenous glucose tolerance tests. *J Clin Endocrinol Metab* 1976;42:222–229.
33. Report of the Expert Committee on the Diagnosis and Classification of Diabetes Mellitus. *Diabetes Care* 1997;20:1183–1197.
34. Ford ES, Giles WH, Dietz WH. Prevalence of the metabolic syndrome among US adults: findings from the Third National Health and Nutrition Examination Survey. *JAMA* 2002;287:356–359.
35. Isomaa B, Almgren P, Tuomi T, et al. Cardiovascular morbidity and mortality associated with the metabolic syndrome. *Diabetes Care* 2001;24:683–689.
36. Stern M. The Insulin Resistance Syndrome. In: Alberti KGMM, Zimmet P, DeFronzo RA, Keen H, eds. *International textbook of diabetes mellitus*, 2nd ed. Chichester, UK: John Wiley & Sons; 1997:255–283.
37. Lebovitz HE. *Clinician's manual on insulin resistance*. London: Science Press; 2002.
38. Aguilar-Bryan L, Bryan J, Nakazaki M. Of mice and men: K_{ATP} channels and insulin secretion. *Recent Prog Horm Res* 2001;56:47–68.
39. Aguilar-Bryan L, Bryan J. Molecular biology of adenosine triphosphate-sensitive potassium channels. *Endocr Rev* 1999;20:101–135.
40. Miki T, Nagashima K, Seino S. The structure and function of the ATP-sensitive K^+ channel in insulin-secreting pancreatic beta-cells. *J Mol Endocrinol* 1999;22:113–123.
41. Ashcroft FM. Mechanisms of the glycaemic effects of sulfonylureas. *Horm Metab Res* 1996;28:456–463.
42. Fuhlendorff J, Rorsman P, Kofod H, et al. Stimulation of insulin release by repaglinide and glibenclamide involves both common and distinct processes. *Diabetes* 1998;47:345–351.
43. Hu S, Wang S, Fanelli B, et al. Pancreatic β-cell KATP channel activity and membrane-binding studies with nateglinide: a comparison with sulfonylureas and repaglinide. *J Pharmacol Exp Ther* 2000;293:444–452.
44. Kahn SE, McCulloch DK, Porte D Jr. Insulin secretion in normal and diabetic humans. In: Alberti KGMM, Zimmet P, DeFronzo RA, Keen H, eds. *International textbook of diabetes mellitus*, 2nd ed. Chichester, UK: John Wiley & Sons, 1997:337.
45. Lebovitz HE. Insulin secretogogues: old and new. *Diabetes Rev* 1999;7: 139–153.
46. Pimenta W, Korytkowski M, Mitrakou A, et al. Pancreatic beta-cell dysfunction as the primary genetic lesion in NIDDM, evidence from studies in normal glucose-tolerant individuals with a first-degree NIDDM relative. *JAMA* 1995;273:1855–1861.
47. Lebovitz HE, Melander A. Sulfonylureas: basic aspects and clinical use. In: Alberti KGMM, Zimmet P, DeFronzo RA, Keen H, eds. *International textbook of diabetes*, 2nd ed. Chichester, UK: John Wiley & Sons, 1997:817.
48. Burge MR, Sood V, Sobhy TA, et al. Sulphonylurea-induced hypoglycaemia in type 2 diabetes mellitus: a review. *Diabetes Obes Metab* 1999;1:199–206.
49. Jennings AM, Wilson RM, Ward JD. Symptomatic hypoglycemia in NIDDM patients treated with oral hypoglycemic agents. *Diabetes Care* 1989;18: 163–183.
50. Campbell IW, Howlett HCS. Worldwide experience of metformin as an effective glucose-lowering agent: a meta-analysis. *Diabetes Metab Rev* 1995;11: S57–S62.
51. Hu S, Wang S, Dunning BE. Tissue selectivity of antidiabetic agent nateglinide: study on cardiovascular and beta-cell KATP channels. *J Pharmacol Exp Ther* 1999;291:1372–1379.
52. Wright A, Burden AC, Paisey RB, et al. Sulfonylurea inadequacy: efficacy of addition of insulin over 6 years in patients with type 2 diabetes in the UK Prospective Diabetes Study (UKPDS 57). *Diabetes Care* 2002;25:330–336.
53. Turner RC, Cull CA, Frighi V, et al. Glycemic control with diet, sulfonylurea, metformin, or insulin in patients with type 2 diabetes mellitus: progressive requirements for multiple therapies (UKPDS 49). *JAMA* 1999;281:2005–2012.
54. Matthews DR, Cull CA, Stratton IM, et al. UKPDS 26: Sulphonylurea failure in non-insulin-dependent diabetic patients over six years. UK Prospective Diabetes Study (UKPDS) Group. *Diabet Med* 1998;15:297–303.
55. Rosenstock J, Schneider J, Samols E, et al. Glimepiride, a new once-daily sulfonylurea. A double-blind placebo-controlled study of NIDDM patients. *Diabetes Care* 1996;19:1194–1199.
56. Chen HH, Oh KY, Terzic A, et al. The modulating actions of sulfonylurea on atrial natriuretic peptide release in experimental acute heart failure. *Eur J Heart Fail* 2000;2:33–40.
57. Cain BS, Meldrum DR, Meng X, et al. Exogenous calcium preconditions myocardium from patients taking oral sulfonylurea agents. *J Surg Res* 1999; 86:171–176.
58. Betteridge DJ, Close L. Diabetes, coronary heart disease and sulphonylureas—not the final word. *Eur Heart J* 2000;21:790–792.
59. Engler RL, Yallon DM. Sulfonylurea K_{ATP} blockade in type 2 diabetics and preconditioning in cardiovascular disease: time for reconsideration. *Circulation* 1996;94:2297–2301.
60. Shapiro ET, Van Cauter E, Tillil H, et al. Glyburide enhances the responsiveness of the beta cell to glucose but does not correct the abnormal patterns of insulin secretion in non-insulin-dependent diabetes mellitus. *J Clin Endocrinol Metab* 1989;69:571–576.
61. Van der Wal PS, Draeger KE, van Iperen AM, et al. Beta cell response to oral glimepiride administration during and following a hyperglycaemic clamp in NIDDM patients. *Diabet Med* 1997;14:556–563.
62. Stenman S, Melander A, Groop PH, et al. What is the benefit of increasing the sulphonylurea dose? *Ann Intern Med* 1993;118:169–172.
63. Wahlin-Boll E, Sartor G, Melander A, et al. Impaired effect of sulfonylurea following increased dosage. *Eur J Clin Pharmacol* 1982;22:21–25.
64. Kawaki J, Nagashima K, Tanaka J, et al. Unresponsiveness to glibenclamide during chronic treatment is induced by reduction of ATP-sensitive K^+ channel activity. *Diabetes* 1999;48:2001–2006.

65. Eliasson L, Renstrom E, Ammala C, et al. PKC-dependent stimulation of exocytosis by sulfonylureas in pancreatic β cells. *Science* 1996;771:813.
66. Clarke BF, Campbell IW. Long-term comparative trial of glibenclamide and chlorpropamide in diet-failed maturity-onset diabetes. *Lancet* 1974;1:246.
67. Muller R, Bauer G, Schroder R, et al. Summary report of clinical investigation of the oral antidiabetic drug HB 419 (glibenclamide). *Horm Metab Res* 1969;1 [Suppl]:88.
68. Dills DG, Schneider J, Glimepiride/Glyburide Research Group. Clinical evaluation of glimepiride versus glyburide in NIDDM in a double-blind comparative study. *Horm Metab Res* 1996;28:426–429.
69. Asplund K, Wiholm BE, Lithner F. Glibenclamide-associated hypoglycaemia: a report on 57 cases. *Diabetologia* 1983;24:412–417.
70. Shorr RI, Wayne RA, Daugherty JR, et al. Incidence and risk factors for serious hypoglycemia in older persons using insulin or sulfonylureas. *Arch Intern Med* 1997;157:1681–1686.
71. Shorr RI, Ray WA, Daugherty JR, et al. Individual sulfonylureas and serious hypoglycemia in older people. *J Am Geriatr Soc* 1996;44:751–755.
72. Van Staa T, Abenhaim L, Monette J. Rates of hypoglycemia in users of sulfonylureas. *J Clin Epidemiol* 1997;50:735–741.
73. Berelowitz M, Schade DS, Fischette C, et al. Comparative efficacy of a once-daily controlled-release formulation of glipizide and immediate release glipizide in patients with NIDDM. *Diabetes Care* 1994;17:1460–1464.
74. Simonson DC, Kourides IA, Fischette CT, et al. Glipizide GITS Study Group. Efficacy, safety, and dose-response characteristics of glipizide gastrointestinal therapeutic system on glycemic control and insulin secretion in NIDDM. Results of two multicenter, randomized, placebo-controlled clinical trials. *Diabetes Care* 1997;20:597–606.
75. Klepzig H, Kober G, Matter C, et al. Sulfonylureas and ischaemic preconditioning. A double-blind, placebo-controlled evaluation of glimepiride and glibenclamide. *Eur Heart J* 1999;20:439–446.
76. Campbell RK. Glimepiride: role of a new sulfonylurea in the treatment of type 2 diabetes mellitus. *Ann Pharmacother* 1998;32:1044–1052.
77. Draeger KE, Wemicke-Panten K, Lomp H-J, et al. Long-term treatment of type 2 diabetic patients with the new oral antidiabetic agent glimepiride (Amaryl): a double-blind comparison with glibenclamide. *Horm Metab Res* 1996;28:419–425.
78. Goldberg RB, Schneider J, Holvey SM, et al. A dose-response study of glimepiride in patients with NIDDM who have previously received sulfonylurea agents. *Diabetes Care* 1996;19:849–856.
79. Langtry HD, Balfour JA. Glimepiride: a review of its use in the management of type 2 diabetes. *Drugs* 1998;55:563–584.
80. Schneider J. An overview of the safety and tolerance of glimepiride. *Horm Metab Res* 1996;28:413–418.
81. Goldberg RB, Damsbo P, Einhorn D, et al. A randomized placebo-controlled trial of repaglinide in the treatment of type 2 diabetes. *Diabetes Care* 1998;21: 1897–1903.
82. Jovanovic L, Dailey G III, Huang W-C, et al. Repaglinide in type 2 diabetes: a 24-week fixed-dose efficacy and safety study. *J Clin Pharmacol* 2000;40: 49–57.
83. Guay DRP. Repaglinide, a novel, short-acting hypoglycemic agent for type 2 diabetes mellitus. *Pharmacotherapy* 1998;18:1195–1204.
84. Damsbo P, Marbury TC, Clauson P, et al. A double-blind randomized comparison of meal-related glycemic control by repaglinide and glyburide in well-controlled type 2 diabetic patients. *Diabetes Care* 1999;22:789–794.
85. Culy CR, Jarvis B. Repaglinide: a review of its therapeutic use in type 2 diabetes mellitus. *Drugs* 2001;61:1625–1660.
86. Marbury T, Huang W-C, Strange P, et al. Repaglinide versus glyburide: a one year comparison trial. *Diabetes Res Clin Pract* 1999;43:155–166.
87. Levien TL, Baker DE, Campbell RK, et al. Nateglinide therapy for type 2 diabetes mellitus. *Ann Pharmacother* 2001;35:1426–1434.
88. Walter YH, Spratt DI, Garreffa S, et al. Mealtime glucose regulation by nateglinide in type-2 diabetes mellitus. *Eur J Clin Pharmacol* 2000;56:129–133.
89. Horton ES, Foley J, Clinkingbeard C, et al. Nateglinide alone and in combination with metformin improves glycemic control by reducing mealtime glucose levels in type 2 diabetes. *Diabetes Care* 2000;23:1660–1665.
90. University Group Diabetes Program. A study of the effects of hypoglycemic agents on vascular complications in patients with adult-onset diabetes. *Diabetes* 1970;19[Suppl 2]:747–830.
91. Noma A. ATP-regulated K^+ channels in cardiac muscle. *Nature* 1983;305: 147–148.
92. Murry CE, Jennings RB, Reimer KA. Preconditioning with ischemia: a delay of lethal cell injury in ischemic myocardium. *Circulation* 1986;74:1124–1136.
93. Daut J, Maier-Rudolph W, vonBeckerath N, et al. Hypoxic dilatation of coronary arteries is mediated by ATP-sensitive potassium channels. *Science* 1990; 247:1341–1344.
94. Cacciapuoti F, Spiezia R, Bianchi U, et al. Effectiveness of glibenclamide on myocardial ischemic ventricular arrhythmias in non-insulin-dependent diabetes mellitus. *Am J Cardiol* 1991;67:843–847.
95. Tomai F, Crea F, Gaspardone A, et al. Molecular and cellular responses: ischemic preconditioning during coronary angioplasty is prevented by glibenclamide, a selective ATP-sensitive K^+ channel blocker. *Circulation* 1994; 90:700–705.
96. Cleveland JC Jr, Meldrum DR, Cain BS, et al. Oral sulfonylurea hypoglycemic agents prevent ischemic preconditioning in human myocardium: two paradoxes revisited. *Circulation* 1997;96:29–32.
97. Garratt KN, Brady PA, Hassinger NL, et al.: Sulfonylurea drugs increase early mortality in patients with diabetes mellitus after direct angioplasty for acute myocardial infarction. *J Am Coll Cardiol* 1999;33:119–124.
98. Brooks RC, Detre KM. Clinical trials of revascularization in diabetics. *Curr Opin Cardiol* 2000;15:287–292.
99. Klamann A, Sarfert P, Launhardt V, et al. Myocardial infarction in diabetic vs non-diabetic subjects. Survival and infarct size following therapy with sulfonylureas (glibenclamide). *Eur Heart J* 2000;21:220–229.
100. Buchanan TA, Xiang AH, Peters RK, et al. Protection from type 2 diabetes persists in the TRIPOD cohort eight months after stopping troglitazone. *Diabetes* 2001;50[Suppl 2]:327PP(abst).
101. Isomaa B, Almgren P, Henricsson M, et al. Chronic complications in patients with slowly progressing autoimmune type 1 diabetes (LADA). *Diabetes Care* 1999;22:1347–1353.
102. Ginsberg HN. Insulin resistance and cardiovascular disease. *J Clin Invest* 2000;6:453–458.
103. Lempiäinen P, Mykkänen L, Pyörälä K, et al. Insulin resistance syndrome predicts coronary heart disease events in elderly nondiabetic men. *Circulation* 1999;100:123–128.
104. Knowler WC, Barrett-Connor E, Fowler SE, et al. Diabetes Prevention Program Group. Reduction in the incidence of type 2 diabetes with lifestyle intervention or metformin. *N Engl J Med* 2002;346:393–403.
105. Bell PM, Hadden DR. Metformin. *Endocrinol Metab Clin North Am* 1997;26: 523–537.
106. Bailey CJ, Turner RC. Drug therapy: metformin. *N Engl J Med* 1996;334: 574–579.
107. Wiernsperger NF, Bailey CJ. The antihyperglycaemic effect of metformin: therapeutic and cellular mechanisms. *Drugs* 1999;58[Suppl 1]:31–39.
108. Makimattila S, Nikkila K, Yki-Jarvinen H. Causes of weight gain during insulin therapy with and without metformin in patients with type 2 diabetes mellitus. *Diabetologia* 1999;42:406–412.
109. Stumvoll M, Nurjhan N, Perriello G, et al. Metabolic effects of metformin in non-insulin-dependent diabetes mellitus. *N Engl J Med* 1995;333:550–554.
110. Kurukulasuriya R, Banerji MA, Chaiden R, et al. Selective decrease in visceral fat is associated with weight loss during metformin treatment in African Americans with type 2 diabetes. *Diabetes* 1999;489[Suppl 1]:A315 (abst).
111. Yu JG, Kruszynska YT, Mulford MI, et al. A comparison of troglitazone and metformin on insulin requirements in euglycemic intensively insulin-treated type 2 diabetic patients. *Diabetes* 1999;48:2414–2421.
112. Hundal RS, Krssak M, Dufour S, et al. Mechanism by which metformin reduces glucose production in type 2 diabetes. *Diabetes* 2000;49:2063–2069.
113. Chu NV, Kong APS, Kim DD, et al. Differential effects of metformin and troglitazone on cardiovascular risk factors in patients with type 2 diabetes. *Diabetes Care* 2002;25:542–549.
114. Glucophage; Glucophage XR prescribing information. Bristol-Myers Squibb Co. Revised October 2000.
115. Garber AJ, Duncan TG, Goodman AM, et al. Efficacy of metformin in type 2 diabetes: results of a double-blind, placebo-controlled, dose-response trial. *Am J Med* 1997;103:491–497.
116. DeFronzo RA, Goodman AM: Efficacy of metformin in patients with non-insulin-dependent diabetes mellitus. *N Engl J Med* 1995;333:541–549.
117. Clarke BF, Campbell IW. Comparison of metformin and chlorpropamide in non-obese, maturity-onset diabetics uncontrolled by diet. *BMJ* 1977;2: 1576–1578.
118. Fisman EZ, Tenenbaum A, Boyko V, et al. Oral antidiabetic treatment in patients with coronary disease: time-related increased mortality on combined glyburide/metformin therapy over a 7.7 year follow-up. *Clin Cardiol* 2001;24:151–158.
119. Olsson J, Lindberg G, Gottsater M, et al. Increased mortality in type 2 diabetic patients using sulphonylurea and metformin in combination: a population-based observational study. *Diabetologia* 2000;43:558–560.
120. Emslie-Smith AM, Boyle DI, Evans JM, et al. Contraindications to metformin therapy in patients with type 2 diabetes—a population-based study of adherence to prescribing guidelines. *Diabet Med* 2001;18:483–488.
121. Saleh YM, Mudaliar SR, Henry RP. Metabolic and vascular effects of the thiazolidinedione troglitazone. *Diabetes Rev* 1999;7:55–76.
122. Watkins PB, Whitcomb RW. Hepatic dysfunction associated with troglitazone. *N Engl J Med* 1998;338:916–917.
123. Gitlin N, Julie NL, Spurr CL, et al. Two cases of severe clinical and histologic hepatotoxicity associated with troglitazone. *Ann Intern Med* 1998;129:36–37.
124. Lebovitz HE, Kreider M, Freed MI. Evaluation of liver function in type 2 diabetic patients during clinical trials: evidence that rosiglitazone does not cause hepatic dysfunction. *Diabetes Care* 2002;25:815–823.
125. Willson TM, Brown PJ, Sternbach DD, et al. The PPARs: from orphan receptors to drug discovery. *J Med Chem* 2000;43:527–550.
126. Willson TM, Lambert MH, Kliewer SA. Peroxisome proliferator-activated receptor γ and metabolic disease. *Annu Rev Biochem* 2001;70:341–367.
127. Kliewer SA, Xu HE, Lambert MH, et al. Peroxisome proliferator-activated receptors: from genes to physiology. *Recent Prog Horm Res* 2001;56:239–264.
128. Lebovitz HE, Banerji MA. Insulin resistance and its treatment by thiazolidinediones. *Recent Prog Horm Res* 2001;56:265–294.
129. Olefsky JM. Treatment of insulin resistance with peroxisome proliferator-activated receptor γ agonists. *J Clin Invest* 2000;106:467–472.
130. Lebovitz HE, Dole JF, Patwardhan R, et al. Rosiglitazone monotherapy is effective in patients with type 2 diabetes. *J Clin Endocrinol Metab* 2001;86:280–288.
131. Aranoff S, Mathisen AL, Rosenblatt S, et al. Pioglitazone hydrochloride

monotherapy improves glycemic control in the treatment of patients with type 2 diabetes. *Diabetes Care* 2000;23:1605–1611.
132. Chao L, Marcus-Samuels B, Mason MM, et al. Adipose tissue is required for the antidiabetic, but not the hypolipidemic effect of thiazolidinediones. *J Clin Invest* 2000;106:1221–1228.
133. Burant CF, Sreenan S, Hirano K, et al. Troglitazone action is independent of adipose tissue. *J Clin Invest* 1997;100:2900–2908.
134. Dresner A, Laurent D, Marcucci M, et al. Effects of free fatty acids on glucose transport and IRS-1-associated phosphatidylinositol 3-kinase activity. *J Clin Invest* 1999;103:253–259.
135. Katsuki A, Murata K, Furuta M, et al. Troglitazone reduces plasma levels of tumour necrosis factor-α in obese patients with type 2 diabetes. *Diabetes Obes Metab* 2000;2:189–191.
136. Steppen CM, Bailey ST, Bhat S, et al. The hormone resistin links obesity to diabetes. *Nature* 2001;409:307–312.
137. Yang W-S, Jeng C-Y, Wu T-J, et al. Synthetic peroxisome proliferator-activated receptor-γ agonists, rosiglitazone, increases plasma levels of adiponectin in type 2 diabetic patients. *Diabetes Care* 2002;25:376–380.
138. Okuno A, Tamemoto H, Tobe K, et al. Troglitazone increases the number of small adipocytes without the change of white adipose tissue mass in obese Zucker rats. *J Clin Invest* 1998;101:1354–1361.
139. Montague CT, O'Rahilly S. The perils of portliness. Causes and consequences of visceral adiposity. *Diabetes* 2000;49:883–888.
140. Adams M, Montague CT, Prins JB, et al. Activators of PPARγ have depot-specific effects on human pre-adipocyte differentiation. *J Clin Invest* 1997;100: 3149–3153.
141. Balfour JA, Plosker GL. Rosiglitazone. *Drugs* 1999;57:921–930.
142. Gillies PS, Dunn CJ. Pioglitazone. *Drugs* 2000;60:333–343.
143. Khan MA, St Peter JV, Xue Jl. A prospective, randomized comparison of the metabolic effects of pioglitazone or rosiglitazone in patients with type 2 diabetes who were previously treated with troglitazone. *Diabetes Care* 2002;25: 708–711.
144. Freed M, Fuell D, Menci L, et al. Effect of combination therapy with rosiglitazone and glibenclamide on PAI-1 antigen, PAI-1 activity, and tPA in patients with type 2 diabetes. *Diabetologia* 2000;43[Suppl 1]:A267(abst).
145. Imano E, Kanda T, Nakatani Y, et al. Effect of troglitazone on microalbuminuria in patients with incipient diabetic nephropathy. *Diabetes Care* 1998;21: 2135–2139.
146. Mayerson AB, Hundal RS, Dufour S, et al. The effects of rosiglitazone on insulin sensitivity, lipolysis, and hepatic and skeletal muscle triglyceride content in patients with type 2 diabetes. *Diabetes* 2002;51:797–802.
147. Lebovitz HE. Rationale for and role of thiazolidinediones in type 2 diabetes. *Am J Cardiol* 2002 *(in press)*.
148. Finegood DT, McArthur MD, Kojwang D, et al. β-Cell mass dynamics in Zucker diabetic fatty rats. Rosiglitazone prevents the rise in net cell death. *Diabetes* 2001;50:1021–1029.
149. Ghazzi M, Perez J, Antonucci T, et al. Cardiac and glycemic benefits of troglitazone treatment in NIDDM. The Troglitazone Study Group. *Diabetes* 1997; 46:433–439.
150. Akazawa S, Sun F, Ito M, et al. Efficacy of troglitazone on body fat distribution in type 2 diabetes. *Diabetes Care* 2000;23:1067–1071.
151. Hsueh WA, Jackson S, Law RE. Control of vascular cell proliferation and migration by PPARγ. *Diabetes Care* 2001;24:392–397.
152. Lebovitz HE. Oral antidiabetic agents. The emergence of α-glucosidase inhibitors. *Drugs* 1992;44[Suppl 3]:21–28.
153. Lebovitz HE. Alpha-glucosidase inhibitors. *Endocrinol Metab Clin North Am* 1997;26:539–551.
154. Chiasson JL, Josse R, Hunt J, et al. The efficacy of acarbose in the treatment of patients with non-insulin dependent diabetes mellitus. *Ann Intern Med* 1994; 121:928–935.
155. Holman RR, Cull CA, Turner RC. A randomized double-blind trial of acarbose in type 2 diabetes shows improved glycemic control over 3 years. *Diabetes Care* 1999;22:960–964.
156. Raskin P, Jovanovic L, Berger S, et al. Repaglinide/troglitazone combination therapy: improved glycemic control in type 2 diabetes. *Diabetes Care* 2000;23: 979–983.
157. Garber A, Davidson J, Mooradian A, et al. Effect of metformin/glyburide tablets on HbA1c in first-line treatment of type 2 diabetes. *Diabetes* 49[Suppl 1]:432-P, 2000(abst).
158. Yki-Jarvinen H, Ryysy L, Nikkila K, et al. Comparison of bedtime insulin regimens in patients with type 2 diabetes mellitus: a randomized, controlled trial. *Ann Intern Med* 1999;130:389–396.
159. Yki-Jarvinen H, Dressler A, Zieman M. Less nocturnal hypoglycemia and better post dinner glucose control with bedtime insulin glargine compared with bedtime NPH insulin during combination therapy in type 2 diabetes. HOE 901/3002 Study Group. *Diabetes Care* 2001;23:1130–1136.
160. Raskin P, Rendell M, Riddle MC, et al. for the Rosiglitazone Clinical Trials Study Group. A randomized trial of rosiglitazone therapy in patients with inadequately controlled insulin-treated type 2 diabetes. *Diabetes Care* 2001;24: 1226–1232.
161. Schwartz S, Raskin P, Fonseca V, et al. Effect of troglitazone in insulin-treated patients with type II diabetes mellitus. *N Engl J Med* 1998;338:861–866.
162. Aviles-Santa L, Sinding J, Raskin P. Effects of metformin in patients with poorly controlled, insulin-treated type 2 diabetes mellitus. A randomized, double-blind, placebo-controlled trial. *Ann Intern Med* 1999;131:182–188.
163. Koshiyama H, Shimono D, Kuwamura N, et al. Inhibitory effect of pioglitazone on carotid arterial wall thickness in type 2 diabetes. *J Clin Endocrinol Metab* 2001;86:3452–3456.

CHAPTER 42

Treatment of the Child and Adolescent with Diabetes

Lori Laffel, Cindy Pasquarello, and Margaret Lawlor

Diabetes in childhood is a chronic metabolic disorder that results in hyperglycemia. In children, as in adults, energy metabolism is altered as a result either of inadequate insulin secretion or of inadequate insulin action, causing aberrant fuel homeostasis, which affects carbohydrate, protein, and fat metabolism. Diabetes is classified into four types: type 1, type 2, gestational, and other types, including secondary diabetes. The approaches to type 1 and type 2 diabetes in children and adolescents will be reviewed. Gestational diabetes does not generally occur in the pediatric population. Many forms of other types of diabetes, due to causes such as pancreatic hypoplasia or pancreatectomy (secondary to hyperinsulinemia or chronic pancreatitis), behave like and are treated similarly to type 1 diabetes. Another common form of secondary diabetes, cystic fibrosis–related diabetes, appears clinically like either type 1 or type 2 diabetes; readers are referred to recent reviews on this subject (1–5).

DIABETES IN CHILDREN AND ADOLESCENTS: INCIDENCE AND PREVALENCE

Although detailed information on the epidemiology of diabetes appears in Chapter 20, we will summarize fundamental statistics about the occurrence of diabetes in youth, because such information is helpful to practicing clinicians in their work with families and the community. In the United States, the incidence rate of type 1 diabetes is approximately 18 per 100,000 (6,7). The age of peak incidence of type 1 diabetes is gender-specific and coincides with the increased insulin demands of puberty (8). In general, the highest incidence is in the 10- to 14-year-old group and the lowest is in the 0- to 5-year-old group for both genders (8,9). Type 1 diabetes is most likely to develop in girls between the ages of 10 and 12, and boys between the ages of 12 and 14. The prevalence of type 1 diabetes is estimated to be 1.7 cases per 1,000 children and adolescents younger than 20 years old.

While the prevalence is lower with 1 in 2,500 children up to 5 years, it is about 1 in 400 children by 5 to 18 years of age. This translates to approximately 123,000 children and adolescents in the United States who have type 1 diabetes (6,7). In children of all age groups, the overall occurrence of type 1 diabetes has been increasing over the past few decades (9). Estimates of the numbers of youth with type 2 diabetes are less clear. Of the approximately 18,000 children in the United States diagnosed with diabetes each year, 8% to 45% appear to have type 2 diabetes in reports from urban centers in the United States during the last decade (10–13). The Diabetes SEARCH Study, currently supported by the Centers for Disease Control and Prevention (CDC) and the National Institute of Diabetes and Digestive and Kidney Diseases (NIDDK) aims to provide national data on both type 1 and type 2 diabetes in children and adolescents (7; http://www.searchfordiabetes.org).

Type 1 Diabetes

Type 1 diabetes is a multifactorial immune-mediated disease characterized by destruction of the pancreatic β-cells by T-cells, leading to a state of insulin deficiency. Type 1 diabetes has long been identified by its previous name, "juvenile diabetes," implying its common, although not exclusive, occurrence during childhood. Current understanding of its etiology includes an interaction between a genetic predisposition to autoimmunity coupled with an external, environmental trigger leading to autoimmune destruction of the insulin-producing β-cells, resulting in total or near-total deficiency of insulin production (see Chapter 23). Environmental factors, including foods (14–17), toxins, and viruses, have been suggested as triggers of the autoimmune process in genetically susceptible persons (18,19). Markers of autoimmunity include the presence of circulating autoantibodies to the β-cells, such as cytoplasmic islet cell antibodies (ICAs), insulin autoantibodies (IAAs), glutamic acid decarboxylase (GAD) antibodies, and 64-kilodalton (IA-2) autoantibodies to tyrosine phosphatases (IS-2 and IA-2β) (20–28). With improvements in the antibody assays, it has been possible to identify antibodies in the sera of more than 90% of patients with newly diagnosed type 1 diabetes. However, these antibodies are neither necessary nor sufficient for the diagnosis of type 1 diabetes. Identifying the presence of these autoantibodies may be helpful in clinical situations in which it is unclear whether the child has type 1 or type 2 diabetes, particularly with the current epidemic of childhood obesity and type 2 diabetes in youth. Screening for pancreatic autoantibodies in family members of patients with type 1 diabetes also is used as a research tool in studies of the prevention of type 1 diabetes (see Chapter 23). Several human leukocyte antigen (HLA) class II genes have been linked to susceptibility to type 1 diabetes, and some have been linked to a reduced risk of diabetes (29–32). It is clear that genetic factors, like environmental factors, do not exclusively account for the pathogenesis of type 1 diabetes. In fact, 80% of families of children with newly diagnosed type 1 diabetes do not report any family history of the disease, and the concordance rate in identical twins is only 30% to 50%. The complex interplay of genetics, environment, and autoimmunity as it relates to the etiology, pathogenesis, and possible prevention of type 1 diabetes is the subject of ongoing research.

With the destruction of the majority of β-cells, insulin deficiency results in the onset of the classic symptoms of type 1 diabetes: polyuria, polydipsia, and polyphagia with accompanying weight loss. The stages are outlined below.

- **Onset:** Symptoms such as increased thirst, increased urination, weight loss despite increased appetite.
- **Honeymoon:** Once insulin therapy is initiated, the residual β-cells regain functional capacity, producing some insulin for a short time.
- **Intensification:** Destruction of β-cells continues, and control of blood glucose becomes more difficult.
- **Total diabetes:** All of the insulin-producing β-cells are destroyed, resulting in total insulin deficiency.

Treatment of type 1 diabetes begins at diagnosis and includes insulin therapy, the development of a meal plan, an activity/exercise plan, training in the use of a blood glucose monitor, and family support. Initial self-management training aims to provide the child or adolescent who has diabetes and his or her family with the knowledge, skills, and problem-solving abilities to manage diabetes on a daily basis. This initial education is followed up by ongoing education evolving with duration of diabetes and the growth and development of the child and adolescent (33–35).

Type 2 Diabetes

Type 2 diabetes in children and adolescents was identified in the late 1970s and has become a growing medical and public health problem as a result of the burgeoning epidemic of childhood obesity (10–13,36,37). Like type 2 diabetes in adults, the increase in youth is the direct result of greater caloric intake with decreased caloric expenditure. Youth commonly have poor eating habits, eating high-calorie, high-fat, "super-sized" fast foods; spend an increased amount of time watching television or using computers or playing video games; and are victims of a reduced emphasis on physical education in schools and physical activity in general (38). Almost all youths with type 2 diabetes are overweight and have a positive family history of type 2 diabetes (10,12,37,39). The increasing prevalence of type 2 diabetes has been most marked in ethnic minority groups, including African Americans, Mexican Americans, Asians, Hispanics, and Native Americans (10,12,13) (see Chapter 29).

The first data on type 2 diabetes in youth are from the Pima Indians, the group with the world's highest prevalence of type 2 diabetes (6). In 1979, the prevalence of type 2 diabetes was 1 in 1,000 children 5 to 14 years of age and 9 in 1,000 youths 15 to 24 years of age (40). By 1996, the prevalence had increased to 22.3 per 1,000 in the 10- to 14-year-old age group and 50.9 per 1,000 in the 15- to 19-year-old group (13). In Northwest Ontario, between 1978 and 1984, the prevalence of type 2 diabetes in Native-American children under the age of 16 years was 2.5 per 1,000, a prevalence higher than that for type 1 diabetes in the white population (11,13,41). In Manitoba, the prevalence of type 2 diabetes among Native-American children studied between 1984 and 1990 was 0.53 per 1,000 children 7 to 14 years of age (11,13,42). In Japanese junior-high-school children, the incidence of type 2 diabetes was recently found to be seven times higher than the incidence of type 1 diabetes (13.9/100,000 vs. 2.07/100,000) and increased more than 30-fold over the past 20 years (43,44).

A study from Cincinnati, Ohio, was the first to document incidence rates of type 2 diabetes in the pediatric population over an extended time (45). One-third of all new cases of diabetes diagnosed between 1982 and 1995 in the 10- to 19-year-old age group were classified as type 2, giving an age-specific incidence of 7.2 per 100,000 per year. In 1992, type 2 diabetes accounted for only 2% to 4% of all newly identified cases of diabetes in patients younger than 19 years of age, but by 1994, 16% of all new cases in children were type 2 diabetes. In the Cincinnati report, 70% of the children with type 2 diabetes were African American, whereas only 10% of the children with type

TABLE 42.1. Risk Factors Associated with the Development of Type 2 Diabetes in Children and Adolescents

- Family history of diabetes
- Body mass index ≥27 kg/m^2; weight for height >85th percentile; >120% ideal body weight
- ≥10 y of age (in mid or late puberty)
- African-American, Hispanic, Asian, and American Indian descent
- Acanthosis nigricans in 41%–92%
- Signs of insulin resistance such as hypertension, hyperlipidemia, and polycystic ovarian syndrome (PCOS)

From the American Diabetes Association Type 2 diabetes in children and adolescents. *Diabetes Care* 2000;23:381–389.

1 diabetes and 14.5% of the general population were African American (45).

In contrast to the similar gender ratio for children with type 1 diabetes, more girls than boys are reported to have type 2 diabetes in studies of type 2 diabetes in children. The ratio of females to males in the Pima Indian population is 2:1; in Ontario Indians, 6:1; in Manitoba Indians, 4:1; and in the predominantly African-American population in Cincinnati, 2:1 (11). Furthermore, diabetes is consistently related to two important variables, obesity and puberty: both states are associated with insulin resistance. Indeed, markers of insulin resistance have recently been identified in 5- to 10-year-old overweight African-American children (46).

Several risk factors are associated with the development of type 2 diabetes: ethnic background, family history of type 2 diabetes, increased blood pressure, increased lipid levels, and obesity (10,12,20,37,45,47,48) (Table 42.1). In addition, acanthosis nigricans, thought to be a cutaneous manifestation of hyperinsulinism, is present in 60% to 70% (vs. the 7% normally seen in this population) of children with type 2 diabetes. These factors are quite similar to the risk factors for type 2 diabetes in adults (10).

A recently convened task force from the NIDDK, CDC, American Diabetes Association (ADA), and the American Academy of Pediatrics recommend testing for diabetes in youth beginning at 10 years of age or at the onset of puberty if earlier. This recommendation includes testing for type 2 diabetes in children and adolescents if they are overweight (defined as weight >120% of ideal body weight, body mass index [BMI] > 85th percentile for age and gender, or weight for height > 85th percentile), *and* have any two of the following:

- Family history of type 2 diabetes in first- or second-degree relative
- Race/ethnicity: African, Hispanic, Asian/South Pacific, and Native-American descent
- Signs of insulin resistance such as hypertension, hyperlipidemia, or polycystic ovary syndrome (PCOS) (10).

Determination of the fasting plasma glucose is the preferred means of testing, with a positive diagnosis when fasting plasma glucose is 126 mg/dL or higher. Testing should be repeated every 2 years (20). The initial treatment of type 2 diabetes in youth is dictated by clinical presentation. Diabetic ketoacidosis (DKA) or severe hyperglycemia with nonketotic hyperosmolar hyperglycemic syndrome (NKHHS) requires emergency management per a DKA protocol. Insulin will likely be needed as therapy in these patients even after their recovery from the acute condition. Others who are not ill at diagnosis can initially be treated with medical nutrition therapy and physical activity (see sections below). Unless there is successful weight loss, most patients will require some form of drug therapy. Previously, insulin was the only drug approved by the U.S. Food and Drug Administration (FDA) for use in children and adolescents. Recently, metformin has been approved for use in adolescents 12 years of age and older. Nonetheless, most pediatric endocrinologists use some of the anti-diabetes oral agents to treat children with type 2 diabetes (10,12). The study of metformin in children and adolescents has recently been published, while investigations of other oral hypoglycemic agents in youth are currently under way (10,49). Markers that aid in the differential diagnosis of type 1 and type 2 diabetes in children and adolescents are outlined in Table 42.2.

While it is apparent that type 2 diabetes is developing in an increasing number of children, as in adults, the prevalence of this disorder is likely underestimated, given the typical lack of symptoms early in the course of the disease. Thus, the emerging epidemic of type 2 diabetes in children and adolescents presents a challenge not only to the diabetes specialist but also to the primary care provider, who plays a pivotal role in screening for risk factors for development of this disease in the general pediatric population (10,50). There are currently NIH-funded multicenter clinical trials under way to examine treatment and prevention strategies of type 2 diabetes in youth.

Maturity-Onset Diabetes of the Young

An important category of other forms of diabetes is maturity-onset diabetes of the young (MODY). MODY is a monogenic (51,52), autosomal dominant, heterogeneous form of diabetes. It is related to a defect in insulin secretion by the β-cells in the pancreas rather than to an impairment of insulin sensitivity (52,53). It is estimated that about 1% to 3% of people with diabetes have MODY. MODY is characterized by early age of onset (10–30 years of age, although it can be as early as 2 to 3 years of

TABLE 42.2. Differential Diagnosis of Type 1 and Type 2 Diabetes in Children and Adolescents

Type 1: immune-mediated diabetes	Type 2: non–immune-mediated diabetes
• Not generally overweight (although as many as one fourth may be overweight)	• Overweight/obese (85%)
• Low endogenous insulin	• Signs of insulin resistance
• Low C-peptide	• High endogenous insulin[a]
• Positive insulin and pancreatic autoantibodies	• High C-peptide levels[a]
• High ketone levels (30%–40% have ketoacidosis)	• Low ketone levels (<33% have ketonuria; 5%–25% have ketoacidosis)

[a]Can be suppressed for 2 to 3 months after diagnosis.

age), treatment with oral anti-diabetes medications versus treatment with insulin, usually an antibody-negative status, and a diagnosis of diabetes in three or more family generations, often with multiple individuals within those generations. The majority of individuals with MODY are not overweight. This diagnosis should be entertained in children and adolescents with a strong family history of diabetes in multiple generations (54). MODY is reviewed extensively in Chapter 26.

THE TEAM APPROACH

In this current era of intensive diabetes control following the release of the Diabetes Control and Complications Trial (DCCT), the team approach to diabetes care remains central to the successful treatment of children and adolescents with diabetes (55–57). Care of youth with either type 1 or type 2 diabetes is complex and time-consuming. In this age of managed care and cost-containment, few primary care physicians, including pediatricians, possess the time to care for these patients and keep up with evolving therapies or new technologies.

The expertise required to deliver the numerous components of the diabetes treatment program resides within a multidisciplinary team that works with the child's family, primary care physician, and school (55,58). The physician-led pediatric diabetes team should be trained in all aspects of pediatric diabetes management and includes a diabetes nurse educator, a dietitian, and a mental health professional—either a social worker or a clinical psychologist. In addition, the team may include an exercise physiologist and subspecialists such as ophthalmologists, podiatrists, nephrologists, gastroenterologists, and others as needed (55). Each team member should appreciate the goals of therapy, the complexities of pediatric diabetes care, the need for individualization, the complications of diabetes, prevention of and early intervention for deteriorating glycemic control, and the impact of the disease on normal childhood and adolescence, as well as on family dynamics.

The process of educating parents and children in diabetes care should begin at the time of diagnosis. Initially, many parents and children or adolescents are overwhelmed and unable to assimilate the extensive body of information of diabetes self-management training. Therefore, it is recommended that self-management training and education be carried out in stages (33–35,59,60).

PATIENT AND PARENT EDUCATION

Today, the child with newly diagnosed diabetes is usually treated as an outpatient or during a very brief inpatient admission. Therefore, education goals need to be tailored to the needs of the individual child or adolescent, the family, and the resources of the healthcare team. These initial goals become an important part of the ongoing process of diabetes follow-up care. Central to successful management and attainment of treatment goals are the child or adolescent with diabetes and his or her family, whose needs should receive priority in planning and implementing the treatment program. The child's primary care provider must be included as a member of the diabetes healthcare team. In addition, caregivers such as day-care providers, teachers, school nurses, coaches, grandparents, and babysitters are integral to successful outcomes (Fig. 42.1). This collaborative approach helps the patient receive optimal diabetes care, taking into account his or her age, day-care or school schedule, eating patterns, personality, temperament, family structure, cultural background, and other medical conditions.

Initial goals are limited to imparting an understanding of the fundamental nature of diabetes and how it is treated. Next, diabetes treatment routines need to be integrated into school, sports activities, day care, and family activities. This occurs through practical experience at home and by frequent contact with the diabetes healthcare team. As time passes, most families are ready to learn the intricate details of diabetes self-management necessary for maintaining optimal glycemic control, while coping with the challenges imposed by such things as physical activity, "picky" or selective eating habits, intercurrent illnesses, and other normal variations in a child or adolescent's daily routine. In addition to imparting facts and teaching prac-

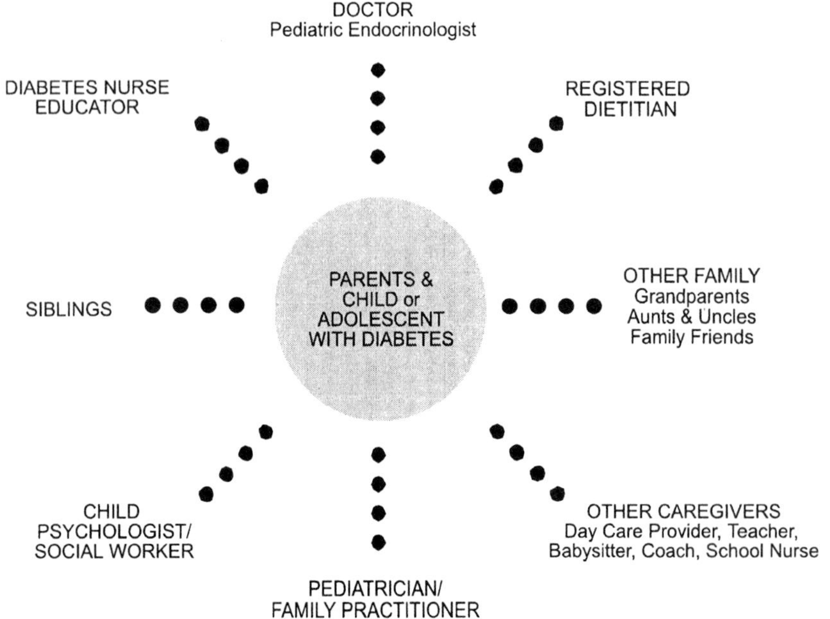

FIG. 42.1. The diabetes healthcare team for the child or adolescent with diabetes.

tical skills, diabetes self-management training and education should attempt to promote desirable health beliefs and attitudes in the young person who has to live with a chronic and incurable disease (33–35).

For the child, this is often best accomplished in an educational setting such as age-appropriate peer education/support groups or summer camps for children with diabetes. The educational program must match the child's level of cognitive development and be adapted to the learning style and intellectual ability of the individual child, adolescent, and family (35,61–63). We urge that parents be fully involved, and we encourage the diabetes healthcare team to supervise, when appropriate, a gradual and flexible transfer of responsibility from parents to the adolescent, facilitating the normal process of separation and attainment of independence that occurs during the teenage years (64–67). Ideally, we encourage cooperation around diabetes tasks between the teen and parent with the goal of developing interdependence, because parent involvement has been consistently associated with better medical and behavioral outcomes for youths with diabetes (64–66,68).

Continued education is necessary during transitions between developmental stages of childhood, such as at school entry, between the school-age years and adolescence, when the adolescent leaves home for college or for independent living, as well as throughout the lifespan. Some families benefit from reinforcement of teaching skills at home with the help of visiting nurse services, either shortly after diagnosis or during challenging family times. We have established a developmental model of care, education, and psychosocial support through our age-based multidisciplinary clinics.

Beginning with the most vulnerable group of youth and their families, the Pediatric and Adolescent Unit of the Joslin Diabetes Center has implemented a comprehensive, family-focused outpatient program of care for children with type 1 diabetes younger than 8 years of age called the Young Children's Program (69,70). It is offered once each month, and approximately 400 families with young children have participated to date. Through a systematic assessment of initial needs, we documented that parents of preschool and early school-age children with diabetes are concerned about the following: collisions between diabetes treatment and normal childhood behavior; differentiating symptoms of hypoglycemia from normal behavior and mood swings; and the impact of diabetes on family relationships (69,70). Fear of hypoglycemia surfaced as a primary concern. One of seven of these very young children experienced severe hypoglycemia (70). Thus, families of young children become extraordinarily reliant upon blood glucose monitoring in these young patients who are unable to identify and communicate hypoglycemic symptoms.

We have implemented a similar comprehensive program for school-age children, 8 to 13 years of age, and their families. This group also meets monthly, with the provision of individualized medical care followed by simultaneous separate support groups for parents and for the youth. Similar to the Young Children's Program, the parent group is facilitated by members of the mental health team, either a child psychologist or social worker, and by members of the medical team, including a physician, a pediatric diabetes specialty nurse, or registered dietitian. Major topics of discussion include transition to middle school, impact of puberty on glycemic control, and review of new technologies along with research updates. An early childhood educator, who coordinates developmentally appropriate activities to insure positive clinic encounters that encourage routine follow-up, supervises the group of youth. Diabetes-specific educational curricula are not routinely discussed.

These comprehensive programs encourage positive interactions between the diabetes healthcare team and the patients along with their families. The positive result of these interactions is evident in our assessment of the Young Children's Program (70). The program evaluation yielded improved follow-up attendance at diabetes care visits for families who participated in the comprehensive Young Children's Program compared with infrequent program attendees (70). In addition, the group of patients with improved follow-up care had significantly fewer children with poor control (glycosylated hemoglobin A_{1c} [HbA_{1c}] >9.9%) than the group with infrequent program attendance and follow-up care ($P < .05$) (70).

Adolescents with diabetes and their families receive multidisciplinary diabetes care as well as medical care and psychosocial support. The program for teens at the Joslin Clinic helps teens and their families devise individualized management programs that fit their lifestyles. Families are helped in the negotiation of acceptable parental involvement in the tasks of diabetes management to sustain adherence to insulin injection routines and blood glucose monitoring (66,71). To provide additional support for the parents as they try to help their adolescents, we initiated a bimonthly evening parent support group facilitated by the multidisciplinary pediatric team. In an initial needs assessment, fear of complications surfaced as a concern in 50% of families, while fear of hypoglycemia was noted by 19%. We stress the importance of continued medical follow-up and frequent blood glucose monitoring for these families to help them overcome these concerns.

We have recently launched a professionally monitored Discussion Board for Teens on the Joslin website. Parents of adolescents also can participate in a Discussion Board specifically for them, as well in the bimonthly discussion group. Parents of adolescents require ongoing help in developing realistic expectations for adolescent blood glucose levels and monitoring behavior, as well as in negotiating an acceptable level of involvement in the diabetes management tasks of their teen. Adolescents with diabetes also require help in developing realistic expectations for blood glucose monitoring and in negotiating with their parents about acceptable levels of involvement in monitoring and insulin routines. The team approach to pediatric diabetes care promotes these goals and remains the accepted standard of care throughout childhood and adolescence (55).

GOALS OF THERAPY

In 1993, the results of the DCCT heralded intensive management or so-called tight control as the standard of care for most patients with type 1 diabetes (56). With scientific evidence showing a marked decrease in the risk of microvascular complications of the eyes, kidneys, and nerves with intensive management, the post-DCCT era emerged (56). Although the study did not enroll patients younger than 13 years of age, there were 195 youth, between the ages of 13 and 17 years old, at entry in the study sample. As a result, diabetes care today utilizes intensive management in the diabetes treatment plans for the majority of children and adolescents with diabetes (72). The theoretical goal of treatment is to restore metabolic function to as near normal as possible while avoiding serious complications of therapy, especially symptomatic hyper- and hypoglycemia. However, the approach to care also incorporates more global goals, such as the normalization of childhood and adolescent development and the maintenance of successful family functioning (34,55,59) (Table 42.3).

TABLE 42.3. Goals of Therapy of the Pediatric and Adolescent Unit of the Joslin Diabetes Center

- Avoidance of symptomatic hyperglycemia and hypoglycemia
- Early intervention for increasing hemoglobin A_{1c} levels
- Prevention of parent/child burnout and isolation
- Prevention of metabolic deterioration of adolescence
- Identification and treatment of behavioral/adjustment dilemmas
- Provision of positive medical experiences
- Provision of realistic expectations for diabetes management
- Integration of diabetes routines into school, day care, and family activities
- Maintenance of normal growth and development

Glycemic goals vary for children and adolescents and reflect developmental differences. Since hypoglycemia can have more of an impact on the neurocognitive function of young children (73–80), the ADA position does not support tight glycemic control for children under the age of 2 years and advises caution for children 8 years old and younger (55). Table 42.4 shows the glycemic control goals for youth with diabetes.

Several studies indicate that children who develop diabetes during infancy and early childhood may be at increased risk for the subsequent development of cognitive impairment (75, 81–84). Such impairment is presumed to be the result of multiple episodes of severe hypoglycemia, which may be more frequent in very young children because of their hypoglycemic unawareness (85–87). Therefore, maintaining very tight control of glucose levels in children with very-early-onset diabetes may be harmful, given the risk of causing recurrent, severe, and potentially debilitating episodes of hypoglycemia that have the potential for neurocognitive sequelae (78,88–90). Care must also be taken to avoid poor glycemic control, as one wants to limit the hyperglycemic exposure that is associated with future complications (91). One report raises the question of a correlation between high long-term HbA_{1c} values and intellectual impairment in boys diagnosed below the age of 6 years (92). Furthermore, fear of hypoglycemia among parents who have witnessed severe hypoglycemia in their young children becomes a major deterrent both to achieving optimal control in these children as they mature and in allowing them to experience many normal activities of childhood that require separation from parents (93–95). A recent publication reports increased parenting stress, in general and in relation to mealtimes, in families with young children with diabetes, which underscores parental fears of hypoglycemia (96).

The prepubertal child may be relatively protected from microvascular complications, although this is still controversial. Signs of eye or kidney disease are extremely rare in the prepubertal child (97). Diabetic nephropathy, for example, with microalbuminuria used as an index of renal glomerular damage, is significantly less prevalent in children younger than 12 years of age than in those older than 12 years of age matched for duration of diabetes (98). Indeed, it is extremely rare to uncover clinically significant microvascular complications in children younger than the age of 10 years (97–99). However, debate continues about the contribution of glycemic control during the prepubertal years to the development of future complications (100). Thus, current clinical care should approach this dilemma by aiming for safe and realistic glycemic targets that limit the occurrence of significant hyperglycemia and hypoglycemia and that match the patient and family's particular needs.

In children and adolescents, as in adults, individualization of the treatment program is important. In highly motivated families, close monitoring of blood glucose and administering multiple insulin injections or utilizing insulin pump therapy using dosage adjustment algorithms are fairly routine. In other families, simplification of the regimen may be the only key to successful management. Thus, while keeping the general therapeutic principles in mind, the diabetes healthcare team must tailor the goals of treatment to the needs and capabilities of each individual child or adolescent with diabetes and his or her family (33–35,59,60).

TYPE 1 DIABETES: GLYCEMIC CONTROL IN THE PEDIATRIC POPULATION AND THE DCCT/EDIC STUDY

Despite multidisciplinary specialty care, glycemic control remains suboptimal in many pediatric diabetes centers worldwide, including our own center. In a recent sample of 300 children with type 1 diabetes, the mean HbA_{1c} was 8.7% ± 1.2%, with 33% achieving an HbA_{1c} level below 8.1% (101). Glycemic control in our population appears quite similar to that reported in other large, cross-sectional studies of pediatric populations (Table 42.5). A multicenter cross-sectional study involving 22 pediatric departments in 18 countries in Europe, Japan, and North America enrolling 2,873 children with type 1 diabetes, reported a mean baseline HbA_{1c} of 8.6 ± 1.7%, with 34% of patients achieving an HbA_{1c} <8.0% (105). Three years later, the mean HbA_{1c} from these centers remained 8.7% ± 1.7% (111). Similarly, a recent cross-sectional nationwide study of 2,579

TABLE 42.4. Goals for Glycemic Control for Children, Adolescents, and Young Adults with Diabetes

	Blood glucose goal range (mg/dL)		
Values by age	Before meals	Bedtime/overnight	HbA_{1c}[a]
Toddlers and preschoolers			7%–9%
Whole blood	90–180	100–200	
Plasma	100–200	110–220	
School age			≤8%
Whole blood	70–180	90–180	
Plasma	80–200	100–200	
Adolescents and young adults			≤7%
Whole blood	70–150	80–160	
Plasma	80–170	90–180	

[a]Reference range, 4%–6%, as the DCCT standard.

TABLE 42.5. Average Glycemic Control in Children and Adolescents Around the World

Study (year) (ref)	Country (city)	N	Mean HbA_{1c} ±SD
Jacobson et al., 1994 (102)	USA (Boston)	61	12.0% ± 2.1% (HbA_1) = 9.68% (HbA_{1c})
Palta et al., 1996 (103)	USA (Madison, WI)	507	11.3% ± 2.9% (GHb) = 9.08 (HbA_{1c})
Tubiana-Rufi et al., 1995 (104)	France	165	8.3% ± 1.6%
DCCT, 1994 (112)[a]	USA and Canada	92/103	8.06% ± 1.25/9.76% ± 1.22%
Rosilio et al., 1998 (105)	France	2,579	8.97% ± 1.98%
Mortensen et al., 1997 (106)	18 countries in Europe, Japan, and North America	2,873	8.6% ± 1.7%
Dorchy et al., 1997 (107)	Belgium	144	6.6% ± 1.2%
Nordfeldt et al., 1997 (108)	Sweden	146	6.9% ± 1.3%
Vanelli et al., 1999 (109)	Italy	201	7.8% ± 1.4%
DIABAUD2, 2001 (110)	Scotland	1,755	9.1% ± 1.5%
Danne et al., 2001 (111)	21 international pediatric centers in 17 countries	2,101	8.74% ± 1.66%
Levine et al., 2001 (101)	USA (Boston)	300	8.7% ± 1.2%

[a]DCCT, N = 92, intensive cohort; N = 103, conventional cohort.

French children with type 1 diabetes reported an overall mean HbA_{1c} of 8.97% ± 1.98%, with 33% of patients achieving an HbA_{1c} less than 8.0% (105). In the DCCT, 83% of the intensively treated patients achieved HbA_{1c} values of 8% or less, compared with only 20% of the patients receiving standard care. Fewer than 5% of the intensively treated patients achieved HbA_{1c} values <6.05% (56).

Intensive insulin therapy, compared with conventional therapy, in the DCCT delayed the onset and slowed the progression of long-term complications in both the adolescent and adult cohorts. The subset of the 195 adolescent patients, ages 13 to 17 years at study entry, randomized to intensive therapy experienced a similar reduction in risk for complications to their adult counterparts (112). In contrast to the adolescent cohorts from the DCCT, the adults in both conventionally and intensively treated groups achieved lower HbA_{1c} values both during the DCCT and during the follow-up Epidemiology of Diabetes Interventions and Complications (EDIC) study (56,112–114). During the DCCT, intensively treated adults achieved HbA_{1c} values of 7.1% compared with values of 8.9% in conventionally treated adults (Fig. 42.2). Among the 195 adolescents, both intensively and conventionally treated adolescent patients had HbA_{1c} values about 1% higher than those of their older counterparts. At the end of the DCCT, all study patients were encouraged to use intensive insulin therapy. During the EDIC follow-up, both groups of adult patients experienced a change in their glycemic control, with HbA_{1c} values in intensively treated adult patients increasing to 7.9% and HbA_{1c} values in the conventionally treated adults decreasing to 8.1%. Nonetheless, the intensively treated adult patients benefited from their initial exposure to intensive insulin therapy, with a sustained risk reduction in the occurrence of retinopathy and nephropathy during the first 4 years of follow-up in the EDIC study (114). This risk reduction has been confirmed after 7 years of follow-up in EDIC (115).

This significant reduction in risk for microvascular complications was sustained in the intensively treated adolescents when they were followed 4 years after the end of the DCCT (113). One hundred seventy-five of the 195 adolescents initially enrolled in the DCCT participated in the follow-up EDIC Study (115). After the release of the results of the DCCT, the conventionally treated patients were invited to receive intensive insulin therapy. During the first 4 years of follow-up, 50% of conventionally treated adolescents selected multiple daily injections, approximately 17% selected insulin pump therapy, while the remainder continued to receive conventional insulin therapy (113). Among the intensively treated youth during the DCCT, 90% elected to continue intensive insulin therapy during the 4 years of follow-up. Despite the difference in diabetes management between the two groups, glycemic control was identical 4 years after the end of the DCCT, with the group assigned to intensive insulin therapy in the DCCT maintaining a mean HbA_{1c} of 8.4% while those who received conventional insulin therapy achieving a mean HbA_{1c} of 8.5%. Despite this equivalence of glycemic control between the two groups, the previous exposure to intensive insulin therapy was associated with a sustained risk reduction for the occurrence of retinopathy and diabetic nephropathy (113,114).

These differences in glycemic control between adult and adolescent patients during the DCCT and EDIC studies underscore the challenges associated with the management of type 1 diabetes in adolescents. This suggests that adolescents and young adults may have particularly challenging metabolic and behavioral factors that warrant additional study in order to devise suc-

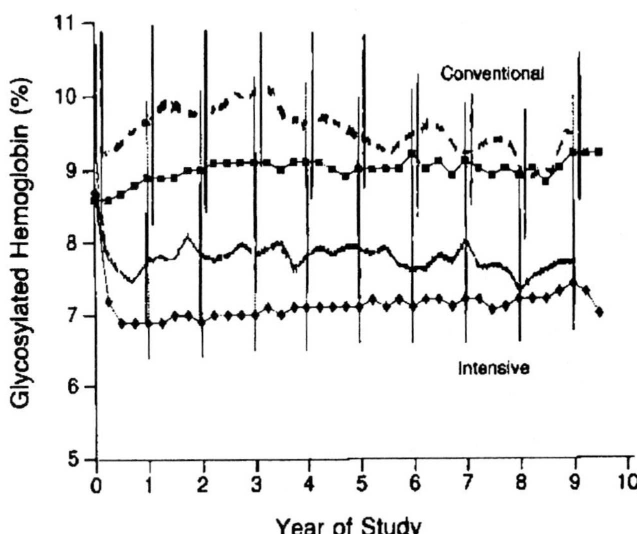

FIG. 42.2. Levels of glycosylated hemoglobin (HbA_{1c}) achieved in the Diabetes Control and Complications Trial. The conventionally and intensively treated (first and third curves from top, respectively) adolescents had higher HbA_{1c} values and more overlap than did their adult counterparts (second and fourth curves, respectively).

cessful treatment programs that can optimize their glycemic control. Issues related to pubertal growth and development, as well as behaviors, likely contribute to these challenges.

Furthermore, achievement of optimal glycemic control remains challenging for most centers caring for youth with type 1 diabetes. A recent follow-up to a large multinational study examining glycemic control reported wide differences in mean glycemic control among specialty centers and values significantly higher than targets achieved in adult population (111). In addition to the long-term risks of late complications that follow long periods of uncontrolled diabetes, youth with poorly controlled diabetes experienced significantly more hospitalizations and emergency room visits compared with youth who achieve HbA_{1c} values of 8% or less (101). For 2 years, we prospectively observed 300 youth, ages 8 to 16 years, with type 1 diabetes. There was a threefold increase in the rate of hospitalizations and emergency room visits among those with average HbA_{1c} values of greater than 9% compared with those with HbA_{1c} values of 8% or less. In addition, the frequency of hypoglycemia was equally high among those with poorly controlled diabetes and those with lower HbA_{1c} values. Despite the lack of optimal control, the occurrence of hypoglycemia in the group with poor control most likely results from the lack of attention to diabetes management tasks (71). Repeatedly, achievement of optimal glycemic control has been found to be significantly related to the frequency of blood glucose monitoring (65,66,71,101). (See section on behavioral factors).

Puberty

Puberty is a challenging period for diabetes management from both physiologic and behavioral standpoints. The hormonal milieu of puberty sets the stage for significant insulin resistance due to increases in the production of growth hormone and sex steroid hormones (115). Amiel and colleagues performed elegant studies of glucose disposal using a hyperinsulinemic clamp in prepubertal, pubertal, and postpubertal individuals (116) (Fig. 42.3). Their investigation confirmed that, despite similar levels of circulating insulin, individuals in the midst of puberty displayed significantly lower (by 30%) glucose disposal than did prepubertal and postpubertal individuals (116). The diminution in glucose disposal was evident in pubertal youth with type 1 diabetes as well as in pubertal normoglycemic control individuals matched for age and gender with the youth with diabetes. Thus, it is quite common for insulin requirements to increase by 50% during pubertal growth and development (116).

An observational study of more than 900 persons at our center who were 15 to 45 years of age, all of whom were diagnosed with type 1 diabetes before the age of 40 years, found significant relationships between HbA_{1c} and age of diabetes onset and attained age (Fig. 42.4). The patients who were the youngest at onset of diabetes had the poorest glycemic control, as expected by the greater severity of their deficit in insulin-producing β-cell capacity (authors' unpublished data). On the other hand, HbA_{1c} was the highest during the late adolescent years, ages 16 to 20, likely reflecting the period of greatest behavioral adjustment and the time when patients experience difficulties with adherence to the diabetes treatment program. These findings suggest that particular attention needs to be focused on older adolescents and young adults, as their glycemic control appears to be deteriorating. Furthermore, patients of this age may be changing their care from pediatric to adult providers and, as a result, may be at great risk for being lost to follow-up. The combination of deteriorating glycemic control and loss to follow-up care places these patients at high risk for the start of microvascular complications (117,118). Together physiologic demands of puberty and behavioral issues add to the challenges of diabetes during this developmental stage (65,66,110,111). The period of adolescence is notable for the need for the rapidly growing and developing youth to experiment and push the limits of his or her environment. These youth are often encouraged to take over much, if not all, of their diabetes tasks. However, with the recognition that puberty is a challenging period for glycemic control, additional parental support and guidance are imperative to prevent excessive glycemic deterioration at this stage. Furthermore, newer studies have confirmed the importance of continued parental guidance to help adolescents avoid deterioration of their schoolwork, to reduce the use of drugs and alcohol, and to reduce the occurrence of teen pregnancy (110). Thus, we promote interdependence between family members and the teen with diabetes that encourages teamwork to support the rigors of diabetes management. This is particularly important in light of the physiologic demands of puberty occurring at a time when the youth is striving for more independence. To help maintain adherence to diabetes tasks, especially to blood glucose monitoring, caregivers must reward the act of monitoring

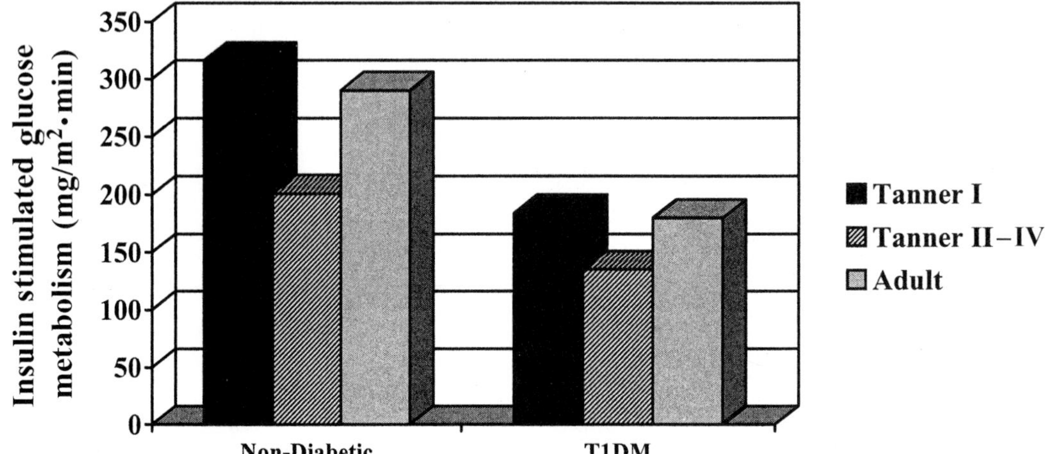

FIG. 42.3. Effect of puberty on insulin-stimulated glucose metabolism in nondiabetic and diabetic subjects. Tanner 1, prepubertal; Tanner 2–4, pubertal; Tanner 5, postpubertal. (Adapted from Amiel SA, Sherwin RS, Simonson D, et al. Impaired insulin action in puberty. A contributing factor to poor glycemic control in adolescents with diabetes. *N Engl J Med* 1986;315:215–219. Copyright © 1986 Massachusetts Medical Society. All rights reserved.)

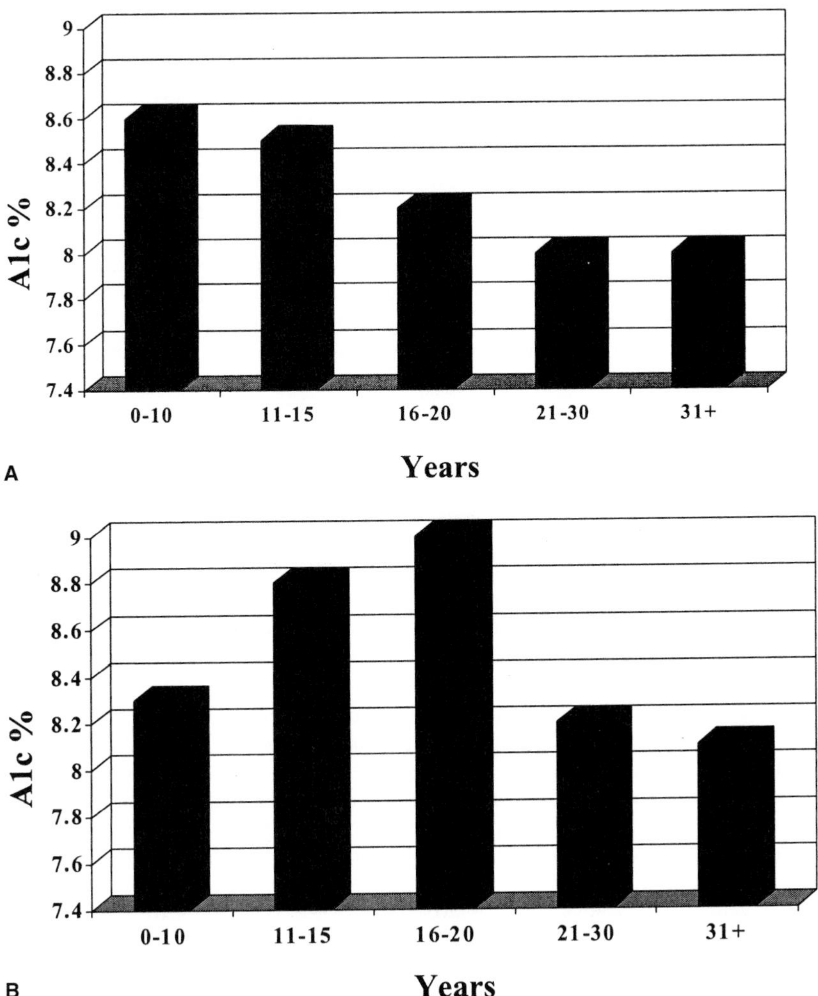

FIG. 42.4. Relationship of HbA_{1c} to age at onset **(A)** and attained age **(B)** among 900 persons at Joslin Diabetes Center with attained age of 15 to 45 years, all of whom were diagnosed with type 1 diabetes before age 40 years (authors' unpublished data).

rather than punish unfavorable blood glucose results (121). (See section on behavioral issues and family studies.)

INSULIN THERAPY

Only the number of insulins currently available and the tools with which to deliver them limit insulin regimens utilized in the management of diabetes in children and adolescents. These regimens can range from the use of a single intermediate- or long-acting insulin (NPH [neutral protamine Hagedorn], lente, ultralente, or glargine) to an intensive program of multiple types of insulins administered through three or four daily injections or aspart/lispro/regular insulin through continuous subcutaneous insulin infusion (CSII) (Table 42.6). The selection of an insulin regimen depends upon many factors, such as type of diabetes, age, glycemic goals, and personal choice. The use of insulin in type 1 diabetes is the main focus of this section.

TABLE 42.6. Insulin Actions by Type of Human Insulins

Insulin type	Onset	Peak	Duration
Insulin aspart	5–10 min	1–3 hr	3–5 hr
Insulin lispro	<15 min	30–90 min	2–4 hr
Regular	30–60 min	2–3 hr	3–6 hr
NPH	2–4 hr	4–10 hr	10–16 hr
Lente	3–4 hr	4–12 hr	12–18 hr
Glargine	1.1 hr	No peak	24 hr
Ultralente	4–6 hr	8–20 hr	20–24 hr
70/30[a]	30 min	2–12 hr	14–24 hr
50/50	30 min	2–3 hr	10–24 hr
75/25	15 min	1.5–3 hr	16–24 hr

[a]70/30 (70% NPH/30% regular), 70/30 (Novolog Mix) (70% insulin aspart protamine suspension/30% insulin aspart); 50/50 (50% NPH/50% regular); 75/25 (75% insulin lispro protamine suspension/25% insulin lispro.

From American Diabetes Association. Health Care Products. Diabetes Forecast. Available at: http://www.diabetes.org/main/community/forecast/jan_2002_insulin.jsp#relative insulins, with permission.

Available insulins are listed by their onset, peak, and duration of action in Table 42.6.

Although there is no one established formula for determining a child's insulin requirement, experience has shown that children with newly diagnosed type 1 diabetes require approximately 0.5 to 0.75 U/kg per day. For children diagnosed before the development of ketonuria, the initial insulin doses may be lower than the 0.5 U/kg per day. With diminished insulin sensitivity associated with DKA, steroid use, puberty, or infection, the initial doses may be as high as 1.0 U/kg per day or more to achieve reasonable glycemic control. Usual subcutaneous daily insulin dose calculations are summarized in Table 42.7. Children younger than 8 years old, often in direct contrast to adolescents, are exquisitely sensitive to insulin. The small insulin needs of infants and toddlers may require insulin diluted to U10, U25, or U50 as opposed to the standard U100 preparations (100 U/mL) to allow for more precise dosing and measurement of insulin in less than 1-unit increments. Diluents are available for specific types of insulins from the insulin manufacturers. Insulin can be diluted either in a pharmacy or at home after parents are taught to dilute the U100 insulin using the diluent specified by the manufacturer for the insulin type.

Although the theoretical goal is to normalize the premeal blood glucose levels to values between 80 and 120 mg/dL and to maintain the middle-of-the-night blood glucose level at 80 mg/dL or above, a number of variables must be considered when establishing individual target blood glucose goals. These variables include, but are not limited to, the stage of diabetes, issues of growth and development (e.g., chronologic age or Tanner stage), activity level, child temperament, family infrastructure, school support, and family fear of hypoglycemia or long-term complications. Adjustments in insulin doses are based on the evaluation of patterns of blood sugars attained over a 3-day period, taking into account the effect of the level of activity as well as the frequency and amount of carbohydrate intake. If there is an emerging pattern of out-of-target blood glucose levels at a consistent time of day, the insulin most responsible for insulin action at that time should be adjusted by 10%. Once that adjustment has been made, ideally it should remain fixed for 2 to 3 days to see the impact of the change before further adjustments are made.

It is not unusual within a period of several weeks after the initiation of insulin therapy for a child's diabetes to enter the honeymoon phase with residual insulin production. During this phase of diabetes, insulin requirements may fall well below the 0.5 U/kg per day generally required to maintain blood glucose targets in the setting of β-cell failure. Children may require only minimal amounts of intermediate- or long-acting insulin, possibly combined with small amounts of aspart, lispro, or regular insulin. Given the autoimmunity of type 1 diabetes, β-cell destruction continues in spite of this honeymoon phase. With the progressive loss of β-cell function, the need for increased exogenous insulin will become readily apparent in the form of increased blood glucose levels. These insulin needs may continue to rise over the ensuing weeks, months, and years as a result of declining β-cell function but also with growth of the child—in both height and weight. Insulin requirements may rise to as much as 1.5 U/kg per day during puberty. As diabetes intensifies, the ability to manage glycemia with a single dose of insulin or with less than 0.5 U/kg becomes virtually impossible. Inadequate overnight dosing of insulin will result in an overproduction of hepatic glucose, resulting in fasting hyperglycemia, occasionally with ketonuria. Most children with diabetes will require, at minimum, a mixture of rapid- and intermediate- or long-acting insulin administered two to three times a day—before breakfast, before the evening meal, and/or at bedtime—to remain free from persistent hyperglycemia and to achieve reasonable 24-hour glucose control. In the adolescent population especially, it is not uncommon for the afternoon snack to consist of more than 15 to 30 g of carbohydrate. That snack may coincide with the waning of the morning NPH. The use of aspart or lispro to cover the added calories of a mid-afternoon snack may be needed to improve the pre-supper blood glucose level.

The newest insulins are called insulin analogues. These "designer" insulins arise from the biochemical alteration of the human insulin molecule. Modifications to the insulin molecule alter its onset, peak, and duration of action, with the goal of creating insulin preparations that mimic insulin action produced by the human β-cells within the pancreatic islets. Clinical trials have shown that these analogues are safe and effective; their advantages include more optimal management of blood glucose levels by the close mimicking of normal physiologic function (123).

The FDA approved the first insulin analogue, lispro (Humalog), in 1996. Lispro has a rapid onset—within 15 minutes of administration—but a duration of action shortened to 2 to 4 hours. The onset, peak, and duration of action of lispro were designed to match the postprandial increase in blood glucose that follows the intake of food. Its rapid onset makes it ideal for administration just before eating. Studies have demonstrated the feasibility of administering lispro after meals in very young children (124). Dosing with lispro after meals allows a care provider to more accurately titrate the insulin doses for an erratic eater, with the goal of matching food intake and insulin more closely and minimizing the potential for hypoglycemia. A diluent for lispro is available, allowing for accurate lispro administration in, for example, 0.1- or 0.25-U increments, making this preparation extremely useful in very young children. Clinical studies have shown that, compared with regular

TABLE 42.7. Usual Subcutaneous Daily Dosages of Insulin in Children and Adolescents with Diabetes

Type	Non-DKA presentation	DKA presentation
Type 1 diabetes		
Child, prepubertal	0.25–0.5 U/kg per day	0.5–0.75 U/kg per day
Adolescent, pubertal	0.5–0.75 U/kg per day	0.75–1.0 U/kg per day
Type 2 diabetes		
Adolescent	20–40 U/day[a]	—

DKA, diabetic ketoacidosis.
[a]Often administered as intermediate-acting insulin as starting dosage. Depending on level of hyperglycemia at presentation, insulin needs can be significantly higher.

insulin, lispro improves HbA_{1c} values, improves postprandial blood glucose levels, results in fewer episodes of hypoglycemia, and enhances hypoglycemia awareness (123,125).

A second rapid-acting insulin, aspart (NovoLog), was recently approved by the FDA and is available for use. Although the onset of action very closely mimics that of lispro, its duration is between 4 to 6 hours. Rapid-acting insulins such as aspart and lispro allow for maximal flexibility of injections at meals versus that of regular insulin, which for maximal effectiveness must be injected 30 to 45 minutes before eating. In a clinical trial comparing the frequency of nocturnal hypoglycemia in an insulin program of regular insulin or a program of aspart, the aspart group had fewer episodes of low blood glucose levels at night, as well as lower HbA_{1c} values (126). Currently, insulin aspart is not approved by the FDA for use in persons younger than 18 years of age. Insulin aspart recently received FDA approval for use in insulin pumps (127). Additional pediatric studies evaluating the effectiveness of aspart are ongoing (126,128).

The third FDA approved insulin analogue is glargine (Lantus). Glargine is the first long-acting insulin analogue to have achieved FDA approval. It appears to be an almost peakless insulin, with a duration of 24 hours or longer. Its pharmacologic action most closely mimics the basal insulin produced by the β-cells when the body is in the fasting state, that is, during the overnight hours. Glargine, a clear U100 insulin preparation, must be injected alone which is unlike the other intermediate- or long-acting insulins, which can be mixed with rapid-acting insulins. The acidic pH of glargine prevents it from being mixed with other insulin preparations. Clinical studies of premeal lispro or regular comparing glargine administered at bedtime with NPH administered either once or twice daily demonstrated that the glargine group experienced lower fasting blood glucose levels with less nocturnal hypoglycemia than the NPH group (129). Glargine has not been approved for use in pediatric patients younger than 6 years of age. Ongoing clinical studies in the pediatric population will define the level of efficacy of this insulin preparation.

Another category of insulin preparations is the group of premixed insulins. One mixture of insulins contains an analogue of lispro with an intermediate-acting insulin called NPL. NPL is a lispro protamine insulin suspension creating a monomeric insulin with an activity profile like that of NPH insulin. The mixture consists of 75% NPL and 25% lispro. There may soon be available a 70/30, as well as a 30/70, preparation of intermediate-acting NPH and insulin aspart.

The use of premixed insulins, i.e., 70/30 (70% NPH/30% regular), 50/50 (50% NPH/50% regular), and 75/25 (75% NPL and 25% lispro), provides ease of administration, but these mixtures are not commonly used in the pediatric population. Premixed insulins are not recommended in the pediatric population unless all other insulin programs have failed. The premixed insulins do not allow for the independent adjustment of either the rapid- or intermediate-acting insulin, as they are in fixed, pre-set ratios that cannot be altered independently of one another. This does not allow a response to increased blood glucose levels or activity without altering the entire insulin program. Premixed insulin may be advantageous for adolescents whose psychosocial needs impair their ability to handle yet one more diabetes related task, that is, the mixing of insulins. Families in which the primary insulin-giver has a learning disability or cannot master the sequencing of steps needed to mix insulins or add together the clear and cloudy doses may benefit from the use of premixed insulins.

A mixed dose of rapid-acting and intermediate-acting insulins administered before breakfast will provide insulin coverage for breakfast and the midday meal, as well as provide early afternoon insulin effect. Because the prebreakfast intermediate insulin effect will have sufficiently waned by late afternoon, the need for a second dose of insulin to provide coverage for the evening meal and overnight hours will become obvious. The peak action of presupper intermediate insulin will occur between midnight and 3 a.m., increasing the risk for nocturnal hypoglycemia. Fasting blood glucose levels may be increased as a result of increasing overnight hepatic production of glucose and overnight release of growth hormone. Increasing the level of presupper intermediate-acting insulin to compensate for the fasting hyperglycemia without monitoring the insulin effect between midnight and 3 a.m. may trigger severe nocturnal hypoglycemia. If the middle-of-the-night blood glucose is 100 mg/dL or less, it is unwise to raise the supper intermediate-acting insulin to correct the fasting hyperglycemia, as the risk for nocturnal hypoglycemia increases. In such instances, a safer approach to managing the fasting hyperglycemia is to administer the rapid-acting insulin alone at dinner and the intermediate- or long-acting insulin at bedtime (approximately 9 p.m.), thus providing more insulin coverage in the hours just before dawn when it is needed. The use of ultralente insulin before supper as a substitute for a bedtime injection in the prepubescent child, maintaining a twice-daily injection program, can occasionally be quite successful (130). The success of this insulin regimen fades rather dramatically with the exuberant hormonal changes in the adolescent, necessitating a multiple daily injection program.

In a common insulin regimen, two thirds of the total daily insulin dose is given before breakfast and the remaining one third, before dinner and/or bedtime. Rapid-acting insulin usually makes up one third of the morning dose, with the remaining two thirds composed of the intermediate-acting insulin. One third to one half of the evening dose is devoted to the rapid-acting insulin, and the remainder is administered as either the supper or bedtime intermediate-acting insulin. Fine-tuning of doses is accomplished through the use of blood glucose monitoring to determine the effectiveness of the insulin program. Families should be encouraged to become active participants in evaluating and self-adjusting insulin doses based on blood glucose levels, anticipated carbohydrate intake, and planned-for activity levels.

Over the past 10 years, since the release of the DCCT results, practitioners worldwide have recognized and accepted the value of aiming to normalize glycemia (56). To achieve this goal, regimens should attempt to mimic the function of the β-cells, using a basal-bolus approach to diabetes management. To date, this is accomplished through either multiple daily injections (using either ultralente or glargine as the basal insulin and lispro, aspart, or regular insulin as the bolus insulin) or through CSII using an insulin pump. Both of these programs have demonstrated advantages over the more conventional insulin programs but are not without distinct disadvantages as well (56). Advantages include greater flexibility around food, with respect to both the timing and amounts; lower risk of hypoglycemia, as the variable peaking of intermediate-acting insulins is eliminated; the ability to "sleep in" without the risk of significant waning of insulin effect by morning with hyperglycemia or the risk of hypoglycemia from lack of calories; and the ability to improve blood glucose levels and glycemic control. Clearly, disadvantages include the need to increase the frequency of blood glucose monitoring to four or more times per day, the required attention to the carbohydrate content of meals/snacks, and the potential for weight gain. The DCCT experience showed that those participants in the intensively managed group were, on average, 10 pounds heavier than those in the conventionally treated group (56). Successful management of diabetes with an intensive insulin program requires a demonstrated comfort level with blood glucose monitoring tools as well as with insulin delivery systems, increased family and school support, proficiency with carbohydrate counting, record-keeping, and more frequent contact with a diabetes healthcare team that can provide 24-hour support. It has been demonstrated that the success of such an insulin program requires that both the child/adolescent and family want this approach and communicate well with each other. Families with major stress, such as conflictual child-parent relationships, major mental illness, or poor adherence to a more conventional treatment program, should defer intensive insulin therapy programs until there has been some resolution to the psychosocial or medical tensions.

INSULIN DELIVERY SYSTEMS

Options for the delivery of insulin are many and varied. They include syringes, pens, pumps, and air injectors.

Traditionally, most pediatric patients receive their insulin by injection with syringes to provide mixing of insulins and flexibility in dosing of both short- and long-acting insulin preparations. Syringes are calibrated to 3/10 cc, 1/2 cc, or 1 cc and have either 29-gauge, 1/2-inch needles or 30-gauge, 5/16-inch needles.

The use of insulin pens with disposable needle tips has long been the delivery system of choice in Europe. The advantage of the insulin pens is that they offer a discrete, rapid way of administering insulin accurately for those children who object to or who feel unsafe carrying a vial of insulin and a syringe. Pens are available as disposable devices holding 300 U of a specified type of insulin or as more-durable equipment that requires replaceable cartridges of either 150 or 300 U of various types of insulins. Currently, it is possible to purchase insulin pens or cartridges of aspart, lispro, NPH, 75/25, or 70/30. The disadvantage of the pen system is that it is not possible to mix insulins together for a single injection with the exception of the above premixed insulin preparations.

Healthcare providers appreciate the challenges associated with intensive insulin therapy. The pharmacokinetics of injected insulin hamper spontaneity of lifestyle and increase the risk of hypoglycemia or hyperglycemia. Since the 1970s, physicians and scientists have investigated alternative insulin delivery systems in an attempt to improve glycemic control and quality-of-life for patients. The use of insulin pumps or CSII therapy provides one approach to intensive insulin therapy that can optimize glycemic control, reduce hypoglycemia, and maintain quality of life (131). Pump use is growing rapidly in the pediatric population.

Insulin pumps offer a continuous infusion of insulin over the course of the day in an effort to replicate basal insulin production by the pancreas. Boluses of insulin are administered at the time of meals or snacks to mimic the normal physiologic peaks of insulin release in response to food intake. Four companies currently make insulin infusion pumps: MiniMed (http://www.minimed.com), Disetronic (http://www.disetronic.com/), Animas (http://www.animascorp.com/), and Deltec (http://www.delteccozmo.com). Although each has individualized features designed to set it apart from its competitors, they have many similarities. See Chapter 39 for additional information on insulin pump therapy.

Each of these battery-run, computerized insulin pumps is about the size of a beeper. They hold a reservoir of insulin and are worn externally, either on a waistband or in a pocket. The pumps are connected by an infusion set of thin plastic tubing that contains most commonly an introducer needle within a Teflon catheter at its end. The catheter, with the aid of the introducer needle, is inserted into the subcutaneous tissue of the abdomen, thigh, or buttocks and is left in place after removal of the introducer needle. Insulin is delivered through the tubing throughout the course of the day and night. The child or adolescent with diabetes or a parent must replace the manually inserted infusion set and the insulin supply every 2 to 3 days.

The ADA's Position Statement on CSII provides recommendations on provider aspects, patient selection, insulin pump choice, and safety (132). Issues related to the use of insulin pumps in the pediatric and adolescent populations are not addressed specifically in the position statement; however, the recommendations have been helpful in the development of center- or practice-specific pump protocols and education programs supporting assessment, initiation, and continued use of CSII in the pediatric population. Table 42.8 presents the advantages and disadvantages of insulin pump therapy. The success of these current insulin delivery systems revolves around the following factors:

- Intensive blood glucose monitoring minimally four to six times a day: none of the available insulin pumps are closed-loop systems able to monitor blood glucose levels and deliver insulin automatically; all pumps must be manually programmed.
- Comfort with and utilization of carbohydrate counting: matching insulin and activity with carbohydrate intake.
- Adult support both at home and in school.
- Access to a diabetes team offering 24-hour/7-day-a-week problem solving and support. The number of decision-making points through the course of the day around fluctuations in blood glucose levels, carbohydrate intake, activity variables, illness, and the presence/absence of ketones makes it imperative that there be adult support in determining insulin doses.

TABLE 42.8. Advantages and Disadvantages of Insulin Pump Therapy

Advantages	Disadvantages
• Greater flexibility around timing of meals • Greater flexibility with portion size of • food • Ability to intensify glycemic control • Fewer severe hypoglycemic episodes • Fewer injections • Immediate access to insulin	• Increased frequency of blood glucose and ketone monitoring • Increased chance of hyperglycemia and DKA due to crimped infusion sets, air bubbles, and dislodged cannula • Potential for skin abscess • Change in hypoglycemic symptoms • Constant attachment to the pump

There is no best, predetermined age to initiate insulin pump therapy. As with all diabetes management issues, individualized treatment plans, after considering the needs of the patient, as well as those of the family, are best. Presently, there are fewer young children than pre-adolescents and adolescents using insulin pumps. Use of insulin pump therapy at nighttime for young children along with daytime insulin injections has been shown to improve glycemia, counterregulatory hormone response, and awareness of hypoglycemia in certain pediatric populations (133,134). We have evaluated pump use in 170 youth with type 1 diabetes. While glycemic control improves after 3 months of pump use, HbA_{1c} values appear to return to baseline by 1 year (135). The worsening of glycemic control after the initial improvement stems from diminished blood glucose monitoring and missed insulin boluses.

At present, there are no clinically approved implantable pumps for children. All of the current pumps are open-loop systems, meaning that the pumps are not able to discern blood glucose levels and automatically deliver insulin. Clearly, the goal of all pump manufacturers is to develop a closed-loop system—an artificial pancreas.

Inhaled insulin therapy may soon be available. Recent reports describe short-term safety and efficacy of inhaled insulin use in patients with type 1 or type 2 diabetes during a 12-week trial (136–138). In addition to receiving inhaled insulin before meals, the experimental group received injected ultralente insulin at bedtime. Additional pediatric studies, as well as long-term trials, are needed to confirm the safety and efficacy of inhaled insulin.

Children should never be forced to self-draw or self-administer insulin before they are either emotionally or physically ready for this responsibility. Although there is no one "right" age at which all children should be taught to prepare and inject insulin or insert pump sets, there are good studies to support the theory that, developmentally, many children may express interest and desire to participate in this responsibility around the age of 10 to 12 (63). Until that time, insulin administration is the responsibility of an adult care provider. All insulin drawn-up and self-administered by a child should be supervised by an adult for accuracy of dosage and technique of injection.

THERAPY FOR TYPE 2 DIABETES IN YOUTH

The treatment goal for youth with type 2 diabetes, similar to that for type 1 diabetes, is normalization of blood glucose values and HbA_{1c}, with a major emphasis on lifestyle change around nutrition and physical activity. Management of related conditions such as hypertension and hyperlipidemia in pediatric patients with type 2 diabetes also is indicated. The overall goal of treatment is to reduce the risk of acute and chronic complications of diabetes. Treatment is aimed at lowering blood glucose levels to near-normal values in all patients with diabetes to avoid (a) acute metabolic decompensation due to DKA or NKHHS; (b) symptoms of polyuria, polydipsia, fatigue, weight loss with polyphagia, blurred vision, recurrent vaginitis/balanitis; (c) the development or progression of complications involving the eyes, kidneys, and nerves; and (d) failure to maintain normal growth and development and a near normal lifestyle.

The initial treatment of type 2 diabetes in youth depends on the clinical presentation (10). Severe hyperglycemia with NKHHS syndrome requires emergency management similar to that for DKA. Insulin will likely be needed as therapy in these patients even after recovery from the acute condition. Others who are not ill at diagnosis can be treated initially with medical nutrition therapy and physical activity (see sections below). Unless there is successful weight loss, most patients will require some form of drug therapy. Insulin was previously the only drug approved by the FDA for use in children. Metformin has recently been approved for the treatment of type 2 diabetes in youth age 12 years and older (139). Nonetheless, most pediatric endocrinologists use some of the oral anti-diabetes agents to treat children with type 2 diabetes, even while there are ongoing studies of many of these agents (46,49).

As with type 1 diabetes, the goal of treatment for youth with type 2 diabetes is normalization of blood glucose values and HbA_{1c}. Management of comorbid conditions such as hypertension and dyslipidemia should be initiated. Macrovascular risk factors such as hypertension and dyslipidemia, when found in a younger individual, have potential for significantly shortening life if diabetes complications begin in early adulthood (140).

Patients who present with DKA or NKHHS should be treated per protocol (see Chapter 53). Indications for initial treatment with insulin include dehydration, ketosis, and acidosis. After stabilization and follow-up, re-evaluation is necessary, as insulin may be tapered and an oral anti-diabetes agent introduced following improvement in metabolic control. Other patients may begin oral anti-diabetes agents along with diet therapy and exercise at diagnosis when the presentation suggests type 2 diabetes and the patient is stable. The consensus statement of the ADA published in March 2000 (10) recommends that metformin be the first oral agent used in pediatric patients with type 2 diabetes. Metformin should not be used in patients with known renal disease, hepatic disease, hypoxemic states, severe infections, or alcohol abuse or with radiocontrast material. In addition, patients of childbearing age should be made aware that metformin may normalize anovulatory cycles in patients with polycystic ovary syndrome, a common condition in adolescent females with type 2 diabetes (49,141,142). Thus, adequate birth control should be addressed in sexually active teens.

If monotherapy with metformin fails to accomplish glycemic goals within 3 to 6 months, additional therapy should be added to the treatment regimen. Supplemental agents include insulin, as well as other oral agents such as a sulfonylurea, other insulin secretagogues such as repaglinide and meglitinide, insulin sensitizers such as thiozolidenediones, or α-glucosidase inhibitors. Insulin can be started either at bedtime alone or twice daily. Frequent blood glucose monitoring should be encouraged, especially aimed at achieving fasting blood glucose levels of less than 126 mg/dL. Frequency of contact with the primary care provider or healthcare team will depend on the therapeutic response to treatment but should occur at least quarterly and more often when therapies are being altered.

MEDICAL NUTRITION THERAPY: NUTRITION EDUCATION

Dissemination of the results of the DCCT brought with it changes in a variety of diabetes self-management tools and recommendations (56,72). Most recently, the ADA's 2002 revision of the Evidence-Based Nutrition Principles and Recommendations increases flexibility in terms of food and meal plans for the child and adolescent with diabetes (143). As a member of the diabetes healthcare team, a registered dietitian provides medical nutrition therapy (MNT) through nutrition assessment, education, and counseling. Patients/families with newly diagnosed type 1 diabetes begin MNT as soon as the patient is medically stable following the diagnosis, and they continue MNT every 3 to 6 months in very young children and every 6 to 12 months in older children and adolescents. Patients with type 2 diabetes also begin MNT at diagnosis and continue as needed to attain weight loss goals. This enables appropriate, ongoing changes to the meal plan reflective of changes in growth and development, and based on family lifestyle and cultural food values.

MNT provides information, motivation, and problem-solving techniques for meal planning and family nutrition for children and adolescents with diabetes. Not surprisingly, children and adolescents with diabetes and their families, as well as professionals, often identify food as the most difficult part of diabetes self-management (100,144). Thus, MNT is an integral component of any successful diabetes self-management plan (143,145).

MNT must be individualized, provide appropriate nutrition, and match the lifestyle of the child or adolescent with diabetes and his or her family. A meal plan is not a diet; it is a guide to choosing healthy, age-appropriate foods in a way that contributes to various positive medical outcomes, such as blood glucose levels, lipid levels, blood pressure, renal function, and normal growth and development in children (143).

Appropriate meal planning should enable patients and families to optimize glycemic control by matching the insulin dose with food and activity. Meal planning is successful when the child or adolescent's meal plan provides flexibility, satiety, satisfaction, and inclusion for the picky eater, partygoer, fast-food lover, and school-lunch or college-cafeteria eater and promotes a sense of normalcy.

MNT provides an individualized prescription of calories and macronutrients for the child or adolescent, which is commonly known as a meal plan. It starts with a nutrition assessment and generates treatment goals (60). The assessment also collects clinical data, dietary history, nutrient intake, and a social history (60). The assessment generates goals for therapy. Goals should be age appropriate, attainable, socially appropriate, and clearly stated. General nutrition goals (143) for children and adolescents with diabetes follow:

- Reach and maintain optimal blood glucose levels
- Achieve optimal lipid and lipoprotein levels
- Maintain normal blood pressure levels
- Prevent and/or treat the complications of diabetes
- Improve general overall health through healthy food choices and an active lifestyle
- Develop a meal plan that takes personal and cultural issues into consideration reflective of the individual/family's wishes and willingness to change
- Provide adequate calories for maintaining or attaining acceptable weight for adolescents and normal growth and development rates for children and adolescents
- For children and adolescents with type 2 diabetes, facilitate lifestyle changes in eating and physical activity.

A team approach by the registered dietitian, physician, nurse educator, and family and child with diabetes is required to achieve nutrition-related goals (145). For children and adolescents who are intensively managed, personal algorithms for therapy adjustment need to be developed (59). Use of blood glucose monitoring results allows for adjustments to the self-management plan. Postprandial blood glucose values help in determining if the present algorithm is working. Knowledge of the child or adolescent's insulin-to-carbohydrate ratio, as well as insulin-sensitivity correction factor, can be important information in calculating the personal algorithm (see Chapter 36).

There are several distinct meal planning systems, such as the exchange system and carbohydrate counting. The DCCT showed that many different approaches to meal planning can be successful (56,72). The outdated "no-concentrated-sweets" approach is very restrictive. The 2002 Nutrition Recommendations offer an expert consensus stating that sucrose (table sugar) and sucrose-containing foods may be eaten but in the context of a healthy diet (143). The no-concentrated-sweets approach ignores important facets of MNT, such as the timing and consistency of meals and snacks. The four general approaches to medical nutrition therapy are (a) general guidelines (146); (b) meal planning (sample menus); (c) exchange lists; and (d) carbohydrate counting.

Both the exchange-list and carbohydrate-counting approaches incorporate flexibility and individualization and strive for optimal glycemic control. The exchange lists have six different exchange groups: bread/starch, protein, milk, fruit, vegetable, and fat. The carbohydrate counting method arises from the 1994 ADA Nutrition Recommendation guidelines, which consider that the total amount of carbohydrate, not the type of carbohydrate, impact on glycemic control (60,145). This allows for the incorporation of all carbohydrate sources, including sucrose, into the meal plan, providing maximum flexibility to patients of all ages. Counting "carbs" is the most common meal planning approach used with pediatric and adolescent populations with diabetes (see Chapter 36 on nutrition for more information on these meal-planning approaches).

MNT requires a caloric and macronutrient prescription. Nutrient requirements for children and adolescents with diabetes appear similar to those for their peers without diabetes. Table 42.9 gives general guidelines for calculating daily calories (60).

The 2002 Nutrition Recommendations allow for the carbohydrate, protein, and fat contents of meal plans to be individualized to achieve optimal metabolic goals. Protein intake of 15% to 20% is adequate for the general population (143). The Recommended Dietary Allowance (RDA) for protein ranges from 2.2 g/kg per day for infants to 0.9 g/kg per day for adolescent males age 15 through 18 years (60). As per the ADA recommendations, carbohydrate and monounsaturated fats combined should make up 60% to 70% of the meal plan (143).

The amount of fat in a meal plan for the child or adolescent over the age of 2 years should not exceed 30% of the total calories, with less than 10% from saturated fat, less than 10% from polyunsaturates; and 10% to 15% from monounsaturates. Dietary cholesterol should be limited to less than 300 mg/day.

Those patients who are of normal weight and have normal lipid levels are encouraged to follow the recommendations of the National Cholesterol Education Program (http://www.nhlbi.nih.gov/about/ncep/). Healthy fat intake can be encouraged by the consumption of lean cuts of red meat, more chicken and turkey without skin, fish and seafood, skim and low-fat milk and milk products, and vegetable proteins (legumes). The results of the Dietary Intervention Study in Children show that there are cholesterol-lowering benefits to a diet reduced in fat

TABLE 42.9. General Guidelines for Calculating Daily Calorie Requirements for Children and Adolescents

Age	Calorie requirements
0–12 y	1,000 kcal for 1st year + 100 kcal/y over age 1 y
12–15 y	
Female	1,500–2,000 kcal + 100 kcal/y over age 12 y
Male	2,000–2,500 kcal + 200 kcal/y over age 12 y
15–20 y	
Female	13–15 kcal/lb (29–33 kcal/kg) desired body weight
Male	15–18 kcal/lb (33–40 kcal/kg) desired body weight

and cholesterol in children with elevated lipid levels. The study shows that a diet low in saturated fat and cholesterol is safe for children and is not a risk for altered growth, nutritional status, or sexual maturation (147). It is important that children and families know the value of a healthy meal plan that incorporates fat and cholesterol in appropriate amounts. As for the use of fat replacers, more research is needed on their role in a child's meal plan. Attention should be directed to the nutrition facts label for any products containing fat replacements, since many such products tend to be higher in carbohydrates than their fat-containing counterparts (143). Following the ADA Nutrition Recommendations becomes important with the epidemic of childhood obesity and type 2 diabetes (11,12,39). Strategies to successfully decrease fat and total calories for children and adolescents with type 2 diabetes need to be developed.

Dietary fiber is a carbohydrate found in such foods as whole grains, breads, cereals, legumes, fruits, and vegetables. Fiber helps in the digestion process, provides satiety, and reduces levels of serum cholesterol and triglycerides. The recommended five-a-day servings of fruits and vegetables is a good guideline to use. Serving children and adolescents foods that provide a source of fiber provides essential vitamins and minerals for health and growth. Grams of fiber are listed on the nutrition label under *Total Carbohydrate*. When calculating the dose of rapid- or fast-acting insulin based on carbohydrate intake, if the serving to be eaten contains 5 or more grams of fiber, the numbers of fiber grams are subtracted from the grams of total carbohydrate. Use of foods containing a large amount of fiber for the treatment of hypoglycemia is *not* recommended.

Sweeteners, such as sucrose, fructose, or aspartame, can all be incorporated into the meal plan of a child or adolescent with diabetes. An individual assessment must be made as to the glycemic impact of these sweeteners. The carbohydrate content of nutritive sweeteners (e.g., sucrose, fructose, and sugar alcohols like sorbitol) must be calculated into the meal plan (143). Ingestion of large amounts of foods containing sugar alcohols like sorbitol, mannitol, and xylitol may cause gastrointestinal upset with flatus or diarrhea, particularly in young children. Choosing nutrient-rich foods is preferable to choosing "sweets" such as cakes and candy that tend to be foods with basically "empty" calories. However, it is important for children and adolescents with diabetes to "fit in" with their peers and share in the food aspects of celebrations, holidays, and parties that tend to include these "treats."

Nonnutritive sweeteners, commonly called "sugar substitutes," are often used in the meal plans of children and adolescents with diabetes. They include saccharin, aspartame, acesulfame potassium, and sucalose. The acceptable daily intake has been determined by the FDA for sweeteners in terms of safety of consumption, with a 100-fold safety factor (145,148). Use of packets and bulk forms of these products, as well as consumption of products such as diet sodas, sugar-free gelatins, and ice pops, will have little effect on blood glucose levels. The major problem is that patients and parents often ignore other components of foods and drinks containing these sweeteners and consume them liberally without calculating their calorie and carbohydrate contents into the meal plan. It is possible to calculate carbohydrates, protein, and fat in such foods from the nutrition-facts label based on the portion size eaten.

What, when, and how much food is eaten by children and adolescents with diabetes are all important. So, too, is where they eat. School is where all children spend the majority of their time; school is where all children have lunch more than 150 times a year. The child or adolescent with diabetes can eat "school lunches." Most school systems post the weekly or monthly school-lunch menu in the newspaper, on community bulletin boards, and, increasingly, on the Internet. School-lunch menus can be calculated to fit the child or adolescent's meal plan as needed for reasons of convenience, sociability, or cost.

Another important issue for the child or adolescent with diabetes is fast food. There are a variety of fast-food guides that provide nutrition information for menu items from most of the major fast-food restaurants. The child or adolescent with diabetes and his or her family benefit from knowledge of the content of carbohydrate, fat, protein, and total calories in fast foods so that they may best match insulin dosage or activity to the meal eaten. Paper copies or information from the Internet can provide this important fast-food nutrition information.

The self-management plan may call for the delivery of a rapid-acting insulin (lispro or aspart) at the end of a meal for some children. Food struggles are not new to parents nor are they specific to diabetes. Post-meal protocols utilizing rapid-acting insulin can help to eliminate some of the food struggles and provide a better match of insulin dose to the food eaten.

Children and adolescents with type 1 diabetes have a slightly increased risk of celiac disease, a common cause of malabsorption in children (149–151). Celiac disease is an autoimmune-mediated disorder that occurs in genetically susceptible individuals. Immune-mediated damage to the mucosa of the small intestine occurs after exposure to the gliadin moiety of gluten, leading to destruction of the absorptive surfaces of the villi of the small intestine. Gluten is found in wheat, rye, barley, and possibly oats (152). Symptoms of celiac disease include diarrhea, weight loss or poor weight gain, growth failure, abdominal pain, chronic fatigue, irritability, an inability to concentrate, malnutrition due to malabsorption, and other gastrointestinal problems (152). Diabetes-specific symptoms may include unexplained hypoglycemia. Diagnosis is based on the results of a blood test [most specific—IgA to tissue transglutaminase (ttg) followed by small bowel biopsy]. At present, the only treatment for celiac disease is a gluten-free diet with the avoidance of the foods listed previously. Children and adolescents with diabetes who also have undiagnosed celiac disease or those diagnosed who do not follow a gluten-free diet often have unpredictable blood sugars with hypoglycemia and deterioration in glycemic control (151). It is very important for families of children with diabetes and celiac disease to work with a registered dietitian who has experience with both diabetes and celiac disease, as gluten-free foods are often very high in carbohydrates.

Eating disorders constitute a challenge in the adolescent population, particularly in females. It is reported that adolescent females with diabetes are twice as likely as adolescent females in general to have an eating disorder or subthreshold eating disorder (153). Insulin omission with the goal of weight loss is the hallmark of eating disorders in the diabetes population (153,154). The resultant adverse health outcomes, such as high HbA_{1c} values, increased hospitalizations, episodes of DKA, and eye and kidney complications, call for identification of and clinical intervention for eating disorders in this population (155–157). Use of such questionnaires as the General Survey of Eating Problems (EAT-26), Eating Disorder Examination (EDE), Children's Eating Disorder Examination, or the Diabetes Eating Problem Survey (DEPS), which is diabetes specific (155), provide tools for screening. As with the general population, more youths with diabetes have subthreshold eating disorders than have DSM-IV–classified eating disorders (158). Little in the literature addresses the problem of eating disorders in the pediatric or adolescent male population; however, practices such as weight gain during football season or weight loss during wrestling season, by way of manipulating insulin doses and food, have been seen in many pediatric and adolescent endocrinology practices. In general, food can be a source of conflict for children and parents. Theories in the literature suggest that those youths with type 1 diabetes who have eating disorders have other underlying psychiatric disorders (159). The emphasis placed on food issues for youths with type 1 diabetes may increase the occurrence of eating disorders in this population (160).

In summary, MNT must be individualized to the family of the child or adolescent with diabetes. The measure of success of the meal plan within the self-management plan is optimal glycemic control with prevention of frequent episodes of hyperglycemia and hypoglycemia.

EXERCISE/PHYSICAL ACTIVITY

All children and adolescents need to be physically active! The Surgeon General's Report on Physical Activity and Health emphasizes the fundamental role of physical activity in promotion of health and prevention of disease (38). Physical activity is necessary for the optimal health for all children and adolescents.

For children and adolescents with diabetes, physical activity plays an added role as a tool in the diabetes treatment plan. For the child or adolescent with type 1 diabetes, a balance of exercise, insulin, and food, using information from blood glucose monitoring, enhances the attainment of optimal blood glucose control. The benefits of exercise for the child or adolescent with type 1 or type 2 diabetes are substantial. With the rise in childhood obesity and sedentary lifestyle, leading to an epidemic of type 2 diabetes in children and adolescents, an increase in physical activity and exercise is necessary. The Kaiser Family Foundation Study reports that the average American child uses electronic media outside of school more than 38 hours a week and that 53% of children 2 to 18 years old have a television in their bedrooms (161).

For the child or adolescent with type 2 diabetes, changes in lifestyle, including aerobic exercise, can result in improved outcomes in terms of glycemic control, weight loss, lipid abnormalities, and hypertension. The benefits of exercise for the child or adolescent with diabetes include:

- Improvement in blood glucose control
- Reduction in dosage of insulin
- Reduction in long-term health risks, including obesity, osteoporosis, hypertension, arteriosclerosis, and cardiovascular disorders
- Appropriate weight gain, weight maintenance, or weight loss
- Improvement in skeletal growth and strength
- Enhancement of muscle development
- Development of self-esteem and social and team building skills
- Development of lifelong healthy habits
- Psychological well-being and improved quality of life
- Stress reduction.

The child or adolescent must enjoy the physical activity, have access to the activity on a regular basis, and find it convenient and fun so that it becomes part of his or her lifestyle. Children and adolescents with diabetes should, like their peers who do not have diabetes, be able to profit from the physical and social benefits of physical activity.

It is important for physical activity to be a part of the family's lifestyle. The child or adolescent with diabetes should not be the only family member encouraged to incorporate physical activity into daily activities: father, mother, and siblings should also be active. Since children and adolescents spend the majority of their time in school and at school-based activities, school personnel and coaches must be aware of the beneficial nature of exercise for all students. Students with diabetes should participate fully in recess, gym classes, and sports. Education and preparation are important. Education for teachers and coaches should include an understanding of signs and symptoms of hypoglycemia and appropriate treatments. Preparation for the student with diabetes would include access to the appropriate supplies for the treatment of hypoglycemia.

The role of physical activity for children and adolescents with type 2 diabetes is paramount. Physical activity uses calories, decreases insulin resistance, and is a tool for weight maintenance or loss (162). Physical activity and dietary modifications are necessary lifestyle changes to improve short- and long-term outcomes for the child or adolescent (10–12,48).

Physical activity can increase the risk of hypoglycemia for children and adolescents who take insulin (163–166) or for those patients with type 2 diabetes who take blood-glucose-lowering oral medications (167). However, the occurrence of hypoglycemia during, immediately following, or hours after physical activity can be minimized. Remember that the child or adolescent is at maximal risk for hypoglycemia for up to 6 to 12 hours following physical activity (168)—the so-called lag effect. Newer management tools such as insulin analogues, insulin delivery devices, and blood glucose monitors can help to prevent and/or manage hypoglycemia. Since physical activity can increase the risk of hypoglycemia, it is necessary to develop individualized exercise/physical activity guidelines for the child or adolescent with type 1 or type 2 diabetes who is treated with insulin. This requires being in tune with individual responses to physical activity, insulin, and carbohydrate intake, arrived at empirically. Checking the blood glucose level before, sometimes during, and after physical activity should be encouraged. Use of blood glucose monitoring is necessary to make appropriate adjustments for physical activity as part of the diabetes treatment plan. These adjustments can decrease the frequency of hypoglycemia.

Children and adolescents with diabetes should always wear diabetes identification—a bracelet, necklace, or shoe tag—in case of hypoglycemic episodes and for a variety of other safety concerns. If the athletic association requires players to remove the identification during practices or games, it is imperative for the coach to be aware of who on his or her team has diabetes, to develop some form of plan (58) to identify when his or her player feels a need to be removed from the game because of symptoms of hypoglycemia, and to have available a source of rapid-acting carbohydrate. Depending on the intensity of the sport and the amount of water lost through dehydration and perspiration, many athletes will prepare their water bottle with a dilute form of fortified sports drink (50% water/50% sports drink) to replenish fluids, electrolytes, and glucose expended during the activity.

Adequate fluid intake is extremely important to avoid dehydration. Dehydration can have an adverse affect on blood glucose levels. Fluid intake before, during, and after exercise is recommended (169). Environmental factors—extremes of heat, humidity, cold, and altitude—can affect blood glucose levels during exercise, and precautions should be taken when exercise or any kind of physical activity is done in any of these environments (169).

Issues of oxygen consumption, muscle uptake, glycogen stores, triglycerides, and free fatty acids affect glycemic control. Maintenance of euglycemia during physical activity in the person with and without diabetes is for the most part hormonally mediated. In the person with type 1 diabetes who is insulin-deficient, excessive release of counterregulatory hormones during physical activity may result in hyperglycemia and the formation of ketone bodies, which can lead to DKA (169).

Physical activity can lower blood glucose levels of patients with diabetes who begin with either normal blood glucose levels or moderate hyperglycemia. With extreme hyperglycemia, physical activity can exacerbate an insulinopenic state, and blood glucose levels may actually increase. It is best to avoid physical activity if ketones are present and/or if the blood glucose level is greater than 300 mg/dL and to treat the ketonuria/hyperglycemia first. If the blood glucose level is less than 100 mg/dL before physical activity, patients should take a carbohydrate snack to avoid hypoglycemia. Patients should be alert to the symptoms and signs of hypoglycemia during physical activity and for several hours thereafter. Patients should have a source of "sugar" (such as glucose tablets or glucose gel) readily available during and after physical activity to treat hypoglycemia. The risks and benefits of physical activity are specific to the individual child or adolescent with diabetes. It is highly recommended that an exercise physiologist, with experience in diabetes, set the physical activity prescription. Necessary adjustments to food and insulin must consider blood glucose levels at the time of physical activity, the type of activity, and the intensity and duration of activity in addition to the timing and dose of insulin, as well as the timing and amount of carbohydrate intake.

A variety of snack bars supply effective carbohydrate sources for the prevention and/or treatment of hypoglycemia. It has been hypothesized that foods containing resistant starch (cornstarch) or foods modified with resistant starch (high amylose cornstarch) may have an effect on postprandial glycemic response, including prevention of hypoglycemia. Thus, a variety of energy bar products are now available that contain resistant starch: uncooked cornstarch. People with diabetes may eat the bars at bedtime to help prevent nocturnal hypoglycemia. Conventional snack bars or energy bars, which contain 15 to 30 g of sugars, are designed to raise blood glucose levels before or during exercise. Some research findings support the utility of both types of products for the prevention of exercise-induced hypoglycemia (170–172). However, there are no published, evidence-based longitudinal studies in subjects with diabetes to prove benefits from the use of resistant starch (143).

The sole use of carbohydrate to treat or prevent an episode of hypoglycemia during physical activity is no longer recommended. For the child or adolescent striving to improve glycemic control or lose weight, the use of additional carbohydrate for physical activity can sabotage desired outcomes. Intensive insulin therapy, either by multiple daily injections or CSII, permits appropriate adjustments in the insulin dose for various activities. Newer insulin analogues and insulin delivery systems coupled with blood glucose monitoring tools allow for adjustments of both insulin and carbohydrates. The amount of adjustment necessary varies from patient to patient and is highly individualized. Individualized physical activity algorithms can be developed from exercise guidelines. In general, however, mild-to-moderate exercise may require that pre-exercise doses be decreased by about 20% for lispro, aspart, or regular insulin and by 10% for intermediate-acting insulin. Heavy exercise may require decreases of 30% to 50% for rapid-acting insulins and 20% to 35% for intermediate-acting insulins. It is difficult to make adjustments in ultralente or glargine insulin for physical activity because of their long duration of action. For patients who use an insulin pump and anticipate 60 minutes or more of exercise, a temporary basal rate may be set by decreasing the current basal rate by 25% to 40%. After the exercise, the pump user may continue with a diminished basal rate, by 25%, for 2 to 4 hours, depending on the intensity of exercise and past experience (59). If activity is strenuous, additional carbohydrates may also be needed. Young children with diabetes often have unpredictable levels of activity, so snacking is often the preferred adjustment, especially for play. Thus, prevention of hypoglycemia due to physical activity necessitates adjustments in both insulin and food. These preventive strategies must take into consideration the type, amount, and duration of the activity, in combination with such variables as the child's age, fitness level, and body mass (173). Although there is no evidence that physical activity in itself can significantly lower HbA_{1c} values, there is evidence of overall health benefits.

A standard recommendation for physical activity includes a 5- to 10-minute warm-up, followed by exercise, followed by a 5- to 10-minute cool-down period (169). This pertains to sports training and other exercises for children, adolescents, and young adults. Most physical activity for young children is spontaneous and is called "play"; for most of this type of physical activity, warm-ups and cool-downs are not necessary. Young individuals in good metabolic control can usually participate safely in most physical activities, including weight training (169). However, the older adolescent and young adult should have formal ophthalmology assessment before unrestricted participation in impact exercises or weight lifting. In addition, cardiac stress testing should be considered for the young adult.

For the most part, children and adolescents with diabetes follow the recommendations for physical activity as stated by the ADA (169). However, children and adolescents with diabetes often experience greater variability in blood glucose levels than do their adult counterparts.

For children, there needs to be a balance between glycemic control and the appropriate tasks of childhood and adolescence. This necessitates planning by parents, school personnel, athletic coaches, other adults, and sometimes even peers. Diabetes self-management training and education on the causes, symptoms, and treatments of hypoglycemia and hyperglycemia; insulin adjustments; nutrition; and physical activity, can make a physically active lifestyle a safe and rewarding experience for children and adolescents with type 1 or type 2 diabetes (169).

MONITORING

The Position Statement of the ADA on tests of glycemia in diabetes stresses the importance of monitoring glycemic status (174). This includes self-monitoring of blood glucose (SMBG) and ketones as well as laboratory measurement of HbA_{1c} and, in certain situations, glycosylated serum protein. The HbA_{1c} has become the standard for assessing glycemic control over a period of approximately 2 to 3 months. The HbA_{1c} should be measured at diagnosis and every 3 months thereafter (174). Goals of therapy using HbA_{1c} data were discussed earlier in this chapter.

As a component of comprehensive self-management training, all children and adolescents with diabetes and their families should receive training in SMBG (33,34). SMBG is necessary for achievement of any of the treatment goals outlined previously. Frequency and timing of monitoring should be individualized to the patient's needs. During periods of acute illness, monitoring frequency should be increased to at least four to six times daily to avoid decompensation (175).

SMBG has made a tremendous impact on how diabetes is managed. Insulin doses, hypoglycemic treatments, physical activity, and general treatment behaviors are based on up-to-the-minute blood glucose results. Intensive therapy, as defined by the DCCT, with its adjustments to treatment regimens, is possible only by utilizing SMBG (56). Widely introduced in the 1980s, blood glucose monitors have become smaller, faster, more accurate, more available, more affordable, and less technique-dependent. Today, more than 30 different monitors are available for home use (176). Healthcare teams make recommendations for monitor use based on the needs of individual patients and families. There are some common features that better accommodate the needs of a pediatric population, such as small size, small blood sample requirement, and short time for results (69). Meter memory and computer download capacity are also important features. "Alternative-site" blood glucose monitors, which allow the use of alternative sites, such as the forearm, upper arm, thigh, calf, and places on the hand, are recent advances in meter technology. Patients report less pain with the use of such alternative sites. However, there have been reports of a lag in the detection of hypoglycemia when using alternative sites compared with fingertips (177). Thus, the FDA has encouraged manufacturers to recommend fingerstick as opposed to alternative-site blood glucose monitoring when hypoglycemia is suspected, in patients with hypoglycemic unawareness, or in very young children who are unable to communicate symptoms. Blood glucose monitoring strips have also been improved for easier blood sampling through capillary-action strips (176).

It is important to note that blood glucose monitoring, whether on fingertips or forearms, with new or old monitors, is about the person with diabetes. It is important to remind patients and their families that they use blood glucose monitoring to provide data and inform management, rather than to criticize diabetes control (175). The diabetes healthcare team can help remove the "blame and shame" of diabetes by reinforcing to children and their parents that blood glucose levels are not "good" or "bad" but instead are "high," "in-range," or "low"; that blood glucose is "checked" not "tested"; and that levels always vary in a person with diabetes so expect some out-of-range results (121). If patients feel blamed by their out-of-range numbers, if they think that blood glucose monitoring takes too much time, or if they do not know what to do with the information, the best and newest technology will not be of clinical value.

Another new monitoring technology involves blood ketone testing rather than traditional urine testing. Recent clinical trials have begun to evaluate the clinical utility of measuring blood ketones (β-hydroxybutyrate) with a home-based monitor (179,180). It is hoped that ongoing clinical research will determine how to use blood β-hydroxybutyrate measurements to better manage sick days, prevent metabolic decompensation, and decrease the economic and human burden of DKA (175). For additional discussion, see section on sick day rules.

Children with type 1 diabetes require monitoring for other diseases, as they are at increased risk for other autoimmune disorders. Clinical management should dictate the frequency with which thyroid function, adrenal function, and laboratory studies to assess gastrointestinal disorders such as celiac disease or inflammatory bowel disease should be monitored. Unexplained glycemic excursions or changes in growth should trigger investigation.

For additional discussions of hypoglycemia, see Chapter 40. Hyperglycemic emergencies and DKA are discussed in Chapter 53.

PREVENTION OF DIABETIC KETOACIDOSIS: SICK-DAY RULES

The cornerstones of sick-day management are (a) never omit insulin, (b) prevent dehydration and hypoglycemia, (c) monitor blood glucose frequently, (d) monitor for ketosis, (e) provide supplemental fast-acting or rapid-acting insulin doses according to guidelines, (f) treat underlying trigger(s), and (g) have frequent contact with the diabetes healthcare team to review clinical status.

Never Omit Insulin. Illness presents specific dilemmas for children and adolescents with diabetes and their families. Insulin must always be administered during illness, even if the child or adolescent is not eating. Infection induces insulin resistance, thereby often necessitating increased or supplemental doses of insulin. Generally, the usually prescribed insulin dosage is supplemented by rapid- or short-acting insulin in the form of lispro, aspart, or regular. The additional or supplemental dose is needed to manage the hyperglycemia and ketosis. The optimal supplemental dosage of insulin is calculated from the blood glucose level and the presence or absence of ketones. Ketones are detected in urine by semiquantitative measurements or with at-home blood monitors that measure β-hydroxybutyrate (3HB). Additional studies are needed to help create and refine sick-day algorithms according to blood 3HB measurements (175,180,181). In general, supplemental insulin dosages, generally 10% to 20% of the total daily insulin dosage, are based on the blood glucose level and the urinary (or blood) ketone results (see Table 42.10 and section on supplemental insulin). Supplements of lispro or aspart may need to be repeated every 2 to 3 hours while regular insulin may need to be administered every 3 to 4 hours. Finally, if the blood glucose level is low, the patient's insulin dosage may be decreased by 20%. Examples of sick-day algorithms using either urine or blood ketone results are shown in Table 42.10.

Prevent Dehydration and Hypoglycemia. Fluid intake to prevent dehydration must be encouraged. Oral hydration is preferred but may be impossible at times of nausea and vomiting. In fact, the presence of vomiting and the inability to hold down orally administered fluids may be the limiting factor for the continued home management of a sick day. If vomiting persists, the healthcare team must be called immediately. Nonetheless, attempts at oral hydration with frequent, small quantities of "clear fluids" are recommended.

The blood glucose level determines whether sugar-containing or sugar-free fluids are used. When the patient is anorexic and usual solid food intake is curtailed or absent, sugar-containing drinks such as regular soda, clear juices, flavored sugar-containing gelatin, or other glucose containing drinks are suggested to provide for usual carbohydrate intake, especially when blood glucose is under 180 to 200 mg/dL. Volumes of 3 to 8 ounces per hour or, for children, 2 mL per pound of body weight per hour or 3 L/m^2 per day should be encouraged. Fluids containing salt and potassium are helpful when gastrointestinal losses from vomiting or diarrhea occur. Fluids such as bouillon, broth, soda, and fruit juices, often in combination, are useful.

Sugar-free drinks are recommended when the patient is able to follow a usual meal plan or take in solids that provide adequate carbohydrates and calories. We suggest that families keep a "sick-day" cupboard stocked with nonperishable items such as gelatins that come as sugar-free and sugar-containing varieties. Antipyretics are important at times of fever in order to reduce any additional insensible fluid losses; in addition to antipyretics for oral use, antipyretics in suppository form are particularly useful at times of nausea and vomiting. Use of antiemetics should be individualized and usually only after consultation with the healthcare team.

Reassessment of hydration status is important to avoid decompensation. Evidence of dehydration such as weight loss, sunken eyes, or dry tongue indicates a need for prompt medical assessment.

TABLE 42.10. Supplemental Insulin Dosages

Based on blood glucose and urine ketone results

Blood glucose level	Ketones (more than a trace)	Suggested extra insulin
80–250 mg/dL	No or yes	None
250–400 mg/dL	No	10% of TDD*
	Yes	20% of TDD*
>400 mg/dL	No or yes	20% of TDD*

- *Total daily dose (TDD) is calculated by adding up all of the insulin administered on a usual day, including rapid- or fast- acting insulin and intermediate/long-acting insulin. Do not include supplements added to the usual dose. In calculating TDD when "sliding scales" are used, select the sliding-scale dose for blood glucose levels of ~150 mg/dL.
- Blood glucose and urine ketones should be monitored every 2–4 hr.
- Supplemental insulin boosters are repeated every 2–3 hr with aspart or lispro, and every 3–4 hr with regular insulin.
- If hyperglycemia and/or urine ketones do not improve after 2 supplemental doses, contact the health-care team. The healthcare team occasionally may recommend intramuscular injection of supplemental regular insulin.
- If hypoglycemia is present (glucose <80 mg/dL) with or without ketones, consider omitting aspart, lispro, or regular and decreasing intermediate/long-acting insulin by 20%; contact healthcare team, especially if patient is vomiting.

Alternative algorithms incorporating more complexity

Blood glucose level	Urine ketones		
	Negative/trace	Small	Moderate/large
<250 mg/dL	No change	0%–5%	0–10%
250–400 mg/dL	5%	10%	15–20%
>400 mg/dL	10%	15%	20%

Future algorithm incorporating results of blood β-hydroxybutyrate (3HB)[a]

Blood glucose level	Blood Ketones (3-HB)				
	0.6–0.9 mM	<1.0 mM	1.0–1.4 mM	≥1.5 mM	≥3.0 mM
<250 mg/dL	Recheck in 1–2 hr	No change	0%–5%	0%–10%	Call healthcare team immediately
250–400 mg/dL		5%	10%	15–20%	
>400 mg/dL		10%	15%	20%	

[a]Sample algorithm awaiting results of clinical trials.

Monitor Blood Glucose Frequently. Self- (or family) monitoring of blood glucose should be performed at least every 2 to 4 hours for sick-day management. More frequent monitoring is recommended if the glucose level is low. Maintaining careful records is helpful for tracking progression of illness and detecting early signs of decompensation prior to progression to frank DKA. Patients and families should be comfortable with the accuracy of their blood glucose meter by utilizing the "check strip" or control solutions periodically and insuring that their supplies are up to date.

Monitor for Ketosis. Traditionally, urine tests for ketones have been an important aspect of monitoring for sick-day management. Recommendations for urine testing for ketones have included testing at 2- to 4-hour intervals during illness, with stress, or whenever the blood glucose is consistently greater than 300 mg/dL (>16.7 mmol/L) (174). However, with the advent of blood monitors that can quantitate blood 3HB, the weaknesses inherent in urine ketone testing become apparent. Blood measurement of 3HB may be a better guide to insulin therapy in the home management of ketosis. A separate, larger issue is whether home use of the 3HB blood test can prove useful in the daily management of type 1 diabetes. Patients and medical staff must be taught how to deal with the new volume of information that they will be collecting. In cases in which both serum glucose levels and ketone levels are elevated or normal, it will be reasonably clear what is required. But what should be done when there is some degree of discordance in the findings, for example, if 3HB levels are elevated in the setting of normal or near-normal glucose values? Clearly, more studies are necessary, and perhaps guidelines for patient self-management of 3HB levels need to be created that are based on the findings of empiric studies. A recent, randomized trial comparing sick-day management using blood 3HB measurements with urine ketone testing suggests reduced need for hospitalization or emergency department assessment with blood ketone versus urine ketone testing (182).

Reinforcement of ketone testing during illness, appropriate storage of supplies, and the use of insulin algorithms based on blood glucose and ketone results are necessary. Supplies for ketone testing must be stored according to the manufacturer's recommendations and replaced at the recommended intervals. Administration of supplemental insulin and hydration are generally adequate interventions for successful treatment of ketosis. If the patient fails to clear ketones within 12 hours, the diabetes healthcare team must be contacted for assessment.

Provide Supplemental Fast-Acting or Rapid-Acting Insulin. During any intercurrent illness, the frequency of monitoring blood glucose and ketone levels should be increased to every 2 to 4 hours. When the blood glucose level is greater than 300 mg/dL on two or more consecutive occasions, patients and families should always monitor for the presence of ketones. Ketones, in general, are markers of insulin deficiency and the need for supplemental insulin (Table 42.10). However, in the setting of gastrointestinal illness with vomiting, diarrhea, increased transit time, and malabsorption, hypoglycemia may prevail in the presence or absence of ketones. Under such circumstances, especially when the blood glucose level is less than 80 mg/dL in the setting of positive ketones, increasing fluid intake with the provision of 10 to15 g of carbohydrates should be encouraged until the blood glucose level increases. Recommendations include the continued administration of fluid until the ketones clear.

Supplemental doses of rapid-acting (lispro or aspart) or fast-acting (regular) insulin should be administered in addition to usual insulin dosages whenever hyperglycemia and ketosis are present. The degree of hyperglycemia and the presence or absence of ketones determines the amount of supplemental insulin. Dosages of supplemental insulin are generally calculated according to weight (0.1–0.3 U/kg), as a percentage of total daily insulin dosage (usually between 10% and 20% of the total daily insulin requirement in the baseline state), or according to team-derived algorithms (Table 42.10) (60). Special algorithms may be required for patients treated with CSII (59). Multidisciplinary team involvement can help to individualize the approach, as particular needs vary according to the patient's insulin sensitivity, the severity and duration of the illness, and the presence of anorexia. If blood glucose levels remain elevated, with or without positive ketones, additional supplemental doses of regular insulin may be needed every 3 to 4 hours. If lispro or aspart insulin is given as the supplemental insulin, dosages may need to be repeated at 2- to 3-hour intervals. Patients (or family members) should continue to monitor blood glucose and urinary or blood ketones every 2 to 4 hours and keep careful records.

Treat Underlying Triggers. Any acute infectious process needs to be evaluated and treated accordingly. Intercurrent viral illnesses, not requiring any specific prescriptive therapy, may still produce elevated glucose levels and ketosis and require sick-day management. Symptomatic treatment with antipyretics and analgesics is beneficial. Patients with a history of recurrent DKA, with known eating disorders or psychosocial problems, and with poor glycemic control are at risk for decompensation and should be advised to call their healthcare team at the earliest symptoms and signs of illness or decompensation (101,183). It is advisable that patients always have access to a phone and transportation for follow-up care.

Frequent Contact with the Medical Team. Patients and family members should be advised to look out for signs that medical attention is needed. These include vomiting that continues for more than 2 to 4 hours; blood glucose levels that exceed 300 mg/dL or persistence of ketones for more than 12 hours; signs of dehydration such as dry mouth, cracked lips, sunken eyes, weight loss, or dry skin; or symptoms that DKA may be developing, such as nausea, abdominal or chest pain, vomiting, ketotic breath, hyperventilation, or altered consciousness. The latter suggests the need for immediate medical attention. If recognized early, milder forms of DKA can be treated in the ambulatory setting, obviating the need for hospitalization (184).

Illness and stress are common. For the child or adolescent with type 1 diabetes, these can be triggers for counterregulation and subsequent metabolic deterioration if no attention is paid to diabetes management tasks. Sick-day management requires increased monitoring of blood glucose and assessment for ketosis. Extensive experience has shown that by assiduously following the guidelines outlined in this protocol, families can successfully manage most intercurrent illnesses in children at home without recourse to a hospital emergency department.

BEHAVIORAL ISSUES

Diabetes care should include careful attention to the educational, developmental, and behavioral issues of childhood and adolescence. (See Chapter 37 for additional discussion.) Since diabetes treatment and self-management training for the child, adolescent, and family with diabetes is time-intensive, copious in content, and evolves over the course of childhood, adolescence, and into adulthood, a team of diverse health providers best accomplishes the goal of optimal diabetes management. This, too, is the position of the ADA's Standards of Medical Care, which calls for a multidisciplinary team approach to the care of the child or adolescent with diabetes (55).

Treatment of diabetes with training in self-management needs to address the overall issues of child and adolescent growth, development, temperament, and behavior, as well as the issues of the natural course of diabetes itself—diagnosis, adaptation, ongoing disease progression, and potential complications. What distinguishes diabetes from many other chronic diseases of childhood are the incessant demands made on patients and families for self-management and the clinical decision-making responsibilities given to parents almost immediately after diagnosis (185). To meet these demands, families need to make adjustments in their lifestyle. The role of the diabetes healthcare team is to help the child or adolescent and his or her family learn, practice, and revise diabetes self-management skills to succeed in balancing the complicated requirements of insulin injection/infusion, meal planning, and physical activity, using the information from frequent blood glucose monitoring. The development of the treatment plan is based on the commonalities of childhood and adolescence and the individualization that takes into account family factors, age, developmental stage, and issues of temperament. As is clear from the preceding discussions in this chapter, diabetes self-management affects many components of family life—eating, physical activity, finances, and time management. One main goal of the diabetes healthcare team is to prevent, predict, or manage behavioral and family complications that arise in response to the pediatric diabetes.

The Psychosocial Therapies Working Group reports that children and adolescents with type 1 or type 2 diabetes face unique demands in dealing with diabetes both because of the nature of their being children and adolescents and because of the chronicity of the disease. The psychosocial challenges include an increased risk for psychiatric disorders, including depression, adjustment and adaptation problems, and eating disorders. All of these disorders can result in poor metabolic control (89). A variety of psychosocial interventions have been shown to be effective in improving metabolic outcomes. As noted previously, this is evident from the outcomes from pediatric behavioral studies and clinical programs carried out at the Joslin Diabetes Center.

Behavioral Risk Factors: Uncontrolled Diabetes and Family Studies

Coping with the unrelenting demands of this chronic incurable disease, for which treatment is complex, difficult, and impacts on the lifestyles of the patient and his or her family, is stressful. It is not surprising, therefore, that emotional difficulties are common. Consequently, an important goal of therapy is the prevention and the identification and treatment of emotional problems and the provision of continuous psychosocial support and encouragement to patients and their families. Despite the previous general description of the goals of therapy, it is critically important to tailor the goals of treatment to the capabilities of the individual patient and family.

Various diabetes treatment tools can significantly help manage and improve glycemic control (186,187). In particular, blood glucose monitoring is central to the successful management of diabetes (65,101,188). However, data suggest that only about 60% of patients with type 1 diabetes routinely perform blood glucose monitoring (189). In a series of studies in the Pediatric and Adolescent Unit at the Joslin Diabetes Center, we have systematically investigated behavioral and family factors that optimize glycemic control and adherence to blood glucose monitoring and other diabetes management tasks in children and adolescents with type 1 diabetes (65–67,101,189a). In summary, frequent blood glucose monitoring is related to better glycemic control; increased family involvement improves adherence to diabetes management tasks; and diabetes-specific family conflict, commonly related to food issues and blood glucose monitoring, hinders control.

Frequent Blood Glucose Monitoring Predicts Better Glycemic Control. In a cohort of young adolescents 10 to 15 years old with type 1 diabetes, the frequency of blood glucose monitoring was significantly associated with HbA_{1c} values, after controlling for gender, duration of diabetes, and pubertal development (Fig. 42.5). This significant association was recently confirmed in a study of 300 youth 7 to 16 years of age with type 1 diabetes at the Joslin Diabetes Center (101).

Parent Involvement in Diabetes Management Tasks Is Related to Increased Monitoring. Parent-adolescent teamwork supports increased adherence to blood glucose monitoring and does not increase family conflict (65). Previous studies have revealed that adherence to diabetes management tasks decreases over the early adolescent years (66,67). This coincides with the predictable decrease in parent involvement during adolescence (64–66). We developed a low-intensity, office-based intervention for 10 to 15 year olds and their parents aimed at maintaining parent involvement in diabetes management tasks over the early adolescent years without the triggering of increased diabetes-related family conflict. This trial demonstrated sustained involvement, diminished family conflict, and better glycemic control. The intervention focused on new ways of communicating about blood glucose monitoring in families that avoided "shame and blame" and promoted realistic parental expectations for blood glucose levels in growing and developing adolescents (65,66).

Realistic Expectations and Blood Glucose Monitoring. We have developed materials focused on blood glucose monitoring for patients of all ages and their family members (121). The *Blood Glucose Monitoring Owners Manual* reviews the importance of monitoring, provides realistic expectations of blood glucose levels for patients and their families, and reinforces the increased flexibility in lifestyle that is possible with increased monitoring. This manual provides a new vocabulary around monitoring that includes the need to *check* (not test) blood glucose and that glucose levels can be *high* or *low* (not bad or good). In a study of 200 at-risk adults with baseline HbA_{1c} 8% or higher, use of this educational tool was significantly associated with more monitoring ($P < .05$) and less-negative attitudes ($P < .05$) (190).

Blood glucose results appear to trigger both negative and positive responses within families. We uncovered from surveys administered to youths ages 8 to 16 years multiple sources of conflict within families around diabetes management tasks. More than half the respondents endorsed conflict around blood glucose monitoring, insulin, and food issues (67) (Fig. 42.6). Decreased conflict within families was associated with increased frequency of blood glucose monitoring. Thus, education focused on positive communication within families around blood glucose results is important and will likely play a critical role with the introduction of the new technologies for frequent or near-continuous monitoring.

Intensive Insulin Therapy and Blood Glucose Monitoring. Our recent experience with insulin pump therapy (CSII) in youth with type 1 diabetes, the fastest-growing group of new pump users, confirms the importance of blood glucose monitoring for

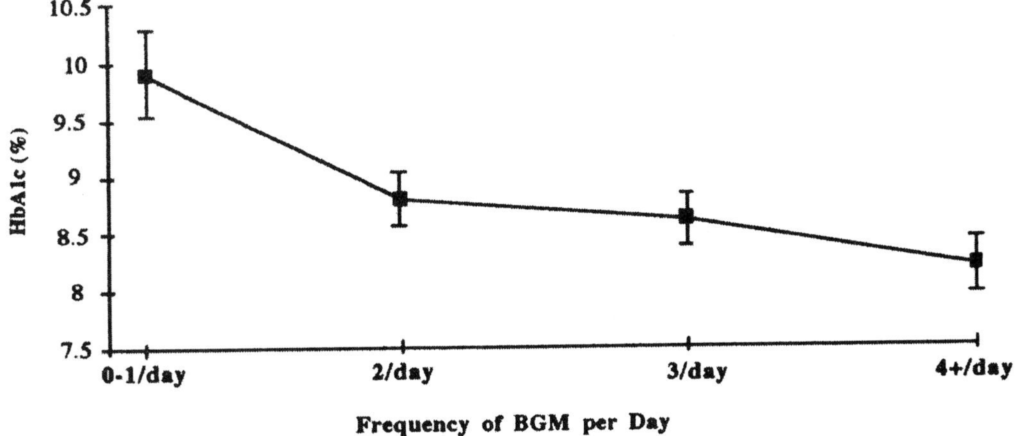

FIG. 42.5. Relationship of frequency of blood glucose monitoring (BGM) and glycemic control (HbA_{1c}) in young adolescents 10 to 15 years old at the Joslin Diabetes Center. (Reprinted from Anderson BJ, Ho J, Brackett J, et al. Parental involvement in diabetes management tasks: relationships to blood glucose monitoring adherence and metabolic control in young adolescents with insulin-dependent diabetes mellitus. *J Pediatr* 1997;130:257–265, copyright 1997 with permission from Elsevier.)

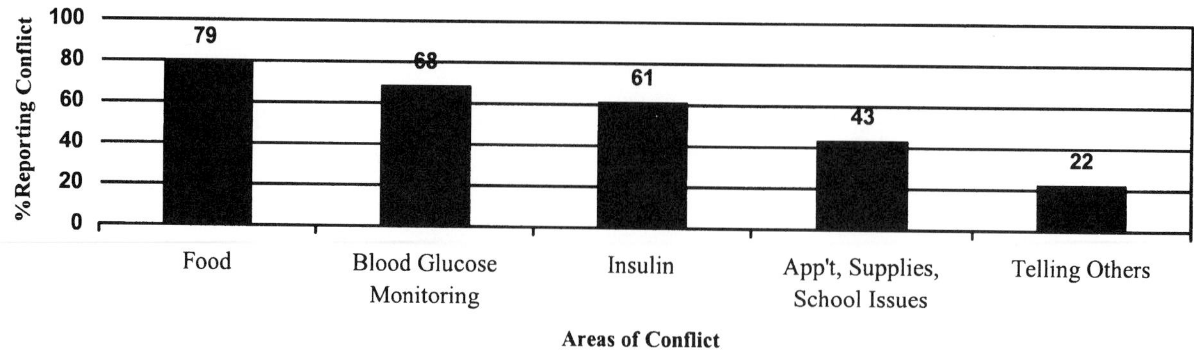

FIG. 42.6. Areas of family conflict reported by youth with type 1 diabetes (personal data).

sustained improvement in glycemic control (191). Evaluation of 109 patients undergoing CSII showed improvement in HbA_{1c} results of about 1% after the first 3 months of pump use (192) (Fig. 42.7). This improvement was associated with a significant increase in blood glucose monitoring, from 3.7 times a day at baseline to 6.1 times a day at 3 months. After 9 months of pump use, there was a decrease in the frequency of monitoring to 4.3 times a day. The decrease in monitoring was associated with a significant increase in HbA_{1c}. Thus, successful pump therapy requires sustained monitoring. With increasing numbers of pediatric patients beginning CSII, there is a need to incorporate family teamwork programs aimed at increasing and sustaining adherence to blood glucose monitoring with pump use (192).

DIABETES IN THE SCHOOL AND DAY-CARE SETTING

Children and adolescents with diabetes are not unlike their peers without diabetes—they spend the majority of their waking hours in school. Because of the need for optimal glycemic control for youth with diabetes, the tasks of diabetes self-management become a necessary part of the school day. The successful integration of diabetes management into the school setting is built on a foundation of good communication between the parent(s), child, school, and healthcare team. Knowledge, understanding, and skill building are necessary for the successful management of diabetes at school.

Laws protect the rights of children with diabetes in the United States, particularly Section 504 of the Rehabilitation Act of 1973, the Individuals with Disabilities Act of 1991, and the Americans with Disabilities Act—ensuring safe and full participation in all school activities. Because diabetes is classified in these laws as a disability, it is illegal to discriminate against a child or adolescent because of diabetes. These laws ensure that the child or adolescent with diabetes is able to monitor blood glucose, inject insulin, follow a meal plan, and participate in physical activities at school, both during the school day and during after-school extracurricular activities. Although children with diabetes are at risk for discrimination at school, great efforts have been made to ensure appropriate care and accommodation in the least restricted environment possible. To this end, the ADA has developed a position statement, "Care of Children With Diabetes in the School and Day Care Setting" (58).

The goal of the position statement is to provide direction for the care of children and adolescents during school. An individ-

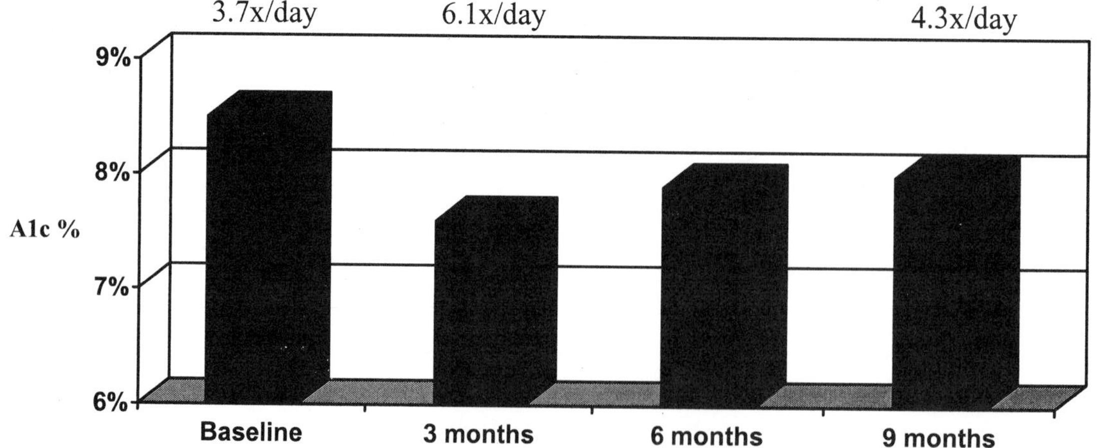

FIG. 42.7. Relationship of frequency of blood glucose monitoring and glycemic control (HbA_{1c}) after the initiation of insulin pump therapy (CSII) in 109 youth with type 1 diabetes. (From Laffel L, Loughlin C, Ramchandani N, et al. Glycemic challenges of pump therapy (CSII) in youth with type 1 diabetes (T1DM). *Diabetes* 2001;50:A66–A67(abst).

ualized care plan provides the framework for addressing the needs of the child with diabetes in a school or day-care environment and states needs, responsibilities, and expectations of the school, the parents, and the child or adolescent during the school day and during school-related extracurricular activities. The development of an individualized diabetes healthcare plan should provide information on the needs of the child or adolescent with diabetes and instructions for blood glucose monitoring, meals and snacks, symptoms and treatment of hypoglycemia, administration of glucagon, symptoms and treatment of hyperglycemia, measurement of ketones, and sick-day rules (58).

School personnel, parents, the diabetes healthcare team, and the child or adolescent with diabetes all have the same goal: to have a healthy, happy student. Through accommodation and support of diabetes self-management tasks at school, the student with diabetes will be afforded the opportunity to safely succeed in diabetes management, academics, and development of evolving social skills.

In summary, pediatric behavioral studies and clinical programs have consistently documented the challenges of achieving optimal metabolic control in youth with diabetes. While new technologies provide hope to our patients and their families, they also increase the burdens placed upon them to achieve a new pattern of normalcy while integrating the rigors of diabetes management into their daily lives. To this end, support from a multidisciplinary diabetes team is important.

REFERENCES

1. Rosenecker J, Eichler I, Barmeier H, et al. Diabetes mellitus and cystic fibrosis: comparison of clinical parameters in patients treated with insulin versus oral glucose-lowering agents. *Pediatr Pulmonol* 2001;32:351–355.
2. Hardin DS, Moran A. Diabetes mellitus in cystic fibrosis. *Endocrinol Metab Clin North Am* 1999;28:787–800.
3. Allen HF, Gay EC, Klingensmith GJ, et al. Identification and treatment of cystic fibrosis-related diabetes. A survey of current medical practice in the U.S. *Diabetes Care* 1998;21:943–948.
4. Cotellessa M, Minicucci L, Diana MC, et al. Phenotype/genotype correlation and cystic fibrosis related diabetes mellitus (Italian Multicenter Study). *J Pediatr Endocrinol Metab* 2000;13:1087–1093.
5. Holl RW, Buck C, Cario H, et al. Diagnosis of diabetes in cystic fibrosis and thalassemia major. *Diabetes Care* 1998;21:671–672.
6. LaPorte RE, Matsushima M, Chang Y. Prevalence and incidence of insulin-dependent diabetes. In: National Diabetes Data Group. *Diabetes in America.* 2nd ed. Bethesda, MD. National Institute of Diabetes and Digestive and Kidney Diseases, 1995:37–46. NIDDK publication 95-1468.
7. American Diabetes Association. Diabetes statistics. In: Raynor J, ed. *Diabetes 2001. Vital statistics.* Alexandria, VA, American Diabetes Association; 2001: 13–27.
8. Karvonen M, Pitkaniemi M, Pitkaniemi J, et al. Sex difference in the incidence of insulin-dependent diabetes mellitus: an analysis of the recent epidemiological data. World Health Organization DIAMOND Project Group. *Diabetes Metab Rev* 1997;13:275–291.
9. Onkamo P, Vaananen S, Karvonen M, et al. Worldwide increase in incidence of type I diabetes—the analysis of the data on published incidence trends. *Diabetologia* 1999;42:1395–1403.
10. Type 2 diabetes in children and adolescents. American Diabetes Association. *Diabetes Care* 2000;23:381–389.
11. Rosenbloom AL, Joe JR, Young RS, et al. Emerging epidemic of type 2 diabetes in youth. *Diabetes Care* 1999;22:345–354.
12. Fagot-Campagna A. Emergence of type 2 diabetes mellitus in children: epidemiological evidence. *J Pediatr Endocrinol Metab* 2000;13[suppl 6]:1395–1402.
13. Fagot-Campagna A, Pettitt DJ, Engelgau MM, et al. Type 2 diabetes among North American children and adolescents: an epidemiologic review and a public health perspective. *J Pediatr* 2000;136:664–672.
14. Karjalainen J, Martin JM, Knip M, et al. A bovine albumin peptide as a possible trigger of insulin-dependent diabetes mellitus. *N Engl J Med* 1992;327: 302–307.
15. Karjalainen J, Saukkonen T, Savilahti E, et al. Disease-associated anti-bovine serum albumin antibodies in type 1 (insulin-dependent) diabetes mellitus are detected by particle concentration fluoroimmunoassay, and not by enzyme linked immunoassay. *Diabetologia* 1992;35:985–990.
16. Vahasalo P, Petays T, Knip M, et al. Relation between antibodies to islet cell antigens, other autoantigens and cow's milk proteins in diabetic children and unaffected siblings at the clinical manifestation of IDDM. The Childhood Diabetes in Finland Study Group. *Autoimmunity* 1996;23:165–174.
17. Gerstein HC. Cow's milk exposure and type 1 diabetes mellitus. A critical overview of the clinical literature. *Diabetes Care* 1994;17:13–19.
18. Laron Z. Lessons from recent epidemiological studies in type 1 childhood diabetes. *J Pediatr Endocrinol Metab* 1999;12[Suppl 3]:733–736.
19. Kraine MR, Tisch RM. The role of environmental factors in insulin-dependent diabetes mellitus: an unresolved issue. *Environ Health Perspect* 1999;107 [suppl 5]:777–781.
20. Report of the Expert Committee on the Diagnosis and Classification of Diabetes Mellitus. *Diabetes Care* 2003;26[Suppl]:S5–S20.
21. Atkinson MA, Kaufman DL, Newman D, et al. Islet cell cytoplasmic autoantibody reactivity to glutamate decarboxylase in insulin-dependent diabetes. *J Clin Invest* 1993;91:350–356.
22. Atkinson MA, Maclaren NK, Riley WJ, et al. Are insulin autoantibodies markers for insulin-dependent diabetes mellitus? *Diabetes* 1986;35:894–898.
23. Atkinson M, Leslie DR. Inverse relation between humoral and cellular immunity to glutamic acid decarboxylase in subjects at risk of insulin-dependent diabetes. *J Endocrinol Invest* 1994;17:581–584.
24. Atkinson MA, Maclaren NK. The pathogenesis of insulin-dependent diabetes mellitus. *N Engl J Med* 1994;331:1428–1436.
25. Atkinson MA, Eisenbarth GS. Type 1 diabetes: new perspectives on disease pathogenesis and treatment. *Lancet* 2001;358:221–229.
26. Kaufman DL, Erlander MG, Clare-Salzler M, et al. Autoimmunity to two forms of glutamate decarboxylase in insulin-dependent diabetes mellitus. *J Clin Invest* 1992;89:283–292.
27. Leslie RD, Atkinson MA, Notkins AL. Autoantigens IA-2 and GAD in type I (insulin-dependent) diabetes. *Diabetologia* 1999;42:3–14.
28. Schott M, Schatz D, Atkinson M, et al. GAD65 autoantibodies increase the predictability but not the sensitivity of islet cell and insulin autoantibodies for developing insulin dependent diabetes mellitus. *J Autoimmun* 1994;7: 865–872.
29. Huang W, Connor E, Rosa TD, et al. Although DR3-DQB1*0201 may be associated with multiple component diseases of the autoimmune polyglandular syndromes, the human leukocyte antigen DR4-DQB1*0302 haplotype is implicated only in beta-cell autoimmunity. *J Clin Endocrinol Metab* 1996;81: 2559–2563.
30. Zimmet PZ, Tuomi T, Mackay IR, et al. Latent autoimmune diabetes mellitus in adults (LADA): the role of antibodies to glutamic acid decarboxylase in diagnosis and prediction of insulin dependency. *Diabet Med* 1994;11:299–303.
31. Deschamps I, Beressi JP, Khalil I, et al. The role of genetic predisposition to type I (insulin-dependent) diabetes mellitus. *Ann Med* 1991;23:427–435.
32. Lazarus A, ed. *Diabetes in the XX1 century, part II: Autoimmunity and beta-cell destruction.* Pawling, NY: Caduceus Medical Publishers; 1994:3–5
33. *Diabetes education goals.* Alexandria, VA: American Diabetes Association, 2002.
34. Mensing C, Boucher J, Cypress M, et al. National standards for diabetes self-management education. Task Force to Review and Revise the National Standards for Diabetes Self-Management Education Programs. *Diabetes Care* 2000;23:682–689.
35. Etzwiler DD. Education of the patient with diabetes. *Med Clin North Am* 1978; 62:857–866.
36. Strauss RS, Pollack HA. Epidemic increase in childhood overweight, 1986-1998. *JAMA* 2001;286:2845–2848.
37. Sinha R, Fisch G, Teague B, et al. Prevalence of impaired glucose tolerance among children and adolescents with marked obesity. *N Engl J Med* 2002;346: 802–810.
38. Physical activity and health: a report of the Surgeon General. S/N 017-023-00196-5. Atlanta, GA: US Department of Health and Human Services, 1996.
39. Young TK, Dean HJ, Flett B, et al. Childhood obesity in a population at high risk for type 2 diabetes. *J Pediatr* 2000;136:365–369.
40. Savage PJ, Bennett PH, Senter RG, et al. High prevalence of diabetes in young Pima Indians: evidence of phenotypic variation in a genetically isolated population. *Diabetes* 1979;28:937–942.
41. Harris SB, Perkins BA, Whalen-Brough E. Non-insulin-dependent diabetes mellitus among First Nations children. New entity among First Nations people of northwestern Ontario. *Can Fam Physician* 1996;42:869–876.
42. Dean HJ, Mundy RL, Moffatt M. Non-insulin-dependent diabetes mellitus in Indian children in Manitoba. *Can Med Assoc J* 1992;147:52–57.
43. Kitagawa T, Owada M, Urakami T, et al. Epidemiology of type 1 (insulin-dependent) and type 2 (non-insulin-dependent) diabetes mellitus in Japanese children. *Diabetes Res Clin Pract* 1994;24[suppl]:S7–S13.
44. Kitagawa T, Owada M, Urakami T, et al. Increased incidence of non-insulin dependent diabetes mellitus among Japanese schoolchildren correlates with an increased intake of animal protein and fat. *Clin Pediatr (Phila)* 1998;37: 111–115.
45. Pinhas-Hamiel O, Dolan LM, Daniels SR, et al. Increased incidence of non-insulin-dependent diabetes mellitus among adolescents. *J Pediatr* 1996;28: 608–615.
46. Freemark M, Bursey D. The effects of metformin on body mass index and glucose tolerance in obese adolescents with fasting hyperinsulinemia and a family history of type 2 diabetes. *Pediatrics* 2000;107:E55.
47. Young-Hyman D, Schlundt DG, Herman L, et al. Evaluation of the insulin resistance syndrome in 5- to 10-year-old overweight/obese African-American children. *Diabetes Care* 2001;24:1359–1364.
48. Pinhas-Hamiel O, Standiford D, Hamiel D, et al. The type 2 family: a setting for development and treatment of adolescent type 2 diabetes mellitus. *Arch Pediatr Adolesc Med* 1999;153:1063–1067.

49. Jones KL, Arslanian S, Peterokova VA, et al. Effect of metformin in pediatric patients with type 2 diabetes: a randomized controlled trial. *Diabetes Care* 2002;25:89–94.
50. Jones KL. Non-insulin dependent diabetes in children and adolescents: the therapeutic challenge. *Clin Pediatr (Phil)* 1998;37:103–110.
51. Thomas H, Jaschkowitz K, Bulman M, et al. A distant upstream promoter of the HNF-4alpha gene connects the transcription factors involved in maturity-onset diabetes of the young. *Hum Mol Genet* 2001;10:2089–2097.
52. Doria A, Plengvidhya N. Recent advances in the genetics of maturity-onset diabetes of the young and other forms of autosomal dominant diabetes. *Curr Opin Endocrinol Diabetes* 2000;7:203–210.
53. Doria A, Yang Y, Malecki M, et al. Phenotypic characteristics of early-onset autosomal-dominant type 2 diabetes unlinked to known maturity-onset diabetes of the young (MODY) genes. *Diabetes Care* 1999;22:253–261.
54. Tattersall R. Maturity-onset diabetes of the young: a clinical history. *Diabet Med* 1998;15:11–14.
55. Standards of medical care for patients with diabetes mellitus. *Diabetes Care* 2002;25[suppl]:S33–S49.
56. DCCT Research Group. The effect of intensive treatment of diabetes on the development and progression of long-term complications in insulin-dependent diabetes mellitus. *N Engl J Med* 1993;329:977–986.
57. Drash AL. The child, the adolescent, and the Diabetes Control and Complications Trial. *Diabetes Care* 1993;16:1515–1516.
58. Care of children with diabetes in the school and day care setting. *Diabetes Care* 2002;25[suppl]:S122–S125.
59. Farkas-Hirsch R, ed. *Intensive diabetes management*. Alexandria, VA: American Diabetes Association, 2001.
60. Skyler JS, ed. *Medical management of type 1 diabetes*. Alexandria, VA: American Diabetes Association, 1998.
61. Grey M, Kanner S, Lacey KO. Characteristics of the learner: children and adolescents. *Diabetes Edu* 1999;25:25–33.
62. Ingersoll GM, Orr DP, Herrold AJ, et al. Cognitive maturity and self-management among adolescents with insulin-dependent diabetes mellitus. *J Pediatr* 1986;108:620–623.
63. Wysocki T, Taylor A, Hough BS, et al. Deviation from developmentally appropriate self-care autonomy. Association with diabetes outcomes. *Diabetes Care* 1996;19:119–125.
64. Anderson BJ, Auslander WF, Jung KC, et al. Assessing family sharing of diabetes responsibilities. *J Pediatr Psychol* 1990;15:477–492.
65. Anderson BJ, Brackett J, Ho J, et al. An office-based intervention to maintain parent-adolescent teamwork in diabetes management. Impact on parent involvement, family conflict, and subsequent glycemic control. *Diabetes Care* 1999;22:713–721.
66. Anderson BJ, Ho J, Brackett J, et al. Parental involvement in diabetes management tasks: relationships to blood glucose monitoring adherence and metabolic control in young adolescents with insulin-dependent diabetes mellitus. *J Pediatr* 1997;130:257–265.
67. Anderson BJ, Vangsness L, Connell A, et al. Family conflict, adherence, and glycemic control in youth with short duration type 1 diabetes (T1DM). *Diabet Med* 2002;50:635–642.
68. Resnick MD, Bearman PS, Blum RW, et al. Protecting adolescents from harm. Findings from the National Longitudinal Study on Adolescent Health. *JAMA* 1997;278:823–832.
69. Lawlor M, Laffel L, Anderson B, et al. *Caring for young children living with diabetes: professional manual*. Boston, MA: Joslin Diabetes Center, 1996.
70. Anderson BJ, Loughlin C, Goldberg E, et al. Comprehensive, family-focused outpatient care for very young children living with chronic disease: lessons from a program in pediatric diabetes. *Child Serv Soc Policy Res Pract* 2001;4: 235–250.
71. Laffel L, Brackett J, Ho J, et al. Changing the process of diabetes care improves metabolic outcomes and reduces hospitalizations. *Qual Manag Health Care* 1998;6:53–62.
72. Rapaport R, Sills IN. Implications of the DCCT for children and adolescents with IDDM. *N J Med* 1994;91:227–228.
73. Rovet JF, Ehrlich RM, Hoppe M. Specific intellectual deficits in children with early onset diabetes mellitus *Child Dev* 1988;59:226–234.
74. Austin EJ, Deary IJ. Effects of repeated hypoglycemia on cognitive function: a psychometrically validated reanalysis of the Diabetes Control and Complications Trial data. *Diabetes Care* 1999;22:1273–1277.
75. Bjorgaas M, Gimse R, Vik T, et al. Cognitive function in type 1 diabetic children with and without episodes of severe hypoglycaemia. *Acta Paediatr* 1997; 86:148–153.
76. Deary IJ, Frier BM. Severe hypoglycaemia and cognitive impairment in diabetes. *BMJ* 1996;313:767–768.
77. Gold AE, Deary IJ, Frier BM. Hypoglycemia and cognitive function. *Diabetes Care* 1993;16:958–959.
78. Kaufman FR, Epport K, Engilman R, et al. Neurocognitive functioning in children diagnosed with diabetes before age 10 years. *J Diabetes Complications* 1999;13:31–38.
79. Matyka KA, Wigg L, Pramming S, et al. Cognitive function and mood after profound nocturnal hypoglycaemia in prepubertal children with conventional insulin treatment for diabetes. *Arch Dis Child* 1999;81:138–142.
80. Strachan MW, Deary IJ, Ewing FM, et al. Recovery of cognitive function and mood after severe hypoglycaemia in adults with insulin-treated diabetes. *Diabetes Care* 2000;23:305–312.
81. Ack M, Miller I, Weil W. Intelligence of children with diabetes mellitus. *Pediatrics* 1961;28:764–770.
82. Ryan C, Vega A, Drash A. Cognitive deficits in adolescents who developed diabetes early in life. *Pediatrics* 1985;75:921–927.
83. Holmes CS, Richman LC. Cognitive profiles of children with insulin-dependent diabetes. *J Dev Behav Pediatr* 1985;6:323–326.
84. Rovet JF, Ehrlich RM, Hoppe M. Intellectual deficits associated with early onset of insulin-dependent diabetes mellitus in children. *Diabetes Care* 1987; 10:510–515.
85. Golden MP, Russell BP, Ingersoll GM, et al. Management of diabetes mellitus in children younger than 5 years of age. *Am J Dis Child* 1985;139:448–452.
86. Grunt JA, Banion CM, Ling L, et al. Problems in the care of the infant diabetic patient. *Clin Pediatr (Phila)* 1978;17:772–774.
87. Ternand C, Go VL, Gerich JE, et al. Endocrine pancreatic response of children with onset of insulin-requiring diabetes before age 3 and after age 5. *J Pediatr* 1982;101:36–39.
88. McCarthy AM, Lindgren S, Mengeling MA, et al. Effects of diabetes on learning in children. *Pediatrics* 2002;109:E9.
89. Delamater AM, Jacobson AM, Anderson B, et al. Psychosocial therapies in diabetes: report of the Psychosocial Therapies Working Group. *Diabetes Care* 2001;24:1286–1292.
90. Northam EA, Anderson PJ, Jacobs R, et al. Neuropsychological profiles of children with type 1 diabetes 6 years after disease onset. *Diabetes Care* 2001; 24:1541–1546.
91. Holl RW, Lang GE, Grabert M, et al. Diabetic retinopathy in pediatric patients with type-1 diabetes: effect of diabetes duration, prepubertal and pubertal onset of diabetes, and metabolic control. *J Pediatr* 1998;132:790–794.
92. Schoenle EJ, Schoenle D, Molinari L, et al. Impaired intellectual development in children with type I diabetes: association with HbA1c, age at diagnosis and sex. *Diabetologia* 2002;45:108–114.
93. Clarke WL, Gonder-Frederick A, et al. Maternal fear of hypoglycemia in their children with insulin dependent diabetes mellitus. *J Pediatr Endocrinol Metab* 1998;11[Suppl 1]:189–194.
94. Marrero DG, Guare JC, Vandagriff JL, et al. Fear of hypoglycemia in the parents of children and adolescents with diabetes: maladaptive or healthy response? *Diabetes Educ* 1997;23:281–286.
95. Green LB, Wysocki T, Reineck BM. Fear of hypoglycemia in children and adolescents with diabetes. *J Pediatr Psychol* 1990;15:633–641.
96. Powers SW, Byars KC, Mitchell MJ, et al. Parent report of mealtime behavior and parenting stress in young children with type 1 diabetes and in healthy control subjects. *Diabetes Care* 2002;25:313–318.
97. Mortensen HB, Vestermark S, Kastrup KW. Metabolic control in children with insulin dependent diabetes mellitus assessed by hemoglobin A1c. *Acta Paediatr Scand* 1982;71:217–222.
98. Dahlquist G, Rudberg S. The prevalence of microalbuminuria in diabetic children and adolescents and its relation to puberty. *Acta Paediatr Scand* 1987;76:795–800.
99. Chase HP, Jackson WE, Hoops SL, et al. Glucose control and the renal and retinal complications of insulin-dependent diabetes. *JAMA* 1989;261: 1155–1160.
100. Holl RW, Lang GE, Grabert M, et al. Diabetic retinopathy in pediatric patients with type-1 diabetes: effect of diabetes duration, prepubertal and pubertal onset of diabetes, and metabolic control. *J Pediatr* 1998;132:790–794.
101. Levine BS, Anderson BJ, Butler DA, et al. Predictors of glycemic control and short-term adverse outcomes in youth with type 1 diabetes. *J Pediatr* 2001; 139:197–203.
102. Jacobson AM, Hauser ST, Lavori P, et al. Family environment and glycemic control: a four-year prospective study of children and adolescents with insulin-dependent diabetes mellitus. *Psychosom Med* 1994;56:401–406.
103. Palta M, Shen G, Allen C, et al. Longitudinal patterns of glycemic control and diabetes care from diagnosis in a population-based cohort with type 1 diabetes. The Wisconsin Diabetes Registry. *Am J Epidemiol* 1996;144:954–961.
104. Tubiana-Rufi N, Moret L, Czernichow P, et al. Risk factors for poor glycemic control in diabetic children in France. *Diabetes Care* 1995;18:1479–1482.
105. Rosilio M, Cotton JB, Wieliczko MC, et al. Factors associated with glycemic control. A cross-sectional nationwide study in 2,579 French children with type 1 diabetes. The French Pediatric Diabetes Group. *Diabetes Care* 1998;21: 1146–1153.
106. Mortensen HB, Hougaard P. Comparison of metabolic control in a cross-sectional study of 2,873 children and adolescents with IDDM from 18 countries. The Hvidore Study Group on Childhood Diabetes. *Diabetes Care* 1997;20: 714–720.
107. Dorchy H, Roggemans MP, Willems P. [Glycosylated hemoglobin in diabetic children 18 years old enrolled in the INAMI study for the purpose of self-monitoring of glucose at home]. *Acta Clin Belg* 1997;52:405–406.
108. Nordfeldt S, Ludvigsson J. Severe hypoglycemia in children with IDDM. A prospective population study, 1992–1994. *Diabetes Care* 1997;20:497–503.
109. Vanelli M, Chiarelli F, Chiari G, et al. Metabolic control in children and adolescents with diabetes: experience of two Italian regional centers. *J Pediatr Endocrinol Metab* 1999;12:403–409.
110. Factors influencing glycemic control in young people with type 1 diabetes in Scotland: a population-based study (DIABAUD2). *Diabetes Care* 2001;24: 239–244.
111. Danne T, Mortensen HB, Hougaard P, et al. Persistent differences among centers over 3 years in glycemic control and hypoglycemia in a study of 3,805

children and adolescents with type 1 diabetes from the Hvidore Study Group. *Diabetes Care* 2001;24:1342–1347.
112. DCCT Research Group. Effect of intensive diabetes treatment on the development of long-term complications in adolescents with insulin-dependent diabetes mellitus. *J Pediatr* 1994;125:177–188.
113. White NH, Cleary PA, Dahms W, et al. Beneficial effects of intensive therapy of diabetes during adolescence: outcomes after the conclusion of the Diabetes Control and Complications Trial (DCCT). *J Pediatr* 2001;139:804–812.
114. The Diabetes Control and Complications Trial/Epidemiology of Diabetes Interventions and Complications Research Group. Retinopathy and nephropathy in patients with type 1 diabetes four years after a trial of intensive therapy. *N Engl J Med* 2000;342:381–389.
115. DCCT/EDIC Research Group. Effect of intensive therapy on the microvascular complications of type 1 diabetes mellitus. *JAMA* 2002;287:2563–2569.
116. Amiel SA, Sherwin RS, Simonson DC, et al. Impaired insulin action in puberty. A contributing factor to poor glycemic control in adolescents with diabetes. *N Engl J Med* 1986;315:215–219.
117. Krolewski AS, Warram JH, Christlieb AR, et al. The changing natural history of nephropathy in type 1 diabetes. *Am J Med* 1985;78:755–798.
118. Jacobson AM, Hauser ST, Willett J, et al. Consequences of irregular versus continuous medical follow-up in children and adolescents with insulin-dependent diabetes mellitus. *J Pediatr* 1997;131:727–733.
119. Anderson BJ, Miller JP, Auslander WF, et al. Family characteristics of diabetic adolescents: relationship to metabolic control. *Diabetes Care* 1981;4:586–594.
120. Johnson PD, White NH, Anderson BJ, et al. *Teenagers with insulin dependent diabetes: a curriculum for adolescents, families, and health professionals.* Ann Arbor, MI: Michigan Diabetes Research and Training Center, University of Michigan; 1992.
121. Lawlor MT, Laffel L, Anderson BJ. *Blood sugar monitoring owner's manual.* Boston: Joslin Diabetes Center, 1997.
122. American Diabetes Association. Health Care Products. Diabetes Forecast. Available at: http:www//diabetes.org/main/community/forecast/jan_2002_insulin.jsp#relativeinsulins.
123. Lando HM: The new "designer" insulins. *Clin Diabetes* 2000;18:154–160.
124. Rutledge KS, Chase HP, Klingensmith GJ, et al. Effectiveness of postprandial Humalog in toddlers with diabetes. *Pedatrics* 1997;100:968–972.
125. Lalli C, Ciofetta M, Del Sindaco P, et al. Long-term intensive treatment of type 1 diabetes with the short-acting insulin analog lispro in variable combination with NPH insulin at mealtime. *Diabetes Care* 1999;22:468–477.
126. Heller S, Kurtzhals P, Verge D, et al. Insulin aspart: promising early results borne out in clinical practice. *Expert Opin Pharmacother* 2002;3:183–195.
127. Bode BW, Strange P. Efficacy, safety, and pump compatibility of insulin aspart used in continuous subcutaneous insulin infusion therapy in patients with type 1 diabetes. *Diabetes Care* 2001;24:69–72.
128. Tamborlane WV, Bonfig W, Boland E. Recent advances in treatment of youth with type 1 diabetes: better care through technology. *Diabet Med* 2001;18: 864–870.
129. Ratner RE, Hirsch IB, Neifing JL, et al. Less hypoglycemia with insulin glargine in intensive insulin therapy for type 1 diabetes. U.S. Study Group of Insulin Glargine in Type 1 Diabetes. *Diabetes Care* 2000;23:639–643.
130. Wolfsdorf JI, Laffel LM, Pasquarello C, et al. Split-mixed insulin regimen with human ultralente before supper and PH (isophane) before breakfast in children and adolescents with IDDM. *Diabetes Care* 1991;14:1100–1106.
131. Boland EA, Grey M, Oesterle A, et al. Continuous subcutaneous insulin infusion. A new way to lower risk of severe hypoglycemia, improve metabolic control, and enhance coping in adolescents with type 1 diabetes. *Diabetes Care* 1999;22:1799–1784.
132. Continuous subcutaneous insulin infusion. *Diabetes Care* 2003;26[Suppl]: S125.
133. Kaufman FR, Halvorson M, Kim C, et al. Use of insulin pump therapy at nighttime only for children 7–10 years of age with type 1 diabetes. *Diabetes Care* 2000;23:579–582.
134. Kanc K, Janssen MM, Keulen ET, et al. Substitution of night-time continuous subcutaneous insulin infusion therapy for bedtime NPH insulin in a multiple injection regimen improves counterregulatory hormonal responses and warning symptoms of hypoglycaemia in IDDM. *Diabetologia* 1998;41: 322–329.
135. Laffel L, Loughlin C, Ramchandani N, et al. Glycemic challenges of insulin pump therapy (CSII) in youth with type 1 diabetes. *Diabetes* 2001;50[suppl 1]:A66–67(abst).
136. Skyler JS, Cefalu WT, Kourides IA, et al. Efficacy of inhaled human insulin in type 1 diabetes mellitus: a randomised proof-of-concept study. *Lancet* 2001; 357:331–335.
137. Cefalu WT, Skyler JS, Kourides IA, et al. Inhaled human insulin treatment in patients with type 2 diabetes mellitus. *Ann Intern Med* 2001;134:203–207.
138. Cefalu WT. Inhaled insulin: a proof-of-concept study. *Ann Intern Med* 2001; 134:795.
139. Jones KL, Arslanian S, Peterokova VA, et al. Effect of metformin in pediatric patients with type 2 diabetes: a randomized controlled trial. *Diabetes Care* 2002;25:89–94.
140. Dean H, Flett B. Natural history of type 2 diabetes diagnosed in children: long-term follow-up in young adult years. *Diabetes* 2002;51[suppl 2]:A-24 (abst).
141. Lewy VD, Danadian K, Witchel SF, et al. Early metabolic abnormalities in adolescent girls with polycystic ovarian syndrome. *J Pediatr* 2001;138:38–44.
142. Palmert MR, Gordon CM, Kartashov AI, et al. Screening for abnormal glucose tolerance in adolescents with polycystic ovary syndrome. *J Clin Endocrinol Metab* 2002;87:1017–1023.
143. Franz MJ, Bantle JP, Beebe CA, et al. Evidence-based nutrition principles and recommendations for the treatment and prevention of diabetes and related complications. *Diabetes Care* 2002;25:148–198.
144. Lockwood D, Frey ML, Gladish NA, et al. The biggest problem in diabetes. *Diabetes Educ* 1986;12:30–33.
145. Franz MJ, Horton ES Sr, Bantle JP, et al. Nutrition principles for the management of diabetes and related complications. *Diabetes Care* 1994;17:490–518.
146. Consumer Information Center: The Food Guide Pyramid. Website. 2001. Available at: http://www/nal.usda.gov:8001/py/pmap.htm.
147. Obarzanek E, Kimm SY, Barton BA, et al. Long-term safety and efficacy of a cholesterol-lowering diet in children with elevated low-density lipoprotein cholesterol: seven-year results of the Dietary Intervention Study in Children (DISC). *Pediatrics* 2001;107:256–264.
148. Nutrition management. In: Kelley DB, ed. *Intensive diabetes management*. 2nd ed. Alexandria, VA: American Diabetes Association; 1998:138–157.
149. Mohn A, Cerruto M, Lafusco D, et al. Celiac disease in children and adolescents with type I diabetes: importance of hypoglycemia. *J Pediatr Gastroenterol Nutr* 2001;32:37–40.
150. Gillett PM, Gillett HR, Israel DM, et al. High prevalence of celiac disease in patients with type 1 diabetes detected by antibodies to endomysium and tissue transglutaminase. *Can J Gastroenterol* 2001;15:297–301.
151. Aktay AN, Lee PC, Kumar V, et al. The prevalence and clinical characteristics of celiac disease in juvenile diabetes in Wisconsin. *J Pediatr Gastroenterol Nutr* 2001;33:462–465.
152. Fasano A. Celiac disease: the past, the present, the future. *Pediatrics* 2001;107: 768–770.
153. Jones JM, Lawson ML, Daneman D, et al. Eating disorders in adolescent females with and without type 1 diabetes: cross sectional study. *BMJ* 2000; 320:1563–1566.
154. Rydall AC, Rodin GM, Olmsted MP, et al. Disordered eating behavior and microvascular complications in young women with insulin-dependent diabetes mellitus. *N Engl J Med* 1997;336:1849–1854.
155. Antisdel J, Laffel LMB, Anderson BJ. Improved detection of eating problems in women with type 1 diabetes using a newly developed survey. *Diabetes* 2001;50:A47(abst).
156. Colton P, Daneman D, Olmsted M, et al. Eating disorders in pre-teen girls with type 1 diabetes mellitus: a case control study. *Diabetes* 200150:A47(abst).
157. Crow SJ, Keel PK, Kendall D. Eating disorders and insulin-dependent diabetes mellitus. *Psychosomatics* 1998;39:233–243.
158. Bryden KS, Neil A, Mayou RA, Peveler RC, Fairburn CG, Dunger DB. Eating habits, body weight, and insulin misuse. A longitudinal study of teenagers and young adults with type 1 diabetes. *Diabetes Care* 1999;22:1956–1960.
159. Daneman D, Olmsted M, Rydall A, et al. Eating disorders in young women with type 1 diabetes. Prevalence, problems and prevention. *Horm Res* 1998;50[suppl 1]:79–86.
160. Marcus M, Wing R. Eating disorders and diabetes. In: Holmes C, ed. Neuropsychological and behavioral aspects of insulin- and non-insulin diabetes mellitus. New York: Springer-Verlag, 1990:102–121.
161. Kaiser Family Foundation. Available at: http://www.kff.org/content/1999/1535.
162. Brownell KD, Kelman JH, Stunkard AJ. Treatment of obese children with and without their mothers: changes in weight and blood pressure. *Pediatrics* 1983; 71:515–523.
163. Schafer LC, Glasgow RE, McCaul KD, et al. Adherence to IDDM regimens: relationship to psychosocial variables and metabolic control. *Diabetes Care* 1983;6:493–498.
164. Riddell MC, Bar-Or O, Ayub BV, et al. Glucose ingestion matched with total carbohydrate utilization attenuates hypoglycemia during exercise in adolescents with IDDM. *Int J Sport Nutr* 1999;9:24–34.
165. Temple MY, Bar-Or O, Riddell MC. The reliability and repeatability of the blood glucose response to prolonged exercise in adolescent boys with IDDM. *Diabetes Care* 1995;18:326–332.
166. Sills IN, Cerny FJ. Responses to continuous and intermittent exercise in healthy and insulin-dependent diabetic children. *Med Sci Sports Exerc* 1983; 15:450–454.
167. Kaufman FR. Diabetes in children and adolescents. Areas of controversy. *Med Clin North Am* 1998;82:721–738.
168. MacDonald MJ. Postexercise late-onset hypoglycemia in insulin-dependent diabetic patients. *Diabetes Care* 1987;10:584–588.
169. Diabetes mellitus and exercise. Physical activity/exercise and diabetes. *Diabetes Care* 2003;26[Suppl]:573–577.
170. Kaufman FR, Halvorson M, Kaufman ND. Evaluation of a snack bar containing uncooked cornstarch in subjects with diabetes. *Diabetes Res Clin Pract* 1997;35:27–33.
171. Kaufman FR, Halvorson M, Kaufman ND. A randomized, blinded trial of uncooked cornstarch to diminish nocturnal hypoglycemia at diabetes camp. *Diabetes Res Clin Pract* 1995;30:205–209.
172. Kaufman FR, Devgan S. Use of uncooked cornstarch to avert nocturnal hypoglycemia in children and adolescents with type I diabetes. *J Diabetes Complications* 1996;10:84–87.
173. *Handbook of exercise in diabetes.* Alexandria, VA: American Diabetes Association, 2002.

174. Tests of glycemia in diabetes. *Diabetes Care* 2003;26[Suppl]:S106–S108.
175. Laffel L. Sick-day management in type 1 diabetes. *Endocrinol Metab Clin North Am* 2000;29:707–723.
176. Grady JC, Kordella T. New products. *Diabetes Forecast* 2003;56;37–40.
177. Jungheim K, Koschinsky T. Glucose monitoring at the arm: risky delays of hypoglycemia and hyperglycemia detection. *Diabetes Care* 2002;25:956–960.
178. Lawlor MT, Laffel L. New technologies and therapeutic approaches for the management of pediatric diabetes. *Curr Diabetes Rep* 2001;1:56–66.
179. Fineberg AE, Bergenstal RM, Bernstein RM, et al. Use of an automated device for alternative site blood glucose monitoring. *Diabetes Care* 2001;24:1217–1220.
180. Laffel L, Kaufman FR, et al. Frequency of elevation in blood B-hydroxybutyrate (B-OHB) during home monitoring and association with glycemia in insulin-treated children and adults. *Diabetes* 2000;49:A92(abst).
181. Kaufman FR, Halvorson M. The treatment and prevention of diabetic ketoacidosis in children and adolescents with type I diabetes mellitus. *Pediatr Ann* 1999;28:576–582.
182. Laffel LMP, Loughlin C, Tovar A, et al. Sick day management (SDM) using blood β-hydroxybutyrate (βOHB) vs urine ketones significantly reduces hospital visits in youth with T1DM: a randomized clinical trial. *Diabetes* 2002;51 [suppl 2]:A105(abst).
183. Polonsky WH, Anderson BJ, Lohrer PA, et al. Insulin omission in women with IDDM. *Diabetes Care* 1994;17:1178–1185.
184. Chase HP, Garg SK, Jelley DH. Diabetic ketoacidosis in children and the role of outpatient management. *Pediatr Rev* 1990;11:297–304.
185. Drash AL, Becker D. Diabetes mellitus in the child: course, special problems, and related disorders. In: Katzen HM, Mahler RJ, eds. *Diabetes, obesity, and vascular disease. Advances in modern nutrition.* Vol 2. New York: Wiley; 1978: 615–643.
186. Nathan DM, McKitrick C, Larkin M, et al. Glycemic control in diabetes mellitus: have changes in therapy made a difference? *Am J Med* 1996;100:157–163.
187. Klein R, Klein BE, Moss SE, et al. The medical management of hyperglycemia over a 10-year period in people with diabetes. *Diabetes Care* 1996;19:744–750.
188. Schiffrin A, Belmonte M. Multiple daily self-glucose monitoring: its essential role in long-term glucose control in insulin-dependent diabetic patients treated with pump and multiple subcutaneous injections. *Diabetes Care* 1982; 5:479–484.
189. Harris MI, Cowie CC, Howie LJ. Self-monitoring of blood glucose by adults with diabetes in the United States population. *Diabetes Care* 1993;16: 1116–1123.
189a. Laffel LMB, Vangsness L, Connell A, et al. Impact of ambulatory, family-focused teamwork intervention on glycemia control in youth with type 1 diabetes. *J Pediatr* 2003;142:409–416.
190. Laffel L, Levine BS, Lawlor M, et al. Ambulatory intervention improves knowledge, monitoring, adherence, and glycemic control: a short-term, randomized trial of high-risk adults with diabetes. *Diabetes* 2000;49:A174(abst).
191. Kaufman FR, Halvorson M, Fisher L, et al. Insulin pump therapy in type 1 pediatric patients. *J Pediatr Endocrinol Metab* 1999;12[Suppl 3]:759–764.
192. Laffel L, Loughlin C, Ramchandani N, et al. Glycemic challenges of pump therapy (CSII) in youth with type 1 diabetes (T1DM). *Diabetes* 2001;50: A66–A67(abst).

CHAPTER 43
Treatment of Older Adults with Diabetes

Caroline S. Blaum and Jeffrey B. Halter

Despite the continual expansion of knowledge about diabetes, including the importance of control of risk factors and glycemia in decreasing the complications of diabetes, much of this knowledge does not specifically address issues in older adults, even though about 50% of people with diabetes in the United States are 60 years and older (1). For example, in the United Kingdom Prospective Diabetes Study (UKPDS), the mean age of participants was 53, although a few older people were enrolled and their number increased during the study. People with significant complications or comorbidities at diagnosis were excluded (2). Therefore, the implications of the results of the UKPDS for the millions of older people with prevalent as well as incident diabetes, many of whom have multiple comorbid conditions, are not yet clear (3).

Clearly, diabetes in older adults is a major health problem (Table 43.1), and older patients with diabetes face major health problems. Those who develop diabetes during middle age will face its debilitating complications as they age or will die prematurely. Those who develop diabetes later in life face an increase in co-occurring risks and complications and comorbidities as they become very old. These older patients and their physicians have no clear clinical guidelines for diabetes management; recommendations must be extrapolated from studies of other age groups. Clinicians confronted with great heterogeneity in the older population and with rapidly changing knowledge about diabetes and its management must understand the similarities and differences in the pathophysiology and management of diabetes in older versus middle-aged adults.

EPIDEMIOLOGY AND DIAGNOSIS OF DIABETES IN OLDER ADULTS

Diabetes is a highly prevalent, and expanding, chronic health problem for older people. The Third National Health and Nutrition Examination Survey (NHANES III), conducted by the National Center for Health Statistics from 1988 through 1994, provided the most recent estimates of the prevalence of diagnosed and undiagnosed diabetes mellitus in the United States among individuals 20 years and older. Among those 60 to 74 and those 75 years and older, respectively, 12.6% and 13.2% had previously diagnosed diabetes and 6.2% and 5.7% had newly diagnosed diabetes according to the criterion for fasting glucose levels established by the American Diabetes Association (ADA). An additional 5% to 6% of people age 60 to 74 met diabetes criteria based only on an oral glucose tolerance test (OGTT) value of more than 200 mg/dL at 2 hours. An overall prevalence of diabetes of approximately 25% among people age 60 to 74 years was confirmed in the Cardiovascular Health Study of older people in the United States and extended to the population over age 75 years. In addition to the high prevalence of diabetes, 20% had impaired glucose tolerance (IGT) by the 1997 ADA diagnostic criteria (4). The incidence of new diagnosis of diabetes mellitus also increased with age until about age 75 and then stabilized. The incidence rate was approximately two per 1,000 among those individuals aged 25 to 44 and increased to approximately five per 1,000 among individuals older than 45 (5).

Most individuals with diabetes who are older than 65 years have type 2 diabetes. However, type 1 diabetes occurs in this age group as well, including some with newly diagnosed diabetes (6). In addition, a small percentage of older individuals who initially have type 2 diabetes become insulin-dependent over time. While the HLA-DR3 allele is more common in older adults who require insulin treatment than in those who do not require insulin, the frequency of antibodies to islet cells in this group is not increased (6).

As in patients with type 2 diabetes in general, atherosclerotic complications are the most significant cause of morbidity and mortality in older patients with diabetes. Observational studies of older adults have suggested that poor glycemic control in

TABLE 43.1. Diabetes: A Key Problem in Older Adults

41% of diabetes population are 65 and older
25% of Medicare expenditures are for diabetes
44% of people 70 and older with diabetes need assistance with one or more activities of daily living
More than 20% of nursing home residents have diabetes

older people with diabetes contributes to excess risk of stroke and cardiovascular events (7,8). Atherosclerotic macrovascular disease accounts for 75% of the mortality among people with diabetes in the United States (9). In the UKPDS, 20% of patients with newly diagnosed diabetes developed macrovascular complications after 9 years, whereas only 9% developed microvascular complications (2).

Microvascular complications are also a significant problem in older adults. In the United States, diabetes is the major cause of renal failure and dialysis in people older than 65 years (10). Diabetic retinopathy is a major cause of visual loss in older adults, and even if it does not lead to blindness, it is associated with disability and depression (11,12). Peripheral neuropathy and peripheral vascular disease are particularly prevalent in older age groups (13). The prevalence of amputations increases with age, as do balance problems, mobility impairment, and chronic pain related to diabetic nerve disorders (14).

The prevalence of disability and functional impairment is greater in older people with diabetes than in older people without diabetes. Older adults with diabetes are about two to three times more likely to have physical limitations (15) and 1.5 times more likely to have ADL (activities of daily living) disability (16) than are those without diabetes. Much of this excess disability is a direct result of complications of diabetes, such as eye disease, stroke, cardiovascular disease, neuropathy, and peripheral vascular disease (15).

Because the hyperglycemia cutoff points for risk of diabetes complications appear to apply similarly to older and younger populations, the ADA diagnostic criteria for diabetes in adults are not modified by the patient's age. Recently, several studies comparing the groups identified by the previous criteria of the World Health Organization (17) versus the ADA fasting glucose criteria (18–21) have been published. Most have found a decreased prevalence of diabetes with the ADA criteria (19,22), although effects have varied in different populations (21). Although this difference in prevalence is small in middle-aged people, it increases with age because older people are more likely to have an elevated 2-hour postchallenge glucose level than an elevated fasting blood glucose level. In addition, the two criteria identify different groups who may have different risks for complications and different outcomes. Studies have suggested that fasting glucose levels may not predict progression to cardiovascular disease or mortality as well as an abnormal postchallenge glucose level (20). Similarly, the ADA category of impaired fasting glucose (IFG) may not predict progression to type 2 diabetes as well as IGT as defined by an OGTT (23). Again this discrepancy may be more pronounced in older adults.

Regardless of the effect of the current diagnostic criteria on determinations of diabetes prevalence in older adults, it is far more common in routine clinical practice to obtain a fasting glucose level than an OGTT. The clinician can use the results of the fasting glucose determination along with a 2-hour glucose level if IFG or other diabetes risk factors are present. It is important to have a high index of suspicion because of the high prevalence of known type 2 diabetes, previously undiagnosed diabetes, and IGT in older people, all of which are associated with excess risk for atherosclerotic disease and mortality. Therefore, *any* elevated fasting blood glucose should be evaluated, and if present on more than one occasion, should mandate the start of patient education regarding glucose intolerance and diabetes, management of associated risks for atherosclerotic disease, and if frank diabetes is present, management of hyperglycemia.

CHANGES IN CARBOHYDRATE METABOLISM WITH AGING

The prevalence of diabetes and glucose intolerance increases with advancing age. These abnormalities in carbohydrate metabolism have features in common, and the glucose intolerance associated with aging increases the risk for development of overt diabetes (24). There is no evidence to suggest that the pathophysiology of type 2 diabetes is any different in older adults than in younger adults. However, physiologic changes that appear to accompany the aging process produce alterations of glucose metabolism even in very healthy older individuals (25). These changes are manifested primarily as an elevation in postprandial blood glucose levels, which may increase by as much as 15 mg/dL (0.8 mmol/L) per decade after the age of 30. The tendency for older adults to have increased postchallenge glucose levels relative to fasting glucose levels has implications for prevalence of diabetes in older adults as defined by the 1997 ADA diagnostic criteria (discussed in previous section).

The pathophysiology of the changes in glucose tolerance associated with aging has been reviewed (25). Glucose absorption following glucose ingestion may be slowed with increasing age, and suppression of hepatic glucose production is delayed (most likely as a result of delayed insulin secretion). A number of age-related changes in regulation of insulin secretion and insulin action have been described.

In addition to intrinsic changes of aging, extrinsic factors may contribute to glucose intolerance. Both the decline in lean body mass and the increase in body fat that accompany aging may contribute to insulin resistance. Levels of physical activity decline with age, and such changes may precipitate or accelerate changes in body composition. Studies of both master athletes and older nonathletes suggest that some of these changes can be either prevented or modified with exercise. Drugs commonly used by older individuals, including diuretics, estrogen, sympathomimetics, glucocorticoids, niacin, phenytoin, and tricyclic antidepressants, can adversely affect glucose metabolism, exacerbating glucose intolerance. Stress states such as myocardial infarction, infection, burns, and surgery can worsen glucose intolerance and precipitate fasting hyperglycemia.

DIABETES AND THE PHYSIOLOGY OF AGING

Many effects of diabetes appear to accelerate age-related physiologic changes. For example, the presence of diabetes confers on diabetic women a risk of cardiovascular disease equal to that for men at the same age (26). Some of the mechanisms presumed to underlie this accelerated vascular aging include effects of diabetes on platelets, increased glycosylation of vascular tissues, and lipoprotein alterations associated with diabetes (27–29).

Changes that occur with diabetes and changes that occur with aging may interact, especially with respect to the general age-related decrease in physiologic reserve in many organ systems. Although most physiologic systems (cardiovascular, renal, pulmonary, central nervous system) in older people function appropriately under normal stable conditions, they may be unable to cope with the increased demands posed by acute illness or injury. Complications of diabetes leading to end-organ damage may further accelerate this loss of physiologic reserve. In addition, the clinical manifestations of diabetes may stress physiologic systems even in the absence of frank pathology. For example, even a mild increase in urine volume in an older diabetic patient with poorly controlled hyperglycemia may exacerbate bladder dysfunction and lead to urinary incontinence. Glycosuria, even without polyuria, can lead to electrolyte imbalance and cardiac arrhythmias.

TREATMENT OF THE OLDER ADULT WITH DIABETES

Determining Treatment Goals

The goals of diabetes management for older patients are not different from those for other patients, and as with patients with diabetes of any age, include far more than treatment of hyperglycemia. These goals are summarized in Table 43.2.

It is important to consider the similarities and differences between older and younger people with diabetes and their impact on diabetes management. Like younger people with diabetes, most older people with diabetes are highly functional and active and deserve the same attention to diabetes management as do younger patients. For both age groups, macrovascular complications are the major causes of morbidity and mortality related to diabetes. For both age groups, co-occurrence of other atherosclerotic risk factors are frequent, and the management of such associated risk factors has been shown to have a favorable impact on morbidity and mortality (30). Finally, the management of diabetes for most people with diabetes, regardless of age, has been shown to be inadequate, with poor physician and patient adherence to published guidelines and recommendations (31–35).

Some key differences between older and younger patients with diabetes can affect management. The older population is very heterogeneous both with respect to their diabetes and their general health status. An older patient with "newly diagnosed" diabetes may truly be a new diabetic patient, with no evidence of diabetes complications and comorbidities; may have had IGT or undiagnosed diabetes for years with complications present at diagnosis; or may have none or many related or unrelated comorbid diseases and disabilities. Some older patients may be more symptomatic from hyperglycemia than are younger patients but are also more prone to complications of treatment. Finally, special evaluation and treatment goals must be devised for frail elderly patients (i.e., those who have multiple comorbidities and disabilities and a significantly impaired physiologic reserve).

TABLE 43.2. Treatment Goals for Older Patients with Diabetes

Alleviation of symptomatic hyperglycemia
Monitoring for and treatment of diabetes complications and related comorbid disease
Prevention of the development or worsening of diabetes complications
Diabetes self-management education and counseling
Identification and treatment of risk factors for atherosclerotic disease
Improved general health, including functional abilities and nutritional status
Identification and management of comorbidity

Because of this complexity and heterogeneity, selecting appropriate management goals for older patients with diabetes should be based on a detailed evaluation. A complete history and physical examination should be done at the time of diagnosis, when control of hyperglycemia and risk factors is inadequate, or when a reassessment of the patient's status is needed. Diabetes complications and the presence of risk factors for diabetic complications, as well as co-occurring diseases and disorders and general functioning, must be assessed.

A key component of the medical history for all patients with diabetes, but especially older patients, is a thorough evaluation of their medications, including prescription and over-the-counter drugs, "alternative medications," and dietary supplements. Older patients commonly take several medications, and drug–drug interactions, drug–disease interactions, and increased expense can be problematic in patients taking multiple drugs.

Laboratory evaluations and subspecialty referrals recommended for older patients with diabetes are not substantially different from those for middle-aged patients with type 2 diabetes, except in unusual circumstances such as severe debilitation or advanced dementia. Laboratory evaluation should include determinations of fasting serum glucose level, glycosylated hemoglobin (HbA_{1c}) (to assess previous level of control and to be used as a baseline), fasting lipid profile, and serum creatinine; urinalysis with examination for proteinuria or microalbuminuria; and an electrocardiogram. The ADA recommends ophthalmologic evaluation at the time of diagnosis and yearly for all patients with type 2 diabetes (12), a recommendation that applies to elderly patients as well, who are at high risk for ocular diseases other than retinopathy.

Recently, the American Geriatrics Society and the California Healthcare Foundation convened a multidisciplinary expert panel to develop evidence-based guidelines to improve diabetes management in older adults (36). A major recommendation was that management be individualized according to health status and preferences of the older diabetes patient. They also recommended that an evaluation of an older diabetes patient include screening and management of geriatric syndromes: polypharmacy, cognitive impairment, depression, falls, urinary incontinence, and pain. Geriatric syndromes are more common in older adults with diabetes than in those without diabetes. (See referenced guidelines for details.)

For many older patients with diabetes, especially those with several comorbid conditions and "geriatric syndromes" and/or problems managing their diabetes, a comprehensive geriatric evaluation, sometimes also referred to as a geriatric or functional assessment, is indicated (36a,37). This is a multifaceted assessment of the patient's capabilities for self-care, including ADL (bathing, grooming, dressing, feeding, toileting, and transferring) and instrumental ADL (e.g., shopping, telephoning, finances, and housework), and indicates the amount of assistance, if any, that the patient needs. It also includes assessment of nutritional status, evaluation for possible depression or cognitive impairment, and evaluation of the patient's social support systems, financial and insurance status, and advance medical directives. Nursing and social-work assistance is invaluable for both geriatric assessment and diabetes teaching and self-management support. These health professionals can help patients and their families access support services available in the community. For some patients, referral to a geriatrician may be necessary.

Symptomatic Hyperglycemia in Older Patients

Aging-related changes and increased comorbid conditions make older patients with diabetes particularly vulnerable to symptoms of hyperglycemia, even if those symptoms are not the "classic" symptoms. Symptoms such as falls, fatigue, dizziness, and increased incontinence may often be traced back to hyperglycemia-associated polyuria. Glycosuria may also be associated with weight loss caused by the loss of calories in the urine. Older people may be at increased risk for depletion of trace nutrients and minerals caused by osmotic diuresis. Magnesium and potassium deficiencies can have deleterious effects on cardiac conduction. Glycosuria can also increase phosphate excretion, which can accelerate calcium loss from bone (38). An impaired central thirst response in older people may contribute to the volume depletion due to osmotic diuresis from hyperglycemia. Clearly, elimination of glycosuria is an important therapeutic goal (blood glucose level approximately 200 mg/dL or 11 mmol/L) in older people with diabetes.

Weight loss caused by uncontrolled hyperglycemia can be a significant problem. Patients with weight loss may be in a constant catabolic state, which can lead to loss of muscle mass, weakness, and potentially to falls and injury. Older patients may not perceive increased hunger, in some cases exacerbating poor nutritional status. The associated catabolic state may predispose to infections and other complications of malnutrition.

An increased concentration of glucose or its metabolites in the lens and aqueous humor of the eye can lead to visual problems. Hyperglycemia may predispose patients to bacterial and fungal infection and increased pain perception (39) and may alter platelet adhesiveness, worsening intermittent claudication. Lipid abnormalities also worsen with poor glycemic control, and high triglyceride levels can predispose to pancreatitis. A careful search for such symptoms of hyperglycemia is clearly indicated in elderly diabetic patients.

In many older patients, symptoms associated with diabetes and hyperglycemia may be atypical. For example, hyperglycemia does not usually lead to dramatic polyuria and polydipsia; more often there will be increased incontinence, a urinary tract infection, or increased lethargy or mental confusion. Similarly, undiagnosed or unmanaged diabetes may manifest as increased bacterial or fungal infections of the skin, unexplained weight loss, increased fatigue, or slow wound healing. Increased paresthesias and weakness, orthostatic hypotension with falls, or decreased vision also should raise suspicion for undiagnosed or inadequately managed diabetes.

The most severe complication of diabetes in older individuals is hyperglycemic hyperosmolar nonketotic coma. This condition is seen almost exclusively in older patients with diabetes. It is often precipitated by a catastrophic event, such as myocardial infarction or stroke, and can sometimes occur in people not previously known to have diabetes. Details of inpatient management are discussed elsewhere in this volume (Chapter 65).

Management of Atherosclerotic Risks and Complications

Findings from the UKPDS and other studies have made it clear that treatment of associated risks for atherosclerotic disease is a major goal of diabetes management (40). A higher proportion of older than younger patients with diabetes have associated hypertension, hyperlipidemia, and atherosclerotic arterial disease (41–45). Although fewer older than younger people smoke cigarettes, smoking-cessation programs should be encouraged for those who do smoke (46). Older patients with diabetes have been shown to benefit as much as or more than patients without diabetes from treatment of hypertension (47). Meta-analysis has shown aspirin use to be beneficial in older patients with diabetes who are at risk for atherosclerosis or have atherosclerosis (48). Treatment of hyperlipidemia in diabetic patients with cardiovascular disease has been shown to be beneficial and may decrease mortality among those who may develop cardiovascular disease; no age limit has been defined (3), although the data available on people older than 75 years are limited. Peripheral vascular occlusive disease and amputations increase with age; therefore, monitoring and evaluation for circulatory problems are indicated. Preventative treatment and monitoring for complications are not appropriate for the few older patients who are in a preterminal state or have advanced dementia. Most older people, even those with comorbidities and disability, will benefit from interventions shown to prevent or slow an increasing burden of illness over a period of several years.

Management of Microvascular Risks and Complications

Many dialysis patients older than 60 have diabetic renal disease, and because of the increasing prevalence of diabetes, the number of older people who have diabetic renal disease is increasing. Currently, treatment of hypertension and hyperglycemia are the major recommended interventions for preventing end-stage renal disease due to diabetes (10). These interventions are appropriate for most older patients with diabetes.

Peripheral neuropathy leading to pain, neuropathic joints, wounds, mobility problems, and amputations contributes to disability and poor quality of life in older patients. The little evidence available suggests that foot care and monitoring may be associated with better outcomes.

Although macular degeneration is the major cause of blindness after age 65, poor vision due to macular edema or other diabetes-related eye disease is highly prevalent among older people with diabetes. Simulations have suggested that few older persons with new-onset diabetes will become blind because of diabetes (49). However, it is important to remember that most older people do not have new-onset diabetes, many have had diabetes for 10 years or more, and the true duration of diabetes is not known for many others. Eye disease either due to or related to diabetes is prevalent in such patients. Therefore, yearly ophthalmologic referral is warranted for most older people with diabetes.

Treatment of Hyperglycemia

While there is broad agreement that symptomatic hyperglycemia should be treated in all older patients regardless of health status, there is much more controversy regarding the benefits of aggressive control of asymptomatic hyperglycemia in older patients. The UKPDS demonstrated that lowering glucose levels reduced risk of microvascular disease (50). Observational studies in older people also suggest that improved glycemic control is associated with improved outcomes—both macrovascular and microvascular. Thus, although the benefits of glycemic control in older diabetes patients have not been demonstrated conclusively, the weight of available evidence suggests it is beneficial. The physician and the older patient must decide when tight glycemic control for potential prevention of long-term complications of diabetes is a reasonable therapeutic goal. If the decision is made to attempt, glycemic goals would be exactly the same as those for middle-aged people.

Several arguments have been made against choosing an aggressive management program for older adults with diabetes. One such argument is that some elderly patients may be less capable than younger patients of carrying out activities requiring the high levels of skill, commitment, and diabetes education necessary to achieving an aggressive treatment goal. However, while methods of learning and memory do change with age, most older individuals are fully capable of learning complicated concepts and tasks (51). To the extent that older adults lead a less hectic, more ordered life than younger adults, it may actually be easier for them to make the type of adjustments in lifestyle necessary for adherence to a good diabetes treatment program. In fact, recent evidence from NHANES III (52) and a community population in Michigan (53) suggest that, on average, glycemic control in older adults may not be any worse than that in younger people with type 2 diabetes.

A common argument against aggressive diabetes management in older adults is based on inaccurate estimates of life expectancy (i.e., why try to prevent complications in someone who is likely to die soon?). However, the median remaining life expectancy for individuals aged 65 is more than 17 years; for those aged 75, 10 years; and for those aged 85, 6 years (54). Furthermore, these median estimates will be exceeded by approximately 50% of the people in a given age cohort. Thus, there is substantial time for the development of diabetes complications in patients whose diagnosis is made during their 60s or 70s.

It is also clear that elderly individuals are susceptible to virtually all of the chronic complications of diabetes. Age and diabetes frequently interact to worsen the risk for many of these complications. For example, creatinine clearance declines with normal aging (55), and age is an independent risk factor for the development of peripheral neuropathy (56,57). Until studies are available demonstrating that the risks of tight glycemic control outweigh the benefits in older adults or that glycemic control does not prevent the development of complications, many elderly patients deserve the same consideration as younger adults regarding aggressive management of their disease.

Some older patients who have a limited life expectancy, multiple chronic diseases, functional or cognitive impairments, poor social support, or who take multiple medications, are clearly not candidates for aggressive management of hyperglycemia (see Frail Older People). For these patients, treatment of symptomatic hyperglycemia and monitoring and managing complications and comorbidities are indicated. One proposed way of deciding about tight glycemic control for a given patient is to consider whether it would be of either no benefit or high risk (30). For older patients, characteristics such as frequent hypoglycemia or severe cognitive impairment would suggest high risk, whereas a preterminal state or advanced disability would suggest that it would not be beneficial.

Once the level of care is decided, subsequent management of older adults becomes clearer. In short, the treatment regimen chosen is the one necessary to achieve treatment goals. The four standard modalities of diabetes therapy—diet, exercise, oral hypoglycemic agents, and administration of insulin—all merit consideration for older adults.

DIET

The role of medical nutritional therapy has been substantially redefined by the ADA (58), and there is no uniformly recommended ADA diet. In general, dietary therapy must be individualized to support the goals of diabetes management; this is true for older as well as younger patients with diabetes. While weight loss in overweight patients with diabetes has many benefits (improved short-term glycemic control, improved blood pressure and lipid profile, and improved glucose tolerance), it has proven difficult for people of any age. Therefore, the goal of dietary therapy is not specifically weight loss. Rather, nutritional therapy should be designed to contribute to optimal glycemic, lipid, and blood pressure management. In obese patients, this may include hypocaloric diets, but it is important to remember that up to one third of older patients with diabetes are not obese and some are undernourished. In these undernourished patients, caloric supplementation and reversal of a catabolic state would be important. The ADA has recognized this fact with special recommendations for institutionalized patients with diabetes that include an increase in caloric intake when appropriate (58).

Older patients with diabetes often have multiple issues to be considered in a nutritional prescription. These include appropriate caloric targets, micronutrient assessment, and the role of dietary management for associated hypertension, hyperlipidemia, and renal disease if present. In addition, older patients may have problems with shopping, finances, or meal preparation that may become evident only during a dietary assessment. Therefore, dietary education and support in nutritional self-management remain important.

EXERCISE

Exercise has been shown to improve glucose tolerance and to be useful in chronic glycemic control in persons with type 2 diabetes (59). However, a much broader consensus regarding the benefits of exercise is emerging—unfortunately without specific clinical recommendations regarding exercise prescriptions for older patients with diabetes. A decrease in the levels of physical activity in the population has been linked to an increase in the prevalence of obesity and type 2 diabetes; the role of exercise as part of lifestyle intervention in the prevention of type 2 diabetes is currently under study (60). In other chronic conditions, including hyperlipidemia, hypertension, atherosclerotic heart disease, and even heart failure, exercise appears to confer therapeutic benefits, although more specific information is needed. Even in frail older patients, resistance and aerobic exercises have been shown to have objective and subjective benefits (61), although such benefits may be short-lived.

Currently, exercise recommendations must be individualized for patients with type 2 diabetes regardless of age. In older patients for whom the goals of treatment include prevention of diabetes complications and glycemic control, an exercise program is part of a diabetes self-care regimen. Clinical judgment is needed regarding exercise recommendations if clinical or preclinical cardiovascular disease is suspected. In frail elderly patients, some forms of exercise may be appropriate and may be directed at conditions other than their diabetes. Unfortunately, despite the many proven or suspected benefits of exercise, there is no clear consensus on precisely what exercise recommendation or what preexercise evaluation is appropriate for any patient with type 2 diabetes, regardless of age or health status.

ORAL MEDICATIONS

Several different classes of medications that work by different mechanisms are currently available for the treatment of hyperglycemia. Most have been tested to some degree in older patients, so benefits and concerns about their use in older people with diabetes have been identified. In older patients with diabetes, combination therapy for hyperglycemia that is based on complementary actions of different drugs can be used. In general, the potential benefit of improved control of hyperglycemia without the use of insulin must be balanced against potential risks associated with a higher prevalence of contraindications to some drugs, polypharmacy, decreased compliance with multidrug therapy, and increased financial burden. At this time, there is no consensus on what constitutes the best approach to pharmacologic therapy for hyperglycemia in older adults.

Sulfonylureas

The sulfonylureas have many advantages for the management of hyperglycemia in older patients with diabetes. First, they are efficacious, with proven ability to decrease HbA_{1c} levels by up to 3% to 5%, and there is no evidence suggesting that these drugs are any less effective in older adults than in younger adults. These drugs have been available for many years, so physicians and patients are familiar with them. They have a good safety profile, an easy dosing schedule, and are much less expensive than newer oral agents. They remain first-line agents for any older patient with diabetes for whom the decision has been made to treat hyperglycemia with medications.

The major risk for older adults treated with sulfonylureas is hypoglycemia. Although hypoglycemic attacks are relatively rare, with attacks leading to hospitalization reported to occur with a frequency of 1.23 cases per 1,000 patient treatment years (62), age alone is a significant risk factor for hypoglycemia. There are multiple factors associated with aging that might increase the risk for hypoglycemia. These include age-associated impairments in hepatic and renal function that alter drug metabolism and excretion. The impairment of hepatic oxidative pathways associated with aging may increase the half-lives of sulfonylureas, which are metabolized extensively by the liver. Renal function, as measured by creatinine clearance, declines with age (55), and insulin clearance has been shown to be reduced (63). Aging also is associated with impairments in the autonomic nervous system (64,65) and reductions in α-adrenergic receptor function (66), suggesting that the sensation of glycemia may not be as acute in older adults as in younger adults. The elderly are frequent users of drugs that are known to increase the risk for hypoglycemia, including α-adrenergic blockers, salicylates, warfarin, sulfonamides, and alcohol. The longer-acting sulfonylureas, glyburide and chlorpropamide, have been reported to cause more episodes of hypoglycemia (67). Hyponatremia has also been seen in older diabetes patients using chlorpropamide, a development that may be related to a drug interaction with thiazide diuretics (68) and intrinsic changes in water metabolism with aging.

Biguanide

Metformin, the only biguanide currently available in the United States, has both advantages and disadvantages for treatment of older patients with diabetes. Chapter 41 has reviewed its characteristics in detail and its proven benefit in obese type 2 diabetes patients (69). A major advantage of metformin for older patients is that, because of its mechanism of action, it does not produce hypoglycemia when used as a single agent. In addition, its association with weight loss is potentially beneficial to obese older patients with diabetes, although up to one third of older diabetes patients, especially the frail elderly and/or those in nursing homes, are not obese and may not be good candidates for metformin. Older patients with hyperlipidemia may benefit from the favorable effects of metformin on lipid profiles.

The major disadvantage of metformin in older patients is its interaction with comorbid conditions, many of which are prevalent in older patients. It is relatively contraindicated in the presence of congestive heart failure, liver disease, and especially renal disease. It should not be used if the serum creatinine exceeds 1.4 mg/dL (124 μmol/L) (women) or 1.5 mg/dL (133 μmol/L) (men). Since the serum creatinine value will overestimate the creatinine clearance in an older patient who has decreased muscle mass, an even lower serum creatinine level may be a cause for concern in such a patient. Therefore, the presence of these conditions, even if asymptomatic, must be carefully assessed in older patients.

Another potential disadvantage of metformin is its gastrointestinal (GI) side effects, generally bloating and flatulence, which may affect older adults more than younger adults. However, it is not known whether older people are more likely than younger people to discontinue metformin because of GI symptoms.

Metformin costs more than the sulfonylurea medications and insulin but less than other oral agents used for treating diabetes.

α-Glucosidase Inhibitors

Acarbose and miglitol are α-glucosidase inhibitors, which delay absorption of sugars through the GI tract. Because postprandial hyperglycemia is particularly common in older people, these agents may merit consideration. They lower HbA_{1c} levels by about 1% (on average) (70). Because of their mechanism of action, they do not cause hypoglycemia, but their use in combination with another hypoglycemic agent may make it more difficult to treat hypoglycemia. The most common side effects are GI. Although they do not cause symptoms of malabsorption, they potentially can lead to weight loss. These drugs are currently more expensive than sulfonylureas or insulin. Although their safety makes them attractive for elderly patients, the potential for weight loss and GI side effects limits their use for older patients with diabetes who are undernourished. These agents can be used as part of combination therapy. Their use in combination with metformin may worsen GI discomfort.

Thiazolidinediones

The thiazolidinediones improve insulin sensitivity and thus could be of particular benefit to older patients with diabetes, who in addition to having diabetes, may have aging-associated insulin resistance. These drugs have moderate potency, lowering HbA_{1c} by up to 2% to 4% (71), although it is not known if this is different in older patients with diabetes. Two thiazolidinediones, pioglitazone and rosiglitazone, are now available. The drugs are currently very expensive, limiting their use for low-income elderly patients. They may be used as part of combination therapy when one agent alone is insufficient to achieve desired control of hyperglycemia.

Meglitinides

Repaglinide is the first of a new class of oral hypoglycemics that enhance insulin secretion, but by a mechanism different from that of the sulfonylureas. Repaglinide acts rapidly to enhance insulin secretion, so it is designed to be used immediately before meals. It is of moderate potency and is currently expensive. No specific information is yet available regarding its use in older patients. If used as additive therapy with sulfonylureas, repaglinide presumably could increase the risk of hypoglycemia. The role of repaglinide in older patients with diabetes awaits further clinical and testing.

D-Phenylalanine Derivative

Nateglinide is the first of a new class of hypoglycemic agent that is a derivative of the amino acid D-phenylalanine. It became available for clinical use in 2001. Nateglinide acts directly on pancreatic β-cells to rapidly stimulate insulin secretion. Because of the rapid onset and short duration of action, it was developed to address mealtime needs for insulin secretion. It is to be taken shortly before a meal at a standard dose of 120 mg, although a 60-mg dose also is available. Because of the glucose-level dependency of its effect on insulin secretion and its short duration of action, its use has been associated with a low rate of hypoglycemia when used alone or in combination with other agents such as metformin. There are currently no known drug interactions, and nateglinide can be used in patients with renal insufficiency.

TABLE 43.3. Combination Oral Therapy of Hyperglycemia in Older Patients: Advantages and Disadvantages

Advantages	Disadvantages
Improved glycemic control	Cost
Potential metabolic benefits due to different drug mechanisms	Increased hypoglycemia risk
May be easier than multidose insulin	May worsen gastrointestinal symptoms
May be safer than multidose insulin	Risk of adverse drug effects due to polypharmacy and comorbidity

Combination Oral Agent Therapy

The many oral hyperglycemic drugs now available have complementary mechanisms of actions, thereby providing a rationale for multidrug therapy to attempt to achieve the desired level of glycemic control in patients without resorting to insulin. In addition, the availability of newer agents brings into the clinical arena physiologic considerations about type 2 diabetes that previously were considered primarily in research settings. However, the clinical importance of specifically targeting insulin resistance, hyperinsulinemia, or "glucose toxicity" remains to be determined. Some advantages and disadvantages of combination oral agent therapy are summarized in Table 43.3.

As with other diabetes management decisions, the choice to use combination therapy to achieve improved glycemic control in older patients requires some special considerations. It is important to reevaluate the glycemic target to see if combination therapy is still appropriate. In those healthy older patients with diabetes in whom the goal is control of hyperglycemia for its potential benefits to decrease future risks, combination oral agent therapy must be carefully monitored to make sure it achieves the treatment goal. In some older patients with diabetes, especially the frailest, problems and difficulties with insulin use are likely, and insulin-induced hypoglycemia may be a greater risk. The use of combination oral agent therapy may be easier and safer for some of these patients, although some oral agent regimens may also cause hypoglycemia.

Several other considerations are especially pertinent to older patients. First, they are much more likely to have a condition or conditions that may be contraindications to the use of some of the drugs in the combination. Second, older patients with comorbidities and diabetes-related complications are likely to be receiving many other medications. Polypharmacy and drug–drug interactions are a major concern, even if all the drugs being used are indicated. Finally, except for insulin and the sulfonylureas, these drugs are very costly and patients may not be able to afford them. Financial considerations can lead to problems in patients either with these medications or with necessary medications for other conditions. Research is clearly needed to assess the safety and efficacy of specific oral-agent combination therapy in older patients with diabetes.

INSULIN

Although the initiation of insulin therapy is sometimes considered to be a difficult and momentous step for an older patient, insulin is indicated for any patient when treatment goals are not being met without it. No studies have demonstrated that elderly patients are unable to use insulin effectively and safely. Insulin therapy can result in euglycemia in those patients for whom this is the goal and should also be used for elderly patients with symptomatic hyperglycemia whose glucose levels cannot be controlled with diet and oral agents. Some advantages and disadvantages of insulin therapy in the population are summarized in Table 43.4.

No special insulin regimens have been identified as being more or less efficacious in older patients. As in younger adults, it is probably difficult to achieve normoglycemia with a single dose of intermediate-acting insulin. Therefore, when aggressive management is indicated, a split-mixed regimen is usually necessary. New rapidly acting insulin analogues offer an opportunity to target postprandial hyperglycemia, which is particularly prevalent in older people. A single dose of insulin may be appropriate, however, to prevent symptomatic hyperglycemia when this is the treatment goal.

Insulin therapy does require some special considerations when used in older adults. Aging alone, or complications secondary to diabetes, may impair vision and the fine-motor skills necessary for insulin administration. Blood glucose monitoring, indicated for patients treated with insulin, requires additional skills that may also be impaired with aging or disease processes. Hyperglycemia and poor diabetes control may be associated with subtle impairments of cognitive function in older adults (72,73). Such impairments, combined with the high prevalence of cognitive disorders in older populations, may adversely affect the ability of an older individual to adhere to a complicated insulin regimen. Older patients with diabetes who live alone without adequate family or support services may be at increased risk for serious sequelae of insulin administration (i.e., hypoglycemia). However, none of these considerations is an absolute contraindication to insulin therapy. If problems are recognized before or at the time of institution of insulin therapy, solutions can usually be found for each. Family members are frequently the most valuable resource. Community support services such as Meals on Wheels, visiting nurse services, and home health aides or homemaker services may be able to provide primary assistance or fill in the gaps.

Hypoglycemia is a potential concern for older patients treated with insulin. Some risk factors for hypoglycemia in this

TABLE 43.4. Insulin Therapy in Older Adults

Advantages	Disadvantages
Glycemic control goals achievable	Requires home blood glucose monitoring
Relatively inexpensive	Injections, often multiple/day
Decreases possible polypharmacy	Overall complexity of regimen
Avoids gastrointestinal symptoms with multiple pills	Risks of hypoglycemia

TABLE 43.5. Risks for Hypoglycemia

Visual impairment
Impaired manual dexterity
Inability to do blood glucose monitoring
Impaired cognitive function
Poor family support

population are summarized in Table 43.5. Hypoglycemia counterregulatory mechanisms are generally intact in otherwise healthy older adults with diabetes mellitus. However, older people on complex medical regimens, who eat meals irregularly, or who have a significant cognitive disorder are likely to be at significant risk. The strategies for prevention of hypoglycemia include appropriate selection of patients for insulin treatment; frequent monitoring of blood glucose levels; adequate diabetes education, with special emphasis on the recognition and treatment of hypoglycemia; dietary assessment and instruction; and the intervention of family, friends, or support services to provide frequent (at least daily) contact for the insulin-treated older adult with diabetes.

Insulin Combined with Oral Agents

A single insulin dose, possibly administered at bedtime, combined with one or more oral agents, may be useful in achieving desired glycemic control in patients with type 2 diabetes (71). As in middle-aged people with diabetes, such a regimen may be reasonable in otherwise healthy and high-functioning older patients with diabetes. However, there is little specific information available about such combination regimens in older adults.

Self-Management Education and General Health Status Counseling

Because diabetes is associated with atherosclerotic risks, comorbidities related to macrovascular and microvascular complications, and increased disability, all of which increase with age in people with and without diabetes, improvement in general health status is an important component of diabetes management in older patients. For older people who may have multiple other conditions associated with their diabetes, it is important to understand how all these conditions affect everyday functioning at home and in society. Key to this is a comprehensive evaluation, as previously discussed. Besides appropriate medical management of diagnosed diseases, it is important to assess an older patient's nutritional status, affective and cognitive status, mobility, and functioning because diabetes has been shown to be associated with impairments in all these conditions. Although approaches to prevention and management of such disabling conditions and disabilities associated with diabetes are in their infancy, it is becoming increasingly important for physicians to learn to identify disabling conditions and functioning difficulties and to apply available management techniques.

Diabetes is fundamentally a self-managed disease. The healthcare provider must educate the patient and family, guide appropriate management choices, manage risks and comorbid conditions, and support the patient's efforts at self-management. Unfortunately, very little is known about self-management in older patients with diabetes. Many older people have other chronic conditions, have friends and family members with chronic conditions, and have retired from work and thus may have the inclination, time, and knowledge base to handle diabetes self-management better than do middle-aged patients with diabetes. However, because some older people may have very poor health and/or be cognitively impaired, the success of diabetes "self-management" will depend on the availability and skills of a caregiver. Future research is urgently needed to clarify the relationships of health status and diabetes self-management in older adults. It is clear, however, that many functioning older people can be expected to manage their diabetes as well as any younger patients with diabetes and should have similar access to education and self-management support.

Management of Older Patients with Diabetes in Special Situations

FRAIL OLDER PEOPLE

The health status of some older patients with diabetes is very poor because of preterminal illnesses, advanced dementia, or significant comorbid problems and functional difficulties. Many such patients also have decreased physiologic reserve and are often termed "frail." Most frail elderly patients live in the community with caregivers, in assisted living facilities, or sometimes alone; others are in nursing homes. For these frail older patients with diabetes, management of their diabetes will be one aspect of the coordinated, multidisciplinary management of their multiple problems. For such patients, a basic diabetes management program may be most appropriate (74). This program would include treatment of symptomatic hyperglycemia, attention to nutritional status (these patients may be malnourished and catabolic), and treatment of diabetes complications and comorbidities directed toward patient comfort, maintenance of function, and prevention of further decline when possible. It is important to remember that findings attributable to hyperglycemia may be substantial and may include infections, worsened mental status, blurred vision, falls, and worsened incontinence. Such patients benefit from geriatric evaluation and multidisciplinary management, and referral to a geriatrician is often appropriate. Research is needed concerning the contribution of diabetes to the frailty syndrome and on the appropriate management of diabetes in this group of patients.

NURSING HOME RESIDENTS

Approximately 3% to 5% of the population over the age of 65 are residing in nursing homes at any given time, and up to one fourth of older people will experience an extended nursing-home stay. The prevalence of diabetes in the nursing-home population is about twice that in the general population. According to the 1987 National Medical Expenditure Survey, diabetic patients in nursing homes had a significantly higher prevalence of diseases associated with diabetes, such as heart disease, hypertension, and kidney failure, than elderly nondiabetic patients in nursing homes; were also more limited in all ADL except feeding; and were more likely to be blind. The frequency of amputations was higher among the diabetic patients in nursing homes, although the difference was not statistically significant (75).

The approach to most nursing-home patients with diabetes should be that of providing basic care with control of hyperglycemia to prevent symptoms and associated acute complications. Tight glycemic control for the prevention of chronic complications may not be appropriate because of the poor health status and reduced life expectancy of most nursing-home patients. Control of hyperglycemia in patients in nursing homes is achieved primarily through the use of diet and medications. Exercise will probably not play a major role in the management of diabetes in these patients. However, patients who are capable of an exercise program should be encouraged to participate to enhance mobility and functional status. Diet is an important therapeutic option, but weight maintenance may be more important than weight reduction for many elderly patients with diabetes who are in nursing homes. One study found that over 20% of patients with diabetes in nursing homes were more than 20% underweight (76), a finding that raises the concern about malnutrition in this population. Thus, a dietitian should evaluate all patients with diabetes at the time of admission to the nursing home. Adjustments in recommended caloric intake should be made for wounds, infections, and level of activity. Patients should be weighed at least monthly, and further dietary adjustments should be made as needed.

As in other situations, the decision regarding use of medications or insulin should be based on the level of glycemic control desired. Often an oral agent is preferred both by the patient and the nursing-home staff, but insulin is needed for those patients for whom glycemic goals cannot be achieved with oral agents. Glucose control may be more easily obtained in the patient with diabetes who is in a nursing home because medications and meals are delivered on a regular schedule. In the nursing-home setting, glucose monitoring may be done more frequently and the response of the physician may be more immediate than in the outpatient setting. In fact, Mooradian et al. (76) found that patients with diabetes in the nursing home had lower levels of HgA_{1c}, fewer episodes of hypoglycemia, and were thinner than a younger group of outpatients with diabetes.

In addition to glycemic control, particular attention should be paid to the prevention of conditions that may be related to, or are exacerbated by, diabetes mellitus. Infections, particularly skin and urinary tract infections, are more common in nursing-home patients with diabetes than in other nursing-home patients. The incidence of urinary tract infections may be reduced by limiting the use of indwelling bladder catheters and by ensuring good urinary output through adequate hydration. Skin infections may be prevented by strict precautions against the development of decubitus ulcers, such as frequent turning of immobilized patients; the use of adequate bed and wheelchair cushioning; and the use of heel protectors. The prevalence of all infections is reduced with good staff hygiene, particularly by the enforcement of strict hand-washing regimens. The use of annual influenza vaccination and one-time pneumococcal vaccination for all nursing-home patients will provide population immunity and protect against epidemics of these illnesses in the nursing home. Immunization and PPD (purified protein derivative) status should be verified and documented for all patients newly admitted to the nursing home. Patients with diabetes who have a positive PPD reaction should be considered for prophylaxis with isoniazid if they have not been treated previously for tuberculosis.

Preventative medicine appropriate for all nursing-home residents, including regular ophthalmologic, dental, and foot care, is especially important for those with diabetes. Many institutions offer these services in the nursing home itself. These interventions will maintain quality of life and, in some circumstances, may serve to detect and ameliorate potentially life-threatening events.

HOSPITALIZED OLDER PATIENTS

The rate of hospitalization among elderly patients with diabetes is 1.7 times the rate among elderly people without diabetes. These include hospitalizations both for diabetes and for other reasons. Regardless of the reason for hospitalization, an appropriate goal for glycemic management should be established for each patient. In general, efforts should emphasize minimizing the likelihood of insulin deficiency, which can contribute to a catabolic state. If this is the primary goal, tight glycemic control is not necessary. Reasonable goals would be a mean plasma glucose level lower than 250 mg/dL (14 mmol/L) and minimal glycosuria. Stressful illnesses such as myocardial infarction, pneumonia, influenza, and stroke or conditions associated with a decline in renal function can exacerbate hyperglycemia and may even precipitate hyperosmolar hyperglycemic nonketotic coma in a patient who is already hospitalized. Thus, older patients with these conditions (including patients previously managed with oral agents or diet alone or even patients not previously recognized as having diabetes) may need to be treated temporarily with insulin. Attention must also be given to fluid status, with the use of appropriate intravenous fluid therapy to prevent dehydration and worsening of hyperglycemia. Frequent glucose monitoring is recommended to prevent wide perturbations in blood glucose levels. Sliding scales of regular insulin can be useful for the acutely ill patient or postoperative patient who is unable to eat. However, once oral intake is adequate, most hospitalized patients are better managed with split-mixed dosing of insulin with adjustments made as needed on the basis of the results of frequent glucose monitoring.

An important risk for the hospitalized older adult with diabetes is hypoglycemia. In general, hypoglycemia in the hospital results from decreased caloric intake or inappropriate changes in insulin dosage (77). Hypoglycemia may be prevented by frequent glucose monitoring, with careful adjustments in the insulin dose as the patient's medical condition changes, and with the establishment of appropriate in-hospital goals for glycemic control.

The basic principles of geriatric medicine apply to the management of hospitalized elderly patients with diabetes. Some general recommendations include strict decubitus precautions, restriction of the use of indwelling catheters, and judicious use of psychoactive drugs [their administration should not be on a "prn" (as required) basis]. Mobility should be encouraged, and physical therapy should begin early in the hospital course, as indicated. Planning for discharge should begin at the time of admission, with input from the social-work service. Involvement of a consultant in geriatric medicine should be considered, particularly if the patient has multiple medical problems and is taking multiple medications, is functionally impaired, and requires or may require home care or nursing-home placement at the time of discharge.

REFERENCES

1. Morley J. An overview of diabetes mellitus in older persons. *Clin Geriatr Med* 1999;15:211–214.
2. Turner RC, Holman RR. The UK prospective diabetes study. *Ann Intern Med* 1996;28:439–444.
3. American Diabetes Association. Clinical practice recommendations 2001. *Diabetes Care* 2001;24[Suppl 1]:28.
4. Harris MI, Flegal KM, Cowie CC, et al. Prevalence of diabetes, impaired fasting glucose, and impaired glucose tolerance in U.S. adults: the Third National Health and Nutrition Examination Survey. *Diabetes Care* 1998;21:518–525.
5. Kenny SJ, Aubert RE, Geiss LS. Prevalence and incidence of non-insulin-dependent diabetes. In: National Diabetes Data Group. *Diabetes in America.* 2nd ed. Bethesda, MD. National Institute of Diabetes and Digestive and Kidney Diseases, 1995:47–68. NIDDKD publication 95-1468.
6. Kilvert A, Fitzgerald MG, Wright AD, et al. Clinical characteristics and aetiological classification of insulin-dependent diabetes in the elderly. *Q J Med* 1986;60:865–872.
7. Kuusisto J, Mykkanen L, Pyorala K, et al. Non-insulin-dependent diabetes and its metabolic control are important predictors of stroke in elderly subjects. *Stroke* 1994;25:1157–1164.
8. Kuusisto J, Mykkanen L, Pyorala K, et al. NIDDM and its metabolic control predict coronary heart disease in elderly subjects. *Diabetes* 1994;43:960–967.
9. Geiss LS, Herman WH, Smith PJ. Mortality in non-insulin-dependent diabetes. In: National Diabetes Data Group. *Diabetes in America*, Bethesda, MD: National Institute of Diabetes and Digestive and Kidney Diseases, 1995: 233–257. NIDDKD publication 95-1468.
10. American Diabetes Association. Position statement: diabetic nephropathy. *Diabetes Care* 2000;23[Suppl 1]:69–72.
11. Klein R, Klein BEK. Vision disorders in diabetes. In: National Diabetes Data Group. *Diabetes in America*, Bethesda, MD: National Institute of Diabetes and Digestive and Kidney Diseases, 1995:293–338. NIDDKD publication 95-1468.

12. American Diabetes Association. Position statement: diabetic retinopathy. *Diabetes Care* 2000:23[Suppl 1]:S73–S76.
13. Palumbo PJ, Melton LJ, III. Peripheral vascular disease and diabetes. In: National Diabetes Data Group. *Diabetes in America*. Bethesda, MD: National Institute of Diabetes and Digestive and Kidney Diseases, 1995:401–408. NIDDKD publication 95-1468.
14. Vinik AI, Park TS, Stansberry KB, et al. Diabetic neuropathies. *Diabetologia* 2000;43:957–973.
15. Gregg EW, Beckles GLA, Williamson DE, et al. Diabetes and physical disability among older U.S. adults. *Diabetes Care* 2000;23:1272–1277.
16. Songer TJ. Disability in diabetes. In: National Diabetes Data Group. *Diabetes in America*. Bethesda, MD: National Institute of Diabetes and Digestive and Kidney Diseases, 1995:259–283. NIDDKD publication 95-1468.
17. World Health Organization. *Diabetes mellitus: report of a WHO study group*. Geneva: World Health Organization; 1985. Technical report series 727.
18. Barzilay J, Spiekerman C, Wahl P, et al. Cardiovascular disease in older adults with glucose disorders: comparison of American Diabetes Association criteria for diabetes mellitus with WHO criteria. *Lancet* 1999;354:622–625.
19. Wahl PW, Savage PJ, Psaty BM, et al. Diabetes in older adults: comparison of 1997 American Diabetes Association classification of diabetes mellitus with 1985 WHO classification. *Lancet* 1998;352:1012–1015.
20. DECODE Study Group. Glucose tolerance and mortality: comparison of WHO and American Diabetes Association diagnostic criteria. *Lancet* 1999;354:617–621.
21. DECODE Study Group. Consequences of the new diagnostic criteria for diabetes in older men and women. *Diabetes Care* 1999;22:1667–1671.
22. Harris MI, Eastman RC, Cowie CC, et al. Comparison of diabetes diagnostic categories in the U.S. population according to the 1997 American Diabetes Association and 1980–1985 World Health Organization diagnostic criteria. *Diabetes Care* 1997;20:1859–1862.
23. Shaw JE, de Courten MP. IGT or IFG for predicting NIDDM: who is right, WHO or ADA? *Diabetes* 1998;47[Suppl]:A150(abst).
24. Edelstein SL, Knowler WC, Bain RP, et al. Predictors of progression from impaired glucose tolerance to NIDDM: an analysis of six prospective studies. *Diabetes* 1997;46:701–710.
25. Halter J. Aging and carbohydrate metabolism. In: Masoro EJ, ed. *Handbook of physiology*. Section 11: Aging. Oxford University Press, 1995:119–145.
26. Vokonas PS, Kannel WB. Diabetes mellitus and coronary heart disease in the elderly. *Clin Geriatr Med* 1996;12:69–78.
27. Betteridge DJ. Diabetic dyslipidemias. *Am J Med* 1994;96[Suppl 6A]:25S–31S.
28. Brownlee M, Cerami A, Vlassara H. Advanced glycosylation end products in tissue and the biochemical basis of diabetic complications. *N Engl J Med* 1988; 318:1315–1321.
29. Lyons TJ. Lipoprotein glycation and its metabolic consequences. *Diabetes* 1992; 42[Suppl 2]:67–73.
30. Vijan S, Stevens DL, Herman WH, et al. Screening, prevention, counseling, and treatment for the complications of type II diabetes mellitus. *J Gen Intern Med* 1997;12:567–580.
31. Weiner JP, Parente ST, Stephen T, et al. Variation in office-based quality: a claims-based profile of care provided to Medicare patients with diabetes. *JAMA* 1995;273:1503–1508.
32. Kell S, Drass J, Bausell R. Measures of disease control in Medicare beneficiaries with diabetes mellitus. *J Am Geriatr Soc* 1999;47:417–422.
33. Kenny SJ, Smith PJ, Goldschmid MG, et al. Survey of physician practice behaviors related to diabetes mellitus in the U.S. *Diabetes Care* 1993;16:1507–1510.
34. Harris MI. Medical care for patients with diabetes: epidemiologic aspects. *Ann Intern Med* 1996;124:117–122.
35. Beckles GL, Engelgau MM, Narayan KM, et al. Population-based assessment of the level of care among adults with diabetes in the U.S. *Diabetes Care* 1998; 21:1432–1438.
36. Brown AF, Mangione CM, Saliba D, Sarkisian CA. California Healthcare Foundation/American Geriatrics Society Panel on Improving Care for Elders with Diabetes. Guidelines for improving the care of the older person with diabetes mellitus. *J Am Geriatr Soc* 2003;51[5 Suppl Guidelines]:S265–280.p

36a. Blaum CS, Halter JB. Diabetes in the elderly. *Drug Therapy* 1994;24:18–30.

37. Stuck AE, Siu AL, Wieland GD, et al. Comprehensive geriatric assessment: a meta-analysis of controlled trials. *Lancet* 1993;342:1032–1036.
38. Morely JE, Kaiser FE. Unique aspects of diabetes mellitus in the elderly. *Clin Geriatr Med* 1990;6:693–719.
39. Morley JE, Mooradian AD, Levine AS, et al. Why is diabetic peripheral neuropathy painful? The effect of glucose on pain perception in humans. *Am J Med* 1984;77:79–83.
40. UK Prospective Diabetes Study Group. Tight blood pressure control and risk of macrovascular and microvascular complications in type 2 diabetes: UKPDS 38. *BMJ* 1998;317:703–713.
41. Applegate W. Hypertension. In: Hazzard WR, Blass JP, Ettinger WH, et al, eds. *Principles of geriatric medicine and gerontology*. 4th ed. New York: McGraw-Hill, 1999:713–720.
42. Moritz DJ, Ostfeld AM, Blazer DI, et al. The health burden of diabetes for the elderly in four communities. *Public Health Rep* 1994;109:782–790.
43. Fillenbaum GG, Pieper CF, Cohen HJ, et al. Comorbidity of five chronic health conditions in elderly community residents: determinants and impact on mortality. *J Gerontol* 2000;55A:M84–M89.
44. Wingard DL, Barrett-Connor E. Heart disease and diabetes. In: National Diabetes Data Group. *Diabetes in America*, 2nd ed. Bethesda, MD. National Institute of Diabetes and Digestive and Kidney Diseases, 1995:429–448. NIDDKD publication 95-1468.
45. Kuller LH. Stroke and diabetes. In: National Diabetes Data Group. *Diabetes in America*. 2nd ed. Bethesda, MD. National Institute of Diabetes and Digestive and Kidney Diseases, 1995:449–456. NIDDKD publication 95-1468.
46. The Agency for Healthcare Policy and Research Smoking Cessation Guideline. *JAMA* 1996;275:1270–1280.
47. Curb JD, Pressel SL, Cutler JA, et al. Effect of diuretic-based antihypertensive treatment on cardiovascular disease risk in older diabetic patients with isolated systolic hypertension. *JAMA* 1996;276:1886–1892.
48. Antiplatelet Trialists' Collaboration. Collaborative overview of randomised trials of antiplatelet therapy: prevention of death, myocardial infarction, and stroke by prolonged antiplatelet therapy in various categories of patients. *BMJ* 1994;308:81–106.
49. Vijan S, Hofer TP, Hayward RA. Cost-utility analysis of screening intervals for diabetic retinopathy in patients with type 2 diabetes mellitus. *JAMA* 2000;283: 889–896.
50. UK Prospective Diabetes Study Group. Intensive blood-glucose control with sulphonylureas or insulin compared with conventional treatment and risk of complications in patients with type 2 diabetes. *Lancet* 1998;352:837–852.
51. Albert M. Cognitive function. In: Albert M, Moss M, eds. *Geriatric neuropsychology*. New York: Guilford Press, 1988:33–53.
52. Shorr R, Franze L, Resnick H, et al. Glycemic control of older adults with type 2 diabetes: findings from the Third National Health and Nutrition Survey, 1988–1994. *J Am Geriatr Soc* 2000;48:264–267.
53. Velez L, Blaum C, Halter JB. Diabetes care practices in community-dwelling patients aged 75 and older: glycemic control and treatment compliance. *J Am Geriatr Soc* 1995;43[Suppl]:SA1(abst).
54. Van Nostrand J, Furner S, Suzman R. *Health data on older Americans: United States, 1992*. Hyattsville, MD: National Center for Health Statistics, Centers for Disease Control and Prevention, 1993.
55. Rowe JW, Andres R, Tobin JD, et al. The effect of age on creatinine clearance in men: a cross-sectional and longitudinal study. *J Gerontol* 1976;31:155–163.
56. Naliboff BD, Rosenthal M. Effects of age on complications in adult onset diabetes. *J Am Geriatr Soc* 1989;37:838–842.
57. Mackenzie RA, Phillips LHD. Changes in peripheral and central nerve conduction with aging. *Clin Exp Neurol* 1981;18:109–116.
58. American Diabetes Association. Position statement: nutrition recommendations and principles for people with diabetes mellitus. *Diabetes Care* 2001;24 [Suppl 1]:44.
59. Exercise and NIDDM. *Diabetes Care* 1990;13:785–789.
60. Eriksson J, Lindstrom J, Valle T, et al. Prevention of type II diabetes in subjects with impaired glucose tolerance: the Diabetes Prevention Study (DPS) in Finland—study design and 1-year interim report on the feasibility of the lifestyle intervention programme. *Diabetologia* 1999;42:793–801.
61. Fiatarone MA, O'Neill EF, Doyle N, et al. The Boston FICSIT study: the effects of resistance training and nutritional supplementation on physical frailty in the oldest old. *J Am Geriatr Soc* 1993;41:333–337.
62. Shorr RI, Ray WA, Daugherty JR, et al. Incidence and risk factors for serious hypoglycemia in older persons using insulin or sulfonylureas. *Arch Intern Med* 1997;157:1681–1686.
63. Minaker KL, Rowe JW, Tonino R, et al. Influence of age on clearance of insulin in man. *Diabetes* 1982;31:851–855.
64. Dorfman LJ, Bosley TM. Age-related changes in peripheral and central nerve conduction in man. *Neurology* 1979;29:38–44.
65. O'Brien IA, O'Hare P, Corrall RJ. Heart rate variability in healthy subjects: effect of age and the derivation of normal ranges for tests of autonomic function. *Br Heart J* 1986;55:348–354.
66. Heinsimer JA, Lefkowitz RJ. The impact of aging on adrenergic receptor function: clinical and biochemical aspects. *J Am Geriatr Soc* 1985;33:184–188.
67. Shorr RI, Ray WA, Daugherty JR, et al. Individual sulfonylureas and serious hypoglycemia in older people. *J Am Geriatr Soc* 1996;44:751–755.
68. Kadowaki T, Hagura R, Kajinuma H, et al. Chlorpropamide-induced hyponatremia: incidence and risk factors. *Diabetes Care* 1983;6:468–471.
69. UK Prospective Diabetes Study Group. Effect of intensive blood-glucose control with metformin on complications in overweight patients with type 2 diabetes (UKPDS 34). *Lancet* 1998;352:854–865.
70. Chiasson JL, Josse RG, Hunt JA, et al. The efficacy of acarbose in the treatment of patients with non-insulin-dependent diabetes mellitus: a multicenter controlled clinical trial. *Ann Intern Med* 1994;121:928–935.
71. DeFronzo RA. Pharmacologic therapy for type 2 diabetes mellitus. *Ann Intern Med* 1999;131:281–303.
72. Reaven G, Thompson LW, Nahm D, et al. Relationship between hyperglycemia and cognitive function in older NIDDM patients. *Diabetes Care* 1990; 13:16–20.
73. U'Ren RC, Riddle MC, Lezak MD, et al. The mental efficiency of the elderly person with type II diabetes mellitus. *J Am Geriatr Soc* 1990;38:505–510.
74. Blaum CS, Halter JB. Diabetes and aging. In: Leahy JL, Clark NG, Cefalu WT, eds. *The medical management of diabetes mellitus*. New York: Marcel Dekker, 2000.
75. Mayfield J, Deb P, Potter DEB. Diabetes and long-term care. In: National Diabetes Data Group. *Diabetes in America*, 2nd ed. Bethesda, MD. National Institute of Diabetes and Digestive and Kidney Diseases, 1995:571–590.
76. Mooradian AD, Osterweil D, Petrasek D, et al. Diabetes mellitus in elderly nursing home patients. A survey of clinical characteristics and management. *J Am Geriatr Soc* 1988;36:391–396.
77. Fisher L, Chesla CA, Bartz RJ, et al. The family and type 2 diabetes: a framework for intervention. *Diabetes Educ* 1998;24:599–607.

CHAPTER 44
Women's Health Issues in Diabetes Mellitus

Julie Lund Sharpless

Several aspects of the female reproductive life cycle are influenced by insulin and the metabolic effects of diabetes. From puberty through childbearing to menopause, women with diabetes may need to make special adjustments in their regimens to maintain optimal control as the reproductive hormones change. Conversely, poor diabetic control can impair normal reproductive function. The waning of reproductive hormones at menopause raises special issues in decisions about hormone replacement therapy in women with diabetes, as well as additional risks for osteoporosis and endometrial cancer.

Most investigations into the effects of diabetes on reproductive function have focused on type 1 insulin-dependent diabetes because this is the most prevalent form in women of reproductive age. Insulin resistance also has reproductive consequences, both in severe forms such as type A insulin resistance and in milder forms as in polycystic ovary syndrome. The changing epidemiology of diabetes in the United States, with an increasing prevalence of obesity and an earlier onset of type 2 diabetes, makes the reproductive consequences of insulin-resistant diabetes more significant. Studies of diabetes in postmenopausal women have focused largely on women with insulin-resistant diabetes. Although issues of cardiovascular disease, hyperlipidemia, and endometrial cancer are important in this population, another classic postmenopausal issue, osteoporosis, is of greater concern for women with type 1 diabetes. Thus, this chapter will review both type 1 and type 2 diabetes and their metabolic effects in women. In many studies, the type of diabetes has not been defined by strict standards such as C-peptide, autoimmune antibodies, or insulin levels; thus, subjects described as insulin-dependent may include persons with either type 1 or type 2 diabetes. In these situations the descriptions "insulin-dependent diabetes mellitus" or "non-insulin-dependent diabetes mellitus" are used as specified in those studies, as the heterogeneity of the populations may help reconcile the results.

MENSTRUAL CYCLES

Menarche

In 1925, Dr. Eliot Joslin observed that "unaided by insulin, no girl in our series developed menstruation after the onset of diabetes" (1). By the mid-20th century, a major series by Bergqvist reported delay in menarche of 15 months associated with diabetes (2). More recently, this observation has been contested by studies showing normal menarche in series of clinic patients (3–6). However, subanalyses in several of these studies showed that those girls with the onset of diabetes before 10 years of age or before menarche still had a delay in menarche, as well as more irregular menses (3,6). The major complications of diabetes have now been shown to correlate with glucose control, as these studies would suggest for age of menarche. Most of these studies, however, did not specifically investigate degree of control in relation to onset of menarche. One indirect clue is available from a study by Yeshaya et al. (6), who found that, among women with diabetes, those with diabetic complications were older at menarche and more likely to have amenorrhea than those without complications, but a direct relationship between menarche and glycemic control has not been established.

Menstrual Dysfunction

Beyond menarche, menstrual periods are often disrupted by diabetes. The major problems are absent menses (amenorrhea) or infrequent menses (oligomenorrhea), but overly frequent menses (polymenorrhea, or more commonly called "dysfunctional uterine bleeding") have also been described. Some type of irregular menses has been reported in 22% to 47% of women with diabetes (3,7). These high prevalence rates likely reflect various definitions of irregularity, as the corresponding incidence in controls ranged from 11% to 35%. The lower figures come from one of the most thorough studies of menstrual cycles in insulin-dependent diabetes by Kjaer et al. (3), using an epidemiologic study of an entire county in Denmark. Kjaer and others (3,8) also have found that the incidence of irregularity correlated inversely with diabetic control and with body weight. Specifically, two groups have shown that the incidence of menstrual disturbances increases with the hemoglobin A_{1c} concentration (HbA_{1c}) and becomes statistically significant with HbA_{1c} values above 10% (3,9).

Regular menstrual function requires the integration of neuronal and hormonal signals between the hypothalamus, the pituitary, the ovaries, and the uterus. Neuronal signals in the hypothalamus trigger the pulsatile release of gonadotropin-releasing hormone (GnRH), which causes the pituitary to release follicle-stimulating hormone (FSH) and luteinizing hormone (LH), which in turn stimulate the development of eggs, estrogen, and progesterone in the ovary. The estrogen fosters proliferation of the endometrium and feeds back to the hypothalamus and pituitary to control its own production. No single mechanism of impairment in diabetes has been established, but abnormalities from the hypothalamus to the ovary have been described.

The most clearly described syndrome of menstrual dysfunction in diabetes is a form of hypothalamic amenorrhea. Hypothalamic amenorrhea (HA) results from lack of stimulation by the hypothalamic GnRH to the pituitary LH and FSH. In HA, serum levels of LH and FSH are low, and studies using frequent sampling show that LH and FSH pulses are decreased or absent and insufficient to stimulate ovulation; thus menses do not occur (10). Women with insulin-dependent diabetes and amenorrhea have been found to have low LH and FSH levels, and decreased LH pulses (8,11) (Fig. 44.1). Various investigators have tried to assess GnRH responsiveness of the pituitary gonadotroph cells by administering a single dose of GnRH to women with diabetes, but results are conflicting and not as informative as those from pulse profiles of LH (12). However, a study by South et al. (11) that showed decreased LH pulses in amenorrheic, diabetic women (as compared with normal cycling nondiabetic women), also noted an increased LH response to GnRH. Both decreased pulses and an increased LH response to GnRH are seen in other forms of hypothalamic amenorrhea. The clinical features of HA in diabetic women are similar to those in the general population. As in women with

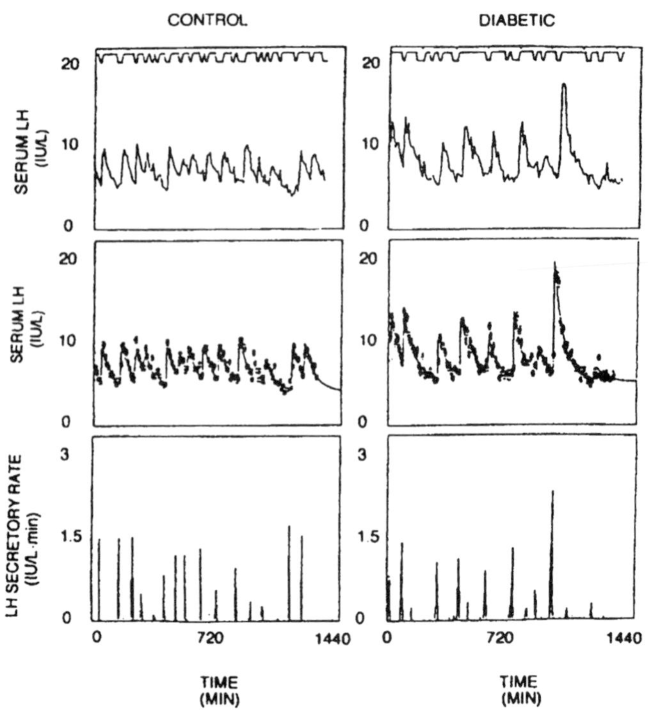

Figure 44.1. Serum luteinizing hormone (LH) pulses in diabetic amenorrhea. Representative profiles of LH concentration versus time series obtained from a eumenorrheic nondiabetic women *(left)* and an amenorrheic diabetic woman *(right)*. (Reprinted from South SA, Asplin CM, Carlson EC, et al. Alterations in luteinizing hormone secretory activity in women with insulin-dependent diabetes mellitus and secondary amenorrhea. *J Clin Endocrinol Metab* 1993;76:1048–1053, with permission. Copyright 1993. The Endocrine Society.)

poorly controlled diabetes, hypothalamic amenorrhea also occurs in nondiabetic women who have inadequate nutrition, frequently as a result of excessive exercise or anorexia nervosa (13). Severe illness can also suppress levels of LH and FSH, as seen in patients hospitalized for other diseases (14). In diabetes, HA may reflect a combination of these factors. Diabetic women with hypothalamic amenorrhea tend to be underweight and/or to have poor glucose control. In the series of HA in diabetes by South et al. (11) and O'Hare et al. (15), women were selected for normal body weight but had elevated mean glycosylated hemoglobin of 12.8% and HbA_{1c} of 11.8%. Djursing et al. (8) included both normal and underweight subjects but did not find a correlation between amenorrhea and glycemic control. An obvious approach to these patients is to improve diabetes control. Unfortunately, after 6 months of improved metabolic control decreasing HbA_{1c} levels from 11.8% to 8.5%, with a concomitant mean weight gain of 4.2 kg, none of six amenorrheic subjects in the series of O'Hare et al. (15) resumed menses, suggesting additional processes contributed to the observed amenorrhea. Women with hypothalamic amenorrhea have an increased risk for estrogen-deficiency osteoporosis (16) and need treatment to restore or replace (i.e., oral contraceptive pills) menstrual cycles to ensure adequate estrogen supplies (17). Although the bone-density response to oral contraceptive pills has not yet been specifically evaluated in diabetes, treatment must be considered because of the additional increased risk of osteoporosis in type 1 diabetes (see discussion below). Other causes of HA, such as eating disorders, which have an increased prevalence in women with diabetes (18), must also be addressed. Even without meeting the full psychiatric DSM III-R criteria for anorexia nervosa or bulimia, 15% to 40% of young women with diabetes disclose disordered eating and underdosing their insulin as a tool for weight loss (19,20). In addition to worsened glycemic control, diabetic patients with eating disorders have an increased incidence of diabetic complications (21,22).

Oligomenorrhea has also been associated with poor glucose control and low body weight in insulin-dependent diabetes (3,8). Some cases of oligomenorrhea in women with diabetes may represent a form fruste of hypothalamic amenorrhea. For research purposes, these studies define hypothalamic amenorrhea as 3 or 6 consecutive months of missed periods and oligomenorrhea as irregular periods occurring nine or fewer times per year. In diabetic women, as in nondiabetic women, the causes of oligomenorrhea are diverse. Oligomenorrhea specific to diabetes has received very little study. Most investigations of oligomenorrhea and diabetes have focused on polycystic ovary syndrome (PCOS) and type 2 diabetes rather than type 1 diabetes. PCOS is defined by oligomenorrhea and hyperandrogenism (such as hirsutism or acne) or hyperandrogenemia (such as elevated serum testosterone concentration or DHEAS). It is often associated with obesity and insulin resistance and carries a high incidence (30%–50%) of subsequent type 2 diabetes (23,24). PCOS is rare in type 1 diabetes with negative C-peptide levels (25). Prelevic et al. (26) found that oligomenorrheic patients with insulin-dependent diabetes who were negative for C-peptide had low androgens and low LH/FSH ratios, while those who were positive for C-peptide had more classic features of PCOS, with elevated androgen levels and LH/FSH ratio and histories of obesity and oligomenorrhea before the diagnosis of diabetes. One recent paper has contested these views, finding a 39% prevalence of PCOS in a group of Spanish patients with insulin-dependent diabetes (27). However, this group did not test C-peptide levels, and controls were excluded if they had signs of hyperandrogenism (hirsutism or acne)—important because normal body hair varies by ethnicity, so higher hirsutism scores are normal in Hispanic women with or without diabetes. Treatment with insulin-sensitizing medications ameliorates the hyperandrogenism of PCOS and has been shown to restore ovulatory cycles (28). Weight loss has also been found to restore regular menses and ovulation, as well as insulin sensitivity in PCOS (29). Because insulin augments LH-driven ovarian androgen synthesis, an elevation in androgens that induces insulin resistance (30) is difficult to distinguish from the elevated insulin levels of insulin resistance that induce hyperandrogenism (31). Blockade of this loop in either direction, by treating the hyperandrogenism (i.e., with the antiandrogens estrogen, flutamide, or spironolactone) or treating the insulin resistance (i.e., with metformin or troglitazone) is effective for PCOS (32).

Oligomenorrhea also is seen in the syndromes of severe insulin resistance. Type A insulin resistance, which is mediated by insulin-receptor defects, and type B insulin resistance, which is mediated by antibodies, share symptom patterns including hirsutism, oligomenorrhea, and hyperandrogenism. Treatment of these syndromes includes the use of antiandrogens, as well as GnRH analogues, to block LH production (33). A defect in the insulin receptor has also been found in some women with PCOS (34).

Ovarian dysfunction is suggested by increased levels of the androgens, including testosterone and androstenedione, in women with insulin-dependent diabetes (35). However, these levels are increased in normally cycling women with insulin-dependent diabetes and are not usually associated with clinical signs of hyperandrogenism such as hirsutism or acne, and the free androgen levels are normal (36). Rather than an ovarian problem, these androgen levels are likely due to the elevated levels of sex hormone–binding globulin (SHBG) stimulated by insulin. This is further supported in a study by Djursing et al. (36) that found that SHBG levels were decreased in the amenorrheic women both with and without diabetes. Thus, hypothalamic, pituitary, and ovarian factors may contribute to menstrual disruption in diabetes.

Carbohydrate Metabolism

Even with regular menstrual cycles, many women with diabetes note changes in their home monitoring of blood glucose results during the cycle. In observational series of women with diabetes, 61% to 70% of patients reported cyclic glucose changes (7,37). Three fourths of these women described higher glucose levels in the luteal phase, especially during the week before menses. A consistent but smaller set report hypoglycemia at the beginning of menses (Fig. 44.2). In Lunt and Brown's study (37), 36% of the women adjusted their insulin to accommodate perimenstrual glucose changes, but this subset did not have better control and even showed a trend toward slightly higher levels of glycosylated hemoglobin. This study did not assess carbohydrate intake or exercise levels but did note that the insulin-adjusting group reported more perimenstrual changes in appetite.

The mechanism behind menstrual glucose changes has been a source of controversy, perhaps because of the heterogeneity of

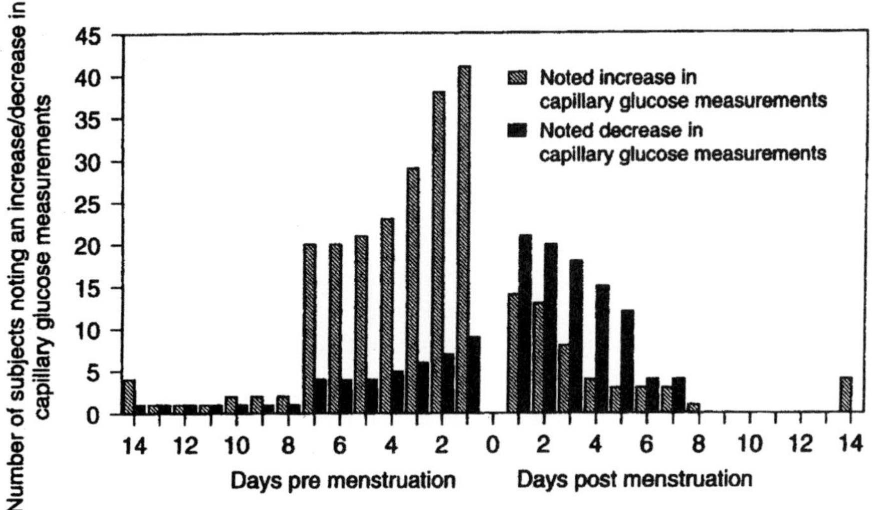

Figure 44.2. Number of subjects noting a perimenstrual change in self-reported capillary glucose measurements. (Reprinted from Lunt H, Brown LJ. Self-reported changes in capillary glucose and insulin requirements during the menstrual cycle. *Diabet Med* 1996;13:525–530, with permission.)

individual responses. In normal cycling, nonobese, nondiabetic women, some (38,39) but not all (40–42), studies of oral glucose tolerance have shown a decline in glucose tolerance during the luteal phase of the menstrual cycle. Progesterone, which increases during the luteal phase, has been implicated as the cause of worsened glucose tolerance because of its ability to induce insulin resistance (43). Intravenous glucose tolerance tests have not, however, shown consistent changes across the menstrual cycle (44). Euglycemic, hyperinsulinemic clamp studies in normal subjects showed no differences in basal levels of glucose, insulin, or glucose turnover during the follicular or luteal phase (45,46). In contrast, in hyperglycemic clamp studies, impaired glucose metabolism is seen in the luteal phase (47). When these same investigators performed hyperglycemic clamp studies in women with insulin-dependent diabetes, they found a heterogeneous response, with no cycle phase differences in some women, and a decrease in luteal-phase insulin sensitivity in others (48). The women who showed cyclic decreases in insulin sensitivity in clamp studies were those who noted premenstrual hyperglycemia; however, they were not different from women without cyclic differences with regard to duration or control of diabetes, age, or body weight. The worsened premenstrual insulin sensitivity was associated with a greater increase in estrogen from the follicular to luteal phase.

The presence or absence of premenstrual syndrome did not affect carbohydrate metabolism assessed by oral glucose tolerance testing in normal subjects across the cycle (41). Premenstrual symptoms in women with diabetes have been correlated only with depression (specifically not hypoglycemia) and do not differ (except the perception by women with diabetes that they were less severe) from those in women without diabetes (7).

SEXUAL DYSFUNCTION

Some surveys have found a high incidence of complaints of sexual dysfunction in women with diabetes, whereas others have reported a similar incidence in women with and without diabetes [reviewed in reference (49)]. The specific components of sexual dysfunction in women are poorly understood. In women as compared with men, sexual function is more variable within an individual and across the life cycle, has a less predictable response to hormones, and is more susceptible to social influences (50). These issues and others have limited research on sexual dysfunction in women, particularly in women with diabetes (51). Extrapolating from research on male sexual dysfunction is not necessarily relevant because of the gender differences in sexual function. For instance, in contrast to studies in men, the first study of sildenafil in women showed no improvement in sexual function (52), although one later study did show some improvement in sexual fantasy and satisfaction (53). Also in contrast to the findings in men, two studies of sexual function in women with diabetes found no correlation between sexual function and glycemic control (with the caveat that the sexual dysfunction predated the diabetes in many of the subjects) (54,55). One study of xerostomia noted that complaints of vaginal dryness were more common in diabetic women who had abnormally low salivary flow rates than in other diabetic women (56). The low salivary flow correlated with higher HbA_{1c} but not with cardiovagal autonomic dysfunction. Thus, although poor diabetic control and extensive vascular and neurologic complications are known to contribute to sexual dysfunction in men (57), few data exist to support parallels in women.

It is important to exclude other comorbid illnesses that can inhibit sexual function. Vulvovaginal candidiasis, which can cause dyspareunia, occurs more frequently in women with poorly controlled diabetes (58,59). Depression, which has an increased prevalence in people with diabetes (60), is also a major cause of sexual dysfunction (61). Treatments for comorbid conditions, particularly depression and hypertension, also can have an impact on sexual function. Treatments for depression, especially selective serotonin reuptake inhibitors, may inhibit sexual function as a side effect but also improve sexual function as the depression is treated (62). Many antihypertensive medications have been implicated in male sexual dysfunction. In women, thiazide diuretics and spironolactone have been noted to decrease vaginal lubrication (49). In summary, diabetes has not yet been shown to be a direct cause of sexual dysfunction in women, but knowledge of the common issues associated with diabetes offers potential therapeutic approaches.

FERTILITY

In women with diabetes who have regular menstrual cycles, the ability to conceive is not affected. Among women with insulin-dependent diabetes diagnosed prior to pregnancy, the cumulative rates of pregnancy (85% in the first year) and of involuntary infertility (17%) were the same as in the control Danish population (63) (Fig. 44.3). In women with menstrual irregularity such as amenorrhea or oligomenorrhea, missed periods represent missed ovulations and therefore decreased opportunity for fertilization. Thus, women with PCOS and diabetes may have decreased fertility (32). Fertility in women with PCOS (studied in nondiabetic patients) is enhanced by weight loss (29) and insulin sensitizers (28). The results of *in vitro* fertilization in a small series of women with insulin-dependent diabetes, in good control as part of the therapy, were not different from the results in women without diabetes (64). Poor glycemic control does not impair the ability to conceive but does impair fertility because of an increase in spontaneous abortion in proportion to the

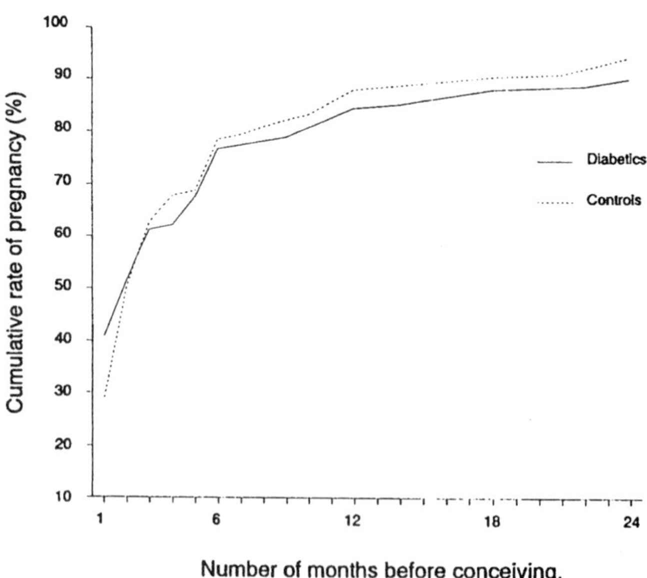

Figure 44.3. Cumulative rate of pregnancy (time to conception) over months for 139 pregnancies in women with diabetes and 199 pregnancies in controls (1959–1989). (Reprinted from Kjaer K, Hagen C, Sando SH. Infertility and pregnancy outcome in an unselected group of women with insulin-dependent diabetes mellitus. *Am J Obstet Gynecol* 1992;166: 1412–1418, copyright 1992, with permission from Elsevier Science.)

increase in HbA_{1c} (65). For women seeking fertility, the first approach should be optimization of glucose control, not only to improve ovulation and decrease the risk of spontaneous abortion but also to decrease the risk of birth defects. The prevalence of fetal malformations is increased when glycemic control is poor during early pregnancy (66) (see Chapter 61).

CONTRACEPTION

Contraception is an essential issue in the care of women with diabetes. Pregnancies must be planned because poor glycemic control during pregnancy leads to an increase in maternal and fetal complications, and good glycemic control reduces that risk (65,66). Nevertheless, most pregnancies in women with diabetes are still unplanned (63). Because of the medical importance of good compliance with the contraceptive regimen in this population, logistical issues are as important as medical effects and side effects associated with various contraceptives (Table 44.1).

For some women with advanced complications of diabetes, contraceptives are necessary for the protection of their own health. Pregnancy may worsen retinopathy (67) and nephropathy (68) and is associated with increased maternal mortality, especially if nephropathy or coronary artery disease is present. For women with these complications who have completed their families, surgical sterilization by tubal ligation should be considered. Women with diabetes need careful counseling on the risks of planned and unplanned pregnancy (see Chapter 61).

Combination Oral Contraceptive Pills

Oral contraceptive pills (OCPs) are the most popular form of reversible contraception and are associated with one of the lowest rates of unintended pregnancy. OCPs combine supraphysiologic doses of estrogen and progesterone and work by several mechanisms, principally by suppressing the hypothalamic and pituitary stimulation of the ovary. A common concern is the potential to worsen glycemic control with OCPs. This stems from reports in which early OCP formulations were used at much higher doses than are currently used. Worsened glucose tolerance was first reported by Waine et al. in 1963 (69), who noted that nondiabetic women treated with a high-dose OCP (containing 100 μg of mestranol) developed impaired glucose tolerance. Women with a history of gestational diabetes mellitus (GDM), a first-degree relative with diabetes, or who are obese or older are at higher risk for the development of impaired glucose tolerance while receiving higher-dose OCPs (70). The impaired glucose tolerance usually reverses within 6 months of discontinuation, except in women with a history of GDM.

Most OCPs currently in use are "low dose" (<50 μg of estradiol) OCPs, which also contain up to a 25-fold lower dose of progesterone and have minimal to no effect on glucose tolerance, even in women with a history of GDM (71–73). In women with pre-existing insulin-dependent diabetes, OCPs can also decrease glucose tolerance, but significant adverse effects on glucose control are very unusual (74). The low-dose OCPs maintain the same contraceptive efficacy as the high-dose OCPs but are associated with a lower risk of some of the other dose-related side effects, such as stroke and cardiovascular disease, effects that have deterred physicians from using OCPs in women with diabetes (75). Not only do changes in the estrogen and progestin doses impact glucose tolerance, so do differences in the particular progestin. The gonane-derived progestins (e.g., norgestrel) produce more hyperinsulinemia (71).

Various OCP formulations can have minor or marked effects on lipids, changes particularly important in women with diabetes who already are at increased cardiovascular risk. In a large study of nine different OCPs used by 1,040 women (without diabetes), compounds with desogestrel increased high-density lipoprotein (HDL) cholesterol and decreased low-density lipoprotein (LDL) cholesterol, compounds with levonorgestrel decreased HDL and increased LDL, and norethindrone had an

TABLE 44.1. Effectiveness of Family-Planning Methods

Effectiveness group	Family-planning method	Pregnancies/100 women in first 12 mo of use (as commonly used)
Always very effective	Norplant implants	0.1
	Vasectomy	0.2
	DMPA and NET-EN injectables	0.3
	Female sterilization	0.5
	TCu-380A intrauterine device	0.8
	Progestogen-only oral contraceptives (during breast-feeding)	1
	Lactational amenorrhea method	2
Effective when used correctly and consistently	Combined oral contraceptives	6–8
	Progestogen-only oral contraceptives (not during breast-feeding)	[a]
	Male condoms	14
Only somewhat effective as commonly used	Coitus interruptus	19
	Diaphragm with spermicide	20
	Fertility awareness–based methods	20
	Female condoms	21
	Spermicides	26
	Cap: nulliparous women	20
	Cap: parous women	40
	No method	85

DMPA, depot medroxyprogesterone acetate.
[a]Outside the context of breast-feeding, progestogen-only contraceptives are somewhat less effective than combined oral contraceptives.
Adapted from World Health Organization. *Improving access to quality care in family planning medical eligibility criteria for contraceptive use,* 2nd ed. WHO/RHR/002. Geneva: World Health Organization, 2000.

intermediate effect (76) (Fig. 44.4). Petersen et al. (77) examined the effects of OCPs with norethisterone, levonorgestrel, and gestodene in 30 diabetic women and found no adverse changes in plasma lipids from any of the compounds. In rare cases, OCPs can induce severe hypertriglyceridemia. This is mostly a risk for women with baseline triglycerides greater than 600 mg/dL (78). Estrogens are contraindicated in patients with any of the familial hypertriglyceridemia syndromes because of the increased risk of pancreatitis. Women with diabetes who are receiving estrogen therapies should have their lipid profiles monitored because poor glycemic control also results in elevated triglycerides. This effect is secondary to the decrease in lipoprotein lipase activity caused by relative insulin deficiency.

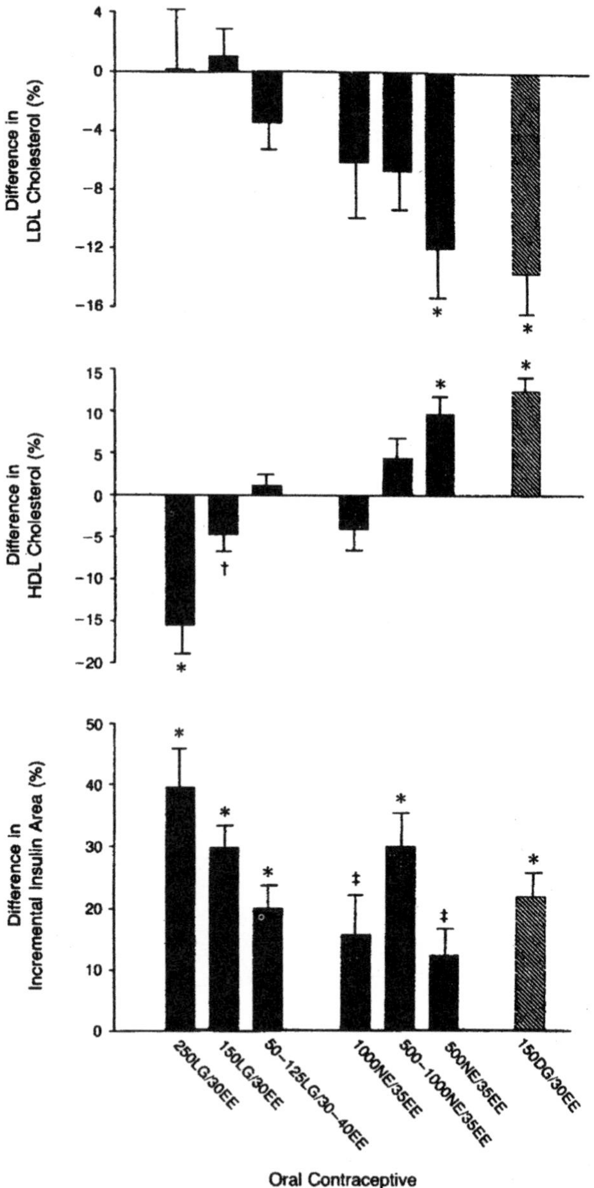

Figure 44.4. Lipid changes in women taking oral contraceptives. Percent differences in HDL and LDL cholesterol levels between women taking one of seven combination oral contraceptives and those not taking oral contraceptives. LG, levonorgestrel; NE, norethindrone; DG, desogestrel; EE, ethinyl estradiol. Numbers denote dosage (μg). (Reprinted from Godsland IF, Crook D, Simpson R, et al. The effects of different formulations of oral contraceptive agents on lipid and carbohydrate metabolism. *N Engl J Med* 1990;323:1375–1381, with permission. Copyright © 1990 Massachusetts Medical Society. All rights reserved.)

Hypertension, another infrequent side effect of OCPs in normal women (79), merits careful attention in the diabetic population. Studies of the use of high-dose OCPs in healthy women demonstrated new hypertension in 4% to 5% and worsening in 9% to 16% of women with pre-existing hypertension (80). This effect may be due to both the estrogen and the progestin components and is reversible with cessation of the OCP. Angiotensinogen production is increased by ethinyl estradiol (81), and progestins may have mineralocorticoid agonist or antagonist effects. Sudden development or worsening of hypertension after starting OCPs should be considered a complication of the medication and mandates discontinuation of the OCP. Few data exist for women with diabetes, except for the lack of problems noted in studies looking at other aspects of OCPs in carefully selected populations. A large (384 women with type 1 diabetes) and reassuring cross-sectional study by Klein et al. (82) showed no association between current or past use of OCPs and severity of hypertension or retinopathy or level of current glycemic control. Another smaller retrospective study also showed that the use of OCPs in women with a mean age of 22.7 years but a mean duration of diabetes of 13.8 years did not increase the risk of their developing early retinopathy or nephropathy (83).

Concern about increased risk of macrovascular complications stems in part from early retrospective observations in a series of diabetic women who were taking high-dose formulations, among whom cerebrovascular thromboses developed in three and myocardial infarction in one of 120 women who used OCPs compared with no such events in the control group who used nonhormonal contraception (84). This increased risk has been supported by subsequent studies demonstrating relative risks from 1.8 to 6.9 in women with diabetes versus nondiabetic OCP users (85,86). However, neither of these studies assessed the relative risk of cerebral or myocardial infarction in women with diabetes not taking OCPs. Another study showed an increased relative risk of stroke in women with diabetes that was the same in users and nonusers of OCPs (87). The risk for cardiovascular events is likely based on thrombotic events, which were increased in women taking OCPs (88), and may be related to the increased clotting factors (factor X, factor II, plasminogen, PAI-1) and decreased platelet aggregation that occur with OCPs (89) and with hyperinsulinemia and hyperglycemia (90,91). Older studies also showed some increased risk among nondiabetic OCP users as compared with nonusers, but the newer (low-dose estrogen and second- and third-generation progestins) OCPs are actually associated with the same or lower risk of cardiovascular disease in nonsmoking, nondiabetic OCP users (88,92,93). It is controversial whether these studies can appropriately account for the excess risk of cardiovascular disease due to smoking, which is high and accounts for the majority of myocardial infarctions in young women (94,95). In nonsmoking women with well-controlled, uncomplicated diabetes, there is probably not an excess risk of cardiovascular disease associated with OCP use, but this has not yet been confirmed in prospective studies. A large retrospective study by Klein et al. (96) did not show any excess mortality in diabetic OCP users. Thus, in otherwise healthy women with diabetes, OCPs decrease health risks by decreasing the risks associated with unintended pregnancy. For women with complications of diabetes, especially vascular disease, or who smoke, these additional risks of estrogen-progestin–based OCPs must be weighed in comparison to the additional risks of pregnancy.

Newly available transdermal forms of estrogen-progestin contraceptives offer the possibility of a lower thrombotic risk based on extrapolation from lower-dose transdermal hormone replacement therapy (97). Another recent therapy is the use of

TABLE 44.2. Lipid Profiles in Women with Diabetes Taking Oral Contraceptive Pills

Type of contraceptive	Fasting glucose	Total cholesterol	Triglycerides	HDL cholesterol	LDL cholesterol
Combined OCPs	↑	↓	↑	↑	↓
DMPA	↑	↑	↔	↓	↑
Norplant	↔	↓	↔	↓	↓
IUD	↓	↓	↔	↔	↓↔

DMPA, depot medroxyprogesterone acetate; HDL, high-density lipoprotein; IUD, intrauterine device; LDL, low-density lipoprotein; OCPs, oral contraceptive pills.
Adapted from Diab KM, Zaki MM. Contraception in diabetic women: comparative metabolic study of Norplant, depot medroxyprogesterone acetate, low dose oral contraceptive pill and CuT380A. *J Obstet Gynaecol Res* 2000; 26:17–26.

OCP tablets taken in extra doses as emergency postcoital contraception. This approach provides higher acute but less chronic exposure to estrogen and progesterone and is more convenient. Unfortunately, it is often poorly tolerated and not as effective as regular OCP use (98). Data are not yet available on the use of these newer contraceptive options in women with diabetes.

Progesterone

A major advantage of progesterone-based contraceptives is the lack of thrombotic or hypertensive effects (75,81). Weight gain and irregular bleeding are, however, common side effects. Progesterone contraceptive options include daily pills, short-term depot injections lasting 3 months (e.g., Depo-Provera), and long-term implants in silastic capsules lasting 5 years (Norplant). Intrauterine devices also may be coated with progesterone. Progesterone-only "mini-pills" are not as effective at suppressing ovulation as are combined OCPs, but they effectively decrease the volume of cervical mucus and increase its viscosity to block implantation (98). Progesterone-only pills have not been studied for their effects on glucose control in women with diabetes, but their high risk of failure is a concern (98). Depot formulations of progesterone do not fail as frequently, but they may increase insulin resistance slightly (99) and are associated with weight gain in some individuals (98). Subdermal levonorgestrel (Norplant) offers the advantage of long-lasting contraception (up to 5 years), which is suitable for many younger women, but requires a minor surgical procedure for insertion. Long-acting progesterone formulations offer good contraception for patients who are unable to comply with daily pills. Emergency contraception can also be accomplished with progesterone alone, using two doses of levonorgestrel ("Plan B"), which would have little metabolic impact on diabetes but is less effective than chronic use (98).

Progesterone contraceptives all worsen glucose tolerance to some degree, which is an issue especially for women at high risk of progressing to type 2 diabetes, such as those with a history of gestational diabetes or PCOS. Kim et al. (100) performed a case-control study of depot medroxyprogesterone acetate (DMPA) users compared with OCP users among Navaho women, a group at very high risk for development of diabetes. They found that the risk of diabetes doubled in women who used DMPA compared with the risk in women with no history of contraceptive use and that the risk increased with longer use. Women gained approximately 3 kg during the first year of use, but the excess risk of developing diabetes persisted even after adjustment for body mass index (BMI) ([weight (kg)]/[height $(m)^2$]). Interestingly, the risk of developing diabetes was lower in the OCP group than in either the control or DMPA groups. In women with preexisting diabetes, changes in glucose tolerance due to progesterone contraceptives, which were greatest with norgestrel, did not necessitate an increase in insulin doses (71). Use of continuous subdermal levonorgestrel was found to increase insulin resistance progressively to a plateau after the first 6 months of use (101). Lipid profiles in women with diabetes showed increased LDL cholesterol and decreased HDL cholesterol with DMPA but decreases in both LDL and HDL with subdermal levonorgestrel or IUD (99) (Table 44.2). Concerns have also been raised about possible decreased bone density in women using DMPA. Prospective studies (in women without diabetes) have now shown that, compared with women using OCPs, women using DMPA lose bone (17,102), but whether this is reversible on cessation of therapy has not been assessed.

Nonhormonal Contraception

Nonhormonal methods, including condoms, IUDs, rhythm methods, and sterilization, have no systemic effects and provide safer contraception for women at high risk for vascular or clotting problems. However, except sterilization, they are associated with high failure rates (98). Male condoms are the only form of contraception offering protection from infectious disease. IUDs, which act principally by a mechanical effect to block implantation, often are coated with progesterone to increase their efficacy. They do not have any disadvantages specific to women with diabetes except for the high rates of unplanned pregnancy at 3.5% and of discontinuation—after 24 months of use, only 57% of women were still using the IUD (103). In studies of IUDs in women with diabetes, side effects were frequent and included expulsion and removal for bleeding or pain but were not different from results in nondiabetic women (103,104). Contraception based on either coitus interruptus or timing of ovulation ("rhythm method") is highly ineffective and is not recommended.

DIABETIC MASTOPATHY

Diabetic mastopathy is a rare complication unique to diabetes. It is a fibro-inflammatory disease of the breast that presents as a firm, nontender breast lump (or lumps) and may be difficult to distinguish from malignancy on physical examination. It occurs mostly in premenopausal women but has been described in men (105). Nearly all reported cases have been in patients with type 1 diabetes; the few patients with type 2 diabetes were taking insulin (106). Diabetic mastopathy is described in women with an average duration of diabetes of 13 (106) to 18 years (107) and occurs in the setting of other diabetic complications, including retinopathy, neuropathy, and nephropathy (106). On mammograms, diabetic mastopathy appears as dense parenchymal changes, while ultrasound also shows nonspecific changes with acoustic shadowing (108). Pathologic specimens show keloidal fibrosis with mononuclear perivasculitis and mononuclear ductitis or lobulitis (106,109). These lesions are benign and are not associated with an increased incidence of neoplasia. In the largest series of 19 cases, four were bilateral and six recurred, highlighting the need for awareness that could spare these women repeated biopsies (110).

MENOPAUSE

Menopause is defined as the permanent cessation of menstrual periods and represents the loss not only of ovarian follicles but also of the elevations of estrogen and progesterone that accompanied the monthly maturation of those follicles. In addition to the loss of menses, the immediate effects of the loss of the steroid hormones are hot flashes and vaginal dryness. In the longer term, the hypogonadism of menopause is associated with increased cardiovascular risk and osteoporosis, both of which are increased in women with diabetes even before menopause.

The age of menopause in women with type 1 diabetes (111) and type 2 diabetes (111,112) has been shown to be the same as that in other women in the same populations. However, the possibility of extensive complications of diabetes secondarily terminating ovarian function was not evaluated in these studies, which included subjects with a mean duration of disease of 9 and 17 years and did not assess complications. One recent report did describe an earlier age of menopause associated with diabetes. In the Familial Autoimmune Diabetes Study, women who were diagnosed before 1964 and had a mean duration of disease of 34 years were a mean of 6 years younger at natural menopause than were their contemporaries who did not have diabetes (113). However, this study includes only 15 women who have reached menopause, five of whom had premature ovarian failure and another autoimmune disease, which can be part of the polyglandular autoimmune syndrome. Data from further follow-up of this cohort will be very interesting.

Premature ovarian failure (POF), defined as menopause before the age of 40, is a component of several uncommon syndromes that also include diabetes (Table 44.3). One of the more frequent of these is polyglandular autoimmune disease, type II. Polyglandular autoimmune syndromes are the associations of multiple destructive autoimmune diseases in endocrine tissues.

TABLE 44.3. Syndromes with Diabetes and Premature Ovarian Failure

Syndrome	Type of diabetes	Type of hypogonadism	Other clinical features	Etiology
Polyglandular autoimmune syndrome	Autoimmune	Primary	Primary hypothyroidism, Addison disease, celiac sprue, pernicious anemia	Destructive lymphocytic infiltration
Hemochromatosis	Insulin resistant or deficient	Primary or secondary	Bronze pigmentation, cirrhosis, dilated cardiomyopathy, loss of body hair	Autosomal dominant defects causing iron overload
Turner's syndrome	Insulin resistant or autoimmune	Primary	Short stature, webbed neck, hearing loss, shield-chest, low hairline, thyroiditis	45 XO karyotype
Down syndrome	Insulin resistant	Primary	Mongoloid facies, cardiac structural abnormalities, mental retardation, shortened phalanges	Trisomy 21
Pseudohypoparathyroidism	Insulin resistant	Primary (resistance to LH, FSH)	Short stature, short metacarpals, round facies, parathyroid hormone resistance	Gαs-inactivating mutations
Crow-Fukase (POEMS) syndrome	Insulin resistant	Primary	Polyneuropathy, organomegaly, endocrinopathies, M-proteins, skin disorder	Plasma cell dyscrasia
Ataxia telangiectasia	Insulin resistant	Primary	Early ataxia, oculocutaneous telangectasia, immunodeficiencies, dysgenetic gonads	Autosomal recessive defect in DNA repair (in ATM helicase)
Fanconi anemia	Insulin resistant	Primary	Short stature, bone marrow hypoplasia, radius malformations, abnormal pigmentation	Autosomal recessive proximal renal tubule dysfunction due to DNA-repair defect
Werner syndrome	Insulin resistant	Primary	Premature aging, atrophic skin, cataracts, early osteopenia, atherosclerosis	Autosomal recessive defect in DNA repair (in Wrn helicase)
Myotonic dystropy	Insulin resistant	Primary or secondary	Muscular dystrophy, mental retardation, premature balding, hypothyroidism	Autosomal dominant trinucleotide repeat in protein kinase DMPK
Prader-Willi syndrome	Insulin resistant	Secondary	Infantile hypotonia, mental retardation, short stature, morbid obesity	Chromosomal deletion in SNRP gene
Kearns-Sayre syndrome	Insulin deficient	Secondary	Ocular myopathy, pigmentary retinopathy, cardiac conduction defects, ataxia	Chromosomal deletions in mitochondrial DNA

FSH, follicle-stimulating hormone; LH, leutenizing hormone.

Type II polyglandular autoimmune disease, or Schmidt syndrome, includes the constellation of autoimmune thyroid disease and Addison disease in association with autoimmune diabetes as redefined by Carpenter in 1964 (114). POF occurs in less than 10% of these patients; other infrequent manifestations are pernicious anemia, celiac sprue, lymphocytic hypophysitis, and vitiligo (115). Schmidt syndrome has incompletely penetrant, autosomal dominant inheritance with onset usually in the 20s or 30s. The individual components may occur in any order. Therefore, in patients with autoimmune diabetes and amenorrhea, thyroid disease and adrenal insufficiency must be considered as reversible causes of menstrual dysfunction. The diagnosis of POF is made by amenorrhea with an increased FSH before the age of 40 years. After the exclusion of other causes (chemotherapy, radiation, or karyotype abnormalities), antiovarian antibodies are present in 27% of patients with POF (116). POF is not reversible, but some ovarian follicles may still be present at diagnosis. For women seeking fertility, careful monitoring may reveal these rare ovulations, and pregnancies have occurred (117,118). Once the diagnosis of premature ovarian failure is established, it is important to screen for thyroid and adrenal failure.

Turner syndrome, which may be less evident in its mosaic form, can include insulin-resistant diabetes and POF due to primary gonadal failure. Hemachromatosis, associated with iron overload in various organs, including the pancreas, liver, and pituitary, may present with diabetes and secondary gonadal failure. Menstrual bleeding reduces the incidence of iron overload in women. Crow-Fukase syndrome (POEMS) is a plasma cell dyscrasia with polyneuropathy, organomegaly, endocrinopathy, M protein, and skin changes. This disease usually has an onset in the sixth decade, so the gonadal failure may not be recognized if a woman is already peri- or postmenopausal. Several more rare diseases such as Kearns-Sayre syndrome (with myopathy) and myotonic dystrophy can present with POF and diabetes. Also, syndromes with impaired DNA repair and/or metabolism such as Werner syndrome (with premature aging), Fanconi anemia (with proximal tubular defects), and ataxia-telangiectasia, are associated with diabetes and gonadal failure. In these entities, other features of the syndrome will signal the diagnosis.

Perimenopausal Symptoms

Despite the various influences of diabetes on menstrual function, little research has been done regarding symptoms at the cessation of menses. No increase in hot flashes is seen in women with diabetes (112). The incidence of vaginal dryness may be increased in relation to HbA_{1c} (56), but genitourinary atrophy at menopause has not been specifically studied. One would expect no differences in short-term hormone replacement therapy for treatment of these symptoms, but this also has not been formally studied. In one study of uncomplicated type 2 diabetes, the incidence of postmenopausal anxiety and depression was slightly increased and was associated with duration of disease and premenopausal depression (119). It is well documented that depression in general is about twice as common in the diabetic population as in the nondiabetic population and that depression is more prevalent in women with diabetes than in men with diabetes (60).

Hormone Replacement Therapy

Estrogen replacement therapy is the prescription of low-dose estrogen in postmenopausal women with the intent of reversing the changes of menopause. In women who have not undergone hysterectomy, the use of progesterone with estrogen is necessary to prevent endometrial cancer. The combination of estrogen and progesterone is termed *hormone replacement therapy* (HRT). Before the need for progesterone was recognized, most women received estrogen alone, and higher doses were used; thus, some older studies of *estrogen replacement therapy* (ERT) show side effects that may be different from those expected if the studies were done with HRT. ERT using the same estrogen doses as HRT is currently appropriate for women who have had a hysterectomy. HRT has been used for short-term treatment of perimenopausal symptoms and long-term reduction of cardiovascular risk and as a major therapy for osteoporosis. Most of the literature on HRT is based on large population studies that include very few women with diabetes. Because of their increased risk for cardiovascular disease, dyslipidemias, and osteoporosis, the risks and benefits of HRT are particularly important for women with diabetes. New prospective data (covered below) have dramatically altered the prescription of HRT for cardiovascular protection, and more data are necessary to apply to decisions for women with diabetes.

Cardiovascular Disease

The cardiovascular benefits of HRT have been the major reason for its use in nondiabetic women. Premenopausal women have a lower risk of heart disease than do men of the same age, but that advantage disappears after menopause. Large-scale epidemiologic studies have shown that restoration of the premenopausal hormones with HRT is associated with a 30% to 50% reduction in death from cardiovascular disease (120–122). Unfortunately, most of the major studies (Rancho-Bernardo, Postmenopausal Estrogen/Progestin Interventions, Framingham, and Nurses' Health) include relatively few women with diabetes. On the basis of these studies, it used to be recommended that most postmenopausal women use HRT to reduce cardiovascular risk. Mortality due to cardiovascular disease is fourfold greater in postmenopausal women with diabetes than in postmenopausal women without diabetes (123). However, premenopausal women with diabetes do not share the lower premenopausal cardiovascular risk in comparison to men that is seen in women without diabetes (124). This suggests that premenopausal women with diabetes may derive less cardiovascular benefit from HRT. Two case-control studies in diabetic women have shown that current users of HRT have no increased risk or a reduced risk of myocardial infarction compared with never-users (96,125).

Several components of the cardiovascular system that may contribute to the estrogen-associated mortality benefits are adversely affected in diabetes, including lipids, carbohydrate metabolism, hemostasis, and vascular function. In addition, the effects of diabetes on the incidence of coronary heart disease are exacerbated by each of the standard risk factors: smoking, hypertension, lipid concentrations, and BMI (126). Short-term studies (6–12 weeks) of ERT and HRT in women with type 2 diabetes have shown improvement in lipid profiles and in glucose control (127,128). These metabolic effects are relevant when HRT is used for any indication.

Lipids

Women's total and LDL cholesterol levels increase after menopause. This change in the lipid profile is associated with an increased risk of cardiovascular disease and is improved with HRT (129). Up to 25% of the benefits of HRT have been attributed to the effects on lipids (122). Diabetes can further exacerbate the postmenopausal lipid profile, and treatment is

TABLE 44.4. Lipid Profiles in Postmenopausal Women with Diabetes

Characteristic	Total cholesterol	Triglycerides	HDL cholesterol	LDL cholesterol
Postmenopausal	↑	↔	↓	↑
Postmenopausal with DM	↑↑	↑↑	↓	↑
Postmenopausal with DM on HRT	↓	↑	↑	↓

DM, diabetes mellitus; HDL, high-density lipoprotein; HRT, hormone replacement therapy; LDL, low-density lipoprotein.

essential because of the already heightened risk of cardiovascular disease in diabetes. In patients with type 1 diabetes, the most common abnormality is an elevation of very-low-density lipoprotein (VLDL) triglycerides, which is correlated with diabetic control (130). This elevation is due to the dependence of triglyceride clearance on the activity of lipoprotein lipase, which is insulin-dependent, as well as to the increase in production of VLDL from the mobilization of free fatty acids. In type 2 diabetes, insulin resistance and obesity combine to cause additional elevations in LDL cholesterol and/or to lower the HDL cholesterol (Table 44.4). Studies of HRT in type 2 diabetes show improvement in LDL cholesterol with little or no change in total cholesterol and a small increase or no change in triglycerides (even in a subset starting with elevated triglycerides) (127,131–134). Although two (127,132) of these studies found an improvement in HDL cholesterol, the others found no change or a small decline. Transdermal HRT regimens do not present the same high dose of estrogen to the liver and do not appear to raise the triglyceride level as much as do oral regimens in women without diabetes. In fact, the one study looking at transdermal estrogen use in type 2 diabetes found a decrease in total cholesterol and triglycerides (97). Because there is also a rare risk of severe hypertriglyceridemia with ERT (78), transdermal estrogens are a better choice for women with moderately elevated triglycerides, but any estrogen is contraindicated in women with markedly elevated triglycerides (>600 mg/dL). Poor glucose control without other metabolic problems typically increases triglyceride concentrations only by twofold to threefold, but in combination with many illnesses and medications that cause hypertriglyceridemia, or in the presence of familial hyperlipoproteinemia syndromes, severe hypertriglyceridemia is more likely to occur.

Glucose Tolerance

Although glucose intolerance was seen in early studies of OCPs and high-dose ERT (100 μg of ethinyl estradiol) (135), current low-dose oral HRT, which has approximately 1/20 the dose of estrogen, has not been shown to adversely affect insulin sensitivity and may improve it. Data from large cohort studies show lower fasting glucose levels in nondiabetic and diabetic women taking estrogen (136,137). Also there is neither a deterioration in glucose tolerance after 12 months of estrogen use in normal women (138) nor an increase in the number of women who develop diabetes after using HRT for several years (139). Decreases in HbA_{1c} have been demonstrated in women with type 2 diabetes taking HRT (128,133,140,141). Brussaard et al. (127) have demonstrated decreases in HbA_{1c}, hepatic glucose production, and waist/hip ratio after 6 weeks use of HRT in type 2 diabetes.

Vascular Effects

A concern about HRT that has been carried over from the experience with OCPs is the risk of hypertension. Fortunately, HRT does not appear to increase the risk of hypertension and has even been shown (in nondiabetic women) to lower blood pressure by a few points (142). One small prospective study looking at HRT in type 2 diabetes saw no change in resting blood pressure (140). Szekacs et al. (143) observed a protective effect of decreased proteinuria without a change in blood pressure.

Vascular changes have also been proposed as a mechanism for decreased cardiovascular morbidity and mortality among women receiving HRT. In nondiabetic women, estrogen has been shown to have a myriad of effects on the vasculature, decreasing plasma fibrinogen and PAI-1 concentrations and stimulating nitric oxide release and vasodilation, as well as long-term genomic effects promoting vasodilation and repair of endothelial cell damage (91). Patients with diabetes have an increased risk of thrombosis, which could be due to vascular dysfunction or altered coagulability but is still poorly understood. Increased levels of fibrinogen, PAI-1, and some of the coagulation factors, as well as abnormalities of platelets and endothelial function, have been found (144). Although levels of some of these factors have been evaluated with HRT in women with diabetes, no correlation has yet been made with absolute risk of clotting. This represents an important area for further study.

Very recently, prospective data that are causing some concern regarding the use of HRT in nondiabetic women are becoming available. The Heart and Estrogen/Progestin Replacement Study (HERS) has shown no clear benefits from HRT for secondary prevention of cardiovascular disease in the first 4 years of treatment (145). The risk of a recurrent coronary heart disease was skewed to a marked increase in the first 4 months of therapy, which tapered down until a relative advantage showed in years 4 and 5. This has been further substantiated by Heckbert et al. (146), who found an increased risk of recurrent myocardial infarction within 60 days of the initiation of HRT, which declined thereafter. These studies highlight the importance of prospective data. Although the above studies of serum markers of cardiovascular risk factors show improvement with HRT in patients with diabetes, it will be several years before definitive evidence of potential mortality benefits of HRT in diabetes becomes available. In the meantime, most guidelines are discouraging the initiation of HRT solely for cardiovascular risk reduction.

OSTEOPOROSIS

The extension of the average life expectancy of people with diabetes that has accompanied improvements in medical care has increased the significance of osteoporosis. Although once controversial, the evidence that bone health is compromised in diabetes is now strong. Bone mineral density (BMD) is lower and the risk of fractures is increased. Several mechanisms have been proposed for diabetes-related osteoporosis and include both the comorbidities of diabetes and more direct pathophysiologic effects of the disease itself.

Fractures

Hip fractures, in particular, are now recognized not only as a major cause of morbidity and mortality but also for their significant impact on economic and social circumstances. Mortality is high in the general population with hip fractures, but the presence of diabetes in a patient with a hip fracture is a risk factor for increased mortality (147). Case-control studies of patients with hip fractures have found an excess of patients with diabetes, suggesting at least a twofold relative risk in all patients with diabetes (148). Women with type 1 diabetes had a 6.9- to 12-fold relative risk of hip fractures compared with women without diabetes (149,150). Data are controversial about the risk of hip and spine fractures in patients with type 2 diabetes. Most studies (148–151) in women with type 2 diabetes also have found an increased risk of hip fractures, with estimates of relative risk almost double the risk in other postmenopausal women. In the Study of Osteoporotic Fractures, women older than 65 years with type 2 diabetes (as defined by excluding those with a diagnosis before the age of 40 years or with a BMI <30), had an increased risk of hip and proximal humerus fractures despite having a higher BMD than women without diabetes (152). There was also a trend toward increased risk of vertebral, forearm, ankle, and foot fractures. In contrast, other investigators have found fewer fractures in women with type 2 diabetes, with a similarly increased BMD at the spine (153,154). The one site with an undisputed increased fracture risk is the foot, which may be related in part to obesity or neuropathy (152,155,156). Focal osteopenia and fractures associated with severe diabetic peripheral neuropathy (Charcot foot) are long recognized as a complication of any type of diabetes.

Bone Density

Although many factors influence the probability of fractures, including number and type of falls, padding of the bony prominences, and geometry of the bone, the most significant factor is the strength of the bone itself. Bone strength is proportional to BMD, which can be measured radiographically. An individual measurement is classified based on the degree of radiographic density in comparison to that in a normal population, with osteopenia defined as 1.0 to 2.5 standard deviations below normal and osteoporosis defined as 2.5 or more standard deviations below normal (157). Bone densitometry techniques have become much more sophisticated in the past two decades, allowing more precise and accurate measurement, as well as measurement at different sites. Based on these changes, more-recent data are more sensitive to differences between groups.

Osteopenia was initially described in adolescents with diabetes, 50% of whom were found to have decreased cortical and trabecular forearm BMD (158). Several subsequent studies found that the forearm BMD in children with only 4 to 6 years of type 1 diabetes was 20% to 50% lower than that in controls (159). One study examining vertebral BMD did not see a difference in children with diabetes (160). Most studies in adults confirm that BMD is lower in patients with type 1 diabetes than in subjects without diabetes (111,161). In contrast, studies in women with type 2 diabetes, controlling for age and obesity, show BMD that is either the same or greater than that in normal subjects (153,154), even in patients treated with insulin (111) (Fig. 44.5). The Rancho Bernardo studies also looked at men with type 2 diabetes and found that their BMD was similar to that in men with normal glucose tolerance, despite the differences the studies found in women (162).

Mechanisms

Is osteoporosis another complication of poor glycemic control? Short-term measures of control such as glucose levels or HbA_{1c} levels would not be expected to reflect cumulative bone damage measured by BMD. Diabetic complications are the cumulative results of long-term poor control. Several investigators have demonstrated an association between BMD and microvascular complications, with the BMD inversely correlated with the presence and extent of microvascular complications in women with normal menstrual cycles (161,163). Mathiassen et al. (164) observed the BMDs of 19 patients with type 1 diabetes (8 women), initially free of complications and found that after 11 years only those who developed retinopathy or proteinuria had worsening of their BMD. The presence of severe peripheral neuropathy in patients with type 1 diabetes has also been found to correlate with decreased BMD at all sites, in comparison to patients with type 1 diabetes without neuropathy and in comparison to healthy subjects (165). Although these were small groups, they were matched for other complications and for activity levels. Using the same paradigm, Forst et al. (166) found a decreased BMD in the cortical bone at the hip and distal limb in association with peripheral neuropathy but normal BMD in the spine of patients with insulin-dependent diabetes. In the Blue Mountain Eye Study in Australia, an association between retinopathy and all fractures was seen in both men and women with all types of diabetes (167). Hypercalciuria has long been noted in patients with poorly controlled insulin-dependent diabetes (168,169) and non–insulin-dependent diabetes (170,171) and has been shown to improve with improved HbA_{1c} (172). Comparably, one study has shown attenuation of bone loss in patients with type 1 diabetes with good glucose control (173). Thus, metabolic control appears to be a major factor in the increased incidence of osteoporosis in patients with diabetes. Poor control, however, would not appear to be the only factor, unless there were also a concomitant compensatory factor to increase BMD in patients with type 2 diabetes.

If the relationship between osteoporosis and diabetes were related only to hyperglycemia, one would expect a similar incidence of osteoporosis in patients with type 1 and type 2 diabetes, but most studies show more osteoporosis in patients with type 1 diabetes (111,174). There may be differences between types of diabetes other than glucose control that impact BMD. Several factors have been investigated, including treatment with insulin, endogenous insulin levels, age of onset, and HbA_{1c}, but the actual mechanism for lower BMD in type 1 diabetes is not known. Osteoporosis is also not associated with exogenous insulin treatment per se. Krakauer et al. (173) and Tuominen et al. (111) separately compared patients with type 1 and type 2 diabetes treated with insulin, showing that insulin is not the cause of the bone loss. Krakauer et al. also found decreased BMD in men and women with type 1 diabetes as compared with those with type 2 diabetes or with controls. Epidemiologic studies at Rancho Bernardo, California, and in Rotterdam, The Netherlands, suggested a correlation between fasting insulin level and BMD in nondiabetic women (175,176). In patients with type 2 diabetes, no consistent association of BMD with endogenous insulin levels, using fasting and 2-hour postchallenge levels, has been found (162,177,178). An autoimmune- or inflammation-mediated process has also been considered because a decrease in BMD has been noted during the first

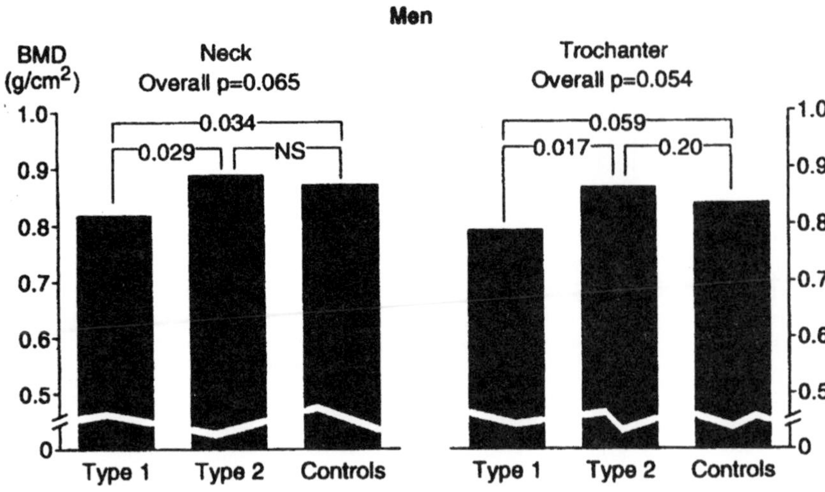

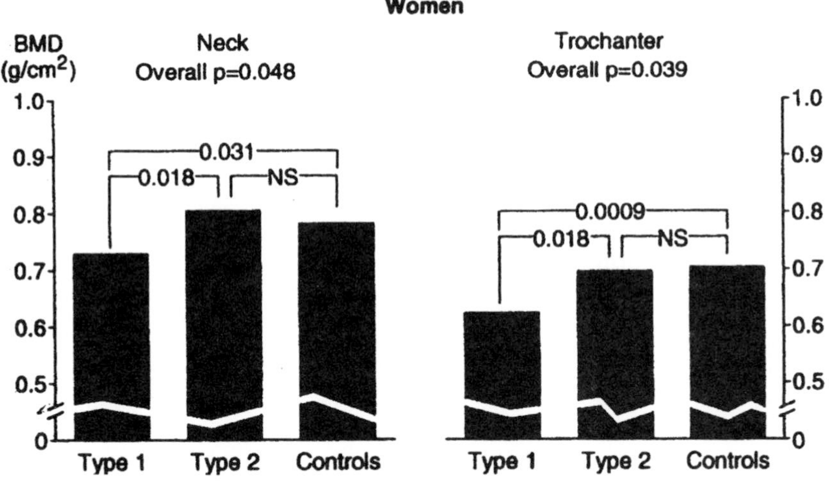

Figure 44.5. Bone density in diabetes. Mean bone mineral density (BMD) (adjusted for age and body mass index) at the proximal femur of subjects with type 1 diabetes (29 men, 27 women), type 2 diabetes (34 men, 34 women), and without diabetes (240 men, 258 women). (Copyright © 1999 American Diabetes Association. From Tuominen JT, Impivaara O, Puuka P, et al. Bone mineral density in patients with type 1 and type 2 diabetes. *Diabetes Care* 1999;22:1196–1200. Reprinted with permission from the American Diabetes Association.)

several years after diagnosis, with an attenuation thereafter (158,164). This suggests an initial insult not specifically related to control, but perhaps to the autoimmune process, similar to that seen in rheumatoid arthritis, in which bone loss is seen in the involved joints. Age of onset of diabetes might be expected to affect either the young adulthood accrual of bone or the age-related loss. However, no correlation between BMD and duration or current glycemic control (by HbA_{1c}) was seen in diabetic children (5.2 years duration, excluded if complications) (160) or postmenopausal women (8.9 years duration, 14 years postmenopausal) (179). Because of the myriad of factors other than diabetes incorporated into BMD over time, as well as the gradual nature of diabetic complications, shorter-term measures of bone metabolism are needed.

Markers of Bone Turnover

Serum and urine markers of bone turnover have been developed to assess short-term changes leading to osteoporosis. Serum levels of alkaline phosphatase and osteocalcin reflect bone formation, while serum levels of collagen cross-links reflect bone resorption. Osteoblast secretion of osteocalcin is decreased by high glucose levels, so bone formation as assessed by osteocalcin is decreased in proportion to diabetic control (180). Thus, in patients with diabetes, this marker is applicable only in limited situations. Similar problems arise with urinary markers such as deoxypyridinoline, which are confounded by glucosuria and thus require very good glycemic control to be useful. Bone resorption measured by deoxypyridinoline after a 12-hour glucose clamp was greater in age- and height-for-age–matched adolescents with diabetes than in controls, suggesting that bone loss in early-onset type 1 diabetes is related to increased turnover (181). This is important because instead of the presumed high turnover rate, as can occur with excess cortisol or with hyperparathyroidism, a low turnover resulting in adynamic bone, also seen in renal failure, is an alternate mechanism for osteoporosis. This possibility is suggested by the observation that fractures take a longer time to heal in persons with diabetes (182). Krakauer et al. (183) have proposed that a low turnover state due to functional hypoparathyroidism and hyperglycemia accounts for the differences between type 1 and type 2 diabetes, but this has yet to be investigated. The heterogeneity of types of diabetes, as well as variable contributions from associated conditions affecting BMD, make it difficult to designate one underlying mechanism for diabetic osteopenia.

Conditions Associated with Diabetes and Osteoporosis

Factors extrinsic to the metabolic changes of diabetes, such as age of onset of type 1 diabetes in relation to stage of bone growth and the lifestyle factors such as obesity and inactivity in type 2 diabetes, have secondary consequences relative to BMD. One such age-related risk for osteoporosis is low peak bone mass. In American women, peak bone mass is achieved by the end of the third decade (184). Thus, to the extent that diabetes may cause osteopenia, women who are young at diabetes onset may never achieve a normal peak bone density and thus reach osteoporotic thresholds earlier in life (Fig. 44.6). Delayed puberty is associated with a lower peak BMD (185); therefore, women with diabetes and delayed menarche may also have a lower peak BMD. In a carefully controlled Finnish study (111), Tuominen et al. defined type 1 diabetes by C-peptide values and therefore were able to use only subjects who had been diagnosed after age 30. Even in these patients, BMD was lower in patients with type 1 diabetes compared with those with type 2 diabetes or with controls, suggesting a secondary loss of bone. Another age-related factor is estrogen status, the major cause of osteoporosis in the general population. Because of their increased risk for menstrual dysfunction, women with type 1 diabetes may also have osteopenia due to estrogen deficiency. Most studies have not assessed the menstrual histories in these women, but one study did find a positive correlation between oral contraceptive use and BMD in women with type 1 diabetes, supporting a component of estrogen deficiency (186). One of the strongest risk factors for osteoporosis is low body weight (187), which is more typical of patients with type 1 diabetes than of those with type 2 diabetes. The obesity commonly present in persons with type 2 diabetes (and often for years before) may have a cumulative protective effect on bone density.

Several other diseases that increase the risk of osteoporosis are particularly relevant in diabetes. Diseases associated with autoimmune diabetes, including Graves disease and celiac sprue, also carry an independent risk for osteoporosis. Treatments for hypertension and hyperlipidemia, which are associated with both types of diabetes, may also affect BMD. Use of loop diuretics to treat hypertension can increase urinary loss of calcium, while thiazides may decrease it. Interesting preliminary case-control studies have suggested that treatment of hyperlipidemia with HMG-CoA reductase inhibitors may increase BMD (188), but these results have not been supported by other studies (189,190) and may represent confounding due to higher BMD in patients with hyperlipidemia (191).

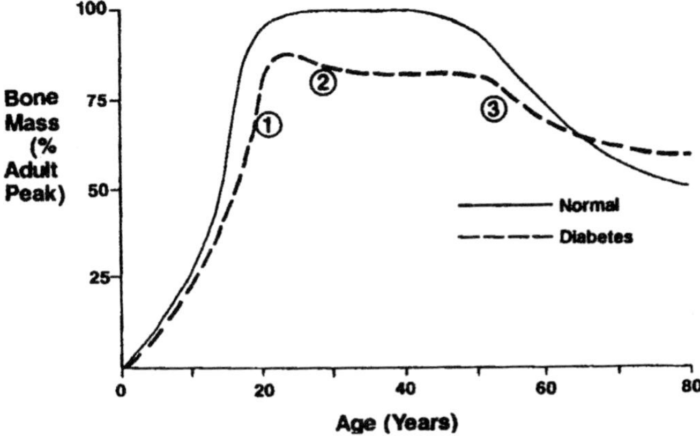

Figure 44.6. Diagram of bone loss. Model for the effects of diabetes on bone mineral density at different times of life. In diabetes, the initial accumulation of bone during adolescence is diminished *(1)*, thus reaching a lower plateau with continued loss associated with hypercalciuria in early adult life *(2)*, followed by later onset and retardation of age-related bone loss *(3)*. Depending on the age of onset, stages 1 and 2 could overlap. (Copyright © 1995 American Diabetes Association. From Krakauer JC, McKenna MJ, Buderer F, et al. Bone loss and bone turnover in diabetes. *Diabetes* 1995;44:775–782. Reprinted with permission from the American Diabetes Association.)

TABLE 44.5. Risk Factors for Osteoporotic Fractures in Diabetes

Risk for osteoporosis
Directly due to diabetes
Type 1 diabetes
Hypoglycemia or hyperglycemia
Nephropathy
Due to complications of diabetes
Nephropathy
Diabetic diarrhea
Due to disease associated with diabetes
Graves disease
Celiac sprue
Risk for falls
Poor vision due to retinopathy or cataracts
Poor balance due to neuropathy
Orthostatic hypotension
Impaired joint motility due to neuroarthropathy

Among women with osteoporosis, almost all hip fractures are due to falls (192). The risk of falling is increased by diabetic complications, including impaired vision due to retinopathy or cataracts and poor balance and orthostatic hypotension due to peripheral and autonomic neuropathy. Acute hypoglycemia and hyperglycemia may also cause impaired vision, incoordination, and muscle weakness. Patients with amputations are at increased risk for falls and immobility-induced osteoporosis because of their limited mobility (Table 44.5).

Treatment

All patients with type 1 diabetes and those with type 2 diabetes and advanced complications should be evaluated for osteoporosis and counseled about modifiable risk factors (getting appropriate exercise, calcium, and vitamin D and avoiding smoking and excessive alcohol). No preventive strategies specific to diabetes are yet known, although as reviewed above, good glycemic control appears to be beneficial. Treatment of osteoporosis in women with diabetes also has not been specifically evaluated and therefore follows guidelines for patients without diabetes. Common comorbid conditions such as nephropathy or gastrointestinal complications require attention. Renal impairment necessitates evaluation of the parathyroid-vitamin D axis as well as dose adjustment of medications. None of the current therapies for osteoporosis have been clinically studied in renal failure. Gastroparesis, malabsorption or sprue, and diabetic diarrhea can all contribute to osteoporosis by interfering with calcium and vitamin D absorption and require separate evaluation and treatment. All patients with diabetes who have extensive neuropathy, amputations, orthostatic hypotension, or impaired vision are at increased risk for falls. In addition to treatments to strengthen bone, these patients need counseling on prevention of falls, including use of walkers, night-lights, muscle-strengthening exercises, and removal of hazards in the home.

ENDOMETRIAL CANCER

A final postmenopausal health issue for women with diabetes is the risk of endometrial cancer. Endometrial cancer is the fourth most common cancer in women, and diabetes has long been considered a risk factor for endometrial cancer. After controlling for body weight, most (193–196) but not all (197) studies have shown that women with diabetes of all types have at least double the risk of endometrial cancer in comparison to the nondiabetic population. The risk directly related to diabetes is controversial because of frequent co-existence of other known risk factors, including obesity, hypertension, and sedentary lifestyle. The confounding of obesity in particular has been evaluated in case-control studies. Shoff and Newcomb (195), studying women in Wisconsin, and Salazar-Martinez et al. (198), studying women in Mexico, found that the additional risk due to diabetes over the risk of body size alone was mostly in obese (BMI >29) women with diabetes. Independent of weight, physical activity greatly decreases the risk of endometrial cancer. In the Swedish Twin Registry of nearly 12,000 women, even "light exercise" such as "walks or gardening" decreased the risk by half, and "hard physical training" reduced the relative risk to one tenth (199). Sturgeon et al. (200) found similar benefits from either recreational or nonrecreational activity and noted that the subjects who were less active also tended to be more obese. Similarly, patients with type 2 diabetes tend to be more obese and less active.

Several potential mechanisms for the risk of endometrial cancer have been postulated. One of the major recognized risk factors for endometrial cancer is unopposed estrogen exposure (201). Recognition of this in the 1970s changed the prescription of estrogen replacement therapy to include progesterone for women with a uterus, a regimen that has eliminated the increased incidence of endometrial cancer seen with estrogen alone. It has been postulated that additional estrogen exposure in obese women, from peripheral conversion in the increased body fat, induces the cancer. Estrogen levels correlate with percentage of ideal body weight in patients with endometrial cancer, and women with diabetes tend to be more obese and have higher levels of estrogens than women without diabetes (202). More directly, Nyholm et al. (203) found that, in comparison to weight-matched controls, women with diabetes had higher levels of total estrogens, although higher levels of sex hormone–binding globulin kept the levels of free estrogen comparable. Because obesity and physical inactivity, as well as type 2 diabetes, are associated with higher insulin levels, investigators have examined the influence of insulin levels in nondiabetic women. C-peptide levels correlated with BMI and estrogen levels, but after adjustment for these factors, no further relationship was seen between C-peptide levels and endometrial cancer (204). Another approach to this issue is to compare the risk in type 1 diabetes versus that in type 2 diabetes, but studies evaluating these variables have also yielded conflicting results (194, 196,205). The heterogeneity of patients with diabetes and of the insulin levels in diabetes has likely obscured these epidemiologic correlations. A long duration of diabetes also was not seen to correlate with the risk of endometrial cancer (195), but insulin levels usually decline with prolonged duration of diabetes. Hyperglycemia, which might be roughly estimated over the long term by incidence of diabetic complications, has not been assessed in relation to endometrial cancer.

SUMMARY

Diabetes has diverse effects on reproductive and postmenopausal health. As with other complications of diabetes, good glucose control may ameliorate some of the problems; others require approaches particular to diabetes. Many of the issues have not been specifically studied, and generalizations can only be made from studies of nondiabetic women. An appreciation of the unique reproductive consequences of diabetes will improve health care for these patients but also highlights the need for further research.

REFERENCES

1. Joslin EP, Root HF, White P. The growth, development and prognosis of diabetic children. *JAMA* 1925;85:420.
2. Bergqvist N. The gonadal function in female diabetics. *Acta Endocrinol* 1954; 19[Suppl]:3–20.
3. Kjaer K, Hagen C, Sando SH, et al. Epidemiology of menarche and menstrual disturbances in an unselected group of women with insulin-dependent diabetes mellitus compared to controls. *J Clin Endocrinol Metab* 1992;75:524–529.
4. Salerno M, Argenziano A, Di Maio S, et al. Pubertal growth, sexual maturation, and final height in children with IDDM. Effects of age at onset and metabolic control. *Diabetes Care* 1997;20:721–724.
5. Schriock EA, Winter RJ, Traisman HS. Diabetes mellitus and its effects on menarche. *J Adolesc Health Care* 1984;5:101–104.
6. Yeshaya A, Orvieto R, Dicker P, et al. Menstrual characteristics of women suffering from insulin-dependent diabetes mellitus. *Int J Fertil Menopausal Studies* 1995;40:269–273.
7. Cawood EH, Bancroft J, Steel JM. Perimenstrual symptoms in women with diabetes mellitus and the relationship to diabetic control. *Diabet Med* 1993;10: 444–448.
8. Djursing H, Hagen C, Nyholm HC, et al. Gonadotropin responses to gonadotropin-releasing hormone and prolactin responses to thyrotropin-releasing hormone and metoclopramide in women with amenorrhea and insulin-treated diabetes mellitus. *J Clin Endocrinol Metab* 1983;56:1016–1021.
9. Schroeder B, Hertweck SP, Sanfilippo JS, et al. Correlation between glycemic control and menstruation in diabetic adolescents. *J Reprod Med* 2000;45:1–5.
10. Perkins RB, Hall JE, Martin KA. Neuroendocrine abnormalities in hypothalamic amenorrhea: spectrum, stability, and response to neurotransmitter modulation. *J Clin Endocrinol Metab* 1999;84:1905–1911.
11. South SA, Asplin CM, Carlsen EC, et al. Alterations in luteinizing hormone secretory activity in women with insulin-dependent diabetes mellitus and secondary amenorrhea. *J Clin Endocrinol Metab* 1993;76:1048–1053.
12. Griffin ML, South SA, Yankov VL, et al. Insulin-dependent diabetes mellitus and menstrual dysfunction. *Ann Med* 1994;26:331–340.
13. Yen SSC. Female hypogonadotropic hypogonadism. Hypothalamic amenorrhea syndrome. *Endocrinol Metab Clin North Am* 1993;22:29–58.
14. Spratt DI, Cox P, Orav J, et al. Reproductive axis suppression in acute illness is related to disease severity. *J Clin Endocrinol Metab* 1993;76:1548–1554.
15. O'Hare JA, Eichold BH 2nd, Vignati L. Hypogonadotropic secondary amenorrhea in diabetes: effects of central opiate blockade and improved metabolic control. *Am J Med* 1987;83:1080–1084.
16. Biller BM, Coughlin JF, Saxe V, et al. Osteopenia in women with hypothalamic amenorrhea; a prospective study. *Obstet Gynecol* 1991;78:996–1001.
17. Hergenroder AC, Smith EO, Shypailo R, et al. Bone mineral changes in young women with hypothalamic amenorrhea treated with oral contraceptives, medroxyprogesterone, or placebo over 12 months. *Am J Obstet Gynecol* 1997;176:1017–1025.
18. Stancin T, Link DL, Reuter JM. Binge eating and purging in young women with IDDM. *Diabetes Care* 1989;12:601–603.
19. Peveler RC, Fairburn CG, Boller I, et al. Eating disorders in adolescents with IDDM. A controlled study. *Diabetes Care* 1992;15:1356–1360.
20. Biggs MM, Basco MR, Patterson G, et al. Insulin withholding for weight control in women with diabetes. *Diabetes Care* 1994;17:1186–1189.
21. Rodin GM, Daneman D. Eating disorders and IDDM. A problematic association. *Diabetes Care* 1992;15:1402–1412.
22. Rydall AC, Rosin GM, Olmsted MP, et al. Disordered eating behavior and microvascular complications in young women with insulin-dependent diabetes mellitus. *N Engl J Med* 1997;336:1849–1854.
23. Dunaif A. Hyperandrogenic anovulation (PCOS): a unique disorder of insulin action associated with an increased risk of non-insulin-dependent diabetes mellitus. *Am J Med* 1995;98[Suppl 1A]:33S–39S.
24. Conn JJ, Jacobs HS, Conway GS. The prevalence of polycystic ovaries in women with type 2 diabetes mellitus. *Clin Endocrinol (Oxf)* 2000;52:81–86.
25. Djursing H. Hypothalamic-pituitary-gonadal function in insulin treated diabetic women with and without amenorrhea. *Dan Med Bull* 1987;34: 139–147.
26. Prelevic GM, Wurzburger MI, Peric LA. The effect of residual beta cell activity on menstruation and the reproductive hormone profile of insulin-dependent diabetics. *Arch Gynecol Obstet* 1989;244:207–213.
27. Escobar-Morreale HF, Rolden B, Barrio R, et al. High prevalence of the polycystic ovary syndrome and hirsutism in women with type 1 diabetes mellitus. *J Clin Endocrinol Metab* 2000;85:4182–4187.
28. Barbieri RL. Induction of ovulation in infertile women with hyperandrogenism and insulin resistance. *Am J Obstet Gynecol* 2000;183:1412–1418.
29. Hoeger K. Obesity and weight loss in polycystic ovary syndrome. *Obstet Gynecol Clin North Am* 2001;28;85–97.
30. Polderman KH, Gooren LJ, Asscheman H, et al. Induction of insulin resistance by androgens and estrogens. *J Clin Endocrinol Metab* 1994;79:265–271.
31. Poretsky L, Kalin MF. The gonadotropic function of insulin. *Endocrinol Rev* 1987;8:132–141.

32. Kalro BN, Loucks TL, Berga SL. Neuromodulation in polycystic ovary syndrome. *Obstet Gynecol Clin North Am* 2001;28:35–62.
33. Corenblum B, Baylis BW. Medical therapy for the syndrome of familial virilization, insulin resistance, and acanthosis nigricans. *Fertil Steril* 1990;53: 421–425.
34. Dunaif A, Wu X, Lee A, et al. Defects in insulin receptor signaling in vivo in the polycystic ovary syndrome (PCOS). *Am J Physiol Endocrinol Metab* 2001;281:E392–E399.
35. Polderman KH, Gooren LJ, Heine RJ. Effects of physiological and supraphysiological doses of insulin on adrenal androgen levels. *Horm Metab Res* 1996;28:152–155.
36. Djursing H, Hagen C, Nyboe Anderson A, et al. Serum sex hormone concentrations in insulin dependent diabetic women with and without amenorrhoea. *Clin Endocrinol (Oxf)* 1985;23:147–154.
37. Lunt H, Brown LJ. Self-reported changes in capillary glucose and insulin requirements during the menstrual cycle. *Diabet Med* 1996;13:525–530.
38. Walsh CH, Malins JM. Menstruation and control of diabetes. *BMJ* 1977;2: 177–179.
39. Sacerdote A, Bleicher SJ. Oral contraceptives abolish luteal phase exacerbation of hyperglycemia in type I diabetes. *Diabetes Care* 1982;5:651–652.
40. Cudworth AG, Veevers A. Carbohydrate metabolism in the menstrual cycle. *Br J Obstet Gynaecol* 1975;82:162–169.
41. Spellacy WN, Ellington AB, Keith G, et al. Plasma glucose and insulin levels during the menstrual cycles of normal women and premenstrual syndrome patients. *J Reprod Med* 1990;35:508–511.
42. Bonora E, Zazaroni I, Alpi O, et al. Influence of the menstrual cycle on glucose tolerance and insulin secretion. *Am J Obstet Gynecol* 1987;157:140–141.
43. Kalkhoff RK. Metabolic effects of progesterone. *Am J Obstet Gynecol* 1982;142: 735–738.
44. Spellacy WN, Carlson KL, Schade SL. Menstrual cycle carbohydrate metabolism. Studies on plasma insulin and blood glucose levels during an intravenous glucose tolerance test. *Am J Obstet Gynecol* 1967;99:382–386.
45. Toth EL, Suthijumroon A, Crockford PM, et al. Insulin action does not change during the menstrual cycle in normal women. *J Clin Endocrinol Metab* 1987; 64:74–80.
46. Diamond MP, Jacob R, Connolly-Diamond M, et al. Glucose metabolism during the menstrual cycle. Assessment with the euglycemic, hyperinsulinemic clamp. *J Reprod Med* 1993;38:417–421.
47. Diamond MP, Simonson DC, DeFronzo RA. Menstrual cyclicity has a profound effect on glucose homeostasis. *Fertil Steril* 1989;52:204–208.
48. Widom B, Diamond MP, Simonson DC. Alterations in glucose metabolism during menstrual cycle in women with IDDM. *Diabetes Care* 1992;15:213–220.
49. Zemel P. Sexual dysfunction in the diabetic patient with hypertension. *Am J Cardiol* 1988;61:27H–33H.
50. Berman JR, Berman LA, Werbin TJ, et al. Female sexual dysfunction: anatomy, physiology, evaluation and treatment options. *Curr Opin Urol* 1999; 9:563–568.
51. Prather RC. Sexual dysfunction in the diabetes female: a review. *Arch Sex Behav* 1988;17:277–284.
52. Kaplan SA, Reis RB, Kohn IJ, et al. Safety and efficacy of sildenafil in postmenopausal women with sexual dysfunction. *Urology* 1999;53:481–486.
53. Caruso S, Intelisano G, Lupo L, et al. Premenopausal women affected by sexual arousal disorder treated with sildenafil: a double-blind, cross-over, placebo-controlled study. *Br J Obstet Gynaecol* 2001;108:623–628.
54. Campbell LV, Redelman MJ, Borkman M, et al. Factors in sexual dysfunction in diabetic female volunteer subjects. *Med J Aust* 1989;151:550–552.
55. Ellenberg M. Diabetes and female sexuality. *Women's Health* 1984;9:75–79.
56. Sreebny LM, Yu A, Green A, et al. Xerostomia in diabetes mellitus. *Diabetes Care* 1992;15:900–904.
57. Herter CD. Sexual dysfunction in patients with diabetes. *J Am Board Fam Pract* 1998;11:327–330.
58. Gibb D, Hockney S, Brown L, et al. Vaginal symptoms and insulin dependent diabetes mellitus. *N Z Med J* 1995;108:252–253.
59. Sobel JD. Epidemiology and pathogenesis of recurrent vulvovaginal candidiasis. *Am J Obstet Gynecol* 1985;152:924–935.
60. Anderson RJ, Freedland KI, Clouse RE, et al. The prevalence of comorbid depression in adults with diabetes: a meta-analysis. *Diabetes Care* 2001;24: 1069–1078.
61. Clayton AH. Recognition and assessment of sexual dysfunction associated with depression. *J Clin Psychiatry* 2001;62[Suppl 3]:5–9.
62. Kroenke K, et al. Similar effectiveness of paroxetine, fluoxetine, and sertraline in primary care: a randomized trial. *JAMA* 2001;286:2947–2955.
63. Kjaer K, Hagen C, Sando SH, et al. Infertility and pregnancy outcome in an unselected group of women with insulin-dependent diabetes mellitus. *Am J Obstet Gynecol* 1992;166:1412–1418.
64. Dicker D, Ben-Rafael Z, Ashkenazi J, et al. In vitro fertilization and embryo transfer in well-controlled, insulin-dependent diabetics. *Fertil Steril* 1992;58: 430–432.
65. Mills JL, Simpson JL, Driscoll SG, et al. Incidence of spontaneous abortion among normal women and insulin-dependent diabetic women whose pregnancies were identified within 21 days of conception. *N Engl J Med* 1988;319: 1617–1623.
66. Hanson U, Persson B, Thunell S. Relationship between haemoglobin A1C in early type 1 (insulin-dependent) diabetic pregnancy and the occurrence of spontaneous abortion and fetal malformation in Sweden. *Diabetologia* 1990; 33:100–104.
67. Klein BE, Moss SE, Klein R. Effect of pregnancy on progression of diabetic retinopathy. *Diabetes Care* 1990;13:34–40.
68. Hayslett JP, Reece EA. Effect of diabetic nephropathy on pregnancy. *Am J Kidney Dis* 1987;9:344–349.
69. Waine H, Frieden EH, Caplan HI, Cole T. Metabolic effects of Enovid in rheumatoid patients. *Arthritis Rheum* 1963;6:796.
70. Harvengt C. Effect of oral contraceptive use on the incidence of impaired glucose tolerance and diabetes mellitus. *Diabetes Metab* 1992;18:71–77.
71. Spellacy WN. Carbohydrate metabolism during treatment with estrogen, progestogen, and low-dose oral contraceptives. *Am J Obstet Gynecol* 1982;142: 732–734.
72. Gupta S. Clinical guidelines on contraception and diabetes. *Eur J Contracept Reprod Health Care* 1997;2:167–171.
73. Skouby SO, Andersen O, Saurbrey N, et al. Oral contraception and insulin sensitivity: in vivo assessment in normal women and women with previous gestational diabetes. *J Clin Endocrinol Metab* 1987;64:519–523.
74. Radberg, Gustafson A, Skryten A, et al. Oral contraception in diabetic women. Diabetes control, serum and high density lipoprotein lipids during low-dose progestogen, combined oestrogen/progestogen and non-hormonal contraception. *Acta Endocrinol (Copenh)* 1981;98:246–251.
75. Kjos SL. Contraception in the diabetic woman. *Clin Perinatol* 1993;20:649–661.
76. Godsland IF, Crook D, Simpson R, et al. The effects of different formulations of oral contraceptive agents on lipid and carbohydrate metabolism. *N Engl J Med* 1990;323:1375–1381.
77. Petersen KR, Skouby SO, Jespersen J. Contraception guidance in women with pre-existing disturbances in carbohydrate metabolism. *Eur J Contracept Reprod Health Care* 1996;1:53–59.
78. Glueck CJ, Lang J, Hamer T, et al. Severe hypertriglyceridemia and pancreatitis when estrogen replacement therapy is given to hypertriglyceridemic women. *J Lab Clin Med* 1994;123:59–64.
79. Woods JW. Oral contraceptives and hypertension. *Hypertension* 1988;11:II11–15.
80. Russell RP, Sullivan MA. The pill and hypertension. *Johns Hopkins Med J* 1970; 127:287–293.
81. Wilson ES, Cruickshank J, McMaster M, et al. A prospective controlled study of the effect on blood pressure of contraceptive preparations containing different types and dosages of progestogen. *Br J Obstet Gynaecol* 1984;91: 1254–1260.
82. Klein BE, Moss SE, Klein R. Oral contraceptives in women with diabetes. *Diabetes Care* 1990;13:895–898.
83. Garg SK, Chase HP, Marshall G, et al. Oral contraceptives and renal and retinal complications in young women with insulin-dependent diabetes mellitus. *JAMA* 1994;271:1099–1102.
84. Steel JM, Duncan LJ. Serious complications of oral contraception in insulin-dependent diabetics. *Contraception* 1978;17:291–295.
85. Jensen G, Nyboe J, Appleyard M, et al. Risk factors for acute myocardial infarction in Copenhagen, II: Smoking, alcohol intake, physical activity, obesity, oral contraception, diabetes, lipids, and blood pressure. *Eur Heart J* 1991; 12:298–308.
86. Croft P, Hannaford PC. Risk factors for acute myocardial infarction in women: evidence from the Royal College of General Practitioners' oral contraception study. *BMJ* 1989;298:165–168.
87. Lidegaard O. Oral contraceptives, pregnancy and the risk of cerebral thromboembolism: the influence of diabetes, hypertension, migraine and previous thrombotic disease. *Br J Obstet Gynaecol* 1995;102:153–159.
88. Porter JB, Hunter JR, Jick H, et al. Oral contraceptives and nonfatal vascular disease. *Obstet Gynecol* 1985;66:1–4.
89. Mammen EF. Oral contraceptives and blood coagulation: a critical review. *Am J Obstet Gynecol* 1982;142:781–790.
90. Meigs JB, Mittleman MA, Nathan DM, et al. Hyperinsulinemia, hyperglycemia, and impaired hemostasis: the Framingham Offspring Study. *JAMA* 2000;283:221–228.
91. Sowers JR. Diabetes mellitus and cardiovascular disease in women. *Arch Intern Med* 1998;158:617–621.
92. Tanis BC, van den Bosch MA, Kemmeren JM, et al. Oral contraceptives and the risk of myocardial infarction. *N Engl J Med* 2001;345:1787–1793.
93. Stampfer MJ, Willett WC, Colditz GA, et al. A prospective study of past use of oral contraceptive agents and risk of cardiovascular diseases. *N Engl J Med* 1988;319:1313–1317.
94. Chasen-Taber L, Stampfer M. Oral contraceptives and myocardial infarction—the search for the smoking gun. *N Engl J Med* 2001;345:1841–1842.
95. Fruzzetti F. Hemostatic effects of smoking and oral contraceptive use. *Am J Obstet Gynecol* 1999;180:S369–S374.
96. Klein BE, Klein R, Moss SE. Mortality and hormone-related exposures in women with diabetes. *Diabetes Care* 1999;22:248–252.
97. Perera M, Sattar N, Petrie JR, et al. The effects of transdermal estradiol in combination with oral norethisterone on lipoproteins, coagulation, and endothelial markers in postmenopausal women with type 2 diabetes: a randomized, placebo-controlled study. *J Clin Endocrinol Metab* 2001;86:1140–1143.
98. World Health Organization. *Improving access to quality care in family planning. Medical eligibility criteria for contraceptive use.* Geneva: WHO Technical Report Service, 2000, WHO/RHR/00.2.
99. Diab KM, Zaki MM. Contraception in diabetic women: comparative metabolic study of Norplant, depot medroxyprogesterone acetate, low dose oral contraceptive pill and CuT380A. *J Obstet Gynaecol Res* 2000;26:17–26.
100. Kim C, Seidel KW, Begier EA, et al. Diabetes and depot medroxyprogesterone contraception in Navajo women. *Arch Intern Med* 2001;161:1766–1771.

101. Konje JC, Otolorin EO, Ladipo OA. The effect of continuous subdermal levonorgestrel (Norplant) on carbohydrate metabolism. *Am J Obstet Gynecol* 1992;166:15–19.
102. Berenson AB, Radecki CM, Grady JJ, et al. A prospective controlled study of the effects of hormonal contraception on bone mineral density. *Obstet Gynecol* 2001;98:576–582.
103. Wiese J. Intrauterine contraception in diabetic women. *Fertil Steril* 1977;28: 422–425.
104. Skouby SO, Molsted-Pedersen L, Kuhl C. Contraception in diabetic women. *Acta Endocrinol Suppl* 1986;277:125–129.
105. Weinstein SP, Conant EF, Orel SG, et al. Diabetic mastopathy in men: imaging findings in two patients. *Radiology* 2001;219:797–799.
106. Seidman JD, Schnaper LA, Phillips LE. Mastopathy in insulin-requiring diabetes mellitus. *Hum Pathol* 1994;25:819–824.
107. Camuto PM, Zetrenne E, Ponn T. Diabetic mastopathy: a report of 5 cases and a review of the literature. *Arch Surg* 2000;135:1190–1193.
108. Garstin WI, Kaufman Z, Michel MJ, et al. Fibrous mastopathy in insulin dependent diabetics. *Clin Radiol* 1991;44:89–91.
109. Tomaszewski JE, Brooks JS, Hicks D, et al. Diabetic mastopathy: a distinctive clinicopathologic entity. *Hum Pathol* 1992;23:780–786.
110. Ely KA, Tse G, Simpson JF, et al. Diabetic mastopathy. A clinicopathologic review. *Am J Clin Pathol* 2000;113:541–545.
111. Tuominen JT, Impivaara O, Puuka P, et al. Bone mineral density in patients with type 1 and type 2 diabetes. *Diabetes Care* 1999;22:1196–1200.
112. Lopez-Lopez R, Huerta R, Malacara JM. Age at menopause in women with type 2 diabetes mellitus. *Menopause* 1999;6:174–178.
113. Dorman JS, Steenkiste AR, Foley TP, et al. Menopause in type 1 diabetic women: is it premature? *Diabetes* 2001;50:1857–1862.
114. Carpenter CCJ, Solomon N, Silverberg S, et al. Schmidt's syndrome (thyroid and adrenal insufficiency): a review of the literature and a report of fifteen new cases including ten instances of coexistent diabetes mellitus. *Medicine* 1964;43:153-180.
115. Weetman AP. Autoimmunity to steroid-producing cells and familial polyendocrine autoimmunity. *Baillieres Clin Endocrinol Metab* 1995;9:157–174.
116. Wheatcroft NJ, Salt C, Milford-Ward A, et al. Identification of ovarian antibodies by immunofluorescence, enzyme-linked immunosorbent assay or immunoblotting in premature ovarian failure. *Hum Reprod* 1997;12:2617–2622.
117. Taylor R, Smith NM, Angus B, et al. Return of fertility after twelve years of autoimmune ovarian failure. *Clin Endocrinol (Oxf)* 1989;31:305–308.
118. Kalantaridou SN, Davis SR, Nelson LM. Premature ovarian failure. *Endocrinol Metab Clin North Am* 1998;27:989–1006.
119. Malacara JM, Huerta R, Rivera B, et al. Menopause in normal and uncomplicated NIDDM women: physical and emotional symptoms and hormone profile. *Maturitas* 1997;28:35–45.
120. Ross RK, Paganini-Hill A, Mack TM, et al. Menopausal oestrogen therapy and protection from death from ischaemic heart disease. *Lancet* 1981;1: 858–860.
121. Beard CM, Kottke TE, Annegers JF, et al. The Rochester Coronary Heart Disease Project: effect of cigarette smoking, hypertension, diabetes, and steroidal estrogen use on coronary heart disease among 40- to 59-year-old women, 1960 through 1982. *Mayo Clin Proc* 1989;64:1471–1480.
122. Bush TL, Barrett-Connor E, Cowan LD, et al. Cardiovascular mortality and noncontraceptive use of estrogen in women: results from the Lipid Research Clinics Program Follow-up Study. *Circulation* 1987;75:1102–1109.
123. Kannel WB, McGee DL. Diabetes and cardiovascular disease. The Framingham study. *JAMA* 1979;241:2035–2038.
124. Kannel WB, Wilson PW. Risk factors that attenuate the female coronary disease advantage. *Arch Intern Med* 1995;155:57–61.
125. Kaplan RC, Heckbert SR, Weiss NS, et al. Postmenopausal estrogens and risk of myocardial infarction in diabetic women. *Diabetes Care* 1998;21:1117–1121.
126. Manson JE, Colditz GA, Stampfer MJ, et al. A prospective study of maturity-onset diabetes mellitus and risk of coronary heart disease and stroke in women. *Arch Intern Med* 1991;151:1141–1147.
127. Brussaard HE, Gevers Leuven JA, Frolich M, et al. Short-term oestrogen replacement therapy improves insulin resistance, lipids and fibrinolysis in postmenopausal women with NIDDM. *Diabetologia* 1997;40:843–849.
128. Andersson B, Mattsson LA, Hahn L, et al. Estrogen replacement therapy decreases hyperandrogenicity and improves glucose homeostasis and plasma lipids in postmenopausal women with noninsulin-dependent diabetes mellitus. *J Clin Endocrinol Metab* 1997;82:638–643.
129. Walsh BW, Schiff I, Rosner B, et al. Effects of postmenopausal estrogen replacement on the concentrations and metabolism of plasma lipoproteins. *N Engl J Med* 1991;325:1196–1204.
130. Lopes-Virella MF, Wohltmann HJ, Loadholt CB, et al. Plasma lipids and lipoproteins in young insulin-dependent diabetic patients: relationship with control. *Diabetologia* 1981;21:216–223.
131. Robinson JG. How HRT alters the lipid profile in women with diabetes. *Medscape Womens Health* 1996;1:4.
132. Lilley SH, Spivey JM, Vadlamudi S, et al. Lipid and lipoprotein responses to oral combined hormone replacement therapy in normolipemic obese women with controlled type 2 diabetes mellitus. *J Clin Pharmacol* 1998;38:1107–1115.
133. Friday KE, Dong C, Fontenot RU. Conjugated equine estrogen improves glycemic control and blood lipoproteins in postmenopausal women with type 2 diabetes. *J Clin Endocrinol Metab* 2001;86:48–52.
134. Manning PJ, Allum A, Jones S, et al. The effect of hormone replacement therapy on cardiovascular risk factors in type 2 diabetes: a randomized controlled trial. *Arch Intern Med* 2001;161:1772–1776.
135. Thom M, Chakravarti S, Oram DH, et al. Effect of hormone replacement therapy on glucose tolerance in postmenopausal women. *Br J Obstet Gynaecol* 1977;84:776–783.
136. Effects of estrogen or estrogen/progestin regimens on heart disease risk factors in postmenopausal women. The Postmenopausal Estrogen/Progestin Interventions (PEPI) Trial. The Writing Group for the PEPI Trial. *JAMA* 1995; 273:199–208.
137. Barrett-Connor E, Laakso M. Ischemic heart disease risk in postmenopausal women. Effects of estrogen use on glucose and insulin levels. *Arteriosclerosis* 1990;10:531–534.
138. Spellacy WN, Buhi WC, Birk SA. Effect of estrogen treatment for one year on carbohydrate and lipid metabolism in women with normal and abnormal glucose tolerance test results. Glucose, insulin, growth hormone, triglycerides, and Premarin. *Am J Obstet Gynecol* 1978;131:87–90.
139. Manson JE, Rimm EB, Colditz GA, et al. A prospective study of postmenopausal estrogen therapy and subsequent incidence of non-insulin-dependent diabetes mellitus. *Ann Epidemiol* 1992;2:665–673.
140. Samaras K, Hayward CS, Sullivan D, et al. Effects of postmenopausal hormone replacement therapy on central abdominal fat, glycemic control, lipid metabolism, and vascular factors in type 2 diabetes: a prospective study. *Diabetes Care* 1999;22:1401–1407.
141. Ferrara A, Karter AJ, Ackerson LM, et al. Hormone replacement therapy is associated with better glycemic control in women with type 2 diabetes: the Northern California Kaiser Permanente Diabetes Registry. *Diabetes Care* 2001; 24:1144–1150.
142. Szekacs B, Vajo Z, Acs N, et al. Hormone replacement therapy reduces mean 24-hour blood pressure and its variability in postmenopausal women with treated hypertension. *Menopause* 2000;7:31–35.
143. Szekacs B, Vajo Z, Varbiro S, et al. Postmenopausal hormone replacement improves proteinuria and impaired creatinine clearance in type 2 diabetes mellitus and hypertension. *Br J Obstet Gynaecol* 2000;107:1017–1021.
144. Banga JD, Sixma JJ. Diabetes mellitus, vascular disease and thrombosis. *Clin Haematol* 1986;15:465–492.
145. Hulley S, Grady D, Bush T, et al. Randomized trial of estrogen plus progestin for secondary prevention of coronary heart disease in postmenopausal women. Heart and Estrogen/progestin Replacement Study (HERS) Research Group. *JAMA* 1998;280:605–613.
146. Heckbert SR, Kaplan RC, Weiss NS, et al. Risk of recurrent coronary events in relation to use and recent initiation of postmenopausal hormone therapy. *Arch Intern Med* 2001;161:1709–1713.
147. Meyer HE, Tverdal A, Falch JA, et al. Factors associated with mortality after hip fracture. *Osteoporos Int* 2000;11:228–232.
148. Meyer HE, Tverdal A, Falch JA. Risk factors for hip fracture in middle-aged Norwegian women and men. *Am J Epidemiol* 1993;137:1203–1211.
149. Forsen L, Sogaard AJ, Meyer HE, et al. Diabetes mellitus and the incidence of hip fracture: results from the Nord-Trondelag Health Survey. *Diabetologia* 1999;42:920–925.
150. Nicodemus KK, Folsom AR. Type 1 and type 2 diabetes and incident hip fractures in postmenopausal women. *Diabetes Care* 2001;24:1192–1197.
151. Paganini-Hill A, Ross RK, Gerkins VR, et al. Menopausal estrogen therapy and hip fractures. *Ann Intern Med* 1981;95:28–31.
152. Schwartz AV, Sellmeyer DE, Ensrud KE, et al. Older women with diabetes have an increased risk of fracture: a prospective study. *J Clin Endocrinol Metab* 2001;86:32–38.
153. van Daele PL, Stolk RP, Burger H, et al. Bone density in non-insulin-dependent diabetes mellitus. The Rotterdam Study. *Ann Intern Med* 1995;122: 409–414.
154. Hirano Y, Kishimoto H, Hagino H, et al. The change of bone mineral density in secondary osteoporosis and vertebral fracture incidence. *J Bone Miner Metab* 1999;17:119–124.
155. Heath H 3rd, Melton LJ 3rd, Chu CP. Diabetes mellitus and risk of skeletal fracture. *N Engl J Med* 1980;303:567–570.
156. Seeley DG, Kelsey J, Jergas M, et al. Predictors of ankle and foot fractures in older women. The Study of Osteoporotic Fractures Research Group. *J Bone Miner Res* 1996;11:1347–1355.
157. World Health Organization. Assessment of fracture risk and its application to screening for postmenopausal osteoporosis. Report of a WHO Study Group. *World Health Organ Tech Rep Ser* 1994;843:1–129.
158. Levin ME, Boisseau VC, Avioli LV. Effects of diabetes mellitus on bone mass in juvenile and adult-onset diabetes. *N Engl J Med* 1976;294:241–245.
159. Selby PL. Osteopenia and diabetes. *Diabet Med* 1988;5:423–428.
160. Roe TF, Mora S, Costin G, et al. Vertebral bone density in insulin-dependent diabetic children. *Metabolism* 1991;40:967–971.
161. Munoz-Torres M, Jodar E, Escobar-Jimenez F, et al. Bone mineral density measured by dual X-ray absorptiometry in Spanish patients with insulin-dependent diabetes mellitus. *Calcif Tissue Int* 1996;58:316–319.
162. Barrett-Connor E, Holbrook TL. Sex differences in osteoporosis in older adults with non-insulin-dependent diabetes mellitus. *JAMA* 1992;268:3333–3337.
163. Kayath MJ, Dib SA, Vieiaa JG. Prevalence and magnitude of osteopenia associated with insulin-dependent diabetes mellitus. *J Diabetes Comp* 1994;8: 97–104.
164. Mathiassen B, Nielsen S, Ditzel J, et al. Long-term bone loss in insulin-dependent diabetes mellitus. *J Intern Med* 1990;227:325–327.

165. Rix M, Andreassen H, Eskildsen P. Impact of peripheral neuropathy on bone density in patients with type 1 diabetes. *Diabetes Care* 1999;22:827–831.
166. Forst T, Pfutzner A, Kann P, et al. Peripheral osteopenia in adult patients with insulin-dependent diabetes mellitus. *Diabet Med* 1995;12:874–879.
167. Ivers RQ, Cumming RG, Mitchell P, et al. Diabetes and risk of fracture: The Blue Mountains Eye Study. *Diabetes Care* 2001;24:1198–1203.
168. Raskin P, Stevenson MR, Barilla DE, et al. The hypercalciuria of diabetes mellitus: its amelioration with insulin. *Clin Endocrinol (Oxf)* 1978;9:329–335.
169. Gertner JM, Tamborlane WV, Horst RL, et al. Mineral metabolism in diabetes mellitus: changes accompanying treatment with a portable subcutaneous insulin infusion system. *J Clin Endocrinol Metab* 1980;50:862–866.
170. Thalassinos NC, Hadjiyann P, Tzanela M, et al. Calcium metabolism in diabetes mellitus: effect of improved blood glucose control. *Diabet Med* 1993; 10:341–344.
171. Nagasaka S, Murakami T, Uchikawa T, et al. Effect of glycemic control on calcium and phosphorus handling and parathyroid hormone level in patients with non-insulin-dependent diabetes mellitus. *Endocrinol J* 1995;42: 377–383.
172. Okazaki R, Totsuki Y, Hamano K, et al. Metabolic improvement of poorly controlled noninsulin-dependent diabetes mellitus decreases bone turnover. *J Clin Endocrinol Metab* 1997;82:2915–2920.
173. Krakauer JC, McKenna MJ, Buderer NF, et al. Bone loss and bone turnover in diabetes. *Diabetes* 1995;44:775–782.
174. Christensen JO, Svendsen OL. Bone mineral in pre- and postmenopausal women with insulin-dependent and non-insulin-dependent diabetes mellitus. *Osteoporos Int* 1999;10:307–311.
175. Barrett-Connor E, Kritz-Silverstein D. Does hyperinsulinemia preserve bone? *Diabetes Care* 1996;19:1388–1392.
176. Stolk RP, Van Daele PL, Pols HA, et al. Hyperinsulinemia and bone mineral density in an elderly population: the Rotterdam study. *Bone* 1996;18:545–549.
177. Kwon DJ, Kim JH, Chung KW, et al. Bone mineral density of the spine using dual energy X-ray absorptiometry in patients with non-insulin-dependent diabetes mellitus. *J Obstet Gynaecol Res* 1996;22:157–162.
178. Haffner SM, Bauer RL. The association of obesity and glucose and insulin concentrations with bone density in premenopausal and postmenopausal women. *Metabolism* 1993;42:735–738.
179. Weinstock RS, Goland RS, Shane E, et al. Bone mineral density in women with type II diabetes mellitus. *J Bone Miner Res* 1989;4:97–101.
180. Rosato MT, Schneider SH, Shapses SA. Bone turnover and insulin-like growth factor I levels increase after improved glycemic control in noninsulin-dependent diabetes mellitus. *Calcif Tissue Int* 1998;63:107–111.
181. Bjorgaas M, Haug E, Johnsen HJ. The urinary excretion of deoxypyridinium cross-links is higher in diabetic than in nondiabetic adolescents. *Calcif Tissue Int* 1999;65:121–124.
182. Loder RT. The influence of diabetes mellitus on the healing of closed fractures. *Clin Orthop* 1988;232:210–216.
183. Krakauer JC, McKenna MJ, Rao DS, et al. Bone mineral density in diabetes. *Diabetes Care* 1997;20:1339–1340.
184. Looker AC, Wahner HW, Dunn WL, et al. Proximal femur bone mineral levels of US adults. *Osteoporos Int* 1995;5:389–409.
185. Finkelstein JS, Klibanski A, Neer RM. A longitudinal evaluation of bone mineral density in adult men with histories of delayed puberty. *J Clin Endocrinol Metab* 1996;81:1152–1155.
186. Lunt H, Florkowski CM, Cundy T, et al. A population-based study of bone mineral density in women with longstanding type 1 (insulin dependent) diabetes. *Diabetes Res Clin Pract* 1998;40:31–38.
187. Ensrud KE, Lipschutz RC, Cauley JA, et al. Body size and hip fracture risk in older women: a prospective study. Study of Osteoporotic Fractures Research Group. *Am J Med* 1997;103:274–280.
188. Meier CR, Schlienger RC, et al. HMG-CoA reductase inhibitors and the risk of fractures. *JAMA* 2000;283:3205–3210.
189. Pedersen TR, Kjekshus J. Statin drugs and the risk of fracture. 4S Study Group. *JAMA* 2000;284:1921–1922.
190. Reid IR, Hague W, Emberson J, et al. Effect of pravastatin on frequency of fracture in the LIPID study: secondary analysis of a randomised controlled trial. Long-term intervention with pravastatin in ischaemic disease. *Lancet* 2001;357:509–512.
191. Adami S, Braga V, Gatti D. Association between bone mineral density and serum lipids in men. *JAMA* 2001;286:791–792.
192. Nevitt MC. Epidemiology of osteoporosis. *Rheum Dis Clin North Am* 1994; 20:535–559.
193. Brinton LA, Berman ML, Mortel R, et al. Reproductive, menstrual, and medical risk factors for endometrial cancer: results from a case-control study. *Am J Obstet Gynecol* 1992;167:1317–1325.
194. La Vecchia C, Negri E, Franceschi S, et al. A case-control study of diabetes mellitus and cancer risk. *Br J Cancer* 1994;70:950–953.
195. Shoff SM, Newcomb PA. Diabetes, body size, and risk of endometrial cancer. *Am J Epidemiol* 1998;148:234–240.
196. Parazzini F, La Vecchia C, Negri E, et al. Diabetes and endometrial cancer: an Italian case-control study. *Int J Cancer* 1999;81:539–542.
197. Kelsey JL, LiVolsi VA, Holford TR, et al. A case-control study of cancer of the endometrium. *Am J Epidemiol* 1982;116:333–342.
198. Salazar-Martinez E, Lazcano-Ponce EC, Lira-Lira GG, et al. Case-control study of diabetes, obesity, physical activity and risk of endometrial cancer among Mexican women. *Cancer Causes Control* 2000;11:707–711.
199. Terry P, Baron JA, Weiderpass E, et al. Lifestyle and endometrial cancer risk: a cohort study from the Swedish Twin Registry. *Int J Cancer* 1999;82:38–42.
200. Sturgeon SR, Brinton LA, Berman ML, et al. Past and present physical activity and endometrial cancer risk. *Br J Cancer* 1993;68:584–589.
201. Smith, DC, Prentice R, Thompson DJ, et al. Association of exogenous estrogen and endometrial carcinoma. *N Engl J Med* 1975;293:1164–1167.
202. Judd HL, Davidson BJ, Frumar AM, et al. Serum androgens and estrogens in postmenopausal women with and without endometrial cancer. *Am J Obstet Gynecol* 1980;136:859–871.
203. Nyholm H, Djursing H, Hagen C, et al. Androgens and estrogens in postmenopausal insulin-treated diabetic women. *J Clin Endocrinol Metab* 1989;69: 946–949.
204. Troisi R, Potischman N, Hoover RN, et al. Insulin and endometrial cancer. *Am J Epidemiol* 1997;146:476–482.
205. Weiderpass E, Persson L, Adami HO, et al. Body size in different periods of life, diabetes mellitus, hypertension, and risk of postmenopausal endometrial cancer (Sweden). *Cancer Causes Control* 2000;11:185–192.

CHAPTER 45

Pancreas and Islet Transplantation

Gordon C. Weir

THE PROBLEM

The devastating complications associated with both type 1 and type 2 diabetes are now clearly linked to hyperglycemia (1–3). The implication of these findings is that normalization of glucose levels with proper treatment early in the course of the disease would prevent the development of the microvascular and neuropathic complications and probably much of the macrovascular disease. The cost of these complications, both in personal and financial terms, is enormous, and the incidence of both forms of diabetes is increasing. Impressive improvements in treatment have been made thanks to self–glucose monitoring, advances in insulin therapy, new oral medications, and higher standards of care, but most people with diabetes continue to develop disabling complications. Although progress is being made in the development of approaches that could prevent autoimmune diabetes, the prospects for preventing type 2 diabetes seems less promising. A mechanical β-cell equivalent consisting of a glucose sensor and an insulin pump could provide patients with normoglycemia, but efforts to develop a satisfactory glucose sensor have been frustrating in spite of many ingenious approaches (4,5). The most obvious solution is to provide patients with the β-cells they are missing, which can be done with pancreas, islet, or β-cell transplants. This appealing concept even was tested clinically as early as 1893 in Bristol, England, when a physician unsuccessfully transplanted pieces of sheep pancreas into the subcutaneous space of a 15-year-old boy with diabetes (6). This conceptually simple goal continues to look like an attractive solution to the problem of diabetes but has turned out to be extraordinarily difficult to accomplish.

β-CELL REPLACEMENT AS A TREATMENT FOR TYPE 1 AND TYPE 2 DIABETES

While it is generally assumed that β-cell–replacement therapy will be useful for people with type 1 diabetes, many fail to appreciate that it could be a very effective treatment for those with type 2 diabetes, thinking that the main problem in type 2 diabetes is insulin resistance, with a deficiency in insulin secretion making only a small contribution. This misses the point that type 2 diabetes develops only when β-cells fail to compensate for insulin resistance (7). The incidence of type 2 diabetes has skyrocketed, largely because of our sedentary Western lifestyle, with its plentiful food, which leads to central obesity with its concomitant insulin resistance. However, to understand the role of the β-cell, it must be appreciated that most people with insulin resistance never become hyperglycemic because their β-cells compensate with increased insulin secretion: hence the key role of β-cell failure in the development of diabetes.

People argue that a prohibitive number of islets would be required for people with type 2 diabetes and that the hyperinsulinemia would be atherogenic. In fact, many people with type 2 diabetes have insulin requirements that are not very different from those of people with type 1 diabetes, in part because of the residual insulin production in the latter. Moreover, the requirement for a large number of islets for so many patients may be solved once ways are found to make insulin-producing cells readily accessible. The health benefits of such transplants would be enormous. The microvascular and neuropathic complications of diabetes should be prevented, and there are reasons to think that the cardiovascular events would be less common. After such a transplant, an individual would still be left with obesity and insulin resistance, with their health consequences, but these would be associated with far less illness than when diabetes is superimposed. There are many approaches that could help with the problem of type 2 diabetes, such as improving insulin sensitivity with new drugs and reducing obesity, but β-cell replacement also could provide major benefits. If one follows the same arguments, β-cell replacement could prevent the hyperglycemia-related complications for almost all forms of diabetes, such as various forms of maturity-onset diabetes of the young (MODY), mitochondrial diabetes, cystic fibrosis, and diabetes secondary to pancreatectomy. In fact, these non–type 1 forms of diabetes may actually be easier targets for β-cell replacement because the transplanted islets would be encountering only allograft rejection and not autoimmunity.

PANCREAS TRANSPLANTATION

Pancreas transplants were first performed on an experimental basis in the 1960s, but the procedure was not widely applied until the mid-1980s (8–11). By the year 2000, more than 1,200 transplants were being performed yearly, with many of these being made possible by an increase in access to insurance coverage. The vast majority of these transplants have been done in the United States and Europe. Improvements in outcome have been due to advances in organ preservation, surgical techniques, and immunosuppressive drugs. The most common transplants and the best results have been obtained with simultaneous kidney/pancreas (SKP) transplants given to patients with type 1 diabetes who have advanced nephropathy. Much less common are pancreas transplants done after a kidney allograft (PAK), which usually require more immunosuppression. Decisions about pancreas transplants often are driven by the availability of a kidney from a living related donor because of the superior outcomes of such transplants compared with dialysis and even transplantation with a cadaveric kidney. Few patients receive a pancreas transplant alone (PTA), although a single center recently reported 225 of these cases (12). Justification of PTA, with its risks of mortality, morbidity, and immunosuppression, requires that patients have serious problems with their diabetes, which might include life-threatening insulin reactions, instability of control, and various psychological problems. A final, even less common, approach is the use of the distal portion of the pancreas provided by a living related donor. There continues to be debate about the efficacy of using only half of the pancreas and the risk of development of either glucose intolerance or frank diabetes in the donors (13).

The excellent results obtainable by simultaneous transplantation of a kidney and pancreas (SPK) are now being experienced by an increasing number of centers, with approximately 85% of the pancreases maintaining euglycemia in the recipient 1 year after transplantation and approximately 50% functioning well after 5 years. The euglycemia means that recipients have normal glucose levels around the clock, are without increased risk of reactive hypoglycemia (14), have normal glycohemoglobin levels, and have no dietary restrictions, even if they are taking medications such as cyclosporine or tacrolimus (FK-506) and glucocorticoids that can inhibit insulin secretion (15,16). Results reported for PAK and PTA have not been as good, but they have been improving steadily (10).

Strategies for drainage of transplanted pancreases have evolved, with most centers now using enteric drainage with a side-to-side anastomosis of the donor duodenum and the recipient ileum (17) (Fig. 45.1). Although this procedure is associated with some risk of infection, it avoids the problems that plagued the use of bladder drainage via the donor duodenum: acidosis, dehydration, infection, and a variety of other problems (18). Bladder drainage was widely used for about 10 years, but many patients who originally had bladder drainage were later converted to enteric drainage. The venous drainage from a transplanted pancreas usually goes directly into the systemic circulation, but some centers are now employing the superior mesenteric vein to allow drainage into the portal vein, which is more physiologically correct but a more technically demanding procedure (19,20).

The most commonly used immunosuppressive therapy in the past has been triple therapy with cyclosporine, azathioprine, and prednisone, but centers are now more likely to use tacrolimus (FK-506), mycophenolate mofetil, and prednisone (21). Antibodies to T cells or the interleukin-2 (IL-2) receptor are usually used during the induction phase. In general, higher doses of immunosuppressive drugs are required for patients who receive pancreas transplants than for those who receive kidney transplants alone, which is worrisome because of the increased risks of infection and malignancy (22). For SKP transplants, kidney rejection is used as a surrogate marker for rejection of the pancreas. Detection of problems with the pancreas is more difficult for PAK and PTA procedures. Some have considered amylase output a useful marker for patients with bladder drainage, but current approaches are more likely to use serum levels of amylase and lipase and pancreas biopsies (23). Immunosuppression is necessary to control not only allograft rejection but also the autoimmunity that originally caused type 1 diabetes in the recipients. The persistent autoimmunity may be especially aggressive, as indicated by SKP transplants performed between identical twins who were not given immunosuppressive medication (24). Neither the exocrine pancreas nor the kidney was rejected, but diabetes recurred, with immune destruction of the islets demonstrated by biopsy. Remarkably, this destruction occurred in only a matter of weeks, which is far more rapid than the normal progression of type 1 diabetes, which typically takes years to produce hyperglycemia (25).

Risk and Benefits of Pancreas Transplantation

Debate continues about how much patients benefit from pancreas transplants (26). This transplantation requires complex surgery and is accompanied by significant mortality and morbidity; patients frequently are hospitalized for extended periods and readmitted for problems such as intraabdominal infection and vascular thrombosis (27). Nonetheless, some studies sug-

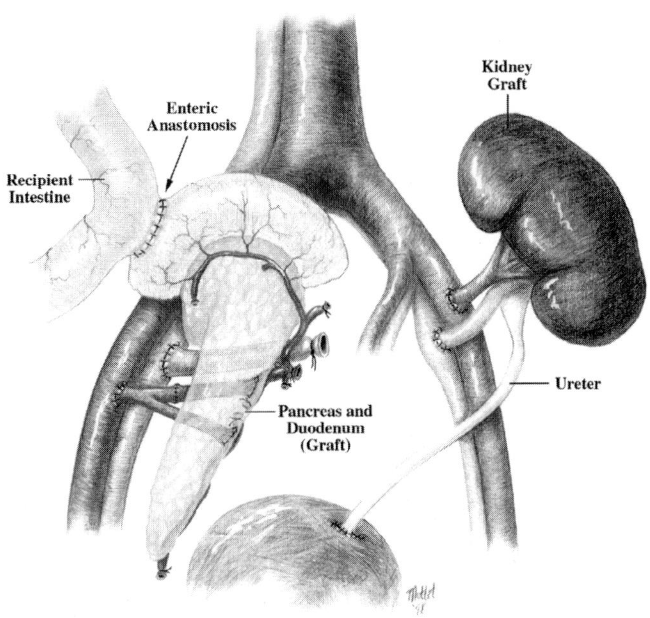

Figure 45.1. Combined pancreas and kidney transplant. The digestive juices of the pancreas are drained into the intestine via an enteric anastomosis between the donor duodenum and the recipient ileum. Venous outflow can be either into the peripheral circulation via the iliac vein as shown or into the portal vein. (Drawing courtesy of Dr. David Sutherland.)

gest that survival is better for patients with SKP transplants than for those with kidney transplants alone (28,29), although it is difficult to find studies with well-matched treatment groups. The impact of these transplants on the complications of diabetes seems to be modest, which is not surprising considering that so many recipients already have advanced abnormalities when they receive the transplant. Various studies have found some stabilization of retinopathy and improvement in nerve conduction velocity, but these changes seem to have little clinical impact (30–32). A recent study found that some histologic improvement of transplanted kidneys can take place after pancreas transplantation (33). Specifically, biopsies of kidneys of patients with PTA that were obtained 5 years after the pancreas transplant showed no benefit, but biopsies at 10 years showed impressive reversal of histologic abnormalities toward normal. A provocative study suggested that patients with autonomic neuropathy before a pancreas transplant have better survival after 7 years than those with failed grafts (34); although encouraging, this finding needs to be confirmed. The most obvious benefit of pancreas transplants is that patients consider their quality of life improved, particularly because of their freedom from insulin injections, hypoglycemic episodes, and food restrictions. It must be remembered that quality of life is a difficult parameter to evaluate (8,26). For example, it has been difficult to show, using standard parameters such as whether patients are more active or perform better at work, that their lives are improved. Nonetheless, the most striking finding, and of undeniable importance, is that patients are very happy to be free of their diabetes.

Debates continue about the risk-to-benefit ratio of pancreas transplantation, particularly with a cost of approximately $100,000 per patient (26). Now that more insurance programs have agreed to cover the costs of this procedure, the demand has increased. There is no prospect for doing large controlled trials of pancreas transplantation, but new knowledge about its value will continue to emerge from smaller studies. Until a major advance occurs in islet transplantation or in the development of some kind of improved insulin delivery system, it seems likely that pancreas transplantation will continue. The use of half of a pancreas might make this form of β-cell replacement therapy available to more patients. The possibility of doing more PTAs may receive more scrutiny, particularly as a procedure for patients with early proteinuria, with its poor prognosis. As renal failure worsens in these individuals, their risk of macrovascular disease and mortality is markedly increased. The Diabetes Control and Complications Trial (DCCT) has proven that improved glycemic control is strongly protective against the development of kidney disease (1); thus, pancreas transplantation could prove valuable for patients headed toward renal failure. This possibility becomes even more attractive because of recent evidence that the progression of diabetic nephropathy might be partially reversible in patients with pancreas transplants (33).

ISLET TRANSPLANTATION

The first successful islet transplants, performed in rodents in the early 1970s (35,36), were made possible by the development of a method of isolating islets from pancreases with collagenase (37), leading to the expectation that such transplants would soon be available to everyone with type 1 diabetes. At the beginning of the 21st century, the failure to meet these expectations has been heartbreaking for countless patients, their friends and families, and the investigators struggling to progress as rapidly as possible. Indeed, there has been much debate about how science should proceed when there are so many opinions about how to balance applied versus basic research (38). The simple explanation for why the problem of islet transplantation has not been solved is that, despite the conceptual simplicity of the task, it has turned out to be extraordinarily difficult. Nonetheless, despite the frustrations and missteps, substantial progress has been made that should provide a foundation for eventual success.

Two Major Barriers to Successful Islet Transplantation

For the sake of simplicity, one can consolidate the problem of islet transplantation into two major barriers: how to provide an adequate supply of insulin-producing cells and how to prevent the processes of transplant rejection and autoimmunity from destroying these cells once transplanted.

Human Islet Allografts

Much work with small and large animal models was necessary before the first serious human islet allografts could be provided in the late 1980s to immunosuppressed patients with kidney transplants (39–43). These early transplants initially used islets obtained from as many as five donor pancreases, with some of these islets being cryopreserved. The islets were injected into the portal vein, using a direct approach with dissection along the umbilical vein; more recently, however, a transhepatic angiographic procedure has gained favor (Fig. 45.2). These islets become wedged in the portal tributaries and engraft, presumably receiving most of their vascular supply from host vessels growing into the islets (44). Portal hypertension, hemorrhage, or thrombosis can occur, but such complications have been rare (45). There were a few early successes, with some recipients being insulin-free for more than 2 years, but then it became apparent that most of these transplants were failures. The initial results were disappointing. Data from the International Islet Transplantation Registry show that between 1990 and 1998, only 33 (12%) of the 267 recipients of islet allografts remained insulin-free for more than 1 week and only 8% maintained that status for over 1 year (45,46). The longest period of independence from insulin was 70 months. About 35% of these allografts had continuing graft function (C-peptide greater than 0.5 ng/mL) after 1 year. However, about 30% of the patients had a marked reduction in C-peptide levels within 1 month, a phenomenon called primary nonfunction. Because such a rapid loss is rarely seen with allografts in the absence of autoimmunity, autoimmune destruction is thought to be largely responsible.

The poor results obtained during the 1990s were very disheartening and discouraged the expansion of clinical trials. Fortunately, the few centers that persisted with transplants made advances that produced important insights (40,45–50). Although very few recipients were freed of their insulin requirements, it became apparent that the function of the grafted islets persisted in some of them, as evidenced by measurable C-peptide production. As is the case with the early stages of type 1 diabetes, residual insulin secretion greatly improved glycemic control even though insulin treatment was still required. Thus, in about 20% to 30% of carefully performed, well-documented islet transplants, C-peptide secretion did persist and appeared to lead to improved glycohemoglobin levels and fewer severe insulin reactions (47).

The Complexities of Islet Allografts

As investigators became more rigorous about details, results began to improve, although they continued to be disappointing. Better results could be obtained if the cold ischemia time of the cadaver pancreases was limited to less than 8 hours before islet isolation and if more than 6,000 islet equivalents per kilogram were transplanted (45,46). Better techniques for islet isolation have evolved. Some find that the new standardized collagenase preparation, Liberase, gives better and more consistent islet yields (51), and efforts have been made to minimize the amount of endotoxin in the reagents. The period immediately after the transplant may be critical. The phenomenon of primary nonfunction, with rapid disappearance of measurable C-peptide, is likely caused by autoimmunity, because such rapid failure virtually never occurs with autotransplants. Other complex events during the early implantation phase must lead to considerable loss of islet mass. For example, there must be some obligatory loss of cells to local hypoxia in nonvascularized clumps of islet tissue (52,53). In addition, a nonspecific inflammatory response (54) and possibly localized clotting (55) may enhance the immune processes of rejection and autoimmunity and activate the innate immune system (56). Hyperglycemia may produce increased oxygen consumption by β-cells, which would further deprive them of oxygen in their local environment, so every effort should be made to maintain euglycemia with aggressive insulin therapy. A case may be made for using intravenous insulin during the first 10 days after the transplant while new vessels from the host enter the islet grafts (44). The hyperglycemic environment appears to have an adverse influence on the outcome of islet transplants (57). There was evidence that the use of anti-thymocyte globulin during the induction period was beneficial (45,50). Some thought the use of nicotinamide, verapamil, pentoxifylline, and vitamin E was valuable (45), but the efficacy of these agents remains to be established.

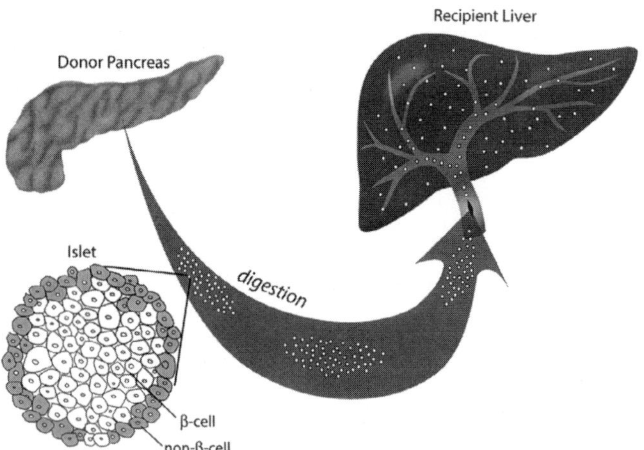

Figure 45.2. Islet transplantation in humans usually is done starting with a cadaver pancreas that is digested with a collagenase/protease mixture. The isolated islets are then introduced into the portal vein either by transhepatic angiography or via laparoscopy. The islets then are carried downstream and wedge in the portal tributaries, whereupon they are vascularized by vessels from the recipient.

Despite these partial successes, the results were far inferior to those of pancreas transplantation, which results in the immediate achievement of normoglycemia in 85% of recipients and in the remaining 15% for at least a year. This indicates that the islets contained in one pancreas should be enough and that both transplant rejection and autoimmunity can be controlled by conventional immunosuppression. Somehow, the islets contained in their normal home in the pancreas must be less vulnerable to immune injury and/or the toxic effects of the immunosuppressive agents. It is also possible that the ability of the pancreas to generate new islets from ducts may be helpful (58). Moreover, the presence of draining lymph nodes contained in the whole pancreas seems to provide a protective effect against autoimmunity (59,60).

A puzzling finding is that the mean time required for the development of insulin independence in the 33 reported successful allograft recipients was 179 ± 24 days (45). One explanation is that insulin independence tended to coincide with the lowering of the doses of immunosuppressive medications such as prednisone, which are diabetogenic, but the actual reason may be much more complex. One might not expect β-cell mass to have increased during this time, but precursor duct cells carried along with the islets (61,62) might have been the source of some new islets. Although host vessels grow into transplanted islets in only 7 to 10 days (44), we have no idea how long it takes the vessels to be fully established. In their normal location in the pancreas, islets have a specialized vasculature; arterioles break into capillaries within the core of the β-cells and then exit through the islet mantle that contains glucagon-secreting α-cells (63,64). When transplanted islets are revascularized, the normal relationship between β- and non–β-cells may not be reestablished, possibly leading to altered β-cell function (65). In addition, reinnervation (66) and topographic remodeling of the islet micro-organs may take a long time. There are other reasons for being concerned that transplanted islets may not function as efficiently as normal islets in the pancreas. It has been found that the oxygen tension of islet grafts situated under the kidney capsule of rodents is considerably lower than that for islets in the pancreas (67), a factor that could result in a reduction in glucose-induced insulin secretion.

Although we now realize that increasing the mass of islets transplanted is helpful, this was not clear in the 1990s. Islets from as many as five donors often failed, while islets from a single pancreas were sometimes sufficient. Another complex variable is islet purity; many of the successful transplants have used islet preparations that had a purity of more than 80%, and others had a purity of 50% or less, raising questions about the influence of non-islet elements such as duct cells. The benefits of immunologic matching of donor and recipient have not been carefully studied, but most successful transplants have been matched only for blood type and not for histocompatibility antigens (45). Measurement of islet autoantibodies prior to transplantation is usually of little help because the titers are typically low, but some have found that the presence of autoantibodies may be associated with a worse outcome (68,69). An approach that may be worth pursuing is the measurement of gene expression of various immune mediators in circulating lymphocytes during the course of transplantation, as this has been found to correlate with kidney allograft rejection (70).

The Edmonton Protocol

Frustrated by the mediocre results of earlier trials, a group of investigators in Edmonton, Alberta, Canada, tried a new approach in 1999 (71). They thought that rapamycin (sirolimus) might be beneficial and that glucocorticoids were toxic to islets. They also did everything possible to improve the quality of their islet preparations and reasoned that more islets would be required than was previously considered necessary. They recruited patients with type 1 diabetes who had serious problems with hypoglycemia, which justified the use of potentially dangerous immunosuppressive agents. In contrast to the procedure for earlier transplants, the islets were used immediately after their isolation rather than being maintained in tissue culture. The immunosuppression regimen included rapamycin (sirolimus) and tacrolimus (FK-506) but no prednisone. For induction, antibody to the IL-2 receptor (daclizumab) was used. Islets were introduced into the liver through the portal vein via transhepatic angiography. Islets from more than one cadaver donor were required, with two sufficing for most of the patients. Normoglycemia was never attained after the first transplant but did occur immediately after the second or third transplant. A total of about 11,000 islet equivalents (IE) per kilogram were used. At the time of this writing, 17 patients have been rendered insulin-free with glycohemoglobin levels in the normal or near normal range. Most of the patients have glucose intolerance, and their stimulated C-peptide release is approximately one third of normal, which suggests that their β-cell mass is marginal or that the grafted β-cells are less efficient than pancreatic β-cells. Some of the patients have maintained normal glycohemoglobin levels without insulin for almost 2 years.

The results of the Edmonton group are spectacularly better than any previous results, but this enthusiasm must be tempered by the reality that patients must receive dangerous immunosuppressive therapy and that two or more cadaver pancreases are required, which means that very few patients will be treated. Nonetheless, this is a true advance that should provide a foundation for future improvements with different protocols. To bring other groups up to the same level, the Immune Tolerance Network funded by the National Institutes of Health, with help from the Juvenile Diabetes Foundation, is funding 10 centers to perform 40 transplants to try to reproduce the Edmonton results. As with the Edmonton trial, the multicenter trial will enroll patients without kidney transplants who have threatening episodes of hypoglycemia; however, patients with severe instability of their control and advancing complications will also be considered.

Allografts in the Absence of Autoimmunity

Insight into the possible problems caused by autoimmunity have been provided by cluster operations for abdominal cancer in which the liver, pancreas, and other organs were removed from the patient, who then received a cadaver liver into which islets isolated from the same cadaver donor were placed, providing a pure allograft situation (46). These islet allografts more often produced normoglycemia than did islets given to patients with type 1 diabetes; patients became insulin-independent 60% of the time, and one patient was insulin-free for 5 years. Although transplantation of the liver may have had some beneficial influence on the immune system, the absence of autoimmunity is suspected to be a major reason for the success. In addition, these recipients are typically unhealthy, so they may require less β-cell mass to accommodate their reduced nutritional intake and weight.

Islet Autografts

Transplantation of islets that do not face immune attack provides important lessons about how well islets can perform in the liver. When pancreases are removed because of painful pancreatitis or some other reason, it is often possible to isolate the islets and transplant them into the liver via the portal vein. These digested pancreatic preparations have typically been relatively impure, containing non-islet pancreatic elements, including duct cells that have the capacity for neogenesis. These patients do remarkably well, with about 70% being insulin-independent at 1 year if they receive more than 300,000 IE (46). Sometimes success can be achieved with even fewer than 200,000 islets—considerably fewer than the usual requirement for successful allografts (72,73). The most obvious explanation for success is that there are no problems with either allorejection or autoimmunity; it must also be remembered, however, that the removal of glucagon by the pancreatectomy and the tendency of these patients to be thin could make them relatively insulin-sensitive.

EFFORTS TO CONTROL TRANSPLANT REJECTION AND AUTOIMMUNITY

Current organ transplants are successful because of immunosuppression, which although more effective than ever, continues to be associated with notable risk, the main threats being susceptibility to infection and the development of malignancy (22). There is great reluctance to use such dangerous drugs in people with type 1 diabetes whose prognosis might otherwise be good. Fortunately, considerable progress is being made in the quest for safer and more effective immunosuppressive drugs. As we learn more about the differences between rejection and autoimmunity, we can expect different approaches to be used for each process. Even different drugs are likely to be required for xenograft rejection.

Induction of Tolerance

A major goal for the transplantation field is to be able to induce tolerance, that is, treatment given only at the time of transplantation will somehow trick the recipient's immune system into accepting transplanted foreign tissue as his or her own. Many different approaches currently being studied could lead to full or operational tolerance (Table 45.1). Tolerance to transplanted tissue has been induced by a variety of techniques in a number of experimental models (74), but many scientific and safety hurdles must be overcome before such approaches can be used in humans. One hopeful example was the islet transplants between different species of nonhuman primates in which anti-CD3 immunotoxin, cyclosporine, and steroids were given only during the peritransplant period, with normoglycemia persisting for more than 100 days in the absence of further immunosuppression (75).

TABLE 45.1. Approaches to the Induction of Tolerance Induction

Graft-based tolerance induction
MHC knockouts (class I or II MHC antigens)
Remove donor antigen-presenting cells (passenger lymphocytes)
Masking of class I MHC antigens by antibodies
Privileged sites (brain, testes, thymus, anterior chamber, other)
Gene transfer to islets (eg, CTLA4Ig, IL-4, TGF-β)
Host response–based tolerance induction
Central tolerance
Clonal deletion: thymic injection of antigen
Clonal inactivation: thymic irradiation
Peripheral tolerance
Anergy
Immune deviation: from Th1 to Th2
Inhibition of co-stimulation (CTLA4Ig, Anti-CD40 ligand)
Peptide-based therapy (parenteral or oral for autoimmunity)
Immunosuppression
Donor-specific transfusion (DST)
Peripheral cell suppression (CD4 subsets)
Clonal deletion of peripheral T cells
Chimerism
Clonal T cells that home to islets and inhibit immune destruction

Adapted from Rossini AA, Greiner DL, Mordes JP. Induction of immunologic tolerance for transplantation. *Physiol Rev* 1999;79:99–141.

Immunosuppression and Immune Modulation

Impressive success with islet allografts in nonhuman primates has been found by blocking co-stimulation with antibodies to CD40 ligand (CD 154) on T cells, which results in inhibition of T-cell activation by antigen-presenting cells. This new agent has produced excellent results in experiments with monkeys and baboons, with normalization of glucose levels and seemingly minimal toxicity (76,77). Unfortunately, trials of this agent in persons with lupus nephritis had to be stopped because of thromboembolic phenomena. Although treatment with anti-CD40 ligand controlled allograft rejection, it is not clear if blockade of co-stimulation will protect against autoimmunity (78).

Another new agent used with some success in nonhuman primate islet allografts has been CTLA4Ig, which also blocks co-stimulation (79). T cells can be inhibited by antibodies in various other ways. An agent in clinical islet transplant trials is a nonmitogenic humanized, Fc receptor–nonbinding OKT3 antibody, which inhibits T-cell activation (80). A variety of other experimental agents could turn out to be useful. FTY720 is an agent that displaces lymphocytes from the peripheral circulation and is effective in various transplantation models (81). Monoclonal antibodies to the transmembrane protein tyrosine kinase phosphatase CD45 have been found to inhibit the rejection of islet allografts (82). The soluble complement receptor 1 (sCR1) TP10 may inhibit the inflammation around newly transplanted islets and may help control primary nonfunction (55). Blockade of the IL-15 receptor with mutated IL-15/Fc can inhibit T-cell expansion and protect islet transplants (83). In other experiments, IL-10/Fc prolonged islet xenografts, possibly by inhibiting macrophage function (84). These are just a few examples of agents that are being developed. Previous experience shows that combination therapy usually provides the best results, so it will be challenging to determine how these new drugs will interact.

Immunologists also are learning more about immunoprivileged sites such as the testes, brain, thymus, and the anterior chamber of the eye, knowledge that may provide insights into possible new strategies (85). Cotransplantation of islets with Sertoli cells has been found to provide some protection against rejection (86). This originally was assumed to be caused by the expression of Fas ligand on Sertoli cells, but recent experiments suggest that the protection is caused by secretion of transforming growth factor-β (TGF-β) (87).

THE SHORTAGE OF INSULIN-PRODUCING TISSUE

At present the only sources of islets for transplantation into humans are cadaver pancreases, which are in very short supply. It is currently not possible to use living donors because not enough islets can be reliably obtained from a donated portion of a pancreas. In the United States, it will be a major challenge to obtain 3,000 usable cadaver pancreases per year, yet the incidence of type 1 diabetes is about 30,000 cases per year (88), and type 2 diabetes develops in more than 10 times as many people. The success of the Edmonton protocol depended on the use of two or more cadaver pancreases. There have been some successes with islets isolated from only one pancreas, but it may be necessary for the donor pancreas to have a large islet mass and for the recipient to be small and insulin-sensitive. Another problem is competition for pancreases with those doing whole-pancreas transplants, particularly because whole-pancreas transplants are presently more often covered by health insurance. This competition is likely to cause problems until islet transplants have been proven to provide superior results. There has been much discussion about the possibility of using human fetal tissue, but despite some advances, this is proving to be a difficult route (89,90). Many transplants of human fetal pancreas have been performed around the world, but no clear benefit has been demonstrated (45). At present, no one has found a way to exploit the growth potential of fetal pancreases; moreover, many ethical and practical issues cloud the future of this approach.

Expansion of Human β-Cells from Stem Cells, Other Precursor Cells, and Cell Lines

It is now appreciated that new β-cells are generated throughout adult life, both from replication of preexisting β-cells and through the formation of new β-cells from precursor cells contained in pancreatic ducts (91). In the presence of hyperglycemia and insulin resistance, β-cell hypertrophy also can contribute to the increase in β-cell mass (92,93). To maintain β-cell mass, birth of new β-cells is balanced by death of β-cells, mainly through apoptosis. There is increasing excitement about the possibility of expanding β-cell number by exploiting the developmental capacity of precursor cells. This could be accomplished with stem cells or other precursor cells by finding new ways to stimulate the replication of existing β-cells or by creating a useful β-cell line.

Stem Cells

The definition of stem cells has become very complex. There are true stem cells, such as hematopoietic or intestinal cells, that have the capacity of unlimited expansion and are capable of generating various cell types. There are embryonic stem cells found in blastocysts that are capable of developing into any specialized cell type. Then there are facultative or functional stem cells that are differentiated cells capable of generating new cells. These can include differentiated pancreatic duct cells that, with the proper stimulus, can change their differentiation and become activated to form new islet and acinar cells (94). It has recently become apparent that stem cells have a much wider capacity for differentiation than has previously been appreciated, with there being examples of hematopoietic stem cells differentiating into liver, nerve, and muscle cells (95). It may also be possible for differentiated cells to turn into cells with characteristics of embryonic stem cells (96).

Recent advances have generated optimism that stem cells might be used to make new β-cells and thus solve the problem of limited β-cell supply. For example, it has recently been shown that duct cells obtained from adult human cadaver pancreases can be expanded *in vitro* and that when these precursor cells (functional stem cells) are stimulated with growth factors and matrix, they form duct cysts from which sprout islets that contain β-cells and the other islet cell types, these being called cultivated human islet buds (CHIBs) (58). At present, not enough CHIBs can be generated to be useful for clinical transplants, but there seems to be potential for further expansion. Although adult pancreatic duct cells have this capacity for islet regeneration, it seems that the process is normally suppressed *in vivo* to accommodate the need for a low rate of neogenesis. With the proper *in vitro* or *in vivo* stimulus, these restraints can be removed, as has been shown to occur after partial pancreatectomy in rats (97,98). These studies raise the hope that a single pancreas could provide enough islets to supply β-cells for more than one recipient. In addition, it might be possible to obtain pancreatic tissue from a person with diabetes and then cultivate new islets, which can be returned in the form of a transplant. For type 1 diabetes, this would mean that allorejection would not be a problem, but autoimmunity would still need to be controlled. For type 2 diabetes, the tantalizing possibility exists that CHIBs could be provided as an autotransplant with no immune rejection. Other workers have obtained considerable expansion of cells obtained from human islets, which unfortunately seem to contain little insulin (99,100). Efforts continue to make these cells differentiate into a β-cell phenotype useful for transplantation.

The possibility of using embryonic stem cells has become more attractive with the demonstration that mouse embryonic stem cells can be grown to form insulin-containing cells capable of curing diabetes in mice with chemically induced diabetes (101). This was accomplished by means of a selection process employing antibiotic resistance genes driven by the insulin promoter. Specialized tissue culture techniques then were applied that produced aggregates of cells containing near-normal amounts of insulin and having the capacity to secrete insulin in response to glucose levels in the physiologic range. This success raises the possibility that human embryonic stem cells might be developed in a similar manner to generate an unlimited supply of β-cells.

Production of Insulin-Producing Cell Lines

Advances in molecular and cell biology have made it theoretically possible to manipulate the differentiation of cells by genetic engineering so that they could be used for transplantation. It has been possible to transform murine insulin-producing cells with the SV40 T antigen, expand these cells, and then turn off the oncogene with a tetracycline response element, with resultant redifferentiation (102). Although such modified murine cells could conceivably be used for transplants into humans if the cells were somehow protected from immune destruction, human cells would be a preferable source. Unfortunately, it has proven difficult to create a comparable human cell line. Another approach would be to create a β-cell equivalent by adding genes or inhibiting the expression of existing genes (103,104). For example, the proinsulin gene can be expressed in cells that normally do not make insulin, with the resulting cells capable not only of making proinsulin and cleaving it to insulin but also of storing and secreting insulin in response to a variety of stimuli. By adding additional genes that influence glucose metabolism, it is even possible to manipulate these cells so that their insulin secretion is partially regulated by glucose. Another approach has been to engineer cells from the intermediate lobe of the pituitary to make insulin (105). These cells are of interest because despite their production of significant quantities of insulin, they are not subject to autoimmune attack. Although these preliminary results are encouraging, it is becoming clear that normal β-cells are remarkably complicated, which means it may be difficult to create near-normal β-cells by altering a few genes. On the other hand, as more is learned about the master switches that control the differentiation of cells, more promising results may emerge. Human insulin-producing cell lines have been derived from β-cells from patients with persistent hyperinsulinemic hypoglycemia of infancy (106). Although these cells can be expanded in tissue culture, they do not contain much insulin and have not yet been engineered to secrete insulin properly in response to physiologic levels of glucose. In considering the potential use of insulin-secreting cells for transplantation, the question remains of whether the non–β-cells of the islet or some equivalent should be contained in the transplanted cell aggregates. It seems that non–β-cells are probably not required, as suggested by experiments in which relatively pure β-cell populations prepared by flow cytometry functioned reasonably well when transplanted into diabetic rodents (107).

Xenotransplantation

Despite increased optimism about the prospects for developing new sources of human β-cells, investigators are still exploring the possibility of using tissue from other species as xenotransplants (Table 45.2). The list of species that are potentially useful include pigs, cows, rabbits, rodents, and even fish. Pigs have had particular appeal because pig insulin has been used in the past for treating people with diabetes, pigs have glucose levels similar to those in humans, pigs are part of the food chain, and people seem to be comfortable about the prospect of using this source. Unfortunately, pig islet tissue is not easy to work with. It continues to be difficult to generate high-quality islets from adult pigs (108,109). Much work is now being done to develop ways of using either fetal or neonatal islet tissue, which are attractive sources because of their growth potential (110–114). One of the problems with this tissue is the immaturity of the cells, which means that it can take weeks or months to normal-

TABLE 45.2. Potential Sources of Insulin-Producing Cells for Islet Transplantation

Human sources
Live donors (probably not an option)
Cadaver pancreata
Fetal pancreata
Expansion of existing human β-cells *in vitro* or *in vivo*
Cultivation of new islets from precursor duct cells *in vitro* or *in vivo*
Stem cells—embryonic and adult
Cell lines
Xenograft sources
Pigs, cows, rodents, rabbits, fish, other
Cell lines
Transgenic pigs (or other species)

ize glucose levels in transplant recipients. Another potential problem is that porcine tissue contains porcine endogenous retroviruses, which can be transferred to human cells in tissue culture (115,116). There is considerable uncertainly about whether this represents a health threat, but in the United States, transplantation of porcine tissue for the treatment of neurologic disease has been allowed to proceed with caution. Thus far, no human recipients of porcine tissue have been reported to carry porcine retroviruses (117).

Immune Attack on Xenogeneic Islets

Rejection of xenografts is a complex and effective process (118–120). There is an early attack called hyperacute rejection mediated by antibodies and complement that can lead to destruction of transplanted organ within minutes. These preformed IgM antibodies recognize a glycoprotein called the Gal-α(1,3)Gal epitope (Gal epitope) that is strongly expressed on the surface of endothelial cells. This is a particular problem for organ transplants because the attack on endothelial cells produces ischemia that leads to rapid death of the organ. Cell transplants may not be as vulnerable to this process. For example, it seems that islet cells from adult pigs have little of this Gal epitope (121). However, even though islet cells might escape hyperacute rejection, they will be subjected to T cell–mediated damage, which seems to be similar to allorejection, and to other insults, such as infiltration with eosinophils and macrophages (118,122). Surprisingly, xenografted tissue may also be susceptible to autoimmune attack, which does not seem to be species-specific (123).

IMMUNOBARRIER TECHNOLOGY

Semipermeable membranes that create an immunobarrier can prevent destructive lymphocytes from killing transplanted islet tissue (124–126). These membranes have openings large enough for glucose, oxygen, and nutrients to reach the encapsulated islets and for insulin to be released to enter the bloodstream. Yet, the holes are small enough to keep white blood cells from penetrating the membrane and reaching the islet cells. Important questions remain about just how permeable the membranes need to be. Recently, it was found that merely maintaining a distance between lymphocytes and islet cells may be enough to prevent autoimmune destruction and allorejection (127,128). Protection of xenotransplants seems to be more difficult because smaller openings might be necessary to limit leakage of shed antigens and to prevent entry of potentially toxic cytokines. It is hoped that immunobarriers, if successful, will make the use of immunosuppressive medication completely unnecessary. Although safe drug treatments that will protect transplanted islet cells may be available in the future, there may be a period during which membrane protection could be clinically useful. The two major approaches are macroencapsulation and microencapsulation.

Macroencapsulation

Macroencapsulation uses devices such as hollow fibers or parallel flat sheets sealed at the edges in which many islets are contained within a single device (125,129–131). Large gel beads or even slabs made of either agarose or alginate can also be considered for macroencapsulation (132). One of the major advantages of such an approach is the possibility of implanting the devices in a variety of locations but of still being able to retrieve or reload them. The main problem with this approach has been the difficulty achieving a practical density, which means that too great a surface area would be required to support the encapsulated islet cells (130). Moreover, questions persist about whether the release of insulin will be rapid enough, particularly from large gel beads, to control blood glucose levels adequately. It is hoped that advances in tissue engineering will improve the potential of macrodevices.

Microencapsulation

Microencapsulation is an approach in which single islets, a small number of islets, or aggregates of cells are contained within a membrane The most commonly used method uses alginate obtained from seaweed, which can form a gel after exposure to calcium or barium in solution (133–137) (Fig. 45.3). Thus, islets can be captured in a small gel bead (less that a millimeter in diameter) that can be coated with a material such as poly-L-lysine that can provide permselectivity. Because poly-L-lysine can generate an inflammatory tissue reaction, an outer layer of alginate usually is added to make the capsules more biocompatible. Recent studies indicate that simple barium alginate microcapsules without a poly-L-lysine coating can successfully protect against autoimmunity and allorejection in mice (128). Agarose has also been used for microcapsules (138), as has alginate mixed with other polymers, such as cellulose sulfate (139). Another approach is to use a polyethylene glycol with photopolymerization to form a coating (140). For a human transplant, probably more than 300,000 islets will need to be encapsulated and placed into the peritoneal cavity, but that can be accommodated, as suggested by a pilot study performed in humans (135).

Although some successes with immunobarrier approaches in both small and large animal models have been reported (126, 133,141), the feasibility and reproducibility of this methodology have still not been established. Many aspects of this technology could be explored to improve the prospects for success. Cooperation between scientists working with polymer chemistry, bioengineering, and islet cell biology needs to be promoted. The field now faces some fundamental questions: how can bio-

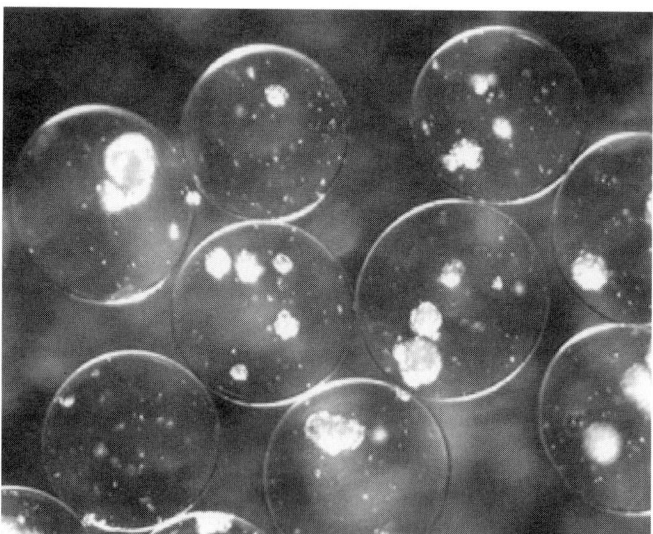

Figure 45.3. Alginate capsules containing porcine neonatal pancreatic cell clusters. Islet cells or aggregates of cells are protected from immune destruction by a semipermeable membrane. A common approach is to use small beads of alginate covered with poly-L-lysine. In some situations the poly-L-lysine is not used. The membrane will prevent penetration by cells and limit the entrance of antibodies. The membrane must be permeable enough to allow the passage of glucose, nutrients, and oxygen to the islets and of insulin out to diffuse into small vessels. (Photograph courtesy of Dr. Abdulkadir Omer.)

incompatibility of the materials be minimized; how thick, dense, and strong should the membranes be; what is the ideal configuration of a device or capsule; should the device be retrievable; and what is the ideal implantation site? Some possibilities are the intraperitoneal space, the omental pouch, the pancreas, a submucosal space in the gut, and a subcutaneous site.

GENE-TRANSFER TECHNOLOGY TO PROTECT ISLETS

Prospects are improving for finding clinically useful vectors that can efficiently transfer genes into cells (142–144), meaning that it will be possible to express genes in islet cells with resultant overproduction or underproduction of designated proteins. Potential vectors for gene transfer include viruses, lipid carriers, or electroporation. An important goal would be to transfer genes so that they would be permanently expressed in all of the insulin-producing cells of an islet. Adenoviral vectors that can transfer genes into islets on a temporary basis are now available; unfortunately, however, their expression cannot be expected to last longer than 80 days. Nonetheless, they can be used for short-term proof-of-principle experiments to learn which genes might be helpful for protecting transplanted islets. Another candidate is the "gutless" adenovirus, which has had so much of its adenovirus structure removed that it should not generate an immune response to the infected cells (145). Another vector that holds attractive promise for efficient gene transfer is the lentivirus, a retrovirus that can transduce genes into the genome of nondividing cells (143,146,147). Permanent transduction can also be obtained with adeno-associated virus vectors (148). It is possible that some way will be found to use synthetic lipid carriers effectively. Yet another possibility is to make transgenic pigs to introduce genes into porcine β-cells using an insulin-promoter construct.

There are many ways by which islets might be protected from either transplant rejection or autoimmune attack. For example, some of the proteins on the outside of a cell, such as class I major histocompatibility (MHC) antigens, might be deleted or changed so that the β-cells would escape recognition by the immune system (149). Another approach is to introduce proteins that might be secreted by transplanted islets and serve as missiles to disable invading lymphocytes. It has already been shown that islets engineered to secrete the small protein CTLA4Ig are more resistant to transplant rejection (150–152). Production of an antibody that would bind to CD40 ligand (CD154) might exert a similar effect. A number of cytokines, such as IL-4, vIL-10, or TGF-β, might exert different kinds of inhibitory influences on attacking lymphocytes. The combination of IL-4 and IL-10 has been able to prevent the development of diabetes in NOD mice, presumably by tilting the immunity away from the destructive Th1 pattern of immune attack (153). Unfortunately, adenoviral expression of IL-10 in transplanted islets has not slowed rejection of rat islets transplanted into mice (154). A recent report suggests islet production of IL-4 was not helpful in preventing allograft rejection (155) but that lentivirus-mediated transduction of islets with IL-4 could protect transplanted islets from insulitis (156). TGF-β can modulate lymphocyte reactions from a Th1 to a Th2 pattern (157,158), but high doses can cause fibrosis, which probably would lead to graft failure. Inhibition of IL-12 with a dominant-negative mutant may also have value for islet transplantation (159). Other potentially valuable peptides that might be secreted by transplanted islets are the IL-1 receptor antagonist protein (IRAP) and soluble type 1 TNF receptors (144). Work is also being carried out with indoleamine 2,3-dioxygenase (IDO), a tryptophane-catabolizing enzyme expressed by the trophoblast that helps inhibit fetal rejection (160).

Another way to improve survival might be to bolster the internal defense mechanisms of β-cells. Various proteins can protect cells against oxidant injury and apoptosis. Thus, one could introduce a gene to make β-cells overexpress catalase or manganese superoxide dismutase, glutathione peroxidase, or heme-oxygenase, which are enzymes that protect against oxidant injury. Alternatively, genes for the anti-apoptotic proteins A20, Bcl2, Bcl-xL, FLIPs, or Myd88 could be used (161–163). Still other genes could provide protection against injury from a combined attack by antibody and complement, which occurs in the early stages of xenograft rejection of organs, but may not be a problem with islets.

It might even be possible to deliver genes to islets *in vivo*, which could be useful for preventing autoimmunity or transplant rejection. One approach is to develop genetically modified lymphocytes that could home to islets through the recognition of islet antigens. A T-cell clone that has been found in mice can home to the islets of NOD mice by recognizing insulin, subduing the autoimmune reaction in the islets, and thereby preventing diabetes (157). This modulation of autoimmunity seems to be exerted by secretion of TGF-β by the T cells. The development of T cells that produce other cytokines, such as IL-4, might also be an attractive strategy. With time, other approaches that could deliver genes to islets *in vivo* are likely to be developed.

PREDICTING THE FUTURE

Attempts to predict the future of islet transplantation have proved hazardous. Unexpected obstacles have plagued this difficult field for decades, and one is not safe predicting anything different for the future. However, with the extraordinary advances occurring in biomedical science, there might be a major breakthrough in the near future; on the other hand, progress might be made in small increments. The results obtained with human allografts should continue to improve as new methods for immunosuppression and immunomodulation are developed that make it possible for more people without kidney transplants to receive islets. There are reasons to be optimistic about the possibility of expansion of human β-cells so that cell supply will no longer be a limiting factor. New approaches to protection from immune destruction are being pursued on many fronts. Even though tolerance is the major goal, it will be necessary to keep working on other approaches, such as better immunosuppressive medications, immunobarrier technology, and gene transfer approaches. Recently, the field of islet transplantation has been infused with new energy and resources that should accelerate the journey to success.

ADDENDUM

Since the initial writing of this chapter, by mid-2004 the Edmonton group transplanted islets to more than 70 patients, using various protocols, and has continued to obtain insulin independence in the vast majority of subjects, although islets from two or more pancreases are still usually required. Other centers in the United States and Europe have been less active, but progress is being made. Two groups have now reported success in obtaining insulin independence from single-donor transplants (164,165). Although encouraging that single-donor islet transplants can succeed, this usually happens only when the recipient has very low insulin requirements and the islet preparation was of excellent quality. It seems likely that the β-cell mass required to normalize glucose levels is proportional to the insulin requirements of the recipient. The Miami and Baylor groups have been successful in coordinating islet transplants between cities, with pancreases flown from Houston to Miami and isolated islets flown back to Houston for implantation (166). This work and that of others show that islets need not be transplanted immediately after isolation, but can be placed in culture and transplanted 1 to 2 days later. To answer the question of whether islets transplanted to individuals with kidney transplants could do as well as the islets-alone Edmonton approach, several groups have had success with a variety of regimens (167–169). A group in Zurich has had comparable success with simultaneous islet kidney transplants (170).

Notable progress has been made in developing immunologic strategies to create tolerance and block autoimmune destruction. This work has been carried out in mice, pigs, and nonhuman primates (171–174).

For further updates on pancreas and islet transplantation, readers are referred to several excellent recent reviews (175–178).

REFERENCES

1. The Diabetes Control and Complications Trial Research Group. The effect of intensive treatment of diabetes on the development and progression of long-term complications in insulin-dependent diabetes mellitus. *N Engl J Med* 1993;329:977–986.
2. UK Prospective Diabetes Study Group. Effect of intensive blood-glucose control with metformin on complications in overweight patients with type 2 diabetes (UKPDS 34). *Lancet* 1998;352:854–865.
3. UK Prospective Diabetes Study Group. Intensive blood-glucose control with sulfonylureas or insulin compared with conventional treatment and risk of complications in patients with type 2 diabetes (UKPDS 33). *Lancet* 1998; 352: 837–853.
4. Palti Y, David GB, Lachov E, et al. Islets of Langerhans generate wavelike electric activity modulated by glucose concentration. *Diabetes* 1996;45: 595–601.
5. Gough DA, Armour JC, Baker DA. Advances and prospects in glucose assay technology. *Diabetologia* 1997;40[Suppl 2]:S102–S107.
6. Williams PW. Notes on diabetes treated with extract and by grafts of sheep's pancreas. *BMJ* 1894;1303–1304.
7. Weir GC, Bonner-Weir S. Insulin secretion in non-insulin-dependent diabetes mellitus. In: LeRoith D, Taylor SI, Olefsky JM, eds. *Diabetes mellitus*, 2nd ed. Philadelphia: Williams and Wilkins, 2000:595–603.
8. Holohan TV. Simultaneous pancreas-kidney and sequential pancreas-after-kidney transplantation. *Health Technol Assess Rep* 1995;4:1–53.
9. Stratta RJ, Weide LG, Sindhi R, et al. Solitary pancreas transplantation. *Diabetes Care* 1997;20:362–368.
10. Sutherland DE. Pancreas and pancreas-kidney transplantation. *Curr Opin Nephrol Hypertens* 1998;7:317–325.
11. Sollinger HW, Odorico JS, Knechtle SJ, et al. Experience with 500 simultaneous pancreas-kidney transplants. *Ann Surg* 1998;228:284–296.
12. Gruessner RW, Sutherland DE, Najarian JS, et al. Solitary pancreas transplantation for nonuremic patients with labile insulin-dependent diabetes mellitus. *Transplantation* 1997;64:1572–1577.
13. Kendall DM, Sutherland DER, Najarian JS, et al. Effects of hemipancreatectomy on insulin secretion and glucose tolerance in healthy humans. *N Engl J Med* 1990;322:898–903.
14. Battezzati A, Bonfatti D, Benedini S, et al. Spontaneous hypoglycaemic after pancreas transplantation in type 1 diabetes mellitus. *Diabet Med* 1998;15: 991–996.
15. Herold KC, Nagamatsu S, Buse JB, et al. Inhibition of glucose-stimulated insulin release from β-TEC3 cells and rodent islets by an analog of FK506. *Transplantation* 1993;55:186–192.
16. Gremlich S, Roduit R, Thorens B. Dexamethasone induces posttranslational degradation of GLUT2 and inhibition of insulin secretion in isolated pancreatic β-cells. *J Biol Chem* 1997;272:3216–3222.
17. Kuo PC, Johnson LB, Schweitzer EJ, et al. Simultaneous pancreas/kidney transplantation—a comparison of enteric and bladder drainage of exocrine pancreatic secretions. *Transplantation* 1997;63:238–243.
18. Bloom RD, Olivares M, Rehman L, et al. Long-term pancreas allograft outcome in simultaneous pancreas-kidney transplantation: a comparison of enteric and bladder drainage. *Transplantation* 1997;64:1689–1695.
19. Stratta RJ, Gaber AO, Shokou-Amiri MH, et al. A prospective comparison of systemic-bladder versus portal-enteric drainage vascularized pancreas transplantation. *Surgery* 2000;127:217–226.
20. Cattral MS, Bigam DL, Heming AW, et al. Portal venous and enteric exocrine drainage versus systemic venous and bladder exocrine drainage of pancreas grafts: clinical outcome of 40 consecutive transplant recipients. *Ann Surg* 2000;232:688–695.
21. Gruessner RW. Tacrolimus in pancreas transplantation: a multicenter analysis. Tacrolimus Pancreas Transplant Study Group. *Clin Transplant* 1997;11: 299–312.
22. London NJ, Farmery SM, Will EJ, et al. Risk of neoplasia in renal transplant patients. *Lancet* 1995;346:403–406.
23. Drachenberg CB, Papdimitriou JC, Klassen DK, et al. Evaluation of pancreas transplant needle biopsy: reproducibility and revision of histologic grading system. *Transplantation* 1997;63:1579–1586.
24. Sutherland DER, Goetz FC, Sibley RK. Recurrence of disease in pancreas transplants. *Diabetes* 1989;38:85–87.
25. Simone EA, Wegmann DR, Eisenbarth GS. Immunologic "vaccination" for the prevention of autoimmune diabetes (type 1A). *Diabetes Care* 1999;22 [suppl 2]:B7–B15.
26. Robertson RP, Holohan TV, Genuth S. Therapeutic controversy: pancreas transplantation for type I diabetes. *J Clin Endocrinol Metab* 1998;83:1868–1874.
27. Manske CL, Wang Y, Thomas W. Mortality of cadaveric kidney transplantation versus combined kidney-pancreas transplantation in diabetic patients. *Lancet* 1995;346:1658–1662.
28. Smets YF, Westendorp RG, van der Piji JW, et al. Effect of simultaneous pancreas-kidney transplantation on mortality of patients with type-1 diabetes mellitus and end-stage renal failure. *Lancet* 1999;353:1915–1919.
29. Becker BN, Brazy PC, Becker YT, et al. Simultaneous pancreas-kidney transplantation reduces excess mortality in type 1 diabetic patients with end-stage renal disease. *Kidney Int* 2000;57:2129–2135.
30. Ramsay RC, Goetz FC, Sutherland DE, et al. Progression of diabetic retinopathy after pancreas transplantation for insulin-dependent diabetes mellitus. *N Engl J Med* 1988;318:208–214.
31. Landgraf R. Impact of pancreas transplantation on diabetic secondary complications and quality of life. *Diabetologia* 1996;39:1415–1424.
32. Navarro X, Sutherland DE, Kennedy WR. Long-term effects of pancreatic transplantation on diabetic neuropathy. *Ann Neurol* 1997;42:727–736.
33. Fioretto P, Steffes MW, Sutherland DER, et al. Reversal of lesions of diabetic nephropathy after pancreas transplantation. *N Engl J Med* 1998;339:69–118.
34. Navarro X, Kennedy WR, Sutherland DER. Autonomic neuropathy and survival in diabetes mellitus: effects of pancreas transplantation. *Diabetologia* 1991;34[Suppl]:S108–S112.
35. Reckard CR, Barker CF. Transplantation of isolated pancreatic islets across strong and weak histocompatibility barriers. *Transplant Proc* 1973;5:761–763.
36. Ballinger WF, Lacy PE. Transplantation of intact pancreatic islets in rats. *Surgery* 1972;72:175–186.
37. Lacy PE, Kostianovsky M. Method for the isolation of intact islets of Langerhans from the rat pancreas. *Diabetes* 1967;16:35–39.
38. Weir GC, Bonner-Weir S. Scientific and political impediments to successful islet transplantation. *Diabetes* 1997;46:1247–1256.
39. Scharp DW, Lacy PE, Santiago JV, et al. Results of our first nine intraportal islet allografts in type 1, insulin dependent diabetic patients. *Transplantation* 1991;51:76–85.
40. Socci C, Falqui L, Davalli AM, et al. Fresh human islet transplantation to replace pancreatic endocrine function in type I diabetic patients. *Acta Diabetol* 1991;28:151–157.
41. Warnock G, Kneteman NM, Ryan EA, et al. Long-term follow-up after transplantation of insulin-producing pancreatic islets into patients with type I (insulin-dependent) diabetes mellitus. *Diabetologia* 1992;35:89–95.
42. Ricordi C, Tzakis AG, Carroll PB, et al. Human islet isolation and allotransplantation in 22 consecutive cases. *Transplantation* 1992;53:407–414.
43. Tzakis AG, Ricordi C, Alejandro R, et al. Pancreatic islet transplantation after upper abdominal exenteration and liver replacements. *Lancet* 1990;336: 402–405.
44. Menger MD, Vajkoczy P, Beger C, et al. Orientation of microvascular blood flow in pancreatic islet isografts. *J Clin Invest* 1994;93:2280–2285.
45. Hering BJ, Ricordi C. Islet transplantation for patients with type 1 diabetes. *Graft* 1999;2:12–27.
46. Brendel MD, Hering BJ, Schultz AO, et al. International Islet Transplant Registry 1999;Newsletter #8:1–20.
47. Alejandro R, Lehmann R, Ricordi C, et al. Long-term function (6 years) of islet allografts in type 1 diabetes. *Diabetes* 1997;46:1983–1989.
48. Oberholzer J, Triponez F, Mage R, et al. Human islet transplantation: lessons from 13 autologous and 13 allogeneic transplantations. *Transplantation* 2000; 69:1115–1123.
49. Secchi A, Socci C, Maffi P, et al. Islet transplantation in IDDM patients. *Diabetologia* 1997;40:225–231.
50. Keymeulen B, Ling Z, Gorus FK, et al. Implantation of standardized beta-cell grafts in a liver segment of IDDM patients: graft and recipient characteristics in two cases of insulin-independence under maintenance immunosuppression for prior kidney graft. *Diabetologia* 1998;41:452–459.
51. Linetsky E, Bottino R, Lehmann R, et al. Improved human islet isolation using a new enzyme blend, Liberase. *Diabetes* 1997;46:1120–1123.
52. Dionne KE, Colton CK, Yarmuch ML. Effect of hypoxia on insulin secretion by isolated rat and canine islets of Langerhans. *Diabetes* 1993;42:12–21.
53. Davalli AM, Scaglia L, Zangen DH, et al. Vulnerability of islets in the immediate posttransplantation period. *Diabetes* 1996;45:1161–1167.
54. Halloran PF, Homik J, Goes N. The "injury response": a concept linking nonspecific injury, acute rejection, and long-term transplant outcomes. *Transplant Proc* 1997;29:79–81.

55. Benent W, Sundberg B, Groth CG, et al. Incompatibility between human blood and isolated islets of Langerhans: a finding with implications for clinical intraportal islet transplantation? *Diabetes* 1999;48:1907–1914.
56. Medzhitov R, Janeway Jr, C. Innate immunity. *N Engl J Med* 2000;343:338–343.
57. Juang J-H, Bonner-Weir S, Wu Y-J, et al. Beneficial influence of glycemic control upon the growth and function of transplanted islets. *Diabetes* 1994;43: 1334–1339.
58. Bonner-Weir S, Taneja M, Weir GC, et al. In vitro cultivation of human islets from expanded ductal tissue. *Proc Natl Acad Sci U S A* 2000;97:7999–8004.
59. Bartlett ST, Chin T, Dirden B, et al. Inclusion of peripancreatic lymph node cells prevents recurrent autoimmune destruction of islet transplants: evidence of donor chimerism. *Surgery* 1995;118:392–397.
60. Uchikoshi F, Yang Z-D, Rostami S, et al. Prevention of autoimmune recurrence and rejection by adenovirus-mediated CTLA4Ig gene transfer to the pancreatic graft in BB rat. *Diabetes* 1999;48:652–657.
61. Lefebvre V, Otonkoski T, Ustinov J, et al. Culture of adult human islet preparations with hepatocyte growth factor and 804G matrix is mitogenic for duct cells but not for beta-cells. *Diabetes* 1998;47:134–137.
62. Kerr-Conte J, Pattou F, Lecomte-Houcke M, et al. Ductal cyst formation in collagen-embedded adult human islet preparations. *Diabetes* 1996;45: 1108–1114.
63. Bonner-Weir S, Orci L. New perspectives on the microvasculature of the islets of Langerhans in the rat. *Diabetes* 1982;31:883–939.
64. Weir GC, Bonner-Weir S. Islets of Langerhans: the puzzle of intraislet interactions and their relevance to diabetes. *J Clin Invest* 1990;85:983–987.
65. Stagner JI, Mokshagundam S, Samols E. Hormone secretion from transplanted islets is dependent upon changes in islet revascularization and islet architecture. *Transplant Proc* 1995;27:3251–3254.
66. Korsgren O, Andersson A, Jansson L, et al. Reinnervation of syngeneic mouse pancreatic islets transplanted into renal subcapsular space. *Diabetes* 1992;41:130–135.
67. Carlsson PO, Palm F, Andersson A, et al. Chronically decreased oxygen tension in rat pancreatic islets transplanted under the kidney capsule. *Transplantation* 2000;69:761–766.
68. Jaeger C, Brendel MD, Hering BJ, et al. Progressive islet graft failure occurs significantly earlier in autoantibody-positive than in autoantibody-negative IDDM recipients of intrahepatic islet allografts. *Diabetes* 1997;46:1907–1910.
69. Braghi S, Bonifacio E, Secchi A, et al. Modulation of humoral islet autoimmunity by pancreas allotransplantation influences allograft outcome in patients with type 1 diabetes. *Diabetes* 2000;49:218–224.
70. Vasconcellos L, Asher F, Schachter D, et al. Cytotoxic lymphocyte gene expression in peripheral blood leukocytes correlates with rejecting renal allografts. *Transplantation* 1998;66:562–566.
71. Shapiro AM, Lakey JR, Ryan EA, et al. Islet transplantation in seven patients with type 1 diabetes mellitus using a glucocorticoid-free immunosuppressive regimen. *N Engl J Med* 2000;27:230–238.
72. Sutherland DER, Gores PF, Hering BJ, et al. Islet transplantation: an update. *Diabetes Metab Rev* 1996;12:137–150.
73. Pyzdroswki KL, Kendall DM, Halter JB, et al. Preserved insulin secretion and insulin independence in recipients of islet autografts. *N Engl J Med* 1992;327: 220–226.
74. Rossini AA, Greiner DL, Mordes JP. Induction of immunologic tolerance for transplantation. *Physiol Rev* 1999;79:99–141.
75. Thomas FT, Ricordi C, Contreras JL, et al. Reversal of naturally occurring diabetes in primates by unmodified islet xenografts without chronic immunosuppression. *Transplantation* 1999;67:846–854.
76. Kenyon NS, Chatzipetrou M, Masetti M, et al. Long-term survival and function of intrahepatic islet allografts in rhesus monkeys treated with humanized anti-CD 154. *Proc Natl Acad Sci U S A* 1999;96:8132–8137.
77. Kenyon NS, Fernandez LA, Lehmann R, et al. Long-term survival and function of intrahepatic islet allografts in baboons treated with humanized andti-CD154. *Diabetes* 1999;48:1473–1481.
78. Markers TG, Serreze DV, Phillips NE, et al. NOD mice have a generalized defect in their response to transplantation tolerance induction. *Diabetes* 1999; 48:967–974.
79. Levisetti M, Padrid PA, Szot GL, et al. Immunosuppressive effects of human CTLA4Ig in non-human primate model of allogeneic pancreatic islet transplantation. *J Immunol* 1997;159:5187–5191.
80. Woodle ES, Xu D, Zivin RA, et al. Phase I trial of a humanized, Fc receptor nonbinding OKT3 antibody, huOKT3gamma1(Ala-Ala) in the treatment of acute renal allograft rejection. *Transplantation* 1999;68:608–616.
81. Quesniaux VF, Menninger K, Kunkler A, et al. The novel immunosuppressant FTY720 induces peripheral lymphodepletion of both T- and B-cells in cynomolgus monkeys when given alone, with cyclosporine neoral or with RAD. *Transplant Immunol* 2000;8:177–187.
82. Basadonna GP, Auersvald L, Khuong CQ, et al. Antibody-mediated targeting of CD45 isoforms: a novel immunotherapeutic strategy. *Proc Natl Acad Sci U S A* 1998;95:3821–3826.
83. Demirci G, Ferrari-Lacraz S, Groves C, et al. IL-15 and IL-2: a matter of life and death for T cells in vivo. *Nat Med* 2001;7:114–118.
84. Feng X, Zheng XX, Yi S, et al. IL-10/Fc inhibits macrophage function and prolongs pancreatic islet xenograft survival. *Transplantation* 1999;68:1775–1783.
85. Selawry HP. Islet transplantation to immunoprivileged sites. In: Lanza RP, Chick WL, eds. *Pancreatic islet transplantation*, Vol. 2. Pittsburgh: R.G. Landes, 1994:75–86.
86. Korbutt GS, Elliott JF, Rajotte RV. Cotransplantation of allogeneic islets with allogeneic testicular cell aggregates allows long-term graft survival without systemic immunosuppression. *Diabetes* 1997;46:317–322.
87. Suarez-Pinzon W, Korbutt GS, Power R, et al. Testicular Sertoli cells protect islet beta-cells from autoimmune destruction in NOD mice by a transforming growth factor-beta1-dependent mechanism. *Diabetes* 2000;49:1810–1818.
88. LaPort RE, Matsushima M, Chang Y-F. Prevalence and incidence of insulin-dependent diabetes. In: *Diabetes in America/National Diabetes Data Group*, 2nd ed. Bethesda, MD: National Institute of Diabetes and Digestive and Kidney Diseases, National Institutes of Health, 1995:37–46.
89. Beattie GM, Otonkoski T, Lopez AD, et al. Functional β-cell mass after transplantation of human fetal pancreatic cells. *Diabetes* 1997;46:244–248.
90. Tuch BE, Simpson AM. Experimental fetal islet transplantation. In: Ricordi C, ed. *Pancreatic islet cell transplantation*. Pittsburgh: R.G. Landes, 1992: 279–290.
91. Bonner-Weir S. Life and death of the pancreatic beta cells. *Trends Endocrinol Metab* 2000;11:375–378.
92. Jonas J-C, Sharma A, Hasenkamp W, et al. Chronic hyperglycemia triggers loss of pancreatic β-cell differentiation in an animal model of diabetes. *J Biol Chem* 1999;274:14112–14121.
93. Montanya E, Nacher V, Biarnes M, et al. Linear correlation between beta-cell mass and body weight throughout the lifespan in Lewis rats: role of beta-cell hyperplasia and hypertrophy. *Diabetes* 2000;49:1341–1346.
94. Zangen DH, Miller CP, Smith FE, et al. Increased islet and ductal insulin promoter-1/idx-1 expression in pancreatic regeneration. *Diabetologia* 1995;38 [suppl.1]:45A.
95. Vogel G. Can old cells learn new tricks? *Science* 2000;287:1418–1419.
96. Kondo T, Raff M. Oligodendrocyte precursor cells reprogrammed to become multipotential CNS stem cells. *Science* 2000;289:1754–1757.
97. Bonner-Weir S, Trent DF, Weir GC. Partial pancreatectomy in the rat and subsequent defect in glucose-induced insulin release. *J Clin Invest* 1983;71:1544–1553.
98. Sharma A, Zangen DH, Reitz P, et al. The homeodomain protein IDX-1 increases after an early burst of proliferation during pancreatic regeneration. *Diabetes* 1999;48:507–513.
99. Ramiya VK, Marraist M, Arfors KE, et al. Reversal of insulin dependent diabetes using islets generated in vitro from pancreatic stem cells. *Nat Med* 2000; 6:278–282.
100. Beattie GM, Itkin-Ansari P, Cirulli V, et al. Sustained proliferation of PDX-1+ cells derived from human islets. *Diabetes* 1999;48:1013–1019.
101. Soria B, Roche E, Berna G, et al. Insulin-secreting cells derived from embryonic stem cells normalize glycemia in streptozotocin-induced diabetic mice. *Diabetes* 2000;49:157–162.
102. Efrat S, Fusco-DeMane D, Lemberg H, et al. Conditional transformation of a pancreatic β-cell line derived from transgenic mice expressing a tetracycline-regulated oncogene. *Proc Natl Acad Sci U S A* 1995;92:3576–3580.
103. Clark SA, Quaade C, Constandy H, et al. Novel insulinoma cell lines produced by iterative engineering of GLUT2, glucokinase, and human insulin expression. *Diabetes* 1997;46:958–967.
104. Hohmeier HE, BeltrandelRio H, Clark SA, et al. Regulation of insulin secretion from novel engineered insulinoma cell lines. *Diabetes* 1997;46:968–977.
105. Lipes MA, Cooper EM, Skelly R, et al. Insulin-secreting non-islet cells are resistant to autoimmune destruction. *Proc Natl Acad Sci U S A* 1996;93: 8596–8600.
106. MacFarlane WM, O'Brien RE, Barnes PD, et al. Sulfonylurea receptor 1 and Kir6.2 expression in the novel human insulin-secreting cell line NES2Y. *Diabetes* 2000;49:953–960.
107. Pipeleers DG, Pipeleers-Marichal M, Hannaert JC, et al. Transplantation of purified islet cells in diabetic rats. I. Standardization of islet cell grafts. *Diabetes* 1991;40:908–919.
108. Davalli AM, Ogawa Y, Scaglia L, et al. Function, mass, and replication of porcine and rat islets transplanted into diabetic nude mice. *Diabetes* 1995;44: 104–111.
109. Brandhorst H, Brandhorst D, Hering BJ, et al. Significant progress in porcine islet mass isolation utilizing Liberase HI for enzymatic low-temperature pancreas digestion. *Transplantation* 1999;68:355–361.
110. Mandel TE, Koulmanda M, Kovarik J, et al. Transplantation of organ cultured fetal pig pancreas in non-obese diabetic (NOD) mice and primates (*Macaca fascicularis*). *Xenotransplantation* 1996;2:128–132.
111. Korsgren O, Andersson A, Sandler S. Pretreatment of fetal porcine pancreas in culture with nicotinamide accelerates reversal of diabetes after transplantation to nude mice. *Surgery* 1993;113:205–214.
112. Tuch BE, Simpson AM, Smith MSR, et al. Basic biology of pig fetal pancreas and its use as an allograft. In: Peterson CM, Jovanovic-Peterson L, eds. *Fetal islet transplantation*. New York: Plenum Press, 1995:51.
113. Korbutt GS, Elliott JF, Ao Z, et al. Large scale isolation, growth, and function of neonatal porcine islets. *J Clin Invest* 1996;97:2119–2129.
114. Yoon K-H, Quickel RR, Tatarkiewicz K, et al. Differentiation and expansion of beta cell mass in porcine neonatal pancreatic cell clusters transplanted into nude mice. *Cell Transplant* 1999;8:673–689.
115. Patience C, Takeuchi Y, Weiss RA. Infection of human cells by an endogenous retrovirus of pigs. *Nat Med* 1997;3:282–286.
116. van der Lean LJ, Lockey C, Griffeth BC, et al. Infection by porcine endogenous retrovirus after islet xenotransplantation in SCID mice. *Nature* 2000;407: 90–94.
117. Paradis K, Langford G, Long Z, et al. Search for cross-species transmission of porcine endogenous retrovirus in patients treated with living pig tissue. *Science* 1999;285:1236–1241.

118. Bach FH, Winkler H, Ferran C, et al. Delayed xenograft rejection. *Immunol Today* 1996;17:379–384.
119. Dorling A, Riesbeck K, Warrens A, et al. Clinical xenotransplantation of solid organs. *Lancet* 1997;349:867–871.
120. Soderlund J, Wennberg L, Castanos-Velez E, et al. Fetal porcine islet-like cell clusters transplanted to cynomolgus monkeys. *Transplantation* 1999;67: 784–791.
121. McKenzie IFC, Koulmanda M, Sandrin MS, et al. Expression of gal(1,3)gal by porcine islet cells and its relevance to xenotransplantation. *Xenotransplantation* 1996;2:139–142.
122. Platt JL, Nagayasu T. Current status of xenotransplantation. *Clin Exp Pharmacol Physiol* 1999;12:1026–1032.
123. Haskins K, Wegmann D. Diabetogenic T-cell clones. *Diabetes* 1996;45: 1299–1305.
124. Colton CK. Implantable biohybrid artificial organs. *Cell Transplant* 1995;4: 415–436.
125. Lacy PE, Hegre OD, Gerasimidi-Vazeou A, et al. Maintenance of normoglycemia in diabetic mice by subcutaneous xenografts of encapsulated islets. *Science* 1991;254:1782–1784.
126. Lanza RP, Jackson R, Sullivan A, et al. Xenotransplantation of cells using biodegradable microcapsules. *Transplantation* 1999;67:1105–1111.
127. Loudovaris T, Jacobs S, Young S, et al. Correction of diabetic NOD mice with insulinomas implanted within Baxter immunoisolation devices. *J Mol Biol* 1999;77:219–222.
128. Duvivier-Kali VF, Omer A, Parent RJ, et al. Complete protection of islets against allorejection and autoimmunity by a simple barium-alginate membrane. *Diabetes* 2001;50:1698–1705.
129. Brauker J, Martinson LA, Young SK, et al. Local inflammatory response around diffusion chambers containing xenografts. *Transplantation* 1996;61: 1671–1677.
130. Suzuki K, Bonner-Weir S, Trivedi N, et al. Function and survival of macroencapsulated syngeneic islets transplanted into streptozocin-diabetic mice. *Transplantation* 1998;66:21–28.
131. Tatarkiewicz K, Hollister-Lock J, Quickel RR, et al. Reversal of hyperglycemia in mice after subcutaneous transplantation of macroencapsulated islets. *Transplantation* 1999;67:665–671.
132. Jain K, Asina SK, Patel SG, et al. Long-term preservation of islets of Langerhans in hydrophilic macrobeads. *Transplantation* 1996;61:532–536.
133. Sun Y, Ma X, Zhou D, et al. Normalization of diabetes in spontaneously diabetic cynomolgus monkeys by xenografts of microencapsulated porcine islets without immunosuppression. *J Clin Invest* 1996;98:1417–1422.
134. De Vos P, De Haan BJ, Wolters GHJ, et al. Improved biocompatibility but limited graft survival after purification of alginate for microencapsulation of pancreatic islets. *Diabetologia* 1997;40:262–270.
135. Soon-Shiong P, Heintz RE, Merideth N, et al. Insulin independence in a type 1 diabetic patient after encapsulated islet transplantation. *Lancet* 1994;343: 950–951.
136. Lanza RP, Chick WL. Transplantation of encapsulated cells and tissues. *Surgery* 1997;121:1–9.
137. Calafiore R. Perspectives in pancreatic and islet cell transplantation for the therapy of IDDM. *Diabetes Care* 1997;20:889–895.
138. Iwata H, Takagi T, Amemiya H, et al. Agarose for a bioartificial pancreas. *J Biomed Mater Res* 1992;26:967–977.
139. Wang T, Lacik I, Brissova M, et al. An encapsulation system for the immunoisolation of pancreatic islets. *Nat Biotechnol* 1997;15:358–362.
140. Cruise GM, Hegre OD, Lamberti FV, et al. In vitro and in vivo performance of porcine islets encapsulated in interfacially photopolymerized poly(ethylene glycol) diacrylate membranes. *Cell Transplant* 1999;8:293–306.
141. Soon-Shiong P, Feldman E, Nelson R, et al. Long-term reversal of diabetes by the injection of immunoprotected islets. *Proc Natl Acad Sci U S A* 1993;90: 5843–5847.
142. Saldeen J, Curiel DT, Eizirik DL, et al. Efficient gene transfer to dispersed human pancreatic islet cells in vitro using adenovirus-polylysine/DNA complexes or polycationic liposomes. *Diabetes* 1996;45:1197-1203.
143. Leibowitz G, Beattie GM, Kafri T, et al. Gene transfer to human pancreatic endocrine cells using viral vectors. *Diabetes* 1999;48:745–753.
144. Giannoukakis N, Rudert WA, Robbins PD, et al. Targeting autoimmune diabetes with gene therapy. *Diabetes* 1999;48:2107–2121.
145. Chen HH. Persistence in muscle of an adenoviral vector that lacks all viral genes. *Proc Natl Acad Sci U S A* 1997;94:1645–1650.
146. Naldini L, Blomer U, Gallay P, et al. In vivo gene delivery and stable transduction of nondividing cells by a lentiviral vector. *Science* 1996;272:263–267.
147. Blomer UL, Naldini L, Kafri T, et al. Highly efficient and sustained gene transfer in adult neurons with a lentivirus vector. *J Virol* 1997;71:6641–6649.
148. Fisher KJ, Jooss K, Alston J, et al. Recombinant adeno-associated virus for muscle directed gene therapy. *Nat Med* 1997;3:306–312.
149. Efrat S, Fejer G, Brownlee M, et al. Prolonged survival of pancreatic islet allografts mediated by adenovirus immunoregulatory transgenes. *Proc Natl Acad Sci U S A* 1995;92:6947–6951.
150. Steurer W, Nickerson PW, Steele AW, et al. Ex vivo coating of islet cell allografts with murine CTLA4/Fc promotes graft tolerance. *J Immunol* 1995;155: 1165–1174.
151. Gainer AL, Korbutt GS, Rajotte RV, et al. Expression of CTLA4-Ig by biolistically transfected mouse islets promotes islet allograft survival. *Transplantation* 1997;63:1017–1021.
152. Feng S, Quickel RR, Hollister-Lock J, et al. Prolonged xenograft survival of islets infected with small doses of adenovirus containing CTLA4Ig. *Transplantation* 1999;67:1607–1613.
153. Rabinovitch A, Suarez-Pinzon WL, Sorensen O, et al. Combined therapy with interleukin-4 and interleukin-10 inhibits autoimmune diabetes recurrence in syngeneic islet-transplanted nonobese diabetic mice. *Transplantation* 1995;60: 368–374.
154. Deng S, Ketchum RJ, Kucher T, et al. IL-10 and TGF-beta gene transfer for xenogeneic islet transplantation: comparison of effect in concordant vs discordant combination. *Transplant Proc* 1997;29:2204–2205.
155. Davies JD, Mueller R, Minson S, et al. Interleukin-4 secretion by the allograft fails to affect the allograft-specific interleukin-4 response in vitro. *Transplantation* 1999;67:1583–1589.
156. Gallichan WS, Kafri T, Krahl T, et al. Lentivirus-mediated transduction of islet grafts with interleukin 4 results in sustained gene expression and protection from insulitis. *Hum Gene Ther* 1998;18:2717–2726.
157. Zekzer D, Wong FS, Wen L, et al. Inhibition of diabetes by an insulin-reactive CD4 T-cell clone in the nonobese diabetic mouse. *Diabetes* 1997;46:1124–1132.
158. King C, Davies J, Mueller R, et al. TGF-beta l alters APC preference, polarizing islet antigen responses toward a Th2 phenotype. *Immunity* 1998;8:601–613.
159. Yasuda H, Nagata M, Arisawa K, et al. Local expression of immunoregulatory IL-12p40 gene prolonged syngeneic islet graft survival in diabetic NOD mice. *J Clin Invest* 1998;102:1807–1814.
160. Mellor AL, Munn DH. Tryptophan catabolism and T-cell tolerance: immunosuppression by starvation? *Immunol Today* 1999;20:469–473.
161. Chao DT, Linette GP, Boise LH, et al. Bcl-XL and Bcl-2 repress a common pathway of cell death. *J Exp Med* 1995;182:821–828.
162. Sarma V, Lin Z, Clark L, et al. Activation of the B-cell surface receptor CD40 induces A20, a novel zinc finger protein that inhibits apoptosis. *J Biol Chem* 1995;270:12343–12346.
163. Rabinovitch LY, Suarez-Pinzon W, Muhkerjee B, et al. Expression of the bcl-2 gene from a defective HSV-1 amplicon vector protects pancreatic beta-cells from apoptosis. *Hum Gene Ther* 1996;7:1719–1726.
164. Hering BJ, Kandaswamy R, Harmon JV, et al. Transplantation of cultured islets from two-layer preserved pancreases in type 1 diabetes with anti-CD3 antibody. *Am J Transplant* 2004;4:390–401.
165. Markmann JF, Deng S, Huang X, et al. Insulin independence following isolated islet transplantation and single islet infusions. *Ann Surg* 2003;237: 749–750.
166. Goss JA, Schock AP, Brunicardi FC, et al. Achievement of insulin independence in three consecutive type-1 diabetic patients via pancreatic islet transplantation using islets isolated at a remote islet isolation center. *Transplantation* 2002;74:1761–1766.
167. Kessler L, Bucher P, Milliat-Guittard L, et al. Influence of islet transportation on pancreatic islet allotransplantation in type 1 diabetic patients within the Swiss-French GRAGIL network. *Transplantation* 2004;77:1301–1304.
168. Fiorina P, Folli F, Bertuzzi F, et al. Long-term beneficial effect of islet transplantation on diabetic macro-microangiopathy in type 1 diabetic kidney-transplanted patients. *Diabetes Care* 2003;26:1129–1136.
169. Cagliero E, Chandraker A, Dea A, et al. Islet cell transplantation in type 1 diabetic patients recipient of renal allografts. *Diabetes* 2004;53:(Suppl 2]A452.
170. Lehmann R, Weber M, Berthold P, et al. Successful simultaneous islet-kidney transplantation using a steroid-free immunosuppression: two-year follow-up. *Am J Transplant* 2004;4:1117–1123.
171. Zheng XX, Sanchez-Fueyo A, Sho M, et al. Favorably tipping the balance between cytopathic and regulatory T cells to create transplantation tolerance. *Immunity* 2003;19:503–514.
172. Nikolic B, Takeuchi Y, Leykin I, et al. Mixed hematopoietic chimerism allows cure of autoimmune diabetes through allogeneic tolerance and reversal of autoimmunity. *Diabetes* 2004;53:376–383.
173. Contreras JL, Jenkins S, Eckhoff DE, et al. Stable alpha- and beta-islet cell function after tolerance induction to pancreatic islet allografts in diabetic primates. *Am J Transplant* 2003;3:128–138.
174. Kamano C, Vagefi PA, Kumagai N, et al. Vascularized thymic lobe transplantation in miniature swine: thymopoiesis and tolerance induction across fully MHC-mismatched barriers. *Proc Natl Acad Sci U S A* 2004;101:3827–3832.
175. Sutherland DE, Gruessner A, Hering BJ. Beta-cell replacement therapy (pancreas and islet transplantation) for treatment of diabetes mellitus: an integrated approach. *Endocrinol Metab Clin North Am* 2004;33:135–148.
176. Oberholzer J, Shapiro AM, Lakey JR, et al. Current status of islet cell transplantation. *Adv Surg* 2003;37:253–282.
177. Shapiro AM, Nanji SA, Lakey JR. Clinical islet transplant: current and future directions towards tolerance. *Immunol Rev* 2003;196:219–236.
178. Robertson RP. Islet transplantation as a treatment for diabetes—a work in progress. *N Engl J Med* 2004;350:694–705.

CHAPTER 46

Diabetes and the Healthcare System: Economic and Social Costs

James L. Rosenzweig

In the United States, the medical costs of diabetes are substantial. As the prototype of the chronic disease involving multiple organ systems, diabetes has presented a great challenge to the health-care system at a time of transition from traditional fee-for-service reimbursement to managed care and capitation. In the United States, a significant proportion of the individuals with diabetes have undiagnosed disease (1). A review of all of the currently accepted performance measures and indicators of quality of care for patients with diabetes shows that goals for care are not being met in the United States and in the world at large (2,3).

In reviewing the management of diabetes mellitus, one must be aware of certain general principles. First of all, diabetes is a complex, chronic disorder. Unlike some other chronic disorders, such as asthma and osteoarthritis, it involves multiple systems. Diabetes is not just an endocrine disease, and control of glycemia, although important, is not the only aim of therapy. Prevention and treatment of the long-term complications of the disease comprise a major part of the overall care of diabetes. Many of the efforts of treatment involve measures that have incremental effects and result in changes in patient behavior that have no perceivable benefit to the patient at the time of intervention but may have significant effects many years later. In accomplishing these goals, the primary caregiver must be able to work in a team with specialists and educators.

PREVALENCE OF DIABETES IN THE UNITED STATES AND IN THE WORLD

Diabetes is one of the most common chronic diseases affecting people in the United States. It is estimated that currently 18.2 million Americans have diabetes, representing 6.3% of the population. This figure includes 13 million individuals with diagnosed diabetes and an estimated 5.3 million people who are currently undiagnosed and untreated. It is estimated that approximately 798,000 new cases of diabetes are diagnosed each year (4). The prevalence of diabetes in the United States increased progressively during the second half of the 20th century, with an approximately 40% increase recorded since the late 1970s. It is clear that the overall burden of diabetes will increase substantially worldwide in the next 20 years.

Several factors have contributed to the increasing burden of diabetes in the United States and worldwide. These include a specific increase in the risk factors for type 2 diabetes, such as increasing obesity (5,6) and lack of adequate physical activity (7), both of which have been shown to increase the likelihood of developing diabetes (8,9). The increased aging of the population worldwide (10) is contributing to the prevalence of a disease associated with aging. In addition, the United States has seen a rapid and proportionately greater growth of those minority populations at the greatest risk for type 2 diabetes and its associated complications (11), as well as of populations throughout the world with increased risk (12). Another factor contributing to the apparent increase in the prevalence of diabetes has been the improvement in surveillance systems for diabetes, which has allowed better assessment of the true burden of diabetes (13).

Many additional new cases probably still go undiagnosed. Data from the National Health Interview Survey indicate that approximately 93% of all people with diabetes have characteristics of type 2 diabetes (14). The prevalence of both diagnosed and undiagnosed diabetes increases progressively with age—from approximately 1.6% of individuals 20 to 39 years of age to approximately 20% of individuals 60 years of age and older. The great majority of individuals older than age 40 years have type 2 diabetes (even a majority of those younger than 40 have type 2 diabetes).

Both diagnosed and undiagnosed diabetes are especially prevalent in minority ethnic populations. When the prevalence is standardized for age and sex, diabetes is 1.6 times more prevalent among non-Hispanic African Americans and 1.9 times more prevalent among Hispanic Americans than among non-Hispanic whites (15). Impaired fasting glucose levels, a condition that is thought to be a precursor to, and to predispose individuals to, type 2 diabetes, is significantly more prevalent in Hispanic-Americans than among non-Hispanic whites and tends to occur at earlier ages in this ethnic population. The incidence and severity of the major secondary complications of diabetes are also greater in these populations than in the general population.

Although the incidence of diabetes will continue to increase substantially in the United States and other developed nations, the rate of increase will be much more rapid in developing countries, which are much less able to handle the financial burden imposed by either conventional or intensive treatment of diabetes. The World Health Organization estimates that the number of people in the world with diabetes may nearly double by the year 2030, approaching 360 million people (16). Enormous increases in diabetes are projected for Southeast Asia, the western Pacific, the eastern Mediterranean, and the Americas. The actual cause of this increasing worldwide epidemic is not entirely clear, but it is likely related to decreased physical activity and changes in diet related to the industrialization in these regions (Fig. 46.1).

IMPACT OF THE COMPLICATIONS OF DIABETES

Diabetes has a major impact on the health of the U.S. population. It is the leading cause of new blindness, end-stage renal disease (ESRD), and non–trauma-related amputations in adults. Care for diabetes and its complications consumes approximately 15% of

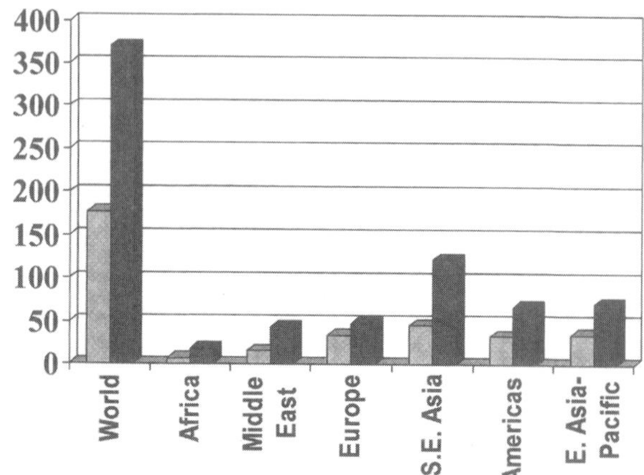

Figure 46.1. Number of persons with diabetes mellitus in the world, by geographic region, in the year 2000, compared with projected estimates by the World Health Organization (WHO) for the year 2030. (Adapted from data from WHO. Available at: http://www.who.int/ncd/dia/databases4.htm. Accessed March 4, 2004.)

the total healthcare expenditures in the country. That figure is out of proportion to the 6% prevalence of diabetes, reflecting the excess morbidity of and medical care required by patients with diabetes.

Diabetes is associated with a substantially increased mortality risk in both men and women. Risk of death is increased threefold to fivefold for persons age 45 to 64 and twofold to threefold for those age 65 to 74. The relative risk declines with advanced age as mortality due to other disease increases. In each age group, women with diabetes have a greater relative mortality risk than do men with diabetes. In the United States, approximately 18% to 20% of those persons who die between the ages of 45 to 74 years have diabetes (17).

People with diabetes are two to four times more likely to experience heart attack or stroke than are people without diabetes (4). People with diabetes younger than age 45 years are 11.5 times more likely to have cardiovascular disease than are people without diabetes. The relative risk of having cardiovascular disease, as well as other comorbidities, which decreases with increasing age, still remains substantially elevated for people with diabetes older than age 65 years (4).

The most common cause of death in people with type 1 or type 2 diabetes is cardiovascular disease, which is the cause of more than 50% of deaths. The acute complications of diabetes, such as ketoacidosis, hyperosmolar coma, and hypoglycemia, are the next most common cause of death, representing about 13%. As individuals with diabetes age, the relative contribution of cardiovascular disease to mortality increases and the contribution of acute complications decreases (18). In the Multiple Risk Factor Intervention Trial, the absolute risk of death related to cardiovascular disease in men with diabetes was substantially increased compared with that in men without diabetes for every age group, ethnic background, and number of additional cardiovascular risk factors (19). The mortality rates for men with diabetes increased steeply as the number of risk factors increased. When patients with diabetes are followed up for 6 years after a myocardial infarction (MI), their mortality risk is increased by 40%, compared with the risk following MI in patients without diabetes (20). The increased risk of post-MI mortality is even more pronounced in women with diabetes than in men with diabetes. Although there has been a substantial decline in mortality due to coronary heart disease in the United States over the past 30 years, this has not been seen in patients with diabetes. In fact, age-adjusted mortality due to heart disease has increased 23% for women with diabetes (21). It is thought that the general decrease in cardiovascular mortality in the general U.S. population is due to a reduction in cardiovascular risk factors and improved methods of treatment of coronary artery disease. These measures have been less effective for patients with diabetes, especially women.

The morbidity associated with the chronic complications of diabetes also represents a significant public health problem. Diabetes is the leading cause of new blindness in adults aged 20 to 74 years (4), accounting for 20% of all new cases of blindness in persons aged 45 to 85 years caused in large part by diabetic retinopathy (22). It is estimated that approximately 90% of these cases can be prevented with improved glycemic control, annual ophthalmologic examinations, and the use of laser treatment if necessary. The prevalence of cataracts is twofold to fourfold higher in patients with type 2 diabetes than in the population without diabetes. Cataracts are a common cause of visual impairment, but not permanent blindness, in older individuals.

Diabetes is also the leading cause of ESRD (4), accounting for 43% of new cases—substantially more than either hypertension or glomerulonephritis. In the United States, the number of new cases of ESRD due to diabetes increased fivefold to sixfold between 1984 and 2001 (23), and the percentage of all cases of ESRD due to diabetes has increased from 28% to 43% (24). A high percentage of these cases could be prevented or substantially delayed with measures aimed at improving glycemic control, more aggressive treatment of hypertension, and early treatment of microalbuminuria with angiotensin-converting enzyme inhibitors.

The risk for amputation in individuals with diabetes is substantially greater than that in people without diabetes; diabetes accounts for greater than 60% of nontraumatic lower-limb amputations in the United States (25). This is due in large part to either peripheral vascular disease or peripheral neuropathy, which occurs in approximately 50% of individuals who have had diabetes 20 years or longer (26). Many of these cases could be prevented by regular foot examinations and treatment, appropriate education in foot self-care, improved control of blood glucose and cholesterol, and smoking cessation.

In the United States, diabetes costs are more than $132 billion annually, with $92 billion related to direct medical costs. In 1992 the cost was $85 billion, and the numbers are increasing each year (27). There is currently no healthcare policy agenda focused on arresting the increase of this chronic disease, which involves 18 million Americans and is the second most expensive disease in the United States. In this country, diabetes is the leading cause of blindness, amputations, ESRD, kidney dialysis, and kidney transplantation (18). The mortality due to type 1 diabetes is 30% higher in the United States than in Europe, and in the United States serious renal disease in all types of diabetes is more than quadruple the rate in Europe (28,29).

GLYCEMIC CONTROL AND MORBIDITY

Poor glycemic control is a major reason for the high incidence of microvascular complications involving the eyes, kidneys, and nerves of people with diabetes. The Diabetes Control and Complications Trial (DCCT) clearly demonstrated the benefits of improved glycemic control in reducing both the incidence and the progression of retinopathy and nephropathy in people with type 1 diabetes (30). Substantial clinical and epidemiologic evidence, especially from the United Kingdom Prospective Diabetes Study (31), the Kumamoto Study (32), and the Wisconsin Epidemiological Study (33), indicates that the same principle applies to patients with type 2 diabetes.

The diagnosis of diabetic ketoacidosis involved approximately 100,000 hospitalizations in the United States between 1989 and 1991 and represented almost 5% of all patients with diabetes admitted to hospitals. Most of these admissions are preventable. Severe hypoglycemia is also a major cause of increased emergency department visits and hospitalizations.

DISABILITY, ABSENTEEISM, AND EMPLOYMENT ISSUES ASSOCIATED WITH DIABETES

Disability affects many persons with diabetes in the United States, with estimates ranging from 20% to 50% of the diabetic population. Individuals with diabetes report rates of disability that are substantially higher than those reported by the general U.S. population. Reported activity limitations were two to three times higher among persons with diabetes than among those without diabetes (34). Patients with type 1 diabetes from the Children's Hospital of Pittsburgh IDDM (insulin-dependent diabetes mellitus) registry were seven times more likely to report work disability than were their nondiabetic siblings.

Impairments for persons with either type 1 or type 2 diabetes increase with age. Disability is more common in minority groups. Disability is proportionately more common in persons with type 2 diabetes than among those with type 1 diabetes (63.5% versus 42.9% report activity limitations), possibly because of the older average age of patients with type 2 diabetes. The major determinant for disability appears to be the presence of the late complications of diabetes.

The effects of disability on the population of persons with diabetes are very extensive. Patients with type 1 diabetes who are disabled have dramatically lower rates of employment than do individuals with diabetes who are not disabled (49% not working versus 12%) and higher rates of absenteeism (13.8 days per year versus 3.0 per year). Disabled individuals with diabetes use healthcare services more frequently, with greater than twice the hospitalization rates and average number of physician visits and a decreased quality of life.

Rates of absenteeism among employees with diabetes are reported as elevated in some studies but not others (35–37). Although there is controversy regarding the importance of absenteeism in persons with diabetes, it is clear that significant rates of absenteeism tend to be limited to a small subset of the population of individuals with diabetes—not more than 30%. Most employees with diabetes have normal work attendance records. There is a suggestion that many of the persons who have high rates of absenteeism may be disabled (34). Disabled people with diabetes tend to be absent more frequently and have longer absences than do people with diabetes who are not disabled.

If the impact of disability in persons with diabetes is similar to that in the general population, disability will have significant effects on their employability. A lower proportion of persons with diabetes than persons without diabetes are currently employed, even after adjustments are made for age (Fig. 46.2), but the proportion of those not employed who are disabled is similar to that in the general population (34).

With a higher degree of unemployment and absenteeism, there is concern that persons with diabetes may face discrimination in the workplace. This has been reported in several studies (38,39). The 1990 Americans with Disabilities Act, however, expanded the opportunities of disabled persons with diabetes. This legislation provides standards in employee hiring and allows for work-rule and work-environment changes to meet the needs of individuals with disabilities. It applies to all employers with at least 15 employees, and diabetes is specifically listed as a disability under the Act. The concept that diabetes is in and of itself a disability is a controversial one, but the legislation makes it illegal to discriminate against an individual just because he or she has diabetes.

Nevertheless, there are specific areas of employment where employment of persons with diabetes continues to be restricted. Persons with diabetes taking insulin have been restricted from being airline pilots, drivers in interstate commerce, drivers of local mass transit, and, until recently, air-traffic controllers. The major concern has been the risk of developing hypoglycemia during situations in which alterations in judgment or consciousness could put the pilot or driver in danger or at risk to others. The availability of self-monitoring of blood glucose, along with a greater variety of insulin regimens in recent years, the ability to adjust doses, and count carbohydrates, has ameliorated this problem somewhat, but the DCCT established that intensified insulin treatment can be associated with an increased risk for severe hypoglycemia (30). Since 1984, the American Diabetes Association has taken the position that "Any person with diabetes, whether insulin dependent or non-insulin dependent, should be eligible for any employment for which he/she is otherwise qualified" (40). It is understood, however, that a small minority of patients with diabetes lack or are unable to recognize the warning signs of hypoglycemia and are at greater risk for alterations in mental function that might lead to confusion or alteration in consciousness. Those individuals who have recurrent episodes of severe hypoglycemia should be individually evaluated and, in some situations, be considered for modification of their employment responsibilities.

OTHER SOCIAL ISSUES IN DIABETES

Driving

It has long been claimed that diabetes is associated with an increased risk of automobile accidents and crashes. Three studies, of drivers in California, Oklahoma, and Washington state, identified increased rates of crashes in drivers with diabetes (41–43). However, it is possible that the drivers with diabetes in these studies were selected because they had more severe disease. In addition, selection bias may have played a role in some of these studies because the drivers with chronic disease were under review for driving offenses. Another study (44) linked the diagnosis of diabetes to an increased risk of hospitalization for driving-related road trauma, but only among younger drivers.

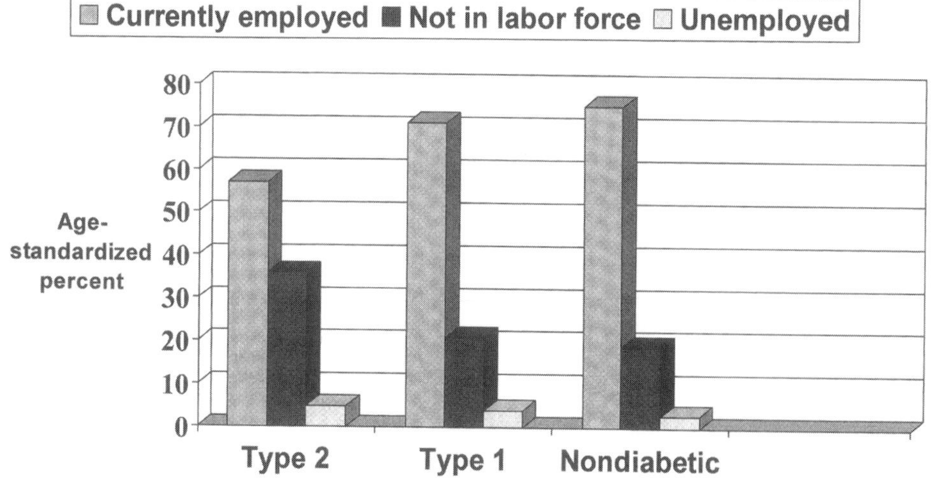

Figure 46.2. The employment status of individuals with type 2 diabetes, with type 1 diabetes, and without diabetes. (From Songer TJ. Disability in diabetes. In: Harris MI, Cowie CC, Stern MP, et al, eds. *Diabetes in America*, 2nd ed. Bethesda, MD: National Institute of Diabetes and Digestive and Kidney Diseases, 1995:259–278. NIDDKD publication no. 95-1468.)

A study of truck-permit holders and commercial drivers in Quebec found an increased relative risk of crashes for drivers with non–insulin-treated diabetes without complications but not for those treated with insulin or with complications (45). Other studies, however, have failed to find an association between driving accidents and diabetes (46–49).

Driving requires complex psychomotor skills, processing of information, and accurate judgment. It is impaired by acute hypoglycemia. Repeated episodes of mild hypoglycemia can be associated with a decreased ability to recognize its symptoms and an increased risk of cognitive impairment. A study of the performance of individuals with diabetes in a driving simulator during induced episodes of mild and moderate hypoglycemia showed that driving performance can be significantly disrupted during relatively mild hypoglycemia, and many individuals fail to take corrective action to treat the hypoglycemia (50). Another study, however, reported that most drivers with hypoglycemia who were cognitively impaired recognized this and reported the perception that they could not drive safely at hypoglycemic levels, but men and middle-aged patients were more likely than women and men under 25 years of age to judge that it was safe for them to drive during hypoglycemia (51). It is important for those with diabetes to have educational reinforcement of safe driving habits and to be encouraged to check glucose levels before driving. Persons whose glucose levels are below 70 mg/dL should be treated before driving. Blood glucose awareness training (BGAT), an 8-week training program that uses behavioral techniques to increase awareness of fluctuations in blood glucose levels, has been associated with fewer and less extreme hypoglycemic events (52) and in follow-up studies has been found to be associated with a reduction in motor vehicle crashes and violations (53).

Because hypoglycemia may be a factor in motor vehicle accidents, most regulatory authorities put restrictions on applicants who have insulin-treated diabetes, whether they have type 1 or type 2 diabetes. However, only individuals with type 1 diabetes appear to be at greater risk for driving mishaps (54). For many years, the U.S. Federal Highway Administration prohibited individuals using insulin from obtaining commercial vehicle driving licenses. However, it had temporarily permitted waivers for some insulin-using drivers (55) but is currently not giving them. Many states are allowing some individuals with insulin-treated diabetes to drive commercial vehicles within state boundaries. The American Diabetes Association has argued for repeal of federal restrictions on commercial drivers with insulin-treated diabetes because of the claim that it is discriminatory and contrary to the Americans with Disabilities Act (56). This remains a complex and contentious issue, in which the justified advocacy for the rights of people with diabetes must be balanced with careful analysis of the risks to public safety.

Travel

The successful management of diabetes requires careful attention to the synchronization of insulin or oral hypoglycemic agents to meals and physical activity. The changes in meals, activity, and time zones that occur with air flight can create unique problems for individuals with diabetes, especially those injecting insulin or using subcutaneous insulin infusion pumps. In addition, travelers to distant countries have to carry syringes and vials of insulin, and the increased security needs of air travel pose special problems. This has become acutely evident since the events of September 11, 2001. Many airlines and countries now require air-travel passengers to carry written documentation of their medical condition and the need to carry syringes, needles, and vials of insulin for injection. Despite these inconveniences, there is no reason why most individuals with diabetes, whether or not they require insulin, should not be able to travel extensively by air across long distances or time zones. Travelers with diabetes should observe the following guidelines, which are modified from the previous edition of this text (57).

1. The patient should review travel plans with his or her care provider and adjust the timing of meals and insulin dosages to the schedule of travel. How this is accomplished is highly individualized for each patient and travel plan. Good communication between patient and care provider is essential.
2. The patient should be supplied with a note from the physician outlining the diagnosis, listing the generic and proprietary names of medications, giving the physician's name and telephone number, and, if possible, listing physicians at the destination who can be consulted in an emergency. Most countries have diabetes associations that can assist international travelers. If the patient carries syringes, lancets, or needles for injection, the note should document the medical necessity for their use.
3. The patient should carry adequate supplies of medications and materials to treat hypoglycemia. He or she should not depend upon the local availability of these materials. These supplies should never be checked in baggage that is not accessible or that might reach a different destination. On some trips, it may be appropriate to carry extra prescriptions for insulin, syringes, and other essential supplies in case of loss or theft.
4. It is important for the insulin-requiring patient to have on his or her person easy identification of diabetes in case of emergency. These individuals should wear medical-alert bracelets or necklaces whether or not they are traveling, but it is especially important for them to wear them during travel to distant places or foreign countries.
5. The patient should conduct frequent glucose monitoring throughout the trip, especially when traveling across time zones and when meal schedules are altered.
6. The patient should take special precautions to avoid motion sickness or travelers' diarrhea, both of which may contribute to hypoglycemia, dehydration, or ketoacidosis, and must be especially careful to have the proper immunizations when traveling abroad.

COSTS OF MEDICAL CARE OF DIABETES

The economic costs of diabetes were reported as $11.6 billion in direct medical costs in 1986 for people with type 2 diabetes (58) and $45.2 billion in direct medical costs in 1992 for all people with a diagnosis of diabetes (59). A study comparing the costs of treatment of patients with and without diabetes in 1992 showed that, on average, the annual per capita health expenditures for patients with diabetes were approximately three and a half times the costs for patients without diabetes. From this it could be calculated that the costs of care of patients with diabetes represented almost 15% of total healthcare expenditures in the United States.

The American Diabetes Association published more extensive analyses of the economic costs of diabetes, calculating that direct medical and indirect expenditures attributable to diabetes totaled $98 billion in 1997 (60) and $132 billion in 2002 (61). Direct costs are those associated with hospitalization, ambulatory care, and medication. Indirect costs represent lost productivity due to morbidity and premature mortality. To this must also be added intangible costs, such as reduced life expectancy and quality of life, for which the assignment of a monetary value is difficult (62,63). The per capita mean costs for persons with diabetes, $13,243 per year, were found to be five times those for persons without diabetes, but this ratio overstates the impact of diabetes because these patients tend to be older, on average (61). The ratio of per capita expenditures between people with and without diabetes was substantially greater for nonwhite patients (4.5:1) than for white patients (3.6:1). Expenditures for outpatient medications were 3.2 times greater for patients with diabetes. The ratio of expenditures between persons with diabetes and persons without diabetes was nearly identical in patients who were younger than 45 years of age (3.2:1) and in those 45 to 64 years of age (3.3:1). This ratio dropped to 1.6:1 for patients 65 years of age and older, as the increased medical costs for nondiabetic elderly patients narrowed the gap.

Direct medical expenditures associated with diabetes totaled $91.8 billion, of which $23.2 billion was related to control of diabetes and blood glucose, $24.6 billion to excess prevalence of the chronic complications of diabetes, and $44.1 billion to excess prevalence of general medical conditions. As expected, the largest proportion of expenditures attributable to diabetes was for inpatient care (43.9%), then for nursing-home care (15.1%), and then for outpatient care (10.9%). Two thirds of the costs for medical care for diabetes are due to care of the elderly. Indirect costs related to diabetes were calculated to be $39.8 billion, of which $7.5 billion was attributed to disability.

The payment for medical services for diabetes is in significant flux. In 1987, 15% of patients were self-paying, whereas in 1991, the number increased to 20%. In 1991, health maintenance organizations (HMOs) became a significant payer group, accounting for 12% of payments for patients with diabetes nationally. This number is now increasing steadily. For some HMOs, diabetes accounts for 15% to 20% of the medical costs, although patients with diabetes account for only 2% of the persons cared for. All patients with diabetes are acutely aware that there is less support for this disease, with regard to education, supplies, and healthcare access.

In 1992, the direct costs of hospitalizations related to diabetes were $37 billion. There has been a decrease in the absolute number of admissions of patients with diabetes—probably approximately 15% during the decade of 1980 to 1990—and a decrease in the primary diagnoses of diabetes by 38% between 1983 and 1990 (64). These data reflect more stringent criteria for hospital admissions. Although the absolute number of admissions of patients with diabetes has decreased, the percentage of diagnoses of diabetes among all discharged patients increased by 27% between 1983 and 1990. These data reflect a relative enrichment of inpatient cases of individuals with diabetes, explaining the increases in hospitalization costs. Diabetes accounted for 8.4% of all hospital admissions during 1989 through 1991, and female patients represented 57% of these admissions. Patients with diabetes are hospitalized 2.4 to 3 times more frequently than are individuals without diabetes. In addition, the duration of their hospital stay is 30% longer on average, exceeding that of patients without diabetes by 1.7 days (65,66). Diseases of the circulatory system were the most frequently listed primary diagnosis: 33% of cases. The proportion of cases in which diabetes was listed as the primary diagnosis declined significantly from 29% in 1980 to 15% in 1990, as treatment of hyperglycemia has shifted from the inpatient to the outpatient setting under managed care in the United States. That trend should be expected to continue. Although hospitalizations for control of glycemia have decreased, the age-adjusted number of hospitalizations per 100 people with diabetes increased 11.7% during 1980 through 1990 (64). It has been estimated that costs associated with the hospitalization of individuals with diabetes in the United States were $37 billion in 1992 and that between 64% and 80% of direct expenditures for people with confirmed diabetes were incurred in the inpatient setting (34,67) (Fig. 46.3).

Diabetes is associated with increased medical care costs in the managed care setting. A comparison of 85,209 patients

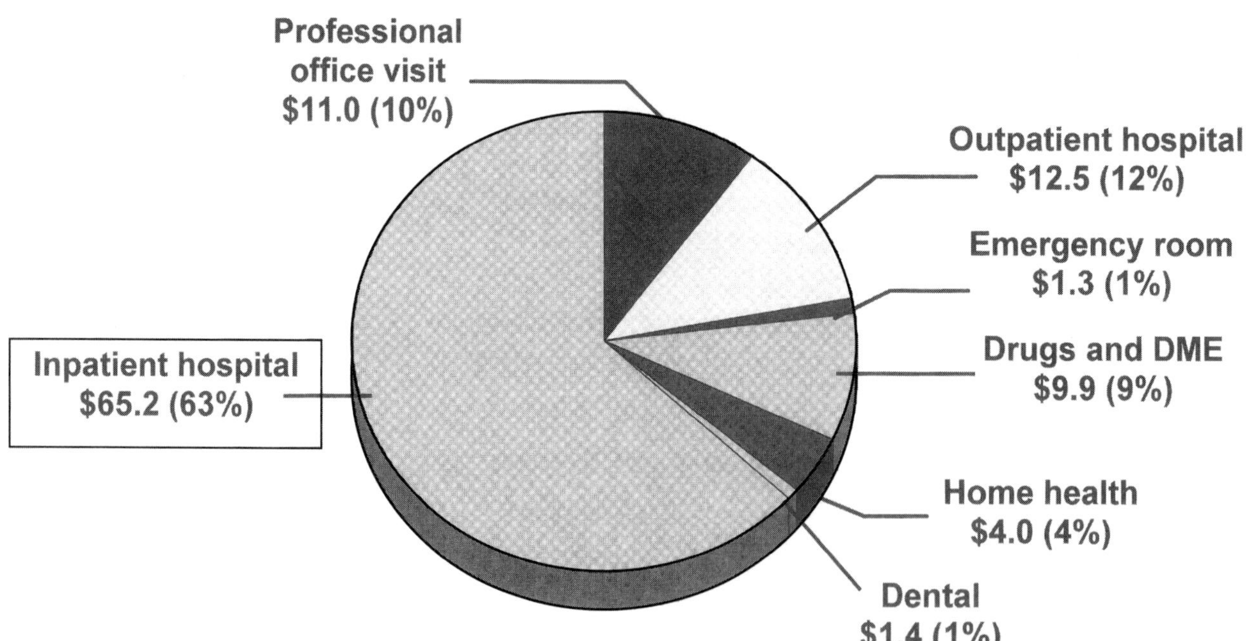

Figure 46.3. Annual healthcare expenditures for patients with diabetes in 1992. Amounts are in $ billions. DME, durable medical equipment. (Data from Rubin RJ, Altman WM, Mendelson DN. Health care expenditures for people with diabetes mellitus, 1992. *J Clin Endocrinol Metab* 1994;78:809A–809F.)

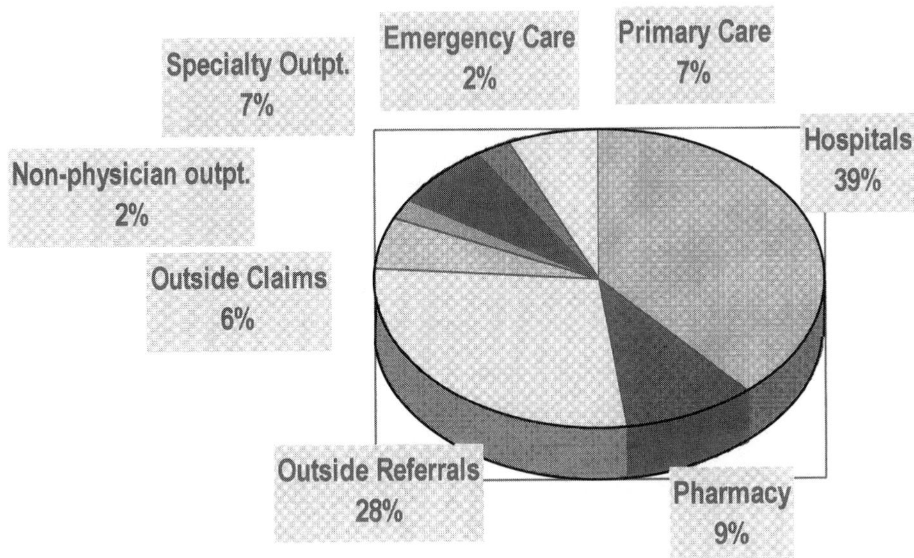

Figure 46.4. Calculation of distribution of excess medical care costs attributable to diabetes in the Kaiser Permanente Health Care System (Data from Selby JV, Zhang D, Ray GT, et al. Excess costs of medical care for patients with diabetes in managed care population. *Diabetes Care* 1997;20:1396–1402.)

with diabetes in the Kaiser Permanente System with age- and sex-matched nondiabetic control subjects showed excess expenditures of $3,494 per person, with per-person expenditures for patients with diabetes 2.4 times those for control patients (68). The largest part of the total excess cost was for inpatient hospital care within the HMO, representing 38.5% of the total. Costs related to primary care in the outpatient setting represented only 6.8% of the total, with specialty outpatient care only 7.2%. (Fig. 46.4). As might be expected, the largest proportion of the total excess charges were related to the treatment of long-term complications of diabetes, principally atherosclerotic heart disease, stroke, and chronic renal failure.

The increased cost of medical care for patients with diabetes is evident from the time of diagnosis. In one study of patients with type 2 diabetes in an HMO setting, medical care costs for the first year after diagnosis were 2.1 times higher than for matched patients without diabetes (69). For the next 8 years after diagnosis, the diabetes-related incremental yearly inpatient, outpatient, and pharmacy medical costs remained relatively constant, averaging $2,257. Although the incremental costs were relatively flat during the course of the study, they did appear to rise in the last 2 years, and it was assumed that they would increase greatly as persons with diabetes developed major chronic complications with longer duration of disease.

From the perspective of the employer, diabetes imposes a substantial economic burden, with respect to both medical care and productivity. In a recent study of the impact of diabetes on the workforce of a large corporation, the incremental costs were substantial (70). The incremental cost of diabetes among employees ranged from $4,671 in the group 18 to 35 years of age to $4,369 in individuals 56 to 64 years of age. Although the largest proportion of the incremental costs were related to medical inpatient care, a substantial amount was related to medically related work loss. It is interesting that the costs related to medically related work loss were higher in the younger group of employees, possibly because after a certain age, the sickest individuals with diabetes may be dropping out of the workforce.

Data have been accumulating that if managed care plans do not improve the overall glycemic control of their patients with diabetes, they, or the healthcare system in general, will be facing higher medical care costs in the long term as the excess costs of care due to complications and comorbidities become manifest. In one study of patients from HealthPartners in Minnesota, 3-year medical care costs were closely correlated with baseline hemoglobin A_{1c} (HbA_{1c}) levels at the start of the measurement period (71). Increases in HbA_{1c} of 1% were associated with a 7% increase in costs. The incremental increases in costs with rising HbA_{1c} were even greater for those patients with hypertension, lipid disorders, and cardiovascular disease.

Recent studies have indicated that efforts to improve glycemic control, although costly in themselves (72), will have long-term benefits, not only in reducing complications but also in reducing costs. An analysis of the DCCT indicated that, if substantial additional resources were invested each year in patients with type 1 diabetes, the increased treatment would be highly cost effective, with an incremental cost of $28,661 per year of life gained. If this is adjusted for improved quality of life, the incremental cost per quality-of-life year gained is $19,998 (73). Marked reductions in cost would be achieved by decreasing ESRD and lower-extremity amputation. Further improvements in cost, life expectancy, and quality of life are achieved if the economics of intensive control are extrapolated over a patient's lifetime (73). Economic modeling of the costs and benefits of intensive control based on the DCCT has been performed and applied to the population of patients with type 2 diabetes in the United States (64). It calculated that the lifetime costs for general and diabetes-related care using intensified treatment for type 2 diabetes would be approximately twice that for standard care. The reduction in lifetime medical costs of complications, however, would largely offset the difference (Table 46.1, reference 74). Although intensive therapy for type 1 and type 2 diabetes is more expensive than conventional therapy in the short run, its long-term cost-effectiveness is comparable to that of pharmacologic treatment of hypertension and elevated cholesterol. This means that from the perspective of public health and the healthcare system, programs to help physicians achieve intensive management of their patients with diabetes would be a worthwhile long-term financial investment (75).

More modest interventions in improving diabetes care have also been shown to improve glycemic control and reduce long-term costs for medical care (76–78). Cost analysis of the care of patients with type 2 diabetes followed in the United Kingdom Prospective Diabetes Study has also shown substantial savings in costs with interventions to control glucose (79,80) and blood pressure (81). Although intensive glucose control in the study increased trial treatment costs by £695 per patient, it reduced the cost of complications by £957 compared with conventional treatment. However, if standard-practice visit patterns were to be assumed rather than trial conditions, the per-patient yearly costs would be lower, at £478. The cost per event-free year of intensive blood glucose control was calculated to be about £1166, indicating that this form of therapy in persons with type 2 diabetes is highly cost effective and supportable economically. Similar economic advantages were found in modeling the results to costs in the Swiss healthcare system (82). In addition, improved glycemic control may also lead to a more productive workforce, reduce the economic burden due to medically related work loss, and improve quality of life (83).

DIABETES, MANAGED CARE, AND DISEASE MANAGEMENT

The burgeoning disease-management concept is rapidly establishing itself as a significant and powerful entity in the healthcare industry for managing chronic diseases. During the past few years, a growing number of disease management vendors have offered a wide variety of programs with multiple incentives for quality improvement and increased cost-effectiveness. The backgrounds and their motivation for providing disease management to healthcare providers can be highly variable. Programs have been developed and are being marketed and implemented by independent disease-management vendors, pharmaceutical corporations, managed care companies, specialized consultants, patient educational services companies, home healthcare companies, and high-technology data management and software companies in what is becoming an exceedingly competitive environment. Many of these companies are joining forces with clinical organizations or other businesses to combine products, skills, and strategies more effectively in the marketplace.

WHAT IS DISEASE MANAGEMENT?

Disease management is a complete and comprehensive method of providing healthcare that focuses on management of care across the continuum for populations of patients with chronic diseases. Disease management is a comprehensive integrated approach to care and reimbursement based fundamentally on the natural course of the disease, with treatment designed to address the illness with maximum effectiveness and efficiency (84). Disease management can be thought of as an approach to care that identifies the optimal processes for care of a patient with a specific condition and implements those processes while measuring the outcome to demonstrate improvement economically, humanistically, and clinically (85). Disease management is oriented toward wellness and prevention. The goals of disease management are to extend the periods of wellness that patients experience, to improve the overall quality of their lives, to prevent occurrence or exacerbation of complications or acute episodes, to direct utilization of services and resources appropriately, and to measure outcomes consistently. In practice, disease management is being implemented as a way to contain costs while maximizing the overall quality of care across an insurance company or employer's population (86,87). Therefore, disease management is being implemented most widely in patients with conditions for which cost savings are most substantial.

WHY IS DISEASE MANAGEMENT NECESSARY?

At least 90 million Americans are diagnosed with one chronic illness; as many as 39 million are diagnosed with more than one chronic illness (88). Research demonstrates that approximately 20% of the population with diabetes incur 80% of healthcare costs (89). This disproportionate utilization is very significant and has the potential to worsen with the aging of the population (88). Traditional healthcare directs efforts at reacting to the acute episode. There is often a lack of continuity of care because of the existence of a healthcare system that provides fragmented and uncoordinated care. Clinical and budgetary priorities are concentrated in conflicting positions, with little common understanding or integration. Disease management provides a responsive, coordinated healthcare system that integrates the activities and priorities of all participants in the delivery of care.

Diabetes is one of the most complex and significant chronic diseases in healthcare. Its emergence as a major cause of clinical

TABLE 46.1. Cost of Treatment, Effectiveness, and Incremental Cost-effectiveness under Standard and Comprehensive Care for Type 2 Diabetes

	Standard care	Comprehensive care	Difference
General medical care and diabetes costs	$32,365	$58,312	$25,947
Eye disease cost	$3,128	$1,536	($1,592)
Renal disease cost	$9,437	$960	($8,477)
Neuropathy, LEA costs	$4,381	$1,469	($2,912)
Coronary artery disease	$13,458	$14,414	$956
Total costs	**$62,769**	**$76,922**	**$13,922**
QALY (undiscounted)	16.04	18.03	1.99
QALY (discounted 3%)	11.43	12.30	0.87
Life years (undiscounted)	17.05	18.37	1.32
Incremental cost/QALY gained			**$16,002**

LEA, lower-extremity amputation; QALY, quality-adjusted life-years.
Data from Eastman RC, Javitt JC, Herman WH, et al. Model of complications of NIDDM: analysis of the health benefits and cost-effectiveness of treating NIDDM with the goal of normoglycemia. *Diabetes Care* 1997;20:735–744.

morbidity and increasing healthcare costs was amply discussed earlier in this chapter. The disease in many people is diagnosed only upon their developing serious and life-threatening complications related to the underlying diabetes. In evaluations of the impact of diabetes on the healthcare system and the effect it has on a population, the facts give a convincing picture of diabetes as an appropriate target for disease management. According to the results of the DCCT, maintaining blood glucose levels as close to normal as possible slows the onset and progression of eye, kidney, and nerve complications related to diabetes (31). The DCCT showed that sustained lowered blood glucose levels had positive effects, even in those patients who had prior histories of poor control. Tighter control also contributed to a lower number of glycemic events that led to hospitalizations. Achieving and maintaining such consistent blood glucose control is extremely challenging both for people with diabetes who are attempting to balance busy lives with management of this disease and for their care providers. Disease management offers an infrastructure for integrating all the key members of the healthcare team with the patients and their significant others, in combination with proactive and comprehensive services to improve the quality and cost-effectiveness of diabetes care.

Notable challenges in the healthcare system affect the ability of clinicians to manage diabetes successfully and support the necessity for disease management as a concept and as a practice. Those challenges include

- The lack of standardized care throughout the continuum of care that has contributed to high variability in physician practice and in resultant patient outcomes
- The lack of accessible and immediately available screening, treatment, prevention, and pharmacologic utilization guidelines and protocols for clinicians in active practice settings
- Lack of resources and systems that provide consistent education and reinforcement for professional care providers
- Inappropriate utilization of services and resources, including hospitalizations and emergency department visits secondary to often preventable glycemic occurrences and events related to acute and/or chronic complications of diabetes
- Lack of consistent systems that can assist clinicians to identify high-risk patients, to institute comprehensive preventive and education programs, and to coordinate appropriate utilization of services
- Absence of systems, formats, and resources for performance and outcome measurement; data collection and analysis; trend analysis; patient identification and risk stratification; tracking and monitoring of patients; and reporting and feedback mechanisms that have strong potential to influence effective healthcare delivery
- Inadequate resources and systems to provide comprehensive patient education and support in long-term self-management
- Inadequate systems for coordinating the care and priorities of multiple participants—the patient, primary care physician, specialists, case managers, nurses, and other care providers—in a focused, concerted, integrated team approach

Diabetes is a disease with multiple stakeholders who have a vested interest in improved systems and outcomes, i.e., patients, providers, employers, community agencies, health plans, health facilities and agencies, and pharmaceutical and other vendors. As a disease state, diabetes presents a combination of high variability in practice and cost, high prevalence of work or school days lost, and significant difficulties in management. However, there is a realistic ability to alter the course of the disease across the continuum of care through implementation of a disease-management program that provides a focused and specific set of goals and interventions, as well as a consistent evaluative process.

ESTABLISHING A DIABETES DISEASE-MANAGEMENT PROGRAM

Several components are necessary for the development and implementation of a successful disease-management program. The purpose of the disease-management program is to provide tools and processes to patients and care providers that integrate the patient as a responsible and empowered partner of the healthcare team.

The objectives of the diabetes disease-management program should encompass clinical standards and expectations, utilization management, patient self-management issues, patient quality of life, staff satisfaction, and the establishment of evaluative processes and tools.

The first objective is to improve clinical outcomes by standardizing care and providing guidelines that have integrated best practice with accreditation criteria for quality and by providing systems that enable clinicians and patients to adhere to the expected standards. Evaluation of improvement is measured by the successful lowering of HbA_{1c} levels across the patient population. Process improvements also include the percentage of patients receiving foot examinations yearly, blood pressure measurements twice a year, comprehensive eye examinations annually, lipid profiles once a year, and urine protein/microalbuminuria screenings once a year.

The second objective is to improve resource utilization by promoting better control over diabetes management as evidenced by reduced number of hospitalizations or emergency department visits, reduced duration of stay related to hypoglycemic or hyperglycemic events, and reduced cardiovascular and lower-extremity complications.

The third objective is to improve patient self-management behaviors and skills by providing patients with accessible and consistent educational programs and behavioral support. Improvement is measured by the increase in the number of patients who self-monitor blood glucose levels daily, check their feet daily, understand how to manage hypoglycemia, and have a sick-day management plan.

A fourth objective is to contribute to a higher quality of life for people with diabetes by providing educational and psychological support during the process of their achieving mastery of self-management and throughout the ongoing experience of living with a chronic illness. Evaluating depression measures and surveying satisfaction levels regarding availability of educational and support mechanisms, access to care, and clinical outcomes are important components of understanding what learning and psychosocial supports are needed. Appropriate support mechanisms are designed to be effective and to have a positive impact on the quality of life. Referral guidelines are designed for individual intervention and follow-up with certified diabetes educators or mental health professionals as needed.

A fifth objective of the disease-management program is to provide evaluative processes and tools for measuring, documenting, analyzing, and reporting patients' compliance rates and responses to treatment, patient outcomes, trends, and overall program effectiveness. Included are the development of risk stratification; tracking and monitoring of clinical, economic, and quality-of-life outcomes; and measurement of key indicators.

A sixth objective is to improve clinician satisfaction by integrating patient and care provider priorities into the overall program structure and by providing ongoing support and feedback.

RECOMMENDED ELEMENTS FOR A DIABETES DISEASE-MANAGEMENT PROGRAM

A diabetes disease-management program should be designed to address the overall needs of the general patient population that has been identified, as well as to target specific activities for patients who have been identified as at high risk for complications. The elements that have been identified as core components for an effective diabetes disease-management program follow:

- Establishment of a collaborative work team
- Development of an assessment process
- Implementation of a risk-management process
- Physician education programs and processes
- Implementation of clinical guidelines
- Educational programs and support mechanisms for professional and office staff
- Programs and tools for patient self-management
- Data management and technological support
- Integration into quality improvement
- Management of care coordination and utilization
- Ongoing support mechanisms

ESTABLISHMENT OF A COLLABORATIVE WORK TEAM

Establishment of a collaborative work team is a key component in the process of providing the foundation for diabetes disease management that promotes and supports the integration and coordination of interdisciplinary members as healthcare teams for management of patient care. The disease-management concept relies on a multidisciplinary methodology for preventing fragmentation and for building a care infrastructure that maximally supports the needs of the patient. The charge of the work team is to tailor the core disease-management program to meet the needs of the patient and care providers and to guide the development, implementation, and evaluation processes. The work team is accountable for developing and maintaining a collaborative process for completing all necessary steps toward achieving a successful program for diabetes disease management. The responsibilities of the work team include the following:

- Assessing the organizational practices and resources, including staffing patterns and skill mix; availability and accessibility of databases; data-management capacity; management systems; and pertinent relationships with patients, families, payers, and referral sources,
- Assessing the current baseline clinical practices and outcomes
- Clarifying the goals and objectives and identification of target areas for improvement
- Modifying the components of the disease-management program as required to address the specific needs of the organization
- Determining the forums, schedules, and materials required for adequate physician and staff educational processes
- Developing and implementing patient educational tools and processes that are appropriate for the general population and for those more intense measures that are specified for high-risk patients
- Planning and developing the steps, conditions, and tools for the implementation phase
- Acting as champions and advisors during the implementation phase
- Providing guidance in the evaluative phase; identifying the most effective and appropriate utilization of the outcomes data and analysis; and directing the information to be used in quality-improvement activities

ASSESSMENT

The assessment process is conducted to determine current baseline clinical and organizational practices. Evaluation of the clinical practices includes determining how well the course of the disease is understood, what the best practice standards are, whether major obstacles to achieving best practice exist and what those barriers are, what the composition of the patient population with diabetes is, and what the specific influences upon compliance and prevention are. The assessment of organizational practice includes determination of the available workforce resources for implementation, as well as technological availability and requirements.

PATIENT IDENTIFICATION

A crucial element in the diabetes disease-management program is the ability to identify all patients within the practice or facility setting who meet criteria for enrollment into the program. Any patient with a diagnosis of diabetes should be considered as a participant in the overall program. The program should be designed to meet the needs and to provide services to all patients with diabetes. In addition to a basic program, other components are designed to target patients who require intensified services, education, and support. Patients can be identified through a variety of sources, i.e., claims data, emergency department data, inpatient admission data, home care admission data, pharmaceutical claims data, physician referrals, and other referrals (e.g., case-management referrals, self-referrals).

In the case that the enrollment is based on a referral system versus inclusion of all patients in a population, referrals can be retrieved from multiple avenues: primary care physicians; nurse practitioners; and staff nurses from a variety of acute inpatient, ambulatory, office, or home care settings.

The role of the primary care physician is very important to the disease-management process. Once the patient has been identified, the primary care physician is contacted to provide a review and approval and to initiate the invitation process to the patient. Whether the enrollment process is automatic inclusion, criteria based, or reliant on referral, once the patient has been identified, he or she becomes an active participant in the program.

RISK STRATIFICATION

A diabetes disease-management program is designed to improve the quality and cost-effectiveness for the entire patient population that has been identified. However, within that larger population there is a group of patients who are considered to be high risk for complications and who account for a significant proportion of resource utilization and medical costs. This subset of patients represents candidates for intensified therapy and intervention.

Risk stratification is a critical process in disease management because it provides a detailed patient profile and identifies those patients who are at risk for developing severe chronic complications (90,91). The risk-stratification information is used as a guide for care providers to enable them to achieve two objectives. The first objective is the development of programs, systems, processes, and tools targeted to the high-risk patient group. Patient educational tools and processes, care coordination, and case-management activities, referrals to certified diabetes educators or specialists, and follow-up regimens are directed by the information that is provided by risk stratification. The second objective is individualization of care based on scientific information that describes the patient's circumstances.

The goals for integrating a risk stratification component into the diabetes disease-management program include (a) prevention or delay of onset of chronic complications or acute events; (b) decrease in the severity of complications that do occur; (c) extension of the patient's life, (d) improvement in the patient's quality of life; (e) decrease in preventable hospitalizations, emergency department visits, or inappropriate utilization of resources; and (f) improvement in patient and care provider satisfaction.

PROFESSIONAL AND OFFICE-STAFF EDUCATIONAL COMPONENT

The complexities and complications inherent in the care and treatment of diabetes have increased the demands on care providers to remain current and competent in the management of this disease. The professional and office staff educational component is designed to maximize the knowledge base, to increase the levels of practical skills, and to expand the level of confidence of care providers in the management of diabetes care. The educational programs are prepared with flexible formats and curriculums to address the scheduling needs of care providers. Programs should be developed that can respond to multiple learning needs at various levels of intensity. The following are suggested types of programs for inclusion in the curriculum.

- Introductory Continuing Medical Education (CME) programs to review the diabetes disease-management program and introduce guidelines or protocols
- Professional staff (certified educational unit; CEU) educational programs for nurses and allied health professionals. These programs include the following:

  Introduction to the disease-management program and clinical guidelines and protocols

  Ongoing educational series about diabetes, including pathophysiology, screening and treatment methodologies, medication management, patient self-management and educational techniques, psychosocial issues, management of acute complications, and prevention and management of chronic complications

  Educational sessions for office staff regarding the administrative components of the disease-management program: formal and informal

  Sessions for training the trainer

  The goal of the diabetes disease-management professional and staff educational component is to provide consistent and continuous learning opportunities that are accessible and meaningful.

PATIENT SELF-MANAGEMENT

Education in self-management of diabetes is a critical element in providing patients with the mechanisms necessary for managing the disease and its subsequent effects on their lives. Empowering patients and helping them acquire the skills for effective self-management are the foundation of the educational process for the patient with diabetes.

For people with diabetes, management of their disease relies on continual treatment and constant balancing of the integral parts of their lives every day. Effective management of diabetes requires vigilance and commitment on a 24-hour-a-day basis and significant lifestyle modifications. Education and self-management play vital roles in guiding the patient toward independent and competent management of diabetes. The goal of the patient educational component of disease management is to facilitate the patient's and the family's ability to increase their diabetes knowledge base for self-management, to increase their confidence in applying the knowledge to practical situations, and to share experiences with other people with diabetes. The effective diabetes disease-management program incorporates multiple individual and group formats, with an emphasis on interactive participation. The healthcare team is provided with standardized patient educational materials so that the patient is receiving consistent information. Technology has enabled care providers to present educational material to patients in a wide range of creative ways, including and not limited to call centers, videos, e-mail, interactive Web sites, and interactive software (88). Curriculums can focus on meaningful topics ranging from survival skills, to meal planning, to intense monitoring of blood glucose, to more in-depth self-management techniques and information. Incentives for maintaining attendance and compliance with educational programs may be a helpful tool for supporting the patient. It is important for the educational programs to address and integrate psychosocial needs and the enormous emotional and psychological toll exacted by living with diabetes. Engaging the patient and family as active partners in the healthcare team and addressing educational needs across the continuum are important attributes for success.

CLINICAL GUIDELINES

Clinical guidelines provide a basis for screening, treatment, evaluation, and pharmacologic management processes in the delivery of care to patients with diabetes. They must be linked to commonly recognized measures of clinician performance (92). Part of every disease-management program entails the development, implementation, and evaluation of disease-specific clinical pathways, which can also encompass care algorithms or protocols. The guidelines must incorporate current knowledge and reference reliable resources. HEDIS (Health Plan Employer Data and Information Set) (93) and American Diabetes Association Clinical Practice Recommendations (3) can be used as important reference elements for the development of guidelines. Consistent reviews for necessary updating and modifications contribute to the credibility of the guidelines. Clinical guidelines that are evidence based, with formal evidence reviews incorporated into their development process, and that have been stringently and authoritatively tested receive much stronger positive responses from physicians and integration into practice (88,94).

Easy accessibility and user-friendly formats for using the guidelines reasonably in a busy practice are often prerequisites to successful implementation (95). Tools that support the guidelines, including documentation forms, physician order sheets, patient surveys, and data collection forms, frequently are developed for use in conjunction with the guidelines. Increased efforts are being made to provide online and Web-based applications. Gaining access to the guidelines can also be combined with the data collection and variance-tracking mechanisms. The objectives of the clinical guidelines are (a) to support optimal clinical practice, (b) to influence clinical behavior to produce improved patient outcomes, and (c) to ensure that patients' expectations are informed and reasonable (3).

If guidelines are developed and implemented by local organizations or care groups, they should be based on the collaboration of an interdisciplinary clinical team that has performed a careful review of current evidence, literature, and reliable clinical practice.

CARE COORDINATION, UTILIZATION MANAGEMENT, AND CASE MANAGEMENT

Care coordination, utilization management, and case management are critical to the implementation of a successful diabetes disease-management program. The population with patients with diabetes encompasses a significant number who are actively experiencing serious or life-threatening complications, have been identified as being in a high-risk category for development of complications, or demonstrate the potential for progression to a high-risk level. In addition, because of the complexity of managing this difficult chronic disease on a daily basis, patients require the intensive support and coordination offered by disease-management programs via care and case management. Patients with diabetes need to have a supportive service available that is geared to assist them toward better self-management and subsequently to an improved quality of life.

The processes of care coordination, utilization management, and case management are closely related in the management of the functions required for ensuring that the patient receives optimal levels of care and services at the right time and in the most appropriate settings. These processes are necessary throughout the continuum of care and have proven to be highly effective in increasing quality and cost-effectiveness of care.

The role of the case manager has expanded beyond the original context of acute, inpatient care and extends into continued management of the patient's care throughout the outpatient and community experience and the coordination with primary care. The case manager supports the disease-management process from the perspective of both the individual patient and the population as a whole. The case manager's responsibilities include the following:

- Coordinating the patient's care throughout the continuum, thereby facilitating the achievement of optimal quality outcomes in clinical care, cost-effectiveness, and patient satisfaction
- Assessing patients to identify specific case-management/care-coordination needs
- Assessing and risk-stratifying patients to identify patients in the high-risk population
- Collaborating with a wide variety of members of a multidisciplinary healthcare team in multiple settings to plan, implement, and evaluate patient care and the related care-delivery systems
- Coordinating multiple services and resources required by the patient and family
- Monitoring and tracking patient response and outcomes to treatment and changes in risk level
- Identifying variances that affect the quality and cost of care and participating in the development and implementation of short- and long-term patient care strategies
- Performing utilization review and management to ensure that appropriate services and resources are provided in a reasonable, high-quality, and cost-effective manner
- Assisting and guiding patients and families in communicating with healthcare providers and in maneuvering through the healthcare system without difficulty
- Assessing and integrating the patient's physical, psychosocial, economic, and lifestyle circumstances into an effective case-management plan
- Analyzing, monitoring, and evaluating complex patient information over significant periods versus concentrating on specific episodes

Quality Improvement

A major purpose of disease-management programs is to support quality-improvement initiatives and to provide a system for outcomes analysis. Within the context of a diabetes disease-management program, the evaluative process that contributes to effective quality improvement is reorganized to encompass entire populations. In this population-based concept, the ability to stratify for risk and identify high-risk patients; to develop and implement "best-practice" protocols, guidelines, interventions, and processes; and to measure patient and system responses and outcomes is increasingly important to the many stakeholders in healthcare delivery.

Integration of valuable data on patient outcome into the quality-improvement program enables care providers to respond to the physical, psychological, functional, and environmental needs of patients in the population with diabetes. Consistent and reliable reporting structures provide a mechanism for utilizing the data in meaningful and productive ways. Including the perspectives of the patient and care provider in the evaluation of quality promotes a comprehensive viewpoint. Prompt response to the data through the development and implementation of plans for improvement or corrective action strengthens the program and increases its credibility.

Some of the indicators measured to evaluate quality and incorporated into the quality-improvement program are level of clinical quality; accessibility to care and services; the patient's quality of life and functional status; levels of satisfaction; and levels of utilization management.

Level of Clinical Quality

The level of clinical quality can be evaluated by assessing patient outcomes, as well as processes. For patients with diabetes, the primary clinical indicator that provides evidence of improvement is the HbA_{1c} level. Other outcomes to measure include physiologic parameters, rates of acute and chronic complications, and mortality rates. Processes to measure for compliance with expected standards of care include foot examinations, comprehensive eye examinations, blood pressure measurements, HbA_{1c} monitoring, lipid-profile monitoring, and urinary protein/microalbumin screening (96,97).

Accessibility to Care and Services

For both patients and care providers, accessibility to prompt, reliable, and comprehensive care and services is of paramount concern. Availability of clinical care and educational and support programs are important to patients with diabetes. Prompt response times and expeditious scheduling promote the sense of security and fortifies the perception of high-quality care.

Quality of Life and Functional Status

Evaluation of quality of life and functional status includes monitoring for improvements in self-care ability, achievements in individual- and population-based goals for self-management and behavior change, treatment and follow-up compliance rates, and patient and family comprehension of self-management.

Satisfaction Levels

To obtain a comprehensive view of how the quality and effectiveness of the diabetes disease management is perceived, assessments need to consider satisfaction levels from the perspectives of multiple stakeholders in the care-delivery process: patients, families, care providers, payers, employers, and others. The indicators for such assessment include levels of satisfaction with the care provided, the accessibility to care and services, and the resultant outcomes of the care provided.

Utilization Management

Utilization management and quality improvement are often very closely linked. Determining and monitoring the appropriateness of care and services and proactively directing care to the most suitable and pertinent settings affect the quality of care from all perspectives. Reductions in unnecessary or preventable hospitalizations and emergency department visits, as well as lost work and school days, decreases in acuity levels, and need for multiple, high-cost services certainly, contribute to a higher level of quality of care and to a lower level of financial risk for the care provider.

DATA MANAGEMENT AND TECHNOLOGY

Advanced technology is essential in the current complicated healthcare industry, with its need for managing enormous amounts of detailed and complex patient information. The establishment of disease management has promoted the need for increasingly powerful and sophisticated technology that can support multiple demands. Technology is an important tool in disease management and has actually become a critical element for achieving the following:

- Establishment of a data-management system with data collection/download capacity and data mining of a multitude of diverse and comprehensive patient databases that allow care providers to collate and analyze multiple types of data, including clinical, insurance claims, utilization, pharmacy, patient survey, referral, and marketing information (88).
- Implementation of a communication network that provides the means for care providers and patients to maintain strong interactive relationships. A communication network may include interactive e-mail, voice mail, Web-based applications, or Internet applications (98).
- Institution of tracking and monitoring systems that alert the care provider when individual patients require attention or intervention.
- Implementation of reliable reporting mechanisms to care providers regarding individual and collective patient information.

Technology can be used to enhance many elements of a diabetes disease-management program but should not be considered the entire program. Technology can accomplish many things:

- Contribute positively to providing a comprehensive network among care providers and patients
- Provide on-time capability for receiving information
- Provide a central database for patient data
- Systematize and automate the data collection, storage, analysis, and reporting functions (98)

Technology should not be used to substitute for the human interaction and personal relationships that exist between patients and care providers but should be integrated into the disease-management program to facilitate and strengthen those components (98).

PHYSICIAN SUPPORT FOR DISEASE MANAGEMENT

Disease-management programs have a significant potential to improve outcomes and reduce costs. However, many physicians remain wary about participating, and physician resistance is one of the top three reasons why disease-management programs are not implemented (94). Several factors influence the physician's perspective. Disease-management programs are built on sophisticated and complex infrastructures that support focused and comprehensive management of a chronic disease and yield positive outcomes. Physicians report that given that same infrastructure without a disease-management vendor they could produce even more impressive improvements in outcome (94). Positive outcomes are based on the physician's commitment to and belief in the disease-management program. If physicians perceive that the disease-management program reduces their control over the management of patient care or dilutes their relationships with their patients, they will not accept the program.

Several success factors that influence physician participation have been identified. First, structuring the program on evidence-based medicine establishes credibility and a more positive response by physicians. Educating the physician about the program, its value to the patient, its support of the physician's role in the coordination of care, and its value to the physician is an important element (94). Maximizing the opportunities for physicians to have input in the development, implementation, and evaluation of the program helps them become more comfortable with the concept of disease management. Modifying the program according to physician input or practices builds support. Demonstrated success of positive outcomes in previous activities encourages physicians to participate. Structuring the program so that the physician truly owns and champions the program is an element for success (98). The impetus of the program should be to support and strengthen the physician-patient relationship. The foundation of an effective disease-management program that will find greater support among physicians is built on a trusting relationship that

- Advocates for the welfare and care of the patient
- Recognizes and values the importance and commitment of the physician to the success of the program
- Upholds the autonomy of the physician and the physician's control over the care of the patient
- Values and incorporates the physician's perspective into the development and implementation of the program
- Provides outcomes that are value-added as identified as important by physicians and patients.

LIFESTYLE MODIFICATIONS AND PSYCHOSOCIAL ISSUES

Diabetes is a chronic disease that affects the patient physically, psychologically, socially, spiritually, cognitively, and economically. It requires a careful balance of activities, 24-hour-a-day management, and significant lifestyle changes. Living well with diabetes means combining a lifelong commitment to maintaining a lifestyle that balances sound nutritional, activity, and overall health habits with adherence to a strict medical-management regimen. Patients with diabetes live with it all day, every day. The person's self-esteem, sense of independence, and self-image all experience enormous strain as his or her lifestyle undergoes significant modifications and alterations. Providing systems, processes, and supports that assist the patient to learn self-management of diabetes is an important factor in the healthcare plan.

Education regarding self-management and lifestyle modification is a critical component in helping patients take control of diabetes and its impact on their lives. Education about managing diabetes is about mastering a wide range of new skills and activities, as well as about adapting to life with a chronic disease (99). Patients are faced with learning self-management skills, including monitoring blood glucose levels, planning meals, scheduling meals and medications, and maintaining exercise programs. They also are faced with the challenge of learning to prioritize commitment to a treatment plan over other activities, to manage unexpected events, to develop contingency plans, to know when to contact supportive resources, and to maintain eternal vigilance to stay well. Effective education in diabetes self-management is associated with many positive outcomes, including improvement in patients' physical and emotional health, improvement in ability to achieve glycemic and metabolic control, a reduction in hospitalizations, a reduction in diabetes-related healthcare costs, and fewer acute and chronic complications.

Patients view diabetes as an integral part in the totality of their lives and not as a separate entity (100). When developing an educational plan, it is important to consider several types of experience in the patients' lives: the emotional experience, the behavioral experience, the ability to make and maintain lifestyle change, and the stage of development.

The emotional experience of a patient is a strong influence on the patient's ability to cope and to learn. A patient's emotional experience encompasses the patient's emotions as related to life events and relationships, as well as the emotional response to having diabetes, and its subsequent effect on life and those events and relationships (101). The emotional response to diabetes encompasses many complex feelings: confusion, grief, anger, denial, ambivalence, and guilt. Patients often feel overwhelmed and out of control. The behavioral experience includes all the actions that the patient needs to employ to deal effectively with diabetes management and all the associated emotions and attitudes. Chronic disease requires a significant adaptation process, and strong coping skills are important tools for the patient (102). Understanding the developmental stage of the patient is critical in developing a plan that addresses the specific needs of the patient.

THE PATIENT'S ROLE IN DIABETES MANAGEMENT

The patient plays the most important role in diabetes management. Patients with diabetes must perceive themselves as active, empowered members of the healthcare team and be able to accept responsibility for self-management and for adhering to treatment plans (100). There must be a commitment to understanding the disease as well as possible and a willingness to continue to learn. The patient's active participation in decision making and planning treatment as a member of the healthcare team contributes substantially to successful self-management. The patient must be able to change behaviors and learn new skills to be able to feel better, to be healthier, and, in some cases, to survive. Working with the team to set goals for treatment and behavior allows the patient to have more immediate control over care that reflects his or her preferences and priorities. The patient needs to make appropriate decisions, multiple times, on a daily basis about self-management and to act on those decisions accordingly (100). The patient must have strong communication skills and a sense of assertiveness to be able to inform the healthcare team when difficulties arise, when circumstances change that impact the treatment plan, or when the goals for glycemic control have not been met.

ISSUES THAT AFFECT PROFICIENT SELF-MANAGEMENT

Changes in behavior and adjustments of lifelong habits and choices are difficult processes. The difficulties of learning new skills, understanding how and why to control a chronic disease, and managing all the associated feelings often lead to frustration and discouragement. Some issues that compound these feelings are stress, burnout, coexisting common psychiatric conditions [e.g., depression (103–105)], physical illness, negative feedback, lack of empowerment, and lack of self-efficacy.

Any of these factors can exert a forceful influence on successful self-care behavior. The more confident a person feels about performing self-care behaviors, the more likely he or she will perform those behaviors (102). Consistent ability to cope with emotional stresses in daily life can be a critical component in a person's success in achieving significant changes in lifestyle. The ability to change and overall behavior are reflections of the person's level of maturity and cognition. A person's capacity to maintain a complicated regimen has an effect on self-care behavior.

ROLE OF THE CARE PROVIDER

The care provider's role is to determine how to support the patient's ability to become a competent self-manager in diabetes care. Several important steps maximize the support a patient needs for learning self-management: (a) performing an accurate and comprehensive patient assessment, (b) developing a mutually trusting relationship, (c) setting reasonable and achievable goals, (d) facilitating an optimal learning experience, and (e) basing the learning experience on empowerment of the patient.

Understanding the impact of the many complex components of a person's life on the learning process is a fundamental element in developing and implementing effective teaching strategies that support each individual. Important information about a person's readiness and ability to learn about self-management can be obtained by a thorough assessment that includes (a) evaluating the patient's current health status; (b) evaluating the patient's psychological status, ability to cope, and emotional well-being; (c) assessing the patient's cognitive skills and literacy level; (d) exploring the patient's life experiences, particularly in managing diabetes; (e) determining the level of understanding the patient has about diabetes and self-care; (f) determining the patient's relationship with care providers; (g) assessing the patient's cultural, social, and economic background and environmental influences; and (h) assessing the patient's priorities and interests.

A relationship based on respect, trust, and understanding supports the learning process. It is the responsibility of the care provider to establish a nonjudgmental, supportive environment that enables the patient to be a motivated, active participant in the learning experience (103). Communication and acceptance of the patient's choices are essential to a productive experience. Incorporating the expectations and values of the patient into the teaching plan provides a base from which the patient can become effective in self-management (106).

Goals provide a framework to guide the patient and the care provider in identifying the specific tasks and activities that need to be achieved. Goals are critical tools in the learning process and should encompass the commitment to behavior change necessary for successful self-management. Patients need to feel accountable for achievement of stated goals, and they respond to goals that are individualized and incorporate their priorities. Setting goals that are measurable, attainable, and action oriented helps the patient to have a clear understanding of what is expected.

An important role for the care provider is to facilitate an optimal learning experience for the patient. A current goal for diabetes education is to provide programs or teaching sessions that integrate the clinical, behavioral, and psychosocial elements of diabetes care and self-management (100). The purpose of diabetes education is not simply to deliver information about the importance of managing diabetes but also to provide information that supports the patient's ability to make informed decisions (99). The learning process is designed to address and incorporate the patient's lived experience with diabetes (100). Education is a continuous and interactive process that assesses and encourages patients to express their concerns and questions, presents information that addresses those issues, and reviews strategies to deal with the behavioral aspects of managing these issues and concerns. Patients are more likely to be engaged participants in a process that is based on their experiences and concerns and is personally relevant. Empowerment is an important concept that requires the redesign of traditional methods for providing patient education. The empowerment model postulates that the patient is responsible for providing and managing the majority of diabetes care and is thus not a passive participant but the center of decision making and control in daily management and treatment (102). As mentioned earlier, the healthcare team is responsible for providing the patient with information enabling the patient to make informed decisions. The patient has both the right and the responsibility to perform in the role of equal partner in the treatment program (101). It is the responsibility of the healthcare team to provide and foster an environment that supports the patient's development or discovery of the capacity to actively solve problems of diabetes care, thus reinforcing the sense of self-efficacy and accountability.

REFERENCES

1. Harris MI, Eastman RC. Early detection of undiagnosed non-insulin–dependent diabetes mellitus. *JAMA* 1996;276:1261–1262.
2. Kenny SJ, Smith PJ, Goldschmid MG, et al. Survey of physician practice behaviors related to diabetes mellitus in the U.S.: physician adherence to consensus recommendations. *Diabetes* 1993;16:1507–1510.
3. American Diabetes Association. Clinical Practice Recommendations 2004. *Diabetes Care* 2004;27[Suppl 1]:S1–S1504.
4. Centers for Disease Control and Prevention. *National diabetes fact sheet: general information and national estimates on diabetes in the United States, 2002.* Atlanta: US Department of Health and Human Services, Centers for Disease Control and Prevention, 2003.
5. Ford ES, Williamson DF, Liu S. Weight change and diabetes incidence: findings from a national cohort of U.S. adults. *Am J Epidemiol* 1997;146:214–222.
6. Bjorntorp P. Obesity. *Lancet* 1997;350:423–426.
7. National Center for Chronic Disease Prevention and Health Promotion. *Physical activity and health: a report of the Surgeon General.* Atlanta: Centers for Disease Control and Prevention, 1996.
8. Leibson CL, O'Brien PC, Atkinson E, et al. Relative contributions of incidence and survival to increasing prevalence of adult-onset diabetes mellitus: a population based study. *Am J Epidemiol* 1997;146:12–22.
9. Diabetes Prevention Program Research Group. Reduction in the incidence of type 2 diabetes with lifestyle modification of metformin. *N Engl J Med* 2002; 346:393–403.
10. Kelly DT. Our future society: a global challenge. *Circulation* 1997;95:2459– 2464.
11. Campbell PR. *Population projections for states by age, sex, race and Hispanic origin, 1995 to 2025.* Washington, DC: Bureau of the Census, 1996.
12. Murray CJL, Lopez AD. Alternative projections of mortality and disability by cause 1990–2020: global burden of disease study. *Lancet* 1997;349:1498–1504.
13. National Center for Chronic Disease Prevention and Health Promotion. *Diabetes surveillance, 1993.* Atlanta: Centers for Disease Control and Prevention, 1993.
14. National Institute of Diabetes and Digestive and Kidney Diseases. *Diabetes statistics.* National Institutes of Health publication no. 98-3926, Nov. 1997, updated Feb. 1998.
15. Harris MI, Flegal KM, Cowie CC, et al. Prevalence of diabetes, impaired fasting glucose, and impaired glucose tolerance in adults. *Diabetes Care* 1998;21: 518–524.
16. World Health Organization. *Diabetes: diabetes estimates.* Available at: http:// www.who.int/ncd/dia/databases/htm. Accessed March 4, 2004.
17. Ford ES, DeStefano F. Risk factors for mortality from all causes and from coronary heart disease among persons with diabetes. *Am J Epidemiol* 1991; 133:1220–1230.
18. Geiss LS, Herman WH, Smith PJ. Mortality in non-insulin-dependent diabetes. In: Harris MI, Cowie CC, Stern MP, et al, eds. National Diabetes Data Group. *Diabetes in America*, 2nd ed. Bethesda, MD: National Institute of Diabetes and Digestive and Kidney Diseases, 1995:233–255. NIDDK publication no. 95-1468.
19. Stamler J, Vaccaro O, Weaton JD, et al. Diabetes, other risk factors, and 12-year cardiovascular mortality for men screened in the Multiple Risk Factor Intervention Trial. *Diabetes Care* 1993;16:434–444.
20. Sprafka JM, Burke GL, Folsom AR, et al. Trends in the prevalence of diabetes in patients with myocardial infarction and effect of diabetes on survival: the Minnesota Heart Survey. *Diabetes Care* 1991;14:1537–1543.
21. Gu K, Cowie CC, Harris MI. Diabetes and decline in heart disease mortality in US adults. *JAMA* 1999;281:1291–1297.
22. Klein R, Klein BEK. Vision disorders in diabetes. In: Harris MI, Cowie CC, Stern MP, et al, eds. *Diabetes in America*, 2nd ed. Bethesda, MD: National Institute of Diabetes and Digestive and Kidney Diseases, 1995:293–331. NIDDKD publication no. 95-1468.
23. CDC Diabetes Public Health Resource. End-stage renal disease. Available at: http://www.cdc.gov/diabetes/statistics/esrd/fig1.htm. Accessed March 4, 2004.
24. National Institute of Diabetes and Digestive and Kidney Diseases. US Renal Data System: 1998 Annual Data Report. Bethesda, MD, July 1998. Available at: http://diabetes.niddk.nih.gov/dm/pubs/statistics/index.htm#13. Accessed March 4, 2004.
25. National Diabetes Fact Sheet. American Diabetes Association. Available at: http:www.diabetes.org/diabetes-statistics/national-diabetes-fact-sheet.jsp. Accessed March 4, 2004.
26. Harris MI, Eastman R, Cowie C. Symptoms of sensory neuropathy in adults with NIDDM in the US population. *Diabetes Care* 1993;16:1446–1452.
27. American Diabetes Association. Economic costs of diabetes in the United States in 2002. *Diabetes Care* 2003;26:917–232.
28. Major cross-country differences in risk of dying for people with IDDM. Diabetes Epidemiology Research International Mortality Study Group. *Diabetes Care* 1991;14:49–54.
29. Lloyd E, Stephenson J, Fuller JH, et al. A comparison of renal disease across two continents: the Epidemiology of Diabetes Complications Study and the EURO-DIAB IDDM Complications Study. *Diabetes Care* 1996;19:219–225.
30. Diabetes Control and Complications Trial Research Group. The effect of intensive treatment of diabetes on the development and progression of long-term complications in insulin-dependent diabetes mellitus. *N Engl J Med* 1994;329:977–986.
31. Stratton IM, Adler AI, Neil HA, et al. on behalf of the UK Prospective Diabetes Study Group. Association of glycaemia with macrovascular and microvascular complications of type 2 diabetes. *BMJ* 2000;321:405–412.
32. Ohkubo Y, Kishikawa H, Araki E, et al. Intensive insulin therapy prevents the progression of diabetic microvascular complications in Japanese patients with non-insulin-dependent diabetes mellitus: a randomized prospective 6-year study. *Diabetes Res Clin Pract* 1995;28:103–117.
33. Klein R, Klein BEK, Moss SE, et al. Relationship of hyperglycemia to the long-term incidence and progression of diabetic retinopathy. *Arch Intern Med* 1994;154:2169–2178.
34. Songer TJ. Disability in diabetes. In: Harris MI, Cowie CC, Stern MP, et al, eds. *Diabetes in America*, 2nd ed. Bethesda, MD: National Institute of Diabetes and Digestive and Kidney Diseases, 1995:259–278. NIDDKD publication no. 95-1468.
35. Brandaleone H, Friedman GJ. Diabetes in industry. *Diabetes* 1953;2:448–453.
36. Pell S, D'Alonzo CA. Sickness absenteeism in employed diabetics. *Am J Public Health* 1967;57:253–260.
37. Pell S, D'Alonzo CA. Sickness and injury experience in employed diabetics. *Diabetes* 1960;9:303–310.
38. Songer TJ, LaPorte RE, Dorman JS, et al. Employment spectrum of IDDM. *Diabetes Care* 1989;12:615–622.
39. Weinstock M, Haft JI. The effect of illness on employment opportunities. *Arch Environ Health* 1974;29:79–83.

40. American Diabetes Association. Clinical Practice Recommendations 2001. *Diabetes Care* 2001;24[Suppl 1]:S118.
41. Waller JA. Chronic medical conditions and medical safety. *N Engl J Med* 1965; 273:1413–1442.
42. Crancer JA, McMurray L. Accident and violation rates of Washington's medically restricted drivers. *JAMA* 1968;205:272–276.
43. Davis TH, Wehling EH, Carpenter RI. Oklahoma's medically restricted drivers: a study of selected medical conditions. *J Okla State Med Assoc* 1973;66: 322–327.
44. DeKlerk NH, Armstrong BK. Admission to hospital for road trauma in patients with diabetes mellitus. *J Epidemiol Community Health* 1983;37:232–237.
45. Laberge-Nadeau C, Dionne G, Ekoe JM, et al. Impact of diabetes on crash risks of truck-permit holders and commercial drivers. *Diabetes Care* 2000;23:612–617.
46. Eadington DW, Frier BM. Type 1 diabetes and driving experience: an eight-year cohort study. *Diabet Med* 1989;6:137–141.
47. Stevens AB, Roberts M, McKane R, et al. Motor vehicle driving among diabetics taking insulin and nondiabetics. *BMJ* 1989;299:591–595.
48. Gislason T, Tomasson K, Reynisdottir H, et al. Medical risk factors amongst drivers in single-car accidents. *J Intern Med* 1997;241:213–219.
49. McGwin G, Sims RV, Pulley L, et al. Diabetes and automotive crashes in the elderly. *Diabetes Care* 1999;22:220–227.
50. Cox DJ, Gonder-Frederick LA, Kovatchev BP, et al. Progressive hypoglycemia's impact on driving simulation performance. *Diabetes Care* 2000;23: 163–170.
51. Weinger K, Kinsley BT, Levy CJ, et al. The perception of safe driving ability during hypoglycemia in patients with diabetes mellitus. *Am J Med* 1999;107: 246–253.
52. Kinsley BT, Weinger K, Bajaj M, et al. Blood glucose awareness training and epinephrine responses to hypoglycemia during intensive treatment in type 1 diabetes. *Diabetes Care* 1999;22:1022–1028.
53. Brunner GA, Semlitch B, Siebenhofer A, et al. Driver's license, driving habits and traffic safety of patients with diabetes mellitus. *Wein Klin Wochenschr* 1996;106:731–736.
54. Cox DJ, Penberthy JK, Zrebiec J, et al. Diabetes and driving mishaps: frequency and correlations from a multinational survey. *Diabetes Care* 2003;26: 2464–2465.
55. Federal Highway Administration. Qualification of drivers. In: *Federal Register*. Washington, DC: Federal Highway Administration, 1992:48011–48015 (49C FR Part 391).
56. Mawby M. Time for law to catch up with life [Editorial]. *Diabetes Care* 1997; 20:1640–1641.
57. Quickel KE. Economic and social costs of diabetes. In: Kahn CR, Weir GC, eds. *Joslin's diabetes mellitus*, 13th ed. Philadelphia: Lippincott Williams & Wilkins, 1994:586–604.
58. Huse DM, Oster G, Killen AR, et al. The economic costs of non-insulin-dependent diabetes mellitus. *JAMA* 1989;262:2708–2713.
59. Ray N, Willis, Thamer M. *Direct and indirect costs of diabetes in the United States in 1992*. Alexandria, VA: American Diabetes Association, 1993.
60. American Diabetes Association. Economic consequences of diabetes mellitus in the U.S. in 1997. *Diabetes Care* 1998;21:196–308.
61. American Diabetes Association. Economic costs of diabetes in the U.S. in 2002. *Diabetes Care* 2003;26:917–932.
62. Jonsson B. The economic impact of diabetes. *Diabetes Care* 1998;21[Suppl 3]: C7–C10.
63. Weisbrod B. *Economics of public health*. Philadelphia: University of Pennsylvania Press, 1961.
64. Aubert RE, Geiss LS, Ballard DJ, et al. Diabetes-related hospitalization and hospital utilization. In: Harris MI, Cowie CC, Reiber G, et al, eds. *Diabetes in America*, 2nd ed. Bethesda, MD: National Institute of Diabetes and Digestive and Kidney Diseases, 1995:553–569. NIDDKD publication no. 95-1468.
65. Peck S, Musco TD, Jejich C. *Diabetes coverage by commercial insurers in the U.S.A.* Washington, DC: Health Insurance Association of America, 1986.
66. Bransum ED. Access to coverage; health insurance for people with diabetes. *Diabetes Spectrum* 1988;1:59–62.
67. Rubin RJ, Altman WM, Mendelson DN. Health care expenditures for people with diabetes mellitus, 1992. *J Clin Endocrinol Metab* 1994;78:809A–809F.
68. Selby JV, Zhang D, Ray GT, et al. Excess costs of medical care for patients with diabetes in managed care population. *Diabetes Care* 1997;20:1936–1402.
69. Brown JB, Glauber HS, Nichols GA, et al. Type 2 diabetes: incremental medical care costs during the first 8 years after diagnosis. *Diabetes Care* 1999;22: 1116–1124.
70. Ramsey S, Summers KH, Leong SA, et al. Productivity and medical costs of diabetes in a large employer population. *Diabetes Care* 2002;25:1–5.
71. Gilmer TP, Manning WG, O'Connor PJ, et al. The cost to health plans of poor glycemic control. *Diabetes Care* 1997;20:1847–1853.
72. The Diabetes Control and Complications Trial Research Group. Resource utilization and costs of care in the Diabetes Control and Complications Trial. *Diabetes Care* 1995;18:1468–1478.
73. The Diabetes Control and Complications Trial Research Group. Lifetime benefits and costs of intensive therapy as practiced in the Diabetes Control and Complications Trial. *JAMA* 1996;276:1409–1415.
74. Eastman RC, Javitt JC, Herman WH, et al. Model of complications of NIDDM: analysis of the health benefits and cost-effectiveness of treating NIDDM with the goal of normoglycemia. *Diabetes Care* 1997;20:735–744.
75. Herman WH, Eastman RC. The effects of treatment on the direct costs of diabetes. *Diabetes Care* 1998;21[Suppl 3]:C19–C24.
76. Greenfield S, Rodgers W, Mangotich M, et al. Outcomes of patients with hypertension and non-insulin-dependent diabetes mellitus treated by different systems and specialties: results of the Medical Outcomes Study. *JAMA* 1995;274:1436–1444.
77. Eckman M, Greenfield S, Mackey W, et al. Foot infections in diabetes patients: decision and cost-effectiveness analysis. *JAMA* 1995;273:712–720.
78. O'Connor P, Rush W, Peterson J, et al. Continuous quality improvement can improve glycemic control for HMO patients with diabetes. *Arch Fam Med* 1996;5:502–506.
79. Gray A, Raikou M, McGuire A, et al. Cost effectiveness of an intensive blood glucose control policy in patients with type 2 diabetes; economic analysis alongside randomised controlled trial (UKPDS 41). *BMJ* 2000;320: 1373–1378.
80. Clarke P, Gray A, Adler A, et al. Cost effectiveness analysis of intensive blood-glucose control with metformin in patients with type II diabetes (UKPDS 51). *Diabetologia* 2001;44:298–304.
81. Gray A, Clarke P, Raikou M, et al. An economic evaluation of atenolol vs. captopril in patients with diabetes (UKPDS 54). *Diabet Med* 2001;18: 438–444.
82. Palmer AJ, Sendi PP, Spinas GA. Applying some UK Prospective Diabetes Study results to Switzerland; the cost-effectiveness of intensive glycaemic control with metformin versus conventional control in overweight patients with type-2 diabetes. *Schweiz Med Wochenschr* 2000;130:1034–1040.
83. Testa MA, Simonson DC. Health economic benefits and quality of life during improved glycemic control in patients with type 2 diabetes mellitus. *JAMA* 1998;280:1490–1496.
84. Zitter M. Disease management: a new approach to health care. *Med Interface* 1995;7(8):70–72,75–76.
85. Moran M. Disease management spreading. *Am Med News* 1999;42(16).
86. Clark CM, Snyder JW, Meek RL, et al. A systematic approach to risk stratification and intervention within a managed care environment improves diabetes outcomes and patient satisfaction. *Diabetes Care* 2001;24:1079–1086.
87. McColloch DK, Price MJ, Hindmarsh M, et al. Improvement in diabetes care using an integrated population-based approach in a primary care setting. *Dis Manag* 2000;2:75–82.
88. Reeder L. Anatomy of a disease management program. *Nurs Manag* April 1999;30:41–45.
89. Selby JV, Karter AJ, Ackerson LM, et al. Developing a predictive rule from automated clinical data bases to identify high-risk patients in a large population with diabetes. *Diabetes Care* 2001;24:1547–1555.
90. Rosenzweig JL, Weinger KL, Poirier-Solomon L, et al. Use of a disease severity index for evaluation of healthcare costs and management of comorbidities of patients with diabetes mellitus. *Am J Manag Care* 2002;8:950–958.
91. Celeste-Harris S, Connor D, Bonsignore P, et al. Diabetes disease management program improves clinical outcomes for inner-city African-American patients. *Diabetes* 2003;52[Suppl 1](abst 258).
92. National Diabetes Quality Improvement Alliance. Available at: http://www.nationaldiabetesalliance.org. Accessed March 4, 2004.
93. NCQA HEDIS® 2005. Overview, comprehensive diabetes care. Available at: http//www/ncqa.org/programs/HEDIS/. Accessed March 4, 2004.
94. Brown J. Physicians support disease management programs with right combination of incentives, education, medical evidence. *Physicians Partnership Report*. Washington, DC: Atlantic Information Services, 1999.
95. Joslin Diabetes Center. *Joslin guidelines for diabetes management*. Available at http://joslin.org/guidelines.shtml. Accessed March 4, 2004.
96. Kiefe CI, Allison JJ, Williams OD, et al. Improving quality improvement using achievable benchmarks for physician feedback. *JAMA* 2001;285:2871–2879.
97. National Diabetes Quality Improvement Alliance Performance Measures Set. Available at: http://nationaldiabetesalliance.org. Accessed March 4, 2004.
98. Special Supplement. Disease management: an industry emerges. *Healthcare Business Roundtable*. Sept/Oct 1999.
99. Clement S. Diabetes self management education. *Diabetes Care* 1999;18:1204–1214.
100. Funnell M, Anderson R. Putting Humpty Dumpty back together again: reintegrating the clinical and behavioral components in diabetes care and education. *Diabetes Spectrum* 1999;12:10–23.
101. Anderson BJ, Rubin RR. Emotional responses to diagnosis. In: Anderson BJ, Rubin RR, eds. *Practical psychology for diabetes clinicians*. Alexandria, VA: America Diabetes Association, 1996:163–173.
102. Peragallo-Dittko V, Godley K, Meyer J. *A core curriculum for diabetes educators*, 2nd ed. Chicago: American Association of Diabetes Educators, 1993.
103. Ciechanowski PS, Katon WJ, Russo JE. Depression and diabetes: impact of depressive symptoms on adherence, function and costs. *Arch Intern Med* 2001;16:3278–3285.
104. Musselman DL, Betan E, Larsen H, et al. Relationship of depression to diabetes type 1 and 2: epidemiology, biology and treatment. *Biol Psychiatry* 2003; 54:317–329.
105. Ciechanowski PS, Katon WJ, Russo JE, et al. The relationship of depressive symptoms to symptom reporting, self-care and glucose control in diabetes. *Gen Hosp Psychiatry* 2003;25:246–252.
106. Poirier L, Maryniuk M, de Groot M. *The Joslin way: a healthcare professional's guide to diabetes patient care*. Boston: Joslin Diabetes Center, 1999.

SECTION VI

Biology of the Complications of Diabetes

CHAPTER 47

Epidemiology of Late Complications of Diabetes: A Basis for the Development and Evaluation of Preventive Programs

Andrzej S. Krolewski and James H. Warram

This chapter reviews the descriptive epidemiology of late complications of diabetes mellitus in the eyes, kidneys, and heart and examines their occurrence in relation to diabetes duration and other risk factors, particularly the level of hyperglycemia. Our intent is to emphasize the findings that are relevant to generating etiologic hypotheses or to developing interventions against these outcomes. To describe their occurrence, we use the indices that were defined in Chapter 20 of this volume: the incidence rate, cumulative risk, and prevalence. For illustrating the natural history of late diabetic complications, we frequently use data from cohort studies carried out in the patient population of the Joslin Clinic. A less selective review of the epidemiology of late diabetic complications can be found in Chapter 35 of the previous edition of *Joslin's Diabetes Mellitus* (1). We first review data for patients with type 1 diabetes and then discuss their similarities and differences to the data for type 2 diabetes.

MEASURE OF DIABETES EXPOSURE

Although conventional hypoglycemic therapies prevent acute metabolic complications in patients with diabetes, they do not restore metabolic homeostasis (2,3). The result of this imperfect treatment is a novel milieu that includes various combinations of metabolic, hormonal, and physiologic alterations. These include hyperinsulinemia, hyperglycemia, hyperlipidemia, abnormalities in blood flow, and the formation of glycation products (2–5), all of which constitute *diabetes exposure*. As a consequence of this exposure, diverse functional and morphologic alterations develop that lead to severe complications affecting the eyes, kidneys, and heart. Despite intensive research, it is not known which components of this collective exposure are responsible for particular complications. Various hypotheses have been proposed, ranging from global hypotheses that invoke a single mechanism and a single component of diabetes exposure as responsible for

TABLE 47.1. Values of Glycosylated Hemoglobin A_{1c} in the Population of the Joslin Clinic according to Age in 1999

		Values of HbA_{1c}[a]		
		Percentile		
Age in 1999/2000	No. of patients	25th	50th	75th
0–9	350	7.5	8.3	9.0
10–19	991	7.8	8.8	9.8
20–29	1114	7.0	8.1	9.5
30–39	1588	7.0	8.0	9.4
40–49	2123	7.1	8.2	9.4
50–59	2564	7.1	8.1	9.3
60–69	2496	6.9	7.9	9.1
70+	2760	6.8	7.6	8.5

[a]Only one measurement (the first in 1999) was used per patient.

all complications, to separate hypotheses for each complication that invoke interactions of diabetes exposures with genetic susceptibility and environmental factors (4–9).

For the purpose of epidemiologic studies, diabetes exposure can be characterized by the level of hyperglycemia or the level of glycosylated hemoglobin (HbA_{1c}). The distribution of the intensity of diabetes exposure as estimated from glycosylated hemoglobin levels ranges widely. For example, in the population of patients who visited the Joslin Clinic in 1999/2000, the distribution of HbA_{1c} levels ranged from 5% to 16% (6% is the upper limit of normal values in the nondiabetic population). The distribution of values varied slightly according to age (Table 47.1). Patients age 20 years and older had slightly lower values than younger patients. The medians for measurements repeated approximately a year later in this same population remained unchanged, and patients tended to maintain their position within the distribution. The majority of those with a high HbA_{1c} level at the first visit in 1999/2000 had a similar value at the second visit 6 to 18 months later. This "tracking" of the level of diabetes control is a notable feature of patients with diabetes (10,11). During follow-up of participants in the Diabetes Control and Complications Trial (DCCT), patients formerly in the intensive treatment group worsened their glycemia within a year so that their distribution of glycosylated hemoglobin A_{1c} (HbA_{1c}) converged with that for the conventionally treated group (12). Interestingly, it became similar to the distribution for patients of the Joslin Clinic (Table 47.1).

EPIDEMIOLOGY OF DIABETIC RETINOPATHY

Cumulative Risk of Retinopathy According to Duration of Diabetes

The most frequent late complication of type 1 diabetes is retinopathy. Following the onset of type 1 diabetes, there is a lag period of about 3 to 4 years before the first cases of nonproliferative retinopathy appear (13–15). The risk then increases exponentially (13–15). For example, during the 5th year of diabetes, nonproliferative retinopathy develops in 1 of 100 patients, whereas in the 14th year, it develops in 11 of 100 patients who have escaped it up to that time (14). By the 15th year of type 1 diabetes, the cumulative risk of nonproliferative retinopathy approaches 100% (Fig. 47.1). Despite its apparent inevitability, the onset of nonproliferative retinopathy can be postponed significantly by improved glycemic control, as was demonstrated by the DCCT (15).

Once patients have developed nonproliferative retinal lesions, they are vulnerable to the development of proliferative retinopathy, the principal cause of blindness in diabetes. The first cases of this advanced stage of diabetic retinopathy appear after 10 years of diabetes and then continue to occur at a constant incidence rate of about 3 per 100 per year regardless of the duration of type 1 diabetes. This constant incidence rate of proliferative retinopathy yields, after 40 years of type 1 diabetes, a cumulative risk of 62% (16), a value supported by several studies (17–19). The absence of a decline in the incidence rate of proliferative retinopathy after most of the population has been affected suggests that almost all patients with type 1 diabetes are susceptible to this complication, just as they are to

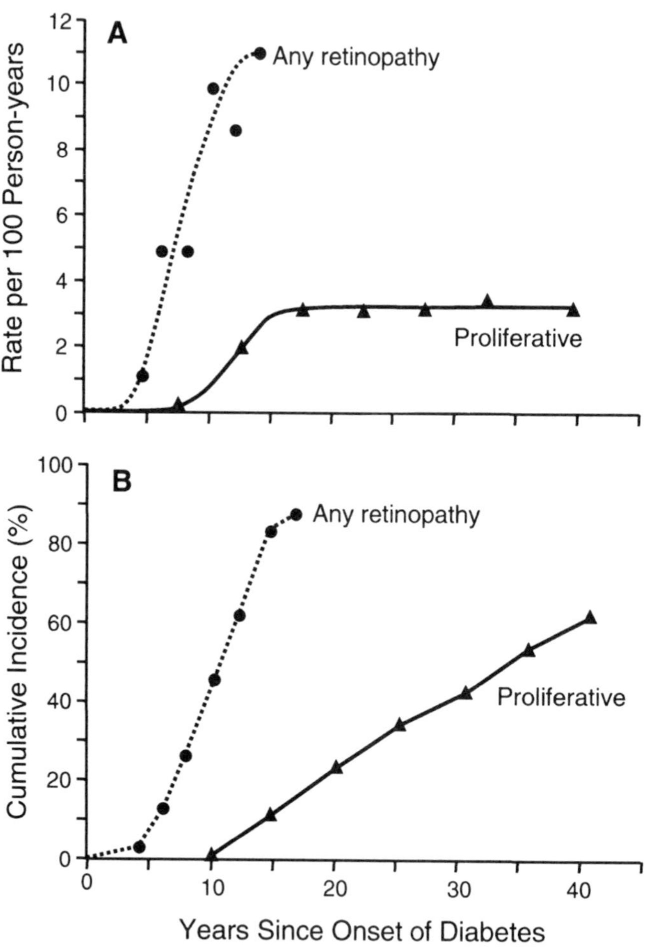

Figure 47.1. Incidence rate and cumulative risk of background and proliferative retinopathy, according to the duration of type 1 diabetes. **A:** The incidence rate of background retinopathy (estimated from Klein et al.) and proliferative retinopathy (adapted from Krolewski et al.), according to the duration of type 1 diabetes. **B:** The cumulative risk of background retinopathy measured by its prevalence (adapted from Klein et al.) and the risk of proliferative retinopathy measured as the cumulative incidence (adapted from Krolewski et al.), according to duration of type 1 diabetes. (Adapted from Klein R, Klein BEK, Moss SE, et al. The Wisconsin Epidemiologic Study of Diabetic Retinopathy. II. Prevalence and risk of diabetic retinopathy when age at diagnosis is less than 30 years. *Arch Ophthalmol* 1984;102:520–526; and copyright © 1986 American Diabetes Association. Krolewski AS, Warram JH, Rand LI, et al. Risk of proliferative diabetic retinopathy in juvenile-onset type I diabetes: a 40-yr follow-up study. *Diabetes Care* 1986;9:443–452. Adapted with permission from the American Diabetes Association.)

nonproliferative retinopathy. However, the contrast between the cumulative risk curve for the onset of retinopathy (exponential) as compared with its progression to proliferative retinopathy (constant) is evidence that the mechanisms underlying these two processes must be different.

Diabetes Exposure and Risk of Retinopathy

Because nonproliferative retinopathy is extremely rare in persons without diabetes but is almost universal in patients with type 1 diabetes, one can infer that this complication is an outcome of diabetes exposure. Many observational studies (20–25) and clinical trials (15,26–28) have demonstrated a relationship between hyperglycemia and the development of various stages of diabetic retinopathy. However, only the results of the DCCT have provided enough data for the evaluation of the dose-response relationship between hyperglycemia and the development of nonproliferative retinopathy and its progression to proliferative retinopathy (15,28).

It appears that high levels of hyperglycemia have an impact on both the onset and progression of retinopathy, whereas low levels have only a moderate impact (15,28). As shown in Figure 47.2, the incidence of retinopathy (development or progression) in the group assigned to intensive diabetes treatment fluctuated around 2.0 per 100 person-years in the nine deciles of the HbA_{1c} distribution below 8.5% and rose to 7.0 per 100 person-years in the highest decile. The results of other follow-up studies showed a similar threshold effect of hyperglycemia on the development and progression of diabetic retinopathy (29,30).

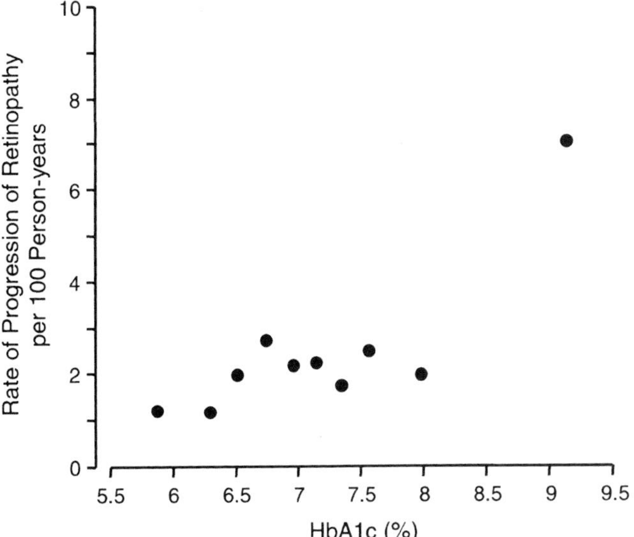

Figure 47.2. Incidence rate of sustained progression of retinopathy according to deciles of the distribution of mean glycosylated hemoglobin A_{1c} (HbA_{1c}) values during the Diabetes Control and Complication Trial (DCCT). Figure was adapted from Figure 5 in DCCT study (15) by omitting the fitted dose-response curve (linear in the log-log scale) to emphasize the pattern of the data. For the first nine deciles, the incidence rate was well approximated by a straight line whose slope coefficient was not statistically significantly different from zero, whereas the incidence rate for the 10th decile lies significantly above the line. This pattern is consistent with a threshold value for HbA_{1c} between the 9th and 10th deciles. (Adapted in 2004 with permission from The Diabetes Control and Complications Trial Research Group. The effect of intensive treatment of diabetes on the development and progression of long-term complications in insulin-dependent diabetes mellitus. *N Engl J Med* 1993;329:977–986. Copyright © 1993 Massachusetts Medical Society. All rights reserved.)

Other Risk Factors for Retinopathy

Several other factors in addition to diabetes exposure are associated with the development of the several stages of diabetic retinopathy. This includes systemic variables such as hypertension, nephropathy, and cardiovascular autonomic neuropathy, as well as ocular variables such as elevated intraocular pressure and myopia.

We reported one of the first prospective observations of the relation between elevated blood pressure and risk of retinopathy (21,31). In that study, the risk of progression of nonproliferative retinopathy was particularly increased in patients with type 1 diabetes with diastolic blood pressure above 70 mm Hg. Subsequently, the Wisconsin Epidemiologic Study of Diabetic Retinopathy showed that systolic blood pressure was associated with the onset of nonproliferative retinopathy, whereas diastolic blood pressure was associated with its progression (32). Data from a clinical trial of sorbinil also demonstrated that elevated diastolic blood pressure was an important risk factor for progression but not for onset of nonproliferative retinopathy (25). Because there has been no clinical trial of blood pressure reduction in the prevention of diabetic retinopathy, the implication of these associations is not clear. Elevated systemic blood pressure may be a risk factor for diabetic retinopathy or just an indicator of microvascular dysfunction, which is also manifested as microalbuminuria and leads to complications in the kidneys as well as the eyes (33).

Previously, it had been supposed that the development of diabetic retinopathy and other late diabetic complications was due to one underlying pathologic process in small vessels (4–6,8,9). However, clinical and epidemiologic studies during the last two decades have provided evidence that the causes of these complications may be different (8,34,35). Still the occurrence of one complication may be a risk factor or indicator for the development of others. For example, the onset of diabetic nephropathy is almost always followed by the development of proliferative retinopathy (16,36,37). Certain aspects of overt proteinuria and declining renal function may accelerate progression of diabetic retinopathy to proliferative retinopathy (36,37). Also, a relation between the presence of autonomic cardiovascular neuropathy and the development of proliferative retinopathy was found. This association, which we demonstrated first in a case-control study (37) and subsequently in a follow-up study (38), was independent of the level of glycemic control, elevated blood pressure, or presence of diabetic nephropathy. However, it is still not clear whether cardiovascular autonomic neuropathy is a risk factor or risk indicator for the development of proliferative diabetic retinopathy.

In addition to these systemic factors, ocular factors seem to modulate the risk of onset and progression of diabetic retinopathy. Higher ocular perfusion pressure predicted the onset and progression of diabetic retinopathy in the Wisconsin Epidemiologic Study (39). This agrees with an earlier study of patients with asymmetric diabetic retinopathy in which lower retinal artery pressure due to carotid occlusion was found on the same side as the eye with less severe retinopathy (40). In a multivariate analysis of the Wisconsin data to adjust for other covariates, the effect of high ocular perfusion pressure remained significant only for the onset of retinopathy. Myopia is another ocular factor that modulates the development of proliferative retinopathy. We were the first to find its protective effect against severe retinopathy in a case-control study of determinants of proliferative diabetic retinopathy in type 1 diabetes (41). This finding has since been confirmed in a prospective study, and several explanations for it have been proposed (39); however, empiric data to distinguish among them are lacking.

Comparison of Risk of Retinopathy in Type 1 and Type 2 Diabetes

The Wisconsin Epidemiologic Study of Diabetic Retinopathy provides the best data to compare the natural history of diabetic retinopathy in whites with type 1 and type 2 diabetes. During a 10-year follow-up, the incidence of retinopathy, the progression of retinopathy, and the development of proliferative retinopathy were highest in patients with type 1 diabetes, intermediate in insulin-treated patients with type 2 diabetes, and lowest in patients with type 2 diabetes treated with oral agents or diet (42). Most of these differences could be accounted for by different levels of glycemic control in the three study groups (24). The contribution of other risk factors to different risk of diabetic retinopathy in type 1 and type 2 diabetes has been less well studied.

Can the Occurrence of Diabetic Retinopathy Be Changed?

As was demonstrated in several clinical trials conducted in highly selected populations of patients with diabetes, improved glycemic control can significantly delay the development of nonproliferative retinopathy and postpone its progression to proliferative retinopathy (15,28,43,44). However, there is less evidence that the natural history of diabetic retinopathy can be changed in the general population of patients with diabetes.

The cumulative risk of proliferative diabetic retinopathy in type 1 diabetes had not changed during the 30-year period between 1950 and 1980. In the cohort study that we conducted at the Joslin Clinic, the cumulative risk of proliferative diabetic retinopathy after 20 years of diabetes was identical in patients who had type 1 diabetes diagnosed in 1939, 1949, and 1959 despite significant differences in the care of these cohorts (16). Similar findings have been reported from Sweden; a secular decline in risk was found for nephropathy but not for proliferative retinopathy over the period from 1970 to 1990 (45,46). Furthermore, in the Wisconsin Epidemiologic Study of Diabetic Retinopathy, no significant change in the incidence of retinopathy was found during 10 years of follow-up despite significant improvement in glycemic control in the study group (24).

EPIDEMIOLOGY OF DIABETIC NEPHROPATHY

Cumulative Risk of Diabetic Nephropathy According to Duration of Diabetes

The natural history of diabetic nephropathy has generally been viewed as a progressive path from normoalbuminuria to end-stage renal disease (ESRD) through intermediate stages marked by microalbuminuria and then overt proteinuria (47). The cumulative risk (estimated by prevalence data) of these stages in patients of the Joslin Clinic with type 1 diabetes according to duration of diabetes is summarized in Figure 47.3. Because several studies have demonstrated that the duration of diabetes before puberty does not contribute to the risk of diabetic nephropathy (48,49), the data in Figure 47.3 are presented according to postpubertal duration of type 1 diabetes. To develop more advanced nephropathy, patients must develop microalbuminuria first, so the top curve can be considered as the cumulative risk of microalbuminuria according to duration of diabetes. Similarly, the height of the intermediate curve indicates the cumulative risk of persistent proteinuria, and the height of the lowest curve traces the cumulative risk of ESRD according to duration of type 1 diabetes.

The cumulative risk of persistent microalbuminuria with duration of diabetes rises at a variable rate (Fig. 47.3). A particularly notable feature is the very early appearance of significant numbers of patients with microalbuminuria: 8% of patients with type 1 diabetes for only 1 to 3 years, a value ten times the 0.8% prevalence among persons without diabetes (50,51). A similarly high prevalence of microalbuminuria in patients with type 1 diabetes with a short duration of diabetes was found in another study (52). The prevalence of microalbuminuria leveled off after 10 years of diabetes (prevalence 20%) and then resumed its steep climb in the second decade, reaching a new

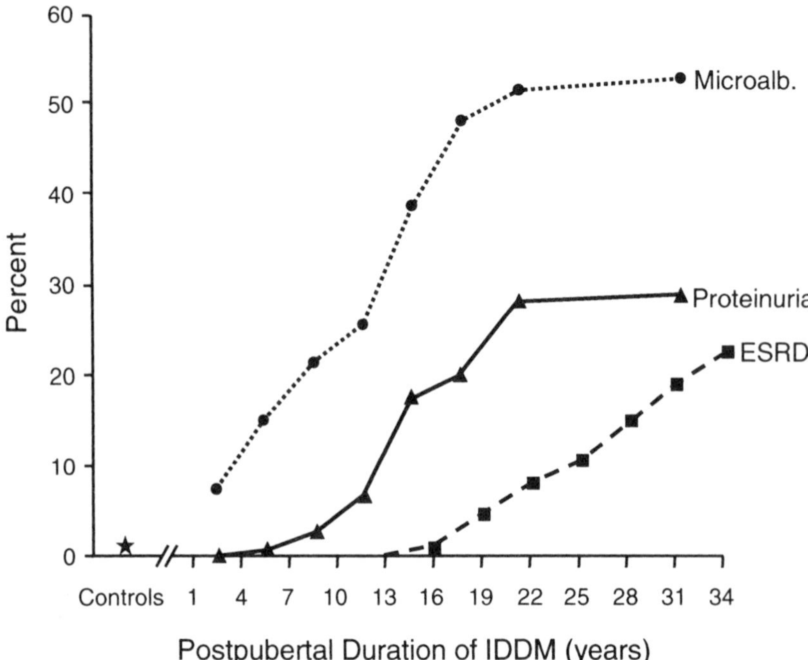

Figure 47.3. Prevalence of stages of diabetic nephropathy according to postpubertal duration of type 1 diabetes (IDDM). Data for microalbuminuria and proteinuria were adapted from Warram et al. Data on end-stage renal disease (ESRD) were adapted from Krolewski et al. For patients with type 1 diabetes diagnosed before age 10 years, postpubertal duration was counted from age 11 years. (Adapted from Warram JH, Gearin G, Laffel LMB, et al. Effect of duration of type 1 diabetes on prevalence of stages of diabetic nephropathy defined by urinary albumin/creatinine ratio. *J Am Soc Nephrol* 1996;7:930–937; and Krolewski M, Eggers PW, Warram JH. Magnitude of end-stage renal disease in type I diabetes: a 35-year follow-up study. *Kidney Int* 1996;50: 2041–2046 with permission from Blackwell Publishing.)

plateau at around 58% prevalence after 30 years of postpubertal duration of diabetes.

The cumulative risks of overt proteinuria and microalbuminuria within the same population can be compared in Figure 47.3. The first cases of overt proteinuria occurred after 5 years' duration, after which the prevalence of overt proteinuria increased abruptly and then leveled off after 21 years, a feature similar to the pattern for microalbuminuria. Following another increase, the prevalence of overt proteinuria leveled off again at around 30% by 30 years of postpubertal duration of type 1 diabetes. This agrees with a 33% cumulative risk of persistent proteinuria after 30 years of diabetes in two previous cohort studies (48,53). The contrast between the 30% cumulative risk for persistent proteinuria and the 58% cumulative risk for microalbuminuria after 30 years of type 1 diabetes has important implications. It indicates that many patients with microalbuminuria, approximately half, may never progress to overt proteinuria (54).

Patients with overt proteinuria are at risk of renal function loss and the development of ESRD. Recently, we determined the cumulative risk of ESRD in a cohort of patients who had type 1 diabetes diagnosed at the Joslin Clinic in 1959 and were followed until 1994 (55). The first case of ESRD occurred after 15 years of postpubertal duration of type 1 diabetes, and the cumulative risk of ESRD reached 22% after 35 years (Fig. 47.3). Because most individuals with persistent proteinuria progress to ESRD (48), one would expect the cumulative risk of ESRD to reach about 30% if followed another 10 years.

Diabetes Exposure and Risk of Diabetic Nephropathy

The level of glycemia seems to be the strongest factor influencing the onset of microalbuminuria. This has been demonstrated in several observational studies (22,51,56–59) as well as in clinical trials (15,26,27,60). In our recent 4-year follow-up study involving 943 normoalbuminuric patients with type 1 diabetes, we determined the shape of the dose-response relationship between the intensity of hyperglycemia and the onset of microalbuminuria (59) and found a nonlinear effect of hyperglycemia on the development of microalbuminuria (Fig. 47.4A). Below HbA_{1c} values of 8.0%, the incidence of microalbuminuria varied little. In contrast, above an HbA_{1c} value of 8.0%, the incidence of microalbuminuria rose steeply with increasing values of HbA_{1c}. For comparison, the risk of microalbuminuria increased almost 20-fold faster between HbA_{1c} values of 8% and 10% than between values of 6% and 8%. This nonlinear pattern of the relationship between level of HbA_{1c} and the risk of microalbuminuria was independent of other risk factors. This finding is consistent with our previous data from a case-control study (51). Evidence of a threshold effect in the relation between HbA_{1c} and microalbuminuria has been reported in DCCT publications, although it was not interpreted as such by the authors (60,61).

In our recent 4-year follow-up study involving 312 patients with microalbuminuria, we examined the relationship between hyperglycemia and progression of microalbuminuria to overt proteinuria (62). The incidence rate of progression increased rapidly between HbA_{1c} values of 6% and 8.5% and then leveled off at higher values, being similar for HbA_{1c} values of 8.5% and 12% (Fig. 47.4B). Since this pattern differs from the dose-response relationship between HbA_{1c} and the onset of microalbuminuria, one may hypothesize that different mechanisms are responsible for the onset of microalbuminuria and its progression to proteinuria.

Using incidence rates from Figure 47.4B, we estimated the cumulative risk of progression of microalbuminuria to overt proteinuria over a 10-year follow-up period according to quartiles of

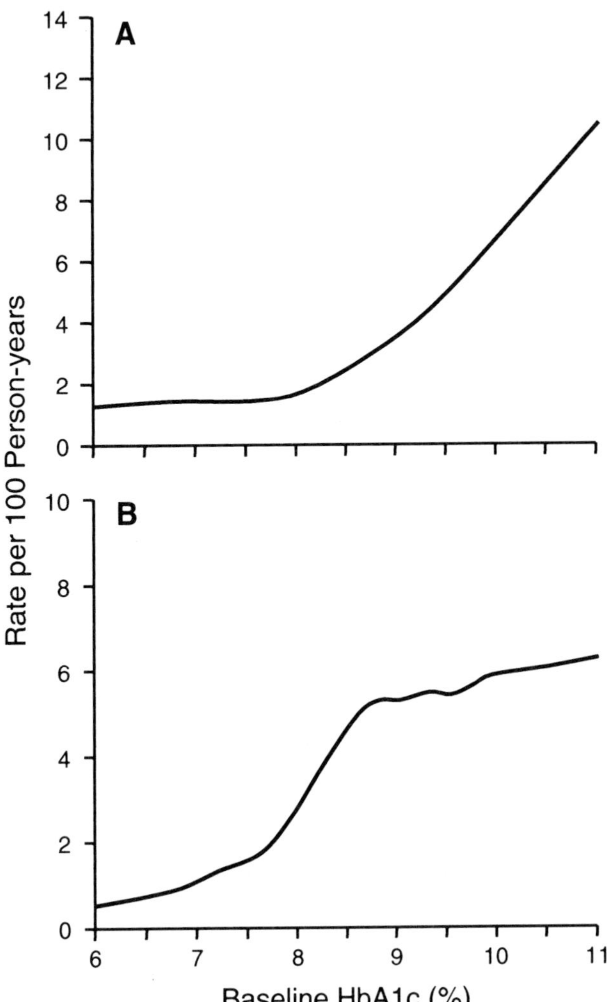

Figure 47.4. A: Dose-response relationship between level of glycosylated hemoglobin A_{1c} (HbA_{1c}) and incidence of microalbuminuria in patients with normoalbuminuria and type 1 diabetes (adapted from Scott et al.) **B:** Dose-response relationship between level of HbA_{1c} and progression to proteinuria in patients with microalbuminuria and type 1 diabetes (adapted from Warram et al.) (Adapted from Scott LJ, Warram JH, Hanna LS, et al. A nonlinear effect of hyperglycemia and current cigarette smoking are major determinants of the onset of microalbuminuria in type 1 diabetes. *Diabetes* 2001;50:2842–2849; and Warram JH, Scott LJ, Hanna LS, et al. Progression of microalbuminuria to proteinuria in type 1 diabetes, *Diabetes* 2000;49: 94–100. Copyright © 2001 and 2000, respectively, American Diabetes Association. Adapted with permission from the American Diabetes Association.)

HbA_{1c} (<8.5%, 8.5% to 9.6%, 9.7% to 10.6%, and >10.7%). The risks were 12%, 46%, 42%, and 50%, respectively. These estimates are similar to data reported by several recent studies (63–66), but are only one half the values reported in the initial publications in the 1980s on the risk associated with microalbuminuria (67–69). This discrepancy is more likely due to an overestimation of the risk of progression in the early studies than to a decline in the risk during the last 15 years.

Confirmation in a clinical trial that good glycemic control reduces the risk of progression of microalbuminuria to overt proteinuria is lacking. Only one very small clinical trial found that improved glycemic control reduced the risk of progression of microalbuminuria to overt proteinuria (70), whereas a larger clinical trial found no relationship between improvement of diabetes control and slower progression of microalbuminuria to overt proteinuria (71).

Patients with diabetes start losing renal function when they have high levels of microalbuminuria or overt proteinuria (50). So far, only a few observational studies have examined the impact of glycemic control on the rate of decline in renal function in patients with type 1 diabetes and proteinuria. Two of them demonstrated a significant association between the HbA_{1c} value and the rate of decline of the glomerular filtration rate (72,73). Interestingly, one study found a dose-response relationship similar to that shown in Figure 47.4B for the association between HbA_{1c} value and progression of microalbuminuria to overt proteinuria (72).

Other Risk Factors for Diabetic Nephropathy

Epidemiologic studies have shown that several factors besides hyperglycemia influence the development of the several stages of diabetic nephropathy. These include predisposition to essential hypertension (74–77), elevated systolic blood pressure (58,76), cigarette smoking (59,78), elevated levels of serum cholesterol and triglycerides (57), and genetic susceptibility to diabetic nephropathy (7). The last seems to play a major role.

The leveling off of the cumulative risk of overt proteinuria after 30 years of diabetes (Fig. 47.3) has previously been reported (48,53) and is evidence that only a subset of individuals are susceptible to the development of this complication (7). The hypothesis about susceptibility to diabetic nephropathy has been strengthened by evidence gained from family studies.

Familial clustering of diabetic nephropathy has been demonstrated in four studies of families with two or more siblings with type 1 diabetes (79–82). In all these studies, if the index sibling had advanced diabetic nephropathy, the other diabetic siblings were more likely to develop nephropathy than if the index sibling did not have nephropathy. The best illustration of the familial clustering of diabetic nephropathy is provided by a study we conducted at the Joslin Diabetes Center in which we attempted to obtain unbiased estimates of familial clustering (81) (Fig. 47.5). The risk of overt proteinuria, expressed as the cumulative incidence after 30 years of type 1 diabetes, was 72% in siblings of affected index cases and 25% in the siblings of unaffected index cases. Adjustment for familial clustering of the level of glycemic control could reduce this difference only slightly. Overall, the conclusion from that study is that susceptibility to overt proteinuria is likely to involve a major gene effect (81). Currently, the search for such a gene is under way using linkage as well as association studies (83).

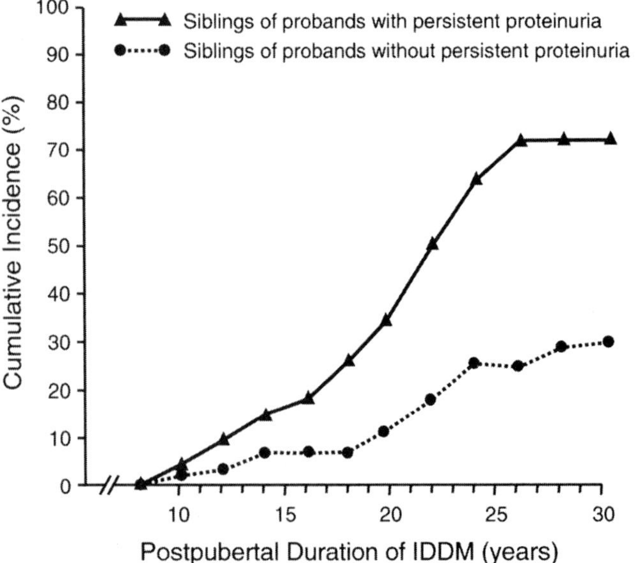

Figure 47.5. Familial occurrence of persistent proteinuria in families with two or more siblings with type 1 diabetes (IDDM): cumulative incidence of persistent proteinuria in the diabetic siblings of the first sibling with diabetes (index case) according to the proteinuria status of the index case. The higher curve is for the diabetic siblings of index cases with proteinuria. The lower curve is for diabetic siblings of index cases without proteinuria despite a long duration of diabetes.

Comparison of Risk of Diabetic Nephropathy in Type 1 and Type 2 Diabetes

Although the risk of diabetic nephropathy in type 2 diabetes seems to be similar to that in type 1 diabetes, the occurrence of this complication in type 2 diabetes is a much larger burden to society because of the 10-times greater frequency of type 2 diabetes than type 1 diabetes. The following is a brief description of some salient features of the natural history of diabetic nephropathy in type 2 diabetes highlighted by pairing them with the features of diabetic nephropathy in type 1 diabetes that were described earlier.

There are no published follow-up studies on the onset and progression of microalbuminuria in patients with type 2 diabetes. However, in a recent cross-sectional study conducted in the population of patients (90% white) attending the Joslin Clinic, the prevalences of persistent microalbuminuria and overt proteinuria according to duration of type 2 diabetes were similar to those for type 1 diabetes (Fig. 47.3) (Krolewski et al., unpublished observation). A similar conclusion can be drawn from comparisons of the results of cohort studies of the natural history of overt proteinuria in type 2 diabetes (84,85) with the corresponding results of studies in type 1 diabetes (48,53). The cumulative risk of persistent proteinuria during long-term follow-up of a cohort of patients with newly diagnosed type 2 diabetes in the population of Rochester, Minnesota, was similar to the cumulative risk of persistent proteinuria in the cohorts of Joslin patients with type 1 diabetes (48,84,85). The first cases of persistent proteinuria occurred after a shorter duration of diabetes in patients with type 2 diabetes than in patients with type 1 diabetes, but the subsequent increases in cumulative risk with duration of diabetes were very similar for the two groups of patients, reaching almost the same cumulative risk after 25 years of diabetes. Similarly, the incidence rate of ESRD in the white U.S. population with diabetes is approximately the same in young patients (mainly type 1 diabetes) as in middle-aged and older patients (predominantly type 2 diabetes) (Fig. 47.6).

Various risk factors were found to have an impact on the occurrence of persistent proteinuria in type 2 diabetes, including the level of glycemic control (84,86). So far, no study has determined the dose-response relationship between the level of hyperglycemia and the risk of diabetic nephropathy in patients with type 2 diabetes that can be compared with that shown for patients with type 1 diabetes in Figure 47.4.

Several studies have demonstrated that the level of systemic blood pressure and predisposition to hypertension are related to the subsequent development of microalbuminuria and overt proteinuria (87,88). Particularly elegant studies of this issue were conducted in Pima Indians with type 2 diabetes (88). Some other reports, however, failed to demonstrate this relationship (84,86). As in type 1 diabetes, many studies demonstrated familial clustering of diabetic nephropathy in patients with type 2 diabetes, in both white (89–92) and minority (93–95) populations.

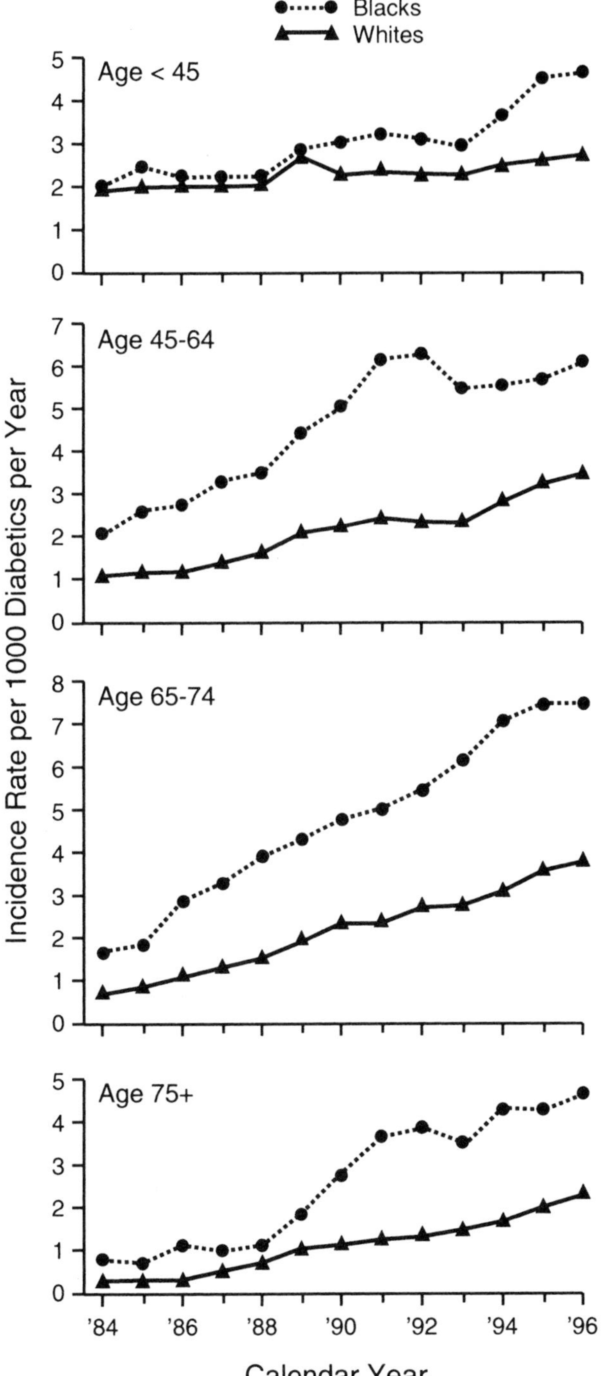

Figure 47.6. Incidence rate of end-stage renal disease in the United States in patients with diabetes according to race, age, and calendar time. (Adapted from Centers for Disease Control and Prevention. Diabetes surveillance 1999. Atlanta, U.S. Department of Health and Human Services, 1999.)

During the past decade, much has been learned about the development and clinical course of diabetic nephropathy in type 2 diabetes in populations such as Asians, blacks, Hispanics, and Native Americans (96–100). In all of these populations, type 1 diabetes is very rare, but type 2 diabetes occurs at a much earlier age than it does in whites. Furthermore, diabetes in these populations is accompanied by a much higher risk of the development of ESRD than it is in white patients (101–105; see also Fig. 47.6). The extent to which this higher risk might be attributable solely to poorer glycemic control is unknown. Higher prevalences of other environmental factors or genetic susceptibilities that interact with hyperglycemia may play important roles.

Can the Occurrence of Diabetic Nephropathy Be Changed?

The natural history of diabetic nephropathy in type 1 diabetes has been changing over the last half-century. We reported the first study documenting this phenomenon and showed that the cumulative incidence of overt proteinuria was significantly lower in patients with type 1 diabetes diagnosed in the late 1940s and 1950s than in those with diabetes diagnosed in the late 1930s (48). As discussed earlier, the cumulative risk of proliferative diabetic retinopathy remained constant in these three cohorts (16). A similar decline in the risk of persistent proteinuria according to calendar time was observed in Denmark (106), and although the mechanisms responsible for the decreased risk are not clear, improved glycemic control during that time interval might have been a factor in both populations. Investigators from Sweden have demonstrated a significant decline in the risk of overt proteinuria in patients with type 1 diabetes followed 10 to 15 years after the implementation of intensified diabetes treatment at the community level (45). Several studies have demonstrated that vigorous antihypertensive treatment might also slow the rate of declining renal function in patients with proteinuria (107,108).

These observations would suggest that a decline in the occurrence of ESRD in patients with diabetes would be evident in recent decades. However, the incidence rates of ESRD in patients with diabetes in the U.S. population showed the opposite trend (109). The incidence rate of ESRD in the U.S. diabetic population during the period from 1984 to 1996 according to age and race is shown in Figure 47.6. Among whites under the age of 45 years with diabetes (mainly type 1 diabetes), the incidence rate increased slightly from 1.9 per 1,000 a year in 1984 to 2.5 per 1,000 a year in 1996. The incidence rates of ESRD increased in an even more dramatic way in the middle-aged and older diabetic population, predominantly with type 2 diabetes. In those aged 45 to 74 years, the incidence rate of ESRD was 0.9 per 1,000 a year in 1984 and has increased steadily every year, reaching 3.5 per 1,000 a year in 1996. Increases also were seen among whites with diabetes in the oldest age group, although the rates were lower than in the three other age categories. In blacks with diabetes, the incidence rate of ESRD was two to three times that in whites with diabetes and the secular trend paralleling that seen in whites (Fig. 47.6).

The secular increase in the incidence of ESRD in the U.S. diabetic population occurred despite the increasing prevalence of antihypertensive treatment in the 1980s and 1990s (110) and the wide use of angiotensin-converting enzyme inhibitors beginning in the early 1990s (111–113). The effect of the latter may not have been evident by 1996, but unpublished data for the years 1997 to 1999 suggest that the incidence rate of ESRD has continued to increase at the same rate as before. At present there is no explanation for the "epidemic" of ESRD among patients with diabetes in the United States and in other countries as well (114).

DIABETES AND CORONARY ARTERY DISEASE

In contrast to eye and kidney complications, which affect patients with diabetes in all populations, coronary artery disease (CAD) is a frequent complication in diabetic patients only in populations in which there is a high risk of CAD in individuals without

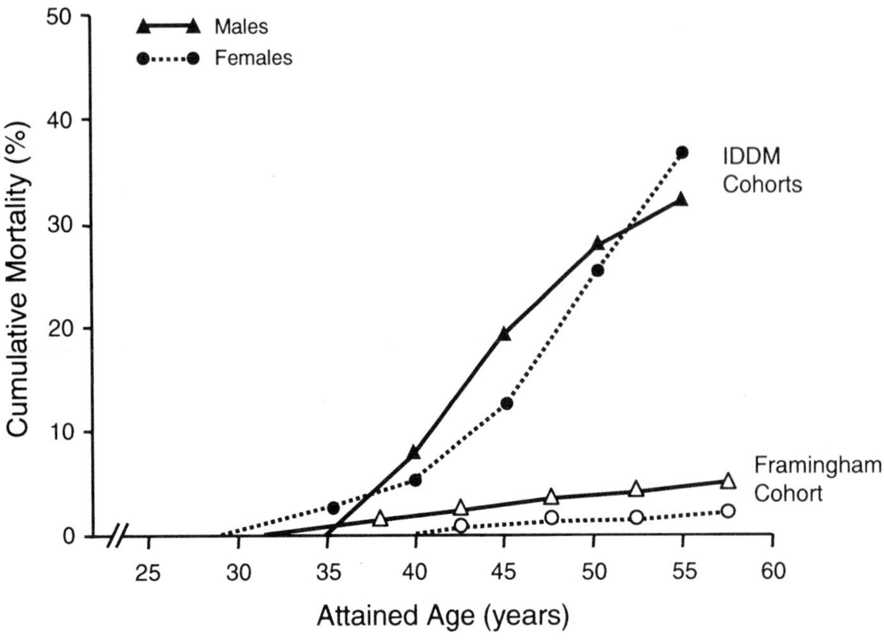

Figure 47.7. Cumulative mortality due to coronary artery disease up to age 55 years in patients with type 1 diabetes (IDDM) and in the nondiabetic participants of the Framingham Heart Study. (Adapted from Krolewski AS, Kosinski EJ, Warram JH, et al. Magnitude and determinants of coronary artery disease in juvenile-onset, insulin-dependent diabetes mellitus. *Am J Cardiol* 1987;59:750–755, copyright 1987, wtih permission from Excerpta Medica.)

diabetes. The excess of CAD in persons with diabetes in these populations is influenced by the conventional CAD risk factors as well as diabetes-specific exposures (115,116). The following review emphasizes data on the role of diabetes-specific exposures on the development of CAD, namely duration of diabetes, level of hyperglycemia, treatment with insulin, insulin resistance, and the presence of diabetic nephropathy.

Risk of Increases in Coronary Artery Disease with Duration of Diabetes and Attained Age

In white populations, the risk of CAD among individuals with diabetes generally increases with the duration of diabetes, but this effect depends on attained age. Figure 47.7 shows the cumulative mortality due to CAD according to attained age in patients who had type 1 diabetes diagnosed before age 21 years and were followed for 20 to 40 years. Also shown for comparison is the cumulative mortality due to CAD in the nondiabetic participants of the Framingham Heart Study. In both groups, the first deaths due to CAD occurred in the fourth decade of life. However, between ages 30 and 55 years, CAD mortality claimed 35% of the group with type 1 diabetes but only 8% of the men and 4% of the women in the nondiabetic group (117). In addition to this excess of CAD deaths, patients who were alive at the end of the 20- to 40-year follow-up had high prevalences of symptomatic and asymptomatic CAD. When all forms of CAD (including CAD deaths) were combined, the cumulative risk of this disease in juvenile-onset type 1 diabetes by age 55 years was about 50% (117). It is notable that the risk of CAD among patients with type 1 diabetes was similar in men and women and increased at the same rate after the age of 30 years, regardless of whether the onset of diabetes had been at age 0 to 9, 10 to 14, or 15 to 20 years (117). These findings suggest that exposure to diabetes before the age of 20 does not contribute to the enormous risk of CAD seen in these patients after age 30. One may postulate, however, that exposure to diabetes after age 20 accelerates the progression of the intermediate stages of coronary atherosclerosis that appear in the general population in the third and fourth decades of life (117–119).

Mortality due to CAD in a cohort of middle-aged white patients with type 2 diabetes is shown in Figure 47.8. Age-adjusted CAD mortality rates during the 24 years following diagnosis of type 2 diabetes are compared with the corresponding rates in nondiabetic individuals followed over the same interval in the Framingham Heart Study (119). From the time of diagnosis of diabetes, the mortality rate in diabetic patients was higher than in the Framingham population, and this excess risk grew larger with increasing duration of diabetes. Other investigators have obtained similar findings (120–123).

Interpretations of these findings vary, however, depending on whether the effect of diabetes is measured as the rate difference or the rate ratio. To illustrate, note that CAD mortality was quite high in diabetic patients in Figure 47.8 (and Figure 47.7 as well) and was the same in men and women. When these rates and the rates in the Framingham population are compared in terms of rate differences (additive scale), the impact of diabetes exposure on CAD mortality increases with diabetes duration in both men and women (Table 47.2). However, when the rates are compared in terms of rate ratios (multiplicative scale), the effect of diabetes exposure does not change with increasing duration in men and diminishes with increasing duration of diabetes in women. These data on mortality among patients with type 1 or type 2 diabetes and in the Framingham population were based on the period 1950 to 1980. Since that time, mortality due to CAD has declined significantly in the general population but not in the diabetic population (see later). As a result of these different trends, the rate differences and rate ratios shown in Table 47.2 may be considered as underestimates.

At present, there is no biologic justification for choosing one scale over the other to estimate the effect of duration of diabetes exposure on the risk of CAD. However, an increasing effect measured on the additive scale has a straightforward interpretation (124–126). It is a measure of CAD risk that is attributable to the cumulative effects of diabetes exposure, which includes both its independent effects and any synergistic effects due to interactions with age-related risk factors. For this reason, a public health perspective is better served by measuring effects on the additive scale (124). Interpretation of the constant or decreasing effects seen on the multiplicative scale, on the other hand, requires

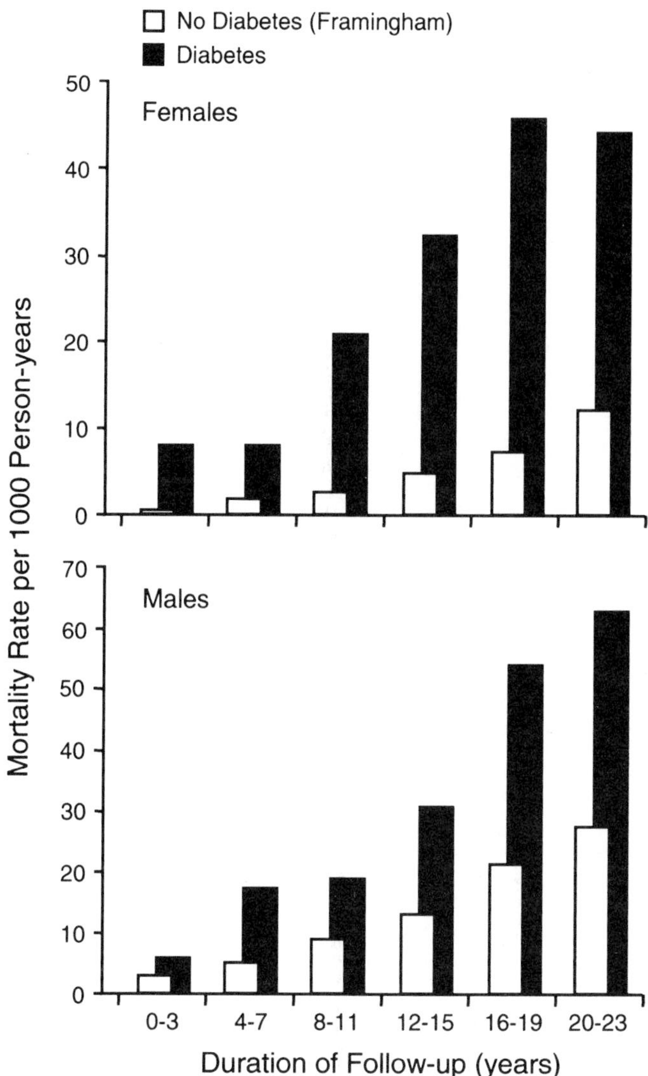

Figure 47.8. Age-adjusted mortality rate due to coronary artery disease in a cohort of patients of the Joslin Diabetes Center whose diabetes was diagnosed between ages 35 and 62 years and who came to the center soon after diagnosis and in the nondiabetic participants of the Framingham Heart Study, according to sex and duration of follow-up. (Adapted from Krolewski AS, Warram JH, Valsania P, et al. Evolving natural history of coronary artery disease in diabetes mellitus. *Am J Med* 1991;90[Suppl 2A]:56S–61S, copyright 1991, with permission from Elsevier Science.)

allowance for the age-related pattern of increasing risk of CAD that occurs independently of diabetes exposure. Uncritical interpretation of such results can be misleading (124–126). For example, some investigators have concluded that the effect of diabetes exposure (127) and other CAD risk factors (128) on the natural history of CAD diminishes with increasing age or duration of diabetes, although most observers would not draw this conclusion from the empiric data displayed in Figures 47.7 and 47.8.

Level of Glycemic Control and Risk of Coronary Artery Disease

At present, data are not adequate to evaluate the relationship between the level of hyperglycemia and risk of CAD in type 1 diabetes. Several observational studies found associations between level of glycemic control and total mortality, and some of the authors of these studies attempted to examine the effect of HbA_{1c} on the risk of CAD specifically (129,130). However, interpretations of negative or positive findings from these studies are confounded by two issues. First, it is not known whether exposure to hyperglycemia has an impact on the early or late stages of CAD. If the first is true one ought to measure HbA_{1c} decades before the CAD event, but if the second is true one ought to measure HbA_{1c} at a time closer to the event. Second, the level of glycemic control determines the risk of diabetic nephropathy, which in turn increases the risk of CAD. Therefore, one cannot dissect the roles of these two factors without a stratified analysis. In patients with type 1 diabetes in the DCCT, there was less CAD among those receiving intensive therapy (better glycemic control) than in those receiving conventional therapy (worse glycemic control), but the difference was not statistically significant (131). If the result had been significant, one would still have to qualify the interpretation in terms of the issues mentioned previously.

The results of observational studies in type 2 diabetes, although less frequently confounded by diabetic nephropathy, are also ambiguous. The results of two cohort studies showed a positive association between the level of hyperglycemia and mortality due to CAD (129,132). However, the findings were confounded by the association of other factors with severe hyperglycemia. The persistence of high levels of glycemia in patients with type 2 diabetes generally leads to the patient being treated with insulin. It was insulin treatment (rather than the severe hyperglycemia) that was associated with the high risk of CAD in several studies (1,120,133–137).

The interpretation of the high CAD risk among patients with type 2 diabetes who are treated with insulin is not clear. Hyperinsulinemia has been implicated in the acceleration of coronary atherosclerosis (138–141). Thus, one can hypothesize that treatment with insulin may contribute to the excess mortality due to CAD. One cannot, however, exclude the possibility that metabolic or cellular abnormalities that underlie insulin resistance and produce the hyperglycemia that requires insulin treatment are the true risk factors for acceleration of atherosclerosis (142–146).

The results of the University Group Diabetes Program (UGDP), conducted in patients with type 2 diabetes and published more than a decade ago, showed that fatal and nonfatal cardiovascular events occurred with equal frequency in patients who received intensive insulin treatment and had good glycemic control and in patients treated with diet and whose average fasting blood glucose level deteriorated from 120 mg/dL at baseline to 160 mg/dL after 3 years of the trial (147). In the recent United Kingdom Prospective Diabetes Study (UKPDS), individuals treated with insulin or a sulfonylurea had slightly less CAD than did individuals treated with diet, although the difference did not reach statistical significance (44).

Other Diabetes-Specific Risk Factors/Indicators of Risk of Coronary Artery Disease

Both type 1 and type 2 diabetes have long preclinical periods. Immunologic abnormalities, which precede by several years the clinical manifestation of type 1 diabetes, do not have an impact on the natural history of atherosclerosis. On the other hand, the metabolic abnormalities associated with low insulin sensitivity, which precede the onset of type 2 diabetes by decades, seem to have an impact on the natural history of coronary atherosclerosis (148,149). In a large cross-sectional study (Insulin Resistance and Atherosclerosis Study, or IRAS), low insulin sensitivity was associated with atherosclerosis in nondiabetic individuals, and this effect was independent of insulin level (150). Interestingly,

TABLE 47.2. Excess Mortality due to Coronary Artery Disease in Patients with Type 2 Diabetes as Compared with That in Nondiabetics, According to Duration of Diabetes, Expressed as the Rate Difference and as the Rate Ratio (Results Adjusted for Age and Type of Diabetes Treatment)

Duration of follow-up (duration of diabetes)	Rate difference[a] (rate/1,000 person-years)		Rate ratio[b] (relative risk)	
	Males	Females	Males	Females
0–3	2.7	7.4	1.9	19.5
4–7	12.2	6.1	3.5	4.6
8–11	10.0	18.6	2.1	8.0
12–15	17.5	27.4	2.3	6.8
16–19	32.6	38.5	2.5	6.4
20–23	35.2	31.7	2.3	3.6

[a]The difference between the standardized mortality rate in the diabetic population and the nondiabetic population. Within each duration stratum, both sets of age-specific rates were standardized to the same age distribution. Within the diabetic population, the treatment-specific rates were standardized to the same distribution within each duration stratum.
[b]The ratio of the standardized mortality rate in the diabetic population to the corresponding rate in the nondiabetic population of Framingham.
Data from Krolewski AS, Warram JH, Valsania P, et al. Evolving natural history of coronary artery disease in diabetes mellitus. *Am J Med* 1991;90 [Suppl 2A]:56S–61S.

the effect appears to be peculiar to whites, being diminished in Hispanics and perhaps absent in blacks. Because low insulin sensitivity is also the strongest risk factor for the development of type 2 diabetes, the IRAS findings can account for the excess CAD in patients with newly diagnosed type 2 diabetes and the excess CAD mortality seen in patients with short-duration diabetes (see Fig. 47.8 and Table 47.2).

Diabetic nephropathy is the most potent risk factor/indicator for CAD in white patients with diabetes. In a large study of patients with type 1 diabetes conducted in Denmark, cardiovascular mortality rates (per 1,000 person-years) in those with proteinuria, in those without proteinuria, and in nondiabetic individuals were 22.1, 2.5, and 0.6, respectively (151). We obtained similar findings in our cohort study conducted in patients of the Joslin Clinic (117). Moreover, in a large multinational study of older diabetic patients, proteinuria was a major predictor of cardiovascular deaths (152). Patients with significant (heavy) proteinuria and type 1 or type 2 diabetes had mortality rates of 42.2 and 27.9 per 1,000 person-years, respectively. The rate in those without proteinuria was 9.4 and 9.2 per 1,000 person-years, respectively. Finally, recent studies in patients with type 2 diabetes found similarly elevated cardiovascular mortality rates in those with overt proteinuria and those with microalbuminuria or normoalbuminuria (153,154).

Several mechanisms can account for the excess of CAD in diabetic patients with proteinuria. First, patients who develop diabetic nephropathy come from families with essential hypertension (74–77) and an excess of CAD (155). Second, the majority of patients with diabetic nephropathy are hypertensive and have lipid abnormalities (56–58,76,156). These abnormalities appear long before the clinical manifestation of diabetic nephropathy. Furthermore, the effect of hypercholesterolemia on CAD mortality is much more potent in patients with diabetic nephropathy than in patients without proteinuria (157,158). Third, patients with diabetic nephropathy and declining renal function have very high plasma levels of advanced glycation end products (159). According to some theories, this could account for accelerating atherosclerosis in these patients (160).

Different Risk of Coronary Artery Disease in Different Diabetic Populations

In some populations of patients with diabetes, CAD is an infrequent complication. The World Health Organization Multinational Study of Vascular Disease in Diabetics documented marked variation in the occurrence of CAD among 14 samples of middle-aged diabetic patients throughout the world. In the cross-sectional part of this study conducted in the 1970s, a high prevalence of indicators of cardiovascular disease, such as electrocardiographic abnormalities and chest-pain symptoms, were found in patients with diabetes from Switzerland, Berlin, and London. A low prevalence of these indices was found in patients with diabetes from Tokyo, Hong Kong, and Native Americans (Pima) in Arizona (161). Similar findings were obtained during the 7-year follow-up study. The CAD mortality rate was highest in the samples of patients with diabetes from Berlin, Switzerland, and London, whereas it was lowest in the patients from Tokyo and Hong Kong and in Pima Indians (162).

The low risk of CAD in the Pima with type 2 diabetes is particularly curious (163). More than half of this population develop type 2 diabetes and most of these patients have poor glycemic control and are insulin-resistant and hyperinsulinemic for most of their lives. Furthermore, renal complications develop as frequently in the Pima with diabetes as in the white population with type 1 diabetes (100). At present there is no explanation for these observations. A similar lack of effect of diabetes exposure on the development of CAD was found among patients with type 2 diabetes in Japan. Figure 47.9 contrasts the mortality rate due to CAD in a cohort of patients with type 2 diabetes patients in Tokyo who were followed for almost 30 years with the mortality rate in a similar cohort of white patients with diabetes followed at the Joslin Clinic (164). Whereas the mortality rates increased steeply with the duration of diabetes in the Joslin cohort, there was minimal CAD mortality in the Tokyo cohort regardless of duration.

In summary, wide variation in the occurrence of CAD among different diabetic populations is consistent with the hypothesis that certain components of prediabetic exposure

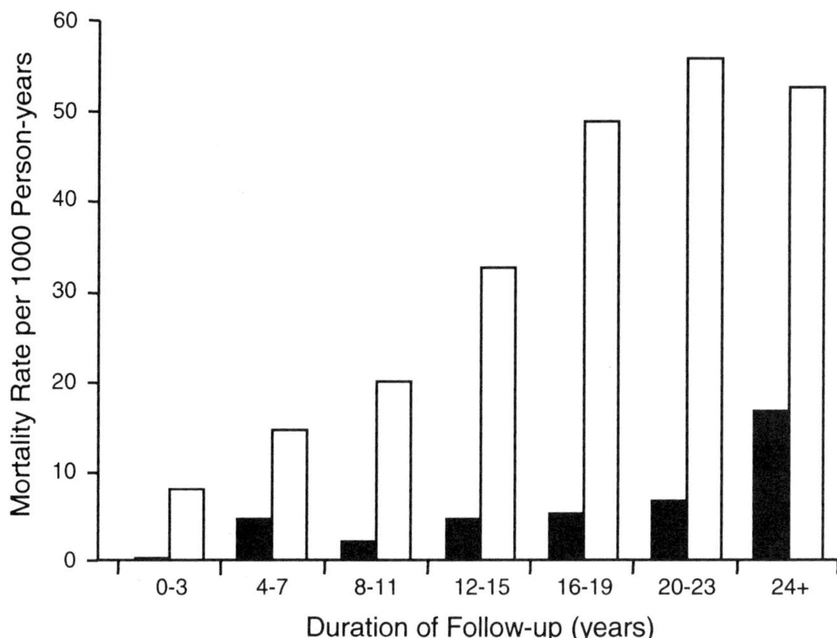

Figure 47.9. Age-adjusted mortality rate due to coronary artery disease in cohorts of patients with type 2 diabetes followed at the Tokyo University in Japan (*shaded bars*) and at the Joslin Clinic in Boston (*open bars*). (Copyright © 1994 American Diabetes Association. Adapted from Matsumoto T, Ohashi Y, Yamada N, et al: Coronary heart disease mortality is actually low in diabetic Japanese by direct comparison with the Joslin cohort. *Diabetes Care* 1994;17:1062–1063, with permission from the American Diabetes Association.)

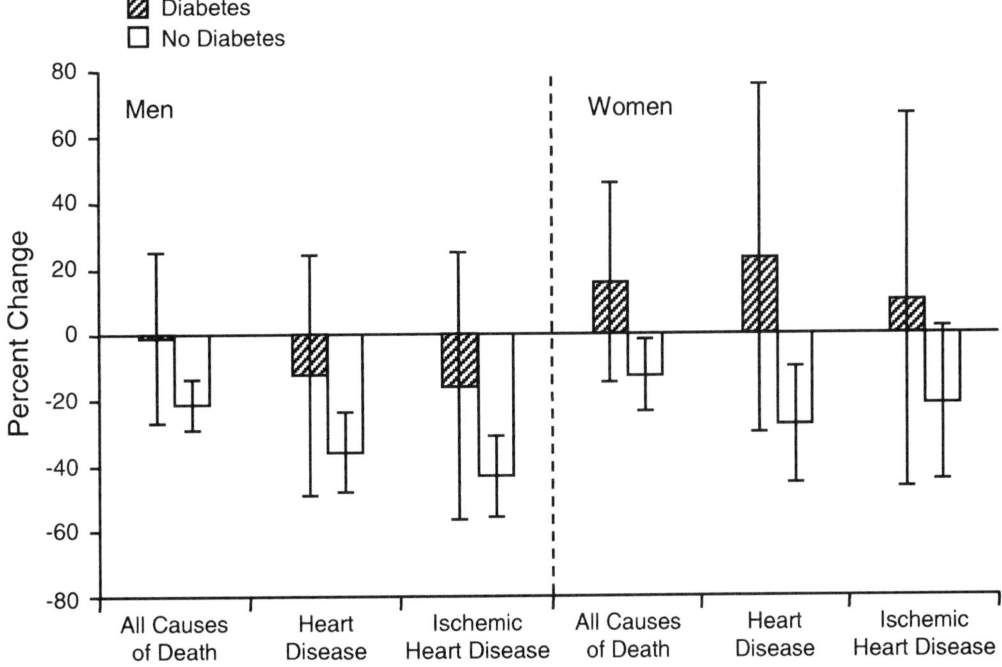

Figure 47.10. Percentage change in age-adjusted mortality rates due to all causes, heart disease, and ischemic heart disease in the general population of the United States between the 1980s and 1990s. Mortality rates were determined during 9 years of follow-up of two representative samples of the U.S. population: the participants of the first National Health and Nutrition Examination Survey (NHANES I) examined between 1971 and 1974 and the participants of the second survey (NHANES II) examined between 1982 and 1984. The former is designated the first cohort and the latter, the second cohort. The change in age-adjusted rates is expressed as a percentage of the rate in the first cohort together with its 95% confidence interval. (Adapted from Gu K, Cowie CC, Harris MI. Diabetes and decline in heart disease mortality in U.S. adults. *JAMA* 1999;281:1291–1297.)

(e.g., insulin resistance and/or hyperinsulinemia), as well as exposures during diabetes, have an impact only on progression of atherosclerotic lesions (117,119). These exposures have no impact on the frequency of atherosclerosis in patients with diabetes from populations in which the initiation of atherosclerosis is infrequent, such as the Pima, Japanese in Tokyo, and Chinese in Hong Kong.

Can the Natural History of Coronary Artery Disease in Patients with Diabetes Be Changed?

Over the past 30 years, there has been a constant decline, about 1% to 2% a year, in mortality due to CAD in the general U.S. population (165,166). This extraordinary phenomenon results from the declining incidence of CAD events as well as improved survival among those who developed CAD. Declining incidence reflects a modification of CAD risk factors, and improving survival reflects improved effectiveness of the treatment of patients with CAD (167–169).

Figure 47.10 shows data from a study that compared mortality in patients with and without diabetes in two cohorts that are representative of the U.S. population—the subjects of the First and Second National Health and Nutrition Examination Surveys (170). One was examined between 1971 and 1974 and the other between 1982 and 1984. The majority of individuals with diabetes in these cohorts had type 2 diabetes. Each cohort was followed for 9 years. Between the two periods, nondiabetic men experienced a 43.8% decline in age-adjusted mortality due to ischemic heart disease, whereas diabetic men experienced only a 16.6% decline. Age-adjusted mortality due to ischemic heart disease declined 20.4% in nondiabetic women but increased 10.7% in diabetic women. Whereas the declines in nondiabetic men and women were highly significant statistically, the changes in individuals with diabetes were not significantly different from 0. The patterns of changes for heart disease mortality as well as all-cause mortality were similar. No other study of the natural history of CAD in individuals with type 2 diabetes has evaluated the change or lack of it over time.

REFERENCES

1. Krolewski AS, Warram JH. Epidemiology of late complications of diabetes. In: Kahn CR, Wier GC, eds. *Joslin's diabetes mellitus*, 13th ed. Philadelphia: Lea & Febiger, 1994:605–619.
2. MacGillivray MH, Voorhess ML, Putnam TI, et al. Hormone and metabolic profiles in children and adolescents with type 1 diabetes mellitus. *Diabetes Care* 1982;5[Suppl 1]:38–47.
3. Sowers JR, Lester MA. Diabetes and cardiovascular disease. *Diabetes Care* 1999;22[Suppl 3]:C14–C20.
4. Parving HH, Viberti GC, Keen H, et al. Hemodynamic factors in the genesis of diabetic microangiopathy. *Metabolism* 1983;32:943–949.
5. Brownlee M, Cerami A, Vlassara H. Advanced glycosylation end products in tissue and the biochemical basis of diabetic complications. *N Engl J Med* 1988;318:1315–1321.
6. Greene D, Lattimer SA, Sima AAF. Sorbitol, phosphoinositides and sodium-potassium-ATPase in the pathogenesis of diabetic complications. *N Engl J Med* 1987;316:599–606.
7. Krolewski AS, Warram JH, Rand LI, et al. Epidemiologic approach to the etiology of type I diabetes mellitus and its complications. *N Engl J Med* 1987;317: 1390–1398.
8. Baynes JW. Role of oxidative stress in development of complications in diabetes. *Diabetes* 1991;40:405–412.
9. King GL, Ishii H, Koya D. Diabetes vascular dysfunctions: a model of excessive activation of protein kinase C. *Kidney Int* 1997;52:S77–S85.
10. Singh BM, McNamara C, Wise PH. High variability of glycated hemoglobin concentrations in patients with IDDM followed for over 9 years. *Diabetes Care* 1997;20:306–308.
11. Antisdel JE, Anderson BJ, Warram JH, et al. Inherent tracking of glycemic control among patients with type 1 diabetes (*submitted for publication*).
12. Retinopathy and nephropathy in patients with type 1 diabetes four years after a trial of intensive therapy. The Diabetes Control and Complications Trial/Epidemiology of Diabetes Interventions of Complications Research Group. *N Engl J Med* 2000;342:381–389.
13. Palmberg P, Smith M, Waltman S, et al. The natural history of retinopathy in insulin-dependent juvenile-onset diabetes. *Ophthalmology* 1981;66:613–618.
14. Klein R, Klein BEK, Moss SE, et al. The Wisconsin Epidemiologic Study of Diabetic Retinopathy. II. Prevalence and risk of diabetic retinopathy when age at diagnosis is less than 30 years. *Arch Ophthalmol* 1984;102:520–526.
15. The Diabetes Control and Complications Trial Research Group. The effect of intensive treatment of diabetes on the development and progression of long-term complications in insulin-dependent diabetes mellitus. *N Engl J Med* 1993;329:977–986.
16. Krolewski AS, Warram JH, Rand LI, et al. Risk of proliferative diabetic retinopathy in juvenile-onset type I diabetes: a 40-yr follow-up study. *Diabetes Care* 1986;9:443–452.
17. Klein R, Klein BEK, Moss SE, et al. The Wisconsin epidemiologic study of diabetic retinopathy. IX. Four-year incidence and progression of diabetic retinopathy when age at diagnosis is less than 30 years. *Arch Ophthalmol* 1989;107:237–243.
18. Orchard TJ, Dorman JS, Maser RE, et al. Pittsburgh epidemiology of diabetes complications study. II. Prevalence of complications in IDDM by sex and duration. *Diabetes* 1990;39:1116–1124.
19. Yokoyama H, Uchigata Y, Otani T, et al. Development of proliferative retinopathy in Japanese patients with IDDM: Tokyo Women's Medical College Epidemiologic Study. *Diabetes Res Clin Pract* 1994;24:113–119.
20. Klein R, Klein BEK, Moss SE, et al. Glycosylated hemoglobin predicts the incidence and progression of diabetic retinopathy. *JAMA* 1988;260:2864–2871.
21. Janka HU, Warram JH, Rand LI, et al. Risk factors for progression of background retinopathy in long-standing IDDM. *Diabetes* 1989;38:460–464.
22. Chase PH, Jackson WE, Hoops SL, et al. Glucose control and the renal and retinal complications of insulin-dependent diabetes. *JAMA* 1989;261:1155–1160.
23. Goldstein DE, Blinder KJ, Ide CH, et al. Glycemic control and development of retinopathy in youth-onset insulin-dependent diabetes mellitus. Results of a 12-year longitudinal study. *Ophthalmology* 1993;100:1125–1132.
24. Klein R, Klein BEK, Moss SE, et al. Relationship of hyperglycemia to the long-term incidence and progression of diabetic retinopathy. *Arch Intern Med* 1994;154:2169–2178.
25. Cohen RA, Hennekens CH, Christen WG, et al. Determinants of retinopathy progression in type 1 diabetes mellitus. *Am J Med* 1999;107:45–51.
26. Wang PH, Lau J, Chalmers TC. Meta-analysis of effects of intensive blood-glucose control on late complications of type I diabetes. *Lancet* 1993;341:1306–1309.
27. Reichard P, Nilsson BY, Rosenqvist U. The effect of long-term intensified insulin treatment on the development of microvascular complications of diabetes mellitus. *N Engl J Med* 1993;329:304–309.
28. Diabetes Control and Complication Trial Research Group. Progression of retinopathy with intensive versus conventional treatment in the diabetes and complications trial. *Ophthalmology* 1995;102:647–661.
29. Warram JH, Manson JE, Krolewski AS. Glycated hemoglobin and the risk of retinopathy in insulin-dependent diabetes mellitus. *N Engl J Med* 1995;332: 1305–1306.
30. Danne T, Weber B, Hartmann R, et al. Long-term glycemic control as a non-linear association to the frequency of background retinopathy in adolescents with diabetes. *Diabetes Care* 1994;17:1390–1396.
31. Janka HU, Ziegler AG, Valsania P, et al. Impact of blood pressure on diabetic retinopathy. *Diabetes Metabol* 1989;15:333–337.
32. Klein R, Klein BEK, Moss SE, et al. Is blood pressure a predictor of the incidence or progression of diabetic retinopathy? *Arch Intern Med* 1989;149:2427–2432.
33. Norgaard K, Feldt-Rasmussen T, et al. Is hypertension a major independent risk factor for retinopathy in type I diabetes? *Diabet Med* 1991;8:334–337.
34. Chavers BM, Mauer SM, Ramsay RC, et al. Relationship between retinal and glomerular lesions in IDDM patients. *Diabetes* 1994;43:441–446.
35. Nathan DM. Long-term complications of diabetes mellitus. *N Engl J Med* 1993;328:1676–1685.
36. Klein R, Moss SE, Klein BEK. Is gross proteinuria a risk factor for the incidence of proliferative diabetic retinopathy? *Ophthalmology* 1993;100:1140–1146.
37. Krolewski AS, Barzilay J, Warram JH, et al. Risk of early-onset proliferative retinopathy in IDDM is closely related to cardiovascular autonomic neuropathy. *Diabetes* 1992;41:430–437.
38. Fong DS, Warram JH, Aiello LM, et al. Cardiovascular autonomic neuropathy and proliferative diabetic retinopathy. *Am J Ophthalmol* 1995;80:1882–1887.
39. Moss SE, Klein R, Klein BEK. Ocular factors in the incidence and progression of diabetic retinopathy. *Ophthalmology* 1994;101:77–83.
40. Gay AJ, Rosenbaum AL. Retinal artery pressure in asymmetric diabetic retinopathy. *Arch Ophthalmol* 1966;75:758–762.
41. Rand LI, Krolewski AS, Aiello LM, et al. Multiple factors in the prediction of risk of proliferative diabetic retinopathy. *N Engl J Med* 1985;313:1433–1438.
42. Klein R, Klein BEK, Moss SE, et al. The Wisconsin Epidemiologic Study of Diabetic Retinopathy. XIV. Ten-year incidence and progression of diabetic retinopathy. *Arch Ophthalmol* 1994;112:1217–1228.
43. Ohkubo Y, Kishikawa H, Araki E, et al. Intensive insulin therapy prevents the progression of diabetic microvascular complications in Japanese patients with non-insulin dependent diabetes mellitus: a randomized prospective 6-year study. *Diabetes Res Clin Pract* 1995;28:103–117.
44. UK Prospective Diabetes Study (UKPDS). Intensive blood glucose control with sulphonylureas or insulin compared with conventional treatment and

risk of complications in patients with type 2 diabetes (UKPDS 33). *Lancet* 1998;352:837–853.
45. Bojestig M, Arnqvist HJ, Hermansson G, et al. Declining incidence of nephropathy in insulin-dependent diabetes mellitus. *N Engl J Med* 1993;330: 15–18.
46. Bojestig M, Arnqvist HJ, Karlberg BE, et al. Unchanged incidence of severe retinopathy in a population of type 1 diabetic patients with marked reduction of nephropathy. *Diabet Med* 1998;15:863–869.
47. Mogensen CE, Christensen CK, Vittinghus E. The stage in diabetic renal disease with emphasis on the stage of incipient diabetic nephropathy. *Diabetes* 1983;32[Suppl 2]:64–78.
48. Krolewski AS, Warram JH, Christlieb AR, et al. The changing natural history of nephropathy in type 1 diabetes. *Am J Med* 1985;78:785–794.
49. Janner M, Knill SE, Diem P, et al. Persistent microalbuminuria in adolescents with type I (insulin-dependent) diabetes mellitus is associated to early rather than late puberty—results of a prospective longitudinal study. *Eur J Pediatr* 1994;153:403–408.
50. Warram JH, Gearin G, Laffel LMB, et al. Effect of duration of type 1 diabetes on prevalence of stages of diabetic nephropathy defined by urinary albumin/creatinine ratio. *J Am Soc Nephrol* 1996;7:930–937.
51. Krolewski AS, Laffel LMB, Krolewski M, et al. Glycated hemoglobin and risk of microalbuminuria in patients with insulin-dependent diabetes mellitus. *N Engl J Med* 1995;332:1251–1255.
52. Stephenson JM, Fuller JH. Microalbuminuria is not rare before 5 years of IDDM. *J Diabetes Complications* 1994;8:166–173.
53. Andersen AR, Christiansen JS, Andersen JK, et al. Diabetic nephropathy in type I (insulin-dependent) diabetes: an epidemiological study. *Diabetologia* 1983;25:496–501.
54. Perkins BA, Ficociello LH, Silva KH, et al. Regression of microalbuminuria in type 1 diabetes. *N Engl J Med* 2003;348:2285–2293.
55. Krolewski M, Eggers PW, Warram JH. Magnitude of end-stage renal disease in type I diabetes: a 35-year follow-up study. *Kidney Int* 1996;50:2041–2046.
56. Mathiesen ER, Ronn B, Storm B, et al. The natural course of microalbuminuria in insulin-dependent diabetes: a 10-year prospective study. *Diabet Med* 1995;12:482–487.
57. Coonrod BA, Ellis D, Becker DJ, et al. Predictors of microalbuminuria in individuals with IDDM. *Diabetes Care* 1993;16:1376–1383.
58. Risk factors for development of microalbuminuria in insulin dependent diabetic patients: a cohort study. Microalbuminuria Collaborative Study Group, United Kingdom. *BMJ* 1993;306:1235–1239.
59. Scott LJ, Warram JH, Hanna LS, et al. A nonlinear effect of hyperglycemia and current cigarette smoking are major determinants of the onset of microalbuminuria in type 1 diabetes. *Diabetes* 2001;50:2842–2849.
60. Effect of intensive therapy on the development and progression of diabetic nephropathy in the Diabetes Control and Complications Trial. The Diabetes Control and Complications (DCCT) Research Group. *Kidney Int* 1995;47: 1703–1720.
61. Krolewski AS, Warram JH. Glycated hemoglobin and risk of microalbuminuria in patients with insulin-dependent diabetes mellitus. *N Engl J Med* 1995; 332:1251–1255.
62. Warram JH, Scott LJ, Hanna LS, et al. Progression of microalbuminuria to proteinuria in type 1 diabetes. *Diabetes* 2000;49:94–100.
63. Forsblom CM, Groop PH, Ekstrand A, et al. Predictive value of microalbuminuria in patients with insulin-dependent diabetes of long duration. *BMJ* 1992;305:1051–1053.
64. Almdal T, Norgaard K, Feldt-Rasmussen B, et al. The predictive value of microalbuminuria in IDDM: a five-year follow-up study. *Diabetes Care* 1994; 17:120–125.
65. Rudberg S, Dahlquist G. Determinants of progression of microalbuminuria in adolescents with IDDM. *Diabetes Care* 1996;19:369–371.
66. Caramori ML, Fioretto P, Mauer M. The need for early predictors of diabetic nephropathy risk. Is albumin excretion rate sufficient? *Diabetes* 2000;49:1399–1408.
67. Parving HH, Oxenboll B, Svendsen PA, et al. Early detection of patients at risk of developing diabetic nephropathy: a longitudinal study of urinary albumin secretion. *Acta Endocrinol* 1982;100:550–555.
68. Viberti GC, Hill RD, Jarrett RJ, et al. Microalbuminuria as a predictor of clinical nephropathy in insulin-dependent diabetes mellitus. *Lancet* 1982;1:1430–1432.
69. Mogensen CE, Christensen CK. Predicting diabetic nephropathy in insulin-dependent patients. *N Engl J Med* 1984;311:89–93.
70. Feldt-Rasmussen B, Mathiesen ER, Deckert T. Effect of two-years of strict metabolic control on progression of incipient nephropathy in insulin-dependent diabetes. *Lancet* 1986;2:1300–1304.
71. Microalbuminuria Collaborative Study Group, United Kingdom. Intensive therapy and progression to clinical albuminuria in patients with insulin dependent diabetes mellitus and microalbuminuria. *BMJ* 1995;311:973–977.
72. Mulec H, Blohme G, Grande B, et al. The effect of metabolic control on rate of decline in renal function in insulin-dependent diabetes mellitus with overt diabetic nephropathy. *Nephrol Dial Transplant* 1998;13:651–655.
73. Hovind P, Rossing P, Tarnow L, et al. Progression of diabetic nephropathy. *Kidney Int* 2001;59:702–709.
74. Viberti GC, Keen H, Wiseman MJ. Raised arterial pressure in parents of proteinuric insulin-dependent diabetics. *BMJ* 1987;295:515–517.
75. Krolewski AS, Canessa M, Warram JH, et al. Predisposition to hypertension and susceptibility to renal disease in insulin-dependent diabetes mellitus. *N Engl J Med* 1988;318:140–145.
76. Barzilay J, Warram JH, Bak M, et al. Predisposition to hypertension: risk factor for nephropathy and hypertension in IDDM. *Kidney Int* 1992;41:723–730.
77. Fagerudd JA, Tarnow L, Jacobsen P, et al. Predisposition to essential hypertension and development of diabetic nephropathy in IDDM patients. *Diabetes* 1998;47:439–444.
78. Sawicki PT, Didjurgeit U, Muhllhauser I, et al. Smoking is associated with progression of diabetic nephropathy. *Diabetes Care* 1994;17:126–131.
79. Seaquist ER, Goetz FC, Rich S, et al. Familial clustering of diabetic kidney disease: evidence for genetic susceptibility to diabetic nephropathy. *N Engl J Med* 1989;320:1161–1165.
80. Borch-Johnsen K, Norgaard K, Hommel E, et al. Is diabetic nephropathy an inherited complication? *Kidney Int* 1992;41:719–722.
81. Quinn M, Angelico MC, Warram JH, et al. Familial factors determine the development of diabetic nephropathy in patients with IDDM. *Diabetologia* 1996;39:940–945.
82. The Diabetes Control and Complications Research Group. Clustering of long-term complications in families with diabetes in the Diabetes Control and Complication Trial. *Diabetes* 1997;46:1829–1839.
83. Krolewski AS. Genetics of diabetic nephropathy: evidence for major and minor gene effects. *Kidney Int* 1999;55:1582–1596.
84. Ballard DJ, Humphrey LL, Melton LJ, et al. Epidemiology of persistent proteinuria in type II diabetes mellitus. Population-based study in Rochester, Minnesota. *Diabetes* 1988;37:405–412.
85. Larson TS, Santanello N, Shahinfar S, et al. Trends in persistent proteinuria in adult-onset diabetes. *Diabetes Care* 2000;23:51–56.
86. Klein R, Klein BEK, Moss SC. Incidence of gross proteinuria in older-onset diabetes: a population-based perspective. *Diabetes* 1993;42:381–389.
87. Nosadini R, Solini A, Velussi M, et al. Impaired insulin-induced glucose uptake by extrahepatic tissue is hallmark of NIDDM patients who have or will develop hypertension and microalbuminuria. *Diabetes* 1994;43: 491–499.
88. Nelson RG, Pettitt DJ, Baird HR, et al. Pre-diabetic blood pressure predicts urinary albumin excretion after the onset of type 2 (non-insulin-dependent) diabetes mellitus in Pima Indians. *Diabetologia* 1993;36:998–1001.
89. Faronato P, Maioli M, Tonolo G, et al. Clustering of albumin excretion rate abnormalities in Caucasian patients with NIDDM. *Diabetologia* 1997;40: 816–823.
90. Canani LH, Gerchman F, Gross JL. Familial clustering of diabetic nephropathy in Brazilian type 2 diabetic patients. *Diabetes* 1999;48:909–913.
91. Fogarty D, Rich SS, Hanna L, et al. Urinary albumin excretion in families with type 2 diabetes is heritable and genetically correlated with blood pressure. *Kidney Int* 2000;57:250–257.
92. Fogarty D, Hanna LS, Wantman M, et al. Segregation analysis of urinary albumin excretion in families with type 2 diabetes. *Diabetes* 2000;49:1057– 1063.
93. Pettitt DJ, Saad MF, Bennett PH, et al. Familial predisposition to renal disease in two generations of Pima Indians with type II (non-insulin-dependent) diabetes mellitus. *Diabetologia* 1990;33:438–443.
94. Imperatore G, Knowler WC, Pettitt DJ, et al. Segregation analysis of diabetic nephropathy in Pima Indians. *Diabetes* 2000;49:1049–1056.
95. Freedman BI, Tuttle AB, Spray BJ. Familial predisposition to nephropathy in African Americans with non-insulin-dependent diabetes mellitus. *Am J Kidney Dis* 1995;25:710–713.
96. Neil A, Hawkins M, Potok M, et al. A prospective population-based study of microalbuminuria as a predictor of mortality in NIDDM. *Diabetes Care* 1993; 16:996–1003.
97 Stephenson JM, Kenny S, Stevens LK, et al. and the WHO Multinational Study Group. Proteinuria and mortality in diabetes: the WHO Multinational Study of Vascular Disease in Diabetes. *Diabet Med* 1995;12:149–155.
98. Nelson RG, Pettitt DJ, Carraher MJ, et al. Effect of proteinuria on mortality in NIDDM. *Diabetes* 1988;1499–1504.
99. Allawi J, Rao PV, Gilbert R, et al. Microalbuminuria in non-insulin-dependent diabetes: its prevalence in Indian compared with Europid patients. *BMJ* 1988;296:462–464.
100. Nelson RG, Kunzelman CL, Pettitt DJ, et al. Albuminuria in type 2 (non-insulin-dependent) diabetes mellitus and impaired glucose tolerance in Pima Indians. *Diabetologia* 1989;32:870–876.
101. Cowie CC. Diabetic renal disease: racial and ethnic differences from an epidemiologic perspective. *Transplant Proc* 1993;25:2426–2430.
102. Pugh JA, Stern MP, Haffner SM, et al. Excess incidence of treatment of end-stage renal disease in Mexican Americans. *Am J Epidemiol* 1988;127:135–144.
103. Cowie CC, Port FK, Wolfe RA, et al. Disparities in the incidence of diabetic end-stage renal disease according to race and type of diabetes. *N Engl J Med* 1989;231:1074–1090.
104. Lee ET, Lee VS, Lu M, et al. Incidence of renal failure in NIDDM. The Oklahoma Indian diabetes study. *Diabetes* 1994;43:572–579.
105. Brancati FL, Whittle JC, Whelton PK, et al. The excess incidence of diabetic end-stage renal disease among blacks. *JAMA* 1992;268:3079–3084.
106. Kofoed-Enevoldsen A, Borch-Johnsen K, Kreiner S, et al. Declining incidence of persistent proteinuria in type I (insulin-dependent) diabetic patients in Denmark. *Diabetes* 1987;36:647–655.
107. Sawicki PT, Muhlhauser I, Didjurgeit U, et al. Effects of intensification of antihypertensive care in diabetic nephropathy. *J Diabetes Complications* 1995;9: 315–317.

108. Parving HH, Jacobsen P, Rossing K, et al. Benefits of long-term antihypertensive treatment on prognosis in diabetic nephropathy. *Kidney Int* 1996;49: 1778–1782.
109. Centers for Disease Control and Prevention. Diabetes surveillance 1999. Atlanta: U.S. Department of Health and Human Services, 1999.
110. Harris MI. Health care and health status and outcomes for patients with type 2 diabetes. *Diabetes Care* 2000;23:754–758.
111. Viberti GC, Mogensen CE, Groop LC, et al. for the European Microalbuminuria Captopril Study Group. Effect of captopril on progression to clinical proteinuria in patients with insulin-dependent diabetes mellitus and microalbuminuria. *JAMA* 1994;271:275–279.
112. Laffel LMB, McGill JB, Gans DJ, on behalf of the North American Microalbuminuria Study Group. The beneficial effect of angiotensin-converting enzyme inhibition with captopril on diabetic nephropathy in normotensive IDDM patients with microalbuminuria. *Am J Med* 1995;99:497–504.
113. Lewis EJ, Hunsicker LG, Bain RP, et al. for the Collaborative Study Group. The effect of angiotensin-converting enzyme inhibition on diabetic nephropathy. *N Engl J Med* 1993;329:1456–1462.
114. Ritz E, Rychlik I, Locatelli F, et al. End-stage renal failure in type 2 diabetes: a medical catastrophe of worldwide dimensions. *Am J Kidney Dis* 1999;34: 795–808.
115. Jarrett RI, Shipley MJ. Mortality and associated risk factors in diabetics. *Acta Endocrinol* 1985;110[Suppl 272]:21–26.
116. Stamler J, Vaccaro O, Neaton JD, et al. Diabetes, other risk factors, and 12-yr cardiovascular mortality for men screened in the multiple risk factor intervention trial. *Diabetes Care* 1993;16:434–444.
117. Krolewski AS, Kosinski EJ, Warram JH, et al. Magnitude and determinants of coronary artery disease in juvenile-onset, insulin-dependent diabetes mellitus. *Am J Cardiol* 1987;59:750–755.
118. Stary HC. Evolution and progression of atherosclerotic lesions in coronary arteries of children and young adults. *Arteriosclerosis* 1989;9[Suppl I]:I19–I32.
119. Krolewski AS, Warram JH, Valsania P, et al. Evolving natural history of coronary artery disease in diabetes mellitus. *Am J Med* 1991;90[Suppl 2A]: 56S–61S.
120. Kleinman JC, Donahue RP, Harris MI, et al. Mortality among diabetics in a national sample. *Am J Epidemiol* 1988;2:389–401.
121. Jarrett RJ, Shipley MJ. Type 2 (non-insulin-dependent) diabetes mellitus and cardiovascular disease—putative association via common antecedents; further evidence from the Whitehall Study. *Diabetologia* 1988;31:737–740.
122. Manson JE, Colditz GA, Stampfer MJ, et al. A prospective study of maturity-onset diabetes mellitus and risk of coronary heart disease and stroke in women. *Arch Intern Med* 1991;151:1141–1147.
123. Fontbonne A, Thibult N, Eschwege E, et al. Body fat distribution and coronary heart disease mortality in subjects with impaired glucose tolerance or diabetes mellitus: the Paris Prospective Study, 15-year follow-up. *Diabetologia* 1992;35:464–468.
124. Walter SD, Holford TR. Additive, multiplicative, and other models for disease risks. *Am J Epidemiol* 1978;108; 341–346.
125. Rothman KJ. Occam's razor pares the choice among statistical models. *Am J Epidemiol* 1978;108:347–349.
126. Silberberg JS. Estimating the benefits of cholesterol lowering: are risk factors for coronary heart disease multiplicative? *J Clin Epidemiol* 1990;43:875–879.
127. Jarrett RJ. Mortality in diabetes. *Q J Med* 1990;76:413–414.
128. Psaty BM, Koepsell TD, Manolio TA, et al. Risk ratios and risk differences in estimating the effect of risk factors for cardiovascular disease in the elderly. *J Clin Epidemiol* 1990;43:961–970.
129. Moss SE, Klein R, Klein BEK, et al. The association of glycemia and cause-specific mortality in a diabetic population. *Arch Intern Med* 1994;154:2473– 2479.
130. Rossing P, Hougaard P, Borch-Johnsen K, et al. Predictors of mortality in insulin dependent diabetes: 10-year observational follow-up study. *BMJ* 1996; 313:779–784.
131. The Diabetes Control and Complications Trial (DCCT) Research Group. Effect of intensive diabetes management on macrovascular events and risk factors in the Diabetes Control and Complications Trial. *Am J Cardiol* 1995;75: 894–903.
132. Kuusisto J, Mykkanen L, Pyorala K, et al. NIDDM and its metabolic control predict coronary heart disease in elderly subjects. *Diabetes* 1994;43:960–967.
133. Vander Zwaag R, Runyan JW, Davidson JK, et al. A cohort study of mortality in two clinic populations of patients with diabetes mellitus. *Diabetes Care* 1983;6:341–346.
134. Hillson RM, Hockaday TDR, Mann JI, et al. Hyperinsulinemia is associated with development of electrocardiographic abnormalities in diabetics. *Diabetes Res* 1984;1:143–149.
135. Janka HU, Ziegler AG, Standl E, et al. Daily insulin dose as a predictor of macrovascular disease in insulin treated non-insulin-dependent diabetics. *Diabetes Metab* 1987;13:359–364.
136. Ronnemaa T, Laakso M, Puukka P, et al. Atherosclerotic vascular disease in middle-aged, insulin-treated, diabetic patients: association with endogenous insulin secretion capacity. *Atherosclerosis* 1988;8:237–244.
137. Liu QZ, Knowler WC, Nelson RG, et al. Insulin treatment, endogenous insulin concentration, and ECG abnormalities in diabetic Pima Indians. Cross-sectional and prospective analyses. *Diabetes* 1992;41:1141–1150.
138. Stout RW. Insulin and atheroma: 20-yr perspective. *Diabetes Care* 1990;13: 631–654.
139. Welborn TA, Wearne K. Coronary heart disease incidence and cardiovascular mortality in Busselton with reference to glucose and insulin concentrations. *Diabetes Care* 1979;2:154–160.
140. Eschwege E, Richard JL, Thibult N, et al. Coronary heart disease mortality in relation with diabetes, blood glucose and plasma insulin levels: The Paris Prospective Study, ten years later. *Horm Metab Res* 1985;15[Suppl]: S41–S46.
141. Yarnel JWG, Sweetnam PM, Marks V, et al. Insulin in ischaemic heart disease: are associations explained by triglyceride concentration? The Caerphilly prospective study. *Br Heart J* 1994;71:293–296.
142. Jarrett RJ. Why is insulin not a risk factor for coronary heart disease? *Diabetologia* 1994;37:945–947.
143. Reaven GM, Laws A. Insulin resistance, compensatory hyperinsulinemia, and coronary heart disease. *Diabetologia* 1994;37:948–952.
144. Fontbonne A. Why can high insulin levels indicate a risk for coronary heart disease? *Diabetologia* 1994;37:953–955.
145. Stern MP. The insulin resistance syndrome: the controversy is dead, long live the controversy! *Diabetologia* 1994;37:956–958.
146. Adler AI, Neil AW, Manley SE, et al. Hyperglycemia and hyperinsulinemia at diagnosis of diabetes and their association with subsequent cardiovascular disease in the United Kingdom Prospective Diabetes Study (UKPDS 47). *Am Heart J* 1999;138:S353–S359.
147. Knatterud GL, Klimt CR, Levin ME, et al. Effects of hypoglycemic agents on vascular complications in patients with adult-onset diabetes. VII. Mortality and selected nonfatal events with insulin treatment. *JAMA* 1978; 240:37–42.
148. Haffner SM, Stern MP, Hazuda HP, et al. Cardiovascular risk factors in confirmed prediabetic individuals. Does the clock for coronary heart disease start ticking before the onset of clinical diabetes? *JAMA* 1990;263:2893–2898.
149. Martin BC, Warram JH, Krolewski AS, et al. Role of glucose and insulin resistance in development of type 2 diabetes mellitus: results of 25-year follow-up study. *Lancet* 1992;340:925–929.
150. Howard G, O'Leary DH, Zaccaro D, et al. Insulin sensitivity and atherosclerosis. The Insulin Resistance Atherosclerosis Study (IRAS) Investigators. *Circulation* 1996;93:1809–1817.
151. Borch-Johnsen K, Kreiner S. Proteinuria: value as predictor of cardiovascular mortality in insulin dependent diabetes mellitus. *BMJ* 1987;294:1651–1654.
152. Stephenson JM, Kenny S, Stevens LK, et al. Proteinuria and mortality in diabetes: the WHO multinational study of vascular disease in diabetes. *Diabet Med* 1995;12:149–155.
153. Gall MA, Borch-Johnsen K, Hougaard P, et al. Albuminuria and poor glycemic control predict mortality in NIDDM. *Diabetes* 1995;44:1303–1309.
154. Valmadrid CT, Klein R, Moss SE, et al. The risk of cardiovascular disease mortality associated with microalbuminuria and gross proteinuria in persons with older-onset diabetes mellitus. *Arch Intern Med* 2000;160:1093–1100.
155. Earle K, Walker J, Hill C, et al. Familial clustering of cardiovascular disease in patients with insulin-dependent diabetes and nephropathy. *N Engl J Med* 1992;326:673–677.
156. Lahdenpera S, Groop PH, Tilly-Kiesi M, et al. LDL subclasses in IDDM patients: relation to diabetic nephropathy. *Diabetologia* 1994;37:681–688.
157. Warram JH, Laffel LMB, Ganda OP, et al. Coronary artery disease is the major determinant of excess mortality in patients with insulin-dependent diabetes mellitus and persistent proteinuria. *J Am Soc Nephrol* 1992;3[Suppl]:S104–S110.
158. Krolewski AS, Warram JH, Christlieb AR. Hypercholesterolemia—a determinant of renal function loss and deaths in IDDM patients with nephropathy. *Kidney Int* 1994;45[Suppl 45]:S125–S131.
159. Makita Z, Radoff S, Rayfield EJ, et al. Advanced glycosylation end products in patients with diabetic nephropathy. *N Engl J Med* 1991;325:836–842.
160. Schwartz CJ, Kelley JL, Valente AJ, et al. Pathogenesis of the atherosclerotic lesion. Implications for diabetes mellitus. *Diabetes Care* 1992;15:1156–1167.
161. Diabetes Drafting Group. Prevalence of small vessel and large vessel disease in diabetic patients from 14 centres. The World Health Organisation Multinational Study of Vascular Disease in Diabetics. *Diabetologia* 1985;28[Suppl]: 615–640.
162. Head J, Fuller JH. International variation in mortality among diabetic patients. The WHO multinational study of vascular disease in diabetics. *Diabetologia* 1990;33:477–481.
163. Nelson RG, Sievers ML, Knowler WC, et al. Low incidence of fatal coronary heart disease in Pima Indians despite high prevalence of non-insulin-dependent diabetes. *Circulation* 1990;81:987–995.
164. Matsumoto T, Ohashi Y, Yamada N, et al. Coronary heart disease mortality is actually low in diabetic Japanese by direct comparison with the Joslin cohort. *Diabetes Care* 1994;17:1062–1063.
165. Stamler J. The marked decline in coronary heart disease mortality rates in the United States, 1968–81. *Cardiology* 1985;72:11–22.
166. Gillum RF. Trends in acute myocardial infarction and coronary heart disease death in the United States. *J Am Coll Cardiol* 1994;23:1273–1277.
167. McGovern PG, Pankow JS, Shahar E, et al. Recent trends in acute coronary heart disease. Mortality, morbidity, medical care and risk factors. *N Engl J Med* 1996;334:884–890.
168. Hunink MG, Goldman L, Tosteson ANA, et al. The recent decline in mortality from coronary heart disease, 1980–1990. The effect of secular trends in risk factors and treatment. *JAMA* 1997;277:535–542.
169. Rosamond WD, Chambless LE, Folsom AR, et al. Trends in the incidence of myocardial infarction and in mortality due to coronary heart disease, 1987–1994. *N Engl J Med* 1998;339:861–867.
170. Gu K, Cowie CC, Harris MI. Diabetes and decline in heart disease mortality in US adults. *JAMA* 1999;281:1291–1297.

CHAPTER 48

Relationship between Metabolic Control and Long-Term Complications of Diabetes

David M. Nathan

For what a man had rather were true, he more readily believes.

—Roger Bacon, 1450

The relationship between metabolic control and development of long-term complications of diabetes mellitus was one of the most contentious issues in medicine (1–5). Whether intensive forms of diabetes therapy, which have as their goal the achievement of near-normal glycemia, would prevent the development and/or ameliorate the progression of diabetes-associated complications (the only testable question in humans) was answered only in the previous decade. This chapter reviews the history of the debate and the human studies that shed light on this relationship. The important clinical trials that finally resolved the debate, including the Diabetes Control and Complications Trial and the United Kingdom Prospective Diabetes Study, are reviewed in detail (6,7).

HISTORY

Although the recognition of diabetes mellitus itself has a venerable history (8), the recognition and description of diabetic complications is relatively new. The first description of retinopathy in diabetes was recorded only 100 years ago (9), and both the occurrence and character of retinal lesions in relation to diabetes were the subject of active debate as recently as 60 years ago (10). The classic lesions of diabetic glomerulosclerosis were described less than 70 years ago (11).

The major reason for the previous lack of clinical appreciation of diabetic complications is related to their dependence on duration of diabetes, the most potent known risk factor for complications (12–18). In the preinsulin era, the limited life span of patients after they developed type 1 diabetes precluded the development of long-term complications. Eight years after the introduction of insulin, diabetic children were described as having "invulnerable" eyes and a future of "limitless hope" (19). Twenty years after insulin became available, however, the results of long-term survival with insulin therapy were noted to include retinopathy, nephropathy, and peripheral and cardiovascular disease (20–22). In a prescient set of observations made more than 50 years ago, Dolger noted that duration of diabetes appeared to be more important than age at onset or type of therapy; that all patients whose diabetes was of sufficient duration developed retinal lesions; that approximately 50% developed proteinuria; and that complications developed in patients whose long-term metabolic control was judged to be good as well as in those whose metabolic control was poor (22). On the other hand, retrospective studies suggested that children with "adequately" controlled diabetes were not vulnerable to growth retardation, cataracts, or retinal hemorrhages (23). Thus, the debate regarding the effects of metabolic control on long-term complications was born.

The history of type 2 diabetes and long-term complications is even murkier. Until the recent extension of the human life span and accompanying increase in the prevalence of obesity led to a dramatic increase in the prevalence of type 2 diabetes (24), type 2 diabetes was a relatively rare disease. Moreover, elderly patients with type 2 diabetes rarely survived the 10 to 20 years after onset of diabetes that are necessary for the development of clinically significant complications. Major advances in general medical care, and especially in cardiac care, now have allowed older patients with type 2 diabetes to live longer. This increased life expectancy has unmasked the risks of long-term complications in type 2 diabetes, much as insulin therapy did for type 1 diabetes. Type 2 diabetes is now widely recognized as a cause of duration-dependent complications similar to those in type 1 diabetes (14,16,25–27). Although the frequency of retinopathy and nephropathy is relatively lower in type 2 than in type 1 diabetes, the 10-fold-greater prevalence of type 2 diabetes makes it the major contributor to vision loss and renal failure secondary to diabetes in the United States (26,28). The association of type 2 diabetes and elevated levels of blood glucose with microvascular complications has been recognized implicitly in the definition of blood glucose criteria for the diagnosis of type 2 diabetes, which are predicated on those glucose levels that are accompanied by microvascular complications (29).

MAJOR ISSUES

Several major questions should be framed before a critical examination of the data are undertaken. The occurrence of retinopathy, nephropathy, and neuropathy as long-term, diabetes-specific complications of all types of diabetes is clear. As noted previously, the diagnostic criteria for type 2 diabetes include glucose levels selected specifically because of the risk they impart for development of long-term complications, specifically retinopathy. (The profound hyperglycemia and absolute requirement for insulin in type 1 diabetes make diagnostic glucose criteria generally unnecessary.) Persons whose glucose levels are elevated but who are not vulnerable to diabetes-specific complications are not considered diabetic but are described nosologically as having impaired glucose tolerance or impaired fasting glucose ("pre-diabetes") (29). Thus, the association of hyperglycemia with certain long-term complications is incorporated into the clinical definition of diabetes, and a glucose threshold for the development of specific complications is implicit in the accepted definition of type 2 diabetes.

The glucose hypothesis, that is, that the long-term complications of diabetes are a consequence of hyperglycemia, is a natural, albeit potentially fallacious, outgrowth of these observations. Although diabetes of diverse etiologies is defined as being related to both hyperglycemia and long-term complications, the conclusion that one leads to the other, although attractive, is not necessarily true. A primary question, therefore, is what relationship exists between the level of hyperglycemia and the occurrence or development of complications.

Even if the relationship between different levels of hyperglycemia and complications is established and delineated, association does not necessarily impute causation. More important, even if hyperglycemia results in the development or progression of complications, the practical questions of whether control of glucose levels will prevent or reverse complications, the extent and duration of the effect, and the costs of such control must be answered.

Important subsidiary questions include the following: (a) Will all diabetes-specific complications respond similarly to changes in glucose level? (b) Is the timing of intervention important, that is, is treatment effective only if instituted before the development of any complications (primary prevention) or is it also effective after the development of complications (secondary intervention)? (c) Does maintenance of a specific glucose level prevent or ameliorate any or all complications? (d) Will different methods (e.g., exogenous administration of insulin vs. pancreatic transplantation) of achieving more normal glycemia have similar effects on complications? (e) Will long-term complications in type 1 and type 2 diabetes respond similarly to therapy? (f) Will nonspecific macrovascular complications, the severity and frequency of which are increased in diabetes, be affected by therapies directed at achieving glucose levels closer to physiologic values?

STUDIES IN ANIMAL MODELS AND OBSERVATIONAL STUDIES IN HUMAN DIABETES

Retinopathy

ANIMAL STUDIES

Although none of the animal models of diabetes and its complications are sufficiently similar to human diabetes to provide more than suggestive evidence, they overwhelmingly support the premise that therapies that normalize blood glucose levels can prevent and/or ameliorate retinopathy, nephropathy, and neuropathy. The animal models fall into three different groups. In one model, animals with chemically induced (with alloxan or streptozotocin) diabetes are treated with insulin with the goal of achieving either tight or loose control of blood glucose levels (30,31). In another model, animals are pancreatectomized and treated with pancreatic or isolated islet cell transplantation (32,33). Finally, animals with genetic diabetes and various degrees of glycemia have been studied (34). Most studies have demonstrated efficacy of intensive therapy aimed at maintaining glucose levels close to the physiologic range in preventing complications. The ability of intensive diabetes therapy to affect complications once they have been initiated is arguable.

Studies by Engerman et al. of dogs with alloxan-induced diabetes are the most compelling of the animal studies (30,31). The diabetic dogs developed microaneurysms and pericyte loss similar to those seen in diabetic humans, changes not generally found in nondiabetic dogs. In an early study, therapy with two daily injections of isophane insulin (NPH insulin) with the goal of aglycosuria ("good control") was initiated soon after the dogs were made diabetic (30). Good control was shown to be associated with fewer microaneurysms than was therapy with one daily injection of isophane insulin ("poor control") over a 5-year period. A later study demonstrated that if dogs with alloxan-induced diabetes were treated with the poor-control regimen for 2.5 years followed by the good-control regimen for 2.5 years, they developed an intermediate number of microaneurysms, suggesting that secondary intervention was not as effective as primary prevention (31). Of note, severe hypoglycemia resulted in the deaths of several dogs in "good control."

HUMAN STUDIES

Type 1 Diabetes. Early studies that examined the relationship of retinopathy to glucose control used relatively insensitive measures of retinopathy and nonquantitative, imprecise measures of chronic glycemia. Knowles reviewed 47 studies of glucose control and development of complications conducted before 1964 and concluded that the studies were hampered by the absence of quantitative methods of evaluating long-term glucose control and complications and by a poor appreciation of clinical-trial methodology (35). In the modern era, nondilated ophthalmoscopy has given way to seven-field stereoscopic fundus photography and fluorescein angiography, and sporadic blood glucose measurements and semiquantitative measures of glycosuria have been supplanted by assays of glycosylated hemoglobin (HbA_{1c}).

Although lacking in these modern innovations, the noninterventional, longitudinal study of Pirart deserves mention, if only for its magnitude (36). Pirart followed a large (4,400) cohort of patients with early- and late-onset diabetes for as long as 25 years. He noted that retinopathy, nephropathy, and neuropathy were more common in patients with a higher glycemic index, a value derived from intermittent measurements of blood and urine glucose levels and other factors. The high attrition rate over time, the lack of objective measures of complications and glycemia, and the possibility that complications led to worsened glucose control—rather than vice versa—detract from this study.

In the modern era, the population-based, observational Wisconsin Epidemiologic Study of Diabetic Retinopathy (WESDR) examined diabetic residents of Wisconsin over time using measurements of HbA_{1c} and seven-field stereoscopic fundus photography. Follow-up over 4 years included more than 90% of the original subjects and revealed a striking association between the incidence of any retinopathy, progression of retinopathy, progression to proliferative retinopathy (37), macular edema (38), and vision loss (39) and the level of HbA_{1c} at baseline. The relationship between levels of HbA_{1c} and retinopathy was continuous; no threshold within the diabetic range for HbA_{1c} with regard to risk of retinopathy was noted. The observed associations remained after the comparisons were controlled for duration of diabetes, age, and baseline retinopathy. Although WESDR subjects were not strictly categorized as having type 1 or type 2 diabetes, the separation by age at onset (<30 years vs. ≥30 years) effectively provided populations of subjects with predominantly type 1 or type 2 diabetes. Other observational studies have confirmed these findings in more-selected type 1 populations (40–43) and have suggested that higher glycemic levels are a risk factor for the development of proliferative retinopathy (18,41,43).

Type 2 Diabetes. An association between retinopathy and glycemia similar to that for type 1 diabetes has been demonstrated for type 2 diabetes. Both the WESDR (14) and a study of type 2 diabetes in an aging population (55–75 years old) (16) showed that the relative risk of developing retinopathy increases as the level of HbA_{1c} increases (Fig. 48.1). Putative risk factors for diabetic retinopathy, other than the level of glycemia, include hypertension (44), pregnancy (45), a family history of diabetic retinopathy (46), and possibly hypercholesterolemia (47), but probably not smoking (48).

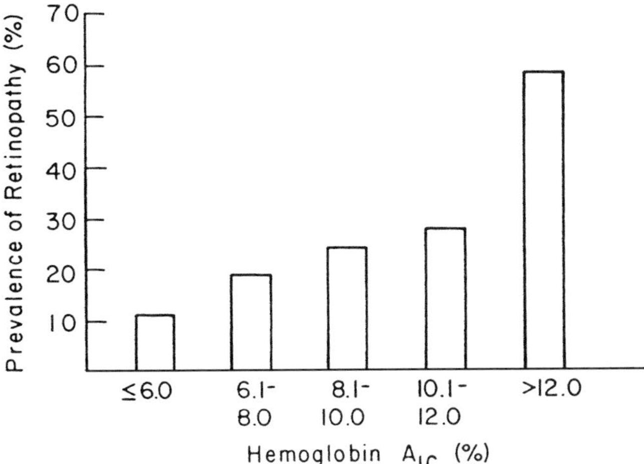

Figure 48.1. Association between mean glucose level as measured by level of glycosylated hemoglobin (HbA_{1c}) and presence of retinopathy in older patients (55 to 75 years) with type 2 diabetes. (Copyright © 1986 American Diabetes Association. From Nathan DM, Singer DE, Godine JE, et al. Retinopathy in older type II diabetics: association with glucose control. *Diabetes* 1986;35:797–801. Reprinted with permission from the American Diabetes Association.)

Nephropathy

ANIMAL STUDIES

Although glomerular lesions in several animal models of diabetes are similar to those seen in diabetic nephropathy in humans, the time course of the development of the lesions is difficult to compare with that in human diabetes. In addition, the contribution of other factors that play important roles in the genesis of human diabetic nephropathy cannot be evaluated in these models. As with retinopathy, studies of nephropathy in animal models can lend support to, but cannot prove, the glucose hypothesis.

Studies in animal models appear to demonstrate that nephropathy can be prevented or even reversed when diabetic animals are treated with pancreatic transplantation or with intensive insulin therapy. Rats with streptozotocin-induced diabetes develop mesangial thickening with immunoglobulin deposition within 6 to 9 months of diabetes onset (32). Successful islet transplantation can prevent the development of such lesions or lead to stabilization and some improvement in established lesions concurrent with normalization of glucose levels (32). Several fundamental problems apply to this model. First, diabetic rats develop a renal lesion (mesangial expansion) that differs from the early lesion of human nephropathy (glomerular basement membrane expansion) and do not develop end-stage renal failure. Second, other potentially important variables that might predict or influence development of nephropathy in humans (e.g., hypertension) cannot be studied in animal models. Third, rats in which transplants of pancreatic islet cells do not succeed in correcting glucose levels also show improvements in renal results (32). Despite these objections, studies in other animal models such as the BB/W (spontaneously diabetic) rat (49) and uninephrectomized, alloxan-treated dog (50) tend to support the role of glucose control in the genesis of nephropathy.

HUMAN STUDIES

Diabetic nephropathy poses several different problems, when compared with retinopathy, regarding the analysis of its association with glucose levels and of the effects of intensive therapy on its development and course. The natural history of diabetic nephropathy, although duration-dependent, extends over many more years than retinopathy before clinical expression becomes evident (51,52). Generally, a minimum of 12 years but usually 15 to 18 years of type 1 diabetes is required before the development of clinical-grade (dipstick-positive, i.e., ≥500 mg per 24 hours) proteinuria, the first incontrovertible sign of developing end-stage renal disease. After the development of clinical-grade proteinuria, a mean of 5 years is required for the decline in creatinine clearance, that terminates in end-stage renal disease, to begin (53). Thus, compared with the time course of diabetic retinopathy, for which signs will appear in 50% of individuals within 5 to 7 years of diabetes onset, the time course for the development of clinical nephropathy (dipstick-positive proteinuria), when it occurs, is much prolonged, requiring a duration of diabetes of approximately 15 years.

With the reluctance to perform kidney biopsies early in the course of diabetes for documentation of microscopic changes in the glomerulus and the less-than-perfect correlation between microscopic changes and clinical course, surrogate markers of evolving nephropathy have tentatively been identified. "Incipient" nephropathy, as demonstrated by microalbuminuria (generally >20–30 mg and <300 mg of urinary albumin per 24 hours), has been identified in retrospective studies of type 1 (54–57) and type 2 (58) diabetes as a predictor or marker for the development of end-stage renal disease. Unfortunately, microalbuminuria can vary considerably in individuals over time, with levels fluctuating from abnormal to normal values. Therefore, a urinary albumin excretion rate of greater than 20 μg per minute (>28 mg per 24 hours) but less than 200 μg per minute (<288 mg per 24 hours) in at least two of three urine collections within a 6-month period has been suggested as a definition of "persistent" microalbuminuria (59). In addition, microalbuminuria may not be a predictor of nephropathy unless hypertension and a decreasing glomerular filtration rate also are present (60). Microalbuminuria can reverse in as many as 58% of affected persons, with lower levels of glycosylated hemoglobin, lower systolic pressure, and lower levels of cholesterol and triglycerides independently associated with regression (61). Finally, most of the data indicating an association between microalbuminuria and nephropathy are retrospective in nature. Whether any intervention that affects this presumed marker for nephropathy also will affect the long-term course of nephropathy has yet to be demonstrated conclusively. Despite these limitations, changes in microalbuminuria have been used as renal endpoints in many controlled trials.

There are several reasons to suspect that the association between glucose control and nephropathy may be more complex than that with retinopathy. The occurrence of nephropathy in no more than 40% of patients with type 1 diabetes and 25% of patients with type 2 diabetes suggests that variables other than glycemia are operant. Hypertension and family history of hypertension (62), smoking (63), and hyperlipidemia (64) have been suggested as possible mediators of nephropathy.

Type 1 Diabetes. The association between levels of glycemia and nephropathy has not been as clearly delineated as that for retinopathy. Although the Pirart study (36) demonstrated an association between the derived glycemic index and an increase in creatinine level over time, cross-sectional or longitudinal studies using objective measurements of glycemia and proteinuria are rare and have not consistently revealed such an association. Only one longitudinal study has demonstrated an association between mean levels of glycosylated hemoglobin, measured over 7 years, and risk of microalbuminuria in type 1 diabetes (65). Although this association persisted when age and duration of diabetes were taken into account, measurements of microalbuminuria at baseline, blood pressure, and other possible confounders were not considered in the analysis.

Potential reasons for the difficulty in establishing a relationship between glycemia and nephropathy, if such a relationship exists, are numerous. First, the development of renal failure may influence glycemic control in a number of ways (e.g., alterations in sensitivity to insulin and development of hypertension and effects of antihypertensive medications on glycemia). Second, uremia, anemia, and transfusions may interfere with or influence the accuracy of measurements of glycosylated hemoglobin. Finally, and most importantly, given the long duration of diabetes necessary before the development of renal failure, it is possible that infrequent measurements of glycosylated hemoglobin, representing a relatively brief period of exposure, may not be predictive of the development of nephropathy. The most convincing data come from the follow-up of long-term clinical trials, such as the DCCT.

Neuropathy

Diabetic neuropathy is protean in nature, with distal, symmetrical, somatosensory neuropathy, autonomic neuropathy, and mononeuropathies. Although electrophysiologic measures of nerve conduction have been available for more than 40 years, their questionable relevance to symptomatic clinical diabetic neuropathy has made the study of glucose control and neuropathy problematic. For example, the early observation that insulin treatment of new-onset type 1 diabetes reversed the slowed motor nerve conduction within 6 weeks in asymptomatic patients supported an acute effect of hyperglycemia on nerve conduction and cast doubt on the role of electrophysiologic testing (66). The absence of histologic data (e.g., sural nerve biopsy) in the vast majority of studies has been a major impediment to our understanding of diabetic neuropathy. A weak association between glycemia and motor and sensory nerve conduction has been documented in type 1 (67) and type 2 (68) diabetes.

CLINICAL TRIALS

Type 1 Diabetes

Although of interest, cross-sectional and longitudinal observational studies can at best only indicate associations between glycemic control (and other confounders) and complications. Randomized, controlled clinical trials examine the effects of treatments designed to achieve near-normal glucose control on the development and progression of complications and can establish causality. The introduction and refinement of methods for self-monitoring of blood glucose levels and of intensive therapies, such as continuous subcutaneous insulin infusion (CSII) with pumps and multiple daily injection (MDI) regimens (69), provided the opportunity to test whether such therapies would have salutary effects. Four well-designed randomized studies (70–73) set the stage for the larger and comprehensive Diabetes Control and Complications Trial (DCCT) (6,74). The first four clinical trials included the multicenter study by the Kroc Collaborative Study Group (70) and studies by the Steno Study Group (71), the Oslo group (72), and the Stockholm Diabetes Intervention Study group (73). All of these trials were secondary intervention studies, including only subjects with retinal lesions at baseline. In addition, the mean duration of diabetes was relatively long. The duration of the trials ranged from 8 to 60 months and included 30 to 100 subjects. (By contrast, the DCCT studied 1,441 subjects with a mean follow-up of 6.5 years.) The total number of patient-years of study was less than 800 in the four previous secondary intervention trials combined. The total number of patient-years for the secondary-intervention component of the DCCT was almost 5,000 at study end in 1993. Except for the Oslo study, which included two intensive-treatment groups, the studies compared subjects with type 1 diabetes randomly assigned to conventional treatment with subjects randomly assigned to CSII (Kroc and Steno) or

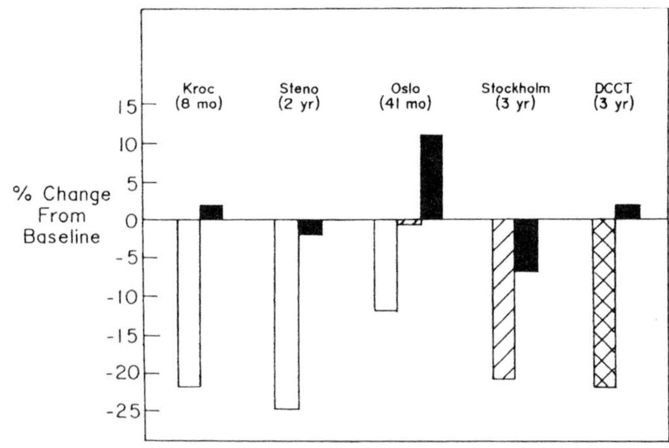

Figure 48.2. Change of glycosylated hemoglobin level from baseline in five controlled clinical trials. *Solid box:* Conventional treatment. *Open box:* Continuous subcutaneous insulin infusion (CSII). *Diagonal:* Multiple daily injections of insulin (MDI). *Hatched:* CSII or MDI. (From Nathan DM. Relationship between metabolic control and long-term complications. In: Kahn DR, Weir GC, eds. *Joslin's diabetes mellitus,* 13th ed. Philadelphia: Lea & Febiger, 1994:620–630. Copyright © 1994 Joslin Diabetes Center.)

MDI (Stockholm). In all the studies the groups receiving intensive treatment maintained significantly lower levels of glycosylated hemoglobin than did those receiving standard treatment (Fig. 48.2). The results of the Kroc (70), Steno (71,75), and Oslo (72,76) studies were similar with regard to retinopathy. In the first 6 to 12 months, a transient worsening of retinopathy occurred in the patients receiving intensive treatment. Only the Stockholm Diabetes Study demonstrated a beneficial effect of intensive therapy over time (73).

DIABETES CONTROL AND COMPLICATIONS TRIAL

In 1993, the DCCT reported the unequivocal salutary effects of intensive diabetes management on the development and progression of the microvascular and neurologic complications of type 1 (insulin-dependent) diabetes (6), ending the 60-year debate regarding the relationship between metabolic control and long-term complications.

Design. The DCCT, initiated in 1983, was designed to answer definitively whether intensive diabetes management would affect the development and/or progression of long-term complications in type 1 diabetes, and at what cost (74). The DCCT provided remarkably clear answers to the following questions: (a) Will intensive therapy aimed at achieving glycemic levels as close to the nondiabetic range as possible prevent the development or slow the progression of complications in patients with type 1 diabetes with no complications at baseline (primary prevention)? (b) Will intensive therapy prevent the progression of complications in patients with type 1 diabetes who already have some evidence of complications at baseline (secondary intervention)? (c) What are the adverse events associated with intensive compared with conventional therapy?

To answer these questions, the DCCT selected two separate cohorts of patients. The primary prevention cohort was 13 to 39 years of age with a duration of diabetes of 1 to 5 years and no evidence of retinopathy or nephropathy. The secondary intervention cohort was of similar age but could have had diabetes for as long as 15 years. They had to have at least one microaneurysm but no more than moderate nonproliferative retinopathy, and they could excrete as much as 200 mg of albumin per 24 hours. The baseline characteristics of the two study cohorts are shown in Table 48.1. Study patients were selected on the basis not only of demographic, clinical, and biochemical cri-

TABLE 48.1. Baseline Characteristics of the Two Study Cohorts of the Diabetic Control and Complications Trial[a]

	Primary prevention		Secondary prevention	
Characteristic	Conventional therapy (n = 378)	Intensive therapy (n = 348)	Conventional therapy (n = 352)	Intensive therapy (n = 363)
Age (y)	26 ± 8	27 ± 7	27 ± 7	27 ± 7
Adolescents, 13–18 y (%)	19	16	9	10
Male sex (%)	54	49	54	53
White race (%)	96	96	97	97
Duration of type 1 diabetes (y)	2.6 ± 1.4	2.6 ± 1.4	8.6 ± 3.7	8.9 ± 3.8
Insulin dose (U/kg of body weight/day)	0.62 ± 0.26	0.62 ± 0.25	0.71 ± 0.24	0.72 ± 0.23
Glycosylated hemoglobin[b] (%)	8.8 ± 1.7	8.8 ± 1.6	8.9 ± 1.5	9.0 ± 1.5
Mean blood glucose[c] (mg/dL)	229 ± 80	234 ± 86	232 ± 78	234 ± 81
Blood pressure (mm Hg)				
Systolic	114 ± 12	112 ± 11	116 ± 12	114 ± 12
Diastolic	72 ± 9	72 ± 9	72 ± 9	72 ± 9
Body weight (% of ideal)	103 ± 14	103 ± 13	105 ± 13	104 ± 12
Current smokers (%)	17	19	19	18
Serum cholesterol (mg/dL)	173 ± 35	176 ± 33	179 ±32	178 ± 33
Serum triglycerides (mg/dL)	77 ± 57	75 ± 41	87 ± 44	87 ± 45
Serum HDL cholesterol (mg/dL)	51 ± 13	52± 13	49 ± 11	49 ± 12
Serum LDL cholesterol (mg/dL)	106 ± 30	109 ± 29	112 ± 28	112 ± 29
Absence of retinopathy (%)	100	100	0	0
Microaneurysms only (%)[d]	0	0	58	67
NPDR(%)[e]				
Mild	0	0	23	18
Moderate	0	0	19	15
Urinary albumin excretion (mg/24 h)	12 ± 8	12 ± 9	19 ± 24	21 ± 25
Creatinine clearance (mL/min)	127 ± 28	128 ± 30	130 ± 30	128 ± 31
Clinical neuropathy (%)[f]	2.1	4.9	9.4	9.4

[a] ± values are means ± SD. To convert values for glucose to millimoles per liter, multiply by 0.05551. To convert values for triglycerides to millimoles per liter, multiple by 0.01129. To convert values for cholesterol, low-density lipoprotein (LDL) cholesterol, and high-density lipoprotein (HDL) cholesterol to millimoles per liter, multiply by 0.02586.

[b] Mean value in nondiabetic persons, 5.05 ± 0.5%.

[c] Based on the mean value of seven determinations during a 24-hour period.

[d] $p = 0.01$ by the Wilcoxon rank-sum test for the difference in the level of retinopathy at baseline between the treatment groups in the secondary intervention trial.

[e] NPDR, nonproliferative diabetic retinopathy. Mild NPDR was defined by the presence of microaneurysms plus mild-to-moderate retinal hemorrhages or hard exudates. Moderate NPDR was defined by the presence of microaneurysms plus any of the following: cotton-wool spots, mild intraretinal microvascular abnormalities or venous beading, or severe retinal hemorrhages.

[f] Defined as a peripheral sensorimotor neuropathy on physical examination by the study neurologist plus either abnormal nerve conduction in two different peripheral nerves or unequivocally abnormal autonomic test results. $P = 0.04$ for the difference between groups in the primary prevention cohort with respect to the baseline prevalence of clinical neuropathy.

TABLE 48.2. Intensive Therapy in the Diabetes Control and Complications Trial

Self-monitoring of blood glucose	≥4 times/day (premeals and prebed) 3 a.m. once/wk for safety (>65 mg/dL) Add postmeal tests if HbA_{1c} goals not met
Glycosylated hemoglobin	HbA_{1c} every 3 mo
Insulin	3 or more injections/day or CSII with external pump Doses adjusted based on ambient glucose (self-monitoring of blood glucose), meal size and content, and anticipated exercise
Supervision	Monthly visits and frequent phone calls Staff included diabetologist, nurse educator, and dietitian

CSII, continuous subcutaneous insulin infusion.

teria but also of an assessment that they would accept random assignment of therapy and of the likelihood that they would continue to participate in a long-term study. On average, these patients were probably more motivated than the usual patient with type 1 diabetes.

DCCT Intensive Treatment and Metabolic Goals. The primary prevention and secondary intervention cohorts were randomly assigned either to conventional therapy (designed to mimic the usual diabetes therapy with one or two daily injections of insulin and daily glucose monitoring) or to intensive therapy (designed to normalize blood glucose control). Conventional therapy had the clinical goals of avoiding any symptoms of hyper- or hypoglycemia but had no specific numeric blood glucose targets. Intensive therapy had the goal of achieving blood glucose control as close to the nondiabetic range as possible, including premeal blood glucose levels between 70 and 120 mg/dL (3.9 to 6.7 mmol/L), peak postprandial levels under 180 mg/dL (10 mmol/L), and HbA_{1c} levels in the nondiabetic range (<6.05%). To reach these goals, patients assigned to intensive therapy used three or more insulin injections per day or insulin pump therapy, guided by frequent self-monitoring of blood glucose levels (Table 48.2). Insulin therapy was adjusted frequently in response to ambient blood glucose levels, diet, and exercise.

DCCT Results. The detailed results of intensive compared with conventional therapy in the DCCT have been reported (6,77–94). The initial report (6) summarized the major results, whereas subsequent reports presented expanded analyses of the effects of intensive therapy on long-term complications, including retinopathy (77–79), nephropathy (80), neuropathy (81–83), and macrovascular disease and its risk factors (84); the effect of intensive therapy on quality of life (85), neurobehavioral outcome (86), and residual insulin secretion (87); the implementation (88) and adverse effects of intensive therapy (89,90); the cost-benefit analysis of intensive therapy compared with conventional therapy (91); the results of intensive therapy in pregnancy (92); and the association among glycemia, long-term complications, and other risk factors (93,94). A long-term follow-up study of the DCCT cohort, the Epidemiology of Diabetes Interventions and Complications (EDIC) study, is under way and is providing further insight into the long-term consequences of intensive therapy (95–99)

Adherence and Metabolic Results. Over the 6.5-year mean follow-up time of the study (range, 3 to 9 years), compliance was excellent, with 99% of the cohort completing the trial (6). In addition, there was virtually no crossover between assigned treatments. Subjects adhered to their assigned treatment more than 97% of the study time. Intensive therapy decreased HbA_{1c} to a nadir of approximately 6.9% by 6 months and maintained a mean HbA_{1c} level during the remainder of the trial that was approximately 2% lower than with conventional treatment (7.2% vs. 9.1%) (Fig. 48.3). Of note, intensive therapy did not lower mean HbA_{1c} to the nondiabetic range.

Retinopathy. Retinopathy was evaluated every 6 months by seven-field stereoscopic fundus photography. The photographs were graded in a central facility, with the graders masked to patient identity. Although many analytic levels of retinopathy were assessed, the principal outcome in the primary prevention study was the development of a sustained (seen on two consecutive exams) three-step or greater progression on a retinopathy severity scale adopted from the Early Treatment of Diabetic Retinopathy Study (ETDRS) (100). Similarly, the principal outcome in the secondary intervention study was a sustained progression of three or more steps from the baseline level. Intensive therapy reduced the development of these end points by 76% in the primary prevention study and by 54% in the secondary intervention study compared with conventional therapy (Fig. 48.4). Other retinopathy outcomes and the effects of intensive therapy are shown in Table 48.3.

The overall effect of intensive therapy was to decrease all stages of retinopathy included in the DCCT. However, intensive therapy was relatively more effective when initiated early in the course of diabetes (shorter vs. longer duration) and when retinopathy was less severe at baseline (77,78). Although intensive therapy reduced the risk for more advanced stages of retinopathy somewhat less than for earlier stages, patients with more advanced retinopathy still benefited from intensive therapy. The beneficial effects of intensive therapy were not seen for the first 3 years of therapy, presumably because of the natural "momentum" of diabetic complications. In addition, intensive therapy was associated with a transient worsening of retinopathy during the first year of therapy. Both of these factors conspired to delay the beneficial effects of intensive therapy, which were similar in almost all subgroups of patients defined by age, gender, and other baseline characteristics.

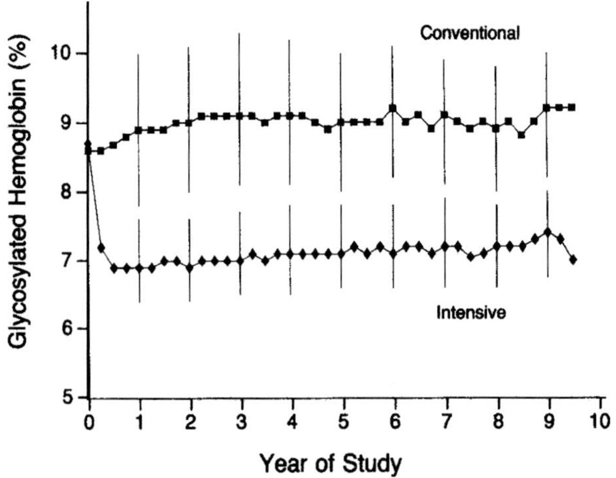

Figure 48.3. Median levels of glycosylated hemoglobin A_{1c} during the Diabetes Control and Complications Trial. (From DCCT Research Group. The effect of intensive treatment of diabetes on the development and progression of long-term complications in insulin-dependent diabetes mellitus. *N Engl J Med* 1993;329:977–986, with permission. Copyright © 1993 Massachusetts Medical Society. All rights reserved.)

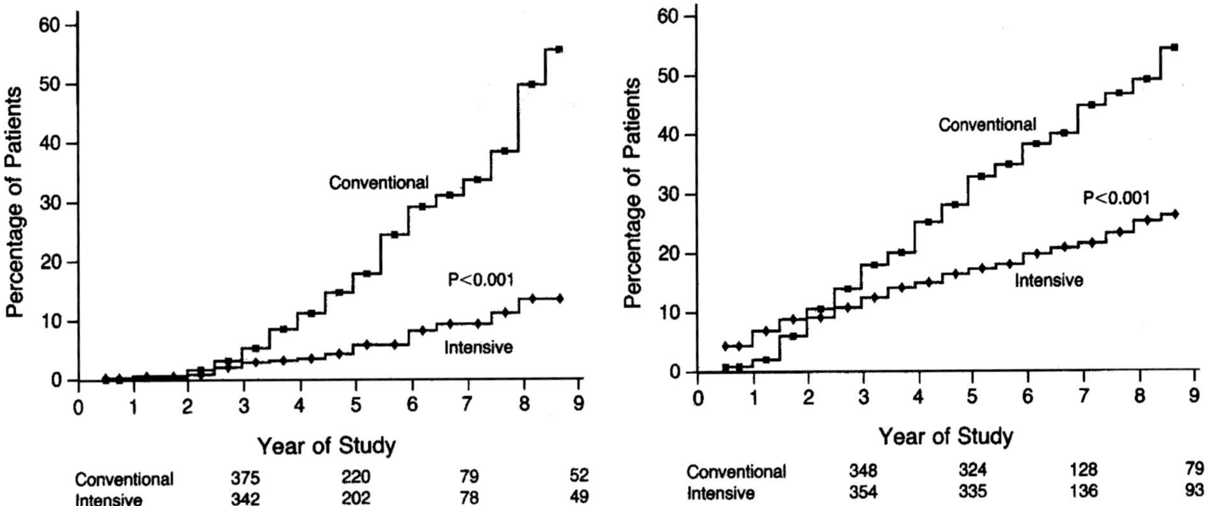

Figure 48.4. Effects of intensive therapy on development **(A)** and progression **(B)** of retinopathy in the Diabetes Control and Complications Trial. (From DCCT Research Group. The effect of intensive treatment of diabetes on the development and progression of long-term complications in insulin-dependent diabetes mellitus. *N Engl J Med* 1993;329:977–986, with permission. Copyright © 1993 Massachusetts Medical Society. All rights reserved.)

The EDIC follow-up has shown further improvement in retinal status in the previous intensive treatment group compared with the previous conventional treatment group (Table 48.3). The difference between the two treatment groups persists, and even expands, 7 years after the end of the DCCT, even though the majority of the previous conventional treatment cohort has changed to intensive therapy and the mean HbA_{1c} levels have drifted closer between the two treatment groups (96,97). The persistent benefit of 6.5 years of intensive therapy during the DCCT further supports the concept of "momentum" with regard to diabetic complications. In addition, the beneficial effects of lower glycemia appear to persist beyond the period of lower glycemia that has been called "imprinting" or "metabolic memory."

The study of families of DCCT volunteers in which there is more than one person with diabetes has revealed clustering of retinopathy within families (101). The tendency for some families with diabetes to develop retinopathy whereas other families do not may be mediated by genetic factors or by some as yet to be identified shared environmental factor. It is interesting that regardless of the cause of clustering, intensive therapy decreased the development and progression of retinopathy in DCCT volunteers who were members of "high-risk" families as well as in DCCT volunteers in low-risk families.

TABLE 48.3 Results of the Diabetes Control and Complications Trial (DCCT) and the Epidemiology of Diabetes Interventions and Complications (EDIC) Study

	Risk reduction with intensive compared with conventional therapy (%)	
Complication	**During DCCT (6.5-y follow-up)**	**During EDIC (4.5-y follow-up after end of DCCT[a])**
Retinopathy		
3-step progression	76	77
Proliferative	64	76
Macular edema	46	72
Laser therapy	56	71
Nephropathy		
Microalbuminuria	35	53
Albuminuria		
≥300 mg/24 h	56	87
Neuropathy	60	

[a]Adjusted for presence of complication at end of DCCT.

Nephropathy. Nephropathy was assessed by measurements of albumin excretion and standard creatinine clearance, based on an annual standardized 4-hour collection and by periodic measurement of iothalamate clearance. The primary analytic end points for nephropathy are shown in Table 48.3 and Figure 48.5. As with retinopathy, the risk for progression of nephropathy was reduced by intensive therapy. This included reduction in the development of microalbuminuria (≥40 mg per 24 hours) and clinical-grade albuminuria (>300 mg per 24 hours). The small number of patients developing clinical nephropathy, defined as a creatinine clearance of less than 70 mL per minute per 1.73 m^2 with albumin excretion greater than 300 mg every 24 hours, precluded a statistically valid analysis of any difference between treatment groups. However, the number of conventionally treated patients who developed this level of renal dysfunction (n = 5) was more than twice the number of intensively treated patients (n = 2). The relatively small number of patients with secondary intervention who had microalbuminuria at baseline (n = 70) made it difficult to demonstrate a benefit of intensive therapy with regard to slowing progression to clinical-grade albuminuria once microalbuminuria had occurred (80). The Steno study had demonstrated such a benefit previously with only 36 patients (71). Their success may have been rooted in the very frequent measurement of repeated 24-hour albumin excretion rates, which decreased the variance of the measurements. The long-term follow-up of the DCCT cohort has reinforced the role of intensive therapy in delaying and perhaps preventing diabetic nephropathy (Table 48.3). During approximately 8 years of post-DCCT follow-up, when HbA_{1c} levels were almost identical, the former intensive therapy group continued to have a markedly reduced risk of microalbuminuria, albuminuria, and more advanced stages of nephropathy (Table 48.3), and had less frequent development of hypertension, compared with the former conventional treatment group (99).

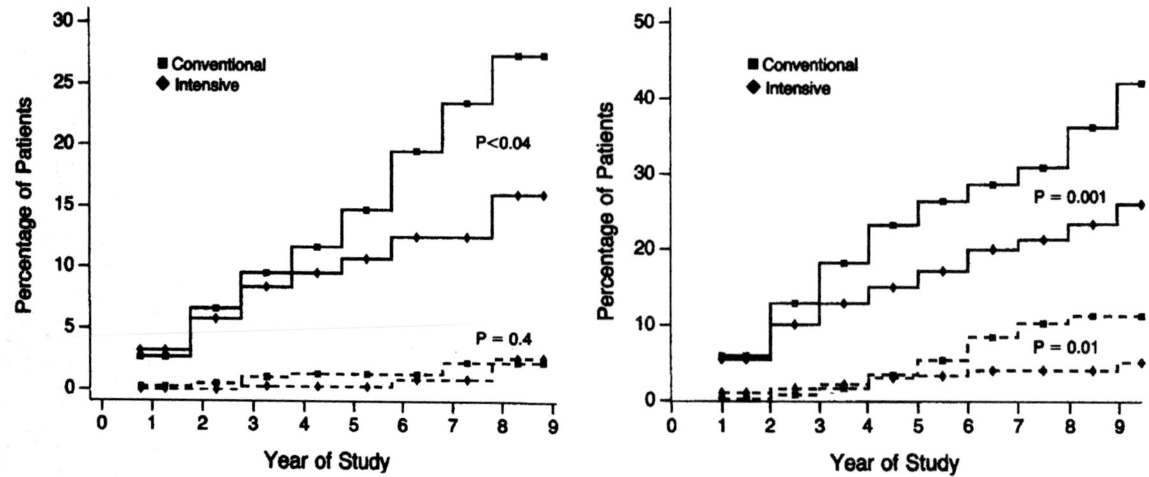

Figure 48.5. Effects of intensive therapy on development of microalbuminuria (≥40 mg/24 h; *solid line*) and clinical albuminuria (≥300 mg/24 h; *dashed line*) in the primary **(A)** and secondary **(B)** Diabetes Control and Complications Trial cohorts. (From DCCT Research Group. The effect of intensive treatment of diabetes on the development and progression of long-term complications in insulin-dependent diabetes mellitus. *N Engl J Med* 1993;329:977–986, with permission. Copyright © 1993 Massachusetts Medical Society. All rights reserved.)

Neuropathy. Confirmed clinical neuropathy was defined as the presence of signs or symptoms of peripheral neuropathy plus either abnormal nerve conduction in at least two peripheral nerves or unequivocally abnormal autonomic nerve testing. Intensive therapy reduced the risk of developing clinical neuropathy 60% in the combined cohorts (Table 48.3) (6,81–83). In addition to the decreased development of confirmed clinical neuropathy, the most stringent of the neurologic outcomes, intensive therapy reduced the risk of deterioration of nerve function, as measured with electrophysiologic methods, that occurred with conventional therapy (81). The decline in autonomic nerve function, assessed with measures of cardiovascular autonomic function, that occurred with conventional therapy was significantly reduced with intensive therapy in the primary prevention, but not in the secondary intervention, cohort (82). There were no significant differences between treatment groups in clinical events secondary to autonomic neuropathy, but the frequency of events was very low in both groups.

Association of Glycemia and Microvascular Complications. The frequent measurements of HbA_{1c} and detection and measurement of microvascular complications using uniform, standardized methods during the mean 6.5 years of the DCCT provided the opportunity to examine the relationship between glycemia and the diabetes-specific complications (93,94). The mathematical modeling of long-term glycemia and complications revealed a continuous relationship between glycemia and retinopathy and nephropathy, with no apparent threshold or breakpoint in the range of diabetic glycemia (Fig. 48.6). The analyses support a continuous benefit of lowering HbA_{1c}, even into the near nondiabetic range. Every 10% decrease in HbA_{1c}, for example, from 10% to 9% or 9% to 8.1%, is associated with a 43% reduction in risk for developing retinopathy. Although the absolute rate of retinopathy decreases in the lower HbA_{1c} range, the relative risk reduction associated with lower HbA_{1c} persists.

Macrovascular Outcomes. The DCCT did not demonstrate a significant difference in major macrovascular outcomes (death from cardiovascular disease, myocardial infarction, and major peripheral vascular events) between treatment groups (84). Although the risk for these combined events was reduced by 41% with intensive therapy, the difference between groups failed

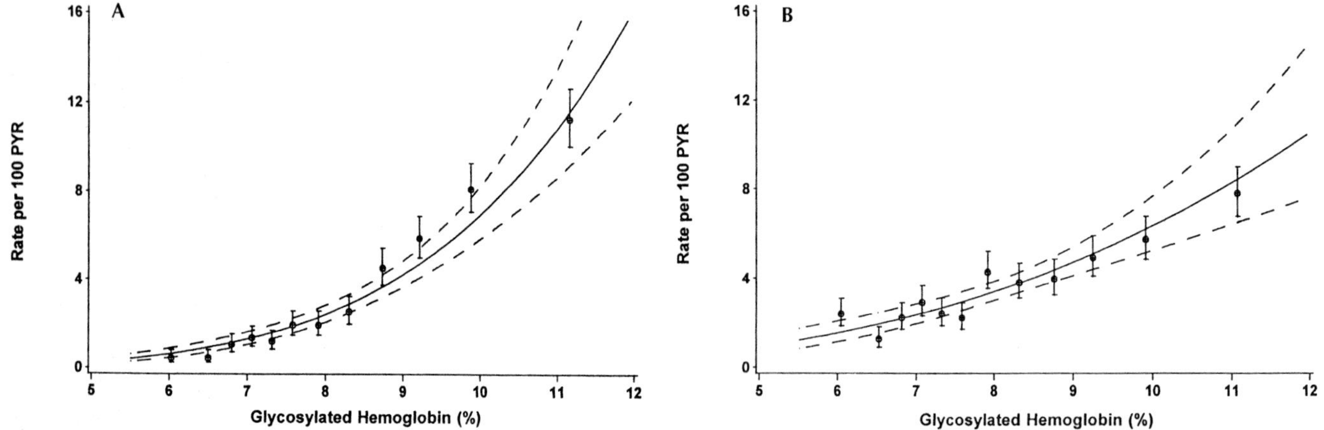

Figure 48.6. Association of mean percentage of glycosylated hemoglobin A_{1c} and sustained retinopathy **(A)** and microalbuminuria **(B)**. (Copyright © 1996 the American Diabetes Association. From The absence of a glycemic threshold for the long-term complication: the perspective of the Diabetes Control and Complications Trial. *Diabetes* 1996;45:1289–1298. Reprinted with permission from the American Diabetes Association.)

to achieve conventional levels of statistical significance ($p = 0.06$). However, several risk factors for cardiovascular disease were improved with intensive therapy, including a 34% reduction in low-density lipoprotein cholesterol ($p = 0.02$). Further study is required to ascertain whether intensive therapy improves the risk of macrovascular disease that accompanies type 1 diabetes. It was reassuring to note that intensive therapy, which included modestly higher insulin doses (0.01 to 0.05 U/kg per day more insulin with intensive than with conventional therapy), did not increase cardiovascular disease. Although the DCCT population being followed long term in the EDIC study remains relatively young and without a large number of cardiovascular events, carotid ultrasound measurements of atherosclerosis (intimal-medial thickness, or IMT) have revealed significant differences between the original intensive and conventional treatment groups, suggesting a beneficial effect of intensive therapy on atherosclerosis (98).

Other Outcomes and Adverse Events. Accompanying the salutary effects of intensive therapy on long-term complications was an approximately threefold increase in severe hypoglycemia, defined as an episode that required assistance to treat (6,89,90). Although the majority of these episodes were clinically benign, the incidence of hypoglycemia resulting in coma and seizures or requiring emergency department treatment was also increased approximately two- to threefold. The more severe hypoglycemic reactions, such as those resulting in seizure or coma, were relatively rare (16 vs. 5 episodes per 100 patient-years in the intensive and conventional treatment groups, respectively). Other adverse events that accompanied intensive therapy included an increased risk for weight gain, secondary in part to the decrease in caloric wasting with decreased glycosuria, and catheter-related infections in patients using insulin pumps. Taken together, none of these adverse events caused significant morbidity or mortality. There were no patient deaths or macrovascular events ascribed to hypoglycemia. Moreover, the increased frequency of hypoglycemia had no adverse effects on neurocognitive function as judged by repeated testing in both treatment groups (86). Finally, despite the demands of intensive therapy, quality of life, measured yearly by self-report (85), did not differ between the two treatment groups.

Imprinting and Metabolic Memory. The long-term follow-up of the DCCT cohort has revealed a persistent effect of the original DCCT intervention even after the differences in HbA_{1c} levels between the two treatment groups have dissipated (96,97). At the end of the DCCT, the subjects in the conventional treatment group were offered instructions in intensive therapy, and all subjects were returned to their own care providers for therapy. HbA_{1c} levels in the original conventional treatment group decreased by approximately 1%, and HbA_{1c} in the original intensive treatment group drifted up so that over the next 5 to 7 years the HbA_{1c} levels were nearly identical. Despite the similar HbA_{1c} levels, the differences in rates of retinopathy and nephropathy continued to expand between the two treatment groups when analyzed on the basis of the original intention-to-treat assignments. This phenomenon has been called "imprinting" and reflects a metabolic memory effect with regard to complications. Whether the apparent long-lasting effects of glycemia are mediated by glycation of proteins that turn over very slowly, or by some other mechanism, is unknown.

Type 2 Diabetes

Until recently, the only clinical trial that examined the impact of glycemic control on long-term complications in type 2 diabetes was the University Group Diabetes Program (UGDP)(102). This multicenter trial compared the effects of five different treatment modalities (diet, diet plus tolbutamide, diet plus phenformin, diet plus standard insulin dose, and diet plus variable-dose insulin) on long-term outcome in patients with newly diagnosed type 2 diabetes. Although the variable-dose insulin regimen maintained mean fasting levels of blood glucose approximately 20% lower than baseline levels, compared with no significant changes from baseline glucose values over time with the other treatment regimens, no significant differences between any of the groups were noted in the degree of retinopathy as measured by fundus photography. The Kumamoto study in Japanese patients with type 2 diabetes, a controlled clinical trial patterned after the DCCT, was the first study to demonstrate convincingly a salutary effect of intensive therapy in type 2 diabetes (103). Although the intensively treated patients had a decrease in retinopathy and nephropathy that paralleled the DCCT results, the Kumamoto study was not considered to be a definitive proof of the glucose hypothesis in type 2 diabetes, in part owing to the clear differences between the Japanese patients with type 2 diabetes and patients with type 2 diabetes in non-Asian societies. The Japanese patients were all relatively thin with small insulin requirements (~0.2 U/kg compared with >0.75 U/kg in the United States).

UNITED KINGDOM PROSPECTIVE DIABETES STUDY

Rationale, Aims, and Design. The United Kingdom Prospective Diabetes Study (UKPDS), which ended in 1997, provided more definitive answers. Originally planned and initiated in 1977 to address the confusion left by the UGDP results, the UKPDS was designed to answer two questions. First, is an "intensive strategy" aimed at achieving fasting glucose levels less than 6 mmol (108 mg/dL) superior to conventional therapy with diet in preventing the complications of diabetes in patients with relatively recent-onset type 2 diabetes (Table 48.4)? Second, are any therapies particularly advantageous with regard to preventing or delaying diabetic complications? The outcomes were aggregated into diabetes-specific complications (combining retinopathy, nephropathy, cataracts, and cardiovascular outcomes), all-cause mortality, and diabetes-related mortality. The study design included stepwise addition of therapies in the conventional and intensive treatment groups if glucose goals were not met. In addition, the intensive therapies were numerous, including three types of sulfonylureas and insulin. The obese subset of patients were also randomly assigned to metformin (104). The results of the UKPDS revealed that metabolic control in type 2 diabetes worsened over time, probably owing to waning β-cell function (105) and requiring the addition of alternative therapies to the originally assigned therapy (Fig. 48.7) (106). Thus, over the course of the study, the majority of subjects

TABLE 48.4. Characteristics of Subjects[a] in the United Kingdom Prospective Diabetes Study (UKPDS) at Baseline

Age (y)	53	Triglycerides (mg/dL)	208
Female (%)	39	Cholesterol (mg/dL)	209
Race (%)		LDL (mg/dL)	135
White	81	HDL (mg/dL)	41
Afro-Caribbean	8	Retinopathy (%)	21
Indian-Asian	10	Proteinuria[b](%)	2
Duration (y)[a]	<1	Neuropathy	12
HbA_{1c} (%)	7.08	Hypertension[c]	24

HDL, high-density lipoprotein; LDL, low-density lipoprotein.
[a] Diagnosed within 1 year.
[b] >300 mg/24 h.
[c] >160/90 mm Hg.

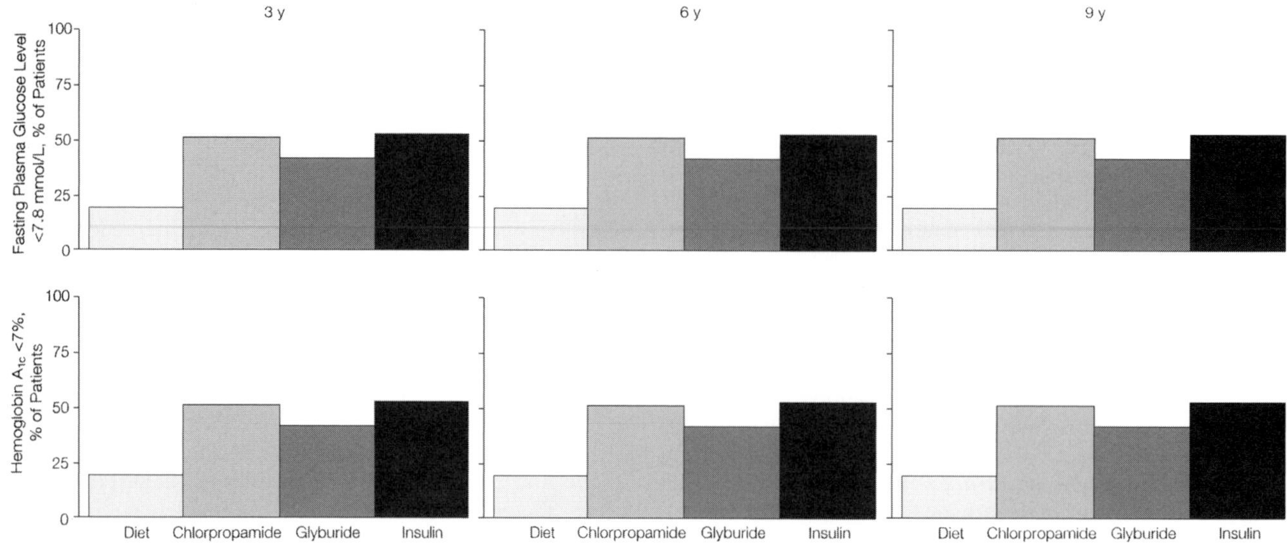

Figure 48.7. Proportion of patients in each therapy allocation. Values are for patients who remained receiving monotherapy and achieved different targets after 3, 6, and 9 years. (From Turner RC, Cull CA, Frighi V, et al. Glycemic control with diet, sulfonylurea, metformin, or insulin I patients with type 2 diabetes mellitus: progressive requirement for multiple therapies (UKPDS). *JAMA* 1999;281:2005–2112, with permission. Copyrighted 1999, American Medical Association.)

receiving conventional treatment had one or more of the intensive therapies added and a substantial fraction (often ≥20%) of the subjects receiving intensive treatment had the alternative intensive therapies added to or substituted for their originally assigned intensive therapy. This design feature, intended to keep glycemia as low as possible in the intensive treatment group, severely undercut the ability to compare the specific intensive therapy modalities (107). Finally, other randomized interventions (early addition of metformin to sulfonylurea therapy, use of acarbose, and intensive vs. conventional hypertension treatment) made the UKPDS protocol byzantine in its complexity.

UKPDS Results. The UKPDS results, analyzed by intention to treat, revealed a benefit of intensive therapy, which resulted in a 1% absolute reduction of HbA_{1c} (11% relative reduction), on the aggregate diabetes outcomes, decreasing the risk by 12% (Table 48.5). This benefit was predicated to a great extent on a beneficial effect on retinopathy and cataracts. There was no significant benefit with regard to cardiovascular disease. The results with metformin were analyzed separately. [The validity of this analysis strategy has been called into question (107)]. Metformin therapy resulted in less weight gain and less hypoglycemia than other intensive therapies. In addition, aggregate diabetes mortality, but not diabetes-related outcomes, were significantly reduced by metformin (104). Early addition of metformin to sulfonylurea, however, resulted in a large and statistically significant increase in cardiovascular mortality. The UKPDS complex design, numerous crossovers, and controversial analytic strategy left many questions. However, the fundamental observation, when combined with the results of the Kumamoto study, that intensive diabetes management improves outcome, specifically microvascular outcomes, is unquestionable.

MACROVASCULAR DISEASE

The multifactorial etiology of cardiovascular disease (CVD) makes it unlikely that the association established between levels of glycemia and complications specific to diabetes, such as retinopathy, will also pertain to CVD. Almost all studies have been in populations with type 2 diabetes or impaired glucose

TABLE 48.5. Major Findings of the United Kingdom Prospective Diabetes Study (UKPDS)

Nonobese + obese	Obese only
Intensive therapy **reduced**[a]	Metformin **reduced**[a]
Aggregate diabetes outcomes by 12% ($p = 0.029$)	Aggregate diabetes outcomes by 32% ($p = 0.003$)
Laser therapy by 29% ($p = 0.003$)	Diabetes-related death by 42% ($p = 0.02$)
Cataract extraction by 24% ($p = 0.046$)	All-cause death by 36% ($p = 0.011$)
Sudden death by 46% ($p = 0.047$)	
Intensive therapy **did not reduce**	Metformin **did not reduce**
Diabetes-related deaths—10% ($p = 0.34$)	Laser therapy—31% ($p = 0.17$)
All-cause mortality—6% ($p = 0.44$)	
Fatal myocardial infarction—6% ($p = 0.63$)	
Nonfatal myocardial infarction—21% ($p = 0.057$)	
Renal failure—27% ($p = 0.45$)	

[a] Compared with conventional therapy.

tolerance (IGT). Although the presence of diabetes (or IGT) increases the prevalence of CVD (108–111), an association between the level of glycemia and the occurrence of CVD had not been easy to demonstrate (112). Recently, however, studies using more accurate measures of long-term glycemia have found a correlation between glycemic levels and prevalence of CVD (11,114). In the Framingham study, level of HbA_{1c} correlated with prevalence of CVD, but only in women (113). Whether diabetes affects CVD directly or through the established risk factors that accompany it, such as hypertension, dyslipidemia, and obesity (in type 2 diabetes), or through other potential risk factors, such as hyperinsulinemia, inflammation, or hemorheologic abnormalities, is not known. The UGDP trial did not demonstrate any impact of glucose control on CVD outcome (108). The UKPDS showed a beneficial impact of metformin therapy, but only when the obese metformin group was compared with the obese controls. The long-term follow-up of the DCCT has demonstrated a beneficial long-term effect of intensive therapy on atherosclerosis, as measured by carotid ultrasonography (98). Studies such as the Diabetes Prevention Program are examining the effects of glycemic control on macrovascular disease and atherosclerosis in the prediabetic population with IGT (115).

CONCLUSIONS: TREATMENT RECOMMENDATIONS

The DCCT Research Group, the UKPDS Research Group, the American Diabetes Association, and other groups have concluded that the significant and consistent effects of intensive therapy in reducing the risk of development and progression of long-term complications of diabetes outweigh its costs, the considerable effort to implement it, and the increased risk for hypoglycemia. Intensive therapy has been endorsed as the treatment of choice for most patients with type 1 or type 2 diabetes. This conclusion is further supported on the basis of the projected economic impact of intensive therapy. Although the annual cost of intensive therapy exceeds the cost of conventional therapy and must be incurred for at least 3 years in type 1 diabetes before a benefit is seen, the long-term benefits of intensive therapy (reducing loss of vision and the need for laser therapy, reducing the incidence of end-stage renal disease and the need for dialysis and transplantation, reducing the number of amputations, and reducing the costs associated with all these problems) make intensive therapy an economically viable therapy (91). The long-term follow-up in EDIC, demonstrating further benefits of intensive therapy even 8 years after the end of the DCCT, supports this conclusion.

Realistically, not all patients with diabetes are able to implement intensive therapy; however, the goal for all patients should be to lower blood glucose levels to as close to the normal range as safety and lifestyle allow. Lower HbA_{1c} levels should translate into an appreciably lower risk for complications (Fig. 48.6).

REFERENCES

1. Cahill GF Jr, Etzwiler DD, Freinkel N. "Control" and diabetes [Editorial]. *N Engl J Med* 1976;294:1004–1005.
2. Siperstein MD, Foster DW, Knowles HC Jr, et al. Control of blood glucose and diabetic vascular disease [Editorial]. *N Engl J Med* 1977;296:1060–1063.
3. Ingelfinger FJ. Debates on diabetes. *N Engl J Med* 1977;296:1228–1230.
4. Siperstein MD. Diabetic microangiopathy and the control of blood glucose. *N Engl J Med* 1983;309:1577–1579.
5. Stern MP, Haffner SM. Prospective assessment of metabolic control in diabetes mellitus: the complications question. *JAMA* 1988;260:2896–2897.
6. The Diabetes Control and Complications Trial Research Group. The effect of intensive treatment of diabetes on the development and progression of long-term complications in insulin-dependent diabetes mellitus. *N Engl J Med* 1993;329:977–986.
7. UK Prospective Diabetes Study (UKPDS) Group. Intensive blood-glucose control with sulphonylureas or insulin compared with conventional treatment and risk of complications in patients with type 2 diabetes (UKPDS 33). *Lancet* 1998;352:837–853.
8. Von Engelhardt D, et al, eds. *Diabetes: its medical and cultural history*. New York: Springer-Verlag, 1989.
9. Nettleship E. Chronic retinitis, with formation of blood-vessels in the vitreous in a patient with diabetes; one eye lost by results of chronic iritis, accompanied by the formation of large vessels in the iris. *Trans Ophthalmol Soc UK* 1888;8:159–161.
10. Ballantyne AJ, Loewenstein A. The pathology of diabetic retinopathy. *Trans Ophthalmol UK* 1943;63:95–115.
11. Kimmelstiel P, Wilson C. Intercapillary lesions in the glomeruli of the kidney. *Am J Pathol* 1936;12:83–97.
12. Palmberg P, Smith M, Waltman S, et al. The natural history of retinopathy in insulin-dependent juvenile-onset diabetes. *Ophthalmology* 1981;88:613–618.
13. Frank RN, Hoffman WH, Podgor MJ, et al. Retinopathy in juvenile-onset type I diabetes of short duration. *Diabetes* 1982;31:874–884.
14. Klein R, Klein BEK, Moss SE, et al. The Wisconsin epidemiologic study of diabetic retinopathy. III. Prevalence and risk of diabetic retinopathy when age at diagnosis is 30 or more years. *Arch Ophthalmol* 1984;102:527–532.
15. Klein R, Klein BEK, Moss SE, et al. The Wisconsin epidemiologic study of diabetic retinopathy. II. Prevalence and risk of diabetic retinopathy when age at diagnosis is less than 30 years. *Arch Ophthalmol* 1984;102:520–526.
16. Nathan DM, Singer DE, Godine JE, et al. Retinopathy in older type II diabetics: association with glucose control. *Diabetes* 1986;35:797–801.
17. Ballard DJ, Melton LJ III, Dwyer MS, et al. Risk factors for diabetic retinopathy: a population-based study in Rochester, Minnesota. *Diabetes Care* 1986; 334–342.
18. Krolewski AS, Warram JH, Rand LI, et al. Risk of proliferative diabetic retinopathy in juvenile-onset type I diabetes: a-40 year follow-up study. *Diabetes Care* 1986;9:443–452.
19. White P. The future of the diabetic child. *JAMA* 1930;95:1160–1162.
20. Joslin EP. Insulin's twenty-fifth anniversary. *Diabetes Abstracts* 1945;5:37.
21. Wagener HP. Retinopathy in diabetes mellitus. *Proc Am Diabetes Assoc* 1943;5:201–216.
22. Dolger H. Clinical evaluation of vascular damage in diabetes mellitus. *JAMA* 1947;134:1289–1291.
23. Boyd JD, Jackson RL, Allen JH. Avoidance of degenerative lesions in diabetes mellitus. *JAMA* 1942;118:694–696.
24. Harris MI, Hadden WC, Knowler WC, et al. Prevalence of diabetes and impaired glucose tolerance and plasma glucose levels in U.S. population aged 20–74 yr. *Diabetes* 1987;36:523–524.
25. Nathan DM, Singer DE, Godine JE, et al. Non-insulin-dependent diabetes in older patients. *Am J Med* 1986;81:837–842.
26. Humphrey LL, Ballard DJ, Frohnert PP, et al. Chronic renal failure in non-insulin-dependent diabetes mellitus: a population based study in Rochester, Minnesota. *Ann Intern Med* 1989;111:788–796.
27. Cowie CC, Port FK, Wolfe RA, et al. Disparities in incidence of diabetic end-stage renal disease according to race and type of diabetes. *N Engl J Med* 1989; 321:1074–1079.
28. Dwyer MS, Melton LJ III, Ballard DJ, et al. Incidence of diabetic retinopathy and blindness: a population based study in Rochester Minnesota. *Diabetes Care* 1985;8:316–322.
29. Report of the Expert Committee on the Diagnosis and Classification of Diabetes Mellitus. *Diabetes Care* 1997;20:1183–1197.
30. Engerman R, Bloodworth JMB Jr, Nelson S. Relationship of microvascular disease in diabetes to metabolic control. *Diabetes* 1977;26:760–769.
31. Engerman RL, Kern TS. Progression of incipient diabetic retinopathy during good glycemic control. *Diabetes* 1987;36:808–812.
32. Mauer SM, Steffes MW, Sutherland DER, et al. Studies of the rate of regression of the glomerular lesions in diabetic rats treated with pancreatic islet transplantation. *Diabetes* 1975;24:280–285.
33. Gray BN, Watkins E Jr. Prevention of vascular complications of diabetes by pancreatic islet transplantation. *Arch Surg* 1976;254–257.
34. Cohen AJ, McGill PD, Rossetti RG, et al. Glomerulopathy in spontaneously diabetic rat. *Diabetes* 1977;36:944–951.
35. Knowles HC Jr. The problem of the relation of the control of diabetes to the development of vascular disease. *Trans Am Clin Climatol Assoc* 1964;76: 142–147.
36. Pirart J. Diabetes mellitus and its degenerative complications: a prospective study of 4,400 patients observed between 1947 and 1973. *Diabetes Care* 1978;1: 168–188;252–266.
37. Klein R, Klein BEK, Moss SE, et al. Glycosylated hemoglobin predicts the incidence and progression of diabetic retinopathy. *JAMA* 1988;260:2864–2871.
38. Klein R, Moss SE, Klein BEK, et al. The Wisconsin epidemiologic study of diabetic retinopathy. XI. The incidence of macular edema. *Ophthalmology* 1989;96:1501–1510.
39. Moss SE, Klein R, Klein BEK. The incidence of vision loss in a diabetic population. *Ophthalmology* 1989;95:1340–1348.
40. Doft BH, Kingsley LA, Orchard TJ, et al. The association between long-term diabetic control and early retinopathy. *Ophthalmology* 1984;91:763–769.
41. McCance DR, Atkinson AB, Hadden DR, et al. Long-term glycaemic control and diabetic retinopathy. *Lancet* 1989;2:824–828.

42. Weber B, Burger W, Hartmann R, et al. Risk factors for the development of retinopathy in children and adolescents with type I (insulin-dependent) diabetes mellitus. *Diabetologia* 1986;29:23–29.
43. Groop LC, Teir H, Koskimies S, et al. Risk factors and markers associated with proliferative retinopathy in patients with insulin-dependent diabetes. *Diabetes* 1986;35:1397–1403.
44. Knowler WC, Bennett PH, Ballintine EJ. Increased incidence of retinopathy in diabetics with elevated blood pressure: a six-year follow-up study in Pima Indians. *N Engl J Med* 1980;302:645–650.
45. Klein BEK, Moss SE, Klein R. Effect of pregnancy on progression of diabetic retinopathy. *Diabetes Care* 1990;13:34–40.
46. Leslie RDG, Pyke DA. Diabetic retinopathy in identical twins. *Diabetes* 1982; 31:19–21.
47. Cohen R, Hennekens CH, Christen CG, et al. Determinants of retinopathy progression in type 1 diabetes mellitus. *Am J Med* 1999;107:45–51.
48. Moss SE, Klein R, Klein BE. Association of cigarette smoking with diabetic retinopathy. *Diabetes Care* 1991;14:119–126.
49. Cohen AJ, McGill PD, Rossetti RG, et al. Glomerulopathy in spontaneously diabetic rat: impact of glycemic control. *Diabetes* 1987;36:944–951.
50. Steffes MW, Buchwald H, Wigness BD, et al. Diabetic nephropathy in the uninephrectomized dog: microscopic lesions after one year. *Kidney Int* 1982; 21:721–724.
51. Andersen AR, Christiansen JS, Andersen JK, et al. Diabetic nephropathy in type I (insulin-dependent) diabetes: an epidemiological study. *Diabetologia* 1983;25:496–501.
52. Rosenstock J, Raskin P. Early diabetic nephropathy: assessment and potential therapeutic interventions. *Diabetes Care* 1986;9:529–545.
53. Kussman MJ, Goldstein HH, Gleason RE. The clinical course of diabetic nephropathy. *JAMA* 1976;236:1861–1863.
54. Viberti GC, Jarrett RJ, Mahmud U, et al. Microalbuminuria as a predictor of clinical nephropathy in insulin-dependent diabetes mellitus. *Lancet* 1982;1: 1430–1432.
55. Parving H-H, Oxenboll B, Svendsen PA, et al. Early detection of patients at risk of developing diabetic nephropathy. A longitudinal study of urinary albumin excretion. *Acta Endocrinol* 1982;100:550–555.
56. Mathiesen ER, Oxenboll B, Johansen K, et al. Incipient nephropathy in type I (insulin-dependent) diabetes. *Diabetologia* 1984;26:406–410.
57. Mogensen CE, Christensen CK. Predicting diabetic nephropathy in insulin-dependent patients. *N Engl J Med* 1984;311:89–93.
58. Mogensen CE. Microalbuminuria predicts clinical proteinuria and early mortality in maturity-onset diabetes. *N Engl J Med* 1984;310:356–360.
59. Feldt-Rasmussen B, Mathieson ER. Validity of urinary albumin excretion in incipient diabetic nephropathy. *Diabet Nephrol* 1984;3:101–104.
60. Chavers BM, Bilous RW, Ellis EN, et al. Glomerular lesions and urinary albumin excretion in type I diabetes without overt proteinuria. *N Engl J Med* 1989;320:966–970.
61. Perkins BA, Ficociello LH, Silva K, et al. Regression of microalbuminuria in type 1 diabetes. *N Engl J Med* 2003;348:2285–2293.
62. Krolewski AS, Canessa M, Warram JH, et al. Predisposition to hypertension and susceptibility to renal disease in insulin-dependent diabetes mellitus. *N Engl J Med* 1988;318:140–145.
63. Rossing P, Hougaard P, Parving HH. Risk factors for development of incipient and overt diabetic nephropathy in type 1 diabetic patients. *Diabetes Care* 2002;25:859–864.
64. Chaturvedi N, Bandinelli S, Mangili R, et al. Microalbuminuria in type 1 diabetes: rates, risk factors and glycemic thresholds. *Kidney Int* 2001;60: 219–227.
65. Chase HP, Jackson WE, Hoops SL, et al. Glucose control and the renal and retinal complications of insulin-dependent diabetes. *JAMA* 1989;261: 1155–1160.
66. Ward JD, Fisher DJ, Barnes CG, et al. Improvement in nerve conduction following treatment in newly diagnosed diabetics. *Lancet* 1971;1:428–430.
67. The DCCT Research Group. Factors in development of diabetic neuropathy. Baseline analysis of neuropathy in feasibility phase of the Diabetes Control and Complications Trial (DCCT). *Diabetes* 1988;37:476–481.
68. Porte D Jr, Graf RJ, Halter JB, et al. Diabetic neuropathy and plasma glucose control. *Am J Med* 1981;70:195–200.
69. Nathan DM. Modern management of insulin-dependent diabetes mellitus. *Med Clin North Am* 1988;72:1365–1378.
70. The Kroc Collaborative Study Group. Blood glucose control and the evolution of diabetic retinopathy and albuminuria: a preliminary multicenter trial. *N Engl J Med* 1984;311:365–372.
71. Lauritzen T, Frost-Larsen K, Larsen H-W, et al. The Steno Study Group: two-year experience with continuous subcutaneous insulin infusion in relation to retinopathy and neuropathy. *Diabetes* 1985;34[Suppl 3]:74–79.
72. Brinchmann-Hansen O, Dahl-Jorgensen K, Hanssen KF, et al. The response of diabetic retinopathy to 41 months of multiple insulin injections, insulin pumps, and conventional insulin therapy. *Arch Ophthalmol* 1988;106:1242–1246.
73. Reichard P, Nilsson B-Y, Rosenqvist U. The effect of long-term intensified insulin treatment on the development of microvascular complications of diabetes mellitus. *N Engl J Med* 1993;329:304–309.
74. The Diabetes Control and Complications Trial (DCCT). Design and methodologic considerations for the feasibility phase. The DCCT Research Group. *Diabetes* 1986;35:530–545.
75. Lauritzen T, Larsen H-W, Larsen K-F, et al., and the Steno Study Group. Effect of 1 year of near-normal blood glucose levels on retinopathy in insulin-dependent diabetics. *Lancet* 1983;1:200–204.
76. Dahl-Jorgensen K, Brinchmann-Hansen O, Hanssen KF, et al. Rapid tightening of blood glucose control leads to transient deterioration of retinopathy in insulin dependent diabetes mellitus: the Oslo study. *BMJ* 1985;290:811–815.
77. The effect of intensive diabetes treatment on the progression of diabetic retinopathy in insulin-dependent diabetes mellitus: The Diabetes Control and Complications Trial. *Arch Ophthalmol* 1995;113:36–51.
78. Diabetes Control and Complications Trial Research Group. Progression of retinopathy with intensive vs conventional therapy in the Diabetes Control and Complications Trial. *Ophthalmology* 1995;102:647–661.
79. The Diabetes Control and Complications Research Group. Early worsening of diabetic retinopathy in the Diabetes Control and Complications Trial. *Arch Ophthalmol* 1998;116:874–886.
80. The Diabetes Control and Complications (DCCT) Research Group. The effect of intensive therapy on the development and progression of diabetic nephropathy in the Diabetes Control and Complications Trial. *Kidney Int* 1995;47:1703–1720.
81. The Diabetes Control and Complications Research Group. The effect of intensive diabetes therapy on the development and progression of neuropathy. *Ann Intern Med* 1995;122:561–568.
82. The effect of intensive diabetes therapy on measures of autonomic nervous system function in the Diabetes Control and Complications Trial (DCCT). *Diabetologia* 1998;41:416–423.
83. The effect of intensive treatment of diabetes on nerve conduction measures in the Diabetes Control and Complications Trial. *Ann Neurol* 1995;38:869–880.
84. The effect of intensive diabetes therapy on macrovascular disease and its risk factors in the Diabetes Control and Complications Trial. *Am J Cardiol* 1995; 75:894–903.
85. Influence of intensive therapy on quality-of-life outcomes in the Diabetes Control and Complications Trial. *Diabetes Care* 1996;19:195–203.
86. Effects of intensive diabetes therapy on neuropsychological function in adults in the Diabetes Complications and Control Trial. *Ann Intern Med* 1996;124;379–388.
87. The Diabetes Control and Complications Trial Research Group. Effect of intensive therapy on residual beta-cell function in patients with type 1 diabetes in the Diabetes Control and Complications Trial. A randomized, controlled trial. *Ann Intern Med* 1998;128:517–523.
88. Implementation of treatment protocols in the Diabetes Control and Complications Trial. *Diabetes Care* 1995;18:361–374.
89. Adverse events and their association with treatment regimens in the Diabetes Control and Complications Trial. *Diabetes Care* 1995;18:1415–1427.
90. The Diabetes Control and Complications Research Group. Hypoglycemia in the Diabetes Control and Complications Trial. *Diabetes* 1997; 46:271–286.
91. The Diabetes Control and Complications Research Group. Lifetime benefits of intensive therapy as practiced in the Diabetes Control and Complications Trial. *JAMA* 1996;276:1409–1415.
92. Pregnancy outcomes in the Diabetes Control and Complications Trial. *Am J Obstet Gynecol* 1996;174:1343–1353.
93. The relationship of glycemic exposure (HbA1c) to the risk of developing retinopathy in the Diabetes Control and Complications Trial. *Diabetes* 1995; 44:968–983.
94. The absence of a glycemic threshold for the development of long-term complications: the perspective of the Diabetes Control and Complications Trial. *Diabetes* 1996;45:1289–1298.
95. Epidemiology of Diabetes Interventions and Complications (EDIC). Design, implementation, and preliminary results of a long-term follow-up of the Diabetes Control and Complications Trial cohort. *Diabetes Care* 1999;22:99–111.
96. The Diabetes Control and Complication Trial/Epidemiology of Diabetes Interventions and Complications Research Group. Retinopathy and nephropathy in patients with type 1 diabetes four years after a trial of intensive therapy. *N Engl J Med* 2000;342:381–389.
97. DCCT/EDIC Research Group. Effect of intensive therapy on the microvascular complications of type 1 diabetes mellitus. *JAMA* 2002;287:2563–2569.
98. The Diabetes Control and Complications Trial/Epidemiology of Diabetes Interventions and Complications Research Group. Intensive diabetes therapy and carotid-intima thickness in type 1 diabetes mellitus. *N Engl J Med* 2003;348:2294–2303.
99. DCCT/EDIC Research Group. Sustained effect of intensive treatment of type 1 diabetes mellitus on development and progression of diabetic nephropathy. The Epidemiology of Diabetes Interventions and Complications Study. *JAMA* 2003;290:2159–2167.
100. Early Treatment Diabetic Retinopathy Study Research Group. Fundus photographic risk factors for progression of diabetic retinopathy. EDTRS Report number 12. *Ophthalmology* 1991;98[5 Suppl]:823–833.
101. Diabetes Control and Complications Research Group. Clustering of long-term complications in families with diabetes in the Diabetes Control and Complications Trial. *Diabetes* 1997;46:1829–1839.
102. A study of the effects of hypoglycemic agents on vascular complications in patients with adult-onset diabetes. VI. Supplementary report on nonfatal events in patients treated with tolbutamide. *Diabetes* 1976;25:1129–1153.
103. Ohkubo Y, Kishikawa H, Araki E, et al. Intensive insulin therapy prevents the progression of diabetic microvascular complications in Japanese patients with non-insulin-dependent diabetes mellitus: a randomized prospective 6-year study. *Diabetes Res Clin Pract* 1995;28:103–117.
104. UK Prospective Diabetes Study (UKPDS) Group. Effect of intensive blood-glucose control with metformin on complications in overweight patients with type 2 diabetes (UKPDS 34). *Lancet* 1998;352:854–865.

105. U.K. Prospective Diabetes Study Group. U.K. Prospective Diabetes Study 16. Overview of 6 years' therapy of type II diabetes, a progressive disease. *Diabetes* 1995;44:1249–1258.
106. Turner RC, Cull CA, Frighi V, et al. Glycemic control with diet, sulfonylurea, metformin, or insulin in patients with type 2 diabetes mellitus: progressive requirement for multiple therapies (UKPDS 49). *JAMA* 1999;281:2005–2112.
107. Nathan DM. Some answers, more controversy, from UKPDS. *Lancet* 1998;352:832–833.
108. Kannel WB, McGee DL. Diabetes and cardiovascular disease. The Framingham Study. *JAMA* 1979;241:2036–2038.
109. Gordon T, Castelli WP, Hjortland MC, et al. Diabetes, blood lipids, and the role of obesity in coronary heart disease risk for women. The Framingham Study. *Ann Intern Med* 1977;87:393–397.
110. Jarrett RJ, McCartney P, Keen H. The Bedford Survey: ten-year mortality rates in newly diagnosed diabetics, borderline diabetics and normoglycemic controls and risk indices for coronary heart disease in borderline diabetics. *Diabetologia* 1982;22:79–84.
111. Wingard DL, Barrett-Connor E, Criqui MH, et al. Clustering of heart disease risk factors in diabetic compared to nondiabetic adults. *Am J Epidemiol* 1983;117:19–26.
112. The International Collaborative Group. Joint discussion. *J Chronic Dis* 1979;32:829–837.
113. Singer DE, Nathan DM, Anderson KM, et al. The association of hemoglobin A_{1c} with prevalent cardiovascular disease in the original cohort of the Framingham Heart Study. *Diabetes* 1992:41:202–208.
114. Stratton IM, Adler AI, Neil HAW, et al. Association of glycemia with macrovascular and microvascular complication of type 2 diabetes (UKPDS 35) Prospective Observational Study. *BMJ* 2000;321:405–419.
115. The Diabetes Prevention Program. Design and methods for a clinical trial in the prevention of type 2 diabetes mellitus. *Diabetes Care* 1999;22:623–634.

CHAPTER 49

Mechanisms of Diabetic Microvascular Complications

Christian Rask-Madsen, Zhiheng He, and George L. King

Patients receiving modern care for diabetes have a dramatically lower risk for developing microvascular complications than they did a few decades ago. In particular, the risk for developing renal disease necessitating dialysis has decreased severalfold. However, diabetes is still the most common cause of blindness and end-stage renal disease and a major reason for peripheral neuropathy. Therefore, there is compelling reason to increase our knowledge about the cellular and molecular mechanisms of these complications so that rational strategies for prevention and treatment can be designed.

Microvascular complications in diabetes have traditionally included retinopathy, nephropathy, and neuropathy. In each of these complications, pathologic changes and cellular dysfunction are seen in nonvascular tissues at early stages and cannot be explained by circulatory changes alone. Thus, in retinopathy and neuropathy, dysfunction of neurons develops in parallel with microvascular pathology. Therefore, these complications cannot be explained entirely as being secondary to microvascular pathology. Nevertheless, this chapter will focus on vascular mechanisms for the development of these complications.

Cardiovascular disease is the major reason for morbidity and mortality among patients with diabetes. Many aspects of heart disease in patients with diabetes are secondary to atherosclerosis, i.e., macrovascular disease. But the mechanisms of some of the myocardial pathologies in diabetes have obvious similarities to mechanisms of complications in other organs, e.g, in the kidney. Therefore, in this chapter we have chosen to describe changes in regulation of vascularization and extracellular matrix in the heart.

Many of the disease mechanisms described below have been demonstrated in several tissues and cell types in diabetes; e.g., oxidative stress, glycation, and activation of protein kinase C (PKC) have been described in all tissues affected by microvascular complications. Therefore, the later sections of this chapter discuss such mechanisms without systematically referring to where they operate. However, one of the biggest challenges in studying these mechanisms is to understand why certain tissues or cell types are preferentially affected by diabetes. For example, even though oxidative stress or activation of PKC occurs in both capillary endothelial cells and pericytes in the retina, there is a pronounced loss of pericytes rather than endothelial cells. Treatment with new drugs, especially those administered systemically, will also have to consider such tissue differences. For example, inhibitors of vascular endothelial growth factor (VEGF) have been proposed as therapy for proliferative retinopathy, but even though increased retinal expression of VEGF may be partly responsible for this complication, decreased expression of VEGF in the heart may be responsible for decreased vascularization of the ischemic myocardium in diabetes (1). Likewise, speculations that inhibition of renal expression of transforming growth factor-β (TGF-β) may prevent renal disease (2,3) should consider the possible importance of TGF-β for the development of collateral vessels to ischemic tissue (4).

The studies discussed below have used many methodologies. When interpreting results from studies in animals or *in vitro*, one should keep certain issues in mind. Animal models of nondiabetic insulin resistance, type 1 diabetes, and type 2 diabetes exist. They may be different from human diabetes for a variety of reasons: species differences; the introduction of hyperglycemia by a diet that is not typical for either the animal or humans (i.e., rich in galactose); induction of diabetes with a toxin given systemically (i.e., streptozotocin); the existence of a monogenic defect (mutations in the gene for leptin or the leptin receptor).

Cell-culture studies have limitations for explaining human disease. However, major advances in the understanding of diabetic complications have derived from the study of differentiated cells that preserve many of their characteristics *in vitro*.

CHANGES IN VASCULAR MORPHOLOGY AND FUNCTION

General Vascular Changes

GROWTH AND APOPTOSIS OF VASCULAR CELLS

In proliferative retinopathy, growth of endothelial cells is evident, whereas in diabetic nephropathy or in the microvessels of the diabetic heart, loss of endothelial cells is observed. On the other hand, the contractile cells of the retinal microvasculature, the retinal capillary pericytes, are lost in diabetic retinopathy, but proliferation of vascular smooth muscle cells (VSMCs) is increased in atherosclerotic lesions.

In retinal capillaries from patients with diabetes, apoptotic pathways are preferentially activated in pericytes rather than in endothelial cells (5,6). Apoptosis in pericytes can be induced by feeding with galactose (7) and by both high glucose concentrations (6) and advanced glycation end-products (AGEs) (8).

In heart biopsy specimens from patients with diabetes, apoptosis of endothelial cells and cardiomyocytes is increased severalfold (9). In endothelial cells cultured in high glucose concentrations, the signaling pathways mediating apoptosis involve hydrogen peroxide (10), nuclear factor-κB (NF-κB) (6), and c-jun N-terminal kinase 1 (JNK1) (10).

BASEMENT MEMBRANE AND EXTRACELLULAR MATRIX

A classic morphologic finding in diabetic microangiopathy is the thickening of basement membranes (11). This phenomenon is generalized and affects both vascular and nonvascular tissues. Basement membranes maintain tissue architecture, modify cellular functions such as proliferation, and provide a filtration barrier. Basement membranes separate cells from the interstitial space or from cells of a different type. In the glomerulus of the kidney, the basement membrane is situated between endothelial cells of the capillaries and epithelial cells of the Bowman capsule; in the retina, the basement membrane separates capillary endothelial cells and pericytes. Basement-membrane proteins are synthesized by several cell types. Thus, renal mesangial matrix proteins are synthesized both by mesangial cells and by endothelial cells. The morphology of the capillary basement membrane varies in different tissues, and its thickness often correlates with the intracapillary pressure. The chemical components of the basement membrane include collagens (mainly type IV), chondroitin, heparan sulfate proteoglycans, and various glycoproteins such as laminin (12–14).

The capillary basement membrane in the retina thickens with age (15) but at an accelerated rate in patients with diabetes and in animal models of diabetes (16). In the retinas of diabetic rats, capillary thickening is more prominent in the inner capillary bed (nerve and ganglion layer) than in the inner and outer plexiform layers (17). In the kidney, increased extracellular matrix manifests as thickening of the glomerular basement membrane, expansion of the mesangium, and tubolointerstitial fibrosis (14). The glomerular basement membrane and the mesangium have been studied most thoroughly. In these tissue compartments, both increased synthesis of extracellular matrix proteins and decreased degradation of matrix protein have been demonstrated. Some extracellular proteins that are not a significant part of normal extracellular matrix are expressed in diabetes. However, most extracellular proteins overexpressed in diabetes are components of the normal mesangium and basement membrane. Collagen type IV and fibronectin are among the proteins most consistently demonstrated to be overexpressed in diabetes (14).

Heparan sulfate proteoglycans constitute a charge barrier to protein diffusion across the glomerular basement membrane. The majority of heparan sulfate anionic sites are in the lamina rara externa of the basement membrane (18). There is a decrease in the heparan sulfate content of the glomerular basement membrane relative to the collagen content (19). Furthermore, the number of anionic sites is decreased (18).

Expression of extracellular matrix protein is increased in diabetes. In the glomeruli, important mediators of this increased production include, among others, angiotensin II (ATII), TGF-β, and connective tissue growth factor (CTGF) (14). The roles of these mediators are discussed below. In addition, degradation of extracellular matrix protein, catalyzed by matrix metalloproteinase (MMP), is decreased. The expression of mRNA of several MMPs is reduced in patients with diabetes and in animal models of diabetes (14). Furthermore, this effect is recapitulated in cell-culture models of a diabetic milieu. For example, expression of MMP2 is decreased in mesangial cells stimulated with ATII (20). The activity of MMP is reduced by several mechanisms. MMP proenzymes are cleaved by plasmin—or in the case of MMP2, by membrane-type MMP1—to yield the active form of the enzyme. The activity of both plasmin and membrane-type MMP1 is reduced in diabetes (21). Furthermore, tissue inhibitor of MMP1 is increased in diabetes (22).

ENDOTHELIAL FUNCTION

Apart from being regulated by the autonomic nervous system and circulating hormones, blood flow is controlled by substances released from the endothelium, acting in a paracrine manner. In both types of diabetes, endothelium-dependent vasodilation is decreased. Endothelial dysfunction can be seen after relatively short periods of elevated concentrations of glucose. Thus, after 6 hours of a high glucose concentration, endothelium-dependent vasorelaxation is decreased in rabbit aorta *ex vivo* (23) or in the forearm of healthy humans (24).

Nitric oxide (NO) is an important mediator of endothelium-dependent vasodilation, but relatively few studies have quantified how much NO contributes to blood flow during basal or stimulated conditions in tissues prone to microvascular complications. When choroidal blood flow in the cat is stimulated by facial nerve stimulation, the increase in blood flow is completely dependent on NO (25). In humans, retinal blood flow at basal conditions and stimulated by flicker is dependent in part on NO (26). Loss of NO-mediated blood flow may underlie the decrease in retinal blood flow observed in diabetes (27). Nerve blood flow in experimental diabetes is associated with a decreased contribution of NO to basal vascular tone (28).

On the other hand, vascular leakage in early streptozotocin-induced diabetes appears dependent on increased production of NO (29). This may be caused by increased expression of endothelial nitric oxide synthase (eNOS) (30–32) or induction of inducible NOS (iNOS) (33). Paradoxically, increased expression of eNOS or iNOS could be associated with decreased bioavailability of NO through the reaction of NO with superoxide, resulting in retinal damage through protein nitration (29,33).

Tissue-Specific Vascular Changes

VASCULAR CHANGES IN THE RETINA

Diabetic retinopathy is the leading cause of blindness in industrialized nations (34). Pathologic changes in retinal microvessel structure and function have been considered the major cause of diabetic retinopathy (35,36). Structural changes include thickening of the capillary basement membrane, increased vessel permeability, loss of retinal pericytes, and formation of capillary microaneurysms. These structural changes are accompanied by decreased retinal blood flow, capillary occlusion, angiogenesis, hemorrhage, fibrotic tissue formation, and tractional retinal detachment. Some of these events, or all of them in combination, can ultimately result in impairment or complete loss of vision (35).

In physiologic states, retinal capillaries consist of contractile pericytes and endothelial cells at an approximate ratio of 1:1, which is lower than the ratio of contractile cells relative to endothelial cells in other vascular beds in the systemic circulation (37,38). This ratio drops to 1:10 in moderate-to-severe stages of nonproliferative retinopathy (39,40). Areas of pericyte loss are generally associated with microaneurysms, where endothelial cells are not supported by pericytes. It has been proposed that there are extensive interactions between pericytes and capillary endothelial cells and that the presence of pericytes is necessary for stabilization of endothelial cells and the maintenance of integrity of the vasculature (41–43). Loss of pericytes causes the formation of microaneurysms and acellular capillaries, further contributing to increased permeability, decreased retinal blood flow, and leukostasis (41–43). The role of pericytes in the integrity of retinal capillaries has been confirmed by studies of mice null for the platelet-derived growth factor-β (PDGF-β) receptor. These animals show loss of pericytes, the formation of microaneurysms, and retinal hemorrhage similar to the changes seen in diabetic retinopathy (44).

Retinal hypoxia increases the expression of a host of angiogenic factors, including, among others, VEGF and placenta growth factor (PIGF), that in turn promote neovascularization. The mechanisms for the altered expression of these growth factors and their molecular effects are discussed in later sections of this chapter.

THE RENAL VASCULATURE IN DIABETES

Acute glomerular hypertrophy occurs early in the course of diabetes (45,46), but with the progressive increase in the mesangial matrix, there is a loss in capillary surface area and thus a decrease in filtration area. Changes in the composition of the basement membrane result in altered permeability and accumulation of glomerular extracellular matrix, eventually leading to glomerular occlusion, fibrosis, and deceased filtering capacity.

The glomerular basement membrane is continuous with the tubular basement membrane via the Bowman capsule. Thickening of basement membrane and expansion of the mesangium are the dominant morphologic features in early diabetic renal disease. Thickening of the glomerular basement membrane was first described by Kimmelstiel and Wilson (47). The hemodynamic factors implicated in the pathogenesis of diabetic nephropathy include increased systemic and intraglomerular pressure. Permeability of the capillaries is altered such that the excretion of proteins with molecular masses of 44 to 150 kDa is increased. Thus, albumin excretion is increased early in diabetes and, like an elevated glomerular filtration rate, can be normalized by intensive insulin treatment (48) or islet cell transplantation (49). This initial alteration in permeability seems to be due primarily to increased filtration pressures across the glomerulus, but altered electrical-charge selectivity of the permeability barrier—changes that permit an increase in the leakage of plasma proteins—may also be involved (50).

Changes in glomerular hemodynamics are mediated in part by circulating or paracrine factors such as ATII and endothelin-1 (ET-1) (51). Similarly, several mediators lead to increased production of extracellular matrix, most notably TGF-β and CTGF. As in changes observed in diabetic retinopathy, increased vascular permeability is also an early manifestation of diabetic nephropathy, with VEGF playing an important role. Signaling pathways operating in diabetic nephropathy are discussed further in subsequent sections.

VASCULAR CHANGES IN NERVES

Diabetic neuropathy is common in diabetic patients, with a prevalence of more than 50% (52). The pathogenesis is multifactorial and considered to be both hyperglycemia-induced pathologic changes intrinsic to neurons (53) and ischemia-induced neuronal damage by decreased neurovascular blood flow (54). Because of the vascular elements, diabetic neuropathy is considered a microvascular complication. Histologically, increases in endothelial cell area and luminar narrowing of capillaries are present in the endoneurium of patients with diabetes (55). Supporting a role for decreased neural blood flow was the finding that, in rats with streptozotocin-induced diabetes, *in vivo* gene transfer of VEGF restored blood flow in the neurotrophic blood vessels and improved nerve function (56). A role for PKC activation in the microvascular changes in diabetic nerve was demonstrated in the same animal model, in which an inhibitor of PKCβ prevented diabetes-induced impairment of nerve blood flow (57,58).

MICROVASCULAR CHANGES IN THE HEART

Patients with diabetes have a high prevalence of chronic heart failure (59) and a high incidence of heart failure and re-infarction after acute myocardial infarction (60); these cannot be explained by more extensive coronary atherosclerosis, a higher prevalence of hypertension, or larger infarcts in this population than in people without diabetes. The causes are likely diastolic dysfunction (61) and insufficient neovascularization during myocardial ischemia (62). Myocardial disease is not a microvascular disease in the traditional sense, yet there are conspicuous similarities in the diabetic heart and traditional microvascular complications, on both pathoanatomic and molecular levels, especially with regard to the production of extracellular matrix as in the diabetic kidney.

An autopsy study showed that the capillary density in nondiabetic patients with a previous myocardial infarction was higher than in normal hearts, but capillary density in diabetic patients with a previous myocardial infarction was lower than in normal hearts (63). Similar observations have been made in animal models of diabetes (64,65), and increased capillary permeability has been reported (66). Cardiac angiogenesis and collateral formation are governed by the balanced action of a wide spectrum of pro-angiogenic and anti-angiogenic factors, including VEGF, fibroblast growth factor (FGF), PDGF, and angiopoietins (67). The altered expression and action of these growth factors is discussed in sections below. Regardless of the individual contribution of these factors to insufficient circulation in diabetic heart disease, clinical trials aimed at treating myocardial ischemia with transfer of certain of these growth factor genes show promise, albeit they have not yet yielded definite results (67).

Diffuse cardiac fibrosis is observed in diabetes (68) and may contribute to diastolic dysfunction. Similar to the pathology of the diabetic kidney, the amount of extracellular matrix is increased in the diabetic heart (69,70).

MECHANISMS FOR MICROVASCULAR PATHOLOGY IN DIABETES

The partial loss of insulin effects—due to dysfunction or destruction of β-cells or to peripheral insulin resistance—and the ensuing hyperglycemia and other disturbances of metabolism have profound consequences on cellular function, extracellular matrix, organ function, and whole-body physiology. The discussion below starts with a description of systemic factors affecting the tissues prone to microvascular complications. On a cellular level, striking similarities exist between many mechanisms thought to be responsible for microvascular complications. Therefore, most of the discussion will be organized according to metabolic pathways or intracellular or extracellular signaling pathways altered by diabetes rather than being divided into sections concerned with the changes characteristic for tissues afflicted by microvascular complications.

Local Changes Caused by Systemic Factors

HYPERTENSION

Microvascular dysfunction and pathology may be initiated by hypertension. For example, the glomerular hyperfiltration observed in diabetes may be caused in part by systemic hypertension. Mechanisms have been described that link mechanical forces to vascular dysfunction, including pressure (71), stretch (72), and shear stress (73). Indirect proof that hypertension in itself may be a cause of microvascular complications is given by clinical trials of antihypertensive drugs that prevent diabetic nephropathy regardless of whether they are diuretics, calcium-channel blockers, or angiotensin-converting enzyme (ACE) inhibitors.

However, hypertension per se is not likely sufficient for the development of microvascular complications. In rats with streptozotocin-induced diabetes or in rats heterozygous for a renin transgene, endothelin receptor and angiotensin receptor 1 (AT1) antagonists both normalized hypertension and partly attenuated declining glomerular filtration rate, but only the AT1 antagonist affected renal pathology as well as expression of TGF-β and type IV collagen messenger RNA (mRNA) (74).

SYMPATHETIC NERVOUS SYSTEM

Overactivity of the sympathetic nervous system can be a participating factor in the development of hypertension in both types of diabetes (75). Furthermore, insulin is thought to have vasoconstrictor effects through activation of the sympathetic nervous system, but insulin-stimulated sympathetic activation is altered in states of insulin resistance (76). During late stages of diabetes, sympathetic denervation may alter vascular responses (76). How sympathetic overactivity, insulin resistance, and autonomic dysfunction quantitatively contribute to integrated vascular function in diabetes is unknown.

ADVANCED GLYCATION END-PRODUCTS

Modification of extracellular and intracellular proteins by sugars can result in the formation of AGEs, which is virtually irreversible (77). This reaction can take place nonenzymatically between glucose and protein through the Amadori product (1-amino-1-deoxyfructose adducts to lysine). However, much faster reactions occur between proteins and intracellularly formed dicarbonyls, including 3-deoxyglucosone, glyoxal, and methylglyoxal. These processes are accelerated by reactive oxygen species (78), perhaps by inhibition of glyceraldehyde-phosphate dehydrogenase (GAPDH), leading to an increase in the formation of triose phosphate, in turn increasing the production of methylglyoxal (79). The most prevalent AGE is carboxymethyl-lysine (80,81). Further nonenzymatic modification results in cross-linking of proteins. Because of their long turnover rate, structural extracellular proteins such as collagen are particularly susceptible to AGE modification. AGEs have been demonstrated in numerous tissues in both types of diabetes, such as the retina (82) and the glomeruli (83).

AGEs may interfere with vascular signaling by facilitating breakdown of NO (84). Furthermore, AGEs may impair the function of intracellular proteins, as in the case of reduced activity of basic fibroblastic growth factor in endothelial cells (85). AGEs also alter the properties of the extracellular matrix. Thus, glycosylation of collagen type IV renders it resistant to degradation by MMP (86). AGE cross-linking of type I collagen expands the packing of collagen molecules (87). Glycosylation of a carboxy-terminal domain of type IV collagen interferes with the normal assembly of collagen networks (88). AGE formation in laminin inhibits assembly of laminin polymers (89) and decreases binding to type IV collagen and heparan sulfate (79). Furthermore, AGE modification alters matrix-cell interactions. For example, modification of type IV collagen decreases endothelial cell adhesion (90). Last, AGE also may act through binding to receptors, the most well characterized being the receptor of AGE (RAGE) (81). It is interesting that stimulation of RAGE can lead to transdifferentiation of renal tubular epithelial cells to myofibroblasts (91), which may be responsible for accumulation of extracellular matrix.

The ability of RAGE signaling to cause diabetic complications was demonstrated directly in a study in which transgenic mice overexpressing iNOS targeted to insulin-producing cells, providing a model for type 1 diabetes, were cross-bred with transgenic mice overexpressing RAGE. Development of glomerular lesions was accelerated in these double-transgenic mice (92) and could be prevented by an AGE inhibitor (92).

AGE formation has effects on numerous vascular signaling molecules. Thus, they reduce the expression of eNOS (93) and increase the expression of ET-1 (94) in endothelial-cell culture. AGEs, through increased production of reactive oxygen species (ROS), activate NF-κB (95), which is responsible for induction of several growth factors. AGEs also increase expression of TGF-β in mesenteric vessels (96) and increase retinal VEGF expression (97). In endothelial-cell culture, AGEs, via RAGE, decrease production of prostacyclin, induce expression of plasminogen activator inhibitor-1 (PAI-1) (98), and induce expression of adhesion molecules in endothelium (99). A soluble receptor for RAGE inhibits barrier function in endothelial cells and vascular permeability in diabetic rats (100).

Many approaches to the pharmacologic inhibition of AGE formation are being attempted. Aminoguanidine, an inhibitor of AGE formation, has shown an effect on preventing nephropathy (101) and retinopathy (102) in animal models of diabetes. Newer agents are being developed, including 2,3-diaminophenazine, an inhibitor of AGE formation (103); ALT-711, which breaks AGE cross-links (104); pyridoxamine; and OBP-9195 (105). It is interesting that treatment with the ACE inhibitor ramipril decreased renal AGE accumulation to the same extent as did an inhibitor of AGE formation, aminoguanidine, perhaps by preventing activation of NAD(P)H oxidase [reduced form of nicotinamide adenine dinucleotide (phosphate)] (106). Results are not yet available from clinical trials with AGE inhibitors for the treatment of diabetic microvascular complications.

VASCULAR INFLAMMATION

Typical elements of inflammatory processes are evident in the vasculature in diabetes (107). Increased expression of vascular adhesion molecules leading to recruitment of leukocytes to the vascular wall is regarded as a pivotal event in early inflammation. Blocking intracellular adhesion molecule-1 (ICAM-1) prevents leukostasis and retinal vascular leakage. The pro-inflammatory cytokine tumor necrosis factor-α (TNF-α) is induced in rats with streptozotocin-induced diabetes (31).

Treatment of such animals with high-dose aspirin; the cyclooxygenase-2 inhibitor meloxicam; or eternacept, which blocks TNF-α actions by competing with its tissue receptors, prevents increased ICAM-1 expression, leukostasis, capillary leakage, and upregulation of eNOS (31). Inflammation may therefore play a role in the development of microvascular complications of diabetes, but current information on this subject is sparse.

Intracellular Consequences of Altered Metabolism

INCREASED INTRACELLULAR GLUCOSE CONCENTRATIONS

Interventional trials of hypoglycemic drug therapy have unequivocally linked hyperglycemia with the development and progression of microvascular complications (108–110). Lowering blood glucose levels has been less successful in preventing atherothrombotic complications, suggesting that factors other than hyperglycemia may be more important for the development of macrovascular complications. The perception of hyperglycemia as the primary cause for microvascular complications explains why the vast majority of studies of the mechanisms responsible have focused on the effects of increased glucose concentrations, even though multiple other metabolic alterations exist in diabetes.

Many of the mechanisms on the cellular level described below involve alteration of cellular homeostasis caused by increased cellular glucose uptake and increased intracellular glucose concentration. This is prevented in part in tissues where insulin resistance decreases cellular glucose uptake. Insulin resistance can thus be viewed as a compensatory mechanism to avoid excessive intracellular glucose concentrations; this has prompted the speculation that tissues that do not have this capability are those prone to diabetic complications (111). Aortic endothelial and smooth muscle cells express GLUT1 (a glucose transport protein not responsive to insulin) but do not express GLUT2 to GLUT5 (112). VSMC can downregulate GLUT1 in response to increasing extracellular glucose concentrations, but endothelial cells cannot (112), thus making endothelial cells more susceptible to the effects of hyperglycemia. Similarly, overexpression of GLUT1, which is not regulated by insulin, in mesangial cells cultured in normal glucose concentrations increased collagen metabolism and accumulation (113).

Characterization of the regulation of glucose transporters in different tissues prone to microvascular complications is not complete, and the dogma given above may not be valid in all tissues. For example, GLUT1, the primary glucose transporter in the retina, is downregulated in diabetes (114). Likewise, insulin stimulates glucose uptake and glycogen synthesis in retinal capillary endothelial cells, but—as expected from the expression of GLUT isoforms—not in aortic endothelial cells (115).

INTRACELLULAR REDOX STATUS AND OXIDATIVE STRESS

Oxidative stress, i.e., an imbalance between ROS and cellular antioxidant defense systems (116,117), may result from alterations of glucose metabolism or be secondary to activation or dysregulation of several enzymes not directly involved in glucose metabolism. In population-based cohorts, vascular oxidative stress, measured by plasma markers, is associated with diabetes, even after adjustments are made for several covariables (118). Furthermore, patients with diabetes have a depletion of the reduced form of intracellular glutathione (119), but an increase in plasma extracellular superoxide dismutase, which is associated with severity of retinopathy and nephropathy (120). Oxidative stress has been demonstrated in organs affected by complications of diabetes; thus, in the vitreous body of the eye of patients with diabetes, lower levels of oxidative metabolites are associated with better blood glucose control (121). On the other hand, intervention against oxidative stress has been shown to prevent organ damage in animal models. For example, transgenic mice overexpressing superoxide dismutase are protected from renal complications of streptozotocin-induced diabetes (122), and long-term treatment of diabetic rodents with antioxidants has had beneficial effects on the development of complications in the retina (123), the kidney (124), and the peripheral nerve (125,126).

In patients with diabetes, smaller trials have shown that dietary supplementation with vitamin E lowers the albumin excretion rate (127,128) and creatinine clearance (128), increases retinal blood flow (128), and improves nerve conduction (129). However, in a substudy of HOPE (Heart Outcomes Prevention Evaluation), currently the largest completed clinical trial of antioxidant therapy, vitamin E supplementation did not decrease the need for retinal laser therapy or improve the urine albumin-creatinine ratio (130).

Oxidative stress may cause cellular dysfunction by promoting formation of AGEs, by inducing DNA strand breaks and activating poly(ADP-ribose) polymerase (PARP) (131,132), by causing dysfunction of eNOS, and by activating p38 and other stress-activated pathways leading to apoptosis. These and other mechanisms are discussed below.

Polyol Pathway. Increased cellular glucose uptake increases the flux of glucose through the polyol pathway (also known as the sorbitol pathway), which consumes NADPH by the aldose reductase reaction and reduces NAD^+ (the oxidized form of nicotinamide adenine dinucleotide) by the sorbitol reductase reaction (133). Activation of the polyol pathway not only may result from increased availability of glucose, the upstream substrate for the pathway, but also may be secondary to inactivation of GAPDH, thus diverting glucose from glycolysis to other pathways of glucose metabolism (132). An overactive polyol pathway will therefore deplete cytosolic NADPH, which is necessary to maintain the primary intracellular antioxidant, glutathione, in its reduced state. Aldose reductase inhibition reduces neuropathy in diabetic dogs (134) and patients with diabetes (135), but although early studies in animal models of diabetes showed promise with regard to an effect on retinopathy or nephropathy, such effects have not been demonstrated in patients with diabetes (134,136).

Pentose Phosphate Pathway. By a different mechanism, increased glucose concentrations may inhibit glucose-6-phosphate dehydrogenase, which catalyzes the first intermediary reaction in the pentose phosphate pathway, the primary source of intracellular NADPH (137–139).

Superoxide Production from Mitochondria. In mitochondria, the citric acid cycle provides NADH and $FADH_2$ (reduced form of flavin adenine dinucleotide), which can act as electron donors for the electron transport chain, creating a proton gradient over the inner mitochondrial membrane. If intracellular glucose concentrations are increased, yielding excessive reducing equivalents for this process, the proton gradient will be high and inhibit the transfer of electrons from reduced coenzyme Q (ubiquinone) to complex III of the electron transport chain (140). Instead, electrons will be transferred to molecular oxygen, producing superoxide.

Vascular NAD(P)H Oxidase. The most important source of superoxide quantitatively in the vascular wall is thought to be an NAD(P)H oxidase that resembles the phagocytic NADPH oxidase but favors NADH as a substrate (141). This oxidase is expressed in endothelial cells (142) and VSMCs (141). Expression and activity of vascular NAD(P)H oxidase is increased in rat models of type 1 (143) and type 2 (144) diabetes. This enzyme may be activated by an increase in the $NADH/NAD^+$ ratio, which in diabetes may be caused by an increased flux through the polyol pathway (see above) or activation of PARP (131). The lactate/pyruvate concentration ratio is an index of cytosolic

NADH/NAD$^+$ ratio, as pyruvate reduces NAD$^+$ in the lactate dehydrogenase reaction. In endothelial-cell cultures, superoxide production is increased by the addition of lactate and decreased by the addition of pyruvate (145). Apart from regulation by cofactor requirements, vascular NAD(P)H oxidase may be regulated by alterations in signaling pathways. Thus, NAD(P)H oxidase activity may be increased by elevated concentrations of glucose and free fatty acids through PKC activation (146), and its expression may be increased by ET-1 (147).

eNOS Dysfunction. Oxidative stress may inhibit NO-mediated endothelial function by degrading NO (148). Alternatively, it may lead to decreased intracellular concentrations of the reduced, active form of BH4, a cofactor for eNOS. The reason for this may be that BH4 either cannot be kept in the reduced form because of decreased NAPDH concentrations (139) or because BH4 is oxidized, preferentially by reaction with peroxynitrite (149). Suboptimal BH4 concentrations lead to "uncoupling" of the oxidase and reductase domain of NO synthase (150), which results in the oxidation of molecular oxygen instead of L-arginine and the synthesis of superoxide instead of NO. Thus, BH4 deficiency may be both cause and effect of vascular oxidative stress (151). Uncoupling of eNOS by peroxynitrate may also be caused by disruption of a zinc-thiolate cluster that stabilizes eNOS as a dimer (152).

In studies of fructose-fed rats, a model of insulin resistance, endothelial BH4 concentrations were reduced and concentrations of oxidized BH4 were increased (153,154). Furthermore, superoxide generation was increased, NO production was decreased, and endothelium-dependent vasorelaxation was impaired. The functional abnormalities were improved by *ex vivo* exposure of vascular tissue to BH4 (153). Oral administration of BH4 increased endothelial BH4 concentrations and improved the functional abnormalities (154). In patients with type 2 diabetes, intrabrachial infusion of BH4 increased forearm endothelium-dependent vasodilation (155).

Tyrosine Nitration. Superoxide reacts with NO with a very high rate constant. The product is the highly reactive intermediate peroxynitrate, which may react with a host of intracellular molecules. One such target is the tyrosine residues of proteins, a reaction that may result in tyrosine nitration (29). Mg-superoxide dismutase (SOD) seems to be a particularly susceptible target for such modification, which decreases its catalytic activity, thus potentially further aggravating oxidative stress (156). Examples of other enzymes modified in this manner include certain metabolic enzymes (157) and prostacyclin synthase (158).

Other Sources of Oxidative Stress. High glucose concentrations may also lead to oxidative stress through activation of xanthine oxidase (159), through glucose autoxidation (160), after formation of ketone bodies (161), or through lipid peroxidation (116).

Antioxidant Defense. Antioxidant defense may be increased in diabetes as a compensatory mechanism to counter the production of ROS, but this mobilization of defense may be inadequate. Thus, in endothelial-cell cultures, high glucose concentrations induce the expression of CuZn-SOD, catalase, and glutathione peroxidase (162), and in patients with diabetes, the plasma concentration of extracellular SOD is increased (120). Accordingly, transgenic mice overexpressing CuZn-SOD are protected from glomerular injury of CuZn-SOD after induction of diabetes (122). However, glutathione synthesis in endothelial cells may be inhibited by high glucose concentrations (163).

HEXOSAMINE PATHWAY AND *O*-LINKED GLYCOSYLATION

Posttranslational modification of nuclear and cytosolic proteins may occur as *O*-linked glycosylation on serine or threonine residues. As with phosphorylation, this may take place as a dynamic modification that modifies protein function (164). *O*-linked glycosylation of certain proteins is increased in diabetes because increased cellular uptake of glucose activates the hexosamine pathway, which results in production of uridine-diphospho-*N*-acetyl-glucosamine, a substrate in the glycosylation reaction (111,165). Activation of the hexosamine pathway is not only a result of increased substrate availability; in patients with diabetes, the expression of glutamine:fructose-6-phosphate amidotransferase (GFAT), the rate-limiting enzyme for the hexosamine pathway, is increased in several tissues prone to complications (166). Little is known about the signaling pathways responsible for GFAT induction, but an example is the activation by ATII of the promoter for GFAT via the AT1 receptor (167). Through activation of the hexosamine pathway, diabetes and high glucose concentrations may lead to *O*-linked glycosylation of eNOS on serine 1177, prohibiting activation of the enzyme by phosphorylation on this residue (168,169). When mesangial cells are grown at high glucose concentrations or with glucosamine or when the cells are transfected with GFAT, *O*-linked glycosylation of p65 NF-κB is increased; this nuclear factor in turn can activate several gene programs, among them pro-inflammatory genes (170). Activation of the hexosamine pathway in mesangial cells also increases the activity of PAI-1 gene transcription (171); this can be mediated through another nuclear factor, Sp1, which may also be glycosylated by high glucose concentrations, leading to increased expression of PAI-1 (172). In glomerular mesangial cells, this is dependent on activation of PKCβ1 and δ (173). Certain growth factors, including TGF-α, are other gene targets for Sp1 activation (174).

Alterations in Intracellular Signal Transduction

ACTIVATION OF PROTEIN KINASE C

In diabetes, PKC is activated in vascular tissue. At least 12 isoforms of PKC exist, and 9 of them are activated by the phospholipid diacylglycerol (DAG). The first described mechanism of PKC activation involves transient receptor-mediated stimulation of phospholipase C, which hydrolyzes inositol phospholipids of the plasma membrane to yield DAG, which again activates PKC after binding to an amino-terminal domain of the enzyme. In diabetes, however, intracellular DAG can also be increased in vascular tissue through *de novo* synthesis from glucose (175) via glyceraldehyde 3-phosphate and phosphatidic acid or from nonesterified fatty acids (176,177). In particular, the β2 isoform of PKC is activated in the retina and renal glomeruli, and treatment with an inhibitor specific for the PKCβ2 isoform partly normalizes retinal blood flow and albuminuria in rats with streptozotocin-induced diabetes (27). Likewise, the same inhibitor decreases mesangial expansion and albuminuria in diabetic db/db mice (178).

Theoretically, PKC may be activated in diabetes independently of DAG synthesis. Thus, *cis*-unsaturated fatty acids may synergistically increase the effect of DAG at basal levels of Ca^{2+} (179,180). Furthermore, superoxide may directly activate PKC by releasing zinc from the zinc finger of the enzyme (181). Whether PKC is activated by such mechanisms in diabetes is unknown. It is interesting that treatment with vitamin E inhibits PKC by lowering vascular DAG concentrations (182), perhaps by increasing the enzymatic breakdown of DAG to phosphatidic acid (183) or by activating protein phosphatase 2A, which will dephosphorylate PKC (184). This may be independent of the antioxidant effects of the vitamin (185).

Vascular PKC activation causes endothelial dysfunction (186). Impaired endothelium-dependent relaxation during high glucose concentrations is prevented by a PKC inhibitor (186). Oral administration of a selective inhibitor of the PKCβ isoform prevents endothelial dysfunction in rats with streptozotocin-induced diabetes (187) or in healthy humans after 6 hours of hyperglycemic clamp (188).

Activation of PKC in the vasculature by high glucose concentrations elicits a host of signaling responses in different vascular cell types. For example, increased concentrations of DAG and PKC activation result in increased expression of ATII in proximal tubular cells (189). Induction of TGF-β in the kidney in diabetic rodents is dependent on PKC. Furthermore, increased permeability of endothelial cells cultured at high glucose concentrations is mediated by PKC (190).

The complexity of the role of PKC in signal transduction pathways important for pathogenesis of microvascular complications is illustrated by the fact that PKC activity may be both upstream and downstream of other mediators such as VEGF and ET-1. Thus, activation of PKC by high glucose may induce VEGF (191) and ET-1 (192), but VEGF-induced proliferation of endothelial cells (193) and retinal neovascularization (194) are dependent on PKC. Furthermore, the induction of ET-1 by PDGF in retinal pericytes (195) and stimulation of mitogen-activated protein kinase (MAPK) by ET-1 in mesangial cells cultured in high concentrations of glucose (196) are dependent on PKC. Other roles for PKC in several signal transduction mechanisms are discussed elsewhere in this chapter.

SELECTIVE VASCULAR INSULIN RESISTANCE

Insulin stimulates skeletal muscle blood flow in healthy, lean individuals (197), but this effect is blunted in people who are obese (197) or who have type 2 diabetes (198). Whether insulin-stimulated blood flow is limiting for insulin-stimulated glucose uptake in skeletal muscle is controversial (199), and vascular effects participating in insulin-stimulated glucose uptake may be represented by insulin-stimulated capillary recruitment rather than by insulin-stimulated blood flow (200,201). Retinal and kidney blood flow also is stimulated during systemic hyperinsulinemia (202,203).

Insulin-stimulated vasorelaxation is a direct effect on blood vessels mediated by endothelium-derived NO and is independent of hormones or activation of the autonomic nervous system (204–206). Regardless of the contribution of vasodilation to glucose uptake during insulin stimulation, insulin-stimulated endothelial NO production may be an important mechanism for vascular homeostasis that is absent in insulin resistance.

Insulin increases endothelial NO production by rapid post-translational mechanisms (207), as well as by induction of eNOS gene expression (208). Both effects are mediated by the 1-phosphatidylinositol 3-kinase (PI3K)–Akt signaling pathway (207,208). However, the MAPK pathway, which mediates the effects of insulin on vascular growth, is intact (209). Thus, a selective insulin resistance to the vascular PI3K-Akt-eNOS signaling pathway exists. Insulin-stimulated insulin receptor substrate (IRS) tyrosine phosphorylation and activation of PI3K and Akt are decreased in the vasculature of Zucker rats (209). But several of these signaling molecules may be affected individually. As an example, *O*-linked glycosylation affects IRS and p85 (169), as well as eNOS itself (168,169). Inhibition of the PI3K pathway may have significance for a variety of stimuli for endothelial NO production, as shear stress, VEGF, and estrogen are also mediated by the PI3K-Akt pathway (210). The cause of vascular insulin resistance has not been described sufficiently but may involve inhibitory effects of ATII on IRS-1 and PI3K (211) or activation of PKC (208).

The physiologic importance of vascular insulin signaling has been demonstrated in knockout animal models. Mice with deletion of the insulin receptor gene in endothelial cells have decreased expression of eNOS in the aorta and in cultured lung endothelial cells (212). Insulin also induces ET-1, and mice with endothelial insulin receptor knockout have decreased vascular expression of ET-1 (212). Moreover, insulin induces VEGF (213), and mice with knockout of the insulin receptor in endothelial cells have decreased retinal neovascularization in the relative hypoxia model as compared with control mice, paralleled with a decreased induction of eNOS, VEGF, and ET-1 (214).

Insulin increases TGF-β secretion by renal proximal tubular cells (215). The effect of insulin on production of growth factors and profibrotic factors may be mediated by MAPK pathways, and to the extent that this insulin-signaling pathway is normal in diabetes (209), hyperinsulinemia may be a cause of microvascular complications.

MITOGEN-ACTIVATED PROTEIN KINASE

Many effects of the diabetic milieu are transduced through the MAPK Erk1/2, p38, and JNK. Inhibition of MAPK, and JNK in particular, is being tested as a treatment for diabetes (216). At high glucose concentrations, JNK is activated in VSMCs (217) and endothelial cells (10), which may lead to apoptosis (10). Under such conditions, activation of p38 MAPK [in VSMCs (217,218)] and Erk1/2 (in mesangial cells [219]) has also been reported.

CELL-CYCLE REGULATION

During cell proliferation, cells have to pass through the G1 phase of the cell cycle and enter the S phase and subsequent phases. The exit from the G1 phase is regulated by heterodimers of cyclins and cyclin-dependent kinases (CDKs), e.g., by phosphorylation of the Rb gene product. This can be modified by CDK inhibitors, among them $p21^{Cip1}$ and $p27^{Kip1}$. There is evidence that the renal pathology in diabetes includes cellular hypertrophy in the glomerulus because cells are arrested in G1 phase, in which synthesis of structural proteins occurs without subsequent DNA synthesis or cell division (220).

Proof of the relevance of such mechanisms for diabetic complications is given in studies of streptozotocin-induced diabetes that caused glomerular expansion because of cellular hypertrophy in wild-type mice but not in mice with knockout of $p21^{Cip1}$ (221). Increased expression of glomerular fibronectin, as well as glomerular and renal hypertrophy, mesangial expansion, and albuminuria during streptozotocin-induced diabetes, is partly prevented in mice with knockout of $p27^{Kip1}$ (222,223).

Such maintenance of glomerular cells in G1 phase may be caused by sustained partial phosphorylation of Rb protein (224). In contrast, proliferating cells in the retina depend on hyperphosphorylation of Rb protein and exit from the G1 phase. Thus, in retinal endothelial cells, the mitogenic action of VEGF is mediated through phosphorylation of Rb by PKCβ2 (194).

Abnormal Regulation of Extracellular Signaling Molecules

GROWTH FACTORS, CYTOKINES, AND OTHER REGULATORS OF CELL GROWTH

The sections below describe selected growth factors separately, although growth factors often act in concert. Description of the cooperative actions of growth factors has begun only recently. A few examples are summarized in the following. Hypoxia and TGF-β, through the transcription factors hypoxia-inducible factor and Smad3, act synergistically to increase VEGF transcription (225). VEGF and PDGF act synergistically to stimulate angiogenesis when VEGFR-1, activated by PDGF, cross-activates VEGFR-2, in turn activated by VEGF (226). Insulin-like growth factor-1 (IGF-1) signaling through its receptor is necessary for the full effects of VEGF on neovascularization (227), and fibroblast growth factor (FGF) and PDGF have superadditive effects on neovascularization (228).

Some growth factors not described below appear to lack major individual effects even though their expression may be altered in diabetes. As an example, fibroblast growth factor-2 (FGF2) concentrations are elevated in patients with diabetic proliferative retinopathy (229,230). Even though FGF can act synergistically with or lead to induction of other growth factors (228,231), transgenic mice overexpressing FGF2 or mice with knockout of the FGF2 gene show no difference in ischemia-associated neovascularization (232), thus arguing against an independent role for FGF in retinopathy.

Vascular Endothelial Growth Factor. VEGF initially was described as a factor mediating vascular permeability. It has since been found to be a potent mediator of angiogenesis (233). In diabetic retinopathy, VEGF is a key regulator of neovascularization and increased vascular permeability, which are key factors for loss of vision. In patients with diabetes, the concentration of VEGF is increased in ocular fluids (234), and its expression, which is rarely detected in normal retinas, is increased in retinas of patients with diabetes, particularly in endothelial cells and perivascular regions (235). Furthermore, retinal VEGF receptors are not detected in nondiabetic animals but are strongly expressed in rats with streptozotocin-induced diabetes (236). VEGF receptors are tyrosine kinase receptors and exist as two types, VEGFR-1 and -2 (previously named Flt-1 and KDR [or Flk-1], respectively) (233). Intravitreous injection of chimeric proteins constructed from the extracellular domain of either receptor joined to IgG showed very high efficiency in preventing ischemia-induced retinal neovascularization (237).

Increased expression of VEGF and its receptors also is found in the kidneys of rats with streptozotocin-induced diabetes (238) and patients with diabetes (239). Renal pathoanatomic changes and function in rats with streptozotocin-induced diabetes (240) or in db/db mice (241) are prevented by treatment with antibodies to VEGF.

Other diabetic complications, however, may result from a decreased angiogenic response and may be responsive to therapy with VEGF. This paradox is well recognized (242). In the heart, local actions of VEGF are needed for normal structure and function, as demonstrated by findings in mice with targeted knockout of VEGF in cardiomyocytes. This genetic manipulation results in several cardiac abnormalities, including fewer cardiac microvessels (243). In diabetes, expression of VEGF and its receptors is decreased in the myocardium even though expression is increased in the retina and glomeruli (1). Several clinical trials have shown an effect of intracoronary VEGF gene transfer to patients with ischemic heart disease (244,245). Similarly, gene VEGF transfer by intramuscular injection of plasmids normalizes the decreased number of blood vessels and reduces nerve blood flow and peripheral neuropathy resulting from streptozotocin- and alloxan-induced diabetes (56). Thus, increased VEGF expression mediates some of the pathology in retinopathy and nephropathy, and treatment strategies aimed at antagonizing VEGF in retinopathy are being evaluated. At the same time, a deficient VEGF response may be present in ischemic heart disease and peripheral ischemia of diabetes and in diabetic neuropathy. Therefore, caution must be taken to ensure the overall success of these therapeutic approaches.

Platelet-Derived Growth Factor. The concentration of PDGF in the vitreous is increased in patients with proliferative retinopathy (246). PDGF acts as a growth factor for retinal endothelial cells through a paracrine/autocrine mechanism (247). PDGF expression is increased in pericytes cultured in high glucose concentrations and in the retina of rats with streptozotocin-induced diabetes (195), and high glucose concentrations increase the expression of PDGF receptor-β in a variety of vascular cells (248). PDGF may upregulate expression of TGF-β protein synergistically with high glucose concentrations through stabilization of TGF-β mRNA (249).

Even though PDGF is upregulated in diabetes, deletion of the PDGF gene paradoxically leads to a phenotype resembling diabetic retinopathy. Thus, PDGF knockout mouse embryos show pericyte loss and endothelial cell proliferation (44), and mice with a heterozygous deletion of the PDGF gene (250) or deletion of PDGF gene targeted to endothelium (251) show pericyte loss and endothelial cell proliferation. It is therefore possible that PDGF upregulation in the diabetic retina is compensating for a postreceptor defect in PDGF signaling, although this remains to be investigated.

Transforming Growth Factor-β. TGF-β, as measured by the Fick principle, is excreted in the kidneys of patients with type 2 diabetes, whereas a net renal extraction is present in the kidneys of healthy people without diabetes (252). Also, among patients with type 2 diabetes, expression of TGF-β mRNA is higher in those with nephropathy (253). In db/db mice, TGF-β shows increased expression in both glomerular and tubular compartments (254).

In mice with streptozotocin-induced diabetes (2) or in db/db mice (3), treatment with neutralizing antibodies to TGF-β prevents glomerular hypertrophy; attenuates increased kidney size (2), mesangial matrix expansion, and increases in plasma creatinine (3); and attenuates induction of TGF-β, type IV collagen, and fibronectin (2,3). In mice with streptozotocin-induced diabetes, treatment with TGF-β antisense oligodeoxynucleotides has the same effects on kidney weight and expression of TGF-β and extracellular matrix proteins (255). The effects of TGF-β on cellular hypertrophy may be caused in part by upregulation of its receptor (256).

Induction of TGF-β may be caused by accumulation of AGE (96). Downstream TGF-β signaling has been described to some extent; e.g., TGF-β mediates expression of type I collagen through Sp1 and Smad3 (257).

In cell cultures, TGF-β is produced by and is acting in a paracrine/autocrine manner on mesangial cells (258), cortical fibroblasts (259), tubular cells (91), and glomerular endothelial cells (260). But TGF-β can be induced by stimuli produced outside the kidney. For example, leptin induces TGF-β1 in glomerular endothelial cells (261) and expression of type II TGF-β receptor (262). Therefore, the quantitatively most important stimulus for TGF-β secretion remains ill-defined, and so do the cell types that represent the source of TGF-β and the target of its actions.

Connective Tissue Growth Factor. As a downstream mediator of some of the effects of TGF-β, CTGF has attracted much attention (263). CTGF has been detected in glomeruli from patients with diabetic nephropathy but not in glomeruli from healthy subjects (264). In mesangial cells, high glucose concentrations induce CTGF expression, and this can be prevented by an antibody to TGF-β (265,266). TGF-β induces CTGF through binding of Smad to the CTGF promotor (267). Apart from TGF-β, CTGF appears to be regulated by PKC (266). TGF-β induction of extracellular matrix proteins, among them fibronectin and collagen isoforms, is dependent on CTGF (14).

It is interesting that the mechanisms described for glomerulosclerosis have a parallel in the mechanisms by which myocardial fibrosis in diabetes is mediated by CTGF. In mice with streptozotocin-induced diabetes or in transgenic mice with overexpression of PKCβ2 targeted to myocardium, TGF-β, CTGF, fibronectin, and type VI collagen are induced as compared with the expression in nondiabetic or wild-type mice (268).

Growth Hormone/Insulin-like Growth Factor. Hypersecretion of growth hormone (GH) occurs in type 1 diabetes (269) and may be a cause of diabetic nephropathy. Thus, transgenic mice overexpressing GH and GH-releasing factor develop glomerular fibrosis (270), and this is accelerated in GH-transgenic mice with streptozotocin-induced diabetes as compared with wild-type diabetic mice (271). Furthermore, transgenic mice overexpressing a dominant-negative GH (271) or mice with knockout of the gene for GH receptor/binding protein (272) are protected from diabetic nephropathy.

Hypersecretion of GH may be a result of decreased plasma concentrations of IGF-1 (269). However, IGF-1 may be overexpressed locally in tissues. Thus, IGF-1 production in the kidney is increased in diabetic animals, and IGF-1 stimulates the production of extracellular matrix proteins from mesangial cells (14).

GH or IGF may also play a role in diabetic retinopathy. In transgenic mice overexpressing a dominant-negative GH mutant gene, or in wild-type mice treated with an inhibitor of GH secretion, ischemia-associated retinal neovascularization was inhibited despite unchanged retinal VEGF expression (273).

THE RENIN-ANGIOTENSIN SYSTEM

A large number of clinical trials have shown that treatment with ACE inhibitors, AT1 receptor blockers, or their combination can prevent the occurrence of renal disease or delay its progression to renal failure (274). Many studies also support the ability of treatment with ACE inhibitors to prevent diabetic retinopathy (274), and one trial showed that nerve electrophysiology parameters, although not clinical parameters, improved after treatment with an ACE inhibitor (275).

Hypertension is an independent risk factor for the presence of nephropathy in patients with type 2 diabetes (276). But the effect of ACE inhibitors on preventing diabetic nephropathy cannot be explained by their antihypertensive effect alone (277). Theoretically, the mechanism for the effect of ACE inhibitors on the prevention of diabetic nephropathy could be as an inhibitor of bradykinin proteolysis. However, a bradykinin B1 receptor antagonist, although efficient at blocking renal bradykinin receptors, did not prevent diabetic nephropathy by itself or affect the beneficial influence of an ACE inhibitor (278).

The demonstration that an ACE inhibitor could prevent increased glomerular capillary pressure (279) was the first indication that ACE inhibition could have renoprotective effects that were not dependent on lowering systemic blood pressure. ATI and ATII are produced locally in the kidney (280). Accordingly, in immortalized proximal tubular cells (189) and mesangial cells (20) grown in high glucose concentrations, ATII secretion is increased. It has been shown that ATII actions may lead to kidney damage through induction of local factors, including extracellular matrix protein synthesis via TGF-β (281). The same mechanism may contribute to cardiac fibrosis (282,283). Apart from promoting extracellular matrix protein synthesis in cardiac fibroblasts (282), ATII also induced myocardial PAI-1 expression, which—by inhibiting metalloproteinases—can inhibit extracellular matrix breakdown (282,284).

Intrarenal production of ATII may explain the low systemic plasma concentrations of renin in diabetes (285), as ATII suppresses renin production as a negative feedback mechanism (286).

ENDOTHELIUM-DERIVED VASODILATING AND VASOCONSTRICTING FACTORS

The most well established endothelium-derived vasomotor substances are NO, prostacyclin, and ET-1. It is important to realize that these factors have effects on several functions other than vasomotion. Endothelium-dependent vasodilating factors may substitute for each other. Thus, prostacyclin (287) and endothelium-derived hyperpolarizing factor (EDHF) (288) may substitute for NO, and decreased vascular NO production in diabetes may be compensated for, in part, by increased production of prostacyclin (289).

Nitric Oxide. Glucose-induced endothelial vasodilator dysfunction seems to be caused to a large extent by ROS. They react directly with NO, causing its degradation, and can be prevented by treatment *in vivo* with probucol, a scavenger of reactive oxygen species, by *in vivo* transfection with the Mn-SOD gene (290), or by antioxidant enzymes *ex vivo* (23).

The mechanisms responsible for decreased NO production are unclear. There are reports of downregulation of eNOS protein (291). Contradicting this finding, other results have shown eNOS mRNA and protein upregulation, accompanied by increased superoxide production, which can degrade NO (143,292). The mechanism *in vivo*, however, seems to be a compensatory increase in eNOS expression secondary to increased breakdown of NO by ROS (293). Regardless of the mechanism, the presence of impaired NO availability is supported by studies showing that *in vitro* transfection of the eNOS gene to aorta (290) and carotid artery (294) of alloxan-treated rabbits prevents impaired endothelium-dependent vasorelaxation. Apart from its role in regulating blood flow, NO may be an intermediary signaling molecule in other pathways. For example, VEGF expression is dependent on NO production (295), and in mesangial cells, NO inhibits glucose-induced expression of fibronectin (296) and collagen (297).

Prostacyclin. In endothelial cells cultured in high glucose concentrations, tyrosine nitration has been shown to decrease the activity of prostacyclin synthase (158,298). This increases apoptosis and expression of adhesion molecules, perhaps by increasing the concentration of prostacyclin precursors such as prostaglandin H_2 (158). Thus, nitration of prostacyclin synthase is associated with upregulation of cyclooxygenase-2 and may be mediated by PKC through activation of NAD(P)H oxidase (299). Prostanoid vasoconstrictors have been shown to be responsible for decreased endothelium-dependent vasodilation in blood vessels from diabetic rabbits (300).

Endothelin-1. Another important aspect of endothelial dysfunction in type 2 diabetes is increased expression of endothelium-derived ET-1, the most potent vasoconstrictor known (301). In obese individuals and in patients with type 2 diabetes, infusion of an ET_A blocker caused a vasoconstriction not seen in healthy, lean individuals, indicating that in insulin-resistant states, ET-1 contributes to basal vasoconstrictor tone (302).

High glucose concentrations activate PKCβ and δ isoforms in endothelial-cell cultures and lead to increased ET-1 expression, which is also dependent on MAPK activity in this situation (192). The downstream mediators of MAPK-regulated ET-1 induction may be the Jun/Fos proteins (303). In diabetes, ET-1 is partly responsible for abnormal retinal hemodynamics (304), and its induction may be mediated through upregulation of PDGF expression (195). Myocardial vascular tone is regulated by ET-1, but more so during rest than during exercise (305).

In endothelial cells, ET-1 expression is increased by insulin (306). The ability of insulin to increase vascular ET-1 production has also been demonstrated in humans (307). The hyperinsulinemia typical for type 2 diabetes in its earlier stages may thus be responsible for ET-1 upregulation, because the MAPK pathway of insulin signaling is not affected by diabetes (209). Apart from acting as a vasoconstrictor, ET-1 promotes fibrosis. ET-1 transgenic mice develop renal interstitial and glomerular fibrosis (308). This occurs in the absence of hypertension (308), which may be explained by a compensatory increase in vascular NO production (309). Renal fibrosis in this animal model may not be identical to that occurring in diabetes, as ET-1 transgenic mice show increased expression of laminin, but not of collagen or fibronectin (310). However, streptozotocin-treated rats show increased expression of fibronectin in retina, renal cortex, and myocardium, and this can be prevented by treatment with an ET-1 receptor antagonist (311). Upregulation of ET-1 expression may be regulated by TGF-β (312).

CONCLUSION

The evolution of our knowledge about altered hormone and cytokine action and of intercellular and intracellular signaling in diabetes has been dramatic. A major limitation of our understanding of the mechanisms leading to microvascular complications is that the sequence of events in altered signaling is often unknown and the overall significance of alteration of an individual signaling parameter often is unclear.

Good glycemic control is difficult to achieve in many patients with diabetes, and diabetic microvascular complications occur even with intensive insulin treatment regimens. In fact, even though good control can be achieved much of the time, intermittent hyperglycemia may be more damaging than constant hyperglycemia to vascular cell homeostasis (313). Although good glycemic control will remain the primary focus of diabetes care, the development of therapy that targets signaling pathways that cause vascular dysfunction and, ultimately, diabetic complications is likely to be important. Further understanding of the mechanisms responsible for the pathogenesis of these complications will ensure a rational approach to their prevention and treatment.

Acknowledgments

Dr. Rask-Madsen is supported by Danish Medical Research Council fellowship 22-01-0498, Dr. He is supported by a Mary K. Iacocca fellowship, and Dr. King is the recipient of National Institutes of Health grant R01 DK53105 and R01 DK59725.

REFERENCES

1. Chou E, Suzuma I, Way KJ, et al. Decreased cardiac expression of vascular endothelial growth factor and its receptors in insulin-resistant and diabetic states: a possible explanation for impaired collateral formation in cardiac tissue. *Circulation* 2002;105:373–379.
2. Sharma K, Jin Y, Guo J, et al. Neutralization of TGF-beta by anti-TGF-beta antibody attenuates kidney hypertrophy and the enhanced extracellular matrix gene expression in STZ-induced diabetic mice. *Diabetes* 1996;45: 522–530.
3. Ziyadeh FN, Hoffman BB, Han DC, et al. Long-term prevention of renal insufficiency, excess matrix gene expression, and glomerular mesangial matrix expansion by treatment with monoclonal antitransforming growth factor-beta antibody in db/db diabetic mice. *Proc Natl Acad Sci U S A* 2000;97: 8015–8020.
4. van Royen N, Hoefer I, Buschmann I, et al. Exogenous application of transforming growth factor beta 1 stimulates arteriogenesis in the peripheral circulation. *FASEB J* 2002;16:432–434.
5. Murata M, Ohta N, Fujisawa S, et al. Selective pericyte degeneration in the retinal capillaries of galactose-fed dogs results from apoptosis linked to aldose reductase-catalyzed galactitol accumulation. *J Diabetes Complications* 2002;16:363–370.
6. Romeo G, Liu WH, Asnaghi V, et al. Activation of nuclear factor-kappaB induced by diabetes and high glucose regulates a proapoptotic program in retinal pericytes. *Diabetes* 2002;51:2241–3348.
7. Pomero F, Allione A, Beltramo E, et al. Effects of protein kinase C inhibition and activation on proliferation and apoptosis of bovine retinal pericytes. *Diabetologia* 2003;46:416–419.
8. Yamagishi S, Amano S, Inagaki Y, et al. Advanced glycation end products-induced apoptosis and overexpression of vascular endothelial growth factor in bovine retinal pericytes. *Biochem Biophys Res Commun* 2002;290:973–978.
9. Frustaci A, Kajstura J, Chimenti C, et al. Myocardial cell death in human diabetes. *Circ Res* 2000;87:1123–1132.
10. Ho FM, Liu SH, Liau CS, et al. High glucose-induced apoptosis in human endothelial cells is mediated by sequential activations of c-Jun NH(2)-terminal kinase and caspase-3. *Circulation* 2000;101:2618–2624.
11. Bergstrand A, Bucht H. The glomerular lesions of diabetes mellitus and their electron-microscope appearances. *J Pathol Bacteriol* 1959;77:231–242.
12. Shimomura H, Spiro RG. Studies on macromolecular components of human glomerular basement membrane and alterations in diabetes. Decreased levels of heparan sulfate proteoglycan and laminin. *Diabetes* 1987;36:374–381.
13. Beisswenger PJ, Spiro RG. Studies on the human glomerular basement membrane. Composition, nature of the carbohydrate units and chemical changes in diabetes mellitus. *Diabetes* 1973;22:180–193.
14. Mason RM, Wahab NA. Extracellular matrix metabolism in diabetic nephropathy. *J Am Soc Nephrol* 2003;14:1358–1373.
15. Nagata M, Katz ML, Robison WG Jr. Age-related thickening of retinal capillary basement membranes. *Invest Ophthalmol Vis Sci* 1986;27:437–440.
16. Robison WG Jr, Kador PF, Kinoshita JH. Retinal capillaries: basement membrane thickening by galactosemia prevented with aldose reductase inhibitor. *Science* 1983;221:1177–1179.
17. Fischer F, Gartner J. Morphometric analysis of basal laminae in rats with long-term streptozotocin diabetes L. II. Retinal capillaries. *Exp Eye Res* 1983; 37:55–64.
18. van den Born J, van Kraats AA, Bakker MA, et al. Reduction of heparan sulphate-associated anionic sites in the glomerular basement membrane of rats with streptozotocin-induced diabetic nephropathy. *Diabetologia* 1995;38: 1169–1175.
19. van den Born J, van Kraats AA, Bakker MA, et al. Selective proteinuria in diabetic nephropathy in the rat is associated with a relative decrease in glomerular basement membrane heparan sulphate. *Diabetologia* 1995;38: 161–172.
20. Singh R, Alavi N, Singh AK, et al. Role of angiotensin II in glucose-induced inhibition of mesangial matrix degradation. *Diabetes* 1999;48:2066–2073.
21. Abdel Wahab N, Mason RM. Modulation of neutral protease expression in human mesangial cells by hyperglycaemic culture. *Biochem J* 1996;320: 777–783.
22. Shankland SJ, Ly H, Thai K, et al. Glomerular expression of tissue inhibitor of metalloproteinase (TIMP-1) in normal and diabetic rats. *J Am Soc Nephrol* 1996;7:97–104.
23. Tesfamariam B, Cohen RA. Free radicals mediate endothelial cell dysfunction caused by elevated glucose. *Am J Physiol* 1992;263:H321–H326.
24. Williams SB, Goldfine AB, Timimi FK, et al. Acute hyperglycemia attenuates endothelium-dependent vasodilation in humans in vivo. *Circulation* 1998;97: 1695–1701.
25. Nilsson SF. The significance of nitric oxide for parasympathetic vasodilation in the eye and other orbital tissues in the cat. *Exp Eye Res* 2000;70:61–72.
26. Dorner GT, Garhofer G, Kiss B, et al. Nitric oxide regulates retinal vascular tone in humans. *Am J Physiol Heart Circ Physiol* 2003;285:H631–H636.
27. Ishii H, Jirousek MR, Koya D, et al. Amelioration of vascular dysfunctions in diabetic rats by an oral PKC beta inhibitor. *Science* 1996;272:728–731.
28. Kihara M, Low PA. Impaired vasoreactivity to nitric oxide in experimental diabetic neuropathy. *Exp Neurol* 1995;132:180–185.
29. El-Remessy AB, Behzadian MA, Abou-Mohamed G, et al. Experimental diabetes causes breakdown of the blood-retina barrier by a mechanism involving tyrosine nitration and increases in expression of vascular endothelial growth factor and urokinase plasminogen activator receptor. *Am J Pathol* 2003;162:1995–2004.
30. Takeda M, Mori F, Yoshida A, et al. Constitutive nitric oxide synthase is associated with retinal vascular permeability in early diabetic rats. *Diabetologia* 2001;44:1043–1050.
31. Joussen AM, Poulaki V, Mitsiades N, et al. Nonsteroidal anti-inflammatory drugs prevent early diabetic retinopathy via TNF-alpha suppression. *FASEB J* 2002;16:438–440.
32. Joussen AM, Poulaki V, Qin W, et al. Retinal vascular endothelial growth factor induces intercellular adhesion molecule-1 and endothelial nitric oxide synthase expression and initiates early diabetic retinal leukocyte adhesion in vivo. *Am J Pathol* 2002;160:501–509.
33. Kowluru RA. Effect of reinstitution of good glycemic control on retinal oxidative stress and nitrative stress in diabetic rats. *Diabetes* 2003;52: 818–823.
34. Thylefors B, Negrel AD, Pararajasegaram R, et al. Global data on blindness. *Bull World Health Organ* 1995;73:115–121.
35. Cai J, Boulton M. The pathogenesis of diabetic retinopathy: old concepts and new questions. *Eye* 2002;16:242–260.
36. Ferris FL 3rd, Davis MD, Aiello LM. Treatment of diabetic retinopathy. *N Engl J Med* 1999;341:667–678.
37. Allt G, Lawrenson JG. Pericytes: cell biology and pathology. *Cells Tissues Organs* 2001;169:1–11.
38. Hirschi KK, D'Amore PA. Pericytes in the microvasculature. *Cardiovasc Res* 1996;32:687–698.
39. Midena E, Segato T, Radin S, et al. Studies on the retina of the diabetic db/db mouse. I. Endothelial cell-pericyte ratio. *Ophthalmic Res* 1989;21:106–111.
40. Agardh CD, Agardh E, Zhang H, et al. Altered endothelial/pericyte ratio in Goto-Kakizaki rat retina. *J Diabetes Complications* 1997;11:158–162.
41. Morisaki N, Watanabe S, Fukuda K, et al. Angiogenic interaction between retinal endothelial cells and pericytes from normal and diabetic rabbits, and phenotypic changes of diabetic cells. *Cell Mol Biol (Noisy-le-grand)* 1999;45: 67–77.
42. Benjamin LE, Hemo I, Keshet E. A plasticity window for blood vessel remodelling is defined by pericyte coverage of the preformed endothelial network and is regulated by PDGF- B and VEGF. *Development* 1998;125: 1591–1598.
43. Benjamin LE, Golijanin D, Itin A, et al. Selective ablation of immature blood vessels in established human tumors follows vascular endothelial growth factor withdrawal. *J Clin Invest* 1999;103:159–165.

44. Lindahl P, Johansson BR, Leveen P, et al. Pericyte loss and microaneurysm formation in PDGF-B-deficient mice. *Science* 1997;277:242–245.
45. Osterby R, Gundersen HJ. Glomerular size and structure in diabetes mellitus. I. Early abnormalities. *Diabetologia* 1975;11:225–229.
46. Osterby R, Gundersen HJ. Fast accumulation of basement membrane material and the rate of morphological changes in acute experimental diabetic glomerular hypertrophy. *Diabetologia* 1980;18:493–500.
47. Kimmelstiel P, Wilson C. Intercapillary lesions in the glomeruli of the kidney. *Am J Pathol* 1936;12:83–98.
48. Wiseman MJ, Saunders AJ, Keen H, et al. Effect of blood glucose control on increased glomerular filtration rate and kidney size in insulin-dependent diabetes. *N Engl J Med* 1985;312:617–621.
49. Steffes MW, Brown DM, Basgen JM, et al. Amelioration of mesangial volume and surface alterations following islet transplantation in diabetic rats. *Diabetes* 1980;29:509–515.
50. Nakamura Y, Myers BD. Charge selectivity of proteinuria in diabetic glomerulopathy. *Diabetes* 1988;37:1202–1211.
51. Cooper ME. Interaction of metabolic and haemodynamic factors in mediating experimental diabetic nephropathy. *Diabetologia* 2001;44:1957–1972.
52. Dyck PJ, Kratz KM, Karnes JL, et al. The prevalence by staged severity of various types of diabetic neuropathy, retinopathy, and nephropathy in a population-based cohort: the Rochester Diabetic Neuropathy Study. *Neurology* 1993;43:817–824.
53. Eichberg J. Protein kinase C changes in diabetes: is the concept relevant to neuropathy? *Int Rev Neurobiol* 2002;50:61–82.
54. Sugimoto K, Murakawa Y, Sima AA. Diabetic neuropathy—a continuing enigma. *Diabetes Metab Res Rev* 2000;16:408–433.
55. Malik RA, Tesfaye S, Thompson SD, et al. Endoneurial localisation of microvascular damage in human diabetic neuropathy. *Diabetologia* 1993;36: 454–459.
56. Schratzberger P, Walter DH, Rittig K, et al. Reversal of experimental diabetic neuropathy by VEGF gene transfer. *J Clin Invest* 2001;107:1083–1092.
57. Nakamura J, Kato K, Hamada Y, et al. A protein kinase C-beta-selective inhibitor ameliorates neural dysfunction in streptozotocin-induced diabetic rats. *Diabetes* 1999;48:2090–2095.
58. Cameron NE, Cotter MA. Effects of protein kinase Cbeta inhibition on neurovascular dysfunction in diabetic rats: interaction with oxidative stress and essential fatty acid dysmetabolism. *Diabetes Metab Res Rev* 2002;18: 315–323.
59. Kannel WB, Hjortland M, Castelli WP. Role of diabetes in congestive heart failure: the Framingham study. *Am J Cardiol* 1974;34:29–34.
60. Stone PH, Muller JE, Hartwell T, et al. The MILIS Study Group. The effect of diabetes mellitus on prognosis and serial left ventricular function after acute myocardial infarction: contribution of both coronary disease and diastolic left ventricular dysfunction to the adverse prognosis. *J Am Coll Cardiol* 1989; 14:49–57.
61. Poirier P, Bogaty P, Garneau C, et al. Diastolic dysfunction in normotensive men with well-controlled type 2 diabetes: importance of maneuvers in echocardiographic screening for preclinical diabetic cardiomyopathy. *Diabetes Care* 2001;24:5–10.
62. Abaci A, Oguzhan A, Kahraman S, et al. Effect of diabetes mellitus on formation of coronary collateral vessels. *Circulation* 1999;99:2239–2242.
63. Yarom R, Zirkin H, Stammler G, et al. Human coronary microvessels in diabetes and ischaemia. Morphometric study of autopsy material. *J Pathol* 1992; 166:265–270.
64. Thompson EW. Quantitative analysis of myocardial structure in insulin-dependent diabetes mellitus: effects of immediate and delayed insulin replacement. *Proc Soc Exp Biol Med* 1994;205:294–305.
65. Warley A, Powell JM, Skepper JN. Capillary surface area is reduced and tissue thickness from capillaries to myocytes is increased in the left ventricle of streptozotocin-diabetic rats. *Diabetologia* 1995;38:413–421.
66. Yamaji T, Fukuhara T, Kinoshita M. Increased capillary permeability to albumin in diabetic rat myocardium. *Circ Res* 1993;72:947–957.
67. Freedman SB, Isner JM. Therapeutic angiogenesis for coronary artery disease. *Ann Intern Med* 2002;136:54–71.
68. Regan TJ, Lyons MM, Ahmed SS, et al. Evidence for cardiomyopathy in familial diabetes mellitus. *J Clin Invest* 1977;60:884–899.
69. Spiro MJ, Crowley TJ. Increased rat myocardial type VI collagen in diabetes mellitus and hypertension. *Diabetologia* 1993;36:93–98.
70. Chen S, Evans T, Mukherjee K, et al. Diabetes-induced myocardial structural changes: role of endothelin-1 and its receptors. *J Mol Cell Cardiol* 2000;32: 1621–1629.
71. Hoyer J, Kohler R, Haase W, et al. Up-regulation of pressure-activated Ca(2+)-permeable cation channel in intact vascular endothelium of hypertensive rats. *Proc Natl Acad Sci U S A* 1996;93:11253–11258.
72. Hamada K, Takuwa N, Yokoyama K, et al. Stretch activates Jun N-terminal kinase/stress-activated protein kinase in vascular smooth muscle cells through mechanisms involving autocrine ATP stimulation of purinoceptors. *J Biol Chem* 1998;273:6334–6340.
73. Chen KD, Li YS, Kim M, et al. Mechanotransduction in response to shear stress. Roles of receptor tyrosine kinases, integrins, and Shc. *J Biol Chem* 1999; 274:18393–18400.
74. Kelly DJ, Skinner SL, Gilbert RE, et al. Effects of endothelin or angiotensin II receptor blockade on diabetes in the transgenic (mRen-2)27 rat. *Kidney Int* 2000;57:1882–1894.
75. Perin PC, Maule S, Quadri R. Sympathetic nervous system, diabetes, and hypertension. *Clin Exp Hypertens* 2001;23:45–55.
76. Scherrer U, Sartori C. Insulin as a vascular and sympathoexcitatory hormone: implications for blood pressure regulation, insulin sensitivity, and cardiovascular morbidity. *Circulation* 1997;96:4104–4113.
77. Brownlee M. Advanced protein glycosylation in diabetes and aging. *Annu Rev Med* 1995;46:223–234.
78. Giardino I, Edelstein D, Brownlee M. BCL-2 expression or antioxidants prevent hyperglycemia-induced formation of intracellular advanced glycation endproducts in bovine endothelial cells. *J Clin Invest* 1996;97:1422–1428.
79. Brownlee M. Biochemistry and molecular cell biology of diabetic complications. *Nature* 2001;414:813–820.
80. Schleicher ED, Wagner E, Nerlich AG. Increased accumulation of the glycoxidation product N(epsilon)-(carboxymethyl)lysine in human tissues in diabetes and aging. *J Clin Invest* 1997;99:457–468.
81. Schmidt AM, Yan SD, Wautier JL, et al. Activation of receptor for advanced glycation end products: a mechanism for chronic vascular dysfunction in diabetic vasculopathy and atherosclerosis. *Circ Res* 1999;84:489–497.
82. Stitt AW, Li YM, Gardiner TA, et al. Advanced glycation end products (AGEs) co-localize with AGE receptors in the retinal vasculature of diabetic and of AGE-infused rats. *Am J Pathol* 1997;150:523–531.
83. Horie K, Miyata T, Maeda K, et al. Immunohistochemical colocalization of glycoxidation products and lipid peroxidation products in diabetic renal glomerular lesions. Implication for glycoxidative stress in the pathogenesis of diabetic nephropathy. *J Clin Invest* 1997;100:2995–3004.
84. Bucala R, Tracey KJ, Cerami A. Advanced glycosylation products quench nitric oxide and mediate defective endothelium-dependent vasodilatation in experimental diabetes. *J Clin Invest* 1991;87:432–438.
85. Giardino I, Edelstein D, Brownlee M. Nonenzymatic glycosylation in vitro and in bovine endothelial cells alters basic fibroblast growth factor activity. A model for intracellular glycosylation in diabetes. *J Clin Invest* 1994;94: 110–117.
86. Mott JD, Khalifah RG, Nagase H, et al. Nonenzymatic glycation of type IV collagen and matrix metalloproteinase susceptibility. *Kidney Int* 1997;52: 1302–1312.
87. Tanaka S, Avigad G, Brodsky B, et al. Glycation induces expansion of the molecular packing of collagen. *J Mol Biol* 1988;203:495–505.
88. Tsilibary EC, Charonis AS, Reger LA, et al. The effect of nonenzymatic glucosylation on the binding of the main noncollagenous NC1 domain to type IV collagen. *J Biol Chem* 1988;263:4302–4308.
89. Charonis AS, Reger LA, Dege JE, et al. Laminin alterations after in vitro nonenzymatic glycosylation. *Diabetes* 1990;39:807–814.
90. Haitoglou CS, Tsilibary EC, Brownlee M, et al. Altered cellular interactions between endothelial cells and nonenzymatically glucosylated laminin/type IV collagen. *J Biol Chem* 1992;267:12404–12407.
91. Oldfield MD, Bach LA, Forbes JM, et al. Advanced glycation end products cause epithelial-myofibroblast transdifferentiation via the receptor for advanced glycation end products (RAGE). *J Clin Invest* 2001;108:1853–1863.
92. Yamamoto Y, Kato I, Doi T, et al. Development and prevention of advanced diabetic nephropathy in RAGE-overexpressing mice. *J Clin Invest* 2001;108: 261–268.
93. Rojas A, Romay S, Gonzalez D, et al. Regulation of endothelial nitric oxide synthase expression by albumin-derived advanced glycosylation end products. *Circ Res* 2000;86:E50–E54.
94. Quehenberger P, Bierhaus A, Fasching P, et al. Endothelin 1 transcription is controlled by nuclear factor-kappaB in AGE-stimulated cultured endothelial cells. *Diabetes* 2000;49:1561–1570.
95. Bierhaus A, Chevion S, Chevion M, et al. Advanced glycation end product-induced activation of NF-kappaB is suppressed by alpha-lipoic acid in cultured endothelial cells. *Diabetes* 1997;46:1481–1490.
96. Rumble JR, Cooper ME, Soulis T, et al. Vascular hypertrophy in experimental diabetes. Role of advanced glycation end products. *J Clin Invest* 1997;99: 1016–1027.
97. Lu M, Kuroki M, Amano S, et al. Advanced glycation end products increase retinal vascular endothelial growth factor expression. *J Clin Invest* 1998;101: 1219–1224.
98. Yamagishi S, Fujimori H, Yonekura H, et al. Advanced glycation endproducts inhibit prostacyclin production and induce plasminogen activator inhibitor-1 in human microvascular endothelial cells. *Diabetologia* 1998;41: 1435–1441.
99. Basta G, Lazzerini G, Massaro M, et al. Advanced glycation end products activate endothelium through signal-transduction receptor RAGE: a mechanism for amplification of inflammatory responses. *Circulation* 2002;105: 816–822.
100. Wautier JL, Zoukourian C, Chappey O, et al. Receptor-mediated endothelial cell dysfunction in diabetic vasculopathy. Soluble receptor for advanced glycation end products blocks hyperpermeability in diabetic rats. *J Clin Invest* 1996;97:238–243.
101. Soulis-Liparota T, Cooper M, Papazoglou D, et al. Retardation by aminoguanidine of development of albuminuria, mesangial expansion, and tissue fluorescence in streptozocin-induced diabetic rat. *Diabetes* 1991;40: 1328–1334.
102. Hammes HP, Martin S, Federlin K, et al. Aminoguanidine treatment inhibits the development of experimental diabetic retinopathy. *Proc Natl Acad Sci U S A* 1991;88:11555–11558.
103. Soulis T, Sastra S, Thallas V, et al. A novel inhibitor of advanced glycation end-product formation inhibits mesenteric vascular hypertrophy in experimental diabetes. *Diabetologia* 1999;42:472–479.

104. Kass DA, Shapiro EP, Kawaguchi M, et al. Improved arterial compliance by a novel advanced glycation end-product crosslink breaker. *Circulation* 2001; 104:1464–1470.
105. Nakamura S, Makita Z, Ishikawa S, et al. Progression of nephropathy in spontaneous diabetic rats is prevented by OPB-9195, a novel inhibitor of advanced glycation. *Diabetes* 1997;46:895–899.
106. Forbes JM, Cooper ME, Thallas V, et al. Reduction of the accumulation of advanced glycation end products by ACE inhibition in experimental diabetic nephropathy. *Diabetes* 2002;51:3274–3282.
107. Adamis AP. Is diabetic retinopathy an inflammatory disease? *Br J Ophthalmol* 2002;86:363–365.
108. The Diabetes Control and Complications Trial Research Group. The effect of intensive treatment of diabetes on the development and progression of long-term complications in insulin-dependent diabetes mellitus. *N Engl J Med* 1993;329:977–986.
109. Ohkubo Y, Kishikawa H, Araki E, et al. Intensive insulin therapy prevents the progression of diabetic microvascular complications in Japanese patients with non-insulin-dependent diabetes mellitus: a randomized prospective 6-year study. *Diabetes Res Clin Pract* 1995;28:103–117.
110. UK Prospective Diabetes Study (UKPDS) Group. Intensive blood-glucose control with sulphonylureas or insulin compared with conventional treatment and risk of complications in patients with type 2 diabetes (UKPDS 33). *Lancet* 1998;352:837–853.
111. Yki-Jarvinen H, Makimattila S. Insulin resistance due to hyperglycaemia: an adaptation protecting insulin-sensitive tissues. *Diabetologia* 1997;40[Suppl 2]:S141–S144.
112. Kaiser N, Sasson S, Feener EP, et al. Differential regulation of glucose transport and transporters by glucose in vascular endothelial and smooth muscle cells. *Diabetes* 1993;42:80–89.
113. Heilig CW, Concepcion LA, Riser BL, et al. Overexpression of glucose transporters in rat mesangial cells cultured in a normal glucose milieu mimics the diabetic phenotype. *J Clin Invest* 1995;96:1802–1814.
114. Badr GA, Tang J, Ismail-Beigi F, et al. Diabetes downregulates GLUT1 expression in the retina and its microvessels but not in the cerebral cortex or its microvessels. *Diabetes* 2000;49:1016–1021.
115. King GL, Buzney SM, Kahn CR, et al. Differential responsiveness to insulin of endothelial and support cells from micro- and macrovessels. *J Clin Invest* 1983;71:974–979.
116. Baynes JW. Role of oxidative stress in development of complications in diabetes. *Diabetes* 1991;40:405–412.
117. Giugliano D, Ceriello A, Paolisso G. Oxidative stress and diabetic vascular complications. *Diabetes Care* 1996;19:257–267.
118. Keaney JF Jr, Larson MG, Vasan RS, et al. Obesity and systemic oxidative stress: clinical correlates of oxidative stress in the Framingham Study. *Arterioscler Thromb Vasc Biol* 2003;23:434–439.
119. Jain SK, McVie R. Effect of glycemic control, race (white versus black), and duration of diabetes on reduced glutathione content in erythrocytes of diabetic patients. *Metabolism* 1994;43:306–309.
120. Kimura F, Hasegawa G, Obayashi H, et al. Serum extracellular superoxide dismutase in patients with type 2 diabetes: relationship to the development of micro- and macrovascular complications. *Diabetes Care* 2003;26:1246–1250.
121. Augustin AJ, Dick HB, Koch F, et al. Correlation of blood-glucose control with oxidative metabolites in plasma and vitreous body of diabetic patients. *Eur J Ophthalmol* 2002;12:94–101.
122. Craven PA, Melhem MF, Phillips SL, et al. Overexpression of Cu2+/Zn2+ superoxide dismutase protects against early diabetic glomerular injury in transgenic mice. *Diabetes* 2001;50:2114–2125.
123. Kowluru RA, Tang J, Kern TS. Abnormalities of retinal metabolism in diabetes and experimental galactosemia. VII. Effect of long-term administration of antioxidants on the development of retinopathy. *Diabetes* 2001;50:1938–1942.
124. Lal MA, Korner A, Matsuo Y, et al. Combined antioxidant and COMT inhibitor treatment reverses renal abnormalities in diabetic rats. *Diabetes* 2000;49:1381–1389.
125. Cameron NE, Cotter MA, Archibald V, et al. Anti-oxidant and pro-oxidant effects on nerve conduction velocity, endoneurial blood flow and oxygen tension in non-diabetic and streptozotocin-diabetic rats. *Diabetologia* 1994;37: 449–459.
126. Nagamatsu M, Nickander KK, Schmelzer JD, et al. Lipoic acid improves nerve blood flow, reduces oxidative stress, and improves distal nerve conduction in experimental diabetic neuropathy. *Diabetes Care* 1995;18:1160–1167.
127. Gaede P, Poulsen HE, Parving HH, et al. Double-blind, randomised study of the effect of combined treatment with vitamin C and E on albuminuria in type 2 diabetic patients. *Diabet Med* 2001;18:756–760.
128. Bursell SE, Clermont AC, Aiello LP, et al. High-dose vitamin E supplementation normalizes retinal blood flow and creatinine clearance in patients with type 1 diabetes. *Diabetes Care* 1999;22:1245–1251.
129. Tutuncu NB, Bayraktar M, Varli K. Reversal of defective nerve conduction with vitamin E supplementation in type 2 diabetes: a preliminary study. *Diabetes Care* 1998;21:1915–1918.
130. Lonn E, Yusuf S, Hoogwerf B, et al. Effects of vitamin E on cardiovascular and microvascular outcomes in high-risk patients with diabetes: results of the HOPE study and MICRO-HOPE substudy. *Diabetes Care* 2002;25:1919–1927.
131. Garcia Soriano F, Virag L, Jagtap P, et al. Diabetic endothelial dysfunction: the role of poly(ADP-ribose) polymerase activation. *Nat Med* 2001;7:108–113.
132. Du X, Matsumura T, Edelstein D, et al. Inhibition of GAPDH activity by poly(ADP-ribose) polymerase activates three major pathways of hyperglycemic damage in endothelial cells. *J Clin Invest* 2003;112:1049–1057.
133. Williamson JR, Chang K, Frangos M, et al. Hyperglycemic pseudohypoxia and diabetic complications. *Diabetes* 1993;42:801–813.
134. Engerman RL, Kern TS, Larson ME. Nerve conduction and aldose reductase inhibition during 5 years of diabetes or galactosaemia in dogs. *Diabetologia* 1994;37:141–144.
135. Greene DA, Arezzo JC, Brown MB. Zenarestat Study Group. Effect of aldose reductase inhibition on nerve conduction and morphometry in diabetic neuropathy. *Neurology* 1999;53:580–591.
136. Sorbinil Retinopathy Trial Research Group. A randomized trial of sorbinil, an aldose reductase inhibitor, in diabetic retinopathy. *Arch Ophthalmol* 1990;108: 1234–1244.
137. Asahina T, Kashiwagi A, Nishio Y, et al. Impaired activation of glucose oxidation and NADPH supply in human endothelial cells exposed to H2O2 in high-glucose medium. *Diabetes* 1995;44:520–526.
138. Zhang Z, Apse K, Pang J, et al. High glucose inhibits glucose-6-phosphate dehydrogenase via cAMP in aortic endothelial cells. *J Biol Chem* 2000;275: 40042–40047.
139. Leopold JA, Cap A, Scribner AW, et al. Glucose-6-phosphate dehydrogenase deficiency promotes endothelial oxidant stress and decreases endothelial nitric oxide bioavailability. *FASEB J* 2001;15:1771–1773.
140. Nishikawa T, Edelstein D, Du XL, et al. Normalizing mitochondrial superoxide production blocks three pathways of hyperglycaemic damage. *Nature* 2000;404:787–790.
141. Griendling KK, Sorescu D, Ushio-Fukai M. NAD(P)H oxidase: role in cardiovascular biology and disease. *Circ Res* 2000;86:494–501.
142. Gorlach A, Brandes RP, Nguyen K, et al. A gp91phox containing NADPH oxidase selectively expressed in endothelial cells is a major source of oxygen radical generation in the arterial wall. *Circ Res* 2000;87:26–32.
143. Hink U, Li H, Mollnau H, et al. Mechanisms underlying endothelial dysfunction in diabetes mellitus. *Circ Res* 2001;88:E14–E22.
144. Kim YK, Lee MS, Son SM, et al. Vascular NADH oxidase is involved in impaired endothelium-dependent vasodilation in OLETF rats, a model of type 2 diabetes. *Diabetes* 2002;51:522–527.
145. Mohazzab KM, Kaminski PM, Wolin MS. NADH oxidoreductase is a major source of superoxide anion in bovine coronary artery endothelium. *Am J Physiol* 1994;266:H2568–H2572.
146. Inoguchi T, Li P, Umeda F, et al. High glucose level and free fatty acid stimulate reactive oxygen species production through protein kinase C-dependent activation of NAD(P)H oxidase in cultured vascular cells. *Diabetes* 2000;49: 1939–1945.
147. Duerrschmidt N, Wippich N, Goettsch W, et al. Endothelin-1 induces NAD(P)H oxidase in human endothelial cells. *Biochem Biophys Res Commun* 2000;269:713–717.
148. Ohara Y, Peterson TE, Harrison DG. Hypercholesterolemia increases endothelial superoxide anion production. *J Clin Invest* 1993;91:2546–2551.
149. Laursen JB, Somers M, Kurz S, et al. Endothelial regulation of vasomotion in apoE-deficient mice: implications for interactions between peroxynitrite and tetrahydrobiopterin. *Circulation* 2001;103:1282–1288.
150. Mayer B, John M, Bohme E. Purification of a Ca2+/calmodulin-dependent nitric oxide synthase from porcine cerebellum. Cofactor-role of tetrahydrobiopterin. *FEBS Lett* 1990;277:215–219.
151. Wever R, Luscher TF, Cosentino F, et al. Atherosclerosis and the two faces of endothelial nitric oxide synthase. *Circulation* 1998;97:108–112.
152. Zou MH, Shi C, Cohen RA. Oxidation of the zinc-thiolate complex and uncoupling of endothelial nitric oxide synthase by peroxynitrite. *J Clin Invest* 2002;109:817–826.
153. Shinozaki K, Kashiwagi A, Nishio Y, et al. Abnormal biopterin metabolism is a major cause of impaired endothelium-dependent relaxation through nitric oxide/O2-imbalance in insulin-resistant rat aorta. *Diabetes* 1999;48:2437–2445.
154. Shinozaki K, Nishio Y, Okamura T, et al. Oral administration of tetrahydrobiopterin prevents endothelial dysfunction and vascular oxidative stress in the aortas of insulin-resistant rats. *Circ Res* 2000;87:566–573.
155. Heitzer T, Krohn K, Albers S, et al. Tetrahydrobiopterin improves endothelium-dependent vasodilation by increasing nitric oxide activity in patients with type II diabetes mellitus. *Diabetologia* 2000;43:1435–1438.
156. MacMillan-Crow LA, Crow JP, Kerby JD, et al. Nitration and inactivation of manganese superoxide dismutase in chronic rejection of human renal allografts. *Proc Natl Acad Sci U S A* 1996;93:11853–11858.
157. Turko IV, Marcondes S, Murad F. Diabetes-associated nitration of tyrosine and inactivation of succinyl-CoA:3-oxoacid CoA-transferase. *Am J Physiol Heart Circ Physiol* 2001;281:H2289–H2294.
158. Zou MH, Shi C, Cohen RA. High glucose via peroxynitrite causes tyrosine nitration and inactivation of prostacyclin synthase that is associated with thromboxane/prostaglandin H(2) receptor-mediated apoptosis and adhesion molecule expression in cultured human aortic endothelial cells. *Diabetes* 2002;51:198–203.
159. Desco MC, Asensi M, Marquez R, et al. Xanthine oxidase is involved in free radical production in type 1 diabetes: protection by allopurinol. *Diabetes* 2002;51:1118–1124.
160. Hunt JV, Dean RT, Wolff SP. Hydroxyl radical production and autoxidative glycosylation. Glucose autoxidation as the cause of protein damage in the experimental glycation model of diabetes mellitus and ageing. *Biochem J* 1988;256:205–212.
161. Jain SK, McVie R, Jackson R, et al. Effect of hyperketonemia on plasma lipid peroxidation levels in diabetic patients. *Diabetes Care* 1999;22:1171–1175.

162. Ceriello A, dello Russo P, Amstad P, et al. High glucose induces antioxidant enzymes in human endothelial cells in culture. Evidence linking hyperglycemia and oxidative stress. *Diabetes* 1996;45:471–477.
163. Urata Y, Yamamoto H, Goto S, et al. Long exposure to high glucose concentration impairs the responsive expression of gamma-glutamylcysteine synthetase by interleukin-1beta and tumor necrosis factor-alpha in mouse endothelial cells. *J Biol Chem* 1996;271:15146–15152.
164. Wells L, Vosseller K, Hart GW. Glycosylation of nucleocytoplasmic proteins: signal transduction and O-GlcNAc. *Science* 2001;291:2376–2378.
165. Schleicher ED, Weigert C. Role of the hexosamine biosynthetic pathway in diabetic nephropathy. *Kidney Int Suppl* 2000;77:S13–S18.
166. Nerlich AG, Sauer U, Kolm-Litty V, et al. Expression of glutamine:fructose-6-phosphate amidotransferase in human tissues: evidence for high variability and distinct regulation in diabetes. *Diabetes* 1998;47:170–178.
167. James LR, Ingram A, Ly H, et al. Angiotensin II activates the GFAT promoter in mesangial cells. *Am J Physiol Renal Physiol* 2001;281:F151–F162.
168. Du XL, Edelstein D, Dimmeler S, et al. Hyperglycemia inhibits endothelial nitric oxide synthase activity by posttranslational modification at the Akt site. *J Clin Invest* 2001;108:1341–1348.
169. Federici M, Menghini R, Mauriello A, et al. Insulin-dependent activation of endothelial nitric oxide synthase is impaired by O-linked glycosylation modification of signaling proteins in human coronary endothelial cells. *Circulation* 2002;106:466–472.
170. James LR, Tang D, Ingram A, et al. Flux through the hexosamine pathway is a determinant of nuclear factor kappaB- dependent promoter activation. *Diabetes* 2002;51:1146–1156.
171. James LR, Fantus IG, Goldberg H, et al. Overexpression of GFAT activates PAI-1 promoter in mesangial cells. *Am J Physiol Renal Physiol* 2000;279:F718–F727.
172. Du XL, Edelstein D, Rossetti L, et al. Hyperglycemia-induced mitochondrial superoxide overproduction activates the hexosamine pathway and induces plasminogen activator inhibitor-1 expression by increasing Sp1 glycosylation. *Proc Natl Acad Sci U S A* 2000;97:12222–12226.
173. Goldberg HJ, Whiteside CI, Fantus IG. The hexosamine pathway regulates the plasminogen activator inhibitor-1 gene promoter and Sp1 transcriptional activation through protein kinase C-beta I and -delta. *J Biol Chem* 2002;277:33833–33841.
174. McClain DA, Paterson AJ, Roos MD, et al. Glucose and glucosamine regulate growth factor gene expression in vascular smooth muscle cells. *Proc Natl Acad Sci U S A* 1992;89:8150–8154.
175. Lee TS, Saltsman KA, Ohashi H, et al. Activation of protein kinase C by elevation of glucose concentration: proposal for a mechanism in the development of diabetic vascular complications. *Proc Natl Acad Sci U S A* 1989;86:5141–5145.
176. Inoguchi T, Xia P, Kunisaki M, et al. Insulin's effect on protein kinase C and diacylglycerol induced by diabetes and glucose in vascular tissues. *Am J Physiol* 1994;267:E369–E379.
177. Yu HY, Inoguchi T, Kakimoto M, et al. Saturated non-esterified fatty acids stimulate de novo diacylglycerol synthesis and protein kinase C activity in cultured aortic smooth muscle cells. *Diabetologia* 2001;44:614–620.
178. Koya D, Haneda M, Nakagawa H, et al. Amelioration of accelerated diabetic mesangial expansion by treatment with a PKC beta inhibitor in diabetic db/db mice, a rodent model for type 2 diabetes. *FASEB J* 2000;14:439–447.
179. Shinomura T, Asaoka Y, Oka M, et al. Synergistic action of diacylglycerol and unsaturated fatty acid for protein kinase C activation: its possible implications. *Proc Natl Acad Sci U S A* 1991;88:5149–5153.
180. Yoshida K, Asaoka Y, Nishizuka Y. Platelet activation by simultaneous actions of diacylglycerol and unsaturated fatty acids. *Proc Natl Acad Sci U S A* 1992;89:6443–6446.
181. Knapp LT, Klann E. Superoxide-induced stimulation of protein kinase C via thiol modification and modulation of zinc content. *J Biol Chem* 2000;275:24136–24145.
182. Kunisaki M, Bursell SE, Umeda F, et al. Normalization of diacylglycerol-protein kinase C activation by vitamin E in aorta of diabetic rats and cultured rat smooth muscle cells exposed to elevated glucose levels. *Diabetes* 1994;43:1372–1377.
183. Koya D, Lee IK, Ishii H, et al. Prevention of glomerular dysfunction in diabetic rats by treatment with d-alpha-tocopherol. *J Am Soc Nephrol* 1997;8: 426–435.
184. Ricciarelli R, Tasinato A, Clement S, et al. alpha-Tocopherol specifically inactivates cellular protein kinase C alpha by changing its phosphorylation state. *Biochem J* 1998;334:243–249.
185. Tasinato A, Boscoboinik D, Bartoli GM, et al. d-alpha-Tocopherol inhibition of vascular smooth muscle cell proliferation occurs at physiological concentrations, correlates with protein kinase C inhibition, and is independent of its antioxidant properties. *Proc Natl Acad Sci U S A* 1995;92:12190–12194.
186. Tesfamariam B, Brown ML, Cohen RA. Elevated glucose impairs endothelium-dependent relaxation by activating protein kinase C. *J Clin Invest* 1991;87:1643–1648.
187. Jack A, Cameron NE, Cotter MA. Treatment with the protein kinase Cβ inhibitor, LY333531, attenuates the development of impaired endothelium-dependent vasodilatation in the mesenteric vasculature of diabetic rats. *Diabetes* 1999(abst 558).
188. Beckman JA, Goldfine AB, Gordon MB, et al. Inhibition of protein kinase Cbeta prevents impaired endothelium-dependent vasodilation caused by hyperglycemia in humans. *Circ Res* 2002;90:107–111.
189. Zhang SL, Filep JG, Hohman TC, et al. Molecular mechanisms of glucose action on angiotensinogen gene expression in rat proximal tubular cells. *Kidney Int* 1999;55:454–464.
190. Hempel A, Maasch C, Heintze U, et al. High glucose concentrations increase endothelial cell permeability via activation of protein kinase C alpha. *Circ Res* 1997;81:363–371.
191. Williams B, Gallacher B, Patel H, et al. Glucose-induced protein kinase C activation regulates vascular permeability factor mRNA expression and peptide production by human vascular smooth muscle cells in vitro. *Diabetes* 1997;46:1497–1503.
192. Park JY, Takahara N, Gabriele A, et al. Induction of endothelin-1 expression by glucose: an effect of protein kinase C activation. *Diabetes* 2000;49:1239– 1248.
193. Xia P, Aiello LP, Ishii H, et al. Characterization of vascular endothelial growth factor's effect on the activation of protein kinase C, its isoforms, and endothelial cell growth. *J Clin Invest* 1996;98:2018–2026.
194. Suzuma K, Takahara N, Suzuma I, et al. Characterization of protein kinase C beta isoform's action on retinoblastoma protein phosphorylation, vascular endothelial growth factor-induced endothelial cell proliferation, and retinal neovascularization. *Proc Natl Acad Sci U S A* 2002;99:721–726.
195. Yokota T, Ma RC, Park JY, et al. Role of protein kinase C on the expression of platelet-derived growth factor and endothelin-1 in the retina of diabetic rats and cultured retinal capillary pericytes. *Diabetes* 2003;52:838–845.
196. Glogowski EA, Tsiani E, Zhou X, et al. High glucose alters the response of mesangial cell protein kinase C isoforms to endothelin-1. *Kidney Int* 1999;55:486–499.
197. Laakso M, Edelman SV, Brechtel G, et al. Decreased effect of insulin to stimulate skeletal muscle blood flow in obese man. A novel mechanism for insulin resistance. *J Clin Invest* 1990;85:1844–1852.
198. Laakso M, Edelman SV, Brechtel G, et al. Impaired insulin-mediated skeletal muscle blood flow in patients with NIDDM. *Diabetes* 1992;41:1076–1083.
199. Yki-Jarvinen H, Utriainen T. Insulin-induced vasodilatation: physiology or pharmacology? *Diabetologia* 1998;41:369–379.
200. Bonadonna RC, Saccomani MP, Del Prato S, et al. Role of tissue-specific blood flow and tissue recruitment in insulin-mediated glucose uptake of human skeletal muscle. *Circulation* 1998;98:234–241.
201. Clark MG, Wallis MG, Barrett EJ, et al. Blood flow and muscle metabolism: a focus on insulin action. *Am J Physiol Endocrinol Metab* 2003;284:E241–E258.
202. Su EN, Yu DY, Alder VA, et al. Direct vasodilatory effect of insulin on isolated retinal arterioles. *Invest Ophthalmol Vis Sci* 1996;37:2634–2644.
203. Schmetterer L, Muller M, Fasching P, et al. Renal and ocular hemodynamic effects of insulin. *Diabetes* 1997;46:1868–1874.
204. Chen YL, Messina EJ. Dilation of isolated skeletal muscle arterioles by insulin is endothelium dependent and nitric oxide mediated. *Am J Physiol* 1996;270:H2120–H2124.
205. Steinberg HO, Brechtel G, Johnson A, et al. Insulin-mediated skeletal muscle vasodilation is nitric oxide dependent. A novel action of insulin to increase nitric oxide release. *J Clin Invest* 1994;94:1172–1179.
206. Duplain H, Burcelin R, Sartori C, et al. Insulin resistance, hyperlipidemia, and hypertension in mice lacking endothelial nitric oxide synthase. *Circulation* 2001;104:342–345.
207. Montagnani M, Chen H, Barr VA, et al. Insulin-stimulated activation of eNOS is independent of Ca2+ but requires phosphorylation by Akt at Ser(1179). *J Biol Chem* 2001;276:30392–30398.
208. Kuboki K, Jiang ZY, Takahara N, et al. Regulation of endothelial constitutive nitric oxide synthase gene expression in endothelial cells and in vivo: a specific vascular action of insulin. *Circulation* 2000;101:676–681.
209. Jiang ZY, Lin YW, Clemont A, et al. Characterization of selective resistance to insulin signaling in the vasculature of obese Zucker (fa/fa) rats. *J Clin Invest* 1999;104:447–457.
210. Govers R, Rabelink T. Cellular regulation of endothelial nitric oxide synthase. *Am J Physiol* 2001;280:F193–F206.
211. Folli F, Kahn CR, Hansen H, et al. Angiotensin II inhibits insulin signaling in aortic smooth muscle cells at multiple levels. A potential role for serine phosphorylation in insulin/angiotensin II crosstalk. *J Clin Invest* 1997;100:2158–2169.
212. Vicent D, Ilany J, Kondo T, et al. The role of endothelial insulin signaling in the regulation of vascular tone and insulin resistance. *J Clin Invest* 2003;111:1373–1380.
213. Poulaki V, Qin W, Joussen AM, et al. Acute intensive insulin therapy exacerbates diabetic blood-retinal barrier breakdown via hypoxia-inducible factor-1 alpha and VEGF. *J Clin Invest* 2002;109:805–815.
214. Kondo T, Vicent D, Suzuma K, et al. Knockout of insulin and IGF-1 receptors on vascular endothelial cells protects against retinal neovascularization. *J Clin Invest* 2003;111:1835–1842.
215. Morrisey K, Evans RA, Wakefield L, et al. Translational regulation of renal proximal tubular epithelial cell transforming growth factor-beta1 generation by insulin. *Am J Pathol* 2001;159:1905–1915.
216. Bennett BL, Satoh Y, Lewis AJ. JNK: a new therapeutic target for diabetes. *Curr Opin Pharmacol* 2003;3:420–425.
217. Natarajan R, Scott S, Bai W, et al. Angiotensin II signaling in vascular smooth muscle cells under high glucose conditions. *Hypertension* 1999;33:378–384.
218. Igarashi M, Wakasaki H, Takahara N, et al. Glucose or diabetes activates p38 mitogen-activated protein kinase via different pathways. *J Clin Invest* 1999;103:185–195.
219. Haneda M, Araki S, Togawa M, et al. Mitogen-activated protein kinase cascade is activated in glomeruli of diabetic rats and glomerular mesangial cells cultured under high glucose conditions. *Diabetes* 1997;46:847–853.

220. Wolf G. Cell cycle regulation in diabetic nephropathy. *Kidney Int Suppl* 2000; 77:S59–S66.
221. Al-Douahji M, Brugarolas J, Brown PA, et al. The cyclin kinase inhibitor p21WAF1/CIP1 is required for glomerular hypertrophy in experimental diabetic nephropathy. *Kidney Int* 1999;56:1691–1699.
222. Awazu M, Omori S, Ishikura K, et al. The lack of cyclin kinase inhibitor p27(Kip1) ameliorates progression of diabetic nephropathy. *J Am Soc Nephrol* 2003;14:699–708.
223. Wolf G, Shankland SJ. P27Kip1: the "rosebud" of diabetic nephropathy? *J Am Soc Nephrol* 2003;14:819–822.
224. Feliers D, Frank MA, Riley DJ. Activation of cyclin D1-Cdk4 and Cdk4-directed phosphorylation of RB protein in diabetic mesangial hypertrophy. *Diabetes* 2002;51:3290–3299.
225. Sanchez-Elsner T, Botella LM, Velasco B, et al. Synergistic cooperation between hypoxia and transforming growth factor-beta pathways on human vascular endothelial growth factor gene expression. *J Biol Chem* 2001;276: 38527–38535.
226. Autiero M, Waltenberger J, Communi D, et al. Role of PlGF in the intra- and intermolecular cross talk between the VEGF receptors Flt1 and Flk1. *Nat Med* 2003;9:936–943.
227. Smith LE, Shen W, Perruzzi C, et al. Regulation of vascular endothelial growth factor-dependent retinal neovascularization by insulin-like growth factor-1 receptor. *Nat Med* 1999;5:1390–1395.
228. Cao R, Brakenhielm E, Pawliuk R, et al. Angiogenic synergism, vascular stability and improvement of hind-limb ischemia by a combination of PDGF-BB and FGF-2. *Nat Med* 2003;9:604–613.
229. Boulton M, Gregor Z, McLeod D, et al. Intravitreal growth factors in proliferative diabetic retinopathy: correlation with neovascular activity and glycaemic management. *Br J Ophthalmol* 1997;81:228–233.
230. Sivalingam A, Kenney J, Brown GC, et al. Basic fibroblast growth factor levels in the vitreous of patients with proliferative diabetic retinopathy. *Arch Ophthalmol* 1990;108:869–872.
231. Seghezzi G, Patel S, Ren CJ, et al. Fibroblast growth factor-2 (FGF-2) induces vascular endothelial growth factor (VEGF) expression in the endothelial cells of forming capillaries: an autocrine mechanism contributing to angiogenesis. *J Cell Biol* 1998;141:1659–1673.
232. Ozaki H, Okamoto N, Ortega S, et al. Basic fibroblast growth factor is neither necessary nor sufficient for the development of retinal neovascularization. *Am J Pathol* 1998;153:757–765.
233. Ferrara N, Gerber HP, LeCouter J. The biology of VEGF and its receptors. *Nat Med* 2003;9:669–676.
234. Aiello LP, Avery RL, Arrigg PG, et al. Vascular endothelial growth factor in ocular fluid of patients with diabetic retinopathy and other retinal disorders. *N Engl J Med* 1994;331:1480–1487.
235. Boulton M, Foreman D, Williams G, et al. VEGF localisation in diabetic retinopathy. *Br J Ophthalmol* 1998;82:561–568.
236. Hammes HP, Lin J, Bretzel RG, et al. Upregulation of the vascular endothelial growth factor/vascular endothelial growth factor receptor system in experimental background diabetic retinopathy of the rat. *Diabetes* 1998;47: 401–406.
237. Aiello LP, Pierce EA, Foley ED, et al. Suppression of retinal neovascularization in vivo by inhibition of vascular endothelial growth factor (VEGF) using soluble VEGF-receptor chimeric proteins. *Proc Natl Acad Sci U S A* 1995;92: 10457–10461.
238. Cooper ME, Vranes D, Youssef S, et al. Increased renal expression of vascular endothelial growth factor (VEGF) and its receptor VEGFR-2 in experimental diabetes. *Diabetes* 1999;48:2229–2239.
239. Bortoloso E, Del Prete D, Gambaro G, et al. Vascular endothelial growth factor (VEGF) and VEGF receptors in diabetic nephropathy: expression studies in biopsies of type 2 diabetic patients. *Ren Fail* 2001;23:483–493.
240. de Vriese AS, Tilton RG, Elger M, et al. Antibodies against vascular endothelial growth factor improve early renal dysfunction in experimental diabetes. *J Am Soc Nephrol* 2001;12:993–1000.
241. Flyvbjerg A, Dagnaes-Hansen F, De Vriese AS, et al. Amelioration of long-term renal changes in obese type 2 diabetic mice by a neutralizing vascular endothelial growth factor antibody. *Diabetes* 2002;51:3090–3094.
242. Duh E, Aiello LP. Vascular endothelial growth factor and diabetes: the agonist versus antagonist paradox. *Diabetes* 1999;48:1899–1906.
243. Giordano FJ, Gerber HP, Williams SP, et al. A cardiac myocyte vascular endothelial growth factor paracrine pathway is required to maintain cardiac function. *Proc Natl Acad Sci U S A* 2001;98:5780–5785.
244. Losordo DW, Vale PR, Hendel RC, et al. Phase 1/2 placebo-controlled, double-blind, dose-escalating trial of myocardial vascular endothelial growth factor 2 gene transfer by catheter delivery in patients with chronic myocardial ischemia. *Circulation* 2002;105:2012–2018.
245. Henry TD, Annex BH, McKendall GR, et al. The VIVA trial: vascular endothelial growth factor in ischemia for vascular angiogenesis. *Circulation* 2003;107:1359–1365.
246. Freyberger H, Brocker M, Yakut H, et al. Increased levels of platelet-derived growth factor in vitreous fluid of patients with proliferative diabetic retinopathy. *Exp Clin Endocrinol Diabetes* 2000;108:106–109.
247. Koyama N, Watanabe S, Tezuka M, et al. Migratory and proliferative effect of platelet-derived growth factor in rabbit retinal endothelial cells: evidence of an autocrine pathway of platelet-derived growth factor. *J Cell Physiol* 1994; 158:1–6.
248. Inaba T, Ishibashi S, Gotoda T, et al. Enhanced expression of platelet-derived growth factor-beta receptor by high glucose. Involvement of platelet-derived growth factor in diabetic angiopathy. *Diabetes* 1996;45:507–512.
249. Fraser D, Wakefield L, Phillips A. Independent regulation of transforming growth factor-beta1 transcription and translation by glucose and platelet-derived growth factor. *Am J Pathol* 2002;161:1039–1049.
250. Hammes HP, Lin J, Renner O, et al. Pericytes and the pathogenesis of diabetic retinopathy. *Diabetes* 2002;51:3107–3112.
251. Enge M, Bjarnegard M, Gerhardt H, et al. Endothelium-specific platelet-derived growth factor-B ablation mimics diabetic retinopathy. *EMBO J* 2002; 21:4307–4316.
252. Sharma K, Ziyadeh FN, Alzahabi B, et al. Increased renal production of transforming growth factor-beta1 in patients with type II diabetes. *Diabetes* 1997; 46:854–859.
253. Iwano M, Kubo A, Nishino T, et al. Quantification of glomerular TGF-beta 1 mRNA in patients with diabetes mellitus. *Kidney Int* 1996;49:1120–1126.
254. Hong SW, Isono M, Chen S, et al. Increased glomerular and tubular expression of transforming growth factor-beta1, its type II receptor, and activation of the Smad signaling pathway in the db/db mouse. *Am J Pathol* 2001;158: 1653–1663.
255. Han DC, Hoffman BB, Hong SW, et al. Therapy with antisense TGF-beta1 oligodeoxynucleotides reduces kidney weight and matrix mRNAs in diabetic mice. *Am J Physiol Renal Physiol* 2000;278:F628–F634.
256. Yang YL, Guh JY, Yang ML, et al. Interaction between high glucose and TGF-beta in cell cycle protein regulations in MDCK cells. *J Am Soc Nephrol* 1998;9: 182–193.
257. Poncelet AC, Schnaper HW. Sp1 and Smad proteins cooperate to mediate transforming growth factor-beta 1-induced alpha 2(I) collagen expression in human glomerular mesangial cells. *J Biol Chem* 2001;276:6983–6992.
258. Ziyadeh FN, Sharma K, Ericksen M, et al. Stimulation of collagen gene expression and protein synthesis in murine mesangial cells by high glucose is mediated by autocrine activation of transforming growth factor-beta. *J Clin Invest* 1994;93:536–542.
259. Han DC, Isono M, Hoffman BB, et al. High glucose stimulates proliferation and collagen type I synthesis in renal cortical fibroblasts: mediation by autocrine activation of TGF-beta. *J Am Soc Nephrol* 1999;10:1891–1899.
260. Chen S, Cohen MP, Lautenslager GT, et al. Glycated albumin stimulates TGF-beta 1 production and protein kinase C activity in glomerular endothelial cells. *Kidney Int* 2001;59:673–681.
261. Wolf G, Hamann A, Han DC, et al. Leptin stimulates proliferation and TGF-beta expression in renal glomerular endothelial cells: potential role in glomerulosclerosis. *Kidney Int* 1999;56:860–872.
262. Han DC, Isono M, Chen S, et al. Leptin stimulates type I collagen production in db/db mesangial cells: glucose uptake and TGF-beta type II receptor expression. *Kidney Int* 2001;59:1315–1323.
263. Gupta S, Clarkson MR, Duggan J, et al. Connective tissue growth factor: potential role in glomerulosclerosis and tubulointerstitial fibrosis. *Kidney Int* 2000;58:1389–1399.
264. Wahab NA, Yevdokimova N, Weston BS, et al. Role of connective tissue growth factor in the pathogenesis of diabetic nephropathy. *Biochem J* 2001; 359:77–87.
265. Riser BL, Denichilo M, Cortes P, et al. Regulation of connective tissue growth factor activity in cultured rat mesangial cells and its expression in experimental diabetic glomerulosclerosis. *J Am Soc Nephrol* 2000;11:25–38.
266. Murphy M, Godson C, Cannon S, et al. Suppression subtractive hybridization identifies high glucose levels as a stimulus for expression of connective tissue growth factor and other genes in human mesangial cells. *J Biol Chem* 1999;274:5830–5834.
267. Chen Y, Blom IE, Sa S, et al. CTGF expression in mesangial cells: involvement of SMADs, MAP kinase, and PKC. *Kidney Int* 2002;62:1149–1159.
268. Way KJ, Isshiki K, Suzuma K, et al. Expression of connective tissue growth factor is increased in injured myocardium associated with protein kinase C beta2 activation and diabetes. *Diabetes* 2002;51:2709–2718.
269. Bereket A, Lang CH, Wilson TA. Alterations in the growth hormone-insulin-like growth factor axis in insulin dependent diabetes mellitus. *Horm Metab Res* 1999;31:172–181.
270. Doi T, Striker LJ, Quaife C, et al. Progressive glomerulosclerosis develops in transgenic mice chronically expressing growth hormone and growth hormone releasing factor but not in those expressing insulinlike growth factor-1. *Am J Pathol* 1988;131:398–403.
271. Chen NY, Chen WY, Bellush L, et al. Effects of streptozotocin treatment in growth hormone (GH) and GH antagonist transgenic mice. *Endocrinology* 1995;136:660–667.
272. Bellush LL, Doublier S, Holland AN, et al. Protection against diabetes-induced nephropathy in growth hormone receptor/binding protein gene-disrupted mice. *Endocrinology* 2000;141:163–168.
273. Smith LE, Kopchick JJ, Chen W, et al. Essential role of growth hormone in ischemia-induced retinal neovascularization. *Science* 1997;276:1706–1709.
274. Gilbert RE, Krum H, Wilkinson-Berka J, et al. The renin-angiotensin system and the long-term complications of diabetes: pathophysiological and therapeutic considerations. *Diabet Med* 2003;20:607–621.
275. Malik RA, Williamson S, Abbott C, et al. Effect of angiotensin-converting-enzyme (ACE) inhibitor trandolapril on human diabetic neuropathy: randomised double-blind controlled trial. *Lancet* 1998;352:1978–1981.
276. Mehler PS, Jeffers BW, Estacio R, et al. Associations of hypertension and complications in non-insulin-dependent diabetes mellitus. *Am J Hypertens* 1997; 10:152–161.
277. Anderson S, Rennke HG, Garcia DL, et al. Short and long term effects of antihypertensive therapy in the diabetic rat. *Kidney Int* 1989;36:526–536.

278. Allen TJ, Cao Z, Youssef S, et al. Role of angiotensin II and bradykinin in experimental diabetic nephropathy. Functional and structural studies. *Diabetes* 1997;46:1612–1618.
279. Zatz R, Dunn BR, Meyer TW, et al. Prevention of diabetic glomerulopathy by pharmacological amelioration of glomerular capillary hypertension. *J Clin Invest* 1986;77:1925–1930.
280. Navar LG, Lewis L, Hymel A, et al. Tubular fluid concentrations and kidney contents of angiotensins I and II in anesthetized rats. *J Am Soc Nephrol* 1994; 5:1153–1158.
281. Kagami S, Border WA, Miller DE, et al. Angiotensin II stimulates extracellular matrix protein synthesis through induction of transforming growth factor-beta expression in rat glomerular mesangial cells. *J Clin Invest* 1994;93: 2431–2437.
282. Kawano H, Do YS, Kawano Y, et al. Angiotensin II has multiple profibrotic effects in human cardiac fibroblasts. *Circulation* 2000;101:1130–1137.
283. Chen MM, Lam A, Abraham JA, et al. CTGF expression is induced by TGF-beta in cardiac fibroblasts and cardiac myocytes: a potential role in heart fibrosis. *J Mol Cell Cardiol* 2000;32:1805–1819.
284. Chen HC, Bouchie JL, Perez AS, et al. Role of the angiotensin AT(1) receptor in rat aortic and cardiac PAI-1 gene expression. *Arterioscler Thromb Vasc Biol* 2000;20:2297–2302.
285. Price DA, Porter LE, Gordon M, et al. The paradox of the low-renin state in diabetic nephropathy. *J Am Soc Nephrol* 1999;10:2382–2391.
286. Schunkert H, Ingelfinger JR, Jacob H, et al. Reciprocal feedback regulation of kidney angiotensinogen and renin mRNA expressions by angiotensin II. *Am J Physiol* 1992;263:E863–E869.
287. Osanai T, Fujita N, Fujiwara N, et al. Cross talk of shear-induced production of prostacyclin and nitric oxide in endothelial cells. *Am J Physiol Heart Circ Physiol* 2000;278:H233–H238.
288. Huang A, Sun D, Smith CJ, et al. In eNOS knockout mice skeletal muscle arteriolar dilation to acetylcholine is mediated by EDHF. *Am J Physiol Heart Circ Physiol* 2000;278:H762–H768.
289. Koltai MZ, Hadhazy P, Posa I, et al. Characteristics of coronary endothelial dysfunction in experimental diabetes. *Cardiovasc Res* 1997;34:157–163.
290. Zanetti M, Sato J, Katusic ZS, et al. Gene transfer of endothelial nitric oxide synthase alters endothelium-dependent relaxations in aortas from diabetic rabbits. *Diabetologia* 2000;43:340–347.
291. Ding Y, Vaziri ND, Coulson R, et al. Effects of simulated hyperglycemia, insulin, and glucagon on endothelial nitric oxide synthase expression. *Am J Physiol Endocrinol Metab* 2000;279:E11–E17.
292. Cosentino F, Hishikawa K, Katusic ZS, et al. High glucose increases nitric oxide synthase expression and superoxide anion generation in human aortic endothelial cells. *Circulation* 1997;96:25–28.
293. Hink U, Li H, Mollnau H, et al. Effects of diabetes mellitus on nitric oxide synthase (NOS III) expression, NOS III mediated superoxide production and vascular nitric oxide bioavailability. *Circulation* 1999;100:I-235(abst).
294. Lund DD, Faraci FM, Miller FJ Jr, et al. Gene transfer of endothelial nitric oxide synthase improves relaxation of carotid arteries from diabetic rabbits. *Circulation* 2000;101:1027–1033.
295. Zhao X, Lu X, Feng Q. Deficiency in endothelial nitric oxide synthase impairs myocardial angiogenesis. *Am J Physiol Heart Circ Physiol* 2002;283:H2371–H2378.
296. Studer RK, DeRubertis FR, Craven PA. Nitric oxide suppresses increases in mesangial cell protein kinase C, transforming growth factor beta, and fibronectin synthesis induced by thromboxane. *J Am Soc Nephrol* 1996;7:999– 1005.
297. Craven PA, Studer RK, Felder J, et al. Nitric oxide inhibition of transforming growth factor-beta and collagen synthesis in mesangial cells. *Diabetes* 1997; 46:671–681.
298. Venugopal SK, Devaraj S, Jialal I. C-reactive protein decreases prostacyclin release from human aortic endothelial cells. *Circulation* 2003;108:1676–1678.
299. Cosentino F, Eto M, De Paolis P, et al. High glucose causes upregulation of cyclooxygenase-2 and alters prostanoid profile in human endothelial cells: role of protein kinase C and reactive oxygen species. *Circulation* 2003;107: 1017–1023.
300. Tesfamariam B, Brown ML, Deykin D, et al. Elevated glucose promotes generation of endothelium-derived vasoconstrictor prostanoids in rabbit aorta. *J Clin Invest* 1990;85:929–932.
301. Hopfner RL, Gopalakrishnan V. Endothelin: emerging role in diabetic vascular complications. *Diabetologia* 1999;42:1383–1394.
302. Mather KJ, Mirzamohammadi B, Lteif A, et al. Endothelin contributes to basal vascular tone and endothelial dysfunction in human obesity and type 2 diabetes. *Diabetes* 2002;51:3517–3523.
303. Lee ME, Dhadly MS, Temizer DH, et al. Regulation of endothelin-1 gene expression by Fos and Jun. *J Biol Chem* 1991;266:19034–19039.
304. Takagi C, Bursell SE, Lin YW, et al. Regulation of retinal hemodynamics in diabetic rats by increased expression and action of endothelin-1. *Invest Ophthalmol Vis Sci* 1996;37:2504–2518.
305. Merkus D, Duncker DJ, Chilian WM. Metabolic regulation of coronary vascular tone: role of endothelin-1. *Am J Physiol Heart Circ Physiol* 2002;283: H1915–H1921.
306. Oliver FJ, de la Rubia G, Feener EP, et al. Stimulation of endothelin-1 gene expression by insulin in endothelial cells. *J Biol Chem* 1991;266:23251–23256.
307. Cardillo C, Nambi SS, Kilcoyne CM, et al. Insulin stimulates both endothelin and nitric oxide activity in the human forearm. *Circulation* 1999;100: 820–825.
308. Hocher B, Thone-Reineke C, Rohmeiss P, et al. Endothelin-1 transgenic mice develop glomerulosclerosis, interstitial fibrosis, and renal cysts but not hypertension. *J Clin Invest* 1997;99:1380–1389.
309. Quaschning T, Kocak S, Bauer C, et al. Increase in nitric oxide bioavailability improves endothelial function in endothelin-1 transgenic mice. *Nephrol Dial Transplant* 2003;18:479–483.
310. Schwarz A, Godes M, Thone-Reineke C, et al. Tissue-dependent expression of matrix proteins in human endothelin-1 transgenic mice. *Clin Sci (Lond)* 2002;103[Suppl]48:39S–43S.
311. Evans T, Deng DX, Chen S, et al. Endothelin receptor blockade prevents augmented extracellular matrix component mRNA expression and capillary basement membrane thickening in the retina of diabetic and galactose-fed rats. *Diabetes* 2000;49:662–666.
312. Rodriguez-Pascual F, Redondo-Horcajo M, Lamas S. Functional cooperation between Smad proteins and activator protein-1 regulates transforming growth factor-beta-mediated induction of endothelin-1 expression. *Circ Res* 2003;92: 1288–1295.
313. Risso A, Mercuri F, Quagliaro L, et al. Intermittent high glucose enhances apoptosis in human umbilical vein endothelial cells in culture. *Am J Physiol Endocrinol Metab* 2001;281:E924–E930.

CHAPTER 50
Pathogenesis of Diabetic Neuropathy

Phillip A. Low

The diabetic neuropathies are those associated with the diabetic state. Although the neuropathies are clearly related to the presence, duration, and severity of hyperglycemia, controversies exist on the types of diabetic neuropathies and their pathogenesis. Diabetic neuropathies have many phenotypes (Table 50.1). *Distal sensory neuropathy* is the most common variety of neuropathy, with mild distal sensory impairment and minimal motor deficits. This category comprises greater than 50% of all diabetic neuropathies. *Distal small fiber neuropathy* is also common; it is characterized paradoxically by a combination of distal positive symptoms, including painfulness and impairment in both pain and temperature perception. Painfulness occurs in many types of diabetic neuropathies. The asymmetric neuropathies are distinctive and are likely due to a combination of microvascular disease, compression injury, and immune-mediated mechanisms. Despite the profusion of manifestations and types of neuropathy, the common garden-variety distal sensory neuropathy is present in essentially all varieties of diabetic neuropathies and comprises the major focus of this chapter.

UNIQUE CHARACTERISTICS OF THE PERIPHERAL NERVE

Because the peripheral nerve axons are extremely long relative to their diameters and are a great distance from their parent cell bodies (in dorsal root ganglion, autonomic ganglion, and motor neurons), their component motor, sensory, and autonomic axons, especially distally, are exquisitely dependent on endoneurial microenvironment for their blood supply, oxygenation, nutrition, and the removal of toxic metabolic products. The peripheral nerve is physiologically unique in several ways, information that has an important bearing on its response as a target to chronic hyperglycemia.

Resistance to Ischemic Fiber Degeneration

The nerve is supplied by a dual system of microvessels. It has an *intrinsic* interconnecting system, connected via arterioles and venules to an epineurial system, the *extrinsic* system (1). The dual system, low energy requirements, and relatively large energy stores together confer on the nerve a large safety factor in its resistance to ischemic fiber degeneration. Earlier experimental data in which peripheral nerve was undercut or the regional supply was ligated demonstrated that nerve fiber degeneration did not occur even when long stretches of nerve were deprived of their intrinsic supply either by arterial ligation (2) or by extensive nerve trunk mobilization with undercutting of connecting blood supply (3).

Lack of Autoregulation

Autoregulation refers to the maintenance of constant blood flow, in spite of changes in blood pressure [within a blood pressure

TABLE 50.1. Types of Diabetic Neuropathies

Symmetric neuropathies
1. Distal sensory neuropathy
2. Large-fiber type of diabetic neuropathy
3. Small-fiber type of diabetic neuropathy
4. Distal small-fiber neuropathy
5. "Insulin" neuritis
6. Proximal diabetic neuropathy (lumbosacral radiculoplexopathy)
7. Chronic inflammatory demyelinating polyradiculoneuropathy (CIDP)

Asymmetric neuropathies
1. Mononeuropathy
2. Mononeuropathy multiplex
3. Radiculopathies
4. Lumbar plexopathy or radiculoplexopathies
5. Proximal diabetic neuropathy (lumbosacral radiculoplexopathy)
6. CIDP

range (the autoregulated range)]. In most tissues, autoregulation is achieved by dynamically varying arteriolar tone and by myogenic rather than neurogenic mechanisms. There is a characteristic blood flow:blood pressure curve, which is flat within the autoregulated range and sloping at either end. We demonstrated a curvilinear relationship of nerve blood flow to blood pressure, a relationship that is explainable on the basis of a passive nonautoregulating system (4). This finding has subsequently been confirmed in anesthetized (5,6) and nonanesthetized rats (7).

Nerve Is a Nutritive-Capacitance Vascular Bed

Another unique characteristic of nerve microvasculature is its *nutritive capacitance* system (5). This is a disadvantaged system where a small change in blood volume results in a disproportionate change in nerve blood flow. The morphologic basis of this system appears to be the large-diameter capillary whose diameter exceeds that of the erythrocyte. The median diameter of the endoneurial capillary is 8 to 9 µm (8), considerably larger than that of erythrocytes (about 7 µm). In other tissues the capillary is smaller than the erythrocytes, resulting in a squeezing action that enhances oxygen release. The large diameter with poorly developed arteriolar smooth muscle (9) results in inefficient oxygen release.

Nerve Can Be Sustained on Anaerobic Metabolism

The peripheral nerve is metabolically unique, being able to function relatively well on anaerobic metabolism and having powerful adaptive mechanisms. Compared with rat brain, the nerve has about 10% of the brain's oxygen requirements but similar energy stores (10,11). When maximally active, the nerve increases its energy demands less than 100%, whereas the brain increases its demands severalfold (11). The relatively large energy stores and the low resting and maximal energy expenditure enable the nerve to function quite well on anaerobically generated high-energy phosphate. It is likely that the low-density capacitance system developed because of the low metabolism of the nerve. We have demonstrated that the nerve will conduct impulses for many additional minutes when energy substrates are increased, as in diabetes (11).

Another strategy of resistance to ischemic conduction failure is a further downregulation of energy-requiring enzymes, a situation that occurs in aging (12) and in chronic hypoxia (13).

UNIQUE CHARACTERISTICS OF HUMAN DIABETIC NEUROPATHY

There are a number of unique characteristics of human and experimental diabetic neuropathy. Four of these are relevant to the pathogenesis of diabetic neuropathy:

- Susceptibility to entrapment/compression neuropathies
- Susceptibility to ischemic fiber degeneration
- Insulin-induced neuritis

Resistance to Ischemic Conduction Failure

When the limb is rendered ischemic, paresthesias develop followed by the loss of sensory then motor functions. The electrophysiologic correlate is a failure of nerve conduction. Both diabetic humans and animals manifest resistance to ischemic conduction failure (RICF) (11,14). Nerve impulses continue to conduct for minutes in diabetic individuals after those in normal individuals have failed to do so. The clinical correlate is that patients are more resistant to paresthesias and retain nerve function for minutes beyond normal subjects.

MECHANISM

The mechanism of RICF likely relates to the unique metabolic characteristics described previously. Diabetic nerves have a severalfold increase in nerve energy substrates (glucose, fructose, glycogen) (11). Their energy requirements are sufficiently low to permit them to continue to conduct impulses on adenosine triphosphate (ATP) derived from anaerobic metabolism (1). Their energy requirements may also be downregulated. The relatively large endoneurial space (relative to brain) results in less susceptibility to lactate- and potassium-induced conduction failure (11).

Susceptibility to Entrapment/ Compression Neuropathies

Diabetic nerve trunks are unduly susceptible to focal neuropathies that occur in a limited number of circumstances (15). Focal neuropathies occur due to repetitive compression, as occurs with leaning on the ulnar nerve at its groove and pressure of the peroneal nerve against the fibular neck (15). Entrapment can occur within the carpal tunnel as with the median nerve, causing carpal tunnel syndrome (15). A third category is the acute onset of focal noncompressive neuropathy, e.g., third cranial nerve.

MECHANISM

The precise pathophysiology is not known. Circumstantial evidence suggests that the combination of ischemia and mechanical susceptibility might be responsible. Evidence for microvascular ischemia clinically includes the acute or subacute onset of, for example, third-nerve palsy in vasculopathic older patients. Pathologic evidence is limited but includes the presence of microinfarcts, multifocal pathology, and fibrinoid change (16). Such changes have been described in two diabetic patients; one died shortly after the onset of oculomotor palsy (17); in the second, a 73-year-old man with diabetes who died shortly after the onset of a focal limb neuropathy, the obturator, femoral, sciatic, and posterior tibial nerves were examined (18). Combined changes of florid round cell infiltration and microvascular changes have been interpreted as being due to a combination of microvascular ischemia and immune-mediated mechanisms. Three sets of findings are consistently found in chronic diabetic neuropathy: first, a thickening of basal lamina (19); second, endothelial-cell and smooth-muscle proliferation (20,21) with increased variance of capillary caliber and the closing of some capillaries (20); third, the tendency of fiber loss to be multifocal rather than diffuse (22,23). The combination of microvascular ischemia, connective tissue changes (24), and myelin alterations could presumably render the nerve trunk susceptible to compression injury.

Excessive Susceptibility to Ischemic Fiber Degeneration of Diabetic Nerves

Ischemia of mild-to-moderate severity is associated with excessive susceptibility to ischemic fiber degeneration. The latter is reported to occur in animals with chronic hyperglycemia in excess of 16 weeks but not with hyperglycemia of shorter duration (25,26). Other studies report excessive susceptibility much earlier in the course of diabetes. Reports include excessive susceptibility to ischemic fiber degeneration in response to epineurial application of endothelin in rats with a duration of hyperglycemia of only 6 to 8 weeks (27), and with the *in vitro* study showing that a medium with increased glucose causes intracellular acidosis with delayed recovery (28).

The human equivalent of susceptibility to ischemic fiber degeneration is not well documented.

Insulin-Induced Neuropathy

Infrequently, an acute painful neuropathy develops within 1 month of the institution of tight glycemic control with insulin therapy in a diabetic patient who previously did not have a neuropathy (29–31). The neuropathy is usually that of a painful distal sensory polyneuropathy, although it also can be a severe generalized neuropathy.

Recent experimental studies provide some insight into the mechanism of insulin neuritis. Insulin administration reproducibly causes acute endoneurial hypoxia by increasing nerve arteriovenous flow and reducing nutritive flow of normal nerves (32). The diabetic state confers resistance to this effect. Within 1 month of commencement of insulin treatment, this susceptibility to the endoneurial hypoxic effect of insulin recurs (32). Endoneurial hypoxia has been demonstrated in experimental and human diabetic neuropathy (33,34). We had suggested that diabetic nerve fibers survive under these hypoxic conditions because of the greatly increased energy substrate stores in experimental and human diabetes (11,35), coupled with the low energy requirements of peripheral nerve (1). Anaerobic metabolism suffices under these circumstances. Insulin treatment causes transient hypoxia in normal but not diabetic nerves (32). With continued insulin treatment, energy substrates are normalized and the susceptibility to insulin-induced endoneurial hypoxia returns in diabetic nerves. The hypoxic tissues with normal energy substrates fare poorly because anaerobic metabolism is inefficient (1), and there may be sufficient hypoxia to result in fiber degeneration.

PATHOGENESIS OF DIABETIC NEUROPATHY

The pathogenesis of the common, garden-variety distal sensory diabetic neuropathy is likely multifactorial. Hyperglycemia is central to any pathogenetic scheme. There are sufficient experimental and observational data to warrant consideration of the following mechanisms in mediating the effects of chronic hyperglycemia:

- Genetic predisposition
- Nerve hypoxia/ischemia
- Oxidative stress
- Overactivity of polyol pathway
- Increased advanced glycation end products
- Deficiency of γ-linolenic acid
- Protein kinase C, especially increase in β-isoform
- Growth factor(s) deficiency
- Dysimmune mechanisms

Genetic Predisposition

One patient with lifelong severe hyperglycemia is free of neuropathy; another has florid neuropathy within a few years of onset of hyperglycemia; another patient with a strong family history of diabetes may actually develop neuropathy before diabetes is diagnosable. Although these types of observations suggest a genetic predisposition to the development of neuropathy, the available data are very limited. Most of the studies to date have focused on the genetics of inheritance of type 1 and type 2 diabetes.

Nerve Ischemia/Hypoxia

EXPERIMENTAL DIABETIC NEUROPATHY

Vasoregulation of nerve microvessels is regulated at the arteriolar, venular, and endothelial cell levels. In the diabetic state, endothelial changes include those of AGE-RAGE-NF-κB [advanced glycosylation end products (AGE)–AGE receptor–nuclear factor κB (NF-κB)], cell adhesion molecules, nitric oxide, and eicosanoids. Experimental diabetic neuropathy results in a reduction in nerve blood flow of about 50% (33,36), which begins by the first week of diabetes (36) and affects the cell body of sensory and sympathetic neurons as well as the axon (37). In diabetes, the combination of increased whole-blood or plasma viscosity, increased aggregability, and reduced red blood cell deformability results in a reduction of blood flow and stagnation hypoxia (1).

Regional nerve blood flow is regulated by systemic blood pressure (4) and the balance between neural vasoconstrictors and vasodilators. Vasoconstriction is known to be mediated by epineurial α-adrenergic (38,39), vasopressin (40), and endothelin receptors (41). The 50% effective concentration (EC_{50}) of endothelin, using identical methodology, is about three orders of magnitude lower, indicating greater potency, than that of adrenoreceptors (41). The EC_{50} of vasopressin is of an order similar to that of endothelin. These potent vasoconstrictor actions are balanced by vasodilatation and are mediated by calcitonin gene–related peptide (42), substance P (42), nitric oxide (NO) (43), and the prostaglandins (44).

Alterations in microvessels in experimental diabetic neuropathy have been reported. These are reported to be excessively sensitive to α-adrenergic agonists (45) and endothelin (46,47). The nerve conduction and blood-flow deficits are prevented by specific antagonists to endothelin (48) and adrenoreceptors (49). Deficits in vasodilators are supported by restoration of blood flow and nerve conduction by an NO donor (50) and vasodilator prostaglandins (51). The reduction of NO is likely the most important in its magnitude and implications (43). The polyol pathway is overactive and competes with nitric oxide synthase for NADPH (reduced form of nicotinamide adenine dinucleotide phosphate). By siphoning off NADPH, chronic hyperglycemia results in a deficiency of NO in nerve endothelium (43,50). Endoneurial NO deficiency has a number of important consequences in the microvasculature. It normally inhibits the expression of P-selectin, intercellular adhesion molecule-1 (ICAM-1), vascular cell adhesion molecule-1 (VCAM-1), and other adhesion molecules (52), a mechanism that is mediated through inhibition of protein kinase C and by preventing the activation of NF-κB (53). NO also inhibits the cytoassembly of NADPH oxidase (54), thereby attenuating the release of superoxide by leukocytes (55). Inhibition of NO, therefore, explains a number of changes seen in experimental diabetic neuropathy (expression of adhesion molecules, activation of NF-κB, expression of cytokines, and generation of superoxide anions).

HUMAN DIABETIC NEUROPATHY

Three main pathologic alterations affect human diabetic peripheral nerve. First, thickening of endoneurial capillary wall and thickening and reduplication of basal lamina have consistently been found (56,57), especially in more recent studies (16,58). Basal lamina thickening, although characteristic, is not specific to the diabetic state, occurring especially with aging and a number of other neuropathies. Second, alterations in capillaries are consistently present. These changes include a reduction in capillary density, reduced capillary area, and capillary closure (16,20,58). Third, the pattern of fiber loss is multifocal, suggestive of ischemic fiber loss (22,23). In a three-dimensional reconstruction of the distribution of fiber loss using autopsy specimens from lumbosacral trunk to sural nerve biopsy specimens, the changes seen in sural nerve manifest the cumulative loss of fibers, whereas multifocal fiber loss is better appreciated in more proximal nerve trunks (59). Although these alterations have been well defined, their specificity has been questioned (60). These studies are all important in attempting to define morphometric abnormalities of endoneurial vessels and fibers. They suffer from their ability to define the results but inability to define the pathogenetic process.

The most concerted and coherent studies of perfusion and oxygenation of human diabetic nerves have been undertaken by the Sheffield group. They were the first to demonstrate reduced oxygen tension in human diabetic neuropathy. They measured endoneurial oxygen tension in exposed sural nerve of 11 patients with diabetic neuropathy (34). Correlative pathologic studies in a separate study were supportive, showing reduced endoneurial capillary density and changes in capillary basement membrane and endothelial cells and in the derived total diffusion barrier that was significantly impaired in the nerves of patients with severe diabetic neuropathy as compared with control subjects (58). Blood flow and oxygen tension recordings in the operating room are not trivial. Recordings using laser Doppler methodology have been reported to show no change or even a slight increase in blood flow and oxygen tension (61). These results are un-interpretable in diabetic neuropathy, because it measures total and not nutritive flow, where shunt flow may actually be increased (62).

A number of innovative approaches have been developed to measure flow and oxygenation. Nerve photography and fluorescein angiography demonstrate delayed fluorescein appearance time and intensity of fluorescence in human diabetic neuropathy (62). These investigators observed direct epineurial arteriovenous shunting in the majority of diabetic neuropathic patients. A novel approach using microlightguide spectrophotometry to measure intravascular oxygen saturation and blood flow in human sural nerve after an intravenous injection of sodium fluorescein has confirmed impaired nerve blood flow and tissue deoxygenation. There was a correlation between rise time, nerve oxygen saturation, glycemic control, and sural nerve sensory conduction velocity (63).

THERAPEUTIC APPLICATIONS

Angiotensin-converting enzyme (ACE) inhibition with lisinopril administered to 13 hypertensive patients with diabetic neuropathy was reported to improve nerve conduction indices and sensory perception thresholds (64). A small, randomized, double-blind, placebo-controlled trial on the effect of the ACE inhibitor trandolapril on 41 normotensive patients with type 1 or type 2 diabetes and mild neuropathy has appeared (65). Changes in the neuropathy symptom and deficit scores, vibration-perception threshold, peripheral-nerve electrophysiology, and cardiovascular autonomic function were assessed at 6 and 12 months. The primary end point was the change in peroneal nerve motor conduction velocity. Peroneal motor nerve conduction velocity ($p = 0.03$) and M-wave amplitude ($p = 0.03$) increased, the F-wave latency ($p = 0.03$) decreased, and sural nerve action potential amplitude increased ($p = 0.04$) significantly after 12 months of treatment with trandolapril as compared with response to placebo.

The study is interesting and has potentially important implications. There is controversy over whether ischemia is a central mechanism or is one of many mechanisms in the production of diabetic neuropathy. In view of the strength of the evidence of the benefits of ACE inhibition on renal function, it might be difficult to set up a specific study on neuropathy, in contrast to a neuropathy piggyback study similar to the Diabetes Control and Complications Trial.

Oxidative Stress

There is considerable evidence of oxidative stress in both experimental and human diabetic neuropathy. We will summarize the evidence in non-neural tissues followed by data on neural tissue. The data on non-neural tissues come from studies of plasma; erythrocytes; and primarily heart, liver, kidney, and pancreas. These studies have focused on evidence of increased lipid peroxidation and alteration in the patterns of glutathione and antioxidant enzymes. Evidence of oxidative stress may be manifested as a reduction or an increase in antioxidant enzymes (66). Not all experts espouse the role of oxidative stress. One view is that the predominant stress is reductive, characterized by an increase in the NADH/NAD$^+$ (reduced form of nicotinamide adenine dinucleotide oxidized form of nicotinamide adenine dinucleotide) ratio (67). Another view, proposed by John Baynes (68), is thoughtful and complicated. He recognizes that increases in glycoxidation and lipoxidation products suggest that oxidative stress is increased in diabetes but that the data are best explained as an increase in carbonyl stress.

OXIDANT STRESS IN HUMAN DIABETES

Oxidative stress refers to a shift in the pro-oxidant:antioxidant status toward the former. Plasma levels of lipid peroxide are increased in human diabetes (69–74) and occur early, even in young persons with diabetes (75). The highest levels were reported in patients with microvascular angiopathy, as manifested as retinopathy or microalbuminuria; lowest in those patients with diabetes without angiopathy (69,76); and normal in patients with well-controlled diabetes (69). The relationship may relate to the observation that low-density lipoproteins of patients with diabetes are significantly more oxidizable than are those of controls, an abnormality that is correctable by 6 weeks of treatment with the antioxidant probucol (77). Presumably, patients with diabetes with angiopathy who have higher levels of low-density lipoproteins will have the greatest lipid peroxidation.

More recent data are more consistent with increased oxidant stress being secondary to metabolic status rather than to complications (78), including a positive correlation with glycosylated hemoglobin and a negative correlation of malondialdehyde with glutathione peroxidase (79). Recent work has focused on combining measurements of lipid peroxidation (increased) with indices of total antioxidant defense (reduced) in diabetes (80,81). Additional emphasis has been placed on evaluation of indices that reflect specific mechanisms and tissues affected by oxidant stress. Measurements include those of increased activation of the oxidative stress–sensitive transcription factor NF-κB (82). Greater importance also is placed on products that specifically reflect neural or DNA damage, such as 4-hydroxynonenal and 8-oxo, 2′-deoxyguanosine in relevant tissue (83). Urinary 8-oxo, 2′-deoxyguanosine excretion and the 8-oxo, 2′-deoxyguanosine content in the mononuclear cells from diabetic patients with complications were higher than those from diabetic patients without complications (84,85).

Glutathione (GSH) is reduced in erythrocytes from patients with type 2 diabetes, with a corresponding increase in oxidized glutathione (GSSG) (86,87). In subsequent studies, this same group additionally demonstrated reductions in the glutathione synthesizing enzyme, γ-glutamylcysteine synthetase, and the transport of thiol [S-(s,4-dintrophenyl)glutathione] in erythrocytes of these patients. These abnormalities were reversible with improved glycemic control. They also demonstrated that a medium high in glucose augments the toxicity of xenobiotics on K562 cells, associated with reduction in both the enzyme and its mRNA (88). Lipid peroxidation is increased and antioxidant enzymes are reduced in the erythrocytes of persons with type 2 diabetes. Changes in GSH and antioxidant enzymes occur early, even at onset of type 1 diabetes (75).

Erythrocyte cuprozinc superoxide dismutase (SOD) is reduced in patients with type 2 diabetes (70,89), and catalase is variably reduced (89). It is suggested that this reduction is mediated by the accumulation of intracellular H_2O_2 (90). Changes in SOD occur early (75).

Levels of α-tocopherol are reported to be reduced in the platelets (90,91) and erythrocytes (92) but not in the plasma of patients with type 1 diabetes. Leukocytes from patients with diabetes were shown to have increased lipid peroxidation, reduced vitamin C levels in 53 patients with type 2 diabetes (93), and reduced cuprozinc SOD (94).

Wolff (95) has emphasized the role of decompartmentalized transitional metals in patients with diabetes, in addition to the effects of hyperglycemia, in producing auto-oxidative lipid peroxidation. Particular emphasis has been placed on copper and iron. Copper levels have been reported to be higher in persons with diabetes than in those without diabetes and are highest in patients with angiopathy (96,97).

OXIDANT STRESS IN EXPERIMENTAL DIABETES

Studies on non-neural tissues have examined plasma, erythrocytes, and tissues such as heart, liver, kidney, and pancreas. These studies have focused on evidence of increased lipid peroxidation, reduction of GSH, and alteration in the patterns of antioxidant enzymes. Evidence of oxidative stress may be associated with a reduction (presumably aggravating stress) or an increase (presumably a compensatory response) in antioxidant enzymes (66). The remainder of this section will focus on changes in nerves, particularly on (a) evidence for reduced free-radical defenses; (b) change in pro-oxidant status; (c) evidence for increased reduced oxygen species; and (d) neural targets.

FREE-RADICAL DEFENSES ARE REDUCED IN PERIPHERAL NERVE

Peripheral nerve has a number of cytosolic and lipophilic antioxidant defenses with closely integrated actions (Table 50.2). These comprise a number of low-molecular-weight and enzymic antioxidant molecules. The key enzymatic scavengers are SOD, catalase, glutathione peroxidase, and glutathione reductase. Glutathione is particularly important in that it is the main scavenger in the blocking of chain propagation (98). The cytosolic and membrane antioxidants work in concert in a well-organized interacting chain. Ample activity of all components is needed to maintain these antioxidants in their reduced state. The literature on free-radical biology is extensive, but information on peripheral nerve, and particularly on the diabetic peripheral nerve, is quite limited.

TABLE 50.2. Some Free-Radical Defenses of Peripheral Nerve

Cytosolic	Membrane
Ascorbate, urate, cysteine, glutathione, transferrin, albumin, β-carotene, ceruloplasmin, reduced glutathione (GSH), glutathione peroxidase, catalase, superoxide dismutase	α-Tocopherol

Free-radical defenses of peripheral nerve are reduced relative to those of brain and liver (99,100). Of great interest is the marked and selective reduction in antioxidant defenses in rodent sciatic nerve (Table 50.3). The activities of GSH and GSH-containing enzyme scavengers (glutathione peroxidase and reductase) are only about 10% that of brain, whereas the activities of other enzymes, such as SOD, are near normal (99). Corresponding enzyme activities of these enzymes in the brain are in turn about half that in the liver (100).

The diabetic state results in additional alterations in these defenses (Table 50.4). Cuprozinc SOD is reduced in sciatic nerve of experimental diabetic neuropathy, and this reduction is improved by insulin treatment (101). Glutathione peroxidase is further reduced in experimental diabetic neuropathy (102), and glutathione peroxidase activity regresses with blood glucose concentration. Plasma and leukocyte ascorbic acid are reduced, and oxidation of this antioxidant is increased (103,104). GSH is reduced in diabetic nerves (105,106).

REDUCED OXYGEN SPECIES ARE INCREASED IN EXPERIMENTAL DIABETIC NEUROPATHY

The potential sources of free-radical generation in diabetes will be briefly considered. Of note is that these mechanisms do not occur in isolation and are best considered as interacting mechanisms that converge to cause lipid peroxidation.

Ischemia/Hypoxia in Experimental Diabetic Neuropathy. A deficit in nerve blood flow of 50% in experimental diabetic neuropathy (107–109) results in the generation of hypoxanthine from ATP, NADPH (the cofactor) and conversion of the inactive enzyme to xanthine oxidase (110,111). The diabetic state and endoneurial ischemia increase lipolysis, resulting in an increase in ω-6 fatty acids such as linoleic acid and arachidonic acid (112), whose peroxidation results in 4-hydroxynonenal (HNE), an aldehydic product of membrane lipid peroxidation, and causes prominent cytotoxic effects in cultured endothelial cells, manifested by morphologic changes, diminished cellular viability, and impaired endothelial barrier function (113). HNE has a relatively long half-life within cells (minutes to hours), allowing for multiple interactions with cellular components (114). It impairs glutamate transport and mitochondrial function in neurons (115) and mediates oxidative stress–induced neuronal apoptosis (116).

Autoxidative Lipid Peroxidation. Hyperglycemia, by a process of autoxidation in the presence of decompartmentalized redox-active trace transitional metals, can generate highly reactive oxidants and result in lipid peroxidation (117). We have demonstrated, using an *in vitro* lipid peroxidation model (ascorbate-iron-EDTA preparation), that a high-glucose medium will result in

TABLE 50.3. Activities of Enzymatic Free-Radical Scavengers in Peripheral Nerve Relative to Brain and Liver

Antioxidant	Nerve	% of Brain	Brain	Liver
GSH-GSSG	261.0 ± 24.0	10	2620.0 ± 124.0	—
GSH-Px (→ H_2O_2)	6.4 ± 2.1	13	48.5 ± 5.5	74.9 ± 7.1
GSH-Px (→ *t*-BOOH)	4.6 ± 1.4	9	50.3 ± 1.4	144.0 ± 16.9
GSSG reductase	2.7 ± 0.3	13	20.5 ± 0.6	56.3 ± 6.1
GST (→ CDNB)	9.4 ± 2.4	4	232.5 ± 14.0	171.3 ± 55.4
GST (→ 4-HNE)	5.4 ± 1.2	5	116.5 ± 10.4	345.2 ± 92.0
DT-diaphorase	9.9 ± 2.2	—	—	208.0 ± 49.9
SOD	93.8 ± 12.4	—	—	171.3 ± 55.4

GSH-GSSG, total glutathione; GSH-Px, glutathione peroxidase; *t*-BOOH, *tert*-butyl-hydroperoxide; GSSG reductase, glutathione disulfide reductase; GST, glutathione transferase; CDNB, 1-chloro-2,4-dinitrobenzene; 4-HNE, 4-hydroxy-2,3-trans-nonenol; SOD, superoxide dismutase. Results are expressed as nmol/min (mg prot, ± SEM.
Modified from Romero FJ, Monsalve E, Hermenegildo C, et al. Oxygen toxicity in the nervous tissue: comparison of the antioxidant defense of rat brain and sciatic nerve. *Neurochem Res* 1991;16:157–161; and Romero FJ, Segura–Aguilar J, Monsalve E, et al. Antioxidant and glutathione-related enzymatic activities in rat sciatic nerve. *Neurotoxicol Teratol* 1990;12:603–605.

lipid peroxidation, *in vitro*, of brain and sciatic nerve. The addition of 20 mM glucose to the incubation medium increased lipid peroxidation fourfold, confirming rapid and marked glucose-mediated auto-oxidative lipid peroxidation (118). These studies confirm the observation of autoxidative glycation/oxidation in plasma (38,119). Glucose autoxidation results in the production of protein-reactive ketoaldehydes, hydrogen peroxide, and other highly reactive oxidants and in the fragmentation of proteins (indicative of free-radical mechanisms).

Advanced Glycosylation End Products (AGE)–AGE Receptor–Nuclear Factor κB (AGE-RAGE-NF-κB). Glycation and the formation of AGE is followed by binding with its receptor (RAGE), the activation of NF-κB (120), and the generation of reactive oxygen species (ROS) and an inflammatory response (121). There is induction of specific DNA binding activity for NF-κB in the VCAM-1 promoter region. The necessity for RAGE and the role of ROS was demonstrated by a block of this induction by anti-RAGE IgG or *N*-acetylcysteine (GSH donor). The application of this finding to humans is supported by the finding that peripheral blood mononuclear cells isolated from patients with diabetic nephropathy show increased activation of NF-κB (82). There is a vicious cycle, with AGE-producing superoxide, superoxide-accelerating AGE generation, and AGE-quenching NO (122).

Overactivity of the Polyol Pathway Generates Reactive Oxygen Species. The overactivity of the polyol pathway generates ROS in a number of ways. Depletion in NADPH results in NO deficiency and an increase in the generation of superoxide anion by leukocytes (see earlier). Because NADPH also is required for the regeneration of GSH, its depletion results in a reduction of GSH (123). Sorbitol dehydrogenase, the second enzyme in the polyol pathway that converts sorbitol to fructose, also contributes to oxidative stress, most likely because depletion of its cofactor NAD^+ leads to the channeling of more glucose through the polyol pathway (123). Overactivity of the polyol pathway results in reductions in myoinositol and taurine. The latter is a potent antioxidant, and its depletion (124) further contributes to oxidative stress.

Protein Kinase C. Although the activity of protein kinase C (PKC) in nerve is uncertain, it is known that inhibition of PKC-β will reduce oxidative stress (125) and will normalize the deficits in blood flow and nerve conduction (126). In endothelial cells, high glucose causes activation of NF-κB. Co-incubation with a selective PKC inhibitor, calphostin C, produced a concentration-dependent inhibition of glucose-induced activation of NF-κB, suggesting that PKC is important at the endothelial cell level in the activation of adhesion molecules and the generation of ROS.

Excessive Lipolysis. The diabetic state and endoneurial ischemia increase lipolysis, resulting in an increase in ω-6 fatty acids, such as linoleic acid and arachidonic acid (112), whose peroxidation results in 4-hydroxynonenal (113) (and discussed earlier). Malondialdehyde also is generated in the cyclooxygenase pathway.

Growth-Factor Deficit. Lipid peroxidation is aggravated by a reduction in nerve growth factor (127). Reduction in nerve growth factor will reduce, and its administration will restore, glutathione peroxidase and catalase (128,129).

Inflammatory Response. The main sources of ROS in mammals are leukocytes and mitochondria. The quantitative roles of the leukocytes, cytokines, and catecholamine oxidation in diabetic nerve are uncertain. Leukocytic infiltration is not a feature in most cases of experimental diabetic neuropathy. In human diabetic neuropathy, there are some suggestions of an immune-mediated process, as suggested by the presence of iritis and inflammatory infiltrates in sympathetic ganglia (130). Some forms of diabetic neuropathy, such as acute autonomic neuropathy and the subacute proximal neuropathies, might be associated with prominent round-cell infiltration. A role of associated ROS and oxidative stress should be considered.

TABLE 50.4. Changes in Antioxidant Defenses in Experimental Diabetes

Antioxidant	Change	Reference(s)
Superoxide dismutase (cuprozinc)	Reduced	101
Glutathione peroxidase	Reduced	102
Ascorbic acid content	Reduced	103,104
Ascorbic oxidation	Reduced	103,104
Reduced glutathione (GSH)	Reduced	105,106

CHANGE IN PRO-OXIDANT STATUS

Altered pro-oxidant status occurs in the diabetic state, with an increase in polyunsaturated fatty acids increasing arachidonic acid (112). With ischemia, superoxide anion is converted to H_2O_2, but its further decomposition, which is mediated by glutathione peroxidase (131), may be compromised if the low content of this enzyme is further reduced. HNE, an aldehydic product of membrane lipid peroxidation, is especially pertinent, in that ischemia, by increasing arachidonic acid, provides a substrate for HNE (114), which mediates neuronal apoptosis (116). Other alterations, especially increases in free iron and copper, have been proposed, but definitive evidence has not yet appeared.

TARGETS OF OXIDANT STRESS

The focus of investigations has been the nerve trunk. Recent emphasis has been based on the realization that human diabetic neuropathy is primarily a distal and sensory neuropathy, and emphasis has shifted to the sensory neuron and nerve terminals. Studies of human skin biopsy specimens of epidermal axons comprising unmyelinated sensory fibers have indeed demonstrated that these alterations precede and are more pronounced than changes seen in nerve trunk. Functional deficits of unmyelinated fibers also occur before deficits are demonstrable in the nerve trunk. Indeed, pathologic alterations of digital nerves have been described, although these changes have been ascribed to local trauma.

Recent studies on spinal roots (132) and dorsal root ganglion (DRG) have demonstrated the presence of prominent myelin alterations of dorsal and ventral roots after 6 months of diabetes. Changes in dorsal root ganglion are prominent (37), consisting of vacuolar degeneration; pigmentary changes are present and are associated with both distal sensory loss (106) and slowing of conduction of proximal nerves (including nerve roots) (133). There is oxidative injury of DRG neurons, with immunolabeling with 8-hydroxydeoxyguanosine, caspase-3, and terminal deoxynucleotidyl transferase–mediated deoxyuridine triphosphate (dUTP) nick and labeling (TUNEL) positivity (133a). A selective loss of the largest neurons is found (133b). Another recent focus is the Schwann cell as a target in hyperglycemic ischemic nerves. The Schwann cell is suggested to be a target of oxidative stress and its apoptosis responsible for delayed ischemic demyelination (134,135).

The specificity of targets needs to be coupled with specificity of mechanisms. HNE is a potent inhibitor of mitochondrial respiration (136). HNE mediates oxidative stress–induced apoptosis of neurons and terminals (116). HNE disrupts neuronal calcium homeostasis and perturbs mitochondrial function, resulting in caspase activation. Activated caspases, in turn, induce activation of c-Jun N-terminal kinase (JNK), resulting in stimulation of the production of transcription factor activator protein-1 (AP-1) DNA-binding protein (137). This action of HNE can be blocked by GSH, which is reduced in diabetes (106). More recently, apoptosis of DRG neurons, neurites, and Schwann cells *in vitro* and *in vivo* in experimental diabetic neuropathy has been reported (138).

THERAPEUTIC APPLICATIONS

Clinical trials with α-lipoic acid are under way. Studies to date have been summarized by Ziegler and Gries (139). The effects of the antioxidant α-lipoic acid have been studied in two multicenter, randomized, double-blind, placebo-controlled trials. In the Alpha-Lipoic Acid in Diabetic Neuropathy Study (ALADIN Study) (140), 328 patients with type 2 diabetes and symptomatic peripheral neuropathy were randomly assigned to treatment with intravenous infusion of α-lipoic acid (ALA) using three doses (ALA 1,200 mg, 600 mg, 100 mg) or placebo over 3 weeks. The total symptom score (TSS) (pain, burning, paresthesia, and numbness) in the feet decreased significantly from baseline to day 19 in the ALA 1,200 and ALA 600 groups compared with the placebo group. Each of the four individual symptom scores was significantly lower in the ALA 600 group than in the placebo group after 19 days (all $p < 0.05$). The total scale of the Hamburg Pain Adjective List (HPAL) was significantly reduced in the ALA 1,200 and ALA 600 groups compared with the placebo group after 19 days (both $p < 0.05$). In the Deutsche Kardiale Autonome Neuropathie Studie (DEKAN Study) (141), patients with type 2 diabetes and cardiac autonomic neuropathy diagnosed by reduced heart-rate variability were randomly assigned to treatment with a daily oral dose of 800 mg of ALA ($n = 39$) or placebo ($n = 34$) for 4 months. Two of four parameters of heart-rate variability at rest were significantly improved in the ALA group compared with the placebo group. A trend toward a favorable effect of ALA was noted for the remaining two indexes. In both studies, no significant adverse events were observed. In conclusion, intravenous treatment with ALA (600 mg/day) over 3 weeks is safe and effective in reducing symptoms of diabetic peripheral neuropathy, and oral treatment with 800 mg/day for 4 months may improve cardiac autonomic dysfunction in type 2 diabetes.

Polyol Pathway Overactivity

Chronic hyperglycemia results in overactivity of the polyol pathway. Aldose reductase converts glucose to sorbitol, and the second enzyme, sorbitol dehydrogenase, converts sorbitol to fructose (141). Endoneurial sugar alcohols (especially sorbitol) are increased in human and experimental diabetes but not to osmotically relevant concentrations (141). Originally, electrophysiologic neuropathy was postulated as being due to the induction of polyol overactivity (142) by myoinositol deficiency (143). Subsequently, acutely reversible slowing of nerve conduction in diabetes has been linked to a myoinositol-related defect in the nerve Na^+,K^+-ATPase (144). This myoinositol-related abnormality in Na^+,K^+-ATPase function is viewed as a cyclic, metabolic defect involving sequential alteration of Na^+-dependent myoinositol uptake, myoinositol content, myoinositol incorporation into membrane phospholipids, and phospholipid-dependent Na^+,K^+-ATPase function in peripheral nerve. Aldose reductase inhibitors have been shown to normalize both nerve myoinositol content and nerve Na^+,K^+-ATPase activity (144). Subsequently, as complexities of the polyol pathway were appreciated, the "sorbitol-myoinositol hypothesis" has been extended to incorporate the complex interactions between hyperglycemia and the vascular, genetic, and environmental variables in the pathogenesis of diabetic complications (145,146). Specifically, competition of aldose reductase with nitric oxide synthase for NADPH results in a deficit of this important endoneurial endothelial vasodilator (43). Abnormalities of this pathway also contribute to oxidant stress (see earlier). The effect of neural polyol pathway activity in diabetes and PKC activity is uncertain. Cytosolic PKC activity was reported to be reduced (147), unchanged (148), or possibly increased (149) in experimental diabetic neuropathy. The improvement in nerve perfusion and conduction with a PKC inhibitor suggests that an increase in PKC is relevant to neuropathy (126,150).

EXPERIMENTAL DIABETIC NEUROPATHY

Studies on experimental diabetic neuropathy have consistently demonstrated efficacy of aldose reductase inhibitors (ARIs) in preventing or ameliorating the conduction deficit. Sorbitol is increased (5- to 10-fold), myoinositol is reduced, and motor conduction is reduced. These biochemical abnormalities are prevented by various ARIs. Sorbinil was reported to partially prevent (151,152) or completely prevent the conduction deficit (153). Sorbinol also was reported to prevent and reverse deficits of the axonal transport of choline acetyltransferase in the cholinergic neurons of the sciatic nerve (154). Similar findings were reported for other ARIs.

The careful electrophysiologic study of Cameron et al. (155) is instructive. They evaluated nerve conduction deficits caused by 2 to 4 months of diabetes in one sensory and six motor nerve branches of mature rats and the effect of the ARI ponalrestat. Diabetes suppressed a maturation-related increase in conduction velocity in the interosseous nerve supplying foot muscles. This was unaffected by any treatment. Large reductions in conduction velocity (22% to 29%) seen for fast nerves supplying four calf muscles and sensory saphenous nerves were prevented by treatment with ponalrestat. In a reversal group, which had 2 months of diabetes followed by 2 months of treatment, restoration of conduction varied among nerves, ranging from 100% in sensory saphenous to 25% in soleus motor branches.

More recent ARIs are more potent. For instance, Cameron et al. (156) reported a potent novel sulfonylnitromethane ARI, Zeneca ZD5522, in experimental diabetic neuropathy, with conduction velocity deficits after 4 months of untreated diabetes rapidly returned to normal within 12 days by treatment with ZD5522. There was a strong correlation between ZD5522-mediated increases in blood flow and conduction velocity. A 37% reduction in endoneurial oxygen tension after 2 months of diabetes was completely prevented by treatment with ZD5522. Similar effects have been reported for other novel ARIs, such as 8′-chloro-2′,3′-dihydrospiro [pyrrolidine-3,6′(5′H)-pyrrolo[1,2, 3-de] [1,4]benzoxazine]-2,5,5′-trione (ADN-138) (157), [5-(3-thienyltetrazol-1-yl)acetic acid (TAT)] (158), and WAY-121,509 (159).

THERAPEUTIC APPLICATIONS

The effect of ARIs has now been studied in large numbers of patients with type 1 and type 2 diabetes. Electrophysiologic improvement occurs relatively early (160), but treatment beyond 3 months has not been shown to confer any additional benefits (161–163). Some improvement of symptoms, especially pain, has been reported (160). Improvement in autonomic indices has been reported (164). Overall, the larger studies have demonstrated only modest or no improvement in clinical neuropathic deficits. The majority of the more positive reports have been published only in abstract form or within supplements. There are encouraging data indicating that chronic users of the drug tolerestat who discontinued treatment demonstrated some worsening of nerve conduction and symptoms and improvement over placebo when they continued the drug for an additional 12 months.

Some caution is necessary in interpreting these negative results. It is my opinion that, while efficacy has not been demonstrated, neither has nonefficacy. For humans, the drug has to be well tolerated yet potent enough to normalize polyol pathway activity. The study needs to be done for a sufficiently long time period. On the basis of what is known about the natural history of progression of diabetic neuropathy, studies will need to be a minimum of 2 years. The severity of neuropathy should not be excessive, so that improvement is possible. These conditions have not been satisfied in the studies to date.

Advanced Glycosylation End Products (AGE)–AGE Receptor–Nuclear Factor-κB

Chronic hyperglycemia has been suggested to cause macro- and microvascular atherogenesis by the generation of AGEs (165). The latter, by increasing macrophage recognition and uptake, stimulates macrophage-derived growth factor, comprising one mechanism suggested to result in the proliferation of smooth muscle and atherogenesis. There is also an AGE-induced increase in low-density lipoproteins in vessel walls and the involvement of other growth factors. Considerable experimental evidence supports this hypothesis (165). These findings also have important implications for treatment. Administration of aminoguanidine hydrochloride results in the formation of unreactive early glycosylation products rather than AGE. These workers have reported that rats treated with aminoguanidine for 10 months did not develop the thickening of renal glomerular basement membrane seen in untreated diabetic animals (165).

As described earlier, AGE binding to its receptor initiates the activation of NF-κB (120), the generation of ROS, and an inflammatory response (121). The quenching action of AGE binding on NO is relevant to nerve ischemia (122). Since AGEs have been suggested to mediate hyperglycemia-induced microvascular atherogenesis and because aminoguanidine prevents their generation, we examined whether aminoguanidine could prevent or ameliorate the physiologic and biochemical indices of experimental diabetic neuropathy. We examined the effects of dose and duration (up to 6 months) of treatment. Experimental diabetic neuropathy caused a 57% reduction in nerve blood flow, abnormal nerve conduction and amplitudes, and a 60% increase in conjugated dienes. Treatment with aminoguanidine normalized nerve blood flow by 8 weeks and significantly improved conduction, in a dose-dependent manner, by 16 and 24 weeks in sciatic-tibial and caudal nerves, respectively (166). Cameron et al. (167) demonstrated that aminoguanidine improved nerve conduction without an effect on polyol pathway metabolites and surmised that the effect was a vascular one.

THERAPEUTIC APPLICATIONS

To my knowledge, no placebo-controlled clinical trials have been published.

Excessive Lipolysis and γ-Linolenic Acid Deficiency

Linoleic acid undergoes desaturation (by δ-6-desaturase) to γ-linolenic acid. In turn, it is elongated to dihomo-γ-linolenic acid, which in turn undergoes desaturation (by δ-5-desaturase enzyme) to arachidonic acid to polyunsaturated fatty acid. A defect at the desaturation step present in diabetic neuropathy can be overcome by the administration of γ-linolenic acid. Efficacy of γ-linolenic acid has been demonstrated in experimental diabetic neuropathy. Two multicenter studies of human diabetic neuropathy are unfortunately inconclusive.

EXPERIMENTAL DIABETIC NEUROPATHY

Dietary supplementation with evening primrose oil, which is rich in γ-linolenic acid, completely prevented the development of the deficit in motor-nerve conduction velocity without affecting levels of sorbitol, fructose, or myoinositol or the deficit in axonal transport of substance P (168,169). In a second experiment, treatment of diabetic rats with evening primrose oil was associated with significant attenuation of the conduction-velocity deficit but not in complete prevention (168). Improvement in conduction occurred *pari passu* with correction of deficits in blood flow and oxygen tension (170). Cameron et al. (171) demonstrated synergism between threshold doses of γ-linoleic acid and ARI and between γ-linoleic acid and antioxidant in reversing the neurovascular and conduction deficits in experimental diabetic neuropathy. They also reported synergism between γ-linoleic acid and ascorbate (172).

THERAPEUTIC APPLICATIONS

Treatment with oral γ-linoleic acid has been reported. A small open study reported improvement in nerve conduction and quantitative sensory indices (173), and improvement also was reported in a small placebo-controlled study involving 12 patients receiving 360 mg and 10 controls receiving placebo (174).

Recently, Keen et al. (175) reported the results of a seven-center double-blind, placebo-controlled study involving 111 patients with mild diabetic neuropathy who were treated with γ-linoleic acid, 480 mg/day, or placebo for 1 year. Indices included motor and sensory conduction, quantitative sensory tests, clinical deficit scores, and a global score. A total of 16 parameters were evaluated and, for all 16 parameters, changes were favorable and reached statistical significance for 13.

A third blinded study has been completed. The study enrolled 291 patients, who were given a dose of γ-linoleic acid of 480 mg/kg. The study was placebo-controlled for the first 12 months. In the subsequent 12 months, both active and placebo groups received γ-linoleic acid. The study largely confirms the findings of the study by Keen et al. (175).

These results are most interesting and await confirmation with a larger study. A major limitations of these studies are the single-center effect and the apparently great deterioration in the placebo group. If the single center were excluded, the studies are clearly negative.

Induction of Protein Kinase C

The effect of hyperglycemia on endothelial cell, retinal, cardiac, and aortic tissue includes the increase of diacylglycerol (176) followed by the sequential activation of PKC and cytosolic phospholipase A_2 (cPLA2), resulting in the liberation of arachidonic acid and increased production of prostaglandin E_2, which are known inhibitors of Na^+,K^+-ATPase (177). The reduction in Na^+,K^+-ATPase activity results in conduction slowing. The relevant PKC is the β-isoform in membrane (178).

Evidence for PKC induction in nerve is indirect. In nerve, inhibition of PKC results in a correction of the deficits in perfusion and nerve conduction (126). The benefits of the inhibitor were blocked by cotreatment with nitric oxide synthase inhibitor (126).

THERAPEUTIC APPLICATIONS

A phase II multicenter clinical trial on the effect of LY333531 on type 1 and type 2 diabetic neuropathy is under way. This is a double-blind, placebo-controlled study of three doses of the drug over 12 months. LY333531 is a specific inhibitor of the β-isoform of PKC; it was synthesized and shown to be a competitive reversible inhibitor of PKC-β_1 and PKC-β_2, with a half-maximal inhibitory constant of approximately 5 nM (179).

Synthesis of Pathogenetic Hypothesis

The above information has been synthesized into a pathogenetic model of diabetic neuropathy (Fig. 50.1). Hyperglycemia results in a reduction in nerve blood flow by altering vasoregulation (at the levels of the endothelial cell and arteriolar smooth muscle) of nerve microvessels and increasing blood viscosity. Microvascular vasoconstrictor tone is increased (increased α-adrenergic and endothelin tone), and vasodilator tone is reduced (reduced endothelial activities of NO, calcitonin gene–related peptide, and substance P. NO deficiency, in addition to reducing microvascular flow, could enhance expression of adhesion molecules, impair the blood–nerve barrier, generate superoxide radicals, and activate PKC and NF-κB. Insulin administration could aggravate hypoxia (by increasing arteriovenous shunt flow and reducing nutritive flow). The ensuing endoneurial ischemia and

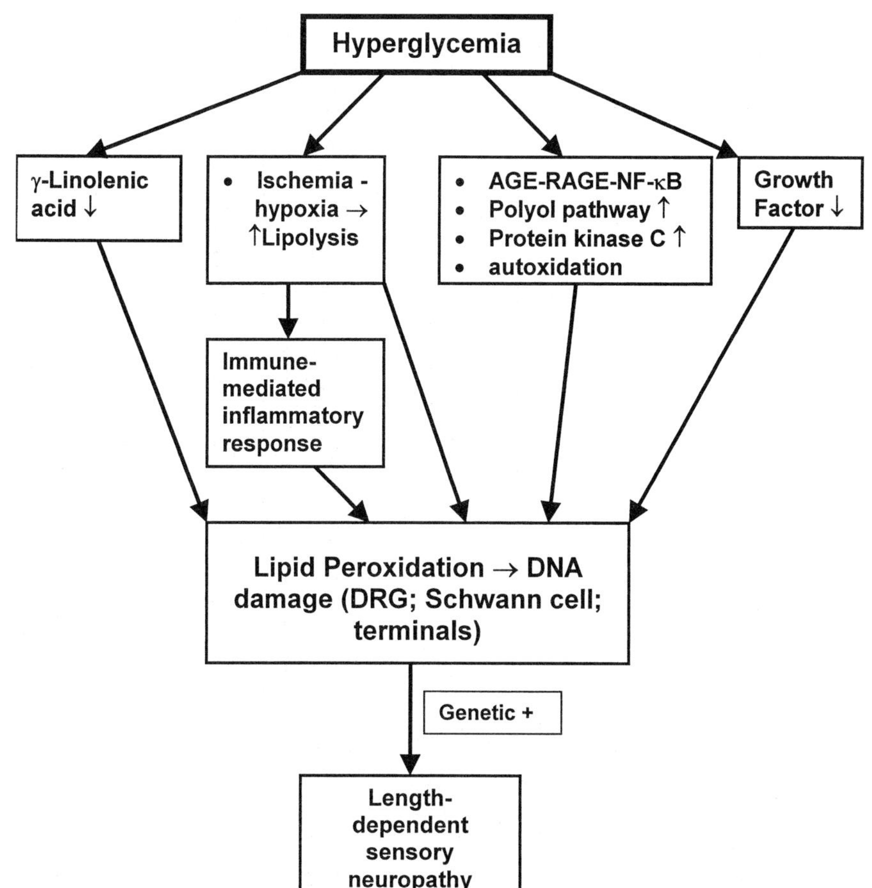

Figure 50.1. Suggested pathogenesis of diabetic neuropathy.

hypoxia, with resultant increased lipolysis, hyperglycemia-induced deficiency in γ-linolenic acid, generation of AGE (with binding to RAGE and activation of NF-κB), overactivity of the polyol pathway and PKC, autoxidation, and deficiency in growth factor result in a lipid peroxidation. The diabetic state exacerbates the inflammatory response to ischemia (180). HNE is particularly important in its ability to cause the apoptosis of neurons, their appendages, and support cells. The pathways in Figure. 50.1 are simplified. The figure depicts all mechanisms as going through oxidative stress and lipid peroxidation. In fact, it is likely that a number of the mechanisms could cause neuropathy by other mechanisms. For instance, PKC increase and polyol pathway overactivity/myoinositol deficiency could work in a significant degree via Na^+,K^+-ATPase deficiency. Growth-factor deficiency could work independently of oxidative stress. The synergism of antioxidants with ARI and with γ-linoleic acid suggests that there are significant interactions and synergism among mechanisms.

The targets of lipid peroxidation are likely multiple. Diabetic neuropathy is primarily a distal sensory neuropathy, so it is not surprising that the dorsal root ganglion appears to be a key target. Dendrites, nerve terminals, Schwann cells, and microvessels could also be important. The DRG has an especially high concentration of mitochondria because of its high energy metabolism. As in all tissues with vigorous oxidative metabolism, there is free-radical generation and a susceptibility to oxidative damage. The mitochondrion is an important micro-target. Impairment in mitochondrial function is manifested as a reduction in membrane potential, opening of the mitochondrial permeability transition pore, and vacuolar and pigmentary degeneration. Mitochondrial DNA is unusually susceptible to oxidative damage. There is normally about 1% leakage of free radicals. Increased free-radical leakage over time leads to increased mutations, as occurs with aging. These dysfunctional mitochondria have increased leakage of reduced oxygen species. A vicious cycle of oxidative damage to inner membrane proteins (of mitochondria) leading to imbalances in the electron transport chain, resulting in increased production of superoxide and hydrogen peroxide, which in turn further damages membrane proteins, is suggested. Leakage of cytochrome *c* leads to activation of the apoptotic cascade, and cells stain positively for activated caspase 3 and TUNEL. The process is slow, with only modest cell loss of large neurons (apoptosis lente). The physiologic alterations (distal sensory neuropathy, reduced sensory threshold, spontaneous firing) in experimental diabetic neuropathy could be due to the sensory neuropathy and radiculopathy described previously.

CONCLUDING THOUGHTS

A number of pathogenetic advances have been made during the past decade and a half. First is the validation that glucose is indeed a neurotoxin and that tight glycemic control will prevent target complications. Second is the appreciation that pathogenetic mechanisms are likely interactive and linked. There is no longer the simplistic view of the metabolic-versus-vascular hypothesis. The major candidate mechanisms are interlaced and may converge. Conversely, synergism appears to exist in methods to treat diabetic neuropathy, for example, antioxidant with ARI and γ-linolenic acid with antioxidant. Third is the evolving improvements in understanding of the targets of glucotoxicity. Evidence is still patchy, but a major target may be the DRG neurons, in addition to the Schwann cell and terminals. Fourth is a better understanding of molecular pathophysiologic mechanisms, especially in apoptosis.

REFERENCES

1. Low PA, Lagerlund TD, McManis PG. Nerve blood flow and oxygen delivery in normal, diabetic, and ischemic neuropathy. *Int Rev Neurobiol* 1989;31: 355–438.
2. Adams WE. The blood supply of nerves. II. The effects of exclusion of its regional sources of supply on the sciatic nerve of the rabbit. *J Anat* 1943;77: 243–250.
3. Lundborg G. Ischemic nerve injury. Experimental studies on intraneural microvascular pathophysiology and nerve function in a limb subjected to temporary circulatory arrest. *Scand J Plast Reconstr Surg* 1970;6:3–113.
4. Low PA, Tuck RR. Effects of changes of blood pressure, respiratory acidosis and hypoxia on blood flow in the sciatic nerve of the rat. *J Physiol* 1984;347: 513–524.
5. Takeuchi M, Low PA. Dynamic peripheral nerve metabolic and vascular responses to exsanguination. *Am J Physiol* 1987;253:E349–E353.
6. McManis PG, Schmelzer JD, Zollman PJ, et al. Blood flow and autoregulation in somatic and autonomic ganglia. Comparison with sciatic nerve. *Brain* 1997;120:445–449.
7. Sundqvist T, Oberg PA, Rapoport SI. Blood flow in rat sciatic nerve during hypotension. *Exp Neurol* 1985;90:139–148.
8. Bell MA, Weddel AGM. A descriptive study of the blood vessels of the sciatic nerve in the rat, man and other mammals. *Brain* 1984;107:871–898.
9. Bell MA, Weddell AG. A morphometric study of intrafascicular vessels of mammalian sciatic nerve. *Muscle Nerve* 1984;7:524–534.
10. Mahalingam R, Wellish M, Wolf W, et al. Latent varicella-zoster viral DNA in human trigeminal and thoracic ganglia. *N Engl J Med* 1990;323:627–631.
11. Low PA, Ward K, Schmelzer JD, et al. Ischemic conduction failure and energy metabolism in experimental diabetic neuropathy. *Am J Physiol* 1985;248: E457–E462.
12. Low PA, Schmelzer JD, Ward KK. The effect of age on energy metabolism and resistance to ischaemic conduction failure in rat peripheral nerve. *J Physiol* 1986;374:263–271.
13. Low PA, Schmelzer JD, Ward KK, et al. Experimental chronic hypoxic neuropathy: relevance to diabetic neuropathy. *Am J Physiol* 1986;250:E94–E99.
14. Horowitz SH, Ginsberg-Fellner F. Ischemia and sensory nerve conduction in diabetes mellitus. *Neurology* 1979;29:695–704.
15. Mulder DW, Lambert EH, Bastron JA, et al. The neuropathies associated with diabetes mellitus: a clinical and electromyographic study of 103 unselected diabetic patients. *Neurology* 1961;11:275–284.
16. Giannini C, Dyck PJ. Basement membrane reduplication and pericyte degeneration precede development of diabetic polyneuropathy and are associated with its severity. *Ann Neur* 1995;37:498–504.
17. Asbury AK, Aldredge H, Hershberg R, et al. Oculomotor palsy in diabetes mellitus: a clinico-pathological study. *Brain* 1970;93:555–566.
18. Raff MC, Sangalang V, Asbury AK. Ischemic mononeuropathy multiplex associated with diabetes mellitus. *Arch Neurol* 1968;18:487–499.
19. Johnson PC, Brendel K, Meezan E. Human diabetic perineurial cell basement membrane thickening. *Lab Invest* 1981;44:265–270.
20. Dyck PJ, Hansen S, Karnes J, et al. Capillary number and percentage closed in human diabetic sural nerve. *Proc Natl Acad Sci U S A* 1985;82:2513–2517.
21. Johnson PC, Doll SC, Cromey DW. Pathogenesis of diabetic neuropathy. *Ann Neurol* 1986;19:450–457.
22. Dyck PJ, Karnes JL, O'Brien P, et al. The spatial distribution of fiber loss in diabetic polyneuropathy suggests ischemia. *Ann Neurol* 1986;19:440–449.
23. Dyck PJ, Lais A, Karnes JL, et al. Fiber loss is primary and multifocal in sural nerves in diabetic polyneuropathy. *Ann Neurol* 1986;19:425–439.
24. Dyck PJ, Giannini C. Pathologic alterations in the diabetic neuropathies of humans: a review. *J Neuropathol Exp Neurol* 1996;55:1181–1193.
25. Nukada H. Increased susceptibility to ischemic damage in streptozocin-diabetic nerve. *Diabetes* 1986;35:1058–1061.
26. Nukada H. Mild ischaemia causes severe pathological changes in experimental diabetic nerve. *Muscle Nerve* 1992;15:1116–1122.
27. Zochodne DW, Cheng C. Diabetic peripheral nerves are susceptible to multifocal ischemic damage from endothelin. *Brain Res* 1999;838:11–17.
28. Wachtler J, Mayer C, Rucker F, et al. Glucose availability alters ischaemia-induced changes in intracellular pH and calcium of isolated rat spinal roots. *Brain Res* 1996;725:30–36.
29. Caravati CM. Insulin neuritis. A case report. *Va Med Monthly* 1933;59:745–746.
30. Ellenberg M. Diabetic neuropathy precipitating after institution of diabetic control. *Am J Med Sci* 1958;236:466–471.
31. Tesfaye S, Malik R, Harris N, et al. Arterio-venous shunting and proliferating new vessels in acute painful neuropathy of rapid glycaemic control (insulin neuritis). *Diabetologia* 1996;39:329–335.
32. Kihara M, Zollman PJ, Smithson IL, et al. Hypoxic effect of exogenous insulin on normal and diabetic peripheral nerve. *Am J Physiol* 1994;266:E980–E985.
33. Tuck RR, Schmelzer JD, Low PA. Endoneurial blood flow and oxygen tension in the sciatic nerves of rats with experimental diabetic neuropathy. *Brain* 1984;107:935–950.
34. Newrick PG, Wilson AJ, Jakubowski J, et al. Sural nerve oxygen tension in diabetes. *BMJ* 1986;293:1053–1054.
35. Dyck PJ, Zimmerman BR, Vilen TH, et al. Nerve glucose, fructose, sorbitol, myo-inositol, and fiber degeneration and regeneration in diabetic neuropathy. *N Engl J Med* 1988;319:542–548.
36. Cameron NE, Cotter MA, Low PA. Nerve blood flow in early experimental diabetes in rats: relation to conduction deficits. *Am J Physiol* 1991;261:E1–E8.

37. Sasaki H, Schmelzer JD, Zollman PJ, et al. Neuropathology and blood flow of nerve, spinal roots and dorsal root ganglia in longstanding diabetic rats. *Acta Neuropathol* 1997;93:118–128.
38. Zochodne DW, Low PA. Adrenergic control of nerve blood flow. *Exp Neurol* 1990;109:300–307.
39. Kihara M, Low PA. Regulation of rat nerve blood flow: role of epineurial alpha-receptors. *J Physiol* 1990;422:145–152.
40. Sasaki H, Low PA. Extreme vasoreactivity of rat epineurial arterioles to vasopressin. *Am J Physiol* 1996;271:H1307–H1313.
41. Zochodne DW, Ho LT, Gross PM. Acute endoneurial ischemia induced by epineurial endothelin in the rat sciatic nerve. *Am J Physiol* 1992;263:H1806–H1810.
42. Zochodne DW, Ho LT. Influence of perivascular peptides on endoneurial blood flow and microvascular resistance in the sciatic nerve of the rat. *J Physiol* 1991;444:615–630.
43. Kihara M, Low PA. Impaired vasoreactivity to nitric oxide in experimental diabetic neuropathy. *Exp Neurol* 1995;132:180–185.
44. Kihara M, Low PA. Vasoreactivity to prostaglandins in rat peripheral nerve. *J Physiol* 1995;484:463–467.
45. Morff RJ. Microvascular reactivity to norepinephrine at different arteriolar levels and durations of streptozocin-induced diabetes. *Diabetes* 1990;39:354–360.
46. Takeda Y, Miyamori I, Yoneda T, et al. Production of endothelin-1 from the mesenteric arteries of streptozotocin-induced diabetic rats. *Life Sci* 1991;48: 2553–2556.
47. Cameron NE, Dines KC, Cotter MA. The potential contribution of endothelin-1 to neurovascular abnormalities in streptozotocin-diabetic rats. *Diabetologia* 1994;37:1209–1215.
48. Cameron NE, Cotter MA. Effects of a nonpeptide endothelin-1 ETA antagonist on neurovascular function in diabetic rats: interaction with the renin-angiotensin system. *J Pharmacol Exp Ther* 1996;278:1262–1268.
49. Cotter MA, Cameron NE, Ferguson K, et al. Effects of chronic alpha-adrenoceptor blockade on nerve function and vascular supply in diabetic rats. *Diabetologia* 1990;33:A92(abst).
50. Cameron NE, Cotter MA. Effects of chronic treatment with a nitric oxide donor on nerve conduction abnormalities and endoneurial blood flow in streptozotocin-diabetic rats. *Eur J Clin Invest* 1995;25:19–24.
51. Cotter MA, Dines KC, Cameron NE. Prevention and reversal of motor and sensory peripheral nerve conduction abnormalities in streptozotocin-diabetic rats by the prostacyclin analogue iloprost. *Naunyn Schmiedebergs Arch Pharmacol* 1993;347:534–540.
52. Davenpeck KL, Gauthier TW, Lefer AM. Inhibition of endothelial-derived nitric oxide promotes P-selectin expression and actions in the rat microcirculation. *Gastroenterology* 1994;107:1050–1058.
53. De Caterina R, Libby P, Peng HB, et al. Nitric oxide decreases cytokine-induced endothelial activation. Nitric oxide selectively reduces endothelial expression of adhesion molecules and proinflammatory cytokines. *J Clin Invest* 1995;96:60–68.
54. Clancy RM, Leszczynska-Piziak J, Abramson SB. Nitric oxide, an endothelial cell relaxation factor, inhibits neutrophil superoxide anion production via a direct action on the NADPH oxidase. *J Clin Invest* 1992;90:1116–1121.
55. Moilanen E, Vuorinen P, Kankaanranta H, et al. Inhibition by nitric oxide-donors of human polymorphonuclear leucocyte functions. *Br J Pharmacol* 1993;109:852–858.
56. Fagerberg SE. Diabetic neuropathy: A clinical and histological study on the significance of vascular affections. *Acta Med Scand* 1959;164[Suppl 345]:1–80.
57. Bischoff A. Die Ultrastruktur peripherer Nerven bei der diabetischen Neuropathie. *Verh Dtsch Ges Inn Med* 1967;72:1138–1141.
58. Malik RA, Newrick PG, Sharma AK, et al. Microangiopathy in human diabetic neuropathy: relationship between capillary abnormalities and the severity of neuropathy. *Diabetologia* 1989;32:92–102.
59. Sugimura K, Dyck PJ. Multifocal fiber loss in proximal sciatic nerve in symmetric distal diabetic neuropathy. *J Neurol Sci* 1982;53:501–509.
60. Llewelyn JG, Thomas PK, Gilbey SG, et al. Pattern of myelinated fibre loss in the sural nerve in neuropathy related to type 1 (insulin-dependent) diabetes. *Diabetologia* 1988;31:162–167.
61. Theriault M, Dort J, Sutherland G, et al. Local human sural nerve blood flow in diabetic and other polyneuropathies. *Brain* 1997;120:1131–1138.
62. Tesfaye S, Harris N, Jakubowski JJ, et al. Impaired blood flow and arterio-venous shunting in human diabetic neuropathy: a novel technique of nerve photography and fluorescein angiography. *Diabetologia* 1993;36: 1266–1274.
63. Ibrahim S, Harris ND, Radatz M, et al. A new minimally invasive technique to show nerve ischaemia in diabetic neuropathy. *Diabetologia* 1999;42: 737–742.
64. Reja A, Tesfaye S, Harris ND, et al. Is ACE inhibition with lisinopril helpful in diabetic neuropathy? *Diabet Med* 1995;12:307–309.
65. Malik RA, Williamson S, Abbott C, et al. Effect of angiotensin-converting enzyme (ACE) inhibitor transdolapril on human diabetic neuropathy: randomised double-blind controlled trial. *Lancet* 1998;352:1978-1981.
66. Ceriello A, dello Russo P, Amstad P, et al. High glucose induces antioxidant enzymes in human endothelial cells in culture. Evidence linking hyperglycemia and oxidative stress. *Diabetes* 1996;45:471–477.
67. Williamson JR, Chang K, Frangos M, et al. Hyperglycemic pseudohypoxia and diabetic complications. *Diabetes* 1993;42:801–813.
68. Baynes JW, Thorpe SR. Role of oxidative stress in diabetic complications: a new perspective on an old paradigm. *Diabetes* 1999;48:1–9.
69. Sato Y, Hotta N, Sakamoto N, et al. Lipid peroxide level in plasma of diabetic patients. *Biochem J* 1979;21:104–107.
70. Matkovics B, Varga SI, Szabo L, et al. The effect of diabetes on the activities of the peroxide metabolism enzymes. *Horm Metab Res* 1982;14:77–79.
71. Kaji H, Kurasaki M, Ito K, et al. Increased lipoperoxide value and glutathione peroxidase activity in blood plasma of type 2 (non-insulin dependent) diabetic women. *Klin Wochenschr* 1985;63:765–768.
72. Ahlskog JE, Uitti RJ, Low PA, et al. No evidence for systemic oxidant stress in Parkinson's or Alzheimer's disease. *Mov Disord* 1995;10:566–573.
73. Jain SK, Krueger KS, McVie R, et al. Relationship of blood thromboxane-B2 (TxB2) with lipid peroxides and effect of vitamin E and placebo supplementation on TxB2 and lipid peroxide levels in type 1 diabetic patients. *Diabetes Care* 1998;21:1511–1516.
74. Nuttall SL, Dunne F, Kendall MJ, et al. Age-independent oxidative stress in elderly patients with non-insulin-dependent diabetes mellitus. *Q J Med* 1999; 92:33–38.
75. Dominguez C, Ruiz E, Gussinye M, et al. Oxidative stress at onset and in early stages of type 1 diabetes in children and adolescents. *Diabetes Care* 1998;21:1736–1742.
76. Collier A, Rumley A, Rumley AG, et al. Free radical activity and hemostatic factors in NIDDM patients with and without microalbuminuria. *Diabetes* 1992;41:909–913.
77. Babiy AV, Gebicki JM, Sullivan DR, et al. Increased oxidizability of plasma lipoproteins in diabetic patients can be decreased by probucol therapy and is not due to glycation. *Biochem Pharmacol* 1992;43:995–1000.
78. Nourooz-Zadeh J, Rahimi A, Tajaddini-Sarmadi J, et al. Relationships between plasma measures of oxidative stress and metabolic control in NIDDM. *Diabetologia* 1997;40:647–653.
79. Ruiz C, Alegria A, Barbera R, et al. Lipid peroxidation and antioxidant enzyme activities in patients with type 1 diabetes mellitus. *Scand J Clin Lab Invest* 1999;59:99–105.
80. Santini SA, Marra G, Giardina B, et al. Defective plasma antioxidant defenses and enhanced susceptibility to lipid peroxidation in uncomplicated IDDM. *Diabetes* 1997;46:1853–1858.
81. Opara EC, Abdel-Rahman E, Soliman S, et al. Depletion of total antioxidant capacity in type 2 diabetes. *Metabolism* 1999;48:1414–1417.
82. Hofmann MA, Schiekofer S, Isermann B, et al. Peripheral blood mononuclear cells isolated from patients with diabetic nephropathy show increased activation of the oxidative-stress sensitive transcription factor NF-kappaB. *Diabetologia* 1999;42:222–232.
83. Toyokuni S. Reactive oxygen species-induced molecular damage and its application in pathology. *Pathol Int* 1999;49:91–102.
84. Hinokio Y, Suzuki S, Hirai M, et al. Oxidative DNA damage in diabetes mellitus: its association with diabetic complications. *Diabetologia* 1999;42:995–998.
85. Krapfenbauer K, Birnbacher R, Vierhapper H, et al. Glycoxidation, and protein and DNA oxidation in patients with diabetes mellitus. *Clin Sci* 1998;95: 331–337.
86. Murakami K, Kondo T, Ohtsuka Y, et al. Impairment of glutathione metabolism in erythrocytes from patients with diabetes mellitus. *Metabolism* 1989;38: 753–758.
87. De Mattia G, Bravi MC, Laurenti O, et al. Reduction of oxidative stress by oral N-acetyl-L-cysteine treatment decreases plasma soluble vascular cell adhesion molecule-1 concentrations in non-obese, non-dyslipidaemic, normotensive patients with non-insulin-dependent diabetes. *Diabetologia* 1998; 41:1392–1396.
88. Yoshida K, Kirokawa J, Tagami S, et al. Weakened cellular scavenging activity against oxidative stress in diabetes mellitus: regulation of glutathione synthesis and efflux. *Diabetologia* 1995;38:201–210.
89. Atalay M, Laaksonen DE, Niskanen L, et al. Altered antioxidant enzyme defences in insulin-dependent diabetic men with increased resting and exercise-induced oxidative stress. *Acta Physiol Scand* 1997;161:195–201.
90. Loven DP, Oberley LW. Free radicals, insulin action and diabetes. In: Oberley LW, ed. *Superoxide dismutase. Vol. III. Disease states.* Boca Raton, FL: CRC, 1985:151–190.
91. Karpen CW, Cataland S, O'Dorisio TM, et al. Interrelation of platelet vitamin E and thromboxane synthesis in type I diabetes mellitus. *Diabetes* 1984;33: 239–243.
92. Gandhi CR, Roychowdhury D. Effect of diabetes mellitus on activities of some glycolytic, hexose monophosphate and other enzymes of erythrocytes of different ages. *Indian J Exp Biol* 1982;20:347–349.
93. Akkus I, Kalak S, Vural H, et al. Leukocyte lipid peroxidation, superoxide dismutase, glutathione peroxidase and serum and leukocyte vitamin C levels of patients with type II diabetes mellitus. *Clin Chim Acta* 1996;244:221–227.
94. Vucic M, Gavella M, Bozikov V, et al. Superoxide dismutase activity in lymphocytes and polymorphonuclear cells in diabetic patients. *Eur J Clin Chem Clin Biochem* 1997;35:517–521.
95. Wolff SP. Diabetes mellitus and free radicals. *Br Med Bull* 1993;49:642–652.
96. Mateo MCM, Bustamante JB, Cantalapiedra MAG. Serum zinc, copper and insulin in diabetes mellitus. *Biomedicine* 1978;29:56–58.
97. Noto R, Alicata R, Sfogliano LA. A study of cupremia in a group of elderly diabetics. *Acta Diabetol Latina* 1983;20:81–85.
98. Niki E. Antioxidants in relation to lipid peroxidation. *Chem Phys Lipids* 1987;44:227–253.
99. Romero FJ, Monsalve E, Hermenegildo C, et al. Oxygen toxicity in the nervous tissue: comparison of the antioxidant defense of rat brain and sciatic nerve. *Neurochem Res* 1991;16:157–161.
100. Romero FJ, Segura–Aguilar J, Monsalve E, et al. Antioxidant and glutathione-related enzymatic activities in rat sciatic nerve. *Neurotoxicol Teratol* 1990;12: 603–605.

101. Low PA, Nickander KK. Oxygen free radical effects in sciatic nerve in experimental diabetes. *Diabetes* 1991;40:873–877.
102. Hermenegildo C, Raya A, Roma J, et al. Decreased glutathione peroxidase activity in sciatic nerve of alloxan-induced diabetic mice and its correlation with blood glucose levels. *Neurochem Res* 1993;18:893–896.
103. Jennings PE, Chirico S, Lunec J, et al. Vitamin C metabolites and microangiopathy in diabetes mellitus. *Diabetes Res* 1987;6:151–154.
104. Som S, Basu S, Mukherjee D, et al. Ascorbic acid metabolism in diabetes mellitus. *Metabolism* 1981;30:572–577.
105. Nickander KK, Schmelzer JD, Rohwer DA, et al. Effect of α-tocopherol deficiency on indices of oxidative stress in normal and diabetic peripheral nerve. *J Neurol Sci* 1994;126:6–14.
106. Nagamatsu M, Nickander KK, Schmelzer JD, et al. Lipoic acid improves nerve blood flow, reduces oxidative stress, and improves distal nerve conduction in experimental diabetic neuropathy. *Diabetes Care* 1995;18:1160–1167.
107. Shupeck M, Ward KK, Schmelzer JD, et al. Comparison of nerve regeneration in vascularized and conventional grafts: nerve electrophysiology, norepinephrine, prostacyclin, malondialdehyde, and the blood-nerve barrier. *Brain Res* 1989;493:225–230.
108. Fealey RD, Low PA, Thomas JE. Thermoregulatory sweating abnormalities in diabetes mellitus. *Mayo Clin Proc* 1989;64:617–628.
109. Schmelzer JD, Low PA. The effect of hyperbaric oxygenation and hypoxia on the blood-nerve barrier. *Brain Res* 1988;473:321–326.
110. Schmelzer JD, Zochodne DW, Low PA. Ischemic and reperfusion injury of rat peripheral nerve. *Proc Natl Acad Sci U S A* 1989;86:1639–1642.
111. Zochodne DW, Ward KK, Low PA. Guanethidine adrenergic neuropathy: an animal model of selective autonomic neuropathy. *Brain Res* 1988;461: 10–16.
112. Yao JK, Low PA. Improvement of endoneurial lipid abnormalities in experimental diabetic neuropathy by oxygen modification. *Brain Res* 1986;362: 362–365.
113. Herbst U, Toborek M, Kaiser S, et al. 4-Hydroxynonenal induces dysfunction and apoptosis of cultured endothelial cells. *J Cell Physiol* 1999;181: 295–303.
114. Keller JN, Mattson MP. Roles of lipid peroxidation in modulation of cellular signaling pathways, cell dysfunction, and death in the nervous system. *Rev Neurosci* 1998;9:105–116.
115. Pedersen WA, Cashman NR, Mattson MP. The lipid peroxidation product 4-hydroxynonenal impairs glutamate and glucose transport and choline acetyltransferase activity in NSC-19 motor neuron cells. *Exp Neurol* 1999;155: 1–10.
116. Kruman I, Bruce-Keller AJ, Bredesen D, et al. Evidence that 4-hydroxynonenal mediates oxidative stress–induced neuronal apoptosis. *J Neurosci* 1997;17: 5089–5100.
117. McEvoy KM, Windebank AJ, Daube JR, et al. 3,4-Diaminopyridine in the treatment of Lambert-Eaton myasthenic syndrome. *N Engl J Med* 1989;321: 1567–1571.
118. Nickander KK, McPhee BR, Low PA, et al. α-Lipoic acid: antioxidant potency against lipid peroxidation of neural tissue in vitro and implications for diabetic neuropathy. *Free Radic Biol Med* 1996;21:631–639.
119. Moy S, Opfer-Gehrking TL, Proper CJ, et al. The venoarteriolar reflex in diabetic and other neuropathies. *Neurology* 1989;39:1490–1492.
120. Schmidt AM, Hori O, Chen JX, et al. Advanced glycation endproducts interacting with their endothelial receptor induced expression of vascular cell adhesion molecule-1 (VCAM-1) in cultured human endothelial cells and in mice. A potential mechanism for the accelerated vasculopathy of diabetes. *J Clin Invest* 1995;96:1395–1403.
121. Khechai F, Ollivier V, Bridey F, et al. Effect of advanced glycation end product–modified albumin on tissue factor expression by monocytes. Role of oxidant stress and protein tyrosine kinase activation. *Arterioscler Thromb Vasc Biol* 1997;17:2885–2890.
122. Bucala R, Tracey KJ, Cerami A. Advanced glycosylation products quench nitric oxide and mediate defective endothelium-dependent vasodilatation in experimental diabetes. *J Clin Invest* 1991;87:432–438.
123. Lee AY, Chung SS. Contributions of polyol pathway to oxidative stress in diabetic cataract. *FASEB J* 1999;13:23–30.
124. Stevens MJ, Lattimer SA, Kamijo M, et al. Osmotically-induced nerve taurine depletion and the compatible osmolyte hypothesis in experimental diabetic neuropathy in the rat. *Diabetologia* 1993;36:608–614.
125. Martinez-Blasco A, Bosch-Morell F, Trenor C, et al. Experimental diabetic neuropathy: role of oxidative stress and mechanisms involved. *Biofactors* 1998;8:41–43.
126. Cameron NE, Cotter MA, Jack AM, et al. Protein kinase C effects on nerve function, perfusion, Na(+), K(+)-ATPase activity and glutathione content in diabetic rats. *Diabetologia* 1999;42:1120–1130.
127. Hellweg R, Hartung HD. Endogenous levels of nerve growth factor (NGF) are altered in experimental diabetes mellitus: a possible role for NGF in the pathogenesis of diabetic neuropathy. *J Neurosci Res* 1990;26:258–267.
128. Nistico G, Cirolo MR, Fiskin K, et al. NGF restores decrease in catalase activity and increases superoxide dismutase and glutathione peroxidase activity in the brain of aged rats. *Free Radic Biol Med* 1992;12:177–181.
129. Sampath D, Jackson GR, Werrbach-Perez K, et al. Effects of nerve growth factor on glutathione peroxidase and catalase on PC12 cells. *J Neurochem* 1994; 62:2476–2479.
130. Low PA, Schmelzer JD, Ward KK, et al. Effect of hyperbaric oxygenation on normal and chronic streptozotocin diabetic peripheral nerves. *Exp Neurol* 1988;99:201–212.
131. Cohen G, Hochstein P. Glutathione peroxidase: the primary agent for the elimination of hydrogen peroxide in erythrocytes. *Biochemistry* 1963;2: 1420–1428.
132. Tamura E, Parry GJ. Severe radicular pathology in rats with longstanding diabetes. *J Neurol Sci* 1994;127:29–35.
133. Sasaki H, Schmelzer JD, Zollman PJ, et al. Neuropathy and blood flow of nerve, spinal roots and dorsal root ganglia in longstanding diabetic rats. *Acta Neuropathol* (Berl) 1997;93:118–128.
133a. Schmeichel AM, Schmelzer JD, Low PA. Oxidative injury and apoptosis of dorsal root ganglion neurons in chronic experimental diabetic neuropathy. *Diabetes* 2003;52(1):165–171.
133b. Kishi M, Tanabe J, Schmelzer JD, et al. Morphometry of dorsal root ganglion in chronic experimental diabetic neuropathy. *Diabetes* 2002;51(3):819–824.
134. Nukada H, McMorran PD. Perivascular demyelination and intramyelinic oedema in reperfusion nerve injury. *J Anat* 1994;185:259–266.
135. Nukada H, van Rij AM, Packer SG, et al. Pathology of acute and chronic ischaemic neuropathy in atherosclerotic peripheral vascular disease. *Brain* 1996;119:1449–1460.
136. Humphries KM, Szweda LI. Selective inactivation of alpha-ketoglutarate dehydrogenase and pyruvate dehydrogenase: reaction of lipoic acid with 4-hydroxy-2-nonenal. *Biochemistry* 1998;37:15835–15841.
137. Camandola S, Poli G, Mattson MP. The lipid peroxidation product 4-hydroxy-2,3-nonenal increases AP-1-binding activity through caspase activation in neurons. *J Biochem* 2000;74:159–168.
138. Russell JW, Sullivan KA, Windebank AJ, et al. Neurons undergo apoptosis in animal and cell culture models of diabetes. *Neurobiol Dis* 1999;6:347–363.
139. Zeigler D, Gries FA. Alpha-lipoic acid in the treatment of diabetic peripheral and cardiac autonomic neuropathy. *Diabetes* 1997;46[Suppl 2]:S62–S66.
140. Ziegler D, Hanefeld M, Ruhnau KJ, et al, the ALADIN Study Group. Treatment of symptomatic diabetic peripheral neuropathy with the antioxidant α-lipoic acid. A 3-week multicentre randomized controlled trial (ALADIN Study). *Diabetologia* 1995;38:1425–1433.
141. Ziegler D, Schatz H, Conrad F, et al. Effects of treatment with the antioxidant alpha-lipoic acid on cardiac autonomic neuropathy in NIDDM patients. A 4-month randomized controlled multicenter trial (DEKAN Study). Deutsche Kardiale Autonome Neuropathy. *Diabetes Care* 1997;20:369–373.
142. Gabbay KH, Merola LO, Field RA. Sorbitol pathway: presence in nerve and cord with substrate accumulation in diabetes. *Science* 1966;151:209–210.
143. Greene DA, Lewis RA, Lattimer SA, et al. Selective effects of myo-inositol administration on sciatic and tibial motor nerve conduction parameters in the streptozocin-diabetic rat. *Diabetes* 1982;31:573–578.
144. Greene DA. A sodium-pump defect in diabetic peripheral nerve corrected by sorbinil administration: relationship to myo-inositol metabolism and nerve conduction slowing. *Metabolism* 1986;35[Suppl 1]:60–65.
145. Greene DA, Lattimer SA, Sima AA. Sorbitol, phosphoinositides, and sodium-potassium-ATPase in the pathogenesis of diabetic complications. *N Engl J Med* 1987;316:599–606.
146. Stevens MJ, Feldman EL, Greene DA. The aetiology of diabetic neuropathy: the combined roles of metabolic and vascular defects. *Diabet Med* 1995;12: 566–579.
147. Kim J, Rushovich EH, Thomas TP, et al. Diminished specific activity of cytosolic protein kinase C in sciatic nerve of streptozocin-induced diabetic rats and its correction by dietary myo-inositol. *Diabetes* 1991;40:1545–1554.
148. Simpson CM, Hawthorne JN. Reduced Na^+-K^+-ATPase activity in peripheral nerve of streptozotocin-diabetic rats: a role for protein kinase C? *Diabetologia* 1988;31:297–303.
149. Kishi Y, Schmelzer JD, Yao JK, et al. α-Lipoic acid: effect on glucose uptake, sorbitol pathway, and energy metabolism in experimental diabetic neuropathy. *Diabetes* 1999;48:2045–2051.
150. Jack AM, Cameron NE, Cotter MA. Effects of the diacylglycerol complexing agent, cremophor, on nerve-conduction velocity and perfusion in diabetic rats. *J Diabetes Complications* 1999;13:2–9.
151. Gillon KR, Hawthorne JN, Tomlinson DR. Myo-inositol and sorbitol metabolism in relation to peripheral nerve function in experimental diabetes in the rat: the effect of aldose reductase inhibition. *Diabetologia* 1983;25:365–371.
152. Cameron NE, Leonard MB, Ross IS, et al. The effects of sorbinil on peripheral nerve conduction velocity, polyol concentrations and morphology in the streptozotocin-diabetic rat. *Diabetologia* 1986;29:168-174.
153. Tomlinson DR, Moriarty RJ, Mayer JH. Prevention and reversal of defective axonal transport and motor nerve conduction velocity in rats with experimental diabetes by treatment with the aldose reductase inhibitor sorbinil. *Diabetes* 1984;33:470-476.
154. Willars GB, Tomlinson DR, Robinson JP. Studies of sorbinil on axonal transport in streptozotocin-diabetic rats. *Metabolism* 1986;35[Suppl 1]:66-70.
155. Cameron NE, Cotter MA, Robertson S. The effect of aldose reductase inhibition on the pattern of nerve conduction deficits in diabetic rats. *Q J Exp Physiol* 1989;74:917–926.
156. Cameron NE, Cotter MA, Dines KC, et al. Aldose reductase inhibition, nerve perfusion, oxygenation and function in streptozotocin-diabetic rats: dose-response considerations and independence from a myo-inositol mechanism. *Diabetologia* 1994;37:651–663.
157. Hirata Y, Fujimori S, Okada K. Effect of a new aldose reductase inhibitor, 8′-chloro-2′,3′-dihydrospiro [pyrrolidine-3,6′ (5′H)-pyrrolo[1,2,3-de] [1,4]benzoxazine]-2,5,5′-trione (AND-138), on delayed motor nerve conduction velocity in streptozotocin-diabetic rats. *Metabolism* 1988;37:159–163.

158. Hotta N, Kakuta H, Fukasawa H, et al. Effect of a potent new aldose reductase inhibitor, (5-(3-thienyltetrazol-1-yl) acetic acid (TAT), on diabetic neuropathy in rats. *Clin Pract* 1995;27:107–117.
159. Cameron NE, Cotter MA, Dines KC, et al. Reversal of defective peripheral nerve conduction velocity, nutritive endoneurial blood flow, and oxygenation by a novel aldose reductase inhibitor, WAY-121,509, in streptozotocin-induced diabetic rats. *J Diabetes Complications* 1996;10:43–53.
160. Judzewitsch RG, Jaspan JB, Polonsky KS, et al. Aldose reductase inhibition improves nerve conduction velocity in diabetic patients. *N Engl J Med* 1983; 308:119–125.
161. Fagius J, Brattberg A, Jameson S, et al. Limited benefit of treatment of diabetic polyneuropathy with an aldose reductase inhibitor: a 24-week controlled trial. *Diabetologia* 1985;28:323–329.
162. Martyn CN, Reid W, Young RJ, et al. Six-month treatment with sorbinil in asymptomatic diabetic neuropathy. Failure to improve abnormal nerve function. *Diabetes* 1987;36:987–990.
163. Sundkvist G, Lilja B, Rosen I, et al. Autonomic and peripheral nerve function in early diabetic neuropathy. Possible influence of a novel aldose reductase inhibitor on autonomic function. *Acta Med Scand* 1987;221:445–453.
164. Giugliano D, Marfella R, Salvatore T, et al. A double-blind controlled study on the effect of tolrestat on diabetic autonomic neuropathy. *Diabetologia* 1991;34[Suppl 2]:A152(abst).
165. Brownlee M, Cerami A, Vlassara H. Advanced glycosylation end products in tissue and the biochemical basis of diabetic complications. *N Engl J Med* 1988; 318:1315–1321.
166. Kihara M, Schmelzer JD, Poduslo JF, et al. Aminoguanidine effects on nerve blood flow, vascular permeability, electrophysiology, and oxygen free radicals. *Proc Natl Acad Sci U S A* 1991;88:6107–6111.
167. Cameron NE, Cotter MA, Dines K, et al. Effects of aminoguanidine on peripheral nerve function and polyol pathway metabolites in streptozotocin-diabetic rats. *Diabetologia* 1992;35:946–950.
168. Tomlinson DR, Robinson JP, Compton AM, et al. Essential fatty acid treatment—effects on nerve conduction, polyol pathway and axonal transport in streptozotocin diabetic rats. *Diabetologia* 1989;32:655–659.
169. Dines KC, Cotter MA, Cameron NE. Effectiveness of natural oils as sources of gamma-linolenic acid to correct peripheral nerve conduction velocity abnormalities in diabetic rats: modulation by thromboxane A2 inhibition. *Prostaglandins Leukot Essent Fatty Acids* 1996;55:159–165.
170. Cameron NE, Cotter MA. Effects of evening primrose oil treatment on sciatic nerve blood flow and endoneurial oxygen tension in streptozotocin-diabetic rats. *Acta Diabetol* 1994;31:220–225.
171. Cameron NE, Cotter MA. Interaction between oxidative stress and gamma-linolenic acid in impaired neurovascular function of diabetic rats. *Am J Physiol* 1996;271:E471–E476.
172. Cameron NE, Cotter MA. Comparison of the effects of ascorbyl gamma-linolenic acid and gamma-linolenic acid in the correction of neurovascular deficits in diabetic rats. *Diabetologia* 1996;39:1047–1054.
173. Jamal GA, Carmichael H, Weir AI. Gamma-linolenic acid in diabetic neuropathy [Letter]. *Lancet* 1986;1:1098.
174. Jamal GA, Carmichael H. The effect of gamma-linolenic acid on human diabetic peripheral neuropathy: a double-blind placebo-controlled trial. *Diabet Med* 1990;7:319–323.
175. Keen H, Payan J, Allawi J, et al. Treatment of diabetic neuropathy with gamma-linolenic acid. The Gamma-Linolenic Acid Multicenter Trial Group. *Diabetes Care* 1993;16:8–15.
176. Inoguchi T, Battan R, Handler E, et al. Preferential elevation of protein kinase C isoform beta II and diacylglycerol levels in the aorta and heart of diabetic rats: differential reversibility to glycemic control by islet cell transplantation. *Proc Natl Acad Sci U S A* 1992;89:11059–11063.
177. Xia P, Kramer RM, King GL. Identification of the mechanism for the inhibition of Na+,K(+)-adenosine triphosphatase by hyperglycemia involving activation of protein kinase C and cytosolic phospholipase A2. *J Clin Invest* 1995;96:733–740.
178. Kunisaki M, Bursell SE, Umeda F, et al. Normalization of diacylglycerol-protein kinase C activation by vitamin E in aorta of diabetic rats and cultured rat smooth muscle cells exposed to elevated glucose levels. *Diabetes* 1994;43: 1372–1377.
179. Ishii H, Jirousek MR, Koya D, et al. Amelioration of vascular dysfunctions in diabetic rats by an oral PKC beta inhibitor. *Science* 1996;272:728–731.
180. Panes J, Kurose I, Rodriguez-Vaca D, et al. Diabetes exacerbates inflammatory responses to ischemia-reperfusion. *Circulation* 1996;93:161–167.

CHAPTER 51
Pathogenesis of Diabetic Nephropathy

Gabriella Gruden and GianCarlo Viberti

The abnormal glycemic milieu of diabetes is closely related to the development of microvascular complications. However, the evidence of a straightforward causal relationship between hyperglycemia and renal disease is less compelling in humans than in animal models. Only about 30% of patients develop clinically overt nephropathy. The majority of subjects with diabetes escape renal failure, and although some histologic damage occurs in their kidneys, their renal function remains essentially normal until they die. It therefore appears that in humans hyperglycemia is necessary, but not sufficient, to cause the renal damage that leads to kidney failure. The risk of developing kidney disease is not linearly correlated to the duration of diabetes; indeed, the incidence peaks after 17 years of type 1 diabetes and then sharply declines, a phenomenon likely due to exhaustion of the subgroup of susceptible subjects (1).

The central question is thus why some diabetic patients are susceptible to and others are protected from renal disease. A diabetic sibling of a person with type 1 diabetes and nephropathy has approximately a 72% cumulative risk of developing renal disease, whereas a diabetic sibling of a person with type 1 diabetes but without nephropathy has only a 25% risk (2). This indicates that inherited factors play an important role in determining susceptibility to diabetic nephropathy but does not provide insight into the nature of these factors.

Family studies have shown that a familial predisposition to raised arterial pressure is an important determinant of susceptibility to renal disease in persons with diabetes. Blood pressure levels are significantly higher in the parents of diabetic subjects with proteinuria than in the parents of diabetic subjects without proteinuria (3). Among Pima Indians with type 2 diabetes, the prevalence of proteinuria is higher in those with hypertensive parents than in those with normotensive parents (4). It has been calculated that the risk of nephropathy among patients with type 1 diabetes is three times higher in those who have at least one parent with a history of hypertension (5). Furthermore, prospective studies have demonstrated that mean blood pressure levels are significantly higher in those patients who progress to microalbuminuria than in those who do not, indicating that high blood pressure plays an important role in the pathogenesis of diabetic kidney disease (6).

Diabetic nephropathy and hypertension are multifactorial disorders that result from interaction between both environmental and genetic factors, making the identification of what confers susceptibility to diabetic kidney disease at the genetic level both difficult and complex. Polymorphisms of genes potentially involved in the genetic predisposition to hypertension, vascular reactivity, and insulin resistance, such as those of the renin-angiotensin system, nitric oxide, aldose reductase, GLUT I, and lipoproteins, have all been investigated in relation to diabetic nephropathy, but studies of candidate genes have, by and large, been inconclusive or, at best, have shown weak associations (7). However, a strong association between a polymorphism in the 5′ end of the aldose reductase gene and the development of diabetic nephropathy in type 1 diabetes has been reported (8) and recently confirmed (9).

Studies of intermediate phenotypic markers of hypertension have provided some insight into the predisposition to diabetic renal disease. The red blood cell sodium-lithium countertransport system is a cell-membrane cation transport system whose activity is both genetically determined and increased in essential hypertension. Sodium-lithium countertransport activity is abnormally high in diabetic patients with proteinuria or microalbuminuria (10,11). High countertransport activity may thus constitute a suitable cell marker for identifying patients at risk of kidney disease. However, sodium-lithium countertransport is not operating *in vivo;* therefore, the pathophysiologic relevance of its abnormalities remains uncertain. The sodium-hydrogen antiport, a ubiquitous transmembrane protein that catalyzes the electroneutral exchange of extracellular sodium for intracellular hydrogen, operates *in vivo* and regulates important cellular events, such as intracellular pH, cell volume, and cell proliferation. Furthermore, at the kidney level, the sodium-hydrogen antiport plays an important role in sodium reabsorption and may thus be involved in the pathogenesis of hypertension. Sodium-hydrogen antiport activity is increased in a number of cell types from patients with type 1 diabetes with microalbuminuria and proteinuria, as well as in subjects with hypertension (12,13). The activity of the sodium-hydrogen antiport is increased by high glucose concentrations in cells from patients with diabetic nephropathy but not in cells from diabetic patients without nephropathy or in cells from healthy controls (13). Furthermore, in prospective studies, the sodium-hydrogen activity of red blood cells predicts the development of proteinuria (14). Cultured skin fibroblasts from siblings of patients with type 1 diabetes show a very close concordance for the sodium-hydrogen antiport activity, indicating that antiport activity is by and large genetically determined (15). However, in both hypertension and diabetic nephropathy, the increased sodium-hydrogen antiport activity is not due to increased expression of the gene encoding for this protein. Alterations in the regulatory pathways of the sodium-hydrogen exchange are more likely to be implicated in its overactivity. Although the pathogenic role of the sodium-hydrogen antiport in diabetic nephropathy remains to be proven, together these studies of intermediate phenotype show that the increased susceptibility to diabetic nephropathy most likely resides in a genetically determined host-cell response to the diabetes environment (16).

In patients with type 2 diabetes, the evidence of a genetically determined susceptibility to the development of diabetic nephropathy is less compelling than in patients with type 1 diabetes. However, there is evidence of a familial clustering of diabetic nephropathy in type 2 diabetes (17–19), and affected sib-pair linkage analyses have identified loci associated with diabetic nephropathy in type 2 diabetes (20–22). Moreover, in patients with type 2 diabetes, nephropathy is associated with cellular markers for hypertension (23), and in families with type 2 diabetes, albumin excretion rate is a heritable trait, with a heritability similar to that for blood pressure (24). Finally, in Pima Indians, blood pressure levels before the onset of diabetes predict the future risk of developing the complication (4).

THE INSULTS: HYPERGLYCEMIA, HYPERTENSION, AND PROTEINURIA

Diabetic nephropathy is characterized histologically by thickening of the glomerular basement membrane, increased fractional mesangial volume, and podocyte abnormalities. Expansion of the glomerular mesangium, which occurs at the expense of the glomerular capillary lumen and filtration surface area, correlates most closely with the decline in renal function and the development of proteinuria (25,26). *Ex vivo* studies have shown that the mesangial expansion is due to both increased production and reduced degradation of extracellular matrix proteins such as type IV and I collagen, laminin, and fibronectin (27).

Although the glomerulus, particularly the mesangium, has been the major focus of interest, tubulointerstitial injury is also a feature of diabetic nephropathy and a predictor of renal dysfunction. Pathologic changes that have been described in association with diabetic nephropathy include thickening of the tubular basement membrane, tubular atrophy, interstitial fibrosis, and arteriosclerosis. Interstitial expansion correlates closely with renal dysfunction, albuminuria, and mesangial expansion. Moreover, the impact of interstitial expansion on renal dysfunction is additive to that of mesangial expansion, suggesting an independent effect (28).

If diabetes-induced abnormalities were sufficient to cause renal disease, all diabetic patients, given time, would develop overt renal disease, and the study of hyperglycemia-induced abnormalities would be sufficient to explain the pathogenesis of these functional or structural abnormalities. But this is not the case. To gain insights into the pathogenic mechanisms of diabetic kidney disease, it is therefore necessary to take into account other insults that either influence the host response to diabetes-induced environmental disturbances, thus conferring susceptibility, or accelerate the progression of kidney damage.

Hyperglycemia

There is no doubt that poor glycemic control is associated with diabetic nephropathy. Levels of hemoglobin A_{1c} (HbA_{1c}) are higher in patients with microalbuminuria and macroalbuminuria than in those with normoalbuminuria (29), and in two longitudinal studies, the glycemic control predicted the future development of microalbuminuria in normotensive type 1 diabetic patients with normoalbuminuria (6,30).

Intervention studies have demonstrated the renoprotective effect of optimal glycemic control in both human and experimental diabetes. In animals, structural glomerular changes and albuminuria can be prevented by the maintenance of normoglycemia by either islet cell transplantation or intensive insulin therapy or can be reversed by transplantation of an affected kidney into a nondiabetic animal (31–33). In humans, the Diabetes Control and Complications Trial (DCCT), a prospective multicenter randomized clinical trial comparing the effect of intensive and conventional insulin therapy on the risk of development and progression of diabetic chronic complications in 1,441 patients with type 1 diabetes, has demonstrated that a sustained improvement in HbA_{1c} reduces the risk of development of diabetic nephropathy (34). Similarly, the United Kingdom Prospective Diabetes Study (UKPDS) has shown that improved glycemic control is effective in the prevention of microalbuminuria in patients with newly diagnosed type 2 diabetes (35). Finally, in a small study of eight patients with type 1 diabetes, pancreatic transplantation and near normoglycemia for 10 years reversed structural abnormalities in the kidney (36).

There is strong evidence that hyperglycemia is necessary in the pathogenesis of diabetic nephropathy, and some of the mechanisms that link hyperglycemia to the functional and structural abnormalities of diabetic kidney disease have been elucidated.

Extracellularly, glucose reacts nonenzymatically with primary amines of proteins, forming glycated compounds. Glucose can also be transported into cells mainly by glucose transporters and can be metabolized to sorbitol via the polyol pathway and to glucosamine in the hexosamine biosynthetic pathway. These biochemical pathways have been implicated in hyperglycemia-induced kidney damage. Furthermore, it has become increasingly clear that excess glucose can exert toxic effects directly by altering intracellular signaling pathways; currently, this is believed to be a major mechanism by which hyperglycemia results in kidney damage.

NONENZYMATIC GLYCOSYLATION

Sustained hyperglycemia leads to nonenzymatic protein glycation, a posttranslation modification that occurs physiologically but is greatly enhanced in hyperglycemic conditions. Glycation results from condensation of reducing sugars with ε-amino groups of lysine residue of proteins. The resulting Schiff base undergoes rearrangement to form relatively stable ketoamines, the Amadori products. These glycated proteins undergo progressive dehydration, cyclization, oxidation, and rearrangement to form advanced glycation end-products (AGEs). Once these AGEs are formed, the reaction is not reversible, and they gradually accumulate over the lifetime of the protein (37).

The hypothesis that AGEs are involved in diabetic kidney disease is based on several observations. In both human and experimental diabetes, AGEs accumulate in renal glomeruli and tubules. This phenomenon is specific, as it does not occur in normal kidneys or in kidneys from patients with glomerulonephritis and without diabetes (38). In normal animals, injection of AGE-modified albumin results in overexpression of matrix molecules, albuminuria, and glomerulosclerosis (39). In diabetic animals, accumulation of AGEs in the kidney is paralleled by the development of albuminuria, mesangial expansion, and thickening of the glomerular basement membrane. Furthermore, administration of aminoguanidine (AGN), an inhibitor of AGE formation, attenuates renal accumulation of AGEs and reduces both albuminuria and mesangial expansion (40).

Ultrastructural and *in vitro* studies have cast light on the mechanisms whereby AGEs can lead to kidney damage. AGEs directly alter the structural and functional properties of extracellular matrix proteins. AGE-mediated protein cross-linking increases matrix rigidity and reduces the susceptibility of protein to enzymatic digestion, thus inducing accumulation and thickening, and favors trapping of plasma proteins, such as low-density lipoprotein (LDL) and immunoglobulin G (IgG). AGN normalizes the defect in matrix degradation that occurs when matrix is incubated in a medium high in glucose, suggesting that the AGN effect in preventing mesangial expansion is in part due to its capacity to normalize mesangial matrix digestion (41). In addition, AGEs can elicit a variety of cellular responses by binding to AGE-specific receptors present on many cell types, including mesangial cells and tubular epithelial cells (42). Interaction of AGE-modified proteins with the AGE receptors serves to degrade AGE proteins but also induces the synthesis and release of cytokines, such as transforming growth factor (TGF-β1), platelet-derived growth factor (PDGF), and insulin-like growth factor (IGF), and results in enhanced production of collagen, laminin, and fibronectin (43,44).

The importance of AGE receptors has recently been given further support by the observation that diabetic animals overexpressing the AGE receptor (RAGE) rapidly develop glomerular lesions similar to those seen in advanced diabetic nephropathy (45). RAGEs are also expressed on tubular epithelial cells, and it has recently been reported that RAGE activation can induce tubular epithelial cell transdifferentiation to myofibroblasts, a key event in the development of tubulointerstitial fibrosis (46).

THE POLYOL PATHWAY

In the polyol pathway, glucose is reduced to sorbitol by the enzyme aldose reductase. In many tissues, the physiologic significance of aldose reductase is difficult to define, but in the renal medullary cells, the primary role of aldose reductase seems to be the formation of sorbitol, an organic osmolyte, in response to the high salinity in the medullary interstitium. It has been argued that, in tissues in which glucose entry into cells is insulin independent, more glucose becomes available for reduction by aldose reductase, resulting in an increased concentration of sorbitol and/or a reduced intracellular concentration of myoinositol. These changes might contribute to diabetic complications via an upset of cellular osmoregulation (47,48). Enhanced activity of the polyol pathway has been demonstrated in diabetic glomeruli in humans (49). However, the initial hypothesis that accumulation of sorbitol and reduction of myoinositol cause tissue damage is unlikely to operate in the kidney because compensatory mechanisms prevent the depletion of inositol in kidney cells (50).

More recently, enhanced AGE production and oxidative stress have been proposed as alternative mechanisms linking the polyol pathway to kidney injury in diabetes. In the polyol pathway, excess sorbitol is oxidized to fructose by the enzyme fructose dehydrogenase. The increased ratio of NADH/NAD (reduced form of nicotinamide adenine dinucleotide/oxidized form of nicotinamide adenine dinucleotide) coupled to the oxidation of sorbitol to fructose can result in cellular oxidative stress. Furthermore, fructose is a reactive sugar that can lead to AGE production (51,52). Recent experiments in cultured bovine aortic endothelial cells have demonstrated that high glucose concentrations increase the production of reactive oxygen species. Further, blockade of the electron transport chain complex II normalizes mitochondrial reactive oxygen species and prevents glucose-induced activation of protein kinase C (PKC), formation of AGEs, accumulation of sorbitol, and activation of the transcription factor nuclear factor-κB (NF-κB) (53).

Various pathophysiologic mechanisms linking activation of the polyol pathway to kidney damage can be postulated. However, to prove that activation of the polyol pathway is not merely an epiphenomenon but a mechanism of renal injury, it is important to have *in vivo* evidence that inhibition of the polyol pathway is beneficial in diabetic nephropathy. To gain this evidence, a series of studies of aldose reductase inhibitors (ARIs) have been carried out in both experimental and human diabetes. Early studies using the ARIs were inconclusive because of dubious compound specificity and drug toxicity. More recently, treatment of diabetic rats for 6 months with the ARI tolrestat resulted in a slight reduction in albumin excretion rate (54), but to date no convincing effect of aldose reductase inhibitors has been reported in controlled studies in humans. This indicates that activation of the polyol pathway is more likely to be an epiphenomenon and that other, more central mechanisms are operating in the pathogenesis of diabetic nephropathy.

HEXOSAMINE BIOSYNTHETIC PATHWAY

Approximately 5% of the glucose entering the cell is metabolized via the hexosamine biosynthetic pathway (HBSP), which converts glucose-6-phosphate into hexosamine-6-phosphate. Glutamine:fructose-6-phosphate aminotransferase (GFAT) is the first and the rate-limiting enzyme of this pathway. In both mesangial cells and NIH-3T3 fibroblasts, GFAT overexpression, which increases the flux through the HBSP, leads to enhanced expression of TGF-β and fibronectin (55,56). Furthermore, high glucose-induced production of TGF-β1 and matrix appears, at least in part, to be mediated by the HBSP because such production is significantly reduced by the GFAT inhibitor azaserine (57). A very low level of expression of GFAT usually is found in glomerular cells, but such expression is significantly enhanced in the glomerular cells of patients with diabetic nephropathy (58), suggesting a potential *in vivo* relevance of the *in vitro* findings. Both high glucose and angiotensin II activate the GFAT promoter in mesangial cells (59), and this provides a potential molecular mechanism of GFAT overexpression in the diabetic glomeruli.

GLUCOTOXICITY

Consistent with the finding in clinical studies that hyperglycemia per se plays a key role in the development of diabetic kidney disease, studies on both kidney cells and isolated glomeruli have confirmed that high glucose concentrations directly alter extracellular matrix deposition.

In mesangial cells, high glucose concentrations induce cell hypertrophy and increase gene expression and protein secretion of extracellular matrix components, such as collagen, laminin, and fibronectin (60). Similarly, levels of type IV and I collagen messenger RNA (mRNA) are enhanced in tubular epithelial cells exposed to high glucose concentrations (28). An additional mechanism whereby high glucose leads to exaggerated matrix deposition is by reducing the activity of metalloproteases, enzymes responsible for extracellular-matrix degradation (61).

Renal cells, similar to cells at other sites of diabetic complications, do not have an absolute requirement of insulin for glucose uptake, so that the intracellular levels of glucose more directly reflect its plasma concentration. The importance of excess glucose entry into mesangial cells is underscored by the observation that glucose-induced effects can be mimicked in normal glucose concentrations by overexpression of the cellular glucose transporter GLUT 1, thus increasing basal glucose uptake (62). This finding also indicates that factors regulating expression of glucose transporter and/or activity can influence glucose uptake and thus glucotoxicity. High glucose concentrations would be expected to reduce glucose transporter expression/activity in order to protect cells from excess glucose entry. However, *in vitro* studies of cultured mesangial cells suggest that exposure to elevated glucose concentrations actually enhances GLUT 1 expression by mesangial cells, triggering a positive feedback mechanism that may result in progressive damage (63). Inhibition of GLUT 1 overexpression prevents overproduction of extracellular matrix molecules in mesangial cells exposed to high glucose (64), providing evidence of a key role of GLUT1 in glucotoxicity (64)

The cellular and intracellular mechanisms whereby high glucose can lead to matrix deposition have been extensively studied since the 1980s, and will be reviewed in depth below.

Hypertension

There is evidence that hypertension plays a critical role in the progression of diabetic nephropathy. Indeed the development of proteinuria is paralleled in most cases by a gradual rise in systemic blood pressure, and there is a significant correlation between the blood pressure levels and the rate of decline in glomerular filtration rate (65). Furthermore, intervention studies in both animals and humans have demonstrated significant renoprotective and antiproteinuric effects of antihypertensive therapy (66–68).

In diabetic nephropathy, hypertension is not merely the result of relentless kidney damage; there is considerable clinical evidence that the elevated arterial pressure is also important in the genesis of the glomerular lesion. In Pima Indians, higher mean blood pressure prior to the onset of diabetes actually predicts an abnormal albumin excretion rate after the diagnosis of diabetes (4). Further, prospective studies in both patients with type 1 and type 2 diabetes and normal albumin excretion have demonstrated that mean arterial pressure levels are significantly higher in those patients who progress to microalbuminuria than in those who do not progress (6,69).

The difference in arterial pressure levels of diabetic patients who develop renal complications and those who do not is numerically small, and the levels in those who develop complications are often in the "normotensive range." However, this difference becomes biologically relevant in the presence of diabetes, which induces loss of autoregulation of glomerular capillary pressure. Under normal conditions, intraglomerular capillary pressure is tightly regulated by precise adjustments in afferent and efferent arteriolar resistance. Hyperglycemia induces vasodilatation, and in diabetes there is a marked reduction in afferent and a lesser reduction in efferent arteriolar resistance. This leads to an increase in levels of glomerular capillary pressure and moreover allows ready transmission of any increase in systemic blood pressure to the glomerular capillary network (70). The metabolic and the hemodynamic insults are thus intimately intertwined in determining altered glomerular hemodynamics.

The notion that enhanced glomerular capillary pressure is involved in diabetic glomerulosclerosis is based on several observations. Conditions known to increase glomerular capillary pressures, such as unilateral nephrectomy, Goldblatt hypertension, and high-protein diet, significantly enhance the extent of glomerular injury in rats with streptozotocin-induced diabetes. Conversely, amelioration of glomerular hypertension slows the rate of progression of the glomerular injury (71,72). Consistent with these animal studies, autopsy studies of diabetic patients with unilateral renal artery stenosis show nodular glomerulosclerosis lesions to be confined to the kidney with the patent renal artery (73). Finally, the greater efficacy of angiotensin-converting enzyme (ACE) inhibitors in their antiproteinuric and renoprotective action as compared with other blood pressure–lowering agents has been in part ascribed to the capacity of ACE inhibitors to reduce glomerular capillary pressure by removing the tonic constrictor effect of angiotensin II on the efferent arteriole (74).

Although increased glomerular capillary pressure has long been associated with the deposition of extracellular matrix, the mechanisms by which the mechanical insult of altered hemodynamics translates into kidney damage have only recently been elucidated. This has followed the demonstration of the unique elastic properties of the glomerular structure and the response of mesangial cells to mechanical stretch in culture.

Glomeruli are highly compliant structures, and when the intraglomerular pressure rises to levels approximating those observed in the diabetic and remnant kidney, glomerular volume increases by about 30%. Volume changes reach their maximum within 3 to 4 seconds following alteration in intraglomerular pressure, thus responding to the most transient variations in intraglomerular pressure. Glomerular expansion is associated with the stretching of its structural components, including the extracellular matrix and the cellular components. Because of the central location of the mesangial regions within the glomerular lobule, mesangial cells experience substantial mechanical stretching. Detailed morphologic studies have demonstrated how numerous cytoplasmic projections emerging from the mesangial cell body extend between adjacent capillaries and firmly attach to the perimesangial regions of the glomerular basement membrane. Therefore, the centrifugal displacement of these regions during glomerular expansion results in marked tridimensional stretching of mesangial cells (75).

Mesangial cells exposed to mechanical stretch in culture undergo alterations in morphology and synthetic activity. Cyclical stretch stimulates the synthesis and deposition of matrix components, such as collagen (I, III, and IV), fibronectin, and laminin, in a manner proportional to the intensity of cellular stretch (76–78). Interestingly, although cyclical stretch stimulates collagen synthesis at all glucose concentrations, net collagen accumulation in the medium can be demonstrated only at high glucose levels (79), the result of catabolic rates that are insufficient to match the increased synthesis in a high-glucose environment. Therefore, the cellular response to a hemodynamic insult can be influenced and exaggerated by high glucose concentration in the milieu. In addition, GLUT1 is overexpressed in an animal model of glomerular hypertension *in vivo*, and stretch enhances glucose uptake by inducing GLUT1 expression in human mesangial cells *in vitro* (80). This suggests that glomerular hypertension may enhance glucotoxicity.

Proteinuria

In diabetic nephropathy and other progressive glomerulopathies, proteinuria is a strong and independent predictor of decline in renal function (81). Excessive protein overload appears to induce tubulointerstitial damage and hence to contribute to the disease progression (82). Specifically, the excessive tubular reabsorption of proteins and the consequent accumulation of proteins in tubular epithelial cells induce the release of vasoactive and inflammatory cytokines, such as endothelin-1, osteopontin, and monocyte chemoattractant protein-1 (MCP-1). These factors in turn lead to overexpression of proinflammatory and fibrotic cytokines and infiltration of mononuclear cells, causing injury of the tubulointerstitium and, ultimately, renal scarring and insufficiency (28,81,83). A vicious cycle is then established in which changes in renal hemodynamics, either primary or in response to nephron loss, induce further proteinuria, perpetuating a mechanism of interstitial scarring and loss of more nephrons. The tubular toxicity of protein raises the possibility that the beneficial effects of ACE inhibitors in diabetic renal disease may reflect their potent antiproteinuric action in addition to the reduction of angiotensin II–mediated effects on growth-factor activation and glomerular hemodynamics (28,81). Limiting protein excretion and the consequent activation of tubular epithelial cell prosclerotic signals thus appears instrumental in protecting the kidney from further damage (Fig. 51.1).

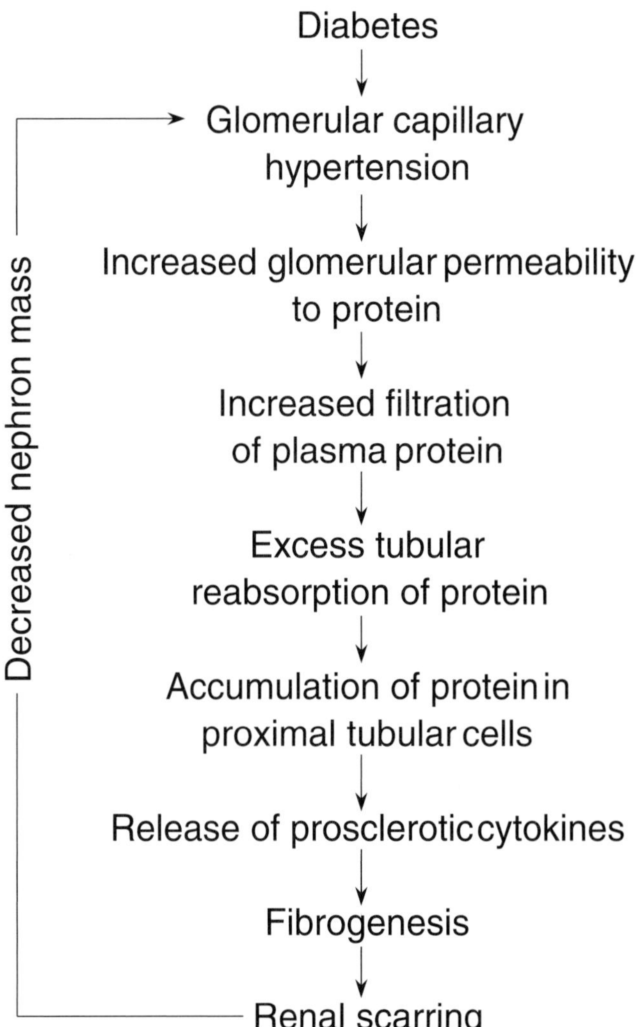

Figure 51.1. Potential mechanisms of proteinuria-induced renal damage. (Modified from Remuzzi G, Bertani T. Pathophysiology of progressive nephropathies. *N Engl J Med* 1998;12:1448–1456.)

MOLECULAR MEDIATORS

To enhance understanding of the pathogenesis of diabetic nephropathy, a number of studies have examined the cellular and molecular mechanisms of kidney damage. These studies have established the critical concept that the insults of hyperglycemia, high blood pressure, and protein overload converge at the cellular level by using similar molecular signaling pathways and influencing the expression of common cytokines (Fig. 51.2).

Transforming Growth Factor-β1

TGF-β is a ubiquitous cytokine that regulates a variety of cellular processes. It exists in three isoforms—TGF-β1, TGF-β2, and TGF-β3—of which TGF-β1 is the best characterized and most highly expressed in the kidney. Glomerular and proximal tubule cells produce TGF-β1 and express both type I and type II TGF-β receptors, which bind to all TGF-β isoforms (84,85).

TGF-β1 has important prosclerotic properties and is a potent inducer of cell hypertrophy and apoptosis. *In vitro,* both glomerular mesangial cells and tubular epithelial cells increase their synthesis of collagen, fibronectin, and laminin in response to TGF-β1. Furthermore, TGF-β1 inhibits the synthesis of collagenases and stimulates production of metalloprotease inhibitors. This results in reduced degradation of extracellular matrix and further contributes to accumulation of matrix (85). Finally, *in vivo,* TGF-β1 induces glomerulosclerosis and proteinuria in healthy animals (86–88).

Numerous studies have explored the role of TGF-β1 in diabetic glomerulosclerosis, and at present there is overwhelming evidence implicating overexpression of TGF-β1 in the pathogenesis of diabetic nephropathy. In both human and experimental diabetes, TGF-β1 gene expression and protein secretion are increased in the glomeruli and tubules (89,90). This effect is sustained in time and closely correlates with the degree of mesangial matrix expansion and with HbA_{1c} levels. The TGF-β type II receptor is also overexpressed in diabetic animals (91), suggesting that the diabetic kidney is hyperresponsive to TGF-β. Finally, and of the greatest importance, in diabetic mice TGF-β blockade significantly reduces overexpression of both type IV collagen and fibronectin and prevents glomerular hypertrophy, glomerulosclerosis, and renal insufficiency (92,93).

The importance of TGF-β1 is further highlighted by *in vivo* and *in vitro* studies showing that the three key insults implicated in the pathogenesis of diabetic nephropathy promote the expression of this cytokine. These studies also suggest that TGF-β1 may have a role in the interaction between metabolic and hemodynamic factors in mediating accumulation of extracellular matrix in the diabetic kidney.

High glucose concentrations induce the expression of TGF-β1 in both mesangial and tubular epithelial cells. Further, inhibition of TGF-β1 prevents glucose-induced hypertrophy of mesangial cells and production of extracellular matrix, indicating that these effects are mediated by TGF-β1 via an autocrine mechanism (94). Exposure of mesangial cells to high glucose concentrations induces overexpression of TGF-β receptors, suggesting that high glucose concentrations may also enhance the response to TGF-β1 (95). On the other hand, TGF-β1 induces the GLUT1 transporter in mesangial cells and can thereby enhance glucotoxicity (96). *In vitro,* AGEs induce TGF-β1 gene expression and protein secretion by mesangial cells (44), and *in vivo* administration of AGEs upregulates TGF-β1 in the kidney (97).

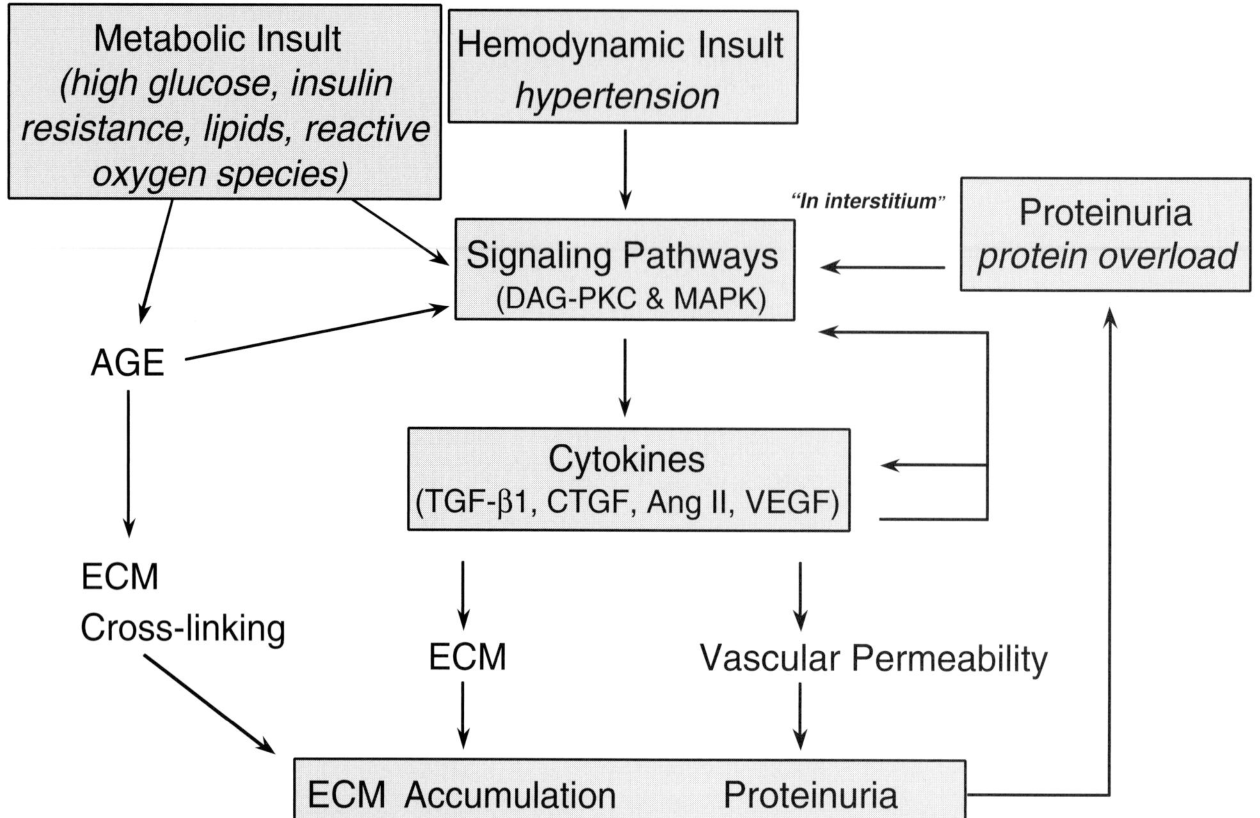

Figure 51.2. Schematic representation of the interaction, at the cellular and intracellular levels, of three insults operating in diabetic nephropathy. AGE, advanced glycation end-product; ECM, extracellular matrix; TGF-β1, transforming growth factor-1β; Ang II, angiotensin II; CTGF, connective tissue growth factor; VEGF, vascular endothelial growth factor; MAPK, mitogen-activated protein kinases; PKC, protein kinase C; DAG, diacylglycerol.

The link between hyperglycemia, TGF-β1, and kidney sclerosis is thus well established.

Recent studies in glomerular epithelial cells have shown that high glucose induces the TGF-β type II receptor without affecting TGF-β1 production. TGF-β mediates high glucose–induced production of fibronectin and collagen type IV (α3 chain) by glomerular epithelial cells, suggesting a role of TGF-β1 in the thickening of the glomerular basement membrane (98,99).

In vivo in the remnant kidney, an animal model of progressive renal injury with many hemodynamic and structural similarities to diabetes, treatment with ACE inhibitors, which normalized glomerular capillary pressure, is associated with reduced expression of TGF-β1 (100). This provides indirect evidence that the hemodynamic insult may affect TGF-β1. This hypothesis has been confirmed *in vitro* by studies showing that cyclic stretch of mesangial cells stimulates TGF-β1 gene expression and protein secretion in an intensity-dependent manner (101) and enhances the expression of the type II TGF-β receptor (102) Further, TGF-β1 mediates, at least in part, stretch-induced overproduction of mesangial matrix (103). Finally, stretch-induced glucose uptake is also mediated by TGF-β1 (80). This suggests a key role of TGF-β1 as final common mediator of sclerosis and glucotoxicity in mesangial cells exposed to metabolic and mechanical perturbations.

In rats with protein-overload nephropathy, inflammatory cells are recruited into the interstitium via a complement-mediated mechanism. These cells are then activated to secrete TGF-β1, which in turn binds to specific receptors on interstitial fibroblasts and induces them to proliferate and secrete matrix components. Thus, TGF-β1 is also crucial in proteinuria-induced interstitial remodeling and scarring (83).

On the basis of this evidence, it is now generally believed that TGF-β1 is the mediator of a final common pathway leading to sclerosis in diabetic nephropathy.

Connective Tissue Growth Factor

Connective tissue growth factor (CTGF) is a novel cytokine that is overexpressed in various sclerotic conditions (104). The importance of CTGF in diabetic nephropathy followed its identification by differential cloning as a gene overexpressed in mesangial cells cultured in high glucose concentrations (105). CTGF is only minimally expressed in the normal kidney, but it is strongly induced in the mesangium in both human and experimental diabetic nephropathy (106,107). AGN diminishes overexpression of both CTGF and intracellular matrix in diabetic mice (108). *In vitro* studies have provided potential mechanisms of CTGF involvement in the pathogenesis of diabetic nephropathy. *In vivo* studies then showed that CTGF is overexpressed in the glomeruli from proteinuric diabetic rats (106) and in the tubulointerstitium in the rat remnant kidney model (109). *In vitro* studies have provided potential mechanisms of CTGF induction in diabetic nephropathy. In mesangial cells, CTGF expression is induced by high glucose concentrations, mechanical stretch, and TGF-β1 (106). Furthermore, CTGF is a crucial downstream mediator of TGF-β1 signaling, but it appears to mediate selectively the TGF-β1 profibrotic effect of increased production of extracellular matrix, whereas it does not have antiproliferative and immunosuppressive activity (110). CTGF also stimulates its own expression, and this capacity of autoinduction has been implicated in the perpetuation of the fibrotic process (106). Recent studies have shown that CTGF binds to IGF-1, TGF-β1, and vascular endothelial growth factor (VEGF) in the extracellular space, whereby modifying their bioactivity. Specifically, CTGF appears to enhance IGF-1 prosclerotic effects, increasing the binding of TGF-β1 to its receptors, and to prevent VEGF binding to the KDR receptor (111). This suggests that CTGF may play a role in the pathogenesis of diabetic nephropathy not only by acting directly on mesangial cells but also by modulating the activity of other cytokines implicated in the pathogenesis of the glomerular damage. In tubular epithelial cells, CTGF is a weak inducer of fibronectin production; however, CTGF may contribute to tubulointerstitial fibrosis by stimulating transdifferentiation of epithelial cells to myofibroblasts (112,113).

Growth Hormone and Insulin-like Growth Factor

IGF-1 is a potent mitogenic polypeptide, under growth hormone (GH) regulation, that binds to a specific receptor (IGF-R1) and to six binding proteins (IGFBPs) that modulate its bioavailability (114). Although circulating IGF-1 levels are normal or reduced in patients with diabetes (115), the local IGF-1 system appears to be upregulated. IGF-1 content of the kidney is increased in experimental diabetes. Furthermore, increases in IGF-R1 and changes in IGFBP expression, leading to enhanced IGF-1 trapping and possibly bioreactivity, have been reported in kidneys from diabetic animals (114). Transgenic animals overexpressing IGF-1 and GH develop glomerular hypertrophy (116). Furthermore, IGF-1 infused in pharmacologic concentrations in humans increases renal plasma flow and the glomerular filtration rate (117). Finally, suppression of the GH/IGF-1 axis prevents the onset of glomerular hyperfiltration and renal hypertrophy in diabetic animals (114,118). IGF is thus believed to play a role in the pathogenesis of early glomerular abnormalities in the diabetic kidney.

IGF-1 stimulates endothelial nitric oxide synthase (eNOS) activity *in vitro* in endothelial cells and induces vasodilation *in vivo,* and this provides a potential link between IGF-1 and glomerular hyperfiltration and hypertrophy (119). In a high-glucose milieu, IGF-1 induces the proliferation of mesangial cells, which also may contribute to the glomerular hypertrophy of early diabetes. In mesangial cells, IGF-1 increases both matrix production and GLUT1 activity (120), suggesting a role of IGF-1 in glomerulosclerotic processes; however, the demonstration that mice transgenic for IGF-1 do not develop glomerulosclerosis has weakened this hypothesis (116).

Vascular Endothelial Growth Factor

VEGF, also known as vascular permeability factor, is a potent inducer of angiogenesis and vascular permeability and dilatation (121). In the adult kidney, VEGF is expressed by both glomerular and tubular epithelial cells, and VEGF receptors are located on the vascular endothelium. However, other glomerular cell types, including mesangial cells, can produce VEGF and express VEGF receptors *in vitro* and in pathologic conditions (122,123). Insults relevant to diabetes, such as high glucose, AGEs, mechanical stretch, angiotensin II, IGF-1, and TGF-β1, have been shown to induce VEGF production *in vitro* in mesangial cells (124–128). Moreover, in glomerular epithelial cells, high glucose induces VEGF in a TGF-β-1–dependent manner, and stretch stimulates both production of VEGF and expression of VEGF receptor (129,130).

Both VEGF and VEGF receptors are overexpressed in the glomeruli *in vivo* in experimental diabetes (131) and in patients with type 2 diabetes (132), and plasma VEGF levels are raised in patients with type 1 diabetes with nephropathy (133). Recent studies in both type 1 and type 2 experimental diabetes have shown that VEGF blockade prevents glomerular hypertrophy and glomerular hyperfiltration and ameliorates proteinuria (134,135), suggesting a role for VEGF in the early glomerular abnormalities of diabetes.

VEGF potently stimulates eNOS expression and activity in cultured endothelial cells (136), and VEGF blockade normalizes eNOS expression by glomerular capillaries (134), providing a potential link between VEGF and both glomerular hyperfiltration and hypertrophy in diabetes. Although VEGF is a potent inducer of permeability of endothelial cells (137), the mechanism linking VEGF to proteinuria remains elusive, as VEGF receptors are expressed primarily on the glomerular endothelium, which plays a minor role in the filtration barrier.

Angiotensin II

Circulating angiotensin II is formed in the blood by the renin-angiotensin system. In addition, there is an intact, independent renin-angiotensin system in the kidney (138) that is abnormally activated in diabetes. Indeed, in diabetic rats, both renin and angiotensinogen gene expression is increased in the kidney. Further, the intensity of ACE immunostaining is enhanced in both glomeruli and renal vessels (139).

ACE inhibitors appear to have a greater efficacy than other blood pressure–lowering agents in their antiproteinuric and renoprotective action. This has been classically ascribed to their effect on glomerular hemodynamics, as suggested by treatments that, by interfering with angiotensin II action, normalize glomerular capillary pressure in diabetic rats (74).

Moreover, in the kidney, angiotensin II can bind to receptors expressed on various renal cell types (140) and exerts important effects, independent of its systemic hemodynamic activity, that may contribute to the progression of renal disease (141). In particular, angiotensin II can directly induce matrix deposition via a TGF-β1–dependent mechanism in both mesangial and tubular cells (142). High glucose induces production of angiotensin II in mesangial cells (143), and stretch magnifies the response of mesangial cells to angiotensin II by upregulating the angiotensin II receptor AT1 (127). Therefore, in mesangial cells the deleterious effects of hyperglycemia and high intraglomerular pressure may result from an enhanced production of and responsiveness to angiotensin II. In glomerular epithelial cells, angiotensin II induces apoptosis via a TGF-β1–dependent mechanism (144), and ACE inhibitors prevent both proteinuria-induced glomerular epithelial-cell damage and overexpression of TGF-β1 (145). This suggests that angiotensin II may be causally implicated in the podocyte abnormalities seen in diabetic nephropathy (146).

In isolated glomeruli, angiotensin II increases glomerular permeability to protein and impairs the size-selective function of the glomerular filter (147,148). The underlying mechanism is still unclear; however, recent studies of human epithelial cells have shown that angiotensin II induces a rapid reduction in the expression of nephrin, a protein of the slit diaphragm implicated in the pathogenesis of proteinuric conditions (149). *In vivo* both angiotensin II receptor antagonists and ACE inhibitors normalize the reduced expression of nephrin that occurs in diabetes (150). Although further studies are required to establish whether reduction in nephrin is a marker of podocyte damage or a mechanism of proteinuria, these recent findings have opened an exciting new area of research. It thus appears that the efficacy of ACE inhibitors and angiotensin II receptor antagonists is due not simply to inhibition of the hemodynamic effects of angiotensin II but also to direct blockade of the cytokine and growth factor action of angiotensin II. On the other hand, exposure of mesangial cells to hemodynamic stretch magnifies their response to angiotensin II via an upregulation of the angiotensin II receptor AT1, making it possible for the deleterious effect of high intraglomerular pressure to result not only from a direct mechanical insult but also from an enhanced angiotensin II effect (127).

TRANSCRIPTION FACTORS AND INTRACELLULAR SIGNALING PATHWAYS

It is important to understand which intracellular mechanisms affect the transcription of the genes coding for extracellular matrix proteins in diabetic nephropathy. Gene transcription is regulated by transcription factors that bind to specific binding sites in the gene promoter region. Cellular responses often result from coordinated activation of sets of genes with binding sites for common transcription factors. Sclerosis is a cellular response to insult, and it is likely to follow this pattern. It is thus critical to identify the transcription factor or factors implicated in matrix overexpression in diabetic nephropathy and to establish which intracellular signaling pathways are involved in induction or activation of these transcription factors.

Nuclear Factor-κB

The transcription factor NF-κB plays a pivotal role in early gene responses by promoting the synthesis of mRNA for various cell-adhesion molecules and cytokines. NF-κB is important in cell survival, and its inhibition has been causally related to apoptosis. Monocytes of patients with diabetic nephropathy have higher NF-κB activity than do monocytes of patients without renal complications (151), and in experimental diabetes, AGEs induce NF-κB activation in the tubuli (152). *In vitro* studies have demonstrated that high glucose, AGEs, angiotensin II, and stretch potently induce NF-κB activation mainly via formation of reactive oxygen species and activation of PKC (153,154), providing potential cellular mechanisms of NF-κB activation in the diabetic kidney. Inhibition of NF-κB reduces interstitial monocyte infiltration in rats with proteinuria, and NF-κB is believed to play a key role in proteinuria-induced tubulointerstitial damage in diabetes (83). Recent studies have shown than NF-κB mediates both stretch and high glucose–induced production of MCP-1 in mesangial cells (155,156), plays a role in apoptosis of glomerular epithelial cells (157), and modulates the TGF-β1 intracellular signaling pathway (158). There is thus preliminary evidence for a role of NF-κB in the pathogenesis of both glomerular and tubular damage in diabetes. Both ACE inhibitors and statins are potent NF-κB inhibitors, and their renoprotective action may be related, at least in part, to the suppression of NF-κB activity.

Fos, Jun, and the AP-1 Transcription Factor

c-fos and *c-jun* are two highly conserved proto-oncogenes. c-Fos and c-Jun proteins combine in homo/heterodimers (c-Fos/c-Jun, c-Jun/c-Jun) to form the AP-1 transcription complex, which binds to and induces genes with AP-1–binding consensus sequences in their promoter regions (159). Genes encoding for TGF-β1, fibronectin, and laminin contain AP-1–binding sites in their promoters; thus, AP-1 may stimulate their transcription and induce expression of extracellular matrix protein genes via direct and indirect mechanisms (160,161).

Increased expression of c-*fos* and c-*jun* mRNA has been demonstrated *in vivo* in rat glomeruli 24 hours after the induction of diabetes (162). In rat mesangial cells *in vitro,* high glucose concentrations induce expression of c-*fos* and c-*jun;* furthermore, c-*fos* is induced after 20 minutes of exposure to mechanical stretch (163,164). There is also evidence *in vitro* that expression of c-*fos* and c-*jun* in mesangial cells induced by high glucose concentrations is associated with increased transcription of target extracellular matrix protein genes via formation of the AP-1 transcription factor (165).

Therefore, the AP-1 transcription factor plays an important role in the cascade leading to excess deposition of matrix deposition. However, which are the signal transduction pathways that cause increased AP-1 expression?

Intracellular Signaling Pathways

PROTEIN KINASE C

PKC, a family of ubiquitous serine-threonine kinases, is important in the transduction of many extracellular signals. There are at least 11 isoforms of PKC; these can be categorized into classical (α, β1, β2, γ), novel (δ, ε, η, θ), and atypical (ζ, λ, μ) on the basis of their common structural features. Both classical and novel PKC isoforms are activated by diacylglycerol (DAG) (166). PKC activation regulates a number of vascular functions, such as vascular permeability, contractility, cellular proliferation, basement membrane synthesis, and signal transduction mechanisms for hormones and cytokines (167). Furthermore, PKC induces expression of c-*fos* and c-*jun* (168,169); thus, PKC can be proposed as a potential candidate responsible for the increased AP-1 expression seen in diabetic nephropathy. This hypothesis is supported by both *in vitro* and *in vivo* data.

In diabetes, DAG levels are increased and PKC is activated in a variety of tissues, including kidney glomeruli (170). The direct role of hyperglycemia in causing these alterations was confirmed by exposing isolated glomeruli and cultured mesangial cells to high glucose concentrations. High glucose concentrations lead to *de novo* DAG synthesis, which is then responsible for PKC activation (171–173). It is interesting that activation of the DAG-PKC pathway in diabetic animals is maintained chronically, and this supports the hypothesis of a role of this system in the pathogenesis of chronic diabetic complications. Furthermore, glycated products and activation of the polyol pathway can also activate the DAG-PKC cascade, suggesting that the activation of DAG-PKC may be a common downstream mechanism by which multiple by-products of glucose exert their adverse effects (174). Recent evidence from studies of cultured bovine endothelial cells suggests that hyperglycemia induces superoxide production by the mitochondrial electron transport chain and that this is the causal link between PKC activation, AGE formation, and sorbitol accumulation (53).

PKC is also a crucial downstream mediator of TGF-β1, angiotensin II, VEGF, and cyclic stretch signaling, indicating that PKC activation is a key intracellular target of both metabolic and hemodynamic insults (175–177).

Multiple cellular and functional abnormalities in the diabetic kidney have been attributed to the activation of the PKC pathway. In mesangial cells *in vitro,* PKC agonists increase production of extracellular matrix components, whereas PKC inhibitors prevent glucose-induced expression of collagen type IV and fibronectin (178); further, many stretch-induced effects have been shown to occur, at least in part, via a PKC-dependent mechanism (78,175). *In vivo,* a specific PKC-β inhibitor prevents the increase in type IV collagen and fibronectin expression in diabetic rat glomeruli and ameliorates albuminuria after 8 weeks of treatment (179–181). In addition, prevention of albuminuria by ramipril in rats with streptozotocin-induced diabetes is associated with the normalization of glomerular PKC (182).

As outlined previously, TGF-β1 is a key mediator of sclerosis in the diabetic kidney, and PKC inhibitors prevent TGF-β1 overexpression in diabetic glomeruli (179). Thus, PKC activation may be responsible for the increased expression of matrix molecules both directly and through TGF-β1 overexpression. The capacity of active PKC to induce c-*fos* and c-*jun* transcription (168,170) and thus to stimulate the formation of the AP-1 transcription factor is believed to be the major underlying mechanism of this combined induction of TGF-β1 and matrix protein genes.

MITOGEN-ACTIVATED PROTEIN KINASES

Extracellular signal–related kinases (ERK), stress-activated protein kinases (JNK), and p38 kinases (p38) are members of the mitogen-activated protein kinase (MAPK) superfamily. These kinases constitute functionally distinct, but structurally related, transduction pathways by which extracellular signals are transmitted to the nucleus to regulate gene expression. Specifically, MAPKs are activated by phosphorylation at specific threonine and tyrosine residues in response to various cytokines and extracellular stresses. Activated MAPKs translocate to the nucleus, where they phosphorylate and transactivate specific transcription factors, which regulate the expression of c-*fos* and c-*jun* genes. Thus, MAPKs may influence extracellular matrix protein genes and TGF-β1 expression via an AP-1–dependent mechanism (183).

Recent *in vitro* and *in vivo* data demonstrate that both ERK and p38 are activated *in vivo* in glomeruli from diabetic rats and *in vitro* in mesangial cells exposed to either high glucose concentrations or mechanical stretch (78,184–188). Furthermore, specific p38 and ERK inhibitors prevent stretch-induced overproduction of matrix (78,188), and PKC inhibition abrogates p38 activation (78,189). This suggests that MAPKs are intracellular mediators leading to matrix overproduction and that they operate downstream of PKC.

In mesangial cells, p38 also is activated by TGF-β1 and mediates TGF-β1–induced fibronectin production; thus, p38 seems to be a key mediator of sclerosis (78). Accordingly, it was recently found that human mesangial cells exposed to stretch show rapid activation of p38, resulting in a direct and independent production of fibronectin and TGF-β1; the latter in turn contributed to the maintenance of long-term p38 activation in a vicious cycle, resulting in the perpetuation of fibronectin accumulation (78) (Fig. 51.3).

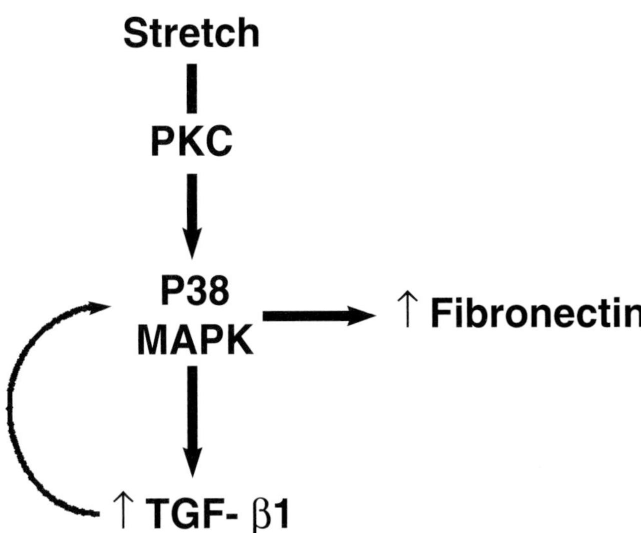

Figure 51.3. Central role of p38 in stretch-induced matrix production in human mesangial cells. Stretch induces p38 mitogen-activated protein kinase (MAPK) activation via a protein kinase C (PKC)–dependent mechanism. p38 mediates stretch-induced transforming growth factor-1β (TGF-β1) and fibronectin production. TGF-β1 in turn maintains activation of p38 and leads to further accumulation of fibronectin. (Modified from Gruden G, Zonca S, Hayward A, et al. Mechanical stretch-induced fibronectin and TGF-β1 production in human mesangial cells is p38 mitogen-activated protein kinase-dependent. *Diabetes* 2000;9:655–661.)

TARGETS FOR PATHOGENESIS-SPECIFIC THERAPY

The combined action of various insults is required to explain the pathogenesis of diabetic nephropathy. Glucose-dependent pathways are clearly relevant, and therefore any therapeutic approach that involves intensification of glycemic control should be considered as part of treatment regimens for diabetic nephropathy. Indeed, in both type 1 and type 2 diabetes, intensified insulin therapy has been shown to retard the development of diabetic kidney disease (34,35). The importance of hemodynamic factors, including systemic and glomerular hypertension, in the pathogenesis of diabetic nephropathy has been underscored by clinical trials of ACE inhibitors and other antihypertensive agents, which have conclusively demonstrated their renoprotective and antiproteinuric effect (66–68). Furthermore, in diabetic nephropathy, proteinuria is a strong and independent predictor of decline in renal function (81). Therefore, the treatment of the diabetic patient at risk of or with established nephropathy requires a concerted approach that aims at optimization of glycemic control, lowering of blood pressure, and reduction of protein excretion either by using antiproteinuric agents or by lowering protein intake.

Formation of AGEs and activation of the polyol pathway have long been proposed as potential mechanisms linking hyperglycemia to kidney damage. However, clinical trials using agents that inhibit these biochemical pathways have so far been either disappointing or inconclusive. In humans, aldose reductase inhibitors have failed to shown any renoprotective effect in controlled studies, and no clinical trial is currently in progress to further test the effect of aldose reductase inhibitors in the prevention and treatment of diabetic nephropathy. AGN, an inhibitor of AGE formation, has been shown to reduce albuminuria and mesangial expansion in animals (40), but preliminary data from the recently completed clinical studies in both type 1 (ACTION 1) and type 2 (ACTION 2) diabetic patients failed to convincingly show a renoprotective effect of AGN and have raised some concern about the safety of this compound. Recently, a new class of compounds that cleave AGE-derived protein cross-links have been synthesized (190). Phenacylthiazolium bromide and other members of this family revert AGE-mediated tissue damage and are effective in the treatment of diabetic subjects with established renal disease (191); however, the role of these compounds in human disease is yet to be explored.

Recently, studies on the cellular and molecular mechanisms involved in the pathogenesis of diabetic nephropathy have provided new targets for therapeutic intervention. TGF-β1 plays a pivotal role in the sclerotic process of the diabetic kidney; therefore, it is an important target for pathogenesis-specific therapy (192,193). However, TGF-β1 has other functions besides promoting fibrosis; most important, TGF-β1 modulates the immune and

TABLE 51.1. Current and Potential Treatment Options of Various Pathogenetic Steps in Diabetic Nephropathy

Mechanism	Treatment
Metabolic insult	
Hyperglycemia	Intensive insulin therapy[a] Agents normalizing mitochondrial reactive oxygen species[b]
AGEs	AGN[c], cross-link breakers[b], glycated albumin antibodies[c]
Polyol	Aldose reductase inhibitors[d]
Hemodynamic insult	
Systemic hypertension	Antihypertensive agents[a]
Glomerular hypertension	ACE inhibitors, low-protein diet[a]
Proteinuria	ACE inhibitors, low-protein diet[a]
Mediators	
TGF-β1	Antibodies[c]
CTGF	Antibodies[b]
Angiotensin II	ACE inhibitors, losartan[a], irbesartan[a]
Signaling pathways	
PKC	PKC-β inhibition (LY333531)[c]
MAPK	MAPK inhibition[b]

AGEs, advanced glycation end products; TGF, transforming growth factor; CTGF, connective tissue growth factor; PKC, protein kinase; MAPK, mitogen-activated protein kinase; AGN, aminoguanidine.
[a]Proven clinically.
[b]Under experimental investigation.
[c]Proven experimentally.
[d]Not proven in humans but effective in animal models.

inflammatory response. Therefore, any attempt at blocking TGF-β1 may lead in the long term to inflammatory, autoimmune, and malignant responses, and this may prevent its use in humans. CTGF, a cytokine recently implicated in the pathogenesis of diabetic nephropathy, is induced by TGF-β1 and seems to mediate TGF-β1 prosclerotic effects exclusively. CTGF is thus a promising therapeutic target, and studies are ongoing to assess the effect of CTGF blockade in experimental diabetes (104).

Activation of PKC is believed to play a key role in diabetic complications. PKC exists in various isoforms (194), and analyses of retina, kidney, and cardiovascular tissues have shown a predominant activation of PKC-β isoforms in the diabetic state with minor increases of other isoforms, suggesting that a specific inhibitor for PKC-β isoforms could be used to circumvent the nonspecificity and *in vivo* toxicity of general PKC inhibition (173). Recent reports demonstrate that a number of *in vivo* abnormalities in diabetic rats can be prevented or normalized with an orally available specific inhibitor of PKC-β isoforms, LY333531. Oral administration of LY333531 to streptozotocin-diabetic rats for 2 weeks prevents changes in the retinal blood flow and glomerular filtration rate and improves the renal albumin excretion rate after 8 weeks of treatment. LY333531 also can prevent the diabetes-induced abnormalities in mRNA expression of TGF-β1, type IV collagen, and fibronectin in the glomeruli and of caldesmon in the aorta (179–182). These findings provide strong evidence that PKC-β blockade can be beneficial in diabetic vascular complications in animals, and clinical trials are currently ongoing to test its safety and efficacy in humans. These studies also suggest that PKC inhibition is a promising therapeutic approach not only for diabetic nephropathy but also for chronic diabetic complications in general. Recent findings indicate that other intracellular signaling molecules, such as ERK and p38, play an important role in the pathogenesis of diabetic vascular complications. Specific p38 inhibitors can be orally administered and have disease-modifying activity in animal models of chronic inflammatory diseases; however, their effect in diabetic complications is yet to be explored. Table 51.1 presents some of the therapeutic targets, either current or potential, along the pathogenic path leading to diabetic kidney disease.

The improvement of gene-transfer techniques, especially vectors for delivering genes, raises the exciting possibility that gene therapy may become a novel therapeutic approach to renal disease. Correction of cellular dysfunction by expressing a deficient gene, addition of a new function by transferring an exogenous gene, and inhibition of unfavorable action by introducing a counteracting gene are potential applications of gene-transfer technology to therapy. It is possible to selectively transfer somatic genes to the kidney using both *in vivo* and *ex vivo* approaches, and it has recently been demonstrated with the HVJ-liposome–mediated gene-transfer method that mesangial matrix expansion of experimental glomerulonephritis can be prevented by antisense oligonucleotides or soluble receptor chimera for TGF-β (195). The potential applications of gene transfer in diabetic nephropathy are enormous, but research in this field has just begun. The advances made in understanding the cellular and intracellular basis of diabetic nephropathy during the past decade can provide specific targets for future gene-transfer therapy.

REFERENCES

1. Cooper ME. Pathogenesis, prevention, and treatment of diabetic nephropathy. *Lancet* 1998;352:213–219.
2. Quinn M, Angelico MC, Warram JH, et al. Familial factors determine the development of diabetic nephropathy in patients with IDDM. *Diabetologia* 1996;39:940–945.
3. Viberti GC, Keen H, Wiseman MJ. Raised arterial pressure in parents of proteinuric insulin dependent dia betics. *BMJ* 1987;295:515–517.
4. Nelson RG. Prediabetic blood pressure predicts urinary albumin excretion after the onset of type 2 diabetes mellitus in Pima Indians. *Diabetologia* 1993;36:998–1001.
5. Krolewski AS. Predisposition to hypertension and susceptibility to renal disease in insulin-dependent diabetes mellitus. *N Engl J Med* 1988;318:140–145.

6. The Microalbuminuria Collaborative Study Group. Predictors of the development of microalbuminuria in patients with type 1 diabetes mellitus: a seven-year prospective study. *Diabet Med* 1999;16:918–925.
7. Marre M. Genetics and the prediction of complications in type 1 diabetes. *Diabetes Care* 1999;22[Suppl 2]:B53-B58.
8. Heesom AE, Hibberd ML, Millward A, et al. Polymorphism in the 5′-end of the aldose reductase gene is strongly associated with the development of diabetic nephropathy in type I diabetes. *Diabetes* 1997;46:287–291.
9. Moczulski DK, Scott L, Antonellis A, et al. Aldose reductase gene polymorphisms and susceptibility to diabetic nephropathy in type 1 diabetes mellitus. *Diabet Med* 2000;17:111–118.
10. Mangili R, Bending JJ, Scott G, et al. Increased sodium-lithium countertransport activity in red cells of patients with insulin-dependent diabetes and nephropathy. *N Engl J Med* 1998;318:146–150.
11. Krolewski AS, Canessa M, Warram JH, et al. Predisposition to hypertension and susceptibility to renal disease in insulin-dependent diabetes mellitus *N Engl J Med* 1998;318:140–145.
12. Trevisan R, Li LK, Messent J, et al. Na^+/H^+ antiport activity and cell growth in cultured skin fibroblasts of IDDM patients with nephropathy. *Diabetes* 1992;1:1239–1246.
13. Ng LL, Davies JE, Siczkowski M, et al. Abnormal sodium-lithium antiporter phenotype and turnover of immortalised lymphoblasts from type 1 diabetic patients with nephropathy. *J Clin Invest* 1994;93:2750–2757.
14. Koren W, Koldanov R, Pronin VS, et al. Enhanced erythrocyte Na^+/H^+ exchange predicts diabetic nephropathy in patients with IDDM. *Diabetologia* 1998;41:201–205.
15. Trevisan R, Fioretto P, Barbosa J, et al. Insulin-dependent diabetic sibling pairs are concordant for Na^+/H^+ antiport activity *Kidney Int* 1999;55:2383–2389.
16. Viberti GC. Why do we have to invoke genetic susceptibility for diabetic nephropathy. *Kidney Int* 1999;55:2526–2527.
17. Canani LH, Gerchman F, Gross JL. Familial clustering of diabetic nephropathy in Brazilian type 2 diabetic patients. *Diabetes* 1999;48:909–913
18. Freedman BI, Tuttle AB, Spray BJ. Familial predisposition to nephropathy in African-Americans with non-insulin-dependent diabetes mellitus. *Am J Kidney Dis* 1995;25:710–713.
19. Fava S, Azzopardi J, Hattersley AT, et al. Increased prevalence of proteinuria in diabetic sibs of proteinuric type 2 diabetic subjects. *Am J Kidney Dis* 2000;35:708–712.
20. Imperatore G, Hanson RL, Pettitt DJ. Sib-pair linkage analysis for susceptibility genes for microvascular complications among Pima Indians with type 2 diabetes. Pima Diabetes Genes Group. *Diabetes* 1998;47:821–830.
21. Vardarli I, Baier LJ, Hanson RL. Gene for susceptibility to diabetic nephropathy in type 2 diabetes maps to 18q22.3-23. *Kidney Int* 2002;62:2176–2183.
22. Bowden DW, Sale M, Howard TD. Linkage of genetic markers on human chromosomes 20 and 12 to NIDDM in Caucasian sib pairs with a history of diabetic nephropathy. *Diabetes* 1997;46:882–886.
23. Herman WH, Prior DE, Yassine MD, et al. Nephropathy in NIDDM is associated with cellular markers for hypertension. *Diabetes Care* 1993; 16:815–818.
24. Fogarty DG, Rich SS, Hanna L, et al. Urinary albumin excretion in families with type 2 diabetes is heritable and genetically correlated to blood pressure. *Kidney Int* 2000;57:250–257.
25. Mauer SM, Steffes MW, Ellis EN, et al. Structural functional relationships in diabetic nephropathy. *J Clin Invest* 1984;74:1143–1155.
26. Fioretto P, Steffes MW, Sutherland DEF, et al. Sequential renal biopsies in IDDM patients: structural factors associated with clinical progression. *Kidney Int* 1995;48:1929–1935.
27. Schleicher ED. Biochemical aspects of diabetic nephropathy. In: Mogensen CE, ed. *The kidney and hypertension in diabetes mellitus.* Boston: Kluwer Academic Publishers, 1997:223–233.
28. Gilbert RE, Cooper ME. The tubulointerstitium in progressive diabetic kidney disease: more than an aftermath of glomerular injury. *Kidney Int* 1999;56:1627–1637.
29. Mathiesen ER, Ronn B, Jensen T, et al. Relationship between blood pressure and urinary albumin excretion in development of microalbuminuria. *Diabetes* 1990;9:245–249.
30. Krolewski AS, Lori L, Krolewski M, et al. Glycosylated haemoglobin and the risk of microalbuminuria in patients with insulin dependent diabetes mellitus. *N Engl J Med* 1995;332:1251–1255.
31. Lee CS, Mauer SM, Brown DM, et al. Renal transplantation in diabetes mellitus in the rat. *J Exp Med* 1974;139:793–800.
32. Maeur SM, Steffes MW, Sutherland DER, et al. Studies of the rate of regression of the glomerular lesions in diabetic rats treated with pancreatic islet transplantation. *Diabetes* 1975;24:280–285.
33. Rasch R. Prevention of diabetic glomerulopathy in streptozotocin diabetic rats. Albumin excretion. *Diabetologia* 1980; 18:413–416.
34. The Diabetes Control and Complications Trial Research Group. The effect of intensive treatment of diabetes on the development and progression of long-term complications in insulin-dependent diabetes mellitus. *N Engl J Med* 1993;329:977–986.
35. UK Prospective Diabetes Study (UKPDS) Group. Intensive blood-glucose control with sulphonylureas or insulin compared with conventional treatment and risk of complications in patients with type 2 diabetes (UKPDS 33). *Lancet* 1998;352:837–853.
36. Fioretto P, Steffes MW, Sutherland DE, et al. Reversal of lesions of diabetic nephropathy after pancreas transplantation. *N Engl J Med* 1998;339:69–75.
37. Raj D, Choudhury D, Welbourne TC, et al. Advanced glycation end products: a nephrologist's prospective. *Am J Kidney Dis* 2000;35:365–380.
38. Makino H, Shikata K, Hironaka K, et al. Ultrastructure of nonenzymatically glycated mesangial matrix in diabetic nephropathy. *Kidney Int* 1995;48:517–526.
39. Vlassara H, Striker LJ, Teichberg S, et al. Advanced glycation end products induce glomerular sclerosis and albuminuria in normal rats. *Proc Natl Acad Sci U S A* 1994;91:11704–11708.
40. Soulis-Liparota T, Cooper ME, Papazoglou D, et al. Retardation by aminoguanidine of development of albuminuria, mesangial expansion, and tissue fluorescence in streptozotocin-induced diabetic rats. *Diabetes* 1991;40: 1328–1334.
41. Lee HB, Cha MK, Song KI, et al. Pathogenic role of advanced glycation end products in diabetic nephropathy. *Kidney Int* 1997;52[Suppl 60]:S60-S65.
42. Soulis T, Thallas V, Youssef S, et al. Advanced glycation end products and the receptor for advanced glycation end products co-localise in organs susceptible to diabetic microvascular injury: immunohistochemical studies. *Diabetologia* 1997;40:619–628.
43. Doi T, Vlassara H, Kirstein M, et al. Receptor-specific increase in extracellular matrix production in mouse mesangial cells by advanced glycosylation end products is mediated via platelet-derived growth factor. *Proc Natl Acad Sci U S A* 1992;89:2873–2877.
44. Pugliese G, Pricci F, Romeo G, et al. Upregulation of mesangial growth factor and extracellular matrix synthesis by advanced glycation end products via a receptor-mediated mechanism. *Diabetes* 1997;46:1881–1887.
45. Yamamoto Y, Kato I, Doi T et al. Development and prevention of advanced diabetic nephropathy in RAGE-overexpressing mice. *J Clin Invest* 2001;108: 261–268.
46. Oldfield MD, Bach LA, Forbes JM, et al Advanced glycation end products cause epithelial-myofibroblast transdifferentiation via the receptor for advanced glycation end products (RAGE). *J Clin Invest* 2001;108:1853–1863.
47. Cogan DG. Aldose reductase and complications of diabetes. *Ann Intern Med* 1984;101:82–91.
48. Kador PF, Robinson WG Jr, Kinoshita JH. The pharmacology of aldose reductase inhibitors. *Annu Rev Pharmacol Toxicol* 1985;25:691–714.
49. Pugliese G, Tilton RG, Speedy A, et al. Modulation of haemodynamics and vascular filtration changes in diabetic rats by dietary myo-inositol. *Diabetes* 1990;39:312–322.
50. Olgemoller B, Schleicher E, Schwaabe S, et al. Up-regulation of myo-inositol transport compensates for competitive inhibition by glucose. *Diabetes* 1993;42:1119–1125.
51. Goldfarb S, Ziyadeh FN, Kern EF, et al. Effects of polyol-pathway inhibition and dietary myo-inositol on glomerular haemodynamic function in experimental diabetes mellitus in rats. *Diabetes* 1991;40:465–471.
52. Hamada Y, Araki N, Horiuchi S, et al. Role of polyol pathway in nonenzymatic glycation. *Nephrol Dial Transplant 1996;* 11:95–98.
53. Nishikawa T, Edelstein D, Du XL, et al. Normalizing mitochondrial superoxide production blocks three pathways of hyperglycaemic damage. *Nature* 2000;404:787–790.
54. McCaleb ML, McKean ML, Hohman TC, et al. Intervention with aldose reductase inhibitor, tolrestat, in renal and retinal lesions of streptozotocin diabetic rats. *Diabetologia* 1991;34:659–701.
55. Weigert C, Brodbeck K, Lehmann R, et al. Overexpression of glutamine: fructose-6-phosphate-amidotransferase induces transforming growth factor-beta1 synthesis in NIH-3T3 fibroblasts. *FEBS Lett* 2001;488:95–99.
56. Burt DJ, Gruden G, Thomas SM, et al. P38 mitogen-activated protein kinase mediates hexosamine-induced TGF β1 mRNA expression in human mesangial cells. *Diabetologia* 2003;46:531–537.
57. Kolm-Litty V, Sauer U, Nerlich A. High glucose-induced transforming growth factor beta1 production is mediated by the hexosamine pathway in porcine glomerular mesangial cells. *J Clin Invest* 1998;101:160–169.
58. Nerlich AG, Sauer U, Kolm-Litty V, et al. Expression of glutamine:fructose-6-phosphate amidotransferase in human tissues: evidence for high variability and distinct regulation in diabetes. *Diabetes* 1998;47:170–178.
59. James LR, Ingram A, Ly H, et al. Angiotensin II activates the GFAT promoter in mesangial cells. *Am J Physiol Renal Physiol* 2001;281(1):F151-F162.
60. Ayo SH, Radnik RA, Glass IIWF, et al. Increased extracellular matrix synthesis and mRNA in mesangial cells grown in high-glucose medium. *Am J Physiol* 1990;260:F185–F191.
61. Birkedal-Hansen H. Proteolytic remodeling of extracellular matrix. *Curr Opin Cell Biol* 1995;7:728–735.
62. Heilig CW, Conception LA, Riser BL, et al. Overexpression of glucose transporters in rat mesangial cells cultured in a normal glucose milieu mimics the diabetic phenotype. *J Clin Invest* 1995;96:1802–1814.
63. Heilig CW, Liu Y, England R, et al. D-glucose stimulates mesangial cell GLUT-1 expression and basal and IGF-I-sensitive glucose uptake in rat mesangial cells. Implication for diabetic nephropathy. *Diabetes* 1997;46:1030–1039.
64. Heilig CW, Kreisberg JI, Freytag S, et al. Antisense GLUT-1 protects mesangial cells from glucose induction of GLUT-1 and fibronectin expression. *Am J Physiol Renal Physiol* 2001;280:F657-F666.
65. Mogensen CE, Christiansen CK. Blood pressure changes and renal function changes in incipient and overt diabetic nephropathy. *Hypertension* 1985;7: II-64-II-73.
66. Zatz R, Dunn BR, Meyer TW, et al. Prevention of diabetic glomerulopathy by pharmacologic amelioration of glomerular capillary pressure. *J Clin Invest* 1986;77:1925–1930.

67. Lewis EJ, Hunsicker LG, Bain RP, et al. The effect of angiotensin-converting-enzyme inhibition on diabetic nephropathy. *N Engl J Med* 1993;329:1456–1462.
68. Viberti GC, Moghensen CE, Groop LC, et al. Effect of captopril on progression to clinical proteinuria in patients with insulin-dependent diabetes mellitus and microalbuminuria. *JAMA* 1994;217:275–279.
69. Ravid M, Brosh D, Ravid-Safran D, et al. Main risk factors for nephropathy in type 2 diabetes mellitus are plasma cholesterol levels, mean blood pressure, and hyperglycemia. *Arch Intern Med* 1998;11:998–1004.
70. Hostetter TH, Rennke HG, Brenner BM. The case for intra-renal hypertension in the initiation and progression of diabetic and other glomerulopathies. *Am J Med* 1982;72:375–380.
71. Zatz R, Meyer TW, Renneke HG, et al. Predominance of hemodynamic rather than metabolic factors in the pathogenesis of diabetic glomerulopathy. *Proc Natl Acad Sci U S A* 1985;2:5963–5967.
72. Mauer SM, Steffes MW, Azar S, et al. The effects of Goldblatt hypertension on development of the glomerular lesions of diabetes mellitus in the rat. *Diabetes* 1978;27:738–744.
73. Thomsen OF, Andersen AR, Christiansen JS, et al. Renal changes in long-term type 1 (insulin-dependent) diabetic patients with and without clinical nephropathy; a light microscopic, morphometric study of autopsy material. *Diabetologia* 1984;26:361–365.
74. Bohlen L, De Courten M, Weidmann P. Comparative study of the effect of ACE-inhibitors and other antihypertensive agents on proteinuria in diabetic patients. *Am J Hypertens* 1994;7:845–92S.
75. Riser BL, Cortes P, Zhao X, et al. Intraglomerular pressure and mesangial stretching stimulate extracellular matrix formation in the rat. *J Clin Invest* 1992;90:1932–1943.
76. Harris RC, Haralson MA, Badr KF. Continuous stretch-relaxation in culture alters rat mesangial cell morphology, growth characteristics, and metabolic activity. *Lab Invest* 1992;66:548–554.
77. Yasuda T, Kondo S, Homma T, et al. Regulation of extracellular matrix by mechanical stress in rat glomerular mesangial cells. *J Clin Invest* 1996;98: 1991–2000.
78. Gruden G, Zonca S, Hayward A, et al. Mechanical stretch-induced fibronectin and TGF-β1 production in human mesangial cells is P38 mitogen-activated protein kinase-dependent. *Diabetes* 2000;9:655–661.
79. Cortes P. Mechanical strain and high glucose-induced alterations in mesangial cell collagen metabolism: role of TGF-β1 *J Am Soc Nephrol* 1998;9:827–836.
80. Gnudi L, Viberti G, Raij L, et al. GLUT-1 overexpression: link between hemodynamic and metabolic factors in glomerular injury? *Hypertension* 2003;42: 19–24.
81. Peterson JC, Adler S, Burkart JM, et al. Blood pressure control, proteinuria and the progression of renal disease: the Modification of Diet in Renal Disease Study. *Ann Intern Med* 1995;123:754–762.
82. Benigni A, Zoja C, Remuzzi G. The renal toxicity of sustained glomerular protein traffic. *Lab Invest* 1995;73:461–468.
83. Remuzzi G, Bertani T. Pathophysiology of progressive nephropathies. *N Engl J Med* 1998;12:1448–1456.
84. Border WA, Noble NA. Transforming growth factor-β in tissue fibrosis. *N Engl J Med* 1994;31:1286–1292.
85. Ziyadeh FN, Han DC. Involvement of TGF-β and its receptors in the pathogenesis of diabetic nephropathy. *Kidney Int* 1997;52[Suppl 60]:S7-S11.
86. Terrell TG, Working PK, Chow CP, et al. Pathology of recombinant human TGF-β1 in rats and rabbits. *Int Rev Exp Pathol* 1993;34B:43–67.
87. Isaka Y, Fuijiwara Y, Ueda N, et al. Glomerulosclerosis induced by *in vivo* transfection of TGF-β or PDGF into rat kidney. *J Clin Invest* 1993;92:2597–2601.
88. Kopp JB, Factor VM, Mozes M, et al. Transgenic mice with increased plasma levels of TGF-β1 develop progressive renal disease. *Lab Invest* 1996;74: 991–1003.
89. Yamamoto T, Nakamura T, Noble NA, et al. Expression of TGF-β is elevated in human and experimental diabetic nephropathy. *Proc Natl Acad Sci U S A* 1993;90:1814–1818.
90. Iwano M, Kubo A, Nishino T, et al. Quantification of glomerular TGF-β 1 mRNA in patients with diabetes mellitus. *Kidney Int* 1996;49:854–859.
91. Hill C, Flyvbjerg A, Gronbaek H, et al. The renal expression of transforming growth factor-beta isoforms and their receptors in acute and chronic experimental diabetes in rats. *Endocrinology* 2000;41:1196–1208.
92. Sharma K, Jin Y, Guo J, et al. Neutralization of TGF-β by anti-TGF-β antibody attenuates kidney hypertrophy and the enhanced extracellular matrix gene expression in streptozotocin-induced diabetic mice. *Diabetes* 1996;45: 522–530.
93. Ziyadeh FN, Hoffman BB, Han DC, et al. Long-term prevention of renal insufficiency, excess matrix gene expression, and glomerular mesangial matrix expansion by treatment with monoclonal anti-transforming growth factor-beta antibody in db/db diabetic mice. *Proc Natl Acad Sci U S A* 2000; 97:8015–8020.
94. Ziyadeh FN, Sharma K, Ericksen M, et al. Stimulation of collagen gene expression and protein synthesis in murine mesangial cells by high glucose is mediated by activation of TGF-β. *J Clin Invest* 1994;93:536–542.
95. Isono M, Mogyorosi A, Han DC, et al. Stimulation of TGF-β type II receptor by high glucose in mouse mesangial cells and in diabetic kidney. *Am J Physiol* 2000;278:F830–F838.
96. Inoki K, Haneda M, Maeda S, et al. TGF-β1 stimulates glucose uptake by enhancing GLUT-1 expression in mesangial cells. *Diabetes* 1999;55:1704–1712.
97. Yang C-W, Vlassara H, Peten EP. Advanced glycation end products upregulate gene expression found in diabetic glomerular disease. *Proc Natl Acad Sci U S A* 1994;91:9436–9440.
98. Iglesias-de la Cruz MC, Ziyadeh FN, Isono M. Effects of high glucose and TGF-β1 on the expression of collagen IV and vascular endothelial growth factor in mouse podocytes. *Kidney Int* 2002;62:901–913.
99. van Det NF, Verhagen NA, Tamsma JT. Regulation of glomerular epithelial cell production of fibronectin and transforming growth factor-beta by high glucose, not by angiotensin II. *Diabetes* 1997;46:834–840.
100. Wu L, Cox A, Roe C. TGF-β1 and renal injury following subtotal nephrectomy in the rats. Role of the renin angiotensin system. *Kidney Int* 1997;51:1553–1567.
101. Riser BL, Cortes P, Heilig C. Cyclic stretch selectively up-regulates transforming growth factor-β isoforms in cultured rat mesangial cells. *Am J Pathol* 1996;148:1915–1923.
102. Gruden G, Thomas S, Burt D, et al. Mechanical stretch induces TGF-β1 and type II-TGF-β receptor in human mesangial cells. *Diabetologia* 1998;41 [Suppl 1]:A38-A144.
103. Hirakata M, Kaname S, Chung U, et al. Tyrosine kinase dependent expression of TGF-β induced by stretch in mesangial cells. *Kidney Int* 1997;51: 1028–1036.
104. Goldschmeding R, Aten J, Ito Y. Connective tissue growth factor CTGF: just another factor in renal fibrosis? *Nephrol Dial Transplant* 2000;15:296–299.
105. Murphy M, Godson C, Cannon S, et al. Suppression subtractive hybridization identifies high glucose levels as a stimulus for expression of connective tissue growth factor and other genes in human mesangial cells. *J Biol Chem* 1999;274:5830–5834.
106. Riser BL, Denichilo M, Cortes P, et al. Regulation of connective tissue growth factor in cultured rat mesangial cells and its expression in experimental diabetic glomerulosclerosis. *J Am Soc Nephrol* 2000;11:25–38.
107. Wahab NA, Yevdokimova N, Weston BS. Role of connective tissue growth factor in the pathogenesis of diabetic nephropathy. *Biochem J* 2001;359 (Pt 1):77–87.
108. Twigg SM, Cao Z, McLennan SV. Renal connective tissue growth factor induction in experimental diabetes is prevented by aminoguanidine. *Endocrinology* 2002; 143:4907–4915.
109. Frazier KS, Paredes A, Dube P, et al. Connective tissue growth factor expression in the rat remnant kidney model and association with tubular epithelial cells undergoing transdifferentiation. *Vet Pathol* 2000;37:328–335.
110. Duncan MR, Frazier KS, Abramson S, et al. Connective tissue growth factor mediates transforming growth factor beta-induced collagen synthesis: down-regulation by cAMP. *FASEB J* 1999;13:1774–1786.
111. Inoki I, Shiomi T, Hashimoto G. CTGF binds vascular endothelial growth factor (VEGF) and inhibits VEGF-induced angiogenesis. *FASEB J* 2002; 16: 219–222.
112. Wang S, Denichilo M, Brubaker C, et al. Connective tissue growth factor in tubulointerstitial injury of diabetic nephropathy. *Kidney Int* 2001; 60:96–105.
113. Gore-Hyer E, Shegogue D, Markiewicz M. TGF-β1 and CTGF have overlapping and distinct fibrogenic effects on human renal cells. *Am J Physiol Renal Physiol* 2002;283:F707 F716.
114. Flyvbjerg A. Putative pathophysiological role of growth factors and cytokines in experimental diabetic kidney disease. *Diabetologia* 2000;43: 1205– 1223.
115. Chestnut RE, Quarmby V. Evaluation of total IGF-I assay methods using samples from type I and type II diabetic patients. *J Immunol Methods* 2002;259: 11–24.
116. Doi T, Striker LJ, Gibson CC, et al. Glomerular lesions in mice transgenic for growth hormone and insulinlike growth factor-I. I. Relationship between increased glomerular size and mesangial sclerosis. *Am J Pathol* 1990;137: 541–552.
117. Giordano M, DeFronzo RA. Acute effect of human recombinant insulin-like growth factor I on renal function in humans. *Nephron* 1995;71:10–15.
118. Landau D, Segev Y, Afargan M, et al. A novel somatostatin analogue prevents early renal complications in the non-obese diabetic mouse. *Kidney Int* 2001;60:505–512.
119. Tsukahara H, Gordienko DV, Tonshoff B, et al. Direct demonstration of insulin-like growth factor-I-induced nitric oxide production by endothelial cells. *Kidney Int* 1994;45:598–604.
120. Schreiber BD, Hughes ML, Groggel GC. Insulin-like growth factor stimulates production of mesangial cell matrix components. *Clin Nephrol* 1995;43:368–374.
121. Ferrara N, David-Smith T. The biology of vascular endothelial growth factor. *Endocrinol Rev* 1997;18:4–25.
122. Thomas S, Vanuystel J, Gruden G, et al. VEGF receptors in human mesangium *in vitro* and in glomerular disease. *J Am Soc Nephrol* 2000;11:1236–1243.
123. Iijima K, Yoshikawa N, Connoly DT, et al. Human mesangial cells and peripheral blood mononuclear cells produce vascular permeability factor. *Kidney Int* 1993;44:959–966.
124. Kim NH, Jung HH, Cha DR. Expression of vascular endothelial growth factor in response to high glucose in rat mesangial cells. *J Endocrinol* 2000;165: 617–624.
125. Yamagishi S, Inagaki Y, Okamoto T. Advanced glycation end product-induced apoptosis and overexpression of vascular endothelial growth factor and monocyte chemoattractant protein-1 in human-cultured mesangial cells. *J Biol Chem* 2002;277:20309–20315.
126. Gruden G, Thomas S, Burt D, et al. Mechanical stretch induces VPF in human mesangial cells: mechanisms of signal transduction. *Proc Natl Acad Sci U S A* 1997;94:12112–12116.

127. Gruden G, Thomas S, Burt D, et al. Interaction of angiotensin II and mechanical stretch on VEGF production by human mesangial cells *J Am Soc Nephrol* 1999;10:730–737.
128. Gruden G, Araf S, Zonca S, et al. IGF-I induces VEGF in human mesangial cells via a Src-dependent mechanism. *Kidney Int* 2003;63:1249–1255.
129. Iglesias-de la Cruz MC, Ziyadeh FN. Effects of high glucose and TGF-β1 on the expression of collagen IV and VEGF in mouse podocytes. *Kidney Int* 2002;62:901–913.
130. Gruden G, Hayward A, Setti G, et al. Stretch up-regulates vascular endothelial growth factor in murine glomerular epithelial cells via a PKC-independent mechanism. *Diabetologia* 2002;45[Suppl 2]:1084(abst).
131. Cooper ME, Vranes D, Youssef S, et al. Increased renal expression of VEGF and its receptor VEGFR-2 in experimental diabetes. *Diabetes* 1999;48:2229–2239.
132. Bortoloso E, Del Prete D, Gambaro G. VEGF and VEGF receptors in diabetic nephropathy: expression studies in biopsies of type 2 diabetic patients. *Ren Fail* 2001;23:483–493.
133. Hovind P, Tarnow L, Oestergaard PB, et al. Elevated vascular endothelial growth factor in type 1 diabetic patients with diabetic nephropathy. *Kidney Int* 2000;57[Suppl 75]:S56–S61.
134. de Vriese AS, Tilton RG, Elger M, et al. Antibodies against VEGF improve early renal dysfunction in experimental diabetes. *J Am Soc Nephrol* 2001;12: 993–1000.
135. Flyvbjerg A, Dagnaes-Hansen F, De Vriese AS. Amelioration of long-term renal changes in obese type 2 diabetic mice by a neutralizing VEGF antibody. *Diabetes* 2002;51:3090–3094.
136. Hood JD, Meininger CJ, Ziche M, et al. VEGF upregulates ecNOS message, protein, and NO production in human endothelial cells. *Am J Physiol* 1998; 274(3 Pt 2):H1054–H1058.
137. Chen J, Braet F, Brodsky S, et al. VEGF-induced mobilization of caveolae and increase in permeability of endothelial cells. *Am J Physiol Cell Physiol* 2002; 282:C1053–01063.
138. Dzau VJ, Ingelfinger JR. Molecular biology and pathophysiology of the intrarenal renin-angiotensin system. *J Hypertens* 1989;7[Suppl 7] :S3-S8.
139. Anderson S, Jung FF, Ingelfinger JR. Renal renin-angiotensin system in diabetes: functional, immunochemical and biological correlations. *Am J Physiol* 1993;265:F477–F486.
140. Chansel D, Czekalski S, Pham P, et al. Characterization of angiotensin II receptor subtypes in human glomeruli and mesangial cells. *Am J Physiol* 1992; 262:F432-F441.
141. Wolf G, Ziladeh FN. The role of angiotensin II in diabetic nephropathy: emphasis on non-hemodynamic mechanisms. *Am J Kidney Dis* 197;29:153–163.
142. Kagami SK, Border WA, Miller DE, et al. Angiotensin II stimulates extracellular matrix protein synthesis through induction of TGF-β expression in rat glomerular mesangial cells. *J Clin Invest* 1994;93:2431–2437.
143. Leehey DJ, Singh AK, Alavi N, et al. Role of angiotensin II in diabetic nephropathy. *Kidney Int Suppl* 2000;77:593-S98.
144. Ding G, Reddy K, Kapasi AA. Angiotensin II induces apoptosis in rat glomerular epithelial cells. *Am J Physiol Renal Physiol* 2002;283(1):F173–F180.
145. Abbate M, Zoja C, Morigi M. TGF-β1 is up-regulated by podocytes in response to excess intraglomerular passage of proteins: a central pathway in progressive glomerulosclerosis. *Am J Pathol* 2002;161:2179–2193.
146. Pagtalunan ME, Miller PL, Jumping-Eagle S. Podocyte loss and progressive glomerular injury in type II diabetes. *J Clin Invest* 1997;99:342–348.
147. Bohrer MP, Deen WM, Robertson CR, et al. Mechanism of angiotensin II-induced proteinuria in the rat. *Am J Physiol* 1977;233:F13–F21.
148. Lapinski R, Perico N, Remuzzi A, et al. Angiotensin II modulates glomerular capillary permselectivity in rat isolated perfused kidney. *J Am Soc Nephrol* 1996;7:653–660.
149. Doublier S, Salvidio G, Lupia E. Nephrin expression is reduced in human diabetic nephropathy: evidence for a distinct role for glycated albumin and angiotensin II. *Diabetes* 2003;52:1023–1030.
150. Bonnet F, Cooper ME, Kawachi H, et al. Irbesartan normalises the deficiency in glomerular nephrin expression in a model of diabetes and hypertension. *Diabetologia* 2001;44:874–877.
151. Hofmann MA, Schiekofer S, Isermann B. Peripheral blood mononuclear cells isolated from patients with diabetic nephropathy show increased activation of the oxidative-stress sensitive transcription factor NF-kB. *Diabetologia* 1999;42:222–232.
152. Morcos M, Sayed AA, Bierhaus A. Activation of tubular epithelial cells in diabetic nephropathy. *Diabetes* 2002;51:3532–3544.
153. Pieper G, Riaz-ul-Haq J. Activation of NFκB in cultured endothelial cells by increased glucose concentration: prevention by calphostin C. *Cardiovasc Pharm* 1997;30:528–532.
154. Lal MA, Brismar H, Eklof AC, et al. Role of oxidative stress in advanced glycation end product-induced mesangial cell activation. *Kidney Int* 2002;61: 2006–2014.
155. Ha H, Yu MR, Choi YJ, et al. Role of high glucose-induced nuclear factor-kappaB activation in monocyte chemoattractant protein-1 expression by mesangial cells. *J Am Soc Nephrol* 2002;13:894–902.
156. Gruden G, Setti G, Hayward A, et al. Rosiglitazone prevents stretch-induced monocyte recruitment by inhibiting the NFkB-MCP-1 pathway in human mesangial cells. *Diabetologia* 2003;46[Suppl 2]:A344(abst).
157. Okado T, Terada Y, Tanaka H, et al. Smad7 mediates transforming growth factor-beta-induced apoptosis in mesangial cells. *Kidney Int* 2002;62:1178–1186.
158. Nagaragan RP, Chen F, Li W, et al. Repression of TGF-β1-mediated transcription by nuclear factor κ. *Biochem J* 2000;348:591–596.
159. Ingram AJ, Scholey JW. Protooncogene expression and diabetic kidney injury. *Kidney Int* 1997;52[Suppl 60]:S70-S76.
160. Kim SI, Angel P, Lavatis R, et al. Autoinduction of TGF-β 1 is mediated by the AP-1 complex. *Mol Cell Biol* 1990;10:1492–1497.
161. Dean DC, McQuillian JJ, Weintraub S. Serum stimulation of fibronectin gene expression appears to result from rapid serum-binding of nuclear proteins to a cAMP response element. *J Biol Chem* 1990;265:3522–3527.
162. Shankland SJ, Scholey JW. Expression of growth related protooncogenes during renal hypertrophy. *Kidney Int* 1995;47:782–788.
163. Kreisberg JI, Radnik RA, Ayo SH, et al. High glucose elevates c-fos and c-jun transcripts and proteins in mesangial cell cultures. *Kidney Int* 1994;46:105–112.
164. Harris RC, Akai Y, Yasuda T, et al. The role of physical forces in alterations of mesangial cell function. *Kidney Int* 1994;45[Suppl 45]:S17-S20.
165. Kreisberg JI, Kreisberg SH. High glucose activates PKC and stimulates fibronectin gene expression by enhancing a cAMP responsive element. *Kidney Int* 1995;48[Suppl 48]:S3–511.
166. Nishizuka Y. Intracellular signalling by hydrolysis of phospholipids and activation of PKC. *Science* 1992;258:607–614.
167. King GL, Ishii H, Koya D. Diabetic vascular dysfunction: a model of excessive activation of protein kinase C. *Kidney Int* 1997;52[Suppl 60]:S77-S85.
168. Messina JL, Standaert ML, Ishizuka T, et al. Role of PKC in insulin's regulation of c-fos transcription. *J Biol Chem* 1992;267:9223–9228.
169. Zhang J, Wang L, Petrin J, et al. Characterization of site-specific mutants altered at protein kinase C β1 isoenzyme autophosphorylation sites. *Proc Natl Acad Sci U S A* 1993;90:6130–6134.
170. Craven PA, DeRubertis FR. Protein kinase C is activated in glomeruli from streptozotocin diabetic rats. *J Clin Invest* 1989;83:1667–1675.
171. Craven PA, Davidson CM, DeRubertis FR. Increase in diacylglycerol mass in isolated glomeruli by high glucose from *de novo* synthesis of glycerolipids. *Diabetes* 1990;39:667–674.
172. Ayo SH, Radnik R, Garoni JA, et al. High glucose increases diacylglycerol mass and activates protein kinase C in mesangial cell cultures. *Am J Physiol* 1991;261:F571-F577.
173. Xia P, Inoguchi T, Kern TS, et al. Characterisation of the mechanism for the chronic activation of diacylglycerol-protein kinase C pathway in diabetes and hypergalactosemia. *Diabetes* 1994;43:1122–1129.
174. Koya D, King GL. Protein kinase C activation and the development of diabetic complications. *Diabetes* 1998;47:859–866.
175. Gruden G, Thomas S, Burt D, et al. Mechanical stretch induces vascular permeability factor in human mesangial cells: mechanisms of signal transduction. *Proc Natl Acad Sci U SA* 1997;94:12112–12116.
176. Weiss RH, Ramirez A. TGF-beta- and angiotensin-II-induced mesangial matrix protein secretion is mediated by protein kinase C. *Nephrol Dial Transplant* 1998; 13:2804–2813.
177. Homma T, Akai Y, Burns KD, et al. Activation of S6 kinase by repeated cycles of stretching and relaxation in rat glomerular mesangial cells. Evidence for involvement of protein kinase C. *J Biol Chem* 1992;267:23129–23135.
178. Studer RK, Craven PA, DeRubertis FR. Role for protein kinase C in the mediation of increased fibronectin accumulation by mesangial cells grown in high-glucose medium. *Diabetes* 1993;42:118–126.
179. Koya D, Jirousek MR, Lin YW, et al. Characterisation of protein kinase C beta isoform activation on the gene expression of transforming growth factor-beta, extracellular matrix components, and prostanoids in the glomeruli of diabetic rats. *J Clin Invest* 1997;100:115–126.
180. Ishii H, Jirousek MR, Koja D, et al. Amelioration of vascular dysfunction in diabetic rats by an oral PKCβ_2 inhibitor. *Science* 1996;222:728–731.
181. Koya D, Haneda M, Nakagawa H, et al. Amelioration of accelerated diabetic mesangial expansion by treatment with PKC-β inhibitor in diabetic db/db mice, a rodent model for type 2 diabetes. *FASEB J* 2000;14:439–447.
182. Osicka TM, Yu Y, Panagiotopoulos S, et al. Prevention of albuminuria by aminoguanidine or ramipril in streptozotocin-induced diabetic rats is associated with the normalization of glomerular protein kinase C. *Diabetes* 2000; 49:87–93.
183. Seger R, Krebs EG. The MAPK signalling cascade. *FASEB J* 1995;9:726–798.
184. Haneda M, Araki S, Togawa M. Mitogen-activated protein kinase cascade is activated in glomeruli of diabetic rats and glomerular mesangial cells cultured under high glucose conditions. *Diabetes* 1997;46:847–853.
185. Dunlop ME, Muggli EE. Small heat shock protein alteration provides a mechanism to reduce mesangial cell contractility in diabetes and oxidative stress. *Kidney Int* 2000;57:464–475.
186. Kang MJ, Wu X, Ly H, et al. Effect of glucose on stress-activated protein kinase activity in mesangial cells and diabetic glomeruli. *Kidney Int* 1999;55:2203–2214.
187. Ingram AJ, Ly H, Thai K, et al. Activation of mesangial cell signaling cascades in response to mechanical stretch. *Kidney Int* 1999;55:476–485.
188. Ishida T, Haneda M, Koya D, et al. Stretch-induced overproduction of fibronectin in mesangial cells is mediated by the activation of mitogen-activated protein kinase. *Diabetes* 1999;48:595–602.
189. Igarashi M, Wakasaki H, Takahara N, et al. Glucose or diabetes activates p38 mitogenactivated protein kinase via differential pathways *J Clin Invest* 1999;103:185–195.

190. Vasan S, Zhang X. An agent cleaving glucose-derived protein cross-linking *in vitro* and *in vivo*. *Nature* 1996;382:275–278.
191. Forbes JM, Soulis T, Thallas V, et al. Renoprotective effects of a novel inhibitor of advanced glycation. *Diabetologia* 2001;44:108–114.
192. Border WA, Noble NA. TGF-β1 in kidney fibrosis: a target for gene therapy. *Kidney Int* 1997;51:1388–1396.
193. Border WA, Noble NA. Evidence that TGF-β1 should be a therapeutic target in diabetic nephropathy. *Kidney Int* 1998;54:1390–1391.
194. Way KJ, Chou E, King GL. Identification of PKC isoform specific biological actions using pharmacological approaches. *Trends Pharmacol Sci* 2000;21: 181–187.
195. Isaka Y, Akagi Y, Ando Y, et al. Gene therapy by TGF-β receptor IgG Fc chimera suppressed extracellular matrix accumulation in experimental glomerulonephritis. *Kidney Int* 1999;55:465–475.

CHAPTER 52

Pathogenesis of Cardiovascular Disease in Diabetes

Edward P. Feener and Victor J. Dzau

Diabetes mellitus is a major independent risk factor for cardiovascular disease (CVD) (1). The increased prevalence of CVD in diabetes has been attributed in large part to the acceleration of coronary atherosclerosis, which occurs at an earlier age and advances more rapidly to clinical cardiovascular events in individuals with diabetes than in those without diabetes (2,3). Patients with diabetes are also prone to arterial thrombosis due to persistently activated thrombogenic pathways and impaired fibrinolysis (4–7). This combination of increased arterial disease and prothrombotic milieu in diabetes is a major underlying cause of acute ischemic coronary heart disease (CHD). Moreover, CHD in diabetes is often diffuse, with an increase in the number of affected vessels and in the incidence of moderate stenosis (3,8). Detection of narrowing of the coronary lumen in patients with diabetes is often impaired by autonomic neuropathy (9,10), which can reduce the symptoms of ischemic CHD, delay its detection, and worsen the prognosis. In addition, diabetic individuals are faced with increased restenosis and mortality rates following revascularization procedures, especially for percutaneous transluminal coronary angioplasty (PTCA) (11). The impact of CHD on myocardial function in diabetes is exacerbated by diabetic cardiomyopathies (12,13), which can impair cardiac contractile function and may accelerate heart failure. Multivariate analyses of a number of large prospective studies with follow-up of 12 to 20 years, including the Framingham Study, the Multiple Risk Factor Intervention Trial, and the Nurses' Health Study, have demonstrated that diabetes is associated with two- to fivefold increases in CHD- and cardiovascular-related death (14–16). This CVD accounts for the majority of premature mortality associated with both type 1 and type 2 diabetes worldwide (17). A combination of factors related to hyperglycemia, hypertension, insulin resistance, dyslipidemia, hypercoagulability, and inflammation contributes to the etiology of CVD associated with diabetes.

HISTOLOGIC CLASSIFICATION OF ATHEROSCLEROSIS

Atherosclerosis is a progressive disease of the arterial wall involving components of inflammation, vascular lipid deposition and remodeling, fibrosis, and thrombosis. The American Heart Association has outlined a histologic classification of atherosclerotic lesions (Table 52.1) (18,19). Initial atherosclerotic lesions and fatty streaks represent the appearance of scattered lipid deposits in the intima associated with increases in macrophages and macrophage foam cells. Although these early lesions are not clinically significant and may regress (20), they also can provide precursors for the formation of advanced complex plaques. Intermediate lesions and atheroma involve increased focal accumulation of lipid within the neointima due to increased levels of foam cells, of both macrophage and vascular smooth muscle cell (VSMC) origin, and the appearance of extracellular lipid droplets, leading to the formation of a lipid-rich plaque core. These intermediate lesions appear to arise from either fatty streaks or preexisting intimal cell masses (21). Fibrous plaques are formed as a cap of connective tissue, mainly involving VSMC in a collagen and proteoglycan matrix, and accumulate between the lipid core and vessel lumen. Thickness of the fibrous cap and its infiltration with macrophages affect the stability of these lesions, such that plaques with thin fibrous caps and those with increased levels of macrophages appear prone to rupture (3,22). Fibrotic lesions also can develop in plaques that do not display a well-defined lipid core. Complicated lesions occur when the plaque becomes disrupted owing to fissure, hemorrhage, or thrombus formation. Recent proposed modifications of this classification have emphasized that fibrous plaques or pathologic intimal thickenings can lead to significant stenosis without thrombi and that luminal thrombosis often occurs in vessels with a less than 50% reduction in diameter (23). Moreover, atherogenesis does not necessarily progress in a uniform manner, but lesion histology instead involves a mosaic of accumulations of lipid, fibrous material, and cellular mass.

Recent analyses of coronary tissue from autopsy studies have indicated that the main causes of coronary sudden death are plaque rupture or erosion, followed by thrombosis and stenosis (23). Plaque rupture is evidenced by contact between the thrombus and the necrotic atheromatous core. Plaque erosion is indicated when the thrombus occurs on a fibrous cap that has lost its luminal endothelium but retains a continuous connective tissue covering the necrotic core. Disruption of the endothelium and fibrous cap can expose the blood to the plaque

TABLE 52.1. Histologic Classification of Atherosclerosis

Lesion classification		Characteristics	Effects of diabetes
Type I	Initial lesions	Atherogenic lipoprotein Increased macrophages Scattered macrophage foam cells	• Impaired endothelial-dependent vasorelaxation
Type II	Fatty streaks	Layers of macrophage foam cells Lipid-laden smooth muscle cells	• Increased monocyte-endothelial cell adherence and infiltration
Type III	Intermediate stage	Scattered extracellular lipid droplets	• Increased production of reactive oxygen species
Type IV	Atheroma	Dense lipid core	• Increased LDL oxidation and glycation
Type V	Fibrous plaque	Fibrous connective tissue Type Va: Fibroatheroma Type Vb: Calcified Type Vc: Lipid core absent or minimal	• Increased LDL uptake by macrophages and SMC foam cells
Type VI	Complicated lesion	Type VIa: Surface disruption (fissure) Type VIb: Hematoma or hemorrhage Type VIc: Thrombosis	• Increased triglycerides • Decreased HDL • Increased small dense LDL • Increased VSMC proliferation • Increased ECM production, glycation, and turnover • Increased calcification • Increased macrophages and alterations in ECM protease and protease inhibitors • Increased levels of acute-phase proteins (CRP and fibrinogen) • Activated thrombogenic pathways and impaired fibrinolysis

LDL, low-density lipoprotein; HDL, high-density lipoprotein; SMC, smooth muscle cells; VSMC, vascular smooth muscle cells; ECM, extracellular matrix; CRP, C-reactive protein.

core rich in tissue factor (24,25), which can trigger the extrinsic coagulation pathway. Moreover, fibrin-rich thrombi may be stabilized by plasminogen activator inhibitor-1 (PAI-1), either circulating or locally released from neointimal smooth muscle cells (SMC) (26,27). Although thrombosis is observed in the majority of cases of coronary sudden death, approximately 20% of these coronary events occur by luminal narrowing without intramural thrombosis (23). Multiple mechanisms lead to narrowing of the coronary lumen, including the progressive expansion of the lesion mass due to lipid accumulation, fibrosis, and neointimal SMC growth; intraplaque hemorrhage; healed plaque erosions and thrombi; and contracture caused by SMC constriction and vascular wound healing (28,29).

CHARACTERISTICS OF CORONARY ATHEROSCLEROTIC LESIONS IN DIABETES

Histopathologic comparison of coronary atherectomy specimens from nondiabetic and diabetic subjects has revealed an increase in the percentage of the total area occupied by lipid-rich atheromatous tissue from 2% ± 1% to 7% ± 2% ($p = 0.01$) and an increase in the incidence of coronary thrombus from 40% to 62% ($p = 0.04$) for nondiabetics and diabetics, respectively (3). Coronary artery atherectomy specimens from subjects with type 2 diabetes have a twofold increase in PAI-1 antigen and a decrease in the level of immunoreactive urokinase plasminogen activator, compared with specimens from age- and gender-matched controls without diabetes (30). Macrophage infiltration was also elevated by nearly twofold ($p = 0.003$) in atherectomy specimens from diabetic subjects (3). In contrast, morphometric analysis of coronary atherectomy specimens from primary lesions has indicated that the relative amounts of collagen-rich and hypercellular plaque components, which comprised approximately 90% of the total lesion area, were similar in diabetic and nondiabetic subjects (3,30). However, given the nature of tissue isolation by directional coronary atherectomy, the cellularity of these specimens in these studies may not represent possible effects of diabetes on SMC hyperplasia at the base or peripheral areas of the stenotic lesions.

Coronary artery calcification in diabetic subjects appears either similar (31) or increased (32,33), compared with that in nondiabetic control subjects. Although plaque calcification can provide a marker of plaque burden and is predictive of future coronary events (34,35), the effects of calcification on the pathophysiology of atherosclerotic lesions are not fully understood. Calcium deposition does not appear to adversely affect plaque mechanical stability (36); however, arterial calcification can increase stiffening, resulting in reduced vascular compliance.

EFFECTS OF DIABETES ON THE PATHOGENESIS OF ATHEROSCLEROSIS

Combinations of pathophysiologic processes contribute to the development of atherosclerosis and its sequel of stenosis and coronary sudden death. As described above, atherosclerotic lesions can arise from fatty streaks or neointimal thickenings. These lesions can expand progressively to reduce luminal diameter and can undergo rupture or erosion, which can trigger thrombosis (23). The atherogenic effects of diabetes and insulin resistance appear to be initiated by a combination of metabolic abnormalities related to hyperglycemia, impaired insulin action or insulin deficiency, a proatherogenic dyslipidemia, and confounding factors such as hypertension and obesity (Fig. 52.1). In addition, vasoactive hormones, cytokines, and growth factors, including angiotensin II (ATII), tumor necrosis factor-α (TNF-α), and vascular endothelial growth factor (VEGF) amplify and in part mediate the adverse vascular effects of these metabolic abnormalities. These metabolic and hormonal imbalances can induce endothelium dysfunction, vascular inflammation, SMC growth, intimal lipid accumulation, fibrosis, and hypercoagulability, leading to atherosclerosis and thrombosis (Fig. 52.1). The effects of diabetes and insulin resistance on a number of these proatherogenic pathways are described further on.

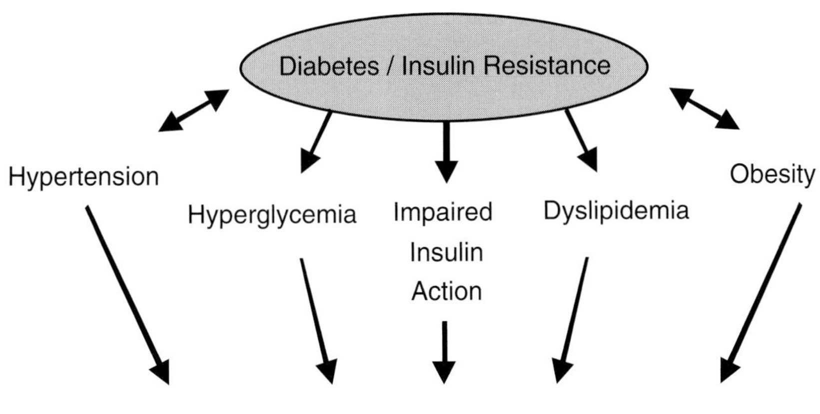

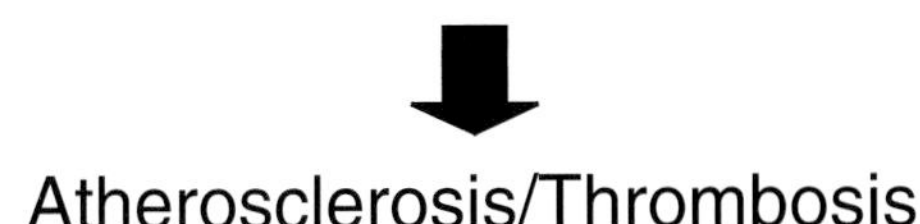

Figure 52.1. Diabetes, insulin resistance, and cardiovascular disease. Diabetes and insulin resistance are associated with a combination of metabolic abnormalities such as hyperglycemia, insulin resistance, insulin deficiency, hyperinsulinemia, hypertriglyceridemia, and reduced high-density lipoprotein that contribute to vascular dysfunctions, atherosclerosis, and thrombosis. In addition, diabetes and insulin resistance often coexist with additional cardiovascular risk factors, including hypertension and obesity, as the insulin resistance syndrome. SMC, smooth muscle cells.

Endothelial-Leukocyte Adhesion

Initial lesions and fatty streaks, also described as intimal xanthoma (23), are characterized by the appearance of macrophage foam cells in the subendothelial area. These foam cells arise from circulating monocytes that have adhered and infiltrated into the vessel wall, differentiated into macrophages, and become lipid laden via the avid uptake of modified low-density lipoprotein (LDL). Diabetes and insulin resistance promote leukocyte infiltration into the arterial wall via several mechanisms. Diabetes and hyperglycemia increase expression of E-selectin, vascular cell adhesion molecule-1 (VCAM-1), and intercellular adhesion molecule-1 (ICAM-1) by endothelial cells (37–39), which bind to leukocyte glycoprotein counterreceptors and integrins, thereby mediating leukocyte tethering, rolling, and firm adhesion (Fig. 52.2). In addition, leukocytes isolated from diabetic subjects display increased adhesiveness to endothelial cells (40,41). Following endothelial-leukocyte adhesion, infiltration of leukocytes to the subendothelial interstitium is stimulated by monocyte chemoattractant protein-1 (MCP-1), which is upregulated in diabetes (42). The infiltrated monocytes differentiate into macrophages, which produce a number of proatherogenic effects by accumulating lipids (43,44) and releasing proinflammatory cytokines and matrix metalloproteinases (45–47). The elaboration of cytokines, growth factors, metalloproteases, and procoagulants from these macrophages likely promotes plaque expansion and generates plaques prone to rupture and thrombosis.

Formation of Lipid-Rich Lesions

Monocyte-derived macrophages endocytose modified LDL via multiple receptors, including both class A and class B scavenger

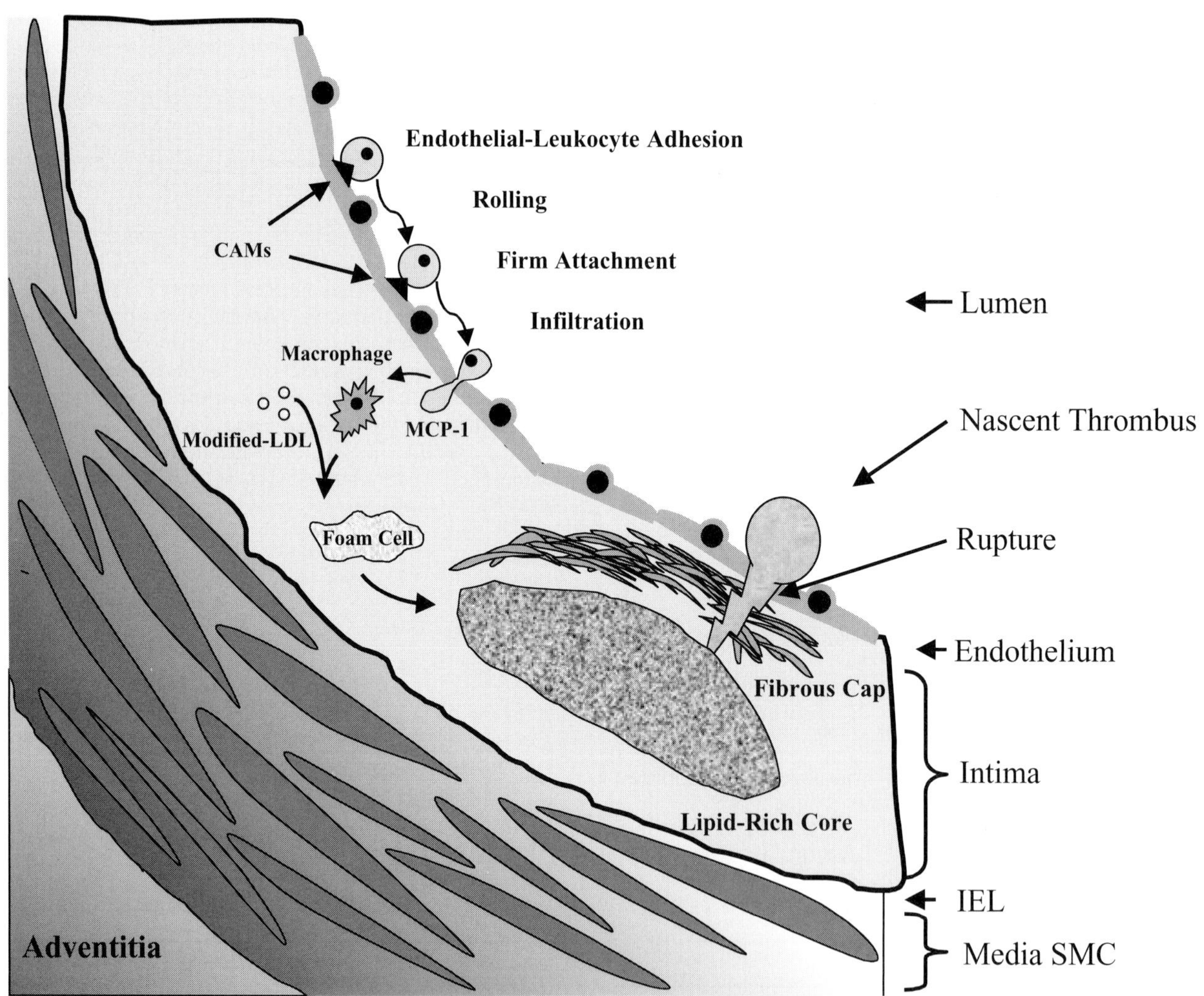

Figure 52.2. Components contributing to the development of fibrous-cap atheroma. Leukocyte binding to endothelial cell adhesion molecules (CAMs) and chemoattraction by monocyte chemoattractant protein-1 (MCP-1) increase the infiltration of monocytes into the subendothelial intima. These monocytes differentiate into macrophages, which release proinflammatory cytokines and endocytose modified low-density lipoprotein to generate foam cells. Focal accumulation of intimal lipid in the form of increased foam cells and extracellular lipid deposits results in the formation of a lipid-rich plaque core, which can become necrotic. Plaques also accumulate fibrotic material consisting of a collagen-proteoglycan matrix and smooth muscle cells (SMC) that have migrated across the internal elastic lamina (IEL). Rupture of this fibrous cap over the lipid core exposes this atheromatous material rich in tissue factor to circulating factors VII and VIIa, which initiates thrombogenic cascades and the formation of a thrombus.

receptors (43,44), lectin-like oxidized LDL receptor-1 (48), and lipoprotein lipase (49). Uptake of lipid in excess of its metabolism results in the formation of macrophage foam cells laden in cholesterol esters. In addition, foam cells can develop similarly from VSMC by the uptake of oxidized LDL via class A and class B scavenger receptors (50,51). Diabetes exacerbates the uptake of modified LDL by foam cells via several mechanisms. First, hyperglycemia increases glucoxidation, resulting in increased levels of oxidized and glycated LDL (52,53), which increase ligand availability for scavenger receptors and lipoprotein lipase. Second, diabetes increases the expression of macrophage class B scavenger receptor CD36 (54), which enhances oxidized LDL endocytosis. Third, diabetes causes a proatherogenic dyslipidemia resulting in reduced high-density lipoprotein (HDL) levels and increased triglycerides, which can reduce reverse cholesterol transport and contribute to increased levels of small dense LDL particles (55). In addition, macrophage foam cells release proinflammatory cytokines, such as TNF-α and interleukin-1, which can induce apoptosis of endothelial cells and VSMC (56). Focal accumulation of foam cells, formation of extracellular lipid droplets, apoptosis of VSMC, and disruption of vascular smooth muscle architecture can result in the formation of a necrotic lipid-rich core (Fig. 52.2).

Fibrous-Cap Formation

Atherosclerotic lesions accumulate fibrous material consisting mainly of VSMC in a collagen-proteoglycan matrix. The fibrous material that separates the plaque core from the luminal surface of the vessel is termed the fibrous cap (Fig. 52.2). Because the atheromatous material is thrombogenic in part attributable to high levels of tissue factor (24,25), the fibrous cap provides a barrier to thrombosis by separating this pool of tissue factor from the blood. The specific effects of diabetes on the composition and stability of the fibrous cap in primary lesions have not yet been described. Diabetes can increase SMC proliferation and extracellular matrix (ECM) production in a porcine atherosclerosis model (57) and increases neointimal hyperplasia and the accumulation of collagen-rich sclerotic tissue in restenotic lesions (58,59). Although these findings suggest that diabetes can promote the accumulation of fibrous material in restenotic lesions, it is unclear whether these findings can be extrapolated to characteristics of the fibrous cap. Several of the effects of diabetes on plaque composition may influence fibrous-cap formation and stability. Increased matrix metalloproteinase activity and macrophage levels in diabetic lesions (60) may shift the proteolytic balance within the cap, leading to the degradation of ECM and weakening of its structural integrity (61), thus increasing susceptibility to rupture or erosion. As described previously, PAI-1 levels are also increased in atherectomy specimens in diabetes. Elevated levels of PAI-1 can reduce SMC migration (62) and thereby might decrease incorporation of SMC into the fibrous cap. Alternatively, increased PAI-1 within lesions also may reduce plasmin-stimulated ECM turnover and thereby promote fibrosis (63). These effects of PAI-1 may lead to the generation of fibrous material with reduced cellularity and increased ECM.

Atherothrombosis

Thrombosis is the major cause of coronary stenosis and sudden death (23). Intramural arterial thrombosis can be triggered by the disruption of complex plaques, which expose the blood to thrombogenic factors that are enriched in the subendothelial area. Tissue factor, the major activator of the extrinsic coagulation pathway, is highly expressed in the plaque core (24,25). Disruption of the plaque surface allows this tissue factor to bind circulating factor VII in blood, resulting in the generation of active VIIa and the formation of tissue factor–VIIa complexes. This complex leads to a cascade involving activation of factor X, formation of prothrombinase complex, generation of thrombin, and cleavage of fibrinogen to fibrin. Elevated levels of tissue factor in vascular tissues in diabetic and obese/insulin-resistant murine models (64,65) may predispose diabetic arteries to the activation of this coagulation cascade. Moreover, increased arterial expression of PAI-1 in diabetes may impair the dissolution of nascent thrombi (30,66). Fibrin-rich thrombi that develop on ruptured plaques can expand to cause occlusion, can spontaneously undergo dissolution, or may become lined with endothelium and incorporated as an expansion of the neointima (28). Although atherosclerotic lesions in diabetes can have attributes (increased PAI-1 and macrophages) that would be expected to promote thrombosis, the direct effects of diabetes on atherothrombosis have not yet been established. A recent report, however, has provided evidence for an increase in healed ruptures in coronary sudden death in diabetes (glucose intolerance) (28), suggesting that diabetes is associated with an increased occurrence of ruptures that contribute to subclinical plaque burden.

Restenosis following Revascularization

The Bypass Angioplasty Revascularization Investigation (BARI) demonstrated that patients with treated diabetes who underwent PTCA or coronary artery bypass graft surgery (CABG) had cardiac-related mortality rates of 20.6% or 5.8%, respectively, after an average follow-up of 5.4 years (67). In contrast, the cardiac mortality rates for other BARI patients receiving PTCA and CABG were 4.8% and 4.7%, respectively. At 7 years of follow-up of BARI patients, the survival of the group with treated diabetes was 76.4% for CABG and 55.7% for PTCA ($p = 0.0011$) compared with survival rates of 86.4% (CABG) and 86.8% (PTCA) for patients without diabetes (11). The basis for the 3.5-fold higher mortality rates for diabetic patients receiving PTCA compared with their nondiabetic counterparts is not fully understood. Serial intravascular ultrasound has indicated that increased restenosis following coronary interventions in diabetes is due to intimal expansion (58). Analysis of coronary atherectomy specimens from restenotic lesions after PTCA revealed that the fraction of collagen-rich sclerotic tissue was increased in lesions from patients with diabetes (59). These results suggest that diabetes increases neointimal fibrosis of arterial lesions resultant from PTCA. Diabetes has also been shown to increase the incidence of restenosis following arterial stenting and saphenous vein graft bypass (68–70).

Animal models have been utilized to examine the effect of diabetes on the neointimal response to balloon catheterization. Balloon catheter–induced injury causes endothelial denudation and arterial stretch, resulting in the formation of a neointima from the proliferative expansion of VSMC, which have migrated across the internal elastic lamina from the vessel media. Streptozotocin (STZ)–induced diabetes in rats has been shown to reduce carotid artery neointimal formation by approximately 50% compared with that in nondiabetic and insulin-treated diabetic controls in this balloon-injury model (71,72). Similarly, alloxan-induced diabetes reduced balloon catheter–induced neointimal formation in rabbits (73). STZ-induced diabetes did not affect the neointimal thickening in response to coronary stent placement in Yucatan miniature swine (74). However, diabetes was associated with increased in-stent thrombosis resulting in sudden death in this porcine model (74). These findings indicate that hyperglycemia caused by STZ-induced diabetes does not increase neointimal hyperplasia but may increase thrombosis in injured vessels. The effects of insulin resistance and type 2 diabetes on the balloon injury–induced neointimal response have been examined in rat obesity models. These studies reveal that neointimal hyperplasia was increased in the type 2 diabetic/insulin-resistant obese Zucker rats and Otsuka Long-Evans Tokushima fatty rats compared with their lean insulin-sensitive controls (72,75,76).

The interpretation of these animal studies is beset with a number of limitations. First, balloon injuries were performed on vessels with little or no preexisting vascular disease. This contrasts with clinical situations, in which revascularization is performed on restenotic vessels with advanced plaque pathologies. Second, most studies that have examined the effect of diabetes on atherosclerosis and neointimal hyperplasia in animal models have utilized the islet β-cell cytotoxins, including STZ or alloxan, to reduce insulin production. Although this approach is effective in generating hyperglycemia resulting from insulin deficiency, these models do not replicate the etiology of type 1 diabetes mediated via autoimmune destruction of β-cells. Third, rat models with obesity-induced insulin resistance have multiple endocrine abnormalities, which may contribute to the exaggerated neointimal response. Although the effects of diabetes on vascular proliferation are not fully understood, neointimal smooth muscle proliferation represents a major component of atherogenesis and an important target for emerging therapeutic strategies (77).

ENDOTHELIAL DYSFUNCTIONS IN DIABETES

The endothelium plays an integral role in vascular structure, hemodynamics, and hemostasis. Diabetes has a number of adverse effects on the vascular endothelium that impair these functions and likely facilitate atherosclerosis and thrombosis. As described above, diabetes increases the expression of leukocyte adhesion molecules that mediate binding and the infiltration of monocytes into the arterial subendothelial space. In addition, diabetes impairs endothelial barrier function, which increases transendothelial permeability and access of circulating molecules to the vascular interstitium. Diabetes also alters endothelial cell synthesis of a host of vasoactive hormones and factors that affect vascular tone, hemodynamics, coagulation, and VSMC physiology. The effects of diabetes on several key endothelial functions are described below.

Permeability of Endothelial Tight Junctions

Increased endothelial permeability is a hallmark of vascular dysfunction in diabetes (78,79). This increased permeability may facilitate penetration of proatherogenic cytokines and lipoproteins into the subendothelial space. Several mechanisms have been postulated to explain the increased transport of molecules across the endothelium in diabetes, including enhanced pinocytosis (78) and increased intercellular diffusion caused by reduced tight-junction formation (80). Diabetes can impair endothelium barrier function via the increased production of VEGF (also called vascular permeability factor) by VSMC. In this pathway, hyperglycemia and hormones, such as ATII, increase synthesis and secretion of VEGF in arterial SMC (81,82). This VEGF can act in a paracrine manner on endothelial cells, where it binds kinase insert domain-containing receptors VEGF-R2 (KDR) and stimulates phosphorylation of tight-junction proteins, such as zonula occluden 1 (83). However, although increased VEGF levels in diabetes have been shown in certain tissues, such as the retina (84), less is known regarding the effects of diabetes on VEGF expression in cardiovascular tissues. In addition, hyperglycemia can exert additional effects on the endothelium via the activation of protein kinase C (PKC) and the increased formation of advanced glycation end-products (AGEs) and reactive oxygen species, which can act directly on endothelial cells to induce hyperpermeability (79,85).

Endothelium-Dependent Vasorelaxation

The vascular endothelium releases several factors that induce vascular smooth muscle relaxation, including nitric oxide (86), prostacyclin I_2, and one or more endothelium-derived hyperpolarizing factors (87). Of these factors, impaired endothelium-dependent vasorelaxation in diabetes has been attributed primarily to the reduced bioavailability of nitric oxide. Nitric oxide production by endothelial nitric oxide synthase (eNOS) is increased in response to shear stress and potent vasodilator hormones such as acetylcholine and bradykinin (86,88) (Fig. 52.3). Nitric oxide emanating from the endothelium acts in a paracrine manner on the vascular smooth muscle, where it binds to soluble guanylyl cyclase and thereby increases the synthesis of cyclic guanosine monophosphate (cGMP) (Fig. 52.3). Elevated cGMP levels activate cGMP-dependent protein kinases, including cGMP kinase I, which play an important role in regulating cytosolic calcium homeostasis. cGMP kinase I phosphorylates the microsomal inositol 1,4,5-trisphosphate (IP_3) receptor complex (89) and thereby inhibits IP_3-stimulated calcium release from intracellular stores, resulting in SMC relaxation.

Reduced vasodilation response to infused acetylcholine (or methacholine, a long-acting muscarinic receptor agonist) and reactive hyperemia have been demonstrated in both type 1 and type 2 diabetes (90–93). Acute hyperglycemia, induced by hyperglycemic clamp, maintained at 300 mg/dL glucose levels for 6 hours, impairs methacholine-induced vasorelaxation in healthy nondiabetic subjects (94). However, although an acute increase in glucose can impair endothelial function, it is unclear whether the mechanism responsible for this effect of acute hyperglycemia is related to the chronic effects of hyperglycemia associated with diabetes. Impaired endothelium-dependent relaxation also occurs in insulin-resistant patients in the absence of overt type 2 diabetes (90,95). Thus, endothelial dysfunction in type 2 diabetes may reflect the combined adverse effects of hyperglycemia and additional metabolic and hormonal abnormalities associated with insulin resistance, such as an increase in free fatty acids and reduced insulin action (96,97). Results from studies of a variety of experimental animal models of type 1 diabetes have demonstrated that reduced endothelium-dependent relaxation occurs in *ex vivo* preparations of coronary, mesenteric, and carotid arteries and aorta (98–101), indicating that this dysfunction is retained in isolated vessels. Because most reports have shown a normal vasodilator response to nitric oxide donors such as sodium nitroprusside (91,102,103), the impairment of vasodilation in diabetes appears to be due mainly to an impairment in endothelium-derived nitric oxide. However, some reports have shown that vasodilator response to nitric oxide donors is also impaired in diabetes and insulin resistance (90,104), suggesting that in certain situations impaired endothelium-dependent vasorelaxation may be superimposed on impaired endothelium-independent relaxation. The mechanism or mechanisms responsible for this resistance to vasorelaxation by nitric oxide donors have not yet been defined. Potential mechanisms could be related to chronic vasoconstriction or oxidant production caused by endothelin-1 or ATII (105–107).

Reductions in both nitric oxide synthesis and stability have been proposed to explain impaired endothelium-dependent

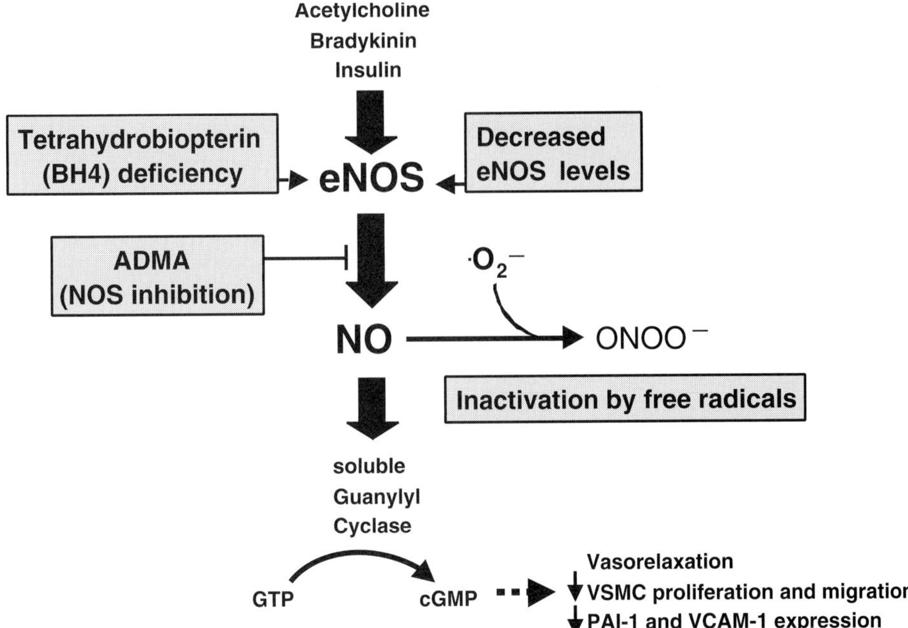

Figure 52.3. Mechanisms responsible for reduced nitric oxide (NO) bioactivity in diabetes. Mechanisms that contribute to reduced NO production include reduced endothelial nitric oxide synthase (eNOS) expression, tetrahydrobiopterin deficiency, and competitive inhibition of eNOS catalytic activity by elevated endogenous asymmetric dimethylarginine (ADMA). In addition, bioactivity of NO can also be reduced by the oxidation of NO to peroxynitrite ($ONOO^-$). VSMC, vascular smooth muscle cells; PAI-1, plasminogen activator inhibitor-1; VCAM-1, vascular cell adhesion molecule-1; GTP, guanosine triphosphate; cGMP, cyclic guanosine monophosphate.

nitric oxide–mediated vasodilation in diabetes. Increased reactive oxygen species in diabetes have been suggested to decrease the half-life of nitric oxide by converting it to peroxynitrite (Fig. 52.3). Consistent with this theory, elevated vascular superoxide production in diabetes via NADPH (reduced form of nicotinamide adenine dinucleotide phosphate) oxidase has been demonstrated 101,108), and antioxidant treatments, including vitamin C, have been shown to improve endothelium-dependent vasorelaxation in diabetes (92,109). Moreover, impairment of endothelial NADPH oxidase activity by the targeted mutation of the *gp91phox* gene has been shown to reduce arterial oxygen-radical formation and enhance endothelium-dependent vasorelaxation (110). Although there is considerable molecular and pharmacologic evidence for a role of vascular oxidants in attenuating endothelium-derived nitric oxide action, potential clinical benefits of antioxidant supplementation, such as vitamin E (RRR-α-tocopheryl acetate at 400 IU/day), for cardiovascular outcomes have not yet been identified (111). However, the potential benefits of substantially higher doses of vitamin E (1,200 IU/day), which may reduce monocyte activity and levels of soluble cell adhesion molecules (112), for cardiovascular complications remain to be examined.

Diabetes has also been reported to reduce vascular nitric oxide synthesis (98). Multiple mechanisms have been proposed to explain the decreased eNOS activity in diabetes and insulin resistance. Reduced eNOS expression has been described in adipose microvessels isolated from obese insulin-resistant Zucker rats and coronary microvessels from alloxan-induced diabetic dogs (98,113), suggesting that reduced protein levels of eNOS may contribute to lower nitric oxide production. In addition, the elevation of circulating levels of asymmetric dimethylarginine, an endogenous NOS inhibitor (114), and a deficiency in tetrahydrobiopterin (115,116), a cofactor for eNOS, have also been implicated in contributing to reduced nitric oxide generation in diabetes and insulin resistance.

The implications of reduced endothelium-derived nitric oxide bioactivity in diabetes goes beyond its hemodynamic effects. Nitric oxide, via cGMP-dependent pathways, has been shown to suppress a number of atherogenic and thrombogenic processes within the vascular wall, including neointimal SMC migration and proliferation and endothelial-leukocyte adhesion (117) (Fig. 52.2). Consistent with these possible antiatherogenic actions of nitric oxide, eNOS deficiency has been reported to increase atherosclerotic lesion size in apolipoprotein E (ApoE)–deficient mice (118). In addition, nitric oxide can also suppress the expression of thrombogenic factors, such as PAI-1 and tissue factor (119,120), which may shift the coagulation balance away from atherothrombosis.

EFFECTS OF DIABETES ON VASCULAR COMPLIANCE AND ARTERIAL STIFFNESS

Arterial stiffness is strongly associated with atherosclerosis (121). The Strong Heart Study (12) and the Atherosclerosis Risk in Communities Study (122) have reported increased arterial stiffness and reduced compliance in subjects with type 2 diabetes. Arterial compliance is also reduced in individuals with type 1 diabetes (123,124). Several theories have been proposed to explain the increased arterial stiffening in diabetes. Increased glycation of ECM proteins, such as collagen and elastin, may increase covalent intermolecular cross-linking and thereby reduce elasticity. Consistent with this theory, treatment with an AGE cross-link "breaker" has been shown to reverse diabetes-induced arterial stiffness (125). Increased arterial stiffness may also result from arterial calcification, arterial-wall thickening, or increased chronic VSMC contraction due to an imbalance in vasoactive hormone activities. Impaired arterial elasticity might contribute to atherogenesis by increasing mechanical strain and shear forces, causing endothelial damage, activation of stretch-activated mechanoreceptors, and increased release of trophic factors (126–128).

EFFECTS OF DIABETES ON COAGULATION AND THROMBOSIS

Diabetes and insulin resistance are associated with a procoagulant milieu (5,6,129,130) that may promote atherothrombosis by facilitating the expansion of nascent thrombi generated by plaque disruption. There is substantial clinical and experimental evidence that diabetes affects multiple coagulation components and pathways, which would be expected to shift the diathesis toward thrombosis. Diabetes is associated with elevated circulating levels of prothrombin fragment 1 + 2 (F1+2) (131), a marker of thrombin generation by the prothrombinase complex, and elevated circulating levels of fibrinopeptide A (130,132), a product of fibrinogen cleavage by thrombin. Diabetes is also associated with persistent platelet activation, as reflected in part by the increases in thromboxane A2 biosynthesis (133), platelet-dependent thrombin generation (134), and spontaneous platelet aggregation (135). Further evidence in support of a procoagulative state in insulin resistance and diabetes is provided by a number of reports showing increases in circulating levels of procoagulant factors and adhesion molecules. The population-based Framingham Offspring Study reported that glucose intolerance was associated with elevated plasma levels of PAI-1, tissue plasminogen activator, and von Willebrand factor (vWf) (136). Similarly, the Insulin Resistance Atherosclerosis Study reported that impaired glucose tolerance was associated with elevated PAI-1 and fibrinogen levels (137). Increased plasma PAI-1, factor VII, and P-selectin were reported in type 1 diabetes (138,139). Similarly, increased circulating levels of PAI-1, VCAM-1, and E-selectin occur in type 2 diabetes (5,140,141). These reports indicate the procoagulant milieu in diabetes is due in large part to the combination of elevated thrombin activation, impaired fibrinolysis, persistently activated platelets, and increased intercellular adhesion.

RISK FACTORS FOR CARDIOVASCULAR DISEASE IN DIABETES

Epidemiologic and clinical studies have identified a number of factors that are associated with the increased incidence of CVD in diabetes. These factors can be grouped into several different categories, including metabolic and lipid-related factors, coagulation and inflammatory factors, and vascular-related factors (Table 52.2). Although some cardiovascular risk factors appear to be associated primarily with diabetes and insulin resistance (such as hyperglycemia and hyperinsulinemia), other risk factors also appear in nondiabetic individuals.

Hyperglycemia

Several large multicenter prospective studies have shown an association between glycemic control and cardiovascular endpoints, including myocardial infarction (MI) and cardiovascular-related mortality. The Diabetes Control and Complications Trial (DCCT) demonstrated that the conventionally treated group had nearly twice as many major macrovascular events as the intensive treatment group, although this difference did not achieve statistical significance (p = 0.08) (142). This study reported that cardiovascular risk factors, including serum cholesterol and triglycerides, were significantly reduced in the intensively treated group. The United Kingdom Prospective Diabetes Study (UKPDS), a prospective study of vascular complications of type 2 diabetes with a mean follow-up of 10 years, demonstrated a 14% reduction in MI for each 1% reduction in glycosylated hemoglobin A_{1c} (143). This study did not detect a threshold for the association between glycemic control and MI. The UKPDS compared the effects of conventional versus intensive glycemic treatment protocols on both microvascular and macrovascular complications. This study showed that intensive control resulted in substantial reductions in microvascular disease, whereas intensive glycemic control resulted in a trend for reduced MI (p = 0.052). In addition, impaired glucose tolerance has also been identified as a risk factor for CVD, suggesting that mildly elevated hyperglycemia in the absence of overt type 2 diabetes may contribute to CVD (144).

Plasma Insulin and Insulin Resistance

Both hyperinsulinemia and insulin resistance have been identified as risk factors for CVD (145,146). The CVD risk associated with insulin has been attributed to an imbalance in the direct effects of insulin action, as well as to the confounding effects of CVD risk factors often associated with the insulin resistance syndrome. The effects of insulin on CVD in diabetes and insulin resistance are related to both systemic metabolic abnormalities and the direct effects of insulin action on the vasculature. With regard to the metabolic effects of insulin, insulin resistance results in glucose intolerance and hypertriglyceridemia, which have adverse cardiovascular effects (146). In addition, the direct actions of insulin on the vasculature have been proposed to mediate a combination of proatherogenic and antiatherogenic effects related to endothelial function and SMC growth (147). Moreover, the insulin resistance syndrome is often associated with a combination of established and emerging CVD risk factors, including hypertension, C-reactive protein (CRP), PAI-1, and fibrinogen (146,148). Hyperinsulinemia or insulin resistance or both may contribute to the elevation of these risk factors either directly in response to changes in insulin action or indirectly via imbalances in metabolites and cytokines that are associated the insulin resistance syndrome.

Lipid and Lipoproteins

Increased atherogenesis in diabetes and insulin resistance has been attributed in large part to a proatherogenic dyslipidemia,

TABLE 52.2. Cardiovascular Risk Factors Associated with Diabetes and Insulin Resistance

Metabolic factors	Coagulation and inflammatory factors	Vascular-related factors
• Hyperglycemia • Insulin resistance • Hyperinsulinemia • Hypertriglyceridemia • Reduced HDL cholesterol • Small dense LDL • Hyperhomocysteinemia	• Increased PAI-1 • Increased platelet activation • Increased fibrinogen • Increased P-selectin, VCAM-1, and ICAM-1 • Increased tissue factor and factor VII • Decreased nitric oxide bioavailability • Increased C-reactive protein	• Hypertension • Impaired endothelium-dependent vasorelaxation • Increased arterial calcification • Decreased arterial compliance

HDL, high-density lipoprotein; LDL, low-density lipoprotein; PAI-1, plasminogen activator inhibitor-1; VCAM-1, vascular cell adhesion molecule-1; ICAM-1, intercellular adhesion molecule-1.

related to hypertriglyceridemia, elevated very-low-density lipoprotein (VLDL), and decreased HDL (146,149). Although total LDL levels are not generally altered, or are only modestly increased, diabetes is associated with alterations in the buoyancy and modification of LDL particles. Insulin resistance results in increased levels of triglyceride-enriched small dense LDL particles, which have been associated with an increased risk of ischemic heart disease (150). Moreover, the combined elevation of fasting insulin, apoprotein B, and small dense LDL particles has been identified as a nontraditional risk factor cluster for ischemic heart disease (151). Additional CVD risk factors associated with diabetic dyslipidemia include increased lipoprotein(a) (152) and nonesterified fatty acids (153).

Lipid-lowering therapies, including HMG-CoA (hydroxymethylglutaryl–coenzyme A) reductase inhibitors and fibrate derivatives, have been shown to reduce coronary events in patients with type 2 diabetes. A subgroup analysis of the Cholesterol and Recurrent Events (CARE) trial revealed that pravastatin reduced total cholesterol by 20% compared with levels in the placebo groups and reduced the relative risk of coronary events in diabetic and nondiabetic patients by 25% ($p = 0.05$) and 23% ($p < 0.001$), respectively (154). Recently, the Heart Protection Study Collaborative Group reported that simvastatin reduced the occurrence of major coronary events by about 25% in diabetic patients and that this response was not dependent on preexisting elevated LDL cholesterol (>116 mg/dL) upon entry into the study (155). The Diabetes Atherosclerosis Intervention Study has shown that treatment of patients with type 2 diabetes with fenofibrate decreased triglycerides, total cholesterol, and LDL cholesterol; increased HDL cholesterol; and reduced coronary artery diameter stenosis compared with values in the placebo group (156). These results provide important clinical evidence that amelioration of the lipid and lipoprotein abnormalities in diabetes can reduce progression of angiographic coronary disease. It should be noted that these drugs could have direct effects on vascular tissues, beyond lipid lowering, that may contribute to their beneficial cardiovascular effects. For example, HMG-CoA inhibition decreases farnesylation and geranylgeranylation of G proteins and ras family proteins and thereby directly inhibits signaling in vascular cells (157).

Circulating Adhesion Molecules

Increased CVD risk in diabetes has been attributed in part to increased circulating levels of adhesion molecules, including vWf, VCAM-1, and E-selectin (141,158–160). The endothelium synthesizes vWf, which is a glycoprotein involved in platelet adhesion and aggregation. VCAM-1 and E-selectin are expressed on the endothelium, where they contribute to leukocyte adherence and recruitment. Circulating levels of these adhesion molecules have been described both as markers of endothelial cell damage and as potential contributors to CVD risk. Although expression of adhesion molecules on the vascular endothelium mediates leukocyte and platelet adherence, the specific functions of soluble adhesion molecules have not yet been fully elucidated. Recent studies have shown that a truncated soluble mutant on P-selectin can increase procoagulant activity (161), providing direct evidence that the soluble fraction of adhesion molecules can play an important role in coagulation.

Plasminogen Activator Inhibitor-1

PAI-1 is the major physiologic regulator of the plasminogen system. Increased PAI-1 inhibits fibrinolysis and thereby reduces thrombus dissolution. An elevation in PAI-1 antigen and activity has been identified as an important risk factor for recurrent MI in both diabetic and nondiabetic subjects (4,162–164). Moreover, the elevated PAI-1 levels that are observed after acute MI are significantly higher in individuals with type 2 diabetes than in subjects without diabetes (165). Increased circulating PAI-1 activity has been correlated with the level of insulin resistance (166–169) and plasma insulin concentration (140,170–172) and has been shown to be elevated in type 2 diabetes (5,140,173,174). A decrease in fibrinolytic activity, due to increased levels of PAI-1, has also been reported in individuals with type 1 diabetes with microalbuminuria (138). The elevation of PAI-1 levels and strong correlation between elevated levels of PAI-1 and MI risk suggest that PAI-1 is an important contributor to coronary events in patients with diabetes.

C-reactive Protein

CRP is an acute-phase protein marker of inflammation that has been associated with an increased risk for CVD (175,176). Increased levels of CRP have been described in both diabetes and insulin resistance (177,178). CRP has been proposed to promote atherosclerosis and atherothrombosis by stimulating chemotactic recruitment of monocytes and upregulating endothelial-leukocyte adhesion molecules and tissue factor expression (179–181). A recent report has shown that transgenic overexpression of CRP accelerates aortic atherosclerosis in ApoE-deficient mice (182), indicating that elevated CRP levels contribute to atherogenesis.

Fibrinogen

Fibrinogen is an acute-phase protein that is elevated in inflammation and provides a number of functions in coagulation. Fibrinogen binds to glycoprotein IIb/IIIa on platelets, thereby promoting platelet aggregation, and is cleaved by thrombin to generate fibrin, a major component of thrombi matrix. Fibrinogen is an abundant plasma protein and a major contributor to blood viscosity. Fibrinogen levels are elevated in diabetes and associated with CVD risk (183–185). Increased fibrinogen levels in diabetes contribute to a procoagulative state and thereby may promote atherothrombosis.

Hyperhomocysteinemia

Homocysteine is a thiol-containing amino acid produced from methionine metabolism. Plasma homocysteine levels are elevated in insulin resistance and type 2 diabetes (186) and are associated with an increased CVD risk in patients with type 2 diabetes (187,188). Homocysteine has been proposed to exert deleterious vascular effects by increasing expression of MCP-1 and tissue factor and impairing endothelium-dependent vasodilation, possibly contributing to monocyte recruitment and thrombosis (189–191). These potential adverse cardiovascular effects of homocysteine in diabetes appear to be related primarily to type 2 diabetes, as hyperhomocysteinemia has not been observed in studies of subjects with type 1 diabetes (192,193).

Endothelium-Dependent Vasodilation

Stimulation of the vascular endothelium with a variety of agonists, such as acetylcholine and hyperemia, stimulates the release of vasorelaxative substances (including nitric oxide) that induce the vasorelaxation of underlying arterial smooth muscle. This endothelium-dependent vasodilation is impaired in type 1 and type 2 diabetes and in insulin resistance (91,92,194). Endothelial vasodilator dysfunction in coronary and brachial arteries has been reported to be a predictive marker for cardiovascular events (195,196).

Hypertension

Hypertension is a major CVD risk factor that often coexists with insulin resistance and diabetes (146). The UKPDS has shown that tight blood pressure control substantially reduces the risk of macrovascular events in patients with type 2 diabetes (197). This study showed that for each 10 mm Hg reduction from ≤160 to <120 mm Hg of systolic blood pressure there was an 11% reduction in MI. Within the range tested, there was no apparent threshold for blood pressure and the reduction of vascular complications. The benefits of blood pressure lowering were observed with both angiotensin-converting enzyme (ACE) inhibitors (captopril) and β-blockers (atenolol), indicating that blood pressure lowering was of primary importance. However, direct beneficial vascular effects of blocking the respective signaling pathways by these therapies cannot be excluded. The Heart Outcomes Prevention Evaluation (HOPE) trial has demonstrated that ACE inhibition can provide protective cardiovascular effects that appear to go beyond blood pressure control. In the HOPE trial, treatment with ramipril similarly reduced a composite of macrovascular outcomes in diabetic and nondiabetic patients (198).

Clustering of Risk Factors for Cardiovascular Disease

Combinations of CVD risk factors (Table 52.2) frequently coexist in individuals with insulin resistance and diabetes. An analysis of a large family study of type 2 diabetes in Finland and Sweden (the Botnia study) indicated that clustering of at least two CVD risk factors, including obesity, hypertension, dyslipidemia, and microalbuminuria, occur in ~10% of individuals with normal glucose tolerance, ~50% of subjects with impaired fasting glucose or impaired glucose tolerance, and up to 80% in subjects with type 2 diabetes (199). The clustering of these metabolic abnormalities and CVD risk factors has been termed the insulin resistance syndrome (also called syndrome X and the metabolic syndrome). The Botnia study reported that cardiovascular-related mortality was elevated sixfold in subjects with this metabolic syndrome (199). The definition of this insulin resistance/metabolic syndrome has been expanded to include both established and emerging CVD risk factors, such as hyperinsulinemia, hyperglycemia, hypertension, central obesity, lipid/lipoprotein abnormalities, impaired endothelial-dependent relaxation, and increased PAI-1, CRP, and fibrinogen (146,148,178). Because these CVD risk factors can develop years before the onset of overt type 2 diabetes, it is likely that the pathogenesis of CVD in patients with type 2 diabetes begins well before the diagnosis of diabetes. Combinations of CVD risk factors, including hyperglycemia, hypertension, hypertriglyceridemia, microalbuminuria, impaired endothelial-dependent relaxation, and increases in circulating coagulation and adhesion molecules, also occur in type 1 diabetes. Although the etiologies of type 1 and type 2 diabetes are markedly different, the specific cardiovascular effects of type 1 diabetes compared with those of type 2 diabetes remain to be elucidated.

Comorbidity of Diabetes and Cardiovascular Disease

In addition to the adverse effects of insulin resistance and diabetes on CVD, there is growing evidence that insulin resistance/diabetes and CVD may share components of a common etiology. For type 2 diabetes and insulin resistance, this has been described as the "common soil" hypothesis, whereby diabetes and CVD may arise from common genetic and environmental antecedents (200). There are a number of molecular mechanisms that may mediate the simultaneous development of diabetes and CVD. For example, TNF-α inhibits insulin receptor signaling and contributes to obesity-induced insulin resistance (201). TNF-α is also a proinflammatory molecule that may contribute to vascular remodeling and atherothrombosis by stimulating VSMC migration and matrix metalloproteinase, tissue factor, and PAI-1 expression (65,202,203). Another example involves the renin-angiotensin system (RAS). Both the HOPE trial (198) and Captopril Prevention Project (204) have reported that treatment with an ACE inhibitor reduced CVD endpoints as well as new diagnoses of diabetes (198,204). Although the effects of ACE inhibition on diabetes were secondary outcomes, these findings are highly suggestive that ACE inhibition can suppress the onset of type 2 diabetes. Additional factors that may independently contribute to both CVD and insulin resistance or type 2 diabetes include free fatty acids and CRP (205,206). Thus, a component of the increased pathogenesis of CVD associated with diabetes could be related to the comorbidity of these diseases, which exist in addition to the downstream effects of diabetes.

Gender

Premenopausal nondiabetic women are at lower risk of developing CVD than are nondiabetic men, and this cardiovascular protection for women is diminished by diabetes. The Rancho Bernardo Study reported that the incidence of fatal ischemic heart disease was similar in men and women with diabetes and corresponded to 1.9- and 3.3-fold increases in CVD risk compared with that in nondiabetic male and female counterparts, respectively (207). The greater relative impact of diabetes on CVD in women also was observed during the 20-year surveillance of the Framingham cohort (14). Subgroup analysis of the Nurse's Health Study at the 20-year follow-up revealed that a relative risk of 9.19 for fatal CHD in young women (<55 years) with diabetes compared with age-matched women without diabetes (16). The basis for the loss of cardiovascular protection in diabetic women is not fully understood but has been attributed in part to greater increases in triglycerides and decreases in HDL cholesterol caused by diabetes in women as compared with those increases in men (208). In addition, premenopausal women have a more robust endothelium-dependent vasodilation than that observed in men, and diabetes causes a greater impairment of this endothelial function in premenopausal women than in men (209).

BIOCHEMICAL MECHANISMS THAT CONTRIBUTE TO VASCULAR COMPLICATIONS

Effects of Hyperglycemia

Substantial evidence from both *in vitro* and *in vivo* studies has demonstrated that hyperglycemia impairs a variety of vascular functions. Exposure of cultured endothelial cells to medium containing high concentrations of glucose (~25 mM), as compared with normal glucose concentrations (~5 mM), has been shown to increase monocyte binding (37,210), endothelin-1 production (105), and intercellular permeability (211) and to decrease eNOS expression (212). Multiple mechanisms have been postulated to explain the adverse effects of glucose on vascular cells (85) (Fig. 52.4).

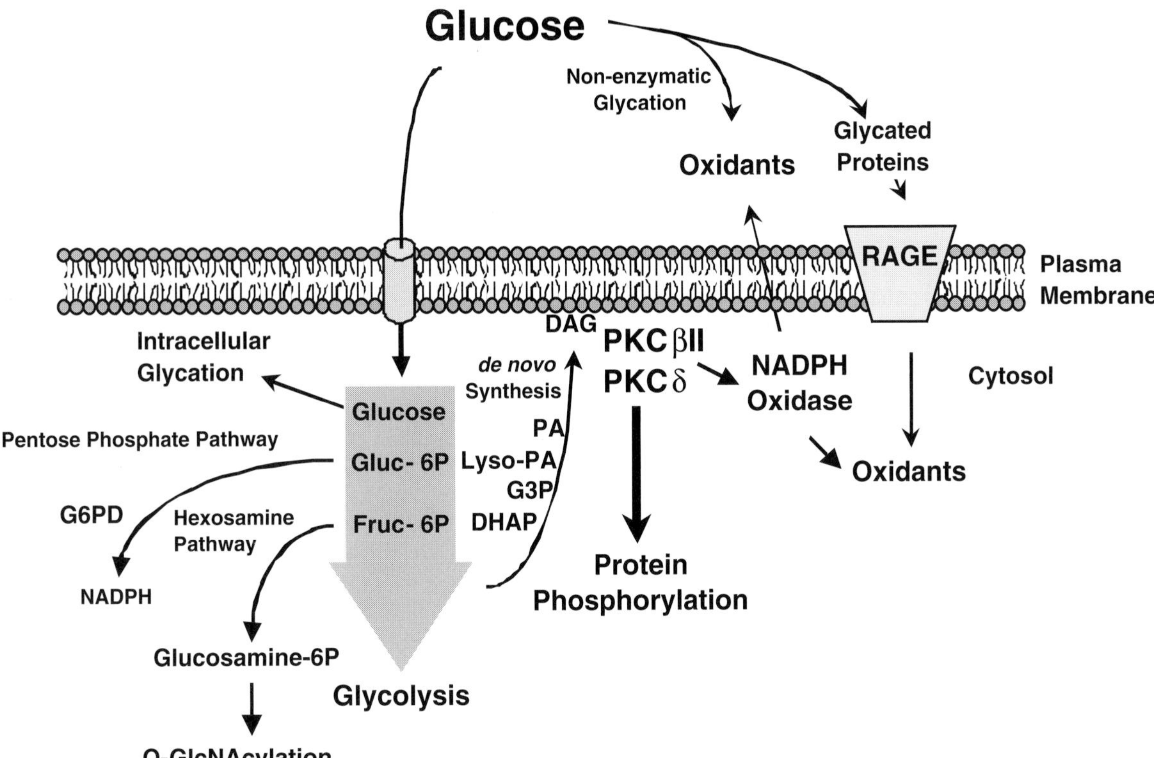

Figure 52.4. Mechanisms contributing to the adverse effects of hyperglycemia on the vasculature. Elevated glucose metabolism via glycolysis generates triose intermediates, which can increase the *de novo* synthesis of diacylglycerol (DAG) and the subsequent activation of protein kinase C (PKC). Glycolytic intermediates can be processed via the pentose phosphate pathway and alter intracellular redox via changes in NADPH (reduced form of nicotinamide adenine dinucleotide phosphate) or can be processed via the hexosamine pathway, leading to increased *O*-linked GlcNAcylation. In addition, hyperglycemia can increase the formation of advanced glycation end-products (AGE), which can generate oxidants and activate cell-surface AGE receptors (RAGE). PA, phosphatidic acid; Lyso-PA, lysophosphatidic acid; G3P, glyceraldehyde 3-phosphate; DHAP, dihydroxyacetone phosphate; G6PD, glucose 6-phosphate dehydrogenase.

One theory proposes that hyperglycemia increases glucose metabolism via glycolysis, resulting in the increased *de novo* synthesis of diacylglycerol (DAG). In this pathway, the glycolytic intermediate glyceraldehyde 3-phosphate is converted to dihydroxyacetone phosphate and then glycerol 3-phosphate, followed by sequential acyl group transfer by acyl-coenzyme A to yield lysophosphatidic acid and phosphatidic acid (Fig. 52.4). DAG is a cofactor for PKC, which increases the translocation to membrane and activation of a subset of PKC isoforms, including PKCβ and PKCδ (213,214). These serine/threonine kinases play an integral role in cellular physiology by phosphorylating cellular targets that regulate cell growth, migration, contraction, gene expression, and metabolism. For example, glucose-induced PKC activation can increase oxygen-radical production mediated by NADPH oxidase (215). This increased oxidant production can affect endothelium function by affecting redox-sensitive signaling pathways and decreasing nitric oxide bioavailability (Fig. 52.3). Hyperglycemia-induced superoxide production in the endothelium results in the activation of poly (ADP-ribose) polymerase, increased protein nitration, and nuclear factor-κB activation (216). Tissue-specific overexpression of PKCβ in the heart induces cardiac fibrosis and contractile abnormalities characteristic of diabetic cardiomyopathies (217). Selective inhibition of the PKCβ isoform has been shown to ameliorate certain renal and retinal vascular dysfunctions and pathologies caused by diabetes (218). Thus, diabetes-induced PKC activation in vascular tissues by hyperglycemia may chronically stimulate protein phosphorylation cascades that contribute to diabetic vasculopathies.

In addition, the increased flux through glycolysis induced by hyperglycemia can increase levels of intermediates, including glucose 6-phosphate and fructose 6-phosphate, which can be metabolized via alternate pathways. Glucose 6-phosphate can enter the pentose phosphate pathway by its oxidation via glucose 6-phosphate dehydrogenase (G6PD) and NADP to yield 6-phosphoglucono-1,5-lactone and NADPH. G6PD is the rate-limiting enzyme in this pathway, and its activity in endothelial cells is reduced in culture media with high glucose concentrations (219). This has been proposed to reduce the availability of NADPH, which is the primary intracellular reducing agent and a cofactor for eNOS. Fructose 6-phosphate can be converted to glucosamine 6-phosphate via glutamine:fructose-6-phosphate amidotransferase, the rate-limiting enzyme in the hexosamine pathway. This pathway leads to the synthesis of UDP-GlcNAc (uridine diphosphate–*N*-acetylglucosamine), which serves as a substrate for *O*-linked GlcNAcylation at serine and threonine residues on both cytosolic and nuclear proteins, including transcription factors such as Sp1 (220). Because *O*-GlcNAcylation of Sp1 inhibits its transcriptional activity, this pathway provides a mechanism for glucose-regulated gene expression (221).

Hyperglycemia can also increase nonenzymatic glycation initiated by Schiff-base formation between glucose and primary amines on proteins and lipids. These Schiff bases undergo spontaneous rearrangements to form Amadori products and AGE. These glycation processes can occur in both extracellular and intracellular milieus (222). Increased glycation induced by high glucose levels has been proposed to adversely affect vascular function via several mechanisms. The process of glycation itself modifies protein structure and spontaneously generates reactive oxygen species. Glycated proteins and lipoproteins can act as agonists to stimulate expression of PAI-1 and tissue factor in vascular cells and monocytes (223,224). In addition, glycation of LDL can facilitate its uptake into macrophages via lipoprotein lipase (49). Reactive glycation moieties generated during rearrangements can form covalent cross-links between proteins, which can decrease the elasticity of ECM proteins. This increased cross-link–induced vascular rigidity can reduce arterial elasticity and compliance in diabetes (125). AGE-modified proteins have been reported to stimulate tissue factor and VCAM-1 expression (224,225); however, the signaling mechanisms that mediate cellular responses to AGE-modified proteins have not been elucidated. AGE-modified proteins can bind to cell-surface receptors for AGE (RAGE), which can increase oxidant stress and lead to the activation of mitogen-activated protein (MAP) kinase pathways (226). However, because glycation reactions and rearrangements can generate a large number of molecular entities, further studies are needed to define the specific molecular structures that constitute ligands for RAGE. Moreover, because RAGE represents a group of receptors including macrophage scavenger receptors (50), the cellular responses to AGE-modified proteins are likely complex. A role of nonenzymatic glycation in vascular dysfunction and pathology in diabetes is supported by a limited number of studies showing that treatment of diabetic rodents with soluble truncated RAGE can improve endothelial barrier function and reduce atherosclerosis in these rodents (79,227). These studies propose that soluble RAGE can scavenge glycated products and thereby reduce their availability to interact with vascular tissues.

Insulin Action on the Vascular Wall

The arterial wall is an insulin-sensitive tissue, which expresses both insulin and insulin-like growth factor I (IGF-I) receptors on endothelial cells and VSMC (228). Activation of the insulin receptor and IGF-I receptor pathways has been shown to affect vascular cell growth, migration, and the production of a variety of vasoactive substances, including hormones and thrombogenic factors (71,105,228–230). Because hyperinsulinemia and insulin resistance are CVD risk factors, changes in plasma insulin or vascular insulin sensitivity may alter vascular insulin action and thereby contribute to vascular dysfunctions and pathologies. Insulin can activate both insulin receptors and IGF-I receptors; however, the affinity of insulin for the IGF-I receptor is 10- to 100-fold less than that for the insulin receptor (228). Although these receptors share structural and signaling characteristics, the IGF-I receptor system appears to exert greater effects on VSMC growth and migration. Normal physiologic concentrations of insulin coincide with the affinity of the insulin receptor, which mediates most insulin actions. However, at high pathophysiologic insulin concentrations associated with hyperinsulinemia, insulin may cross-react with IGF-I receptors, thereby stimulating VSMC migration and proliferation (Fig. 52.5).

The insulin/IGF-I receptor pathways also may provide protective vascular effects. Activation of the IGF-I pathway can protect VSMC from apoptosis and thereby may contribute to plaque stability (231). Insulin also provides antiapoptosis effects for endothelial cells (232). In addition, insulin action on the endothelium may provide antiatherogenic effects by increasing eNOS expression and nitric oxide production. Infusion of insulin has been shown to induce vasodilation of brachial and femoral arteries via a nitric oxide–dependent pathway (97,233). Insulin also increases nitric oxide production in endothelial cells (229). Thus, under normal physiologic insulin concentrations, the effects of insulin in promoting increased endothelial nitric oxide production may contribute to vasorelaxation and suppress atherogenesis.

Recent findings suggest that vascular tissues can display selective insulin resistance. *Ex vivo* studies have shown that insulin-stimulated eNOS expression is impaired in vascular tissue preparations from obese insulin-resistant Zucker rats (113). In this model, insulin-induced activation of the phosphoinositide 3-kinase (PI 3-kinase) pathway is impaired, whereas insulin stimulation of the MAP kinase pathways is normal (234). These findings suggest that vascular tissues develop selective insulin resistance related to activation by insulin of the PI 3-kinase/eNOS pathway. Because eNOS-derived nitric oxide provides mainly antiatherogenic effects, insulin resistance in endothelial cells leading to impairment in the eNOS/nitric oxide pathway is likely to be proatherogenic. Although insulin can also increase potentially proatherogenic factors, such as PAI-1 and endothelin-1 (230,235), the effects of the balance of hyperinsulinemia and vascular insulin resistance on the expression of these genes in endothelial cells remain to be established. Moreover, because nitric oxide can suppress these genes (119), the effects of insulin on nitric oxide may add a confounding factor to the regulation of proatherogenic gene expression in the vascular wall.

Recent studies have begun to identify mechanisms that regulate insulin signaling in vascular cells. Insulin action in the vasculature is mediated by the insulin receptor–stimulated tyrosine of insulin receptor substrate (IRS) proteins, which are adapter molecules that couple the activated insulin receptor to downstream signaling pathways (Fig. 52.5). Both ATII and endothelin-1 have been shown to inhibit insulin signaling that leads to PI 3-kinase activation in VSMC (236,237). Similarly, TNF-α has been shown to inhibit insulin signaling in endothelial cells (238). The mechanisms that inhibit insulin signaling involve the inhibition of insulin receptor–stimulated IRS-1 tyrosine phosphorylation and the subsequent docking of IRS proteins with the p85 regulatory subunit of PI 3-kinase (Fig. 52.5). The insulin-stimulated PI 3-kinase pathway has been shown to activate and upregulate eNOS in endothelial cells (229,239). Although IRS-1– and IRS-2–deficient mice display impaired endothelium-dependent vasorelaxation and enhanced neointimal expansion in response to vascular injury (240,241), it is not known whether these abnormalities are due to the absence of IRS protein expression in the vascular wall or to circulating factors associated with systemic insulin resistance. Evidence for a direct role of insulin action in the endothelium in vascular homeostasis is provided by studies showing that endothelial cell–specific insulin receptor knockout decreases both eNOS and endothelin-1 expression (242).

Renin-Angiotensin System

Although insulin resistance, insulin deficiency, hyperglycemia, and dyslipidemia likely represent the primary determinants that initiate the adverse effects of diabetes on CHD, a host of vascular hormones, cytokines, and growth factors play key roles in accelerating the progression of coronary atherosclerosis by promoting vascular remodeling, inflammation, fibrosis, and thrombosis. The role of the RAS in CVD has received considerable attention related to its systemic effects on blood pressure control and to its proinflammatory effects within plaques. The RAS involves the proteolytic processing of the protein precursor angiotensinogen to angiotensin I by renin, followed by its

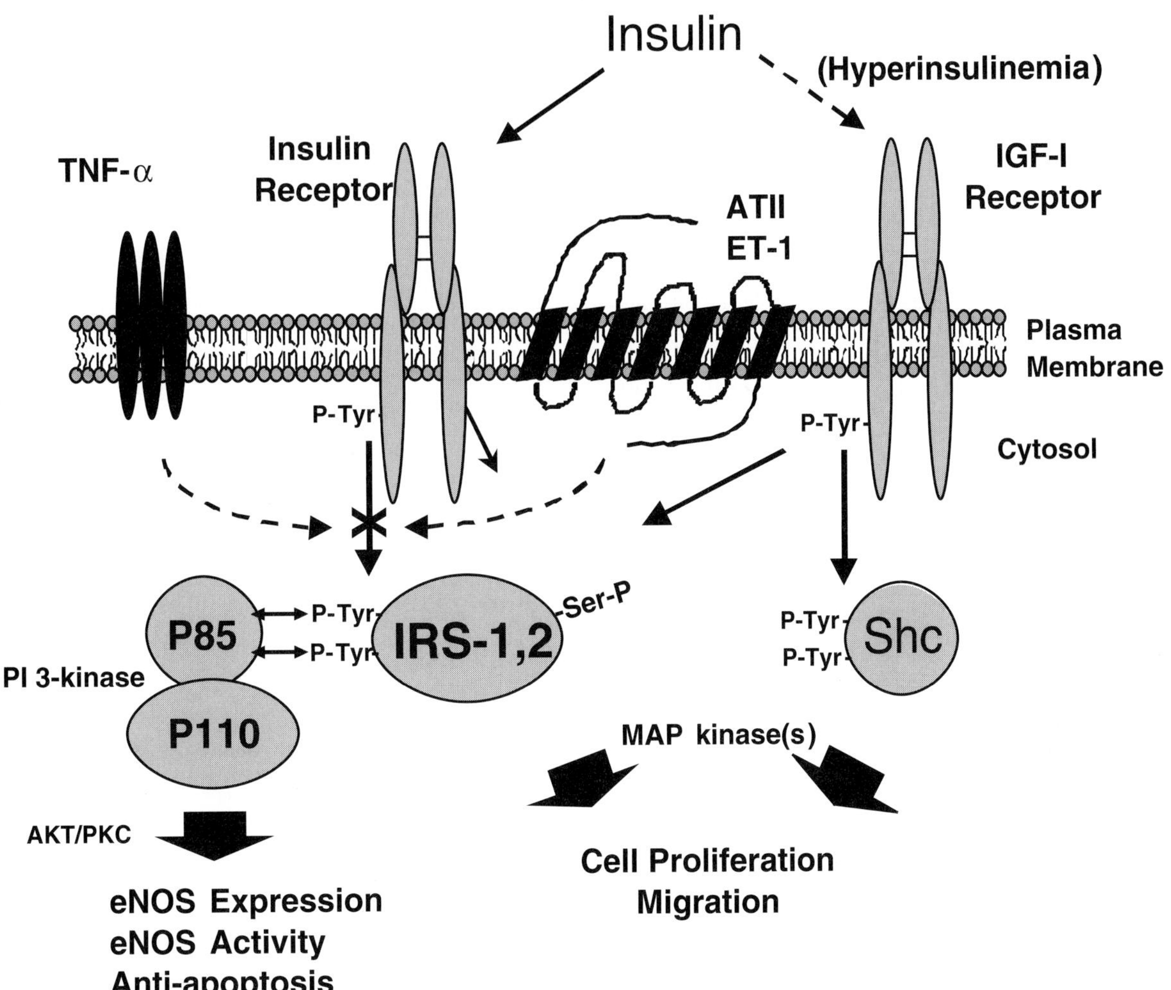

Figure 52.5. Insulin signaling, action, and mechanisms of insulin resistance in the vasculature. Insulin at normal physiologic concentrations activates the insulin receptor tyrosine kinase, which induces the phosphorylation of adapter proteins such as insulin receptor substrate (IRS)-1, -2, and Shc. Metabolic insulin resistance results in hyperinsulinemia, resulting in insulin concentrations capable of activating the insulin-like growth factor (IGF)-1 receptor. Insulin receptor signaling in vascular cells can be inhibited by tumor necrosis factor α (TNF-α), angiotensin II (ATII), and endothelin-1 (ET-1). These cytokines and hormones induce serine phosphorylation of IRS proteins and thereby can inhibit insulin receptor-activity and/or insulin receptor-IRS docking. PI 3-kinase, phosphoinositide 3-kinase; MAP kinase, mitogen-activated protein kinase; AKT, protein kinase B; PKC, protein kinase C; eNOS, endothelial nitric oxide synthase.

subsequent cleavage, primarily by ACE (dipeptidyl carboxypeptidase), to generate the octapeptide ATII. ATII signaling via the ATI receptor has been attributed to the majority of RAS action in the vasculature. The RAS plays an integral role in blood pressure regulation via a combination of mechanisms, including vasoconstriction, stimulation of renal tubular sodium resorption, and effects on the central and sympathetic nervous tissues. Inhibition of the RAS by ACE inhibitors and AT1 antagonists is widely used in the management of hypertension and its related adverse cardiovascular impact (197). In addition, there is considerable evidence that ATII is generated locally within plaques (46,243), where it may locally promote atherosclerosis and thrombosis (244,245).

Clinical trials have demonstrated that suppression of the RAS by ACE inhibitors reduces the onset and/or progression of cardiovascular complications of diabetes (197,246–249). Recent results of the HOPE trial have shown that treatment of patients at high risk for cardiovascular events with the ACE inhibitor ramipril provided protective effects against cardiovascular outcomes in diabetic patients, even in the absence of hypertension (198,248). Although the basis for these beneficial effects has not yet been fully elucidated, a substudy of the HOPE trial that measured carotid ultrasound changes has shown that the ACE inhibitor–treated group had a reduced rate of progression in carotid intimal-medial thickness (250), consistent with a reduction in atherosclerosis. In addition, ACE inhibition can also reduce vascular PAI-1 and tissue factor expression (26,251,252), which may shift the coagulation diathesis away from thrombosis. The HOPE trial has shown that ACE inhibition provides protective cardiovascular effects for both diabetic and nondiabetic patients but does not eliminate the excessive cardiovascular risk associated with diabetes.

CONCLUSION

Although the results of the DCCT and UKPDS have shown that intensive glycemic control in type 1 and type 2 diabetes can reduce cardiovascular complications, current therapies to normalize insulin action and glycemic control in diabetes do not eradicate its deleterious impact on the cardiovascular system. Moreover, because insulin resistance, type 2 diabetes, and CVD may arise from common genetic, metabolic, inflammatory, and hormonal antecedents, treatments to ameliorate the excessive CVD burden for diabetic patients will likely need to target the underlying causes of the metabolic syndrome. Diabetes and insulin resistance cause a combination of both systemic and intravascular abnormalities in metabolism, oxidation, inflammation, and hormone and cytokine actions that are proatherogenic and prothrombotic. In addition to intensive management of hyperglycemia, dyslipidemia, and insulin action, additional targets to slow or reverse the pathogenesis of cardiovascular disease in diabetes include strategies to preserve endothelium function, suppress vascular inflammation, reduce intravascular oxidative stress, and normalize metabolically coupled signaling cascades. The optimal use of these therapies will likely need to begin before the onset of vascular remodeling and clinical symptoms of CHD. Moreover, given the increased prevalence of obesity, insulin resistance, and type 2 diabetes, which are increasingly occurring in adolescents and young adults, strategies to preserve cardiovascular health in these individuals will need to begin in their early decades of life.

REFERENCES

1. Grundy SM, Benjamin IJ, Burke GL, et al. Diabetes and cardiovascular disease: a statement for healthcare professionals from the American Heart Association. *Circulation* 1999;100:1134–1146.
2. Natali A, Vichi S, Landi P, et al. Coronary atherosclerosis in type II diabetes: angiographic findings and clinical outcome. *Diabetologia* 2000;43:632–641.
3. Moreno PR, Murcia AM, Palacios IF, et al. Coronary composition and macrophage infiltration in atherectomy specimens from patients with diabetes mellitus. *Circulation* 2000;102:2180–2184.
4. Gray RP, Yudkin JS, Patterson DL. Plasminogen activator inhibitor: a risk factor for myocardial infarction in diabetic patients. *Br Heart J* 1993;69:228–232.
5. McGill JB, Schneider DJ, Arfken CL, et al. Factors responsible for impaired fibrinolysis in obese subjects and NIDDM patients. *Diabetes* 1994;43:104–109.
6. Colwell JA. Vascular thrombosis in type II diabetes mellitus. *Diabetes* 1993;42: 8–11.
7. Garcia Frade LJ, de la Calle H, Torrado MC, et al. Hypofibrinolysis associated with vasculopathy in non insulin dependent diabetes mellitus. *Thromb Res* 1990;59:51–59.
8. Henry P, Makowski S, Richard P, et al. Increased incidence of moderate stenosis among patients with diabetes: substrate for myocardial infarction? *Am Heart J* 1997;134:1037–1043.
9. Ziegler D. Cardiovascular autonomic neuropathy in type 1 diabetes. *J Diabetes Complications* 2001;15:14.
10. Castells I, Salinas I, Rius F, et al. Inducible myocardial ischaemia in asymptomatic type 2 diabetic patients. *Diabetes Res Clin Pract* 2000;49:127–133.
11. Seven-year outcome in the Bypass Angioplasty Revascularization Investigation (BARI) by treatment and diabetic status. *J Am Coll Cardiol* 2000;35:1122–1129.
12. Devereux RB, Roman MJ, Paranicas M, et al. Impact of diabetes on cardiac structure and function: the Strong Heart Study. *Circulation* 2000;101:2271–2276.
13. Spector KS. Diabetic cardiomyopathy. *Clin Cardiol* 1998;21:885–887.
14. Kannel WB, McGee DL. Diabetes and cardiovascular disease. The Framingham Study. *JAMA* 1979;241:2035–2038.
15. Stamler J, Vaccaro O, Neaton JD, et al. Diabetes, other risk factors, and 12-yr cardiovascular mortality for men screened in the Multiple Risk Factor Intervention Trial. *Diabetes Care* 1993;16:434–444.
16. Hu FB, Stampfer MJ, Solomon CG, et al. The impact of diabetes mellitus on mortality from all causes and coronary heart disease in women: 20 years of follow-up. *Arch Intern Med* 2001;161:1717–1723.
17. Morrish NJ, Wang SL, Stevens LK, et al. Mortality and causes of death in the WHO Multinational Study of Vascular Disease in Diabetes. *Diabetologia* 2001;44[Suppl 2]:S14–S21.
18. Stary HC, Chandler AB, Glagov S, et al. A definition of initial, fatty streak, and intermediate lesions of atherosclerosis. A report from the Committee on Vascular Lesions of the Council on Arteriosclerosis, American Heart Association. *Circulation* 1994;89:2462–2478.
19. Stary HC, Chandler AB, Dinsmore RE, et al. A definition of advanced types of atherosclerotic lesions and a histological classification of atherosclerosis. A report from the Committee on Vascular Lesions of the Council on Arteriosclerosis, American Heart Association. *Arterioscler Thromb Vasc Biol* 1995; 15:1512–1531.
20. Strong JP, Malcom GT, McMahan CA, et al. Prevalence and extent of atherosclerosis in adolescents and young adults: implications for prevention from the Pathobiological Determinants of Atherosclerosis in Youth Study. *JAMA* 1999;281:727–735.
21. Ikari Y, McManus BM, Kenyon J, et al. Neonatal intima formation in the human coronary artery. *Arterioscler Thromb Vasc Biol* 1999;19:2036–2040.
22. Moreno PR, Bernardi VH, Lopez-Cuellar J, et al. Macrophage infiltration predicts restenosis after coronary intervention in patients with unstable angina. *Circulation* 1996;94:3098–3102.
23. Virmani R, Kolodgie FD, Burke AP, et al. Lessons from sudden coronary death: a comprehensive morphological classification scheme for atherosclerotic lesions. *Arterioscler Thromb Vasc Biol* 2000;20:1262–1275.
24. Wilcox JN, Smith KM, Schwartz SM, et al. Localization of tissue factor in the normal vessel wall and in the atherosclerotic plaque. *Proc Natl Acad Sci U S A* 1989;86:2839–2843.
25. Toschi V, Gallo R, Lettino M, et al. Tissue factor modulates the thrombogenicity of human atherosclerotic plaques. *Circulation* 1997;95:594–599.
26. Hamdan AD, Quist WC, Gagne JB, et al. Angiotensin-converting enzyme inhibition suppresses plasminogen activator inhibitor-1 expression in the neointima of balloon-injured rat aorta. *Circulation* 1996;93:1073–1078.
27. Hasenstab D, Lea H, Clowes AW. Local plasminogen activator inhibitor type 1 overexpression in rat carotid artery enhances thrombosis and endothelial regeneration while inhibiting intimal thickening. *Arterioscler Thromb Vasc Biol* 2000;20:853–859.
28. Burke AP, Kolodgie FD, Farb A, et al. Healed plaque ruptures and sudden coronary death: evidence that subclinical rupture has a role in plaque progression. *Circulation* 2001;103:934–940.
29. Burke AP, Farb A, Malcom GT, et al. Plaque rupture and sudden death related to exertion in men with coronary artery disease. *JAMA* 1999;281: 921–926.
30. Sobel BE, Woodcock-Mitchell J, Schneider DJ, et al. Increased plasminogen activator inhibitor type 1 in coronary artery atherectomy specimens from type 2 diabetic compared with nondiabetic patients: a potential factor predisposing to thrombosis and its persistence. *Circulation* 1998;97:2213–2221.
31. Simon A, Giral P, Levenson J: Extracoronary atherosclerotic plaque at multiple sites and total coronary calcification deposit in asymptomatic men. Association with coronary risk profile. *Circulation* 1995;92:1414–1421.
32. Mielke CH, Shields JP, Broemeling LD. Coronary artery calcium, coronary artery disease, and diabetes. *Diabetes Res Clin Pract* 2001;53:55–61.
33. Schurgin S, Rich S, Mazzone T. Increased prevalence of significant coronary artery calcification in patients with diabetes. *Diabetes Care* 2001;24:335–338.
34. Keelan PC, Bielak LF, Ashai K, et al. Long-term prognostic value of coronary calcification detected by electron-beam computed tomography in patients undergoing coronary angiography. *Circulation* 2001;104:412–417.
35. Lehto S, Niskanen L, Suhonen M, et al. Medial artery calcification. A neglected harbinger of cardiovascular complications in non-insulin-dependent diabetes mellitus. *Arterioscler Thromb Vasc Biol* 1996;16:978–983.
36. Huang H, Virmani R, Younis H, et al. The impact of calcification on the biomechanical stability of atherosclerotic plaques. *Circulation* 2001;103: 1051–1056.
37. Kim JA, Berliner JA, Natarajan RD, et al. Evidence that glucose increases monocyte binding to human aortic endothelial cells. *Diabetes* 1994;43:1103–1107.
38. Richardson M, Hadcock SJ, DeReske M, et al. Increased expression in vivo of VCAM-1 and E-selectin by the aortic endothelium of normolipemic and hyperlipemic diabetic rabbits. *Arterioscler Thromb* 1994;14:760–769.
39. Morigi M, Angioletti S, Imberti B, et al: Leukocyte-endothelial interaction is augmented by high glucose concentrations and hyperglycemia in a NF-kB-dependent fashion. *J Clin Invest* 1998;101:1905–1915.
40. Kunt T, Forst T, Fruh B, et al. Binding of monocytes from normolipidemic hyperglycemic patients with type 1 diabetes to endothelial cells is increased in vitro. *Exp Clin Endocrinol Diabetes* 1999;107:252–256.
41. Carantoni M, Abbasi F, Chu L, et al. Adherence of mononuclear cells to endothelium in vitro is increased in patients with NIDDM. *Diabetes Care* 1997;20:1462–1465.
42. Takahara N, Kashiwagi A, Nishio Y, et al. Oxidized lipoproteins found in patients with NIDDM stimulate radical-induced monocyte chemoattractant protein-1 mRNA expression in cultured human endothelial cells. *Diabetologia* 1997;40:662–670.
43. Gough PJ, Greaves DR, Suzuki H, et al. Analysis of macrophage scavenger receptor (SR-A) expression in human aortic atherosclerotic lesions. *Arterioscler Thromb Vasc Biol* 1999;19:461–471.
44. Kapinsky M, Torzewski M, Buchler C, et al. Enzymatically degraded LDL preferentially binds to CD14(high) CD16(+) monocytes and induces foam cell formation mediated only in part by the class B scavenger-receptor CD36. *Arterioscler Thromb Vasc Biol* 2001;21:1004–1010.
45. Inoue M, Itoh H, Ueda M, et al. Vascular endothelial growth factor (VEGF) expression in human coronary atherosclerotic lesions: possible pathophysiological significance of VEGF in progression of atherosclerosis. *Circulation* 1998;98:2108–2116.
46. Schieffer B, Schieffer E, Hilfiker-Kleiner D, et al. Expression of angiotensin II and interleukin 6 in human coronary atherosclerotic plaques: potential implications for inflammation and plaque instability. *Circulation* 2000;101: 1372–1378.

47. Sukhova GK, Schonbeck U, Rabkin E, et al. Evidence for increased collagenolysis by interstitial collagenases-1 and -3 in vulnerable human atheromatous plaques. *Circulation* 1999;99:2503–2509.
48. Kataoka H, Kume N, Miyamoto S, et al. Expression of lectinlike oxidized low-density lipoprotein receptor-1 in human atherosclerotic lesions. *Circulation* 1999;99:3110–3117.
49. Zimmermann R, Panzenbock U, Wintersperger A, et al. Lipoprotein lipase mediates the uptake of glycated LDL in fibroblasts, endothelial cells, and macrophages. *Diabetes* 2001;50:1643–1653.
50. Ohgami N, Nagai R, Ikemoto M, et al. Cd36, a member of the class b scavenger receptor family, as a receptor for advanced glycation end products. *J Biol Chem* 2001;276:3195–3202.
51. Mietus-Snyder M, Gowri MS, Pitas RE. Class A scavenger receptor up-regulation in smooth muscle cells by oxidized low density lipoprotein. Enhancement by calcium flux and concurrent cyclooxygenase-2 up-regulation. *J Biol Chem* 2000;275:17661–17670.
52. Lyons TJ, Baynes JW, Patrick JS, et al. Glycosylation of low density lipoprotein in patients with type 1 (insulin-dependent) diabetes: correlations with other parameters of glycaemic control. *Diabetologia* 1986;29:685–689.
53. Bucala R, Makita Z, Koschinsky T, et al. Lipid advanced glycosylation: pathway for lipid oxidation in vivo. *Proc Natl Acad Sci U S A* 1993;90:6434–6438.
54. Griffin E, Re A, Hamel N, et al. A link between diabetes and atherosclerosis: glucose regulates expression of CD36 at the level of translation. *Nat Med* 2001;7:840–846.
55. Sibley SD, Hokanson JE, Steffes MW, et al. Increased small dense LDL and intermediate-density lipoprotein with albuminuria in type 1 diabetes. *Diabetes Care* 1999;22:1165–1170.
56. Geng YJ, Wu Q, Muszynski M, et al. Apoptosis of vascular smooth muscle cells induced by in vitro stimulation with interferon-gamma, tumor necrosis factor-alpha, and interleukin-1 beta. *Arterioscler Thromb Vasc Biol* 1996;16: 19–27.
57. Suzuki LA, Poot M, Gerrity RG, et al. Diabetes accelerates smooth muscle accumulation in lesions of atherosclerosis: lack of direct growth-promoting effects of high glucose levels. *Diabetes* 2001;50:851–860.
58. Kornowski R, Mintz GS, Kent KM, et al. Increased restenosis in diabetes mellitus after coronary interventions is due to exaggerated intimal hyperplasia. A serial intravascular ultrasound study. *Circulation* 1997;95:1366–1369.
59. Moreno PR, Fallon JT, Murcia AM, et al. Tissue characteristics of restenosis after percutaneous transluminal coronary angioplasty in diabetic patients. *J Am Coll Cardiol* 1999;34:1045–1049.
60. Uemura S, Matsushita H, Li W, et al. Diabetes mellitus enhances vascular matrix metalloproteinase activity: role of oxidative stress. *Circ Res* 2001;88: 1291–1298.
61. Aikawa M, Rabkin E, Okada Y, et al. Lipid lowering by diet reduces matrix metalloproteinase activity and increases collagen content of rabbit atheroma: a potential mechanism of lesion stabilization. *Circulation* 1998;97:2433-2444.
62. Redmond EM, Cullen JP, Cahill PA, et al. Endothelial cells inhibit flow-induced smooth muscle cell migration: role of plasminogen activator inhibitor-1. *Circulation* 2001;103:597-603.
63. Kaikita K, Fogo AB, Ma L, et al. Plasminogen activator inhibitor-1 deficiency prevents hypertension and vascular fibrosis in response to long-term nitric oxide synthase inhibition. *Circulation* 2001;104:839–844.
64. Kislinger T, Tanji N, Wendt T, et al. Receptor for advanced glycation end products mediates inflammation and enhanced expression of tissue factor in vasculature of diabetic apolipoprotein E-null mice. *Arterioscler Thromb Vasc Biol* 2001;21:905–910.
65. Samad F, Pandey M, Loskutoff DJ. Tissue factor gene expression in the adipose tissues of obese mice. *Proc Natl Acad Sci U S A* 1998;95:7591–7596.
66. Pandolfi A, Cetrullo D, Polishuck R, et al. Plasminogen activator inhibitor type 1 is increased in the arterial wall of type II diabetic subjects. *Arterioscler Thromb Vasc Biol* 2001;21:1378–1382.
67. The Bari Investigators. Influence of diabetes on 5-year mortality and morbidity in a randomized trial comparing CABG and PTCA in patients with multivessel disease. *Circulation* 1997;96:1761–1769.
68. Ahmed JM, Hong MK, Mehran R, et al. Influence of diabetes mellitus on early and late clinical outcomes in saphenous vein graft stenting. *J Am Coll Cardiol* 2000;36:1186–1193.
69. Abizaid A, Costa MA, Centemero M, et al. Clinical and economic impact of diabetes mellitus on percutaneous and surgical treatment of multivessel coronary disease patients: insights from the Arterial Revascularization Therapy Study (ARTS) trial. *Circulation* 2001;104:533–538.
70. Elezi S, Kastrati A, Pache J, et al. Diabetes mellitus and the clinical and angiographic outcome after coronary stent placement. *J Am Coll Cardiol* 1998;32: 1866–1873.
71. Indolfi C, Torella D, Cavuto L, et al. Effects of balloon injury on neointimal hyperplasia in streptozotocin- induced diabetes and in hyperinsulinemic non-diabetic pancreatic islet-transplanted rats. *Circulation* 2001;103: 2980–2986.
72. Park SH, Marso SP, Zhou Z, et al. Neointimal hyperplasia after arterial injury is increased in a rat model of non-insulin-dependent diabetes mellitus. *Circulation* 2001;104:815–819.
73. Schiller NK, McNamara DB. Balloon catheter vascular injury of the alloxan-induced diabetic rabbit: the role of insulin-like growth factor-1. *Mol Cell Biochem* 1999;202:159–167.
74. Carter AJ, Bailey L, Devries J, et al. The effects of uncontrolled hyperglycemia on thrombosis and formation of neointima after coronary stent placement in a novel diabetic porcine model of restenosis. *Coron Artery Dis* 2000;11:473–479.
75. Ridray S, Heudes D, Michel O, et al. Increased SMC proliferation after endothelial injury in hyperinsulinemic obese Zucker rats. *Am J Physiol* 1994; 267:H1976–H1983.
76. Tamura K, Kanzaki T, Tashiro J, et al. Increased atherogenesis in Otsuka Long-Evans Tokushima fatty rats before the onset of diabetes mellitus: association with overexpression of PDGF beta-receptors in aortic smooth muscle cells. *Atherosclerosis* 2000;149:351–358.
77. Dzau VJ, Braun-Dullaeus RC, Sedding DG. Vascular proliferation and atherosclerosis: new perspectives and therapeutic strategies. *Nat Med* 2002;8:1249–1256.
78. Yamaji T, Fukuhara T, Kinoshita M. Increased capillary permeability to albumin in diabetic rat myocardium. *Circ Res* 1993;72:947–957.
79. Wautier JL, Zoukourian C, Chappey O, et al. Receptor-mediated endothelial cell dysfunction in diabetic vasculopathy. Soluble receptor for advanced glycation end products blocks hyperpermeability in diabetic rats. *J Clin Invest* 1996;97:238–243.
80. Antonetti DA, Barber AJ, Khin S, et al. Vascular permeability in experimental diabetes is associated with reduced endothelial occludin content: vascular endothelial growth factor decreases occludin in retinal endothelial cells. Penn State Retina Research Group. *Diabetes* 1998;47:1953–1959.
81. Natarajan R, Bai W, Lanting L, et al. Effects of high glucose on vascular endothelial growth factor expression in vascular smooth muscle cells. *Am J Physiol* 1997;273:H2224–H2231.
82. Williams B, Baker AQ, Gallacher B, et al. Angiotensin II increases vascular permeability factor gene expression by human vascular smooth muscle cells. *Hypertension* 1995;25:913–917.
83. Antonetti DA, Barber AJ, Hollinger LA, et al. Vascular endothelial growth factor induces rapid phosphorylation of tight junction proteins occludin and zonula occluden 1. A potential mechanism for vascular permeability in diabetic retinopathy and tumors. *J Biol Chem* 1999;274:23463–23467.
84. Aiello LP, Avery RL, Arrigg PG, et al. Vascular endothelial growth factor in ocular fluid of patients with diabetic retinopathy and other retinal disorders. *N Engl J Med* 1994;331:1480–1487.
85. Koya D, King GL. Protein kinase C activation and the development of diabetic complications. *Diabetes* 1998;47:859–866.
86. Palmer RM, Ferrige AG, Moncada S. Nitric oxide release accounts for the biological activity of endothelium-derived relaxing factor. *Nature* 1987;327: 524–526.
87. Brandes RP, Schmitz-Winnenthal FH, Feletou M, et al. An endothelium-derived hyperpolarizing factor distinct from NO and prostacyclin is a major endothelium-dependent vasodilator in resistance vessels of wild-type and endothelial NO synthase knockout mice. *Proc Natl Acad Sci U S A* 2000;97: 9747–9752.
88. Dimmeler S, Fleming I, Fisslthaler B, et al. Activation of nitric oxide synthase in endothelial cells by Akt-dependent phosphorylation. *Nature* 1999;399: 601–605.
89. Schlossmann J, Ammendola A, Ashman K, et al. Regulation of intracellular calcium by a signalling complex of IRAG, IP3 receptor and cGMP kinase Ibeta. *Nature* 2000;404:197–201.
90. Caballero AE, Arora S, Saouaf R, et al. Microvascular and macrovascular reactivity is reduced in subjects at risk for type 2 diabetes. *Diabetes* 1999; 48: 1856–1862.
91. Johnstone MT, Creager SJ, Scales KM, et al. Impaired endothelium-dependent vasodilation in patients with insulin-dependent diabetes mellitus. *Circulation* 1993;88:2510–2516.
92. Ting HH, Timimi FK, Boles KS, et al. Vitamin C improves endothelium-dependent vasodilation in patients with non-insulin-dependent diabetes mellitus. *J Clin Invest* 1996;97:22–28.
93. Clarkson P, Celermajer DS, Donald AE, et al. Impaired vascular reactivity in insulin-dependent diabetes mellitus is related to disease duration and low density lipoprotein cholesterol levels. *J Am Coll Cardiol* 1996;28:573–579.
94. Williams SB, Goldfine AB, Timimi FK, et al. Acute hyperglycemia attenuates endothelium-dependent vasodilation in humans in vivo. *Circulation* 1998; 97: 1695–1701.
95. Vehkavaara S, Seppala-Lindroos A, Westerbacka J, et al. In vivo endothelial dysfunction characterizes patients with impaired fasting glucose. *Diabetes Care* 1999;22:2055–2060.
96. Steinberg HO, Tarshoby M, Monestel R, et al. Elevated circulating free fatty acid levels impair endothelium-dependent vasodilation. *J Clin Invest* 1997; 100:1230–1239.
97. Steinberg HO, Brechtel G, Johnson A, et al. Insulin-mediated skeletal muscle vasodilation is nitric oxide dependent. A novel action of insulin to increase nitric oxide release. *J Clin Invest* 1994;94:1172–1179.
98. Zhao G, Zhang X, Smith CJ, et al. Reduced coronary NO production in conscious dogs after the development of alloxan-induced diabetes. *Am J Physiol* 1999;277:H268–H278.
99. Diederich D, Skopec J, Diederich A, et al. Endothelial dysfunction in mesenteric resistance arteries of diabetic rats: role of free radicals. *Am J Physiol* 1994;266:H1153–H1161.
100. Meraji S, Jayakody L, Senaratne MP, et al. Endothelium-dependent relaxation in aorta of BB rat. *Diabetes* 1987;36:978–981.
101. Lund DD, Faraci FM, Miller FJJ, et al. Gene transfer of endothelial nitric oxide synthase improves relaxation of carotid arteries from diabetic rabbits. *Circulation* 2000;101:1027–1033.

102. O'Driscoll G, Green D, Rankin J, et al. Improvement in endothelial function by angiotensin converting enzyme inhibition in insulin-dependent diabetes mellitus. *J Clin Invest* 1997;100:678–684.
103. O'Driscoll G, Green D, Maiorana A, et al. Improvement in endothelial function by angiotensin-converting enzyme inhibition in non-insulin-dependent diabetes mellitus. *J Am Coll Cardiol* 1999;33:1506–1511.
104. Calver A, Collier J, Vallance P. Inhibition and stimulation of nitric oxide synthesis in the human forearm arterial bed of patients with insulin-dependent diabetes. *J Clin Invest* 1992;90:2548–2554.
105. Park JY, Takahara N, Gabriele A, et al. Induction of endothelin-1 expression by glucose: an effect of protein kinase C activation. *Diabetes* 2000;49:1239–1248.
106. Cheetham C, O'Driscoll G, Stanton K, et al. Losartan, an angiotensin type I receptor antagonist, improves conduit vessel endothelial function in type II diabetes. *Clin Sci* (Lond) 2001;100:13–17.
107. Horio D, Clermont AC, Abiko A, et al. Angiotensin AT(1) receptor antagonism normalizes retinal blood flow and acetylcholine-induced vasodilatation in normotensive diabetic rats. *Diabetologia* 2004;47:113–123.
108. Guzik TJ, West NE, Black E, et al. Vascular superoxide production by NAD(P)H oxidase: association with endothelial dysfunction and clinical risk factors. *Circ Res* 2000;86:E85–E90.
109. Timimi FK, Ting HH, Haley EA, et al. Vitamin C improves endothelium-dependent vasodilation in patients with insulin-dependent diabetes mellitus. *J Am Coll Cardiol* 1998;31:552–557.
110. Gorlach A, Brandes RP, Nguyen K, et al. A gp91phox containing NADPH oxidase selectively expressed in endothelial cells is a major source of oxygen radical generation in the arterial wall. *Circ Res* 2000;87:26–32.
111. Yusuf S, Dagenais G, Pogue J, et al. Vitamin E supplementation and cardiovascular events in high-risk patients. The Heart Outcomes Prevention Evaluation Study Investigators. *N Engl J Med* 2000;342:154–160.
112. Devaraj S, Jialal I. Low-density lipoprotein postsecretory modification, monocyte function, and circulating adhesion molecules in type 2 diabetic patients with and without macrovascular complications: the effect of alpha-tocopherol supplementation. *Circulation* 2000;102:191–196.
113. Kuboki K, Jiang ZY, Takahara N, et al. Regulation of endothelial constitutive nitric oxide synthase gene expression in endothelial cells and in vivo: a specific vascular action of insulin. *Circulation* 2000;101:676–681.
114. Fard A, Tuck CH, Donis JA, et al. Acute elevations of plasma asymmetric dimethylarginine and impaired endothelial function in response to a high-fat meal in patients with type 2 diabetes. *Arterioscler Thromb Vasc Biol* 2000;20: 2039–2044.
115. Meininger CJ, Marinos RS, Hatakeyama K, et al. Impaired nitric oxide production in coronary endothelial cells of the spontaneously diabetic BB rat is due to tetrahydrobiopterin deficiency. *Biochem J* 2000;349:353–356.
116. Heitzer T, Krohn K, Albers S, et al. Tetrahydrobiopterin improves endothelium-dependent vasodilation by increasing nitric oxide activity in patients with type II diabetes mellitus. *Diabetologia* 2000;43:1435–1438.
117. Janssens S, Flaherty D, Nong Z, et al. Human endothelial nitric oxide synthase gene transfer inhibits vascular smooth muscle cell proliferation and neointima formation after balloon injury in rats. *Circulation* 1998;97:1274–1281.
118. Knowles JW, Reddick RL, Jennette JC, et al. Enhanced atherosclerosis and kidney dysfunction in eNOS(-/-)Apoe(-/-) mice are ameliorated by enalapril treatment. *J Clin Invest* 2000;105:451–458.
119. Bouchie JL, Hansen H, Feener EP. Natriuretic factors and nitric oxide suppress plasminogen activator inhibitor-1 expression in vascular smooth muscle cells. Role of cGMP in the regulation of the plasminogen system. *Arterioscler Thromb Vasc Biol* 1998;18:1771–1779.
120. Yang Y, Loscalzo J. Regulation of tissue factor expression in human microvascular endothelial cells by nitric oxide. *Circulation* 2000;101:2144–2148.
121. van Popele NM, Grobbee DE, Bots ML, et al. Association between arterial stiffness and atherosclerosis: the Rotterdam Study. *Stroke* 2001;32:454–460.
122. Salomaa V, Riley W, Kark JD, et al. Non-insulin-dependent diabetes mellitus and fasting glucose and insulin concentrations are associated with arterial stiffness indexes. The ARIC study. Atherosclerosis Risk in Communities Study. *Circulation* 1995;91:1432–1443.
123. Berry KL, Skyrme-Jones RA, Cameron JD, et al. Systemic arterial compliance is reduced in young patients with IDDM. *Am J Physiol* 1999;276:H1839–H1845.
124. Lambert J, Smulders RA, Aarsen M, et al. Carotid artery stiffness is increased in microalbuminuric IDDM patients. *Diabetes Care* 1998;21:99–103.
125. Wolffenbuttel BH, Boulanger CM, Crijns FR, et al. Breakers of advanced glycation end products restore large artery properties in experimental diabetes. *Proc Natl Acad Sci U S A* 1998;95:4630–4634.
126. Chen KD, Li YS, Kim M, et al. Mechanotransduction in response to shear stress. Roles of receptor tyrosine kinases, integrins, and Shc. *J Biol Chem* 1999;274:18393–18400.
127. Hoyer J, Kohler R, Haase W, et al. Up-regulation of pressure-activated Ca(2+)-permeable cation channel in intact vascular endothelium of hypertensive rats. *Proc Natl Acad Sci U S A* 1996;93:11253–11258.
128. Ohno M, Cooke JP, Dzau VJ, et al. Fluid shear stress induces endothelial transforming growth factor beta-1 transcription and production. Modulation by potassium channel blockade. *J Clin Invest* 1995;95:1363–1369.
129. Carr ME. Diabetes mellitus: a hypercoagulable state. *J Diabetes Complications* 2001;15:44–54.
130. el Khawand C, Jamart J, Donckier J, et al. Hemostasis variables in type I diabetic patients without demonstrable vascular complications. *Diabetes Care* 1993;16:1137–1145.
131. Myrup B, Rossing P, Jensen T, et al. Procoagulant activity and intimal dysfunction in IDDM. *Diabetologia* 1995;38:73–78.
132. Ford I, Singh TP, Kitchen S, et al. Activation of coagulation in diabetes mellitus in relation to the presence of vascular complications. *Diabet Med* 1991;8: 322–329.
133. Davi G, Gresele P, Violi F, et al. Diabetes mellitus, hypercholesterolemia, and hypertension but not vascular disease per se are associated with persistent platelet activation in vivo. Evidence derived from the study of peripheral arterial disease. *Circulation* 1997;96:69–75.
134. Aoki I, Shimoyama K, Aoki N, et al. Platelet-dependent thrombin generation in patients with diabetes mellitus: effects of glycemic control on coagulability in diabetes. *J Am Coll Cardiol* 1996;27:560–566.
135. Menys VC, Bhatnagar D, Mackness MI, et al. Spontaneous platelet aggregation in whole blood is increased in non-insulin-dependent diabetes mellitus and in female but not male patients with primary dyslipidemia. *Atherosclerosis* 1995;112:115–122.
136. Meigs JB, Mittleman MA, Nathan DM, et al. Hyperinsulinemia, hyperglycemia, and impaired hemostasis: the Framingham Offspring Study. *JAMA* 2000;283:221–228.
137. Festa A, D'Agostino R Jr, Mykkanen L, et al. Relative contribution of insulin and its precursors to fibrinogen and PAI-1 in a large population with different states of glucose tolerance. The Insulin Resistance Atherosclerosis Study (IRAS). *Arterioscler Thromb Vasc Biol* 1999;19:562–568.
138. Gruden G, Cavallo-Perin P, Bazzan M, et al. PAI-1 and factor VII activity are higher in IDDM patients with microalbuminuria. *Diabetes* 1994;43:426–429.
139. Jilma B, Fasching P, Ruthner C, et al. Elevated circulating P-selectin in insulin dependent diabetes mellitus. *Thromb Haemost* 1996;76:328–332.
140. Juhan-Vague I, Roul C, Alessi MC, et al. Increased plasminogen activator inhibitor activity in non insulin dependent diabetic patients—relationship with plasma insulin. *Thromb Haemost* 1989;61:370–373.
141. Kado S, Nagata N. Circulating intercellular adhesion molecule-1, vascular cell adhesion molecule-1, and E-selectin in patients with type 2 diabetes mellitus. *Diabetes Res Clin Pract* 1999;46:143–148.
142. Effect of intensive diabetes management on macrovascular events and risk factors in the Diabetes Control and Complications Trial. *Am J Cardiol* 1995;75: 894–903.
143. Stratton IM, Adler AI, Neil HA, et al. Association of glycaemia with macrovascular and microvascular complications of type 2 diabetes (UKPDS 35): prospective observational study. *BMJ* 2000;321:405–412.
144. Haffner SM. Impaired glucose tolerance, insulin resistance and cardiovascular disease. *Diabet Med* 1997;14[Suppl 3]:S12–S18.
145. Despres J-P, Lamarche B, Mauriege P, et al. Hyperinsulinemia as an independent risk factor for ischemic heart disease. *N Engl J Med* 1996;334:952–957.
146. Zavaroni I, Bonora E, Pagliara M, et al. Risk factors for coronary artery disease in healthy persons with hyperinsulinemia and normal glucose tolerance. *N Engl J Med* 1989;320:702–706.
147. Feener EP, King GL. Vascular dysfunction in diabetes mellitus. *Lancet* 1997;350:SI9–SI13.
148. Haffner SM, Mykkanen L, Festa A, et al. Insulin-resistant prediabetic subjects have more atherogenic risk factors than insulin-sensitive prediabetic subjects: implications for preventing coronary heart disease during the prediabetic state. *Circulation* 2000;101:975–980.
149. Koivisto VA, Stevens LK, Mattock M, et al. Cardiovascular disease and its risk factors in IDDM in Europe. EURODIAB IDDM Complications Study Group. *Diabetes Care* 1996;19:689–697.
150. Lamarche B, Tchernof A, Moorjani S, et al. Small, dense low-density lipoprotein particles as a predictor of the risk of ischemic heart disease in men. Prospective results from the Quebec Cardiovascular Study. *Circulation* 1997;95:69–75.
151. Lamarche B, Tchernof A, Mauriege P, et al. Fasting insulin and apolipoprotein B levels and low-density lipoprotein particle size as risk factors for ischemic heart disease. *JAMA* 1998;279:1955–1961.
152. Hiraga T, Kobayashi T, Okubo M, et al. Prospective study of lipoprotein(a) as a risk factor for atherosclerotic cardiovascular disease in patients with diabetes. *Diabetes Care* 1995;18:241–244.
153. Forsblom CM, Sane T, Groop PH, et al. Risk factors for mortality in type II (non-insulin-dependent) diabetes: evidence of a role for neuropathy and a protective effect of HLA-DR4. *Diabetologia* 1998;41:1253–1262.
154. Goldberg RB, Mellies MJ, Sacks FM, et al. Cardiovascular events and their reduction with pravastatin in diabetic and glucose-intolerant myocardial infarction survivors with average cholesterol levels: subgroup analyses in the cholesterol and recurrent events (CARE) trial. The Care Investigators. *Circulation* 1998;98:2513–2519.
155. Collins R, Armitage J, Parish S, et al. MRC/BHF Heart Protection Study of cholesterol-lowering with simvastatin in 5963 people with diabetes: a randomised placebo-controlled trial. *Lancet* 2003;361:2005–2016.
156. Effect of fenofibrate on progression of coronary-artery disease in type 2 diabetes: the Diabetes Atherosclerosis Intervention Study, a randomised study. *Lancet* 2001;357:905–910.
157. Essig M, Nguyen G, Prie D, et al. 3-Hydroxy-3-methylglutaryl coenzyme A reductase inhibitors increase fibrinolytic activity in rat aortic endothelial cells. Role of geranylgeranylation and Rho proteins. *Circ Res* 1998;83:683–690.

158. Steiner M, Reinhardt KM, Krammer B, et al. Increased levels of soluble adhesion molecules in type 2 (non-insulin dependent) diabetes mellitus are independent of glycaemic control. *Thromb Haemost* 1994;72:979–984.
159. Jager A, van Hinsbergh VW, Kostense PJ, et al. Increased levels of soluble vascular cell adhesion molecule 1 are associated with risk of cardiovascular mortality in type 2 diabetes: the Hoorn study. *Diabetes* 2000;49:485–491.
160. Otsuki M, Hashimoto K, Morimoto Y, et al. Circulating vascular cell adhesion molecule-1 (VCAM-1) in atherosclerotic NIDDM patients. *Diabetes* 1997;46: 2096–2101.
161. Andre P, Hartwell D, Hrachovinova I, et al. Pro-coagulant state resulting from high levels of soluble P-selectin in blood. *Proc Natl Acad Sci U S A* 2000; 97:13835–13840.
162. Hamsten A, Walldius G, Szamosi A, et al. Plasminogen activator inhibitor in plasma: risk factor for recurrent myocardial infarction. *Lancet* 1987;2:3–9.
163. Paramo JA, Colucci M, Collen D. Plasminogen activator inhibitor in the blood of patients with coronary artery disease. *BMJ* 1985;291:573–574.
164. Wiman B, Hamsten A. Correlation between fibrinolytic function and acute myocardial infarction. *Am J Cardiol* 1990;66:54G–56G.
165. Gray RP, Patterson DL, Yudkin JS. Plasminogen activator inhibitor activity in diabetic and nondiabetic survivors of myocardial infarction. *Arterioscler Thromb* 1993;13:415–420.
166. Potter van Loon BJ, Kluft C, Radder JK, et al. The cardiovascular risk factor plasminogen activator inhibitor type 1 is related to insulin resistance. *Metabolism* 1993;42:945–949.
167. Juhan-Vague I, Jespersen TJ. Involvement of the hemostatic system in the insulin resistance syndrome. A study of 1500 patients with angina pectoris. *Arterioscler Thromb* 1993;13:1865–1873.
168. Landin K, Stigendal L, Eriksson E, et al. Abdominal obesity is associated with an impaired fibrinolytic activity and elevated plasminogen activator inhibitor-1. *Metabolism* 1990;39:1044–1048.
169. Juhan-Vague I, Alessi MC, Vague P. Increased plasma plasminogen activator inhibitor 1 levels. A possible link between insulin resistance and atherothrombosis. *Diabetologia* 1991;34:457–462.
170. Juhan-Vague I, Alessi MC, Joly P, et al. Plasma plasminogen activator inhibitor-1 in angina pectoris. Influence of plasma insulin and acute-phase response. *Atherosclerosis* 1989;9:362–367.
171. Vague P, Juhan-Vague I, Aillaud MF, et al. Correlation between blood fibrinolytic activity, plasminogen activator inhibitor level, plasma insulin level, and relative body weight in normal and obese subjects. *Metabolism* 1986;35: 250–253.
172. Landin K, Tensborn L, Smith U. Elevated fibrinogen and plasminogen activator inhibitor (PAI-1) in hypertension are related to metabolic factors for cardiovascular disease. *J Intern Med* 1990;227:273–278.
173. Jokl R, Laimins M, Klein RL, et al. Platelet plasminogen activator inhibitor 1 in patients with type II diabetes. *Diabetes Care* 1994;17:818–823.
174. Auwerx J, Bouillon R, Collen D, et al. Tissue-type plasminogen activator antigen and plasminogen activator inhibitor in diabetes mellitus. *Arteriosclerosis* 1988;8:68–72.
175. Koenig W, Sund M, Frohlich M, et al. C-reactive protein, a sensitive marker of inflammation, predicts future risk of coronary heart disease in initially healthy middle-aged men: results from the MONICA (Monitoring Trends and Determinants in Cardiovascular Disease) Augsburg Cohort Study, 1984 to 1992. *Circulation* 1999;99:237–242.
176. Ridker PM, Hennekens CH, Buring JE, et al. C-reactive protein and other markers of inflammation in the prediction of cardiovascular disease in women. *N Engl J Med* 2000;342:836–843.
177. Schalkwijk CG, Poland DC, van Dijk W, et al. Plasma concentration of C-reactive protein is increased in type I diabetic patients without clinical macroangiopathy and correlates with markers of endothelial dysfunction: evidence for chronic inflammation. *Diabetologia* 1999;42:351–357.
178. Festa A, D'Agostino RJ, Howard G, et al. Chronic subclinical inflammation as part of the insulin resistance syndrome: the Insulin Resistance Atherosclerosis Study (IRAS). *Circulation* 2000;102:42–47.
179. Torzewski M, Rist C, Mortensen RF, et al. C-reactive protein in the arterial intima: role of C-reactive protein receptor-dependent monocyte recruitment in atherogenesis. *Arterioscler Thromb Vasc Biol* 2000;20:2094–2099.
180. Pasceri V, Willerson JT, Yeh ET. Direct proinflammatory effect of C-reactive protein on human endothelial cells. *Circulation* 2000;102:2165–2168.
181. Cermak J, Key NS, Bach RR, et al. C-reactive protein induces human peripheral blood monocytes to synthesize tissue factor. *Blood* 1993;82:513–520.
182. Paul A, Ko KW, Li L, et al. Reactive protein accelerates the pression of atherosclerosis in apolipoprotein E-deficient mice. *Circulation* 2004;109:645–655.
183. Kannel WB, Wolf PA, Castelli WP, et al. Fibrinogen and risk of cardiovascular disease. The Framingham Study. *JAMA* 1987;258:1183–1186.
184. Howard BV, Cowan LD, Go O, et al. Adverse effects of diabetes on multiple cardiovascular disease risk factors in women. The Strong Heart Study. *Diabetes Care* 1998;21:1258–1265.
185. Stec JJ, Silbershatz H, Tofler GH, et al. Association of fibrinogen with cardiovascular risk factors and cardiovascular disease in the Framingham Offspring Population. *Circulation* 2000;102:1634–1638.
186. Meigs JB, Jacques PF, Selhub J, et al. Fasting plasma homocysteine levels in the insulin resistance syndrome: the Framingham offspring study. *Diabetes Care* 2001;24:1403–1410.
187. Hoogeveen EK, Kostense PJ, Jakobs C, et al. Hyperhomocysteinemia increases risk of death, especially in type 2 diabetes: 5-year follow-up of the Hoorn Study. *Circulation* 2000;101:1506–1511.
188. Soinio M, Marniemi J, Laakso M, et al. Elevated plasma homocystein level is an independent predictor of coronary heart disease events in patients with type 2 diabetes mellitus. *Ann Intern Med* 2004;140:94–1000.
189. Sung FL, Slow YL, Wang G, et al. Homocysteine stimulates the expression of monocyte chemoattractant protein-1 in endothelial cells leading to enhanced monocyte chemotaxis. *Mol Cell Biochem* 2001;216:121–128.
190. Khajuria A, Houston DS. Induction of monocyte tissue factor expression by homocysteine: a possible mechanism for thrombosis. *Blood* 2000;96:966–972.
191. Chao CL, Kuo TL, Lee YT. Effects of methionine-induced hyperhomocysteinemia on endothelium-dependent vasodilation and oxidative status in healthy adults. *Circulation* 2000;101:485–490.
192. Pavia C, Ferrer I, Valls C, et al. Total homocysteine in patients with type 1 diabetes. *Diabetes Care* 2000;23:84–87.
193. Cronin CC, McPartlin JM, Barry DG, et al. Plasma homocysteine concentrations in patients with type 1 diabetes. *Diabetes Care* 1998;21:1843–1847.
194. Steinberg HO, Chaker H, Leaming R, et al. Obesity/insulin resistance is associated with endothelial dysfunction. Implications for the syndrome of insulin resistance. *J Clin Invest* 1996;97:2601–2610.
195. Schachinger V, Britten MB, Zeiher AM. Prognostic impact of coronary vasodilator dysfunction on adverse long- term outcome of coronary heart disease. *Circulation* 2000;101:1899–1906.
196. Perticone F, Ceravolo R, Pujia A, et al. Prognostic significance of endothelial dysfunction in hypertensive patients. *Circulation* 2001;104:191–196.
197. UK Prospective Diabetes Study Group. Tight blood pressure control and risk of macrovascular and microvascular complications in type 2 diabetes: UKPDS 38. *BMJ* 1998;317:703–713.
198. Yusuf S, Sleight P, Pogue J, et al. Effects of an angiotensin-converting-enzyme inhibitor, ramipril, on cardiovascular events in high-risk patients. The Heart Outcomes Prevention Evaluation Study Investigators. *N Engl J Med* 2000;342: 145–153.
199. Isomaa B, Almgren P, Tuomi T, et al. Cardiovascular morbidity and mortality associated with the metabolic syndrome. *Diabetes Care* 2001;24:683–689.
200. Stern MP. Diabetes and cardiovascular disease: the "common soil" hypothesis. *Diabetes* 1995;44:369–374.
201. Hotamisligil GS, Peraldi P, Budavari A, et al. IRS-1-mediated inhibition of insulin receptor tyrosine kinase activity in TNF-α and obesity-induced insulin resistance. *Science* 1996;271:665–668.
202. Rajavashisth TB, Xu XP, Jovinge S, et al. Membrane type 1 matrix metalloproteinase expression in human atherosclerotic plaques: evidence for activation by proinflammatory mediators. *Circulation* 1999;99:3103–3109.
203. Goetze S, Xi XP, Kawano Y, et al. TNF-alpha-induced migration of vascular smooth muscle cells is MAPK dependent. *Hypertension* 1999;33:183–189.
204. Hansson L, Lindholm LH, Niskanen L, et al. Effect of angiotensin-converting-enzyme inhibition compared with conventional therapy on cardiovascular morbidity and mortality in hypertension: the Captopril Prevention Project (CAPPP) randomised trial. *Lancet* 1999;353:611–616.
205. Dresner A, Laurent D, Marcucci M, et al. Effects of free fatty acids on glucose transport and IRS-1-associated phosphatidylinositol 3-kinase activity. *J Clin Invest* 1999;103:253–259.
206. Pradhan AD, Manson JE, Rifai N, et al. C-reactive protein, interleukin 6, and risk of developing type 2 diabetes mellitus. *JAMA* 2001;286:327–334.
207. Barrett-Connor EL, Cohn BA, et al. Why is diabetes mellitus a stronger risk factor for fatal ischemic heart disease in women than in men? The Rancho Bernardo Study. *JAMA* 1991;265:627–631.
208. Walden CE, Knopp RH, Wahl PW, et al. Sex differences in the effect of diabetes mellitus on lipoprotein triglyceride and cholesterol concentrations. *N Engl J Med* 1984;311:953–959.
209. Steinberg HO, Paradisi G, Cronin J, et al. Type II diabetes abrogates sex differences in endothelial function in premenopausal women. *Circulation* 2000; 101:2040–2046.
210. Patricia MK, Kim JA, Harper CM, et al. Lipoxygenase products increase monocyte adhesion to human aortic endothelial cells. *Arterioscler Thromb Vasc Biol* 1999;19:2615–2622.
211. Hempel A, Maasch C, Heintze U, et al. High glucose concentrations increase endothelial cell permeability via activation of protein kinase C alpha. *Circ Res* 1997;81:363–371.
212. Ding Y, Vaziri ND, Coulson R, et al. Effects of simulated hyperglycemia, insulin, and glucagon on endothelial nitric oxide synthase expression. *Am J Physiol Endocrinol Metab* 2000;279:E11–E17.
213. Inoguchi T, Battan R, Handler E, et al. Preferential elevation of protein kinase C isoform beta II and diacylglycerol levels in the aorta and heart of diabetic rats: differential reversibility to glycemic control by islet cell transplantation. *Proc Natl Acad Sci U S A* 1992;89:11059–11063.
214. Igarashi M, Wakasaki H, Takahara N, et al. Glucose or diabetes activates p38 mitogen-activated protein kinase via different pathways. *J Clin Invest* 1999; 103:185–195.
215. Inoguchi T, Li P, Umeda F, et al. High glucose level and free fatty acid stimulate reactive oxygen species production through protein kinase C-dependent activation of NAD(P)H oxidase in cultured vascular cells. *Diabetes* 2000;49: 1939–1945.
216. Garcia SF, Virag L, Jagtap P, et al. Diabetic endothelial dysfunction: the role of poly(ADP-ribose) polymerase activation. *Nat Med* 2004;140:94–100.
217. Wakasaki H, Koya D, Schoen FJ, et al. Targeted overexpression of protein kinase C beta2 isoform in myocardium causes cardiomyopathy. *Proc Natl Acad Sci U S A* 1997;94:9320–9325.

218. Ishii H, Jirousek MR, Koya D, et al. Amelioration of vascular dysfunctions in diabetic rats by an oral PKC beta inhibitor. *Science* 1996;272:728–731.
219. Zhang Z, Apse K, Pang J, et al. High glucose inhibits glucose-6-phosphate dehydrogenase via cAMP in aortic endothelial cells. *J Biol Chem* 2000;275: 40042–40047.
220. Du XL, Edelstein D, Rossetti L, et al. Hyperglycemia-induced mitochondrial superoxide overproduction activates the hexosamine pathway and induces plasminogen activator inhibitor-1 expression by increasing Sp1 glycosylation. *Proc Natl Acad Sci U S A* 2000;97:12222–12226.
221. Yang X, Su K, Roos MD, et al. O-linkage of N-acetylglucosamine to Sp1 activation domain inhibits its transcriptional capability. *Proc Natl Acad Sci U S A* 2001;98:6611–6616.
222. Shinohara M, Thornalley PJ, Giardino I, et al. Overexpression of glyoxalase-I in bovine endothelial cells inhibits intracellular advanced glycation endproduct formation and prevents hyperglycemia-induced increases in macromolecular endocytosis. *J Clin Invest* 1998;101:1142–1147.
223. Zhang J, Ren S, Sun D, et al. Influence of glycation on LDL-induced generation of fibrinolytic regulators in vascular endothelial cells. *Arterioscler Thromb Vasc Biol* 1998;18:1140–1148.
224. Khechai F, Ollivier V, Bridey F, et al. Effect of advanced glycation end product-modified albumin on tissue factor expression by monocytes. Role of oxidant stress and protein tyrosine kinase activation. *Arterioscler Thromb Vasc Biol* 1997;17:2885–2890.
225. Schmidt AM, Hori O, Chen JX, et al. Advanced glycation endproducts interacting with their endothelial receptor induce expression of vascular cell adhesion molecule-1 (VCAM- 1) in cultured human endothelial cells and in mice. A potential mechanism for the accelerated vasculopathy of diabetes. *J Clin Invest* 1995;96:1395–1403.
226. Taguchi A, Blood DC, del Toro G, et al. Blockade of RAGE-amphotericin signalling suppresses tumour growth and metastases. *Nature* 2000;405:354–360.
227. Park L, Raman KG, Lee KJ, et al. Suppression of accelerated diabetic atherosclerosis by the soluble receptor for advanced glycation endproducts. *Nat Med* 1998;4:1025–1031.
228. King GL, Goodman AD, Buzney S, et al. Receptors and growth-promoting effects of insulin and insulinlike growth factors on cells from bovine retinal capillaries and aorta. *J Clin Invest* 1985;75:1028–1036.
229. Zeng G, Quon MJ. Insulin-stimulated production of nitric oxide is inhibited by wortmannin. *J Clin Invest* 1996;98:894–898.
230. Nordt TK, Sawa H, Fujii S, et al. Augmentation of arterial endothelial cell expression of the plasminogen activator inhibitor type-1 (PAI-1) gene by proinsulin and insulin in vivo. *J Mol Cell Cardiol* 1998;30:1535–1543.
231. Patel VA, Zhang QJ, Siddle K, et al. Defect in insulin-like growth factor-1 survival mechanism in atherosclerotic plaque-derived vascular smooth muscle cells is mediated by reduced surface binding and signaling. *Circ Res* 2001;88: 895–902.
232. Hermann C, Assmus B, Urbich C, et al. Insulin-mediated stimulation of protein kinase Akt: A potent survival signaling cascade for endothelial cells. *Arterioscler Thromb Vasc Biol* 2000;20:402–409.
233. Scherrer U, Randin D, Vollenweider P, et al. Nitric oxide release accounts for insulin's vascular effects in humans. *J Clin Invest* 1994;94:2511–2515.
234. Jiang ZY, Lin YW, Clemont A, et al. Characterization of selective resistance to insulin signaling in the vasculature of obese Zucker (fa/fa) rats. *J Clin Invest* 1999;104:447–457.
235. Oliver FJ, de la Rubia G, Feener EP, et al. Stimulation of endothelin-1 gene expression by insulin in endothelial cells. *J Biol Chem* 1991;266:23251–23256.
236. Folli F, Kahn CR, Hansen H, et al. Angiotensin II inhibits insulin signaling in aortic smooth muscle cells at multiple levels. A potential role for serine phosphorylation in insulin/angiotensin II crosstalk. *J Clin Invest* 1997;100:2158–2169.
237. Jiang ZY, Zhou QL, Chatterjee A, et al. Endothelin-1 modulates insulin signaling through phosphatidylinositol 3-kinase pathway in vascular smooth muscle cells. *Diabetes* 1999;48:1120–1130.
238. Kim F, Gallis B, Corson MA. TNF-alpha inhibits flow and insulin signaling leading to NO production in aortic endothelial cells. *Am J Physiol Cell Physiol* 2001;280:C1057–C1065.
239. Zeng G, Nystrom FH, Ravichandran LV, et al. Roles for insulin receptor, PI3-kinase, and Akt in insulin-signaling pathways related to production of nitric oxide in human vascular endothelial cells. *Circulation* 2000;101:1539–1545.
240. Abe H, Yamada N, Kamata K, et al. Hypertension, hypertriglyceridemia, and impaired endothelium-dependent vascular relaxation in mice lacking insulin receptor substrate-1. *J Clin Invest* 1998;101:1784–1788.
241. Kubota T, Kubota N, Moroi M, et al. Lack of insulin receptor substrate-2 causes progressive neointima formation in response to vessel injury. *Circulation* 2003;107:3073–3080.
242. Vicent D, Ilany J, Kondo T, et al. The role of endothelial insulin signaling in the regulation of vascular tone and insulin resistance. *J Clin Invest* 2003;111: 1373–1380.
243. Diet F, Pratt RE, Berry GJ, et al. Increased accumulation of tissue ACE in human atherosclerotic coronary artery disease. *Circulation* 1996;94:2756–2767.
244. Morishita R, Gibbons GH, Ellison KE, et al. Evidence for direct local effect of angiotensin in vascular hypertrophy. In vivo gene transfer of angiotensin converting enzyme. *J Clin Invest* 1994;94:978–984.
245. Feener EP, Northrup JM, Aiello LP, et al. Angiotensin II induces plasminogen activator inhibitor-1 and -2 expression in vascular endothelial and smooth muscle cells. *J Clin Invest* 1995;95:1353–1362.
246. Zuanetti G, Latini R, Maggioni AP, et al. Effect of the ACE inhibitor lisinopril on mortality in diabetic patients with acute myocardial infarction data from the GISSI-3 study. *Circulation* 1997;96:4239–4245.
247. Gustafsson I, Torp-Pedersen C, Kober L, et al. Effect of the angiotensin-converting enzyme inhibitor trandolapril on mortality and morbidity in diabetic patients with left ventricular dysfunction after acute myocardial infarction. Trace Study Group. *J Am Coll Cardiol* 1999;34:83–89.
248. Heart Outcomes Prevention Evaluation Study Investigators. Effects of ramipril on cardiovascular and microvascular outcomes in people with diabetes mellitus: results of the HOPE study and MICRO-HOPE substudy. *Lancet* 2000;355:253–259.
249. Tatti P, Pahor M, Byington RP, et al. Outcome results of the Fosinopril Versus Amlodipine Cardiovascular Events Randomized Trial (FACET) in patients with hypertension and NIDDM. *Diabetes Care* 1998;21:597–603.
250. Dagenais GR, Yusuf S, Bourassa MG, et al. Effects of ramipril on coronary events in high-risk persons: results of the Heart Outcomes Prevention Evaluation study. *Circulation* 2001;104:522–526.
251. Chen HC, Bouchie JL, Perez AS, et al. Role of the angiotensin AT(1) receptor in rat aortic and cardiac PAI-1 gene expression. *Arterioscler Thromb Vasc Biol* 2000;20:2297–2302.
252. Zaman AK, Fujii S, Sawa H, et al. Angiotensin-converting enzyme inhibition attenuates hypofibrinolysis and reduces cardiac perivascular fibrosis in genetically obese diabetic mice. *Circulation* 2001;103:3123–3128.

SECTION VII

Diabetic Complications: Clinical Aspects

CHAPTER 53
Diabetic Ketoacidosis and Hyperosmolar Hyperglycemic State

Jennifer Wyckoff and Martin J. Abrahamson

DEFINITIONS

Hyperosmolar hyperglycemic state (HHS) and diabetic ketoacidosis (DKA) represent two distinct metabolic derangements manifested by insulin deficiency and severe hyperglycemia. HHS occurs when insulin deficiency relative to insulin requirements causes hyperglycemia, which in turn leads to dehydration, ultimately resulting in a severe hyperosmolar state. DKA occurs in the setting of more severe insulin deficiency, when low circulating levels of insulin lead not only to hyperglycemia and dehydration but also to the production of ketone bodies and acidosis. DKA is defined as the presence of all three of the following: (i) hyperglycemia (glucose >250 mg/dL), (ii) ketosis, and (iii) acidemia (pH <7.3) (1). HHS is characterized by severe hyperglycemia and hyperosmolarity. HHS and DKA are not mutually exclusive but rather two conditions that both result from some degree of insulin deficiency. They can and often do occur simultaneously. In fact, one third of patients admitted for hyperglycemia exhibit characteristics of both HHS and DKA (2).

EPIDEMIOLOGY

In one of the largest studies of the epidemiology of DKA, Faich et al. (3) reported an annual incidence of DKA in Rhode Island of 46 cases per 10,000 persons with diabetes and of 1.4 cases per 10,000 persons in the general population. Nationally, DKA contributes to approximately 100,000 hospital admissions per year (1,4–6) and accounts for 2% to 9% of hospital admissions in persons with diabetes (1,3,7,8).

More than 20% of patients admitted for DKA had previously undiagnosed diabetes (3,9,10). Another 15% of admissions were of patients with multiple admissions for DKA (3). Several studies reported that the average age of patients admitted for DKA was 40 to 50 years (3,4), but that the risk decreased with age (10). Some studies have reported a female predominance (3,6, 9,10), possibly because young women were more likely to have repeated episodes of DKA (9,11). A slight increase in cases during the winter months has also been cited (3,9).

DKA is the leading cause of death of patients with diabetes who are younger than 24 years old, accounting for about one half of the deaths in this population group (5). Before the discovery of insulin in 1922, the mortality due to DKA was virtually 100% (12). By 1932, mortality decreased to 29% (12). By the 1950s, the reported mortality was 15%, with the improvement credited primarily to the widespread use of antibiotics, the introduction of intravenous potassium replacement, and the use of norepinephrine for blood pressure support (13). Mortality rates ranging from 2.5% to 9% among patients admitted with DKA have been reported in more recent studies (3,5,9,12). The studies reporting all-cause in-hospital mortality reported higher mortality rates than studies that reported mortality due to DKA alone and excluded deaths attributable to the factors that precipitated the DKA (11). Mortality among patients with DKA has been related to age, level of consciousness on admission, severity of acidosis, degree of hyperosmolarity, severity of azotemia, and nursing home residence (2,3,10). In addition to short-term mortality, there appears to be an increased risk of microvascular complications of diabetes with long-term follow-up of survivors of DKA (10).

One of the most interesting aspects of the epidemiologic study of hyperglycemic states is the epidemiology of DKA in various ethnic groups. In a retrospective chart review of adults with DKA admitted between 1994 and 1995 to a Texas hospital, 80% of whites admitted with DKA were classified as having type 1 diabetes (14). In contrast, only 53% of African Americans and 34% of Hispanic patients who were admitted with DKA had type 1 diabetes. By definition, patients who required insulin from the time of diagnosis of diabetes were considered to have type 1 diabetes, and patients who had prolonged treatment with either diet or oral hypoglycemic agents were considered to have type 2 diabetes. No difference was found in serum electrolytes, renal function, glucose, pH, anion gap, osmolality, or level of ketosis between those classified as having type 1 diabetes and those classified as having type 2 diabetes. Despite the conventional wisdom that DKA in type 2 diabetes usually is triggered by extreme physiologic stress, in the majority of these cases, no precipitating event could be identified.

PATHOPHYSIOLOGY

Understanding the clinical manifestations of DKA and HHS requires a thorough knowledge of the pathophysiology of these two closely related disturbances. In both DKA and HHS, relative insulin deficiency is the critical underlying defect. In both DKA and HHS, inadequate levels of circulating insulin relative to insulin requirements lead to hyperglycemia, which in turn leads to dehydration. Hyperglycemia can lead to progressive dehydration and hyperosmolarity and ultimately to HHS. If insulin deficiency is severe enough, ketosis and ultimately acidosis develop (Fig. 53.1).

Relative insulin deficiency—not absolute insulin deficiency—is necessary for the development of both DKA and HHS. Even patients with type 2 diabetes and "normal" insulin levels may develop DKA if the level of insulin resistance causes a large enough increase in insulin requirements. Insulin resistance is mediated by several factors, including the underlying pathophysiology of type 2 diabetes and an increase in the levels of counterregulatory hormones, including cortisol, glucagon, epinephrine, and growth hormone (Table 53.1).

There is an extensive literature exploring the relative importance of insulin deficiency and insulin resistance due to counterregulatory hormones to the development of DKA (15–24). The facts that the incidence of DKA has decreased dramatically since the introduction of insulin in the 1920s and that insulin administration is the mainstay of therapy for DKA demonstrate the central role of insulin deficiency in the development of DKA (15). Early studies supporting insulin deficiency as the primary cause of DKA demonstrated low levels of insulin or C-peptide or both in the face of hyperglycemia (15,16). Withdrawal of insulin from patients with type 1 diabetes results in hyperglycemia and increased levels of ketone bodies within a matter of hours, as well as in elevations in some counterregulatory hormones (17).

Despite this evidence, the impact of increased insulin resistance due to the counterregulatory hormones in the promotion of DKA and HHS must not be underestimated. Clinicians appreciate the increased risk of DKA that occurs with any physiologic stress in the patient with type 1 diabetes. Elevated levels of counterregulatory hormones have been observed during episodes of DKA (18–21). Furthermore, the severity of DKA appears to be decreased in conditions in which there is a deficiency of counterregulatory hormones (22,23).

Nevertheless, in the absence of insulin deficiency, elevated levels of counterregulatory hormones alone do not cause DKA. Gerich et al. (24) studied the effects of infusing counterregulatory hormones into insulin-dependent patients. Neither glucagon

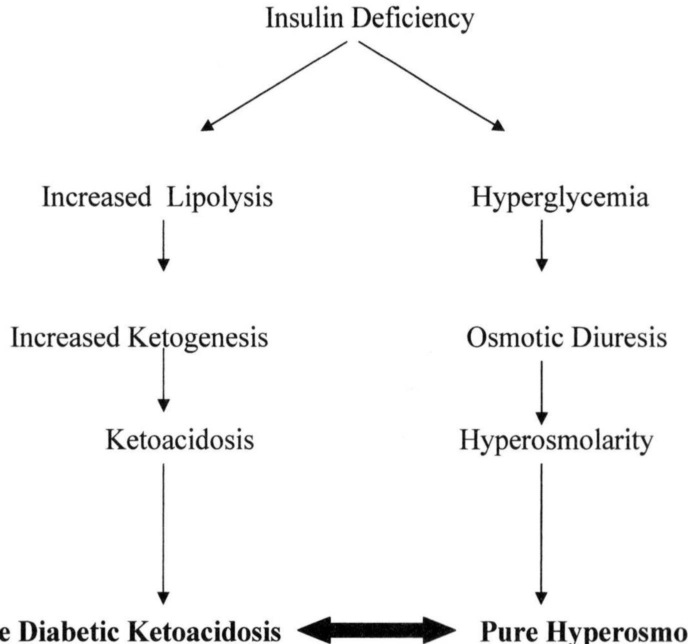

Figure 53.1. Hyperglycemic states.

TABLE 53.1. Regulation of Ketogenesis and Glucose Metabolism

	Ketogenesis	Gluconeogenesis	Glycogenolysis	Glycolysis	Glycogen synthesis
Insulin	↓	↓	↓	↑	↑
Glucagon	↑	↑	↑	↓	↓
Cortisol	↑	↑	↑	↓	↓
Growth hormone	↑	↑	↑	↓	↓
Catecholamines	↑	↑	↑	↓	↓

From Kreisberg R. Diabetic ketoacidosis. In: Rifkin H, Porte D, eds. *Diabetes mellitus: theory and practice*, 4th ed. New York: Elsevier Science, 1990:591–603.

infusion nor growth hormone infusion produced an elevation in free fatty acids or ketone bodies until insulin was withdrawn.

HYPERGLYCEMIA

Hyperglycemia occurs in both HHS and DKA. Hyperglycemia results from increased glucose production (gluconeogenesis and glycogenolysis) and decreased peripheral utilization (glycolysis, lipogenesis, and glycogen synthesis). Figure 53.2 gives an overview of these processes. Cox and Nelson (25) provide an excellent comprehensive review of the biochemistry involved in hyperglycemia.

Gluconeogenesis refers to the production of glucose from pyruvate or oxaloacetate. Glycolysis refers to the inverse—the breakdown of glucose to pyruvate. Glycolysis and gluconeogenesis utilize many, but not all, of the same enzymes; therefore, only one of these processes can occur in a tissue at any one time.

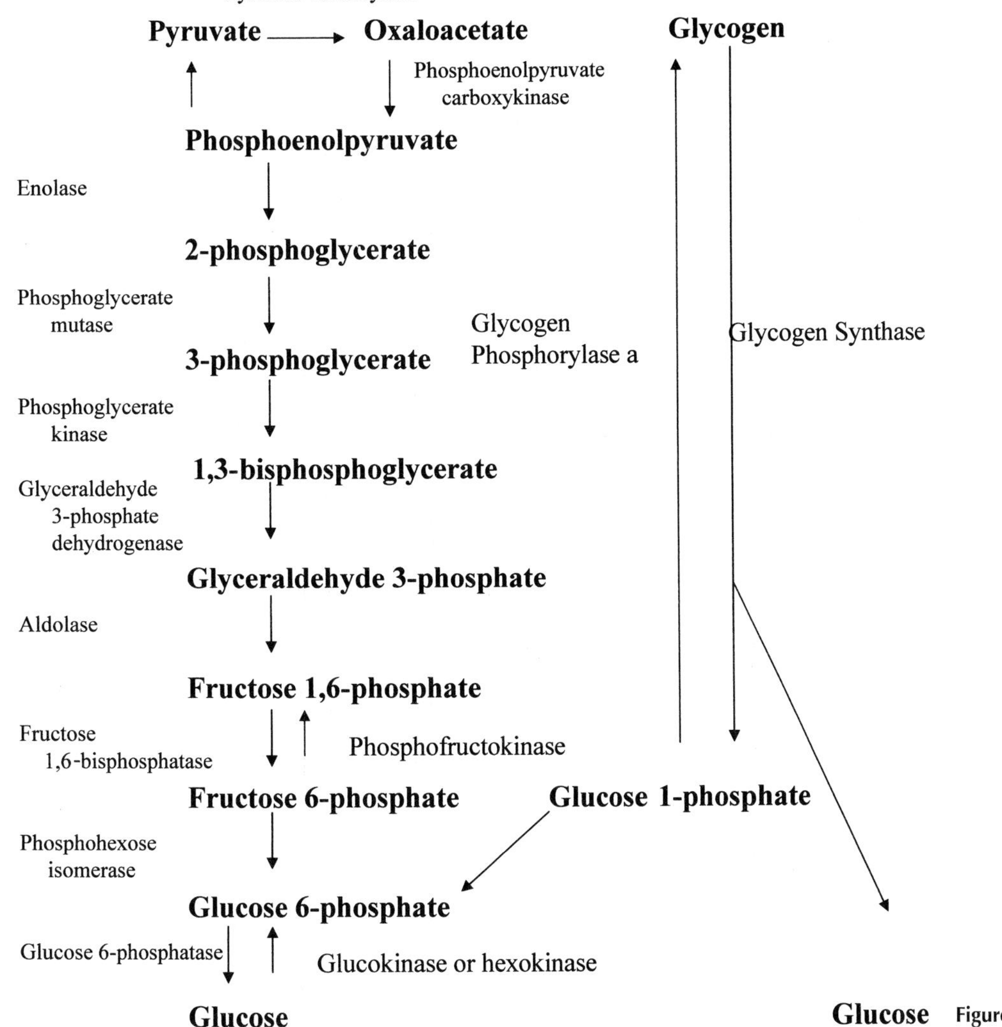

Figure 53.2. Ketogenesis.

Although the two pathways act in a reciprocal manner and share enzymes, each also utilizes unique enzymes. It is these unique enzymes that are critical to the control of these two pathways.

Gluconeogenesis occurs primarily in the liver. In this pathway, pyruvate is converted to oxaloacetate and then ultimately to glucose. The enzymes unique to gluconeogenesis are pyruvate carboxylase, fructose 1,6-bisphosphatase, and glucose 6-phosphatase. The pathway begins in the mitochondrion, where pyruvate is converted to oxaloacetate by pyruvate carboxylase, the first rate-limiting enzyme in the pathway. Pyruvate carboxylase is regulated by levels of acetyl-CoA (coenzyme A), which is required as a positive effector. Oxaloacetate is then reduced to malate by malate dehydrogenase and transported into the cytosol of the hepatocyte. There, malate is reoxidized into oxaloacetate. The oxaloacetate is then converted to phosphoenolpyruvate by phosphoenolpyruvate carboxykinase, another important enzyme in gluconeogenesis. Phosphoenolpyruvate is then converted to fructose 1,6-bisphosphate through a series of reactions catalyzed by enzymes shared with the glycolytic pathway.

Fructose 1,6-bisphosphate is converted to fructose 6-phosphate by another enzyme unique to gluconeogenesis, fructose 1,6-bisphosphatase. Next, fructose 6-phosphate is converted to glucose 6-phosphate by phosphohexose isomerase. Fructose 1,6-bisphosphatase is the second rate-limiting enzyme. It is induced by high levels of acetyl-CoA and suppressed by high levels of glucose 6-phosphate. Fructose 1,6-bisphosphatase is also regulated by fructose 2,6-bisphosphate. Fructose 2,6-bisphosphate is the regulator through which glucagon inhibits fructose 1,6-bisphosphatase. Glucose 6-phosphate is then dephosphorylated by glucose 6-phosphatase to glucose in the last rate-limiting step. The activity of this enzyme is suppressed by insulin.

Glycolysis occurs in cells throughout the body. The first step in the metabolism of glucose is entry of the glucose into the cytoplasm of the cell. Glucose uptake is largely insulin mediated, particularly in muscle and adipose tissue. Without insulin, cellular uptake and therefore glycolysis are greatly reduced. Once in the cytoplasm, glucose is phosphorylated by hexokinase (or glucokinase in the liver) into glucose 6-phosphate. This is the first rate-limiting step in glycolysis. Hexokinase is inhibited by its product, glucose 6-phosphate, and is induced by insulin.

Glucose 6-phosphate is converted to fructose 6-phosphate by phosphohexose isomerase. Then fructose 6-phosphate is converted to fructose 1,6-bisphosphate by phosphofructokinase-1. The activity of phosphofructokinase-1, the next rate-limiting enzyme, is regulated by glucagon through fructose 2,6-bisphosphate. Then, fructose 1,6-bisphosphate is converted through a series of reactions to phosphoenolpyruvate. In the last step, phosphoenolpyruvate is transformed by pyruvate kinase.

Glycogen synthesis and glycogenolysis occur primarily in liver and muscle. The key step in glycogenolysis is catalyzed by the enzyme glycogen phosphorylase a. Glycogen synthase is the key enzyme in glycogen synthesis. Glucagon and epinephrine act to inactivate glycogen synthase and activate glycogen phosphorylase, thereby inducing glycogenolysis and inhibiting glycogen synthesis.

DEHYDRATION AND HYPEROSMOLARITY

In both HHS and DKA, hyperglycemia results in an osmotic diuresis, which leads to dehydration. Hyperosmolarity develops, as the urine is relatively hypo-osmolar. Initially, the glycosuria causes an increase in the glomerular filtration rate. Once hypovolemia becomes significant, the glomerular filtration rate decreases and renal glucose losses may decrease as well. As renal clearance of glucose declines, hyperglycemia and hyperosmolarity worsen.

KETOGENESIS AND ACIDOSIS

Although the same mechanisms cause hyperglycemia and dehydration in both DKA and HHS, DKA is distinguished by ketogenesis (Fig. 53.3). Laffel (26) provides an excellent review of

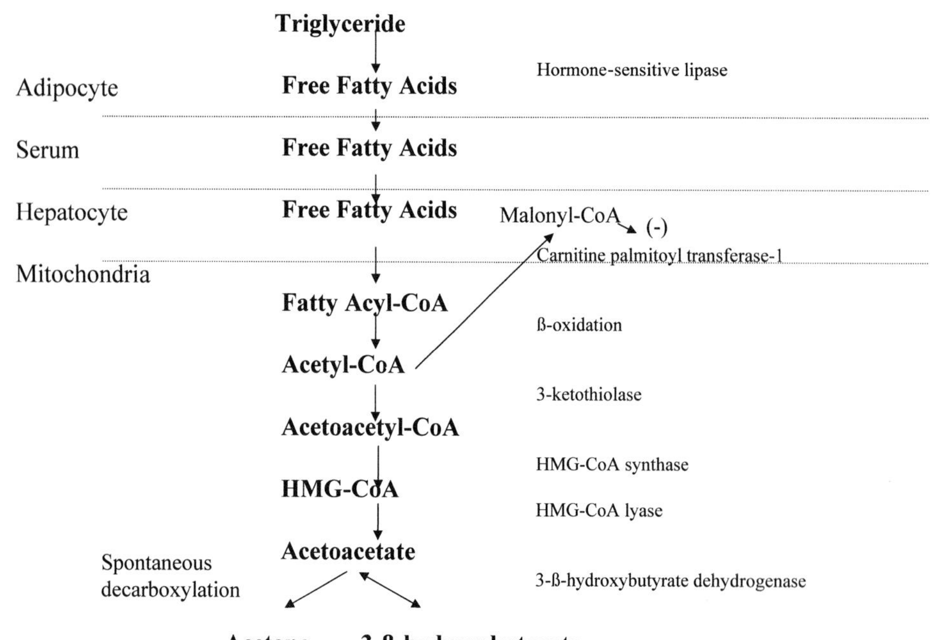

Figure 54.3. Glucose metabolism. HMG-CoA, hydroxymethylglutaryl–coenzyme A.

ketone metabolism. In the adipocyte, hormone-sensitive lipase converts triglycerides into diglycerides, which are then converted into free fatty acids. Hormone-sensitive lipase is stimulated by counterregulatory hormones and inhibited by insulin.

Free fatty acids are converted in the cytoplasm of the hepatocyte to fatty acyl-CoA. Fatty acyl-CoA is transported into the mitochondria of the hepatocyte by the carnitine shuttle. Glucagon inhibits the enzyme acetyl-CoA carboxylase, which leads to reduced levels of malonyl-CoA. Malonyl-CoA normally inhibits carnitine palmitoyl transferase-1 (CPT-1), the rate-limiting step in the carnitine shuttle (26). Once in the mitochondrion, the fatty acyl-CoA undergoes β-oxidation to acetyl-CoA. Acetyl-CoA is then converted in the mitochondrion to acetoacetate. The rate-limiting step is HMG-CoA (hydroxymethylglutaryl–coenzyme A) synthase. Acetoacetate, in turn, is then either spontaneously decarboxylated into acetone or converted to 3-β-hydroxybutyrate by 3-β–hydroxybutyrate dehydrogenase. Under normal circumstances, the ratio of 3-β-hydroxybutyrate to acetoacetate is about 1:1. Acetone is present in much lower quantities. In DKA, although levels of all three ketone bodies increase, the level of 3-β-hydroxybutyrate increases dramatically relative to that of acetoacetate, with ratios that may reach 10:1 (27).

Normally, ketone bodies increase insulin release from the pancreas; the insulin in turn suppresses ketogenesis. In the insulin-deficient state, the pancreatic β-cells are unable to respond, and ketogenesis proceeds unchecked.

Ketolysis occurs in the mitochondria of organs, which can use ketone bodies as an alternative energy source. Ketone bodies provide an important source of energy for the central nervous system during periods of starvation. However, skeletal muscle is probably the largest contributor to ketolysis. Acetoacetate is converted back to acetoacetyl-CoA by succinyl-CoA oxoacid transferase (SCOT). This is the rate-limiting step in ketolysis. Acetoacetyl-CoA is then converted to acetyl-CoA by methylacetoacetyl-CoA thiolase (MAT). Some ketones are also eliminated via the urine. Acetoacetate and 3-β-hydroxybutyrate are strong organic acids, which dissociate readily and account for the acidosis of DKA. Acetone does not dissociate and therefore does not worsen acidosis. It is excreted slowly via the lungs.

PRECIPITATING CAUSES OF DIABETIC KETOACIDOSIS AND HYPEROSMOLAR HYPERGLYCEMIC STATE

Infection remains the most common precipitating cause of DKA and HHS and accounts for 20% to 40% of all cases of DKA and HHS (28). The most common infections remain those of the urinary tract and lungs. Even though patients' caloric intake is decreased during intercurrent illness, most of them need to increase their insulin dose and fail to do so. Elderly patients with diabetes often neglect the increases in polyuria and polydipsia that are associated with increasing glucose concentrations during periods of intercurrent illness and present for medical attention at a more advanced stage of their illness. Up to 20% of individuals with newly diagnosed cases of type 1 diabetes, and even some with cases of type 2 diabetes, present with DKA. Some subjects with type 2 diabetes who present with DKA as the first manifestation of the disease are able to stop insulin and take oral antidiabetic agents once blood sugars have stabilized. Other precipitating causes of DKA and HHS include cerebrovascular accidents, myocardial infarction, pancreatitis, and alcohol abuse. These causes account for about 10% of all cases of DKA and HHS. Omission of insulin remains a common cause of DKA in the adolescent population, many of whom utilize this as an opportunity to control their weight (29). This is also a common cause of DKA in African Americans (30). Drugs also may precipitate DKA and HHS, with most frequent offenders being steroids, sympathomimetic agents (dobutamine and terbutaline), and thiazides. Recently, newer antipsychotic drugs (e.g., clozapine, olanzapine, and risperidone) have been associated with the development of hyperglycemia, and patients have presented with DKA as the first manifestation of their diabetes (31–37). Therapy with interferon-α and ribavirin has been associated with the development of DKA in a patient with hepatitis C (38). DKA has been reported in association with the use of protease inhibitors and pentamidine therapy, and recreational use of cocaine and "ecstasy" has also been reported to precipitate DKA (39–43). In some patients, no obvious precipitating cause can be found.

DIAGNOSIS

History and Physical Examination

DKA usually evolves over a shorter period (usually less than 24 hours) than HHS, which tends to evolve over a few days. The symptoms of uncontrolled diabetes may be present for a number of days prior to the development of the acute metabolic decompensation. In some situations, e.g., in patients with type 1 diabetes who are using continuous subcutaneous insulin infusion pumps with regular insulin or short-acting insulin analogues, the symptoms of DKA can evolve much more rapidly—over 4 to 12 hours—if insulin delivery is disrupted. The pathophysiologic consequences of hyperglycemia, hyperketonemia, and insulin deficiency account for many of the classic symptoms and physical findings seen in DKA and HHS. High glucose levels lead to an osmotic diuresis, dehydration, and ultimately hypotension. The high ketone concentrations are responsible for the metabolic acidosis and also cause an osmotic diuresis because the renal threshold for ketones is low and ketones are osmotically active substances. The anionic charge on the ketones leads to excretion of positively charged ions, including sodium, potassium, calcium, and magnesium, to maintain electrical neutrality. The high solute excretion further impairs reabsorption of water from the renal tubule and loop of Henle, resulting in further loss of water and electrolytes. Insulin per se promotes reabsorption of water and sodium from the renal tubules. Insulin deficiency promotes further loss of water and electrolytes. The average amounts of electrolytes and fluids lost in patients with DKA are shown in Table 53.2. Losses of potassium and phosphate are further exacerbated by the acidosis, which leads to loss of intracellular potassium and phosphate. This may complicate therapy (see below). Ketone production by the liver leads to the metabolic acidosis. Hyperglycemia leads to an increase in serum osmolality, which in

TABLE 53.2. Average Fluid and Electrolyte Losses in Diabetic Ketoacidosis and Hyperosmolar Hyperglycemic State

Sodium	500 mEq
Chloride	350 mEq
Potassium	300–1000 mEq
Calcium	50–100 mmol
Phosphate	50–100 mmol
Magnesium	25–50 mmol

turn causes a further shift of fluid out of cells and leads to intracellular dehydration (44,45).

On the basis of the above pathophysiology, patients with DKA and HHS present with increasing polyuria and polydipsia, loss of weight, nausea, vomiting, increasing malaise, and dehydration. Patients with HHS tend to be more dehydrated at the time of presentation than patients with DKA. Abdominal pain is a common symptom in patients with DKA and may be due to the ketosis per se (with no evidence of intraabdominal pathology) or sometimes may be related to the cause of DKA. Fever is often present but may be absent even in the presence of infection because of the vasodilation that accompanies a metabolic acidosis. Patients may be alert at the time of presentation, but changes in mental status are common and may vary from drowsiness to coma. It is important to inquire about symptoms of the precipitating cause of the acute metabolic decompensation, such as symptoms of a urinary tract infection; the presence of cough, fever, or chills; the recent introduction of new medications; or chest pain. All women of reproductive age should be asked about possible pregnancy and have a pregnancy test at the time of presentation.

On examination, patients usually are dehydrated and have evidence of Kussmaul respiration if there is underlying acidosis. Assessment of the degree of dehydration is important. Decreased tissue turgor suggests 5% dehydration. An orthostatic change in pulse alone suggests that there has been loss of approximately 10% of extracellular fluid volume (~2 L), whereas an orthostatic change in pulse and blood pressure (>15/10 mm Hg) suggests a 15% to 20% fluid deficit (3 to 4 L). Supine hypotension, when present, suggests either severe dehydration and a decrease in extracellular fluid volume of more than 20% or underlying sepsis. Assessment of degree of dehydration may be difficult in the elderly and those with underlying autonomic neuropathy, who may have orthostatic hypotension at baseline. Fever may be present in those who have an underlying infection. The absence of fever, however, does not rule out infection—acidosis is associated with vasodilation and may lead to hypothermia. Hypothermia is an ominous finding and represents a poor prognostic sign. At the time of presentation, patients may be alert or have various degrees of change in mental status, ranging from drowsiness to stupor to coma. The level of consciousness correlates more closely with the underlying serum osmolality than with the degree of acidemia. Up to 25% of patients with DKA and HHS complain of vomiting at the time of presentation. Some of these patients have acute gastritis and may be vomiting brown-colored fluid or blood when they are seen in the emergency department. Diffuse abdominal pain and tenderness may be present. It is important to differentiate this as a manifestation of DKA from other causes of acute abdominal pain that may have precipitated the acute metabolic illness. Neck stiffness may be present even in the absence of underlying meningitis. When underlying meningeal infection is a possibility, examination of the CSF is essential. Examination for signs of the precipitating illness is important; this includes thorough examination of the skin, throat, and chest for infection. Table 53.3 summarizes the important clinical features that need to be reviewed when assessing a patient with severe hyperglycemia.

TABLE 53.3. Initial Evaluation of the Patient with Suspected Diabetic Ketoacidosis and Hyperosmolar Hyperglycemic State

- History of diabetes, medications, and symptoms
- History of diabetes-related complications
- Utilization of medications
- Social and medical history (including alcohol use)
- Vomiting and ability to take fluids by mouth
- Identify precipitating event leading to elevated glucose (pregnancy, infection, omission of insulin, myocardial infarction, central nervous system event)
- Assess hemodynamic status
- Examine for presence of infection
- Assess volume status and degree of dehydration
- Assess presence of ketonemia and acid–base disturbance

Laboratory Investigations

Initial laboratory evaluations of the patient with DKA or HHS must include plasma glucose, electrolytes, blood urea nitrogen (BUN) and creatinine, CO_2, serum and urine ketones, calculation of the anion gap, arterial blood gas (for DKA), complete blood count and differential, and electrocardiogram. Cultures of urine, blood, and throat should be done if clinically indicated, and a chest radiograph should be obtained if there is any concern about an underlying cardiopulmonary problem. Measurement of glycosylated hemoglobin (HbA_{1C}) may provide information about the underlying degree of metabolic control. The initial laboratory investigations that should be performed on patients with DKA or HHS are summarized in Table 53.4.

The serum sodium level may be low or normal. It may even be elevated in patients who are severely dehydrated even though total body sodium is depleted. The acidosis leads to a shift of potassium out of the cells. Serum potassium levels at presentation may be high, normal, or low even though total body potassium may be depleted. Unless the initial serum potassium is elevated above 5.5 mEq/L or the patient is in acute renal failure or oliguric, potassium replacement is required when treatment is initiated, because resolution of the acidosis will lead to cellular reuptake of potassium and the potential for hypokalemia and the risk of cardiac arrhythmia.

Calculations for determining the effective serum osmolality and anion gap are presented in Table 53.5. As noted above, the level of consciousness correlates more closely with serum osmolality than with pH (45). Coma in an individual whose serum osmolality is less than 320 mOsm/kg warrants further evaluation for other causes of the coma.

Serum amylase and lipase levels may be elevated even in the absence of pancreatitis. In a recent study, serum amylase and lipase levels were nonspecifically elevated in 16% to 25% of cases of DKA (46). The cause of this elevation is not known.

TABLE 53.4. Laboratory Evaluation of the Patient with Suspected Diabetic Ketoacidosis and Hyperosmolar Hyperglycemic State

- SMA 7
- Complete blood count
- Serum ketones
- Calculate serum osmolality and anion gap based on glucose and clinical findings
- Measure osmolar gap if ingestion of osmotically active substances other than glucose suspected
- Urinalysis and urine culture
- Consider blood culture
- Consider chest radiograph
- Consider measuring HCG
- Acid–base assessment if indicated by clinical findings
- HbA_{1c}

HCG, human chorionic gonadotropin; HbA_{1c}, glycosylated hemoglobin.

TABLE 53.5. Commonly Used Calculations in the Evaluation of Patients with Severe Hyperglycemia

- Calculation of effective serum osmolality:

$$2[\text{Na} + \text{K}] + \frac{(\text{glucose in mg/dL})}{18} + \frac{\text{BUN}}{2.8} + \frac{\text{ETOH}}{4.6}$$

- Calculation of the anion gap:

$$[\text{Na}] - [\text{Cl} + \text{HCO}_3]$$

- Correction of serum sodium:

$$\text{Corrected Na} = [\text{Na}] + 1.6 \times \frac{[\text{glucose in mg/dL}] - 100}{100}$$

- Uncomplicated metabolic acidosis:

$$\Delta \text{ anion gap}: \Delta \text{ bicarbonate} = 1$$

- Metabolic acidosis and metabolic alkalosis:

$$\Delta \text{ anion gap}: \Delta \text{ bicarbonate} = <1$$

BUN, blood urea nitrogen; ETOH = ethyl alcohol.

Although serum lipase measurement is more specific for the diagnosis of pancreatitis, this is not true in DKA, and elevations of either amylase or lipase to more than three times normal do not confirm the diagnosis of pancreatitis in these situations. It should be noted, too, that coexisting acute pancreatitis may be present in 10% to 15% of patients with DKA (47).

Leukocytosis may occur in DKA in the absence of infection, thereby making it more difficult to diagnose infection. The mechanism for this finding is not clearly understood.

Differential Diagnosis

Other causes of ketoacidosis need to be considered when patients with diabetes present with ketosis. These include starvation ketosis and alcoholic ketoacidosis. Starvation does not usually cause acidosis. Pregnant patients are more likely to develop ketoacidosis due to starvation because pregnancy is associated with an accelerated state of starvation and lipolysis and ketogenesis may be more accentuated and start within 6 hours of fasting (48). Alcohol may be associated with ketoacidosis. In this condition, plasma glucose levels are not always elevated. Serum ketones as measured by the nitroprusside reaction are not always significantly positive, because there is increased production of β-hydroxybutyrate in alcoholic ketosis and this is not measured in the nitroprusside reaction.

Other causes of an anion gap metabolic acidosis need to be considered in the differential diagnosis of DKA. These include lactic acidosis, uremia, and drugs (salicylates, methanol, ethylene glycol, and paraldehyde). Table 53.6 summarizes the salient findings in patients with other causes of ketosis and an anion gap acidosis.

Unusual Clinical and Laboratory Findings

Although the majority of people presenting with DKA and HHS have plasma glucose levels above 250 mg/dL, some patients may have lower plasma glucose levels at the time of presentation. "Euglycemic ketoacidosis" was originally described in situations in which the plasma glucose concentration was less than 300 mg/dL and the plasma bicarbonate concentration was 10 mEq/L or lower, but serum glucose levels lower than this have been reported (49). Euglycemic ketoacidosis has been reported in patients using continuous subcutaneous insulin infusion pumps, which contain short-acting insulin (regular- or short-acting analogues lispro or aspart). In these patients, interruption of insulin delivery results in the rapid development of ketosis, as patients become profoundly insulin deficient within 2 to 4 hours of cessation of insulin delivery. Euglycemic DKA has also been reported during pregnancy and in subjects using "conventional" insulin regimens (50,51). In these patients, the excretion of larger amounts of glucose in the urine or lower rates of hepatic glucose production may account for the relatively "normal" glucose concentrations. These patients are usually alert and, if they are not vomiting, can sometimes be managed with frequent administration of subcutaneous insulin rather than intravenous insulin infusions (see below).

Serum ketones may be negative in some situations, such as alcoholic ketoacidosis or DKA associated with hypoxia. In

TABLE 53.6. Differential Diagnosis of Ketosis and Anion Gap Acidosis

	Starvation ketosis	Pregnancy ketosis	Diabetic ketoacidosis	Alcoholic ketoacidosis	Lactic acidosis	Uremic acidosis	Salicylate intoxication	Methanol or ethylene glycol ingestion
pH	Normal	Normal or decreased	Decreased	Decreased	Decreased	Slight decrease	Decreased or increased	Decreased
Plasma glucose	Normal	Normal or increased	Increased	Normal	Normal	Normal	Normal	Normal
Anion gap	Normal	Normal to increased	Increased	Increased	Increased	Increased	Increased	Increased
Serum ketones	Slight increase	Slight increase	Increased	Normal to increased[a]	Normal to slight increase	Normal	Normal	Normal
Serum osmolality	Normal	Normal	Increased	Normal	Normal	Increased	Normal	Increased markedly Measure serum levels

[a]β-hydroxybutyrate is increased.

these circumstances, the nitroprusside reaction fails to detect β-hydroxybutyrate, which is the dominant ketone present. Under "normal" conditions, the ratio of β-hydroxybutyrate to acetoacetate is 3:1. This increases to 8:1 in alcoholic ketoacidosis or DKA associated with severe hypoxia.

Serum creatinine may be spuriously elevated in DKA; the ketones interfere with the measurement of creatinine when measured by the alkaline picrate (Jaffe) assay, resulting in a falsely elevated level (51). Treatment of the ketoacidosis leads to resolution of the problem.

Although the most common acid–base disturbance seen in DKA is an uncomplicated, partially compensated metabolic acidosis, other abnormalities of acid–base status may occur (52). These can range from a hyperchloremic acidosis (associated with no anion gap) to a metabolic alkalosis associated with vomiting. In the typical patient with DKA, the increase in the anion gap (ΔAG) is usually equivalent to the decrease in the serum bicarbonate concentration (ΔCO_2). The ratio of the ΔAG to ΔCO_2 (Δ:Δ ratio) is equal to 1 in uncomplicated DKA. Hyperchloremic acidosis may occur at any stage during the course of DKA but is more likely to occur during treatment with fluids that include saline. Loss of ketoanions in the urine is associated with a decrease in the serum bicarbonate concentration. During treatment, large amounts of fluid and NaCl are administered. Chloride is reabsorbed to maintain electrical neutrality. This may lead to excess chloride and a hyperchloremic acidosis, which is associated with a normal anion gap. The Δ:Δ ratio in this situation is not equal to 1 (44). Excessive vomiting in DKA may lead to excess loss of hydrogen ions and a metabolic alkalosis, which is characterized by a decrease in the chloride concentration and a normal serum bicarbonate level. Once again the Δ:Δ ratio is not equal to 1 (see Table 53.5) (53,54).

TREATMENT

Treatment of both DKA and HHS is based on correcting the underlying pathophysiologic defects, correcting the fluid and electrolyte imbalance, normalizing the blood glucose, correcting the acid–base disturbance, treating the precipitating cause, and determining what factors need to be addressed to prevent a recurrence. The fluid and electrolyte abnormalities are treated with saline, water, and potassium; the hyperglycemia is treated with insulin; and the acidosis is treated with insulin and sometimes bicarbonate.

Fluids

Fluid and electrolyte losses are considerable in most patients with DKA or HHS. Initially, fluid replacement is aimed at correcting the volume deficit rather than restoring serum osmolality to normal. Restoration of intravascular volume lowers blood sugar (independent of insulin) and decreases the counterregulatory hormones, improving insulin sensitivity. Normal saline (osmolar concentration, 308 mOsm/kg) is recommended for initial fluid therapy. Even though this fluid is isotonic, it is relatively hypotonic compared with the osmolality of the patient's serum. If the patient is in shock or has an inadequate blood pressure response to normal saline, colloid may sometimes be used together with normal saline (55). The initial rate of fluid administration depends on the degree of volume depletion and the patient's underlying cardiac status and ranges from 2 to 4 L during the first hour of therapy to 1 L per hour (15 to 20 mL/kg per hour). There is some debate concerning the optimal time to change from normal saline to 0.45% normal saline. Once the corrected sodium is normal or elevated and most of the initial volume deficit is replaced, most clinicians would change treatment to 0.45% normal saline. The rate of fluid replacement must take into account ongoing urinary losses and be administered at a rate that will correct the fluid deficits in 24 hours (56). Osmolality should be corrected at a rate of approximately 3 mOsm/kg per hour. Once serum glucose has dropped to less than 250 mg/dL, dextrose-containing fluids should be used (5% dextrose in 0.45% saline) and the insulin infusion rate adjusted to maintain blood glucose levels in the 120 to 180 mg/dL range.

Fluids are administered to children at a rate of 10 to 20 mL/kg per hour during the first hour of treatment, usually not exceeding 50 mL/kg during the first 4 hours of therapy. The rate of fluid replacement is calculated so that the fluid deficit is replaced over 48 hours. Too-rapid correction of the fluid deficit or osmolality does not appear to increase the risk for the development of cerebral edema, a rare but devastating complication of DKA, which is more common in children (57).

Potassium replacement is started as soon as the initial serum potassium is known, providing that it is less than 5.5 mEq/L and the patient is passing urine and not in acute renal failure. Guidelines for fluid correction are provided in Table 53.7.

Insulin

For many years there has been debate about the optimal method and dose of insulin administration for patients with DKA or HHS. There is clear evidence that patients with DKA are insulin resistant and require supraphysiologic doses of insulin to ensure suppression of lipolysis and hepatic gluconeogenesis. Intravenously administered insulin has a half-life of 4 to 5 minutes, whereas regular insulin administered via the intramuscular or subcutaneous route has a half-life of ~2 or 4 hours, respectively.

After the discovery of insulin, patients with DKA were treated with small, frequent doses of intravenous or intramuscular insulin, but this soon gave way to "high-dose" bolus insulin therapy. It was later realized that even "low" doses of insulin administered by intravenous infusion (doses of 4 to 8 units per hour) were sufficient to suppress lipolysis and hepatic gluconeogenesis by 100% and were associated with serum insulin levels of approximately 100 μU/mL, concentrations significantly higher than those in the average nondiabetic person. Large doses of insulin given intravenously intermittently

TABLE 53.7. Suggested Fluid Replacement in Patients with Diabetic Ketoacidosis and Hyperosmolar Hyperglycemic State[a]

Administer NS as indicated to maintain hemodynamic status, then follow general guidelines:

- NS for first 4 hr.
- Consider half NS thereafter.
- Change to D5 half NS when blood glucose ≤250 mg/dL.

Hours	Volume
1st half-hour to 1 hour	1 L
2nd hr	1 L
3rd hr	500 mL–1 L
4th hr	500 mL–1 L
5th hr	500 mL–1 L
Total 1st 5 hr	3.5–5 L
6th–12th hr	250–500 mL/hr

[a]May need to adjust type and rate of fluid administration in the elderly and in patients with congestive heart failure or renal failure.
NS, normal saline; D5, 5% dextrose in water.

TABLE 53.8. Guidelines for Insulin Management in Diabetic Ketoacidosis and Hyperosmolar Hyperglycemic State

- Regular insulin 10 U i.v. stat (for adults) or 0.15 U/kg i.v. stat.
- Start regular insulin infusion 0.1 U/kg per hour or 5 U per hour.
- Increase insulin by 1 U per hour every 1–2 hr if less than 10% decrease in glucose or no improvement in acid–base status.
- Decrease insulin by 1–2 U per hour (0.05–0.1 U/kg per hour) when glucose ≤250 mg/dL and/or progressive improvement in clinical status with decrease in glucose of >75 mg/dL per hour.
- Do not decrease insulin infusion to <1 U per hour.
- Maintain glucose between 140 and 180 mg/dL.
- If blood sugar decreases to <80 mg/dL, stop insulin infusion for no more than 1 hr and restart infusion.
- If glucose drops consistently to <100 mg/dL, change i.v. fluids to D10 to maintain blood glucose between 140 and 180 mg/dL.
- Once patient is able to eat, consider change to s.c. insulin:

  Overlap short-acting insulin s.c. and continue i.v. infusion for 1–2 hr.
  For patients with previous insulin dose: return to prior dose of insulin.
  For patients with newly diagnosed diabetes: full-dose s.c. insulin based on 0.6 U/kg per day.

every hour lead to much higher peak insulin levels that wane within approximately 30 minutes of the administration of insulin and result in minimal biologic effects for at least 15 minutes every hour. Thus, continuous infusion of "low-dose" insulin has become the standard of treatment in most medical centers. Such treatment is associated with fewer metabolic complications (i.e., hypoglycemia, hypokalemia, hypophosphatemia, hypomagnesemia, hyperlactatemia, and osmotic dysequilibrium) than is therapy with large, intermittent doses. Intermittent low-dose intramuscular insulin (5 units) given every hour or every 2 hours after an initial intramuscular loading dose of 20 units is also acceptable treatment for DKA, especially in centers where it is difficult to monitor low-dose intravenous infusions, and is associated with serum insulin levels of 60 to 90 μU/mL. With this treatment regimen, the initial decline in glucose is usually not as rapid as with intravenous insulin. Subcutaneous insulin can also be used in DKA, but because it takes longer to achieve peak insulin concentrations, it is associated with a less rapid initial decline in glucose concentrations and may cause late hypoglycemia more frequently than intramuscular insulin.

Therefore, for the majority of patients, insulin is given simultaneously with intravenous fluids, starting with an intravenous loading dose of 0.15 U/kg body weight (usually 10 U in adults), followed by a continuous infusion of insulin at a rate of 0.1 U/kg per hour (usually 5 to 7 U per hour in adults) (58). If the patient is in shock or the initial serum potassium level is less than 3.3 mEq/L, resuscitation with intravenous fluids or potassium replacement or both is instituted before commencing the insulin infusion. An insulin infusion of 5 to 7 U per hour should lower serum glucose concentrations by 50 to 75 mg/dL per hour and is usually sufficient to inhibit lipolysis, stop ketogenesis, and suppress hepatic gluconeogenesis (59–67). The insulin infusion rate should be continually reassessed and increased if the rate of decrease in glucose is less than 50 mg/dL per hour, providing that other causes for the lack of response to therapy have been excluded. These include worsening of the acidosis and inadequate hydration. Once the serum glucose has decreased to less than 250 mg/dL, the rate of infusion may often be decreased to 0.05 to 0.1 U/kg per hour until the patient is able to take fluids and food by mouth. At this stage, a subcutaneous insulin regimen can be commenced, ensuring that the intravenous infusion is continued for at least 1 to 2 hours after the subcutaneous administration of short-acting insulin. Recommendations for insulin administration are summarized in Table 53.8.

Milder forms of DKA and HHS can be treated with subcutaneous or intramuscular insulin. Comparison of intravenous, subcutaneous, and intramuscular regimens for treatment of mild DKA has shown no significant difference in outcomes except for a more rapid decrease in ketones and glucose during the first 2 hours of treatment with intravenous insulin (68–74).

Potassium

Most patients with DKA and HHS have already lost considerable amounts of potassium at the time of presentation. Despite this, total body losses of serum potassium may be low, normal, or elevated (75,76). Intracellular dehydration and the metabolic acidosis lead to intracellular depletion of potassium, which is largely an intracellular cation. Correction of the fluid deficit and acidosis in combination with insulin therapy leads to a shift of potassium back into the cells and a decrease in the serum potassium concentration. To prevent hypokalemia, potassium supplementation is started if the initial serum potassium is less than 5.5 mEq/L and urine output is adequate. Guidelines for potassium replacement are shown in Table 53.9. Usually 20 to 30 mEq of potassium is added to each liter of fluid. Some authors prefer to use potassium chloride, and others use two-thirds potassium chloride and one-third potassium phosphate. Larger concentrations of potassium are used if the serum potassium drops below 3.5 mEq/L. If the initial serum potassium is less than 3.3 mEq/L, potassium replacement is required before initiating the insulin infusion, which is started only when the potassium has risen to above 3.5 mEq/L.

Bicarbonate

The serum insulin concentrations achieved with the low-dose insulin infusion during treatment of DKA usually are sufficient to suppress lipolysis and reverse ketogenesis. In most situations, treatment with insulin results in resolution of the acid–base abnormality. No studies to date have shown any benefit of bicarbonate therapy in patients with DKA whose pH is between 6.9 and 7.1 (77–79). Severe acidosis, however, is associated with a number of adverse vascular effects, including hypotension, decreased cardiac output, decreased peripheral vascular resistance, increased pulmonary arterial resistance, bradycardia, and arrhythmias. It also causes renal and mesenteric ischemia, cerebral vasodilatation, increased cerebrospinal

TABLE 53.9. Guidelines for Potassium Replacement in Diabetic Ketoacidosis and Hyperosmolar Hyperglycemic State

- Do not administer potassium if serum potassium >5.5 mEq/L or patient is anuric.
- Use KCl but alternate with KPO_4 if there is severe phosphate depletion and patient is unable to take phosphate by mouth.
- Add i.v. potassium to each liter of fluid administered unless contraindicated.

Serum K (mEq/L)	Additional K required
<3.5	40 mEq/L
3.5–4.5	20 mEq/L.
4.5–5.5	10 mEq/L
>5.5	Stop K infusion

fluid pressure, and coma; decreases the buffer reserve considerably; and also may increase insulin resistance (80). Potential adverse effects of bicarbonate therapy, on the other hand, include an overshoot alkalosis, paradoxical cerebrospinal fluid acidosis, hypokalemia, volume overload, alteration in tissue oxygenation, and overproduction of ketoacids. Thus, treatment with bicarbonate should be considered only in patients whose pH is less than 7.0 unless some of the adverse clinical manifestations of acidemia are present. Usually 100 mL of sodium bicarbonate is mixed with 400 mL sterile water and administered at a rate of 200 mL per hour intravenously. The venous pH should be checked 30 minutes later and treatment repeated if the pH remains below 7.0 (Table 53.10).

Phosphate

Phosphate depletion is common in DKA and HHS. Intracellular phosphate is lost, and renal phosphate excretion is increased. During treatment with insulin, phosphate is taken up intracellularly with resultant hypophosphatemia (81). Hypophosphatemia is associated with a number of clinical sequelae, including decreased cardiac output, respiratory muscle weakness, rhabdomyolysis, central nervous system depression, seizures and coma, acute renal failure, and hemolysis. Intravenous phosphate therapy may lead to hypocalcemia. Thus, the degree of phosphate replacement and type of phosphate treatment required in DKA and HHS remain controversial. Most studies have not shown any obvious benefit of routine phosphate replacement in DKA (82). Phosphate replacement, therefore, should be reserved for those with severe hypophosphatemia of 1.5 mg/dL or less and in whom serum calcium concentrations are normal. The use of small amounts of potassium phosphate with potassium chloride given intravenously appears to be safe and effective. Oral phosphate repletion is always preferable to intravenous repletion and should be commenced as soon as patients are able to take food by mouth.

TABLE 53.10. Guidelines for Bicarbonate Therapy in Diabetic Ketoacidosis

- Use clinical judgment in deciding if bicarbonate therapy is indicated.
- If pH is <7.0, give 100 mL $NaHCO_3$ over 45 min.
- Check acid–base status 30 min later and repeat if pH remains <7.0.

Ongoing Monitoring

Successful management of DKA and HHS requires frequent clinical and laboratory reassessment. Blood glucose should be checked hourly (either fingerstick capillary blood glucose or venous plasma glucose), and electrolytes and acid–base status should be reviewed every 2 to 4 hours as indicated. Measurement of venous pH is acceptable for those in whom there is no need to assess arterial P_{O_2} or P_{CO_2}. The venous pH is approximately 0.03 unit less than the arterial pH (83). BUN and creatinine should be checked every 4 hours. Frequent measurement of serum or urine ketones is usually not necessary, providing that the patient is responding to treatment. During treatment of the acidosis, β-hydroxybutyrate is converted to acetoacetate, which may result in an apparent increase in the ketone concentration. Thus, frequent measurement of ketones (measuring acetoacetate) may be misleading. Bedside patient blood ketone testing that measures β-hydroxybutyrate has recently become available. Measurement of the rate of decline of β-hydroxybutyrate with this technique may facilitate treatment (84). Use of a flow chart documenting clinical status (blood pressure, intake and output of fluids, and level of consciousness if indicated), serum glucose, electrolytes, and anion gap is recommended. An example of a flow chart is shown in Table 53.11. If pneumonia is suspected and the initial chest radiograph shows no evidence of consolidation, a repeat chest radiograph should be performed after at least 4 L of fluid has been administered. Pregnancy testing should be considered for women of reproductive age because of the potential deleterious consequences of DKA and uncontrolled diabetes on fetal well-being.

Once the patient is able to tolerate oral fluids and start eating, the shift from intravenous to subcutaneous insulin should be undertaken. When changing to subcutaneous insulin, the intravenous infusion of insulin should be continued for 1 to 2 hours after the subcutaneous insulin has been administered, and the dextrose infusion should be continued until the patient has eaten a meal. The initial dose of subcutaneous insulin should contain some short- or rapid-acting insulin. Stopping the insulin infusion for more than 30 to 60 minutes without administering short- or rapid-acting subcutaneous insulin should be avoided because the half-life of intravenous insulin is 2 to 4 minutes and ketoacidosis may recur rapidly in the absence of exogenous insulin.

Complications of Therapy

Hypoglycemia and hypokalemia remain common complications of therapy. Both can be avoided by ensuring appropriate glucose and potassium administration as recommended earlier

TABLE 53.11. Suggested Flow Chart for Use in Management of Diabetic Ketoacidosis/Hyperosmolar Hyperglycemic State

Date Time	Mental status	Blood pressure	Pulse	Glucose	Na	K	Cl	HCO_3	Ca	PO_4	Anion gap	Ketones	Blood gas	Insulin dose units/hr	IV fluids	Urine output

in the chapter. Hypophosphatemia may occur during therapy. There are no data supporting the use of intravenous potassium phosphate routinely during treatment of DKA and HHS. Intravenous phosphate should be given judiciously, but oral phosphate repletion should commence as soon as the patient is able to tolerate food and fluids by mouth. Persistent acidosis that does not respond to therapy may be caused by hypophosphatemia, sepsis, and inadequate insulin administration.

Hyperchloremia and hyperchloremic acidosis may occur during treatment of DKA. Chloride losses are less than sodium losses during DKA. Because replacement solutions have equal parts of sodium and chloride, relative hyperchloremia will occur during treatment. This is usually of no clinical consequence, and normalization of the anion gap during treatment with persistent reduction of bicarbonate is not an unexpected finding during the course of treatment.

Hypocalcemia may occur during treatment, especially during therapy with phosphate. Serum calcium levels should be checked before phosphate supplementation is started.

Pulmonary edema or respiratory distress syndrome or both may occur during treatment of DKA and HHS. Elderly patients are at risk for this complication, which may be caused by excessive fluid replacement, left ventricular dysfunction, or a capillary leak syndrome. Ongoing assessment of oxygen saturation and fluid balance, sometimes with invasive hemodynamic monitoring, is critical during treatment.

Cerebral edema is a rare complication of treatment of DKA. Clinically significant cerebral edema is more likely to occur in children, affecting approximately 1% of all children with DKA, but it is very rare in adults (85). Children at risk for the development of cerebral edema include those with lower P_{CO_2} and high BUN concentrations at presentation, those whose serum sodium level rises more slowly during therapy, and those who require bicarbonate therapy. The rate of fluid administration and rate of decline of glucose concentrations do not appear to be associated with the development of cerebral edema in children (57). Sudden deterioration of level of consciousness in a child being treated for DKA should arouse clinical suspicion for cerebral edema. Hyperosmolar therapy remains the treatment of choice for these situations.

Venous thrombosis and pulmonary embolism are rare "complications" of DKA and HHS (85). Patients presenting with dehydration and electrolyte imbalance are in a hypercoagulable state. Prophylaxis for venous thromboembolism should be considered in those most at risk, including the elderly and obese patients.

PREVENTION

DKA and HHS are preventable disorders. Infection and inadequate insulin administration (inappropriate reduction or omission of insulin and noncompliance with insulin regimens) remain the most common causes of DKA and HHS. Patient education and 24-hour access to advice and care remain the cornerstone of preventative therapy. Patients should be taught how to manage their diabetes during periods of stress or intercurrent infection ("sick-day" rules) and should understand the importance of frequent monitoring of blood glucose concentrations, urine ketones, temperature, and, if necessary, blood pressure, pulse, and weight during these times. They should have access to healthcare providers who are trained to manage diabetes during these periods and who are familiar with guidelines for referral to an emergency department, should home management be unsuccessful or should vomiting develop. Education programs have been shown to reduce the rate of episodes and admissions for DKA in susceptible groups of patients.

The elderly patient living in a nursing home, who is unable to keep up with fluid losses or is unaware of fluid losses during intercurrent illness, is particularly at risk for the development of HHS. Education of caregivers who should learn to recognize signs and symptoms of increasing hyperglycemia will reduce the incidence of severe HHS. These people should also know when to increase the frequency of blood glucose monitoring in those at risk and should have access to specialty care if indicated.

REFERENCES

1. Kitabchi A, Umpierraz G, Murphy M, et al. Management of hyperglycemic crises in patients with diabetes. *Diabetes Care* 2001;24:131–153.
2. Wachtel T, Tetu-Mouradjian L, Goldman D, et al. Hyperosmolarity and acidosis in diabetes mellitus: a three year experience in Rhode Island. *J Gen Intern Med* 1991;6:495–502.
3. Faich G, Fishbein H, Ellis S. The epidemiology of diabetic acidosis: a population-based study. *Am J Epidemiol* 1983;117:551–558.
4. Kreisberg R. Diabetic ketoacidosis. In: Rifkin H, Porte D, eds. *Diabetes mellitus: theory and practice*, 4th ed. New York: Elsevier Science, 1990:591–603.
5. White N. Diabetic ketoacidosis in children. *Endocrinol Metab Clin North Am* 2001;29:657–682.
6. Javor K, Kotsanos J, McDonald R, et al. Diabetic ketoacidosis charges relative to medical charges of adult patients with type I diabetes. *Diabetes Care* 1997;20: 349–354.
7. Murphy C, Faulkenberry E, Rumpel J, et al. The use of county hospital emergency room by diabetic patients. *Diabetes Care* 1985;8:48–51.
8. Scott R, Brown L, Clifford P. Use of health services by diabetic persons. II. Hospital admissions. *Diabetes Care* 1985;8:43–47.
9. Ellemann K, Soerensen J, Pedersen L, et al. Epidemiology and treatment of diabetic ketoacidosis in community population. *Diabetes Care* 1984;7:528–532.
10. Johnson D, Palumbo P, Chu C. Diabetic ketoacidosis in a community-based population. *Mayo Clin Proc* 1980;55:83–88.
11. DeFronzo R, Matsuda M, Barrett E. Diabetic ketoacidosis: a combined metabolic-nephrologic approach to therapy. *Diabetes Rev* 1984;2:209–238.
12. Kitabchi AE, Fisher JN, Murphy MB, et al. Diabetic ketoacidosis and the hyperglycemic, hyperosmolar nonketotic state. In: Kahn CR, Weir GC, eds. *Joslin's diabetes mellitus*, 13th ed. Philadelphia: Lippincott Williams & Wilkins, 1994:739–765.
13. Skillman T, Wilson R, Knowles H. Mortality of patients with diabetic acidosis in a large city hospital. *Diabetes* 1958;7:109–113.
14. Balasubramanyam A, Zern J, Hyman D, et al. New profiles of diabetic ketoacidosis. Type I vs type 2 diabetes and effect of ethnicity. *Arch Intern Med* 1999;159:2317–2322.
15. Schade D, Eaton R. Pathogenesis of diabetic ketoacidosis: a reappraisal. *Diabetes Care* 1979;2:296–306.
16. Chupin M, Charbonnel B, Chupin F. C-peptide blood levels in keto-acidosis and in hyperosmolar non-ketotic diabetic coma. *Acta Diabetol Lat* 1981;18: 123–128.
17. Matteri R, Murphy M, Kitabachi A. Metabolic dysfunction during pump withdrawal in brittle diabetics. *Diabetes* 1982;31:68A(abst).
18. Schade D, Eaton R, Standefer J. Glucocorticoid regulation of plasma ketone body concentration in insulin deficient man. *J Clin Endocrinol Metab* 1977;44: 1069–1079.
19. Alberti K, Hockaday T. Diabetic coma: serum growth hormone before and during treatment. *Diabetologia* 1973;9:13–19.
20. Muller W, Faloona G, Unger R. Hyperglucagonemia in diabetic ketoacidosis: its prevalence and significance. *Am J Med* 1973;54:52–57.
21. Christiansen N. Plasma norepinephrine and epinephrine in untreated diabetics during fasting and after insulin administration. *Diabetes* 1974;23:1–8.
22. Barnes A, Bloom S, Alberti K, et al. Ketoacidosis in the pancreatectomized man. *N Engl J Med* 1977;296:1250–1253.
23. Barnes A, Kohner E, Bloom S, et al. Importance of pituitary hormones in the aetiology of diabetic ketoacidosis. *Lancet* 1978;1:1171–1174.
24. Gerich J, Lorenzi M, Bier D, et al. Effects of physiologic levels of glucagon and growth hormone on human carbohydrate and lipid metabolism: studies involving administration of exogenous hormone during suppression of endogenous hormone secretion of somatostatin. *J Clin Invest* 1976;57:875–974.
25. Cox M, Nelson D. Glycolysis and the catabolism of hexoses. In: *Lehninger principles of biochemistry*, 3rd ed. New York: Worth, 2000:527–566.
26. Laffel L. Ketone bodies: a review of physiology, pathophysiology and application of monitoring to diabetes. *Diabetes Metab Res Rev* 1999;15:412–426.
27. Cox M, Nelson D. Carbohydrate biosynthesis. In: *Lehninger principles of biochemistry*, 3rd ed. New York: Worth, 2000:722–733.
28. Polonsky W, Anderson B, Lohrer P, et al. Insulin omission in women with IDDM. *Diabetes Care* 1994;17:1178–1185.
29. Musey V, Lee J, Crawford R, et al. Diabetes in urban African-Americans. I. Cessation of insulin therapy is the major precipitating cause of diabetic ketoacidosis. *Diabetes Care* 1995;18:483–489.
30. Wirshing D, Spellberg B, Erhart S, et al. Novel antipsychotics and new onset diabetes. *Soc Biol Psychiatry* 1998;44:778–783.
31. Selva K, Scott S. Diabetic ketoacidosis associated with olanzapine in an adolescent patient. *J Pediatr* 2001;138:936–938.
32. Croarkin P, Jacobs K, Bain B. Diabetic ketoacidosis associated with risperidone treatment? *Psychosomatics* 2000;41:369–370.
33. Goldstein L, Sporn J, Brown S, et al. New-onset diabetes mellitus and diabetic ketoacidosis associated with olanzapine treatment. *Psychosomatics* 1999;40: 438–443.
34. Gatta B, Rigalleau V, Gin H. Diabetic ketoacidosis with olanzapine treatment. *Diabetes Care* 1999;22:1002–1003.
35. Ai D, Roper T, Riley J. Diabetic ketoacidosis and clozapine. *Postgrad Med J* 1998;74:493–494.
36. Lindenmayer J, Patel R. Olanzapine-induced ketoacidosis with diabetes mellitus. *Am J Psychiatry* 1999;156:1471.
37. Bhatti A, McGarrity T, Gabbay R. Diabetic ketoacidosis induced by alpha interferon and ribavirin treatment in a patient with hepatitis C. *Am J Gastroenterol* 2001;96:604–605.
38. Besson C, Jubault V, Viard J, et al. Ketoacidosis associated with protease inhibitor therapy. *AIDS* 1998;12:1399–1400.
39. Kan V, Nylen E. Diabetic ketoacidosis in an HIV patient: a new mechanism of HIV protease inhibitor-induced glucose intolerance. *AIDS* 1999;13:1987–1989.
40. Lu C, Wu H, Chuang L, et al. Pentamidine-induced hyperglycemia and ketosis in acquired immunodeficiency syndrome. *Pancreas* 1995;11:315–316.
41. Warner E, Greene G, Buchsbaum M, et al. Diabetic ketoacidosis associated with cocaine use. *Arch Intern Med* 1998;158:1799–1802.
42. Seymour H, Gilman D, Quin J. Severe ketoacidosis complicated by 'ecstasy' ingestion and prolonged exercise. *Diabet Med* 1996;13:908–909.
43. Fulop M, Tannenbaum H, Dreyer N. Ketotic hyperosmolar coma. *Lancet* 1973; 22:635–639.
44. Yadav D, Nair S, Norkus E, et al. Nonspecific hyperamylasemia and hyperlipasemia in diabetic ketoacidosis: incidence and correlation with biochemical abnormalities. *Am J Gastroenterol* 2000;95:3123–3128.
45. Nair S, Yadav D, Pitchumoni C. Association of diabetic ketoacidosis and acute pancreatitis: observations in 100 consecutive episodes of DKA. *Am J Gastroenterol* 2000;95:2795–2800.
46. Mahoney C. Extreme gestational starvation ketoacidosis: case report and review of pathophysiology. *Am J Kidney Dis* 1992;20:276–280.
47. Munro J, Campbell I, McCuish A, et al. Euglycaemic diabetic ketoacidosis. *BMJ* 1973;9:578–580.
48. Franke B, Carr D, Hatem M. A case of euglycaemic diabetic ketoacidosis in pregnancy. *Diabet Med* 2001;18:858–859.
49. De P, Child D. Euglycaemic diabetic ketoacidosis—is it on the rise? *Pract Diab Int* 2001;18:239–240.
50. Kemperman F, Weber J, Gorgels J, et al. The influence of ketoacids on plasma creatinine assays in diabetic ketoacidosis. *J Intern Med* 2000;248:511–517.
51. Adrogue HJ, Wilson H, Boyd AE 3rd, et al. Plasma acid-base patterns in diabetic ketoacidosis. *N Engl J Med* 1982;307:1603–1610.
52. Cronin J, Kroop S, Diamond J, et al. Alkalemia in diabetic ketoacidosis. *Am J Med* 1984;77:192–194.
53. Jimenez J, Daminano A, Fernandez E, et al. Metabolic alkalosis in diabetic ketosis. *JAMA* 1975;233:1193–1194.
54. Hillman K. Fluid resuscitation in diabetic emergencies—a reappraisal. *Intensive Care Med* 1987;13:4–8.
55. Adrogue H, Barrero J, Eknoyan G. Salutary effects of modest fluid replacement in the treatment of adults with diabetic ketoacidosis. Use in patients without extreme volume deficit. *JAMA* 1989;262:2108–2113.
56. Gebara B. Risk factors for cerebral edema in children with diabetic ketoacidosis. *N Engl J Med* 2001;344:1556.
57. Alberti K. Low-dose insulin in the treatment of diabetic ketoacidosis. *Arch Intern Med* 2001;137:1367–1376.
58. Harrower A. Treatment of diabetic ketoacidosis by direct addition of insulin to intravenous infusion. A comparison of "high dose" and "low dose" techniques. *Br J Clin Pract* 1079;33:85–86.
59. Fort P, Waters S, Lifshitz F. Low-dose insulin infusion in the treatment of diabetic ketoacidosis: bolus versus no bolus. *J Pediatr* 1980;96:36–40.
60. Piters K, Kumar D, Pei E, et al. Comparison of continuous and intermittent intravenous insulin therapies for diabetic ketoacidosis. *Diabetologia* 1977;13: 317–321.
61. Butkiewicz E, Leibson C, O'Brien P, et al. Insulin therapy for diabetic ketoacidosis. Bolus insulin injection versus continuous insulin infusion. *Diabetes Care* 1995;18:1187–1190.
62. Kitabchi A. Low-dose insulin therapy in diabetic ketoacidosis: fact or fiction? *Diabetes Metab Rev* 1989;5:337–363.
63. Morris L, Kitabchi A. Efficacy of low-dose insulin therapy for severely obtunded patients in diabetic ketoacidosis. *Diabetes Care* 1980;3:53–56.
64. Genuth S. Constant intravenous insulin infusion in diabetic ketoacidosis. *JAMA* 1973;223:1348–1351.
65. Semple P, White C, Manderson W. Continuous intravenous infusion of small doses of insulin in treatment of diabetic ketoacidosis. *BMJ* 1974;2:694–698.
66. Kitabchi A, Fisher J, Matteri R, et al. The use of continuous insulin delivery systems in treatment of diabetes mellitus. *Adv Intern Med* 1983;28:449–490.
67. Kitabchi A, Ayyagari V, Guerra S. The efficacy of low-dose versus conventional therapy of insulin for treatment of diabetic ketoacidosis. *Ann Intern Med* 1976;84:633–638.
68. Heber D, Molitch M, Sperling M. Low-dose continuous insulin therapy for diabetic ketoacidosis. Prospective comparison with "conventional" insulin therapy. *Arch Intern Med* 1977;137:1377–1380.
69. Martin A, Martin M. Continuous infusion of insulin vs repeated S.C. injections in the treatment of diabetic ketoacidosis in children. *Acta Diabetol Lat* 1978;15: 81–87.
70. Fisher J, Shahshahani M, Kitabchi A. Diabetic ketoacidosis: low-dose insulin therapy by various routes. *N Engl J Med* 1977;297:238–241.
71. Sacks H, Shahshahani M, Kitabchi A, et al. Similar responsiveness of diabetic ketoacidosis to low-dose insulin by intramuscular injection and albumin-free infusion. *Ann Intern Med* 1979;90:36–42.
72. Alberti K, Hockaday T, Turner R. Small doses of intramuscular insulin in the treatment of diabetic "coma." *Lancet* 1973;2:515–522.

73. Drop S, Duval-Arnould J, Gober A, et al. Low-dose intravenous insulin infusion versus subcutaneous insulin injection: a controlled comparative study of diabetic ketoacidosis. *Pediatrics* 1977;59:733–738.
74. Beigelman P. Potassium in severe diabetic ketoacidosis. *Am J Med* 1973;54:419–420.
75. Adrogue H, Lederer E, Suki W, et al. Determinants of plasma potassium levels in diabetic ketoacidosis. *Medicine* (Baltimore) 1986;65:163–172.
76. Morris L, Murphy M, Kitabchi A. Bicarbonate therapy in severe diabetic ketoacidosis. *Ann Intern Med* 1986;105:836–840.
77. Viallon A, Zeni F, Lafond P, et al. Does bicarbonate therapy improve the management of severe diabetic ketoacidosis? *Crit Care Med* 1999;27:2690–2693.
78. Gamba G, Oseguera J, Castrejon M, et al. Bicarbonate therapy in severe diabetic ketoacidosis. A double blind, randomized, placebo controlled trial. *Rev Invest Clin* 1991;43:234–238.
79. Kraut J, Kurtz I. Use of base in the treatment of severe acidemic states. *Am J Kidney Dis* 2001;38:703–727.
80. Bohannon N. Large phosphate shifts with treatment for hyperglycemia. *Arch Intern Med* 1989;149:1423–1425.
81. Fisher J, Kitabchi A. A randomized study of phosphate therapy in the treatment of diabetic ketoacidosis. *J Clin Endocrinol Metab* 1983;57:177–180.
82. Brandenburg M, Dire D. Comparison of arterial and venous blood gas values in the initial emergency department evaluation of patients with diabetic ketoacidosis. *Ann Emerg Med* 1998;31:459–465.
83. Wallace T, Meston N, Gardner S, et al. The hospital and home use of a 30-second hand-held blood ketone meter: guidelines for clinical practice. *Diabet Med* 2001;18:640–645.
84. Edge J, Hawkins M, Winter D, et al. The risk and outcome of cerebral oedema developing during diabetic ketoacidosis. *Arch Dis Child* 2001;85:16–22.
85. Quigley R, Curran R, Stagl R, et al. Management of massive pulmonary thromboembolism complicating diabetic ketoacidosis. *Ann Thorac Surg* 1994;57:1322–1324.

CHAPTER 54

Ocular Complications of Diabetes Mellitus[1]

Lloyd M. Aiello, Lloyd Paul Aiello, and Jerry D. Cavallerano

> Ocular complications in diabetes are frequent, distressing and destined to become one of the challenging problems of the future.

These prophetic words of Dr. Howard Root opened the chapter on ocular complications in the 1935 edition of Joslin's *The Treatment of Diabetes Mellitus* (1). Indeed, as insulin increased the life span of persons with diabetes, diabetic retinopathy became a major cause of severe visual loss in the United States and in other industrialized countries of Europe and the Americas. By the 1960s, diabetic retinopathy was recognized as the leading cause of new, severe visual loss in the United States among persons 21 to 74 years old. Diabetic retinopathy is still neither preventable nor curable.

Dedicated efforts by researchers and patients, however, have established treatment and surgical modalities that can reduce the 5-year risk of severe visual loss (visual acuity 5/200 or worse) from proliferative diabetic retinopathy (PDR) to less than 2% and the 5-year risk of moderate visual loss (a doubling of the visual angle; e.g., 20/20 reduced to 20/40) from diabetic macular edema to 12% or less.

Ongoing research efforts continue to hold promise that diabetic retinopathy eventually will be curable or preventable. Presently, however, clinical goals must concentrate on identifying eyes at risk of visual loss and ensuring that appropriate and timely laser surgery is offered. If patients with diabetes receive currently recommended care, remarkable preservation of vision can be achieved.

SIGNIFICANCE OF APPROACHING/REACHING HIGH-RISK PROLIFERATIVE DIABETIC RETINOPATHY AND CLINICALLY SIGNIFICANT MACULAR EDEMA

In 1969, the first evidence of the effectiveness of scatter (panretinal) laser photocoagulation surgery in the treatment of dia-

[1]The reports of the Early Treatment Diabetic Retinopathy Study (17–39), which form the basis of the discussion of diabetic retinopathy, and other key retinopathy studies are widely quoted and paraphrased and set the standards of care for patients with diabetic retinopathy. Frequently used terms and abbreviations are given in Table 54.1. Portions of this chapter appear in *Principles and Practices of Ophthalmology: The Harvard System*, 2nd ed. Philadelphia: WB Saunders, 2000, and the *Journal of the American Optometric Association* 1990;61:533–543.

TABLE 54.1. Abbreviations of Commonly Used Terms

CSME	Clinically significant macular edema
DRS	Diabetic Retinopathy Study
DRVS	Diabetic Retinopathy Vitrectomy Study
ETDRS	Early Treatment Diabetic Retinopathy Study
FPD	Fibrous proliferations on or within 1 disc diameter of disc margin
FPE	Fibrous proliferations elsewhere—not FPD
H/Ma	Hemorrhages and/or microaneurysms
HE	Hard exudates
IRMA	Intraretinal microvascular abnormalities
MVL	Moderate visual loss: a doubling of the visual angle (e.g., 20/40 to 20/80 at two consecutive, completed 4-month follow-up visits)
NPDR	Nonproliferative diabetic retinopathy
NVD	Neovascularization of the disc: new vessels on or within 1 disc diameter of disc margin
NVE	Neovascularization elsewhere: new vessels elsewhere in the retina outside of disc and more than 1 disc diameter from disc margin
PDR	Proliferative diabetic retinopathy
SE	Soft exudates (cotton-wool spots)
SVL	Severe visual loss: visual acuity equal to or less than 5/200 at two consecutive, completed 4-month follow-up visits
VB	Venous beading

betic retinopathy was promulgated in the ophthalmologic and medical communities (2). Since these promising beginnings, dramatic strides have been made in treating diabetic retinopathy and macular edema through the effective use of scatter (panretinal) laser and other surgical techniques. The value of these techniques has received strong support from the findings of three major nationwide, randomized, and controlled clinical trials in the United States: the Diabetic Retinopathy Study (DRS) (3–16), the Early Treatment Diabetic Retinopathy Study (ETDRS) (17–39), and the Diabetic Retinopathy Vitrectomy Study (DRVS) (40–44). With proper diagnosis and treatment, the 5-year risk of severe visual loss from PDR could be virtually eliminated. Additionally, clinical trials in the United States (45–52), Japan (53), and the United Kingdom (54,55) have demonstrated that intensive control of diabetes, as measured by glycosylated hemoglobin (HbA_{1c}) levels, can reduce the risk of onset and progression of diabetic retinopathy.

Nevertheless, diabetic retinopathy remains a leading cause of blindness in the United States for persons between the ages of 20 and 74 years (56–58). This blindness usually results from nonresolving vitreous hemorrhage, traction retinal detachment, or diabetic macular edema. However, the 5-year risk of severe visual loss can be reduced to less than 2% if a person with diabetic retinopathy approaching or just reaching high-risk proliferative retinopathy, as defined below, undergoes scatter (panretinal) laser photocoagulation surgery (59,60). Furthermore, people with clinically significant diabetic macular edema (CSME) can reduce the risk of moderate visual loss by 50% or more, to approximately 12% or less, if they receive appropriate focal laser surgery (17). Because diabetic retinopathy is often asymptomatic in its most treatable stages, early detection of diabetic retinopathy through regularly scheduled ocular examination is critical.

This chapter reviews prognostic implications of the lesions of diabetic retinopathy and the risks of progression of retinopathy, placing particular emphasis on identifying patients at risk of visual loss and in need of laser surgery. The laser treatment techniques are described in only general terms in this chapter but are carefully detailed in ETDRS reports 3 and 4 (19,20). Nonretinal ocular complications of diabetes mellitus and alterations in visual function also are discussed.

EPIDEMIOLOGY OF DIABETIC RETINOPATHY

An estimated 16 to 17 million Americans have diabetes mellitus (diabetes), but approximately 6 million of these cases have not been diagnosed (61). Among the American population with diabetes, 5% to 10% have type 1 diabetes (insulin-dependent diabetes), which is usually diagnosed before the age of 40 years. The majority of diabetic patients, however, have type 2 diabetes (non–insulin-dependent diabetes), which is usually diagnosed after the age of 40 years; these patients may or may not be treated with insulin. While those with type 1 diabetes experience a high incidence of severe ocular complications and are more likely to develop significant ocular problems during their lifetimes, those with type 2 diabetes account for the majority of clinical cases of diabetic eye disease because of their larger overall number.

TABLE 54.2. Medical Problems Presenting Significant Risk for Development of Diabetic Retinopathy or Affecting Its Course

Condition	Comment
RISK INDICATORS OF DIABETIC RETINOPATHY	
Joint contractures	Association of retinopathy and contractures has been established. Eye examination is indicated. Care of joint contractures is important.
Neuropathy	Peripheral neuropathy may result in difficulty in handling contact lenses. Neuropathy in lower extremities may alter mobility; therefore, restoration and maintenance of as much vision as possible is important.
CONDITIONS THAT MAY AFFECT COURSE OF DIABETIC RETINOPATHY	
Hypertension	Appropriate medical treatment is indicated for prevention of cardiovascular disease, stroke, and death. Hypertension itself may result in hypertensive retinopathy superimposed on diabetic retinopathy.
Elevated lipids	Appropriate management to normalize lipids is important. Proper diet and drug treatment may result in less retinal vessel leakage and hard exudate.
Proteinuria; elevated creatinine level	Aggressive management of renal disease is indicated to avoid renal retinopathy, which may increase risk of progression of diabetic retinopathy and of neovascular glaucoma.
Cardiovascular disease	Increased risk of peripheral vascular disease, particularly coronary vascular disease, is often associated with an increase in the attenuation and arteriosclerotic closure of the arterial system of the retina. A decreased risk of hemorrhage into the vitreous may result, but there also may be a decrease in retinal function with associated decrease in vision. Aggressive management of cardiovascular risk factors theoretically could relieve some of the ischemic process in the retina.

Diabetic retinopathy is a highly specific vascular complication of both type 1 and type 2 diabetes, and the duration of diabetes is a significant risk factor for the development of retinopathy (62). After 20 years of diabetes, nearly all patients with type 1 diabetes and more than 60% of those with type 2 diabetes have some degree of retinopathy. Laser surgery and other surgical modalities help minimize the risk of moderate and severe visual loss from diabetes mellitus and, in some cases, restore useful vision for those who have suffered visual loss. These surgical modalities, particularly laser surgery, are most effective if initiated when a person approaches or just reaches high-risk PDR or before a person has lost visual acuity from diabetic macular edema (26).

The 5-year risk of severe visual loss from high-risk PDR may be as high as 60%, and the risk of moderate visual loss from CSME may be as high as 30%. Because PDR and macular edema may cause no ocular or visual symptoms when the retinal lesions are most amenable to treatment, a major clinical goal is to identify eyes at risk of visual loss and ensure that patients are referred for laser surgery at the appropriate time. Even minor errors in diagnosis of the level of retinopathy can result in a significant increase in a person's risk of visual loss.

Furthermore, collateral health and medical problems present a significant risk for the development and progression of diabetic retinopathy (Table 54.2) (63). These factors include pregnancy (64–66), chronic hyperglycemia (45–55,67–70), hypertension (54,71), renal disease (69), and hyperlipidemia (37,72). Patients with these conditions require careful medical evaluation and follow-up for the progression of diabetic retinopathy and optimization of their medical status.

CLINICAL TRIALS OF DIABETIC RETINOPATHY: SCIENTIFIC BASIS FOR MANAGEMENT

In the United States, the results of four nationwide randomized clinical trials have determined in large part the strategies for appropriate clinical management of patients with diabetic retinopathy. The United Kingdom Prospective Diabetes Study (UKPDS) adds significant information to supplement the findings of the studies in the United States.

Diabetic Retinopathy Study

The DRS (3–16) (Table 54.3) conclusively demonstrated that scatter (panretinal) photocoagulation significantly reduces the risk of severe visual loss from PDR, particularly when high-risk PDR is present.

Early Treatment Diabetic Retinopathy Study

The ETDRS (17–39) provided valuable information concerning the timing of scatter (panretinal) laser surgery for advancing diabetic retinopathy and conclusively demonstrated that focal photocoagulation for CSME reduces the risk of moderate visual loss by 50% or more (Table 54.4). Furthermore, the ETDRS demonstrated that both early scatter (panretinal) laser surgery (before high-risk PDR) and deferral of treatment "until and as soon as high-risk PDR developed" are effective in reducing the risk of severe visual loss. Scatter laser surgery, therefore, should be considered as an eye approaches the high-risk stage and "usually should not be delayed if the eye has reached the high-risk proliferative stage" (26). For patients with type 2 diabetes mellitus or type 1 diabetes mellitus of long standing, early photocoagulation should be considered.

Diabetic Retinopathy Vitrectomy Study

The DRVS (40–44) provided guidelines for the most opportune time for vitrectomy surgery for patients with type 1 and type 2 diabetes who suffered from vitreous hemorrhage (40,41,44) or from severe PDR in eyes with useful vision (Table 54.5) (42,43). In these early years of *pars plana* vitrectomy, early vitrectomy for eyes with recent severe vitreous hemorrhage and a visual acuity of less than 5/200 was beneficial, especially for patients with type 1 diabetes. Furthermore, the chance of achieving visual acuity of 10/20 or better was increased by early vitrectomy in eyes with severe proliferating neovascular retinopathy, again especially for patients with type 1 diabetes. However, surgical tools and techniques for vitrectomy in patients with diabetic retinopathy have evolved significantly over the past two decades, making precise prediction of clinical outcome for the DRVS data potentially less applicable and present surgical outcomes probably more favorable.

Diabetes Control and Complications Trial

The Diabetes Control and Complications Trial (DCCT) (45–52) conclusively demonstrated that intensive control of glycemic levels, as reflected by measurements of HbA_{1c}, significantly reduces the risk of onset of diabetic retinopathy, progression of preexisting retinopathy, and the need for laser surgery for persons with type 1 diabetes. Intensive therapy reduced the risk of

TABLE 54.3. Diabetic Retinopathy Study

Major eligibility criteria
- Visual acuity ≥20/100 in each eye
- PDR in at least one eye or severe NPDR in both eyes
- Both eyes suitable for photocoagulation

Major design features
- One eye of each patient assigned randomly to photocoagulation [scatter (panretinal), local (direct confluent treatment of surface new vessels)]; other eye assigned to follow-up without photocoagulation
- The eye assigned to treatment then randomly assigned to argon laser or xenon arc

Major conclusions
- Photocoagulation reduced risk of SVL by ≥50% (SVL = visual acuity ≤5/200 at two consecutively completed 4-month follow-up visits)
- Modest risks of decrease in visual acuity (usually only one line) and constriction of visual field (risks greater with xenon than argon)
- Treatment benefit outweighs risks for eyes with high-risk PDR (50% 5-year rate of SVL in such eyes without treatment reduced to 20% by treatment)

For abbreviations, see Table 54.1.
Table prepared by Matthew D. Davis, M.D., and the ETDRS Research Group for the Diabetes 2000 Program of the American Academy of Ophthalmology.

TABLE 54.4. Early Treatment Diabetic Retinopathy Study

Major eligibility criteria
- Visual acuity ≥20/40 (≥20/400 if reduction caused by macular edema)
- Mild NPDR to non–high-risk PDR, with or without macular edema
- Both eyes suitable for photocoagulation

Major design features
- One eye of each patient assigned randomly to early photocoagulation and the other to deferral (careful follow-up and photocoagulation if high-risk PDR develops)
- Patients assigned randomly to aspirin or placebo

Major conclusions
- Focal photocoagulation (direct laser for focal leaks and grid laser for diffuse leaks) reduced risk of MVL (doubling of the visual angle) by ≥50% and increased the chance of a small improvement in visual acuity
- Both early scatter with or without focal photocoagulation and deferral followed by low rates of severe visual loss (5-year rates in deferral subgroups 2%–10%; in early photocoagulation groups, 2%–6%)
- Focal photocoagulation should be considered for eyes with CSME
- Scatter photocoagulation not indicated for mild to moderate NPDR but should be considered as retinopathy approaches high-risk PDR and usually should not be delayed when this high-risk stage is present

Aspirin had no effect on progression of retinopathy, frequency of vitreous hemorrhage, or cataract development

For abbreviations, see Table 54.1.
Table prepared by Matthew D. Davis, M.D., and the ETDRS Research Group for the Diabetes 2000 Program of the American Academy of Ophthalmology.

onset of retinopathy by 76% and resulted in a 63% reduction in the risk of progression of retinopathy. There was a 47% reduction in the risk of developing severe nonproliferative diabetic retinopathy (NPDR) or PDR, a 23% reduction in the risk of developing clinically significant macular edema, and a 56% reduction in the risk of requiring laser surgery for those on intensive therapy. Significantly, these benefits persisted for 4 years after the period of intensive control, despite convergence of glycemic control for both groups after 4 years (52). Similar reduction of risks was identified for other microvascular complications of diabetes, such as renal disease and neuropathy.

United Kingdom Prospective Diabetes Study

The UKPDS (54,55) and studies in Japan (53) demonstrated similar reduction in risk for onset and progression of diabetic retinopathy for persons with type 2 diabetes. The UKPDS enrolled 3,867 patients with newly diagnosed type 2 diabetes. Intensive therapy to control blood glucose, using either sulfonylureas or insulin, resulted in a 17% risk reduction for progression of diabetic retinopathy, a 29% risk reduction in the need for laser photocoagulation surgery, a 23% risk reduction for the development of vitreous hemorrhage, and a 16% risk reduction in legal blindness.

TABLE 54.5. Diabetic Retinopathy Vitrectomy Study

RECENT SEVERE VITREOUS HEMORRHAGE (GROUP H)
- Major eligibility criteria
  - Visual acuity ≥5/200
  - Vitreous hemorrhage consistent with visual acuity, duration 1–6 months
  - Macula attached by ultrasound
- Major design features
  - In most patients, only one eye eligible
  - Eligible eye(s) assigned randomly to early vitrectomy or conventional management (vitrectomy if center of macula detaches or if vitreous hemorrhage persists for 1 year; photocoagulation as needed and as possible)
- Major conclusions
  - Chance of recovery of visual acuity ≥10/20 increased by early vitrectomy, at least in patients with type 1 diabetes, who were younger and had more severe PDR (in most severe PDR group, ≥10/20 at 4 years in 50% of early vitrectomy group vs. 12% in conventional management group)

VERY SEVERE PDR WITH USEFUL VISION (GROUP NR)
- Major eligibility criteria
  - Visual acuity ≥10/200
  - Center of macula attached
  - Extensive, active, neovascular or fibrovascular proliferations
- Major design features
  - Same as group H (except conventional management included vitrectomy after a 6-month waiting period in eyes that developed severe vitreous hemorrhage)
- Major conclusions
  - Chance of visual acuity ≥10/20 increased by early vitrectomy, at least for eyes with very severe new vessels

Note: The DRVS was conducted prior to the advent of several surgical advances such as endolaser, now commonly used during vitreoretinal surgery in patients with diabetic retinopathy. Caution is therefore warranted if extrapolating DRVS results to patients receiving such current therapeutic modalities. For abbreviations, see Table 54.1.
Table prepared by Matthew D. Davis, M.D., and the ETDRS Research Group for the Diabetes 2000 Program of the American Academy of Ophthalmology.

DIAGNOSIS, CLASSIFICATION, AND MANAGEMENT OF DIABETIC RETINOPATHY

Retinal Lesions

The processes by which diabetes mellitus results in retinopathy and maculopathy are not fully understood. It is apparent in studies with laboratory animals, however, that hyperglycemia itself, even in animals not genetically diabetic, is sufficient to cause diabetic retinopathy (73). The elevated blood glucose level is thought to induce structural, physiologic, and hormonal changes that affect the retinal capillaries. The retinal capillary mural cells become less functional and endothelial cell dysfunction results (74–76). Alteration in retinal blood flow is observed early in the course of diabetes (77,78).

Basic pathophysiologic processes in the development of diabetic retinopathy include (a) loss of pericytes associated with retinal capillaries, (b) thickening of the basement membrane, (c) changes in retinal blood flow, (d) outpouching of capillary walls to form microaneurysms, (e) closure of retinal capillaries and arterioles leading to retinal nonperfusion, (f) breakdown of the blood/retinal barrier with increased vascular permeability of retinal capillaries, (g) proliferation of new retinal and/or iris vessels, (h) development of fibrovascular tissue, and (i) contraction of vitreous and fibrous proliferation with subsequent vitreous hemorrhage and/or retinal detachment as a result of traction.

HEMORRHAGES AND/OR MICROANEURYSMS

The various diabetic retinal lesions and their severity, both alone and in aggregate, are excellent predictors of the risk of progression of retinopathy and visual loss (Table 54.6) (29). The development of the various lesions of diabetic retinopathy is believed to result from the occurrence of various pathologic processes and interactions during the course of diabetes and development of diabetic eye disease. The retinal pericytes, which are intimately associated within the basement membrane of the retinal endothelial cells, are normally present in a one-to-one ratio with the endothelial cells themselves. This is a ratio higher than that found anywhere else in the body. This finding and other cell-culture data have suggested that the retinal pericytes are critical supporting cells for the retinal capillaries (79,80). The loss of the retinal pericytes is thought, therefore, to be a factor contributing to the development of endothelial cell dysfunction and weakness of the retinal capillary wall, possibly contributing to the formation of microaneurysms, which, along with venous dilatation, is one early clinical sign of diabetic retinopathy (15,19,20).

TABLE 54.6. Proliferative Diabetic Retinopathy at 1-Year Visit, By Severity of Individual Lesion

Lesion	Grade	PDR in 1 year, %
H/Ma	Present in 2–5 fields	9
	Very severe	57
IRMA	None	9
	Moderate in 2–5 fields	57
VB	Absent	15
	Present in 2–5 fields	59

See Table 54.1 for abbreviations.
From Early Treatment Diabetic Retinopathy Study Research Group. Fundus photographic risk factors for progression of diabetic retinopathy: ETDRS report no. 12. *Ophthalmology* 1991;98[Suppl 5]:823–833.

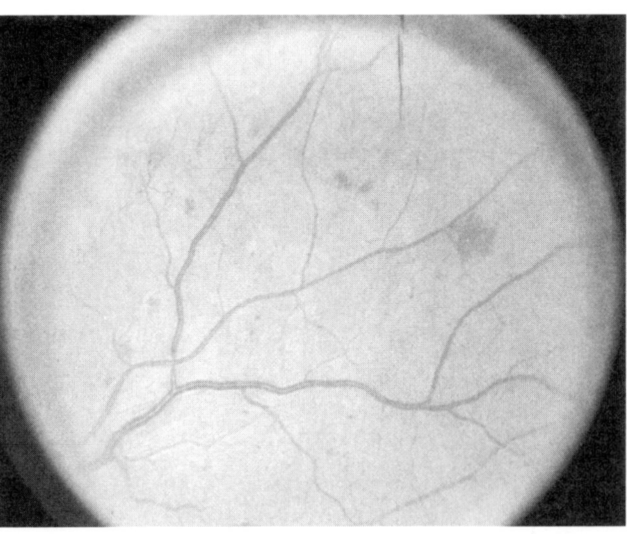

Figure 54.1. Standard photograph 2A of the modified Airlie House classification of diabetic retinopathy demonstrating a moderate degree of hemorrhage and/or microaneurysms.

The early clinical signs of diabetic retinopathy are microaneurysms, which are saccular outpouchings of retinal capillaries (Fig. 54.1). Ruptured microaneurysms, leaking capillaries, and intraretinal microvascular abnormalities can result in intraretinal hemorrhages. The clinical appearance of these hemorrhages reflects the retinal architecture at the retinal level of the hemorrhage. Hemorrhages in the nerve-fiber layer assume a more flame-shaped appearance, coinciding with the structure of the nerve-fiber layer that runs parallel to the retinal surface. Hemorrhages deeper in the retina, where the arrangement of cells is approximately perpendicular to the surface of the retina, assume a pinpoint or dot shape and are more characteristic of diabetic retinopathy.

The term "dot/blot hemorrhages" has been used to describe these small intraretinal hemorrhages characteristic of diabetic retinopathy. Because it is very difficult, if not impossible, to distinguish small dot/blot hemorrhages from microaneurysms, and because critical evaluation of these lesions has determined that little additional clinically significant information is obtained by differentiating these two lesions, they are classically evaluated together and referred to as "hemorrhages and microaneurysms."

VENOUS CALIBER ABNORMALITIES

Venous caliber abnormalities (Fig. 54.2) are early indicators of diabetic retinopathy and are often indicators of severe retinal hypoxia. These abnormalities can be venous dilatation, beading, or loop formation. These venous changes usually occur where there are large areas of nonperfusion adjacent to the veins. Treatment with scatter (panretinal) photocoagulation may cause these abnormal veins to become more normal in appearance over time.

INTRARETINAL MICROVASCULAR ABNORMALITIES

Intraretinal microvascular abnormalities (IRMAs) (Fig. 54.3) are preexisting vessels with endothelial cell proliferation that some consider new vessel growth within the retina that become "shunts" through areas of nonperfusion. IRMAs may be seen adjacent to cotton-wool spots, which result from microinfarcts in the nerve-fiber layer of the retina. IRMAs are often associated with a severe stage of nonproliferative retinopathy, and frank

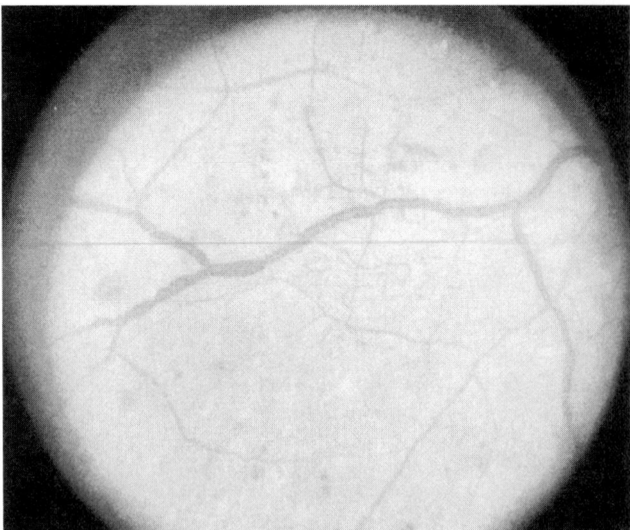

Figure 54.2. Standard photograph 6B of the modified Airlie House classification of diabetic retinopathy demonstrating venous beading.

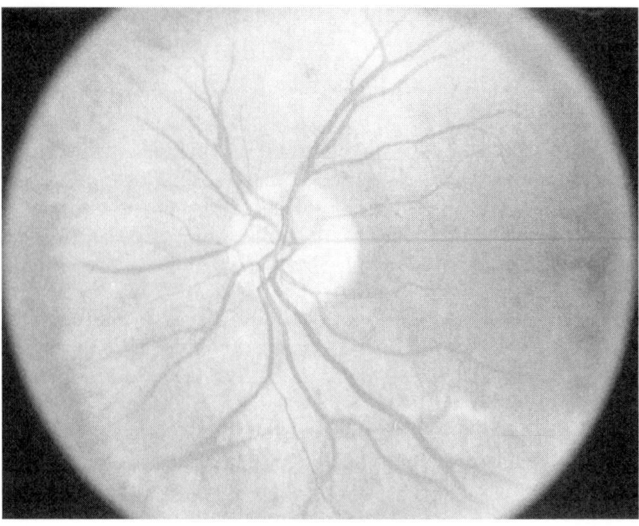

Figure 54.4. Standard photograph 10A of the modified Airlie House classification of diabetic retinopathy demonstrating neovascularization of the optic disc covering approximately one fourth to one third of the disc area.

neovascularization is likely to appear on the surface of the retina or optic disc within a short time.

RETINAL NEOVASCULARIZATION

PDR (Fig. 54.4) is marked by the development of new, abnormal retinal vessels. The rate of growth of these new vessels is variable. These vessels grow either at or near the optic disc [neovascularization of the disc (NVD)] or elsewhere on the surface of the retina [neovascularization elsewhere (NVE)]. Translucent fibrous tissue is often associated with the new vessels. This fibroglial tissue appears opaque and becomes adherent to the adjacent vitreous.

Patients with high-risk PDR require immediate scatter laser photocoagulation. High-risk PDR is characterized by any one or more of the following lesions: (a) NVD approximately one fourth to one third the disc area or more in size (i.e., greater than or equal to NVD in ETDRS standard photo 10A) (9,27) (Fig. 54.4); (b) NVD less than one fourth the disc area in size if fresh vitreous or preretinal hemorrhage is present; or (c) NVE greater than or equal to one half the disc area in size if fresh vitreous or preretinal hemorrhage is present (Fig. 54.5). Because identification of high-risk characteristics is critical for determining delivery of sight-saving care, careful attention must be paid to the presence or absence of new vessels, the location of new vessels, the severity of new vessels, and the presence or absence of preretinal or vitreous hemorrhage (5).

Levels of Diabetic Retinopathy

Scatter (panretinal) laser photocoagulation surgery should be considered as retinopathy approaches or reaches the high-risk stage of PDR. An eye is considered to be approaching the high-risk stage when there are retinal signs of severe or very severe NPDR or new vessels not fulfilling the definition of high-risk PDR (see Proliferative Diabetic Retinopathy), especially if associated with very severe NPDR. The baseline level of retinopathy

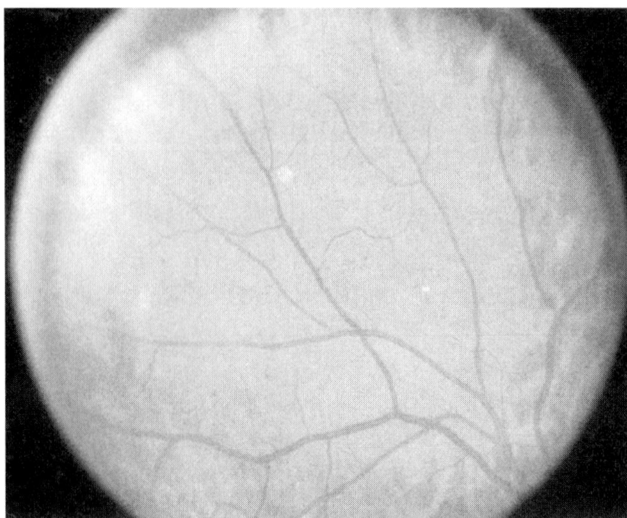

Figure 54.3. Standard photograph 8A of the modified Airlie House classification of diabetic retinopathy demonstrating intraretinal microvascular abnormalities.

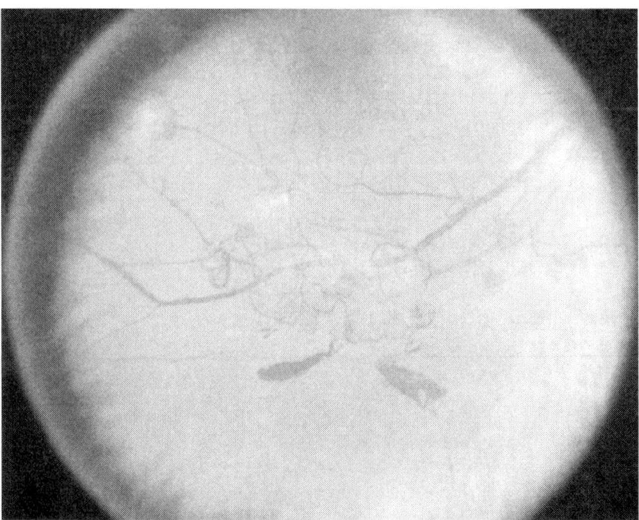

Figure 54.5. Standard photograph 7 of the modified Airlie House classification of diabetic retinopathy demonstrating neovascularization elsewhere in the retina greater than one half disc area with fresh hemorrhage present.

TABLE 54.7. Levels of Retinopathy

NONPROLIFERATIVE DIABETIC RETINOPATHY
- A. Mild NPDR
  - At least one microaneurysm
  - Definition not met for B, C, D, E, or F (see below)
- B. Moderate NPDR
  - H/Ma greater than standard photograph 2A (Fig. 54.1) or SE, VB, or IRMA definitely present
  - Definition not met for C, D, E, or F (see below)
- C. Severe NPDR
  - H/Ma greater than standard photograph 2A (Fig. 54.1) in all four quadrants or VB in two or more quadrants (Fig. 54.3) or
  - IRMA greater than standard photograph 8A (Fig. 54.2) in at least one quadrant
- D. Very severe NPDR
  - Any two or more of C above
  - Definition not met for E or F

PROLIFERATIVE DIABETIC RETINOPATHY (PDR)
- Composition of PDR (at least one of the following)
  - NVD or NVE
  - Preretinal or vitreous hemorrhage
  - Fibrous tissue proliferation
- E. Early PDR
  - New vessels
  - Definition not met for F
- F. High-risk PDR
  - NVD ≥ ¼–⅓ disc area (Fig. 54.4) or
  - NVD and vitreous or preretinal hemorrhage or
  - NVE ≥ ½ disc area and preretinal or vitreous hemorrhage (Fig. 54.5)

CLINICALLY SIGNIFICANT DIABETIC MACULAR EDEMA
- Thickening of the retina located ≤500 μm from the center of the macula or
- HE located ≤500 μm from the center of the macula with thickening of the adjacent retina or
- A zone of retinal thickening, one disc area or larger in size, with any portion located ≤1 disc diameter from the center of the macula

See Table 54.1 for abbreviations.
From Early Treatment Diabetic Retinopathy Study Research Group. Early photocoagulation for diabetic retinopathy: ETDRS report no. 9. *Ophthalmology* 1991;98[Suppl 5]:766–785; and Early Treatment Diabetic Retinopathy Study Research Group. Classification of diabetic retinopathy from fluorescein angiograms: ETDRS report no. 11. *Ophthalmology* 1991;98 [Suppl 5]:807–822, with permission.

is a strong indicator of the risk of progression from the NPDR stage to both early PDR and high-risk PDR (Tables 54.6, 54.7, and 54.8) (29).

NONPROLIFERATIVE DIABETIC RETINOPATHY

Diabetic retinopathy is broadly classified as NPDR and PDR. Diabetic macular edema can occur with either NPDR or PDR and is discussed separately. Accurate diagnosis of a patient's "diabetic retinopathy level" is critical because the risk of progression to PDR and high-risk PDR varies and is closely correlated with the specific level of NPDR (Table 54.8, Fig. 54.6).

Mild NPDR is marked by at least one retinal microaneurysm, but hemorrhages and microaneurysms are less than those in ETDRS standard photograph 2A (Fig. 54.1) in all four retinal quadrants (Fig. 54.1 and Table 54.7). No other retinal lesions or abnormalities associated with diabetes are present. Those with mild NPDR have a 5% risk of progression to PDR within 1 year and a 15% risk of progression to high-risk PDR within 5 years (Table 54.8).

Moderate NPDR (Table 54.7) is characterized by hemorrhages and/or microaneurysms (H/Ma) greater than those pictured in ETDRS standard photograph 2A in at least one quadrant but in less than four retinal quadrants, with or without venous beading and IRMA to a mild degree. The risk of progression to PDR within 1 year is 12% to 27%, and the risk of progression to high-risk PDR within 5 years is 33% (Table 54.8).

Patients with mild or moderate NPDR generally are not candidates for scatter (panretinal) laser surgery and can be followed safely at 6- to 12-month intervals as determined by the examiner. The presence of macular edema, even with mild or moderate degrees of NPDR, requires follow-up in a shorter period. If CSME is present, focal laser treatment is advisable (Table 54.8). Coincident medical problems or pregnancy will necessitate more frequent reevaluation.

Severe NPDR is based on the severity of H/Ma, IRMA, and/or venous beading and is determined by any one of the following lesions (Table 54.7): (a) H/Ma greater than ETDRS standard photo 2A (Fig. 54.1) in four quadrants, (b) venous beading (Fig. 54.2) in two or more quadrants, or (c) IRMA greater than ETDRS standard photo 8A (Fig. 54.3) in at least one quadrant.

Eyes with severe NPDR have a 52% risk of developing PDR within 1 year and a 60% risk of developing high-risk PDR within 5 years. These patients require follow-up evaluation in 2- to 4-month intervals. Because the clinical effectiveness of laser photocoagulation for clinically significant macular edema in the presence of PDR may be reduced compared with treatment of clinically significant macular edema alone, treatment of clinically significant macular edema in patients with severe or very severe NPDR is indicated because of a high risk of developing PDR and requiring scatter (panretinal) laser surgery in a relatively short time. In addition, scatter (panretinal) laser surgery can worsen macular edema—another reason for optimizing the macular edema status of these patients who are likely to require scatter (panretinal) laser photocoagulation in the near term (Table 54.8).

Eyes with *very severe NPDR* (Table 54.7) have two or more lesions of severe NPDR but no frank neovascularization. These eyes have a 75% risk of developing PDR within 1 year. Patients with severe or very severe NPDR may be candidates for scatter (panretinal) laser surgery, particularly those with type 2 diabetes, and macular edema, if present, often requires treatment. Frequent reevaluation at 2- to 3-month intervals is important for these eyes (Table 54.8).

PROLIFERATIVE DIABETIC RETINOPATHY

Diabetic retinopathy marked by new vessel growth on the optic disc (NVD) or elsewhere (NVE) on the retina or by fibrous-tissue proliferation is designated PDR. Early PDR does not meet the definition of high-risk PDR (Table 54.7). Eyes with early PDR (less than high risk) have a 75% risk of developing high-risk PDR within a 5-year period. These eyes may require scatter (panretinal) laser surgery. Macular edema, even if not clinically significant, may benefit from focal treatment before scatter is initiated, as discussed above (nonproliferative diabetic retinopathy) (Table 54.8).

In patients with early PDR (less than high-risk PDR), early scatter (panretinal) laser surgery should be considered if any of the associated findings are present: (a) any new vessels accompanied by severe or very severe NPDR, (b) elevated new vessels, (c) or NVD. In the presence of macular edema, patients with severe NPDR or worse should be considered for focal treatment of macular edema whether or not the macular edema is clinically significant, in preparation for the impending future need of scatter laser photocoagulation (Table 54.8).

In patients with severe or very severe NPDR or early PDR, the patient's type of diabetes is important. It has been demonstrated in the ETDRS that patients with type 2 diabetes have their risk of severe visual loss or vitrectomy surgery reduced by 50% if scatter (panretinal) laser surgery is initiated prior to the development of high-risk PDR. In contrast, patients with type 1

TABLE 54.8. General Management Recommendations

	Natural course/ Rate of progression to		Evaluation		Treatment strategies		
	PDR 1 y	HRC 1 y	Color fundus photo	FA	PRP	Focal	F/U (mo)
1. Mild NPDR	5%	15%	—	—	—	—	—
No macular edema	—	—	No	No	No	No	12
Macular edema	—	—	Yes	Occ	No	No	4–6
CSME	—	—	Yes	Yes	No	Yes	2–4
2. Moderate NPDR	12%–27%	33%	—	—	—	—	—
No macular edema	—	—	Yes	No	No	No	6–8
Macular edema	—	—	Yes	Occ	No	No	4–6
CSME	—	—	Yes	Yes	No	Yes	2–4
3. Severe NPDR	52%	60%	—	—	—	—	—
No macular edema	—	—	Yes	No	Consider	No	3–4
Macular edema	—	—	Yes	Occ	Consider	Occ	2–3
	—	—	—	—	AF	—	—
CSME			Yes	Yes	Consider	Yes	2–3
			—	—	AF	—	—
4. Very severe NPDR	75%	75%	—	—	—	—	—
No macular edema	—	—	Yes	No	Consider	No	2–3
Macular edema[a]	—	—	Yes	Occ	Consider	Occ	2–3
	—	—	—	—	AF	—	—
CSME	—	—	Yes	Yes	Consider	Yes	2–3
	—	—	—	—	AF	—	—
5. Non–high-risk PDR	—	75%	—	—	—	—	—
No macular edema	—	—	Yes	No	Consider	No	2–3
Macular edema[a]	—	—	Yes	Occ	Consider	Occ	2–3
	—	—	—	—	AF	—	—
CSME	—	—	Yes	Yes	Consider	Yes	2–3
	—	—	—	—	AF	—	—
6. High-risk PDR	—	—	—	—	—	—	—
No macular edema	—	—	Yes	No	Yes	No	2–3
Macular edema[a]	—	—	Yes	Yes	Yes	Usually	1–2
CSME	—	—	—	Yes	Yes	Yes	1–2

HRC, high-risk characteristics; FA, fluorescein angiogram; PRP, scatter (panretinal photocoagulation); F/U, follow-up; Occ, occasionally; AF, after focal. For all other abbreviations, see Table 54.1.
[a]Not CSME.

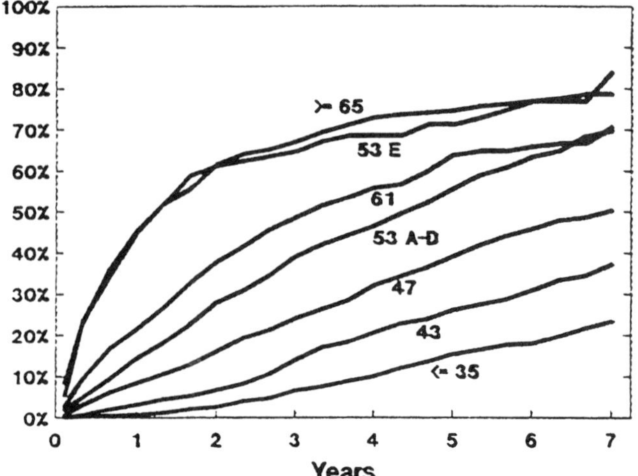

Figure 54.6. Life-table cumulative event rates of high-risk proliferative retinopathy by level of retinopathy severity at baseline in eyes assigned to deferral of photocoagulation in the ETDRS: level ≤35, mild NPDR; level 43, moderate NPDR; level 47, moderate to severe NPDR; level 53 A–D, severe NPDR; level 53 E, very severe NPDR; level 61, early PDR; level ≥65, PDR less than high-risk PDR (27). See Table 54.1 for abbreviations.

diabetes showed no significant difference in the risk of severe visual loss or vitrectomy if laser surgery is delayed until the development of PDR with high-risk characteristics (59,60).

Diabetic Macular Edema

Diabetic macular edema may be present at any level of retinopathy (Table 54.8). Alterations in the structure of the macula observed in diabetes include (a) macular edema (a collection of intraretinal fluid in the macula with or without lipid exudates and with or without cystoid changes); (b) nonperfusion of parafoveal capillaries with or without intraretinal fluid; (c) traction in the macula by fibrous-tissue proliferation causing dragging of the retinal tissue, surface wrinkling, or detachment of the macula; (d) intraretinal or preretinal hemorrhage in the macula; (e) lamellar or full-thickness retinal hole formation; (f) various combinations of the above.

The clinical definition of macular edema is retinal thickening within two disc diameters of the center of the macula. This definition is not based on the presence of fluorescein leakage. Retinal thickening or hard exudates with adjacent retinal thickening that threaten or involve the center of the macula are considered to be clinically significant. CSME as defined by the ETDRS includes any one of the following lesions (Table 54.7): (a) retinal thickening at or within 500 μm from the center of the macula (Fig. 54.7), (b) hard exudates at or within 500 μm from the cen-

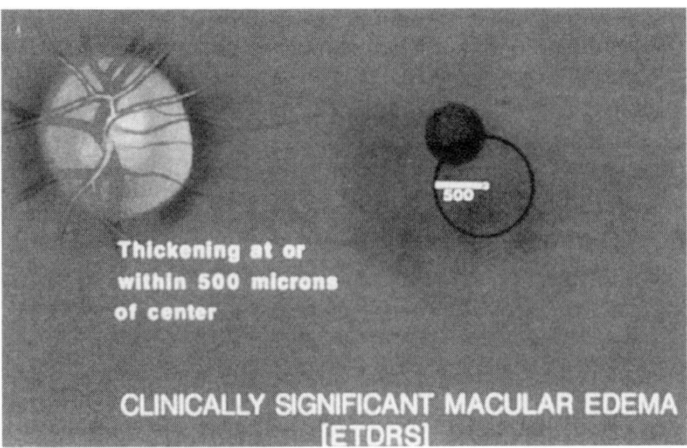

Figure 54.7. Schematic showing clinically significant macular edema with thickening of the macular less than 500 μm from the center of the macula. (Schematic courtesy of Robert Murphy, M.D., with permission.)

ter of the macula if there is thickening of the adjacent retina (Fig. 54.8), or (c) an area or areas of retinal thickening at least one disc area in size, at least part of which is within one disc diameter of the center of the macula (Fig. 54.9).

In managing CSME, there are particular retinal lesions identified on fluorescein angiography that are amenable to treatment. These "treatable lesions" associated with macular edema include (a) focal leaks more than 500 μm from the center of the macula thought to be causing retinal thickening and/or hard exudates (Fig. 54.10); (b) focal leaks 300 to 500 μm from the center of the macula thought to be causing retinal thickening and/or hard exudates, if the treating ophthalmologist does not believe that treatment is likely to destroy the remaining perifoveal capillary network (Fig. 54.11), and visual acuity is 20/40 or worse; (c) areas of diffuse macular leakage (Fig. 54.12) from extensive numbers of microaneurysms or from many IRMAs; or (d) avascular zones other than the normal foveal avascular zone, not previously treated (Fig. 54.12B).

Focal laser surgery for CSME consists of "direct" laser treatment, "grid" laser treatment, or "combination" focal laser and grid laser treatment. These treatment methods are described in detail elsewhere (18,20). Table 54.8 summarizes the management recommendations for CSME at the various retinopathy levels.

International Classification of Diabetic Retinopathy

While the classification of diabetic retinopathy used in the ETDRS is evidence-based and unparalleled for clinical research involving diabetic retinopathy, this classification is at times challenging to employ, especially clinically. In order to simplify classification and standardize communication between retinal specialists and ophthalmologists and other healthcare providers worldwide, in 2001 the American Academy of Ophthalmology initiated a project to establish a consensus International Classification of Diabetic Retinopathy and Diabetic Macular Edema (80a,b). The consensus panel included 31 participants from 16 countries. The consensus panel relied on evidence-based studies, including the Early Treatment Diabetic Retinopathy Study (ETDRS) and the Wisconsin Epidemiologic Study of Diabetic Retinopathy. This International Classification of Diabetic Retinopathy and Diabetic Macular Edema described five clinical levels of diabetic retinopathy: *no apparent retinopathy* (no abnormalities), *mild NPDR* (microaneurysms only), *moderate NPDR* (more than microaneurysms only but less than severe NPDR), *severe NPDR* (any of the following: >20 intraretinal hemorrhages in each 4 quadrants, definite VB in 2+ quadrants, prominent IRMA in 1+ quadrant and no PDR), and *PDR* (one or more of retinal neovascularization, vitreous hemorrhage, or preretinal hemorrhage). Table 54.9 compares levels of DR in the International Classification of DR with ETDRS levels of DR.

Additionally, the International Classification identified two broad levels of diabetic macular edema (DME): *macular edema apparently absent* (no apparent retinal thickening or hard exudates [HE] in the posterior pole) and *macular edema apparently present* (some apparent retinal thickening or HE in the posterior pole); if present, macular edema was subclassified as *mild DME* (some retinal thickening or HE in the posterior pole but distant from the center of the macula), *moderate DME* (retinal thickening or HE approaching the center of the macula but not involv-

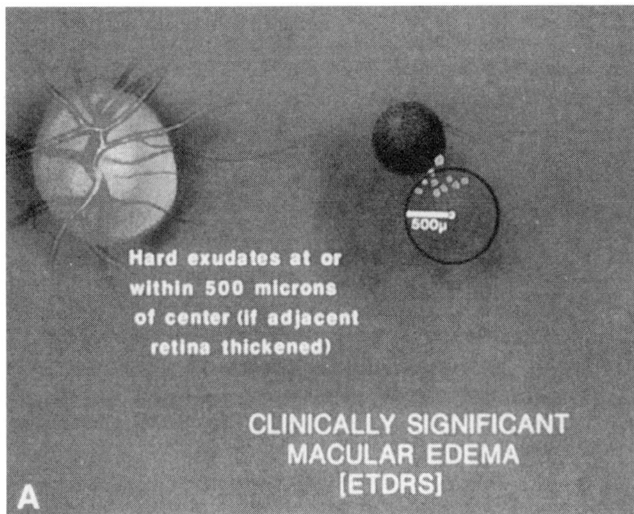

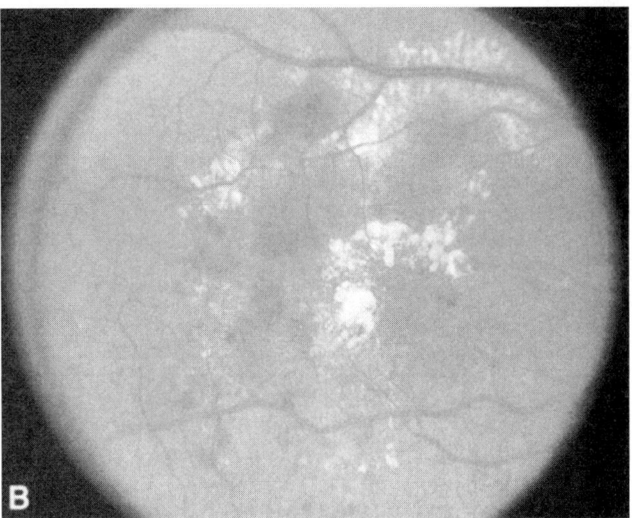

Figure 54.8. A: Schematic showing clinically significant macular edema (CSME) with hard exudates at or within 500 μm from the center of the macula, with thickening of the retina adjacent to the exudates (Schematic courtesy of Robert Murphy, M.D., with permission.) **B:** Clinical appearance of hard exudates less than 500 μm from the center of the macula. There is thickening of the adjacent retina, not appreciated without stereoscopic observation.

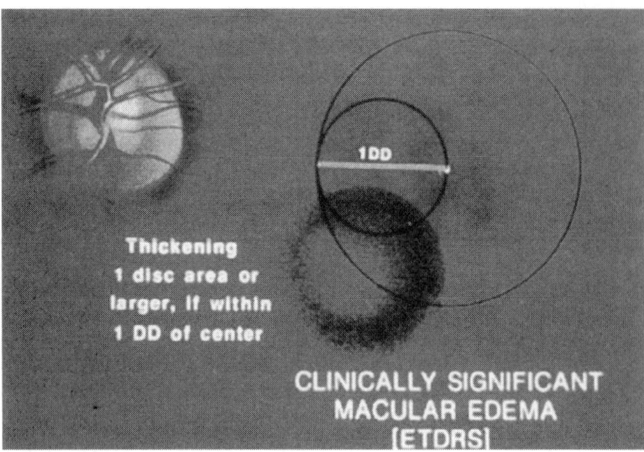

Figure 54.9. Schematic showing area of thickening one disc area in size, part of which is within one disc diameter of the center of the macula. (Schematic courtesy of Robert Murphy, M.D., with permission.)

TABLE 54.9. International Clinical Diabetic Retinopathy Scale Compared with Early Treatment Diabetic Retinopathy Study Levels of Diabetic Retinopathy

International classification level of DR	ETDRS level of DR
No apparent retinopathy	Level 10: DR absent
Mild NPDR	Level 20: very mild NPDR
Moderate NPDR	Levels 35, 43, 47: moderate NPDR
Severe NPDR	Levels 53A–E: severe to very severe NPDR
PDR	Levels 61, 65, 71, 75, 81, 85: PDR, high-risk PDR, very severe or advanced PDR

DR, diabetic retinopathy; NPDR, nonproliferative diabetic retinopathy; PDR, proliferative diabetic retinopathy.
Data from Wilkinson CP, Ferris FL III, Klein RE, et al. Proposed international clinical diabetic retinopathy and diabetic macular edema disease severity scales. *Ophthalmology* 2003;110:1677–1682; Early Treatment Diabetic Retinopathy Study Research Group. Fundus photographic risk factors for progression of diabetic retinopathy: ETDRS report no. 12. *Ophthalmology* 1991:98[Suppl 5]:823–833; and Early Treatment Diabetic Retinopathy Study Research Group. Grading diabetic retinopathy from stereoscopic color fundus photographs—an extension of the modified Airlie House classification: ETDRS report no. 10. *Ophthalmology* 1991;98[Suppl 5]:786–806.

ing the center), or *severe DME* (retinal thickening or HE involving the center of the macula). Table 54.10 (page 913) compares levels of DME in the International Classification with ETDRS levels of DME.

Overall, the International Classification of Diabetic Retinopathy and Diabetic Macular Edema reduces the number of levels of DR, simplifies descriptions of the categories, and describes the levels without relying on reference to the standard photographs of the Airlie House Classification of DR. While the classification does simplify clinical levels of DR, the International Classification of Diabetic Retinopathy and Diabetic Macular Edema is not a replacement for ETDRS levels of DR in large-scale clinical trials or studies in which precise retinopathy classification is required.

Role of Clinical Fluorescein Angiography in Management of Diabetic Retinopathy

Fluorescein angiography of the macula in the presence of CSME is valuable for the detection of treatable lesions, as previously described. However, its use for identifying lesions such as NVE or feeder vessels on NVD is usually not necessary because the lesions are clinically evident and scatter (panretinal) laser surgery is the method of choice for the treatment of diabetic retinopathy as it approaches or reaches the high-risk stage.

Angiographic risk factors for progression of NPDR to PDR have been identified (28,30). Analysis of data for the untreated (deferred) eyes in the ETDRS indicates that the following lesions are independently related to outcome: (a) fluorescein leakage, (b) capillary loss on fluorescein angiography, (c) capillary dilatation on fluorescein angiography, and (d) the following color fundus photographic risk factors: IRMA, venous beading, and H/Ma. Hard and soft exudates have an inverse relationship to progression. It is widely accepted that capillary loss as documented on fluorescein angiography is a risk factor for progression of NPDR to PDR (28,30,74–76). However, capillary dilatation on fluorescein angiography, fluorescein leakage,

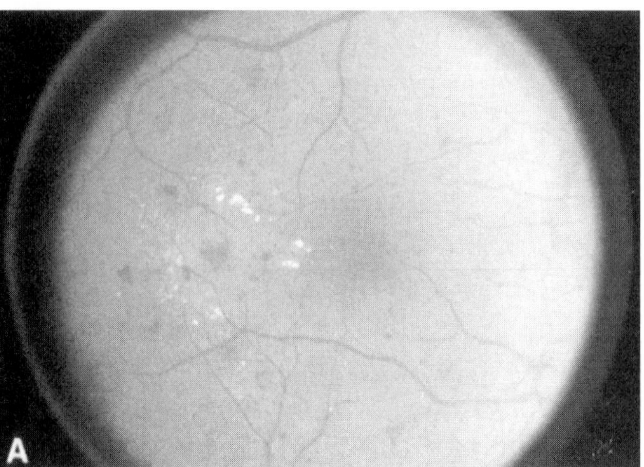

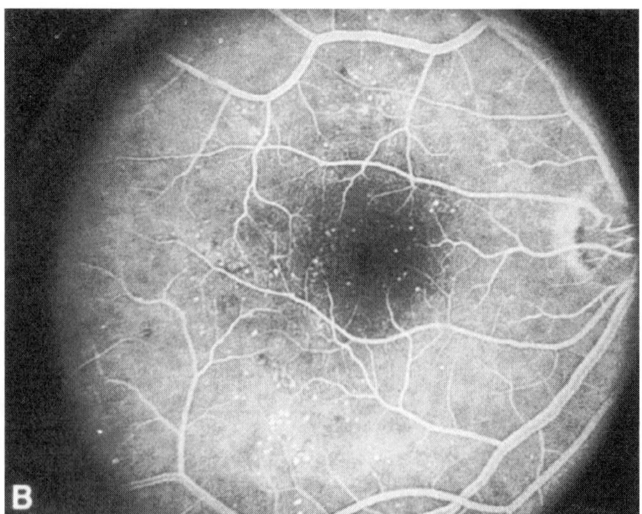

Figure 54.10. A: Clinical picture showing macular edema more than 500 μm from the center of the macula (edema not appreciated without stereoscopic evaluation). **B:** Fluorescein angiogram showing focal leaks from microaneurysms more than 500 μm from the center of the macula.

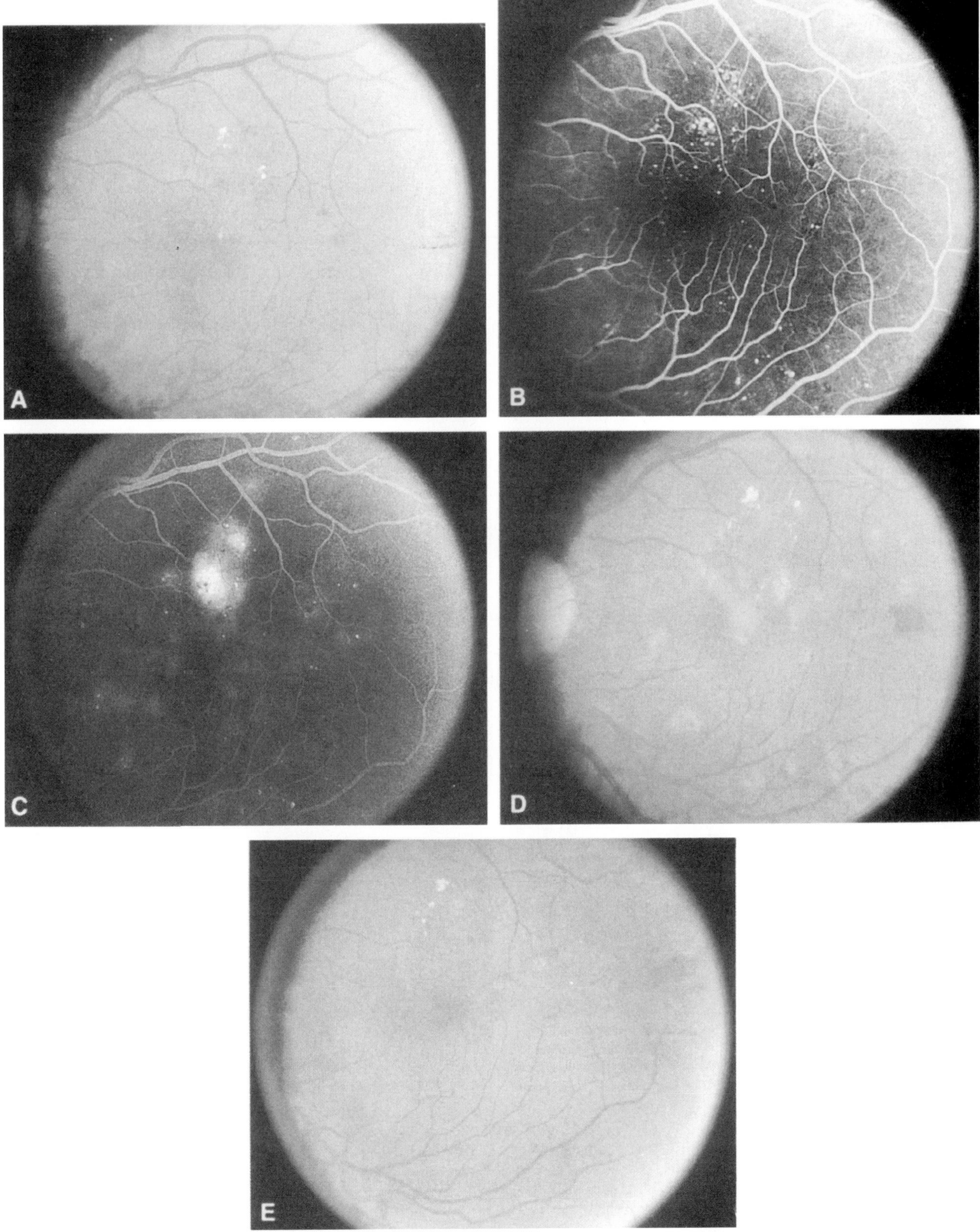

Figure 54.11. A: There is a small area of retinal thickening just above the center of the macula (poorly appreciated without stereopsis), detectable monocularly because of blurring of the choroidal pattern. Several microaneurysms are visible within the thickened area. There is a little hard exudate around the edges of the edematous patch, some of which extends almost to the center of the macula. Thickening extends to within 500 μm of the center of the macula (clinically significant macular edema). Visual acuity was 20/15. **B:** In the 17- to 18-second phase of the fluorescein angiogram, microaneurysms and slightly dilated capillaries are visible in the area of thickening. **C:** The 7-minute phase of the angiogram shows leakage into the retina from the two groups of microaneurysms noted in **B**. **D:** Treatment has been applied to most of the microaneurysms. **E:** Four months later the appearance of the retina is satisfactory, with flattening of the center of the macula and disappearance of the thickening noted before the treatment. Visual acuity remains at 20/15.

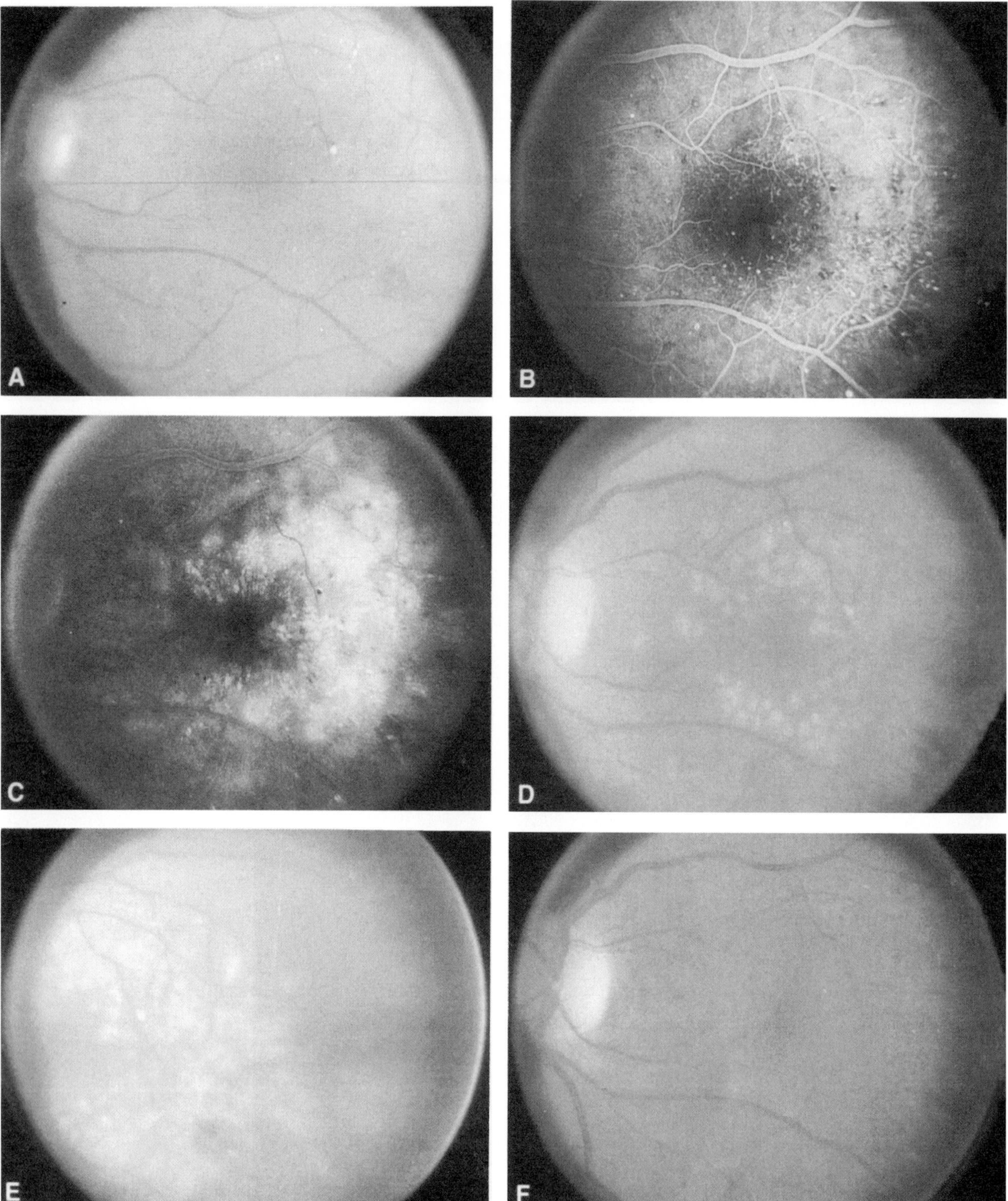

Figure 54.12. A: Clinical picture showing retinal thickening temporal to the center of the macula extending just to the center. Visual acuity is 20/40. **B:** Early phase of the angiogram shows capillary loss adjacent to the foveal avascular zone, capillary dilatation, and scattered microaneurysms. **C:** The 7-minute phase of the angiogram shows extensive small cystoid spaces temporal to the center of the macula and above and below it. The center appears uninvolved. **D:** The microaneurysms have been treated focally and, in addition, laser burns have been applied in a grid pattern in the areas of diffuse leakage. **E:** The temporal extent of the grid laser treatment. **F:** Four months after treatment, hemorrhages and hard exudates have decreased and the retinal thickening can no longer be detected. Visual acuity was 20/25.

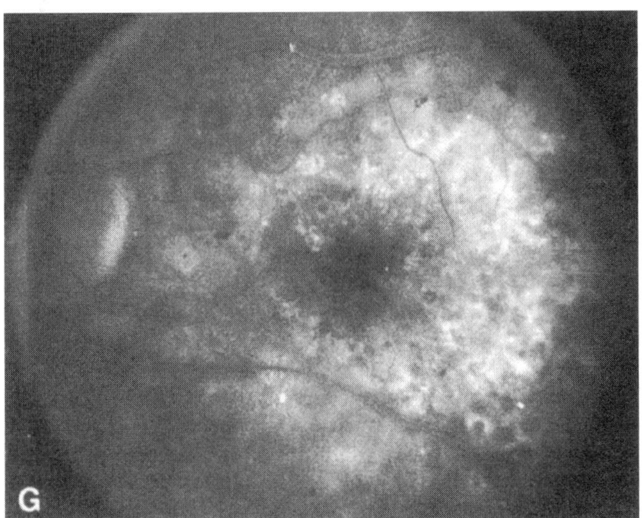

Figure 54.12. *(continued)* **G:** The 7-minute phase of the angiogram showing disappearance of most of the cystoid space visible in **C**.

capillary loss on fluorescein angiography, and the ETDRS color fundus photographic retinopathy are all closely correlated. Although the fluorescein angiography abnormalities provide additional prognostic information, the color fundus photographic grading of retinopathy levels of both eyes gives the same prognostic results (29,30). Therefore, the increase in power to predict progression from NPDR to PDR by fluorescein angiography is "not of significant clinical importance to warrant routine fluorescein angiography" (30).

Periodic follow-up retinal examinations, however, are necessary. The appropriate interval can be determined by skillful grading of seven standard-field stereo color fundus photographs and/or retinal evaluation by an examiner experienced in the management of diabetic eye disease. Because the level of diabetic retinopathy as derived from color fundus photography or retinal ophthalmic evaluation is closely correlated with the rate of progression of diabetic retinopathy, the accurate determination of the level of retinopathy becomes of paramount clinical importance and determines the appropriate retinal reevaluation interval. Also, since fluorescein angiography classification cannot "identify all cases destined to progress," and because initiation of scatter (panretinal) laser photocoagulation should be considered as diabetic retinopathy approaches (before or just as it reaches) the high-risk stage, "periodic follow-up of all patients with diabetic retinopathy continues to be of fundamental clinical importance" (30). Table 54.8 summarizes the appropriate use of fundus photography and fluorescein angiography in monitoring and treating diabetic retinopathy and macular edema.

LASER PHOTOCOAGULATION

Timing of Photocoagulation

In the ETDRS, the 3-year risk of moderate visual loss from macular edema without focal laser treatment was 30%. Focal laser surgery for CSME reduced this risk to 15% or less (17), a reduction in risk of approximately 50%, and focal treatment also increased the chance of improvement in visual acuity of one line or more. On the other hand, scatter (panretinal) laser surgery was not effective in managing diabetic macular edema and in some cases may have had a deleterious effect on the progression of macular edema.

Eyes with CSME and retinopathy approaching high-risk PDR are best treated first with focal photocoagulation for the macular edema 6 to 8 weeks before initiating scatter (panretinal) laser surgery. Eyes with mild or moderate NPDR and CSME respond best to prompt focal photocoagulation, with scatter treatment delayed unless severe or very severe NPDR or PDR occurs. Delaying scatter photocoagulation while focal treatment is being completed is unlikely to increase the risk of severe visual loss, provided the retinopathy is not progressing rapidly and careful follow-up can be maintained. Delaying scatter photocoagulation while focal treatment is completed in eyes with high-risk PDR usually is not advisable, and the macular edema will usually be treated at the first treatment session of scatter photocoagulation.

Focal treatment was not attended by adverse effects on central visual field or color vision in comparison with eyes assigned to deferral of focal treatment in the ETDRS (18). Any harmful effects of early photocoagulation as reflected by constriction of the peripheral visual fields seem to be due mostly to scatter photocoagulation. Because the principal benefit of treatment is the prevention of a further decrease in visual acuity, focal laser surgery should be considered in all eyes with CSME, especially if the center of the macula is threatened or involved, even if visual acuity is normal. However, it should be noted that macular edema that is not particularly extensive may resolve

TABLE 54.10. International Clinical Diabetic Macular Edema Scale Compared with Early Treatment Diabetic Retinopathy Study Where Noted

Disease severity level	Findings	DME vs. ETDRS scale
DME apparently absent	No apparent retinal thickening or hard exudates (HE) in posterior pole	
DME apparently present	Some apparent retinal thickening or HE in posterior pole	Mild DME: some retinal thickening or HE in posterior pole but distant from center of the macula **(ETDRS: DME but not CSME)** Moderate DME: retinal thickening or HE approaching the center but not involving the center **(ETDRS: CSME)** Severe DME: retinal thickening or HE involving the center of the macula **(ETDRS: CSME)**

DME, diabetic macular edema; HE, hard exudates; CSME, clinically significant macular edema.
Data from Wilkinson CP, Ferris FL III, Klein RE, et al. Proposed international clinical diabetic retinopathy and diabetic macular edema disease severity scales. *Ophthalmology* 2003;110:1677–1682; and Early Treatment Diabetic Retinopathy Study Research Group. Photocoagulation for diabetic macular edema; Early Treatement Diabetic Retinopathy Study report no. 1. *Arch Ophthalmol* 1985;103:1796–1806.

spontaneously in as many as 30% of patients. Thus, in cases where visual acuity is excellent, the fovea is not particularly threatened by edema, hard exudates, or subretinal fibrosis, the likelihood for requiring scatter (panretinal) photocoagulation in the near future is low, and the patient demonstrates excellent compliance with follow-up evaluations, the edema may, at the discretion of the patient and the treating physician, be monitored carefully without immediate focal photocoagulation. However, should the visual acuity show signs of deterioration, the macular edema show signs of progression, or the level of retinopathy advance to a stage where scatter (panretinal) laser photocoagulation is likely in the near future, prompt focal laser surgery for the macular edema is indicated.

The DRS demonstrated in 1976 that scatter (panretinal) photocoagulation was effective in reducing the risk of severe visual loss from high-risk PDR (3). Because the DRS did not provide a clear choice between prompt treatment or deferral of treatment unless there was progression to high-risk PDR, one question of concern for the ETDRS was whether earlier scatter photocoagulation, before the development of high-risk PDR, justified the side effects and risks of laser surgery (Table 54.11).

In the ETDRS, early treatment, compared with "deferral" of photocoagulation until the development of high-risk PDR (26), was associated with a small reduction in the incidence of severe visual loss; however, the 5-year rates of severe visual loss were low for both the early-treatment group and the group assigned to "deferral" of treatment (2.6% and 3.7%, respectively). Provided that careful follow-up can be maintained, scatter laser surgery is not recommended for eyes with mild or moderate NPDR (26). When retinopathy is more severe (i.e., severe or very severe NPDR and early PDR), scatter photocoagulation should be "considered and usually should not be delayed if the eye has reached the high-risk proliferative stage" (26).

As retinopathy approaches the high-risk stage (very severe NPDR or early PDR), the benefits and risks of early photocoagulation may be roughly balanced. Initiating scatter photocoagulation early in at least one eye seems particularly appropriate when both of the patient's eyes are approaching the high-risk stage, as optimal timing of photocoagulation may be difficult if both eyes require photocoagulation simultaneously. Also, prompt scatter photocoagulation of the retina should be considered for eyes with neovascularization in the anterior chamber angle, whether or not high-risk PDR is present (26). It has been demonstrated in the ETDRS that patients with type 2 diabetes have their risk of severe visual loss or vitrectomy surgery reduced by 50% if scatter (panretinal) laser surgery is initiated prior to the development of high-risk PDR. In contrast, patients with type 1 diabetes showed no difference in the risk of severe visual loss or vitrectomy if laser surgery was delayed until the development of high-risk PDR (59,60).

Treatment Program

The treatment program (Table 54.8) for diabetic retinopathy consists of (a) initial scatter laser photocoagulation surgery as the diabetic retinopathy approaches or reaches the high-risk stage, (b) careful follow-up at 3- to 4-month intervals following the treatment, (c) re-treatment of persistent or recurrent treatable lesions, and (d) focal laser photocoagulation treatment for macular edema prior to scatter (panretinal) photocoagulation to reduce the risk of progression of macular edema secondary to scatter photocoagulation (see above).

As high-risk PDR is reached, the major threat for severe visual loss (SVL; visual acuity ≤ 5/200 at two consecutive, completed 4-month follow-up visits) is traction retinal detachment. A lesser threat of persistent visual loss, but a more common complication, is vitreous hemorrhage. The primary goal of the scatter laser surgery is the prevention of traction retinal detachment, particularly involving the macula.

TABLE 54.11. Complications and Side Effects of Scatter (Panretinal) Laser Photocoagulation

Side effects
- Peripheral field constriction
- Nyctalopia (night blindness)
- Internal ophthalmoplegia
- Mild color vision changes

Complications
- Foveal burn
- Macular edema (secondary to scatter laser photocoagulation or heavy focal burn)
- Foveal traction
- Serous and/or choroidal detachment
- Acute angle–closure glaucoma
- Cornea and lens burns
- Retrobulbar hemorrhage due to retrobulbar anesthesia injection (rarely used today)
- Secondary retinal hole and rhegmatogenous retinal detachment
- Retinopathy progression to traction retinal detachment

Various strategies are involved in follow-up treatment. The ocular lesions to be considered for follow-up photocoagulation include new flat neovascularization or elevated neovascularization and new, persistent, or recurrent CSME. The treatment methods include additional scatter laser treatment, local laser to NVE, focal laser for CSME, *pars plana* vitrectomy for recurrent hemorrhages with fibrovascular proliferation causing traction, and, when appropriate, continued observation. Further scatter treatment may be placed between previously placed laser scars as long as these scars do not become confluent and the extent of the scatter treatment is not such as to totally destroy retinal function.

Although laser surgery often is considered painless, some patients may experience discomfort in association with the treatment. There usually is some discomfort or pain in all patients when the peripheral retina is treated. Complications and side effects of laser photocoagulation are summarized in Table 54.11.

In summary, scatter treatment significantly reduces the risk of severe visual loss from PDR. Both early scatter treatment prior to development of high-risk PDR and deferral of treatment until the development of high-risk PDR reduce the risk of severe visual loss. The rates of severe visual loss are low for each group after treatment. Consequently, it is recommended that scatter laser treatment not be used for mild to moderate NPDR. For severe NPDR and early PDR, scatter treatment is appropriate when close follow-up is unlikely, the disease process is progressing rapidly, or in patients with type 2 diabetes.

NONRETINAL OCULAR COMPLICATIONS

Clinical Significance

The potentially devastating effects of diabetes on the retina and the attendant threat of visual loss are generally well recognized (81). All structures of the eye, however, are susceptible to the deleterious effects of diabetes (Table 54.12). Some of these effects are of little consequence and go unnoticed by both the patient and the physician. Other effects, while not sight-threatening, result in uncomfortable vision or other symptoms interfering with normal visual function. Still other effects, while perhaps most prevalent with diabetes, require evaluation to rule out potentially life-threatening underlying causes other than diabetes.

Complications

MONONEUROPATHIES

Mononeuropathies of the third, fourth, or sixth cranial nerves may arise in association with diabetes (81,82) (see Chapter 56). These nerve palsies are usually of serious concern to the patient and present a significant diagnostic challenge, because misdiagnosis may keep a life-threatening lesion from being treated. On the other hand, a full neurologic evaluation, including computed tomography, magnetic resonance imaging, and other tests, may prove unwarranted and unnecessary. In one review of cranial nerve palsies treated in a diabetic patient population in 1967, 42% of mononeuropathies were not diabetic in origin (82). This finding underscores the danger of routinely attributing mononeuropathies, even in a diabetic person, to the diabetic condition itself without carefully ruling out other potential causes. The percentage of all extraocular muscle palsies attributable to diabetes mellitus is estimated at 4.5% to 6% (83–85).

Histopathologic studies of diabetic third-nerve palsies suggest that they are secondary to ischemic infarction of the nutrient vessels to the oculomotor nerve within the cavernous sinus or subarachnoid space (86,87). By extension, vascular infarct with resulting ischemia to any of the cranial nerves serving the extraocular muscles is generally accepted as the cause of diabetes-related cranial-nerve palsies.

The trochlear or fourth cranial nerve is the least likely to be affected by diabetes (81,82,84) (Table 54.13). Palsies of the oculomotor or third cranial nerve are more frequent and are usually accompanied by a ptosis of the affected eye, which may block or mask a horizontal and vertical diplopia. The ptosis itself, however, is usually sufficient to cause a person to seek medical evaluation. Characteristically, the affected eye has an exotropic and hypotropic posture (down and out). Pain may be associated with the onset of the palsy, which is usually acute (82,88–91). The pupil is usually unaffected or spared in diabetic third-nerve palsy, although there may be pupillary involvement in up to 20% of diabetes-induced third-nerve palsies (92,93). Pupillary involvement suggests external pressure on the nerve by a mass lesion or aneurysm and is sufficient reason to arrange immediate consultation for neurologic evaluation. In one series, 19.2% of all oculomotor-nerve palsies were associated with diabetes (94).

Paralysis of the abducens or sixth cranial nerve occurs at least as often as third-nerve palsies in diabetes (81,83,84). Patients with sixth-nerve palsies usually complain of horizontal diplopia, sometimes only on extreme lateral gaze to the side of the affected eye. The affected eye is generally esotropic and frequently cannot be moved past the midline. The sixth cranial nerve has a lengthy path, and there are many causes of abducens nerve insult, some of which are life-threatening.

Mononeuropathies also may be the initial presenting sign of new-onset diabetes. Diabetes should therefore be considered in the differential diagnosis of any mononeuropathy affecting the extraocular muscles, even in patients who do not claim a history of diabetes. Diabetes-induced third-, fourth-, and sixth-nerve palsies are usually self-limited and should resolve spontaneously in 2 to 6 months, although more or less time may be needed and the palsies may recur or subsequently develop in the contralateral eye.

Treatment involves patching one eye to eliminate diplopia, if symptoms warrant, and a mild analgesic if needed. In monocular patients, or in patients with poor vision in one eye, the maintenance of vision, especially when ptosis obstructs the visual axis of the eye with better sight, may present a challenge. Taping of the lid or the use of a ptosis crutch may be required, although the problems of corneal drying associated with diabetes-induced corneal hypoesthesia and poor epithelial adhesions are significant.

PERIORBITAL AND ORBITAL STRUCTURES

Waite and Beetham (81) reported a slightly higher frequency of xanthelasma in their diabetic patients than in their nondiabetic patients. The xanthelasma are usually of no clinical significance. A far more serious complication is orbital infection, usually at the apex of the orbit, with fungi of the order Mucorales (see Chapter 60). Although rare, mucormycosis (also called phycomycosis) is a fungal infection that develops in the adjacent periorbital sinuses in predisposed persons (95,96). Schwartz and coworkers found that 80% of their patients with the disorder had diabetes; most had diabetic ketoacidosis (96). The condition is frequently fatal, and prompt diagnosis is crucial. The patient typically has internal and external ophthalmoplegia, as well as decreased vision, proptosis, and ptosis. Treatment of the diabetic condition and aggressive treatment of the infectious

TABLE 54.12. Nonretinal Complications of Diabetes Mellitus

Structure	Complication	Management
Extraocular muscles	Mononeuropathy	1. Examination to rule out other causes 2. Consultation with internist or diabetologist 3. Neurologic referral 4. Patient education 5. Follow-up at 6 weeks or as indicated
Cornea	Decreased sensitivity Recurrent erosion Poor reepithelialization Abrasion Ulceration	1. Artificial tears 2. Patient education 3. Careful contact lens–patient selection
Iris	Iris neovascularization (rubeosis iridis) Neovascular glaucoma	1. Referral for possible panretinal photocoagulation 2. Management of glaucoma
Lens	Diabetic cataract Premature cataract Refractive fluctuations	1. Optimal refractive correction 2. Surgical referral 3. Control of blood glucose level

TABLE 54.13. Diabetic Nerve Palsies

Cranial nerve	Symptoms and signs
III (oculomotor)	Complete or partial ptosis Horizontal and vertical diplopia Affected eye "down and out" Possible supraorbital pain Pupillary sparing (80% of cases) Decreased sursumduction and adduction
IV (trochlear)	Vertical diplopia with associated esotropia Vertical deviation increases in downward gaze or when head is tilted to side of affected muscle Vertical deviation decreases with abduction of the affected eye Esotropia increases with downward gaze
VI (abducens)	Lateral or horizontal diplopia Esotropia of the affected eye Decreased abduction Possible head turn in the direction of the affected eye

organism with amphotericin B may result in recovery, although the survival rate still remains at only 57% (97,98).

CONJUNCTIVA AND LACRIMAL SYSTEM

Changes in the microcirculation of the bulbar conjunctiva of diabetic persons have been identified. In one series, microaneurysms of the bulbar conjunctiva were observed before cataract surgery in 63.6% of 22 eyes of diabetic patients (99). Histologically, these conjunctival microaneurysms show a thickened basement membrane, proliferation of endothelium, and lamellated hyaline deposits similar to the retinal microaneurysms in diabetic retinopathy (100). Diurnal variations in the dilation of conjunctival veins have also been noted (101). Insulin use itself appears to affect the composition of tears, sometimes resulting in a decrease in their lysozyme content (102).

Conjunctivitis and other disorders of the conjunctiva and lacrimal system need to be treated aggressively. Mild infections or marginal dry-eye syndromes potentially can cause serious ocular injuries, particularly in the presence of neuropathies or compromised corneal integrity.

CORNEA

The cornea of the diabetic person is often more susceptible to injury and slower to heal after injury than is the cornea of a nondiabetic person. A potential threat to corneal integrity is the measured reduction of corneal sensitivity in the diabetic individual (103). In animal studies, measured corneal sensitivity was significantly lower in dogs with poorly controlled diabetes than in nondiabetic dogs and diabetic dogs with good blood glucose control (104). The decrease in corneal sensitivity was also more marked with increased duration of diabetes in the dogs with poorly controlled diabetes.

The reduction of corneal sensitivity results in elevated tactile corneal thresholds (105). This reduction usually affects both eyes symmetrically and is the result of diffuse polyneuropathy of the trigeminal nerve and its branches. Other studies have suggested that panretinal photocoagulation can reduce corneal sensitivity caused by inadvertent thermal injury to the sensory nerves to the cornea between the choroid and the sclera (106). The reduction of corneal sensitivity may predispose a person to the development of neurotrophic corneal ulcerations (107). Furthermore, there is mounting evidence supporting the clinical impression that once corneal abrasions develop, the cornea in the diabetic patient is slower to heal than the cornea in the nondiabetic patient, presumably due to alterations in the basement membrane of the epithelium in patients with diabetes (108–110).

Waite and Beetham (81) found disorders in the deeper layers of the cornea as well, and subsequent research has verified the presence of these wrinkles in Descemet membrane layer in persons with diabetes (111,112). Subsequent studies demonstrated increased corneal thickness in diabetic individuals compared with that in nondiabetic control individuals (113,114), changes representing minimal corneal swelling, possibly as the result of increased corneal hydration.

Potential corneal complications affect contact-lens wear for diabetic patients. The person with diabetes may be a poor candidate for contact lenses, because discomfort from a poorly fitting or damaged lens may be absent because of a reduction in corneal sensitivity. Corneal abrasions or minor erosions that may be detected in an otherwise healthy cornea may develop into significant ulcerations. Long-term (1 week) extended-wear contact lenses should be used with extreme caution and careful monitoring and reserved only for patients with optimal conditions and specific needs, such as aphakia. All diabetic users of contact lenses should be properly educated about potential problems, early signs of lens rejection and infection, and corneal abrasion. The risk of corneal abrasion and the delay of corneal wound healing apparent in diabetic persons because of irregularities in the corneal basement epithelium dictate careful and selective contact-lens wear, although diabetes itself is not a contraindication for the use of either rigid or soft contact lenses. Many of the programmed-replacement or flexible-wear lenses provide adequate safeguards for successful adaptation to contact-lens wear.

The tendency for corneal abrasion may necessitate the use of artificial tears, particularly in dry environments. In chronic cases not remedied by tear replacement therapy, punctal plugs or punctal cauterization may be indicated. Patients with diabetes should be alerted to the potential side effects of contact lenses, and follow-up evaluations need to be frequent and thorough. The necessity of wearing safety glasses and goggles for appropriate work and sport environments should be emphasized. For ocular examination and treatment, care must be exercised to avoid corneal insult when treating or examining the retina with a corneal contact fundus lens, particularly if the patient has had a corneal abrasion in the past.

There have been no studies evaluating the risk of keratorefractive surgery to reduce myopia or hyperopia for persons with diabetes; however, diabetic persons should be evaluated carefully prior to undergoing LASIK (laser-assisted *in situ* keratomileusis), PRK (photoreactive keratectomy), or other keratorefractive surgical techniques.

IRIS

Diabetic complications affecting the iris have been well documented and the subject of much study. Glycogen deposits in the pigment epithelial cells of the iris can cause thickening of ocular tissue and depigmentation of the epithelial layer of the iris (81). Similar glycogen deposition occurs in the retina, optic nerve, epithelium of the lens capsule, and ciliary body (81,115,116). The most serious diabetic complication affecting the iris is neovascularization of the iris (NVI) or *rubeosis iridis*, a growth of new blood vessels on the iris (Fig. 54.13). Usually these vessels are first observed at the pupillary border and may resemble grape clusters. Neovascularization may already exist in the filtration angle without evidence of neovascularization at the pupillary border or on the iris surface. If NVI progresses, a fine network of vessels may grow over the iris tissue and into the filtration angle of the eye. Fibrous tissue accompanying the new vessels may contract and pull the underlying pigmented layer of the iris forward through the pupillary opening, resulting in ectropion uveae. Fibrovascular growth in the filtration angle may result in peripheral anterior synechiae. Closure of the angle by the fibrovascular network results in neovascular glaucoma, although intraocular pressure may be elevated prior to angle involvement because of protein and cellular leakage from the proliferating vessels (117,118). Neovascular glaucoma is difficult to manage and requires aggressive treatment. Usually NVI is first seen around the pupillary margin, although the vessels can grow initially in or near the filtration angle. Evaluation with a slit-lamp biomicroscope is necessary to observe and evaluate these vessels. The development of neovascular glaucoma in one eye is strongly correlated with the development of the same condition in the patient's other eye.

Diabetes is the second leading cause of neovascular glaucoma, accounting for 32.2% of cases, as opposed to 36.1% of cases resulting from retinal venous obstructive disease (119–122). This neovascularization of the anterior segment occurs in 4% to 7% of diabetic eyes and may be present in up to 40% to 60% of eyes with proliferative retinopathy that have not been treated with scatter laser photocoagulation (95–97).

Treatment for NVI and neovascular glaucoma includes scatter (panretinal) laser photocoagulation; goniophotocoagulation with a green or yellow laser; topical antiglaucoma medications; systemic antiglaucoma medications; antiglaucomatous filtration surgery, including Molteno valve implants; or, usually, a combination of one or more of the above therapies (2,123–127).

GLAUCOMA

Open-angle glaucoma is 1.4 times more common in the diabetic population than in the nondiabetic population (128–131). The prevalence of glaucoma increases with age and duration of diabetes, but medical therapy for open-angle glaucoma is generally effective. Choice of treatment of open-angle glaucoma in diabetic individuals must be influenced by the patient's general medical condition. Caution must be exercised with the use of topical β-adrenergic blockers in masking hypoglycemic symptoms or affecting concurrent cardiovascular disease. Systemic acetazolamide or other carbonic anhydrase inhibitors (CAIs) may be used if needed, but since these medications can cause metabolic acidosis, electrolyte monitoring should be done more frequently. The presence of renal disease may influence how these and other pressure-lowering drugs may be used, and close cooperation with the internist is important. Topical CAIs and recently available antiglaucoma eye drops have added safe additional medication for the treatment of glaucoma. Argon laser trabeculoplasty may normalize intraocular pressures in some if medical therapy proves ineffective.

Narrow-angle glaucoma and acute angle-closure glaucoma are comparatively rare. Narrow-angle glaucoma does not seem to be more common in persons with diabetes than in the general population, but investigations suggest that the shallower the anterior chamber of the patient's eye, the more likely the patient is to respond abnormally to an oral glucose-tolerance test (132). The postulated mechanism for this association is autonomic dysfunction within the anterior segment of the eye resulting in a hypersensitivity to both sympathetic and parasympathetic autonomic mediators, with the iris-lens diaphragm moving forward and closing the angle. Anterior chambers generally become shallower with age.

In acute angle-closure glaucoma, the outflow angle in the anterior chamber of the eye formed by the iris plane and the posterior corneal surface becomes closed, blocking outflow to the outflow channels of the trabecula meshwork. The result is a dramatic and rapid rise in intraocular pressure, with ocular pain, decreased vision, colored halos around lights, and, fre-

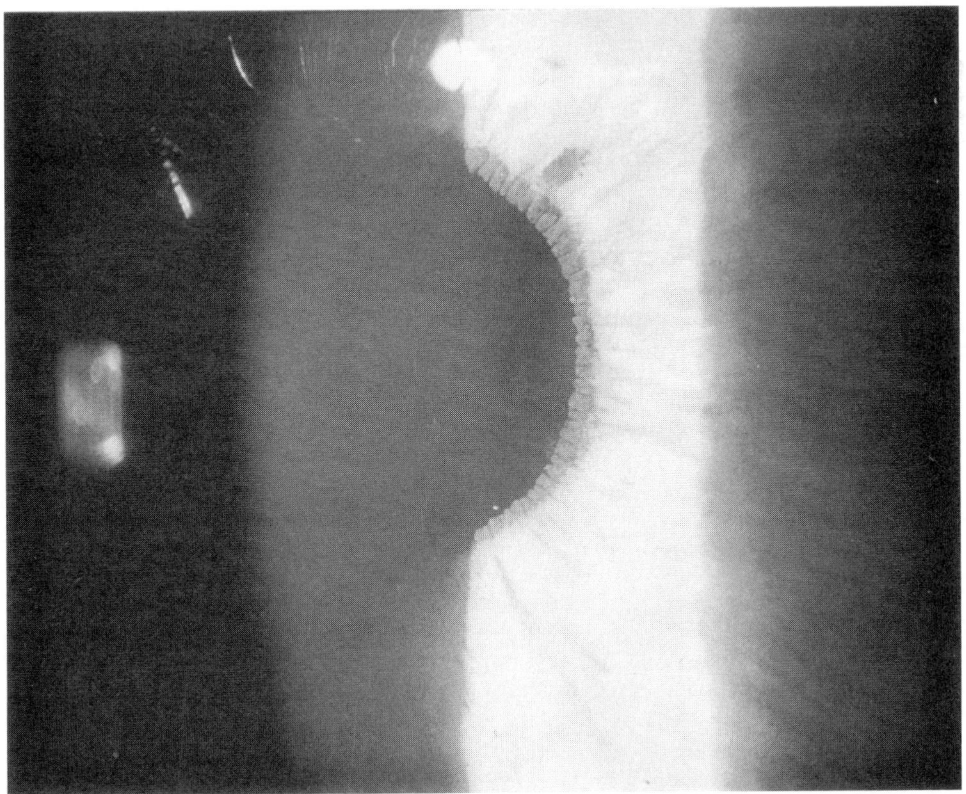

Figure 54.13. Neovascularization of the iris (rubeosis iridis) around the pupillary margin.

quently, nausea and vomiting. Angle-closure glaucoma should be considered as part of the differential diagnosis for a diabetic patient presenting with nausea and vomiting.

Angle-closure glaucoma is considered a medical emergency. Treatment consists of attempts to break the angle closure medically with miotic drops and to lower the pressure with either systemic or topical medications. A peripheral iridectomy or laser iridotomy can restore the normal aqueous outflow and prevent future episodes of angle closure. Because pupil dilation can trigger an angle-closure attack, care needs to be exercised before dilation of any pupil.

LENS

Diabetic effects on the crystalline lens can result in transitory refractive changes and cataracts.

Refractive Changes

Refractive changes related to fluctuation of blood glucose levels are readily acknowledged by all clinicians, and diabetes has also been found to affect accommodation ability.

Blood Glucose Levels

The mechanism of such refractive changes due to fluctuations in blood glucose levels is only poorly understood. Myopic or hyperopic shifts with changes of blood glucose levels or as an initial symptom or sign of undiagnosed diabetes are common in the phakic eye (81). These refractive shifts can be of several diopters or more and are thought to be the result of osmotic swelling of the crystalline lens. Rapid shifting of blood glucose levels may result in uncorrectable blurring of vision.

Sudden refractive shifts are frequently the presenting symptom for a person with new diabetes. Patients who were able to see clearly at a distance either with or without their glasses may complain that their distance vision is now blurry. On the other hand, those who required reading glasses or who were experiencing difficulty with close work may now find they can read more easily without their glasses, misinterpreting the change as "an improvement" in their eyes. Patients with uncontrolled or poorly controlled blood glucose levels should be encouraged to postpone the purchase of eyeglasses until their blood glucose levels have stabilized. This stabilization may take 4 to 6 weeks to occur, although the effects of a rise in blood glucose level on refractive state are generally recognized as being more sudden. Any coexisting physical condition that impacts on blood glucose level, such as infection or stress, is reason not to prescribe glasses, especially if a person recognizes recent or sudden fluctuations in vision.

The proposed cause of such refractive shifts in phakic eyes involves fluid absorption by the crystalline lens. The galactitol and sorbitol pathways have been implicated, and rat models have shown that osmotic changes caused by the accumulation of galactitol in the lenses of rats fed with galactose leads to lens swelling and premature cataract development (133–140). The sorbitol pathway, however, is most likely beneficial in protecting the lens against glucose-generated osmotic changes (138).

Accommodation

While discussions of refractive changes associated with diabetes most frequently are directed to refractive shifts related to elevated blood glucose levels, there is evidence that diabetes alters accommodative ability. Waite and Beetham (81) demonstrated transitory paresis of accommodation in 21% of the diabetic patients in their study. This paresis was most predominant in the 20- to 50-year-old group and resolved with improvement of the diabetic condition. Transient accommodative paralysis accompanied with hyperopia may be associated with either a rise or fall in blood glucose levels, most frequently after insulin treatment has been started, and may be present even in young individuals (140).

Reduced accommodative ability and diminished pupillary response have been demonstrated following heavy panretinal argon laser photocoagulation (141). It is postulated that this internal ophthalmoplegia following heavy panretinal laser photocoagulation is the result of direct or indirect injury to the parasympathetic motor fibers to the ciliary body and the iris. These fibers enter the globe at the posterior pole and course forward between the sclera and the choroid. As the fibers course forward, the choroid becomes thinner, providing less protection against the heat generated in the retinal pigment epithelium from the laser surgery. Unlike the paresis of accommodation associated with uncontrolled diabetes, the internal ophthalmoplegia associated with scatter (panretinal) photocoagulation surgery is generally irreversible, since the laser burns cause permanent damage to the underlying parasympathetic nerve fibers.

Diabetic persons frequently demonstrate presbyopia at an earlier age than nondiabetic persons, and the loss of accommodative ability frequently progresses more rapidly for diabetic persons. Consequently, it is not uncommon for myopic contact-lens wearers, who need to accommodate more through contact lenses than through spectacle lenses, or hyperopic individuals to demonstrate difficulty in reading or in close tasks. Identifying these problems may be difficult because of refractive changes secondary to fluctuation in blood glucose levels. These changes in accommodation are irreversible with age.

Cataracts

Cataracts occur earlier in life and progress more rapidly in the presence of diabetes (137–142). Cataracts are 1.6 times more common in people with diabetes than in those without diabetes (142–144). Incidence of cataract surgery in the nondiabetic population in the Beaver Dam Eye Study (150) was one-fifth to one-half the incidence of cataract in the Wisconsin Epidemiologic Study of Diabetic Retinopathy in each age stratum studied (145). This increased risk of cataract development for the diabetic person occurs both in persons with earlier-onset diabetes and those with later-onset diabetes. In persons diagnosed with diabetes at age 30 years or older, cataract is the most common cause of visual impairment. Several studies suggested that aspirin use can reduce the risk of cataract for persons with diabetes (146–149). Other studies do not support this finding (148,149). The ETDRS results do not support the use of 650 mg of aspirin per day to reduce the risk of cataract development in the ETDRS patient population (32). In the Beaver Dam Eye Study, persons with older-onset diabetes were significantly more likely to have cortical lens opacities or prior cataract surgery than persons without diabetes in the same age group (150). Many factors are correlated with cataract development, including duration of diabetes and retinopathy status in the patient with earlier-onset diabetes, the use of diuretics, and the HbA_{1c} level (139). In patients with later-onset diabetes, age of the patient, severity of retinopathy, use of diuretics, lower intraocular pressure, smoking, and lower diastolic blood pressure may be risk factors (150,151).

Fortunately, cataract extraction is 90% to 95% successful in restoring useful vision, but the surgery is not without potential complications unique to diabetes, such as delayed wound healing, acceleration of diabetic retinopathy, iris or retinal neovascularization, and macular edema. Cataracts obscuring retinal examination may need to be removed surgically to permit retinal examination and, in some cases, appropriate laser photocoagulation surgery. Diabetic patients undergoing simultaneous kidney/pancreas transplantation are at an increased risk of developing all types of cataract, independent of the use of corticosteroids after transplantation (152).

Reversible lenticular opacities related to diabetes mellitus have also been reported (153–160). These reversible cataracts can occur in different layers of the lens and are most frequently related to poor metabolic control of diabetes. The so-called true diabetic cataracts are usually bilateral and are characterized by dense bands of white, subcapsular spots that are snowflake in appearance or fine, needle-shaped opacities (161) (Fig. 54.14). Because these diabetic cataracts are related to prolonged periods of severe hyperglycemia and untreated diabetes mellitus, they are only rarely now seen in the United States and other industrialized countries.

Management of diabetic cataract involves the same treatment strategies as those for age-related cataracts. For visual impairment not requiring surgery, optimal refractive correction is beneficial. Glare-control lenses and the use of sunglasses may relieve cataract-induced visual symptoms. Surgically, intraocular lens implants provide the most natural postsurgical refractive correction, depending on retinopathy status (162). Both phacoemulsification and extracapsular cataract extraction provide appropriate surgical approaches to cataract extraction and intraocular lens implantation; however, in one study, phacoemulsification was generally associated with better postoperative visual acuity, less postoperative inflammation, and reduced need for capsulotomy (163). A retrospective review of 150 eyes of 119 diabetic patients comparing phacoemulsification surgery to other surgical techniques did not demonstrate significant differences in postoperative visual acuity or rate of progression of diabetic retinopathy (164). In each study, the principal determinant of postoperative vision and progression of retinopathy was related to the preoperative presence of diabetic macular edema and level of nonproliferative diabetic retinopathy.

VITREOUS

Problems with the vitreous in the diabetic patient are intimately related to retinal disease (165–174). PDR is associated with an increased incidence of posterior vitreous detachment, although frequently a partial vitreous detachment, rather than a total posterior vitreous detachment, is present (166). Partial vitreous detachment may result in vitreous hemorrhage, an increase in retinal neovascularization, and tractional retinal detachment (174).

OPTIC DISC

Although the optic disc usually is discussed only in relation to PDR and neovascularization at the disc, it can be affected in a variety of other ways by diabetes. Optic disc edema unrelated to anterior ischemic optic neuropathy or other neurologic disorders can occur with diabetes mellitus (175,176). The condition seems to be related to a vasculopathy of the most superficial layer of capillaries of the optic disc (177) and is more common in younger patients with type 1 diabetes. Although transient optic disc edema usually leaves little or no lasting effect on visual acuity or visual fields, especially in younger patients, some residual disc pallor may follow resolution of the disc edema. One or both eyes may be affected.

Diabetic papillopathy must be distinguished from other causes of disc swelling, such as true papilledema from increased intracranial pressure; pseudopapilledema, such as optic nerve head drusen; toxic optic neuropathies; neoplasm of the optic nerve; and hypertension (178).

Optic disc pallor can occur following spontaneous remission of proliferative retinopathy or remission following scatter (panretinal) laser photocoagulation (179). This disc pallor does not result in a change of the cup/disc ratio. Since diabetes poses an increased risk for the development of open-angle glaucoma and anterior ischemic optic neuropathy, the disc pallor following remission of retinopathy or panretinal photocoagulation must

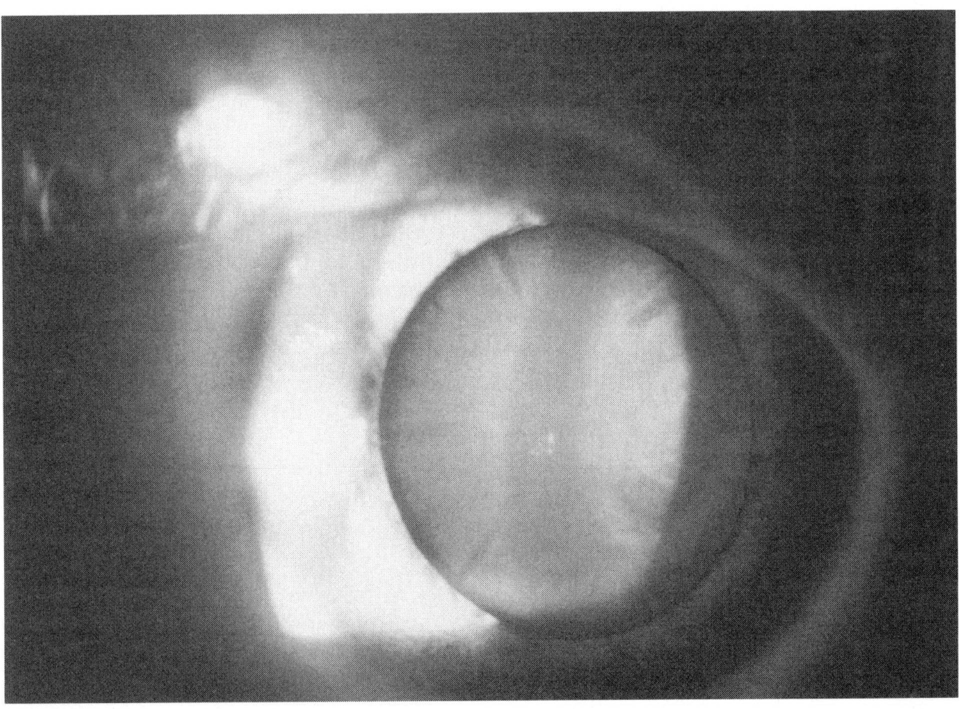

Figure 54.14. Diabetic cataract in a 16-year-old girl.

be considered when evaluating the optic-nerve head for open-angle glaucoma or low-tension glaucoma (179).

FUTURE HORIZONS

Molecular and Cellular Advances

Over the past several decades, remarkable advances in our understanding of the basic mechanisms underlying diabetes and diabetic retinopathy have been achieved. These new insights into the processes underlying the fundamental molecular and cellular changes ultimately resulting in sight-threatening complications of diabetic retinopathy are permitting the development of new interventional approaches. These new therapeutic modalities hold great promise for further reducing or eliminating the complications of diabetic eye disease. Advances have been made in understanding many areas, including the changes in the sorbitol pathway, the development of oxidative stress, the production of advanced glycosylation end-products (AGEs), and the activation of protein kinase C. Each of these various pathways has been associated with a variety of the complications of diabetes, and they are often intimately related.

An area of substantial study has been the increased flux through the sorbitol pathway in cells exposed to a hyperglycemic environment. Consequently, aldose reductase inhibitors have been evaluated extensively for their potential use in ameliorating diabetic retinopathy. A multicenter clinical trial, the Sorbinil Retinopathy Trial (180,181), tested whether a daily dose of sorbinil could reduce the complications of diabetes mellitus. Over a 3-year period, the drug had no clinically important effect on the course of diabetic retinopathy in adults with type 1 diabetes of moderate duration (180,181). However, the group taking sorbinil did show a slight lowering in the number of microaneurysms. Unfortunately, there were complications in nearly 7% of the initial 202 participants taking the drug. These adverse reactions included toxic epidermal necrolysis, erythema multiforme, and Stevens–Johnson syndrome. Because of this lack of efficacy in humans and the associated side effects, no aldose reductase inhibitors are currently being used on a routine clinical basis for the treatment of diabetic retinopathy.

A variety of studies has also looked at antioxidants as a potential ameliorator of oxidative stress present under the diabetic condition. Preliminary data on antioxidants such as vitamin E have been promising with regard to preventing or reversing early changes in retinal circulation in animals and in correcting the abnormal retinal blood flow present in patients with short-duration diabetes and minimal diabetic retinopathy (78,182,183).

When proteins are exposed to high levels of glucose for extended periods, AGEs may be formed (184). Recent studies have suggested that these AGEs can cause a variety of changes in cellular processes and may contribute to diabetic ocular complications. Inhibitors of AGEs are being evaluated for clinical usefulness.

A promising area of research involves the activation of protein kinase C by diabetes (185). Activation of this enzyme can result in wide-ranging effects underlying endothelial dysfunction in the eye and other organs. In addition, protein kinase C is a key mediator of signaling processes induced by other growth factors involved in retinal neovascularization, diabetic macular edema, and perhaps earlier stages of diabetic retinopathy as well. A particular isoform (the β isoform) of protein kinase C appears to specifically mediate many of the complications arising in the eye. Consequently, inhibitors of protein kinase C β have been evaluated in animal models, with documented ability to normalize retinal blood flow, suppress retinal permeability, prevent retinal neovascularization, and normalize retinal blood flow in patients with no or mild nonproliferative retinopathy. These agents are currently in clinical trials to determine whether they can prevent or slow the progression of diabetic retinopathy and/or diabetic macular edema. Results from these studies are expected in the next few years.

Another promising area of investigation is the evaluation of the various growth factors mediating the later-stage complications of diabetic retinopathy. Numerous angiogenic agents, such as vascular endothelial growth factor, have been identified as key modulators of the retinal neovascular response and the increase in retinal vascular permeability. Several inhibitors of these agents have been developed with very promising results observed in animal models and over the next few years may add significantly to our therapeutic armamentarium. In addition, preliminary results from small uncontrolled studies suggest that intravitreal administration of steroids may have a significant effect in reducing diabetic macular edema and may actually improve vision in a subset of these patients. Currently, a number of these agents are in clinical trials.

Patient Access to Eye Care

Despite demonstrated methods of reducing vision loss from diabetes, many patients are deprived of sight-saving care. Enhanced and facilitated access to quality eye care can have a substantial impact on preserving human vision and eliminating blindness as a complication of diabetes. In addition to saving of vision, substantial savings in health costs would also be achieved. There are many barriers to quality eye care, including ignorance of the importance of such care, a shortage in caregivers, geographic isolation and distances, socioeconomic challenges, and cultural patterns.

Telemedicine initiatives hold great theoretical potential for surmounting these barriers. One system that has been studied is the Joslin Vision Network (JVN), a telemedicine-enabling technology for remote-site diagnosis and management of chronic-disease care of diabetes mellitus within the Joslin Diabetes Eye Health Care Model (186–188). Evaluation for level of diabetic retinopathy using the JVN compares favorably with evaluation using the current gold standard, 35-mm stereoscopic color slide of seven standard retinal fields as used in the ETDRS. Such validated systems are uniquely positioned to provide efficient, cost-effective eye examination and medical intervention strategies for persons with diabetes, increasing access to quality eye care and treatment and providing a database warehouse for clinical trials, treatment outcomes, and population-based studies (186–188).

Deployment of this type of technology in a community-based and community-owned program enhances the potential to reach patients who do not have access to specialty eye care. This approach can be implemented in culturally sensitive diabetes healthcare programs in geographically diverse communities. These programs would screen for undiagnosed diabetes in the general population, access the retina at appropriate intervals to diagnose the level of diabetic retinopathy for timely medical and surgical treatment as necessary, manage diabetes medically, and collect data for population-based studies and clinical research.

GUIDELINES

Until modalities are in place to prevent or cure diabetic retinopathy and other complications, the clinical emphasis must be placed on identification, careful follow-up, and timely laser photocoagulation for patients with diabetic retinopathy and diabetic eye disease. Proper care will result in reduction of personal suffering, as well as in a substantial cost savings for the individuals with diabetes, their families, and society in general (189–191). Therefore, strict guidelines have been established for the ocular care of people with diabetes (Tables 54.8 and 54.14).

All patients with diabetes should be informed of the likelihood of developing retinopathy and the associated threat of visual loss. The natural course and treatment of diabetic retinopathy should be discussed, including the asymptomatic nature of early disease and the importance of routine examination. Patients should be informed of the relationship between glycemic control and the risk of developing ocular and other medical complications. Patients must be made aware that diabetic nephropathy, as manifest by proteinuria, requires aggressive early treatment with proper diet and blood pressure control, especially with angiotensin-converting enzyme (ACE) inhibitors, to reduce renal disease and avoid superimposed renal retinopathy (and the possible associated risk of neovascular glaucoma). The association of joint contractures, hypertension, cardiovascular disease, elevated lipid levels, and neuropathy with onset and progression of diabetic retinopathy should be discussed.

Women with diabetes who are contemplating pregnancy should have a complete eye examination before they conceive. Pregnant women with diabetes should ideally have their eyes examined early in each trimester of their pregnancy or more frequently, as indicated by level of retinopathy, and 6 weeks after delivery. Because pregnancy may exacerbate existing retinopathy and be associated with hypertension, careful medical and ocular observation during pregnancy is crucial. In women with PDR, cesarean delivery may be considered in some cases rather than vaginal delivery to reduce the risk of vitreous hemorrhage. Close communication among the various members of the healthcare team is essential.

Patients with diabetic retinopathy, even in its mildest form, must be informed of the availability and benefits of early and timely laser photocoagulation therapy in reducing the risk of visual loss. The management program outlined in Table 54.8 is fundamental. Furthermore, patients with visual impairment of any degree, legal blindness, or total blindness should be informed of the availability of visual, vocational, and psychosocial rehabilitation programs.

CONCLUSIONS

In its earliest stages, diabetic retinopathy usually causes no symptoms. Visual acuity may be very good at the time of diagnosis of diabetic retinopathy, even when significant ocular disease is present. It is crucial at this stage for a patient's physician to initiate a careful program of education and medical and ocular follow-up.

As retinal disease progresses, visual acuity may become compromised by macular edema, episodes of vitreous hemorrhage, macular nonperfusion, or traction retinal detachment. The resulting loss of visual acuity can cause significant difficulties in the work or home environment. This loss often puts extreme psychologic stress on patients with diabetes and their families. The healthcare provider should identify some stresses, and appropriate support for the patients should be offered. In many cases, the patient will experience a significant drop in visual acuity for a period of time. Although in many cases excellent vision can ultimately be obtained and retained for many decades, the period during which the patient experiences this visual decline can lead to great uncertainty and anxiety.

It is of critical importance that the level of ocular disease be monitored carefully and appropriate observation, laser treatment, vitreoretinal surgery, or other intervention be applied promptly when indicated. If these approaches are followed, most patients can now retain excellent vision with many decades of stable ocular status once the diabetic retinopathy has become quiescent. New therapies on the horizon promise even better outcomes.

Thus, it is obvious that a very close interaction between the patient and a diverse healthcare team is essential. The healthcare team will commonly require services of both the ophthalmologist and internist, as well as the diabetologist, nurse practitioner, diabetes educator, dietician, psychosocial worker, and many other specialties, depending on the particular situation. With such access, careful lifelong and routine ophthalmic follow-up, optimization of glycemic and systemic medical control, and timely laser photocoagulation, the risk of blindness in persons with diabetes mellitus can essentially be eliminated.

REFERENCES

1. Joslin EP. *The treatment of diabetes mellitus*, 5th ed. Philadelphia: Lea & Febiger, 1935:411.
2. Aiello LM, Beetham WP, Balodimos MC, et al. Ruby laser photocoagulation in treatment of diabetic proliferating retinopathy: preliminary report. In: Goldberg MF, Fine SL, eds. *Symposium on the treatment of diabetic retinopathy.* US Public Health Service. Publication no. 1890. Washington, DC: US Government Printing Office, 1969:437–463.
3. The Diabetic Retinopathy Study Research Group. Preliminary report on effects of photocoagulation therapy. *Am J Ophthalmol* 1976;81:383–396.
4. The Diabetic Retinopathy Study Research Group. Photocoagulation treatment of proliferative diabetic retinopathy: the second report of Diabetic Retinopathy Study findings. *Ophthalmology* 1978;85:82–106.
5. The Diabetic Retinopathy Study Research Group. Four risk factors for severe visual loss in diabetic retinopathy: the third report from the Diabetic Retinopathy Study. *Arch Ophthalmol* 1979;97:654–655.
6. The Diabetic Retinopathy Study Research Group. *Photocoagulation treatment of proliferative diabetic retinopathy: a short report of long range results.* Diabetic Retinopathy Study (DRS) report no. 4. Amsterdam: Excerpta Medica, 1980.
7. Diabetic Retinopathy Study Research Group. Photocoagulation treatment of proliferative diabetic retinopathy: relationship of adverse treatment effects to retinopathy severity: Diabetic Retinopathy Study report no. 5. *Dev Ophthalmol* 1981;2:248–261.

TABLE 54.14. Eye Examination Schedule

Type of diabetes mellitus	Recommended initial eye examination	Routine follow-up[a]
Type 1	5 years after onset or during puberty	Yearly
Type 2	At time of diagnosis	Yearly
Pregnancy with preexisting diabetes	Prior to pregnancy for counseling	• Early in first trimester • Each trimester or more frequently as indicated • 6 weeks postpartum

[a]Abnormal findings will dictate more frequent follow-up examinations (see Table 54.8).

8. Diabetic Retinopathy Study Report Research Group. Report 6: design, methods, and baseline results. *Invest Ophthalmol Vis Sci* 1981;21:149–209.
9. Diabetic Retinopathy Study Research Group. Report 7. A modification of the Airlie House classification of diabetic retinopathy. *Invest Ophthalmol Vis Sci* 1981;21:210–226.
10. The Diabetic Retinopathy Study Research Group. Photocoagulation treatment of proliferative diabetic retinopathy: clinical application of Diabetic Retinopathy Study (DRS) findings, DRS report no. 8. *Ophthalmology* 1981;88: 583–600.
11. Diabetic Retinopathy Study Research Group. Report 9: assessing possible late treatment effects in stopping clinical trials early: a case study by F Ederer, MJ Podgor. *Controlled Clin Trials* 1984;5:373–381.
12. Rand LI, Prud'homme GJ, Ederer F, Canner PL, Diabetic Retinopathy Research Group. Factors influencing the development of visual loss in advanced diabetic retinopathy: Diabetic Retinopathy Study report no. 10. *Invest Ophthalmol Vis Sci* 1985;26:983–991.
13. Kaufman SC, Ferris FL III, Swartz M, Diabetic Retinopathy Study Research Group. Intraocular pressure following panretinal photocoagulation for diabetic retinopathy: Diabetic Retinopathy report no. 11. *Arch Ophthalmol* 1987; 105:807–809.
14. Ferris FL III, Podgor MJ, Davis MD, the Diabetic Retinopathy Study Research Group. Macular edema in diabetic retinopathy study patients: Diabetic Retinopathy Study report number 12. *Ophthalmology* 1987;94:754–760.
15. Kaufman SC, Ferris FL III, et al, the DRS Research Group. Factors associated with visual outcome after photocoagulation for diabetic retinopathy: Diabetic Retinopathy Study report #13. *Invest Ophthalmol Vis Sci* 1989;30:23–28.
16. The Diabetic Retinopathy Study Research Group. Indications for photocoagulation treatment of diabetic retinopathy: Diabetic Retinopathy Study report no. 14. *Int Ophthalmol Clin* 1987;27:239–253.
17. Early Treatment Diabetic Retinopathy Study Research Group. Photocoagulation for diabetic macular edema; Early Treatment Diabetic Retinopathy Study report no. 1. *Arch Ophthalmol* 1985;103:1796–1806.
18. Early Treatment Diabetic Retinopathy Study Research Group. Treatment techniques and clinical guidelines for photocoagulation of diabetic macular edema: Early Treatment Diabetic Retinopathy Study report no. 2. *Ophthalmology* 1987;94:761–774.
19. The Early Treatment Diabetic Retinopathy Study Research Group. Techniques for scatter and local photocoagulation treatment of diabetic retinopathy: Early Treatment Diabetic Retinopathy Study report no. 3. *Int Ophthalmol Clin* 1987;27:254–264.
20. The Early Treatment Diabetic Retinopathy Study Research Group. Photocoagulation for diabetic macular edema: Early Treatment Diabetic Retinopathy Study report no. 4. *Int Ophthalmol Clin* 1987;27:265–272.
21. The Early Treatment Diabetic Retinopathy Study Research Group. Case reports to accompany Early Treatment Diabetic Retinopathy Study reports 3 and 4. *Int Ophthalmol Clin* 1987;27:273–333.
22. Kinyoun J, Barton F, Fisher M, et al, the ETDRS Research Group. Detection of diabetic macular edema: ophthalmoscopy versus photography—Early Treatment Diabetic Retinopathy Study report no. 5. *Ophthalmology* 1989;96: 746–751.
23. Prior MJ, Prout T, Miller D, et al. C-peptide and the classification of diabetes patients in the Early Treatment Diabetic Retinopathy Study. Report no. 6. The ETDRS Research Group. *Ann Epidemiol* 1993;3:9–17.
24. Early Treatment Diabetic Retinopathy Study Research Group. Early Treatment Diabetic Retinopathy Study design and baseline patient characteristics: ETDRS report no. 7. *Ophthalmology* 1991;98[Suppl 5]:741–756.
25. Early Treatment Diabetic Retinopathy Study Research Group. Effects of aspirin treatment on diabetic retinopathy: ETDRS report no. 8. *Ophthalmology* 1991;98[Suppl 5]:757–765.
26. Early Treatment Diabetic Retinopathy Study Research Group. Early photocoagulation for diabetic retinopathy: ETDRS report no. 9. *Ophthalmology* 1991;98[Suppl 5]:766–785.
27. Early Treatment Diabetic Retinopathy Study Research Group. Grading diabetic retinopathy from stereoscopic color fundus photographs—an extension of the modified Airlie House classification: ETDRS report no. 10. *Ophthalmology* 1991;98[Suppl 5]:786–806.
28. Early Treatment Diabetic Retinopathy Study Research Group. Classification of diabetic retinopathy from fluorescein angiograms: ETDRS report no. 11. *Ophthalmology* 1991;98[Suppl 5]:807–822.
29. Early Treatment Diabetic Retinopathy Study Research Group. Fundus photographic risk factors for progression of diabetic retinopathy: ETDRS report no. 12. *Ophthalmology* 1991;98[Suppl 5]:823–833.
30. Early Treatment Diabetic Retinopathy Study Research Groups. Fluorescein angiographic risk factors for progression of diabetic retinopathy: ETDRS report no. 13. *Ophthalmology* 1991;98[Suppl 5]:834–840.
31. Early Treatment Diabetic Retinopathy Study Research Group. Aspirin effects on mortality and morbidity in patients with diabetes mellitus. ETDRS report no. 14. *JAMA* 1992;268:1292–1300.
32. Early Treatment Diabetic Retinopathy Study Research Group. Aspirin effects on the development of cataracts in patients with diabetes mellitus. ETDRS report no. 16. *Arch Ophthalmol* 1992;110:339–342.
33. Flynn HW, Chew EY, Simons BD, et al. Early Treatment Diabetic Retinopathy Study Research Group. Pars plana vitrectomy in the early treatment diabetic retinopathy study. ETDRS report no. 17. *Ophthalmology* 1992;99:1351–1357.
34. Davis MD, Fisher MR, Gangnon RE, et al. Risk factors for high-risk proliferative diabetic retinopathy and severe visual loss: Early Treatment Diabetic Retinopathy Study report # 18. *Invest Ophthalmol Vis Sci* 1998;39:233–252.
35. Early Treatment Diabetic Retinopathy Study Research Group. Focal photocoagulation treatment of diabetic macular edema: relationship of treatment effect to fluorescein angiographic and other retinal characteristics at baseline. EDDRS report no. 19. *Arch Ophthalmol* 1995;113:1144–1155.
36. Chew EY, Klein ML, Murphy RP, et al. Effects of aspirin on vitreous/preretinal hemorrhage in patients with diabetes mellitus. Early Treatment Diabetic Retinopathy Study report no. 20. *Arch Ophthalmol* 1995;13:52–55.
37. Chew EY, Klein ML, Ferris FL 3rd, et al. Association of elevated serum lipid levels with retinal hard exudates in diabetic retinopathy. Early Treatment Diabetic Retinopathy Study (ETDRS) report no. 22. *Arch Ophthalmol* 1996;114: 1079–1084.
38. Fong DS, Segal PP, Myers F, et al. Subretinal fibrosis in diabetic macular edema: Early Treatment Diabetic Retinopathy Research Group. ETDRS report 23. *Arch Ophthalmol* 1997;115:873–877.
39. Fong DS, Ferris FL 3rd, Davis MD, et al. Causes of severe visual loss in the early treatment diabetic retinopathy study: ETDRS report no. 24. Early Treatment Diabetic Retinopathy Study Research Group. *Am J Ophthalmol* 1999;127: 137–141.
40. The DRVS Research Group. Two-year course of visual acuity in severe proliferative diabetic retinopathy with conventional management: Diabetic Retinopathy Vitrectomy Study (DRVS) report no. 1. *Ophthalmology* 1985;92: 492–502.
41. The Diabetic Retinopathy Vitrectomy Study Research Group. Early vitrectomy for severe vitreous hemorrhage in diabetic retinopathy: two-year results of a randomized trial: Diabetic Retinopathy Vitrectomy Study report no. 2. *Arch Ophthalmol* 1985;103:1644–1652.
42. The Diabetic Retinopathy Vitrectomy Study Research Group. Early vitrectomy for severe proliferative diabetic retinopathy in eyes with useful vision: results of a randomized trial—Diabetic Retinopathy Vitrectomy Study report no. 3. *Ophthalmology* 1988;95:1307–1320.
43. The Diabetic Retinopathy Vitrectomy Study Research Group. Early vitrectomy for severe proliferative diabetic retinopathy in eyes with useful vision: clinical application of results of a randomized trial—Diabetic Retinopathy Vitrectomy Study report no. 4. *Ophthalmology* 1988;95:1321–1334.
44. The Diabetic Retinopathy Vitrectomy Study Research Group. Early vitrectomy for severe vitreous hemorrhage in diabetic retinopathy: four-year results of a randomized trial: Diabetic Retinopathy Study report no. 5. *Arch Ophthalmol* 1990;108:958–964.
45. Diabetes Control and Complications Trial Research Group. Are continuing studies of metabolic control and microvascular complications in insulin-dependent diabetes mellitus justified? *N Engl J Med* 1988;318:246–250.
46. The Diabetes Control and Complications Trial Research Group. The relationship of glycemic exposure (HbA_{1c}) to the risk of development and progression of retinopathy in the Diabetes Control and Complications Trial. *Diabetes* 1995;44:968–983.
47. The Diabetes Control and Complications Trial Research Group. Progression of retinopathy with intensive versus conventional treatment in the Diabetes Control and Complications Trial. *Ophthalmology* 1995;102:647–661.
48. The Diabetes Control and Complications Trial Research Group. Hypoglycemia in the Diabetes Control and Complications Trial. *Diabetes* 1997;46: 271–286.
49. The Diabetes Control and Complications Trial Research Group. Lifetime benefits and costs of intensive therapy as practiced in the Diabetes Control and Complications Trial. *JAMA* 1996;276:1409–1415.
50. The Diabetes Control and Complications Trial Research Group. The effect of intensive treatment of diabetes on the development and progression of long-term complications in insulin dependent diabetes mellitus. *N Engl J Med* 1993;329:977–986.
51. The Diabetes Control and Complications Trial Research Group. The relationship of glycemic exposure (HbA_{1c}) to the risk of development and progression of retinopathy in the Diabetes Control and Complications Trial. *Diabetes* 1995;44:968–983.
52. Diabetes Control and Complications Trial/Epidemiology of Diabetes Intervention and Complications Research Group. Retinopathy and nephropathy in patients with type 1 diabetes four years after a trial of intensive therapy. *N Engl J Med* 2000;342:381–389.
53. Ohkubo Y, Kishikawa H, Araki E, et al. Intensive insulin therapy prevents the progression of diabetic microvascular complications in Japanese patients with non-insulin-dependent diabetes mellitus: a randomized prospective 6-year study. *Diabetes Res Clin Pract* 1995;28:103–117.
54. Kohner EM, Aldington SJ, Stratton IM, et al. United Kingdom Prospective Diabetes Study, 30: diabetic retinopathy at diagnosis of non-insulin-dependent diabetes mellitus and associated risk factors: *Arch Ophthalmol* 1998;116: 297–303.
55. UK Prospective Diabetes Study Group. Effect of intensive blood-glucose control with sulphonylureas or insulin compared with conventional treatment and risk of complications in patients with type 2 diabetes (UKPDS 33). *Lancet* 1998;352:837–853.
56. Klein R, Klein BEK, Moss SE, et al. The Wisconsin Epidemiologic Study of Diabetic Retinopathy, II: prevalence and risk of diabetic retinopathy when age at diagnosis is less than 30 years. *Arch Ophthalmol* 1984;102:520–526.
57. Klein R, Klein BEK, Moss SE, et al. The Wisconsin Epidemiologic Study of Diabetic Retinopathy, III: prevalence and risk of diabetic retinopathy when age at diagnosis is 30 or more years. *Arch Ophthalmol* 1984;102:527–532.
58. Klein R, Klein BEK. Vision disorders in diabetes. In: *Diabetes in America.* National Institutes of Health, National Institute of Diabetes and Digestive and Kidney Diseases. NIH publication no. 95-1468, 1995:293–336.

59. Ferris FL III. Early photocoagulation in patients with either type I or type II diabetes. *Trans Am Ophthalmol Soc* 1996;94:505–537.
60. Ferris FL. How effective are treatments for diabetic retinopathy? *JAMA* 1993; 269:1290–1291.
61. Harris MI. Classification, diagnostic criteria, and screening for diabetes. In: *Diabetes in America.* National Institutes of Health, National Institute of Diabetes and Digestive and Kidney Diseases. NIH publication no. 95-1468, 1995: 15–36.
62. Rand LI, Krolewski AS, Aiello LM, et al. Multiple factors in the prediction of risk of proliferative diabetic retinopathy. *N Engl J Med* 1985;313:1433–1438.
63. Aiello LP, Cahill MT, Wong JS. Systemic considerations in the management of diabetic retinopathy. *Am J Ophthalmol* 2001;132:760–766.
64. Moloney JBM, Drury MI. The effect of pregnancy on the natural course of diabetic retinopathy. *Am J Ophthalmol* 1982;93:745–756.
65. Serup L. Influence of pregnancy on diabetic retinopathy. *Acta Endocrinol Suppl* 1986;277:122–124.
66. Phelps RL, Sakol P, Metzger BE, et al. Changes in diabetic retinopathy during pregnancy: correlations with regulation of hyperglycemia. *Arch Ophthalmol* 1986;104:1806–1810.
67. The Kroc Collaborative Study Group. Blood glucose control and the evolution of diabetic retinopathy and albuminuria: a preliminary multicenter trial. *N Engl J Med* 1984;311:365–372.
68. Grunwald JE, Riva CE, Martin DB, et al. Effect of an insulin-induced decrease in blood glucose on the human diabetic retinal circulation. *Ophthalmology* 1987;94:1614–1620.
69. Chase HP, Jackson WE, Hoops SL, et al. Glucose control in the renal and retinal complications of insulin-dependent diabetes. *JAMA* 1989;261:1155–1160.
70. Brinchmann-Hansen O, Dahl-Jørgensen K, Hanssen KF, et al. Effects of intensified insulin treatment on various lesions of diabetic retinopathy. *Am J Ophthalmol* 1985;100:644–653.
71. Krolewski AS, Canessa M, Warram JH, et al. Predisposition to hypertension and susceptibility to renal disease in insulin-dependent diabetes mellitus. *N Engl J Med* 1988;318:140–145.
72. Stern MP, Patterson JK, Haffner SM, et al. Lack of awareness and treatment of hyperlipidemia in type II diabetes in a community survey. *JAMA* 1989;262: 360–364.
73. Engerman RL, Kern TS. Is diabetic retinopathy preventable? *Int Ophthalmol Clin* 1987;27:225–229.
74. Bresnick GH. Background diabetic retinopathy. In: Ryan SJ, ed. *Retina.* Vol 2. Medical retina. St Louis: Mosby, 1989:327–366.
75. Shimizu K, Kobayashi Y, Muraoka K. Midperipheral fundus involvement in diabetic retinopathy. *Ophthalmology* 1981;88:601–612.
76. Niki T, Muraoka K, Shimizu K. Distribution of capillary nonperfusion in early-stage diabetic retinopathy. *Ophthalmology* 1984;91:1431–1439.
77. Bursell SE, Clermont AC, Kinsley BT, et al. Retinal blood flow changes in patients with insulin-dependent diabetes mellitus and no diabetic retinopathy. *Invest Ophthalmol Vis Sci* 1996;37:886–897.
78. Feng D, Bursell SE, Clermont AC, et al. Von Willebrand factor and retinal circulation in early-stage retinopathy of type 1 diabetes. *Diabetes Care* 2000:23: 1694–1698.
79. Antonelli-Orlidge A, Saunders KB, Smith SR, et al. An activated form of transforming growth factor beta is produced by cocultures of endothelial cells and pericytes. *Proc Natl Acad Sci U S A* 1989;86:4544–4548.
80. Orlidge A, D'Amore PA. Inhibition of capillary endothelial cell growth by pericytes and smooth muscle cells. *J Cell Biol* 1987;105:1455–1462.
80a. Wilkinson CP, Ferris FL III, Klein RE, et al. Proposed international clinical diabetic retinopathy and diabetic macular edema disease severity scales. *Ophthalmology* 2003;110:1677–1682.
80b. Chew EY. A simplified diabetic retinopathy scale. *Ophthalmology* 2003;110: 1675–1676.
81. Waite JH, Beetham WP. The visual mechanism in diabetes mellitus: a comparative study of 2002 diabetics and 457 non-diabetics for control. *N Engl J Med* 1935;212:367–379, 429–443.
82. Zorrilla E, Kozak GP. Ophthalmoplegia in diabetes mellitus. *Ann Intern Med* 1967;67:968–976.
83. Rucker CW. Paralysis of the third, fourth, and sixth cranial nerves. *Am J Ophthalmol* 1958;46:787–794.
84. Rush JA, Younge BR. Paralysis of cranial nerves III, IV, and VI: cause and prognosis in 1,000 cases. *Arch Ophthalmol* 1981;99:76–79.
85. Rucker CW. The causes of paralysis of the third, fourth, and sixth cranial nerves. *Am J Ophthalmol* 1966;61:1293–1298.
86. Asbury AK, Aldredge H, Hershberg R, et al. Oculomotor palsy in diabetes mellitus: a clinico-pathological study. *Brain* 1970;93:555–566.
87. Weber RB, Daroff RB, Mackey EA. Pathology of oculomotor nerve palsy in diabetics. *Neurology* 1970;20:835–838.
88. Jackson WPU. Ocular nerve palsy with severe headache in diabetics. *BMJ* 1955;408–409.
89. Waind APB. Ocular nerve palsy associated with severe headache. *BMJ* 1956; 1:901–902.
90. Lincoff HA, Cogan DG. Unilateral headache and oculomotor paralysis not caused by aneurysm. *Arch Ophthalmol* 1957;57:181–189.
91. King FP. Paralyses of the extraocular muscles in diabetes. *Arch Intern Med* 1959;104:318–322.
92. Goldstein JE, Cogan DG. Diabetic ophthalmoplegia with special reference to the pupil. *Arch Ophthalmol* 1960;64:592–600.
93. Eareckson VO, Miller JM. Third-nerve palsy with sparing of pupil in diabetes mellitus: a subsequent identical lesion of the opposite eye. *Arch Ophthalmol* 1952;47:607–610.
94. Green WR, Hackett ER, Schlezinger NS. Neuro-ophthalmologic evaluation of oculomotor nerve paralysis. *Arch Ophthalmol* 1964;72:154–167.
95. Baum JL. Rhino-orbital mucormycosis: occurring in an otherwise apparently healthy individual. *Am J Ophthalmol* 1967;63:335–339.
96. Schwartz JN, Donnelly EH, Klintworth GK. Ocular and orbital phycomycosis. *Surv Ophthalmol* 1977;22:3–28.
97. Blitzer A, Lawson W, Meyers BR, et al. Patient survival factors in paranasal sinus mucormycosis. *Laryngoscope* 1980;90:635–648.
98. Fleckner RA, Goldstein JH. Mucormycosis. *Br J Ophthalmol* 1969;53:542–548.
99. Funahashi T, Fink AI. The pathology of the bulbar conjunctiva in diabetes mellitus, I: microaneurysms. *Am J Ophthalmol* 1963;55:504–511.
100. Henkind P. The eye in diabetes mellitus: signs, symptoms, and their pathogenesis. In: Mausolf FA, ed. *The eye and systemic disease*, 2nd ed. St Louis: Mosby, 1980:187–203.
101. Ditzel J, Beaven DW, Renold AE. Early vascular changes in diabetes mellitus. *Metabolism* 1960;9:400–407.
102. Moses RA, ed. *Adler's physiology of the eye: clinical applications*, 6th ed. St Louis: Mosby, 1975:22.
103. Ishida N, Rao GN, del Cerro M, et al. Corneal nerve alterations in diabetes mellitus. *Arch Ophthalmol* 1984;102:1380–1384.
104. MacRae SM, Engerman RL, Hatchell DL, et al. Corneal sensitivity and control of diabetes. *Cornea* 1982;1:223–226.
105. Schwartz DE. Corneal sensitivity in diabetics. *Arch Ophthalmol* 1974;91: 174–178.
106. Rogell GD. Corneal hypesthesia and retinopathy in diabetes mellitus. *Ophthalmology* 1980;87:229–233.
107. Hyndiuk RA, Kazarian EL, Schultz RO, et al. Neurotrophic corneal ulcers in diabetes mellitus. *Arch Ophthalmol* 1977;95:2193–2196.
108. Hatchell DL, Pederson HJ, Faculjak ML. Susceptibility of the corneal epithelial basement membrane to injury in diabetic rabbits. *Cornea* 1982;1:227–231.
109. Kenyon K, Wafai Z, Michels R, et al. Corneal basement membrane abnormality in diabetes mellitus. *Invest Ophthalmol Vis Sci* 1978;17[Suppl]:245 (abst).
110. Khodadoust AA, Silverstein AM, Kenyon KR, et al. Adhesion of regenerating corneal epithelium: the role of basement membrane. *Am J Ophthalmol* 1968;65: 339–348.
111. Henkind P, Wise GN. Descemet's wrinkles in diabetes. *Am J Ophthalmol* 1961; 52:371–374.
112. Pardos GJ, Krachmer JH. Comparison of endothelial cell density in diabetics and a control population. *Am J Ophthalmol* 1980;90:172–174.
113. Busted N, Olsen T, Schmitz O. Clinical observations on the corneal thickness and the corneal endothelium in diabetes mellitus. *Br J Ophthalmol* 1981;65: 687–690.
114. Olsen T, Busted N. Corneal thickness in eyes with diabetic and nondiabetic neovascularisation. *Br J Ophthalmol* 1981;65:691–693.
115. Hoffmann M. Concerning diseases of the ocular nerves in diabetes mellitus. *Arch Ophthalmol* 1914;43:39–49.
116. Yanoff M, Fine BS, Berkow JW. Diabetic lacy vacuolation of iris pigment epithelium: a histopathologic report. *Am J Ophthalmol* 1970;69:201–210.
117. Gartner S, Henkind P. Neovascularization of the iris (rubeosis iridis). *Surv Ophthalmol* 1978;22:291–312.
118. Zirm M. Protein glaucoma—overtaxing of flow mechanisms? Preliminary report. *Ophthalmologica* 1982;184:155–161.
119. Brown GC, Magargal LE, Schachat A, et al. Neovascular glaucoma: etiologic considerations. *Ophthalmology* 1984;91:315–320.
120. Pavan PR, Folk JC. Anterior neovascularization. *Int Ophthalmol Clin* 1984;24: 61–70.
121. Madsen PH. Rubeosis of the iris and haemorrhagic glaucoma in patients with proliferative diabetic retinopathy. *Br J Ophthalmol* 1971;55:368–371.
122. Ohrt V. The frequency of rubeosis iridis in diabetic patients. *Acta Ophthalmol* (Copenh) 1971;49:301–307.
123. Krill AE, Archer D, Newell FW. Photocoagulation in complications secondary to branch vein occlusion. *Arch Ophthalmol* 1971;85:48–60.
124. Wand M, Dueker DK, Aiello LM, et al. Effects of panretinal photocoagulation on rubeosis iridis, angle neovascularization, and neovascular glaucoma. *Am J Ophthalmol* 1978;86:332–339.
125. Pavan PR, Folk JC, Weingeist TA, et al. Diabetic rubeosis and panretinal photocoagulation: a prospective, controlled, masked trial using iris fluorescein angiography. *Arch Ophthalmol* 1983;101:882–884.
126. Simmons RJ, Dueker DK, Kimbrough RL, et al. Goniophotocoagulation for neovascular glaucoma. *Trans Am Acad Ophthalmol Otolaryngol* 1977;83:80–89.
127. Aiello LM, Wand M, Liang G. Neovascular glaucoma and vitreous hemorrhage following cataract surgery in patients with diabetes mellitus. *Ophthalmology* 1983;90:814–820.
128. Armstrong JR, Daily RK, Dobson HL, et al. The incidence of glaucoma in diabetes mellitus: a comparison with the incidence of glaucoma in the general population. *Am J Ophthalmol* 1960;50:55–63.
129. Cristiansson J. Glaucoma simplex in diabetes mellitus. *Acta Ophthalmol* 1965; 43:224–234.
130. Becker B, Bresnick G, Chevrette L, et al. Intraocular pressure and its response to topical corticosteroids in diabetes. *Arch Ophthalmol* 1966;76:477–483.
131. Klein BEK, Klein R, Moss SE. Intraocular pressure in diabetic persons. *Ophthalmology* 1984;91:1356–1360.
132. Mapstone R, Clark CV. Prevalence of diabetes in glaucoma. *BMJ* 1985;291: 93–95.

133. Gwinup G, Villarreal A. Relationship of serum glucose concentration to changes in refraction. *Diabetes* 1976;25:29–31.
134. Kinoshita JH, Merola LO, Satoh K, et al. Osmotic changes caused by the accumulation of dulcitol in the lenses of rats fed with galactose. *Nature* 1962;194: 1085–1087.
135. Chylack LT Jr, Kinoshita JH. A biochemical evaluation of a cataract induced in a high-glucose medium. *Invest Ophthalmol* 1969;8:401–412.
136. Kinoshita JH. Mechanisms initiating cataract formation. *Invest Ophthalmol Vis Sci* 1974;13:713–724.
137. Harding RH, Chylack LT Jr, Tung WH. The sorbitol pathway as a protector of the lens against glucose-generated osmotic stress. *Invest Ophthalmol Vis Sci* 1981;20[Suppl]:34(abst).
138. Bursell S-E, Karalekas DP, Craig MS. The effect of acute changes in blood glucose on lenses in diabetic and non-diabetic subjects using quasi-elastic light scattering spectroscopy. *Curr Eye Res* 1989;8:821–833.
139. Bursell S-E, Baker RS, Weiss JN, et al. Clinical photon correlation spectroscopy evaluation of human diabetic lenses. *Exp Eye Res* 1989;49:241–258.
140. Marmor MF. Transient accommodative paralysis and hyperopia in diabetes. *Arch Ophthalmol* 1973;89:419–421.
141. Rogell GD. Internal ophthalmoplegia after argon laser panretinal photocoagulation. *Arch Ophthalmol* 1979;97:904–905.
142. Klein BEK, Klein R, Moss SE. Prevalence of cataracts in a population-based study of persons with diabetes mellitus. *Ophthalmology* 1985;92:1191–1196.
143. Ederer F, Hiller R, Taylor HR. Senile lens changes and diabetes in two population studies. *Am J Ophthalmol* 1981;91:381–395.
144. Epstein DL. Reversible unilateral lens opacities in a diabetic patient. *Arch Ophthalmol* 1976;94:461–463.
145. Klein R, Klein BEK, Moss SE. Visual impairment in diabetes. *Ophthalmology* 1984:91:1–9.
146. Cotlier E. Senile cataract: evidence for acceleration by diabetes and deceleration by salicylate. *Can J Ophthalmol* 1981;16:113–118.
147. Harding JJ, Van Heyningen R. Drugs, including alcohol, that act as risk factors for cataract, and possible protection against cataract by aspirin-like analgesics and cyclopenthiazide. *Br J Ophthalmol* 1988;72:809–814.
148. West SK, Munoz BE, Newland HS, et al. Lack of evidence for aspirin use and prevention of cataracts. *Arch Ophthalmol* 1987;105:1229–1231.
149. Klein BEK, Klein R, Moss S. Is aspirin use associated with lower rates of cataracts in diabetic individuals? *Diabetes Care* 1987;10:495–499.
150. Klein BE, Klein R, Wang Q, Moss SE. Older-onset diabetes and lens opacities. The Beaver Dam Eye Study. *Ophthalmic Epidemiol* 1995;2:49–55.
151. Klein BE, Klein R, Moss SE. Incidence of cataract surgery in the Wisconsin Epidemiologic Study of Diabetic Retinopathy. *Am J Ophthalmol* 1995;119: 295–300.
152. Pai RP, Mitchell P, Chow VC, et al. Posttransplant cataract: lessons from kidney-pancreas transplantation. *Transplantation* 2000;69:1108–1114.
153. Lawrence RD, Oakley W, Barne IC. Temporary lens changes in diabetic coma and other dehydrations. *Lancet* 1942;2:63–65.
154. Lawrence RD. Temporary cataracts in diabetes. *Br J Ophthalmol* 1946;30:78–81.
155. Roberts W. Rapid lens changes in diabetes mellitus. *Am J Ophthalmol* 1950;33: 1283–1285.
156. Neuberg HW, Griscom JH, Burns RP. Acute development of diabetic cataracts and their reversal: a case report. *Diabetes* 1958;7:21–26.
157. Jackson RC. Temporary cataracts in diabetes mellitus. *Br J Ophthalmol* 1955; 39:629–631.
158. Turtz CA, Turtz AI. Reversal of lens changes in early diabetes. *Am J Ophthalmol* 1958;46:219–220.
159. Brown CA, Burman D. Transient cataracts in a diabetic child with hyperosmolar coma. *Br J Ophthalmol* 1973;57:429–433.
160. O'Brien CS, Molsberry JM, Allen JH. Diabetic cataract: incidence and morphology in 126 young diabetic patients. *JAMA* 1934;103:892–897.
161. Rosen E. Diabetic needles. *Br J Ophthalmol* 1945;29:645–653.
162. Straatsma BR, Pettit TH, Wheeler N, et al. Diabetes mellitus and intraocular lens implantation. *Ophthalmology* 1983;90:336–343.
163. Dowler JG, Hykin PG, Hamilton AM. Phacoemulsification versus extracapsular cataract extraction in patients with diabetes. *Ophthalmology* 2000;107: 457–462.
164. Borrillo JL, Mittra RA, Dev S, et al. Retinopathy progression and visual outcomes after phacoemulsification in patients with diabetes mellitus. *Trans Am Ophthalmol Soc* 1999;97:435–445.
165. Jalkh A, Takahashi M, Topilow HW, et al. Prognostic value of vitreous findings in diabetic retinopathy. *Arch Ophthalmol* 1982;100:432–434.
166. Tagawa H, McMeel JW, Furukawa H, et al. Role of the vitreous in diabetic retinopathy, I: vitreous changes in diabetic retinopathy and in physiologic aging. *Ophthalmology* 1986;93:596–601.
167. Tagawa H, McMeel JW, Trempe CL. Role of the vitreous in diabetic retinopathy, II: active and inactive vitreous changes. *Ophthalmology* 1986;93: 1188–1192.
168. Nasrallah FP, Jalkh AE, van Coppenolle FV, et al. The role of the vitreous in diabetic macular edema. *Ophthalmology* 1988;95:1335–1339.
169. Smith JL. Asteroid hyalitis: incidence of diabetes mellitus and hypercholesteremia. *JAMA* 1958;168:891–893.
170. Bard LA. Asteroid hyalitis: relationship to diabetes and hypercholesterolemia. *Am J Ophthalmol* 1964;58:239–242.
171. Smith JL. Asteroid hyalitis and diabetes mellitus. *Trans Am Acad Ophthalmol Otolaryngol* 1965;69:269–278.
172. Luxenberg M, Sime D. Relationship of asteroid hyalosis to diabetes mellitus and plasma lipid levels. *Am J Ophthalmol* 1969;67:406–413.
173. Davis MD. Viterous contraction in proliferative diabetic retinopathy. *Arch Ophthalmol* 1965;74:741–751.
174. Tolentino FI, Lee P-F, Schepens CL. Biomicroscopic study of vitreous cavity in diabetic retinopathy. *Arch Ophthalmol* 1966;75:238–246.
175. Lubow M, Makley TA Jr. Pseudopapilledema of juvenile diabetes mellitus. *Arch Ophthalmol* 1971;85:417–422.
176. Pavan PR, Aiello LM, Wafai MZ, et al. Optic disc edema in juvenile-onset diabetes. *Arch Ophthalmol* 1980;98:2193–2195.
177. Appen RE, Chandra SR, Klein R, et al. Diabetic papillopathy. *Am J Ophthalmol* 1980;90:203–209.
178. Barr CC, Glaser JS, Blankenship G. Acute disc swelling in juvenile diabetes: clinical profile and natural history of 12 cases. *Arch Ophthalmol* 1980;98: 2185–2192.
179. Johns KJ, Leonard-Marti T, et al. The effect of panretinal photocoagulation on optic nerve cupping. *Ophthalmology* 1989;96:211–216.
180. The Sorbinil Retinopathy Trial Research Group. A randomized trial of sorbinil, an aldose reductase inhibitor in diabetic retinopathy. *Arch Ophthalmol* 1990;108:1234–1244.
181. The Sorbinil Retinopathy Trial Research Group. The sorbinil retinopathy trial: neurology results. *Neurology* 1993;43:1141–1149.
182. Kunisaki M, Bursell S-E, Clermont AC, et al. Vitamin E treatment prevents diabetes-induced abnormality in retinal blood flow via the diacylglycerol-protein kinase C pathway. *Am J Physiol* 1995;269:E239–E246.
183. Bursell SE, Clermont AC, Aiello LP, et al. High-dose vitamin E supplementation normalizes retinal blood flow and creatinine clearance in patients with type I diabetes. *Diabetes Care* 1999;22:1245–1251.
184. de la Rubia Sanchez G, Oliver-Pozo J, et al. Modulation of endothelin-1 (ET-1) receptor on retinal pericytes by elevated glucose levels. *Invest Ophthalmol Vis Sci* 1991;32[Suppl 4]:1302(abst).
185. Shiba T, Bursell S-E, Clermont A, et al. Protein kinase C (PKC) activation is a causal factor for the alteration of retinal blood flow in diabetes of short duration. *Invest Ophthalmol Vis Sci* 1991;32(4)[Suppl]:75(abst).
186. Bursell S-E, Cavallerano JD, Cavallerano AA, et al. Stereo nonmydriatic digital-video color retinal imaging compared with Early Treatment Diabetic Retinopathy Study seven standard field 35-mm stereo color photos for determining level of diabetic retinopathy. *Ophthalmology* 2001;108:572–585.
187. Aiello LM, Cavallerano J, Cavallerano A, et al. The Joslin Vision Network (JVN) Innovative Telemedicine Care for Diabetes. *Ophthalmol Clin North Am* 2000;13:213–224.
188. Aiello LM, Bursell S-E, Cavallerano J, et al. Joslin Vision Network Validation Study: pilot image stabilization phase. *J Am Optom Assoc* 1998;69:699–710.
189. Javitt JC, Aiello LP, Bassi LJ, et al. Detecting and treating retinopathy in patients with Type I diabetes mellitus: savings associated with improved implementation of current guidelines. *Ophthalmology* 1991;98:1565–1574.
190. Awh CC, Cupples HP, Javitt JC. Improved detection and referral of patients with diabetic retinopathy by primary care physicians: effectiveness of education. *Arch Intern Med* 1991;151:1405–1408.
191. Huse DM, Oster G, Killen AR, et al. The economic costs of non-insulin-dependent diabetes mellitus. *JAMA* 1989;262:2708–2713.

CHAPTER 55
Management of Diabetic Kidney Disease

Mark E. Williams and Robert C. Stanton

The management of patients with diabetic nephropathy has become both increasingly complex and increasingly rewarding in the past 10 years. The elucidation of at least some of the underlying mechanisms has led to a number of therapeutic interventions that, when applied aggressively, will lead to a highly significant reduction in the number of patients who progress to end-stage renal disease (ESRD). Although these approaches have not led to either the complete prevention or cure of diabetic nephropathy, they have produced dramatic improvements in patients' quality of life and mortality rates and have decreased healthcare costs. Much research remains to be done, but the promise of even more effective therapeutic approaches is on the horizon. This chapter reviews the current approaches to treatment and briefly anticipates future therapies.

The seriousness of diabetic nephropathy is demonstrated by the following. First, patients with diabetic nephropathy have a reduced life span. Second, diabetic patients with nephropathy have more comorbid events (such as worse cardiac and peripheral vascular disease) than do diabetic patients without nephropathy, events that significantly affect the patient's lifestyle and ability to work. Third, diabetic nephropathy is now the major cause of ESRD in the United States and throughout most of the world (1). Fourth, the financial costs of caring for these patients are rapidly increasing, as treatment of ESRD (dialysis and transplantation) is paid for by national healthcare systems such as Medicare in the United States (2). Thus, for reasons of quality of life, morbidity and mortality, and financial costs, the prevention or slowing of the progression of diabetic nephropathy will significantly benefit both the patient and public heath.

In this chapter, we will review the current approaches to therapy. Although we cover all therapeutic interventions, our focus is primarily on hypertension and the use of medications that block the actions of angiotensin. The approach to hypertension and the use of angiotensin-blocking drugs has had a dramatic impact on the progression of both type 1 and type 2 diabetes. The use of these drugs in providing optimal treatment of diabetic nephropathy has increased in importance and complexity. Thus, a detailed analysis of these drugs follows.

DIAGNOSIS, SCREENING, AND NATURAL HISTORY

Diabetic kidney disease takes years to develop. It is rare to see diabetic nephropathy earlier than 3 years after the diagnosis of diabetes; it usually is seen after 5 to 15 years in patients with type 1 diabetes (2). For patients with type 1 diabetes, this time course is well understood because these patients present with very clear symptoms at diagnosis. The natural history of kidney disease in type 2 diabetes is less well understood, as patients can have relatively mild symptoms for quite some time before a diagnosis is made. It is likely, however, that in type 2 diabetes, as in type 1 diabetes, kidney disease develops only after a number of years of diabetes. From the physician's standpoint, the practical difference is that screening for kidney disease is not necessary before at least 3 years and usually not until 5 years after the diagnosis in patients with type 1 diabetes but should begin at the time of diagnosis in patients with type 2 diabetes because the duration of their disease is unknown.

The earliest known manifestation of diabetic kidney disease is the presence of small amounts of albumin in the urine, called microalbuminuria (3). Protein excretion in the urine normally does not exceed 100 to 200 mg per 24 hours. Much of this protein comes from the tubules, but a percentage is filtered through the glomeruli. Studies done 20 years ago showed that urinary excretion of albumin, which is normally excreted in amounts of less than 30 mg per 24 hours, increases even before total urinary protein levels increase (4). This very important insight allowed physicians to detect diabetic nephropathy much earlier than they had in the past, thus permitting earlier therapeutic interventions to prevent progression. Microalbuminuria is the presence in the urine of 30 to 300 mg of albumin per 24 hours. When albumin levels exceed 300 mg per 24 hours, this condition is called proteinuria or overt nephropathy. Microalbuminuria has been called "early diabetic nephropathy" or "incipient nephropathy," which to some suggests early, possibly insignificant, disease that does not require therapeutic intervention. It must be stressed, however, that microalbuminuria is the earliest marker we are aware of. Clearly, mechanistic changes over a number of years in the glomeruli of the kidney are now being expressed as the presence of albumin in the urine. An ideal situation would be to look at renal glomeruli during the course of diabetes to detect changes even before microalbuminuria is present (as ophthalmologists can detect early retinal pathology). Because this is not possible, we use as a marker a point at which the glomerular filter has been sufficiently damaged to permit the passage of albumin. The point is that microalbuminuria *is* kidney disease that needs to be treated and not simply monitored. It should be noted that not all patients with microalbuminuria progress to overt proteinuria and renal failure. Although a variety of attempts have been made to find markers (both genetic and physiologic) that can determine who will progress to overt proteinuria and kidney failure and who will not, there is not yet a standard that lets us ascertain this. Thus, at this time we strongly recommend treating all patients who have microalbuminuria as if they are going to progress to more severe kidney disease because preventing it from worsening has clear benefits and the treatments are all reasonably safe and prudent.

As previously noted, patients with type 1 diabetes should be screened 3 to 5 years after diagnosis, and patients with type 2 diabetes should be screened at the time of diagnosis. Patients should be tested yearly by examining the urine for albumin. At this time, we recommend using the albumin/creatinine ratio in a spot urine test, as this accurately reflects 24-hour total excretion in most circumstances. Although a 24-hour urine test for albumin can be done, it has a few drawbacks, including inconvenience for the patient and the possibility of an incomplete collection. The ratio has been shown to be quite accurate for both diagnosis and follow-up (3). The albumin/creatinine ratio is normally less than 30 μg of albumin per milligram of creatinine. A ratio of more than 30 μg of albumin per milligram of creatinine is abnormal. The current recommendation is to repeat the albumin measurement on two more occasions during a 3- to 6-month period; if microalbuminuria persists, the patient has diabetic nephropathy (5). Some causes of transient increases in albuminuria include exercise, dietary intake, pregnancy, drugs, and other factors that can alter both protein delivery and glomerular hemodynamics. Although transient increases of up to 300 mg of albumin in 24 hours have been seen, levels of greater than 150 to 200 mg per 24 hours usually remain elevated after one or two more measurements. Of note, dipsticks used in standard urinalysis for the determination of protein in urine are not sensitive enough to measure albumin excretion of greater than 300 μg per milligram of creatinine and thus are not sufficiently sensitive to measure levels of microalbuminuria of 30 to 300 μg per milligram of creatinine.

The diagnosis of diabetic nephropathy is usually quite evident in the appropriate clinical setting, but it is important to be aware of associations that support the diagnosis or suggest the possibility of another diagnosis for a patient with diabetes and renal disease. A diagnosis of diabetic kidney disease is supported by the following. First, a large majority of patients have albuminuria. It has been suggested that up to 100% of patients with diabetic nephropathy have albuminuria; however, this is clearly not the case. The absence of albuminuria should certainly prompt a search for an alternate diagnosis, but in the absence of clear signs to seek an alternate diagnosis, there is usually nothing else to consider. Second, the urinary sediment is characteristically unremarkable—i.e., there are usually no casts, no white blood cells, and no red blood cells—although red blood cells (2 to 15 per high-power field) may be seen in up to 30% of patients. Third, the majority of patients have retinopathy before the onset of diabetic kidney disease. Fourth, as previously noted, the duration of the disease is also important; it is relatively unusual to diagnose diabetic nephropathy before 5 years of diabetes. Deviations from any of the above associations should prompt a search for alternate diagnoses in a patient with diabetes and kidney disease. It is rarely, if ever, necessary to obtain a renal biopsy to make a diagnosis of diabetic nephropathy. Renal biopsy in a patient with diabetes is used principally when there is a question about whether the kidney disease is due to a disorder other than diabetes.

EPIDEMIOLOGY

Diabetic nephropathy occurs in 30% to 50% of patients with type 1 or type 2 diabetes (5). In the past, except in select ethnic populations, the incidence and prevalence of nephropathy have been lower in patients with type 2 diabetes than in those with in type 1 diabetes. In recent years, however, the incidence and prevalence of diabetic nephropathy have been steadily increasing, so that the percentage of patients with type 2 diabetes who have nephropathy is approaching that seen in patients with type 1 diabetes (6). ESRD due to hypertension and glomerulonephritis is relatively unchanged, but there has been an inexorable increase in the cases of ESRD due to diabetic nephropathy such that almost 50% of all cases of ESRD are caused by diabetes. The increasing incidence of diabetic nephropathy in patients with type 2 diabetes is in part the result of the greater success in decreasing mortality due to type 2 diabetes. Improved management of the cardiovascular complications of type 2 diabetes through better control of lipids and improved and more stringent blood pressure control has significantly increased life expectancy and has allowed time for other complications to develop. The increased prevalence of diabetic nephropathy is due in part to the current worldwide epidemic of diabetes.

Specific ethnic populations are at unusually high risk for developing diabetic nephropathy. Native Americans (e.g., the Pima Indians of the southwestern United States) (7) and African Americans have a high prevalence of diabetes and diabetic nephropathy (8,9). The reasons for the increased risk have not been clearly identified. It is likely that there is a very strong genetic basis for the observed susceptibility. But factors such as hypertension and diet also may play a role. In any event, a concerted effort to understand the specific susceptibility of these groups is of great importance to the prevention of the increased morbidity and mortality associated with the onset of diabetic nephropathy.

In general, the incidence of diabetic nephropathy follows a pattern of increase about 5 years after diagnosis, with the highest incidence 5 to 15 years after diagnosis of type 1 diabetes. There is a gradual decline in the incidence of diabetic nephropathy with increased duration of type 1 diabetes so that by 20 to 25 years after the diagnosis the incidence of diabetic nephropathy decreases. The natural history of diabetic nephropathy in type 2 diabetes is less well characterized because of the indefinite start of the disease.

WHO IS GOING TO PROGRESS FROM MICROALBUMINURIA TO MORE SEVERE RENAL DISEASE?

A major question surrounding therapy is who will progress from microalbuminuria to frank proteinuria (>300 mg/24 hours) and to ESRD. Because not all patients progress, perhaps not all of them need to be treated aggressively. Although this is an important question, the answer is not clear. A few studies have tried to determine markers for progression. A recent study by Caramori et al. (10) suggested that the rate of increase of albuminuria was predictive; i.e., a rapid rate was predictive of subsequent progression of disease. However, although the correlation is good, the albumin excretion rate was too variable to be used routinely for clinical decision making. Also, Thomas and colleagues (11) reviewed data from the Diabetes Complication and Control Trial (DCCT) to evaluate the relationship between an increase in blood pressure and progression to albuminuria. The retrospective analysis showed that an increase in albumin excretion routinely preceded an increase in blood pressure to a hypertensive range (140/90 mm Hg). They concluded that an increase in blood pressure was not a good marker for progression. Interestingly, this relationship was observed only in the conventionally treated group; in the intensively treated group, an increase in blood pressure preceded an increase in albuminuria. Thus, at this time there are no clear markers for progression, and even the intensity of treatment may affect markers. Considering the potential seriousness of worsening disease and the negative effect of increased albuminuria and frank proteinuria on cardiovascular and renal outcomes, we recommend very aggressive treatment of any patient with established microalbuminuria or frank proteinuria. The study by Thomas et al. (11) also illustrates the important point that the changing treatments for diabetes are possibly altering the phenotypic expression of diabetic nephropathy. For example, diabetic nephropathy (biopsy proven) with no albuminuria and no preceding retinopathy is now being diagnosed in more patients.

CREATININE CLEARANCE SHOULD BE ESTIMATED IN PATIENTS WITH KIDNEY DISEASE TO ACCURATELY ASSESS KIDNEY FUNCTION

An important consideration when evaluating patients with diabetic nephropathy is the relation between serum creatinine and the actual glomerular filtration rate (GFR). The creatinine clearance overestimates the actual GFR because a percentage of the creatinine is secreted into the tubule rather than filtered. Nevertheless, the creatinine clearance offers a highly useful approximation of GFR. A 24-hour urine test to determine creatinine clearance can be done, but a number of formulas use a combination of weight (as a marker of muscle mass), age, sex, and other factors to estimate creatinine clearance (12). An excellent and relatively simple formula is the Cockcroft-Gault calculation of the estimate of creatinine clearance.

$$\text{Estimated CrCl} = (140 - \text{age})/(\text{Serum Cr}) \times (\text{wt in kg}/72) \times 0.85 \text{ (if female)}$$

This formula often provides surprises to non-nephrologists, as the creatinine clearance determined is considerably lower than expected (especially in older women). For example, the clearance for a 70-year-old woman with a serum creatinine of 1.5 mg/dL and a weight of 50 kg is

$$\text{Estimated CrCl} = (140 - 70)/1.5 \times (50/72) \times 0.85 = 27.5 \text{ mL/min}$$

Determining the creatinine clearance is important for evaluating the severity of diabetic kidney disease and knowing with certainty that the patient is receiving proper dosages of drugs. For example, treatment with metformin is not recommended for patients with creatinine clearances of less than 50 mL per minute, and the dosages of many medications need to be adjusted for patients with impaired renal function.

As noted above, the creatinine clearance (measured either by 24-hour urine assessment or by a formula) is quite useful but overestimates the GFR. The overestimate may be greater for patients with diabetic kidney disease than for patients with nondiabetic kidney disease. The reason for this difference is unclear (although it may be due to a reduction in muscle mass and thus in the production of creatinine in patients with diabetes as compared with that in nondiabetic patients). In any event, it is important to be aware of the relationship between serum creatinine and GFR, as some patients with apparently "normal" serum creatinine values actually have significantly impaired renal function.

TREATMENTS

Control of Blood Glucose Levels

For many years, controversy existed over how stringent blood glucose control should be to prevent the development or progression of diabetic nephropathy. A number of studies have illustrated that intensive control of blood glucose levels is beneficial to kidney function. But the landmark DCCT study definitively demonstrated that tight control of the blood glucose significantly reduced the development of diabetic nephropathy and slowed progression of type 1 diabetes (13). In that study, 1,441 patients with type 1 diabetes were evaluated for a mean of 6.5 years and assigned either to a conventional therapy group [median hemoglobin A_{1c} (HbA_{1c}) of 9.1%] or to an intensive therapy group (median HbA_{1c} of 7.2%). Intensive therapy led to a decrease in the presentation of microalbuminuria (defined as >40 mg per 24 hours) by 39% and led to a decrease in progression to albuminuria (defined as >300 mg per 24 hours) by 54% (Fig. 55.1). This dramatic reduction in the development and progression of diabetic nephropathy was achieved by diet, use of an external insulin pump, and/or the injection of three or more daily insulin injections associated with frequent monitoring of blood glucose level. A recent publication studied the same group of patients 4 years after the DCCT study to determine whether benefits of the DCCT persisted after completion of the trial (14). At the end of the DCCT, the patients in the conventional therapy group were offered intensive therapy, and the care of all patients was transferred to their own physicians. Nephropathy was evaluated on the basis of urine specimens obtained from 1,302 patients, approximately half from each group, during the third or fourth year. The median HbA_{1c} values of the conventional therapy group (8.2%) and intensive therapy group (7.9%) were closer than in the original DCCT study. The authors reported that microalbuminuria was detected for the first time in 11% of 573 patients in the former

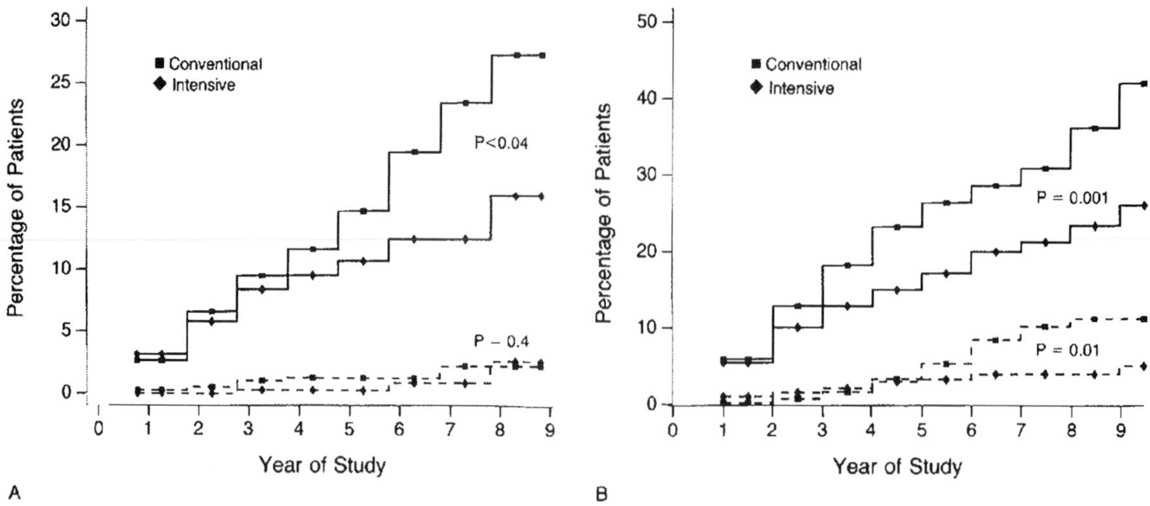

Figure 55.1. Changes in albuminuria in group receiving intensive treatment versus group receiving conventional treatment for primary prevention of albuminuria **(A)** and for secondary prevention of progression to overt albuminuria **(B)**. (Reprinted from The Diabetes Control and Complications Trial Research Group. *N Engl J Med* 1993;329:977–986, with permission. Copyright © 1993 Massachusetts Medical Society. All rights reserved.)

conventional therapy group as compared with 5% of 601 patients in the former intensive therapy group, representing a 53% odds reduction. The risk of new albuminuria was reduced by 86% in the intensive therapy group. Although blood glucose control worsened in the intensive therapy group, the importance of intensive control was still evident. Two significant observations can be made about these studies: Control of blood glucose to levels as close to normal as possible (without causing repeated hypoglycemic events) is beneficial; worsening of blood glucose control over years of diabetes therapy is quite common. This worsening of blood glucose control likely reflects a combination of increasing ineffectiveness of insulin due to multiple factors (e.g., changing metabolic requirements, resistance to effects of injected insulin, difficulty in maintaining the strict intensive regimen, age of the patient, genetic factors, and other as yet unanticipated factors). Thus, target blood glucose and HbA_{1c} levels should be aimed for but may not be achieved. The chief adverse events associated with intensive therapy were a twofold to threefold increase in episodes of severe hypoglycemia and weight gain. In any event, the data strongly support the aggressive pursuit of close-to-normal blood glucose levels through an intensive mixture of diet, exercise, and insulin therapy in order so slow the progression of renal disease.

For type 2 diabetes, control of the blood glucose is also critical. A number of studies have shown he benefit of tight control of blood glucose in patients with type 2 diabetes with diabetic nephropathy (15). The large, comprehensive UK Prospective Diabetes Study Group (UKPDS) trial is of great importance (16). Patients in the conventional therapy group had an average HbA_{1c} of 7.9%, whereas the average was 7.0% in the intensively treated group. In the intensively treated group, the reduction in risk for developing microalbuminuria was 11%, and the risk reduction for progression of microalbuminuria to proteinuria was 3.5%. Although these reductions are modest, the number of patients studied was large and the improvements were highly significant. The change in HbA_{1c} was also relatively modest, and it is likely that greater reductions would have a greater protective effect on kidney function. The recommendation for blood glucose control in diabetic nephropathy in both type 1 and type 2 diabetes is to aim for HbA_{1c} values of less than 7%.

Considering the central importance of hyperglycemia to the development of diabetic complications, it would appear that intensive control of blood glucose alone should be adequate to protect against the development or progression of diabetic kidney disease, but that is clearly not the case. Blood glucose control is only part of the management profile; blood pressure control is of paramount importance. In patients with type 2 diabetes in the UKPDS, controlling blood pressure was more important than lowering glucose levels in protecting the kidney. The next sections discuss in depth the management of hypertension, an essential part of treating a patient with diabetic nephropathy.

Management of Hypertension

More than 11 million people in the United States have coexistent diabetes mellitus and hypertension; however, hypertension in patients with diabetes remains underrecognized and undertreated. Hypertension and the risk of nephropathy form a continuum (17), so that all diabetic persons with hypertension, and even those with high normal blood pressure, are in a high-risk category (18). In addition, hypertension and diabetes combined are devastating to the cardiovascular system.

Hypertension is particularly prevalent in diabetic patients with nephropathy. Hypertension is now considered an early abnormality, not a late complication, of nephropathy. In patients with type 1 diabetes, a rise in systemic pressure may precede or predict the presence of diabetic nephropathy. In patients with type 2 diabetes, hypertension is common even without nephropathy, so that many patients with microalbuminuria and most of those with proteinuria are hypertensive (19) or are receiving treatment for hypertension (Table 55.1).

Several factors contribute to hypertension in type 1 and type 2 diabetes (20) (Fig. 55.2). The role of genetic factors in the clinical management of the diabetic patient with nephropathy has not yet been adequately defined.

Of further clinical importance is the link between hypertension and cardiovascular disease. Although diabetes and hypertension are both independent risk factors for cardiovascular disease, more than doubling the risk of cardiovascular mortality,

TABLE 55.1. Prevalence of Arterial Hypertension in Patients with Diabetes Mellitus

Type of diabetes	Stage	Number of patients	Prevalence of hypertension,[a] % (mean)	Prevalence of antihypertensive treatment,[b] %
1	Normoalbuminuria	562	42	8
	Microalbuminuria	215	52	12
	Proteinuria	180	79	48
2	Normoalbuminuria	323	71	30
	Microalbuminuria	151	90	39
	Proteinuria	75	93	65

[a]Hypertension is defined according to The Sixth Report of the Joint National Committee on Prevention, Detection, Evaluation, and Treatment of High Blood Pressure (JNC-VI) as blood pressure ≥140/90 mm Hg.
[b]Rates of antihypertensive treatment are relatively low.
Modified from Deedwania PC. Hypertension and diabetes: new therapeutic options. *Arch Intern Med* 2000;160:1585–1594, with permission. Copyright 2000, American Medical Association.

the risk is even greater when nephropathy is present. Cardiovascular causes account for more than half of the mortality associated with nephropathy (21). The diabetic patient with hypertension is already burdened with a greater prevalence of cardiovascular risk factors, such as dyslipidemia, hyperuricemia, thrombotic tendency, and left ventricular hypertrophy. The additional cardiovascular risk attributed to nephropathy is not adequately understood. However, aggressive therapy provides the opportunity to reduce excessive deaths due to cardiovascular disease (19).

Effective antihypertensive therapy is generally regarded as the best inhibitor of diabetic nephropathy (22,23) almost regardless of the class of agent used (24,25). Convincing data now strongly support a role of hypertension in the progression of diabetic renal insufficiency, both for type 1 and for type 2 diabetes (26,27), as well as the benefit of early control of hypertension (Figs. 55.3 to 55.5). Although many studies of type 1 diabetic nephropathy have clearly demonstrated the benefit of controlling hypertension, the benefit in type 2 diabetes is not as clear. In a recent meta-analysis of 100 controlled and uncontrolled trials, about one third of the studies included only patients with type 2 diabetes. Overall, each 10 mm Hg decrease in mean arterial pressure was associated with an increase in GFR of about 4 mL per minute, which otherwise declined by 8 mL per minute (28). Angiotensin-converting enzyme (ACE) inhibitors were used in almost half of the groups. However, the duration of the study was greater than 1 year in only 13% of the study groups.

Hypertension, which exacerbates all the vascular complications of diabetes, worsens albuminuria and accelerates the decline in GFR. Because the afferent arteriole fails to autoregulate normally in patients with diabetic nephropathy, any increase in mean systemic pressure can be transmitted to the glomeruli (29). Further increases in glomerular capillary pressure derive from the effect of the increase in efferent arteriolar resistance by angiotensin (30).

Important management decisions that clinicians now face concerning the hypertensive diabetic patient with nephropathy include the following three questions (31,32):

1. *When should treatment be initiated following the JNC-VI (Sixth Report of the Joint National Committee on Prevention, Detection, Evaluation, and Treatment of High Blood Pressure) guidelines, in which hypertension is still defined as 140/90 mm Hg?*

   The blood pressure levels of diabetic patients need to be lower than those generally recommended to maximize the reduction in risk of renal disease. The JNC-VI recommended that all diabetic patients with blood pressure in excess of 130/85 mm Hg (mean arterial pressure, 100 mm Hg) be treated with both lifestyle modifications and drugs (Table 55.2). These guidelines were based on clinical trial results available in 1997 and have been supported by additional trials since the

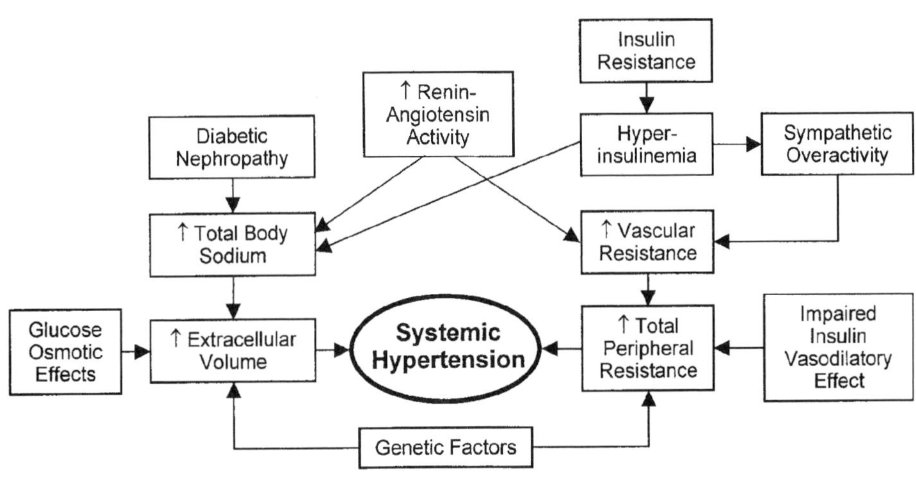

Figure 55.2. Important factors contributing to hypertension in type 1 and type 2 diabetes. Established nephropathy is associated with sodium retention. (Adapted from Arau-Pacheco C, Raskin P. Hypertension in diabetes mellitus. *Endocrinol Metab Clin North Am* 1996;25:401–423. Copyright 1996, with permission from Elsevier Science.)

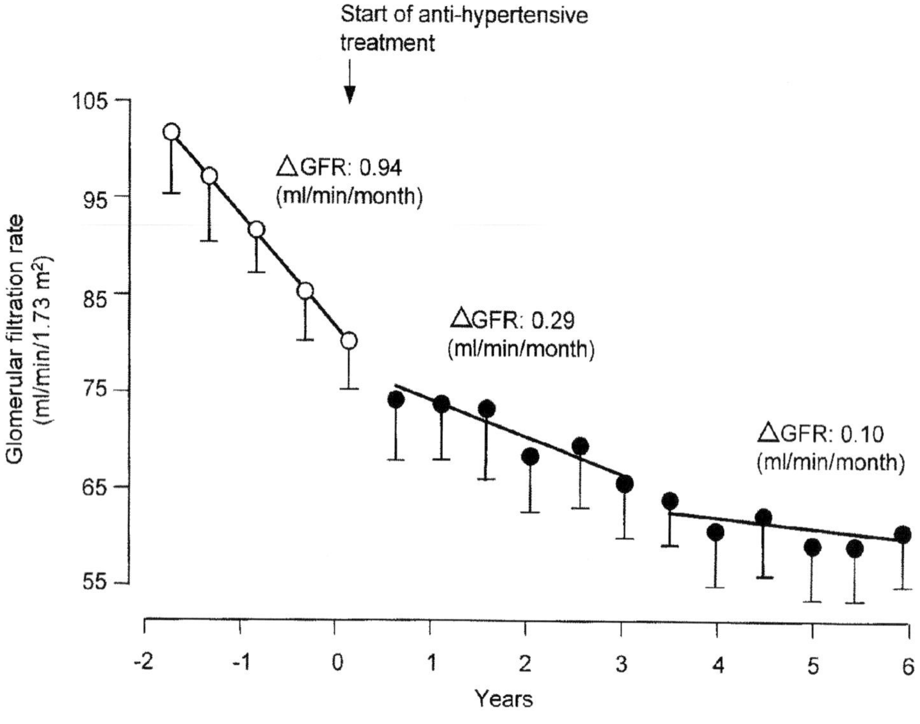

Figure 55.3. Course of change in glomerular filtration rate (GFR) in diabetic nephropathy during effective treatment for hypertension. (Reprinted from Parving HH. Renoprotection in diabetes: genetic and non-genetic risk factors and treatment. *Diabetologia* 1998;41:745–759, with permission. Copyright 1998 by Springer-Verlag.)

guidelines were issued (33). Patients with hypertension and diabetes should be treated as if they already have target organ damage. Convincing studies conducted over more than two decades show that hypertension should be corrected at all levels of kidney function because aggressive control of hypertension is of key importance in slowing the loss of renal function. The effectiveness of blood pressure control appears to be related to the blood pressure achieved. A measurable decrease in proteinuria, a likely sign of renal protection, is also achievable by a reduction in systemic blood pressure.

2. *What should the target blood pressure be?*

Although the unique sensitivity of diabetic nephropathy to systemic pressure has gained acceptance, the target blood pressure is still a source of some confusion (34). The primary goal is to lower blood pressure to the desired target levels. Guidelines of the JNC-VI (The 1997 report) reduced the target blood pressure for patients with diabetes to 130/85 mm Hg, values below those for nondiabetic hypertensive patients. Furthermore, recent treatment recommendations by a working group of the National Kidney Foundation based on subsequent tests have urged a slightly lower target blood pressure, 130/80 mm Hg, to better preserve kidney function.

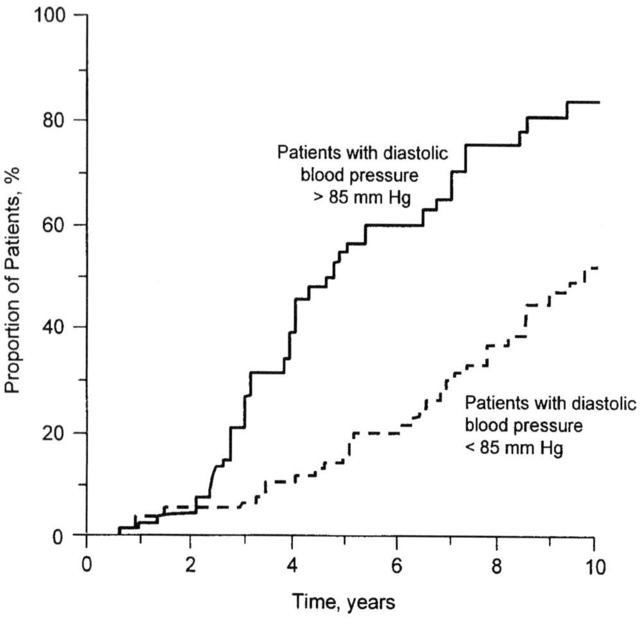

Figure 55.4. Benefit of aggressive blood pressure control in diabetic nephropathy. Renal endpoint (loss of 40% of glomerular filtration rate) was less likely when diastolic blood pressure was lower than 85 mm Hg. (Reprinted from Ismail N, Becker B, Strzelczyk P, et al. Renal disease and hypertension in non-insulin-dependent diabetes mellitus. *Kidney Int* 1999;55:1–28, with permission.) Data are from [32].

TABLE 55.2. Risk Stratification and Treatment of Diabetic Patients with Nephropathy[a]

Blood pressure stages (mm Hg)	Diabetes, with or without other risk factors (part of risk group C)
High-normal (130–139/85–89)	Lifestyle modification and drug therapy
Stage 1 (140–159/90–99)	Lifestyle modification and drug therapy
Stages 2 and 3 (>160/>100)	Lifestyle modification and drug therapy

[a]By JNC-VI (Sixth Report of the Joint National Committee). All patients with diabetes and/or renal insufficiency should be instructed on lifestyle modification. All those with blood pressure >130/>85 mm Hg should also be started on drug therapy.
Adapted from the Sixth Report of Joint National Committee on Prevention, Detection, Evaluation, and Treatment of High Blood Pressure. *Arch Intern Med* 2000;160:1277–1283.

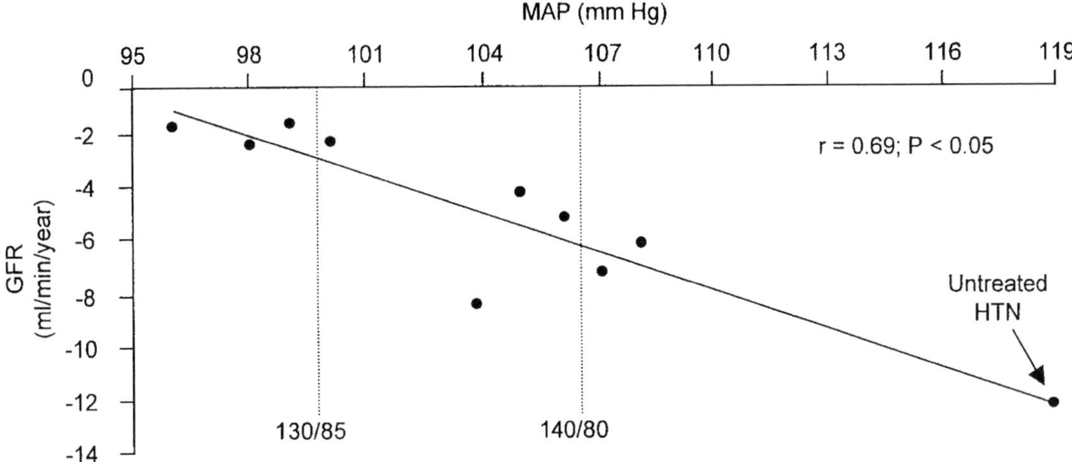

Summary of studies on nephropathy progression used in figure:

- Parving HH et al. *Br Med J*, 1989
- Viberti GC et al. *JAMA*, 1993
- Klaur S et al. *N Eng J Med*, 1983*
- Hebert L et al. *Kidney Int*, 1994
- Lebovitz H et al. *Kidney Int*, 1994
- Moschio G et al. *N Eng J Med*, 1996*
- Bakris GL et al. *Kidney Int*, 1996
- Bakris GL *Hypertension*, 1997
- GISEN Group, *Lancet*, 1997*

Figure 55.5. Relationship between achieved blood pressure and reduction in glomerular filtration rate (GFR) in clinical trials. Six of the nine trials were of patients with diabetic renal disease. Trials marked by an asterisk are of patients with nondiabetic renal disease. MAP, mean arterial pressure; HTN, hypertension. (Reprinted from Bakris GL, Williams M, Dworkin L, et al. Preserving renal function in adults with hypertension and diabetes: a consensus approach. National Kidney Foundation Hypertension and Diabetes Executive Committees Working Group. *Am J Kidney Dis* 2000;36:646–661, with permission.)

Adults with proteinuria of greater than 1 g per 24 hours should maintain pressure goals as low as 125/75 mm Hg in the absence of contraindications (35). Clinical trial data confirm that the mean arterial pressure should be lowered to at least 92 mm Hg (corresponding to a blood pressure of about 130/70 mm Hg) for optimal renal protection (36). The lower the pressure, as tolerated, the greater the potential for preservation of renal function. Data from the Modification of Diet in Renal Disease (MDRD) study (37), the Hypertension Optimal Treatment (HOT) trial (38), the UKPDS (39), and the Appropriate Blood Pressure Control in Diabetes (ABCD) trial (40) have demonstrated that reducing the target blood pressures can preserve renal function or reduce cardiovascular events. (However, no trials that target the lower values of 125/75 mm Hg have been completed.) Concern for increased cardiovascular risk at lower blood pressures (J-curve) has so far not been supported by evidence (41,42). In fact, although recommendations for target blood pressure have been based on the effect of lowering systemic pressure on renal function, it is now evident that reductions in blood pressure decrease associated cardiovascular morbidity and mortality (43). In the diabetic subgroup of the HOT study, for example, the groups with the lowest target blood pressure (diastolic ≤80 mm Hg) had the lowest rate of cardiovascular events (38). Tight control of blood pressure also reduced the overall rate of complications in the UKPDS study, in which tight blood pressure control (144/82 mm Hg) was associated with a 37% reduction in microvascular endpoints and a 44% reduction in the rate of stroke (39).

3. *Which classes of drugs are preferable?*

Successful blood pressure correction is more important than the specific treatment used. However, agents in specific classes of antihypertensive drugs have been investigated in clinical trials involving patients with type 1 and type 2 diabetes with various stages of diabetic nephropathy. Treatment with ACE inhibitors, calcium antagonists, and β-blockers may have similar effects on mean arterial pressure (29) (see following discussion), with no class having a greater antihypertensive effect than other classes (Fig. 55.6), and all are effective in reducing cardiovascular events (43). Most patients will require an "antihypertensive cocktail" that includes several drugs. Nonetheless, the quality of blood pressure control remains poor (44,45), and adequate control is seldom achieved, with only a minority of patients achieving the lower blood pressure goals for diabetic patients with nephropathy (46). Among the barriers that must be overcome to achieve target levels include cultural, emotional, and economic issues contributing to noncompliance by the patient (47); insufficient knowledge base and time limitations among physicians; and the inadequacy of blood pressure measurement outside the medical setting (48). Many hypertensive patients with persistent proteinuria should be referred to a nephrologist.

The subsequent sections will review ACE inhibitors and comparable therapies (49). Blood pressure reduction can be achieved by several classes of drugs. There are many special considerations in selecting antihypertensive therapy for the patient with diabetes (Table 55.3). Therapy with a diuretic, although no longer justified as monotherapy for the diabetic patient, is frequently required for the hypertensive diabetic with nephropathy. Loop diuretics are necessary for patients with impaired renal function. Potential side effects limit their benefit, including deleterious metabolic effects on lipids, glucose, and electrolytes. In addition to these unwanted

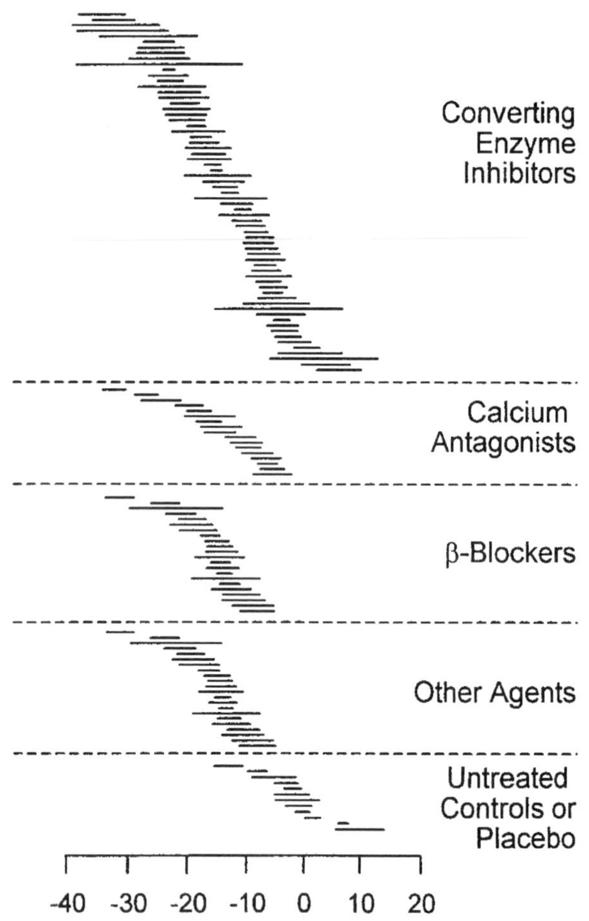

Figure 55.6. Meta-analysis of blood pressure–lowering effects of different antihypertensive agents in type 1 and type 2 diabetes. Blood pressure reductions with ACE inhibitors, calcium antagonists, and β-blockers were similar, as were reductions with different ACE inhibitors (not shown). (Reprinted from Kasiske BL, Kalil RS, Ma JZ, et al. Effect of antihypertensive therapy on the kidney in patients with diabetes: a meta-regression analysis. *Ann Intern Med* 1993;118:129–138, with permission.)

TABLE 55.3. Special Considerations in Selecting Antihypertensive Therapy for the Diabetic Patient with Nephropathy

Drug class	Special considerations
Diuretic	Edema common in diabetic nephropathy; thiazides not effective in renal insufficiency
Angiotensin-converting enzyme (ACE) inhibitor	Treatment of choice Reduce proteinuria and protect from progression Risk of hyperkalemia Risk of worsening renal function No adverse effects on glucose or lipid levels Avoid in renal failure
Angiotensin receptor blocker	Alternative to ACE inhibitor
Calcium-channel blocker	May use in combination with ACE inhibitor Variable effects on diabetic nephropathy
β-Blocker	No long-term data on diabetic nephropathy Increased risk of hypoglycemia May mask warning signs of hypoglycemia Use if history of myocardial infarction or tachycardia
α-Blockers	Never shown to reduce disease progression Neutral effect on proteinuria Orthostatic hypotension Neutral on lipids and glucose intolerance Recent concern about congestive heart failure

side effects, diuretics could also cause reactive stimulation of the renin-angiotensin system (RAS). Potassium-sparing diuretics are contraindicated in the presence of impaired renal function because of the risk of hyperkalemia. Adequate long-term data are not available on protection from diabetic complications such as nephropathy with other classes of antihypertensive drugs, such as α-blockers, central α-agonists, and β-blockers. Although their use in diabetic patients is discouraged, the effectiveness of β-blockers (50) is supported by the UKPDS study, in which atenolol was as effective as captopril in lowering blood pressure and protecting against microvascular complications (39). A recently suggested algorithm for reaching blood pressure goals in diabetic patients with renal insufficiency is shown if Figure 55.7.

Antihypertensive agents that both lower blood pressure and decrease proteinuria (see further on) include ACE inhibitors, angiotensin-receptor blockers, nondihydropyridine calcium–channel blockers, and β-blockers (51). High sodium intake reduces the antiproteinuric effect of both ACE inhibitors and calcium-channel blockers (33). Furthermore, ACE inhibitors, angiotensin-receptor blockers, and nondihydropyridine calcium-channel blockers attenuate both the abnormal permeability of the glomerular basement membrane and the morphologic damage associated with diabetic nephropathy. ACE inhibitors attack a fundamental abnormality in the hypertensive diabetic—capillary vasoconstriction—and pro-vide nearly uniform renal protective effects that surpass those of blood pressure control along (51,53). ACE inhibitors should be titrated to moderate or high doses as tolerated.

Many diabetic patients will tolerate angiotensin-receptor blockers better than they do ACE inhibitors. Several studies, primarily in patients without diabetes, have indicated that the renal protective effects of angiotensin-receptor blockers are similar to those of ACE inhibitors in reducing proteinuria. At present, comparative studies with ACE inhibitors are incomplete.

The ability of conventional antihypertensive agents to lower proteinuria is intermediate between that of ACE inhibitors and no therapy (Fig. 55.8), and conventional agents may have no effect on proteinuria independent of that due to blood pressure reduction. Renal protection provided by calcium-channel blockers is less uniform (see further on); first-generation dihydropyridine calcium-channel blockers, for example, may increase renal progression despite blood pressure control, and their use is more controversial because of safety concerns (40,54). The selection of additional agents will depend on the presence of extracellular volume expansion, in which case diuretics should be added, and on secondary issues such as metabolic profiles, drug safety, and comorbid conditions (43). ACE inhibitors (55), non-dihydropyridine calcium-channel blockers (56), and probably

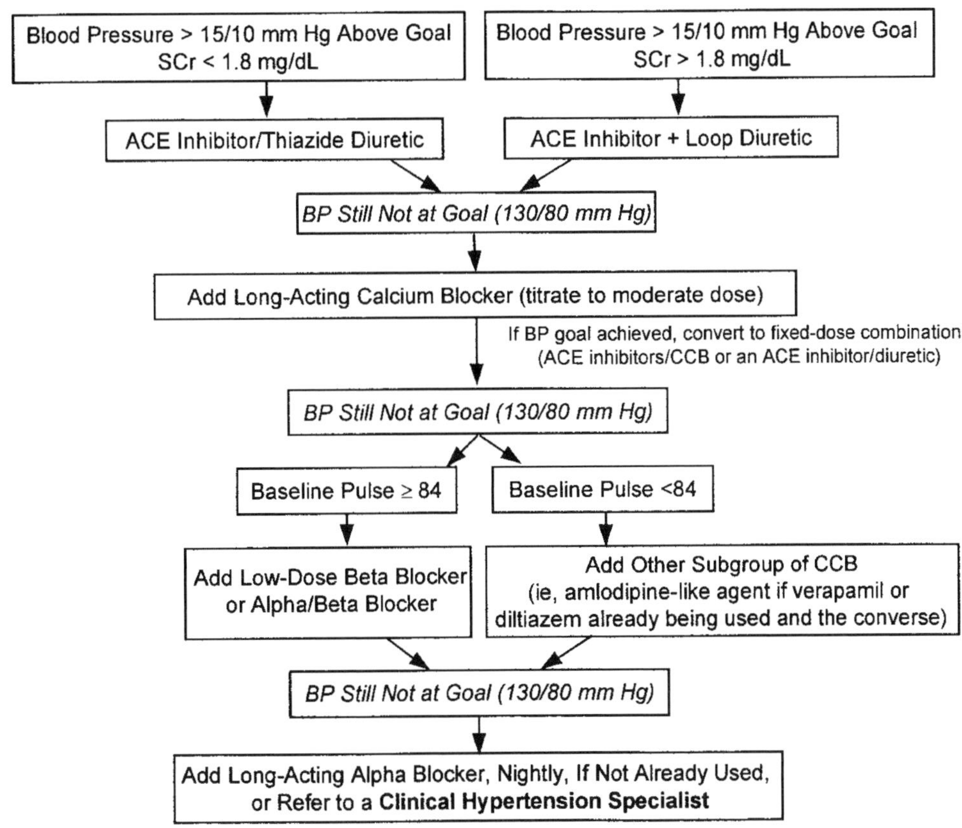

Figure 55.7. Treatment algorithm for patients with renal insufficiency and diabetes. SCr, serum creatinine; ACE, angiotensin-converting enzyme; BP, blood pressure; CCB, calcium-channel blocker. (Adapted from Bakris GL, Williams M, Dworkin L, et al. Preserving renal function in adults with hypertension and diabetes: a consensus approach. National Kidney Foundation Hypertension and Diabetes Executive Committees Working Group. *Am J Kidney Dis* 2000;36:646–61, with permission.)

angiotensin-receptor blockers do not adversely affect glucose or lipid metabolism, which might worsen microvascular and macrovascular complications. Combination therapy will generally be required and can be more effective than monotherapy (57). The lower blood pressure goals recommended by JNC-VI not only may be effective in slowing renal progression and cardiovascular events but also may be cost-effective in the long run (46).

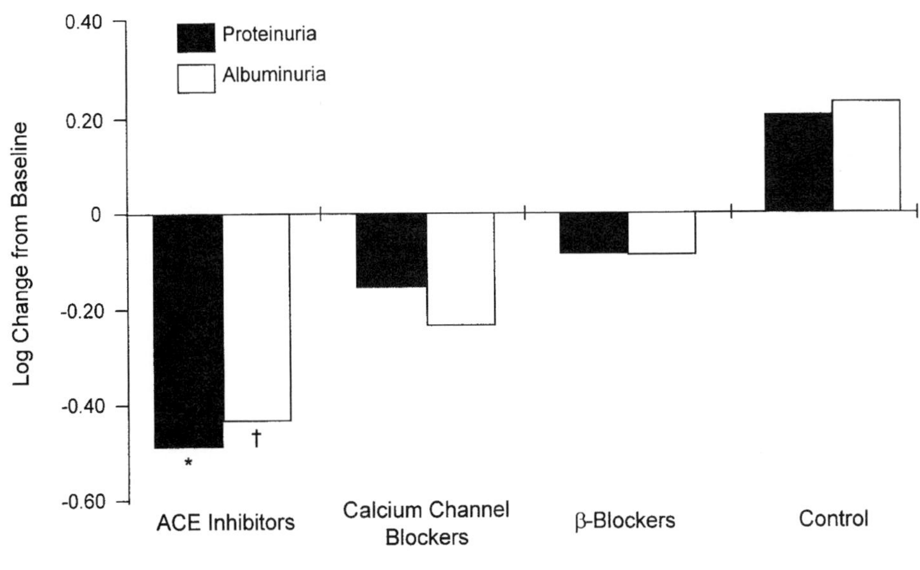

Figure 55.8. Meta-analysis indicating the effect of various antihypertensive agents on proteinuria and albuminuria in type 1 and type 2 diabetes. ACE, angiotensin-converting enzyme. (Reprinted from Deedwania PC. Hypertension and diabetes: new therapeutic options. *Arch Intern Med* 2000;160:1585–1594, with permission. Copyrighted 2000, American Medical Association.) Data are from [28].

Angiotensin-Converting Enzyme Inhibitors

The optimal drug management of diabetic nephropathy is still evolving (58–60). ACE inhibitors have, in recent years, gained widespread acceptance as first-line therapy to improve the prognosis for hypertensive diabetic patients with early or advanced nephropathy (5,61,62). Several lines of evidence, including animal models and human clinical trials, have led to the conclusion that ACE inhibitors, a class that includes more than 20 comparable compounds, provide selective protection in diabetic nephropathy independent of their ability to lower systemic blood pressure. Furthermore, the benefit of ACE inhibitors in patients with diabetes appears to exceed that in patients without diabetes. In contrast, other antihypertensive agents have little or no effect after beneficial influences on blood pressure are accounted for (28,63).

Nonetheless, several unresolved issues remain. The more definitive ACE inhibitor trials have generally been placebo controlled rather than comparisons with other available agents, although additional drugs frequently were necessary for blood pressure control. Not all patients will benefit equally from therapy with an ACE inhibitor (64,65), and questions about the accuracy of the assumption that all ACE inhibitors are equivalent remain unanswered (66,67). Critical review suggests that these agents may merely postpone ESRD rather than prevent it indefinitely. As a result, multiple interventions are likely to be necessary, particularly with current low blood pressure targets, and an individualized approach is necessary for maximum benefit to slow long-term progression. Furthermore, although three large trials in patients without progressive renal disease [ABCD (40), Captopril Prevention Project (CAPPP) (68), and Fosinopril versus Amlodipine Cardiovascular Events Randomized Trial (FACET) (54)] suggest a special advantage of ACE inhibitors for cardiovascular events, the most common determinants in diabetic patients with nephropathy (68), the overall long-term efficacy and safety profiles of ACE inhibitors in diabetic patients with nephropathy have not been determined.

Studies continue to elaborate on the complex role of angiotensin in diabetic glomerulosclerosis. As the key player in the pathophysiology of diabetic nephropathy, angiotensin II (ATII) has important hemodynamic and nonhemodynamic actions (70). The direct effects of ATII on increasing systemic vascular resistance and vascular tone have a unique role when applied to renal hemodynamics, in which vasoconstriction of the outgoing efferent glomerular arteriole causes increased glomerular capillary pressure. Brenner (71) proposed that the resulting glomerular hypertension is the basis for renal damage and glomerular proteinuria in diabetic nephropathy. Angiotensin also has direct structural and functional effects independent of those on renal hemodynamics. Exposure of proximal tubular, mesangial, and smooth muscle cells to ATII stimulates matrix molecular synthesis and cell hypertrophy, predominantly in response to increased production of transforming growth factor-β (TGF-β) by ATII itself. Angiotensin also stimulates filtration of proteins across the glomerular capillary wall. Metabolically, angiotensin may help reduce blood glucose levels by serving as an insulin-sensitizing vasoactive hormone (72).

These effects occur despite the apparent suppression of the circulating RAS in diabetes. However, the kidney may be exposed to excessive intrarenal actions by ATII through compartmental localization of the intrarenal RAS (73). Significant angiotensin may also be generated by pathways alternative to the ACE pathway; in patients with diabetes, more than one third of ATII formation may occur through these alternative routes.

These complex effects suggest that the actions of ACE inhibitors, the most important clinical innovation for slowing the progression of diabetic nephropathy, are complicated (Table 55.4). The benefits, clarified in experimental and animal studies, are due not only to control of blood pressure but also to renal hemodynamic and cellular effects. ACE inhibitors are known to decrease levels of ATII and inhibit actions mediated by the ATII receptor. ACE inhibitors block circulating and tissue levels of ATIIs. Systemically, ACE inhibitors decrease vascular resistance by antagonizing ATII–mediated vasoconstriction, potentiating the vasodepressor kinin system, and inhibiting effects of the sympathetic nervous system. Although the renal effects of ACE inhibitors may not be completely understood (74), ACE inhibitors, more than other antihypertensive drugs, complement their systemic hypotensive action by lowering the high intraglomerular pressure that is fundamental to diabetic nephropathy. ACE inhibitors also inhibit the effects of ATII on renal cells independent of hemodynamics. They retard glomerular basement membrane thickening (75) and tubular interstitial injury (76) in diabetic rats without hypertension, modulate intrinsic properties of the glomerular basement membrane (68) such as functional clearance of neutral dextran molecules, and ameliorate glomerular size-selective dysfunction. Nonhemodynamic benefits also include the blocking of the growth factor properties of ATII (77) and morphologic protection (78) through reduced matrix protein synthesis, decreased formation of matrix collagen, and decreased glomerular cytokine release (TGF-β, platelet-derived growth factor, and endothelin). Recent laboratory data indicate that activation of TGF-β may mediate some of the hypertrophic and proliferative effects of ATII on the diabetic kidney (79). Data also suggest that reduction in the production of TGF-β by ACE inhibitors may mediate some of these beneficial effects (80). In animal models of nephropathy, ACE inhibitors reduce glomerular production of TGF-β coincident with slowing the progression of renal disease. In patients with type 1 diabetes, ACE inhibitors–related reduction in serum levels of TGF-β correlate with long-term renal protection (79). Of particular importance for diabetic patients, ACE inhibitors may improve insulin sensitivity.

Experimental studies in animal models preceded important clinical trials in patients with type 1 and type 2 diabetes (82). Early studies by Zatz et al. (83) clearly established a beneficial effect of ACE inhibitors in experimental diabetes. Other data have shown that ACE inhibitors decrease the detrimental

TABLE 55.4. Differences between the Clinical Effects of Angiotensin-Converting Enzyme Inhibitors and Angiotensin II (type 1) Receptor Blockers

Effect	ACE inhibitors	AR blockers
Inhibit ACE and angiotensin II synthesis	Yes	No
Blockade of AR	No	Yes
Increased plasma renin levels	Yes	Yes
Effect on angiotensin II formed by alternate pathways	No	Yes
Increased bradykinin levels	Yes	No
Approved for hypertension	Yes	Yes
Approved for diabetic nephropathy	Yes (captopril)	Yes
Cough, urticaria, angioedema	Yes	Less likely
Hyperkalemia	Yes	Milder
Deterioration of renal function	Potential	Potential
Contraindication in pregnancy	Yes	Yes

ACE, angiotensin-converting enzyme; AR, angiotensin II receptor.

effects of ATII in the kidney (84) and ameliorate functional and structural changes that produce clinical renal failure.

Human interventional trials, the largest of which have used the ACE inhibitors captopril and enalapril, are best classified by the type of diabetes and stage of nephropathy. Long-term trials have recently increased the emphasis on the significance of reductions in proteinuria as a surrogate renal outcome, which may correlate with conventional outcome measures such as creatinine clearance or GFR. Proteinuria is now considered to be an independent risk factor for progression of renal disease. Although it has yet to be proven that a reduction in proteinuria indicates a better a long-term prognosis in diabetic nephropathy, proteinuria is increasingly accepted as a promoter of progressive loss of renal function by directly damaging the kidneys (85) through tubular cell injury and interstitial damage. Proteinuria increases over time in untreated patients. Higher levels of proteinuria correlate with decreased GFR in diabetic patients (86).

Serving as a sign of earlier renal disease, microalbuminuria predicts the development of persistent proteinuria and a later decline in renal function. Data suggest that microalbuminuria may progress to proteinuria in about half of patients (4), especially if microalbuminuria develops within the first 10 years of diabetes (87). Studies suggest that reduction in proteinuria is an indicator of therapeutic response. Infrequently, nonproteinuric renal disease occurs in diabetes, usually with a nonglomerular microvascular pathology.

Agents to reduce proteinuria are now essential components in the treatment of chronic renal failure (88,89) (Fig. 55.9). Reductions in microalbuminuria or proteinuria are consistent effects of therapy with ACE inhibitors. Compared with conventional

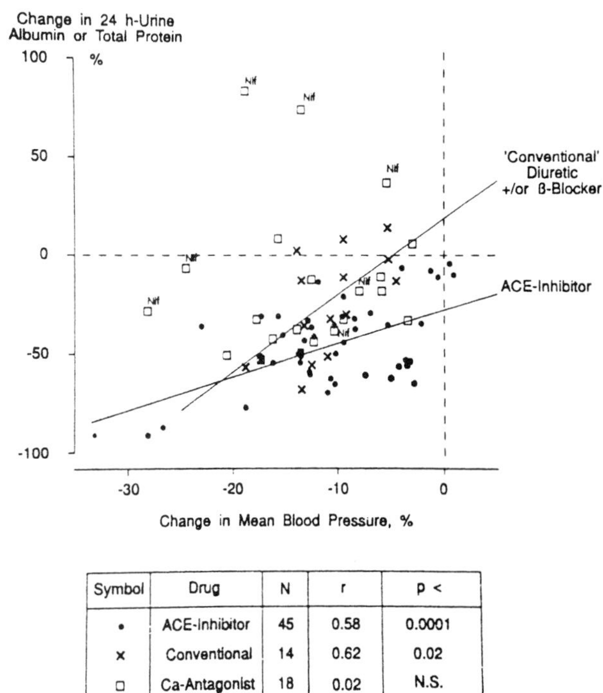

Symbol	Drug	N	r	p <
•	ACE-Inhibitor	45	0.58	0.0001
x	Conventional	14	0.62	0.02
□	Ca-Antagonist	18	0.02	N.S.

Figure 55.10. Meta-analysis showing relationship of reduction in blood pressure to percent changes in albuminuria on total protein excretion in patients with diabetes on different antihypertensive regimens. Even without blood pressure lowering, angiotensin-converting enzyme (ACE) inhibitors reduced proteinuria. With other agents, proteinuria diminished only after blood pressure was reduced. (Reprinted from Weidmann P, Boehlen LM, de Courten M. Effects of different antihypertensive drugs on human diabetic proteinuria. *Nephrol Dial Transplant* 1993;8:582–584, with permission.)

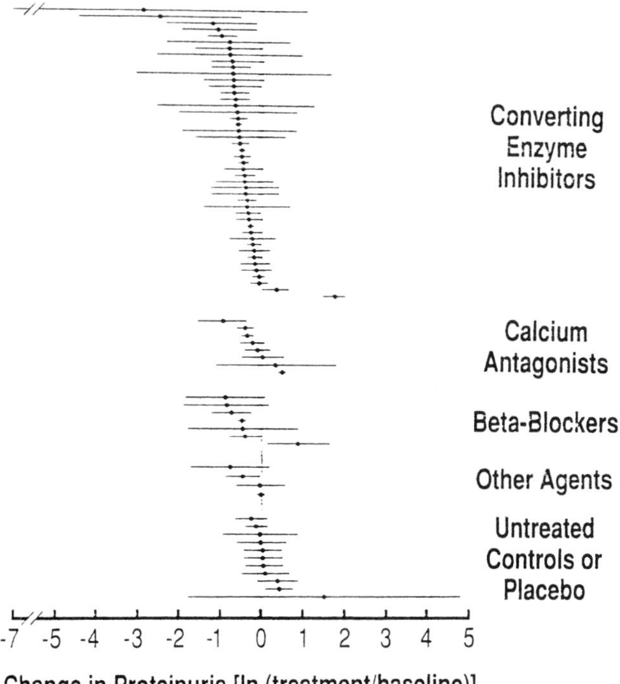

Figure 55.9. Regression analysis showing effects of antihypertensive agents on proteinuria. Effects of calcium antagonists, β-blockers, and other agents in the analysis were intermediate between those of angiotensin-converting enzyme inhibitors and no treatment. (Reprinted from Kasiske BL, Kalil RS, Ma JZ, et al. Effect of antihypertensive therapy on the kidney in patients with diabetes: a meta-regression analysis. *Ann Intern Med* 1993;118:129–138, with permission.)

diuretic therapy with or without a β-blocker, ACE inhibitors produce the greatest reduction in urinary protein excretion, independent of mean arterial pressure reduction (Fig. 55.10). Proteinuria is reduced even before systemic pressure is lowered significantly, and patients with the most severe proteinuria appear to benefit the most from ACE inhibitor therapy. The attributes of ACE inhibitors that reduce urinary protein losses include reductions in systemic pressure, in filtration of proteins across the glomerular capillary wall (90), and in glomerular membrane permeability (74). The renal protective effect appears to be present for all agents in the ACE inhibitor class. A recent meta-analysis found no significant difference among ACE inhibitors in the reduction of proteinuria (28). Potential clinical differences might derive from decreased compliance in patients receiving short-acting agents or differences in tissue penetration among ACE inhibitors.

DIABETIC NEPHROPATHY IN PATIENTS WITH TYPE 1 DIABETES

Patients without Microalbuminuria. Treating patients with type 1 diabetes who have normal urinary albumin excretion and normal systemic pressure with ACE inhibitors for primary prevention is premature. Only about one third of patients with type 1 diabetes will develop nephropathy, and those at risk are difficult to identify. Although available studies were not adequately designed or powered to answer this question, stratified analysis in a large trial by the EUCLID (EURODIAB Controlled Trial of Lisinopril in Insulin Dependent Diabetes) Study Group suggested that those whose albumin excretion rate is within the higher range of normal, who are at risk for progression to microalbuminuria, might benefit from early initiation of therapy (91). A small difference in blood pressure in the ACE inhibitor group, also seen in many other trials, could have accounted for some of the reduction in albuminuria.

Patients with Microalbuminuria. Because the risk of progression of microalbuminuria (incipient nephropathy) to overt nephropathy is significant, several organizations, including the American Diabetes Association, now recommend ACE inhibitor therapy for all patients with type 1 diabetes with microalbuminuria, even if their blood pressure is not elevated above normal (92–94). This is especially true when the patient's microalbuminuria is worsening despite having achieved strict glycemic control.

Patients with type 1 diabetes are almost always normotensive if their urinary albumin excretion is normal. Blood pressure usually begins to rise subtly within the normal range after the onset of microalbuminuria. The incidence of overt hypertension is approximately 20% among all patients with type 1 diabetes with microalbuminuria (increasing as the patient progresses to overt nephropathy). A minority will be expected to develop hypertension each year. Increases in microalbuminuria are closely related to increases in blood pressure (35). Along with glycemic control, several studies have shown reversal of microalbuminuria with early antihypertensive treatment (95). Glycemic control and hypertension are the dominant clinical factors predicting the risk of progression of microalbuminuria. The natural course of albumin excretion is to increase by 10% to 30% each year. Response to therapy would be evident by stabilization or even reduction in microalbuminuria rates.

A number of studies support the recommendation to use ACE inhibitors in normotensive patients with microalbuminuria to attenuate expected increases in albuminuria over 1 (96), 2 (97, 98), or 4 years (99). Although ACE inhibitors are effective in reducing microalbuminuria levels in normotensive patients with type 1 diabetes (25), the guidelines have been based largely on studies comparing ACE inhibitors with placebo and with alternative antihypertensive therapy. The one available study, by Crepaldi et al. (100), did not resolve the question of whether ACE inhibitors have specific renal protective effect in microalbuminuria.

Reduction of risk of progression tends to occur during the first year or so of therapy. Because renal function does not clearly decline when microalbuminuria is stable, no benefits with regard to long-term functional loss have been reported. In a recent report of normotensive patients with microalbuminuria, only those progressing to overt proteinuria showed a decline in GFR after several years, but functional benefit was not specific to treatment with an ACE inhibitor (101).

Additional analysis suggests limitations in studies of ACE inhibitor therapy. In the microalbuminuria subgroup of patients in the EUCLID Study, lisinopril lowered urinary albumin excretion by 49% over 2 years. Blood pressure was significantly lower in the treated group, and the reduction in albuminuria in the treatment group did not reach statistical significance in subgroup analysis. In studies by the North American Microalbuminuria Study Group (98), captopril prevented an increase in albuminuria and produced a small but significant decrease in blood pressure relative to changes with placebo. In the European Microalbuminuria Study Group, both lisinopril and nifedipine caused a 53% reduction in risk of progression from microalbuminuria to clinical proteinuria that persisted after statistical adjustment was made for blood pressure differences (100). It is essential that study groups have similar blood pressure levels because of the influence of systemic pressure on both proteinuria and preservation of renal function.

In hypertensive patients with microalbuminuria, the therapeutic advantage of an ACE inhibitor probably diminishes as hypertension is corrected (102). Interventional trials show the same effect of ACE inhibitors and placebo at lower mean arterial pressures. Several large clinical trials have documented that patients with microalbuminuria and hypertension respond to antihypertensive therapy with a reduction in risk of progression to overt nephropathy (see above section).

A meta-analysis has strengthened the case for the use of ACE inhibitors in patients with microalbuminuria (49). Nine trials (seven in patients with type 1 diabetes) were identified that evaluated (Fig. 55.11) the progression to proteinuria from microalbuminuria in patients with diabetic nephropathy with at least 1 year of follow-up. In about half of the studies, patients were hypertensive at baseline. For individuals treated with an

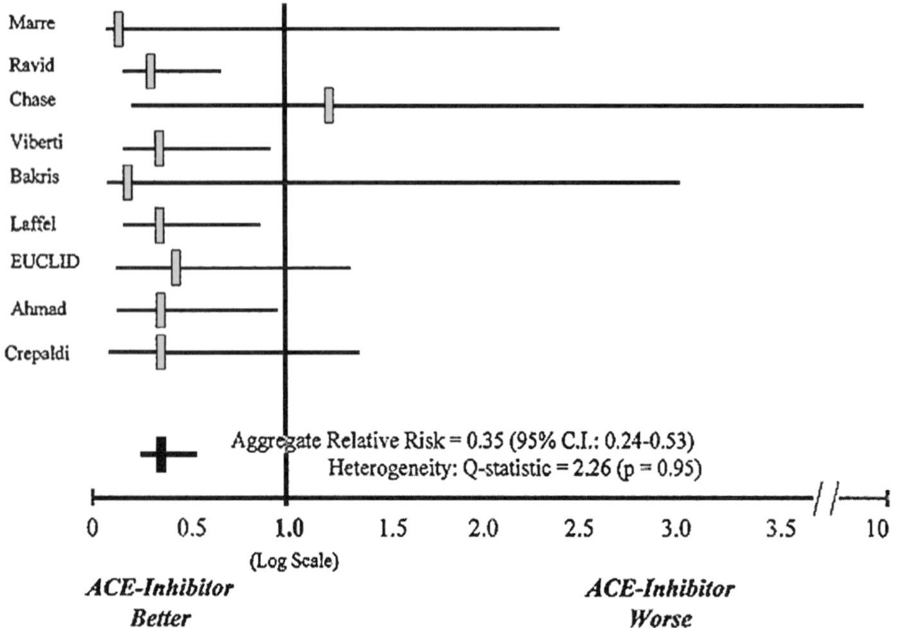

Figure 55.11. Meta-analysis of angiotensin-converting enzyme (ACE) inhibitors in seven trials in patients with type 1 diabetes with renal disease. (The studies of patients with type 2 diabetes reported in the meta-analysis are omitted.) Only one study failed to show a reduction in risk to progression to microalbuminuria with ACE inhibitor compared with placebo. EUCLID, EURODIAB Controlled Trial of Lisinopril in Insulin Dependent Diabetes. (Modified from Kshirsagar AV, Joy MS, Hogan SL, et al. Effect of ACE inhibitors in diabetic and nondiabetic chronic renal disease: a systematic overview of randomized placebo-controlled trials. *Am J Kidney Dis* 2000;35:695–707, with permission.)

ACE inhibitor (captopril, enalapril, or lisinopril), the relative risk of progression from microalbuminuria to proteinuria was 0.35 compared with those treated with placebo. However, in eight of nine trials reviewed, mean arterial pressures were slightly lower in the group treated with an ACE inhibitor at the end of therapy.

In response to ACE inhibitor therapy, urinary albumin excretion typically falls during the first 3 months and then remains constant. Doses of ACE inhibitors should be increased if albumin excretion rates remain elevated but only if the systemic blood pressure is not low and hyperkalemia or worsening renal function tests do not necessitate a dosage reduction or cessation of therapy.

Cigarette smoking has also been associated with the development and progression of microalbuminuria (95), and patients should be encouraged to discontinue smoking.

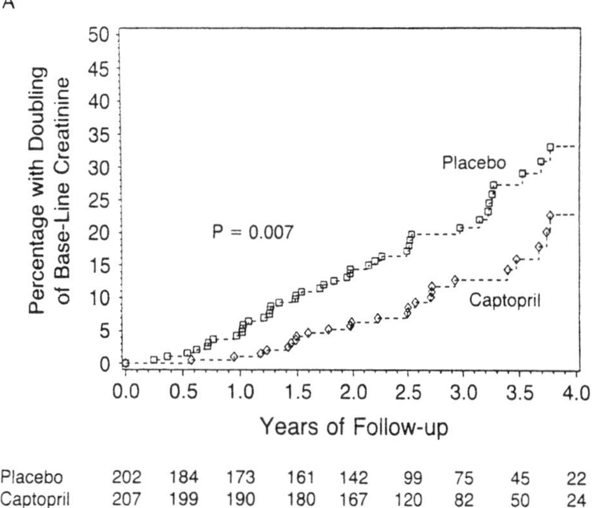

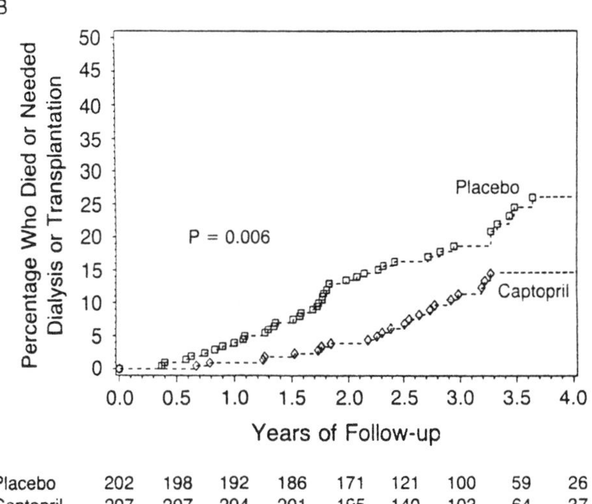

Figure 55.12. Effect of angiotensin-converting enzyme inhibitor (captopril, 25 mg t.i.d.) on retarding loss of renal function in type 1 diabetic nephropathy. Cumulative incidence curves for primary endpoint **(A)** and secondary endpoint **(B)** are shown according to baseline serum creatinine level. *P* values are captopril versus placebo. (Reprinted from Lewis EJ, Hunsicker LG, Bain RP, et al. The effect of angiotensin-converting-enzyme inhibition on diabetic nephropathy. *N Engl J Med* 1993;329:1456–1462, with permission. Copyright © 1993 Massachusetts Medical Society. All rights reserved.)

Patients with Overt Nephropathy. The Collaborative Study Group trial, published by Lewis et al. in 1999 (36), was the definitive randomized trial of ACE inhibitors in adult patients with type 1 diabetes with overt nephropathy. In this frequently cited study, 409 patients with proteinuria and mild renal dysfunction were randomized to captopril or placebo. Treatment with captopril was associated with a 40% reduction in risk of progression in renal dysfunction (i.e., doubling of serum creatinine) and a 50% reduction in the defined endpoints of kidney dialysis, transplantation, or death (Fig. 55.12). Slowing of the rate of loss of kidney function was achieved during roughly the first year of exposure, with little apparent benefit thereafter. Previously hypertensive patients did not attain lower blood pressures with captopril during the trial, whereas the average blood pressures of the one fourth who were normotensive at entry were 5 mm Hg lower with ACE inhibitor therapy. The median reduction in the proteinuria was ~3 g per 24 hours. Hyperkalemia was not significant in the group receiving an ACE inhibitor. The group who entered the trial with near-normal renal function (serum creatinine <1.5 mg/dL) did show a significant benefit from therapy with an ACE inhibitor. A separate cost-benefit model of the trial results indicated that captopril would result in an absolute cost savings of $32,550 per patient with type 1 diabetic nephropathy over the course of a lifetime (103).

As noted above, results indicating an advantage of ACE inhibitor therapy in general have been partly confounded by the lower blood pressure results compared with placebo groups. In addition, data on enhancement of life expectancy have been limited (68). One recent small prospective trial, however, showed a cumulative death rate of 11% 10 years after onset of nephropathy in patients receiving ACE inhibitors, compared with an expected mortality of 50% to 75% from historical data (86).

DIABETIC NEPHROPATHY IN PATIENTS WITH TYPE 2 DIABETES

For several reasons, the optimal therapy for patients with type 2 diabetes with nephropathy, including the use of ACE inhibitors, is less clear than that for patients with type 1 diabetes with nephropathy. In patients with type 2 diabetes, the course of renal dysfunction is more heterogeneous (104), and the natural progression less well characterized than in patients with type 1 diabetic nephropathy. The transition from normal albumin excretion to microalbuminuria is less certain in patients with type 2 diabetes, although levels similar to those in patients with type 1 diabetes are considered clinically significant. Progression from microalbuminuria to overt nephropathy and ESRD in type 2 diabetic nephropathy is more variable compared with the uniformly high proportion of progression in type 1 diabetic nephropathy.

Proteinuria, especially at low levels, may be a less specific finding in type 2 diabetic nephropathy. Nonetheless, recent recognition of the importance of microalbuminuria in type 2 diabetic nephropathy has emerged. Several consensus groups have recommended screening for microalbuminuria in patients with type 2 diabetes as a preventive strategy (94). Although microalbuminuria is not as predictive of progression to overt nephropathy in type 2 diabetes as in type 1 diabetes, it has additional benefits as an independent marker of atherosclerotic disease and premature death in patients with type 2 diabetes (105). Microalbuminuria is frequently associated with mild elevations in cholesterol and triglycerides, recognized risk factors for cardiovascular disease. In addition, the development of microalbuminuria may be linked to systemic abnormalities in glucose and lipid metabolism, hemostasis, and coagulation.

In addition, the relationship between renal structure and function is less secure in type 2 than type 1 diabetic nephropathy.

Recent data suggest that the majority of patients with type 2 diabetes with microalbuminuria have nonspecific changes in biopsy specimens or even normal-appearing glomeruli (106). Only subsets of patients with microalbuminuria or proteinuria have structural damage limited to diabetic nephropathy. Glomerular histology is often atypical for diabetic nephropathy, with more advanced arterial and/or tubulointerstitial lesions.

The benefits of ACE inhibitors are less well substantiated than in type 1 diabetic nephropathy, and the level of renal protection appears to be lower in type 2 diabetic nephropathy (107). One effect of ACE inhibitor therapy in type 1 diabetic nephropathy, the improvement in glomerular size-selective dysfunction, is not reproduced in type 2 diabetic nephropathy, even when pure diabetic-type glomerular lesions are present (108). Nonetheless, ACE inhibitors are considered desirable in several stages of nephropathy.

Patients without Microalbuminuria. Observational data suggest that patients with type 2 diabetes without albuminuria who are treated with an ACE inhibitor are less likely to progress to microalbuminuria than are those treated with conventional therapy. Data on the advantage of ACE inhibitors in slowing the development (as opposed to progression) of microalbuminuria in type 2 diabetes are limited. Ravid et al. (109) evaluated patients without either hypertension or microalbuminuria in a prolonged trial published in 1998. One hundred fifty-six patients with type 2 diabetes with normal blood pressure and mean urine albumin losses of only 12 mg per day received either enalapril 10 mg daily or a placebo over 6 years. Enalapril limited the increase in microalbuminuria to 12 to 16 mg per day as compared with an increase of 11 to 27 mg per day in the placebo group. Three times as many (19%) in the placebo group crossed the threshold to microalbuminuria. The fall-off in renal function was small in the placebo group (14 mL per minute in >6 years), but even less (9 mL per minute) in the ACE inhibitor group. After 6 years, renal function was better preserved and proteinuria was lower in patients treated with the ACE inhibitor than in those treated with placebo, although the absolute reduction in risk of microalbuminuria was a modest 12.5%. This low-risk population did not provide data on risk reduction for progression to overt nephropathy.

A recent computerized model of medical decision analysis indicated that routine ACE inhibitor therapy in all Pima Indians with type 2 diabetes, who have an extremely high rate of ESRD, would provide more cost-savings than would screening for microalbuminuria (110). The simple strategy of treating all patients with type 2 diabetes with an ACE inhibitor, based on a model of patients who are 50 years of age with diagnosed type 2 diabetes and a prevalence of microalbuminuria of 11% and proteinuria of 3%, provided increased quality-adjusted life expectancy at a modest cost (111).

Patients with Microalbuminuria. Early ACE inhibitor therapy at the onset of microalbuminuria has been recommended, even in patients with type 2 diabetes. Prospective controlled trials indicate that, as in patients with type 1 diabetes, progression to overt proteinuria is reduced. However, this is an even smaller subset in patients with type 2 diabetes, because most are hypertensive. In an extended placebo-controlled trial versus enalapril 10 mg daily, a steady, gradual increase in levels of microalbuminuria occurred over 5 years in the placebo group, for an overall increase of 2.5-fold and a 13% increase in plasma creatinine levels (112). In contrast, levels of microalbuminuria in the group treated with enalapril remained stable, as did renal function (Fig. 55.13). In the enalapril group, the risk of progression to overt proteinuria was reduced to one-third that in the placebo group (12% versus 42%). Mean blood pressure remained normal. When 2 years of unblinded follow-up were included, ACE inhibitor therapy resulted in an absolute risk reduction of 42%. On the basis of these data, ACE inhibitors are preferred therapy in microalbuminuric patients with type 2 diabetes even in the absence of hypertension.

The benefits of early intervention have also been shown in hypertensive patients with type 2 diabetes with subclinical proteinuria. During two and a half years of maintenance enalapril therapy, patients with an initial baseline urinary albumin excretion rate of less than 300 mg per 24 hours demonstrated better

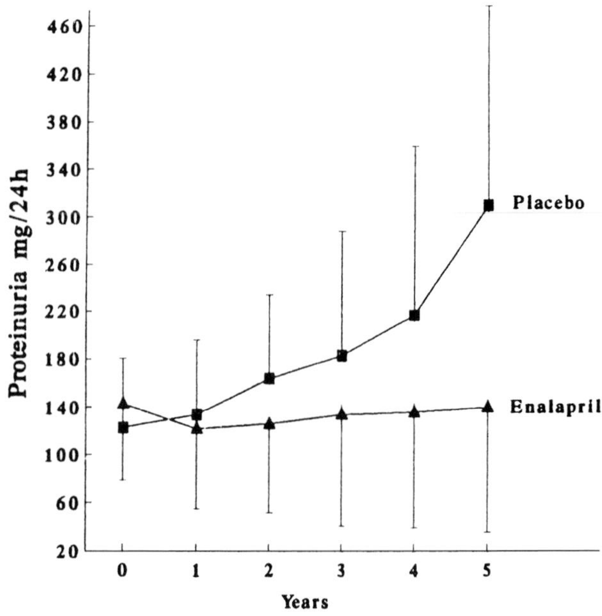

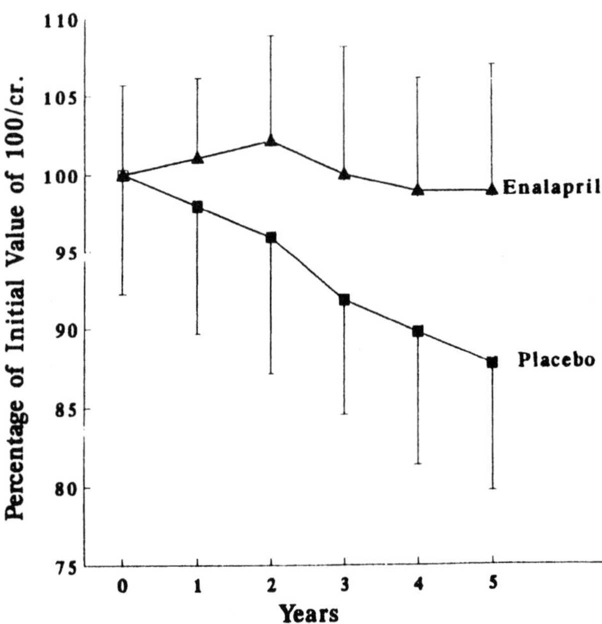

Figure 55.13. Effect of angiotensin-converting enzyme (ACE) inhibitor (enalapril, 10 mg daily) on stabilizing proteinuria **(top)** and renal function **(bottom)** in a 5-year period in normotensive patients with type 2 diabetes with microalbuminuria. The risk of progression to overt proteinuria was also reduced. Kidney function declined by 13% in the placebo group and remained stable in the ACE inhibitor group. (Reprinted from Ravid M, Savin H, Jutrin I, et al. Long-term stabilizing effect of angiotensin-converting enzyme inhibition on plasma creatinine and on proteinuria in normotensive type II diabetic patients. *Ann Intern Med* 1993;118:577–581, with permission.)

preservation of renal function than did those receiving an antihypertensive regimen that excluded an ACE inhibitor, although, as in several other clinical trials, the mean systemic blood pressure was lower in the enalapril group (110). Another prospective trial of hypertensive type 2 patients included a subset with overt albuminuria. In patients with microalbuminuria, the rate of deterioration in renal function was better stabilized in those treated with enalapril than in those treated with nifedipine (114).

Patients with Overt Nephropathy. No adequate prospective controlled study has documented a benefit from therapy with an ACE inhibitor using accepted renal endpoints in patients with type 2 diabetes with overt nephropathy (proteinuria >300 mg per 24 hours). One small study compared lisinopril and atenolol in patients with type 2 diabetes with overt nephropathy and hypertension. The study, which was double blinded for only 12 months, showed that the loss of glomerular rate was slowed by about half in both groups after the first 6 months, while the ACE inhibitor produced greater reductions in proteinuria (115). Although a meta-analysis of several independent clinical trials [ABCD (40), CAPPP (68), and FACET (54)] has shown significant cardiovascular benefits of ACE inhibitor therapy in hypertensive patients with type 2 diabetes, no trial in patients with nephropathy has provided adequate information.

RISKS

Although as a class ACE inhibitors have a relatively safe adverse event profile, concerns about safety and tolerability may account for the use of relatively low doses in clinical practice. Cough and angioedema are not primarily dose related. The most common adverse outcomes are hyperkalemia and increased azotemia.

Hyperkalemia, a well-recognized complication of ACE inhibitor therapy (116), results when levels of serum aldosterone decrease and potassium clearance by the kidney is diminished. Previous studies indicate that ACE inhibitors in general raise serum potassium levels by about 15% (117). Patients with impaired renal function are at particular risk because the adaptive increase in potassium excretion by surviving nephrons is mediated in part by increased adrenal production of aldosterone. Aldosterone levels are acutely suppressed by ACE inhibitors, but the reduction in serum aldosterone levels with an ACE inhibitor throughout the course of therapy is variable. Differences in pharmacokinetic properties of ACE inhibitors may account for this variability.

The most common cause of renal deterioration in patients receiving an ACE inhibitor is relative hypotension, which results in impaired renal perfusion. The effect is compounded in diabetic patients with renal impairment because the function of the nephrons is not maximized when perfusion pressure falls. In the presence of advanced renal insufficiency, aggressive blood pressure control may lead to a critical increase in serum creatinine levels (118). The decline in renal function is more slowly reversible when ACE inhibitor therapy is halted. Severe deterioration may occur in the added presence of volume depletion or the use of nonsteroidal antiinflammatory drugs. More severe deterioration in renal function, i.e., a greater than 50% increase in serum creatinine level, also occurs when renal perfusion is already further stressed in patients with underlying chronic renal failure or renal artery stenosis.

Angiotensin-Receptor Blockers

The angiotensin-receptor (AR) blockers are currently being evaluated as alternatives to ACE inhibitors for managing diabetic nephropathy (119). Although AR blockers may be broadly similar to ACE inhibitors, there are significant clinical differences (Table 55.4). Clinical trials have demonstrated the efficacy of AR blockers in reducing blood pressure (120), with a potency equal to that of ACE inhibitors, calcium-channel blockers, and β-blockers (121).

It is reasonable to expect that these agents might reproduce the beneficial renal effects of ACE inhibitors (74) and broaden the therapeutic options for the physician. In fact, by blocking ATII activity at the ATI receptor site responsible for all the known clinical actions of ATII (122), AR blockers could more effectively block the RAS, because more than one third of ATII formation is generated by pathways alternative to the ACE pathway. Although ACE inhibitors also result in accumulation of bradykinin by inactivating a kinin-degrading enzyme, data suggest that kinins do not contribute to renal protection in a diabetic model. AR blockers may antagonize the effects of ATII generated by any pathway, while having no effect on bradykinin metabolism.

Although no long-term comparative trials with ACE inhibitors have been completed, AR blockers are known to be similar to ACE inhibitors in their effects on renal hemodynamics and proteinuria. Data suggest that AR blockers may produce greater renal vasodilatation than ACE inhibitors, suggesting more complete inhibition of angiotensin. Whether this is a class effect is unknown. AR blockers are known to diminish glomerulosclerosis in diabetic rats (123), blocking the development of albuminuria and hypertension (124) and protecting against glomerular histologic injury (125,126). AR blockers, similar to ACE inhibitors, also affect glomerular permeability. Several small studies have shown that AR blockers reduce proteinuria unrelated to diabetes as effectively as do ACE inhibitors and have similar effects on glomerular size-selective functions that are mediated by ATII. AR blockers do not appear to duplicate the acute hemodynamic benefit of ACE inhibitors in diabetic hyperfiltration. However, a crossover trial comparing AR blockers with ACE inhibitors in patients with type 1 diabetes with overt nephropathy and hypertension that was published in 2000 revealed similar reductions in proteinuria and systemic blood pressure (125). Renal function, with an average baseline GFR of 90 mL per minute, remained stable with both treatments. The ACE inhibitor group showed a slight increase in serum potassium, although still within the normal range.

In short-term trials in humans, AR blockers appear to have beneficial renal effects in type 2 diabetic nephropathy. A 12-week pilot study of 47 hypertensive patients with type 2 diabetes with nephropathy who were treated with irbesartan indicated a mild increase in creatinine clearance and a reduction in proteinuria as compared with the group treated with the calcium-channel blocker amlodipine (126). A second small and short-duration trial demonstrated a reduction by about half in levels of microalbuminuria. A longer-term clinical study in early type 2 diabetic nephropathy (most with microalbuminuria) compared the effects of the ATI receptor antagonist losartan with those of the ACE inhibitor enalapril. During 52 weeks of active treatment, both were effective in reducing clinical and ambulatory blood pressure, although the former fell short of currently recommended target blood pressures. Both treatments reduced urinary albumin excretion significantly—by about one half. Renal function declined by about 10% in each group. Fourteen percent of the enalapril group, but none of the losartan group, developed a cough (127). These results have formed the basis of three large placebo controlled clinical trials, the ABCD-V2 trial, the Irbesartan Diabetic Nephropathy Trial, and the Losartan Renal Protection Study (58).

The appropriate blood pressure control in diabetes, the second part of the ABCD trial (ABCD-V2), is a continuation of the completed ABCD trial and uses valsartan as the initial antihypertensive treatment. The Irbesartan Diabetic Nephropathy Trial (IDNT) compared irbesartan, amlodipine, and a placebo in hypertensive patients with type 2 diabetes with nephropathy (128). The Losartan Renal Protection Study (RENAAL) (129) compared losartan with placebo in patients with type 2 diabetes with nephropathy. The results of these trials were reported in 2001 (130–132). Treatment with losartan (130) and irbesartan (131,132) significantly reduced progression of renal disease, as evaluated by increasing proteinuria, doubling of serum creatinine level, and ESRD. These results strongly support the use of AR blockers in patients with type 2 diabetes with kidney disease. It is likely that ACE inhibitors and AR blockers are equally effective in patients with type 1 and type 2 diabetes with diabetic kidney disease. The larger studies will not be done because of a confluence of economic and political factors preventing a head-to-head trial comparing ACE inhibitors with AR blockers. Recent evidence also suggests that the use of an ACE inhibitor and an AR blocker in combination offers a further benefit in reducing proteinuria.

The increasing use of AR blockers for renal protection is based on expectations not only of benefits comparable to those with ACE inhibitors but also of a more favorable side-effect profile (133,134). Clinical trials support the remarkable safety of AR blockers. Kinin-associated cough is avoided, and angioedema has rarely been reported. The comparative risk of causing renal dysfunction is probably similar to that of ACE inhibitors. The risk of hyperkalemia appears to be comparable to or lower than that with ACE inhibitors. Previous data indicated that AR blockers raised the serum potassium levels by less than 10% over a 1-month period in hypertensive patients with renal disease (135). A recent randomized crossover trial comparing hemodynamically equipotent doses of valsartan and lisinopril reported that, in the presence of renal insufficiency, the AR blocker did not raise serum potassium to the same degree as did the ACE inhibitor (136). The trial apparently did not include patients with diabetes, however. Like ACE inhibitors, AR blockers are contraindicated during pregnancy. The AR blocker losartan has a uricosuric effect that lowers serum uric acid levels, but this is of uncertain benefit. AR blockers have been used in combination with other agents, such as calcium-channel blockers. In general, AR blockers in combination with ACE inhibitors would provide better inhibition of the RAS and less elevation of bradykinin levels than either one alone.

Calcium-Channel Blockers

Supplemental or alternative therapy is frequently required in patients treated with ACE inhibitors or AR blockers. Either may produce an insufficient decline in blood pressure, particularly with the current low blood pressure goals for hypertensive patients with diabetes. Other patients will require alternative therapy because of hyperkalemia, drug intolerance, or refractory proteinuria, or for cardiac indications.

With the predominance of ACE inhibitor and AR blocker therapy in recent years, there has been a shift away from β-blockers and toward calcium-channel blockers (137,138). Some calcium-channel blockers can even be given as alternatives to ACE inhibitors (139). More commonly, calcium-channel blockers are used in combination therapy. However, unlike the ACE inhibitors, their efficacy in preventing progressive renal dysfunction is controversial (140), and their effects on the kidney are not uniform within the class (141).

Two subclasses of calcium-channel blockers have reached the stage of clinical use, the dihydropyridines, such as nifedipine and related agents; and the nondihydropyridines, consisting of phenylalylkamines (such as verapamil) and benzothiazepines (such as diltiazem) (142). These calcium-channel blockers have in common the blockade of voltage-operated calcium channels, including those involving postreceptor effects of ATII itself (143). By preventing calcium entry, calcium-channel blockers prevent some actions of ATII. Calcium is known to be an important intracellular messenger.

Calcium-channel blockade in vascular smooth muscle results in vasodilatation and blood pressure reduction. In the kidney, experimental blockage of calcium-dependent mechanisms in animals and humans may result in inhibition of the vasoconstrictive and hypertrophic effects of angiotensin. The predominant effect of calcium-channel blockade in experimental animals, however, is the preferential vasodilatory action on the afferent arteriole. All calcium-channel blockers appear to dilate the afferent arteriole, but their effects on the efferent arteriole may vary (142).

The calcium-channel blocking agents differ with regard to their duration of action, activation of the sympathetic nervous system, and interactions with voltage-operated membrane channels; the potential impact of subclass differences among calcium-channel blockers has best been demonstrated by experimental kidney micropuncture studies in animal models. Afferent arteriolar vasodilatation is shared by calcium-channel blockers of different subclasses, resulting in potential impairment of renal autoregulation. As a result, as systemic pressure is reduced, the desired lowering of intraglomerular pressure may not occur unless efferent arteriolar resistance is also decreased (Table 55.5).

Decreased efferent tone has been shown in diabetic animal models treated with diltiazem or verapamil (143). Other studies have shown no effect of the dihydropyridine nifedipine on efferent arteriolar resistance (144). Additional renal effects, such

TABLE 55.5. Comparison of Systemic and Renal Hemodynamic Effects of Commonly Used Calcium-Channel Blockers and the Angiotensin-converting Enzyme Inhibitor Class of Antihypertensive Drugs

Agents	Subclass	Blood pressure	Afferent arteriole resistance	Efferent arteriole resistance	Glomerular capillary pressure	Proteinuria
Diltiazem	NDHP	↓	↓	↓	↓	↓
Verapamil	NDHP	↓	↓	↓	↓	↓
Nifedipine	DHP	↓	↓	—	—	Variable
ACE inhibitors	—	↓	↓	↓	↓	↓

ACE, angiotensin-converting enzyme; NDHP, nondihydropyridine; DHP, dihydropyridine.

as changes in permeability of the glomerular basement membrane or histologic damage from diabetes, may also differ among subclasses of calcium-channel blockers.

These different renal effects are most relevant to the renal protective reduction in proteinuria, a surrogate marker of renal disease progression. Early studies revealed differences between the antiproteinuric effects of certain calcium-channel blockers (the nondihydropyridines verapamil and diltiazem) compared with the neutral or worsening effects of others (the dihydropyridine nifedipine), unrelated to the extent of blood pressure control (145). Hemodynamic disturbances in autoregulation, allowing direct transmission of systemic blood pressure to the glomerulus, would favor proteinuria, whereas a hemodynamic reduction in glomerular pressure or permeability or a reduction in glomerular hypertrophy (146) would minimize glomerular injury and proteinuria.

These complex actions account for conflicting effects on proteinuria and support the confirmations by recent clinical trials that nondihydropyridines reduce proteinuria and the dihydropyridines do not. The renal effects of nondihydropyridines such as diltiazem and verapamil more closely resemble those of ACE inhibitor therapy. A number of comparative trials in both type 1 and type 2 diabetic nephropathy have been reported.

Data on the use of calcium-channel blockers in patients with type 1 diabetes with incipient nephropathy are limited. The decrease in blood pressure and microalbuminuria with nifedipine was comparable to that with the ACE inhibitor perindopril over 12 months in a mixed population of nonhypertensive and hypertensive patients with type 1 and type 2 diabetes (145). A short-term randomized trial in normotensive microalbuminuric patients with type 1 diabetes reported a slight decline in systemic pressure with either nifedipine or captopril. Nonetheless, urinary albumin excretion rate increased 40% with nifedipine but decreased 40% with the ACE inhibitor. No significant changes in renal function occurred (146). In patients with type 1 diabetes with overt nephropathy, several agents, including nifedipine, nisoldipine, and isoldipine, failed to reduce proteinuria despite blood pressure reductions similar to those with ACE inhibitors (142). No studies have demonstrated a reduction in rate or loss of function in the long -term.

More trials in patients with type 2 diabetes have been reported. Both dihydropyridine and nondihydropyridine calcium-channel blockers may be useful in type 2 diabetic nephropathy. In several studies, nondihydropyridines and ACE inhibitors reduced the urinary albumin excretion to a similar extent. However, dihydropyridine calcium-channel blockers failed to reduce proteinuria levels in patients with type 2 diabetes and overt nephropathy.

In several studies, nondihydropyridines appear to be effective in patients with type 2 diabetes with overt nephropathy. Treatment with diltiazem resulted in a 30% reduction of proteinuria in nephrotic patients with type 2 diabetes with nephropathy in a 6-week crossover trial, similar to a group treated with lisinopril (147). The first long-term trial of calcium-channel blockers versus other antihypertensive therapies reported that nondihydropyridines slowed renal progression similarly to the ACE inhibitor and more than a β-blocker (148). Slowing of progression of renal disease correlated with reductions in proteinuria (Fig. 55.14).

A trial by Bakris et al. published in 1998 (149) indicated that the combination of the nondihydropyridine verapamil and the ACE inhibitor trandolapril had additive effects compared with either agent alone, despite similar levels of blood pressure reduction. Of note, one study (150) has addressed the issue of

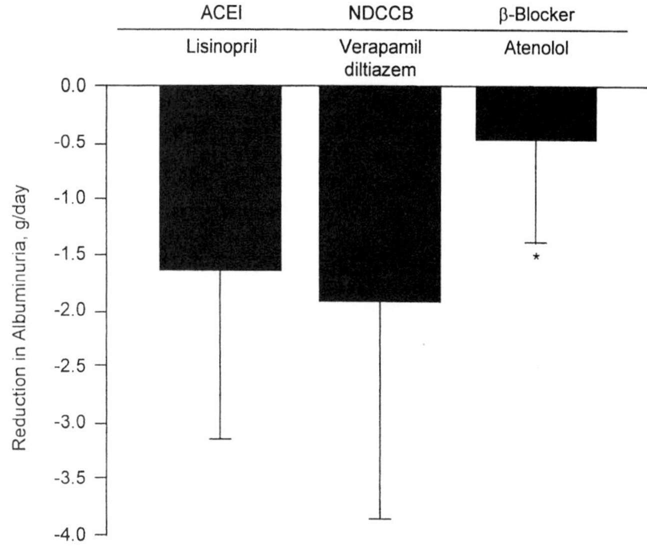

Figure 55.14. Similar sustained reduction (63 months) of albuminuria with the nondihydropyridine calcium-channel blockers (NDCCBs) verapamil and diltiazem and the angiotensin-converting enzyme inhibitor (ACEI) lisinopril in type 2 diabetic nephropathy. NDCCBs and the ACE inhibitor also had similar effects on slowing the decline in renal function. Despite similar blood pressure, the β-blocker atenolol was less effective. **P* < 0.01 compared with other groups. (Reprinted from Bakris GL, Copley JB, Vicknair N, et al. Calcium-channel blockers versus other antihypertensive therapies on progression of NIDDM associated nephropathy. *Kidney Int* 1996;50:1641–1650, with permission.)

underrepresentation of African Americans with type 2 diabetes in clinical trials, particularly because calcium-channel blockers may be more effective than ACE inhibitors for treating hypertension in African Americans (151). Over 6 months, proteinuria worsened by 50% in patients treated with isradipine compared with a 30% reduction in those treated with captopril; these changes were not related to changes in systemic hemodynamics or renal function. Caution is indicated when calcium-channel blockers are used in African Americans.

The safety of calcium-channel blockers in diabetic patients has been widely debated. In 1995, a meta-analysis indicated that short-acting dihydropyridine calcium-channel blockers might be harmful, particularly in patients with hypertension and diabetes, by increasing the rate of myocardial infarction (152). At the premature termination of the ABCD trial, increased cardiovascular morbidity and rates of myocardial infarction in hypertensive patients with type 2 diabetes treated with nisoldipine relative to those in patients treated with enalapril were reported (40). The FACET study also was terminated owing to reported increases in cardiovascular events in a group of patients with type 2 diabetes treated with a dihydropyridine calcium-channel blocker (54). In contrast, the Syst-Eur Trial reported reduced cardiovascular events with the long-acting calcium-channel blocker nitrendipine (153), and the HOT trial reported an association of felodipine with a reduction in cardiovascular events (38). Although the cardiovascular risk is of concern, the above trials have not established the degree of this risk associated with calcium-channel blockers, which remains uncertain (154). Slow-acting formulations of calcium-channel antagonists may be safer (140). No changes in the recommended use of calcium-channel blockers has yet emerged from these trials (142).

Role of Diet in Slowing Progression of Diabetic Nephropathy

Diet clearly has a role in nephropathy by improving glycemic control. Moreover, as weight loss contributes to improved glycemic control, the value of the diet cannot be overstated. In addition, dietary changes can improve blood pressure regulation by reducing sodium intake and possibly be resulting in a more balanced diet. The role of other specific diets in preventing progression is more controversial. In particular, a low-protein diet has been advocated as being of particular importance in slowing progression of diabetic nephropathy. Animal and human studies have shown that the institution of a low-protein diet slowed the progression of both diabetic and nondiabetic kidney disease (155–157). The rationale is that increased protein intake leads to an increased GFR and increased glomerular hydrostatic pressure. Reducing this pressure (as ACE inhibitors do) by reducing protein in the diet should be protective for the kidney. Although studies in humans have been apparently successful, however, in practice it is quite difficult for a patient to stay on a low-protein diet. The recommendations at this time are for patients not to eat less than 0.6 g of protein per kilogram daily to avoid malnutrition. In general, less than 0.8 g/kg daily is considered a low-protein diet. At this time we recommend reviewing a patient's diet with a nutritional expert, and if the diet is quite high in protein, to suggest reducing the protein content. Possibly a low-protein diet should be used only by patients for whom other interventions cannot be done or are inadequate.

MANAGEMENT OF END-STAGE RENAL DISEASE

The above-discussed treatments represent the evolution of management of diabetic nephropathy over the past few years; however, eventual progression to ESRD may still be expected in many patients with type 1 or type 2 diabetes. Despite recent advances from clinical trials outlined above, in the United States diabetes has risen from a common cause of new cases of ESRD to being the largest single cause (Fig. 55.15). In the United States, the increase in incidence of ESRD due to diabetes continues to exceed all other major causes. The high incidence of ESRD due to diabetes extends globally (Fig. 55.16).

TABLE 55.6. Comparison of Dialysis Options for the Uremic Diabetic Patient

	Hemodialysis	Peritoneal dialysis
Advantages	Very efficient Closer medical surveillance Ease of EPO administration Less protein loss IDPN available	Better tolerated Easy access Cardiovascular tolerance Intraperitoneal insulin Avoids heparin Potassium control Less hypoglycemia Less hypertension IDPN available
Disadvantages	Need vascular access Inconvenient Cardiac stress Hypotension Hyperkalemia Hypoglycemia	Peritonitis Must be trainable Time commitment Technical failure Withdrawal More GI complaints Orthostatic hypotension

EPO, erythropoietin; IDPN, intradialytic parenteral nutrition; GI, gastrointestinal.

The ESRD population is growing by 10% per year. Summary statistics from the 1999 United States Renal Data Systems (USRDS) report show 84,076 diabetics receiving dialysis and 18,350 with transplants at year-end 1997, comprising 33% of the total Medicare ESRD population. More than 33,000 diabetic patients, or nearly 42% of all new patients, initiated treatment under the Medicare program that year (2,158).

The incidence rates of reported therapy for ESRD have risen from 48 to 124 per million population over the past reported decade. About one half of the patients are older than 64 years of age, and only 2% are younger than 20. Much of the increase is due to older type 2 diabetic patients, so that the mean age of diabetic patients with ESRD is now over 60. About two thirds have type 2 diabetes.

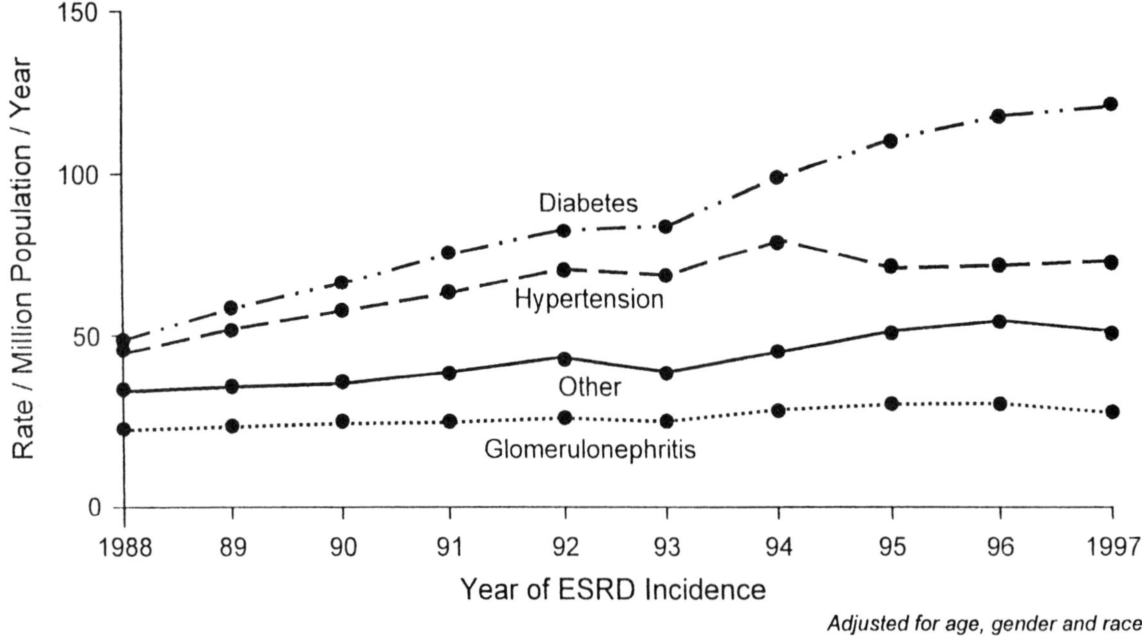

Figure 55.15. Incidence rates of end-stage renal disease (ESRD) in the United States by primary diagnosis for the years 1988 through 1997.

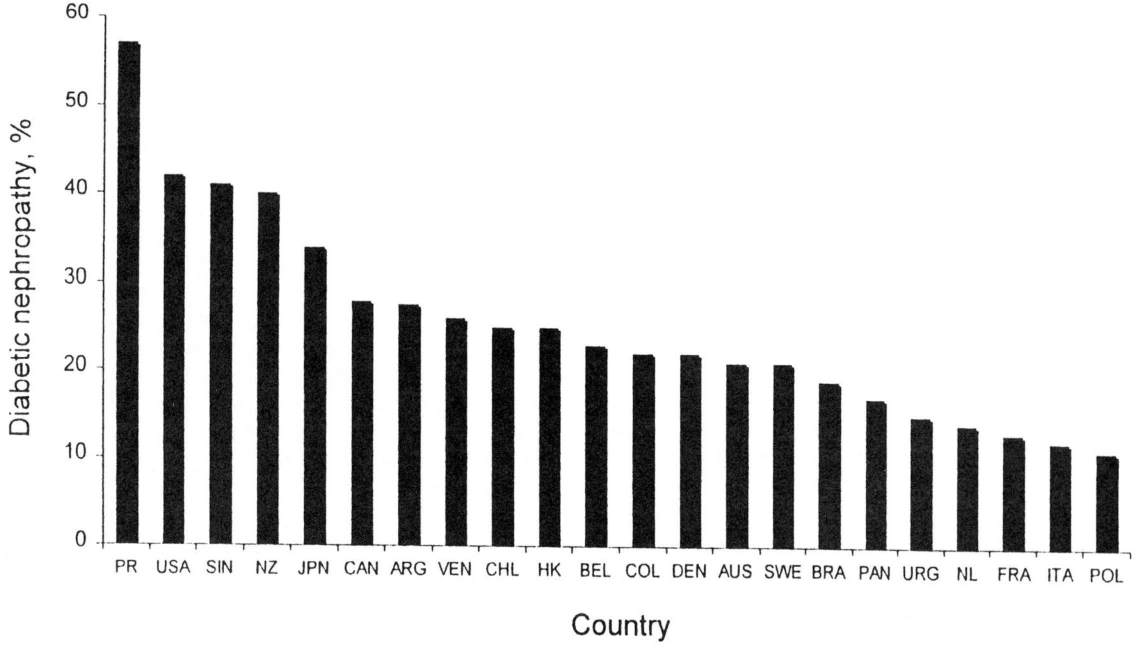

Figure 55.16. High global incidence of end-stage renal disease due to diabetes. PR, Puerto Rico; USA, United States of America; SIN, Singapore; NZ, New Zealand; JPN, Japan; CAN, Canada; ARG, Argentina; VEN, Venezuela; CHL, Chile; HK, Hong Kong; BEL, Belgium; COL, Colombia; DEN, Denmark; AUS, Austria; SWE, Sweden; BRA, Brazil; PAN, Panama; URG, Uruguay; NL, The Netherlands; FRA, France; ITA, Italy; POL, Poland. (Reprinted from Williams ME. Management of the diabetic transplant. *Kidney Int* 1995;48:1660–1669, with permission.)

ESRD in patients with diabetes reflects the demographics of diabetes itself (159). About 70% of diabetic patients with ESRD are white and 30% are black. The predominant cause is type 1 diabetes in whites and type 2 diabetes in blacks (160).

Dialysis options for the diabetic patient receiving dialysis are shown in Table 55.6. In the United States, patients with diabetes are somewhat more likely than those without diabetes to be managed with chronic hemodialysis and less likely to have a functioning transplant. Whatever the modality, the treatment of patients with diabetes is considerably more costly than that of patients without diabetes: Compared with an average of $42,853 spent annually for all patients, the cost for each patient with diabetes was greater by more than $8,000 regardless of modality. The number of hospital admissions is one-fifth higher, and the number of days hospitalized is one-fourth greater than for patients without diabetes (2).

TABLE 55.7 End-Stage Renal Disease Problems for the Patient with Diabetes

Problem	Evaluation
Vascular access	Preservation of vasculature and early assessment for native fistula
Glycemic control	Hemoglobin A_{1c}, home glucose monitoring
Angina, myocardial infarction	Exercise tolerance test, P-thallium, echocardiogram, catheterization
Visual impairment	Ophthalmology evaluation
Foot ulcers	Podiatry evaluation
Peripheral vascular disease, limb amputation	Doppler flow studies
Gastroparesis	Gastric emptying study
Neuropathic problems	Electromyography, neurologist
Malnutrition	Serum albumin, dietary counseling, physical exam

Diabetic patients with ESRD are also those at greatest risk for complications and more likely to have other comorbid conditions. Only a multidisciplinary team of healthcare providers, including the nephrologist, ophthalmologist, vascular surgeon, transplant specialist, cardiologist, podiatrist, renal nutrition expert, and social worker, can provide optimal management to address the list of problems in the diabetic patient with ESRD (Table 55.7). As the transition from renal failure to ESRD occurs, new complexities in management emerge. For example, insulin requirements decrease, retinopathy progresses, hypertension (161) and fluid retention worsen, and gastroparesis becomes refractory to medication. Complications are severe in one half of the patients: One third are blind, one third have diagnosed coronary artery disease, and one in five have had a myocardial infarction. In turn, other uremic problems may be worsened by the presence of diabetes, including nausea, vomiting, impotence, neuropathy, and vascular disease. The functionally dependent diabetic patient with ESRD with multiple comorbid conditions requires increased care by the dialysis provider (162).

Although the optimal time to initiate dialysis has yet to be defined, dialysis needs to be initiated earlier in uremic diabetic patients, to avoid life-threatening events and acceleration of retinopathy. Goals of management include preservation of vascular access, control of hyperglycemia and hypoglycemia, reduction in cardiac mortality, maintenance of vision, avoidance of foot ulcers and limb amputation, and prevention of malnutrition.

Good glycemic management continues to be a priority when the diabetic patient reaches ESRD (163). Recent data suggest a high mortality risk associated with large weight gains resulting from hyperglycemia in diabetic patients receiving dialysis (165). Glycemic control may retard complications of microvascular disease (165), limit hyperkalemia (166), prevent catabolism, and minimize infection. It may also be associated with shorter hospitalizations, improved gastroparesis and orthostatic hypotension, decreased myocardial infarction, and higher serum albumin levels.

TABLE 55.8. Consequences of Hyperglycemia in Patients with Diabetes on Hemodialysis

- Thirst, excessive fluid intake, weight gains between dialysis, hypertension
- Pulmonary edema
- Increased weight gains
- Severe hyperkalemia
- Diabetic ketoacidois
- Shifts in serum osmolality
- Anorexia, nausea, vomiting, weakness
- Increased risk of infection

Signs and symptoms of hyperglycemia are modified in the patient undergoing dialysis (167,168) (Table 55.8). Anorexia, nausea, vomiting, weakness, worsened gastroparesis, and altered mental status may also occur. Sustained severe hyperglycemia may produce only vague, nonspecific symptoms (169). However, insulin dosing and glucose regulation are more complex when diabetic patients become dependent on dialysis (170). Lower doses of insulin may suffice, and oral agents or even insulin may be discontinued in some patients. Alternatively, hypoglycemia is a potentially serious complication feared by diabetic patients receiving dialysis (171). Severe episodes cause significant morbidity, including new retinal hemorrhages and coronary ischemia or even death, and make tight glycemic control almost impossible. Mechanisms of hypoglycemia include decreased insulin clearance, causing inappropriate elevations of insulin levels, lack of gluconeogenesis by failed kidneys, and impaired sympathetic counterregulatory responses. Additional hypoglycemic factors are shown in Table 55.9.

In a recent review (172), 4% of admissions of patients with ESRD (one third of them were nondiabetics) were for hypoglycemia. Almost one half of admissions due to hypoglycemia were drug-related, but more than one third were due to sepsis. Hypoglycemia was often fatal if associated with sepsis or malnutrition. Drugs that are important causes of drug-induced hypoglycemia include sulfonylureas and nonselective β-blockers. Prolonged sulfonylurea–induced hypoglycemia may occur in diabetic patients with ESRD and cause hypoglycemic coma and brain damage (173). Renal failure is a well-recognized risk factor for hypoglycemia. Additional risk factors include reduced oral intake, previous hypoglycemic episodes, and long duration of diabetes. Biguanides and acarbose should be avoided. Glyburide carries a risk comparable to that of the first-generation sulfonylurea chlorpropamide and greater than that of other currently popular oral hypoglycemic agents because its weak metabolites are cleared by the kidneys. Avid binding to pancreatic islets by glyburide may be associated with a sustained insulin response. Acceptable oral hypoglycemic agents in ESRD include glipizide, newer thiazolidenediones, and possibly meglitimide. Diverse symptoms caused by hypoglycemia in chronic renal failure are predominantly neuroglycopenic and include headaches, nausea, vomiting, confusion, drowsiness, lethargy, tremors, seizures, and unconsciousness. Angina (174), silent myocardial infarction, and elevated systemic blood pressure may also occur. Hypoglycemic unawareness is frequent.

TABLE 55.9. Risk Factors for Hypoglycemia in End-stage Renal Disease

- Oral hypoglycemic agents
- Reduced intake
- Malnutrition
- Liver disease
- Alcohol ingestion
- Longer-duration diabetes
- Other drugs

According to USRDS data for 1997, almost 24,000 diabetic patients with ESRD died. There were 270 deaths per 1,000 patient years, compared with 200 for nondiabetic patients with ESRD. Over the past few years, survival of diabetic patients receiving dialysis has remained constant or has even increased, despite the overall aging of the ESRD population with diabetes (175). However, by every account, morbidity and mortality remain significantly higher than for nondiabetic patients with ESRD (176). The worse prognosis for patients with diabetes receiving dialysis is due in large part to progression of comorbid conditions. The overall mortality risk is increased about 1.5-fold in diabetic versus nondiabetic patients with ESRD. Survival of patients with diabetes is slightly reduced at 1 year (Fig. 55.17) but falls to roughly one half at 5 years compared with patients with ESRD due to all other causes. Most of the excess mortality in diabetes is due to associated cardiovascular disease, which is greater in patients with type 1 or type 2 diabetes. A growing number of studies have reported predictors of survival in ESDR. As in patients without diabetes, the survival of patients with diabetes is affected by comorbid conditions (177). The number of preexisting comorbid conditions at the start of dialysis is greater for patients with diabetes than for patients without diabetes.

Ischemic heart disease poses the major threat to sustained survival of the patient with diabetes who is receiving dialysis. The risk of coronary artery disease is dramatically increased in patients with type 1 diabetes and nephropathy (178,179). In a recent study of more than 400 ESRD patients followed from the start of therapy for ESRD, diabetes independently predicted cardiac death over a mean follow-up of 41 months (180). Management must address individual coronary risk factors (181). With ESRD, high cholesterol levels tend to remit, whereas triglyceride levels, which are weaker coronary risk factors, worsen. In addition, the ApoB/ApoA1 (apolipoprotein B/apolipoprotein A1) ratio, an atherogenic index of uremia, is more elevated in patients with diabetes undergoing dialysis (182), as is lipoprotein (A), Lp(A), a recently emphasized risk factor (183). Finally, limited data support an inverse relationship between the frequency and duration of dialysis and coronary risk in diabetic patients.

Clinical strategies to achieve better cardiac outcomes must improve preventive measures and therapy for coronary disease. However, the efficacy of coronary preventive measures in the diabetic patient with ESRD is unclear. Because coronary risk is high, aggressive diagnostic testing for coronary artery disease is appropriate. Unfortunately, diabetes itself is associated with an increased rate of coronary restenosis following percutaneous transluminal coronary angioplasty (PTCA) (184,185) and of subsequent progression of coronary disease. Long-term outcomes have been relatively poor in dialysis patients receiving PTCA, in whom repeat procedures can be anticipated (186).

The management of hypertension in the uremic patient with diabetes is complicated by the presence of renal disease and renal replacement therapy. Calcium-channel blockers and ACE inhibitors are primary treatments. ACE inhibitors are underutilized because of the fear of hyperkalemia. Factors that need to be considered when hypertension is uncontrolled include poor drug absorption (in the presence of gastroparesis), dialyzability (atenolol, methyldopa, captopril), cost (methyldopa

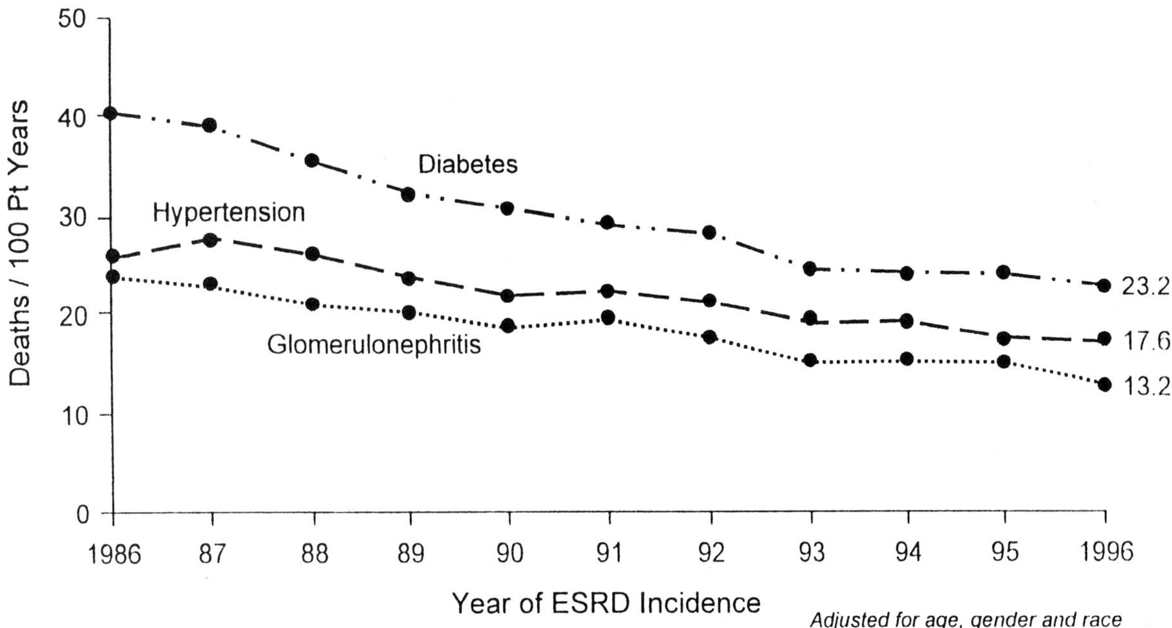

Figure 55.17. Adjusted 1-year mortality rates for diabetes versus other common causes of end-stage renal disease (ESRD) over a 10-year period in the United States. Adjusted by age, race, and gender. (Source: US Renal Data Systems.)

and clonidine are relatively inexpensive), and side effects. Long-term aggressive correction of hypertension in patients with diabetes may reduce the risk of coronary artery disease (187). However, the effects of antihypertensive regimens on cardiovascular disease or other diabetic complications in patients with uremia have not been adequately studied. Overtreatment of hypertension in diabetic patients with uremia who are at risk for coronary ischemia may be dangerous, especially because intradialytic hypotension is more likely in patients with diabetes.

Diabetes is the leading cause of blindness in uremic patients. The ocular complications in type 1 and type 2 diabetes are similar. Progression of retinopathy is a major problem for the diabetic patient receiving dialysis, although ophthalmologic screening programs can prevent vision loss and are cost effective (188). Almost all patients with type 1 diabetes have background or proliferative retinopathy when they start dialysis; 75% have visual disturbances, and 50% have significant visual loss (189). About half as many patients with type 2 diabetes are affected. With current technology, dialysis itself does not appear to exacerbate vision loss (190). The visual prognosis for uremic patients with diabetes has improved because of the collaboration among the nephrologist, diabetologist, and ophthalmologist. The stage of retinopathy determines the ophthalmologic treatment (191). Early intervention is mandatory. Visual acuity may be improved by resolution of macular edema following correction of anemia with erythropoietin (192). Raising the red cell mass by treatment with erythropoietin may also improve retinal hard exudates (193). With aggressive eye management, diabetic patients undergoing dialysis can achieve a visual prognosis similar to that of diabetic patients who have received a kidney transplant (194).

Amputations of the lower extremities are a major source of morbidity for diabetic patients receiving dialysis (195). Uremic diabetic patients with lower-limb disability make poor psychosocial adjustments to illness and should be psychologically prepared for long periods of convalescence (196).

Many clinicians advocate the use of peritoneal dialysis as an alternative to hemodialysis for uremic diabetic patients. Nonetheless, peritoneal dialysis is the treatment option for less than one in four adults with diabetes in the United States (2). Although peritoneal dialysis has several potential advantages, actual data supporting an advantage of this type of dialysis in diabetic patients are limited but do suggest that techniques and patient survival have improved. Fewer than half of the patients on peritoneal dialysis remain on that modality after 2 years of treatment.

Glycemic control in patients receiving peritoneal dialysis is a desirable therapeutic goal. Intraperitoneal administration of insulin eliminates the need for injections, provides more consistent insulin absorption, lowers peripheral insulin levels, lessens the risk of hypoglycemia, and provides constant basal insulin dosing. The major benefit of intraperitoneal administration of insulin is improved glycemic control (197). Although significant clinical benefit has not been proven in clinical trials, intraperitoneal insulin is preferred in most patients receiving peritoneal dialysis (198). Hypoglycemic reactions are fewer and milder than in patients receiving hemodialysis (199). Survival data for patients receiving peritoneal dialysis are similar to those for patients receiving hemodialysis, as are the prevalent causes of mortality.

NOVEL APPROACHES TO TREATMENT OF DIABETIC NEPHROPATHY

Trials of a number of novel approaches to therapy are in the planning stages or are under way. All of these therapies are aimed at interfering with one or more of the mechanisms of diabetic nephropathy.

Protein kinase C (PKC) is a serine/threonine kinase that has been shown to play important roles in normal cell growth, cancerous cell growth, and a number of other intracellular processes. Studies, especially those of King and associates (200), have shown that hyperglycemia leads to activation of isoforms of PKC, especially PKCβ. It has been suggested that PKCβ plays an important pathophysiologic role in the development of vascular, retinal, and other complications of diabetes mellitus. Using an inhibitor that specifically blocks PKCβ (LY333531), King and colleagues showed, in diabetic rats, that both retinopathy and nephropathy improved in animals treated with the PKCβ inhibitor. In particular, the GFR and albumin excretion rate improved. These intriguing results have led to a worldwide trial of the PKCβ inhibitor for retinopathy. Nephropathy trials will start in the near future, suggesting that PKC inhibitors may play an important role in future treatments for diabetic nephropathy.

As discussed in Chapter 51, oxidant stress in thought to be a critical factor in the development of diabetic nephropathy. Koya and colleagues studied the utility of vitamin E in reducing the progression of nephropathy (201) and found that the increase in albuminuria and GFR in rats was significantly reduced by vitamin E. Currently, a number of studies are aimed at determining whether antioxidants such as vitamin E have a therapeutic role in the treatment of diabetic nephropathy. So far, results have been equivocal with a variety of antioxidants, but trials of various agents and dosing regimens are ongoing.

Advanced glycation end-products (AGEs) are proteins that have reacted with glucose nonenzymatically. Although they exist normally, the number of AGEs increases significantly in patients with diabetic nephropathy. AGEs have been implicated in the development of the complications of diabetes (202). In particular, AGEs can cause collagen cross-linking and, by binding to specific receptors, can lead to the production of oxidants and to cellular damage. Administration of AGEs to animals can cause a number of changes seen in animals with diabetes. A number of ongoing trials of inhibitors of AGEs are attempting to determine whether these drugs can both help patients with established nephropathy and prevent diabetic nephropathy.

POSSIBLE APPROACHES TO THE COMPLETE PREVENTION OR CURE OF DIABETIC NEPHROPATHY

At this time there is no clear approach to the complete prevention or cure of diabetic nephropathy. Suggested approaches include the treatment of all patients with diabetes with ACE inhibitors or AR blockers as a preventive measure and islet cell/pancreatic transplantation (203). The suggestion of using blockers of ATII action is based on the idea that angiotensin plays a critical role in the development of diabetic nephropathy, although at this time, there is no evidence for this or for any effect of these drugs on the development of diabetic nephropathy. Considering that as many as 60% to 70% of patients with diabetes will not develop nephropathy, we believe that it is not appropriate for all patients to take these drugs until sufficient positive studies have been completed. On the other hand, if a patient with diabetes has hypertension, the use of ACE inhibitors or AR blockers makes sense, as they will lower blood pressure and possibly have other therapeutic benefits.

Pancreatic transplants have been shown to actually slow and reverse lesions of diabetic nephropathy. Mauer and colleagues studied patients up to 10 years after pancreatic transplantation and showed by renal biopsy that there was a clear regression of disease (203). Although this is very exciting, pancreatic transplantation is not widely used because the risks of immunosuppression and because the relative scarcity of pancreases make this approach useful only in a select number of patients. Of promise, however, is the new field of islet cell transplantation. In theory, successful islet cell transplants should be as effective as pancreatic transplants.

SUMMARY OF RECOMMENDATIONS

- Screening of patients:
  - Patients with type 1 diabetes should be screened for microalbuminuria yearly 5 years after diagnosis. Patients with type 2 diabetes should be screened early, starting at the time of diagnosis. The preferred screening method is the albumin/creatinine ratio.
- For patients with established microalbuminuria (>30 mg per 24 hours) or proteinuria (>300 mg per 24 hours):
  - Tight control of blood glucose is desirable (aim for HbA_{1c} of <7%).
  - Tight control of blood pressure is desirable (aim for 130/80 mm Hg; if proteinuria >1 g per 24 hours, aim for blood pressure of 125/75 mm Hg).
  - Use ACE inhibitors or AR blockers in all patients (including normotensive patients).
  - Use above approaches to reduce proteinuria levels (goals, 50% reduction, aiming for <500 mg per 24 hours or as near to the normal range as possible). Prevention of increases in proteinuria is a main goal.
  - Evaluate diet and reduce protein if excessive. Consider low-protein diets in select circumstances.
  - Evaluate lipids and aim for control as near as possible to recommended, healthy ranges.
  - Encourage patient to stop smoking.

Last, much evidence suggests that a team approach that provides intensive follow-up is optimal. The patient and the health-care team need to become partners in care. Thus internists, diabetologists, nephrologists, nurses, educators, dietitians, exercise physiologists, and the patient form a critical team that will provide the patient with the best possible outcome.

REFERENCES

1. Ritz E, Rychlik I, Locatelli F, et al. End-stage renal failure in type 2 diabetes: a medical catastrophe of worldwide dimensions. *Am J Kidney Dis* 1999;34: 795–808.
2. US Renal Data System, USRDS 1999 Annual Data Report. Bethesda, MD: National Institutes of Health, National Institute of Diabetes and Digestive and Kidney Diseases, April 1999.
3. Schwab SJ, Dunn, FL, Feinglos, MN. Screening for microalbuminuria. A comparison of single sample methods of collection and techniques of albumin analysis. *Diabetes Care* 1992;15:1581–1584.
4. Mogensen CE. Microalbuminuria as a predictor of clinical diabetic nephropathy. *Kidney Int* 1987;31:673–684.
5. American Diabetes Association. Diabetic nephropathy. *Diabetes Care* 2003;26 [Suppl 1]:S94–S98.
6. Ritz E, Orth SR. Nephropathy in patients with type 2 diabetes mellitus. *N Engl J Med* 1999;341:1127–1133.
7. Nelson RG, Knowler WC, Pettitt DJ, et al. Diabetic kidney disease in Pima Indians. *Diabetes Care* 1993;16[Suppl 1]:335–341.
8. Brancati FL, Whittle JC, Whelton PK, et al. The excess incidence of diabetic end-stage renal disease among blacks. A population-based study of potential explanatory factors. *JAMA* 1992;268:3079.
9. Smith SR, Svetkey LP, Dennis VW. Racial differences in the incidence and progression of renal diseases. *Kidney Int* 1991;40:815–822.
10. Caramori ML, Fioretto P, Mauer M. The need for early predictors of diabetic nephropathy risk. Is albumin excretion rate sufficient? *Diabetes* 2000;49:1399–1408.
11. Thomas W, Shen Y, Molitch ME, et al. Rise in albuminuria and blood pressure in patients who progressed to diabetic nephropathy in the Diabetes Control and Complications Trial. *J Am Soc Nephrol* 2001;12:333–340.
12. Levy AS, et al. Clinical practice guidelines for chronic kidney disease. *Am J Kidney Dis* 2002;39[Suppl 1]:S82–S86.
13. The Diabetes Control and Complications Trial Research Group. The effect of intensive treatment of diabetes on the development and progression of long-term complications in insulin-dependent diabetes mellitus. *N Engl J Med* 1993;329:977–986.

14. The Diabetes Control and Complications Trial Research Group. Retinopathy and nephropathy in patients with type 1 diabetes four years after an intensive trial with insulin. *N Engl J Med* 2000;342:381–389.
15. Ohkubo Y, Kishikawa H, Araki E, et al. Intensive insulin therapy prevents the progression of diabetic microvascular complications in Japanese patients with non-insulin-dependent diabetes mellitus: a randomized prospective 6-year study. *Diabetes Res Clin Pract* 1995;28:103.
16. UK Prospective Diabetes Study Group. Intensive blood-glucose control with sulphonylureas or insulin compared with conventional treatment and risk of complications in patients with type 2 diabetes (UKPDS 33). *Lancet* 1998;352: 837–853.
17. Friedman EA. Renal syndromes in diabetes. *Endocrinol Metab Clin North Am* 1996;25:293–324.
18. Mailloux LU, Leavy AS. Hypertension in patients with chronic renal disease. *Am J Kidney Dis* 1998;32[Suppl 3]:S120–S141.
19. Ritz E, Rychlik I, Miltenberger-Miltenyi G. Optimizing antihypertensive therapy in patients with diabetic nephropathy. *J Hypertens Suppl* 1998;16:S17–S22.
20. Ribeiro AB. Abnormalities of systemic blood pressure in diabetes mellitus. *Kidney Int* 1992;42:1470–1483.
21. Pyorala K, Laakso M, Uusitupa M. Diabetes and atherosclerosis: an epidemiologic view. *Diabetes Metab Rev* 1987;3:463–524.
22. Parving HH, Andersen AR, Smidt UM, et al. Early aggressive antihypertensive treatment reduces rate of decline in kidney function in diabetic nephropathy. *Lancet* 1983;1:1175–1179.
23. Mogensen CE. Progression of nephropathy in long-term diabetics with proteinuria and effect of initial anti-hypertensive treatment. *Scand J Clin Lab Invest* 1976;36:383–388.
24. Arauz-Pacheco C, Raskin P. Hypertension in diabetes mellitus. *Endocrinol Metab Clin North Am*, 1996;25:401–423.
25. Mogensen CE. Management of early nephropathy in diabetic patients. *Annu Rev Med* 1995;46:79–93.
26. Ismail N, Becker B, Strzelczyk P, et al. Renal disease and hypertension in non-insulin-dependent diabetes mellitus. *Kidney Int* 1995;55:1–28.
27. Hasslacher C, Bostedt-Kiesel A, Kempe HP, et al. Effect of metabolic factors and blood pressure on kidney function in proteinuric type 2 (non-insulin-dependent) diabetic patients. *Diabetologia* 1993;36:1051–1056.
28. Kasiske BL, Kalil RS, Ma JZ, et al. Effect of antihypertensive therapy on the kidney in patients with diabetes: a meta-regression analysis. *Ann Intern Med* 1993;118:129–138.
29. Hostetter T. Pathogenesis of diabetic glomerular hypertension: hemodynamic considerations. *Semin Nephrol* 1990;10:219–227.
30. Bakris GL, Smith A. Effects of sodium intake on albumin excertion in patients with diabetic nephropathy treated with long-acting calcium antagonists. *Ann Intern Med* 1996;125:201–204.
31. Cooper ME, Johnston CI. Optimizing treatment of hypertension in patients with diabetes. *JAMA* 2000;283:3177–3179.
32. Bjorck S. Clinical trials in overt diabetic nephropathy. In: Mogensen CE, ed. *The kidney and hypertension in diabetes mellitus*. Boston: Kluwer Academic Publishers, 1998;409–428.
33. Bakris GL, Williams M, Dworkin L, et al. Preserving renal function in adults with hypertension and diabetes: a consensus approach. National Kidney Foundation Hypertension and Diabetes Executive Committees Working Group. *Am J Kidney Dis* 2000;36:646–661.
34. Fox C. Diabetes and hypertension: an era of clarity or confusion. *J Hum Hypertens* 1999;13[Suppl 2]:S9–S17.
35. Keane WF, Eknoyan G. Proteinuria, albuminuria, risk, assessment, detection, elimination (PARADE): a position paper of the National Kidney Foundation. *Am J Kidney Dis* 1999;33:1004–1010.
36. Lewis JB, Berl T, Bain RP, et al. Effect of intensive blood pressure control on the course of type 1 diabetic nephropathy. Collaborative Study Group. *Am J Kidney Dis* 1999;34:809–817.
37. Peterson JC, Adler S, Burkart JM, et al. Blood pressure control, proteinuria, and the progression of renal disease. The Modification of Diet in Renal Disease Study. *Ann Intern Med* 1995;123:754–762.
38. Hansson L, Zanchetti A, Carruthers SG, et al. Effects of intensive blood-pressure lowering and low-dose aspirin in patients with hypertension: principal results of the Hypertension Optimal Treatment (HOT) randomised trial. HOT Study Group. *Lancet* 1998;351:1755–1762.
39. UK Prospective Diabetes Study Group. Tight blood pressure control and risk of macrovascular and microvascular complications in type 2 diabetes: UKPDS 38. *BMJ* 1998;317:703–713.
40. Estacio RO, Jeffers BW, Hiatt WR, et al. The effect of nisoldipine as compared with enalapril on cardiovascular outcomes in patients with non-insulin-dependent diabetes and hypertension. *N Engl J Med* 1998;338:645–652.
41. Pickering TG. Advances in the treatment of hypertension. *JAMA* 1999;281: 114–116.
42. Fletcher AE, Bulpitt CJ. How far should blood pressure be lowered? *N Engl J Med* 1992;326:251–254.
43. Grossman E, Messerli FH, Goldbourt U. High blood pressure and diabetes mellitus: are all antihypertensive drugs created equal? *Arch Intern Med* 2000;160:2447–2452.
44. Berlowitz DR, Ash AS, Hickey EC, et al. Inadequate management of blood pressure in a hypertensive population. *N Engl J Med* 1998;339:1957–1963.
45. Tarnow L, Rossing P, Gall MA, et al. Prevalence of arterial hypertension in diabetic patients before and after the JNC-V. *Diabetes Care* 1994;17:1247–1251.
46. Elliott WJ, Weir DR, Black HR. Cost-effectiveness of the lower treatment goal (of JNC VI) for diabetic hypertensive patients. Joint National Committee on Prevention, Detection, Evaluation, and Treatment of High Blood Pressure. *Arch Intern Med* 2000;160:1277–1283.
47. Sowers JR, Williams M, Epstein M, et al. Hypertension in patients with diabetes. Strategies for drug therapy to reduce complications. *Postgrad Med* 2000; 107:47–4, 60.
48. Sever PS. Blood pressure control for the hypertensive patients: what can we do better? *Am J Hypertens* 1997;10(7 Pt 2):128S–130S.
49. Kshirsagar AV, Joy MS, Hogan SL, et al. Effect of ACE inhibitors in diabetic and nondiabetic chronic renal disease: a systematic overview of randomized placebo-controlled trials. *Am J Kidney Dis* 2000;35:695–707.
50. Bell DSH. β-adrenergic blockage agents in patients with diabetes—friend and foe. *Endocr Pract* 1999;5:51–53.
51. Weidmann P, Boehlen LM, de Courten M. Effects of different antihypertensive drugs on human diabetic proteinuria. *Nephrol Dial Transplant* 1993;8: 582–584.
52. Heeg JE, de Jong PE, van der Hem GK, et al. Efficacy and variability of the antiproteinuric effect of ACE inhibition by lisinopril. *Kidney Int* 1989;36: 272–279.
53. Lewis EJ, Hunsicker LG, Bain RP, et al. The effect of angiotensin-converting-enzyme inhibition on diabetic nephropathy. The Collaborative Study Group. *N Engl J Med* 1993;329:1456–1462.
54. Tatti P, Pahor M, Byington RP, et al. Outcome results of the Fosinopril Versus Amlodipine Cardiovascular Events Randomized Trial (FACET) in patients with hypertension and NIDDM. *Diabetes Care* 1998;21:597–603.
55. Peters AL, Hsueh W. Antihypertensive agents in diabetic patients: great benefits, special risks. *Arch Intern Med* 1999;159:541–542.
56. Freis ED. Improving treatment effectiveness in hypertension. *Arch Intern Med* 1999;159:2517–2521.
57. Marks JB, Raskin P. Nephropathy and hypertension in diabetes. *Med Clin North Am* 1998;82:877–907.
58. Schrier RW. Treating high-risk diabetic hypertensive patients with comorbid conditions. *Am J Kidney Dis* 2000;36[3 Suppl 1]:S10–S17.
59. Dunfee TP. The changing management of diabetic nephropathy. *Hosp Pract* 1995;30:45–49, 53–555.
60. Sawicki PT. Do ACE inhibitors offer specific benefits in the antihypertensive treatment of diabetic patients? 17 years of unfulfilled promises. *Diabetologia* 1998;41:598–602.
61. Parving HH. Renoprotection in diabetes: genetic and non-genetic risk factors and treatment. *Diabetologia* 1998;41:745–759.
62. Williams ME. Angiotensin converting enzyme inhibitors in the prevention of diabetic renal diseases. *Curr Opin Endocrinol Diabetes* 1997;4:10–15.
63. Deedwania PC. Hypertension and diabetes: new therapeutic options. *Arch Intern Med* 2000;160:1585–1594.
64. Cook DJ, Guyatt GH. Interpreting, integrating, and individualizing evidence about the prevention of diabetic nephropathy. *Ann Intern Med* 1999;131: 707–708.
65. Wang PH. When should ACE inhibitors be given to normotensive patients with IDDM? *Lancet* 1997;349:1782–1783.
66. Furberg CD, Herrington DM, Psaty BM. Are drugs within a class interchangeable? *Lancet* 1999;354:1202–1204.
67. Pitt B. Use of 'Xpril' in patients with chronic heart failure. A paradigm or epitaph for our times? *Circulation* 1994;90:1550–1551.
68. Hansson L, Lindholm LH, Niskanen L, et al. Effect of anglotensin-converting-enzyme inhibition compared with conventional therapy on cardiovascular morbidity and mortality in hypertension: the Captopril Prevention Project (CAPPP) randomized trial. *Lancet* 1999;353:611–616.
69. Sawicki PT, Muhlhauser I, Didjurgeit U, et al. Intensified antihypertensive therapy is associated with improved survival in type 1 diabetic patients with nephropathy. *J Hypertens* 1995;13:933–938.
70. Allen AM, Zhuo J, Mendelsohn FA. Localization of angiotensin AT1 and AT2 receptors. *J Am Soc Nephrol* 1999;10:S23–S29.
71. Brenner BM. Hemodynamically mediated glomerular injury and the progressive nature of kidney disease. *Kidney Int* 1983;23:647–655.
72. Morris AD, Donnely R. Clinical review 79: angiotensin II: an insulin-sensitizing vasoactive hormone? *J Clin Endocrinol Metab* 1996;81:1303–1306.
73. Harris RC, Inagam T. Molecular biology and pharmacology of angiotensin receptor subtypes in hypertension, physiology, diagnosis and management. In: 2nd ed. Brenner BM, eds. New York: Raven Press, 1995:1721–1738.
74. Gansevoort RT, de Zeeuw D, de Jong PE. Is the antiproteinuric effect of ACE inhibition mediated by interference in the renin-angiotensin system? *Kidney Int* 1994;45:861–867.
75. Allen TJ, Cao Z, Youssef S, et al. Role of angiotensin II and bradykinin in experimental diabetic nephropathy. Functional and structural studies. *Diabetes* 1997;46:1612–1618.
76. Gilbert RE, Cox A, Wu LL, et al. Expression of transforming growth factor-beta1 and type IV collagen in the renal tubulointerstitium in experimental diabetes: effects of ACE inhibition. *Diabetes* 1998;47:414–422.
77. Vranes D, Cooper ME, Dilley RJ. Angiotensin-converting enzyme inhibition reduces diabetes-induced vascular hypertrophy: morphometric studies. *J Vasc Res* 1995;32:183–189.
78. Sassy-Prigent C, Heudes D, Jouquey S, et al. Morphometric detection of incipient glomerular lesions in diabetic nephropathy in rats. Protective effects of ACE inhibition. *Lab Invest* 1995;73:64–71.

79. Wolf G, Ziyadeh FN. The role of angiotensin II in diabetic nephropathy: emphasis on nonhemodynamic mechanisms. *Am J Kidney Dis* 1997;29:153–163.
80. Sharma K, Eltayeb BO, McGowan TA, et al. Captopril-induced reduction of serum levels of transforming growth factor-beta1 correlates with long-term renoprotection in insulin-dependent diabetic patients. *Am J Kidney Dis* 1999; 34:818–823.
81. Gerstein HC. Cardiovascular and metabolic benefits of ACE inhibition: moving beyond blood pressure reduction. *Diabetes Care* 2000;23:882–823.
82. Anderson S, Meyer TW, Rennke HG, et al. Control of glomerular hypertension limits glomerular injury in rats with reduced renal mass. *J Clin Invest* 1985;76:612–619.
83. Zatz R, Dunn BR, Meyer TW, et al. Prevention of diabetic glomerulopathy by pharmacological amelioration of glomerular capillary hypertension. *J Clin Invest* 1986;77:1925–1930.
84. Maki DD, Ma JZ, Louis TA, et al. Long-term effects of antihypertensive agents on proteinuria and renal function. *Arch Intern Med* 1995;155:1073–1080.
85. Remuzzi G. Renoprotective effect of ACE inhibitors: dissecting the molecular clues and expanding the blood pressure goal. *Am J Kidney Dis* 1999;34:951–954.
86. Parving HH, Rossing P, Hommel E, et al. Angiotensin-converting enzyme inhibition in diabetic nephropathy: ten years' experience. *Am J Kidney Dis* 1995;26:99–107.
87. Warram JH, Gearin G, Laffel L, et al. Effect of duration of type I diabetes on the prevalence of stages of diabetic nephropathy defined by urinary albumin/creatinine ratio. *J Am Soc Nephrol* 1996;7:930–937.
88. Heeg JE, de Jong PE, van der Hem GK, et al. Reduction of proteinuria by angiotensin converting enzyme inhibition. *Kidney Int* 1987;32:78–83.
89. Maschio G, Alberti D, Janin G, et al. Effect of the angiotensin-converting-enzyme inhibitor benazepril on the progression of chronic renal insufficiency. The Angiotensin-Converting-Enzyme Inhibition in Progressive Renal Insufficiency Study Group. *N Engl J Med* 1996;334:939–945.
90. Hansen PM, Mathiesen ER, Kofoed-Enevoldsen A, et al. Possible effect of angiotensin-converting enzyme inhibition on glomerular charge selectivity. *J Diabetes Complications* 1995;9:158–162.
91. The EUCLID Study Group. Randomised placebo-controlled trial of lisinopril in normotensive patients with insulin-dependent diabetes and normoalbuminuria or microalbuminuria. *Lancet* 1997;349:1787–1792.
92. American Diabetes Association. Consensus development conference on the diagnosis and management of nephropathy in patients with diabetes mellitus. American Diabetes Association and the National Kidney Foundation. *Diabetes Care* 1994;17:1357–1361.
93. Mogensen CE, Keane WF, Bennett PH, et al. Prevention of diabetic renal disease with special reference to microalbuminuria. *Lancet* 1995;346:1080–1084.
94. Bennett PH, Haffner S, Kasiske BL, et al. Screening and management of microalbuminuria in patients with diabetes mellitus: recommendations to the Scientific Advisory Board of the National Kidney Foundation from an ad hoc committee of the Council on Diabetes Mellitus of the National Kidney Foundation. *Am J Kidney Dis* 1995;25:107–112.
95. Marré M, Leblanc H, Suarez L, et al. Converting enzyme inhibition and kidney function in normotensive diabetic patients with persistent microalbuminuria. *BMJ* 1987;294:1448–1452.
96. Marré M, Chatellier G, Leblanc H, et al. Prevention of diabetic nephropathy with enalapril in normotensive diabetics with microalbuminuria. *BMJ* 1988; 297:1092–1095.
97. Viberti G, Mogensen CE, Group LC, et al. Effect of captopril on progression to clinical proteinuria in patients with insulin-dependent diabetes mellitus and microalbuminuria. European Microalbuminuria Captopril Study Group. *JAMA* 1994;271:275–279.
98. Laffel LM, McGill JB, Gans DJ. The beneficial effect of angiotensin-converting enzyme inhibition with captopril on diabetic nephropathy in normotensive IDDM with microalbuminuria. North American Microalbuminuria Study Group. *Am J Med* 1995;99:497–504.
99. Mathiesen ER, Hommel E, Giese J, et al. Efficacy of captopril in postponing nephropathy in normotensive insulin dependent diabetic patients with microalbuminuria. *BMJ* 1991;303:81–87.
100. Crepaldi G, Carta Q, Deferrari G, et al. Effects of lisinopril and nifedipine on the progression to overt albuminuria in IDDM patients with incipient nephropathy and normal blood pressure. The Italian Microalbuminuria Study Group in IDDM. *Diabetes Care* 1998;21:104–110.
101. Mathiesen ER, Hommel E, Hansen HP, et al. Randomised controlled trial of long term efficacy of captopril on preservation of kidney function in normotensive patients with insulin dependent diabetes and microalbuminuria. *BMJ* 1999;319:24–25.
102. Mogensen CE. Microalbuminuria, blood pressure and diabetic renal disease: origin and development of ideas. *Diabetologia* 1999;42:263–285.
103. Rodby RA, Firth LM, Lewis EJ. An economic analysis of captopril in the treatment of diabetic nephropathy. The Collaborative Study Group. *Diabetes Care* 1996;19:1051–1061.
104. Gambara V, Mecca G, Remuzzi G, et al. Heterogeneous nature of renal lesions in type II diabetes. *J Am Soc Nephrol* 1993;3:1458–1466.
105. Alzaid AA. Microalbuminuria in patients with NIDDM: an overview. *Diabetes Care* 1996;19:79–89.
106. Fioretto P, Mauer M, Brocco E, et al. Patterns of renal injury in NIDDM patients with microalbuminuria. *Diabetologia* 1996;39:1569–1576.
107. American Diabetes Association. Diabetic nephropathy. *Diabetes Care* 1997;20 [Suppl 1]:524–527.
108. Ruggenenti P, Mosconi L, Sangalli F, et al. Glomerular size-selective dysfunction in NIDDM is not ameliorated by ACE inhibition or by calcium channel blockade. *Kidney Int* 1999;55:984–994.
109. Ravid M, Brosh D, Levi Z, et al. Use of enalapril to attenuate decline in renal function in normotensive, normoalbuminuric patients with type 2 diabetes mellitus. A randomized, controlled trial. *Ann Intern Med* 1998;128:982–988.
110. Kiberd BA, Jindal KK. Should all Pima Indians with type 2 diabetes mellitus be prescribed routine angiotensin-converting enzyme inhibition therapy to prevent renal failure? *Mayo Clin Proc* 1999;74:559–564.
111. Golan L, Birkmeyer JD, Welch HG. The cost-effectiveness of treating all patients with type 2 diabetes with angiotensin-converting enzyme inhibitors. *Ann Intern Med* 1999;131:660–667.
112. Ravid M, Savin H, Jutrin I, et al. Long-term stabilizing effect of angiotensin-converting enzyme inhibition on plasma creatinine and on proteinuria in normotensive type II diabetic patients. *Ann Intern Med* 1993;118:577–581.
113. Lebovitz HE, Wiegmann TB, Cnaan A, et al. Renal protective effects of enalapril in hypertensive NIDDM: role of baseline albuminuria. *Kidney Int Suppl* 1994;45:S150–S155.
114. Chan JC, Ko GT, Leung DH, et al. Long-term effects of angiotensin-converting enzyme inhibition and metabolic control in hypertensive type 2 diabetic patients. *Kidney Int* 2000;57:590–600.
115. Nielsen FS, Rossing P, Gall MA, et al. Long-term effect of lisinopril and atenolol on kidney function in hypertensive NIDDM subjects with diabetic nephropathy. *Diabetes* 1997;46:1182–1188.
116. Keilani T, Schlueter W, Battle D. Selected aspects of ACE inhibitor therapy for patients with renal disease: impact on proteinuria, lipids and potassium. *J Clin Pharmacol* 1995;35:87–97.
117. Reardon LC, Macpherson DS. Hyperkalemia in outpatients using angiotensin-converting enzyme inhibitors. How much should we worry? *Arch Intern Med* 1998;158:26–32.
118. Bakris GL, Weir MR. Angiotensin-converting enzyme inhibitor-associated elevations in serum creatinine: is this a cause for concern? *Arch Intern Med* 2000;160:685–693.
119. Ichikawa I. Angiotensin receptors: what is new? *Am J Kidney Dis* 2000;35: LVIII–LVIX.
120. Weir MR. Angiotensin-II receptor antagonists: a new class of antihypertensive agents. *Am Fam Physician* 1996;53:589–594.
121. Grossman E, Messerli FH, Neotal JM. Angiotensin II receptor blockers: equal or preferred substitutes for ACE inhibitors? *Arch Intern Med* 2000;160: 1905–1911.
122. Midran A, Ripstein J. Angiotensin receptor blockers: pharmacology and clinical significance. *J Am Soc Nephrol* 1999;10[Suppl 12]:S273–S277.
123. O'Donnell MP, Carry GS, Oda H, et al. Irbesartan lowers blood pressure and ameliorates renal injury in experimental non-insulin-dependent diabetes mellitus. *Kidney Int Suppl* 1997;63:S218–S220.
124. Remuzzi A, Perc N, Amuchastegui CS, et al. Short- and long-term effect of angiotensin II receptor blockade in rats with experimental diabetes. *J Am Soc Nephrol* 1993;4:40–49.
125. Andersen S, Tarnow L, Rossing P, et al. Renoprotective effects of angiotensin II receptor blockade in type 1 diabetic patients with diabetic nephropathy. *Kidney Int* 2000;57:601–606.
126. Pohl M, Cooper M, Ulrey J, et al. Safety and efficacy of irbesartan in hypertensive patients with type 2 diabetes and proteinuria. *Am J Hypertens* 1997;10: 105A(abst).
127. Lacourciere Y, Belanger A, Godin C, et al. Long-term comparison of losartan and enalapril on kidney function in hypertensive type 2 diabetics with early nephropathy. *Kidney Int* 2000;58:762–769.
128. Porush JG, Berl T, Anzalone DA, et al. Multi-center collaborative trial of angiotensin II receptor antagonism on morbidity, mortality, and renal function in hypertensive type II diabetic patients with nephropathy. *Am J Hypertens* 1998;11:73(abst).
129. Dasbach EJ, Shahinfar S, Santarello NC, et al, for the RENAAL Investigators. Quality of life in patients with NIDDM and nephropathy at baseline: The Losartan Renal Protection Study (RENAAL). *Diabetes* 1999;48:A389(abst).
130. Brenner BM, Cooper ME, de Zeeuw D, et al. Effects of losartan on renal and cardiovascular outcomes in patients with type 2 diabetes and nephropathy. *N Engl J Med* 2001;345:861–869.
131. Lewis EJ, Hunsicker LG, Clarke WR, et al. Renoprotective effect of the angiotensin-receptor antagonist irbesartan in patients with nephropathy due to type 2 diabetes. *N Engl J Med* 2001;345:851–860.
132. Parving HH, Lehnert H, Bröchner-Mortensen J, et al. The effect of irbesartan on the development of diabetic nephropathy in patients with type 2 diabetes. *N Engl J Med* 2001;345:870–878.
133. Pitt B, Segal R, Martinez FA, et al. Randomised trial of losartan versus captopril in patients over 65 with heart failure (Evaluation of Losartan in the Elderly Study, ELITE). *Lancet* 1997;349:747–752.
134. Mackenzie HS, Ziai F, Omer SA, et al. Angiotensin receptor blockers in chronic renal disease: the promise of a bright clinical future. *J AM Soc Nephrol* 1999;10[Suppl 12]:S283–S286.
135. Gansevoort RT, de Zeeuw D, Shahinfar S, et al. Effects of the angiotensin II antagonist losartan in hypertensive patients with renal disease. *J Hypertens Suppl* 1994;12[Suppl 2]:S37–S42.
136. Bakris GL, Siomos M, Richardson D, et al. ACE inhibition or angiotensin receptor blockade: impact on potassium in renal failure. VAL-K Study Group. *Kidney Int* 2000;58:2084–2092.

137. Epstein M. Calcium antagonists and diabetic nephropathy. *Arch Intern Med* 1991;151:2361–2364.
138. Epstein M. A symposium: calcium antagonists and the diabetic patient: recent controversies and future perspectives. *Am J Cardiol* 1998; 82:1R–3R.
139. Slataper R, Vicknair N, Sadler R, et al. Comparative effects of different antihypertensive treatments on progression of diabetic renal disease. *Arch Intern Med* 1993;153:973–980.
140. Nielsen B, Flyvbjerg A. Calcium channel blockers—the effect on renal changes in clinical and experimental diabetes: an overview. *Nephrol Dial Transplant* 2000;15:581–585.
141. Valentino VA, Wilson MD, Weart W, et al. A perspective on converting enzyme inhibitors and calcium channel antagonists in diabetic renal disease. *Arch Intern Med* 1991;151:2367–2372.
142. Kloke HJ, Branten AJ, Huysmans FT, et al. Antihypertensive treatment of patients with proteinuric renal diseases: risks or benefits of calcium channel blockers? *Kidney Int* 1998;53:1559–1573.
143. Epstein M. Calcium antagonists and renal disease. *Kidney Int* 1998;54:1771–1784.
144. Dworkin LD, Benstein JA, Parker M, et al. Calcium antagonists and converting enzyme inhibitors reduce renal injury by different mechanisms. *Kidney Int* 1993;43:808–814.
145. Melbourne Diabetic Nephropathy Study Group. Comparison between perindopril and nifedipine in hypertensive and normotensive diabetic patients with microalbuminuria. *BMJ* 1991;302:210–216.
146. Mimran A, Insua A, Ribstein J, et al. Contrasting effects of captopril and nifedipine in normotensive patients with incipient diabetic nephropathy. *J Hypertens* 1988;6:919–923.
147. Bakris GL. Effects of diltiazem or lisinopril on massive proteinuria associated with diabetes mellitus. *Ann Intern Med* 1990;112:707–708.
148. Bakris GL, Copley JB, Vicknair N, et al. Calcium channel blockers versus other antihypertensive therapies on progression of NIDDM associated nephropathy. *Kidney Int* 1996;50:1641–1650.
149. Bakris GL, Weir MR, DeQuattro V, et al. Effects of an ACE inhibitor/calcium antagonist combination on proteinuria in diabetic nephropathy. *Kidney Int* 1998;54:1283–1289.
150. Guasch A, Parham M, Zayas CF, et al. Contrasting effects of calcium channel blockade versus converting enzyme inhibition no proteinuria in African Americans with non-insulin-dependent diabetes mellitus and nephropathy. *J Am Soc Nephrol* 1997;8:793–798.
151. Saunders E, Weir MR, Kong BW, et al. A comparison of the efficacy and safety of a beta-blocker, a calcium channel blocker, and a converting enzyme inhibitor in hypertensive blacks. *Arch Intern Med* 1990;150:1707–1713.
152. Furberg CD, Psaty BM, Meyer JV. Nifedipine. Dose-related increase in mortality in patients with coronary heart disease. *Circulation* 1995;92:1326–1331.
153. Tuomilehto J, Rastenyte D, Birkenhager WH, et al. Effects of calcium-channel blockade in older patients with diabetes and systolic hypertension. Systolic Hypertension in Europe Trial Investigators. *N Engl J* Med 1999;340:677–684.
154. Cutler JA. Calcium-channel blockers for hypertension—uncertainty continues. *N Engl J Med* 1998;338:679–681.
155. Effects of dietary protein restriction on the progression of moderate renal disease in the Modification of Diet in Renal Disease Study. *J Am Soc Nephrol* 1996;7:2616–2626.
156. Brenner BM, Lawler EV, Mackenzie HS. The hyperfiltration theory: a paradigm shift in nephrology. *Kidney Int* 1996;49:1774–1777.
157. Pedrini MT, Levey AS, Lau J, et al. The effect of dietary protein restriction on the progression of diabetic and nondiabetic renal diseases: a meta-analysis. *Ann Intern Med* 1996;124:627–632.
158. Williams ME. Management of the diabetic transplant recipient. *Kidney Int* 1995;48:1660–1669.
159. Benhamou PY, Marwah T, Balducci F, et al. Classification of diabetes in patients with end-stage renal disease. *Clin Nephrol* 1992;38:239–244.
160. Perneger TV, Brancati FL, Whelton PK, et. End-stage renal disease attributable to diabetes mellitus. *Ann Intern Med* 1994;121:912–918.
161. Arauz-Pacheco C, Raskin P. Hypertension in diabetes mellitus. *Endocrinol Metab Clin North Am* 1996;25:401–423.
162. Sankarasubbaiyan S, Holley JL. An analysis of the increased demands placed on dialysis health care team members by functionally dependent hemodialysis patients. *Am J Kidney Dis* 2000;35:1061–1067.
163. Williams ME. Insulin management of a diabetic patient on hemodialysis. *Semin Dial* 1992;5:69.
164. Ifudu O, Dulin AL, Friedman EA. Interdialytic weight gain correlates with glycosylated hemoglobin in diabetic hemodialysis patients. *Am J Kidney Dis* 1994;23:686–691.
165. Gray H, O'Rahilly S. Toward improved glycemic control in diabetes. What's on the horizon? *Arch Intern Med* 1995;155:1137–1142.
166. Montoliu J, Revert L. Lethal hyperkalemia associated with severe hyperglycemia in diabetic patients with renal failure. *Am J Kidney Dis* 1985;5:47–48.
167. Al-Kudsi RR, Daugirdas JT, Ing JS, et al. Extreme hyperglycemia in dialysis patients. *Clin Nephrology* 1982;17:228–231.
168. Goldfarb S, Cox M, Singer I, et al. Acute hyperkalemia induced by hyperglycemia: Hormonal mechanisms. *Ann Intern Med* 1976:84:426–432.
169. Williams ME. What are the clinically important consequences of ESRD-associated endocrine dysfunction? *Semin Dial* 1997;10:11.
170. Mujais SK, Fadda G. Carbohydrate metabolism in end-stage renal disease. *Semin Dial* 1989;2:46.
171. Rodriguez VO, Arem R, Adrogue HJ. Hypoglycemia in dialysis patients. *Semin Dial* 1995;8:95.
172. Haviv YS, Sharkia M, Safardi R. Hypoglycemia in patients with renal failure. *Ren Fail* 2000;22:219–223.
173. Krepinsky J, Ingram AJ, Clase C. prolonged sulfonylurea-induced hypoglycemia in diabetic patients with end-stage renal disease. *Am J Kidney Dis* 2000;35:500–505.
174. Duh E, Feinglos M. Hypoglycemia-induced angina pectoris in a patient with diabetes mellitus. *Ann Intern Med* 1994;121:945–946.
175. Friedman EA. How can care of the diabetic ESRD patients be improved? *Semin Dial* 1991;4:13.
176. Blau A, Ben-David A, Eliahou HE. High short-term mortality of diabetic patients entering dialysis. *Isr J Med Sci* 1994;30:528–530.
177. Collins AJ, Hanson G, Umen A, et al. Changing risk factor demographics in end-stage renal disease patients entering hemodialysis and the impact of long-term mortality. *Am J Kidney Dis* 1990;15:422–432.
178. Manske CL. Coronary artery disease in diabetic patients with nephropathy. *Am J Hypertens* 1993;6:367S–374S.
179. Krolewski AS, Kosinski EJ, Warram JH, et al. Magnitude and determinants of coronary artery disease in juvenile-onset, insulin-dependent diabetes mellitus. *Am J Cardiol* 1987;59:750–755.
180. Foley RN, Parfrey PS, Harnett JD, et al. Clinical and echocardiographic disease in patients starting end-stage renal disease therapy. *Kidney Int* 1995;47:186–192.
181. Ma KW, Greene EL, Raij L. Cardiovascular risk factors in chronic renal failure and hemodialysis populations. *Am J Kidney Dis* 1992;19:505–513.
182. Sakurai T, Oka T, Hasegawa H, et al. Comparison of lipids, apoprotein and associated activities between diabetic and nondiabetic end-stage renal disease. *Nephron* 1992;61:409–414.
183. Hirata K, Kikuchi S, Saku K, et al. Apolipoprotein (A) phenotypes and serum lipoprotein (A) levels in maintenance hemodialysis patients with/without diabetes mellitus. *Kidney Int* 1993;44:1062–1070.
184. Ahmed WH, Shubrooks SJ, Gibson CM, et al. Complications and long-term outcome after percutaneous coronary angioplasty in chronic hemodialysis patients. *Am Heart J* 1994;128:252–255.
185. Aronson D, Bloomgarden Z, Rayfield EJ. Potential mechanisms promoting restenosis in diabetic patients. *J Am Coll Cardiol* 1996;27:528–532.
186. Kahn JK, Rutherford BD, McConahay, et al. Short- and long-term outcome of percutaneous transluminal coronary angioplasty in chronic dialysis patients. *Am Heart J* 1990;119:484–489.
187. Caldwell BV. Treating hypertension in the diabetic patient: therapeutic goals and the role of calcium channel blockers. *Clin Ther* 1993;15:618–636.
188. Javitt JC, Aiello LP. Cost-effectiveness of detecting and treating diabetic retinopathy. *Ann Intern Med* 1996;124:164–169.
189. Watanabe Y, Yuzawa Y, Mizumoto D, et al. Long-term follow up study of 268 diabetic patients undergoing haemodialysis, with special attention to visual acuity and heterogeneity. *Nephrol Dial Transplant* 1993;8:725–734.
190. Diaz-Buxo JA, Burgess WP, Greenman WP, et al. Visual function in diabetic patients undergoing dialysis: comparison of peritoneal and hemodialysis. *Int J Artif Organs* 1984;7:257–262.
191. Berman DH, Garcia CA. Diabetic retinopathy: a review. *Semin Dial* 1989;2:226.
192. Friedman EA, Brown CD, Berman DH. Erythropoietin in diabetic macular edema and renal insufficiency. *Am J Kidney Dis* 1995;26:202–208.
193. Berman DH, Friedman EA. Partial absorption of hard exudates in patients with diabetic end-stage renal disease and severe anemia after treatment with erythropoietin. *Retina* 1994;14:1–5.
194. Berman DH, Friedman EA, Lundin AP. Aggressive ophthalmological management in diabetic end-stage renal disease: a study of 31 consecutively referred patients. *Am J Nephrol* 1992;12:344–350.
195. Shaw JE, Boulton AJ, Gokal R. Management of foot problems in diabetes. *Perit Dial Int* 1996;16[Suppl 1]:S279–S282.
196. Carrington AL, Mandsley SK, Morley M, et al. Psychological status of diabetic people with or without lower limb disability. *Diabetes Res Clin Pract* 1996;32:19–25.
197. Khanna R. Peritoneal dialysis in diabetic end-stage renal disease. In: Gokal R, Nolph KD, eds. *The textbook of peritoneal dialysis*. Dordrecht: Kluwer Academic, 1994:639.
198. Johnston JR. Maintaining diabetic patients on long-term peritoneal dialysis. *Semin Dial* 1995;8:390.
199. Tzamaloukas AH, Murata GH, Eisenberg B, et al. Hypoglycemia in diabetics on dialysis with poor glycemic control: hemodialysis versus continuous ambulatory peritoneal dialysis. *Int J Artif Organs* 1992;15:390–392.
200. Ishii H, Jirousek MR, Koya D, et al. Amelioration of vascular dysfunction in diabetic rats by an oral PKC beta inhibitor. *Science* 1996;272:728–731.
201. Koya D, Haneda M, Kikkawa R, et al. d-alpha-tocopherol treatment prevents glomerular dysfunctions in diabetic rats through inhibition of protein kinase C-diacylglycerol pathway. *Biofactors* 1998;7:69–76.
202. Abdel-Rahman E, Bolton WK. Pimagedine: a novel therapy for diabetic nephropathy. *Expert Opin Investig Drugs* 2002;11:565–574.
203. Fioretto P, Steffes MW, Sutherland DE, et al. Reversal of lesions of diabetic nephropathy after pancreas transplantation. *N Engl J Med* 1998;339:69–75.

CHAPTER 56

The Nervous System and Diabetes

Roy Freeman

Most recognized neurologic complications associated with diabetes involve the peripheral nervous system, and it is these that will be emphasized in this chapter. The diabetic neuropathies include several distinctive clinical syndromes with differing clinical manifestations, anatomic distributions, clinical courses, and possibly underlying pathophysiologies.

Disorders of the nervous system associated with diabetes have long been recognized. Rollo is credited with having recorded this association in 1798, and until the middle of the 19th century, diabetes itself was attributed to a primary disorder of the central nervous system. It was Marchal de Calvi in 1864 who first suggested that diabetes might be the cause rather than the effect of neuropathy (1,2). Pavy's (3) description in 1885 of neuropathic symptoms is noteworthy for its completeness.

> The usual account given by these patients is that they cannot feel properly in their legs, that their feet are numb, that their legs seem too heavy—as one expressed it, "as if he had 20 pound weights on his legs, and a feeling as if his boots were a good deal too large for his feet." Darting or "lightening" pains are often complained of. Or there may be hyperesthesia, so that a mere pinching of the skin gives rise to great pain; or, it might be, the patient is unable to bear the contact of the seam of a dress against the skin on account of the suffering it causes. Not infrequently there is deep-seated pain, located, as the pain describes it, in the marrow of the bones, which are tender on being grasped; and I have noticed that these pains are generally worse at night. With this there is the usual loss or impairment of the patellar tendon reflex.

CLASSIFICATION

There are several diabetic neuropathies. The most commonly used classification is based on the clinical presentation. Because the understanding of the etiology and pathophysiology of the diabetic peripheral neuropathies is incomplete, current classifications are based primarily on clinical manifestations. Many patients do not manifest a single type of diabetic neuropathy but rather a mixture of neuropathic features often dominated by one or another subtype.

Historical classifications begin with Leyden (4) who described hyperesthetic, paralytic, and ataxic forms of neuropathy. Jordan (5), on the basis of observations of patients treated at the Joslin Clinic, recognized three types of neuropathy: (a) a "hyperglycemic" type dominated by sensory symptoms, without neurologic signs, that was usually reversed by treatment of diabetes; (b) a chronic "circulatory-degenerative" type with advanced sensory, motor, and reflex abnormalities associated with arterial insufficiency of the legs; and (c) a "neuritic" type characterized by more-acute neuropathic symptoms and signs. In a similar classification Treusch (6) described (a) diabetes with pain in which control of diabetes improved symptoms, (b) ischemic neuropathy, (c) diabetic polyneuritis, and (d) visceral neuritis. Goodman et al. (7) listed (a) function neuropathy with uncontrolled diabetes without neurologic deficit, (b) organic neuropathy with neurologic signs and, (c) posttreatment neuropathy. These classifications all have the disadvantage of mixing clinical and uncertain pathophysiologic criteria. Locke (8) proposed a simpler anatomic classification system in which lesions of nerve roots produce radiculopathy; lesions of mixed nerves produce *polyneuropathy*.

More recent classifications continue to emphasize topographic body distribution (9) and are summarized by Dyck's classification (10) into (a) symmetric distal polyneuropathy with sensory, or sensorimotor motor involvement; (b) symmetric proximal lower limb neuropathy; (c) asymmetric focal neuropathy including cranial, truncal, limb plexus, multifocal entrapment, and ischemic neuropathies; (d) asymmetric neuropathy combined with symmetric distal polyneuropathy; and (e) mixed forms.

Perhaps the simplest and most widely used classification was initially proposed by Thomas (11). This approach divides the diabetic neuropathies into diffuse, generalized, or symmetric polyneuropathies (sensory, motor, and autonomic) and focal neuropathies (mononeuropathy, mononeuropathy multiplex, plexopathy, radiculopathy, and cranial neuropathy). A modification of this classification is shown in Table 56.1.

TABLE 56.1. Classification of Diabetic Neuropathy

A. Symmetric neuropathies
  1. Distal symmetric sensorimotor polyneuropathy
  2. Autonomic neuropathy
  3. Acute painful neuropathy
  4. Hyperglycemic neuropathy
  5. Treatment-induced neuropathy
  6. Symmetric proximal lower extremity neuropathy
B. Focal and multifocal neuropathy
  1. Cranial neuropathy
  2. Thoracoabdominal neuropathy
  3. Focal limb neuropathy
  4. Diabetic amyotrophy

SYMMETRIC NEUROPATHIES

Generalized Polyneuropathy

EPIDEMIOLOGY

Predominately sensory or sensorimotor distal polyneuropathy is the most common of the diabetic neuropathies. Epidemiologic studies suggest that the prevalence of diabetic peripheral neuropathy ranges from 5% to 100%. This large range is in part a consequence of variations in the study population, patient selection, the diagnostic criteria for the diagnosis of diabetes, the sensitivity of methods used to detect peripheral neuropathy, and the duration of diabetes in the study cohort. Diabetic peripheral neuropathy is more prevalent in tertiary care centers and diabetes clinic populations, where patients are more likely to have complications than are patients in the community. Similarly, prevalence is typically higher if ascertainment is based on electrophysiologic measurements, autonomic testing, or quantitative sensory testing and lower if it is based on subjective symptoms and physical findings. The prevalence of neuropathy also increases with age and increasing duration of diabetes.

In a large population-based epidemiologic study, Pirart (12) followed a cohort of 4,400 patients from 1947 to 1978 and, using clinical criteria, found evidence of neuropathy in 7.5% of patients at the time of diagnosis. The prevalence of neuropathy increased to 50% after 25 years of follow-up. In a controlled, longitudinal study of 132 patients with type 2 diabetes, Partenen et al. (13) documented the progression of polyneuropathy diagnosed using clinical criteria (pain and paresthesias) and electrodiagnostic studies. The prevalence of nerve-conduction abnormalities in the legs and feet increased from 8.3% at baseline to 16.7% after 5 years and to 41.9% after 10 years. The decline in sensory and motor action potential amplitudes was more prominent than the slowing of nerve-conduction velocity. After 10 years, more than 40% of patients no longer had ankle reflexes and 20% had vibration loss.

Several cross-sectional studies have examined the prevalence of diabetic polyneuropathy. In the Rochester diabetic neuropathy cohort, the prevalence was 54% in patients with type 1 diabetes and 45% in patients with type 2 diabetes (14). In the EURODIAB IDDM Complications Study, the prevalence of peripheral neuropathy in 3,250 randomly selected patients with insulin-dependent diabetic was 28% (15). Similar prevalences were reported in the Pittsburgh Epidemiology of Diabetes Complications Study (16), the multicenter, diabetic clinic-based study on the prevalence of diabetic neuropathy in Italy (17), and in a multicenter study of diabetic patients in the United Kingdom who were attending hospital-based diabetic clinics (18).

RISK FACTORS

Hyperglycemia is now well established as a risk factor in both patients with type 1 diabetes (19,20) and patients with type 2 diabetes (13). Other correlates and associations include age, duration of diabetes, quality of metabolic control, height, the presence of background or proliferative diabetic retinopathy, cigarette smoking, high-density lipoprotein cholesterol, and the presence of cardiovascular disease (15,16,18,21).

CLINICAL FEATURES

Numbness and paresthesia begin in the toes and gradually and insidiously ascend to involve the feet and lower legs. Sensory deficit usually occurs symmetrically in the distal territory of overlapping nerves, but not infrequently, asymmetric patterns of sensory loss in root or nerve distribution may be superimposed on this distal symmetric pattern of sensory loss. Because the distal portion of longer nerves are affected first, the feet and lower legs are involved before the hands, producing the typical "stocking-and-glove" pattern of sensory deficit. In most patients, the symptoms of polyneuropathy are mild and consist of numbness or paresthesia of the toes and sensory disturbances often described as "like walking on pebbles" or "having cotton bunched up under the toes." In some patients, "positive" symptoms are present. These include superficial burning, paresthesia, deep aching pains, dysesthesia, contact-induced discomfort, and paroxysmal jabbing pains. These symptoms are typically more severe at night. In more severe cases, distal portions of thoracic intercostal nerves are affected, producing an asymptomatic midline sensory loss in a teardrop distribution over the anterior thorax and abdomen that gradually spreads laterally (22). A similar pattern of deficits that gradually increase in size may occur on the vertex of the scalp and the central aspect of the face. This thoracic and abdominal sensory loss differs from focal thoracic truncal radiculopathy (23–25) in that it manifests as a painless, bilateral, symmetrical, and persistent form of neuropathy. Impaired touch and two-point discrimination in the fingertips may interfere with the reading of Braille (26). Sensory symptoms and signs are commonly accompanied by mild distal weakness and features of autonomic neuropathy.

Both lightly myelinated and unmyelinated small nerve fibers and the myelinated large nerve fibers are affected (Table 56.2). Dysfunction of small and large fibers occurs in varying combinations; however, in most cases the earliest deficits involve the small nerve fibers. Features characteristic of a small-fiber peripheral neuropathy include deficits in pain and temperature perception, paresthesias and dysesthesias, pain, deficits in the perception of visceral pain, dysautonomia, and predisposition to foot ulceration. Proprioception and deep tendon reflexes are relatively preserved. Nerve-conduction studies may be normal or minimally abnormal when small-fiber features dominate since these measurements are dependent on conduction in the surviving large, myelinated nerve fibers. This presentation, which resembles the dissociated sensory deficits that accompany as syrinx, has been described as pseudosyringomyelic. In contrast, features characteristic of large-fiber

TABLE 56.2. Features of Small- and Large-Fiber Neuropathy

Small-fiber dysfunction	Large-fiber dysfunction
Burning or lancinating pain	Loss of position and vibration sensation
Hyperesthesia	Areflexia
Paresthesia	Nerve-conduction abnormalities
Loss of pain and temperature sensation	
Dysautonomia	
Foot ulceration	
Loss of visceral pain	

peripheral neuropathy include loss of position and vibration perception sense and loss of deep-tendon reflexes. Nerve-conduction studies are usually abnormal. This presentation, which has features in common with the pattern of deficits that are associated with tabes dorsalis, has been termed pseudotabetic.

Marked distal muscle weakness with sparing of sensation occasionally occurs but often is due to mononeuropathy multiplex involving the peroneal or ulnar nerves. A pure or predominant motor polyneuropathy with few or no sensory symptoms or signs is rarely due to diabetes and should trigger a search for alternative causes of weakness, such as motor neuron disease, primary muscle disease, spinal cord disease, or other potentially treatable causes of peripheral neuropathy, such as chronic inflammatory demyelinating polyneuropathy (27). Once established, sensory and sensorimotor distal neuropathy is a permanent condition; although the course of painful manifestations is highly variable: It may last for months to years and may be exacerbated by intercurrent illness, infection, and depression. In one report, 36 patients with pain for at least 12 months showed no significant change in symptoms over a mean follow-up period of 4.7 years (28).

Although selected large-fiber neuropathies might be expected to cause muscle weakness, painless loss of vibration and position sense, and impaired tendon reflexes, pathologic (29,30), clinical (31), and quantitative sensory studies (32) have not demonstrated pure loss of large fibers in diabetic peripheral neuropathy (33). However, patients with disproportionate large-fiber involvement may manifest muscle weakness, atrophy of the intrinsic foot muscles, and weakness of the extensors and flexors of the toes and ankles with foot drop. When these deficits are combined with proprioceptive deficit in the toes and feet, a "pseudotabetic" gait ataxia may result. Neuropathy of this severity often coexists with diabetic retinopathy and neuropathy.

FOOT ULCERATION

Foot ulceration and neuropathic arthropathy are two of the more dreaded neurologic complications of diabetic neuropathy. Foot ulcers usually occur in patients with either small- or large-fiber neuropathy. Painless ulcers in weight-bearing areas occur on a background of insensitivity to pain, impaired proprioception, atrophy of intrinsic foot muscles, and the consequent maldistribution of weight-bearing, disturbed sweating, impaired capillary blood flow caused by autonomic neuropathy, and noninflammatory edema. Deformity of the foot due to muscle weakness and atrophy produces a maldistribution of weight-bearing and results in callus formation (34–37). The importance of a careful neurologic examination with careful attention to foot sensation cannot be overemphasized (38). The foot that is at risk for ulceration may be determined simply using the Semmes–Weinstein monofilaments (39).

Neuropathic arthropathy (Charcot joint or diabetic osteoarthropathy) is a rarer complication. This occurs primarily in the metatarsophalangeal and metatarsal–tarsal joints and is believed to be due to a combination of impaired deep pain, proprioceptive sensibility, and autonomic neuropathy. A good blood supply appears critical to the development of this complication (40). Trauma, even of a minor nature, or foot surgery may precipitate a Charcot joint. In addition, recurrent trauma may cause pathologic fractures of metatarsal bones with progressive external rotation and eversion deformities of the foot (35,41).

Acute Painful Neuropathy

Acute painful neuropathy (42) is a variant of sensory polyneuropathy in which severe burning pain of the extremities is combined with deep aching pain in proximal muscles, jabs of pain radiating from the feet to the legs, and striking hypersensitivity or allodynia of the extremities and trunk to touch, clothing, or bed sheets that is often likened to sunburn. Objective sensory deficit is surprisingly mild in comparison with the painful paresthesia and dysesthesia. Nerve-conduction velocities are frequently normal or minimally abnormal.

Anorexia, weight loss, and depression are often so prominent that the term "diabetic neuropathic cachexia" as coined by Ellenberg (43) to describe this syndrome. This syndrome often correlates poorly with severity of diabetes or presence of other diabetic microangiopathic complications. Prognosis may be good in some patients, with gradual recovery over a period of months (42), particularly if the onset of symptoms follows a metabolic disturbance (44). The condition appears more commonly in males (45). Recurrent episodes may occur infrequently (46).

Treatment-Induced Neuropathy

Sensory neuropathy sometimes appears for the first time coincident with treatment with insulin or oral hypoglycemic agents (47,48) and has been referred to as a treatment-induced neuropathy (49). Although the cause is unknown, it has been suggested that improved glycemic control may initiate regenerating axonal sprouts, which generate ectopic nerve impulses (49). Alternately, it has been proposed that the pain is due to changes in the epineurial vasculature, such as arterial attenuation and tortuosity, arteriovenous shunting, and neovascular proliferation (50). There is usually gradual improvement as treatment continues and glycemic control is maintained.

Hyperglycemic Neuropathy

"Hyperglycemic" neuropathy refers to widespread paresthesias of the extremities and trunk that occasionally occur in patients with newly diagnosed or poorly controlled diabetes and that rapidly improve with control of hyperglycemia. The unique reversibility of this form of neuropathy and the diffuse rather than distal distribution of paresthesias suggest a pathophysiologic basis different from that for later-appearing diabetic sensory neuropathy. In an experimental model of diabetes, acute hyperosmolar hyperglycemia was associated with reduced nerve-conduction velocity and axon shrinkage (51).

Chronic Inflammatory Demyelinating Polyneuropathy

Several investigators have drawn attention to the association between chronic inflammatory demyelinating polyneuropathy (CIDP) and diabetes. The typical presentation of patients with superimposed CIDP includes symmetric weakness with demyelination and conduction block on electromyography and demyelination on nerve biopsy. The clinical progression is characteristically more rapid than that of diabetic polyneuropathy, weakness may be more prominent and there is often a satisfactory clinical response to immune modulation (51a–51d).

The differentiation from patients with diabetic polyneuropathy is not easily accomplished owing to several features in common. An elevated cerebrospinal fluid protein is present in both conditions, as are demyelinating changes on nerve conduction studies. The presence of conduction block on nerve conduction studies, however, is more suggestive of CIDP. The prevalence of conduction block appears similar in CIDP patients with and without diabetes mellitus (51b).

The characteristic nerve biopsy in both CIDP and diabetic polyneuropathy shows axonal and demyelinating changes (51a,51e). While a prominent inflammatory infiltrate on nerve biopsy may indicate CIDP, inflammation is only rarely seen in CIDP, and, furthermore, inflammation may also be present on nerve biopsies of patients with a generalized diabetic peripheral neuropathy (51f,51g).

ASYMMETRIC NEUROPATHIES

Cranial Neuropathy

Cranial neuropathies also belong to the category of mononeuropathies. The majority of diabetic cranial neuropathies affect the third and sixth cranial nerves (52,53), whereas the fourth cranial nerve is rarely affected alone (52). Onset of diplopia is followed by complete ophthalmoplegia within several days. In cases of third-nerve involvement, there may be complete ptosis but the pupil is typically spared. Weakness involves all extraocular muscles except the lateral rectus and superior oblique muscles. The pain, which is characteristically in the frontal and periorbital region, accompanies ophthalmoplegia in about 50% of cases. Unlike painful ophthalmoplegia associated with temporal arteritis (54), eye muscle weakness occurs in a specific nerve distribution rather than from ischemic muscle involvement. The suggestion that pain may be due to involvement of the first and second divisions of the trigeminal nerve in the cavernous sinus is supported by the occasional presence of sensory impairment in the distribution of the trigeminal nerve (52). However, a more likely explanation is that pain originates from ischemia or pain-sensitive terminals in the sheath of the third nerve (55). Differentiation from a neoplastic or vascular lesion in the orbital fissure, cavernous sinus, infarction at the base of the brain, or focal midbrain infarction (56) should be made with brain imaging studies such as magnetic resonance imaging (MRI). Sparing of the pupil may be a consequence of the relatively intact peripherally located pupillomotor fibers supplied by cavernous sinus blood and spared by the centrally placed nerve lesion. However, compressive lesions of the third nerve within the cavernous sinus also may spare the pupil (57) and should be excluded by brain imaging studies. Recovery without residual weakness always occurs and is usually complete within 3 months, supporting the notion that focal demyelination without axonal destruction is the responsible lesion (58).

Convincing evidence that other cranial nerve palsies occur with increased frequency in diabetes is lacking. In one uncontrolled study, impaired olfaction was reported in 35 of 58 patients with diabetes who showed no evidence of abnormalities of the nasal mucosa (59).

Optic disc edema indistinguishable in appearance from papilledema with associated hemorrhages of the nerve fiber layer and cotton-wool spots has been described in juvenile-onset diabetes (60,61). This usually is associated with only mild impairment in visual acuity and a favorable prognosis. This condition is of obscure etiology but is believed to be due to vasculopathy of the most superficial capillary layer of the disc and adjacent retina (60,61). Anterior ischemic optic neuropathy may occur in diabetes but is more closely associated with hypertension. This is an ischemic infarction of the anterior optic nerve that produces acute edema of the optic disc, profound visual loss, and subsequent development of optic atrophy. Optic atrophy and nerve deafness are associated with diabetes in Wolfram syndrome.

Facial paralysis due to seventh nerve palsy may occur with increased frequency in patients with diabetes (62), and the prognosis for recovery may be worse than in patients without diabetes (63). In view of the high frequency of this neuropathy in the general population, its designation as a diabetic mononeuropathy remains uncertain.

Proximal Motor Neuropathy

Diabetic amyotrophy was originally described by Bruns (64) in 1890 and again by Garland and Taverner (65) in 1953 as *diabetic myelopathy*. Because clinical and pathologic evidence for spinal cord involvement was not forthcoming, this syndrome was subsequently designated *diabetic amyotrophy* (66), a deliberately noncommittal term with regard to localization of the disease process. An array of terms have subsequently been used for this syndrome, including *femoral neuropathy* (67,68), *asymmetric motor neuropathy* (69), *subacute proximal diabetic neuropathy* (70, 71), *proximal mononeuropathy multiplex* (72), *diabetic polyradiculopathy* (73), and *diabetic lumbosacral radiculoplexus neuropathy* (74). Asbury (75) has recommended that the term *diabetic amyotrophy* be dropped because of its ambiguity and that the term *proximal motor neuropathy* be used instead.

This neuropathy typically occurs with a peak incidence in the fifth or sixth decade in patients with type 2 diabetes. Many patients have mild or unrecognized diabetes at the time of diagnosis. In a recent series, diabetic amyotrophy was the presenting manifestation of diabetes in one third of the subjects (76). Some authors have emphasized an association with poor glycemic control (66,77,78).

The clinical picture is one of acute or subacute pain, weakness, and atrophy of the pelvic girdle and thigh musculature. The iliopsoas and quadriceps are usually involved, producing weakness of hip flexion and knee stabilization within several weeks of onset of pain. As a result, buckling of the knee and difficulty climbing stairs are typical symptoms. In some cases, coexistent weakness of the glutei, hamstrings, thigh adductors, and, less commonly, the peroneal and tibial muscles is present, indicative of the more widespread distribution of the disorder. Symptoms may have a monophasic or stepwise progression (77,79–83). Symptoms begin unilaterally but extend to the opposite extremity within weeks or months (74). Most patients have weight loss, and some appear cachectic. The extent of the weight loss highlights the systemic nature of the disorder. The weight loss may be compounded by anorexia caused by reactive depression or the use of narcotic analgesics.

Despite its designation as a motor neuropathy, subtle sensory symptoms and signs are commonly present in the form of paresthesias and sensory disturbance in the anterior thigh and anteromedial aspects of the lower leg typically in the anterior femoral cutaneous and saphenous nerve distribution. The knee jerk is nearly always reduced or absent on the affected side, whereas ankle jerks may be preserved unless compromised by a coexistent distal polyneuropathy.

Deep, aching pain is prominent and is localized to the hip, buttock, and anterior thigh. Pain is unrelieved by rest, is typically worse at night than during the day, and is not increased with straight leg raising or other mechanical maneuvers. The process is typically unilateral in onset, but subsequent involvement of the opposite leg often occurs within 3 to 4 months.

Despite early reports to the contrary (66), signs of myelopathy are absent and plantar responses are usually flexor. Pain, sensory abnormalities, and weakness in thoracic root distribution occasionally occur concomitantly (25), but isolated shoulder-girdle involvement is distinctly uncommon (73) and, when present, usually occurs in patients with marked leg weakness (70,78,79).

Differentiation from compressive lumbar nerve-root disease and neoplastic infiltration of lumbosacral plexus may be difficult, and laminectomies and laparotomies have occasionally been carried out in such patients in search of a structural cause. As originally pointed out by Root and Rogers (84), and more recently discussed by Hirsh (85), the absence of mechanical signs and symptoms, lack of back pain, prominent nocturnal pain with failure to respond to bed rest, and muscular atrophy and weakness involving more than one lumbar root usually distinguishes proximal motor neuropathy from nerve-root compression.

The prognosis is usually good, with most patients showing resolution of pain followed later by gradual return of strength over a period of 6 to 18 months (73,77,78). Patients with unilateral and relatively focal pain and weakness seem to improve more rapidly and completely than patients with more widespread involvement. Because of the severe pain and disability associated with this syndrome, the ability to reassure affected patients of a favorable prognosis provides them great psychological relief.

There has been considerable debate concerning the etiology and proper classification of proximal motor neuropathy (75). Subramony and Wilbourn (86) have emphasized the heterogenicity of the syndrome, in that some patients with proximal motor neuropathy have clinical and electromyographic evidence of distal polyneuropathy whereas others appear to have a more localized process. The finding of slow nerve-conduction velocities in femoral and distal nerves (81,86–89) and of features of demyelination in nerve biopsy specimens in these patients indicates that "diabetic amyotrophy" is a form of diabetic neuropathy with a predilection for proximal nerves rather than a primary disorder of anterior horn cells of muscle. On the basis of extensive clinical electrophysiologic experiences, Bastron and Thomas (73) at the Mayo Clinic concluded that the disorder is a polyradiculopathy. Electromyography of patients with diabetic amyotrophy characteristically displays abundant fibrillations in the affected limb muscles and the paraspinal muscles. Nerve-conduction studies are unable to differentiate patients with diabetic amyotrophy from those with a generalized polyneuropathy.

Recent studies have emphasized the likelihood that this disorder has a vascular basis (90,91). A vascular etiology was first proposed for the more acute case of diabetic amyotrophy by Raff and Asbury (72,75), who documented occlusion of intrafascicular artery of the obturator nerve and numerous small-vessel infarcts in the lumbosacral plexus and proximal nerve trunks of the patient who exhibited the rapid appearance of painful proximal asymmetric leg weakness.

The possibility that this disorder has an inflammatory etiology has led to the use of immune-modulating therapies. Intravenous immunoglobulins, plasmapheresis, and corticosteroids have all been used in open-label, uncontrolled studies (71,90,92). While preliminary results suggest some clinical benefit, the need for blinded, placebo-controlled trials is highlighted by the patient of Said et al. (91), who had a spontaneous remission shortly after biopsy and prior to the initiation of corticosteroid therapy (92a).

Thoracic Radiculopathy

This entity, also known as thoracoabdominal neuropathy, did not gain attention in the English-language literature until the late 1970s (23,24). Similar to painful proximal motor neuropathies of the legs, this disorder usually occurs in middle-aged patients and often in those who have relatively mild diabetes. In many cases, patients with this syndrome have had previous or concomitant painful lumbar root syndromes in the lower extremities.

Onset of pain is usually acute, and the pain may be located in the back, chest, or abdomen. The character of the pain resembles that of herpes zoster and is usually deep and aching with some elements of superficial sharp or burning pain. Changes in pain with alterations of position or physical activity are variable. Paresthesia and cutaneous hypersensitivity are usually present but may be mild or absent, sometimes resulting in failure to recognize the neuropathic basis for pain. The pain is usually unilateral but is sometimes bilateral, may be distributed over more than one dermatomal segment, and often does not have a classic girdling radicular distribution. There may be an accompanying area of sensory loss or dysesthesia in the distribution of one or more adjacent intercostal nerves, the dorsal or ventral rami, or their branches (93). Impairment in light touch and hypersensitivity to pin stimulation, however, are often absent. In severe cases, weakness and laxity of segmental paraspinal and abdominal muscles are present and abdominal hernia may even occur (94,95). Electromyography of paraspinal, intercostal, and abdominal muscles is diagnostically helpful and usually shows changes of acute denervation (24,25,96,97). As with proximal lower-extremity motor neuropathy, weight loss may be prominent, and because of the frequent absence of definite neuropathic symptoms and signs, exhaustive, unfruitful searches for an intrathoracic or intraabdominal neoplasm often are undertaken. The finding of electromyographic abnormalities usually leads to the correct diagnosis. Cases in which the distribution of symptoms and signs conforms to a single thoracic root should be evaluated with x-ray and MRI studies of the thoracic spine to exclude a compressive radiculopathy. The prognosis is usually better for the lower extremity radiculopathies, with a gradual recovery within a matter of months to a year (23).

Similar to other diabetic mononeuropathies and radiculopathies, the etiology of thoracic radiculopathy is obscure, although the acute onset and spontaneous recovery suggest a focal ischemic process. The observation that thoracic radiculopathy, proximal asymmetric motor neuropathy, and cranial mononeuropathy occur among middle-aged patients with type 2 diabetes, often appear in the same patient, improve spontaneously, and have a tendency to recur suggests a common physiologic mechanism. Although no pathologic studies of patients with thoracic radiculopathy have been published, postmortem studies of patients with diabetic polyneuropathy do show axonal and demyelinative lesions of nerve roots (81,98). Skin biopsies of patients with thoracic radiculopathy have shown a marked reduction in dermal and epidermal nerve fibers in the affected dermatome (98a).

Limb Mononeuropathy

Mononeuropathy is particularly common in persons with diabetes and may occur on the basis of focal ischemia, entrapment, compression, or trauma to superficially placed nerves (99). Any of the major peripheral nerves may be affected. Symptoms may present suddenly or gradually. When several nerves are involved simultaneously, the disorder is referred to as mononeuropathy multiplex. Many patients with diabetic polyneuropathy have electrophysiologic or clinical evidence of superimposed focal mononeuropathy at various common sites of entrapment or nerve injury, such as the median nerve at the wrist, ulnar nerve at the elbow, peroneal nerve at the fibular head, radial nerve above the elbow, and lateral cutaneous nerve of the thigh (99). This may be because nerves affected by segmental demyelination are known to be particularly sensitive to the effects of compression and anoxia. Differential diagnosis of mononeuropathy or mononeuropathy multiplex include vasculitis, paraproteinemic neuropathy, amyloidosis, acromegaly, hypothyroidism, sarcoidosis, Lyme disease, and bleeding into peripheral nerves caused by coagulation defects.

Carpal tunnel syndrome caused by median-nerve entrapment in the wrist is particularly common among persons with diabetes. A recent study report neurophysiologic evidence consistent with a carpal tunnel syndrome in 23% of patients with mild diabetic neuropathy. The carpal tunnel syndrome usually produces symptoms and signs similar to those in persons without diabetes. Occasionally, however, distal median-nerve mononeuropathy may occur in the absence of the usual pain and sensory symptoms of carpal tunnel syndrome. Although entrapment is still possible in such cases, coexistent distal ulnar neuropathy and bilateral involvement may suggest distal polyneuropathy rather than nerve entrapment (100). Nerve-conduction studies showing prolonged distal latencies in multiple nerves rather than limited to the median nerve will serve to distinguish distal polyneuropathy from entrapment.

Peroneal mononeuropathy typically produces sudden painless foot drop and, in addition to vascular factors, may be due to trauma because of the superficial location of the nerve at the fibular head. Ulnar mononeuropathy is probably also related to the vulnerable position of the nerve at the elbow. In this case, symptoms usually appear insidiously and may be due to chronic trauma rather than to acute injury or entrapment. Phrenic neuropathy, resulting in diaphragmatic paralysis, may occur rarely in patients with diabetes (101).

PATHOLOGY OF PERIPHERAL NEUROPATHY

Pathogenesis of Symmetric Neuropathies

The pathophysiologic basis of diabetic distal polyneuropathy remains uncertain. The two major prevailing theories relate the metabolic effects of chronic hyperglycemia and the effects of ischemia on peripheral nerves to the pathogenesis of this disorder (102,103). Alterations in neurotrophic factors and immunologic mechanisms also may play a pathogenetic role. It is likely that multiple interacting factors play a role in the pathogenesis of this disorder.

METABOLIC

The metabolic hypothesis proposes that hyperglycemia produces several metabolic derangements, including increased tissue levels of sorbitol and fructose (104,105), decreased concentrations of nerve *myo*-inositol and taurine (106), decreased Na^+/K^+ adenosine triphosphatase (ATPase) activity (104,105), nonenzymatic glycosylation of proteins, altered fatty acid metabolism, and abnormalities of axonal flow. Some or all of these factors may be responsible for functional and structural changes in nerve fibers.

Polyol Pathway Abnormalities

The polyol pathway may play a role in several of these metabolic changes. The hyperglycemic milieu results in activation of the polyol pathway and, in a reaction catalyzed by the enzymes aldose reductase and sorbitol dehydrogenase, leads to the conversion of glucose to the polyol sugars sorbitol and fructose. The accumulation of sorbitol results in reduced intracellular levels of *myo*-inositol and taurine, which in turn reduce Na^+/K^+ ATPase and contribute to the structural and functional changes (104).

Decreased levels of intracellular *myo*-inositol lead to reduced phosphoinositide synthesis and decreased production of diacylglycerol. This in turn impairs protein kinase C activation and may lead to decreased Na^+/K^+ ATPase activity. Impaired Na^+/K^+ ATPase activity results in abnormal decreased nodal Na^+ membrane potentials, increased intraaxonal Na^+, and possible nodal swelling and other structural change. Activation of the polyol pathway also may promote oxidative stress by depleting NADPH, a cofactor for both aldose reductase and glutathione reductase, which leads to a decrease in reduced glutathione and increase in oxidized glutathione (104).

Endoneurial concentrations of sorbitol and fructose are increased in the alloxan and streptozotocin model of diabetes. Aldose reductase inhibition reduces endoneurial sorbitol and restores Na^+/K^+ ATPase activity and *myo*-inositol and taurine levels in somatic and autonomic nerves (106,107). Treatment with aldose reductase inhibitors also leads to improved nerve-conduction velocities in these diabetic rat models.

These metabolic abnormalities may not perfectly replicate human diabetic neuropathy. While sorbitol levels are elevated in nerve biopsy specimens (and appear to be associated with loss of myelinated fibers), a concomitant decrease in *myo*-inositol levels has not been demonstrated (108,109).

Myo-*Inositol*

Myo-inositol and inositol levels are reduced within the peripheral nerve in the streptozotocin model of diabetes. Dietary supplementation with *myo*-inositol reverses the slowing of nerve-conduction velocity and reduction in intracellular Na^+/K^+ ATPase that occurs in this experimental model of diabetic peripheral neuropathy (104,110). This, however, has not been replicated in human diabetic peripheral neuropathy. As noted above, a reduction in endoneurial *myo*-inositol is not apparent in human diabetic nerves (108,109,111).

Taurine

Osmoregulation, in order to maintain the intracellular milieu, may also result in endoneurial metabolic changes in diabetic neuropathy. The increase in intracellular osmolality due to shunting of glucose into the polyol pathway and the consequent accumulation of sorbitol may lead to compensatory depletion of the endoneurial osmolytes taurine and *myo*-inositol to maintain osmotic balance (106).

Abnormal Lipid Metabolism

Diabetes also results in alterations in the metabolism of essential fatty acids and prostaglandin. Hyperglycemia leads to inhibition of δ-6-desaturase, the enzyme that converts dietary linoleic acid to γ-linolenic acid. γ-Linolenic acid is a precursor of arachidonic acid that provides the substrate for several vasoactive prostanoids, including prostacyclin. In addition, γ-linolenic acid metabolites play a role in the nerve membrane structure, nerve blood flow, and nerve conduction (112).

Several studies in streptozotocin-diabetic rats have revealed that the deficits in nerve conduction can be reversed by a dietary supplement of evening primrose (113,114). This effect was attenuated by the cyclooxygenase inhibition with flurbiprofen (115).

Oxidative Stress

Oxidative stress also is implicated in the etiology of diabetic neuropathy. There is evidence that activity of oxygen-free radicals is enhanced in diabetes. Indices of increased oxidative stress such as malondialdehyde, conjugated dienes, and lipid hydroperoxides are increased in experimental diabetic neuropathy.

Furthermore, diabetes compromises antioxidant defense mechanisms. There are documented reductions in scavengers of oxygen free radicals, such as reduced glutathione, superoxide dismutase, catalase, ascorbic acid, and α-tocopherol (116).

Antioxidant therapy with a number of agents, including probuchol (117), vitamin E (117,118), glutathione (119), carvedilol (120), butylated hydroxytoluene (121), transitional metal chelating agents (122), and α-lipoic acid (123), have improved measures of nerve function in experimental diabetic peripheral neuropathy.

Advanced Glycosylation End Products

The reducing sugars glucose, fructose, and galactose react with the free amino groups of proteins to form early reversible Schiff bases and Amadori products. These in turn undergo a chemical rearrangement to form advanced glycosylation end products. In the setting of prolonged hyperglycemia, nonenzymatic glycosylation of proteins occurs, which results in structural changes to the components of the extracellular matrix (124,125).

These structural changes may lead to functional neural and vascular abnormalities. Advanced glycosylated end products also may quench nitric oxide, thereby attenuating endothelium-mediated vasodilatation (126). Aminoguanidine may inhibit the formation of advanced glycosylated end products and improve nerve and vascular function (124–128). There have been no reports of human trials with this agent.

Protein Kinase C Activation

Hyperglycemia leads to increased synthesis of diacylglycerol, which leads to activation of protein kinase C. Protein kinase C may also be activated by oxidative stress and advanced glycosylated end products. Protein kinase C activation causes increased vascular permeability, impaired nitric oxide synthesis, and changes in blood flow (129).

There is some evidence that impaired protein kinase C activity may contribute to reduced Na^+/K^+ ATPase activity. Recently data have emerged suggesting that there is increased protein kinase C activity in the retina, kidney, and the vasculature of nerve tissue.

Protein kinase C elevations compromise nerve regeneration in experimental models of diabetic peripheral neuropathy (130,131). In experimental models of diabetes, treatment with nonspecific (132) and β-specific protein kinase C inhibitors normalized the observed neurophysiologic abnormalities (132a).

Poly (ADP-Ribose) Polymerase

There is increasing evidence that poly (ADP-ribose) polymerase (PARP) plays a critical role in mediating several pathways of hyperglycemia-induced damage (activation of PKC isoforms, hexosamine pathway flux, and AGE formation). This most likely occurs by inhibiting GAPDH activity. DNA strand breaks due to oxidative stress are a major cause of PARP activation (132b, 132c). In streptozotocin-induced diabetic rats, the PARP inhibitors, 3-aminobenzamide and 1,5-isoquinolinediol, reversed deficits in nerve blood flow and conduction (132c).

Neurotrophic Factors

The neurotrophins are proteins that promote the growth, maintenance, survival, and differentiation of specific populations of neurons. There is evidence that failure of neurotrophic support is in part responsible for the pathogenesis of diabetic polyneuropathy. Nerve growth factor (NGF), the prototypical growth factor, has been particularly well studied, because it is necessary for the growth maintenance and survival of the sympathetic and small sensory nerve fibers. NGF also regulates the expression of the neuropeptides substance P and calcium gene–related peptides in dorsal root ganglion sensory neurons and sympathetic nerves.

Retrograde axonal transport from the target tissues to the neuronal cell body is impaired in diabetes (133,134). There is evidence of decreased expression of NGF in skin, sympathetic ganglia, and submandibular glands in experimental diabetic neuropathy. This reduction is attenuated or prevented by NGF. When administered to streptozotocin-induced diabetic rats, NGF maintained the response to thermal noxious stimulation (the tail-flick threshold) and prevented the observed reduction in levels of the neuropeptides substance P and calcitonin gene–related peptide measured from cervical dorsal root ganglia (135). Differential dosage effects may be present, as a recent report documented dystrophic changes in the sympathetic ganglia following the administration of NGF in an experimental model of diabetic autonomic neuropathy (136).

Neurotrophin-3 (NT-3) supports the survival and differentiation of large-fiber sensory neurons. Expression of NT-3 may also be reduced in diabetes. Tomlinson and coworkers reported that NT-3 messenger RNA (mRNA) is deficient in leg muscle from diabetic rats (137). Administration of recombinant NT-3 to diabetic rats increased the conduction velocity of sensory nerves. The motor conduction velocity was unaffected (137).

VASCULAR FACTORS

Hyperglycemia-related metabolic alterations produce interposed changes in tissues and the microvasculature that are then responsible for ischemic pathologic changes in nerve fibers. Animal models of diabetic neuropathy have demonstrated that the neuropathy is accompanied by reduced endoneurial blood flow, increased endoneurial vascular resistance, and reduced endoneurial oxygen tension (138,139). Therapy with vasodilators (140,141) or oxygen supplementation (142,143) may improve the conduction-velocity slowing/electrophysiologic and biochemical abnormalities that occur in these experimental models of diabetic neuropathy.

Microangiopathy

Early investigators emphasized macrovascular findings in peripheral nerves and, on the basis of studies of limbs amputated for arteriosclerotic gangrene, attributed the neuropathic changes to arteriosclerotic occlusive disease of the vasa nervorum (143). Fagerberg (145,146) described the presence of material positive for periodic acid–Schiff staining stenosis and hyalinization of intraneural vessels. Other authors have suggested the possible role of microvascular changes in capillary endothelial basement membranes, with thickening of the perivascular space, which is known to be more frequent in diabetic neuropathy than in other acquired neuropathies (147,148). Timperley et al. (149) described endothelial cell hyperplasia in endoneurial blood vessels of the sural nerve, with plugging of the vascular lumen by necrotic cellular material in patients with severe diabetic neuropathy.

Dyck and colleagues (150,151) observed thickening of capillary walls and documented capillary closure and platelet thrombi occlusions in the small arteries and arterioles that supply peripheral nerves that was more pronounced in patients with diabetic neuropathy than in age-matched controls. Malik and colleagues (152,153) also documented basement-membrane thickening, reduced capillary number (152), and endothelial hyperplasia (152,153).

Giannini and Dyck (154,155) recently confirmed the presence of a significant increase in reduplicated basement membranes with pericyte degeneration in diabetic sural nerves that resulted in an increase in mural area. In these studies, the number of endoneurial microvessels per square millimeter and the average luminal area and size distribution of these microvessels were not significantly different in the sural nerves of patients with diabetes mellitus compared with those of control subjects. Intravascular thrombi and vascular occlusions could not be confirmed in these studies. The most consistently reported ultrastructural microvascular abnormalities in diabetic neuropathy are thus basement-membrane thickening and endothelial-cell hyperplasia. Several studies have established a correlation between ultrastructural microvascular disease in peripheral nerve and severity of diabetic neuropathy (151,152,155,156).

Spatial Distribution of Nerve-Fiber Loss

Dyck (157) systematically studied the spatial distribution of pathologic abnormalities along the length of peripheral nerve in a population of diabetic patients and nondiabetic controls (157). In postmortem studies, nerve tissue was obtained from the fifth lumbar roots; segmental nerves in lumbar and sacral plexus; and proximal and distal portions of sciatic, tibial, peroneal, and sural nerves of patients with diabetic neuropathy and control subjects to determine the proximal-to-distal pattern of nerve-fiber damage. The number of myelinated fibers was counted in each level of nerve. In patients with diabetic neuropathy, a pattern of multifocal nerve-fiber loss was found to begin in proximal segmental nerves and to worsen distally. Dorsal roots were more affected than ventral roots.

These findings were felt to correlate best with a multifocal pathologic process of nerve beginning proximally and affecting multiple levels of nerve. Distal worsening of nerve-fiber degeneration was attributed to the cumulative effect of multiple random lesions along the course of the nerve (157). The strong similarity of this pattern of nerve-fiber loss to previously described patterns in necrotizing vasculitis and experimental studies of microsphere embolization (158,159) suggested that ischemia plays an important role in diabetic neuropathy.

Llewelyn and coworkers (160), however, compared the pattern of fiber loss in sural nerve biopsies of patients with type 1 diabetes, patients with hereditary sensory and motor neuropathy, and controls. They noted that a patchy, nonuniform pattern of fiber loss also was present in the biopsies obtained from patients with hereditary neuropathies—disorders unlikely to have a vascular basis, although the extent of the multifocal fiber loss was less than that reported by Dyck and coworkers.

Axonal and Demyelinating Features

At one time considerable debate existed concerning whether segmental demyelination or axonal degeneration is the primary abnormality in diabetic neuropathy. Some investigators (161,162) suggested a primary degeneration of motor and sensory nerve cell bodies with secondary degeneration of peripheral nerve and nerve root axons and centripetal degeneration of the posterior columns in spinal cord. According to this scheme, dysfunction of the nerve cell body causes the initial manifestations to appear at the periphery because of a "dying-back" process that begins distally and spreads proximally (29,163).

Chopra and colleagues (148,164) held that segmental demyelination, presumably the result of a metabolic disturbance of Schwann cell function, was the primary abnormality. Thomas and Lascelles (165), in studies of teased-fiber preparations, emphasized segmental demyelination and remyelination as the main pathologic change but also identified axonal degeneration in severe cases. Said et al. (29), found evidence of both primary and secondary demyelination, whereas Behse et al. (147), finding loss of large and small myelinated fibers and unmyelinated fibers, concluded that axonal degeneration and Schwann cell damage proceed independently of each other. Vital and coworkers (166,167) reported that both axonal degeneration and demyelination were present in nerve biopsy specimens (166,167), whereas Dyck and colleagues confirmed that a reduction in the number of myelinated fibers is the characteristic finding in the diabetic peripheral nerve but is a secondary response to axonal degeneration rather than part of a primary process of demyelination and remyelination (30,151).

Pathogenesis of Asymmetric Neuropathies

On the basis of the careful study of a very small number of cases, the pathologic basis of diabetic mononeuropathy and mononeuropathy multiplex is presumed to be ischemic infarction of nerve. Raff and Asbury (72) described a patient with an acute and rapidly progressive asymmetric neuropathy who was found to have numerous microinfarcts in the proximal portions of the obturator, femoral, sciatic, and tibial nerves. The occurrence of infarcts in bridging interfascicular bundles was similar to the distribution of microinfarcts in other ischemic mononeuropathies (168).

In a more recent study, biopsy of intermediate cutaneous nerve of thigh in ten patients with type 2 diabetes with diabetic amyotrophy revealed the presence of an inflammatory infiltrate in the epineurium, perineurium, and endoneurium. In select cases, vasculitis of the epineurial and perineurial blood vessels has been observed (90,91).

Dyck and Windebank (168a) reported the pathology in distal cutaneous nerves (the majority sural nerves) of 33 patients with a diabetic lumbosacral radiculoplexus neuropathy. Common findings included multifocal fiber loss, perineurial thickening, neovascularization, and abortive regeneration of nerve fibers forming microfasciculi. In addition there was evidence of mural and perivascular inflammation, separation and fragmentation of mural smooth muscle layers of microvessels, and hemosiderin-laden macrophages. The pathologic findings are suggestive of an immune-mediated microvasculitis leading to ischemic injury.

A vascular cause of diabetic ophthalmoplegia is strongly supported by postmortem studies (56,167,168) in which focal swelling together with axonal and demyelinative lesions were identified in the precavernous or cavernous sinus portions of the third nerve. Extensive hyaline thickening of nutrient vessels of the third nerve without vascular occlusion was found in all three cases. Subclinical oculomotor nerve injury may be present in diabetes (171).

Pathogenesis of Diabetic Autonomic Neuropathy

The pathologic basis of diabetic autonomic neuropathy is not completely understood. A number of investigators have identified abnormalities in paravertebral sympathetic ganglia, including neurons distended by lipid-rich material (172–174), vacuolar degeneration of neurons produced by dilation of endoplasmic reticulum (174), and mononuclear cell infiltration of autonomic nerve bundles and ganglia (174). Loss of myelinated nerve fibers has been described in sympathetic communicating rami (175,176), vagus nerves (175,177,178), splanchnic nerves (176), and nerves to the bladder wall (179).

MANAGEMENT OF DIABETIC NEUROPATHY

Treatment of Hyperglycemia

Management of diabetic neuropathy, whether painful or painless, begins with treatment of hyperglycemia. Although the precise relationship between poor diabetic control and peripheral neuropathy is uncertain, there is unequivocal evidence, based on multicenter, randomized, controlled trials, supporting strict control of blood glucose levels in patients with or without diabetic neuropathy (180–186). These conclusions are supported by experimental models of diabetes produced by streptozotocin or alloxan; reductions in nerve conduction velocity occur acutely and can, at least in early stages, be restored by treatment with insulin (187).

It is of historic interest that, as recently as 1986, a review of the existing literature regarding the relationship of the development and severity of neuropathy to glycemic control, conducted by the American Neurological Association Committee on Health Care issues, could not definitively support the concept that rigorous control of blood sugar prevents or ameliorates diabetic peripheral neuropathy (188).

Several uncontrolled retrospective studies had demonstrated that patients with poor diabetic control develop all diabetic complications, including neuropathy, earlier and more severely than do patients with better control (12,189). In addition, severity of hyperglycemia measured by fasting glucose and glycosylated hemoglobin levels in patients with newly diagnosed diabetes was inversely correlated with motor but not conduction velocity (190). Finally, in patients with newly diagnosed diabetes, improvement in blood glucose and glycosylated hemoglobin levels after treatment with oral hypoglycemic agents (191) or insulin (192) was associated with an improvement in motor but not sensory nerve conduction velocities.

In a groundbreaking study, the Diabetes Control and Complications Trial (DCCT) unquestionably established the necessity of meticulous control of hyperglycemia. Two cohorts of patients with type 1 diabetes were studied: a primary prevention group who had diabetes for 1 to 5 years without retinopathy or microalbuminuria and a secondary intervention cohort who had diabetes for 1 to 15 years and mild to moderate nonproliferative retinopathy and an albumin excretion rate less than 200 mg per 24 hours. A total of 1,441 patients were enrolled into the two cohorts at 29 centers between 1983 and 1989. When the study terminated in June 1993, the duration of follow-up ranged from 3 to 9 years (mean, 6.5 years). The subjects were randomized to two treatment arms: conventional therapy and intensive therapy. Conventional therapy was designed to prevent symptoms of hyperglycemia and hypoglycemia with one to two insulin injections per day whereas intensive treatment was designed to maintain blood glucose levels as close as possible to normal range and consisted of three or more insulin injections per day or insulin pump treatment. Within 6 months of enrollment, the mean levels of glycosylated hemoglobin A_{1c} decreased from 9% to 7% and this level of reduction was maintained throughout the trial (180).

In the DCCT, peripheral neuropathy was an exclusion criterion if "sufficiently severe to merit treatment." A confirmed clinical neuropathy (i.e., abnormal history, physical examination, or both confirmed by unequivocally abnormal neurophysiologic studies) was present at baseline in 3.5% of patients in the primary-prevention cohort and in 9.4% of patients in the secondary-intervention cohort. Intensive therapy significantly reduced the development of confirmed clinical neuropathy by 64% in the combined cohorts after 5 years of follow-up; 5% of the intensive-therapy group developed a confirmed clinical neuropathy compared with 13% of the conventional-therapy group. The prevalence of nerve-conduction abnormalities was reduced by 44%; 26% of the intensive-treatment group developed abnormal nerve conductions compared with 46% of the conventional-treatment group. Nerve-conduction velocities remained relatively stable in the intensively treated cohort but decreased significantly in the cohort treated with conventional therapy (19,180,193).

There are also data supporting the benefits of meticulous control of hyperglycemia in type 2 diabetes. A similar, albeit considerably smaller, trial was conducted in Kamamoto, Japan. One hundred ten Japanese patients with type 2 diabetes were randomly assigned to receive multiple or conventional insulin injections. The primary-prevention cohort comprised 55 patients without retinopathy and a urinary albumin excretion rate less than 30 mg per 24 hours, whereas the 55 patients in the secondary-intervention cohort had uncomplicated retinopathy and a urinary albumin excretion rate less than 300 mg per 24 hours. The appearance and the progression of retinopathy, nephropathy, and neuropathy were assessed every 6 months. After 6 years, the intensively treated cohort showed significant improvement in nerve-conduction velocities, whereas the conventionally treated group showed significant deterioration in the median nerve-conduction velocities and vibration threshold. This study relied on surrogate measures of neuropathy; symptoms and quality of life were not evaluated (182).

These studies show that it is feasible to maintaining meticulous control of blood sugars; however, it is not a risk-free endeavor. In the DCCT, 3,788 episodes of hypoglycemia occurred that were severe enough to necessitate assistance. Of these episodes, 1,027 were associated with coma and/or seizure. Hypoglycemia occurred almost twice as frequently in the intensively treated group than in the conventionally treated group (65% vs. 35%). The overall rate of severe hypoglycemia was 61.2 per 100 patient-years in the intensive group versus 18.7 in the conventionally treated group per 100 patient-years, a relative risk of 3.28. The relative risk for coma and/or seizure was 3.02 for intensive therapy.

PANCREATIC TRANSPLANTATION

Pancreatic transplantation in humans and animal models of diabetes restores the euglycemic state and obviates the need for exogenous insulin. In streptozotocin-induced experimental diabetic neuropathy, pancreatic transplantation reverses the nerve-conduction abnormalities and autonomic defects (194,195). Several centers have consistently reported that pancreatic transplantation, in patients with well-established diabetes, improves nerve-conduction velocities, small- and large-fiber sensory thresholds, and measures of somatosensory and autonomic function (196–202). The degree of improvement in these studies has been quite modest. This is most likely due to the severity of the peripheral neuropathy at the time of transplantation.

Treatment of Metabolic Abnormalities

Based on our understanding of the pathogenesis of diabetic peripheral neuropathy, a number of different agents from diverse chemical classes have entered clinical trial. While some of these agents have shown promise in clinical trials, none are yet approved for clinical use.

ALDOSE REDUCTASE INHIBITORS

Specific treatment with aldose reductase inhibitors, which is directed at the presumed pathophysiologic basis of diabetic neuropathy, has been under investigation for a number of years. Alrestatin was the first aldose reductase inhibitor to be used in humans, but it produced equivocal results and a high incidence of adverse reactions (203). Sorbinil, a longer-acting aldose reductase inhibitor, underwent a more thorough clinical investigation. Results in these studies were equivocal, with some studies showing improvement in electrophysiologic and clinical parameters (204–206), whereas others were negative (207–209). Unfortunately, sorbinil was associated with a high frequency of hypersensitivity reactions, with rash, fever, lymphadenopathy, and abnormal liver chemistries occurring in approximately 10% of patients. The aldose reductase inhibitors, zenarestat and tolrestat also cause side effects, while trials with the aldose reductase inhibitors ponalrestat and zopolrestat failed to demonstrate effectiveness (209a).

The optimistic results obtained with aldose reductase inhibitors in preclinical studies have thus not been replicated in large human trials. While this may reflect inadequacies in the animal models of diabetes, several other factors are also likely to play a role in the failure of these clinical trials. As noted above, side effects, insufficient drug potency, and inadequate nerve penetration have limited other trials. It is possible that the trials were too short to demonstrate a difference between active drug and the control group, that the neuropathy had progressed beyond reversibility, or that the study end points did not reflect improvement in nerve structure or function. Trials with this class of agents are still in progress.

MYO-INOSITOL

Myo-inositol is an important component of the phospholipids that make up cell membranes and other cellular structures. The concentration of *myo*-inositol is reduced in peripheral nerves of diabetic animals and is normalized by aldose reductase inhibitors and *myo*-inositol supplementation (210). Improved function in experimental and human diabetic nerves following treatment with aldose reductase inhibitors has been attributed in part to increased *myo*-inositol concentrations. However, despite an earlier report of reduced levels of *myo*-inositol in patients with diabetic neuropathy (211), more recent biochemical and pathologic studies have indicated that the nerve *myo*-inositol concentration is not reduced in diabetic patients with or without neuropathy (108,109,111). Furthermore, in controlled clinical trials, *myo*-inositol supplementation has not appeared to improve the features of diabetic peripheral neuropathy (210).

EVENING PRIMROSE OIL

Human studies, particularly in type 1 diabetes, replicate the deficient conversion of linoleic acid to γ-linolenic acid. There is preliminary evidence, based on small placebo-controlled trials of short duration, that treatment with γ-linolenic acid for 6 to 12 months improves or delays the progression of the clinical and neurophysiologic abnormalities of diabetic peripheral neuropathy. A typical dose of evening primrose oil used in these studies was 6 g, which contains approximately 480 mg of γ-linolenic acid (212–214).

α-LIPOIC ACID

The effects of the antioxidant α-lipoic acid (thioctic acid) were studied in two multicenter, randomized, double-blind placebo-controlled trials. In a 3-week trial, 328 patients with type 2 diabetes who had symptomatic peripheral neuropathy were treated with an intravenous infusion of α-lipoic acid using three doses (1,200 mg, 600 mg, 100 mg) or placebo. There was a symptomatic improvement in patients treated with the two higher doses of α-lipoic acid (215). A meta-analysis of more than 1,000 patients treated for 3 weeks with 600 mg per day, given intravenously, showed decreased symptoms of pain, paresthesias, and numbness (215a). In a placebo-controlled trial, 73 patients with type 2 diabetes with reduced heart-rate variability were randomized to receive a daily oral dosage of 800 mg of α-lipoic acid or placebo for 4 months. The root-mean-square successive difference and spectral power in the low-frequency band improved in the patients treated with α-lipoic acid. Seventeen patients failed to complete the study (216). A large 4-year multicenter trial is currently in progress.

NEUROTROPHINS

NGF is the neurotrophin most widely studied in humans. In a phase 2 trial of recombinant human (rh) NGF in 250 patients with diabetic polyneuropathy, improvements in signs and symptoms were seen after treatment with either 0.1 or 0.3 mg of rhNGF per kilogram administered subcutaneously three times a week for 6 months (217). The occurrence of local injection-site pain in over 90% of subjects receiving NGF may have unblinded this study. In a larger phase 3 trial, 1,019 subjects were randomly assigned to receive either placebo or 0.1 mg of rhNGF per kilogram by subcutaneous injection three times a week for 48 weeks. This trial failed to replicate the findings of the earlier trial. This may be related to the rhNGF manufacturing process, which differed in the two studies (218). There are no reported studies of NT-3 in the treatment of diabetic neuropathy. Insulin growth factor has not been tested in human clinical trials.

PROTEIN KINASE C β INHIBITION

In phase 2 trials, treatment with the specific protein kinase C β inhibitor roboxistaurin (32 and 64 mg) improved symptoms and signs of peripheral neuropathy. Multicenter phase 3 trials are currently in progress.

AUTONOMIC NEUROPATHY

With the arguable exception of pain, the autonomic manifestations of diabetes are responsible for the most troublesome and disabling features of diabetic peripheral neuropathy and result in a significant proportion of the mortality and morbidity associated with the disease. A broad constellation of symptoms occur that affect cardiovascular, urogenital, gastrointestinal, pupillomotor, regulatory, and sudomotor functions. This topic has been covered in detail in a recent review (219). The impairment is usually gradual and progressive, although severe autonomic dysfunction occurs shortly after the diagnosis of type 1 diabetes in rare cases (220). The availability of sensitive, specific, and reproducible noninvasive tests of autonomic function has enhanced our understanding of the prevalence, pathophysiology, and clinical manifestations of this disorder (221). Estimates of the prevalence of diabetic autonomic neuropathy are dependent on the criteria used for diagnosis and the specific population under study. Few studies of diabetic autonomic neuropathy are without referral or selection bias. A community-based population study in Oxford, England, showed a prevalence of autonomic neuropathy, defined by the presence of one or more abnormal heart-rate-variability test results, of 16.7% (222). The prevalence of symptomatic visceral autonomic neuropathy was 5.5% in a population-based study of diabetic patients in Rochester, Minnesota (14). The prevalence of symptoms of autonomic dysfunction and abnormal tests of autonomic nervous system function in diabetic clinic-based populations and tertiary referral centers is considerably higher.

Cardiovascular System

The cardiovascular autonomic neuropathy has diverse manifestations. An increased resting heart rate is observed frequently in diabetic patients; most likely this is due to the vagal cardiac neuropathy that results in unopposed cardiac sympathetic nerve activity. The tachycardia may be followed by a decrease in heart rate and, ultimately, a fixed heart rate due to the progressive dysfunction of the cardiac sympathetic nervous system (223–225).

Orthostatic hypotension, the most incapacitating manifestation of autonomic failure, is a common feature of diabetic cardiovascular autonomic neuropathy. This is a consequence of efferent sympathetic vasomotor denervation that causes reduced vasoconstriction of the splanchnic and other peripheral vascular beds. Diminished cardiac acceleration and cardiac output, particularly in association with exercise, also may play a role in the presentation of this disorder.

Several authors have drawn attention to the association between increased mortality and cardiovascular autonomic dysfunction in patients with diabetes. Estimates of the mortality associated with cardiovascular autonomic neuropathy range from 27% to 56% over 5 to 10 years. There is also an increased frequency of sudden death in patients with autonomic neuropathy. Proposed mechanisms by which the autonomic nervous system may result in sudden death or influence the outcome of patients with diabetes who have cardiovascular disease include absent or altered perception of myocardial ischemia and infarction; deficient hemodynamic response to cardiovascular stresses such as surgery, infection and anesthesia; increased predisposition to cardiac arrhythmias due to QT interval dispersion; and alterations in sympathetic–parasympathetic cardiac innervation balance (197,226–229a).

Urogenital System

Symptoms of bladder dysfunction have been observed in 37% to 50% of patients with diabetes, and physiologic evidence of bladder dysfunction is present in 43% to 87% of patients with type 1 diabetes (230–231). Bladder symptoms associated with autonomic neuropathy include hesitancy, poor stream, increased intervals between micturition, and a sense of inadequate bladder emptying. These symptoms may be followed by urinary retention and overflow incontinence (230,233,238).

Erectile dysfunction is a frequent and disturbing symptom in male diabetic patients. Reported incidence has ranged from 30% to 75% (235–238). Impotence may be the earliest symptom of diabetic autonomic neuropathy, although vascular, hormonal, and psychogenic etiologies, alone or in combination, may also be implicated. Nitric oxide is an important mediator of noncholinergic nonadrenergic corpus cavernosum relaxation (239). *In vivo* studies of isolated corpus cavernosum tissue from men with diabetes have demonstrated functional impairment in autonomic- and endothelial-dependent relaxation of corpus cavernosum smooth muscle (240). Impotence due to autonomic neuropathy progresses gradually but is usually permanent 2 years after onset. Sympathetically mediated ejaculatory failure may precede the appearance of impotence, although impotence can occur with retained ability to ejaculate and experience orgasm. Retrograde ejaculation will occur if the bladder neck fails to close. This function is also controlled by the sympathetic nervous system (241,242). There are few studies of genital autonomic neuropathy in female patients with diabetes (243).

Gastrointestinal System

Autonomic dysfunction occurs throughout the gastrointestinal tract, producing several specific clinical syndromes. Gastric emptying is delayed in 30% to 50% of both patients with type 1 diabetes and patients with type 2 diabetes (243,245). The term "gastroparesis diabeticorum" was first introduced by Kassander (246) to describe the altered gastrointestinal motility in diabetics. Food residue is retained in the stomach as a result of absent or decreased gastric peristalsis compounded by lower intestinal dysmotility (247). Diabetic gastroparesis may manifest as nausea, postprandial vomiting, bloating, abdominal distention and pain, belching, loss of appetite, and early satiety. Many patients, however, are asymptomatic despite impaired gastric motility (245). A gastric splash may be elicited on clinical examination. Gastroparesis is also associated with the development of bezoars (248) and bacterial overgrowth of the stomach and small intestine, esophagitis, gastric ulcers, and gastritis (249). Gastroparesis may impair the establishment of adequate glycemic control by mismatching plasma glucose and insulin levels. The absorption of orally administered drugs may also be affected (246,250). Recent studies have implicated hyperglycemia as a cause of impaired gastric and small intestinal motility during fasting and after food intake.

Diarrhea and other lower gastrointestinal tract symptoms also may occur. Diabetic diarrhea manifests as a profuse, watery, typically nocturnal diarrhea that can last for hours or days and that frequently alternates with constipation. Abdominal discomfort is commonly associated with diabetic diarrhea. The pathogenesis of diabetic diarrhea includes reduced gastrointestinal motility, reduced receptor-mediated fluid absorption, bacterial overgrowth, pancreatic insufficiency, coexistent celiac disease, and abnormalities in the metabolism of bile salts (251–253). Fecal incontinence, due to anal sphincter incompetence or reduced rectal sensation, is another manifestation of diabetic intestinal neuropathy (254,255). Incontinence is often exacerbated by diarrhea.

Sudomotor System

Sudomotor dysfunction is a common feature of diabetic autonomic neuropathy. This generally manifests as anhidrosis of the extremities, which may be accompanied by hyperhidrosis in the trunk. Initially, patients display a loss of thermoregulatory sweating in a glove-and-stocking distribution, which, with progression of autonomic neuropathy, extends from the lower to the upper extremities and to the anterior abdomen, conforming to the length dependency of diabetic neuropathy. This process ultimately may result in global anhidrosis (256).

Hyperhidrosis may also accompany diabetic autonomic neuropathy. Excessive sweating may occur as a compensatory phenomenon involving proximal regions such as the head and trunk that are spared in a dying-back neuropathy. Gustatory sweating, the abnormal production of sweat that appears over the face, head, neck, shoulders and chest after eating even nonspicy foods, is occasionally observed (257). In contrast to truncal hyperhidrosis, which does not occur in response to eating, gustatory hyperhidrosis is not likely to be a compensatory response to anhidrosis (258).

TREATMENT OF AUTONOMIC DYSFUNCTION

Treatment of Orthostatic Hypotension

The removal of potential reversible causes of orthostatic hypotension is the first and most important management step. Medications such as diuretics, antihypertensive agents, antianginal agents, and antidepressants are the most common offending agents.

Numerous agents from diverse pharmacologic groups have been implemented in the treatment of orthostatic hypotension. 9-α-Fluorohydrocortisone (fludrocortisone acetate), a synthetic mineralocorticoid, is the medication of first choice for most patients with orthostatic hypotension. Treatment is initiated with a 0.1-mg tablet and can be increased to 0.5 mg daily. Treatment may unfortunately be limited by supine hypertension. Other side effects include ankle edema, hypokalemia, and, rarely, congestive heart failure. Potassium supplementation usually is required, particularly when higher dosages are used.

A sympathomimetic agent can be added to fludrocortisone acetate should the patient remain symptomatic. The peripherally acting selective α-agonist midodrine, which recently has been approved by the U.S. Food and Drug Administration (FDA) to treat orthostatic hypotension, is the most widely used of these pressors. Patient sensitivity to this agent varies, and the dose should be titrated from 2.5 mg to 10 mg three times a day. Potential side effects of this agent include pilomotor reactions, pruritus, supine hypertension, gastrointestinal complaints, and urinary retention. Other sympathomimetic agents used are ephedrine and pseudoephedrine (259).

Treatment of Gastroparesis Diabeticorum

Frequent small meals and pharmacotherapy are standard treatments for this disorder. The dopamine agonist metoclopramide continues to be the first line of therapy for this gastroparesis. Given in doses ranging from 5 to 20 mg orally, 30 minutes before meals and at bedtime, metoclopramide accelerates gastric emptying and has a central antiemetic action. It also may release acetylcholine from intramural cholinergic neurons or directly stimulate antral muscle (260–262). Domperidone (10 to 20 mg four times a day), a peripheral D_2-receptor antidopaminergic agent, is frequently helpful in the treatment of this disorder (263–267). Erythromycin and related macrolide compounds may have motilin-agonist properties. Intravenous and oral erythromycin (250 mg three times a day) improves gastric emptying time in diabetic patients with gastroparesis (268).

Gastric antisecretory agents such as the H_2 antagonists and proton-pump inhibitors may be used as supplementary agents to treat the symptoms of gastroesophageal reflux. Most patients can be treated with these medical interventions, and placement of a jejunostomy tube is rarely necessary. Patients with severe cases with intractable vomiting may benefit from nasogastric suctioning.

Treatment of Erectile Dysfunction

Medications influencing autonomic function such as psychotropic and antihypertensive agents should be discontinued. Oral therapy with the selective phosphodiesterase 5 inhibitors is now the first-line therapy for male erectile dysfunction. These agents enhance blood flow to the corpora cavernosa with sexual stimulation. The most extensively used of these agents is sildenafil (50 mg) (269). Tadalafil (20 mg) (269a) and vardenafil (20 mg) (269b) are also effective in more than 60% of diabetic patients with erectile dysfunction. Unfortunately, some men with diabetes do not respond satisfactorily to this intervention. Furthermore, the medication is contraindicated in patients treated with nitrates and agents that compete with or inhibit the cytochrome P450 system. Angina, hypertension requiring treatment with multiple medications, and congestive heart failure are also contraindications (270,271). Other therapies include the injection of vasoactive substances such as papaverine, phentolamine, and prostaglandin E_1 into the corpus cavernosum; transurethral delivery of vasoactive agents (272–276); and the use of mechanical devices such as the vacuum erection device or constricting rings (277). Penile prosthetic implants may be used if these therapies fail or are not tolerated by the patient.

Treatment of Hyperhidrosis

This socially embarrassing phenomenon may be treated with anticholinergic agents such as trihexyphenidyl, propantheline, or scopolamine. High doses of these agents are usually required, and therapy is usually limited by other anticholinergic side effects, such as dry mouth, urinary retention, and constipation. Gustatory sweating may respond to topical anticholinergic agents (277a) and to injections of botulinum toxin type A (277b).

PAINFUL DIABETIC NEUROPATHY

Pain is one of the more distressing and difficult-to-manage symptoms of diabetic neuropathy and occurs in both focal neuropathy and symmetric polyneuropathy. In polyneuropathy, the incidence, severity, and duration of pain are quite variable, whereas in focal mononeuropathy and radiculopathy, pain is usually more severe but temporary.

The pathophysiologic basis for the pain of diabetic neuropathy has not been established. Several investigators have attempted to define the structural basis of painful diabetic polyneuropathy. Morphologic abnormalities that have been associated with neuropathic pain include axonal sprouting, acute axonal degeneration, active degeneration of myelinated fibers, and disproportionate loss of large-caliber nerve fibers. Recent controlled studies, however, have failed to support these associations.

Brown et al. (278) described axonal degeneration and nerve-fiber sprouting predominantly involving small myelinated and unmyelinated fibers in sural nerve biopsies of two patients with painful distal diabetic neuropathy. Because small myelinated and unmyelinated fibers mediate pain sensation, it was proposed that pain results from increased ectopic activity in the regeneration of small-fiber nerve sprouts. In a later study that provided some support for this hypothesis, Said et al. (29) noted severe loss of unmyelinated and small myelinated axons with axonal sprouting in five patients with clinical features of small-fiber sensory diabetic neuropathy, autonomic dysfunction, and plantar ulceration. Three of these patients had painful manifestations.

This hypothesis has not been supported by all studies. Dyck et al. (279) found that painful diabetic neuropathy was correlated with acute breakdown of myelinated nerve fibers. There was no evidence of differential involvement of small and large nerve fibers. Archer et al. (42) found acute degeneration with regeneration in nerve fibers of all diameters in three patients with acute and severe painful polyneuropathy.

Britland et al. (280) found uniform degeneration and regeneration in large and small myelinated fibers and in small unmyelinated fibers in patients with either acute or chronic painful neuropathy, as well as in patients with painless neuropathy and neurotrophic foot ulcers. There were no differences in the extent of unmyelinated fiber pathology or acute axonal degeneration in patients with and without pain, but fibers with disproportionately large Schwann cells relative to axon diameter occurred exclusively in patients with painful neuropathy, raising the possibility that axonal atrophy may play a role in pain production.

Llewelyn and colleagues (281) noted that the presence of pain did not correlate with active degeneration of myelinated fibers or with regenerative activity in myelinated or unmyelinated axons, whereas Malik and colleagues (282) reported, based on morphologic data derived from 30 diabetic sural nerves, that there was no difference in myelinated and unmyelinated fiber pathology between patients with painless and patients with painful neuropathy. Sprouting of unmyelinated fibers was no more common in patients with painful neuropathy than patients with painless neuropathy.

TREATMENT OF PAINFUL NEUROPATHY

Treatment of pain requires attempts at strict control of blood glucose levels, as there is evidence that hyperglycemia may reduce the pain threshold. Because painful diabetic neuropathy may persist for months and occasionally for years, continued use of opiates should be avoided. When non-opiate analgesics are effective, they should be taken on a carefully timed, regular basis throughout the day, as in the management of cancer pain, not after the pain has been allowed to build in repeated crescendo fashion. Since the pain of diabetic neuropathy is characteristically worse at night, regular dosing of an analgesic in the early evening and again before sleep may improve sleep. A variety of agents from diverse pharmacologic classes, the so-called adjuvant analgesics, have been used to treat neuropathic pain (Table 56.3).

Tricyclic and Other Antidepressants

The tricyclic antidepressants and anticonvulsants are the agents used as first-line therapy for the treatment of neuropathic pain. The tertiary amine amitriptyline is the best studied of these agents and has been shown in several randomized, blinded clinical trials to significantly improve neuropathic pain

TABLE 56.3. Pharmacotherapy for Neuropathic Pain

Agent	Initial dose	Dose increment	Effective dose
Gabapentin	100–300 mg qd	100–200 q 3–5 d	300–1800 mg tid
Tricyclic antidepressants	10–25 mg qd	10–25 mg/wk	25–150 mg
Pregabalin	50–75 mg bid	25–150 q 3 d	50–200 mg tid
Lamotrigine	25 mg qd	25–50 mg/wk	200–400 mg bid
Topiramate	50 mg qd	50 mg qd	200 mg bid
Carbamazepine	100–200 mg bid	100–200 mg q 2 d	200–400 mg tid
Tramadol	50 mg qd	50 mg qd	50–100 mg qid
Duloxetine	60 mg qd	30–60 mg	60 mg bid
Venlafaxine	37.5 mg qd	37.5 q 3–5 d	75 mg bid
Capsaicin	0.075% qid	—	0.075% qid
Mexiletine	150 mg	150 mg qd	150–300 mg tid

qd, once a day; bid, twice a day; tid, three times a day; qid, four times a day.

(283–285). Side effects include drowsiness, constipation, dry mouth, weight gain, and orthostatic hypotension. The secondary amines nortriptyline and desipramine have a less troublesome side-effect profile (284–286). A meta-analysis of antidepressant use in randomized placebo-controlled trials revealed that tricyclic agents provided at least a 50% reduction in pain intensity in 30% of individuals with neuropathic pain (287).

Current data suggest that selective serotonin reuptake inhibitors are not as effective as tricyclic agents in the management of diabetic neuropathic pain (285,288). The selective norepinephrine and serotonin reuptake inhibitors venlafaxine and duloxetine may prove useful in the treatment of painful diabetic polyneuropathy. These agents inhibit reuptake of serotonin and norepinephrine with the muscarinic, histaminic, and adrenergic side effects that accompany use of the tricyclics (288a,288b).

Anticonvulsants

Anticonvulsants from several classes have been used to treat painful diabetic neuropathy. Gabapentin is currently the most frequently prescribed anticonvulsant for the treatment of neuropathic pain. In blinded, randomized, placebo-controlled trials, this agent demonstrated effectiveness in the treatment of painful diabetic neuropathy (289). Gabapentin is well absorbed and not metabolized. It is not bound to plasma proteins. There is no hepatic metabolism, and the agent is excreted unchanged by kidneys. The clearance of gabapentin is reduced in patients with impaired creatinine clearance, and dose adjustment is required. Gabapentin does not compete for or inhibit the cytochrome P-450 system. Side effects include drowsiness, dizziness, and fatigue (290).

Pregabalin has shown effectiveness in alleviating pain associated with diabetic peripheral neuropathy. In a randomized, double-bind, placebo-controlled, parallel-group, multicenter, 8-week trial, 146 patients were randomized to receive placebo or pregabalin, 300 mg per day. Pregabalin produced significant improvements versus placebo for mean pain scores, mean sleep interference scores, and measures of quality of life. Pregabalin has similar pharmacokinetic features to gabapentin, but, in contrast, displays linear pharmacokinetics (291).

The mechanism of the analgesic action of these agents is not fully elucidated. Pregabalin and gabapentin are structurally related to the neurotransmitter gamma-aminobutyric acid (GABA), although there is no evidence that they bind directly to GABA receptors or that they influence the uptake or breakdown of GABA. A proposed mechanism of action, based on the observation that gabapentin binds to the $\alpha_2\delta$ subunit of the voltage-dependent calcium channel, is that gabapentin modulates neurotransmission in the presynaptic dorsal horn neurons (291a–291d).

Carbamazepine was first used to treat trigeminal neuralgia and is approved by the FDA for this indication. This agent has also been used successfully to treat diabetic peripheral neuropathy (292). Side effects include dizziness; drowsiness; balance difficulties; skin rash; and rarely leukopenia, thrombocytopenia, and hepatic damage. Other anticonvulsants that may be effective for the treatment of neuropathic pain include phenytoin (293), lamotrigine (294), and topiramate (294a,b).

Antiarrhythmics

The class 1b antiarrhythmic agent mexiletine, a sodium-channel blocker, has been studied for the treatment of diabetic peripheral neuropathy (295–299). The rationale for sodium-channel blockers in the treatment of diabetic peripheral neuropathy is that they inhibit neuron depolarization and thereby impair spontaneous firing of regenerating fibers that have a low threshold for depolarization. The results with this anesthetic antiarrhythmic agent, which is structurally similar to lidocaine, have been inconsistent. Some have suggested that responsiveness to this agent may be predicted on the basis of the response to intravenous lidocaine (300). Side effects of this agent are frequent and include gastrointestinal disturbance, headache, dizziness, and tremor. Use of this agent is contraindicated in patients with second- or third-degree heart block. It may worsen cardiac arrhythmias.

Topical Agents

The use of topical agents to treat diabetic painful neuropathy offers several theoretical advantages. There are minimal systemic side effects, no drug interactions, and usually no need for drug titration. Also, the pharmacotherapeutic effect is applied directly to the site of pain generation, although chronic neuropathic pain usually results in changes at more proximal sites in the peripheral and central nervous system. Capsaicin, an extract of chili peppers, is the most widely used of these agents and is available in cream form. This neurotoxin initially activates and then depletes substance P from the terminals of unmyelinated C fibers. There is some evidence that the application of capsaicin produces degeneration followed by reinnervation of epidermal nerve fibers (301). The results of treatment trials with this agent have been inconsistent (302–304). Side effects include cutaneous burning, erythema, and sneezing. Several local anesthetic creams are also available and may prove to be of benefit in the treatment of diabetic neuropathic pain (305).

Opiate and Atypical Opiate Analgesics

There is evidence that the "nonnarcotic" analgesic tramadol may be effective in the treatment of painful diabetic peripheral neuropathy (306). This agent, which is a mixed-opioid agonist, exhibits low-affinity binding to the μ opiate receptor. It is biochemically distinct from other opioids in that analgesia is only partially antagonized by naloxone. Tramadol inhibits reuptake of norepinephrine and serotonin. Side effects of this medication include dizziness, nausea, constipation, and drowsiness. This agent has a low potential for abuse but should be avoided in opiate-dependent patients and patients with a tendency to abuse drugs. The use of opioids to treat neuropathic pain remains controversial.

REFERENCES

1. Marchal de Calvi CJ. *Recherches sur les accidents diabetiques*. P Asselin, 1894.
2. Marton MM. Diabetic neuropathy: a clinical study of 150 cases. *Brain* 1953;76:594–624.
3. Pavy FW. Introductory address to the discussion on the clinical aspect of glycosuria. *Lancet* 1885;2:1033–1035.
4. Leyden E. Beitrage zur Klinik des Diabetes Mellitus. *Wein Med Wochenschr* 1893;43:926.
5. Jordan WR. Neuritic manifestations in diabetes mellitus. *Arch Intern Med* 1936;57:307–366.
6. Treusch JV. Diabetic neuritis: a tentative working classification. *Proc Mayo Clin* 1945;20:393–402.
7. Goodman JI, Barmoel S, Frankel L. *The diabetic neuropathies*. Springfield, MA: Charles C Thomas Publisher, 1953.
8. Locke S. The peripheral nervous system in diabetes mellitus. *Diabetes* 1964;13:307–311.
9. Bruyn GW, Garland H. Neuropathies of endocrine origin. In: Vinken PJ, Bruyn GW, eds. *Handbook of clinical neurology*. Amsterdam: North-Holland Publishing, 1970:29–71.
10. Dyck PJ, Karnes J, O'Brien PC. Diagnosis, staging, and classification of diabetic neuropathy and association with other complications. In: Dyck PJ, Thomas PK, Asbury AK, eds. *Diabetic neuropathy*. Philadelphia: WB Saunders, 1987:36–44.
11. Thomas PK, Tomlinson DR. Diabetic and hypoglycemic neuropathy. In: Dyck PJ, Thomas EH, Lambert RB, eds. *Peripheral neuropathy*. Philadelphia: WB Saunders, 1993:1219–1250.
12. Pirart J. [Diabetes mellitus and its degenerative complications: a prospective study of 4,400 patients observed between 1947 and 1973 (3rd and last part) (author's transl)]. [French]. *Diabete Metab* 1977;3:245–256.
13. Partanen J, Niskanen L, Lehtinen J, et al. Natural history of peripheral neuropathy in patients with non-insulin-dependent diabetes mellitus. *N Engl J Med* 1995;333:89–94.
14. Dyck PJ, Kratz KM, Karnes JL, et al. The prevalence by staged severity of various types of diabetic neuropathy, retinopathy, and nephropathy in a population-based cohort: the Rochester Diabetic Neuropathy Study. *Neurology* 1993;43:817–824.
15. Tesfaye S, Stevens LK, Stephenson JM, et al. Prevalence of diabetic peripheral neuropathy and its relation to glycaemic control and potential risk factors: the EURODIAB IDDM Complications Study. *Diabetologia* 1996;39:1377–1384.
16. Maser RE, Steenkiste AR, Dorman JS, et al. Epidemiological correlates of diabetic neuropathy. Report from Pittsburgh Epidemiology of Diabetes Complications Study. *Diabetes* 1989;38:1456–1461.
17. Fedele D, Comi G, Coscelli C, et al. A multicenter study on the prevalence of diabetic neuropathy in Italy. Italian Diabetic Neuropathy Committee. *Diabetes Care* 1997;20:836–843.
18. Young MJ, Boulton AJ, Macleod AF, et al. A multicentre study of the prevalence of diabetic peripheral neuropathy in the United Kingdom hospital clinic population. *Diabetologia* 1993;36:150–154.
19. Effect of intensive diabetes therapy on the development and progression of neuropathy in the Diabetes Control and Complications Trial. The Diabetes Control and Complications Trial (DCCT) Research Group. *Ann Intern Med* 1995;122:561–568.
20. Reichard P, Pihl M, Rosenqvist U, Sule J. Complications in IDDM are caused by elevated blood glucose level: the Stockholm Diabetes Intervention Study (SDIS) at 10-year follow up. *Diabetologia* 1996;39:1483–1488.
21. Veglio M, Sivieri R. Prevalence of neuropathy in IDDM patients in Piemonte, Italy: the Neuropathy Study Group of the Italian Society for the Study of Diabetes, Piemonte Affiliate. *Diabetes Care* 1993;16:456–461.
22. Waxman SG, Sabin TD. Diabetic truncal polyneuropathy. *Arch Neurol* 1981; 38:46–47.
23. Ellenberg M. Diabetic truncal mononeuropathy: a new clinical syndrome. *Diabetes Care* 1978;1:10–13.
24. Longstreth GF, Newcomer AD. Abdominal pain caused by diabetic radiculopathy. *Ann Intern Med* 1977;86:166–168.
25. Sun SF, Streib EW. Diabetic thoracoabdominal neuropathy: clinical and electrodiagnostic features. *Ann Neurol* 1981;9:75–79.
26. Heinrichs RW, Moorhouse JA. Touch-perception thresholds in blind diabetic subjects in relation to the reading of Braille type. *N Engl J Med* 1969;280:72–75.
27. Stewart JD, McKelvey R, Durcan L, et al. Chronic inflammatory demyelinating polyneuropathy (CIDP) in diabetics. *J Neurol Sci* 1996;142(1–2):59–64.
28. Boulton AJ, Armstrong WD, Scarpello JH, et al. The natural history of painful diabetic neuropathy—a 4-year study. *Postgrad Med J* 1983;59:556–559.
29. Said G, Slama G, Selva J. Progressive centripetal degeneration of axons in small fibre diabetic polyneuropathy. *Brain* 1983;106:791–807.
30. Dyck PJ, Lais A, Karnes JL, et al. Fiber loss is primary and multifocal in sural nerves in diabetic polyneuropathy. *Ann Neurol* 1986;19:425–439.
31. Young RJ, Zhou YQ, Rodriguez E, et al. Variable relationship between peripheral somatic and autonomic neuropathy in patients with different syndromes of diabetic polyneuropathy. *Diabetes* 1986;35:192–197.
32. Gruener G, Dyck PJ. Quantitative sensory testing: methodology, applications, and future directions. *J Clin Neurophysiol* 1994;11:568–583.
33. Dyck PJ, Bushek W, Spring EM, et al. Vibratory and cooling detection thresholds compared with other tests in diagnosing and staging diabetic neuropathy. *Diabetes Care* 1987;10:432–440.
34. Edmonds ME. The diabetic foot: pathophysiology and treatment. *Clin Endocrinol Metab* 1986;15:889–916.
35. Boulton AJ. The pathogenesis of diabetic foot problems: an overview. *Diabet Med* 1996;13[Suppl 1]:S12–S16.
36. Reiber GE. The epidemiology of diabetic foot problems. *Diabet Med* 1996;13 [Suppl 1]:S6–S11.
37. Reiber GE, Vileikyte L, Boyko EJ, et al. Causal pathways for incident lower-extremity ulcers in patients with diabetes from two settings. *Diabetes Care* 1999;22:157–162.
38. Boulton AJ, Kubrusly DB, Bowker JH, et al. Impaired vibratory perception and diabetic foot ulceration. *Diabet Med* 1986;3:335–337.
39. Kumar S, Fernando DJ, Veves A, et al. Semmes-Weinstein monofilaments: a simple, effective and inexpensive screening device for identifying diabetic patients at risk of foot ulceration. *Diabetes Res Clin Pract* 1991;13:63–67.
40. Shapiro SA, Stansberry KB, Hill MA, et al. Normal blood flow response and vasomotion in the diabetic Charcot foot. *J Diabetes Complications* 1998;12: 147–153.
41. Klenerman L. The Charcot joint in diabetes. *Diabet Med* 1996;13[Suppl 1]: S52–S54.
42. Archer AG, Watkins PJ, Thomas PK, et al. The natural history of acute painful neuropathy in diabetes mellitus. *J Neurol Neurosurg Psychiatry* 1983;46:491–499.
43. Ellenberg M. Diabetic neuropathic cachexia. *Diabetes* 1974;23:418–423.
44. Young RJ, Ewing DJ, Clarke BF. Chronic and remitting painful diabetic polyneuropathy. Correlations with clinical features and subsequent changes in neurophysiology. *Diabetes Care* 1988;11:34–40.
45. Blau RH. Diabetic neuropathic cachexia: report of a woman with this syndrome and review of the literature. *Arch Intern Med* 1983;143:2011–2012.
46. Jackson CE, Barohn RJ. Diabetic neuropathic cachexia: report of a recurrent case. *J Neurol Neurosurg Psychiatry* 1998;64:785–787.
47. Caravati CM. Insulin neuritis: a case report. *Va Med Monthly* 1933;59:745–746.
48. Ellenberg M. Diabetic neuropathy precipitating after institution of diabetic control. *Am J Med Sci* 1958;236:466.
49. Llewelyn JG, Thomas PK, Fonseca V, et al. Acute painful diabetic neuropathy precipitated by strict glycemic control. *Acta Neuropathol* (Berl) 1986;72: 157–163.
50. Tesfaye S, Malik R, Harris N, et al. Arterio-venous shunting and proliferating new vessels in acute painful neuropathy of rapid glycaemic control (insulin neuritis). *Diabetologia* 1996;39:329–335.
51. Dyck PJ, Lambert EH, Windebank AJ, et al. Acute hyperosmolar hyperglycemia causes axonal shrinkage and reduced nerve conduction velocity. *Exp Neurol* 1981;71:507–514.

51a. Stewart JD, McKelvey R, Duran L, et al. Chronic inflammatory demyelinating polyneuropathy (CIDP) in diabetics. *J Neurol Sci* 1996;142:59–64.

51b. Gorson KC, Ropper AH, Adelman LS, Weinberg DH. Influence of diabetes mellitus on chronic inflammatory demyelinating polyneuropathy. *Muscle Nerve* 2000;23:37–43.

51c. Haq RU, Pendlebury WW, Fries TJ, Tandan R. Chronic inflammatory demyelinating polyradiculoneuropathy in diabetic patients. *Muscle Nerve* 2003;27:465-470.

51d. Sharma KR, Cross J, Farronay O, et al. Demyelinating neuropathy in diabetes mellitus. *Arch Neurol* 2002;59:758–765.

51e. Krendel DA, Costigan DA, Hopkins LC. Successful treatment of neuropathies in patients with diabetes mellitus [See comments]. *Arch Neurol* 1995;52:1053–1061.

51f. Younger DS, Rosoklija G, Hays AP, et al. Diabetic peripheral neuropathy: a clinicopathologic and immunohistochemical analysis of sural nerve biopsies. *Muscle Nerve* 1996;19:722–727.

51g. Uncini A, De Angelis MV, Di Muzio A, et al. Chronic inflammatory demyelinating polyneuropathy in diabetics: motor conductions are important in the differential diagnosis with diabetic polyneuropathy. *Clin Neurophysiol* 1999;110:705–711.

52. Zorrilla E, Kozak GP. Ophthalmoplegia in diabetes mellitus. *Arch Intern Med* 1967;67:968–976.
53. Ross AT. Recurrent cranial nerve palsies in diabetes mellitus. *Neurology* 1962;12:180–185.
54. Barricks ME, Traviesa DB, Glaser JS, et al. Ophthalmoplegia in cranial arteritis. *Brain* 1977;100:209–221.
55. Asbury AK, Fields HL. Pain due to peripheral nerve damage: an hypothesis. *Neurology* 1984;34:1587–1590.
56. Breen LA, Hopf HC, Farris BK, et al. Pupil-sparing oculomotor nerve palsy due to midbrain infarction. *Arch Neurol* 1991;48:105–106.
57. Nadeau SE, Trobe JD. Pupil sparing in oculomotor palsy: a brief review. *Ann Neurol* 1983;13:143–148.
58. Asbury AK, Aldredge H, Hershberg R, et al. Oculomotor palsy in diabetes mellitus: a clinicopathological study. *Brain* 1970;93:555–566.
59. Jørgensen MB, Buch NH. Studies on the sense of smell and taste in diabetics. *Acta Otolaryngol* 1961;53:539–545.
60. Pavan PR, Aiello LM, Wafai MZ, et al. Optic disc edema in juvenile-onset diabetes. *Arch Ophthalmol* 1980;98:2193–2195.
61. Lubow M, Makley TA, Jr. Pseudopapilledema of juvenile diabetes mellitus. *Arch Ophthalmol* 1971;85:417–422.
62. Korczyn AD. Bell's palsy and diabetes mellitus. *Lancet* 1971;1:108–109.
63. Adour KK, Wingerd J. Idiopathic facial paralysis (Bell's palsy): factors affecting severity and outcome in 446 patients. *Neurology* 1974;24:1112–1116.
64. Bruns L. Ueber neuritische Lähmungen beim Diabetes Mellitus. *Berl Klin Wochenschr* 1890;27:509–515.
65. Garland H, Taverner D. Diabetic myelopathy. *BMJ* 1953;1:1405–1413.
66. Garland JT. Diabetic amyotrophy. *BMJ* 1955;2:1287–1290.
67. Coppack SW, Watkins PJ. The natural history of diabetic femoral neuropathy. *Q J Med* 1991;79:307–313.
68. Calverley JR, Mulder DW. Femoral neuropathy. *Neurology* 1960;10:963–967.
69. Sullivan JF. The neuropathies of diabetes. *Neurology* 1958;8:243–249.
70. Williams IR, Mayer RF. Subacute proximal diabetic neuropathy. *Neurology* 1976;26:108–116.
71. Pascoe MK, Low PA, Windebank AJ, et al. Subacute diabetic proximal neuropathy. *Mayo Clin Proc* 1997;72:1123–1132.
72. Raff MC, Asbury AK. Ischemic mononeuropathy and mononeuropathy multiplex in diabetes mellitus. *N Engl J Med* 1968;279:17–21.
73. Bastron JA, Thomas JE. Diabetic polyradiculopathy: clinical and electromyographic findings in 105 patients. *Mayo Clin Proc* 1981;56:725–732.
74. Dyck PJ, Norell JE, Dyck PJ. Microvasculitis and ischemia in diabetic lumbosacral radiculoplexus neuropathy. *Neurology* 1999;53:2113–2121.
75. Asbury AK. Proximal diabetic neuropathy. *Ann Neurol* 1977;2:179–180.
76. Barohn RJ, Sahenk Z, Warmolts JR, et al. The Bruns-Garland syndrome (diabetic amyotrophy): revisited 100 years later. *Arch Neurol* 1991;48:1130–1135.
77. Casey EB, Harrison MJ. Diabetic amyotrophy: a follow-up study. *BMJ* 1972;1:656–659.
78. Hamilton CR, Jr., Dobson HL, Marshall J. Diabetic amyotrophy: clinical and electron microscopic studies in six patients. *Am J Med Sci* 1968;256:81–90.
79. Locke S, Lawrence DG, Legg MA. Diabetic amyotrophy. *Am J Med* 1963; 34:775–785.
80. Chokroverty S, Reyes MG, Rubino FA, et al. The syndrome of diabetic amyotrophy. *Ann Neurol* 1977;2:181–194.
81. Chokroverty S. Proximal nerve dysfunction in diabetic proximal amyotrophy: electrophysiology and electron microscopy. *Arch Neurol* 1982;39:403–407.
82. Chokroverty S. AAEE case report 13: diabetic amyotrophy. *Muscle Nerve* 1987;10:679–684.
83. Chokroverty S, Sander HW. AAEM case report 13: diabetic amyotrophy. *Muscle Nerve* 1996;19:939–945.
84. Root HF, Rogers MH. Diabetic neuritis with paralysis. *N Engl J Med* 1930; 202:1049–1053.
85. Hirsh LF. Diabetic polyradiculopathy simulating lumbar disc disease: report of four cases. *J Neurosurg* 1984;60:183–186.
86. Subramony SH, Wilbourn AJ. Diabetic proximal neuropathy: clinical and electromyographic studies. *J Neurol Sci* 1982;53:293–304.
87. Gilliatt RW, Willison RG. Peripheral nerve conduction in diabetic neuropathy. *J Neurol Neurosurg Psychiatry* 1962;25:11–18.
88. Chopra JS, Hurwitz LJ. Femoral nerve conduction in diabetes mellitus and chronic occlusive vascular disease. *Electroencephalogr Clin Neurophysiol* 1968; 25:399.
89. Lamontagne A, Buchthal F. Electrophysiological studies in diabetic neuropathy. *J Neurol Neurosurg Psychiatry* 1970;33:442–452.
90. Said G, Goulon-Goeau C, Lacroix C, et al. Nerve biopsy findings in different patterns of proximal diabetic neuropathy. *Ann Neurol* 1994;35:559–569.
91. Said G, Elgrably F, Lacroix C, et al. Painful proximal diabetic neuropathy: inflammatory nerve lesions and spontaneous favorable outcome. *Ann Neurol* 1997;41:762–770.
92. Krendel DA, Costigan DA, Hopkins LC. Successful treatment of neuropathies in patients with diabetes mellitus. *Arch Neurol* 1995;52:1053–1061.
92a. Dyck PJ, Windebank AJ. Diabetic and nondiabetic lumbosacral radiculoplexus neuropathies: new insights into pathophysiology and treatment. *Muscle Nerve* 2002;25(4):477–491.
93. Stewart JD. Diabetic truncal neuropathy: topography of the sensory deficit. *Ann Neurol* 1989;25:233–238.
94. Boulton AJ, Angus E, Ayyar DR, et al. Diabetic thoracic polyradiculopathy presenting as abdominal swelling. *BMJ* (Clin Res Ed) 1984;289:798–799.
95. Parry GJ, Floberg J. Diabetic truncal neuropathy presenting as abdominal hernia. *Neurology* 1989;39:1488–1490.
96. Kikta DG, Breuer AC, Wilbourn AJ. Thoracic root pain in diabetes: the spectrum of clinical and electromyographic findings. *Ann Neurol* 1982;11:80–85.
97. Streib EW, Sun SF, Paustian FF, et al. Diabetic thoracic radiculopathy: electrodiagnostic study. *Muscle Nerve* 1986;9:548–553.
98. Dolman CL. The morbid anatomy of diabetic neuropathy. *Neurology* 1963;13: 135–142.
98a. Lauria G, McArthur JC, Hauer PE, et al. Neuropathological alterations in diabetic truncal neuropathy: evaluation by skin biopsy. *J Neurol Neurosurg Psychiatry* 1998;65:762–766.
99. Fraser DM, Campbell IW, Ewing DJ, et al. Mononeuropathy in diabetes mellitus. *Diabetes* 1979;28:96–101.
100. Jung Y, Hohmann TC, Gerneth JA, et al. Diabetic hand syndrome. *Metabolism* 1971;20:1008–1015.
101. de Carvalho MA, Matias T, Evangelista T, et al. Bilateral phrenic nerve neuropathy in a diabetic patient. *Eur J Neurol* 1996;3:481–482.
102. Low PA. Recent advances in the pathogenesis of diabetic neuropathy. *Muscle Nerve* 1987;10:121–128.
103. Cameron NE, Cotter MA. Metabolic and vascular factors in the pathogenesis of diabetic neuropathy. *Diabetes* 1997; 46[Suppl 2]:S31–S37.
104. Greene DA, Lattimer SA. Impaired rat sciatic nerve sodium-potassium adenosine triphosphatase in acute streptozocin diabetes and its correction by dietary myo-inositol supplementation. *J Clin Invest* 1983; 72:1058–1063.
105. Greene DA, Yagihashi S, Lattimer SA, et al. Nerve Na^+-K^+-ATPase, conduction and myoinositol in the insulin deficient BB-rat. *Am J Physiol* 1984; 247:E534–E539.
106. Stevens MJ, Lattimer SA, Kamijo M, et al. Osmotically-induced nerve taurine depletion and the compatible osmolyte hypothesis in experimental diabetic neuropathy in the rat. *Diabetologia* 1993;36:608–614.
107. Greene DA, Mackway AM. Decreased myo-inositol content and Na^+-K^+-ATPase activity in superior cervical ganglion of STZ-diabetic rat and prevention by aldose reductase inhibition. *Diabetes* 1986;35:1106–1108.
108. Dyck PJ, Zimmerman BR, Vilen TH, et al. Nerve glucose, fructose, myo-inositol, and fiber degeneration and regeneration in diabetic neuropathy. *N Engl J Med* 1988;319:542–548.
109. Dyck PJ, Sherman WR, Hallcher LM, et al. Human diabetic endoneurial sorbitol, fructose, and myo-inositol related to sural nerve morphometry. *Ann Neurol* 1980;8:590–596.
110. Greene DA, Lewis RA, Lattimer SA, et al. Selective effect of myo-inositol administration on sciatic and tibial motor nerve conduction parameters in the streptozotocin-diabetic rat. *Diabetes* 1983;31:573–578.
111. Hale PJ, Nattrass M, Silverman SH, et al. Peripheral nerve concentrations of glucose, fructose, sorbitol and myoinositol in diabetic and non-diabetic patients. *Diabetologia* 1987;30:464–467.
112. Horrobin DF. Essential fatty acids in the management of impaired nerve function in diabetes. *Diabetes* 1997;46[Suppl 2]:S90–S93.
113. Cameron NE, Cotter MA, Robertson S. Essential fatty acid diet supplementation: effects on peripheral nerve and skeletal muscle function and capillarization in streptozocin-induced diabetic rats. *Diabetes* 1991;40:532–539.
114. Julu PO. Essential fatty acids prevent slowed nerve conduction in streptozotocin diabetic rats. *J Diabet Complications* 1988;2:185–188.
115. Cameron NE, Cotter MA, Dines KC, et al. The effects of evening primrose oil on nerve function and capillarization in streptozotocin-diabetic rats: modulation by the cyclo-oxygenase inhibitor flurbiprofen. *Br J Pharmacol* 1993;109:972–979.
116. Low PA, Nickander KK, Tritschler HJ. The roles of oxidative stress and antioxidant treatment in experimental diabetic neuropathy. *Diabetes* 1997;46 [Suppl 2]:S38–S42.
117. Cameron NE, Cotter MA, Archibald V, et al. Anti-oxidant and pro-oxidant effects on nerve conduction velocity, endoneurial blood flow and oxygen tension in non-diabetic and streptozotocin-diabetic rats. *Diabetologia* 1994;37: 449–459.
118. Cotter MA, Love A, Watt MJ, et al. Effects of natural free radical scavengers on peripheral nerve and neurovascular function in diabetic rats. *Diabetologia* 1995;38:1285–1294.
119. Bravenboer B, Kappelle AC, Hamers FP, et al. Potential use of glutathione for the prevention and treatment of diabetic neuropathy in the streptozotocin-induced diabetic rat. *Diabetologia* 1992;35:813–817.
120. Cotter MA, Cameron NE. Neuroprotective effects of carvedilol in diabetic rats: prevention of defective peripheral nerve perfusion and conduction velocity. *Naunyn Schmiedebergs Arch Pharmacol* 1995;351:630–635.
121. Cameron NE, Cotter MA, Maxfield EK. Anti-oxidant treatment prevents the development of peripheral nerve dysfunction in streptozotocin-diabetic rats. *Diabetologia* 1993;36:299–304.
122. Cameron NE, Cotter MA. Neurovascular dysfunction in diabetic rats. Potential contribution of autoxidation and free radicals examined using transition metal chelating agents. *J Clin Invest* 1995;96:1159–1163.
123. Nagamatsu M, Nickander KK, Schmelzer JD, et al. Lipoic acid improves nerve blood flow, reduces oxidative stress, and improves distal nerve conduction in experimental diabetic neuropathy. *Diabetes Care* 1995;18:1160–1167.
124. Brownlee M. Glycation products and the pathogenesis of diabetic complications. *Diabetes Care* 1992;15:1835–1843.
125. Brownlee M. Nonenzymatic glycosylation of macromolecules: prospects of pharmacologic modulation. *Diabetes* 1992;41[Suppl 2]:57–60.
126. Bucala R, Tracey KJ, Cerami A. Advanced glycosylation products quench nitric oxide and mediate defective endothelium-dependent vasodilatation in experimental diabetes. *J Clin Invest* 1991;87:432–438.
127. Edelstein D, Brownlee M. Mechanistic studies of advanced glycosylation end product inhibition by aminoguanidine. *Diabetes* 1992;41:26–29.

128. Tilton RG, Chang K, Hasan KS, et al. Prevention of diabetic vascular dysfunction by guanidines: inhibition of nitric oxide synthase versus advanced glycation end-product formation. *Diabetes* 1993;42:221–232.
129 Sheetz MJ, King GL. Molecular understanding of hyperglycemia's adverse effects for diabetic complications. *JAMA* 2002;288:2579–2588.
130. Kim J, Rushovich EH, Thomas TP, et al. Diminished specific activity of cytosolic protein kinase C in sciatic nerve of streptozocin-induced diabetic rats and its correction by dietary myo-inositol. *Diabetes* 1991;40:1545–1554.
131. Roberts RE, McLean WG. Protein kinase C isozyme expression in sciatic nerves and spinal cords of experimentally diabetic rats. *Brain Res* 1997;754:147–156.
132. Cameron NE, Cotter MA, Jack AM, et al. Protein kinase C effects on nerve function, perfusion, Na(+),K(+)- ATPase activity and glutathione content in diabetic rats. *Diabetologia* 1999;42:1120–1130.
132a. Nakamura J, Kato K, Hamada Y, et al. A protein kinase C–beta-selective inhibitor ameliorates neural dysfunction in streptozotocin-induced diabetic rats. *Diabetes* 1999;48:2090–2095.
132b. Du X, Matsumura T, Edelstein D, et al. Inhibition of GAPDH activity by poly(ADP-ribose) polymerase activates three major pathways of hyperglycemic damage in endothelial cells. *J Clin Invest* 2003;112:1049–1057.
132c. Obrosova IG, Li F, Abatan OI, et al. Role of poly(ADP-ribose) polymerase activation in diabetic neuropathy. *Diabetes* 2004;53:711–720.
133. Hellweg R, Hartung HD. Endogenous levels of nerve growth factor (NGF) are altered in experimental diabetes mellitus: a possible role for NGF in the pathogenesis of diabetic neuropathy. *J Neurosci Res* 1990;26:258–267.
134. Jakobsen J, Brimijoin S, Skau K, et al. Retrograde axonal transport of transmitter enzymes, fucose-labeled protein, and nerve growth factor in streptozotocin-diabetic rats. *Diabetes* 1981;30:797–803.
135. Apfel SC, Arezzo JC, Brownlee M, et al. Nerve growth factor administration protects against experimental diabetic sensory neuropathy. *Brain Res* 1994; 634:7–12.
136. Schmidt RE, Dorsey DA, Beaudet LN, et al. Effect of NGF and neurotrophin-3 treatment on experimental diabetic autonomic neuropathy. *J Neuropathol Exp Neurol* 2001;60:263–273.
137. Tomlinson DR, Fernyhough P, Diemel LT. Role of neurotrophins in diabetic neuropathy and treatment with nerve growth factors. *Diabetes* 1997;46[Suppl 2]:S43–S49.
138. Tuck RR, Schmelzer JD, Low PA. Endoneurial blood flow and oxygen tension in the sciatic nerves of rats with experimental diabetic neuropathy. *Brain* 1984;107:935–950.
139. Cameron NE, Cotter MA, Low PA. Nerve blood flow in early experimental diabetes in rats: relation to conduction deficits. *Am J Physiol* 1991;261:E1–E8.
140. Cameron NE, Cotter MA, Ferguson K, et al. Effects of chronic alpha-adrenergic receptor blockade on peripheral nerve conduction, hypoxic resistance, polyols, Na(+)-K(+)-ATPase activity, and vascular supply in STZ-D rats. *Diabetes* 1991;40:1652–1658.
141. Cameron NE, Cotter MA, Robertson S. Rapid reversal of a motor nerve conduction deficit in streptozotocin-diabetic rats by the angiotensin converting enzyme inhibitor lisinopril. *Acta Diabetol* 1993;30:46–48.
142. Low PA, Tuck RR, Dyck PJ, et al. Prevention of some electrophysiologic and biochemical abnormalities with oxygen supplementation in experimental diabetic neuropathy. *Proc Natl Acad Sci U S A* 1984;81:6894–6898.
143. Yao JK, Low PA. Improvement of endoneurial lipid abnormalities in experimental diabetic neuropathy by oxygen modification. *Brain Res* 1986;362: 362–365.
144. Woltman HW, Wilder RM. Diabetes mellitus: pathologic changes in the spinal cord and peripheral nerves. *Arch Intern Med* 1929;44:576–603.
145. Fagerberg S-E. Diabetic neuropathy. *Acta Med Scand* 1959;164[Suppl 345]: 1–81.
146. Fagerberg S-E. Neuropathie diabétique. *World Neurol* 1961;2:509–519.
147. Behse F, Buchthal F, Carlsen F. Nerve biopsy and conduction studies in diabetic neuropathy. *J Neurol Neurosurg Psychiatry* 1977;40:1072–1082.
148. Chopra JS, Hurwitz LJ, Montgomery DA. The pathogenesis of sural nerve changes in diabetes mellitus. *Brain* 1969;92:391–418.
149. Timperley WR, Boulton AJ, Davies-Jones GA, et al. Small vessel disease in progressive diabetic neuropathy associated with good metabolic control. *J Clin Pathol* 1985;38:1030–1038.
150. Dyck PJ, Hansen S, Karnes J, et al. Capillary number and percentage closed in human diabetic sural nerve. *Proc Natl Acad Sci U S A* 1985;82:2513–2517.
151. Yasuda H, Dyck PJ. Abnormalities of endoneurial microvessels and sural nerve pathology in diabetic neuropathy. *Neurology* 1987;37:20–28.
152. Malik RA, Veves A, Masson EA, et al. Endoneurial capillary abnormalities in mild human diabetic neuropathy. *J Neurol Neurosurg Psychiatry* 1992;55: 557–561.
153. Malik RA, Tesfaye S, Thompson SD, et al. Endoneurial localisation of microvascular damage in human diabetic neuropathy. *Diabetologia* 1993;36: 454–459.
154. Giannini C, Dyck PJ. Ultrastructural morphometric abnormalities of sural nerve endoneurial microvessels in diabetes mellitus. *Ann Neurol* 1994;36: 408–415.
155. Giannini C, Dyck PJ. Basement membrane reduplication and pericyte degeneration precede development of diabetic polyneuropathy and are associated with its severity. *Ann Neurol* 1995;37:498–504.
156. Malik RA, Newrick PG, Sharma AK, et al. Microangiopathy in human diabetic neuropathy: relationship between capillary abnormalities and the severity of neuropathy. *Diabetologia* 1989;32:92–102.
157. Dyck PJ, Karnes JL, O'Brien P, et al. The spatial distribution of fiber loss in diabetic polyneuropathy suggests ischemia. *Ann Neurol* 1986;19:440–449.
158. Dyck PJ, Conn DL, Okazaki H. Necrotizing angiopathic neuropathy. Three-dimensional morphology of fiber degeneration related to sites of occluded vessels. *Mayo Clin Proc* 1972;47:461–475.
159. Dyck PJ, Benstead TJ, Conn DL, et al. Nonsystemic vasculitic neuropathy. *Brain* 1987;110:843–853.
160. Llewelyn JG, Thomas PK, Gilbey SG, et al. Pattern of myelinated fibre loss in the sural nerve in neuropathy related to type 1 (insulin-dependent) diabetes. *Diabetologia* 1988;31:162–167.
161. Greenbaum D, Richardson PC, Salmon MV, et al. Pathological observations on six cases of diabetic neuropathy. *Brain* 1964;87:201–214.
162. Olsson Y, Säve-Söderbergh J, Sourander P, et al. A patho-anatomical study of the central and peripheral nervous system in diabetes of early onset and long duration. *Pathol Eur* 1968;3:62–79.
163. Coërs C, Hildebrand J. Latent neuropathy in diabetes and alcoholism: electromyographic and histological study. *Neurology* 1965;15:19–38.
164. Chopra JS, Sawhney BB, Chakravorty RN. Pathology and time relationship of peripheral nerve changes in experimental diabetes. *J Neurol Sci* 1977;32:53–67.
165. Thomas PK, Lascelles RG. The pathology of diabetic neuropathy. *Q J Med* 1966;35:489–509.
166. Vital C, Le Blanc M, Vallat JM, et al. [Ultrastructural study of peripheral nerve in 16 diabetics without neuropathy. Comparisons with 16 diabetic neuropathies and 16 non-diabetic neuropathies (author's transl)] [French]. *Acta Neuropathol* (Berl) 1974;30:63–72.
167. Vital C, Vallat JM, Le Blanc M, et al. [Peripheral neuropathies caused by diabetes mellitus. Ultrastructural study of 12 biopsied cases] [French]. *J Neurol Sci* 1973;18:381–398.
168. Asbury AK, Johnson PC. Pathology of peripheral nerve. *Major Probl Pathol* 1978;9:1–311.
168a. Dyck PJ, Windebank AJ. Diabetic and nondiabetic lumbosacral radiculoplexus neuropathies: new insights into pathophysiology and treatment. *Muscle Nerve* 2002;25:477–491.
169. Dreyfus PM, Hakim S, Adams RD. Diabetic ophthalmoplegia: report of case, with postmortem study and comments on vascular supply of human oculomotor nerve. *Arch Neurol Psychiatry* 1957;77:337–349.
170. Weber RB, Daroff RB, Mackey EA. Pathology of oculomotor nerve palsy in diabetics. *Neurology* 1970;20:835–838.
171. Smith BE, Dyck PJ. Subclinical histopathological changes in the oculomotor nerve in diabetes mellitus. *Ann Neurol* 1992;32:376–385.
172. Appenzeller O, Richardson EP Jr. The sympathetic chain in patients with diabetic and alcoholic polyneuropathy. *Neurology* 1966;16:1205–1209.
173. Hensley GT, Soergel KH. Neuropathologic findings in diabetic diarrhea. *Arch Pathol* 1968;85:587–597.
174. Duchen LW, Anjorin A, Watkins PJ, et al. Pathology of autonomic neuropathy in diabetes mellitus. *Ann Intern Med* 1980;92:301–303.
175. Olsson Y, Sourander P. Changes in the sympathetic nervous system in diabetes mellitus: a preliminary report. *J Neurovasc Relat* 1968;31:86–95.
176. Low PA, Walsh J: C, Huang CY, et al. The sympathetic nervous system in diabetic neuropathy: a clinical and pathological study. *Brain* 1975;98:341–356.
177. Kristensson K, Nordborg C, Olsson Y, et al. Changes in the vagus nerve in diabetes mellitus. *Acta Pathol Microbiol Scand* 1971;79[A]:684–685.
178. Britland ST, Young RJ, Sharma AK, et al. Vagus nerve morphology in diabetic gastropathy. *Diabetic Med* 1990;7:780–787.
179. Faerman I, Glocer L, Celener D, et al. Autonomic nervous system and diabetes: histological and histochemical study of the autonomic nerve fibers of the urinary bladder in diabetic patients. *Diabetes* 1973;22:225–237.
180. The effect of intensive treatment of diabetes on the development and progression of long-term complications in insulin-dependent diabetes mellitus: the Diabetes Control and Complications Trial Research Group. *N Engl J Med* 1993;329:977–986.
181. The effect of intensive diabetes therapy on measures of autonomic nervous system function in the Diabetes Control and Complications Trial (DCCT). *Diabetologia* 1998;41:416–423.
182. Ohkubo Y, Kishikawa H, Araki E, et al. Intensive insulin therapy prevents the progression of diabetic microvascular complications in Japanese patients with non-insulin-dependent diabetes mellitus: a randomized prospective 6-year study. *Diabetes Res Clin Pract* 1995;28:103–117.
183. Reichard P, Britz A, Carlsson P, et al. Metabolic control and complications over 3 years in patients with insulin dependent diabetes (IDDM): the Stockholm Diabetes Intervention Study (SDIS). *J Intern Med* 1990;228:511–517.
184. Reichard P, Berglund B, Britz A, et al. Intensified conventional insulin treatment retards the microvascular complications of insulin-dependent diabetes mellitus (IDDM): the Stockholm Diabetes Intervention Study (SDIS) after 5 years. *J Intern Med* 1991;230:101–108.
185. Reichard P, Nilsson BY, Rosenqvist U. The effect of long-term intensified insulin treatment on the development of microvascular complications of diabetes mellitus. *N Engl J Med* 1993;329:304–309.
186. Gaede P, Vedel P, Parving HH, et al. Intensified multifactorial intervention in patients with type 2 diabetes mellitus and microalbuminuria: the Steno type 2 randomised study. *Lancet* 1999;353:617–622.
187. Eliasson SG. Properties of isolated nerve fibres from alloxanized rats. *J Neurol Neurosurg Psychiatry* 1969;32:525–529.
188. Does improved control of glycemia prevent or ameliorate diabetic polyneuropathy? Committee on Health Care Issues, American Neurological Association. *Ann Neurol* 1986;19:288–290.

189. Gregersen G. Diabetic neuropathy: influence of age, sex, metabolic control, and duration of diabetes on motor conduction velocity. *Neurology* 1967;17: 972–980.
190. Graf RJ, Halter JB, Halar E, et al. Nerve conduction abnormalities in untreated maturity-onset diabetes: relation to levels of fasting plasma glucose and glycosylated hemoglobin. *Ann Intern Med* 1979;90:298–303.
191. Porte D Jr, Graf RJ, Halter JB, et al. Diabetic neuropathy and plasma glucose control. *Am J Med* 1981;70:195–200.
192. Ward JD, Barnes CG, Fisher DJ, et al. Improvement in nerve conduction following treatment in newly diagnosed diabetics. *Lancet* 1971;1:428–430.
193. Anonymous. Effect of intensive diabetes treatment on nerve conduction in the Diabetes Control and Complications Trial. *Ann Neurol* 1995;38:869–880.
194. Schmidt RE, Plurad SB, Olack BJ, et al. The effect of pancreatic islet transplantation and insulin therapy on experimental diabetic autonomic neuropathy. *Diabetes* 1983;32:532–540.
195. Schmidt RE, Plurad SB, Olack BJ, et al. The effect of pancreatic islet transplantation and insulin therapy on neuroaxonal dystrophy in sympathetic autonomic ganglia of chronic streptozocin-diabetic rats. *Brain Res* 1989;497: 393–398.
196. Kennedy WR, Navarro X, Goetz FC, et al. Effects of pancreatic transplantation on diabetic neuropathy. *N Engl J Med* 1990;322:1031–1037.
197. Navarro X, Kennedy WR, Loewenson RB, et al. Influence of pancreas transplantation on cardiorespiratory reflexes, nerve conduction, and mortality in diabetes mellitus. *Diabetes* 1990;39:802–806.
198. Navarro X, Sutherland DE, Kennedy WR. Long-term effects of pancreatic transplantation on diabetic neuropathy. *Ann Neurol* 1997;42:727–736.
199. Nusser J, Scheuer R, Abendroth D, et al. Effect of pancreatic and/or renal transplantation on diabetic autonomic neuropathy. *Diabetologia* 1991;34 [Suppl 1]:S118–S120.
200. Solders G, Wilczek H, Gunnarsson R, et al. Effects of combined pancreatic and renal transplantation on diabetic neuropathy: a two-year follow-up study. *Lancet* 1987;2:1232–1235.
201. Solders G, Tyden G, Persson A, et al. Improvement in diabetic neuropathy 4 years after successful pancreatic and renal transplantation. *Diabetologia* 1991; 34[Suppl 1]:S125–S127.
202. Trojaborg W, Smith T, Jakobsen J, et al. Effect of pancreas and kidney transplantation on the neuropathic profile in insulin-dependent diabetics with end-stage nephropathy. *Acta Neurol Scand* 1994;90:5–9.
203. Fagius J, Jameson S. Effects of aldose reductase inhibitor treatment in diabetic polyneuropathy: a clinical and neurophysiological study. *J Neurol Neurosurg Psychiatry* 1981;44:991–1001.
204. Jaspan J, Maselli R, Herold K, et al. Treatment of severely painful diabetic neuropathy with an aldose reductase inhibitor: relief of pain and improved somatic and autonomic nerve function. *Lancet* 1983;2:758–762.
205. Judzewitsch RG, Jaspan JB, Polonsky KS, et al. Aldose reductase inhibition improves nerve conduction velocity in diabetic patients. *N Engl J Med* 1983;308:119–125.
206. Young RJ, Ewing DJ, Clarke BF. A controlled trial of sorbinil, an aldose reductase inhibitor, in chronic painful diabetic neuropathy. *Diabetes* 1983;32: 938–942.
207. Lewin IG, O'Brien IA, Morgan MH, et al. Clinical and neurophysiological studies with the aldose reductase inhibitor, sorbinil, in symptomatic diabetic neuropathy. *Diabetologia* 1984;26:445–448.
208. Martyn CN, Reid W, Young RJ, et al. Six-month treatment with sorbinil in asymptomatic diabetic neuropathy: failure to improve abnormal nerve function. *Diabetes* 1987;36:987–990.
209. O'Hare JP, Morgan MH, Alden P, et al. Aldose reductase inhibition in diabetic neuropathy: clinical and neurophysiological studies of one year's treatment with sorbinil. *Diabet Med* 1988;5:537–542.
209a. Pfeifer MA, Schumer MP, Gelber DA. Aldose reductase inhibitors: the end of an era or the need for different trial designs [Review]? *Diabetes* 1997;46 [Suppl 2]:S82–S89.
210. Gregersen G. Myoinositol supplementation. In: Dyck PJ, Thomas PK, Asbury AK, et al., eds. *Diabetic neuropathy*. Philadelphia: WB Saunders, 1987:188–189.
211. Mayhew JA, Gillon KR, Hawthorne JN. Free and lipid inositol, sorbitol and sugars in sciatic nerve obtained post-mortem from diabetic patients and control subjects. *Diabetologia* 1983;24:13–15.
212. Jamal GA, Carmichael H. The effect of gamma-linolenic acid on human diabetic peripheral neuropathy: a double-blind placebo-controlled trial. *Diabet Med* 1990;7:319–323.
213. Jamal GA. The use of gamma linolenic acid in the prevention and treatment of diabetic neuropathy. *Diabet Med* 1994;11:145–149.
214. Keen H, Payan J, Allawi J, et al. Treatment of diabetic neuropathy with gamma-linolenic acid. The Gamma-Linolenic Acid Multicenter Trial Group. *Diabetes Care* 1993;16:8–15.
215. Zeigler D, Hanefeld M, Ruhnau KJ, et al. Treatment of symptomatic diabetic peripheral neuropathy with the anti-oxidant alpha-lipoic acid: a 3-week multicentre randomized controlled trial (ALADIN). *Diabetologia* 1995;38: 1425–1433.
215a. Ziegler D, Nowak H, Kempler P, et al. Treatment of symptomatic diabetic polyneuropathy with the antioxidant alpha-lipoic acid: a meta-analysis. *Diabet Med* 2004;21:114–121.
216. Zeigler D, Schatz H, Conrad F, et al. Effects of treatment with the antioxidant alpha-lipoic acid on cardiac neuropathy in NIDDM patients: a 4-month randomized controlled multicenter trial (DEKAN Study). Deutsche Kardiale Autonome Neuropathie. *Diabetes Care* 1997;20:369–373.
217. Apfel SC, Kessler JA, Adornato BT, et al. and the NGF Study Group. Recombinant human nerve growth factor in the treatment of diabetic polyneuropathy. *Neurology* 1998;51:695–702.
218. Apfel SC, Schwartz S, Adornato BT, et al. Efficacy and safety of recombinant human nerve growth factor in patients with diabetic polyneuropathy: a randomized controlled trial. *JAMA* 2000;284:2215–2221.
219. Vinik AI, Maser RE, Mitchell BD, Freeman R. Diabetic autonomic neuropathy. *Diabetes Care* 2003;26(5):1553–1579.
220. Said G, Goulon-Goeau C, Slama G, et al. Severe early-onset polyneuropathy in insulin–dependent diabetes mellitus: a clinical and pathological study. *N Engl J Med* 1992;326:1257–1263.
221. Ewing DJ, Clarke BF. Diabetic autonomic neuropathy: present insights and future prospects. *Diabetes Care* 1986;9:648–665.
222. Neil HA, Thompson AV, John S, et al. Diabetic autonomic neuropathy: the prevalence of impaired heart rate variability in a geographically defined population. *Diabet Med* 1989;6:20–24.
223. Lloyd-Mostyn RH, Watkins PJ. Defective innervation of heart in diabetic autonomic neuropathy. *BMJ* 1975;3:15–17.
224. Bennett T, Hosking DJ, Hampton JR. Cardiovascular control in diabetes mellitus. *BMJ* 1975;2:585–587.
225. Ewing DJ, Campbell IW, Clarke BF. Heart rate changes in diabetes mellitus. *Lancet* 1981;1:183–186.
226. Ewing DJ, Campbell IW, Clarke BF. The natural history of diabetic autonomic neuropathy. *Q J Med* 1980;49:95–108.
227. O'Brien IA, McFadden JP, Corrall RJ. The influence of autonomic neuropathy on mortality in insulin-dependent diabetes. *Q J Med* 1991; 79:495–502.
228. Rathmann W, Ziegler D, Jahnke M, et al. Mortality in diabetic patients with cardiovascular autonomic neuropathy. *Diabet Med* 1993;10:820–824.
229. Sampson MJ, Wilson S, Karagiannis P, et al. Progression of diabetic autonomic neuropathy over a decade in insulin-dependent diabetics. *Q J Med* 1990;75:635–646.
229a. Maser RE, Mitchell BD, Vinik AI, Freeman R. The association between cardiovascular autonomic neuropathy and mortality in individuals with diabetes: a meta-analysis. *Diabetes Care* 2003;26:1895–1901.
230. Frimodt-Moller C, Mortensen S. Treatment of diabetic cystopathy. *Ann Intern Med* 1980;92:327–328.
231. Ellenberg M. Development of urinary bladder dysfunction in diabetes mellitus. *Ann Intern Med* 1980;92:321–323.
232. Ioanid CP, Noica N. Incidence and diagnostic aspects of the bladder disorders in diabetics. *Eur Urol* 1981;7:211–214.
233. Bradley WE. Diagnosis of urinary bladder dysfunction in diabetes mellitus. *Ann Intern Med* 1980;92:323–326.
234. Appell RA, Whiteside HV. Diabetes and other peripheral neuropathies affecting lower urinary tract function. In: Krane RJ, Siroky MB, eds. *Clinical neurourology*. Boston: Little, Brown and Company, 1992:365–373.
235. McCulloch DK, Campbell IW, Wu FC, et al. The prevalence of diabetic impotence. *Diabetologia* 1980;18:279–283.
236. Ellenberg M. Impotence in diabetes: the neurologic factor. *Ann Intern Med* 1971;75:213–219.
237. Kaiser FE, Korenman SG. Impotence in diabetic men. *Am J Med* 1988;85 [Suppl 5A]:147–152.
238. Hakim LS, Goldstein I. Diabetic sexual dysfunction. *Endocrinol Metab Clin North Am* 1996;25:379–400.
239. Rajfer J, Aronson WJ, Bush PA, et al. Nitric oxide as a mediator of relaxation of the corpus cavernosum in response to nonadrenergic, noncholinergic neurotransmission. *N Engl J Med* 1992;326:90–94.
240. de Tejada IS, Goldstein I, Azadzoi K, et al. Impaired neurogenic and endothelium-mediated relaxation of penile smooth muscle from diabetic men with impotence. *N Engl J Med* 1989;320:1025–1030.
241. DeGroat WC, Booth AM. Physiology of male sexual function. *Ann Intern Med* 1980;92:329–331.
242. Krane RJ, Siroky MB. Neurophysiology of erection. *Neurol Clin North Am* 1981;8:91–102.
243. Ellenberg M. Sexual function in diabetic patients. *Ann Intern Med* 1980;92: 331–333.
244. Wegener M, Borsch G, Schaffstein J, et al. Gastrointestinal transit disorders in patients with insulin-treated diabetes mellitus. *Dig Dis* 1990;8:23–36.
245. Horowitz M, Harding PE, Maddox AF, et al. Gastric and oesophageal emptying in patients with type 2 (non-insulin-dependent) diabetes mellitus. *Diabetologia* 1989;32:151–159.
246. Kassander P. Asymptomatic gastric retention in diabetics (gastroparesis diabeticorum). *Ann Intern Med* 1958;48:797–812.
247. Vogelberg KH, Rathmann W, Helbig G. Sonographic examination of gastric motility in diabetics with autonomic neuropathy. *Diabetes Res* 1987; 5:175–179.
248. Brady PG, Richardson R. Gastric bezoar formation secondary to gastroparesis diabeticorum. *Arch Intern Med* 1977;137:1729.
249. Parkman HP, Schwartz SS. Esophagitis and gastroduodenal disorders associated with diabetic gastroparesis. *Arch Intern Med* 1987;147:1477–1480.
250. Loo FD, Palmer DW, Soergel KH, et al. Gastric emptying in patients with diabetes mellitus. *Gastroenterology* 1984;86:485–495.
251. Ogbonnaya KI, Arem R. Diabetic diarrhea: pathophysiology, diagnosis, and management. *Arch Intern Med* 1990;150:262–267.
252. Valdovinos MA, Camilleri M, Zimmerman BR. Chronic diarrhea in diabetes mellitus: mechanisms and an approach to diagnosis and treatment. *Mayo Clin Proc* 1993;68:691–702.

253. Lysy J, Israeli E, Goldin E. The prevalence of chronic diarrhea among diabetic patients. *Am J Gastroenterol* 1999;94:2165–2170.
254. Schiller LR, Santa Ana CA, Schmulen AC, et al. Pathogenesis of fecal incontinence in diabetes mellitus: evidence for internal-anal-sphincter dysfunction. *N Engl J Med* 1982;307:1666–1671.
255. Fedorak RN, Field M, Chang EB. Treatment of diabetic diarrhea with clonidine. *Ann Intern Med* 1985;102:197–199.
256. Fealey RD, Low PA, Thomas JE. Thermoregulatory sweating abnormalities in diabetes mellitus. *Mayo Clin Proc* 1989;64:617–628.
257. Watkins PJ. Facial sweating after food: a new sign of diabetic autonomic neuropathy. *BMJ* 1973;1:583–587.
258. Stuart DD. Diabetic gustatory sweating. *Ann Intern Med* 1978;89:223–224.
259. Freeman R. Treatment of orthostatic hypotension. *Semin Neurol* 2003;23: 435–442.
260. Snape WJ, Jr., Battle WM, Schwartz SS, et al. Metoclopramide to treat gastroparesis due to diabetes mellitus: a double-blind, controlled trial. *Ann Intern Med* 1982;96:444–446.
261. Longstreth GF, Malagelada J-R, Kelly KA. Metoclopramide stimulation of gastric motility and emptying in diabetic gastroparesis. *Ann Intern Med* 1977; 86:195–196.
262. Perkel MS, Moore C, Hersh T, et al. Metoclopramide therapy in patients with delayed gastric emptying: a randomized, double-blind study. *Dig Dis Sci* 1979;24:662–666.
263. Horowitz M, Harding PE, Chatterton BE, et al. Acute and chronic effects of domperidone on gastric emptying in diabetic autonomic neuropathy. *Dig Dis Sci* 1985;30:1–9.
264. Watts GF, Armitage M, Sinclair J, et al. Treatment of diabetic gastroparesis with oral domperidone. *Diabet Med* 1985;2:491–492.
265. Patterson D, Abell T, Rothstein R, et al. A double-blind multicenter comparison of domperidone and metoclopramide in the treatment of diabetic patients with symptoms of gastroparesis. *Am J Gastroenterol* 1999;94: 1230–1234.
266. Farup CE, Leidy NK, Murray M, et al. Effect of domperidone on the health-related quality of life of patients with symptoms of diabetic gastroparesis. *Diabetes Care* 1998;21:1699–1706.
267. Barone JA. Domperidone: a peripherally acting dopamine 2-receptor antagonist. *Ann Pharmacother* 1999;33:429–440.
268. Janssens J, Peeters TL, Vantrappen G, et al. Improvement of gastric emptying in diabetic gastroparesis by erythromycin: preliminary studies. *N Engl J Med* 1990;322:1028–1031.
269. Rendell MS, Rajfer J, Wicker PA, Smith MD. Sildenafil for treatment of erectile dysfunction in men with diabetes: a randomized controlled trial. Sildenafil Diabetes Study Group. *JAMA* 1999;281:421–426.
269a. Saenz DT, Anglin G, Knight JR, Emmick JT. Effects of tadalafil on erectile dysfunction in men with diabetes. *Diabetes Care* 2002;25:2159–2164.
269b. Goldstein I, Young JM, Fischer J, et al. Vardenafil, a new phosphodiesterase type 5 inhibitor, in the treatment of erectile dysfunction in men with diabetes: a multicenter double-blind placebo-controlled fixed-dose study. *Diabetes Care* 2003;26:777–783.
270. Jackson G, Benjamin N, Jackson N, et al. Effects of sildenafil citrate on human hemodynamics. *Am J Cardiol* 1999;83:13C–20C.
271. Kloner RA, Zusman RM. Cardiovascular effects of sildenafil citrate and recommendations for its use. *Am J Cardiol* 1999;84:11N–17N.
272. Virag R. Intracavernous injection of papaverine for erectile failure. *Lancet* 1982;2:938.
273. Zorgniotti AW, LeFleur RS. Auto-injection of the corpus cavernosum with a vasoactive drug combination for vasculogenic impotence. *J Urol* 1985;133:39–41.
274. Stackl W, Hasun R, Marberger M. Intracavernous injection of prostaglandin E1 in impotent men. *J Urol* 1988;140:66–68.
275. Zentgraf M, Baccouche M, Junemann KP. Diagnosis and therapy of erectile dysfunction using papaverine and phentolamine. *Urol Int* 1988;43:65–75.
276. Linet OI, Ogrinc FG. Efficacy and safety of intracavernosal alprostadil in men with erectile dysfunction: the Alprostadil Study Group. *N Engl J Med* 1996; 334:873–877.
277. Witherington R. Suction device therapy in the management of erectile impotence. *Urol Clin North Am* 1988;15:123–128.
277a. Shaw JE, Abbott CA, Tindle K, et al. A randomised controlled trial of topical glycopyrrolate, the first specific treatment for diabetic gustatory sweating. *Diabetologia* 1997; 40:299–301.
277b. Restivo DA, Lanza S, Patti F, et al. Improvement of diabetic autonomic gustatory sweating by botulinum toxin type A. *Neurology* 2002:59:1971–1973.
278. Brown MJ, Martin JR, Asbury AK. Painful diabetic neuropathy: a morphometric study. *Arch Neurol* 1976;33:164–171.
279. Dyck PJ, Lambert EH, O'Brien PC. Pain in peripheral neuropathy related to rate and kind of fiber degeneration. *Neurology* 1976;28:466–471.
280. Britland ST, Young RJ, Sharma AK, C et al. Association of painful and painless diabetic polyneuropathy with different patterns of nerve fiber degeneration and regeneration. *Diabetes* 1990;39:898–908.
281. Llewelyn JG, Gilbey SG, Thomas PK, et al. Sural nerve morphometry in diabetic autonomic and painful sensory neuropathy: a clinicopathological study. *Brain* 1991;114:867–892.
282. Malik RA. The pathology of human diabetic neuropathy. *Diabetes* 1997;46 [Suppl 2]:S50–S53.
283. Max MB, Culnane M, Schafer SC, et al. Amitriptyline relieves diabetic neuropathy pain in patients with normal or depressed mood. *Neurology* 1987;37: 589–596.
284. Max MB, Kishore-Kumar R, Schafer SC, et al. Efficacy of desipramine in painful diabetic neuropathy: a placebo-controlled trial. *Pain* 1991;45:3–9.
285. Max MB, Lynch SA, Muir J, et al. Effects of desipramine, amitriptyline, and fluoxetine on pain in diabetic neuropathy. *N Engl J Med* 1992;326:1250–1256.
286. Sindrup SH, Gram LF, Skjold T, et al. Clomipramine vs desipramine vs placebo in the treatment of diabetic neuropathy symptoms: a double-blind cross-over study. *Br J Clin Pharmacol* 1990;30:683–691.
287. Sindrup SH, Jensen TS. Pharmacologic treatment of pain in polyneuropathy. *Neurology* 2000;55:915–920.
288. Sindrup SH, Gram LF, Brosen K, et al. The selective serotonin reuptake inhibitor paroxetine is effective in the treatment of diabetic neuropathy symptoms. *Pain* 1990;42:135–144.
288a. Sindrup SH, Bach FW, Madsen C, et al. Venlafaxine versus imipramine in painful polyneuropathy: a randomized, controlled trial. *Neurology* 2003; 60:1284–1289.
288b. Rowbotham MC, Goli V, Kunz NRT, Lei D. Venlafaxine extended release in the treatment of painful diabetic neuropathy: a double-blind, placebo-controlled study. *Pain* 2004:110:697–706.
289. Backonja M, Beydoun A, Edwards KR, et al. Gabapentin for the symptomatic treatment of painful neuropathy in patients with diabetes mellitus: a randomized controlled trial. *JAMA* 1998;280:1831–1836.
290. McLean MJ. Gabapentin. *Epilepsia* 1995;36[Suppl 2]:S73–S86.
291. Rosenstock J, Tuchman M, LaMoreaux L, Sharma U. Pregabalin for the treatment of painful diabetic peripheral neuropathy: a double-blind, placebo-controlled trial. *Pain* 2004:110:628–638.
291a. Gee NS, Brown JP, Dissanayake VU, et al. The novel anticonvulsant drug, gabapentin (Neurontin), binds to the alpha2delta subunit of a calcium channel. *J Biol Chem* 1996;217:5768–5776.
291b. Field MJ, Hughes J, Singh L. Further evidence for the role of the alpha(2)delta subunit of voltage dependent calcium channels in models of neuropathic pain. *Br J Pharmacol* 2000:131:282–286.
291c. Taylor CP, Gee NS, Su TZ, et al. A summary of mechanistic hypotheses of gabapentin pharmacology. *Epilepsy Res* 1998; 29:233–249.
291d. Fehrenbacher JC, Taylor CP, Vasko MR. Pregabalin and gabapentin reduce release of substance P and CGRP from rat spinal tissues only after inflammation or activation of protein kinase C. *Pain* 2003;105:133–141.
292. Rull JA, Quibrera R, Gonzalez-Millan H, et al. Symptomatic treatment of peripheral diabetic neuropathy with carbamazepine (Tegretol): double blind crossover trial. *Diabetologia* 1969;5:215–218.
293. Saudek CD, Werns S, Reidenberg MM. Phenytoin in the treatment of diabetic symmetrical polyneuropathy. *Clin Pharmacol Ther* 1977;22:196–199.
294. McCleane GJ. Lamotrigine in the management of neuropathic pain: a review of the literature. *Clin J Pain* 2000;16:321–326.
294a. Thienel U, Neto W, Schwabe SK, Vijapurkar U. Topiramate in painful diabetic polyneuropathy: findings from three double-blind placebo-controlled trials. *Acta Neurol Scand* 2004;110:221–231.
294b. Barbano RL, Herrmann DN, Hart-Gouleau S, et al. Effectiveness, tolerability, and impact on quality of life of the 5% lidocaine patch in diabetic polyneuropathy. *Arch Neurol* 2004:61:914–918.
295. Dejgard A, Petersen P, Kastrup J. Mexiletine for treatment of chronic painful diabetic neuropathy. *Lancet* 1988;1:9–11.
296. Jarvis B, Coukell AJ. Mexiletine: a review of its therapeutic use in painful diabetic neuropathy. *Drugs* 1998;56:691–707.
297. Oskarsson P, Ljunggren JG, Lins PE. Efficacy and safety of mexiletine in the treatment of painful diabetic neuropathy: the Mexiletine Study Group. *Diabetes Care* 1997;20:1594–1597.
298. Stracke H, Meyer UE, Schumacher HE, et al. Mexiletine in the treatment of diabetic neuropathy. *Diabetes Care* 1992;15:1550–1555.
299. Wright JM, Oki JC, Graves L. Mexiletine in the symptomatic treatment of diabetic peripheral neuropathy. *Ann Pharmacother* 1997;31:29–34.
300. Galer BS, Harle J, Rowbotham MC. Response to intravenous lidocaine infusion predicts subsequent response to oral mexiletine: a prospective study. *J Pain Symptom Manage* 1996;12:161–167.
301. Simone DA, Nolano M, Johnson T, et al. Intradermal injection of capsaicin in humans produces degeneration and subsequent reinnervation of epidermal nerve fibers: correlation with sensory function. *J Neurosci* 1998;18:8947–8959.
302. Treatment of painful diabetic neuropathy with topical capsaicin. A multicenter, double-blind, vehicle-controlled study. The Capsaicin Study Group. *Arch Intern Med* 1991;151:2225–2229.
303. Capsaicin Study Group. Effect of treatment with capsaicin on daily activities of patients with painful diabetic neuropathy. *Diabetes Care* 1992;15:159–165.
304. Tandan R, Lewis GA, Badger GB, et al. Topical capsaicin in painful diabetic neuropathy. Effect on sensory function. *Diabetes Care* 1992;15:15–18.
305. Raskin P, Donofrio PD, Rosenthal NR, et al. Topiramate vs placebo in painful diabetic neuropathy: analgesic and metabolic effects. *Neurology* 2004; 63:865–873.
306. Harati Y, Gooch C, Swenson M, et al. Double-blind randomized trial of tramadol for the treatment of the pain of diabetic neuropathy. *Neurology* 1998;50: 1842–1846.

CHAPTER 57
Hypertension in Diabetes Mellitus

Samy I. McFarlane, Jonathan Castro, Dmitri Kirpichnikov, and James R. Sowers

Hypertension is a very common comorbid condition in diabetes and accounts for up to 85% of excess cardiovascular disease (CVD) risk. Conversely, patients with hypertension are more prone to diabetes than are normotensive patients. Hypertension substantially increases the risk for coronary heart disease (CHD), stroke, retinopathy, and nephropathy. When hypertension coexists with diabetes, the risk of stroke or CVD is doubled and the risk for developing end-stage renal disease is increased five to six times compared with the risk for hypertensive patients without diabetes. In type 2 diabetes, hypertension usually clusters with the other components of the cardiometabolic syndrome, such as microalbuminuria, central obesity, insulin resistance, dyslipidemia, hypercoagulation, increased inflammation, left ventricular hypertrophy (LVH), and hyperuricemia. In type 1 diabetes, hypertension is usually a manifestation of diabetic nephropathy, and hypertension and nephropathy appear to exacerbate each other.

Hypertension in individuals with diabetes has characteristic features, including volume expansion, increased salt sensitivity, isolated systolic hypertension, loss of the nocturnal dipping of blood pressure and pulse, and increased propensity toward orthostatic hypotension and albuminuria.

To maximize the CVD risk reduction in this high-risk population, they should be treated with aspirin and have their low-density lipoprotein (LDL)-cholesterol lowered to less than 100 mg/dL and their blood pressure lowered to a target of 130/80 mm Hg. Combination of two or more drugs is usually necessary to achieve the target blood pressure of 130/80 mm Hg. Thiazide diuretics, angiotensin-converting enzyme (ACE) inhibitors and angiotensin-receptor (AR) blockers, β-blockers, and calcium-channel blockers are beneficial in reducing the incidence of CVD and stroke incidence in patients with diabetes.

RELATIONSHIP BETWEEN HYPERTENSION AND DIABETES

The major cause of mortality in patients with diabetes is CVD (1). Risk factors for CVD that cluster in diabetes (Table 57.1) include hypertension, central obesity, dyslipidemia, microalbuminuria, coagulation abnormalities, loss of nocturnal dipping of blood pressure and pulse, and LVH (2). Among those risk factors, hypertension is approximately twice as frequent in patients with diabetes as in those without diabetes and accounts for up to 85% of the CVD risk. Conversely, patients with hypertension are more prone to diabetes than are normotensive persons (2). In a large prospective study of 12,550 adults, type 2 diabetes was almost 2.5 times as likely to develop in patients with hypertension as in their normotensive counterparts after adjustment for age, sex, race, education, adiposity, family history with respect to diabetes, physical activity level, and other health-related behavior (3). The association between hypertension and insulin resistance, and the resultant hyperinsulinemia, is well established. In untreated patients with essential hypertension, fasting and postprandial insulin levels were higher than in normotensive controls, regardless of the body mass index (BMI), with a direct correlation between plasma insulin concentrations and blood pressure. On the basis of these results, the authors concluded in this study that essential hypertension is an insulin-resistance state (4). Another study of 24 adults documented that patients with hypertension, whether treated or untreated, are insulin resistant, hyperglycemic, and hyperinsulinemic compared with a well-matched control group (5). Insulin resistance and hyperinsulinemia are also present in rats with genetic hypertension, such as Dahl hypertensive and spontaneously hypertensive rat strains (6,7). On the other hand,

TABLE 57.1. Metabolic Disorders Associated with Hypertension and Diabetes

Central obesity
Microalbuminuria
Low HDL-cholesterol levels
High triglyceride levels
Small, dense LDL-cholesterol particles
Hyperinsulinemia/insulin resistance
Endothelial dysfunction
Increased apolipoprotein B levels
Increased fibrinogen levels
Increased PAI-1 levels
Increased C-reactive protein and other inflammatory markers
Absent nocturnal dipping of blood pressure and pulse
Left ventricular hypertrophy
Increased uric acid levels
Premature coronary artery disease

HDL, high-density lipoprotein; LDL, low-density lipoprotein; PAI-1, plasma-activator inhibitor-1.

the association of insulin resistance and essential hypertension does not occur in secondary hypertension (8). These data suggest a common genetic predisposition for essential hypertension and insulin resistance, a concept that is also supported by the finding of altered glucose metabolism in normotensive offspring of hypertensive patients (9,10).

HEMODYNAMIC AND METABOLIC CHARACTERISTICS OF HYPERTENSION IN DIABETES

Hypertension in patients with diabetes, compared with hypertension in those without diabetes, has unique features, such as increased salt sensitivity, volume expansion, loss of nocturnal dipping of blood pressure and pulse, increased propensity to proteinuria and orthostatic hypotension, and isolated systolic hypertension (2). Most of these features are considered risk factors for CVD (Table 57.1) and are particularly important for selecting the appropriate antihypertensive medication, for example, low-dose diuretics for treatment of volume expansion and ACE inhibitors or AR blockers for proteinuria.

Salt Sensitivity and Volume Expansion

Alterations in sodium balance and extracellular fluid volume have heterogeneous effects on blood pressure in both normotensive and hypertensive subjects (11). Increased salt intake does not raise blood pressure in all hypertensive subjects, and sensitivity to dietary salt intake is greatest in the elderly; those with diabetes, renal insufficiency, and low renin status; and African Americans (12,13). Studies demonstrated that salt sensitivity in normotensive subjects is associated with a greater age-related increase in blood pressure (14). This is particularly important to consider in the management of hypertension in patients with diabetes, especially elderly persons, since the prevalence of both diabetes and salt sensitivity increases with age. Thus, a decreased salt intake along with other aspects of diet such as reductions in fat and free carbohydrates and an increase in potassium are important to institute in these patients (2).

Loss of Nocturnal Decline in Blood Pressure

Normotensive individuals and most patients with hypertension have a reproducible circadian pattern to blood pressure and heart rate during 24-hour ambulatory monitoring (15). Typically, the blood pressure is highest while the patient is awake and lowest during sleep, a pattern called "dipping," in which blood pressure decreases by 10% to 15%. Patients with loss of nocturnal decline in blood pressure, "non-dippers," have a less than 10% decline in blood pressure during the night compared with their daytime blood pressure values (16). Patients with diabetes and many of those with the cardiometabolic syndrome have a loss of nocturnal dipping, as demonstrated by 24-hour ambulatory monitoring of blood pressure. This is particularly important since the loss of nocturnal dipping conveys excessive risk for stroke and myocardial infarction. In fact, ambulatory blood pressure has been reported to be superior to office blood pressure in predicting target-organ involvement such as LVH (17,18). About 30% of episodes of myocardial infarction and 50% of strokes occur between 6:00 a.m. and noon. This is particularly important in deciding strategies for the optimal dosing of antihypertensive medications, for which drugs that provide consistent and sustained 24-hour blood pressure control will be advantageous (19).

Microalbuminuria

There is considerable evidence that hypertension in type 1 diabetes is a consequence, rather than a cause, of renal disease and that nephropathy precedes the rise in blood pressure (20). Persistent hypertension in patients with type 1 diabetes is often a manifestation of diabetic nephropathy, as indicated by an elevation of urinary albumin at the diagnosis of the disease (20). Hypertension and nephropathy appear to exacerbate each other. In type 2 diabetes, microalbuminuria is associated with insulin resistance (21), salt sensitivity, loss of nocturnal dipping, and LVH (22). Elevated systolic blood pressure is a significant determining factor in the progression of microalbuminuria (23,24). Indeed, there is increasing evidence that microalbuminuria is an integral component of the metabolic syndrome associated with hypertension (21,22). This concept is important to consider in selecting pharmacologic therapy for hypertension in patients with diabetes, for which medications that decrease both proteinuria and blood pressure, such as ACE inhibitors and AR blockers, have evolved as increasingly important tools for reducing the progression of nephropathy. Further, aggressive blood pressure lowering, often requiring several drugs, is very important in controlling the progressive diabetic renal disease.

Isolated Systolic Hypertension

With the progression of atherosclerosis in patients with diabetes, the larger arteries lose elasticity and become rigid. The systolic blood pressure increases disproportionately because the arterial system is incapable of expansion for any given volume of blood ejected from the left ventricle, leading to isolated systolic hypertension, which is more common and occurs at a relatively younger age in patients with diabetes (2,25).

Orthostatic Hypotension

Pooling of blood in dependent veins when an individual rises from a recumbent position normally leads to a decrease in stroke volume and systolic blood pressure with concomitant increases in systemic vascular resistance, diastolic blood pressure, and heart rate. In patients with diabetes and autonomic dysfunction, excessive venous pooling can cause immediate or delayed orthostatic hypotension that might cause a reduction in cerebral blood flow, leading to intermittent lightheadedness, fatigue, unsteady gait, and syncope (26–28). This is important to recognize in patients with diabetes and concomitant hypertension because it has several diagnostic and therapeutic implications; for example, discontinuation of diuretic therapy and volume repletion might be necessary for the treatment of chronic orthostasis. Also, in the subset of patients with "hyperadrenergic" orthostatic hypertension, as manifested by excessive sweating and palpitation, the use of low-dose clonidine might be necessary to blunt an excess sympathetic response (29). Furthermore, increased propensity for orthostatic hypertension in patients with diabetes renders β-adrenergic receptor blockers less desirable and second-line agents for these patients. In addition, doses of all antihypertensive agents must be titrated more carefully in patients with diabetes, who have greater propensity for orthostatic hypertension while having a high supine blood pressure.

TARGET BLOOD-PRESSURE LEVELS IN PATIENTS WITH DIABETES

The Hypertension Optimal Treatment (HOT) (30) and the United Kingdom Prospective Diabetes Study (UKPDS) (31) demonstrated improved outcomes, particularly in preventing stroke, in patients assigned to lower blood pressure targets. In the HOT trial, improved outcomes were achieved in the group assigned to a target diastolic blood pressure of less than 80 mm Hg (30). Epidemiologic studies also suggest an increase in CVD events and mortality with a blood pressure of greater than 120/70 mm Hg, and a target blood pressure of less than 130/80 mm Hg is currently recommended by the Seventh Joint National Committee on Prevention, Detection, Evaluation, and Treatment of High Blood Pressure (JNC-VII) (32) and the American Diabetes Association (ADA) (33). The treatment algorithm (Fig. 57.1) reflects the new JNC-VII treatment goal of blood pressure less than 130/80 mm Hg as well as the latest recommendations regarding drug therapy and reflects the results

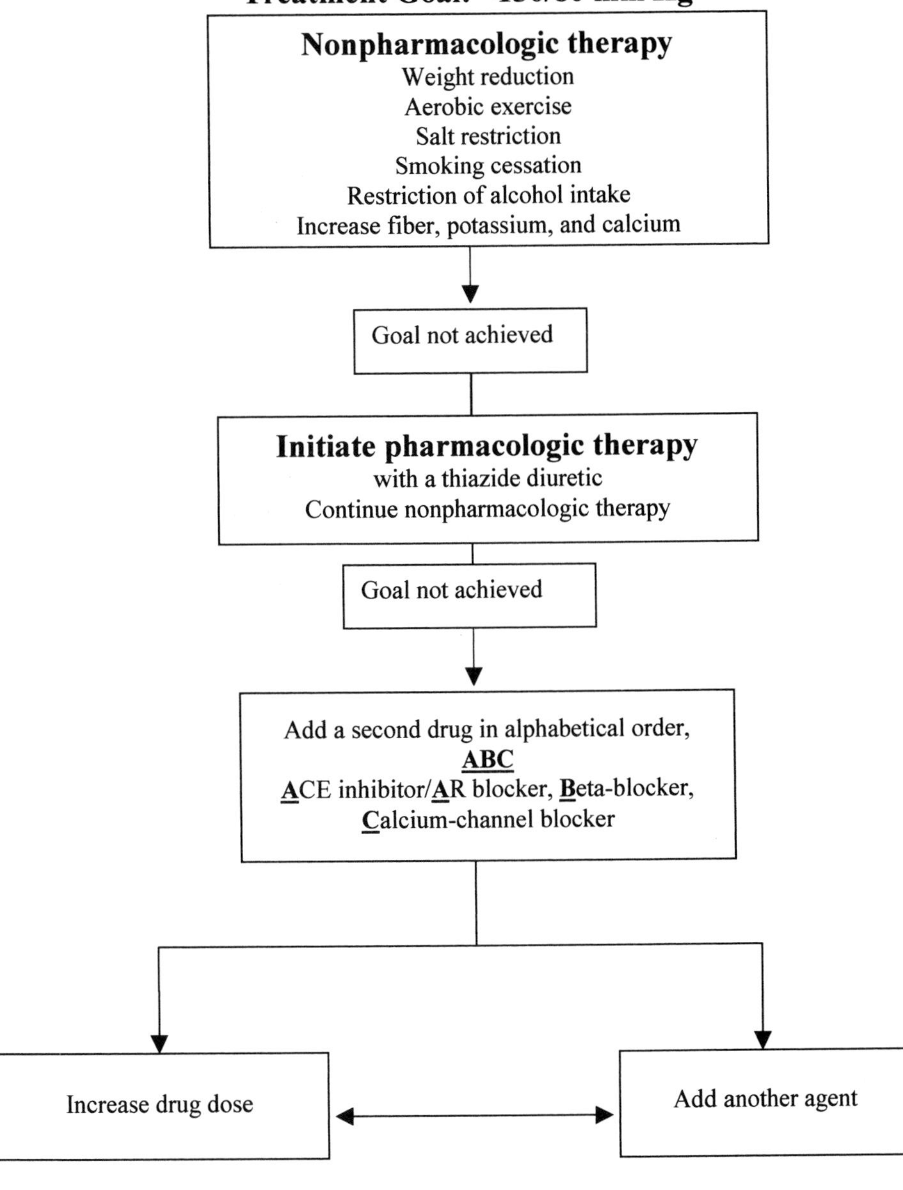

Figure 57.1. Treatment of hypertension in patients with diabetes. *In patients with >1 g proteinuria and renal insufficiency, blood pressure goal is <125/75 mm Hg. ACE, angiotensin-converting enzyme; AR, angiotensin receptor.

of the Antihypertensive and Lipid-Lowering Treatment to Prevent Heart Attack (ALLHAT) study (34,35).

TREATMENT OF HYPERTENSION IN PATIENTS WITH DIABETES

Dietary and Lifestyle Modifications

Both JNC-VII and ADA recommend lifestyle and dietary modifications as an integral part of the management of hypertension in patients with diabetes. Addressing other CVD risk factors such as smoking, inactivity, and elevated LDL-cholesterol is also emphasized (32,34). Dietary and lifestyle modifications recommended for patients with hypertension are listed in Table 57.2. Based on the results of the Dietary Approaches to Stop Hypertension (DASH) study (36), both the reduction of sodium intake to levels below the current recommendation of 100 mmol per day and the DASH diet lower blood pressure substantially, with greater effects when the combination is used (37). Dietary management and exercise in patients with diabetes should be integrated in the overall nutritional and lifestyle management of these patients.

Pharmacologic Therapy for Hypertension in Patients with Diabetes

ANGIOTENSIN-CONVERTING ENZYME INHIBITORS

ACE inhibitors were first introduced in the early 1980s as antihypertensive agents. Subsequently, their ability to attenuate albuminuria and the progression of renal disease led to their use as renoprotective agents in diabetic nephropathy (38,39); more recently, randomized controlled trials have shown that ACE inhibitors provide cardiovascular and microvascular benefits and may also improve insulin resistance and prevent the development of diabetes (40–42). These cardiovascular benefits are greater than those attributable to the decrease in blood pressure, per se, and are particularly pronounced in people with diabetes (42). In patients with type 1 diabetes and proteinuria, treatment with an ACE inhibitor was associated with a 50% reduction in the risk of the combined endpoints of death, dialysis, and transplantation (38). Furthermore, ACE inhibitors provide considerable benefits in diabetic patients with heart failure. In the Studies of Left Ventricular Dysfunction (SOLVD) trial, ACE inhibitors reduced left ventricular mass and left ventricular dilation and significantly reduced mortality and hospitalization for heart failure (43).

Treatment with ACE inhibitors is associated with cough in a substantial minority of patients (up to 15%) (44) and is probably due to the accumulation of bradykinin and related substances.

TABLE 57.2. Dietary and Lifestyle Modification in the Management of Hypertension

1. Weight loss [maintain normal body weight (BMI, 18.5–24.9)]
2. Exercise (aerobic physical activity) 30–45 min at least three times per week
3. Reduced sodium intake to 100 mmol (2.4 g) per day
4. Smoking cessation
5. Adequate intake of dietary potassium, calcium, and magnesium
6. Reduced alcohol intake to <1 oz of ethanol (24 oz of beer) per day
7. Diet rich in fruits and vegetables but low in fat

BMI, body mass index.

Angioedema is rare and unpredictable but a potentially life-threatening adverse effect, particularly if the upper airway is involved. It requires immediate discontinuation of the drug and supportive care, including airway protection (45). ACE inhibitors reduce aldosterone secretion and may cause hyperkalemia, especially at the initiation of therapy (46). This is of particular concern in patients with diabetes and in those receiving potassium-sparing diuretics. Concomitant use of thiazide or loop diuretics and dietary modification of potassium intake should allow the use of ACE inhibitors without inducing hyperkalemia. It is also important to note that, in patients with normal renal function, ACE inhibitors have little effect on glomerular filtration. However with reduction in renal function, these agents might precipitate uremia. Because of the high risk of renal failure, ACE inhibitors are also contraindicated in patients with bilateral renal-artery stenosis and unilateral stenosis in those with one kidney.

ANGIOTENSIN II RECEPTOR BLOCKERS

There are at least four types of angiotensin II receptors (ARs) (47). Of these, the AT1 receptors mediate most of the effects of angiotensin II, including vasoconstriction, aldosterone release, increased sympathetic outflow, and stimulation of sodium resorption. AR blockers selectively inhibit the binding of angiotensin II to the AT1 receptors; therefore they are also called AT1 receptor blockers (48). Unlike ACE inhibitors, AR blockers have no effects on the bradykinin system and therefore are very well tolerated, with a lower incidence of side effects such as cough (49). Angioedema may occur rarely but much less commonly than with ACE inhibitors. Although there are no specific recommendations, AR blockers should not be used in patients who developed angioedema while receiving ACE inhibitors, since angioedema is a potentially life-threatening condition (50,51). In addition, because of inhibition of aldosterone release by AR blockers, hyperkalemia is a concern, especially in those with renal insufficiency; as with ACE inhibitors, progressive azotemia and renal failure might occur in those with bilateral renal artery stenosis or those with one kidney and unilateral stenosis of the renal artery.

The JNC-VII recommended the use of AR blockers as one of several alternative first-line therapies for patients with hypertension who cannot tolerate or do not respond to the recommended first-line medications (32). In addition, AR blockers were also recommended as an initial therapy for those who could not tolerate ACE inhibitors (usually because of cough) and in whom ACE inhibitors are recommended (52), such as patients with diabetes and proteinuria, heart failure, systolic dysfunction, postmyocardial infarction, and mild renal insufficiency. However, three major studies, the Reduction of Endpoints in NIDDM with the Angiotensin II Antagonist Losartan (RENAAL) study (53), the Irbesartan Microalbuminuria Type 2 Diabetes in Hypertensive Patients (IRMA II) study (54), and the Irbesartan in Diabetic Nephropathy Trial (IDNT) (55), showed that AR blockers are effective in reducing the progression of renal disease in patients with type 2 diabetes and hypertension. Blood pressure control was similar in the placebo- and AR blocker–treated groups, indicating that AR blockers protect the kidney independent of blood pressure reduction. In the RENAAL trial, the risk of the primary endpoint (a composite of doubling of serum creatinine, end-stage renal disease, or death from any cause) was reduced by 16% with losartan. The risk of doubling of serum creatinine was reduced by 25% and the risk of end-stage renal disease was reduced by 28% over a follow-up period of 3.4 years (53). The study also documented reduction in the initial hospitalization for heart failure. In the Losartan Intervention for Endpoint Reduction in Hypertension (LIFE trial) study (56), losartan resulted in a statistically greater reduction in CVD morbidity and mortality in diabetic patients with hypertension and LVH than did atenolol. Losartan especially reduced the incidence of fatal and nonfatal strokes by 25%, major causes of death and disability in diabetic patients. Finally, in the LIFE trial, losartan reduced the new onset of diabetes by 25% compared with atenolol. These benefits were above and beyond those attributable to blood pressure reduction alone. On the basis of this evidence and because of the better tolerability, AR blockers are recommended as a first-line therapy for patients with diabetes and hypertension, along with ACE inhibitors.

β-BLOCKERS

β-Blockers are very useful antihypertensive agents in the treatment of hypertension in patients with diabetes (2). In the UKPDS study, atenolol reduced microvascular complications of diabetes by 37%, strokes by 44%, and death related to diabetes by 32%. In that study the efficacy of the β-blocker atenolol was equal to that of the ACE inhibitor captopril in reducing the microvascular and macrovascular complications of diabetes, most probably secondary to their ability to modulate the renin-angiotensin-aldosterone system. In a nonrandomized study, hypertensive patients receiving a β-blocker had a 28% higher risk of diabetes than did those receiving no medication. In contrast, patients with hypertension who received thiazide diuretics, ACE inhibitors, or calcium-channel blockers were found to be at no greater risk for subsequent development of diabetes than were patients receiving no medication (3). However increased risk for the development of diabetes with β-blocker therapy was not found in other randomized studies (57). Despite the potentially adverse metabolic effects of β-blockers, they have proved to have significant long-term favorable effects on CVD in hypertensive patients with diabetes and, therefore, should be used in patients with diabetes, particularly those with coronary disease.

CALCIUM-CHANNEL BLOCKERS

For patients to achieve a target blood pressure of 130/80 mm Hg, clinical studies suggest that at least 65% of them require two or more different antihypertensive agents (58–60). In patients with diabetes, additional therapies beside ACE inhibitors and diuretics may include a long-acting calcium-channel blocker (CCB) (25). A nondihydropyridine CCB such as verapamil or diltiazem may have greater beneficial effects on proteinuria than a dihydropyridine CCB such as nifedipine (61). However, with the use of an ACE inhibitor (or an AR blocker) as a first-line treatment, together with a diuretic, the addition of a long-acting dihydropyridine such as amlodipine, nifedipine, or felodipine will reduce both proteinuria and the rate of CVD events. If the blood pressure goal is still not achieved, a low-dose β-blocker or an α/β-blocker can be added. It is important to note that the Appropriate Blood Pressure Control in Diabetes (ABCD) trial demonstrated that ACE inhibitors were superior to CCBs in reducing CVD events; however, these differences are likely the result of the beneficial effects of ACE inhibitors rather than a negative effect of the CCBs, and the use of these agents is particularly helpful in achieving the target blood pressure, especially in patients with isolated systolic blood pressure not responding to the addition of a low-dose diuretic (62).

DIURETICS

The Antihypertensive and Lipid-Lowering Treatment to Prevent Heart Attack Trial (ALLHAT) was designed to determine whether treatment with a CCB or an ACE inhibitor lowers the incidence of coronary heart disease (CHD) or other CVD events compared with treatment with a diuretic (35). Of a total of 33,357 participants aged 55 years or older with hypertension and at least one other CHD risk factor, 15,297 had diabetes (36.0% of the entire cohort) (63). Of these individuals, 50.2% were male, 39.4% were African American, and 17.7% were Hispanic. The diabetic cohort in ALLHAT provided valuable information about the treatment of hypertension in older diabetic patients at risk for incident CVD. Thiazide-type diuretics were effective as part of combined therapy that reduced stroke. Therefore, they are recommended as preferred antihypertensive therapy (Fig. 57.1). Diuretics have generally been shown to prevent CVD complications and usually enhance the antihypertensive efficacy of a multidrug regimen, as indicated in Figure 57.1.

FIXED-DOSE COMBINATIONS

The use of fixed-dose combination therapy has the potential of enhancing compliance and reducing side effects and the cost of medications (64). Several diuretic-based combinations are available, including one with a β-blocker, one with an ACE inhibitor, and one with an AR blocker. The use of these agents is increasing (65). Other useful fixed-dose combinations include ACE inhibitors and calcium antagonists. These combination medications have the potential to improve control and compliance (2,64,65).

NEED FOR MULTIPLE MEDICATIONS

To achieve the recommended target blood pressure of 130/80 mm Hg, patients with hypertension and diabetes will need two or more drugs. Data from our group and others indicate that multiple medications are usually necessary to achieve such a goal (58–60). Addition of a second drug from a different class should be initiated when use of a single drug in adequate doses fails to achieve the blood pressure goal. The JNC-VII recommends initiation of therapy with two drugs when blood pressure is 20/10 mm Hg above goal (32). This will probably increase the likelihood of achieving the blood pressure goal.

REFERENCES

1. Haffner SM, Lehto S, Ronnemaa T, et al. Mortality from coronary heart disease in subjects with type 2 diabetes and in nondiabetic subjects with and without prior myocardial infarction. *N Engl J Med* 1998;339:229–234.
2. Sowers JR, Epstein M, Frohlich ED. Diabetes, hypertension, and cardiovascular disease: an update. *Hypertension* 2001;37:1053–1059.
3. Gress TW, Nieto J, Shahar E, et al. Hypertension and antihypertensive therapy as risk factors for type 2 diabetes mellitus. *N Engl J Med* 2000;342:905–912.
4. Ferrannini E, Buzzigoli G, Bonadonna R, et al. Insulin resistance in essential hypertension. *N Engl J Med* 1987;317:350–357.
5. Shen DC, Shieh SM, Fuh MM, et al. Resistance to insulin-stimulated-glucose uptake in patients with hypertension. *J Clin Endocrinol Metab* 1988;66:580–583.
6. Kotchen TA, Zhang HY, Covelli M, et al. Insulin resistance and blood pressure in Dahl rats and in one-kidney, one-clip hypertensive rats. *Am J Physiol* 1991;261:E692–E697.
7. Reaven GM, Chang H. Relationship between blood pressure, plasma insulin and triglyceride concentration, and insulin action in spontaneous hypertensive and Wistar-Kyoto rats. *Am J Hypertens* 1991;4:34–38.
8. Sechi LA, Melis A, Tedde R. Insulin hypersecretion: a distinctive feature between essential and secondary hypertension. *Metabolism* 1992;41:1261–1266.
9. Beatty OL, Harper R, Sheridan B, et al. Insulin resistance in offspring of hypertensive parents. *BMJ* 1993;307:92–96.
10. Grunfeld B, Balzareti M, Romo M, et al. Hyperinsulinemia in normotensive offspring of hypertensive parents. *Hypertension* 1994;23:I12–I15.
11. Semplicini A, Ceolotto G, Massimino M, et al. Interactions between insulin and sodium homeostasis in essential hypertension. *Am J Med Sci* 1994;307 [Suppl 1]:S43–S46.
12. Weinberger MH. Salt sensitive human hypertension. *Endocr Res* 1991;17:43–51.
13. Luft FC, Miller JZ, Grim CE, et al. Salt sensitivity and resistance of blood pressure. Age and race as factors in physiological responses. *Hypertension* 1991; 7:I102–I108.
14. Weinberger MH, Fineberg NS. Sodium and volume sensitivity of blood pressure. Age and pressure change over time. *Hypertension* 1991;18:67–71.
15. Verdecchia P, Porcellati C, Schillaci G, et al. Ambulatory blood pressure. An independent predictor of prognosis in essential hypertension. *Hypertension* 1994;24:793–801.

16. Nakano S, Kitazawa M, Tsuda S, et al. Insulin resistance is associated with reduced nocturnal falls of blood pressure in normotensive, nonobese type 2 diabetic subjects. *Clin Exp Hypertens* 2002;24:65–73.
17. Nielsen FS, Hansen HP, Jacobsen P, et al. Increased sympathetic activity during sleep and nocturnal hypertension in type 2 diabetic patients with diabetic nephropathy. *Diabet Med* 1999;16:555–562.
18. Ohkubo T, Hozawa A, Yamaguchi J, et al. Prognostic significance of the nocturnal decline in blood pressure in individuals with and without high 24-h blood pressure: the Ohasama study. *J Hypertens* 2002;20:2183–2189.
19. White WB. A chronotherapeutic approach to the management of hypertension. *Am J Hypertens* 1996;9:29S–33S.
20. Arun CS, Stoddart J, Mackin P, et al. Significance of microalbuminuria in long-duration type 1 diabetes. *Diabetes Care* 2003;26:2144–2149.
21. McFarlane SI, Banerji M, Sowers JR. Insulin resistance and cardiovascular disease. *J Clin Endocrinol Metab* 2001;86:713–718.
22. Mitchell TH, Nolan B, Henry M, et al. Microalbuminuria in patients with non-insulin-dependent diabetes mellitus relates to nocturnal systolic blood pressure. *Am J Med* 1997;102:531–535.
23. Mogensen CE. Microalbuminuria and hypertension with focus on type 1 and type 2 diabetes. *J Intern Med* 2003;254:45–66.
24. Tagle R, Acevedo M, Vidt DG. Microalbuminuria: is it a valid predictor of cardiovascular risk? *Cleve Clin J Med* 2003;70:255–261.
25. McFarlane SI, Farag A, Sowers J. Calcium antagonists in patients with type 2 diabetes and hypertension. *Cardiovasc Drug Rev* 2003;21:105–118.
26. Streeten DH, Anderson GH Jr. The role of delayed orthostatic hypotension in the pathogenesis of chronic fatigue. *Clin Auton Res* 1998;8:119–124.
27. Streeten DH, Auchincloss JH Jr, Anderson GH Jr, et al. Orthostatic hypertension. Pathogenetic studies. *Hypertension* 1985;7:196–203.
28. Jacob G, Costa F, Biaggioni I. Spectrum of autonomic cardiovascular neuropathy in diabetes. *Diabetes Care* 2003;26:2174–2180.
29. Streeten DH. Pathogenesis of hyperadrenergic orthostatic hypotension. Evidence of disordered venous innervation exclusively in the lower limbs. *J Clin Invest* 1990;86:1582–1588.
30. Hansson L, Zanchetti A, Carruthers SG, et al. Effects of intensive blood-pressure lowering and low-dose aspirin in patients with hypertension: principal results of the Hypertension Optimal Treatment (HOT) randomised trial. HOT Study Group. *Lancet* 1998;351:1755–1762.
31. Tight blood pressure control and risk of macrovascular and microvascular complications in type 2 diabetes: UKPDS 38. UK Prospective Diabetes Study Group. *BMJ* 1998;317:703–713.
32. Chobanian AV, Bakris GL, Black HR, et al. The Seventh Report of the Joint National Committee on Prevention, Detection, Evaluation, and Treatment of High Blood Pressure: the JNC 7 report. *JAMA* 2003;289:2560–2572.
33. Arauz-Pacheco C, Parrott MA, Raskin P. Treatment of hypertension in adults with diabetes. *Diabetes Care* 2003;26[Suppl 1]:S80–S82.
34. Bakris GL, Williams M, Dworkin L, et al. Preserving renal function in adults with hypertension and diabetes: a consensus approach. National Kidney Foundation Hypertension and Diabetes Executive Committees Working Group. *Am J Kidney Dis* 2000;36:646–661.
35. Major outcomes in high-risk hypertensive patients randomized to angiotensin-converting enzyme inhibitor or calcium channel blocker vs diuretic: The Antihypertensive and Lipid-Lowering Treatment to Prevent Heart Attack Trial (ALLHAT). *JAMA* 2002;288:2981–2997.
36. Sacks FM, Svetkey LP, Vollmer WM, et al. Effects on blood pressure of reduced dietary sodium and the Dietary Approaches to Stop Hypertension (DASH) diet. DASH-Sodium Collaborative Research Group. *N Engl J Med* 2001;344:3–10.
37. Conlin PR, Chow D, Miller ER 3rd, et al. The effect of dietary patterns on blood pressure control in hypertensive patients: results from the Dietary Approaches to Stop Hypertension (DASH) trial. *Am J Hypertens* 2000;13:949–955.
38. Lewis EJ, Hunsicker LG, Bain RP, et al. The effect of angiotensin-converting-enzyme inhibition on diabetic nephropathy. The Collaborative Study Group. *N Engl J Med* 1993;329:1456–1462.
39. Bakris GL, Sowers JR. Microalbuminuria in diabetes: focus on cardiovascular and renal risk reduction. *Curr Diab Rep* 2002;2:258–262.
40. McFarlane SI, Kumar A, Sowers JR. Mechanisms by which angiotensin-converting enzyme inhibitors prevent diabetes and cardiovascular disease. *Am J Cardiol* 2003;91:30H–37H.
41. McFarlane SI, Shin JJ, Rundek T, et al. Prevention of type 2 diabetes. *Curr Diab Rep* 2003;3:235–241.
42. Heart Outcomes Prevention Evaluation Study Investigators. Effects of ramipril on cardiovascular and microvascular outcomes in people with diabetes mellitus: results of the HOPE study and MICRO-HOPE substudy. *Lancet* 2000;355:253–259.
43. Shindler DM, Kostis JB, Yusuf S, et al. Diabetes mellitus, a predictor of morbidity and mortality in the Studies of Left Ventricular Dysfunction (SOLVD) trials and registry. *Am J Cardiol* 1996;77:1017–1020.
44. Malini PL, Strocchi E, Fiumi N, et al. ACE inhibitor-induced cough in hypertensive type 2 diabetic patients. *Diabetes Care* 1999;22:1586–1587.
45. Sabroe RA, Black AK. Angiotensin-converting enzyme (ACE) inhibitors and angio-oedema. *Br J Dermatol* 1997;136:153–158.
46. McFarlane SI, Sowers JR. Cardiovascular endocrinology: 1. Aldosterone function in diabetes mellitus: effects on cardiovascular and renal disease. *J Clin Endocrinol Metab* 2003;88:516–523.
47. Unger T, Chung O, Csikos T, et al. Angiotensin receptors. *J Hypertens Suppl* 1996;14:S95–S103.
48. Stanton A. Potential of renin inhibition in cardiovascular disease. *J Renin Angiotensin Aldosterone Syst* 2003;4:6–10.
49. Rake EC, Breeze E, Fletcher AE. Quality of life and cough on antihypertensive treatment: a randomised trial of eprosartan, enalapril and placebo. *J Hum Hypertens* 2001;15:863–867.
50. Gavras I, Gavras H. Are patients who develop angioedema with ACE inhibition at risk of the same problem with AT1 receptor blockers? *Arch Intern Med* 2003;163:240–241.
51. MacLean JA, Hannaway PJ. Angioedema and AT1 receptor blockers: proceed with caution. *Arch Intern Med* 2003;163:1488–1489.
52. Kendall MJ. Therapeutic advantages of AT1 blockers in hypertension. *Basic Res Cardiol* 1998;93[Suppl 2]:47–50.
53. Brenner BM, Cooper ME, de Zeeuw D, et al. Effects of losartan on renal and cardiovascular outcomes in patients with type 2 diabetes and nephropathy. *N Engl J Med* 2001;345:861–869.
54. Parving HH, Lehnert H, Brochner-Mortensen J, et al. The effect of irbesartan on the development of diabetic nephropathy in patients with type 2 diabetes. *N Engl J Med* 2001;345:870–878.
55. Lewis EJ, Hunsicker LG, Clarke WR, et al. Renoprotective effect of the angiotensin-receptor antagonist irbesartan in patients with nephropathy due to type 2 diabetes. *N Engl J Med* 2001;345:851–860.
56. Lindholm LH, Ibsen H, Dahlof B, et al. Cardiovascular morbidity and mortality in patients with diabetes in the Losartan Intervention For Endpoint reduction in hypertension study (LIFE): a randomised trial against atenolol. *Lancet* 2002;359:1004–1010.
57. Kaplan NM. Management of hypertension in patients with type 2 diabetes mellitus: guidelines based on current evidence. *Ann Intern Med* 2001;135:1079–1083.
58. McFarlane SI, Jacober SJ, Winer N, et al. Control of cardiovascular risk factors in patients with diabetes and hypertension at urban academic medical centers. *Diabetes Care* 2002;25:718–723.
59. Cushman WC, Ford CE, Cutler JA, et al. Success and predictors of blood pressure control in diverse North American settings: the Antihypertensive and Lipid-Lowering Treatment to Prevent Heart Attack Trial (ALLHAT). *J Clin Hypertens* (Greenwich) 2002;4:393–405.
60. Black HR, Elliott WJ, Neaton JD, et al. Baseline characteristics and early blood pressure control in the CONVINCE trial. *Hypertension* 2001;37:12–18.
61. Staessen JA, Wang JG, Thijs L. Calcium-channel blockade and cardiovascular prognosis: recent evidence from clinical outcome trials. *Am J Hypertens* 2002;15:85S–93S.
62. Schrier RW, Estacio RO. Additional follow-up from the ABCD trial in patients with type 2 diabetes and hypertension. *N Engl J Med* 2000;343:1969.
63. Barzilay JI, Jones CL, Davis BR, et al. Baseline characteristics of the diabetic participants in the Antihypertensive and Lipid-Lowering Treatment to Prevent Heart Attack Trial (ALLHAT). *Diabetes Care* 2001;24:654–658.
64. Bakris GL, Weir MR. Achieving goal blood pressure in patients with type 2 diabetes: conventional versus fixed-dose combination approaches. *J Clin Hypertens* (Greenwich) 2003;5:202–209.
65. Law MR, Wald NJ, Morris JK, et al. Value of low dose combination treatment with blood pressure lowering drugs: analysis of 354 randomised trials. *BMJ* 2003;326:1427.

CHAPTER 58

Diabetes Mellitus and Heart Disease

Michael T. Johnstone and Richard Nesto

Heart disease was thought to be associated with diabetes as early as 1883, when Vergeley recommended testing the urine of patients with angina for glucose (1). However, as more patients with diabetes survived following the discovery of insulin and improvements in treatments for renal failure and infection, there was a marked increase in morbidity and mortality from cardiovascular disease. Diabetes is the seventh leading cause of death in the United States, with much of that mortality a result of cardiovascular disease (2). However, because these statistics are based on the underlying cause of death, they underestimate the true impact of diabetes on mortality.

Ultimately, atherosclerosis accounts for 65% to 80% of all deaths among North American patients with diabetes, compared with one third of all deaths in the general North American population (3–5). A two- to fourfold excess in mortality due to coronary artery disease (CAD) among individuals with diabetes has been noted in a number of prospective studies encompassing a variety of ethnic and racial groups (6). Diabetes also increases the likelihood of severe carotid atherosclerosis (7,8), and mortality from stroke is increased almost threefold in patients with diabetes (9). Both type 1 and type 2 diabetes are therefore powerful and independent risk factors for CAD, stroke, and peripheral arterial disease (3,9,10). Furthermore, when patients with diabetes develop clinical events, they sustain a worse prognosis than patients without diabetes (11). Coupled with these macrovascular complications are such microvascular complications as retinopathy, neuropathy, and nephropathy, all of which account for most of the morbidity and mortality associated with diabetes mellitus. Although diabetes may be a problem of glucose metabolism, the American Heart Association (AHA) has recently stated that "diabetes is a cardiovascular disease" (3).

EPIDEMIOLOGY

More than 10 million Americans carry the diagnosis of diabetes mellitus, and another 5 million are estimated to have undiagnosed diabetes (3). The prevalence of type 2 diabetes, which accounts for 90% of all cases of diabetes, is increasing in the United States and around the world because of the advancing age of the population, improved screening and detection, and the increase in risk factors such as obesity and physical inactivity. A growing ethnic diversity in the United States, including ethnic groups particularly susceptible to type 2 diabetes such as Hispanics, blacks, and South Asians, also contribute to the increasing prevalence of type 2 diabetes (3,12). The obesity epidemic will result in an increasing number of patients with diabetes. In 1998, obesity affected 18% of the U.S. population (13). The problem of obesity is anticipated to grow with the increasing weight of the U.S. population. Between 1991 and 1998, the body weight of the American male increased by 3% and that of the American female increased by 5%.

Diabetes and Cardiovascular Mortality

A meta-analysis of several studies estimated the risk of death from CAD in patients with diabetes at 2.58 in men and 1.85 in women (14). These values are in contrast with those from the Rancho Bernardo Study (15), which followed subjects aged 40 to 79 for 14 years and found that while death rates were also increased in subjects with diabetes, the risk factor–adjusted relative odds were 3.3 in women and 1.9 in men. Factors associated with an increase in mortality rates among those with diabetes include male gender, black race, longer duration of diabetes, and insulin use (16). Overall, cardiovascular disease, which includes coronary artery and cerebrovascular disease, accounts for 65% of all deaths among persons with diabetes. Although much of these data are based on findings in patients with type 2 diabetes, patients with type 1 diabetes have similar causes of death, including CAD and renal failure (17,18).

Life expectancy is shortened, with diabetic males living, on average, 9.1 years less and diabetic females living 6.7 years less than their nondiabetic counterparts (19). Haffner and colleagues examined the mortality among 1,000 persons with type 2 diabetes and 1,300 subjects without diabetes and found that the mortality of those with diabetes was similar to that for those without diabetes who had a myocardial infarction (MI) (20) (Fig. 58.1). These data suggest that caregivers should treat individuals with type 2 diabetes as if they had experienced an MI. Mukamal et al. (21) studied 1,935 patients hospitalized with an acute MI and found that the mortality among those with diabetes in the short-term period was similar to that of the patients without diabetes who had an MI previously and twice that of patients without diabetes who had suffered their first acute coronary event. Malmberg et al. (22) evaluated the findings of the OASIS (Organization to Assess Strategies for Ischemic Syndromes) registry and found that patients with diabetes hospitalized for unstable angina or non–Q-wave MI had the same long-term morbidity and mortality as patients without diabetes with established cardiovascular disease.

Over the past three decades, there have been significant decreases in cardiovascular mortality in the United States. However, the effect on mortality in patients with diabetes has lagged well behind that in the general population (23). The death rate among nondiabetic men with CAD decreased by 36.4% as compared to a decrease of 13.1% for diabetic men, and the death rate among nondiabetic women decreased by 27% as compared to an increase of 23% among diabetic women (23).

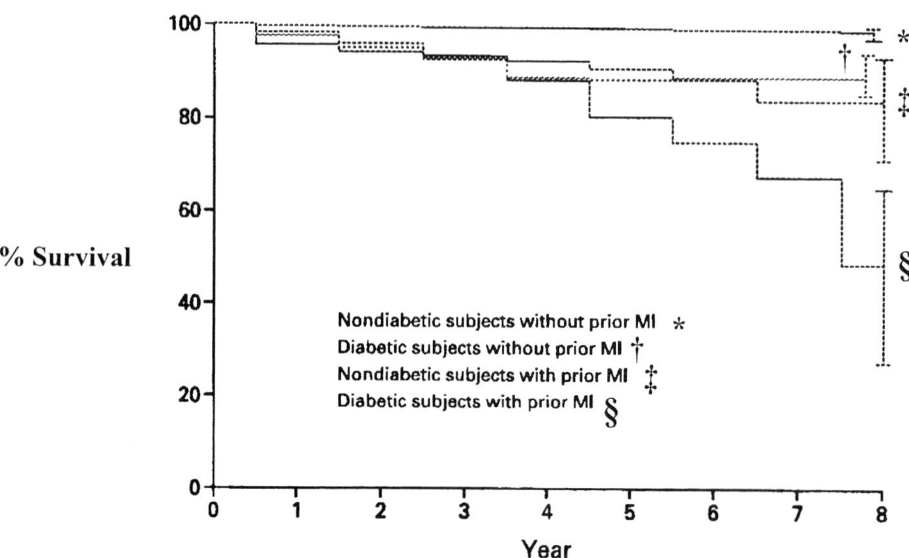

Figure 58.1. Kaplan-Meier estimates of the probability of death from coronary heart disease in 1,059 subjects with type 2 diabetes and 1,378 nondiabetic subjects with and without prior myocardial infarction (MI). Error bars denote 95% confidence intervals. (From Haffner SM, Lehto S, Ronnemaa T, et al. Mortality from coronary heart disease in subjects with type 2 diabetes and in nondiabetic subjects with and without prior myocardial infarction. *N Engl J Med* 1998; 339:229–324, with permission. Copyright © 1998 Massachusetts Medical Society. All rights reserved.)

Prevalence and Risk Factors for Coronary Artery Disease in Type 1 Diabetes

Long-term follow-up of patients with type 1 diabetes has demonstrated that the first cases of clinically manifest CAD occur late in the third decade or in the fourth decade of life regardless of whether diabetes developed early in childhood or during late adolescence. CAD risk increases rapidly after the age of 40, and by the age of 55 years, 35% of men and women with type 1 diabetes die of CAD (18) compared with 8% of those without diabetes. Women with type 1 diabetes lose most of the inherent protection from CAD observed in women without diabetes (18,24,25). The occurrence of severe coronary atherosclerosis before the age of 55 in a subset of patients with type 1 diabetes regardless of whether diabetes developed in childhood or adolescence suggests that diabetes mainly accelerates the progression of early atherosclerotic lesions that commonly occur, even in the absence of diabetes, at a young age in the general population (18).

Diabetic nephropathy, which develops in approximately 30% to 40% of patients with type 1 diabetes, dramatically increases the prevalence of CAD (18,26). Patients with persistent proteinuria who were followed in the Steno Memorial Hospital had a 37-fold increased mortality from cardiovascular disease relative to that of the general population, while patients without proteinuria had a cardiovascular mortality that was only 4.2 times higher (26). Patients with type 1 diabetes followed from the onset of microalbuminuria developed CAD eight times more frequently than patients without microalbuminuria (27). Krolewski et al. (17) reported that the risk of development of CAD in patients with persistent proteinuria was 15 times higher than the risk among those without proteinuria. Angiographic studies have shown that almost all patients with diabetic nephropathy older than age 45 have one or more clinically significant coronary stenoses (28). Microalbuminuria in type 1 diabetes is therefore not only a marker for renal disease but also a potent marker of CAD risk.

Several mechanisms contribute to the atherosclerotic process in the presence of diabetic nephropathy, including hypertension, lipid abnormalities, fibrinolysis, and coagulation alterations, all of which are detectable in the early stages of diabetic nephropathy when renal function is still normal (29). Hypertension is frequently present in patients with diabetic nephropathy even when the creatinine concentrations remain normal and can intensify CAD in patients with type 1 diabetes. Diabetic nephropathy is associated with an atherogenic lipoprotein profile that includes elevated levels of low-density lipoprotein (LDL) and very-low-density lipoprotein (VLDL), decreased levels of high-density lipoprotein (HDL), and elevated [Lp(a)] levels of lipoprotein a (30–32). Furthermore, a hypercoagulable state characterized by increased levels of plasminogen-activator inhibitor-1 (PAI-1), factor VII, and (plasma) fibrinogen, has been described in microalbuminuric patients with type 1 diabetes (33). Finally, reduced renal function leads to the accumulation of advanced glycosylation end products (AGEs) in the circulation and tissue (34,35).

The risk for the development of diabetic nephropathy is only partially determined by glycemic control and is highly influenced by genetic susceptibility (26,27). Several studies have established that a genetic susceptibility contributes to the high prevalence of CAD among patients with type 1 diabetes with nephropathy. CAD is twice as common a cause of death among parents of diabetic patients with nephropathy than among parents of diabetic patients without nephropathy. Among patients with diabetes with nephropathy, those who had a cardiovascular event are six times more likely than patients who did not have such an event to have a familial history of cardiovascular disease. A history of cardiovascular disease in both parents or in the father of a patient with type 1 diabetes increases the risk of nephropathy in the offspring tenfold and threefold, respectively (36). Parents of diabetic offspring with nephropathy also have higher blood pressure than parents whose diabetic offspring do not have diabetic nephropathy (37).

Interestingly, recent studies have shown that an association between the angiotensin-converting enzyme insertion/deletion (ACE I/D) polymorphism, potentially affecting the level of angiotensins and kinins in the kidney, can affect the development of renal disease in patients with type 1 diabetes (38). The same polymorphism has been linked to MI in patients without diabetes (39), as well as in patients with type 1 diabetes (40,41) and type 2 diabetes (42).

Prevalence and Risk Factors for Coronary Artery Disease in Type 2 Diabetes

Type 2 diabetes increases relative risk of cardiovascular disease two- to fourfold compared with the risk in the general population (43–46). The increase in cardiovascular risk is particularly high in women. The protection against atherosclerosis in premenopausal women is almost completely lost in women with diabetes (47,48).

While traditional risk factors play an important role in the development of atherosclerosis in subjects with diabetes, the rate of cardiovascular mortality and morbidity in persons with diabetes exceeds by 50% the rate predicted by these risk factors. Several other risk factors may account for this discrepancy. Possible nontraditional risk factors include insulin resistance, insulin levels, and hyperglycemia.

Many of these patients with type 2 diabetes have several of these risk factors for CAD. The term *metabolic syndrome* was first used by Gerald Reaven in 1988 (49) to describe this clustering of risk factors including hypertension, dyslipidemia, hyperglycemia, and insulin resistance. The National Cholesterol Education Program Adult Treatment Panel III (ATPIII) guidelines for cholesterol management in 2001 recognized that the metabolic syndrome is a collection of the risk factors mentioned above, as well as abdominal obesity (50).

PATHOPHYSIOLOGY OF DIABETIC CARDIOVASCULAR COMPLICATIONS

The increased risk of cardiovascular disease in individuals with diabetes is explained in part by the clustering of risk factors, including dyslipidemia, hypertension, hyperglycemia, hyperinsulinemia, and prothrombotic factors. Some of these risk factors are described in detail subsequently.

Insulin Levels, Insulin Resistance, and Hyperglycemia

Insulin resistance that is present many years or more before the clinical onset of overt diabetes resistance is associated with other atherogenic risk factors, such as hypertension, lipid abnormalities, and a procoagulant state (51–57) (Table 58.1) that promotes atherosclerosis many years before overt hyperglycemia ensues (58,59). Indeed, several studies have shown an inverse correlation between insulin sensitivity and atherosclerosis (60–62). Investigators using the Bruneck Study database suggest (63) that these risk factors are present in 84% of patients with type 2 diabetes. Thus, an increased prevalence of CAD is apparent in patients with impaired glucose tolerance (44,46,64)

TABLE 58.1. Cardiovascular Risk Factors Associated with Insulin Resistance

Hypertension (51,52)
Abdominal obesity (53,57)
Dyslipidemia (54–56,281)
  Increased very-low-density lipoprotein–triglyceride
  Decreased high-density lipoprotein
  Small dense atherogenic low-density lipoprotein particles
  Postprandial lipemia
Elevated PAI-1 activity (58)

PAI-1, plasminogen activator inhibitor-1.
From Aronson D, Johnstone MT. Coronary artery disease in diabetes. In: Johnstone MT, Veves A. *Diabetes and cardiovascular disease.* Totowa, NJ: Humana Press, 2001. Reprinted with permission from Humana Press.

and in those with newly diagnosed type 2 diabetes (65,66). The duration of insulin resistance among hyperglycemic and diabetic individuals probably contributes to the development of atherosclerosis. However, no obvious association between the extent or severity of macrovascular complications and the duration or severity of type 2 diabetes (24,67) has been found, most likely because the duration of insulin resistance is often unknown.

Another possibility is that the serum insulin level and not insulin resistance has direct cardiovascular effects. Despres and colleagues (68) followed 2,000 diabetic men without clinically overt CAD for 5 years and found that those who had a cardiovascular event had serum insulin levels that were 18% higher than those in controls.

Serum glucose levels may be an important risk factor for cardiovascular disease. Andersson and Svardsudd (69) demonstrated that fasting serum glucose levels are independently related to all-cause and cardiovascular mortality. The San Antonio Heart Study (70) showed similar findings for subjects in the highest quartile of fasting glucose levels, who had a 4.7 times greater risk of cardiovascular disease than did those in the first two quartile levels combined.

The direct relationship between glucose levels and cardiovascular disease also is seen in patients with type 1 diabetes. A 1% increase in levels of glycosylated hemoglobin doubled the increase in cardiovascular disease (71). Several studies have shown a direct relationship with the serum glucose levels on clinical events, including MI and strokes, with glucose levels ranging from an abnormal glucose tolerance test to frank diabetes (72–74). This graded effect of serum glucose levels on clinical events may be due in part to a direct effect on the vasculature, as evidenced by a similar direct relationship of serum glucose levels to the intima-media thickness of the carotid (as a marker for the presence and degree of atherosclerosis). The Atherosclerosis Risk in Communities (ARIC) study demonstrated that fasting glucose tolerance was directly related to carotid wall thickness in individuals free of symptomatic cardiovascular disease (8).

The level of chronic hyperglycemia, as determined by measurements of glycosylated hemoglobin, may also be an independent risk factor for coronary heart disease, particularly in women (75,76). Recent prospective studies demonstrated that microalbuminuria in patients with type 2 diabetes is also an independent predictor of increased cardiovascular mortality (77,78). Insulin resistance may play an important role as a risk factor in the development of diabetic cardiovascular disease. Hyperinsulinemia may be the mechanism by which the effect of hyperglycemia results in atherosclerosis. Insulin level is elevated in patients with the metabolic syndrome. The possibility that insulin resistance could result in an increase in cardiovascular disease was first demonstrated in population studies that showed an association between fasting insulin levels and cardiovascular mortality (60,79–81). In the Insulin Resistance Atherosclerosis Study, subjects were evenly divided among patients with normal serum glucose, hyperglycemia with normal glucose tolerance, and diabetes. The relationship of insulin levels and cardiovascular disease is further strengthened by basic research studies that showed the effect of insulin on various possible mediators for the development of atherosclerosis, specifically the increase in PAI-1 and the mitogenic effect on smooth muscle cells *in vitro* (82).

Dyslipidemia

An important mechanism for the development of diabetic atherosclerosis is dyslipidemia. The central feature of diabetic dyslipidemia is increased levels of VLDL due both to increased production of VLDL and to decreased catabolism of triglyceride-rich lipoproteins, including chylomicrons. The increase in hepatic production of VLDL occurs in response to increased delivery of fatty acids from (a) decreased free fatty acid uptake from the striated muscle and (b) increased delivery of the free fatty acids from the increased adipose tissue associated with central obesity.

The increase in triglyceride-rich lipoproteins accumulates not only because of increased VLDL production but also because of decreased catabolism of triglyceride lipoproteins. Lipoprotein lipase, which plays an important role in the metabolism of triglyceride-rich lipoproteins and in particular chylomicrons, is decreased in uncontrolled type 2 diabetes.

The increased level of triglyceride-rich lipoproteins provides an increase in substrate for the cholesterol ester transfer protein. This promotes the flux of cholesterol from HDL particles, which results in decreased HDL levels, a common finding in type 2 diabetes. Yet other mechanisms must be involved, because low HDL levels can occur in the absence of hypertriglyceridemia. The degree of HDL reduction is not related to the degree of control of diabetes or to the mode of treatment in type 2 diabetes. One mechanism of the protective effect of HDL against atherosclerosis may be its ability to prevent oxidation of LDL. There may be qualitative differences in HDL from patients with poorly controlled diabetes that may make it a less effective antioxidant than HDL from normal individuals (83).

Although the dyslipidemia of diabetes is not characterized by marked elevations of LDL, there are differences in the LDL type found in patients with type 2 diabetes. Specifically, the LDL is smaller and denser than typical LDL particles (84). These smaller, denser LDL particles have a greater tendency to undergo oxidation, which accelerates the atherosclerotic process.

Increased Oxidative Stress in Diabetes

There is recent evidence that increased oxidative stress in diabetes contributes to the development of diabetic complications (85). This increased stress may be due in part to the decreased availability of antioxidants such as ascorbic acid, vitamin E, uric acid, and glutathionine. In addition, there may be an increase in lipid peroxidation products and superoxide anion products, which may lead to altered vascular function (85–87).

The increase in oxidative stress may be the result of several pathways, including advanced glycation end product (AGE) production; small, dense LDL formation; altered polyol activity; or imbalance in the redox state (88). The activation of this polyol pathway is due to the conversion of glucose to sorbitol via aldolase reductase, which has been associated with microvascular complications (89,90).

The recent data from the Heart Outcomes Prevention Evaluation (HOPE) study have shown that treatment with the antioxidant vitamin E at 400 IU per day for a mean of 4.5 years had no apparent effect on cardiovascular morbidity or mortality in both diabetics and nondiabetics (91). King's group has had rather intriguing results demonstrating that therapy with high doses of vitamin E (1800 IU per day) normalizes retinal hemodynamic abnormalities and improves renal function without improving glycemic control in patients with type 1 diabetes of short duration (92). Whether this effect is via antioxidant-dependent or -independent pathways remains to be elucidated.

Oxidative stress also precedes the formation of some AGEs, including pentosidine and *N*-ε-carboxymethyllysine (CML), and the activation of the diacylglycerol–protein kinase C (DAG-PKC) pathway.

Advanced Glycation End Products in Diabetes

AGEs occur as a result of the nonenzymatic glycation of both lipids and proteins. Initially, a labile covalent bond develops between the aldehyde of the glucose molecule and the amino acid side chain on both sugars and lipids. Specifically, glucose is covalently bound mainly to lysine residues in proteins, forming fructose-lysine residues. This reaction results in the development of a Schiff base, which, in turn, undergoes another chemical reaction to form a ketoamine, termed an Amadori product. These products result in cumulative oxidative damage to proteins. These products include CML (93) and pentosidine (94). The increased levels of pentosidine and CML correlate with the severity of diabetic complications, including nephropathy, retinopathy, and vascular disease. One such Amadori product is glycated (or glycosylated) hemoglobin A_{1c} (HbA_{1c}), which is commonly used to monitor glycemic control in diabetic patients. Since both free-radical oxidation and glycation are involved, these substances are also called glyoxidation products.

AGEs cross-link to the proteins composing the extracellular matrix and vascular basement membrane, which results in reduced solubility and decreased enzymatic digestion (95,96). AGE formation also prevents proper assembly of basement proteins, thereby altering their function. This in turn may alter the ability of cells to bind to their substrates.

AGEs are derived from oxidation of lipids (97,98). The side chains of unsaturated fatty acids undergo oxidation, which yields reactive carbonyl-containing fragments [malondialdehyde (MDA), glyoal 4-hydroxynonenal (4-HNE)] and then react with amino groups, mainly lysine residues.

Enhanced glycation, oxidation, and glyoxidation of lipoproteins have been postulated as a possible cause for the development of diabetic macrovascular disease. Certainly there are increased levels of AGE-modified LDL-apoprotein and LDL-lipid in persons with diabetes relative to levels in persons without diabetes (99). This would suggest that even in the face of similar glycemic control and other cardiovascular risk factors, the development of diabetic vascular complications would depend on differences of oxidative stress as well as on the tissue level of antioxidants.

The evidence for this possible role of these altered lipoproteins includes the presence of oxidized lipoproteins in the vessel wall (100,101) and the demonstration of lesion regression with antioxidants (102). One study (103) showed that the susceptibility of LDL to oxidation was correlated with the degree of atherosclerosis in 35 male survivors of an MI.

Vlassara and colleagues (104) identified a specific receptor for AGEs on monocyte/macrophages, termed RAGE (receptor for AGEs). The subsequent interaction with the AGE and its receptor may induce the release of the cytokines tumor necrosis factor (TNF) and interleukin-1 (105). Other cytokines that have been demonstrated include the synthesis and release of procoagulant activity and platelet-activating factor (PAF) by endothelial cells (106,107), as well as the induction of platelet-derived growth factor (PDGF-AA), which can be indirectly responsible for fibroblast and smooth muscle proliferation (108). Furthermore, increased AGE-receptor interaction has been shown to result in the enhanced expression of vascular cell adhesion molecule (VCAM) (109–111), which in turn results in increased atherogenesis.

The important role of the AGE receptor in the development of atherosclerosis was further strengthened by the demonstration that atherosclerosis was less severe in the usually atherosclerotic apolipoprotein E-knockout mice when they were administered an antibody-fragment that neutralized RAGE (112). This effect was seen without any effect on glycemic control or lipoprotein profile.

Thrombosis and Fibrinolysis in Diabetes

Plaque disruption with overlying thrombosis is a major cause of acute coronary syndromes, including MI, sudden death, and stroke. Because patients with type 1 and type 2 diabetes, particularly those with type 2 diabetes, have higher rates of acute coronary syndromes than the population without diabetes, heightened arterial prothrombotic reactivity may play a pivotal role in the development of these macrovascular complications.

There are three underlying mechanisms for this prothrombosis: heightened platelet reactivity, increased procoagulant activity, and decreased antithrombotic and fibrinolytic activity. The principal components of a thrombus are platelets and fibrin. The coagulation is initiated by the exposure of tissue factor within the arterial plaque at the time of plaque disruption. This results in the activation of factor VII/VIIa, which forms the "tenase complex" with factors X and V, resulting in the activation of thrombin. Thrombin stimulates platelet reactivity and the conversion of fibrinogen to fibrin, producing a thrombus.

The platelets of diabetic individuals appear to have an increased adherence to the vessel wall and increased circulating platelet mass (113). Platelet aggregometry studies that measure *in vitro* platelet reactivity have demonstrated increased aggregation of platelets in response to the agonists ADP, collagen, and thrombin and even spontaneous aggregation of platelets without any agonist (114–118). Assessment of platelet reactivity *in vivo* by measurement of blood or urine metabolites released from activated platelets such as thromboxane B_2 has shown increased reactivity relative to that of normal healthy controls (114,115).

Patients with diabetes have increased concentrations of fibrinogen, von Willebrand factor, and factor VII (119–121). Although the mechanisms of the increased concentrations of these factors have yet to be elucidated, the level of serum fibrinogen correlates with the levels of proinsulin and insulin in the blood (122). However, neither the plasma level of fibrinogen control nor the level of the plasma prothrombin fragment 1+2, a cleavage product of prothrombin, is reduced with improved metabolic control.

Several reports indicate that the activity of antithrombotic factors, including protein C and antithrombins, are decreased in subjects with diabetes, which further potentiates the hypercoagulable state (123–126).

Fibrinolysis is also impaired in individuals with diabetes, particularly those with type 2 diabetes (127,128). This impairment may be due to the increased activity of PAI-1 in the blood, which counteracts the action of native tissue plasminogen activator (t-PA) to induce fibrinolysis. PAI-1 is elevated not only in resting states but also in response to physiologic stimuli. The serum level of PAI-1 may be elevated as a result of several factors, including elevated serum levels of insulin, lipids, and glucose (129). The impairment of the fibrinolytic system can potentially exacerbate the development and persistence of thrombi, resulting in an increased risk of vascular occlusion.

Endothelial Function and Diabetes

Alterations in endothelial function may play an important role in the development of diabetic complications. Decreased blood flow in many organs has been reported, including the kidney, retina, and peripheral retinal nerves. Patients with recent diabetes have decreased retinal blood flow, as indicated by increased vascular resistance. The mechanism of this increased vascular resistance is probably partly due to the increase in the intercellular signal transduction kinase, protein kinase C (PKC) (130–133). This increase in PKC may result in an increase in endothelin-1. It has been documented that abnormalities in hemodynamic profiles precede diabetic nephropathy. This increase in glomerular filtration is probably due to the effect of hyperglycemia on arteriolar resistance.

The vascular endothelium has been shown to be important in modulating blood cell–vessel wall interaction, regulating blood flow, angiogenesis, lipoprotein metabolism, and vasomotion. An important mediator in maintaining vascular homeostasis is endothelium-derived relaxing factor (EDRF) (134), which has since been found to be nitric oxide (135). The release of nitric oxide activates soluble guanylate cyclase, resulting in the formation of cyclic guanosine monophosphate (cGMP), which, in turn, activates cGMP–dependent protein kinases, resulting in relaxation of vascular smooth muscle (136–139). Alterations in the expression, release, or activity of EDRF may play an important role in the initiation and progression of both micro- and macrovascular disease. Several studies have shown that endothelial-dependent vasodilator function is impaired in patients with type 1 diabetes without hypertension and dyslipidemia (140). This impairment is in contrast to that in patients with type 2 diabetes, who have an impairment of both endothelial-dependent and endothelial-independent (smooth muscle) vasodilator function (141,142).

Although the mechanism is unknown, several possibilities are present. Acute hyperglycemia impairs endothelial-dependent vasodilation in both macro- and microvessels (143). Insulin also may play a role. Insulin results in vasodilation due in part to nitric oxide production. Glucose-clamp experiments with insulin infusion have shown that subjects with type 2 diabetes have little improvement in endothelial-dependent vasodilation relative to that in subjects without diabetes (143). As stated previously, there appears to be an increase in oxygen-derived free radicals in the diabetic state. Several studies have shown that high doses of vitamin C can improve endothelial-dependent vasodilation in patients with both type 1 and type 2 diabetes (144,145). Intensive lipid lowering by statin therapy does not improve vasoreactivity in patients with type 2 diabetes, suggesting that mechanisms other than dyslipidemia are responsible for endothelial dysfunction (146).

Another possible culprit for this impairment of endothelial function found in individuals with diabetes may be the endogenous competitive inhibitor of nitric oxide synthase, asymmetric dimethylarginine (ADMA) (147). ADMA has been found to be elevated in subjects with diabetes (148,149).

CLINICAL FEATURES OF CARDIOVASCULAR DISEASE IN DIABETES

Angiographic Features of Coronary Artery Disease in Patients with Diabetes

Autopsy, angiographic, and angioscopic studies have documented the severe and diffuse nature of the atherosclerotic coronary involvement in patients with diabetes. Early autopsy data have shown that patients with diabetes have a greater number of coronary vessels involved, with more diffuse distribution of atherosclerotic lesions (150,151). Large angiographic studies comparing patients with diabetes to matched controls in the setting of acute MI (152) or elective angioplasty (153) or prior to coronary bypass surgery (154) have all shown that diabetes is associated with significantly more severe proximal and distal CAD (Table 58.2). An important finding with regard to the pathogenesis of acute coronary syndromes is the autopsy (155) and angioscopic (156) evidence suggesting a significant increase in plaque ulceration and thrombosis in diabetic compared with nondiabetic patients.

Silent Ischemia

The propensity of patients with diabetes to present with either silent or unrecognized MI is well established (157,158). Atypical symptoms such as confusion, dyspnea, fatigue, or nausea and vomiting were the presenting complaint in 32% to 42% of patients with diabetes with MI compared with 6% to 15% of patients without diabetes (157,159). Several groups have reported that the detection of silent ischemia by various noninvasive techniques, including treadmill exercise testing (160,161), ambulatory Holter monitoring (162), and exercise thallium scintigraphy (163–166), is more common in patients with diabetes than in those without diabetes. This finding, however, is not supported by all studies (167,168).

A plausible explanation for painless infarction and ischemic episodes in patients with diabetes is autonomic neuropathy with involvement of the sensory supply to the heart. In autopsies of patients with diabetes who died of silent MIs, typical diabetic neuropathic changes were found in the intracardiac sympathetic and parasympathetic fibers (169), and several studies correlated abnormalities in autonomic function in patients with silent ischemia (160,162,164,170). The anginal perceptual threshold—the time from the onset of myocardial ischemia (assessed by ST segment depression) to the onset of chest pain during exercise testing—is prolonged in patients with diabetes compared with those without diabetes. This delay in the perception of pain may be related to the impairment of autonomic nervous function (170).

Acute Coronary Syndromes in Patients with Diabetes

Acute ischemic events represent a major cause of death in the diabetic population (65). Diabetic patients who suffer an MI have a higher mortality than nondiabetic patients both in the acute phase and on long-term follow-up. Numerous studies have shown that in-hospital mortality rates from MI in patients with diabetes are 1.5- to 2-fold higher than in patients without diabetes (152,171–174). Diabetes remains an independent predictor for a poor prognosis in the thrombolytic era. In the Thrombolysis and Angioplasty in Myocardial Infarction (TAMI) trials, the in-hospital mortality rate was nearly twice as high in patients with diabetes, with more congestive heart failure and twice the rate of clinically recognized reinfarction (152). In the

TABLE 58.2. Angiographic Studies in Patients with Diabetes[a]

Study (reference)	No. of patients		Patients with multivessel disease(%)[b]		p Value
	Diabetic	Nondiabetic	Diabetic	Nondiabetic	
TAMI (152)	148	923	65[c]	46	<0.0001
TIMI II (379)	439[d]	2,900	40.8	26.8	<0.001
Orlander et al. (180)	236	348	58.2	41.6	<0.001
Stein et al. (153)	1,133	9,300	32.4[e]	28.2	<0.004
BARI (228)	353	1,476	46	40	<0.05
NHLBI (247)	281	1,833	27.7	17.7	<0.01
CASS (154)	317	1,843	85.8	77.7	<0.001

[a]Because most patients undergoing initial angioplasty have single-vessel disease, they have milder coronary artery disease than patients with acute myocardial infarction, who have an array of single-, double-, and triple-vessel disease, or patients undergoing coronary bypass grafting, who usually have double- and triple-vessel disease.
[b]Multivessel disease is defined by the presence of two or more vessels with at least one stenosis <75%.
[c]For men. Correspondending values for women are 63% and 41%, respectively.
[d]Not all patients underwent angiography.
[e]Patients were selected for angioplasty, and therefore this study includes a larger proportion of patients with single-vessel disease.
TAMI, Thrombolysis and Angioplasty in Myocardial Infarction; TIMI, Thrombolysis in Myocardial Infarction; BARI, Bypass Angioplasty Revascularization Investigation; NHLBI, National Heart, Lung and Blood Institute; CASS, Coronary Artery Surgery Study.

Global Utilization of Streptokinase and Tissue Plasminogen Activator for Occluded Coronary Arteries (GUSTO-I) trial, mortality at 30 days was highest among patients with diabetes treated with insulin (12.5%) compared with patients with diabetes not treated with insulin (9.7%) and nondiabetic (6.2%) patients (p <0.001) (175). Similar results have been reported from the other large studies (176–178). Diabetes is also a risk factor for cardiogenic shock in the setting of acute ischemic syndromes (179). Overall, despite the overall improvement in survival from an acute MI with thrombolysis, the in-hospital mortality rates in patients with diabetes remain 1.5 to 2 times higher than in patients without diabetes (175,178).

This increased in-hospital mortality among patients with diabetes with acute MI is due predominantly to an increase in the incidence of congestive heart failure (172,174,180,181), although increases in the incidence of reinfarction, infarct extension, and recurrent ischemia have also been reported (172–174,181,182).

Studies using serial determinations of total creatine kinase activity (180,181), radionuclide ventriculography (183), or echocardiography have found no evidence that patients with diabetes sustain more extensive infarctions than their nondiabetic counterparts (184). Thus, congestive heart failure and cardiogenic shock are more common and more severe in subjects with diabetes than would be expected from the size of the index infarction (178,180,181,183,185,186). The observation that clinical manifestations of heart failure occur in patients with diabetes despite a modest decrease in left ventricular ejection fraction (EF) led to the suggestion that preexisting diastolic dysfunction is a major culprit in the congestive symptoms (174). Indeed, subclinical diabetic cardiomyopathy, which is characterized by diastolic dysfunction (187), is likely to be an important factor in this setting.

It should be emphasized, however, that reductions in both left ventricular EF (183,188) and the regional EF of the noninfarcted myocardium (152,183,187) have been well documented in patients with diabetes following MI as compared with patients without diabetes. For example, early angiography in the TAMI trials has demonstrated worse ventricular function in the noninfarcted zone in patients with diabetes (152).

The performance of the left ventricle following MI is determined largely by the extent of coronary disease (189) and the quality of collateral circulation. Thus, the diffuse nature of coronary atherosclerosis (Table 58.2) in diabetes may contribute to systolic dysfunction of the noninfarcted myocardium. Moreover, a recent study has shown that patients with diabetes have a reduced ability to develop collateral blood vessels in the presence of CAD (190), a finding that also may explain the more frequent occurrence of postinfarction angina and infarct extension (173,174,182,184).

Patients with diabetes surviving MI also suffer higher late mortality rates than patients without diabetes (174,182, 191–193). Late mortality is related primarily to both recurrent MI and the development of new congestive heart failure (176, 178,184,192–194).

MEDICAL THERAPY FOR CORONARY ARTERY DISEASE IN PATIENTS WITH DIABETES

Diabetes exerts a deleterious effect on the short- and long-term course following MI through diverse mechanisms, some of which (e.g., cardiomyopathy) cannot be modified at the time of presentation. Because patients with diabetes are at greater risk, application of effective preventive and treatment measures may result in a particularly large survival benefit.

Insulin

One possible mechanism for the increased mortality among diabetic patients with acute MI may be the altered metabolism of the myocardium. The diabetic state results in increased fatty acid metabolism, compromising glycolysis in both ischemic and nonischemic territories. Free fatty acids and their intermediates may potentiate ischemic injury. One way to attenuate free fatty acid oxidation is by the intravenous infusion of insulin-glucose. It was that rationale that led Malmberg and colleagues (195) to evaluate the effect of insulin-glucose infusion followed by multidose insulin treatment in patients with diabetes [Diabetes Mellitus Insulin-Glucose Infusion in Acute Myocardial Infarction (DIGAMI) Study] (Fig. 58.2). Patients with diabetes with an acute MI within the previous 24 hours were randomized to two separate arms. Insulin-glucose infusion was given for the first 24 hours and until stable normoglycemia in the experimental arm. Then subcutaneous multidose insulin was given to maintain normoglycemia for a 3-month period. Control patients received standard coronary care unit care and did not receive insulin unless clinically indicated.

The 3-month mortality was not significantly different for the control and experimental groups. However, the 1-year mortality was 18.6% in the experimental group and 26% in the control group, or a relative risk reduction of approximately 30%. This improvement in mortality continued for a total of 3.4 years, with an absolute reduction of mortality of 11% (196).

Aspirin

Studies have shown an increased platelet adhesiveness and aggregability (197), with a concomitant increased release of thromboxane A_2 (115) in subjects with diabetes. On the basis of these data, several authors stated that patients with diabetes may require larger doses of aspirin to suppress the synthesis of thromboxane A_2 (115,198). Furthermore, in the Second International Study of Infarct Survival (ISIS-2) study, there was no reduction in mortality in subjects with diabetes receiving 160 mg of aspirin daily (199).

The Antiplatelet Trialists' Collaboration meta-analysis quantified the benefit of aspirin in patients with diabetes who had had a previous cardiovascular event (200). The relative benefit on vascular events was 17% in the patients with diabetes and 22% in those without diabetes. Although the number was lower for patients with diabetes than for patients without diabetes in terms of percentage benefit, the absolute number of events prevented was similar in the two groups (38 ± 12 per 1,000 compared with 36 ± 3 per 1,000, respectively), probably because of the higher event rates in patients with diabetes.

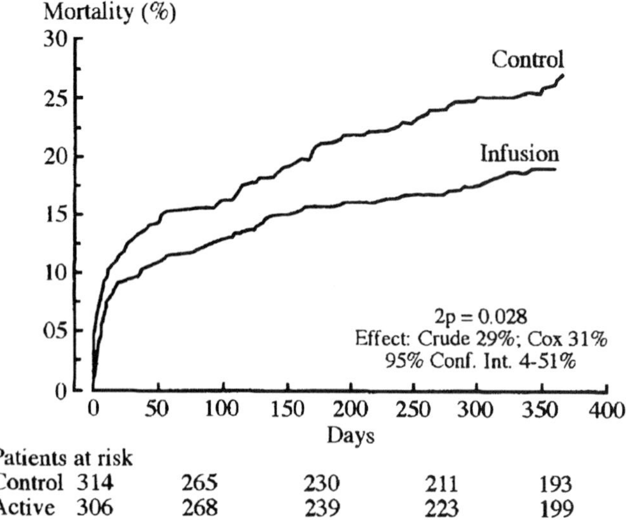

Figure 58.2. Actuarial mortality curves in the patients receiving insulin-glucose infusion and in the control group of the present Diabetes Mellitus Insulin-Glucose Infusion in Acute Myocardial Infarction (DIGAMI) study during 1 year of follow-up. Numbers below graph, number of patients at different times of observation; Active, patients receiving infusion; Conf. Int, confidence interval. (Reprinted from Malmberg K, Ryden L, Efendic S, et al. Randomized trial of insulin-glucose infusion followed by subcutaneous insulin treatment in diabetic patients with acute myocardial infarction (DIGAMI study): effects on mortality at 1 year. *J Am Coll Cardiol* 1995; 26:57–65, with permission. Copyright 1995, with permission from Excerpta Medica.)

Data from the U.S. Physicians' Health Study and the Early Treatment Diabetic Retinopathy Study (ETDRS) indicate that aspirin may also be efficacious as primary prevention in patients with diabetes (201).

A major risk of aspirin therapy is gastric mucosal injury and gastrointestinal hemorrhage. These effects are dose related and are reduced to placebo levels when enteric-coated preparations of 75 to 325 mg are used once daily (202). The ETDRS established, using serial retinal photography, that aspirin therapy is not associated with an increased risk of retinal or vitreous hemorrhage.

The American Diabetes Association (ADA) recommends the use of aspirin therapy (81 to 325 mg/day) as secondary prevention in any patient with evidence of large-vessel disease. Aspirin is also recommended as primary prevention in patients with diabetes with the following: (a) family history of CAD, (b) cigarette smoking, (c) hypertension, (d) obesity, (e) albuminuria, (f) LDL >130 mg/dL, (g) HDL <40 mg/dL, or (h) triglycerides >250 mg/dL (202).

β-Blockers

β-Blockers are effective in reducing reinfarction and sudden death in patients with diabetes, perhaps to a greater extent than in patients without diabetes. Early treatment of MI with β-blockers resulted in a 37% reduction in mortality in patients with diabetes compared with a 13% reduction in mortality in all patients, whereas reduction in long-term mortality was 48% and 33% in diabetics and all patients, respectively (203).

In a controlled study evaluating the use of atenolol in patients with, or at risk for, CAD who had noncardiac surgery, diabetes was the strongest predictor of death after 2 years of follow-up, with twice the mortality compared with that in patients without diabetes (204). Compared with patients without diabetes, patients with diabetes receiving atenolol had no increased risk of death, whereas those given placebo had a fourfold increase in risk (204). It should be emphasized that the deterioration in glycemic control or blunted counterregulatory response to hypoglycemia is seldom a serious clinical problem, especially when cardioselective β_1-blockers are used (203,205).

Angiotensin-Converting Enzyme Inhibition

Inhibition of the angiotensin-converting enzyme (ACE) is now unequivocally associated with a substantial mortality reduction in patients surviving MI with left ventricular dysfunction (EF <40%) (206). The investigators of the Third Gruppo Italiano per lo Studio della Streptochinasi nell'Infarto Miocardico (GISSI-3) compared the effect of early administration (within 24 hours of admission) of lisinopril in patients with and without diabetes presenting with MI (207). Compared with placebo, lisinopril dramatically reduced both 6-week (30% vs. 5%) and 6-month (20% vs. 0%) mortality in patients with diabetes versus those without diabetes. These findings are corroborated by subgroup analysis of the Survival and Ventricular Enlargement (SAVE) study (208). A retrospective analysis using data from the Trandolapril Cardiac Evaluation (TRACE) study, a randomized, double-blind, placebo-controlled trial evaluating trandolapril in patients after acute MI who had an EF less than or equal to 35%, has shown a 36% reduction of death from any cause and a 62% reduction in the risk of progression to severe heart failure (209). Recently, the HOPE study has shown that ramipril substantially lowers the risk of death, MI, stroke, coronary revascularization, heart failure, and complications related to diabetes in a high-risk group of patients with preexisting vascular disease (210,211) (Fig. 58.3).

ACE inhibitors have become the primary agents of choice for the treatment of hypertension associated with diabetes because they do not adversely affect the glycemic control and lipid profile (212,213). In fact, ACE inhibitors may actually enhance insulin sensitivity in patients with type 2 diabetes, with or without hypertension (214–216). ACE inhibitors are especially desirable in patients with evidence of diabetic nephropathy.

Serum potassium and creatinine should be monitored closely in the first few weeks of therapy. A rapid decline in renal function can occur in patients with bilateral renal artery stenosis, which is more common in patients with diabetes. Hyporeninemic hypoaldosteronism is frequently associated with diabetes and predisposes the patients to clinically significant hyperkalemia when ACE inhibitors are initiated.

Glycoprotein IIb/IIIa Antagonists

Glycoprotein IIb/IIIa (GpIIb/IIIa) antagonists, which are antiplatelet agents, have become an important therapeutic modality in the treatment of unstable angina and non–Q-wave MIs. In particular, these agents have been shown to be of equal, if not greater, benefit in the diabetic population than in its nondiabetic counterpart. The Platelet Receptor Inhibition in Ischemic Syndrome Management in Patients Limited by Unstable Signs and Symptoms (PRISM-PLUS) study (217,218) compared heparin with heparin plus the GpIIb/IIIa inhibitor tirofiban in 1,208 patients, with 362 patients having diabetes. The cumulative endpoint at 7 days of death, MI, refractory angina, or rehospitalizations for unstable angina was reduced to 21.4% in patients receiving heparin alone and to 14.8% in those receiving heparin plus tirofiban in the diabetic group; and to 16.7% in patients receiving heparin alone and to 12.4% in those receiving heparin plus tirofiban in the nondiabetic group. There was no difference in the ability of the standard dose of tirofiban required to result in an inhibition in platelet aggregation of over 80% after a 12-hour infusion in the patients with and without diabetes, despite the hyperaggregability of platelets in patients with diabetes.

The EPILOG study (219), which evaluated percutaneous coronary angioplasty plus the GpIIb/IIIa antagonist abciximab versus angioplasty alone, found no significant difference in acute events, while the longer term follow-up revealed a higher rate of subsequent revascularization involving the target vessel in the subjects with diabetes. The Evaluation of Platelet IIb/IIIa Inhibitor for Stenting (EPISTENT) Trial (220), which evaluated coronary stenting plus abciximab and heparin versus stenting plus heparin alone, demonstrated a marked decrease of target vessel revascularization in patients with diabetes. The rate of target vessel revascularization in patients with diabetes randomized to stenting and heparin was 16.6%, whereas the rate among those randomized to stenting and abciximab was 8.1%, a 50% decrease. One recent study (221) did not demonstrate a difference in efficacy of two glycoprotein IIb/IIIa receptor inhibitors, abciximab and tirofiban, when used in patients with diabetes undergoing percutaneous coronary intervention.

Thrombolytic Therapy

Thrombolytic therapy is of substantial benefit in patients with diabetes. In the Global Utilization of Streptokinase and t-PA for Occluded Coronary Arteries (GUSTO-I) angiographic substudy, early infarct-related artery patency [TIMI (Thrombolysis in Myocardial Infarction) flow grade 3] and reocclusion rates were similar among diabetics and nondiabetics (222,379).

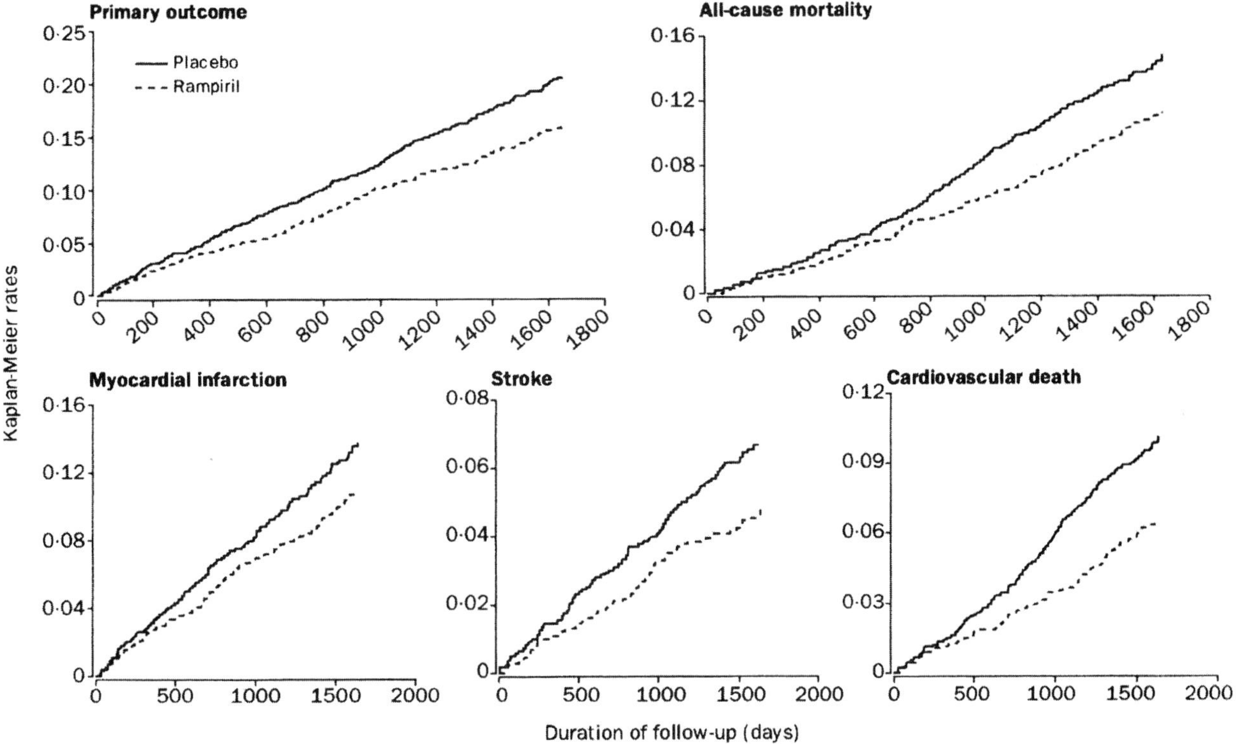

Figure 58.3. Kaplan-Meier survival curves for study participants with diabetes in the HOPE study comparing the use of ramipril (----) vs. placebo (——). (Reprinted from Heart Outcomes Prevention Evaluation Study [HOPE] Investigators. Effects of ramipril on cardiovascular and microvascular outcomes in people with diabetes mellitus: results of the HOPE study and MICRO-HOPE substudy. *Lancet* 2000;355:253–259, with permission. Copyright 2000, with permission from Elsevier.)

Patients with diabetes treated with various fibrinolytic agents benefit by the same mortality reduction as nondiabetic patients (152,223) (Table 58.3). In an overview of fibrinolytic trials in patients with MI, the relative reduction in 35-day mortality was slightly, but not significantly, greater in patients with diabetes than in nondiabetic patients (21.7% vs. 14.3%) (223). In these trials, no increase in serious bleeding complications or stroke was observed in patients with diabetes. Retinal bleeding is an extremely uncommon complication of thrombolytic therapy in patients with diabetes. In the GUSTO-1 study, 300 of 6,011 patients with diabetes had proliferative retinopathy, but none developed intraocular hemorrhage (224). It is unlikely that thrombolytic therapy would increase vitreous hemorrhage, which is due to vitreous detachment in patients with diabetic retinopathy. Thus, the concern that many clinicians have with regard to thrombolytic therapy in patients with diabetic retinopathy is not supported by the results of large clinical trials. It is probably unjustified to deny these patients the proven life-saving benefit of thrombolysis.

REVASCULARIZATION PROCEDURES IN PATIENTS WITH DIABETES

Because CAD is a major health problem in patients with diabetes, the need for a revascularization procedure frequently arises. Therefore, many patients with diabetes require some form of revascularization procedure. A significant and increasing proportion of patients undergoing angioplasty are diabetic. In the 1977 to 1981 National Heart, Lung and Blood Institute (NHLBI) registry, 9% of patients undergoing angioplasty had diabetes (225). More recent large trials suggest that the prevalence of diabetes among patients undergoing angioplasty increased to approximately 17% to 19% (226,227). The influence of diabetes on outcome after revascularization procedures received attention following the results of the Bypass Angioplasty Revascularization Investigation (BARI) study, which suggested that patients with diabetes with significant CAD involving the left anterior descending coronary artery had improved mortality if they underwent coronary artery bypass grafting (CABG) (228). The results of the Coronary Angioplasty versus Bypass Revascularization Investigation (CABRI) investigators (229) demonstrated that the mortality among patients with diabetes is double that of patients without diabetes, independent of the means of revascularization, be it CABG or percutaneous transluminal coronary angioplasty (PTCA). Among patients with and without diabetes, there was no significant mortality difference between PTCA and CABG, although there was a trend favoring CABG, especially in the diabetic population (229).

Angioplasty

Angioplasty provides effective relief of angina in most patients and is performed with similar success in patients with and without diabetes (153). However, increased restenosis rates in patients with diabetes greatly limit long-term benefits from angioplasty. The importance of diabetes as a clinical risk factor for restenosis after percutaneous interventions has been demonstrated in multiple studies. The initial report from the NHLBI Angioplasty Registry indicated that the angiographic restenosis rate in patients with diabetes was 47%, as compared with 32% in patients without diabetes (230), and subsequent studies have reported restenosis rates of 49% to 71% among patients with diabetes (231–236).

TABLE 58.3. Effect of Thrombolytic Therapy in Patients with Diabetes

Study (reference)	Thrombolytic agent	No. of patients		In-hospital/short-term mortality (%)		*p* Value
		Diabetic	Nondiabetic	Diabetic	Nondiabetic	
ISIS-2 (199)	SK	15,694	1,287	8.9	11.8[a]	NR
FTT Collaborative Group (223)	SK, rt-PA, UK, APSAC	38,814	4,529	8.7	13.6[b]	NR
TAMI (152)	rt-PA, UK	923	148	6	11	<0.02
International t-PA/ Streptokinase Mortality Trial (176)	rt-PA, SK	8,055	833	7.5[c]	11.8	<0.001[d]
GISSI-2 (178)	rt-PA, SK	8,069	1,266	5.8[e]	8.7	NR
TIMI (379)	rt-PA	2,900	439	4.1	10.2	<0.001[f]
GUSTO (222)	rt-PA, SK	34,705	6,125	6.2	10.6	<0.0001[g]

[a]Five-week mortality rate in the streptokinase vs. placebo group.
[b]The 35-day mortality.
[c]For type 2 diabetes. In-hospital mortality for those with type 1 diabetes was 16.9%.
[d]After multivariate analysis, only the mortality for patients with diabetes for >10 years remained significant.
[e]For type 2 diabetes. In-hospital mortality for patients with type 1 diabetes was 10.1%.
[f]The 42-day mortality.
[g]The 30 day mortality.
FTT, Fibrinolytic Therapy Trialists; GISSI, Gruppo Italiano per lo Studio della Streptochinasi nell'Infarto Miocardico; GUSTO, Global Utilization of Streptokinase and t-PA for Occluded Coronary Arteries; ISIS-2, Second International Study of Infarct Survival; SK, streptokinase; TAMI, Thrombolysis and Angioplasty in Myocardial Infarction; rt-PA, recombinant tissue plasminogen activator; UK, urokinase; APSAC, anisoylated plasminogen-streptokinase activator complex; NR, not reported; TIMI, Thrombolysis in Myocardial Infarction.
From Aronson D, Johnstone MT. Coronary artery disease in diabetes. In: Johnstone MT, Veves A. *Diabetes and cardiovascular disease.* Totowa, NJ: Humana Press, 2001. Reprinted with permission from Humana Press.

New angioplasty devices also have failed to have any major impact on the restenosis rate among patients with diabetes. Diabetes is associated with a twofold increase in recurrent clinical events after directional coronary atherectomy (237–239), and diabetic patients have higher restenosis rates after excimer laser angioplasty (240). Recently, intracoronary stents have been shown to decrease restenosis as compared with rates with PTCA (241). Several groups have reported that, even with stents, patients with diabetes have higher restenosis rates than patients without diabetes (242–245), although this finding is debated (246).

The full impact of the higher rates of restenosis following angioplasty on the cardiovascular morbidity of patients with diabetes is significant. Numerous studies have shown that patients with diabetes experience a greater need for repeat revascularization (angioplasty or CABG), a higher rate of cardiac events, and lower overall survival rates following coronary angioplasty compared with their nondiabetic counterparts (153,237,239,247–250). Recent data from the EPISTENT and other studies (251) suggest that the combination of stenting with platelet glycoprotein IIb/IIIa blockade may decrease the incidence of death, MI, and target vessel revascularization among patients with diabetes (252).

Although vessel recoil also may contribute to loss of luminal size, the increased restenosis rate in patients with diabetes following stent placement underscores the role of enhanced proliferation of smooth muscle cells as the major mechanism for restenosis in these patients, because coronary artery stenting decreases elastic recoil and vascular spasm at the treated site (244). A study using intravascular ultrasound found exaggerated intimal proliferation in patients with diabetes at the site of angioplasty-induced arterial injury, and this proliferative response was particularly striking in restenotic lesions (253). Thus, the diabetic state promotes proliferation of smooth muscle cells and deposition of extracellular matrix following arterial injury. Surprisingly, the possibility that strict glycemic control may reduce restenosis rates among patients with diabetes (254) has not been addressed clinically or experimentally. Ongoing studies are examining means of reducing the restenosis rate, including the use of beta-radiation [Anti-Proliferative Effect of Beta-Radiation on Restenosis Prevention in Diabetic Patients after Coronary Stent Implantation (ANTIPODES)].

Subjects with diabetes with restenosis following percutaneous intervention have less intimal hypercellular tissue in the restenotic lesion relative to that in subjects without diabetes (255). Sobel's group has found an increase in the intramural synthesis of PAI-1 in the vessel walls of rabbits subjected to experimental angioplasty (256,257). PAI-1 synthesis is stimulated by insulin. In turn, PAI-1 may inhibit the remodeling and proteolysis that normally occurs after PTCA, resulting in the accumulation of the extracellular matrix and lipid, with a relative decrease in the relative amount of migration and proliferation of smooth muscle cells. One recent development has suggested that haptoglobin phenotype may determine which patients with diabetes may develop restenosis after coronary stent implantation (258).

Coronary Artery Bypass Surgery

CABG is as effective in relieving anginal symptoms in patients with diabetes as in patients without diabetes (154). Diabetes is not associated with increased perioperative mortality during bypass graft surgery, although wound infections and the average hospital stay are increased (259,260). With respect to vein grafts, several reports have noted decreased survival of vein grafts in patients with diabetes (261–263). Intimal proliferation that causes luminal loss in the first years following bypass surgery with venous conduit may be accelerated in patients with diabetes (264). In contrast, the benefit of internal mammary artery conduits is well documented among patients with diabetes (263,265). Data from the Duke registry indicate that the long-term benefit of one internal mammary artery graft is at least as great in patients with diabetes as in those without diabetes (265). Nonetheless, the long-term survival rate after bypass surgery remains consistently lower in patients with diabetes than in those without diabetes (265–267).

Angioplasty versus Coronary Artery Bypass Surgery in Multivessel Coronary Artery Disease

Coronary angioplasty has been widely accepted as the initial revascularization procedure for treatment of most single-vessel CAD, whereas CABG has been the standard form of revascularization for multivessel disease. However, in the past decade, angioplasty has been proposed and evaluated as an alternative to CABG in patients with multivessel disease.

The influence of diabetes on outcome after PTCA for patients with multivessel disease received attention following the results of the BARI study (228). The BARI study enrolled 1,829 patients (including 353 patients with diabetes [19%] with angiographically documented multivessel CAD and either clinically severe angina or objective evidence of marked myocardial ischemia requiring revascularization. Cause of death was classified as cardiac if it occurred less than 1 hour after onset of cardiac symptoms or within 1 hour to 30 days after a documented or probable MI or as a result of intractable congestive heart failure, cardiogenic shock, or another documented cardiac cause.

A review of 5-year all-cause mortality rates showed a near doubling of mortality among patients with diabetes receiving insulin or oral therapy assigned to multivessel angioplasty compared with those assigned to surgery (35% vs. 19%, $p = 0.003$). In contrast, the 5-year mortality among patients without diabetes and patients with diabetes not receiving drug treatment was 9% with both revascularization strategies. Cause-specific 5.4-year cardiac mortality rates were 3.5 times higher in the PTCA group (20.6% vs. 5.8%) (228). These results raised concern about selection of revascularization procedures in patients with diabetes with multivessel CAD and prompted a clinical alert by the NHLBI stating that CABG should be the preferred initial revascularization choice in medically treated patients with diabetes who have multivessel CAD (268).

A subsequent report from the BARI investigators indicated that the survival benefit of CABG is limited to patients with diabetes receiving an internal mammary artery (IMA) graft. Cardiac mortality after 5.4 years was 2.9% when IMA was used and 18.2% when only saphenous vein graft conduits were used. The latter rate was similar to that for patients receiving PTCA (20.6%) (269). The mortality benefit afforded by IMA was most apparent in those experiencing MI during follow-up (an effect seen also in patients without diabetes). As an IMA graft is less susceptible to atherosclerosis, it may provide an alternative source of perfusion to maintain ventricular function in regions of hypoperfusion resulting from coronary occlusion.

Three recent studies examined the effect of revascularization strategies in patients with diabetes. In a large prospective cohort of 3,220 patients with multivessel disease, of whom 770 (24%) had diabetes, Barsness and associates evaluated the relationship between diabetes and survival after revascularization with either PTCA or CABG (270). Although diabetes was strongly associated with a worse long-term prognosis, the 5-year survival for patients with diabetes undergoing PTCA was 76%, whereas the rate for those without diabetes was 88%. Similarly, in the group of patients undergoing CABG, 5-year survival was 74% in those with diabetes and 86% in those without diabetes. Unlike other studies, however, no significant differential effect of diabetes was seen on outcome between patients treated with PTCA and those treated with CABG. In a similar study, Weintraub and associates (271), using an observational database, prospectively compared the outcome of PTCA (n = 834) and CABG (n = 1,805) in patients with diabetes with multivessel coronary disease. Correcting for baseline differences, they found no difference in survival for the group as a whole. However, in the insulin-requiring subgroup, 5- and 10-year survival rates were 68% and 36% after PTCA and 75% and 47% after CABG, respectively.

Gum et al. (248) performed a retrospective outcome analysis of 525 patients with diabetes who underwent coronary revascularization. Overall, actuarial survival curves showed a nonsignificant trend favoring the CABG group for survival at 6 years (30% vs. 37%; $p = 0.08$).

A crucial question is why CABG may be superior to PTCA in patients with diabetes in the setting of multivessel disease. The only difference between the diabetic groups in the BARI study was the revascularization procedure chosen. Hence, the difference in prognosis is likely to be related to the relative efficacy of these revascularization procedures.

The major advantage of CABG over PTCA is the ability to achieve complete revascularization (272,273). The superiority of CABG over angioplasty in providing complete revascularization is exemplified in the BARI study itself. In the BARI population, 3.1 grafts were placed per patient undergoing CABG (274), whereas the mean number of successfully treated lesions in the PTCA group was 2.0 (269). Similar numbers are reported by other studies comparing multivessel angioplasty and CABG (248,270,271).

Previous CABG studies have emphasized that complete revascularization is essential for obtaining survival benefit in patients with multivessel disease (273). If complete revascularization (which is accomplished almost exclusively through CABG surgery) is essential for survival benefit, the successful application of multivessel angioplasty (which entails a strategy that selectively targets high-priority lesions) requires that a comparable proportion of myocardium supplied through high-priority lesions be revascularized by each of the two strategies. Because multiple treatment sites can result in restenosis independently when multivessel angioplasty is performed (243), it is likely that this goal is frequently not achieved in patients with diabetes, given their high restenosis rates (Table 58.2). Thus, the worse outcome of patients with diabetes undergoing PTCA may be mediated in part by the frequent occurrence of incomplete revascularization (248). Van Belle and colleagues suggest that restenosis, especially in its occlusive form, is a major determinant of long-term mortality in patients with diabetes after coronary angioplasty. When these investigators studied 604 patients with diabetes who underwent angioplasty, followed by a 6-month follow-up angiogram and long-term follow-up, they found that the group that had no restenosis had a 10-year mortality of 24% compared with a 35% mortality in the group with nonocclusive restenosis and a 59% mortality in the group that had occlusive restenosis ($p<0.0001$) (256,275). The impact of incomplete revascularization may be more pronounced in view of the more diffuse and distal CAD (154,247) and worse coronary vasodilatory reserve in patients with diabetes (276). Thus PTCA may fail to alter the aggressive natural course of CAD in patients with diabetes rather than leading to increased mortality (269).

MANAGEMENT OF RISK FACTORS

It is important to identify the risk factors of an individual patient in order to develop a plan for risk reduction. The goals for risk reduction are summarized in Table 58.4, which is adapted from a recent review from an AHA executive summary (277).

Cholesterol Reduction

The Scandinavian Simvastatin Survival Study (4S) has demonstrated the effectiveness of cholesterol-lowering therapy

TABLE 58.4. Goals for Management of Risk Factors in Patients with Diabetes

Risk factor	Goal of therapy	Recommending body
Cigarette smoking	Complete cessation	ADA
Blood pressure	<130/85 mm Hg	JNC VI (NHLBI)
	<130/80 mm Hg	ADA
LDL cholesterol	<100 mg/dL	ATP III (NHLBI), ADA
Triglycerides 200–499 mg/dL	Non-HDL cholesterol <130 mg/dL	ATP III (NHLBI)
HDL cholesterol <40 mg/dL	Raise HDL (no set goal)	ATP III (NHLBI)
Prothrombotic state	Low-dose aspirin therapy (patients with CHD and other high-risk patients)	ADA
Glucose	Hemoglobin A_{1c} <7%	ADA
Overweight and obesity (BMI ≥25 kg/m^2	Lose 10% of body weight in 1 yr	OEI (NHLBI)
Physical inactivity	Exercise prescription dependent on patient status	ADA
Adverse nutrition	See text	ADA, AHA, and NHLBI's ATP III, OEI, and JNC VI

ADA, American Diabetes Association; JNC VI, Sixth Report of the Joint National Committee on Prevention, Detection, Evaluation, and Treatment of High Blood Pressure; NHLBI, National Heart, Lung and Blood Institute; ATP III, National Cholesterol Education Program Adult Treatment Panel III; HDL, high-density lipoprotein; CHD, coronary heart disease; OEI, Obesity Education Initiative Expert Panel on Identification, Evaluation, and Treatment of Overweight and Obesity in Adults, AHA, American Heart Association.
From Grundy SM, Garber A, Goldberg R, et al. Prevention Conference VI: Diabetes and Cardiovascular Disease: executive summary. *Circulation* 2002;105:2231–2239, with permission from Lippincott Williams & Wilkins.

(278,279) for secondary prevention of death and morbidity in patients with angina or prior infarction. Compared with the placebo group, the relative total mortality and cardiovascular mortality were 0.57 and 0.64, respectively.

Subjects in the 4S study had relatively high LDL-cholesterol levels at baseline (~185 mg/dL). However, the majority of patients with coronary disease (including those with diabetes) have lower LDL-cholesterol levels. The Cholesterol and Current Events (CARE) study, which included 586 patients with diabetes, determined the effect of cholesterol-lowering therapy in patients with coronary disease with average cholesterol levels (mean, 139 mg/dL). In the 586 subjects with diabetes and CAD, 40 mg of pravastatin was associated with a 25% decrease in coronary events and revascularization procedures, similar to a 23% decrease observed in patients without diabetes (280).

These results strongly suggest that cholesterol lowering improves the prognosis of diabetic patients with CAD. The absolute clinical benefit achieved by cholesterol lowering may be greater in diabetic patients than in nondiabetic patients with CAD because patients with diabetes have a higher absolute risk of recurrent CAD, higher case-fatality rates (184), and more atherogenic LDL-cholesterol (58,99,281,282).

Several recent publications have argued against the relevance of the traditional classification to primary and secondary prevention in the setting of diabetes (20). The rationale for this approach stems from both the high event rates in patients with diabetes without clinical evidence of CAD (presumably due to the very high rates of subclinical atherosclerosis) (20), as well as to the worse prognosis in patients who have had a clinical event compared with nondiabetic subjects (184). These data suggest that LDL-cholesterol should be lowered to less than 100 mg/dL even in diabetic subjects without prior CAD.

Tight glycemic control is the cornerstone of therapy for diabetic dyslipidemia. HMG CoA reductase inhibitors reduce coronary risk even when the LDL level lies within the average range in individuals with type 2 diabetes (283,284). However, tight glycemic control does not completely reverse the lipid profile in patients with type 2 diabetes. Tan and colleagues (285) found that patients with excellent control of their glucose levels (average HbA_{1c} <6.6%) continued to have a low HDL level and a predominance of small dense LDL particles.

The target level of LDL-cholesterol should be 100 mg/dL. This can first be achieved by diet with the addition of statins if necessary. If the triglyceride level is greater than 200 mg/dL even in the face of an LDL less than 100 mg/dL, fibrate therapy should be considered. The recent Veterans Affairs High-density Lipoprotein Cholesterol Intervention Trial demonstrated that the fibrate gemfibrozil reduced both coronary events and strokes (286). Recent data suggest that when the LDL level is less than 125 mg/dL, the triglyceride and HDL levels are significantly stronger predictors of recurrent cardiac events than when the LDL levels are greater than 125 mg/dL (287). This only strengthens the rationale for treating patients with low HDL or elevated triglyceride levels.

Nicotinic acid can both lower triglyceride levels and raise HDL levels. However, its beneficial effect on lipids in the patient with diabetes is offset by its tendency to worsen hyperglycemia, making it relatively contraindicated in such patients.

Treatment of Hypertension

Hypertension is about twice as frequent in patients with diabetes as in the general population (288,289). Isolated systolic hypertension is considerably more common in patients with diabetes. The combined presence of hypertension and diabetes considerably accelerates the development of both macrovascular and microvascular diabetic complications. However, the most significant manifestation of this combination of diseases is that they confer a greater risk of ischemic heart disease, stroke, and peripheral vascular disease in affected individuals. The high cardiovascular risk associated with the coexistence of hypertension and diabetes led the Joint National Committee on Prevention, Detection, Evaluation, and Treatment of High Blood Pressure to include hypertensive patients with diabetes in the same risk group as hypertensive patients who have clinically manifest cardiovascular disease (290). These patients should be considered for prompt pharmacologic therapy even if they have high-normal blood pressure.

Current evidence suggests that, for the prevention of cardiovascular events, ACE inhibitors (291,292) and low-dose diuretics (293) are the preferred first-line agents for hypertensive patients with diabetes, whereas a controversy exists with regard to the efficacy of calcium antagonists in preventing cardiovascular complications (294). In the Appropriate Blood Pressure Control in Diabetes (ABCD) trial, patients in the nisoldipine group had a fivefold higher risk of fatal and nonfatal acute MI than did the enalapril group (291). In the Fosinopril versus Amlodipine Cardiovascular Events Randomized Trial (FACET), patients receiving fosinopril had half the risk of the combined outcome of acute MI, stroke, or hospitalized angina than did those receiving amlodipine (295). However, the combined therapy resulted in a lower incidence of cardiovascular events than either treatment alone and could be interpreted as evidence that combination therapy is the preferred strategy (295). Control of hypertension is unlikely to be achieved by monotherapy in patients with diabetes, as demonstrated in the ABCD trial (291).

The Systolic Hypertension in Europe (Syst-Eur) compared outcomes of treatments with nitrendipine versus placebo in patients with isolated systolic hypertension. Endpoint reduction achieved by active treatment was significantly larger in the subgroup with diabetes (69% vs. 26% cardiovascular events), indicating a remarkable benefit from first-line treatment with a calcium antagonist (296). Similarly, the results of the Hypertension Optimal Treatment (HOT) trial showed a reduction in the rate of MI events in patients with diabetes (n = 1,501, representing the largest trial of a calcium antagonist in patients with diabetes) with the long-acting dihydropyridine calcium antagonist felodipine (297).

The evidence for aggressive antihypertensive treatment in patients with type 1 diabetes, hypertension, and nephropathy is now overwhelming (298,299). ACE inhibitors are particularly useful in this population, with clear evidence that these agents reduced the progression of kidney dysfunction and the number of patients who will develop end-stage renal failure (215,216).

The HOPE study (and the MICRO-HOPE substudy) (Fig. 58.3) demonstrated that ramipril significantly reduced the rates of MI, stroke, and deaths in patients with diabetes without overt cardiovascular disease and one other risk factor (211). The importance of blocking the renin-angiotensin system was further strengthened by the results of the Losartan Intervention for Endpoint Reduction in Hypertension (LIFE) study (300). These results demonstrated that lorsartan reduced total and cardiovascular mortality more than did atenolol in patients with diabetes with hypertension and left ventricular hypertrophy.

The Sixth Report of the Joint National Committee on Prevention, Detection, Evaluation, and Treatment of High Blood Pressure (JNC-VI) has incorporated these principles for the treatment of hypertension in the presence of diabetes and has included a more aggressive program of blood pressure reduction, aiming for a target of less than 135/85 mm Hg in patients with type 1 and type 2 diabetes (290). The ADA aims for the lower target blood pressure of 130/80 mm Hg (289).

In addition, the ADA guidelines included a target of 125/75 mm Hg in patients with proteinuria of greater than 1 g per day. ACE inhibitors are recommended as the initial antihypertensive drug of choice in patients with diabetes (290,298,299).

Glycemic Control

A central issue in the treatment of patients with diabetes is whether tight glycemic control will reduce CAD morbidity and mortality. The Diabetes Control and Complications Trial (DCCT) conclusively showed that the greater the average blood glucose in patients with type 1 diabetes (as assessed by HbA_{1c}), the greater the risk of developing retinopathy, neuropathy, and nephropathy (301). Although the number of combined major macrovascular events was almost twice as high in the conventionally treated group as in the intensively treated group, the differences were not statistically significant ($p = 0.08$) because patients participating in this study were young and early in the course of their disease (301,302). However, hyperglycemic animals develop fatty streaks resembling those of human type II atherosclerotic lesions in the absence of hyperinsulinemia (303), and data from the Stockholm Diabetes Intervention Study indicate that, in patients with type 1 diabetes, tight control retards the development of atherosclerosis, as measured by the development of carotid intima-media thickening (304). Thus, tight control is indicated in patients with type 1 diabetes for prevention of both microvascular and macrovascular complications. It is noteworthy that the average total insulin dose in the intensive-treatment group of the DCCT trial was less than 10% higher than in the conventional-treatment group. Thus, unless acceleration of atherosclerosis is exquisitely sensitive to small differences in exogenous insulin dose, it is unlikely that this form of therapy increases the risk for cardiovascular disease.

The United Kingdom Prospective Diabetes Study (UKPDS) was a prospective, randomized intervention trial aimed at determining whether patients with type 2 diabetes can clinically benefit from intensive glycemic control. In this study, 3,867 patients with newly diagnosed type 2 diabetes were randomly assigned to an intensive-treatment policy or to a conventional-treatment policy. Compared with the conventional-treatment group, the intensive-treatment group demonstrated a 16% reduction in risk ($p = 0.052$) for fatal and nonfatal MI, but all-cause mortality did not differ between these two groups (305). In this study, intensive therapy resulted in a 0.9% difference in median HbA_{1c} between the intensive (7.0%) and conventional (7.9%) groups over 10 years. Alternatively, as recent data from the DCCT indicate, for all microvascular complications (306), there is probably a continuous relative-risk reduction relationship over the range of HbA_{1c} for CAD (307).

The current recommendations of the ADA set the goal for glycemic control in patients with type 2 diabetes at a fasting (preprandial) glucose level of less than 120 mg/dL and an HbA_{1c} level of less than 7% (normal range 4% to 6%) (308). It is reasonable to believe that the mechanisms by which hyperglycemia promotes atherosclerosis and cardiovascular events are operative in all individuals with hyperglycemia. Because the major morbidity and mortality in patients with type 2 diabetes is a consequence of accelerated atherosclerosis, improved glycemic control is likely to result in a reduction of macrovascular events and probably in a reduction in mortality.

Specific metabolic abnormalities induced by diabetes can adversely affect mechanical performance or increase the myocardial vulnerability to ischemic insults. Thus, insulin administration and improved metabolic control during the acute phase of MI may reduce myocardial damage, improve contractility, and decrease mortality (184). In one study, insulin-glucose infusion in the immediate period after infarction resulted in a significant decline in mortality (309). However, this approach has not been proven to be useful in the *acute* phase of MI in other studies (195,196).

In a recent study, intensive glycemic control in patients with diabetes with MI was associated with a 52% reduction in the 1-year mortality rate (196), and the survival advantage was maintained for up to 5 years (310,311). These findings demonstrate that glycemic control may be valuable even in patients with diabetes with established CAD. More studies are needed to better delineate the importance of metabolic derangements in patients with diabetes during myocardial ischemia.

The Metabolic Syndrome

The ATPIII guidelines present an opportunity for physicians to identify patients with the metabolic syndrome who are at increased risk for developing CAD. The Diabetes Prevention Program demonstrated that either a rigorous regimen of diet and exercise or metformin can prevent or delay diabetes (312). Diagnosing the metabolic syndrome in these patients would allow earlier treatment and thereby reduce the likelihood of their developing CAD (Fig. 58.4).

CONGESTIVE HEART FAILURE AND DIABETES

Paralleling the incidence of CAD in patients with diabetes is the incidence of heart failure. Heart failure is a frequent clinical manifestation of the end stage of cardiovascular complications that afflicts patients with diabetes. The Framingham Study was the first study that showed the risk of symptomatic heart failure was increased 2.4-fold in men with diabetes and fivefold in women with diabetes (313). Population-based studies have revealed that 15% to 25% of patients with heart failure are diabetic, as are 25% to 30% of patients hospitalized for heart failure (314–316).

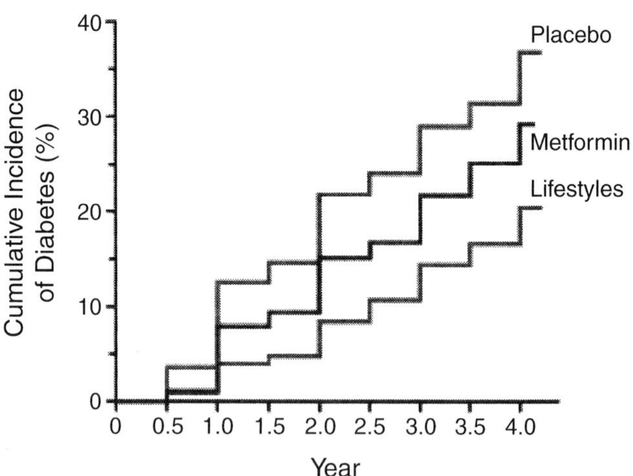

Figure 58.4. Cumulative incidence of diabetes according to study group. The incidence of diabetes differed significantly among the three groups ($p < 0.001$ for each comparison). (From Knowler WC, Barrett-Connor E, Fowler SE, et al. Reduction in the incidence of type 2 diabetes with lifestyle intervention or metformin. *N Engl J Med* 2002;346:393–403, with permission.)

However, these epidemiologic studies do not reveal the frequency of diabetic cardiomyopathy. Whether diabetic cardiomyopathy exists as a separate entity is controversial. The diagnosis of diabetic cardiomyopathy is defined as heart failure in the absence of an identifiable etiology. The presence of congestive heart failure in the person with diabetes in the absence of CAD and hypertension is uncertain.

In the Framingham Study (313), few patients with heart failure did not have CAD, hypertension, or rheumatic disease. The presence of CAD was diagnosed solely on the basis of clinical symptoms and electrocardiographic evidence and not by noninvasive testing or coronary angiography. Therefore, CAD that did not manifest symptoms or typical electrocardiographic changes may have led to the development of heart failure. Patients with diabetes are more prone to silent MIs, accounting for nearly 30% of cases (317). CAD is the most common cause of congestive heart failure in the overall U.S. (318) and diabetic (31) populations. Diffuse CAD can lead to nontransmural infarction with patchy necrosis and myocardial fibrosis, resulting in an impairment of systolic function. Myocardial ischemia may result not only in systolic dysfunction but also in diastolic dysfunction (319,320). In the setting of an acute MI, patients with diabetes have been reported in some studies to develop heart failure up to 50% of the time (321). The GUSTO-1 trial demonstrated that heart failure developed in 27% of the subjects with type 1 diabetes compared with 20% of those with type 2 diabetes and 15% of those in the nondiabetic group. This amounts to the occurrence of heart failure almost twice as frequently in the diabetic population relative to the nondiabetic population (174). Persons with diabetes are also almost twice as likely as those without diabetes to develop heart failure as a result of an acute coronary syndrome (7.2% vs. 3.8%).

Not surprisingly, the presence of heart failure in the diabetic population is associated with a poorer long-term prognosis. The GUSTO-1 study demonstrated that cardiac mortality at 30 days in the subjects with type 1 diabetes was 12.5% compared with 9.7% in those with type 2 diabetes and 6.2% in those without diabetes. This poorer outcome was not the result of a larger MI but may have been due to response of the noninfarcted myocardium to the infarct. The MILIS database demonstrated that the prognosis of patients with diabetes was worse relative to that of patients without diabetes (4-year cardiac mortality rates of 25.9% in those with diabetes and 14.5% in those without diabetes), despite the presence of smaller infarcts [as measured by peak creatine phosphokinase (CPK) or area under the curve] and fewer Q-wave infarcts (174). The GUSTO-1 study also found that vessel patency after MI did not explain this worse prognosis either, since there were similar degrees of infarct-related patency at 90 minutes in the patients with and without diabetes (221). Compensatory hyperkinesis of the noninfarcted walls, which is frequently found in the subject without diabetes immediately after MI, is often blunted in the patient with diabetes (221). This may account for the increased incidence of heart failure.

As discussed earlier in this chapter, hypertension occurs in 40% to 60% of patients with type 2 diabetes (322). Hypertension is the most common cause of heart failure in persons with diabetes after CAD, accounting for 24% of the cases. Diabetes increases the likelihood of development of heart failure 1.8-fold in hypertensive men and 3.7-fold in hypertensive women (322).

DIABETIC CARDIOMYOPATHY

The question whether diabetes itself, distinct from CAD and hypertension, results in a dilated cardiomyopathy, remains controversial. The term diabetic cardiomyopathy was first coined by Rubler in 1972 (323). In the 35- to 64-year-old Framingham cohort, diabetes increased the risk of congestive heart failure in men fourfold and in women eightfold, even after adjustment for blood pressure, age, cholesterol, weight, and a history of CAD (313). The more recent Washington DC Dilated Cardiomyopathy Study used case-controlled analyses to determine that there was an association between diabetes and idiopathic cardiomyopathy (324,325).

Persons with diabetes, and especially women, have greater left ventricular mass and higher heart rates than their nondiabetic counterparts. Some studies report that patients with diabetes may have an abnormal exercise response, with an attenuation of augmentation of left ventricular EF relative to that of healthy persons without diabetes (326–330). Furthermore, various groups have reported diastolic abnormalities using various parameters, including prolonged isovolumic relaxation time (331–333), decreased rates of left ventricular diastolic filling (334–336), and abnormal transmitral flow velocities (187, 336–339). Increased echo density has also been reported despite normal wall thicknesses, which could suggest increased collagen deposition present in the myocardium (340).

Pathologically, postmortem studies of patients with diabetic cardiomyopathy have revealed that they have features similar to those of patients with other forms of nonischemic cardiomyopathy. This includes myocyte hypertrophy, interstitial fibrosis, and infiltration with periodic acid-Schiff–positive materials, with coronary arterioles having thickened basement membranes, as well as the presence of intramyocardial microangiopathy (341–343).

Theories abound regarding the possible mechanism or mechanisms underlying diabetic cardiomyopathy. These include both cellular and molecular perturbations, as well as metabolic abnormalities. Insulin may play a central role in the cellular and mo-lecular mechanisms of diabetic cardiomyopathy. Studies with a line of transgenic mice in which the gene for the insulin-regulated glucose transporter GLUT4 has been deleted demonstrate hyperinsulinemia and cardiomyopathy (344,345). Calcium homeostasis may be altered and has been reported in various animal models of diabetes, suggesting a diminished but prolonged increase in intracellular calcium concentration (346). Hyperglycemia increases calcium-activated signaling through protein kinase C, which may in turn result in cardiac dysfunction. Abnormalities in myofibrillar proteins, including altered phosphorylation of troponin I and myosin light chains, also may play a role in diabetes-associated impairment of contractile function (347,348). Advanced glycosylation results in abnormal collagen cross-linking, which may contribute to decreased compliance and, in turn, to diastolic dysfunction (349).

Several metabolic perturbations may contribute to the development of diabetic cardiomyopathy. Glucose contributes 10% to 15% of the energy of the heart under normal conditions. However, during insulin stimulation, increased workload, and ischemia, the metabolism of glucose is increased. Studies using diabetic animal models have demonstrated that diabetic hearts have a blunted uptake of basal and insulin-stimulated myocardial glucose (350). The glucose that is transported into the heart of a diabetic animal is often shunted to glycogen because of increased fatty acid utilization (351,352). Increased fatty acid uptake and oxidation itself may decrease cardiac function. Ketoacidosis may occur in diabetes. The ketones produced are avidly taken up by the diabetic heart and reduce coenzyme A, which in turn inhibits the citric acid cycle, thereby reducing the energy capability of the muscle and resulting in myocardial dysfunction (353,354).

DIABETIC AUTONOMIC NEUROPATHY

Autonomic neuropathy is a common complication of both type 1 and 2 diabetes. Common clinical manifestations of diabetic autonomic neuropathy (DAN) include orthostatic hypotension, gastroparesis, and resting tachycardia (355). Cardiovascular autonomic neuropathy (CAN) of diabetes confers both an increased risk for the development of cardiovascular disease and a poorer prognosis for those individuals once they develop clinically apparent CAD (356–359). The symptoms of CAN include postural hypotension and resting tachycardia described previously, as well as painless myocardial ischemia. Patients with diabetes with CAN do not have the morning increase in MIs and acute cardiovascular disease events ("circadian variation") found in the patients without diabetes but rather show an even distribution of such events throughout the day (360–362). Parasympathetic nerve fibers are affected first, leading to a relative increase in sympathetic tone that results in a resting tachycardia and attenuation of the expected increase in heart rate and blood pressure with exercise (363,364). The decrease of parasympathetic tone may be responsible for the exaggerated coronary vasoconstriction, which may result in worsening ischemia (365,366). Postural hypotension is a principal clinical manifestation of sympathetic dysfunction (367).

The development of CAN parallels the occurrence of end-organ damage, including retinopathy and nephropathy, and generally occurs in those patients with diabetes of long duration with poorer glycemic control. However, subclinical CAN may occur relatively early in the disease. An important method for early detection is reduced heart-rate variability, which is measured over a 24-hour period (368,369). Alternative methods for early detection of CAN include cardiac radionuclide imaging using the norepinephrine analogue metaiodobenzylguanidine (MIBG), which evaluates cardiac sympathetic activity. The activity is reduced in patients with diabetes with CAN, suggesting reduced sympathetic activity (370).

The estimates of the prevalence of CAN vary depending on the methods used to diagnose its presence and the population studied. In a series of patients with newly diagnosed type 1 diabetes, the incidence of CAN was 8% (368), whereas in a large series including patients with type 1 and type 2 diabetes, the incidence of reduced heart-rate variability was 50% (369). In one small series, 75% of patients with diabetes for 10 years and no significant CAD had evidence of adrenergic denervation as determined by MIBG imaging (370).

As stated earlier, the diagnosis of CAN is a harbinger for serious cardiovascular complications and increased mortality in individuals with diabetes (357–359). The 5-year mortality in a cohort of individuals with type 1 diabetes and CAN was fivefold greater than that in individuals with type 1 diabetes without CAN (358). Although the presence of CAN in patients with type 2 diabetes is not as well characterized as that in patients with type 1 diabetes, one study did show that those individuals with type 2 diabetes with CAN 5 years after being diagnosed with diabetes had a higher cardiovascular mortality in the subsequent 5 years than those with type 2 diabetes who were free of CAN (356).

Numerous experimental and clinical studies have shown that the perturbations in autonomic activity may be important in the development of cardiac arrhythmias. The demonstration of restricted heart-rate variability in persons with diabetes has been shown to be associated with the development of both cardiac arrhythmias and sudden cardiac death, particularly in post-MI patients with left ventricular dysfunction (371–373). The severity of the autonomic dysfunction has been shown to be associated with a higher incidence of arrhythmias. Because individuals with symptomatic clinical CAN usually have had diabetes for a longer time and have poorer glucose control, this may represent a subgroup with more advanced disease and more cardiovascular complications, including previous MIs.

The mechanisms for the increased morbidity and mortality associated with CAN include increased risk of ventricular arrhythmia, silent myocardial ischemia, impaired coronary vasomotor regulation, and increased resting heart rate. Sudden cardiac death has long been known to be associated with diabetes in the absence of cardiovascular disease (357). Transient decreases in heart-rate variability preceded the onset of ST-segment shift and precipitated life-threatening arrhythmias in a group of diabetic patients with CAD who were survivors of sudden cardiac arrest (374). The Honolulu Heart Program also demonstrated that diabetes was independently associated with the risk of sudden cardiac death (375). Prolongation of the QT interval in individuals with diabetes has been shown to correlate with the degree of autonomic neuropathy (376) and may be a method to screen for those persons with diabetes at risk for sudden cardiac death. One group used QT dispersion as a means to evaluate for the presence and degree of autonomic neuropathy. QT dispersion was defined as the longest corrected QT interval minus the shortest corrected QT interval. These investigators found that the greater the QT dispersion, the greater the risk for ventricular arrhythmias and that increased dispersion was more likely in diabetic individuals with CAN (376).

It has long been recognized that patients with diabetes have less severe anginal pain or no pain at all associated with myocardial ischemia (160,169,170,377). Patients with diabetes may present with rather atypical symptoms, including shortness of breath, diaphoresis, gastrointestinal complaints, or profound fatigue. This blunted or altered pain response to myocardial ischemia in patients with diabetes has been attributed to CAN. Zarich and colleagues (361) showed that 90% of ischemic episodes were asymptomatic in a group of patients with diabetes with documented CAD who underwent ambulatory electrocardiographic (ECG) monitoring.

The altered anginal response is further complicated by the resting tachycardia, which alters the threshold for myocardial ischemia. Myocardial oxygen demand is determined largely by the heart rate–blood pressure product. The resting tachycardia, as a result of parasympathetic denervation, increases myocardial oxygen demand. Therefore any activity puts the diabetic patient with CAD closer to his or her ischemic threshold. Cardiac autonomic neuropathy also can affect coronary blood flow independent of the altered endothelial function (365). One study evaluated the cold pressor test in patients with diabetes and found that the increase in flow in response to cold was lower in those with sympathetic nerve dysfunction compared with those without sympathetic nerve dysfunction (366).

The presence of autonomic neuropathy results in a twofold to threefold increase in cardiac morbidity and mortality in patients with diabetes undergoing noncardiac surgery. This increased risk of general anesthesia in this group of patients with diabetes may be due in part to the relative hemodynamic instability that often occurs (378).

SCREENING FOR THE PRESENCE OF CORONARY ARTERY DISEASE

Little is known about the appropriate screening tests for CAD in patients with no clear evidence of CAD. The American Diabetes Association/American College of Cardiology (ADA/ACC) (311) have developed a consensus as to which patients are at increased risk for cardiac events; which patients should be screened; and what is the appropriate follow-up to a positive test result. The potential benefit of diagnosing CAD in patients with diabetes allows for the initiation of both preventive measures and anti-ischemic therapy, including medication or revascularization therapy. Although no evidence exists for risk intervention in patients with diabetes and asymptomatic CAD, aggressive therapy has been shown to reduce cardiovascular mortality in diabetic individuals with known CAD (as discussed earlier in this chapter). Thus, the identification of CAD in asymptomatic patients is important in order to institute aggressive secondary preventive measures.

Although stress testing is clearly indicated for those diabetic individuals who have established CAD, it is not clear what test would be appropriate in patients who do not have known CAD. Table 58.5 lists those indications set by the ADA/ACC Consensus Panel (311). Stress testing is warranted if the patient has typical or atypical cardiac symptoms. Silent ischemia is a frequent occurrence in diabetic individuals. A resting ECG showing evidence of an infarction or ischemia warrants stress testing. The presence of peripheral or carotid occlusive arterial disease is strongly associated with CAD. Therefore, any diabetic individual with evidence of peripheral vascular disease should undergo stress testing. Multiple risk factors in the same patient increase the possibility of identifying significant CAD. The addition of two other risk factors to diabetes increases the cardiovascular death rate by threefold. Autonomic neuropathy has been strongly associated with cardiac morbidity and mortality; however, data are insufficient regarding whether this is an independent risk factor and enough to warrant stress testing. Microalbuminuria is also an important risk factor for cardiovascular mortality, and therefore warrants stress testing.

Asymptomatic patients with diabetes and one or no risk factors along with a normal ECG do not require cardiac testing. Those patients with carotid or peripheral vascular disease, beginning a vigorous exercise program, with minor ST-T wave changes on ECG, or with two or more risk factors should undergo an exercise stress test. If these patients are limited by an inability to exercise, they should undergo a pharmacologic (dobutamine) stress echo or persantine thallium nuclear test. If these patients have a baseline ECG making a proper assessment of an ECG stress test difficult, they should undergo nuclear or echocardiographic stress testing. Patients with clear evidence of an MI or who have ischemia on their ECG, should also undergo stress perfusion imaging or a stress echo test.

TABLE 58.5. Indications for Cardiac Testing in Patients with Diabetes

1. Typical or atypical cardiac symptoms
2. Resting electrocardiographic findings suggestive of ischemia or infarction
3. Peripheral or carotid occlusive arterial disease
4. Sedentary lifestyle, age 35 years, and plans to begin a vigorous exercise program
5. Two or more of the risk factors listed below in addition to diabetes:
   a. Total cholesterol ≥240 mg/dL, LDL cholesterol ≥160 mg/dL, or HDL cholesterol <35 mg/dL
   b. Blood pressure >140/90 mm Hg
   c. Smoking
   d. Family history of premature coronary artery disease
   e. Positive micro-/macroalbumininuria test

 From the Consensus Development Conference on the Diagnosis of Coronary Heart Disease in People with Diabetes. *Diabetes Care* 1998;21:1551–1559. Reprinted with permission from the American Diabetes Association.

A negative test at a high workload, defined as completing 9 minutes or stage 3 of a Bruce treadmill protocol, should provide some reassurance of a favorable prognosis with regard to cardiovascular disease. However, these patients must be routinely followed and, should their symptoms change, undergo a repeat stress test. Those individuals who have mildly positive tests [defined as 1- to 1.5-mm ST depression at a moderate to high exercise level (Bruce stage 3)] are also in a low-risk group. These patients may require perfusion imaging or a stress echo test to determine if this is a false-positive result, especially since many of these patients underwent stress testing prior to beginning a vigorous exercise program. If either of these tests is negative, these patients can have regular clinical evaluations and have a repeat stress-testing every 2 years or when they develop new symptoms. A moderately positive test in an asymptomatic person with diabetes should warrant a stress echo or cardiac nuclear test, since a large perfusion defect indicates a significant risk for cardiac events in the next 1 to 2 years. If the defect is moderate or large, as determined by echo or perfusion testing, the threshold for having the patients undergo cardiac catheterization should be low. A markedly positive stress test is defined as hypotension with exercise, a positive test at a heart rate of less than 120 beats per minute, an exercise capacity of less than 6 minutes, and greater than 2-mm ST depression. The asymptomatic patient with diabetes who has such a test should undergo cardiac catheterization.

EVALUATION OF RISK FACTORS

Table 58.5 (277) reviews the evaluation of the risk factors in such patients with diabetes. In summary, to develop a plan for risk reduction, it is important to identify the risk factors of an individual patient. To evaluate for risk factors in patients with diabetes, it is important for the patient to have a careful medical history and physical examination along with certain laboratory tests. Such tests include a lipoprotein analysis to evaluate not only the LDL level but also the levels of HDL and triglycerides. Predisposing risk factors need to be assessed, including family history, degree of obesity, and level of physical activity. This assessment should also include an evaluation of the renal status, including the determination for the presence of microalbuminuria or macroalbuminuria. The presence of microalbuminuria in the patient with type 2 diabetes signifies an increased risk for cardiovascular disease. Patients with proteinuria of greater than 1 g per day may require more aggressive goals (<125/75 mm Hg) for blood pressure control. ACE inhibitors frequently are regarded as the initial antihypertensive drug of choice in patients with diabetes (290,298,299).

The medical management of patients with clinical cardiovascular disease includes risk reduction and can be defined as secondary prevention. However, a significant portion of the diabetic population has no overt evidence of cardiovascular disease. Such evidence would make it necessary to institute less aggressive management of cardiovascular risk factors for primary prevention.

In patients with type 2 diabetes, the years of insulin resistance can result in atherogenesis long before the onset of hyperglycemia. Clinical evidence of insulin resistance includes abdominal obesity, high-normal blood pressure, high-normal triglycerides (150 to 250 mg/dL), reduced HDL (<40 mg/dL in men; <50 mg/dL in women), borderline high-risk LDL (130 to 159 mg/dL), and in some patients, impaired fasting glucose (110 to 126 mg/dL). The detection of impaired fasting glucose is a strong risk factor for type 2 diabetes. Therefore, it becomes important to follow the guidelines in Table 58.4 not only to reduce the risk of cardiovascular disease but also to delay the onset of type 2 diabetes.

Recent evidence suggests that either lifestyle intervention or treatment with metformin also can reduce the development of diabetes in persons at high risk (312). It is presumed that measures that reduce the development of diabetes also will reduce the incidence of diabetes' most important sequela, cardiovascular disease.

REFERENCES

1. Vergely P. De l'angine de poitrine dans ses rapports avec le diabete. *Gaz Hebd Med Chir* (Paris) (Series 2) 1883:20:364–368.
2. Trends in diabetes mortality. *MMWR Morb Mortal Wkly Rep* 1988;37:769–773.
3. Grundy SM, Benjamin IJ, Burke GL, et al. Diabetes and cardiovascular disease: a statement for healthcare professionals from the American Heart Association. *Circulation* 1999;100:1134–1146.
4. Barrett-Connor E, Orchard T. Diabetes and heart disease. In: National Diabetes Data Group, Diabetes Data Compiled 1984. Washington, DC: U.S. Department. of Health and Human Services, 1985:XVI-1–XVI-41.
5. American Diabetes Association. Consensus statement: role of cardiovascular risk factors in prevention and treatment of macrovascular disease in diabetes. *Diabetes Care* 1993;16:72–78.
6. Pyorala K, Laakso M, Uusitupa M. Diabetes and atherosclerosis: an epidemiologic view. *Diabetes Metab Rev* 1987;3:463–524.
7. O'Leary DH, Polak JF, Cronmal RA, et al. Distribution and correlates of sonographically detected carotid artery disease in the Cardiovascular Health Study. The CHS Collaborative Research Group. *Stroke* 1992;23:1752–1760.
8. Folsom AR, Eckfeldt JH, Weitzman S, et al. Relation of carotid artery wall thickness to diabetes mellitus, fasting glucose and insulin, body size, and physical activity. Atherosclerosis Risk in Communities (ARIC) Study Investigators. *Stroke* 1994;25:66–73.
9. Stamler J, Vaccaro O, Neaton JD, et al. Diabetes, other risk factors, and 12-yr cardiovascular mortality for men screened in the Multiple Risk Factor Intervention Trial. *Diabetes Care* 1993;16:434–444.
10. Schwartz CJ, Valente AJ, Sprague EA, et al. Pathogenesis of the atherosclerotic lesion. Implications for diabetes mellitus. *Diabetes Care* 1992;15:1156–1167.
11. Aronson D. Pharmacologic modulation of autonomic tone: implications for the diabetic patient. *Diabetologia* 1997;40:476–481.
12. Carter JS, Pugh JA, Monterrosa A. Non-insulin-dependent diabetes mellitus in minorities in the United States. *Ann Intern Med* 1996;125:221–232.
13. Mokdad AH, Serdula MK, Dietz WH, et al. The spread of the obesity epidemic in the United States, 1991–1998. *JAMA* 1999;282:1519–1522.
14. Lee WL, Cheung AM, Cape D, et al. Impact of diabetes on coronary artery disease in women and men: a meta-analysis of prospective studies. *Diabetes Care* 2000;23:962–968.
15. Barrett-Connor EL, Cohn BA, Wingard DC, et al. Why is diabetes mellitus a stronger risk factor for fatal ischemic heart disease in women than in men? The Rancho Bernardo Study [published erratum appears in *JAMA* 1991;265: 3249]. *JAMA* 1991;265:627–631.
16. Gu K, Cowie CC, Harris MI. Mortality in adults with and without diabetes in a national cohort of the U.S. population, 1971–1993. *Diabetes Care* 1998;21: 1138–1145.
17. Krolewski AS, Kosinski EJ, Warram JH, et al. Magnitude and determinants of coronary artery disease in juvenile-onset, insulin-dependent diabetes mellitus. *Am J Cardiol* 1987;59:750–755.
18. Krolewski AS, Warram JH, Rand LI, et al. Epidemiologic approach to the etiology of type I diabetes mellitus and its complications. *N Engl J Med* 1987; 317:1390–1398.
19. Bale GS, Entmacher PS. Estimated life expectancy of diabetics. *Diabetes* 1977; 26:434–438.
20. Haffner SM, Lehtol S, Ronnemaa T, et al. Mortality from coronary heart disease in subjects with type 2 diabetes and in nondiabetic subjects with and without prior myocardial infarction. *N Engl J Med* 1998;339:229–234.
21. Mukamal KJ, Nesto RW, Cohen MC, et al. Impact of diabetes on long-term survival after acute myocardial infarction: comparability of risk with prior myocardial infarction. *Diabetes Care* 2001;24:1422–1427.
22. Malmberg K, Kusuf S, Gerstein HC, et al. Impact of diabetes on long-term prognosis in patients with unstable angina and non-Q-wave myocardial infarction: results of the OASIS (Organization to Assess Strategies for Ischemic Syndromes) Registry. *Circulation* 2000;102:1014–1019.
23. Gu K, Cowie CC, Harris MI. Diabetes and decline in heart disease mortality in U.S. adults. *JAMA* 1999;281:1291–1297.
24. Donahue RP, Orchard TJ. Diabetes mellitus and macrovascular complications. An epidemiological perspective. *Diabetes Care* 1992;15:1141–1155.
25. Maser RE, Wolfson SK Jr, Ellis D, et al. Cardiovascular disease and arterial calcification in insulin-dependent diabetes mellitus: interrelations and risk factor profiles. Pittsburgh Epidemiology of Diabetes Complications Study-V. *Arterioscler Thromb* 1991;11:958–965.
26. Borch-Johnsen K, Norgaard K, Hommel E, et al. Is diabetic nephropathy an inherited complication? *Kidney Int* 1992;41:719–722.
27. Jensen T, Borch-Johnsen K, Kofoed-Enevoldsen A, et al. Coronary heart disease in young type 1 (insulin-dependent) diabetic patients with and without diabetic nephropathy: incidence and risk factors. *Diabetologia* 1987;30:144–148.
28. Manske CL, Wang Y, Rector T, et al. Coronary revascularisation in insulin-dependent diabetic patients with chronic renal failure. *Lancet* 1992;340: 998–1002.
29. Deckert T, Kofoed-Enevoldsen A, Norgaard K, et al. Microalbuminuria. Implications for micro- and macrovascular disease. *Diabetes Care* 1992;15: 1181–1191.
30. Jensen T, Stender S, Deckert T. Abnormalities in plasmas concentrations of lipoproteins and fibrinogen in type 1 (insulin-dependent) diabetic patients with increased urinary albumin excretion. *Diabetologia* 1988;31:142–145.
31. Jones SL, Close CF, Mattock MB, et al. Plasma lipid and coagulation factor concentrations in insulin dependent diabetics with microalbuminuria. *BMJ* 1989;298:487–490.
32. Winocour PH, Durrington PN, Bhatnagar D, et al. Influence of early diabetic nephropathy on very low density lipoprotein (VLDL), intermediate density lipoprotein (IDL), and low density lipoprotein (LDL) composition. *Atherosclerosis* 1991;89:49–57.
33. Gruden G, Cavallo-Perin P, Bazzen M, et al. PAI-1 and factor VII activity are higher in IDDM patients with microalbuminuria. *Diabetes* 1994;43:426–429.
34. Makita Z, Radoff S, Rayfield EJ, et al. Advanced glycosylation end products in patients with diabetic nephropathy. *N Engl J Med* 1991;325:836–842.
35. Makita Z, Bucala R, Rayfield EJ, et al. Reactive glycosylation endproducts in diabetic uraemia and treatment of renal failure. *Lancet* 1994;343:1519–1522.
36. Earle K, Walker J, Hill C, et al. Familial clustering of cardiovascular disease in patients with insulin-dependent diabetes and nephropathy. *N Engl J Med* 1992;326:673–677.
37. Krolewski AS, Caness M, Warra JH, et al. Predisposition to hypertension and susceptibility to renal disease in insulin-dependent diabetes mellitus. *N Engl J Med* 1988;318:140–145.
38. Marre M, Jeunemaitre X, Gallois Y, et al. Contribution of genetic polymorphism in the renin-angiotensin system to the development of renal complications in insulin-dependent diabetes: Genetique de la Nephropathie Diabetique (GENEDIAB) study group. *J Clin Invest* 1997;99:1585–1595.
39. Cambien F, Poirier O, Lecerf L, et al. Deletion polymorphism in the gene for angiotensin-converting enzyme is a potent risk factor for myocardial infarction. *Nature* 1992;359:641–644.
40. Tarnow L, Cambien F, Rossing P, et al. Insertion/deletion polymorphism in the angiotensin-I-converting enzyme gene is associated with coronary heart disease in IDDM patients with diabetic nephropathy. *Diabetologia* 1995;38: 798–803.
41. Ruiz J, Blanche H, Cohen N, et al. Insertion/deletion polymorphism of the angiotensin-converting enzyme gene is strongly associated with coronary heart disease in non-insulin-dependent diabetes mellitus. *Proc Natl Acad Sci U S A* 1994;91:3662–3665.
42. Keavney BD, Dudley CR, Stratton IM, et al. UK prospective diabetes study (UKPDS) 14: association of angiotensin-converting enzyme insertion/deletion polymorphism with myocardial infarction in NIDDM. *Diabetologia* 1995;38: 948–952.
43. Kannel WB, McGee DL. Diabetes and cardiovascular disease. The Framingham Study. *JAMA* 1979;241:2035–2038.
44. Jarrett RJ, McCartney P, Keen H. The Bedford survey: ten year mortality rates in newly diagnosed diabetics, borderline diabetics and normoglycaemic controls and risk indices for coronary heart disease in borderline diabetics. *Diabetologia* 1982;22:79–84.
45. Jarrett RJ, Shipley MJ. Type 2 (non-insulin-dependent) diabetes mellitus and cardiovascular disease—putative association via common antecedents; further evidence from the Whitehall Study. *Diabetologia* 1988;31:737–740.
46. Fontbonne A, Eschwege E, Cambient F, et al. Hypertriglyceridaemia as a risk factor of coronary heart disease mortality in subjects with impaired glucose tolerance or diabetes. Results from the 11-year follow-up of the Paris Prospective Study. *Diabetologia* 1989;32:300–304.
47. Nathan DM. Long-term complications of diabetes mellitus. *N Engl J Med* 1993;328:1676–1685.
48. Barrett-Connor E, Wingard DL. Sex differential in ischemic heart disease mortality in diabetics: a prospective population-based study. *Am J Epidemiol* 1983;118:489–496.
49. Reaven G. Syndrome X: 10 years after. *Drugs* 1999;58[Suppl 1]:19–20.
50. Executive Summary of the Third Report of the National Cholesterol Education Program (NCEP). Expert Panel on Detection, Evaluation, and Treatment of High Blood Cholesterol in Adults (Adult Treatment Panel III). *JAMA* 2001;285:2486–2497.
51. Ferrannini E, Buzzigoli G, Bonadonna R, et al. Insulin resistance in essential hypertension. *N Engl J Med* 1987;317:350–357.
52. Zavaroni I, Bonora E, Pagliara M, et al. Risk factors for coronary artery disease in healthy persons with hyperinsulinemia and normal glucose tolerance. *N Engl J Med* 1989;320:702–706.
53. Larsson B, Svardsudd K, Welin L, et al. Abdominal adipose tissue distribution, obesity, and risk of cardiovascular disease and death: 13 year follow up of participants in the study of men born in 1913. *BMJ (Clin Res Ed)* 1984;288: 1401–1404.
54. Laakso M, Barrett-Connor E. Asymptomatic hyperglycemia is associated with lipid and lipoprotein changes favoring atherosclerosis. *Arteriosclerosis* 1989;9:665–672.

55. Laws A, King AC, Haskell WL, et al. Relation of fasting plasma insulin concentration to high density lipoprotein cholesterol and triglyceride concentrations in men. *Arterioscler Thromb* 1991;11:1636–1642.
56. Modan M, Halkin H, Lusky A, et al. Hyperinsulinemia is characterized by jointly disturbed plasma VLDL, LDL, and HDL levels. A population-based study. *Arteriosclerosis* 1988;8:227–236.
57. Peiris AN, Sothmany S, Hoffman RG, et al. Adiposity, fat distribution, and cardiovascular risk. *Ann Intern Med* 1989;110:867–872.
58. Reaven GM. Role of insulin resistance in human disease (syndrome X): an expanded definition. *Annu Rev Med* 1993;44:121–131.
59. Reaven GM, Laws A. Insulin resistance, compensatory hyperinsulinaemia, and coronary heart disease. *Diabetologia* 1994;37:948–952.
60. Howard G, O'Leary DH, Zaccaro D, et al. Insulin sensitivity and atherosclerosis. The Insulin Resistance Atherosclerosis Study (IRAS) Investigators. *Circulation* 1996;93:1809–1817.
61. Laakso M, Sarlund H, Salonen R, et al. Asymptomatic atherosclerosis and insulin resistance. *Arterioscler Thromb* 1991;11:1068–1076.
62. Agewall S, Wikstrand J, Dahlof C, et al. Urinary albumin excretion is associated with the intima-media thickness of the carotid artery in hypertensive males with non-insulin-dependent diabetes mellitus. *J Hypertens* 1995;13: 463–469.
63. Bonora E, Kiechl S, Williet J, et al. Prevalence of insulin resistance in metabolic disorders: the Bruneck Study. *Diabetes* 1998;47:1643–1649.
64. Fuller JH, Shipley MJ, Rose G, et al. Coronary-heart-disease risk and impaired glucose tolerance. The Whitehall Study. *Lancet* 1980;1:1373–1376.
65. Morrish NJ, Stevens LK, Head J, et al. A prospective study of mortality among middle-aged diabetic patients (the London Cohort of the WHO Multinational Study of Vascular Disease in Diabetics) II: Associated risk factors [published erratum appears in *Diabetologia* 1991;34:287]. *Diabetologia* 1990;33:542–548.
66. Uusitupa M, Siitoneno, Pyorala K, et al. The relationship of cardiovascular risk factors to the prevalence of coronary heart disease in newly diagnosed type 2 (non-insulin-dependent) diabetes. *Diabetologia* 1985;28:653–659.
67. Head J, Fuller JH. International variations in mortality among diabetic patients: the WHO Multinational Study of Vascular Disease in Diabetics. *Diabetologia* 1990;33:477–481.
68. Despres JP, Lamarch B, Mauriege P, et al. Hyperinsulinemia as an independent risk factor for ischemic heart disease. *N Engl J Med* 1996;334:952–957.
69. Andersson DK, Svardsudd K. Long-term glycemic control relates to mortality in type II diabetes. *Diabetes Care* 1995;18:1534–1543.
70. Wei M, Gaskill SP, Haffner SM, et al. Effects of diabetes and level of glycemia on all-cause and cardiovascular mortality. The San Antonio Heart Study. *Diabetes Care* 1998;21:1167–1172.
71. Klein R, Klein BE, Moss SE. The Wisconsin Epidemiologic Study of Diabetic Retinopathy. XVI. The relationship of C-peptide to the incidence and progression of diabetic retinopathy. *Diabetes* 1995;44:796–801.
72. Wingard DL, Barrett-Connor EL, Scheidt-Nave C, et al. Prevalence of cardiovascular and renal complications in older adults with normal or impaired glucose tolerance or NIDDM. A population-based study. *Diabetes Care* 1993; 16:1022–1025.
73. Kuusisto J, Mykkanen L, Pyorala K, et al. Non-insulin-dependent diabetes and its metabolic control are important predictors of stroke in elderly subjects. *Stroke* 1994;25:1157–1164.
74. Rodriguez BL, Lau N, Burchfiel CM, et al. Glucose intolerance and 23-year risk of coronary heart disease and total mortality: the Honolulu Heart Program. *Diabetes Care* 1999;22:1262–1265.
75. Singer DE, Nathan DM, Anderson KM, et al. Association of HbA1c with prevalent cardiovascular disease in the original cohort of the Framingham Heart Study. *Diabetes* 1992;41:202–208.
76. Kuusisto J, Mykkanen L, Pyorala K, et al. NIDDM and its metabolic control predict coronary heart disease in elderly subjects. *Diabetes* 1994;43:960–967.
77. Mattock MB, Morrish NJ, Viberti G, et al. Prospective study of microalbuminuria as predictor of mortality in NIDDM. *Diabetes* 1992;41:736–741.
78. Neil A, Hawkins M, Potok M, et al. A prospective population-based study of microalbuminuria as a predictor of mortality in NIDDM. *Diabetes Care* 1993;16:996–1003.
79. Ducimetiere P, Eschwege T, Papoz L, et al. Relationship of plasma insulin levels to the incidence of myocardial infarction and coronary heart disease mortality in a middle-aged population. *Diabetologia* 1980;19:205–210.
80. Pyorala K. Relationship of glucose tolerance and plasma insulin to the incidence of coronary heart disease: results from two population studies in Finland. *Diabetes Care* 1979;2:131–141.
81. Welborn TA, Wearne K. Coronary heart disease incidence and cardiovascular mortality in Busselton with reference to glucose and insulin concentrations. *Diabetes Care* 1979;2:154–160.
82. Stout RW. Insulin and atheroma: 20-yr perspective. *Diabetes Care* 1990;13:631–654.
83. Gowri MS, van der Westhuyzen DR, Bridges SR, et al. Decreased protection by HDL from poorly controlled type 2 diabetic subjects against LDL oxidation may be due to the abnormal composition of HDL. *Arterioscler Thromb Vasc Biol* 1999;19:2226–2233.
84. Tsai EC, Hirsch IB, Brunzell JD, et al. Reduced plasma peroxyl radical trapping capacity and increased susceptibility of LDL to oxidation in poorly controlled IDDM. *Diabetes* 1994;43:1010–1014.
85. Baynes JW, Thorpe SR. Role of oxidative stress in diabetic complications: a new perspective on an old paradigm. *Diabetes* 1999;48:1–9.
86. Ceriello A, Quatraro A, Caretta F, et al. Evidence for a possible role of oxygen free radicals in the abnormal functional arterial vasomotion in insulin dependent diabetes. *Diabete Metab* 1990;16:318–322.
87. Kilhovd BK, Berg TJ, Birkeland KJ, et al. Serum levels of advanced glycation end products are increased in patients with type 2 diabetes and coronary heart disease. *Diabetes Care* 1999;22:1543–1548.
88. Baynes JW. Role of oxidative stress in development of complications in diabetes. *Diabetes* 1991;40:405–412.
89. King GL, Shiba T, Oliver J, et al. Cellular and molecular abnormalities in the vascular endothelium of diabetes mellitus. *Annu Rev Med* 1994;45:179–188.
90. Gabbay KH. The sorbitol pathway and the complications of diabetes. *N Engl J Med* 1973;288:831–836.
91. Yusuf S, Dagenais G, Pogue J, et al. Vitamin E supplementation and cardiovascular events in high-risk patients. The Heart Outcomes Prevention Evaluation Study Investigators. *N Engl J Med* 2000;342:154–160.
92. Bursell SE, Clermont AC, Aiello LM, et al. High-dose vitamin E supplementation normalizes retinal blood flow and creatinine clearance in patients with type 1 diabetes. *Diabetes Care* 1999;22:1245–1251.
93. Ahmed MU, Thorpe SR, Baynes JW. Identification of *N*-epsilon-carboxymethyllysine as a degradation product of fructoselysine in glycated protein. *J Biol Chem* 1986;261:4889–4894.
94. Sell DR, Monnier VM. Structure elucidation of a senescence cross-link from human extracellular matrix. Implication of pentoses in the aging process. *J Biol Chem* 1989;264:21597–21602.
95. Baron AD. Insulin and the vasculature—old actors, new roles. *J Invest Med* 1996;44:406–412.
96. Moncada S. Eighth Gaddum Memorial Lecture. University of London Institute of Education, December 1980. Biological importance of prostacyclin. *Br J Pharmacol* 1982;76:3–31.
97. Fu MX, Requena JR, Jenkins AJ, et al. The advanced glycation end product, *N*-epsilon-(carboxymethyl)lysine, is a product of both lipid peroxidation and glycoxidation reactions. *J Biol Chem* 1996;271:9982–9986.
98. Requena JR, Fu MX, Ahmed MU, et al. Quantification of malondialdehyde and 4-hydroxynonenal adducts to lysine residues in native and oxidized human low-density lipoprotein. *Biochem J* 1997;322:317–325.
99. Bucala R, Makita Z, Koschinsky T, et al. Lipid advanced glycosylation: pathway for lipid oxidation in vivo. *Proc Natl Acad Sci U S A* 1993;90:6434–6438.
100. Haberland ME, Fong D, Cheng L. Malondialdehyde-altered protein occurs in atheroma of Watanabe heritable hyperlipidemic rabbits. *Science* 1988;241: 215–218.
101. Rosenfeld ME, Palinski W, Yla-Herttuala S, et al. Distribution of oxidation specific lipid-protein adducts and apolipoprotein B in atherosclerotic lesions of varying severity from WHHL rabbits. *Arteriosclerosis* 1990;10:336–349.
102. Carew TE, Schwenke DC, Steinberg D. Antiatherogenic effect of probucol unrelated to its hypocholesterolemic effect: evidence that antioxidants in vivo can selectively inhibit low density lipoprotein degradation in macrophage-rich fatty streaks and slow the progression of atherosclerosis in the Watanabe heritable hyperlipidemic rabbit. *Proc Natl Acad Sci U S A* 1987;84:7725–7729.
103. Regnstrom J, Nilsson J, Tomvall P, et al. Susceptibility to low-density lipoprotein oxidation and coronary atherosclerosis in man. *Lancet* 1992;339:1183–1186.
104. Vlassara H, Brownlee M, Cerami A. Novel macrophage receptor for glucose-modified proteins is distinct from previously described scavenger receptors. *J Exp Med* 1986;164:1301–1309.
105. Vlassara H, Brownlee M, Manogue KR, et al. Cachectin/TNF and IL-1 induced by glucose-modified proteins: role in normal tissue remodeling. *Science* 1988;240:1546–1548.
106. Bevilacqua MP, Pober JS, Majeau GR, et al. Interleukin 1 (IL-1) induces biosynthesis and cell surface expression of procoagulant activity in human vascular endothelial cells. *J Exp Med* 1984;160:618–623.
107. Breviario F, Bertocchi F, Dejana E, et al. IL-1-induced adhesion of polymorphonuclear leukocytes to cultured human endothelial cells. Role of platelet-activating factor. *J Immunol* 1988;141:3391–3397.
108. Raines EW, Dower SK, Ross R. Interleukin-1 mitogenic activity for fibroblasts and smooth muscle cells is due to PDGF-AA. *Science* 1989;243:393–396.
109. O'Brien KD, Allen KD McDonald TO, et al. Vascular cell adhesion molecule-1 is expressed in human coronary atherosclerotic plaques. Implications for the mode of progression of advanced coronary atherosclerosis. *J Clin Invest* 1993; 92:945–951.
110. Beekhuizen H, van Furth R. Monocyte adherence to human vascular endothelium. *J Leukoc Biol* 1993;54:363–378.
111. Pohlman TH, Stanness KA, Beatly PG, et al. An endothelial cell surface factor(s) induced in vitro by lipopolysaccharide, interleukin 1, and tumor necrosis factor-alpha increases neutrophil adherence by a CDw18-dependent mechanism. *J Immunol* 1986;136:4548–4553.
112. Park L, Raman KG, Lee KJ, et al. Suppression of accelerated diabetic atherosclerosis by the soluble receptor for advanced glycation endproducts. *Nat Med* 1998;4:1025–1031.
113. Brown AS, Hong AS, De Belder A, et al. Megakaryocyte ploidy and platelet changes in human diabetes and atherosclerosis. *Arterioscler Thromb Vasc Biol* 1997;17:802–807.
114. Winocour PD, Watala C, Kinglough-Rathbone RL. Membrane fluidity is related to the extent of glycation of proteins, but not to alterations in the cholesterol to phospholipid molar ratio in isolated platelet membranes from diabetic and control subjects. *Thromb Haemost* 1992;67:567–571.

115. Davi G, Catalano I, Averna M, et al. Thromboxane biosynthesis and platelet function in type II diabetes mellitus. *N Engl J Med* 1990;322:1769–1774.
116. Ishii H, Umeda F, Nawata H. Platelet function in diabetes mellitus. *Diabetes Metab Rev* 1992;8:53–66.
117. Hendra T, Betteridge DJ. Platelet function, platelet prostanoids and vascular prostacyclin in diabetes mellitus. *Prostaglandins Leukot Essent Fatty Acids* 1989;35:197–212.
118. Menys VC, Bhatnagar D, Mackness MI, et al. Spontaneous platelet aggregation in whole blood is increased in non-insulin-dependent diabetes mellitus and in female but not male patients with primary dyslipidemia. *Atherosclerosis* 1995;112:115–122.
119. Kannel WB, D'Agostino RB, Wilson PW, et al. Diabetes, fibrinogen, and risk of cardiovascular disease: the Framingham experience. *Am Heart J* 1990;120: 672–676.
120. Lufkin EG, Fass DN, O'Fallon WM, et al. Increased von Willebrand factor in diabetes mellitus. *Metabolism* 1979;28:63–66.
121. Kannel WB, Wolf PA, Castelli WP, et al. Fibrinogen and risk of cardiovascular disease. The Framingham Study. *JAMA* 1987;258:1183–1186.
122. Eliasson M, Roder ME, Dinesen B, et al. Proinsulin, intact insulin, and fibrinolytic variables and fibrinogen in healthy subjects. A population study. *Diabetes Care* 1997;20:1252–1255.
123. Ceriello A, Dello Russo P, Zuccotti C, et al. Decreased antithrombin III activity in diabetes may be due to non-enzymatic glycosylation—a preliminary report. *Thromb Haemost* 1983;50:633–634.
124. Brownlee M, Vlassara H, Cerami A. Inhibition of heparin-catalyzed human antithrombin III activity by nonenzymatic glycosylation. Possible role in fibrin deposition in diabetes. *Diabetes* 1984;33:532–535.
125. Ceriello A, Giugliano D, Quatraro A, et al. Daily rapid blood glucose variations may condition antithrombin III biologic activity but not its plasma concentration in insulin-dependent diabetes. A possible role for labile non-enzymatic glycation. *Diabetes Metab* 1987;13:16–9.
126. Ceriello A, Quatraro A, Dello Russo P, et al. Protein C deficiency in insulin-dependent diabetes: a hyperglycemia-related phenomenon. *Thromb Haemost* 1990;64:104–107.
127. Auwerx J, Bouillon R, Collen D, et al. Tissue-type plasminogen activator antigen and plasminogen activator inhibitor in diabetes mellitus. *Arteriosclerosis* 1988;8:68–72.
128. McGill JB, Schneider DJ, Arfken CL, et al. Factors responsible for impaired fibrinolysis in obese subjects and NIDDM patients. *Diabetes* 1994;43: 104–109.
129. Nordt TK, Schneider DJ, Sobel BE. Augmentation of the synthesis of plasminogen activator inhibitor type-1 by precursors of insulin. A potential risk factor for vascular disease. *Circulation* 1994;89:321–330.
130. Small KW, Stefansson E, Hatchell DL. Retinal blood flow in normal and diabetic dogs. *Invest Ophthalmol Vis Sci* 1987;28:672–675.
131. Clermont AC, Brittis M, Shiba T, et al. Normalization of retinal blood flow in diabetic rats with primary intervention using insulin pumps. *Invest Ophthalmol Vis Sci* 1994;35:981–990.
132. Bursell SE, Clermont AC, Kinsley BT, et al. Retinal blood flow changes in patients with insulin-dependent diabetes mellitus and no diabetic retinopathy. *Invest Ophthalmol Vis Sci* 1996;37:886–897.
133. Miyamoto K, Ogura Y, Nishiwaki H, et al. Evaluation of retinal microcirculatory alterations in the Goto-Kakizaki rat. A spontaneous model of non-insulin-dependent diabetes. *Invest Ophthalmol Vis Sci* 1996;37:898–905.
134. Furchgott RF, Zawadzki JV. The obligatory role of endothelial cells in the relaxation of arterial smooth muscle by acetylcholine. *Nature* 1980;288:373–376.
135. Palmer RM, Ferrige AG, Moncada S. Nitric oxide release accounts for the biological activity of endothelium-derived relaxing factor. *Nature* 1987;327:524–526.
136. Ignarro LJ, Buga GM, Wood KS, et al. Endothelium-derived relaxing factor produced and released from artery and vein is nitric oxide. *Proc Natl Acad Sci U S A* 1987;84:9265–9926.
137. Dinerman JL, Lowenstein CJ, Snyder SH. Molecular mechanisms of nitric oxide regulation. Potential relevance to cardiovascular disease. *Circ Res* 1993;73:217–222.
138. Lincoln TM, Cornwell TL, Taylor AE. cGMP-dependent protein kinase mediates the reduction of Ca^{2+} by cAMP in vascular smooth muscle cells. *Am J Physiol* 1990;258(Pt 1):C399–C407.
139. Collins P, Chappell SP, Griffith TM, et al. Differences in basal endothelium-derived relaxing factor activity in different artery types. *J Cardiovasc Pharmacol* 1986;8:1158–1162.
140. Johnstone MT, Creager SJ, Scales KM, et al. Impaired endothelium-dependent vasodilation in patients with insulin-dependent diabetes mellitus. *Circulation* 1993;88:2510–2516.
141. McVeigh GE, Brennan GM, Roddy MA, et al. Impaired endothelium-dependent and independent vasodilation in patients with type 2 (non-insulin-dependent) diabetes mellitus. *Diabetologia* 1992;35:771–776.
142. Williams SB, Cusco JA, Roddy MA, et al. Impaired nitric oxide–mediated vasodilation in patients with non-insulin-dependent diabetes mellitus. *J Am Coll Cardiol* 1996;27:567–574.
143. Steinberg HO, Chaker H, Leaming R, et al. Obesity/insulin resistance is associated with endothelial dysfunction. Implications for the syndrome of insulin resistance. *J Clin Invest* 1996;97:2601–2610.
144. Ting HH, Timimi FK, Boles KS, et al. Vitamin C improves endothelium-dependent vasodilation in patients with non-insulin-dependent diabetes mellitus. *J Clin Invest* 1996;97:22–28.
145. Timimi FK, Ting H, Haley EA, et al. Vitamin C improves endothelium-dependent vasodilation in patients with insulin-dependent diabetes mellitus. *J Am Coll Cardiol* 1998;31:552–557.
146. van Etten RW, De Koning EJ, Honing MI, et al. Intensive lipid lowering by statin therapy does not improve vasoreactivity in patients with type 2 diabetes. *Arterioscler Thromb Vasc Biol* 2002;22:799–804.
147. Cooke JP. Does ADMA cause endothelial dysfunction? *Arterioscler Thromb Vasc Biol* 2000;20:2032–2037.
148. Fard A, Tuck C, Di Tullio MR, et al. Plasma asymmetric dimethylarginine is elevated and endothelial function is impaired after a high fat meal in type 2 diabetics. *Circulation* 1999;100[Suppl II]:3700(abst).
149. Asagami T, Li W, Abbasi FA, Tsao PS et al. Metformin attenuates plasma asymmetric dimethylarginine and monocyte adhesion in type 2 diabetes. *Circulation* 1999;102[Suppl II]:1129(abst).
150. Vigorita VJ, Moore GW, Hutchins GM. Absence of correlation between coronary arterial atherosclerosis and severity or duration of diabetes mellitus of adult onset. *Am J Cardiol* 1980;46:535–542.
151. Waller BF, Palumbo PJ, Lie JT, et al. Status of the coronary arteries at necropsy in diabetes mellitus with onset after age 30 years. Analysis of 229 diabetic patients with and without clinical evidence of coronary heart disease and comparison to 183 control subjects. *Am J Med* 1980;69:498–506.
152. Granger CB, Califf RM, Young S, et al. Outcome of patients with diabetes mellitus and acute myocardial infarction treated with thrombolytic agents. The Thrombolysis and Angioplasty in Myocardial Infarction (TAMI) Study Group. *J Am Coll Cardiol* 1993;21:920–925.
153. Stein B, Weintraub WS, Gebhart SP, et al. Influence of diabetes mellitus on early and late outcome after percutaneous transluminal coronary angioplasty. *Circulation* 1995;91:979–989.
154. Barzilay JI, Kronmal RA, Bittner V, et al. Coronary artery disease and coronary artery bypass grafting in diabetic patients aged > or = 65 years (report from the Coronary Artery Surgery Study [CASS] Registry). *Am J Cardiol* 1994; 74:334–339.
155. Davies MJ, Bland JM, Hangartner JR, et al. Factors influencing the presence or absence of acute coronary artery thrombi in sudden ischaemic death. *Eur Heart J* 1989;10:203–208.
156. Silva JA, Escobar A, Collins TJ, et al. Unstable angina. A comparison of angioscopic findings between diabetic and nondiabetic patients. *Circulation* 1995;92:1731–1736.
157. Bradley RF, Schonfeld A. Diminished pain in diabetic patients with acute myocardial infarction. *Geriatrics* 1962;17:322–326.
158. Margolis JR, Kannel WS, Feinleib M, et al. Clinical features of unrecognized myocardial infarction—silent and asymptomatic. Eighteen year follow-up: the Framingham Study. *Am J Cardiol* 1973;32:1–7.
159. Soler NG, Bennett MA, Pentecost BL, et al. Myocardial infarction in diabetics. *Q J Med* 1975;44:125–132.
160. Marchant B, Umanchandran V, Stevenson R, et al. Silent myocardial ischemia: role of subclinical neuropathy in patients with and without diabetes. *J Am Coll Cardiol* 1993;22:1433–1437.
161. Hume L, Oakley GD, Boulton AJ, et al. Asymptomatic myocardial ischemia in diabetes and its relationship to diabetic neuropathy: an exercise electrocardiography study in middle-aged diabetic men. *Diabetes Care* 1986;9:384–388.
162. O'Sullivan J, Conroy RM, MacDonald K, et al. Silent ischaemia in diabetic men with autonomic neuropathy. *Br Heart J* 1991;66:313–315.
163. Nesto RW, Phillips RT, Kett KG, et al. Angina and exertional myocardial ischemia in diabetic and nondiabetic patients: assessment by exercise thallium scintigraphy [published erratum appears in *Ann Intern Med* 1988; 108:646]. *Ann Intern Med* 1988;108:170–175.
164. Abenavoli T, Rubler S, Fisher VJ, et al. Exercise testing with myocardial scintigraphy in asymptomatic diabetic males. *Circulation* 1981;63:54–64.
165. Langer A, Freeman MR, Josse RG, et al. Detection of silent myocardial ischemia in diabetes mellitus. *Am J Cardiol* 1991;67:1073–1078.
166. Milan Study on Atherosclerosis and Diabetes (MiSAD) Group. Prevalence of unrecognized silent myocardial ischemia and its association with atherosclerotic risk factors in noninsulin-dependent diabetes mellitus. *Am J Cardiol* 1997;79:134–139.
167. Callaham PR, Froelicher VF, Klein J, et al. Exercise-induced silent ischemia: age, diabetes mellitus, previous myocardial infarction and prognosis. *J Am Coll Cardiol* 1989;14:1175–1180.
168. Caracciolo EA, Chaitman BR, Forman SA, et al. Diabetics with coronary disease have a prevalence of asymptomatic ischemia during exercise treadmill testing and ambulatory ischemia monitoring similar to that of nondiabetic patients. An ACIP database study. ACIP Investigators. Asymptomatic Cardiac Ischemia Pilot Investigators. *Circulation* 1996;93:2097–2105.
169. Faerman I, Faccio E, Milei J, et al. Autonomic neuropathy and painless myocardial infarction in diabetic patients. Histologic evidence of their relationship. *Diabetes* 1977;26:1147–1158.
170. Ambepityia G, Kopelman PG, Ingram D, et al. Exertional myocardial ischemia in diabetes: a quantitative analysis of anginal perceptual threshold and the influence of autonomic function. *J Am Coll Cardiol* 1990;15:72–77.
171. Jaffe AS, Spadaro JJ, Schechtman K, et al. Increased congestive heart failure after myocardial infarction of modest extent in patients with diabetes mellitus. *Am Heart J* 1984;108:31–37.
172. Savage MP, Krolewski AS, Kenien GG, et al. Acute myocardial infarction in diabetes mellitus and significance of congestive heart failure as a prognostic factor. *Am J Cardiol* 1988;62(10 Pt 1):665–669.

173. Malmberg K, Ryden L. Myocardial infarction in patients with diabetes mellitus. *Eur Heart J* 1988;9:259–264.
174. Stone PH, Muller JE, Hartwell T, et al. The effect of diabetes mellitus on prognosis and serial left ventricular function after acute myocardial infarction: contribution of both coronary disease and diastolic left ventricular dysfunction to the adverse prognosis. The MILIS Study Group. *J Am Coll Cardiol* 1989;14:49–57.
175. Mak KH, Molitemo DJ, Granger CB, et al. Influence of diabetes mellitus on clinical outcome in the thrombolytic era of acute myocardial infarction. GUSTO-I Investigators. Global Utilization of Streptokinase and Tissue Plasminogen Activator for Occluded Coronary Arteries. *J Am Coll Cardiol* 1997;30: 171–179.
176. Barbash GI, White HD, Modan M, et al. Significance of diabetes mellitus in patients with acute myocardial infarction receiving thrombolytic therapy. Investigators of the International Tissue Plasminogen Activator/Streptokinase Mortality Trial. *J Am Coll Cardiol* 1993;22:707–713.
177. Lee KL, Woodlief LH, Topol EJ, et al. Predictors of 30-day mortality in the era of reperfusion for acute myocardial infarction. Results from an international trial of 41,021 patients. GUSTO-I Investigators. *Circulation* 1995;91:1659–1668.
178. Zuanetti G, Latini R, Maggioni A, et al. Influence of diabetes on mortality in acute myocardial infarction: data from the GISSI-2 study. *J Am Coll Cardiol* 1993;22:1788–1794.
179. Holmes DR Jr, Berger PB, Hochman JS, et al. Cardiogenic shock in patients with acute ischemic syndromes with and without ST-segment elevation. *Circulation* 1999;100:2067–2073.
180. Orlander PR, Goff DC, Morrissey M, et al. The relation of diabetes to the severity of acute myocardial infarction and post-myocardial infarction survival in Mexican-Americans and non-Hispanic whites. The Corpus Christi Heart Project. *Diabetes* 1994;43:897–902.
181. Lehto S, Pyorala K, Miettinen H, et al. Myocardial infarct size and mortality in patients with non-insulin-dependent diabetes mellitus. *J Intern Med* 1994; 236:291–297.
182. Ulvenstam G, Aberg A, Bergstrand R, et al. Long-term prognosis after myocardial infarction in men with diabetes. *Diabetes* 1985;34:787–792.
183. Iwasaka T, Takahashi N, Nakamura S, et al. Residual left ventricular pump function after acute myocardial infarction in NIDDM patients. *Diabetes Care* 1992;15:1522–1526.
184. Aronson D, Rayfield EJ, Chesebro JH. Mechanisms determining course and outcome of diabetic patients who have had acute myocardial infarction. *Ann Intern Med* 1997;126:296–306.
185. Fava S, Azzopardi J, Muscat HA, et al. Factors that influence outcome in diabetic subjects with myocardial infarction. *Diabetes Care* 1993;16:1615–1618.
186. Gwilt DJ, Petri M, Lewis PW, et al. Myocardial infarct size and mortality in diabetic patients. *Br Heart J* 1985;54:466–472.
187. Zarich SW, Arbuckle BB, Cohen LR, et al. Diastolic abnormalities in young asymptomatic diabetic patients assessed by pulsed Doppler echocardiography. *J Am Coll Cardiol* 1988;12:114–120.
188. Takahashi N, Iwasaka T, Sugiura T, et al. Left ventricular regional function after acute anterior myocardial infarction in diabetic patients. *Diabetes Care* 1989;12:630–635.
189. The GUSTO Angiographic Investigators. The effects of tissue plasminogen activator, streptokinase, or both on coronary-artery patency, ventricular function, and survival after acute myocardial infarction. *N Engl J Med* 1993;329: 1615–1622.
190. Abaci A, Oguzhan A, Kahraman S, et al. Effect of diabetes mellitus on formation of coronary collateral vessels. *Circulation* 1999;99:2239–2242.
191. Herlitz J, Malmberg K, Karlson BW, et al. Mortality and morbidity during a five-year follow-up of diabetics with myocardial infarction. *Acta Med Scand* 1988;224:31–38.
192. Capone RJ, Pawitan Y, el-Sherif N, et al. Events in the cardiac arrhythmia suppression trial: baseline predictors of mortality in placebo-treated patients. *J Am Coll Cardiol* 1991;18:1434–1438.
193. Gilpin E, Ricou F, Dittrich H, et al. Factors associated with recurrent myocardial infarction within one year after acute myocardial infarction. *Am Heart J* 1991;121(2 Pt 1):457–465.
194. Taylor GJ, Moses HW, Katholi RE, et al. Six-year survival after coronary thrombolysis and early revascularization for acute myocardial infarction. *Am J Cardiol* 1992;70:26–30.
195. Malmberg K, Ryden L, Efendic S, et al. Randomized trial of insulin-glucose infusion followed by subcutaneous insulin treatment in diabetic patients with acute myocardial infarction (DIGAMI study): effects on mortality at 1 year. *J Am Coll Cardiol* 1995;26:57–65.
196. Malmberg K. Prospective randomised study of intensive insulin treatment on long term survival after acute myocardial infarction in patients with diabetes mellitus. DIGAMI (Diabetes Mellitus, Insulin Glucose Infusion in Acute Myocardial Infarction) Study Group. *BMJ* 1997;314:1512–1515.
197. Tschoepe D, Roesen P, Schweppert B, et al. Platelets in diabetes: the role in the hemostatic regulation in atherosclerosis. *Semin Thromb Hemost* 1993;19: 122–128.
198. DiMinno G, Silver MJ, Cerbone AM, et al. Trial of repeated low-dose aspirin in diabetic angiopathy. *Blood* 1986;68:886–891.
199. Randomised trial of intravenous streptokinase, oral aspirin, both, or neither among 17,187 cases of suspected acute myocardial infarction: ISIS-2. ISIS-2 (Second International Study of Infarct Survival) Collaborative Group. *Lancet* 1988;2:349–360.
200. Antiplatelet Trialists' Collaboration. Collaborative overview of randomized trials of antiplatelet therapy. I. Prevention of death, myocardial infarction, and stroke by prolonged antiplatelet therapy in various categories of patients. *BMJ* 1994;308:81–106.
201. Colwell JA. Aspirin therapy in diabetes. *Diabetes Care* 1997;20:1767–1771.
202. Aspirin therapy in diabetes. American Diabetes Association. *Diabetes Care* 1997;20:1772–1773.
203. Kendall MJ, Lynch KP, Hjalmarson A, et al. Beta-blockers and sudden cardiac death. *Ann Intern Med* 1995;123:358–367.
204. Mangano DT, Layug EL, Wallace A, et al. Effect of atenolol on mortality and cardiovascular morbidity after noncardiac surgery. Multicenter Study of Perioperative Ischemia Research Group [published erratum appears in *N Engl J Med* 1997;336:1039]. *N Engl J Med* 1996;335:1713–1720.
205. Shorr RI, Ray WA, Daugherty JR, et al. Antihypertensives and the risk of serious hypoglycemia in older persons using insulin or sulfonylureas. *JAMA* 1997;278:40–43.
206. Pfeffer MA. ACE inhibitors in acute myocardial infarction: patient selection and timing. *Circulation* 1998;97:2192–2194.
207. Zuanetti G, Latini R, Maggioni AP, et al. Effect of the ACE inhibitor lisinopril on mortality in diabetic patients with acute myocardial infarction: data from the GISSI-3 study. *Circulation* 1997;96:4239–4245.
208. Moye LA, Pfeffer MA, Wun CC, et al. Uniformity of captopril benefit in the SAVE Study: subgroup analysis. Survival and Ventricular Enlargement Study. *Eur Heart J* 1994;15[Suppl B]:2–8.
209. Gustafsson I, Torp-Pedersen C, Kober L, et al. Effect of the angiotensin-converting enzyme inhibitor trandolapril on mortality and morbidity in diabetic patients with left ventricular dysfunction after acute myocardial infarction. Trace Study Group. *J Am Coll Cardiol* 1999;34:83–89.
210. Yusuf S, Sleight P, Pogue J, et al. Effects of an angiotensin-converting-enzyme inhibitor, ramipril, on cardiovascular events in high-risk patients. The Heart Outcomes Prevention Evaluation Study Investigators. *N Engl J Med* 2000;342: 145–153.
211. Heart Outcomes Prevention Evaluation Study (HOPE) Investigators. Effects of ramipril on cardiovascular and microvascular outcomes in people with diabetes mellitus: results of the HOPE study and MICRO-HOPE substudy. Heart Outcomes Prevention Evaluation Study Investigators. *Lancet* 2000;355: 253–259.
212. Torlone E, Rambotti AM, Periello G, et al. ACE-inhibition increases hepatic and extrahepatic sensitivity to insulin in patients with type 2 (non-insulin-dependent) diabetes mellitus and arterial hypertension. *Diabetologia* 1991;34: 11–25.
213. Pollare T, Lithell H, Berne C. A comparison of the effects of hydrochlorothiazide and captopril on glucose and lipid metabolism in patients with hypertension. *N Engl J Med* 1989;321:868–873.
214. Bak JF, Gerdes LU, Sorensen NS, et al. Effects of perindopril on insulin sensitivity and plasma lipid profile in hypertensive non-insulin-dependent diabetic patients. *Am J Med* 1992;92[Suppl 4B]:69S–72S.
215. Lewis EJ, Hunsicker LG, Bain RP, et al. The effect of angiotensin-converting-enzyme inhibition on diabetic nephropathy. The Collaborative Study Group [published erratum appears in *N Engl J Med* 1993;330:152]. *N Engl J Med* 1993; 329:1456–1462.
216. Ravid M, Savin H, Jutrin I, et al. Long-term stabilizing effect of angiotensin-converting enzyme inhibition on plasma creatinine and on proteinuria in normotensive type II diabetic patients. *Ann Intern Med* 1993;118:577–581.
217. Inhibition of the platelet glycoprotein IIb/IIIa receptor with tirofiban in unstable angina and non-Q-wave myocardial infarction. Platelet Receptor Inhibition in Ischemic Syndrome Management in Patients Limited by Unstable Signs and Symptoms (PRISM-PLUS) Study Investigators. *N Engl J Med* 1998;338:1488–1497.
218. Steinhubl SR, Kottke-Marchant K, et al. Attainment and maintenance of platelet inhibition through standard dosing of abciximab in diabetic and non-diabetic patients undergoing percutaneous coronary intervention. *Circulation* 1999;100:1977–1982.
219. Platelet glycoprotein IIb/IIIa receptor blockade and low-dose heparin during percutaneous coronary revascularization. The EPILOG Investigators. *N Engl J Med* 1997;336:1689–1696.
220. Randomised placebo-controlled and balloon-angioplasty-controlled trial to assess safety of coronary stenting with use of platelet glycoprotein IIb/IIIa blockade. The EPISTENT Investigators. Evaluation of Platelet IIb/IIIa Inhibitor for Stenting. *Lancet* 1998;352:87–92.
221. Roffi M, Moliterno DJ, Meler B, et al. Impact of different platelet glycoprotein IIb/IIIa receptor inhibitors among diabetic patients undergoing percutaneous coronary intervention: Do Tirofiban and ReoPro Give Similar Efficacy Outcomes Trial (TARGET) 1-year follow-up. *Circulation* 2002;105:2730–2736.
222. Woodfield SL, Lundergan CF, Reiner JS, et al. Angiographic findings and outcome in diabetic patients treated with thrombolytic therapy for acute myocardial infarction: the GUSTO-I experience. *J Am Coll Cardiol* 1996;28:1661–1669.
223. Fibrinolytic Therapy Trialists' (FTT) Collaborative Group: indications for fibrinolytic therapy in suspected acute myocardial infarction: collaborative overview of early mortality and major morbidity results from all randomized trials of more than 1000 patients. *Lancet* 1994;343:311–322.
224. Mahaffey KW, Granger CB, Toth CA, et al. Diabetic retinopathy should not be a contraindication to thrombolytic therapy for acute myocardial infarction: review of ocular hemorrhage incidence and location in the GUSTO-1 trial. Global Utilization of Streptokinase and t-PA for Occluded Coronary Arteries. *J Am Coll Cardiol* 1997;30:1606–1610.

225. Detre K, Holubkov R, Kelsey S, et al. Percutaneous transluminal coronary angioplasty in 1985–1986 and 1977–1981. The National Heart, Lung, and Blood Institute Registry. *N Engl J Med* 1988;318:265–270.
226. Adelman A, Cohen EA, Kimball BP, et al. A comparison of directional atherectomy with balloon angioplasty for lesions of the left anterior descending coronary artery. *N Engl J Med* 1993;329:228–233.
227. Parisi A, Folland E, Hartigan P. A comparison of angioplasty with medical therapy in the treatment of single-vessel coronary artery disease. *N Engl J Med* 1993;326:10–16.
228. The Bypass Angioplasty Revascularization Investigation (BARI) Investigators. Comparison of coronary bypass surgery with angioplasty in patients with multivessel disease. *N Engl J Med* 1996;335:217–225.
229. Kurbaan AS, Bowker TJ, Ilsley CD, et al. Difference in the mortality of the CABRI diabetic and nondiabetic populations and its relation to coronary artery disease and the revascularization mode. *Am J Cardiol* 2001;87:947–950 (abst 3).
230. Holmes DJ, Vlietstra RE, Smith HC, et al. Restenosis after percutanous transluminal coronary angioplasty (PTCA): a report from the PTCA Registry of the National Heart, Lung, and Blood Institute. *Am J Cardiol* 1984;53:77C–81C.
231. Weintraub W, Kosinski AS, Brown CL 3rd, et al. Can restenosis after coronary angioplasty be predicted from clinical variables. *J Am Coll Cardiol* 1993; 21:6–14.
232. Vandormael MG, Deligonul U, Kern MJ, et al. Multilesion coronary angioplasty: clinical and angiographic follow-up. *J Am Coll Cardiol* 1987;10:246–252.
233. Quigley PJ, Hlatky MA, Hinohara T, et al. Repeat percutaneous transluminal coronary angioplasty and predictors of recurrent restenosis. *Am J Cardiol* 1989;63:409–413.
234. Rensing BJ, Hermans WR, Vos J, et al. Luminal narrowing after percutaneous transluminal coronary angioplasty. A study of clinical, procedural, and lesional factors related to long-term angiographic outcome. Coronary Artery Restenosis Prevention on Repeated Thromboxane Antagonism (CARPORT) Study Group. *Circulation* 1993;88:975–985.
235. Bach R, Jung R, Kohsiek I, et al. Factors affecting the restenosis rate after percutaneous transluminal coronary angioplasty. *Thromb Haemost* 1994;74 [Suppl1]:S55–S77.
236. Lambert M, Bonan R, Cote G, et al. Multiple coronary angioplasty: a model to discriminate systemic and procedural factors related to restenosis. *J Am Coll Cardiol* 1988;12:310–314.
237. Popma JJ, Mintz GS, Satler LF, et al. Clinical and angiographic outcome after directional coronary atherectomy. A qualitative and quantitative analysis using coronary arteriography and intravascular ultrasound. *Am J Cardiol* 1993;72:55E–64E.
238. Warth D, Leon MB, O'Neill W, et al. Rotational atherectomy multicenter registry: acute results, complications and 6-month angiographic follow-up in 709 patients. *J Am Coll Cardiol* 1994;24:641–648.
239. Levine GN, Jacobs AK, Keeler GP, et al. Impact of diabetes mellitus on percutaneous revascularization (CAVEAT-I). CAVEAT-I Investigators. Coronary Angioplasty Versus Excisional Atherectomy Trial. *Am J Cardiol* 1997;79:748–755.
240. Rabbani L, Edelman ER, Ganz P, et al. Relation of restenosis after excimer laser angioplasty to fasting insulin levels. *Am J Cardiol* 1994;73:323–327.
241. Fischman DL, Leon MB, Balm DS, et al. A randomized comparison of coronary-stent placement and balloon angioplasty in the treatment of coronary artery disease. Stent Restenosis Study Investigators. *N Engl J Med* 1994;331: 496–501.
242. Kastrati A, Schomig A, Elezi S, et al. Predictive factors of restenosis after coronary stent placement. *J Am Coll Cardiol* 1997;30:1428–1436.
243. Kastrati A, Schomig A, Elezi S, et al. Interlesion dependence of the risk for restenosis in patients with coronary stent placement in multiple lesions. *Circulation* 1998;97:2396–2401.
244. Carrozza J, Kuntz RE, Fishman RF, et al. Restenosis after arterial injury caused by coronary stenting in patients with diabetes mellitus. *Ann Intern Med* 1993;118:344–349.
245. Wang N, Gundry SR, Van Arsdell G, et al. Percutaneous transluminal coronary angioplasty failures in patients with multivessel disease. Is there an increased risk? *J Thorac Cardiovasc Surg* 1995;110:214–221.
246. Van Belle E, Bauters C, Hubert E, et al. Restenosis rates in diabetic patients: a comparison of coronary stenting and balloon angioplasty in native coronary vessels. *Circulation* 1997;96:1454–1460.
247. Kip KE, Faxon DP, Detre KM, et al. Coronary angioplasty in diabetic patients. The National Heart, Lung, and Blood Institute Percutaneous Transluminal Coronary Angioplasty Registry. *Circulation* 1996;94:1818–1825.
248. Gum P, O'Keefe JH Jr, Borken AM, et al. Bypass surgery versus coronary angioplasty for revascularization of treated diabetic patients. *Circulation* 1997;96[Suppl 9]:II–7–10.
249. Ellis CJ, French JK, White HD, et al. Results of percutaneous coronary angioplasty in patients <40 years of age. *Am J Cardiol* 1998;82:135–139.
250. Dauerman HL, Baim DS, Cutlip DE, et al. Mechanical debulking versus balloon angioplasty for the treatment of diffuse in-stent restenosis. *Am J Cardiol* 1998;82:277–284.
251. Walton BL, Mum K, Taniuchi M, et al. Diabetic patients treated with abciximab and intracoronary stenting. *Catheter Cardiovasc Interv* 2002;55:321–325.
252. Marso SP, Lincoff AM, Ellis SG, et al. Optimizing the percutaneous interventional outcomes for patients with diabetes mellitus: results of the EPISTENT (Evaluation of Platelet IIb/IIIa Inhibitor for Stenting Trial) diabetic substudy. *Circulation* 1999;100:2477–2484.
253. Kornowski R, Mintz GS, Kent KM, et al. Increased restenosis in diabetes mellitus after coronary interventions is due to exaggerated intimal hyperplasia. A serial intravascular ultrasound study. *Circulation* 1997;95:1366–1369.
254. Aronson D, Bloomgarden Z, Rayfield EJ. Potential mechanisms promoting restenosis in diabetic patients. *J Am Coll Cardiol* 1996;27:528–535.
255. Moreno PR, Murcia AM, Palacios IF, et al. Coronary composition and macrophage infiltration in atherectomy specimens from patients with diabetes mellitus. *Circulation* 2000;102:2180–2184.
256. Sobel BE. Acceleration of restenosis by diabetes: pathogenetic implications. *Circulation* 2001;103:1185–1187.
257. Sobel BE. Increased plasminogen activator inhibitor-1 and vasculopathy. A reconcilable paradox. *Circulation* 1999;99:2496–2498.
258. Roguin A, Ribichini F, Ferrero V, et al. Haptoglobin phenotype and the risk of restenosis after coronary artery stent implantation. *Am J Cardiol* 2002;89: 806–810.
259. Fietsam R Jr, Bassett J, Glover JL. Complications of coronary artery surgery in diabetic patients. *Am Surg* 1991;57:551–557.
260. Slaughter MS, Olson MM, Lee JT Jr, et al. A fifteen-year wound surveillance study after coronary artery bypass. *Ann Thorac Surg* 1993;56:1063–1068.
261. Palac RT, Meadows WR, Hwang MH, et al. Risk factors related to progressive narrowing in aortocoronary vein grafts studied 1 and 5 years after surgery. *Circulation* 1982;66(2 Pt 2):I40-I44.
262. Lytle BW, Loop FD, Cosgrove DM, et al. Long-term (5 to 12 years) serial studies of internal mammary artery and saphenous vein coronary bypass grafts. *J Thorac Cardiovasc Surg* 1985;89:248–258.
263. Hirotani T, Kameda T, Kumamoto T, et al. Effects of coronary artery bypass grafting using internal mammary arteries for diabetic patients. *J Am Coll Cardiol* 1999;34:532–538.
264. Davies M, Kim JH, Klyachkin ML, et al. Diabetes mellitus and experimental vein graft structure and function. *J Vasc Surg* 1994;19:1031–1043.
265. Morris JJ, Smith LR, Jones RH, et al. Influence of diabetes and mammary artery grafting on survival after coronary bypass. *Circulation* 1991;84 [5 Suppl]:III275–III284.
266. Herlitz J, Brandrup-Wognsen G, Haglid M, et al. Mortality and morbidity during a period of 2 years after coronary artery bypass surgery in patients with and without a history of hypertension. *J Hypertens* 1996;14:309–314.
267. Lawrie GM, Morris GC Jr, Glaeser DH. Influence of diabetes mellitus on the results of coronary bypass surgery. Follow-up of 212 diabetic patients ten to 15 years after surgery. *JAMA* 1986;256:2967–2971.
268. Ferguson J. NHLBI BARI clinical alert on diabetics treated with angioplasty. *Circulation* 1995;92:3371.
269. The Bypass Angioplasty Revascularization Investigation (BARI). Influence of diabetes on 5-year mortality and morbidity in a randomized trial comparing CABG and PTCA in patients with multivessel disease. *Circulation* 1997;96: 1761–1769.
270. Barsness GW, Peterson ED, Ohman EM, et al. Relationship between diabetes mellitus and long-term survival after coronary bypass and angioplasty. *Circulation* 1997;96:2551–2556.
271. Weintraub W, Stein B, Kosinski A, et al. Outcome of coronary bypass surgery versus coronary angioplasty in diabetic patients with multivessel coronary artery disease. *J Am Coll Cardiol* 1998;31:10–19.
272. Zhao XQ, Brown BG, Stewart DK, et al. Effectiveness of revascularization in the Emory Angioplasty versus Surgery Trial. A randomized comparison of coronary angioplasty with bypass surgery. *Circulation* 1996;93:1954–1962.
273. Bell MR, Gersh BJ, Schaff HV, et al. Effect of completeness of revascularization on long-term outcome of patients with three-vessel disease undergoing coronary artery bypass surgery. A report from the Coronary Artery Surgery Study (CASS) Registry. *Circulation* 1992;86:446–457.
274. Schaff HV, Rosen AD, Shemin RJ, et al. Clinical and operative characteristics of patients randomized to coronary artery bypass surgery in the Bypass Angioplasty Revascularization Investigation (BARI). *Am J Cardiol* 1995;75: 18C–26C.
275. Van Belle E, Kotelers R, Bauters C, et al. Patency of percutaneous transluminal coronary angioplasty sites at 6-month angiographic follow-up: a key determinant of survival in diabetics after coronary balloon angioplasty. *Circulation* 2001;103:1218–1224.
276. Nahsar P, Brown RE, Oskarsson H, et al. Maximal coronary flow reserve and metabolic coronary vasodilation in patients with diabetes mellitus. *Circulation* 1995;91:635–640.
277. Grundy SM, Garber A, Goldberg R, et al. Prevention Conference VI: Diabetes and Cardiovascular Disease: executive summary: conference proceeding for healthcare professionals from a special writing group of the American Heart Association. *Circulation* 2002;105:2231–2239.
278. Scandinavian Simvastatin Survival Study Group. Randomized trial of cholesterol lowering in 4444 patients with coronary heart disease: Scandinavian Simvastatin Survival Study (4S). *Lancet* 1994;334:1383–1389.
279. Pyorala K, Pedersen TR, Kjekshus J, et al. Cholesterol lowering with simvastatin improves prognosis of diabetic patients with coronary heart disease. A subgroup analysis of the Scandinavian Simvastatin Survival Study (4S). *Diabetes Care* 1997;20:614–620.
280. Sacks FM, Moye LA, Davis BR, et al. Relationship between plasma LDL concentrations during treatment with pravastatin and recurrent coronary events in the Cholesterol and Recurrent Events Trial. *Circulation* 1998;97: 1446–1452.
281. Selby JV, Austin MA, Newman B, et al. LDL subclass phenotypes and the insulin resistance syndrome in women. *Circulation* 1993;88:381–387.
282. Lyons TJ. Glycation and oxidation: a role in the pathogenesis of atherosclerosis. *J Cardiol* 1993;71:26B–31B.

283. Goldberg RB, Mellies MJ, Sacks FM, et al. Cardiovascular events and their reduction with pravastatin in diabetic and glucose-intolerant myocardial infarction survivors with average cholesterol levels: subgroup analyses in the cholesterol and recurrent events (CARE) trial. The CARE Investigators. *Circulation* 1998;98:2513–2519.
284. Haffner SM. Epidemiological studies on the effects of hyperglycemia and improvement of glycemic control on macrovascular events in type 2 diabetes. *Diabetes Care* 1999;22[Suppl 3]:C54–C56.
285. Tan CE, Chew LS, Chio LF, et al. Cardiovascular risk factors and LDL subfraction profile in type 2 diabetes mellitus subjects with good glycaemic control. *Diabetes Res Clin Pract* 2001;51:107–114.
286. Rubins HB, Robins SJ, Collins D, et al. Gemfibrozil for the secondary prevention of coronary heart disease in men with low levels of high-density lipoprotein cholesterol. Veterans Affairs High-Density Lipoprotein Cholesterol Intervention Trial Study Group. *N Engl J Med* 1999;341:410–418.
287. Sacks FM, Tonkin AM, Craven T, et al. Coronary heart disease in patients with low LDL-cholesterol: benefit of pravastatin in diabetics and enhanced role for HDL-cholesterol and triglycerides as risk factors. *Circulation* 2002; 105:1424–1428.
288. National High Blood Pressure Education Program Working Group Report on Hypertension and Diabetes. *Hypertension* 1994;23:145–158.
289. American Diabetes Association. Consensus statement on the treatment of hypertension in diabetes. *Diabetes Care* 1993;16:1394–1401.
290. The Sixth Report of the Joint National Committee on Prevention, Detection, Evaluation, and Treatment of High Blood Pressure. *Arch Intern Med* 1997;157: 2413–2446.
291. Estacio RO, Jeffers BW, Hiatt WR, et al. The effect of nisoldipine as compared with enalapril on cardiovascular outcomes in patients with non-insulin-dependent diabetes and hypertension. *N Engl J Med* 1998;338:645–652.
292. Tatti P, Pahor M, Byington RP, et al. Outcome results of the Fosinopril Versus Amlodipine Cardiovascular Events Randomized Trial (FACET) in patients with hypertension and NIDDM. *Diabetes Care* 1998;21:597–603.
293. Curb JD, Pressel SL, Cutler JA, et al. Effect of diuretic-based antihypertensive treatment on cardiovascular disease risk in older diabetic patients with isolated systolic hypertension. Systolic Hypertension in the Elderly Program Cooperative Research Group [published erratum appears in *JAMA* 1997; 277:1356]. *JAMA* 1996;276:1886–1892.
294. Pahor M, Psaty BM, Furberg CD. Treatment of hypertensive patients with diabetes. *Lancet* 1998;351:689–690.
295. Sowers JR. Comorbidity of hypertension and diabetes: the Fosinopril versus Amlodipine Cardiovascular Events Trial (FACET). *Am J Cardiol* 1998;82[9B]: 15R–19R.
296. Tuomilehto J, Rastenyte D, Birkenhager WH, et al. Effects of calcium-channel blockade in older patients with diabetes and systolic hypertension. Systolic Hypertension in Europe Trial Investigators. *N Engl J Med* 1999;340:677–684.
297. Hansson L, Zanchetti A, Carruthers SG, et al. Effects of intensive blood-pressure lowering and low-dose aspirin in patients with hypertension: principal results of the Hypertension Optimal Treatment (HOT) randomised trial. HOT Study Group. *Lancet* 1998;351:1755–1762.
298. Cooper ME. Pathogenesis, prevention, and treatment of diabetic nephropathy. *Lancet* 1998;352:213–219.
299. Parving HH. Renoprotection in diabetes: genetic and non-genetic risk factors and treatment. *Diabetologia* 1998;41:745–759.
300. Lindholm LH, Ibsen H, Dahlof B, et al. Cardiovascular morbidity and mortality in patients with diabetes in the Losartan Intervention for Endpoint Reduction in Hypertension Study (LIFE): a randomised trial against atenolol. *Lancet* 2002;359:1004–1010.
301. The effect of intensive treatment of diabetes on the development and progression of long-term complications in insulin-dependent diabetes mellitus. The Diabetes Control and Complications Trial Research Group. *N Engl J Med* 1993;329:977–986.
302. Effect of intensive diabetes management on macrovascular events and risk factors in the Diabetes Control and Complications Trial. *Am J Cardiol* 1995;75: 894–903.
303. Kunjathoor VV, Wilson DL, LeBoeuf RC. Increased atherosclerosis in streptozotocin-induced diabetic mice. *J Clin Invest* 1996;97:1767–1773.
304. Jensen-Urstad KJ, Reichard PG, Rosfors JS, et al. Early atherosclerosis is retarded by improved long-term blood glucose control in patients with IDDM. *Diabetes* 1996;45:1253–1258.
305. UK Prospective Diabetes Study (UKPDS) Group. Intensive blood-glucose control with sulphonylureas or insulin compared with conventional treatment and risk of complications in patients with type 2 diabetes (UKPDS 33). *Lancet* 1998;352:837–853.
306. The absence of a glycemic threshold for the development of long-term complications: the perspective of the Diabetes Control and Complications Trial. *Diabetes* 1996;45:1289–1298.
307. Klein R, Klein BE, Moss SE, et al. Glycosylated hemoglobin in a population-based study of diabetes. *Am J Epidemiol* 1987;126:415–428.
308. Consensus statement. The pharmacological treatment of hyperglycemia in NIDDM. *Diabetes Care* 1995;18:1510–1518.
309. Clark RS, English M, McNeill GP, et al. Effect of intravenous infusion of insulin in diabetics with acute myocardial infarction. *BMJ (Clin Res Ed)* 1985; 291:303–305.
310. Malmberg K, Norhammar A, Wedel H, et al. Glycometabolic state at admission: important risk marker of mortality in conventionally treated patients with diabetes mellitus and acute myocardial infarction: long-term results from the Diabetes and Insulin-Glucose Infusion in Acute Myocardial Infarction (DIGAMI) study. *Circulation* 1999;99:2626–2632.
311. Consensus Development Conference on the Diagnosis of Coronary Heart Disease in people with diabetes: 10–11 February 1998, Miami, FL. American Diabetes Association. *Diabetes Care* 1998;21:1551–1559.
312. Knowler WC, Barrett-Connor E, Fowler SE, et al. Reduction in the incidence of type 2 diabetes with lifestyle intervention or metformin. *N Engl J Med* 2002; 346:393–403.
313. Kannel WB, Hjortland M, Castelli WP. Role of diabetes in congestive heart failure: the Framingham Study. *Am J Cardiol* 1974;34:29–34.
314. Croft JB, Giles WH, Pollard RA, et al. National trends in the initial hospitalization for heart failure. *J Am Geriatr Soc* 1997;45:270–275.
315. Polanczyk CA, Rohde LE, Dec GW, et al. Ten-year trends in hospital care for congestive heart failure: improved outcomes and increased use of resources. *Arch Intern Med* 2000;160:325–332.
316. Reis SE, Holubkov R, Edmundowicz D, et al. Treatment of patients admitted to the hospital with congestive heart failure: specialty-related disparities in practice patterns and outcomes. *J Am Coll Cardiol* 1997;30:733–738.
317. Butler R, MacDonald TM, Struthers AD, et al. The clinical implications of diabetic heart disease. *Eur Heart J* 1998;19:1617–1627.
318. Garcia MJ, McNamara PM, Gordon T, et al. Morbidity and mortality in diabetics in the Framingham population. Sixteen-year follow-up study. *Diabetes* 1974;23:105–111.
319. Hamby RI, Zoneraich S, Sherman L. Diabetic cardiomyopathy. *JAMA* 1974; 229:1749–1754.
320. Litwin SE, Grossman W. Diastolic dysfunction as a cause of heart failure. *J Am Coll Cardiol* 1993;22[Suppl 4A]:49A–55A.
321. Timmis AD. Diabetic heart disease: clinical considerations. *Heart* 2001;85: 463–469.
322. Hypertension in Diabetes Study (HDS): II. Increased risk of cardiovascular complications in hypertensive type 2 diabetic patients. *J Hypertens* 1993;11: 319–325.
323. Rubler S, Dlugash J, Yuceoglu YZ, et al. New type of cardiomyopathy associated with diabetic glomerulosclerosis. *Am J Cardiol* 1972;30:595–602.
324. Coughlin SS, Pearle DL, Baughman KL, et al. Diabetes mellitus and risk of idiopathic dilated cardiomyopathy. The Washington DC Dilated Cardiomyopathy Study. *Ann Epidemiol* 1994;4:67–74.
325. Coughlin SS, Tefft MC. The epidemiology of idiopathic dilated cardiomyopathy in women: the Washington DC Dilated Cardiomyopathy Study. *Epidemiology* 1994;5:449–455.
326. Mildenberger RR, Bar-Shlomo B, Druck MN, et al. Clinically unrecognized ventricular dysfunction in young diabetic patients. *J Am Coll Cardiol* 1984;4: 234–238.
327. Vered A, Battler A, Segal P, et al. Exercise-induced left ventricular dysfunction in young men with asymptomatic diabetes mellitus (diabetic cardiomyopathy). *Am J Cardiol* 1984;54:633–637.
328. Zola B, Kahn JK, Juni JE, et al. Abnormal cardiac function in diabetic patients with autonomic neuropathy in the absence of ischemic heart disease. *J Clin Endocrinol Metab* 1986;63:208–214.
329. Mustonen JN, Uusitupa MI, Tahvanainen K, et al. Impaired left ventricular systolic function during exercise in middle-aged insulin-dependent and noninsulin-dependent diabetic subjects without clinically evident cardiovascular disease. *Am J Cardiol* 1988;62:1273–1279.
330. Arvan S, Singal K, Knapp R, et al. Subclinical left ventricular abnormalities in young diabetics. *Chest* 1988;93:1031–1034.
331. Rynkiewicz A, Semetkowska-Jurkiewicz E, Wyrzykowski B. Systolic and diastolic time intervals in young diabetics. *Br Heart J* 1980;44:280–283.
332. Shapiro LM, Howat AP, Calter MM, et al. Left ventricular function in diabetes mellitus. II: Relation between clinical features and left ventricular function. *Br Heart J* 1981;45:129–132.
333. Shapiro LM, Howat AP, Calter MM. Left ventricular function in diabetes mellitus. I: Methodology, and prevalence and spectrum of abnormalities. *Br Heart J* 1981;45:122–128.
334. Sanderson JE, Brown DJ, Rivellese A, et al. Diabetic cardiomyopathy? An echocardiographic study of young diabetics. *BMJ* 1978;1:404–407.
335. Hausdorf G, Rieger U, Koepp P. Cardiomyopathy in childhood diabetes mellitus: incidence, time of onset, and relation to metabolic control. *Int J Cardiol* 1988;19:225–236.
336. Danielsen R. Factors contributing to left ventricular diastolic dysfunction in long-term type I diabetic subjects. *Acta Med Scand* 1988;224:249–256.
337. Takenaka K, Sakamoto T, Amano K, et al. Left ventricular filling determined by Doppler echocardiography in diabetes mellitus. *Am J Cardiol* 1988;61: 1140–1143.
338. Bouchard A, Sanz N, Botvinick EH, et al. Noninvasive assessment of cardiomyopathy in normotensive diabetic patients between 20 and 50 years old. *Am J Med* 1989;87:160–166.
339. Paillole C, Dahan M, Paycha F, et al. Prevalence and significance of left ventricular filling abnormalities determined by Doppler echocardiography in young type I (insulin-dependent) diabetic patients. *Am J Cardiol* 1989;64: 1010–1016.
340. Di Bello V, Talarico L, Picaro E, et al. Increased echodensity of myocardial wall in the diabetic heart: an ultrasound tissue characterization study. *J Am Coll Cardiol* 1995;25:1408–1415.
341. Factor SM, Borczuk A, Charron MJ, et al. Myocardial alterations in diabetes and hypertension. *Diabetes Res Clin Pract* 1996;31[Suppl]:S133–S142.

342. van Hoeven KH, Factor SM. A comparison of the pathological spectrum of hypertensive, diabetic, and hypertensive-diabetic heart disease. *Circulation* 1990;82:848–855.
343. Hardin NJ. The myocardial and vascular pathology of diabetic cardiomyopathy. *Coron Artery Dis* 1996;7:99–108.
344. Katz EB, Stenbit AE, Hatton K, et al. Cardiac and adipose tissue abnormalities but not diabetes in mice deficient in GLUT4. *Nature* 1995;377:151–155.
345. Stenbit AE, Tsao TS, Li J, et al. GLUT4 heterozygous knockout mice develop muscle insulin resistance and diabetes. *Nat Med* 1997;3:1096–1101.
346. Lagadic-Gossmann D, Buckler KH, Le Prigent K, et al. Altered Ca^{2+} handling in ventricular myocytes isolated from diabetic rats. *Am J Physiol* 1996; 270(5 Pt 2):H1529–H1537.
347. Liu X, Takeda N, Dhalla NS. Troponin I phosphorylation in heart homogenate from diabetic rat. *Biochim Biophys Acta* 1996;1316:78–84.
348. Liu X, Takeda N, Dhalla NS. Myosin light-chain phosphorylation in diabetic cardiomyopathy in rats. *Metabolism* 1997;46:71–75.
349. Norton GR, Candy G, Woodiwiss AJ. Aminoguanidine prevents the decreased myocardial compliance produced by streptozotocin-induced diabetes mellitus in rats. *Circulation* 1996;93:1905–1912.
350. Barrett EJ, Schwartz RG, Young LH, et al. Effect of chronic diabetes on myocardial fuel metabolism and insulin sensitivity. *Diabetes* 1988;37:943–948.
351. Laughlin MR, Taylor J, Chesnick AS, et al. Nonglucose substrates increase glycogen synthesis in vivo in dog heart. *Am J Physiol* 1994;267(1 Pt 2): H219–H223.
352. Russell RR 3rd, Cline GW, Guthrie PH, et al. Regulation of exogenous and endogenous glucose metabolism by insulin and acetoacetate in the isolated working rat heart. A three tracer study of glycolysis, glycogen metabolism, and glucose oxidation. *J Clin Invest* 1997;100:2892–2899.
353. Taegtmeyer H. On the inability of ketone bodies to serve as the only energy providing substrate for rat heart at physiological work load. *Basic Res Cardiol* 1983;78:435–450.
354. Russell RR 3rd, Taegtmeyer H. Coenzyme A sequestration in rat hearts oxidizing ketone bodies. *J Clin Invest* 1992;89:968–973.
355. Spallone V, Menzinger G. Autonomic neuropathy: clinical and instrumental findings. *Clin Neurosci* 1997;4:346–358.
356. Toyry JP, Niskanen LK, Mantysaari MJ, et al. Occurrence, predictors, and clinical significance of autonomic neuropathy in NIDDM. Ten-year follow-up from the diagnosis. *Diabetes* 1996;45:308–315.
357. Sampson MJ, Chambers JB, Sprigings DC, et al. Abnormal diastolic function in patients with type 1 diabetes and early nephropathy. *Br Heart J* 1990;64:266–271.
358. O'Brien IA, McFadden JP, Corrall RJ. The influence of autonomic neuropathy on mortality in insulin-dependent diabetes. *Q J Med* 1991;79:495–502.
359. Orchard TJ, Lloyd CE, Maser RE, et al. Why does diabetic autonomic neuropathy predict IDDM mortality? An analysis from the Pittsburgh Epidemiology of Diabetes Complications Study. *Diabetes Res Clin Pract* 1996;34 [Suppl]:S165–S171.
360. Muller JE, Tofler GH, Stone PH. Circadian variation and triggers of onset of acute cardiovascular disease. *Circulation* 1989;79:733–743.
361. Zarich S, Waxman S, Freeman RT, et al. Effect of autonomic nervous system dysfunction on the circadian pattern of myocardial ischemia in diabetes mellitus. *J Am Coll Cardiol* 1994;24:956–962.
362. Bernardi L, Ricordi L, Lazzari P, et al. Impaired circadian modulation of sympathovagal activity in diabetes. A possible explanation for altered temporal onset of cardiovascular disease. *Circulation* 1992;86:1443–1452.
363. Kahn JK, Zola B, Juni JE, et al. Decreased exercise heart rate and blood pressure response in diabetic subjects with cardiac autonomic neuropathy. *Diabetes Care* 1986;9:389–394.
364. Hilsted J, Galbo H, Christensen NJ. Impaired cardiovascular responses to graded exercise in diabetic autonomic neuropathy. *Diabetes* 1979;28:313–319.
365. Di Carli MF, Tobes MC, Mangner T, et al. Effects of cardiac sympathetic innervation on coronary blood flow. *N Engl J Med* 1997;336:1208–1215.
366. Di Carli MF, Bianco-Batlles D, Landa ME, et al. Effects of autonomic neuropathy on coronary blood flow in patients with diabetes mellitus. *Circulation* 1999;100:813–819.
367. Spallone V, Menzinger G. Diagnosis of cardiovascular autonomic neuropathy in diabetes. *Diabetes* 1997;46[Suppl 2]:S67–S76.
368. Ziegler D, Dannehl K, Volksu D, et al. Prevalence of cardiovascular autonomic dysfunction assessed by spectral analysis and standard tests of heart-rate variation in newly diagnosed IDDM patients. *Diabetes Care* 1992;15:908–911.
369. Ewing DJ, Neilson JM, Shapiro CM, et al. Twenty-four-hour heart rate variability: effects of posture, sleep, and time of day in healthy controls and comparison with bedside tests of autonomic function in diabetic patients. *Br Heart J* 1991;65:239–244.
370. Kreiner G, Wolzt M, Fasching P, et al. Myocardial m-[^{123}I]iodobenzylguanidine scintigraphy for the assessment of adrenergic cardiac innervation in patients with IDDM. Comparison with cardiovascular reflex tests and relationship to left ventricular function. *Diabetes* 1995;44:543–549.
371. Kleiger RE, Miller JP, Bigger JT Jr, et al. Decreased heart rate variability and its association with increased mortality after acute myocardial infarction. *Am J Cardiol* 1987;59:256–262.
372. Farrell TG, Bashir Y, Cripps T, et al. Risk stratification for arrhythmic events in postinfarction patients based on heart rate variability, ambulatory electrocardiographic variables and the signal-averaged electrocardiogram. *J Am Coll Cardiol* 1991;8:687–697.
373. Bigger JT Jr, Fleiss JL, Steinman RC, et al. Frequency domain measures of heart period variability and mortality after myocardial infarction. *Circulation* 1992;85:164–171.
374. Pozzati A, Pancaldi LG, Di Pasquale G, et al. Transient sympathovagal imbalance triggers "ischemic" sudden death in patients undergoing electrocardiographic Holter monitoring. *J Am Coll Cardiol* 1996;27:847–852.
375. Curb JD, Rodriguez BL, Burchfiel CM, et al. Sudden death, impaired glucose tolerance, and diabetes in Japanese American men. *Circulation* 1995;91:2591–2595.
376. Kahn JK, Sisson JC, Vinik AI. QT interval prolongation and sudden cardiac death in diabetic autonomic neuropathy. *J Clin Endocrinol Metab* 1987;64:751–754.
377. Burgos LG, Ebert TJ, Asiddao C, et al. Increased intraoperative cardiovascular morbidity in diabetics with autonomic neuropathy. *Anesthesiology* 1989; 70:591–597.
378. Keyl C, Lemberger P, Palitzsch KD, et al. Cardiovascular autonomic dysfunction and hemodynamic response to anesthetic induction in patients with coronary artery disease and diabetes mellitus. *Anesth Analg* 1999;88:985–991.
379. Mueller HS, Cohen LS, Braunwald E, et al. Predictors of early morbidity and mortality after thrombolytic therapy of acute myocardial infarction. Analyses of patient subgroups in the Thrombolysis in Myocardial Infarction (TIMI) trial, phase II. *Circulation* 1992;85:1254–1264.

CHAPTER 59
Erectile Dysfunction and Diabetes

Ricardo Munarriz, Abdulmaged Traish, and Irwin Goldstein

Male sexual dysfunctions are classified into dysfunctions of libido, problems with emission/ejaculation/orgasm, impotence, and priapism. Erectile dysfunction (ED) or impotence is the most common of the various sexual dysfunctions, and because multiple advances have been realized in understanding the physiologic and biochemical mechanisms involving penile erection and in clinical techniques of improving ED, this chapter will be devoted primarily to the sexual dysfunction of impotence.

Erectile dysfunction or impotence is the consistent inability to achieve or sustain an erection of sufficient rigidity to permit satisfactory sexual intercourse (1). It has been estimated from data collected in 1948 that 10 million American males, or approximately 1 in 10 men, have impotence (1,2). New epidemiologic research in a random, community-based population of aging men suggests that the prevalence of impotence among men 39 to 70 years of age is greater than 50% (3). Contemporary studies indicate that impotence afflicts over 30 million American men.

The prevalence of impotence is particularly high in certain groups of patients. In the previous study (3), aging, treated hypertension, treated heart disease, and treated diabetes were among several physiologic variables found to strongly predict impotence. The prevalence of self-assessed complete impotence was more than three times higher among men with diabetes than among men without diabetes. Impotence is an age-dependent disorder (2,4,5) that affects the diabetic male an average of 10 to 15 years earlier than it does his nondiabetic counterpart. Other studies have demonstrated this higher prevalence of impotence among men with diabetes than in the general male population. Depending on the investigators and the study population, the reported prevalence of impotence in diabetic men has ranged from 35% to 75% (6–12).

Impotence in men with diabetes develops insidiously over a period of months or years (9). Patients frequently describe diminished penile rigidity and reduced ability to sustain an erection. Impotence, however, is not always a late progressive complication of the disease but can occur early in its natural history. Libido may persist despite poor erectile performance (8,9).

ANATOMY OF THE PENIS

The penis has two paired corpora cavernosa and a corpus spongiosum, which surrounds the urethra and distally forms the glans penis. Each corpus cavernosum is surrounded by a thick fibrous sheath, the tunica albuginea, which is composed of wavy collagen and elastin that allows erectile tissue to expand and elongate. Formation of tunica plaques (Peyronie disease) can result in loss of tunica compliance, penile curvature, and veno-occlusion dysfunction (4). The erectile tissue consists of multiple, interconnected lacunae lined by vascular endothelium. The walls of the lacunae, the trabeculae, are composed of thick bundles of smooth muscle and a fibroelastic frame (5).

The internal pudendal artery enters the perineum through the Alcock canal and gives rise to four terminal branches (dorsal artery, cavernosal artery, bulbar artery, and the scrotal artery). Along with the nerves that run within the Alcock canal (pudendal nerves), the blood vessels in this region are vulnerable to compression injuries such as those that may occur during bicycle riding (13). It has been recently demonstrated that the dorsal artery interconnects with the cavernosal artery (14). This communication is responsible for the success of microvascular penile bypass surgery between the inferior epigastric artery (donor vessel) and the dorsal artery (recipient vessel) in patients with cavernosal artery occlusion. Last, accessory pudendal arteries provide additional blood flow to the corpora cavernosa. Injury to these arteries during radical retropubic prostatectomy may explain why some patients experience ED following successful nerve-sparing procedures (15).

Multiple muscular helicine arteries branch off each cavernosal artery and open directly into the lacunar spaces. Blood drains from the corporal bodies through subtunica venules located between the periphery of the erectile tissue and the tunica albuginea. Subtunica venules coalesce to form larger emissary veins that pierce the tunica albuginea (16,17).

The peripheral innervation of the penis consists of sympathetic nerves arising from the 11th thoracic to the second lumbar spinal cord segments and from parasympathetic and somatic nerves arising from the second, third, and fourth sacral spinal cord segments. Somatic innervation is via the pudendal nerve, which is composed of efferent fibers innervating the striated musculature of the perineum and of afferent fibers from the penile and perineal skin (18).

PHYSIOLOGY OF ERECTION

Central Mechanism of Erection

Penile erections are elicited by local sensory stimulation of the genital organs (reflexogenic erections) and by central psychogenic stimuli received by or generated within the brain (psychogenic erections) (18,19). Recently, specific regions of the brain (inferior temporal cortex, right insula, right inferior frontal cortex, and left anterior cingulated cortex) activated by visual evoked sexual arousal have been identified by positron emission tomography (20). The medial preoptic area and the paraventricular nucleus within the hypothalamus appear to integrate visual (occipital area), tactile (thalamus), olfactory (rhinencephalon), and imaginative (limbic system) input and send neural projections to the thoracolumbar sympathetic and sacral parasympathetic centers of the spinal cord (21). Dopamine and oxytocin are thought to play important roles in mediating the pre-erectile response in the medial preoptic area and the paraventricular nucleus respectively (22). In contrast, the nucleus paragigantocellularis (nPGi) in the brainstem exerts an inhibitory effect on sexual arousal (23). Nerves from the nPGi project to sacral segments of the spinal cord and release serotonin. This has been postulated as the reason specific serotonin reuptake inhibitors (SSRIs) depress sexual function. Because men treated with SSRI drugs most commonly exhibit delayed or blocked ejaculation, cases of premature ejaculation have also been successfully managed with SSRI treatment. The locus ceruleus also exerts inhibitory input via sympathetic nerves that interface with hypothalamic nuclei as well as with the spinal cord. Withdrawal of sympathetic input due to suppressed activity of the locus caeruleus during rapid eye movement (REM) sleep is thought to lead to episodes of nocturnal penile tumescence (22,24). The pudendal nerve, which is the afferent limb for reflexogenic erections, collects somatic sensation from the genital skin. The autonomic nerve fibers that arise from the sacral parasympathetic center (S2–S4) make up the efferent limb for this reflex, innervating the penile smooth muscle. Reflexogenic and psychogenic erectile mechanisms probably act synergistically in the control of penile erection (18,25–31).

Erection follows relaxation of arterial and trabecular smooth muscle (32). Dilation of the cavernosal and helicine arteries increases blood flow into the lacunar spaces. Relaxation of the trabecular smooth muscle dilates the lacunar spaces, accommodating a larger volume of blood and thus engorging the penis. The expansion of the relaxed trabecular walls against the tunica albuginea compresses the plexus of subtunica venules (16,33,34). This results in increased resistance to the outflow of blood with increased lacunar space pressure, making the penis rigid. The reduction of venous outflow by the mechanical compression of subtunica venules is known as the corporal veno-occlusive mechanism (Fig. 59.1).

Contraction of penile smooth muscle results in detumescence. Activation of sympathetic constrictor nerves causes an increase in the tone of the smooth muscle of the helicine arteries and the trabeculae, resulting in a reduction of arterial inflow, a collapse of the lacunar spaces with decompression of subtu-

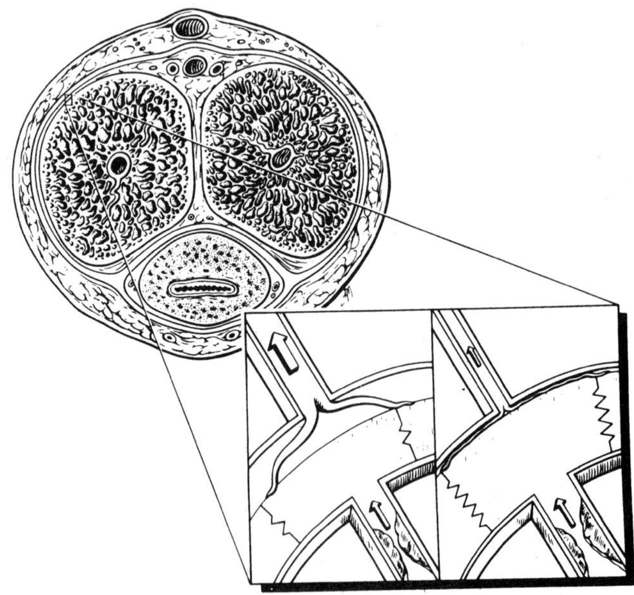

Figure 59.1 Schematic cross-section of the penis including two corporal bodies and a corpus spongiosum. **Insets:** Enlargements of the subtunica space between the trabeculae and the tunica albuginea. Drainage from erection tissue passes via subtunica venules into emissary veins that drain through the tunica. When the penis is in the flaccid state **(left inset)**, the contracted corporal smooth muscle allows blood to drain from the erectile tissue to the subtunica venules under conditions of low outflow resistance. When the penis is in the erect state **(right inset)**, following activation of efferent autonomic nerves, the elevated pressure in the lacunar space expands the trabecular structures against the tunica albuginea. The expanded volume of the corporal tissue both mechanically compresses and physically stretches the subtunica venules, greatly increasing the resistance to flow through these venous channels. The resultant restriction of venous outflow through the subtunica venules is called the corporal veno-occlusive mechanism.

nica venules (16,33,34), an increase in venous outflow from the lacunar space, and a return of the penis to the flaccid state.

Peripheral Mechanisms of Erection

NEUROGENIC REGULATION OF PENILE ERECTION

Erectile function in the penis is regulated by autonomic (parasympathetic and sympathetic) and somatic (sensory and motor) pathways to the erectile tissues and perineal striated muscles. Three sets of peripheral nerves innervate the penis, the sympathetic nerves, the parasympathetic nerves, and the pudendal nerves.

The sympathetic nerves (T10–L2), which are responsible for detumescence and maintenance of flaccidity, project to the corpora, as well as to the prostate and bladder neck via the hypogastric nerves. Postganglionic noradrenergic fibers pass posterolateral to the prostate in the so-called nerves of Walsh to enter the corpora cavernosa medially. Adrenergic tone is crucial in initiating detumescence and in maintaining the flaccid state of the penis, because the smooth muscle of the arteries and cavernosal trabeculae must remain actively contracted. Contraction of cavernosal trabecular smooth muscle in response to norepinephrine is mediated by α_1-adrenergic receptors. Prejunctional α_2-adrenergic receptors on adrenergic nerves inhibit neurotransmission and provide a self-regulating negative feedback loop for secreted norepinephrine. Cholinergic nerves act on prejunctional muscarinic receptors to also inhibit adrenergic nerve activity.

It is possible that adrenergic imbalance toward vasoconstriction impairs erection. While specific factors that contribute to this imbalance remain unknown, aging and/or associated disease states may cause selective upregulation of specific adrenergic receptor subtypes, resulting in higher efficacy for norepinephrine action. Since norepinephrine is a key modulator of erectile function, it is plausible that α-adrenergic receptor antagonists may prove useful in the treatment of ED. Clinical experience with drugs such as yohimbine and phentolamine have had varying efficacy in men with ED. The role of α-adrenergic receptors in the physiology of penile erection is reviewed more completely elsewhere (35,36).

The parasympathetic nerves, originating in the intermediolateral nuclei of the S2 to S4 spinal cord segments, provide the major excitatory input to the penis and are responsible for vasodilation of the penile vasculature and subsequent erection. Exiting through the sacral foramina, these nerves pass forward lateral to the rectum as the pelvic nerve and synapse in the pelvic plexus with postganglionic nonadrenergic, noncholinergic (NANC) nerve fibers, which travel within the cavernous nerves to the corpora cavernosa. Vasoactive intestinal peptide (VIP) and nitric oxide (NO) are two NANC neurotransmitters that are often co-localized in the same nerves in penile tissue. However, the role of VIP as a modulator of penile erection remains unclear because the experimental results with this peptide on erectile function are inconsistent. Intracavernosal administration of VIP in animals and humans has yielded varying results, ranging from no effect to partial tumescence to full erection. Furthermore, the lack of specific and effective antagonists for VIP hinders experimental investigation concerning its role in erectile function.

The primary mediator of NANC parasympathetic input is NO. The ability of NO, a highly reactive and unstable gas, to regulate a wide array of physiologic functions in mammals has become evident only within the last two decades. Along with carbon monoxide, NO is a unique primary effector molecule with the characteristics of an intracellular second messenger that defies previous classification schemes. It is apparently synthesized on demand with little or no storage, and it directly activates a soluble enzyme (guanylate cyclase) rather than a "traditional" receptor molecule. NO is produced by nitric oxide synthase (NOS), which uses the amino acid L-arginine and molecular oxygen as substrates to produce NO and L-citrulline. NO can readily cross plasma membranes to enter target cells, where it binds the heme component of soluble guanylate cyclase. This activation of guanylate cyclase stimulates the production of cyclic guanosine monophosphate (cGMP), with the resultant activation of the cGMP-dependent protein kinase, which regulates the intracellular events, leading to relaxation of trabecular smooth muscle. The levels of cGMP also are regulated by phosphodiesterases, which break down cGMP and terminate signaling. Sildenafil (Viagra) is a potent, selective, and reversible inhibitor of phosphodiesterase type 5, the major enzyme responsible for cGMP hydrolysis in penile erectile tissue (37). Inhibition of this enzyme leads to the increase in levels of intracellular cGMP and enhancement of the relaxation of smooth muscle in response to stimuli that activate the NO/cGMP pathway. This activity may explain the success of sildenafil in the treatment of male ED (38).

Recently, it has become evident that NO interacts directly with other cellular targets, including receptors, ion channels, and pumps, that may modulate the contractility of smooth muscle cells, independently of the cGMP pathway (39–41). Thus, NO has intracellular targets in addition to guanylate cyclase that may play a role in the regulation of vascular and trabecular smooth muscle contractility.

The activity of NANC nerves may be modulated by cholinergic nerves, which facilitate NANC relaxation by stimulating the synthesis and release of NO and other vasodilatory neurotransmitters such as VIP. Thus, the release of acetylcholine may coordinate withdrawal of adrenergic input and increase of NANC input by binding to prejunctional muscarinic receptors on adrenergic and NANC nerves (24). In certain disease states, such as diabetes, the ability of the corpus cavernosum to synthesize and release acetylcholine is diminished (42). Such processes may be responsible in part for the compromised erectile function associated with diabetes. Parasympathetic nerves are also vulnerable during surgical procedures, such as abdominoperineal resection of the rectum and radical prostatectomy (15,43).

The pudendal nerves comprise motor efferent and sensory afferent fibers innervating the ischiocavernous and bulbocavernous muscles as well as the penile and perineal skin. Pudendal motor neuron cell bodies are located in the Onuf nucleus of the S2 to S4 segments. The pudendal nerve enters the perineum through the lesser sciatic notch at the posterior border of the ischiorectal fossa and runs in the Alcock canal (pudendal canal) toward the posterior aspect of the perineal membrane. At this point, the pudendal nerve gives rise to the perineal nerve, with branches to the scrotum and the rectal nerve supplying the inferior rectal region. The dorsal nerve of the penis emerges as the last branch of the pudendal nerve. It then turns distally along the dorsal penile shaft, lateral to the dorsal artery. Multiple fascicles fan out distally, supplying proprioceptive and sensory nerve terminals to the dorsum of the tunica albuginea and the skin of the penile shaft and glans penis.

NON-NEURONAL MODULATORS OF PENILE ERECTION

In addition to neurogenic mechanisms, local paracrine/autocrine factors, with vasoactive and/or trophic effects, profoundly influence the function of the smooth muscle in the penis. These include endothelins, prostanoids, NO, and oxygen.

Endothelin-1 (ET-1), a member of the endothelin family of peptides, is one of the most potent vasoconstrictors known at this time. Similar to NO, the release of endothelin from the intimal lining of vascular compartments can be induced by shear stress. However, little is known about the physiologic or cellular mechanisms that regulate its production. In human corpus cavernosum, ET-1 is synthesized by the endothelium and elicits strong, sustained contractions of corpus cavernosum smooth muscle. Both major subtypes of endothelin receptors (ET_A and ET_B) have been identified in penile corpus cavernosum and are distributed on both the endothelium and the smooth muscle. It has also been suggested that endothelin may exert vasodilatory effects at low concentrations through a "super-high" affinity form of the ET_B receptor potentially by stimulating NO production. However, the significance of this mechanism in penile erection remains unclear. In rabbit models of disease, ET_B receptors in penile corpus cavernosum were upregulated in alloxan-induced diabetic rabbits and downregulated in hypercholesterolemic Watanabe rabbits. Additionally, elevated plasma endothelin levels have been reported in both diabetic and nondiabetic men with ED. Thus, endothelin may contribute to the maintenance of penile flaccidity by providing sustained tone to the trabecular smooth muscle, and alterations in endothelin production may result in impaired erectile function. Several selective antagonists of endothelin receptor subtypes have been developed, but their efficacy and safety in the treatment of ED have not been fully evaluated.

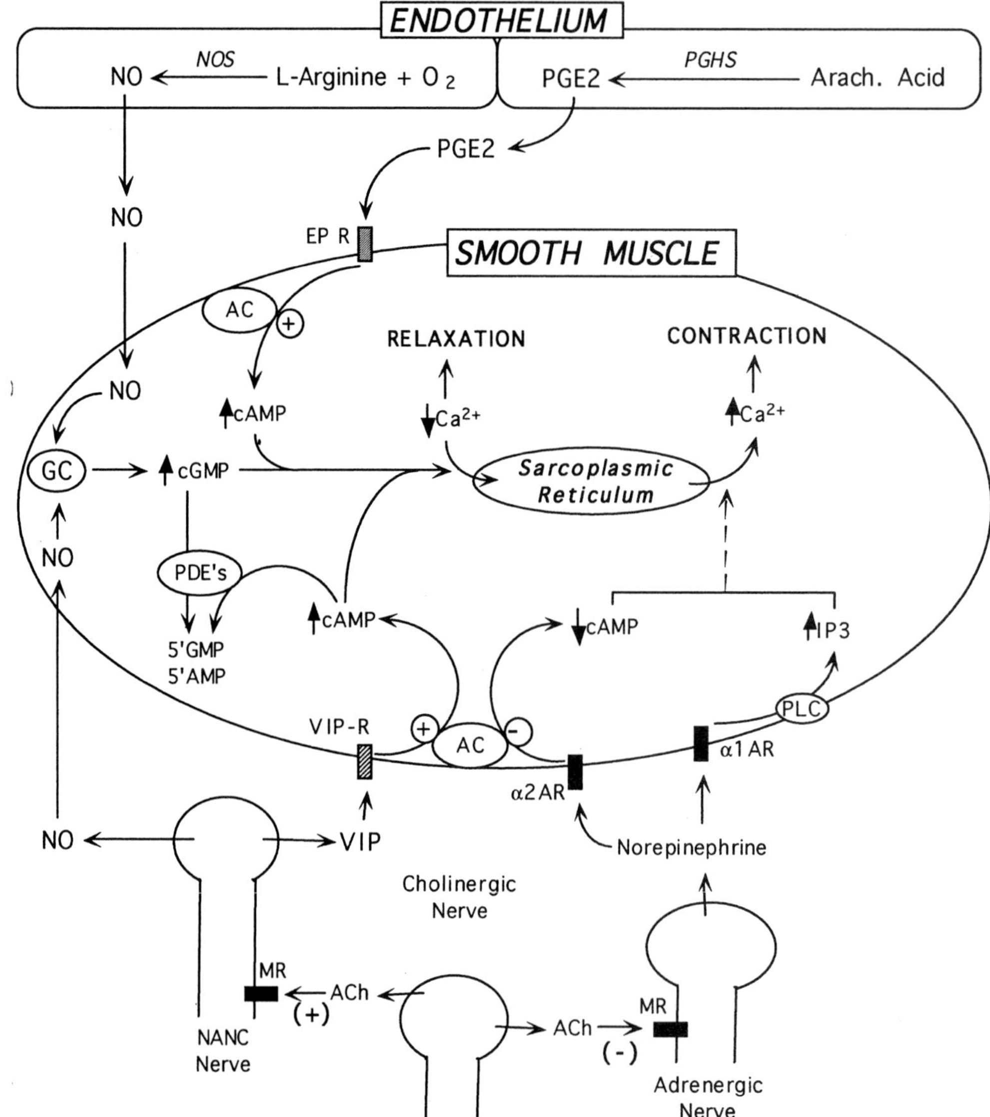

Figure 59.2. Schematic diagram of the neurogenic and endothelium-derived mechanisms that exert local control of corporal smooth muscle tone. Neurogenic mechanisms involve three neuroeffector systems: adrenergic (constrictor) using norepinephrine as a neurotransmitter; cholinergic (dilator) using acetylcholine (AC) and/or vasoactive intestinal polypeptide (VIP) as a neurotransmitter; and nonadrenergic, noncholinergic (NANC) (dilator) using nitric oxide (NO) as a neurotransmitter. Endothelium-derived vasoactive substances such as NO (dilator), prostaglandins (PGs) (both constrictor and dilator), and endothelin (constrictor) also may contribute to the control of trabecular smooth muscle tone. AC, adenylate cyclase; Ach, acetylcholine; AR, adrenergic receptor; cAMP, cyclic adenosine monophosphate; cGMP, cyclic guanosine monophosphate; EP R, PGE receptor; GC, guanylate cyclase; IP3, inositol trisphosphate; MR, muscarinic receptor; NOS, nitric oxide synthase; PDE, phosphodiesterase; PGHS, prostaglandin G/H synthase; PLC, phospholipase C.

Nitric oxide is synthesized and released not only by the NANC nerves but also by the vascular endothelium. Vasodilators such as acetylcholine and bradykinin act by binding their respective membrane receptors and increasing intracellular Ca^{2+} within endothelial cells. Physical stimuli, such as shear stress, are also known to enhance NO production in endothelium. In the penis, shear-induced NO production by endothelium is most likely to occur during the onset of erection, when blood flow into the cavernosal bodies is rapidly increased. The mode of action of endothelium-derived NO is identical to that of nerve-derived NO, as described in the previous section (Fig. 59.2).

Prostaglandins (PG) are prostanoids (as are eicosanoids), which are 20-carbon derivatives produced by the action of cyclooxygenases on the common precursor arachidonic acid in both endothelial and smooth muscle cells of the corpora cavernosa. Prostanoids act locally and exert both trophic and tonic effects in an autocrine and paracrine manner. Although the precise physiologic role of prostaglandins in penile erection remains poorly defined, experimental evidence indicates that they may play an important role in the regulation of the production of extracellular matrix. Further, the antiplatelet-aggregating effects of PGI_2 (prostacyclin), similar to those of NO, may be important in preventing coagulation of blood, since blood flow within the cavernosal bodies is negligible during full penile tumescence. The five primary active prostanoid compounds in the penis are the prostaglandins PGD_2, PGE_2, $PGF_{2\alpha}$, PGI_2, and thromboxane A_2 (TXA_2). Prostanoids can induce both relaxation and contraction in penile corpus cavernosum. PGE is the only endogenous prostaglandin that appears to elicit relaxation of human trabecular smooth muscle; the others cause constriction or have no effect on smooth muscle tone. There are five major groups of prostanoid receptors, termed DP, EP, FP, IP, and TP, which mediate the effects of PGD, PGE, PGF, PGI, and thromboxane, respectively. The multifunctional, dose-dependent effects of prostanoids may be explained by the coupling of receptor subtypes and isoforms to different second messenger systems. Clinically, PGE_1 (alprostadil) has been developed as the first U.S. Food and Drug Administration (FDA)-approved intracavernosal injectable drug for the treatment of ED.

Oxygen tension plays an active role in regulating penile erection. Measurements of cavernosal blood Po_2 in human volunteer subjects indicate that oxygen tensions change rapidly from venous (~35 mm Hg) to arterial (~100 mm Hg) levels during the transition of the penis from the flaccid to the erect state. Maintenance of constant oxygen tension is a critical imperative in most tissues of the body. The penis is the only organ that changes from venous to arterial oxygen tensions during the course of its normal function. This transition is the basis of a unique regulatory mechanism that takes advantage of key synthetic enzymes that utilize molecular oxygen as a cosubstrate. NO synthase and prostaglandin synthase are two well-studied examples of a class of enzymes known as dioxygenases. At low oxygen tension, measured in the flaccid state of the penis, the synthesis of NO is inhibited, preventing relaxation of trabecular smooth muscle. This inhibition of NO production is probably necessary for the maintenance of penile flaccidity. Following vasodilation of the resistance arteries, the increase in arterial flow raises oxygen tension. In the oxygen-enhanced environment, autonomic dilator nerves and the endothelium are able to synthesize NO, mediating relaxation of trabecular smooth muscle. The synthesis of prostanoids is similarly regulated in the flaccid versus the erect state. Therefore, oxygen tension may regulate the types of vasoactive substances present in the vascular bed. At low oxygen tension, norepinephrine- and endothelin-induced contraction may predominate, while at high oxygen tension, NO and prostaglandins are produced because of the availability of molecular oxygen required for their synthesis.

PATHOPHYSIOLOGY OF DIABETES-RELATED ERECTILE DYSFUNCTION

Although impotence in men with diabetes may be primarily psychogenic, several reports have documented that a primarily organic origin is more common (8,9). In patients with diabetes, the erectile disorder is rarely reversible, lending support to an organic cause (11,44). Organic impotence can be differentiated from psychogenic impotence by monitoring nocturnal erections associated with REM. Men with diabetes have been found to have a decrease in such REM-associated erections (45), lending support to an organic basis of their impotence.

Vasculopathy and neuropathy are common complications associated with the natural history of diabetes mellitus. It is hypothesized that cavernosal artery insufficiency, corporal veno-occlusive dysfunction, and/or autonomic neuropathy are the major organic pathophysiologic mechanisms leading to persistent erectile impairment in men with diabetes mellitus (46). The role of hormonal abnormalities in the pathophysiology of organic-based impotence is controversial.

Neurogenic Erectile Dysfunction

Penile autonomic neuropathy has a major role in the pathophysiology of ED in men with diabetes. The incidence of peripheral and autonomic neuropathy is significantly higher in impotent than in potent men with diabetes (8,47). Erectile failure is a common feature of diabetic autonomic neuropathy (48) and may precede the appearance of neuropathy (49).

Until recently, clinical tests of the integrity of the autonomic nerves to the corpora have been performed exclusively by indirect testing, such as tests of nocturnal penile tumescence. Since patients with diabetes commonly have associated hemodynamic abnormalities, indirect testing is not reliable as a technique for accurate documentation of cavernosal nerve integrity (50).

The presence of bladder areflexia and bladder or bowel dysfunction provides indirect support for the impairment of the motor efferent autonomic cavernosal nerves, since the bladder and penis receive autonomic innervation from a common origin (8,51). Ellenberg (8) found that 82% of impotent patients with diabetes had evidence of neuropathic bladder by cystometric diagnosis, whereas only 10% of age-matched potent patients with diabetes had bladder involvement. Vascular reflexes such as beat-to-beat variation in heart rate provide another indirect measurement of autonomic parasympathetic neuropathy. Several studies have also documented abnormal vascular reflexes in the impotent patient with diabetes (52).

The possibility of direct testing of the autonomic innervation of the corpora is now being investigated by recording the electrical activity of the corporal smooth muscle with the use of intracavernosal electromyographic needles or surface electrodes on the penile shaft (53). With use of single-potential analysis, waveforms of a defined duration, amplitude, and polyphasicity can be recorded in healthy subjects (54). In patients with peripheral neuropathy secondary to diabetes, the single-potential analysis of cavernous electrical activity may reveal potentials that are of abnormal duration and amplitude (54,55). Because this technique is at the initial development phase and is available in only a few centers, further investigations will be needed for its validation as a test of the autonomic nervous system.

Several tests are used in the evaluation of the presence of neuropathy in the sensory afferent nerves from the penile skin and the motor efferent nerves to the perineal skeletal musculature. These tests include perineal electromyography, sacral latency testing, evaluation of dorsal nerve somatosensory-evoked potential, and testing of vibration-perception sensitivity (56–59). An abnormal result in somatic testing may suggest, but does not prove, the co-existence of autonomic neuropathy in the corpora cavernosa. Faerman et al. (60) reported morphologic alterations in the unmyelinated nerves in the corpus cavernosum of impotent men with diabetes. Ultrastructural studies of penile nerves in rats with long-term streptozotocin-induced diabetes reveal axonal degeneration with loss of axonal filaments, tubules, and mitochondria (61). The most prominent finding we observed in the penile nerves of impotent patients with diabetes was a thickening of the Schwann and perineurial cell basement membranes (62).

The nerves in patients with diabetes can exhibit biochemical abnormalities, which are subject to some degree of improvement with strict glycemic control (63). Excessive nonenzymatic glycosylation of myelin proteins and polyol pathway activity and abnormal metabolism of myoinositol and its phospholipid derivatives have been proposed as possible biochemical mechanisms in the pathogenesis of diabetic neuropathy (64). In addition, neural ischemic insult has been proposed as a possible mechanism for diabetic polyneuropathy (65). It is now known that hyperglycemia induces decreases in endoneurial blood flow and nerve conduction velocities (66).

Melman et al. (67) were the first to report diminished levels of norepinephrine in the tissues of patients with diabetes. Norepinephrine depletion was most severe in patients with insulin-dependent diabetes. These results were corroborated by Lincoln et al. (68), who also found diminished levels of norepinephrine and a marked reduction in acetylcholinesterase-positive fibers in corpus cavernosum tissue of patients with diabetes. These findings suggest the possibility of a depletion in the number of cholinergic nerves in corpus cavernosum of patients with diabetes. Impotent men with diabetes have a functional impairment of the neurogenic dilator mechanism of penile smooth muscle (69) (Fig. 59.3). Corporal tissue from impotent men with diabetes accumulates and releases less acetylcholine than does corporal tissue from impotent men without diabetes (70). Because relaxation of penile smooth muscle is necessary for erection and the cholinergic neuroeffector system facilitates this smooth muscle relaxation, the dysfunction of penile cholinergic nerves may be contributory to the development of impotence in men with diabetes. The duration of diabetes is negatively correlated to the ability of the cholinergic nerves to synthesize acetylcholine (70). Therefore, patients with long-standing diabetes are more likely to present with penile autonomic neuropathy.

Several studies have reported a decrease in the tissue levels of VIP and the number of VIP-like immunoreactive fibers in human corpus cavernosum from patients with diabetes (68,71). Findings are similar in rats with streptozotocin-induced diabetes (72).

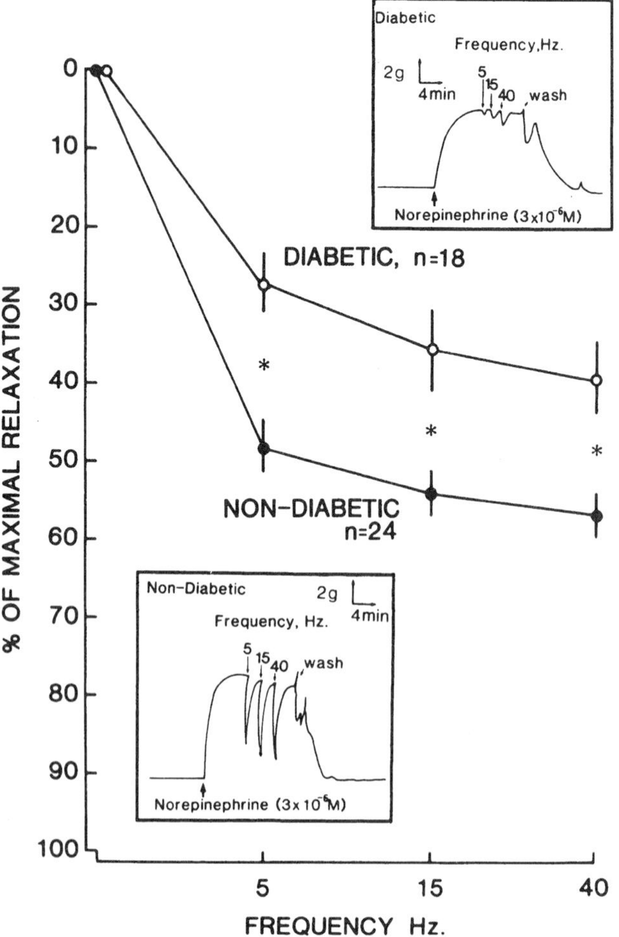

Figure 59.3. Human corporal erectile tissue from diabetic impotent patients reveals electrical field stimulation relaxation responses to 5, 15, and 40 Hz that average 28% to 35% of maximal relaxation, responses that are significantly diminished in comparison to those in nondiabetic tissues. This finding suggests a functional impairment of the neurogenic dilator mechanism of penile smooth muscle in diabetic impotent men.

Vasculogenic Erectile Dysfunction

Vascular disease, of either large or small vessels, is a major contributor to the morbidity and mortality of diabetes (73,74). Diabetic microangiopathy produces alterations and decompensation of local microvascular blood flow (75). There is progressive venule dilation, periodic arteriolar vasoconstriction, and sclerosis of the walls of the arterioles, capillaries, and venules (76). Endothelial cell metabolism and function, thickness of the basement membrane of the vessel wall, oxygen transport, blood-flow properties, and hemostasis also are altered in diabetic microangiopathy (77). Similarly, large-vessel disease is strongly associated with diabetes. Intimal, medial, and luminal changes observed in obliterative atherosclerosis have been well-documented (78). There is growing evidence supporting a role of hyperglycemia in increasing levels of diacylglycerol (79,80), which induces activation of protein kinase C (PKC) (79,81). Activation of this enzyme leads to vascular dysfunction by disrupting NO signaling, which is thought to be a factor contributing to the vascular and neural abnormalities seen in patients with diabetes. In addition, hyperglycemia induces decrease in Na^+-K^+-ATPase activity (82). A reduction in the activity of this enzyme may enhance vascular smooth muscle vasoconstriction and impaired veno-occlusion. PKC activation has been postulated to mediate the hyperglycemia-induced decrease in Na^+-K^+-ATPase activity. Finally, PKC activation may increase the expression of vascular endothelial growth factor (VEGF) and vascular permeability factor (VPF). These factors have been implicated in the pathogenesis of diabetic macular edema and diabetic retinopathy (79,81).

Atherosclerotic vascular disease and ED are strongly related. Arteriosclerosis is the most common organic disorder leading to impotence (83). Among men with clinically significant peripheral arterial disease, 40% to 50% complain of impotence, and in 80% of these cases, the primary cause of the impotence is organic (84). ED develops when more than 50% of the major arterial supply to the penis is involved in atherosclerotic occlusive disease (85). Atherosclerosis has also been observed to have an adverse effect on the ultrastructure of corpus cavernosum in 40% to 45% of men with diabetic impotence; as the smooth muscle cell content decreases, the severity of symptoms and clinical findings increases (86–89).

Postmortem examinations of impotent diabetic men have revealed numerous penile arterial vascular abnormalities, including fibrous proliferation of the intima, medial fibrosis, calcification, narrowing, and obliteration of the lumen. Such vascular alterations in the penile arteries impede blood flow to the cavernous bodies at the time of erection and are thus in part responsible for the ED (90).

Impotent men with diabetes may also have associated vascular risk factors, such as cigarette smoking, hypertension, and hyperlipidemia (1). Cigarette smoking is a statistically significant independent risk factor in the development of angiographically confirmed atherosclerotic arterial occlusive disease to the hypogastric-cavernous arterial bed. Five, ten, and twenty pack-year (1 pack, or 20 cigarettes, per day for 1 year) histories of exposure to cigarette smoking are associated with 15%, 30%, and 70% incidence, respectively, of arterial occlusive disease within the common penile artery (90,91). Hypertension also was noted in 45% of impotent men, while hyperlipidemia or other disturbances of lipid metabolism were found in 40% to 50% of impotent men (84).

Diabetes-associated vascular disease affects the physiology of erection by many routes—at the level of large inflow vessels, the penile microvasculature, the lacunar space endothelium, and the penile fibroelastic frame. One mechanism of diabetes-induced, atherosclerosis-associated ED is the lowering of arterial perfusion pressure and arterial inflow to the lacunar spaces of the corpora cavernosa (92–94). The clinical consequences of these hemodynamic changes are a diminished rigidity of the erect penis and a prolongation of the time to maximal erection. Another mechanism is interference with corporal veno-occlusion. In all men with organic impotence, the incidence of corporal veno-occlusive dysfunction may be as high as 86% (95).

Corporal veno-occlusive dysfunction associated with diabetes can be due to a structural alteration in the fibroelastic components of the trabeculae (1). Loss of compliance of the fibroelastic frame of the penis may be the result of altered synthesis of collagen or elastin, altered tissue cellularity (96–98), or alterations in the reactivity of the smooth muscle of the corpus cavernosum and the endothelial cells of the lacunar space (99). Activation of PKC has been implicated in the hyperglycemia-induced increases in expression of transforming growth factor β (TGF-β), a potent prosclerotic cytokine that facilitates accumulation of extracellular matrix protein in the corpus cavernosum, which reduces penile compliance and impairs veno-occlusion in patients with diabetes (100). Functional studies in isolated human corporal tissue have demonstrated decreased endothelium-dependent relaxation of the penile smooth muscle and loss of compliance of the penile fibroelastic frame. These may result in an inability of the trabeculae to expand against the tunica albuginea and compress the subtunica venules. The clinical consequences of such hemodynamic alterations are excessive outflow of lacunar blood, which prevents the attainment of adequate penile rigidity and duration of erection.

Endocrinologic Erectile Dysfunction

Studies in the 1940s through the 1960s demonstrated abnormal endocrinologic factors, primarily hypogonadotropic hypogonadism, in association with diabetic impotence. These conclusions were based on the presence of both pituitary gonadotropin and 17-ketosteroids in the urine and on the documentation of infiltration of testicular interstitial matrix with collagen-like material and abnormalities in the seminiferous tubules in testicular biopsy material (7).

Endocrine studies of men with diabetes that have been carried out since the advent of radioimmunoassay analyses have had variable results (8,9,60,101,102). Total serum testosterone values are not consistently altered in impotent men with diabetes. In some series, values were normal or low or the magnitude of the increase following stimulation with human chorionic gonadotropin was attenuated in men with diabetes. In one series, a deficit of gonadal function was inferred from high urinary excretion of luteinizing hormone and free testosterone levels in serum. In another study (103), a decrease in concentration of luteinizing hormone followed a lowering of the blood sugar level in impotent men with diabetes but not in potent controls, suggesting that hyperglycemia may be responsible for these endocrine abnormalities.

The etiologic significance of the hypothalamic-pituitary-testicular axis in ED is unclear. Androgens influence the growth and development of the male reproductive tract and secondary sexual characteristics (104). Their effect on libido and sexual behavior is well established (105), but the effect of androgens on normal erectile physiology is poorly understood. Androgen-receptor sites have been demonstrated in the sacral parasympathetic nucleus and on neurons of the hypothalamus and limbic system, suggesting possible hormonal regulation of these centers involved in erection. In animals castration has also been found to reduce the size of some motor neurons, dendritic length, number of chemical synapses onto the somatic and dendritic membranes, and gap junctions between motor neurons in the spinal nuclei (106–108).

Patients with castration levels of testosterone can achieve erections comparable in quality to those achieved by men with normal levels of testosterone in response to visual sexual stimulation (109). This observation suggests that the neurovascular mechanisms that control erection are functional in the presence of low levels of androgens. On the other hand, it has been shown that hypogonadal men have decreased nocturnal penile erectile activity and show improved activity when they receive androgen replacement (105).

Thyroid disease, pituitary disorders, adrenal disease, and hyperprolactinemia, in addition to hypogonadism, may all be associated with ED in men with diabetes. One study found serum prolactin to be similar in normal and diabetic patients, while another study reported an above-average incidence of hyperprolactinemia in diabetic patients (101,110). Declining libido and impotence can be seen as early symptoms in patients with hyperprolactinemia. Hyperprolactinemia is associated with low circulating levels of testosterone, which appear to be secondary to the inhibition by elevated levels of prolactin of normal pulsation of gonadotropin-releasing hormone. In approximately one-half of impotent patients with hyperprolactinemia and low levels of testosterone, potency is not restored by normalization of serum testosterone levels, implying that prolactin may have an antagonistic effect on the peripheral action of testosterone (1). Hyperthyroid states are commonly associated with diminished libido and, less frequently, with impotence. Impotence associated with hypothyroid states has been reported and may be secondary to associated low levels of testosterone secretion and elevated levels of prolactin (110). Although endocrine-related impotence does not play a major role in the overall pathogenesis of diabetic impotence, a recognized hormonal abnormality may be amenable to medical treatment; thus, endocrine screening is recommended for impotent patients with diabetes.

EVALUATION OF ERECTILE FUNCTION IN PATIENTS WITH DIABETES

The process of care model for the evaluation and treatment of erectile dysfunction was developed with input from a multidisciplinary panel of experts in family medicine, internal medicine, endocrinology, psychiatry, psychology, and urology to advance new guidelines for the diagnosis and treatment of ED in the primary care setting (111). These guidelines begin the management of patients with ED with the identification and diagnosis of the problem. ED is the persistent or repeated inability, for a duration of at least 3 months, to attain and/or maintain an erection sufficient for satisfactory sexual performance (112), and the diagnosis is based on the patient's self-report in conjunction with a clinical evaluation. In some cases, it may be necessary for physicians to carefully inquire about sexual functioning, paying special attention to the sensitivity of the topic and to the patient's comfort level. Validated sexual questionnaires, such as the International Index of Erectile Function (IIEF), may be helpful tools in the evaluation of erectile function (113). The cornerstone of the patient evaluation is a comprehensive and detailed sexual, medical, and psychosocial history; physical examination; and focused laboratory testing. Specialized diagnostic tests, such as nocturnal tumescence, biothesiometry, and penile vascular studies (duplex Doppler ultrasound, dynamic infusion cavernosometry, and cavernosography), although not always indicated, may corroborate the impressions discovered on the initial evaluation. As a general rule, for the diabetic patient with ED, sophisticated invasive testing should be considered only under unusual conditions. It should be stressed that the secondary psychologic reaction to these organic factors must not be ignored. Successful treatment of the impotent patient with diabetes who has primary organic and secondary psychologic impotence demands attention to both dysfunctions.

Sexual, Medical, and Psychosocial History

A detailed and comprehensive sexual history should include past and present assessment of sexual desire (libido), orgasms, ejaculatory function, and erectile capabilities (rigidity, spontaneity, sustaining capabilities) during both sexual and nonsexual circumstances (nocturnal erections). In addition to physiologic erectile responses, overall sexual satisfaction should also be assessed.

The medical history should include focused questions on medical illness (chronic/medical illness; e.g., diabetes, anemia, renal failure), neurologic illness (e.g., spinal cord injury, multiple sclerosis, lumbosacral disk disease), endocrinologic illness (e.g., hypogonadism, hyperprolactinemia, thyroid disorders), atherosclerotic vascular risk factors (e.g., hypercholesterolemia, hypertension, diabetes, smoking, family history), medications/recreational drug use (e.g., antihypertensives, antidepressants, alcohol, cocaine), pelvic/perineal/penile trauma (e.g., bicycling injury), surgical (e.g., radical prostatectomy, laminectomy, vascular bypass surgery), and psychiatric history (e.g., depression, anxiety).

Given the personal, interpersonal, social, and occupational implications of sexual problems, a brief psychosocial history is mandatory for every patient. Current psychological state, self-esteem, and history of sexual trauma/abuse, as well as past and present relationships and social and occupational performance, should be addressed.

Physical Examination

A routine physical examination with special emphasis on the genitourinary vascular and neurologic systems may confirm aspects of the medical history (e.g., penile curvature, neuropathies) and occasionally may reveal unsuspected physical findings such as penile plaques (Peyronie disease) and small testes (hypogonadism) responsible for the patient's ED.

Laboratory Testing

Laboratory testing is strongly recommended. Standard serum chemistries, complete blood cell count and lipid profiles may elucidate vascular risk factors such as hypercholesterolemia, diabetes, and renal failure. Determinations of serum prostate-specific antigen (PSA) following the American Urological Association guidelines and serum thyroid-stimulating hormone (TSH) may be indicated in select cases.

The integrity of the hypothalamic-pituitary-gonadal axis should be examined in every patient with ED. It is unclear which testosterone assay (total, free, and bioavailable) is the best; however, there is a consensus that at least one of these assays should be performed. Although pituitary adenomas are a rare cause of sexual dysfunction, this potentially life-threatening disease and reversible cause of ED should not be forgotten. Abnormalities in any of these tests may correlate clinically with diminished sexual desire and with atrophic testis on physical examination

Patient/Partner Education

Patient and partner education is a critical component in the diagnosis of ED and should be carried out whenever possible. The results of the history, physical examination, laboratory testing, and the need for additional diagnostic testing should be reviewed in detail with the patient and his partner, and if indicated, appropriate referrals should be made. Patient and partner education not only facilitates physician-patient-partner communication it enhances patient compliance and treatment adherence.

Specialized Diagnostic Testing

The introduction of sildenafil in 1998 dramatically changed the need for specialized testing. Diagnostic modalities such as duplex Doppler ultrasound, cavernosometry, caversonography, and selective pudendal arteriogram expand the physician's and patient's understanding of the pathophysiologic mechanisms, but disadvantages such as invasiveness, cost, and the associated risks and complications have reduced the indications for specialized testing.

Nocturnal penile tumescence testing is one of the most common specialized diagnostic tests performed today, but its ability to evaluate axial rigidity is poor. The use of this popular diagnostic tool should be limited to the discrimination between organic and psychogenic ED (114).

Penile biothesiometry, a noninvasive specialized diagnostic modality that measures vibratory thresholds, provides further understanding of the somatosensory pathway and has proved helpful in the management of diabetic patients with ED.

Noninvasive and invasive vascular testing of diabetic patients with ED has been reported in numerous series (115,116). These include office intracavernosal injection testing, duplex Doppler ultrasound, studies of the penile brachial index, penile plethysmography, cavernosal artery systolic occlusion pressure in the erect state, recordings of the change in the diameter of the cavernosal artery in the flaccid and erect state, and selective internal pudendal arteriography in the erect state. The incidence of suspected vascular pathology by such vascular testing is 33% to 87% (4).

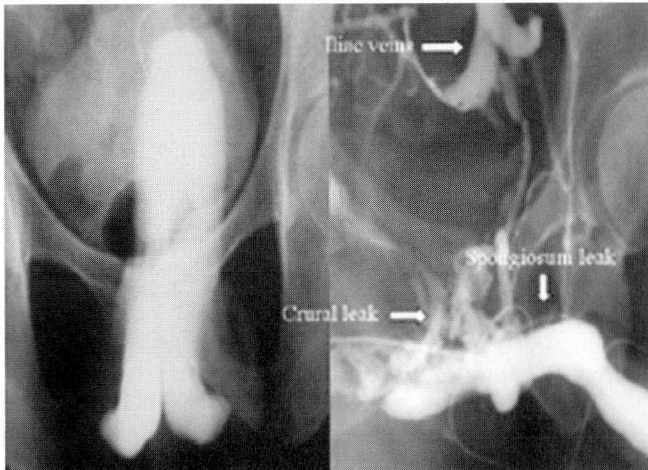

Figure 59.4. Pharmacocavernosography following administration of intracavernosal vasoactive agents in an impotent nondiabetic patient with normal corporal veno-occlusion **(left)** and in an impotent diabetic patient with abnormal "diffuse" corporal veno-occlusion **(right)**. In the nondiabetic patient, no veins draining the corporal body are visualized. In the diabetic patient, numerous veins draining the corporal body are visualized.

Pharmacocavernosography of diabetic men with ED typically shows a diffuse pattern of venous leaking (50,117,118), including the dorsal, cavernosal and crural veins; corpus spongiosum; and glans penis. It has been inferred from the diffuse pattern of abnormal vein visualization seen in patients with diabetes that the primary basis of the pathology is a pancavernosal pathosis such as poor compliance or abnormal smooth muscle function (Fig. 59.4). The diffuse diabetic pattern is different from the pharmacocavernosographic pattern of abnormal visualization of veins in impotent patients with Peyronie disease (119), following trauma (50), or as a consequence of a penile fracture (120). The focal cavernosal pathology of these latter disorders is reflected by the focal site-specific abnormalities seen on pharmacocavernosography.

Indications for Referral

Primary care physicians should manage the vast majority of patients with ED. However, there are several indications for referrals:

1. Young patients with presumed pure cavernosal artery insufficiency secondary to pelvic/perineal trauma. These patients may be candidates for curative vascular reconstruction.
2. Patients with significant penile curvature (e.g., Peyronie disease or congenital penile deformity). Surgical correction may be necessary to facilitate sexual intercourse.
3. Patients with aortic aneurysm or bulbosacral disc disease that requires vascular or neurosurgical intervention.
4. Patients with complicated endocrinopathies such as hypogonadism and pituitary adenoma.
5. Patients with complicated psychiatric or psychosexual disorders (e.g., refractory depression, and transsexualism).
6. Patient or physician request for specialized evaluation.
7. Medical or legal reasons (occupational or iatrogenic injuries).

Modifying Reversible Causes

Health professionals should work with patients to modify reversible causes of ED such as psychogenic ED, hypogonadism, hyperprolactinemia, specific drug-related ED, and cavernosal artery insufficiency secondary to blunt perineal trauma.

Diabetic men with ED who are determined to be hypogonadotropic on the basis of several repeat determinations of low serum testosterone levels in early morning specimens should receive hormonal therapy. In these cases, testosterone replacement is used to maintain normal serum levels of testosterone and to restore potency and libido. Because of the relatively unpredictable serum levels of testosterone obtained following oral administration of testosterone and its poor efficacy and associated hepatic side effects (121), testosterone enanthate administered intramuscularly in doses of 200 to 300 mg every 2 to 3 weeks is preferred. The amount and frequency of administration will vary with the individual and can be titrated (122). Newer topical preparations (patch or gel) are better tolerated and more efficacious and have a significantly better side effect profile.

Testosterone may induce a marked increase in libido without exerting a positive effect on erectile capabilities in patients with diabetes who do not have hypogonadal disorders. Testosterone is contraindicated in patients with adenocarcinoma of the prostate, because testosterone may increase the rate of growth of the adenocarcinoma of the prostate (123). In addition, testosterone replacement should be used with caution in patients with a history of bladder outlet obstruction or with coronary artery disease.

Before testosterone replacement therapy is initiated, it is recommended that a digital rectal examination be performed and that determinations of serum levels of PSA, liver function, and lipid profile be carried out. This practice should be repeated regularly.

The treatment of hyperprolactinemia in patients with diabetes consists of (a) the cessation of medication causing hyperprolactinemia (e.g., estrogens, α-methyldopa), (b) the administration of bromocriptine, or (c) the surgical ablation or extirpation of a pituitary prolactin-secreting tumor. Treatment with exogenous testosterone to supplement the diminished levels of serum testosterone usually seen with this disorder does not appear to reverse the ED (124,125).

Sexual therapy alone or in conjunction with therapy with vasoactive agents has been proven efficacious in the treatment of psychogenic ED.

Thiazide diuretics and β-blockers are the antihypertensive agents most commonly associated with ED. α-Adrenergic blockers are perhaps least likely to cause erectile difficulties. Digoxin, a Na^+-K^+-ATPase inhibitor, appears to be commonly associated with ED. Psychotropic agents such as SSRIs, neuroleptics, and antipsychotics, have been associated with ED and with ejaculatory, orgasmic, and sexual desire difficulties. Luteinizing hormone–releasing hormone agonists and antiandrogens, commonly used in the treatment of advanced prostate carcinoma, also are associated with ED and diminished sexual desire.

Patients with destructive behaviors, alcoholism, cigarette smoking, and recreational drug use should be counseled on the potential etiologic role of these factors in ED.

Pure cavernosal artery insufficiency, secondary to blunt perineal trauma, is a reversible cause of ED. In consequence, a small and selected group of young patients may benefit from microvascular arterial bypass surgery, which was introduced in the early 1970s. The aim of arterial reconstructive surgery for impotence is to increase blood flow to the penis by bypassing arterial obstruction. These procedures showed that bringing a new source of blood to the corporal tissue could restore potency.

Contemporary procedures of penile microvascular arterial bypass surgery involve anastomosis of the inferior epigastric

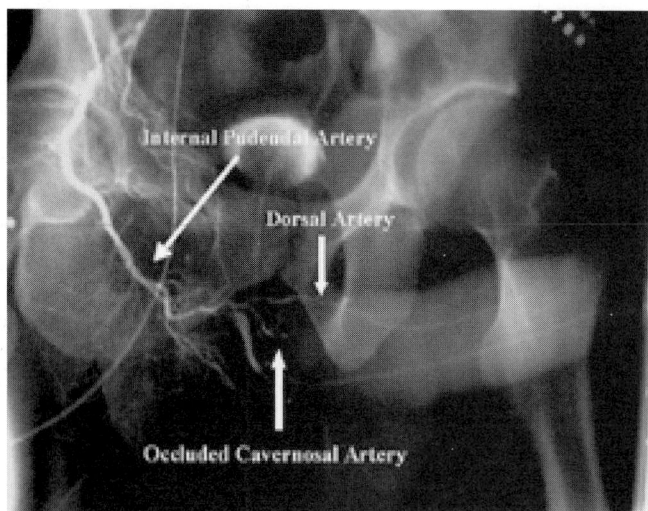

Figure 59.5. Selective internal pudendal arteriograms showing a focal cavernosal artery occlusion at the level of the Alcock canal.

artery to a dorsal artery (126). It appears that patient selection for these procedures is most critical and strongly influences the results of the surgery. The best candidates appear to be younger men with discrete lesions in the pudendal artery, the common penile artery, or both as a result of pelvic or perineal trauma (Fig. 59.5), rather than older men with more generalized arteriosclerotic occlusive disease involving the hypogastric system (126–128). Surgical technique and adherence to principles of vascular and microvascular surgery, especially those that result in preservation of endothelium, are also essential for anastomotic patency.

Patients with diabetes are thus only rarely considered good candidates for this procedure. Those who are considered should have undergone duplex Doppler ultrasound, as well as dynamic infusion cavernosometry caversonography (invasive diagnostic modality that provides quantitative assessment of the cavernosal arterial system and the veno-occlusive mechanism) and selective internal pudendal arteriography.

FIRST-LINE THERAPY

First-line interventions, characterized by ease of administration, reversibility, noninvasive nature, and low cost, include oral erectogenic agents (e.g., sildenafil, apomorphine, oral phentolamine), vacuum erection devices, and psychosexual or couples therapy.

Oral Erectogenic Agents

The introduction of *sildenafil* in 1998 revolutionized the management of men with ED (38). Sildenafil not only has allowed patients and health care professionals to openly discuss human sexuality it has also increased the number of patients using other therapeutic modalities, such as intracavernosal injections and penile prostheses.

Sildenafil, a potent (50% inhibitory concentration [IC_{50}] = 3.5 nM) and selective inhibitor of phosphodiesterase type 5 (PDE 5), which blocks the hydrolysis of cGMP, enhances the accumulation of cGMP, and potentiates the relaxant effects of NO. The absorption of this drug is rapid, and the availability is 40% after oral administration. Peak of plasma concentration is 30 to 120 minutes, with a mean of 60 minutes (129,130). Fatty foods decrease the maximal concentration to 29% (129,131). Sildenafil is metabolized in the liver by the cytochrome P450 and is excreted in feces (80%) and urine (13%) (129,131). Sildenafil is used on demand (prn), and the recommended initial dose is 50 mg taken 1 hour before sexual activity. The dose can be adjusted based on efficacy and tolerability. The maximum recommended dose is 100 mg, no more than once per day, independent of the dosage used. In general terms, the vast majority of patients (75%) use 100 mg, and only 2% of patients use 25 mg (38). The initial dose in patients older than 65 years of age, in patients with renal or liver insufficiency, or in patients receiving drugs that inhibit cytochrome P450 (erythromycin, cimetidine) is 25 mg.

Sildenafil is contraindicated in patients taking nitroglycerine. The most recent package label update recommended use of sildenafil under careful medical supervision, in patients who have suffered a cardiovascular accident, myocardial infarction, or severe arrhythmia within the previous 6 months; or in patients with hypotension (< 90/50 mm Hg), severe hypertension (> 170/110 mm Hg), cardiac insufficiency, unstable angina, or retinitis pigmentosa. The American College of Cardiologists and the American Heart Association (ACC/AHA) also recommended the use of sildenafil with caution in patients receiving complex antihypertensive regimens; with coronary artery disease, borderline blood pressure, or renal or liver insufficiency; or who use drugs that inhibit cytochrome P450 (130).

The rate of discontinuation of this agent is extremely low (0.4% to 1.2%) (132), most likely because of its low side effect profile and high efficacy. The most common side effects of sildenafil are headaches (16%), facial flushing (10%), dyspepsia (7%), nasal congestion (4%), and diarrhea (3%) (131). In addition, at the 100-mg dose, 2% to 3% of men may experience transient alterations in color vision.

Sildenafil is effective in treating ED caused by many different factors (133–136), including diabetes. Recently, a study of 268 diabetic patients (type 1, 21%; type 2, 79%) showed that sildenafil improved erectile function in 57% of patients, compared with 10% in the placebo group, with a successful rate of sexual activity of 48% versus 12% for the placebo group (137).

Yohimbine hydrochloride, an α_2-adrenergic blocking agent, has long been considered an aphrodisiac. Reports of its efficacy in ED were first published 30 years ago (138). In a prospective, double-blind, placebo-controlled study in patients with predominantly organic disease, including patients with diabetes-related impotence, the rate of response to yohimbine was not statistically increased over that to placebo. However, 21% of the patients who received yohimbine achieved a complete response (139,140).

Phentolamine is an α_1- and α_2-adrenergic antagonist that decreases adrenergic tone, thus facilitating erectile function and delaying detumescence. Oral phentolamine is absorbed rapidly, with the peak plasma concentrations achieved in 30 to 60 minutes and a half-life of 5 to 7 hours (141). A prospective, double-blind, and placebo-controlled efficacy and safety trial of oral phentolamine (60 mg) reported a 36.7% success rate compared with 13.4% for placebo (142). The most common side effects were nasal congestion (10%), headache (3%), dizziness (3%), tachycardia (3%), and nausea (1%) (141). This moderately efficacious drug has recently been recently withdrawn from FDA review, but it is available in some countries in Europe and Central and South America.

Apomorphine is a central dopamine agonist known to induce mild to moderate penile erection in men (143). When administered sublingually, apomorphine has a very rapid rate of absorption and onset of action (20–30 minutes). Two recent phase 3 clinical trials involving 977 men with mild to moderate ED treated with sublingual apomorphine reported the achievement of erections firm enough for sexual intercourse (144).

However, significant side effects such as nausea (25%–44%), headache (12%–19%), dizziness (5%–16%), and yawning (10%–16%) were reported during the first 4 weeks of treatment. In addition, occasional episodes of syncope at the higher doses (5–6 mg) also were noted. The efficacy and tolerability of apomorphine in diabetic patients with ED was evaluated in a multicenter, double-blind, crossover study (145). The percentage of attempts resulting in erections firm enough for sexual intercourse varied from 18% to 45% compared with 18% to 26% for placebo. The most common side effect was nausea (16%) with doses of 2, 4, 5, or 6 mg. Despite a significant placebo effect, the investigators concluded that apomorphine is an efficacious and safe treatment for ED in patients with diabetes. Apomorphine HCL has recently been withdrawn from FDA review.

Vardenafil, a potent (IC_{50} 0.7 nM) and selective PDE 5 inhibitor, is currently in clinical trials. Preliminary reports of a multicenter, randomized, double-blind, placebo-controlled phase 3 trial in patients with diabetes mellitus and ED showed a statistically significant improvement in the rate of erection of 72% for the 20-mg group compared with the placebo group ($P < .0001$). Vardenafil also improved IIEF (International Index of Erectile Function) scores and rates of successful penetration when compared with those for placebo ($P < .0001$). The success rates were dose-related and the side effects generally mild or moderate.

Cialis is also a potent and selective PDE 5 inhibitor, but it has a long half-life. A European multicenter, double blind, placebo-controlled study to assess the efficacy and safety of daily Cialis in men with mild to moderate ED (n = 294) showed statistically significant increases in all domain scores of the IIEF ($P \leq .002$) (146). Responses to IIEF question 3 and question 4 were significantly increased with all doses of Cialis compared with placebo ($P = .001$). Both the percentage of successful intercourse attempts and the number of satisfying intercourse attempts were increased with Cialis. It was well tolerated with no significant changes in blood pressure, laboratory values, or electrocardiogram. The most common adverse events were headache, back pain, myalgia, and dyspepsia. Interestingly, no color vision alterations were observed.

Protein kinase C b inhibitors are being studied as possible agents for treatment of ED. It has been postulated that activation of PKC-β may be responsible for the deleterious effects of hyperglycemia on neurovascular structure and function. Some of the physiopathologic mechanisms involve decreased NO activity, enhanced expression of TGF-β, and modulation of VEGF/VPF signal transduction. In preclinical models of diabetes, inhibitors of PKC-β prevented or reversed hyperglycemia-induced vascular and neurogenic dysfunction (66). A phase 3 study of efficacy of a PKC-β inhibitor in males with diabetes and ED is ongoing.

The simplicity, noninvasiveness, and safety of topical administration make vasoactive agents ideal for the treatment of patients with sexual dysfunction. Recently, a double-blind, placebo-controlled study of *Topiglan* (1% alprostadil in a formulation with 5% SEPA [soft enhancer of percutaneous absorption]) reported significant changes in penile rigidity with minimal side effects (skin erythema, mild warmth or burning) when applied to the glans penis in patients with mild to moderate ED in an office-based setting (147). In contrast, when Topiglan is applied to the entire penis, the rates of penile erythema and discomfort were higher. Further research is needed before this agent can be established as a first-line therapy agent.

Vacuum Constrictive Devices

The use of vacuum constrictive devices, a well-established noninvasive first-line therapy recently approved by the FDA for over-the-counter distribution, is a viable therapeutic option for diabetic patients with ED because of the absence of significant complications associated with the use of these devices and their high degree of acceptance among patients who elect to use them (148–150). A variety of external penile appliances are now available for the management of diabetic impotence. The majority have three common components: a vacuum chamber, a vacuum pump that creates negative pressure within the chamber, and a constrictor or tension band that is applied to the base of the penis after erection is achieved. While standing, the patient places his penis in the chamber, which is attached to a pump mechanism that can produce a negative pressure within the chamber. The negative pressure draws blood into the penis to produce an erection-like state. When adequate tumescence and rigidity have been achieved, the patient transfers a constrictor band at the base of the chamber to the base of the penis, thereby "trapping" blood within the penis (Fig. 59.6).

Vacuum-induced erection is significantly different from a physiologically induced erection. The latter is achieved by the initial relaxation of the corporal smooth musculature, thus allowing for engorgement of blood into the lacunar spaces. With vacuum-induced erection, corporal smooth muscle relaxation does not occur initially and blood is simply trapped in both the intracorporeal and extracorporeal compartments of the

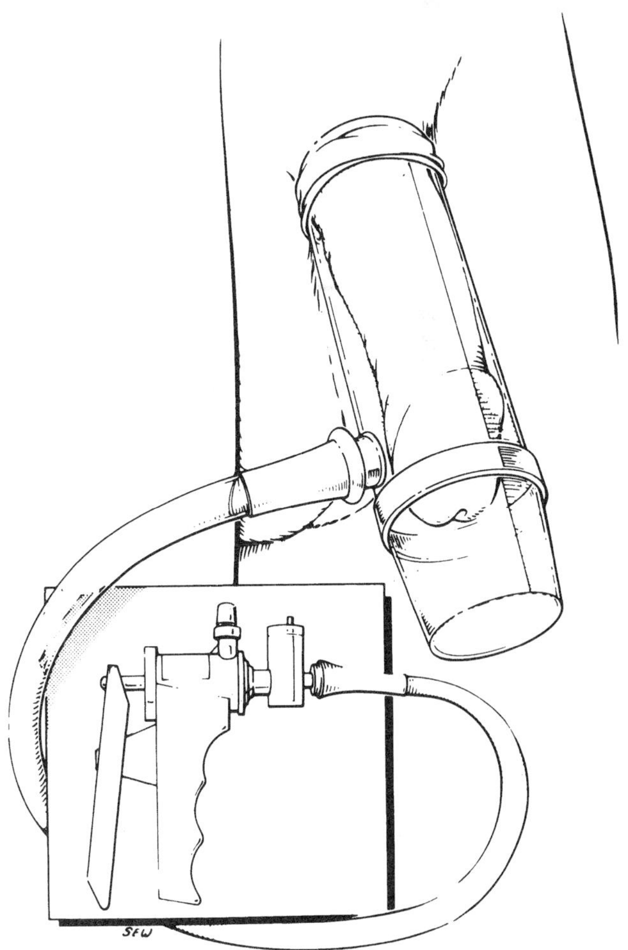

Figure 59.6. Although many different devices are manufactured, the majority have three components in common: a vacuum chamber, a vacuum pump that creates negative pressure within the chamber, and a constrictor or tension band that is applied to the base of the penis after erection is achieved.

penis. Venous stasis and decreased arterial inflow are observed from the constricting band at the base of the penis to the glans penis distally. This may result in penile distension, edema, and cyanosis if the device is used for too long. In most cases, manufacturers recommend that the vacuum-induced erection be maintained for less than 30 minutes. Second, a physiologically induced erection will cause rigidity along the entire length of the corpora, whereas a vacuum-induced erection causes rigidity only distal to the constricting band, permitting the penis to pivot at its base.

In monkeys, increases in cross-sectional corporal area secondary to vacuum-induced erections were found to be only 50% of those induced by intracavernosal papaverine (see below). This limited corporal expansion may be secondary to the continued smooth muscle contraction of the corpora (151). In humans, vacuum constrictive devices may induce an expansion of penile diameter equal to or greater than that attained during a physiologically induced erection, presumably secondary to the entrapment of blood in extracorporeal tissues. Venous drainage from the corpora proximal to the constrictor device is not altered (152).

Theoretically, in almost all men with ED, the vacuum constrictor devices should create penile rigidity sufficient for vaginal penetration. Men with diabetic ED who have had a penile prosthesis explanted may also be treated successfully with a vacuum constrictor device (153). However, patients with significant intracorporeal scarring, such as those with severe Peyronie disease, after priapism, or previously infected penile implants, may not be able to develop adequate rigidity. Patients who do not obtain sufficient penile rigidity with intracavernosal pharmacotherapy alone could be candidates for a vacuum constrictor device used in conjunction with self-injection therapy.

To date the complications from the use of these devices have been minor and self-limited (148–150,154). They have included difficulty with ejaculation, penile pain, ecchymoses, hematomas, and petechiae. Patients taking aspirin or warfarin are more likely to develop vascular complications. Many of the devices manufactured have a valve that limits the vacuum pressure (<250 mm Hg), a feature that might decrease the complication rate. Patient acceptance and satisfaction with vacuum constrictive devices in all types of impotence, including diabetic impotence, has been reported to be 68% to 83%. The reasons for discontinuation of this treatment have included premature loss of penile tumescence and rigidity, penile pain, pain during ejaculation, and inconvenience (155).

Sexual Therapy: Individual or Couples

Sexual therapy addressing relationship distress, sexual performance concerns, and dysfunctional communication patterns is likely to enhance sexual functioning. It is recommended that both patient and partner participate in the sexual therapy.

Sexual therapy is also indicated and beneficial in patients or couples who desire to resume sexual activity after a prolonged period of abstinence. Last, sexual therapy is effective in addressing psychological reactions to the medical or surgical treatment.

SECOND-LINE THERAPY

Second-line therapy is indicated in cases of partial or minimal response to first-line therapy or when the associated side effects are not well tolerated. In addition, a small group of patients may prefer more invasive but efficacious or reliable therapies.

Intraurethral Alprostadil

Intraurethral alprostadil, an FDA-approved medication for the treatment of men with ED, is shaped in the form of a semisolid pellet. This compound is the same as that used for intracavernosal injection, but the doses required are significantly larger (125–1,000 μg). A double-blind, placebo-controlled study of 1,511 men, 27 to 88 years of age, with ED of various etiologies showed that, when tested in an office setting, 65.9% of patients had erections sufficient for intercourse, and that 50% achieved successful intercourse in the home situation (156). The most common side effect was penile pain (10.8%), with hypotension-related symptoms the next most common (3.3%). No patients had priapism or penile fibrosis. Intraurethral application of alprostadil is a relatively safe and moderately effective second-line therapy for the treatment of ED.

Intracavernosal Self-Injection

One of the most important advances in the treatment of impotence during the past decade has been that of self-administration by intracavernosal injection of vasoactive agents that either relax the corporal smooth musculature directly or block adrenergic tone of the corporal smooth muscle (157). The pioneering work in this area involved the use of papaverine hydrochloride (158), a direct smooth-muscle relaxant, or phenoxybenzamine (159) or phentolamine mesylate (160), both α-adrenergic blocking agents. As the clinical use of these agents became more widespread, several issues became apparent. Intracavernosal injection of phentolamine alone was not as effective as injection of papaverine in producing an erection. In addition, injection of papaverine alone was not as effective as injection of papaverine and phentolamine together. More recently, the FDA approved two synthetic formulations of PGE_1: alprostadil sterile powder and alprostadil alfadex for intracavernosal administration. They are identical with respect to pharmacology, efficacy, and safety. The majority of responders (85%) required 20 μg or less. A variety of solutions containing the above agents are presently being used in clinical practice (161,162).

The mechanism of action of papaverine hydrochloride and prostaglandin El (PGE_1) is that of direct relaxation of smooth muscle. Therefore, injected intracavernosally, they will maximize arterial inflow as well as corporal veno-occlusion by relaxing the arterial and trabecular smooth musculature, respectively. Phentolamine, on the other hand, blocks adrenergically induced muscle tone and therefore does not, by itself, initiate erections but does prolong the erectile response (163).

Intracavernosal injections will work best in patients with diabetic ED whose arterial inflow and corporal veno-occlusion mechanism are normal. These would include diabetic patients with purely neurogenic ED or those with psychogenic impotence. Patients with diabetic ED caused by arterial insufficiency also may respond by virtue of the long-acting and maximal dilator effects provided by this therapy. Diabetic patients with ED caused by significant corporal veno-occlusive dysfunction, however, would be those least likely to respond to such therapy (164).

In general, intracavernosal pharmacotherapy, like vacuum constrictor therapy, can be offered to most patients with organic diabetic impotence. Those diabetic patients with poor manual dexterity, poor visual acuity, morbid obesity, or for whom a transient hypotensive episode may have deleterious consequences (e.g., patients with unstable cardiovascular disease and transient ischemic attacks) should be offered this option only after careful consideration. Diabetic patients taking aspirin or warfarin have been treated successfully with intracavernosal injections. Patients with significant psychiatric disease or who might misuse or abuse this therapy should be excluded from treatment. Once patients are offered intracavernosal pharmacotherapy, they should be informed of the risks and complications of this form of therapy and informed that it will not affect orgasm or ejaculation and that it is used solely for restoration of erectile capabilities. The usual therapeutic goal is for the patient to achieve a rigid erection lasting 30 minutes to 1 hour that is rigid enough for satisfactory vaginal penetration (164).

Diabetic patients who enter a program for pharmacologic treatment of inadequate erectile response should first be asked to read and sign a detailed informed-consent form that clearly states the known complications of this treatment and discusses the possibility of long-term side effects. A dosage-determination phase defines the lowest dose required for the achievement of an appropriate erectile response. Diabetic patients with purely neurogenic ED would first be given an extremely low dose since they are the patients most likely to respond. Patients with vascular disease will usually start with a higher dose, which is subsequently increased by increments. To minimize pain and bleeding, an insulin syringe with a 27- to 30-gauge needle usually is used. Patients also are taught to compress the site of injection for 3 minutes following injection. After an appropriate dose has been determined, the patient is instructed in proper injection techniques. When patients are in the more sexually stimulating home environment, it is very common for them to decrease the dose from that determined in the office. The patient also is instructed in sterile technique. Patients are told not to administer an injection more frequently than once a day.

Follow-up information has been obtained on approximately 4,000 impotent patients throughout the world, including many with diabetic impotence, who have been treated with papaverine alone or in combination with phentolamine (165). Reported side effects have included hematomas, burning pain after injection, urethral damage, cavernositis or local infections, fibrotic changes of the corpora cavernosa, curvature, and prolonged erections or priapism. Cavernositis or infection has been extremely rare. Burning pain at the time of injection has been most common with PGE_1 and appears to be less of a problem when PGE_1 is mixed with other agents. Hematomas were noted in a small percentage of patients undergoing self-injection therapy; these usually resolve within a few days without any permanent sequelae.

The two most important complications are prolonged erections and localized fibrotic changes of the corpora cavernosum. Prolonged erections usually occur during the dosage-determination phase and have been reported in 2.3% to 15% of all patients treated. Patients must be cautioned to call their physician if an erection persists for 4 hours or longer. In the majority of patients, detumescence of these prolonged erections will occur without medical intervention; however, some patients will require an intracavernosal injection of an α-adrenergic agonist such as epinephrine, phenylephrine, or metaraminol. An initial intracavernosal injection of 200 μg of phenylephrine has been successful and may be repeated as necessary until detumescence (166). Following the dosage-determination phase, the complication of prolonged erection is quite rare (less than 1% of injections) and, if treated according to the protocol described previously, should not produce any permanent sequelae.

The most frequent side effect (reported in 1.5% to 60% of patients treated for 1 year) of intracavernosal pharmacologic therapy is the formation of painless fibrotic nodules within the corpora cavernosa, which sometimes leads to penile curvature. In one series, the development of fibrotic nodules was related to the frequency of injection and the duration of treatment (166). The complications of corporal fibrosis and prolonged erections have been seen less frequently in men treated with PGE_1 alone. We feel that the formation of cavernosal fibrotic nodules is to some extent secondary to trauma and bleeding within the corpus and for this reason stress the importance of application of compression over the injection site for 3 minutes.

In addition, attempts to decrease the amount of fluid injected are encouraged. The goal of therapy is the injection of less than 0.5 mL of drug mixture intracavernosally. Diabetic patients injecting 1 mL or more of the papaverine and phentolamine mixture can reduce this volume by adding PGE_1—thus the use of a three-drug mixture.

There have been several cases of diffuse fibrosis of the corpora following intracavernosal injections. These have almost invariably been associated with the development of ischemic priapism. Theoretically, these patients should not respond to intracavernosal therapy, but there are several reports in the literature that documented successful treatment of ED due to corporal fibrosis with intracavernosal injection of a combination of papaverine and phentolamine (168). Therefore, the degree of corporal scarring and fibrosis required to obviate the positive results of intracavernosal pharmacotherapy has not been determined.

Systemic side effects of this treatment have included vasovagal episodes and syncope, which are probably related to hypotension. These side effects are infrequent and usually occur during the dosage-determination phase. It would be expected that diabetic patients with significant corporal veno-occlusive dysfunction would exhibit an increase in systemic distribution of intracavernosal agents and therefore be more susceptible to this side effect. As mentioned previously, diabetic patients for whom transient hypotensive episodes may have significant deleterious effects should be carefully evaluated before receiving this therapy. Intracavernosal pharmacotherapy with papaverine has been associated with hepatotoxicity. In the first 201 patients we treated, only three cases (1.5%) of abnormal liver function tests were reported during a mean follow-up period of 26 months (166). Others have seen essentially no changes in liver function during this therapy, while one series reported at least one chemical abnormality of liver function in 40% of patients.

Forskolin, a naturally occurring alkaloid that directly activates the catalytic domain of adenylate cyclase, has demonstrated efficacy as an auxiliary vasoactive agent in a preliminary study of patients who had previously failed high-volume, high-concentration injection therapy (169). Forskolin is especially useful in patients with diabetes or post-radical prostatectomy ED who develop significant corporal pain with the use of intracavernosal PGE_1 as FDA-approved Caverject and EDEX or as standard three-agent pharmacotherapy (papaverine, phentolamine, and PGE_1). The mechanism of PGE_1-induced pain in such patients is related, in part, to the development of diabetic or postoperative penile autonomic neuropathy, lowering the threshold of nociceptive (pain) nerve fibers to mechanical stimulation causing a hyperalgic effect. Preliminary reports on the use of intracavernosal forskolin, papaverine, and phentolamine as a salvage tri-mix in the management of post-radical prostatectomy ED when PGE_1 alone or standard three-agent pharmacotherapy results in clinically significant penile pain showed that 83% of patients had satisfactory and sustained axial rigidity for sexual intercourse. None of these patients experienced corporal pain.

Although penile self-injection therapy is highly effective (70%–90%), the average dropout rate is 64% (range, 46%–80%) (170,171). A recent study demonstrated that keeping the cost of therapy low and ensuring patient and partner education and continued support throughout treatment reduces dropout rates (172).

THIRD-LINE THERAPY

Surgical Prostheses

Third-line treatment interventions are highly invasive, irreversible, and associated with multiple devastating complications such as device infection, erosion, and malfunction. Penile prostheses should be viewed only as a last-resort therapy in patients with treatment-refractory ED. Despite their significant cost and potential invasiveness, penile prostheses have been associated with high rates of patient satisfaction in several studies.

The urologic subspecialty of ED developed in the early 1970s, following the development of an intracorporeal penile prosthesis by Small and Carrion (173) and Scott et al. (174). Through the 1970s and early 1980s, the development of penile prostheses proceeded along two distinct lines: the malleable or rigid prosthesis and the multicomponent inflatable prosthesis. Self-contained inflatable devices were introduced more recently. Last, modifications of the three-piece inflatable device subsequently led to the introduction of a two-piece inflatable device.

Initially, the postoperative complication rate following placement of malleable devices was relatively low and implantation was relatively simple. Therefore, the rates of component failure and re-operation were kept to a minimum. With these devices, the length and girth of the penis do not change in the "tumescent" and "detumescent" phases, which at times results in an aesthetically less desirable "tumescent" phase. The inflatable devices, unlike the malleable devices, are based on hydraulic principles, thus allowing the patient to inflate and deflate the device to simulate tumescent and nontumescent phases. This provided an improved aesthetic result, especially in the "detumescent" phase, but initially was coupled with a relative increase in component failure and reoperation. Activation of the multicomponent inflatable device allows for an increase in penile girth during the "tumescent" phase (50).

Subsequent improvements of inflatable devices have markedly reduced the likelihood of re-operation and component failure (Fig. 59.7). Self-contained inflatable devices have been designed to preserve the aesthetic qualities of an inflatable device and combine them with ease of surgical implantation and a potential decrease in component failure. Further ease of implantation of an inflatable device was attained with the introduction of two-piece inflatable devices. The second- and third-generation prostheses have been designed to increase aesthetic results, increase penile girth at times, decrease the likelihood for component failure, and, when possible, facilitate implantation.

Contemporary data indicate that surgical success with inflatable penile prosthesis is 95% to 97% (175,176), but surgical success does not always represent patient satisfaction. To answer this important question, we performed a phase 2, multiinstitutional, large-scale, retrospective study, with independently analyzed medical records and questionnaire data from consecutive eligible patients of seven physician investigators (177). Among those who returned the questionnaire, 89% of patients with Mentor Alpha-1 answered that it fulfilled their expectations as a therapy for ED, including 28% who claimed fulfillment as expected, 31% better than expected, and 30% much better than expected. Satisfaction responses of 80% or greater were noted with regard to intercourse ability and confidence, device rigidity, and function. Interestingly, implantation of inflatable penile prosthesis did not result in 80% or greater satisfaction responses in changes in partner relationship (as judged by the patient), feelings of the partner about the relationship (as judged by the patient), or increased confidence in social activities and work. Such information is important when providing preoperative counseling to patients so that postoperative expectations will be appropriate.

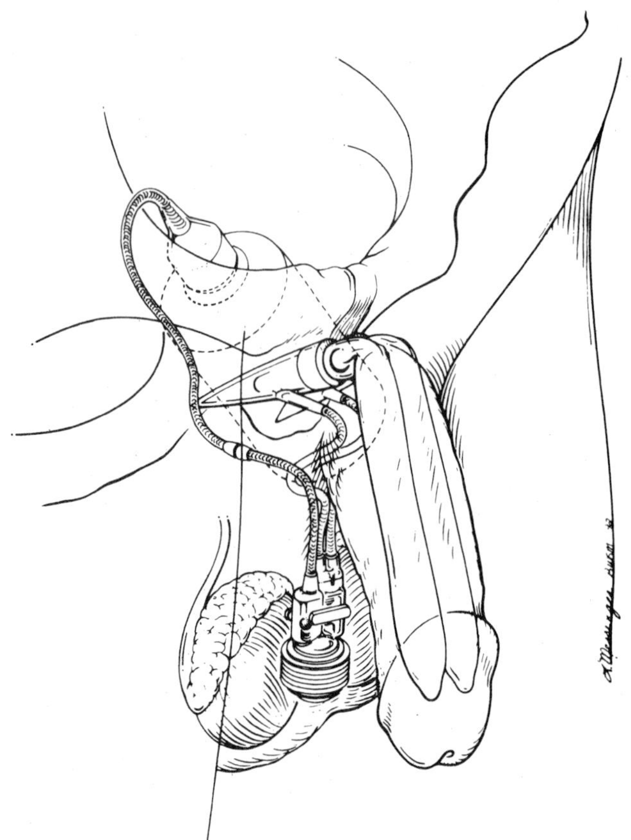

Figure 59.7. Inflatable devices are based on hydraulic principles, thus allowing the patient to inflate and deflate the device to simulate tumescent and nontumescent phases. The multicomponent device depicted, a Mentor Alpha-1, allows for an increase in penile girth during the simulated tumescent phase. The three components consist of a reservoir placed in the retropubic space, two penile cylinders placed in the corpora cavernosa, and a pump apparatus with inflate and deflate mechanisms placed in the scrotum. The advantage of this device is its lack of connectors or connector components between the pump and the cylinders, the known high-pressure portion of a hydraulic device.

With the advent of newer and more effective first- and second-line therapies such as sildenafil, intracavernosal pharmacotherapy, and vacuum erection devices, many physicians now consider the implantation of a penile prosthesis the last treatment option for ED. Thus, penile implantation is offered to diabetic patients with organic impotence after other, nonsurgical, forms of therapy have been attempted and failed. Patients whose ED is thought to be psychogenic, who have not responded to appropriate psychological or behavioral sex therapy, and who have no psychological contraindications for therapy may be treated in the same manner.

Certainly, appropriate counseling of diabetic patients before implantation of a prosthesis is essential to the success of this surgery. The purpose of the prosthesis is to simulate an erection by providing penile rigidity sufficient for intercourse. The ability of the patient to ejaculate and have an orgasm is not altered by the implantation of a prosthesis but in some cases may be restored. In addition, diabetic patients undergoing the surgery should be informed of the potential complications of prosthetic surgery, as well as of their consequences and sequelae. The postoperative complications of penile implant surgery usually are relegated to those of component failure, postoperative infection, or device erosion. Probably the most significant complication of prosthetic surgery is infection. The best defense against infection is prophylaxis. We request that patients scrub their genitalia and perineum for 10 minutes each day for 7 days with chlorhexidine digluconate soap (e.g., Hibiclens), before the surgery (50). In addition, oral quinolones are prescribed for 3 days before the surgery. Patients also are given intravenous perioperative antibiotics (vancomycin and gentamicin), and surgical technique must be meticulous. The incidence of infections following penile prosthetic surgery ranges between 1% and 9% (178).

Following implantation, the time frame for the presentation of infection will vary depending on the organism involved. Infections with more virulent and aggressive bacteria will usually present within the first few postoperative days, with the patient presenting with fever, pain, and swelling overlying the prosthesis accompanied by purulent wound drainage. However, a group of patients will complain of prolonged pain overlying the device but will have not obvious purulent drainage from the wound. Prolonged pain, fixation of the pump or tubing to the overlying scrotal skin, elevated white blood cell count and sedimentation rate, and hyperglycemia in diabetic patients may all be helpful in diagnosing a possible infection by less virulent organisms. Duplex Doppler ultrasound may also be helpful in cases in which clinical findings are not conclusive (179).

The re-operative rate for penile prosthetic surgery has been reported to be between 3% and 44%, with newer series showing a markedly lower rate (180). Penile prostheses have been accepted by patients and physicians worldwide, with over 80% of patients reporting satisfaction after prosthetic surgery (50).

Should penile prosthesis insertion be indicated, the Mentor alpha-1 inflatable penile prosthesis is the device that provides the widest diameter penile erection during inflation and the lowest mechanical failure rate (1.3%). The Bioflex material has an increased abrasion resistance and higher tensile strength than do silicone-based devices. The superior outcome data in terms of mechanical reliability have remained durable over the past 10 years.

Venous Surgery

At present, most diabetic patients who show evidence of corporal veno-occlusive dysfunction by pharmacocavernosometry and cavernosography should not be considered for surgical and/or radiologic options to increase venous outflow resistance (181,182). In diabetic patients, the dysfunction may be related to a pancavernosal alteration in corporal tissue compliance. In such patients, cavernosography may reveal a more generalized corporal veno-occlusive dysfunction with visualization of the glans, corpus spongiosum, dorsal vein, and cavernosal vein. The available procedures (crural plication, ligation, or excision of the deep dorsal vein of the penis; ligation of cavernosal veins; spongiolysis; or a combination of the above, including the radiologic administration of coils or sclerosing agents), have not demonstrated long-term success in impotent diabetic patients (181,182). Complications reported from the various procedures, especially those involving proximal penile dissection, include diminished penile sensation and shortened penile length.

REFERENCES

1. Krane RJ, Goldstein I, Saenz de Tejada I. Impotence. *N Engl J Med* 1989;321: 1648–1659.
2. Kinsey AC, Pomeroy W, Martin C. Age and sexual outlet. In: Kinsey AC, Pomeroy W, Martin C, eds. *Sexual behavior in the human male*. Philadelphia: WB Saunders, 1948:218.
3. Goldstein I. The effect of AIDS-related diseases on the development of impotence. In: *Proceedings and Abstracts of the National Institutes of Health Consensus Development Conference on Impotence*, Bethesda, MD, December 7–9, 1992(abst).
4. Akkus E, Carrier S, Baba K, et al. Structural alterations in the tunica albuginea of the penis: impact of Peyronie's disease, ageing and impotence. *Br J Urol* 1997;79:47–53.
5. Goldstein AMB, Meehan JP, Zakhary R, et al. New observations on microarchitecture of corpora cavernosa in man and possible relationship to mechanism of erection. *Urology* 1982;20:259–266.
6. Rubin A, Babbott D. Impotence and diabetes mellitus. *JAMA* 1958;168: 498–500.
7. Schöffling K, Federlin K, Ditschuneit H, et al. Disorders of sexual function in male diabetics. *Diabetes* 1963;12:519–527.
8. Ellenberg M. Impotence in diabetes: the neurologic factor. *Ann Intern Med* 1971;75:213–219.
9. Kolodny RC, Kahn CB, Goldstein HH, et al. Sexual dysfunction in diabetic men. *Diabetes* 1974;23:306–309.
10. Renshaw DC. Impotence in diabetics. *Dis Nerv Syst* 1975;36:369–371.
11. McCulloch DK, Campbell IW, Wu FC, et al. The prevalence of diabetic impotence. *Diabetologia* 1980;18:279–283.
12. Lester E, Grant AJ, Woodroffe FJ. Impotence in diabetic and non-diabetic hospital outpatients. *BMJ* 1980;281:354–355.
13. Oberpenning F, Roth S, Leusmann DB, et al. The Alcock syndrome: temporary penile insensitivity due to compression of the pudendal nerve within the Alcock canal. *J Urol* 1994;151:423-425.
14. Hakim LS, Nehra A, Kulaksizoglu H, et al. Penile microvascular arterial bypass surgery. *Microsurgery* 1995;16:296–308.
15. Breza J, Aboseif SR, Orvis BR, et al. Detailed anatomy of penile neurovascular structures: surgical significance. *J Urol* 1989;141:437–443.
16. Lue TF, Tanagho EA. Functional anatomy and mechanism of penile erection. In: Tanagho EA, Lue TF, McClue RD, eds. *Contemporary management of impotence and infertility*. Baltimore: Williams & Wilkins, 1988:39–50.
17. Puech-Leao P, Reis JMSM, Glina S, et al. Leakage through the crural edge of corpus cavernosum: diagnosis and treatment. *Eur Urol* 1987;13:163–165.
18. de Groat WC, Steers WD. Neuroanatomy and neurophysiology of penile erection. In: Tanagho EA, Lue TF, McClue RD, eds. *Contemporary management of impotence and infertility*. Baltimore: Williams & Wilkins, 1988:3–27.
19. Weiss HD. The physiology of human penile erection. *Ann Intern Med* 1972; 76:793–799.
20. Stoleru S, Gregoire MC, Gerard D, et al. Neuroanatomical correlates of visually evoked sexual arousal in human males. *Arch Sex Behav* 199;28:1–21.
21. Giuliano F, Bernabe J, Brown K, et al. Erectile response to hypothalamic stimulation in rats: role of peripheral nerves. *Am J Physiol* 1997;273:R1990–R1997.
22. Giuliano F, Rampin O. Central neural regulation of penile erection. *Neurosci Biobehav Rev* 2000;24:517–533.
23. Marson L, McKenna KE. The identification of a brainstem site controlling spinal sexual reflexes in male rats. *Brain Res* 1990;515:303–308.
24. Saenz de Tejada I, Kim NN, Goldstein I, et al. Regulation of pre-synaptic alpha adrenergic activity in the corpus cavernosum. *Int J Impot Res* 2000;12[suppl 1]:S20–S25.
25. Weiss HD. The physiology of human penile erection. *Ann Intern Med* 1972; 76:793–799.
26. Hart BL, Leedy MG. Neurological bases of male sexual behavior: a comparative analysis. In: Adler N, Pfaff D, Goy RW, eds. *Handbook of behavioral neurobiology*, Vol 7. *Reproduction*. New York: Plenum, 1985:373–422.
27. MacLean PD, Ploog DW. Cerebral representation of penile erection. *J Neurophysiol* 1962;25:29–55.
28. MacLean PD, Denniston RH, Dua S. Further studies on cerebral representation of penile erection: caudal thalamus, midbrain, and pons. *J Neurophysiol* 1963;26:274–293.
29. Dua S, MacLean PD. Localization for penile erection in medial frontal lobe. *Am J Physiol* 1964;207:1425–1434.
30. Saper CB, Loewy AD, Swanson LW, et al. Direct hypothalamo-autonomic connections. *Brain Res* 1976;117:305–312.
31. Swanson LW, Sawchenko PE. Hypothalamic integration: organization of the paraventricular and supraoptic nuclei. *Annu Rev Neurosci* 1983;6:269–324.
32. Saenz de Tejada I, Goldstein I, Blanco R, et al. Smooth muscle of the corpora cavernosae: role in penile erection. *Surg Forum* 1985;36:623–624.
33. Blanco R, Saenz de Tejada I, Goldstein I, et al. Cholinergic neurotransmission in human corpus cavernosum. II. Acetylcholine synthesis. *Am J Physiol* 1988;254:H468–H472.
34. Ignarro LJ, Bush PA, Buga GM, et al. Nitric oxide and cyclic GMP formation upon electrical field stimulation cause relaxation of corpus cavernosum smooth muscle. *Biochem Biophys Res Comm* 1990;170:843–850.
35. Traish AM, Kim NN, Goldstein I, et al. Alpha adrenergic receptors in the penis. *J Androl* 1999;20:671–682.
36. Traish AM, Kim NN, Moreland RB, Goldstein I, eds. Proceedings of the International Symposium on Alpha Blockade in Sexual Dysfunction. *Int J Impot Res* 2000;12[suppl 1]:S1–S88.
37. Moreland RB, Goldstein I, Kim NN, Traish A. Sildenafil citrate, a selective phosphodiesterase type 5 inhibitor: research and clinical implications in erectile dysfunction. *Trends Endocrinol Metab* 1999;10:97–104.
38. Goldstein I, Lue TF, Padma-Nathan H, et al. Oral sildenafil in the treatment of erectile dysfunction. Sildenafil Study Group. *N Engl J Med* 1998;338: 1397–1404.

39. Gupta S, Moreland RB, Munarriz R, et al. Possible role of Na^+-K^+-ATPase in the regulation of human corpus cavernosum smooth muscle contractility by nitric oxide. *Br J Pharmacol* 1995;116:2201–2206.
40. Stamler JS. Redox signaling: nitrosylation and related target interactions of nitric oxide. *Cell* 1994;78:931–936.
41. Schmidt HHHW, Walter U. NO at work. *Cell* 1994;78:919–925.
42. Blanco R, Saenz de Tejada I, et al. Dysfunctional penile cholinergic nerves in diabetic impotent men. *J Urol* 1990;144:278–280.
43. Lue TF, Zeineh SJ, Schmidt RA, et al. Neuroanatomy of penile erection: its relevance to iatrogenic impotence. *J Urol* 1984;131:273–280.
44. Jensen SB. Sexual dysfunction in insulin-treated diabetics: a six-year follow-up study of 101 patients. *Arch Sex Behav* 1986;15:271–283.
45. Karacan I, Salis PJ, Catesby J, et al. Nocturnal penile tumescence and diagnosis in diabetic impotence. *Am J Psychiatry* 1978;135:191–197.
46. Saenz de Tejada I, Goldstein I. Diabetic penile neuropathy. *Urol Clin North Am* 1988;15:17–22.
47. Campbell IW. Diabetic autonomic neuropathy. *Br J Clin Pract* 1976;30:153.
48. Fairburn CG, McCulloch DK, Wu FC. The effects of diabetes on male sexual function. *Clin Endocrinol Metab* 1982;11:749–767.
49. McCullock DK, Young RJ, Prescott RS. The natural history of impotence in diabetic men. *Diabetologia* 1980;18:279.
50. Goldstein I, Krane RJ. Diagnosis and therapy of erectile dysfunction. In: Walsh PC, Retik AB, Stamey TA, Vaughan ED Jr, eds. *Campbell's urology*, 6th ed. Philadelphia: WB Saunders, 1992:3033–3072.
51. Faerman I, Vilar O, Rivarola MA, et al. Impotence and diabetes: studies of androgenic function in diabetic impotent males. *Diabetes* 1972;21:23–30.
52. Nisen HO, Alfthan OS, Lindstrom BL, et al. Single breath beat-to-beat variation testing in the diagnosis of autonomic neuropathy in impotence. *Int J Impot Res* 1990;2[suppl 2]:136.
53. Wagner G, Gerstenberg T, Levin RJ. Electrical activity of corpus cavernosum during flaccidity and erection of the human penis: a new diagnostic method. *J Urol* 1989;142:723–725.
54. Stief CG, Djamilian M, Schaebsdau F, et al. Single potential analysis of cavernous electric activity—a possible diagnosis of autonomic impotence? *World J Urol* 1990;8:75.
55. Buvat J, Quittelier E, Lemaire A, et al. Electromyography of the human penis, including single potential analysis during flaccidity and erection induced by vasoactive agents. *Int J Impot Res* 1990;2[suppl 2]:85.
56. Ertekin C, Akjürekli Ö, Gürses AN, et al. The value of somatosensory-evoked potentials and bulbocavernosus reflex in patients with impotence. *Acta Neurol Scand* 1985;71:48–53.
57. Newman HF. Vibratory sensitivity of the penis. *Fertil Steril* 1970;21:791–793.
58. Goldstein I. Electromyography: evoked-response evaluations. In: Barrett DM, Wein AJ, eds. *Controversies in neuro-urology*. New York: Churchill Livingstone, 1984;3D:117–129.
59. Padma-Nathan H, Goldstein I. Neurologic assessment of the impotent male. In: Montague DK, ed. *Disorders of male sexual functions*. Chicago: Year Book Medical Publications, 1987:86–94.
60. Faerman I, Glocer L, Fox D, et al. Impotence and diabetes: histological studies of the autonomic nervous fibers of the corpora cavernosa in impotent diabetic males. *Diabetes* 1974;23:971–976.
61. Fani K, Lundin AP, Beyer MM, et al. Pathology of the penis in long-term diabetic rats. *Diabetologia* 1983;25:424–428.
62. Saenz de Tejada I, Andry C, Blanco R, et al. Ultrastructural studies of autonomic nerves within the corpus cavernosum of impotent diabetic patients. In: Virag H, Virag R, eds. *Proceedings of the First World Meeting on Impotence*. Paris: Les Editions du Ceri, 1986:210–214.
63. Porte D Jr, Graf RJ, Halter JB, et al. Diabetic neuropathy and plasma glucose control. *Am J Med* 1981;70:195–200.
64. Clements RS Jr. Peripheral nerve biochemistry in diabetes. *Clin Physiol* 1985;5[suppl 5]:19–22.
65. Dyck P. Hypoxic neuropathy: does hypoxia play a role in diabetic neuropathy? *Neurology* 1989;39:111–118.
66. Cameron N, Cotter M, Jack A, et al. Inhibition of protein kinase C corrects nerve conduction and blood flow deficits in diabetic rats. *Diabetologia* 40: A31(abst).
67. Melman A, Henry DP, Felten DL, et al. Effect of diabetes upon penile sympathetic nerves in impotent patients. *South Med J* 1980;73:307–309.
68. Lincoln J, Crowe R, Blacklay PF, et al. Changes in the VIPergic, cholinergic and adrenergic innervation of human penile tissue in diabetic and non-diabetic impotent males. *J Urol* 1987;137:1053–1059.
69. Saenz de Tejada I, Goldstein I, Azadzoi K, et al. Impaired neurogenic and endothelium-mediated relaxation of penile smooth muscle from diabetic men with impotence. *N Engl J Med* 1989;320:1025–1030.
70. Blanco R, Saenz de Tejada I, Goldstein I, et al. Dysfunctional penile cholinergic nerves in diabetic impotent men. *J Urol* 1990;144:278–280.
71. Gu J, Polak JM, Lazarides M, et al. Decrease of vasoactive intestinal polypeptide (VIP) in the penises from impotent men. *Lancet* 1984;2:315–318.
72. Crowe R, Lincoln J, Blacklay PF, et al. Vasoactive intestinal polypeptide-like immunoreactive nerves in diabetic penis: a comparison between streptozotocin-treated rats and man. *Diabetes* 1983;32:1075–1077.
73. Ruzbarsky V, Michal V. Morphologic changes in the arterial bed of the penis with aging: relationship to the pathogenesis of impotence. *Invest Urol* 1977;15:194–199.
74. Herman A, Adar R, Rubinstein Z. Vascular lesions associated with impotence in diabetic and nondiabetic arterial occlusive disease. *Diabetes* 1978;27:975–981.
75. Jager E. *Beitrage zur Pathologie des Auges*. Vienna 1855.
76. Ashton N. Vascular changes in diabetes with particular reference to the retinal vessels: preliminary report. *Br J Ophthalmol* 1949;33:407–420.
77. McMillan DE. Deterioration of the microcirculation in diabetes. *Diabetes* 1975;24:944–957.
78. Colwell JA, Halushka PV, Sarji KE, et al. Vascular disease in diabetes: pathophysiological mechanisms and therapy. *Arch Intern Med* 1979;139:225–230.
79. Craven PA, DeRubertis FR. Protein kinase C is activated in glomeruli from streptozotocin diabetic rats. Possible mediation by glucose. *J Clin Invest* 1989;83:1667–1675.
80. Craven PA, Davidson CM, DeRubertis FR. Increase in diacylglycerol mass in isolated glomeruli by glucose from de novo synthesis of glycerolipids. *Diabetes* 1990;39:667–674.
81. Inoguchi T, Battan R, Handler E, et al. Preferential elevation of protein kinase C isoform β2 and diacylglycerol levels in the aorta and heart of diabetic rats: differential reversibility to glycemic control by islet cell transplantation. *Proc Natl Acad Sci U S A* 1992;89:11059–11063.
82. Xia P, Kramer RM, King GL. Identification of the mechanism for the inhibition of Na^+,K^+ adenosine triphosphatase by hyperglycemia involving activation of protein kinase C and cytosolic phospholipase A2. *J Clin Invest* 1995;96:733–740.
83. Jünemann K-P, Persson-Jünemann C, Alken P. Pathophysiology of erectile dysfunction. *Semin Urol* 1990;8:80–93.
84. Virag R, Bouilly P, Frydman D. Is impotence an arterial disorder? A study of arterial risk factors in 440 impotent men. *Lancet* 1985;1:181–184.
85. Rosen MP, Greenfield AJ, Walker TG, et al. Arteriogenic impotence: findings in 195 impotent men examined with selective internal pudendal angiography. *Radiology* 1990;174:1043–1048.
86. Wetterauer U, Stief CG, Kulvelis F, et al. Ultrastructural changes of the cavernous tissue in erectile dysfunction. In: *Proceedings of the Sixth Biennial International Symposium on Corpus Cavernosum Revascularization and Third Biennial World Meeting on Impotence*. Boston, October 1988:11(abst).
87. Persson C, Diederichs W, Lue TF, et al. Correlation of altered penile ultrastructure with clinical arterial evaluation. *J Urol* 1989;142:1462–1468.
88. Jevtich MJ, Khawand NY, Vidic B. Clinical significance of ultrastructural findings in the corpora cavernosa of normal and impotent men. *J Urol* 1990;143:289–293.
89. Mersdorf A, Goldsmith PC, Diederichs W, et al. Ultrastructural changes in impotent penile tissue: a comparison of 65 patients. *J Urol* 1991;145:749–758.
90. Michal V, Pospíchal J. Phalloarteriography in the diagnosis of erectile impotence. *World J Surg* 1978;2:239–248.
91. Rosen MP, Greenfield AJ, Walker TG, et al. Cigarette smoking: an independent risk factor for atherosclerosis in the hypogastric-cavernous arterial bed of men with arteriogenic impotence. *J Urol* 1991;145:759–763.
92. Mottonen M, Nieminen K. Relation of atherosclerotic obstruction of the arterial supply of corpus cavernosum to erectile dysfunction. In: *Proceedings of the Sixth Biennial International Symposium on Corpus Cavernosum Revascularization and Third Biennial World Meeting on Impotence*. Boston, October 1988:12(abst).
93. Aboseif SR, Breza J, Orvis BR, et al. Erectile response to acute and chronic occlusion of the internal pudendal and penile arteries. *J Urol* 1989;141: 398–402.
94. Takagane H, Matsuzaka J, Aoki H, et al. Hemodynamic studies of penile erection in dogs: blood flow changes in the corpus cavernosum caused by arterial ligation. In: *Proceedings of the Sixth Biennial International Symposium on Corpus Cavernosum Revascularization and Third Biennial World Meeting on Impotence*. Boston, October 1988:13(abst).
95. Rajfer J, Rosciszewski A, Mehringer M. Prevalence of corporeal venous leakage in impotent men. *J Urol* 1988;140:69–71.
96. Fischer GM, Swain ML, Cherian K. Increased vascular collagen and elastin synthesis in experimental atherosclerosis in the rabbit: variation in synthesis among major vessels. *Atherosclerosis* 1980;35:11–20.
97. Pietilä K, Nikkari T. Enhanced synthesis of collagen and total protein by smooth muscle cells from atherosclerotic rabbit aortas in culture. *Atherosclerosis* 1980;37:11–19.
98. Ehrhart LA, Holderbaum D. Aortic collagen, elastin and non-fibrous protein synthesis in rabbits fed cholesterol and peanut oil. *Atherosclerosis* 1980;37: 423–432.
99. Azadzoi KM, Saenz de Tejada I. Hypercholesterolemia impairs endothelium-dependent relaxation of rabbit corpus cavernosum smooth muscle. *J Urol* 1991;146:238–240.
100. Nehra A, Hall SJ, Basil G, et al. Systemic sclerosis and impotence: a clinicopathological correlation. *J Urol* 1993;153:1140–1146.
101. Jensen SB, Hagen C, Frøland A, et al. Sexual function and pituitary axis in insulin treated diabetic men. *Acta Med Scand Suppl* 1979;624:65–68.
102. Murray FT, Wyss HU, Thomas RG, et al. Gonadal dysfunction in diabetic men with organic impotence. *J Clin Endocrinol Metab* 1987;65:127–135.
103. Ziedler A, Gelfand R, Tamagna E, et al. Pituitary gonadal function in diabetic male patients with and without impotence. *Andrologia* 1982;14:62–68.
104. Wilson JD, George FW, Griffin JE. The hormonal control of sexual development. *Science* 1981;211:1278–1284.
105. Kwan M, Greenleaf WJ, Mann J, et al. The nature of androgen action on male sexuality: a combined laboratory-self-report study on hypogonadal men. *J Clin Endocrinol Metab* 1983;57:557–562.
106. Sar M, Stumpf WE. Androgen concentration in motor neurons of cranial nerves and spinal cord. *Science* 1977;197:77–79.
107. Sar M, Stumpf WE. Distribution of androgen target cells in the rate forebrain and pituitary after [3H]-dihydrotestosterone administration. *J Steroid Biochem* 1977;8:1131–1135.
108. Murray FT, Klimberg IW. Organic impotence. In: Bardin CW, ed. *Current ther-*

apy in endocrinology and metabolism, Vol 3. Philadelphia: BC Decker, 1988: 252–262.
109. Bancroft J, Wu FCW. Changes in erectile responsiveness during androgen replacement therapy. *Arch Sex Behav* 1983;12:59–66.
110. Mooradian AD, Morley JE, Billington CJ, et al. Hyperprolactinaemia in male diabetics. *Postgrad Med J* 1985;61:11–14.
111. The process of care model for the evaluation and treatment of erectile dysfunction. The Process of Care Consensus Panel. *Int J Impot Res* 1999;11(2):59–74.
112. NIH Consensus Development Panel on Impotence. *JAMA* 1993;270:83–90.
113. Rosen RC, Riley A, Wagner G, et al. The International Index of Erectile Function (IIEF): a multidimensional scale for assessment of erectile dysfunction. *Urology* 1977;49(6):822–830.
114. Udelson D, Park K, Sadeghi-Nejad H, et al. Axial penile buckling forces vs. Rigidscan radial rigidity as a function of intracavernosal pressure: why Rigidscan does not predict functional erections in individual patients. *J Impot* 1999;11:327–336.
115. Abelson D. Diagnostic value of the penile pulse and blood pressure: a Doppler study of impotence in diabetics. *J Urol* 1975;113:636–639.
116. Karacan I. Diagnosis of erectile impotence in diabetes mellitus: an objective and specific method. *Ann Intern Med* 1980;92:334–337.
117. Goldstein I, Siroky MB, Krane RJ. Impotence in diabetes mellitus. In: Krane RJ, Siroky MB, Goldstein I, eds. *Male sexual dysfunction*. Boston: Little, Brown, 1983:77–86.
118. Goldstein I, Krane RJ, Greenfield AJ, et al. Vascular diseases of the penis: impotence and priapism. In: Pollack HM, ed. *Clinical urography*, Vol 3. Philadelphia: WB Saunders, 1990:2231–2252.
119. Gasior BL, Levine FJ, Howannesian A, et al. Plaque-associated corporal veno-occlusive dysfunction in idiopathic Peyronie's disease: a pharmacocavernosometric and pharmacocavernosographic study. *World J Urol* 1990;8:90–96.
120. Penson DF, Seftel AD, Krane RJ, et al. The hemodynamic pathophysiology of impotence following blunt trauma to the erect penis. *J Urol* 1992;148:1171–1180.
121. Wilson JD, Griffin JE. The use and misuse of androgens. *Metabolism* 1980;29: 1278–1295.
122. Snyder PJ, Lawrence DA. Treatment of male hypogonadism with testosterone enanthate. *J Clin Endocrinol Metab* 1980;51:1335–1339.
123. Jackson JA, Waxman J, Spiekerman AM. Prostatic complications of testosterone replacement therapy. *Arch Intern Med* 1989;149:2365–2366.
124. Carter JN, Tyson JE, Tolis G, et al. Prolactin-secreting tumors and hypogonadism in 22 men. *N Engl J Med* 1978;299:847–852.
125. Franks S, Jacobs HS, Martin N, et al. Hyperprolactinaemia and impotence. *Clin Endocrinol* 1978;8:277–287.
126. Levine FJ, Goldstein I. Vascular reconstructive surgery in the management of erectile dysfunction. *Int J Impot Res* 1990;2:59–78.
127. Levine FJ, Greenfield AJ, Goldstein I. Arteriographically determined occlusive disease within the hypogastric cavernous bed in impotent patients following blunt perineal and pelvic trauma. *J Urol* 1990;144:1147–1153.
128. Levine FJ, Greenfield AJ, Goldstein I. Arteriographically determined occlusive disease within the hypogastric cavernous bed in impotent patient following blunt perineal and pelvic trauma. *J Urol* 1990;144:1147–1153.
129. Pfizer: NDA submission, 1997, and Viagra labeling, update Dec. 1998.
130. Cheitlin MD, Hutter AM, Jr, Brindis RG, et al. ACC/AHA expert document. Use of sildenafil (Viagra) in patients with clinical risk from cardiovascular disease. American College of Cardiology/American Hearth Association, 1998.
131. Boolell M, Allen MJ, Ballard SA, et al: Sildenafil: an orally active type 5 cyclic GMP-specific phosphodiesterase inhibitor for the treatment of penile erectile dysfunction. *Int J Impot Res* 1996;8:47–52.
132. Morales A, Gingell C, Collins M, et al: Clinical safety of sildenafil citrate (Viagra) in the treatment of erectile dysfunction. *Int J Impot Res* 1998;10:69–73.
133. Wagner G, Maytom M, Smith M, et al: Analysis of the efficacy of sildenafil (Viagra) in the treatment of erectile dysfunction in elderly patients. *J Urol* 1998;159[5S]:S239(abst).
134. Steers WD and the Sildenafil Study Group. Meta-analysis of the efficacy of sildenafil (Viagra) in the treatment of severe erectile dysfunction. *J Urol* 1998; 159[5S]:S238(abst).
135. Holgren E, Giuliano F, Hulting C, et al: Sildenafil in the treatment of erectile dysfunction caused by spinal cord injury: a double-blind placebo-controlled flexible-dose 2-way crossover study. *Neurology* 1998;50:A127(abst).
136. Padma-Nathan H and the Sildenafil Study Group. Efficacy of Viagra (sildenafil citrate) in the treatment of erectile dysfunction in men with transurethral or radical prostatectomy. *J Urol* 1999 (abst).
137. Rendell MS. Sildenafil improves intercourse success in patients with erectile dysfunction and diabetes. In: *Program and Abstracts of the 34th Annual Meeting of the EASD*, Barcelona, Spain, 1998(abst 300).
138. Margolis R, Prieto P, Stein L, et al. Statistical summary of 10,000 male cases using Afrodex in treatment of impotence. *Curr Ther Res* 1971;13:616–622.
139. Morales A, Condra M, Owen JA, et al. Is yohimbine effective in the treatment of organic impotence? Results of a controlled trial. *J Urol* 1987;137:1168–1172.
140. Morales A, Condra MS, Owen JE, et al. Oral and transcutaneous pharmacologic agents in the treatment of impotence. *Urol Clin North Am* 1988;15:87–93.
141. Goldstein I, Carson C, Rosen R, et al. Vasomax for the treatment of male erectile dysfunction. *World J Urol* 2001;19(1):51–56.
142. Becker AJ, Stief CG, Machtens S, et al. Oral phentolamine as treatment for erectile dysfunction. *J Urol* 1998;159:1214–1215.
143. Morales A, Heaton J, Johnston B, et al. Oral and topical treatment of erectile dysfunction: present and future. *Urol Clin North Am* 1995;22:879–886.
144. Padma-Nathan H, Auerbach S, Lewis R, et al: Efficacy and safety of apomorphine SL vs placebo for male erectile dysfunction. *J Urol* 161(4):214.
145. Dula E, Nuys V, Auerbach S, Buttler S, et al. Efficacy and safety of apomorphine Sl vs placebo for erectile dysfunction in diabetic patients. In: *Program and Abstracts of the Second Fall Meeting of the Society for the Study of Impotence*, Cleveland, OH, 2000(abst B5).
146. Porst H, Giuliano F, Meuleman E, et al. Daily IC 351 treatment of ED. In: *Program and Abstracts of the Second Fall Meeting of the Society for the Study of Impotence*, Cleveland, OH, 2000(abst B13).
147. Goldstein I, Payton T, Schechter PJ. A double-blind, placebo-controlled, efficacy and safety study of topical gel formulation 1% alprostadil (Topiglan) for the in-office treatment of erectile dysfunction. *Urology* 2001;57:301–305.
148. Nadig PW, Ware JC, Blumoff R. Noninvasive device to produce and maintain an erection-like state. *Urology* 1986;27:126–131.
149. Nadig PW. Vacuum erection devices. A review. *World J Urol* 1990;8:114–117.
150. Witherington R. External penile appliances for management of impotence. *Semin Urol* 1990;8:124–128.
151. Diederichs W, Kaula NF, Lue TF, et al. The effect of subatmospheric pressure on the simian penis. *J Urol* 1989;142:1087–1089.
152. Wespes E, Schulman CC. Hemodynamic study of the effect of vacuum device on human erection. *Int J Impot Res* 1990;2[suppl 2]:337(abst).
153. Moul JW, McLeod DG. Negative pressure devices in the explanted penile prosthesis population. *J Urol* 1989;142:729–731.
154. Witherington R. Vacuum constriction device for management of erectile impotence. *J Urol* 1989;141:320–322.
155. Sidi AA, Becher EF, Zhang G, et al. Patient acceptance of and satisfaction with an external negative pressure device for impotence. *J Urol* 1990;144:1154–1156.
156. Padma-Natham H, Hellstrom WJ, Kaiser FE, et al. Treatment of men with erectile dysfunction with transurethral alprostadil. Medicated urethral system for erection. *N Engl J Med* 1997;336:7.
157. Juenemann K-P, Lue TF, Fournier GR Jr, et al. Hemodynamics of papaverine- and phentolamine-induced penile erection. *J Urol* 1986;136:158–161.
158. Virag R. Intracavernous injection of papaverine for erectile failure [letter]. *Lancet* 1982;2:938.
159. Brindley GS. Pilot experiments on the actions of drugs injected into the human corpus cavernosum penis. *Br J Pharmacol* 1986;87:495–500.
160. Zorgniotti AW, Lefleur RS. Auto-injection of the corpus cavernosum with a vasoactive drug combination for vasculogenic impotence. *J Urol* 1985;133: 39–41.
161. Stackl W, Hasun R, Marberger M. Intracavernous injection of prostaglandin E1 in impotent men. *J Urol* 1988;140:66–68.
162. Lee LM, Stevenson RWD, Szasz G. Prostaglandin EI versus phentolamine/papaverine for the treatment of erectile impotence: a double-blind comparison. *J Urol* 1989;141:549–550.
163. Azadzoi KM, Payton T, Krane RJ, et al. Effects of intracavernosal trazodone hydrochloride: animal and human studies. *J Urol* 1990;144:1277–1282.
164. Padma-Nathan H, Goldstein I, et al. Intracavernosal pharmacotherapy: the pharmacologic erection program. *World J Urol* 1987;5:160–165.
165. Zentgraf M, Baccouche M, Jünemann KP. Diagnosis and therapy of erectile dysfunction using papaverine and phentolamine. *Urol Int* 1988;43:65–75.
166. Padma-Nathan H, Goldstein I, Krane RJ. Treatment of prolonged or priapistic erections following intracavernosal papaverine therapy. *Semin Urol* 1986; 4:236–238.
167. Levine SB, Althof SE, Turner LA, et al. Side effects of self-administration of intracavernous papaverine and phentolamine for the treatment of impotence. *J Urol* 1989;141:54–57.
168. Lakin MM, Montague DK. Intracavernous injection therapy in post-priapism cavernosal fibrosis. *J Urol* 1988;140:828–829.
169. Mulhall JP, Daller M, Traish AM, et al. Intracavernosal forskolin: role in management of vasculogenic impotence resistant to standard 3-agent pharmacotherapy. *J Urol* 1997;158:1768–1769.
170. Fallon B. Intracavernous injection therapy for male erectile dysfunction. *Urol Clin North Am* 1995;22:833.
171. Mulhall JP. Intracavernosal injection therapy: a practical guide. *Tech Urol* 1997;3:129.
172. Mulhall JP, Jahoda AE, Cairney M, et al. The causes of patient dropout from penile self-injection therapy for impotence. *J Urol* 1999;162:1291–1294.
173. Small MP, Carrion HM. A new penile prosthesis for treating impotence. *Contemp Surg* 1975;7(2):29–33.
174. Scott FB, Bradley WE, Timm GW. Management of erectile impotence: use of implantable inflatable prosthesis. *Urology* 1973;2:80–82.
175. Merril DC: Mentro inflatable penile prosthesis. *Urol Clin North Am* 1989;16:51–66.
176. Furlow WL, Motley RC: The inflatable penile prosthesis: clinical experience with a new controlled expansion cylinder. *J Urol* 1988;139:945–946.
177. Goldstein I, Newman L, Baum N, et al. Safety and efficacy outcome of Mentor Alpha-1 inflatable penile prosthesis implantation for impotence treatment. *J Urol* 1997;157:833–839.
178. Carson CC. Infections in genitourinary prostheses. *Urol Clin North Am* 1989;16:139–147.
179. Kessler R. Surgical experience with the inflatable penile prosthesis. *J Urol* 1980;124:611–612.
180. McAuley I, Munarriz RM, Maitland S, et al. In: *Program and Abstracts of the Second Fall Meeting of the Society for the Study of Impotence*, Cleveland, OH. 2000 (abst A44).
181. Sharlip ID. The role of vascular surgery in arteriogenic and combined arteriogenic and venogenic impotence. *Semin Urol* 1990;8:129–137.
182. Bar-Moshé O, Vandendris M. Treatment of impotence due to perineal venous leakage by ligation of crura penis. *J Urol* 1988;139:1217–1219.

CHAPTER 60

Infection and Diabetes

Deborah E. Sentochnik and George M. Eliopoulos

It is commonly believed that the incidence of infection is higher in persons with diabetes mellitus and that such infections result in complications and death more frequently than would be anticipated in otherwise healthy individuals (1,2). Older studies, upon which much of this information is based, focus particularly on infections of the urinary tract, the respiratory tree, and the extremities and derive their data from autopsy cases. However, in these studies the degree to which infection at these sites actually contributed to the cause of death is frequently not clear, and control groups are typically lacking. More recent studies, while documenting excess mortality among patients with diabetes, have ascribed this largely to cardiovascular disease rather than to uncontrolled infection (3,4).

In diabetes mellitus, a number of factors greatly complicate efforts to assess risk of infection and resulting complications. The most basic is the problem of determining an appropriate estimate of the population at risk, which may be difficult to obtain for diabetes and is rarely if ever presented. Furthermore, in diabetes, as in other chronic diseases in which the natural history for any individual may span decades, historical controls are of limited utility, given the expected improvements in the general health of a population, the development of more effective diagnostic techniques, earlier medical intervention, and the availability of expanded therapeutic options, including more active and better tolerated antimicrobial agents. A number of variables, including duration of illness, severity of noninfectious complications, concurrent illnesses, level of glucose control, and even degree of medical supervision, result in a very heterogeneous group of individuals at risk even within a more narrowly defined time frame. Finally, some infections that may be particular to diabetics, such as emphysematous cholecystitis, are so uncommon that information regarding risk factors and management options is limited.

Despite these limitations, much is known both about those uncommon infections that occur predominantly in patients with diabetes mellitus and about the more common infections that, while not restricted to those with diabetes, will often complicate the general management of this group of patients. To acknowledge such limitations in advance is to underscore the need for careful individualization in the approach to diagnosis and therapy for any diabetic patient with suspected or proven infection.

DIABETES AND THE IMMUNE SYSTEM

Defining altered host responses in diabetes has long been hampered both by the complexity of the systems in question and by the rather limited availability of techniques to study these responses. *In vivo* the various arms of the immune system are highly dynamic and interdependent. It is thus simplistic to study any single component of it *in vacuo*. Historically, however, methodologic constraints did in fact limit such studies to individual aspects of host defenses, such as leukocyte adherence or phagocytosis, exclusive of other components of the system. Even more recent has been the increase in the appreciation of complex interactions, not only among the various cellular elements of the immune system itself but also among the elements of the immune system and other body components such as the vascular endothelium. As the approaches to the investigation of these issues evolve, it becomes increasingly more difficult to compare studies. It is for these reasons that, even after decades of investigation, questions remain about whether diabetes itself results in specific immunologic defects and how such defects might predispose to infection (5).

Function of Polymorphonuclear Leukocytes

MOBILIZATION AND CHEMOTAXIS

Using the Rebuck skin window technique, which was to remain the standard for many years, Perillie et al. (6) studied polymorphonuclear leukocyte (PMN) chemotaxis in ten patients with well-controlled diabetes, six patients with diabetic ketoacidosis, four patients with nondiabetic uremic acidosis, and ten healthy controls. An abrasion was created on the volar forearm, and sterile coverslips were serially applied over the next several hours. Mobilization of PMNs to the area of inflammation was graded by microscopic examination of the coverslip after staining. The PMNs of all acidotic patients had a diminished early (24 hour) response. This response time became normal in the four patients with diabetes whose acidosis was corrected. In an ambitious analysis of leukocyte function, Brayton et al. (7) examined chemotaxis with use of a modified Rebuck technique in 18 patients with fairly well-controlled diabetes, five of whom were acidotic at the time of study. At 2 and 4 hours, mobilization of the PMNs of all diabetic subjects was diminished. However, at later time points, no differences were seen between the mobilization responses of the PMNs of diabetic subjects and those of healthy controls. The PMNs of acidotic uremic patients had a chemotactic response similar to that of controls at all time points.

Mowat and Baum (8), in an *in vitro* study using a modified tissue-culture chamber, studied chemotaxis of PMNs from 31 diabetic patients with various degrees of glycemic control. A chemotactic index was derived by comparing the original number of PMNs with the number that had completely crossed a filter barrier in response to chemoattractants. The PMNs of all patients with diabetes had a lower chemotactic index (i.e., diminished response), without any correlation between chemotactic index and type of therapy or fasting blood glucose levels. Incubation of the PMNs from 11 controls with glucose at concentrations of 100 to 900 mg/dL did not change the chemotactic index of the PMNs. Incubation of the PMNs of diabetic patients with insulin at concentrations of 10 to 100 μU/mL improved the chemotactic index of PMNs of the diabetic patients if glucose was also present. Molenaar et al. (9) used a bacterial factor from *Escherichia coli* as a chemoattractant and found a lower chemotactic index for the PMNs of 52 first-degree relatives of 15 patients with diabetes as compared with the chemotactic index for the PMNs of controls. Not all the subjects with diabetes had PMNs with a depressed chemotactic index, but the average chemotactic index was lower than that for the PMNs of their relatives. A later study (10) that used a similar technique (Boyden modified chamber) with cells washed free of plasma found no difference in the chemotactic index of the PMNs of control subjects and those of patients with insulin-dependent diabetes mellitus (IDDM) with various degrees of glucose control or duration of disease.

Shortly after the above studies were conducted, there was a shift to the subagarose technique for assaying chemotaxis. This technique yielded more reproducible results and corrected for chemokinetic movement. Measurements are made of the migration from a center well in an agarose plate toward a chemoattractant (zymogen-activated plasma) and of random migration toward a control well. With this technique, the average chemotactic index of the PMNs of 58 patients with diabetes was found to be depressed (11). Chemically defined chemotactic activity of PMNs under agarose was investigated by Naghibi et al. (12) for 26 patients receiving oral hyperglycemic agents, daily insulin injections, or continuous insulin infusion before an intensive control regimen and in 11 of these patients after institution of the intensive regimen. Chemotaxis of the PMNs of all groups was comparable to that of control PMNs.

PHAGOCYTOSIS

Bybee and Rogers (13) studied leukocyte phagocytosis in 31 patients with well-controlled diabetes, seven patients with diabetic acidosis, and a control group. Washed PMNs and an equal number of *Staphylococcus aureus* or *Staphylococcus epidermidis* were incubated together for 60 minutes in 10% human serum. Phagocytosis was considered to be present if at least one bacterium was ingested. There was no quantitation of the number of organisms engulfed per cell. Only the PMNs of ketotic diabetic patients were found to exhibit diminished phagocytosis. This defect was corrected if acidosis was reversed but not if the cells were incubated with normal serum. Control PMNs functioned normally if they were incubated with serum from acidotic diabetic patients. However, serum factors may have been diluted out, given that a 10% concentration of serum was used.

Bagdade et al. (14) used a similar system, but with 90% serum, to examine phagocytosis of *Streptococcus pneumoniae* type 25 by leukocytes from eight patients who were not acidotic but had poorly controlled diabetes. Decreased phagocytosis was especially notable when fasting blood glucose levels were higher than 250 mg/dL. After the patients' glucose levels were controlled, phagocytic activity improved but did not attain control values. In contrast to the findings of Bybee and Rogers (13), the activity of control PMNs was diminished when the cells were incubated with serum from patients with diabetes, whereas the activity of PMNs from patients with diabetes was increased when the cells were incubated with normal serum. The work of Rayfield et al. (15) supported the possibility of an opsonization defect affecting PMNs of individuals with diabetes. Normal PMNs had decreased uptake of radiolabeled *E. coli* or *S. aureus* in the presence of serum from patients with diabetes.

Using the lysostaphin assay technique, which allows differentiation between phagocytosis and intracellular killing, Tan et al. (16) demonstrated a defect in phagocytosis of *S. aureus* by the PMNs of 31 patients with adult-onset diabetes. The presence of the defect showed no correlation with level of glycemic control or history of recurrent infections. The addition of normal serum had no effect. Using shorter observation periods, Nolan et al. (17) found that PMNs from 17 patients with poorly controlled diabetes ingested a smaller proportion of an inoculum of 10^6 *S. aureus* after 20 minutes (the interval during which most engulfment takes place under normal physiologic conditions) than did control PMNs. This difference vanished at 60 minutes. Davidson et al. (18) measured engulfment of *Candida guilliermondii* over a 45-minute period by PMNs from 11 patients with moderately well-controlled diabetes. The ratio of white cells to organisms was such that 90% of the control cells would have ingested at least one yeast cell in 30 minutes. Phagocytosis was diminished in the PMNs of the patients with diabetes, regardless of levels of glycosylated hemoglobin 1C (HbA_{1c}). A defect in opsonization was suggested, since preopsonized yeast particles added to serum from diabetic patients with PMNs from control subjects were engulfed at normal levels. Alexiewicz et al. (19) demonstrated impaired phagocytic ability of PMNs from patients with newly diagnosed, non-IDDM, which correlated inversely with fasting serum glucose level. Both phagocytosis and glucose control improved significantly after 3 months of therapy with glyburide. The authors also demonstrated an inverse relationship between cytosolic calcium concentrations in PMNs and phagocytic function and postulated that the functional defect may relate to the high calcium levels.

ADHERENCE

Comparatively few papers have specifically addressed the question of adherence by the leukocytes of patients with diabetes. Peterson et al. (20) found that the PMNs of six of seven patients with poorly controlled diabetes exhibited impaired adherence to a glass-wool column. Adherence improved 1 to 2 months later when glycemic control had improved. However, no control patients were examined. Bagdade et al. (21) showed an enhancement of adherence of PMNs to a nylon-fiber column following an improvement in the control of blood glucose levels. Adherence increased from 53% to 74% of control values. In another study, Bagdade and Walters (22) demonstrated a direct relationship between degree of glucose control and PMN adherence.

Andersen et al. (23) pointed the study of adhesion in a dramatic new direction by devising a more physiologic system. Noting that vascular endothelium is not a passive participant in the inflammation cascade, they examined the ability of PMNs from 26 patients with diabetes and from age-matched controls to bind to bovine aortic endothelium. The PMNs of 60% of the patients with diabetes had severely depressed function that did not correlate with HbA_{1c} levels. PMN–PMN aggregation was not defective. No quantitative defect in fibronectin was seen, but a qualitative defect could not be excluded.

BACTERICIDAL ACTIVITY

Early studies, such as that of Dziatkowiak et al. (24), compared the number of live *S. aureus* bacteria in a granulocyte with the total number engulfed to calculate the proportion of organisms killed. Several studies (16) demonstrated diminished killing by the PMNs of patients with diabetes while others did not. Repine et al. (25) took a more quantitative and functional approach. Instead of using a single low ratio of bacteria to PMNs, they used five different ratios (1:1 to 100:1). Study patients included infected and noninfected individuals with and without diabetes. Cells were incubated with *S. aureus* for 1 hour, after which colonies were counted. The rates of intracellular killing of bacteria by PMNs from uninfected controls and by PMNs of persons with well-controlled diabetes were comparable. PMNs from uninfected patients with poorly controlled diabetes functioned less well, especially when the higher ratios of bacteria to white cells were used. Although the functioning of PMNs from infected patients with well-controlled diabetes was on a par with the functioning of those from uninfected controls, the PMNs from the infected patients with diabetes did not display the increase in killing activity seen in the PMNs of infected patients without diabetes. The bactericidal function of PMNs from infected patients with poorly controlled diabetes was the lowest of all the groups. Naghibi et al. (12), using a single low ratio of bacteria to PMNs, found depressed bactericidal function of the PMNs of patients against *Pseudomonas aeruginosa*, but they did not study any infected patients. Serum from patients with diabetes had an inhibitory effect on PMNs from both normal controls and diabetic subjects before and after intensive glucose management. Bactericidal activity of PMNs from the patients with diabetes remained depressed even after intensive management.

Stimulated PMNs display a burst of oxidative metabolism that produces superoxide anions and other oxygen-derived species implicated in bacterial killing. These reactions produce chemiluminescence, a sensitive indicator of oxidative metabolism that correlates with antimicrobial activity. Shah et al. (26) looked at the production of superoxide anion and chemiluminescence of PMNs from patients with diabetes, examining the cells in both the resting state and in response to soluble and particulate stimuli. In resting PMNs from patients with diabetes, the chemiluminescence of cells placed in serum from patients with diabetes was comparable to that of cells placed in control serum. Superoxide production was higher in autologous serum from patients with diabetes than in normal serum. The significance of these findings taken together was unclear. When stimulated, the PMNs from patients with diabetes showed a blunted response with regard to both superoxide production and chemiluminescence. Cross-incubation serum studies effected no change, suggesting that an intracellular defect rather than an inhibitory serum factor might have been present. The precise role of defective *in vitro* bactericidal activity of PMNs, associated with impaired superoxide production, as a predisposing factor for infection is uncertain, however. Such defects can be demonstrated in patients with diabetes who have not been subject to recurrent or particularly serious infections (27).

Sato et al. (28) reported improvement in chemoluminescence measurements related to O_2^- and OCl^- production by PMNs of patients with diabetes after 4 weeks of therapy with an aldose reductase inhibitor, although levels did not reach those of PMNs from healthy controls. This observation could not be attributed to improvement in glucose control, as both the postprandial glucose and HbA_{1c} levels were unchanged. It has been suggested that advanced glycation products associated with diabetes may bind to specific motifs common to lactoferrin, lysozyme, and other antimicrobial proteins found in PMNs and interfere with the antimicrobial function of these host defense molecules (29).

The PMNs of patients with diabetes have shown a decreased prostaglandin E and thromboxane B_2 response to stimulation by zymosan or killed *S. aureus* (30). The synthesis and release of leukotriene B_4 by these cells also were diminished compared with those of the PMNs of sex- and age-matched controls (31). The significance of these findings is not known.

Monocyte Function in Diabetes

Geisler et al. (32) found a decrease in the total number of circulating monocytes in 14 patients with diabetes. These cells displayed diminished phagocytosis of *Candida albicans* but not of latex particles or sheep red blood cells. Glass et al. (33) proposed that monocytes from patients with diabetes have a diminished activity of "lectinlike" receptors necessary for the recognition of cell-wall components of microorganisms. Attachment of *S. epidermidis* to these monocytes was impaired, but attachment to coated sheep red blood cells, which are recognized by the Fc receptor, was normal. It could not be assessed whether the proportion of monocytes with the lectinlike receptors was reduced, each receptor had a lower affinity, or each monocyte had fewer receptors. Katz et al. (34) described subpopulations of monocytes with a reduced ability to phagocytose *Listeria monocyto-*

genes. Impaired monocyte chemotaxis has also been reported (35). Monocytes from patients with diabetes have been found to exhibit increased adhesion to fibronectin. Although this property may play a role in the genesis of atherosclerosis (36), its relationship to antimicrobial function is not known. The metabolic activity in response to the ingestion of zymosan particles by the monocytes from patients with diabetes is increased, as reflected by higher levels of chemiluminescence, superoxide production, and hexose monophosphate shunt activity than those exhibited by control monocytes (37). The consequences of this increased activity have not been evaluated. Studies of monocytes from patients with diabetes report upregulated secretion of inflammatory mediators such as tumor necrosis factor-α (TNF-α), interleukin-1β (IL-1β), and prostaglandin E_2 (38).

Cell-Mediated Immunity

Reports of defects of cell-mediated immunity *in vitro* in patients with diabetes abound. Unfortunately, results are piecemeal both because of the complex interrelationships involved in the cell-mediated immune system and because of the evolution of study techniques over time.

MacCuish et al. (39) found that lymphocyte transformation in response to the mitogen phytohemagglutinin (PHA) was diminished in patients with poorly controlled diabetes. Meanwhile, Casey et al. (40,41) determined that the transformation of lymphocytes of patients with diabetes in response to PHA was normal regardless of the patient's glycemic control but that the response to a staphylococcal antigen was decreased. These authors did not mention any ketotic patients. In a study by Speert and Silva (42), the lymphocytes of children with diabetic ketoacidosis had a decreased mitogenic response that reverted to normal when metabolic derangements were corrected. There may be a diminished release of migration-inhibition factor by T lymphocytes from patients with diabetes (43,44). T-lymphocyte subsets have been studied with regard to the possibility of an autoimmune basis of diabetes. While alterations of CD4-to-CD8 lymphocyte ratios during the evolution and progression of diabetes have been noted (45–47), no relationship of these changes to infection has been detected. No agreement has been reached as to whether the number and function of T and B cells in patients with diabetes is increased, decreased, or normal as compared with those in controls (10).

An acquired defect in the production of IL-2 by T cells has been demonstrated in patients with IDDM (48), as have increased levels of receptors for this cytokine (49). Decreased responsiveness to interferon of natural killer cells from patients with IDDM has been observed (50). The implications of these abnormalities with regard to defense against infection remain speculative at the present time.

Miscellaneous Factors

Abnormalities in the microvascular circulation of individuals with diabetes may result in decreased tissue perfusion (51). While it is intuitively understandable that such abnormalities might facilitate the acquisition of infection and impair response to therapy, it is unclear what role microvascular defects actually play in the pathogenesis of infections relatively specific for patients with diabetes, such as mucormycosis, malignant external otitis, and emphysematous cholecystitis. Reviews of these topics often mention the arteriolar narrowing seen on pathologic examination, but comparisons with control specimens have not been reported. It appears that the white blood cells of patients with diabetes may play a role in producing damage to the capillary and venular endothelium (52,53).

INFECTIONS STRONGLY ASSOCIATED WITH DIABETES

Mucormycosis

THE ORGANISM AND HOST RESPONSE

The term *mucormycosis* connotes a variety of infections caused by fungi belonging to the order Mucorales, members of the class Zygomycetes (54,55). *Zygomycosis* and *phycomycosis* are synonyms that have been rendered obsolete by ongoing reclassification. *Rhizopus* species (especially *Rhizopus oryzae* and *Rhizopus arrhizus*) are the most commonly isolated pathogens, followed by *Mucor* organisms. *Cunninghamella* (56) and other species have also been found to cause disease. These molds produce large, thick-walled, nonseptate hyphae that branch at more-or-less right angles. Ubiquitous in the environment, these organisms are most often found in decaying matter. Humans commonly inhale the spores, which have a low virulence potential. The ability of the spores to germinate successfully is dependent on specific host factors. Most information regarding pathogenesis comes from studies in rabbit and mouse models. After inhalation of spores, normal animals do not become ill, whereas diabetic animals develop a rapidly progressive pulmonary disease (57). Alveolar macrophages from normal mice, but not those from diabetic mice, will ingest the spores and inhibit their germination into the invasive hyphal forms. Experimentally, neither hyperglycemia nor metabolic acidosis alone is sufficient to permit infection (58), despite the propensity for the development of certain mucormycosis syndromes among acidotic patients with diabetes. In contrast to normal human serum, the serum of patients with diabetes with ketoacidosis does not inhibit the growth of *R. oryzae* (59). It has been proposed that acidosis disrupts the ability of transferrin to bind iron, a deficiency that results in the release of free iron into the serum and perhaps to an interference in the host defenses against *Rhizopus* (60), an iron-requiring organism (61). Credence has been lent to the proposed role of iron regulation in host defense by the increasing recognition of the occurrence of deferoxamine-associated mucormycosis in patients undergoing dialysis. In this situation, it appears that *Rhizopus* organisms may be able to use the iron mobilized by the chelating agent, a capability that has been demonstrated in other organisms (61).

CLINICAL SYNDROMES

Mucormycosis may present as a rhinocerebral, pulmonary, cutaneous, gastrointestinal, or disseminated form of the disease. Rhinocerebral mucormycosis was first recognized more than 50 years ago (62). It occurs primarily in persons with diabetes, although other immunocompromised patients may be affected, and is one of the most fulminant forms of fungal disease affecting that population. The typical patient presents with ketoacidosis. Fungal elements gain entry through the nasopharynx, where tissue invasion may result in nasal discharge that may be tinged with blood. Close inspection of the infected region may reveal necrotic areas with black eschar involving the nasal mucosa or hard palate. The patient is likely to have a fever and to remain lethargic even after metabolic derangements have been corrected. Commonly, by the time the diagnosis is suspected, headache and/or facial pain already reflect extension of the process into the paranasal sinuses and possibly into the orbit of the eye. Occasional patients present with a dramatic, rapid onset of ocular proptosis and vision loss caused by invasion of the orbit. Rapid progression of clinical findings is the result of invasion of blood vessels, with vascular occlusion and subsequent necrosis of tissues dependent on the affected vessels. Progression of thrombosis can include the cavernous sinus

(63) and the internal carotid artery (64). Invasion of the brain results in meningoencephalitis and/or abscess formation with deterioration of neurologic function.

Progression usually occurs over a matter of hours to days and is invariably fatal if the patient is not treated early. Diagnosis must be established by demonstration of characteristic invasion of tissues by hyphal elements in biopsy specimens. A careful search for evidence of vascular invasion must be conducted. Culture results will often be negative. Spinal fluid findings are nonspecific (65). Sinus films may show mucosal thickening and clouding with some spotty destruction of the orbit (66). Computed tomography (CT) scans, with special orbital views, can help define the extent of involvement, although the extent estimated by this method may underestimate the actual extent of involvement determined at surgery (67). Angiography has been used to define the degree of large-vessel involvement. Magnetic resonance imaging offers the potential to provide useful information on the extent of infection, including assessment of soft tissue and vascular structures. Extension beyond the orbit carries a poor prognosis.

Aggressive surgical management is mandatory in all situations; radical debridement sometimes necessitates orbital exenteration. Repeated debridement may be necessary. Concomitantly, underlying metabolic disorders must be addressed. Amphotericin B remains the standard antifungal therapy and must be used in conjunction with surgery (54,68,69). Aggressive antifungal therapy should be used, and although the exact duration of treatment and the total dosage administered have not been well defined, it is reasonable to aim for a total dosage of at least 2 g. The currently approved azole antifungal agents have no defined role in therapy (70). Repeated imaging is necessary to follow the response to treatment, and repeated biopsy may be necessary (71). With optimal therapy, mortality remains at 50%, despite some reports of more encouraging results (72). The nature of the almost universal neurologic residua depends on the anatomic structures that have already been compromised by the time the infection is brought under control.

The remaining forms of mucormycosis do not have a predilection for a specific host, although the pulmonary disease may have a distinctive presentation in patients with diabetes. In contrast to the fatal pneumonia and extensive thrombosis that is typical in immunocompromised patients, diabetic patients have been noted to develop endobronchial and large-airway lesions that may follow a less fulminant course. The main complication of pulmonary mucormycosis is massive hemoptysis. Lesions may respond to aggressive local resection in combination with intravenous therapy with amphotericin B (73–76).

Malignant External Otitis

In 1968, Chandler (77) described a series of patients with a disorder termed *malignant external otitis* (MEO). Occasionally referred to as *progressive, invasive,* or *necrotizing external otitis,* these names attest to the destructive nature of the process. These terms connote a slowly progressive cellulitis that begins in the soft tissues of the external auditory canal. As it penetrates more deeply into the subcutaneous tissue, this process may spread via the fissures of Santorini (clefts in the cartilaginous floor of the external canal) into the mastoid air cells. Access to the temporal bone (osteomyelitis) occurs through the cartilaginous/osseous junction in the outer ear canal (78). The great majority of cases are due to *P. aeruginosa* even though this is not a normal colonizer of the ear in any patient group (79). Most patients are elderly, and 75% to 90% have diabetes. There does not appear to be a distinct relationship between MEO and ketoacidosis or the magnitude of hyperglycemia (80).

Typically, patients will present with a 2- to several-week history of external otitis unresponsive to local therapy. The evolution into MEO, with localized invasion of soft tissue and osseous structures, is heralded by unrelenting, severe otalgia often accompanied by purulent discharge (81). It is unusual for patients to appear systemically ill or to have a fever and an elevated white blood cell count. One of the hallmarks of MEO that distinguishes it from simple external otitis is the finding of granulation tissue, usually at the junction of the cartilaginous and osseous portion of the canal, in more than 90% of cases. A swollen, reddened, moist-appearing canal is usual. The tympanic membrane is normal in the rare cases in which it can be visualized. The extent to which the process has progressed toward the base of the skull is reflected clinically by progressive involvement of cranial nerves. The facial nerve may be impaired at presentation in up to 50% of cases (78,82), the result of swelling of the soft tissue surrounding the styloid foramen where the nerve exits the skull or of direct invasion of the bone at the foramen itself. The function of cranial nerves IX, X, and XI can be affected next as the jugular foramen becomes involved (82,83). Finally, the hypoglossal canal can be destroyed. In the most extreme cases, contralateral cranial nerves are compromised as the destructive process erodes the base of the skull. Meningitis may result by extension into the subarachnoid space.

Plain films of the ear canal are of limited sensitivity and specificity for this condition. While technetium scanning is highly sensitive, it is of low specificity, as is gallium scanning. CT scanning, with special views, is a useful imaging modality (84), although tumors cannot be reliably distinguished from MEO. Magnetic resonance imaging provides excellent detail and is, perhaps, the most widely used modality for the initial assessment of patients suspected of having this disorder.

In Chandler's original series (77), the mortality rate from MEO was 50%. A 1981 review of this entity cited a mortality rate of 20% (80). Cure rates since 1985 may have reached 90% (85). The improvement in survival may be attributable in part to the development of more effective antipseudomonal antibiotics. As important, however, is the likelihood that increased awareness by physicians of this entity has led to earlier recognition of affected patients and thus to the possible control of infection with antibiotic therapy and local debridement and to a diminished need for the more radical surgical procedures necessitated by more advanced disease.

Standard antibiotic regimens for treatment of MEO due to *P. aeruginosa* previously consisted of an antipseudomonal penicillin plus an aminoglycoside for a prolonged period (4 to 6 weeks or more) (82,86). With the advent of newer, potentially less-toxic antipseudomonal agents, new regimens have evolved. Monotherapy with the antipseudomonal third-generation cephalosporin, ceftazidime, for 4 to 6 weeks, much of it as home therapy, realized a rate of favorable response of 92% in a series of 20 patients, 30% of whom presented with ipsilateral facial palsy (87). Follow-up at 1 year showed no recurrences. While the results are encouraging, it is of note that two of the patients in this series did not even need debridement, indicating that some presented with the extreme of mild disease. In another study, 21 of 23 patients with MEO were successfully treated with 6 weeks of oral therapy with ciprofloxacin (88). However, only 65% of the patients in this study had diabetes. At present, therapy with an antipseudomonal fluoroquinolone—which may permit oral administration—appears to be an acceptable approach in most patients with a susceptible organism. However, close medical supervision is necessary, as repeated debridement may be required (89). While emergence of resistance has not been a frequent problem in studies using monotherapy (or combination therapy), this possibility should be considered in patients for whom therapy fails.

Emphysematous Pyelonephritis

Severe bacterial urinary tract infection in the patient with diabetes may result in emphysematous pyelonephritis. The precise definition of this rare entity varies among authors. The most rigorous definition includes a requirement for the presence of gas within the renal parenchyma, which may enter the perinephric space by extension. Gas can occur in the calices, collecting system, or bladder, but if it is limited to these sites, these entities are distinct from true emphysematous pyelonephritis and carry different prognoses. The differential diagnosis includes iatrogenic manipulation with introduction of air and fistula formation arising from the digestive system. The first reference to emphysematous pyelonephritis is usually cited as 1898 (90), although in retrospect, it appears that this patient probably had gas only in the collecting system. A number of cases have been reported, but the disorder is rare (91–95). Between 85% and 100% of patients have had diabetes mellitus. Up to 40% of patients may have had concomitant obstruction, which is present in almost all nondiabetic patients with emphysematous pyelonephritis. At presentation, it is not possible clinically to distinguish emphysematous from uncomplicated acute pyelonephritis unless gas has spread beyond the bounds of perirenal tissues to cause subcutaneous crepitation. Pneumaturia is distinctly unusual.

Plain radiographs (96) ultrasound, or abdominal CT scans will reveal gas within the renal parenchyma. A plain x-ray film may show a mottled renal parenchyma with gas bubbles, often in a radial distribution. As the infection advances, gas may be seen outside the renal cortex either outlining the kidney or forming thin crescents, although this classic finding is unusual. Abdominal CT scanning is especially useful for documenting the spread of gas beyond the Gerota fascia. About 10% of patients have bilateral involvement (93). Radiologic evaluation should be undertaken if a suspected case of acute pyelonephritis does not respond to adequate antibiotic therapy within a few days. CT scans may also uncover previously unsuspected abscesses.

The usual causative organisms are typical urinary pathogens, including *E. coli, Klebsiella pneumoniae, Proteus mirabilis,* and *Enterobacter aerogenes.* There are case reports implicating other organisms, including *Candida* species (97); typically, anaerobes are not found. It is not clear why the microbes involved produce gas in a specific clinical situation. The presence of glycosuria, while providing a substrate for production of gas by fermentation, is clearly not the sole factor, given the rarity of emphysematous pyelonephritis and the frequency of glycosuria.

While it is clear that therapy with antibiotics directed at the offending organisms and management of underlying diabetes are imperative, the role of surgical intervention is much less well defined. The lack of prospective, controlled studies is understandable given the rarity of the syndrome. Obstruction should always be sought and relieved as necessary. Some authors suggest following the resolution of gas radiographically and proceeding with nephrectomy only if the patient fails to respond to appropriate antibiotics (93). Others have recommended total nephrectomy as soon as the diagnosis is made, citing the possibility of rapid clinical deterioration in some patients (92). A reasonable approach in an otherwise relatively stable patient might be to try medical management with potent antibiotics, relieve any obstruction, undertake percutaneous drainage as appropriate, and consider nephrectomy if clinical improvement does not occur. Nephrectomy may be especially appropriate if the affected kidney is shown to be nonfunctioning, as occurs in about one half of the patients (94). However, clinical decisions are often not straightforward, as in the case of bilateral emphysematous pyelonephritis or disease in a solitary functioning kidney.

The duration of antibiotic therapy is not addressed in various reviews, but a several-week course would appear prudent. Reported mortality rates range from 10% to 40% (92,93,98). At autopsy, 50% of 42 patients had severe acute and chronic necrotizing pyelonephritis with multiple cortical abscesses, 20% had papillary necrosis, and 20% had intrarenal vascular thrombi (95). In one fourth of the cases, the kidney could not even be identified. Currently, this rare entity may carry a better prognosis if a high index of clinical suspicion is maintained to ensure early imaging studies.

Emphysematous Cholecystitis

Emphysematous cholecystitis is a rare complication of acute cholecystitis in which air is found in the lumen and wall of the gallbladder, with possible extension to the pericholecystic space. It was first diagnosed at surgery in 1908, with the first preoperative diagnosis made by abdominal roentgenography in 1931 (99). In 1975, Mentzer et al. (100) published their comprehensive study, which encompassed the 161 cases reported to date in the literature and three cases of their own. More than one third of the patients in this series had diabetes. In contrast to acute cholecystitis, for which almost three fourths of the patients are female, males account for three fourths of the cases of emphysematous cholecystitis. Perforation and gangrene of the gallbladder are 30 times and three times more common, respectively, and mortality is ten times higher in patients younger than 60 years old but only twice as high for those older than 60 years than in patients with acute cholecystitis. Diabetes does not appear to be an independent factor relative to a worse prognosis. Cholelithiasis is present about one half of the time.

Patients present with pain in the right upper quadrant, nausea and vomiting, and fever. During the next 48 hours, gas develops within the gallbladder lumen and wall, with progression into the surrounding tissues in the next 48 hours (101). Even during this time, one cannot reliably distinguish acute uncomplicated cholecystitis from emphysematous cholecystitis at the bedside. Diagnosis is established by radiographic documentation of gas in the aforementioned areas. On plain films, one may initially see a globular shadow representing the air-filled gallbladder. Soon afterwards, intramural—usually submucosal—air may be visualized (99). Air may sometimes be seen only in the biliary radicles (102). Air under the diaphragm suggests perforation and is a poor prognostic sign (99). Differential diagnosis of these radiographic findings includes the presence of enterovesicular fistula. Ultrasonography has proven a useful tool, although plain films must still be obtained to rule out a porcelain gallbladder or a heavily calcified stone as the source of high-density echoes (103,104). CT is another useful modality in making the diagnosis.

Given the high complication rate of emphysematous cholecystitis, it is important to consider this diagnosis early in the patient with diabetes who is suspected of having acute cholecystitis. It has been recommended that cholecystectomy be performed as soon as the diagnosis is established (101). Typically, a crepitant gangrenous gallbladder is found at surgery. Cultures are positive 50% to 90% of the time, a frequency much higher than that for simple acute cholecystitis. *Clostridium perfringens* is isolated from 25% to 50% of positive cultures, along with more typical enteric organisms such as *E. coli.* Antibiotic coverage should include anaerobes as well as both gram-positive and gram-negative facultative organisms.

The issue of elective cholecystectomy for asymptomatic gallstones in patients with diabetes has been a source of controversy. Because of the perceived increased risk of mortality or severe complications among diabetic patients with acute cholecystitis, for many years it was recommended that those with cholelithiasis undergo prophylactic cholecystectomy. However, complications appear to be uncommon when diabetic patients with asymptomatic stones are followed without surgery. Del Favero et al. (105) followed 47 non–insulin-requiring diabetic patients with asymptomatic gallstones over 5 years; only 15% developed any symptoms, and only two patients developed acute cholecystitis or jaundice. A retrospective controlled study suggested that diabetes alone was not correlated with a higher mortality rate during an episode of acute cholecystitis (106). In a decision-analysis model, it was found—under a broad range of assumptions—that, when managed expectantly (i.e., observed without surgery), diabetic patients with asymptomatic gallstones did no worse than nondiabetic patients (107). Other work suggests a higher rate of infectious complications following cholecystectomy for acute cholecystitis among diabetic than nondiabetic patients (108). In treatment of acute cholecystitis, the trend has been toward expeditious (within 24 hours) surgery (101). The outcome of this approach, in contrast to that of surgery following a "cooling-off" period, has not been rigorously examined in relation to patients with diabetes. Nevertheless, while severe complications are infrequent when diabetic patients with asymptomatic gallstones are observed expectantly, laparoscopic techniques have also reduced the morbidity of cholecystectomy. Therefore, decisions regarding benefits of elective cholecystectomy can be made on a case-by-case basis (109).

INFECTIONS CAUSED BY THERAPEUTIC INTERVENTIONS

Insulin Therapy

Standard self-administered insulin injections result in abscesses remarkably rarely. Preservatives added to insulin have antibacterial activity. Before the 1970s, glass syringes stored in methylated industrial spirit were used. The inadvertent substitution of surgical spirit, which contains a larger number of additives, was more often, although still rarely, associated with abscess formation (110,111). Disposable syringes have largely replaced glass syringes. Manufacturers and many medical practitioners recommend discarding plastic syringes after a single use. However, repeated use of syringes for a month or more has not been reported to result in an increased rate of infection if the syringe is refrigerated between uses, if the needle is wiped with alcohol, or if the syringe–needle unit is soaked in alcohol between uses (112).

In an investigation of the actual insulin injection practices of a group of patients with diabetes, no injection-site infections or significant bacterial contamination of equipment was found. This was despite a lack of "traditional practices" such as wiping the vial and skin or even washing the hands before injection (112,113). Half the patients reused their syringes many times. In a study of jet insulin injectors, for which cleaning every 2 weeks was recommended, no significant growth was seen in cultures of any of the injectors from 19 patients (114). On the other hand, continuous subcutaneous insulin infusion (CSII) has been more commonly associated with infectious complications, typically in the form of abscesses at the needle site (115,116). This is among the most common reasons cited by patients for discontinuing this form of therapy (117). No association between the staphylococcal carrier state and infection at the injection site has been shown (118).

Penile Implants

Men with diabetes make up one fourth to one third of the approximately 17,000 patients each year who undergo penile implant procedures for impotence. The implant apparatuses available range from rigid rods placed in the paired corpora cavernosa to the new, more commonly used, inflatable devices (119,120). Included among the inflatable implants are those with multiple components placed in the scrotum, abdominal wall, and corpora cavernosa that have been available since 1973 and several similar types of succeeding units. The most recent implants are contained entirely in the corpora cavernosa. All types are inserted with a single incision. There is no correlation between the type of prosthesis or incision and the rate of infection (119,120). The infection rate ranges from 0.8% to 8%, with most series having an average of 2% to 3%. This is an improvement from the 15% rate seen before antibiotic prophylaxis became routine. In several series, no increased incidence of infection in patients with diabetes was noted (121,122). *S. epidermidis* is the infecting organism in 40% to 80% of the infections, with coliforms being isolated in most of the others. Infection is thought to originate at the time of surgery primarily as a result of contamination with microorganisms of the skin or colorectal area. Rarely, late infection caused by hematogenous seeding has been reported (122).

Evidence of infection is seen 2 weeks to 2 years after implantation, with the gram-negative organisms tending to present in the earlier part of the range. Systemic signs and symptoms are usually absent. The degree of local findings can be subtle, such as tenderness with manipulation, mechanical malfunction, mild hyperemia or erosion over the mechanism, or formation of periprosthetic adhesive tissue. More dramatic evidence of infection, such as pain, swelling, induration, fistula formation, or extrusion of the device, tends to occur with infections with gram-negative organisms, although not exclusively. Findings at surgical exploration can range from minor adhesions to gross purulence. Immediate therapy consists of removal of the prosthesis, therapy with broad-spectrum intravenous antibiotics, and postoperative drainage. The rate of infection is increased for implants after the first procedure.

Prevention of infection of penile prostheses focuses on the time of surgery. As with all procedures incorporating prosthetic material, concurrent infection, particularly of the urinary tract, is a contraindication to surgery. Antibiotic prophylaxis, an appropriately clean operating room environment, extensive skin preparation, and copious intraoperative irrigation have all been recommended as means of decreasing the chance of infection (120).

Organ Transplantation

Renal transplantation is an option for a number of diabetic patients with end-stage renal disease. For patients receiving a living-related kidney allograft, 1-year patient and graft survival rates are approximately 97% and 90%, respectively (123). Although immunosuppression methods have improved greatly over the years, permitting the use of lower doses of immunosuppressive drugs, infection is still a significant problem in this population. The sources of infection can be the endogenous flora, reactivated latent infection, infection with opportunistic pathogens, or primary transmission from the donor allograft (124,125). Kontoyiannis and Rubin (126) proposed a now-classic timetable for infections that occur in renal transplant recipients. Although exceptions occur, this timetable serves as a useful tool in thinking about likely infections at various time points following transplantation. In the first month following transplantation, these patients present with the same kinds of infectious complications seen in any postoperative patient (i.e., wound, urinary tract, pulmonary, and intravenous catheter bacterial infections). The most serious opportunistic infections are unlikely during the early part of this period. Cumulative immunosuppression is at its height 1 to 6 months after transplantation, and it is during this period that the patient is at greatest risk of opportunistic infections, such as those due to cytomegalovirus, *Pneumocystis carinii,* and *Aspergillus* species, among others. After these first 6 months, the recipient is susceptible to chronic forms of viral disease contracted earlier in his or her course, some opportunistic infections, and diseases found in the community. For further information, the reader is directed to in-depth reviews of the large body of data on this topic (123,126,127).

Since the course of immunosuppression for pancreatic transplantation follows essentially the same pattern as that for renal transplantation, it would be expected that the time frame for infectious complications of the two would be similar. Urinary tract infection is the most common cause of readmission to the hospital in this population (128,129). A study of heart transplantation in carefully selected patients with diabetes revealed no increased risk of infection (130).

Infections Associated with Dialysis

CONTINUOUS AMBULATORY PERITONEAL DIALYSIS

Various forms of ambulatory peritoneal dialysis constitute a common modality of therapy for end-stage renal disease in patients with diabetes. Like any indwelling foreign body, dialysis catheters inserted into the peritoneum carry a risk of infection. For continuous ambulatory peritoneal dialysis (CAPD), one to two episodes of catheter-related peritonitis per patient per year, on average, can be anticipated, although it appears that some patients suffer multiple episodes whereas others have fewer than the expected number (131–133). The rate of CAPD-related infection does not appear to be greater in diabetic than nondiabetic patients (134,135). This is also true for patients receiving chronic intermittent peritoneal dialysis (136) for whom the overall risk of infection is lower than that for patients receiving CAPD.

The source of infection (132) can be intraluminal, from touch contamination of the apparatus at insertion, a break in the tubing or attachment site that permits ingress of bacteria, or contamination at bag changes caused by poor technique. Contamination of dialysate is another potential route of entry of microorganisms. Infection also can occur by the periluminal route, for the skin never makes a complete seal with the catheter at the exit site. Both these routes can result in infection with organisms of the endogenous skin flora. Coagulase-negative staphylococci account for 40% of the cases of peritonitis in patients undergoing CAPD (137), and other gram-positive organisms, such as *S. aureus* and streptococci, are responsible for another 30%. Gram-negative organisms are seen in almost 30% of cases, often reflecting a third route of infection (i.e., contamination of the peritoneum and then the catheter from an intestinal source). Such contamination can occur without an overt disruption in the bowel mucosa. A bowel source is suggested by findings of multiple organisms or anaerobes in the dialysate. It is uncommon for blood cultures to be positive as the result of CAPD peritonitis. The risk of septicemia of all causes among patients undergoing peritoneal dialysis was estimated to be approximately 1% per year in a recent study (138). Positive blood cultures should prompt a search for a source that has led to hematogenous seeding. Fungi, especially *Candida* species, account for almost 5% of cases of CAPD-associated peritonitis, with the rate no higher in patients with diabetes. *Mycobacterium tuberculosis* is seen in fewer than 3% of cases. A number of unusual causes of CAPD peritonitis have been seen (139).

Patients with exit-site infections may be unaware of any problems until an examiner notes erythema at the site. Serous or purulent discharge may be present. Infections in the subcutaneous tunnel can be very difficult to diagnose, especially when no concurrent exit-site infection is present, because signs may be absent early in the course of infection. Ultrasound imaging may be helpful in finding a localized collection around the tunnel, but one may not be present. Either an exit-site or a tunnel infection may exist without causing peritonitis, but each increases the risk of peritoneal infection. Patients with peritonitis may have very mild symptoms of abdominal discomfort with or without a low-grade fever, but almost all will note a cloudy dialysate. Some individuals may present with acute illness and appear septic, particularly if they have *S. aureus* infection. Regardless of patient presentation, CAPD peritonitis is documented by noting more than 100 cells/mm^3 (mostly PMNs) in the dialysate, which normally contains 50 to 100 cells/mm^3 with a predominance of macrophages. For infection to be documented definitively, an organism must be demonstrated in the dialysate, either by Gram staining or culture (133). Culture of large volumes of dialysate (50 to 100 mL) can greatly improve yield. The Gram stain is positive in fewer than 50% of cases, even when concentrated dialysis fluid is examined. Noninfectious causes of cloudy dialysate should not result in increased cell counts. With treatment, patients should improve clinically, culture results become negative, and cell counts fall dramatically in 4 to 5 days. It should be kept in mind that cell counts can vary with the time that dialysate is permitted to dwell within the peritoneum. Sequential sampling for evaluation of cellular response should be performed at comparable time points of the dialysis cycle. If resolution of infection is delayed, a tunnel infection or other complicating factor should be ruled out. If cultures remain negative and the patient is not improving, the possibility of tuberculosis should be considered.

The route of delivery, type of antibiotic, and duration of therapy have not been studied in a prospective, controlled manner, and conventional regimens can vary by institution. Empiric initial coverage should include both gram-positive and gram-negative organisms. A number of antibiotics can be mixed directly into the dialysate and given intraperitoneally (140). Oral or intravenous therapy is sometimes used. Catheter removal is generally included in the treatment for fungal and mycobacterial peritonitis (131). The traditional approach of removal of the catheter for patients with pseudomonal infection has not been reevaluated since the advent of more effective and less toxic antipseudomonal agents. Catheter removal may be needed in other cases of infection that are refractory to treatment with appropriate antibiotics alone.

HEMODIALYSIS

Many diabetic patients with end-stage renal disease undergo hemodialysis, which may be carried out with a vascular catheter intended for either temporary or long-term use. In the latter case, catheters are tunneled subcutaneously and cuffed to permit anchoring of the catheter to the tissues (141). The attendant risks and the principles of management of infections of these lines are analogous to those for any deep intravascular access lines.

Permanent access for hemodialysis can be attained with an arteriovenous fistula, which can be accomplished in several ways. If vessels are of sufficient caliber and patency, an autologous graft can be surgically created between the radial artery and the cephalic vein (or other suitable vessels). A bovine heterograft can be placed between the vessels, or prosthetic material such as polytetrafluoroethylene (PTFE) can be used as a graft. Vascular access–related infections are more frequent with temporary or permanent catheters than with grafts or native fistulas (142,143).

Standard vascular surgery prophylaxis is used for placement of fistulas. The expected 1% of fistulas that become infected perioperatively typically has only a delay in maturation. The true incidence of late infections is difficult to determine because many series focus on hospitalized patients, whereas many of these infections are successfully treated on an outpatient basis. Localized graft infections typically manifest as tenderness, warmth, and erythema over the graft—perhaps with exudate. Findings may, however, be much more subtle, consisting of hemorrhage or mechanical malfunction caused by infection-related destruction of the anastomotic site. As many as one third of patients who present with bacteremia caused by access-site infection have an unremarkable fistula on examination. Blood cultures (not obtained through the access site) and cultures of any pus are the keys to bacteriologic diagnosis. Grafts can also be infected by hematogenous spread of microorganisms from a distant site of infection.

S. aureus is estimated to cause up to 80% of graft infections (144), with gram-negative organisms and coagulase-negative staphylococci being responsible for much of the remainder. Endocarditis, osteomyelitis, or septic pulmonary emboli caused by distant seeding increase mortality and the rate of primary treatment failure (145,146). Mortality rates among patients with grafts are also higher if the identifiable focus for the bacteremia is other than the graft (144). It is generally agreed that patients with *S. aureus* bacteremia related to graft infection should receive a prolonged course of antibiotic therapy (e.g., 6 weeks) (132,144). The use of transesophageal echocardiography to detect cardiac vegetations increases the likelihood of identifying patients with endocarditis who might benefit most from prolonged antibiotic therapy (147). However, high rates of focal infection of bones, joints, or other sites in hemodialysis patients with *S. aureus* bacteremia often mandate prolonged courses of antimicrobial therapy even if echocardiographic evidence of endocarditis is lacking. How to manage the graft itself, particularly if it is prosthetic, is controversial. While excision of the graft is the approach most likely to prove curative, the desire to preserve the graft is often paramount. In selected cases with localized infection of access grafts, it appears that bypass of the involved segment, with removal of the focally infected material, can be accomplished successfully, with salvage of the graft (148).

INFECTIONS POSSIBLY RELATED TO DIABETES

Urinary Tract Disease

BACTERIURIA

An association between urinary tract infection and diabetes mellitus was noted in autopsy series in the 1940s (149). Since then, numerous studies have been published regarding the prevalence of bacteriuria in persons with diabetes. The number of studies documenting an increased prevalence and the number that have not are approximately equal. Those studies that did demonstrate an increase found it almost exclusively in adult women. Reports have varied regarding presence and/or type of controls, clinical setting, definition of diabetes, and definition of infection, making it difficult to compare studies. Three papers examining the prevalence of asymptomatic bacteriuria in outpatients with diabetes found a prevalence of approximately 9% in women (i.e., two- to fourfold higher than that in controls) (149–151). It is of note that these investigations can remark only on *prevalence,* as subjects were tested at one point in time. Therefore, it cannot be determined whether women with diabetes are more prone to episodes of bacteriuria or if they simply experience the same frequency of bacteriuria as nondiabetic women but that episodes persist for more prolonged periods.

Lower urinary tract disease in patients with diabetes is of concern because of the perception that these patients have more-complicated infections of the upper urinary tract. The incidence of bacteremia due to the Enterobacteriaceae also is increased in patients with diabetes, presumably because of the increased incidence of urinary tract infections (152). Information relating disease in the urinary tract specifically to asymptomatic or symptomatic bacteriuria is lacking. It is also not known how often asymptomatic bacteriuria progresses to symptomatic bacteriuria. Thus, the benefit, if any, of treating asymptomatic episodes in this population is not clear. Some of the presumed predisposing factors that have been examined include age, neurogenic bladder, duration of diabetes, and degree of glycemic control. Results do not all agree, and since several of the conditions may be closely interrelated, it is often not possible to demonstrate definitively any independent associations. Although it might appear intuitive that the presence of a large postvoiding residual volume of urine would predispose an individual to bacteriuria, there is no consistent evidence of such a causal relationship (152). A neurogenic bladder can predispose to infection because of the high likelihood of instrumentation for diagnosis and/or therapy in these patients. It is not known whether the risk of infection posed by instrumentation is higher than usual in patients with diabetes. The distribution of organisms found in the urine of patients with diabetes is similar to that in other populations. Diabetes was found not to be a risk factor for recurrent urinary tract infections in postmenopausal women (153).

PYELONEPHRITIS AND RENAL PAPILLARY NECROSIS

While the precise incidence of pyelonephritis in individuals with diabetes as compared with that in persons without diabetes is not well documented, patients with diabetes have been shown to be at increased risk for renal papillary necrosis, which is often, although not always, a result of pyelonephritis. One study has shown that diabetic patients with proteinuria are more apt to develop infections with P-fimbriated strains of *E. coli,* which are more likely than nonfimbriated strains to cause ascending infection (154). There is a suggestion from work done in a diabetic rat model that polyuria facilitates the ascent of bacteria from the bladder by creating vesicoureteral reflux (155).

Infection may be both a cause and an effect of renal papillary necrosis. Most patients who are symptomatic for this entity have concomitant pyelonephritis (156). In addition to the colicky flank pain that is possible from the passing of a papillary fragment, there may be fever, chills, flank tenderness, and pyuria. Renal papillary necrosis should be suspected in patients with diabetes who have frequently relapsing or difficult-to-eradicate pyelonephritis as well as in those who have a particularly fulminant presentation of pyelonephritis accompanied by hematuria. Diabetes is estimated to be present in 30% to 50% of patients with renal papillary necrosis. Of note is evidence for other risk factors, such as analgesic use, in these patients (157,158). Autopsy series of persons with diabetes have noted renal papillary necrosis in about 5% (156). A study of diabetic outpatients with and without asymptomatic bacteriuria found mild or moderate papillary necrosis by intravenous pyelography in 18 of 76 patients, but in none of 34 nondiabetic control subjects (156). The percentage of patients who had experienced more than three urinary tract infections was higher in those with papillary necrosis. Women account for 80% of patients with papillary necrosis among both diabetic and nondiabetic patients.

Eradication of infection is a requirement for effective treatment. Catheter drainage or percutaneous nephrostomy may be required for obstruction and pyelonephrosis. Debris may be dislodged with irrigation or direct urologic manipulations (157). The appropriate duration of antibiotic therapy, which should be directed at usual urinary pathogens, has not been clearly established.

RENAL ABSCESSES

It has been stated that renal abscesses occur with twice the frequency in persons with diabetes as in persons without diabetes (159,160). However, controls have often been compiled retrospectively or merely extrapolated from diagnoses at discharge. Renal parenchymal abscesses can be divided into renal carbuncles (cortical abscesses) and corticomedullary abscesses. Carbuncles are formed from multiple interconnecting cortical microabscesses. More than 90% of them are due to *S. aureus*, and almost all result from hematogenous seeding of the kidney from a distant focus. Only rarely are they due to ascending urinary tract infection (162). Corticomedullary abscesses are typically associated with some underlying abnormality of the urinary tract such as reflux or obstruction, often in association with instrumentation (159). Bacteriologic studies usually reveal the involvement of gram-negative enteric organisms that commonly cause urinary tract infections, such as *E. coli*, *Klebsiella* species, and *Proteus* species. Patients with parenchymal abscesses can present with flank pain, fever, chills, or abdominal pain. Nausea and vomiting are common. Dysuria may be absent, and urinalysis may reveal no abnormalities. A flank mass can be palpated about half the time. Blood cultures may be positive. CT is a useful modality for diagnosing and following parenchymal abscesses (162). Ultrasound can also be helpful. There is a chance that these abscesses will resolve with antibiotic therapy alone, but if no clinical improvement is seen within a few days, if a collection is large, or if obstructive uropathy is present, prompt drainage is required (161). Drainage may initially be attempted with a percutaneous catheter. A prolonged course of antibiotic therapy is generally required. Open incision and drainage may be needed for those who do not respond to closed drainage.

PERINEPHRIC ABSCESS

Diabetes is routinely mentioned as a major contributing factor in perinephric abscess. Various series report that 14% to 75% of patients with perinephric abscess also have diabetes (161). Frequently, however, many patients in these series have also had previous urinary tract infection, undergone urologic surgery, or had other risk factors, and it cannot be determined which of these individuals have had concomitant diabetes.

A perinephric abscess consists of purulent material between the Gerota fascia and the capsule of the kidney and most often results from rupture of a renal parenchymal abscess. Rarely, it may be the result of contiguous extension of a local process such as osteomyelitis or intraabdominal infection. The bacteria isolated from the abscess thus reflect the source of the infection. *S. aureus* (usually from a renal carbuncle) and gram-negative enteric organisms (as from rupture of a corticomedullary abscess) are the most common. As with any abscess, presentation may be fulminant or the course may be indolent and the presentation delayed (163,164). Fever and flank tenderness are the most common signs. Urinalysis can reveal abnormalities if ascending urinary tract infection is the underlying cause. A high clinical suspicion is usually needed to make the diagnosis. Often a patient with undiagnosed perinephric abscess will be treated for pyelonephritis without the symptoms resolving within 4 to 5 days. This delay in response should prompt radiographic evaluation, preferably with an abdominal CT scan, which can reveal suggestive or even characteristic findings. Perinephric abscesses can track along any of several fascial planes, leading to peritoneal, retroperitoneal, or pleural space collections. The utility of CT scanning in the diagnosis of perinephric abscesses may be responsible for a recent decrease in the mortality rate from 50% to one of 0% to 5% (163). In contrast to parenchymal abscesses, perinephric abscesses mandate drainage in combination with a prolonged course of antibiotics. Placement of a catheter for closed drainage, often under CT guidance, may suffice, but open drainage may be needed for collections that are slow to resolve or multiloculated or if the patient is failing to improve with closed drainage of the abscess.

Fungal Infections

ORAL CANDIDIASIS

Although persons with diabetes are often said to experience an increased incidence of oral candidiasis (165), most papers address the issue of colonization only. Hill et al. (166) using the direct swab technique, found that a level of HbA_{1c} of 12% or greater correlated with yeast colonization. Analyzing a much larger group of patients (412 patients), Fisher et al. (167) found no correlation between level of glycemic control and yeast colonization as determined by the oral rinse technique. Both these studies and others have documented an increased rate of candidal carriage as well as an overall increase in colony counts in patients with diabetes who wear dentures as compared with those who do not. A study of the incidence of overt denture stomatitis failed to show any difference between the incidence in diabetic and nondiabetic persons with dentures (168). Bartholomew et al. (165) examined cytologically the oral mucosa of a group of 60 diabetic inpatients and 57 age- and sex-matched controls, none of whom had clinically apparent oral candidiasis. Almost 75% of the patients with diabetes, versus 35% of controls, were colonized. Although no difference was found between the incidence of antibiotic usage in patients with diabetes who were colonized and those who were not, there were no control patients receiving antibiotics.

Treatment of clinically overt oral candidiasis in patients with diabetes is the same as that for nondiabetic patients. Clotrimazole troches offer an alternative to nystatin solutions. For refractory cases, oral systemic therapy is an option. Fluconazole has proven useful for treatment of even severe candidal mucositis such as that seen in chronic mucocutaneous candidiasis, which in rare cases is associated with diabetes mellitus, and for treatment of oral candidiasis associated with AIDS (169).

VULVOVAGINAL CANDIDIASIS

Although there is an often-repeated anecdotal association between diabetes and vulvovaginal candidiasis, no prospective controlled trials have addressed the issue, and the confounding effect of concomitant antibiotic use has not been factored out in most studies. A study of the vaginal microbial flora of diabetic and nondiabetic women showed no difference in the isolation of *C. albicans* (170). Most experts agree with the statement of Sobel (171) that vulvovaginal candidiasis is "unlikely to be the only manifestation of occult diabetes"; none of 85 women with recurrent vaginal candidiasis who were referred to that author for evaluation of diabetes mellitus had an abnormal 2-hour glucose tolerance test (171). The incidence of candidal vulvovaginitis increases during pregnancy, a change that may be due to an estrogenic effect that results in an increase in vaginal glycogen stores. This change in ambient glycogen levels has also been postulated to occur in persons with diabetes (172). Various azoles are available for intravaginal use. Therapy with intravaginally administered miconazole results in a 90% cure rate after 1 week. Oral fluconazole therapy may be useful in some cases (140).

FUNGAL URINARY TRACT INFECTION

C. albicans and, less commonly, *Candida* (formerly *Torulopsis*) *glabrata,* are found in the urine of a small percentage of healthy women (173). The use of antibiotics or the presence of an indwelling urinary catheter are conditions frequently predisposing to increased colonization with these fungi. Although there is debate concerning how many colonies are indicative of urinary tract infection, 10^5 colonies/mL of urine is generally considered significant, although true infection can occur with even lower colony counts. Lower urinary tract infection is typically antecedent to ascending infection. Most patients have the previously mentioned risk factors and/or an abnormal urinary tract. It is not clear precisely what role diabetes itself plays. A review of *C. glabrata* infections noted that three of nine patients with "significant urinary tract infections" had undergone urologic surgery and, oftentimes, had been treated with antibiotics (174). Discontinuation of antibiotics or removal of an indwelling catheter may be sufficient to clear candidal organisms from the urine. More often, however, because many of these patients have residual urinary tract abnormalities that may hinder clearance, therapy may be required. In the past, local instillation of amphotericin B into the bladder, either intermittently or with constant irrigation, was favored. More recently, fluconazole has been preferred for treatment of infection due to susceptible *Candida* species in most circumstances because it can be administered orally and high concentrations are achieved in the urine.

Pyelonephritis due to candidal organisms can result from hematogenous spread in systemic candidiasis (175), for which diabetes is not a risk factor. Manifestations of upper urinary tract disease related to initial cystitis, with infection ascending to the upper tract, can manifest as fungus balls (176), which are aggregates of pseudohyphae that can be found in the renal pelvis or ureters and appear as irregular, radiolucent filling defects (177). Fungus balls may be found more frequently in patients with diabetes. Removal of the obstructing mass, either by closed methods such as with a basket or by an open surgical procedure, is required. The antifungal therapy in this situation must be individualized. Bladder irrigation alone is not adequate because the upper tract is not reached. Systemic antifungal therapy with azoles or amphotericin B is required for parenchymal upper tract disease.

A form of fungal ball that is particularly unusual and difficult to deal with is the renal aspergilloma (178). Several of the reported patients have had diabetes, sometimes in conjunction with other possible predisposing conditions such as immunosuppression. Patients typically give no evidence of disseminated aspergillosis and present with symptoms suggestive of renal colic associated with kidney stones or sloughed renal papillae. Retrograde pyelography is the most informative radiologic test. The recovery of aspergillus from fungal urine cultures is higher than the recovery when routine (bacterial) culture techniques are used. The cornerstone of therapy is the removal of the obstructing mass. The means by which the fungal ball is removed can range from spontaneous evacuation by the patient to multiple open procedures, and possibly even nephrectomy when the mass is not expelled or otherwise removed. Amphotericin B has been used in this setting, but the precise role of amphotericin therapy and the optimal regimens for its use are still unclear.

STAPHYLOCOCCUS AUREUS INFECTIONS

It has generally been maintained that the frequency of carriage of *S. aureus* by persons with diabetes, particularly those who use daily insulin injections, is higher than that in diabetic subjects using oral hypoglycemic agents and in nondiabetic subjects. However, studies addressing this issue are often difficult to evaluate and even more difficult to compare because of the lack of consistent control groups and stratification of patients. Smith and O'Connor (179) found a 75% rate of nasal carriage in diabetic children as compared with a 44% rate in hospitalized nondiabetic children. Healthy adults and patients with diabetes receiving oral hypoglycemic agents had a 35% carriage rate, whereas patients with diabetes using insulin had a 53% carriage rate. The idea that the use of needles could be an important factor was examined by Tuazon et al. (180), who found a 35% rate of carriage of *S. aureus* in both intravenous drug abusers and insulin-using diabetic patients but an 11% rate in diabetic patients receiving only oral hypoglycemic therapy and in nondiabetic subjects who did not receive injections. Chandler and Chandler (181) reported a higher rate of carriage of *S. aureus* in patients with diabetes than in subjects without diabetes, but statistical analysis was minimal; all of the patients with diabetes being considered as one entity regardless of therapy, which ranged from dietary therapy alone to daily insulin injections. A population-based study by Boyko et al. (182) did not demonstrate an increased prevalence of *S. aureus* carriage among patients with non–insulin-dependent diabetes, regardless of the form of therapy they were receiving. Lipsky et al. (183) considered a number of factors, including recent hospitalizations, level of glycemic control, type of therapy, age, and recent antibiotic use, in a group of diabetic outpatients. Of the 44 controls, 11% had nasal colonization with *S. aureus,* whereas 30.5% of the 59 patients with diabetes were colonized. The rate of colonization was no different for those who injected insulin and those who did not. However, the level of glycemic control was inversely related to *S. aureus* colonization (i.e., the higher the glucose levels, the higher the rate of colonization). This factor has typically not been looked at as a distinct variable in earlier studies. Overall, one of the few definitive statements that can be made regarding this issue is that certain groups of persons with diabetes may have an increased rate of staphylococcal carriage and that this increase may be related to the level of glycemic control or to injection therapy. Suspicion regarding a role for the latter is based on evidence for higher carriage rates among intravenous drug abusers and patients undergoing hemodialysis. It may well be, however, that use of injections is simply a confounding factor when studying the diabetic population.

What are the consequences of an increased rate of carriage of *S. aureus*? In all populations, the rate of postoperative wound infection may be higher among carriers (184). Although patients with diabetes often are categorized as being at high risk for staphylococcal infection in general, investigations of this issue are not abundant. For many years, the "definitive" work was that of Greenwood (185), who in 1927 found a 2.4% rate of erysipelas, furuncles, and carbuncles in a diabetic population. His study included neither cultures nor controls. A paper published in 1942 documented no increased rate of infection (186). Although extensive reviews of staphylococcal infections may include a number of patients with diabetes (187), the insufficiency of the data presented makes it impossible to derive a denominator for the number of patients with diabetes at risk. A study of the rate of *S. aureus* carriage in a population of patients undergoing CAPD noted a 77% carriage rate among those with diabetes as compared with a 36% rate among those without diabetes (188). All carriers had a higher rate of exit-site infections, but only patients with diabetes had a higher rate of tunnel infections.

While many series have examined the incidence and outcome of staphylococcal bacteremia (189), it is again impossible to draw conclusions about the proportional risk in the diabetic population. Studies are often retrospective and without controls (190). For the same reason, it is difficult to determine the role of diabetes as a risk factor for the development of endocarditis in the setting of staphylococcal bacteremia. Diabetes often is found as a comorbid condition in those who appear more likely to have a poor outcome with endocarditis (191). Cooper and Platt (192) did not find an increased mortality among diabetic patients with diabetes with *S. aureus* endocarditis as compared with nondiabetic patients with *S. aureus* endocarditis or with diabetic patients with *S. aureus* bacteremia without endocarditis. Of note is that all cases of endocarditis due to a primary focus of infection occurred in the diabetic group. Five of six of the diabetic patients with endocarditis had chronic infection with *S. aureus* in an extremity—in distinction to the situation in which the primary focus is an intravenous catheter, which is usually quickly identified as the source and removed and for which a short course (2 to 3 weeks) of intravenous therapy is often adequate. The risk for diabetic patients with bacteremia related to a promptly removed focus is not known, and a conservative course of therapy (4 to 6 weeks) is reasonable.

Soft-Tissue Infections

Consideration of soft-tissue infections is complicated by confusing nomenclature and a lack of uniform terminology (193,194). One approach has been to use definitions based on the anatomic structures (tissues and tissue planes) involved, but this cannot always be ascertained reliably unless surgical exploration is undertaken. In addition, because of the close relationship of various tissues and potential spaces of the soft tissues, various designations often reflect progressive stages of a single infection. Classification by causative organisms has also been used, but any organism may cause a variety of clinical syndromes, depending on what other microbes are present and what level of tissue is infected. Progress in culture techniques has revealed that polymicrobial infection with a broader spectrum of organisms than has previously been appreciated is often present. The issue is further confounded by the frequent use of eponyms. In recent years there has been debate about the utility of any of the present designations. Obviously, the point of classification should be to organize in a rational fashion the features of an illness to permit accurate communication and judgments about progression, prognosis, and intervention. An attempt has been made here to use the most common terms found in the literature. The reader is referred to any standard surgery or infectious disease text for additional information on this extensive topic.

NECROTIZING FASCIITIS

In several series (195–198), 20% to 80% of patients with necrotizing fasciitis had diabetes. In the most general terms, necrotizing fasciitis is any necrotizing soft-tissue infection that spreads along fascial planes, either with or without overlying cellulitis. It is sometimes categorized bacteriologically as type 1 or type 2, with type 1 referring to an infection involving at least one anaerobe and one or more facultative anaerobes such as streptococci or Enterobacteriaceae (basically, organisms of the intestinal flora) and type 2 referring specifically to an infection with group A streptococci alone or in combination with *S. aureus*. Persons with diabetes are prone to type 1 infection. It is most common on the extremities, especially the legs, but can also affect the perineum, abdominal wall, and perianal region. It can also occur almost anywhere as a postoperative wound infection. At presentation, patients are almost universally febrile with systemic signs of moderate to severe toxicity. Initially, examination of the involved site may reveal only edema, warmth, and tenderness. However, as the infection progresses, causing necrosis of the subcutaneous tissues, the vessels supplying the overlying skin become thrombotic, resulting in overlying bullae, gangrene, ulcerations, or discoloration accompanied by anesthesia. Sometimes a small area of overt skin injury belies a large area of underlying fascial necrosis. Underlying musculature becomes involved less frequently (myonecrosis) because of its richer blood supply. Crepitation is reported in about 50% of patients. Necrotizing fasciitis due to group A streptococci may be associated with streptococcal toxic shock syndrome, a dramatic and often fatal condition. A description of this syndrome and a discussion of pathophysiology and recent concepts in treatment are presented elsewhere (199).

The cornerstone of management of necrotizing fasciitis is a high index of clinical suspicion and prompt surgical exploration, with debridement of all the tissues found to be involved. Repeated explorations and ensuing debridement are usually necessary (194–196,199). Grafting may ultimately be necessary. Antibiotic coverage should be aimed at enteric gram-negative organisms, anaerobes, and streptococci. Antistaphylococcal therapy is appropriate when these organisms are suspected. The diagnosis carries a high mortality rate that worsens with delay in surgical intervention and when underlying disease is present.

FOURNIER'S GANGRENE

Fournier's gangrene, first described in 1883, is a rare, anatomically based subclassification of necrotizing fasciitis that occurs around the male genitalia (200–202). It is generally associated with some form of perirectal or urologic disease, often in combination with diabetes. Infection in the periurethral area can spread through the vascular corpus spongiosum to penetrate the tunica albuginea, thus spreading to involve Buck's fascia of the penis. It can then progress along dartos fascia of the scrotum and penis, a direct extension of Colles scrotal fascia, which in turn is an extension of Scarpa's fascia of the anterior abdominal wall. Perirectal infections can have their entry point at Colles fascia and then follow the same tract. Penetration of Colles fascia can result in spread to the buttocks and thigh (201). The typical bacteriologic finding is a mixture of gram-negative bacteria, anaerobes, and possibly streptococci, again reflecting intestinal organisms. Cellulitis is evident relatively early because of the lack of subcutaneous tissue in the penis and scrotum. There is much pain, with swelling, erythema, crepitation, and possible breakdown of the skin with overlying bullae, along with signs of systemic toxicity. Progression is rapid, particularly if the abdominal fascial planes become involved. The testicles are spared because they have a blood supply separate from the fascial and cutaneous circulation of the scrotum. Wide surgical debridement of devitalized tissue is necessary, whereas orchiectomy is not (201,202). Fortunately, the scrotal skin has excellent regenerative properties, and skin grafting may not be necessary. The mortality rate is high, remaining in the range of 40% to 50% even with aggressive management. Incidence of diabetes mellitus in series (there are only about 400 cases in the literature) ranges from 0 to 40%. Whether diabetes increases the risk of death from this syndrome is unknown.

The counterpart of Fournier's gangrene in the female carries no eponym and is less well described, but it involves the vulva and perineum (203). Predisposing factors may include diabetes and pelvic surgical procedures, including episiotomy and pudendal block. Early recognition and surgical debridement are again paramount.

SYNERGISTIC NECROTIZING CELLULITIS

Some sources consider synergistic necrotizing cellulitis as a distinct category of necrotizing soft-tissue infection that preferentially affects patients with diabetes (204). Several authors suggest it may be the severe end of the spectrum of type 1 necrotizing fasciitis that occurs in those with underlying illnesses. The flora is generally made up of one or more species of gram-negative aerobic (or facultative) bacteria and an obligate or facultative anaerobe. A "synergistic" relationship between the infecting organisms has been postulated, given the occurrence of two organisms with differing oxygen requirements. However, the flora may simply reflect the source of the cellulitis, such as the bowel. The role of anaerobes in typical necrotizing fasciitis has come to be appreciated more in the last 10 years. Swartz (205) considers synergistic necrotizing cellulitis to be a variant of necrotizing fasciitis with prominent involvement of skin and muscle as well as of the subcutaneous tissues and fascia. There is classically thin, brown, and malodorous "dishwater pus" seen coming from small ulcers in the skin with surrounding blue–gray gangrene. Normal-appearing skin between the ulcers belies extensive necrosis of underlying muscles and intervening tissue. Early recognition and therapy with broad-spectrum antibiotics combined with wide surgical debridement, including debridement of necrotic muscle, are imperative (204,205). As might be surmised from the aggressive nature of this infection, mortality rates are higher than those for a typical necrotizing fasciitis.

NONCLOSTRIDIAL ANAEROBIC CELLULITIS

Although clostridial infection of soft tissue does not occur with increased frequency in the diabetic population, nonclostridial cellulitis (206), which can present in a similar fashion, does. Many non–spore-forming anaerobes have been found mixed with facultative bacteria such as streptococci, enteric gram-negative organisms, or staphylococci. Although the bacteriologic composition of the infection is comparable to that of synergistic necrotizing cellulitis, nonclostridial anaerobic cellulitis sharply contrasts with this entity in its lack of muscle involvement. The cellulitis typically occurs around a lower-extremity wound. Extensive gas is found on radiologic examination, and crepitation is typically palpable. Other skin findings are minimal. There is moderate systemic toxicity. Antibiotic therapy is aimed at a mixed anaerobic and aerobic infection. Surgical debridement of necrotic tissue with exploration to exclude involvement of deeper tissues is undertaken as necessary.

Tuberculosis

The purported relationship between diabetes and tuberculosis dates back to Roman times. Autopsies in the 18th and 19th centuries were supportive of this association as well, although the tubercle bacillus was not discovered until 1882 (207). However, as in so many conditions frequently thought to be associated with diabetes, the actual increased risk is difficult to assess because of the lack of controlled prospective studies. In addition, studies have tended to draw from populations that may, for other reasons, have a higher incidence of tuberculosis. Such groups at increased risk might include clinic populations and hospitalized patients. In an extensive recent review of the epidemiology of tuberculosis, Rieder et al. (208) drew on three large surveys from the 1950s that included some form of control group and/or information on the population. The combined data suggest a relative risk of tuberculosis in individuals with diabetes that is 2.0 to 3.6 times the risk in those without diabetes. In Papua New Guinea, the frequency of occurrence of tuberculosis in patients with diabetes was found to be 11 times the expected rate in the general population (209). An association between tuberculosis and diabetes has been noted recently in the United States as well. In a case–control study using hospital discharge data from California, diabetes was identified as an independent risk factor for tuberculosis in Hispanic and, to a lesser extent, non-Hispanic white patients (210). The Centers for Disease Control and Prevention (CDC) still identifies diabetes mellitus as a medical condition that increases the risk of tuberculosis and justifies tuberculin skin-test screening of affected individuals (211).

GENERAL CARE OF THE DIABETIC PATIENT WITH REGARD TO INFECTION AND IMMUNIZATION

Generally speaking, the selection of antibiotics for the treatment of infections in patients with diabetes is influenced by the same factors that affect the choice of drugs for any other individual. An extra measure of caution should be applied when considering potentially nephrotoxic drugs. Because many patients with diabetes have or are at risk for diabetic nephropathy, it would be especially desirable to prevent the added insult of toxic injury. When such drugs must be used, careful attention should be directed to measures of renal function, drug dosing, and measurement of serum levels of drug if applicable. By the same token, consideration should be given to possible difficulties arising from the use of potentially ototoxic (auditory and/or vestibular) antibiotics in patients with visual loss due to diabetic retinopathy. In this group, difficulties with hearing or balance may have greater significance than in the general population. When orally administered antibiotics are used in patients with diabetic gastroenteropathy, the possibility of unreliable drug absorption should be kept in mind.

Immunizations

Patients with diabetes should receive immunizations according to the guidelines set forth by the CDC (212). None of the available toxoids or vaccines is contraindicated solely on the basis of diabetes (212). There are two vaccines for which diabetics should be given special consideration: the influenza vaccine and the pneumococcal vaccine (213). Immunization of individuals with diabetes, who are at risk of serious complications from influenza and pneumococcal disease, is a national public health objective in the United States (214). The influenza vaccine, a combination of inactivated viral strains that is modified annually (215), is 70% to 90% effective if the circulating virus is homologous to the vaccine strains. Immunization with influenza vaccine is particularly important for the elderly, who experience excess morbidity and mortality from the complications of influenza (216). In one study, when patients with diabetes who had influenza were stratified by age into those older and those younger than 45 years, those older than 45 years had excess morbidity and mortality if they also had cardiovascular disease (217). Good antibody responses have been documented in individuals with well-controlled diabetes (218) receiving either insulin or oral therapy (219,220). Immunization with influenza vaccine can substantially reduce hospital admissions of individuals with diabetes during influenza outbreaks (221).

The pneumococcal vaccine available since 1984 is a 23-valent vaccine containing capsular polysaccharide antigens of at least 85% to 90% of those strains responsible for invasive disease (222). The vaccine appears to be effective in individuals with diabetes (223). While the techniques of measuring antibody responses to pneumococcal vaccine have been controversial (224), it appears that people with diabetes do have an adequate antibody response (225). It is not clear whether diabetes alone increases the risk of pneumococcal disease or its complications. Diabetes has often been present in patients with serious pneumococcal infection, but usually as a comorbid condition (225). Diabetic patients with cardiac disease may be at some increased risk for serious pneumococcal infection, and pneumococcal vaccination is suggested in these cases as for patients with cardiopulmonary disease in general (212,213,223,226).

The hepatitis B vaccine is worth noting in connection with diabetes in that questions had been raised about whether adequate antibody levels are achieved after the usual dosing schedule of 0, 1, and 6 months (227–229). It appears that most young diabetic individuals do respond to a standard regimen with adequate antibody titers (230). Further studies may determine which populations, if any, might benefit from booster doses of this vaccine.

Perioperative Glucose Control

Intriguing new information suggests that good control of blood glucose levels in the immediate perioperative period may reduce the risk of postoperative infection in patients with diabetes. Data supporting this concept have derived from studies of patients undergoing cardiac (231–233) or major intraabdominal (233) surgical procedures. Although it is conceivable that early postoperative hyperglycemia merely reflects infection or extensive tissue injury that may predispose to infection, evidence is pointing to the likelihood that hyperglycemia itself is a likely risk factor for serious infection in the postoperative period (234).

REFERENCES

1. Robbins SL, Tucker AW Jr. The cause of death in diabetes: a report of 307 autopsied cases. *N Engl J Med* 1944;231:865–868.
2. Seymour A, Phear D. The causes of death in diabetes mellitus. A study of diabetic mortality in the Royal Adelaide Hospital from 1956 to 1960. *Med J Aust* 1963;1:890–894.
3. Sasaki A, Horiuchi N, Hasegawa K, et al. Mortality and causes of death in type 2 diabetic patients: a long-term follow-up study in Osaka District, Japan. *Diabetes Res Clin Pract* 1989;7:33–40.
4. Kessler II. Mortality experience of diabetic patients: a twenty-six year follow-up study. *Am J Med* 1971;51:715–724.
5. van der Meer JWM. Defects in host defense mechanisms. In: Rubin RR, Young LS, eds. *Clinical approach to infection in the compromised host,* 3rd ed. New York: Plenum Medical Book Company, 1994:33–66.
6. Perillie PE, Nolan JP, Finch SC. Studies of the resistance to infection in diabetes mellitus: local exudative cellular response. *J Lab Clin Med* 1962;59: 1008–1015.
7. Brayton RG, Stokes PE, Schwartz MS, et al. Effect of alcohol and various diseases on leukocyte mobilization phagocytosis and intracellular bacterial killing. *N Engl J Med* 1970;282:123–128.
8. Mowat AG, Baum J. Chemotaxis of polymorphonuclear leukocytes from patients with diabetes mellitus. *N Engl J Med* 1971;284:621–627.
9. Molenaar DM, Palumbo PJ, Wilson WR, et al. Leukocyte chemotaxis in diabetic patients and their nondiabetic first-degree relatives. *Diabetes* 1976;25: 880–883.
10. Valerius NH, Eff C, Hansen NE, et al. Neutrophil and lymphocyte function in patients with diabetes mellitus. *Acta Med Scand* 1982;211:463–467.
11. Tater D, Tepaut B, Bercovicl JP, et al. Polymorphonuclear cell derangements in type I diabetes. *Horm Metab Res* 1987;19:642–647.
12. Naghibi M, Smith RP, Baltch AL, et al. The effect of diabetes mellitus on chemotactic and bactericidal activity of human polymorphonuclear leukocytes. *Diabetes Res Clin Pract* 1987;4:27–35.
13. Bybee JD, Rogers DE. The phagocytic activity of polymorphonuclear leukocytes obtained from patients with diabetes mellitus. *J Lab Clin Med* 1964;64: 1–13.
14. Bagdade JD, Root RK, Bulger RJ. Impaired leukocyte function in patients with poorly controlled diabetes. *Diabetes* 1974;23:9–15.
15. Rayfield EJ, Ault MJ, Keusch GT, et al. Infection and diabetes: the case for glucose control. *Am J Med* 1982;72:439–450.
16. Tan JS, Anderson JL, Watanakunakorn C, et al. Neutrophil dysfunction in diabetes mellitus. *J Clin Lab Med* 1975;85:26–33.
17. Nolan CM, Beaty HN, Bagdade JD. Further characterization of the impaired bactericidal function of granulocytes in patients with poorly controlled diabetes. *Diabetes* 1978;27:889–894.
18. Davidson J, Sowden JM, Fletcher J. Defective phagocytosis in insulin controlled diabetics: evidence for a reaction between glucose and opsonizing proteins. *J Clin Pathol* 1984;37:783.
19. Alexiewicz JM, Kumar D, Smogorzewski M, et al. Polymorphonuclear leukocytes in non-insulin-dependent diabetes mellitus: abnormalities in metabolism and function. *Ann Intern Med* 1995;123:919-924.
20. Peterson CM, Jones RL, Koenig RJ, et al. Reversible hematologic sequelae of diabetes mellitus. *Ann Intern Med* 1977;86:425–429.
21. Bagdade JD, Stewart M, Walters E. Impaired granulocyte adherence: a reversible defect in host defense in patients with poorly controlled diabetes. *Diabetes* 1978;27:677–681.
22. Bagdade JD, Walters E. Impaired granulocyte adherence in mildly diabetic patients: effects of tolazamide treatment. *Diabetes* 1980;29:309–311.
23. Andersen B, Goldsmith GH, Spagnuolo PJ. Neutrophil adhesive dysfunction in diabetes mellitus: the role of cellular plasma factors. *J Lab Clin Med* 1980;111:275–285.
24. Dziatkowiak H, Kowalska M, Denys A. Phagocytic and bactericidal activity of granulocytes in diabetic children. *Diabetes* 1982;31:1041–1043.
25. Repine JE, Clawson CC, Goetz FC. Bactericidal function of neutrophils from patients with acute bacterial infections and from diabetics. *J Infect Dis* 1980; 142:869–875.
26. Shah SV, Wallin JD, Eilen SD. Chemiluminescence and superoxide anion production by leukocytes from diabetic patients. *J Clin Endocrinol Metab* 1983;57: 402–409.
27. Wykretowicz A, Wierusz-Wysocka B, Wysocki J, et al. Impairment of the oxygen-dependent microbicidal mechanism of polymorphonuclear neutrophils in patients with type 2 diabetes is not associated with increased susceptibility to infection. *Diabetes Res Clin Pract* 1993;19:195–201.
28. Sato N, Kashima K, Uehara Y, et al. Epalrestat, an aldose reductase inhibitor, improves an impaired generation of oxygen-derived free radicals by neutrophils from poorly controlled NIDDM patients. *Diabetes Care* 1997;20: 995–998.
29. Li YM. Glycation ligand binding motif in lactoferrin: implications in diabetic infection. *Adv Exp Med Biol* 1998;443:57–63.
30. Qvist R, Larkins RG. Diminished production of thromboxane B_2 and prostaglandin E by stimulated polymorphonuclear leukocytes from insulin treated diabetic subjects. *Diabetes* 1983;32:622–626.
31. Jubiz W, Draper RE, Gale J, et al. Decreased leukotriene B_4 synthesis by polymorphonuclear leukocytes from male patients with diabetes mellitus. *Prostaglandins Leukotrienes Med* 1984;14:305–311.
32. Geisler G, Almdal T, Bennedsen J, et al. Monocyte functions in diabetes mellitus. *Acta Pathol Microbiol Immunol Scand* 1982;90C:33–37.
33. Glass EJ, Stewart J, Matthews DM, et al. Impairment of monocyte "lectin-like" receptor activity in type I (insulin-dependent) diabetic patients. *Diabetologia* 1987;30:228–231.
34. Katz S, Klein B, Elian I, et al. Phagocytic activity of monocytes from diabetic patients. *Diabetes Care* 1983;6:479–482.
35. Hill HR, Augustine NH, Rallison ML, et al. Defective monocyte chemotactic response in diabetes mellitus. *Clin Immunol* 1983;3:70–77.
36. Setiadi H, Wautier J-L, Courilon-Mallet A, et al. Increased adhesion to fibronectin and MO-I expression by diabetic monocytes. *J Immunol* 1987;138: 3230–3234.
37. Kitahara M, Eyre HJ, Lynch RE, et al. Metabolic activity of diabetic monocytes. *Diabetes* 1980;29:251–256.
38. Offenbacher S, Salvi GE. Induction of prostaglandin release from macrophages by bacterial endotoxin. *Clin Infect Dis* 1999;28:505–513.
39. MacCuish AC, Urbaniak SJ, Campbell CJ, et al. Phytohemagglutinin transformation and circulating lymphocyte subpopulations in insulin-dependent diabetic patients. *Diabetes* 1974;25:908–912.
40. Casey JI, Heeter BJ, Klyshevich KA. Impaired response of lymphocytes of diabetic subjects to antigen of *Staphylococcus aureus. J Infect Dis* 1987;136: 495–501.
41. Casey J, Sturm C Jr. Impaired response of lymphocytes from non-insulin-dependent diabetics to staphage lysate and tetanus antigen. *J Clin Microbiol* 1982;15:109–114.
42. Speert DP, Silva J Jr. Abnormalities of *in vitro* lymphocyte response to mitogens in diabetic children during acute ketoacidosis. *Am J Dis Child* 1978;132: 1014–1017.
43. Kolterman OG, Olefsky JM, Kurahara C, et al. A defect in cell-mediated immune function in insulin-resistant diabetic and obese subjects. *J Lab Clin Med* 1980;96:535–543.
44. Topliss D, How J, Lewis M, et al. Evidence for cell-mediated immunity and specific suppressor T-lymphocyte dysfunction in Graves' disease and diabetes mellitus. *J Clin Endocrinol Metab* 1983;57:700–705.
45. Pozzilli P, Visalli N, Cavallo MG, et al. Normalization of the CD4/CD8 lym-

phocyte ratio and increased B lymphocytes in long standing diabetic patients following therapy with thymopentin. *Diabetes Res* 1987;6:51–56.
46. Faustman D, Eisenbarth G, Daley J, et al. Abnormal T-lymphocyte subsets in type I diabetes. *Diabetes* 1989;38:1462–1468.
47. Fisher BM, Smith JG, McCruden DC, et al. Responses of peripheral blood cells and lymphocyte subpopulations to insulin-induced hypoglycaemia in human insulin-dependent (type I) diabetes. *Eur J Clin Invest* 1987;17:208–213.
48. Kaye WA, Adri MN, Soelder JS, et al. Acquired defect in interleukin-2 production in patients with type I diabetes mellitus. *N Engl J Med* 1986;315: 920–924.
49. Giordano C, Galluzzo A, Marco A, et al. Increased soluble interleukin-2 receptor levels in the sera of type I diabetic patients. *Diabetes Res* 1988;8:135–138.
50. Negishi K, Gupta S, Chandy KG, et al. Interferon responsiveness of natural killer cells in type I human diabetes. *Diabetes Res* 1988;7:49–52.
51. McMillan DE. The microcirculation: changes in diabetes mellitus. *Mayo Clin Proc* 1988;63:517–520.
52. Vermes I, Steinmetz ET, Zeyen LJJM, et al. Rheological properties of white blood cells are changed in diabetic patients with microvascular complications. *Diabetologia* 1987;30:434–436.
53. Williamson JR, Tilton RG, Chang K, Kilo C. Basement membrane abnormalities in diabetes mellitus: relationship to clinical microangiopathy. *Diabetes Metab Rev* 1988;4:339–370.
54. Lehrer RI (moderator-UCLA conference). Mucormycosis. *Ann Intern Med* 1980;93:93–108.
55. Rippon JW. Zygomycosis. In: *Medical mycology: the pathogenic fungi and the pathogenic* Actinomycetes. Philadelphia: WB Saunders, 1988:681–713.
56. Brennan RO, Crain BJ, Proctor AM, et al. *Cunninghamella*: a newly recognized cause of rhinocerebral mucormycosis. *Am J Clin Pathol* 1983;80:98–102.
57. Waldorf AR, Ruderman N, Diamond RD. Specific susceptibility to mucormycosis in murine diabetes and bronchoalveolar macrophage defense against *Rhizopus*. *J Clin Invest* 1984;74:150–160.
58. Waldorf AR. Host-parasite relationship in opportunistic mycoses. *Crit Rev Microbiol* 1986;13:133–172.
59. Gale GR, Welch AM. Studies of opportunistic fungi; inhibition of *Rhizopus oryzae* by human serum. *Am J Med Sci* 1961;241:604–612.
60. Artis WM, Fountain JA, Delcher HK, et al. A mechanism of susceptibility to mucormycosis in diabetic ketoacidosis: transferrin and iron availability. *Diabetes* 1982;31:1109–1114.
61. Daly AL, Velazquez LA, Bradley SF, et al. Mucormycosis: association with deferoxamine therapy. *Am J Med* 1989;87:468–471.
62. Gregory JE, Golden A, Haymaker W. Mucormycosis of the central nervous system: a report of three cases. *Bull Johns Hopkins Hosp* 1943;73:405–419.
63. Marr TJ, Traismann HS, Davis T, et al. Rhinocerebral mucormycosis and juvenile diabetes mellitus: report of a case with recovery. *Diabetes Care* 1978;1: 250–251.
64. Lowe JT Jr, Hudson WR. Rhinocerebral phycomycosis and carotid internal artery thrombosis. *Arch Otolaryngol* 1975;101:100–103.
65. Rubin RH. Fungal infection in the compromised host. In: Rubin RH, Young LS, eds. *Clinical approach to infection in the compromised host*. New York: Plenum Medical Book Co, 1988:203–204.
66. Oakley LA, Fisher JF, Dennison JH. Bread mold infection in diabetes: the life-threatening condition of rhinocerebral zygomycosis. *Postgrad Med* 1986;80: 93–96.
67. Greenberg MR, Lippman SM, Grinnell VS, et al. Computed tomographic findings in orbital mucor. *West J Med* 1985;143:102–103.
68. Abramson E, Wilson D, Arky RA. Rhinocerebral phycomycosis, in association with diabetic ketoacidosis: report of two cases and a review of clinical and experimental experience with amphotericin B therapy. *Ann Intern Med* 1967;66:735–742.
69. Tierney MR, Baker AS. Infections of the head and neck in diabetes mellitus. *Infect Dis Clin North Am* 1995;9:195–216.
70. Saag MS, Dismukes WE. Azole antifungal agents: emphasis on new triazoles. *Antimicrob Agents Chemother* 1988;32:1–8.
71. Hamill R, Oney LA, Crane LR. Successful therapy for rhinocerebral mucormycosis with associated bilateral brain abscesses. *Arch Intern Med* 1983;143:581–583.
72. Parfrey NA. Improved diagnosis and prognosis of mucormycosis: a clinicopathologic study of 33 cases. *Medicine* (Baltimore) 1986;65:113–123.
73. Koziel H, Koziel MJ. Pulmonary complications of diabetes mellitus. Pneumonia. *Infect Dis Clin North Am* 1995;9:65–96.
74. Bigby TD, Serota ML, Tierney LM Jr, et al. Clinical spectrum of pulmonary mucormycosis. *Chest* 1986;89:435–439.
75. Johnson GM, Baldwin JJ. Pulmonary mucormycosis and juvenile diabetes [Letter]. *Am J Dis Child* 1981;135:567–568.
76. Donohue JF. Endobronchial mucormycosis [Letter]. *Chest* 1983;83:585.
77. Chandler JR. Malignant external otitis. *Laryngoscope* 1968;78:1257–1294.
78. Zaky DA, Bentley DW, Lowy K, et al. Malignant external otitis: a severe form of otitis in diabetic patients. *Am J Med* 1976;61:298–302.
79. Salitt IE, Miller B, Wigmore M, et al. Bacterial flora of the external canal in diabetics and non-diabetics. *Laryngoscope* 1982;92:672–673.
80. Doroghazi RM, Nadol JP Jr, Hyslop NE Jr, et al. Invasive external otitis: report of 21 cases and review of the literature. *Am J Med* 1981;71:603–613.
81. Pelton SI, Klein JO. The draining ear. Otitis media and externa. *Infect Dis Clin North Am* 1988;2:117–129.
82. Rubin J, Yu VL. Malignant external otitis: insights into pathogenesis clinical manifestations: diagnosis and therapy. *Am J Med* 1988;85:391–398.
83. Corey JP, Levandowski RA, Panwalker AP. Prognostic implications of therapy for necrotizing external otitis. *Am J Otol* 1985;6:353–358.
84. Gherini SG, Brackmann DE, Bradley WG. Magnetic resonance imaging and computerized tomography in malignant external otitis. *Laryngoscope* 1986;96: 542–548.
85. Babiatzki A, Sandé J. Malignant external otitis. *J Laryngol Otol* 1987;101: 205–210.
86. Kraus DH, Rehm SJ, Kinney SE. The evolving treatment of necrotizing external otitis. *Laryngoscope* 1988;98:934–939.
87. Johnson MP, Ramphal R. Malignant external otitis: report on therapy with ceftazidime and review of therapy and prognosis. *Rev Infect Dis* 1990;12: 173–180.
88. Lang R, Goshen S, Kitzes-Cohen R, et al. Successful treatment of malignant external otitis with oral ciprofloxacin: report of experience with 23 patients. *J Infect Dis* 1990;161:537–540.
89. Leggett JM, Prendergast K. Malignant external otitis: the use of oral ciprofloxacin. *J Laryngol Otol* 1988;102:53–54.
90. Kelly HA, MacCallum WG. Pneumaturia. *JAMA* 1898;31:375.
91. Freiha FS, Messing EM, Gross DM. Emphysematous pyelonephritis. *JCE Urol* 1979;18:9.
92. Ahlering TE, Boyd SD, Hamilton CL, et al. Emphysematous pyelonephritis: a 5-year experience with 13 patients. *J Urol* 1985;134:1086–1088.
93. Zabbo A, Montie JE, Popowniak KL, et al. Bilateral emphysematous pyelonephritis. *Urology* 1985;25:293–296.
94. Michaeli J, Mogle P, Perlberg S, et al. Emphysematous pyelonephritis. *J Urol* 1984;131:203–208.
95. Cook DJ, Achong MR, Dobranowski J. Emphysematous pyelonephritis: complicated urinary tract infection in diabetes. *Diabetes Care* 1982;12:229–232.
96. Ouellet LM, Brook MP. Emphysematous pyelonephritis: an emergency indication for the plain abdominal radiograph. *Ann Emerg Med* 1988;17:722–724.
97. Hildebrand T-S, Nibbe L, Frei U, et al. Bilateral emphysematous pyelonephritis caused by *Candida* infection. *Am J Kidney Dis* 1999;33:E10.
98. Lowe FC, Walther JM. Case profile: emphysematous pyelonephritis. *Urology* 1986;28:532–533.
99. Sarmiento RV. Emphysematous cholecystitis: report of four cases and review of the literature. *Arch Surg* 1966;93:1009–1014.
100. Mentzer RM Jr, Golden GT, Chandler JG, et al. A comparative appraisal of emphysematous cholecystitis. *Am J Surg* 1975;129:10–15.
101. Schwartz SI. Gallbladder and extrahepatic biliary system. In: Schwartz SI, Shires GT, Spencer FC, et al., eds. *Principles of surgery*, 5th ed. New York: McGraw Hill, 1989:1381–1412.
102. Ruby ST, Gladstone A, Treat M, et al.. Emphysematous cholecystitis: a case report. *JAMA* 1983;249:248–249.
103. Nemcek AA Jr, Gore RM, Vogelzang RL, et al. The effervescent gallbladder: a sonographic sign of emphysematous cholecystitis. *AJR Am J Roentgenol* 1980;150:575–593.
104. Hunter ND, Macintosh PK. Acute emphysematous cholecystitis: an ultrasonic diagnosis. *AJR Am J Roentgenol* 1980;134:592–593.
105. Del Favero G, Caroli A, Meggiato T, et al. Natural history of gallstones in non-insulin-dependent diabetes mellitus: a prospective 5-year follow-up. *Dig Dis Sci* 1994;39:1704–1707.
106. Ransohoff DF, Miller GL, Forsythe SB, et al. Outcome of acute cholecystitis in patients with diabetes mellitus. *Ann Intern Med* 1987;106:829–832.
107. Friedman LS, Roberts MS, Brett AS, et al. Management of asymptomatic gallstones in the diabetic patient: a decision analysis. *Ann Intern Med* 1988;109: 913–919.
108. Hickman MS, Schwesinger WH, Page CP. Acute cholecystitis in the diabetic: a case-control study of outcome. *Arch Surg* 1988;123:409–411.
109. Schwesinger WH, Diehl AK. Changing indications for laparoscopic cholecystectomy. Stones without symptoms and symptoms without stones. *Surg Clin North Am* 1996;76:493–504.
110. Insulin injections and infections [Editorial]. *BMJ* 1981;282:340.
111. Swift PGF, Hearnshaw JR. Insulin injections and infections [Letter]. *BMJ* 1981;282:1323.
112. Borders LM, Bingham PR, Riddle MC. Traditional insulin-use practices and the incidence of bacterial contamination and infection. *Diabetes Care* 1984;7: 121–127.
113. Poteet GW, Reinert B, Ptak HE. Outcome of multiple usage of disposable syringes in the insulin-requiring diabetic. *Nurs Res* 1987;36:350–352.
114. Price JP, Kruger DF, Saravolatz LD, et al. Evaluation of the insulin jet injector as a potential source of infection. *Am J Infect Control* 1989;17:258–263.
115. Brink SJ, Stewart C. Insulin pump treatment in insulin-dependent diabetes mellitus: children, adolescents, and young adults. *JAMA* 1986;255:617–621.
116. Chantelau E, Lange G, Sonnenberg GE, et al. Acute cutaneous complications and catheter needle colonization during insulin-pump treatment. *Diabetes Care* 1987;10:478–482.
117. Bell DS, Ackerson C, Cutter G, et al. Factors associated with discontinuation of continuous subcutaneous insulin infusion. *Am J Med Sci* 1988;295:23–28.
118. van Faassen I, Razenberg PPA, Simoons-Smit AM, et al. Carriage of *Staphylococcus aureus* and inflamed infusion sites with insulin pump therapy. *Diabetes Care* 1989;12:153–155.
119. Carson CC. Infections in genitourinary prostheses. *Urol Clin North Am* 1989; 16:139–147.
120. Blum MD. Infections of genitourinary prostheses. *Infect Dis Clin North Am* 1989;3:259–274.
121. Montague DK. Periprosthetic infections. *J Urol* 1987;138:68–69.

122. Carson CC, Robertson CN. Late hematogenous infection of penile prostheses. *J Urol* 1988;139:50–52.
123. Rubin RH. Infection in the organ transplant recipient. In: Rubin RH, Young LS, eds. *Clinical approach to infection in the compromised host,* 3rd ed. New York: Plenum Press, 1994:629–705.
124. Gottesdiener KM. Transplanted infections: donor-to-host transmission with the allograft. *Ann Intern Med* 1989;110:1001–1016.
125. Bowen PH II, Lobel SA, Caruana RJ, et al. Transmission of human immunodeficiency virus (HIV) by transplantation: clinical aspects and time course analysis of viral antigenemia and antibody production. *Ann Intern Med* 1988; 108:46–48.
126. Kontoyiannis DP, Rubin RH. Infection in the organ transplant recipient: an overview.*Infect Dis Clin North Am* 1995;9:811–822.
127. Basgoz N, Rubin RH. Antimicrobial prophylaxis in patients undergoing solid organ transplantation. *Curr Clin Top Infect Dis* 1995;15:344–364.
128. Sudan D, Sudan R, Stratta R. Long-term outcome of simultaneous kidney-pancreas transplantation: analysis of 61 patients with more than 5 years follow-up. *Transplantation* 2000;69:550–555.
129. Smets YF, van der Pijl JW, van Dissel JT, et al. Infectious disease complications of simultaneous pancreas kidney transplantation. *Nephrol Dial Transplant* 1997;12:764–771.
130. Rheuman MJ, Rheuman B, Icenogle T, et al. Diabetes and heart transplantation. *J Heart Transplant* 1988;7:356–358.
131. Peterson PK, Keane WF. Infections in chronic peritoneal dialysis patients. *Curr Clin Top Infect Dis* 1985;6:239.
132. Steigbigel RT, Cross AS. Infections associated with hemodialysis and chronic peritoneal dialysis. *Curr Clin Top Infect Dis* 1984;5:124–145.
133. Vas SI. Infections of continuous ambulatory peritoneal dialysis catheters. *Infect Dis Clin North Am* 1989;3:301–328.
134. Amair P, Khanna R, Leibel B, et al. Continuous ambulatory peritoneal dialysis in diabetics with end-stage renal disease. *N Engl J Med* 1982;306:625–630.
135. Madden MA, Zimmerman SW, Simpson DP. Continuous ambulatory peritoneal dialysis in diabetes mellitus: the risks and benefits of intraperitoneal insulin. *Am J Nephrol* 1982;2:133–139.
136. Kraus ES, Spector DA. Characteristics and sequelae of peritonitis in diabetics and nondiabetics receiving chronic intermittent peritoneal dialysis. *Medicine* (Baltimore) 1983;62:52–57.
137. Vas SI, Law L. Microbiological diagnosis of peritonitis in patients on continuous ambulatory peritoneal dialysis. *J Clin Microbiol* 1985;21:522–523.
138. Powe NR, Jaar B, Furth SL, et al. Septicemia in dialysis patients: incidence, risk factors, and prognosis. *Kidney Int* 1999;55:1081–1090.
139. Arfania D, Everett D, Nolph K, Rubin J. Uncommon causes of peritonitis in patients undergoing peritoneal dialysis. *Arch Intern Med* 1981;141:61–64.
140. Gilbert DN, Moellering RC Jr, Sande MA, eds. *The Sanford guide to antimicrobial therapy,* 13th ed. Hyde Park, VT: Antimicrobial Therapy, 2000.
141. Schwab SJ, Beathard G. The hemodialysis catheter conundrum: hate living with them, but can't live without them. *Kidney Int* 1999;56:1–17.
142. Vas SI. Infections associated with peritoneal and hemodialysis. In: Bisno AL, Waldvogel FA, eds. *Infections associated with indwelling medical devices* . Washington DC: American Society for Microbiology, 1989:215–248.
143. Stevenson KB, Adcox MJ, Mallea MC, et al. Standardized surveillance of hemodialysis vascular access infections: 18-month experience at an outpatient, multifacility hemodialysis center. *Infect Control Hosp Epidemiol* 2000; 21:200–203.
144. Quarles LD, Rutsky EA, Rostand SG. *Staphylococcus aureus* bacteremia in patients on chronic hemodialysis. *Am J Kidney Dis* 1985;6:412–419.
145. Cross AS, Steigbigel RT. Infective endocarditis and access site infections in patients on hemodialysis. *Medicine* (Baltimore) 1976;55:453–466.
146. Francioli P, Masur H. Complications of *Staphylococcus aureus* bacteremia: occurrence in patients undergoing long-term hemodialysis. *Arch Intern Med* 1982;142:1655–1658.
147. Marr KA, Kong L, Fowler VG, et al. Incidence and outcome of *Staphylococcus aureus* bacteremia in hemodialysis patients. *Kidney Int* 1998;54:1684–1689.
148. Schwab DP, Taylor SM, Cull DL, et al. Isolated arteriovenous dialysis access graft segment infection: the results of segmental bypass and partial graft excision. *Ann Vasc Surg* 2000;14:63–66.
149. Bryan CS, Reynolds KL, Metzger WT. Bacteremia in diabetic patients: comparison of incidence and mortality with nondiabetic patients. *Diabetes Care* 1985;8:244–249.
150. Keane EM, Boyko EJ, Reller LB, et al. Prevalence of asymptomatic bacteriuria in subjects with NIDDM in San Luis Valley of Colorado. *Diabetes Care* 1988; 11:708–712.
151. Schmitt JK, Fawcett CJ, Gullickson G. Asymptomatic bacteriuria and hemoglobin A1. *Diabetes Care* 1986;9:518–520.
152. Sawers JS, Todd WA, Kellett HA, et al. Bacteriuria and autonomic nerve function in diabetic women. *Diabetes Care* 1986;9:460–464.
153. Raz R, Gennesin Y, Wasser J, et al. Recurrent urinary tract infections in postmenopausal women. *Clin Infect Dis* 2000;30:152–156.
154. Brauner A, Östenson CG. Bacteremia with P-fimbriated *Escherichia coli* in diabetic patients: correlation between proteinuria and non-P-fimbriated strains. *Diabetes Res* 1987;6:61–65.
155. Levison ME, Pitsakis PG. Effect of insulin treatment on the susceptibility of the diabetic rat to *Escherichia coli*–induced pyelonephritis. *J Infect Dis* 1984; 150:554–560.
156. Groop L, Laasonen L, Edgren J. Renal papillary necrosis in patients with IDDM. *Diabetes Care* 1989;12:198–202.
157. Eknoyan G, Qunibi WY, Grissom RT, et al. Renal papillary necrosis: an update. *Medicine* (Baltimore) 1982;61:55–73.
158. Mujais SK. Renal papillary necrosis in diabetes mellitus. *Semin Nephrol* 1984; 4:40–47.
159. Saiki J, Vaziri ND, Barton C. Perinephric and intranephric abscesses: a review of the literature. *West J Med* 1982;136:95–102.
160. Plevin SN, Balodimos MC, Bradley RF. Perinephric abscess in diabetic patients. *J Urol* 1979;103:539–543.
161. Patterson JE, Andriole VT. Renal and perirenal abscesses. *Infect Dis Clin North Am* 1987;1:907–926.
162. Bova JG, Potter JL, Arevalos E, et al. Renal and perirenal infection: the role of computerized tomography. *J Urol* 1985;133:375–378.
163. Hutchison FN, Kaysen GA. Perinephric abscess: the missed diagnosis. *Med Clin North Am* 1988;72:993–1014.
164. Edelstein H, McCabe RE. Perinephric abscess: modern diagnosis and treatment in 47 cases. *Medicine* (Baltimore) 1988;67:118–131.
165. Bartholomew GA, Rodu B, Bell DS. Oral candidiasis in patients with diabetes mellitus: a thorough analysis. *Diabetes Care* 1987;10:607–612.
166. Hill LVH, Tan MH, Pereira LH, et al. Association of oral candidiasis with diabetic control. *J Clin Pathol* 1989;42:502–505.
167. Fisher BM, Lamey P-J, Samaranayake LP, et al. Carriage of *Candida* species in the oral cavity in diabetic patients: relationship to glycaemic control. *J Oral Pathol* 1987;16:282–284.
168. Phelan JA, Levin SM. A prevalence study of denture stomatitis in subjects with diabetes mellitus or elevated plasma glucose levels. *Oral Surg Oral Med Oral Pathol* 1986;62:303–305.
169. Vazquez JA, Sobel JD. Fungal infections in diabetes. *Infect Dis Clin North Am* 1995;9:97–116.
170. Williams DN, Knight AH, King H, et al. The microbial flora of the vagina and its relationship to bacteriuria in diabetic and non-diabetic women. *Br J Urol* 1975;47:453–457.
171. Sobel JD. Vulvovaginal candidiasis—what we do and do not know [editorial]. *Ann Intern Med* 1984;101:390–392.
172. Rein MF, Holmes KK. Nonspecific vaginitis vulvovaginal candidiasis and trichomoniasis. *Curr Clin Top Infect Dis* 1983;4:281.
173. Roy JB, Geyer JR, Mohr JA. Urinary tract candidiasis: an update. *Urology* 1984;23:533–537.
174. Frye KR, Donovan JM, Drach GW. Torulopsis glabrata urinary infections: a review. *J Urol* 1988;139:1245–1249.
175. Frangos DN, Nyberg LM Jr. Genitourinary fungal infections. *South Med J* 1986;79:455–459.
176. Fisher J, Mayhall G, Duma R, et al. Fungus balls of the urinary tract. *South Med J* 1979;72:1281–1284.
177. Urinary tract candidosis. *Lancet* 1988;2:1000–1002.
178. Bibler MR, Gianis JT. Acute ureteral colic from an obstructing renal aspergilloma. *Rev Infect Dis* 1987;9:790–794.
179. Smith JA, O'Connor JJ. Nasal carriage of *Staphylococcus aureus* in diabetes mellitus. *Lancet* 1966;2:776–777.
180. Tuazon CU, Perez A, Kishaba T, et al. *Staphylococcus aureus* among insulin-injecting diabetic patients: an increased carrier rate. *JAMA* 1975;231:1272.
181. Chandler PT, Chandler SD. Pathogenic carrier rate in diabetes mellitus. *Am J Med Sci* 1977;273:259–263.
182. Boyko EJ, Lipsky BA, Sandoval R, et al. NIDDM and prevalence of nasal *Staphylococcus aureus* colonization: San Luis Valley diabetes study. *Diabetes Care* 1989;12:189–192.
183. Lipsky BA, Pecoraro RE, Chen MS, et al. Factors affecting staphylococcal colonization among NIDDM outpatients. *Diabetes Care* 1987;10:483–486.
184. Tuazon CU. Skin and skin structure infections in the patient at risk: carrier state of *Staphylococcus aureus*. *Am J Med* 1984;76[Suppl 5A]:166–171.
185. Greenwood AM. A study of the skin in five hundred cases of diabetes. *JAMA* 1927;89:774–779.
186. Williams JR. Does diabetes mellitus predispose the patient to the pyogenic skin infections? A study of the etiologic relationship of furunculosis and carbuncle. *JAMA* 1942;118:1357.
187. Musher DM, McKenzie SO. Infections due to *Staphylococcus aureus*. *Medicine* (Baltimore) 1977;56:383–409.
188. Luzar MA, Coles GA, Faller, et al. *Staphylococcus aureus* nasal carriage and infection in patients on continuous ambulatory peritoneal dialysis. *N Engl J Med* 1990;322:505–509.
189. Mylotte JM, McDermott C, Spooner JA. Prospective study of 114 consecutive episodes of *Staphylococcus aureus* bacteremia. *Rev Infect Dis* 1987;9:891–907.
190. Cluff LE, Reynolds RC, Page DL, et al. Staphylococcal bacteremia and altered host resistance. *Ann Intern Med* 1968;69:859–873.
191. Watanakunakorn C, Baird IM. Prognostic factors in *Staphylococcus aureus* endocarditis and results of therapy with a penicillin and gentamicin. *Am J Med Sci* 1977;273:133–139.
192. Cooper G, Platt R. *Staphylococcus aureus* bacteremia in diabetic patients: endocarditis and mortality. *Am J Med* 1982;73:658–662.
193. Sentochnik DE. Deep soft-tissue infections in diabetic patients. *Infect Dis Clin North Am* 1995;9:53–164.
194. Dellinger EP. Severe necrotizing soft-tissue infections: multiple disease entities requiring a common approach. *JAMA* 1981;246:1717–1721.
195. Rouse TM, Malangoni MA, Schulte WJ. Necrotizing fasciitis: a preventable disaster. *Surgery* 1982;92:765–770.
196. Ahrenholz DH. Necrotizing soft-tissue infections. *Surg Clin North Am* 1968; 68:199–214.

197. Gozal D, Ziser A, Shupak A, et al. Necrotizing fasciitis. *Arch Surg* 1986;121: 233–235.
198. Freeman HP, Oluwole SF, Ganepola GAP, et al. Necrotizing fasciitis. *Am J Surg* 1981;142:377–383.
199. Stevens DL. Streptococcal toxic shock syndrome associated with necrotizing fasciitis. *Annu Rev Med* 2000;51:271–288.
200. O'Dell K, Shipp J. Fournier's syndrome in a ketoacidotic diabetic patient after intrascrotal insulin injections because of impotence. *Diabetes Care* 1983; 6:601–603.
201. Spirnak JP, Resnick MI, Hampel N, et al. Fournier's gangrene: report of 20 patients. *J Urol* 1984;131:289–291.
202. Lamb RC, Juler GL. Fournier's gangrene of the scrotum: a poorly defined syndrome or a misnomer? *Arch Surg* 1983;118:38–40.
203. Addison WA, Livengood CH III, Hill GB, et al. Necrotizing fasciitis of vulvar origin in diabetic patients. *Obstet Gynecol* 1984;63:473–479.
204. Stone HH, Martin JD Jr. Synergistic necrotizing cellulitis. *Ann Surg* 1972; 175:702–711.
205. Swartz MN. Subcutaneous tissue infections and abscesses. In: Mandell GL, Douglas RG Jr, Bennett JE, eds. *Principles and practice of infectious disease*, 3rd ed. New York: Churchill Livingstone, 1990:808–818.
206. Bessman AN, Wagner W. Nonclostridial gas gangrene: report of 48 cases and review of the literature. *JAMA* 1975;233:958–963.
207. Oscarsson PN, Silwer H. Incidence of pulmonary tuberculosis among diabetics: search among diabetics in the county of Kristianstad. *Acta Med Scand Suppl* 1958;335:23–48.
208. Rieder HL, Cauthen GM, Comstock GW, et al. Epidemiology of tuberculosis in the United States. *Epidemiol Rev* 1989;11:79–98.
209. Patel MS. Bacterial infections among patients with diabetes in Papua New Guinea. *Med J Aust* 1989;150:25–28.
210. Pablos-Mendez A, Blustein J, Knirsch CA. The role of diabetes mellitus in the higher prevalence of tuberculosis among Hispanics. *Am J Public Health* 1997; 87:574–579.
211. Centers for Disease Control. Screening for tuberculosis and tuberculosis infection in high-risk populations: recommendations of the Advisory Committee for Elimination of Tuberculosis. *MMWR* 1995;44:18–34.
212. General recommendations on immunization. Recommendations of the Advisory Committee on Immunization Practices (ACIP). *MMWR Morb Mortal Wkly Rep* 1994;43(RR-1):1–38.
213. ACP Task Force on Adult Immunization. *Guide for adult immunization*, 2nd ed. Philadelphia: American College of Physicians, 1990.
214. Centers for Disease Control and Prevention. Influenza and pneumococcal vaccination rates among persons with diabetes mellitus—United States, 1997. *MMWR Morb Mortal Wkly Rep* 1999;48:961–967.
215. Centers for Disease Control. Prevention and control of influenza. Recommendations of the Immunization Practices Advisory Committee (ACIP). *MMWR Morbid Mortal Wkly Rep* 1990;39:1–15.
216. Barker WH, Mullooly JP. Pneumonia and influenza deaths during epidemics: implications for prevention. *Arch Intern Med* 1982;142:85–89.
217. Diepersloot RJA, Bouter KP, Beyer WEP, et al. Humoral immune response and delayed type hypersensitivity to influenza vaccine in patients with diabetes mellitus. *Diabetologica* 1987;30:397–401.
218. Lederman MM, Rodman HM, Schacter BZ, et al. Antibody response to pneumococcal polysaccharides in insulin-dependent diabetes mellitus. *Diabetes Care* 1982;5:3–96.
219. Pozzilli P, Gale EAM, Visalli N, et al. The immune response to influenza vaccination in diabetic patients. *Diabetologica* 1986;29:850–884.
220. Feery BJ, Hartman LJ, Hampson AW, Proietto J. Influenza immunization in adults with diabetes mellitus. *Diabetes Care* 1983;6:475–478.
221. Colquhoun AJ, Nicholson KG, Botha JL, et al. Effectiveness of influenza vaccine in reducing hospital admissions in people with diabetes. *Epidemiol Infect* 1997;119:335–341.
222. Fedson DS. Pneumococcal vaccine. In: Plotkin SA, Mortimer EA Jr, eds. *Vaccines*. Philadelphia: WB Saunders, 1988:271–299.
223. Butler JC, Breiman RF, Campbell JF, et al. Pneumococcal polysaccharide vaccine efficacy. An evaluation of current recommendations. *JAMA* 1993;270: 1826–1831.
224. Spika JS, Fedson DS, Facklam RR. Pneumococcal vaccination: controversies and opportunities. *Infect Dis Clin North Am* 1990;4:11–27.
225. Beam TR Jr, Crigler ED, Goldman JK, et al. Antibody response to polyvalent pneumococcal polysaccharide vaccine in diabetics. *JAMA* 1980;244: 2621–2624.
226. Centers for Disease Control. Pneumococcal polysaccharide vaccine. *MMWR Morbid Mortal Wkly Rep* 1989;38:64–68,73–76.
227. Centers for Disease Control. Protection against viral hepatitis. Recommendations of the Immunization Practices Advisory Committee (ACIP). *MMWR* 1990;39:1–26.
228. Pozzilli P, Arduini P, Visalli N. Reduced protection against hepatitis B virus following vaccination in patients with type I (insulin-dependent) diabetes. *Diabetologia* 1987;30:817–819.
229. Hadler SC. Vaccines to prevent hepatitis B and hepatitis A virus infections. *Infect Dis Clin North Am* 1990;4:29–46.
230. Marseglia GL, Scaramuzza A, d'Annunzio G, et al. Successful immune response to a recombinant hepatitis B vaccine in young patients with insulin-dependent diabetes mellitus. *Diabet Med* 1996;13:630–633.
231. Golden SH, Peart-Vigilance C, Kao WH, et al. Perioperative glycemic control and the risk of infectious complications in a cohort of adults with diabetes. *Diabetes Care* 1999;22:1408–1414.
232. Furnary AP, Zerr KJ, Grunkemeier GL, et al. Continuous intravenous insulin infusion reduces the incidence of deep sternal wound infection in diabetic patients after cardiac surgical procedures. *Ann Thorac Surg* 1999; 67:352–360.
233. Pomposelli JJ, Baxter JK 3rd, Babineau TJ, et al. Early postoperative glucose control predicts nosocomial infection rate in diabetic patients. *J Parenter Enteral Nutr* 1998;22:77–81.
234. Khaodhiar L, McCowen K, Bistrian B. Perioperative hyperglycemia, infection or risk? *Curr Opin Clin Nutr Metab Care* 1999;2:79–82.

CHAPTER 61
Diabetes and Pregnancy

Florence M. Brown and Allison B. Goldfine

Pregnancy may be complicated by diabetes in two distinct forms: gestational and pregestational diabetes. Gestational diabetes typically is diagnosed during the second half of pregnancy and occurs when the β-cell reserve is unable to counterbalance the insulin resistance caused by placental hormones. Although gestational diabetes mellitus usually is asymptomatic, the consequences may be substantial. Fetal complications include stillbirth, macrosomia, increased risk of birth trauma, and neonatal hyperbilirubinemia and/or hypoglycemia. In the United States, the definition of gestational diabetes is based on the results of the 3-hour 100-g oral glucose tolerance test. The interpretation of this test remains controversial, in part because the diagnostic thresholds define future risk of type 2 diabetes rather than fetal outcomes and because laboratory techniques for measuring glucose have changed over time (1). At this time, the American College of Obstetrics and Gynecology (ACOG) accepts two different diagnostic criteria for gestational diabetes (2), one of which is recommended by the American Diabetes Association (ADA) (3) (Table 61.1). To complicate matters, the World Health Organization (WHO) defines gestational diabetes on the basis of the 2-hour 75-g glucose tolerance test (4). The use of multiple diagnostic criteria used in the United States and worldwide underscores the lack of outcome data from randomized clinical trials.

Diabetes that antedates pregnancy is called pregestational diabetes. Because of differences in the age-specific incidence rates of the two diseases in relation to the childbearing years, most of the patients in the population at the Joslin Clinic with pregestational diabetes have type 1 rather than type 2 diabetes. However, the prevalence of obesity in childhood and adulthood has resulted in a higher prevalence of type 2 diabetes and its onset at younger ages. Many centers are seeing increasing rates of pregestational type 2 diabetes, especially in Hispanic and Native American communities (5). In addition, as women delay childbearing into their fourth and fifth decades, type 2 diabetes is seen during pregnancy with increasing frequency in these women. Often women do not seek medical attention until they become pregnant, so it may rest with the obstetrician to make the diagnosis of diabetes and determine the type of process underlying the diagnosis. The importance of the ADA recommendation to screen the population at high risk for "gestational diabetes" as soon as feasible during pregnancy cannot be overemphasized. In fact, the purpose of early screening in high-risk patients is to identify undiagnosed pregestational type 2 diabetes (6). Features that identify patients at high risk are discussed in the specific section on gestational diabetes.

Pregnancies complicated by pregestational diabetes, either type 1 or type 2, carry additional risks to both the mother and the fetus beyond the effects on fetal growth and development in midpregnancy and late pregnancy that occur with gestational diabetes. Metabolic derangements present at the time of conception and during blastogenesis and organogenesis increase the risk of spontaneous abortions and congenital malformations. Placental vasculopathy in patients with diabetic complications may adversely affect the necessary flow of oxygen and nutrients to the fetus later in pregnancy.

This chapter discusses these two categories of diabetes and pregnancy: gestational diabetes and pregestational diabetes. Discussion of the management of pregestational diabetes focuses on defining and reducing fetal and maternal risks. The pathogenesis, diagnosis, and treatment of gestational diabetes are reviewed. We first will consider the management of women with pregestational diabetes.

PREGESTATIONAL DIABETES

Most women with diabetes hope and expect to be able to bear children, and for only a few of them is pregnancy absolutely contraindicated. Yet there is a broad range of risk to both the mother

TABLE 61.1. Two Diagnostic Criteria for Gestational Diabetes

	Plasma glucose levels (mg/dL) after 100 mg oral glucose	
	Carpenter and Coustan	National Diabetes Data Group
Fasting	≤95	≤105
1 h	≤180	≤190
2 h	≤155	≤165
3 h	≤140	≤145

American Diabetes Association recommends Carpenter and Coustan criteria (3). American College of Obstetrics and Gynecology accepts both criteria (2). In either case, two or more venous plasma samples must exceed diagnostic levels to be positive.

and the fetus within this group of women. Concurrent conditions or complications, including retinopathy, nephropathy, neuropathy, hypoglycemia unawareness, hypertension, hypercholesterolemia, maternal age, obesity, and behaviors such as smoking and poor glycemic control, may impact risk. Thus, an assessment of risk should be made for every woman *prior* to pregnancy, and her individual risk should be discussed with her and with her spouse or partner. All attempts should be made to optimize any modifiable risk factors. To accomplish this, during their reproductive years, all women should be educated by their primary care physicians and/or diabetes healthcare provider on the importance of pregnancy planning to ensure the most successful pregnancy possible. The infants of patients who receive preconception counseling incur fewer congenital malformations and lower healthcare costs (7).

More than 50 years ago at the Joslin Clinic, Priscilla White devised a classification system to stratify fetal and maternal risk in pregnant women with diabetes (8). The White classification of diabetes during pregnancy was defined by duration of diabetes, age of onset, and concurrent complications. The premise of the White classification was that younger age at diagnosis and longer duration of diabetes increase the risk of microvascular and macrovascular complications and that these complications affect maternal and fetal outcomes. An updated version of the White classification is shown in Table 61.2 (9).

Table 61.2. White Classification of Diabetes During Pregnancy (Revised)

Gestational diabetes	Abnormal glucose tolerance test, but euglycemia maintained by diet alone or diet alone insufficient, insulin required
Class A	Diet alone sufficient, any duration or age of onset
Class B	Age at onset ≥20 y and duration <10 y
Class C	Age at onset 10–19 y or duration 10–19 y
Class D	Age at onset <10 y or duration ≥20 y or background retinopathy or hypertension (not preeclampsia)
Class R	Proliferative retinopathy or vitreous hemorrhage
Class F	Nephropathy with proteinuria >500 mg/dL
Class RF	Criteria for both classes R and F coexist
Class H	Arteriosclerotic heart disease clinically evident
Class T	Prior renal transplantation

Women in classes below A require insulin therapy. Women in classes R, F, RF, H, and T have no criteria for age at diabetes onset or duration of diabetes but usually have long-term diabetes. The development of a complication moves the patient to the next class.

In current medical practice, almost all women with preexisting diet-controlled diabetes will require insulin during their pregnancies because the goals for fasting and postprandial glucose levels have been lowered since the original classification system was first devised. Thus, the women who would previously have been in "class A," defined by preexisting diet-controlled diabetes at any age of onset or duration, would now be assigned to class B or below, defined as age of onset at 20 years of age or younger and a duration of less than 10 years. Class C is defined by age of onset at 10 to 19 years of age or duration of 10 to 19 years. Class D includes women with age of onset at less than 10 years of age or duration of 20 years or more or women with a shorter duration of diabetes or with older age of onset who also have background retinopathy or hypertension. Hypertension caused by preeclampsia is not included in class D diabetes. Class F indicates the presence of diabetic nephropathy as defined by proteinuria of greater than 500 mg per day or albuminuria of greater than 300 mg per day. A normal spot urine microalbumin value of less than 20 μg per milligram of creatinine has increased both the sensitivity and the specificity of ruling out diabetic nephropathy and eliminated the need for a baseline 24-hour urine (10). Class R includes women who have proliferative retinopathy or vitreous hemorrhage. Class RF patients meet criteria for both R and F. Class T includes patients with prior renal transplantation. Patients in class H have clinically apparent coronary artery disease.

Studies from the Joslin Clinic (11,12) and other institutions demonstrate very little difference in outcomes in classes B, C, and D, whereas class F diabetes increases the risk of maternal hypertensive complications and fetal intrauterine growth retardation and prematurity (12–21), with reduced perinatal survival ranging from 89% to 100% but averaging approximately 95% in a series of 10 different studies compiled by Reece and colleagues (21). Microalbuminuria has been shown to be a risk factor for preeclampsia. Of 158 normotensive women with microalbuminuria as defined by urinary excretion of 190 to 499 mg of protein per 24 hours, 31% developed preeclampsia. In patients with hypertension *plus* microalbuminuria, the incidence of preeclampsia was 50% (22–24). A lower-case "f" could be used to distinguish this additional risk in classes B, C, D, and R. For example, a 30-year-old woman who has had diabetes for 8 years and has microalbuminuria would be defined as "Bf." If this woman also has hypertension, she would be classified as "Df" (although additional studies are needed to evaluate the risk from lower levels of microalbuminuria). Changes in the classification system would require consensus but could provide additional useful clinical information.

Fetal Risk

CONGENITAL MALFORMATIONS AND SPONTANEOUS ABORTIONS

In the 1940s, just 20 years after the discovery of insulin, congenital malformations accounted for about 15% of the 20% to 30% perinatal mortality rate among infants of mothers with diabetes (25). Advances in medical and obstetric care, including home blood glucose monitoring, fetal monitoring to detect fetal distress, and the ability to assess fetal lung maturity, have reduced the incidence of stillbirth and respiratory distress syndrome due

TABLE 61.3. Congenital Malformations in Infants of Diabetic Mothers

Anomaly	Ratio of incidences[a]	Gestational age after ovulation (weeks)
Caudal regression	252	3
Spina bifida, hydrocephalus, or other CNS defect	2	4
Anencephalus	3	4
Heart anomalies	4	
Transposition of great vessels		5
Ventricular septal defect		6
Atrial septal defect		6
Anal/rectal atresia	3	6
Renal anomalies	5	
Agenesis	6	5
Cystic kidney	4	5
Ureter duplex	23	5
Situs inversus	84	4

[a]Ratio derived from Kucera's equation (27): (number of cases of anomaly in diabetic group *divided by* the total diabetic group)/(number of cases of this anomaly in control group *divided by* the total control group).

to prematurity. More recently, the perinatal mortality rate for infants of diabetic women remains elevated, at approximately 3%, compared with 1.5% in the general population. However, 50% of perinatal deaths in infants of diabetic women are due to lethal fetal anomalies, which now account for most of the excess perinatal mortality.

An increased incidence of congenital malformations in diabetic pregnancies was first suggested in the 1940s by Priscilla White and others (8,18,26). In 1971, Kucera pooled data from 47 reports published between 1945 and 1965 that included different geographic areas and ethnic populations. Of 7,101 infants born to diabetic mothers, 4.8% had congenital malformations compared with 0.65% of 431,764 reported in the general population by WHO (27). More recent studies report incidences of 5% to 9% in clinics treating women with pregestational diabetes (28) as compared with approximately 2% in the general population. Ten malformations have been identified with a higher frequency in infants of diabetic women than in infants of the general population (27) (Table 61.3). The malformations most commonly associated with diabetes, including neural tube, renal, and cardiac defects, occur before the 7th week after conception (29). The finding of multiple associated anomalies suggests a "hit" during blastogenesis that occurs during the first 4 weeks of fetal development. Anomalies during blastogenesis tend to be more severe than those that occur during organogenesis (weeks 4 to 5 after conception) and may increase the risk of spontaneous abortions (30). Thus, interventions to control glycemia and reduce the risk of malformations must begin before conception and continue through the first 7 weeks after conception.

The suggestion that maternal hyperglycemia was associated with anomalies was made by Leslie et al. (31), who reported three affected infants among a total of five infants of diabetic mothers with poor metabolic control as defined by levels of hemoglobin A_{1c} (HbA_{1c}). Miller et al. (32) reported that for patients with HbA_{1c} levels of 8.5% of less, the incidence of malformations was 3.4% as compared with an incidence of 22.4% in patients with HbA_{1c} levels greater than 8.5%. Although one study suggested a threshold for increased malformations as 12 standard deviations (SD) above the mean (33), a continuum of risk may be present with more modest elevations (34) (Table 61.4). Furthermore, an increased incidence

Table 61. 4. Association of Major Malformations in Infants of Mothers with Established Diabetes with Initial Maternal Glycohemoglobin Level

		Degree of elevation of glycohemoglobin (malformations/infants)[a]		
Author, date (ref.)	*n*	Moderate	High	Highest
Miller et al., 1981 (32)	106	<7 (2/48 [4.2])	7–9.8 (8/35 [22.9])	≥10 (5/23 [21.7])
Ylinen et al., 1984 (35)	142	<6 (2/63 [3.2])	6–9.8 (5/62 [8.1])	≥10 (4/17 [23.5])
Reid et al., 1984 (36)	127	<6 (2/58 [3.4])	6–9.9 (5/44 [11.4])	≥10 (6/25 [24.0])
Key et al., 1987 (37)	61	<5.8 (2/45 [4.4])	5.8–9.4 (4/13 [30.8])	≥9.5 (3/3 [100])
Greene et al., 1989 (33)	250	<6 (3/99 [3.0])	6–12 (6/123 [4.9])	≥12 (11/28 [39.3])
Hanson et al., 1990 (38)	491	<6 (3/429 [0.7])	6–7.9 (2/31 [6.5])	≥8 (5/31 [16.1])
Rosenn et al., 1994 (39)	228	<4 (4/95 [4.2])	4.0–9.9 (7/121 [5.8])	≥10 (3/12 [25.0])
Total	1405	(18/837 [2.2])	37/429 [8.6])	(37/139 [26.6])

[a]Data are SD above normal mean [*n/n* (%)].

of spontaneous abortions also has been reported in patients with elevated HbA_{1c} levels (28).

Because congenital malformations occur early in the first trimester of pregnancy, studies have been focused on improving glycemic control beginning before conception. For ethical reasons, these studies are not randomized, and patients who present for preconception counseling tend to be a self-motivated group. These studies reveal a 2% to 3% risk of malformations in infants of the subjects who receive preconception counseling, compared with a 6% to 10% risk in infants of patients who present for diabetes management after conception (40–48). These findings are consistent with the belief that optimization of blood glucose levels before conception can reduce this risk of malformations to a level near that of the general population. Despite the potential benefit of preconception counseling, fewer than 50% of diabetic pregnancies are planned. Women who plan their pregnancies tend to be married, nonsmokers, and white; have higher income and education levels; and report supportive relationships with their healthcare providers. Of note, women whose doctors discourage pregnancy are more likely to have unplanned pregnancies than are women who are encouraged and supported (49).

MACROSOMA AND CESAREAN SECTION

Large-for-gestational age infants are defined as those greater than the 90th percentile weight for gestational age. The incidence of macrosomia has been reported to be 28.5% among infants of patients with type 1 diabetes as compared with 13.1% among infants of controls without diabetes (50). Macrosomic infants experience increased rates of birth trauma, neonatal hypoglycemia, hyperbilirubinemia, respiratory distress, erythrocytosis, and hypertrophic cardiomyopathy. A relationship between maternal glycemic control in one or more trimesters of pregnancy and macrosomia has been noted in many (50–54) but not all (55,56) studies. Fasting glucose level appears to have less effect than nonfasting glucose level on macrosomia. Greater maternal weight gain during pregnancy has also been associated with higher infant birth weight. Factors inversely related to infant birth weight include maternal blood pressure higher than 140/90 mm Hg at any time during pregnancy and class F or RF diabetes.

A likely mechanism underlying the relationship between maternal hyperglycemia and infant birth weight was first proposed by Pederson et al. (57) in the 1950s. Maternal transfer of glucose and other substrates across the placenta causes fetal pancreatic hyperplasia and hypersecretion of insulin by fetal β-cells. This results in fetal anabolism and increased fetal adiposity. Hypersecretion of insulin by hyperplastic β-cells after delivery may result in neonatal hypoglycemia (defined as plasma glucose <40 mg/dL) and occurs when the maternal source of glucose to the fetus has been eliminated and relative fetal hyperinsulinemia persists.

NEONATAL HYPOGLYCEMIA

The incidence of neonatal hypoglycemia was approximately 30% in one large study, ranging from 25% in infants of class B mothers to 38% in infants of class D and R mothers (58). Neonates of women who achieve mean preprandial capillary glucose levels of less than 110 mg/dL during the second and third trimesters may have a lower incidence of moderate-to-severe hypoglycemia (<30 mg/dL) than neonates whose mothers have mean capillary glucose levels higher than 110 mg/dL (18.6% vs. 40.6%, respectively) (59). Achieving mean intrapartum glucose levels of less than 100 mg/dL can also decrease the incidence of neonatal hypoglycemia (60).

PREMATURITY AND PERINATAL SURVIVAL

Prematurity occurs with greater frequency in infants of diabetic mothers, especially when diabetes is complicated by renal disease. In most cases, preeclampsia or fetal distress with or without intrauterine growth retardation is present. The incidence of prematurity depends on the definition. Delivery before the 34th week of gestation occurs in approximately 25% of class F or RF pregnancies and before the 37th week of gestation in 50% of pregnancies. Morbidities, including predelivery intrauterine growth retardation and postdelivery respiratory distress syndrome of varying severity, occur in approximately 20% of pregnancies (61).

Variations in the incidence of preeclampsia at different centers arise in part because of the difficulty in distinguishing preeclampsia from the worsening proteinuria and hypertension typical of the late second trimester and the third trimester of pregnancy in patients with chronic diabetic nephropathy. Clinical signs that suggest preeclampsia, such as hemolysis, thrombocytopenia, and transaminase elevations, may not always be present. On the basis of this indistinct clinical picture, the obstetrician is in the difficult position of balancing a poorly defined maternal risk with potential neonatal risks from early delivery.

Most infants of class F and RF pregnancies and many infants of class B through D pregnancies require monitoring in a neonatal intensive care unit. Therefore, these infants should be delivered in tertiary care hospitals where such services are available. Monitoring in neonatal intensive care units is expensive, particularly when infants require lengthy stays, but may be critical to ensure good outcomes for the newborn. Despite the high incidence of short-term morbidity, the overall perinatal survival in class F and RF infants is greater than 95% (21). There are fewer data regarding long-term outcomes for these infants. Pooled data from three separate studies involving 80 children evaluated, on average, at 38 months of age (range, 8 to 78 months) demonstrated psychomotor impairment in 6% (range, 3.7% to 9%) (62).

Maternal Risk

HYPOGLYCEMIA

Hypoglycemia is the most pervasive risk that women with uncomplicated diabetes face during their pregnancies. Severe hypoglycemia occurs in up to 40% of these pregnancies (63). The most severe hypoglycemia occurs during the first half of pregnancy and may be the result of several factors, including emphasis on strict blood glucose control, inconsistent dietary intake associated with morning sickness, and relative insulin sensitivity as compared with that during the second half of pregnancy (64).

Although rats that sustain severe, prolonged hypoglycemia during organogenesis have an increased incidence of congenital malformations, severe hypoglycemia does not seem to be teratogenic in humans. The difference between animal models and humans is not clear but may be related to a dose or duration effect relative to the duration of gestation.

Women whose only symptoms of hypoglycemia are related to neuroglycopenia are at increased risk of severe hypoglycemia. To reduce the risk of severe hypoglycemia, they should assess their blood glucose levels more frequently, including before and after meals, before and after exercise, and before driving. Newer techniques providing continuous glucose sensing may prove to be protective. Hypoglycemia should be treated immediately with 15 g of fast-acting carbohydrate. The finger-stick blood glucose level should be rechecked in 15 minutes and an additional 15 g of carbohydrate given until symptoms have resolved or the blood glucose level is greater than 80 mg/dL. Treating hypoglycemia with unrestricted carbohydrate may result in rebound hyperglycemia. Family and friends should be ready to assist in the case of severe hypoglycemia. Designated family members and friends should be taught how to use the Glucagon Emergency Kit®.

To improve glycemic control and to ensure the appropriate temporal relationship between caloric ingestion and insulin pharmacokinetics, meals and snack times should be consistent. Many patients use carbohydrate counting in association with short-acting insulin given before meals, with the insulin dose based on a predetermined insulin/carbohydrate ratio and the amount of carbohydrate ingested at a particular meal. This approach allows for flexibility with dietary intake. In the nonpregnant population with diabetes, two insulin analogues, insulin lispro and insulin aspart, have been shown to effectively reduce postprandial hyperglycemia (65–70). Given the shortened duration of action of these insulin analogues, they cause less premeal and nocturnal hypoglycemia than does regular human insulin. Data regarding the use of short-acting insulin analogues in pregnancy are limited, but there are no clear adverse effects (71,72). Because pregnancy is a physiologic state associated with exaggerated postmeal hyperglycemia and premeal hypoglycemia, short-acting insulin analogues may be useful therapeutic agents. The new basal insulin analogue insulin glargine, with its long duration of action, has not been studied in pregnancy. The potential effects on the fetus of its binding to the insulin-like growth factor (IGF) receptor with 6.5 times the avidity of human insulin have not been evaluated (73). Insulin lispro has a Food and Drug Administration pregnancy safety rating of B, whereas insulin aspart and insulin glargine have ratings of C.

HYPERTENSIVE DISORDERS

Patients with preexisting diabetes are at increased risk of hypertensive complications during pregnancy. According to the National High Blood Pressure Education Program Working Group Report on High Blood Pressure in Pregnancy 2000, hypertensive disorders are classified as (a) chronic hypertension; (b) preeclampsia–eclampsia; (c) preeclampsia–eclampsia superimposed on chronic hypertension; and (d) gestational hypertension (74). Chronic hypertension is defined as a blood pressure greater than 140/90 mm Hg that is noted before pregnancy or up to the 20th week of gestation. The definition also includes hypertension that is diagnosed during pregnancy and persists beyond 12 weeks post partum. Preeclampsia usually occurs after 20 weeks' of gestation and is defined by blood pressure higher than 140/90 mm Hg associated with proteinuria of greater than 0.3 g of protein per 24-hour urine specimen. Preeclampsia–eclampsia may be superimposed on chronic hypertension, as patients with chronic hypertension are at increased risk of preeclampsia. This condition is associated with a sudden increase in blood pressure, new-onset proteinuria, development of HELLP syndrome (hemolytic anemia, elevated liver enzymes, low platelet counts), or a sudden increase in proteinuria if present in early gestation. Gestational hypertension is diagnosed after 20 weeks of gestation when there are no associated signs of preeclampsia in patients without chronic hypertension.

The ADA supports the goal of maintaining blood pressure under 130/80 mm Hg in nonpregnant patients with diabetes (75). Antihypertensive treatment decreases the rate of progression of diabetic nephropathy and reduces both proteinuria and the decline in the glomerular filtration rate (GFR). It reduces mortality from 94% to 45% and the need for dialysis and transplantation from 73% to 31% 16 years after the development of overt nephropathy. No randomized controlled studies have evaluated the effect of antihypertensive therapy during pregnancy on microvascular and macrovascular complications. The effect of antihypertensive therapy on maternal and fetal endpoints in the general pregnant population has been evaluated. Maternal endpoints include the development of proteinuria, cesarean section, and placental abruption. Fetal outcomes include perinatal mortality, prematurity, small for gestational age, and/or admission to special-care nurseries. Two recent meta-analyses suggest that reduction in mean arterial pressure by antihypertensive medications is associated with an increased odds ratio for small-for-gestational age infants (76,77). It is interesting that the risk of respiratory distress syndrome may be decreased in patients receiving antihypertensive therapy. The Working Group Report recommends initiation of antihypertensive therapy for blood pressures exceeding 150 to 160 mm Hg systolic or 100 to 110 mm Hg diastolic, or lower in the case of risk factors such as renal disease (74).

Because of the lack of supporting data, there are no guidelines regarding initiation of antihypertensive therapy in the hypertensive diabetic gravida. Given the increased risk of end-organ damage in this population, the Joslin Clinic and others recommend initiating therapy when the blood pressure during pregnancy is at or above 130/80 mm Hg, especially if microalbuminuria or diabetic nephropathy is present (62). A broad range of choices of antihypertensive agents are available, including α-methyldopa and labetalol (77); however, it is important to note that angiotensin-converting enzyme inhibitors and angiotensin II–receptor blockers are contraindicated in the second and third trimesters of pregnancy (78).

Complications of Diabetes during Pregnancy

NEPHROPATHY

One third of patients with type 1 diabetes will develop nephropathy during their lifetime (79), with the peak onset 16 to 18 years after the diagnosis of diabetes. Thus, it is not surprising that 5% to 10% of pregnant women with type 1 diabetes have coexistent nephropathy. This complication imparts higher maternal and fetal risk because of the association with hypertensive complications of pregnancy, including chronic hypertension, preeclampsia, and consequent need for early delivery.

Conversely, the physiologic changes of pregnancy may affect renal function. Increases in GFR, urinary albumin excretion, and mean arterial pressure in pregnancies complicated by nephropathy may worsen preexisting nephropathy. Glomerular hyperfiltration is thought to be one of the initial insults to the diabetic kidney, and some studies have demonstrated an association between increased GFR and higher albumin excretion rates (80,81). During normal pregnancy, the GFR increases by 40% to 60%. There is cause for concern that the pregnant state is an intrinsic environmental exposure to hyperfiltration. Furthermore, albumin excretion increases during the last few weeks of normal pregnancy and peaks 1 week post partum. This physiologic response is exaggerated in women with type 1 diabetes, including those who have normal albumin excretion rates at the beginning of pregnancy. Nevertheless, 6 weeks after delivery, urinary excretion returns to normal for both groups of women (82).

Studies involving women with class F diabetes demonstrate that a majority of these patients develop proteinuria in the nephrotic range by the third trimester of pregnancy. Creatinine clearance remains unchanged throughout pregnancy; however, this actually represents abnormal renal function, because GFR normally rises during pregnancy (18,62). A review by Reece et al. (21) demonstrates an overall incidence of maternal complications such as chronic hypertension and preeclampsia in 42% and 41% of these pregnancies, respectively. The frequency of fetal complications in women with class F diabetes is also increased, with intrauterine growth retardation in 15%, preterm delivery in 25%, and neonatal respiratory distress syndrome in 20%. Nevertheless, overall perinatal survival is 95%. Most studies suggest that pregnancy does not alter the natural history of declining renal function with time, particularly in patients with mild nephropathy. However, some studies do suggest that a subgroup of patients with moderate-to-severe nephropathy, as defined by a creatinine clearance of less than 90 mL per minute and 24-hour urinary protein excretion of greater than 1 g, at the beginning of pregnancy may have a more rapid long-term postpartum decline of GFR as a result of pregnancy, but these data are limited by small sample size (18). One small study suggested that treatment with captopril, started 6 months before conception and stopped after a missed menstrual period and positive pregnancy test, resulted in prolonged reduction in proteinuria during all trimesters of pregnancy compared with baseline values (83).

RETINOPATHY

Risk of progression of diabetic retinopathy is increased as a result of pregnancy (84). This risk is influenced by several factors; in particular, the severity of baseline retinopathy and elevation of the HbA_{1c} more than 6 SD above normal at the first prenatal visit contribute to this risk. The Diabetes in Early Pregnancy Study revealed a two-step progression of retinopathy in 10% of patients with no retinopathy, in 20% of patients with mild nonproliferative retinopathy, and in 55% of patients with moderate nonproliferative retinopathy. Risk of progression to proliferative retinopathy occurred in 6% of patients with mild retinopathy and in 30% of those with moderate retinopathy (84). The Diabetes Control and Complications Trial (DCCT) demonstrated a 1.63-fold risk of progression of retinopathy in the pregnant intensively treated group as compared with their risk before pregnancy. In the conventionally treated group, this risk was 2.4 times greater in the pregnant group than in the nonpregnant group (85). At the end of the DCCT, however, there was no difference in level of retinopathy in patients who had become pregnant as compared with patients who never became pregnant, suggesting no long-term risk of pregnancy for retinopathy.

Management of Diabetes in Pregnancy

PRECONCEPTION COUNSELING

All women of childbearing age with preexisting type 1 or type 2 diabetes, whether or not they are planning a pregnancy, should be educated about the importance of achieving near-normal blood glucose control before conception to reduce the risk of congenital anomalies and spontaneous abortions.

Women with preexisting diabetes who express a desire to conceive should be referred, if possible, to a specialized diabetes and pregnancy program. Preconception counseling should include an assessment of maternal and fetal risk and guidance in achieving preconception management goals. Maternal risk assessment also should include a formal dilated funduscopic examination and clearance for pregnancy by an ophthalmologist. Daily folic acid, 1 mg taken orally, or a prenatal vitamin containing folic acid, 1 mg taken orally, to decrease the risk of neural tube defects should be recommended. Folic acid may be started before conception to prevent neural tube defects, although it has not clearly been demonstrated to reduce events associated specifically with diabetes. Metabolic goals should be established prior to conception (86). Self-management skills should be reviewed. Nutrition counseling to establish an individualized meal plan should be provided. Many patients with type 1 diabetes benefit from implementation of carbohydrate counting and the establishment of an empirically determined insulin/carbohydrate ratio. Mental health professionals should be available for consultations or ongoing management. Preconception blood glucose goals are shown in Table 61.5.

TABLE 61.5. Preconception Treatment Goals

Goal	Plasma (mg/dL)	Whole blood (mg/dL)
Fasting and premeal glucose	80–110	70–100
2-h postprandial glucose	100–155	90–140
Hemoglobin A_{1c}	<7%; normal if possible	
Avoid hypoglycemia		

ASSESSMENT OF RENAL FUNCTION

A spot urine microalbumin/creatinine ratio and serum creatinine measurement should be obtained. A protein/creatinine ratio should be obtained if the urine microalbumin is elevated.

CARDIAC EVALUATION

Cardiac evaluation should be considered for women 35 years or older who have one or more additional risk factors for coronary artery disease, including hypertension (blood pressure >130/80 mm Hg), smoking, positive family history, hypercholesterolemia (low-density liproprotein ≥100 mg/dL, high-density lipoprotein ≤40 mg/dL), or renal disease (microalbuminuria or nephropathy) (87,88). Testing may include one or more of the following: electrocardiogram, echocardiogram, and exercise tolerance testing (89), with the recognition that the resting electrocardiogram is the least sensitive of these tests.

MANAGEMENT OF HYPERTENSION AND/OR MICROALBUMINURIA

Angiotensin-converting enzyme inhibitors and angiotensin II–receptor blockers should be stopped either before pregnancy or early in the first trimester. Alternative antihypertensive agents include α-methyldopa, hydralazine, β-blockers (e.g., metoprolol and labetalol), and calcium channel blockers (e.g., diltiazem and nifedipine), if necessary. Blood pressure should be managed aggressively.

MANAGEMENT OF HYPERLIPIDEMIA

All cholesterol-lowering agents, including statins, are contraindicated during pregnancy. They should be discontinued before conception. Pregnancy is a risk factor for pancreatitis caused by hypertriglyceridemia. Several cases of pancreatitis associated with hypertriglyceridemia are described in the literature, along with approaches for treatment, including caloric restriction, supplementation with medium-chain triglycerides, and use of intravenous heparin (90–92).

Treatment of Diabetes during Pregnancy

Home blood glucose monitoring is a critical component of diabetes management during pregnancy. Home blood glucose monitoring is performed a minimum of four times daily, including before breakfast, 2 hours after meals, before driving, and with signs or symptoms of hypoglycemia. Premeal and middle-of-the-night testing may be necessary in some patients. First-void urine samples are tested for ketones.

TABLE 61.6. Postconception Treatment Goals

Goal	Plasma (mg/dL)	Whole blood (mg/dL)
Fasting and premeal glucose	70–106	60–95
1-h postmeal glucose	100–155	90–140
2-h postmeal glucose	90–130	80–120
Urinary ketones	Negative	
Normalization of hemoglobin A_{1c}		
Avoidance of severe hypoglycemia		
Blood sugar goals must be relaxed for patients with hypoglycemia unawareness		

METABOLIC GOALS DURING PREGNANCY

The metabolic goals during pregnancy have received a great deal of attention and most authorities accept the guidelines in Table 61.6 (3).

Multiple daily insulin injections or continuous subcutaneous insulin infusion (CSII) are almost always required during pregnancy in women with type 1 diabetes to achieve therapeutic goals. The therapy for type 2 diabetes associated with pregnancy is more variable and ranges from medical nutrition therapy to intensive insulin therapy. Modern approaches to intensive insulin therapy utilize the so-called basal-bolus approach. This method uses the concept of meeting both resting (basal) insulin needs and meal-time (bolus) insulin needs in the most physiologic manner possible. Intermediate- to long-acting insulin may be used for basal coverage. Premeal short-acting insulin analogues are used for bolus insulin requirements. Alternatively, CSII uses short-acting insulin for both basal and bolus needs. Patients may need to be seen every 1 to 4 weeks for diabetes management, depending on the sophistication of their self-management skills and the complexity of their medical problems. Intensive insulin therapy should be considered the standard of care during pregnancy.

Fetal Monitoring

Evaluations for neural tube defects and other congenital malformations begin with triple-screen testing at approximately 15 to 21 weeks of gestation. A fetal anatomic survey is performed at 18 weeks of gestation. Fetal echocardiography may be performed at 20 to 22 weeks of gestation to screen for cardiac defects that might not be detected on the 18-week ultrasound scan. Ultrasound is used at 28 weeks of gestation to evaluate fetal growth and the quantity of amniotic fluid. Fetal surveillance, including nonstress test and biophysical profile as well as maternal monitoring of fetal activity (2), is initiated in the third trimester to reduce the risk of stillbirth. The timing and frequency of fetal surveillance depend on diabetes control, coexistence of diabetic nephropathy or hypertension, and fetal growth as shown on ultrasound.

Labor and Delivery

The method of delivery is based on the usual obstetric indications, as well as on fetal weight and the presence or absence of active retinal changes. Infants of diabetic mothers are more likely to be macrosomic. Furthermore, the distribution of adiposity is such that, compared with infants of nondiabetic mothers of the same weight, infants of diabetic mothers have a greater shoulder and chest-to-head disproportion, which increases the risk of shoulder dystocia during delivery of the macrosomic infant. Cesarean sections are recommended for fetuses of an estimated weight greater than 4,500 g. This guideline may be individualized to account for prior obstetric history and adequacy of pelvic size. However, ultrasound remains an imprecise measure of fetal weight and can result in cesarean delivery of normal-weight infants.

It is important to maintain euglycemia during labor or prior to a scheduled cesarean section. Patients are instructed to take their usual bedtime insulin the night before delivery. A small dose of intermediate-acting insulin, such as one third of the preconception dose, may be given the morning of induction. Alternatively, intermediate-acting insulin can be withheld and an intravenous insulin infusion begun and titrated to achieve and maintain normoglycemia. Patients with insulin pumps may continue their basal infusion if the infusion set is inserted in the thigh or hip. Basal rates are decreased if the glucose levels drop below 80 mg/dL. If the blood glucose levels rise above 110 mg/dL, the pump may be stopped and an intravenous insulin drip initiated and titrated to maintain blood glucose levels in the range of 80 to 110 mg/dL.

For prolonged labor, 5% dextrose administered intravenously at a rate of 100 to 125 mL per hour will prevent starvation ketosis. If there is concern about volume overload in the setting of preeclampsia, a 10% dextrose drip at 50 mL per hour may be started. Boluses of intravenous glucose should never be given unless absolutely necessary to correct severe maternal hypoglycemia because the elevated maternal blood glucose levels increase the risk of neonatal hypoglycemia, hypoxia, and acidosis.

Postpartum Management

Marked insulin sensitivity frequently occurs immediately post partum, and insulin requirements routinely drop to below preconception levels. Patients should be aware that stringent blood glucose control is no longer necessary immediately post partum. To decrease the risk of severe hypoglycemia, one third to one half of the preconception insulin dose is given during the first 24 hours post partum. Insulin dosing should be titrated daily toward the preconception dose as necessary. Patients with thyroid insufficiency should resume preconception doses of L-thyroxine. Because patients are usually discharged before stabilization of blood glucose, frequent communication between the patient and healthcare providers remains necessary. By 2 weeks post partum, insulin requirements have stabilized, making this a good time for a postpartum visit focusing on glucose management. Between 2 and 6 weeks post partum, patients carefully adjust their diabetes regimen. Serial fasts may be necessary to reestablish appropriate basal insulin rates for patients using insulin pumps. Preprandial and postprandial blood glucose readings and carbohydrate records will help determine insulin-to-carbohydrate ratios in some patients. Insulin requirements may remain low in breastfeeding mothers. Access to carbohydrate should be readily available to prevent hypoglycemia during nursing. Glycemic data should be reviewed again at the 6-weeks postpartum visit, at which time management of complications and concurrent medical problems should be addressed. Urine microalbumin, thyroid function, and HbA_{1c} should be reevaluated. The American Academy of Pediatrics considers the angiotensin-converting enzyme inhibitors captopril and enalapril safe for use by the breastfeeding mother and are resumed in patients with nephropathy, microalbuminuria, and hypertension (93). Plans for future medical, diabetes, and ophthalmologic care are discussed with the patient. Both contraception and the importance of planning future pregnancies should also be reviewed during the 6-week postpartum visit. Contraception is particularly important in women with diabetes, who must delay future pregnancies until they are medically stable and have achieved near euglycemia. The choice of contraception is individualized, taking into account desire for additional children, presence or absence of vasculopathy, ease of compliance, inherent failure rates, number of sexual partners, smoking history, and age (94).

GESTATIONAL DIABETES

Definition and Incidence

Gestational diabetes is defined as carbohydrate intolerance of any degree with onset or first recognition during pregnancy (95). This definition does not preclude the possibility that diabetes antedated conception but remained unrecognized until medical visits during pregnancy. Furthermore, the definition applies regardless of whether diet or insulin is used to manage glycemia during pregnancy and whether or not disordered carbohydrate metabolism persists post partum. Diagnosis of gestational diabetes is important to identify both infants at risk of adverse outcomes and women at risk of subsequent development of diabetes. Reports of adverse events date back to at least 1882, when Duncan (96) reported fetal death in 13 of 19 pregnancies in 15 women and maternal death within 1 year of delivery in 9 of the cases. In addition to fetal demise, gestational diabetes has been linked to the complications of large for gestational age; macrosomia; birth trauma, such as increased maternal lacerations and neonatal shoulder dystocia; increased need for cesarean section; and neonatal metabolic disorders such as hypoglycemia, hyperbilirubinemia, and disordered calcium balance. Accurate diagnosis and improved management have favorably altered perinatal outcomes in this condition. For the mother, there is increased risk of subsequent development of diabetes.

The frequency of gestational diabetes depends on both the population studied and the diagnostic criteria used, resulting in a range of prevalence between 1% and 14%. The prevalence of gestational diabetes tends to be higher in populations with high rates of type 2 diabetes. The prevalence in the general U.S. population is about 4% (97), whereas the prevalence in non-Hispanic white women is lower, at about 2% (98).

Pathogenesis

Glucose metabolism deteriorates to some degree in all pregnant women (99), although only a minority of women develop gestational diabetes. In rare circumstances, a woman can develop type 1 diabetes coincident with pregnancy; however, this is uncommon. In populations at greater risk of type 1 diabetes, diabetes of pregnancy may identify risk of development of type 1 disease (100). In most studies, the frequencies of human leukocyte antigens HLA-DR2, DR3, and DR4 that confer risk for type 1 diabetes are similar in women with gestational diabetes and in healthy pregnant women, and the prevalence of autoimmune markers of β-cell destruction in women with gestational diabetes is low. Rather, the pathogenesis of the vast majority of cases of gestational diabetes more closely resembles that of type 2 diabetes.

Fasting plasma insulin levels increase gradually during pregnancy, and during the third trimester, may be double those during the nonpregnant state. Fasting insulin levels are not lower in women with gestational diabetes; however, both the first-phase insulin response and the insulin response to a given glycemic stimulus is lower in women with gestational diabetes than in women with normal glucose tolerance (101,102). Peak plasma insulin levels are achieved later during oral glucose tolerance tests in women with gestational diabetes than in women with normal glucose tolerance. Elevated proinsulin levels are seen early in the gestational diabetic pregnancy (103) and may persist post partum (104), providing further evidence that a defect in β-cell insulin secretion in addition to insulin resistance underlies this disorder.

Screening and Diagnosis

Although the importance of diagnosis and treatment of carbohydrate intolerance during pregnancy is evident, the procedures used to screen pregnant women and the diagnostic criteria are widely disputed. In 1964, O'Sullivan and Mahan (1) evaluated 752 pregnant women with a 3-hour oral glucose tolerance test with 100 g of glucose; 2 SD above the mean threshold for each hour assessed was established to be abnormal based on the future risk of diabetes to the mother in a second group of 1,013 women also tested during pregnancy and followed for a subsequent 5 to 10 years post partum. If two glucose values were exceeded, 22% of women developed diabetes within 7 to 8 years. In the years that followed, the "O'Sullivan and Mahan" criteria became widely accepted for the diagnosis of gestational diabetes. These studies used venous whole blood samples. So when most laboratories shifted to plasma venous samples in 1979 the National Diabetes Data Group (NDDG) recommended conversion by an upward adjustment of 15% to account for the difference in sample measurement (105). Subsequently to account for both changes in laboratory techniques of glucose measurement from the older Somogyi-Nelson assay to the newer enzymatic assays, and the switch from whole blood to plasma venous samples, Carpenter and Coustan (106) again revised the diagnostic criteria in 1982. It is important to note that all of these criteria are based on the original work of O'Sullivan and Mahan and that these were validated on the basis of predictive value of subsequent risk of diabetes in the mother and not specifically to determine maternal or fetal risk during pregnancy.

In much of the world, however, a 75-g 2-hour oral glucose tolerance test is administered, and gestational diabetes is diagnosed according to WHO criteria for the diagnosis of diabetes outside of pregnancy (4). The WHO diagnostic criteria are less stringent than those discussed above. In centers where WHO criteria of impaired glucose tolerance are used to identify women with gestational diabetes, a higher proportion of pregnancies are diagnosed as abnormal than when the other criteria are employed. WHO criteria were not developed specifically for use during pregnancy, nor are thresholds set for detection of either maternal or fetal complications.

Performance of either the 75-g 2-hour or the 100-g 3-hour oral glucose tolerance test evaluates the fasting (between 8 and 14 hours) glucose level and the value at 1 and 2 hours after the glucose load. The 100-g test includes an additional glucose assessment at 3 hours. Normal values based on Carpenter and Coustan criteria include a fasting plasma glucose level of 95 mg/dL or less (5.3 mmol/L); 1 hour, 180 mg/dL or less (10.0 mmol/L); 2 hour, 155 mg/dL or less (8.6 mmol/L); and for the 100-g load 3 hour, 140 mg/dl or less (7.8 mmol/L) (107). Normal values based on NDDG criteria include a fasting plasma glucose level of 105 mg/dL or less (5.8 mmol/L); 1 hour, 190 mg/dL or less (10.6 mmol/L); 2 hour, 165 mg/dL or less (9.2 mmol/L); and 3 hour, 145 g/dL or less (8.0 mol/L). In either test, *two* or more of the venous plasma concentrations must be exceeded to be positive.

In addition to the cost of three or four glucose assessments, the glucose tolerance test is difficult to administer, as it requires women to fast overnight before testing and takes several hours. Screening of women between 24 and 28 weeks of gestation with a plasma or serum glucose level obtained 1 hour following a 50-g glucose load (glucose load test), administered at any time of day without regard to the time since the last meal, has become a well validated and widely applied screening procedure. A value of 140 mg/dL or higher (7.8 mmol/L) identifies 80% of women with gestational diabetes, and a value of 130 mg/dL or higher (7.2 mmol/L) increases sensitivity to 90% (108). Because of the test's high sensitivity (low false-negative rates), women with normal values on this test do not require more extensive testing. However, because of the test's lower specificity (high false-positive rates), between 78% and 87% for the 140 and 130 mg/dL threshold, respectively, women with elevated values require the performance of a diagnostic glucose tolerance test.

Although universal screening of women for gestational diabetes was previously recommended, a series of identifying factors place a woman at lower risk for this complication of pregnancy. These factors include age younger than 25 years, normal body weight, absence of a first-degree relative with diabetes, no history of abnormal glucose metabolism or poor obstetric outcome, *and* not being of a racial or ethnic group with a high prevalence of diabetes. Risk assessment should occur at the first prenatal visit. If a woman meets *all* of these criteria, testing for carbohydrate intolerance during pregnancy may be discretionary (107). Women with multiple risk factors, thus those at high risk, should undergo screening procedures as soon as feasible. If their glucose tolerance is normal early in pregnancy, testing should be repeated between 24 and 28 weeks of gestation, the interval recommended for women at moderate risk.

There is substantial evidence that criteria for diagnosis of gestational diabetes are arbitrary. The relationship between maternal carbohydrate tolerance and rate of macrosomia, need for neonatal special care, and cesarean section may be linear or curvilinear with no threshold value at which a change in risk can be demonstrated (109–111). As such, any abnormal glucose value on diagnostic testing may not be classified as gestational diabetes but may be associated with increased maternal or fetal risk. Threshold values in the future could become subject to evaluation of the cost and effectiveness of intervention.

Management

Although glucose is not the only metabolic fuel that is abnormal during a diabetic pregnancy, because of the ease of assessment, it is the focus of the medical management of the pregnancy. Tight glycemic control can reduce fetal risks (112). However, excessively stringent target levels put the mother at risk of hypoglycemic events, and some evidence suggests that this may also put the infant at risk of being small for gestational age (113). Although glycemic targets have remained somewhat controversial and there have not been universal adjustments of targets for meters that report whole blood levels as compared with plasma glucose levels, current ADA recommendations are to maintain fasting whole blood glucose levels lower than 95 mg/dL (5.3 mmol/L), 1-hour postprandial levels lower than 140 mg/dL (7.8 mmol/L), and/or 2-hour postprandial levels lower than 120 mg/dL (6.7 mmol/L) (6). Glycemic response to the diagnostic carbohydrate load may be abnormal even when the excursions to a mixed meal are maintained. Home glucose monitoring allows for precise assessment of both the need for and the response to more extensive interventions. Despite the emotional burden of increased monitoring, these techniques allow immediate patient feedback of the physiologic response to foods and can be effective in demonstrating the need for dietary compliance. Many women will have improved glucose profiles when medical nutritional therapy is begun. Although medical nutritional therapy is central in the management of gestational diabetes, the ideal diet remains controversial. Nutritional recommendations are affected by the woman's body habitus, physical activity, and weight gain, but goals are to achieve glycemic targets without being so restrictive as to promote either ketonemia or ketonuria. For patients who are not underweight, modest caloric restriction may be appropriate. A starting plan may provide about 30 kcal per kilogram of actual body weight for the woman who has ideal body weight, 40 kcal/kg for the woman who is less than 80% of ideal body weight, 25 kcal/kg for the woman who is 120% to 150% of ideal body weight, and limited to as low as 12 kcal/kg for the patient who is over 150% ideal body weight (114). In all groups, adjustments are based on assessment of weight gain and the presence of urine ketones. Limiting carbohydrate to 35% to 45% of total calories (with the balance 20% to 25% protein and 35% to 40% fat) can reduce postprandial glucose levels. Interestingly, women with gestational diabetes may demonstrate their greatest carbohydrate intolerance after the breakfast meal and may improve with more strict carbohydrate restriction solely at that meal. The balance between simple carbohydrate foods (high glycemic index) and complex carbohydrates (low glycemic index) is also likely to be important to the maternal glycemic excursions (115). Iron and other nutritional supplements should be administered if necessary.

About 50% of women initially treated with diet alone will require additional therapy, and insulin therapy usually is recommended. Although both insulin-sensitizing agents, biguanide and thiazolidendiones, have been demonstrated to increase rates of ovulation in insulin-resistant women with ovulatory dysfunction, after conception most women are then switched to insulin for glycemic management. Likewise, sulfonylureas rarely are used during pregnancy for concern about teratogenicity and neonatal hypoglycemia. However, in one study of 404 women randomly assigned to glyburide or insulin between 11 and 33 weeks of gestation, use of a sulfonylurea was not associated with any difference in infant rates of large for gestational age, macrosomia, lung complications, hypoglycemia, neonatal intensive care admissions, or fetal anomalies (116).

Insulin management must be individualized, but most pregnant women require about 0.7 units/kg daily, divided into three doses. As in nonpregnant women, about two thirds of the insulin is administered in the morning and one third is administered in the evening, with a 1:2 ratio of short- to intermediate- (or long-) acting insulin. Insulin requirements increase by about 50% from 20 to 24 weeks to around 30 to 32 weeks of gestation, at which time insulin needs often stabilize. The ultra–short-acting insulin analogues insulin lispro and insulin aspart have been reported to improve postprandial glucose in women with type 1 or type 2 diabetes; thus, they could be advantageous during pregnancy and, in limited studies, lispro appears to be safe and effective for the management of gestational diabetes (70,71).

There remains some controversy regarding the current recommendations of strict adherence to glycemic targets for all women with gestational diabetes, as only a minority of the infants are at risk for perinatal morbidity over the range of glycemia commonly encountered during the pregnancy complicated by gestational diabetes. Home glucose monitoring and often insulin use thus could be viewed as being prescribed to many women whose infants are not at risk of complications. Several studies suggest alternate management strategies based on careful assessment of fetal growth using the ultrasound measurement of fetal abdominal circumference to identify those infants at highest risk (117), with intensive intervention reserved for the patient whose fetal abdominal circumference measures greater than the 70th percentile (118). However, until further studies are performed using such treatment decision tools, strict glycemic management for all women with gestational diabetes remains advisable.

Although antenatal care focuses on glycemic management, the woman with gestational diabetes requires close monitoring for the development of hypertension, proteinuria, edema, and preeclampsia or eclampsia, all of which are more common than in the nondiabetic pregnancy. Goals of obstetrical management include the prevention of stillbirth or compromised fetal health at delivery, achievement of lung maturity, and prevention of birth trauma. especially in the macrosomic infant prone to shoulder dystocia. Weekly biophysical profiles are frequently begun at 36 weeks of gestation. A sonographic evaluation is frequently performed at 38 weeks, with induction of labor for the large-for-gestational age infant and cesarean delivery for the macrosomic infant. The infant judged appropriate in size for gestational age may be managed expectantly until 40 weeks, at which time evaluation may include reassessment of size, cervical ripeness, and lung maturity, with induction of labor upon favorable evaluation. Most obstetrical protocols recommend delivery for all women between 40 and 41 weeks (119).

Labor and Delivery

The diagnosis of gestational diabetes impacts not only on the prenatal monitoring of maternal glucose and fetal size and activity but also on the method of delivery. In the Toronto Tri-Hospital Gestational Diabetes Project, women with gestational diabetes with untreated borderline hyperglycemia had a 29% rate of fetal macrosomia, more than double that for the treated women with gestational diabetes (10%) or healthy control subjects (14%). However, despite the smaller birth size in the treated women with gestational diabetes, the rates of cesarean delivery were similar in the group with borderline hyperglycemia and in the treated group (120). The increased cesarean rate in the group with gestational diabetes could be due to the increased likelihood of the physician's performing a cesarean section in a woman diagnosed with gestational diabetes regardless of fetal size.

If the woman does not require insulin during the prenatal period, labor and delivery can likely proceed without special attention to maternal glycemia. If insulin is required, and labor and delivery are to be scheduled, it is preferable to schedule for the morning hours. In this case, the usual insulin dose can be administered the evening before the scheduled delivery, and the morning dose can be held. If the induction procedure is judged likely to be lengthy, a fraction between 25% and 30% of the usual morning insulin dose may be administered, especially if the mother will be allowed meals during early labor. If the maternal glucose rises above 110 mg/dL, an insulin drip should be considered, as maternal hyperglycemia may cause neonatal hyperinsulinemia and hypoglycemia post partum. If the mother took insulin and spontaneous labor ensues, a dextrose infusion with the rate adjusted to a target glucose of 80 to 110 mg/dL may be required to prevent maternal hypoglycemia.

Postpartum

SPECIFIC TO THE MOTHER

In most cases, the glucose intolerance that first arises during pregnancy resolves immediately post partum, and insulin, if required during pregnancy, is no longer required. The earlier in pregnancy the diabetes develops and the more extreme the insulin requirement, the less likely the condition is to resolve post partum. It is prudent to make a single glucose check in the hospital before the patient is discharged to ensure that the glucose level has returned to the normal range. Women who have been performing home glucose monitoring can repeat a measurement after discharge. The most information is gained if this check is performed 1 or 2 hours postprandially. Women with elevated values should present for early postpartum glucose tolerance testing. Otherwise, a 75-g glucose tolerance test performed about 2 months post partum will identify women with persistent diabetes or impaired glucose tolerance. At this time, a test of glycosylated hemoglobin (Hb_{A1} or HbA_{1c}) is not an adequate test, because this value depends both on the level of hyperglycemia and on the life span of red cells. The bleeding associated with delivery produces a reticulocytosis that falsely lowers the glycosylated hemoglobin value during the postpartum period. If glucose levels are elevated, insulin therapy is indicated in the lactating woman, as oral agents may be excreted in the breast milk. Because about 50% of women who have had gestational diabetes will go on to develop diabetes over the next 20 years, an evaluation of glycemia should occur annually. In the woman who develops impaired glucose tolerance or type 2 diabetes, additional cardiac risk factors should be identified and may require treatment. In all women with a history of gestational diabetes, medications that increase insulin resistance should be avoided whenever possible.

Because abnormal glucose levels in early conception are associated with congenital defects, women with a history of gestational diabetes who are planning a future pregnancy should have glucose assessments before conception (121) and should receive counseling regarding this during the postpartum period. If impaired glucose tolerance or type 2 diabetes is found, adequate glycemic control appears more important in prevention of congenital malformations in future pregnancies than is the type of drug used to maintain glucose control (122). Ideally, women on oral medications should be switched to insulin before conception.

In planning postpartum contraception, the estrogen-progesterone combination type of hormonal therapy should be used if this is the contraception method chosen, because in a limited study, progesterone-only therapy was associated with increased rate of development of type 2 diabetes (123). In most cases, the desire to have additional offspring is a very strong and complex one. However, a careful study of the Latino population with previous gestational diabetes indicates an increased risk of progression to type 2 diabetes conferred by additional pregnancies (124).

Given the high risk of future type 2 diabetes in these patients, they would be well served with interventions that delay or prevent diabetes. The Finnish Diabetes Prevention Study Group (125) and the Diabetes Prevention Program (126) demonstrated that aggressive lifestyle management involving nutrition therapy and daily exercise can reduce the onset of type 2 diabetes by nearly 60% as compared with the rates in a nonintervention control group of patients with impaired glucose tolerance, including, but not limited to, patients with previous gestational diabetes. Use of medications has also been demonstrated to reduce the risk of future diabetes in high-risk populations. In the Diabetes Prevention Program, use of metformin reduced the onset of type 2 diabetes by 35% compared with that in the control population (126). Similarly, acarbose resulted in a 25% decrease in conversion of patients with impaired glucose tolerance to type 2 diabetes (127). In women with prior gestational diabetes, use of troglitazone resulted in a more than 50% reduction in the incidence of diabetes in high-risk Hispanic women in the Troglitazone in Prevention of Diabetes (TRIPOD) study (128). Although troglitazone is no longer on the market, pioglitazone and rosiglitazone may have similar protective benefits and need to be studied. However, lifestyle management of diet and exercise offers the most favorable reduction in progression to diabetes and has no risk of adverse effects that can be associated with medical therapies. These data support the importance of insurance coverage for postpartum nutrition and exercise counseling and monitoring of metabolic status in women who have had gestational diabetes.

SPECIFIC TO THE INFANT

The newborn infant is at greater risk of several metabolic complications, the most frequent of which is hypoglycemia. This likely is due to hyperinsulinemia, which develops *in utero* in response to the increased maternal fuel. At delivery, the infant's physiology changes from one of continuous feeding to one of fasting and feeding. The infant is at greatest risk of hypoglycemia in the first hours after birth, before the first feeding. The infant should also be assessed for lung maturity and for bilirubin and calcium balance, and a careful physical examination should be performed to assess for birth defects.

The long-term effects of the intrauterine environment on the growth and development of the child have not been exhaustively studied. Clearly, given the genetic predisposition for diabetes, children of diabetic parents are at increased risk of ultimately developing diabetes as compared with children having no family history of diabetes. Few studies have addressed the additional risk of maternal hyperglycemia to the offspring. Careful epidemiologic data have been collected since the mid-1960s among the Pima Indians of Arizona, a group with an increased overall risk of type 2 diabetes. By age 10 to 14 years of age, the 2-hour post–75-g-load glucose level in children was shown to increase based on the 2-hour postload glucose level measured during the mother's pregnancy. In addition, the prevalence of diabetes in the offspring was higher in the cohort born from a diabetic pregnancy than in those who were not (129). Among the Pima, there is a U-shaped distribution of the prevalence of diabetes such that both small- and large-for-gestational-age infants are at increased risk of subsequent development of diabetes. Interestingly, there was some protective effect of breastfeeding for 2 months or more, as compared with the prevalence among children who had not been breastfed as infants (130). Although the duration of follow-up evaluation is not as long as in the Pima Indians, similar investigations are ongoing in the largely white cohort in the Northwestern University Diabetes in Pregnancy Study, in which longitudinal studies have been ongoing since the late 1970s. These studies also demonstrate an increased body mass index starting between the ages of 4 and 6 years in the offspring of women with gestational diabetes, as compared with healthy term infants in the Chicago metropolitan area, and an increased risk of impaired glucose tolerance during adolescence (131,132). Additional recommendations for the offspring born from the diabetic pregnancy may evolve as our understanding of the impact of the maternal milieu develops.

REFERENCES

1. O'Sullivan J, Mahan CM. Criteria for the oral glucose tolerance test in pregnancy. *Diabetes* 1964;13:278–285.
2. ACOG Practice Bulletin. Clinical management guidelines for obstetrician-gynecologists. Number 30, September 2001 (replaces Technical Bulletin no. 200, December 1994). Gestational diabetes. *Obstet Gynecol* 2001;98:525–538.
3. American Diabetes Association. Gestational diabetes mellitus. *Diabetes Care* 2004;27[Suppl 1]:S88–S90.
4. World Health Organization: WHO Expert Committee on Diabetes Mellitus. Second Report. Technical Report Series, no. 646. Geneva: World Health Organization, 1980.
5. Mokdad AH, Ford ES, Bowman BA, et al. Diabetes trends in the U.S.: 1990–1998. *Diabetes Care* 2000;23:1278–1283.
6. Metzger BE, Coustan DR. Summary and recommendations of the Fourth International Workshop-Conference on Gestational Diabetes Mellitus. The Organizing Committee. *Diabetes Care* 1998;21[Suppl 2]:B161–B167.
7. Elixhauser A, Weschler JM, Kitzmiller JL, et al. Cost-benefit analysis of preconception care for women with established diabetes mellitus. *Diabetes Care* 1993;16:1146–1157.
8. White P. Pregnancy complicating diabetes. *Am J Med* 1949;7:609–616.
9. Hare J, White P. Gestational diabetes and the White classification. *Diabetes Care* 1980;3:394.
10. Warram J, Krolewski AS. Use of the albumin/creatinine ratio in patient care and clinical studies. In: Morgens CE, ed. *The kidney and hypertension in diabetes mellitus.* Boston: Kluwer Academic Publishers, 1998:85–96.
11. Kitzmiller JL, Brown ER, Phillippe M, et al. Diabetic nephropathy and perinatal outcome. *Am J Obstet Gynecol* 1981;141:741–751.
12. Greene MF, Hare JW, Krache M, et al. Prematurity among insulin-requiring diabetic gravid women. *Am J Obstet Gynecol* 1989;161:106–111.
13. Reece EA, Coustan DR, Hayslett JP, et al. Diabetic nephropathy: pregnancy performance and fetomaternal outcome. *Am J Obstet Gynecol* 1988;15:56–66.
14. Dunne F, Chowdhur TA, Hartland A, et al. Pregnancy outcome in women with insulin-dependent diabetes mellitus complicated by nephropathy. *Q J Med* 1999;92:451–454.
15. Grenfell A, Brudenell JM, Doddridge MC, et al. Pregnancy in diabetic women who have proteinuria. *Q J Med* 1986;59:379–386.
16. Rosenn B, Miodovnik M, Khoury JC. Outcome of pregnancy in women with diabetic nephropathy. *Am J Obstet Gynecol* 1997;176:S179.
17. Kimmerle R, Zass RP, Cupisti S, et al. Pregnancies in women with diabetic nephropathy: long-term outcome for mother and child. *Diabetologia* 1995;38: 227–235.
18. Gordon M, Landon MB, Samuels P, et al. Perinatal outcome and long-term follow-up associated with modern management of diabetic nephropathy. *Obstet Gynecol* 1996;87:401–409.
19. Reece EA, Leguizamon G, Homko C. Stringent controls in diabetic nephropathy associated with optimization of pregnancy outcomes. *J Matern Fetal Med* 1998;7:213–216.
20. Rosenn BM, Miodovnik M. Medical complications of diabetes mellitus in pregnancy. *Clin Obstet Gynecol* 2000;43:17–31.
21. Reece EA, Leguizamon G, Homko C. Pregnancy performance and outcomes associated with diabetic nephropathy. *Am J Perinatol* 1998;15:413–421.
22. Combs CA, Rosenn B, Kitzmiller JL, et al. Early-pregnancy proteinuria in diabetes related to preeclampsia. *Obstet Gynecol* 1993;82:802–807.
23. Ekbom P. Pre-pregnancy microalbuminuria predicts pre-eclampsia in insulin-dependent diabetes mellitus. Copenhagen Pre-eclampsia in Diabetic Pregnancy Study Group. *Lancet* 1999;353:377.
24. Schroder W, Heyl W, Hill-Grasshoff B, et al. Clinical value of detecting microalbuminuria as a risk factor for pregnancy-induced hypertension in insulin-treated diabetic pregnancies. *Eur J Obstet Gynecol Reprod Biol* 2000;91: 155–158.
25. Centers for Disease Control. Perinatal mortality and congenital malformations in infants born to women with insulin-dependent diabetes mellitus—United States, Canada, and Europe, 1940–1988. *JAMA* 1990;264:437–441.
26. Lawrence R, Oakle W. Pregnancy and diabetes. *Q J Med* 1942;11:45–75.
27. Kucera J. Rate and type of congenital anomalies among offspring of diabetic women. *J Reprod Med* 1971;7:73–82.
28. Greene MF. Prevention and diagnosis of congenital anomalies in diabetic pregnancies. *Clin Perinatol* 1993;20:533–547.
29. Mills JL, Baker L, Goldman AS. Malformations in infants of diabetic mothers occur before the seventh gestational week. Implications for treatment. *Diabetes* 1979;28:292–293.
30. Opitz JM. Blastogenesis and the "primary field" in human development. *Birth Defects Original Article Series* 1993;29:3–37.
31. Leslie R, Pyke DA, John PN, et al. Hemoglobin A1 in diabetic pregnancy. *Lancet* 1978;2:958–959.
32. Miller E, Hare JW, Cloherty JP, et al. Elevated maternal hemoglobin A1c in early pregnancy and major congenital anomalies in infants of diabetic mothers. *N Engl J Med* 1981;304:1331–1334.
33. Greene M, Hare JW, Cloherty JP, et al. First trimester hemoglobin A1 and risk for major malformations. *Teratology* 1989;39:225–331.
34. Kitzmiller JL, Buchanan TA, Kjos S, et al. Pre-conception care of diabetes, congenital malformations, and spontaneous abortions. *Diabetes Care* 1996;19: 514–541.
35. Ylinen K, Aula P, Stenman UH, et al. Risk of minor and major fetal malformations in diabetics with high haemoglobin A1c values in early pregnancy. *BMJ (Clin Res Ed)* 1984;289:345–346.
36. Reid M, Hadden D, Harley JM, et al. Fetal malformations in diabetics with high haemoglobin A1c in early pregnancy [Letter]. *BMJ (Clin Res Ed)* 1984;289: 1001.
37. Key TC, Giuffrida R, Moore TR. Predictive value of early pregnancy glycohemoglobin in the insulin-treated diabetic patient. *Am J Obstet Gynecol* 1987; 156:1096–1100.
38. Hanson U, Persson B, Thunell S. Relationship between haemoglobin 1Ac in early type 1 (insulin-dependent) diabetic pregnancy and the occurrence of spontaneous abortion and fetal malformation in Sweden. *Diabetologia* 1990; 33:100–104.
39. Rosenn BM, Miodovnik M, Combs CA, et al. Glycemic thresholds for spontaneous abortion and congenital malformations in insulin-dependent diabetes mellitus. *Obstet Gynecol* 1994;84:515–520.

40. Fuhrmann K, Reiher H, Semmler K, et al. Prevention of congenital malformations in infants of insulin-dependent diabetic mothers. *Diabetes Care* 1983; 6:219–223.
41. Fuhrmann K, Reiher H, Semmler K, et al. The effect of intensified conventional insulin therapy before and during pregnancy on the malformation rate in offspring of diabetic mothers. *Exp Clin Endocrinol* 1984;83:173–177.
42. Goldman JA, Dicker D, Feldberg D, et al. Pregnancy outcome in patients with insulin-dependent diabetes mellitus with preconceptional diabetic control: a comparative study. *Am J Obstet Gynecol* 1986;155:293–297.
43. Damm P, Molsted-Pedersen L. Significant decrease in congenital malformations in newborn infants of an unselected population of diabetic women. *Am J Obstet Gynecol* 1989;161:1163–1167.
44. Steel JM, Johnstone FD, Hepburn DA, et al. Can prepregnancy care of diabetic women reduce the risk of abnormal babies? *BMJ* 1990;301:1070–1074.
45. Kitzmiller JL, Gavin LA, Gin GD, et al. Preconception care of diabetes. Glycemic control prevents congenital anomalies. *JAMA* 1991;265:731–736.
46. Rosenn B, Miodovnik M, Combs CA, et al. Pre-conception management of insulin-dependent diabetes: improvement of pregnancy outcome. *Obstet Gynecol* 1991;77:846–849.
47. Tchobroutsky C, Vray MM, Altman JJ. Risk/benefit ratio of changing late obstetrical strategies in the management of insulin-dependent diabetic pregnancies. A comparison between 1971–1977 and 1978–1985 periods in 389 pregnancies. *Diabete Metab* 1991;17:287–294.
48. Willhoite MB, Bennert HW Jr, Palomaki GE, et al. The impact of preconception counseling on pregnancy outcomes. The experience of the Maine Diabetes in Pregnancy Program. *Diabetes Care* 1993;16:450–455.
49. Holing EV, Beyer CS, Brown ZA, et al. Why don't women with diabetes plan their pregnancies? *Diabetes Care* 1998;21:889–895.
50. Jovanovic-Peterson L, Peterson CM, Reed GF, et al. Maternal postprandial glucose levels and infant birth weight: the Diabetes in Early Pregnancy Study. The National Institute of Child Health and Human Development—Diabetes in Early Pregnancy Study. *Am J Obstet Gynecol* 1991;164(1 Pt 1):103–111.
51. Rey E, Attie C, Bonin A. The effects of first-trimester diabetes control on the incidence of macrosomia. *Am J Obstet Gynecol* 1999;181:202–206.
52. Gold AE, Reilly R, Little J, et al. The effect of glycemic control in the preconception period and early pregnancy on birth weight in women with IDDM. *Diabetes Care* 1998;21:535–538.
53. Peck RW, Price DE, Lang GD, et al. Birthweight of babies born to mothers with type 1 diabetes: is it related to blood glucose control in the first trimester? *Diabet Med* 1991;8:258–262.
54. Schwartz R, Gruppuso PA, Petzold K, et al. Hyperinsulinemia and macrosomia in the fetus of the diabetic mother. *Diabetes Care* 1994;17:640–648.
55. Small M, Cameron A, Lunan CB, et al. Macrosomia in pregnancy complicated by insulin-dependent diabetes mellitus. *Diabetes Care* 1987;10:594–599.
56. Combs CA, Gunderson E, Kitzmiller JL, et al. Relationship of fetal macrosomia to maternal postprandial glucose control during pregnancy. *Diabetes Care* 1992;15:1251–1257.
57. Pederson J. Weight and length at birth of infants of diabetic mothers. *Acta Endocrinol* 1954;16:330–342.
58. Cordero L, Treuer SH, Landon MB, et al. Management of infants of diabetic mothers. *Arch Pediatr Adolesc Med* 1998;152:249–254.
59. Landon MB, Gabbe SG, Piana R, et al. Neonatal morbidity in pregnancy complicated by diabetes mellitus: predictive value of maternal glycemic profiles. *Am J Ostet Gynecol* 1987;156:1089–1095.
60. Curet LB, Izquierdo LA, Gilson GJ, et al. Relative effects of antepartum and intrapartum maternal blood glucose levels on incidence of neonatal hypoglycemia. *J Perinatol* 1997;17:113–115.
61. Combs CA, Kitzmiller JL. Diabetic nephropathy and pregnancy. *Clin Obstet Gynecol* 1991;34:505–515.
62. Leguizamon G, Reece EA. Effect of medical therapy on progressive nephropathy: influence of pregnancy, diabetes and hypertension. *J Matern Fetal Med* 2000;9:70–78.
63. Kimmerle R, Heinemann L, Delecki A, et al. Severe hypoglycemia incidence and predisposing factors in 85 pregnancies of type I diabetic women. *Diabetes Care* 1992;15:1034–1047.
64. Rosenn BM, Miodovnik M, Holcberg G, et al. Hypoglycemia: the price of intensive insulin therapy for pregnant women with insulin-dependent diabetes mellitus. *Obstet Gynecol* 1995;85:417–422.
65. Anderson JH Jr, Brunelle RL, Koivisto VA, et al. Reduction of postprandial hyperglycemia and frequency of hypoglycemia in IDDM patients on insulin-analog treatment. Multicenter Insulin Lispro Study Group. *Diabetes* 1997;46: 265–270.
66. Brunelle BL, Llewelyn J, Anderson JH Jr, et al. Meta-analysis of the effect of insulin lispro on severe hypoglycemia in patients with type 1 diabetes. *Diabetes Care* 1998;21:1726–1731.
67. Del Sindaco P, Ciofetta M, Lalli C, et al. Use of the short-acting insulin analogue lispro in intensive treatment of type 1 diabetes mellitus: importance of appropriate replacement of basal insulin and time-interval injection-meal. *Diabet Med* 1998;15:592–600.
68. Ebeling P, Jansson PA, Smith U, et al. Strategies toward improved control during insulin lispro therapy in IDDM. Importance of basal insulin. *Diabetes Care* 1997;20:1287–1289.
69. Colombel A, Murat A, Krempf M, et al. Improvement of blood glucose control in type 1 diabetic patients treated with lispro and multiple NPH injections. *Diabet Med* 1999;16:319–324.
70. Hermansen K, Colombo M, Storgaard H, et al. Improved postprandial glycemic control with biphasic insulin aspart relative to biphasic insulin lispro and biphasic human insulin in patients with type 2 diabetes. *Diabetes Care* 2002;25:883–888.
71. Jovanovic L, Ilic S, Pettitt DJ, et al. Metabolic and immunologic effects of insulin lispro in gestational diabetes. *Diabetes Care* 1999;22:1422–1227.
72. Pettitt DJ, Ospina P, Kolaczynski JW, et al. Comparison of an insulin analog, insulin aspart, and regular human insulin with no insulin in gestational diabetes mellitus. *Diabetes Care* 2003;26:183–186.
73. Kurtzhals P, Schaffer L, Sorensen A, et al. Correlations of receptor binding and metabolic and mitogenic potencies of insulin analogs designed for clinical use. *Diabetes* 2000;49:999–1005.
74. Report of the National High Blood Pressure Education Program Working Group on High Blood Pressure in Pregnancy. *Am J Obstet Gynecol* 2000;183(1): S1–S22.
75. Summary of Revisions for the 2001 Clinical Practice Recommendations. *Diabetes Care* 2001;24[Suppl 1]:S3.
76. von Dadelszen P, Ornstein MP, Bull SB, et al. Fall in mean arterial pressure and fetal growth restriction in pregnancy hypertension: a meta-analysis. *Lancet* 2000;355:87–92.
77. Magee LA, Elran E, Bull SB, et al. Risks and benefits of beta-receptor blockers for pregnancy hypertension: overview of the randomized trials. *Eur J Obstet Gynecol Reprod Biol* 2000;88:15–26.
78. Briggs CG, Freeman RK, Yafee SJ. *Drugs in pregnancy and lactation.* Vol. 6. Philadelphia: Lippincott Williams & Wilkins, 2002:174–181, 469–476.
79. Krolewski AS, Warram JH, Christlieb AR, et al. The changing natural history of nephropathy in type I diabetes. *Am J Med* 1985;78:785–794.
80. Zatz R, Meyer TW, Rennke HG, et al. Predominance of hemodynamic rather than metabolic factors in the pathogenesis of diabetic glomerulopathy. *Proc Natl Acad Sci U S A* 1985;82:5963–5967.
81. Mogensen CE. Early glomerular hyperfiltration in insulin-dependent diabetics and late nephropathy. *Scand J Clin Lab Invest* 1986;46:201–206.
82. McCance DR, Traub AI, Harley JM, et al. Urinary albumin excretion in diabetic pregnancy. *Diabetologia* 1989;32:236–239.
83. Hod M, van Dijk DJ, Karp M, et al. Diabetic nephropathy and pregnancy: the effect of ACE inhibitors prior to pregnancy on fetomaternal outcome. *Nephrol Dial Transplant* 1995;10:2328–2333.
84. Chew EY, Mills JL, Metzger BE, et al. Metabolic control and progression of retinopathy. The Diabetes in Early Pregnancy Study. National Institute of Child Health and Human Development Diabetes in Early Pregnancy Study. *Diabetes Care* 1995;18:631–637.
85. The Diabetes Control and Complications Trial Research Group. Effect of pregnancy on microvascular complications in the diabetes control and complications trial. *Diabetes Care* 2000;23:1084–1091.
86. American Diabetes Association. Clinical practice recommendations. Preconception care of women with diabetes. *Diabetes Care* 2004;27[Suppl]: S76–S78.
87. Brown FM, Hare JW. Diabetic neuropathy and coronary heart disease. In: Reece EA, Coustan DR, eds. *Diabetes mellitus in pregnancy. Principles and practice.* New York: Churchill Livingstone, 1995:345–351.
88. Krolewski AS, Kosinski EJ, Warram JH, et al. Magnitude and determinants of coronary artery disease in juvenile-onset, insulin-dependent diabetes mellitus. *Am J Cardiol* 1987;59:750–755.
89. Consensus Development Conference on the Diagnosis of Coronary Heart Disease in People with Diabetes: 10-11 February 1998, Miami, Florida. American Diabetes Association. *Diabetes Care* 1998;21:1551–1559.
90. Hsia SH, Connelly PW, Hegele RA. Successful outcome in severe pregnancy-associated hyperlipemia: a case report and literature review. *Am J Med Sci* 1995;309:213–218.
91. Loo CC, Tan JY. Decreasing the plasma triglyceride level in hypertriglyceridemia-induced pancreatitis in pregnancy: a case report. *Am J Obstet Gynecol* 2002;187:241–242.
92. Mizushimat T, Ochi K, Matsumura N, et al. Prevention of hyperlipidemic acute pancreatitis during pregnancy with medium-chain triglyceride nutritional support. *Int J Pancreatol* 1998;23:187–192.
93. ACOG Practice Bulletin. Chronic hypertension in pregnancy. *Obstet Gynecol* 2001;98:177–184.
94. Kjos SL. Postpartum care of the woman with diabetes. *Clin Obstet Gynecol* 2000;43:75–86.
95. Metzger BE. Summary and recommendations of the Third International Workshop-Conference on Gestational Diabetes Mellitus. *Diabetes* 1991;40 [Suppl 2]:197–201.
96. Duncan M. On puerperal diabetes. *Trans Obstet Soc Lond* 1882;256–285(24).
97. Engelgau MM, Herman WH, Smith PJ, et al. The epidemiology of diabetes and pregnancy in the U.S., 1988. *Diabetes Care* 1995;18:1029–1033.
98. Green JR, Pawson IG, Schumacher LB, et al. Glucose tolerance in pregnancy: ethnic variation and influence of body habitus. *Am J Obstet Gynecol* 1990;163 (1 Pt 1):86–92.
99. Kuhl C. Glucose metabolism during and after pregnancy in normal and gestational diabetic women. 1. Influence of normal pregnancy on serum glucose and insulin concentration during basal fasting conditions and after a challenge with glucose. *Acta Endocrinol* (Copenh) 1975;79:709–719.
100. Damm P, Kuhl C, Bertelsen A, et al. Predictive factors for the development of diabetes in women with previous gestational diabetes mellitus. *Am J Obstet Gynecol* 1992;167:607–616.

101. Catalano PM, Tyzbir ED, Wolfe RR, et al. Carbohydrate metabolism during pregnancy in control subjects and women with gestational diabetes. *Am J Physiol* 1993;264(1 Pt 1):E60–E67.
102. Bowes SB, Hennessy TR, Umpleby AM, et al. Measurement of glucose metabolism and insulin secretion during normal pregnancy and pregnancy complicated by gestational diabetes. *Diabetologia* 1996;39:976–983.
103. Swinn RA, Wareham NJ, Gregory R, et al. Excessive secretion of insulin precursors characterizes and predicts gestational diabetes. *Diabetes* 1995;44: 911–915.
104. Kuhl C. Serum proinsulin in normal and gestational diabetic pregnancy. *Diabetologia* 1976;12:295–300.
105. National Diabetes Data Group. Classification and diagnosis of diabetes mellitus and other categories of glucose intolerance. *Diabetes* 1979;18:1039–1057.
106. Carpenter MW, Coustan DR. Criteria for screening tests for gestational diabetes. *Am J Obstet Gynecol* 1982;144:768–773.
107. ADA Expert Committee on the Diagnosis and Classification of Diabetes Mellitus, Report of the Expert Committee on the Diagnosis and Classification of Diabetes Mellitus, Clinical Practice Recommendations 2000. *Diabetes Care* 2000[Suppl 1]:S4–S19.
108. Coustan DR, Nelson C, Carpenter MW, et al. Maternal age and screening for gestational diabetes: a population-based study. *Obstet Gynecol* 1989;73: 557–561.
109. Berkus MD, Langer O. Glucose tolerance test: degree of glucose abnormality correlates with neonatal outcome. *Obstet Gynecol* 1993;81:344–348.
110. Sermer M, Naylor CD, Farine D, et al. The Toronto Tri-Hospital Gestational Diabetes Project. A preliminary review. *Diabetes Care* 1998;21[Suppl 2]: B33–B42.
111. Moses RG, Calvert D. Pregnancy outcomes in women without gestational diabetes mellitus related to the maternal glucose level. Is there a continuum of risk? *Diabetes Care* 1995;18:1527–1533.
112. Drexel H, Bichler A, Sailer S, et al. Prevention of perinatal morbidity by tight metabolic control in gestational diabetes mellitus. *Diabetes Care* 1988;11: 761–768.
113. Langer O, Levy J, Brustman L, et al. Glycemic control in gestational diabetes mellitus—how tight is tight enough: small for gestational age versus large for gestational age? *Am J Obstet Gynecol* 1989;161:646–653.
114. Jovanovic-Peterson L. *Medical management of pregnancy complicated by diabetes*, 2nd ed. Alexandria, VA: American Diabetes Association, 1995.
115. Clapp JF 3rd. Maternal carbohydrate intake and pregnancy outcome. *Proc Nutr Soc* 2002;61:45–50.
116. Langer O, Conway DL, Berkus MD, et al. A comparison of glyburide and insulin in women with gestational diabetes mellitus. *N Engl J Med* 2000;343: 1134–1138
117. Bochner CJ, Medearis AL, Williams J 3rd, et al. Early third-trimester ultrasound screening in gestational diabetes to determine the risk of macrosomia and labor dystocia at term. *Am J Obstet Gynecol* 1987;157:703–708.
118. Buchanan TA, Kjos SL, Montoro MN, et al. Use of fetal ultrasound to select metabolic therapy for pregnancies complicated by mild gestational diabetes. *Diabetes Care* 1994;17:275–283.
119. Hod M, Bar J, Peled Y, et al. Antepartum management protocol. Timing and mode of delivery in gestational diabetes. *Diabetes Care* 1998;21[Suppl 2]: B113–B117.
120. Naylor CD, Sermer M, Chen E, et al. Cesarean delivery in relation to birth weight and gestational glucose tolerance: pathophysiology or practice style? Toronto Trihospital Gestational Diabetes Investigators. *JAMA* 1996;275:1165–1170.
121. Schaefer-Graf UM, Buchanan TA, Xiang A, et al. Patterns of congenital anomalies and relationship to initial maternal fasting glucose levels in pregnancies complicated by type 2 and gestational diabetes. *Am J Obstet Gynecol* 2000;182: 313–320.
122. Towner D, Kjos SL, Leung B, et al. Congenital malformations in pregnancies complicated by NIDDM. *Diabetes Care* 1995;18:1446–1451.
123. Kjos SL, Peters RK, Xiang A, et al. Contraception and the risk of type 2 diabetes mellitus in Latina women with prior gestational diabetes mellitus. *JAMA* 1998;280:533–538.
124. Peters RK, Kjos SL, Xiang A, et al. Long-term diabetogenic effect of single pregnancy in women with previous gestational diabetes mellitus. *Lancet* 1996;347:227–230.
125. Tuomilehto J, Lindstrom J, Eriksson JG, et al. Prevention of type 2 diabetes mellitus by changes in lifestyle among subjects with impaired glucose tolerance. *N Engl J Med* 2001;344:1343–1350.
126. Knowler WC, Barrett-Connor E, Fowler SE, et al: Diabetes Prevention Program Research Group. Reduction in the incidence of type 2 diabetes with lifestyle intervention or metformin. *N Engl J Med* 2002;346:393–403.
127. Chiasson JL, Josse RG, Gomis R, et al. Acarbose for prevention of type 2 diabetes mellitus: the STOP-NIDDM randomised trial. *Lancet* 2002;359:2072–2077.
128. Buchanan TA, Xiang AH, Peters RK, et al. Preservation of pancreatic beta-cell function and prevention of type 2 diabetes by pharmacological treatment of insulin resistance in high-risk Hispanic women. *Diabetes* 2002;51:2796–2803.
129. Pettitt DJ, Bennett PH. In: Reece EA, Coustan DR, eds. *Diabetes mellitus in pregnancy: principles and practice.* Churchill Livingstone: New York, 1995: 379–388.
130. Forman MR, Hoffman HJ, Harley EE, et al. The Pima infant feeding study: the role of sociodemographic factors in the trend in breast- and bottle-feeding. *Am J Clin Nutr* 1982;35:1477–1486.
131. Silverman BL, Landsberg L, Metzger BE. Fetal hyperinsulinism in offspring of diabetic mothers. Association with the subsequent development of childhood obesity. *Ann N Y Acad Sci* 1993;699:36–45.
132. Silverman BL, Metzger BE, Cho NH, et al. Impaired glucose tolerance in adolescent offspring of diabetic mothers. Relationship to fetal hyperinsulinism. *Diabetes Care* 1995;18:611–617.

CHAPTER 62
Cutaneous Manifestations of Diabetes Mellitus

Mark H. Lowitt and Jeffrey S. Dover

Patients with diabetes mellitus commonly suffer from a wide variety of cutaneous maladies. Estimates of the frequency of skin disease in people with diabetes range from 30% overall (1) to 71% of patients with type 1 diabetes mellitus (2). While several skin conditions are specific to diabetes, most of them also occur in individuals without diabetes. The clinical manifestations and complications of skin disease are frequently more severe in the setting of diabetes. The pathophysiology of most cutaneous disorders in the patient with diabetes remains poorly understood. Recent advances in genetic research may soon answer some longstanding questions. For example, results from a recent study indicate that the G82S polymorphism of the *RAGE* gene (receptor for advanced glycosylation end products) is associated with microangiopathic skin conditions in patients with type 2 diabetes (3). In this chapter, we describe the characteristic skin conditions associated with diabetes, incorporating discussion of clinical presentation, pathology, pathogenesis, and treatment (Table 62.1).

CUTANEOUS INFECTIONS IN DIABETES

Candidiasis

Candidal infections of mucosal membranes, genitalia, and nails are more prevalent in patients with poorly controlled diabetes than in the population without diabetes (4–7). Women are more prone to these infections than are men (5). Although yeast infections may be the initial presentation of diabetes, they generally occur in patients already known to have diabetes (6). In indi-

TABLE 62.1. Skin Manifestations of Diabetes

Cutaneous infections
- Candidiasis
- Dermatophytosis
- Phycomycosis
- Erythrasma
- Malignant external otitis

Neurologic lesions
- Charcot joint
- Compensatory hyperhidrosis
- Neuropathic ulcer

Disorders of collagen
- Necrobiosis lipoidica
- Granuloma annulare
- Scleredema diabeticorum
- Waxy skin
- Sclerodermalike change of the hand

Metabolic diseases
- Porphyria cutanea tarda
- Yellow skin
- Xanthomatosis
- Hemochromatosis
- Glucagonoma syndrome
- Generalized pruritus

Skin conditions with strong but unexplained association with diabetes
- Acquired ichthyosis
- Diabetic dermopathy
- Diabetic bullae
- Rubeosis
- Vitiligo
- Acanthosis nigricans
- Finger "pebbles"
- Perforating disorders

Cutaneous reactions to diabetes therapy
- Insulin-induced disorders
  - Insulin allergy
  - Insulin lipodystrophy
  - Insulin-induced lipohypertrophy
- Hypoglycemic agents
  - Hypersensitivity reactions
  - Disulfiram reactions

From Fine JD, Moschella S. Diseases of nutrition and metabolism. In: Moschella SL, Hurley HJ, eds. *Dermatology.* Philadelphia: WB Saunders Company, 1985.

viduals with diabetes, the ratio of epidermal glucose to blood glucose is higher than in persons without diabetes (8), a situation that may produce an environment that is more favorable for the growth of yeast and fungi (9).

ORAL MUCOSAL CANDIDIASIS

Distinctive forms of oral mucosal candidiasis include thrush (curdlike white colonies) over intra-oral surfaces; atrophic candidiasis, which manifests as bright red atrophy of the hard palate or tongue; sore mouth; and angular cheilitis (perlèche), which presents as superficial or deep erosions along the labial commissures. Antifungal creams or troches usually are required to eradicate infection.

CANDIDAL PARONYCHIA

The frequency of candidal paronychia, the inflammation surrounding the nail that is caused by a candidal infection, is increased in persons with diabetes. In one study of 250 women with diabetes, 9.6% had clinical evidence of candidal paronychia as compared with 3.4% of 500 controls without diabetes (10). Typical candidal paronychia begins with erythema, swelling, and pain at the lateral nail fold, leading to its separation from the nail margin. The proximal nail fold then becomes involved, and the cuticle may separate from the nail plate (11). Purulent drainage may be mistaken for bacterial infection. Candidal paronychia is characterized by intermittent exacerbations with episodic indolent periods, a course that may result in a rippled appearance of the nail plate. Patients with occupations in which the hands are frequently immersed in water are more prone to this condition (12). Practical treatment includes keeping the hands as dry as possible. The wearing of cotton gloves under rubber or vinyl gloves can protect hands during dishwashing. Topical antifungal solutions usually are adequate for treatment; however, patients with refractory cases may require oral therapy with an imidazole.

CANDIDAL VULVITIS

Candidal vulvovaginitis is characterized by pruritus, vulvar erythema, and occasionally fissuring and pustules (11). Glycosuria may promote growth of *Candida* species. Certain case studies have shown that the severity of pruritus is proportional to the degree of glycosuria and hyperglycemia (13). Broad-spectrum antibiotics, birth-control pills, and topical corticosteroids are also common causes of candidal vulvovaginitis. Antifungal vaginal suppositories or oral imidazole antifungal agents are necessary to eradicate infection. Non–*Candida albicans* species of *Candida* are now being recognized as pathogens in vulvovaginitis, particularly in women with diabetes. These organisms are often resistant to standard oral antifungal agents (13). Oral nystatin solution may be beneficial in reducing the reservoir of *Candida* organisms in the gastrointestinal tract.

CANDIDAL BALANITIS

Men with candidal balanitis present with diffuse or focal erythema of the glans penis, often in association with pain or pruritus. White discharge in association with erosions or pustules is commonly seen, particularly under the foreskin of uncircumcised patients. Men with balanitis and phimosis, especially if middle-aged or elderly, should be evaluated for diabetes. In one retrospective study, among 100 men requiring circumcision for phimosis, 35% had diabetes. For most of these patients, diabetes had not been diagnosed previously (7). Administration of topical or oral imidazoles is the treatment of choice. If phimosis is present, a cotton-tipped applicator may be used to gently introduce the anticandidal preparation underneath the foreskin (11).

Dermatophyte Infections

Tinea pedis (athlete's foot) is more prevalent in persons with diabetes than in the general population (4). Although innocuous in most people, tinea can create fissures and portals of entry that may lead to severe bacterial infections in those with diabetes. Web spaces are pruritic, scaly, erythematous, and macerated. Vesicles and pustules may also be present. A "moccasin" distribution of scaling extending from the soles onto the lateral feet is another variant of tinea pedis. Long-standing tinea pedis may involve the nails, which develop a thick, yellowish brown roughened nail plate and subungual debris. Potassium hydroxide (KOH) scraping identifies branching, septate hyphae (12). Patients who have tinea involving their hands or fingernails may inoculate other body sites as well.

Topical antifungal agents are the mainstays of treatment for these infections. For severe fungal infections of skin, hair, or nails, administration of an oral imidazole (such as itraconazole) or an allylamine antifungal agent (such as terbinafine) is the treatment of choice. Blood counts and liver function tests must be monitored during treatment, and drug interactions between imidazole antibiotics and other drugs metabolized by the hepatic cytochrome P450 system must be anticipated. Preventive foot care, including careful drying, wearing of cotton socks, and wearing of sandals in public shower facilities may help prevent infection. Topical ciclopirox administered as a nail lacquer is a welcome recent therapeutic option.

Phycomycetes Infections

The phycomycetes are a group of fungi found on decaying vegetation and foods with a high sugar content. Although rarely pathogenic, the genera most commonly involved in human infection include *Rhizopus*, *Mucor*, and *Absidia* (14). In the clinical setting, all diseases caused by these organisms are referred to as mucormycosis.

Several major clinical syndromes, involving the rhinocerebral, thoracic, gastrointestinal and cutaneous systems are described (15). Of these, rhinocerebral disease is most closely associated with diabetes. The fungal organism colonizes the nasal turbinates and sinuses but can invade the orbit and brain, particularly in the setting of diabetic ketoacidosis. Characteristically black crusty or purulent material is present on the turbinates, septa, or palate, and mucormycosis may initially be mistaken for bacterial sinusitis. Cutaneous mucormycosis occurs when the organism colonizes burned or skin-grafted tissues or nonhealing leg ulcers in patients with diabetes (16).

The diagnosis can be confirmed by skin biopsy or a KOH tissue preparation of sputum or skin, which may demonstrate the large, broad, nonseptate hyphae characteristic of phycomycetes (14). Debridement of necrotic tissue, intravenous administration of amphotericin B, correction of acid–base imbalance, and control of hyperglycemia are the necessary components of treatment (17). The more invasive forms of disease frequently are fatal.

Bacterial Infections

Although patients with well-controlled diabetes do not have increased susceptibility to most bacterial infections, evidence suggests that patients with poorly controlled diabetes may develop more frequent or severe bacterial infections than experienced by the rest of the population (18). Several authors have described abnormalities in leukocyte function associated with diabetes, including diminished chemotaxis (19), depressed phagocytosis (20,21), decreased bacteriocidal activity, (22–25), decreased leukocyte migration (25), and an altered early granulocyte phase of the local cellular inflammatory response (26).

Bacterial infections of the lower extremities are a particular risk for patients with diabetes who have vascular disease or neuropathy (18). Careful foot care and early treatment of dermatophytosis are essential in minimizing potential bacterial portals of entry. A recent review of predisposing factors in hospitalized patients with cellulitis identified diabetes, prior history of cellulitis, edema, dry feet, and evidence of tinea pedis as the most important risk factors (27) (also see Chapter 66).

MALIGNANT EXTERNAL OTITIS

Malignant external otitis is a severe necrotizing bacterial infection that occurs almost exclusively in patients with diabetes (28). Beginning in the external auditory canal, the infection invades local soft tissues and ultimately leads to osteomyelitis of the temporal bone, occasionally progressing to fatal meningitis. *Pseudomonas aeruginosa* is the causative agent in virtually all cases. Symptoms can include unremitting ear pain, purulent otic discharge, and cranial nerve palsies. A tender ear and mastoid area with granulation tissue or polyps in the external auditory canal are typical physical findings. More than 20% of patients have bilateral disease (29). Extended therapy with antipseudomonal agents is necessary, and surgical debridement may also be required.

ERYTHRASMA

Erythrasma is a superficial infection usually affecting intertriginous areas of the skin that is caused by *Corynebacterium minutissimum*. Carriage of fluorescent diphtheroids on clinically normal skin is more common in patients with poorly controlled diabetes than in persons without diabetes. Obesity may be an additional contributing factor, especially in those with adult-onset diabetes (30).

Reddish brown, slightly scaly patches typically occur in the intertriginous areas such as the axillae, groin, and web spaces and can be pruritic or asymptomatic. Erythrasma is commonly limited to the toe webs, manifesting with white discoloration and maceration. Frequently, the diagnosis is missed, and not infrequently toe-web involvement is misdiagnosed as tinea pedis. The characteristic coral red fluorescence using a Wood light is diagnostic. The red glow seen is from a porphyrinlike substance produced by the bacteria (31). Gram stain or culture of affected skin scrapings shows gram-positive rods and threadlike filaments traversing the stratum corneum (32). Topical imidazole antifungal agents, topical antibiotics, and systemic erythromycin or tetracycline each provide effective treatment for the disorder. Fusidic acid in a topical preparation is a recent addition to the therapeutic armamentarium (33).

NEUROPATHIC AND ISCHEMIC DIABETIC SKIN DISEASES

Diabetic Polyneuropathy

Diabetic neuropathy is usually bilateral and more severe in the lower extremities than in the upper extremities (34). Dry shiny skin and ulceration on pressure points, particularly on structurally deformed feet, are common. Skin hypoesthesia is one of the most important signs of polyneuritis (34). Lack of thermal sensitivity may lead to burns, calluses, and subsequent ulceration (35). Abnormalities of motor function are much less obvious than sensory defects. Paralysis of the intrinsic muscles of the feet, the most common motor alteration, results in atrophy of the interosseus muscles, which is demonstrated by the "fan sign"—the inability to separate the toes. Such alteration in motor alteration causes the foot to adopt unusual positions, resulting in claw toe or hammer toe deformities or the Charcot joint. In the latter, the tarsal and metatarsal bones are gradually destroyed and joint spaces are obliterated (34,36). As autonomic neuropathy develops and progresses, sweat glands become inactivated. Patients with diabetes may exhibit a compensatory hyperhidrosis of the trunk or face in response to anhidrosis of the lower body (37). Dry and thickened skin of the anhidrotic diabetic foot is prone to fissures, which may serve as portals of entry for bacteria and fungi. Unperceived chronic pressure to the toenails results in thickening, abnormal curvature, and hypertrophy of the nail plate. Ingrown toenails may lead to secondary bacterial infection (12).

Peripheral Vascular Disease

Peripheral vascular disease (PVD) in patients with diabetes can be diffuse and early in onset. The predilection for atherosclerosis and microangiopathy plays a role in the vessel occlusion that occurs in diabetes (38). Some authors consider that microangiopathy plays a part in diabetic vascular disease, while others disagree (38,39). The skin of the lower extremities in patients with diabetes who have PVD is thin, smooth, cold, and often mottled in the dependent position (40,41). Hair is either sparse or absent. Other signs of PVD include pallor or cyanosis with elevation, dependent rubor, and delayed capillary refill.

Diabetic Ulcers

Among the 16 million patients with diabetes in the United States, 1,200 amputations are performed every week (42). This shocking figure indicates the grave importance of identification and treatment of the myriad of causes of cutaneous ulceration in patients with diabetes.

Neuropathic ulcers develop most frequently in areas of high pressure and repeated trauma such as the toes, heels, and metatarsal heads (35) (Fig. 62.1; see also color plate). The patient may present with pain, paresthesia, or anesthesia of the legs and feet. Only occasionally is the ulcer completely asymptomatic in presentation (36).

Venous ulcers tend to occur on the medial malleoli in association with superficial varicosities and yellow–brown discoloration of the skin and are seldom painful. Rest and elevation of the leg ease venous ulcers by controlling edema and reducing venous hypertension.

Arterial ulcers are typically painful (except when accompanied by neuropathy) and occur more distally, on the tips of the toes and on the heel (41). Ulcers of arterial origin may respond to control of hypertension and diabetes as well as to increased exercise, which promotes collateral circulation. Cessation of smoking can be critical. Aggressive treatment of infection, administration of antiplatelet agents or anticoagulants, and surgical revascularization are important treatment modalities in severe cases. Advances in wound healing offer new effective treatments. A recent series of ten patients with diabetic ulcers demonstrated complete healing in seven of ten with the use of sharp debridement and application of a bilayered human-skin equivalent (a construct of live human keratinocytes on a type I collagen dermal matrix, both derived from human fetal foreskin) (42).

A recent study examined the proliferative capacity and ultramicroscopic appearance of fibroblasts taken from leg ulcers of patients with diabetes as compared with fibroblasts taken from nonulcerated skin of patients with diabetes and from control subjects without diabetes (43). Fibroblasts from cutaneous ulcers in individuals with diabetes were found to proliferate at a significantly slower rate than fibroblasts from either control group. Electron microscopic evaluation of fibroblasts from lesional and nonlesional skin in patients with diabetes revealed a large dilated endoplasmic reticulum, a lack of microtubular structures, and multiple lamellar and vesicular bodies. These abnormalities were not seen in the fibroblasts from the control subjects.

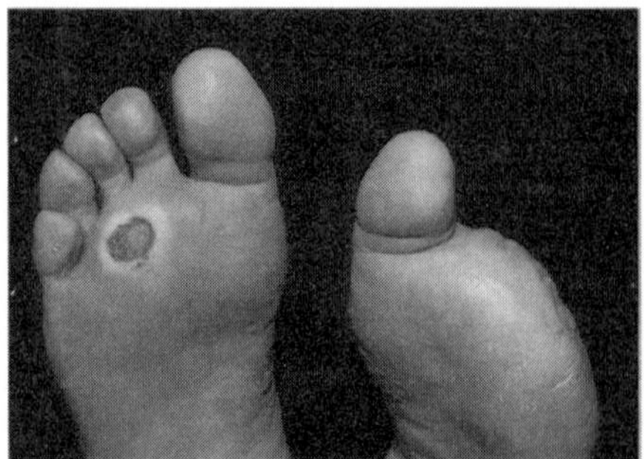

Figure 62.1. (See also color plate.) Acute neuropathic ulcer in a 34-year-old man with diabetes who has had previous amputations for osteomyelitis secondary to ulceration.

DISORDERS OF COLLAGEN

Necrobiosis Lipoidica

Necrobiosis lipoidica is an unusual skin disorder that is strongly associated with diabetes mellitus. The entity was first described in 1929 (44) and was named *necrobiosis lipoidica diabeticorum* (NLD) in 1932 (45). Because of the significant minority of cases of this condition that are associated with diabetes, most investigators now choose to call this condition simply *necrobiosis lipoidica* (NL).

Typical lesions of NL occur on the pretibial skin as irregular ovoid plaques with a violaceous indurated periphery and a yellow central atrophic area (Figs. 62.2 and 62.3; see also color plate). Overlying superficial telangiectasia and scattered hyperkeratotic plugs often are noted (46). The lesions can start as small firm reddish brown papules, which slowly enlarge. They are usually multiple and bilateral, with ulceration seen in approximately 35%. Ulcers often are secondary to minor trauma or are iatrogenically induced by intralesional injection of corticosteroids. It is curious that the ulcers only rarely lead to infection. Patients may complain of pruritus, dysesthesia, or pain at the site of lesions. More frequently, however, the lesions of NL are asymptomatic, and it is the cosmetic disability that is of greatest concern to the patient. Although most commonly found on the lower legs (85% of cases involve only the legs), other locations include the hands, fingers, forearms, face, and scalp (47). Lesions in these locations are often annular, erythematous, or brown and can coalesce to form larger serpiginous plaques, which demonstrate little or no atrophy.

Muller and Winkelmann's classic papers in 1966 (47,48) demonstrate the close association between NL and diabetes. Of their 171 patients with NL, 65% had diabetes. Of the remainder available for study, 42% (8 of 19) demonstrated abnormal glucose tolerance with abnormal oral glucose tolerance tests or cortisone glucose tolerance tests. Among those with normal glucose tolerance, 55% had family histories of glucose intolerance. Despite the high prevalence of diabetes in patients with NL, it is relatively uncommon; the reported prevalence being 3 per

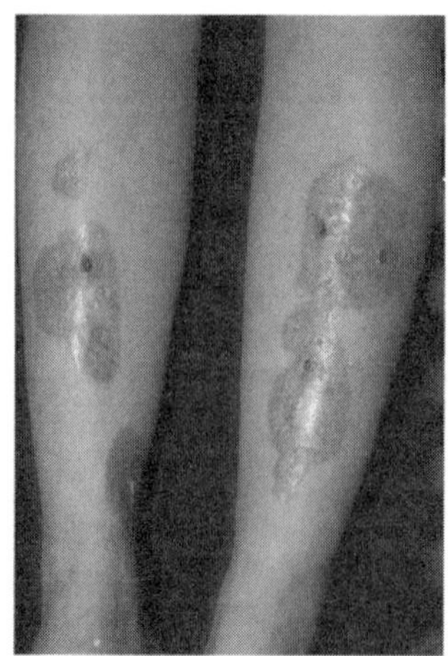

Figure 62.2. (See also color plate.) Necrobiosis lipoidica in a 24-year-old patient with type 1 diabetes.

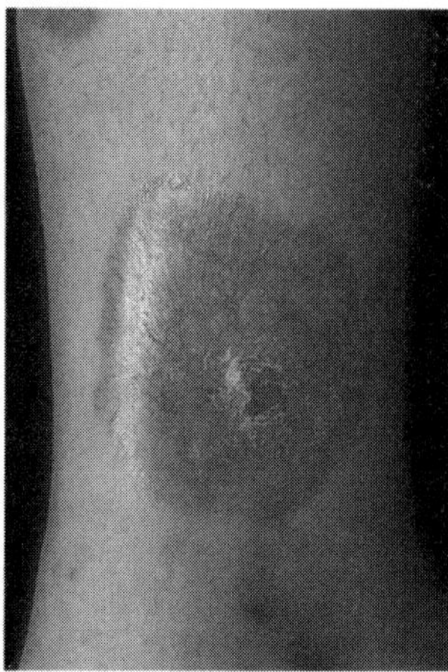

Figure 62.3. (See also color plate.) Necrobiosis lipoidica in a 24-year-old patient with type 1 diabetes.

1,000 patients with diabetes. The female-to-male ratio is 3:1, with an average age of onset of 30 years in patients with diabetes. Fifty percent of patients with NL demonstrate other diabetes-related end-organ damage (47).

Despite extensive investigation, the etiology of NL remains largely unknown. Evidence suggests that NL and glycemic control are not related (49) and that genetic factors do not play a large role (50). Vascular etiologies have been entertained; however, vascular changes are absent in one third of biopsy samples. A link with diabetic microangiopathy has been suggested, yet the caliber of the affected vessels in NL is usually larger than the caliber of vessels affected in diabetes. The abnormal collagen found in NL has invited speculation on a direct etiologic relationship of NL to the collagen itself, as a result of accelerated aging of collagen in diabetes, (51) abnormal collagen cross-linking, or overhydrated collagen produced in response to osmotic effects generated by the end products from the aldose reductase (polyol) pathway (52). Abnormal leukocyte mobility has also been implicated (53). Immune-complex disease has been considered as a cause of NL. Ullman and Dahl (54) reported deposition of C3, fibrinogen, and immunoglobulin around dermal blood vessels in nine of 12 patients with NL, but subsequent reports only partially confirm these results. A review of NL addresses these theories in greater detail (55).

Clinically, early NL can be difficult to distinguish from granuloma annulare. As the lesions enlarge, however, NL becomes more distinct, with the epidermal change, atrophy, and yellow color seen developing. Other conditions included in the differential diagnosis for NL are listed in Table 62.2.

A consistently effective treatment for NL has yet to be found. Potent topical corticosteroids applied to the inflammatory rim of lesions are thought to help control disease progression. Other agents used, with variable results, include fibrinolytic agents such as stanozolol, pentoxifylline, and aspirin and dipyridamole, ticlopidine, nicotinamide, and clofazimine, but none have ever been demonstrated to be effective in blinded studies. Ulcerative NL usually responds to routine ulcer treatment, but surgical intervention occasionally becomes necessary. Recent reports described the resolution of extensive ulcerative NL with oral cyclosporine (56) and mycophenolate mofetil (57).

TABLE 62.2. Clinical Differential Diagnosis for Necrobiosis Lipoidica

Diabetic dermopathy
Rheumatoid nodules
Granuloma annulare
Stasis dermatitis
Morphea
Erythema nodosum

Granuloma Annulare

Granuloma annulare (GA) is characterized by an annular configuration of flesh-colored or pale red papules and plaques that occur in a localized or generalized (disseminated) pattern (Fig. 62.4; see also color plate). Most studies find no association between diabetes and localized GA (58–60) but a link between disseminated GA and diabetes has repeatedly been demonstrated (61,62). In one study, 21% of 100 patients with generalized GA were found to have diabetes (62).

The lesions of GA may vary in size from a few millimeters to 5 cm (64). Localized GA is most characteristically located on the dorsa of the hands and feet. A single lesion is present in one half of patients with GA (65). The papules develop and enlarge slowly in a centrifugal fashion over a period of months to years. Only 15% of patients develop more than ten lesions. Generalized GA is characterized by a symmetrical eruption of hundreds of tiny papules, which can occur all over the body surface. Localized GA eventually undergoes spontaneous resolution—usually within 2 years. Lesions often recur at the same site, however. Resolution in patients with generalized GA is less likely (65). Ulceration and scar formation are rare (64).

Localized GA appears most commonly in children and young adults, affecting twice as many females as males. Generalized GA is, however, more likely to occur in older women (64). The etiology of GA is unknown. Immunoglobin G (IgG) and C3 have been found in blood vessels of involved skin, suggesting an immunologic role. The differential diagnosis includes tinea corporis, sarcoidosis, NL, secondary or tertiary syphilis, annular lichen planus, and insect bites.

Treatment of GA is often unsatisfactory, but fortunately the disease is usually asymptomatic and self-limited. Topical or intralesional corticosteroids are sometimes of benefit in the treatment of localized disease. Treatment of disseminated GA is difficult. Therapy can include the use of systemic corticosteroids, potassium iodide, antimalarials, nicotinic acid, and dapsone, although controversy exists regarding their efficacy (65). One study reported complete clearance of disease in all five patients treated with oral psoralens plus ultraviolet A (PUVA) irradiation (66).

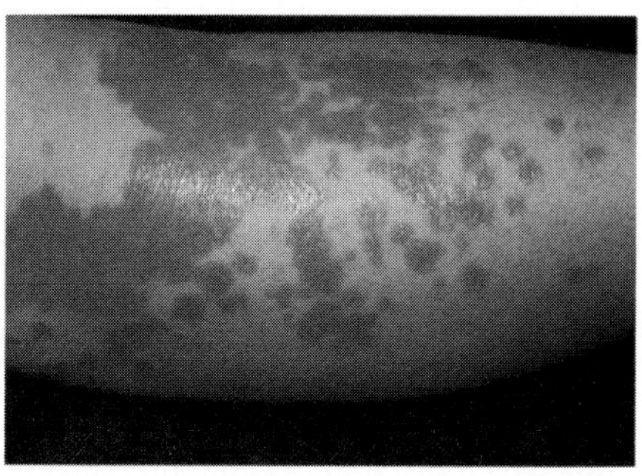

Figure 62.4. (See also color plate.) Disseminated granuloma annulare.

Scleredema Diabeticorum

Scleredema diabeticorum is a diffuse, nonpitting induration of skin characteristically occurring on the upper back, neck, and shoulders. In one study of 484 patients with diabetes, 2.5% were affected (67). Erythema and induration typically begin on the posterior and lateral neck and may extend to the upper back and extremities, including the hands, resulting in extreme limitation of movement. The indurated areas are typically erythematous and finely papular. Patients may perceive decreased light touch and pain in the involved areas. In one report, eight of 13 patients with scleredema diabeticorum had persistent disease lasting up to 20 years (68).

In contrast, another form of scleredema occurs in younger patients without diabetes after streptococcal infection. This subset of scleredema tends to resolve spontaneously within a period of months in 85% of patients (32).

Males are more often affected than are women (ratio 4:1, respectively) (69). Most patients are middle-aged. Both patients with type 1 diabetes and those with type 2 diabetes are affected, but in most instances, diabetes is long-standing. Patients are generally obese, exhibiting a high frequency of diabetic retinopathy, neuropathy, hypertension, and ischemic heart disease. The etiology of scleredema diabeticorum is unknown (70).

The differential diagnosis for scleredema includes scleroderma, eosinophilic fasciitis, eosinophilia myalgia syndrome, and lymphedema. No uniformly effective treatment exists (71). Although scleredema is not generally considered to respond to increased glycemic control (69), a case report documents temporary improvement of rapidly progressive scleredema with improved glycemic control and intravenous prostaglandin E (72). Scleredema associated with paraproteinemia has been treated with photopheresis (73).

Waxy Skin

Persons with juvenile-onset type 1 diabetes can develop waxy, tight skin, also known as diabetic thick skin, in association with limited joint mobility. Rosenbloom et al. (74,75) studied more than 300 patients with type 1 diabetes and found 30% to have elements of this syndrome. Biopsies of wrist skin reveal a markedly thickened dermis, with sparse glands and hair follicles. Increased collagen cross-linking, perhaps related to elevated nonenzymatic glycosylation, has been offered as an explanation (76,77). Some resolution of skin findings has been reported in association with improved glycemic control (78,79).

Plantar Hyperkeratosis

Thickening of scale on the plantar surfaces has been described in association with obesity (80). The prevalence of this skin finding was 35% in 156 obese persons with diabetes and individuals without diabetes whose body mass indices were 27 to 51. The excessive keratin production and retention are theorized to occur in response to direct pressure due to excess weight. This finding may therefore be more likely related to obesity than to diabetes directly.

Acquired Ichthyosis

In a study of 238 people with type 1 diabetes, ichthyosiform skin changes of the skins were noted in 48% of patients (2). Acquired ichthyosis was the most common skin abnormality in the patients described in this report.

METABOLIC DISEASES

Porphyria Cutanea Tarda

Porphyria cutanea tarda (PCT) is a disorder of heme synthesis characterized by a sporadic cutaneous eruption and uroporphyrinuria. It is estimated that 25% of men between the ages of 45 and 75 years who have PCT have diabetes (81). Men are more frequently affected than are women. The classic clinical picture includes vesicles, bullae, and erosions over the dorsal hands and arms and other sun-exposed areas. The primary lesions heal slowly, leaving scarring and milia (tiny epidermal inclusion cysts). Patients also are noted to exhibit skin fragility and hypertrichosis. The enzymatic defect, a deficiency of uroporphyrinogen decarboxylase, leads to excessive serum uroporphyrins, which accumulate in tissues. These compounds are excreted in the urine, which fluoresces pink under a Wood light. The iron concentration in serum is frequently increased. Uroporphyrinogen decarboxylase deficiency occurs both in a familial (autosomal dominant) form and a sporadic/induced form, which is triggered by alcohol, estrogens, or any of several hepatotoxic aromatic hydrocarbons. Treatments of choice include avoidance of alcohol, serial phlebotomy, and administration of antimalarial agents (82).

Yellow Skin

As many as 10% of patients with diabetes may have yellow discoloration of the skin. The yellow color may be caused by the concentration of carotene in areas of prominent sebaceous activity (face, forehead, and axilla) and areas of thick stratum corneum (palms, soles, and bony prominences). These patients, unlike those with jaundice of hyperbilirubinemia, do not exhibit scleral icterus (83).

Early reports linked hypercarotenemia with diabetes, citing elevated carotene levels in more than 50% of patients with diabetes (84). These studies may have been conducted at a time when the recommended diabetes diet included large amounts of foods high in carotene. Hoerner et al. (85) used spectrophotometry to compare skin color and levels of serum carotene in individuals with and without diabetes. They found that the skin of the group with diabetes was yellower than the skin of the group without diabetes but found no correlation between skin color and carotene level. The explanation for a higher incidence of yellow skin among patients with diabetes is unclear and remains controversial.

Xanthomatosis

ERUPTIVE XANTHOMA

Eruptive xanthomas occur in one per 1000 patients with diabetes (84). Lesions are small, firm, nontender, pinkish yellow papules, most commonly occurring in crops on the knees, elbows, back, buttocks, and trunk (Fig. 62.5; see also color plate). Persistent papules may coalesce to form larger plaques.

In patients with significant insulin deficiency, decreased lipoprotein lipase activity results in elevated serum triglyceride levels. Cutaneous eruptive xanthomas form when the serum triglyceride level rises above 1000 mg/dL (84). Lipids accumulated in the serum may be deposited extracellularly in the form of cholesterol or triglycerides in the dermis or subcutaneous tissue. This deposition creates a cutaneous xanthoma.

Lesions are indistinguishable from those in other conditions producing hypertriglyceridemia. Chronic biliary cirrhosis, nephrotic syndrome, chronic pancreatitis, and myxedema may

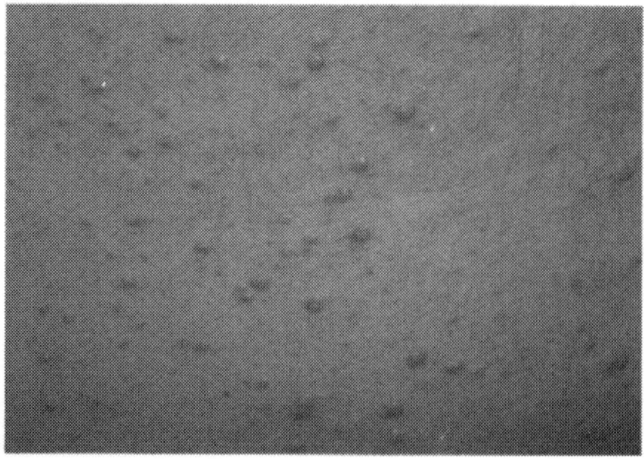

Figure 62.5. (See also color plate.) Eruptive xanthomata of the abdomen in a 45-year-old patient with uncontrolled type 1 diabetes.

cause secondary eruptive xanthomas. Prompt control of hyperlipidemia can result in disappearance of the papules. Weight reduction, carbohydrate restriction, and antilipemic agent therapy may be necessary. Aggressive insulin therapy and good glycemic control are important in patients with diabetes to help resolve the cutaneous manifestations of the hypertriglyceridemia.

XANTHELASMA

Xanthelasma is a distinctive type of xanthoma that occurs on the eyelids. Lesions begin as small yellow–orange macules, which thicken to form oval foamy plaques. Xanthelasma is most common in middle-aged women and is particularly associated with hyperlipoproteinemia, hepatobiliary disorders, and diabetes. Although 50% or more of patients may be normolipemic, it is considered appropriate to obtain serum lipid profiles in these patients. Surgical removal is frequently successful, although recurrences are common. Ablation with cryosurgery (86), laser surgery (87), and bichloracetic acid (88) have been reported as safe and effective. Xanthelasma does not usually regress when diabetes is controlled (18); however, one study documents regression in xanthelasma in 50% of 36 patients treated with the lipid-lowering agent probucol (89).

Hemochromatosis

Hemochromatosis is a disorder of iron storage in which increased gastrointestinal absorption of iron leads to deposition of excessive iron in tissues. The most significant complications result from deposition in the liver, heart, joints, pancreas, and skin. Diabetes is found in 65% of patients, particularly those with family histories of diabetes. In 90% of patients, skin involvement is manifested by diffuse bronzed hyperpigmentation, which is due to cutaneous deposition of melanin and hemosiderin. Therapy includes phlebotomy and use of iron-chelating agents (90). Hematochromatosis is an important secondary cause of diabetes (see Chapter 27).

Lipodystrophy

Progressive lipodystrophy, a rare disorder characterized by complete absence of subcutaneous fat, is associated with diabetes (91). Most cases involve the face, back, upper trunk, and upper extremities. Onset is insidious and discomfort is absent. In the most common partial type, the cheeks are hollowed with prominent malar eminences. Muscles and veins are prominent in affected areas (91). Approximately 20% of these patients develop diabetes (92). Generalized lipodystrophy is an autosomal recessive disorder with onset at puberty and results in an acromegalic appearance (93). Decreased binding of insulin to its receptor has been shown (94), but the complete molecular basis for the insulin resistance is unknown and involves insulin resistance of postreceptor signal transduction pathway. Patients with progressive lipodystrophy and diabetes frequently are insulin-resistant or require high doses of insulin. Diabetic control does not improve or alter lipodystrophy. Autologous fat transplantation has been reported to be successful in some cases. Familial partial lipodystrophy of the Dunnigan type (FPLD; Mendelian Inheritance in Man 151660), demonstrates autosomal dominant inheritance. Loss of subcutaneous fat from the extremities and trunk begins in puberty. The predisposition to diabetes and its complications is greater in affected women than in affected men (95).

Glucagonoma Syndrome

In 1942, Becker et al. (96) first described the characteristic eruption of glucagonoma in a patient with an islet-cell type of pancreatic carcinoma. Their report represents the classic clinical presentation of the syndrome with its symmetric confluent areas of macular, erythematous, and vesicular eruptions with exfoliation and superficial necrosis. It was not until 1966 that McGavran et al. (97) documented the hyperglucagonemia and consequent hyperglycemia, resulting from a functioning islet-cell tumor. Wilkinson (98) later called the characteristic skin changes of this glucagon secreting α-cell carcinoma "necrolytic migratory erythema." The eruption occurs most severely in intertriginous and periorificial areas. Individual lesions last from 7 to 14 days, heal centrally, and are found in various stages of development. Other associated cutaneous findings include glossitis, conjunctivitis, periorbital crusting, ridging and thickening of nails, and paronychia (99).

Approximately two thirds of patients with glucagonoma have cutaneous abnormalities, and approximately 67% have fasting hyperglycemia. Neither the presence nor the severity of hyperglycemia appears to be related to the degree of skin manifestations. Anemia and weight loss are frequent (100).

The eruption may precede by years all other symptoms of pancreatic islet-cell tumors (101). Removal of the carcinoma prior to metastasis results in complete cure and clearing of cutaneous symptoms (102,103). Unfortunately, most glucagonomas have already metastasized at the time of clinical diagnosis. The cutaneous eruption, which may wax and wane spontaneously, is typically misdiagnosed and resembles many dermatoses, including pemphigus foliaceus, bullous pemphigoid, vasculitis, and psoriasis (100).

Extreme fasting hyperglucagonemia (>500 pg/mL) is present in most cases. Hypoaminoacidemia occurs, in part secondary to the consumption of large quantities of amino acids by enhanced gluconeogenesis. Initial workup includes a determination of fasting plasma glucagon concentration by radioimmunoassay, followed by abdominal imaging. Celiac and hepatic arteriography may also be required (100).

Hyperglucagonemia or the presumed secondary hypoaminoacidemia may be responsible for the skin changes, a possibility suggested by the improvement of cutaneous lesions following systemic administration of amino acids (100,104). Various chemotherapeutic agents have been used when surgery has failed or was not an option; the agents have included streptozotocin and phenoxybenzamine.

OTHER SKIN CONDITIONS STRONGLY ASSOCIATED WITH DIABETES

Diabetic Dermopathy

The lesions of diabetic dermopathy (DD), also known as pigmented pretibial patches or shin spots, are by some reports the most common cutaneous finding in diabetes (105). Early lesions are small, flat-topped, dull, red papules that are typically painless. Over several weeks, the lesions progress to atrophic hyperpigmented irregular patches approximately 5 to 12 mm in diameter. Lesions can be linear, grouped, or individual and frequently appear in crops. Individual lesions resolve over 1 to 2 years, but the emergence of new lesions makes the course appear stationary (18). The lesions are most commonly located on the anterior shins, as well as on the forearms, anterior thighs, and feet, with a propensity to appear over bony prominences (8).

Melin (106) found DD in 50% of male patients and in 29% of female patients with diabetes who were older than 50 years of age. There is controversy as to whether DD is more common with increasing duration and severity of diabetes. The lesions are not specific to diabetes, however. Similar lesions have been noted in 1.5% of medical students and in 30% of randomly selected endocrinology patients (107). The etiology is unknown. Because of the appearance of DD over bony prominences, trauma is thought to play a role. In a study of 19 patients with preexisting DD treated with local heat or cold, 16 developed new lesions (108). Melin could not, however, reproduce the disease with repetitive blows from a rubber mallet. Generally, no treatment other than the protection of susceptible areas from repetitive trauma is indicated.

Diabetic dermopathy has been associated with diabetic retinopathy, neuropathy, and nephropathy (109). A recent study of white subjects with type 2 diabetes and diabetic dermopathy revealed the association of this skin disease with the G82S polymorphism of the gene coding for the receptor for advanced glycosylation end products (the *RAGE* gene) (110).

Diabetic Bullae

Spontaneous bullous formation is a rare but distinct cutaneous sign of diabetes. Known as diabetic bullae, bullous diabeticorum, or idiopathic bullae of diabetes, it is a diagnosis made by exclusion. Kramer (111), in 1930, described asymptomatic blisters on the extremities of patients with diabetes. Diabetic bullae generally are found bilaterally on the extremities of patients with diabetes, particularly those with neuropathy and/or retinopathy (112). The locations of the blisters in a recent series of 12 patients with type 2 diabetes included the toes (5 of 12), heel (2 of 12), and anterior tibial area (2 of 12) (113). The lesions are typically asymptomatic and nonhemorrhagic, ranging in size from vesicles to 3- to 5-cm bullae. Notably, there is no surrounding erythema.

The etiology of diabetic bullae is unclear. Proposed causes include mechanical trauma, ultraviolet light, immune-mediated vasculitis (32), and altered calcium and magnesium levels related to renal failure, changes leading to facilitated epidermal and dermal separation with trauma. The histology of this disorder is not well defined, as both epidermal and subepidermal blistering have been reported. A recent case report documents the presence of hyalinosis of cutaneous blood vessels, which may support an underlying vascular etiology (114). Diabetic bullae may represent more than one entity, a diversity that may explain different histologic presentations.

The differential diagnosis includes localized bullous pemphigoid, porphyria cutanea tarda, drug-induced blistering, and blisters of renal failure. Direct immunofluorescence of perilesional skin is normal in diabetic bullae, distinguishing it from bullous pemphigoid. It is essential to make this distinction to avoid the unnecessary use of glucocorticoids in patients with diabetes (115). Treatment is symptomatic, with compresses or incision and drainage if necessary. Lesions generally resolve spontaneously within several weeks.

Rubeosis

Rubeosis is a descriptive term for the rosy facial coloration found in many patients with diabetes. This appearance tends to be more pronounced in lighter-skinned individuals. The cause remains unknown, but erythema may result from the decreased ability of the thickened dermal vessels to vasoconstrict (116). Some authors believe that improved diabetes control may lessen the erythema. Protection from the sun and avoidance of topical irritants and dietary vasodilators such as alcohol or substances causing facial flushing by their increased temperature, such as coffee or tea, may be helpful.

Vitiligo

Vitiligo is an acquired condition of skin characterized by symmetrical circumscribed macular depigmentation in a localized or generalized pattern. Lesions occur typically around the nostrils, mouth, genitals, and the extensor surface of the hands. Other frequent locations include axillae, nipples, shins, and elbows. Dermatomal patterns occur rarely. Overlying hair can be white or normally pigmented. The amelanotic macules progressively enlarge, and skin depigmentation can be almost complete. In 50% of cases, onset is before the age of 20 years.

Vitiligo is associated with diabetes mellitus. Dawber et al. (117) found vitiligo present in 4.8% of patients with adult-onset diabetes, as compared with 0.7% to 1% of the general population. An increased frequency in patients with type 1 diabetes has been reported as well. Of 2,000 patients with vitiligo, however, 3.1% had diabetes.

The pathogenesis of vitiligo is unclear, but there is substantial evidence implicating an autoimmune process. Vitiligo can occur in association with states of polyglandular hypofunction, including Addison disease, Hashimoto thyroiditis, hypoparathyroidism, gonadal failure, diabetes mellitus, pernicious anemia, celiac sprue, and myasthenia gravis. Elevated titers of antithyroid, antiadrenal, and antigastric antibody activity have been found in children with diabetes and vitiligo (118). It is therefore surprising that the prevalence would be increased in individuals with adult-onset diabetes, which is not thought to be an autoimmune disease, although some patients classified as having type 2 diabetes actually may have slowly progressing autoimmune diabetes.

The condition is asymptomatic but can be very difficult for the patient emotionally. Management includes the use of cosmetics to cover depigmented areas and the avoidance of exposure to the sun, although minimal spontaneous repigmentation in sun-exposed areas has been reported. PUVA therapy has been used successfully for repigmentation, although more than 200 treatments may be needed, for an improvement rate of 50% to 70% (119). In exceptional cases, and only with diffuse involvement, bleaching agents may be applied to surrounding skin. This treatment is irreversible, prolonged, and requires thorough evaluation of potential psychosocial ramifications for the patient. The course of vitiligo associated with diabetes is not affected by glycemic control.

Acanthosis Nigricans

Acanthosis nigricans is a cutaneous condition characterized by the presence of confluent areas of mid- to dark-brown epidermal thickening with a characteristic "velvety" texture. The lesions appear most commonly in the axillae, neck, groin, and intertriginous areas but also may appear over extensor surfaces like the knees, elbows, and knuckles.

In a recent study of 216 patients newly diagnosed with type 2 diabetes (119a), 31% were found to have acanthosis nigricans at the time of presentation. These patients require higher insulin doses than those without this cutaneous finding. A childhood form of the condition, which often occurs during adolescence, usually is benign. In adulthood the condition can be associated with obesity, endocrinopathies, insulin resistance, and malignancy. Acanthosis nigricans associated with obesity is usually benign but indicates the presence of insulin resistance. The lesions may reverse with weight loss. Familial acanthosis nigricans with autosomal dominant inheritance has been reported as well (120). A recent study of 397 people in 33 Mexican-American families demonstrated evidence of very high heritability of acanthosis nigricans. The condition was highly correlated with diabetes mellitus, obesity, and increased fasting insulin levels in patients without diabetes (121). Several endocrine disorders, including Addison disease, polycystic ovarian disease, Cushing disease, acromegaly, and diabetes mellitus are associated with benign acanthosis nigricans. Kahn et al. (122) described two syndromes linking diabetes mellitus, glucose intolerance, and insulin resistance with acanthosis nigricans. In type "A" insulin resistance, the resistance is due to a reduction in the number of cellular insulin receptors, whereas in type "B" insulin resistance, the basis of the resistance is thought to be the presence of antibodies to the insulin receptor. Acanthosis nigricans also occurs in association with certain drugs, including diethylstilbestrol, nicotinic acid, and corticosteroids. When acanthosis nigricans occurs out of the setting of any of the previous conditions, underlying malignancy must be suspected (123). The most commonly associated tumors are adenocarcinoma, particularly of gastric origin. Squamous cell carcinoma, undifferentiated carcinoma, and lymphoma have also been associated with acanthosis nigricans. In two thirds of cases, the lesions of acanthosis nigricans parallel the course of the malignancy.

Treatment of acanthosis nigricans is directed primarily at identification and treatment of the underlying condition, if known. Locally, the lesions can be peeled with 5% to 10% salicylic acid in petrolatum, but no treatments are uniformly effective. A recent review states that metformin, octreotide, retinoids, and topical vitamin D3 analogues can be beneficial (123a).

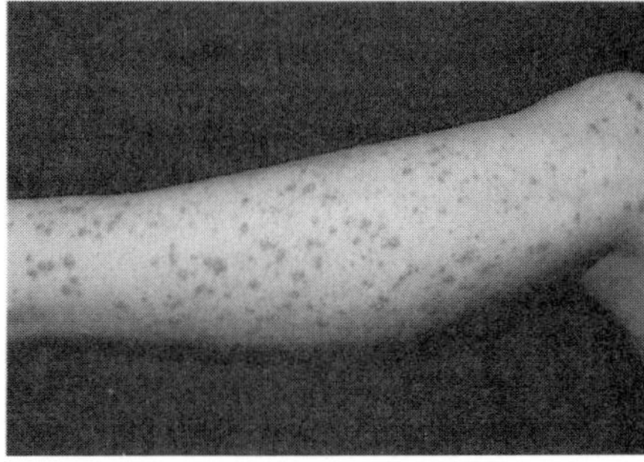

Figure 62.6. (See also color plate.) Perforating folliculitis in a 50-year-old patient with diabetes with retinopathy and nephropathy.

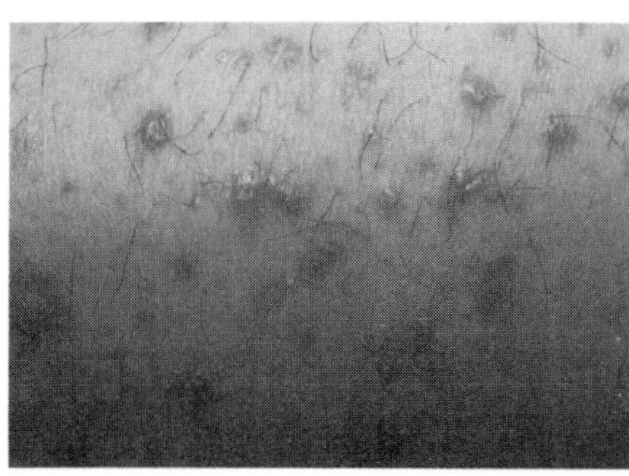

Figure 62.7. (See also color plate.) Perforating folliculitis in a 50-year-old patient with diabetes with retinopathy and nephropathy.

Finger "Pebbles"

Huntley (124) described distinctive tiny skin-colored grouped papules and thickening over the extensor surfaces of the fingers in 75% of patients with diabetes mellitus, as compared with 21% of control patients without diabetes. The finding was recently reported again (125). Because of the similarity in the appearance of these papules with acanthosis nigricans, some physicians interpret these cutaneous findings as a variant of acanthosis nigricans.

Perforating Disorders

The perforating disorders are a group of diseases in which dermal material perforates through the epidermis out to the surface of the skin. The four classic members of this group are reactive perforating collagenosis, Kyrle disease, perforating folliculitis, and elastosis perforans serpiginosa. All but the last appear to be associated with diabetes, occurring most commonly in patients with coexisting nephropathy. These diseases are occasionally seen in patients with renal disease without diabetes and are rarely noted in healthy individuals.

Reactive perforating collagenosis is characterized by follicular plugs over the extremities, particularly the knees and elbows (126). Kyrle disease affects a similar subpopulation of older patients with severe diabetes and renal disease. Keratin plugs are surrounded by erythema and are found in various stages of development (Figs. 62.6 and 62.7; see also color plate). Lesions preferentially occur on the extremities, buttocks, and sacral region (127). Perforating folliculitis produces similar, but slightly smaller, more numerous lesions, most often on the extremities. Pruritus, the most common complaint, can be extremely resistant to treatment.

Generalized Pruritus

The frequency of generalized pruritus in diabetes is unknown; however, many believe that it is increased in diabetes. Pruritus without primary lesions in a patient with diabetes requires a thorough workup to rule out known causes of pruritus. Patients with systemic disease (renal disease, liver disease, hypo- or hyperthyroidism, iron-deficiency anemia), or lymphoreticular malignancies (e.g., Hodgkin disease) may present initially with pruritus. Each of these, as well as a primary dermatologic cause of itching, should first be ruled out before the pruritus is attributed to diabetes.

CUTANEOUS REACTIONS TO THERAPY FOR DIABETES

Insulin-Induced Disorders

The incidence of cutaneous reactions to insulin has diminished considerably since the introduction of recombinant human insulin. Insulin allergy may be secondary to the insulin molecule, additives, or protein contaminants in the commercial preparation (128,129). Local reactions to insulin include erythema, pruritus, induration at the injection site, edema, subcutaneous nodules, or urticaria (130). Serious immediate generalized reactions such as angioedema, serum sickness, bronchial constriction, dyspnea, cardiovascular collapse, and anaphylaxis have occurred but are rare and necessitate discontinuation of insulin therapy in type 2 diabetes and aggressive desensitization techniques in type 1 diabetes (128,131). Delayed reactions, which are usually local at the site of injection, occur approximately 2 weeks after initiation of treatment. Injections that are too superficial may cause cutaneous reactions. Occasional cases of insulin allergy have occurred in association with human (128) and recombinant insulin (132).

Insulin-induced lipoatrophy is now rare (132, 133). Atrophy of subcutaneous fat may occur, resulting in atrophic plaques at insulin injection sites 6 to 24 months after initiation of therapy. Insulin-induced lipohypertrophy is more common in males than in females and is caused by repetitive injections into the same site, a presumed local anabolic effect of insulin (131).

Hypoglycemic Agents

The most common adverse effects of hypoglycemic drugs, which contain sulfa-based components, are gastrointestinal and dermatologic (134). Cutaneous hypersensitivity reactions are similar for the various oral hypoglycemic drugs. Serious cutaneous reactions include a diffuse exfoliative dermatitis; erythema multiforme, which may progress to Stevens–Johnson syndrome; and toxic epidermal necrolysis (135). Cross-reactivity with other sulfonylurea agents may occur, as well as with other sulfa-containing drugs such as thiazides, furosemide, and some antibiotics. Thus, when substitution is necessary, it must be done cautiously. Topically applied preparations may act to sensitize a person to sulfonamides. Fisher (136) reported two cases of a widespread contact dermatitis in patients receiving oral hypoglycemic agents who had previously been sensitized with topical agents containing the *para*-amino group. A disulfiramlike reaction may result from the ingestion of alcohol in patients receiving a first-generation sulfonylurea agent (134) and occurs in as many as 10% to 30% of patients taking an oral sulfonylurea. Chlorpropamide is the most common offending agent (137,138).

Among the many new oral therapies for diabetes and insulin resistance, most have not yet been reported to cause cutaneous adverse effects. The α-glucosidase inhibitor acarbose, however, was recently reported to cause erythema multiforme after 2 weeks of therapy (139).

REFERENCES

1. Halprin KM, Ohkawara A. Glucose entry into the human epidermis, I: the concentration of glucose in the human epidermis. *J Invest Dermatol* 1967;49:559–560.
2. Yosipovitch G, Hodak E, Vardi P, et al. The prevalence of cutaneous manifestations in IDDM patients and their association with diabetes risk factors and microvascular complications. *Diabetes Care* 1998;21:506–509.
3. Kankova K, Vasku A, Hajek D, et al. Association of G82S polymorphism in the *RAGE* gene with skin complications in type 2 diabetes. *Diabetes Care* 1999;22:1745.
4. Alteras I, Saryt E. Prevalence of pathogenic fungi in the toe-webs and toenails of diabetic patients. *Mycopathologia* 1979;67:157–159.
5. Sonck CE, Somersalo O. The yeast flora of the anogenital region in diabetic girls. *Arch Dermatol* 1962;88:846–852.
6. Muller SA. Dermatologic disorders associated with diabetes mellitus. *Mayo Clin Proc* 1966;41:689–703.
7. Cates JI, Finestone A, Bogash M. Phimosis and diabetes mellitus. *J Urol* 1973;110.406–407.
8. Petarka ES, Fusaro RM. Cutaneous carbohydrate studies, III: comparison of the fasting glucose content of the skin of the back, arm, abdomen and thigh. *J Invest Dermatol* 1966;47:410–411.
9. Knight L, Fletcher J. Growth of *Candida albicans* in saliva: stimulation by glucose associated with antibiotics, corticosteroids and diabetes mellitus. *J Infect Dis* 1971;123:371–377.
10. Stone OJ, Mullins JF. Incidence of chronic paronychia. *JAMA* 1962;186:71–73.
11. Huntley AC. The cutaneous manifestations of diabetes mellitus. *J Am Acad Dermatol* 1982;7:427–455.
12. Greene RA, Scher RK. Nail changes associated with diabetes mellitus. *Dermatology* 1987;16:1015–1021.
13. Goswami R, Dadhwal V, Tejaswi S, et al. Species-specific prevalence of vaginal candidiasis among patients with diabetes mellitus and its relation to their glycaemic status. *J Infect* 2000;41:162–166.
14. Utz JP, Shadomy HJ. Deep fungal infections. In: Fitzpatrick TB, Eisen AZ, Wolff K, et al, eds. *Dermatology in general medicine.* Vol 2. New York: McGraw-Hill, 1987:2248–2275.
15. Rippon JW. Systemic mycosis. In: Rose NR, Barron AL, Crane LR, et al, eds. *Microbiology: basic principles and clinical application.* New York: MacMillan, 1983:299–310.
16. Tomford JW, Whittlesey D, Ellner JJ, et al. Invasive primary cutaneous phycomycosis in diabetic leg ulcers. *Arch Surg* 1980;115:770–771.
17. Bennett JE. Fungal infection. In: Wilson JD, Braunwald K, Isselbacher KJ, et al, eds. *Harrison's principles of internal medicine.* Vol 2. 12th ed. New York: McGraw-Hill, 1991:2063–2081.
18. Freinkel RK, Freinkel N. Cutaneous manifestations of endocrine disorders. In: Fitzpatrick TB, Eisen AZ, Wolff K, et al, eds. *Dermatology in general medicine.* New York: McGraw-Hill, 1987.
19. Mowat AG, Baum J. Chemotaxis of polymorphonuclear leukocytes from patients with diabetes mellitus. *N Engl J Med* 1971;284:621–627.
20. Davidson J, Swoden JM, Fletcher J. Defective phagocytosis in insulin controlled diabetes: Evidence for a reaction between glucose and opsonizing proteins. *J Clin Pathol* 1984;37:783–786.
21. Rayfield EJ, Ault MJ, Keusch GT, et al. Infection and diabetes: the case for glucose control. *Am J Med* 1982;72:439–450.
22. Repine JE, Clawson CC, Goetz FC. Bacterial function of neutrophils from patients with acute bacterial infections and from diabetes. *J Infect Dis* 1980;142:869–875.
23. Bagdade JD, Root RK, Bulger RJ. Impaired leukocyte function in patients with poorly controlled diabetes. *Diabetes* 1974;23:9–15.
24. Nolan CN, Beaty HN, Bagdade JD. Further characterization of the impaired bacterial function of granulocytes in patients with poorly controlled diabetes. *Diabetes* 1978;27:889–894.
25. Kontras SB, Bodenbender MT. Studies of the inflammatory cycle in juvenile diabetes. *Am J Dis Child* 1968;116:130–134.
26. Perillie PE, Nolan JP, Finch SC: Studies of the resistance to infection in diabetes mellitus: local exudative cellular response. *J Lab Clin Med* 1962;59: 1008–1015.
27. Koutkia P, Mylonakis E, Boyce J. Cellulitis: evaluation of possible predisposing factors in hospitalized patients. *Diagn Microbiol Infect Dis* 1999;34:325–327.
28. Harter DH, Petersdorf RG. Bacterial meningitis and brain abscess. In: Wilson JD, Braunwald K, Isselbacher KJ, et al, eds. *Harrison's principles of internal medicine.* Vol 2. 12th ed. New York: McGraw-Hill, 1991:2023–2031.
29. Zaky DA, Bentley DW, Lowy K, et al. Malignant external otitis: a severe form of otitis in diabetic patients. *Am J Med* 1976;61:298–302.
30. Somerville DA, Lancaster-Smith M. The aerobic cutaneous microflora of diabetic subjects. *Br J Dermatol* 1973;89:395–400.
31. Gilgor RS. Cutaneous infections in diabetes mellitus. In: Jelinek JE, ed. *The skin in diabetes.* Philadephia: Lea & Febiger, 1986.
32. Sibbald RG, Schachter RK. The skin and diabetes mellitus. *Int Dermatol* 1984;23:567–584.
33. Wilkinson JD. Fusidic acid in dermatology. *Br J Dermatol* 1998;139[Suppl] 53:37–40.
34. Faerman I, Jadzinsky M, Podolsky S. Diabetic neuropathy and sexual dysfunction. In: Podolsky S, ed. *Clinical diabetes: modern management.* New York: Appleton-Century-Crofts, 1980.
35. Phillips TJ, Dover JS. Leg ulcers. *J Am Acad Dermatol* 1991;25:965–987.
36. Levin M, O'Neal ME. *The diabetic foot.* St. Louis: Mosby, 1988.
37. Hurley HJ. The eccrine sweat glands. In: Moschella SL, Hurley HJ, eds. *Dermatology.* Vol 2. 2nd ed. Philadelphia: WB Saunders, 1985.
38. Danowski TS, Bahl VK, Fisher ER. Macrovascular and microvascular disease and their prevention. In: Podolsky S, ed. *Clinical diabetes and modern management.* New York: Appleton-Century-Crofts, 1980.
39. Logerfo FW, Coffman JD. Vascular and microvascular disease of the foot in diabetes. *N Engl J Med* 1984;311:25;1615–1618.
40. Haroon TS. Diabetes and skin—a review. *Scott Med J* 1974;19:257–267.
41. Edwards EA, Coffman JD. Cutaneous changes in peripheral vascular disease. In: Fitzpatrick TB, Eisen AZ, Wolff K, et al, eds. *Dermatology in general medicine.* Vol 2. 3rd ed. New York: McGraw-Hill, 1987:1997–2022.

42. Brem H, Balledux J, Bloom T, et al. Healing of diabetic foot ulcers and pressure ulcers with human skin equivalent: a new paradigm in wound healing. *Arch Surg* 2000;135:627–634.
43. Loots MA, Lamme EN, Mekkes JR, et al. Cultured fibroblasts from chronic diabetic wounds on the lower extremity (non-insulin-dependent diabetes mellitus) show disturbed proliferation. *Arch Dermatol Res* 1999;291:93–99.
44. Oppenheim M. Eigentumlich disseminierte Degeneration des Bindegewebes der haut bie einem Diabetiker. *Zentralbl Haut Geschlechtskr* 1929–1930;32: 179.
45. Urbach E. Beitrage zu einer Physiologischen und Pathologischin chemi der haut: Eine neue diabetische Stoffwechseldermatose, Nekrobiosis Lipoidica Diabeticorum. *Arch Dermatol Syph* 1932;166:273–285.
46. Lever WF, Shaumburg-Lever G. *Histopathology of the skin,* 6th ed. Philadephia: JB Lippincott Co., 1990.
47. Muller SA, Winkelmann RK. Necrobiosis lipoidica diabeticorum: a clinical and pathological investigation of 171 cases. *Arch Dermatol* 1966;93:272–281.
48. Muller SA, Winkelmann RK. Necrobiosis lipoidica diabeticorum: results of glucose-tolerance tests in nondiabetic patients. *JAMA* 1966;195:433–436.
49. Dandona P, Freedman D, Barter S, et al. Glycosylated haemoglobin in patients with necrobiosis lipoidica and granuloma annulare. *Clin Exp Dermatol* 1981;6:299–302.
50. Soler NG, McConnachie PR. HLA antigens and necrobiosis lipoidica diabeticorum—a comparison between insulin-dependent patients with diabetes with and without necrobiosis. *Postgrad Med J* 1983;59:759–762.
51. Hamlin CR, Kohn RR, Luschin JH: Apparent accelerated aging of human collagen in diabetes mellitus. *Diabetes* 1975;24:902–904.
52. Eaton RP. The collagen hydration hypothesis: a new paradigm for the secondary complications of diabetes mellitus. *J Chronic Dis* 1986;39:763–766.
53. Gange RW, Black MM, Carrington P. Defective neutrophil migration in granuloma annulare, necrobiosis lipoidica, and sarcoidosis. *Arch Dermatol* 1979;115:32–35.
54. Ullman S, Dahl MV. Necrobiosis lipoidica: an immunofluorescence study. *Arch Dermatol* 1977;113:1971–1973.
55. Lowitt MH, Dover JS: Necrobiosis lipoidica. *J Am Acad Dermatol* 1991;25: 735–748.
56. Darvay A, Acland KM, Russel-Jones R. Persistent ulcerated necrobiosis lipoidica responding to treatment with cyclosporin. *Br J Dermatol* 1999; 141:725–727.
57. Reinhard G, Lohmann F, Uerlich M, et al. Successful treatment of ulcerated necrobiosis lipoidica with mycophenolate mofetil. *Acta Derm Venereol* 2000; 80:312–313.
58. Mobaken H, Gisslen H, Johannisson G. Granuloma annulare: cortisone-glucose tolerance test in a nondiabetic group. *Acta Derm Venereol* 1970;50: 440–444.
59. Meier-Ewert H, Allenby CF. Granuloma annulare and diabetes mellitus. *Arch Dermatol Res* 1971;241:194–198.
60. Williamson DM, Dykes JRW. Carbohydrate metabolism in granuloma annulare. *Int J Dermatol* 1972; 58:400–404.
61. Haim S, Friedman-Birnbaum R, Haim N, et al: Carbohydrate tolerance in patients with granuloma annulare: study of fifty-two cases. *Br J Dermatol* 1973;88:447–451.
62. Eng AM: Erythematous generalized granuloma annulare. *Arch Dermatol* 1979;115:1210–1211.
63. Dabski K, Winkelmann RK. Generalized granuloma annulare: histopathology and immunopathology. Systematic review of 100 cases and comparison with localized granuloma annulare. *J Am Acad Derm* 1989;20:28–46.
64. Wells RS, Smith MA. The natural history of granuloma annulare. *Br J Dermatol* 1963;75:199–205.
65. Dahl MV, Goltz RW. Granuloma annulare. In: Fitzpatrick TB, Eisen AZ, Wolff K, et al, eds. Dermatology in general medicine, Vol 2. 3rd ed. New York: McGraw-Hill, 1987:1018–1022.
66. Kerker BJ, Huang CP, Morison WL. Photochemotherapy of generalized granuloma annulare. *Arch Dermatol* 1990;126:359–361.
67. Cole GW, Headley J, Skowsley R. Scleroderma diabeticorum: a common and distinct cutaneous manifestation of diabetes mellitus. *Diabetes Care* 1983;6: 189–192.
68. Cohn BA, Wheeler CE, Griggaman RA. Scleredema adultorum of Buschke and diabetes mellitus. *Arch Dermatol* 1970;101:27–35.
69. Fleischmajer R, Faludi G, Krol S. Scleredema and diabetes mellitus. *Arch Dermatol* 1970;101:21–26.
70. Jelinek JE. Collagen disorders in which diabetes and cutaneous features coexist. In: Jelinek JE, ed. *The skin in diabetes*. Philadelphia: Lea & Febiger, 1988.
71. Parker SC, Kenton DA, Black MM. Scleredema. *Clin Exp Dermatol* 1989;14: 385–386.
72. Ikeda Y, Suehiro T, Abe T, et al. Severe diabetic scleredema with extension to the extremities and effective treatment using prostaglandin E1. *Intern Med* 1998;37:861–864.
73. Stables GI, Taylor PC, Highet AS. Scleredema associated with paraproteinaemia treated by extracorporeal photopheresis. *Br J Dermatol* 2000;142: 781–783.
74. Rosenbloom AL, Silverstein JH, Kubilis PS, et al. Limited joint mobility (LJM) in insulin-dependent diabetes mellitus high risk for microvasculopathy (MVP). *Pediatr Res* 1980;14:580(abst).
75. Barta L. Flexion contractures in a diabetic child (Rosenbloom syndrome). *Eur J Pediatr* 1980;135:101–102.
76. Chang KF, Uitto J, Rowold EA, et al. Increased cross linkages in experimental diabetes. *Diabetes* 1980;29:778–781.
77. Schnider SL, Kohn RR. Effects of age and diabetes mellitus on the solubility and nonenzymatic glucosylation of human skin collagen. *J Clin Invest* 1981;67:1630–1635.
78. Lieberman LS, Rosenbloom AL, Riley WK, et al. Reduced skin thickness with pump administration of insulin. *N Engl J Med* 1980;303:940–941.
79. Haustein UF. Scleroderma-like lesions in insulin-dependent diabetes mellitus. *J Eur Acad Dermatol Venerol* 1999;13:50–53.
80. Garcia-Hidalgo L, Orozco-Topete R, Gonzalez-Barranco J, et al. Dermatoses in 156 obese adults. *Obes Res* 1999;7:299–302.
81. Grossman ME, Poh-Fitzpatrick MB. Porphyria cutanea tarda: diagnosis and management. *Med Clin North Am* 1980;64:807–827.
82. Poh-Fitzpatrick MB. Prophyrin-sensitized cutaneous photosensitivity: pathogenesis and treatment. *Clin Dermatol* 1985;3:41–82.
83. Leung AKC. Carotenemia. *Adv Pediatr* 1987;34:223–248.
84. Huntley AC. Diabetes mellitus and miscellaneous metabolic conditions affecting the skin. In: Jelinek JE, ed. *The skin in diabetes*. Philadelphia: Lea & Febiger, 1986.
85. Hoerner E, Dreyfuss F, Herzberg M. Carotenemia, skin color and diabetes mellitus. *Acta Diabetol Lat* 1975;12:202–207.
86. Hawk JL. Cryotherapy may be effective for eyelid xanthelasma. *Clin Exp Dermatol* 2000;25:351.
87. Raulin C, Schoenermark MP, Werner S, et al. Xanthelasma palpebrarum: treatment with the ultrapulsed CO_2 laser. *Lasers Surg Med* 1999;24:122–127.
88. Haygood LJ, Bennett JD, Brodell RT. Treatment of xanthelasma palpebrarum with bichloracetic acid. *Dermatol Surg* 1998;24:1027–1031.
89. Fujita M, Shirai K. A comparative study of the therapeutic effect of probucol and pravastatin on xanthelasma. *J Dermatol* 1996;23:598–602.
90. Powell LW, Isselbacher KJ. Hemochromatosis. In: Wilson JD, Braunwald E, Isselbacher KJ, et al, eds. *Harrison's principles of internal medicine.* Vol 2. 12th ed. New York: McGraw-Hill, 1991:1834–1835.
91. Taylor WB, Honeycutt WM. Progressive lipodystrophy and lipoatrophic diabetes. *Arch Dermatol* 1961;84:31–36.
92. Murray I. Lipodystrophy. *BMJ* 1952;2:1236–1239.
93. Fine J, Moschella SL. Diseases of nutrition and metabolism. In: Moschella SL, Hurley HJ, eds. *Dermatology* .Vol 2. 2nd ed. Philadelphia: WB Saunders, 1985.
94. Oseid S, Beck-Nielson H, Pederson O, et al. Decreased binding of insulin to its receptor in patients with congenital generalized lipodystrophy. *N Engl J Med* 1977;296:245–248.
95. Garg A. Gender differences in the prevalence of metabolic complications in familial partial lipodystrophy (Dunnigan variety). *J Clin Endocrinol Metab* 2000;85:1776–1782.
96. Becker SW, Kahn D, Rothman S. Cutaneous manifestations of internal malignant tumors. *Arch Dermatol Syph* 1942;45:1069–1080.
97. McGavran MH, Unger RH, Recant L, et al. A glucagon-secreting alpha-cell carcinoma of the pancreas. *N Engl J Med* 1966;274:1408–1413.
98. Wilkinson DS. Necrolytic migratory erythema with carcinoma of the pancreas. *Trans St. John's Hosp Dermatol Soc* 59:244–250.
99. Leichter SB. Clinical and metabolic aspects of glucagonoma. *Medicine* (Baltimore) 1980;59:100–113.
100. Stacpoole PW. The glucagonoma syndrome: clinical features, diagnosis and treatment. *Endocrinol Rev* 1984;2:347–361.
101. Domen JA, Schroeter AL, Rogers RS III. *Arch Intern Med* 1980;140:262–263.
102. Kahan RS, Perez-Figaredo RA, Neimans A. Necrolytic migratory erythema. *Arch Dermatol* 1977;113:792–797.
103. Sweet RD. A dermatosis specifically associated with a tumor of pancreatic alpha cells. *Br J Dermatol* 1974;90:301–308.
104. Norton JA, Kahn CR, Schiebinger R, et al. Amino acid deficiency and the skin rash associated with glucagomona. *Ann Intern Med* 1979;91:213–215.
105. Bernstein JE, Medenica M, Soltani K, et al. Bullous eruption of diabetes mellitus. *Arch Dermatol* 1979;115:324–325.
106. Melin H. An atrophic circumscribed skin lesion in the lower extremities of patients with diabetes. *Acta Med Scand* 1964;176[Suppl 423]:1–75.
107. Danowski TS, Sabeh G, Sarver ME, et al. Skin spots and diabetes mellitus. *Am J Med Sci* 1966;251:570–575.
108. Lithner F. Cutaneous reaction of the extremities of patients with diabetes to local thermal trauma. *Acta Med Scand* 1975;198:319–325.
109. Shemer A, Bergman R, Linn S, et al. Diabetic dermopathy and internal complications in diabetes mellitus. *Int J Dermatol* 1998;37:113–115.
110. Kankova K, Blazkova M, Marova I. Genetic polymorphism of *RAGE* and diabetic late skin complications. *Pathophysiology* 1998;5[Suppl 1]:175(abst).
111. Kramer DW. Early or warning signs of impending gangrene in diabetes. *Med J Rec* 1930;132:338–342.
112. Kurwa A, Roberts P, Whitehead R. Concurrence of bullous and atrophic skin lesions in diabetes mellitus. *Arch Dermatol* 1971;103:670–675.
113. Lipsky BA, Baker PD, Ahroni JH. Diabetic bullae: 12 cases of a purportedly rare cutaneous disorder. *Int J Dermatol* 2000;107:209–210.
114. Derighetti M, Hohl D, Krayenbuhl BH, et al. Bullosus diabeticorum in a newly discovered type 2 diabetes mellitus. *Dermatology* 2000;200:366–367.
115. Jelinek JE. Cutaneous markers of diabetes mellitus and the role of microangiopathy. In: Jelinek JE, ed. *The skin in diabetes*. Philadelphia: Lea & Febiger, 1986.
116. Ditzel J. Functional microangiopathy in diabetes mellitus. *Diabetes* 1968;17:388–397.
117. Dawber RPR, Bleehen SS, Vallance-Owen J. Vitiligo and diabetes mellitus. *Br J Dermatol* 1971;84:600.
118. Macaron C, Winter RJ, Traisman HS, et al. Vitiligo and juvenile diabetes mellitus. *Arch Dermatol* 1977;113:1515–1517.

119. Parrish JA, Fitzpatrick TB, Shea C, et al. Photochemotherapy of vitiligo: use of orally administered psoralens and a high-intensity longwave ultra-violet system. *Arch Dermatol* 1976;112:1531–1534.
119a. Litonjua P, Pinero-Pilona A, Aviles-Santa L, Raskin P. Prevalence of acanthosis nigricans in newly-diagnosed type 2 diabetes. *Endocr Pract* 2004;10: 101–106.
120. Tasjian D, Jarratt M. Familial acanthosis nigricans. *Arch Dermatol* 1984;120: 1351–1354.
121. Burke JP, Duggirala R, Hale DE, et al. Genetic basis of acanthosis nigricans in Mexican Americans and its association with phenotypes related to type 2 diabetes. *Hum Genet* 2000;200:366–367.
122. Kahn CR, Flier JS, Bar RS, et al. The syndromes of insulin resistance and acanthosis nigricans: insulin-receptor disorders in man. *N Engl J Med* 1976; 294:739–745.
123. Haynes HA. Cutaneous manifestations of internal malignancy. In: Braunwald E, Isselbacher KJ, Petersdorf RG, et al, eds. *Harrison's principles of internal medicine.* Vol 2. 4th ed. New York: McGraw-Hill, 1987:1588–1593.
123a. Hermanns-Le T, Scheen A, Pierard GE. Acanthosis nigricans associated with insulin resistance: pathophysiology and management. *Am J Clin Dermatol* 2004;5:199–203.
124. Huntley AC. Finger pebbles: a common finding in diabetes mellitus. *J Am Acad Dermatol* 1986;14:612–617.
125. Hollister DS, Brodell RT. Finger "pebbles": a dermatologic sign of diabetes mellitus. *Postgrad Med* 2000;41:39–41.
126. Poliak SC, Lebwohl MG, Parris A, et al. Reactive perforating collagenosis associated with diabetes mellitus. *N Engl J Med* 1982;306:81–84.
127. Wolff-Schreiner EC. Kyrle'e disease. In: Fitzpatrick TB, Eisen AZ, Wolff K, et al, eds. *Dermatology in general medicine.* Vol 1. 3rd ed. New York: McGraw-Hill, 1987:541–545.
128. Shore RN, Shelley WB, Kyle GC. Chronic urticaria from isophane insulin therapy: sensitivity associated with non-insulin components in commercial preparations. *Arch Dermatol* 1975;111:947.
129. Grammer LC, Chen PY, Patterson R. Evaluation and management of insulin allergy. *J Allergy Clin Immunol* 1983;71:2:250–254.
130. Lieberman P, Patterson R, Metz R, et al. Allergic reactions to insulin. *JAMA* 1971;215:1106–1112.
131. Gilgor RS, Lazarus GS. Skin manifestations of diabetes mellitus. In: Ellenberg M, Rifkin H, eds. *Diabetes mellitus: theory and practice,* 3rd ed. New Hyde Park, NY: Medical Examination Publishing, 1983:879–893.
132. Murao S, Hirata K, Ishida T, et al. Lipoatrophy induced by recombinant human insulin injection. *J Intern Med* 1998;37:1031–1033.
133. Valenta LJ, Elias AN. Insulin-induced lipodystrophy in diabetic patients resolved by treatment with human insulin. *Ann Intern Med* 1985;102:6: 790–791.
134. Peters AL, Davidson MB. Use of sulfonyluric agents in older diabetic patients. *Clin Geriatr Med* 1990;6:903–921.
135. Bruinsma W. *A guide to drug reactions.* Amsterdam: Excerpta Medica, 1973:99.
136. Fisher AA. Systemic contact dermatitis from Orinase and Diabinese in diabetic with para-amino hypersensitivity. *Cutis* 1982;29:551–565.
137. Fitzgerald MG, Gaddie R, Malins JM, et al: Alcohol sensitivity in patients with diabetes receiving chlorpropamide. *Diabetes* 1962;11:40–43.
138. Groop L, Eriksson CJP, Huipponen R, et al. Roles of chlorpropamide, alcohol and acetaldehyde in determining the chlorpropamide-alcohol flush. *Diabetologia* 1984;26:34–38.
139. Kono T, Hayami M, Iobayashi H, et al. Acarbose-induced generalised erythema multiforme. *Lancet* 1999;31:396–397.

CHAPTER 63

Joint and Bone Manifestations of Diabetes Mellitus

M. Elaine Husni, Susan F. Kroop, and Lee S. Simon

As modern therapeutics have helped decrease the mortality and morbidity of diabetes mellitus, increased musculoskeletal symptoms may be discovered as these patients lead longer and more active lives. It is important to recognize the various joint and bone manifestations of diabetes. Although the other complications of diabetes are better recognized as causes of morbidity and mortality, the musculoskeletal syndromes associated with it may be very debilitating. Overall, changes in the connective tissue of patients with diabetes are probably due to disturbances in the structural macromolecules of the extracellular matrix. Many of these rheumatologic manifestations of diabetes mellitus have been reviewed in the last several years (1–3). A wide range of musculoskeletal syndromes have been described in association with diabetes (Table 63.1). In general, these are syndromes commonly or uniquely associated with diabetes mellitus. There are also common rheumatic diseases with an increased incidence in the diabetic population.

RHEUMATIC SYNDROMES UNIQUELY OR COMMONLY ASSOCIATED WITH DIABETES MELLITUS

Adhesive Capsulitis of the Shoulder

Adhesive capsulitis of the shoulder is a common problem manifested by diffuse shoulder pain associated with a loss of motion in all directions and little or no evidence of intraarticular disease (4). The joint capsule is thickened and adherent to the humeral head. Arthroscopy reveals a marked reduction in the volume of the glenohumeral joint. Increased uptake of ^{99m}Tc-methylene diphosphonate by the periarticular tissue has been demonstrated, suggesting the presence of inflammation (5). Bone demineralization follows. Although patients may recover spontaneously within 3 years, the syndrome may recur, and some patients with severe disease may become disabled (3).

The association of adhesive capsulitis and diabetes mellitus has been well documented. Bridgman (6) identified adhesive capsulitis in 11% of 800 diabetic patients as compared with an incidence of 2.5% in 600 control patients. Alternatively, abnormal glucose tolerance tests were seen in 28% of patients with adhesive capsulitis compared with 12% of age- and sex-matched controls attending a rheumatology clinic (6). Arkkila et al. (7) found an overall cumulative prevalence of shoulder capsulitis of 14% in patients with diabetes mellitus. The prevalence was 10% in patients with type 1 diabetes and 22% in patients with type 2 diabetes. Furthermore, adhesive capsulitis is associated with age in patients with type 1 and type 2 diabetes and with duration of diabetes in patients with type 1 diabetes only. Pal et al. (8) found adhesive capsulitis in 20.4% of patients with type 1 diabetes, in 18.3% of patients with type 2 diabetes, and in 5.3% of normal control subjects.

The treatment of patients is directed toward increasing the range of motion of the tightened joint. Early physical therapy, including exercises, heat, and ultrasound, may be helpful. Splinting may lead to further restriction of motion and is contraindicated. Treatment of pain during physical therapy is important. Treatment includes the use of nonsteroidal antiinflammatory drugs (NSAIDs) as both antiinflammatory agents and analgesics. In addition, opioids may occasionally be necessary. Although there are no long-term studies concerning the use of local glucocorticoid injections in this setting, intraarticular injections may occasionally be useful in decreasing pain and increasing motion. In our experience, full recovery of motion may take as long as 6 months. Rarely, patients may require manipulation of the shoulder while they are under

TABLE 63.1. Musculoskeletal Syndromes Associated with Diabetes Mellitus

Rheumatic syndromes uniquely or commonly associated with diabetes mellitus
Adhesive capsulitis
Shoulder-hand syndrome
Diabetic hand syndrome
Dupuytren's disease
Neuroarthropathy
Hyperostosis
Common rheumatic diseases associated with diabetes mellitus
Osteoarthritis
Gout and hyperuricemia
Calcium pyrophosphate deposition arthropathy
Osteopenia
Osteolysis of forefoot
Migratory osteolysis of hip and knee

general anesthesia to increase the range of motion. In severe cases of adhesive capsulitis, the patient may not recover full motion and may become disabled.

Shoulder-Hand Syndrome

Shoulder-hand syndrome (SHS) is characterized by adhesive capsulitis of the shoulder associated with pain, swelling, tenderness, dystrophic skin, and vasomotor instability in the hand. It is one of a family of disorders that includes reflex sympathetic dystrophy syndrome, major and minor causalgia, Sudeck atrophy, and algodystrophy. Doury et al. (9) described these syndromes as consisting of severe pain disproportionate to the findings of the physical examination in association with articular or periarticular swelling. Steinbrocker and Argyros (10,11) described three stages of this syndrome. During the first stage, which lasts 3 to 6 months, there is pain, tenderness, swelling, and vasomotor changes, including temperature and color changes in the affected hand. The second stage, which also may last 3 to 6 months, is characterized by trophic skin changes characterized by shiny skin with loss of normal wrinkling. The final stage is characterized by atrophy of skin and subcutaneous tissue, tendon contractures, and progressive osteopenia. Spontaneous improvement may occur, although without treatment the patient may lose function of the affected limb permanently.

Trauma is the most common condition predisposing to SHS, but diabetes; cerebrovascular disease; myocardial infarction; post-thoracotomy state; hyperthyroidism; hyperlipidemia; electrocution; medications, including barbiturates, isoniazid, ethionamide, and cycloserine; and previous exposure to radioiodine, have all been associated with the onset of this syndrome (3). In one study of 108 patients with SHS or related conditions, 7.4% had diabetes (9). The prevalence of diabetes actually may be greater in patients with this syndrome, since glucose tolerance tests were not performed in all cases.

Radiographic findings in SHS typically include a diffuse, patchy osteopenia. Measurements of bone mineral density demonstrate loss of up to one third of the bone mass. Three-phase bone scintigraphy reveals asymmetric uptake and increased blood flow and, in most cases, pooling in phases 1 and 2. The phase-3 images are characterized by increased uptake in the periarticular tissues. A small percentage of patients may show decreased uptake on bone scintigraphs.

Treatment of patients with SHS is most effective when begun early in the development of the syndrome. Analgesic medication and range-of-motion exercises should be prescribed. If these are ineffective, systemic glucocorticoid therapy or sympathetic blockade should be considered. In patients with diabetes, regional sympathetic-ganglion block with a long-acting anesthetic agent, performed by an anesthesiologist, is the preferred treatment method since the use of systemic glucocorticoids may cause difficulties in the maintenance of glucose control. Steinbrocker and Argyros (11) reviewed 146 patients with SHS and found some improvement in up to 80% treated with glucocorticoids or regional sympathetic blockade. Intraarticular steroids may also be used, but no controlled trials exist and experience with this technique is limited. Patients are candidates for surgical sympathectomy if the above approaches provide only temporary relief of symptoms. Recently, interest has increased in the use of α-adrenergic blockade and other vasoactive drugs in the treatment of SHS.

Diabetic Hand Syndrome

Diabetic hand syndrome (DHS), also termed cheiropathy, stiff-hand syndrome, diabetic stiff hand, diabetic contractures, or syndrome of limited joint mobility, was first described by Jung et al. (12) in adults with diabetes and by Grgic et al. (13) in a pediatric population with diabetes and short stature (see reference 14 for a comprehensive review of this syndrome). The syndrome has since been described in juveniles with type 1 diabetes and normal stature and in adults with type 1 or type 2 diabetes (15–19). The reported prevalence of DHS in diabetes ranges from 8% to 53% (20–27). Most studies suggest a prevalence of about 35% in patients with diabetes (28–31). It is more common in patients with type 1 diabetes and may be associated with duration of disease. The onset of DHS may not be related to the patient's sex or insulin dosage. It is unclear whether the onset of cheiropathy is related to metabolic control. Silverstein et al. (32) have shown that poor long-term glycemic control, as measured by elevated hemoglobin A_{1c} levels, does increase the risk of earlier onset of hand symptoms in patients with type 1 diabetes. Clinically, patients complain of stiffness, loss of dexterity, and weakness of their hands. The skin on the hands is typically thick, tight, and waxy, and changes may appear compatible with scleredema. There is evidence of recurrent tenosynovitis and decreased range of motion of the small joints of the hands. The patient may exhibit the prayer sign, that is, when asked to hold the palms of the hands together, the patient is unable to bring the fingers and palms together because of flexor tendon contractures. Limitation of flexion and extension occurs predominantly in the proximal interphalangeal and metacarpophalangeal joints. Decreased grip strength results. Sclerodactyly and thick skin may be present.

Much has been reported about the relationship of DHS with the age of the patient, the duration of diabetes, and the presence of diabetic retinopathy (12,29,33,35). In general, DHS is more common in patients with long-standing diabetes and microvascular disease. The presence of DHS may indicate that the patient is at high risk for microvascular disease. In patients with diabetes for 16 years, the prevalence of observed microvascular lesions was three- to fourfold higher in those with hand contractures than in those without contractures (29,33–36). There is some evidence that joint contractures in patients with diabetes are linked with delayed median-nerve conduction and intrinsic hand-muscle wasting (37–39).

In addition, a form of restrictive lung disease has been described in patients with DHS in which total and vital lung capacity is decreased (20,24–26). These patients are usually asymptomatic but may experience dyspnea secondary to hypoxemia. It is likely that in some instances similar abnormalities in connective tissue occur in the hand and the lung.

The limitation of joint movement probably results from dermal and subcutaneous sclerosis (30,40–41). In addition, the fibrous thickening of the flexor tendon sheaths contributes to the loss of mobility. The pathogenesis of these altered connective tissues remains obscure. Pathologically, a biopsy of the thickened skin reveals dermal fibrosis with increased collagen deposition in the dermis and loss of sebaceous glands and other secondary skin appendages (29,31). Raynaud phenomenon, digital ulcers, or other systemic manifestations of scleroderma or other autoimmune diseases are not present. Laboratory evaluation is unrevealing, and radiographs of the hands may be normal or show diffuse osteopenia. Some investigators have documented increased cross-linking of collagen, which leads to increased resistance to collagenase and the resultant decrease in turnover (42–44). Increased nonenzymatic glycosylation of collagen, which might increase intermolecular cross-linking, has also been demonstrated (45–51). Other possible factors include increased hydration of collagen, swelling of the connective tissue through the aldose reductase pathway, and microangiopathy leading to increased collagen synthesis.

Importantly, the role of sorbitol has been hypothesized as possibly contributing to the microvascular complications in patients with diabetes. Hyperglycemia promotes increases in the amount of sorbitol accumulating in cells. In cells, glucose is converted to sorbitol via the enzyme aldose reductase, which may be responsible for an increase in cell osmolality, decreased cell myoinositol, and other factors that may promote collagen and connective tissue abnormalities (52–54). Thus, if sorbitol plays a major role in collagen dysregulation or tissue damage, the use of aldose reductase inhibitors in patients with diabetes may decrease the accumulation of sorbitol and subsequently decrease the microvascular and collagen complications of diabetes. Clinical trials of aldose reductase inhibitors have not shown consistent improvement in the microvascular complications, such as retinopathy, neuropathy, and nephropathy (52–54). There is one report of three patients with contractures who demonstrated a reversal of hand symptoms with aldose reductase inhibitors (55).

Another proposed mechanism is the accumulation of advanced glycosylated end products (AGEs) that may predispose to collagen abnormalities and tissue injury (56,57). Hyperglycemia provides an environment of enhanced glucose availability that accelerates the deposition of AGEs into tissues. This may lead to a stronger cross-linking potential of collagen *in vivo* and vascular injury, as endothelial cells have receptors for AGEs. Clinical trials are now being conducted on aminoguanidine, an agent that prevents the deposition of AGEs in tissue, for the prevention of diabetic nephropathy (58). Perhaps future studies will be undertaken for DHS.

Therapy for the diabetic hand syndrome should include dynamic splinting and an attempt to increase range of motion through exercise. It is unclear without prospective studies whether an increase in exercise will prevent the onset of limited joint mobility or will restore joint mobility that has been lost. Aspirin, NSAIDs, or opiate analgesics for those who are not responding to local modalities may be helpful in controlling pain and stiffness. There are case reports in the literature suggesting that better glycemic control may lead to a decrease in skin thickness (59).

Dupuytren Disease

Dupuytren disease is common in the general population and increases in incidence as the population ages (3,60). It causes a focal flexion contracture with a thickened band of palmar fascia. Flexion deformities along with tethering of the skin are noted. Knuckle pads (Garrod pads), as well as heel-pad nodules, may be noted (3). Pain and loss of motion result. Dupuytren contracture, in which a low-grade inflammatory reaction producing nodularity may occur, often is associated with diabetes. Contractures may involve the third, fourth, or fifth flexor tendons.

It has been suggested that 25% of patients with Dupuytren contractures have diabetes (2,61). In addition, studies have shown that 21% to 63% of patients with diabetes have the contractures, in contrast to 5% to 22% of the normal population (2). Noble et al. (62) reported the development of this complication in more than 50% of patients with diabetes and an increase in incidence with duration of diabetes and also demonstrated that a high proportion—as high as 16% of adults with diabetes—have Dupuytren contracture at the time of diagnosis of diabetes.

The pathogenesis of Dupuytren disease remains unknown. Occasionally, a history of occupational or other trauma may precede its onset. Investigators have described the occurrence of modified fibroblasts (myofibroblasts) that resemble smooth muscle cells and are contractile within tendon nodules (63,64). Proliferation of these cells with subsequent contraction might subject neighboring fascial structures to intermittent tension, resulting in hypertrophy. These same cells have also been reported in the nodules of patients with Ledderhose disease and may be present in the abnormal tissues of patients with Peyronie disease (65,66).

In addition, studies have documented the deposition of increased amounts of type III collagen in the palmar aponeurosis and in diseased fascia. It appears that as more type III collagen is deposited, the disease becomes more severe. The greatest proportion of type III collagen is found in the nodules. It is unknown whether onset is linked to impaired glucose tolerance (67–69) or whether good glucose control in the diabetic patient will limit onset of this problem (70–73). The presence of $CD3^+$ lymphocytes in tissue and expression of major histocompatibility complex class II proteins may implicate a T cell–mediated autoimmune disorder (74–76).

Treatment includes aggressive physical therapy, including dynamic splinting and exercises. NSAIDs or other analgesics may be helpful in decreasing pain. Intralesional glucocorticoid injections may provide relief of pain as well as increased range of motion. Occasionally, surgical release of the contracture is necessary.

Neuroarthropathy

Diabetes mellitus is one of the major causes of Charcot joints. The usual presentation is that of a patient with long-standing diabetes, often complicated by hypertension, proteinuria, and retinopathy, who develops joint swelling or deformity after the age of 50. The foot is most commonly involved, followed in frequency by the ankle and knee. Rarely, upper extremity joints are involved. Unilateral painless foot swelling is the most common presentation. Warmth and erythema may be present. When they are present, the differential diagnosis includes gout, pseudogout, osteomyelitis, or septic arthritis. Typically, there are few systemic symptoms and no documented fever and leukocytosis. Radiographically, there are destructive changes of the tarsometatarsal and metatarsophalangeal joints. Involvement of the tarsal and proximal metatarsal bones may occur and lead to osteoporosis, osteolysis, and bone fragmentation (77,78).

Another physical examination finding of neuropathic joint is termed "claw toe." This arises as chronic motor neuropathy affects the small intrinsic muscles of the feet. When the larger muscles of the anterior tibial compartment are unopposed, subluxation of the proximal interphalangeal metatarsal joints may result, leading to a claw-toe appearance. This may lead to excessive pressure on the metatarsal heads and thus the tendency to form skin ulcers.

Patients with diabetic peripheral sensory neuropathy have a loss of pain and proprioceptive sensations distally. This loss of the normal afferent signals reduces the protection of the joint from microtrauma, which may result in progressive joint destruction (2,3). In addition, ischemia secondary to both large- and small-vessel disease may play an etiologic role. Whitehouse and Wechstein (77) have suggested that this osteopathy represents a healing phase of local osteomyelitis.

Management of diabetic neuroarthropathy is difficult. Lumbar sympathectomy, arthrodesis, immobilization, and special footwear have been of little value. Minimizing trauma, maintenance of good muscle strength, use of appropriate shoes, and regular inspection of the skin and nails to avoid secondary infection may be helpful. Splinting may exacerbate the problem and may lead to skin ulceration, perforation, and secondary osteomyelitis.

Spinal neuroarthropathy characterized by usually symmetric extensive new bone formation (hyperostosis) also occurs. The vertebral changes include sclerosis and altered bony trabeculae. These changes result in an inability of the vertebrae to withstand normal stresses, with resultant collapse. Typically, local pain and tenderness may occur in association with irritation of the nerve root.

Although not a true neuroarthropathy, the carpal tunnel syndrome (CTS) is a frequent cause of hand pain in patients with diabetes. Entrapment of the median nerve within the carpal tunnel results in hand pain and numbness in the second to fourth fingers, particularly at night. Diabetes mellitus is one of the systemic diseases most frequently associated with CTS. In one study, diabetes was present in 16.6% of patients with CTS (3). Other sensory peripheral neuropathies, such as ulnar neuropathy, may coexist with CTS and may be associated with the diabetic hand syndrome discussed previously. Therapy for CTS includes the use of NSAIDs and splinting. If these are ineffective, local glucocorticoid injection or surgical release of the retinaculum may be indicated.

Hyperostosis

Although patients with type 1 diabetes have a tendency to develop osteopenia (78) (see later section), patients with type 2 diabetes seem to make more bone or to develop hyperostosis. In one study of 428 diabetic patients, 25% had hyperostosis of different areas, including spine involvement, hyperostosis frontalis interna, calcification of the pelvic ligaments, and osteitis condensans ilii (3). New bone formation around the hips, knees, and wrists has also been noted (25,79). In Morgagni syndrome, hyperostosis frontalis interna is accompanied by type 2 diabetes (3).

The most common form of new bone formation in diabetes is disseminated idiopathic skeletal hyperostosis (DISH) or ankylosing hyperostosis of the spine. This syndrome occurs in 2% to 4% of the normal population over the age of 40; in contrast, the prevalence is 13% in patients with diabetes (80,81). In patients with diabetes between the ages of 60 and 69, the prevalence increases to more than 20% (81). The presence of DISH is also associated with obesity, independent of diabetes. No correlation has been found between the degree of diabetic control and the extent of the hyperostosis.

Typically, a patient with DISH may complain of some mild back pain and stiffness, but range of motion is preserved. Occasionally, the abnormality may be an incidental radiographic finding. Sparing of the posterior spinal joints probably accounts for the preservation of good back motion (82). The syndrome is characterized by asymmetric osteophytes or bony outgrowths that extend vertically along the anterolateral surface of the vertebral bodies, particularly on the right. Anterior bridges between vertebrae and sclerosis of the underlying bony cortex are seen. Unlike patients with ankylosing spondylitis, these patients rarely complain of early-morning stiffness and loss of back motion. In addition, the sacroiliac joints are spared. Radiographically, the vertebral body osteoporosis seen in ankylosing spondylitis is absent. Although early reports suggested an association between DISH and the histocompatibility antigen HLA-B27, this has not been confirmed (2,83,84). The thoracic spine is most commonly involved in DISH, followed by the cervical spine and the lumbar spine. If extensive involvement of the anterior cervical spine occurs, it may result in dysphagia and disturbance of esophageal function.

In addition to the spinal involvement of DISH, widespread osseous changes may be detected elsewhere. These changes are most common around the acetabulum and where fluffy new bone is formed, but similar changes around the knees and wrists have been documented. In addition, some of the changes in the spine can be internal within the canal as well as external. Changes have been noted around the apophyseal joints; these changes may impinge on emerging nerve roots, while the intervertebral discs may be relatively normal. Thus, there may be symptoms of radicular irritation as well as mild localized pain. Degenerative arthritis of the hips has frequently been noted. However, this is a common occurrence in this particular age group with or without DISH. It is unclear whether a progressive degenerative disease of the hip is a unique phenomenon in this syndrome or is just an associated clinical event.

The explanation for the association of diabetes and new bone formation is unclear. Levels of growth hormone are normal in these patients. An abnormal or exaggerated serum insulin response to glucose challenge has been documented in some patients with ankylosing hyperostosis without diabetes (85,86). It is probable that insulin and/or insulin-like growth factors may be important in promoting new bone formation in patients with adult-onset diabetes, obesity, or both of these disorders.

COMMON RHEUMATIC DISEASES ASSOCIATED WITH DIABETES MELLITUS

Osteoarthritis

Osteoarthritis, or degenerative joint disease, is the most common rheumatic disease in the general population. It may be asymptomatic or mild, but severe involvement leads to pain, stiffness, and limitation of motion in the affected joints, most commonly involving the knees, hips, and spine, and may be a source of major disability and morbidity. It is difficult to establish a relationship between common diseases such as osteoarthritis and diabetes, but several studies have documented a positive correlation (3). Several investigators have suggested that the prevalence of osteoarthritis is higher in young and middle-aged diabetic patients and that joint damage starts at an earlier age and is much more severe in diabetic than in control patients (3).

Insulin has been demonstrated to stimulate cartilage growth and proteoglycan biosynthesis. These effects are likely mediated through somatomedin (insulin-like growth factor-1) (87–94). Although insulin may alter the extracellular matrix present in bone and cartilage, the significance of such changes, particularly as a cause of osteoarthritis, has not been determined. Treatment of osteoarthritis is directed toward the control of pain with acetaminophen or NSAIDs, as well as physical therapy–guided exercise programs for the strengthening of muscles and tendons.

Gout and Hyperuricemia

Gout is a heterogeneous disorder characterized by hyperuricemia and arthritis induced by the accumulation of urate crystals. Acute gouty arthritis is characterized by severe joint pain, redness, warmth, and tenderness usually affecting a lower extremity joint. Gout is a recognized but relatively uncommon complication of diabetic ketoacidosis (3). Patients with diabetes who have uncontrolled glucose metabolism associated with ketoacidosis will develop hyperuricemia as a result of competitive inhibition of tubular excretion of urate in the kidney by organic acids. Dehydration and increased protein catabolism also play a role. In addition, many patients with advanced diabetes have nephropathy, which may lead to renal transplantation. Transplant patients require immunosuppressive therapy to prevent rejection of the transplanted kidney. Antirejection drugs such as cyclosporine may increase serum uric acid levels, leading to gouty flares and tophaceous gout.

There is also a possible correlation between chronically stable diabetes and onset of gout symptoms (95,96). Previous studies have demonstrated an increased incidence of hyperuricemia in individuals with stable diabetes and of hyperglycemia in patients with gout. It is likely that a significant proportion of this latter group are patients with gout who are obese with relative states of insulin resistance leading to abnormal glucose tolerance. In addition, many of these studies did not make age correlations. It is now known that glucose tolerance decreases with age. Thus, age may be a link between gout and diabetes. Unfortunately, no prospective studies with age-, sex-, and weight-matched controls have been performed, but it appears that the risk of gout in nonobese patients with diabetes is no greater than that in the normal population (3). Paradoxically, the new onset of frank diabetes has been accompanied by a decrease in serum urate levels and a reduction in the frequency and severity of attacks in patients with preexisting gout (3,97). In general, obesity may be the most important factor linking hyperglycemia with hyperuricemia, as obesity is known to precipitate hyperglycemia, hyperuricemia, and hyperlipidemia (98,99).

Acute gouty attacks may be treated with indomethacin, other NSAIDs, or colchicine. Long-term prophylaxis with allopurinol or a uricosuric agent may be necessary in some clinical settings.

Calcium Pyrophosphate Deposition Disease

Pseudogout is an inflammatory arthritis caused by the deposition of calcium pyrophosphate dihydrate crystals in synovial structures. It may present as an acute monoarticular arthritis, chronic polyarticular inflammatory arthritis, or asymptomatic chondrocalcinosis, defined as linear deposition of calcium pyrophosphate crystals in cartilage, which appear calcified on plain radiographs. Calcium pyrophosphate deposition disease (CPPD) arthropathy is suggested by the radiologic finding of chondrocalcinosis in a patient with acute or chronic inflammatory arthritis and the identification by polarizing light microscopy of weakly positive birefringent rhomboid-shaped crystals in synovial fluid. Acute inflammatory arthritis secondary to CPPD, or pseudogout, without radiographic evidence of chondrocalcinosis, has been reported, particularly in the small joints (2).

In 1974, McCarty et al. (101) demonstrated the apparent clinical association of CPPD arthropathy with diabetes. However, this observation has not been confirmed (100). Alexander et al. (100) were unable to document the association in 105 consecutive patients with CPPD arthropathy. The incidence of CPPD arthropathy in diabetic patients has been reported to range between 8% and 73% (3) compared with an incidence of 0.2% in the normal population (101). This discrepancy must be attributable to variations in the diagnostic criteria used in the studies as well as to intervening variables such as age and osteoarthritis.

It is possible that the simultaneous occurrence of CPPD arthropathy and diabetes represents no more than the chance association of two relatively common abnormalities in elderly patients. Alternatively, it is also possible that diabetic patients with chondrocalcinosis are more susceptible than diabetic patients to symptomatic articular disease such as pseudogout. Certainly, an elderly patient presenting with CPPD arthropathy should be tested for subclinical diabetes. The corollary is true as well; pseudogout should be considered in each diabetic patient who presents with articular symptoms.

Symptomatic CPPD arthropathy may be managed with systemic antiinflammatory drugs such as NSAIDs, colchicine, or prednisone. Aspiration of the affected joints alone and/or the intraarticular injection of glucocorticoids may also be effective. McCarty et al. (101,102) suggested that control of hyperglycemia in diabetic patients did not appear to influence the frequency or severity of recurrent attacks of CPPD arthropathy.

Osteopenia

There is controversy about the incidence of osteopenia and osteoporosis in patients with diabetes. Several studies support the relationship between type 1 diabetes and reduced bone mass (103–108). In children, objective measurements of forearm bone mineral density reveal an 8% reduction in cortical bone density and a 14% reduction in trabecular bone density in children with diabetes compared with these values in age- and sex-matched controls (104). A similar reduction in bone mass occurs in adults (106). The decrease in bone density is detectable early in the disease (104). In adults, the rate of bone loss is maximal at or soon after diagnosis of diabetes and is correlated with the serum level of endogenous insulin (109). As insulin levels fall, the incidence of osteopenia increases. However, the relationship between the degree of metabolic control in patients with type 1 diabetes and the degree of osteopenia has not been well documented. In patients with type 2 diabetes, results of forearm bone density studies are conflicting (103,110–112). As discussed previously, hyperostosis, not osteopenia, may occur in this patient population.

Although patients with diabetes may have osteopenia, the evidence regarding the consequences of this osteopenia is confusing. The incidence of diabetes among patients with femoral neck fractures appears to be greater than expected by chance, the relative risk values reported being 1.16 to 3.4 (113–117). However, there is no good evidence about the incidence of vertebral compression fractures in patients with diabetes (118).

The role of insulin in normal bone turnover remains a puzzle. Insulin is an anabolic hormone, and the effects of insulin and insulin-like growth factors have been well documented (119–126). Insulin stimulates nucleotide synthesis by osteoblasts *in vitro*, promotes the intracellular accumulation of amino acids in membranous bone, and can restore levels of circulating somatomedin in experimental diabetes (122–124). Insulin-like growth factors have also been shown to promote synthesis of bone collagen (119,120,123,125) and to increase the deposition of calcium in the skeleton (121,126). These findings suggest that when circulating levels of insulin are decreased, the synthesis of a good bone matrix will be inadequate and the bone will not calcify. It is possible that in type 2 diabetes, with its insulin resistance, hyperinsulinemia will stimulate bony overgrowth. This suggestion is supported by recent data demonstrating that bone mineral density is increased, not decreased, in patients with type 2 diabetes who have increased levels of endogenous insulin but decreased sensitivity to insulin (127).

Osteolysis of Forefoot

A distinct clinical syndrome has been described in patients with diabetes that is characterized by patchy or generalized osteoporosis of the distal metatarsal and proximal phalanges in association with variable amounts of pain and erythema (3,128–130). Because of the appearance of the forefoot, both cellulitis and osteomyelitis need to be considered in the differential diagnosis and excluded by laboratory, radiographic, and microbiologic data. Diabetic patients with this syndrome do not necessarily have small-vessel vascular disease or neuropathy. Osteopenia may be accompanied by juxtaarticular erosions mimicking rheumatoid arthritis or gout (128,129). Articular surfaces are initially spared, but progressive osteolysis may cause disappearance of adjacent bone. At any stage during this process, the syndrome may resolve spontaneously and normal bony architecture may be partially or completely restored. The cause of this condition is unknown. Severe disease with osteoporosis and subsequent fracture or fragmentation of the bone may be confused with neuropathic joint disease. Because the syndrome resolves spontaneously, no specific treatment is recommended.

Migratory Osteolysis of Hip and Knee

The syndrome of migratory osteolysis of the hip and knee is characterized by local areas of decreased bone density or osteopenia associated with significant local pain. The pain may last for up to 1 year and usually resolves without sequelae. Typically, the patient is a woman over 50 years of age who presents with severe pain initially involving one joint in the lower extremity. The painful joint is usually a large weight-bearing joint, but any joint can be affected. The pain is out of proportion to the physical findings. There are few signs of inflammation, although an effusion may be present. However, the joint fluid is usually not inflammatory when aspirated. There may be a recent history of pain similar in type that may have affected a different joint in the lower extremity and resolved spontaneously. Blood tests are usually not helpful. Radiographs of the joint may reveal a small localized area of osteopenia, but the bone scan will show significantly increased uptake over the affected area.

The etiology of this syndrome remains obscure. In a study of 34 patients with involvement of the hip, five were diabetic and all had an exaggerated serum triglyceride response following alcohol ingestion (3). Doury et al. (9) made an association between diabetes and migratory osteolysis of the knee; however, both of these syndromes are typically seen in patients older than 50 years, the age at which the incidence of type 2 diabetes increases. Patients are typically remarkably sensitive to low-dose glucocorticoid treatment, which may exacerbate the insulin resistance and thus worsen the diabetes. In Europe the use of calcitonin has gained popularity. However, because calcitonin induces a decrease in the output of endogenous insulin *in vitro*, this therapy should be used with caution (3).

REFERENCES

1. Gray RG, Gottlieb NL. Rheumatic disorders associated with diabetes mellitus: literature review. *Semin Arthritis Rheum* 1976;6:19–34.
2. Holt PJL. Rheumatological manifestations of diabetes mellitus. *Clin Rheum Dis* 1981;7:723–746.
3. Crisp AJ, Heathcoate JG. Connective tissue abnormalities in diabetes mellitus. *J R Coll Physicians* 1984;18:132–141.
4. Bruckner FE. Frozen shoulder (adhesive capsulitis) [editorial]. *J R Soc Med* 1982;75:688–689.
5. Stodell MA, Nicholson R, Scott J, et al. Radioisotope scanning in the painful shoulder. *Rheumatol Rehabil* 1980;19:163–166.
6. Bridgman JF. Periarthritis of the shoulder and diabetes mellitus. *Ann Rheum Dis* 1972;31:69–71.
7. Arkkila P, Dnatola I, Biidari J, et al. Shoulder capsulitis in type I and II diabetic patients: association with diabetic complications and related diseases. *Ann Rheum Dis* 1996;55:907–914.
8. Pal B, Anderson, J, Dick WC, et al. Limitation of joint mobility and shoulder capsulitis in insulin and non insulin dependent diabetes mellitus. *Br J Rheumatol* 1986:25:147–151.
9. Doury P, Dirheimer Y, Pattin S. *Algodystrophy: diagnosis and therapy of a frequent disease of the locomotor apparatus.* Berlin: Springer-Verlag, 1981.
10. Steinbrocker O. The shoulder-hand syndrome: associated painful homolateral disability of the shoulder and hand with swelling and atrophy of the hand. *Am J Med* 1947;3:402–407.
11. Steinbrocker O, Argyros TG. The shoulder-hand syndrome: present status as a diagnostic and therapeutic entity. *Med Clin North Am* 1958;42:1533–1553.
12. Jung Y, Hohmann TC, Gerneth JA, et al. Diabetic hand syndrome. *Metabolism* 1971;20:1008–1015.
13. Grgic A, Rosenbloom AL, Weber FT, et al. Joint contractures—common manifestation of childhood diabetes mellitus. *J Pediatr* 1976;88:584–588.
14. Kapoor A, Sibbitt WL Jr. Contractures in diabetes mellitus: the syndrome of limited joint mobility. *Semin Arthritis Rheum* 1989;18:168–180.
15. Lundbaek K. Stiff hands in long-term diabetes. *Acta Med Scand* 1957;158: 447–451.
16. Pastan RS, Cohen AS. The rheumatologic manifestation of diabetes mellitus. *Med Clin North Am* 1978;62:829–839.
17. Campbell RR, Hawkins SJ, Maddison PJ, et al. Limited joint mobility in diabetes mellitus. *Ann Rheum Dis* 1985;44:93–97.
18. Slama G, Letanoux M, Thibult N, et al. Quantification of early subclinical limited joint mobility in diabetes mellitus. *Diabetes Care* 1985;8:329–332.
19. Eaton RP. The collagen hydration hypothesis: a new paradigm for the secondary complications of diabetes mellitus. *J Chronic Dis* 1986;39:763–766.
20. Schuyler MR, Niewoehner DE, Inkley SP, et al. Abnormal lung elasticity in juvenile diabetes. *Am Rev Respir Dis* 1976;113:37–41.
21. Eversmeyer WH. Digital sclerosis in adult insulin-dependent diabetes [letter]. *Arthritis Rheum* 1983;26:932.
22. Rosenbloom AL, Silverstein JH, Riley WJ, Maclaren NK. Limited joint mobility in childhood diabetes: family studies. *Diabetes Care* 1983;6:370–373.
23. Rosenbloom AL. Skeletal and joint manifestations of childhood diabetes. *Pediatr Clin North Am* 1984;31:569–586.
24. Buckingham BA, Uitto J, Sandborg C, et al. Sclerodermalike changes in insulin-dependent diabetes mellitus: clinical and biochemical studies. *Diabetes Care* 1984;7:163–169.
25. Buckingham B, Perejda AJ, Sandborg C, et al. Skin, joint and pulmonary changes in type I diabetes mellitus. *Am J Dis Child* 1986;140:420–423.
26. Schnapf BM, Banks RA, Silverstein JH, et al. Pulmonary function in insulin-dependent diabetes mellitus with limited joint mobility. *Am Rev Respir Dis* 1984;130:930–932.
27. Larkin JG, Frier BM. Limited joint mobility and Dupuytren's contracture in diabetic, hypertensive, and normal populations. *BMJ* 1986;292:1494.
28. Traisman HS, Traisman ES, Marr TJ, et al. Joint contractures in patients with juvenile diabetes and their siblings. *Diabetes Care* 1978;1:360–361.
29. Rosenbloom AL, Silverstein JH, Lezotte DC, et al. Limited joint mobility in childhood diabetes mellitus indicates increased risk for microvascular disease. *N Engl J Med* 1981;305:191–194.
30. Seibold JP. Digital sclerosis in children with insulin dependent diabetes mellitus. *Arthritis Rheum* 1982;25:1357–1361.
31. Starkman H, Brink S. Limited joint mobility of the hand in type I diabetes mellitus. *Diabetes Care* 1982;5:534–536.
32. Silverstein JH, Gordon G, Pollock BH, et al. Long-term glycemic control influences the onset of limited joint mobility in type 1 diabetes. *J Pediatr* 1998; 132: 944–947.
33. Lawson PM, Maneschi F, Kohner EM. The relationship of hand abnormalities to diabetes and diabetic retinopathy. *Diabetes Care* 1983;6:140–143.
34. Rosenbloom AL, Silverstein JH, Lezotte DC, et al. Limited joint mobility in diabetes mellitus of childhood: natural history and relationship to growth impairment. *J Pediatr* 1982;101:874–878.
35. Fitzcharles MA, Duby S, Waddell RW, et al. Limitation of joint mobility (cheiroarthropathy) in adult noninsulin-dependent diabetic patients. *Ann Rheum Dis* 1984;43:251–257.

36. Starkman HS, Gleason RE, Rand LI, et al. Limited joint mobility (LJM) of the hand in patients with diabetes mellitus: relation to chronic complications. *Ann Rheum Dis* 1986;45:130–135.
37. Aljahlan M, Lee K, Toth E. Limited joint mobility in diabetes: diabetic cheiroarthropathy may be a clue to more serious complications. *Postgrad Med* 1999;105:99–106.
38. Gamstedt A, Holm-Glad J, Ohlson CG, et al. Hand abnormalities are strongly associated with the duration of diabetes mellitus. *J Intern Med* 1993; 234:189–193.
39. Chaudhuri KR, Davidson AR, Morris IM. Limited joint mobility and carpal tunnel syndrome in insulin-dependent diabetes. *Br J Rheumatol* 1989;28:191–194.
40. Robertson JR, Earnshaw PM, Campbell IW. Tenolysis in juvenile diabetic cheiroarthropathy. *BMJ* 1979;2:971–972.
41. Sherry DD, Rothstein RRL, Perty RE. Joint contractures preceding insulin-dependent diabetes mellitus. *Arthritis Rheum* 1982;11:1362–1364.
42. Harris ED Jr, Farrell ME. Resistance to collagenase: a characteristic of collagen fibrils cross-linked by formaldehyde. *Biochim Biophys Acta* 1972;278:133–141.
43. Vater CA, Harris ED Jr, Siegel RC. Native cross-links in collagen fibrils induce resistance to human synovial collagenase. *Biochem J* 1979;181:639–645.
44. Chang K, Uitto J, Rowold EA, et al. Increased collagen cross-linkages in experimental diabetes: reversal by β-aminopropionitrile and D-penicillamine. Diabetes 1980;29:778–781.
45. Berenson GS, Radhakrishnamurthy B, Dalferes ER Jr, et al. Connective tissue macromolecular changes in rats with experimentally induced diabetes and hyperinsulinism. *Diabetes* 1972;21:733–743.
46. Sharma C, Dalferes ER Jr, Radhakrishnamurthy B, et al. Glycoprotein biosynthesis during inflammation in normal and streptozotocin-induced diabetic rats. *Inflammation* 1985;9:273–283.
47. Tenni R, Tavella D, Donnelly P, et al. Cultured fibroblasts of juvenile diabetics have excessively soluble pericellular collagen. *Biochem Biophys Res Comm* 1980;92:1071–1075.
48. Rosenberg H, Modrak JB, Hassing JM, et al. Glycosylated collagen. *Biochem Biophys Res Comm* 1979;91:498–501.
49. Schnider SL, Kohn RR. Glucosylation of human collagen in aging and diabetes mellitus. *J Clin Invest* 1980;66:1179–1181.
50. Schnider SL, Kohn RR. Effects of age and diabetes mellitus on the solubility and nonenzymatic glycosylation of human skin collagen. *J Clin Invest* 1981; 67:1630–1635.
51. Perejda AJ, Uitto J. Nonenzymatic glycosylation of collagen and other proteins: relationship to development of diabetic complications. *Coll Relat Res* 1982;2: 81–88.
52. Freidman, E. Aldose reductase inhibitor in prevention of diabetic complications. In: Rose BD, ed. *UpToDate*. Wellesley, MA: 2003. Available at: www.uptodate.com
53. Macleod AF, Boulton AJ, Owens DR, et al. A multicentre trial of the aldose-reductase inhibitor tolrestat, in patients with symptomatic diabetic peripheral neuropathy. North European Tolrestat Study Group. *Diabetes Metab* 1992; 18:14–20.
54. Frank RN. The aldose reductase controversy. *Diabetes* 1994;43:169–172.
55. Eaton RP, Sibbitt WL Jr, Harsh A. The effect of an aldose reductase inhibiting agent on limited joint mobility in diabetic patients. *JAMA* 1985;253:1437–1440.
56. Brownlee M. Glycation and diabetic complications. *Diabetes* 1994;43:836–841.
57. Weiss, MF. Pathogenic role of advanced glycation end products (AGEs): an overview. *Perit Dial Int* 1999:19[Suppl 2]:S47.
58. Freidman, E. Aminoguanidine in the prevention of diabetic complications. In: Rose BD, ed. *UpToDate*. Wellesley, MA: 2003. Available at: www.uptodate.com
59. Lieberman LS, Rosenbloom AL, Riley WJ, et al. Reduced skin thickness with pump administration of insulin [letter]. *N Engl J Med* 1980;303:940–941.
60. Mikkelsen OA. The prevalence of Dupuytren's disease in Norway: a study in a representative population sample of the municipality of Haugesund. *Acta Chir Scand* 1972;138:695–700.
61. Davies JS, Finesilver EM. Dupuytren's contracture—with a note on the incidence of the contracture in diabetes. *Arthritis Surg* 1932;24:933–989.
62. Noble J, Heathcote JG, Cohen H. Diabetes mellitus in the aetiology of Dupuytren's disease. *J Bone Joint Surg* [Br] 1984;66B:322–325.
63. Gabbiani G, Majno G. Dupuytren's contracture: fibroblast contraction? An ultrastructural study. *Am J Pathol* 1972;66:131–146.
64. Gabbiani G, Majno G, Ryan GB. The fibroblast as a contractile cell: the myofibroblast. In: Kulonen E, Pikkarainen J, eds. *Biology of fibroblast*. New York: Academic Press, 1973:139–154.
65. Luck JV. Dupuytren's contracture: a new concept of the pathogenesis correlated with surgical management. *J Bone Joint Surg*[Am] 1959;41A:635–664.
66. Somers KD, Dawson DM, Wright GL Jr, et al. Cell culture of Peyronie's disease plaque and normal penile tissue. *J Urol* 1982;127:585–588.
67. Revach M, Cabilli C. Dupuytren's contracture and diabetes mellitus. *Isr J Med Sci* 1972;8:774–775.
68. Spring M, Fleck H, Cohen BD. Dupuytren's contracture: warning of diabetes? *N Y State J Med* 1970;70:1037–1041.
69. Ravid M, Dinzi Y, Sohar E. Dupuytren's disease in diabetes mellitus. *Acta Diabetol Lat* 1977;14:170–174.
70. Bazin S, Le-Lous M, Duance VC, et al. Biochemistry and histology of the connective tissue of Dupuytren's disease lesions. *Eur J Clin Invest* 1980;10:9–116.
71. Brickley-Parsons D, Glimcher MJ, Smith RJ, et al. Biochemical changes in the collagen of the palmar fascia in patients with Dupuytren's disease. *J Bone Joint Surg* [Am] 1981;63A:787–797.
72. Ehrlich HP, Brown H, White BS. Evidence for type V and I trimer collagens in Dupuytren's contracture palmar fascia. *Biochem Med* 1982;28:273–284.
73. Aumailley M, Krieg T, Razaka G, et al. Influence of cell density on collagen biosynthesis in fibroblast cultures. *Biochem J* 1982;206:505–510.
74. Baird KS, Alwan WH, Croscan JF, et al. T cell mediated response in Dupuytren's disease. *Lancet* 1993;342:366.
75. Hordon L. Diabetic neuropathic arthropathy. In: Rose BD, ed. *UpToDate*. Wellesley, MA: 2003. Available at: www.uptodate.com
76. Sheon RP, Anderson BC. Dupuytren's contracture. In: Rose BD, ed. *UpToDate*. Wellesley, MA: 2003. Available at: www.uptodate.com
77. Whitehouse FW, Wechstein M. On diabetic osteopathy: a radiographic study of 21 patients. *Diabetes Care* 1978;1:303–304.
78. Forgács S, Rosinger A, Vertes L. Diabetes mellitus and osteoporosis. *Endokrinologie* 1976;67:343–350.
79. Teotia SPS, Teotia M, Singh RK, et al. Hyperostosis and diabetes mellitus. *J Indian Med Assoc* 1978;71:117–118.
80. Julkunen H, Heinonen OP, Knekt P, et al. The epidemiology of hyperostosis of the spine together with its symptoms and related mortality in a general population. *J Scand Rheumatol* 1975;4:23–27.
81. Julkunen H, Kärävä R, Viljanen V. Hyperostosis of the spine in diabetes mellitus and acromegaly. *Diabetologia* 1966;2:123–126.
82. Vernon-Roberts B, Pirie CJ, Trenwith V. Pathology of the dorsal spine in ankylosing hyperostosis. *Ann Rheum Dis* 1974;33:281–288.
83. Forgács S, Halmos T, Salamon F. Bone changes in diabetes mellitus. *Isr J Med Sci* 1972;8:782–783.
84. Resnick D, Shapiro RF, Wiesner KE, et al. Diffuse idiopathic skeletal hyperostosis (DISH). *Semin Arthritis Rheum* 1978;7:153–187.
85. Julkunen H, Heinonen OP, Pyörälä K. Hyperostosis of the spine in an adult population: its relation to hyperglycaemia and obesity. *Ann Rheum Dis* 1971; 30:605–612.
86. Littlejohn GO, Smythe HA. Marked hyperinsulinemia after glucose challenge in patients with diffuse idiopathic skeletal hyperostosis. *J Rheumatol* 1981;8: 965–968.
87. Phillips LS, Young HS. Nutrition and somatomedin. II. Serum somatomedin activity and cartilage growth activity in streptozotocin-diabetic rats. *Diabetes* 1976;25:516–527.
88. Weiss RE, Reddi AH. Influence of experimental diabetes and insulin on matrix-induced cartilage and bone differentiation. *Am J Physiol* 1980;238: E200–E207.
89. Weiss RE, Gorn AH, Nimni ME. Abnormalities in the biosynthesis of cartilage and bone proteoglycans in experimental diabetes. *Diabetes* 1981;30:670–677.
90. Axelsson I, Lorentzon R, Pita JC. Biosynthesis of rat growth plate proteoglycans in diabetes and malnutrition. *Calcif Tissue Int* 1983;35:237–242.
91. Caterson B, Baker JR, Christner JE, et al. Diabetes and osteoarthritis. *Ala J Med Sci* 1980;17:292–299.
92. Stuart CA, Furlanetto RW, Lebovitz HE. The insulin receptor of embryonic chicken cartilage. *Endocrinology* 1979;105:1293–1302.
93. Foley TP Jr, Nissley SP, Stevens RL, et al. Demonstration of receptors for insulin and insulin-like growth factors on swarm rat chondrosarcoma chondrocytes: evidence that insulin stimulates proteoglycan synthesis through the insulin receptor. *J Biol Chem* 1982;257:633–639.
94. Axelsson I, Pita JC, Howell DS, et al. Kinetics of proteoglycans and cells in growth plate of normal, diabetic, and malnourished rats. *Pediatr Res* 1990;27: 41–44.
95. Whitehouse FW, Cleary WJ Jr. Diabetes mellitus in patients with gout. *JAMA* 1966;197:73–76.
96. Boyle JA, McKiddie M, Buchanan KD, et al. Diabetes mellitus and gout: blood sugar and plasma insulin responses to oral glucose in normal weight, overweight, and gouty patients. *Ann Rheum Dis* 1969;28:374–378.
97. Herman JB, Goldbourt U. Uric acid and diabetes: observations in a population study. *Lancet* 1982;2:240–245.
98. Yano K, Rhoads GG, Kagan A. Epidemiology of serum uric acid among 8000 Japanese-American men in Hawaii. *J Chronic Dis* 1977;30:171–184.
99. Berkowitz D. Gout, hyperlipidemia, and diabetes interrelationships. *JAMA* 1966:197:77–80.
100. Alexander GM, Dieppe PA, Doherty M, et al. Pyrophosphate arthropathy: a study of metabolic associations and laboratory data. *Ann Rheum Dis* 1982;41: 377–381.
101. McCarty DJ, Silcox DC, Coe F, et al. Diseases associated with calcium pyrophosphate dihydrate crystal deposition: a controlled study. *Am J Med* 1974;56:704–714.
102. McCarty DJ, Silcox DC. Gout and pseudogout. *Geriatrics* 1973;28(June):110–120.
103. Levin ME, Boisseau VC, Avioli LV. Effects of diabetes mellitus on bone mass in juvenile and adult onset diabetes. *N Engl J Med* 1976;294:241–245.
104. Shore RM, Chesney RW, Mazess RB, et al. Osteopenia in juvenile diabetes. *Calcif Tissue Int* 1981;33:455–457.
105. Rosenbloom AL, Lezotte DC, Weber FT, et al. Diminution of bone mass in childhood diabetes. *Diabetes* 1977;26:1052–1055.
106. McNair P, Madsbad S, Christiansen C, et al. Osteopenia in insulin treated diabetes mellitus: its relation to age at onset, sex, and duration of disease. *Diabetologia* 1978;15:87–89.
107. Wiske PS, Wentworth SM, Norton JA Jr, et al. Evaluation of bone mass and growth in young diabetics. *Metabolism* 1982;31:848–854.
108. Selby PL. Osteopenia and diabetes. *Diabet Med* 1988;5:423–428.

109. McNair P, Christiansen C, Christensen MS, et al. Development of bone mineral loss in insulin-treated diabetes: a 1½ years follow-up study in sixty patients. *Eur J Clin Invest* 1981;11:55–59.
110. Meema HE, Meema S. The relationship of diabetes mellitus and body weight to osteoporosis in elderly females. *Can Med Assoc J* 1967;96:132–139.
111. De Leeuw I, Abs R. Bone mass and bone density in maturity-type diabetics measured by the ^{125}I photonabsorption technique. *Diabetes* 1977;26:1130–1135.
112. Ishida H, Seino Y, Matsukura Y, et al. Diabetic osteopenia and circulating levels of vitamin D metabolites in type 2 (noninsulin-dependent) diabetes. *Metabolism* 1985;34:797–801.
113. Paganini-Hill A, Ross RK, Gerkins VR, et al. Menopausal estrogen therapy and hip fractures. *Ann Intern Med* 1981;95:28–31.
114. Gallagher JC, Melton LJ, Riggs BL. Examination of prevalence rates of possible risk factors in a population with a fracture of the proximal femur. *Clin Orthop* 1980;153:158–165.
115. Hutchinson TA, Polansky SM, Feinstein AR. Post-menopausal oestrogens protect against fractures of hip and distal radius: a case-control study. *Lancet* 1979;2:705–709.
116. Menczel J, Makin M, Robin G, et al. Prevalence of diabetes mellitus in Jerusalem: its association with presenile osteoporosis. *Isr J Med Sci* 1972;8:918–919.
117. Alffram P-A. An epidemiologic study of cervical and trochanteric fractures of the femur in an urban population. *Acta Orthop Scand Suppl* 1964;65:9–109.
118. Nabarro JDN. Compression fractures of the dorsal spine in hypoglycaemic fits in diabetes. *BMJ* 1985;291:1320.
119. Canalis E. The hormonal and local regulation of bone formation. *Endocrinol Rev* 1983;4:62–77.
120. Raisz LG, Kream BE. Regulation of bone formation. *N Engl J Med* 1983;309:29–35, 83–89.
121. Locatto ME, Fernández MC, Abranzón H, et al. Calcium metabolism of rats with varying degrees of insulinopenia. *Bone Miner* 1990;8:119–130.
122. Puche RC, Romano MC, Locatto ME, et al. The effect of insulin on bone resorption. *Calcif Tissue Res* 1973;12:8–15.
123. Hahn TJ, Downing SJ, Phang JM. Insulin effects on amino acid transport in bone: dependence on protein synthesis and Na^+. *Am J Physiol* 1971;220:1717–1723.
124. Phillips LS, Orawski AT. Nutrition and somatomedin. III. Diabetic control, somatomedin, and growth in rats. *Diabetes* 1977;26:864–869.
125. Canalis E. Effect of hormones and growth factors on alkaline phosphatase activity and collagen synthesis in cultured rat calvariae. *Metabolism* 1983;32:14–20.
126. Dixit PK, Stern AMK. Effect of insulin on the incorporation of citrate and calcium into the bones of alloxan-diabetic rats. *Calcif Tissue Int* 1979;27:227–232.
127. Weinstock RS, Goland RS, Shane E, et al. Bone mineral density in women with type II diabetes mellitus. J Bone Miner Res 1989;4:97–101.
128. Schwarz GS, Berenyi MR, Siegel MW. Atrophic arthropathy and diabetic neuritis. *Am J Roentgenol* 1969;106: 523–529.
129. Clouse ME, Gramm HF, Legg M, et al. Diabetic osteoarthropathy: clinical and roentgenographic observations in 90 cases. *J Am Roentgenol* 1974;121:22–34.
130. Lithner F, Hietala S-O, Steen L. Skeletal lesions and arterial calcifications of the feet in diabetics. *Acta Med Scand Suppl* 1984;687:47–54.

CHAPTER 64

Effects of Diabetes Mellitus on the Digestive System

Hiroshi Mashimo, Roger J. May[†], and Raj K. Goyal

In 1936, Bargen (1) first described diarrhea and steatorrhea as complications of diabetes. It is now clear that all parts of the digestive system are affected by diabetes, and digestive system dysfunction is an important contributor to the morbidity of this disease (2–4). Digestive symptoms related to diabetes are reported to be common. Feldman and Schiller (3) questioned 136 unselected patients at a hospital diabetes clinic about the presence of gastrointestinal (GI) symptoms. Three fourths of all

[†]Deceased.

patients had digestive symptoms. Frequent GI symptoms were constipation (60%), abdominal pain (34%), nausea and vomiting (29%), diarrhea (22%), and fecal incontinence (20%). Moreover, digestive symptoms in persons with diabetes may lead to clinically significant decreases in quality-of-life scores (5). A more recent U.S. national survey of upper GI symptoms, including heartburn, also showed significantly more upper GI symptoms in persons with diabetes (50% vs. 38% in controls) (6). However, it is unclear whether such GI symptoms are significantly different in the diabetic population than in the nondiabetic population except for decreased heartburn and increased use of laxatives (7). Regardless, asymptomatic abnormalities of gut function frequently occur in these patients.

PATHOGENESIS OF DIGESTIVE SYSTEM DYSFUNCTION

The digestive system dysfunction in diabetes may result from diabetes itself or, more often, from diabetes-associated complications. Diabetic neuropathy plays an important role in motor and secretory abnormalities in the GI tract, in nausea, vomiting, and the syndrome of abdominal pain. Diabetic angiopathy and vascular complications play a role in the pathogenesis of intestinal ischemia, in the severity and outcome of cholecystitis and biliary tract surgery, and in the nerve and muscle dysfunction of diabetic gastroenteropathy. Defects in immune mechanisms in diabetes are related to an increased incidence of esophageal candidiasis, and decreased resistance to infection accounts for the many pyogenic complications in the digestive tracts of these patients.

Some of the digestive system abnormalities in diabetes may not be causally related to diabetes but may reflect a common association of diabetes with these abnormalities. For example, the increased incidence of gallstones and fatty liver is due to associated obesity and hyperlipidemia in patients with type 2 diabetes, and the incidence of celiac disease is increased because of a common gene that predisposes to both conditions. Similarly, gastric parietal cell antibodies are found in human leukocyte antigen (HLA) haplotypes that are prevalent in patients with type 1 diabetes (8).

Hormonal Changes in Diabetes

Other hormonal changes described in patients with diabetes play important roles in the pathogenesis of many digestive disorders. For example, increased postprandial hormone release of glucagon and pancreatic peptide in patients with diabetes may exacerbate the disturbed motility in subjects with type 2 diabetes (9). Amylin, a peptide hormone cosecreted with insulin by the pancreatic β-cells, is deficient in patients with type 1 diabetes and elevated in patients in the early stages of type 2 diabetes. Patients in the later stages of type 2 diabetes have reduced amylin secretion that appears before reduced insulin secretion. Amylin and its analogue pramlintide delay gastric emptying (10). Activity of the gastric inhibitory peptide (GIP) that normally inhibits gastric emptying is almost completely lost in patients with type 2 diabetes, although glucagon-like peptide-1 (GLP-1), expressed mainly by the gut L-cells after feeding, maintains its ability to stimulate insulin secretion in these patients, even long after sulfonylurea secondary failure, and may be an important therapeutic alternative in diabetes (11). Ghrelin, a novel peptide hormone synthesized primarily in the stomach, has potent insulin-releasing, appetite-promoting, and gastric promotility effects. This hormone is decreased in the serum of persons with type 2 diabetes (12).

Enteric Neuropathy in Diabetes

The GI tract is richly innervated by nerves, which can be divided into intrinsic and extrinsic nerves (13). The intrinsic nerves constitute the enteric nervous system (ENS). The extrinsic nerves contain sensory (afferent) and motor (efferent) fibers and are carried along sympathetic, parasympathetic, and somatic pathways to the central nervous system (CNS) (Fig. 64.1). In diabetes, any

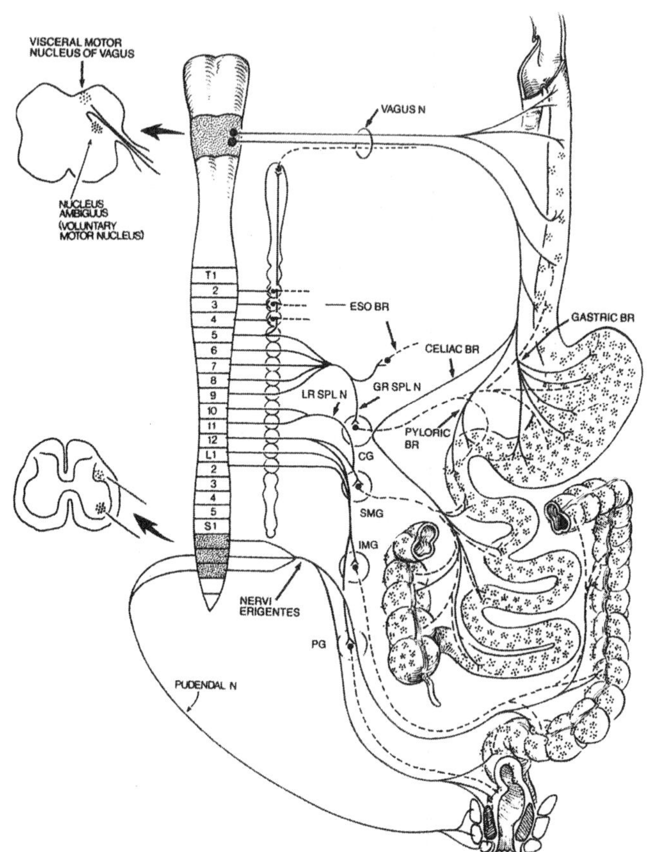

Figure 64.1. Efferent innervation of the gastrointestinal tract. The α motor neurons innervate skeletal muscle at either end of the gut. The α motor neurons to the pharynx and upper esophagus are present in the nucleus ambiguus, and their axons are carried in the vagus nerve. The α motor neurons to the external anal sphincter are present in Onuf's nucleus, and their axons are carried in the pudendal nerve. The sympathetic pathway consists of cell bodies of preganglionic neurons located in spinal cord segments T2 through L2. The preganglionic fibers are carried in the greater splanchnic nerve (GR SPL N), lesser splanchnic nerve (LR SPL N), and smallest splanchnic nerve (not labeled) to terminate in the celiac ganglion (CC), superior mesenteric ganglion (SMG), inferior mesenteric ganglion (IMG), and pelvic ganglion (PC). The postganglionic sympathetic neurons are distributed in a segmental fashion to the gastrointestinal tract. The parasympathetic pathway consists of vagal and sacral outflows. The vagal pathway consists of preganglionic parasympathetic axons whose cell bodies are present in the dorsal motor nucleus of vagus. The vagal parasympathetic fibers supply the gastrointestinal tract up to the right half of the colon. Sacral preganglionic parasympathetic fibers arising from neurons in spinal cord segments S2 to S4 (nervi erigentes) supply the left half of the colon, including the rectum and the internal anal sphincter. The postganglionic parasympathetic nerves and fibers are present intramurally in the gut wall. Sympathetic and parasympathetic nerves make extensive contacts with neurons in the enteric nervous system. In diabetes mellitus one or more components of efferent or afferent innervation (not shown) may be involved (see text). (From Goyal RK, Crist J. Neurology of the gut. In: Sleisenger MH, Fordtran JS, eds. *Gastrointestinal disease: pathophysiology, diagnosis, management.* Philadelphia: WB Saunders, 1989:21–52, with permission.)

one or several of the various components of the nerve elements that control gut function may be involved. The extent of neuropathy appears related to the duration of diabetes (14) and the age of patients (15). Diabetic enteric neuropathy is responsible for many of the GI abnormalities in these patients. The wide spectrum of possible enteric neuropathies may explain the wide range of GI dysfunction in the patient with diabetes.

PARASYMPATHETIC INNERVATION

The vagal efferents provide parasympathetic innervation to the entire gut down to the right half of the transverse colon. The left half of the colon and the rectum are innervated by sacral parasympathetic efferents. Parasympathetic preganglionic efferents are thinly myelinated or unmyelinated cholinergic axons. It is now clear that there are two parallel pathway vagal fibers that terminate on excitatory and inhibitory postganglionic neurons, respectively, in the enteric plexuses. The parasympathetic influence on the gut includes precise and localized motor and secretory control activity. The vast majority (>80%) of the vagal fibers are low-threshold afferents that are involved in nonnoxious sensations and primarily mediate reflex activities, including nausea, vomiting, and satiety.

Morphologic studies of vagal abnormalities in diabetes have had variable results. Diani et al. (16) reported marked abnormalities in the vagus nerve in nonketonuric and ketonuric diabetic Chinese hamsters. Analysis of axons from the ventral division of the vagus nerve demonstrated that in the diabetic animals the number of nonmyelinated axons and the numerical and volume density of myelinated fibers were markedly decreased. In an autopsy study of patients with diabetes, Smith (17) demonstrated sparse changes in the vagus nerve. Sections obtained at both the cervical and the diaphragmatic levels of the vagus showed that a small number of fibers had undergone segmental demyelination. A larger number of fibers showed wallerian changes of degeneration. Duchen et al. (18) described more severe pathologic changes of the vagus nerve in an autopsy study of four patients with prolonged diabetes. Guy et al. (19) described pathologic changes in a segment of the abdominal vagus removed during gastric surgery from a patient with severe gastroparesis. These changes included a marked reduction in unmyelinated axons; the remaining axons were characterized by a small diameter with an associated increase in surrounding collagen. In contrast to the above findings, Yoshida et al. (20) found no abnormalities on morphologic analysis of sections of the abdominal vagus nerve in five patients with diabetes, two of whom had symptomatic gastroparesis.

Functional studies provide evidence of parasympathetic efferent denervation of the gut in diabetes. Patients with longstanding diabetes have been found to have an impairment of the cephalic phase of gastric acid secretion. In such patients, sham feeding or insulin-induced hypoglycemia is associated with a diminished secretory response, a finding indicative of decreased vagal influence on the stomach. Moreover, the rise in serum levels of pancreatic polypeptide with sham feeding is also impaired in patients with advanced diabetes, indicating deficient parasympathetic innervation of the pancreas (21).

Of note, vagal or autonomic neuropathy does not uniformly affect innervation to all visceral organs. Similarly, there is no direct correlation between the presence of peripheral neuropathy and autonomic neuropathy. Autonomic neuropathy involving the heart is not predictive of GI dysmotility or of its extent (22).

SYMPATHETIC INNERVATION

The preganglionic neurons of sympathetic efferents are located in the spinal cord (T5 to L3), and the corresponding postganglionic neurons are located in the various sympathetic ganglia. The sympathetic efferent fibers entering the gut are postganglion adrenergic fibers that exert most of their actions indirectly via the enteric neurons. The sympathetic efferents exert inhibitory effects on the gut except in the sphincters, which are contracted by the sympathetic nerves.

In a pathologic study of autopsy findings in diabetic patients, Duchen et al. (18) found several abnormalities in the pattern of sympathetic innervation. In the intermediolateral columns of the spinal cord, where the sympathetic neurons arise, cell numbers appeared reduced at several thoracic levels. In addition, in the cervical and celiac sympathetic ganglia, neurons were distended or vacuolated with enlarged club-shaped neural processes. Chang et al. (23) demonstrated that rats with experimentally induced diabetes have a deficiency in adrenergic-mediated absorption of fluid and electrolyte in the ileum and colon, presumably secondary to deficient sympathetic innervation.

Sympathetic afferents carry visceral nociceptive information to the CNS. They also are involved in many sympathetic reflexes, including nausea and vomiting. It is possible that sympathetic afferent stimulation in neuropathy may be involved in the syndrome of abdominal pain, nausea, and vomiting, and the loss of afferent activity may lead to impaired perception of visceral pain.

ENTERIC NERVOUS SYSTEM

The enteric plexus, which consists of the myenteric and submucous plexuses, forms the ENS, which is the "local brain" of the gut. The ENS resembles the CNS in that it contains sensory, motor, and integrating-command interneurons and program generators. Moreover, ENS neurons, like CNS neurons, employ a large variety of neurotransmitters. These include acetylcholine, neuropeptides such as cholecystokinin (CCK), galanin, calcitonin gene-related peptide (CGRP), gastrin-releasing peptide (GRP), enkephalins, somatostatin, substance P, vasoactive intestinal polypeptide (VIP), purines such as adenosine triphosphate (ATP) and adenosine, and possibly amino acids such as γ-aminobutyric acid (GABA), and nitric oxide (NO). The major inhibitory neurotransmitters are VIP and NO, and the main excitatory neurotransmitters are acetylcholine and substance P.

Previous pathologic studies of diabetic patients in which conventional sections were used found the morphology of the myenteric plexus to be normal. More recent pathologic studies that used tangential sections demonstrated mild abnormalities in these patients. Smith (17) described the myenteric plexus of the esophagus as being mostly normal, with only a small number of neurons with swollen irregular processes. She also described the lymphocytic infiltration of a large number of nonneuronal cells in the plexus. Duchen et al. (18) confirmed this finding in sections from a wider distribution of the gut. Duchen also described infiltration of the ganglia with inflammatory cells, especially around unmyelinated axons. In contrast, Yoshida et al. (20), who prepared extensive sections from the stomachs of patients with diabetes, described the myenteric plexus as being completely normal with no evidence of morphologic change or inflammatory infiltrate.

Rats with streptozotocin-induced diabetes show distinctive and contrasting changes in the nerves in the ileum and proximal colon (24–26). In the ileum, immunohistochemical studies show degeneration of adrenergic and serotonin-containing nerves, intact cholinergic nerves, decreased stores of CGRP, increase in VIP and neuropeptide Y, and normal stores of substance P. In contrast, in the proximal colon, the local stores of all these neurotransmitters are either normal or increased. It is noteworthy that the diabetic rats had diarrhea (23). The diminished adrenergic innervation of the ileum might well have contributed to the diarrhea by impairing fluid and electrolyte absorption in this segment. Mouse models of diabetes also show structural changes in the interstitial cells of Cajal, which are thought to generate electrical pacemaker activity and mediate motor neurotransmission in the stomach. These cells were greatly reduced in the distal stomach, and the normally close associations between these cells and enteric nerve terminals were infrequent in nonobese diabetic (NOD) mice. These observations suggest that damage to interstitial cells of Cajal may play a key role in the pathogenesis of diabetic gastropathy (27).

Functional studies also suggest defects in cholinergic innervation in diabetic rats. Nowak et al. (28) measured the contraction of longitudinal and circular strips of intestine in response to electrical field stimulation in rats with streptozotocin-induced diabetes. Among the three groups of rats, significant differences were seen only in strips of longitudinal muscle from the ileum. The amplitude of contraction was highest in control rats, lowest in diabetic rats, and intermediate in insulin-treated diabetic rats. These changes were seen in the atropine-sensitive contractions, suggesting impaired cholinergic neuromuscular transmission in the distal small bowel in diabetic rats. The relaxatory neuropeptide VIP was found to be increased in immunohistochemical studies of a streptozotocin-treated rat model of diabetes, but electron microscopy revealed degeneration of nerve fibers containing this peptide (29,30). Tissue stores of VIP and its basal release were also decreased in the same diabetic rat model and were partly reversible with insulin therapy (31).

Studies have also shown that nitrergic inhibitory neurotransmission is impaired in diabetics. Decrease in neuronal nitric oxide synthase (nNOS), an enzymatic source of NO, was noted in a number of diabetic animal models, including spontaneously diabetic rats and genetic (nonobese diabetic) and toxin-elicited (streptozotocin) models of diabetes in mice (32–34). Watkins et al. (33) demonstrated defects in gastric emptying and nonadrenergic, noncholinergic relaxation of pyloric muscle that resembled defects in mice with a deletion of the nNOS gene. The diabetic mice manifested a pronounced reduction in pyloric nNOS protein and messenger RNA (mRNA). The decline of nNOS in diabetic mice did not result from loss of myenteric neurons. Expression of nNOS and pyloric function were restored to normal levels by insulin treatment. Thus, diabetic gastropathy in mice reflected an insulin-sensitive reversible loss of nNOS. In diabetic animals, delayed gastric emptying could be reversed with a phosphodiesterase inhibitor, sildenafil (33). However, it has also been demonstrated that sildenafil delays gastric emptying of liquids in rats (35). These findings have implications for novel therapeutic approaches and may clarify the etiology of diabetic gastropathy.

SOMATIC INNERVATION

Each end of the GI tube (pharynx, upper esophagus, and external anal sphincter) is composed of striated muscle fibers that are innervated by somatic nerves. Moreover, the parietal peritoneum and abdominal wall receive somatic sensory innervation. Both sensory and motor neuropathies are well-known complications of diabetes. They may cause, on one hand, abnormalities in pharyngeal swallowing and, on the other, external anal sphincter dysfunction during defecation. Sensory neuropathy and radiculopathy may also be responsible for unexplained abdominal pain in patients with diabetes.

The pathogenesis of diabetic neuropathies is not fully understood. Recent revelations of the pathogenesis of diabetic neuropathy may have great bearing on the future prevention of this complication. Biological changes leading to neuropathy that occur with hyperglycemia in patients with diabetes include increased production of advanced glycosylation end products, increased activity of the polyol pathway, disturbance in metabolism of myoinositol and its phospholipid derivatives, elevation of endothelial angiotensin and abnormal permeability of the small blood vessels, impaired neurotrophic support, and impaired resistance to oxidative stress. Currently, treatment of diabetic neuropathy consists of achievement of better glycemic control and treatment of symptoms related to neuropathy. Specific treatments capable of preventing or curing neuropathy are being studied. With the introduction of potent aldose reductase inhibitors, the role of increased activity of the polyol pathway (and related abnormalities in myoinositol metabolism) in the pathogenesis of diabetes-associated complications may be clarified. Despite interesting results obtained with aldose reductase inhibitors in animal studies, initial results in patients with diabetes are less encouraging (36). Other metabolic approaches, such as antioxidants and γ-linolenic acid supplementation, seem promising (37). Clearly, early detection of diabetic neuropathy is required, because at present a preventive approach is the most effective way to avoid or postpone debilitating complications. More research is needed to make effective curative treatments of diabetic neuropathy available.

Gut Smooth Muscle in Diabetes

In general, the intestinal smooth muscle in diabetes is normal and functionally intact. Although the primary disorder of gut motility appears to be one of hypomotility or even atony, experimental observations strongly argue that these changes are the result of deficient innervation. When cholinergic agonists are administered, contractions are of normal amplitude (38). In an extensive review of many sections obtained from all parts of the stomach, Yoshida et al. (20) demonstrated normal smooth muscle without evidence of degeneration or vacuolation. In contrast, Duchen et al. (18) and Guy et al. (19), in a small number of patients, described morphologic abnormality of intestinal smooth muscle. Both groups of investigators observed eosinophilic or hyaline-like bodies (rounded or club shaped) lying in or replacing smooth muscle cells. The extensive autopsy studies of Duchen et al. (18) described the presence of these smooth muscle bodies throughout the GI tract and, in addition, in the smooth muscle of the bladder. The significance of these hyaline bodies is unclear, but the preponderance of clinical data indicates that the intestinal smooth muscle is functionally healthy. Histologic changes in gastric smooth muscle were also reported in overt gastroparetic patients with longstanding type 1 diabetes, including smooth muscle degeneration and fibrosis, with eosinophilic inclusion bodies (M-bodies), which appear to be unique to this condition (39).

There are also electrophysiologic changes in the gut smooth muscle with diabetes. In rat models of type 2 diabetes, for example, the gastric fundus shows functional impairment of neuromuscular transmission, reduced maximum activity of the electrogenic pump, increased sensitivity of muscarinic receptors, reduced sensitivity of adrenoreceptors, and reduced myogenic activity in gastric smooth muscles. These alterations in the properties of smooth muscle may be involved in diabetes-induced gastroparesis (40). The colonic smooth muscle also shows changes, including a more depolarized membrane and a reduction in reactivity of adrenoreceptors to noradrenaline. However, there is also notable attenuation of nonadrenergic noncholinergic inhibitory transmission, suggesting that the constipation appearing with diabetes involves dysfunction of both the enteric autonomic nerves and the smooth muscles in the colon (41).

Microangiopathic Changes in Diabetes

Microangiopathic changes in the GI tract of patients with diabetes are frequently mentioned in the clinical literature. De Las Casas and Finley (42) reported pathologic studies documenting these changes in duodenal biopsies from a patient with longstanding type 1 diabetes and chronic diarrhea. They described striking histopathologic findings of diabetic microangiopathy, including prominent mural thickening and luminal narrowing of blood vessels within the duodenum secondary to accumulation of hyaline material, which was periodic acid–Schiff positive and intensely stained with monoclonal antibodies to type IV collagen. Potential mechanisms for diabetes-specific microvasculature disease, including decreased vasodilators such as NO, increased vasoconstrictors such as angiotensin II and endothelin-1, and increased permeability factors such as vascular endothelial growth factor have recently been reviewed (43).

ABDOMINAL PAIN IN DIABETES

Both acute and chronic abdominal pain can present rather uniquely in patients with diabetes. Syndromes of acute and chronic abdominal pain can masquerade as disorders of intraabdominal or pelvic pathology and must be recognized to permit the institution of appropriate therapy.

Acute Abdominal Pain

Acute abdominal pain, tenderness, and vomiting have long been recognized as frequent in patients presenting with diabetic ketoacidosis (44). Unexplained abdominal pain in the setting of diabetic metabolic decompensation tends to be generalized or epigastric in location. The mechanism of acute abdominal pain is not clear. Hyperamylasemia can occur but is not correlated with the presence of pancreatitis. It has been suggested that abdominal pain and vomiting might be due to the gastric dilatation and intestinal ileus that can occur secondary to the metabolic acidosis. Theoretically, the pain could be due to a stretching of the hepatic capsule in response to hepatic steatosis; abrupt hepatic distention, however, is unlikely to be due to steatosis. Finally, acute pain may simply be due to activation of nociceptors in response to metabolic derangements.

Campbell et al. (44) reviewed the clinical findings and outcome in 211 episodes of metabolic decompensation in 140 patients with diabetes over an 8-year period. Forty-four patients experienced severe abdominal pain and tenderness that necessitated diagnostic evaluation. In 17 patients, the abdominal pain could be attributed to an underlying disorder (e.g., pyelonephritis or appendicitis) considered to have precipitated the metabolic decompensation. In the other 29 patients, the abdominal pain remained unexplained and was attributed to the ongoing ketoacidosis. Patients with unexplained abdominal pain were younger than 40 years of age and, with only three exceptions, had a plasma bicarbonate level of less than 10 mEq/L. The authors suggested that acute abdominal pain in patients with diabetes older than 40 years of age or with plasma bicarbonate levels greater than 10 mEq/L should not be attributed to the metabolic decompensation and that a search should be undertaken for an underlying abdominal or pelvic disorder. In all patients, GI, renal, and pelvic diseases should be excluded, especially in those with fever, localized abdominal pain or tenderness, or abnormal laboratory findings. The acute abdominal pain associated with diabetic ketoacidosis resolves with correction of the metabolic abnormalities. It is important to recognize this entity to avoid unnecessary and harmful exploration laparotomy in these patients.

Chronic Abdominal Pain

Chronic abdominal pain can occur as a result of diabetic sensory neuropathy and can masquerade as serious intraabdominal pathology, especially when it is associated with weight loss. Thoracic polyradiculopathy is an important cause of chronic pain in patients with diabetes. Longstreth (45) described the syndrome of chronic abdominal pain and weight loss caused by thoracic radiculopathy in 10 middle-aged or elderly patients with type 2 diabetes. Some of these patients initially underwent investigations focused on possible malignancy. Some had even undergone laparotomy in a search for possible carcinoma of the pancreas. In the affected patients, the pain tended to be asymmetric rather than bilateral and most often affected the left upper abdomen and often radiated into or from the lower thoracic spine. At times both the upper abdomen and the lower chest were involved in the pattern of symptoms. The pain was described as a pressure discomfort or sharp pain and at times had neuropathic qualities such as "burning" or "stabbing." The pain was often worse at night and aggravated by light pressure. The onset of the pain was gradual, being at first intermittent, later more frequent, and finally constant. It is especially noteworthy that the pain was not brought on or affected by either eating or defecation, a possible clue that the pain did not originate from the GI tract. Marked weight loss—up to 19 kg—occurred in some of the patients and presumably was caused by pain-induced anorexia. The diagnosis of thoracic radiculopathy secondary to diabetes was confirmed by electromyographic demonstration of either unilateral or bilateral denervation of the paraspinal muscles in the middle thoracic to upper lumbar region in seven of the patients. Nine patients recovered spontaneously, but two had recurrent polyradiculopathy. A combination of nonsteroidal antiinflammatory drugs and tricyclic antidepressants has been used in other syndromes of radiculopathy and/or peripheral neuropathy and is worth a trial in this syndrome.

PHARYNX AND ESOPHAGUS IN DIABETES

Pharyngeal and esophageal motor abnormalities are frequently found in persons with diabetes and are more prevalent in patients with peripheral or autonomic neuropathy. However, these motor abnormalities rarely produce significant symptoms. Thus, dysphagia and chest pain should be thoroughly evaluated and not ascribed to the diabetes. The incidence of reflux esophagitis and candida esophagitis may be increased in patients with diabetes.

Pharyngeal Motility

In barium studies, Borgstrom et al. (46) evaluated "swallowing complaints" in 18 patients with diabetes, 16 of whom had evidence of autonomic neuropathy. Videofluoroscopy of the pharynx demonstrated motor abnormalities in 14 patients. These included defective epiglottic mobility, defective closure of the laryngeal vestibule, and weakness of the pharyngeal musculature. When symptoms of pharyngeal dysphagia are present, swallowing therapy may be helpful in the management of these patients.

Esophageal Motility

Several prospective studies have demonstrated that abnormalities of esophageal motility and transit are quite common among diabetic patients with neuropathy but are usually asymptomatic. Horowitz et al. (47) performed scintigraphic studies of esophageal emptying of a solid bolus and found delayed emptying in 42% of patients with type 1 diabetes and in 30% of patients with type 2 diabetes who were receiving oral hypoglycemic agents. Other groups have reported similar results (48,49).

Manometric studies of esophageal motility are an even more sensitive measure of esophageal motor dysfunction. Hollis et al. (50) studied esophageal motility in patients with diabetes and found that 56% had abnormal esophageal motility. Abnormalities were more common in patients with diabetic neuropathy. Among those with evidence of peripheral sensory neuropathy but not of autonomic neuropathy, 80% had abnormalities in esophageal motility. All four patients in this study who had evidence of autonomic neuropathy showed abnormalities of esophageal motility. In patients with peripheral neuropathy alone, esophageal motility showed (a) contractions of low or normal amplitude, (b) some decrease in velocity of peristalsis, (c) an increased frequency of dropped swallows, and (d) a mild delay of transit. Nevertheless, in patients with peripheral neuropathy alone, the majority of swallows are associated with normal peristalsis. Diabetic patients with autonomic neuropathy have an increased frequency of multipeaked and simultaneous contractions. Huppe et al. (51) and Loo et al. (52) reported similar abnormalities. Correlating scintigraphic studies of esophageal transit to manometric studies, Keshavarzian et al. (53) found that multipeaked contractions usually are associated with normal esophageal transit but that simultaneous contractions are associated with delayed transit. Another group showed that, in type 1 diabetes, retarded esophageal transit usually reflects either peristaltic failure or focal low-amplitude pressure. In these studies, as in others, the overwhelming majority of patients were free of esophageal symptoms. Even patients with motility patterns compatible with diffuse esophageal spasm were usually asymptomatic. Chest pain was a rare symptom (54).

The mechanism of the esophageal motor abnormalities in diabetes remains unclear. Loo et al. (52) reported that the administration of atropine inhibited the development of the second esophageal peak. It has been suggested that the presumed loss of vagal innervation of the esophagus is the mechanism of abnormal peristalsis, although experimental demonstration of this theory has not been documented. In one study, disorder of motor nerve conduction velocity correlated with esophageal motility disorders, but no significant correlation could be found between esophageal dysfunction and diabetic autonomic neuropathy, as measured by coefficient of variation of cardiac R-R intervals (55).

Clouse et al. (56) suggested that the esophageal motor abnormalities observed in patients with diabetes were due to coincident psychiatric disease (depression and anxiety disorders) rather than to neuropathy. Psychiatric illness, as defined by testing, was present in 87% of those diabetic patients with motor abnormalities but in only 21% of those with normal motility. This association was independent of neuropathy. In this study, the vast majority of patients were without esophageal symptoms.

Reflux Esophagitis

In patients without esophageal symptoms, abnormal gastroesophageal reflux on ambulatory pH testing was significantly more prevalent in insulin-dependent diabetics (28% more) compared with healthy persons without diabetes. Moreover, reflux was associated with cardiovascular autonomic neuropathy (abnormal reflux = 38.7% in diabetic patients with cardiovascular autonomic neuropathy and 10.5% in diabetic patients without autonomic neuropathy) (57). In patients with symptomatic diabetic gastroparesis, the combination of gastric distention and increased gastric residual volume may make gastroesophageal reflux a more common occurrence. Jackson et al. (58) compared 24-hour esophageal pH, autonomic function testing, and electrogastrography (EGG) in two patient groups with symptoms of gastroesophageal reflux disease: one group with diabetes and one without diabetes. In this study, those with diabetes frequently had normal 24-hour pH but abnormal autonomic functioning. In contrast, those without diabetes had abnormal 24-hour pH but normal autonomic function. The two groups had identically abnormal mean EGG values. In patients with diabetes, the lower esophageal sphincter generally demonstrates normal pressures and relaxation (50). Therefore, it is unclear whether gastroesophageal reflux is more frequent in diabetic individuals than in normal controls, although the symptom of heartburn is less frequent in the patients with diabetes (7). The decreased symptoms of heartburn may be related to sensory impairment in these patients. The treatment of reflux esophagitis in patients with diabetes is no different from that in patients without diabetes (4).

Candida Esophagitis

An important esophageal complication of diabetes is candida esophagitis. Impaired immunity associated with diabetes is believed to increase susceptibility to this disorder. Moreover, stasis of esophageal contents associated with abnormal motor function could contribute to the susceptibility to candida infection. Extensive esophageal candidiasis may be asymptomatic or may be associated with symptoms of odynophagia (pain on swallowing) or dysphagia. Presence or absence of oral candidiasis has no reliable predictive value for esophageal candidiasis. The technique of barium swallow is relatively insensitive for detecting this disorder; with advanced esophageal candidiasis, a single- or double-contrast barium swallow may demonstrate extensive mucosal abnormalities suggestive of esophagitis. Fiberoptic esophagoscopy is much more sensitive and often demonstrates innumerable scattered white plaques over variable lengths of the esophagus. Esophageal brushings obtained through the endoscope can confirm the diagnosis.

Therapy for affected diabetic persons with otherwise intact immunity most commonly consists of nystatin suspension, 1 to 3 million units administered orally four times per day, or 10 mg of clotrimazole troches given orally five times per day, which are equally effective. More effective is fluconazole, 200 mg on day 1, followed by 100 mg once a day for a minimum of 3 weeks and at least 2 weeks after symptom resolution to prevent recurrence. If the patient is unresponsive, swish and swallow of itraconazole solution, 200 mg per day, for 2 weeks after symptom resolution, for a total of 3 weeks, is often prescribed. Ketoconazole may be somewhat less effective but is only one-third the cost of itraconazole. However, potential for hepatotoxicity has been recognized. The absorption of either itraconazole or ketoconazole is significantly decreased with antacids, and the two should not be administered concomitantly. Relapse is common and often occurs 2 to 4 months after clinical cure. Refractory esophageal candidiasis due to drug resistance may require systemic therapy with amphotericin B. Newer antifungal drugs being developed for fluconazole-resistant *Candida* include rilopirox (59) and voriconazole (60). Immunologic treatments being developed include vaccines and antibodies to *Candida*.

Dysphagia in Diabetes

Although minor pharyngeal and esophageal motor abnormalities are quite common in diabetes, they are usually asymptomatic (46). Because this is a disorder associated with few, if any, symptoms, specific therapy is generally not needed. In general, prokinetic agents (metoclopramide or domperidone), which have been shown to enhance esophageal contractions, have not been shown to improve esophageal transit in patients with delayed transit, as demonstrated by scintigraphic techniques. In one study, acute administration of oral cisapride improved esophageal transit in patients with baseline slowing of transit (61). Orally administered erythromycin has also been shown to improve esophageal transit after 2 weeks of therapy (62). After 1 year of treatment with tolrestat, an aldose-reductase inhibitor, patients with type 2 diabetes with asymptomatic diabetic neuropathy showed significant improvement in esophageal transit time on scintigraphy (63).

It is not known if the relative lack of esophageal symptoms in patients with diabetes is due to changes in sensory threshold caused by associated sensory neuropathy involving the esophagus. Feldman and Schiller (3) reported that 27% of unselected patients with diabetes complained of some dysphagia. In general, significant dysphagia in a patient with diabetes should not be explained by the diabetic pharyngeal or esophageal motility abnormalities, and a search for another associated cause of dysphagia should be undertaken.

STOMACH IN DIABETES

Gastric Motor Activity

The stomach normally performs four distinct functional motor activities. It (a) acts as a reservoir to accommodate the volume of solids and liquids of a meal; (b) pulverizes solids and mixes them with gastric acid to reduce the particle size for optimal digestion; (c) empties liquids and pulverized solids into the duodenum during the postprandial digestive period; and (d) empties the remaining food residues, including indigestible material, during the interdigestive period. These actions are achieved in different functional compartments of the stomach, i.e., the proximal stomach, the distal stomach, and the pyloric sphincter region (Fig. 64.2). In diabetes, all of these functions may be impaired (Table 64.1).

PROXIMAL STOMACH

The proximal stomach consists of the fundus and the orad third of the gastric body. The proximal stomach exhibits tonic contractions, producing prolonged elevations in pressure lasting 1 to 6 minutes. These contractions press gastric contents aborally toward the distal stomach and the duodenum and play an important role in gastric emptying. They are stimulated by excitatory fibers in the vagus and by hormones such as motilin. Normally, the proximal stomach relaxes with each swallow ("receptive relaxation") and also as the volume of swallowed food builds up ("accommodation"). With receptive relaxation and accommodation, the stomach can hold increasing volumes without increasing gastric pressure, which enhances its function as a reservoir. Receptive relaxation is mediated by inhibitory fibers in the vagus nerve, whereas accommodation is mediated by inhibitory neurohormonal influences. The resting tone of the fundus in patients with diabetes is comparable to that in healthy subjects, but fundic contractions, as measured by a motility index, are reduced in patients with diabetes (64). The status of the receptive relaxation or accommodation in patients with diabetes is poorly characterized, but these inhibitory responses are thought to be impaired owing to the loss of inhibitory nerves in patients with diabetes.

TABLE 64.1. Gastric Motor Abnormalities in Diabetes Mellitus

Gastric contractions
1. Reduced amplitude of fundic contractions
2. Reduced amplitude of antral contractions
3. Reduced frequency of antral contractions
4. Absence of antral interdigestive migrating motor complex (IMMC)
5. Periods of sustained high-frequency, nonpropagated contractions
6. Pylorospasm
Electrogastrographic findings
1. Tachygastria
2. Bradygastria
3. Flat pattern
4. Absence of postprandial increase in strength of slow waves
Delay in gastric emptying
1. Liquids: variable
2. Digestible solids: frequent
3. Indigestible solids: very frequent

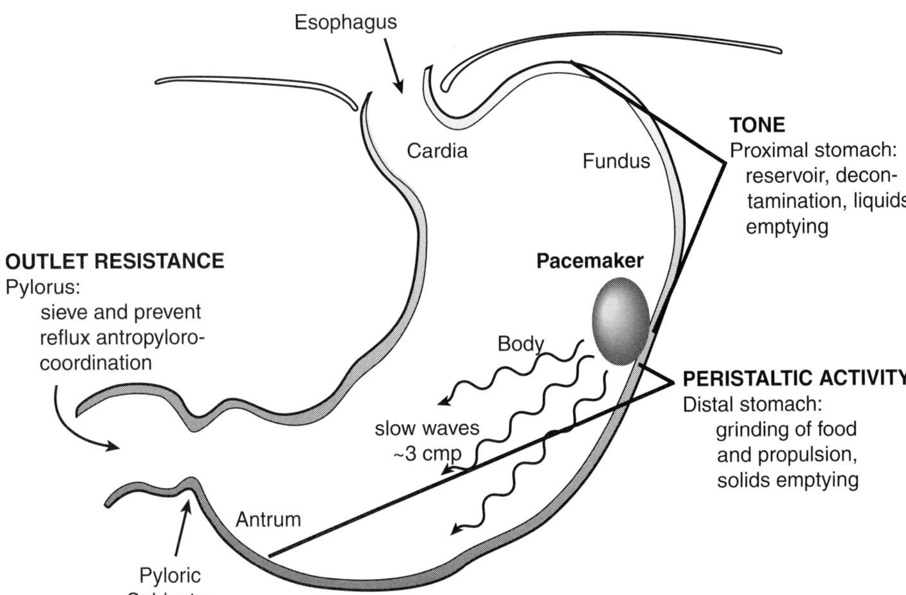

Figure 64.2. Functional integration of different parts of the stomach. The proximal stomach serves as a reservoir that actively accommodates increasing volumes of food during a meal. Its tone creates a pressure gradient to the pylorus, which largely influences the emptying of liquids from the stomach. The more distal regions of the gut actively grind the food into smaller sizes until it can pass through the sieve created by the pylorus. The timing and placement of the contraction waves are determined by "pacemaker" cells scattered in the body of the stomach, which create a rhythmic wave of electrical activity (slow waves) that marches distally to the pylorus at three cycles per minute. (Adapted from Koch KL. Diabetic gastropathy: gastric neuromuscular dysfunction in diabetes mellitus: a review of symptoms, pathophysiology, and treatment [Review]. *Dig Dis Sci* 1999;44:1061–1075.)

DISTAL STOMACH

In the distal two thirds of the stomach, contraction waves arise proximally and distally to the gastroduodenal junction, carrying part of the gastric contents ahead of the wave. In the interdigestive (fasting) period, four phases of variable motor activity occur in a cyclic fashion (65). During phase I, few, if any, contractions occur in the stomach. During phase II, intermittent random contractions are propagated distally over short distances. This is followed by phase III, which is a brief complex of rhythmic (three cycles per minute), strong propulsive contractions. Phase III originates in the proximal stomach and migrates through the distal stomach. This succession of cycles has been termed the interdigestive migrating motor complex (IMMC), and the period of an entire cycle is approximately 100 minutes. In the digestive (postmeal) period, the phase III activity, if present, is abolished and replaced by the phase II–like activity. The rate of contractions in the distal stomach always occurs at a predictable time that is a multiple of three or four, such that maximal rate of the phasic contractions in the distal stomach is never more than three or four per minute. This rhythm of the peristaltic contractions is paced by the underlying intrinsic electrical waves (called slow waves) that arise from pacemaker cells identified as the interstitial cells of Cajal. These slow waves occur at a rate of about three or four cycles per minute. These cycles originate in a region of the greater curvature of the gastric body (gastric pacemaker) and move distally toward the pylorus at an accelerating rate of 0.5 to 4 cm per second.

Gastric slow waves can be recorded by surface electrodes; this recording is called an electrogastrogram (EGG, Fig. 64.3). When the depolarizations become large, they are superimposed by action potentials, causing gastric contractions (Fig. 64.4). On the other hand, when the amplitude of slow-wave depolarizations decreases, no action potentials are triggered and no contractions occur. The slow-wave rhythm also influences the strength of their depolarizations. The decreased amplitude of depolarization results from abnormal rhythms (dysrhythmia) of gastric slow waves such as tachygastria (increased slow-wave frequency), bradygastria (decreased slow-wave frequency), or gastric arrhythmia (irregular slow-wave frequencies) (Fig. 64.5) (66,67). Gastric slow-wave frequencies and amplitude of depolarizations (also described as power of the slow waves) can be monitored with cutaneous EGGs.

Some patients with diabetic gastroparesis have gastric dysrhythmia. In one study, nine of ten patients with diabetic gastroparesis had runs of tachygastria as compared with only one subject from a comparable control group (67). Similarly, in another study of six patients with diabetic gastroparesis, one had tachygastria, two had bradygastria, and the remaining three had flat-line patterns on cutaneous gastrograms (68). In yet another study, patients with diabetic gastroparesis had normal slow-wave cycles but lacked the normal postprandial increase in strength of the slow waves (9). Such electrogastrographic abnormalities could also be demonstrated in a high proportion of children with insulin-dependent diabetes, which correlated with both poor hyperglycemic control and delayed gastric emptying (69). Patients with diabetic gastroparesis may show decreased or normal cycle numbers, decreased or normal amplitudes, and peristaltic or nonperistaltic contractions in any permutation and combination (70,71). The motility index, which is the product of amplitude and number of contractions over time, does not take into account the peristaltic behavior of the contractions. Therefore, the clinical importance of changes in the motility index in diabetes is limited. Fischer et al. (9) observed that the normal postprandial increase in antral motility and myoelectrical activity was missing in patients with diabetes with symptomatic gastroparesis. Malagelada et al. (72) demonstrated that patients with diabetes with symptomatic gastroparesis had no antral IMMCs but had normal IMMCs in the duodenum. In patients with diabetes without symptoms of gastroparesis, IMMC activity was present in both the antrum and the duodenum, whereas symptomatic patients with diabetic gastroparesis had no IMMC activity in the antrum and, for some, in the duodenum (73). In contrast to the general pattern of decreased gastric motor activity, occasional patients with diabetes demonstrate fasting patterns of ectopic and aberrant antral motility. In some patients, episodes of sustained high-frequency activity (three cycles per minute) that is neither propagated nor associated with IMMC activity have been observed in the antrum. These motor abnormalities may also cause gastric stasis. This phenomenon has been related to intestinal motor aberrations created by sympathetic denervation (74).

In diabetes, changes in gastric slow waves and contractions may be due to several factors, including changes in innervation and metabolic abnormalities. Vagal innervation plays a very

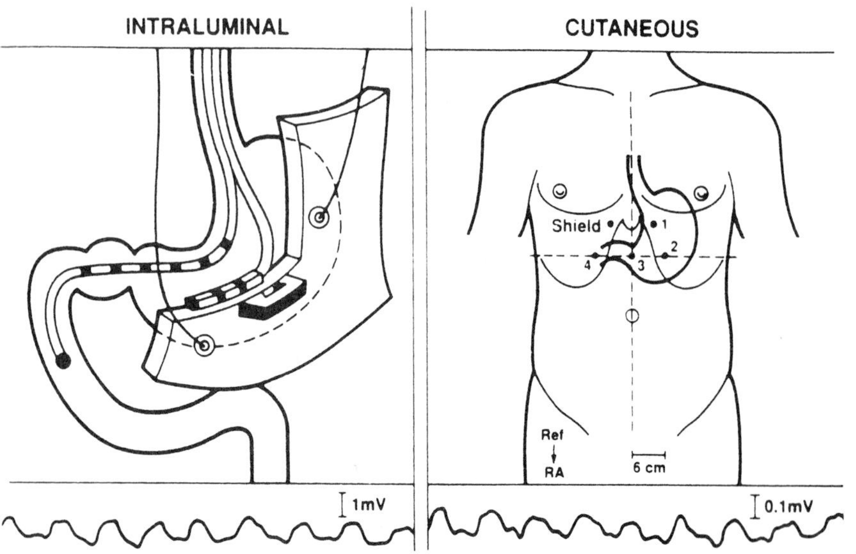

Figure 64.3. Recording of gastric electrical activity by electrographic techniques. Intraluminal electrogastrographic techniques use an internal electrode system that is apposed to the stomach wall by an external magnet placed on the abdominal wall. Cutaneous techniques involve placement of skin electrodes over the region of the stomach. Each technique records a sinusoidal waveform, but the intraluminal signal is ten times stronger than the cutaneous signal. (From Hasler W, Owyang C. Peptide-induced gastric arrhythmias: a new cause of gastroparesis. *Regul Pept Lett* 1990;2:6–12, with permission.)

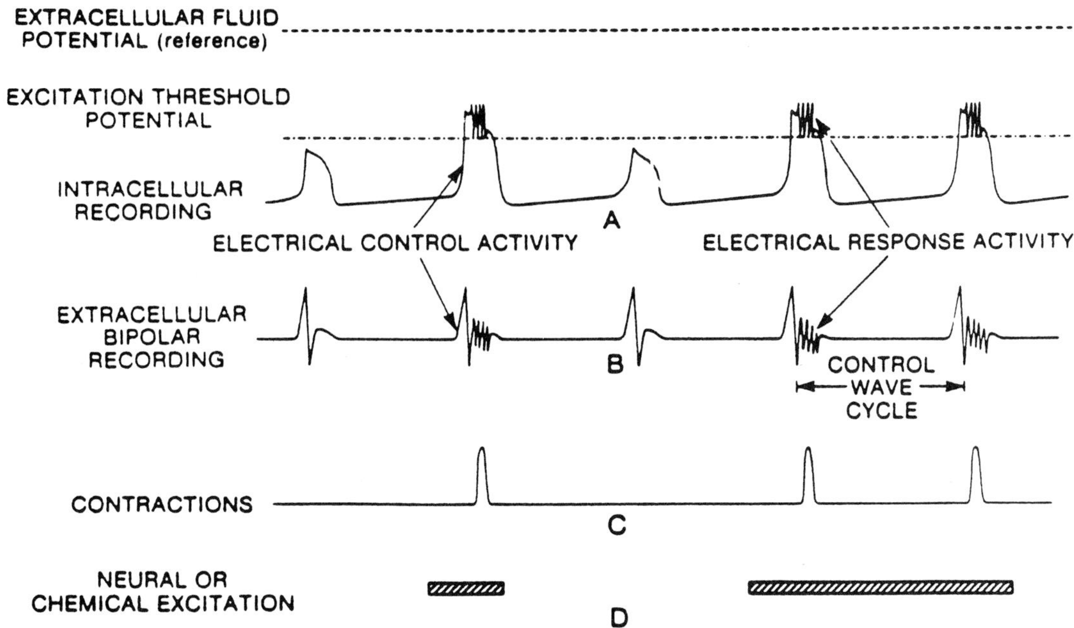

Figure 64.4. Relationship between intracellular and extracellular electrical activities and contractile activity. Resting membrane potential in intracellular recordings is negative with respect to extracellular fluid potential. Intracellularly recorded monophasic depolarizations are recorded as biphasic or triphasic depolarizations by extracellular bipolar electrodes. In intracellular recordings, bursts of electrical response activity appear during depolarized phase of control potential, but in extracellular recordings, they appear after initial large depolarization of control potential. However, their temporal relationship to contractile activity is the same in both types of recordings. Membrane potential depolarizations that do not exceed the excitation threshold level are not superimposed with a bout of electrical response activity and are not accompanied by a contraction. Neurochemical stimulation (*rectangles*) increases the amplitude of electrical control activity oscillation and results in a burst of electrical response activity and a contraction during depolarization. An understanding of the electromechanical relationships of the gastrointestinal smooth muscle is necessary for evaluation of the importance of abnormalities in electromyographic studies of the gastrointestinal tract in diabetes mellitus. (From Sarna SK. In vivo myoelectric activity: methods, analysis and interpretation. In: *Handbook of physiology. The gastrointestinal system.* Vol 1. *Motility and circulation.* Bethesda: American Physiological Society, 1989:817–863, with permission.)

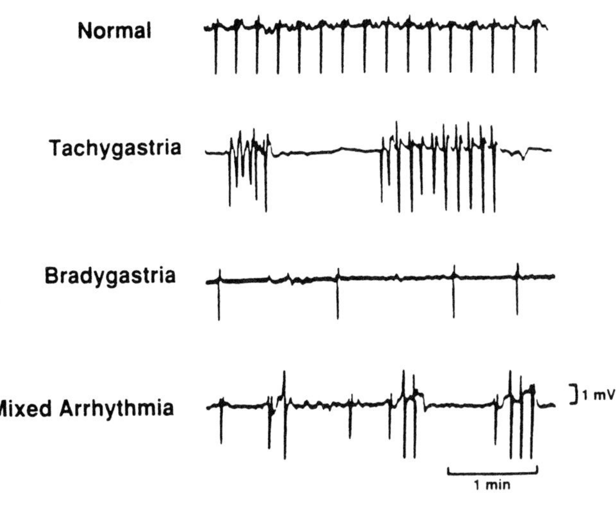

Figure. 64.5. Examples of normal and dysrhythmic slow wave recordings using serosally placed electrodes on canine stomach. Similar patterns of dysrhythmic slow waves are observed on external electrogastrographs in patients with diabetes (see text). (From Hasler W, Owyang C. Peptide-induced gastric arrhythmias: a new cause of gastroparesis. *Regul Pept Lett* 1990;2:6–12, with permission.)

important role in determining the rate, rhythm, and propagation of slow waves and, therefore, in the number, rate, and peristaltic behavior of contractions. Vagal innervation of the stomach is essential for interdigestive cyclic motor activity. With vagotomy, fasting motor activity in the stomach is abolished and the IMMC originates in the duodenum distal to the stomach (65). The cyclic release of motilin from endocrine cells in the duodenum and jejunum plays an important role in initiating IMMCs in the stomach. This cyclic motilin release is mediated by vagal cholinergic influences in the dog but perhaps not in humans. Fox and Behar (38) suggested that this decreased activity in the distal stomach is due to decreased cholinergic transmission; when such patients were treated with parenteral bethanechol, the amplitude and frequency of contractions increased to normal levels.

Acute changes in blood glucose concentration can have major effects on GI motor function. Barnett and Owyang (75) demonstrated that experimentally induced hyperglycemia in normal subjects reduced antral motor activity and abolished the gastric component of the IMMC. With increasing hyperglycemia, levels of serum motilin fell. Because motilin is postulated to be a physiologic regulator of gastric IMMC activity, the authors suggested that the hyperglycemic reduction in motor activity might be due in part to a hyperglycemic reduction in the levels of serum motilin. The investigators noted, however, that gastric IMMC activity was reduced at levels of blood glucose that had no effect on the serum motilin level. Hence they suggested that hyperglycemia per se might also decrease antral motor activity independent of changes in serum motilin levels. Serum motilin levels were also elevated in patients with diabetes, suggesting therefore that the absence of gastric IMMC activity in these patients was not due to a deficiency of circulating serum motilin (75,76). The group also showed that hyperglycemia causes gastric slow-wave dysrhythmias that could be prevented by administration of indomethacin in healthy volunteers (77). Subsequently, others have shown that hyperglycemia attenuates the stimulation of antral pressures and propagates antral sequences by the motilin receptor agonist erythromycin (78) and attenuates the expected acceleration of both solid and liquid emptying with erythromycin treatment (79,80). Yet others have implicated the role of dopamine stimulation in hyperglycemic disturbance of gastric motility (81,82).

Regardless of the motility changes ascribed to hyperglycemia, the impact of chronically elevated blood glucose concentrations on the rate of gastric emptying remains unclear. An inverse relationship between rate of gastric emptying and blood glucose levels has been reported: Gastric emptying is slower during hyperglycemia and faster during hypoglycemia (83). However, there is also contrary evidence for delayed gastric emptying with hypoglycemia (84). Moreover, Holzapfel et al. (85) reported that there was no relation between emptying and fasting blood glucose concentration, its postprandial increase, or their reduction to euglycemic values in patients with type 2 diabetes. These data did not support a major role of hyperglycemia in gastric stasis.

Fischer et al. (9) proposed that higher-than-normal postprandial blood levels of glucagon may, at least in part, be responsible for disturbed gastric motility in patients with type 2 diabetes. Frank et al. (86) indeed found higher postprandial levels of glucagon and lower insulin concentrations in the nonneuropathic patients with type 2 diabetes in their study. Meanwhile, entry of ingested glucose into the blood and the levels of other various enteropeptides (CCK, glucose-dependent insulinotropic polypeptide, neurotensin, and peptide YY) were similar to that in subjects without diabetes, suggesting that the postprandial hyperglycemia was from hepatic release.

PYLORUS

The gastric pylorus is a narrow channel that can actively change the size of its opening under the influence of excitatory and inhibitory nerves. The pylorus is not a usual sphincter, because under basal conditions its resting pressure is not elevated (65). The opening size of the pylorus determines not only the rate of gastric emptying but also the size of the food particles that are permitted to leave the stomach. Soon after a meal, as the peristaltic waves in the stomach and antrum carry pieces of food toward it, the pylorus opens partially so that only liquids or small particles pass through, and solid chunks of food are trapped in the antrum to be ground by powerful antral contractions. If the pylorus does not open or relax, gastric emptying of liquids, as well as of ground and unground solids, is inhibited and gastric stasis occurs. It has been reported that luminal contents in the small bowel may inhibit gastric emptying by enhancing pyloric closure via neurohormonal reflexes (65). Wider opening of the pylorus is also essential for movement of large pieces of food during the IMMC.

Careful manometric studies have shown that patients with diabetes have increased fasting and postprandial pyloric motor activity. In addition, these patients demonstrate episodes of "pylorospasm" characterized by prolonged periods of increased tonic and phasic motor activity in this region (87). It has been suggested that pyloric motor activity and pylorospasm could act as a "brake" on gastric emptying and hence could contribute to the morbidity and disability of gastroparesis. The increased pyloric motor activity might be due to an increase in cholinergic or noncholinergic excitatory nerve activity or to a decrease in adrenergic or nonadrenergic (VIPergic and nitrergic) activity with resultant decreased pyloric inhibition.

DUODENUM

Normally, duodenal activity is coordinated with antral and pyloric activity. During the period of enhanced gastric emptying, the duodenal and pyloric activities are inhibited with each antral peristalsis. The inhibition is followed by contractions that form a peristaltic sequence with antral contractions. Such a duodenal inhibition can be called receptive relaxation of the duodenum and is due to inhibitory neural influences. Impairment of this duodenal relaxation results in antroduodenal incoordination, and this acts to inhibit gastric emptying. However, the importance of antroduodenal incoordination in diabetic gastroparesis is unclear. Duodenal mucosal afferent nerves also play an important role in reflex modulation of gastric emptying of liquids based on the composition of a liquid meal emptied from the stomach (65). Liquid meals of high caloric densities, high fat content, high osmolality, and acid pH stimulate duodenal receptors to inhibit gastric emptying. No information is available on duodenogastric reflexes in diabetic gastroparesis.

Gastric Emptying

The motor activities of various parts of the stomach are well designed to regulate the emptying of different physical constituents of food, so that the liquid and digestible solid components are emptied in the digestive period (within 2 to 3 hours after ingestion) and indigestible solids are emptied from the stomach during the interdigestive period (2 to 3 hours after a meal). In diabetic gastroparesis, gastric emptying of all these components is affected to varying degrees, depending upon the stage of the disease and the underlying pathophysiologic defects. Figure 64.6 shows patterns of gastric emptying of liquids and solids in one patient with diabetic gastroparesis and in a normal control.

EMPTYING OF LIQUIDS

Gastric emptying of liquids is normally influenced by the composition of the liquid meal, whose characteristics—e.g., acidity, caloric and nutritional content, and osmolality—elicit different responses from duodenal receptors and, in turn, from reflexes responsible for emptying (65). Hence, the liquid emptying varies in different studies because of the use of meals ranging from simple solutions (water, 10% dextrose, and orange juice) to complex nutritional solutions that truly justify the term "liquid meal." However, even with a standardized meal, gastric emptying of liquids in patients with diabetes is variable. Keshavarzian and Iber (88) demonstrated rapid emptying of liquids in patients with diabetes and suggested that it was due to diminished receptive relaxation in the diabetic stomach. In contrast, Loo et al. (89) and Wright et al. (90) demonstrated normal emptying of liquids in patients with diabetes. Others have demonstrated delayed emptying of liquids in patients with diabetes (91–93). The delayed emptying of liquids may be due to reduced fundic motor activity and antral motility. Another factor that could affect liquid gastric emptying is hyperglycemia. Induced hyperglycemia in normal subjects is associated with a slowing of the gastric emptying of liquid meals containing fat and protein; hyperglycemia may cause a reflex decrease in vagal excitatory tone of the stomach with a resulting delay in gastric emptying (94). There was no correlation between the degree of delay of emptying of liquids and the delay in emptying of solids (91).

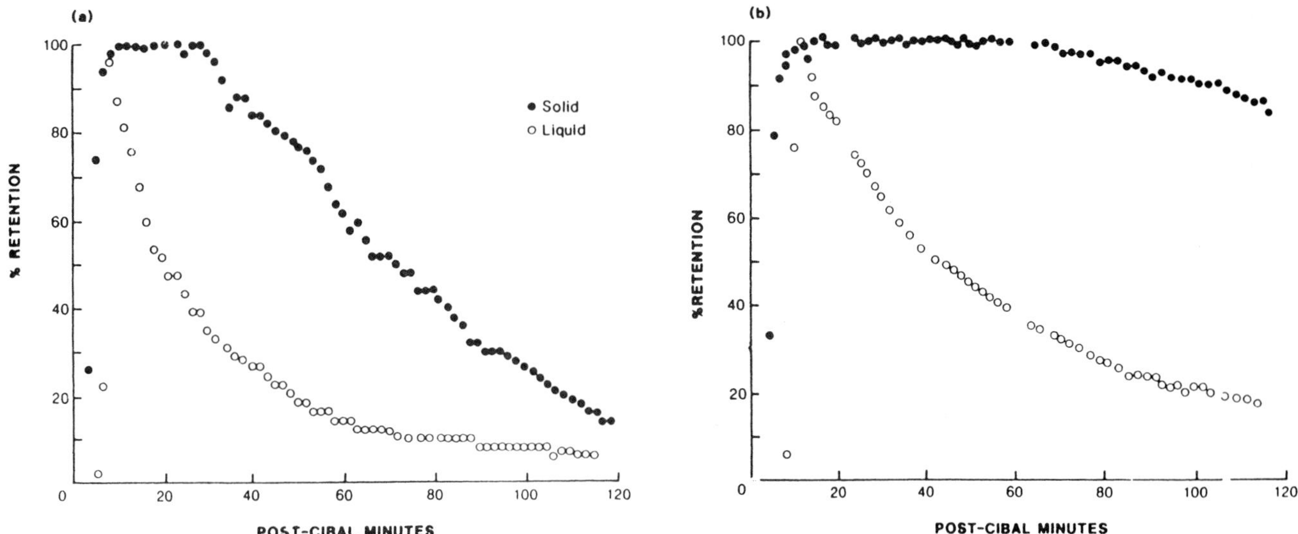

Figure. 64.6. Gastric emptying of solids and liquids in one control subject **(A)** and a diabetic patient with autonomic neuropathy **(B).** Note that emptying of solids is slower than that of liquids and both solid and liquid emptying are slower in the diabetic patient. (From Horowitz M, Harding PE, Chatterton BE, et al. Acute and chronic effects of domperidone on gastric emptying in diabetic autonomic neuropathy. *Dig Dis Sci* 1985;30:1–9, with permission.)

EMPTYING OF DIGESTIBLE SOLIDS

Normally, in the postprandial period, digestible solids are emptied more slowly than liquids because solids must be pulverized to a size (<2 mm) sufficient to pass through the sieve created by the contracted pyloric sphincter. In patients with diabetes, the gastric emptying of solids is frequently delayed. Horowitz et al. (47) studied gastric emptying among unselected patients with diabetes. Emptying of solids was delayed among 58% of patients with type 1 diabetes (61) and 30% of patients with type 2 diabetes.

EMPTYING OF INDIGESTIBLE SOLIDS

Indigestible solids, such as dietary fiber, normally do not empty during the postprandial period of motor activity because of the functional sieving produced by the pyloric sphincter (65). Such ingredients of food are emptied during the interdigestive period by phase III activity of the IMMC. Since gastric IMMC activity is impaired and often absent in symptomatic patients with diabetes, the emptying of indigestible solids from the stomach is delayed in these patients.

Feldman et al. (95) studied the emptying of indigestible solids in normal and diabetic subjects. Normal subjects emptied all of the ingested markers within 6 hours, a rate faster than that of the patients with diabetes (Fig. 64.7). A gastric-emptying study using a radiopaque marker identified patients with diabetes with symptoms of gastroparesis more accurately than did a scintigraphic technique using a meal of ^{99}Tc-labeled scrambled eggs. Similar radiopaque markers have been validated by other groups in the diagnosis of diabetic gastroparesis (96,97).

Radiopaque-marker gastric-emptying studies measure both lag time at which the interdigestive motor pattern reappears after a meal and the efficacy with which phase III motor activity empties the indigestible markers. Patients who lack IMMC activity in the stomach and have delayed gastric emptying of radiopaque markers are more likely to have abnormal gastric emptying of dietary fiber and would be more susceptible to the formation of gastric bezoars. If the pyloric sphincter fails to open widely because of either a motility abnormality or partial mechanical stenosis, gastric stasis of indigestible food would occur. However, a recent study cast doubt on the relationship of antral phase III activity in emptying indigestible markers as established from animal studies. Radiopaque markers (1.5-mm, 3-mm, and 7-mm cubes) were given with a test meal and followed by fluoroscopy with simultaneous antral manometry in normal subjects. None of the subjects had an antral phase III before all markers were emptied from the stomach. Instead, the typical irregular postprandial pressure activity was present in all subjects until the emptying was completed, and the highest postprandial motility index during the emptying study was comparable to the motility index during late phase II. Contrary to common opinion, the occurrence of gastric emptying of indigestible solids after a meal can be unrelated to the antral phase III, at least up to a particle size of 3 mm and perhaps even 7 mm (98).

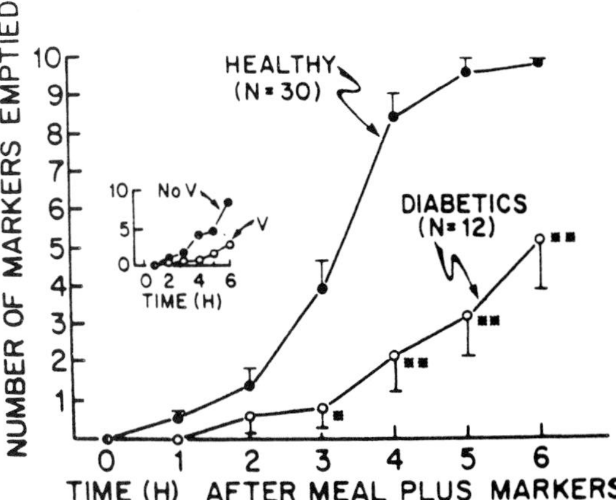

Figure 64.7. Emptying of solid radiopaque markers in 30 healthy subjects and 12 patients with diabetes. Emptying of solid radiopaque markers was significantly delayed in diabetic patients ($p < 0.01$ vs. controls at 3 hours; $p < .001$ at 4, 5, and 6 hours). The insert shows that emptying of solid markers was slower in seven patients with diabetes with vomiting (V) than in five patients with diabetes with no vomiting (no V) ($p < 0.05$ at 6 hours). (From Feldman M, Smith HJ, Simon TR. Gastric emptying of solid radiopaque markers: studies in healthy subjects and patients with diabetes. *Gastroenterology* 1984;87:895–902, with permission.)

Diabetic Gastropathy

Diabetic gastropathy is defined as a symptom complex with functional, contractile, electrical, and sensory dysfunction of the stomach associated with diabetes. In its classical form, called diabetic gastroparesis, it is associated with delayed gastric emptying. However, many patients with dyspeptic symptoms have normal or even enhanced gastric emptying. Thus even the definition of what constitutes a clinically relevant abnormality of gastric motility remains unclear.

DIABETIC GASTROPARESIS

Delayed emptying of solid or nutrient meals is found in up to 50% of patients with type 1 diabetes and in 30% of patients with type 2 diabetes (94). However, the degree of delay for various constituents of food, i.e., liquids, digestible solids, and indigestible solids, is not the same. Simultaneous assessment of gastric emptying of liquids and digestible solids using dual markers (^{99}Tc-labeled solid phase and ^{111}In-labeled liquid phase) showed that indigestible solids are particularly delayed in persons with diabetes (96,99). Figure. 64.6 shows patterns of gastric emptying of liquids and solids in one patient with diabetic gastroparesis and in a healthy control.

There is a wide range of symptoms in diabetic gastroparesis, and the degree of delayed gastric emptying correlates poorly with severity of symptoms. Many patients with abnormal gastric emptying have no specific symptoms and may be found to have a gastric bezoar or a largely dilated stomach with retained contents. Frequently, however, these patients have symptoms of anorexia, early satiety, and postprandial abdominal fullness and discomfort that resemble simple dyspepsia. Vomiting of old food, however, is indicative of gastroparesis. Nausea and vomiting are common when gastric distention is associated with obstruction and vigorous gastric contractions. In some patients, atonic dilation of the stomach, even when massive, may not be associated with nausea or vomiting. Nausea and reflex vomiting may be elicited by the stimulation of the gastric afferents carried via vagal and sympathetic nerves to the vomiting center in the brainstem. If gastric stasis and distention are primary causes of nausea and vomiting in diabetic gastroparesis, these symptoms should respond to gastric decompression by either vomiting or by insertion of a nasogastric tube.

Severe nausea and vomiting can limit oral nutrition and be a contributor to morbidity. Gastroparesis also may lead to poor glucose control because of both unpredictable oral intake and poor absorption of nutrients from delayed gastric emptying. When nausea and vomiting are prominent symptoms, some determination should be made regarding whether or not gastroparesis is the primary cause of these symptoms. Although some patients may develop vague upper abdominal discomfort from excessive gastric dilation, when patients complain of marked upper abdominal or midabdominal pain, a search should be made for other GI and abdominal diseases.

Kong et al. (100) studied the natural history of diabetic gastroparesis in a cohort of 86 outpatients with diabetes followed 9 to 14 years later. Of the 86 patients, solid gastric emptying was delayed in 56% and liquid emptying was delayed in 28%. At follow-up, the 21 patients who had died had a greater duration of diabetes and a higher score for autonomic neuropathy than did patients who were alive, but there were no differences in gastric emptying or esophageal transit between the two groups and no evidence that gastroparesis was associated with a poor prognosis overall. Autonomic neuropathy rather than myopathy has long been considered the cause of gastroparesis. However, autonomic dysfunction does not necessarily predict the presence of gastroparesis in patients with type 1 diabetes (101).

In some patients with diabetes, gastric emptying may fluctuate between normal and delayed. In some patients, nausea and vomiting are associated with episodes of pyloric spasm (87). These abnormalities may cause gastric stasis and the symptoms of nausea and vomiting intermittently. Such patients would be expected to respond to treatments that inhibit abnormal contractions, such as anticholinergic agents, rather than to prokinetic agents (Fig. 64.8). In still other patients with diabetes, nausea and vomiting may be due to an unknown cause unrelated to gastroparesis, and nausea and vomiting may cause, rather than result from, delayed gastric emptying. The vomiting reflex, regardless of activation by central or peripheral mechanisms, produces dysrhythmia of gastric slow waves and inhibition of antral contractions and characteristic retropropulsive motor activities in the small bowel. It is well known that stimulation of the vestibular system by circular vection involving rotation of a drum with alternating dark and light vertical stripes around a subject placed inside the drum leads to development of symptoms of motor sickness. Such a stimulation also causes tachygastria (68). Tachygastria is associated with weakened contractions and delayed gastric emptying (67). If delayed gastric emptying represents a GI motor response to nausea and vomiting, treatment should be directed toward searching for and treating the underlying cause of nausea and vomiting and primary use of antiemetics (Fig. 64.8).

DIABETIC GASTROPATHY WITHOUT DELAYED GASTRIC EMPTYING

Many patients with diabetes manifest symptoms of gastropathy without associated delayed gastric emptying. The symptoms of

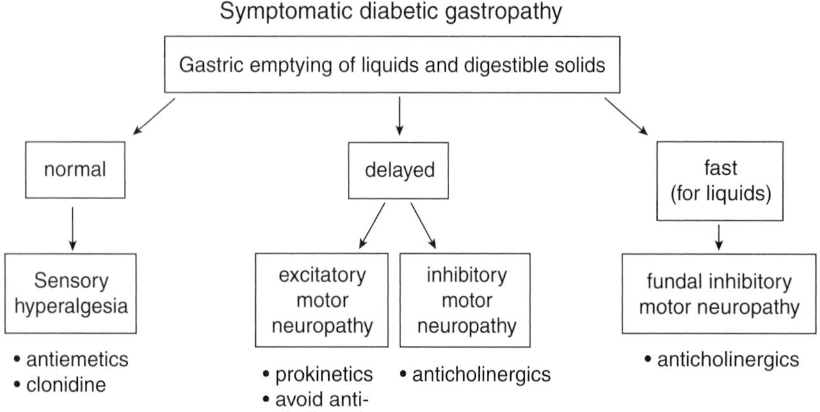

Figure. 64.8. Treatment rationale in symptomatic diabetic gastropathy.

this group of patients do not distinguish them from those with delayed gastric emptying. Some patients with diabetes, and particularly obese patients with type 2 diabetes, may complain of early satiety but have accelerated gastric emptying. These patients show no evidence of autonomic neuropathy (102). However, this symptom complex is thought to be due to loss of nitrergic innervation of the gastric fundus in patients with diabetes, which impairs receptive relaxation and accommodation reflexes. Nausea and vomiting are also common complaints in patients with diabetes, occurring in almost one third (72). Nausea and vomiting are common symptoms during acute ketoacidosis, and in most patients they subside with treatment of the acute metabolic abnormality. Sometimes they occur in a chronic pattern of daily symptoms that wax and wane in severity. In a minority of symptomatic patients with diabetes, the pattern is paroxysmal; such patients may have varying periods with minimal or no symptoms, only to be unexpectedly disabled by the sudden onset of severe nausea and vomiting, necessitating hospitalization for dehydration and ketoacidosis.

Even without ketoacidosis, patients with diabetes experience nausea and vomiting that correlate poorly with delayed gastric emptying (22). Several physiologic factors may play a role, including decreased compliance of the proximal stomach, which may account for an increased perception of gastric distention in patients with type 1 diabetes (103). Moreover, blood glucose concentrations appear to affect the perception of sensations arising from the GI tract; during hyperglycemia, gastric distention in healthy subjects produced more intense nausea and fullness (104,105). However, it is unclear whether physiologic changes in blood glucose levels directly alter sensation.

DIAGNOSIS OF DIABETIC GASTROPATHY

The presenting symptoms of diabetic gastropathy are nonspecific and also could be caused by mechanical obstruction of the gut, peptic ulcer disease, gastroesophageal reflux, chronic cholecystitis, pancreatitis, or metabolic conditions such as uremia, hypercalcemia, hypokalemia, hypocortisolemia, hypothyroidism, or pregnancy. Abdominal pain is generally not considered a significant feature of the clinical presentation of diabetic gastropathy. The relative lack of symptoms in patients with diabetes has been attributed, in part, to afferent neuropathy (106). However, one study showed that abdominal pain was a feature in almost 90% of patients with diabetic gastroparesis. The pain was described as burning, vague, or crampy. Only 36% localized to the upper abdomen. In all, 60% of patients complained of postprandial pain, whereas 80% complained of nocturnal pain that interfered with sleep. Generally, pain responded poorly or not at all to prokinetic agents (107). Nausea or vomiting in the morning, particularly with cranial neurologic symptoms, is an important indicator for considering central nervous system and metabolic disorders. A number of medications, including antidepressants with anticholinergic properties, can also slow gastric emptying. Eating disorders such as anorexia nervosa may be present, particularly in adolescents. Vomiting of old food suggests either gastroparesis or gastric outlet obstruction. An approach to the evaluation of patients with suspected diabetic gastropathy is detailed in Table 64.2.

Delayed gastric emptying is the hallmark test of diabetic gastroparesis. A number of different methods are used for measuring gastric emptying in humans. The method of choice depends on whether solid or liquid meals are to be studied, the level of precision required, the degree of invasiveness that the subject or patient will tolerate, ethical considerations, and the local facilities and expertise available. Simple studies such as a plain abdominal film and an upper GI series help identify patients with gastric bezoar and major problems of gastric stasis. Barium studies and esophagogastroduodenoscopy help exclude mechanical causes of gastric outlet obstruction. Gastric emptying of indigestible solids can be determined by studying the emptying of radiopaque markers from the stomach with serial abdominal radiographs (96).

TABLE 64.2. Investigations in Suspected Diabetic Gastropathy[a]

Blood examination: glucose, electrolytes, TSH, HCG, ANA, ?drug levels
Upper endoscopy: rule out *Helicobacter pylori* infection, mechanical obstruction, mucosal disease
Radiographic upper gastrointestinal study: rule out obstruction
Abdominal ultrasound: rule out gallbladder and pancreatic disease
Response to prokinetic agent 2–4 wk
CT scan in selected patients
Gastric emptying of liquids and digestible solids
Gastric emptying of solid markers
Gastric tone, compliance, and motility studies
Gastric sensitivity testing
Electrogastrography
Stress level/psychiatric factors evaluation

TSH, thyroid-stimulating hormone; HCG, human chorionic gonadotropin; ANA, antinuclear antibody; CT = computed tomography.
[a]Possible investigations for patients with suspected diabetic gastropathy. Besides appropriate blood examination and ruling out obstruction, further investigations are based on the clinical scenario.

There is no true "gold standard" in this field, but scintigraphy, with appropriate labeling of the test-meal components and appropriate corrections applied to the obtained images, is still the choice and most widely used diagnostic tool in the clinical setting. Emptying of both solid and liquid meals can be assessed simultaneously with the use of dual markers: a ^{99}Tc-labeled solid phase and an ^{111}In-labeled liquid phase (99). Most other techniques are compared with this method, but its application is limited by the need to restrict exposure to ionizing radiation. Clinically, a variety of different meals are used to measure gastric emptying of solids. Because both the physical state of the labeled meal and its nutritional composition determine the rate of emptying in control subjects, the degree of sensitivity of different test meals in detecting abnormalities in diabetes varies.

The most sensitive technique for the measurement of gastric emptying involves the use of chicken liver labeled with ^{99}Tc-sulfur colloid by either *in vivo* or *in vitro* methods (61). The labeled liver is then cooked and incorporated into a complex meal. This technique appears to yield the most stable bonding of the radionuclide to solids. In healthy subjects, the labeled meal is emptied in two phases, a lag phase, which appears to correlate with antral grinding of the meal, and a postlag phase of emptying, which represents the passage of the dispersed chyme from the stomach. However, the more involved process of preparing the meal and issues of palatability have perhaps hindered its wide acceptance. More commonly, a less sensitive technique is used that binds the ^{99}Tc-sulfur colloid with cooked eggs, either scrambled or in an egg salad sandwich (70). This test meal usually empties in a single linear phase, because the binding of label to solid is not as stable, and some of the label begins emptying early with the liquid phase.

Gastric emptying is highly variable in patients with diabetes. Some patients with diabetes—particularly those with nausea and vomiting—have evidence of delayed gastric emptying, whereas other patients with diabetes may in fact exhibit accelerated gastric emptying. Presence or absence of symptoms of upper GI dysfunction correlated poorly with objective measures of gastric emptying in subjects with type 1 diabetes. Nowak et al. (108) studied 21 patients with type 1 diabetes by solid-phase gastric-emptying scintiscan. Thirteen patients had symptoms of GI dysfunction (nausea, vomiting, early satiety, or constipation), and eight patients had no GI symptoms. Eleven patients had orthostatic hypotension. As a group, the patients with diabetes showed gastric emptying that was not significantly different from that of 12 healthy control subjects. Those patients with diabetes without GI symptoms and without orthostatic hypotension, however, showed a gastric emptying half-time that was significantly faster than that of the control subjects. Conversely, those patients with diabetes with nausea, vomiting, and early satiety (or early satiety alone) showed emptying times that were significantly greater than those of the patients with diabetes without these symptoms. No correlation was found between the gastric emptying and the duration of diabetes, the fasting blood glucose at the time of the study, or the respiratory variation in heart rate. These observations indicate that highly variable rates of gastric emptying occur in patients with type 1 diabetes and that accelerated gastric emptying may occur in patients with diabetes who have no symptoms of GI dysfunction.

Alternatives to scintigraphy are tracer methods that indirectly measure gastric emptying by assessing the time it takes for ingested marker substance to appear in either the blood or the breath, such as following the appearance in blood of paracetamol (109) or octanoin (110). These methods assume that there is no barrier either to the absorption of the tracer or to its metabolism and require normal intestinal absorption, liver metabolism, and lung function (for breath testing). Such techniques may be useful for screening in large populations, but they require sampling over several hours, are cumbersome, require complicated calculations, and possibly are too inaccurate for clinical use. However, a simplified nonradioactive assessment of solid gastric emptying has recently been proposed that uses a [^{13}C]*Spirulina platensis* breath test that results in a half-life for solids comparable with those obtained by scintigraphy (110).

The double-sampling gastric aspiration technique is used mainly for physiologic investigations in the research laboratory. It allows serial measurements of the composition of the gastric contents and of the volume and composition of gastric secretions but can be used only with liquid meals. Other imaging tools such as ultrasonography and epigastric impedance measurements produce results that correlate well with those obtained by scintigraphy or aspiration. The main advantage of ultrasonography is that it is noninvasive and does not require radioactive isotopes. It can provide information on gastric emptying rate, on antral diameter, and in duplex mode, on motility and transpyloric flow, particularly of liquids. However, it is time consuming, less accurate in obese patients or for solid emptying, and requires a skilled operator. Moreover, the presence of large amounts of gas in the stomach may hinder the study (111). Epigastric impedance to electrical current increases after drinking liquid with low conductance, such as water. Subsequent decline in impedance reflects the duration of gastric emptying. Although electrical impedance measures are noninvasive, they cannot be used for solid or semisolid meals and are sensitive to body movements. Nevertheless, impedance has been applied to documenting improvement in gastric emptying with metoclopramide and may help in confirming or ruling out the presence of gastroparesis (112). Magnetic resonance imaging (MRI) allows the physician to follow the rate of gastric emptying while simultaneously observing any morphologic abnormalities that may contribute to abnormal gastric function. However, this assessment is time consuming and expensive and remains an investigative research tool (113).

Other noninvasive tools include breath hydrogen testing (114) and the potato-lactulose breath test (115), which have been reported to identify patients with diabetic gastroparesis. A metal-detector test has also identified transit disorders in different GI segments of patients with diabetes mellitus. (116).

Regardless of the method used, the clinician must be aware of the intersubject variability for each test in healthy individuals and of the factors known to influence the gastric pattern.

TREATMENT OF DIABETIC GASTROPATHY

Treatment of diabetic gastropathy entails improving gastric emptying, when abnormal, and improving symptoms. The principles of treatment are (a) acute management; (b) dietary adjustments; (c) use of gastric prokinetic agents that enhance gastric emptying; (d) treatment of associated conditions; and in severe cases, possibly (e) feeding jejunostomy or surgery.

Acute Management

In situations in which severe episodes of protracted vomiting are associated with dehydration and diabetic ketoacidosis, hospitalization is mandatory. In such cases, it is essential that the patient be fasted, and the passage of a nasogastric tube may be necessary. Intravenous fluid should be administered, and insulin should be given as indicated by the serum levels of glucose and ketones.

Dietary Adjustments

Dietary adjustments should be made in all patients with symptomatic gastroparesis. A standard American Diabetes Association diet may be poorly tolerated. The recommended diet should be low in fiber and fat and administered in frequent, small feedings (117). It may be necessary to obtain caloric counts to determine the adequacy of nutritional intake. If caloric intake is inadequate, the diet can be supplemented with high-calorie liquid supplements. Because liquids are emptied more easily from the gastroparetic stomach, these will be better tolerated. Some patients may even find it more practical to ingest the majority of their nutrition as liquid supplements. A three-step dietary program has been advocated (Table 64.3) (70).

Gastric Prokinetic Agents

Gastric prokinetic agents are a group of drugs characterized by their ability to enhance gastric emptying and reduce gastric stasis. The pharmacology of these drugs, including the mechanisms of receptor interaction and prokinetic action, is not yet

TABLE 64.3. Three-step Program in Treatment of Severe Gastroparesis

Step 1: Rehydration Day 1–2
- Sip Gatorade or salty bouillon solution to ingest goal 1–1.5L over 24 hours, multiple vitamins
- Avoid citrus or highly sweetened drinks

Step 2: Advance diet to soups
- Soups with noodles/rice and crackers, 6 small-volume meals per day, goal 1,500 cal/day and maintain/gain weight
- Avoid fatty foods

Step 3: Introduction of more solid foods
- Starches (require less electrocontractile work), chicken, fish
- At least 6 small-volume meals/day
- Multivitamins
- Avoid red meat, fresh vegetables, fiber

From Koch KL. Diabetic gastropathy: gastric neuromuscular dysfunction in diabetes mellitus: a review of symptoms, pathophysiology, and treatment [Review]. *Dig Dis Sci* 1999;44:1061–1075.

fully defined. A variety of pharmacologic agents may have gastric prokinetic effects. For patients with severe acute gastroparesis, the present treatment consists of mainly intravenous erythromycin and oral dopamine antagonists. Substituted benzamides remain the best option for chronic maintenance therapy. Currently under investigation are a number of serotonergic receptor agonists, macrolides devoid of antibiotic activity, and CCK antagonists.

Metoclopramide. Metoclopramide is lipid soluble and readily crosses the blood–brain barrier. It has powerful central antiemetic and peripheral gastric prokinetic actions.

Pharmacology. Metoclopramide is a dopamine D_2-receptor antagonist, a 5-HT_3 (5-hydroxytryptamine-3) receptor antagonist, an acetylcholine releaser, and a cholinesterase inhibitor. It also has some local anesthetic and antiarrhythmic properties and has direct stimulating action on smooth muscle. Its prokinetic activities in the gut are thought to reflect a combination of an antagonism of the inhibitory effects of dopamine on gastric motility and an enhancement of cholinergic activity in the gastroduodenum that can be blocked by anticholinergic agents (118). When administered parenterally or orally, metoclopramide can increase the amplitude and frequency of fundic and antral contractions (72) and induce associated pyloric and duodenal coordination.

This drug may not initiate gastric IMMC activity. Achem-Karam et al. (73) observed that parenteral administration of metoclopramide initiated gastric IMMC activity in patients with diabetes if it was given more than 30 minutes after the previous cycle of IMMC activity. Malagelada et al. (72) could not induce such activity with metoclopramide in patients with diabetes. Chaussade et al. (119) also failed to initiate such activity with metoclopramide, although they administered metoclopramide less than 30 minutes after the previous cycle of IMMC activity. The IMMC-like activity produced by metoclopramide does not show the full distal migration characteristic of the normal IMMC.

In clinical studies, metoclopramide enhances the rate of gastric emptying of both solids and liquids (89) and reduces symptoms in patients with diabetes. However, there is poor correlation between the reduction of symptoms and enhancement of gastric emptying (70). Even some patients with complete relief of nausea and vomiting may not demonstrate improvement in gastric emptying. For example, Snape et al. (93) reported that with metoclopramide the rate of liquid emptying at 60 minutes in patients with diabetes increased from 32.8% to 56.8%; control subjects emptied 79.4% of the meal in this period. Seventy percent of the patients were symptomatically improved with metoclopramide treatment, and 50% experienced complete relief of symptoms with only minimal changes in the rate of emptying. Moreover, tolerance to stimulation of gastric emptying may develop after a month of therapy, whereas symptomatic relief persists with long-term therapy. This phenomenon may reflect the beneficial antiemetic effects of metoclopramide independent of its prokinetic activity (120).

Pharmacokinetics. The onset of action of metoclopramide is 1 to 30 minutes after intravenous injection, 10 to 15 minutes after intramuscular injection, and 30 to 60 minutes after oral or rectal intake. The duration of action is 1 to 2 hours (120). The bioavailability is not significantly altered in chronic versus acute therapy (121).

Dosage and Administration. Metoclopramide is available as 5- and 10-mg tablets, as an injectable solution containing 5 mg/mL, and as rectal suppositories (121). The usual dose is 10 mg taken orally 15 to 30 minutes before meals and at bedtime. It is also available as syrup for use in children. Oral therapy may not be effective in acute stages of the disease. In such circumstances, it can be administered by slow intravenous injection, intramuscularly, subcutaneously, or rectally (122). Higher doses may be used if tolerated. Patients with renal failure require downward adjustment of the dose.

Side Effects and Drug Interactions. As a dopamine antagonist that is capable of crossing into the CNS, metoclopramide is associated with many CNS adverse effects, which are seen in up to 20% of subjects, thus limiting its use. These effects include drowsiness, restlessness, anxiety, and depression. Dystonic symptoms, including tardive dyskinesia, oculogyric crises, opisthotonos, trismus, and torticollis, may occur. Parkinson-like symptoms, including tremor, rigidity, and akinesia, may be produced. Metoclopramide therapy may increase the risk of seizures in patients with underlying seizure disorders. In addition, its antidopaminergic activity enhances the release of prolactin and, in female patients, can lead to breast enlargement, nipple tenderness, galactorrhea, and amenorrhea. It also raises levels of aldosterone and thyrotropin and reduces levels of luteinizing hormone, follicle-stimulating hormone, and growth hormone. This drug should not be used in patients with pheochromocytoma, parkinsonism, or seizure disorder. It should be used with care and in smaller doses in children and the elderly because of the greater incidence of side effects in these patients. Metoclopramide enhances the side effects of other D_2-receptor antagonists, such as the phenothiazines, and its prokinetic effects are annulled by the concomitant use of drugs with antimuscarinic properties. It enhances the effects of monoamine oxidase inhibitors.

Domperidone. Domperidone is a benzimidazole derivative (123). Its use remains investigational in the United States, but it is available for clinical practice in both Canada and Europe.

Pharmacology. Domperidone is a D_2-receptor antagonist, but unlike metoclopramide it may not release acetylcholine from cholinergic nerves. However, it is a cholinesterase inhibitor. It does not cross as readily as metoclopramide into the CNS and hence is associated with a lower incidence of neurologic side effects (124,125). Domperidone enhances the frequency and amplitude of antral and duodenal contractions, improves antroduodenal coordination, and enhances the rate of gastric emptying of both solids and liquids. In clinical studies of patients with diabetes with gastroparesis, treatment with domperidone was associated with an improvement in both the rate of gastric emptying and the severity of clinical symptoms. However, as with metoclopramide, there was no correlation between the degree of improvement in symptoms and the magnitude of enhancement of gastric emptying. Moreover, after 4 weeks of oral administration, domperidone had no significant effect on solid emptying, although improved liquid emptying and decrease in symptoms could still be observed (124). Koch et al. (68) studied the effect of domperidone treatment on symptoms of gastroparesis, the rate of gastric emptying of a radionuclide-labeled solid meal, and gastric electrical activity as assessed by EGG. After 6 months of treatment with domperidone, all six patients studied reported improvement in their symptoms. However, the mean rate of gastric emptying was not significantly improved, and two patients showed no change or even a decrease in the rate. It is interesting that all six patients demonstrated a normalization of the gastric electrical activity on EGG. In some trials, symptomatic improvement and toleration has been observed with domperidone for as long as 12 years (126).

Pharmacokinetics. Peak plasma concentrations of domperidone are reached within 10 to 30 minutes after oral or intramuscular administration and from 1 to 3 hours after insertion of a rectal suppository. The bioavailability of intramuscularly administered domperidone is 90%, in contrast to 15% for the orally administered drug (123).

Dosage and Administration. The recommended dose of domperidone is 20 to 40 mg taken orally 60 minutes before meals and at bedtime. The usual total dose is 40 to 120 mg per day. It is also available as suppositories. However, its intravenous use is not recommended in view of reports of associated cardiac arrhythmias.

Adverse Effects. Because domperidone does not cross the blood–brain barrier and enter the CNS as readily as metoclopramide, the incidence of neurologic side effects is much lower with domperidone than with metoclopramide (124). However, because both the chemoreceptor trigger zone and the site of prolactin release are located outside the blood–brain barrier, it acts as an antiemetic and causes hyperprolactinemia. In 10% to 15% of female patients, it causes breast enlargement, nipple tenderness, galactorrhea, and amenorrhea. Other side effects include dry mouth, skin rash, itching, headache, diarrhea, and nervousness, and neuroleptic malignant syndrome has also been reported in a diabetic patients with gastroparesis. Cardiac arrhythmias have been reported with intravenous administration. Domperidone is useful for the treatment of gastroparesis in patients with coincident Parkinson disease, as it does not exacerbate the extrapyramidal symptoms of Parkinson disease (127).

Other Dopaminergic Drugs. Levosulpiride, which is related to metoclopramide, has been demonstrated to have an accelerating effect on the emptying of solids from the stomach of patients with diabetic gastroparesis. The drug is also effective in relieving upper GI symptoms in patients whose gastric emptying times remain very slow (81). Alizapride, another D_2-receptor antagonist, has been helpful in relieving nausea and vomiting for a variety of causes, but its prokinetic effects in the upper GI tract are uncertain (128).

Cisapride. Cisapride is a benzamide derivative that is chemically distinct from domperidone and metoclopramide. The drug is no longer available in the United States except for investigational or compassionate use but is available for clinical therapy in both Canada and Europe.

Pharmacology. Cisapride has no antidopaminergic properties but enhances the release of acetylcholine in the intestinal myenteric plexus. It also has 5-HT_3 receptor antagonistic and 5-HT_4 agonistic properties. It enhances the amplitude of contractions throughout the gut, including the stomach and small and large bowels, and therefore its prokinetic effect extends through the entire gut. The increased gastroduodenal activity is associated with enhanced gastroduodenal coordination (129). Rapid MRI studies of patients with diabetic gastroparesis showed that antral contraction frequency, amplitude, and velocity were unchanged after cisapride administration, and cisapride-induced acceleration of liquid gastric emptying in diabetic gastroparesis may be related to changes in proximal gastric tone or gastric outlet resistance (114). At therapeutic doses, cisapride has no effect on gastric acid secretion. In patients with diabetes, it improves the rate of gastric emptying of both digestible and indigestible solids and liquids (61,130,131). Generally, there is no correlation between the degree of cisapride-mediated improvement in clinical symptoms and the magnitude of enhancement of gastric emptying. In contrast to the time-dependent deterioration of the beneficial effect of metoclopramide and domperidone, chronic therapy with cisapride is associated with continued enhancement of gastric emptying (129). Horowitz and Roberts (132) studied the effects of acute and chronic treatment with cisapride on the rates of gastric emptying of both solids and liquids in patients with diabetes (61). With acute therapy, cisapride not only reduced clinical symptoms but also improved the rate of emptying of both solids and liquids. With chronic therapy with cisapride over 4 weeks, the pattern of symptomatic improvement continued; moreover, the enhanced rate of gastric emptying persisted even after 14 months of use. Of interest is the inverse relationship of the magnitude of improvement of gastric emptying to the rate of emptying with placebo; i.e., the patients who showed the greatest degree of improvement with cisapride were those with the slowest rate of emptying at baseline.

Side Effects and Drug Interactions. Cisapride is associated with a low incidence of side effects. Because this drug lacks antidopaminergic properties, it does not have neurologic side effects. Infrequently reported side effects include headache, abdominal cramps, and diarrhea, reflecting effects on the distal bowel (120). Prokinetic effects on the gut are blocked by agents with antimuscarinic properties. Cisapride is associated in a dose-dependent manner with prolongation of QT interval (133) and cardiac arrhythmias. Patients with recurrent severe hypoglycemia or renal impairment may be at increased risk of cisapride-related cardiotoxicity.

Pharmacokinetics. The half-life of cisapride after intravenous administration is 19.4 hours. Bioavailability after oral administration is 35% to 40%. Plasma levels after ingestion of a 10-mg tablet peak at 1.5 to 2.0 hours (120).

Dosage and Administration. Cisapride is available in Europe and Canada as 10-mg tablets for oral use. It is not available as suppositories or for parenteral use. The recommended dosage is 10 to 20 mg three times a day taken 30 to 60 minutes before meals (120).

Motilin Agonists and Erythromycin (Motilides). Erythromycin is a macrolide antibiotic.

Pharmacology. Erythromycin is known to have many GI side effects. Itoh et al. (134) observed that in the dog stomach, erythromycin in doses 2,000 times smaller than the usual antibacterial doses induced typical phase II and phase III contractions that migrated to the duodenum and upper jejunum. The contractile pattern induced by erythromycin was similar to a spontaneous or motilin-induced migrating motor-activity front. Erythromycin also caused endogenous release of motilin in the dog; therefore, the authors suggested that the action of erythromycin in inducing IMMCs is mediated indirectly by release of motilin. Subsequent studies of isolated rabbit duodenum showed that erythromycin is a motilin agonist, interacting directly with motilin receptors (135). Moreover, Lin et al. (136) observed that when dogs were treated with intravenous erythromycin, there was an increase in inadequately triturated food particles (>0.5 mm) in the duodenum. Whether this abnormality in gastric emptying affects digestion and absorption remains unknown. Sato et al. (137) have identified erythromycin derivatives, EM523, EM536, and EM574, that have no antibiotic activity but are up to 3,000 times more potent than erythromycin in inducing IMMCs in the dog.

Erythromycin and various macrolide derivatives have been found to induce migrating motor complexes in humans (138). Otterson and Sarna (139) further found that erythromycin initiated IMMCs only when administered in very small doses (1 mg/kg intravenously) and not with larger doses. Larger doses (up to 25 mg/kg intravenously) initiated retrograde giant contractions and "vomiting complexes," periods of generalized inhibition of all activity, and giant peristaltic contractions. These higher doses also produced increased coordinated antroduodenal activity. Cineradiography confirmed this enhanced antrobulbar activity (140). Various other groups have shown improved gastric emptying in patients with diabetes treated with erythromycin (62,141–144). Petrakis et al. (79,80) and others (78) showed that intravenous erythromycin–induced acceleration of gastric emptying in patients with diabetes was related to the plasma glucose level. The induced hyperglycemia reduced the erythromycin-induced acceleration of both solid- and liquid-phase gastric emptying. In spite of the inhibitory effect of induced hyperglycemia on gastric emptying, erythromycin was still able to accelerate the emptying rate.

DiBaise et al. (145) studied the role of prolonged intravenous erythromycin in the ambulatory setting as a treatment for severe gastroparesis in 11 patients; one received no benefit, two had complete responses, and all others reported some benefit. Antibiotic resistance or secondary infections were not encountered. Intravenous motilin is also able to increase gastric emptying in patients with diabetes with gastroparesis (146).

To date, there are no controlled studies documenting a beneficial effect of intravenous or oral erythromycin therapy on symptoms of gastroparesis. Only a few anecdotal reports attest to possible beneficial activity. It is not clear if the lack of efficacy of oral therapy is related to the failure of absorption of erythromycin because of gastroparesis or to the occurrence of tachyphylaxis with chronic therapy.

Pharmacokinetics. After intravenous administration of erythromycin lactobionate, peak serum levels are reached 15 to 30 minutes after initiation of the infusion. The peak action following intravenous administration lasts for about 1 hour. Oral erythromycin succinate does not achieve as high a serum level as erythromycin stearate.

Dosage and Administration. Erythromycin is available for oral use as erythromycin stearate and erythromycin ethylsuccinate and for intravenous use as erythromycin lactobionate. The lactobionate is administered as an infusion over a 30-minute period as a dose of 200 mg diluted in normal saline. Lower doses (60 to 100 mg) may be effective. For oral use, erythromycin stearate is used at dosages of 250 mg administered three times a day 30 to 60 minutes before each meal.

Adverse Effects. Erythromycin administration has been associated with nausea, vomiting, and abdominal cramping in 80% to 95% of healthy subjects.

New Serotonergic Agonists. Tegaserod, a 5-HT_4 receptor partial agonist (Novartis) (147), and prucalopride, a 5-HT_4 receptor complete agonist (Janssen) (148), have been introduced for human use as potent promotility agents with significant pharmacologic effects on the mid and distal gut. Their potential use in delayed gastric emptying is being evaluated.

Cholecystokinin Receptor Agonists. The effect of recently developed CCK-A–specific receptor antagonists—namely, loxiglumide and its dextroisomer—dexloxiglumide—on improving gastric emptying was studied in the rat (149). This has become available for human use and is currently under study (150).

TREATMENT OF BEZOARS

If gastric bezoar is present, it can be disrupted with a forceful pulsating jet of water during endoscopy (151). Alternatively, the patient is instructed to consume 1 to 2 L of clear liquids or a cellulase solution (0.5 g/dL of water) over a 24-hour period for 2 days or is administered an infusion of metoclopramide, 40 mg, over a 24-hour period for 3 days (152, 153).

FEEDING JEJUNOSTOMY

The endoscopic placement of both percutaneous gastrostomies and jejunostomies may be useful in some patients with diabetes with gastroparesis and malnutrition. These procedures are successful if the tubes are carefully placed and maintained. It should be recognized that feeding jejunostomies, whether surgically or endoscopically placed, are useful palliative measures that can greatly improve hydration and nutrition. These devices relieve the patient of the need to eat and drink and thereby reduce the clinical symptoms of gastroparesis (154).

SURGERY

In general, surgery is of no proven benefit in diabetic gastroparesis. The reported conservative gastric operations, such as loop gastroenterostomy and vagotomy and pyloroplasty, have been unsuccessful. Guy et al. (19), who reported on two patients with gastroparesis, stressed that these patients were the only patients with diabetes to have undergone elective surgery for gastroparesis in a 10-year period at their institution. In these two patients, clinical improvement, but not complete relief of symptoms, was observed only after extensive operations resulting in subtotal gastrectomy, truncal vagotomy, and Roux-en-Y gastrojejunostomy. Reardon et al. (155) reported their experience with surgery in a single patient This individual failed to respond to a pyloroplasty but did seem to benefit from the placement of both a surgical gastrostomy, which aided in decompressing the stomach, and a jejunostomy, which was successfully employed for enteral feedings. These experiences coincide with the observations of others who suggest that the surgical management of states of gastric retention (postsurgical, idiopathic, and diabetic) likely require a subtotal or near-total gastrectomy with Roux-en-Y gastrojejunostomy (39,156). In general, such surgery for diabetic gastroparesis should be avoided.

TREATMENT OF SYMPTOMS ASSOCIATED WITH DIABETIC GASTROPATHY

Most of the symptoms of diabetic gastropathy that do not resolve with the improvement of gastric emptying with prokinetic agents or those that occur without delayed gastric emptying require consideration of following approaches.

Antidepressants

Some patients with diabetic gastroparesis have associated depression. These patients need sympathetic support, psychotherapy, and, if appropriate, antidepressant therapy. Because of the negative effects of drugs with anticholinergic properties on both gastroparesis and the action of prokinetic agents, antidepressive agents should be carefully selected and should include agents with minimal anticholinergic properties, such as desipramine (Norpramin), trazodone (Desyrel), and serotonergic reuptake inhibitors such as fluoxetine (Prozac), paroxetine (Paxil), sertraline (Zoloft), and citalopram (Celexa).

Anticholinergic Agents

Anticholinergic agents worsen delayed gastric emptying and are contraindicated in patients with overt gastroparesis. However, in certain patients having diabetic gastropathy without delayed gastric emptying with selective deficiency of the inhibitory innervation and unopposed excitatory cholinergic innervation, a therapeutic trial of short-acting anticholinergics may be indicated (Fig. 64.8).

Clonidine

Clonidine, an α_2-adrenergic receptor agonist and antihypertensive agent, reduces perception of gastric distention in normal volunteers. No dose effect of clonidine was observed on gastric emptying. Clonidine relaxes the stomach and reduces gastric sensation without inhibiting accommodation or emptying (157). In a small uncontrolled study involving patients with diabetic gastroparesis, subjects showed improvement in both gastric emptying and symptom scores while taking clonidine, and this effect was maintained for 6 to 56 weeks of follow-up (158). These findings suggest that adrenergic influences play a role in the pathophysiology of diabetic gastroparesis and that clonidine may be a useful alternative for treating patients with this condition.

Behavioral Therapy

In an analysis by Soykan et al. (159) of patients with gastroparesis, 26% of whom had diabetes, the majority of diabetic patients responded well to pharmacologic agents; however, patients with predominant abdominal pain and also a history of physical and sexual abuse had poorer outcome with prokinetic agents. Such patients may benefit from behavioral therapy.

Accustimulation and Gastric Electrical Stimulation

Nondrug treatments of the nausea and vomiting related to gastroparesis have included accustimulation and direct gastric electrical stimulation. The accustimulation at P6 Neiguan point, a traditional Chinese acupuncture site, has been reported to reduce nausea in the first trimester of pregnancy, after surgery, and after chemotherapy (160). The mechanism of this action is unknown, and physiologic studies are necessary. A portable stimulation wristband has been introduced (ReliefBand, Woodside Biomedical, Carlsbad, CA), which is intended to stimulate this accustimulation site (161).

Direct electrical stimulation of the stomach using a surgically implantable stimulator (Enterra therapy, Medtronic, Minneapolis, MN) is being used experimentally, particularly in patients who are refractory to drug treatments and have lost weight despite nutritional support (162). Preliminary evidence supports the conclusion that the stimulators improve nausea, without consistent improvement in gastric emptying. In contrast to gastric electrical stimulation, gastric pacing of the human stomach has been evaluated only for short intervals, and no clear-cut therapeutic applications have been established (163).

HELICOBACTER PYLORI IN DIABETES

From the pediatric literature, there appears to be increased incidence of *Helicobacter pylori* in persons with diabetes compared with those without diabetes. In one study of 88 children with type 1 diabetes and 42 healthy control children, 55.6% of the children with diabetes and 30.9% of the control children were positive for anti-*H. pylori* immunoglobulin G (IgG). *H. pylori* status was not related to gastric emptying time (164). The literature about adults is conflicting. Some studies report a higher frequency of *H. pylori* infection in adult patients affected with type 2 diabetes than in subjects without diabetes (165) and a nearly twofold higher frequency of nonulcer, nongastritis dyspepsia in those with diabetes as compared with those without diabetes (166). Autonomic neuropathy was associated with increased occurrence and recurrence of *H. pylori* infection (167). In contrast, another study consisting of a validated questionnaire for GI symptoms and blood enzyme-linked immunosorbent assay (ELISA) for *H. pylori* showed that the seroprevalence of *H. pylori* was 33% and 32%, respectively, in patients with diabetes and in controls. Although patients with diabetes had a significantly higher prevalence of early satiety, fullness, and bloating than did controls, none of these symptoms correlated with presence or absence of *H. pylori*. Thus, *H. pylori* infection appeared not to be associated with diabetes or upper GI symptoms in diabetes (168). From a practical standpoint, patients with diabetic gastropathy should be evaluated and treated if *H. pylori* is present.

SMALL BOWEL IN DIABETES

Motor and Electrical Activity

Normally, the fasting pattern of small-bowel motility is characterized by the presence of the cyclic IMMC. In the small bowel, as in the stomach, the IMMC is characterized by periods of motor silence (phase I), random motor activity (phase II), and intense motor activity (phase III). In the small bowel, phase III activity consists of high-frequency (10 to 12 contractions per minute) complexes that are propagated distally through the entire small intestine. The highest frequency of contractions is determined by the rate of slow waves (pace-setter potential) in the small bowel. In healthy subjects approximately 80% of phase III activity originates in the stomach, whereas 10% to 20% originates in the duodenum. In each case the initiated complex then travels distally. After a meal, small-bowel motility consists of randomly occurring nonpropulsive or segmental contractions. Interspersed among the segmental contractions are some peristaltic contractions that propagate aborally for several centimeters and cause periodic slow shifts of intestinal contents distally. Another type of small-bowel contraction is called a "giant contraction," as it is 1.5 to 2 times the amplitude and 4 to 6 times the duration of a normal contraction of the small bowel. The giant contractions occur without regard to the intestinal slow waves. Normally, these giant contractions are present only in the distal small bowel. Abnormally, retrogradely propagated giant contractions occur during nausea and vomiting, and antegradely propagated giant contractions occur with a variety of pharmacologic manipulations that cause diarrhea (169).

Camilleri and Malagelada (74) analyzed GI motility by manometric studies in 14 patients with diabetes with gastroparesis but no diarrhea. All of the patients had long histories of type 1 diabetes. The following abnormalities of both fasting and fed motor activity in the small bowel were observed. (a) Migrating motor complexes were noted in the small bowel in most of the patients, although 60% of the observed phase III complexes did not have an antral component; among control subjects, only 8% of phase III complexes failed to originate in the antrum. (b) In 28% of the patients, the amplitude and frequency of duodenal and jejunal contractions were decreased. (c) In addition, 64% of the patients had striking periods of marked phasic pressure activity that were not propagated; these complexes consisted of both short bursts and long periods of high-frequency (10 to 12 contractions per minute) activity that were often isolated and not propagated distally as is characteristic of phase III activity. (d) After the test meal, 50% of the patients failed to develop the typical fed motor pattern; instead, the long and short bursts of high-frequency activity persisted. The appearance of abnormal complexes was thought to be due to sympathetic denervation that might result in the loss of an inhibitory "brake," thus allowing the appearance of ectopic and uncoordinated high-frequency motor activity. The small-bowel motor patterns observed in the patients with diabetes were similar to those observed in dogs following experimental ganglionectomy of the celiac and superior mesenteric plexuses (170).

Dooley et al. (171) studied fasting GI motility in 12 patients with diabetes who had unexplained diarrhea and evidence of autonomic neuropathy. In 16%, phase III activity was completely absent at all levels of the antrum, duodenum, and jejunum. In 81%, phase III activity had no antral component, whereas in 62.5% the proximal duodenum was not involved by the complex. In 12.5% of the patients, the observed phase III activity originated in the jejunum without antral or duodenal components. Furthermore, in three patients, phase III activity was abnormally propagated; in one, phase III activity appeared simultaneously in the small-bowel leads, and in the other two, the complex was conducted at an excessively rapid rate.

There is no adequate functional test of the small bowel that is analogous to solid-phase gastric emptying studies of the stomach. A diagnosis of intestinal dysmotility generally relies on symptoms, plain abdominal radiographs, barium studies, and intestinal manometry. Studies using hydrogen or hydrogen-lactulose breath tests to measure oral-cecal transit time cannot distinguish the contribution of delayed gastric emptying unless the latter is measured independently (98), and an early increase in exhaled hydrogen can result from bacterial overgrowth. A noninvasive metal-detector test to study intestinal transit has been described (118). As in gastric dysmotility, mechanical obstruction must be ruled out in the evaluation of patients with symptoms of intestinal dysmotility.

Small-Bowel Transit and Bacterial Overgrowth

Bacterial overgrowth in the small intestine and autonomic neuropathy seem to play a major role in the genesis of chronic diarrhea in patients with diabetes. Dooley et al. (171), using the lactulose-hydrogen breath test, studied oral-cecal transit times. Transit was prolonged in patients with diabetes (173 ± 20 minutes) compared with the time in control subjects (93 ± 10 minutes), but it is unclear how much of the prolonged transit reflected delayed gastric emptying as opposed to delayed small-bowel transit. In patients with diabetes with delayed transit, there was no correlation between abnormal motility and individual transit times. Twenty-five percent of the patients with diabetes who had diarrhea had evidence of bacterial overgrowth of the small bowel and improved clinically with antibiotic therapy. Two of the three patients who had bacterial overgrowth did have phase III activity. However, conduction of the complexes through the entire jejunum and ileum was not studied.

Wegener et al. (172) incorporated lactulose into a radionuclide-labeled meal so that they could measure gastric emptying and small-bowel transit simultaneously. Of the 43 patients with type 1 diabetes who had been hospitalized for various diabetic complications, 60% had clinical evidence of autonomic neuropathy, 30% had vomiting, and 14% complained of diarrhea. The oral-cecal transit times of the patients with diabetes were not significantly different from those of a large number of control subjects. However, more patients with diabetes than control subjects had delayed small-bowel transit (23% vs. 3.6%), and even when patients with delayed gastric emptying were excluded, this trend among patients with diabetes persisted. Although all six patients with diarrhea had delayed gastric emptying and evidence of autonomic neuropathy, there was no consistent pattern of rapid or delayed transit in these patients. Keshavarzian and Iber (88) examined oral-cecal transit by the hydrogen breath-test technique in patients with diabetes with and without peripheral neuropathy and autonomic neuropathy. Of the 25 patients studied, 12% had diarrhea and 16% had nausea without vomiting. In both the diabetic and control subjects, the transit of a liquid meal to the cecum was more rapid than that of a solid meal. There was no significant difference between the transit times in controls and patients with diabetes for either meal. No significant differences in transit times were seen in patients with diabetes with and without autonomic neuropathy and peripheral neuropathy. Sixteen percent of patients demonstrated rapid transit and 16% demonstrated slow transit, and there was no striking correlation between the clinical complaint of diarrhea and abnormal transit.

Virally-Monod et al. (173) demonstrated the high prevalence of small intestinal bacterial overgrowth by glucose-hydrogen breath testing and the success of antibiotic treatment in a population of patients with diabetes with chronic diarrhea. In the 35 patients with diabetes studied, 15 (43%) had small-intestinal bacterial overgrowth syndrome and 20 had no bacterial overgrowth. Age, duration of diabetes, level of glycosylated hemoglobin A_{1c}, and presence of autonomic neuropathy did not differ between the patients with and without bacterial overgrowth. However, those identified with bacterial overgrowth had longer duration of diarrhea, higher number of stools, and more frequent GI symptoms. There was dramatic clinical improvement in most patients with bacterial overgrowth treated with antibiotics.

Gluten-sensitive Enteropathy

Diabetes per se has no demonstrable effect on mucosal morphology or absorption in the small bowel. However, gluten-sensitive enteropathy (GSE) can coexist with diabetes and may be a cause of or contributor to diarrhea in such patients. Shanahan et al. (174) undertook HLA subtyping in patients with type 1 diabetes, GSE, and both disorders. HLA haplotypes B8 and DR3 were more prevalent in patients with GSE alone and in patients with both diabetes and GSE. Therefore, some patients are at increased risk for developing both type 1 diabetes and GSE as a result of autoimmune features associated with their HLA status. In this study of 24 patients with both disorders, the diagnosis of GSE was made after the onset of clinical diabetes in more than one half of the patients.

A Swedish study tested children and adolescents with a new diagnosis of type 1 diabetes for prevalence of IgA-antiendomysial and IgA-antigliadin autoantibodies. They found that in this population, prevalence of GSE at diagnosis of type 1 diabetes was 6% to 8% and suggest that screening for celiac disease is justified among patients with newly diagnosed type 1 diabetes (175).

Various serologic markers can be used to screen for GSE. Immunoglobulin A antiendomysial antibody (IgA-EMA) has been shown in North American children with type 1 diabetes to have a sensitivity of 94% and specificity of 91% for IgA-sufficient patients (176). The recent discovery that the autoantigen responsible for the endomysial pattern is tissue transglutaminase has led to the development of automated enzyme immunoassays for autoantibody quantitation. These commercial tests for tissue transglutaminases are simpler to perform and also comparably sensitive. In either test, positive results should be confirmed by intestinal biopsy, and false-positive results require serial follow-up. Symptomatic children require biopsy regardless of their serology.

Intestinal Fluid Secretion

In streptozotocin-treated diabetic rats, net secretion of fluid and electrolytes by the intestine is increased. This increase is thought to be due to sympathetic denervation (23). Sympathetic nerves release norepinephrine, which acts on α_2-adrenergic receptors present on the enterocytes. The villous enterocyte responds to stimulation of the α_2-adrenergic receptor by stimulating intracellular calcium-mediated electroneutral NaCl absorption, and the crypt enterocyte responds to stimulation of the α_2-adrenergic receptor by stimulating intracellular calcium-mediated chloride secretion. However, the adrenergic influences cause net fluid absorption. In the absence of adrenergic influence, a net secretion of fluid and electrolytes occurs in the small bowel, particularly in the postprandial state. In some patients with diabetic diarrhea, this secretory defect may be corrected by an agonist receptor α_2-adrenergic such as clonidine (177).

Treatment of Intestinal Dysmotility

Treatment of intestinal dysmotility includes a low-fat diet, antibiotics, and prokinetic agents. Although clinical trials have not been done, it is common practice to use a different antibiotic for 7 to 10 days each month to avoid drug resistance. Typically, doxycycline, 100 mg twice a day, metronidazole, 500 mg three times a day, ciprofloxacin, 500 mg twice a day, or double-strength trimethoprim-sulfamethoxazole twice a day is used. In general, prokinetic agents such as cisapride and erythromycin are less effective in treating intestinal dysmotility than gastroparesis (178). In refractory or intermittent but severe intestinal dysmotility, a venting jejunostomy is helpful. However, attempts should first be made to use the small bowel for nutrition. Trial infusions of liquid formulas, including elemental preparations, are warranted. Octreotide was initially shown to inhibit intestinal secretion and induce small-bowel activity similar to the interdigestive motor complex. Patients given the drug for up to 15 days seemed to improve (179). However, further studies suggest that the induced contractile activity is not well coordinated and is often simultaneous or very rapidly propagating. In healthy individuals, low doses (50 µg three times a day) inhibit small-bowel transit and ileocolonic bolus transfers, suggesting that octreotide may be helpful in treating diarrheal states but not conditions that cause small-bowel stasis and bacterial overgrowth (180). The role of octreotide in treatment of diabetic intestinal dysmotility needs further studies. Total parenteral nutrition may be required with bowel failure. Intestinal transplantation and pacing are still experimental.

COLON IN DIABETES

Colonic involvement in diabetes usually causes constipation but may sometimes also cause diarrhea.

Colonic Motility

Normal colonic motor activity consists of short-duration contractions (<10 seconds), long-duration contractions (>1 minute), and peristaltic contractions (duration >1 minute and amplitude two to three times larger than other colonic contractions). The short-duration contractions occur as a result of spikes associated with colonic slow waves. They occur irregularly at a frequency of 3 to 12 per minute, corresponding to the frequency of colonic slow waves. Long-duration contractions and giant contractions occur without regard to slow waves or spikes. The short- and the long-duration contractions occur singly or in trains and may be propagated or nonpropagated (segmental). The propagated wave may be propagated antegrade (peristaltic) or retrograde (retroperistaltic). Segmental and retropulsive contractions form the main activity of the right colon. An increase in segmental contractions in the left side of the colon is associated with constipation, and a decrease is associated with diarrhea. Peristaltic short-and long-duration contractions are responsible for slow caudal shifts of colonic contents. Giant peristaltic contractions propagate at velocities of 2 to 3 cm per second and are responsible for rapid shifts of large volumes of colonic contents. These movements are called "mass movements." Giant peristaltic contractions occur that sweep over the entire colon during defecation, but they also occur without associated defecation when they travel over a small segment of the colon. Mass movements are induced in the left side of the colon as a reflex response to stimulation such as eating (gastrocolonic reflex). These reflexes, mediated by neurohormonal influences and parasympathetic nerves, play an important role in giant peristaltic contractions and associated mass movements (181).

Information available on colonic electrical activity and motility in diabetics is limited. Battle et al. (182) studied colonic myoelectric and motor activity in the sigmoid colon in 12 patients with type 1 diabetes; although 11 of the patients had clinical evidence of autonomic neuropathy, 6 had no or mild constipation

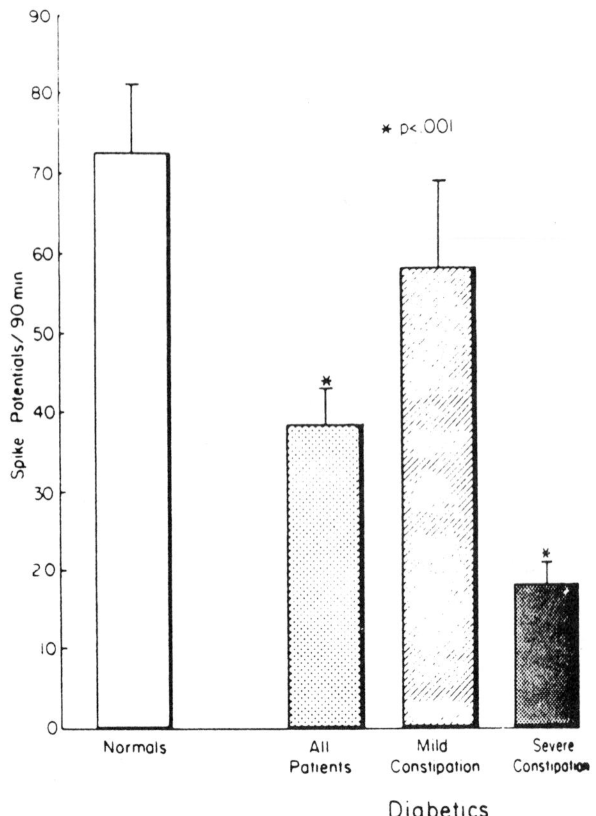

Figure. 64.9. Effect of a meal on sigmoid colon activity in patients with diabetes. Note that the cumulative spike potential response after ingestion of a 1,000-calorie meal is decreased in patients with diabetes mellitus. This decrease is most marked in patients who have severe constipation. Asterisk indicates significant ($p < 0.001$) decrease in response in various patient groups as compared with healthy controls. (From Battle WM, Snape WI Jr, Alavi A, et al. Colonic dysfunction in diabetes mellitus. *Gastroenterology* 1980;79:1217–1221, with permission.)

and 6 patients had severe constipation as defined by a stool frequency of two or fewer stools per week. After subjects consumed a standardized meal, both the myoelectric spike activity and the motor response were greater in the control than in the diabetic subjects (Fig. 64.9). Those patients with severe constipation had no postprandial response, whereas the six patients with mild constipation had a distinct but reduced postprandial response. In these latter patients with diabetes, the myoelectric response was delayed until 60 to 90 minutes after the meal, in contrast to the physiologic response, which occurred during the first 30 minutes after the meal. Wegener et al. (172) report delayed whole-gut transit in 26% of diabetics; they used a carmine red method, but this assay cannot distinguish the contributions of different segments of the gut. Metal detectors have also been used to assess colonic transit, showing normal or prolonged transit, which did not necessarily correlate to complaint of constipation, in both in type 1 and type 2 diabetic patients compared with controls (116).

Constipation and Colonic Dilation

Constipation is a symptom, rather than a disease, and is characterized by decreased frequency of defecation, increased stool hardness, and/or difficulty passing fecal matter. Constipation is common in the diabetic population (183) and is considered to be a complication of autonomic dysfunction of the gut. A sweat test devised to detect autonomic neuropathy in patients with diabetes has been shown to correlate with the presence of chronic constipation (184). Overall, persons with diabetes had slower colonic transit than did those without diabetes, and those with diabetes who experience constipation or use laxatives have a greater prevalence of delayed colonic transit or evacuatory dysfunction than do community controls (185).

The treatment of constipation in patients with diabetes is similar to that for the general population. In clinical practice, constipation in a diabetic patient is treated conservatively with the usual methods using bulking agents (such as psyllium) and stool softeners. If these agents fail, laxatives used prudently can be quite helpful (182).

There are anecdotal reports of roles for additional agents in patients with diabetes who do not respond to conventional treatments. Intramuscular administration of the cholinesterase inhibitor neostigmine has been shown to stimulate colonic myoelectric activity to a normal level in patients with diabetes. Whereas the administration of neostigmine and metoclopramide is associated with increased colonic motor activity, neither agent has been shown to consistently improve the clinical pattern of constipation, probably because they increase the frequency of segmental contractions but do not promote overall colonic transit. Some patients with diabetes with both gastroparesis and constipation may experience an improvement in constipation during treatment with metoclopramide. Whether this beneficial effect reflects a direct action of metoclopramide on the colon or an indirect effect by increasing oral intake and promoting colonic bulk remains unclear (182). Cisapride was shown to have prokinetic properties in some, but not all, patients with idiopathic or diabetic constipation (186) but currently is limited to investigational and compassionate use. Tegaserod, a 5-HT_4 receptor agonist, increases colonic transit in animals and healthy subjects and is being introduced for the treatment of constipation-predominant irritable bowel syndrome (187). It may soon find a place as a prokinetic agent in the future treatment of constipation associated with diabetes. Domperidone and alizapride are D_2-receptor antagonists, which antagonize the constipatory effects of opiates in rats (128). Promotility effects on human colon have yet to be established. There are also anecdotal reports of improved chronic constipation in patients with diabetes taking the aldose reductase inhibitor epalrestat (188). This and other members of its class hold promise in reversing some of the complications of autonomic neuropathy.

Infrequently, colonic dysfunction in patients with diabetes may lead to more severe colonic disorders. Berenyi and Schwarz (189) described 13 patients with autonomic dysfunction and marked sigmoid dilation. Surprisingly, the majority of these patients experienced diarrhea. Diabetes was present in 9 of the 13 patients and was thought to be the underlying cause of the observed autonomic dysfunction.

Diabetes and Colon Cancer

A number of studies have suggested a potential modest increase in colorectal cancer risk in patients with type 2 diabetes (190–193), even though these patients may be less likely to be screened for colorectal cancer (194). Among proposed biological mechanisms to account for this epidemiologic correlation are the observations that higher levels of insulin in patient with type 2 diabetes, analogous to insulin-like growth factor (as in acromegaly) (195), may influence cell proliferation and apoptosis (196) and thus play a role in carcinogenesis (197). Delayed stool transit and elevated fecal bile acid concentrations, associated with hyperglycemia and diabetic neuropathy, have also been suggested as factors contributing to the development of colon cancer. Earlier studies of the contribution of diabetes to colorectal cancer incidence and mortality are compromised by small sample sizes and failure to adjust for covariates. The 1959 to 1972 Cancer Prevention Study, with more than 1 million respondents, showed that persons with diabetes were indeed more likely to develop colorectal cancer during the 13-year follow-up period than were persons without diabetes. After adjustment for colorectal cancer risk factors, such as race, educational level, body mass index, smoking, alcohol use, dietary intake, aspirin use, physical activity, and family history of colorectal cancer, the incidence density ratio comparing colorectal cancer in those with diabetes and those without diabetes was 1.30 (95% confidence interval, 1.03 to 1.65) for men and 1.16 (95% confidence interval, 0.87 to 1.53) for women. However, diabetes was not associated with a greater case-fatality rate (198).

DIABETIC DIARRHEA

Clinical Features

By definition, "diabetic diarrhea" is a clinical syndrome that occurs in patients with diabetes without an identifiable underlying GI disorder and is therefore a diagnosis of exclusion (199). The clinical characteristics vary in different patients, presumably because the underlying pathogenetic mechanisms are numerous and heterogeneous. Hence not all patients respond to a common treatment. Most patients with this disorder have longstanding diabetes with its associated complications (200). Almost all have evidence of both peripheral and autonomic neuropathy, and autonomic neuropathy is thought to be an underlying mechanism. Examination of the rectal mucosa from symptomatic patients showed a significant decrease in substance P, but not in VIP or somatostatin, compared with that in diabetic patients with normal bowel habits or in nondiabetic controls (201). In the majority of affected patients, the pattern of diarrhea is intermittent, lasting weeks to months, with intervening periods of either normal stool frequency or constipation. Although early reports emphasized a predominantly nocturnal pattern of diarrhea, later series described a variable pattern, with the majority of patients experiencing a persistent or predominantly daytime pattern commonly associated with fecal incontinence (200). In diabetic diarrhea, stool weight can vary from 200 to 1,600 g per day. Coincident steatorrhea can occur in 40% to 50% of patients, is usually mild, and generally does not cause progressive weight loss. In a diabetic patient, the documentation of steatorrhea does not exclude the diagnosis of diabetic diarrhea but should prompt a careful exclusion of underlying jejunal and pancreatic disease (202).

Pathogenesis

Proposed mechanisms of diabetic diarrhea include pancreatic exocrine insufficiency, altered intestinal motility, bacterial overgrowth, altered composition of the bile-salt pool and bile-salt excretion, and increased intestinal secretion as a result of autonomic neuropathy. A review of medical records of patients with diabetes and diarrhea seen at a tertiary referral practice revealed that diarrhea was often due to celiac sprue, bacterial overgrowth in the small bowel, or fecal incontinence in conjunction with anorectal dysfunction. However, these causes could be excluded in about half of the patients, and abnormal intestinal motility or secretion was deemed to be the likely cause of diarrhea in these patients (203). Oral hypoglycemic agents have been associated with chronic diarrhea, and one report suggested that metformin but not sulfonylurea was independently associated with chronic diarrhea and with fecal incontinence (204).

ROLE OF EXOCRINE PANCREATIC INSUFFICIENCY

Given the high incidence of impaired pancreatic exocrine function in patients with type 1 diabetes, exocrine insufficiency in steatorrhea would seem to be a possible mechanism of diabetic diarrhea. Because of the high capacity for enzyme secretion of the exocrine pancreas, however, the observed 50% to 60% reduction in bicarbonate and enzyme secretion does not impair luminal digestion and hence does not result in steatorrhea (205). In patients with diabetic diarrhea, duodenal intubation studies have demonstrated little or no reduction in exocrine function (200). Furthermore, empiric trials of pancreatic enzyme supplements have routinely been ineffective in reducing the volume of diarrhea in these patients.

ROLE OF ABNORMAL SMALL-BOWEL MOTILITY AND BACTERIAL OVERGROWTH

Abnormal small-bowel motility in diabetes may be associated with bowel stasis and bacterial overgrowth (173). Clearance of luminal bacteria by normal small-bowel motility generally prevents the development of pathologic concentrations of bacteria. Normally, bacteria are present in the proximal small bowel in very low concentrations, but the concentration increases with the stasis caused by obstruction or motility disorders. The IMMC is absent in the intestine of some patients with diabetic diarrhea.

In clinical studies, the prevalence of bacterial overgrowth in patients with diabetes with diarrhea has ranged from 20% to 43% (202,206). In one study, however, none of 11 patients had clinically significant bacterial overgrowth (207). In patients with bacterial overgrowth, steatorrhea often is present as a result of impaired micelle formation caused by bacterial deconjugation and hydroxylation of bile salts (207). The presence of bacterial overgrowth can be documented by (a) culture of jejunal contents (206), (b) [^{14}C]glycocholate (208) or [^{14}C]xylose breath tests (207), or (c) glucose- or lactulose-hydrogen breath tests (207). In clinical practice, one may alternatively observe the effect of an empiric trial of antibiotics (tetracycline or metronidazole). In patients with bacterial overgrowth resistant to empiric antibiotic therapy, jejunal intubation studies may be performed so that accurate antibiotic sensitivity determinations can be done.

Autonomic neuropathy, by causing alterations in small-bowel motility, might result in rapid intestinal transit, which in turn may lead to diarrhea in affected patients with diabetes. However, careful studies suggest that transit through the small intestine in patients with diabetic diarrhea is delayed—not accelerated (171). This slowing of transit has been documented both by breath tests (171) and by luminal sampling via multilumen tubes (202). Although small-bowel motility is abnormal in patients with diabetes with diarrhea, no specific pattern of abnormal motility was found to correlate with rapid or delayed transit (171). It seems unlikely that diabetic diarrhea is due to rapid intestinal transit, and presumably slow intestinal transit in this population is the likely basis for the increased incidence of bacterial overgrowth.

BILE-SALT MALABSORPTION

Altered bile-salt circulation and kinetics through the gut have been suggested as possible factors in diabetic diarrhea (209). Bile salts usually are absorbed efficiently in the terminal ileum, and the passage of increased amounts of bile salts into the colon results in increased colonic secretion of fluid and electrolytes. Observations in diabetic subjects suggest that increased amounts of bile salts escape ileal absorption and pass into the colon. Studies of kinetics and turnover of the bile-salt pool in patients with diabetes with diarrhea indicate that metabolism of endogenous bile salts by intestinal bacteria is increased (209). Although these results could be caused by abnormal contact between the bile salts and bacteria in the small bowel as a result of overgrowth, they more likely reflect the action of colonic bacteria on bile salts. In addition, the size of the bile-salt pool has been described as reduced, and the fraction of the bile-salt pool that is excreted has been found to be increased (208). Although bile-salt malabsorption does occur in diabetic patients with diarrhea, this phenomenon does not appear to be the mechanism of the diarrhea. For example, Schiller et al. (209) found that increased fecal excretion of bile salts is a nonspecific finding in several forms of both clinical and experimental diarrhea and does not prove a pathogenetic basis of the bile-salt excretion in the diarrhea. Indeed, there are no clinical data attesting to the efficacy of agents that bind bile salts (e.g., cholestyramine) in halting diabetic diarrhea.

IMPAIRED INTESTINAL ABSORPTION OF FLUID

Diarrhea in patients with diabetes might also result from impaired intestinal absorption of fluid and electrolytes secondary to autonomic neuropathy. In experimental studies, Chang et al. (177) demonstrated that a component of fluid and electrolyte absorption in the ileum and colon is mediated by α_2-adrenergic receptors. Adrenergic-mediated fluid and electrolyte transport does not play a physiologic role in jejunal absorption. Studying the pathogenesis of diarrhea in rats with streptozotocin-induced chronic diabetes, Chang et al. (23) demonstrated a decrease in sympathetic tone in the ileal and colonic mucosa that was presumably secondary to sympathetic denervation caused by autonomic neuropathy. The resulting reduction in absorption of fluid and electrolytes in these segments of the intestine produced clinical diarrhea. *In vitro* studies also demonstrated that the impaired sympathetic tone in the ileum and colon was accompanied by adrenergic-denervation hypersensitivity, presumably as a result of an increase in the number of α_2-adrenergic receptors. In the diabetic rat, administration of clonidine, an α_2-adrenergic agonist, can correct this defect in ileal and colonic absorption (23).

Few clinical studies have directly examined intestinal fluid and electrolyte absorption in patients with diabetes. Whalen et al. (203) studied fluid and electrolyte absorption in the jejunum and ileum of 13 patients with diabetes with unexplained diarrhea. Under fasting conditions, the absorption of fluid and electrolytes in the jejunum and ileum of these patients was comparable to that of controls. Following the administration of a test meal, however, the volume of the test meal in the ileum was greater in diabetic than control subjects, suggesting that the ileal absorption of the fluid from the test meal was impaired. Indirect evidence of impaired sympathetic innervation of the gut in diabetic subjects with diarrhea also comes from the observation that therapy with clonidine strikingly reduced the volume of diarrhea, presumably by stimulating intestinal adrenergic receptors (210). The prevalence of these different pathogenetic disorders (including impaired absorption) in a population of patients with diabetes with diarrhea is not known. However, at least some fraction of patients with diabetes appear to experience diarrhea related to the impaired fluid and electrolyte absorption in the ileum and colon caused by sympathetic denervation.

Diagnostic Studies

Patients with diabetes with chronic intermittent or persistent diarrhea should undergo a careful evaluation. Investigators at the Mayo Clinic suggest three sequential assessments. First, blood tests should assess glucose control, electrolyte balance, evidence of malabsorption or anemia, thyroid status, antinuclear antibody, and possible drug levels. Stool specimens should be sent for culture and, in the appropriate setting, for parasitology. Flexible sigmoidoscopy should also be part of the initial workup to rule out mucosal disease in the distal colon. In the second step, small-bowel aspirate and biopsy are advocated if the results of initial blood or stool tests are abnormal. Patients with steatorrhea need to have disorders of jejunal malabsorption and pancreatic insufficiency carefully excluded. Anorectal function tests are suggested if initial blood and stool tests are normal. In the third step, if the outlined evaluation fails to identify a definite source of diarrhea, it is likely that increased fecal-fluid excretion is due to impaired intestinal absorption of fluid and electrolytes. In these patients, measurement of GI transit or therapeutic trials with opioids, clonidine hydrochloride, and, rarely, cholestyramine resin or octreotide acetate (or both methods) are recommended (202).

Therapy

If the evaluation identifies a specific cause of the diarrhea, directed therapy should be undertaken. If diagnostic studies for the presence of bacterial overgrowth are not available, it is reasonable to undertake an empiric trial of antibiotics. In patients for whom diagnostic studies are unrevealing and antibiotic therapy is unhelpful, trials of symptomatic therapy with diphenoxylate/atropine or loperamide are reasonable. Because diarrhea in these patients is episodic, symptomatic therapy can be used during periods of symptoms and later discontinued. In patients for whom symptomatic therapy is unsuccessful, a trial of clonidine is reasonable (210,212,213). However, there are few data to suggest the proper dosage and schedule of clonidine. Moreover, no data exist on the rate of success of clonidine therapy in patients with diabetes with unexplained diarrhea. Fedorak et al. (210) reported good results with high doses of clonidine (0.5 to 0.6 mg) administered every 12 hours, but these were associated with increased risk for excessive sedation. Experimental studies suggest that a state of adrenergic hypersensitivity may exist. As such, lower doses may be effective and better tolerated. In patients with diabetes with coincident diarrhea, autonomic neuropathy, and orthostatic hypotension, clonidine therapy does not appear to exacerbate the orthostatic hypotension, presumably because of the underlying neuropathy. There are also reports of topical administration of clonidine with a transdermal preparation (215).

If diarrhea is severe and unresponsive to clonidine, the somatostatin analogue octreotide should be considered. Although the specific mechanism of somatostatin action in diabetic diarrhea is unknown, this drug may reduce intestinal mucosal secretion and enhance mucosal absorption under physiologic conditions and, anecdotally, in diabetic diarrhea (216–219). Octreotide must be administered parenterally, either subcutaneously in divided doses or intravenously through a constant infusion pump. When administered in this fashion, octreotide has been demonstrated to produce striking reductions in the volume of diabetic diarrhea in a small number of patients (220,221). Of interest, in this setting octreotide was also helpful in the management of refractory orthostatic hypotension. There have been anecdotal reports of successful treatment of severe diabetic diarrhea with octreotide (216) and with ondansetron, a selective 5-HT_3 antagonist (222).

ANORECTAL FUNCTION IN DIABETES

Fecal Incontinence

CLINICAL FEATURES

Fecal incontinence denotes the inability to retain stool and prevent its involuntary passage, which can occur with or without the patient's knowledge. Although a small percentage of patients experience incontinence even with solid stool, the majority of affected individuals suffer this problem with liquid stool. The prevalence of fecal incontinence among patients with diabetes is approximately 20% (3), and the incidence and severity appear to correlate with duration of diabetes and with evidence of microangiopathy or neuropathy (223). This is likely an underestimate, because many embarrassed patients complain of diarrhea rather than incontinence. Patients with diabetes frequently have both diarrhea and fecal incontinence. Almost one third of affected patients have mild steatorrhea, which does not correlate with the volume of the diarrhea. Most patients with diabetes with fecal incontinence have normal or only moderately increased daily stool volumes but also exhibit multiple abnormalities of anorectal sensory and motor functions that are not present in continent patients with diabetes (252). Among patients with diabetes, the frequency of incontinence varies from several episodes daily to a few episodes yearly and worsens during periods of diarrhea. On physical examination, both continent and incontinent patients with diabetes appear to have reduced resting and squeeze pressures in the anal canal. It should be recognized that the subjective assessment of sphincter function on rectal examination correlates poorly with actual manometric measurements of sphincter pressure (224).

QUANTIFICATION

Schiller et al. (225) assessed the anal continence mechanism for liquids and solids in diabetes. The continence mechanism for liquids was assessed by determining the volume of saline infused into the rectum that a person could hold without leaking. Both the intrarectal saline volume at which the first leak occurred and the total volume retained were much lower in incontinent patients with diabetes than in continent patients with diabetes or in control subjects. Moreover, the volume at first leak showed a better correlation with clinical continence than did the strength of anal sphincter squeeze measured manometrically. The anal continence mechanism for solids was determined by measuring the applied weight required to pull a solid sphere through the contracted sphincter. Patients with diabetes with fecal incontinence expelled the spheres at lower applied weights than did control subjects (Table 64.4).

PATHOGENESIS

At the junction of the distal rectum and the pelvic floor, the anal canal extends as a slit-like lumen 2.5 to 5.0 cm through the diaphragm of the pelvis musculature. One of the muscles of the diaphragm, the puborectalis, forms a sling of fibers that originates from both sides of the pubis symphysis and passes backward to the posterior wall of the anorectal junction. This sling of voluntary striated muscle is innervated by branches of the sacral nerve (S3, S4), and its tonic contraction creates a relatively acute angle of 80 to 100 degrees at the anorectal junction (anorectal angle) that is thought to be a major contributor to the continence of solid stool.

The internal anal sphincter consists of a thickening of the rectal circular muscle that extends the length of the anal canal. It is composed of involuntary smooth muscle whose tonic contraction is due to intrinsic myogenic activity and a variety of neurohormonal influences. Sympathetic innervation via the hypogastric nerve (L5) results in contraction of the sphincter. Parasympathetic innervation via the pelvic nerves (S1, S2, and S3) exerts both excitatory and inhibiting influences. The excitatory neurons are both cholinergic and noncholinergic. The inhibitory neurons are nonadrenergic and noncholinergic, and possibly involve NO and vasoactive intestinal peptide as neurotransmitters. It is estimated that the tonic contraction of the internal anal sphincter results in approximately 80% of the resting closure of the anal canal. With rectal distention the sphincter relaxes transiently (anorectal inhibitory reflex). Although the inhibitory reflex could "allow" incontinence of stool, sensation mediated by rectal distention results in both reflex and voluntary contraction of the external anal sphincter, resulting in closure of the anal canal.

TABLE 64.4. Effect of Diabetes on Anal Sphincter Pressure and Anal Continence: Incontinent Diabetic Patients Have Sphincter Hypotension, Decreased Squeeze-pressure Increment, and Marked Incontinence of Liquids

	Nondiabetic controls (*n* = 35)	Incontinent diabetics (*n* = 16)	Continent diabetics (*n* = 14)
Basal pressure (mm Hg)	63 ± 4	37 ± 4	54 ± 5
Squeeze increment (mm Hg)	111 ± 13	75 ± 10	99 ± 18
Continence of solid sphere			
Weight held with sphincter relaxed (g)	685 ± 32	532 ± 52	624 ± 48
Weight held with sphincter contracted (g)	1065 ± 37	799 ± 64	951 ± 55
Continence of infused saline			
Saline infused before first leak (mL)	1253 ± 71	410 ± 107	1222 ± 424
Total saline held (ml)	1423 ± 39	715 ± 115	1328 ± 86

Data from Schiller LR, Santa Ana CA, Schmulen AC, et al. Pathogenesis of fecal incontinence in diabetes mellitus: evidence for internal-anal-sphincter dysfunction. *N Engl J Med* 1982;307:1666–1671.

The external anal sphincter consists of at least three bundles of striated muscle that surround the anal canal and act as a single unit. It is a voluntary muscle with innervation by the pudendal nerve (S2, S3, S4). Whereas the external sphincter demonstrates some tonic activity at rest (contributing to closure), its voluntary contraction is a major mechanism for continence of stool and flatus. The fibers of the pudendal nerve are cholinergic and exert their effect at the motor end plate via nicotinic receptors. With rectal distention, the external anal sphincter contracts reflexively to close the anal canal (sphincteric reflex). Rectal sensation is mediated by afferent pelvic splanchnic fibers passing to the sacral cord (S2, S3) and alerts the subject to rectal distention produced by stool or flatus. The stimulus of rectal distention causes conscious or reflexive contraction of the external anal sphincter and puborectalis.

Under physiologic conditions, the internal anal sphincter provides resting closure of the anal canal and some protection against rectal leakage and fecal stress incontinence. As stool passes into the rectum, distention of the rectum alerts one to contract both the external anal sphincter, which tightens the closure of the anal canal, and the puborectalis, which further closes the anorectal angle. Contractions of the external anal sphincter and puborectalis nullify the relaxation of the internal sphincter associated with rectal distention. These mechanisms maintain continence until defecation is appropriate.

In various patients with diabetes with fecal incontinence, anorectal testing has demonstrated (a) decreased resting and squeeze anal pressures, (b) decreased sensation to rectal distention, (c) an elevated threshold for the external anal sphincteric reflex, and (d) impaired anocutaneous reflex. Decreased threshold of sensation to distention and to electrical stimulation noted particularly in the upper anal canal has been suggested as an early abnormality in the development of diabetic incontinence (226). The rectoanal inhibitory reflex involving the internal anal sphincter has been described as normal by some groups (227,228) but diminished in patients with longstanding diabetes and fecal incontinence (223,225) (Fig. 64.10). Prolonged pudendal nerve terminal latency has also been correlated with diabetic patients having fecal incontinence (229) and may explain the decreased squeeze pressure, because this is generated by the skeletal external anal sphincter muscle, which is indirectly innervated by the pudendal nerve.

At least in some patients with diabetes, instability of the internal anal sphincter plays a major role in fecal incontinence. During basal recording, some patients with diabetes demonstrated oscillations in anal electrical activity and pressure. Some patients also exhibited spontaneous transient anal relaxations, and fecal leakage occurred as the anal pressure fell below the rectal pressure (230).

The observed basal hypotonia of the anal canal is presumably caused by dysfunction of the internal anal sphincter secondary to diabetic autonomic neuropathy. Patients with diabetes with fecal incontinence not only show evidence of autonomic neuropathy but also suffer from diarrhea, suggesting a distinctive pattern of sympathetic denervation of the gut that results in both impaired fluid absorption and dysfunction of the internal sphincter.

Altered rectal sensation in patients with diabetes is presumably a manifestation of sensory neuropathy and is not observed in patients with fecal incontinence related to other disorders. Because rectal sensation mediates the afferent limb of the sphincteric reflex, it is not surprising that the threshold for reflex contraction of the external anal sphincter is also elevated. In patients with diabetes, however, the threshold for anorectal inhibitory reflex is comparable to that for control subjects (227). In this setting, fecal incontinence can occur because an amount of rectal distention that will induce relaxation of the internal sphincter may fail either to initiate reflex contraction of the external sphincter or to alert the subject to contract the sphincter voluntarily.

The etiology of fecal incontinence in diabetes is multifactorial, including dysfunction of the internal anal sphincter, decreased sensation of the rectal vault, impaired fluid absorption, dysfunction of the external anal sphincter, and impaired "sampling" function of the anal canal. As in other regions of the upper GI tract, these physiologic measures correlate poorly with the extent of autonomic neuropathy.

TREATMENT

In patients with diabetes, fecal incontinence usually occurs in relation to liquid stool. Because the success of attempts to develop continence is much greater if the patient has solid stools, every effort should be made to identify and treat the underlying cause of diarrhea. In some patients, trials of clonidine can be undertaken to control so-called diabetic diarrhea. In patients with functional diarrhea, the use of antidiarrheal agents, such as loperamide and diphenoxylate/atropine, is

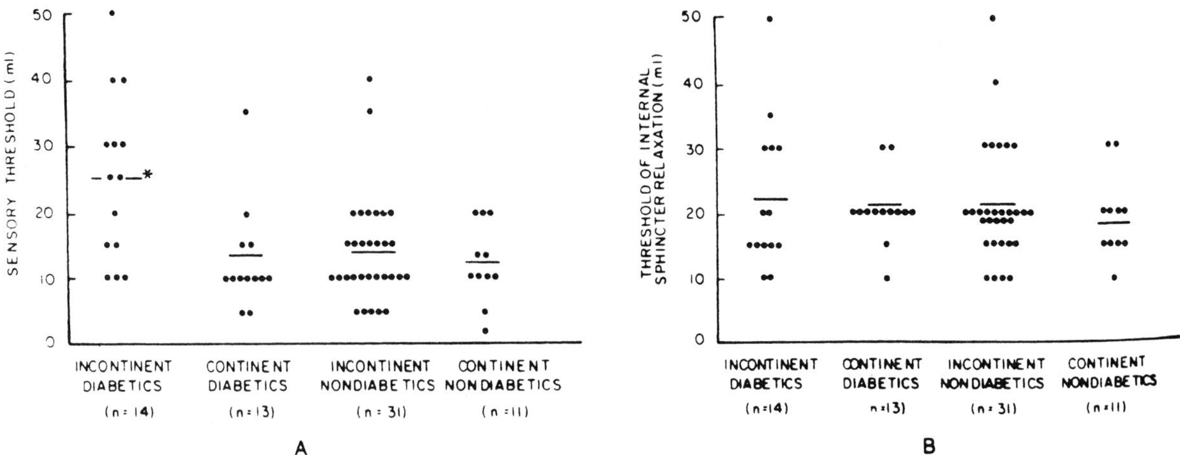

Figure 64.10. Anorectal sensory thresholds and thresholds of internal anal sphincter relaxation in four groups of subjects. The mean threshold of rectal sensation **(A)** was significantly higher in the incontinent patients with diabetes than in the other three groups of patients ($p < 0.02$), as indicated by the asterisk. There were no significant differences in thresholds of internal sphincter relaxation **(B).** Note that in all groups except the incontinent patients with diabetes the sensory threshold was lower than the threshold for internal anal sphincter relaxation. These observations suggest that fecal incontinence in patients with diabetes may be due to an increase in the sensory threshold above that for internal anal sphincter relaxation. (From Wald A, Tunuguntla AK. Anorectal sensorimotor dysfunction in fecal incontinence and diabetes mellitus: modification with biofeedback therapy. *N Engl J Med* 1984;310:1282–1287, with permission. Copyright © 1984 Massachusetts Medical Society. All rights reserved.)

helpful. If these measures are unsuccessful in achieving fecal continence, the performance of anorectal manometry is recommended. Basal anal canal pressure, sensory threshold pressure for rectal distention, and internal anal sphincter relaxation and external anal sphincter contraction responses to rectal distention should be studied. If manometric studies demonstrate an elevated sensory threshold for rectal distention, biofeedback training can be helpful in obtaining symptomatic relief (228).

Biofeedback training in incontinent patients with diabetes employs a balloon catheter to achieve both rectal sensory and external sphincter conditioning (Fig. 64.11). Using this technique, Wald and Tunuguntla (228) noted improvement in 73% of

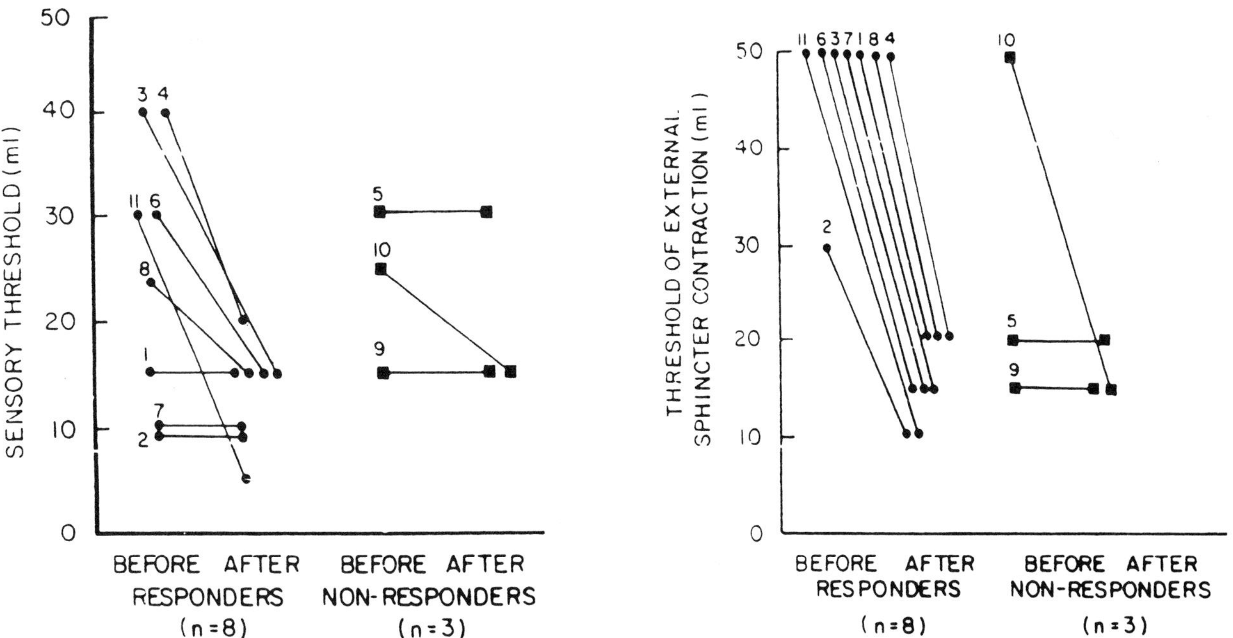

Figure 64.11. Effect of biofeedback conditioning of rectal sensation on anorectal sensory threshold and threshold of external anal sphincter contraction in eight responders (decreased frequency of fecal continence) and three nonresponder patients with diabetes. **Left:** Normalization of rectal sensory thresholds to less than 20 mL occurred in all but one patient with thresholds above 20 mL. No improvement in the sensory threshold was noted in patient 5. **Right:** Thresholds of external sphincter contraction showing strong association between improvement of the external sphincter response and reestablishment of bowel control. (Reprinted from Wald A, Tunuguntla AK. Anorectal sensorimotor dysfunction in fecal incontinence and diabetes mellitus: modification with biofeedback therapy. *N Engl J Med* 1984;310:1282–1287, with permission. Copyright © 1984 Massachusetts Medical Society. All rights reserved.)

patients with diabetes, who achieved a reduction in fecal soiling without any striking change in stool frequency. Improvement in fecal control correlated with the ability to improve both the sensory threshold and the threshold for phasic external sphincter contraction. Most important, the manometric improvements did result in clinically meaningful enhancements in lifestyle, as patients experienced a greater freedom of activity once the risk and frequency of rectal incontinence were reduced. Long-term testing demonstrated that the improvements in sensory and sphincter thresholds were sustained during periods of follow-up exceeding 1 year. Presumably, enhancement of sensory perception results from recruitment of adjacent neurons that mediate rectal sensation. By relearning the appropriate physiologic response to rectal distention, patients thereby regain improved control over rectal function.

BILIARY SYSTEM IN DIABETES

Cholelithiasis is common in patients with diabetes, especially in women with type 2 diabetes (231,232). Patients with diabetes may have physiologic reasons for being at increased risk for the formation of cholesterol gallstones. First, in these patients, total body cholesterol synthesis is increased independently of obesity, which may lead to more lithogenic bile. Second, patients with diabetes have larger gallbladders (233) and possibly diminished gallbladder motility, which could result in enhanced formation of cholesterol crystals. Despite these physiologic factors, recent studies suggest that diabetes alone may not significantly increase the risk for gallstones. Earlier studies did not differentiate the effects of obesity, hypertriglyceridemia, and other cofactors known to contribute to increased risk of gallstones.

Lithogenic Bile

Under physiologic conditions, the liver secretes bile that is unsaturated with respect to cholesterol, and the relative amounts of bile salts and lecithin in the bile are capable of maintaining cholesterol in a stable solution (234). Pathologic disorders that result in either a decrease in bile-salt secretion or an increase in cholesterol secretion will result in the formation of bile that is supersaturated with respect to cholesterol. Cholesterol crystals and eventually gallstones can develop from such lithogenic bile. Risk factors leading to the secretion of lithogenic bile include (a) increasing age, (b) obesity, (c) hypertriglyceridemia, and (d) decreased size of the bile-salt pool (235).

Haber and Heaton (236) examined the lipid composition of bile in patients with diabetes and in controls matched for obesity. Patients with type 1 or type 2 diabetes were matched to nondiabetic control subjects by age, gender, and obesity index. The analyses demonstrated no significant difference between the cholesterol saturation of bile in patients with diabetes and that of appropriately matched control subjects. The bile of patients with type 1 diabetes was unsaturated with respect to cholesterol. Patients with type 2 diabetes had a higher body mass index and more saturated bile than did patients with type 1 diabetes. Thus, the risk of lithogenic bile is greater in patients with type 2 diabetes than in those with type 1 diabetes and is related to concurrent obesity rather than to diabetes itself. Other studies have also suggested that diabetes per se does not predispose to secretion of abnormal bile (235). Similarly, there was no significant correlation of diabetes with type of stone, i.e., pigment or cholesterol, when corrected for other variables such as age and presence of cirrhosis (237).

Gallbladder Emptying

Studies using radiographic cholecystography have suggested that the emptying of the gallbladder is delayed or impaired in patients with diabetes. Other studies using ultrasonography and scintigraphy have yielded contradictory results. Stone et al. (238) used radionuclide cholescintigraphy to analyze gallbladder emptying in response to intravenous cholecystokinin octapeptide. Stimulated gallbladder emptying was lower in patients with diabetes than in controls (55% vs. 74%). Furthermore, the most severe impairment of gallbladder emptying occurred in patients with diabetes with associated autonomic neuropathy. Similar results were described by other groups using ultrasonography (239). With ultrasonography, Keshavarzian et al. (240) found contrasting results in an examination of fasting gallbladder volume and postprandial emptying. Among patients with diabetes, both fasting and postprandial gallbladder volumes were comparable to the respective values in controls. No effect of autonomic neuropathy on gallbladder emptying could be demonstrated. In patients with type 1 diabetes of less than 10 years' duration, no differences in emptying could be discerned, although the authors suggested that a dilated gallbladder at rest may correlate with autonomic neuropathy and the increased likelihood of stone formation (241). It is difficult to reconcile the differences in gallbladder motor function reported in these studies. Although differences in methodology may be a factor, a consistent pattern of gallbladder motor dysfunction has not been established in patients with diabetes.

Gallstones

PREVALENCE

In keeping with these contrasting observations about gallbladder function among patients with diabetes, studies on the prevalence of gallstones in this population have also yielded contradictory results. The findings of both autopsy studies (242,243) and epidemiologic studies (244) have conflicted. A large case-control study from Canada failed to find any association between cholesterol cholelithiasis and clinical diabetes (245). Epidemiologic studies based in Italy showed that multiple risk factors, including hyperinsulinemia, are associated with the formation of gallstones (246). More recent studies suggested that diabetes is associated with gallstones on univariate analysis but not on multivariate analysis (247) and that obesity and age, which are associated with type 2 diabetes, are stronger risk factors for the development of gallstones than is the presence of type 2 diabetes (248). Hence, if diabetes does affect the prevalence of gallstones, the effect is small.

TREATMENT

The surgical approach to the management of asymptomatic gallstones has been changing. As pointed out by Pellegrini (249), several observations have discouraged the routine use of surgery in patients without diabetes with asymptomatic gallstones. Among such patients, relatively few develop symptoms during periods of follow-up as long as 20 years. In addition, life-threatening complications of gallstone disease are rarely the first manifestation. Milder symptoms of biliary colic usually arise first and prompt a timely surgical referral before the appearance of acute cholecystitis and cholangitis. Furthermore, long-term follow-up of many patients with mild symptoms indicates that the majority remain free of serious complications. Finally, autopsy studies indicate that more than 90% of patients with gallstone disease die of an unrelated cause.

The role of surgery in patients with diabetes with asymptomatic gallstones has been controversial. In the past, it was believed that patients with diabetes with cholelithiasis should undergo surgery, even if asymptomatic, to avoid the increased morbidity and mortality presumed to occur in patients with diabetes. This aggressive perspective perhaps originated with Rabinowitch in 1932, who suggested that patients with diabetes and cholecystitis fared worse than patients without diabetes (250). In 1961, Turrill et al. (251) reported that the mortality rate after surgery for gallstones was fivefold higher in patients with diabetes. Deaths in that series occurred primarily in patients with diabetes who were undergoing emergency surgery. When the analysis was limited to patients in the fifth and sixth decades of life who underwent emergency cholecystectomy, the mortality among patients with diabetes was reported to be 20-fold higher than that among patients without diabetes. Others have also reported increased morbidity and mortality associated with emergency surgery for gallstones among patients with diabetes and recommended elective surgery for gallstones when possible, because the mortality among patients with diabetes with elective surgery was comparable to that among patients without diabetes (78,86,250). Both Turrill et al. (251) and Mundth (252) even recommended that all patients with diabetes undergo screening with oral cholecystography and that all with gallstones undergo elective surgery. Yet other authors report similar increases in morbidity and mortality for acute cholecystitis and suggest early surgery but believe that this is not necessarily an indication for cholecystectomy in asymptomatic patients (75,253).

Further analyses of the morbidity and mortality of gallstone surgery among patients with diabetes criticized the conclusions of earlier studies with respect to several issues: First, modern morbidity and mortality rates are much lower as a result of the use of antibiotics and improvements in medical and surgical care; second, earlier studies did not report the prevalence of concurrent medical disorders among the patients with diabetes (e.g., atherosclerosis) that might affect the rate of postoperative complications independent of diabetes; and finally, studies, including that of Mundth (252), did not include a contemporary control group that was analyzed over a comparable period (254). Several retrospective studies more critically examined the morbidity and mortality among patients with diabetes with surgical gallstone disease (255). Patients with diabetes undergoing surgery tended to be older than patients without diabetes and to have more concurrent medical disorders, especially cardiovascular disease. There was a trend toward increased surgical mortality among the patients with diabetes, but this difference was statistically significant in only one study. It is interesting that in a review of a 21-year period at one institution, the case-fatality rate among patients with diabetes with surgical gallstone disease decreased over the course of the study, presumably as a result of improvements in medical and surgical care (256).

In both patients with diabetes and those without diabetes, morbidity and mortality were increased in the setting of emergency cholecystectomy and with preoperative evidence of cardiovascular and renal disease. In none of the studies was diabetes per se a risk factor for increased operative mortality. Analyses indicated that the presence of preoperative concurrent medical disorders predicted postoperative morbidity and mortality more accurately than did the presence of diabetes. In reviewing earlier surgical studies, Walsh et al. (257) suggested that 50% to 80% of the patients with diabetes in those studies showed evidence of occlusive vascular disease, which might have accounted for the observed increase in morbidity and mortality independent of diabetes.

There was a trend toward increased postoperative complications among patients with diabetes, but it is unclear whether this risk is related to diabetes or to concurrent medical disorder. Hickman et al. (255) observed that with emergency cholecystectomy the incidence of postoperative infectious complications was higher in patients with diabetes, an increase that could not be explained by any pattern of concurrent medical disorders. In contrast, Sandler et al. (258), applying regression analysis, demonstrated that the twofold higher rate of postoperative complications in patients with diabetes was related to coincident medical problems rather than to diabetes per se (80). Furthermore, the increased incidence of postoperative complications among patients with diabetes occurred with both emergency and elective cholecystectomy (38).

In summary, the current data do not support elective cholecystectomy in patients with diabetes with asymptomatic gallstones. Nevertheless, because emergency cholecystectomy for acute cholecystitis is associated with increased morbidity and possibly increased mortality, one should consider elective surgery in those patients with diabetes with concurrent biliary symptoms, especially if serious medical disorders do not coexist. Laparoscopic cholecystectomy may provide a safer and preferable alternative to abdominal cholecystectomy (259).

EXOCRINE PANCREAS AND DIABETES

Diabetes in Pancreatic Disease

Primary disorders of the exocrine pancreas can affect islet cell function and result in states of glucose intolerance or in overt diabetes. For example, with acute pancreatitis of any etiology, hyperglycemia can result and is recognized as a prognostic sign of severity of pancreatitis (260). In this setting, hyperglycemia is thought to be secondary to increased circulating levels of glucagon and epinephrine rather than to islet destruction with actual insulin deficiency. Indeed, individuals who are not diabetic before an episode of acute pancreatitis will again achieve normal glucose control after resolution of the episode. In contrast, both diabetes and glucose intolerance are recognized complications of advanced chronic pancreatitis. The advanced stages of pancreatic injury and fibrosis result in damage to the islets, with resulting insulin deficiency and chronic diabetes (261).

Exocrine Pancreas in Diabetes

Well-recognized changes in pancreatic exocrine morphology and function have been identified in idiopathic diabetes mellitus. In type 1 diabetes, there is widespread islet atrophy and fibrosis with associated atrophy and fibrosis in the surrounding exocrine tissue (262). Careful studies of pancreatic histology in patients who died shortly after initial presentation of type 1 diabetes showed that the effects of diabetes on the endocrine and exocrine pancreas are halted at a relatively early stage. In parts of the diabetic pancreas where the islets remain intact and concentrations of insulin in β-cells determined immunohistochemically are normal, the surrounding exocrine tissue appears normal. In contrast, in those areas where the islets have atrophied, the surrounding acinar tissue also is atrophied. These observations support the hypothesis that insulin and other islet cell peptides have trophic effects on the surrounding acinar cells and are consistent with a microcirculatory architecture of the pancreas (263). Blood traveling through islet capillaries supplies surrounding exocrine tissue and exposes the acinar cells to high concentrations of islet cell peptides. Both insulin and pancreatic polypeptide appear to have trophic effects on acinar glands, whereas glucagon and somatostatin may have inhibitory effects. By this theory, islet dysfunction resulting in either decreased levels of trophic hormones or increased levels of inhibitory peptides could result in exocrine dysfunction (264).

In type 2 diabetes, the changes in the islets are less extensive, with variable reduction of the β-cells; there is hyalinosis of the islets of varying extent and severity. The associated changes in the surrounding exocrine tissue are less extensive than those seen in type 1 diabetes but are easily demonstrated nevertheless. As indicated by ultrasound examination, the overall size of the pancreas is smaller than in control subjects (264). On histologic study, the reduction in gland size correlates with atrophy and fibrosis of exocrine tissue.

Careful studies of pancreatic exocrine function in diabetes have demonstrated a surprisingly high prevalence of dysfunction (203,265). Vagal cholinergic and peptidergic neurons are involved in stimulating exocrine secretion. VIP increases water and bicarbonate secretion, whereas acetylcholine and GRP increase enzyme secretion. However, the role of diabetic autonomic neuropathy in pancreatic exocrine dysfunction remains unclear. Exocrine function has traditionally been measured by duodenal intubation and collection of pancreatic secretions following stimulation of the gland with both cholecystokinin and secretin. Exocrine function can also be measured indirectly by assessing serum levels of immunoreactive trypsin, which were shown to correspond to exocrine secretions into the duodenal lumen (266). Both direct (203,265) and indirect (266) measures of exocrine function identify moderate degrees of exocrine deficiency in 65% to 80% of patients with type 1 diabetes. With direct studies, both amylase secretion and bicarbonate secretion were found to be reduced 55% to 65% (203,265). Despite the marked reduction in exocrine function in a large fraction of the diabetic population, steatorrhea caused by exocrine insufficiency is quite rare owing to the large secretory capacity of the exocrine pancreas. Both direct and indirect studies of exocrine function found a significant correlation between the declining endogenous insulin secretion, as measured by C-peptide concentration, and amylase and bicarbonate output (265,266). In some studies the reduction in exocrine function worsened with time and corresponded to the progressive decline in concentrations of C-peptide (265). This correlation is thought to represent the causal effect of insulin deficiency on exocrine function and would support the hypothesis of the trophic effects of insulin on exocrine function. Hence, with a decline in the release of endogenous insulin in type 1 diabetes, the surrounding acinar cells atrophy, with resulting exocrine dysfunction. In type 2 diabetes for which insulin therapy is not required, there is also a demonstrable decrease in exocrine secretion but of a magnitude smaller than that observed in type 1 diabetes and insulin-dependent type 2 diabetes (265).

Although the presence of autonomic neuropathy could reduce pancreatic exocrine secretion as a result of reduced secretomotor action, careful secretory studies have suggested that this is not the case (203). In diabetic patients requiring insulin, the decreased exocrine secretion cannot be corrected with supramaximal concentrations of cholecystokinin and secretin. In addition, when bethanechol was administered simultaneously with cholecystokinin and secretin, the additional cholinergic stimulation also failed to correct the decrease in exocrine secretion. These data are seen to indicate a reduction in or atrophy of the acinar cell mass rather than an alteration in the secretomotor activity of the nerves or hormones on the pancreas.

Hyperamylasemia and Pancreatitis

Hyperamylasemia has been reported in 46% to 79% of patients with diabetic ketoacidosis (267). Abdominal pain and tenderness occur in up to 45%, and a history of vomiting exists in up to 73% (267). In the past, this constellation of symptoms and findings was attributed to acute pancreatitis. However, more recent careful analyses have indicated that acute pancreatitis is rarely present in diabetic ketoacidosis and hence is not a common cause of the abdominal symptoms and hyperamylasemia (268). Hyperamylasemia is often not present at the initial presentation with ketoacidosis but can develop later during hospitalization (267). The magnitude of serum amylase elevation is variable, but the level reaches up to six times higher than normal, which is an elevation often considered specific for acute pancreatitis. However, there is no correlation between hyperamylasemia and the abdominal symptoms, and hyperamylasemia occurs with equal frequency in patients with and without these symptoms. In the vast majority of patients with ketoacidosis and hyperamylasemia, isoamylase testing has demonstrated that the major contributor to the elevation is a salivary-type, rather than a pancreatic, isoamylase. Simultaneous lipase levels are usually normal. The source of the salivary-type isoamylase is unclear, because all forms of isoamylase other than pancreatic isoamylase are assayed as the salivary-type isoenzyme. Hyperamylasemia may be a consequence of acidemia and serum hyperosmolality per se rather than a specific consequence of diabetic acidosis. Eckfeldt et al. (269) collected serum from 33 patients with metabolic or respiratory acidosis in the absence of diabetic acidosis or renal failure. The total serum amylase level was elevated in 36% of these patients, and five patients had marked elevations in a range usually considered diagnostic of acute pancreatitis. There was a trend toward a greater prevalence of hyperamylasemia with worsening acidosis, but the difference was not statistically significant. As in other studies of hyperamylasemia, the majority of patients had a salivary-type isoamylase of unknown origin, and almost all affected patients had normal lipase levels. More recent studies showed that nonspecific hyperamylasemia and hyperlipasemia in diabetic ketoacidosis are common, occurring in 16% to 25% of cases, and elevations of amylase correlated with pH and serum osmolality, but lipase elevation correlated with serum osmolality alone (270,271). From such studies, diagnosis of acute pancreatitis, based solely on elevated amylase or lipase, even if more than three times normal, does not seem justifiable.

The cause of the abdominal symptoms in diabetic ketoacidosis remains uncertain but is likely not related to pancreatitis. Alternate explanations for the pain have included intestinal ileus or gastric dilatation caused by the underlying acidosis. In patients presenting with diabetic ketoacidosis and hyperamylasemia for whom a reasonable question exists regarding the presence of pancreatitis, examination of the lipase level and studies of pancreatic morphology by abdominal imaging should be helpful.

Although there is no known association between diabetes mellitus and pancreatitis, two important associations should be recognized. First, the incidence of gallstones may be increased in type 2 diabetes because of coincident obesity. In this setting, acute pancreatitis secondary to the passage of gallstones can occur (235). Second, type IV hyperlipoproteinemia occurs more frequently in type 2 diabetes. In susceptible patients, high dietary fat intake might turn type IV hyperlipoproteinemia into type V hyperlipoproteinemia, which is associated with an increased risk of acute pancreatitis.

Pancreatic Cancer and Diabetes

In population-based case-control studies of pancreatic cancer conducted in the United States, diabetes was a risk factor for pancreatic cancer (272,273), as well as a possible complication of the tumor (273). A significant positive trend in risk with increasing years prior to diagnosis of pancreatic cancer was apparent, with persons with diabetes diagnosed at least 10 years prior to diagnosis having a significant 50% increased risk. Use of insulin or duration of insulin use did not correlate with risk of developing pancreatic cancer. However, increased insulin level has been proposed as a possible "unifying concept" in the increased risk of various cancers seen in persons with diabetes (274). Patients with abnormal glucose metabolism, as determined by elevated serum glucose levels 1 hour after an oral glucose challenge, were found to have an increased risk of developing pancreatic carcinoma even if patients who died of that disease during the first 5 years of follow-up were excluded from consideration (275).

LIVER IN DIABETES

Increased Hepatic Glycogen

It is surprising that hepatic glycogen is increased in some patients with diabetes, because adequate serum levels of insulin are necessary to stimulate glycogen synthesis. Nevertheless, in some patients with type 1 diabetes, increased hepatic glycogen does occur and results in or contributes to clinical hepatomegaly (276). Among these patients, the disorder is observed with increased frequency in patients with "brittle" diabetes who are prone to hypoglycemia. In these patients, intermittent excesses in insulin therapy appear to achieve the serum levels necessary to stimulate glycogen synthesis in the liver. Although increased hepatic glycogen can cause hepatomegaly, it does not produce clinical liver dysfunction as typified by abnormal laboratory testing or clinical symptoms (15,277).

Diabetic Fatty Liver

Hepatic steatosis is defined as the accumulation of lipid by the liver, usually in the form of triglyceride, such that the weight of lipid exceeds 5% of the total weight of the liver (278,279). Histologic studies indicate that diabetic hepatic steatosis can produce either microvesicular or macrovesicular deposition of fat. In general, with marked fatty infiltration, there is macrovesicular fatty deposition with some hepatocellular destruction. Hepatocyte necrosis is usually mild and is not associated with an inflammatory infiltrate.

It is difficult to estimate accurately the incidence of this lesion in diabetes because a percutaneous liver biopsy is necessary for proper identification. The medical literature reports a wide range in incidence, differences that are probably due to the large variation in body weight of patients, as well as to the effect of the type of diabetes on this disorder. In type 1 diabetes the incidence of hepatic steatosis is low (4% to 17%) (279). In these patients, hepatic steatosis is related to inadequate serum levels of insulin and hence to poor diabetic control. Increased mobilization of fatty acids from peripheral adipose tissue results in an increased hepatic concentration of fatty acids and enhanced hepatic synthesis of triglyceride and very-low-density lipoprotein (VLDL) (278). Both hyperlipidemia and hepatic steatosis are readily reversible with appropriate insulin therapy. Because of this reversibility, the incidence of hepatic steatosis in type 1 diabetes remains relatively low.

In type 2 diabetes, the incidence of hepatic steatosis is high (21% to 78%) and is related primarily to concurrent obesity rather than to the duration of the diabetes or the adequacy of control (279). It is difficult to differentiate the effect of diabetes from that of obesity in the pathogenesis of fatty liver in this setting. In patients with morbid obesity, without coincident diabetes, the incidence of fatty liver can be as high as 94% (281).

In type 2 diabetes, the pathogenesis of hepatic steatosis is multifactorial (279,282). Increased serum and hepatic fatty acids found in these patients result in an increased rate of hepatic triglyceride synthesis that exceeds a relatively normal rate of hepatic secretion of VLDL. In type 2 diabetes, hepatic steatosis is less readily reversible and is managed more effectively by the introduction of a low-calorie, low-carbohydrate diet with achievement of weight loss.

The role of peroxisome proliferator-activated receptor γ (PPARγ), which is an important regulator of genes involved in glucose and lipid metabolism, in the liver has generally not been appreciated because, in contrast to PPARα or PPARδ, PPARγ is not abundantly expressed in the liver under normal conditions. However, in several murine models of obesity and type 2 diabetes mellitus, there is increased expression of PPARγ in the liver. Moreover, treatment of diabetic mice with selective PPARγ ligands and with the activators thiazolidinediones resulted in the development of severe hepatic centrilobular steatosis. In light of reports that troglitazone has been associated with rare but serious hepatotoxicity in patients, further insight into PPARγ-mediated versus non–PPARγ-mediated effects of thiazolidinediones in humans is needed (283).

In general, the hepatic steatosis of diabetes produces asymptomatic hepatomegaly and few, if any, clinical symptoms. The results of laboratory studies of hepatic function and injury tend to be normal. Mild elevations of these test values have been documented in up to 18% of unselected patients with either type 1 or type 2 diabetes, particularly of alkaline phosphatase and γ-glutamyltranspeptidase (284,285). Diagnostic imaging studies can document the presence of hepatic steatosis; an abdominal computed tomographic (CT) scan can show decreased hepatic density caused by fatty infiltration, and abdominal ultrasonography demonstrated a reflective or "bright" pattern in 23% of unselected patients in one series (286).

The natural history of hepatic steatosis of diabetes is controversial. In general, this lesion is benign and not prone to progression to a more severe hepatic injury. Indeed, it is rare to document actual cirrhosis as a consequence of hepatic steatosis, although epidemiologically there is a correlation between diabetes and hepatitis C infection, which is the leading cause of chronic liver disease in the United States (277).

Diabetic Steatonecrosis

A more severe histologic lesion has been described in some patients with diabetic fatty liver. Steatonecrosis ("nonalcoholic steatohepatitis" or "fatty liver hepatitis") produces histologic changes similar to those seen in alcoholic hepatitis or following ileojejunal bypass in obese patients (279,282,287), consisting of moderate steatosis with macrovesicular fatty change. Fibrosis may be both periportal and pericentral. Hepatocellular degeneration and necrosis may occur, with intracellular hyaline bodies identical to Mallory bodies. Although chronic inflammatory cells may infiltrate the portal areas, there is no infiltration by polymorphonuclear cells, a finding that may distinguish this lesion from that of alcoholic hepatitis. Infiltration by polymorphonuclear cells is common and almost pathognomonic for alcoholic hepatitis in the setting of the other histologic findings.

In some patients with diabetic steatonecrosis, bridging fibrosis between portal tracts and central veins may exist.

As might be expected, steatonecrosis is more common in patients with type 2 diabetes, particularly in middle-aged, obese women (277). Although it usually presents as asymptomatic hepatomegaly with abnormal values in liver function tests, rarely the patient presents with complaints of fatigue and with ascites. Laboratory studies may demonstrate marked elevations of the sedimentation rate, as well as mild-to-moderate elevations in alkaline phosphatase and γ-glutamyltranspeptidase levels; elevations of transaminases tend to be mild. In general, the levels of bilirubin, albumin, and globulin are normal.

The finding of pericentral fibrosis raised concerns in the past regarding the progression of this lesion to more severe liver disease. In other disorders, sclerosis of the terminal hepatic venules suggests progressive liver injury that may be a harbinger of eventual cirrhosis (284). In steatonecrosis, however, progression to more severe liver disease seems less common. In one study, bridging fibrosis was found in those patients with diabetes of longer duration (282), but actual cirrhosis proved to be rare. In a study that provided long-term follow-up of 35 patients with nonalcoholic steatohepatitis, the hepatic histology in 91% of the patients remained stable or changed only slowly (288). Only 9% of the patients demonstrated deterioration of the histologic lesion, and cirrhosis was found in only two patients.

Steatonecrosis in a patient with type 1 diabetes has been reported (287). Although this patient presented with mild jaundice and hepatosplenomegaly, liver biopsy did not demonstrate cirrhosis. With improved diabetic control, the liver function test became normal, hepatosplenomegaly resolved, and serial imaging studies by abdominal CT scan demonstrated a return of hepatic density to near-normal values.

Primary Liver Cancer

A Swedish population-based study showed increased risk of developing primary liver cancer and biliary tract cancers among patients with diabetes (273). Selection bias was minimized by excluding patients in whom liver and biliary tract cancers were diagnosed during the first year of follow-up. Overall standardized incidence ratios (SIRs) adjusted for age, sex, and calendar year for comparison during the 1 to 24 years of follow-up was 2.5. The risk was higher in men (SIR = 3.2) than in women (SIR = 2.0), and the incidence of primary liver cancer alone was increased fourfold (SIR = 4.1). After exclusion of patients with diabetes with concomitant diseases that predispose to primary liver cancer, such as alcoholism, cirrhosis, and hepatitis, the persistence of an approximately threefold excess risk was observed. Similar increased association of liver cancer and diabetes has been noted in Japan (289), Italy (290), and the United States (291), although the latter did not show increased risk in the absence of viral or alcoholic cirrhosis.

REFERENCES

1. Bargen JA, Bollmann J, Kepler E. The diarrhea of diabetes and steatorrhea of pancreatic insufficiency. *Proc Mayo Clin* 1936;11:737–742.
2. Folwaczny C, Riepl R, Tschop M, et al. Gastrointestinal involvement in patients with diabetes mellitus: Part I (first of two parts). Epidemiology, pathophysiology, clinical findings [Review]. *Z Gastroenterol* 1999;37:803–815.
3. Feldman M, Schiller L. Disorders of gastrointestinal motility associated with diabetes mellitus. *Ann Intern Med* 1983;98:378–384.
4. Verne GN, Sninsky CA. Diabetes and the gastrointestinal tract [Review]. *Gastroenterol Clin North Am* 1998;27:861–874.
5. Talley NJ, Young L, Bytzer P, et al. Impact of chronic gastrointestinal symptoms in diabetes mellitus on health-related quality of life. *Am J Gastroenterol* 2001;96:71–76.
6. Ricci JA, Siddique R, Stewart WF, et al. Upper gastrointestinal symptoms in a U.S. national sample of adults with diabetes. *Scand J Gastroenterol* 2000;35:152–159.
7. Maleki D, Locke GR, Camilleri M, et al. Gastrointestinal tract symptoms among persons with diabetes mellitus in the community. *Arch Intern Med* 2000;160:2808–2816.
8. DeBlock C, DeLeeuw I, Rooman R, et al. Gastric parietal cell antibodies are associated with glutamic acid decarboxylase-65 antibodies and the HLA DQA1*0501-DQB1*0301 haplotype in Type 1 diabetes mellitus. Belgian Diabetes Registry. *Diabet Med* 2000;17:618–622.
9. Fischer H, Heidemann T, Hengst K, et al. Disturbed gastric motility and pancreatic hormone release in diabetes mellitus. *J Physiol Pharmacol* 1998;49:529–541.
10. Vella JS, Camilleri M, Szarka LA, et al. Effects of pramlintide, an amylin analogue, on gastric emptying in type 1 and type 2 diabetes mellitus. *Neurogastroenterol Motil* 2002;14:123–131.
11. Nauck MA. Glucagon-like peptide 1 (GLP-1): a potent gut hormone with a possible therapeutic perspective [Review]. *Acta Diabetol* 1998;35:117–129.
12. Poykko SM, Kellokoski E, Horkko S, et al. Low plasma ghrelin is associated with insulin resistance, hypertension, and the prevalence of type 2 diabetes. *Diabetes* 2003;52:2546–2553.
13. Goyal RK, Hirano I. The enteric nervous system. *N Engl J Med* 1996;334:1106–1115.
14. Dyrberg T, Benn J, Christiansen JS, et al. Prevalence of diabetic autonomic neuropathy measured by simple bedside tests. *Diabetologia* 1981;20:190–194.
15. Jeyarajah R, Samarawickrama P, Jameel MM. Autonomic function tests in non-insulin dependent diabetic patients and apparently healthy volunteers. *J Chronic Dis* 1986;39:479–484.
16. Diani A, West C, Vidmar T, et al. Morphometric analysis of the vagus nerve in nondiabetic and ketonuric diabetic Chinese hamsters. *J Comp Pathol* 1984;94:495–504.
17. Smith B. Neuropathology of the oesophagus in diabetes mellitus. *J Neurol Neurosurg Psychiatry* 1974;37:1151–1154.
18. Duchen LW, Anjorin A, Watkins PJ, et al. Pathology of autonomic neuropathy in diabetes mellitus. *Ann Intern Med* 1980;92:301–303.
19. Guy RJ, Dawson JL, Garrett JR, et al. Diabetic gastroparesis from autonomic neuropathy: surgical considerations and changes in vagus nerve morphology. *J Neurol Neurosurg Psychiatry* 1984;47:686–691.
20. Yoshida MM, Schuffler MD, Sumi SM. There are no morphologic abnormalities of the gastric wall or abdominal vagus in patients with diabetic gastroparesis. *Gastroenterology* 1988;94:907–914.
21. Buysschaert M, Donckier J, Dive A, et al. Gastric acid and pancreatic polypeptide responses to sham feeding are impaired in diabetic subjects with autonomic neuropathy. *Diabetes* 1985;34:1181–1185.
22. Annese V, Bassotti G, Caruso N, et al. Gastrointestinal motor dysfunction, symptoms, and neuropathy in noninsulin-dependent (type 2) diabetes mellitus. *J Clin Gastroenterol* 1999;29:171–177.
23. Chang EB, Bergenstal RM, Field M. Diarrhea in streptozocin-treated rats. Loss of adrenergic regulation of intestinal fluid and electrolyte transport. *J Clin Invest* 1985;75:1666–1670.
24. Belai A, Lincoln J, Milner P, et al. Differential effect of streptozotocin-induced diabetes on the innervation of the ileum and distal colon. *Gastroenterology* 1991;100:1024–1032.
25. Eaker EY, Sallustio JE, Marchand SD, et al. Differential increase in neuropeptide Y-like levels and myenteric neuronal staining in diabetic rat intestine. *Regul Pept* 1996;61:77–84.
26. Lincoln J, Bokor JT, Crowe R, et al. Myenteric plexus in streptozotocin-treated rats. Neurochemical and histochemical evidence for diabetic neuropathy in the gut. *Gastroenterology* 1984;86:654–661.
27. Ordog T, Takayama I, Cheung WK, et al. Remodeling of networks of interstitial cells of Cajal in a murine model of diabetic gastroparesis. *Diabetes* 2000;49:1731–1739.
28. Nowak TV, Harrington B, Kalbfleisch JH, et al. Evidence for abnormal cholinergic neuromuscular transmission in diabetic rat small intestine. *Gastroenterology* 1986;91:124–132.
29. Belai A, Lincoln J, Milner P, et al. Enteric nerves in diabetic rats: increase in vasoactive intestinal polypeptide but not substance P. *Gastroenterology* 1985;89:967–976.
30. Loesch A, Belai A, Lincoln J, et al. Enteric nerves in diabetic rats: electron microscopic evidence for neuropathy of vasoactive intestinal polypeptide-containing fibres. *Acta Neuropathol* 1986;70:161–168.
31. Nowak TV, Chey WW, Chang TM, et al. Effect of streptozotocin-induced diabetes mellitus on release of vasoactive intestinal polypeptide from rodent small intestine. *Dig Dis Sci* 1995;40:828–836.
32. Takahashi T, Nakamura K, Itoh H, et al. Impaired expression of nitric oxide synthase in the gastric myenteric plexus of spontaneously diabetic rats. *Gastroenterology* 1997;113:1535–1544.
33. Watkins CC, Sawa A, Jaffrey S, et al. Insulin restores neuronal nitric oxide synthase expression and function that is lost in diabetic gastropathy. *J Clin Invest* 2000;106:373–384.
34. Mashimo H, Kjellin A, Goyal RK. Gastric stasis in neuronal nitric oxide synthase-deficient knockout mice. *Gastroenterology* 2000;119:766–773.
35. de Rosalmeida MC, Saraiva LD, da Graca JR, et al. Sildenafil, a phosphodiesterase-5 inhibitor, delays gastric emptying and gastrointestinal transit of liquid in awake rats. *Dig Dis Sci* 2003;48:2064–2068.

36. Pfeifer MA, Schumer MP, Gelber DA. Aldose reductase inhibitors: the end of an era or the need for different trial designs? [Review]. *Diabetes* 1997;6 [Suppl 2]:S82–S89.
37. Vinik AI. Diabetic neuropathy: pathogenesis and therapy [Review]. *Am J Med* 1999;107[2B]:17S–26S.
38. Fox S, Behar J. Pathogenesis of diabetic gastroparesis: a pharmacologic study. *Gastroenterology* 1980;78:757–763.
39. Ejskjaer NT, Bradley JL, Buxton-Thomas MS, et al. Novel surgical treatment and gastric pathology in diabetic gastroparesis. *Diabet Med* 1999;16:488–495.
40. Xue L, Suzuki H. Electrical responses of gastric smooth muscles in streptozotocin-induced diabetic rats. *Am J Physiol* 1997;272:G77–G83.
41. Imaeda K, Takano H, Koshita M, et al. Electrical properties of colonic smooth muscle in spontaneously non-insulin-dependent diabetic rats. *J Smooth Muscle Res* 1998;34:1–11.
42. De Las Casas LE, Finley JL. Diabetic microangiopathy in the small bowel. *Histopathology* 1999;35:267–270.
43. Brownlee M. Biochemistry and molecular cell biology of diabetic complications. *Nature* 2001;414:813–820.
44. Campbell IW, Duncan LJ, Innes JA, et al. Abdominal pain in diabetic metabolic decompensation. Clinical significance. *JAMA* 1975;233:166–168.
45. Longstreth GF. Diabetic thoracic polyradiculopathy: ten patients with abdominal pain. *Am J Gastroenterol* 1997;92:502–505.
46. Borgstrom PS, Olsson R, Sundkvist G, et al. Pharyngeal and oesophageal function in patients with diabetes mellitus and swallowing complaints. *Br J Radiol* 1988;61:817–821.
47. Horowitz M, Harding PE, Maddox AF, et al. Gastric and oesophageal emptying in patients with type 2 (non-insulin-dependent) diabetes mellitus. *Diabetologia* 1989;32:151–159.
48. Sundkvist G, Hillarp B, Lilja B, et al. Esophageal motor function evaluated by scintigraphy, video-radiography and manometry in diabetic patients. *Acta Radiol* 1989;30:17–19.
49. Karayalcin B, Karayalcin U, Aburano T, et al. Esophageal clearance scintigraphy, in diabetic patients—a preliminary study. *Ann Nucl Med* 1992;6:89–93.
50. Hollis JB, Castell DO, Braddom RL. Esophageal function in diabetes mellitus and its relation to peripheral neuropathy. *Gastroenterology* 1977;73:1098–1102.
51. Huppe D, Tegenthoff M, Faig J, et al. Esophageal dysfunction in diabetes mellitus: is there a relation to clinical manifestation of neuropathy? *Clin Investig* 1992;70:740–747.
52. Loo FD, Dodds WJ, Soergel KH, et al. Multipeaked esophageal peristaltic pressure waves in patients with diabetic neuropathy. *Gastroenterology* 1985;88:485–491.
53. Keshavarzian A, Iber FL, Nasrallah S. Radionuclide esophageal emptying and manometric studies in diabetes mellitus. *Am J Gastroenterol* 1987;82:625–631.
54. Holloway RH, Tippett MD, Horowitz M, et al. Relationship between esophageal motility and transit in patients with type I diabetes mellitus. *Am J Gastroenterol* 1999;94:3150–3157.
55. Kinekawa F, Kubo F, Matsuda K, et al. Relationship between esophageal dysfunction and neuropathy in diabetic patients. *Am J Gastroenterol* 2001;96: 2026–2032.
56. Clouse RE, Lustman PJ, Reidel WL. Correlation of esophageal motility abnormalities with neuropsychiatric status in diabetics. *Gastroenterology* 1986;90:1146–1154.
57. Lluch I, Ascaso JF, Mora F, et al. Gastroesophageal reflux in diabetes mellitus. *Am J Gastroenterol* 1999;94:919–924.
58. Jackson AL, Rashed H, Cardoso S, et al. Assessment of gastric electrical activity and autonomic function among diabetic and nondiabetic patients with symptoms of gastroesophageal reflux. *Dig Dis Sci* 2000;45:1727–1730.
59. Nenoff P, Taneva E, Pfeil B, et al. In vitro activity of rilopirox against fluconazole-susceptible and fluconazole-resistant Candida isolates from patients with HIV infection. *Mycoses* 1999;42:55–60.
60. Ally R, Schurmann D, Kreisel W, et al. Esophageal Candidiasis Study Group. A randomized, double-blind, double-dummy, multicenter trial of voriconazole and fluconazole in the treatment of esophageal candidiasis in immunocompromised patients. *Clin Infect Dis* 2001;33:1447–1454.
61. Horowitz M, Maddox A, Harding PE, et al. Effect of cisapride on gastric and esophageal emptying in insulin-dependent diabetes mellitus. *Gastroenterology* 1987;92:1899–1907.
62. Kao CH, Wang SJ, Pang DY. Effects of oral erythromycin on upper gastrointestinal motility in patients with non-insulin-dependent diabetes mellitus. *Nucl Med Commun* 1995;16:790–793.
63. Fabiani F, De Vincentis N, Staffilano A. Effect of Tolrestat on oesophageal transit time and cholecystic motility in type 2 diabetic patients with asymptomatic diabetic neuropathy. *Diabete Metab* 1995;21:360–364.
64. Samsom M, Smout AJ. Abnormal gastric and small intestinal motor function in diabetes mellitus [Review]. *Dig Dis* 1997;15:263–274.
65. Sarna SK. In vivo myoelectric activity: methods, analysis, and interpretation. In: *Handbook of physiology: the gastrointestinal system*, Vol 1. Bethesda, MD: American Physiological Society, 1989:817–863.
66. Hasler W, Owyang C. Peptide-induced gastric arrythmias: a new cause of gastroparesis. *Regul Pept Lett* 1990;2:6–12.
67. Koch KL. Electrogastrography: physiological basis and clinical application in diabetic gastropathy [Review]. *Diabetes Technol Ther* 2001;3:51–62.
68. Koch KL, Stern RM, Stewart WR, et al. Gastric emptying and gastric myoelectrical activity in patients with diabetic gastroparesis: effect of long-term domperidone treatment. *Am J Gastroenterol* 1989;84:1069–1075.
69. Cucchiara S, Franzese A, Salvia G, et al. Gastric emptying delay and gastric electrical derangement in IDDM. *Diabetes Care* 1998;21:438–443.
70. Koch KL. Diabetic gastropathy: gastric neuromuscular dysfunction in diabetes mellitus: a review of symptoms, pathophysiology, and treatment [Review]. *Dig Dis Sci* 1999;44:1061–1075.
71. Pfaffenbach B, Wegener M, Adamek RJ, et al. Antral myoelectric activity, gastric emptying, and dyspeptic symptoms in diabetics. *Scand J Gastroenterol* 1995;30:1166–1171.
72. Malagelada JR, Rees WD, Mazzotta LJ, et al. Gastric motor abnormalities in diabetic and postvagotomy gastroparesis: effect of metoclopramide and bethanechol. *Gastroenterology* 1980;78:286–293.
73. Achem-Karam SR, Funakoshi A, Vinik AI, et al. Plasma motilin concentration and interdigestive migrating motor complex in diabetic gastroparesis: effect of metoclopramide. *Gastroenterology* 1985;88:492–499.
74. Camilleri M, Malagelada JR. Abnormal intestinal motility in diabetics with the gastroparesis syndrome. *Eur J Clin Invest* 1984;14:420–427.
75. Barnett JL, Owyang C. Serum glucose concentration as a modulator of interdigestive gastric motility [erratum appears in *Gastroenterology* 1988;95:262]. *Gastroenterology* 1988;94:739–744.
76. Hasler WL, Soudah HC, Dulai G, et al. Mediation of hyperglycemia-evoked gastric slow-wave dysrhythmias by endogenous prostaglandins. *Gastroenterology* 1995;108:727–736.
77. Kawagishi T, Nishizawa Y, Okuno Y, et al. Effect of cisapride on gastric emptying of indigestible solids and plasma motilin concentration in diabetic autonomic neuropathy. *Am J Gastroenterol* 1993;88:933–938.
78. Rayner CK, Su YC, Doran SM, et al. The stimulation of antral motility by erythromycin is attenuated by hyperglycemia. *Am J Gastroenterol* 2000;95: 2233–2241.
79. Petrakis IE, Chalkiadakis G, Vrachassotakis N, et al. Induced-hyperglycemia attenuates erythromycin-induced acceleration of hypertonic liquid-phase gastric emptying in type-I diabetic patients. *Dig Dis* 1999;17:241–247.
80. Petrakis IE, Vrachassotakis N, Sciacca V, et al. Hyperglycaemia attenuates erythromycin-induced acceleration of solid-phase gastric emptying in idiopathic and diabetic gastroparesis. *Scand J Gastroenterol* 1999;34:396–403.
81. Mansi C, Savarino V, Vigneri S, et al. Gastrokinetic effects of levosulpiride in dyspeptic patients with diabetic gastroparesis. *Am J Gastroenterol* 1995;90: 1989–1993.
82. Quigley EM. Pharmacotherapy of gastroparesis [Review]. *Expert Opin Pharmacother* 2000;1:881–888.
83. Bjornsson ES, Urbanavicius V, Eliasson B, et al. Effects of hyperglycemia on interdigestive gastrointestinal motility in humans. *Scand J Gastroenterol* 1994;29:1096–1104.
84. Berne C. Hypoglycaemia and gastric emptying [published erratum appears in *Diabet Med* 1996;13:846]. *Diabet Med* 1996;13[Suppl 5]:S28–S30.
85. Holzapfel A, Festa A, Stacher-Janotta G, et al. Gastric emptying in type II (non-insulin-dependent) diabetes mellitus before and after therapy readjustment: no influence of actual blood glucose concentration. *Diabetologia* 1999;42:1410–1412.
86. Frank JW, Saslow SB, Camilleri M, et al. Mechanism of accelerated gastric emptying of liquids and hyperglycemia in patients with type II diabetes mellitus. *Gastroenterology* 1995;109:755–765.
87. Mearin F, Camilleri M, Malagelada JR. Pyloric dysfunction in diabetics with recurrent nausea and vomiting. *Gastroenterology* 1986;90:1919–1925.
88. Keshavarzian A, Iber FL. Gastrointestinal involvement in insulin-requiring diabetes mellitus. *J Clin Gastroenterol* 1987;9:685–692.
89. Loo FD, Palmer DW, Soergel KH, et al. Gastric emptying in patients with diabetes mellitus. *Gastroenterology* 1984;86:485–494.
90. Wright RA, Clemente R, Wathen R. Diabetic gastroparesis: an abnormality of gastric emptying of solids. *Am J Med Sci* 1985;289:240–242.
91. Horowitz M, Fraser R. Disordered gastric motor function in diabetes mellitus [Review]. *Diabetologia* 1994;37:543–551.
92. Lyrenas EB, Olsson EH, Arvidsson UC, et al. Prevalence and determinants of solid and liquid gastric emptying in unstable type I diabetes. Relationship to postprandial blood glucose concentrations. *Diabetes Care* 1997;20:413–418.
93. Snape WJJ, Battle WM, Schwartz SS, et al. Metoclopramide to treat gastroparesis due to diabetes mellitus: a double-blind, controlled trial. *Ann Intern Med* 1982;96:444–446.
94. Kong MF, Horowitz M. Gastric emptying in diabetes mellitus: relationship to blood-glucose control [Review]. *Clin Geriatr Med* 1999;15:321–338.
95. Feldman M, Smith HJ, Simon TR. Gastric emptying of solid radiopaque markers: studies in healthy subjects and diabetic patients. *Gastroenterology* 1984;87:895–902.
96. Kikuchi K, Kusano M, Kawamura O, et al. Measurement and evaluation of gastric emptying using radiopaque barium markers. *Dig Dis Sci* 2000;45: 242–247.
97. Iida M, Ikeda M, Kishimoto M, et al. Evaluation of gut motility in type II diabetes by the radiopaque marker method. *J Gastroenterol Hepatol* 2000;15: 381–385.
98. Stotzer PO, Abrahamsson H. Human postprandial gastric emptying of indigestible solids can occur unrelated to antral phase III. *Neurogastroenterol Motil* 2000;12:415–419.
99. Hornbuckle K, Barnett JL. The diagnosis and work-up of the patient with gastroparesis. *J Clin Gastroenterol* 2000;30:117–124.
100. Kong MF, Horowitz M, Jones KL, et al. Natural history of diabetic gastroparesis. *Diabetes Care* 1999;22:503–507.

101. Clouse RE, Lustman PJ. Gastrointestinal symptoms in diabetic patients: lack of association with neuropathy. *Am J Gastroenterol* 1989;84:868–872.
102. Bertin E, Schneider N, Abdelli N, et al. Gastric emptying is accelerated in obese type 2 diabetic patients without autonomic neuropathy. *Diabetes Metab* 2001;27:357–364.
103. Samsom M, Salet GA, Roelofs JM, et al. Compliance of the proximal stomach and dyspeptic symptoms in patients with type I diabetes mellitus. *Dig Dis Sci* 1995;40:2037–2042.
104. Hebbard GS, Sun WM, Dent J, et al. Hyperglycaemia affects proximal gastric motor and sensory function in normal subjects. *Eur J Gastroenterol Hepatol* 1996;8:211–217.
105. Lingenfelser T, Sun W, Hebbard GS, et al. Effects of duodenal distension on antropyloroduodenal pressures and perception are modified by hyperglycemia. *Am J Physiol* 1999;276:G711–G718.
106. Rathmann W, Enck P, Frieling T, et al. Visceral afferent neuropathy in diabetic gastroparesis. *Diabetes Care* 1991;14:1086–1089.
107. Hoogerwerf WA, Pasricha PJ, Kalloo AN, et al. Pain: the overlooked symptom in gastroparesis. *Am J Gastroenterol* 1999;94:1029–1033.
108. Nowak TV, Johnson CP, Kalbfleisch JH, et al. Highly variable gastric emptying in patients with insulin dependent diabetes mellitus. *Gut* 1995;37:23–29.
109. van Wyk M, Sommers DK, Snyman JR, et al. The proportional cumulative area under the curve of paracetamol used as an index of gastric emptying in diabetic patients with symptoms of gastroparesis. *Clin Exp Pharmacol Physiol* 1995;22:637–640.
110. Lee JS, Camilleri M, Zinsmeister AR, et al. A valid, accurate, office based non-radioactive test for gastric emptying of solids. *Gut* 2000;46:768–773.
111. Darwiche G, Almer LO, Bjorgell O, et al. Measurement of gastric emptying by standardized real-time ultrasonography in healthy subjects and diabetic patients. *J Ultrasound Med* 1999;18:673–682.
112. Gilbey SG, Watkins PJ. Measurement by epigastric impedance of gastric emptying in diabetic autonomic neuropathy. *Diabet Med* 1987;4:122–126.
113. Borovicka J, Lehmann R, Kunz P, et al. Evaluation of gastric emptying and motility in diabetic gastroparesis with magnetic resonance imaging: effects of cisapride. *Am J Gastroenterol* 1999;94:2866–2873.
114. Burge MR, Tuttle MS, Violett JL, et al. Breath hydrogen testing identifies patients with diabetic gastroparesis. *Diabetes Care* 2000;23:860–861.
115. Burge MR, Tuttle MS, Violett JL, et al. Potato-lactulose breath hydrogen testing as a function of gastric motility in diabetes mellitus. *Diabetes Technol Ther* 2000;2:241–248.
116. Folwaczny C, Hundegger K, Volger C, et al. Measurement of transit disorders in different gastrointestinal segments of patients with diabetes mellitus in relation to duration and severity of the disease by use of the metal-detector test. *Z Gastroenterol* 1995;533:517–526.
117. Nompleggi D, Bell SJ, Blackburn GL, et al. Overview of gastrointestinal disorders due to diabetes mellitus: emphasis on nutritional support [Review]. *JPEN J Parenter Enteral Nutr* 1989;13:84–91.
118. Albibi R, McCallum RW. Metoclopramide: pharmacology and clinical application. [Review]. *Ann Intern Med* 1983;98:86–95.
119. Chaussade S, Grandjouan S, Couturier D. Motilin and diabetic gastroparesis: effect of MTC. *Gastroenterology* 1986;90:2039–2040.
120. Brown CK, Khanderia U. Use of metoclopramide, domperidone, and cisapride in the management of diabetic gastroparesis [Review]. *Clin Pharm* 1990;9:357–365.
121. O'Connell ME, Awni WM, Goodman M, et al. Bioavailability and disposition of metoclopramide after single- and multiple-dose administration in diabetic patients with gastroparesis. *J Clin Pharmacol* 1987;27:610–614.
122. Trapnell BC, Mavko LE, Birskovich LM, et al. Metoclopramide suppositories in the treatment of diabetic gastroparesis. *Arch Intern Med* 1986;146: 2278–2279.
123. Barone JA. Domperidone: a peripherally acting dopamine2-receptor antagonist [Review]. *Ann Pharmacother* 1999;33:429–440.
124. Dumitrascu DL, Weinbeck M. Domperidone versus metoclopramide in the treatment of diabetic gastroparesis. *Am J Gastroenterol* 2000;95:316–317.
125. Patterson D, Abell T, Rothstein R, et al. A double-blind multicenter comparison of domperidone and metoclopramide in the treatment of diabetic patients with symptoms of gastroparesis. *Am J Gastroenterol* 1999;4:1230–1234.
126. Horowitz M, Harding PE, Chatterton BE, et al. Acute and chronic effects of domperidone on gastric emptying in diabetic autonomic neuropathy. *Dig Dis Sci* 1985;30:1–9.
127. Day JP, Pruitt RE. Diabetic gastroparesis in a patient with Parkinson's disease: effective treatment with domperidone. *Am J Gastroenterol* 1989;84:837–838.
128. Dhasmana KM, Banerjee AK, Zhu YN, et al. Role of dopamine receptors in gastrointestinal motility. *Res Commun Chem Pathol Pharmacol* 1989;64:485–488.
129. Chang CS, Lien HC, Yeh HZ, et al. Effect of cisapride on gastric dysrhythmia and emptying of indigestible solids in type-II diabetic patients. *Scand J Gastroenterol* 1998;33:600–604.
130. Feldman M, Smith HJ. Effect of cisapride on gastric emptying of indigestible solids in patients with gastroparesis diabeticorum. A comparison with metoclopramide and placebo. *Gastroenterology* 1987;92:171–174.
131. Annese V, Lombardi G, Frusciante V, et al. Cisapride and erythromycin prokinetic effects in gastroparesis due to type 1 (insulin-dependent) diabetes mellitus. *Aliment Pharmacol Ther* 1997;11:599–603.
132. Horowitz M, Roberts AP. Long-term efficacy of cisapride in diabetic gastroparesis. *Am J Med* 1990;88:195–196.
133. Wang SH, Lin CY, Huang TY, et al. QT interval effects of cisapride in the clinical setting. *Int J Cardiol* 2001;80:179–183.
134. Itoh Z, Suzuki T, Nakaya M, et al. Structure-activity relation among macrolide antibiotics in initiation of interdigestive migrating contractions in the canine gastrointestinal tract. *Am J Physiol* 1985;248:G320–G325.
135. Omura S, Tsuzuki K, Sunazuka T, et al. Macrolides with gastrointestinal motor stimulating activity. *J Med Chem* 1987;30:1941–1943.
136. Lin HC, Sanders SL, Gu YG, et al. Erythromycin accelerates solid emptying at the expense of gastric sieving. *Dig Dis Sci* 1994;39:124–128.
137. Sato F, Marui S, Inatomi N, et al. EM574, an erythromycin derivative, improves delayed gastric emptying of semi-solid meals in conscious dogs. [erratum appears in *Eur J Pharmacol* 2000;404:397]. *Eur J Pharmacol* 2000;395: 165–172.
138. Tomomasa T, Kuroume T, Arai H, et al. Erythromycin induces migrating motor complex in human gastrointestinal tract. *Dig Dis Sci* 1986;31:157–161.
139. Otterson MF, Sarna SK. Gastrointestinal motor effects of erythromycin. *Am J Physiol* 1990;259:G355–G363.
140. Boiron M, Dorval E, Metman EH, et al. Erythromycin elicits opposite effects on antrobulbar and duodenal motility: analysis in diabetics by cineradiography. *Arch Physiol Biochem* 1997;105:591–595.
141. Ishii M, Nakamura T, Kasai F, et al. Erythromycin derivative improves gastric emptying and insulin requirement in diabetic patients with gastroparesis. *Diabetes Care* 1997;20:1134–1137.
142. Erbas T, Varoglu E, Erbas B, et al. Comparison of metoclopramide and erythromycin in the treatment of diabetic gastroparesis. *Diabetes Care* 1993;16: 1511–1514.
143. Desautels SG, Hutson WR, Christian PE, et al. Gastric emptying response to variable oral erythromycin dosing in diabetic gastroparesis. *Dig Dis Sci* 1995;40:141–146.
144. Janssens J, Peeters TL, Vantrappen G, et al. Improvement of gastric emptying in diabetic gastroparesis by erythromycin. Preliminary studies. *N Engl J Med* 1990;322:1028–1031.
145. DiBaise JK, Quigley EM. Efficacy of prolonged administration of intravenous erythromycin in an ambulatory setting as treatment of severe gastroparesis: one center's experience. *J Clin Gastroenterol* 1999;28:131–134.
146. Peeters TL, Muls E, Janssens J, et al. Effect of motilin on gastric emptying in patients with diabetic gastroparesis. *Gastroenterology* 1992;102:97–101.
147. Degen L, Matzinger D, Merz M, et al. Tegaserod, a 5-HT4 receptor partial agonist, accelerates gastric emptying and gastrointestinal transit in healthy male subjects. *Aliment Pharmacol Ther* 2001;15:1745–1751.
148. Briejer MR, Bosmans JP, Van Daele P, et al. The in vitro pharmacological profile of prucalopride, a novel enterokinetic compound. *Eur J Pharmacol* 2001;423:71–83.
149. Scarpignato C, Kisfalvi I, D'Amato M, et al. Effect of dexloxiglumide and spiroglumide, two new CCK-receptor antagonists, on gastric emptying and secretion in the rat: evaluation of their receptor selectivity in vivo. *Aliment Pharmacol Ther* 1996;10:411–419.
150. Scarpignato C, Pelosini I. Management of irritable bowel syndrome: novel approaches to the pharmacology of gut motility [Review]. *Can J Gastroenterol* 1999;13[Suppl]:50A–65A.
151. Lange V. Gastric phytobezoar: an endoscopic technique for removal. *Endoscopy* 1986;18:195–196.
152. Smith BH, Mollot M, Berk JE. Use of cellulase for phytobezoar dissolution. *Am J Gastroenterol* 1980;73:257–259.
153. Delpre G, Kadish U, Glanz I. Metoclopramide in the treatment of gastric bezoars. *Am J Gastroenterol* 1984;79:739–740.
154. Fontana RJ, Barnett JL. Jejunostomy tube placement in refractory diabetic gastroparesis: a retrospective review. *Am J Gastroenterol* 1996;91:2174–2178.
155. Reardon TM, Schnell GA, Smith OJ, et al. Surgical therapy of diabetic gastroparesis. *J Clin Gastroenterol* 1989;11:204–207.
156. Karlstrom L, Kelly KA. Roux-Y gastrectomy for chronic gastric atony. *Am J Surg* 1989;157:44–49.
157. Thumshirn M, Camilleri M, Choi MG, et al. Modulation of gastric sensory and motor functions by nitrergic and alpha2-adrenergic agents in humans. *Gastroenterology* 1999;116:573–585.
158. Rosa E, Silva L, Troncon LE, et al. Treatment of diabetic gastroparesis with oral clonidine. *Aliment Pharmacol Ther* 1995;9:179–183.
159. Soykan I, Lin Z, Sarosiek I, et al. Gastric myoelectrical activity, gastric emptying, and correlations with symptoms and fasting blood glucose levels in diabetic patients. *Am J Med Sci* 1999;317:226–231.
160. Dundee JW. Belfast experience with P6 acupuncture antiemesis. *Ulster Med J* 1990;59:63–70.
161. Bertolucci LE, DiDario B. Efficacy of a portable accustimulation device in controlling seasickness. *Aviat Space Environ Med* 1995;66:1155–1158.
162. GEMS Study Group. GEMS Study Group: Report of a multicenter study on electrical stimulation for the treatment of gastroparesis. *Gastroenterology* 1997;112:A735(abst).
163. Forster J, Sarosiek I, Delcore R, et al. Gastric pacing is a new surgical treatment for gastroparesis. *Am J Surg* 2001;182:676–681.
164. Arslan D, Kendirci M, Kurtoglu S, et al. *Helicobacter pylori* infection in children with insulin dependent diabetes mellitus. *J Pediatr Endocrinol Metab* 2000;13:553–556.
165. Quatrini M, Boarino V, Ghidoni A, et al. *Helicobacter pylori* prevalence in patients with diabetes and its relationship to dyspeptic symptoms. *J Clin Gastroenterol* 2001;32:215–217.
166. Marrollo M, Latella G, Melideo D, et al. Increased prevalence of *Helicobacter pylori* in patients with diabetes mellitus. *Dig Liver Dis* 2001;33:21–29.

167. Gentile S, Turco S, Oliviero B, et al. The role of autonomic neuropathy as a risk factor of *Helicobacter pylori* infection in dyspeptic patients with type 2 diabetes mellitus. *Diabetes Res Clin Pract* 1997;42:41–48.
168. Xia HH, Talley NJ, Kam EP, et al. *Helicobacter pylori* infection is not associated with diabetes mellitus, nor with upper gastrointestinal symptoms in diabetes mellitus. *Am J Gastroenterol* 2001;96:1039–1046.
169. Otterson MF, Sarr MG. Normal physiology of small intestinal motility [Review]. *Surg Clin North Am* 1993;73:1173–1192.
170. Marlett JA, Code CF. Effects of celiac and superior mesenteric ganglionectomy on interdigestive myoelectric complex in dogs. *Am J Physiol* 1979;237: E432–E443.
171. Dooley CP, el Newihi HM, Zeidler A, et al. Abnormalities of the migrating motor complex in diabetics with autonomic neuropathy and diarrhea. *Scand J Gastroenterol* 1988;23:217–223.
172. Wegener M, Borsch G, Schaffstein J, et al. Gastrointestinal transit disorders in patients with insulin-treated diabetes mellitus. *Dig Dis* 1990;8:23–36.
173. Virally-Monod M, Tielmans D, Kevorkian JP, et al. Chronic diarrhoea and diabetes mellitus: prevalence of small intestinal bacterial overgrowth. *Diabetes Metab* 1998;24:530–536.
174. Shanahan F, McKenna R, McCarthy CF, et al. Coeliac disease and diabetes mellitus: a study of 24 patients with HLA typing. *Q J Med* 1982;51:329–335.
175. Carlsson AK, Axelsson IE, Borulf SK, et al. Prevalence of IgA-antiendomysium and IgA-antigliadin autoantibodies at diagnosis of insulin-dependent diabetes mellitus in Swedish children and adolescents. *Pediatrics* 1999;103:1248–1252.
176. Fraser-Reynolds KA, Butzner JD, Stephure DK, et al. Use of immunoglobulin A-antiendomysial antibody to screen for celiac disease in North American children with type 1 diabetes. *Diabetes Care* 1998;21:1985–1989.
177. Chang EB, Field M, Miller RJ. Enterocyte alpha 2-adrenergic receptors: yohimbine and p-aminoclonidine binding relative to ion transport. *Am J Physiol* 1983;244:G76–G82.
178. Camilleri M. Appraisal of medium- and long-term treatment of gastroparesis and chronic intestinal dysmotility [Review]. *Am J Gastroenterol* 1994;89: 1769–1774.
179. Edmunds MC, Chen JD, Soykan I, et al. Effect of octreotide on gastric and small bowel motility in patients with gastroparesis. *Aliment Pharmacol Ther* 1999;12:167–174.
180. von der Ohe MR, Camilleri M, Thomforde GM, et al. Differential regional effects of octreotide on human gastrointestinal motor function. *Gut* 1995;36:743–748.
181. Sarna SK. Colonic motor activity [Review]. *Surg Clin North Am* 1993;73: 1201–1223.
182. Battle WM, Snape WJ Jr, Alavi A, et al. Colonic dysfunction in diabetes mellitus. *Gastroenterology* 1980;79:1217–1221.
183. Bytzer P, Talley NJ, Leemon M, et al. Prevalence of gastrointestinal symptoms associated with diabetes mellitus: a population-based survey of 15,000 adults. *Arch Intern Med* 2001;161:1989–1996.
184. Altomare D, Pilot MA, Scott M, et al. Detection of subclinical autonomic neuropathy in constipated patients using a sweat test. *Gut* 1992;33:1539–1543.
185. Maleki D, Camilleri M, Burton DD, et al. Pilot study of pathophysiology of constipation among community diabetics. *Dig Dis Sci* 1998;43:2373–2378.
186. Demol P, Ruoff HJ, Weihrauch TR. Rational pharmacotherapy of gastrointestinal motility disorders [Review]. *Eur J Pediatr* 1989;148:489–495.
187. Camilleri M. Review article: tegaserod. *Aliment Pharmacol Ther* 2001;15: 277–289.
188. Nakamura T, Okano R, Uchiyama H, et al. Effectiveness of aldose reductase inhibitors for diabetic gastroenteropathy with constipation. *Intern Med* 1997;36:479–483.
189. Berenyi MR, Schwarz GS. Megasigmoid syndrome in diabetes and neurologic disease. Review of 13 cases. *Am J Gastroenterol* 1967;47:311–320.
190. Le Marchand L, Wilkens LR, Kolonel LN, et al. Associations of sedentary lifestyle, obesity, smoking, alcohol use, and diabetes with the risk of colorectal cancer. *Cancer Res* 1997;57:4787–4794.
191. Nishii T, Kono S, Abe H, et al. Glucose intolerance, plasma insulin levels, and colon adenomas in Japanese men. *Jpn J Cancer Res* 2001;92:836–840.
192. Steenland K, Nowlin S, Palu S. Cancer incidence in the National Health and Nutrition Survey I. Follow-up data: diabetes, cholesterol, pulse and physical activity. *Cancer Epidemiol Biomarkers Prevention* 1995;4:807–811.
193. La Vecchia C, Negri E, Decarli A, et al. Diabetes mellitus and colorectal cancer risk. *Cancer Epidemiol Biomarkers Prevention* 1997;6:1007–1100.
194. Bell RA, Shelton BJ, Paskett ED. Colorectal cancer screening in North Carolina: associations with diabetes mellitus and demographic and health characteristics. *Prev Med* 2001;32:163–167.
195. Ma J, Pollak MN, Giovannucci E, et al. Prospective study of colorectal cancer risk in men and plasma levels of insulin-like growth factor (IGF)-I and IGF-binding protein-3. *J Natl Cancer Inst* 1999;91:620–625.
196. Tran TT, Medline A, Bruce WR. Insulin promotion of colon tumors in rats. *Cancer Epidemiol Biomarkers Prevention* 1996;5:1013–1015.
197. Giovannucci E. Insulin, insulin-like growth factors and colon cancer: a review of the evidence [Review]. *J Nutr* 2001;131[11 Suppl]:3109S–3120S.
198. Calle EE, Terrell DD. Utility of the National Death Index for ascertainment of mortality among cancer prevention study II participants. *Am J Epidemiol* 1993;137:235–241.
199. Nakamura T, Suda T, Kon M. Pathophysiology and treatment of diabetic diarrhea. [Review]. *J Smooth Muscle Res* 1996;32:27–42.
200. Ogbonnaya KI, Arem R. Diabetic diarrhea. Pathophysiology, diagnosis, and management [Review]. *Arch Intern Med* 1990;150:262–267.
201. Lysy J, Karmeli F, Sestieri M, et al. Decreased substance P content in the rectal mucosa of diabetics with diarrhea and constipation. *Metabolism* 1997;46:730–734.
202. Valdovinos MA, Camilleri M, Zimmerman BR. Chronic diarrhea in diabetes mellitus: mechanisms and an approach to diagnosis and treatment [Review]. *Mayo Clin Proc* 1993;68:691–702.
203. Whalen GE, Soergel KH, Geenen JE. Diabetic diarrhea. A clinical and pathophysiological study. *Gastroenterology* 1969;56:1021–1032.
204. Bytzer P, Talley NJ, Jones MP, et al. Oral hypoglycaemic drugs and gastrointestinal symptoms in diabetes mellitus. *Aliment Pharmacol Ther* 2001;15:137–142.
205. el Newihi H, Dooley CP, Saad C, et al. Impaired exocrine pancreatic function in diabetics with diarrhea and peripheral neuropathy. *Dig Dis Sci* 1988; 33:705–710.
206. Goldstein F, Wirts CW, Kowlessar OD. Diabetic diarrhea and steatorrhea. Microbiologic and clinical observations. *Ann Intern Med* 1970;72:215–218.
207. Simon GL, Gorbach SL. *Intestinal flora and gastrointestinal function. Physiology of the gastroinestinal tract,* 2nd ed. New York: Raven Press, 1987.
208. Molloy AM, Tomkin GH. Altered bile in diabetic diarrhoea. *BMJ* 1978;2: 1462–1463.
209. Schiller LR, Bilhartz LE, Santa Ana CA, et al. Comparison of endogenous and radiolabeled bile acid excretion in patients with idiopathic chronic diarrhea. *Gastroenterology* 1990;98:1036–1043.
210. Fedorak RN, Field M, Chang EB. Treatment of diabetic diarrhea with clonidine. *Ann Intern Med* 1985;102:197–199.
211. Gattuso JM, Kamm MA. Adverse effects of drugs used in the management of constipation and diarrhoea [Review]. *Drug Safety* 1994;10:47–65.
212. Roof LW. Treatment of diabetic diarrhea with clonidine. *Am J Med* 1987;83:603–604.
213. Chang EB, Fedorak RN, Field M. Experimental diabetic diarrhea in rats. Intestinal mucosal denervation hypersensitivity and treatment with clonidine. *Gastroenterology* 1986;91:564–569.
214. Sacerdote A. Topical clonidine for diabetic diarrhea. *Ann Intern Med* 1986;105:139.
215. Murao S, Hirata K, Ishida T, et al. Severe diabetic diarrhea successfully treated with octreotide, a somatostatin analogue. *Endocr J* 1999;46:477–478.
216. Nakabayashi H, Fujii S, Miwa U, et al. Marked improvement of diabetic diarrhea with the somatostatin analogue octreotide. *Arch Intern Med* 1994;154: 1863–1867.
217. Walker JJ, Kaplan DS. Efficacy of the somatostatin analog octreotide in the treatment of two patients with refractory diabetic diarrhea. *Am J Gastroenterol* 1993;88:765–776.
218. Mourad FH, Gorard D, Thillainayagam AV, et al. Effective treatment of diabetic diarrhoea with somatostatin analogue, octreotide. *Gut* 1992;33: 1578–1580.
219. Tsai ST, Vinik AI, Brunner JF. Diabetic diarrhea and somatostatin. *Ann Intern Med* 1986;104:894.
220. Dudl RJ, Anderson DS, Forsythe AB, et al. Treatment of diabetic diarrhea and orthostatic hypotension with somatostatin analogue SMS 201-995. *Am J Med* 1987;83:584–588.
221. Bossi A, Baresi A, Ballini A, et al. Ondansetron in the treatment of diabetic diarrhea. *Diabetes Care* 1994;17:453–454.
222. Epanomeritakis E, Koutsoumbi P, Tsiaoussis I, et al. Impairment of anorectal function in diabetes mellitus parallels duration of disease. *Dis Colon Rectum* 1999;42:1394–1400.
223. Scarpello JH, Hague RV, Cullen DR, et al. The 14C-glycocholate test in diabetic diarrhoea. *BMJ* 1976;2:673–675.
224. Read NW, Harford WV, Schmulen AC, et al. A clinical study of patients with fecal incontinence and diarrhea. *Gastroenterology* 1979;76:747–756.
225. Schiller LR, Santa Ana CA, Schmulen AC, et al. Pathogenesis of fecal incontinence in diabetes mellitus: evidence for internal-anal-sphincter dysfunction. *N Engl J Med* 1982;307:1666–1671.
226. Aitchison M, Fisher BM, Carter K, et al. Impaired anal sensation and early diabetic faecal incontinence. *Diabet Med* 1991;8:960–963.
227. Wald A. Incontinence and anorectal dysfunction in patients with diabetes mellitus. [Review]. *Eur J Gastroenterol Hepatol* 1995;7:737–739.
228. Wald A, Tunuguntla AK. Anorectal sensorimotor dysfunction in fecal incontinence and diabetes mellitus. Modification with biofeedback therapy. *N Engl J Med* 1984;310:1282–1287.
229. Pinna Pintor M, Zara GP, Falletto E, et al. Pudendal neuropathy in diabetic patients with faecal incontinence. *Int J Colorectal Dis* 1994;9:105–109.
230. Sun WM, Katsinelos P, Horowitz M, et al. Disturbances in anorectal function in patients with diabetes mellitus and faecal incontinence. *Eur J Gastroenterol Hepatol* 1996;8:1007–1012.
231. Misciagna G, Leoci C, Guerra V, et al. Epidemiology of cholelithiasis in southern Italy. Part II: Risk factors. *Eur J Gastroenterol Hepatol* 1996;8:585–593.
232. Chapman BA, Wilson IR, Frampton CM, et al. Prevalence of gallbladder disease in diabetes mellitus. *Dig Dis Sci* 1996;41:2222–2228.
233. Chapman BA, Chapman TM, Frampton CM, et al. Gallbladder volume: comparison of diabetics and controls. *Dig Dis Sci* 1998;43:344–348.
234. Moseley RH. Function of the normal liver. In: O'Grady JG, Lake JR, Howdle PD, eds. *Comprehensive clinical hepatology*. New York: Mosby, 2000:3.1–3.16.
235. Shoda J, He BF, Tanaka N, et al. Increase of deoxycholate in supersaturated bile of patients with cholesterol gallstone disease and its correlation with de novo syntheses of cholesterol and bile acids in liver, gallbladder emptying, and small intestinal transit. *Hepatology* 1995;21:1291–1302.

236. Haber GB, Heaton KW. Lipid composition of bile in diabetics and obesity-matched controls. *Gut* 1979;20:518–522.
237. Diehl AK, Schwesinger WH, Holleman DR, et al. Clinical correlates of gallstone composition: distinguishing pigment from cholesterol stones. *Am J Gastroenterol* 1995;90:967–972.
238. Stone BG, Gavaler JS, Belle SH, et al. Impairment of gallbladder emptying in diabetes mellitus. *Gastroenterology* 1988;95:170–176.
239. Dhiman RK, Arke L, Bhansali A, et al. Cisapride improves gallbladder emptying in patients with type 2 diabetes mellitus. *J Gastroenterol Hepatol* 2001;16: 1044–1050.
240. Keshavarzian A, Dunne M, Iber FL. Gallbladder volume and emptying in insulin-requiring male diabetics. *Dig Dis Sci* 1987;32:824–828.
241. Arslanoglu I, Unal F, Sagin F, et al. Real-time sonography for screening of gallbladder dysfunction in children with type 1 diabetes mellitus. *J Pediatr Endocrinol Metab* 2001;14:61–69.
242. Newman H, Northup J. The autopsy incidence of gallstones. *Int Abstr Surg* 1959;109:1–13.
243. Zahor Z, Sternby MH, Kagan A, et al. Frequency of cholelithiasis in Prague and Malmo: an autopsy study. *Scand J Gastoenterol* 1974;9:3–7.
244. Strom BL, Tamragouri RN, Morse ML, et al. Oral contraceptives and other risk factors for gallbladder disease. *Clin Pharmacol Ther* 1986;39:335–341.
245. Honore LH. The lack of a positive association between symptomatic cholesterol cholelithiasis and clinical diabetes mellitus: a retrospective study. *J Chronic Dis* 1980;33:465–469.
246. Misciagna G, Guerra V, Di Leo A, et al. Insulin and gallstones: a population case control study in southern Italy. *Gut* 2000;47:144–147.
247. Attili AF, Capocaccia R, Carulli N, et al. Factors associated with gallstone disease in the MICOL experience. Multicenter Italian Study on Epidemiology of Cholelithiasis. *Hepatology* 1997;26:809–818.
248. Pacchioni M, Nicoletti C, Caminiti M, et al. Association of obesity and type II diabetes mellitus as a risk factor for gallstones. *Dig Dis Sci* 2000;45:2002–2006.
249. Pellegrini CA. Asymptomatic gallstones. Does diabetes mellitus make a difference? *Gastroenterology* 1986;91:245–247.
250. Rabinowitch IM. On the mortality resulting from the surgical treatment of chronic gallbladder disease in diabetes mellitus. *Ann Surg* 1932;96:70–74.
251. Turrill FL, McCarron MM, Mikkelson WP. Gallstones and diabetes: an ominous association. *Am J Surg* 1961;102:184–190.
252. Mundth ED. Cholecystitis and diabetes mellitus. *N Engl J Med* 1962;267: 642–646.
253. Landau O, Deutsch AA, Kott I, et al. The risk of cholecystectomy for acute cholecystitis in diabetic patients. *Hepatogastroenterology* 1992;39:437–438.
254. Del Favero G, Caroli A, Meggiato T, et al. Natural history of gallstones in non-insulin-dependent diabetes mellitus. A prospective 5-year follow-up. *Dig Dis Sci* 1994;39:1704–1707.
255. Hickman MS, Schwesinger WH, Page CP. Acute cholecystitis in the diabetic. A case-control study of outcome. *Arch Surg* 1988;123:409–411.
256. Ransohoff DF, Miller GL, Forsythe SB, et al. Outcome of acute cholecystitis in patients with diabetes mellitus. *Ann Intern Med* 1987;106:829–832.
257. Walsh DB, Eckhauser FE, Ramsburgh SR, et al. Risk associated with diabetes mellitus in patients undergoing gallbladder surgery. *Surgery* 1982;91:254–257.
258. Sandler RS, Maule WF, Baltus ME. Factors associated with postoperative complications in diabetics after biliary tract surgery. *Gastroenterology* 1986;91: 157–162.
259. Wetter LA, Way LW. Surgical therapy for gallstone disease [Review]. *Gastroenterol Clin North Am* 1991;20:157–169.
260. Ranson JH, Rifkind KM, Roses DF, et al. Prognostic signs and the role of operative management in acute pancreatitis. *Surg Gynecol Obstet* 1974;139: 69–81.
261. Foulis AK. The pathology of the endocrine pancreas in type 1 (insulin-dependent) diabetes mellitus [Review]. *APMIS* 1996;104:161–167.
262. Foulis AK, Liddle CN, Farquharson MA, et al. The histopathology of the pancreas in type 1 (insulin-dependent) diabetes mellitus: a 25-year review of deaths in patients under 20 years of age in the United Kingdom. *Diabetologia* 1986;29:267–274.
263. Henderson JR, Daniel PM, Fraser PA. The pancreas as a single organ: the influence of the endocrine upon the exocrine part of the gland [Review]. *Gut* 1981;22:158–167.
264. Fonseca V, Berger LA, Beckett AG, et al. Size of pancreas in diabetes mellitus: a study based on ultrasound. *Br Med J Clin Res Ed* 1985;291:1240–1241.
265. Frier BM, Saunders JH, Wormsley KG, et al. Exocrine pancreatic function in juvenile-onset diabetes mellitus. *Gut* 1976;17:685–691.
266. Dandona P, Freedman DB, Foo Y, et al. Exocrine pancreatic function in diabetes mellitus. *J Clin Pathol* 1984;37:302–306.
267. Vinicor F, Lehrner LM, Karn RC, et al. Hyperamylasemia in diabetic ketoacidosis: sources and significance. *Ann Intern Med* 1979;91:200–204.
268. Vantyghem MC, Haye S, Balduyck M, et al. Changes in serum amylase, lipase and leukocyte elastase during diabetic ketoacidosis and poorly controlled diabetes. *Acta Diabetol* 1999;36:39–44.
269. Eckfeldt JH, Leatherman JW, Levitt MD. High prevalence of hyperamylasemia in patients with acidemia. *Ann Intern Med* 1986;104:362–363.
270. Nair S, Yadav D, Pitchumoni CS. Association of diabetic ketoacidosis and acute pancreatitis: observations in 100 consecutive episodes of DKA. *Am J Gastroenterol* 2000;95:2795–2800.
271. Yadav D, Nair S, Norkus EP, et al. Nonspecific hyperamylasemia and hyperlipasemia in diabetic ketoacidosis: incidence and correlation with biochemical abnormalities. *Am J Gastroenterol* 2000;95:3123–3128.
272. Calle EE, Murphy TK, Rodriguez C, et al. Diabetes mellitus and pancreatic cancer mortality in a prospective cohort of United States adults. *Cancer Causes Control* 1998;9:403–410.
273. Gullo L. Diabetes and the risk of pancreatic cancer. *Ann Oncol* 1999;10 [Suppl 4]:79–81.
274. Strickler HD, Wylie-Rosett J, Rohan T, et al. The relation of type 2 diabetes and cancer [Review]. *Diabetes Technol Ther* 2001;3:263–274.
275. DeMeo MT. Pancreatic cancer and sugar diabetes [Review]. *Nutr Rev* 2001;59:112–115.
276. Baig NA, Herrine SK, Rubin R. Liver disease and diabetes mellitus [Review]. *Clin Lab Med* 2001;21:193–207.
277. Manderson WG, McKiddie MT, et al. Liver glycogen accumulation in unstable diabetes. *Diabetes* 196;17:13–16.
278. Stone BG, Van Thiel DH. Diabetes mellitus and the liver [Review]. *Semin Liver Dis* 1985;5:8–28.
279. Foster KJ, Griffith AH, Dewbury K, et al. Liver disease in patients with diabetes mellitus. *Postgrad Med J* 1980;56:767–772.
280. Drew SI, Joffe B, Vinik A, et al. The first 24 hours of acute pancreatitis. Changes in biochemical and endocrine homeostasis in patients with pancreatitis compared with those in control subjects undergoing stress for reasons other than pancreatitis. *Am J Med* 1978;64:795–803.
281. Reid AE. Nonalcoholic steatohepatitis [Review]. *Gastroenterology* 2001;121: 710–723.
282. Falchuk KR, Fiske SC, Haggitt RC, et al. Pericentral hepatic fibrosis and intracellular hyalin in diabetes mellitus. *Gastroenterology* 1980;78:535–541.
283. Boelsterli UA, Bedoucha M. Toxicological consequences of altered peroxisome proliferator-activated receptor gamma (PPARgamma) expression in the liver: insights from models of obesity and type 2 diabetes [Review]. *Biochem Pharmacol* 2002;63:1–10.
284. Worner TM, Lieber CS. Perivenular fibrosis as precursor lesion of cirrhosis. *JAMA* 1985;254:627–630.
285. Silverman JF, O'Brien KF, Long S, et al. Liver pathology in morbidly obese patients with and without diabetes. *Am J Gastroenterol* 1990;85:1349–1355.
286. Pamilo M, Sotaniemi EA, Suramo I, et al. Evaluation of liver steatotic and fibrous content by computerized tomography and ultrasound. *Scand J Gastroenterol* 1983;18:743–747.
287. Lenaerts J, Verresen L, Van Steenbergen W, et al. Fatty liver hepatitis and type 5 hyperlipoproteinemia in juvenile diabetes mellitus. Case report and review of the literature. *J Clin Gastroenterol* 1990;12:93–97.
288. Powell EE, Cooksley WG, Hanson R, et al. The natural history of nonalcoholic steatohepatitis: a follow-up study of forty-two patients for up to 21 years. *Hepatology* 1990;11:74–80.
289. Fujino Y, Mizoue T, Tokui N, et al. Prospective study of diabetes mellitus and liver cancer in Japan. *Diabetes Metab Res Rev* 2001;17:374–379.
290. La Vecchia C, Negri E, Decarli A, et al. Diabetes mellitus and the risk of primary liver cancer. *Int J Cancer* 1997;73:204–207.
291. El-Serag HB, Richardson PA, Everhart JE. The role of diabetes in hepatocellular carcinoma: a case-control study among United States Veterans. *Am J Gastroenterol* 2001;96:2462–2470.

CHAPTER 65
Treatment of Diabetes in the Hospitalized Patient

Howard A. Wolpert

Diabetes-related hospitalizations in the United States totaled 13.9 million days in 1997 (1). The advances made in anesthesia and perioperative cardiovascular monitoring in recent years have led to a dramatic improvement in the outcome following major surgery in patients with diabetes (2). Too often, however, inattention to the metabolic management of the patient with diabetes will lead to complications in the hospital course and prolong hospital stay. Illness and surgery trigger counterregulatory hormone responses that counteract insulin action and can lead to metabolic instability and decompensation. In the hospitalized patient, host defenses against infection are compromised by disruption of the mucocutaneous barriers by endotracheal tubes, catheters, and surgical procedures. Furthermore, hyperglycemia directly inhibits immune function, adding to the risk for nosocomial infection. It is hoped that current trends toward the use of standardized treatment protocols to improve and expedite hospital care will have a positive impact on inpatient diabetes management.

TREATMENT CONSIDERATIONS: GOALS

Prevention of Metabolic Decompensation

The prevention of metabolic decompensation from the "stress" of illness and surgery is a key goal in the management of diabetes in the hospitalized patient. Surgery and illness induce a metabolic response that is characterized by increased secretion of epinephrine, glucagon, cortisol, and growth hormone (3,4). These counterregulatory hormones lead to a state of insulin resistance, with accelerated lipolysis and protein catabolism (5). In nondiabetic patients, there is a compensatory increase in insulin secretion that, in addition to maintaining glucose homeostasis, will counteract the catabolism and tissue breakdown. In the patient with diabetes, these counterregulatory changes can lead to metabolic decompensation with severe hyperglycemia and osmotic diuresis accompanied by dehydration and electrolyte disturbances. In patients with marked insulin deficiency, the increased levels of epinephrine and glucagon will trigger a state of accelerated lipolysis and ketogenesis that can culminate in diabetic ketoacidosis. The fundamental goal in the management of diabetes in the hospitalized patient is to ensure that there is sufficient circulating insulin to counteract this catabolic state.

Promotion of Wound Healing

The catabolic state that develops during injury and surgery can compromise the nutritional state of the patient and delay wound healing (6). Insulin has a key anabolic role in the physiologic responses that restrain tissue catabolism during injury. Studies in animal models of diabetes indicate that hyperglycemia and insulin deficiency attenuate the process of wound healing (7). The administration of insulin to injured nondiabetic patients markedly attenuates protein breakdown and urea generation (8,9). In addition, insulin therapy in the injured patient reduces the efflux of amino acids from skeletal muscle (10). Although there are no definitive data demonstrating that tight glycemic control improves wound healing in patients with diabetes, the weight of evidence showing that insulin blunts protein catabolism provides a strong physiologic rationale for ensuring that the hospitalized diabetic patient has adequate insulin (11).

Minimizing Infection Risk

The answer to the question of how tightly to control hyperglycemia in the hospitalized patient depends on several considerations. Hyperglycemia has direct effects on immune function that can increase susceptibility to infection (12). Furthermore, the impaired phagocytic and bactericidal function of neutrophils from patients with poorly controlled diabetes is reversed with intensive glycemic control (13,14). Data from the Beth Israel Deaconess Medical Center, affiliated with the Joslin Clinic, clearly indicate that early postoperative glucose control is an important predictor of serious nosocomial infections such as bacteremia, pneumonia, and surgical wound infections (15). One hundred consecutive diabetic patients undergoing elective surgery over a 4-month period were prospectively followed for the development of postoperative infections. Patients with hyperglycemia (defined as at least one serum glucose measurement > 220 mg/dL) on postoperative day 1 had an infection rate 2.7 times that noted in diabetic patients whose serum glucose measurements were all ≤220 mg/dL. Remarkably, when urinary tract infections were excluded from the analysis, hyperglycemia on postoperative day 1 was associated with a 5.8-fold increase in rates of nosocomial infection. These findings have been confirmed in an analysis from the Johns Hopkins institutions of postoperative infection rates in diabetic patients undergoing coronary bypass grafting (16). Postoperative glucose levels in the cohort were divided into quartiles and, independent of other factors, including underlying comorbidity and the severity of illness during the recovery, the patients in the lowest quartile (mean glucose level, 121 to 206 mg/dL) had lower infection rates.

Evidence from the Bypass Angioplasty Revascularization Investigation (BARI) (17) that patients with diabetes and multivessel coronary artery disease who receive internal mammary grafts have superior long-term survival compared with those who receive saphenous vein grafts or percutaneous transluminal coronary angioplasty has important implications with respect to perioperative diabetes management. Coronary bypass with internal mammary grafts has become the procedure of choice in patients with diabetes and multivessel coronary artery disease; however, this surgery is associated with a markedly higher incidence of postoperative deep sternal wound infections compared with saphenous vein grafting. In patients undergoing internal mammary grafting, the incidence approaches 11.5% to 14.3% (18,19), and there is a significant correlation between postoperative blood glucose levels and infection rates (20,21). Retrospective data from the St. Vincent Medical Center in Portland, Oregon, show that the implementation of a perioperative insulin infusion protocol in 1991 resulted in more than a 50% reduction in deep sternal wound infections (21). Mean blood glucose levels with the continuous insulin infusion protocol were significantly lower than those achieved prior to 1991 with subcutaneous insulin (199 ± 1.4 vs. 241 ± 1.9 mg/dL on the operative day; 176 ± 0.8 vs. 206 ± 1.2 mg/dL on postoperative day 1). During the period of analysis, the rate of deep sternal wound infections in the nondiabetic patient population remained constant, suggesting a causal link between the improved perioperative glucose control and reduced infection risk.

There is no definitive evidence from randomized controlled clinical trials demonstrating that tight glycemic control reduces rates of perioperative infection. However, the evidence that hyperglycemia directly impairs immune function and the weight of the empiric data showing a link between perioperative glycemic control and risk of infection provide support for a policy of aiming for blood glucose levels of less than 200 to 220 mg/dL in the surgical patient.

Risks of Hypoglycemia

The goal of avoiding hyperglycemia needs to be balanced against the increased risk of hypoglycemia associated with tight glycemic control. In the hospitalized patient with diabetes, the major concern related to hypoglycemia is the potential triggering of ventricular arrhythmias. Circumstantial evidence links hypoglycemia with sudden death in patients with diabetes, and experimental clamp studies have demonstrated that the epinephrine surges that occur with hypoglycemia can be accompanied by alterations in ventricular repolarization and ectopy (22,23). However, data from the Diabetes Mellitus Insulin Glucose Infusion in Acute Myocardial Infarction (DIGAMI) study suggest that the risks from hypoglycemia in the hospitalized diabetic patient are minimal. In this study, 306 patients with type 2 diabetes presenting with myocardial infarction (MI) were randomized to an intensive treatment protocol with an intravenous insulin-glucose infusion. Fifteen percent of these patients had at least one episode of hypoglycemia [predefined as a blood glucose level <3 mmol/L (54 mg/dL)], and none of these episodes were associated with any direct harmful effects (24).

Outcome Following Myocardial Infarction

The importance of intensive glycemic control in improving outcome following MI remains controversial. Patients with diabetes who have blood glucose concentrations ≥11 mmol/L at presentation of MI are at greater risk for in-hospital mortality (25). Although stress hyperglycemia may simply be a marker of the severity of illness, several plausible biologic mechanisms could account for this association. The relative insulin deficiency underlying the hyperglycemia will limit myocardial glucose uptake, and energy generation becomes increasingly dependent on free fatty acids, which are toxic to the ischemic myocardium (26). Moreover, the insulin deficiency will trigger lipolysis, thereby increasing circulating levels of free fatty acids. In addition, insulin deficiency leads to increased activity of plasminogen activator inhibitor type-1 (PAI-1), with a resultant impairment in fibrinolysis (27). In the DIGAMI study, the patients presenting with MI randomized to the intensive-treatment protocol with intravenous insulin had an improved outcome. However the subset analysis revealed that only those patients in the intensive-treatment arm who were categorized as low risk and who were not receiving insulin at presentation demonstrated this benefit (28). This raises the possibility that it was not the intensive management but rather the withdrawal of other diabetes therapies (such as sulfonylureas) that led to the improved survival after MI (29). Although the DIGAMI data do not unequivocally demonstrate that the tight peri-MI glycemic control per se accounted for the improved outcome, the intensive treatment regimen did not lead to any harmful complications in the study (24). The physician should consider use of an intravenous insulin infusion to maintain tight glycemic control if the MI patient is in a coronary care unit where intense monitoring allows the safe implementation of this regimen.

CONSIDERATIONS IN CLINICAL DECISION MAKING

Clinical decisions about how to manage diabetes in the hospitalized patient rest on several considerations.

Risks of Oral Agents in the Hospitalized Patient

Lactic acidosis is a rare, but serious, complication of metformin therapy, and this agent should be withheld from at-risk patients (30). The recommendation to withhold metformin includes the following conditions: radiologic procedures with dye loads (risk of renal impairment with delayed drug clearance), major surgery (risk of hypoperfusion with anaerobic metabolism and lactate generation), general anesthesia in patients with autonomic neuropathy (high risk of hypotension) (31), ischemic limbs (anaerobic metabolism and lactate generation), hepatic disease (impaired lactate metabolism), and cardiorespiratory failure with hypoxia.

Sulfonylureas are associated with an increased risk for prolonged drug-induced hypoglycemia in the patient with reduced caloric intake, renal disease, and a previous history of hypoglycemia (32), and these agents should be used judiciously in the hospitalized patient with these characteristics.

The use of sulfonylurea agents to manage diabetes in the patient presenting with acute MI is controversial. Sulfonylureas block the adenosine triphosphate (ATP)–sensitive potassium channels present in the myocardium and coronary vasculature, and this action impairs ischemic preconditioning and the coronary vasodilatory response to ischemia (33). Retrospective data from the Mayo Clinic showed a significantly higher in-hospital mortality following coronary angioplasty treatment for acute MI in those patients with diabetes treated with sulfonylurea agents (34). Subset analysis from the DIGAMI study also points to a possible deleterious effect of sulfonylurea therapy on post-MI outcome (28). However, no relationship between treatment with sulfonylureas and adverse outcome following MI was noted in a recent analysis of the Health Care Financing Administration database of 64,171 elderly patients with diabetes (35).

Type of Diabetes

In patients with type 2 diabetes controlled with oral agents, the major consideration of the physician deciding on initial therapy is whether the patient is likely to have sufficient β-cell insulin secretory capacity to counteract the insulin resistance that develops with hospitalization. In the absence of adequate β-cell reserve, insulin therapy is necessary. The patient with well-controlled diabetes receiving submaximal dosages of oral agents usually will manage to maintain satisfactory perioperative glycemic control without the medications when taking no calories in orally. In contrast, the patient with poorly controlled diabetes receiving maximal oral therapy will probably not have sufficient β-cell reserve to compensate for the insulin resistance and will need to have insulin therapy initiated.

Despite the insulin resistance associated with illness/injury, the obese patient with insulin-requiring type 2 diabetes often will need considerably less insulin when placed on a controlled diet during hospitalization. The initial response to insulin administered in the hospital often predicts whether the patient is likely to require a reduction in insulin dosage.

Metabolic Response to Hospitalization

Several potential factors and mechanisms contribute to the development of insulin resistance in the hospitalized patient. This includes inactivity, starvation, use of medications such as steroids and dobutamine (36), and the release of counterregulatory hormones triggered by the stress of illness, surgery, and anesthesia. Consideration of all of these factors will help the physician decide whether the patient with type 2 diabetes is likely to need insulin therapy and to anticipate changes in insulin requirements during the hospital course.

Metabolic and hormonal responses will vary depending on the type of anesthesia and surgery. Barker et al. (37) compared the impact of local versus general anesthesia in patients with type 2 diabetes controlled with diet and oral agents who were undergoing cataract extraction. The patients who received local anesthesia had stable perioperative glucose levels despite omission of the diabetes medications on the morning of surgery. In contrast, the patients who had general anesthesia had significant increases in both the blood glucose and serum cortisol levels, with the glucose rising from a fasting level of 6.6 mmol/L to 8.6 mmol/L 2 hours after the procedure. Thomas et al. (38) have noted that patients with type 1 diabetes undergoing coronary artery bypass grafting require considerably higher rates of intravenous insulin infusion to maintain stable glycemic control than those required by similar patients undergoing general surgery.

The glucose infusion rates typically used in clinical practice do not cover basal energy requirements and are insufficient to suppress starvation ketosis. An infusion of 10% dextrose at 100 cc per hour would provide only 2.2 $mg{\cdot}kg^{-1}{\cdot}min^{-1}$ for a 70-kg person, whereas Wolfe and Peters (39) have demonstrated that fasting normal volunteers require infusions of 4 $mg{\cdot}kg^{-1}{\cdot}min^{-1}$ to suppress lipolysis. Although most fasting patients have reduced insulin requirements, the catabolic state induced by fasting can lead to insulin resistance. Ljungqvist et al. (40) pretreated a cohort of nondiabetic patients with a high-dose glucose infusion (5 $mg{\cdot}kg^{-1}{\cdot}min^{-1}$) overnight before abdominal surgery. Compared with control patients who underwent the same operation in the fasted state, the fed patients had a substantial improvement in insulin sensitivity during the 24-hour period following the abdominal surgery. This catabolism-related insulin resistance is a major factor underlying the marked glucose elevations that often will develop in the hospitalized diabetic patient with relatively modest intravenous glucose loads.

The administration of Ringer lactate to the patient with diabetes undergoing surgery can markedly increase glucose levels. Lactate is a gluconeogenic precursor, and in situations of stress such as surgery the rate of gluconeogenesis may be enhanced. Thomas and Alberti (41) noted that the mean plasma glucose concentration in a group of patients with type 2 diabetes undergoing major surgery who received 1 to 1.5 L of Ringer lactate increased from 8.5 to 16.0 mmol/L, whereas the glucose concentration in the diabetic control group who did not receive intravenous fluids perioperatively increased only by 2.1 mmol/L.

The importance of the perioperative metabolic state of the patient on the postoperative course has received little attention in clinical care. Nygren et al. (42) subjected a cohort of nondiabetic patients scheduled for elective hip replacement to euglycemic hyperinsulinemic clamps [to induce a state of physiologic hyperinsulemia (serum insulin levels 58 ± 3 to 64 ± 4 μU/mL)] for 4 to 5 hours before the surgery and throughout the operation. The perioperative insulin and glucose infusion blunted the normal stress response to surgery, as reflected by significant attenuation of postoperative changes in plasma levels of free fatty acid, serum cortisol levels, and fat oxidation, and there was an associated normalization of postoperative insulin sensitivity. In addition to blunting the catabolic response to surgery, the insulin-glucose infusion may have a positive impact on anabolic changes during the recovery from surgery. Levels of insulin-like growth factor 1 (IGF-1) declined less after surgery in the subjects receiving the infusion than in the control subjects. In addition, levels of IGF-binding protein-1 more than halved following the infusion, whereas levels in the control subjects more than doubled. Although IGF-1 activity was not measured directly, these contrasting changes in the two study groups would lead to a marked difference in the bioavailability of IGF-1 that could have an impact on healing and recovery following surgery. Further studies are required to determine whether implementation of this treatment protocol would lead to improved clinical endpoints and shorter hospital stays.

The insulin clamp studies of Nygren et al. (42) suggest that the postoperative deterioration in glucose tolerance is related primarily to a decrease in glucose uptake by the insulin-sensitive tissues rather than to an impairment in insulin-mediated suppression of endogenous glucose production. This has relevance to clinical decision making: When adjusting insulin replacement regimens in the postoperative patient who is hyperglycemic, the physician should give initial consideration to increasing insulin coverage during the day to enhance disposal of consumed glucose by the insulin-sensitive tissues rather than to increasing overnight insulin coverage.

Other Considerations

When making insulin adjustments for the patient receiving glucocorticoid therapy, the physician needs to consider the pharmacokinetic action and dosage schedule of the steroid. For example, prednisone taken at breakfast will lead to insulin resistance in the afternoon that can usually be covered by prebreakfast intermediate insulin. Patients receiving high-dose prednisone will require proportionately larger insulin doses, and some patients will develop late-morning hypoglycemia due to the onset of the intermediate insulin, an effect that can be obviated by having the patient take this insulin midmorning. Patients receiving prednisone in the morning will often have relative adrenal insufficiency overnight, and bedtime insulin coverage will need to be reduced accordingly.

Nutritional supplements given to the hospitalized will often contain substantial amounts of carbohydrate despite their being labeled "no added sugar." For the hospitalized diabetic patient with marked glycemic excursions, the physician needs to exclude carbohydrate-containing nutritional supplements as a contributing factor.

The accuracy of bedside glucose monitors will be affected by the hematocrit level. Anemia (with hematocrits in the range of 20%) will result in an overestimation of the glucose level, and this can mask the diagnosis of true hypoglycemia (43). Consumption of high doses of ascorbic acid by the patient will lead to the overestimation of glucose levels by the Accu-Chek and Precision devices. Therapeutic acetaminophen and dopamine concentrations will also interfere with the accuracy of some bedside glucose monitors (44).

TREATMENT GUIDELINES

Several comprehensive reviews (3,45–47) present specific guidelines for inpatient diabetes management. Figure 65.1 shows an algorithm commonly used by staff at the Joslin Clinic in the care of the diabetic surgical patient. Tracer studies have shown that major surgery has no effect on the absorption rates of subcutaneously injected neutral protamine Hagedorn (NPH) insulin (48). It is our practice to give intravenous glucose from midnight onward to patients who are in the hospital the evening before surgery. These patients generally receive their usual evening dose of intermediate insulin. For patients admitted to the hospital the morning of surgery, we recommend that the dose of intermediate insulin in the preceding evening be reduced by 10% to 20%. This minimizes the risk for hypoglycemia during the early morning activity involved in coming to the hospital. Previous recommendations (3) that the evening intermediate insulin be withheld were based on the use of animal insulins that have a longer duration of action than biosynthetic human insulin.

Insulin sliding scales have an important role in the inpatient management of diabetes. The assertion by Queale et al. (49) that sliding scales are of no benefit in this setting is not valid because this conclusion was based on a retrospective analysis of severely ill patients whose sliding-scale dosages were not appropriately individualized. Moreover, many patients examined did not have basal insulin coverage. "Corrective" sliding scales that start at glucose levels greater than 175 to 200 mg/dL have an important role in preventing severe hyperglycemia in the hospitalized patient. However, with the exception of patients whose diabetes is readily controlled by diet or modest dosages of oral agents, sliding scales alone usually do not provide adequate diabetes control for the hospitalized patient. Patients whose diabetes is well controlled out of the hospital with submaximal doses of oral agents usually will require corrective sliding-scale insulin coverage in addition to their usual diabetes medications when hospitalized with a medical illness. In contrast, patients whose diabetes is poorly controlled with maximal oral therapy usually do not have the β-cell reserve to compensate for the insulin resistance associated with illness; these patients, like patients with type 1 diabetes, will require basal coverage with intermediate- or long-acting insulin formulations in addition to the sliding scale.

In writing insulin orders for the hospitalized patient, the physician should make a distinction between sliding scales used to "correct" hyperglycemia and "anticipatory" premeal sliding scales required in patients with absent or markedly impaired β-cell function to provide fast-acting insulin to cover anticipated carbohydrate intake. Anticipatory sliding scales should provide premeal insulin coverage even if the premeal glucose level is in the desired physiologic range. Typically, the patient who receives morning and bedtime intermediate insulin will require anticipatory prebreakfast and predinner sliding-scale insulin and compensatory coverage before lunch and at bedtime. The patient whose basal insulin requirements are covered by ultralente or insulin glargine will lack the lunchtime insulin coverage provided by the morning intermediate insulin and will require anticipatory insulin coverage before breakfast, lunch, and dinner with compensatory coverage at bedtime. The physician will need to review the patient's response to administered insulin to assess if dosages require adjustment: the initial sliding scale written usually provides for additive increases in the insulin dosages as the glucose level increases; however, because of hyperglycemia-induced insulin resistance, many patients will require relatively greater insulin dosages at high glucose levels and the sliding scale coverage in the upper range will need to be disproportionately greater.

Although there have been no comprehensive studies of continuous subcutaneous insulin infusion (CSII) during surgery, in our experience CSII provides good metabolic control perioperatively. At our institution most patients receiving CSII continue it during surgery. Patients receiving CSII who are undergoing major surgery for which there may be hemodynamic instability and concern about potential problems with absorption of subcutaneous insulin will usually be given CSII perioperatively. Basal CSII rates are generally left unchanged from usual settings. Provided that the glucose level before the surgical procedure level is in the target range, the levels after the procedure are generally within acceptable limits. During the preoperative period, the patient should go through the formal process of ensuring that the basal-rate settings are correct by skipping meals. The patient should change the infusion catheter the day

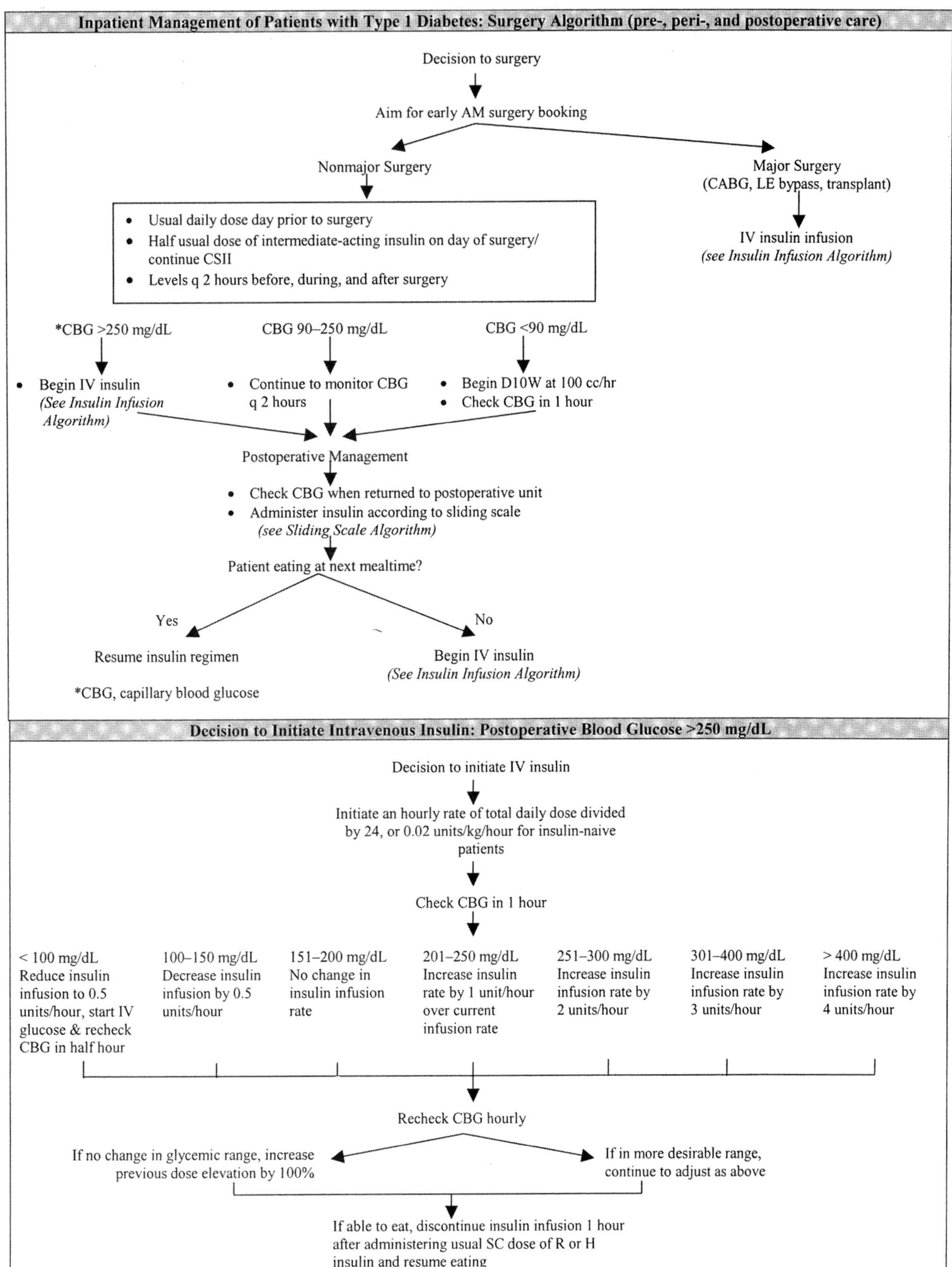

Figure 65.1. Inpatient management of patients with type 1 diabetes: surgery algorithm (pre-, peri-, and postoperative care).

before, and it is important to ensure that the catheter is placed in a site that does not interfere with the surgical field and that the cannula and tubing are securely fastened.

Intravenous insulin is the most precise means of managing diabetes perioperatively, and several different regimens have been recommended. Alberti has been a proponent of the use of glucose-insulin-potassium infusion (45,50). With this regimen, fixed concentrations of glucose, insulin, and potassium are mixed up in a single bag and the infusion rate is adjusted according to the perioperative blood glucose measurements. The proportion of insulin to glucose (expressed as units per g) in the infusate mixture prepared before surgery will be varied depending on the patient's condition and the planned procedure: liver disease, 0.5–0.6; obesity, 0.4–0.6; severe infection 0.6–0.8; steroid therapy, 0.5–0.8; cardiopulmonary bypass, 0.8–1.2; and other circumstances, 0.3–0.4.

Although studies have established the efficacy of the glucose–insulin–potassium infusion in perioperative diabetes management (51,52), this approach is limited by the need to mix up a new bag with a different proportion of insulin and glucose every time the glucose level is out of the target range. The use of a separate glucose infusion and a variable-rate insulin infusion gets around this problem. The starting insulin infusion rate will need to be individualized depending on several considerations, including the patient's usual insulin requirements, the blood glucose level, and identifiable factors that affect insulin sensitivity.

Because of the short half-life of intravenous insulin, interruption of the infusion rapidly leads to metabolic decompensation. Some authors (48) have suggested that this problem might be prevented by also giving a subcutaneous depot of intermediate insulin to patients receiving continuous intravenous insulin. Patients who are sedated or under anesthesia are at particular risk for developing unrecognized hypoglycemia, and the patient receiving CSII to maintain tight glycemic control requires frequent glucose monitoring.

CONCLUSION

Improvements in anesthesia and perioperative care have markedly improved the outlook for the patient with diabetes. There are no definitive data from randomized clinical trials indicating that tight glycemic control will shorten hospital stays or improve wound healing and the outcome for the hospitalized patient. However, the weight of evidence indicates that the metabolic state of the patient is an important determinant of prognosis and that risks from hypoglycemia in the hospitalized patient are minimal. Treatment plans and goals will obviously need to be individualized. However, if available resources permit, the physician should strive to ensure tight metabolic control in the hospitalized patient.

REFERENCES

1. American Diabetes Association. Economic consequences of diabetes mellitus in the U.S. in 1997. *Diabetes Care* 1998;21:296–309.
2. Hjortrup A, Sorensen C, Dyremose E, et al. Influence of diabetes mellitus on operative risk. *Br J Surg* 1985;72:783–785.
3. Hirsch IB, McGill JB, Cryer PE, et al. Perioperative management of surgical patients with diabetes mellitus. *Anesthesiology* 1991;74:346–359.
4. Traynor C, Hall GM. Endocrine and metabolic changes during surgery: anaesthetic implications. *Br J Anaesth* 1981;53:153–160.
5. Nygren JO, Thorell A, Soop M, et al. Perioperative insulin and glucose infusion maintains normal insulin sensitivity after surgery. *Am J Physiol* 1998;275: E140–E148.
6. Ziegler TR, Gatzen C, Wilmore DW. Strategies for attenuating protein-catabolic responses in the critically ill. *Annu Rev Med* 1994;45:459–480.
7. Yue DK, McLennan S, Marsh M, et al. Effects of experimental diabetes, uremia and malnutrition on wound healing. *Diabetes* 1987;36:295–299.
8. Hinton P, Littlejohn S, Allison SP, et al. Insulin and glucose to reduce catabolic response to injury in burned patients. *Lancet* 1971;1:767–769.
9. Woolfson AMJ, Heatley RV, Allison SP. Insulin to inhibit protein catabolism after injury. *N Engl J Med* 1979;300:14–17.
10. Brooks DC, Bessey PQ, Black PR, et al. Insulin stimulates branched chain amino acid uptake and diminishes nitrogen flux from skeletal muscle of injured patients. *J Surg Res* 1986;40:395–405.
11. McMurry JF Jr. Wound healing with diabetes: better glucose control for better wound healing. *Surg Clin North Am* 1984;64:769–778.
12. Pozzilli P, Leslie RDG. Infections and diabetes: mechanisms and prospects for prevention. *Diabet Med* 1994;11:935–941.
13. Nolan CM, Beaty HN, Bagdade JD. Further characterization of the impaired bactericidal function of granulocytes in patients with poorly controlled diabetes. *Diabetes* 1978;27:889–894.
14. Rassias AJ, Marrin CAS, Arruda J, et al. Insulin infusion improves neutrophil function in diabetic cardiac surgery patients. *Anesth Analg* 1999;88:1011–1016.
15. Pomposelli JJ, Baxter JK III, Babineau TJ, et al. Early postoperative glucose control predicts nosocomial infection rate in diabetic patients. *J Parenter Enteral Nutr* 1998;22:77–81.
16. Golden SH, Peart-Vigilance C, Kao WHL, et al. Perioperative glycemic control and the risk of infectious complications in a cohort of adults with diabetes. *Diabetes Care* 1999;22:1408–1414.
17. The BARI Investigators. Seven-year outcome in the Bypass Angioplasty Revascularization Investigation (BARI) by treatment and diabetic status. *J Am Coll Cardiol* 2000;35:1122–1229.
18. Grossi EA, Esposito R, Harris LJ, et al. Sternal wound infections and use of internal mammary artery grafts. *J Thorac Cardiovasc Surg* 1991;102:342–347.
19. Borger MA, Rao V, Weisel RD, et al. Deep sternal wound infection: risk factors and outcome. *Ann Thorac Surg* 1998;65:1050–1056.
20. Zerr KJ, Furnary AP, Grunkemeier GL, et al. Glucose control lowers the risk of wound infection in diabetics after open heart operations. *Ann Thorac Surg* 1997;63:356–361.
21. Furnary AP, Zerr KJ, Grunkemeier GL, et al. Continuous intravenous insulin infusion reduces the incidence of deep sternal wound infection in diabetic patients after cardiac surgical procedures. *Ann Thorac Surg* 1999;67:352–362.
22. Marques JL, George E, Peacey SR, et al. Altered ventricular repolarization during hypoglycaemia in patients with diabetes. *Diabet Med* 1997;14:648–654.
23. Lindstrom T, Jorfeldt L, Tegler L, et al. Hypoglycaemia and cardiac arrhythmias in patients with type 2 diabetes mellitus. *Diabet Med* 1992;9:536–541.
24. Malmberg K, McGuire DK. Diabetes and acute myocardial infarction: the role of insulin therapy. *Am Heart J* 1999;138:S381–S386.
25. Capes SE, Hunt D, Malmberg K, et al. Stress hyperglycaemia and increased risk of death after myocardial infarction in patients with and without diabetes: a systematic overview. *Lancet* 2000;355:733–738.
26. Oliver MF, Opie LH. Effects of glucose and fatty acids on myocardial ischemia and arrhythmias. *Lancet* 1994;343:155–158.
27. Jain SK, Nagi DK, Slavin BM, et al. Insulin therapy in type 2 diabetic patients suppresses plasminogen activator inhibitor-1 activity and proinsulin-like molecules independently of glycaemic control. *Diabet Med* 1993;10:27–32.
28. Malmberg K. Prospective randomised study of intensive insulin treatment on long term survival after acute myocardial infarction in patients with diabetes mellitus. *BMJ* 1997;314:1512.
29. Nattrass M. Managing diabetes after myocardial infarction. *BMJ* 1997;314:1497.
30. Mercker SK, Maier C, Neumann G, et al. Lactic acidosis as a serious perioperative complication of antidiabetic biguanide medication with metformin. *Anesthesiology* 1997;87:1003–1005.
31. Burgos LG, Ebert TJ, Asiddao C, et al. Increased intraoperative cardiovascular morbidity in diabetics with autonomic neuropathy. *Anesthesiology* 1989;70: 591–597.
32. Krepinsky J, Ingram AJ, Clase CM. Prolonged sulphonylurea-induced hypoglycemia in diabetic patients with end-stage renal disease. *Am J Kidney Dis* 2000;35:500–505.
33. Cleveland JC Jr., Meldrum DR, Cain BS, et al. Oral sulphonylurea hypoglycemic agents prevent ischemic preconditioning in human myocardium: two paradoxes revisited. *Circulation* 1997;96:29–32.
34. Garratt KN, Brady PA, Hassinger NL, et al. Sulphonylurea drugs increase early mortality in patients with diabetes mellitus after direct angioplasty for acute myocardial infarction. *J Am Coll Cardiol* 1999;33:119–124.
35. Jollis JG, Simpson RJ Jr, Cascio WE, et al. Relation between sulphonylurea therapy, complications, and outcome for elderly patients with acute myocardial infarction. *Am Heart J* 1999;138:S376–S380.
36. Wood SM, Milne JR, Evans SF, et al. Effect of dobutamine on insulin requirements in a patient with ketoacidosis. *BMJ* 1981;282:946–947.
37. Barker JP, Robinson PN, Vafidis GC, et al. Metabolic control of on-insulin-dependent diabetic patients undergoing cataract surgery: comparison of local and general anaesthesia. *Br J Anaesth* 1995;74:500–505.
38. Thomas DJB, Hinds CJ, Rees GM. The management of insulin dependent diabetes during cardiopulmonary bypass and general surgery. *Anaesthesia* 1983;38:1047–1052.
39. Wolfe RR, Peters EJ. Lipolytic response to glucose infusion in human subjects. *Am J Physiol* 1987;252:E218–E223.
40. Ljungqvist O, Thorell A, Gutniak M, et al. Glucose infusion instead of preoperative fasting reduces postoperative insulin resistance. *J Am Coll Surg* 1994; 178:329–336.

41. Thomas DJB, Alberti KGMM. Hyperglycaemic effects of Hartmann's solution during surgery in patients with maturity onset diabetes. *Br J Anaesth* 1978; 50:185–188.
42. Nygren J, Thorell A, Efendic S, et al. Site of insulin resistance after surgery: the contribution of hypocaloric nutrition and bed rest. *Clin Sci* 1997;93:137–146.
43. Louie RF, Tang Z, Sutton DV, et al. Point-of-care glucose testing: effects of critical variables, influence of reference instruments, and a modular glucose meter design. *Arch Pathol Lab Med* 2000;124:257–266.
44. Tang Z, Du X, Louie RF, et al. Effects of drugs on glucose measurements with handheld glucose meters and a portable glucose analyzer. *Am J Clin Pathol* 2000;113:75–86.
45. Alberti KGMM, Gill GV, Elliott MJ. Insulin delivery during surgery in the diabetic patient. *Diabetes Care* 1982;5[Suppl 1]:65–77.
46. Gavin LA. Perioperative management of the diabetic patient. *Endocrinol Metab Clin North Am* 1992;21:457–475.
47. Hirsch IB, Paauw DS, Brunzell J. Inpatient management of adults with diabetes. *Diabetes Care* 1995;18:870–878.
48. Hjortrup A, Madsbad S, Andersen M, et al. Effect of major surgery on absorption rate of NPH insulin injected s.c. *Br J Anaesth* 1990;64:741–742.
49. Queale WS, Seidler AJ, Brancati FL. Glycemic control and sliding scale insulin use in medical inpatients with diabetes mellitus. *Arch Intern Med* 1997;157: 545–552.
50. Alberti KGMM. Diabetes and surgery. *Anesthesiology* 1991;74:209–211.
51. Thai AC, Husband DJ, Gill GV, et al. Management of diabetes during surgery: a retrospective study of 112 cases. *Diabete Metab* 1984;10:65–70.
52. Christiansen CL, Schurizek BA, Malling B, et al. Insulin treatment of the insulin-dependent diabetic patient undergoing minor surgery. *Anaesthesia* 1988;43:533–537.

CHAPTER 66
The Diabetic Foot: Strategies for Treatment and Prevention of Ulcerations

John M. Giurini

Diabetic foot disease affects nearly 2 million patients with diabetes in the United States annually (1). This places an inordinate social and economic burden not only on the United States healthcare system but also on the families of these patients. It is estimated that almost $200 million is spent annually strictly for the care of the diabetic foot (2). This represents only the direct costs of hospitalization, medications, and surgery. Indirect costs such as lost employment, disability, and stress on the family unit cannot even be estimated. More amputations are performed in patients with diabetes than any other group of patients.

The management of diabetic foot disease is focused primarily on avoiding amputation of lower extremities. This goal is carried out through three main strategies: identification of the "at-risk" foot, treatment of the acutely diseased foot, and prevention of further problems. Vital to the success of any program is education of the patient and family members. A comprehensive program of diabetic foot management must include each of these aspects for successful salvage of limbs.

These goals are best met by the establishment of a dedicated limb-salvage team. The members of this team must be dedicated to meeting the challenge of the patient with diabetes whose fears of limb loss are rivaled by fears of blindness and kidney failure (3,4). Members of this team most commonly include a podiatrist, an endocrinologist, a vascular surgeon, and a pedorthist. The team also may include plastic surgeons, infectious disease specialists, orthopedic surgeons, and diabetes teaching nurses. All players must know their role and be available in a timely fashion for consultation.

Several systems exist for grading the at-risk foot (5–7). The main purpose of any classification system is to standardize descriptions of lesions and to formulate algorithms for treatment. While each system claims to be complete, all have pitfalls. Identifying the patient with diabetes at risk for ulceration requires examination of the feet, including the vascular and neurologic systems, skin condition, and foot structure.

IDENTIFICATION OF RISK FACTORS

While certain clinical features are known to increase the risk for lower-extremity amputation, peripheral sensory neuropathy has been identified as the major risk for diabetic foot ulceration (8). Pecoraro et al. (9) placed peripheral sensory neuropathy in the face of unperceived trauma at the entrance to the pathway to ulceration and amputation (Fig. 66.1). The inability of a patient with diabetes to feel pain places him or her at significant risk for future foot problems. Knowledge of this condition and education on preventive measures are critical to the patient's ability to avoid ulcerations. However, even with appropriate preventive measures, ulcerations will develop. Unperceived or unintentional trauma occurs that results in breaks in the skin and inoculation by bacteria.

Clinically significant peripheral sensory neuropathy can be detected by using a 128-millihertz (mHz) tuning fork and a 5.07 Semmes–Weinstein monofilament wire as screening tools to identify at-risk patients (10–12). While loss of vibratory sensation is the initial step in the development of clinically significant neuropathy, grading with a tuning fork is often a subjective exercise without scientifically established norms. A biothesiometer provides more objective documentation of a patient's ability to perceive vibratory sensation. Clinical studies have determined a vibratory perception threshold of 25 mHz as identifying patients at risk for ulceration (13). This instrument, how-

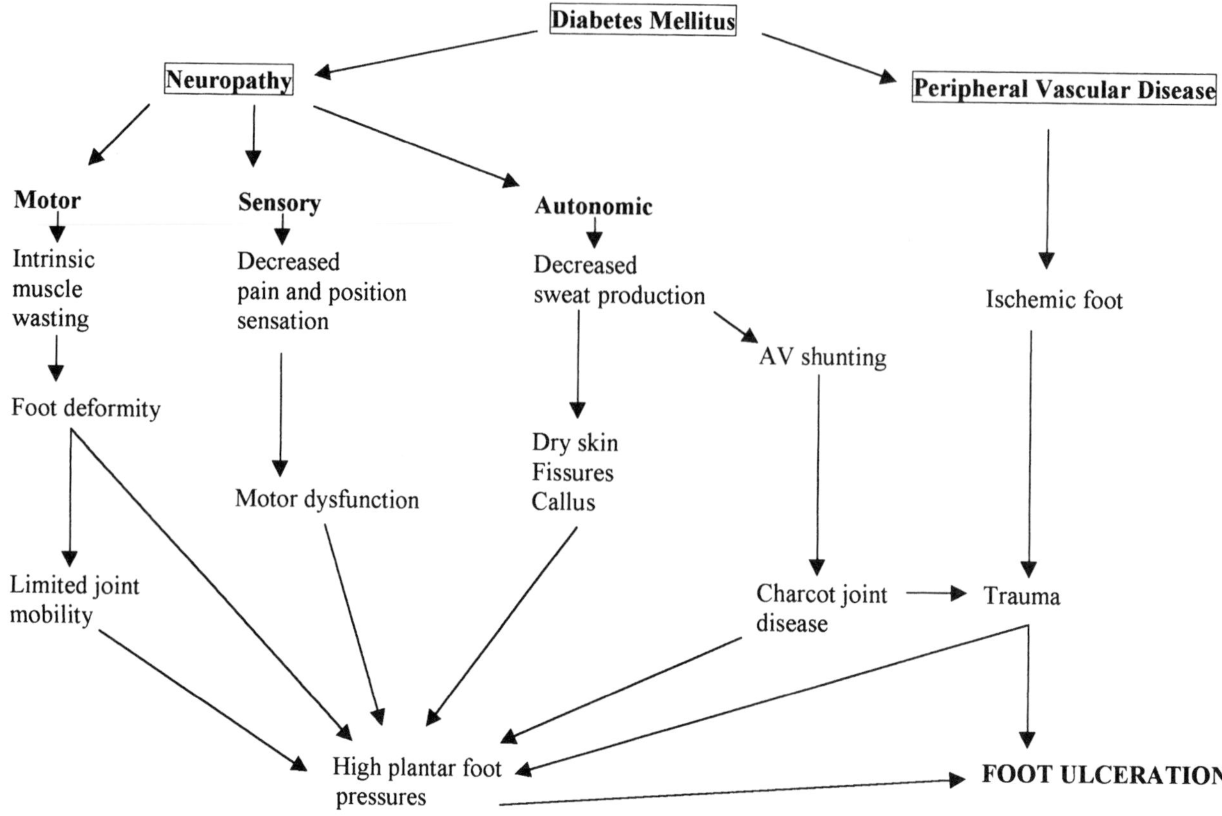

Figure 66.1. Clinical pathways leading to foot ulceration.

ever, is not readily available to the practicing clinician. It is used primarily in clinical trials where documentation of the degree of sensory neuropathy is important in stratifying groups.

The 5.07 (10 g) Semmes–Weinstein monofilament wire is an effective and inexpensive device to identify the patient at risk for foot ulceration. Several clinical trials have demonstrated that patients with diabetes who are unable to perceive this gauge of monofilament wire are at a statistically significant higher risk for development of ulceration than are patients who are able to detect the wire (12). Proper use of the wire requires application of the wire against the foot with enough force to gently bend the wire (Fig. 66.2). Inability to feel the wire implies lack of adequate protective sensation. By testing different sites on the foot, areas of insensitivity can be mapped and identified to the patient. These patients then must be educated on the significance of sensory neuropathy and the steps to preventing foot ulcerations. Regular evaluation by a foot care specialist is recommended for these individuals.

Formal nerve conduction studies in patients with diabetes have not been shown to alter treatment planning. Nerve conduction studies are rarely helpful or necessary for the evaluation of neuropathy. Many patients with type 2 diabetes have clinically significant neuropathy at the time of diagnosis, and nerve conduction studies will be abnormal in the majority of these patients.

Motor neuropathy can produce foot deformities that put the foot at risk for ulceration (Fig. 66.3). Loss of innervation of the

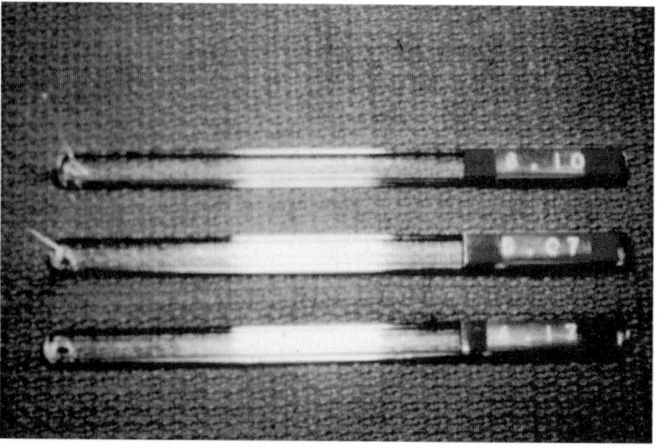

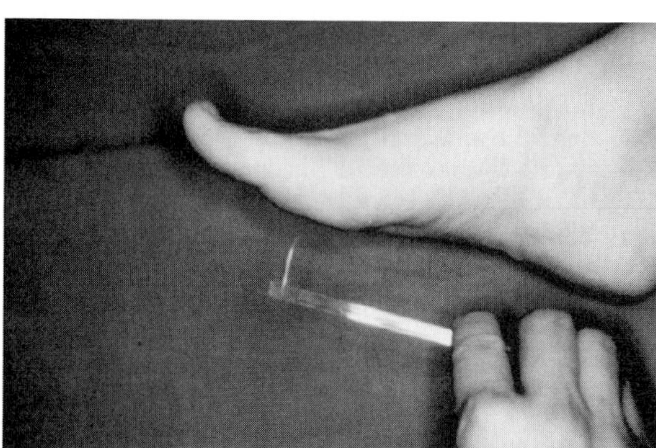

Figure 66.2. Proper use of the monofilament wire requires application of just enough pressure to bend the monofilament.

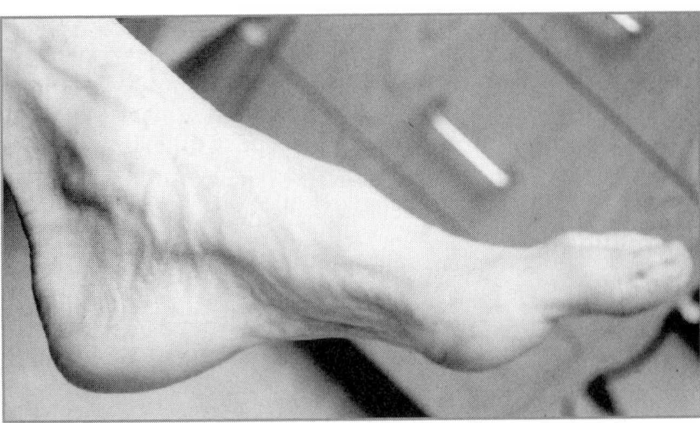

Figure 66.3. The intrinsic minus foot is particularly vulnerable to ulceration as a result of the digital and plantarflexion deformities that may occur.

intrinsic musculature of the foot can lead to common foot deformities such as hammer toes, claw toes, and plantar-flexed metatarsals. Plantarly prominent metatarsal heads result in areas of high focal pressures that have been shown to increase risk for foot ulceration. Digital deformities can be irritated dorsally by shoe gear, resulting in corns or even ulcerations.

Autonomic neuropathy, although less common than peripheral sensory neuropathy, can also affect the feet. Most commonly, autonomic neuropathy affects local temperature regulation and the function of sweat glands. Loss of sweat production can lead to dry skin (14). Untreated this can lead to cracking and fissuring, especially in the heel, creating a portal of entry for bacteria.

Peripheral vascular disease by itself is responsible for only a small percentage of diabetic foot ulcerations. Only 15% of all diabetic foot ulcers are purely ischemic (15). However, arterial insufficiency can lead to nonhealing of ulcerations once they have developed. The single most important indicator of adequate perfusion is the presence of palpable pedal pulses. Additional clinical maneuvers to assess vascular status should include measurement of the venous filling time and evaluation for dependent rubor and pallor on elevation. The presence of a slowly or nonhealing ulceration in the face of absent pulses warrants further evaluation. This may be in the form of noninvasive arterial studies. Pulse volume recordings and the character of the distal pulses on Doppler evaluation (monophasic vs. triphasic) can provide valuable information on the patient's ability to heal the ulceration. Although ankle–brachial indices (ABIs) are measured, they are of limited usefulness in the patient with diabetes. The ABIs often are artifactually elevated due to medial calcinosis of pedal vessels. Assessment of a patient's ability to heal should not be based solely on this measurement. The presence of a nonhealing ulceration with clinical or objective evidence of arterial insufficiency warrants a prompt referral to a vascular surgeon (16).

The areas under the metatarsal heads are the most vulnerable areas for plantar ulcerations. These areas have been identified as having high focal pressures in patients with diabetes (17–19). A symptom of these high pressures is the presence of callus tissue under a metatarsal head. This most commonly results from plantarly prominent metatarsal heads, as occurs in the intrinsic minus foot and when the plantar fat pad atrophies (20,21). More recently, an association between limited joint mobility and high plantar foot pressures has been discussed as a risk factor for foot ulcerations (22,23). Other causes of high foot pressures include developmental foot deformities such as bunions, hammer toes, or rocker-bottom deformities from Charcot joint disease.

Quantitation of plantar foot pressures in the form of vertical load is possible with various computerized pressure-sensing equipment (24). These devices are expensive for most private practitioners and are most useful as a research tool. A Harris mat (ink-impregnated foil that demonstrates pressure points in static stance), however, is a simple, inexpensive tool that can be helpful in identifying areas of high plantar foot pressures.

CLASSIFICATION OF ULCERATIONS

As previously noted, several classification systems for grading ulcerations exist (6). Classification systems have two primary purposes: (a) to provide healthcare professionals with a common language to describe and understand common conditions, in this case diabetic ulcerations; and (b) to help direct the management and treatment of these conditions. While these are noble and useful purposes, there are also notable deficiencies in each of these grading systems. Some neglect the importance of ischemia, others are too complex to remember, and others are not completely applicable to diabetic ulcers but are more appropriate to pressure or decubitus ulcers. Nevertheless, for the purposes of this book, the Wagner classification has been selected for the discussion of ulcerations and their management, as it is the simplest, best known, and most widely used system. One should, however, by aware of its shortcomings. The Wagner classification system is based strictly on ulcer description and depth. It ignores the importance of ischemia and infection in determining the severity of the ulceration. In other words, although a Wagner grade 1 or 2 ulceration in a patient with adequate blood flow can often be managed with little to no complications, a similar condition in patients with poor perfusion can be a limb-threatening condition.

Grade 0 Foot

The Wagner grade 0 foot is the diabetic foot without ulceration but with one or more risk factors. Clinically significant sensory neuropathy as described above is one such risk factor. Other risk factors include bony deformities, atrophic fat pad, plantarflexed metatarsals, peripheral vascular disease, and Charcot joint disease. Dermatologic conditions also may pose risks to the grade 0 foot. Such conditions include dry, scaly skin with fissures, or thickened, discolored nail plates as seen in chronic onychomycosis. Although peripheral sensory neuropathy is the primary component cause for ulceration, the predictive index for ulceration increases significantly with each additional component cause identified (25). This constellation or grouping of risk factors is referred to as sufficient causes for ulceration (i.e., two or more component causes equal a sufficient cause for ulceration) (25).

Appropriate evaluation of this foot should include a careful neurologic examination using the 5.07 Semmes–Weinstein monofilament wire (26). Mapping of insensate areas helps the patient and the physician identify vulnerable areas. The foot should be closely inspected for corns or calluses, because these areas will identify focal pressures or irritation that may lead to ulceration. The vascular examination should include palpation of pedal pulses and observation for pallor with elevation or rubor on dependency. The physician should inspect for fissures either on the heels or in the interdigital spaces.

Management of the grade 0 foot centers on a program of education and prevention. Patients should be educated about the risks associated with the neuropathic foot and instructed on the early signs of inflammation, irritation, and infection and the initial treatment of these conditions. They should also be edu-

TABLE 66.1. Advantages of Changing Shoes

Prevents accumulation of pressure in any one area
Maintains support from the upper
Maintains shock absorption from the outer sole
Allows inspection of the foot

cated on the importance of good glycemic control in the management of foot disease.

Disease prevention in this patient population may include shoe-gear modification to decrease plantar foot pressures and to accommodate foot deformities and the use of orthotic devices and padded hosiery to further decrease plantar foot pressures (27,28). The simple habit of changing shoes every 4 hours can also help modify plantar foot pressures. This simple technique has several advantages in ulcer prevention: (a) it prevents the accumulation of pressure over any one area of the foot for extended periods; (b) it reduces loss of shock absorption and support functions of the outer soles and leather uppers, which occur the longer a shoe is worn; (c) it provides the patient with the opportunity to inspect his or feet frequently, allowing earlier detection of potential foot lesions (Table 66.1).

Regular visits to the foot specialist are recommended as part of a program of education and prevention. Depending on the patient's risk category, these visits should be scheduled annually, semiannually, or more frequently. Pulses should be palpated and any lesion should be noted at each visit. Corns and calluses should be debrided (29–31). The patient should be instructed on the proper care of the nails and skin. Moisturizing creams should be prescribed for application to the bottom of the foot for dry, scaly skin to avoid fissures. The interdigital spaces should also be inspected for fissures or evidence of tinea pedis.

The single most important aspect of preventive self-care is for the patient to inspect his or her feet daily. In those situations in which patients are unable to perform this function themselves, a family member should receive instruction on how to do this properly. Proper inspection involves inspecting the bottom of the foot visually and feeling it for lesions such as blisters, loose skin, or open sores. Patients also should note any areas of unexplained swelling or redness. The interdigital spaces are particularly problematic areas. They should be inspected and kept dry to prevent maceration, which may lead to athlete's foot and secondary bacterial infection.

Grade 1 Foot

The grade 1 ulceration implies the presence of two or more risk factors: peripheral sensory neuropathy and at least one other risk factor, such as bony deformities, plantarly prominent metatarsal heads with distally displaced fat pad, limited joint mobility, or ill-fitting shoes. The grade 1 ulceration extends to the dermis but not beyond (5). The evaluation of ulcerations should include a search for risk factors and an underlying cause. Ulcerations themselves should be evaluated for size, depth, and location. Knowledge of the anatomic structures involved, as well as the presence of any infection, will help direct treatment. The presence and type of drainage should also be noted. Cultures are of limited usefulness at this stage as the ulceration likely will be colonized with multiple organisms representing primarily skin flora (32).

Treatment most commonly requires soft-tissue debridement and elimination of all pressure from the site of ulcerations (8). Ulcerations most commonly will have some degree of hyperkeratosis surrounding the ulcer bed. In many cases, this callus tissue will overhang the margins of the ulcer, thus preventing ulcer healing from the "inside out." Therefore, all exuberant hyperkeratotic tissue must be debrided to a healthy granular bed that will support further granulation. Debridement has the added advantage of promoting dependent drainage and perhaps stimulating growth factors. Studies have suggested that ulcers that have undergone aggressive debridement may heal faster (33).

The second important concept of wound healing is off-loading, the technique by which pressure at the site of the ulceration is eliminated or reduced. There are various means of accomplishing this. The most effective is total non–weight-bearing on the affected extremity by means of crutches or a walker. This is often impractical for most patients, making compliance a serious issue. Therefore, techniques such as the total-contact cast and felted foam dressings have been devised as a compromise to relieve pressure, increase compliance, and improve the chances for healing (34–37).

Dressings are changed daily to provide a moist wound environment, which has been shown to be conducive to wound healing. Normal saline, hydrogels, and growth factors are acceptable choices for superficial ulcerations without active drainage or infection. Harsh, undiluted chemicals should be avoided, as they can be toxic to granulation tissue (38). Topical antibiotics have limited usefulness in this setting (39). If an infection is suspected, it is best treated with systemic antibiotics. Oral antibiotics are recommended only when clinical signs of infection are present (i.e., erythema, purulent drainage). Overuse of oral antibiotics may lead to superinfection or development of resistant strains. Exceptions to this rule include patients with severe peripheral vascular disease, in whom development of infection may be limb-threatening, or in patients receiving immunosuppressive medications, as in kidney or kidney/pancreas transplant recipients.

Repeated ulcerations may warrant consideration of surgical correction of any underlying structural deformity. Metatarsal osteotomies, digital arthroplasties, and metatarsal-head resections have all proven useful in the prevention of recurrent ulcerations (40–45).

Grade 2 Foot

Failure to adequately off-load grade 1 lesions likely will lead to deepening ulcerations beyond the level of the dermis (5). Deeper structures such as tendons or joint capsule may often be involved (grade 2). Appropriate management of these ulcerations depends on the accurate assessment of ulcer depth and the structures involved.

The most accurate and cost-effective method for assessing ulcer depth is to probe the ulcer base gently with a stainless-steel blunt probe. This technique can detect undermining of the ulceration, presence of any penetrating sinus tract, and involvement of deeper structures (Fig. 66.4). The ability to probe bone with this simple technique has an 89% specificity for the diagnosis of osteomyelitis. This compares favorably with more expensive and invasive tests such as labeled white blood cell (WBC) scans and magnetic resonance imaging (MRI) (46). Bone, joint, or tendon involvement should alert the clinician to the possible need for hospitalization, complete bed rest, surgical debridement, and broad-spectrum intravenous antibiotics (47).

Areas of undrained infection should be opened and drained dependently. Although most of these debridements can be performed at the bedside in severely neuropathic patients, if the infection is expected to be extensive, the patient should be brought to the operating room for a thorough debridement. The wound is then packed open (47). All nonviable, necrotic tissue

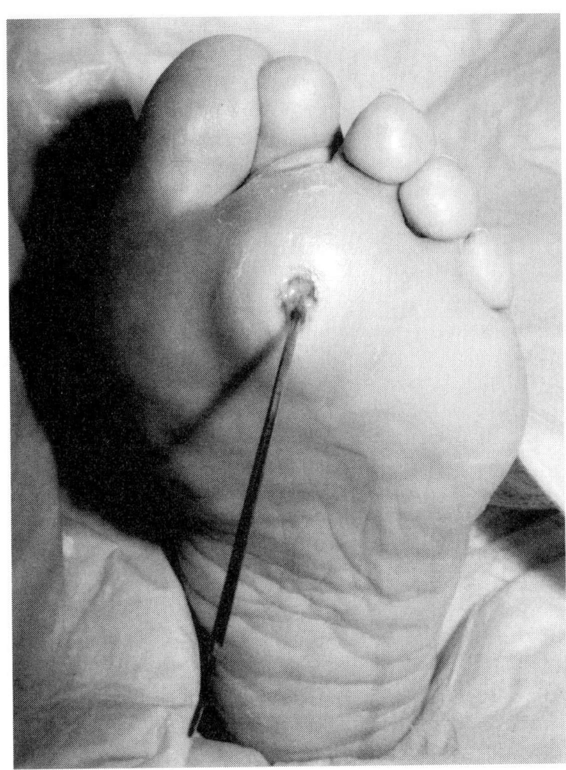

Figure 66.4. A blunt stainless steel probe is a clinically cost-effective tool for diagnosing osteomyelitis.

should be sharply debrided. This may often require the removal of infected tendon and/or bone. Antibiotics are adjusted to cover the offending organisms. The choice of antibiotics should be based on deep cultures taken at the time of surgery (48).

The clinician often may delay or avoid the aggressive debridement of the infected foot in patients with ischemia. Such delay may actually lead to further tissue loss and potential limb loss. The infection should be controlled first by debridement. Once this is accomplished, an arteriogram and lower extremity revascularization should be performed in the patient with an ischemic limb to prevent further tissue loss and to salvage the limb (49). Recent advances in vascular surgery and anesthesia have made this option safe and successful in patients with diabetes (49).

Although radiographs are not always sensitive enough to make the diagnosis of osteomyelitis, they should be performed on all long-standing, full-thickness ulcerations to evaluate for osteomyelitis. Bone scans, labeled WBC scans, MRIs, and bone biopsies have been recommended as more sensitive studies for diagnosing osteomyelitis (50–54). However, any of these modalities can result in false-positive and false-negative diagnoses. Once again, the ability to probe bone with a blunt, sterile probe is both reliable and cost-effective in diagnosing osteomyelitis (46).

Not all patients with grade 2 ulcerations require hospitalization (16). Outpatient treatment of these lesions must follow the same principles as those applied to treating grade 1 ulcerations, namely strict adherence to non–weight-bearing if healing is expected to occur. Although rare, ulcerations over exposed tendon and capsule have the ability to granulate. The same strategies to off-load grade 1 ulcerations (e.g., felted foam dressings, total-contact cast) should be applied to grade 2 ulcerations. Dressings typically are changed twice daily because of the increased drainage that commonly occurs with these ulcerations. It is best if dressings are changed by a healthcare professional, such as a visiting nurse, trained in recognition of early signs of infection. Oral antibiotics, while often not necessary in grade 1 ulcerations, are more commonly prescribed in grade 2 ulcerations because of the depth of the ulcerations, the vital structures involved, and the presence of drainage, creating an ideal environment for bacterial growth. First-generation cephalosporins are often a good initial choice as they provide broad-spectrum coverage and good coverage of staphylococci (55,56). Any changes in antibiotics should be based on deep wound cultures and sensitivity as well as the clinical response of the wound.

The care of the foot following complete healing is just as important as the care provided to rid the foot of infection. Regular patient follow-up is essential to ensure proper wound healing and assess the effectiveness of any orthotic device and shoegear modification. This is especially important in cases in which metatarsal heads have been resected, either single or multiple. One can expect that additional pressure will be transferred to adjacent metatarsal heads (57). It is therefore important for the foot to be protected with an appropriate orthotic device. These patients will also require education on selection of appropriate shoe gear. Conventional jogging shoes fitted with an orthotic device are appropriate for most patients with diabetes. However, patients with more severe foot deformities need specialized shoe gear. Extra-depth shoes that have a deep toe box may be required (Fig. 66.5). In some cases custom-molded shoes may be necessary. Patients also need to be educated on the care of the foot. Daily care should consist of daily inspection, especially between the toes, and the daily use of an appropriate moisturizing cream on the heel and the sole of the foot to avoid fissures. Both the inside and the outside of the shoes should also be

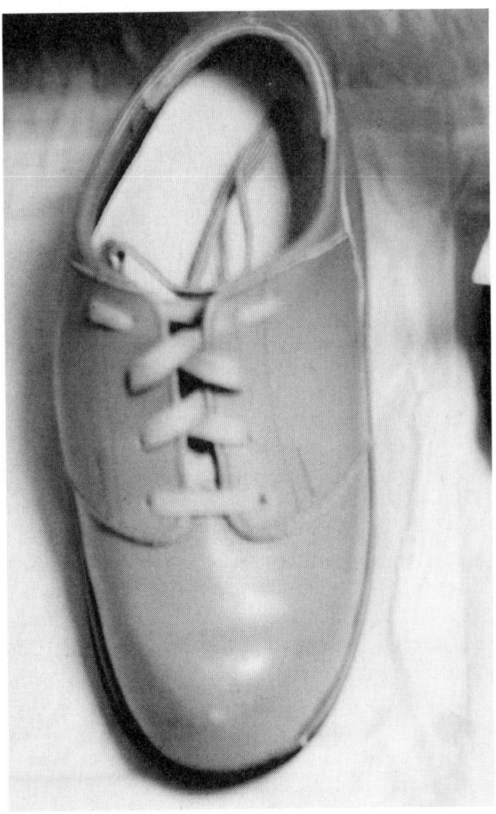

Figure 66.5. The rounded, deeper toe box of an extra-depth shoe is helpful in accommodating deformities such as bunions and hammer toes.

inspected every day. The patient should understand the need for regular visits to a foot specialist for continued monitoring.

Grade 3 Foot

Grade 3 ulcerations typically result from grade 2 ulcerations that have not responded to local care or have been neglected. Less common causes include particularly aggressive bacteria that result in early and rapid tissue necrosis and puncture wounds that lead to direct inoculation of underlying bony structures. Invariably, these ulcerations involve bone. Therefore, hospitalization and surgical debridement often is necessary.

The key to managing grade 3 ulcerations is to perform an adequate incision and drainage procedure of any underlying infection (47). Any sinus tract discovered must be explored. Any abscess must be drained, and all devitalized tissue must be debrided. In some cases, open amputations may be required to control the spread of infection and achieve limb salvage. This should be performed initially without regard to the vascular status of the limb.

After the infection has been cleared and healthy granulation tissue is seen, thought can be given to surgical reconstruction of the wound and foot. This may involve simple delayed primary closure or more complicated reconstructive surgery, including additional bone resections, tissue flaps, or skin grafts (58). No single technique can be applied to all wounds. A flexible approach to wound closure will maximize limb salvage. These lesions will make maximum use of all members of the diabetic foot team (49,59).

Because ablative surgery is common in the grade 3 foot, pressure is often transferred to adjacent areas of the foot, increasing the risk of chronic ulcerations. The long-term management of the grade 3 foot must emphasize prevention of transfer ulcerations. Prevention of recurrent ulcerations requires knowledge of orthoses and footwear. These at-risk patients should be encouraged to schedule regular visits to their podiatrist for the purpose of preventive diabetic foot care, education, and evaluation of orthoses and footwear. When orthoses and shoe gear are worn out, they should be replaced immediately. The goal of these interventions is to distribute plantar foot pressure evenly and avoid concentrating pressure in any one area.

Grade 4 Foot

Diabetic patients with grade 4 lesions may pose several challenges, including a variety of underlying risk factors. The cooperation and involvement of a dedicated limb-salvage team will often be required to help manage the various issues encountered in this particular group of patients. The team may include vascular surgeons, podiatrists, plastic and reconstructive surgeons, and orthopedic surgeons. The primary goal is to limit the amount of tissue loss and maintain a functional extremity.

Gangrenous changes in the lower extremity can commonly occur in one of two ways. Minor injury to the foot can result in gangrenous changes of the skin when severe arterial insufficiency is present (9). Injuries such as puncture wounds, superficial abrasions, or heel fissures may appear minor. Yet, they can have devastating consequences in the patient with arterial insufficiency. The arteries below the level of the popliteal artery are most commonly affected. This results in lack of adequate perfusion and oxygenation. Initially, there may be a focal area of necrosis. If not corrected, tissue loss will increase, leading to dry gangrene. The second potential cause of gangrene is overwhelming infection. In this case, occlusion of digital arteries can occur as a result of marked edema of the local tissue or an infective vasculitis (60). The clinical findings described as "wet gangrene" result from infective vasculitis. It is therefore imperative to identify the underlying cause in the hope of minimizing further tissue loss. When gangrene results from arterial insufficiency, an immediate vascular assessment should be instituted and lower-extremity revascularization performed where possible (61). If infection is the primary cause, selection of an appropriate antibiotic and aggressive debridement with adequate incision and drainage is the treatment of choice.

The vessels most commonly affected by diabetic vascular disease are the anterior and posterior tibial arteries. A significant clinical feature of the diabetic foot is that the foot vessels (i.e., dorsalis pedis) are often spared (62,63). This is significant because it makes distal arterial bypass procedures possible and effective. This contradicts the concept of "small-vessel disease," which has been associated with the diabetic foot since the late 1950s. It previously was believed that lack of healing of diabetic foot ulcers was due to occlusive disease of the digital arteries (64). Several investigators have shown that this does not occur (65). Most vascular surgeons and individuals who deal with the diabetic foot on a regular basis believe that small-vessel disease is not a major issue in the diabetic foot.

Adequate preoperative evaluation for arterial insufficiency requires visualization of the pedal arteries. The current standard of care dictates the use of digital subtraction angiography (DSA) to assess the level of revascularization accurately (49). Once revascularization has been performed, an amputation at the most distal level that will support healing should be performed with consideration to preserving as much of the weight-bearing surface of the foot as possible. This will allow more efficient ambulation, better distribution of plantar pressures, and easier shoeing of the foot.

When gangrene results from extensive or overwhelming infection, immediate incision and drainage must be performed, because any delay in treatment may lead to systemic toxicity, including a substantial risk of mortality. This may necessitate open amputation and should be performed even in the face of arterial insufficiency. Once control of the infection has been established and the patient is stable, thought should turn to foot salvage. This may require revascularization or reconstructive surgery of the foot and ankle.

Grade 5 Foot

The only treatment for extensive necrosis of the foot is primary amputation. Arterial occlusion and lack of arterial inflow are the main causes of gangrene. Even in these advanced cases, patients should undergo vascular assessment in the form of DSA and, if possible, revascularization so that the most distal level of amputation that will support healing is performed. It should be remembered that oxygen consumption increases dramatically with more-proximal amputations, increasing work and energy expenditure by the patient during ambulation. Because many of these patients already have some compromise of cardiac function, this becomes an important factor in their postoperative recuperation and in their ability to function independently (66).

CARE OF THE AMPUTATED FOOT

One of the risk factors for recurrent ulcerations is prior foot surgery, either reconstructive or ablative. The partially amputated foot poses special problems due to the loss of the weight-bearing surface (67). In basic terms, the same weight-bearing forces that acted before the amputation are at work after the amputation. However, those forces are now distributed over a

TABLE 66.2. Preferred Characteristics of a Shoe

Soft leather upper for accommodation
Rigid heel counter for support
Cushioned outer sole such as crepe or Vibram for shock absorption
Laces rather than slip-ons
Change shoes every 4 hours

smaller area. Consequently, the pressure over any one area is increased. In addition, certain types of amputations may lead to muscle imbalances and contractures (68). This can lead to an abnormal gait and further changes in plantar pressures.

Proper protection of these feet requires the use of orthotic devices and, very often, specially designed therapeutic shoes. Custom-molded orthoses should be made of a soft, closed-celled material that will allow for good shock absorption and accommodation of any lesions or deformities. These must be inspected regularly, because they do fatigue and collapse, thus losing their accommodative properties. Shoe-gear modification is almost always necessary for these at-risk feet. Basic recommendations for shoe gear should include a soft upper with a deep or rounded toe box to accommodate deformities such as bunions or hammer toes. The outer sole should be made of a soft shock-absorbing material such as EVA (ethylvinylacetate), crepe, or Vibram. These typically wear well and are the best shock absorbers. Patients should also be encouraged to wear shoes with laces as opposed to loafers, because a better, more supportive fit is provided by a laced shoe. Finally, patients should be encouraged to change their shoes every 3 to 4 hours to avoid pressure points, to maintain the support and stability of the shoe, and to allow patients the opportunity to inspect their feet during the course of the day (Table 66.2). When the patient has severe foot deformities, as those seen with Charcot joint disease, a custom-molded shoe may be the patient's best alternative.

Regular examination by a podiatrist is an important part of preventive care. The role of the podiatrist is to detect early warning signs of impending trouble. The presence of corns or calluses is a sign of focal pressure, from either weight-bearing forces or shoe irritation. The myth that calluses are protective and should not be trimmed has proven to be false (29–31). Any corn or callus should be trimmed by a podiatrist. Nails should be inspected for proper growth and care. Patients with diabetes should be instructed on the importance of avoiding "bathroom surgery" for the self-care of ingrown nails. While cutting nails straight across may be desired, few patients' nails allow this. Current convention dictates that nails should be trimmed according to the contour of the nail. Diabetic patients with profound sensory neuropathy or evidence of peripheral vascular disease should not be allowed to trim their own nails and should seek professional care. Diabetic patients should have their orthoses and shoes evaluated regularly for increased wear and loss of support. When this occurs they should be replaced immediately.

FOOT SURGERY FOR THE DIABETIC PATIENT

Not so long ago, patients with diabetes were advised to avoid foot surgery at all cost. Small-vessel disease and the risk of infections were cited as factors that impaired healing. This misinformation and misconception prevented many patients with diabetes from undergoing potentially limb-sparing foot procedures. Today, a more aggressive approach to the diabetic foot, including earlier surgical intervention, to prevent major amputations has been advocated by various centers (40–45,49,69).

Local surgical intervention may be advised where bony deformities exist, which are known to pose risk for ulceration, or where chronically recurrent ulcerations have failed to heal. Hammer toes and plantar-flexed metatarsals are known risks for ulceration, as they are often areas of high focal pressures. Arthroplasties and metatarsal osteotomies have been shown to be effective surgical treatments to allow primary healing of the ulcer and to decrease the risk of recurrence (41,65). Local surgical procedures such as metatarsal head resections can be performed to resect localized osteomyelitic bone (70,71). Multiple metatarsal head resections can be performed as an alternative to distal amputation and still leave a functional foot capable of efficient ambulation (42,43). Furthermore, maintaining as much of the plantar weight-bearing surface as possible allows better weight distribution.

In recent years, there has been increased discussion on the role of prophylactic surgery in the diabetic patient. Some groups define prophylactic surgery as surgery performed to correct an underlying deformity even in the absence of a history of ulceration (40,69). Other groups subscribe to a narrower definition of prophylactic surgery: surgery performed on those deformities that have a history of ulceration to prevent further ulceration and possible amputation (44).

When surgery is being considered, proper patient selection and preoperative evaluation are tantamount to success. A thorough history and physical examination should be performed, with special emphasis on the cardiac and vascular examination. Whenever possible, surgery should be performed with the patient under local anesthesia with mild sedation to minimize stress on the heart. Many of these surgical procedures are amenable to this type of anesthesia because of the patients' sensory neuropathy (72).

CHARCOT JOINT DISEASE

It is estimated that one in 680 patients with diabetes have Charcot joint disease (73). However, this may be an underestimate, as many cases go undetected until the late stages. Classically, Charcot joint disease presents as unexplained swelling and erythema of the foot. Although there is often a history of trauma prior to the development of the Charcot joint, the trauma may be so insignificant that patients are unable to recall a specific injury. It is often believed that profound sensory neuropathy makes this a painless process. In fact, patients may complain of mild to moderate discomfort. The pain, however, is not in proportion to the degree of bone and joint destruction seen on radiographs (74). Charcot joint disease is one of the most misdiagnosed entities involving the diabetic foot. Common misdiagnoses include osteomyelitis, tendinitis, gout, or acute sprain. It is important to maintain a high index of suspicion when encountering diabetic patients with unexplained painless swelling. In these patients, in the absence of a portal of entry, a diagnosis of Charcot joint disease should be considered until proven otherwise.

Initial evaluation of a suspected Charcot joint should begin with plain radiographs. In most circumstances, no further diagnostic studies are necessary, as the bone destruction is often quite obvious. Computed tomography (CT) scans and MRIs are rarely necessary to make the diagnosis of Charcot joint. CT scans may be useful for preoperative planning if surgical correction of the deformity is being contemplated. Although any joint of the foot can be affected, the most common location is the tarsometatarsal articulations (Lisfranc joint) (73). Charcot joint disease is characterized by three clinical phases: acute, coalescence, and reconstruction or remodeling. The acute phase is characterized by edema, localized warmth, erythema, and joint crepitus with range-of-motion examination. Radiographically, this phase is characterized by osseous debris, fragmentation, and possible subluxations of joints. The degree of fragmentation is variable and most often is related to the particular joints involved and continued ambulation on the fractures.

Once appropriate treatment is instituted, edema and erythema reduce rapidly. As the Charcot joint progresses to the next phase of coalescence, skin temperature begins to equilibrate and joint crepitus diminishes. Plain radiographs will show resorption of osseous fragments and the laying down of new bone. The reconstructive or remodeling phase occurs over a period of months and years. During this phase, the joints further stabilize and remodel by way of increased trabeculations and new bone growth. This can eventually lead to a stable foot devoid of significant motion. Unfortunately, in many cases, the foot can be severely deformed, with obvious bony prominences susceptible to ulceration (e.g., the rocker-bottom foot) (74) (Fig. 66.6).

Treatment for the acute Charcot foot is directed at eliminating weight-bearing forces that may lead to further destruction and deformity. This is best achieved by the use of crutches, a walker, or in the event of bilateral involvement, a wheelchair. A walking cast in acute Charcot joint disease is not appropriate treatment. Noncompliance with non–weight-bearing in the early stages of this disease will cause further fragmentation of bone, resulting eventually in greater deformity (Fig. 67.6). Casts, splints, or braces may be used for immobilization and to provide stability to the involved joints but not for weight-bearing initially (75). Our preference is the use of a removable bivalved cast brace that will allow regular inspection of the insensate skin (Fig. 66.7). Adjunctive therapies, such as biphosphonates or electrical bone stimulation, have been discussed as means to enhance healing (76,77). While isolated reports appear to favor these modalities, further clinical trials are needed for objective documentation of their effectiveness.

No weight-bearing is allowed as long as crepitus across joints and elevated skin temperature persist. Lack of attention to these clinical parameters will result in reexacerbation of the disease. Protected weight-bearing can be instituted when the clinical examination and serial radiographs show gradual resolution of the inflammatory process and healing of the involved joints. When appropriate, weight-bearing is instituted in a gradual manner and with protection. Weight-bearing is begun with a protective brace and with 15 to 20 lb of pressure. This can be increased in 10-lb increments per week as long as there are no signs of reactivation. Should reactivation occur, the patient should be returned to non–weight-bearing until resolution of these symptoms. As weight-bearing progresses, the patient is eventually allowed to ambulate short distances without assistive devices.

Long-term management of chronic Charcot joint often involves accommodation of any resultant foot deformity to avoid ulceration. Whenever possible, conventional shoe gear is preferred over custom-molded shoes. All shoes should be fitted with a well-molded Plastizote orthotic device that will support and cushion the foot. If severe foot deformity develops, there may be no alternative to a custom-molded shoe that matches the shape of the foot (78).

There has been much recent discussion in the surgical literature of surgical reconstruction foot rendered deformed or unstable by Charcot joint disease (79–81). Severe deformity and instability is not uncommon when destruction involves the

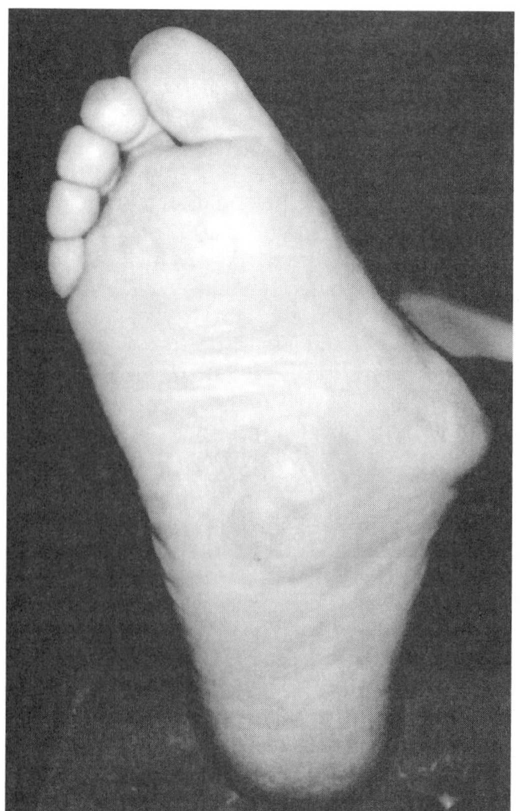
A

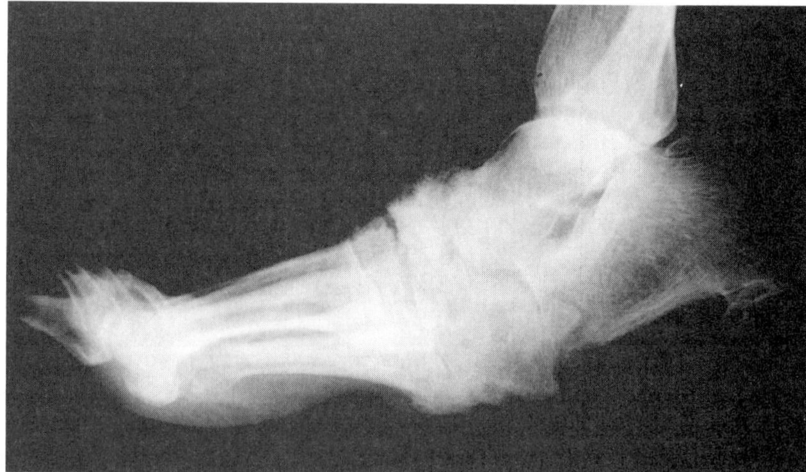
B

Figure 66.6. Photograph and radiograph showing the rocker-bottom deformity of advanced Charcot joint disease.

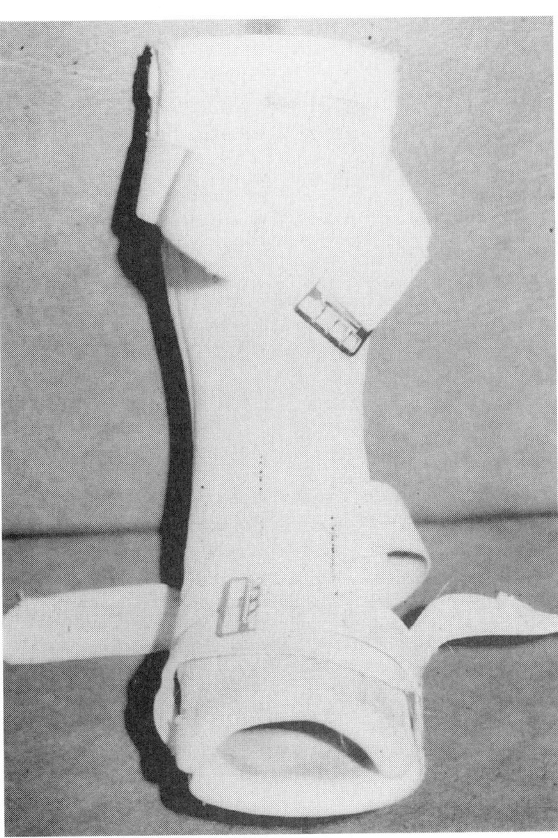

Figure 66.7. A lined bivalved fiberglass cast brace for the treatment of Charcot joint disease.

midtarsal, subtalar, or ankle joints. This can lead to a high likelihood for ulceration or difficulty with ambulation. Arthrodesis of the involved joints can provide a stable platform for ambulation and resistance to further ulcerations. Patients who elect to undergo these procedures must be advised as to the need for prolonged immobilization and non–weight-bearing—in some cases as long as 6 months. Strict adherence to the principles of internal fixation is required if success and limb salvage is expected.

FUTURE OF DIABETIC FOOT MANAGEMENT

The amount of interest in the diabetic foot has increased tremendously over the past 5 years. One only has to look at the numbers of wound-care centers that have sprouted up nationwide as evidence (82,83). The major impetus for this interest is the financial burden of caring for the diabetic foot. In 1980, more than $200 million was spent in direct hospital costs alone for the treatment of diabetic-foot complications and amputations (2). While current cost estimates for the United States are not available, one can only assume that they are significantly higher and will only get higher as the population continues to age and the incidence of diabetes continues to increase.

Most research has centered on treatment of foot ulcers and identification of those factors important in wound healing. Such research has increased our knowledge of the mechanism of wound healing and the identification of various growth factors and their roles in wound healing (84,85) From this research, autologous platelet-derived wound healing factor was introduced as a topical dressing to help promote wound healing. State-of-the-art research has recently made platelet-derived growth factor available as a topical gel for use on diabetic foot ulcerations (86). Recombinant DNA technology is used to produce this factor in the laboratory. Early experience with this product has been favorable. Other factors potentially conducive to wound healing are currently being developed in the laboratory using similar technology and should be available for clinical trials within the next 5 years.

The newest area of promise involves the use of bioengineered living-skin equivalents. These products have previously been approved for use in venous stasis ulcerations. Recently, one product, Apligraf, received US Food and Drug Administration approval for use in diabetic foot ulcerations. This product is a dermal/epidermal composite graft grown from neonatal foreskin. It is grown into large sheets on mesh in culture media. It is applied to a properly prepared ulcer bed in the same way that a skin graft is applied. The clinical trials that led to the approval of this product showed a higher percentage of healed ulcerations and a faster healing rate compared with controls (87).

There continues to be great interest in the treatment and prevention of sensory neuropathy. Earlier studies involving aldose reductase inhibitors had to be suspended before any useful clinical results could be evaluated because of a high incidence of adverse effects. However, the available data suggested that these agents might have some usefulness. Controversy exists concerning the potential role of these agents in the management of diabetic peripheral neuropathy. Recently, there has been renewed interest in these agents, which have been modified to reduce the risk of adverse effects. Tolrestat and γ-linoleic acid have been studied intensively, with promising, but inconclusive, results (88–90).

Diabetic neuritis or painful neuropathy remains one of the most frustrating conditions for the patient and for the clinician. The cause of this condition is not well understood. It is often believed that poor glycemic control may be responsible for exacerbations of this condition, although this is not universally accepted. Treatment often consists of trial and error using various agents. Most commonly, the combination of an analgesic with a tricyclic antidepressant has proven most effective, albeit not universally successful (91). Gabapentin is being used with increasing frequency. While it appears to be relatively safe, there have been conflicting reports on its efficacy (92–94).

Diabetic neuroarthropathy (Charcot joint) is another area fertile for investigation. The underlying cause of Charcot joint has not been clearly elucidated. Further, medications that may modulate the Charcot process have been studied on a small scale (77). Prospective, randomized trials are needed to determine whether these medications have any role in the treatment of Charcot joint disease. Anecdotal reports have claimed a role for the use of electrical bone stimulation to achieve more rapid consolidation (76,95). These studies have looked at small numbers of patients and have suffered from being neither randomized nor blinded trials. A large, randomized, double-blinded multicenter trial is needed to determine the efficacy of this modality of treatment.

SUMMARY

The impact of sensory neuropathy and vascular insufficiency of the foot in patients with diabetes can be reduced by frequent surveillance, patient education, and aggressive early intervention for addressing foot lesions. The coordination of care between physicians and podiatrists in dealing with the diabetic foot has the potential to save limbs and improve the quality of life for patients with diabetes.

REFERENCES

1. Reiber GE, Boyko EJ, Smith DG. Lower extremity foot ulcers and amputations in diabetes. National Diabetes Data Group, ed. *Diabetes in America,* 2nd ed. Bethesda, MD. National Institutes of Health, 1995:409–428. NIH publication 95-1468.
2. Kozak GP, Rowbotham JL, Gibbons GW. Diabetic foot disease: a major problem. In Kozak GP, et al. *Management of diabetic foot problems.* Philadelphia: WB Saunders, 1995:1–9.
3. Thomson FJ, Veves A, Ashe H, et al. A team approach to diabetic foot care—the Manchester experience. *Foot* 1991;1:75–82.
4. Edmonds ME, Blundell MP, Morris HE, et al. Improved survival of the diabetic foot: the role of the specialist foot clinic. *Q J Med* 1986;232:763–771.
5. Wagner FW Jr. The dysvascular foot: a system for diagnosis and treatment. *Foot Ankle* 1981;2:64–122.
6. Armstrong DG, Lavery LA, Harkless LB. Treatment-based classification system for assessment and care of diabetic feet. *J Am Podiatr Med Assoc* 1996;86:311–316.
7. Lavery LA, Armstrong DG, Harkless LB. Classification of diabetic foot wounds. *J Foot Ankle* 1996;35:528–531.
8. Young MJ, Veves A, Boulton AJM. The diabetic foot: aetiopathogenesis and management. *Diabetes Metab Rev* 1993;9:109–127.
9. Pecoraro RE, Reiber GE, Burgess EM. Pathways to diabetic limb amputation: basis for prevention. *N Engl J Med* 1994;331:854–860.
10. Kumar S, Fernando DJS, Veves A, et al. Semmes–Weinstein monofilaments: a simple, effective and inexpensive screening device for identifying diabetic patients at risk of foot ulceration. *Diabetes Res Clin Pract* 1991;13:63–68.
11. Sosenko JM, Kato M, Soto R, et al. Comparison of quantitative sensory-threshold measures for their association with foot ulceration in diabetic patients. *Diabetes Care* 1990;13:1057–1061.
12. Pham H, Armstrong DG, Harvey C, et al. Screening techniques to identify people at high risk for diabetic foot ulceration: a prospective multicenter trial. *Diabetes Care* 2000;23:606–611.
13. Young MJ, Manes C, Boulton AJM. Vibration perception predicts foot ulceration: a prospective study. *Diabet Med* 1992;9[Suppl 2]:P75.
14. Ewing DJ, Martyn CN, Young RJ, et al. The value of cardiovascular autonomic function tests: 10 years experience in diabetes. *Diabetes Care* 1995;8:491–498.
15. Murray HJ, Boulton AJM. The pathophysiology of diabetic foot ulceration. *Clin Podiatr Med Surg* 1995;12:1–17.
16. Caputo GM, Cavanagh PR, Ulbrecht JS, et al. Assessment and management of foot disease in patients with diabetes. *N Engl J Med* 1994;331:854–860.
17. Young MJ, Taylor PM, Boulton AJM. A new, non-invasive technique to predict foot ulcer risk. *Diabetes* 1993;42[Suppl 1]:A632(abst).
18. Tovey FI. The manufacture of diabetic footwear. *Diabet Med* 1984;l1:69–71.
19. Tovey FI, Moss MJ. Specialist shoes for the diabetic foot. In: Connor H, Boulton AJM, Ward JD, eds. *The foot in diabetes.* Chichester: John Wiley, 1987: 97–108.
20. Rosen RC, Davids MS, Bohanski LM. Hemorrhage into plantar callus and diabetes mellitus. *Cutis* 1985;35:339–341.
21. Harkless LB, Dennis KJ. You see what you look for and recognize what you know. *Clin Podiatr Med Surg* 1987;4:331–339.
22. Delbridge L, Perry P, Marr S, et al. Limited joint mobility in the diabetic foot: relationship to neuropathic ulceration. *Diabet Med* 1988;5:333–337.
23. Fernando DJS, Masson EA, Veves A, et al. Relationship of limited joint mobility to abnormal foot pressures and diabetic foot ulceration. *Diabetes Care* 1991; 14:8–11.
24. Veves A, Fernando DJS, Walewski P, et al. A study of plantar pressures in a diabetic clinic population. *Foot* 1991;1:89–92.
25. Reiber GE, Vileikyte L, Boyko EJ, et al. Causal pathways for incident lower-extremity ulcers in patients with diabetes from two settings. *Diabetes Care* 1999;22:157–162.
26. Olmos PR, Cataland S, O'Dorisio TM, et al. The Semmes–Weinstein monofilament as a potential predictor of foot ulceration in patients with noninsulin-dependent diabetes. *Am J Med Sci* 1995;309:76–82.
27. Veves A, Masson EA, Fernando DJS, et al. Use of experimental padded hosiery to reduce foot pressures in diabetic neuropathy. *Diabetes Care* 1989;12:653–655.
28. Veves A, Masson EA, Fernando DJS, et al. Studies of experimental hosiery in diabetic neuropathic patients with high foot pressures. *Diabet Med* 1990;7: 324–326.
29. Young MJ, Cavanagh PR, Thomas G, et al. The effect of callus removal on dynamic plantar pressures in diabetic patients. *Diabet Med* 1992;9:55–57.
30. Murray HJ, Young MJ, Hollis S, et al. The association between callus formation, high pressures and neuropathy in diabetic foot ulceration. *Diabet Med* 1996;13:979–982.
31. Pitei DL, Foster A, Edmond. M. The effect of regular callus removal on foot pressures. *J Foot Ankle Surg* 1999;38:251–256.
32. Joseph WS, Axler DA. Microbiology and antimicrobial therapy of diabetic foot infections. *Clin Podiatr Med Surg* 1990;7:467–481.
33. Steed DL, Donohoe D, Webster MW, et al. Effect of extensive debridement and treatment on the healing of diabetic foot ulcers. *J Am Coll Surg* 1996;183:61–64.
34. Pollard JP, LeQuesne LP. Methods of healing diabetic forefoot ulcers. *BMJ* 1983;286:436–437.
35. Burden AC, Jones GR, Jones R, et al. Use of the Scotchcast boot in treating diabetic foot ulcers. *BMJ* 1983;286:1555–1557.
36. Coleman WC, Brand PW, Birke JA. The total contact cast: a therapy for plantar ulcerations on insensitive feet. *J Am Podiatry Assoc* 1984;74:548–552.
37. Mueller MJ, Diamond JE, Sinacore DR. Total contact casting in treatment of diabetic plantar ulcers. *Diabetes Care* 1989;12:384–388.
38. Kucan JO, Robson MC, Heggers JP, et al. Comparison of silver sulfadiazine, povidone-iodine and physiologic saline in the treatment of chronic pressure ulcers. *J Am Geriatr Soc* 1981;29:232–235.
39. Lineweaver W, Howard R, Soucy D, et al. Topical antimicrobial activity. *Arch Surg* 1985;120:267–270.
40. Gudas CJ. Prophylactic surgery in the diabetic foot. *Clin Podiatr Med Surg* 1987;4:445–458.
41. Tillo TH, Giurini JM, Habershaw GM, et al. Review of metatarsal osteotomies for the treatment of neuropathic ulcerations. *J Am Podiatr Med Assoc* 1990;80: 211–217.
42. Jacobs RL. Hoffman procedure in the ulcerated diabetic neuropathic foot. *Foot Ankle* 1982;3:142–149.
43. Giurini JM, Basile P, Chrzan JS, et al. Panmetatarsal head resection: a viable alternative to the transmetatarsal amputation. *J Am Podiatr Med Assoc* 1993;83: 101–107.
44. Giurini JM, Rosenblum BI. The role of foot surgery in patients with diabetes. *Clin Podiatr Med Surg* 1995;12:119–127.
45. Rosenblum BI, Giurini JM, Chrzan JS, et al. Preventing loss of the great toe with the hallux interphalangeal joint arthroplasty. *J Foot Ankle Surg* 1994;33: 557–560.
46. Grayson ML, Gibbons GW, Balogh K, et al. Probing to bone in infected pedal ulcers: a clinical sign of underlying osteomyelitis in diabetic patients. *JAMA* 1995;273:721–723.
47. Gibbons GW. The diabetic foot: amputations and drainage of infection. *J Vasc Surg* 1987;5:791–793.
48. Wheat LJ, Allen SD, Henry M, et al. Diabetic foot infections: bacteriologic analysis. *Arch Intern Med* 1986;146:1935–1940.
49. LoGerfo FW, Gibbons GW, Pomposelli FB Jr, et al. Trends in the care of the diabetic foot: expanded role of arterial reconstruction. *Arch Surg* 1992;127: 617–621.
50. Newman LG, Waller J, Palestro CJ, et al. Unsuspected osteomyelitis in diabetic foot ulcers: diagnosis and monitoring by leukocyte scanning with indium in 111 oxyquinoline. *JAMA* 1991;266:1246–1251.
51. Keenan AM, Tindel NL, Alavi A. Diagnosis of pedal osteomyelitis in diabetic patients using current scintigraphic techniques. *Arch Intern Med* 1989;149: 2262–2266.
52. Hetherington VJ. Technetium and combined gallium and technetium scans in the neurotrophic foot. *J Am Podiatr Assoc* 1982;72:458–463.
53. Morrison WB, Schweitzer ME, Wapner KL, et al. Osteomyelitis in feet of diabetics: clinical accuracy, surgical utility, and cost-effectiveness of MR imaging. *Radiology* 1995;196:557–564.
54. Yuh WTC, Corson JD, Baraniewski HM, et al. Osteomyelitis of the foot in diabetic patients: evaluation with plain film, 99mTc-MDP bone scintigraphy, and MR imaging. *AJR Am J Roentgenol* 1989;152:795–800.
55. Jones EW, Edwards R, Finch R, et al. A microbiological study of diabetic foot lesions. *Diabet Med* 1984;2:212–215.
56. Lipsky BA, Pecoraro RE, Wheat LJ. The diabetic foot: soft tissue and bone infection. *Infect Dis Clin North Am* 1990;4:409–432.
57. Ulbrecht JS, Perry J, Hewitt FG, et al. Controversies in footwear for the diabetic foot at risk. In: Kominsky SJ, ed. *Medical and surgical management of the diabetic foot.* Boston: Mosby–Year Book, 1994:441–453.
58. Attinger CE. Use of soft tissue techniques for the salvage of the diabetic foot. In: Kominsky SJ, ed. *Medical and surgical management of the diabetic foot.* Boston: Mosby–Year Book, 1994:323–366.
59. Gibbons GW, Marcaccio EJ Jr, Burgess AM, et al. Improved quality of diabetic foot care, 1984 vs 1990: reduced length of stay and costs, insufficient reimbursement. *Arch Surg* 1993;128:576–581.
60. Edmonds M, Foster A, Greenhill M, et al. Acute septic vasculitis not diabetic microangiopathy leads to digital necrosis in the neuropathic foot. *Diabet Med* 1992;9[Suppl 1]:P85.
61. Klamer TW, Towne JB, Bandyk DF, et al. The influence of sepsis and ischemia on the natural history of the diabetic foot. *Am Surg* 1987;53:490–494.
62. Pomposelli FB Jr, Jepsen SJ, Gibbons GW, et al. A flexible approach to infrapopliteal vein grafts in patients with diabetes mellitus. *Arch Surg* 1991; 126:724–729.
63. Pomposelli FB Jr, Jepsen SJ, Gibbons GW, et al. Efficacy of the dorsalis pedis bypass for limb salvage in diabetic patients: short term observations. *J Vasc Surg* 1990;11:745–752.
64. Goldenberg SG, Allen M, Joshi RA, et al. Nonatheromatous peripheral vascular disease of the lower extremity in diabetes mellitus. *Diabetes* 1959;8:201.
65. LoGerfo FW, Coffman JD. Vascular and microvascular disease in the diabetic foot: implications for foot care. *N Engl J Med* 1984;311:1615–1619.
66. Pinzur MS, Gold J, Schwartz D, et al. Energy demands for walking in dysvascular amputees as related to the level of amputation. *Orthopaedics* 1992;15: 1033–1037.
67. Golner MG. The fate of the second leg in the diabetic amputee. *Diabetes* 1960; 9:100–103.
68. Chang BB, Bock DE, Jacobs RL, et al. Increased limb salvage by the use of unconventional foot amputations. *J Vasc Surg* 1994;19:341–349.
69. Armstrong DG, Lavery LA, Stern S, et al. Is prophylactic diabetic foot surgery dangerous? *J Foot Ankle Surg* 1996;35:585–589.
70. Rosenblum BI, Pomposelli FB, Giurini JM. Maximizing foot salvage by a combined approach to foot ischemia and neuropathic ulceration in patients with diabetes mellitus: a five year experience. *Diabetes Care* 1994;17:983–987.

71. Martin JD, Delbridge L, Reeve TS, et al. Radical treatment of mal perforans in diabetic patients with arterial insufficiency. *J Vasc Surg* 1990;12:264–268.
72. Frykberg R, Giurini J, Habershaw G, et al. Prophylactic surgery in the diabetic foot. In: Kominsky SJ, ed. *Medical and surgical management of the diabetic foot.* Boston: Mosby–Year Book, 1994:399–439.
73. Sinha S, Munichoodappa C, Kozak GP: Neuroarthropathy (Charcot joints) in diabetes mellitus: clinical study of 101 cases. *Medicine* 1972;52:191–210.
74. Sanders LJ, Frykberg RG. Diabetic neuropathic osteoarthropathy: the Charcot foot. In: Frykberg RG, ed. *The high risk foot in diabetes mellitus.* New York: Churchill Livingstone, 1991:297–338.
75. Lesko P, Maurer PC. Talonavicular dislocations and midfoot arthropathy in neuropathic diabetic feet: natural course and principles of treatment. *Clin Orthop* 1989;240:226–231.
76. Bier RR, Estersohn HS. A new treatment for Charcot joint in the diabetic foot. *J Am Podiatr Med Assoc* 1987;77:63–69.
77. Selby PL, Young MJ, Boulton AJM. Bisphosphonates: a new treatment for diabetic Charcot neuroarthropathy? *Diabet Med* 1994;11:28–31.
78. Janisse DJ. Prescription insoles and footwear. *Clin Podiatr Med Surg* 1995;12: 41–61.
79. Banks AS, McGlamry ED. Charcot foot. *J Am Podiatr Med Assoc* 1989;79:213–235.
80. Bono JV, Rogers DJ, Jacobs RL. Surgical arthrodesis of the neuropathic foot: a salvage procedure. *Clin Orthop Rel Res* 1993;296:14–20.
81. Papa J, Myerson M, Girard P. Salvage, with arthrodesis, in intractable diabetic neuropathic arthropathy of the foot and ankle. *J Bone Joint Surg Am* 1993;75: 1056–1066.
82. Knighton DR, Fylling CP, Fiegel VD, et al. Amputation prevention in an independently reviewed at-risk diabetic population using a comprehensive wound care protocol. *Am J Surg* 1990;160:466–472.
83. Steed DL, Edington H, Moosa HH, et al. Organization and development of a university multidisciplinary wound care clinic. *Surgery* 1993;114:775–779.
84. Bennett NT, Schulz GS. Growth factors and wound healing biomechanical properties of growth factors and their receptors. *Am J Surg* 1993;165:728–737.
85. Bennett NT, Schulz GS. Growth factors and wound healing, II: role in normal wound and chronic wound healing. *Am J Surg* 1993;166:74–81.
86. Steed DL. Clinical evaluation of recombinant human platelet-derived growth factor for the treatment of lower extremity diabetic ulcers. Diabetic Ulcer Study Group. *J Vasc Surg* 1995;21:71–81.
87. Pham HT, Rosenblum BI, Lyons TE, et al. Evaluation of a human skin equivalent for the treatment of diabetic foot ulcers in a prospective, randomized, clinical trial. *Wounds* 1999;11:79–86.
88. Boulton AJM, Levin S, Comstock J. A multicentre trial of the aldose reductase inhibitor, tolrestat, in patients with symptomatic diabetic neuropathy. *Diabetologia* 1990;33:431–437.
89. Sima AAF, Brill V, Nathaniel T, et al. Regeneration and repair of myelinated fibers in sural nerve biopsy specimens from patients with diabetic neuropathy treated with sorbinil. *N Engl J Med* 1988;319:548–555.
90. Keen H, Payan J, Allawi J, et al. Treatment of diabetic neuropathy with γ-linolenic acid. *Diabetes Care* 1992;16:8.
91. Young RJ, Clarke BF. Pain relief in diabetic neuropathy: the effectiveness of imipramine and related drugs. *Diabet Med* 1985;2:262.
92. Nicholson B. Gabapentin use in neuropathic pain syndromes. *Acta Neurol Scand* 2000;101:359–371.
93. Backonja MM. Gabapentin monotherapy for the symptomatic treatment of painful neuropathy: a multicenter, double-blind, placebo-controlled trial in patients with diabetes mellitus. *Epilepsia* 1999;40[Suppl 6]:S57–S59.
94. Morello CM, Leckband SG, Stoner CP, et al. Randomized double-blind study comparing the efficacy of gabapentin with amitriptyline on diabetic peripheral neuropathy pain. *Arch Intern Med* 1999;159:1931–1937.
95. Grady JF, O'Connor KJ, Axe TM, et al. Use of electrostimulation in the treatment of diabetic neuroarthropathy. *J Am Podiatr Med Assoc* 2000;90:287–294.

CHAPTER 67

Vascular Disease of the Lower Extremities in Diabetes Mellitus: Etiology and Management

Cameron M. Akbari and Frank W. LoGerfo

Problems of the diabetic foot are the most common causes of hospitalization in patients with diabetes, with an annual health care cost of more than $1 billion (1). The prospect of possible amputation terrifies patients with diabetes and justifiably so: diabetes mellitus is a contributing factor in half of all lower extremity amputations in the United States, and the relative risk for leg amputation is 40 times greater among persons with diabetes than among those without diabetes (1,2). Moreover, up to 50% of diabetic amputees will undergo a second leg amputation within 5 years of the initial amputation. Foot ulceration will affect 15% of all individuals with diabetes during their lifetime, with an annual incidence of 3% in patients with diabetes, and is clearly a significant risk factor in the pathway to limb loss (3).

THE DIABETIC FOOT: FUNDAMENTAL CONSIDERATIONS

The principal pathogenic mechanisms in diabetic foot disease are ischemia, neuropathy, and infection; acting together they contribute to the sequence of tissue necrosis, ulceration, and gangrene. Fundamentally, limb salvage strategies are focused on a clear understanding of these abnormalities in patients with diabetes, which subsequently allows for improved prevention and treatment in this population.

Although discussed in greater detail elsewhere in this book, a brief discussion of neuropathy is warranted here, since it afflicts as many as 50% to 60% of all patients (4,5) and is present in more than 80% of diabetic patients with foot lesions (6). Broadly classified as focal and diffuse neuropathies, the latter are more common and include the autonomic and chronic sensorimotor polyneuropathies, which both contribute to foot ulceration.

Sensorimotor neuropathy initially involves the distal lower extremities, progresses centrally, and is typically symmetric. Sensory nerve-fiber involvement leads to loss of the protective sensation of pain, whereas motor-fiber destruction results in small-muscle atrophy in the foot. Consequently, the metatarsals are flexed with metatarsal head prominence and "clawing" of the toes. This causes abnormal pressure points to develop on the bony prominences without sensation, with subsequent erosion and ulceration. Meanwhile, autonomic neuropathy in the foot causes loss of sympathetic tone, which results in increased arteriovenous shunting and inefficient nutrient flow. Autonomic denervation of oil and sweat glands leads to cracking of dry skin, which further predisposes the diabetic foot to skin breakdown and ulceration (7).

The spectrum of infection in diabetic foot disease ranges from superficial ulceration to extensive gangrene with fulminant sepsis. The majority of infections are polymicrobic, with the most common pathogens being staphylococci and streptococci. The more complicated wounds, such as deep ulcers or those with associated abscesses, may harbor anaerobes and gram-negative bacilli. Potential sources of diabetic foot infection include a simple puncture wound or ulcer, the nail plate, and the interdigital web space. Untreated cellulitis can lead to the spread of bacteria along tendon sheaths and to deep-space plantar infection, with eventual destruction of the interosseous

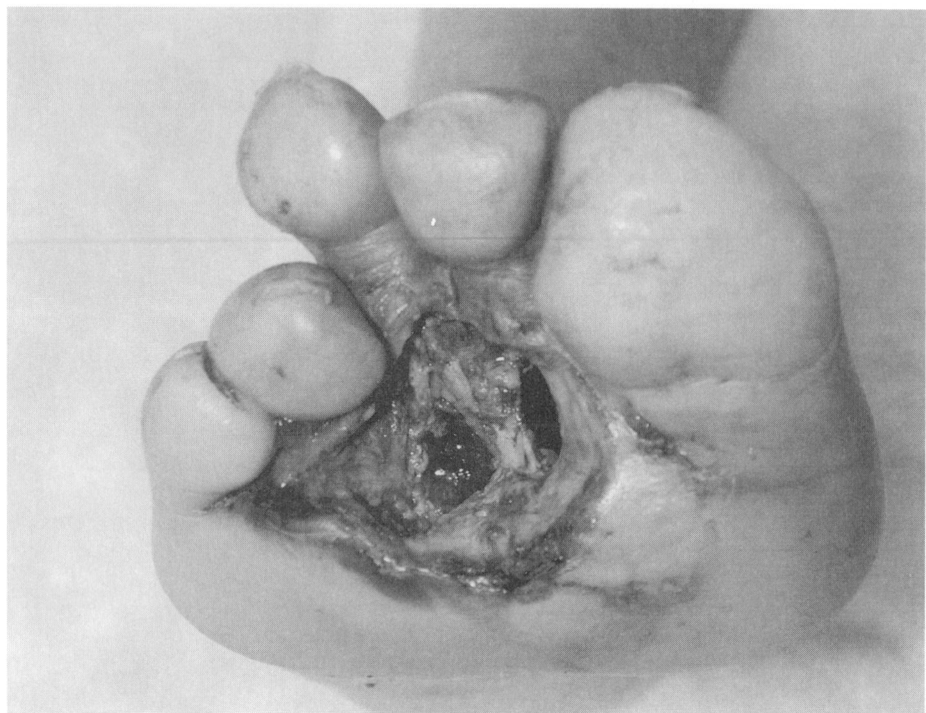

Figure 67.1. This 57-year-old man with diabetes and significant sensorimotor neuropathy underwent a metatarsal head resection for a "neuropathic" ulcer. Pedal pulses were not palpable. Subsequent appearance of the wound is shown, with clearly ischemic edges and complete failure of healing.

fascia and spread to the foot dorsum. With worsening infection, edema is also commonly seen, which leads to elevated compartmental pressures, with resultant capillary thrombosis and further impairment of nutrient blood flow.

Evaluation for ischemia may begin once the infection has begun to resolve and signs of systemic toxicity have disappeared. The decision to perform arteriography and vascular reconstruction should be made during this waiting period, which is usually no longer than 5 days. Further delays may lead to loss of opportunity to salvage the foot (8). A proper evaluation for underlying vascular disease is essential for limb salvage in patients with diabetic foot ulceration, even when neuropathy and infection are present. *All* limb salvage efforts will fail unless ischemia has been recognized and corrected (Fig. 67.1). Most important, consideration should be given to the unique pathophysiology of diabetes and vascular disease and the need to tailor treatment decisions in diabetic patients with lower extremity vascular disease.

PATHOPHYSIOLOGY OF VASCULAR DISEASE IN DIABETES MELLITUS

Microvascular Abnormalities

Many of the complications of diabetes may best be characterized as alterations in vascular structure and function, with subsequent end-organ damage and death (9). Specifically, two types of vascular disease are observed in patients with diabetes, a nonocclusive microcirculatory impairment involving the capillaries and arterioles of the kidneys, retina, and peripheral nerves and a macroangiopathy characterized by atherosclerotic lesions of the coronary and peripheral arterial circulation (10–13). The former is relatively unique to diabetes, whereas the latter lesions are morphologically and functionally similar in nondiabetic and diabetic patients.

One of the greatest impediments to understanding and treating vascular disease in patients with diabetes is the misconception that they have an untreatable occlusive lesion in the microcirculation, which has fostered the belief that arterial reconstruction is futile. This idea originated from an uncontrolled histologic study demonstrating the presence of periodic acid-Schiff-positive material occluding the arterioles in amputated limb specimens from diabetic patients (14). However, subsequent prospective anatomic staining and arterial casting studies (15) have demonstrated the *absence* of an arteriolar occlusive lesion (16). Further evidence comes from physiologic studies of femoro-popliteal bypass grafts in diabetic and nondiabetic patients in which direct vasodilator administration into these grafts demonstrates a comparable fall in peripheral resistance between the two groups (17), again supporting the absence of a distal occlusive arteriolar lesion. Dispelling the notion of "small-vessel disease" is fundamental to the principles of limb salvage in patients with diabetes, since arterial reconstruction is almost always possible and successful in these patients.

While there is no occlusive lesion in the diabetic microcirculation, other structural changes do exist, most notably thickening of the capillary basement membrane. However, these changes do not lead to narrowing of the capillary lumen, and arteriolar blood flow may be normal or even increased despite these changes (18). Thickening of the capillary basement membrane is a structural change observed in both diabetic retinopathy and nephropathy.

In the diabetic foot, thickening of the basement membrane theoretically may impair the migration of leukocytes and the hyperemic response following injury and thus may increase the susceptibility of the diabetic foot to infection (19,20). Although resting total skin microcirculatory flow is similar in diabetic and nondiabetic patients, the capillary blood flow is reduced in patients with diabetes, indicating a maldistribution and functional ischemia of the skin (21). Moreover, studies of skin microvascular flow have demonstrated a reduced maximal hyperemic response in patients with diabetes, suggesting that a *functional* microvascular impairment is a major contributing factor to diabetic foot problems (22). All of these changes result in an inability to vasodilate and achieve maximal blood flow following injury.

Diabetes also affects the axon reflex (23). Normally, injury directly stimulates nociceptive C fibers, which results in both orthodromic conduction to the spinal cord and antidromic conduction to adjacent C fibers and other axon branches. One function of this axon reflex is neuropeptide secretion, such as substance P and calcitonin gene–related peptide, which directly and indirectly (through release of histamine by mast cells) causes vasodilation and increased permeability. This neurogenic vasodilatory response is impaired in diabetes, further reducing the hyperemic response when it is most needed—under conditions of injury and inflammation (24).

Endothelial dysfunction is seen in the earliest stages of atherogenesis and is characterized *in vivo* by an impaired endothelium-dependent vasodilatory response. Normally, endothelium-derived nitric oxide allows for arterial vasodilation in response to either a pharmacologic (e.g., acetylcholine) or a physiologic (e.g., increased shear stress) stimulus. Both type 1 and type 2 diabetes are characterized by an abnormal endothelium-dependent vasodilation (25,26), possibly due to the effects of prolonged hyperglycemia or insulin resistance on both the micro- and macrocirculation (27).

Macrovascular Abnormalities

Lower extremity arterial disease is more common among patients with diabetes than among those without diabetes. The presence of diabetes is associated with a two- to threefold excess risk of intermittent claudication compared with its absence (28). Despite significant advances in the prevention and treatment of peripheral vascular disease, diabetes continues to be the single strongest cardiovascular risk factor for the development of critical leg ischemia and limb loss (29).

Unlike microvascular disease, which is unique to diabetes and its metabolic alterations, the cause of lower extremity ischemia is similar in diabetic and nondiabetic patients and is due to accelerated atherosclerosis. One notable difference between these populations is the pattern and location of the occlusive atherosclerotic lesion. As noted earlier, there is no evidence for an occlusive lesion at the arteriolar level ("small-vessel disease") in patients with diabetes. However, patients with diabetes are more likely to have atherosclerotic disease affecting the infrapopliteal (tibial) arteries, with *sparing* of the foot arteries (30), which allows for successful arterial reconstruction to these distal vessels. Conversely, the superficial femoral or popliteal artery is less likely to be affected by the occlusive process, allowing these vessels to serve as a possible inflow source for bypass grafting (Fig. 67.2).

Because the foot vessels are often patent in the patient with diabetes and because of the success of bypass grafting to these vessels, an appropriate evaluation for ischemia is essential in patients with diabetes. The complex milieu of motor and sensory neuropathy, thickening of the capillary basement membrane, loss of the neurogenic inflammatory response, and the wide spectrum of microcirculatory and endothelial abnormalities all result in a biologically compromised foot. Unless ischemia is recognized and corrected, limb salvage efforts with the diabetic foot will fail, even if infection and neuropathy have been appropriately treated.

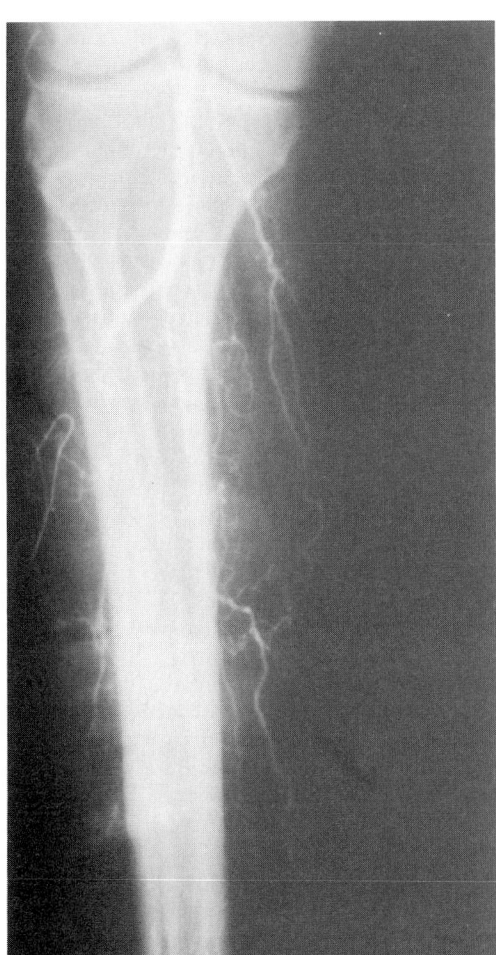

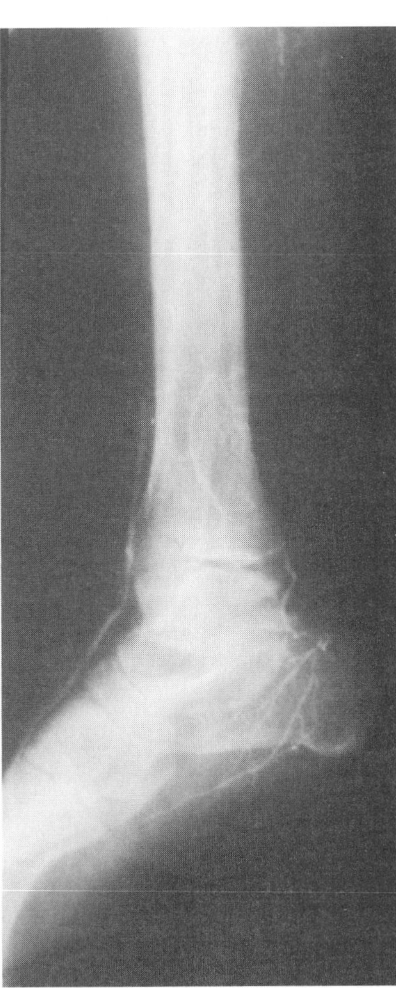

Figure 67.2. Angiogram demonstrating the characteristic pattern of lower extremity vascular disease in diabetes, with atherosclerotic occlusion of the tibial arteries and sparing of the foot vessels. Note the normal appearance of the popliteal artery, another characteristic finding.

DIAGNOSIS

As with any other disease process, evaluation should begin with a detailed history and physical examination. In the patient with a diabetic foot ulcer, it is helpful to consider the duration of the ulcer, the type of treatments used, and any past history of foot ulceration and treatment. Although nocturnal rest pain in the foot is strongly suggestive of lower extremity arterial disease in the nondiabetic patient, the variable effects of neuropathy make pain more difficult to evaluate in the diabetic limb. Similarly, claudication symptoms may be entirely absent in the patient with an ischemic diabetic foot ulcer. Long-standing foot ulceration, coexisting cardiac disease (such as angina or heart failure), and sensorimotor neuropathy may all limit the ability to ambulate sufficiently to manifest claudication symptoms.

Physical examination should be directed toward the underlying pathophysiology of foot ulceration. Neuropathy may easily be evaluated: observation may reveal the morphologic motor abnormalities such as "claw foot" or Charcot's osteoarthropathy, while monofilament testing will assess the degree of sensory neuropathy. Noting the location of the ulcer may also be helpful, since purely ischemic lesions typically occur in the most distal parts of the foot, such as the toes, forefoot, or heel, in contrast to the neuropathic ulcers seen on weight-bearing areas.

All ulcers, including those with a significant neuropathic component, should be assessed for an ischemic component. The peripheral pulses at all levels should be palpated. Although patients with diabetes have a propensity for development of atherosclerotic occlusion of the tibial arteries, it is not unusual to encounter atherosclerosis of the aortoiliac region (evidenced by diminished femoral pulses) or other vessels of the lower extremity. Similarly, the examination should not end with the popliteal pulse: 40% of diabetic patients presenting with ischemic ulceration or gangrene of the lower extremity have palpable popliteal pulses. In fact, recognition of the anatomic pattern of diabetic vascular disease leads to the *single* most important aspect of the physical examination: the presence or absence of a palpable foot pulse. In simplest terms, if the foot pulses are not palpable, the presence of occlusive vascular disease can be assumed.

A variety of noninvasive arterial tests may be ordered in an effort to quantify the degree of ischemia. However, in the presence of diabetes, *all* of these tests have significant limitations. Although Doppler-derived pressure measurements have proved to be reliable in localizing the degree and level of arterial occlusive disease in nondiabetic patients, their use is limited in the presence of diabetes. Medial arterial calcinosis occurs frequently in patients with diabetes and is characterized by a *nonobstructive* calcification of the vessel wall at the media layer; its presence can result in noncompressible arteries with artifactually high segmental systolic pressures and ankle-brachial indices. Medial calcification should be suspected whenever the ankle pressure greatly exceeds arm pressure or when the Doppler signal at the ankle cannot be obliterated with greater than 250 mm Hg pressure. Lower levels of calcification in the toe vessels support the use of toe systolic pressure measurements as a more reliable indicator of arterial flow to the foot (31). However, the use of toe pressures is often limited by the proximity of the foot ulcer to the cuff site, the size of the cuff itself, and other extrinsic variables.

Segmental Doppler waveforms and pulse volume recordings are unaffected by medial calcification. A normal Doppler waveform is triphasic; with proximal obstruction, the waveform becomes monophasic (Fig. 67.3). Pulse volume recordings rely on plethysmographic recordings of the change in volume that occurs with each pulsation. A sharp upstoke, narrow peak, and dicrotic notch characterize a normal recording. With increasing levels of arterial insufficiency, the waveform loses the dicrotic notch, followed by loss of amplitude and blunting of the waveform (Fig. 67.4). Since neither of these tests relies on obliterating flow within a vessel (unlike Doppler-derived pressures), they may prove useful in the diabetic patient with suspected arterial insufficiency. However, significant limitations exist in their use, and caution should be exercised when interpreting their results. Evaluation of these waveforms is primarily qualitative and not quantitative. A flat forefoot tracing is a convincing demonstration of ischemia, but it is difficult to make clinical decisions based on the magnitude of the waveform. Similarly, severity of arterial insufficiency cannot be accurately interpreted, since no reliable quantitative scoring exists (Fig. 67.5). In addition, the quality of the waveforms is affected by peripheral edema, cuff size, and motion artifact. Finally, the presence of ulceration, especially at the forefoot level, often precludes accurate cuff placement.

Regional transcutaneous oximetry ($TcPo_2$) measurements are also unaffected by medial calcinosis, and recent studies have noted its reliability in predicting healing of ulcers and amputation levels (32). Limitations, including a lack of equipment standardization, user variability, and a large "gray area" of values, preclude its applicability. Furthermore, $TcPo_2$ measurements are

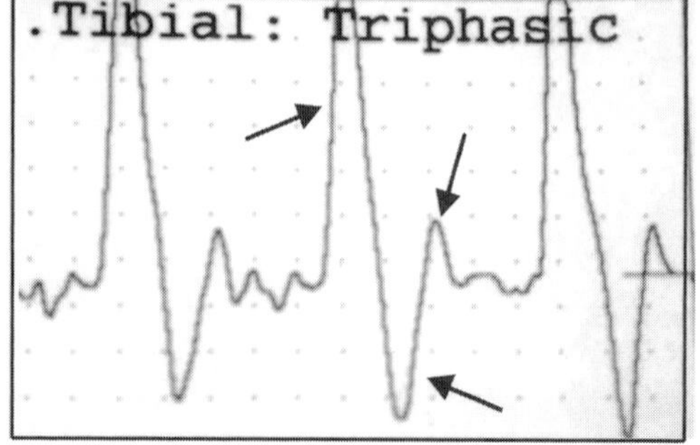

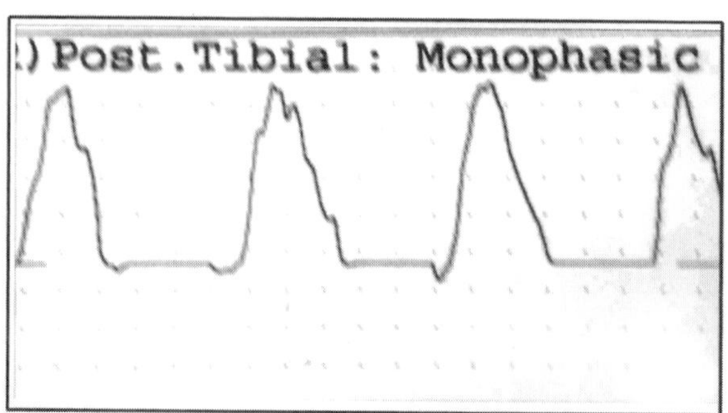

Figure 67.3. Left, The normal Doppler tracing illustrates a triphasic flow pattern, with forward flow in systole (*first arrow*), a reversal of flow in early diastole (*second arrow*), and a secondary forward flow in late diastole *(third arrow)*. **Right,** With proximal arterial obstruction, the waveform becomes monophasic with loss of the reverse flow component and blunting of the systolic peak.

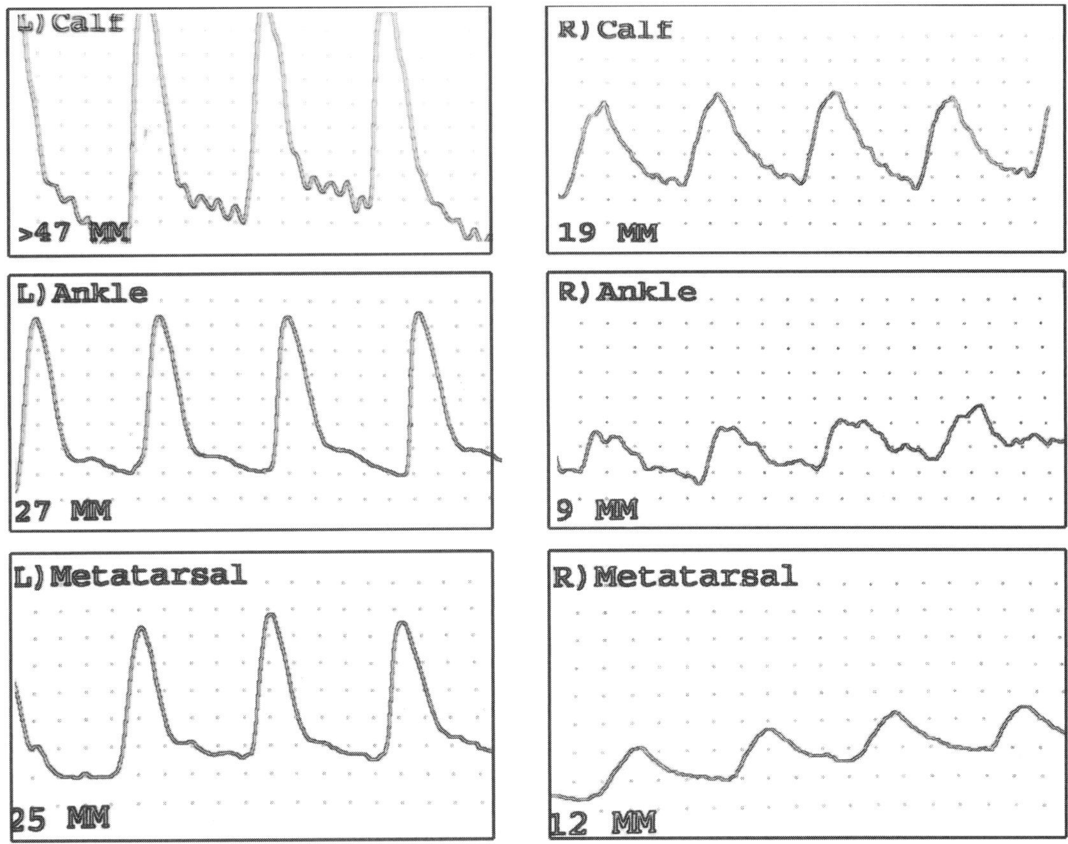

Figure 67.4. Left, Normal pulse volume recordings (PVRs) illustrate a brisk, sharp rise to the systolic peak, with a dicrotic notch. **Right,** With increasing levels of proximal arterial obstruction, the waveform loses the dicrotic notch, the peak becomes more rounded, and the downslope is prolonged. Severe occlusive disease produces a flattened waveform with a slow upstroke and downstroke.

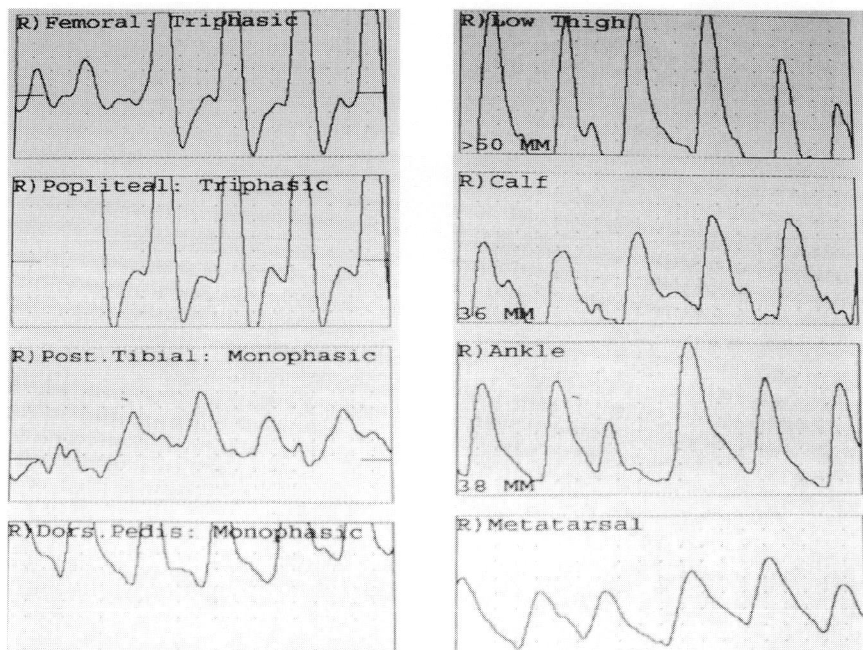

Figure 67.5. Noninvasive lower extremity arterial studies of the patient shown in Figure 67.1. On the basis of the ankle and metatarsal pulse volume recording waveforms, these results were interpreted as "mild tibial disease."

higher in diabetic patients with foot ulcers than in the nondiabetic population, which further limits the ability of this test to predict ischemia (33).

The limitations of noninvasive vascular testing in diabetic patients with foot ulceration emphasize the continued importance of a thorough bedside evaluation and clinical judgment. To reiterate, the status of the foot pulse is the most important aspect of the physical examination. In simplest terms, it can be assumed that occlusive disease is present if the foot pulses are not palpable. This finding alone is an indication for contrast arteriography in the clinical setting of tissue loss, poor healing, or gangrene, even if neuropathy may have been the antecedent cause of skin breakdown or ulceration.

Concern for contrast-induced renal failure should not mitigate against a high-quality angiogram of the circulation in the entire lower extremity. The incidence of contrast nephropathy is not higher in the diabetic patient without preexisting renal disease, even with the use of ionic contrast (34,35). The more costly nonionic agents should be reserved for the diabetic patient with compromised renal function. Even in this group, the concern for contrast nephropathy should not delay arteriography, as it seldom requires dialysis for treatment. More recently, attention has focused on the roles of magnetic resonance angiography, carbon dioxide angiography, and duplex scanning as replacements for contrast arteriography. However, each has its limitations, and although we have selectively used these modalities, we continue to rely heavily on a high-quality contrast arteriogram for most of our patients requiring distal arterial reconstruction.

Whatever preoperative imaging modality is chosen prior to arterial reconstruction, it is mandatory that consideration be given to the pattern of lower extremity vascular disease in patients with diabetes. Because the foot vessels are often spared by the atherosclerotic occlusive process, even when the tibial arteries are occluded, it is essential that arteriograms not be terminated at the midtibial level. The complete infrapopliteal circulation should be incorporated, including the foot vessels (Fig. 67.6). The advent of digital subtraction angiography, which allows for subtraction of the bones from the final images, has greatly helped in visualizing these distal vessels (Fig. 67.7). These principles, namely preangiographic hydration, the use of selective femoral and/or digital subtraction arteriography, and demonstration of the foot arteries even when the leg arteries are occluded, are fundamental considerations for lower extremity arteriography in patients with diabetes.

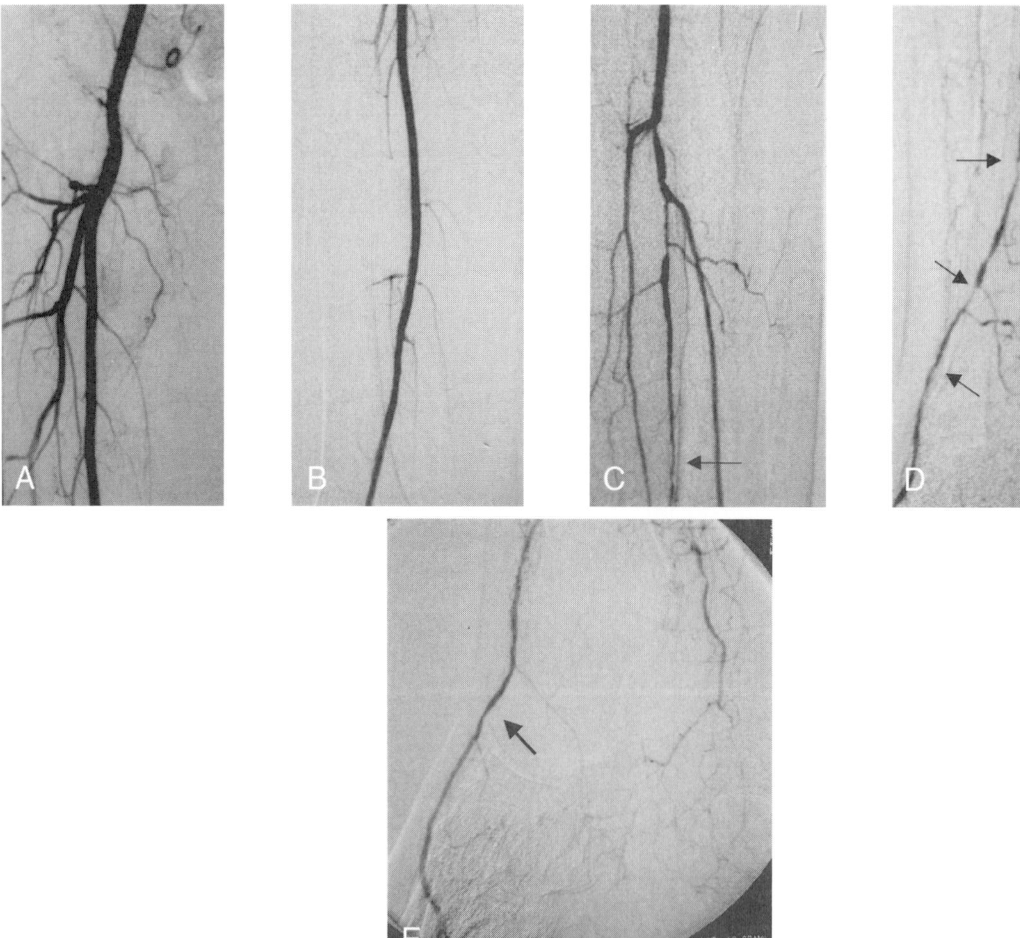

Figure 67.6. Digital subtraction angiogram of the patient shown in Figure 67.1. Note the normal appearance of the femoral and popliteal arteries (**A** and **B**). At the tibial level, however, there are occlusions of the peroneal (**C,** *arrow*), anterior tibial (**D,** *multiple arrows*), and posterior tibial (**D,** *single arrow*) arteries. **E,** Demonstration of the importance of visualization of the foot arteries, showing a patent dorsalis pedis artery (*arrow*). A popliteal-to-dorsalis pedis bypass was subsequently performed which allowed for successful limb and foot salvage.

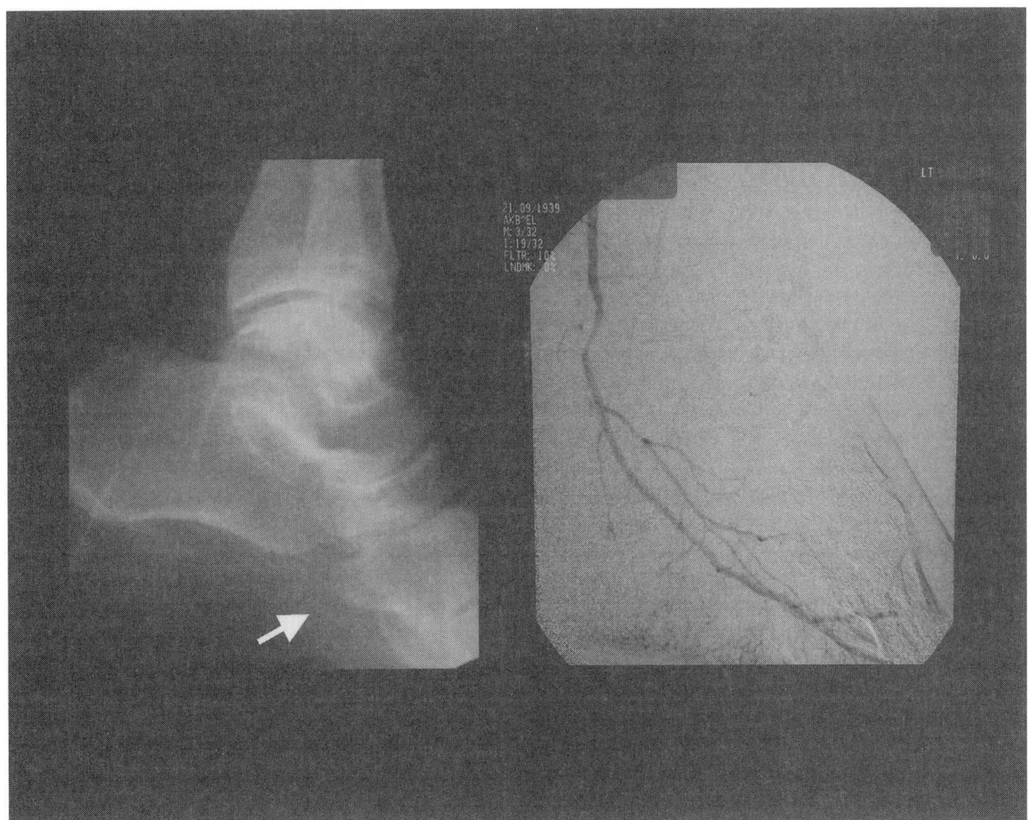

Figure 67.7. Two arteriograms of the foot in the same patient with a heel ulcer. **Left:** A conventional angiogram showing only a minimally opacified plantar artery (*white arrow*). The posterior tibial artery is not well visualized due to overlying bony structures. Because no target outflow artery was available, amputation was recommended. **Right:** Repeat arteriogram using digital subtraction techniques, illustrating a patent distal posterior tibial artery. Successful bypass was performed.

PRINCIPLES OF ARTERIAL RECONSTRUCTION IN THE DIABETIC FOOT

The concept of ischemia must be modified in making decisions about arterial reconstruction in the diabetic foot, since the biologically compromised foot requires *maximal* circulation to heal an ulcer. This leads to three significant principles: (a) all diabetic foot ulcers should be evaluated for an ischemic component; (b) correction of a moderate degree of ischemia will improve healing in the biologically compromised diabetic foot; and (c) whenever possible, the arterial reconstruction should be designed to restore normal arterial pressure to the target area. These three concepts form the basis of a critical difference in the approach to arterial reconstruction in diabetic and nondiabetic patients. In patients without diabetes, more proximal arterial reconstructions to the profunda or popliteal artery may restore perfusion adequate to obtain wound healing, in contrast to the diabetic patient, who mandates normal pulsatile pressure to the foot ulcer.

A complete arteriogram facilitates choosing an outflow artery that will restore a palpable foot pulse. Proximal bypass to the popliteal or tibioperoneal arteries may restore foot pulses. More often, however, because of the pattern of occlusive disease in the diabetic patient, bypass grafting to the popliteal or even tibial arteries cannot accomplish this goal because of more distal obstruction. Similarly, although excellent results have been reported with peroneal artery bypass (36), the peroneal artery is not in continuity with the foot vessels and may not achieve maximal flow, particularly to the forefoot, to achieve healing.

Restoration of the foot pulse is a fundamental goal of revascularization in the diabetic foot. Specifically, autogenous vein grafting to the dorsalis pedis, distal posterior tibial, and plantar arteries incorporates our knowledge of the anatomic pattern of diabetic vascular disease and provides durable and effective limb salvage. The choice of outflow artery should be based on availability of conduit, the location of the foot ulcer, and the quality of the outflow vessel.

The dorsalis pedis bypass represents the single most important advance in our management plan for diabetic limb salvage (37,38). Fundamental to the success of the dorsalis pedis bypass is meticulous technique and its appropriate use. The principal indication for the pedal graft is the absence of any other vessel that has continuity with the foot, particularly in cases with tissue loss. Dorsalis pedis bypass is unnecessary when a more proximal bypass will restore foot pulses and should not be done if there is an inadequate length of autogenous vein. In addition, if the dorsum of the foot is extensively infected and the peroneal artery is of good quality on the preoperative arteriogram, preference should be given to peroneal artery bypass.

Our initial report of dorsalis pedis arterial bypass demonstrated technical feasibility and short-term durability of the procedure, with patency and limb salvage rates approaching 90%

at 3 years (39). We subsequently reported on a more extensive 8-year experience encompassing 384 vein grafts to the dorsalis pedis artery in 367 patients (40). Ninety-five percent of the patients had diabetes, and all procedures were performed for limb-threatening ischemia. Twenty-nine grafts (7.5%) failed within the first 30 days, but 19 were successfully revised when a correctable technical problem was found at reoperation. The perioperative in-hospital mortality rate was 1.8%, and the actuarial primary and secondary patency rates were 68% and 82% at 5 years' follow-up. Furthermore, the limb salvage rate was 87% at 5 years, again attesting to the durability of the dorsalis pedis graft.

The distal location of the dorsalis pedis artery theoretically necessitates a long venous conduit, which is often not attainable. However, by using the popliteal or distal superficial femoral artery as an inflow site, a shorter length of vein may be used, with excellent long-term patency (41). This is particularly true in the patient with diabetes, again due to the pattern of atherosclerotic disease. In the authors' institutional experience of 384 pedal bypasses over a 7-year period, 60% of grafts used the more distal inflow site, usually the popliteal artery. This avoids dissection in the groin and upper thigh, a common location for wound complications, and also obviates the need for foot extension of the vein harvest incision. The approach is flexible, in that the vein graft to the dorsalis pedis artery can be prepared as an *in situ*, reversed, or nonreversed vein graft, without any significant difference in outcome (42). With the *in situ* or nonreversed graft, the valves may be lysed blindly, or preferably, cut under direct vision with an angioscope. This also allows for concomitant angioscopic assessment of the vein to detect any intraluminal abnormalities (43).

Active infection in the foot is commonly encountered in the complicated ischemic diabetic foot. However, it is not a contraindication to dorsalis pedis bypass, as long as the infectious process is controlled and located remotely from the proposed incision. Adequate control implies resolution of cellulitis, lymphangitis, and edema, especially in areas of proposed incisions required to expose the distal artery or saphenous vein. At the authors' institution, the results of 56 vein bypasses to the dorsal pedal artery in patients with ischemic foot lesions complicated by infection were recently reviewed (44). This included 15 patients with severe gangrene, osteomyelitis, and/or deep-space abscess. The average duration between admission and bypass was 10 days. Although there was a 12% wound infection rate, the primary graft patency was 92% at 36 months' follow-up. This aggressive approach to revascularization in the ischemic and infected foot resulted in a rate of limb salvage of 98% at the end of 3 years.

In the patient with an ischemic heel ulcer or gangrene, first consideration should be given to the posterior tibial or plantar arteries if they are patent by preoperative imaging. However, the absence of a patent posterior tibial artery is not a contraindication to arterial bypass and limb salvage. Our large experience with dorsalis pedis artery bypass has allowed us to examine its role and efficacy in the treatment of ischemic heel lesions (45). Over a 6-year period at our institution, 96 patients underwent pedal bypass for heel ulceration. When compared with a similar cohort of 336 patients with forefoot lesions undergoing dorsalis pedis bypass, there were no differences at 5 years with respect to primary patency, secondary patency, or limb salvage. More important, dorsalis pedis bypass accomplished complete healing in 87% (84 of 96) of heel lesions, with healing rates being independent of the presence or absence of an intact pedal arch, and it allowed for a limb salvage rate of almost 90% at 5 years.

Despite the technical success of lower extremity bypass in patients with diabetes, there continues to be a guarded optimism about long-term patient function and survival. In an effort to dispel concerns regarding *late* graft patency, limb salvage, and survival among patients with diabetes, we recently reviewed our experience with lower extremity revascularization in a largely diabetic population of almost 1,000 patients followed 5 years or longer (46). A total of 962 vein grafts were performed on 843 patients, of which 83% (795 grafts) were in patients with diabetes. Minimum follow-up was 5 years and extended up to 9 years. The dorsalis pedis or plantar/tarsal arteries served as the outflow artery in 271 (35%) of the patients with diabetes. Cumulative 5-year primary graft patency was 74.7% overall, with no difference among patients with and without diabetes (diabetic, 75.6% vs. nondiabetic, 71.9%). The secondary graft patency rate was 76.2% for the entire cohort and was also similar in the diabetic and nondiabetic groups (diabetic, 77% vs. nondiabetic, 73.6%). Most important, 5-year limb salvage and survival rates were virtually identical in diabetic and nondiabetic patients. The overall limb salvage rate was 87.1% (diabetic, 87.3% vs. nondiabetic, 85.4%). Survival at 5 years was 58.1% in the entire cohort (diabetic, 58.2% vs. nondiabetic, 58.0%). These data strongly emphasize that concern for *long-term* mortality, limb loss, and graft patency in diabetic patients is unwarranted and should not prevent aggressive attempts at distal bypass required for limb salvage.

ADJUNCTIVE PROCEDURES IN THE DIABETIC FOOT

It must be remembered that ischemia is only one component of the total problem. Prompt recognition and control of infection assumes first priority in the consideration of any diabetic foot problem. Recognizing that a benign-appearing superficial ulcer may rapidly progress to a potentially fatal infection underscores the importance of a thorough evaluation for infection in these patients. Therefore a complete examination of the infected areas is mandatory, and the wound should be thoroughly inspected, including unroofing of all encrusted areas, to determine the extent of involvement. Immediate incision and drainage of all infected tissue planes and abscesses is mandatory. The incision must be long enough, wide enough, and deep enough to ensure complete drainage of pus or débridement of necrotic tissue. Drains and small stab incisions do not provide dependent drainage and are not used. Dressings should consist of gauze sponges moistened with normal saline or 0.25% povidone-iodine solution. Full-strength astringents, hot compresses, and whirlpools lead to more harm than good.

Following successful revascularization, secondary procedures may be performed for both limb *and* foot salvage. Previous surgical débridements or amputations may be revised, and chronic ulcerations may be treated by ulcer excision, arthroplasty, or hemiphalangectomy. In the patient with extensive tissue loss, both local flaps and free flaps may be used. Due to the architecture of the diabetic foot, underlying bony structural abnormalities are often the cause of ulceration and may be corrected by metatarsal head resection or osteotomy. Heel ulcers may be treated by partial calcanectomy and local (e.g., flexor tendon) or even free-flap coverage.

Once the diabetic foot has healed, attention should be turned to lifelong foot care and preventive maintenance. While daily bathing and inspection should be emphasized, soaking should be discouraged. Because of sensory neuropathy, water should always be hand-tested for temperature to avoid scalding. Liberal use of moisturizer is encouraged to prevent calluses and cracks in dry skin. Self-treatment of calluses and corns, or so-called bathroom surgery, is never permitted, and in most instances, the diabetic individual should seek a qualified podiatrist for foot and nail maintenance. Footwear and stockings should fit well (without folds, wrinkles, or seams), be comfortable, and, to avoid pressure points, be changed daily. Again, the advice and care of a qualified podiatrist is indispensable for the diabetic individual who is prone to developing foot problems (47).

CONCLUSION

Our knowledge of the pathophysiology of lower extremity vascular disease in patients with diabetes has allowed us to incorporate it into our overall treatment plan of the diabetic foot, with improved limb and foot salvage. This is reflected in a recent report from our institution, which has seen a significant reduction in every category of lower limb amputation since 1984 (38). For the primary physician caring for the diabetic patient, limb salvage should be the rule rather than the exception. This can only be possible with a thorough understanding of diabetic peripheral vascular disease, an awareness of the complex physiology of the diabetic foot, and a logical treatment plan based on our current knowledge of the disease process.

REFERENCES

1. Grunfeld C. Diabetic foot ulcers: etiology, treatment, and prevention. *Adv Intern Med* 1991;37:103–132.
2. Nathan DM. Long-term complications of diabetes mellitus. *N Engl J Med* 1993;328:1676–1685.
3. Reiber GE, Boyko EJ, Smith DG. Lower extremity foot ulcers and amputations in diabetes. In: National Diabetes Data Group, ed. *Diabetes in America*, 2nd ed. Washington, DC: National Institutes of Health, 1995:409–428.
4. Factors in the development of diabetic neuropathy: Baseline analysis of neuropathy in the feasibility phase of the Diabetes Control and Complications Trial (DCCT). The DCCT Research Group. *Diabetes* 1988;37:476–481.
5. Dyck PJ, Kratz KM, Karnes JL, et al. The prevalence by staged severity of various types of diabetic neuropathy, retinopathy, and nephropathy in a population-based cohort: the Rochester Diabetic Neuropathy Study. *Neurology* 1993;43:817–824.
6. Caputo GM, Cavanagh PR, Ulbrecht JS, et al. Assessment and management of foot disease in patients with diabetes. *N Engl J Med* 1994;331:854–860.
7. Young MJ, Veves A, Boulton AJM. The diabetic foot: aetiopathogenesis and management. *Diabetes Metab Rev* 1993;9:109–127.
8. Akbari CM, Pomposelli FB, Jr. The diabetic foot. In: Perler B, Becker G, eds. *A clinical approach to vascular intervention*. New York: Thieme Medical Publishers, 1998:211–218.
9. Akbari CM, LoGerfo FW. Diabetes and peripheral vascular disease. *J Vasc Surg* 1999;30:373–384.
10. Cameron NE, Cotter MA. The relationship of vascular changes to metabolic factors in diabetes mellitus and their role in the development of peripheral nerve complications. *Diabetes Metab Rev* 1994;10:189–224.
11. LoGerfo FW, Coffman JD. Vascular and microvascular disease of the foot in diabetes. *N Engl J Med* 1984;311:1615–1619.
12. Williamson JR, Tilton RG, Chang K, et al. Basement membrane abnormalities in diabetes mellitus: Relationship to clinical microangiopathy. *Diabetes Metab Rev* 1988;4:339–370.
13. LoGerfo FW. Vascular disease, matrix abnormalities, and neuropathy: implications for limb salvage in diabetes mellitus. *J Vasc Surg* 1987;5:793–796.
14. Goldenberg SG, Alex M, Joshi RA, et al. Nonatheromatous peripheral vascular disease of the lower extremity in diabetes mellitus. *Diabetes* 1959;8:261–273.
15. Strandness DE Jr, Priest RE, Gibbons GE. Combined clinical and pathologic study of diabetic and nondiabetic peripheral arterial disease. *Diabetes* 1964;13:366–372.
16. Conrad MC. Large and small artery occlusion in diabetics and nondiabetics with severe vascular disease. *Circulation* 1967;36:83–91.
17. Barner HB, Kaiser GC, Willman VL. Blood flow in the diabetic leg. *Circulation* 1971;43:391–394.
18. Parving HH, Viberti GC, Keen H, et al. Hemodynamic factors in the genesis of diabetic microangiopathy. *Metabolism* 1983;32:943–949.
19. Flynn MD, Tooke JE. Aetiology of diabetic foot ulceration: a role for the microcirculation? *Diabet Med* 1992;8:320–329.
20. Rayman G, Williams SA, Spencer PD, et al. Impaired microvascular hyperaemic response to minor skin trauma in type I diabetes. *BMJ* 1986;292:1295–1298.
21. Jorneskog G, Brismar K, Fagrell B. Skin capillary circulation severely impaired in toes of patients with IDDM, with and without late diabetic complications. *Diabetologia* 1995;38:474–480.
22. Akbari CM, LoGerfo FW. The micro- and macrocirculation in diabetes mellitus. In: Veves A, ed. *A clinical approach to diabetic neuropathy*, 1st ed. New York: Humana Press, 1998:319–331.
23. Veves A, Akbari CM, Primavera J, et al. Endothelial dysfunction and the expression of endothelial nitric oxide synthetase in diabetic neuropathy, vascular disease, and foot ulceration. *Diabetes* 1997;47:457–463.
24. Parkhouse N, LeQueen PM. Impaired neurogenic vascular response in patients with diabetes and neuropathic foot lesions. *N Engl J Med* 1988; 318:1306–1309.
25. Williams SB, Cusco JA, Roddy M, et al. Impaired nitric oxide–mediated vasodilation in patients with non-insulin-dependent diabetes mellitus. *J Am Coll Cardiol* 1996;27:567–574.
26. Johnstone MT, Creager SJ, Scales KM, et al. Impaired endothelium-dependent vasodilation in patients with insulin-dependent diabetes mellitus. *Circulation* 1993;88:2510–2516.
27. Akbari CM, Saouaf R, Barnhill DF, et al. Endothelium-dependent vasodilatation is impaired in both microcirculation and macrocirculation during acute hyperglycemia. *J Vasc Surg* 1998;28:687–694.
28. Brand FN, Abbott RD, Kannel WB. Diabetes, intermittent claudication, and risk of cardiovascular events. The Framingham Study. *Diabetes* 1989;38: 504–509.
29. Dormandy J, Heeck L, Vig S. Predicting which patients will develop chronic critical leg ischemia. *Semin Vasc Surg* 1999;12:138–141.
30. Menzoian JO, LaMorte WW, Paniszyn CC, et al. Symptomatology and anatomic patterns of peripheral vascular disease: differing impact of smoking and diabetes. *Ann Vasc Surg* 1989;3:224–228.
31. Young MJ, Adams JE, Anderson GF, et al. Medial arterial calcification in the feet of diabetic patients and matched non-diabetic control subjects. *Diabetologia* 1993;36:615–621.
32. Ballard JL, Eke CC, Bunt TJ, et al. A prospective evaluation of transcutaneous oxygen measurements in the management of diabetic foot problems. *J Vasc Surg* 1995;22:485–492.
33. Wyss CR, Matsen FA III, Simmons CW, et al. Transcutaneous oxygen tension measurements on limbs of diabetic and nondiabetic patients with peripheral vascular disease. *Surgery* 1984;95:339–346.
34. Parfrey PS, Griffiths SM, Barrett BJ, et al. Contrast material–induced renal failure in patients with diabetes mellitus, renal insufficiency, or both. A prospective controlled study. *N Engl J Med* 1989;321:395–397.
35. Schwab SJ, Hlatky MA, Pieper KS, et al. Contrast nephrotoxicity: a randomized controlled trial of a nonionic and ionic contrast agent. *N Engl J Med* 1989;320:149–153.
36. Plecha EJ, Seabrook GR, Bandyk DF, et al. Determinants of successful peroneal artery bypass. *J Vasc Surg* 1993;17:97–106.
37. LoGerfo FW, Gibbons GW, Pomposelli FB Jr, et al. Trends in the care of the diabetic foot: expanded role of arterial reconstruction. *Arch Surg* 1992;127:617–621.
38. Akbari CM, LoGerfo FW. Distal bypasses in the diabetic patient. In: Yao JST, Pearce WH, eds. *Current techniques in vascular surgery*. New York: McGraw-Hill, 2001:285–296.
39. Pomposelli FB Jr, Jepsen SJ, Gibbons GW, et al. Efficacy of the dorsal pedis bypass for limb salvage in diabetic patients: short-term observations. *J Vasc Surg* 1990;11:745–752.
40. Pomposelli FB Jr, Marcaccio EJ, Gibbons GW, et al. Dorsalis pedis arterial bypass: durable limb salvage for foot ischemia in patients with diabetes mellitus. *J Vasc Surg* 1995;21:375–384.
41. Veith FJ, Gupta SK, Samson RH, et al. Superficial femoral and popliteal arteries as inflow sites for distal bypasses. *Surgery* 1981;90:980–990.
42. Pomposelli FB Jr, Jepsen SJ, Gibbons GW, et al. A flexible approach to infrapopliteal vein grafts in patients with diabetes mellitus. *Arch Surg* 1991;126:724–729.
43. Akbari CM, LoGerfo FW. Saphenous vein bypass to pedal arteries in diabetic patients. In: Yao JST, Pearce WH, eds. *Techniques in vascular and endovascular surgery*. Norwalk, CT: Appleton & Lange, 1998:227–232.
44. Tannenbaum GA, Pomposelli FB Jr, Marcaccio EJ, et al. Safety of vein bypass grafting to the dorsal pedal artery in diabetic patients with foot infections. *J Vasc Surg* 1992;15:982–990.
45. Berceli SA, Chan AK, Pomposelli FB Jr, et al. Efficacy of dorsal pedal artery bypass in limb salvage for ischemic heel ulcers. *J Vasc Surg* 1999;30:4 99–508.
46. Akbari CM, Pomposelli FB Jr, Gibbons GW, et al. Lower extremity revascularization in diabetes: late observations. *Arch Surg* 2000;135:452–456.
47. Akbari CM, Pomposelli FB Jr. Diabetes and diseases of the foot. *Intern Med* 2000;21:10–17.

CHAPTER 68
Diabetes Mellitus and Wound Healing

Parham A. Ganchi and Elof Eriksson

Diabetes mellitus, the most common endocrine disease, is a complex systemic disorder with a broad range of effects on nearly every organ system. It ranks in the top ten causes of death in the United States and encompasses a heterogeneous and progressive group of abnormalities with a wide spectrum of severity (1). Although difficult to determine precisely because of inconsistent standards of diagnosis, the prevalence of diabetes in the United States is probably between 1% and 2%, with a range as high as 11% (2). Generally, it is clear that both morbidity and mortality are increased in this population. However, the effects of diabetes on wound healing remain controversial and the mechanism underlying altered wound healing is poorly understood.

Diabetes itself is one of the earliest described diseases. The Ebers Papyrus dating back to 1500 B.C. lists some of the symptoms and possible treatments for this ailment (3). The gangrenous foot wound is clearly described in biblical writings, although its association with diabetes was likely unknown. In 1887, Pryce describes the chronic painless foot ulcer associated with diabetic neuropathy (4). The diabetic foot ulcer continues to be a significant healthcare problem and a major source of morbidity for the diabetic patient. In fact, ulcers of the leg and foot are the most common complications of diabetes (5). Furthermore, there are estimates that diabetic ulcers will increase by 14% per year (6). Fifteen percent of all patients with diabetes will develop a nonhealing foot wound during their lifetime despite meticulous glucose and dietary control (7,8). Diabetic patients have a 15-fold higher risk of lower-extremity amputation and account for at least 50% of the more than 50,000 nontraumatic amputations performed in the United States each year (9,10). The financial cost of the diabetic foot wound to society is formidable. An estimated $500 million is spent annually, with amputations costing about $25,000 in the United States (11). In one study, successful conservative management of a diabetic foot ulcer led to a savings of 80% compared with the cost of amputation (12). Furthermore, these estimates do not include financial and psychological losses incurred by the diabetic patient, his or her family, and society as a result of the limitations imposed by the amputation.

The cliché that postoperative wound complications are increased in patients with diabetes is not entirely supported by the literature (13). If patients are matched for age, sex, weight, and comorbidities, several studies show that diabetic patients have no significant increase in postoperative wound complications as compared with nondiabetic patients (14,15). In fact, no increase has been found in postoperative cardiopulmonary, vascular, or infectious wound complications after major vascular or abdominal surgery (16–20). This is in sharp contrast to a number of animal and *in vitro* studies that clearly document that optimal glycemic control leads to optimal wound healing in diabetes (21–25). Hyperglycemia and insulin deficiency are linked to decreased formation of granulation tissue and collagen, poor deep-wound tensile strength, deficient capillary ingrowth, and defective immune function, among other deficiencies (22,26–32). Whether these laboratory findings have clinical significance remains to be shown.

The wound classically associated with diabetes is the nonhealing foot ulcer (Fig. 68.1). Wounds in other locations are rarely as challenging clinically, and few data exist to support an association between diabetes and wounds other than the foot ulcer. Elimination of the diabetic foot ulcer would reduce the number of in-hospital days for the diabetic patient more than the elimination of any other problem associated with diabetes. It is one of the most common and morbid complications of diabetes, and a great deal of literature has been written on this subject. To review the effects of diabetes on clinically relevant derangements in wound healing, we will examine the pathophysiology of the foot ulcer. Specifically, we will review the triad of neuropathy, ischemia, and infection, all common complications of diabetes and all culprits in the pathogenesis of the nonhealing foot ulcer.

NEUROPATHY

Neuropathy in the diabetic patient can take many forms. They range from the "classic" chronic progressive distal symmetric neuropathies to the acute mononeuropathies to the pressure palsies most often affecting the median and ulnar nerves (33,34). The distal symmetric neuropathy is the most common symptomatic neuropathy associated with diabetes mellitus (35). It is a diffuse neuropathy with sensory loss predominating over motor deficits. The symptoms start distally and progress proximally in a stocking distribution, with the longest nerves affected first (36,37). Pathologically, there is a distal dying back of the axons (33,36). Mainly large myelinated fibers are lost,

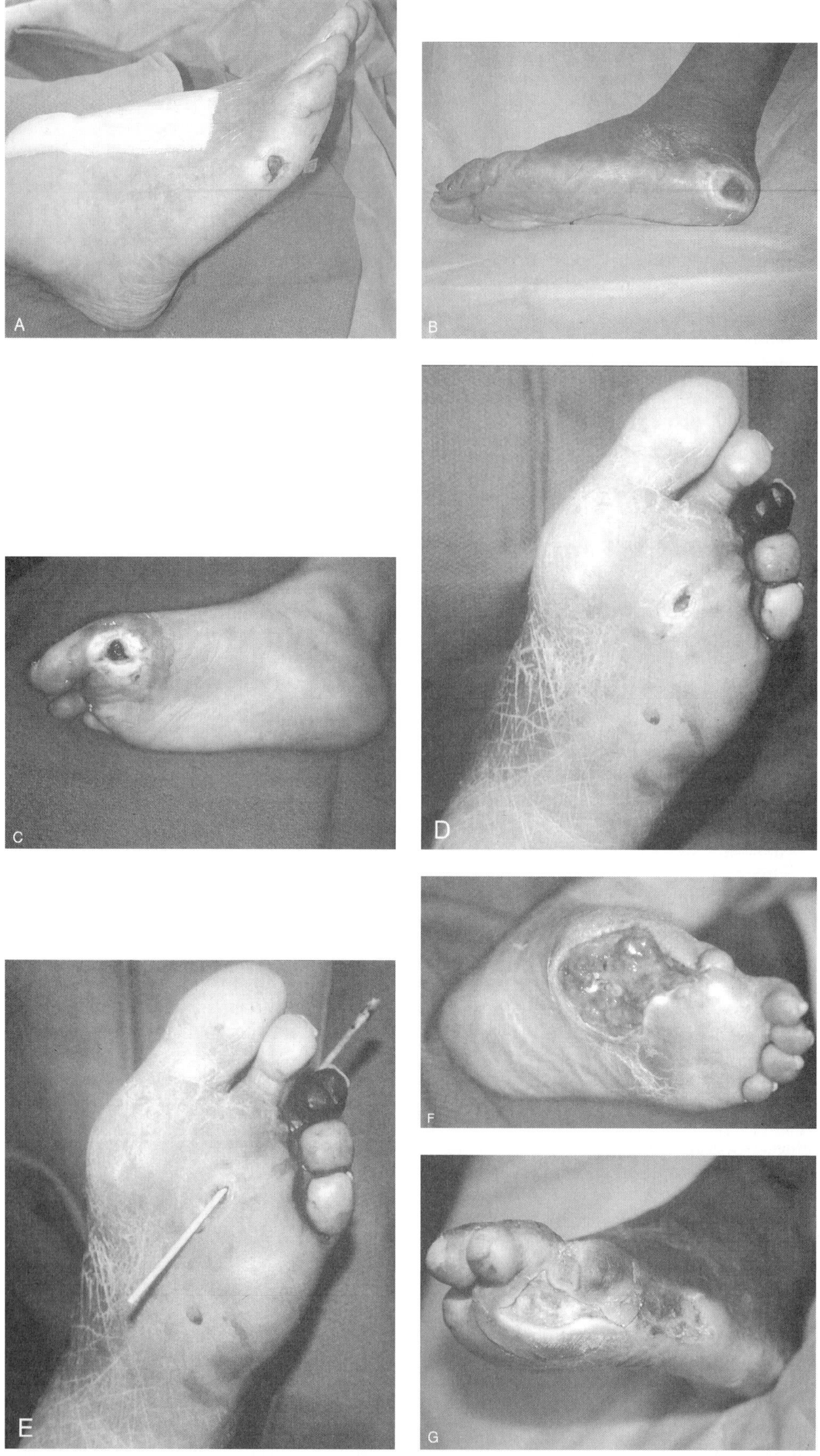

Figure 68.1. Typical diabetic foot ulcers. **A:** Early neuropathic ulcer over fifth metatarsal prominence. **B:** Chronic heel ulcer. **C:** Neuropathic forefoot ulcer over first metatarsal head with callus formation. **D, E:** Deceptively small metatarsal head ulcer with necrotic toe. Note true extent of ulcer, penetrating the foot to the dorsum. **F, G:** Advanced diabetic ulcers with extensive soft tissue and bone loss. Note clawing of toes.

with variable loss of small unmyelinated fibers (38–40). There is focal demyelination and regeneration with slowing of conduction velocities, elevation in sensory thresholds, and slowing of axonal transport (33,41–43). Signs and symptoms vary with the nerve fibers involved (44). Loss of large sensory fibers can lead to diminished light touch and proprioception, and damage to large motor fibers, though less common, may result in unsteadiness and weakness of the intrinsic muscles of the foot. Injury to small fibers results in increased pain thresholds and an inability to recognize temperature changes. These abnormalities predispose to repeated foot injuries and eventually to ulceration.

The prevalence of neuropathy in the diabetic population has been difficult to determine, with estimates ranging from 10% to 90% (45–49). The Diabetes Control and Complications Trial (DCCT) quoted a 50% prevalence of significant neuropathy among their population, although a range of 20% to 30% represents more closely those patients who have symptoms or findings on examination (45,50). Generally, the incidence of neuropathy seems to increase with duration of disease and severity of hyperglycemia (51–53). One large study found an incidence of neuropathy of 8% at diagnosis of diabetes that increased to 50% at 25 years after diagnosis (54). However, this association is far from perfect. Many studies have shown a correlation between neuropathy and height, age independent of duration of diabetes, and smoking (45,51,54,55). Furthermore, the DCCT failed to find a correlation between neuropathy and levels of glycosylated hemoglobin (45).

Autonomic neuropathy also plays a role in diabetic foot ulceration and closely parallels the incidence of somatic neuropathy. Like somatic neuropathy, the incidence of autonomic neuropathy seems to increase with duration of disease. One study found a 4% incidence at the time of diagnosis of diabetes. This increased to 28% after 5 years (56). Others have shown a prevalence of 50% in unselected diabetic populations (57). Abnormal autonomic function tests were shown in 20% to 40% of various groups of patients with diabetes, with up to 20% having cardiovascular abnormalities and 12% having postural hypotension (58–60). However, although almost all patients with sensory neuropathy have an associated autonomic neuropathy, the autonomic abnormality is rarely symptomatic.

Many studies show a clear correlation between diabetic neuropathy and foot ulceration, with up to 80% of patients with foot ulcers having a clinically significant neuropathy (61–64). The positive predictive value of a clinically detectable neuropathy was shown in a prospective study, in which an increased vibration perception threshold was associated with a sevenfold increased risk of ulceration over 4 years (65). A more clinically useful examination, the Semmes-Weinstein nylon monofilament test, has also been shown to identify those at increased risk for ulceration (61,66–68). The inability to feel the 10-g filament greatly increases the patient's risk of developing an ulcer. Undoubtedly, neuropathy plays a considerable role in the development of diabetic foot ulcers.

Sensory neuropathy is by far the major contributor to ulcer formation. Specifically, loss of pain sensation typically leads to repetitive trauma from walking, usually with poorly fitting shoes or from a foreign body in the patient's shoe that the patient does not feel. This is compounded by loss of proprioception, which can lead to abnormal foot posture and amplified trauma from walking. Additionally, autonomic neuropathy can lead to sudomotor abnormalities, resulting in decreased sweating and dry skin that is prone to cracking. These breaks in the skin are portals for infection and further ulcer formation.

As autonomic neuropathy progresses, there is sympathetic denervation of the foot, resulting in loss of vasoconstrictor tone and peripheral vasodilation. As arteriovenous shunts open, there is, on average, a fivefold increase in blood flow to the skin, even in the absence of other signs of neuropathy (69–72). Clinically, the skin is deceptively warm and healthy appearing, with bounding pulses, marked venous distention, and an elevated venous PO_2 secondary to shunting of blood (73). Increased capillary pressure may result in neuropathic edema that can further compromise tissue integrity (74). It has been suggested that shunting may bypass capillary beds, resulting in compromised flow of nutrients and oxygen to the bypassed tissues (75). However, it has been shown that nutritive capillary flow is not only normal but often increased (71). Blood flow to bone is also increased and may be responsible for the osteopenia of advanced disease, predisposing the patient to the development of Charcot neuroarthropathy (76).

Neuropathy alone is not sufficient to cause ulceration. Clearly trauma of some form is necessary. With time, loss of pain sensation in the foot can be compounded by structural abnormalities (34). Damage to motor nerves, specifically the tibial nerve, can lead to weakness and wasting of the intrinsic muscles of the foot. This leads to an imbalance between the flexor and extensor forces, deforming the shape of the foot itself. The metatarsal heads become more prominent, with unopposed dorsiflexion of the metatarsophalangeal joints; exaggerated interphalangeal joint plantarflexion results in clawing of the toes. The weight of the body is shifted onto a smaller surface, mainly the metatarsal heads and heel. In the early phases, the patient has a red, swollen foot with a clear sensory deficit on examination. As the neuropathy progresses, daily activities in the absence of adequate protective proprioceptive and nociceptive function lead to joint erosions, unrecognized fractures, and demineralization and devitalization of bones. Neuroarthropathy or Charcot joints develop as the foot collapses, the longitudinal arch flattens, and a rocker bottom deformity with weight bearing on the distal tarsal row develops, leaving the patient with an insensate misshapen foot (Fig. 68.2). Deformity becomes a constant source of abnormal pressure that in synergy with sensory dysfunction leads to ulceration. In one study, neuropathic feet with abnormally distributed pressures resulted in a 28% ulceration rate over 2.5 years as compared with no ulcers in neuropathic feet with normal pressures (77).

Sites of high pressure loading, such as the metatarsal heads and heel, are prone to callus formation as exuberant keratin production is stimulated by high shear forces (Fig. 68.1B,C) (78). Callus buildup itself leads to further increases in pressure loading, which eventually results in foci of hemorrhage, liquefaction necrosis, and ulcer formation. Callus over a weight-bearing area is strongly predictive of ulcer formation, whereas callus removal decreases local pressures and the risk of ulceration (79,80). Clearly, the combination of neuropathy and altered pressure loading is a major risk factor for foot ulceration in the patient with diabetes. Deformity leads to altered pressure loading, which leads to callus formation and ultimately to ulceration. Repeated and continuous trauma disrupts the orderly sequence of cellular events necessary for wound healing and results in a nonhealing wound. Unchecked, these processes can result in a vicious cycle of further deformity, abnormal pressure loading, and progression of tissue breakdown.

The etiology of neuropathy in the patient with diabetes is complex and likely multifactorial. The ravages of neuropathy begin distally and are most likely to affect longer nerves first, such as those in the feet. This may be the result of the cumulative effect of multiple insults, both biochemical and vascular in nature, or increased capillary hydrostatic pressure, which is relatively unique to the feet and lower extremities (33,53). The association between hyperglycemia and worsening neuropathy is convincing and has been demonstrated by several groups (51–54). Furthermore, strict glucose control using continuous subcutaneous insulin infusion or pancreas transplantation can

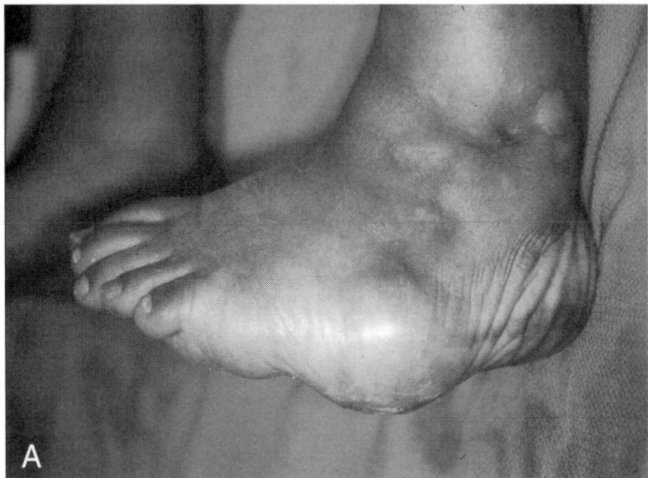

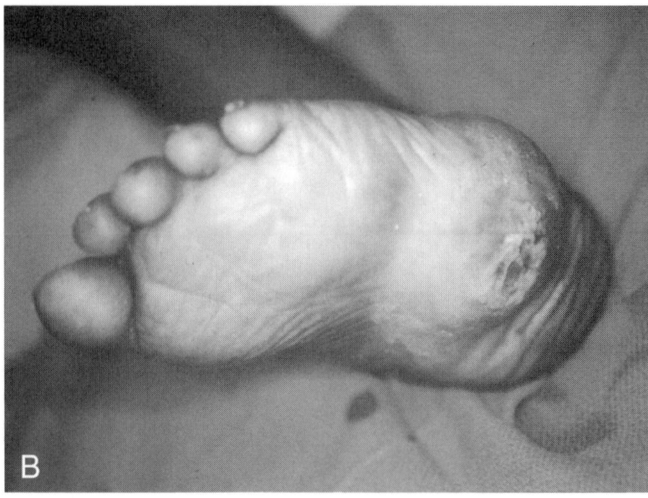

Figure 68.2. A, B: Charcot foot. Note ulcer forming over area of abnormally high pressure in this misshapen foot.

slow or even halt the progression of neuropathic changes (45,81,82). The DCCT showed that intense glucose control led to a 69% reduction in subclinical neuropathy and a 57% reduction in clinically evident neuropathy (83). Some of the more convincing data regarding the pathogenesis of diabetic neuropathy implicate activation of the sorbitol pathway, the formation of advanced glycation end products, and increased oxidative stress (84–93). Animal models show that hyperglycemia can augment the sorbitol pathway in peripheral nerves. The products of this pathway can either directly or indirectly lead to nerve damage. Unfortunately, these animal data are not easily reproduced in human studies (94–97).

Glucose uptake in peripheral nerves occurs independently of insulin. As a result, serum hyperglycemia leads to intracellular hyperglycemia and activation of the enzyme aldose reductase, stimulating the production of sorbitol (33,98). The concentrations of the intracellular osmolytes sorbitol, myoinositol, and taurine normally respond to changes in extracellular osmolality, buffering the intracellular environment (99–101). However, as hyperglycemia artificially drives the sorbitol pathway, intracellular accumulation of the osmolyte sorbitol leads to compensatory depletion of myoinositol and taurine (84,85,102,103). Initially, nerve damage was attributed to the intracellular accumulation of sorbitol and the resultant increased influx of water. This increased water content was shown in both diabetic animal and human nerves and was found to be reversible with aldose reductase inhibitors (104). However, the magnitude of the osmotic change was believed to be too small to account for significant peripheral neuropathy. Alternatively, the depletion of myoinositol, a significant component of phosphoinositide metabolism and a key determinant in the Na^+-K^+-ATPase that maintains nerve membrane potential, may become limiting for phosphoinositide signaling. Taurine depletion can exacerbate oxidative stress and lead to dysregulation of neuronal hyperexcitability and neurotransmitter release (85,102,105–110). The nerves of diabetic rats were found to have decreased myoinositol levels. The severity of myoinositol depletion correlated with decreased Na^+-K^+-ATPase activity and slowing of nerve conduction velocity. Furthermore, both defects were corrected with myoinositol supplementation or aldose reductase inhibitors (111–116). Although these data are intriguing, not all the evidence is supportive (117–120).

Activation of the sorbitol pathway consumes NADPH (reduced form of nicotinamide adenine dinucleotide phosphate), a cofactor necessary for the function of glutathione reductase and nitric oxide synthase activity, leading to depletion of both reduced glutathione and nitric oxide (92,121–125). Glutathione is a potent antioxidant and a critical element in the cellular defense against oxidative stress. Although direct evidence is lacking, oxidative tissue damage in diabetes has been attributed to NADPH consumption and the resultant depletion of reduced glutathione (121,126). Nitric oxide is a potent endothelium-derived mediator of vasodilation and neurotransmission (122,127). Aldose reductase–mediated depletion of NADPH can hinder nitric oxide synthase activity, which is NADPH dependent. Decreased nitric oxide production by the endothelial cells of the vasa nervorum can lead to limited vasodilation and impaired blood flow in the endoneurium of peripheral nerves, leading to local ischemia and neuronal dysfunction (92,98,121,123–125,128,129).

Activity of the sorbitol pathway can generate highly reactive sugar moieties that can glycate proteins, forming advanced glycation end products (AGE) (33,130). In general, high glucose concentrations can lead to the nonspecific glycation of both intracellular and extracellular proteins. Insulin-independent tissues such as peripheral nerves are particularly prone to hyperglycemia-induced glycation of intracellular proteins. Glycation of tubulin, a component of microtubules in nerves, can interfere with axonal transport, and AGE can nonspecifically consume nitric oxide, quenching its local vasodilatory effects and predisposing to neural ischemia (121,131). Aminoguanidine, an inhibitor of AGE formation, can reverse nerve conduction and blood flow abnormalities in diabetic rats (130,132,133). Finally, extracellular AGE are felt to play a role in the development of large-vessel atherosclerosis and ischemia in the patient with diabetes. AGE-induced abnormalities in the extracellular matrix have been shown to alter the structure and function of the vasculature, decreasing elasticity in large vessels and increasing permeability across the carotid artery in rats (130). By blocking the cytostatic effect of nitric oxide on vascular smooth muscle, accumulation of AGE is thought to contribute to the premature and accelerated evolution of atherosclerosis and large-vessel occlusive disease in the diabetic patient (130).

ISCHEMIA

Ischemia and its complications are responsible for some of the most devastating ravages of diabetes mellitus. Patients with diabetes are at an increased risk of developing atherosclerotic disease of both large and small vessels and do so at an earlier age and at an accelerated rate (134,135). More than 80% have vascular disease 20 years after diagnosis of their diabetes, and 75% of patients with diabetes die of vascular disease or its complications (136). Ischemia clearly plays a role in diabetic foot ulcers as well. Tissue hypoxia as measured by a reduction in dorsal foot transcutaneous oxygen tension has been shown to be an independent predictor of foot ulceration in the diabetic patient (137). However, purely ischemic ulcers are relatively uncommon, representing only 10% to 15% of diabetic foot ulcers (63,138,139). Most of these ulcers are neuropathic or neuroischemic in nature (54,75,134,140,141). Certainly, the metabolic requirements of a wound are greater than those of uninjured tissues (142). Therefore, a diabetic foot with adequate tissue perfusion may become ischemic once it is wounded if it is unable to augment blood flow to the injured tissues. Vascular occlusive disease in combination with an abnormal autonomic response secondary to neuropathy may limit the ability to augment flow. This creates the vicious cycle of a wound leading to ischemia, leading to a larger wound, which, if uninterrupted, often leads to amputation.

The patient with diabetes has a 20-fold increased risk of developing atherosclerosis of the lower extremities (134). The process starts at a younger age, is accelerated, and has less male bias than in the nondiabetic patient. The risk of developing an occluded artery in the lower extremity is almost twice as high in the diabetic than in the nondiabetic patient, and the distribution of disease tends to be more diffuse (143). Vascular occlusive disease is associated with almost two thirds of nonhealing diabetic foot ulcers and is an etiologic factor in almost half of all amputations (62). The Framingham Study showed a 50% higher incidence of nonpalpable pedal pulses in women with diabetes and a 25% higher rate in men with diabetes compared with their nondiabetic counterparts (135). Although the frequency of proximal disease involving the iliac and femoral vessels tends to parallel that of the general population, patients with diabetes have a unique tendency for significant involvement of the tibial and peroneal vessels between the knee and ankle (Fig. 68.3) (1,3,144–146). It is interesting that the vessels in the foot tend to be spared. In fact, the vessels in the feet of diabetic patients may be less involved with atherosclerosis than are the pedal vessels in nondiabetic patients (147,148). As a result, patients with diabetes are often good candidates for bypass surgery, with the vast majority having surgically correctable disease with excellent long-term results (149–152).

One of the impediments to aggressive revascularization of the diabetic foot had been the myth of small-vessel disease. This

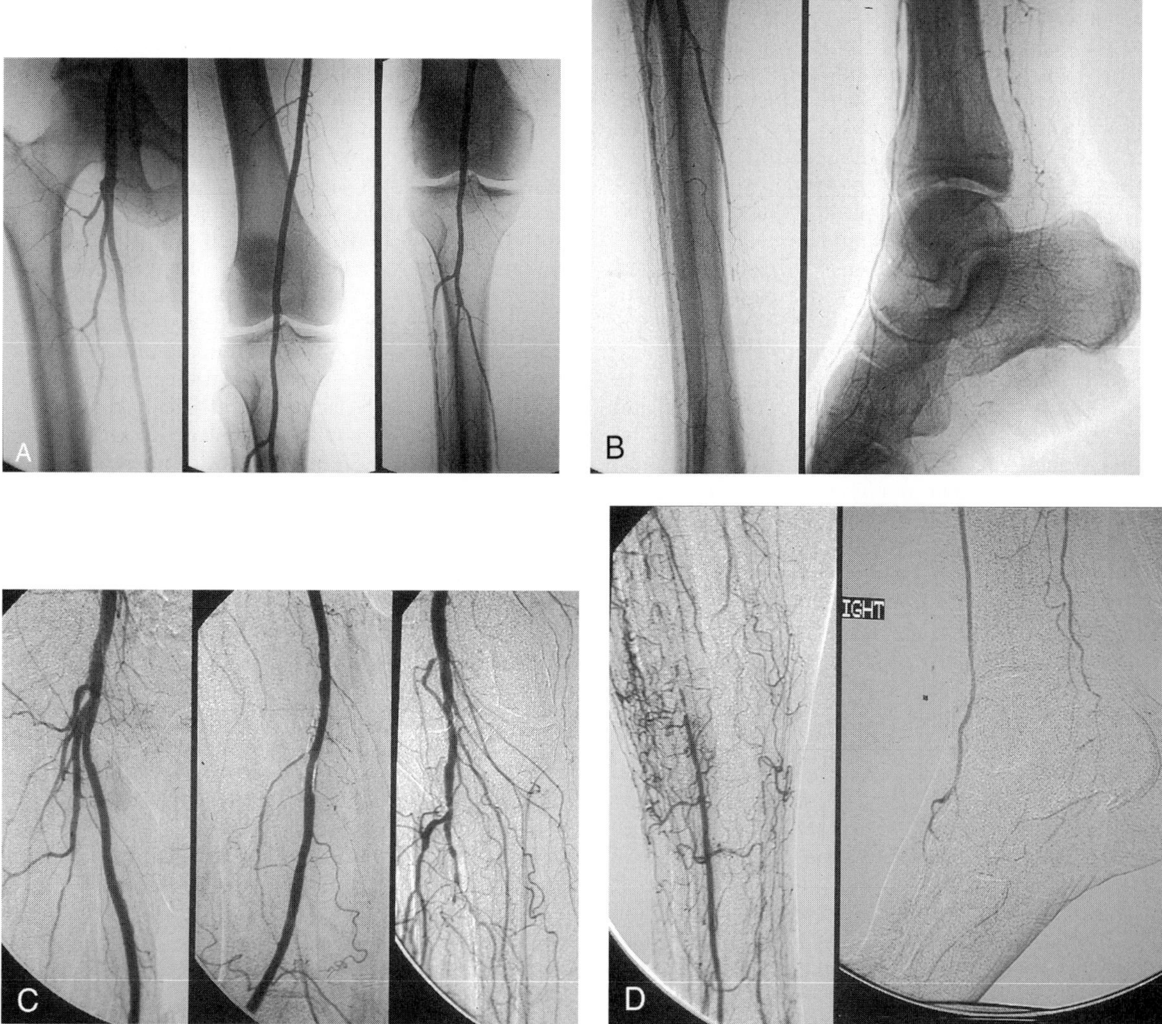

Figure 68.3. Two patients (**A, B** and **C, D**) with typical diabetic lower extremity vascular occlusive disease. Note predominantly infrapopliteal involvement with relative sparing of the foot.

myth was promoted to explain the apparent dilemma of the nonhealing diabetic foot ulcer in the presence of palpable pedal pulses. Unfortunately, this was given some credibility by a retrospective, unblinded study of amputation specimens in 1959 (153). Periodic acid-Schiff–positive staining material seen in small vessels on histologic sections was interpreted as proof of small-vessel occlusive disease specific to the diabetic foot. However, since then, multiple studies have failed to confirm these findings. No difference in occlusive disease was found in arterial casts of amputation specimens of diabetic and nondiabetic patients (147). Strandness and colleagues (148) repeated the 1959 study of Goldenberg et al. (153) and were unable to confirm their findings. A study of diabetic and nondiabetic patients after femoropopliteal bypass surgery showed no difference in arteriolar resistance or reactivity to papaverine treatment (154). Wyss et al. (155) were unable to show a significant difference in transcutaneous oxygen tension in the extremities of patients with peripheral vascular disease with and without diabetes. Finally, there was no difference in the oxygen gradient between arterial blood and pedal skin in diabetic patients with ulcers compared with those without ulcers and those without diabetes (156). Although it has been shown that the basement membrane of muscle capillaries in diabetic feet is thickened, there is little evidence that microvascular disease contributes to ischemia or foot ulceration (157).

Abnormal hemorheology is one factor that can contribute to localized microvascular occlusion and ischemia. The combination of increased plasma viscosity, increased aggregability, and reduced red blood cell deformability in the diabetic patient can lead to stagnation of blood flow, hypoxia, and ischemia (158,159). The red blood cell is stiff and unable to deform to pass through the small capillary channels. This stiffness occurs during the hyperglycemic state and is a result of nonenzymatic glycation of the red blood cell membrane protein spectrin (160–162). This process not only renders the red blood cell stiff but also increases aggregability, which leads to increased blood viscosity (163). Increased viscosity leads to increased resistance and, in order to maintain flow, to increased perfusion pressures. This increased pressure leads to increased transudation and, paradoxically, higher viscosity. Because of the thixotropic nature of blood, as flow slows, it becomes more and more resistant to acceleration of flow (163). This increases shear stress to the microvascular wall, leading to increased permeability and extravasation of plasma proteins. The resultant stagnation within the microcirculation leads to occlusion, hypoxia, and finally ischemia (163,164). Interestingly, the stiffness of the red blood cell membrane can be reversed within 24 hours if normoglycemia is maintained (165,166).

Another functional defect in oxygen delivery involves hemoglobin itself. Under hyperglycemic conditions, hemoglobin is glycosylated, resulting in a shift in the oxygen-hemoglobin dissociation curve to the left (15,167). Glycosylated hemoglobin has a higher affinity for oxygen and releases less oxygen to tissues (15,168). As a result, under hyperglycemic conditions, oxygen delivery is hampered in two ways. The red blood cell is rendered stiff and more likely to aggregate, resulting in increased blood viscosity and poor microperfusion, and hemoglobin is glycosylated, preventing the efficient release of oxygen at the tissue level. However, it is notable that both conditions are reversed with good glucose control. A diabetic foot wound clearly has higher metabolic needs and oxygen requirements than unwounded skin (142,169,170). Baseline ischemia is therefore amplified in the face of a healing wound. Thus, it is critical to optimize blood flow and oxygen delivery to the foot. In the patient with nonpalpable pedal pulses, a vascular workup is a must. Most occlusive lesions in this population are amenable to surgical bypass with excellent long-term results. Although not yet shown in clinical studies, optimizing blood glucose control may improve the local microvascular hemorheology and allow for better oxygen release by hemoglobin at the tissue level. Furthermore, minimizing edema with leg elevation and wrapping is also beneficial to local nutrient delivery and wound healing.

INFECTION AND INFLAMMATION

Although infection is not the instigator of ulceration in the diabetic foot, it can clearly be a major impediment to healing. Once an ulcer is established through a combination of neuropathy, ischemia, and repetitive trauma, it can become chronic and unable to heal secondary to superimposed infection. In fact, infection complicating ischemia often leads to amputation in the patient with diabetes, with infection playing a significant role in two thirds of lower-extremity amputations in this population (9,62,171). In general, patients with diabetes are at an increased risk of acquiring an infection and of developing a more severe variant when compared with their nondiabetic counterparts (172,173). Several studies have showed an increased risk of postoperative wound infections in patients with diabetes (134,174–180). Diabetes is an independent risk factor for postoperative wound infection in patients undergoing cardiac surgery, cholecystectomy, vascular surgery, and hip arthroplasty (174–177,181–185). Glucose control may lower this risk after open-heart surgery (178). However, many of the early studies showing increased postoperative morbidity in patients with diabetes have not stood up to the scrutiny of correcting for age, weight, sex, and comorbid conditions (17–20,174–180). These conflicting results stand in sharp contrast to the clearly hostile environment of the diabetic foot in wound healing. Surgical and traumatic wounds in other locations may or may not be at increased risk of developing complications. There is no doubt, however, that wound healing in the diabetic foot is often highly compromised. Some of the factors that hinder wound healing in the foot include lack of prompt and appropriate wound care secondary to the patient's inability to feel (neuropathy) or see (retinopathy) an early ulcer, abnormally high pressures and continued trauma to a deformed foot, ischemia as a result of large-vessel occlusive disease or abnormal hemorheology, or more likely, a combination of the above.

Breaks in the skin, whether they are imperceptible cracks, fissures in calluses, or large wounds, are portals of entry for bacteria. In the diabetic foot wound, this initial bacterial inoculum is not eliminated efficiently. As a result, the normal repair processes are delayed or halted altogether. The most common aerobe in diabetic foot wounds is *Staphylococcus aureus*, followed by streptococci and gram-negative bacilli such as *Escherichia coli*. Almost all infected diabetic foot wounds also harbor anaerobes and are polymicrobial in nature (152,186–189). Unlike the patient without diabetes, the patient with diabetes is often unable to respond to infection with increased blood flow. Rather, vascular occlusive disease impairs the delivery of much-needed oxygen and antibiotics. Autonomic neurogenic vascular responses are rendered ineffective by neuropathy. Microthrombi form in small arterioles, compounding any existing ischemia (3). The increased oxygen and nutrient requirements of an infected open wound, together with the inability to meet these requirements, result in a vicious cycle that can ultimately lead to massive tissue necrosis and sepsis.

Many studies have documented immune deficiencies directly related to the metabolic derangements caused by poorly controlled diabetes. As a result, the World Health Organization has classified diabetes as a secondary immunodeficiency disease

(190). Specifically, a great deal of research on wound healing in diabetes has focused on leukocyte function. In the early inflammatory phase of wound healing, the neutrophil is a critical line of defense against bacteria and debris and is necessary to the orderly progression of the healing cascade. In the patient with diabetes, deep wounds were found to be relatively deficient in neutrophils (24,191,192). This may explain the failure of these wounds to progress and heal.

Although it is assumed that individuals with diabetes are more prone to infection than are those without diabetes, most of the data documenting immune dysfunction in the presence of hyperglycemia are based on *in vitro* models. *In vitro* studies of neutrophils from subjects with poorly controlled diabetes have revealed defects in chemotaxis, adherence, phagocytosis, diapedesis, intracellular killing, and complement function (28–32,193–203). It appears that most of these defects are corrected when normoglycemia is attained. However, this is somewhat controversial, with some studies suggesting a defect in the patient's serum and not in the neutrophil itself (29,201,204,205). Others note that although phagocytosis and intracellular killing are improved with normoglycemia, overall granulocyte function remains abnormal, suggesting additional defects (206,207). The thickened capillary basement membrane of patients with diabetes may act as yet another impediment to the migration of activated leukocytes. Granulocytes accumulate in the microvasculature, further impairing the passage of red blood cells already compromised by abnormal hemorheology and macrovascular occlusive disease. There is increased edema and local ischemia is accentuated, leading to further deterioration. Although there appears to be clear *in vitro* evidence for immune dysfunction in the patient with diabetes, the clinical significance of these findings and the benefits of normoglycemia to wound healing in the diabetic patient remain unclear.

Multiple groups have shown deficient wound healing in diabetic animal models. Hyperglycemic obese mice have delayed wound closure as compared with normoglycemic controls (169). There is decreased accumulation of collagen and fewer myofibroblasts in these wounds, delaying closure by contraction. Slow or inadequate granulocyte influx into diabetic wounds has been associated with deficient protocollagen and collagen synthesis in deep surgical wounds (24,191,192,201,208). These wounds have poor tensile strength (22,25). Experiments with subcutaneous cylinders have shown decreased production of hydroxyproline, a key component of collagen (23). Other findings include poor capillary ingrowth and inadequate fibroblast proliferation (208,209). Most of these defects are corrected with insulin administration or reduction in glucose concentrations or both.

In sharp contrast to the abnormalities encountered with deep surgical wounds, healing of superficial corneal wounds in diabetic rats and humans was equivalent to that in their nondiabetic counterparts (210,211). Both groups showed minimal leukocyte infiltration, suggesting that granulocytes are not an important part of epithelialization. Rather, granulocyte function seems to be intimately related to the healing of deep wounds, whereas collagen formation is critical to tissue restoration. Other studies have shown that wound healing in experimental diabetes is improved with zinc supplementation or with large doses of vitamin A (212,213). Insulin administration, independent of glucose concentrations, was found to be necessary for satisfactory capillary ingrowth into healing wounds in diabetic animals (208). Poor intracellular glucose levels correlated with fewer granulocytes and fibroblasts in the early phases of wound healing, leading to deficient collagen deposition and poor tensile strength. Interestingly, the timing of insulin administration also was found to be important. Only if insulin was given immediately after wounding did the formation of granulation tissue return to normal, suggesting compromise of an early event in wound healing (191,214). This corresponds to the phase when neutrophil function is crucial to wound healing. On the other hand, others report that insulin neither prevents nor corrects the multiple tissue defects associated with diabetes (215,216).

TREATMENT

Diabetic foot ulcers, like all chronic wounds, will heal only if the underlying pathology is corrected (217). Most of these chronic wounds will heal with proper local care. However, the recurrence rates are quite high. Furthermore, patients who suffer recurrent ulcers are those at highest risk for amputation (62). Unlike acute wounds that sustain a transient external insult, chronic wounds are exposed to both physical and biochemical stressors for a prolonged period. This leads to a sustained inflammatory state, with increased local tissue damage and ineffective healing. In the patient with diabetes, the typical foot ulcer is a result of chronic recurrent trauma resulting from a combination of neuropathy and a misshapen foot. This can be aggravated by ischemia and superimposed infection.

The key to the management of diabetic foot ulcer is early, aggressive care (218,219). This has been shown to improve prognosis and reduce the risk of amputation. There are some basic guidelines for managing the chronic diabetic foot ulcer. Initially, it is important to establish the true extent of the wound. Often, the external appearance of the ulcer does not betray the true severity of the injury (Fig. 68.1D,E). Therefore, a close examination is critical. Any necrotic or marginally viable tissues, including bone, should be débrided until only healthy tissues are left (188). There is nothing more expedient, effective, and cost-effective as sharp surgical débridement for cleaning a wound. The goal is to remove all necrotic tissues and foreign bodies from the wound, drain abscesses or deep infections, and keep the bacterial count to a minimum. For deep wounds, a radiograph of the foot can be helpful in determining the extent of bony involvement. Deep infections should be treated with broad-spectrum antibiotics initially. Most infections in this population are polymicrobial, involving gram-positive, gram-negative, and anaerobic organisms (152,186–189). An abscess or contained deep infection can be cultured and the antibiotic coverage tailored to the culture results. Cultures of superficial open wounds are rarely helpful, as most of these wounds are colonized with a multitude of organisms. Antibiotic use in these superficial open wounds is usually unnecessary.

For the most part, topical treatments are of little benefit to the management of diabetic foot ulcers. The long and growing list of topical agents is a testament to their lack of efficacy. No topical débriding agent can substitute for surgical débridement. Topical antimicrobials such as povidone-iodine (Betadine), acetic acid, Dakin solution, and hydrogen peroxide not only destroy surface bacteria but also destroy cellular elements critical to wound healing (3,220,221). Antibiotic ointments are safe and effective at reducing surface bacteria and should be used as an adjunct to and not a substitute for surgical débridement. They also maintain a moist environment, which promotes wound healing (222,223). Recent experimental studies with wound chambers have demonstrated accelerated wound healing in a wet environment (222). The potential benefits of wet treatments in diabetic wounds still remain to be explored. One of the only topical agents shown to be of any benefit in treating diabetic foot ulcers is platelet-derived growth factor (224–229). Once again, this growth factor accelerates healing in a clean wound and is not a substitute for adequate surgical débridement.

Once the wound itself has been optimized with débridement, drainage, and appropriate antibiotics, local conditions must be enhanced for healing to occur (203). First and foremost, tissue oxygenation must be adequate for wound healing to take place. Diabetic foot ulcers are most commonly found on the forefoot overlying the metatarsal heads or the interphalangeal joint of the great toe. Approximately 30% of these plantar forefoot ulcers are associated with significant atherosclerosis of the tibioperoneal vessels, which contribute to their poor healing (Fig. 69.3) (1,3,144–146). A pulse examination is a must in all patients with wounds in the foot. In the absence of palpable pedal pulses, a vascular workup is obligatory. Segmental pressure measurements, pulse volume recordings, transcutaneous oxygen pressures, and various diffusion clearing techniques can be used to assess the blood supply to the foot (3,230,231). It has been noted that successful treatment of an ulcer is better predicted by the degree of ischemia than by the extent of the ulcer itself (231). Another group looked at a number of variables and concluded that the local transcutaneous P_{O_2} is the critical physiologic determinant of healing in a diabetic ulcer (230). Furthermore, although atherosclerotic occlusive disease of the lower extremities is quite common in patients with diabetes, it is usually very amenable to reconstructive bypass surgery. Once the diagnosis is made, a vascular surgery consultation should be obtained (149–152).

Other local impediments to wound healing include edema and dry, inelastic skin. Edema is usually at its peak when the patient presents with an acutely inflamed, often infected, wound. Simple elevation and gentle compression will minimize edema and facilitate the diffusion of oxygen, nutrients, antibiotics, leukocytes, and fibroblasts to the healing wound. Elevation and compression should be gently balanced in the patient with occlusive vascular disease, as too much of either can further limit perfusion to an already ischemic wound. Optimizing cardiac and renal function, strict glucose control, eliminating infection, and maximizing nutrition will all aid in minimizing edema (152). Nutrition is often overlooked. A serum albumin of less than 3.0 g/dL is a poor prognostic sign and should be treated appropriately (232). Soaking the feet has been taught traditionally but has been shown to be of little benefit (233). In fact, soaking can lead to maceration of previously healthy tissues with progression of infection. In the insensate foot of the neuropathic patient, hot water may lead to further tissue damage. Instead, moisturizers are a safe alternative and can be used to keep the skin more pliable and, therefore, more resistant to cracking. Calluses should be removed proactively to minimize local pressure and shear (79,80).

Abnormally high local pressures are one of the main sources of diabetic foot ulcers. The insensate, misshapen diabetic foot is subjected to poorly distributed pressures without effective feedback. The result is chronic repetitive trauma, which culminates in an ulcer. Once the ulcer has been débrided, infections drained, and adequate blood supply confirmed, the patient must not bear weight on the wound for it to heal. Because these ulcers do not hurt, most patients continue to walk on them. The result is progression of the ulcer, not healing. Some have advocated the use of crutches and wheelchairs. However, most diabetic patients with significant neuropathy are somewhat ataxic, and the use of crutches can be dangerous (3,234).

One of the best techniques for optimizing conditions for wound healing, minimizing pressure on the ulcer, and allowing the patient to remain somewhat ambulatory is the total contact cast (3,75,234–239). The bony prominences of the foot are gently padded, a hydrocolloid or similar dressing is applied to the wound, and a below-knee plaster cast is applied. This redistributes pressures across the foot, minimizing point loading. Extending the cast to below the knee also minimizes shear, translating it into forward motion instead. A rocker bottom reduces forefoot loading on toe-off. A relatively occlusive environment is maintained to augment wound healing. The total contact cast is most effective in patients with adequate blood supply; an open, well-drained wound; no systemic signs of infection; and close follow-up (3,235–237,240). It has been shown that even locally infected wounds, including localized osteomyelitis, can be effectively treated with the occlusive cast (238,239). Excellent results have been reported with the total contact cast (241–246). Generally, 80% to 90% of ulcers are healed within 1 to 2 months. Smaller forefoot ulcers usually heal within 1 month. Larger ulcers and more posterior plantar ulcers tend to take longer. Even with the cast in place, weight bearing should be limited in this latter subgroup.

Once an ulcer has healed, the challenge of preventing a recurrence remains. Most recurrences happen in the first month, when the newly formed scar is most tenuous (237). Often this is attributed to infection, but usually the real culprit is shear. Careful examination will reveal the early preulcerative changes, including blistering, petechiae, erythema, and localized warmth. Protection from repeated stress is the key to prevention. Edmonds et al. (139,141) demonstrated how important proper footwear can be in preventing recurrence. Patients who returned to wearing their own shoes after an ulcer had healed had a recurrence rate of 83% as compared with a recurrence rate of 26% for those who were given specially designed protective shoes. The goal is to distribute the stresses of walking evenly over the entire plantar surface of the foot. This can be accomplished with a soft insole, a molded insole, or a rigid-soled rocker bottom shoe. Patients must be educated so that they understand the problem and will make a real attempt to alter their lifestyles. Walking habits need to be altered to minimize shear stress. Shear is greatest during fast walking, quick starts and stops, and with long strides (247).

Areas that cannot be addressed with a well-designed shoe need to be addressed surgically. It is almost impossible to maintain a healed ulcer in the face of a persistent bony deformity. Correction of clawing at the metatarsophalangeal joints and interphalangeal joints, arthrodesis of the interphalangeal joint of the great toe, resection of prominent metatarsal heads, and even lengthening of the Achilles tendon may all be necessary to maintain a healed ulcer (3,237). Interestingly, percutaneous lengthening of the Achilles tendon may be the single best treatment for a recurrent plantar forefoot ulcer in the face of an adequate blood supply. This improves ankle dorsiflexion, minimizing abnormal pressure on the forefoot during walking. Along with proper shoes or braces, significant decreases in recurrence are noted. The callus is another benign-appearing fixed deformity that must be dealt with aggressively in this population (3,217,234,237). All calluses should be viewed as preulcerative lesions, especially in the neuropathic foot with altered sympathetic function. These hyperkeratotic deformities in the context of a dry, insensate foot create severe localized shear and compressive stresses, creating the perfect milieu for ulcer formation. Calluses and unyielding bony prominences should be removed, the foot should be padded with custom-designed shoes and insoles, and skin cleansing and care with moisturizers should be emphasized. The patient must have a good appreciation of the problem and, together with an experienced and diligent clinician, work toward preventing these highly morbid wounds.

Acknowledgments

We would like to thank Dr. Julian Pribaz, Dr. Michael Conte, Ann Crowley, RNC, Christine Gallagher, Leyla Ganchi, and Guyon Ganchi for their contributions to this work.

REFERENCES

1. Morain W, Colen L. Wound healing in diabetes mellitus. *Clin Plast Surg* 1990;17:493–501.
2. Foster D. Diabetes mellitus. In: Fauci A, Braunwald E, Isselbacher K, et al., eds. *Harrison's principles of internal medicine*, 15th ed. New York: McGraw-Hill, 1998:2060.
3. Levin M. Pathogenesis and management of diabetic foot lesions. In: Levin M, O'Neal L, Bowker J, eds. *The diabetic foot*. St. Louis: Mosby–Year Book, 1993:17.
4. Pryce T. A case of perforating ulcers of both feet associated with diabetes and ataxic symptoms. *Lancet* 1887;2:11.
5. Bild D, Teutsch S. The control of hypertension in persons with diabetes: a public health approach. *Public Health Rep* 1987;102:522–529.
6. Stevens P. *Growth and innovation strategies*. Colleyville, TX, 2000.
7. Chittenden S, Shami S. Microangiopathy in diabetes mellitus: causes, prevention and treatment. *Diabetes Res* 1991;17:105–114.
8. Palumbo P, Melton L. Peripheral vascular disease and diabetes. In: National Diabetes Data Group, ed. *Diabetes in America*. Washington, DC: US Government Printing Office, 1985:1468.
9. Reiber G, Pecoraro R, Koepsell T. Risk factors for amputation in patients with diabetes mellitus. A case-control study. *Ann Intern Med* 1992;117:97–105.
10. Most R, Sinnock P. The epidemiology of lower extremity amputation in diabetic individuals. *Diabetes Care* 1983;87.
11. Reiber G. Diabetic foot care: financial implications and practical guidelines. *Diabetes Care* 1992;15[Suppl 1]:29–31.
12. Apelqvist J, Ragnarson-Tennvall G, Persson U, et al. Diabetic foot ulcers in a multi-disciplinary setting: an economic analysis of primary healing and healing with amputation. *J Intern Med* 1994;235:463–471.
13. Casey J, Flinn W, Yao J, et al. Correlation of immune and nutritional status with wound complications in patients undergoing vascular surgery. *Surgery* 1983;93:822–827.
14. Hjortrup C, Rasmussen B, Kehlet H. Morbidity in diabetic and non-diabetic patients after major vascular surgery. *BMJ* 1983;287:1107–1108.
15. Silhi N. Diabetes and wound healing. *J Wound Care* 1998;7:47–51.
16. Palmisano J. Surgery and diabetes. In: Kahn JR, Weir GC, eds. *Joslin's diabetes mellitus*, 13th ed. Philadelphia: Lea & Febiger, 1994:955–961.
17. Lawrie G, Morris G, Glaeser D. Influence of diabetes mellitus on the results of coronary bypass surgery: follow-up of 212 patients ten to 15 years after surgery. *JAMA* 1986;256:2967–2971.
18. Walsh D, Eckhauser F, Ramsburgh S, et al. Risk associated with diabetes mellitus in patients undergoing gallbladder surgery. *Surgery* 1982;91:254–257.
19. Hjortrup A, Sorensen C, Dyremose E. Influence of diabetes mellitus on operative risk. *Br J Surg* 1985;72:783–785.
20. Clement R, Rousou J, Engelman R, et al. Perioperative morbidity in diabetics requiring coronary artery bypass surgery. *Ann Thorac Surg* 1988;46:321–323.
21. Taitelman U, Reece E, Bessman A. Insulin in the management of the diabetic surgical patient, continuous intravenous infusion vs subcutaneous administration. *JAMA* 1977;237:658–660.
22. Gottrup F, Andreassen T. Healing of incisional wounds in stomach and duodenum: the influence of experimental diabetes. *J Surg Res* 1981;31: 61–68.
23. Goodson W, Hunt T. Wound healing and the diabetic patient. *Surg Gynecol Obstet* 1979;149:600.
24. Goodson W, Hunt T. Deficient collagen formation by obese mice in a standard wound model. *Am J Surg* 1979;138:692–694.
25. McMurry J. Wound healing with diabetes mellitus. *Surg Clin North Am* 1984;64:769–778.
26. Yue D, McLennan S, Marsh M, et al. Effects of experimental diabetes, uremia and malnutrition on wound healing. *Diabetes* 1987;36:295–299.
27. Yue D, Swanson B, McLennan S, et al. Abnormalities of granulation tissue and collagen formation in experimental diabetes, uremia and malnutrition. *Diabet Med* 1986;3:221–225.
28. Robertson H, Polk H. The mechanism of infection in patients with diabetes mellitus: a review of leukocyte malfunction. *Surgery* 1974;75:123–128.
29. Bagdade J, Stewart M, Walters E. Impaired granulocyte adherence: a reversible defect in host defense in patients with poorly controlled diabetes. *Diabetes* 1978;27:677–681.
30. Molenaar D, Palumbo P, Wilson W, et al. Leukocyte chemotaxis in diabetic patients and their nondiabetic first-degree relatives. *Diabetes* 1976;25 [Suppl 2]:880–883.
31. Mowat A, Baum J. Chemotaxis of polymorphonuclear leukocytes from patients with diabetes mellitus. *N Engl J Med* 1971;284:621–627.
32. Hostetter M. Handicaps to host defense: effects of hyperglycemia on C3 and *Candida albicans*. *Diabetes* 1990;39:271–275.
33. Ward J, Tesfaye S. Pathogenesis of diabetic neuropathy. In: Pickup J, Williams G, eds. *Textbook of diabetes*. London: Blackwell Sciences, 1997:49.1.
34. Greene D, Feldman E, Stevens M. Neuropathy in the diabetic foot: new concepts in etiology and treatment. In: Levin M, O'Neal L, Bowker L. eds. *The diabetic foot*. St. Louis: Mosby–Year Book, 1993:135.
35. Melton L, Dyck P. Epidemiology. In: Dyck P, Thomas P, Asbury A, eds. *Diabetic neuropathy*, Philadelphia: WB Saunders, 1987.
36. Watkins P, Edmonds M. Clinical features of diabetic neuropathy. In: Pickup J, Williams G, eds. *Textbook of diabetes*. London: Blackwell Sciences, 1997; 50.1.
37. Thomas P, Brown P. Diabetic polyneuropathy. In: Dyck P, Thomas P, Asbury A, eds. *Diabetic neuropathy*. Philadelphia: WB Saunders, 1987.
38. Dyck P, Sherman W, Hallcher L. Human diabetic endoneurial sorbitol, fructose, and myo-inositol related to sural nerve morphometry. *Ann Neurol* 1980;8:590–596.
39. Brown M, Martin J, Asbury A. Painful diabetic neuropathy: a morphometric study. *Arch Neurol* 1976;33:164–167.
40. Dyck P, Hansen S, Karnes J, et al. Capillary number and percentage closed in human diabetic sural nerve. *Proc Natl Acad Sci U S A* 1985;52:2513–2517.
41. Hill M, Colen L, Vinik A. Microvascular and compression mechanisms in the etiology of diabetic neuropathy. In: LeRoith D, Taylor S, Olefsky J, eds. *Diabetes mellitus*. Philadelphia: Lippincott-Raven Publishers, 1996:759.
42. Llewelyn J, Gilbey S, Thomas B, et al. Sural nerve morphometry in diabetic autonomic and painful sensory neuropathy: a clinicopathological study. *Brain* 1991;44:867–892.
43. Simmons DA. Pathogenesis of diabetic neuropathy. In: Kahn CR, Weir GC, eds. *Joslin's diabetes mellitus*, 13th ed. Philadelphia: Lea & Febiger, 1994: 665–690.
44. Greene D, Sima A, Albers J. Diabetic neuropathy. In: Rifkin H, Porte D, eds. *Diabetes mellitus, theory and practice*. St. Louis: Mosby–Year Book, 1990.
45. Boulton A, Knight G, Drury J, et al. The prevalence of symptomatic diabetic neuropathy in an insulin treated population. *Diabetes Care* 1985;8:125–128.
46. Lehtinen J, Uusitupa M, Siitonen O, et al. Prevalence of neuropathy in newly diagnosed NIDDM and nondiabetic control subjects. *Diabetes* 1989;38:1307–1313.
47. Maser R, Steenkiste A, Dorman J, et al. Epidemiological correlates of diabetic neuropathy. *Diabetes* 1989;8:1456–1461.
48. Neil H, Thompson A, John S, et al. Prevalence of diabetic neuropathy in a community. *Diabet Med* 1989;6:20.
49. Young M, Boulton A, MacLeod A, et al. A multicentre study of the prevalence of diabetic peripheral neuropathy in the United Kingdom Hospital clinic population. *Diabetologia* 1993;36:150–153.
50. Newrick P, Boulton A, Ward J. The distribution of diabetic neuropathy in a British clinic population. *Diabetes Res Clin Pract* 1986;2:263.
51. DCCT Research Group. Factors in development of diabetic neuropathy. Baseline analysis of neuropathy in feasibility phase of Diabetes Control and Complications Trial (DCCT). *Diabetologia* 1988;37:476–481.
52. Porte D, Graf R, Halter J, et al. Diabetic neuropathy and plasma glucose control. *Am J Med* 1981;70:195–200.
53. Thomas P. Diabetic neuropathy: models, mechanisms and mayhem. *Can J Neurol Sci* 1992;19:1–7.
54. Pirart J. Diabetes mellitus and its degenerative complications: a prospective study of 4400 patients observed between 1947 and 1973. *Diabetes Care* 1978; 1:168.
55. Harati Y. Frequently asked questions about diabetic peripheral neuropathies. *Neurol Clin* 1992;10:783–807.
56. Canal N, Comi G, Saibene V. The relationship between peripheral and autonomic neuropathy in insulin dependent diabetes: a clinical and instrumental evaluation. In: Canal N, Pozza G, eds. *Peripheral neuropathies*. Amsterdam: Elsevier, 1978:247.
57. Fernandez-Castaner M, Mendola G, Levy I. The prevalence and clinical aspects of the cardiovascular autonomic neuropathy in diabetic patients [in Spanish]. *Med Clin* (Barc) 1984;84:215.
58. Ewing D, Clarke B. Diabetic autonomic neuropathy: present insights and future prospects. *Diabetes Care* 1986;9:648–665.
59. O'Brien I, O'Hare J, Lewin I, et al. The prevalence of autonomic neuropathy in insulin-dependent diabetes mellitus: a controlled study based on heart rate variability. *Q J Med* 1986;61:957–967.
60. Krolewski A, Warram J, Cupples A, et al. Hypertension, orthostatic hypotension and the microvascular complications of diabetes. *J Chronic Dis* 1985;38:319–326.
61. Caputo G, Cavanagh P, Ulbrecht J, et al. Assessment and management of foot disease in patients with diabetes. *N Engl J Med* 1994;331:854–521.
62. Pecoraro P, Reiber G, Burgess E. Pathways to diabetic limb amputation: basis for prevention. *Diabetes Care* 1990;13:513–521.
63. Boulton A. The diabetic foot: neuropathic in aetiology? *Diabet Med* 1990; 7:852–858.
64. Boulton A. Peripheral neuropathy and the diabetic foot. *The Foot* 1992;2:67.
65. Young M, Breddy J, Veves A, et al. The prediction of neuropathic foot ulceration using vibration perception thresholds. *Diabetes Care* 1994;17:557–560.
66. Sosenko J, Kato M, Sozo R, et al. Comparison of quantitative sensory-threshold measures for their association with foot ulceration in diabetic patients. *Diabetes Care* 1990;13:1057–1061.
67. Birke J, Sims D. Plantar sensory threshold in the ulcerative foot. *Lepr Rev* 1986;57:261.
68. Klenerman L, McCabe C, Cogley D, et al. Screening for patients at risk of diabetic foot ulceration in a general diabetic outpatient clinic. *Diabet Med* 1996;13:561–563.
69. Edmonds M, Roberts V, Watkins P. Blood flow in the diabetic neuropathic foot. *Diabetologia* 1982;22:9–15.
70. Watkins P, Edmonds M. Sympathetic nerve failure in diabetes. *Diabetologia* 1983;25:73–77.
71. Flynn M, Edmonds M, Tooke J, et al. Direct measurement of capillary blood flow in the diabetic neuropathic foot. *Diabetologia* 1988;31:652–656.
72. Archer A, Watkins P, Roberts V. Blood flow patterns in painful diabetic neuropathy. *Diabetologia* 1984;27:563–567.
73. Boulton A, Scarpello J, Ward J. Venous oxygenation in the diabetic neuropathic foot: evidence of arteriovenous shunting? *Diabetologia* 1982;22:6–8.

74. Edmonds M, Archer A, Watkins P. Ephedrine: a new treatment for diabetic neuropathic oedema. *Lancet* 1;1983;548–551.
75. Boulton A. Foot problems in patients with diabetes mellitus. In: Pickup J, Williams G, eds. *Textbook of diabetes*. London: Blackwell Sciences, 1997:58.1.
76. Edmonds M, Clarke M, Newton S, et al. Increased uptake of bone radio-pharmaceutical in diabetic neuropathy. *Q J Med* 1985;57:843–855.
77. Veves A, Murray H, Young M, et al. The risk of foot ulceration in diabetic patients with high foot pressure: a prospective study. *Diabetologia* 1992;35: 660–663.
78. Macfarlane R, Jeffcoate W. Factors contributing to the presentation of diabetic foot ulcers. *Diabet Med* 1997;14:867–870.
79. Young M, Cavanagh P, Thomas G, et al. Effect of callus removal on dynamic foot pressures in diabetic patients. *Diabet Med* 1992;9:55–57.
80. Murray H, Young M, Boulton A. Relationship between callus formation, pressures and neuropathy in diabetic foot ulceration. *Diabet Med* 1994;11 [Suppl 2]:5.
81. Service F, Rizza R, Daube J. Near normoglycaemia: improved nerve conduction and vibration sensation in diabetic neuropathy. *Diabetologia* 1985;28:722–727.
82. Kennedy W, Navarro X, Goetz F, et al. Effects of pancreatic transplantation on diabetic neuropathy. *N Engl J Med* 1990;322:1031–1037.
83. The Diabetes Control and Complications Trial Research Group. The effect of intensive treatment of diabetes on the development and progression of long-term complications in insulin-dependent diabetes mellitus. *N Engl J Med* 1993;329:977–986.
84. Greene D, Sima A, Stevens M, et al. Complications: neuropathy, pathogenetic considerations. *Diabetes Care* 1992;15:1902–1925.
85. Greene D, Lattimer S, Sima A. Sorbitol, phosphoinositides and sodium-potassium-ATPase in the pathogenesis of diabetic complications. *N Engl J Med* 1987;316:599–606.
86. Dvornik D. Hyperglycemia in the pathogenesis of diabetic complications. In: Porte D, ed. *Aldose reductase inhibition: an approach to the prevention of diabetic complications*. New York: McGraw-Hill, 1987:69.
87. Tuck R, Schmelzer J, Low P. Endoneurial blood flow and oxygen tension in the sciatic nerve of rats with experimental diabetic neuropathy. *Brain* 1984;107:935.
88. Cameron N, Cotter M, Low P. Nerve blood flow in early experimental diabetes in rats: relation to conduction deficits. *Am J Physiol* 1991;261:E1.
89. Cameron N, Cotter M, Ferguson K. Effects of chronic alpha-adrenergic receptor blockade on peripheral nerve conduction, hypoxic resistance, polyols, Na/K-ATPase activity, and vascular supply in STZ-D rats. *Diabetes* 1991;40:1652–1658.
90. Brownlee M. Glycation products and the pathogenesis of diabetic complications. *Diabetes Care* 1992;15:1835.
91. Richard S, Tamas C, Sell D, et al. Tissue-specific effects of aldose reductase inhibition on fluorescence and cross-linking of extracellular matrix in chronic galactosemia. Relationship to pentosidine cross-links. *Diabetes* 1991;40:1049–1056.
92. Moncada S, Palmer R, Higg E. Nitric oxide: physiology, pathophysiology and pharmacology. *Pharmacol Rev* 1991;43:109–142.
93. Gryglewski R, Palmer R, Moncada S. Superoxide anion is involved in the breakdown of endothelium-derived vascular relaxing factor. *Nature* 1986;320: 454–456.
94. Bertelsmann F, Faes T, de Weerdt O. Treatment of diabetic autonomic neuropathy with the aldose reductase inhibitor Statil. *Diabetologia* 1991;34[Suppl 2]:A37.
95. Boulton A, Levin S, Comstock JA. multicentre trial of the aldose-reductase inhibitor, tolrestat, in patients with symptomatic diabetic neuropathy. *Diabetologia* 1990;33:431–437.
96. Christensen J, Varnek L, Gregersen G. The effect of an aldose reductase inhibitor (sorbinil) on diabetic neuropathy and neural function of the retina: a double-blind study. *Acta Neurol Scand* 1985;71:164–167.
97. Young R, Ewing D, Clark B. A controlled trial of sorbinil, an aldose reductase inhibitor, in chronic painful diabetic neuropathy. *Diabetes* 1983;32:938–942.
98. Greene D, Stevens M. The sorbitol-osmotic and sorbitol-redox hypotheses. In: LeRoith S, Taylor S, Olefsky J, eds. *Diabetes mellitus*. Philadelphia: Lippincott-Raven Publishers, 1996:801.
99. Moriyama T, Garcia-Perez A, Burg M. High extracellular NaCl stimulates synthesis of aldose reductase, an osmoregulatory protein, in renal medullary cells. *Kidney Int* 1989;35:499.
100. Kwon MH, Yamauchi A, Uchida S. Renal Na-myo-inositol cotransporter mRNA expression in Xenopus oocytes: regulation by hypertonicity. *Am J Physiol* 1991;260:F258–F263.
101. Burg M, Kador P. Sorbitol, osmoregulation, and the complications of diabetes. *J Clin Invest* 1988;81:635–640.
102. Tomlinson D. Polyols and myoinositol in diabetic neuropathy—of mice and men. *Mayo Clin Proc* 1989;64:1030–1033.
103. Stevens M, Lattimer S, Kamijo M. Osmotically induced nerve taurine depletion and the compatible osmolyte hypothesis in experimental diabetic neuropathy in the rat. *Diabetologia* 1993;36:608–614.
104. Griffey R, Eaton R, Sibbitt R. Diabetic neuropathy: structural analysis of nerve hydration by magnetic resonance spectroscopy. *JAMA* 1988;260:2872–2878.
105. Huxtable R. From heart to hypothesis: a mechanism for the calcium modulatory effects on actions of taurine. In: Huxtable R, Franconi F, Giotti A, eds. *The biology of taurine: methods and mechanisms*. New York: Plenum Press, 1987:371.
106. Malone J, Lowitt S, Cook W. Nonosmotic diabetic cataracts. *Pediatr Res* 1990;27:293–296.
107. Lombardi J. Effects of taurine on calcium ion uptake and protein phosphorylation in rat retinal membrane preparations. *J Neurochem* 1985;45:268.
108. Nakamura J, Del Monte M, Shewach D. Inhibition of phosphatidylinositol synthase by glucose in human retinal pigment epithelial cells. *Am J Physiol* 1992;262:E417–E426.
109. Cheung W. Calmodulin plays a pivotal role in cellular regulation. *Science* 1980;207:19–27.
110. Nestler E, Greengard P. Protein phosphorylation in the brain. *Nature* 1983; 305:583.
111. Greene D, De Jesus P, Winegrad A. Effects of insulin and dietary myoinositol on impaired peripheral motor nerve conduction velocity in acute streptozotocin diabetes. *J Clin Invest* 1975;55:1326–1336.
112. Greene D, Lattimer S, Ulbrecht J, et al. Glucose-induced alterations in nerve metabolism: current perspective on the pathogenesis of diabetic neuropathy and future directions for research and therapy. *Diabetes Care* 1985;8:290–299.
113. Greene D, Lattimer S. Action of sorbinil in diabetic peripheral nerve. Relationship of polyol (sorbitol) pathway inhibition to a myo-inositol-mediated defect in sodium-potassium ATPase activity. *Diabetes* 1984;33:712–714.
114. Tomlinson D, Sidenius P, Larsen JR. Slow component-a of axonal transport, nerve myo-inositol and aldose reductase inhibition in streptozotocin-diabetic rats. *Diabetes* 1986;35:398–402.
115. Tomlinson D, Mayer J. Reversal of deficits in axonal transport and nerve conduction velocity by treatment of streptozotocin diabetic rats with myo-inositol. *Exp Neurol* 1985;89:420–427.
116. Finegold D, Lattimer S, Nolle S. Polyol pathway activity and myo-inositol metabolism: a suggested relationship in the pathogenesis of diabetic neuropathy. *Diabetes* 1983;32:988.
117. Lambourne J, Tomlinson D, Brown A, et al. Opposite effects of diabetes and galactosaemia on adenosine triphosphatase activity in rat nervous tissue. *Diabetologia* 1987;30:360–362.
118. Llewelyn J, Patel N, Thomas P. Sodium, potassium adenosine triphosphatase activity in peripheral nerve tissue of galactosaemic rats. Effects of aldose reductase inhibition. *Diabetologia* 1987;30:971–972.
119. Hale P, Nattrass M, Silverman S. Peripheral nerve concentrations of glucose, fructose, sorbitol and myoinositol in diabetic and non-diabetic patients. *Diabetologia* 1987;30:464–467.
120. Dyck P, Zimmerman B, Vilen T, et al. Nerve glucose, fructose, sorbitol, myo-inositol, and fibre degeneration and regeneration in diabetic neuropathy. *N Engl J Med* 1988;319:542–548.
121. Cameron N, Cotter M. The relationship of vascular changes to metabolic factors in diabetes mellitus and their role in the development of peripheral nerve complications. *Diabetes Metab Rev* 1994;10:189–224.
122. Moncada S, Palmer R, Higgs E. Biosynthesis of nitric oxide from L-arginine: a pathway for the regulation of cell function and communication. *Biochem Pharmacol* 1989;38:1709–1715.
123. Durante W, Sen A, Sunahara F. Impairment of endothelium-dependent relaxation in aorta from spontaneously diabetic rats. *Br J Pharmacol* 1988;94:463–468.
124. Kamata K, Miyata N, Kasuya Y. Impairment of endothelium-dependent relaxation and changes in levels of cyclic GMP in aorta from streptozotocin-induced diabetic rats. *Br J Pharmacol* 1989;97:614–618.
125. Vallance P, Collier J, Moncada S. Effects of endothelium-derived nitric oxide on peripheral arterial tone in man. *Lancet* 1989;2:997–1000.
126. Carroll P, Thornton B, Greene D. Glutathione redox state is not the link between polyol pathway activity and diminished (Na, K)-ATPase activity in experimental diabetic neuropathy. *Diabetes* 1986;35:1282–1285.
127. Garthwaite J, Charles S, Chess-Williams R. Endothelium-derived relaxing factor release on activation of NMDA receptors suggests role as intercellular messenger in the brain. *Nature* 1988;336:385–388.
128. Stevens M, Dananberg J, Feldman E, et al. The linked roles of nitric oxide, aldose reductase and (Na, K)-ATPase in the slowing of nerve conduction in the streptozotocin diabetic rat. *J Clin Invest* 1994;94:853–859.
129. Rapoport R, Murad F. Agonist-induced endothelium-dependent relaxation in the rat thoracic aorta may be mediated through cGMP. *Circ Res* 1983;52: 352–357.
130. Hammes H-P, Brownlee M. Advanced glycation end products and the pathogenesis of diabetic complications. In: LeRoith D, Taylor, Olefsky J, eds. *Diabetes mellitus: a fundamental and clinical text*. Philadelphia: Lippincott-Raven Publishers, 1996:810.
131. Cullum N, Mahon J, Stringer K, et al. Glycation of rat sciatic nerve tubulin in experimental diabetes mellitus. *Diabetologia* 1991;34:387–389.
132. Kihara M, Schmelzer M, Poduslo J, et al. Aminoguanidine effects on nerve blood flow, vascular permeability, electrophysiology and oxygen free radicals. *Proc Natl Acad Sci U S A* 1991;88:6107–6111.
133. Cameron N, Cotter M, Dines K, et al. Effects of aminoguanidine on peripheral nerve function and polyol pathway metabolites in streptozotocin-diabetic rats. *Diabetologia* 1992;35:946–950.
134. Laing P. The development and complications of diabetic foot ulcers. *Am J Surg* 1998;176[Suppl 2A]:11S.
135. Abbott R, Brand F, Kannel W. Epidemiology of some peripheral arterial findings in diabetic men and women: experiences from the Framingham Study. *Am J Med* 1990;88:376–381.
136. Wellman K, Volk B. Historical review. In: Volk B, Wellman K, ed. *The diabetic pancreas*. New York: Plenum Press, 1977:1.
137. McNeely M, Boyko E, Ahroni J, et al. The independent contributions of diabetic neuropathy and vasculopathy in foot ulceration. How great are the risks? *Diabetes Care* 1995;18:216–219.

138. Thompson F, Veves A, Ashe H. A team approach to diabetic foot care: the Manchester experience. *The Foot* 1991;1:75.
139. Edmonds M. Experience in a multi-disciplinary diabetic foot clinic. In: Connor H, Boulton A, Ward J, eds. *The foot in diabetes*. Chichester: John Wiley and Sons, 1987:121.
140. Holewski J, Moss K, Sless R. Prevalence of foot pathology and lower extremity complications in a diabetic outpatient clinic. *J Rehabil Res Dev* 1989; 26:35.
141. Edmonds M, Blundell M, Morris H. The diabetic foot: impact of a foot clinic. *Q J Med* 1986;232:763.
142. Caldwell M, Shearer J, Morris A, et al. Evidence for aerobic glycolysis in lambda-carrageenan wounded skeletal muscle. *J Surg Res* 1984;37:63–68.
143. MacKaay A, Beks P, Dur A, et al. The distribution of peripheral vascular disease in a Dutch caucasian population: comparison of type II diabetic and non-diabetic subjects. *Eur J Vasc Endovasc Surg* 1995;9:170–175.
144. Janka H, Standl E, Mehnert H. Peripheral vascular disease in diabetes mellitus and its relation to cardiovascular risk factors: screening with Doppler ultrasonic technique. *Diabetes Care* 1980;3:207–213.
145. Levin M, Sicard G. Evaluating and treating diabetic peripheral vascular disease: part I. *Clin Diabetes* 1987;5:62.
146. Logerfo F, Gibbons G. Vascular disease of the lower extremities in diabetes mellitus: etiology and management. In: Kahn CR, Weir GC, eds. *Joslin's diabetes mellitus*, 13th ed. Philadelphia: Lea & Febiger, 1994: 970–975.
147. Conrad M. Large and small artery occlusion in diabetics and nondiabetics with severe vascular disease. *Circulation* 1967;36:83–91.
148. Strandness D, Priest R, Gibbons G. Combined clinical and pathologic study of diabetic and nondiabetic peripheral arterial disease. *Diabetes* 1964;13:366–372.
149. Cantelmo N, Snow J, Menzoian J, et al. Successful vein bypass in patients with an ischemic limb and a palpable popliteal pulse. *Arch Surg* 1986;121: 217–220.
150. Stonebridge P, Tsoukas A, Pomposelli F, et al. Popliteal-to-distal bypass grafts for limb salvage in diabetics. *Eur J Vasc Surg* 1991;5:265–269.
151. Auer A, Hurley J, Binnington H, et al. Distal tibial vein grafts for limb salvage. *Arch Surg* 1983;118:597–602.
152. Reiber G, Lipsky B, Gibbons G. The burden of diabetic foot ulcers. *Am J Surg* 1998;176[Suppl 2A]:5S.
153. Goldenberg S, Alex M, Joshi R. Nonatheromatous peripheral vascular disease of the lower extremity in diabetes mellitus. *Diabetes* 1959;8:261–273.
154. Barner H, Kaiser G, Willman V. Blood flow in the diabetic leg. *Circulation* 1971;43:391–394.
155. Wyss C, Matsen F, Simmons C, et al. Transcutaneous oxygen tension measurements on limbs of diabetic and nondiabetic patients with peripheral vascular disease. *Surgery* 1994;95:339–346.
156. Krahenbuhl B, Mossaz A. On vascular non-disease of the foot in diabetes. *N Engl J Med* 1985;312:1190–1191.
157. LoGerfo F, Coffman J. Current concepts: vascular and microvascular disease of the foot in diabetes: implications for foot care. *N Engl J Med* 1984;311: 1615–1619.
158. McMillan D. The microcirculation in diabetes. *Microcirc Endothel Lymph* 1984;1:3.
159. Isogai Y, Iida A, Michizuki K, et al. Hemorheological studies on the pathogenesis of diabetic microangiopathy. *Thromb Res* 1976;8[Suppl 2]:17–24.
160. McMillan D, Utterback N, LaPuma J. Reduced erythrocyte deformity in diabetes. *Diabetes* 1982;31[Suppl 3]:64.
161. Maeda N, Kon K, Imiazumi I. Alteration of rheological properties of human erythrocytes by crosslinking of membrane proteins. *Biochim Biophys Acta* 1983;735:104–112.
162. Bridges J, Dalby A, Millar J. An effect of D-glucose on platelet stickiness. *Lancet* 1965;1:75.
163. Thomas P, Eliason S. Diabetic neuropathy. In: Dyck P, Thomas P, Lambert E, eds. *Peripheral neuropathy*. Philadelphia: WB Saunders, 1984:1173.
164. Simpson L. Intrinsic stiffening of red blood cells as the fundamental cause of diabetic nephropathy and microangiopathy: a new hypothesis. *Nephron* 1985;39:344–351.
165. Juhan L, Bunoacare M, Jouve R. Abnormalities of erythrocyte deformability and platelet aggregation in insulin-dependent diabetics corrected by insulin in vivo and in vitro. *Lancet* 1982;1:535.
166. Schmid-Schonbein H, Wells R, Goldstone J. Influence of deformability of human red cells upon blood viscosity. *Circ Res* 1969;25:131–143.
167. Ditzel J. Changes in red cell oxygen release capacity in diabetes mellitus. *Fed Proc* 1979;38:2484–2488.
168. McDonald M, Bleichman M, Bunn H, et al. Functional properties of the glycosylated minor components of human hemoglobin. *J Biol Chem* 1979;254: 702–707.
169. Goodson W, Hunt T. Wound collagen accumulation in obese hyperglycaemic mice. *Diabetes* 1986;35:491–495.
170. Flynn M, Tooke J. Aetiology of diabetic foot ulceration: a role for the microcirculation? *Diabet Med* 1992;8:320–329.
171. Klamer T, Towne J, Bandyk D. The influence of sepsis and ischemia on the natural history of the diabetic foot. *Am Surg* 1987;53:490–494.
172. Cruse P, Foord R. A five-year prospective study of 23,649 surgical wounds. *Arch Surg* 1973;107:206.
173. Boyko E, Lipsky B. Infection and diabetes mellitus. In: National Diabetes Data Group. *Diabetes in America,* 2nd ed. Bethesda, MD: National Institute of Diabetes and Digestive and Kidney Diseases, 1995:485. NIDDKD publication 95-1468.
174. Spelman D, Russo P, Harrington G, et al. Risk factors for surgical wound infection and bacteremia following coronary artery bypass surgery. *Aust N Z J Surg* 2000;70:47–51.
175. Carpino P, Khabbaz K, Bojar R, et al. Clinical benefits of endoscopic vein harvesting in patients with risk factors for saphenectomy wound infections undergoing coronary artery bypass grafting. *J Thorac Cardiovasc Surg* 2000; 119: 69–75.
176. Allen K, Griffith G, Heimansohn D, et al. Endoscopic versus traditional saphenous vein harvesting: a prospective randomized trial. *Ann Thorac Surg* 1998;66:26–31.
177. Borger M, Rao V, Weisel R, et al. Deep sternal wound infection: risk factors and outcomes. *Ann Thorac Surg* 1998;65:1050–1056.
178. Zerr K, Furnary A, Grunkemeier G, et al. Glucose control lowers the risk of wound infection in diabetics after open heart operations. *Ann Thorac Surg* 1997;63:356–361.
179. Shpitz B, Sigal A, Kaufman Z, et al. Acute cholecystitis in diabetic patients. *Am Surg* 1995;61:964–967.
180. Babineau T, Bothe A. General surgery considerations in the diabetic patient. *Infect Dis Clin North Am* 1995;9:183–193.
181. Grossi E, Esposito R, Harris L, et al. Sternal wound infections and use of internal mammary artery grafts. *Cardiovasc Surg* 1991;102:342–346.
182. Hickman M, Schwesinger W, Page C. Acute cholecystitis in the diabetic: a case-control study of outcome. *Arch Surg* 1988;123:409–411.
183. Josephs L, Cordts P, DiEdwardo C, et al. Do infected inguinal lymph nodes increase the incidence of postoperative groin wound infection? *J Vasc Surg* 1993;17:1077–1080.
184. Wymenga A, van Horn J, Theeuwes A, et al. Perioperative factors associated with septic arthritis after arthroplasty. Prospective multicenter study of 362 knee and 2,651 hip operations. *Acta Orthop Scand* 1992;63:665–671.
185. Robison J, Ross J, Brothers T, et al. Distal wound complications following pedal bypass: analysis of risk factors. *Ann Vasc Surg* 1995;9:53.
186. Lipsky B, Pecoraro R, Wheat J. The diabetic foot: soft tissue and bone infection. *Infect Dis Clin North Am* 1990;4:409–432.
187. Frykberg R, Veves A. Diabetic foot infections. *Diabetes Metab Rev* 1996;12: 255–270.
188. Lipsky B, Pecoraro R, Ahroni J. Foot ulceration and infections in elderly diabetics. *Clin Geriatr Med* 1990;6:747–769.
189. Sapico F, Witte J, Canawati H, et al. The infected foot of the diabetic patient: quantitative microbiology and analysis of clinical features. *Rev Infect Dis* 1984;6[Suppl 1]:S171–S176.
190. Pozzilli P, Leslie R. Infections and diabetes: mechanisms and prospects for prevention. *Diabet Med* 1994;11:935–941.
191. Goodson W, Hunt T. Wound healing in experimental diabetes mellitus, importance of early insulin therapy. *Surg Forum* 1978;29:95–98.
192. Goodson W, Hunt T. Studies of wound healing in experimental diabetes mellitus. *J Surg Res* 1987;22:221.
193. Nolan C, Beaty H, Bagdade J. Further characterization of the impaired bactericidal function of granulocytes in patients with poorly controlled diabetes. *Diabetes* 1978;27:889–894.
194. Bybee J, Rogers D. The phagocytic activity of polymorphonuclear leukocytes obtained from patients with diabetes mellitus. *J Lab Clin Med* 1964;64:1.
195. Bagdade J, Walters E. Impaired granulocyte adherence in mildly diabetic patients: effects of tolazamide treatment. *Diabetes* 1980;29:309–311.
196. Bagdade J, Root R, Bugler R. Impaired leukocyte function in patients with poorly controlled diabetes. *Diabetes* 1974;23:9–15.
197. Tan J, Anderson J, Watanakunakorn D, et al. Neutrophil dysfunction in diabetes mellitus. *J Lab Clin Med* 1975;85:26–33.
198. Ainsworth S, Allison F. Studies on the pathogenesis of acute inflammation: the inflammatory response induced by thermal injury to ear chambers of rabbits. *J Clin Invest* 1970;49:433–441.
199. Brayton R, Stokes P, Schwarz M. Effect of alcohol and various diseases on leukocyte mobilization, phagocytosis and intracellular bacterial killing. *N Engl J Med* 1970;282:123–128.
200. Stadelmann W, Digenis A, Tobin G. Impediments to wound healing. *Am J Surg* 1998;176[Suppl 2A]:39S.
201. Bagdade J, Nielson K, Bulger R. Reversible abnormalities in phagocytic function in poorly controlled diabetes. *Am J Med Sci* 1972;263:451–456.
202. Caricco T, Mehrhof A, Cohen I. Biology of wound healing. *Surg Clin North Am* 1984;64:721–733.
203. Rosenberg C. Wound healing in the patient with diabetes mellitus. *Nursing Clin North Am* 1990;25:247–261.
204. Pecoraro R, Chen M. Ascorbic acid in diabetes mellitus. *Ann N Y Acad Sci* 1987;498:248–256.
205. Miller M, Baker L. Leukocyte functions in juvenile diabetes mellitus: humoral and cellular aspects. *J Pediatr* 1972;81:979–982.
206. Repine J, Clawson C, Goetz F. Bactericidal function of neutrophils from patients with acute bacterial infection and from diabetics. *J Infect Dis* 1980; 142:869–875.
207. Gin H, Brottier E, Aubertin J. Influence of glycaemic normalisation on phagocytic and bactericidal functions of granulocytes in insulin dependent diabetes patients. *J Clin Pathol* 1984;37:1029–1031.
208. Weringer E, Kelso J, Tamai I. The effect of insulin 2-deoxyglucose-induced hyperglycemia and starvation on wound healing in normal mice. *Diabetes* 1981;30:407–410.
209. Arquilla E, Weringer E, Nakajo M. Wound healing: a model for the study of diabetic angiopathy. *Diabetes* 1976;25[Suppl 2]:811–819.

210. Snip RC, Thoft R, Tolentino F. Similar epithelial healing rates of the corneas of diabetic and nondiabetic patients. *Am J Ophthalmol* 1980;90:463–468.
211. Fowler S. Wound healing in the corneal epithelium in diabetic and normal rats. *Exp Eye Res* 1980;31:167–179.
212. Seifter E, Rettura G, Padawer J, et al. Impaired wound healing in streptozotocin diabetes, prevention by supplemental vitamin A. *Ann Surg* 1981;194: 42–50.
213. Engel E, Erlick N, Davis R. Diabetes mellitus: impaired wound healing from zinc deficiency. *J Am Podiatry Assoc* 1981;71:536–544.
214. Kohn R, Hensse S. Abnormal collagen in cultures of fibroblasts from diabetic patients. *Biochem Biophys Res Comm* 1978;76:765.
215. Grotendorst G, Martin G, Pencev D, et al. Stimulation of granulation tissue formation by platelet-derived growth factor in normal and diabetic rats. *J Clin Invest* 1985;76:2323–2329.
216. Alberti K, Press C. The biochemistry of the complications of diabetes mellitus. In: Keen H, Jarrett J, ed. *Complications of diabetes*. London: Edward Arnold, 1992.
217. Reiber G, Vileikyte L, Boyko E, et al. Causal pathways for incident lower-extremity ulcers in patients with diabetes from two settings. *Diabetes Care* 1999;22:157–162.
218. Griffiths G, Wieman T. Meticulous attention to foot care improves the prognosis in diabetic ulceration. *Surg Gynecol Obstet* 1992;174:49.
219. Dyck P. New understanding and treatment of diabetic neuropathy. *N Engl J Med* 1992;326:1287–1288.
220. Lineaweaver W, Howard R, Soucy D, et al. Topical antimicrobial toxicity. *Arch Surg* 1985;120:267–270.
221. Oberg M, Lindsey D. Do not put hydrogen peroxide or povidone iodine in wounds! *Am J Dis Child* 1987;141:27–28.
222. Svensjo T, Pomahac B, Yao F, et al. Accelerated healing of full-thickness skin wounds in a wet environment. *Plast Reconstr Surg* 2000;106:602–612.
223. Field C, Kerstein M. Overview of wound healing in a moist environment. *Am J Surg* 1993;167[Suppl 1A]:2S–6S.
224. Smiell J. Clinical safety of becaplermin (rhPDGF-BB) gel. Becaplermin Study Group. *Am J Surg* 1998;176[Suppl 2A]:68S–73S.
225. Smiell J, Wieman T, Steed D, et al. Efficacy and safety of becaplermin (recombinant human platelet-derived growth factor-BB) in patients with nonhealing, lower extremity diabetic ulcers: a combined analysis of four randomized studies. *Wound Repair Regen* 1999;7:335–346.
226. Wieman T. Clinical efficacy of becaplermin (rhPDGF-BB) gel. Becaplermin Gel Study Group. *Am J Surg* 11998;76[Suppl 2A]:74S–79S.
227. Embil J, Papp K, Sibbald G, et al. Recombinant human platelet-derived growth factor-BB (becaplermin) for healing chronic lower extremity ulcers: an open-label clinical evaluation of efficacy. *Wound Repair Regen* 2000;8: 162–168.
228. Temple M, Nahata M. Pharmacotherapy of lower limb diabetic ulcers. *J Am Geriatr Soc* 2000;48:822–828.
229. Ladin D. Becaplermin gel (PDGF-BB) as topical wound therapy. Plastic Surgery Educational Foundation DATA Committee. *Plast Reconstr Surg* 2000; 105:1230–1231.
230. Pecoraro R, Ahroni J, Boyko E, et al. Chronology and determinants of tissue repair in diabetic lower-extremity ulcers. *Diabetes* 1991;40:1305–1313.
231. Sage R, Doyle D. Surgical treatment of diabetic foot ulcers: a review of forty-eight cases. *J Foot Surg* 1984;23:102–111.
232. Dickhaut S, Delee J, Page C. Nutritional status: importance in predicting wound-healing after amputation. *J Bone Joint Surg* 1984;66:71–75.
233. Levin M, Spratt I. To soak or not to soak. *Clin Diabetes* 1986;4:44.
234. Laing P. Diabetic foot ulcers. *Am J Surg* 1994;167[Suppl 1A]:31S–36S.
235. Mueller M, Diamond J, Sinacore D, et al. Total contact casting in the treatment of diabetic plantar ulcers: controlled clinical trial. *Diabetes Care* 1989;12:384–388.
236. Burden A, Jones G, Jones R, et al. Use of the "Scotchcast boot" in treating diabetic foot ulcers. *BMJ* 1983;286:1555–1557.
237. Coleman W, Brand P. The diabetic foot. In: Porte D, Sherwin R, eds. *Diabetes mellitus*. Stamford, CT: Appleton & Lange, 1997:1159.
238. Orr H. The principles involved in the treatment of osteomyelitis and compound fractures. *Lancet* 1934;54:622.
239. Trueta J. Treatment of war wounds and fractures. *BMJ* 1942;1:616.
240. Brand P. *Insensitive feet: a practical handbook on foot problems in leprosy*. London: The Leprosy Mission, 1977.
241. Sinacore D, Mueller M, Diamond J, et al. Diabetic plantar ulcers treated with total-contact casting: a clinical report. *Phys Ther* 1987;67:1543–1549.
242. Walker S, Helm P, Pullium G. Total-contact casting and chronic diabetic neuropathic foot ulcerations: healing rates by wound location. *Arch Phys Med Rehabil* 1987;68:217–221.
243. Laing P, Cogley D, Klenerman L. Neuropathic foot ulceration treated by total contact casts. *J Bone Joint Surg* [Br] 1991;4:133.
244. Husband M, Carr J. A simplified method of total contact casting for diabetic foot ulcers. *Contemp Orthop* 1993;26:143.
245. Helm P, Walker S, Pullium G. Total contact casting in diabetic patients with neuropathic foot ulcerations. *Arch Phys Med Rehabil* 1984;65:691–693.
246. Myerson M, Papa J, Eaton K, et al. The total-contact cast for management of neuropathic ulceration of the foot. *J Bone Joint Surg* 1992;74:261–263.
247. Edmonds M, Blundell M, Morris M, et al. Improved survival of the diabetic foot: the role of a specialized foot clinic. *Q J Med* 1986;60:763–771.

SECTION

VIII

Hypoglycemia and Islet Cell Tumors

CHAPTER 69
Hypoglycemia

Benjamin Glaser and Gil Leibowitz

Hypoglycemia, simply defined as a low blood glucose level, is a laboratory finding that may or may not be associated with significant pathology. Pathologic hypoglycemia may be caused by a large spectrum of entities, which vary depending on the age at onset and the presence of other, related symptoms. In this chapter we will provide a systematic approach to the diagnosis and treatment of hypoglycemic disorders in adults and children.

REGULATION OF GLUCOSE LEVELS (GLUCOSE HOMEOSTASIS)

The central nervous system (CNS) is dependent on the oxidation of glucose as its primary source of energy. Lack of an adequate glucose supply results in brain dysfunction (neuroglycopenia) and, if prolonged, in irreversible neuronal damage and death. In the healthy adult, the glucose requirements of the brain have been estimated at about 1 mg/(kg · min), corresponding to about 100 g/day in a 70-kg man. Uptake of glucose by the CNS is facilitated by two glucose transporters, GLUT1 and GLUT3, neither of which is regulated by insulin. During hypoglycemia, this glucose transport system is rate-limiting. Chronic hypoglycemia is associated with upregulation of glucose transport, a phenomenon that may be important in the development of hypoglycemia unawareness (see below).

In the fasting state, the brain can utilize ketone bodies (β-hydroxybutyrate and acetoacetate) as alternate energy sources. The uptake of ketone bodies by the brain is proportional to their concentration in the blood. Oxidation of ketone bodies can provide a significant energy source only when circulating levels are elevated, as in the case of a prolonged fast. Therefore, when glucose levels are low, but ketone levels are very high, the brain is partially protected from the deleterious effects of hypoglycemia. However, when both glucose and ketone levels are low, as in insulin-induced hypoglycemia and disorders of fatty acid oxidation, the brain is particularly vulnerable to metabolic damage.

Given the importance of glucose for neural function, it is not surprising that redundant mechanisms have evolved to prevent hypoglycemia. The circulating glucose concentration is determined by the balance between glucose input (absorption plus production) and glucose utilization. During fasting, glucose production is dependent on the availability of the substrates and the metabolic machinery required for glycogenolysis and gluconeogenesis. Glucose utilization is determined by insulin-stimulated glucose uptake as well as by the availability of alternative energy sources, particularly for muscle (1).

The major mechanisms responsible for prevention of hypoglycemia are shown in Figure 69.1. In the postabsorptive state, insulin levels fall, resulting in decreased uptake of glucose by the liver, muscle, and fat and relieving the insulin-mediated suppression of glycogenolysis, gluconeogenesis, and lipolysis. Hepatic glycogenolysis provides most of the glucose requirements during the first 12 to 24 hours of fasting (2), provided that the glycogen stores are adequate and that the uptake of glucose by muscle and fat is not excessive. During more prolonged fasting, after liver glycogen stores are depleted, lipolysis and protein breakdown supply a steady stream of fatty acids, glycerol, and amino acids. The fatty acids are used by muscle as an energy source and by the liver to produce ketone bodies, which can then be used as an energy source by most tissues of the body. Glycerol and amino acids are taken up by the liver and kidney and used as substrates for gluconeogenesis. A recent study demonstrated that net glucose production in healthy males was about 1.8 mg/(kg · min) during a fast lasting up to 40 hours. The contribution of gluconeogenesis to this basal glucose production increased from 41% after 12 hours to 92% after 40 hours of fasting (3). In prolonged fasting, the kidney produces 25% or more of the total glucose requirement, achieved primarily through gluconeogenesis from glutamine, lactate, and glycerol (4). The importance of renal glucose production is emphasized by the finding that severe chronic renal insufficiency may be associated with fasting hypoglycemia (see below).

If glucose levels dip below the threshold of hypoglycemia, counterregulatory hormones are released, resulting in a further increase in glucose production (see below). This threshold has been estimated at 67 mg/dL (i.e., just below the normal glucose level in the postabsorptive state and above the level at which neuroglycopenic symptoms usually occur) (5). The ventromedial hypothalamus appears to be of primary importance in initiating the counterregulatory response (6). The counterregulatory hormones can be divided into two major groups: the rapid-acting hormones (catecholamines and glucagon) and the slow-acting hormones (growth hormone and cortisol).

The catecholamines (epinephrine and norepinephrine) act by further suppressing insulin release while directly stimulating hepatic and renal gluconeogenesis, inhibiting peripheral utiliza-

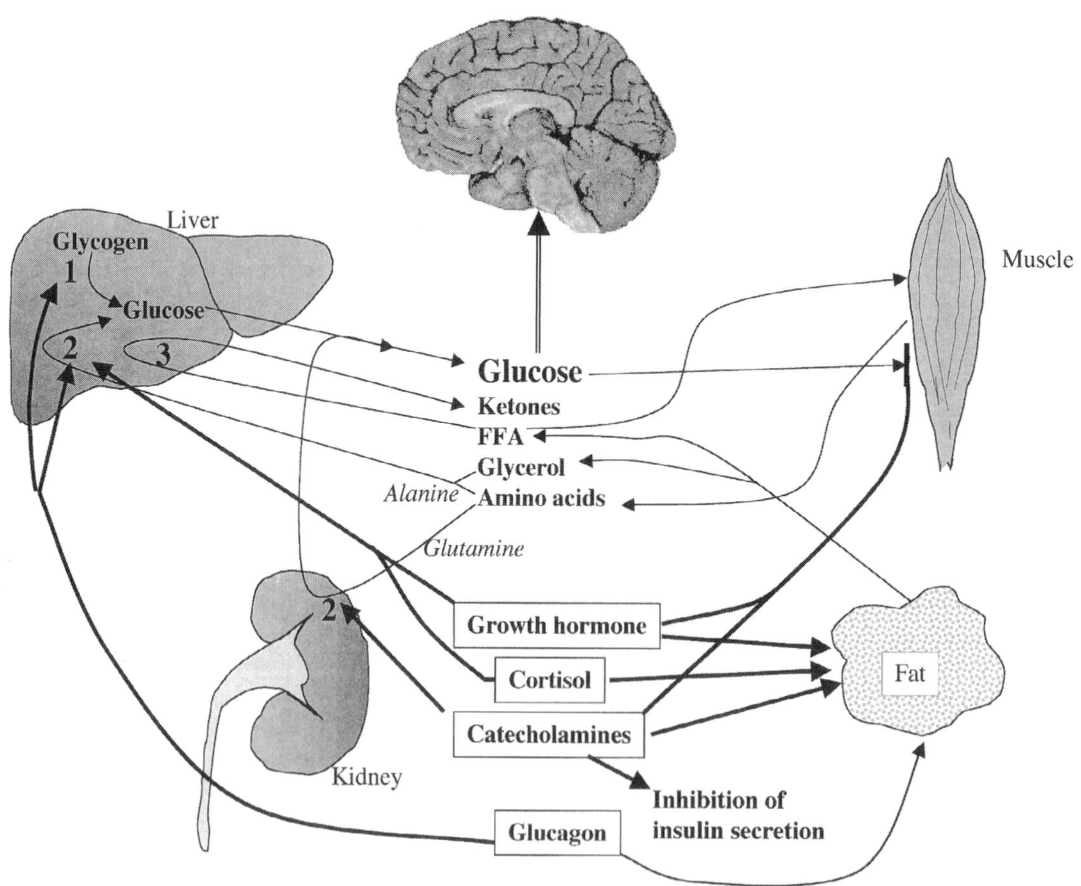

Figure 69.1. Schematic diagram showing the major pathways by which plasma glucose concentrations are maintained in the fasting state. Glucose uptake by the brain is obligatory and constant and is not dependent on hormonal action. During short-term fasting, hepatic glycogen is broken down to glucose by the glycogenolysis pathway *(1)*. During longer fasts, the breakdown of muscle and fat provides the liver with the necessary substrates for gluconeogenesis *(2)* and ketogenesis *(3)*. Hepatic gluconeogenesis *(2)* depends primarily on the availability of alanine, whereas renal gluconeogenesis uses glutamine as its primary substrate. Glucagon prevents hypoglycemia, primarily by stimulating hepatic glycogenolysis and gluconeogenesis. Catecholamines stimulate both hepatic and renal gluconeogenesis, while stimulating lipolysis, inhibiting glucose uptake by muscle, and directly inhibiting insulin secretion. Cortisol and growth hormone stimulate both hepatic gluconeogenesis and lipolysis, whereas growth hormone also suppresses peripheral utilization of glucose.

tion of glucose, and stimulating lipolysis. The latter provides both substrate for glyconeogenesis (glycerol) and an alternative energy source for muscle (fatty acids and ketone bodies). Glucagon acts primarily by stimulating hepatic glucose production, having little or no effect on peripheral glucose utilization or renal glucose production. Although glucagon stimulates lipolysis and thus ketogenesis, it appears to have a minimal net effect on the mobilization of gluconeogenic precursors from fat (7). Catecholamines and glucagon act independently, and both are required for an adequate glycemic response. Failure of either will significantly impair the glycemic response to hypoglycemia (8).

The counterregulatory effects of cortisol and growth hormone take several hours to become evident. Therefore, these hormones play a small role in the prevention of acute hypoglycemia but are important in the prevention of hypoglycemia during prolonged fasting. Cortisol stimulates both hepatic gluconeogenesis and lipolysis, resulting in increased levels of free fatty acids and glycerol. Growth hormone has a similar effect on lipolysis and gluconeogenesis, while simultaneously suppressing peripheral utilization of glucose. Both of these hormones rely on increased lipolysis to provide substrates for gluconeogenesis, as well as free fatty acids and ketone bodies, which are used as alternative energy sources. These are in effect glucose sparing in that they decrease the dependence of muscle and other non-neural tissues on glucose. This emphasizes the importance of the lipolytic and ketogenic pathways in the prevention of hypoglycemia. If levels of fatty acids or ketone bodies fail to increase, either because of inadequate fat stores or because of metabolic defects that prevent their production, utilization of glucose by muscle will increase, as will the risk of hypoglycemia, even if the remaining counterregulatory mechanisms function normally.

Therefore, despite the multiple redundant mechanisms that have evolved to prevent hypoglycemia, malfunction of any one of them will place the patient at risk of developing hypoglycemia. The specific nature of the malfunction will determine the associated clinical syndrome, with some defects resulting in profound, treatment-resistant hypoglycemia and others causing only mild hypoglycemia during prolonged fasting. In this chapter we review the common and rare causes of hypoglycemia. Because of the complexity of this problem in the developing child, and because of recent major advances in this field, a separate section is devoted to causes and treatment of hypoglycemia in the newborn and infant.

MEASUREMENT OF CIRCULATING GLUCOSE LEVELS

Accurate measurement of the circulating concentration of glucose is crucial to making the diagnosis of hypoglycemia. Appropriate reference standards must be used, because levels differ depending on whether whole blood or plasma is measured and if the sample is obtained from an artery, vein, or capillary. Most reference ranges are based on venous plasma samples. Arterial glucose concentrations are higher than venous glucose concentrations because of substantial glucose extraction across the forearm during hyperinsulinemic conditions. Glucose concentrations in whole blood are lower than those in plasma because glucose is metabolized by the glycolytic pathway in red blood cells and leukocytes, resulting in unequal distribution of glucose between intracellular and extracellular fluid. Whole-blood glucose measurements may be spuriously high in severe anemia and low in polycythemia vera or in the presence of excessive leukocytosis. Spuriously low glucose measurements due to glycolysis in blood cells *in vitro* (pseudohypoglycemia) should be avoided by transferring plasma rapidly to the laboratory for centrifugation. If delay is anticipated, chilling on ice will decrease the rate of *in vitro* glycolysis. Alternatively, this artifact can be minimized by collecting the blood in a tube containing inhibitors of glycolysis, such as oxalate and fluoride.

Glucose values frequently are measured in capillary blood obtained by a fingerstick and applied to a reagent strip for analysis by visual inspection or by a glucose meter. Visual inspection of a reagent strip to which blood has been applied is not a reliable way to distinguish normal from low glucose values. Glucose-meter measurements may be subject to artifacts resulting from poor technique of the patient or the medical staff performing the test or from technical problems with the glucose meter. Moreover, most glucose meters are calibrated to measure high glucose values and thus may be inaccurate in the hypoglycemic range. Therefore, although glucose meters may be very useful for screening patients to determine if symptoms correlate with low glucose measurements, thus excluding hypoglycemia when levels are high, the definitive diagnosis of hypoglycemia must always be based on an appropriately calibrated, standard chemical test in the laboratory.

DEFINITION OF HYPOGLYCEMIA

The diagnosis of hypoglycemia is most convincingly based on the Whipple triad: symptoms consistent with hypoglycemia, a low plasma glucose concentration, and relief of symptoms after the plasma glucose level is raised to normal by administration of exogenous glucose (9). However, the cutoff glucose concentration for defining hypoglycemia is controversial. A review of the literature reveals that glucose concentrations that have been proposed range from 45 to 75 mg/dL (2.5 to 4.2 mmol/L). This controversy stems from the fact that hypoglycemia can be defined in several ways, including the normal response to fasting, the level at which clinical neuroglycopenic symptoms appear, and the level at which a physiologic counterregulation response is triggered. Thus, the glucose level at which hypoglycemia is diagnosed depends primarily on the definition used. According to the first criterion, glucose concentrations in venous plasma obtained after an overnight fast are considered abnormal if they are lower than 60 mg/dL (3.3 mmol/L). However, if hypoglycemia is defined as the clinical pathophysiologic state characterized by autonomic and neuroglycopenic symptoms, then glucose concentrations below 54 mg/dL (3.0 mmol/L) should be defined as pathologic (10).

Defining hypoglycemia is further complicated by the fact that the normal plasma glucose response to prolonged fasting is different in adult men and women. In adult men, the normal fasting plasma glucose level is above 55 mg/dL (3.1 mmol/L) at 24 hours and 50 mg/dL (2.8 mmol/L) at 48 and 72 hours. In normal premenopausal women, fasting plasma glucose levels may dip as low as 35 mg/dL (1.9 mmol/L) at 24 hours, whereas more prolonged fasts may drive glucose levels to as low as 30 mg/dL (1.7 mmol/L) and, rarely, even below this (Fig. 69.2) (11). Responses of counterregulatory hormones to lowered blood glucose are reduced in healthy young women, which may explain these low fasting plasma glucose levels (12). Because the normal glucose response to fasting may vary according to the age and gender of the patient, the appearance of neuroglycopenic symptoms is an important indication that the measurement of a low plasma glucose concentration is indeed true hypoglycemia. In the healthy adult, prolonged fasting results in the formation of ketone bodies that can be used as an alternative fuel for brain metabolism; therefore, neuroglycopenia may not occur at glucose levels that under other conditions would cause severe symptoms. In contrast, hypoglycemia induced by insulin or insulin-like factors is associated with sup-

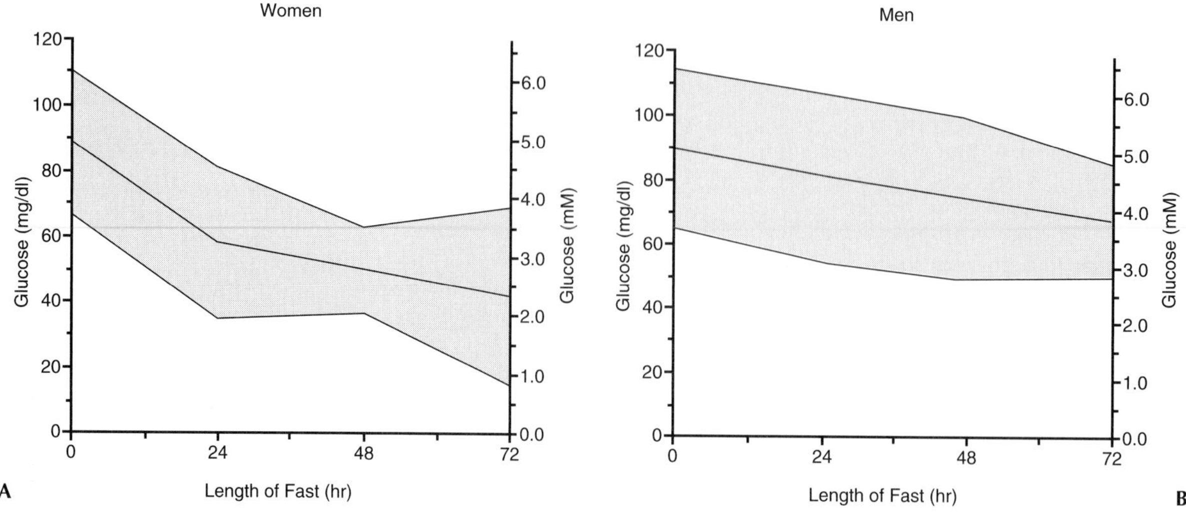

Figure 69.2. Glycemic response to a 72-hour fast in nonobese adult women **(A)** and men **(B)**. Plasma glucose levels were measured by the glucose oxidase method and are presented as the mean ± 2 standard deviations. (Data from Merimee TJ, Tyson JE. Stabilization of plasma glucose during fasting: normal variations in two separate studies. *N Engl J Med* 1974;291:1275–1278.)

pression of ketosis, and the brain may therefore be sensitive to moderate reductions in glucose levels.

An alternative approach is to define hypoglycemia on the basis of the physiologic counterregulatory hormone response to lowering of plasma glucose. Insulin secretion is suppressed at glucose levels of 76 to 72 mg/dL (4.2 to 4.0 mmol/L), and glucose-counterregulatory hormones are released at glucose levels of 70 to 65 mg/dL (3.9 to 3.6 mmol/L) (1).

In practice, the definition of hypoglycemia should be adjusted to the clinical situation. Although there is no well-defined glucose concentration for defining hypoglycemia, venous glucose concentrations between 45 and 60 mg/dL (2.5 and 3.3 mmol/L) strongly suggest hypoglycemia, and those below 45 mg/dL (2.5 mmol/L) are usually indicative of important pathology. If the low glucose level is associated with neurologic symptoms, the clinical suspicion for hypoglycemia is high and prompt evaluation to identify the cause is required. In patients with diabetes treated with insulin, glucose levels should be maintained above 75 mg/dL (4.2 mmol/L) to prevent symptomatic hypoglycemia and hypoglycemia unawareness (see Chapter 40).

SIGNS AND SYMPTOMS OF HYPOGLYCEMIA

Signs and symptoms of hypoglycemia result from neuronal glucose deprivation and can be divided into two categories: autonomic and neuroglycopenic (Table 69.1). The former result from the activation of the autonomic nervous system, with release of epinephrine from the adrenal medulla into the circulation and of norepinephrine from sympathetic postganglionic nerve terminals within the target tissues. Under normal circumstances, the glycemic threshold for catecholamine release is higher than that for induction of neuroglycopenic symptoms. Therefore, the autonomic symptoms precede the neuroglycopenic symptoms. Symptoms and signs related to catecholamine release include tremulousness, pallor, palpitations, tachycardia, widened pulse pressure, and anxiety. Sweating, hunger, and paresthesias are also common and are mediated by acetylcholine. In adults, sweating is often very prominent and is thought to be mediated by sympathetic cholinergic postganglionic neurons (13).

Neuroglycopenic symptoms are the result of glucose deprivation in the brain. Because glucose is the main fuel of metabolism in brain tissue, reduced levels of glucose may be insufficient to supply the brain with its energy requirements. Thus, the symptoms of neuroglycopenia and those of hypoxia are virtually indistinguishable. They include nonspecific complaints, such as weakness, fatigue and dizziness, headache, behavioral changes, and confusion. Affected persons often show poor judgment, perform their activities in an automatic, repetitive manner, and become uncooperative. They may become lethargic, irritable, and occasionally even aggressive. There is variable impairment of cognitive functions, including difficulty in think-

TABLE 69.1. Signs and Symptoms of Hypoglycemia in the Adult

Autonomic		Neuroglycopenic	
Symptoms	**Signs**	**Symptoms**	**Signs**
Hunger	Pallor	Weakness, fatigue	Cortical blindness
Sweating	Tachycardia	Dizziness	Hypothermia
Anxiety	Widened pulse pressure	Headache	Seizures
Paresthesias		Confusion	Coma
Palpitations		Behavioral changes	
Tremulousness		Cognitive dysfunction	
		Blurred vision, diplopia	

ing and concentration, aphasia, and slurred speech. In addition, hypoglycemia may cause blurred vision, cortical blindness, paresthesias, hemiplegia, hypothermia, and eventually coma, seizures, and death. Symptoms are less specific in the neonate than in the older child and adult and may include irritability, jitteriness, changes in tone, cyanosis, tachypnea, lethargy, and frank coma or seizures (see section on neonatal hypoglycemia).

The glycemic threshold for the appearance of counterregulatory hormone response and for neuroglycopenic symptoms is dynamic. It shifts to higher glucose concentrations following sustained hyperglycemia in patients with poorly controlled diabetes (14) and to lower glucose concentrations in patients with recurrent episodes of hypoglycemia (15). Even a single episode of hypoglycemia can blunt catecholamine response to subsequent hypoglycemia (16). The shift in glycemic thresholds following recurrent hypoglycemia results from an adaptive increase in uptake of glucose by the brain, probably due to increased cerebral blood flow (17) and enhanced extraction of glucose induced by upregulation of the brain glucose transporters GLUT1 and GLUT3 (18). In addition to depending on the previous glycemic environment, the response to hypoglycemia depends on the availability of alternative fuels for the brain, such as ketone bodies and lactate (19).

Cerebral energy requirements, the adaptive changes in glucose extraction, and the ability to utilize alternative fuels are not uniform in all the regions of the brain. Thus, enhanced uptake of glucose in response to recurrent hypoglycemia can maintain normal metabolism and function in some regions of the brain, while other regions may remain susceptible to hypoglycemia-induced dysfunction. From the clinical standpoint, a patient with recurrent hypoglycemia may fail to develop warning symptoms of hypoglycemia and may not be able to react quickly enough to avert severe neuroglycopenia and coma when the glucose concentration reaches a critical threshold. Therefore, enhanced uptake of glucose by the brain following recurrent hypoglycemia is potentially dangerous and should be considered maladaptive (18).

Severe and prolonged hypoglycemic episodes may cause neuronal cell death, resulting in permanent impairment of brain function. However, if the hypoglycemia is treated effectively, apparent full recovery is the rule even after severe episodes of hypoglycemia. There are concerns that recurrent hypoglycemia may result in permanent damage to intellectual capacity, although in adults there is no conclusive evidence to support this notion. Prospective studies of patients with diabetes at risk for recurrent severe hypoglycemia show no effect on long-term cognitive function (20,21). In contrast, children younger than 5 years of age do show a permanent impairment in IQ after recurrent events of hypoglycemia (22). Thus, hypoglycemia is harmful to the developing brain during the first years of life.

CLASSIFICATION OF HYPOGLYCEMIC DISORDERS

The differential diagnosis of hypoglycemia is broad (Fig.69.3). The various hypoglycemic disorders can be classified on the basis of glucose kinetics (increased glucose utilization vs. defi-

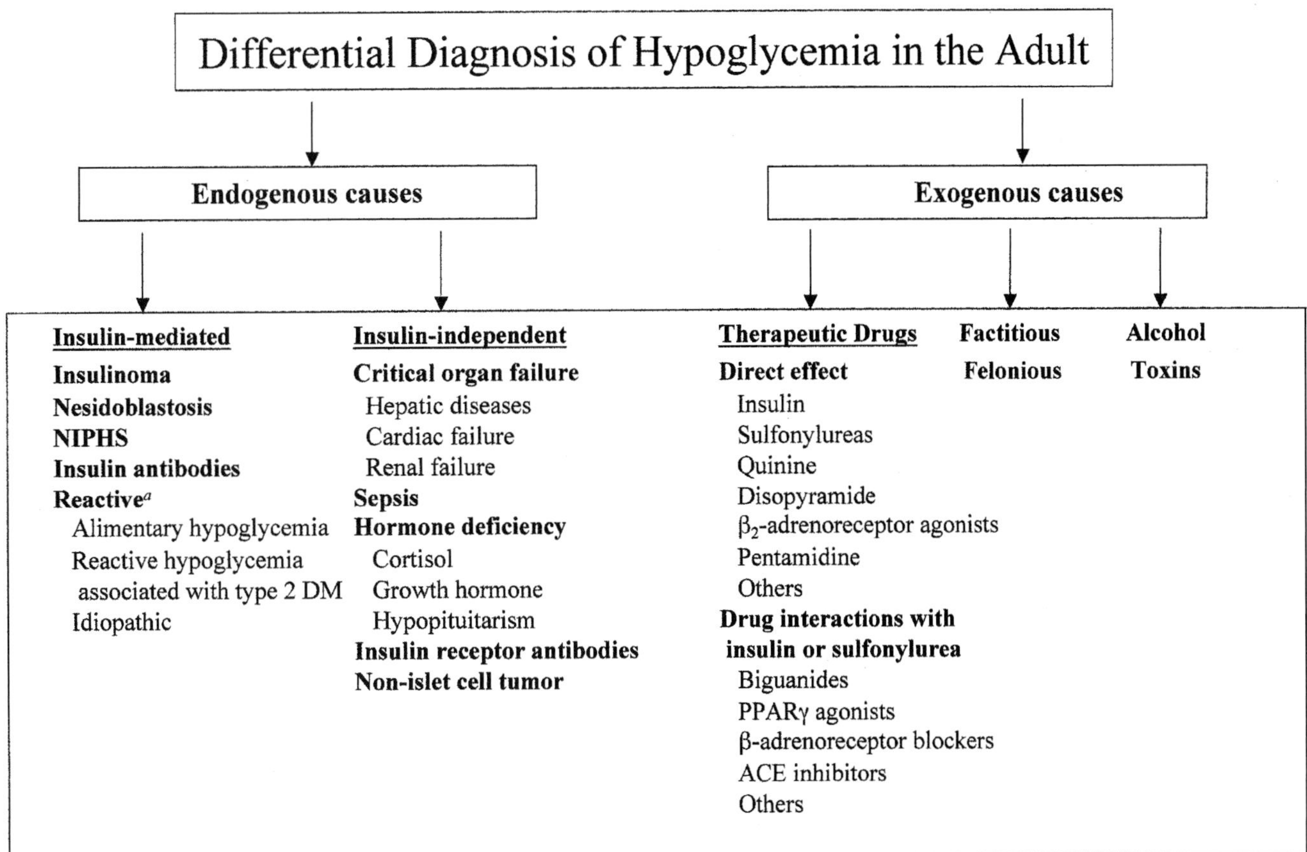

Figure 69.3. The major causes of hypoglycemia in the adult are grouped according to mechanism. NIPHS, noninsulinoma pancreatogenous hypoglycemia; PPAR-γ, peroxisome proliferator-activated receptor-γ; ACE, angiotensin-converting enzyme. [a]Postprandial symptoms are common but usually not associated with hypoglycemia.

cient glucose production), insulin mediation (hyperinsulinemic vs. hypoinsulinemic), etiology (endogenous vs. exogenous causes), age (adults vs. infants and children), and the clinical characteristics of the patient (appears healthy or ill) (23).

From a clinical standpoint, it is common to classify hypoglycemic disorders as fasting or reactive. Reactive hypoglycemia refers to the occurrence of hypoglycemia in the postprandial state, not during fasting, and usually does not imply a serious underlying disorder. However, this term describes the timing of hypoglycemia and has no implication regarding mechanism or etiology. For example, postprandial hypoglycemia may be the predominant finding in some patients with insulinoma (23). Moreover, the majority of patients referred for evaluation of postprandial symptoms do not have low plasma glucose levels at all. Therefore, true functional/reactive hypoglycemia is not common (24,25).

In this chapter, we refer to hypoglycemic disorders based on the age group of the patients. In adults, hypoglycemia may be caused by drugs, systemic disease, abnormalities in counterregulatory hormones, or tumors. Hypoglycemia arising as a consequence of the therapeutic use of insulin or oral hypoglycemic agents in patients with diabetes, the most common exogenous cause of hypoglycemia, is considered elsewhere in this volume (see Chapters 40 and 41). In infants and nondiabetic children, hypoglycemia often results from inborn genetic defects in proteins important for regulating insulin secretion or substrate metabolism. In recent years, there has been an explosion of information on the human genome, leading to better classification and characterization of different hypoglycemic disorders. Thus, the etiologies of hypoglycemia in this age group are discussed separately.

EXOGENOUS CAUSES OF HYPOGLYCEMIA

Drug-Induced Hypoglycemia

Many drugs have been associated with hypoglycemia (Table 69.2); however, a cause-and-effect relationship has not been established for many of these agents. Factors predisposing to drug-induced hypoglycemia include very young and very old age, impaired renal and liver functions, and poor nutrition (26). Drugs may cause hypoglycemia by several mechanisms: (a) by increasing release of insulin secondary to activation of the insulin secretion machinery or secondary to a direct toxic effect to pancreatic islets resulting in nonregulated insulin release; (b) by increasing uptake and utilization of glucose in the peripheral tissue; and (c) by decreasing production of glucose by the liver. In addition, drugs may interact with sulfonylurea agents and insulin and potentiate their hypoglycemic effects. In these cases it may be difficult to assess the role of the individual drugs in the development of hypoglycemia.

Many of the drugs that have been associated with hypoglycemia are in very common use, and patients, particularly the elderly, are frequently receiving multiple drugs. Therefore, iatrogenic hypoglycemia should always be included in the differential diagnosis. Doing so may facilitate diagnosis and treatment and prevent unnecessary diagnostic and therapeutic procedures. The most common causes of drug-induced hypoglycemia are alcohol and treatment with a sulfonylurea or insulin in patients with diabetes. The latter is discussed in Chapter 41.

DRUGS AND TOXINS THAT INCREASE INSULIN RELEASE

Quinine and Related Drugs

The antimalarial drug quinine and its antiarrhythmic derivative quinidine have been shown to induce hyperinsulinemic hypoglycemia. Quinine-related substances stimulate insulin secretion from pancreatic β-cells and cause a mild decrease in blood glucose levels that is usually not sufficient to induce symptoms of hypoglycemia in healthy subjects. The hypoglycemic effect of quinine may become more prominent in the presence of renal failure, since drug clearance is reduced and the concentration of quinine in the blood is higher. In addition to quinine-induced hyperinsulinemia, acutely ill patients with malaria are prone to development of hypoglycemia because of consumption of glucose by the malarial parasites. In patients with malaria falci-

TABLE 69.2. Hypoglycemia-Causing Drugs

Increased insulin	Increased insulin sensitivity[a]	Decreased hepatic glucose output	Autoimmune mechanism	Miscellaneous and unknown mechanisms[b]
Insulin (common)	β-adrenergic blockers	Alcohol (common)	Hydralazine	Sulfonamides
Sulfonylureas (common)	ACE inhibitors	Unripe akee fruit	Procainamide	Salicylates
Disopyramide	Biguanides	—	Isoniazid	Anticoagulants (dicumarol, warfarin)
Quinine	PPARγ agonists	—	Interferon-α	Analgesic and antiinflammatory drugs (indomethacin, colchicine, paracetamol phenylbutazone)
Pentamidine	—	—	Sulfhydryl-containing drugs (methimazole, penicillamine, captopril, gold thioglucose)	Antipsychotic drugs (haloperidol, chlorpromazine, lithium)
Ritodrine	—	—	—	Ketoconazole
Isoniazid[c]	—	—	—	Selegiline (antiparkinsonian agent)
Chloroquine[c]	—	—	—	Octreotide
				Phenytoin

ACE, angiotensin-converting enzyme; PPARγ, peroxisome proliferator-activated receptor-γ.
[a]These drugs very rarely cause hypoglycemia by themselves but may exacerbate hypoglycemia in patients treated with oral hypoglycemic agents or insulin.
[b]Most of these drugs are in very common use and only rarely have been reported to be associated with hypoglycemia. Furthermore, in many cases, the direct cause-and-effect relationship was not proven.
[c]Appear to cause hypoglycemia by decreasing insulin clearance.

parum who are treated with quinine, hypoglycemia may be overlooked because the neurologic symptoms may be attributed to cerebral malaria. Therefore, blood glucose should be carefully monitored and a glucose supplement administered to prevent dangerous hypoglycemia (27,28).

Disopyramide

Disopyramide, used clinically as an antiarrhythmic agent, has been shown to increase insulin secretion from pancreatic β-cells, resulting in hyperinsulinemic hypoglycemia. The drug causes closure of the β-cell K_{ATP} channel, binding to the channel at a site distinct from the sulfonylurea binding site (29). Disopyramide often is used in elderly patients, who may also suffer from impaired renal function and who appear to be particularly susceptible to the glucose-lowering effect of the drug (30). A recent study found that the use of disopyramide did not affect the risk of hypoglycemia in an ambulatory patient population, suggesting that this side effect may be minor in the general population and may be of clinical importance only in selected patients at particular risk (31). It has been claimed that, although rare in absolute terms, disopyramide is one of the most common causes of drug-induced hypoglycemia in nondiabetic patients (32).

β_2-Adrenoreceptor Agonists

Ritodrine therapy to delay premature delivery during pregnancy can stimulate insulin secretion and cause hypoglycemia in the newborn and rarely in the mother (33). Therapeutic doses of β_2-adrenoreceptor agonists administered to patients with bronchial asthma were not reported to induce hypoglycemia; however, albuterol overdose was reported to cause hypoglycemia in a young child (34).

Pentamidine

Pentamidine is used for the treatment of *Pneumocystis carinii* pneumonia in patients with AIDS and for parasitic infections, including trypanosomiasis and leishmaniasis. The drug is toxic to pancreatic β-cells, resulting in unregulated release of insulin from the damaged β-cells and leading to hypoglycemia followed by hyperglycemia and even permanent diabetes mellitus. The toxicity to the β-cells is more common and severe following systemic administration and is related to the cumulative dose of the drug (35,36).

DRUGS THAT INCREASE INSULIN SENSITIVITY

Biguanides and Peroxisome Proliferator-Activated Receptor-γ Agonists

Metformin and the glitazones do not usually cause hypoglycemia when taken alone. Over 10 years of follow-up among patients with type 2 diabetes taking metformin in the UK Prospective Diabetes Study (UKPDS), the proportion of patients per year who had one or more episodes of hypoglycemia was 4.2%, none of whom developed severe hypoglycemia (37). The biguanides and glitazones may augment hypoglycemia caused by sulfonylureas and insulin by increasing the uptake and utilization of glucose (38). Metformin also decreases hepatic production of glucose and decreases intestinal absorption of glucose.

Angiotensin-Converting Enzyme Inhibitors

The association between angiotensin-converting enzyme (ACE) inhibitors and hypoglycemia in patients with diabetes treated with sulfonylureas or insulin is controversial. One study reported that 14% of all hospital admissions for hypoglycemia might be attributable to ACE inhibitors (39). The association between ACE inhibitors and hypoglycemia was not explained by potential confounding factors, such as the type of diabetes treatment and congestive heart failure (40). ACE inhibitors can intensify the glucose-lowering effect of insulin or sulfonylureas. A study using a hyperinsulinemic euglycemic clamp protocol found that captopril improved sensitivity to insulin in healthy volunteers with normal blood pressure. With enalapril, however, the increase in insulin sensitivity was less pronounced and did not achieve statistical significance (41,42). ACE inhibitors may indirectly increase insulin sensitivity by increasing circulating kinins, leading to vasodilatation and increased uptake of glucose in muscle tissue. Nevertheless, large series of patients with diabetes treated with ACE inhibitors, including the UKPDS, show that these are safe and that the risk of hypoglycemia is very low (43).

β-Adrenergic Receptor Blocking Agents

Nonselective β-adrenergic receptor blocking agents, such as propranolol, have been associated with hypoglycemia in otherwise healthy children but not in healthy adults (44). Most of the cases of hypoglycemia associated with these agents were in patients with diabetes receiving insulin or sulfonylureas. Thus, it is difficult to prove a cause-and-effect relationship between therapy with β-blockers and hypoglycemia (45). β-Blockers can increase glucose uptake in skeletal muscle by antagonizing the effects of catecholamines on glucose uptake and lipolysis (46). Suppression of lipolysis with reduction of nonesterified free fatty acids in plasma improves insulin sensitivity and indirectly reduces gluconeogenesis. β-Blockers decrease insulin secretion from pancreatic β-cells. Therefore, insulin-treated patients with diabetes may be more susceptible to the glucose-lowering effects of β-blockers, whereas patients with type 2 diabetes treated with oral medications or diet may have exacerbations of hyperglycemia rather than hypoglycemia. Similar to ACE inhibitors, β-blockers were not associated with a higher frequency of hypoglycemic episodes in large series of patients with type 2 diabetes, including the UKPDS (43). β-Blockers may block the adrenergic response to hypoglycemia, leading to hypoglycemia unawareness and a predominance of the neuroglycopenic symptoms. Moreover, β-blockers may delay the recovery from hypoglycemia because of inhibition of catecholamine-mediated glucose counterregulation. Catecholamines are not required for prompt recovery from hypoglycemia in patients with intact islet-cell function; however, β-blockade may become critical in glucagon-deficient patients with type 1 diabetes. The risk for severe hypoglycemia in insulin-treated patients with diabetes can be reduced by using one of the relatively selective β_1-adrenergic antagonists (47).

DRUGS THAT DECREASE HEPATIC GLUCOSE PRODUCTION

Hypoglycemia resulting from suppressed hepatic production of glucose may occur in the setting of acute drug intoxication, which may result in metabolic inhibition of gluconeogenesis, such as with alcohol or in hepatic necrosis, as may occur after paracetamol poisoning. Hypoglycemia may be exacerbated if acute renal failure occurs concomitantly with hepatic toxicity.

Alcohol-Induced Hypoglycemia

The most common cause of drug-induced hypoglycemia secondary to suppressed gluconeogenesis is alcohol overdose. Alcohol-induced hypoglycemia may occur in persons of all ages and in all classes of society. It is more common in men than in women and in malnourished persons on a low-calorie diet. Young children are especially susceptible to the hypoglycemic effects of alcohol. Therefore, accidental consumption of even modest amounts of alcohol may result in hypoglycemia in infants and young children (48). Fewer than 1% of patients with alcohol intoxication presenting to the emergency room have hypoglycemia. However, because of the very high incidence of alcohol intoxication relative to the incidence of all other causes of hypoglycemia, alcohol can be implicated in 18% to 52% of patients admitted to the emergency department because of sustained hypoglycemia (26). This variation in the incidence of alcohol-induced hypoglycemia in different series probably reflects social, ethnic, and cultural differences in alcohol consumption among the populations studied. Symptoms of alcohol intoxication may be very similar to those of neuroglycopenia, making clinical differentiation difficult. Thus, immediate routine determination of blood glucose is recommended for all intoxicated patients in the emergency department to guarantee rapid identification of those with significant hypoglycemia. A delay in the diagnosis may result in permanent brain damage and death. The mortality rate among hospitalized patients with alcohol-induced hypoglycemia may be as high as 10% (26).

Ethanol is usually still detectable in the blood at the time the patient presents with hypoglycemia but may not be markedly elevated and may correlate poorly with the glucose concentration. Characteristically, the patient with alcohol-induced hypoglycemia is an alcoholic with a history of moderate to excessive consumption of alcohol and little or no protein or carbohydrate intake during the preceding hours or days. The patient often is referred to the hospital in a comatose state and also may suffer from hypothermia. Most patients do not experience autonomic response to alcohol-induced hypoglycemia, and some chronic alcoholics can tolerate low blood glucose levels without symptomatic neuroglycopenia. The diminished neuronal response to hypoglycemia may result from recurrent subclinical episodes of hypoglycemia that reduce the glycemic threshold for the appearance of counterregulatory hormone response and for neuroglycopenic symptoms. There may also be a direct effect of alcohol on the activation of the hypothalamic–adrenal axis in response to hypoglycemia. In addition, plasma ketone bodies are often high and can be used as an alternative fuel for brain metabolism. Some patients present with alcoholic ketoacidosis, which may occur several days following alcohol ingestion and resembles diabetic ketoacidosis. In these patients, plasma glucose levels are usually normal or high; however, some patients may present with severe hypoglycemia. Both the pathogenesis of this condition and the reason certain patients develop hypoglycemia while others become hyperglycemic are unknown. This medical emergency should be treated with intravenous glucose injection preceded by thiamine injection to prevent the development of Wernicke encephalopathy.

Alcohol causes hypoglycemia by inhibiting gluconeogenesis. Ethanol is metabolized in the liver by alcohol dehydrogenase to acetaldehyde and then to acetic acid by aldehyde dehydrogenase. The enzymatic reactions generate free hydrogen ions, with subsequent reduction of nicotinamide dinucleotide (NAD) to NADH. The depletion of hepatic NAD stores inhibits the metabolism of precursors in the gluconeogenic pathway, including the conversion of lactate to pyruvate, several steps in the tricarboxylic acid cycle, and the conversion of glycerol to glucose (49). Ethanol does not inhibit glycogenolysis. Thus, well-nourished obese patients and those who have had significant carbohydrate intake within 12 to 24 hours are likely to have adequate hepatic glycogen stores, which partially protect them from hypoglycemia.

Ethanol also inhibits the release of corticotropin, cortisol, and growth hormone in response to hypoglycemia. The glucagon and epinephrine responses to hypoglycemia may also be delayed, although this is controversial. The failure to activate a counterregulatory hormone response may contribute to the development of fasting hypoglycemia (50).

In addition to inducing fasting hypoglycemia, alcohol may increase the risk for reactive hypoglycemia. Moderate alcohol consumption was shown to increase insulin secretion in response to glucose stimulation. Thus, a mixture of alcohol and sucrose may induce postprandial reactive hypoglycemia due to insulin excess. For example, 10% to 20% of healthy volunteers who consumed a gin and tonic (a sucrose-rich alcoholic beverage) on an empty stomach and did not eat for several hours afterwards developed symptomatic reactive hypoglycemia (51).

Interaction Between Alcohol and Antidiabetic Drugs

The effect of alcohol on insulin-induced hypoglycemia is controversial. In one study, blood glucose levels were similar after administration of insulin and ethanol together or insulin alone (52). However, alcohol does inhibit gluconeogenesis (see above) and has been reported to be commonly involved in admissions to the hospital for hypoglycemia resulting from insulin overdose (53). Furthermore, there are concerns that alcohol consumption may exacerbate the brain-damaging effects of hypoglycemia. There is very limited information on the interaction between sulfonylureas and the hypoglycemic effects of alcohol. In one large series of patients with drug-induced hypoglycemia, a few patients with diabetes developed hypoglycemia following administration of both sulfonylureas and alcohol (54).

Hypoglycin A

Hypoglycemia may occur after the ingestion of the unripe akee fruit. The akee fruit is commonly consumed in Jamaica, and if eaten unripe may cause severe weakness, vomiting, convulsions, coma, and eventually death. The symptoms are associated with severe hypoglycemia resulting from the toxin hypoglycin A, which inhibits fatty acid oxidation and thus causes a metabolic syndrome very similar to that caused by inborn errors of fatty acid metabolism (see section on hypoglycemia in the neonate) (55). Both ketogenesis and hepatic gluconeogenesis are inhibited, causing both hypoglycemia and lowered ketone bodies, a combination that may be particularly neurotoxic.

OTHER DRUGS

Many drugs cause hypoglycemia by various mechanisms, some of which have not yet been completely defined. Some drugs, such as sulfonamide, dicumarol, and phenylbutazone, interact with sulfonylureas to enhance their hypoglycemic activity. Other drugs, including isoniazid and synthetic antimalarial drugs such as chloroquine, may rarely induce hypoglycemia in patients with diabetes by reducing the clearance of insulin from the blood. A large dose of salicylates may induce hypoglycemia in young children, but rarely in adults. The mechanism of salicylate-induced hypoglycemia is unknown but may be related to increased peripheral utilization of glucose, suppression of hepatic gluconeogenesis, or augmentation of insulin release (26). Recent studies have shown that salicylates can enhance insulin sensitivity by inhibiting the IκB kinase (56).

Factitious Hypoglycemia

Most cases of factitious hypoglycemia are caused by the deliberate administration of insulin or oral hypoglycemic agents by the patient, although accidental administration or administration by a caregiver may occur as well. The prevalence of factitious hypoglycemia is unknown. It was suggested that it is more common in women than in men, although this has not been confirmed (57). The typical patient is young, aged 15 to 40 years, and has access to insulin or oral hypoglycemic agents such as sulfonylureas. The patient may be a medical or paramedical worker or a family member of a person with diabetes treated with oral hypoglycemic agents or insulin and may know the effects of the abused medication and the symptoms of hypoglycemia. Most patients seem to be "mentally healthy" and provide detailed description of their "illness," obviously omitting the fact that hypoglycemic drugs were abused. Similar to other factitious diseases, use of hypoglycemic drugs is usually denied. When confronted with this possibility, the patient may respond in an aggressive manner, blaming the physician for not trusting him or her. These patients may be very sophisticated in concealing self-administration of hypoglycemic drugs, and episodes of hypoglycemia may occur even during close supervision in the hospital. The history of episodes of hypoglycemia may extend over periods of many years, sometimes with intervals of remission explained by irregular administration of the drugs. The history may suggest the presence of an insulinoma, and failure to diagnose the cause of hyperinsulinism may result in an unnecessary laparotomy and even pancreatectomy.

Accidental administration of insulin or oral hypoglycemic agents may produce "factitious" hypoglycemia. Inadvertent administration of insulin to the wrong patient in a hospital is a rare cause of hypoglycemia. Unintended use of oral hypoglycemic agents may result from a prescribing error by a physician or a pharmacist or by substitution of an oral hypoglycemic for another medication by the patient or by a family member. Insulin and drug-induced factitious hypoglycemia may also be the result of attempted suicide or homicide.

The diagnosis of factitious hypoglycemia should be considered in all patients with hyperinsulinemic hypoglycemia. The initial history may provide clues suggesting the presence or absence of factitious hypoglycemia; however, each patient must be fully evaluated regardless of initial impression. We recently evaluated a young soldier with a highly suggestive history of insulinoma, no apparent access to insulin or drugs, and no suggestion of secondary gain, who was subsequently proven to have ingested glibenclamide. Another patient, with a clinical history highly suspicious of factitious hypoglycemia and easy access to medical personnel and medication, was subsequently proven to have a benign insulinoma.

The biochemical diagnosis of insulin-induced factitious hypoglycemia is relatively simple if blood is collected during an episode of hypoglycemia for glucose, insulin, and C-peptide measurement. Plasma insulin is high, with discordant low levels of C-peptide, reflecting the suppression of endogenous insulin secretion by low glucose levels. If insulin and C-peptide measurements are discordant, the presence of antibodies to insulin should be excluded. Insulin antibodies may cause spuriously high or low insulin measurements, depending on the method used in the insulin assay. The presence of circulating antibodies should also be excluded by direct measurement using specific assays and by measuring insulin levels on serial dilutions of plasma samples. Nonlinear correlation between measured insulin and plasma dilution indicates the presence of a substance that interferes with the insulin assay. In the past, the presence of insulin antibodies was thought to be *prima facie* evidence of exogenous insulin administration. However, modern, highly purified, recombinant human insulin rarely causes clinically significant antibody production, and it is now clear that antibodies may also occur in rare patients with autoimmune hypoglycemia and prior to the clinical onset of type 1 diabetes. Therefore, detection of insulin antibodies should not be regarded as a specific and sensitive assay for the diagnosis of factitious hypoglycemia. In the past, all commercially available insulin was obtained from beef or porcine pancreas. Thus, species-specific assays could be developed to prove the exogenous origin of circulating insulin. Today, most commercial insulin is of human origin, making these assays obsolete; however, the increasing use of insulin analogues may cause a revival of this approach.

In contrast to surreptitious administration of insulin, secretagogue-induced hypoglycemia is associated with elevation of both insulin and C-peptide levels. Plasma levels of C-peptide fail to be suppressed in response to the insulin hypoglycemia test, and the response to different stimuli, such as glucagon and glucose, may be excessive, similar to the findings in patients with insulinoma. Therefore, the diagnosis of factitious hypoglycemia due to insulin secretagogues is usually a difficult challenge. For confirmation or exclusion of the diagnosis, blood levels of some of the relevant drugs should be measured during hypoglycemia in an experienced toxicology laboratory. The increasing number of drugs available that stimulate insulin secretion is making this task progressively more difficult.

On certain occasions, when there is strong clinical suspicion of factitious hypoglycemia, it may be necessary to search the hospital room of a patient to find insulin vials, syringes, needles, or drug tablets to confirm the diagnosis of factitious hypoglycemia. A room search is considered by some to be unethical and should be performed only after careful consideration and approval of the appropriate hospital authorities.

The treatment of factitious hypoglycemia is the same whether it is mediated by insulin or sulfonylurea and includes immediate relief of hypoglycemia by intravenous glucose followed by psychiatric intervention to prevent recurrent episodes of hypoglycemia. Management involves a supportive confrontation followed by long-term psychiatric care. Factitious hypoglycemia is a serious psychiatric disturbance. Although some patients admit that the motive is to gain attention, sympathy, or some other secondary gain, in the majority insight is limited and the long-term prognosis is poor. Hypoglycemia may recur or may be followed by other psychosomatic symptoms or drug abuse. Some patients may later commit suicide (58).

ENDOGENOUS CAUSES OF HYPOGLYCEMIA

Hypoglycemia Due to Critical-Organ Failure

Sepsis and diseases that cause severe hepatic, cardiac, or renal failure are common causes of hypoglycemia among hospitalized patients. Patients with malnutrition or with failure of more than one critical organ are more susceptible to severe hypoglycemia.

HEPATIC DISEASES

Hepatic glycogenolysis and gluconeogenesis play critical roles in the maintenance of postabsorptive blood glucose. Since the normal liver has a very large capacity for glucose production, hypoglycemia will occur only in the face of massive destruction of the liver parenchyma or in the presence of accelerated utilization of glucose. Accelerated utilization of glucose may be present in several clinical conditions, including treatment with insulin or oral medications and during sepsis. Hypoglycemia has been reported in patients with severe liver failure due to toxic hepatitis, fulminant viral hepatitis, fatty liver, or hepatitis associated with alcohol administration and cholangitis. In the latter, sepsis complicating biliary obstruction may contribute to the development of hypoglycemia. Hypoglycemia is uncommon in patients with cirrhosis. Plasma levels of insulin may be relatively high because of the presence of portal-systemic shunts and reduced hepatic insulin extraction (59).

CARDIAC FAILURE

Occasionally, hypoglycemia may occur in patients with severe congestive heart failure. The primary mechanism causing hypoglycemia in these patients is not known but may be the combination of cachexia, lack of gluconeogenic substrate, and liver dysfunction due to hepatic hypoxia and congestion. Patients admitted to intensive care units may develop ischemic hepatitis resulting from episodes of acute heart failure and hypotension. A retrospective study of patients with ischemic hepatitis showed that hypoglycemia is common, occurring in one third of the patients (60).

RENAL FAILURE

Renal insufficiency may be associated with hypoglycemia, particularly in patients with end-stage renal disease (61). In one retrospective study, 3.6% of patients with end-stage renal failure admitted to the hospital had hypoglycemia (62). The most common associated pathologies were drug-induced hypoglycemia and sepsis. Severe malnutrition was associated with 7% of hypoglycemic episodes in these patients. Hypoglycemia associated with either sepsis or malnutrition was associated with a particularly high mortality.

Diabetic and nondiabetic patients undergoing either hemodialysis or peritoneal dialysis can develop spontaneous hypoglycemia during or immediately after dialysis (63). This is thought to be caused by increased insulin secretion induced by a high glucose concentration in the dialysis fluid combined with reduced renal insulin clearance. In addition, hypoglycemia may occur when the patients are dialyzed with a glucose-free dialysis fluid. Patients with an initially low plasma glucose level and those who do not eat during dialysis are particularly at risk for hypoglycemia. The hormonal response to hypoglycemia is blunted, and hypoglycemia unawareness is common (64).

The pathogenesis of hypoglycemia in renal failure involves multiple mechanisms, including reduced supply of substrate for gluconeogenesis, especially in patients with severe cachexia, malnutrition with decreased carbohydrate intake, resistance to the hyperglycemic effect of glucagon, and inhibition of gluconeogenesis (65). In healthy volunteers, renal glucose production accounts for 25% of systemic glucose appearance in the postabsorptive state. Furthermore, epinephrine infusion, which increased plasma epinephrine to levels observed during hypoglycemia, increased the renal release of glucose nearly twofold so that, at the end of the infusion, renal glucose release accounted for 40% of systemic glucose production and essentially all of the increase due to adrenergic stimulation (66). Thus, renal glucose production may have an important role in glucose homeostasis in the postabsorptive state and during hypoglycemia. Patients with renal failure are therefore more susceptible to hypoglycemia (67). A considerable number of patients with end-stage renal failure have diabetes. These patients may develop hypoglycemia as a result of decreased clearance of hypoglycemic drugs or insulin.

Sepsis

Sepsis frequently is associated with hypoglycemia in hospitalized patients. In experimental animals, there are several metabolically distinct phases. In the early phase of sepsis, glucose production and utilization are increased and the animals may be hyperglycemic. Hyperglycemia is followed by a hypoglycemic phase in which hepatic glucose production is decreased. This phase is characterized by a rapid depletion of hepatic glycogen content, impaired glycogenesis, and depressed gluconeogenesis, combined with increased peripheral utilization of glucose (68). Regulation of glucose metabolism by the liver is a complicated process that includes several hormonal regulatory factors, such as insulin, glucagon, and catecholamines. Transcriptional and posttranscriptional regulation of β_2-adrenergic receptor gene expression may be responsible for the altered hepatic glucose metabolism during the progression of sepsis (69). Increased utilization of glucose during sepsis is explained by increased use of glucose by macrophage-rich tissues such as liver, spleen, and lung (70). The muscle and fat cells make only a only modest contribution to the increase in glucose utilization. Cytokines such as interleukin-1, interleukin-6, and tumor necrosis factor-α released during sepsis can increase insulin secretion and stimulate glucose transport, leading to imbalance between glucose production and utilization (71,72). Some of these factors have also been implicated in induction of insulin resistance in states of sepsis.

Endocrine Deficiency Disorders and Hypoglycemia

Decreased secretion of multiple glucoregulatory hormones secondary to recurrent hypoglycemia in patients with insulinoma or type 1 diabetes may exacerbate hypoglycemia and prevent prompt recovery of glucose levels. However, in the adult, hormone deficiencies alone are rarely directly responsible for spontaneous hypoglycemia, since insulin secretion is suppressed in response to hypoglycemia and the counterregulatory mechanisms are partially redundant.

Glucagon and Catecholamine Deficiency

Glucagon and epinephrine are important in the counterregulatory response to short-term hypoglycemia. Glucagon increases endogenous glucose production by stimulating hepatic glycogenolysis and gluconeogenesis. In contrast to glucagon, which exclusively affects glucose production, catecholamines have multiple effects on glucose homeostasis, including suppression of endogenous insulin secretion, stimulation of gluconeogenesis and glycogenolysis, and inhibition of glucose utilization. The relative importance of glucagon compared with catecholamines in the physiologic response to hypoglycemia is controversial; however, deficiency of both glucagon and epinephrine in the presence of insulin may result in severe hypoglycemia (73). In clinical practice, isolated deficiency of glucagon and/or epinephrine in patients without diabetes is extremely rare. There are very few case reports of children with hypoglycemia that was presumed to be due to selective deficiency of epinephrine or glucagon (74,75). In some patients with presumed glucagon or epinephrine deficiency, other causes of hypoglycemia, such as hyperinsulinism, were not excluded and the secretion of other glucoregulatory hormones was not studied. Hypoglycemia does not occur in patients receiving glucocorticoid and mineralocorticoid replacement therapy after bilateral adrenalectomy and in patients treated with adrenoreceptor blockers (73). Thus, isolated deficiencies of epinephrine or glucagon rarely, if ever, cause spontaneous hypoglycemia in the absence of hyperinsulinism or an additional factor that decreases glucose levels.

GROWTH-HORMONE AND CORTISOL DEFICIENCIES

In contrast to the rapid-acting hormones glucagon and epinephrine, growth hormone and cortisol are more important in the late response to hypoglycemia. The counterregulatory effects of these hormones are evident after more than 3 hours of hypoglycemia. Growth hormone and cortisol increase plasma levels of free fatty acids and glycerol, resulting in suppression of glucose utilization and an increase in gluconeogenesis. In addition, cortisol increases gluconeogenesis by induction of hepatic gluconeogenic enzymes (1). The major glucoregulatory effects of growth hormone and cortisol are on hepatic gluconeogenesis. Therefore, deficient growth hormone and/or cortisol may cause hypoglycemia, especially after a prolonged fast when hepatic glycogen stores are depleted. The problem may be compounded when both hormones are deficient, as seen in patients with hypopituitarism.

In clinical practice, however, most adults with growth-hormone and/or cortisol deficiency do not develop spontaneous hypoglycemia. Fasting plasma glucose concentrations of patients with primary adrenal insufficiency and patients with corticotropin deficiency are similar to those in normal controls (76). Plasma glucose concentrations after prolonged insulin infusion were lower in patients with panhypopituitarism; however, the recovery from hypoglycemia was intact (77), and the risk of hypoglycemia is not higher compared with that in patients with isolated deficiency of growth hormone or corticotropin. When present, the tendency to develop hypoglycemia following prolonged fasting can be corrected by glucocorticoid replacement, whereas growth-hormone replacement has minimal effect on fasting glucose (77). Adults with hypopituitarism may develop hypoglycemia when glucose production is decreased, as during alcohol ingestion or sepsis, or when glucose utilization is increased, such as during vigorous exercise or pregnancy. Newborns and young children with hypopituitarism are more susceptible to hypoglycemia. Thus, cortisol and growth hormone are probably more important in glucose counterregulation in early life. This hypothesis is supported by experimental data showing that glucocorticoid-deficient newborn mice develop hypoglycemia more frequently during fasting than do adult mice (78).

Immune Hypoglycemia

Hypoglycemia may rarely result from autoantibodies directed against insulin or the insulin receptor. The antibodies disrupt the synchronous coupling between changes in blood glucose and insulin action, thus leading to hypoglycemia.

HYPOGLYCEMIA CAUSED BY ANTIBODIES TO INSULIN

The most common cause for the presence of circulating insulin antibodies is the administration of insulin to patients with diabetes. The antibodies may reduce the levels of free insulin postinjection, resulting in higher postprandial levels of glucose, but may also increase the half-life of insulin (79). Theoretically, a prolonged half-life of insulin causes late hypoglycemia after a bolus injection of insulin. In practice, however, the antibodies do not have a major effect on glycemic control and the incidence of severe hypoglycemia (80). Antibodies to insulin also may develop in patients with recent-onset type 1 diabetes before insulin treatment, relatives of patients with type 1 diabetes or other autoimmune disorders, and occasionally in otherwise healthy subjects (81).

In rare patients, insulin antibodies may be a primary cause of hypoglycemia. The majority of patients with hypoglycemia induced by antibodies to insulin are Japanese. The higher prevalence of autoimmune hypoglycemia in the Japanese population is probably explained by the higher prevalence of specific HLA class 2 alleles that are strongly associated with the disease in this population (82). Hypoglycemia is often postprandial, although fasting hypoglycemia may also occur. Patients often develop hyperglycemia immediately after a meal or glucose load followed by hypoglycemia 2 to 3 hours later. The severity of hypoglycemia varies, and the presentation may be of severe neuroglycopenia with symptoms of confusion, cognitive dysfunction, and even coma. Patients may have other autoimmune diseases, such as Graves disease, systemic lupus erythematosus, or rheumatoid arthritis (80). Exposure to sulfhydryl-containing medications, especially methimazole, was reported for almost half of the patients (82). Interferon-α and medications that cause drug-induced lupus, such as hydralazine, procainamide, and isoniazid, also may cause the development of insulin antibodies and hypoglycemia. Several patients with plasma-cell dyscrasias were reported to have hypoglycemia due to monoclonal insulin-binding antibodies with a low affinity for insulin and a high binding capacity (80). Insulin levels in patients with insulin antibodies causing hypoglycemia usually are high (>100 μU/mL). The endogenous insulin antibodies may interfere with the insulin assay, leading to spurious high or low results, depending on the insulin assay used. C-peptide levels are not fully suppressed because insulin is endogenously secreted. In contrast, surreptitious insulin injection leads to high plasma insulin levels together with complete suppression of C-peptide secretion. The presence of insulin antibodies can be confirmed by high binding of radioactively labeled insulin to polyethylene glycol–precipitated serum samples or by enzyme-linked immunosorbent assay (81). Insulin autoantibodies associated with hypoglycemia cannot be distinguished from those found in insulin-treated patients with diabetes.

The pathogenesis of hypoglycemia caused by insulin antibodies reflects the equilibrium between bound and free insulin, leading to inappropriate release of free insulin that dissociates from the antibodies while the blood glucose concentration is already decreased. Other possible mechanisms, including enhancement of insulin binding to its receptor resulting from cross-linking by the insulin antibodies or direct stimulation of insulin secretion by insulin antibodies, may be operative in some patients (80).

Most patients with autoimmune hypoglycemia due to insulin antibodies experience spontaneous remission (82). If autoimmune hypoglycemia is precipitated by a medication, it should be discontinued and the problem of hypoglycemia will resolve. Patients with recurrent nonremitting hypoglycemia may benefit from frequent low-carbohydrate meals to reduce postprandial hyperglycemia and insulin secretion. Medications that reduce glucose absorption or insulin secretion, such as acarbose, diazoxide, and octreotide, have also been used; however, the results are not consistent. Finally, glucocorticoid therapy and plasmapheresis have also been tried, with the goal of lowering the titer of insulin antibodies (80).

HYPOGLYCEMIA CAUSED BY ANTIBODIES TO INSULIN RECEPTOR

Most patients with hypoglycemia caused by antibodies to the insulin receptor are women. A history of concomitant autoimmune disease is common, and several patients with Hodgkin disease have been reported. The hypoglycemia may be fasting or postprandial and often presents with severe symptoms of neuroglycopenia. Hypoglycemia may be preceded by a phase of severe insulin resistance associated with acanthosis nigricans and hyperglycemia in some patients, whereas others present only with hypoglycemia. The reason for the versatility in the biologic function of the insulin receptor antibodies, even in the same patient at different time points, is not clear. It may be related to the possibility that the polyclonal antibodies to insulin receptor are composed of different subpopulations of immunoglobulins, some activating the insulin receptor and others inhibiting insulin action. Thus, variation in the titer of different antibody populations over time may determine whether the patient presents with insulin resistance or hypoglycemia. The titer of the insulin-receptor antibodies also may affect the clinical presentation. Low antibody titer with partial occupation of the insulin receptor may induce maximal stimulation of the insulin receptor, leading to hypoglycemia. However, a high titer of insulin antibodies may increase the degradation of the insulin receptor and decrease the number and function of the receptors, leading to insulin resistance and hyperglycemia. It also was suggested that the appearance of low-affinity insulin receptors that are resistant to the inhibitory effects of insulin-receptor antibodies may contribute to the switch from insulin resistance and hyperglycemia to hypoglycemia in some patients with insulin-receptor antibodies (80).

Insulin levels are usually higher than expected for the glucose concentration and may suggest the presence of an insulinoma. However, C-peptide levels are usually partially or completely suppressed. The cause of the nonsuppressed insulin levels is not known and may be related to decreased clearance of circulating insulin by receptor-mediated endocytosis and/or activation of the insulin receptors on pancreatic β-cells, which may augment insulin production (83). The prognosis of hypoglycemia associated with antibodies to insulin receptor is poor, with a high mortality rate due to severe concomitant autoimmune disease or malignancy and potentially severe hypoglycemia. Hypoglycemia may respond to a high-dose glucocorticoid therapy. Plasmapheresis and cytotoxic drugs such as cyclophosphamide can also be used to reduce the titer of antibodies to insulin receptor; however, the clinical effect is inconsistent and the experience with these therapies for hypoglycemia induced by insulin-receptor antibody is limited (80).

Tumor-Associated Hypoglycemia

INSULINOMA

Insulin-producing islet-cell tumors occur with an incidence of 4 per 1 million person-years. The onset is usually insidious. About 94% of the tumors are sporadic, while the rest occur as part of the multiple endocrine neoplasia type 1 syndrome [MEN1; Mendelian Inheritance in Man (MIM) no. 131100; at http://www.ncbi.nlm.nih.gov/Omim/]. Between 5% and 10% of tumors are malignant (84). Diagnosis is made by submitting the patient to a prolonged fast, which is terminated either when neuroglycopenia is demonstrated or after 72 hours. The definitive diagnosis is based on the Whipple triad, combined with levels of nonsuppressed insulin, C-peptide, and proinsulin. A recent publication suggests that a 48-hour fast may be sufficient to confirm the diagnosis in almost all cases (85). It is of critical importance to differentiate tumor hyperinsulinism from factitious hyperinsulinism caused by surreptitious injection of insulin or by ingestion of β-cell–stimulating drugs (see above). Insulinomas are discussed in more detail in Chapter 70.

NON–ISLET CELL TUMOR HYPOGLYCEMIA

Hypoglycemia may rarely occur in association with non–islet cell tumors. The majority are large mesenchymal and epithelial tumors such as sarcoma, mesothelioma, fibroma, hemangiopericytoma, and hepatoma. Two thirds of the tumors are either retroperitoneal or abdominal; most of the rest are in the thorax. Other common cancers occasionally associated with hypoglycemia include cancer of the lung, breast, kidney, and the gastrointestinal tract and endocrine tumors such as carcinoid and adrenocortical carcinoma. Patients with hematologic malignancies such as leukemia and lymphoma may rarely develop hypoglycemia. In these patients, tumor-associated hypoglycemia must be distinguished from pseudohypoglycemia caused by *in vitro* glucose metabolism by the markedly elevated white blood cells (see above). Rarely, hypoglycemia may be the presenting symptom in patients with non–islet cell tumors, although it is more common for it to develop in a patient with a known malignant tumor.

The clinical symptoms resemble those of an insulinoma, with neuroglycopenia being the prominent feature. Glucose utilization is markedly increased, and patients may require large quantities of intravenous glucose to maintain normal plasma glucose concentrations. Hypoglycemia may be severe and refractory to medical treatment. When possible, complete surgical resection will ameliorate the hypoglycemia. Patients for whom complete resection is not feasible may benefit from partial removal of the tumor, which can be associated with prolonged remission of hypoglycemia.

The pathogenesis of non–islet cell tumor hypoglycemia (NICTH) is complex, and multiple factors may be involved. The tumor itself utilizes large amounts of glucose; however, glucose uptake by peripheral tissues is also increased and hepatic glucose production is inhibited, suggesting increased insulin-like activity (86,87). Levels of circulating insulin, C-peptide, and proinsulin are suppressed.

The presence of a humoral factor that mediates the tumor-induced hypoglycemia has been studied extensively. Insulin-like growth factor II (IGF-II), a protein with high homology to proinsulin, is expressed and secreted from mesenchymal tumors that cause hypoglycemia (87,88). IGF-II can bind to the insulin receptor, causing insulin-like activity in the absence of insulin. Circulating levels of IGF-II are modestly increased in some but not all patients with tumor-induced hypoglycemia and return to normal after surgical resection of the tumor and resolution of hypoglycemia (89). Overproduction of an incompletely processed form of IGF-II with a higher molecular weight ("big" IGF-II) is found in most patients with non–β-cell tumors and hypoglycemia (90,91).

Under physiologic conditions, IGF-II forms a 150-kDa complex together with insulin-like growth factor–binding protein 3 (IGFBP-3) and an acid-labile subunit (ALS). Normally, the majority of the circulating IGF-II is transported as part of the 150-kDa complex, only 25% being in a free form. The large complex crosses the capillary bed very poorly; thus, only a small fraction of IGF-II can bind to insulin receptors in the target tissues and exert its hypoglycemic effect. In some patients with tumor-induced hypoglycemia, big IGF-II forms smaller complexes and the 150-kDa complex is absent or decreased. The cause of this failure to form the "normal" 150-kDa complex is not clear and may vary in different patients. Abnormal glycosylation of big-IGF-II has been proposed, but it is not certain that this is responsible for the abnormal complex formation (92,93). Other possible mechanisms include defects in the secretion of the ALS and preferential binding of the big IGF-II to proteins other than IGFBP-3 and ALS. Baxter et al. (94) suggested that big IGF-II itself may inhibit acid-labile subunit binding to the IGFBP-3 directly, thus preventing the formation of the 150-kDa complex. Regardless of the mechanism involved, failure to form the 150-kDa complex causes a larger fraction of IGF-II to be transported in small complexes or as a free protein that is more readily available for binding to insulin receptors. Therefore, although total IGF-II may be normal or only mildly elevated, the levels of the bioactive IGF-II are typically increased (90–92).

Patients with NICTH frequently have low serum levels of growth hormone, which may further decrease hepatic glucose production and exacerbate the hypoglycemia (89). Although insulin and total IGF-I levels are typically low in patients with NICTH, free IGF-I levels in plasma recently were shown to be markedly elevated, suggesting a possible mechanism to explain the low levels of growth hormone seen in these patients (91). The diagnosis of NICTH is suggested when hypoglycemia is found in combination with suppressed insulin, C-peptide, and total IGF-I concentrations. IGF-II levels may be elevated, but the measurement of big IGF-II may be superior for the definitive diagnosis of NICTH.

Ectopic insulin secretion in non–islet cell tumors is exceedingly rare. It was convincingly shown in one recent case report of a patient with carcinoma of the uterine cervix (95). Relative hyperinsulinemia was demonstrated in a few other patients; however, ectopic insulin secretion by the tumor was not proven (96,97).

NONINSULINOMA, PANCREATOGENOUS HYPOGLYCEMIA SYNDROME

Hyperinsulinemic hypoglycemia not caused by an insulinoma was described in five patients evaluated at the Mayo Clinic (98). All patients had neuroglycopenic symptoms 2 to 4 hours after a meal but not during a prolonged (72 hour) fast. No insulinoma was found during operation by palpation and intraoperative ultrasound. All patients had a positive response to arterial calcium stimulation and underwent gradient-guided partial pancreatectomy. There was no recurrence of symptoms during prolonged follow-up after surgery. Pancreatic tissue from all patients showed islet hyperplasia and nesidioblastosis. No insulinoma was found in the resected pancreatic tissue. Mutations in the *SUR1* and *Kir6.2* genes that are common in patients with familial persistent hyperinsulinemic hypoglycemia of infancy were not identified in these patients. This syndrome is rare, as there were only nine adult patients with histologic findings of nesidioblastosis among 300 patients who underwent surgery for suspected insulinoma at the Mayo Clinic. The precise etiology of this entity, which may represent a novel mechanism of hypoglycemia, is not known. Previous studies have described rare cases of hypoglycemia due to "nesidioblastosis" in adults, but the genetic studies were not done at the time (99,100).

Rarely, patients with hyperinsulinism due to mutations of glutamate dehydrogenase, glucokinase, or of either of the β-cell K_{ATP}-channel genes (see below) may have mild disease that only comes to medical attention during adulthood. A complete medical history may reveal episodes of idiopathic epilepsy or other signs of neuroglycopenia after prolonged fast or during intercurrent illness in the neonatal period or during childhood.

Reactive Hypoglycemia

Reactive hypoglycemia refers to disorders in which hypoglycemia occurs exclusively after meals and not in the postabsorptive state. All the disorders that cause postabsorptive hypoglycemia also can produce hypoglycemia in the postprandial state. Thus, the term "reactive hypoglycemia" does not have any implication regarding the etiology, and the presence of a syndrome causing postabsorptive hypoglycemia should always be considered in patients with postprandial hypoglycemia.

Congenital defects in carbohydrate metabolism, such as galactosemia and hereditary fructose intolerance, cause postprandial hypoglycemia in children (see below). In adults reactive hypoglycemia can be subdivided into three categories: (a) hypoglycemia after surgery of the upper gastrointestinal tract (alimentary hypoglycemia), (b) hypoglycemia in patients with elevated glucose in an oral glucose tolerance test (early diabetes hypoglycemia), and (c) idiopathic functional hypoglycemia.

ALIMENTARY HYPOGLYCEMIA

Alimentary hypoglycemia occurs in some patients after gastrectomy with or without gastric drainage procedure and rarely in the absence of gastrointestinal surgery (101). The hypoglycemia results from accelerated movement of ingested food into the small intestine, followed by rapid absorption of glucose that stimulates insulin secretion. Stimulation of enteric hormone secretion may further augment insulin secretion. The hypoglycemic effect of the secreted insulin persists after the glucose load is cleared from the circulation, thus leading to hypoglycemia. Typically, hyperglycemia develops within half an hour, followed by hypoglycemia approximately 1.5 to 3 hours after food ingestion. Symptoms may be severe, including seizures, coma, and even death. Alimentary hypoglycemia should be distinguished from the dumping syndrome that may cause similar symptoms within 1 hour after eating in the absence of hypoglycemia. The dumping syndrome is caused by contraction of the plasma volume due to fluid shift into the gastrointestinal tract (23). Both dumping syndrome and alimentary hypoglycemia have become very rare, since most patients with peptic ulcer disease are now treated medically.

REACTIVE HYPOGLYCEMIA ASSOCIATED WITH EARLY DIABETES MELLITUS

Reactive hypoglycemia was reported to be an early manifestation of type 2 diabetes more than four decades ago (102). Diabetic patients with reactive hypoglycemia usually have mild hyperglycemia and develop symptoms of hypoglycemia 3 to 5 hours after a meal. It was suggested that the hyperglycemia provokes a gradual increase in insulin secretion, which may persist after the disposal of the ingested glucose, leading to the late hypoglycemia. The prevalence and significance of reactive hypoglycemia in patients with diabetes is controversial. Type 2 diabetes is a common disease; however, spontaneous postprandial hypoglycemia has been documented in very few patients. Moreover, in some patients the diagnosis was based on an oral glucose tolerance test (OGTT) that showed elevated blood glucose levels within the first 2 hours after glucose load, followed by glucose levels below 50 mg/dL. The correlation between low blood glucose concentrations several hours after an oral glucose load and postprandial hypoglycemia is poor. For example, only 5% of patients with early diabetes and hypoglycemia after an oral glucose load had symptoms of hypoglycemia after meals (103). It is possible that patients frequently develop asymptomatic hypoglycemia during the early stages of diabetes; however, there are no data to support this hypothesis.

IDIOPATHIC FUNCTIONAL HYPOGLYCEMIA

Symptoms suggestive of hypoglycemia several hours after a meal are common. The appearance of postprandial autonomic symptoms is commonly diagnosed as "reactive hypoglycemia"; however, blood glucose concentrations are not usually measured during such "hypoglycemic" episodes and when measured are usually normal. Most patients with autonomic symptoms after meals evaluated for hypoglycemia have been found to have psychoneurotic disturbances with frequent somatic complaints (104,105). An effort to document the correlation between glycemia and symptoms was made by measuring blood glucose in 28 patients during a total of 132 reported episodes of symptomatic hypoglycemia. Only six (5%) of these episodes were associated with blood glucose levels below 50 mg/dL (2.8 mmol/L), and these occurred in five (18%) different patients. Relief of symptoms by ingesting food was more often associated with low than with normal blood glucose levels (24). In another study of 118 patients with suspected postprandial hypoglycemia, only five (4%) were found to have hypoglycemia after a glucose load and after meals (106).

In many patients, low glucose levels during an OGTT are used to diagnose reactive hypoglycemia because it may be difficult to document glucose levels during symptomatic episodes. However, when critically evaluated, no correlation was found between plasma glucose levels measured after oral glucose administration and glucose levels measured during symptoms. Furthermore, most patients with low blood glucose levels after an oral glucose load have normal glucose levels after a mixed meal (23). In a large study of 650 healthy subjects who remained asymptomatic during a 100-g OGTT, 25% had a circulating glucose nadir below 54 mg/dL, 10% below 47 mg/dL, 5% below 43 mg/dL, and 2.5% below 40 mg/dL (106). The fact that approximately 10% of the general healthy population has nadir glucose levels lower than 50 mg/dL indicates that a low glucose level on OGTT is not a reliable criterion for the diagnosis of reactive hypoglycemia, and thus this test should not be used for this purpose. Establishment of the diagnosis of reactive hypoglycemia requires documentation of low blood glucose levels during spontaneous symptomatic episodes. Although true idiopathic reactive hypoglycemia probably exists, it is rare even in a referral population.

The pathogenesis of true idiopathic reactive hypoglycemia is unknown. Insulin sensitivity is increased in patients with idiopathic reactive hypoglycemia (107). The changes in insulin sensitivity are probably not explained by increased binding of insulin to its receptor, and there is no evidence that insulin secretion is increased. A reduced glucagon response may play a role in the development of late hypoglycemia after glucose ingestion; however, there are few data that support this hypothesis (108).

TREATMENT

Low-carbohydrate or high-fiber diets, avoidance of simple sugars that are rapidly absorbed, and the use of multiple small meals are recommended for patients with reactive hypoglycemia. A high-protein diet is often administered to patients with reactive hypoglycemia; however, this diet is also high in fat and its clinical efficacy is unknown. Therefore, it should no longer be recommended. Cornstarch, doxepin, α-glucosidase inhibitors, biguanides, and anticholinergic agents have been successful in some patients with reactive hypoglycemia. The efficacy and the precise role of such treatments in the management of reactive hypoglycemia need to be determined in larger studies (23).

DIAGNOSTIC AND THERAPEUTIC APPROACH TO THE HYPOGLYCEMIC PATIENT

The symptoms and signs of hypoglycemia are nonspecific; therefore, the first step in the evaluation of a patient with suspected hypoglycemia is always to document low blood glucose when the patient experiences spontaneous symptoms. The demonstration that symptoms are relieved by an increase in blood glucose level following ingestion of food or glucose further supports the diagnosis of hypoglycemia (Whipple triad). Repeated normal blood glucose measurements during the occurrence of symptoms exclude the possibility of hypoglycemia, and no further evaluation is required for this diagnosis. In some patients, documentation of blood glucose during spontaneous symptoms may be difficult because the symptomatic episodes are infrequent, the duration of symptoms is short, and the patient is far from a medical facility. Glucosemeter measurements of capillary blood glucose can be used to correlate patient symptoms with blood glucose levels and to exclude hypoglycemia as the cause of the symptoms. However, the results should be interpreted with caution because the measurement of blood glucose may be technically poor because it is performed by an inexperienced patient suffering from autonomic and potentially neuroglycopenic symptoms.

A careful history of the occupation of the patient; the existence of family members with diabetes being treated with sulfonylureas or insulin; and alcohol abuse, predisposing illnesses, and medications taken by the patient is crucial to making the correct diagnosis. The patient should be asked about the frequency and duration of symptomatic episodes, the presence of neuroglycopenia and/or autonomic symptoms, whether they are relieved by ingestion of glucose, and when the symptoms occur (fasting vs. postprandial). Patients who develop hypoglycemia only during the postprandial period may have idiopathic reactive hypoglycemia. However, other hypoglycemic disorders, including insulinoma, may present as postprandial hypoglycemia, and therefore prompt evaluation of other causes of hypoglycemia should be performed.

If hypoglycemia is confirmed or the clinical suspicion for hypoglycemia is high but measuring blood glucose during spontaneous symptoms is not feasible, the patient should be admitted for further testing (Fig. 69.4). The next diagnostic step is to measure insulin, C-peptide, and, if possible, proinsulin levels. Alcohol and medications known to cause hypoglycemia should always be considered and discontinued before the patient is evaluated. This may prevent unnecessary, time-consuming, and expensive tests. If the episodes of hypoglycemia are infrequent, it may be necessary to provoke hypoglycemia by a prolonged 48- to 72-hour fast or by insulin infusion to test C-peptide suppression. Relatively high levels of insulin, C-peptide, and proinsulin during spontaneous or induced hypoglycemia and the failure to suppress C-peptide secretion in response to insulin-induced hypoglycemia suggest the diagnosis of insulinoma (see Chapter 70 on islet-cell tumors). Blood levels of oral insulin secretagogues should always be measured during hypoglycemia to exclude surreptitious administration of drugs. Rare patients with insulin antibody–mediated hypoglycemia may also have hyperinsulinemic hypoglycemia with nonsuppressed C-peptide. Hypoglycemia associated with high levels of insulin and suppressed C-peptide suggests surreptitious administration of insulin; however, patients with autoimmune antibodies to insulin receptor may also present with inappropriately high levels of insulin and suppressed C-peptide during hypoglycemia. Suppression of both insulin and C-peptide levels during hypoglycemia suggests the diagnosis of tumor-induced hypoglycemia, and determination of plasma IGF-II and appropriate imaging studies should be performed. Deficiencies in glucoregulatory hormones, including cortisol and growth hormone, should always be excluded, although deficiencies in glucoregulatory hormones alone in otherwise healthy subjects will rarely cause hypoglycemia under normal conditions.

The acutely ill patient suffers from multisystem disease, and multiple factors may cause hypoglycemia. Organ failure, including renal, hepatic, and cardiac failure, is common. These patients are at risk for iatrogenic hypoglycemia (e.g., insulin added to total parenteral nutrition or pentamidine-induced hypoglycemia in patients with pneumocystis pneumonia). Sepsis and inanition are common contributing factors. Some of the acutely ill patients admitted to the hospital suffer from underlying malignancy that may cause tumor hypoglycemia (NICTH). Treatment of the underlying acute illness, improvement in critical-organ function, and careful monitoring of the drugs administered to the patient result in resolution of hypoglycemia, and extensive hormonal evaluation is usually not required.

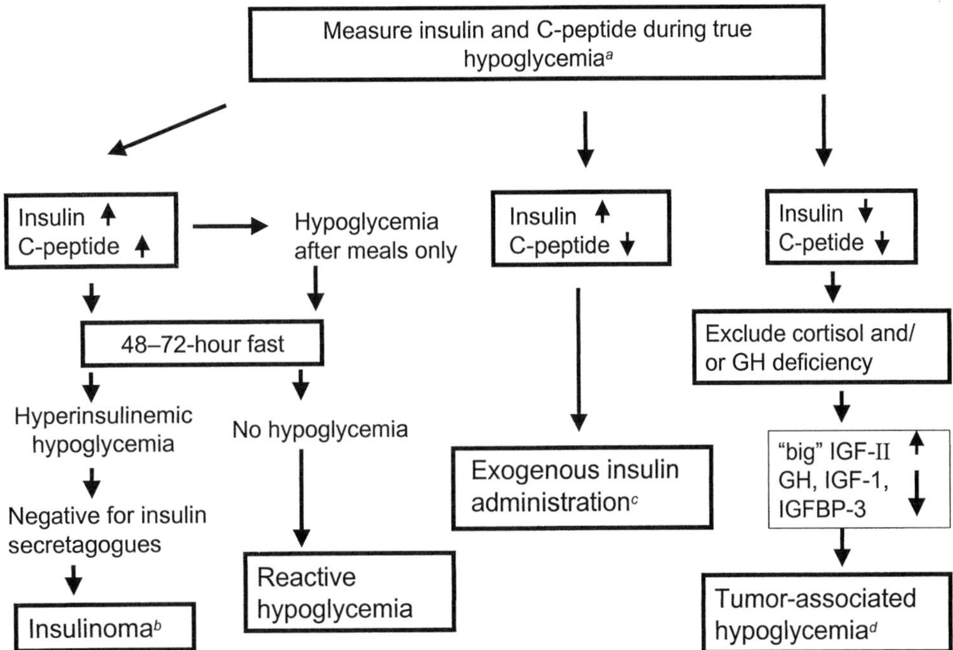

Figure 69.4. Workup of hypoglycemia in the non–acutely ill patient. [a]See text for definition of true hypoglycemia. [b]Rare patients with insulin antibody–mediated hypoglycemia may also have hyperinsulinemic hypoglycemia with nonsuppressed C-peptide. The endogenous insulin antibodies may interfere with the insulin assay, leading to spuriously high or low results, depending on the insulin assay used. Measurement of antibodies to insulin is not part of the routine workup of hypoglycemia; however, it should be considered in some patients. [c]Patients with autoimmune antibodies to insulin receptor may also present with inappropriately high levels of insulin and suppressed C-peptide during hypoglycemia. Measurement of antibodies to insulin receptor is not part of the routine workup of hypoglycemia; however, it should be considered in some patients. [d]Ethanol and other medications that inhibit gluconeogenesis may lead to suppression of endogenous insulin production secondary to hypoglycemia.

HYPOGLYCEMIA IN NEONATES AND INFANTS

A separate discussion of hypoglycemia in the young child is appropriate since the problem in this age group differs from that in adults in several important ways. Neonatal hypoglycemia frequently is caused by a specific genetic defect. In some cases, the precise genetic etiology is known, whereas in others, the information presently available is limited. Our understanding of the genetic etiology of disease is expanding at an exponential rate, and the latest information is constantly being updated in the online version of MIM (http://www.ncbi.nlm.nih.gov/Omim/). For this reason, whenever possible, we have included the MIM numbers of specific genetic entities in parentheses. The reader is encouraged to consult the MIM Web site for the latest genetic information and updated clinical references on these diseases.

Glucose Homeostasis in Infants and Children

The basic mechanisms of glucose homeostasis in the neonate are similar to those of the adult, although some critical differences make the neonate more prone to hypoglycemia. Glucose requirements of the neonate are considerably higher than those of the adult, primarily because of the increased ratio of brain to body mass. Premature infants require 5 to 6 mg/(kg · min) and full-term neonates require 3 to 5 mg/(kg · min), whereas adults require only 2 to 3 mg/(kg · min) (3,109). The fetus receives the glucose it needs as a constant supply from the placenta. As soon as the umbilical cord is cut, the neonate must suddenly rely on oral intake, glycogenolysis, and gluconeogenesis. However, the healthy breastfeeding infant gets little oral nutrition immediately after birth. Glycogen stores are relatively low and are rapidly depleted. The gluconeogenic pathway may be immature, since in the fetus of a well-nourished mother, glycogenolysis and gluconeogenesis are virtually absent. All of the gluconeogenic enzymes except phosphoenolpyruvate carboxykinase (PEPCK) are expressed early in fetal development. PEPCK, the rate-limiting enzyme in the gluconeogenesis pathway, is not expressed in the mammalian fetus but appears immediately after birth. The rapid decline in insulin and the surge in plasma glucagon appear to be responsible for induction of its transcription and activation. Stable-isotope studies in healthy humans have shown that both gluconeogenesis and ketogenesis are active 12 to 24 hours after birth (110,111). Both of these, however, require a steady supply of substrates. In infants who are small for gestational age, or in infants of mothers with inadequate nutrition, adequate supplies of these substrates may not be available.

Therefore, normal neonates are at risk of hypoglycemia from the moment of birth. Blood glucose levels fall naturally, and significant hypoglycemia is avoided only if all of the necessary mechanisms function properly and rapidly. The precise level at which this normal decline in glucose endangers neurologic development is not known; therefore, the need for therapeutic intervention is still controversial. Congenital defects in any of the mechanisms required to maintain euglycemia will result in more severe and persistent hypoglycemia. Rapid diagnosis and effective treatment of these disorders will have a profound impact on long-term prognosis.

Defining Hypoglycemia in the Newborn Period

The definition of hypoglycemia in the newborn has been the subject of controversy for the last several decades. Even today, there is no clear consensus on how hypoglycemia should be defined in each specific category of patient. The subject has recently been extensively reviewed (112,113).

METHODOLOGIC ISSUES

Accurate laboratory determination of circulating glucose levels is not a trivial problem, even as we enter the 21st century. Bedside capillary glucose determinations are designed primarily for use by persons with diabetes and are therefore calibrated to differentiate between euglycemia and hyperglycemia. Although some of these determinations may be adequate as screening aids, none are sufficiently accurate or sensitive to reliably confirm the diagnosis of hypoglycemia. Reliable and sensitive laboratory analyses are required before the diagnosis of hypoglycemia can be confirmed, and any method used must be validated at glucose concentrations below 40 to 50 mg/dL (2.2 to 2.8 mmol/L) (112,113).

DEFINITION

Pathologic hypoglycemia can be defined in several ways, including (a) glucose levels less than 2 standard deviations below the mean for age-matched controls, (b) glucose levels causing clinically evident symptoms of hypoglycemia, (c) the glucose threshold for acute symptoms of neuroglycopenia determined in healthy neonates, and (d) the glucose threshold below which irreversible brain damage may occur. Clearly, the latter definition is the most important in terms of long-term prognosis; however, it is also the most difficult to delineate. The degree of neurologic damage is related not only to the glucose level achieved but also to the frequency and duration of hypoglycemia. In addition, factors other than glucose play important roles in determining the neurotoxic potential of any particular glucose level. One of the most important among these factors is the availability of alternative fuels such as ketone bodies. The infant brain is capable of utilizing ketone bodies as a partial source of energy. Therefore, the same level of hypoglycemia may be less damaging in the presence of elevated ketone bodies. For this reason, hypoketotic hypoglycemia due to hyperinsulinism or defects in fatty acid metabolism may be particularly damaging.

Comparison with Healthy Control Populations

Population surveys in the 1960s and 1980s have established the range and standard deviations of glucose values for different categories of neonates (Table 69.3) (113). While these studies provide normative data, they do not necessarily define the threshold for irreversible brain damage and do not take into consideration the duration of hypoglycemia. Therefore, although they provide a useful reference range, they have limited impact on the clinical decision-making process.

Clinical Definition

The classical definition of hypoglycemia is based on the Whipple triad as defined above. In the adult or the older child, symptoms of adrenergic stimulation and neuroglycopenia can usually be readily identified (Table 69.1). In the newborn, however, signs may be nonspecific, including cyanosis, apnea, irritability, poor feeding, or hypothermia. Therefore, the rapid diagnosis of symptomatic neonatal hypoglycemia requires a high index of suspicion on the part of the treating physician.

Neuroglycopenia

More recently, there has been an attempt to correlate glucose levels with objective measures of neural function. In 1988, Koh et al. (114) observed abnormal auditory evoked potentials in neonates with glucose levels ranging from 25 to 47 mg/dL (1.4 to 2.6 mmol/L). Pryds et al. (115) measured cerebral blood flow and plasma catecholamine levels in hypoglycemic infants [glucose <30 mg/dL (1.7 mmol/L)] and normoglycemic controls and demonstrated an increase in cerebral blood flow and concentrations of epinephrine. The recent development of methods for the microanalysis of hormones and substrates, along with the availability of methods permitting *in vivo* measurements of cerebral blood flow, glucose uptake, and high-energy phosphate content, will open up the way to more accurate assessments of the effects of hypoglycemia on neural function.

TABLE 69.3. Proposed Definitions of Hypoglycemia in Neonates

	Blood glucose values by birthweight class (mg/dL in serum or plasma)		
Basis for definition	**Term AGA**	**LBW**	**VLBW**
Population survey (2 SD below population means)			
<48 h old	<35	<25	<25
>48 h old	<45	<45	<45
Functional correlations (brain electrophysiology, counterregulatory responses, and cerebral blood flow)	<30	—	—
Adverse long-term outcome	—	47	—
Proposed treatment guidelines			
<24 h old	45	45	45
24–72 h old	50	50	50
>72 h old	60	60	60

AGA, average for gestational age; LBW, low body weight; VLBW, very low body weight.
Modified from Cornblath M, Ichord R. Hypoglycemia in the neonate. *Semin Perinatol* 2000;24:136–149.
The reader is referred to this publication for a more detailed description of the criteria.

Long-Term Outcome Data

None of the methods outlined above answer the cardinal question: At what glucose level does irreversible brain damage occur? Most studies have tried to answer this question retrospectively by correlating neurologic status of older children with hypoglycemic events in infancy. Lucas et al. (116) determined that, in infants with a birth weight less than 1,850 g, glucose levels lower than 47 mg/dL (2.6 mmol/L) on 5 or more days correlated positively with abnormal neurologic and developmental outcome at 18 months. However, this appeared to be at least partially reversible, because by 7 to 8 years of age, the neurologic deficit appeared to be much milder. More recently, Duvanel et al. (117) demonstrated that recurrent episodes of hypoglycemia were strongly correlated with persistent neurologic and developmental deficits at the age of 5 years. In fact, infants with recurrent, moderate hypoglycemia had a poorer neurologic outcome than did those with a single, severe episode of hypoglycemia. A prospective, randomized trial of alternative treatment regimens is still needed to establish the policy that assures the best possible long-term neurologic outcome in premature and small-for-gestational-age infants.

Operational Definition of Hypoglycemia

In view of the limited data available for long-term implications of hypoglycemia, Cornblath et al. (112) have proposed an "operational threshold" of hypoglycemia to be used as an indication for action but not necessarily diagnostic of pathology. They recommended that the operational threshold be defined as a plasma glucose level lower than 30 to 36 mg/dL (1.7 to 2 mmol/L) during the first 24 hours of life in a healthy full-term or preterm (24 to 27 weeks of gestation) formula-fed infant. If the level persists after feeding or recurs, treatment should be initiated to maintain a glucose level above 45 mg/dL (2.5 mmol/L). In sick, low-birth-weight, or premature infants, this threshold may be increased to 45 to 50 mg/dL (2.5 to 2.8 mmol/L), because these infants may have increased glucose requirements due to sepsis, hypoxia, or other systemic disease. After the first 24 hours, an operational threshold of 40 to 50 mg/dL (2.2 to 2.8 mmol/L) is recommended. Below these values, therapy should be initiated to increase levels above the threshold, although this alone should not be taken as diagnostic of neuroglycopenia or neurologic damage. Infants of any age with confirmed glucose levels below 20 to 25 mg/dL (1.1 to 1.4 mmol/L) should be treated rapidly and aggressively with parenteral glucose. If hypoglycemia persists or recurs beyond the first week of life, then a full diagnostic evaluation is indicated.

Transient Neonatal Hypoglycemia

As soon as the fetus is disconnected from the constant glucose supply through the umbilical cord, it becomes dependent on an immediate endogenous supply of glucose to maintain its energy needs. This is initially supplied by the liver through glycogenolysis and soon thereafter by gluconeogenesis using substrates supplied by fat and muscle. Any prenatal problem that limits the availability of either of these substrates puts the newborn at risk for hypoglycemia. The liver begins to store glycogen in the ninth week of gestation, but most of the glycogen stores are accumulated during the last weeks of gestation. Adequate stores are dependent on adequate delivery of substrate from the mother, which may be deficient in fetuses with retardation of intrauterine growth and in infants who are postterm. Therefore, all premature (gestation less than 38 weeks), small-for-gestational age, and postterm infants are at risk of having inadequate glycogen stores and hence of having hypoglycemia immediately after birth. In all of these cases, oral or parenteral replacement of glucose at rates similar to normal neonatal glucose requirements will prevent hypoglycemia. Once adequate intake is established and adequate glycogen and fat stores are available, hypoglycemia resolves and does not recur.

ASPHYXIA

Perinatal asphyxia may cause hypoglycemia and in some cases transient hyperinsulinism. Initially, it may be difficult to differentiate between apnea due to hyperinsulinemic hypoglycemia and hyperinsulinism secondary to asphyxia, because insulin levels and parameters of glucose metabolism may be similar. However, the latter is transient, and spontaneous resolution of the hyperinsulinism within a few days is expected. The pathophysiology of asphyxia-induced hyperinsulinism is not known (118–122).

INFANT OF DIABETIC MOTHER

Infants born to diabetic mothers are at high risk for developmental anomalies, macrosomia, respiratory distress syndrome, and neonatal hypoglycemia. Although the precise mechanisms have not yet been defined for all of these defects, it is clear that maternal glycemic control has an important impact on all of them. The macrosomia is thought to be caused by intrauterine hyperinsulinism due to chronic fetal exposure to high glucose levels from the mother. This hyperglycemic stimulus may also result in β-cell hyperplasia and hyperresponsiveness, resulting in hyperinsulinemic hypoglycemia when the supply of maternal glucose is abruptly interrupted. This clinical picture is essentially identical to the initial presentation of infants with hyperinsulinism of infancy (see below), confirming the importance of prenatal hyperinsulinism. Not uncommonly, neonates with hyperinsulinism of infancy are misdiagnosed as being infants of diabetic mothers if a careful prenatal history is not obtained.

Good glycemic control during the first 9 to 12 weeks of pregnancy greatly decreases the incidence of birth defects, while good glycemic control during the last 3 months of pregnancy decreases the incidence and severity of macrosomia and postnatal hypoglycemia (see Chapter 61).

BECKWITH–WIEDEMANN SYNDROME

Beckwith–Wiedemann syndrome (BWS; MIM no. 130650) is associated with macrosomia, macroglossia, and abdominal wall defects. Hypoglycemia is present in 30% to 50% of the patients and is usually mild and transient, resolving within the first few days of life. Rarely, hypoglycemia may be more severe and persistent, requiring continued medical treatment or even partial pancreatectomy. Insulin levels may be high or inappropriately elevated for the prevailing glucose level. Prompt glycemic response to glucagon during hypoglycemia confirms that the primary etiology of the hypoglycemia is hyperinsulinism.

Although the genetic etiology of BWS has not been confirmed in all cases, the syndrome may be caused by any of several different genetic mutations on chromosome 11p15.5. This chromosomal region contains at least three imprinted genes, including *IGFII*, which is expressed only from the paternal allele, and *H19* and $p57^{kip2}$, which are expressed only from the maternal allele. IGF-II is an important growth factor, particularly during fetal development. In transgenic animals, overexpression of *IGFII* by β-cells results in islet hyperplasia (123). H19 is an untranslated RNA molecule thought to be an important regulator of levels of IGF-II mRNA (124), and $p57^{kip2}$ (CDKN1C, MIM no. 600856) is an important inhibitor of several G_1 cyclin/Cdk complexes and thus is involved in cell-cycle arrest in terminally differentiated cells (125).

Mutations associated with BWS mutations include duplication of the paternally derived allele or loss of imprinting, resulting in expression of the maternally derived *IGFII* allele (126). Both of these defects would be expected to result in increased *IGFII* expression, and in fact, overexpression of this growth factor has been documented in approximately 20% of cases. Although *IGFII* overexpression may explain the generalized overgrowth seen in this syndrome, and perhaps the β-cell hyperplasia, it is not clear that it explains the hyperinsulinism and hypoglycemia, since the hyperplastic β-cells should still be normally regulated. Recently, patients have been identified who have maternally inherited mutations in the cyclin-dependent kinase inhibitor $p57^{kip2}$ (127). As with the abnormalities of *IGFII* expression, underexpression of this growth-regulating gene could explain the overgrowth phenomena and β-cell hypertrophy, but it is not clear how this alone causes unregulated insulin secretion.

In the focal form of hyperinsulinism of infancy (see below), somatic loss of the maternal allele at this locus is associated with β-cell adenomatous hyperplasia. However, these patients have severe, diazoxide-unresponsive hypoglycemia, which appears to be caused by a concomitant mutation on the paternal allele of one of the two subunits of the β-cell K_{ATP} channel. Therefore, the transient, diazoxide-responsive, hyperinsulinemic hypoglycemia seen in 30% to 50% of patients with BWS has not yet been entirely explained. The 5% of patients with BWS who have severe, drug-unresponsive hypoglycemia may have concomitant mutations on the K_{ATP}-channel genes (128).

HYPOGLYCEMIA IN ERYTHROBLASTOSIS FETALIS

Transient hyperinsulinemic hypoglycemia has been reported in association with erythroblastosis fetalis (EF), although the precise etiology and pathophysiology is still unclear. The incidence of hypoglycemia appears to correlate with severity of EF, ranging from 17% to 31% in patients with severe disease to as low as 2% in patients with milder disease. Insulin levels are usually inappropriately elevated, and elevated pancreatic insulin content with hypertrophy and hyperplasia of the pancreatic islets has been reported. Although hypoglycemia may be present before exchange transfusions are initiated, it may appear or be further exacerbated 1 to 2 hours after the transfusions. Because early feeding does not prevent the hypoglycemia in all cases, glucose levels should be monitored in all EF patients, and if hypoglycemia is diagnosed, intravenous glucose supplementation should be given until oral feedings are well established and provide adequate caloric intake (129–132).

Endocrine Deficiency Disorders

Both growth hormone and cortisol deficiency result in decreased hepatic gluconeogenesis and decreased availability of gluconeogenic substrates. Although symptomatic hypoglycemia is rarely associated with deficiency of either or both of these hormones in the adult (see above), in the neonate and small child, hypoglycemia is common, particularly if both hormones are deficient. Pituitary hormone deficiencies can be single or multiple (MIM nos. 173110 and 601538) (133,134) and can occur either as isolated entities or as part of a syndrome of midline defects such as microphallus or septooptic dysplasia (MIM no. 182230). Primary adrenal insufficiency may be due to congenital adrenal hyperplasia (MIM no. 201910, no. 202010, no. 202110) or primary adrenal hypoplasia (MIM no. 240200, no. 300200) (135).

Patients typically present with ketotic hypoglycemia, suppressed insulin levels, and blunted glycemic response to glucagon. At initial presentation, patients with isolated growth-hormone deficiency may have low plasma levels of ketone bodies and may not have ketonuria. The diagnosis is made by measuring growth hormone and cortisol during spontaneous or induced hypoglycemia. Treatment is based on immediate correction of the hypoglycemia with intravenous glucose, followed by appropriate hormone replacement. Another stimulatory test may be indicated to confirm the diagnosis. Recurrent hypoglycemia per se may secondarily blunt the cortisol response to acute hypoglycemia (136). Therefore, an isolated, blunted cortisol response in the face of recurrent hypoglycemia must be interpreted with caution.

Although a decreased epinephrine response to hypoglycemia has been reported in patients with recurrent hypoglycemia, this is unlikely to be a primary defect and is more likely secondary to recurrent hypoglycemia, very much like the hypoglycemia unawareness syndrome seen in some patients with diabetes.

Ketotic Hypoglycemia

Ketotic hypoglycemia, also called substrate-limited hypoglycemia, is claimed to be the most common form of childhood hypoglycemia. Ketotic hypoglycemia usually presents between the ages of 18 months and 2 years and typically resolves in mid childhood. It is more common in boys than in girls and is associated with decreased muscle mass and body fat. Affected children develop hypoglycemia with ketonemia and ketonuria upon fasting or during periods of caloric restriction or high caloric requirements, such as intercurrent illnesses. The precise etiology is still unknown, but alanine levels tend to be low, implying a defect in protein catabolism or amino acid efflux from skeletal muscle. The response of counterregulatory hormones to hypoglycemia is normal, except for that of epinephrine, which tends to be low. This is unlikely to be a primary defect, however, and is more likely due to recurrent mild hypoglycemia. Treatment is based on the avoidance of fasting and the careful monitoring of urinary ketone levels during intercurrent illness. Fluids high in carbohydrates should be given in situations of increased caloric requirement, and intravenous glucose is necessary if oral feeding must be interrupted for any reason (137).

Inborn Errors of Intermediate Metabolism

Many enzymatic defects may lead to hypoglycemia by interfering with glycogenesis, glycogenolysis, or gluconeogenesis. The defect may block one or more critical metabolic steps directly or may exert its effect indirectly by limiting the availability of necessary substrates. Alternatively, specific defects may prevent the production of alternative energy sources so that the glucose requirement surpasses the normal production capacity. We have classified the major metabolic defects that are typically associated with clinically relevant hypoglycemia according to the major metabolic pathway disrupted (Fig. 69.5).

GLYCOGEN STORAGE DISEASES

The glycogen storage diseases are a class of diseases caused by mutations in any of several enzymes responsible for the generation or breakdown of glycogen (137,138). Because glycogen is the major source of glucose during a short fast, these diseases are characterized by fasting hypoglycemia, the severity of which depends on the specific gene mutated and the nature of the specific mutation (Fig. 69.5).

Glycogen synthase catalyzes the conversion of glucose-6-phosphate to glycogen. Deficiency of this enzyme (glycogen storage disease type 0, MIM no. 240600) is extremely rare, but it results in a severe decrease in glycogen stores. Because hepatic

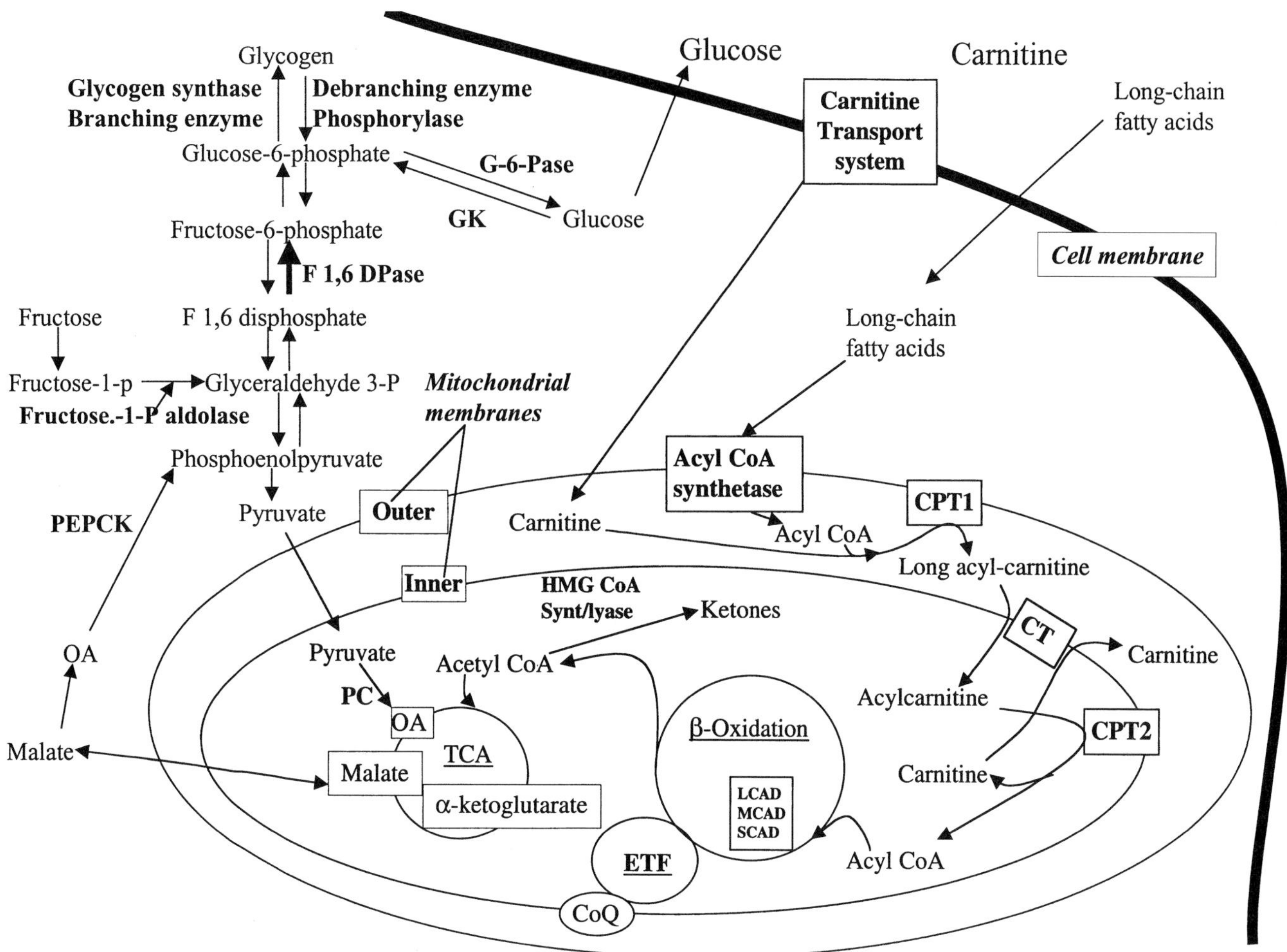

Figure 69.5. Schematic diagram showing the major pathways of glucose synthesis and fatty acid oxidation. Defects in any of many steps in the process (in bold type) can cause hypoglycemia. G-6-Pase, glucose-6-phosphatase; F 1,6 DPase, fructose-1,6-diphosphatase; PEPCK, phosphoenolpyruvate carboxykinase; PC, pyruvate carboxylase; HMG-CoA synt/lyase, 3-hydroxy-3-methylglutaryl CoA synthase and lyase; CPT-1, CPT-2, carnitine palmitoyl transferase 1 and 2; CT, carnitine translocase; LCAD, MCAD, and SCAD, long-, medium- and short-chain acyl-CoA dehydrogenases; ETF, electron-transport-flavoproteins; OA, oxaloacetate.

glycogen is the major source of glucose during the first 12 to 24 hours of a fast, patients typically present with hypoglycemia after an overnight fast. Blood levels of ketones are markedly elevated, whereas levels of alanine and lactate are low. Glycogen is also the major repository for the excess glucose during the postprandial period. Therefore, it is not surprising that patients with glycogen synthase deficiency have postprandial hyperglycemia. Recently, mutations have been documented in the glycogen synthase gene (*GYS2*) in several patients with this clinical syndrome (139,140).

Glucose-6-phosphatase catalyzes the conversion of glucose-6-phospate to glucose, the final step in both glycogenolysis and gluconeogenesis. The enzyme system consists of the enzyme itself and three translocase systems that allow the entry of glucose-6-phosphate into the endoplasmic reticulum (ER), and the exit of phosphate and glucose from the ER. Defective enzyme activity (glycogen storage disease type I, MIM no. 232200, no. 232220, and no. 232240) can be caused by mutations in the enzyme itself (type IA) or in any of the translocase systems (types IB–D) and is usually associated with severe hypoglycemia presenting shortly after birth. Hypoglycemia occurs after short periods of fasting and is associated with mild ketosis, lactic acidosis, and severe hyperlipidemia. The latter leads to eruptive xanthomas and pancreatitis. Accumulation of glycogen in the liver results in severe hepatomegaly, and hepatic adenomas usually develop later in life. In addition to the features of glycogen storage disease type IA, patients with types IB and IC may also have neutropenia, recurrent infection (mainly skin abscess), and inflammatory bowel disease. The diagnosis is suspected when hypoglycemia is associated with increased lactate and lipid levels. Glucagon administration results in little or no increase in plasma glucose, differentiating this class of diseases from hyperinsulinemic hypoglycemia. The definitive diagnosis is made by enzyme analysis of liver biopsy tissue. Treatment is based on the continued supply of glucose throughout the day. Initially, this is accomplished by frequent feedings during the day and continuous nasogastric feeding at night. Raw cornstarch has been effectively used throughout the day to provide a steady supply of glucose. Liver transplantation has been attempted successfully in recent years (137).

Other enzymatic defects of glycogenesis or glycogenolysis can produce a similar clinical picture, although the hypoglycemia is typically less severe because the gluconeogenesis pathway is intact. These include debrancher enzyme deficiency (glycogen storage disease type III, MIM no. 232400), brancher enzyme deficiency (glycogen storage disease type IV, MIM no. 232500), and phosphorylase deficiency (glycogen storage disease type VI).

DISORDERS OF GLUCONEOGENESIS

Mutations in any of several of the enzymes in the gluconeogenesis pathway can result in hypoglycemia. Fructose 1,6-diphosphatase deficiency (MIM no. 229700) is similar to glycogen storage disease type I, presenting with lactic acidosis and hypoglycemia (141). Hypoglycemia is less severe, occurring primarily during fasting or intercurrent illness. Glucose response to glucagon can be normal in the postprandial period, emphasizing the importance of performing the glucagon test during fasting hypoglycemia, when glycogen stores are depleted in the absence of circulating hyperinsulinism. Treatment consists of a high carbohydrate diet, avoidance of fasting, and intravenous glucose during catabolic situations.

Pyruvate carboxylase deficiency (MIM no. 266150) causes severe mental retardation and subacute encephalomyelopathy, whereas hypoglycemia is not common.

HEREDITARY FRUCTOSE INTOLERANCE (MIM NO. 229600)

The enzyme fructose-1-phosphate aldolase catalyzes the cleavage of fructose-1-phosphate to form dihydroxyacetone phosphate and D-glyceraldehyde. Deficiency of the enzyme, caused by any of a number of genetic mutations, results in the inability to metabolize fructose and the inhibition of gluconeogenesis and glycogenolysis by the accumulation of fructose-1-phosphate. Infants present with failure to thrive, recurrent vomiting, and hepatomegaly and renal Fanconi syndrome. Hypoglycemia worsens after fructose-containing feedings, and administration of intravenous fructose can be fatal. These patients are entirely asymptomatic until fructose is introduced into the diet in the form of fruits or sucrose. Avoidance of fructose in the diet prevents the hypoglycemia and other symptoms.

GALACTOSEMIA

Deficiency of the enzyme galactose-1-phosphate uridyl transferase results in accumulation of galactose-1-phosphate, which inhibits glycogenolytic enzymes. Although hypoglycemia may occur, it is uncommon, and patients more typically present with vomiting, diarrhea, jaundice, and sepsis precipitated by inclusion of galactose in the diet. Long-term effects, thought to be caused by elevated circulating levels of galactose-1-phosphate, include intellectual impairment, cataracts, hepatic dysfunction, renal tubular disease, cerebellar syndrome, and ovarian dysfunction. A galactose-restricted diet prevents the acute symptoms, but long-term side effects may persist.

MAPLE SYRUP URINE DISEASE

Autosomal recessive mutations in any of the subunits of branch-chain α-ketoacid dehydrogenase results in accumulation of the branched-chain amino acids (BCAA), leucine, isoleucine, and valine. A common mutation in the E1α subunit has been found in the Mennonite population in the United States. Classical maple syrup urine disease (MSUD; MIM no. 248600, no. 248610, and no. 248611) manifests between 5 and 15 days of life with decreased feeding, vomiting, and progressive encephalopathy. During acute decompensation, hypoglycemia and ketosis are common. The mechanism causing hypoglycemia is not clear but may be due to decreased availability of amino acids, particularly alanine, as substrates for gluconeogenesis. Magnetic resonance imaging of the brain shows a unique pattern of edema that eventually evolves to cerebellar atrophy and ataxia. Inadequate adjustment of the diet may result in a typical dermatitis, scalded-skin syndrome, caused by isoleucine deficiency. The urine has a characteristic odor, which should raise suspicion of the disease. The diagnosis can be made by plasma amino acid analysis by either high-performance liquid chromatography or tandem mass spectrometry. The enzyme activity can be measured in leukocytes or fibroblasts. Treatment of acute decompensation consists of removing the metabolic toxins by hemodialysis or hemofiltration, followed by total parenteral nutrition with glucose, insulin, and amino acid mixtures free of BCAA. Chronic treatment consists of BCAA-free formula. The prognosis is variable, but normal or near-normal growth and development can be achieved with early diagnosis and aggressive treatment.

PROPIONIC ACIDEMIA AND METHYLMALONIC ACIDEMIA

Both propionic acidemia and methylmalonic acidemia disrupt the metabolic pathway that converts propionyl-CoA to succinyl-CoA. The former is a rare disorder occurring in nonconsanguineous populations at an incidence of one in 500,000 or less. It is a severe disorder with a poor prognosis. Presentation is within the first week of life, with chronic vomiting and anorexia. Patients are immunocompromised and may present first with the presumptive diagnosis of immune deficiency. Laboratory findings include hyperammonemia and ketoacidosis with mildly elevated lactic acid levels. Neutropenia may be present during crisis. Treatment includes dietary manipulations and metronidazole to reduce propionate production by the gut bacteria.

Methylmalonic acidemia is more common than propionic acidemia, with an incidence of one in 48,000 to 61,000 births, and can be caused be a variety of defects of the conversion of methylmalonyl-CoA to succinyl-CoA, a process that requires cobalamin (vitamin B_{12}). The disease can be caused by mutations in methylmalonyl-CoA mutase itself; defects in the cytoplasmic, lysosomal, or mitochondrial processing of cobalamin; or severe vitamin B_{12} deficiency. Cobalamin-related defects usually produce relatively mild disease, and in the majority of cases, there is a significant clinical response to treatment with pharmacologic doses of vitamin B_{12}. Infants of strict vegetarians may present with methylmalonic acidemia, megaloblastic anemia, and homocystinuria with normal or low plasma methionine levels as a result of a severe deficiency in dietary vitamin B_{12} (142). The mechanism causing hypoglycemia, which is usually mild to moderate, is not clear.

DISORDERS OF FATTY ACID OXIDATION

Fatty acid β-oxidation is an important energy source, particularly during fasting and times of metabolic stress such as acute illness. Disorders of fatty acid oxidation are rare but are important causes of hypoglycemia in the infant. Recent molecular genetic studies have identified the precise etiology of several distinct clinical entities. We will review the salient features of this class of disorders, providing additional details on the most common forms. For more detailed information, the reader is referred to two recent comprehensive reviews (137,143).

The process of fatty acid β-oxidation is complex and involves a cascade of enzymes, transporters, and cofactors (Fig. 69.5). Fatty acids enter the cell and form fatty acyl-CoA, with the reaction catalyzed by acyl-CoA synthase. Long-chain acyl-CoAs are transferred into the mitochondria by the carnitine shuttle. In the mitochondria, fatty acyl-CoA undergoes β-oxidation repetitively by transferring electrons to flavoprotein-linked dehydrogenases and then to the mitochondrial respiratory chain. The process is catalyzed by a series of enzymes, including acyl-CoA dehydrogenases, which act on short-, medium-, or long-chain acyl-CoAs; 3-hydroxy-acyl-CoA; and a mitochondrial trifunctional protein. The final product of fatty acid oxidation is acetylCoA, which is then used to produce acetoacetate and β-hydroxybutyrate (ketone bodies), which are released into the circulation.

Disruption of this process at any level will result in failure to metabolize fatty acids, leading to loss of a critical energy source and failure to produce ketone bodies. During prolonged aerobic exercise, fasting, or any intercurrent illness, fatty acid oxidation accounts for a major part of oxygen consumption by muscle. In contrast, energy requirements of the brain are supplied primarily by glucose and secondarily by oxidation of ketone bodies. Patients with disorders in fatty acid oxidation have both hypoglycemia and hypoketonemia and are thus particularly prone to neurologic damage. In a recent review of 50 patients with long-chain 3-hydroxy-acyl-CoA dehydrogenase deficiency, hypoketotic hypoglycemia was the presenting symptom in 78%. Lactic acidosis was a common feature of metabolic crisis. Mortality was high (38%), and surviving patients continued to suffer from recurrent metabolic crises despite medical treatment. Interestingly, 86% of the patients had chronic, nonspecific symptoms prior to metabolic decompensation that could have led to earlier diagnosis had the index of clinical suspicion been higher. Early diagnosis appears to be associated with improved survival and long-term prognosis (144).

The mechanism by which these disorders cause hypoglycemia is unclear and is thought to be due the combined effect of at least two factors: Increased peripheral utilization of glucose due to the absence of fatty acids and ketone bodies as alternative energy sources may rapidly deplete glycogen stores and overtax the gluconeogenesis machinery. Hepatic gluconeogenesis may be further inhibited nonspecifically because of a decrease in energy sources needed to drive the process or specifically by inhibition of pyruvate carboxylase, the first gluconeogenic enzyme, since this enzyme requires acetyl-CoA for optimal activity (145).

The clinical presentations of most disorders of fatty acid oxidation are similar. The diagnosis is suspected clinically when fasting hypoketotic hypoglycemia is found in the absence of hyperinsulinism. Metabolic derangement typically associated with Reye syndrome, such as encephalopathy with hyperammonemia, metabolic acidosis, and elevated transaminases, may be present. It has been suggested that since the incidence of true Reye syndrome is decreasing, the majority of children presenting with this constellation of symptoms in fact have an inherited metabolic disorder (146). Myopathy and/or cardiomyopathy may also be prominent features. Acute symptoms are typically precipitated by fasting or by acute intercurrent illness.

The diagnosis can be made by analysis of urine for organic acids and measurement of plasma carnitine and acylcarnitines. Electrospray tandem mass spectrometry can be used to obtain an acylcarnitine profile, which is usually diagnostic for specific defects. This analysis can be performed on a dried blood spot, and it is currently being investigated for use in routine neonatal screening (147–149). The definitive enzymatic defect can be identified by direct enzyme assays on cultured fibroblasts or the identification of specific genetic defects.

Carnitine Deficiency

Carnitine is required for the transfer of long-chain fatty acids into the mitochondria for oxidation. Primary carnitine deficiency is caused by a defect in the plasma membrane carnitine transporter in the kidney and muscle (MIM no. 212140). Recessive mutations in this transporter result in urinary carnitine wasting and decreased intracellular levels of carnitine. Patients presenting before the age of 1 year typically present with hypoketotic hypoglycemia, liver failure, and acute encephalopathy, whereas older patients present with skeletal or cardiac myopathy. Free carnitine and acylcarnitine levels in plasma are very low, and patients respond to dietary supplements. Defects in carnitine palmitoyl transferase 1 (CPT-1; MIM no. 255120) and carnitine-acylcarnitine translocase (MIM no. 212138) result in a similar clinical picture with variable severity, depending on the specific defect. Each has a typical carnitine/acylcarnitine plasma profile. In contrast, carnitine palmitoyl transferase 2 (CPT-2; MIM no. 255220) frequently presents in adolescents or young adults with predominantly muscle involvement, although a more severe neonatal form and an intrauterine malformative form also exist. The age at onset and severity seem to correlate with the specific mutation inherited and with the level of residual enzyme activity. Patients suffering from other organic acid disorders frequently have secondary carnitine deficiency, presumably due to excretion of large quantities of acylcarnitines in the urine, and dietary carnitine supplementation may be beneficial (150).

Medium-Chain Acyl-CoA Dehydrogenase Deficiency

Medium-chain acyl-CoA dehydrogenase (MCAD; MIM no. 201450) deficiency is one of the most common organic acidemias and is also one of the first to be described. Although more than 25 mutations have been described, a single founder mutation (A985G) is responsible for about 90% of cases (151). MCAD is responsible for the first step in the oxidation of fatty acyl-CoA esters of chain length C4 to C12, and the diagnosis can be made by finding increased urinary excretion of C6 to C8 dicarboxylic acids and their glycine conjugates. The disease presents in early childhood with Reye syndrome–like symptoms, including hypoglycemia, coma, and fatty liver, usually associated with febrile disease or other metabolic stress. This disease may be one cause of sudden infant death syndrome. Symptoms may develop rapidly and result in death before intervention can be initiated. Recent studies have suggested that the severity and relative frequency of this disease may justify routine neonatal screening (148,152,153).

Multiple Acyl-CoA Dehydrogenase Deficiency

Multiple acyl-CoA dehydrogenase deficiency (MADD; glutaric aciduria type 2) is a rare organic acidemia that can be caused by mutations in any one of three molecules: either subunit of the electron transfer flavoprotein or electron transfer flavoprotein dehydrogenase. This enzyme system is involved in the transfer of electrons from acyl-CoA dehydrogenases to coenzyme Q of the mitochondrial electron transport chain. The clinical severity of the disease correlates with the severity of the metabolic defect. The severe form (MADD:S) is associated with severe neonatal acidosis and hypoglycemia, as well as multiple congenital malformations similar to those observed in the intrauterine, lethal form of CPT-2 deficiency. Most patients do not survive the neonatal period. Milder disease may be diagnosed later in life, usually during childhood or adolescence, and frequently after a metabolic stress such as febrile illness. The mechanism by which MADD causes its associated metabolic abnormalities emphasizes the complex interaction between different metabolic pathways. The enzyme complex is responsible for the oxidation of short-, medium-, and long-chain fatty acids, as well as for the oxidation of glutaryl-CoA, a degradation product of lysine. Blockage of the latter reaction results in the hallmark finding of glutaric aciduria. Hyperammonemia probably is caused by decreased availability of acetyl-CoA, resulting in decreased synthesis of *N*-acetylglutamate, which is required for the first step of the urea cycle. Hypoglycemia is caused by increased utilization of glucose and decreased gluconeogenesis, as with other disorders of fatty acid oxidation. Glutaryl-CoA may interfere with the malate shuttle, further compromising mitochondrial function. Heart, liver, and muscle damage are caused by accumulation of acylcarnitine. Binding of CoA esters to carnitine causes a secondary carnitine deficiency that further exacerbates the metabolic defect. Treatment consists primarily of prevention of catabolic states. Supplementation with riboflavin and carnitine may be of benefit to patients with mild disease. The diagnosis is made by typical acylcarnitine profile on tandem mass spectrometry and can be confirmed by enzyme analysis in fibroblasts (144,154–156).

DEFECTS OF KETOGENESIS

Ketones are an important source of energy for extrahepatic tissues. They are generated almost exclusively in the liver by conversion of acetyl- and acetylacetyl-CoA to acetoacetate, a process that requires the mitochondrial enzymes 3-hydroxy-3-methylglutaryl-CoA (HMG-CoA) synthase and lyase. A mitochondrial HMG-CoA synthase mutation was recently reported in a 6-year-old patient with severe hypoketotic hypoglycemic coma and normal levels of carnitine and urinary organic acids. This case demonstrates the importance of the mitochondrial form of this enzyme in ketone production and the importance of ketone bodies in the prevention of hypoglycemia during prolonged fasting (157).

HMG-CoA lyase also catalyzes the final step in leucine degradation; however, its main role in the liver is to cleave HMG-CoA to acetoacetic acid and acetyl-CoA. Deficiency of this enzyme (MIM no. 246450) causes severe hypoketotic hypoglycemia with metabolic acidosis and increased excretion of organic acids (158). The clinical picture is more severe than in HMG-CoA synthase deficiency, but decompensation can be avoided by glucose supplementation during catabolic stress. Restriction of leucine intake does not appear to be particularly helpful, because the primary metabolic defect is ketone deficiency and not the accumulation of toxic metabolites. Secondary carnitine deficiency may develop, and dietary supplementation may be beneficial.

Hyperinsulinism of Infancy

Hyperinsulinism of infancy (HI) has been referred to by a number of names, including "nesidioblastosis," β-cell dysmaturation syndrome, persistent hyperinsulinemic hypoglycemia of infancy, and others (MIM no. 256450). The pathogenesis of this disease has just recently begun to be elucidated. However, our current knowledge is still limited and is only beginning to affect the clinical diagnosis and treatment of patients with this devastating disease. For a more complete discussion on the etiology, diagnosis, and treatment of this syndrome, the reader is referred to a number of recent comprehensive reviews (159–162). Given the rapidity of progress over the last few years, it is likely that our understanding of the disease will continue to grow rapidly and that the diagnostic and treatment approaches to these patients will evolve quickly over the next few years.

DIAGNOSIS

The biochemical diagnosis of hypoglycemia secondary to insulin hypersecretion is based on documentation of inappropriately elevated insulin levels in the presence of symptomatic hypoglycemia (163,164). Grossly elevated insulin levels can usually be readily demonstrated in patients with severe disease that appears shortly after birth. In milder cases, however, fasting insulin levels may fluctuate greatly, and it may be difficult to convincingly demonstrate the presence of pathologically elevated concentrations of insulin. Surrogate measurements of insulin action, including inappropriate hypoketonemia, exaggerated glycemic response to glucagon, and a markedly elevated glucose requirement to prevent hypoglycemia, are particularly useful in such patients. Mildly to moderately elevated serum levels of ammonia suggest the presence of the recently discovered hyperinsulinism/hyperammonemia syndrome (165–167). A systematic approach to the diagnosis of HI has recently been reviewed in detail (167).

TABLE 69.4. Initial Diagnostic Evaluation of Infant with Hypoglycemia

1. ***Hormones and intermediate metabolites to be measured at the time of spontaneous or induced hypoglycemia***

Blood	Urine
Glucose	Ketone bodies
Insulin	Reducing substances
C-peptide	Organic acids
Free fatty acids	
Ketone bodies	
Lactate/pyruvate	
Amino acids	
Total/free carnitine	
Acyl-carnitine profile	
Ammonia	
Growth hormone	
Cortisol	
T_4, T_3, TSH	

T_4, thyroxine; T_3, triidothyronine; TSH, thyrotropin.

2. ***Glucagon stimulation test***
   A glucose response of >39 mg/dL (>1.7 mmol/L) after intravenous glucagon excludes a primary hepatic or metabolic defect.
3. ***Calculate glucose requirement (enteral + parenteral)***
   Total glucose requirements >15 mg/(kg · min) are highly suggestive of hyperinsulinism.

Although the clinical diagnosis may be difficult, for most patients the definitive diagnosis can be made rapidly if the appropriate blood and urine samples are obtained during an episode of spontaneous hypoglycemia (Table 69.4) and adequate attention is paid to the glucose dose required to prevent recurrent hypoglycemia (159,168). However, if the index of suspicion is not sufficiently high, the diagnosis may be missed in patients with relatively mild disease.

ETIOLOGY

Mutations in any of at least five different genes can cause HI. Two of these, the sulfonylurea-receptor gene, *SUR1* (ABCC8), and the potassium-channel gene *Kir6.2* (KCNJ11), code for subunits of the β-cell K_{ATP} channel. Two other genes code for glucokinase and glutamate dehydrogenase, which are enzymes important for the regulation of β-cell metabolism. The fifth gene codes for mannose phosphate isomerase. The mechanism by which mutations in this gene cause hypoglycemia is not yet understood. Each genetic etiology has its own specific clinical characteristics that affect the treatment approach and make genetic counseling complex.

Hyperinsulinism Due to Mutations in K_{ATP}-Channel Genes (HI-K_{ATP}) (MIM no. 256450)

The β-cell K_{ATP} channels are open in the resting state, allowing free passage of potassium ions out of the cell and maintaining the cell membrane in a hyperpolarized state. Metabolism of glucose and other fuels results in an increase in the adenosine triphosphate/adenosine diphosphate (ATP/ADP) ratio, which causes the K_{ATP} channel to close. This results in membrane depolarization, opening of the voltage-gated calcium channels, an influx of calcium into the cell, and ultimately insulin secretion. Thus, the K_{ATP} channel "senses" the intracellular metabolic state and uses this information to regulate insulin secretion (Fig. 69.6).

The K_{ATP} channel is made up of two subunits. The first, the sulfonylurea receptor (SUR-1), is the regulatory subunit of the channel, having two nucleotide binding domains and domains that bind channel openers such as diazoxide, and channel closers such as drugs of the sulfonylurea class. An endogenous regulator of this subunit, endosulfine, was recently cloned, but its physiologic significance is not yet known (169). The second subunit (Kir6.2) creates the ion-specific pore. The functional channel is a hetero-octamer, made up of four molecules of SUR1 and four of Kir6.2. The genes for these two subunits are located adjacent to each other on the short arm of chromosome 11, about 30 centimorgan (cM) centromeric to the insulin gene.

Genetic mutations that decrease the function of either of these two subunits will cause defective K_{ATP} channels, resulting in membrane depolarization and unregulated insulin secretion. To date, more than 50 different mutations have been reported, three in the *Kir6.2* gene and the remainder in the *SUR1* gene. The vast majority of these mutations are recessive, meaning that channel function will be compromised only if there are mutations in both alleles. However, the structure of the channel suggests that dominant mutations are also possible, and indeed, the first dominant *SUR1* mutation in humans was recently reported in an isolated Finnish population. Patients with this mutation have relatively mild, diazoxide-sensitive hyperinsulinism. All patients inherited their mutation on the maternal allele, a finding that cannot be readily explained (170).

Most patients with HI have diffuse pancreatic involvement (diffuse-HI), with all β-cells showing large nuclei and abundant cytoplasm, histologic evidence of metabolic hyperactivity. In these cases, the HI is caused by genomic mutations that affect all β-cells equally. Patients may be homozygous for a single mutation or compound heterozygous for two different recessive *SUR1* or *Kir6.2* mutations.

In about 30% to 40% of patients with HI, however, a limited region of their pancreases shows a distinct histologic finding of β-cell hyperplasia. B-Cells within the lesion show the typical features of metabolic hyperactivity, whereas β-cells throughout the remainder of the pancreas are small, with small nuclei and sparse cytoplasm, suggesting a metabolic resting state (162). It was recently discovered that these are clonal lesions in which the precursor cell has undergone somatic loss of the maternal

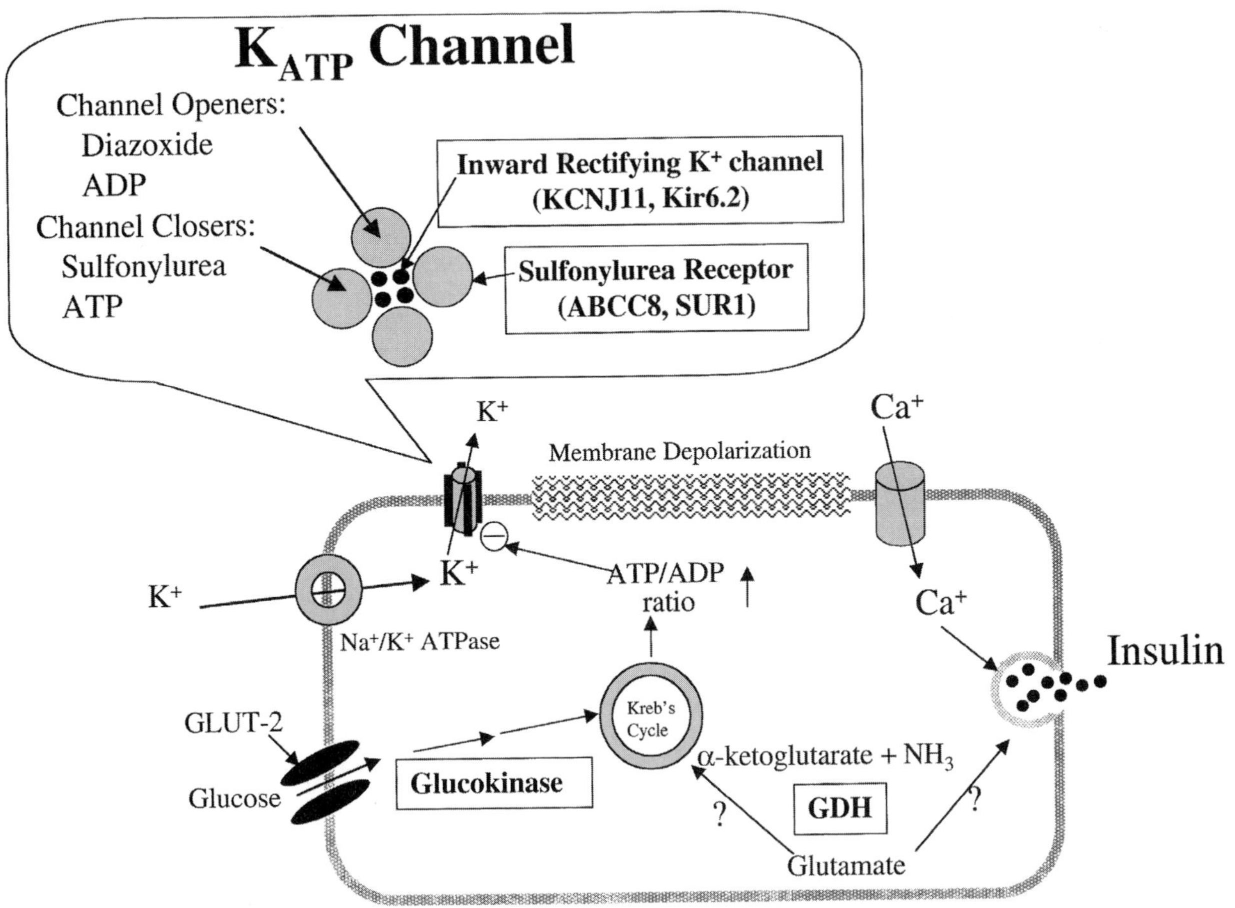

Figure 69.6. Schematic diagram showing the major pathway of glucose-regulated insulin secretion. The K_{ATP} channel is composed of four molecules of SUR1 and four molecules of Kir.6.2, as shown in the box in the upper left corner. Glucokinase is the rate-limiting step in glucose metabolism, and glutamate dehydrogenase (GDH) catalyzes the conversion of the amino acid glutamine to α-ketoglutarate. Hyperinsulinism of infancy can be caused by mutations in any of the four proteins highlighted by boxes. The mechanism by which activating GDH mutations cause hyperinsulinism is controversial. (Modified from Glaser B. Hyperinsulinism in the newborn. *Semin Perinatol* 2000;24:150–163.)

allele of chromosome 11p15, the region containing the K_{ATP}-channel genes as well as imprinted genes such as *IGFII*, *p57^{kip2}*, and *H19* (171). IGF-II is a growth-stimulating factor expressed only from the paternal allele. *H19* and *p57^{kip2}* inhibit proliferation through different mechanisms and are expressed exclusively from the maternal allele. These patients are also heterozygous for a genomic, recessive *SUR1* or *Kir6.2* mutation that is always located on the paternal allele (172,173). Therefore, β-cells within the lesion carry only mutant K_{ATP}-channel genes, express the growth factor, and lack expression of the two inhibitors of proliferation. The result is clonal proliferation of β-cells that release insulin in an unregulated manner, resulting in a syndrome of diazoxide-unresponsive severe hyperinsulinemic hypoglycemia. Resection of the hyperplastic region results in cure of hyperinsulinism and the return of normal insulin secretory dynamics (174). As discussed below, it is important to differentiate between the diffuse and focal forms of HI, since the treatment considerations are different. Since the genetic differentiation of these two forms of disease is not yet feasible, a number of clinical tests are being developed to differentiate between focal and diffuse HI (175–177).

Hyperinsulinism Due to Mutations in the Glutamate Dehydrogenase Gene (MIM no. 138130)

In 1996 a clinical syndrome of hyperinsulinemic hypoglycemia with mild to moderate hyperammonemia (HI/HA) was described (165). It was subsequently demonstrated that most cases are due to dominant gain-of-function mutations in the regulatory domain of the mitochondrial enzyme glutamate dehydrogenase (GDH) (Fig. 69.6). This enzyme catalyzes the reversible conversion of glutamate to α-ketoglutarate. The exact mechanism by which this results in unregulated insulin secretion is still controversial (166,178,179). The associated hyperammonemia is thought to be caused by increased activity of the same enzyme in the liver, where the conversion of glutamate to α-ketoglutarate is accompanied by the production of ammonia. GDH overactivity causes depletion of glutamate, resulting in a decrease of *N*-acetylglutamate, a regulator of carbamoylphosphate synthase, the first enzyme in the pathway of NH_3 detoxification. Thus, hyperammonemia is caused by a combination of increased production and decreased metabolism of NH_3.

Patients with HI/HA tend to suffer from both fasting and postprandial hypoglycemia, which becomes evident after a few months of age (180). They may be very sensitive to high-protein meals, and indeed this may be the etiology of the entity "leucine-sensitive hyperinsulinism" described in the 1970s. In most patients, the hypoglycemia responds well to treatment with diazoxide, and therefore surgical intervention is rarely needed (see below). The hyperammonemia appears to be benign, with no apparent neurologic manifestations. HI/HA appears to be responsible for disease in 3% to 5% of hyperinsulinemic infants. In some of these, no GDH mutations have been identified, suggesting that mutations in other genes may cause this phenotype.

Hyperinsulinism Due to Mutations in the Glucokinase Gene (MIM no. 602485)

We recently described a family with fasting and postprandial hypoglycemia caused by a dominant mutation in the glucokinase gene (181). *In vitro* studies documented that the mutation increased the affinity of the enzyme for glucose and decreased the glucose threshold for insulin secretion, consistent with the clinical findings in the affected patients. Mutations that have the opposite effect on glucokinase affinity for glucose have been previously reported to cause one form of maturity-onset diabetes of the young (MODY) (182). These findings provided further evidence that glucokinase is the β-cell "glucose sensor." Despite extensive genetic testing, very few patients with hyperinsulinism due to mutations in the glucokinase gene (HI-GCK) have been reported.

Hyperinsulinism Due to Mutations in the Mannose Phosphate Isomerase Gene (MIM no. 602579)

Mutations in the mannose phosphate isomerase (*MPI*) gene cause a novel variant of the carbohydrate-deficient glycoprotein syndrome, designated CDGS type 1b. The syndrome manifestations include protein-losing enteropathy with chronic diarrhea, hepatic disease, and coagulopathy. Neurologic manifestations that characterize CDGS type 1a, which is caused by mutations in the mannose phosphate mutase gene, are notably absent. Recently, four cases of CDGS type 1b with hypoglycemia were reported, and in two, absolute or relative hyperinsulinism was documented. The mechanism by which MPI mutations cause hyperinsulinism is not known, but diazoxide treatment appears to be effective. Diagnosis requires a high level of clinical suspicion, because the routine biochemical evaluation may be identical to that found in HI due to other genetic etiologies, and gastrointestinal symptoms are common in HI-K_{ATP}. The biochemical diagnosis is made by documenting protein hypoglycosylation, usually by isoelectric focusing of serum transferrin. Definitive diagnosis can be made by determining enzyme activity in lymphocytes or fibroblasts, or by genetic evaluation. Precise diagnosis is critical, since patients respond well to mannose therapy (183,184).

Other Causes of Hyperinsulinemic Hypoglycemia

Despite extensive genetic evaluation, in about 40% of patients with clinical evidence of HI, no mutation can be identified in any of the five genes described above. Some mutations could have been missed, because the mutation-detection methods used were only 85% to 90% sensitive and intronic mutations and deletions were not systematically sought. However, it seems likely that the clinical syndrome may be more heterogeneous than previously suspected. Evidence for multiple other genetic etiologies for hyperinsulinemic hypoglycemia comes from numerous recent publications reporting hyperinsulinism as part of several, apparently unrelated clinical syndromes, including Kabuki syndrome (185), short-chain 3-hydroxyacyl-CoA dehydrogenase deficiency (186), and exercise-induced hyperinsulinism (187). It seems likely, therefore, that the coming years will witness a flurry of publications documenting novel genetic forms of hyperinsulinism.

TREATMENT

Treatment can be divided into several phases. After the initial diagnostic blood samples are obtained (Table 69.4), the hypoglycemia must be corrected immediately using intravenous glucose at a dose sufficient to prevent further hypoglycemia and thus prevent irreversible brain damage. This dose may be very high [>15 mg/(kg · min)] and frequently requires central venous access.

Until recently, the next phase of treatment was entirely empiric. Attempts are made to decrease and stop parenteral glucose requirement by adding a combination of medical therapies, which include diazoxide, somatostatin analogue (188), nifedipine (189), and glucagon (190). Additional pharmacologic interventions have been proposed, including recombinant IGF-I, which has been shown to suppress insulin secretion in patients with HI (191); glucocorticoids, which induce resistance to endogenous insulin and correct the inadequate cortisol response sometimes seen in these patients; and growth hormone given in combination with somatostatin analogue to counteract the suppression of growth hormone by somatostatin. However, the clinical utility of these interventions has yet to be critically assessed. The definition of what is adequate glucose control has been the subject of considerable discussion. Most investigators recommend maintaining all glucose levels above 60 mg/dL (3.3 mmol/L), a level that leaves a sufficient margin of error to prevent frequent episodes of neuroglycopenia (192). In only a minority of cases can this goal be attained with medical therapy alone without concomitant intensive dietary intervention.

Once stabilized, and the diagnosis of HI confirmed, a decision must be made regarding the need for surgical intervention and the extent of such intervention. It is generally accepted that those patients who respond well to medical treatment can be treated chronically without undue risk of long-term complications. Surgery must be considered for patients who do not respond adequately to medical treatment. Patients with focal disease can be readily and successfully treated by localized resection of the hyperplastic region, whereas patients with diffuse disease require extensive pancreatic resection (80% to 95%) and are at risk for persistent hypoglycemia postoperatively and/or insulin-requiring diabetes later in childhood. The decision to proceed to surgery is complicated by the finding that medically treated patients tend to improve with time and that even those requiring very intensive medical management during the newborn period may enter clinical remission after several months or years of medical management. Although no consensus has been reached, the current trend is to consider early surgery for patients with focal disease, because the surgical results are excellent, whereas to attempt intensive long-term medical treatment for patients with diffuse disease and to opt for surgery only if this is not successful.

GENETIC COUNSELING

The genetic heterogeneity of HI makes genetic counseling extremely complex. The fact that in many cases the precise genetic etiology of disease is not known makes it even harder. In patients with HI/HA or HI-GK, the disease is transmitted as an autosomal dominant trait. If one parent is affected, subsequent siblings have a 50% chance of having the disease. If the disease is caused by a spontaneous mutation in the patient, the risk to subsequent children appears to be negligible. In patients with HI-K_{ATP} and diffuse disease, the disease is most probably transmitted as an autosomal recessive trait, and thus subsequent children would have a 25% risk of developing the disease. However, as described above, dominant mutations in this gene are possible and must be considered in individual cases. In patients with focal disease due to paternally inherited *SUR1* or *Kir6.2* mutations, the risk to subsequent siblings is determined by the incidence of somatic mutations causing loss of the maternal allele of Ch11p in β-cell precursors. This risk is not known; however, analysis of siblings of patients with known *SUR1* mutations suggests that the risk for disease in a sibling inheriting one mutation on the paternal allele is very small—probably less than 2% to 3%. More data are needed to provide a more accurate risk estimate.

Diagnostic Approach to the Hypoglycemic Infant

Cost-effectiveness analyses may not support routine glucose testing in all neonates. However, the index of suspicion must be high, and glucose measurements should be made if the infant presents with any of the nonspecific symptoms possibly associated with neonatal hypoglycemia. In addition, infants at particular risk for hypoglycemia, such as those who are small or large for gestational age or who are premature, should be monitored for the first 24 to 48 hours or longer if necessary. While bedside glucometer testing has improved considerably, confirmation with laboratory measurements is required to convincingly diagnose or exclude hypoglycemia (see above).

Persistent hypoglycemia, defined as glucose levels less than 40 to 50 mg/dL (2.2 to 2.8 mmol/L) beyond the first 48 hours of life, requires more complete evaluation. Because it may take time to obtain results from many of the laboratory tests, early and complete laboratory evaluation will greatly facilitate rapid accurate diagnosis and hence more effective treatment. If the clinical situation allows, performance of a glucagon stimulation test during hypoglycemia will have both diagnostic and therapeutic significance. The dosage of glucagon is controversial and dosages ranging from 0.03 mg/kg to a 1-mg total dose have been recommended (159,168). A glycemic response over 30 mg/dL (1.7 mmol/L) is considered highly suggestive of hyperinsulinism and excludes primary defects in glycogen synthesis or glycogenolysis. It also provides an indication of whether glucagon can be useful in the specific patient as an emergency treatment of hypoglycemia should the need arise in the future.

If the performance of a glucagon test is technically not possible, if the results are negative, or if hypoglycemia recurs, immediate resuscitation with glucose is necessary. In the asymptomatic and otherwise healthy infant, 30 to 60 mL of 5% glucose in water given orally may be sufficient. It is necessary to perform serial glucose measurements every 15 to 30 minutes. If the infant is symptomatic, or in preterm neonates, intravenous treatment should be initiated with a 2-mL/kg bolus of 10% dextrose solution ($D_{10}W$), followed by a continuous infusion of glucose that approximates the normal glycemic requirement of the newborn [5 to 6 mg/(kg · min)]. Recurrent episodes of hypoglycemia should be treated with repeated doses of 2 mL/kg $D_{10}W$ followed by increases in the glucose infusion rate by increments of 2 mg/(kg · min). Glucose requirements above the normal hepatic glucose uptake are highly suggestive of increased peripheral glucose utilization secondary to hyperinsulinism. In these patients, glucose requirement may be extremely high—greater than 20 mg/(kg · min). Requirements greater than 12 mg/(kg · min) require central venous access to avoid vascular damage and to guarantee uninterrupted infusion.

Once stabilization has been accomplished, the specific diagnosis must be established (Fig. 69.7). Low levels of ketone bodies, low levels of free fatty acids, absence of reducing substances, and normal lactic acid levels suggest either hyperinsulinism or a fatty acid disorder. Determination of serum carnitine/acylcarnitine profile will provide the specific diagnosis.

The presence of appropriate ketotic response without hepatomegaly suggests ketotic hypoglycemia or counterregulatory hormone (growth hormone or cortisol) deficiency. Hepatomegaly in the presence of ketosis suggests a defect in glycogenolysis. The presence or absence of lactic acidosis will further narrow the diagnostic possibilities since deficiencies in pyruvate carboxylase, PEPCK, glucose-6-phosphatase, or fructose-1,6-diphosphatase will result in high lactate levels, whereas in glycogen storage disease types III and VI, lactate levels will be normal.

In many cases, the definitive diagnosis cannot be made during episodes of spontaneous hypoglycemia, and a diagnostic fast is needed. Because fasting can be particularly dangerous in patients with defects in fatty acid oxidation, and because the fast is of little diagnostic value in these patients, it is recommended that a carnitine/acylcarnitine profile be obtained before a diagnostic fast is attempted. If a disorder of fatty acid oxidation is suspected, definitive testing should be accom-

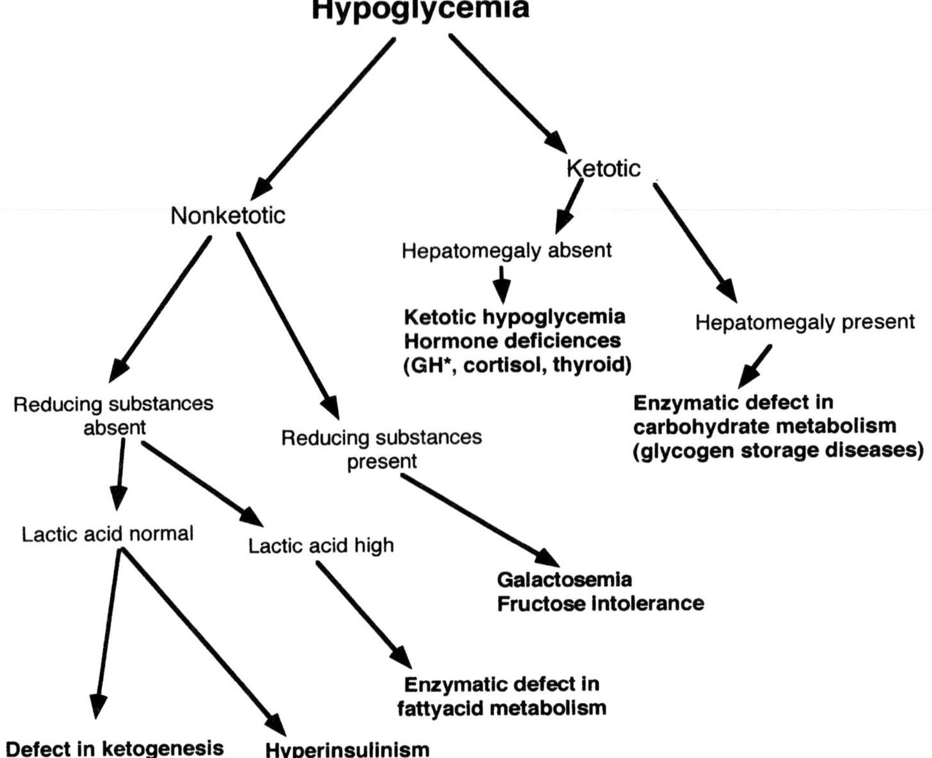

Figure 69.7. Schematic approach to the differential diagnosis of hypoglycemia. *Ketones may be temporarily absent in infants deficient in growth hormone (GH). (Data from Glaser B, Landau H, Permutt MA. Neonatal hyperinsulinism. *Trends Endocrinol Metab* 1999;10:55–61.)

plished and any form of fasting should be scrupulously avoided.

Once the initial clinical/biochemical diagnosis is made, specific treatment should be initiated as outlined above for each of the specific diagnoses. Further testing may be needed to define the specific enzyme defect. At this point, it is highly recommended that referral to a tertiary care center specializing in the specific class of defects identified be considered. This is particularly true for patients with hyperinsulinism (159). Medical management of these patients is particularly challenging because of the technical difficulties involved in maintaining the very high rates of glucose administration, the volatility of glucose control, and the vulnerability to unexpected and unpredictable severe hypoglycemia. If pancreatic surgery is required, localization studies such as pancreatic venous sampling or intraarterial calcium infusions may be indicated, and these are rarely available except in highly specialized tertiary care centers.

In terms of long-term prognosis, neonatal hypoglycemia can be divided into two major groups. The first consists of the transient hypoglycemia frequently seen in small-for-gestational age or premature infants. The precise definition of hypoglycemia in these infants has not been determined, and the long-term consequences of treatment have not been prospectively studied. However, correlations with poor neurologic outcome have been made (116). Therefore, given the severe, life-long consequences of inadequate treatment and the relative ease of correction of hypoglycemia in these infants, it seems prudent to treat them with the goal of restoring glucose values to the normal physiologic range (113).

In the second group of patients, those with clear metabolic defects resulting in moderate to severe persistent hypoglycemia, there is no doubt that success of treatment correlates directly with ultimate neurologic outcome. This is particularly true of hyperinsulinism, in which inadequate treatment routinely results in severe neurologic damage or even death, whereas successful prevention of severe recurrent hypoglycemia is almost always associated with normal on near-normal neurologic outcome (193).

Acknowledgments

The authors thank Drs. Orly Elpeleg and Erol Cerasi for their critical review of the manuscript and for their many helpful suggestions.

REFERENCES

1. Bolli GB, Fanelli CG. Physiology of glucose counterregulation to hypoglycemia. *Endocrinol Metab Clin North Am* 1999;28:467–493.
2. Rothman DL, Magnusson I, Katz LD, et al. Quantitation of hepatic glycogenolysis and gluconeogenesis in fasting humans with 13C NMR. *Science* 1991;254:573–576.
3. Katz J, Tayek JA. Gluconeogenesis and the Cori cycle in 12-, 20-, and 40-h-fasted humans. *Am J Physiol* 1998;275:E537–E542.
4. Stumvoll M, Meyer C, Perriello G, et al. Human kidney and liver gluconeogenesis: evidence for organ substrate selectivity. *Am J Physiol* 1998;274: E817–E826.
5. Schwartz NS, Clutter WE, Shah SD, et al. Glycemic thresholds for activation of glucose counterregulatory systems are higher than the threshold for symptoms. *J Clin Invest* 1987;79:777–781.
6. Borg WP, Sherwin RS, During MJ, et al. Local ventromedial hypothalamus glucopenia triggers counterregulatory hormone release. *Diabetes* 1995;44: 180–184.
7. Cherrington AD. Banting Lecture 1997. Control of glucose uptake and release by the liver *in vivo*. *Diabetes* 1999;48:1198–1214.

8. De Feo P, Perriello G, Torlone E, et al. Evidence against important catecholamine compensation for absent glucagon counterregulation. *Am J Physiol* 1991;260:E203–E212.
9. Whipple AO. The surgical therapy of hyperinsulinism. *J Int Chir* 1938;3: 237–276.
10. Cryer PE. Symptoms of hypoglycemia, thresholds for their occurrence, and hypoglycemia unawareness. *Endocrinol Metab Clin North Am* 1999;28: 495–500.
11. Merimee TJ, Tyson JE. Stabilization of plasma glucose during fasting: normal variations in two separate studies. *N Engl J Med* 1974;291:1275–1278.
12. Davis SN, Cherrington AD, Goldstein RE, et al. Effects of insulin on the counterregulatory response to equivalent hypoglycemia in normal females. *Am J Physiol* 1993;265:E680–E689.
13. Towler DA, Havlin CE, Craft S, et al. Mechanism of awareness of hypoglycemia. Perception of neurogenic (predominantly cholinergic) rather than neuroglycopenic symptoms. *Diabetes* 1993;42:1791–1798.
14. Boyle PJ, Schwartz NS, Shah SD, et al. Plasma glucose concentrations at the onset of hypoglycemic symptoms in patients with poorly controlled diabetes and in nondiabetics. *N Engl J Med* 1988;318:1487–1492.
15. Amiel SA, Sherwin RS, Simonson DC, et al. Effect of intensive insulin therapy on glycemic thresholds for counterregulatory hormone release. *Diabetes* 1988;37:901–907.
16. Heller SR, Cryer PE. Reduced neuroendocrine and symptomatic responses to subsequent hypoglycemia after 1 episode of hypoglycemia in nondiabetic humans. *Diabetes* 1991;40:223–226.
17. Boyle PJ, Nagy RJ, O'Connor AM, et al. Adaptation in brain glucose uptake following recurrent hypoglycemia. *Proc Natl Acad Sci U S A* 1994;91: 9352–9356.
18. Boyle PJ. Alteration in brain glucose metabolism induced by hypoglycaemia in man. *Diabetologia* 1997;40[Suppl 2]:S69–S74.
19. Amiel SA. Hypoglycaemia in diabetes mellitus—protecting the brain. *Diabetologia* 1997;40[Suppl 2]:S62–S68.
20. The effect of intensive treatment of diabetes on the development and progression of long-term complications in insulin-dependent diabetes mellitus: the Diabetes Control and Complications Trial Research Group. *N Engl J Med* 1993;329:977–986.
21. Reichard P, Britz A, Rosenqvist U. Intensified conventional insulin treatment and neuropsychological impairment. *BMJ* 1991;303:1439–1442.
22. Rovet JF, Ehrlich RM, Hoppe M. Intellectual deficits associated with early onset of insulin-dependent diabetes mellitus in children. *Diabetes Care* 1987; 10:510–515.
23. Service FJ. Classification of hypoglycemic disorders. *Endocrinol Metab Clin North Am* 1999;28:501–517.
24. Palardy J, Havrankova J, Lepage R, et al. Blood glucose measurements during symptomatic episodes in patients with suspected postprandial hypoglycemia. *N Engl J Med* 1989;321:1421–1425.
25. Snorgaard O, Binder C. Monitoring of blood glucose concentration in subjects with hypoglycaemic symptoms during everyday life. *BMJ* 1990;300: 16–18.
26. Marks V, Teale JD. Drug-induced hypoglycemia. *Endocrinol Metab Clin North Am* 1999;28:555–577.
27. Phillips RE, Looareesuwan S, White NJ, et al. Hypoglycaemia and antimalarial drugs: quinidine and release of insulin. *BMJ (Clin Res Ed)* 1986;292: 1319–1321.
28. White NJ, Warrell DA, Chanthavanich P, et al. Severe hypoglycemia and hyperinsulinemia in falciparum malaria. *N Engl J Med* 1983;309:61–66.
29. Hayashi S, Horie M, Tsuura Y, et al. Disopyramide blocks pancreatic ATP-sensitive K+ channels and enhances insulin release. *Am J Physiol* 1993; 265:C337–C342.
30. Hasegawa J, Mori A, Yamamoto R, et al. Disopyramide decreases the fasting serum glucose level in man. *Cardiovasc Drugs Ther* 1999;13:325–327.
31. Takada M, Fujita S, Katayama Y, et al. The relationship between risk of hypoglycemia and use of cibenzoline and disopyramide. *Eur J Clin Pharmacol* 2000;56:335–342.
32. Cacoub P, Deray G, Baumelou A, et al. Disopyramide-induced hypoglycemia: case report and review of the literature. *Fundam Clin Pharmacol* 1989;3:527–535.
33. Caldwell G, Scougall I, Boddy K, et al. Fasting hyperinsulinemic hypoglycemia after ritodrine therapy for premature labor. *Obstet Gynecol* 1987; 70:478–480.
34. Wasserman D, Amitai Y. Hypoglycemia following albuterol overdose in a child. *Am J Emerg Med* 1992;10:556–557.
35. Bouchard P, Sai P, Reach G, et al. Diabetes mellitus following pentamidine-induced hypoglycemia in humans. *Diabetes* 1982;31:40–45.
36. Waskin H, Stehr-Green JK, Helmick CG, et al. Risk factors for hypoglycemia associated with pentamidine therapy for pneumocystis pneumonia. *JAMA* 1988;260:345–347.
37. Effect of intensive blood-glucose control with metformin on complications in overweight patients with type 2 diabetes (UKPDS 34): UK Prospective Diabetes Study (UKPDS) Group. *Lancet* 1998;352:854–865.
38. Horton ES, Whitehouse F, Ghazzi MN, et al. Troglitazone in combination with sulfonylurea restores glycemic control in patients with type 2 diabetes: the Troglitazone Study Group. *Diabetes Care* 1998;21:1462–1469.
39. Herings RM, de Boer A, Stricker BH, et al. Hypoglycaemia associated with use of inhibitors of angiotensin converting enzyme. *Lancet* 1995;345: 1195–1198.
40. Thamer M, Ray NF, Taylor T. Association between antihypertensive drug use and hypoglycemia: a case-control study of diabetic users of insulin or sulfonylureas. *Clin Ther* 1999;21:1387–1400.
41. Lind L, Pollare T, Berne C, et al. Long-term metabolic effects of antihypertensive drugs. *Am Heart J*1994;128:1177–1183.
42. Heise T, Heinemann L, Kristahn K, et al. Insulin sensitivity in patients with essential hypertension: no influence of the ACE inhibitor enalapril. *Horm Metab Res* 1999;31:418–423.
43. Efficacy of atenolol and captopril in reducing risk of macrovascular and microvascular complications in type 2 diabetes: UKPDS 39—UK Prospective Diabetes Study Group. *BMJ* 1998;317:713–720.
44. Kolter MN, Berman L, Rubenstein AH. Hypoglycemia precipitated by propranolol. *Lancet* 1966;2:1389–1390.
45. Hesse B, Pedersen JT. Hypoglycaemia after propranolol in children. *Acta Med Scand* 1973;193:551–552.
46. Jenkins DJ. Propranolol and hypoglycemia. *Lancet* 1967;1:164.
47. Cryer PE, White NH, Santiago JV. The relevance of glucose counterregulatory systems to patients with insulin-dependent diabetes mellitus. *Endocr Rev* 1986;7:131–139.
48. MacLaren NK, Valman HB, Levin B. Alcohol-induced hypoglycaemia in childhood. *BMJ* 1970;1:278–280.
49. Madison LL, Lochner A, Wulff J. Ethanol-induced hypoglycemia, II: mechanism of suppression of hepatic gluconeogenesis. *Diabetes* 1967;16:252–258.
50. Berman JD, Cook DM, Buchman M, et al. Diminished adrenocorticotropin response to insulin-induced hypoglycemia in nondepressed, actively drinking male alcoholics. *J Clin Endocrinol Metab* 1990;71:712–717.
51. Flanagan D, Wood P, Sherwin R, et al. Gin and tonic and reactive hypoglycemia: what is important—the gin, the tonic, or both? *J Clin Endocrinol Metab* 1998;83:796–800
52. Kolaczynski JW, Ylikahri R, Harkonen M, et al. The acute effect of ethanol on counterregulatory response and recovery from insulin-induced hypoglycemia. *J Clin Endocrinol Metab* 1988;67:384–388.
53. Hart SP, Frier BM. Causes, management and morbidity of acute hypoglycaemia in adults requiring hospital admission. *Q J Med* 1998;91:505–510.
54. Seltzer HS. Drug-induced hypoglycemia: a review of 1418 cases. *Endocrinol Metab Clin North Am* 1989;18:163–183.
55. Schulz H. Inhibitors of fatty acid oxidation. *Life Sci* 1987;40:1443–1449.
56. Kim JK, Kim YJ, Fillmore JJ, et al. Prevention of fat-induced insulin resistance by salicylate. *J Clin Invest* 2001;108:437–446.
57. Marks V, Teale JD. Hypoglycemia: factitious and felonious. *Endocrinol Metab Clin North Am* 1999;28:579–601.
58. Grunberger G, Weiner JL, Silverman R, et al. Factitious hypoglycemia due to surreptitious administration of insulin: diagnosis, treatment, and long-term follow-up. *Ann Intern Med* 1988;108:252–257.
59. Arky RA. Hypoglycemia associated with liver disease and ethanol. *Endocrinol Metab Clin North Am* 1989;18:75–90.
60. Fuchs S, Bogomolski-Yahalom V, Paltiel O, et al. Ischemic hepatitis: clinical and laboratory observations of 34 patients. *J Clin Gastroenterol* 1998;26: 183–186.
61. Fischer KF, Lees JA, Newman JH. Hypoglycemia in hospitalized patients. Causes and outcomes. *N Engl J Med* 1986;315:1245–1250.
62. Haviv YS, Sharkia M, Safadi R. Hypoglycemia in patients with renal failure. *Ren Fail* 2000;22:219–223.
63. Greenblatt DJ. Fatal hypoglycaemia occurring after peritoneal dialysis. *BMJ* 1972;2:270–271.
64. Jackson MA, Holland MR, Nicholas J, et al. Occult hypoglycemia caused by hemodialysis. *Clin Nephrol* 1999;51:242–247.
65. Arem R. Hypoglycemia associated with renal failure. *Endocrinol Metab Clin North Am* 1989;18:103–121.
66. Stumvoll M, Chintalapudi U, Perriello G, et al. Uptake and release of glucose by the human kidney: postabsorptive rates and responses to epinephrine. *J Clin Invest* 1995;96:2528–2533.
67. Stumvoll M, Meyer C, Mitrakou A, et al. Important role of the kidney in human carbohydrate metabolism. *Med Hypotheses* 1999;52:363–366.
68. Naylor JM, Kronfeld DS. *In vivo* studies of hypoglycemia and lactic acidosis in endotoxic shock. *Am J Physiol* 1985;248:E309–316.
69. Yang J, Dong LW, Tang C, et al. Transcriptional and posttranscriptional regulation of beta(2)-adrenergic receptor gene in rat liver during sepsis. *Am J Physiol* 1999;277:R132–R139.
70. Meszaros K, Lang CH, Bagby GJ, et al. *In vivo* glucose utilization by individual tissues during nonlethal hypermetabolic sepsis. *FASEB J*1988;2:3083–3086.
71. Mathison JC, Wolfson E, Ulevitch RJ. Participation of tumor necrosis factor in the mediation of gram negative bacterial lipopolysaccharide-induced injury in rabbits. *J Clin Invest* 1988;81:1925–1937.
72. Lee MD, Zentella A, Vine W, et al. Effect of endotoxin-induced monokines on glucose metabolism in the muscle cell line L6. *Proc Natl Acad Sci U S A* 1987; 84:2590–2594.
73. Cryer PE. Glucose counterregulation in man. *Diabetes* 1981;30:261–264.
74. Kollee LA, Monnens LA, Cecjka V, et al. Persistent neonatal hypoglycaemia due to glucagon deficiency. *Arch Dis Child* 1978;53:422–424.
75. Kerr DS, Brooke OG, Robinson HM. Fasting energy utilization in the smaller of twins with epinephrine-deficient hypoglycemia. *Metabolism* 1981;30:6–17.
76. Malerbi D, Liberman B, Giurno-Filho A, et al. Glucocorticoids and glucose metabolism: hepatic glucose production in untreated Addisonian patients and on two different levels of glucocorticoid administration. *Clin Endocrinol (Oxf)* 1988;28:415–422.

77. Boyle PJ, Cryer PE. Growth hormone, cortisol, or both are involved in defense against, but are not critical to recovery from, hypoglycemia. *Am J Physiol* 1991;260:E395–E402.
78. Muglia L, Jacobson L, Dikkes P, et al. Corticotropin-releasing hormone deficiency reveals major fetal but not adult glucocorticoid need. *Nature* 1995; 373:427–432.
79. Van Haeften TW. Clinical significance of insulin antibodies in insulin-treated diabetic patients. *Diabetes Care* 1989;12:641–648.
80. Redmon JB, Nuttall FQ. Autoimmune hypoglycemia. *Endocrinol Metab Clin North Am* 1999;28:603–618.
81. Dean BM, McNally JM, Bonifacio E, et al. Comparison of insulin autoantibodies in diabetes-related and healthy populations by precise displacement ELISA. *Diabetes* 1989;38:1275–1281.
82. Uchigata Y, Eguchi Y, Takayama-Hasumi S, et al. Insulin autoimmune syndrome (Hirata disease): clinical features and epidemiology in Japan. *Diabetes Res Clin Pract* 1994;22:89–94.
83. Kulkarni RN, Bruning JC, Winnay JN, et al. Tissue-specific knockout of the insulin receptor in pancreatic beta cells creates an insulin secretory defect similar to that in type 2 diabetes. *Cell* 1999;96:329–339.
84. Grant CS. Surgical aspects of hyperinsulinemic hypoglycemia. *Endocrinol Metab Clin North Am* 1999;28:533–554.
85. Hirshberg B, Livi A, Bartlett DL, et al. Forty-eight-hour fast: the diagnostic test for insulinoma. *J Clin Endocrinol Metab* 2000;85:3222–3226.
86. Moller N, Blum WF, Mengel A, et al. Basal and insulin stimulated substrate metabolism in tumour induced hypoglycaemia; evidence for increased muscle glucose uptake. *Diabetologia* 1991;34:17–20.
87. Eastman RC, Carson RE, Orloff DG, et al. Glucose utilization in a patient with hepatoma and hypoglycemia. Assessment by a positron emission tomography. *J Clin Invest* 1992;89:1958–1963.
88. Daughaday WH, Emanuele MA, Brooks MH, et al. Synthesis and secretion of insulin-like growth factor II by a leiomyosarcoma with associated hypoglycemia. *N Engl J Med* 1988;319:1434–1440.
89. Ron D, Powers AC, Pandian MR, et al. Increased insulin-like growth factor II production and consequent suppression of growth hormone secretion: a dual mechanism for tumor-induced hypoglycemia. *J Clin Endocrinol Metab* 1989; 68:701–706.
90. Zapf J, Futo E, Peter M, et al. Can "big" insulin-like growth factor II in serum of tumor patients account for the development of extrapancreatic tumor hypoglycemia? *J Clin Invest* 1992;90:2574–2584.
91. Frystyk J, Skjaerbaek C, Zapf J, et al. Increased levels of circulating free insulin-like growth factors in patients with non-islet cell tumour hypoglycaemia. *Diabetologia* 1998;41:589–594.
92. Daughaday WH, Trivedi B, Baxter RC. Serum "big insulin-like growth factor II" from patients with tumor hypoglycemia lacks normal E-domain O-linked glycosylation, a possible determinant of normal propeptide processing. *Proc Natl Acad Sci U S A* 1993;90:5823–5827.
93. Hizuka N, Fukuda I, Takano K, et al. Serum high molecular weight form of insulin-like growth factor II from patients with non-islet cell tumor hypoglycemia is O-glycosylated. *J Clin Endocrinol Metab* 1998;83:2875–2877.
94. Baxter R, Holman S, Corbould A, et al. Regulation of the insulin-like growth factors and their binding proteins by glucocorticoid and growth hormone in non—islet cell tumor hypoglycemia. *J Clin Endocrinol Metab* 1995;80: 2700–2780.
95. Seckl MJ, Mulholland PJ, Bishop AE, et al. Hypoglycemia due to an insulin-secreting small-cell carcinoma of the cervix. *N Engl J Med* 1999;341:733–736.
96. Lyall SS, Marieb NJ, Wise JK, et al. Hyperinsulinemic hypoglycemia associated with a neurofibrosarcoma. *Arch Intern Med* 1975;135:865–867.
97. Kiang DT, Bauer GE, Kennedy BJ. Immunoassayable insulin in carcinoma of the cervix associated with hypoglycemia. *Cancer* 1973;31:801–805.
98. Service FJ, Natt N, Thompson GB, et al. Noninsulinoma pancreatogenous hypoglycemia: a novel syndrome of hyperinsulinemic hypoglycemia in adults independent of mutations in *Kir6.2* and *SUR1* genes. *J Clin Endocrinol Metab* 1999;84:1582–1589.
99. Harness JK, Geelhoed GW, Thompson NW, et al. Nesidioblastosis in adults: a surgical dilemma. *Arch Surg* 1981;116:575–580.
100. Fong TL, Warner NE, Kumar D. Pancreatic nesidioblastosis in adults. *Diabetes Care* 1989;12:108–114.
101. Permutt MA, Kelly J, Berstein R, et al. Alimentary hypoglycemia in the absence of gastrointestinal surgery. *N Engl J Med* 1973;288:1206–1210.
102. Seltzer HS, Fajans SS, Conn JW. Spontaneous hypoglycemia as an early manifestation of diabetes mellitus. *Diabetes* 1956;5:437–442.
103. Faludi G, Bendersky G, Gerber P. Functional hypoglycemia in early latent diabetes. *Ann N Y Acad Sci* 1968;148:868–874.
104. Anthony D, Dippe S, Hofeldt FD, et al. Personality disorder and reactive hypoglycemia: a quantitative study. *Diabetes* 1973;22:664–675.
105. Ford CV, Bray GA, Swerdloff RS. A psychiatric study of patients referred with a diagnosis of hypoglycemia. *Am J Psychiatry* 1976;133:290–294.
106. Lev-Ran A, Anderson RW. The diagnosis of postprandial hypoglycemia. *Diabetes* 1981;30:996–999.
107. Tamburrano G, Leonetti F, Sbraccia P, et al. Increased insulin sensitivity in patients with idiopathic reactive hypoglycemia. *J Clin Endocrinol Metab* 1989; 69:885–890.
108. Foa PP, Dunbar JC, Jr., Klein SP, et al. Reactive hypoglycemia and A-cell ("pancreatic") glucagon deficiency in the adult. *JAMA* 1980;244:2281–2285.
109. Ogata ES. Carbohydrate metabolism in the fetus and neonate and altered neonatal glucoregulation. *Pediatr Clin North Am* 1986;33:25–45.
110. Bougneres PF. Stable isotope tracers and the determination of fuel fluxes in newborn infants. *Biol Neonate* 1987;52:87–96.
111. Denne SC, Kalhan SC. Glucose carbon recycling and oxidation in human newborns. *Am J Physiol* 1986;251:E71–E77.
112. Cornblath M, Hawdon JM, Williams AF, et al. Controversies regarding definition of neonatal hypoglycemia: suggested operational thresholds. *Pediatrics* 2000;105:1141–1145.
113. Cornblath M, Ichord R. Hypoglycemia in the neonate. *Semin Perinatol* 2000;24:136–149.
114. Koh TH, Aynsley-Green A, Tarbit M, et al. Neural dysfunction during hypoglycaemia. *Arch Dis Child* 1988;63:1353–1358.
115. Pryds O, Christensen NJ, Friis-Hansen B. Increased cerebral blood flow and plasma epinephrine in hypoglycemic, preterm neonates. *Pediatrics* 1990;85: 172–176.
116. Lucas A, Morley R, Cole TJ. Adverse neurodevelopmental outcome of moderate neonatal hypoglycaemia. *BMJ* 1988;297:1304–1308.
117. Duvanel CB, Fawer CL, Cotting J, et al. Long-term effects of neonatal hypoglycemia on brain growth and psychomotor development in small-for-gestational-age preterm infants. *J Pediatr* 1999;134:492–498.
118. Abraham CS, Temesvari P, Kovacs J, et al. Plasma and cerebrospinal fluid hyperinsulinism in asphyxiated piglets. *Biol Neonate* 1996;70:296–303.
119. Bhowmick SK, Lewandowski C. Prolonged hyperinsulinism and hypoglycemia in an asphyxiated, small for gestation infant: case management and literature review. *Clin Pediatr (Phila)* 1989;28:575–578.
120. Collins JE, Leonard JV. Hyperinsulinism in asphyxiated and small-for-dates infants with hypoglycaemia. *Lancet* 1984;2:311–313.
121. Klenka HM, Seager J. Hyperinsulinism in asphyxiated and small-for-dates infants with hypoglycaemia [Letter]. *Lancet* 1984;2:975.
122. Schultz K, Soltesz G. Transient hyperinsulinism in asphyxiated newborn infants. *Acta Paediatr Hung* 1991;31:47–52.
123. Petrik J, Pell JM, Arany E, et al. Overexpression of insulin-like growth factor-II in transgenic mice is associated with pancreatic islet cell hyperplasia. *Endocrinology* 1999;140:2353–2363.
124. Li YM, Franklin G, Cui HM, et al. The H19 transcript is associated with polysomes and may regulate IGF2 expression in *trans*. *J Biol Chem* 1998;273: 28247–28252.
125. Matsuoka S, Edwards MC, Bai C, et al. *p57KIP2*, a structurally distinct member of the p21CIP1 Cdk inhibitor family, is a candidate tumor suppressor gene. *Genes Devel* 1995;9:650–662.
126. Weksberg R, Shen DR, Fei YL, et al. Disruption of insulin-like growth factor 2 imprinting in Beckwith-Wiedemann syndrome. *Nat Genet* 1993;5:143–150.
127. Hatada I, Ohashi H, Fukushima Y, et al. An imprinted gene *p57KIP2* is mutated in Beckwith-Wiedemann syndrome. *Nat Genet* 1996;14:171–173.
128. DeBaun MR, King AA, White N. Hypoglycemia in Beckwith-Wiedemann syndrome. *Semin Perinatol* 2000;24:164–171.
129. Barrett CT, Oliver TK Jr. Hypoglycemia and hyperinsulinism in infants with erythroblastosis fetalis. *N Engl J Med* 1968;278:1260–1262.
130. From GL, Driscoll SG, Steinke J. Serum insulin in newborn infants with erythroblastosis fetalis. *Pediatrics* 1969;44:549–553.
131. Raivio KO, Osterlund K. Hypoglycemia and hyperinsulinemia associated with erythroblastosis fetalis. *Pediatrics* 1969;43:217–225.
132. Driscoll SG, Steinke J. Pancreatic insulin content in severe erythroblastosis. *Pediatrics* 1967;39:448–450.
133. Wu W, Cogan JD, Pfaffle RW, et al. Mutations in *PROP1* cause familial combined pituitary hormone deficiency. *Nat Genet* 1998;18:147–149.
134. Tatsumi K, Miyai K, Notomi T, et al. Cretinism with combined hormone deficiency caused by a mutation in the *PIT1* gene. *Nat Genet* 1992;1:56–58.
135. Peter M, Viemann M, Partsch CJ, et al. Congenital adrenal hypoplasia: clinical spectrum, experience with hormonal diagnosis, and report on new point mutations of the *DAX-1* gene. *J Clin Endocrinol Metab* 1998;83:2666–2674.
136. Hussain K, Hindmarsh P, Aynsley-Green A. Neonatal hyperinsulinism (HI) is associated with abnormal cortisol responses to hypoglycaemia (HY). *Horm Res* 2000;53[Suppl 2]:26.
137. Lteif AN, Schwenk WF. Hypoglycemia in infants and children. *Endocrinol Metab Clin North Am* 1999;28:619–646.
138. Chen YT, Burchel A. Glycogen storage diseases. In: Scriver CR, Beaudet AL, Sly WS, et al., eds. *The metabolic and molecular basis of inherited disease*, 7th ed. New York: McGraw Hill, 1995:935–965.
139. Aynsley-Green A. Hepatic glycogen synthetase deficiency. *Arch Dis Child* 1977;52:573.
140. Orho M, Bosshard NU, Buist NR, et al. Mutations in the liver glycogen synthase gene in children with hypoglycemia due to glycogen storage disease type 0. *J Clin Invest* 1998;102:507–515.
141. Rallison ML, Meikle W, Zigrang W. Hypoglycemia and lactic acidosis associated with fructose-1,6-diphosphatase deficiency. *J Pediatr* 1979;9:933.
142. Burlina AB, Bonafe L, Zacchello F. Clinical and biochemical approach to the neonate with a suspected inborn error of amino acid and organic acid metabolism. *Semin Perinatol* 1999;23:162–173.
143. Ozand PT. Hypoglycemia in association with various organic and amino acid disorders. *Semin Perinatol* 2000;24:172–193.
144. Den Boer ME, Wanders RJ, Morris AA, et al. Long-chain 3-hydroxylacyl-CoA dehydrogenase deficiency: clinical presentation and follow-up of 50 patients. *Pediatrics* 2002;109:99–104.
145. Gonzalez-Manchon C, Martin-Requero A, Ayuso MS, et al. Role of endogenous fatty acids in the control of hepatic gluconeogenesis. *Arch Biochem Biophys* 1992;292:95–101.

146. Burton BK. Inborn errors of metabolism in infancy: a guide to diagnosis. *Pediatrics* 1998;102:E69.
147. Vreken P, van Lint AE, Bootsma AH, et al. Quantitative plasma acylcarnitine analysis using electrospray tandem mass spectrometry for the diagnosis of organic acidaemias and fatty acid oxidation defects. *J Inherit Metab Dis* 1999; 22:302–306.
148. Rashed MS, Rahbeeni Z, Ozand PT. Application of electrospray tandem mass spectrometry to neonatal screening. *Semin Perinatol* 1999;23:183–193.
149. Rashed MS, Ozand PT, Bucknall MP, et al. Diagnosis of inborn errors of metabolism from blood spots by acylcarnitines and amino acids profiling using automated electrospray tandem mass spectrometry. *Pediatr Res* 1995;38:324–331.
150. Scaglia F, Longo N. Primary and secondary alterations of neonatal carnitine metabolism. *Semin Perinatol* 1999;23:152–161.
151. Zhang Z, Kolvraa S, Zhou Y, et al. Three RFLPs defining a haplotype associated with the common mutation in human medium-chain acyl-CoA dehydrogenase (MCAD) deficiency occur in Alu repeats. *Am J Hum Genet* 1993;52:1111–1121.
152. Clayton PT, Doig M, Ghafari S, et al. Screening for medium chain acyl-CoA dehydrogenase deficiency using electrospray ionisation tandem mass spectrometry. *Arch Dis Child* 1998;79:109–115.
153. Naylor EW, Chace DH. Automated tandem mass spectrometry for mass newborn screening for disorders in fatty acid, organic acid, and amino acid metabolism. *J Child Neurol* 1999;14[Suppl 1]:S4–S8.
154. Wilson GN, de Chadarevian JP, Kaplan P, et al. Glutaric aciduria type, II: review of the phenotype and report of an unusual glomerulopathy. *Am J Med Genet* 1989;32:395–401.
155. Poplawski NK, Ranieri E, Harrison JR, et al. Multiple acyl-coenzyme A dehydrogenase deficiency: diagnosis by acylcarnitine analysis of a 12-year-old newborn screening card. *J Pediatr* 1999;134:764–766.
156. Rhead WJ, Wolff JA, Lipson M, et al. Clinical and biochemical variation and family studies in the multiple acyl-CoA dehydrogenation disorders. *Pediatr Res* 1987;21:371–376.
157. Thompson GN, Hsu BY, Pitt JJ, et al. Fasting hypoketotic coma in a child with deficiency of mitochondrial 3-hydroxy-3-methylglutaryl-CoA synthase. *N Engl J Med* 1997;337:1203–1207.
158. Barash V, Mandel H, Sella S, et al. 3-Hydroxy-3-methylglutaryl-coenzyme A lyase deficiency: biochemical studies and family investigation of four generations. *J Inherit Metab Dis* 1990;13:156–164.
159. Aynsley-Green A, Hussain K, Hall J, et al. Practical management of hyperinsulinism in infancy. *Arch Dis Child Fetal Neonatal Ed* 2000;82:F98–F107.
160. Glaser B, Thornton P, Otonkoski T, et al. Genetics of neonatal hyperinsulinism. *Arch Dis Child Fetal Neonatal Ed* 2000;82:F79–F86.
161. Rahier J, Guiot Y, Sempoux C. Persistent hyperinsulinaemic hypoglycaemia of infancy: a heterogeneous syndrome unrelated to nesidioblastosis. *Arch Dis Child Fetal Neonatal Ed* 2000;82:F108–F112.
162. Shepherd RM, Cosgrove KE, O'Brien RE, et al. Hyperinsulinism of infancy: towards an understanding of unregulated insulin release. *Arch Dis Child Fetal Neonatal Ed* 2000;82:F87–F97.
163. Aynsley-Green A, Polak JM, Bloom SR, et al. Nesidioblastosis of the pancreas: definition of the syndrome and the management of the severe neonatal hyperinsulinaemic hypoglycaemia. *Arch Dis Child* 1981;56:496–508.
164. Landau H, Perlman M, Meyer S, et al. Persistent neonatal hypoglycemia due to hyperinsulinism: medical aspects. *Pediatrics* 1982;70:440–446.
165. Zammarchi E, Filippi L, Novembre E, et al. Biochemical evaluation of a patient with a familial form of leucine-sensitive hypoglycemia and concomitant hyperammonemia. *Metabolism* 1996;45:957–960.
166. Stanley CA, Lieu YK, Hsu BY, et al. Hyperinsulinism and hyperammonemia in infants with regulatory mutations of the glutamate dehydrogenase gene. *N Engl J Med* 1998;338:1352–1357.
167. Weinzimer SA, Stanley CA, Berry GT, et al. A syndrome of congenital hyperinsulinism and hyperammonemia. *J Pediatr* 1997;130:661–664.
168. Glaser B, Landau H, Permutt MA. Neonatal hyperinsulinism. *Trends Endocrinol Metabol* 1999;10:55–61.
169. Héron L, Virsolvy A, Apiou F, et al. Isolation, characterization, and chromosomal localization of the human *ENSA* gene that encodes alpha-endosulfine, a regulator of beta-cell K(ATP) channels. *Diabetes* 1999;48:1873–1876.
170. Huopio H, Reimann F, Ashfield R, et al. Dominantly inherited hyperinsulinism caused by a mutation in the sulfonylurea receptor type 1. *J Clin Invest* 2000;106:897–906.
171. de Lonlay P, Fournet JC, Rahier J, et al. Somatic deletion of the imprinted 11p15 region in sporadic persistent hyperinsulinemic hypoglycemia of infancy is specific of focal adenomatous hyperplasia and endorses partial pancreatectomy. *J Clin Invest* 1997;100:802–807.
172. Ryan FD, Devaney D, Joyce C, et al. Hyperinsulinism: the molecular aetiology of focal disease. *Arch Dis Child* 1998;79:445–447.
173. Verkarre V, Fournet JC, de Lonlay P, et al. Paternal mutation of the sulfonylurea receptor (*SUR1*) gene and maternal loss of 11p15 imprinted genes lead to persistent hyperinsulinism in focal adenomatous hyperplasia. *J Clin Invest* 1998;102:1286–1291.
174. de Lonlay-Debeney P, Poggi-Travert F, Fournet JC, et al. Clinical features of 52 neonates with hyperinsulinism. *N Engl J Med* 1999;340:1169–1175.
175. Dubois J, Brunelle F, Touati G, et al. Hyperinsulinism in children: diagnostic value of pancreatic venous sampling correlated with clinical, pathological and surgical outcome in 25 cases. *Pediatr Radiol* 1995;25:512–516.
176. Ferry RJ, Kelly A, Grimberg A, et al. Calcium-stimulated insulin secretion in diffuse and focal forms of congenital hyperinsulinism. *J Pediatr* 2000;137: 239–246.
177. Grimberg A, Ferry RJ, Kelly A, et al. Dysregulation of insulin secretion in children with congenital hyperinsulinism due to sulfonylurea receptor mutations. *Diabetes* 2001;50:322–328.
178. Maechler P, Wollheim CB. Mitochondrial glutamate acts as a messenger in glucose-induced insulin exocytosis. *Nature* 1999;402:685–689.
179. MacDonald MJ, Fahien LA. Glutamate is not a messenger in insulin secretion. *J Biol Chem* 2000;275:34025–34027.
180. Stanley CA, Fang J, Kutyna K, et al. Molecular basis and characterization of the hyperinsulinism/hyperammonemia syndrome: predominance of mutations in exons 11 and 12 of the glutamate dehydrogenase gene: HI/HA Contributing Investigators. *Diabetes* 2000;49:667–673.
181. Glaser B, Kesavan P, Heyman M, et al. Familial hyperinsulinism caused by an activating glucokinase mutation. *N Engl J Med* 1998;338:226–230.
182. Froguel P, Zouali H, Vionnet N, et al. Familial hyperglycemia due to mutations in glucokinase. Definition of a subtype of diabetes mellitus. *N Engl J Med* 1993;328:697–702.
183. Babovic-Vuksanovic D, Patterson MC, Schwenk WF, et al. Severe hypoglycemia as a presenting symptom of carbohydrate-deficient glycoprotein syndrome. *J Pediatr* 1999;135:775–781.
184. de Lonlay P, Cuer M, Vuillaumier-Barrot S, et al. Hyperinsulinemic hypoglycemia as a presenting sign in phosphomannose isomerase deficiency: a new manifestation of carbohydrate-deficient glycoprotein syndrome treatable with mannose. *J Pediatr* 1999;135:379–383.
185. Bereket A, Turan S. Kabuki syndrome: two cases presenting with endocrine problems. *Horm Res* 2000;53[Suppl 2]:164.
186. Hussain K, Clayton PE, Krywawych S, et al. Hyperinsulinism (HI) in childhood associated with a defect in short chain 3-hydroxyacyl CoA dehydrogenase deficiency (SCHAD): a new syndrome linking abnormal fatty acid metabolism and HI. *Horm Res* 2000;53[Suppl 2]:9.
187. Meissner T, Otonkoski T, Feneberg R, et al. Exercise-induced hypoglycemic hyperinsulinism. *Arch Dis Child* 2001;84:254–257.
188. Glaser B, Landau H, Smilovici A, et al. Persistent hyperinsulinaemic hypoglycemia of infancy: long-term treatment with the somatostatin analogue Sandostatin. *Clin Endocrinol* 1989;31:71–80.
189. Lindley K, Dunne M, Kane C, et al. Ionic control of beta cell function in nesidioblastosis: a possible therapeutic role for calcium channel blockade. *Arch Dis Child* 1996;74:373–378.
190. Grimberg A, Weinzimer S, Baker L. Long-term treatment of congenital hyperinsulinism with subcutaneous infusion of combined octreotide and glucagon. *Horm Res* 1997;48[Suppl 2]:36.
191. Katz LE, Ferry RJ Jr, Stanley CA, et al. Suppression of insulin oversecretion by subcutaneous recombinant human insulin-like growth factor I in children with congenital hyperinsulinism due to defective beta-cell sulfonylurea receptor. *J Clin Endocrinol Metab* 1999;84:3117–3124.
192. Baker L, Thornton PS, Stanley CA. Management of hyperinsulinism in infants. *J Pediatr* 1991;119:755–757.
193. Gross-Tsur V, Shalev RS, Wertman-Elad R, et al. Neurobehavioral profile of children with persistent hyperinsulinemic hypoglycemia of infancy. *Dev Neuropsychol* 1994;10:153–163.

CHAPTER 70

Endocrine Tumors of the Pancreas

Maha T. Barakat, Houman Ashrafian, and Stephen R. Bloom

Pancreatic endocrine tumors make up only 1% to 2% of all tumors of the pancreas but form an important group in that they tend to be more benign and treatable than the common exocrine tumors. Although the identification of the menin gene has provided some insights into the tumorigenesis of the rare familial form of pancreatic endocrine tumors, the heterogeneity of phenotypes and the absence of menin mutations in some cases remain unexplained. With the advent of technological advances facilitating the retrieval and analysis of large data sets, such as gene expression microarray profiling and multivariate analysis of complex traits (1), we are now poised to identify subsequent molecular events and use the information to prognosticate and risk stratify patients with the menin gene mutation. In addition, these techniques will permit comparison of the findings in patients with multiple endocrine neoplasia type 1 (MEN1) with those in patients with the more common sporadic form of disease in whom no menin mutation is apparent and to relate the pathogenesis of these potentially distinct but related tumor entities. To maximize the power of these basic science techniques, this analysis of the complex pathways in relation to tumor behavior will necessitate ever more rigorous clinical assessment of phenotype definitions. Indeed, gene-expression data have already been shown to provide invaluable prognostic information with regard to breast carcinoma (2,3), prostate carcinoma (4), and diffuse large B-cell lymphoma (5) and can predict imminent metastatic behavior in malignant melanoma (6).

Pancreatic endocrine tumors are derived from the diffuse neuroendocrine system of the gastrointestinal tract (7) and were formerly classified as apudomas (tumors of the *a*mine *p*recursor *u*ptake and *d*ecarboxylation system). These neuroendocrine cells can produce a myriad of hormones, many of which are also present in the brain. The hormones provide a complex network of communication, each having endocrine, paracrine, autocrine, or neurotransmitter functions crucial to the finely tuned functioning and regulation of the gastroenteropancreatic system.

INCIDENCE

Although the annual incidence of neuroendocrine pancreatic tumors is about 3.5 to 4 per million population, there is a vast discrepancy between the clinical incidence and that found post mortem, suggesting an abundance of asymptomatic disease. Pancreatic endocrine tumors have been detected in 0.3% to 1.6% of unselected autopsies in which only a few sections of the pancreas were examined, whereas they were found in up to 10% when the whole pancreas was examined systematically (8). Unlike neuroendocrine tumors of the gut, carcinoid tumors rarely occur in the pancreas and will not be covered in this chapter.

ETIOLOGY

The etiology of pancreatic endocrine tumors has many similarities to tumorigenesis in the better-studied colorectal carcinoma model. The similarities will be discussed in this section, and this

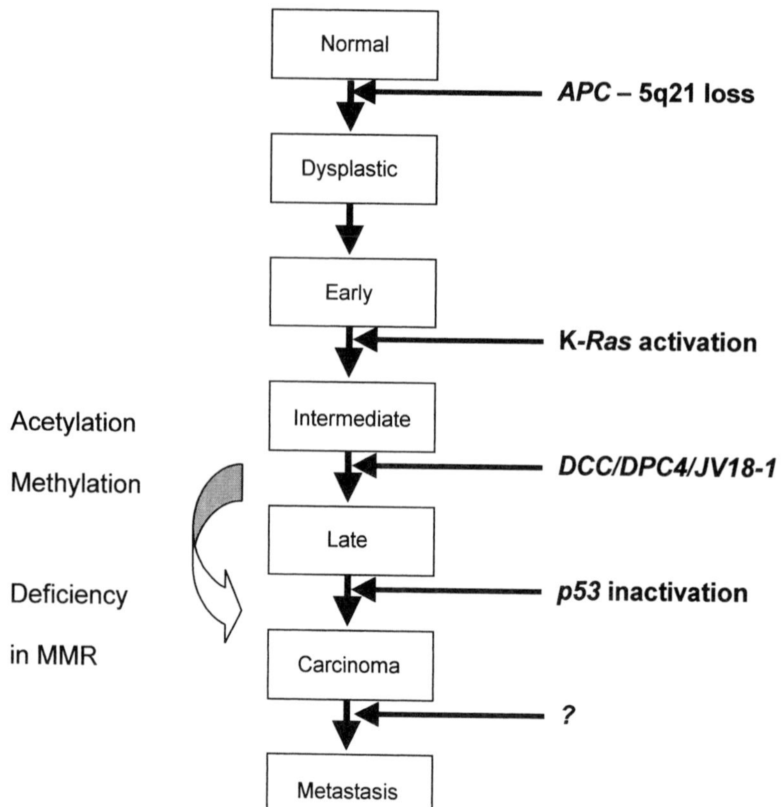

Figure 70.1. Genetic changes associated with colorectal tumorigenesis. Mutations in the adenomatous polyposis gene (*APC*) initiate tumorigenesis, and tumor progression results from mutations in the other genes indicated. MMR, mismatch pair. (Adapted from Fearon ER, Vogelstein B. A genetic model for colorectal tumorigenesis. *Cell* 1990;61:759–767; and Kinzler KW, Vogelstein B. Lessons from hereditary colorectal cancer. *Cell* 1996;87:159–170; with additional data from Shannon BA, Iacopetta BJ. Methylation of the hMLH1, p16, and MDR1 genes in colorectal carcinoma: associations with clinicopathological features. *Cancer Lett* 2001;167:91–97.)

analogy will help in understanding the development of pancreatic endocrine tumors.

Genetic Model from Colorectal Tumorigenesis

It is becoming increasingly clear that tumorigenesis involves a series of multiple genetic alterations leading to activation of oncogenes and/or inactivation of tumor suppressor genes and ultimately to loss of apoptosis. The genetic basis of colorectal neoplasia has provided a salient model for this sequential process (9). The transition from healthy colonic epithelia through increasingly dysplastic adenoma to colorectal cancer involves the acquisition of mutations in specific genes, including *APC*, K-*ras*, *DCC*, and *p53* [Fig. 70.1; data also from (10)]. Furthermore, although the total accumulation of genetic alterations is important, the exact sequence of events is critical for determining the phenotype, as illustrated by the early loss of *Lkb1*, rendering the cells resistant to oncogene-induced transformation, in Peutz-Jeghers syndrome (11).

Mutations in the adenomatous polyposis gene (*APC*) occur both in autosomal dominant familial adenomatous polyposis (FAP) and sporadically. The initiation of tumorigenesis requires a two-hit process, as outlined in Knudson's model (12). In the case of germline mutations, the first hit to the *APC* gene is inherited with the germline, thus being identical in all cells. Alternatively, in somatic mutations the first hit can occur as a rare event in a particular somatic cell. A second hit in both germline and somatic cases inactivates the unaffected allele, resulting in loss of heterozygosity (LOH) and initiates tumorigenesis.

The *APC* gene, located on chromosome 5q21, encodes a 312-kDa tumor suppressor protein with many possible protein/protein interactions, including binding sites for β-catenin, end-binding protein-1 (EB1), and axin (13). It is termed a "gatekeeper" gene, because in normal human colonic cells, the APC/axin protein complex facilitates the phosphorylation and subsequent degradation of β-catenin, thus preventing β-catenin–stimulated transcriptional activation and cell proliferation (Fig. 70.2) (14). It is therefore highly relevant that the majority of *APC* mutations in FAP result in the deletion of the carboxyterminal end, including the β-catenin and axin binding sites (15). This then initiates cell proliferation and tumorigenesis. Indeed, in addition to colorectal neoplasia, *APC* mutations have been associated with small-bowel tumors, desmoid tumors, and medulloblastomas.

To a certain extent, there seems to be some correlation between genotype and phenotype in mutations affecting *APC*. Depending on the region of the gene affected, the resulting phenotype may be attenuated polyposis, classic polyposis, congenital hypertrophy of the retinal pigment epithelium (CHRPE), or Gardner syndrome (mandibular osteomas and desmoid tumors) (15). The resultant phenotype is determined by the functional consequences of the different mutations in *APC* and downstream modifying events.

Application of the Model to Pancreatic Endocrine Tumors

Although there is currently no direct evidence, it is likely that the process of tumorigenesis of pancreatic endocrine neoplasia follows the model of sequential accumulation of mutations, analogous to colonic neoplasia. In fact, there are many similarities between the two types of tumors. The familial form of pancreatic endocrine tumors is the autosomal dominant type MEN1, in which the other features include anterior pituitary tumors (27%); parathyroid hyperplasia (90%); and, more rarely, foregut carcinoid (14%), adrenocortical tumors (5%), and pheochromocytoma (<1%) (16). Nonendocrine tumors include angiofibroma (85%), collagenoma (70%), lipoma (30%), and

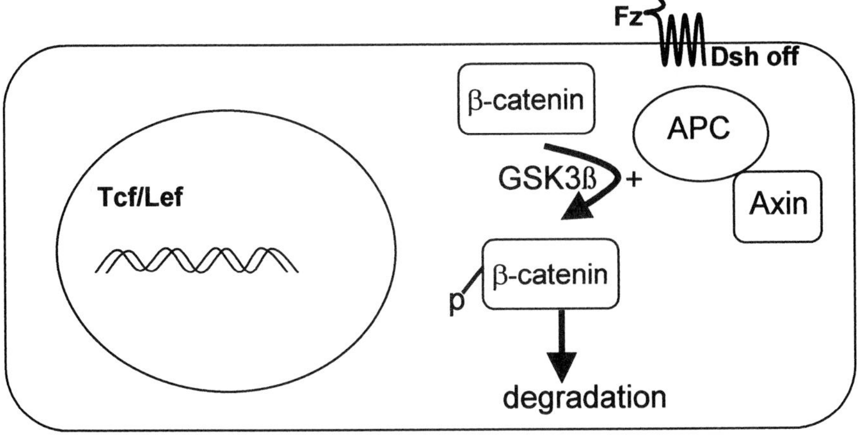

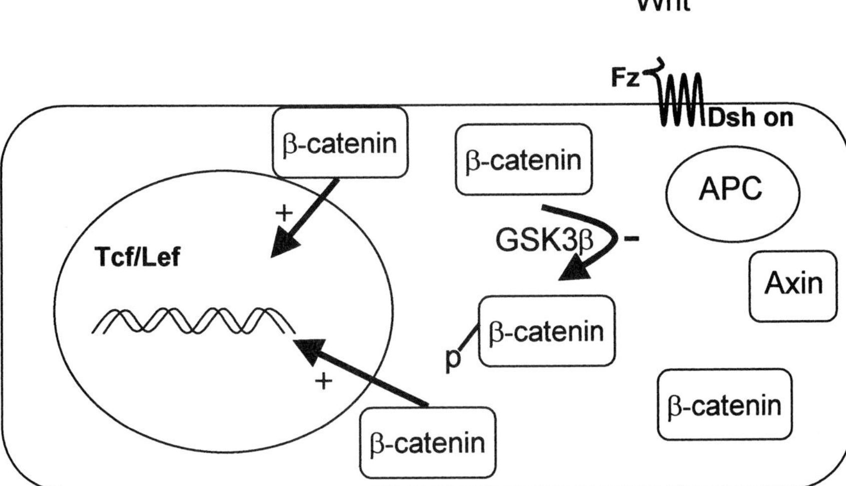

Figure 70.2. The APC/axin β-catenin "destruction pathway" and regulation of transcription. The APC/axin complex modulates the activity of GSK3β (glycogen synthase kinase 3β) and facilitates the phosphorylation of β-catenin, leading to the degradation of β-catenin. When the cells are exposed to Wnt (wingless and integration activated gene product), which acts on cell surface receptors of the frizzled family (Fz), the APC/axin complex is inactivated by an unknown mechanism requiring disheveled protein (Dsh), and β-catenin accumulates in the cell. This enters the nucleus and interacts with Tcf/Lef (T-cell factor/lymphoid enhancer binding factor) DNA-binding protein to activate new gene expression. An analogous situation occurs with inactivating mutations in *APC*. APC, adenomatous polyposis. (Adapted from Peifer M, Polakis P. Wnt signaling in oncogenesis and embryogenesis—a look outside the nucleus. *Science* 2000;287:1606–1609; and Kinzler KW, Vogelstein B. Lessons from hereditary colorectal cancer. *Cell* 1996;87:159–170.)

ependymoma (<1%). Pancreatic endocrine tumors can, however, also occur sporadically.

In 1988, Larsson and colleagues localized the *MEN1* gene to chromosome 11q13 (17). Germline-inactivating mutations in this gene have been found in 95% of patients with familial MEN1, whereas in sporadic cases somatic mutations were found in a smaller proportion of patients: 21% of those with parathyroid adenoma, 33% with gastrinomas, 17% with insulinoma, 36% with bronchial carcinoids, and 50% to 70% with sporadic thymic and duodenal carcinoid (16,18–21). *MEN1* is known to be a tumor suppressor, and it is likely that the transition from normal cells to neuroendocrine neoplasia in familial MEN1 requires a series of sequential genetic alterations starting with *MEN1* [Fig. 70.3; data from (22–26)]. It is possible that, where there is no detectable *MEN1* mutation (for instance, in the 5% of familial and in the majority of sporadic cases), the mutation cannot be detected given current techniques or that *MEN1* is inactivated by mechanisms other than mutation, e.g., alterations in promoter methylation. It is interesting that the 5′-region of *MEN1* contains a CpG-rich area, and hypermethylation of similar regions in the promoter of the *VHL* and the *hMLH1* genes has been shown to be a frequent cause of somatic second hit in tumorigenesis in von Hippel–Lindau disease and colorectal carcinoma, respectively (27–29).

Similar to colorectal neoplasia, the initiation of tumorigenesis from the *MEN1* tumor suppressor gene requires a two-hit process [Knudson's model (12,23)]. In germline mutations, the first hit to the *MEN1* gene is inherited and only one more hit is required for loss of heterozygosity, whereas in somatic mutations of sporadic cases, two hits are required to result in tumorigenesis (17,30,31). In the mouse model with the homologue *Men1* germline mutation, the remaining wild-type *Men1* allele was retained until tumor formation, when somatic loss of this wild-type allele occurred in all tumors developed by the mice (22). The clinical features of familial MEN1 differ from somatic *MEN1* mutations, in that age of onset of tumor expression is usually earlier (in keeping with the Knudson's hypothesis) and that there is tumor multiplicity in terms of both multiple organs affected and also multiple tumors in one organ (16).

Menin, a 610-amino-acid protein, is the product of the *MEN1* gene, and the native form has been shown to bind to and inhibit JunD, an activator protein-1 (AP-1) transcription factor (32). In addition, menin suppresses p65-mediated transcriptional activation on NF-κB sites (33), interacts with Smad3, facilitating transforming growth factor β (TGF-β)–mediated inhibition of cell growth (34), and may be important in the activity of a tumor metastasis suppressor nm23 (26), further suggestive of a tumor-suppressor role for menin (Fig. 70.4). Native menin has also been shown to inhibit insulin promoter activity and secretion and, when cotransfected into INS-1 insulinoma cells, results in inhibition of cell proliferation (35).

Despite the similarities of the etiologies of pancreatic neuroendocrine tumors and the colorectal tumorigenesis model, several differences need to be highlighted. First, the slower rate

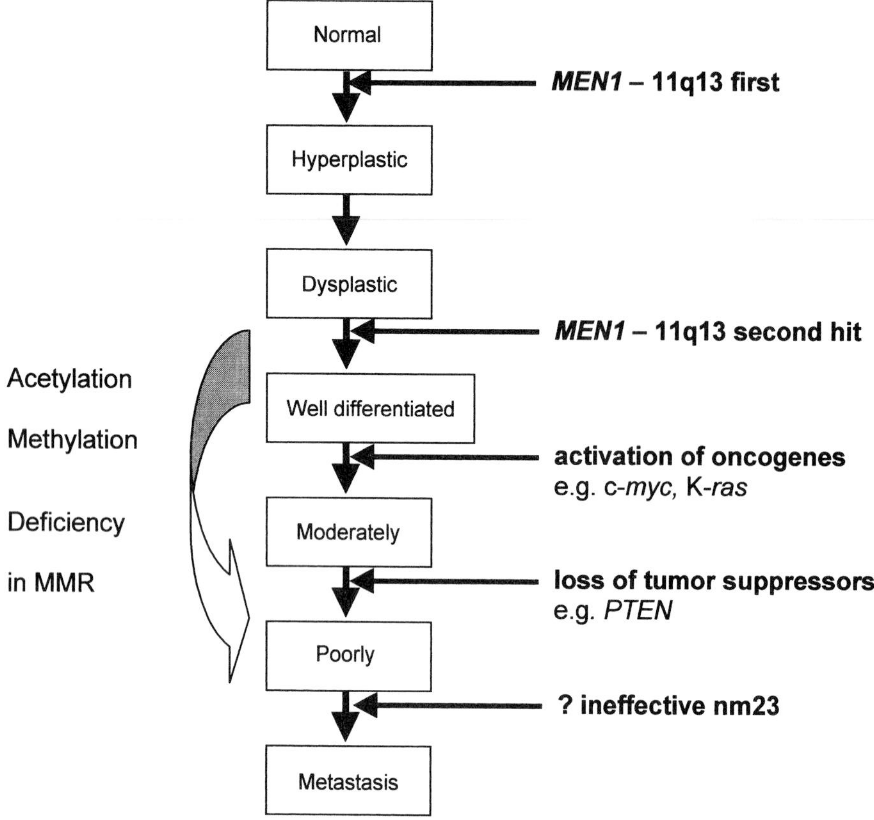

Figure 70.3. A model of genetic changes associated with pancreatic endocrine tumorigenesis. nm23 is a putative tumor metastasis suppressor. MEN1, multiple endocrine neoplasia type 1; MMR, mismatch pair; PTEN, phosphatase and tensin homologue. (Data from Crabtree JS, Scacheri PC, Ward JM, et al. A mouse model of multiple endocrine neoplasia, type 1, develops multiple endocrine tumors. *Proc Nath Acad Sci U S A* 2001;98:1118–1123; Pannett AA, Thakker RV. Somatic mutations in MEN type 1 tumors, consistent with the Knudson "two-hit" hypothesis. *J Clin Endocrinol Metab* 2001;86:4371–4374; Pelengaris S, Khan M. Oncogenic co-operation in beta-cell tumorigenesis. *Endocr Relat Cancer* 2001;8:307–314; Wang L, Ignat A, Axiotis CA. Differential expression of the PTEN tumor suppressor protein in fetal and adult neuroendocrine tissues and tumors: progressive loss of PTEN expression in poorly differentiated neuroendocrine neoplasms. *Appl Immunohistochem Mol Morphol* 2002;10:139–146; and Yaguchi H, Ohkura N, Tsukada T, et al. Menin, the multiple endocrine neoplasia type 1 gene product, exhibits GTP-hydrolyzing activity in the presence of the tumor metastasis suppressor nm23. *J Biol Chem* 2002; 277:38197–38204.)

of growth of neuroendocrine tumors and in many cases a more benign progression exists, and this may be due intrinsically to more signaling blocks and to less exposure to carcinogens. Second, there seems to be very little in the way of genotype-phenotype correlation in *MEN1* mutations (36). The development of, for instance, an insulinoma rather than a gastrinoma may be determined by local factors such as the number of pancreatic β-cells and their baseline proliferation rate. Most patients with familial MEN1 will develop nonfunctioning pancreatic tumors, whereas 40% will develop gastrinoma; 10%, insulinoma; and 2%, other functioning pancreatic tumors, such as glucagonoma, VIPoma (VIP, vasoactive intestinal polypeptide), and somatostatinoma (16).

Similarly, there is a wide spectrum in the aggressiveness of different pancreatic neuroendocrine tumors. The tumor phenotype will be determined by many factors (the particular *MEN1* mutation itself and many other downstream effects). As previously mentioned, familial MEN1 tends to result in a more aggressive tumor phenotype (earlier onset and multiplicity) compared with somatic mutations. The loss of expression of the phosphatidylinositol 3′-phosphatase and tumor suppressor gene *PTEN* (phosphatase and tensin homologue) on chromosome 10 has been shown in 54% (7 of 13) of poorly differentiated neuroendocrine tumors, whereas the two moderately differentiated neuroendocrine tumors in the series retained PTEN immunostaining (25). *PTEN* may be only one of many downstream factors that determine phenotype.

PHYSIOLOGY

There is a complex relationship between cells and enteric neurons in the gastroenteropancreatic system. This is orchestrated by a vast number of regulatory peptides secreted from neuroendocrine cells, which act in an autocrine, paracrine, and endocrine manner as well as an neurocrine manner, in which the peptides behave as neurotransmitters and neuromodulators (7,37–40).

CLINICAL FEATURES

Despite the plethora of known gut hormones, it is possible that some still cannot be detected by current techniques. When a neuroendocrine tumor is diagnosed histologically, if no circulating gut hormone is found, it is termed "nonfunctioning." However, it may just be that the secreted hormone is as yet undetectable. The patients tend to be asymptomatic initially and to develop symptoms from tumor bulk at later stages of disease progression (41). On the other hand, for those "functioning" tumors that secrete detectable hormones (e.g., insulin or gastrin), the clinical picture is very much dependent on the nature of the secreted hormone, each giving a defined syndrome [Table 70.1; data from (40,42–45)], rather than on tumor bulk. Indeed, it is common for more than one hormone to be co-secreted at presentation or even for a tumor to dedifferentiate and start producing multiple hormones. This is particularly the case with MEN1. Genetic testing for MEN1 is now readily available, and screening of family members is recommended once a germline *menin* mutation is found.

IMMUNOCYTOCHEMICAL AND BASELINE BIOCHEMICAL MARKERS

The neuroendocrine tumors share certain general immunocytochemical markers, including the secretory granules chromogranins, neuron-specific enolase (NSE), pancreatic polypeptide, human chorionic gonadotropin (hCG) subunits, and peptide histidine-methionine (46–48). Chromogranins A, B, and C (CgA, CgB, CgC) are located alongside specific hormones in large

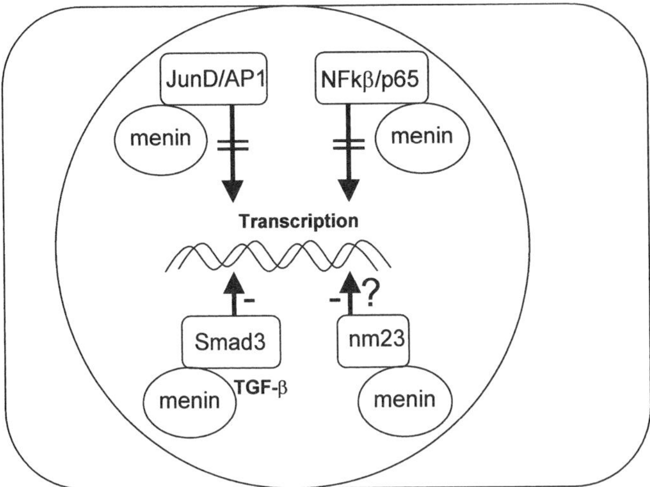

Figure 70.4. Interactions of native menin in its tumor-suppressor role. JunD is a member of the Jun family of proteins that dimerize with themselves or with Fos members to form the AP-1 (activator protein-1) transcriptional factor; menin binds JunD and inhibits JunD-mediated transcriptional activation. Menin also represses p65 (NF-κβ protein)–mediated transcriptional activation. Smad3, a downstream component of the transforming growth factor β (TGF-β) signaling pathway, interacts with menin to alter transcription, leading to inhibition of cell growth. Finally, in the presence of the putative tumor metastasis suppressor nm23, menin attains atypical GTPase activity, and this may affect transcription. (Data from Yaguchi H, Ohkura N, Tsukada T, et al. Menin, the multiple endocrine neoplasia type 1 gene product, exhibits GTP-hydrolyzing activity in the presence of the tumor metastasis suppressor nm23. *J Biol Chem* 2002;277: 38197–38204; Agarwal SK, Guru SC, Heppner C, et al. Menin interacts with the AP1 transcription factor JunD and represses JunD-activated transcription. *Cell* 1999;96:143–152; Heppner C, Bilimoria KY, Agarwal SK, et al. The tumor suppressor protein menin interacts with NF-kappaB proteins and inhibits NF-kappaB-mediated transactivation. *Oncogene* 2001;20: 4917–4925; and Kaji H, Canaff L, Lebrun JJ, et al. Inactivation of menin, a Smad3-interacting protein, blocks transforming growth factor type beta signaling. *Proc Natl Acad Sci U S A* 2001;98:3837–3842.)

dense-core vesicles of neuronal and neuroendocrine cells, with CgA being the most widely distributed (49). With the exceptions of the lactotrophs of the pituitary and some pancreatic β-cell tumors, which show positive staining for CgB, CgA-positive tumors include anterior pituitary, parathyroid, medullary thyroid, gastroenteropancreatic, ectopic ACTH (adrenocorticotropic hormone), ganglioneuromas, neuroblastomas, pheochromocytoma, and small-cell lung and prostate tumors.

Some of the above-mentioned tissue markers can be detectable in plasma. Plasma CgA is elevated in 94% of pancreatic endocrine tumors, whereas pancreatic polypeptide is elevated in 74% (50). CgA, however, seems to be the best marker for metastatic carcinoid, whereas plasma CgB appears better for detecting benign insulinomas. A fragment of CgB termed GAWK (CgB-420-493) is a 74-amino-acid peptide originally isolated from human pituitaries, and high plasma concentrations are found in various neuroendocrine tumors, including pancreatic, pheochromocytoma, medullary carcinoma of the thyroid, and ACTH-producing lung tumors. GAWK is particularly elevated in pancreatic endocrine tumors, making it a useful marker (51). In another study of pancreatic endocrine tumors, pancreastatin was elevated in 33% of patients, whereas GAWK was elevated in 50% (52).

In addition to the general hormones associated with neuroendocrine tumors, the "functioning" tumors will also secrete specific hormones, e.g., gastrin, glucagon, pancreatic polypeptide, somatostatin, neurotensin, or VIP, which should be measured in the fasting state. Other baseline hormones, such as parathyroid hormone–related peptide (PTHrP), can be measured in the nonfasting state; the next section will discuss hormones requiring provocative testing for interpretation (e.g., insulin). Not uncommonly, tumors secrete multiple hormones (53). For instance, as many as 62% of patients have elevated gastrin despite only 30% presenting with peptic ulcer disease.

The diagnosis of gastrinoma requires an elevated fasting gastrin level in the presence of increased basal gastric acid output. The latter is required to make the diagnosis, because there are other causes of elevated gastrin, including proton pump inhibitors, H_2-antagonists, atrophic gastritis, hypercalcemia, and renal impairment. The fasting gastrin should be measured with the patient off proton pump inhibitors for at least 2 weeks and off H_2-blockers for at least 3 days. However, in view of the high risk of peptic ulcer perforation in gastrinoma, caution should be exercised before cessation of therapy, particularly when the clinical suspicion is high (e.g., family history of MEN1, hypercalcemia, or negative *Helicobacter pylori* status). Indeed, even with the patient on proton pump inhibitors, the fasting gastrin level may be interpretable in that very high levels (>500 pg/mL or >250 pmol/L) are highly suggestive of gastrinoma and should be followed by localization imaging rather than by repeat measurement of gastrin levels with the patient off therapy (54). Studies of basal gastric acid output often are required to distinguish primary from secondary hypergastrinemia, in which spontaneous basal acid (proton) outputs of 20 to 25 mmol per hour are almost diagnostic and >10 mmol per hour suspicious. The measurement of basal acid output is not readily available in many centers, and an alternative is the dynamic secretin test. This is particularly useful when the gastrin level during treatment is not high enough to be diagnostic and discontinuation of pharmacologic treatment for repeat gastrin testing is not feasible.

The diagnosis of insulinoma requires the measurements of insulin and C-peptide in the presence of hypoglycemia. This therefore requires the provocative test of a 3-day fast and is covered in the next section.

BIOCHEMICAL ASSAYS: DYNAMIC TESTS

Whereas a normal response to intravenous secretin is a decline in serum gastrin levels, an increase of more than 200 pg/mL (100 pmol/L) offers a sensitivity of 80% to 85% for the presence of gastrinoma (55,56). The diagnosis of insulinoma requires the measurement of insulin and C-peptide in the presence of hypoglycemia [glucose ≤2.2 mmol/L (40 mg/dL)]. The hypoglycemia is achieved with a 3-day fast, allowing free access to noncaloric fluids. By 24 hours, 66% of patients with insulinomas develop hypoglycemia, and by 48 hours, more than 95% of insulinomas can be diagnosed (57). If no hypoglycemia is achieved at the end of the 3-day fast, the patient's exercising for 15 minutes can further increase the sensitivity of the test. If hypoglycemia occurs, simultaneous plasma and urine samples need to be taken for sulfonylurea analysis to exclude drug-induced hypoglycemia. In the presence of hypoglycemia and a negative sulfonylurea screen, inappropriately elevated insulin and C-peptide are highly suggestive of an insulinoma. The finding of ketones on urinalysis during the fast is against the diagnosis.

An alternative diagnosis to insulinoma, giving the same results at the end of a 3-day fast, is nesidioblastosis. This is a condition in which nesidioblasts differentiate from pancreatic duct epithelium and form endocrine cells that are separate from the true islets, resulting in hyperinsulinism and hypoglycemia (58).

TABLE 70.1. Tumor Syndromes of Pancreatic Endocrine Tumors

Tumor type	% of pancreatic endocrine tumors	Malignancy (%)	% with familial MEN1	Tumor location	Syndrome
Insulinoma	70–75	<10	4–5	Pancreas >99%	Hypoglycemia Weight gain
Gastrinoma	20–25	>50	20–25	Duodenum 70% Pancreas 25%	Abdominal pain Diarrhea Peptic ulceration
VIPoma	3–5	>50	6	Pancreas 90%	Secretory diarrhea Hypokalemia Achlorhydria Metabolic acidosis Flushing
Glucagonoma	1–2	>70	1–20	Pancreas 100%	Necrolytic migratory erythema Diabetes Cachexia Thromboembolic disease
PPoma	<1	>60	18–44	Pancreas 100%	Pain Weight loss Diarrhea
Somatostatinoma	<1	>50	45	Pancreas 55% Duodenum + jejunum 44%	Steatorrhea Diabetes Gallstones Weight loss
Carcinoid	<1 Mostly extrapancreatic	90	Rare	Midgut 75–87% Foregut 2–33% Hindgut 1–8% Unknown 2–15%	Classical carcinoid Flushing Diarrhea Wheeze Cardiac fibrosis Pellagra dermatosis
ACTHoma CRFoma	<1	>99	Rare	Pancreas 4–14% (of all ectopic ACTH)	Cushing syndrome Pigmentation
PTHrPoma	<1	>99	Rare	Pancreas	Hypercalcemia Nephrolithiasis Nephrocalcinosis Osteoporosis
Calcitoninoma	<1	>80	16	Pancreas	Diarrhea, flushing
GRFoma	<1	50	16	Pancreas 30% Lung 54% Jejunum 7%	Acromegaly
"Nonfunctioning"	<1	>80	18–44	Pancreas + gastrointestinal tract	Symptoms of tumor bulk Weight loss

VIP, vasoactive intestinal polypeptide; PP, pancreatic polypeptide; ACTH, adrenocorticotropic hormone; CRF, corticotropin-releasing factor; PTHrP, parathyroid hormone–related peptide; GRF, growth hormone–releasing factor. Data from Taheri S, Ghatei MA, Bloom SR. Gastrointestinal hormones and tumor syndromes. In: De Groot LJ, Jameson JL, eds. *Endocrinology*. Philadelphia: WB Saunders, 2001:2547–2558; Aldridge MC, Williamson RCN. Surgery of endocrine tumours of the pancreas. In: Lynn J, Bloom SR, eds. *Surgical endocrinology*. Oxford: Butterworth-Heinemann, 1993:503–520; Arnold R, Simon B, Wied M. Treatment of neuroendocrine GEP tumours with somatostatin analogues: a review. *Digestion* 2000;62[Suppl 1]:84–91; Schindl M, Kaczirek K, Kaserer K, et al. Is the new classification of neuroendocrine pancreatic tumors of clinical help? *World J Surg* 2000;24:1312–1318; and Jensen RT. Endocrine tumors of the gastrointestinal tract and pancreas. In: Braunwald E, Fauci AS, Kasper DL, et al, eds. *Harrison's principles of internal medicine*. New York: McGraw-Hill, 2001:593–603.

Histologically, hyperplasia of islet-like cells is seen, with no adenoma. In the neonate, this gives rise to persistent hyperinsulinemic hypoglycemia of infancy (PHHI), but adult-onset nesidioblastosis is being increasingly recognized (59). The mutations known to result in nesidioblastosis are inactivation of the sulfonylurea receptor gene 1 (*SUR1*), inactivation of the inward rectifying K^+ channel subunit of the ATP-sensitive K^+ channel (*Kir6.2*), activation of the glucokinase gene, and activation of the glutamate dehydrogenase gene (16,60). There seems to be no recognized susceptibility to malignancy with germline mutations in these tissue-selective genes.

LOCALIZATION BY IMAGING

Pancreatic surgery is fraught with difficulty, and accurate localization of pancreatic lesions is essential to guide the surgeon. There are four useful imaging modalities: dedicated pancreatic computed tomographic (CT) scanning, endoscopic

TABLE 70.2. The Proposed Classification into Benign, Uncertain, and Malignant Gastroenteropancreatic Tumors (85)

Risk factor	Benign phenotype	Uncertain phenotype	Malignant phenotype
Size (cm)	≤2	>2	>2
Local infiltration	No	Yes	Yes
Angioinvasion	No	Yes	Yes
Atypia	No	Yes	Yes
Gross invasion	No	No	Yes
Metastasis	No	No	Yes

Data from Rindi G, Capella C, Solcia E. Cell biology, clincopathological profile; and classification of gastro-enteropancreatic endocrine tumors. *J Mol Med* 1998;76:413–420.

ultrasonography (EUS), pancreatic magnetic resonance imaging (MRI), and somatostatin-receptor scintigraphy (SRS). EUS has received much attention recently and has been shown to have a sensitivity of 80% to 90% for detecting pancreatic neuroendocrine tumors (61–65) and lower sensitivities for detecting extrapancreatic tumors (66–68). In one study, in fact, EUS showed the highest sensitivity in localizing insulinomas (94%) compared with SRS (12%), transabdominal ultrasound (12%), CT (29%), and MRI (13%) (65). The smallest lesion detectable by EUS was a 5-mm tumor in the pancreatic head. Intraoperative ultrasound is also useful in identifying small tumors that may not have been well defined preoperatively.

Another useful imaging modality is SRS, which has a sensitivity of up to 90% and a specificity of 80% for detecting functioning and nonfunctioning tumors of the pancreas, excluding insulinoma (69–71). Unlike other neuroendocrine tumors, insulinomas rarely express somatostatin receptors, thereby limiting the sensitivity of SRS to 10% to 50% (72,73). The exception is malignant insulinomas, which tend to express somatostatin receptors, and SRS is recommended for staging.

With very small tumors (<5 mm), or when multiple tumors can be seen, selective angiography with calcium gluconate (or secretin) injection into the main pancreatic arteries provides biochemical localization for functioning neuroendocrine tumors. The procedure involves cannulation of the gastroduodenal, inferior pancreaticoduodenal, superior mesenteric, splenic, and hepatic arteries in turn. The territory of each of these arteries is studied for the presence of a vascular blush, and then the secretagogue calcium gluconate (or secretin) is injected into each artery in turn. Venous samples are taken at 30-second intervals from the hepatic vein. The normal response to intraarterial calcium gluconate is a reduction in secretion of pancreatic neuroendocrine hormones; in the presence of neuroendocrine tumor, however, there is a doubling in neuroendocrine hormone release. This can be detected in the hepatic vein at 30 seconds (74–78). We find this technique invaluable at our institution because, first, it informs the surgeon of which artery supplies the territory of the tumor; second, it offers a biochemical diagnosis even before the tumor is large enough to be seen on imaging; third, where two types of tumors coexist (e.g., both insulinoma and gastrinoma in MEN1), they can be differentiated; and finally, since the hepatic artery is also injected with secretagogue, the technique provides biochemical evidence of the presence or lack of liver metastases.

Positron-emission tomography has also been applied to neuroendocrine tumors, and the use of such tracers as the monoamine oxidase inhibitor harmine for localization of nonfunctioning neuroendocrine tumors seems particularly promising (79). MIBG ([I123]-metaiodobenzyl guanidine) scanning, on the other hand, is not useful diagnostically for gastroenteropancreatic neuroendocrine tumors, because they derive from endoderm, not neuroectoderm, and catecholamine synthesis is rarely found (80).

Finally, intraoperative and gamma probes provide the last form of imaging for the surgeon. These probes are able to detect accumulation of the tracer (indium-111-DTPA-D-Phe1)-pentetreotide more efficiently (>90%) than SRS (68% to 77%), including lesions less than 5 mm in size, and radioguided surgery has been found to identify 57% more lesions than detected by the "palpating finger" (81).

CLINICOPATHOLOGIC CLASSIFICATION

In 1963 Williams and Sandler (82) were the first to classify gut neuroendocrine tumors, and subsequently numerous nomenclature systems have appeared. Most recently, a new classification of neuroendocrine gastroenteropancreatic tumors based on clinicopathologic patterns has been devised (83–85). The proposed classification into benign, uncertain, and malignant gastroenteropancreatic tumors is summarized in Table 70.2 (85). In the case of functioning pancreatic endocrine tumors, the biological behavior of the tumor is dependent as much on its pathologic features as on the endocrine hyperfunction syndrome present (Table 70.1) (86,87).

TREATMENT

Curative Surgery

RESECTION OF THE PRIMARY LESION

A primary pancreatic lesion should be resected if surgically possible, particularly if no metastases have developed. These tumors are often very slow growing, but the main problems with functioning tumors result from the secreted hormone rather than from tumor bulk. This is particularly the case with insulinomas, which can result in sudden death from inappropriate insulin secretion rather than from tumor bulk or metastases. In fact, approximately 90% of insulinomas can be enucleated from the pancreas without the need to perform local pancreatic resection.

RESECTION OF LIVER METASTASES

With improved liver surgery techniques, curative hepatic surgery is considered with increasing frequency if the primary tumor has been resected or is potentially resectable, if the liver can withstand the resection, and if there are no extrahepatic metastases. The outcome in recent studies show a 4- to 5-year survival of 70% to 85% with curative surgery (88–92). Best outcomes are achieved when there are fewer than four metastases (46 months median disease–free survival) (92).

LIVER TRANSPLANTATION

In exceptional cases in which the liver metastases are unresectable, a liver transplant may be considered. A meta-analysis of liver transplantation for neuroendocrine tumors with 30 cases (13 foregut and 15 pancreatic primaries) showed a survival of 52% after 1 year (93). The complication rate of the surgery was high, and 6 of the 12 patients who died within the first year died as a consequence of the transplant procedure itself. At our institution, a patient with a pancreatic PTHrPoma who underwent resection of the primary pancreatic tumor 17 years ago and a liver transplant for metastases 10 years ago remains alive. She has recently developed pleural and peritoneal metastases and is being treated with radiolabeled octreotide.

Medical

The medical treatments for the various endocrine hyperfunction syndromes are summarized in Table 70.3. These treatments should be put into operation pending curative surgery or if surgery is not possible. As can be seen, somatostatin analogues are frequently required.

SOMATOSTATIN ANALOGUES

Somatostatin analogues are effective for symptomatic control in many functioning neuroendocrine pancreatic tumors (94,95). Somatostatin is widely expressed throughout the body, and neuroendocrine tumors are frequently somatostatin positive (96). The longer-acting analogues of somatostatin (lanreotide and octreotide; Figure 70.5) preferentially bind the somatostatin 2 receptors (sstr2), and to a lesser extent, somatostatin 5 receptors (sstr5) (97,98).

Octreotide and lanreotide have been shown to have effects on hormone secretion and antiproliferative effects mainly via sstr2 (73,97–99). Although most gastroenteropancreatic neuroendocrine tumors express all five somatostatin receptors, those lacking somatostatin 2 [such as 50% to 90% of insulinomas (72,73)] are unresponsive to lanreotide and octreotide.

Both *in vitro* and *in vivo* experiments have indicated that somatostatin and its analogues have an antiproliferative effect, and there have been case reports of tumor regression (100–104). However, phase II trials of the effects of octreotide and lanreotide in patients with metastatic neuroendocrine tumors showed partial tumor regression in only 3% to 5% of patients treated with high-dose analogues, whereas stabilization of tumor was the best outcome, occurring in 36% to 70% of patients (105–108).

In nonfunctioning neuroendocrine tumors, somatostatin analogues should be used if the SRS scan is positive and the tumor is aggressive, with greater than 25% tumor growth in 1 year or evidence of high mitotic rate from histology (using the Ki67 value, CD44 expression, or somatostatin-receptor content) (80).

TABLE 70.3. Medical Treatments for Specific Pancreatic Endocrine Tumor Syndromes

Endocrine tumor	Treatment options
Insulinoma	Dietary changes Diazoxide Guar gum Intravenous dextrose to cover fasting Somatostatin analogue if SRS scan positive
Gastrinoma	Proton pump inhibitor
Glucagonoma	Somatostatin analogue Anticoagulation Insulin if diabetes mellitus
VIPoma	Rehydration Potassium supplementation Somatostatin analogue Bicarbonate in acute attacks
Somatostatinoma	Pancreatic enzyme replacement Insulin if diabetes mellitus
PTHrPoma	Rehydration Biphosphonates Somatostatin analogue
Nonfunctioning	Somatostatin analogue if SRS scan positive and aggressive phenotype

SRS, somatostatin-receptor scintigraphy; PTHrP, parathyroid hormone–related peptide; VIP, vasoactive intestinal polypeptide.

INTERFERON-α

Interferon-α (IFN-α) was first introduced for the treatment of carcinoid tumors for its ability to stimulate natural killer cells and control hormone secretion, symptoms, and tumor growth (109). Numerous series have used INF-α in malignant neuroendocrine tumors, and the largest studies have shown a 42% biochemical and 14% tumor response in carcinoid tumors and a 51% biochemical and 12% tumor response in neuroendocrine pancreatic tumors (110,111). However, side effects are common and include flu-like symptoms, weight loss, fatigue, and depression. The use of INF-α is limited now to metastatic carcinoid tumors, particularly when the tumor is not somatostatin analogue (112). Finally, the combination of octreotide and INF-α has been compared with monotherapies, and no difference in the antiproliferative response was found (80,112).

CHEMOTHERAPY

The slow growth rate of many neuroendocrine tumors (<25% in 1 year) would imply that chemotherapy should not be the treatment of choice except in the most aggressive tumors. However, well-differentiated pancreatic endocrine tumors (particularly VIPomas) seem to respond to streptozotocin combined with either 5-fluorouracil (5-FU) or adriamycin (with response rates of 40% to 69% and median survival 2.2 years) compared with metastatic carcinoid tumors (response rates around 20%) (113).

The chemosensitivity of undifferentiated and highly aggressive neuroendocrine tumors, on the other hand, is similar to that of small-cell carcinoma of the lung, and a response rate of 50% to 67% (median survival 9 months to 1.75 years) has been shown with a combination of etoposide (VP16) and cisplatin (CDDP) (114,115). The greatest benefit was seen in patients with undifferentiated pancreatic endocrine tumors and foregut carcinoid tumors. Not surprisingly, this combination was not effective in differentiated neuroendocrine tumors.

Interventional Radiology

HEPATIC ARTERY EMBOLIZATION

The liver is the most common site of metastases from gastroenteropancreatic neuroendocrine tumors. In the case of functioning tumors, these metastases will produce symptoms according to the hormone hyperfunction syndrome (Table 70.1). Should these metastases be unresectable, hepatic arterial embolization offers a therapeutic option. This is possible because the liver has a dual blood supply, receiving 20% to 25% of blood from the hepatic artery and 75% to 80% from the hepatic portal vein. It is crucial to ensure prior to the procedure that the portal vein is patent.

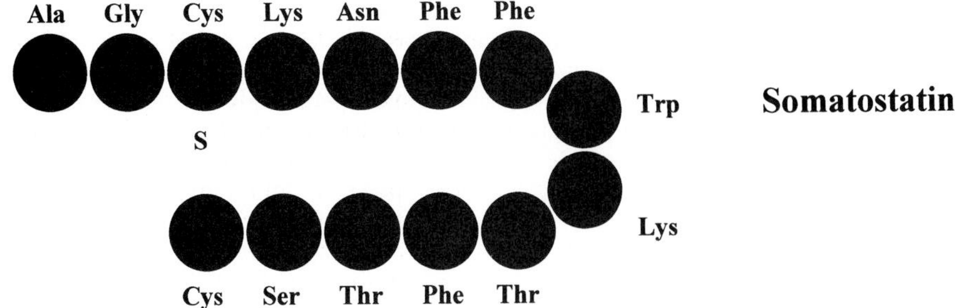

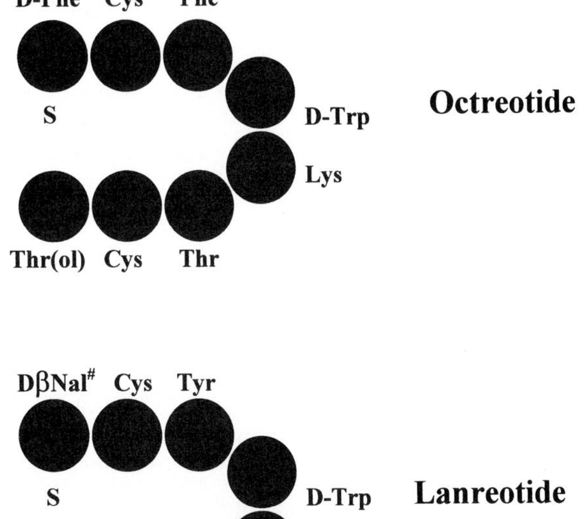

Figure 70.5. Secondary structure of somatostatin and its analogues octreotide and lanreotide. DβNal#, β-(2-naphthyl)alanine.

Selective hepatic arterial embolization has been shown to reduce both hormonal symptoms and tumor burden in patients with pancreatic neuroendocrine tumors and carcinoid tumors (116–118). The symptomatic and biochemical response rates are impressive (40% to 90%), with a median duration of response between 10 and 15 months. The radiologic response rate, however, is lower, at 15% to 40%; this may reflect the fact that, although the metastasis may not have changed in size, it may have undergone central necrosis. Patients undergoing hepatic embolization need to be monitored closely for at least 1 week in the hospital, because the procedure has a high rate of postembolic syndrome, including pain, fever, nausea, leukocytosis, and derangements in liver enzymes (in 50% to 90%). More severe complications, including renal failure, hepatic abscess, liver necrosis, and gallbladder necrosis, occur in 10% of patients, with a mortality of 3% to 7%.

Formal hospital protocols for managing embolization procedures are essential, and include preembolization intravenous methylprednisolone; central venous pressure monitoring; intravenous octreotide, aprotinin, and broad-spectrum antibiotics; and oral allopurinol. With carcinoid, additional oral cyproheptadine and nicotinamide are required, whereas with insulinoma, careful monitoring of the blood glucose is necessary.

CHEMOTHERAPY COMBINED WITH HEPATIC ARTERIAL OCCLUSION

Systemic chemotherapy with 5-FU–streptozotocin alternated with adriamycin-dacarbazine has been combined with hepatic arterial embolization in the treatment of neuroendocrine tumors. In a large retrospective analysis, the response rate to this regimen was 20% higher and the time of tumor growth control increased from 4 to 22 months for pancreatic neuroendocrine tumors and from 10 to 24 months for the carcinoid tumors as compared with hepatic arterial occlusion alone (119). However, the patients were not randomized and patient groups were different.

CHEMOEMBOLIZATION AND RADIOEMBOLIZATION

Hepatic arterial occlusion can be combined with local cytotoxic chemotherapy—termed chemoembolization (120,121). Chemoembolization has recently been compared with curative hepatic resections and provided a median survival time after treatment of 32 months (range, 7 to 63 months) and an actuarial 5-year survival of 40% (92). As with hepatic arterial occlusion, chemoembolization is only palliative but has great functional benefits for patients with hypersecreting tumors. A comparison of chemoembolization, hepatic arterial occlusion alone, and hepatic artery occlusion followed by systemic chemotherapy has not yet been reported.

More experimentally, the procedure of radioembolization, involving the injection of microspheres labeled with a radioisotope (such as yttrium-90) into the arterial branches supplying hepatic metastases, has been devised (122). This results in simultaneous hepatic embolization and local irradiation (brachyradiotherapy). The procedure is still experimental but may offer some advantages in the future.

Hepatic Cryosurgery

Hepatic cryosurgery involves placing a cryoprobe into hepatic metastases, which induces cellular damage and subsequent tumor destruction. It is, however, contraindicated when the tumor occupies greater than 40% of the liver. It has been used in a small series of eight patients with neuroendocrine tumors, giving a symptom-free survival time of 12 months (median) and overall survival with disease of 25 months (median) (123). Further studies and comparisons with other treatment options, such as radiofrequency ablation (RFA), are needed.

Palliative (Cytoreduction) Surgery

In earlier series, palliative cytoreductive surgery did not prolong survival in patients with gastroenteropancreatic neuroendocrine tumors (124,125). With improved surgical techniques, more recent studies have shown better outcomes. Among 34 patients who underwent hepatic resections, 15 were potentially curative and 19 were palliative (90). The median survival had not been reached, but the estimated 5-year survival was 85% in the patients with complete resections, compared with 63% for patients with palliative resections.

Radiolabeled Somatostatin Analogues

Trials with radiolabeled somatostatin analogue therapy for SRS-scan–positive neuroendocrine tumors are ongoing. Currently, indium-111–and yttrium-90–labeled octreotide and lanreotide compounds are being used. In fact, yttrium-90-DOTA-DPhe1-Tyr3-octreotide has been developed with high specificity for sstr2. In ten patients, this resulted in tumor volume reduction in two and partial remission or stable disease in two (126). More recently, 27 patients (24 carcinoid and 3 pancreatic endocrine tumors) were treated with two doses of indium-111–pentetreotide, and this resulted in symptom improvement in 62%, biochemical improvement in 81%, and a decrease in Hounsfield units on CT scanning in 27%, with a partial radiographic response in 8% of patients (127).

This form of therapy is the most exciting development in the field of neuroendocrine tumors, and we eagerly await the results of the major trials.

PROGNOSIS

There is a wide spectrum of tumor behavior within neuroendocrine tumors; some are well differentiated and slow growing, and others are very aggressive and metastasize. Prognosis is related not only to tumor behavior but also to the endocrine hyperfunction syndrome present. For instance, a slow-growing, well-differentiated 1-cm insulinoma can cause sudden death from hypoglycemia, and similarly, a small gastrinoma can cause a life-threatening gastrointestinal bleed.

Clearly, the best prognosis is achieved if the primary tumor is resected before it metastasizes, with 5- and 10-year survival rates exceeding 50%. In unresectable tumors, the presence or development of liver metastases, the degree of differentiation, and the particular endocrine hyperfunction syndrome determine survival.

REFERENCES

1. Phillips TJ, Belknap JK. Complex-trait genetics: emergence of multivariate strategies. *Nat Rev Neurosci* 2002;3:478–485.
2. Hedenfalk I, Duggan D, Chen Y, et al. Gene-expression profiles in hereditary breast cancer. *N Engl J Med* 2001;344:539–548.
3. van't Veer LJ, Dai H, van de Vijver MJ, et al. Gene expression profiling predicts clinical outcome of breast cancer. *Nature* 2002;415:530–536.
4. Dhanasekaran SM, Barrette TR, Ghosh D, et al. Delineation of prognostic biomarkers in prostate cancer. *Nature* 2001;412:822–826.
5. Alizadeh AA, Eisen MB, Davis RE, et al. Distinct types of diffuse large B-cell lymphoma identified by gene expression profiling. *Nature* 2000;403:503–511.
6. Clark EA, Golub TR, Lander ES, et al. Genomic analysis of metastasis reveals an essential role for RhoC. *Nature* 2000;406:532–535.
7. Polak JM, Bloom SR. Regulatory peptides of the gastrointestinal and respiratory tracts. *Arch Int Pharmacodyn Ther* 1986;280:16–49.
8. Kimura W, Kuroda A, Morioka Y. Clinical pathology of endocrine tumors of the pancreas. Analysis of autopsy cases. *Dig Dis Sci* 1991;36:933–942.
9. Fearon ER, Vogelstein B. A genetic model for colorectal tumorigenesis. *Cell* 1990;61:759–767.
10. Shannon BA, Iacopetta BJ. Methylation of the hMLH1, p16, and MDR1 genes in colorectal carcinoma: associations with clinicopathological features. *Cancer Lett* 2001;167:91–97.
11. Bardeesy N, Sinha M, Hezel AF, et al. Loss of the Lkb1 tumour suppressor provokes intestinal polyposis but resistance to transformation. *Nature* 2002;419:162–167.
12. Knudson AG Jr. Mutation and cancer: statistical study of retinoblastoma. *Proc Natl Acad Sci U S A* 1971;68:820–823.
13. Rubinfeld B, Albert I, Porfiri E, et al. Loss of beta-catenin regulation by the APC tumor suppressor protein correlates with loss of structure due to common somatic mutations of the gene. *Cancer Res* 1997;57:4624–4630.
14. Peifer M, Polakis P. Wnt signaling in oncogenesis and embryogenesis—a look outside the nucleus. *Science* 2000;287:1606–1609.
15. Kinzler KW, Vogelstein B. Lessons from hereditary colorectal cancer. *Cell* 1996;87:159–170.
16. Marx SJ, Agarwal SK, Kester MB, et al. Multiple endocrine neoplasia type 1: clinical and genetic features of the hereditary endocrine neoplasias. *Recent Prog Horm Res* 1999;54:397–438.
17. Larsson C, Skogseid B, Oberg K, et al. Multiple endocrine neoplasia type 1 gene maps to chromosome 11 and is lost in insulinoma. *Nature* 1988;332: 85–87.
18. Marx SJ, Agarwal SK, Kester MB, et al. Germline and somatic mutation of the gene for multiple endocrine neoplasia type 1 (MEN1). *J Intern Med* 1998;243: 447–453.
19. Lubensky IA, Debelenko LV, Zhuang Z, et al. Allelic deletions on chromosome 11q13 in multiple tumors from individual MEN1 patients. *Cancer Res* 1996;56:5272–5278.
20. Jakobovitz O, Nass D, DeMarco L, et al. Carcinoid tumors frequently display genetic abnormalities involving chromosome 11. *J Clin Endocrinol Metab* 1996; 81:3164–3167.
21. Emmert-Buck MR, Lubensky IA, Dong Q, et al. Localization of the multiple endocrine neoplasia type I (MEN1) gene based on tumor loss of heterozygosity analysis. *Cancer Res* 1997;57:1855–1858.
22. Crabtree JS, Scacheri PC, Ward JM, et al. A mouse model of multiple endocrine neoplasia, type 1, develops multiple endocrine tumors. *Proc Natl Acad Sci U S A* 2001;98:1118–1123.
23. Pannett AA, Thakker RV. Somatic mutations in MEN type 1 tumors, consistent with the Knudson "two-hit" hypothesis. *J Clin Endocrinol Metab* 2001;86:4371–4374.
24. Pelengaris S, Khan M. Oncogenic co-operation in beta-cell tumorigenesis. *Endocr Relat Cancer* 2001;8:307–314.
25. Wang L, Ignat A, Axiotis CA. Differential expression of the PTEN tumor suppressor protein in fetal and adult neuroendocrine tissues and tumors: progressive loss of PTEN expression in poorly differentiated neuroendocrine neoplasms. *Appl Immunohistochem Mol Morphol* 2002;10:139–146.
26. Yaguchi H, Ohkura N, Tsukada T, et al. Menin, the multiple endocrine neoplasia type 1 gene product, exhibits GTP-hydrolyzing activity in the presence of the tumor metastasis suppressor nm23. *J Biol Chem* 2002;277:38197–38204.
27. Herman JG, Latif F, Weng Y, et al. Silencing of the VHL tumor-suppressor gene by DNA methylation in renal carcinoma. *Proc Natl Acad Sci U S A* 1994; 91:9700–9704.
28. Prowse AH, Webster AR, Richards FM, et al. Somatic inactivation of the VHL gene in Von Hippel-Lindau disease tumors. *Am J Hum Genet* 1997;60:765–771.
29. Herman JG, Umar A, Polyak K, et al. Incidence and functional consequences of hMLH1 promoter hypermethylation in colorectal carcinoma. *Proc Natl Acad Sci U S A* 1998;95:6870–6875.

30. Thakker RV, Bouloux P, Wooding C, et al. Association of parathyroid tumors in multiple endocrine neoplasia type 1 with loss of alleles on chromosome 11. *N Engl J Med* 1989;321:218–224.
31. Bystrom C, Larsson C, Blomberg C, et al. Localization of the MEN1 gene to a small region within chromosome 11q13 by deletion mapping in tumors. *Proc Natl Acad Sci U S A* 1990;87:1968–1972.
32. Agarwal SK, Guru SC, Heppner C, et al. Menin interacts with the AP1 transcription factor JunD and represses JunD-activated transcription. *Cell* 1999; 96:143–152.
33. Heppner C, Bilimoria KY, Agarwal SK, et al. The tumor suppressor protein menin interacts with NF-kappaB proteins and inhibits NF-kappaB-mediated transactivation. *Oncogene* 2001;20:4917–4925.
34. Kaji H, Canaff L, Lebrun JJ, et al. Inactivation of menin, a Smad3-interacting protein, blocks transforming growth factor type beta signaling. *Proc Natl Acad Sci U S A* 2001;98:3837–3842.
35. Sayo Y, Murao K, Imachi H, et al. The multiple endocrine neoplasia type 1 gene product, menin, inhibits insulin production in rat insulinoma cells. *Endocrinology* 2002;143:2437–2440.
36. Kouvaraki MA, Lee JE, Shapiro SE, et al. Genotype-phenotype analysis in multiple endocrine neoplasia type 1. *Arch Surg* 2002;137:641–647.
37. Polak JM, Bloom SR. The diffuse neuroendocrine system in gastroenterology. *Biochem Soc Trans* 1980;8:19–22.
38. Bloom SR, Polak JM. Gut hormones in disease. *Scand J Gastroenterol Suppl* 1983;82:1–5.
39. Polak JM, Bloom SR. Some aspects of neuroendocrine pathology. *J Clin Pathol* 1987;40:1024–1041.
40. Taheri S, Ghatei MA, Bloom SR. Gastrointestinal hormones and tumor syndromes. In: De Groot LJ, Jameson JL, eds. *Endocrinology*. Philadelphia: WB Saunders, 2001:2547–2558.
41. Legaspi A, Brennan MF. Management of islet cell carcinoma. *Surgery* 1988; 104:1018–1023.
42. Aldridge MC, Williamson RCN. Surgery of endocrine tumours of the pancreas. In: Lynn J, Bloom SR, eds. *Surgical endocrinology*. Oxford: Butterworth-Heinemann, 1993:503–520.
43. Arnold R, Simon B, Wied M. Treatment of neuroendocrine GEP tumours with somatostatin analogues: a review. *Digestion* 2000;62[Suppl 1]:84–91.
44. Schindl M, Kaczirek K, Kaserer K, et al. Is the new classification of neuroendocrine pancreatic tumors of clinical help? *World J Surg* 2000;24:1312–1318.
45. Jensen RT. Endocrine tumors of the gastrointestinal tract and pancreas. In: Braunwald E, Fauci AS, Kasper DL, et al, eds. *Harrison's principles of internal medicine*. New York: McGraw-Hill, 2001:593–603.
46. Tapia FJ, Polak JM, Barbosa AJ, et al. Neuron-specific enolase is produced by neuroendocrine tumours. *Lancet* 1981;1:808–811.
47. Hamid QA, Bishop AE, Sikri KL, et al. Immunocytochemical characterization of 10 pancreatic tumours, associated with the glucagonoma syndrome, using antibodies to separate regions of the pro-glucagon molecule and other neuroendocrine markers. *Histopathology* 1986;10:119–133.
48. Yiangou Y, Williams SJ, Bishop AE, et al. Peptide histidine-methionine immunoreactivity in plasma and tissue from patients with vasoactive intestinal peptide-secreting tumors and watery diarrhea syndrome. *J Clin Endocrinol Metab* 1987;64:131–139.
49. Winkler H, Fischer-Colbrie R. The chromogranins A and B: the first 25 years and future perspectives. *Neuroscience* 1992;49:497–528.
50. Eriksson B, Arnberg H, Lindgren PG, et al. Neuroendocrine pancreatic tumours: clinical presentation, biochemical and histopathological findings in 84 patients. *J Intern Med* 1990;228:103–113.
51. Sekiya K, Ghatei MA, Salahuddin MJ, et al. Production of GAWK (chromogranin-B 420-493)-like immunoreactivity by endocrine tumors and its possible diagnostic value. *J Clin Invest* 1989;83:1834–1842.
52. Yasuda D, Iguchi H, Funakoshi A, et al. Comparison of plasma pancreastatin and GAWK concentrations, presumed processing products of chromogranin A and B, in plasma of patients with pancreatic islet cell tumors. *Horm Metab Res* 1993;25:593–595.
53. Wood SM, Polak JM, Bloom SR. Gut hormone secreting tumours. *Scand J Gastroenterol Suppl* 1983;82:165–179.
54. Ashrafian H, Taylor-Robinson SD, Calam J, et al. Once you start, you can't stop. *Lancet* 2002;359:226.
55. McGuigan JE, Wolfe MM. Secretin injection test in the diagnosis of gastrinoma. *Gastroenterology* 1980;79:1324–1331.
56. Frucht H, Howard JM, Slaff JI, et al. Secretin and calcium provocative tests in the Zollinger-Ellison syndrome. A prospective study. *Ann Intern Med* 1989; 111:713–722.
57. Friesen SR. Update on the diagnosis and treatment of rare neuroendocrine tumors. *Surg Clin North Am* 1987;67:379–393.
58. Aynsley-Green A, Polak JM, Bloom SR, et al. Nesidioblastosis of the pancreas: definition of the syndrome and the management of the severe neonatal hyperinsulinaemic hypoglycaemia. *Arch Dis Child* 1981;56:496–508.
59. Witteles RM, Straus II FH, Sugg SL, et al. Adult-onset nesidioblastosis causing hypoglycemia: an important clinical entity and continuing treatment dilemma. *Arch Surg* 2001;136:656–663.
60. Zumkeller W. Nesidioblastosis. *Endocr Relat Cancer* 1999;6:421–428.
61. Glover JR, Shorvon PJ, Lees WR. Endoscopic ultrasound for localisation of islet cell tumours. *Gut* 1992;33:108–110.
62. Lightdale CJ, Botet JF, Woodruff JM, et al. Localization of endocrine tumors of the pancreas with endoscopic ultrasonography. *Cancer* 1991;68:1815–1820.
63. Palazzo L, Roseau G, Salmeron M. Endoscopic ultrasonography in the preoperative localization of pancreatic endocrine tumors. *Endoscopy* 1992;24 [Suppl 1]:350–353.
64. Rosch T, Lightdale CJ, Botet JF, et al. Localization of pancreatic endocrine tumors by endoscopic ultrasonography. *N Engl J Med* 1992;326:1721–1726.
65. Zimmer T, Scherubl H, Faiss S, et al. Endoscopic ultrasonography of neuroendocrine tumours. *Digestion* 2000;62[Suppl 1]:45–50.
66. Thompson NW, Czako PF, Fritts LL, et al. Role of endoscopic ultrasonography in the localization of insulinomas and gastrinomas. *Surgery* 1994;116:1131–1138.
67. Ruszniewski P, Amouyal P, Amouyal G, et al. Localization of gastrinomas by endoscopic ultrasonography in patients with Zollinger-Ellison syndrome. *Surgery* 1995;117:629–635.
68. de Kerviler E, Cadiot G, Lebtahi R, et al. Somatostatin receptor scintigraphy in forty-eight patients with the Zollinger-Ellison syndrome. GRESZE: Groupe d'Etude du Syndrome de Zollinger-Ellison. *Eur J Nucl Med* 1994;21: 1191–1197.
69. Krenning EP, Kwekkeboom DJ, Bakker WH, et al. Somatostatin receptor scintigraphy with [111In-DTPA-D-Phe1]- and [123I-Tyr3]-octreotide: the Rotterdam experience with more than 1000 patients. *Eur J Nucl Med* 1993;20: 716–731.
70. Termanini B, Gibril F, Reynolds JC, et al. Value of somatostatin receptor scintigraphy: a prospective study in gastrinoma of its effect on clinical management. *Gastroenterology* 1997;112:335–347.
71. Lebtahi R, Cadiot G, Sarda L, et al. Clinical impact of somatostatin receptor scintigraphy in the management of patients with neuroendocrine gastroenteropancreatic tumors. *J Nucl Med* 1997;38:853–858.
72. Modlin IM, Tang LH. Approaches to the diagnosis of gut neuroendocrine tumors: the last word (today). *Gastroenterology* 1997;112:583–590.
73. Wulbrand U, Wied M, Zofel P, et al. Growth factor receptor expression in human gastroenteropancreatic neuroendocrine tumours. *Eur J Clin Invest* 1998; 28:1038–1049.
74. Doppman JL, Miller DL, Chang R, et al. Gastrinomas: localization by means of selective intraarterial injection of secretin. *Radiology* 1990;174:25–29.
75. Doppman JL, Miller DL, Chang R, et al. Insulinomas: localization with selective intraarterial injection of calcium. *Radiology* 1991;178:237–241.
76. Fedorak IJ, Ko TC, Gordon D, et al. Localization of islet cell tumors of the pancreas: a review of current techniques. *Surgery* 1993;113:242–249.
77. O'Shea D, Rohrer-Theurs AW, Lynn JA, et al. Localization of insulinomas by selective intraarterial calcium injection. *J Clin Endocrinol Metab* 1996;81:1623–1627.
78. Goldstone AP, Scott-Coombes DM, Lynn JA. Surgical management of gastrointestinal endocrine tumours. *Baillieres Clin Gastroenterol* 1996;10:707–736.
79. Eriksson B, Bergstrom M, Orlefors H, et al. Use of PET in neuroendocrine tumors. In vivo applications and in vitro studies. *Q J Nucl Med* 2000;44:68–76.
80. Role of somatostatin analogues in oncology. European Neuroendocrine Tumor Network (ENET). February 24-27, 2000, Innsbruck, Austria. Round Table Discussion. *Digestion* 2000;62[Suppl 1]:98–107.
81. Adams S, Baum RP. Intraoperative use of gamma-detecting probes to localize neuroendocrine tumors. *Q J Nucl Med* 2000;44:59–67.
82. Williams ED, Sandler M. The classification of carcinoid tumors. *Lancet* 1963;1: 238–239.
83. Kloppel G, Heitz PU. Classification of normal and neoplastic neuroendocrine cells. *Ann N Y Acad Sci* 1994;733:19–23.
84. Capella C, Heitz PU, Hofler H, et al. Revised classification of neuroendocrine tumors of the lung, pancreas and gut. *Digestion* 1994;55[Suppl 3]:11–23.
85. Rindi G, Capella C, Solcia E. Cell biology, clinicopathological profile, and classification of gastro-enteropancreatic endocrine tumors. *J Mol Med* 1998; 76:413–420.
86. Kloppel G, Heitz PU. Pancreatic endocrine tumors. *Pathol Res Pract* 1988; 183: 155–168.
87. Solcia E, Sessa F, Rindi G, et al. Classification and histogenesis of gastroenteropancreatic endocrine tumours. *Eur J Clin Invest* 1990;20[Suppl 1]:S72–S81.
88. Que FG, Nagorney DM, Batts KP, et al. Hepatic resection for metastatic neuroendocrine carcinomas. *Am J Surg* 1995;169:36–42.
89. Chen H, Hardacre JM, Uzar A, et al. Isolated liver metastases from neuroendocrine tumors: does resection prolong survival? *J Am Coll Surg* 1998;187: 88–92.
90. Chamberlain RS, Canes D, Brown KT, et al. Hepatic neuroendocrine metastases: does intervention alter outcomes? *J Am Coll Surg* 2000;190:432–445.
91. Jaeck D, Oussoultzoglou E, Bachellier P, et al. Hepatic metastases of gastroenteropancreatic neuroendocrine tumors: safe hepatic surgery. *World J Surg* 2001;25:689–692.
92. Yao KA, Talamonti MS, Nemcek A, et al. Indications and results of liver resection and hepatic chemoembolization for metastatic gastrointestinal neuroendocrine tumors. *Surgery* 2001;130:677–682.
93. Bechstein WO, Neuhaus P. Liver transplantation for hepatic metastases of neuroendocrine tumors. *Ann N Y Acad Sci* 1994;733:507–514.
94. Anderson JV, Bloom SR. Neuroendocrine tumours of the gut: long-term therapy with the somatostatin analogue SMS 201-995. *Scand J Gastroenterol Suppl* 1986;119:115–128.
95. Wynick D, Bloom SR. Clinical review 23: The use of the long-acting somatostatin analog octreotide in the treatment of gut neuroendocrine tumors. *J Clin Endocrinol Metab* 991;73:1–3.
96. Polak JM, Bloom SR. Somatostatin localization in tissues. *Scand J Gastroenterol Suppl* 1986;119:11–21.

97. Reisine T, Bell GI. Molecular biology of somatostatin receptors. *Endocr Rev* 1995;16:427–442.
98. Patel YC, Srikant CB. Subtype selectivity of peptide analogs for all five cloned human somatostatin receptors (hsstr 1-5). *Endocrinology* 1994;135: 2814–2817.
99. Buscail L, Esteve JP, Saint-Laurent N, et al. Inhibition of cell proliferation by the somatostatin analogue RC-160 is mediated by somatostatin receptor subtypes SSTR2 and SSTR5 through different mechanisms. *Proc Natl Acad Sci U S A* 1995;92:1580–1584.
100. Sharma K, Srikant CB. Induction of wild-type p53, Bax, and acidic endonuclease during somatostatin-signaled apoptosis in MCF-7 human breast cancer cells. *Int J Cancer* 1998;76:259–266.
101. Kraenzlin ME, Ch'ng JC, Wood SM, et al. Can inhibition of hormone secretion be associated with endocrine tumour shrinkage? *Lancet* 1983;2:1501.
102. Clements D, Elias E. Regression of metastatic vipoma with somatostatin analogue SMS 201-995. *Lancet* 1985;1:874–875.
103. Shepherd JJ, Senator GB. Regression of liver metastases in patient with gastrin-secreting tumour treated with SMS 201-995. *Lancet* 1986;2:574.
104. Wiedenmann B, Rath U, Radsch R, et al. Tumor regression of an ileal carcinoid under the treatment with the somatostatin analogue SMS 201-995. *Klin Wochenschr* 1988;66:75–77.
105. Arnold R, Trautmann ME, Creutzfeldt W, et al. Somatostatin analogue octreotide and inhibition of tumour growth in metastatic endocrine gastroenteropancreatic tumours. *Gut* 1996;38:430–438.
106. di Bartolomeo M, Bajetta E, Buzzoni R, et al. Clinical efficacy of octreotide in the treatment of metastatic neuroendocrine tumors. A study by the Italian Trials in Medical Oncology Group. *Cancer* 1996;77:402–408.
107. Eriksson B, Renstrup J, Imam H, et al. High-dose treatment with lanreotide of patients with advanced neuroendocrine gastrointestinal tumors: clinical and biological effects. *Ann Oncol* 1997;8:1041–1044.
108. Faiss S, Rath U, Mansmann U, et al. Ultra-high-dose lanreotide treatment in patients with metastatic neuroendocrine gastroenteropancreatic tumors. *Digestion* 1999;60:469–476.
109. Oberg K, Funa K, Alm G. Effects of leukocyte interferon on clinical symptoms and hormone levels in patients with mid-gut carcinoid tumors and carcinoid syndrome. *N Engl J Med* 1983;309:129–133.
110. Oberg K, Eriksson B. The role of interferons in the management of carcinoid tumors. *Acta Oncol* 1991;30:519–522.
111. Eriksson B, Oberg K. An update of the medical treatment of malignant endocrine pancreatic tumors. *Acta Oncol* 1993;32:203–208.
112. Oberg K. Interferon in the management of neuroendocrine GEP-tumors: a review. *Digestion* 2000;62[Suppl 1]:92–97.
113. Rougier P, Mitry E. Chemotherapy in the treatment of neuroendocrine malignant tumors. *Digestion* 2000;62[Suppl 1]:73–78.
114. Moertel CG, Kvols LK, O'Connell MJ, et al. Treatment of neuroendocrine carcinomas with combined etoposide and cisplatin. Evidence of major therapeutic activity in the anaplastic variants of these neoplasms. *Cancer* 1991; 68:227–232.
115. Fjallskog ML, Granberg DP, Welin SL, et al. Treatment with cisplatin and etoposide in patients with neuroendocrine tumors. *Cancer* 2001;92:1101–1107.
116. Ajani JA, Carrasco CH, Charnsangavej C, et al. Islet cell tumors metastatic to the liver: effective palliation by sequential hepatic artery embolization. *Ann Intern Med* 1988;108:340–344.
117. Carrasco CH, Chuang VP, Wallace S. Apudomas metastatic to the liver: treatment by hepatic artery embolization. *Radiology* 1983;149:79–83.
118. Eriksson BK, Larsson EG, Skogseid BM, et al. Liver embolizations of patients with malignant neuroendocrine gastrointestinal tumors. *Cancer* 1998;83: 2293–2301.
119. Moertel CG, Johnson CM, McKusick MA, et al. The management of patients with advanced carcinoid tumors and islet cell carcinomas. *Ann Intern Med* 1994;120:302–309.
120. Wallace S, Ajani JA, Charnsangavej C, et al. Carcinoid tumors: imaging procedures and interventional radiology. *World J Surg* 1996;20:147–156.
121. Stokes KR, Stuart K, Clouse ME. Hepatic arterial chemoembolization for metastatic endocrine tumors. *J Vasc Interv Radiol* 1993;4:341–345.
122. Andrews JC, Walker SC, Ackermann RJ, et al. Hepatic radioembolization with yttrium-90 containing glass microspheres: preliminary results and clinical follow-up. *J Nucl Med* 1994;35:1637–1644.
123. Bilchik AJ, Sarantou T, Foshag LJ, et al. Cryosurgical palliation of metastatic neuroendocrine tumors resistant to conventional therapy. *Surgery* 1997;122: 1040–1047.
124. McEntee GP, Nagorney DM, Kvols LK, et al. Cytoreductive hepatic surgery for neuroendocrine tumors. *Surgery* 1990;108:1091–1096.
125. Soreide O, Berstad T, Bakka A, et al. Surgical treatment as a principle in patients with advanced abdominal carcinoid tumors. *Surgery* 1992;111:48–54.
126. de Jong M, Bakker WH, Krenning EP, et al. Yttrium-90 and indium-111 labelling, receptor binding and biodistribution of [DOTA0,d-Phe1,Tyr3] octreotide, a promising somatostatin analogue for radionuclide therapy. *Eur J Nucl Med* 1997;24:368–371.
127. Anthony LB, Woltering EA, Espenan GD, et al. Indium-111-pentetreotide prolongs survival in gastroenteropancreatic malignancies. *Semin Nucl Med* 2002;32:123–132.

Index

Note: Page numbers in *italics* indicate figures; page numbers followed by "t" indicate a table concerning the subject.

D

T